Small Animal Clinical Pharmacology & Therapeutics

Second Edition

Small Animal Clinical Pharmacology & Therapeutics

Dawn Merton Boothe, DVM, MS, PhD, DACVIM, DACVP
Professor
Department of Physiology and Pharmacology
College of Veterinary Medicine
Director
Clinical Pharmacology Laboratory
Auburn University
Auburn, Alabama

ELSEVIER
SAUNDERS

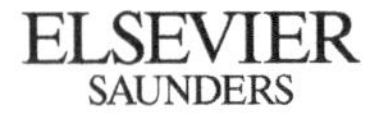
SAUNDERS

3251 Riverport Lane
St. Louis, Missouri 63043

SMALL ANIMAL CLINICAL PHARMACOLOGY AND THERAPEUTICS
ISBN: 978-0-7216-0555-5

Notice

Knowledge and best practice in this field are constantly changing. As new research and experience broaden our understanding, changes in research methods, professional practices, or medical treatment may become necessary.

Practitioners and researchers must always rely on their own experience and knowledge in evaluating and using any information, methods, compounds, or experiments described herein. In using such information or methods they should be mindful of their own safety and the safety of others, including parties for whom they have a professional responsibility.

With respect to any drug or pharmaceutical products identified, readers are advised to check the most current information provided (i) on procedures featured or (ii) by the manufacturer of each product to be administered, to verify the recommended dose or formula, the method and duration of administration, and contraindications. It is the responsibility of practitioners, relying on their own experience and knowledge of their patients, to make diagnoses, to determine dosages and the best treatment for each individual patient, and to take all appropriate safety precautions.

To the fullest extent of the law, neither the Publisher nor the authors, contributors, or editors, assume any liability for any injury and/or damage to persons or property as a matter of products liability, negligence or otherwise, or from any use or operation of any methods, products, instructions, or ideas contained in the material herein.

Library of Congress Cataloging-in-Publication Data

Small animal clinical pharmacology and therapeutics / [edited by] Dawn Merton Boothe. -- 2nd ed.
p. ; cm.
Rev. ed. of: Small animal clinical pharmacology and therapeutics / Dawn Merton Boothe. c2001.
Includes bibliographical references and index.
ISBN 978-0-7216-0555-5 (pbk. : alk. paper) 1. Dogs--Diseases--Treatment. 2. Cats--Diseases--Treatment. 3. Veterinary pharmacology.
I. Boothe, Dawn Merton. II. Boothe, Dawn Merton. Small animal clinical pharmacology and therapeutics.
[DNLM: 1. Dog Diseases--drug therapy. 2. Cat Diseases--drug therapy. 3. Veterinary Drugs. SF 991]
SF991.B676 2012
636.7'0895--dc22
2011004138

Vice President and Publisher: Linda Duncan
Acquisitions Editor: Heidi Pohlman
Senior Developmental Editor: Shelly Stringer
Publishing Services Manager: Julie Eddy
Senior Project Manager: Celeste Clingan
Design Direction: Margaret Reid

Printed in the United States of America

Last digit is the print number: 9 8 7 6

Contributors

Paul R. Avery, VMD, PhD
Associate Professor
Department of Microbiology, Immunology and Pathology
College of Veterinary Medicine
Colorado State University
Fort Collins, Colorado
Biologic Response Modifiers: Interferons, Interleukins, Recombinant Products, and Liposomal Products

E. Murl Bailey, Jr., DVM, MS, PhD, DABVT
Professor of Toxicology
Department of Veterinary Physiology and Pharmacology
College of Veterinary Medicine and Biomedical Sciences
Texas A&M University
College Station, Texas

Ellen N. Behrend, VMD, PhD, DACVIM
Professor
Department of Clinical Sciences
College of Veterinary Medicine
Auburn University
Auburn, Alabama
Drug Therapy for Endocrinopathies

Harry W. Boothe, DVM
Professor
Department of Clinical Sciences
College of Veterinary Medicine
Auburn University
Auburn, Alabama
Disinfectants, Antiseptics, and Related Biocides

Janice L. Cain, DVM, DACVIM
Staff Veterinarian
Bishop Ranch Veterinary Center
San Ramon, California
Rational Use of Reproductive Hormones

Tanya D. Civco, DVM, DACVIM
Associate Professor
Department of Clinical Sciences
College of Veterinary Medicine
Auburn University
Auburn, Alabama
Drug Therapy for Endocrinopathies

Tad B. Coles, DVM
Institutional Animal Care and Use Committee Veterinarian
Research and Graduate Studies
Kansas University
Lawrence, Kansas
Freelance Medical Writing and Regulatory Consulting
Overland Park, Kansas
Drugs for the Treatment of Helminth Infections – Anthelmintics

Autumn P. Davidson, DVM, MS, DACVIM
Clinical Professor
Department of Medicine and Epidemiology
School of Veterinary Medicine
University of California
Davis, California
Staff Internist
Department of Internal Medicine
VCA Animal Care Center of Sonoma
Rohnert Park, California
Rational Use of Reproductive Hormones

Reid P. Groman, DVM, DACVIM, DACVECC
Department of Clinical Studies
School of Veterinary Medicine
University of Pennsylvania
Philadelphia, Pennsylvania
Fluids, Electrolytes, and Acid-Base Therapy

Sophie A. Grundy, BVSc (Hons), MACVSc, DACVIM
Graduate Student Researcher
Department of Population Health and Reproduction
University of California
Davis, California
Veterinarian
Internal Medicine and Reproduction
VCA Sacramento Animal Medicine Group
Carmichael, California
Rational Use of Reproductive Hormones

Robert A. Kennis, DVM, MS, DACVD
Associate Professor
Department of Clinical Sciences
College of Veterinary Medicine
Auburn University
Auburn, Alabama
Dermatologic Therapy

India F. Lane, DVM, MS, EdD
Associate Professor of Medicine
Director of Educational Enhancement
Department of Small Animal Clinical Sciences
College of Veterinary Medicine
The University of Tennessee
Knoxville, Tennessee
Internist
W.W. Armistead Veterinary Teaching Hospital
College of Veterinary Medicine
The University of Tennessee
Knoxville, Tennessee
Treatment of Urinary Disorders

Randy C. Lynn, DVM, MS, DACVP
Director
Professional Services Group
IDEXX Pharmaceuticals, Inc.
Greensboro, North Carolina
Drugs for the Treatment of Protozoal Infections
Drugs for the Treatment of Helminth Infections – Anthelmintics

Elizabeth A. Martinez, DVM, DACVA
Associate Professor
Department of Small Animal Clinical Sciences
College of Veterinary Medicine
Texas A&M University
College Station, Texas
Anesthetic Agents
Muscle Relaxants

Katrina L. Mealey, DVM PhD, DACVIM, DACVCP
Professor
Department of Veterinary Clinical Sciences
College of Veterinary Medicine
Washington State University
Pullman, Washington
Pharmacogenetics
Antiinflammatory Drugs
Glucocorticoid and Mineralocorticoids

Jennifer E. Stokes, DVM, DACVIM
Clinical Associate Professor
Small Animal Clinical Sciences
College of Veterinary Medicine
University of Tennessee
Knoxville, Tennessee
Treatment of Urinary Disorders

Michael D. Willard, DVM, MS, DACVIM
Professor
Department of Small Animal Clinical Sciences
College of Veterinary Medicine
Texas A&M University
College Station, Texas
Fluids, Electrolytes, and Acid-Base Therapy

Heather Wilson, DVM
Assistant Professor
Department of Small Animal Clinical Sciences
College of Veterinary Medicine and Biomedical Sciences
Texas A&M University
College Station, Texas
Chemotherapy

Dedication

To the Lisa Howes and Dougie MacIntires of our profession; those unnamed heroes whose never-ending desire to do what is right and good for animals and their owners—and their willingness to act on that desire—ensures that veterinary medicine remains among the most giving and most respected of professions.

Are not two sparrows sold for a cent? And yet not one of them will fall to the ground apart from your Father. But the very hairs of your head are all numbered. So do not fear; you are more valuable than many sparrows.
Matthew: 10:29-31, New International Version

A righteous man cares for the needs of his animal
Prov: 12:10, New International Version

Acknowledgments

As with any textbook, there are many persons to thank for their contributing efforts. Included would be the contributing authors whose expertise was critical, and the editorial staff at Elsevier for their patience during this 10-year lapse in editions. Special thanks for direct help are extended to Mrs. Debbie Allgood who assisted with the task of typing and collating references. Harry Boothe (once again) read and re-read each chapter for editorial and content purposes, a fitting task for a detailed-oriented surgeon. More importantly, he constantly provided the encouragement to persevere in the completion of this second edition, despite cross-country moves, new jobs, children and the lesser important, but nonetheless never-ending distractions. I would woefully fail in my acknowledgments if I neglected to recognize my laboratory manager, Jameson Sofge, for his day-to-day willingness, flexibility, and readiness to help in any task that might reduce my distractions. I also thank the manager before him, Tiffany Finch, who accompanied me as I moved from Texas A&M University to Auburn and ensured the persistence of the Clinical Pharmacology Laboratory. The American College of Veterinary Clinical Pharmacology—including the newer, younger and remarkably motivated diplomates—are recognized for their continued efforts to expand the discipline and reveal its importance to the practice of veterinary medicine, whether to the veterinary patient or its owner. Finally and foremost, my thanks to our Lord for providing the motivation, materials, and support to finish what seemed to be a never-ending task.

Preface

Ten years have lapsed between the first and second editions of *Small Animal Clinical Pharmacology and Therapeutics*. An increased recognition of the importance and benefits of the human–companion animal bond by the profession has contributed to the remarkable changes that have occurred in the provision of health care to dogs and cats. Many private specialty practices now supersede academic veterinary teaching hospitals in terms of cases, clinicians, facilities, and diagnostic or therapeutic interventions. Corporate veterinary medicine has become an influential force in the provision of health care to dogs and cats. Electronic media and pharmacy services are simultaneously a blessing and a bane; discriminating between the two can be difficult. "Natural" products are increasingly perceived by consumers as the safer and preferred approach to prevention or treatment of diseases. The decade has seen a focus on public health in terms of antimicrobial resistance, bioterrorism, and translational medicine. Excitingly, an appreciation of the importance of naturally occurring diseases in dogs and cats as translational models for the same disease in humans has emerged in human and veterinary medicine, paving the way for integrated clinical research. The client's expectation of better care for their pet contributes to an urgency in the provision of quality care to our canine and feline patients. It has been accompanied by an explosion of information, scientific and otherwise, that must be used judiciously.

Among the goals of this second edition is the provision of information that will facilitate this judicious use. Pharmacology is directed physiology; as such, it is a dose away from toxicology (the dose *does* make the poison). With every therapeutic intervention we implement in our patient, our intent is to supersede signals that the patient's body has put in place to maintain normal physiology or correct pathophysiology. Each dose increases the risk of adversity as a result of therapeutic failure, medication error, or an adverse drug reaction. It is only with an accurate assessment of what we know, and a deep respect of and acknowledgement for what we don't know, that we should approach the use of drugs in our patients. Yet, today's veterinary curriculum often do not provide the education needed to promote judicious drug use, inadvertently promoting a more cavalier approach based on formulary-derived recipes rather than literature-based science. Today's pharmaceutical market provides fewer approved drugs, leading to increased use of drugs and preparations (e.g., compounded products) that are not approved for use—and thus not scientifically studied—in the target species. Surveillance of adverse drug events or medication errors is paramount to safe drug use in the patient. Yet, the availability of such data to the veterinary profession is hampered by limitations in practitioner reporting, user-friendly reporting sites, and the ability of regulatory or other agencies to analyze and to report the data to the profession in a timely and effective fashion. Accordingly, this edition continues to emphasize the basic principles of pharmacology, factors that impact plasma drug concentrations and the nuances of the individual patient that mandate an individualized approach to drug therapy. For newer drugs or therapeutic approaches in particular, the intent is to encourage judicious use through discussion of the physiology of the target organ, the pathophysiology of the target disease, and the clinical pharmacology of the drugs of interest. The second edition includes an increased emphasis on rational antimicrobial use, pharmacogenetics, and, in each chapter, expansion of tabular data that summarizes drug use and the addition of key points to emphasize major concepts.

Among the most time consuming efforts made toward improvement of the second edition is an assessment of the evidentiary basis for the therapeutic intent of each drug. This is manifested in part by a transition from a non-referenced to a reference-based textbook. Many time-honored therapeutic interventions are based on anecdotal evidence or standard of care expressed by experts; such information is difficult to reference. Indeed, dosing regimens offer an excellent example in that regimens for the same drug may vary widely. Multiple texts or formularies were consulted for dosing regimens provided in this table. For some dosing regimens, consensus could be determined; for others, an attempt was made to represent the diversity. The nature of scientific evidence is also diverse. For some therapeutic interventions, case reports are cited. For others, systematic reviews (often largely based on human data) are cited. However, the last decade has seen a marked increase in the report of clinical trials (not a sufficient number to allow meta-analyses), and an attempt has been made to identify and summarize the relevance of these studies to drug use in dogs or cats. Randomized, placebo-controlled (cross-over or parallel) blinded studies are the minimum criteria for a well-designed clinical trial attempting to demonstrate a treatment effect in sample populations. When possible, whether the study succeeded in minimizing bias and selecting a representative patient sample population is addressed. Among the more common assessments was the validity of statements regarding treatment effects. Most clinical trials are designed to minimize the risk of identifying a difference as real rather than from probability (a Type I error). However, failing to identify a true treatment effect (a Type II error) also is important, and it is this error (the power of the study) that is most negatively impacted by a small sample size. Readers and investigators tend to over-interpret the failure of a study to demonstrate a significant difference. The assumption is made that such failure is evidence that a treatment does not have an effect, or worse, that treatments have equal effects. Accordingly, for many of the clinical trials reviewed in this text that did not demonstrate a treatment effect, the assessment includes a statement as to whether the investigators cited the power of the study to detect a significant difference. A related concern is the issue of *statistical* versus *clinical* differences among treatment groups. The commonly chosen p value of 0.05 is not sacrosanct; as clinicians, a p value of 0.1 (the probability that the different response between groups would occur despite no treatment effect is ≤10% rather than ≤5%) may be just as relevant to our patient. On the other hand, even a statistical difference may not justify a therapeutic intervention if the magnitude of differential response between the treatment groups is not clinically relevant.

This text focuses on evidenced-based therapeutic interventions. Among the limitations of texts such as these is the risk that important, clinically relevant information was potentially missed despite exhaustive data base reviews. Nonetheless, it is with pleasure, humility, and honor that I offer the updated second version of this text. My hope is that it provides helpful evidence-based assessment of therapeutic interventions that can be provided to the canine and feline patient through the practitioner.

Contents

SECTION FIVE
Drugs Targeting Inflammation or Immunomodulation, 1045

APPENDICES

Principles of Drug Therapy

Dawn Merton Boothe

1

Chapter Outline

The intent of drug therapy is to induce a desired pharmacologic response for a sufficiently long period of time while preventing adverse drug events (see Chapter 4). For most drugs the magnitude of pharmacologic response is proportionately related to the (log of) drug concentration at the tissue (receptor) site (Figure 1-1). Understanding the relationship among dose, drug concentration, and response requires an understanding of the pharmacodynamics (i.e., the science of drug action), or the physiologic and biochemical effects of a drug and their relationship to the drug's mechanism of actions. Most commonly, the response is measured in the animal but may also occur in a microbe or parasite.[1] Pharmacodynamics may be studied *in vitro* (isolated cells or tissue), *ex vivo* (isolated cells or tissues after exposure to the drug in the intact animal), or *in vivo* (exposure and study occurs in the whole animal). Pharmacodynamics ultimately should be integrated with the science of pharmacokinetics, that is drug movements through the body.

DOSE–RESPONSE RELATIONSHIP

Pharmacodynamic responses occur at many levels, ranging from single molecules to whole animals. Drugs induce their responses through a number of mechanisms, most of which involve direct or indirect interactions with cell macromolecules and generally proteins. Direct interactions with nonprotein molecules are less common, but examples include nucleic acids (e.g., cancer chemotherapeutic agents), metal chelating drugs, or antacids used to chemically neutralize gastric acid. Drug responses more commonly reflect the interaction of the drug, acting as a **ligand,** with **receptors** (Figure 1-2). A receptor most commonly is a large protein macromolecule (e.g., structural, enzymatic, carrier, or ion channel proteins) responsible for cellular signaling. Receptors may be located on or in the cell membrane, in the cytosol, or within an intracellular structure (i.e., nucleus). Physiologic functions of the body generally are regulated by multiple receptor-mediated mechanisms, each responding to different molecular stimuli. Examples of target receptor categories include hormones, neuromodulatory receptors, and neurotransmitters.

Interaction between a drug and its receptor generally results in activation (either directly or indirectly) of cellular biochemical processes (e.g., ion conductance, protein phosphorylation, or DNA transcription) by way of a transduction pathway that ultimately brings about the pharmacologic effect.[1] A time lag may be associated with transduction (Figure 1-2). Activation reflects the drug's mechanism of action, whereas the sequelae of the stimulation at the molecular, cellular, or tissue level reflect the drug's pharmacodynamic effects. Secondary intracellular messenger molecules are often activated by drug–receptor interaction; they subsequently set in motion a cascade of events that eventually causes the response. Among the most common receptors are transmembrane receptors linked to guanosine triphosphate–binding proteins (G proteins). These then activate second messenger systems such as adenylyl cyclase (e.g., beta-adrenoceptors), the cytosolic

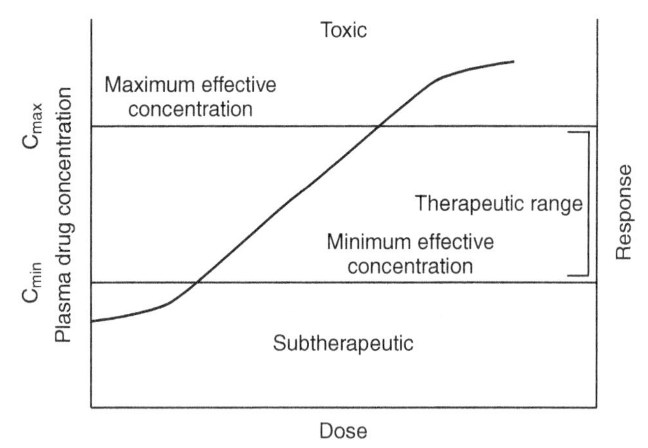

Figure 1-1 The relationship among log plasma or tissue drug concentration and dose and response generally can be considered linear within the concentrations used therapeutically. Ideally, plasma drug concentration will fall within the therapeutic range (between C_{max} and C_{min}) throughout most of the dosing interval. A representative concentration versus response curve generally yields a sigmoidal shape. At lower (20% response) and higher concentrations (>80% response), larger dose increases are required to stimulate a response. Therapeutic doses should target the linear portion of the curve, between 20% and 80% of the maximal effect. Above that point increasingly larger doses again are needed to generate a change in response, and the risk of toxicity increases, although the dosing interval may be prolonged for safe drugs.

inositol triphosphate pathway (e.g., alpha-adrenoceptors), or membrane-bound diacylglycerol (DAG).

Two properties describe drug-receptor interactions: affinity, or the capacity of a drug to bind to a receptor, and intrinsic efficacy (or activity), or the capacity of a drug to activate or inactivate a receptor. The latter is a complex relationship dependent on drug concentration, receptor activation, and cellular response. *Affinity* is usually mathematically defined as the reciprocal of the dissociation constant of the drug for the receptor.[1] A receptor often is characterized by multiple types (e.g., alpha- and beta-adrenergics; mu, kappa, and delta opioid receptors) and subtypes (e.g., alpha 1 and 2, beta 1, 2, or 3; mu 1 or 2). The selectivity of a drug action generally reflects the specificity of the drug for the target receptor binding. Drugs often target multiple receptors, although interactions may be concentration dependent or may result in blocking rather than activating specific receptors. Receptor characteristics (e.g., numbers and affinities) are influenced by both external and intracellular conditions. Tissues vary in receptor numbers and subtypes; indeed, proper physiologic responses are dependent on this variability. The relationship between a drug and pharmacologic response was at one time assumed to be directly proportional to the number of receptors occupied by the drug, with a maximal response reflecting 100% occupancy and activation (i.e., the drug receptor theory). However, the interactions are much more complex than that described by a simple linear relationship. Different kinetic relationships (linear, log-linear,

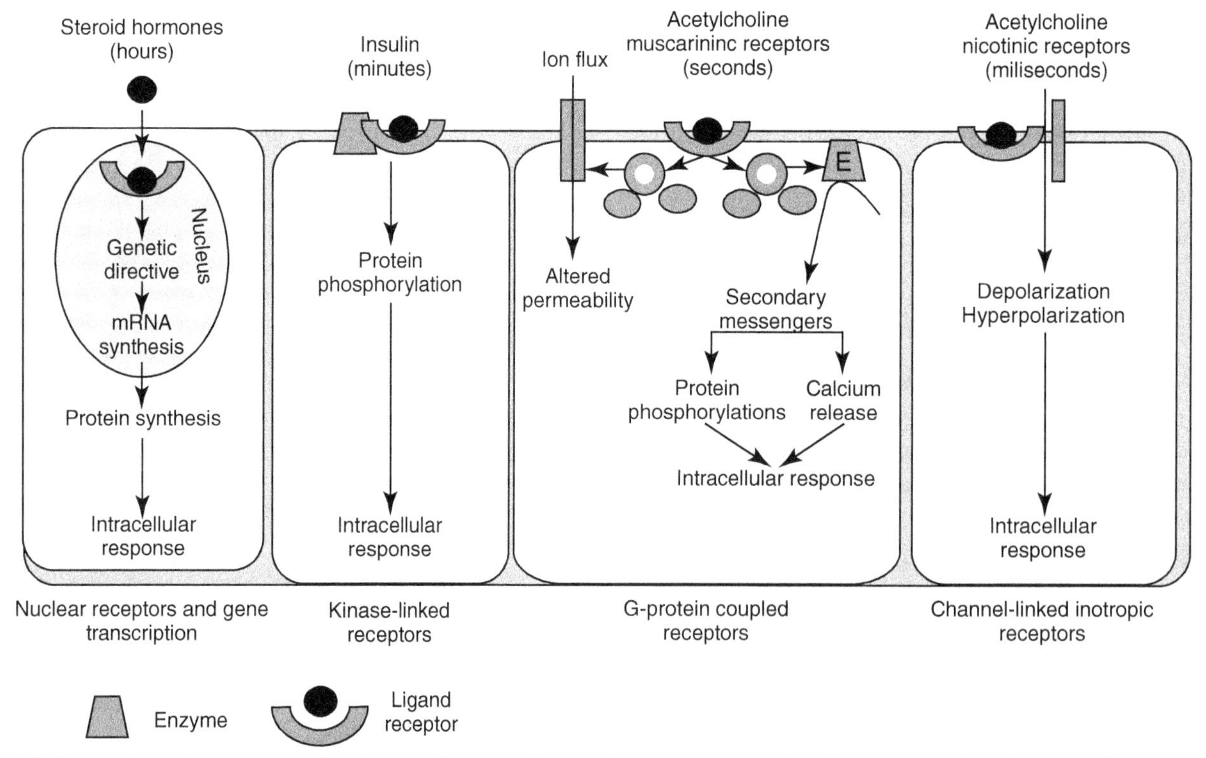

Figure 1-2 Examples of drug–receptor interactions at the cell membrane, cytosol or organelle site, and the secondary amplification cascades that ultimately result in the pharmacodynamic response.

polynomial), multiple activation states, (active, inactive, resting), cell amplification of the drug-receptor signal, and existence of spare receptors are some examples of the complexities that determine the relationship between drug concentration and response. The scientific description, examination, and ultimate prediction of drug–receptor interactions are often accomplished by generation of dose–response curves; the graphic representation most generally is represented by a sigmoidal curve (Figure 1-3; see also Fig. 1-1). The curve indicates that increasing drug concentration at the receptor site increases the number of bound receptors and thus drug effect. If concentration–response curves are plotted on a logarithmic (x) axis, the portion of the curve that lies between 20% and 80% of the maximal response is generally linear. This is the portion most relevant to therapeutic concentrations and thus encompasses the therapeutic range. Increasing a drug dose within this range generally results in a proportional increase in response. However, once the 80% mark is passed, as receptors become saturated, a much larger increase in concentration (dose) is necessary to increase response. Although this may increase the risk of adverse effects, for drugs which are safe, it may also prolong the dosing interval since the response will not change much as concentrations decline to the 80% level. At that point, drug concentration declines exponentially (generally first order), and response will also decline log-linearly with time (e.g., 50% decline with one half-life). Note that for some drugs (i.e., drugs that irreversibly interact with receptors, drugs with active metabolites,), response may not be related to plasma (tissue) drug concentrations.

The interaction of a drug with a receptor is similar to that between a substrate binding to the active site of an enzyme. As such, similar equations and parameters are used to describe the relationship between dose and response. The **effective dose** (ED) is the quantity of administered drug that will produce the (desired) effects for which it is administered. The median effective dose (ED_{50}) is the dose that produces the desired effect in 50% of a population. However, *dose* is a less accurate descriptor of what is happening at the receptor than is *effective concentration (EC)*. The affinity of the drug for the receptor is described by the (effective concentration) EC_{50}, the drug concentration that yields 50% of the maximal response (see Figure 1-3, *A*). The different actions of a drug, such as therapeutic and adverse effects, are often due to the drug binding to different receptors with different EC_{50} values. Ideally, the EC_{50} for an adverse event is higher than that of a therapeutic response. The ratio of adverse event EC_{50} to the therapeutic effect EC_{50} is the **therapeutic index** and provides some indication of drug safety in that the larger the index, the safer the drug. *Efficacy* and *potency* are two terms used to describe the relationship among drug, concentration, and response. **Efficacy** refers to the maximum effect (E_{max}) a drug can have ($e = 1$ indicates a full response), whereas **potency** is a comparative term that describes the concentration of two drugs necessary to induce the same magnitude of response. Generally, plots describing efficacy and potency are based on log $_{10}$ concentration versus percent response curve. (see Figure1-3, *A*). Drugs are considered equal in efficacy if they can cause the same magnitude of response; the more potent drug will cause an EC_{50} at a lower concentration. As such, the dose of a less potent drug may simply need to be increased to achieve the same effect of the more potent drug.

Drug–receptor interactions do not always yield the maximal response. Receptor interaction with a drug that acts as an **agonist** (generally, a structural analog of the targeted receptor) results in some level of activation. The occupation theory of drug–receptor interaction indicates that the magnitude of the response produced by an agonist is directly proportional to the number of receptors occupied.[1] Pharmacodynamic antagonism occurs when one drug inhibits the agonistic effects of another

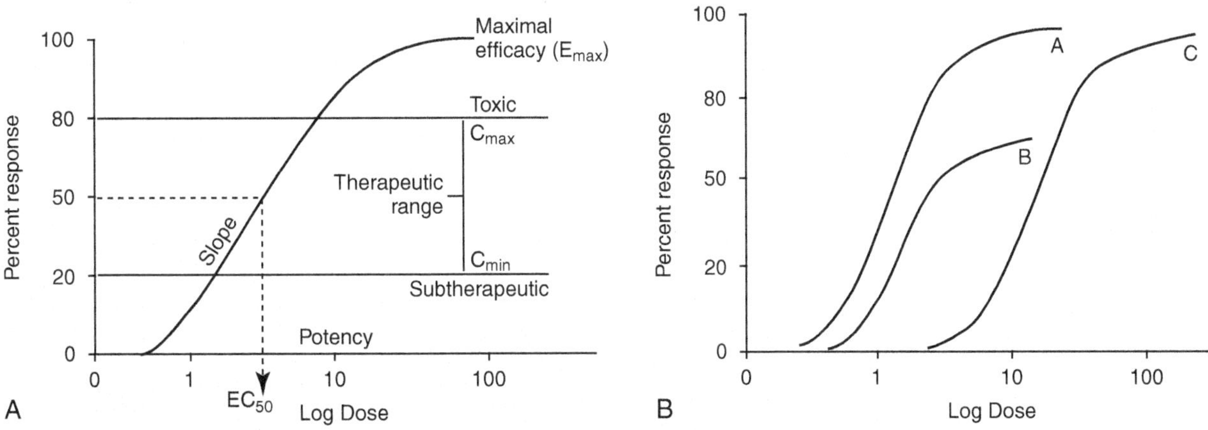

Figure 1-3 Drugs that are equally effective will cause the maximum response but may not be equally potent, i.e., they may not have the same relationship between dose (concentration) and response (**A**). Because drugs A and C result in the same maximum response (E_{max}), they are equally effective, whereas drug B is less effective (**B**). However, drug B is more potent than drug C, and drug A is more potent than both because the dose or concentration of A necessary to achieve a 50% maximum response (ED_{50} or EC_{50}) is less than that for B or C. A similar set of curves can be used to describe competitive and noncompetitive inhibition. A drug that noncompetitively inhibits another drug will prevent it from reaching its maximum effect, and thus decrease the E_{max} (plot B, with noncompetitive drug present, plot A without it). In contrast, a drug that competitively inhibits another drug will not alter its E_{max}, but will increase the concentration of the drug necessary to achieve it (plot C represents a drug with a competitor present; plot A, drug without competitor).

through actions at the same pathway, although this does not have to occur at the receptor. Like an agonist, an **antagonist** interacts selectively with receptors, but it lacks intrinsic efficacy and thus is able to block or reduce the action of an agonist at the receptor. Drugs that target opioid receptors (at least three types, with mu receptors having at least two subtypes) offer an example of the different sequelae of drug–receptor interactions. The "**full**" agonist (e.g., fentanyl) results in the maximal effect (e.g., at mu receptors). A drug that acts as a "**reversal**" agent would reduce the effect of an exogenous agonist (e.g., naloxone reverses the effects of fentanyl) whereas a "**blocking**" drug antagonizes endogenous agonists (e.g., catecholamines targeted by beta- or alpha-blockers). Drugs might have dual agonist and antagonist properties at the same receptor (although to variable degrees in different tissues). Because the response is not maximal, they are referred to as **partial (low-efficacy) agonists**; buprenorphine is a partial agonist opioid at mu receptors. Drugs might also act as an agonist at some receptors and an antagonist at other receptors. Butorphanol is a **mixed agonist/antagonist** (at kappa and mu receptors, respectively).

The relationship between an antagonist and receptor can be described as competitive or noncompetitive. Competition between compounds occurs at the same receptors and can be reversible or irreversible. **Reversible** antagonists easily dissociate from the receptor, whereas **irreversible** antagonists form a stable chemical bond with the receptor (e.g., in alkylation). If the interaction is reversible, an agonist present at sufficiently high concentrations can displace an antagonist. As such, reversal of the agonist or the response may require a higher dose (or a repeat dose) of the antagonist (see Figure 1-3, *B*). In contrast, an irreversible antagonist cannot be displaced from the receptor. As such, the cellular response can not occur until the receptor is replaced (duration dependent on rate of receptor turnover) and any remaining unbound antagonist has been removed from the body. The presence of a reversible competitive inhibitor will decrease the potency of a drug because a higher concentration will be necessary to induce the same pharmacologic response.

In contrast, the presence of an irreversible competitive inhibitor will decrease the efficacy of the drug by preventing the maximal possible response. In contrast to competitive antagonists, noncompetitive antagonists interact with receptors at a site different from the agonist–receptor interaction site. The interaction often involves a site in the transduction pathway between the receptor and the pharmacodynamic response.[1] Noncompetitive interactions are generally, but not always, reversible. Note that three other types of antagonism, in addition to pharmacodynamic, can occur between drugs: chemical antagonism results from a direct chemical interaction between two drugs (i.e., a weak acid and weak base), physiologic antagonism occurs when two drugs act in the same physiologic system but act on different receptors or pathways, and pharmacokinetic antagonism occurs when one drug alters the response to another drug through changes in disposition (see Chapter 2).

Pharmacodynamic responses are also influenced by the presence of drugs beyond activation. Receptor upregulation and downregulation is an adaptive mechanism that may affect clinical response. Sequelae may include but are not limited to **tachyphylaxis,** a rapidly decreasing response to a drug after administration of only a few doses; **tolerance**, a decreasing response to repeated constant doses of a drug that will necessitate a concentration and thus dose increase, if the response is to be maintained; and **withdrawal,** the syndrome of often painful physical and psychological symptoms that occurs when an addictive substance is discontinued.

The pharmacodynamic response to a drug ideally will occur with any given dose within a therapeutic range. The therapeutic range provides a target for the dosing regimen. It consists of a minimum effective plasma drug concentration (PDC) (**trough** or C_{min}), below which therapeutic failure is likely to occur, and a maximum effective PDC (**peak** or C_{max}), above which a type A adverse reaction (see Chapter 4) is more likely to occur (see Figures 1-1 and 1-3).[2,3] Dosing regimens are composed of a dose (e.g., mg/kg) and an interval (e.g., every 8 hours) for each route. The dose of the regimen generally is designed to achieve and maintain PDC within the therapeutic range throughout most of the dosing interval. Thus targeted peak PDCs often approximate but do not exceed C_{max}, whereas trough concentrations approximate but generally do not drop below C_{min}. However, a **therapeutic range** is a population statistic that describes the concentrations between which most animals will exhibit the (desired) pharmacodynamic response; each animal will respond (therapeutically or adversely) at a different point in the range. Although most animals will respond at some point within the range (the majority in the middle of the range), a small percentage will respond above or below the range. Therapeutic drug monitoring (see Chapter 5) is used to establish where in the therapeutic range the individual animal will respond; in other words, it will establish the patient's therapeutic range. Ideally, studies that determine the dosing regimen in a target species reflect integration of pharmacokinetic and pharmacodynamic studies in that species.[4] Two primary components of a dosing regimen are dose interval. In general, dose, which ultimately determines PDC, is influenced primarily by the tissue that dilutes the drug (i.e., volume of distribution), whereas interval is influenced by elimination of the drug (i.e., half-life). Unfortunately, studies that describe the time course of a drug in animals are limited and, when available, generally focus on healthy rather than diseased animals. As such, clinicians are faced with individualizing dosing regimens in the patient according to the principles of clinical pharmacology—that is, the study of drugs[5] and their behavior (disposition)[6] in animals.

DETERMINANTS OF DRUG DISPOSITION

Mechanisms of Drug Movement

Drugs move through the body by two major mechanisms: bulk flow and passive diffusion. The cardiovascular system is the primary determinant of bulk flow; glomerular filtration is one of the more important specific examples. The chemical nature of the drug does not affect bulk flow. Most drugs are characterized by a molecular weight (MW) of 350 or less, ensuring movement of unbound drug between endothelial cells despite the presence of protein filters in the endothelial gaps. Exceptions are made for those tissues whose capillaries are not fenestrated, because endothelial cell junctions are tight. Drug movement for these tissues must occur across cell membranes. Drugs can move through cells directly through the lipid layers of the cell (e.g., passive diffusion), through aqueous pores formed by aquaporins (proteins) that span the width of the membrane, by combination with transmembrane carrier proteins, and by pinocytosis. Of these, transmembrane (passive) diffusion and carrier-mediated movement are most important.

KEY POINT 1-1 Passive diffusion is the most common method by which compounds move through the body. It is most influenced by the concentration gradient of diffusible drug across the membrane to be diffused.

Passive diffusion occurs independent of any other mechanism of drug movement and requires no energy. Passive diffusion through cell membranes depends on a number of factors. The single most important factor is concentration of diffusible drug, which is most easily manipulated by increasing the dose. Additionally, host and drug factors will also influence the concentration of diffusible drug. Host determinants of passive diffusion are subject to change and include thickness of the membrane to be traversed (inversely proportional; e.g., edematous compared with normal tissues), surface area (directly proportional; e.g., small intestine versus stomach), environmental pH (see ionization), and temperature (directly proportional). In contrast, drug characteristics influencing passive diffusion are not subject to change, and thus cannot be easily manipulated. They largely influence lipid solubility of the drug.[2,3] Lipid solubility is, in turn, influenced by a number of drug characteristics, including the inherent chemical structure of a drug, such as molecular weight (smaller molecules diffuse more easily) and **partition coefficient** (PC). The PC is an experimental measure of relative lipid solubility as influenced by the chemical structure of the drug. The ratio is determined by mixing the drug in a combination of water and an organic solvent (e.g., octanyl). The difference in drug concentration between the two solvents once mixing is complete reflects, in part, the inherent lipid versus water solubility of the drug. Measurement of the concentration of drug in each solvent generates an octanyl:water coefficient or PC, which might be useful for predicting the ability of a drug to pass through cell membranes. A ratio greater than 1 suggests greater distribution to the organic phase, indicating lipid solubility. For example, in regards to providing analgesia, fentanyl (PC of 717) is both more potent and more rapid acting, but shorter in duration, compared to morphine (PC of 0.7), presumably because it can move more rapidly through the blood–brain barrier (Figure 1-4). Benzene rings, carbon double bonds and methyl groups tend to make a drug more lipid soluble, whereas polar compounds such as amine or hydroxyl groups contribute to drug-water solubility.

In addition to lipid solubility, drug pKa and environmental (host) pH will also influence distribution of drug into body compartments. The Henderson-Hasselbalch equation describes the pH partition theory (Figure 1-5). Assuming a drug is sufficiently lipid soluble to cross cell membranes, a steady-state equilibrium will be reached when the amount of drug moving from one area equals the amount moving in the opposite direction and the concentration of diffusible drug will be equivalent on either side of a membrane. However, in its ionized form, a drug is not diffusible, cannot traverse lipid membranes, and becomes trapped and thus "partitioned" by the pH in its surrounding environment. Although the concentration of the nonionized (diffusible) portion on each side of the membrane will be equal (assuming a steady state equilibrium is reached), the total concentration on either side may differ if the pH on either side of the membrane is different (Figure 1-5). The difference depends on the pKa of the drug and the environmental pH on either side of the membrane. Drugs will be trapped by ionization when present in an "unlike" environment. Drug pKa (the pH at which the drug is 50% ionized and 50% nonionized; ratio 1:1), and its behavior as a weak acid or base defines the degree of ionization. For a weak acid, as local pH decreases (becoming more "like"), the nonionized and thus diffusible proportion will increase. In contrast, for a weak acid, an increase in pH ("unlike") will increase the ionized proportion. The opposite is true for a weak base: increasing pH will increase the nonionized or diffusible proportion, whereas a pH decrease will increase the ionized, nondiffusible portion (Box 1-1).

KEY POINT 1-2 A drug will be more nonionized and more likely to diffuse into tissues when present in a "like" environment—that is, acidic drugs in an acidic environment.

Although less common, drug movements other than passive diffusion and bulk flow influence PDC. Carrier-mediated transport includes both facilitated diffusion (nonactive) or active transport. An example important transport system is the **P-glycoprotein** system, an MDR-1 gene product best known for imparting multidrug resistance to cancer cells (and to microbes).[7] However, this transport system occurs in several tissues in the body, including renal tubular brush borders and bile canniculi (responsible for drug excretion from the body); the brain or other "sanctuaries" (responsible for keeping exogenous componds out of critical tissues); characterized by a blood–tissue barrier; and in portals of entry, including the lower gastrointestinal tract (reducing oral drug bioavailability).[8] Pinocytosis is a rare drug movement exemplified by the uptake of vitamin B_{12} in the ileum and aminoglycosides by renal tubular cells.

Plasma Drug Concentrations

Although response to a drug reflects concentrations at the tissue (or cellular level), because tissue samples cannot be collected easily, drug concentrations at the tissue site are approximated by measuring PDCs. After administration of a fixed dose of a drug, several drug movements act in concert to determine PDC (Figure 1-6).[2,3,6,9] These movements largely, but not exclusively, depend on passive diffusion of the drug and include absorption (A) from the site of administration to

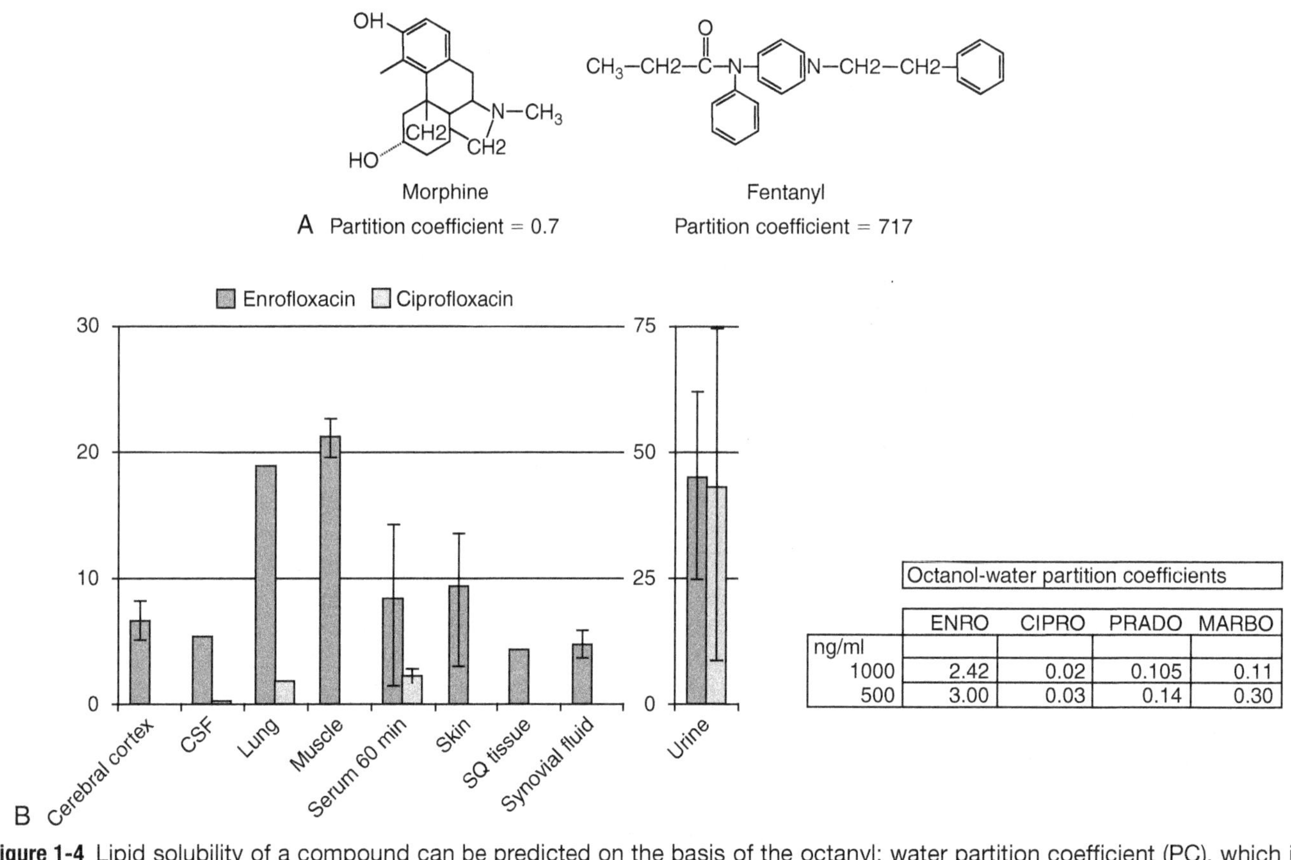

Octanol-water partition coefficients				
ng/ml	ENRO	CIPRO	PRADO	MARBO
1000	2.42	0.02	0.105	0.11
500	3.00	0.03	0.14	0.30

Figure 1-4 Lipid solubility of a compound can be predicted on the basis of the octanyl: water partition coefficient (PC), which in turn depends on chemical structure. **A,** Morphine and fentanyl both reach the central nervous system in sufficient quantity to provide analgesia. However, fentanyl is much more lipid soluble, as is supported by its octanyl:water partition coefficient of 717 compared with that of morphine (0.7). Fentanyl is much more potent and more rapid acting, but it also has a shorter duration of effect. **B,** The PC among the fluorinated quinolones suggests that enrofloxacin would have better tissue distribution than ciprofloxacin. This is supported by the relative concentrations of enrofloxacin versus ciprofloxacin in serum compared with tissues 60 minutes after administration of 20 mg/kg intravenous enrofloxacin in dogs. Although PC is an important determinant of lipid solubility, it may vary with surrounding pH. (ENRO, enrofloxacin; CIPRO, ciprofloxacin; PRADO, pradofloxacin; MARBO, marbofloxacin.)

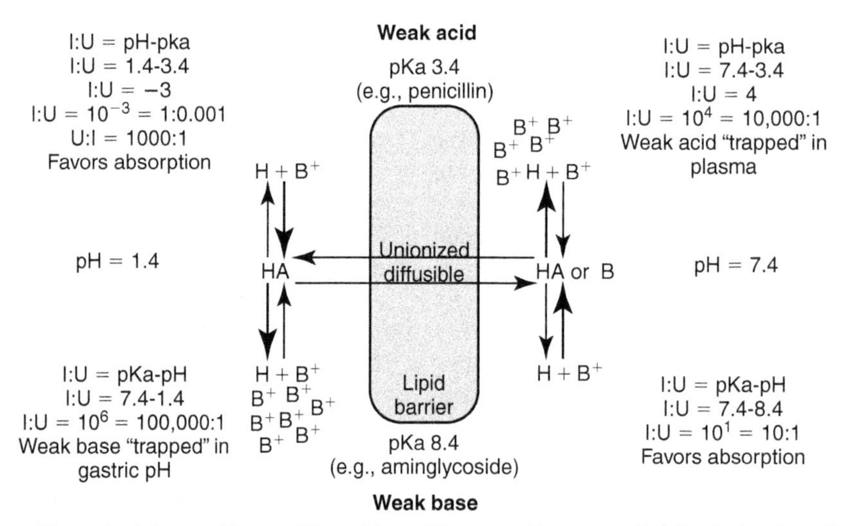

Figure 1-5 The Henderson-Hasselbalch equation and the pH partition hypothesis predict the behavior of an ionizable compound on the basis of its pKa and the ambient pH. A weak base (bottom) will be predominantly ionized in an acidic environment (i.e., gastric pH), and thus is likely to be trapped. It is less likely to be ionized in a higher pH and thus is more diffusible (i.e., plasma). In contrast, a weak acid (top) is likely to be nonionized in the acidic environment and thus is more likely than the weak base to move across the lipid membrane and be absorbed. However, in the plasma the higher pH will increase the proportion of ionized drug, limiting its diffusion from plasma into cells. (see Box 1-1.)

Box 1-1

The pH Partition Hypothesis

The **pH partition hypothesis** is the ratio of ionized:nonionized drug and is based on pH (of the environment) and pKa (of the drug) (see Figure 1-5). The proportion of ionized to unionized drug is described by the Henderson-Hasselbalch equation. For acids, the ratio (ionized:nonionized) is 10^n, and for a weak base the ratio is 10^{-n}. The ratio of the ionized:nonionized (I:U) drug can be useful for predicting movement between tissues. A drug is considered significantly ionized if the ratio (I:U) is greater than 100. Thus for a weak acid the drug is considered ionized in an environmental pH that is 2 or more higher than its pK_a (pH – pKa = 2; $10^n = 10^2 = 100$ I : 1 U) A weak base is considered ionized if the pH is or 2 or more below its pK_a.. (pH – pKa = -2; $10^{-n} = 10^{-(-2)} = 10^2 = 100$). Ideally, for drug movement to occur by passive diffusion, the pH will be no more than 2 pH units above the pKa for the acid and no more than 2 pH units below the pKa for the base. The gastrointestinal tract (pH 6.0) offers an example of how pH partition influences drug movement. Orally administered aminoglycosides (weak bases with pK_a approximating 7 to 9) are ionized at a ratio of approximately 1000:1 ($6 - 9 = -3$, $10^{-n} = 10^{-(-3)}$, = 10^3 = 1000:1 [I:U]. Thus there is only one nonionized or diffusible ion for each 1000 ionized amikacin molecules. The ionized molecules will be trapped and will not be absorbed, limiting absorption of this water-soluble drug. In contrast, the proportion of the ionized weak acid penicillin (pKa about 2) would be 0.0001:1 ($2 - 6 = 10^{-4}$); for every ionized molecule, 10,000 molecules would be nonionized (the inverse of 0.0001:1). As such, if other factors are supportive (e.g., the drug is not destroyed by the gastric acidity), penicillin should be well absorbed from the gastrointestinal tract. The urine is another site where pH partition may influence drug movement. Penicillin located in urine with a pH of 7 would be ionized at a ratio of 10,000:1 (10^5), whereas the aminoglycoside would be ionized at a ratio of only 100:1. If the urine pH was 8, the ratio of I:U would be 10 for the aminoglycoside, which is not considered significant to preclude drug movement. In either pH the aminoglycoside would be more likely than the penicillin to be passively resorbed and to penetrate microbial membranes. Drug that is partitioned by ionization acts as a reservoir, replacing nonionized drug that may leave the other side of the membrane in an open system. Eventually, assuming the nonionized side remains "open," both sides of the membrane will eventually be depleted of drug.

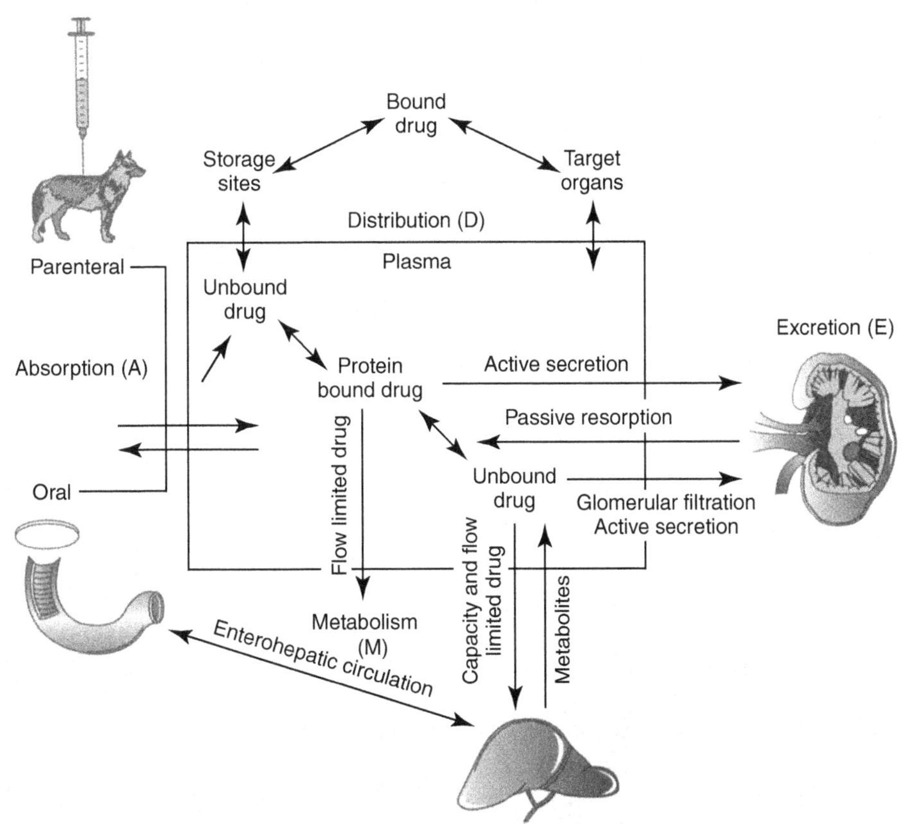

Figure 1-6 The determinants of plasma drug concentration (ADME) act in concert after administration of a fixed dose. The drug must first be absorbed, most commonly from the gastrointestinal tract (Absorption–A). Orally administered drug passes through the liver before reaching systemic circulation (not shown). Once in circulation, drug not bound to plasma proteins (free drug) is distributed into tissues (Distribution–D), where it can be bound to tissues or distributed back to circulation. Elimination of the drug from the body occurs by hepatic metabolism (Metabolism–M) and renal or biliary excretion (Excretion—E) of the drug or its metabolites. Drugs that are protein bound will not be filtered by the kidney or metabolized by the liver unless actively secreted in the kidneys and or characterized by flow-limitation in the liver. Excreted drugs can be passively reabsorbed by the kidney or following biliary excretion after deconjugation in the gastrointestinal drug (enterohepatic circulation). (Adapted from Ettinger SJ, Feldman EF, editors: *Textbook of veterinary internal medicine,* ed 5, Philadelphia, 2000, Saunders.)

systemic circulation, defined as the major vessels and well-perfused organs; distribution (D) of the drug from systemic circulation to tissues (target and nontarget) and back again; and elimination of the drug from the body by metabolism (M) and excretion (E). These drug movements are dynamic, occurring simultaneously, and their net effects determine PDC at any time during the dosing interval after administration of a fixed dose. Because passive diffusion is the major determinant of each drug movement, each in turn is influenced by a number of other factors. The impact of these factors on the drug movements and the time course of drug in the body as a result of these movements can be described or modeled mathematically, leading to the study of pharmacokinetics. Each drug movement is influenced by host and drug factors that may affect therapeutic success (see Chapter 2).

KEY POINT 1-3 Plasma drug concentrations at any point in time after administration of a dose reflect the combined effects of four dynamic drug movements: absorption, distribution, metabolism, and excretion.

Absorption

Bioavailability, extent, and rate of absorption. The percentage of an administered dose of drug that reaches systemic circulation and is thus able to induce a response is referred to as **bioavailability** (F).[2,3,9,10] Bioavailability (see Pharmacokinetics section) is used to predict drug efficacy after different routes of administration or administration of different formulations of the same drug. Absolute bioavailability or extent of absorption is the actual bioavailability and can be determined only by comparing the appearance of the drug preparation to that after intravenous administration of the drug. In contrast, relative bioavailability of two different preparations or by two routes of administration of the same drug can be evaluated by comparing their area under the curve (AUC).[10] The area under the concentration versus time curve (AUC) describes the entire time course of the drug. Because its magnitude depends on maximum drug concentration and rate of elimination, it is influenced by several drug movements, including absorption. The AUC is used to calculate several other pharmacokinetic parameters; clinically, it is useful for determining response to certain drugs, particularly antimicrobials.[11,12]

KEY POINT 1-4 Absolute bioavailability of a drug preparation can be determined only by comparing its appearance to 100% availability, which occurs only after intravenous administration.

The greater the bioavailability, or extent of absorption of a drug, the greater the anticipated pharmacologic response. However, pharmacologic response of two different drug preparations or the same drug given by different routes may vary even if equally bioavailable; two products are considered bioequivalent only if neither their rate nor their extent of absorption differ. Differences in the rate of absorption (e.g., absorption half-life [see Pharmacokinetics section]) may cause different time to onset, as well as lower peak concentrations, although the duration of effect may be longer.

Factors impacting drug absorption are most profound for orally administered drugs. Factors impacting other routes are addressed under "Routes of Administration."

Oral absorption. Most orally administered drugs reach systemic circulation after absorption from the small intestine. The rate and extent of drug absorption in the gastrointestinal tract depend on a number of host factors, most of which affect passive diffusion (Figure 1-7).[9] These include gastrointestinal pH, which favors absorption of weak acids; surface area, which favors absorption in the small intestine compared with the stomach; motility, which mixes the drug, the concentration of diffusible drug at the site of movement; permeability and thickness of the mucosal epithelium; and intestinal blood flow, which maintains the concentration gradient across the mucosal epithelium. The latter factor of blood flow is important only for drugs capable of rapid transfer across the epithelium.

In general, the intestinal surface area is so large that changes seldom are of sufficient magnitude to effect absorption (see Chapter 2). However, changing particle size of the drug preparation may cause differences in the rate or extent of absorption and markedly different bioequivalences. Drug preparations often are specifically designed to alter rates of absorption by manipulation of particle size.

Bioavailability of an orally administered drug also is influenced by factors after it passes into the gastrointestinal epithelium. Bioavailability is decreased if the drug is metabolized by intestinal epithelial cells, microbes, or by the liver. Additionally, enterocytes can decrease oral bioavailability of a drug by causing its efflux from enterocytes, in part because of the presence of active transport proteins located on enterocyte cell membranes.[13]

Transport membranes may act alone or in concert with one another; for some drugs, one transporter may predominate, but for others, none may. Identifying the role of each transporter protein is complicated and difficult to study. Several families have been identified. (1) Transporters located on the apical cell membrane include the family of organic anion-transporting polypeptides (OATPs); these proteins are also located in the liver, kidney, and brain and influence distribution and excretion. These proteins transport a large number of amphipathic drugs (e.g., digoxin, steroids) and endogenous compounds (e.g., steroids, thyroid hormones). (2) Proton-dependent oligopeptide transporters (POTs), driven by a proton gradient, are present in the kidney, brain, and the gastrointestinal tract, where their activity appears to increase from the duodenum to the ileum. Among the drugs influenced by these transporters are beta-lactam antimicrobials, ACE-inhibitors, and prodrugs of selected antivirals. (3) The family of ATP-binding cassette (ABC) superfamily of transporters includes the P-glycoproteins. These include multidrug resistance protein (MRP1) and a multispecific organic anion transporter (MOAT) also located in other tissues. An efflux transporter, P-glycoprotein is characterized by broad substrate specificity. Because it is abundant in enterocytes, it can profoundly decrease the oral bioavailability

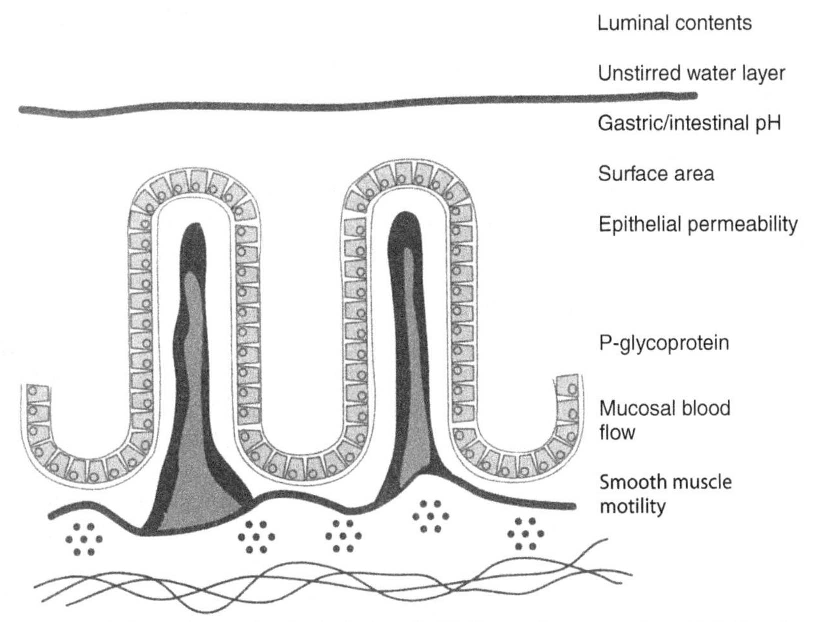

Figure 1-7 The determinants of oral drug absorption include local pH, the surface area to which the dissolved drug is presented, epithelial permeability, mucosal blood flow (particularly for drugs very rapidly absorbed), and smooth muscle motility. The drug must be diffusible, and thus must be in the dissolved state (to establish a concentration gradient). Most drugs are absorbed in the small intestine because of its larger surface area. The drug transport system, P-glycoprotein, decreases bioavailability through drug efflux from the intestinal epithelial cell.

of target drugs. It is associated and shares substrate specificity with selected cytochrome-P450 enzymes (most notably, CYP3A), which decreases drug that is not effluxed from the cell by the transporter (see Chapter 2).[13]

Hepatic metabolism also can profoundly affect the PDC of an orally administered drug. After gastrointestinal absorption, drugs enter the portal vein and then the liver (Figure 1-8). As such, an orally administered drug is exposed to hepatocytes before it enters the systemic circulation. Drugs characterized by a high hepatic extraction ratio (>70% extracted) are almost completely removed from the blood by hepatocytes during the first passage of blood through the liver. As a result, after oral administration, drugs that undergo first-pass metabolism may not reach systemic circulation in concentrations sufficiently high to cause a pharmacologic response. Despite good to excellent oral absorption, such drugs are characterized by poor bioavailability and are administered either parenterally (e.g., lidocaine) or in oral doses high enough to compensate for first-pass metabolism by the liver. Examples of drugs that are orally administered yet undergo significant hepatic first-pass metabolism include selected cardiac drugs (e.g., propranolol and other beta-blockers, diltiazem in some species, hydralazine, nitroglycerin), diazepam, and opioid analgesics. The negative effects of first-pass metabolism on pharmacologic response may be reduced if the drug metabolites (e.g., propranolol and diazepam) are also pharmacologically active.

Distribution

Once a drug reaches the systemic circulation, it must be distributed from the central (blood) compartment to peripheral tissues to impart a pharmacologic effect. Further, drug

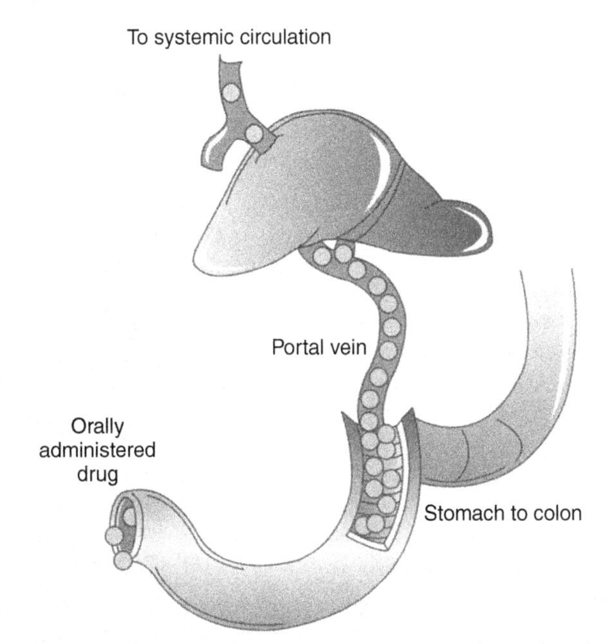

Figure 1-8 First-pass metabolism occurs as drug absorbed from the gastrointestinal tract (from the stomach to the lower colon) enters the portal vein and flows to the liver. Once in the liver, drugs that are characterized by a high extraction are removed rapidly from the blood before entering systemic circulation. Plasma concentrations of such drugs may not reach therapeutic concentrations unless the dose is increased to compensate for first-pass metabolism. The amount of drug removed on the first pass from the liver differs among species and ages and according to the presence or absence of disease. First-pass metabolism can be avoided by transmucosal absorption in the oral cavity, or rectal absorption.

in tissues will be distributed back into plasma so that it can be eliminated. The major factors that determine drug distribution to and from tissues include drug lipid solubility and its ability to penetrate cell membranes, the degree to which the drug is bound to plasma or tissue proteins, and regional (organ) blood flow. The presence of transport proteins (p-glycoprotein, OATPs, and POTs) also influence drug distribution, particularly in "sanctuary" tissues characterized by tissue–blood barriers (e.g., brain, cerebrospinal fluid, placenta).[13]

Binding of lipid-soluble drugs to plasma proteins facilitates their circulation. Drug binding to proteins may influence several determinants of drug movement, including distribution.[14] Weakly acidic drugs tend to bind to albumin, whereas weakly basic drugs tend to bind to α_1-glycoproteins.[15] The large molecular weight of protein precludes movement of bound drug from circulation into tissues. As such, the protein-bound drug is not pharmacologically active; cannot be filtered in the normal glomerulus, and for some drugs (i.e., capacity-limited, discussed later), cannot reach drug metabolizing enzymes in the hepatocyte (or other organ). Presumably, drugs that are highly protein bound may be more likely to be involved in adverse reactions early in the dosing regimen because displacement of only a small proportion of drug from the protein (e.g., due to competition with other protein-bound drugs or hypoalbuminemia) can increase the total amount of free, active drug (Figure 1-9).[2,3] A drug is considered significantly (highly) protein bound if 80% or more bound; for a drug bound less than 80%, displacing enough drug to significantly increase the unbound proportion is difficult. For example, displacement of only 1% of a drug that is 99% protein bound (e.g., nonsteroidal antiinflammatories) can double the concentration of pharmacologically active drug. In contrast, to double the pharmacologically active form of a drug that is only 80% bound (i.e., going from 20% to 40% unbound) would require displacement of 25% of the bound drug, which is clinically difficult to achieve. Yet even with highly protein-bound drugs, the clinical relevance of displacement and increased concentrations of unbound drug is questionable: in the face of normal renal and hepatic function, clearance of the freed drug by these organs will increase such that "extra" drug is rapidly removed.[16] However, it is not clear that clearance will increase sufficiently in the face of organ dysfunction (e.g., renal or liver disease). Further, the package insert for Converia, which is highly protein bound, indicates that the plasma drug concentration of several other highly protein bound drugs increased with co-administration.

KEY POINT 1-6 If a protein-bound drug is displaced from its binding protein, the increase in concentration of free and thus active drug is likely to be short-lived as the free drug is cleared more rapidly in the normal animal, thus potentially offsetting any risk associated with increased concentration.

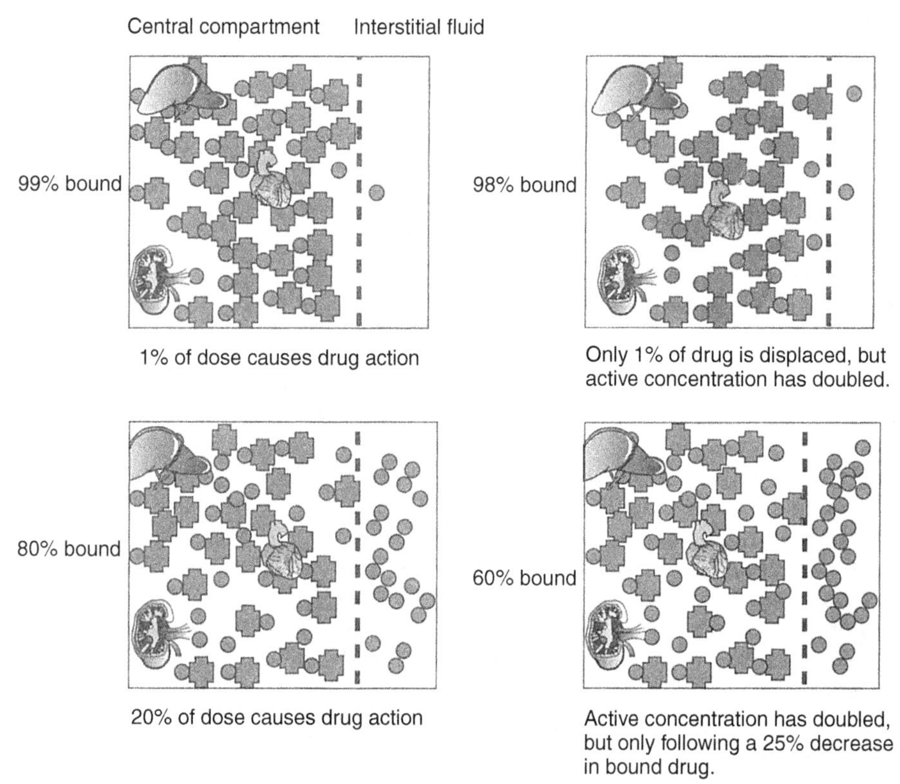

Figure 1-9 Displacement of drug from protein-binding sites becomes significant only if a drug is greater than 80% protein bound. Displacement of only 1% of a drug that is 99% protein bound doubles the pharmacologically active form of the drug (top two diagrams). For a drug that is 80% protein bound, however, 20% of the dose is responsible for pharmacologic actions. Displacement of 25% of the drug is necessary to double the pharmacologically active drug. However, because unbound drug will be cleared more rapidly (assuming normal organ function), displacement of highly bound drugs may not be clinically important.

In addition to its ability to reach target tissues and organs of elimination, distribution of a drug is important because of its influence on PDC and drug elimination. The amount of tissue to which a drug is distributed, often estimated by the theoretical parameter, **volume of distribution** (Vd) of the drug, directly but inversely influences PDC.[2,3,17] Because it is theoretical, Vd is generally referred to as *apparent* Vd. The Vd of a drug also describes the ease with which the drug leaves the plasma. Simplistically, volume of distribution is also the volume to which a drug would have to be distributed if it were present throughout the body in the same concentration as that measured in the plasma after intravenous (IV) administration of a known dose. It can be exemplified by adding 5 g of dextrose (considered the dose) to each of two beakers containing a different but unknown volume of water. The dextrose is allowed to distribute equally throughout the beaker (no membranes are present in the beaker) and then the concentration is measured. If the concentration in beaker A is 5% (50 mg/mL or 5 g/100 mL), then the volume of water in the beaker must be 100 mL. If the concentration in beaker B is 2.5% (25 mg/mL or 25 g/100 mL), the volume must be 200 mL. The Vd in beaker A is twice that in beaker B. The Vd of a drug in an animal is determined essentially the same way: a known dose is given intravenously to ensure that all the drug reaches the site being measured, the drug is allowed to distribute until equilibrium (or pseudo-equilibrium) is reached, and the peak drug concentration is determined. The Vd is then calculated by dividing the dose by the peak concentration (the y intercept, Co, A or B): Vd = Dose/Co (see the Pharmacokinetics section).

The PDC (and response to) a drug at a known dose varies inversely with Vd. Vd differences among species and ages (pediatric versus geriatric) can dramatically affect PDC (see Chapter 2). In addition, diseases associated with fluid retention or obesity are likely to increase the Vd of many drugs (and thus decrease PDC), whereas dehydration or weight loss is likely to decrease Vd and thus increase PDC (see Chapter 2). The impact depends upon whether the drug is distributed to total body water (i.e., a lipid-soluble drug) or extracellular fluid (i.e., a water-soluble drug). Because the distribution of a drug to peripheral tissues removes drugs from organs of drug clearance, Vd also directly and proportionately influences elimination half-life (Figure 1-10). Thus any factor that increases Vd will tend to decrease PDC but prolong the elimination half-life and thus the presence of the drug in the body.

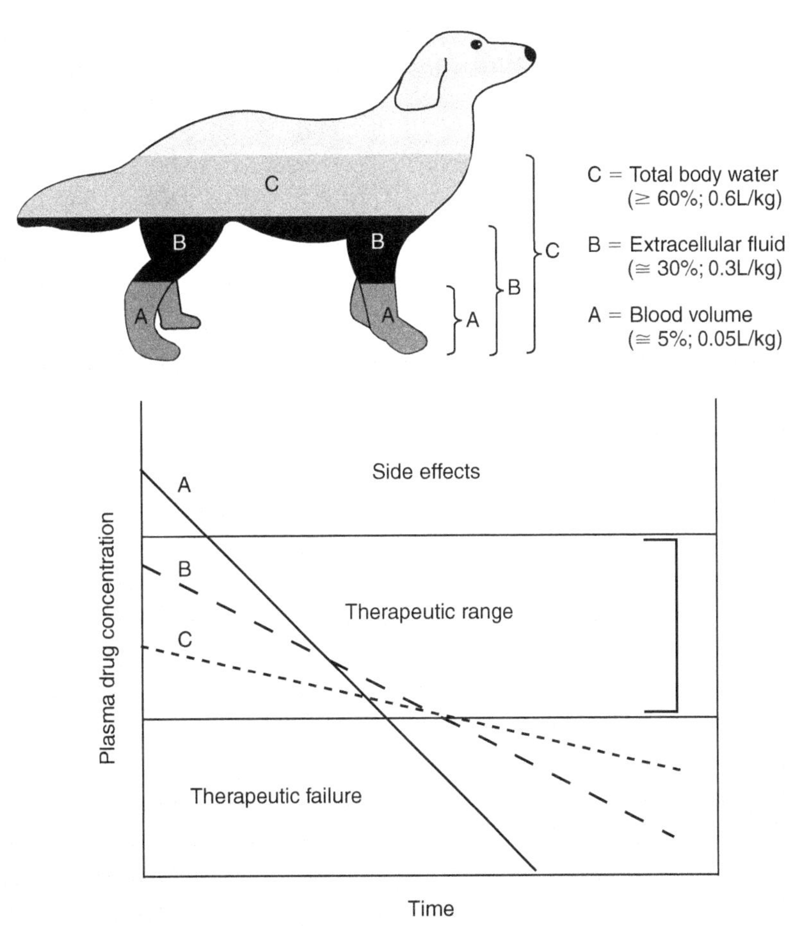

Figure 1-10 Despite its theoretical nature, the size of the apparent volume of distribution (Vd) may indicate the body compartment to which the drug is distributed. These include **(A)** the blood compartment (i.e., a drug tightly bound to plasma proteins), **(B)** extracellular fluid (e.g., a water-soluble drug), or **(C)** total body water (i.e., a liphophilic drug that penetrates cell membranes). Increasingly larger volumes represented by these compartment inversely affect plasma drug concentration (PDC) and the slope of the elimination (k_{el}) curve. This curve determines elimination half-life, which changes directly with Vd.

If a semipermeable membrane divided the beakers used to exemplify Vd into two compartments, distribution of the dextrose throughout each beaker would have taken longer than if the membrane were not present. At distribution equilibrium, (the amount of drug moving from one side equals the amount of drug moving from the other side. Further, at equilibrium, although the amount of drug passing between the two compartments is equal, membrane or fluid characteristics result in different concentrations of drug on each side of the membrane after equilibrium has been reached. Thus both the rate (i.e., distribution half-life) and extent of drug distribution may be affected by membranes. The body contains many membranes whose characteristics are sufficiently complex that multiple compartments may be formed. Extracellular and intracellular compartments (which together make up total body water) are major compartments to which drugs distribute. Most capillaries are fenestrated and present no barrier to passage of unbound drugs from plasma to interstitial fluid. Hence water-soluble drugs tend to be distributed to extracellular fluid (ECF; 20% to 30% of body weight) and thus are often characterized by a Vd of 0.1 to 0.3 L/kg. Lipid-soluble drugs tend to cross cell membranes and thus distribute into both ECF and intracellular fluid (ICF; i.e., total body water [TBW]) and as such, generally have a larger Vd (>0.6 L/kg). The Vd of highly protein-bound drugs reflects the plasma compartment, and as such is very small (0.05% of the body weight, or 0.05 L/kg). Such drugs may appear to distribute to their total volume almost instantaneously, resulting in a PDC versus time described by a single component, or a one compartment model (see the pharmacokinetics section). However, it is the Vd of the unbound or pharmacologically active drug that is more descriptive of the disposition and pharmacologic effects of a highly bound drug.

Capillaries of selected organs, including the brain, cerebrospinal fluid, eye, testis, and prostate, are not fenestrated, and drugs must diffuse through the capillary endothelium to penetrate these tissues.[18,19] For treatment of such organs, lipid-soluble drugs (i.e., Vd >0.6 L/kg) are more likely than water-soluble drugs to penetrate the endothelial barrier and achieve therapeutic concentrations. However, simply because a drug has a Vd that equals or exceeds the volume of TBW does not assure lipid solubility nor does it guarantee sufficient tissue distribution. Drug distribution to various tissues differs with drug chemistry, and intracellular accumulation may occur for many reasons. Ion trapping was previously discussed; drugs also can bind to intracellular proteins (i.e., Na+ K+ ATPase of digoxin), bone (e.g., Ca^{2+} or Mg^{+} by tetracyclines) or other macromolecules (e.g., lysozymes by aminoglycosides). Bound drug is generally not active (unless binding occurs to target ligands), but bound drug may act as a reservoir for interstitial and plasma drug concentration (e.g., the antimicrobial cefovecin). Ion trapping or binding of a drug will remove it from plasma; as such, as PDC decreases, for any given dose, the Vd will increase. The Vd of a drug characterized by such multicompartments may result in a Vd that is greater than the volume of the animal (e.g., >1 L/kg). Such a drug exemplifies the theoretical nature of Vd in that it simply (mathematically) describes the amount of tissue that is diluting the drug if the concentrations measured in plasma were the same throughout the body. Although Vd is a useful parameter, particularly for calculating drug dose, it should not be used to indicate where (i.e., ECF, ICF, TBW, or selected tissues) a drug has distributed. Further, because the rate and extent of drug distribution to tissues varies, the time to equilibrium also will vary. Calculations for Vd (and determining peak PDC) generally should not occur until distribution equilibrium has been reached.

KEY POINT 1-5 Volume of distribution is used to calculate the dose by estimating the volume of tissue that will dilute the drug after its intravenous administration. It is theoretical because it provides no information regarding the site of distribution. However, it proportionately impacts plasma drug concentration (inversely) and elimination half-life (directly).

The term **distribution equilibrium,** or steady-state equilibrium, is often used to refer to the state in which the amount of drug leaving plasma for tissues is equivalent to the amount of drug leaving tissues for plasma. The reality is that distribution equilibrium may not ever be achieved because drugs are characterized by an "open" system—that is, drug is continually being eliminated. Hence, the term *pseudoequilibrium* is more appropriate. Distribution equilibrium is less likely to be achieved for drugs with a short half-life, particularly when administered at a long dosing interval. Drugs that accumulate (given at a dosing interval that is shorter than the half-life; see later discussion) are more likely to reach a state of equilibrium between doses, although the actual concentrations may fluctuate between C_{max} and C_{min} during a dosing interval.

Documenting the extent to which a drug distributes to a specific site is difficult because techniques are required that allow collection of interstitial versus intracellular tissue. Measurement of drug in interstitial fluid or ICF might confirm the site of drug distribution. However, collecting a sample of sufficient size using methods that are not traumatic (and thus do not impact drug movement) is difficult. Several techniques have been developed to collect fluid representative of ECF. Examples include tissue cage models; "wick" methods; and more recently and perhaps most appropriately, the use of microfiltration systems that collect directly from ECF using a microprobe. A less representative method of reporting tissue concentrations is measurements of drug in homogenized tissues; this measures both extracellular and intracellular drug. Drugs bound (trapped) inside a cell (e.g., as a result of binding to proteins, or ionization) may markedly increase drug concentrations in homogenized tissue, but the drug may not be pharmacologically active or available to interstitial tissues. However, intracellular drug may act as a reservoir, providing continued input to interstitial fluid even as PDCs decline. Drug-void cells, on the other hand, will artificially dilute actual drug concentrations in the ECF.

Thiobarbiturates and propofol undergo a phenomenon of **redistribution**, relevant only for drugs for which an immediate effect can be realized (i.e., general anesthetics). After a rapid intravenous bolus administration of these drugs, they distribute first into a "central blood pool" composed of low-volume, high-blood-flow organs such as the brain. Anesthetic

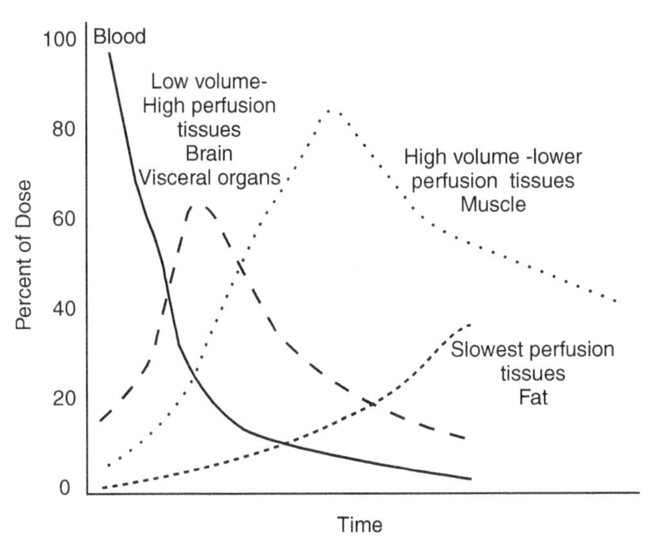

Figure 1-11 The phenomenon of redistribution involves the rapid distribution of drugs to a central blood pool composed of low-volume, high-blood-flow organs such as the brain followed by rapid redistribution to lean tissues. Further redistribution to fatty tissues further reduces plasma drug concentration and thus the pharmacologic effect. Sight hounds tend to have a prolonged recovery with these drugs because redistribution to the fat compartment is less. The effects of these drugs are also magnified in the presence of hypovolemic shock because a higher percentage of blood containing the drug flows to the brain and heart.

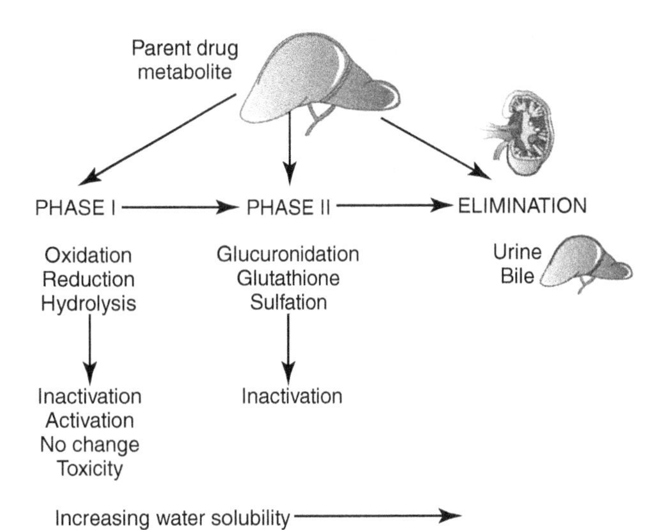

Figure 1-12 Hepatic metabolism can occur in one, two, or multiple phases. Phase I reactions are oxidative, most often accomplished by cytochrome-P450 (hepatic microsomal) enzymes. Phase I metabolites may be subjected to either phase I or phase II metabolism. Although phase I metabolites may be inactivated, they may also be the only active form of the drug (prodrugs). Metabolites may also exhibit similar, less, or more activity compared to the parent compound. Finally, they can also be an important source of drug-induced toxicity. Phase II metabolism generally inactivates the drug. The rate and extent of both phases of metabolism vary among species, ages, and disease states.

effects occur rapidly. However, the drug effect rapidly terminates, primarily because of redistribution from the brain to lean tissues such as muscle (Figure 1-11). Continued redistribution to fatty tissues further reduces PDC and thus the pharmacologic effect; sight hounds (which lack body fat) tend to have a prolonged recovery with these drugs. The effects of these drugs are also magnified in the presence of hypovolemic shock because a higher percentage of blood containing the drug flows to the brain and heart.

Drugs that distribute to TBW may take longer than distribution to ECF. Clinically, peak PDC (C_{max}) cannot be assessed until distribution has reached equilibrium (or pseudo-equilibrium). If PDCs are being monitored in a patient, blood samples for peak drug concentrations should not be collected until this time. For orally administered drugs, distribution occurs during absorption and sampling should occur after absorption is complete, generally within 1 to 2 hours after administration.

Metabolism

The rate at which a drug is excreted from the body is the final determinant of PDC. Most drugs are eliminated by hepatic metabolism, renal excretion, or both.[2,3] Lipid-soluble drugs require conversion to a water-soluble form before they can be eliminated by the kidney; otherwise, their passive resorption in the renal tubules would preclude excretion. A single change in the molecular structure of a lipid-soluble drug to a more water-soluble form may reduce a half-life of weeks or months to only a few hours. Metabolism can occur in two phases (Figure 1-12). Drugs or their metabolites may undergo both phases or only phase II metabolism. In general, phase I metabolism chemically changes the drug so that it is more water soluble and thus more susceptible to phase II metabolism; phase II metabolism generally renders the drug sufficiently water soluble to be renally excreted. An exception is made for some phase II metabolites (e.g., selected acetylated compounds) that may not only remain reactive but also may be more lipid soluble than the conjugated metabolite.

KEY POINT 1-7 Perhaps more so than any other factor affecting drug disposition, drug metabolism is complicated by physiologic, pharmacologic, and pathologic factors.

The majority of drug metabolism occurs in the liver. However, the liver is not the only site of drug-metabolizing enzymes; other organs with substantial metabolic capacity attributable to CYP or other enzymes include the kidney and portals of entry (i.e., lungs, skin, and gastrointestinal tract). Most drug-metabolizing enzymes are located in the smooth endoplasmic reticulum (SER) of the hepatocyte; others are located in the cytosol of the cell. Those located in the SER generally consist of a protein (cytochrome) with an iron central core (pigmented like hemoglobin, hence "P") that, when bound to carbon monoxide, absorbs light at 450 nm; as such, the isozymes are referred to as *cytochrome P450 enzymes (CYP450* or simply *CYP).* When the liver is subjected to homogenization and special centrifugation procedures, the SER forms vesicles or microsomes that contain drug-metabolizing enzymes; hence these enzymes also are referred to as *microsomal drug-metabolizing enzymes.* These enzymes are actually an enzyme system that can be identified genetically as a superfamily containing several families of enzymes.[20-23] Classification and nomenclature of CYP450 is based on gene sequence similarity. The importance of enzymes in humans and the proportion of drugs metabolized by the respective enzyme are 1A2 (13%), 2A6 (4%), 2B6 (1%), 2C (18%), 2D6 (1.5%), 2E1 (7%), and 3A4 (30%). All CYP-mediated drug metabolic reactions involve the addition of a single atom of oxygen onto the substrate; as such the CYP drug-metabolizing system is actually an electron-transport system, and oxygen radicals are generated during the metabolic process. Iron serves as a mechanism for separating molecules of oxygen; a lipid environment, (NADP reductase serves as the electron donor) and oxygen are required for CYP-catalyzed metabolism to occur. Not surprisingly, overlap among drug substrates for the different isozymes is among the reasons that isoenzyme activity can not be predictably extrapolated among species. Inducers and inhibitors differ in normal animals, among species, breeds, ages and gender, as well as tissue. Different concentrations of the various isoenzymes in tissues contribute to tissue specificities of some drug toxicities. The patterns of drug metabolism are complex, and the sequelae of the reactions variable. Drugs can be metabolized through several pathways, and metabolites often are further metabolized; metabolic pathways can also go backward to previous metabolites.

The major phase I drug-metabolizing reactions include oxidation (addition of oxygen across a carbon double bond [including on a benzene ring], addition of oxygen to a carbon chain, or deamination), hydrolysis (addition of water), and reduction (addition of hydrogen) (Figure 1-13).

The sequela of phase I metabolism commonly is drug inactivation (e.g., phenobarbital). However, phase I metabolites often are equally, more (i.e., primidone or prodrugs, which must be activated such as enalapril), or less (e.g., diazepam, cyclosporine) active than the parent compound. More problematic, phase I metabolites often are reactive

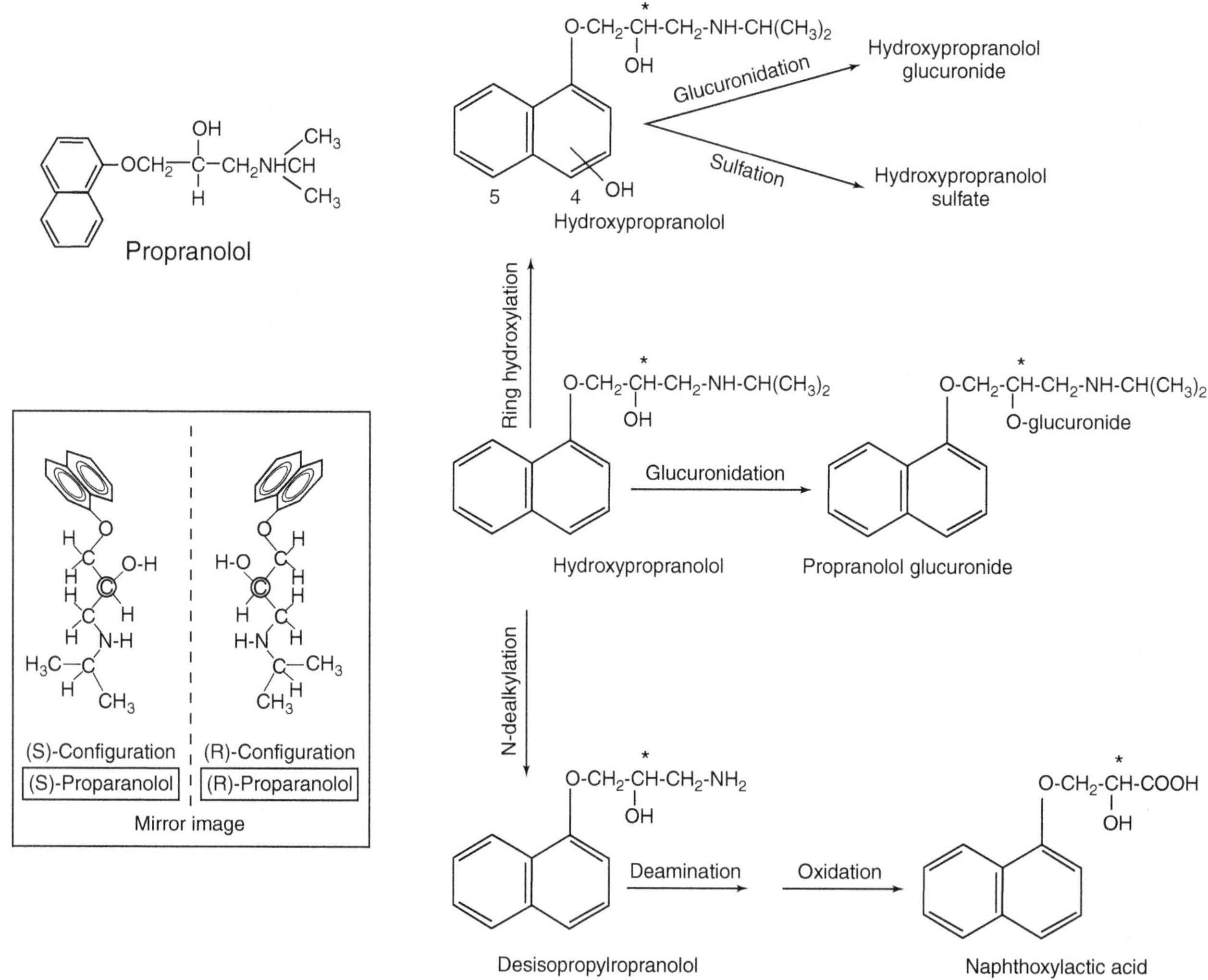

Figure 1-13 Propranolol offers an example of complex metabolism. Hepatic metabolism of propranolol follows multiple pathways, including both phase I (formation of hydroxyl propranolol) and phase II (glucuronidation). Propranolol contains a chiral carbon *(asterisk)* resulting in enantiomers *(inset).* Each will potentially be metabolized by different pathways.

(e.g., oxygen radicals) and thus are more toxic (e.g., acetaminophen) than the parent compound (see Chapter 3).[23,24] In such instances, phase II metabolism is critical to protecting the liver (or other metabolizing tissue) from metabolic products.

Phase II metabolism, also known as **conjugation,** occurs when a large water-soluble molecule is chemically added to either the parent drug or its phase I metabolite; this phase is often referred to as *synthetic* (see Figure 1-13). Generally, with the exception of glutathione transferase, phase II reactions require energy. As with phase I enzymes, families of enzymes catalyze each of the synthetic reactions. Glucuronidation is the most common phase II reaction; common substrates include OH and COOH functional groups (see Figure 1-13). The cat is deficient in some (but not all) glucuronide synthetic enzymes and as such does not eliminate phenols or carboxylic acids well (see Chapter 2). Glucuronide conjugates are eliminated in the urine and bile; degradation in the gastrointestinal tract and reabsorption of the substrate results in enterohepatic circulation. The glutathione transferase system targets electrophiles (compounds seeking electrons) and as such has several different roles in the body, including detoxification of radical metabolites. However, the enzyme can be rapidly depleted, which increases the risk of liver, red blood cell, or other tissue damage; n-acetylcysteine is a precursor for glutathione that can be used to replenish the system. Sulfonation targets hydroxyl groups and as such compensates somewhat for glucuronide deficiencies in cats. Acetylation is a less common synthetic reaction; sulfonamides are common substrates. The dog is a poor acetylator (see Chapter 2). With rare exceptions, phase II metabolites are inactive. The most common exception is with acetylation, which may result in formation of active metabolites (e.g., procainamide). Most hepatic drug metabolites are excreted in the urine, although some conjugated drugs undergo biliary excretion. Such drugs are potentially subject to enterohepatic circulation. Species (and no doubt breed) differences in both phase I and phase II metabolism are well recognized but insufficiently described (see Chapter 2).

Exogenous products are not the only substrates for drug-metabolizing enzymes. Many metabolic reactions are critical to formation or degradation of endogenous substances. Important noncytochrome metabolic enzymes include those that oxidize aldehydes or alcohols (esterases: e.g., acetylcholinesterases), monoamine oxidases (responsible for metabolism of endogenous catecholamines, dopamine, and related molecules) and dehydrogenases (alcohol and aldehyde) responsible for many endogenous reactions.

Factors that can affect hepatic drug metabolism include the amount and activity of drug-metabolizing enzymes and, if the drug is characterized by a high extraction ratio (>70%, a flow-limited drug), and hepatic blood flow. For flow-limited drugs, removal by drug-metabolizing enzymes is so rapid that the only limitation to the rate of elimination is blood flow. In contrast, extraction of capacity-limited drugs is slow. Protein binding directly decreases the clearance and thus rate of elimination of capacity-limited, but not flow-limited, drugs. Disease, drug interactions, and species differences can have a profound impact on drug metabolism and thus drug elimination (see Chapter 2).

Enantiomers and Drug Disposition

Whenever a carbon atom has four different structures bonded to it, two different molecules can be formed. Stereoisomers are chemical compounds with the same molecular formula that differ only by the orientation of functional groups in space around the central atom (e.g., carbon). Enantiomers are stereoisomers that differ due to orientation of four different groups around a single carbon (or phosphorous or nitrogen) atom and are nonsuperimposable mirror images of one another (Figure 1-14). The center atom around which the asymmetry occurs is referred to as the *chiral molecule.* The enantiomers are differentiated as to either D (dextrorotatory) or L (levorotatory). More commonly, they are defined by the direction in which they rotate light. As such, they are "optical isomers": if one enantiomer rotates light to the left (S, or sinister [counterclockwise]), the other will rotate it to the right (R, rectus [clockwise]) the same number of degrees. The only physical difference between enantiomers is the direction in which they rotate light. However, although the physical characteristics of enantiomers are similar, the pharmacodynamics (including both potency and efficacy) and pharmacokinetics (all phases of disposition) may be profoundly different for each isomer. Most enantiomeric drugs are sold as racemic mixtures (generally 50:50), and administration of such drugs represents polypharmacy.[25] Further complicating enantiomer disposition is the potential for each enantiomer to be converted to the other after administration. Species differences are likely to be profound. Unfortunately, analysis of enantiomers in tissue samples is difficult: they are so physically similar that their physical separation and thus quantitation from one another is difficult. Examples of drugs that exist as enantiomers include selected anthelmintics, verapamil, ketamine, inhalant anesthetics (isoflurane), selected cardiac drugs (e.g., beta blockers, including propranolol [see Figure 1-13], albuterol, and others), and a number of nonsteroidal antiinflammatories (e.g., the profens [ketoprofen, carprofen]). Occasionally, the name of a drug indicates it is a sole isomer (e.g., levofloxacin is the L isomer of ofloxacin.)

Excretion

Renal excretion is the most important route of drug elimination for both parent (especially water soluble) drugs and their metabolites (Figure 1-15).[2,3,26,27] Host factors that determine renal excretion include renal blood flow (including glomerular filtration rate), active tubular secretion, and tubular (generally passive) reabsorption. The kidney is also capable of metabolizing some drugs (e.g., imipenem), although this capacity is only occasionally of clinical importance.

Glomerular filtration is a passive process. Drugs enter the glomerulus by bulk flow, being excluded if too large (> 60,000 MW) as occurs for highly protein-bound drug if the glomerulus is healthy. In contrast, active transport of drugs in the proximal tubules is very efficient, rapid, and insensitive to protein binding. However, it is susceptible to competition among drugs. Separate active transport (p-glycoprotein,

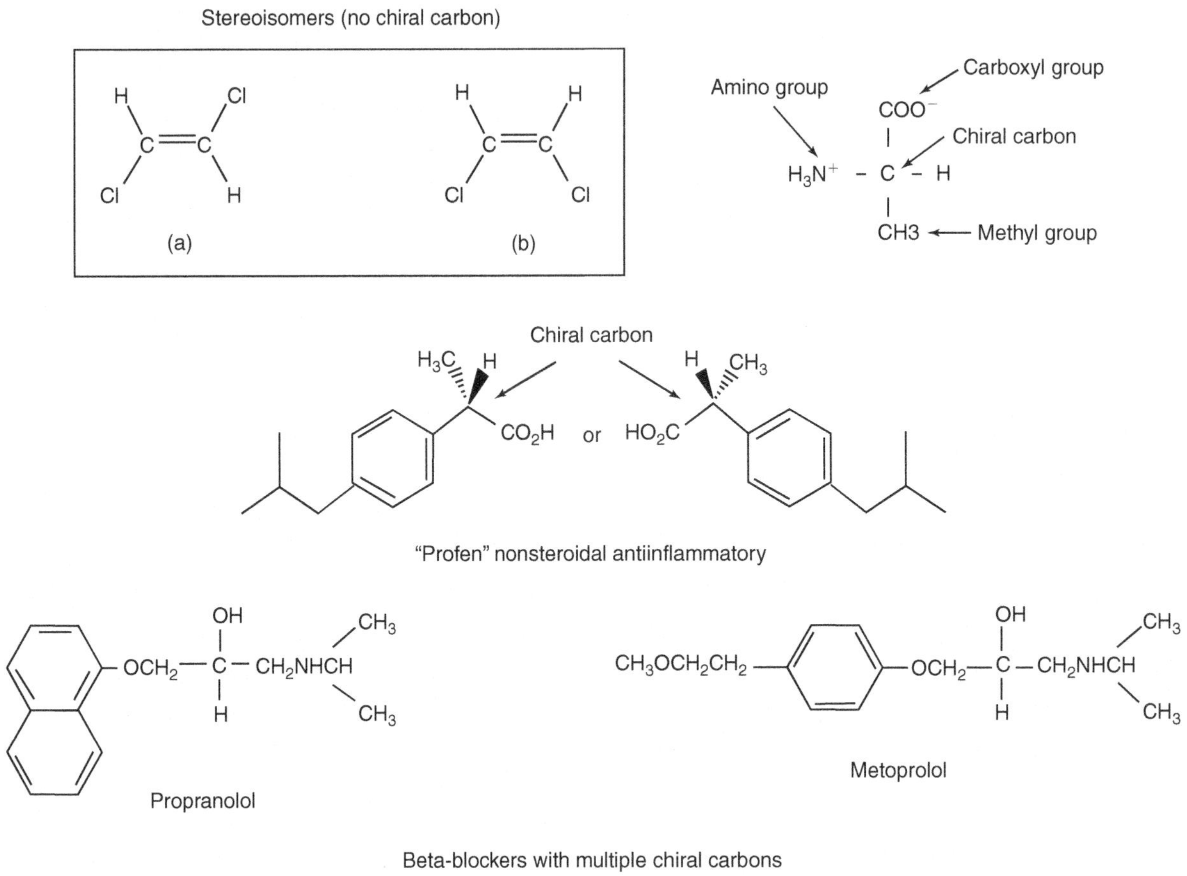

Stereoisomers (no chiral carbon)

(a) (b)

Amino group, Carboxyl group, Chiral carbon, Methyl group

Chiral carbon

"Profen" nonsteroidal antiinflammatory

Propranolol

Metoprolol

Beta-blockers with multiple chiral carbons

Figure 1-14 Enantiomers are stereoisomers that exist as mirror images that are not superimposable because of the presence of a chiral carbon *(top)*. Rotation of the four groups attached to the chiral carbon results in either S or R isomers (depending on the rotation of light by each molecule). Although they are similar in MW and chemistry, the body often responds to and handles enantiomers differently. Most products are manufactured as racemic (1:1). Some compounds contain more than one chiral compound, complicating disposition. Further, interconversion among species contributes to the complexities that characterize the pharmacokinetics and thus predictability of disposition of these compounds. Examples of compounds that exist as stereoisomers include many nonsteroidal antiinflammatories *(middle)* or beta-blockers *(bottom)*. Commercial products often contain mixtures of both enantiomers of a drug. However, some drugs are marketed as only the active enantiomer and are often named to indicate as such (e.g., "levo" as in levetiracetam or "dextro" as in dextromethorphan).

OATPs, POTs) systems exist for acid, basic, and neutral drugs. Probenecid has been used clinically to compete with and thus inhibit the renal excretion of other weakly acidic drugs such as expensive beta-lactam antimicrobials (e.g., penicillin historically and imipenem more recently), thus prolonging therapeutic PDC. Reabsorption of drugs from renal tubules into peritubular capillaries slows renal excretion. The extent to which a drug is reabsorbed depends on its lipid solubility and its ionization. Weakly acidic drugs are more likely to be reabsorbed in acidic urine but are trapped and excreted in alkaline urine. Urinary pH can be therapeutically altered such that the renal excretion rate of a drug can be modified, particularly in cases of overdose or toxicity. Drugs excreted in the urine that do not undergo passive reabsorption will be progressively concentrated in the renal tubule. Tubular cells may be exposed to higher concentrations of drugs, which may increase the risk of nephrotoxicity. Drug concentration in the urine can be of therapeutic benefit in some situations, such as bacterial cystitis. Most antibacterials excreted in the urine achieve concentrations that exceed plasma at least tenfold (see Chapter 6); for such drugs, culture and susceptibility data and, in particular, minimum inhibitory concentrations based on PDC may underestimate efficacy if infection is limited to the urine.

In contrast to renal excretion, biliary excretion is very slow and much less clinically important. Drugs are eliminated in the bile by at least three active transport (p-glycoprotein) systems: one each for organic acids, organic bases, and organic neutral compounds. Characteristics that determine biliary excretion of drugs include chemical structure, polarity, and MW, with the latter being one of the major determinants (generally drugs >600 MW in size). Drugs excreted in the bile are in greater contact with the intestine and its flora compared with other drugs and are thus more likely to cause adverse reactions in the gastrointestinal tract. In addition, conjugated (phase II) drugs excreted by this route may undergo enterohepatic circulation (Figure 1-16) if intestinal bacteria unconjugate the drug or metabolite, allowing intestinal absorption to occur. Enterohepatic circulation prolongs drug elimination half-life and further exposes the gastrointestinal tract to drug.

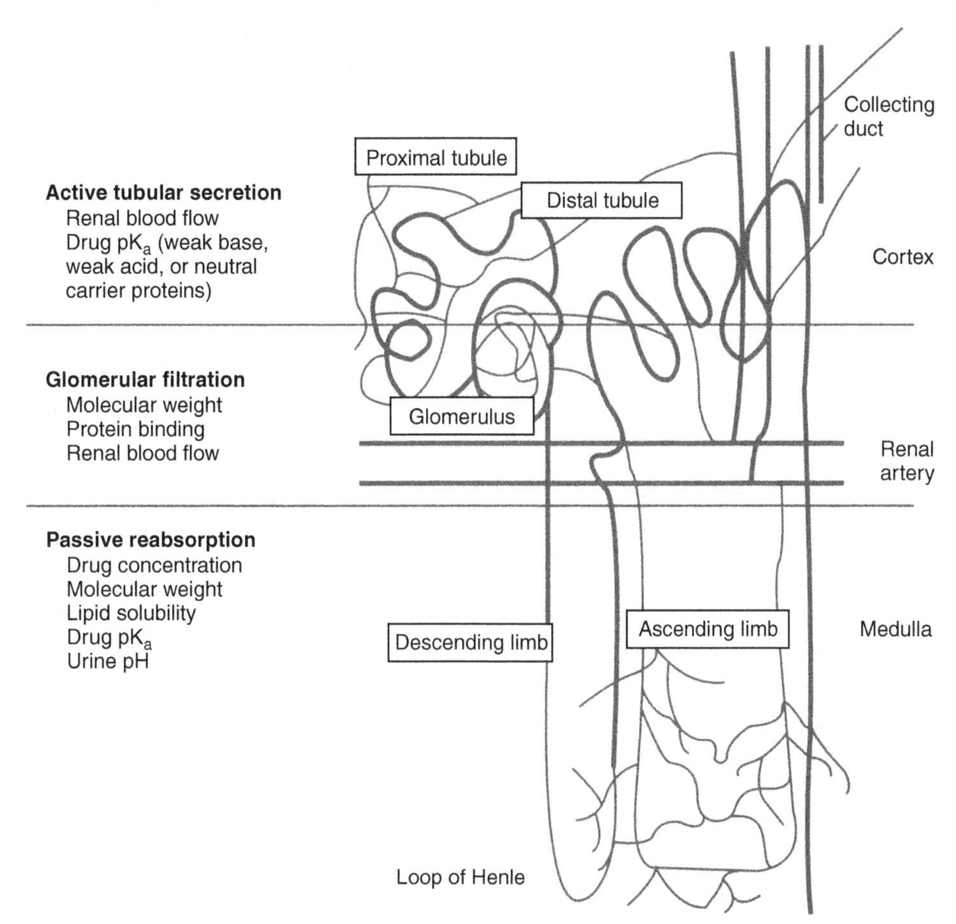

Figure 1-15 Renal excretion is the most common route of elimination of drugs and their metabolites. Three drug movements determine the rate of renal excretion. Active tubular secretion in the proximal tubule is a rapid process not limited by protein binding. Glomerular filtration is a passive process; protein-bound drugs cannot be filtered through the glomerulus. The rates of both active tubular secretion and glomerular filtration both depend on renal blood flow. Nonionized drugs that are sufficiently lipid soluble may be passively resorbed. Because urine drug concentration increases, passive resorption should also increase the concentration.

Elimination and Clearance

The combined effects of hepatic metabolism and renal and biliary excretion, as well as other routes of elimination not discussed (e.g., pulmonary, sweat), irreversibly remove or clear the drug from the body. Elimination refers to the disappearance of drug from plasma. Elimination half-life is among the more clinically relevant and the most often reported pharmacokinetic parameters. It is defined as the time necessary for plasma or blood concentrations to decline by 50%.[28] Elimination half-life, however, is also dependent on Vd. Along with the therapeutic range, the elimination half-life should be the basis for an appropriate dosing interval. The amount of fluctuation in drug concentrations during a chosen dosing interval depends on the elimination half-life of the drug. Further, drug elimination half-life determines the time to steady state when either a drug (or new dose) is begun or discontinued. For example, at one drug elimination half-life, 50% of the dose has been eliminated; by five drug elimination half-lives, more than 97% of the drug has been eliminated (Figure 1-17, Table 1-1, and Box 1-2). Finally, the elimination half-life, along with the dosing interval, also determines the amount of drug that accumulates with each dose as steady-state equilibrium is reached (see the discussion of accumulation later in this chapter). This reflects first-order elimination, which might be considered a protective mechanism to ensure rapid elimination of potentially toxic substances.

Clearance is a parameter often used to assess the excretory capacity and thus physical well-being of an organ. Plasma clearance (CL) is the volume of plasma irreversibly cleared of the drug per unit time and represents the sum total of organ clearance (Figure 1-18) [2,3,30,31] As such, it is the most important of the pharmacokinetic parameters.[32] Clearance differs from elimination because it is a volume per unit time, not a rate constant (amount per unit time). If the drug is cleared exclusively by one organ (e.g., renal clearance of aminoglycosides or hepatic clearance of caffeine), then plasma CL also represents clearance of the specific organ and can be used to evaluate the function of the organ. With first-order elimination, the volume of blood cleared per unit time by an organ is independent of PDC—that is, the same volume of blood will be irreversibly cleared of drug by an organ regardless of how much drug is in the blood. The exception occurs only if so much drug is present in the blood that the organ of clearance becomes saturated such that zero-order elimination emerges.

Although clearance is the reason that PDC ultimately declines (thus is physiologically independent of any other factor), pharmacokinetically it is obtained or calculated from the volume to which the drug is distributed (Vd) and the rate at which the drug is eliminated from the volume (k_{el} or half-life). Clearance can be calculated on the basis of compartmental modeling, or from AUC based on noncompartmental analysis (see the pharmacokinetics section). Despite its importance, practically, clearance is minimally useful in the design of dosing regimens other than through its impact on elimination half-life unless calculating a constant rate infusion. In contrast, half-life is the clinically useful estimate of how long a drug stays in the body. Yet, while half-life is the pharmacokinetic parameter measured directly from the PDC versus time curve, physiologically, it is a "hybrid" parameter in that it is affected by both distribution (Vd) and clearance (CL) (Box 1-3). The more rapidly a drug is cleared by an organ, the shorter the drug half-life. However, if a drug is distributed to a large tissue volume, PDC will be lower. Thus, although clearance (which is concentration independent) does not change, the volume cleared per unit time contains less drug and elimination decreases. If the Vd is much smaller, PDC is higher, more drug is in the volume of blood that is cleared. (see Figure 1-10). As such, the rate of elimination decreases. Thus drug elimination half-life changes directly and proportionately with Vd but inversely and proportionately with CL. The clinical significance of the relationship among Vd, CL, and half-life is exemplified in a patient who has renal disease and eventually becomes dehydrated as a result of uncompensated chronic renal disease. Initially, as renal function declines, a smaller volume of blood goes through the kidney, which thus clears less blood. Drug elimination half-life decreases. However, as the patient becomes dehydrated, blood and ECF volume contracts, and the Vd decreases. As a result, PDC increases such that more drug is in each volume of blood

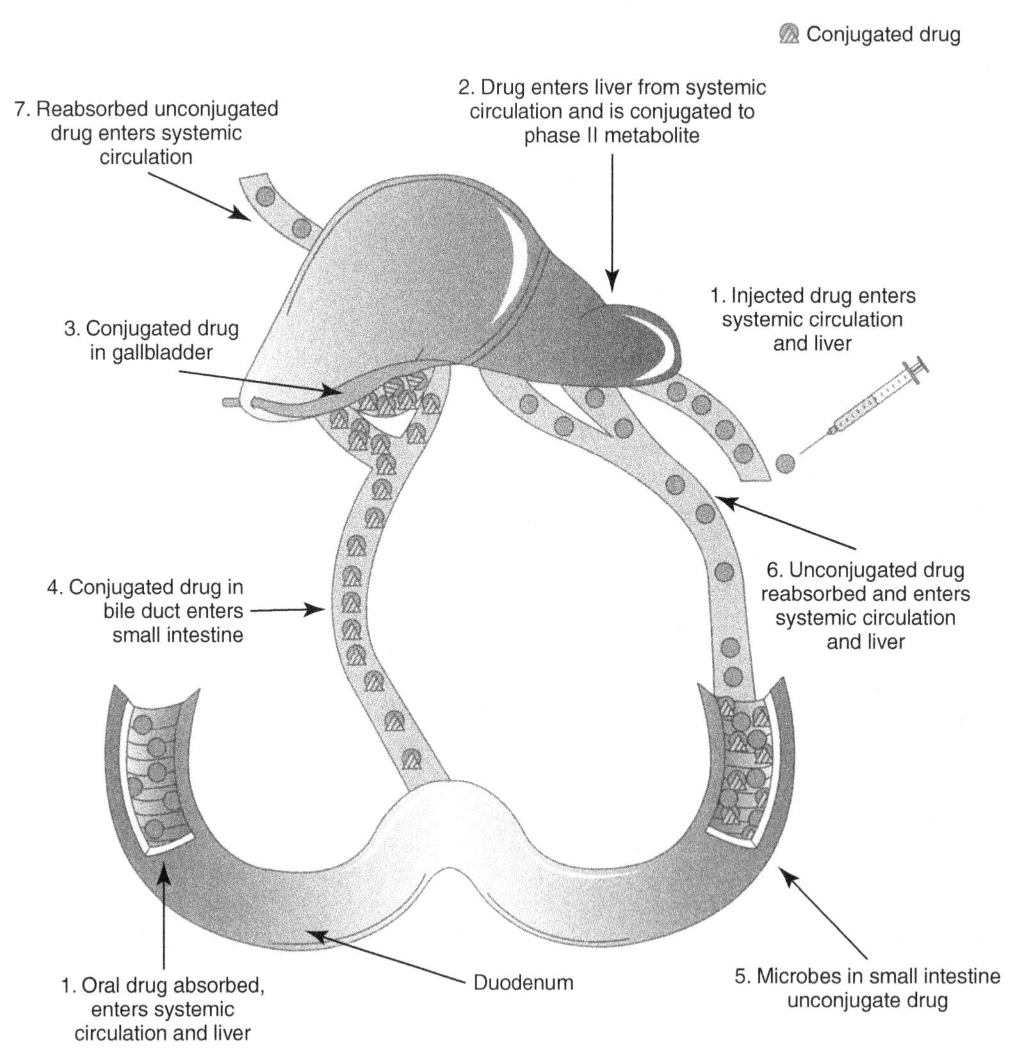

Figure 1-16 Enterohepatic circulation can prolong the elimination half-life of a drug. After oral or parenteral administration, the drug is conjugated in the liver and eliminated in the bile. The drug travels from the duodenum to the lower small intestine and colon. Bacterial degradation results in deconjugation of the drug, which can then be reabsorbed.

as it is cleared. Thus in the patient with both fluid volume contraction (half-life decreases) and compromised renal function (half-life increases), drug half-life may not change from normal even though renal function may be impaired. With volume replacement (i.e., fluid therapy), Vd will increase, causing half-life to increase because less drug is now in the smaller volume that is being cleared.

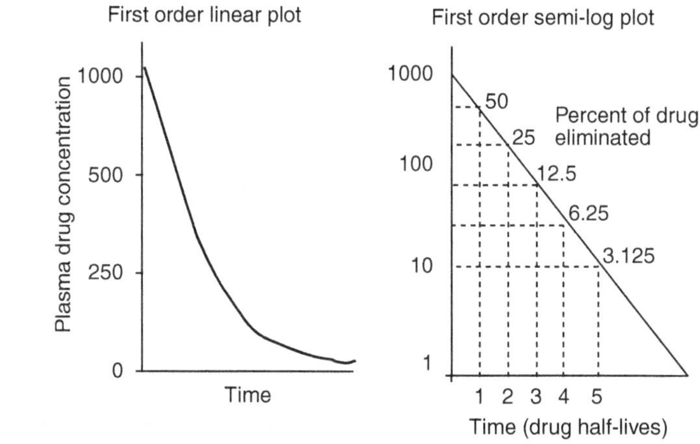

Figure 1-17 Drug elimination half-life can be derived from the plasma drug concentration versus time plot. Because most drugs are eliminated in a first order process (a constant fraction is eliminated per unit time), the amount of drug eliminated is concentration dependent. The relationship between concentration and time is linear when plotted on semilogarithmic paper but curvilinear when plotted on linear paper. The opposite is true for zero-order elimination (i.e., a constant amount is eliminated per unit time): The plot is linear on linear paper but curvilinear on semilogarithmic paper. For first-order elimination, if a line is drawn between two points (such as might be obtained from a peak and trough concentration), the line can be extrapolated to the *y* axis. The half-life is the time that elapses as plasma drug concentration decreases by half. Calculation of half-life is described in Box 1-3.

FIXED DOSING REGIMENS

Dose

A fixed dosing regimen comprises a route, a dose, and an interval (or frequency)(see Box 1-3). The dose necessary to achieve a specified target PDC (e.g., C_{max}) following a single dose depends on the volume of tissue that will dilute the dose administered, estimated by Vd:[2,3]

$$\text{Dose} = [C_{max}]\,[Vd]$$

The dose of drug must be increased or decreased proportionately with changes in Vd to achieve the same target PDC

Box 1-2

Zero- Versus First-Order Elimination

The importance of first-order (constant fraction) versus zero-order (constant amount; see Figure 1-17)[29] elimination can be appreciated best in the context of the elimination rate constant. Assume an animal has ingested several aspirin to the point that the plasma drug concentration has surpassed the therapeutic range of 100 to 500 mg/mL and has achieved the toxic concentration of 2000 mg/mL. The half-life of aspirin in the dog is about 9 hours. First-order elimination results in a concentration of 1000 ng/mL by 9 hours and 500 ng/mL at 18 hours. Thus by 18 hours, the drug is back into the therapeutic range, and by 36 hours, it approximates the low therapeutic range. For zero-order elimination a constant amount is eliminated per unit time. For example, if 100 ng/mL of aspirin is eliminated every 9 hours, by the time 36 hours has elapsed, concentrations will have declined to only 1600 ng/mL.

Table 1-1 Impact of Half Life and Dosing Interval on Fluctuation in or Accumulation of Plasma Drug Concentrations

FLUCTUATION				*ACCUMULATION*		
At 4-Hour Half-Life, If Interval (h) Is	Ratio of Interval to Half-Life	Ratio of C_{max} to C_{min}	Decline During Dosing Interval by (%)	If the Half-Life is 72 Hours and the Interval (h) Is	Ratio of Dosing Interval to Half-Life	Ratio of PDC After First Dose Compared with Steady State
2	0.5	0.71	29.3	1	0.01	104.03
4	1	0.50	50.0	3	0.04	35.01
6	1.5	0.35	64.6	4	0.06	26.38
8	2	0.25	75.0	6	0.08	17.76
12	3	0.125	87.5	10	0.14	10.86
16	4	0.063	93.7	12	0.17	9.14
24	6	0.016	98.4	18	0.25	6.27
				24	0.33	4.83
				36	0.50	3.40
				72	1	2.00

PDC, Plasma drug concentration.

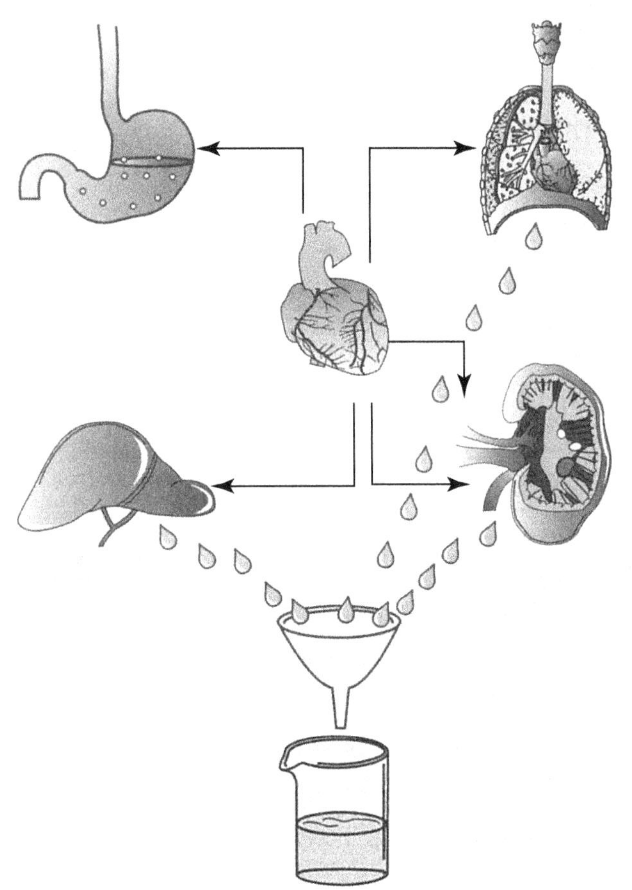

Figure 1-18 The clearance of drug from the body (plasma) is the sum total from each of the organs of clearance. Several organs not shown are also capable of drug clearance, most notably the skin.

Box 1-3

Half-Life Calculation

Half-life of any drug movement can be determined in several ways. Half-life can be directly determined from a drug concentration versus time graph by measuring the distance on the X axis (time) that occurs as PDC (Y axis) decreases by 50% (see Figures 1-20 and 1-23). More often, half-lives for each component of a drug concentration versus time curve are determined from each slope, or rate constant, k_i: At one half-life ($t_2 - t_1 = t_{1/2}$), the drug concentration declines by 50%. Thus at t_2- t_1, $C_1/C_2 = 2$. However, because drug concentrations (Y axis) are natural logs, C_1/C_2 becomes the natural log (ln) of 2 = 0.693. Thus the rate constant or slope of any line $k_i = 0.693/t_{1/2}$. Conversely, if the rate constant is known, $t_{1/2} = 0.693/k_i$. In the same manner, half-life also might be calculated from peak and trough concentrations collected from a patient (see Chapter 5). The slope, or k_i, is simply the rise/run, or $(C_1 - C_2)/(t_2 - t_1)$ where C is the concentration of sample 1 or 2 and t is the time that samples 1 and 2 were collected (see Figure 1-20). Because concentration is logarithmic, the actual equation becomes

$$K_i, = \ln [C_1 / C_2] / t_2 - t_1$$

For example, if gentamicin samples collected at 2 hours and 12 hours after an intravenous dose were 10.5 and 2.0 mg/mL, respectively, the k_{el} for gentamicin in this animal would be 0.17 h^{-1} and the elimination half-life would be calculated at 4.2 hours.

(or C_0 or C_{max})(see Figures 1-10 and 1-19). Often, the dose is not intended to reach C_{max} but rather C_{min} (e.g., phenobarbital) or midway between the two extremes of the therapeutic range. The concentration within a therapeutic range that is selected as the target depends on the drug efficacy and safety. The Vd of a drug is the sole determinant of PDC for single doses of an intravenously administered drug. With multiple dosing the relationship between elimination half-life and dosing interval also may influence PDC (see later discussion). For extravascular drugs, bioavailability also must be considered, with the dose inversely but proportionately influenced by bioavailability:

$$\text{Dose} = [C_{max}]\,[\text{Vd}]\,/\,F\,.$$

By definition, with intravenous administration, F= 1, or 100% bioavailability.

Interval

The relationship between elimination half-life and dosing interval determines the amount of fluctuation in PDC during a dosing interval. This relationship has several clinical implications (see Table 1-1 and Figures 1-20 and 1-21). The shorter the elimination half-life compared with the dosing interval, the greater the fluctuation. The dosing interval for a drug is based on the time (T_{max}) it takes for PDC to decline from the peak concentration achieved after dosing (C_{max}) to the lowest concentration that occurs during the

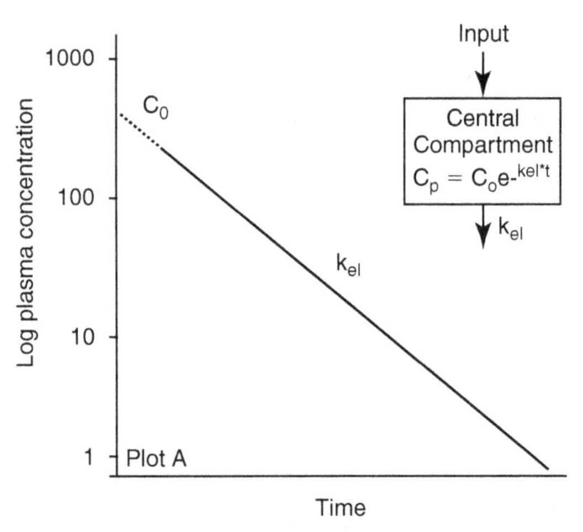

Figure 1-19 Plasma drug concentration (PDC) versus time curves after intravenous administration. This drug could be described by a one-compartment open model because it plots as a single straight line (one slope) on semilogarithmic paper. There is no initial distribution phase, and the volume of distribution is based on PDC extrapolated *(dotted line)* from the first concentration measured back to time zero (C_0). The equation for this single component curve would be $C_p = C_o e^{-kt}$ where C_p is the plasma drug concentration at any time and t and k are the elimination rate constants (slope) of the curve. Such behavior is unusual for a drug because it implies instantaneous distribution from plasma to tissues or failure to leave circulation. The latter might happen if a drug is very tightly bound to plasma proteins and total, rather than unbound drug, is measured.

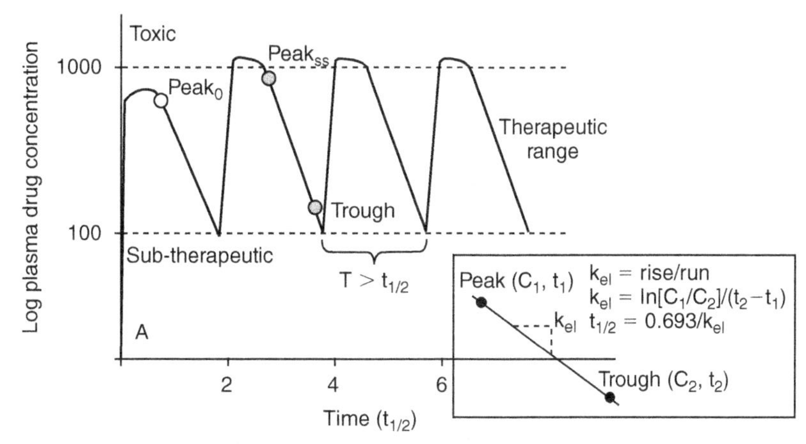

Figure 1-20 Plasma drug concentration versus time curves after multiple extravascular dosing for a drug that is administered at a dosing interval substantially longer than the elimination half-life. Such a drug is less likely to accumulate because most of the drug will be eliminated during a dosing interval. For such drugs equilibrium between tissue and plasma concentrations is never reached and steady state is not really relevant. The risk of toxicity and therapeutic failure is a potential concern with each dose, unless the dosing interval is shortened such that fluctuation during the dosing interval is minimized. For monitoring, a peak and trough concentration may be necessary. The *inset* demonstrates how the half-life of a drug might be calculated from drug concentrations measured at two time points after administration of a dose.

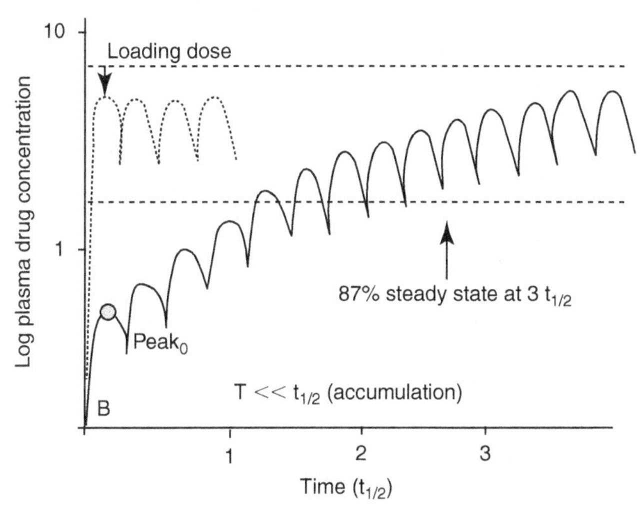

Figure 1-21 Plasma drug concentration versus time curves following multiple extravascular dosing for a drug that is administered at a dosing interval substantially shorter than the elimination half-life (see also Figure 1-16). The amount that the drug accumulates as steady state is reached determines the drug concentration at steady state and is based on the magnitude of difference between dosing interval (T) and drug half-life ($t_{1/2}$). Such a drug will accumulate because most of the drug from the previous dose is still in the body by the next dose. Although equilibrium may not be truly reached, steady-state (characterized by the same C_{max} and C_{min} at each dosing interval) occurs after three to five drug half-lives have elapsed after administration at the same dose, interval and route. For some drugs, if a rapid therapeutic response is desired, a loading dose can be given. Note, however, that steady state has not been reached and plasma drug concentration may increase or decrease as steady-state is reached if the maintenance dose is not correct. When monitoring is done for such drugs, generally a single sample collected at any time during the dosing interval is sufficient to reflect the whole dosing interval.

dosing interval (C_{min}) (see Figures 1-20 through 1-22). Thus the interval depends on the amount of fluctuation in PDC allowed during the dosing interval and the half-life of the drug, or its inverse ($0.693/t_{1/2}$), the elimination rate constant (k_{el}). If C_{min} for a drug is close to half of C_{max}, then approximately one drug half-life (i.e., $T_{max} = t_{1/2}$) can elapse before the next dose should be administered. A more appropriate interval can be calculated with k_{el} if C_{min} does not approximate half of C_{max}:

$$T_{max} = [\ln C_{max} / C_{min}] / k_{el}$$

The longer the elimination half-life of a drug, or the wider the difference between C_{max} and C_{min}, the longer the possible interval (or T_{max}) between doses. Understanding the relationship between dosing interval and elimination half-life can help determine which aspect of the dosing regimen (i.e., close or interval) should be changed when trying to improve drug response by either increasing PDCs or minimizing fluctuation during the interval. Through altered kinetics in the patient, two scenarios are offered.

The first scenario is dosing with a drug at an interval that is close to or longer than the drug elimination half-life. With this scenario, prolonging a dosing interval (e.g., for convenience) may allow drug concentrations to fluctuate excessively during the dosing interval and may result in either adverse events as C_{max} is approached with each dose or therapeutic failure as C_{min} is approached just before each subsequent dose. Note that wide fluctuation between C_{max} and C_{min} may not necessarily be undesirable. For example, if the drug is effective despite nondetectable drug concentrations, the interval can be longer than the half-life might dictate. Examples include concentration-dependent antimicrobials (e.g., aminoglycosides), drugs that accumulate in tissues (e.g., omeprazole), drugs such as diazepam whose metabolites are active (some with drug half-lives longer than that of the

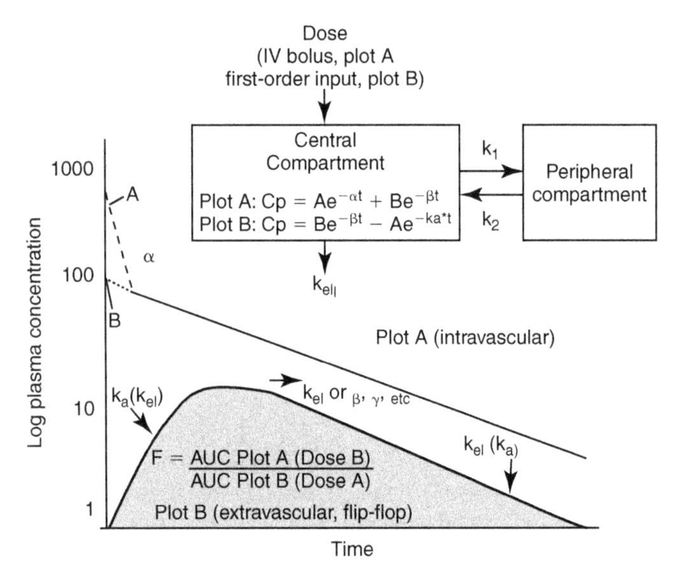

Figure 1-22 After intravenous administration, a drug distributed to peripheral tissues generally is characterized by at least two components or phases when plotted on semilogarithmic paper. According to compartmental modeling, the plasma drug concentration (PDC) declines in the first phase (component) due to both distribution into tissues and back and elimination (excretion) from the body. Once a distribution equilibrium (pseudo-equilibrium) has been reached, PDC decline is caused only by elimination (second phase or component of the curve). The two phases can be separated by stripping and residual analysis, or linear regression. The first (stripped and subsequently fitted) component of the curve *(coarse dotted line)* is understand to represent distribution, and the slope *(α)* is the distribution rate constant. The slope of the second phase of the curve is the elimination rate constant (k_{el}). The equation for the curve represented by plot B (two components) can be used to determine the concentration of drug in plasma (or the tissue being sampled) at any time (t) by the equation: $C_p = Ae^{-\alpha t} + Be^{-\beta t}$. The volume of distribution (Vd) for this drug is ideally based on PDC after distribution, usually determined by extrapolating *(fine dotted line)* the terminal or elimination phase of the PDC versus time curve (*B* on plot A) yielding Vd area or Vd extrapolation. The Vd based on the extrapolated concentration for the first component of the line (*A* on Plot A) might be used to calculate the central volume (Vc) to which the drug is immediately distributed. The second PDC versus time curve (Plot B) reflects extravascular (e.g., oral) administration of the same dose of drug. The upswing of the PDC versus time curve reflects the simultaneous movements of absorption, distribution and elimination from the body, all occurring during first-order input (a constant fraction moves per unit time). As each movement reaches pseudoequilibrium (amount moving either way is the same), remaining movements that have not yet reached equilibrium emerge. Of the movements, elimination from the body will not reach equilibrium (open model) and as such, emerges as the terminal movement or component. The absorption rate constant (k_a) can be derived from the upswing of the curve but only after the elimination component of the curve has been mathematically stripped. Generally, the distribution phase of nonintravenous doses is masked by the absorptive phase. The equation of extravascular PDC versus time curves follows the general equation: $C_p = Be^{-\beta t} - Ae^{-ka\,t}$ where A is the extrapolated drug concentration from the absorptive phase of the curve; it is subtracted from the overall equation because it represents the area that is "missing" from the curve as the drug is being absorbed. The elimination rate constant of a drug should be the same, regardless of the route of elimination. However, in some cases the rate of absorption is so slow that it limits the rate of elimination. As such, the absorption rate constant determines the slope of the terminal curve (i.e., k_a and k_{el} are "flip-flopped," as is demonstrated in the figure). A flip-flop model should be suspected if the elimination rate constant after extravascular administration is significantly less than that after IV administration. As such, a flip-flop model can be ascertained only if the drug is give intravenously. If IV administration is not done to affirm the terminal slope as k_{el} , it should be reported as the disappearance rate constant, k_d. IV administration is also necessary to determine Vd,CL and absolute bioavailabililty (F) of a drug. (see Box 1-6.)

parent compound), and drugs whose effects are irreversible (e.g., receptors or enzymes are destroyed (e.g., aspirin and thromboxane synthetase).

On the other hand, if the drug is characterized by a narrow therapeutic window, fluctuation should be minimized and a shorter interval may be indicated. To add one half-life to the dosing interval, the dose must be doubled; however, to add subsequent half-lives, the dose must be doubled each time. Thus to add three half-lives to a dosing interval, the dose must be increased eightfold (2^3) (e.g., time dependent drugs or anticonvulsants). Some drug half-lives are short on the order of minutes (e.g., epinephrine). Constant rate infusion may be indicated if an intravenous preparation is available such that therapeutic concentrations can be maintained for a clinically relevant period while avoiding the negative consequences of undesirable fluctuations in PDC that might occur with convenient dosing intervals (see later discussion). Manufacturers have provided an alternative approach to maintenance of PDCs for drugs with a short half-life by formulating the drug in a preparation characterized by slowed absorption (e.g., extended release preparations) or (less commonly) distribution. However, even if absorption is prolonged, once the drug enters circulation, it's elimination half-life is the same. Absorption of a drug might be slowed by several methods. Examples of parenteral slow-release preparations include drug-esters (drug is released by esterases at the site of administration) or liposomal or other products that release drug as the product is degraded. Oral methods include extended- or delayed-release products consisting of capsules that degrade at different rates. Note, however, that absorption may be so slow that therapeutic concentrations are never reached. Many preparations used in animals have been formulated for humans, and the release kinetics may vary substantially in animals.. A less common mechanism of constant drug input is slow release from circulating plasma proteins for a drug that is highly protein bound (e.g., cefovecin).

A second scenario is a drug administered at an interval that is much shorter than the half-life. For such drugs, little drug may be eliminated during the dosing interval, and shortening the interval will be beneficial only if an additional dose is added (rather than dividing the same daily dose into more dosing periods). For example, assume the half-life of phenobarbital approximates an average of 72 hours. Dividing the dose into 8- rather than 12-hour intervals offers no advantage because 3 days must lapse for 50% of the drug to be eliminated. Indeed, a 24-hour dosing interval may be sufficient for most patients, unless induction of drug-metabolizing enzymes causes the half-life to markedly decrease (see Chapter 2). For drugs with very long half-lives, depending on the C_{max} and C_{min} of the drug, dosing intervals generally can be correspondingly long. However, a dosing interval that is too long might result in too much fluctuation in PDC during a dosing interval, which may be problematic for drugs characterized by a narrow therapeutic window. It also might lead to noncompliance if the owner forgets to medicate. In both situations the recommended dosing interval is often shorter than the drug elimination half-life. In such instances the drug will accumulate, and the concept of steady state and the potential need for a loading dose must be addressed (see below).

Accumulation

If a drug is administered at an interval that is approximately three half-lives, most (87.5%) of the drug will be eliminated between each dose. However, if the interval is shorter, some drug from the previous dose will still be present in the plasma when the next dose is given. Indeed, if the drug is administered at an interval that equals the half-life, 50% of the previous dose is still in the body when the next dose is given. Thus if each subsequent dose of drug is administered at an interval (T) that is equal to or shorter than the drug half-life, most of the previous dose is still in the body, and the drug accumulates with multiple doses (see Figures 1-17 and 1-21).[2,3] Eventually, a steady state is reached such that the amount of drug administered with each dose equals the amount eliminated during the dosing interval. As with drug elimination, approximately three to five drug half-lives must elapse following a fixed dosing regimen before steady state is reached. Note that steady state is a relevant issue only for drugs that accumulate—that is, the drug is administered at a dosing interval that is shorter than the drug elimination half-life. The amount of accumulation can be described by the accumulation ratio (R), which describes the magnitude of the drug concentration following the first dose compared with that at steady state (Css); the ratio can be applied to C_{min}, C_{max}, or $C_{average}$ ($R = Css/C^{1st}$).

Just as the amount of fluctuation between C_{min} and C_{max} depends on the relationship between half-life and interval (i.e., for a drug dosed at an interval shorter than the half-life), the accumulation ratio also depends on the relationship between dose and interval, being logarithmically proportional to the difference between the two: $R = 1/1- e^{-kel^{*} T}$ where R = the accumulation ratio, T = the dosing interval and k_{el} = the elimination rate constant (see Figure 1-21 and Tables 1-1 and 1-2). The dosing regimen of drugs that accumulate is generally designed so that drug concentrations will be in the therapeutic range at steady state. If the elimination half-life is equal to the dosing interval, although PDC will fluctuate twofold between doses, the drug will also accumulate twofold (i.e., C_{max} at first dose:C_{max} at steady state = 2) as steady-state is reached.The greater the half-life compared with the dosing interval, the more the drug will accumulate (see Table 1-2). Using the example of phenobarbital, as drug is begun, the elimination half-life may approximate 72 hours (k_{el}=0.693/72 h). When the seventh dose is given 72 hours later, 50% of the first dose still remains. Based on a 72-hour half-life and 12-hour dosing interval, an accumulation ratio of 9 is expected. Thus if peak PDC following the first dose of 3.5 mg/kg was 2 µg/mL, concentrations of 18 µg/mL would be expected at steady state 9 to 14 days later. Because drug concentrations fluctuate very little for drugs that accumulate, missed doses should present minimal risk of therapeutic failure. The missed dose can simply be given with the next dose. However, to change PDCs substantially, multiple doses (i.e., a "miniloading" dose) must be given. When monitoring, a single sample collected at any time during the dosing interval should accurately reflect PDC throughout the dosing interval because concentrations change minimally during the interval.

Table 1-2 Rate of Drug Accumulation Based on the Length of the Dosing Interval (T) Compared with Elimination Half-Life ($t_{1/2}$)

Dosing Interval (Hours)	Elimination Half-Life (Hours)	T: $t_{1/2}$ Ratio	Accumulation*
6	24	0.25	6.2
8	24	0.33	4.8
12	24	0.5	3.4
24	24	1	2
48	24	2	1.3
72	24	3	1.14
96	24	4	1.0

*Accumulation is the ratio of peak plasma drug concentration following the dose at steady state compared with that following the first dose ($Cmax_{ss}$: $Cmax_{first\ dose}$).

With a 21-day half-life in dogs, bromide offers an extreme example of accumulation when dosed once daily. At steady state, bromide concentrations will be 35 times what they were after the first dose. Likewise, during a 24-hour dosing interval, fluctuations in PDC will be so small that they should not be detectable. Levetiracetam, on the other hand, offers an example at the other end of the spectrum: With a 2-hour half-life, 87% of the drug may be eliminated during an 8-hour dosing interval. Missed doses may put the patient at risk for therapeutic failure, and monitoring might best include both a peak and trough sample. If only one sample can be collected, a trough sample might be sufficient because the drug is so safe. However, if side or adverse effects are of concern with the drug (e.g., clorazepate), both a peak and trough sample might be collected for drugs with a short half-life compared with the dosing interval.

Clinically, drugs that accumulate present another problem not encountered with drugs administered at an interval that precludes accumulation. Maximum therapeutic efficacy is not realized until steady-state concentrations are reached, which may be an unacceptable time for some patients (e.g., epileptics receiving potassium bromide [KBr]) (see Figure 1-21). In such situations a loading dose can be administered with the intent of achieving therapeutic concentrations with a single dose or, in the case of bromide, several days of dosing. Note, however, that a loading dose **does not** achieve steady state. Steady state is achieved only after the drug is administered at the same dose for three to five drug half-lives. As such, although a properly calculated loading dose will result in PDCs immediately achieving the therapeutic range, the maintenance dose must be designed to maintain these concentrations. A loading dose should be considered only when therapeutic response depends on steady-state concentrations and the time to this point is unacceptable (i.e., three to five drug half-lives). The benefits of loading (i.e., a rapid response) should be weighed against the risk of adverse events that will be increased if the body does not have time to accommodate to high drug concentrations. Further, pet owners are not likely to understand the concept of loading and may either forget to modify or intentionally continue a loading dose, the latter because they wrongly assume that a higher dose can be tolerated longer.

A loading dose always is accompanied by a maintenance dose; the maintenance would be the same regardless of whether a loading dose is administered concurrently because it also is designed to achieve therapeutic concentrations at steady state. The maintenance dose should "match" the loading dose—that is, it should be designed to maintain what the loading dose achieved. The maintenance dose, not the loading dose, determines PDC at steady state: By the time steady state is reached (three to five half-lives), the loading dose will have been eliminated. However, at one half-life, while 50% of the loading dose will have been eliminated, 50% of steady-state concentrations will have been achieved. If the maintenance dose fails to maintain what the loading dose achieved, PDC will either decline (maintenance dose too small) or increase (dose too great) as steady state is achieved. Either miscalculation can lead to therapeutic failure. The greatest decrease (or increase) will occur during the first elimination half-life after loading is completed; as such, inappropriate patient response may occur at one half-life.

The loading dose is calculated according to the (apparent) Vd at steady state (Vd_{ss}) of the drug and the targeted PDC at steady state, C_{ss} (mg/mL). Thus for drugs with 100% bioavailability (e.g., intravenously administered drugs):

$$\text{Loading dose } (D_L\,;\ \text{mg/kg}) = Vd_{ss} \times C_{ss}$$

The dose can be adjusted for less than 100% bioavailability by:

$$D_L = Vd_{ss} \times C_{ss} / F \text{ where F is the bioavailability (fraction of the drug absorbed)}$$

Using bromide as an example, the minimum effective concentration (C_{min}) is 1 mg/mL (1 gm/L). With a Vd of 0.3 L/kg, and near 100% oral bioavailability, a loading dose intended to achieve the minimum therapeutic range would be C_{min}* Vd/F or (0.3 l/kg) * (1 gm/L)/1 or 300 mg/kg. Because potassium bromide is only 69% bromide (potassium MW = 35; bromide MW = 79), the dose of potassium bromide necessary to achieve 1 mg/mL is 300 mg/kg/0.69 = 433 (rounded up to 450 mg/kg). Note that he loading dose of bromide that targets 1 mg/ml at steady-state is much higher than the daily maintenance dose (approximately 30 mg/kg per day) that would achieve 1 mg/mL at steady state (approximately 2.5 months of dosing). The difference between the loading dose of a drug and its maintenance dose reflects the difference between the elimination half-life and the dosing interval. Simplistically, the loading dose should reflect all the doses that would be given as the drug reaches steady state, less the amount eliminated during that same time period. The longer the elimination half-life, the larger the loading dose compared to the maintenance dose.

Constant-rate infusion (CRI) offers an example of a drug that is administered at an interval that is much shorter than the half-life (Box 1-4). For CRI the rate is infinitely small. The rate of infusion (ROI or k_o) should result in an input that equals the output. Output will be described by (total body) clearance (CL; ml/kg/hr) of the drug: ROI (mg/kg/h) = CL × C_{ss} (see pharmacokinetics section). Because clearance, in turn, reflects the volume of blood from which drug is eliminated per unit time (CL = Vd * k_{el}), then ROI = Css * Vd * k_{el}. Further, because k_{el} can be calculated from half-life, then ROI = Css * Vd * (0.693/$t_{1/2}$). When calculating CRI, care must be taken to ensure that units are converted such that they match. Note that increasing the ROI will increase the total concentration achieved at steady state but will not increase or decrease the time to steady state. As with any other dosing scheme, steady state will not be achieved with a CRI until three to five elimination half-lives have elapsed, which may be unacceptably long. As such, a loading dose may be indicated when administering a CRI if patient response time is too long. Note, however, that a sufficient clinical response may occur well before maximum drug concentrations are achieved at steady-state. Likewise, the time for drug concentrations to decline after a CRI is discontinued will be based on the same elimination rate constant: Three to five drug half-lives must elapse before the drug is eliminated from the body, although clinical response may resolve well before all the drug is entirely eliminated.

Box 1-4

Calculation of a Constant-Rate Infusion for Fentanyl

In normal dogs, the volume of distribution (Vd) of fentanyl ranges from 4 to 10 L/kg and its $t_{1/2}$ ranged from 2.5 to 6 h. Using an average Vd or 7 L/kg and 3h as the $t_{1/2}$, then k_{el} = 0.693/3 = 0..35 hr^{-1} and clearance (CL) becomes (0.173 $hour^{-1}$ * 7 L/kg) = 2.45 L/kg/h (2450 mL/kg/h to match units). To target C_{min} or 1 ng/mL (or 1 µg/L) of fentanyl at steady state (9-15 hours), the rate of infusion (ROI or Ro) = ([1 ng/mL] * 2450 mL/kg/h) = 2450 ng/kg/h (2.45 µg/kg/h) or 0.04 µg/kg/min. If the half-life is 3 hours, steady-state concentrations should be reached in approximately 9 to 15 hours. Although analgesic relief may not require steady-state concentrations, safety of the constant-rate infusion cannot be fully assessed until steady state is reached. If the time to steady state is too long, 1 ng/mL (C_{min}) can be immediately reached by an administration of a loading dose (DL): DL = C_{ss} * Vd = (5 L/kg * 1 µg/L) or 5 µg/kg, which can be administered as an intravenous bolus.

Extrapolation of dosing regimens among species for drugs that accumulate is more difficult than for drugs that do not. For drugs that do not accumulate, dose is largely based on Vd and, if not administered intravenously, bioavailability (which can be difficult to extrapolate among species). However, for drugs that accumulate, if the drug is given in multiple doses, both Vd and elimination half-life must be taken into account for intravenous drugs, along with bioavailability for nonintravenous drugs.

PHARMACOKINETICS

The quantitative description of drug movements in the body is referred to as *pharmacokinetics*. Pharmacokinetic modeling is used to predict the behavior of a drug in the body. Generally, the drug of interest is given at the desired route of administration as a single dose, and drug concentrations are collected over time, preferably for at least three elimination half-lives to ensure that all phases of drug movement are identified. For bioavailability studies, the drug should be given intravenously (100%) as well as by the route of interest, ideally using a randomized crossover paired design. For drugs intended for multiple dosing, particularly chronically, pharmacokinetic analysis also should take place across the intended duration of therapy to detect changes in drug disposition over time. Several methods of pharmacokinetic modeling are used to study drug movements; the most common described in the veterinary literature are either compartmental or noncompartmental analysis; population pharmacokinetics represents an emerging variation.[2,3,9,33] Boxes 1-3 to 1-6 provide some useful pharmacokinetic equations.

Compartmental Analysis

Compartments

Plotting of PDC versus time data on semilogarithmic paper linearizes the data for most drugs because drug movements follow first-order kinetics—that is, a constant fraction rather than a constant amount (zero order) of drug moves (is absorbed, distributed, or excreted) per unit time. For first-order behavior, the amount of drug per unit time varies with the concentration of drug, whereas with zero-order elimination (as might occur when metabolism enzymes are saturated), the amount eliminated per unit time is concentration independent. Theoretically, after administration, each movement to which the drug is subjected occurs at a different rate: absorption and distribution are generally faster than elimination. Each movement results in a change in the slope of the curve, with each slope thus reflecting a different drug movement or combination of movements. Intravenous drug administration yields a PDC versus time curve that begins with the highest PDC (see Figures 1-19 and 1-22).

After intravenous administration (no absorption), data described by a single component (i.e., only one slope or rate; see Figure 1-19) is interpreted to indicate that only one compartment or drug movement occurs, which is elimination from the body (excretion Such a behavior might describe a drug whose distribution is either instantaneous (or occurs before the first sample is collected) or is limited to plasma (i.e., highly protein bound drug). The model is described as a one-compartment open (meaning drug can move into or out of compartments) model. More commonly, two drug movements characterize the time course of the drug in the body (see Figure 1-22, plot A). For such drugs, PDCs initially decline because of the combined effects of two drug movements: distribution to (and from) tissues and excretion (elimination) from the body. Because distribution is generally more rapid, elimination emerges after distribution equilibrium (pseudo-equilibrium) is reached (i.e., the amount of drug moving into tissue equals the amount of drug leaving the tissue). Beyond that point, less drug is leaving the plasma because changes in PDC reflect only one drug movement, excretion (elimination from the body). The elimination is slower (the slope is flatter). Data for such drugs is characterized as a two-compartment open model.[2,3,9] More than two compartments may emerge as drug behavior is modeled. Drugs also can be bound to peripheral tissues. For such drugs the time to distribution to well perfused tissues may reach equilibrium more rapidly than to the deeper peripheral tissues, and the PDC versus time curves may be composed of three or more components: the terminal component presumably reflecting elimination from the body, the next component potentially reflecting distribution to a "deep" compartment, and the initial component reflecting distribution to "peripheral" compartments.

If a drug is given via an extravascular route (e.g., orally, intramuscularly, subcutaneously), the initial change in PDC is characterized by an increase (see Figure 1-22, plot B; nonintravenous). Once absorption is complete, drug concentrations decline as elimination becomes the primary drug movement (see Figure 1-22, plot B; nonintravenous). Because absorption generally is slower than distribution, the latter is often "masked" by the absorptive phase and can not be mathematically determined. Thus, extravascular administration may be characterized only by two drug movements, absorption and elimination (one compartment open model with first order input). It is important to note that the assignment of each component or compartment of the PDC versus curve to a specific drug movement is theoretical. While conceptually, this approach to modeling makes sense, other models also can describe the data without compartmentalization (e.g., physiologic).

Mathematical Description

In order to pharmacokinetically describe or model drug behavior, thus allowing prediction of drug concentrations at any time, the time course of drug movements is reduced to one equation that best describes, or "fits" the data. If the data are best described by multiple compartments, each component should be described uniquely in the equation. Thus to distinguish the rate constant and Y intercept of one movement from those of another, each slope must be separated or "stripped" from the combined curve. Each component of PDC can be manually separated from the previous component. To do so, the terminal-most component is first extrapolated to the Y axis, and the "predicted" Y values on that line are subtracted from the "actual" data on the PDC versus time curve. The residuals (predicted) are plotted at the same time points, and a new line is drawn to represent the next (proximal) component of the curve. The process is repeated for each component until the initial component has been identified. The process of residual analysis is tedious; as such, computer-generated programs generally strip the data and identify the components. Each component that results from stripping is then subjected to linear regression to determine the equation that best describes each component of the time versus PDC relationship. Thus, one of the disadvantages of compartmental analysis is that predicted data, rather than actual data, may be the basis for determining pharmacokinetic parameters. This does not represent a problem unless the predicted data are not a good "fit"; poorly fitting data will contribute to the variability of the data. Scientific papers that describe the pharmacokinetics of a drug on the basis of compartmental analysis should provide an assessment (e.g., sum of residuals) of how well the actual data fit the "best" predictive line resulting from linear regression, thus providing an indication of the relevance of the predicted parameters to actual parameters. The advantage of compartmental analysis is that each component may reflect a different drug movement (absorption, distribution, or elimination), thus elucidating drug behavior. However, no matter how good the fit, the labeling of a component of the curve with a drug movement is theoretical and may not actually reflect what occurs in the body. Further, the labeling of each of the components of the curve with a drug movement, although routinely done, is theoretical: modeling does not assure the first component is distribution, the next elimination, etc.

Once separated, each component of the PDC versus time curve is described by a Y intercept (Co if one compartment [see Figure 1-19], A and B if two compartments [see Figure 1-22, plot A], or A, B, and C for three compartments, and so forth) and a rate constant (k_{el} for one compartment or α, β, or γ, and so forth, for multiple compartments). The Y intercept for each component is determined by extrapolation of the line of each component (beginning with the terminal-most) back to the Y axis. For a one-compartment model, the extrapolated Y intercept is generally referred to as *Co* to indicate plasma drug concentrations at time 0. For multiple components each succeeding component is not extrapolated until that portion of the line has been stripped from the distal component. The units of PDC as extrapolated to Y are weight/volume (i.e., μg/mL, mg/mL, mg/L, and so on). The rate constant (or slope) describes the percentage change per unit time for each component. The rate constant of the terminal-most component is generally referred to as k_{el} but also referred to as β if a two-component curve, γ with three components, and so on. Alternatively, the slopes or rate constant may simply be referred to as λ (lambda; i.e., λ_1, λ_2, λ_z, etc with λ_z being the terminal component) as a reminder that assignment of movements is theoretical. The units of rate constants are the inverse of time ($time^{-1}$, e.g., min^{-1}). The rate constant of the initial component of the curve following intravenous administration is generally referred to as α and the distribution rate constant.

Box 1-5

Parameters for Compartmental Analysis

Plasma drug concentrations (Cp), at any time (t) after administration. For open model, after intravenous administration:

One compartment: $Cp = Coe^{-kt}$ (Figure 1-19)

Two compartment: $Cp = Ae^{-\alpha t} + Be^{-\beta t}$ (Figure 1-22)

Three compartment: $Cp = Ae^{-\alpha t} + Be^{-\beta t} + Ce^{-\gamma t}$.

For first order input (extravascular): $Cp = Be^{-kel*t} - Ae^{-ka*t}$

Area under the curve (AUC): One compartment: $AUC = A/\alpha$; (or Co/k_{el}). Two compartment: $AUC = A/\alpha + B/\beta$: three compartment: $AUC = A/\alpha + B/\beta + C/\gamma$. Units for AUC are reflected in its determinants: plasma drug concentrations represented by the respective Y intercepts Co, A B, C, and so on, reported in weight/volume (e.g., mg/L or μg/mL), and the respective rate constants (α, β, γ, and so on for intravenous administration and k_a for the absorptive phase of extravascular administration; reported in inverse time or $time^{-1}$[e.g., min^{-1}]).

Area under the moment curve (AUMC): A/α^2 for one compartment; $A/\alpha^2 + B/\beta^2$ for a two-compartment model, and so on).

(Apparent) Volume of Distributions (Vd): Vc (volume of the central compartment), Vd_B, Vd area, and Vd_{ss}; $> Vd_B >$ Vd area $> Vd_{ss} >$ Vc.): Units of volume/mass (e.g., L/kg) reflect the dose (generally mg/kg) and extrapolated drug concentration (C_0 or B). The Vd of a drug can be determined only after intravenous administration because bioavailability = 100 %; if F is known, Vd can be calculated substituting D * F for D in each of the equations.

One compartment: Vd = Dose/Co

Two compartment: V_c = Dose/A

Vd_B = Dose/B (Figure 1-22, Figure 1-23)

Vd area = Dose/(AUC * β)

Vdss: (D × AUMC)/AUC^2

Dose (D) (units generally mass/mass, e.g., mg/kg):

Intravenous administration: D = Co * Vd

Extravascular administration: D = Co * Vd/F

Clearance (CL): The CL of a drug represents the fraction of the Vd of a drug that is cleared per unit time (k_{el}). Thus if the Vd and k_{el} (or half-life) of a drug are known, the CL of the drug can also be determined: $CL = Vd \bullet k_{el}$ Because CL is calculated from Vd, it can be determined only after intravenous administration of a drug (unless F is known).

Volume or weight units must match for all calculations.

Once the Y intercept and slope of each curve is identified, the PDC versus time curve, regardless of the number of components, can be described by the following basic equation: $(Cp) = Coe^{-kt}$, where Cp is the plasma drug concentration at any time, t; Co is the instantaneous plasma drug concentration (before distribution or elimination have occurred, extrapolated from the appropriate component of the curve), and k is the respective elimination rate constant (slope of the line). This equation is simply the semilogarithmic (because movements are first order) version of the equation for a line, Y= mx + B where Y is the concentration (Cp) at any time X (t), m is the (logarithmic) slope of the line (e^{-k}), and B is the Y intercept (Co) (Box 1-5).

A similar approach to modeling is taken for extravascular data, which must be described by at least two components. The slope of the upswing of the PDC versus time curve (once stripped from the distribution or elimination components of the curve) describes the absorption rate constant, designated k_a; the Y intercept must be determined after all other components of the curve are stripped (see Figure 1-22). For extravascular administration, the model would be referred to as a *one-compartment open model with first-order input,* indicating that the rate of absorption, like the rate of elimination, is first order. If the decline in PDC after the absorptive phase revealed two slopes, the model would be two compartments, with the first compartment or component possibly representing distribution that was slower than absorption. For some drugs (including extended- or delayed-release preparations), the rate of absorption is slower than the rate of elimination. For such drugs, absorption is reflected in the terminal-most, rather than initial, component of the PDC versus time curve and the elimination rate constant for such drugs is determined from the upswing of the PDC versus time curve. Such drugs are generally said to follow a "flip-flop" model and can be identified only after intravenous administration because it is only through this route that the effects of absorption are removed from the terminal component of the curve (see Figure 1-22). Drugs exhibiting a flip-flop behavior are characterized by a terminal rate constant following intravenous administration that is statistically shorter than the terminal rate constant measured after non-IV administration.

Area under the Curve (AUC)

Once the equation of the PDC versus time curve of a drug has been established, a number of parameters can be determined to further describe or explore drug behavior (see Box 1-5). Among the more important parameters generated from pharmacokinetic analysis is the **AUC**, a parameter that indicates duration and extent of exposure of a drug after administration of a specific dose. Following compartmental analysis, AUC is calculated by dividing the Y intercept of each slope by the rate constant of the slope; for multiple compartments the terms are additive. Thus, for a one-compartment model, AUC = A/α; (or Co/ k_{el}); for a two-compartment model, AUC = $A/\alpha + B/\beta$, and so on (see Figure 1-22). The units for AUC are reflected in its determinants: PDC (Co, A, B, and so on) of mg/mL (or weight/volume) and a rate constant (inverse time or time^{-1}: min^{-1}). An example would be an AUC of 546 mg * min/mL.

AUC is used to calculate several other parameters important to the description of drug behavior. Area under the moment curve (**AUMC**: A/α^2 for one-compartment model, $A/\alpha^2 + B/\beta^2$ for a two-compartment model, and so on) is a parameter with little physiologic relevance, but it is used to calculate other parameters. Among the more important parameters based on AUC is bioavailability, the percentage of a drug that reaches systemic circulation. Absolute bioavailability is determined by measuring the AUC after nonintravenous administration (see shaded area of plot B in Figure 1-22) and comparing it with the AUC measured after intravenous administration (100% absorption), with differences in doses adjusted for as needed. Rather than presented as a percentage, bioavailability is often presented as a ratio (F) and, as such, is unit-less. If the AUC for both curves is equal, bioavailability is 100% (F = 1) (Box 1-6).

Box 1-6

Bioavailability Calculation

Bioavailability (F, unitless) is the percentage of a drug that reaches systemic circulation. **Absolute** bioavailability is determined by measuring the area under the curve (AUC) after nonintravenous administration and comparing it with the AUC measured after intravenous administration (100% absorption), with differences in doses adjusted for as needed (see Figure 1-22): F = [AUC $_X$] * [Dose $_{IV}$] / [AUC $_{IV}$] * [Dose $_X$], where X is the nonintravenous route of administration (Figure 1-22). **Relative** bioavailability can be compared between different nonintravenous routes in the same manner.

Rate Constants and Half-lives

Generally, because each component of the curve is associated with a specific drug movement, the half-life is also associated with that movement (e.g., absorption, distribution, or elimination [disappearance] half-lives), each referring to the time necessary for 50% of the respective drug movement to be complete (or reach equilibrium). Of the drug movements, elimination from the body is generally the slowest. As such, the elimination half-life is represented by the slope of the terminal, or final component, of the PDC versus time curve. However, this assignment can only be confirmed with IV administration since the terminal component of non-IV administration may reflect absorption (i.e., a flip-flop model). If an intravenous dose is not studied, the terminal component may be referred to as a *disappearance rate constant* or *half-life*. The distribution half-life is generally calculated from the initial component of the curve (generally referred to as α) following intravenous administration; the distribution component of the curve is often masked with oral administration. Absorption half-life is derived from the k_a unless a flip-flop model has been identified. Note that the faster the absorption half-life, the higher C_{max} and shorter T_{max}, the time to the maximum concentration. Because half-life is calculated from the inverse of k_{el} ($t_{1/2} = 0.693/k_{el}$) (see Box 1-4), half-life from a sample population cannot be normally distributed. As such, reports providing descriptive statistics should be reported as harmonic mean (derived from averaging the inverse of each half-life, [1/HL + 1/HL...] and reinversing the mean) and pseudo standard deviation is generally reported.

Volume of Distribution

The dose of a drug is based on the target concentration and the volume of tissue to which the drug appears to be distributed. The actual volume of tissue distribution cannot be calculated. However, the Vd is a theoretical volume to which the drug is distributed (or the volume of tissue that dilutes a drug), assuming that the drug concentration throughout the body is the same as that measured in plasma. Because this is unlikely, and because it is mathematically derived, the Vd of a drug is referred to as *apparent*. The Vd of a drug is calculated by administering a known dose intravenously and dividing it by the maximum PDC that occurs after the drug is distributed but before any elimination occurs: Vd = Dose/PDC (Co)

(Figure 1-23). Because dose is generally in milligrams per kilogram and C_0 (or B) is generally milligrams per milliliter (the same as grams per liter), Vd is generally reported as liters per kilogram. The Vd of a drug can be determined only after intravenous administration in order to ensure that all drug reaches systemic circulation (i.e., bioavailability = 100 %). Occasionally, if a drug is not given intravenously, scientific articles or drug package inserts might report Vd/F, indicating the Vd corrected for bioavailability that is less than 100% (F<1). However, the clinical relevance of this parameter largely depends on knowledge of bioavailability.

The Vd of a drug is primarily used to calculate the dose of the drug (see Box 1-5). Three different Vds are reported in the literature. Because the PDC cannot be measured immediately (before distribution and elimination influence the curve), the PDC used to determine Vd must be derived after the terminal component is extrapolated to the Y intercept (see Figure 1-22). If the plasma elimination curve yields only one component (e.g., distribution from plasma does not occur or is instantaneous), PDC is extrapolated to time 0 or C_0, yielding the volume of the central compartment (Vc). This volume can be used to determine the initial concentration of a drug (e.g., to assess potential toxicity) or to estimate plasma volume. However, for many drugs distribution is not instantaneous and the PDC versus time curve is multicomponent. To remove the effects of elimination that occur during distribution, the terminal component of the PDC is then extrapolated to the Y axis. Generally referred to as *B* if the model is two-compartment, this PDC theoretically reflects peak PDC after distribution has reached equilibrium (pseudo-equilibrium) but prior to elimination. The Vd after distribution has reached pseudo-equilibrium then becomes Vd = Dose/B, often referred to as *Vd area, Vd extrapolated,* or *Vdβ*. For multicomponent curves, Vc can still be determined using the extrapolated initial component of the curve using A (or C_0): Vc = Dose/C_0 or Dose/A (see Figure 1-22).[2,3,12,30,34,35] Because Vd area is influenced by clearance (it is based on extrapolation of the terminal elimination curve), it tends to overestimate the true volume. It is useful to predict the amount of drug that remains to be excreted at any time point during elimination.[17] The third Vd is that which occurs at steady state, when equilibrium has been reached (Vdss). True equilibrium can be reached only if clearance does not occur, or if input equals output, as might occur with CRI.[17] As such, Vdss is independent of clearance and more accurately reflects the true volume diluting the drug. (see Box 1-5).

The Vd, although a calculated parameter, is used to calculate **clearance,** which is the physiologic action that is responsible for the elimination of drug (see Box 1-5). As with Vd, CL/F may be reported in studies for which an intravenous drug was not administered. However, this is not a clinically relevant parameter unless bioavailability has been demonstrated to be 100% for the animals in the study in question or unless bioavailability is known. Although generally calculated, clearance can be measured. However, collection requires repeated sample of the tissue into which drug is cleared. Plasma clearance of a drug that is cleared exclusively through the urine can be determined by sequentially sampling urine rather than plasma or, as with creatinine clearance, collecting a volume of urine into which the drug has cleared and plasma samples containing the drug at the beginning and end of the sampling time. Determining clearance of a drug excreted in the bile would require biliary catheterization.

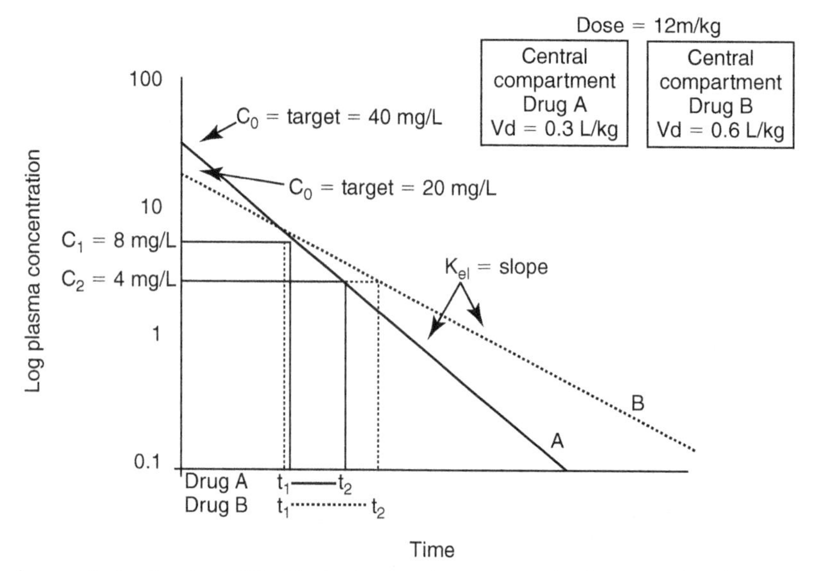

Figure 1-23 Changes in volume of distribution (Vd) affect plasma drug concentration and the slope of the elimination (k_{el}) curve that determines elimination half-life. The former is impacted because movement of drug into tissues removes it from plasma and thus organs of elimination. Plot A represents PDC versus time following administration of a dose of drug in an animal with a Vd that is half of that represented in plot B (compartment size increased in the latter). Note that the slope of the plasma elimination curves for animal B is flatter. As such, elimination half-life also will be longer. Drug half-life can be determined by measuring the time (t_2 - t_1) necessary for PDC to decrease drop 50% (C_1 to C_2).

Noncompartmental Analysis

All models are, by definition, incorrect. Thus, a disadvantage of compartmental analysis is that data (particularly poor fitting data) is forced to fit the "best" equation that mathematically describes the data (Box 1-7). The more variable the data, the more inaccurate compartmental analysis is because the greater the deviation of actual data from predicted data. Noncompartmental analysis often is used in lieu of compartmental analysis, particularly if rate constants are not necessary to describe the behavior of a drug in the body. Further, no attempt is made to relate noncompartmental pharmacokinetic parameters with physiologic processes, thus reducing confusion or bias that might occur with interpretation. For noncompartmental analysis the primary parameter determined is AUC. This parameter can be determined in a variety of ways, but the most common (for noncompartmental analysis) is the trapezoidal method (Figure 1-24).[33,34] For this method a series of sequential trapezoids are drawn, each defined by a line drawn between two subsequent data points in the PDC versus time curve. The remainder of the trapezoid is determined by dropping the lines from each data point on the line to the X axis. The area for each trapezoid is determined, and areas are summed to generate AUC. The last trapezoid can end at either the last actual time point measured or be extrapolated "to infinity" based on the slope of the terminal component of the data. As with compartmental analysis, the elimination rate constant (terminal component of the curve) and thus half-life is based on the best-fit analysis. However, all other remaining parameters are based on AUC. As such, mean residence time, **MRT,** is a comparable, more physiologically descriptive and thus preferred parameter to elimination half-life. Based on AUC, MRT describes the average time a molecule is in the body (or the time necessary for 63.2% of a drug to be eliminated). The difference between MRT after intravenous versus extravascular administration is the mean absorption time, **MAT**, providing a noncompartmental method for assessment of the absorptive phase of the drug.

Box 1-7

Parameters for Noncompartmental Analysis

Mean residence time: MRT = AUC/AUMC (area under the curve/area under the moment curve)

Clearance (intravenous only): CL = dose/AUC

Extravascular: CL and volume of distribution (Vd) must be corrected for bioavailability by multiplying by D * F. For extravascular administration, mean absorption time (MAT) describes the absorptive phase of the drug movement; however, it can be determined only if the drug is also studied intravenously (MAT = MRT_{EV}- MRT_{IV} where EV = extravascular).

Vd at steady state (intravenous only): Vd_{ss} = Vdss: (D × AUMC)/ AUC^2 (* Extravascular: Vdss: (D * F x AUMC)/AUC^2)

Volume or weight units must match for all calculations.

(From Martinez MN: Special series: use of pharmacokinetics in veterinary medicine, Article II: volume, clearance, and half-life, *J Am Vet Med Assoc* 213:1122-1127, 1998.)

Alternative Pharmacokinetics

Pharmacokinetic studies generally are implemented in a sample population of the target species by administration of a dose via the intended route and subsequent intermittent collection of tissues (generally blood, representing the central compartment, but occasionally specific tissues representing peripheral/compartments), that are subjected to quantitative analysis of the drug and or its metabolites. The number of animals and samples from each animal must be sufficient for accurate

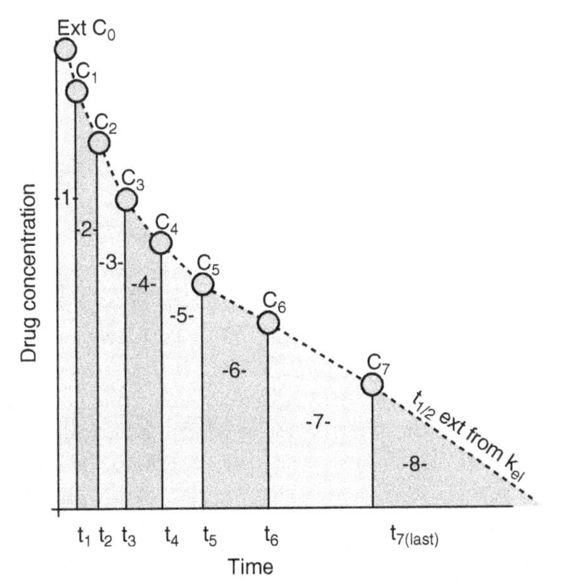

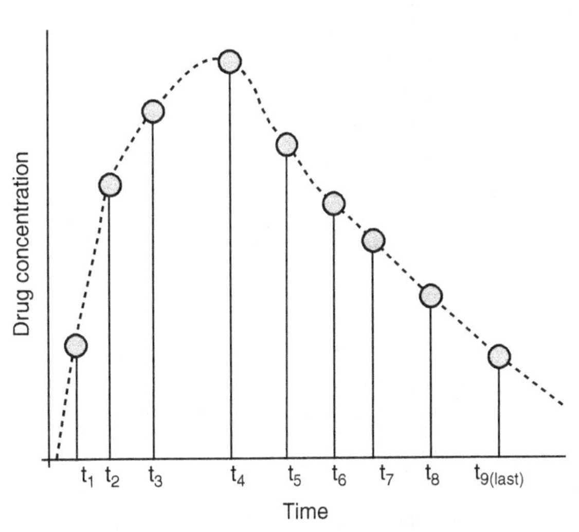

Figure 1-24 For noncompartmental analysis the area under the curve is determined by adding the area calculated for the trapezoids formed by two adjacent data points. If AUC is determined to infinity, the terminal component is based on the slope of the terminal time points as determined by linear regression. The advantage of noncompartmental analysis is that actual data points are used rather than predicted data. As with compartmental analysis, the more data points, the more accurately the data is likely to represent the actual time course.

description of the time course of drug concentrations in the sampled tissue. The more the data points, the better the data represents the population. The approval process for animal drugs does not necessarily require pharmacokinetic modeling of drugs; if required, generally the studies are performed in normal animals. Pharmacokinetics for human drugs are performed in humans, with studies involving dogs most often focusing on toxicity. Data often are available only through Freedom of Information Act publications. *Population pharmacokinetics* study the sources of variability in drug concentrations among patients, and as such the science takes advantage of multiple studies that differ in study design or subjects. Further, population pharmacokinetics can take advantage of data collected in patients, which generally is restricted because of ethical considerations that might limit the study to small sample numbers.[35] With limitations, a pharmacokinetic profile of a drug might also be generated for the individual patient using this approach (Chapter 5).

OTHER CONSIDERATIONS

Dosing Based on Allometric Scaling and Body Surface Area

Allometry refers to the phenomenon of changes in shape that result from changes in size. Allometric scaling attempts to predict a change in physiologic response based on a change in another physiologic parameter. Over 34 anatomic, physiologic (including heart rate, blood volume, and glomerular filtration), and biochemical parameters correlate with body weight across species; not surprisingly, body weight has been extensively examined as a method of allometrically scaling for species differences in physiologic processes. Using the allometric equation $Y = a\ W^b$, many physiologic parameters (Y) do appear to be predicted by weight (W) adjusted with an allometric exponent (b) of 0.67 to 1. The usefulness of adjusting doses on the basis of body weight scaled according to body surface area ($BSA = 10 - W^{2/3}$) was initially realized in children receiving drugs characterized by a narrow therapeutic index.[37,38]

As with children, the simplest method of dosing based on body weight, tends to underdose small animals and overdose larger animals, and the use of BSA should improve accuracy of dosing. Because animals differ so much in body shape as well as size, the equation can be further normalized by the addition of the shape constant K: $BSA = K \bullet 10 - W^{2/3}$. The formula is most commonly applied to cancer chemotherapeutic drugs, with the supposition that large-breed dogs would benefit most (thus preventing the relative overdosing they received compared with smaller dogs). However, because the incidence of adverse reactions to cancer chemotherapeutic drugs increased in smaller dogs compared with larger dogs using this approach, the method needs to be reassessed. Several observations made by Price and associates[36] help support the need to re-examine the application of the method to all animals. First, studies have suggested that the mass exponent used to correct weight (⅔ or 0.67) is incorrect. Other studies have shown that the exponent may vary as a function of age. This and other factors suggest that a range of mass exponents should be applied to animals within the same species. Second, although studies have shown that the allometric scaling of doses does help normalize doses among species, normalization using the same shape constant (K) within species has not been documented. Although a single K may be appropriate for the domestic cat, marked differences should be expected for the dog. Indeed, previous literature reveals that a number of shape constants have been used in dogs, ranging from 9.9 to 12.3 (Appendix 2), with the smaller value being applied to smaller or more compact dogs. It may be necessary to apply different constants to growing animals.

Using allometric scaling based on body weight or BSA, even adjusted for body shape, as a method of predicting dose (which incorporates both pharmacodynamics and pharmacokinetics) is likely to be difficult; many aspects of drug disposition seemingly are not related to BSA or body weight. These include protein binding; effects of pH on drug movement; actions of p-glycoprotein (i.e., active tubular secretion in renal tubular cells); differences in the composition of body compartments; and, most dramatically, differences in the rate, extent, and type of drug-metabolizing enzymes among the species. One study evaluated the allometric relationship between body weight and drug elimination half-life. Because half-life is equally affected by Vd and clearance, it serves as a good parameter to assess the overall relationship. Not surprisingly, those drugs whose half-lives are most likely to be predicted by allometric scaling tended to be minimally protein bound, characterized by a Vd indicative of distribution to ECF and excreted renally in the unchanged but also undergoing flow-limited hepatic extraction;[38] many antimicrobials meet these criteria. Half-life tended to be less correlated allometrically with body weight for drugs that were highly protein bound, distributed to specialized body compartments, or metabolized by the liver in a capacity-limited fashion.[37,38] Additional studies are needed to identify the most appropriate factors to be used to allometrically scale dosing regimens. To date, use of weight adjusted to BSA appears to be the most reasonable method for smaller animals.

Routes of Administration

Choice of the route and technique of administration is generally based on several factors, including the physicochemical properties of the drug, formulation to be used, therapeutic indication, pathophysiology of the disease, and the target species. The manufacturer's recommendations should always be followed carefully unless it is explicitly known that a proposed deviation will not adversely alter the activity or kinetic fate of the principal ingredients. Note that regardless of the dosage form used, it is imperative to have an appreciation of the makeup of the pharmaceutical formulation, the factors that may alter the efficacy of the product, and the best way to derive optimal therapeutic benefit from the agent without jeopardizing its bioavailability or pharmacologic action.

KEY POINT 1-8 The route of administration might influence the rate and extent of absorption but should not influence distribution or clearance. As such, elimination half-life should not differ.

Oral Administration

The United States Pharmacopeia provides an excellent source of currently accepted dosing forms.[38] Common oral dosage forms include tablets, capsules, boluses, powders, granules, syrups, solutions, suspensions, and pastes. Oral bioavailability of oral dosing forms may profoundly differ. Other specialized delivery systems are also available, including enteric-coated tablets and sustained-action or controlled-release preparations. However, if designed for human use, their behavior in animals may be substantially different, particularly if orally administered. The advantages of oral dosing are that it is usually convenient and safe, sterility is not a requirement, and the danger of acute drug reaction is not as great as with intravenous administration. The disadvantages include a slower onset of action and unpredictability and inconsistency of absorption, including the sequela of exposing the drug to the unstable gastrointestinal tract. Additionally, dosing may be difficult in fractious animals, poor technique or dysphagia may lead to intratracheal delivery and subsequent bronchopneumonia, and inactivation may occur within the gastrointestinal tract. Some drugs may cause esophageal damage, particularly in cats.

Parenteral Administration

The most common parenteral dosage form is a stable aqueous solution. Less frequently, the active components may be dissolved in an inert vegetable oil, which delays absorption. Other kinds of prolonged-release preparations include subcutaneous implants of solid dosage forms and relatively insoluble salts and esters as suspensions in various vehicles. It is important to appreciate the basic differences between these and standard pharmaceutical preparations. First, accidental intravenous administration can lead to serious and even fatal effects related to microembolism. Second, persistent drug residues in racing or other show animals may have ethical and legal ramifications. The stability of solutions intended for parenteral administration often is delicate, depending on pH, temperature, and the presence of stabilizers, solubilizers, and preservatives. Indiscriminate mixing of such products for the sake of convenience (e.g., single versus multiple injections) should be avoided unless proof exists that the formulations are physically and chemically compatible. Several novel approaches for the parenteral delivery of drugs are being developed, including microspheres, microcapsules, liposomes, microsponges, resealed carrier erythrocytes, and projectile biodegradable missiles. Additionally, monoclonal antibodies have been used to carry highly selective, bound drugs to specific target tissues or even cells. Implantable controlled-release drug delivery systems include pellets (composed of various polymeric forms) and silicone capsules. Several implantable devices also have been introduced that permit constant systemic delivery of a drug within the body; these include osmotically or propellant-driven pumps and mini pumps. The advent of nanotechnology is likely to markedly improve drug delivery to targeted tissues. Liposomes are the earliest example of drug delivery systems based on nanotechnology; more current products include polymer-drug conjugates.

The most frequently used parenteral routes are intravenous (IV), intramuscular (IM), and subcutaneous (SC). Common but less frequently used routes include epidural, intradermal, intratracheal, and intraperitoneal (IP). Occasional routes of injection include intraarterial, intramedullary, intrathecal, intrathoracic, subarachnoid, intracardiac, subconjunctival, and intratesticular. Intralesional injection is a way of attaining high concentrations of a drug at the target site. In all cases solutions for injection must be sterile, techniques must be aseptic, and the dose must be accurate; a painful reaction is a possibility. For the IV route, aqueous solutions are preferable, which lead immediately to predictably high blood levels with a rapid onset of action. Irritating and nonisotonic solutions can be injected intravenously if done slowly and carefully. Usually, but not always, drugs given intravenously can be given intramuscularly or subcutaneously, but injection may be painful (e.g., arginine vehicles, or other basic or acidic solutions). Further, IM absorption of some IV drugs (e.g., diazepam) is not predictable. The IM route can be used for aqueous or oleaginous suspensions, solutions, and other depot preparations. Absorption occurs either hematogenously or by way of lymphatics and usually is fairly rapid except in the case of long-acting preparations. The addition of esters can variably prolong absorption depending on the rate of hydrolysis. Acetate salts are more slowly hydrolyzed than succinate salts (e.g., glucocorticoids); benzathine salts are more slowly hydrolyzed than procaine salts (e.g., penicillin). Moderately irritating preparations can be injected intramuscularly, but tissue reaction and necrosis may become evident with time. The duration of drug action is longer than for IV injection but most often is slightly shorter than for SC administration; however, this is not always predictable. A disadvantage of the IM route is the possibility of improper deposition in nerves, blood vessels, fat, or between muscle bundles in connective tissue sheaths. The advantages of the SC route are similar to those of the IM route, although irritant preparations and oily vehicles should be avoided due to possible undesirable reactions. The rate of absorption from SC injection sites may be unpredictable and depends on several factors. The most important of these is blood flow, and the presence of vasoconstrictors or vasodilators can substantially alter rates of absorption. Usually, the rate of absorption is slightly slower than from IM sites.

Miscellaneous Parenteral Routes

The other parenteral routes of administration are generally used for the following purposes: epidural and subarachnoid for spinal analgesia and myelography; intradermal testing for hypersensitivity and for vaccination; intratracheal treatment of respiratory tract infections; intraarterial with simultaneous venous constriction, with the latter causing high concentrations of drug in the dependent area for a short time (occasionally necessary in cancer chemotherapy and special radiographic or other imaging techniques); intramedullary (blood transfusion or fluid therapy directly into the bone marrow) when other routes are awkward, as in neonates; intrathecal (cisterna magna) for treatment of meningoencephalitis and myelography; intrathoracic (intrapleural or intrapulmonary and); and intracardiac for emergencies, especially cardiac arrest.

Inhalation (pulmonary route). Gases, volatile agents, and fine particles usually are rapidly absorbed from the airways and alveoli into the pulmonary circulation. Delivery into the respiratory passages is done by standard anesthetic machines in the case of inhalation anesthetics or by vaporization or nebulization for the local delivery of expectorants, bronchodilators, and antiinfective agents. Drugs in the gaseous state readily reach the alveolar surfaces, whereas only particles less than 2 μm (produced by nebulization) are inspired into the terminal ducts and alveoli. Particles less than 5 μm may reach the respiratory bronchioles, and those 5 to 10 μm in size may reach the upper respiratory tract and larger airways. Because the depth of airway penetration is influenced by depth of respiration (directly) and respiratory rate (inversely) as well as the tortuosity of the airways, aerosolization generally should not be the sole route of administration of drugs in animals. Aqueous solutions of antibacterial drugs intended for injection may be delivered intratracheally. Absorption of drugs may occur after topical administration in the respiratory tract.

Topical administration (local application). Drugs can be applied topically to the skin and its adnexa or to a variety of mucous membranes. The routes that may be used include sublingual, intranasal, intravaginal, intrauterine, intracystic, rectal, preputial, ocular, and aural. Many dosage forms have been developed to deliver active principles to the site of application to produce local effects. However, in many instances absorption into the systemic circulation also occurs. A wide variety of preparations are available for dermal application, including ointments, creams, pastes, dusting powders, lotions, sprays, liniments, and poultices. Systemic effects may occur as a result of the animal licking at the applied medication or due to percutaneous drug absorption, which often occurs, especially when the skin is damaged or inflamed (e.g., burns, ulcers, wounds, dermatitis). Absorption through the skin can also be enhanced by occlusive dressings, inunction, or the use of dimethyl sulfoxide (DMSO) as a carrier. Several drugs are deliberately applied to the skin with the anticipation of systemic effects after transdermal absorption—for example, transdermal gels, ectoparasiticides available as "pour-on" formulations, nitroglycerin ointment, and scopolamine in a transdermal patch device as well as iontophoresis devices. Of these the pluronic-lecithin transdermal gels, which are generated through compounding pharmacies, appear to be minimally effective for all but a few drugs and their use is not recommended unless specifically supported by scientific studies.

Transmucosal administration. **Transmucosal** or buccal drug administration represents a variation of oral administration (see previous discussion of topical administration). Drugs are given by mouth with the intent of absorption occurring through the mucosa of the mouth. A major advantage of this route of administration is avoidance of first-pass metabolism, which occurs with drugs that are swallowed. Convenience may be an additional reason. In contrast to the skin, mucosal tissues do not contain a stratum corneum, and therefore drugs are not presented with a significant barrier to movement into vascular tissues. Several methods of transmucosal delivery have been studied in dogs, including transmucosal gels (often with carboxymethylcellulose as the carrier), sprays, and patches. Among the difficulties associated with transmucosal administration in animals is maintaining contact time between drug and surface.

REFERENCES

1. Lees P, Cunningham FM, Elliott J: Principles of pharmacodynamics and their applications in veterinary pharmacology, *J Vet Pharmacol Ther* 27:397–414, 2004.
2. Ritschel WA, Kearns GL: *Handbook of basic pharmacokinetics including clinical applications*, ed 5, Philadelphia, 1999, Hamilton Drug Intelligence Publications.
3. Rollins DE: Pharmacokinetics and drug excretion in bile. In Benet LZ, Massoud N, Rowland M, editors: *Clinical pharmacokinetics: concepts and applications*, Philadelphia, 1989, Lea & Febiger.
4. Toutain PL, Lees P: Integration and modeling of pharmacokinetic and pharmacodynamic data to optimize dosage regimens in veterinary medicine, *J Vet Pharmacol Ther* 27:467–477, 2004.
5. Beal SL, Benet LZ, Benowitz NL, et al: *Pharmacokinetic basis for drug treatment*, New York, 1984, Raven Press.
6. Baggott JD: Principles of drug disposition in domestic animals. In Baggott JD, editor: *The basis of veterinary clinical pharmacology*, Philadelphia, 1977, Saunders, pp 73–112.
7. Kim RB: Drugs as p-glycoprotein substrates, inhibitors and inducers, *Drug Metab Rev* 34:47–54, 2002.
8. Mealey KL: Therapeutic implications of the MDR-1 gene, *J Vet Pharmacol Ther* 27:257–264, 2004.
9. Notari RE: *Biopharmaceutics and clinical pharmacokinetics: an introduction*, ed 4, New York, 1987, Marcel Dekker.
10. Toutain PL, Bousquet-Mélou A: Bioavailability and its assessment, *J Vet Pharmacol Ther* 27:455–466, 2004.
11. Schentag JJ: Correlation of pharmacokinetic parameters to efficacy of antibiotics: relationships between serum concentrations, MIC values, and bacterial eradication in patients with gram-negative pneumonia, *Scand J Infect Dis* 74(Suppl):218–234, 1991.
12. Martinez MN: Special series: use of pharmacokinetics in veterinary medicine, Article IV: clinical application of pharmacokinetics, *J Am Vet Med Assoc* 213:1418–1420, 1998.
13. Kunta JR, Sinco PJ: Intestinal drug transporters: in vivo function and clinical importance, *Curr Drug Metab* 5:109–124, 2004.
14. Craig WA, Ebert SC: Protein binding and its significance in antibacterial therapy, *Infect Dis Clin North Am* 3:407–414, 1989.
15. Belpaire FM, DeRick A, Dello C, et al: Alpha 1-acid glycoprotein and serum binding of drugs in healthy and diseased dogs, *J Vet Pharmacol Ther* 10:43–48, 1987.
16. Toutain PL, Bousquet-Mélou A: Free drug fraction vs. free drug concentration: a matter of frequent confusion, *J Vet Pharmacol Ther* 25:460–463, 2002.
17. Toutain PL, Bousquet-Mélou A: Volumes of distribution, *J Vet Pharmacol Ther* 27:441–453, 2004.
18. Bergan T: Pharmacokinetics of tissue penetration of antibiotics, *Rev Infect Dis* 3:45–66, 1981.
19. LeFrock JL, Prince RA, Richards ML: Penetration of antimicrobials into the cerebrospinal fluid and brain. In Ristuccia AM, Cuhna BA, editors: *Antimicrobial therapy*, New York, 1984, Raven Press, pp 397–413.
20. Schenkman JP, Kupfer D: *Hepatic cytochrome P-450 monooxygenase system*, New York, 1982, Pergamon Press, pp 99-156.
21. Parkinson A: Biotransformation of xenobiotics. In Klaassen CD, editor: *Casarett and Doull's toxicology: the basic science of poisons*, ed 5, New York, 1996, McGraw-Hill, pp 113–186.

22. Bogaards JJP, Bertrandoe M, Jacsonoe P: Determining the best animal model for human cytochrome P450 activities: a comparison of mouse, rat, rabbit, dog, micropig, monkey and man, *Xenobiotica* 30:1131–1152, 2000.
23. Guengerich FP: Cytochrome P450 and chemical toxicology, *Chem Res Toxicol* 21:70–83, 2008.
24. Mitchell JR, Smith CV, Lauferburg BH, et al: Reactive metabolites and the pathophysiology of acute lethal cell injury. In Mitchell JR, Homing MG, editors: *Drug metabolism and drug toxicity*, New York, 1984, Raven Press, pp 301–318.
25. Landoni MF, Soraci AL, Delatour P, et al: Enantioselective behavior of drugs used in domestic animals: a review, *J Vet Pharmacol Ther* 20:1–16, 1997.
26. Somogyi A: New insight into the renal secretion of drugs, *Trends Pharmacol Sci* 8:354–357, 1987.
27. Bekersky I: Renal excretion, *J Clin Pharmacol* 27:447–449, 1989.
28. Toutain PL, Bousquet-Mélou A: Plasma terminal half-life, *J Vet Pharmacol Ther* 27:427–439, 2004.
29. Dayton PG, Cucinell SA, Weiss N, et al: Dose-dependence of drug plasma level decline in dogs, *J Pharmacol Exp Ther* 158:305–316, 1967.
30. Martinez MN: Special series: use of pharmacokinetics in veterinary medicine, Article II: volume, clearance, and half-life, *J Am Vet Med Assoc* 213:1122–1127, 1998.
31. Martinez MN: Special series: use of pharmacokinetics in veterinary medicine, Article V: clinically important errors in data interpretation, *J Am Vet Med Assoc* 213:1564–1569, 1998.
32. Toutain PL, Bousquet-Mélou A: Plasma clearance, *J Vet Pharmacol Ther* 27:415–425, 2004.
33. Nestorov I: Whole-body physiologically based pharmacokinetic models, *Expert Opin Drug Metab Toxicol* 3(2):235–249, 2007.
34. Gabrielsson J, Weiner D: *Pharmacokinetic and Pharmacodynamic Data Analysis: Concepts and Applications*, Stockholm, 2000, Swedish Pharmaceutical Press, Sweden.
35. Guidance for Industry: Population Pharmacokinetics. Accessed May 05, 2010. http://www.fda.gov/downloads/Drugs/GuidanceComplianceRegulatoryInformation/Guidances/ucm072137.pdf
36. Price GS, Frazier DL: Use of body surface area (BSA)-based dosages to calculate chemotherapeutic drug dose in dogs, I. Potential problems with current BSA formulae, *J Vet Intern Med* 12:267–271, 1998.
37. Riviere JE, Martin-Jimenez T, Sudlof S, et al: Interspecies allometric analysis of the comparative pharmacokinetics of 44 drugs across veterinary and laboratory animal species, *J Vet Pharmacol Therap* 20:453–463, 1997.
38. United States Pharmacopeia, National Formulary, General Chapter 1151.

2 Factors Affecting Drug Disposition

Dawn Merton Boothe

Chapter Outline

Ideally, fixed dosing regimens are based on scientific studies performed with the drug of interest in the target species. Often, however, the dose for a drug used in dogs or cats is extrapolated from other species, especially humans to dogs and humans or dogs to cats, rather than based on scientific studies. For those drugs backed by scientific evidence, sample numbers are often too small, resulting in marked variability in the pharmacokinetic parameters. Further, as in human medicine, animals in which pharmacokinetic studies are performed are generally healthy and may not represent the state of disease in the animals treated with the drug. A number of factors can alter plasma drug concentrations (PDCs) in the patient due to changes in drug disposition, thereby increasing the risk of therapeutic failure. Many of these can be anticipated, allowing for adjustments in the dosing regimen. In addition to the disposition of a drug, these factors might also alter patient response to the drug. These factors might be categorized as physiologic factors such as species and age; pathologic factors, particularly cardiac, renal, or hepatic disease; and pharmacologic factors that occur when one drug alters the kinetics or response to another drug (Box 2-1).

PHYSIOLOGIC FACTORS

Age-Induced Differences

Drug Disposition in the Geriatric Animal

This discussion focuses on some of the clinically important changes that are likely to alter response to drug therapy in geriatric patients (Table 2-1) and on actions that can be implemented to compensate or reduce the sequelae of these changes. Age is associated with changes both in pharmacokinetics (gerontokinetics) and pharmacodynamics, with changes generally compared with those of the young adult.[1-3] Data in animals are limited, but in general, disposition pattern changes described for humans appear to extrapolate adequately to dogs and cats.[4] Geriatric animals are at a greater risk for therapeutic failure because of normal aging changes in physiology, an increased incidence of disease, and the likelihood of polypharmacy in response to disease; moreover, a decrease in normal organ protective mechanisms may increase the risk of adverse events. The age at which body functions shift from a period of growth to a period of decay (16 to 18 years in humans) has not been established in dogs and cats. The age probably differs among canine breeds. Aging is accompanied by permanent loss of up to 30% of body cells, with a parallel loss in oxygen consumption. Body composition changes, as do regional blood flow rates. Physiologic functions generally decline steadily with increasing age. In humans basal metabolic rate decreases by 0.4% per year[2]; according to the National Research Council,[5] energy requirements of dogs decrease as they age. Changes among the body systems can influence all four drug movements.

KEY POINT 2-1 As the geriatric animal ages, organ mass reduces in size and function by approximately 25%, resulting in corresponding changes in drug disposition.

Cardiovascular. As animals age, cardiac output decreases and circulation transit time increases. In humans cardiac output decreases by about 1% per year for a total decline of 30% to

Box 2-1

Examples of Factors that Affect Drug Disposition

Pharmacologic Factors

Pharmaceutical interactions
- Therapeutical inequivalence
- Direct drug–drug interactions
- Drug–diet interactions

Pharmacokinetic interactions
Pharmacodynamic interactions

Pathologic Factors

Gastrointestinal disease
Hepatic disease
Renal disease
Cardiovascular disease
Pulmonary disease
Neurologic disease
Metabolic disease

Physiologic Factors

Route of administration
Species variations
Genetic (breed) factors
Age
Sex
Body weight and surface area
Pregnancy and lactation
Diet and nutrition
Temperament
Environment
Circadian rhythms

40% in the aged. Regional and organ blood flow rates similarly decrease.[2] The net effect of these changes depends on the state of disease but can influence each drug movement. Absorption, metabolism, and excretion are likely to decrease, whereas distribution may increase or decrease depending on the state of vascular responses or fluid retention.[2,6,7] As cardiac function decreases, secondary compensatory responses can lead to further risks of adverse reaction.[7] Blood flow is preferably redistributed to the brain and heart, increasing the risk of toxicity of drugs toxic to these tissues.

Central and peripheral nervous systems. As the geriatric patient ages, brain weight and peripheral fiber numbers decrease. Connective tissue infiltrates peripherally.[2] Oxygen consumption and cerebral blood flow decrease. In addition, decreased amounts of selected neurotransmitters have been documented. Morita and coworkers[8] reported alterations in the blood–brain barrier in elderly dogs.

Respiratory. In human geriatric patients, residual lung volume decreases by 50% with accompanying decreases in vital capacity, arterial oxygen pressure (PO_2), and maximum oxygen uptake. In addition, the central response to hypoxia and hypercapnia, such as that induced by opioid analgesics, decreases.[2] Anesthetic or other sedating agents must be used more cautiously.

Gastrointestinal. As animals age, deglutition decreases as a result of decreased salivation and pharyngeal and esophageal motility. Gastric function is characterized by atrophy of the mucosa with a reduction of hydrochloric acid secretion and a subsequent increase in gastric pH. Gastrointestinal motility is generally reduced. The intestinal macrovilli and microvilli also atrophy, increasing the risk of bacterial overgrowth. These sequelae tend to reduce the absorption and thus the PDC of orally administered drugs. Changes in gastrointestinal function (including reduction of gastroprotective effects) may also predispose the geriatric patient to adverse effects induced by toxic drugs such as chemotherapeutic agents and nonsteroidal antiinflammatory drug (NSAID) analgesics. The latter should be used with caution; the clinician should anticipate and be prepared to treat toxicities. Digestibility of key nutrients, such as fat, tends to decrease in elderly cats.[9] As with humans, the intestinal microbiota population shifts in elderly dogs and cats, with lactobacilli decreasing and clostridia increasing in dogs[10] and bifidobacteria decreasing in cats.[11] In addition to response to antimicrobials, these changes might influence enterohepatic circulation of bile acids and thus, potentially, some drugs.[12]

Hepatic. Changes in hepatic function are important to the geriatric animal because of the liver's role in the metabolism of drugs.[13] Hepatocyte number and function decrease, as do hepatic and splanchnic blood flow, hepatic oxidation, and cytochrome P450 content (the primary drug-metabolizing enzyme). Both flow-limited and capacity-limited drugs are affected. For example, hepatic clearance of both opioid analgesics (which are characterized by first-pass metabolism; i.e., flow limited) and nonsteroidal analgesics (eliminated principally by hepatic metabolism; i.e., capacity limited) is decreased in geriatric patients. Increased response of human geriatric patients to opioid analgesics—they require 60% to 75% less drug than younger patients do—has been attributed to changes in drug elimination.[14,15] Changes in hepatic function, oxygenation, and nutrition may also predispose the liver to drug-induced hepatotoxicity. Because of reduced hepatic function, the geriatric patient may be less able to generate endogenous hepatoprotectant agents, increasing the risk of drug-induced hepatotoxicity (Chapter 4).

Urinary. As renal blood flow decreases, the glomerular filtration rate and active secretory capacity of the nephron unit progressively decrease with age. Both result in a similar decline in renal clearance. Renal excretion is the major route of elimination of many drugs. Changes in renal clearance tend to prolong the elimination and thus increase PDCs in the geriatric patient. Changes in renal function also render the geriatric patient more susceptible to adverse drug reactions such as those induced by aminoglycosides, angiotensin-converting enzyme inhibitors, and NSAID analgesics.

Body weight and composition. Changes in body composition may be among the most complex in the geriatric animal. Like humans, dogs tend to lose lean body mass and accumulate body fat as they age (Figure 2-1).[16] In male humans, fat increases from approximately 18% in young adults up to 50% in the aged.[2] Increased proportion of body

Table 2-1 The Impact of Age-Related Differences in Physiology on Xenobiotic Disposition

	Absorption	Distribution	Metabolism	Excretion
Geriatric				
	Decreased gastric motility prolongs time to peak effect	Increased fat mass and decreased lean body weight results in decreased distribution, higher concentration, and shorter half-life of water-soluble drugs	Decreased hepatic mass and drug metabolizing enzymes (phases I and II)	Decreased GFR, decreased renal clearance
	Increased risk of bacterial overgrowth	Increased body fat increasing distribution and prolonging half-life of lipid-soluble drugs	Decreased hepatic blood flow, decreased clearance of flow-limited drugs, increased absorption of drugs that undergo first-pass metabolism	Decreased renal clearance and longer half-life
	Generally decreased absorption	Decreased protein binding compensated for by clearance of free compound (?)	Decreased hepatic clearance and prolonged half-life	Decreased renal protection
	Decreased gastroprotection	Increased distribution to heart and brain as cardiac function declines	Decreased hepatoprotection	
		Decreased distribution of water-soluble drugs resulting in increased drug concentrations, shorter half-life	Higher plasma drug concentration	
Pediatric				
≤ 12 weeks	Increased absorption for first 24 hours (during colostrum absorption)	Increased volume of distribution, reduced plasma concentrations	Decreased phase I metabolism, being absent for first weeks and reaching adult levels at 3 to 4 months	Decreased renal clearance until 2 to 3 months
	Decreased acidity leading to decreased absorption of weak acids	Greater proportion of extracellular fluid reducing plasma concentrations of water-soluble compounds	Increased bioavailability of drugs that normally undergo first-pass metabolism	Prolonged half-life
	Decreased rate (not extent) of absorption of most drugs	Longer half-life	Decreased response to compounds that must be metabolized to active state	
	Milk possibly binding to luminal contents	Decreased distribution of compounds that accumulate in fat	Decreased peripheral metabolism of compounds	
	Reduced absorption of fat-soluble drugs	Decreased protein binding possibly increasing distribution		
		Increased blood flow to brain and heart		
		Increased permeability of blood–brain barrier		

GFR, Glomerular filtration rate.

fat is accompanied by a decrease in total body water and cell mass. Although extracellular fluid does not change in total amount, the relative proportion of total body water that it makes up increases. Thus the proportion of intracellular to extracellular fluid decreases. The sequelae of these changes depend on the drug. As distribution of water-soluble drugs decreases with total body water, PDCs tend to increase. The distribution of lipid-soluble drugs increases as the proportion of body fat increases, however, which tends to decrease PDCs unless the patient is dosed on a mg/kg basis. The impact of aging on body composition in dogs varies with breeds. For example, in one study body fat increased with age in Great Danes but not Labrador Retrievers or Papillons,[17] although this did occur within 1 year of death in

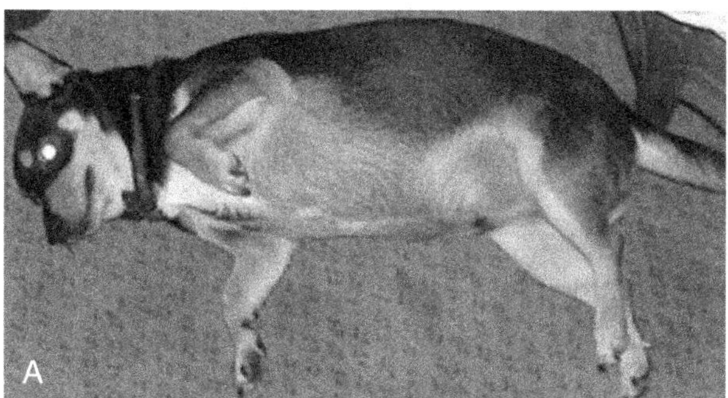

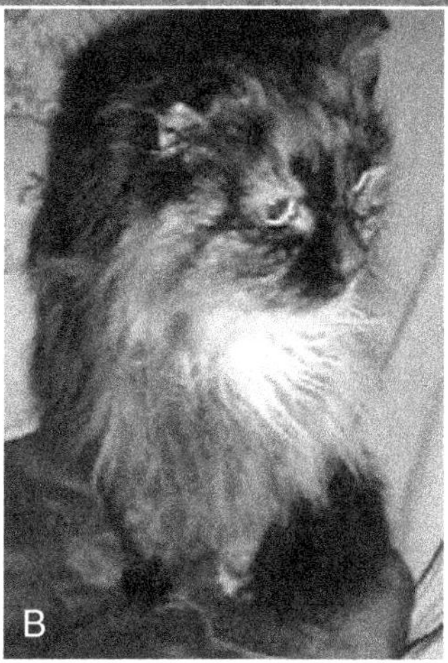

Figure 2-1 The geriatric dog and cats may represent two extremes in regard to the impact of aging on disposition. Body mass frequently increases in dogs **(A)** but decreases in geriatric cats **(B)**. Mass loss in cat reflects lean tissue and fat. In contrast to the geriatric animal, adult cats, like dogs, may be characterized by marked differences in body composition, as is exemplified by the obese cat or dog. Water-soluble drugs generally do not distribute to fat, and dosing of water-soluble drug on the basis of total body weight may result in overdose. Dosing on lean body weight is more prudent. Distribution of a lipid-soluble drug to the fat compartment, on the other hand, may increase the volume of distribution, decreasing drug concentrations. For such animals dosing on total body weight (per kg) is more reasonable.

elderly Labrador Retrievers in another study.[16] Although middle-aged cats tend to be overweight, geriatric cats often become thin.[9] Thus PDCs of water-soluble compounds might be expected to be higher in older animals compared with those of young adults, even if dosing on an mg/kg body weight basis, whereas for lipid soluble drugs, dosing on an mg/kg body weight basis might compensate for potential changes in plasma concentrations.

Serum albumin. Although total serum plasma protein content probably remains the same in the geriatric animal, the proportion represented by albumin decreases and that by gamma globulins increases. Changes in serum albumin can be clinically important to patients receiving highly protein-bound drugs, such as NSAIDs. Decreased albumin can result in a greater proportion of free drug: Most NSAIDs are close to 99% protein bound. A decrease of only 1% (i.e., 99% to 98% binding) doubles the concentration of a pharmacologically active drug. The sequelae of increased PDC may be offset by a compensatory increased clearance, because only unbound drugs are generally conducive to hepatic or renal clearance. However, this balance might be minimized if organs of clearance are negatively affected.

Receptor sensitivity and pharmacodynamics. Geriatric patients respond differently to some drugs, which suggests that tissue receptor sensitivity to the drugs is altered. Changes in receptor number or responsiveness have been implicated but not documented.[2,3] Physiologic changes such as altered neurotransmission or intracellular constituents have also been suggested. For example, geriatric patients are less likely to perceive, appreciate, or express pain. Thus the need for analgesic therapy is often not detected. In addition, geriatric patients are less able to respond to many analgesic drugs.

Disease. Aged animals are more likely to be suffering from diseases that affect not only drug disposition but also tissue receptivity to drugs and organ protection.[15] The immune system of the geriatric patient is not as effective as that of the adult,[18] leading to the use of bactericidal antimicrobials and minimizing the use of immunosuppressive drugs. In addition, the geriatric patient is more likely to be receiving multiple drugs, which increases the likelihood of drug interactions. Finally, diseases of selected organs may predispose these organs to drug-induced toxicity.

Drug Disposition in the Pediatric Animal

With regard to dogs and cats, *pediatric* generally refers to the first 12 weeks of life.[19] Important developmental changes occurring within this time spectrum, however, justify further staging into neonatal (0 to 2 weeks), infant (>2 to 6 weeks), and pediatric (>6 to 12 weeks) periods of growth. Changes associated with each of these periods cause accompanying changes in drug disposition, thus rendering the pediatric patient more susceptible to drug-induced adverse reactions. All four determinants of drug disposition (i.e., absorption, distribution, metabolism, and excretion) undergo dramatic changes as the neonate matures (see Table 2-1).[20,21] However, the clinical significance of these sequelae varies.

KEY POINT 2-2 Drug clearance generally does not reach adult capacity until approximately 3 months of age.

Absorption. Young kittens have decreased energy, carbohydrate, and organic matter digestibility compared with kittens older than 19 weeks of age.[22] However, because the surface area of the small intestine is large, even in neonates, the extent of drug absorption probably does not clinically differ between normal pediatric and adult animals. The rate of absorption tends to be slower in pediatric animals, however, probably because of decreased gastric emptying and irregular intestinal peristalsis. As a result, peak PDCs may be lower in pediatric patients. The decreased rate of absorption might actually protect against toxic drug concentrations.[23,24] However, protection may not be present before absorption of colostrum. During this period the permeability of the intestinal mucosa is increased, leading to increased rate and extent of drug absorption. Occasionally, drugs that normally are not absorbed from the gastrointestinal tract (e.g., aminoglycosides, carbenicillin, and other acid-sensitive beta-lactams and enteric sulfonamides) can reach systemic circulation. Intestinal permeability decreases rapidly after the ingestion of colostrum,[24,25] possibly because of the endogenous release of hydrocortisone or adrenocorticotropic hormone. Exogenous supplementation of either of these hormones by the 24-hour prepartum mother prevents increased permeability and colostrum absorption in the neonate.

A number of other factors may alter small intestinal drug absorption in pediatric patients. Gastric pH is neutral in the newborn; adult levels are not reached until sometime after birth, depending on the species.[23,25] Increased gastric pH (achlorhydria) may decrease the absorption of many drugs that require disintegration and dissolution or are ionized in a less acidic environment (e.g., weak acids such as penicillins). Milk diets can reduce drug absorption by either decreasing gastric emptying or directly interacting with drugs (e.g., milk can impair absorption of tetracyclines). The "unstirred water layer" adjacent to the surface area of the mucosal cells is thicker in the neonate than in the older pediatric patient and may limit the rate of absorption of some drugs. As biliary function matures, the absorption of fat-soluble drugs (e.g., griseofulvin and fat-soluble vitamins) increases. Microbial colonization of the gastrointestinal tract may alter response to antimicrobial drugs, extrahepatic metabolism, or enterohepatic circulation.[26,27]

Absorption from the rectal mucosa is rapid. Rectal administration of drugs or fluids can be used for pediatric patients when venous catheterization is difficult, to reduce complications associated with intravenous administration (e.g., sedation, anesthesia), or when oral administration is undesirable (e.g., antiemetics). Several pediatric drugs intended for systemic effects are available as rectal suppositories. Limited data from studies of human infants indicate that peak plasma concentrations after rectal administration may be higher than those obtained by other routes.[26]

Absorption of drugs administered parenterally to pediatric animals also varies from that of adults. The rate of absorption after intramuscular administration changes with age as muscle mass and its accompanying blood flow increase and as vasomotor responses mature.[26] Because muscle mass is small, subcutaneous administration is frequently preferred for pediatric patients. Again, variability in subcutaneous absorption rates can be anticipated with age. Less fat but greater water may result in faster absorption compared with that in adults.[28] Environmental temperature probably influences subcutaneous absorption, particularly in newborns whose thermoregulatory mechanism functions poorly. Cold environments are likely to reduce subcutaneous drug absorption if the neonate is not kept warm. The same is true for patients in a state of hypothermia. Intraperitoneal administration can be a lifesaving route of blood and fluid administration, particularly for the newborn with inaccessible central veins. Isotonic fluids are rapidly absorbed, and up to 70% of red blood cells are absorbed in 48 to 72 hours.[29] Blood and fluids can also be administered into the medullary cavity of large bones.[30,31]

Absorption of volatile anesthetics from the pediatric respiratory tract is rapid because minute ventilation is greater.[19] Thus young animals are more sensitive to the effects of gas anesthetics. Although not a common route of drug administration, percutaneous absorption of drugs is likely to be greater in pediatric patients. Percutaneous absorption is directly related to skin hydration, which is greatest in neonates. Topical administration of potentially toxic lipid-soluble drugs (e.g., hexachlorophene and organophosphates) is not recommended.

Distribution. The most important factors contributing to differences in drug distribution in pediatric patients are differences in body fluid compartments and drug binding to serum proteins. Body fluid compartments undergo profound changes with the growth of the neonate. Both the percentage of total body water and the ratio of compartmental volumes change with maturation. The percentage of total body water decreases with age, but the decrease is more substantial in the extracellular versus the intracellular compartment (see Table 2-1; Figure 2-2).[32] Daily fluid requirements are greater in neonatal and pediatric patients, in part because a larger proportion of their body weight is represented by body water (see Figure 2-2). The sequelae of these body compartment differences depend on the normal distribution of the drug. Most water-soluble drugs are distributed to extracellular fluids. In pediatric patients the volume to which these drugs is distributed is therefore higher than in adults; PDCs correspondingly decrease. Thus it may be necessary to increase doses to prevent therapeutic failure. A different pattern might be expected for lipid-soluble drugs because they tend to be distributed to total body water. Such drugs should be dosed according to body weight (e.g., mg/kg). Although decreased PDCs resulting from increased distribution may protect the pediatric patient from potentially toxic drug concentrations,[33] a poor therapeutic response may result from failure to generate therapeutic drug concentrations of water-soluble drugs. The disposition of several antimicrobials in neonatal animals has been reviewed by Baggott,[34] with differences in disposition generally found to be similar to those described for humans. Ampicillin is characterized by volumes that are larger in puppies and kittens (threefold to fourfold higher) compared with adults, resulting in clinically significant lower drug concentrations.[35,36] Distribution of enrofloxacin, a lipid-soluble drug, is somewhat unpredictable and age dependent in kittens, being smaller at 2 to 4 weeks but greater at 4 to 6 weeks.[37] Changes in the half-life of each drug parallel changes in distribution. Because many drugs are distributed to a larger volume in pediatric patients, a longer half-life should be anticipated, and it may be necessary to prolong the dosing interval. However, for enrofloxacin in kittens this effect was balanced by increased clearance at 6 weeks.[37]

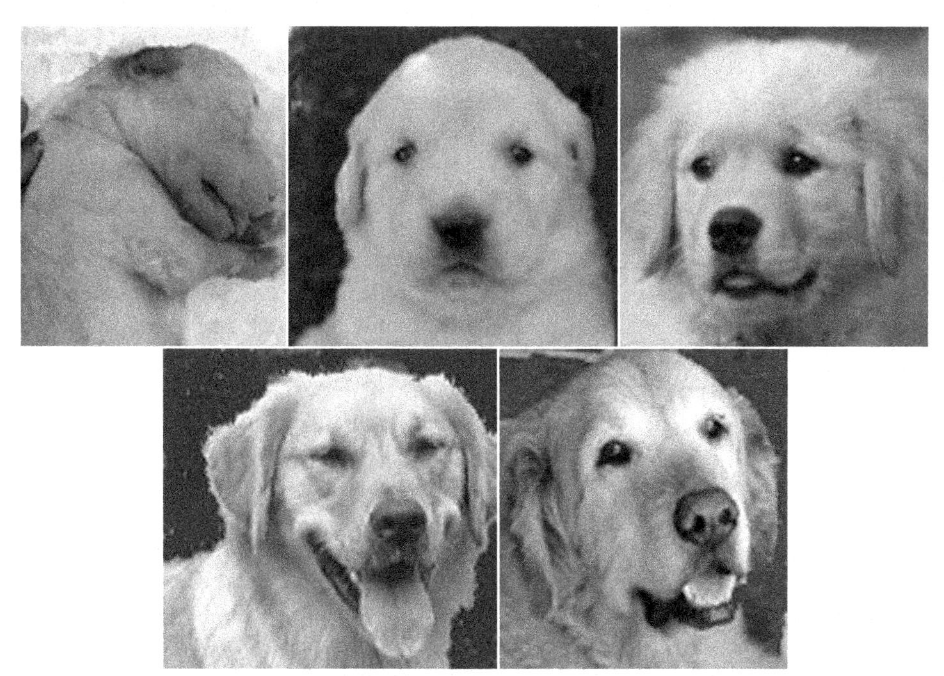

Figure 2-2 Differences in body composition can be appreciated between the two age extremes by following changes as the animal ages. The extracellular compartment and total body water of dogs and cats is greatest in the neonate and gradually decreases toward adult proportions as the animal ages. Increased extracellular fluid and increased total body water result in larger volumes of distribution of most drugs in neonates or pediatric animals, which may decrease plasma drug concentrations and prolong half-life. As the adult ages, fluid content declines, especially in the geriatric cat. The impact of these changes might be greater on water-soluble drugs because the extracellular component represents a greater proportion of total body water in the young animal.

Because the proportion of body fat is smaller in pediatric patients, the distribution of lipid-soluble drugs that accumulate in fat (e.g., organophosphates, chlorinated hydrocarbons, ultrashort thiobarbiturates) may be proportionately decreased. Although drug half-life would decrease, PDCs may become toxic. Many lipid-soluble drugs have a high affinity for and are bound by plasma proteins, thus facilitating their movement through the body. Binding, however, limits their distribution to tissues. Predicting the distribution of highly protein-bound drugs is complicated in the pediatric patient. Serum concentrations of both serum albumin, the protein to which most drugs are bound, and α_1-glycoproteins (to which basic drugs preferentially bind) are decreased in pediatric patients.[38] Protein binding of drugs may also be reduced because of differences in albumin structure or because drugs compete with endogenous substrates (e.g., bilirubin) for binding sites.[24,39] As drugs are displaced, the concentration of free, pharmacologically active drugs and the risk of adverse reactions increases. These changes are significant, however, only if the drug is highly (i.e., >80%) protein bound and characterized by a small therapeutic index. Although the concentration of free drug increases, that of total drug in the plasma tends to decrease because unbound drug is free to distribute into tissue.[39] Consequently, drug half-life may increase, and longer dosing intervals may be indicated for potentially toxic drugs. Increased clearance of unbound drug may ultimately normalize a half-life that has been lengthened by an increased volume of distribution.

Differences in regional organ blood flow might cause clinically important changes in drug disposition in pediatric animals. Differences in renal blood flow have been documented[40,41] and result in clinically important differences in drug excretion. Blood flow to vessel-rich tissues of the body (i.e., heart and brain) is greater and faster;[19] the pediatric patient is thus more susceptible to drug-induced cardiac and central nervous system (CNS) toxicity. The potential for CNS toxicity is further increased because the blood–brain barrier is poorly developed immediately after birth. Increased permeability protects the neonatal brain from a deficiency of nutritional fuels in stressful states (e.g., hypoglycemia, hypoxia, acidosis) by allowing the movement of oxidizable substrates such as lactate into brain cells.[42] The status of efflux proteins is not yet established. Drugs normally incapable of reaching the adult brain are, however, also able to reach brain cells, which are very susceptible to their effects, thus increasing the risk of CNS toxicity.[43,44]

Metabolism. Drug elimination, including both hepatic metabolism and renal excretion, is limited in neonatal and pediatric patients. Thus many drugs administered to the young animal are characterized by decreased clearance.[20,24] In contrast to human infants, hepatic metabolism of drugs is incompetent in the near-term and neonatal puppy.[45-47] Both phase I (e.g., oxidative) and phase II (e.g., glucuronidation) reactions are reduced. The various pathways of metabolism mature at different rates. Phase I activity may not occur in the neonatal puppy and may not be evident until day 9 if it does. Activity appears to progressively increase after day 25, not reaching adult levels until 135 days postpartum.[46] Drug metabolism in pediatric patients, however, is quite complex. For example, Ecobichon and coworkers[48] found that in Beagle puppies, phase I metabolites decreased with age, and for phase II metabolism, glucuronidation was the most predominant, with sulfonation decreasing as puppies got older.

Generally, decreased hepatic drug metabolism is reflected as decreased plasma clearance, increased plasma half-life, and potentially toxic PDCs. Dose reduction, dose prolongation of intervals, or both may be indicated for some drugs. Oral bioavailability of drugs characterized by significant first-pass metabolism in adults (e.g., propranolol) is probably greater in puppies and kittens. Response to prodrugs (e.g., primidone; prednisone; enalapril; and, potentially, methylprednisolone) may be reduced because of decreased formation of active drug products. Pediatric hepatic drug-metabolizing enzymes do appear to be inducible by phenobarbital and other drugs. Nonhepatic drug-metabolizing enzymes also appear to be decreased in pediatric patients. For example, pediatric lower plasma cholinesterase can result in increased sensitivity to organophosphates, succinylcholine, and procaine.

Excretion. Reduced renal excretion, characteristic of the pediatric puppy, results in decreased clearance of renally excreted parent drugs and products of phase II drug metabolism. Although the number of glomeruli remains constant throughout pediatric development, both glomerular filtration and renal tubular function progressively increase.[41,49] Adult values may not be reached until approximately 2.5 months of age. In contrast to glomerular filtration and secretion, renal tubular reabsorption in puppies appears to be similar to that in adults as long as body fluids and electrolytes are maintained.[50,51] The sequelae of developmental changes in pediatric renal function include decreased clearance and prolonged half-life of drugs (primarily water soluble) excreted by the kidneys. Such a pattern has been shown for several drugs. Compared with current recommendations for adults, pediatric patients may require a higher dose (owing to increased volume of distribution) and longer intervals (owing to increased distribution and decreased clearance) for gentamicin administration. More important, modifications should be anticipated in the gentamicin dosing regimen of unhealthy puppies because they are likely to be affected by conditions that increase the potential for gentamicin-induced nephrotoxicity (e.g., dehydration). However, underdeveloped glomeruli may actually protect the pediatric patient from aminoglycoside-induced nephrotoxicity.[21] Further investigations are needed to establish safe yet effective doses of gentamicin for the neonatal puppy or kitten.

Specific Drug Therapy for the Pediatric Patient

Fluid therapy. Pediatric patients are predisposed to dehydration because extracellular fluid is increased, renal capacity to conserve water is decreased, the ratio of surface area to body weight is large, and fluid loss through immature skin is greater.[52] Fluids can be administered by several routes. Crystalloids administered rectally should be isotonic; rapid rectal absorption of hyperosmolar solutions can lead to life-threatening hyperosmolarity. Subcutaneous administration may be an acceptable route if small volumes of isotonic fluids are administered in patients with normal hydration. Intraosseous fluid administration is an acceptable route of administration if a central vein is not accessible.[53] Oral rehydration is recommended as the preferred therapy for dehydration caused by diarrhea in human pediatric patients.[54]

Antimicrobial therapy. As for adults, an appreciation of the chemotherapeutic triangle (i.e., relationship among host, drug, and microorganism) is necessary for the appropriate use of antimicrobials with pediatric patients. Several antimicrobials are not recommended for pediatric patients. These include chloramphenicol, tetracyclines, doxycycline, and other drugs that undergo enterohepatic circulation (e.g., clindamycin) and thus are more likely to disrupt the normal colonization of the alimentary tract in pediatric patients.

Beta-lactam antibiotics are generally the drugs of choice for pediatric patients whenever possible. Although drug half-lives are likely to be prolonged, they tend to be safe because they are characterized by a wide therapeutic index. Higher doses may be necessary to achieve desired peak PDCs because their distribution is greater. The time interval of administration can be prolonged to compensate for the longer half-life. Therapeutic drug monitoring should be used to improve the safety and efficacy of aminoglycosides whenever possible. Higher doses and longer intervals may be necessary to achieve recommended peak and trough concentrations. Amikacin, which is potentially less nephrotoxic (and more effective against *Pseudomonas* spp.) than gentamicin, might be preferred. Quinolones are very effective and, for most patients, safe antimicrobials. They are characterized by excellent tissue distribution. However, these drugs are not appropriate for large-breed pediatric animals because they can cause destructive lesions in the cartilage of long bones. Thus the author does not recommend these drugs as first choice for any pediatric patient. The use of disease-modifying agents containing glucosamine should be encouraged in any animal in which cartilage is growing (or repairing). The combination of a sulfonamide with trimethoprim or ormetroprim tends to be safe and effective for kittens and puppies. Oral tetracyclines should be avoided in nursing animals and before tooth extraction. Therapeutic indications for lincosamides and macrolides are limited for pediatric patients. Because both groups of drugs undergo extensive biliary secretion and enterohepatic circulation, they should not be used as first-choice antimicrobials. An exception should be made for *Mycoplasma* infections for which tylosin is the drug of choice. Metronidazole is the drug of choice for *Giardia* infections in dogs and cats, and it is often used for the treatment of anaerobic infections. Decreased clearance and prolonged half-life should be anticipated in kittens and puppies; lower doses and longer intervals may be necessary to prevent CNS toxicity. Enrofloxacin is one of the few drugs that has been studied well in neonatal to pediatric kittens.[37] After oral administration, bioavailability of enrofloxacin (5 mg/kg) was at least 33% at 2 weeks of age, increasing to 50% at 4 and 70% at 6 and 8 weeks of age. Following intravenous and subcutaneous administration, the area under the curve compared to adult cats varied with the age of the kittens and route of administration. Neonates (younger than 2 weeks of age) presented as most "different," with area under the curve at least twofold higher than that of any other age (4, 6, or 8 weeks), although elimination half-life was similar among the groups studied. In general, volume of distribution (Vd) was greater (up to twofold) at 4 and 6 weeks compared with the younger age groups and adults, indicating the need for a higher dose; because clearance was faster as well, elimination half-life was actually shorter than with adults.

Sedation, anesthesia, and analgesia. Opioid agonists are the preferred sedative, premedicant, or analgesic of some veterinary clinicians for pediatric patients.[19] Although associated with marked cardiac and respiratory depression, the effects of opioid agonists are largely reversible with opioid antagonists. Bradycardia can be prevented in older pediatric patients by premedication with atropine or glycopyrrolate. Whereas the duration of fentanyl analgesia (nontransdermal patch) is generally too short to justify its use for adult patients, some clinicians prefer it for short-term intraoperative analgesia for pediatric patients because it minimally affects the cardiovascular system. Ketamine can be administered subcutaneously, intramuscularly, or intravenously for the restraint and immobilization of young cats. Response to ultrashort barbiturates such as thiopental and methohexital or similar agents (e.g., propofol) should be exaggerated in young animals because of decreased body fat and hepatic clearance. Dilution to a 1% to 2% solution is indicated to prevent over-administration.

Complications associated with intravenous administration can be reduced by rectal administration of either thiopental or methohexital in human pediatric patients. As a class the benzodiazepines can probably be used safely in pediatric patients. Elimination occurs primarily by hepatic metabolism and is likely to be slower in pediatric patients. Benzodiazepines are, however, characterized by a wide therapeutic index. Midazolam, the newest member of this group, is more potent, has a faster onset of action, and is more rapidly eliminated than diazepam. Although not approved for use in human pediatric patients, it has been used in this age group successfully to induce sedation.[55] Inhalant anesthetics are preferred for maintenance anesthesia in veterinary pediatric patients. Halothane, methoxyflurane, enflurane, and isoflurane, and to a lesser degree, sevoflurane have been used. Hypotension is a complication of all gas anesthetics, however, and variable patient response necessitates close monitoring.

Pregnancy and Lacation

Maternal–Fetal–Placental Unit

Even the most simple pharmacokinetic representation of the maternal–fetal system is complex, being composed of at least three compartments: maternal, placental, and fetal. The pharmacokinetics of each compartment is determined, in turn, by its own rate of absorption, distribution, metabolism, and elimination.[56-58] Pregnancy is further complicated by its dynamic nature, with dramatic changes in placental and fetal growth and in the physiology of the pregnant animal. All pharmacokinetic processes change in concert with the progression of pregnancy.

KEY POINT 2-3 Assuming that most drugs administered to the pregnant or lactating bitch or queen will reach the offspring is prudent. Water-soluble drugs should be chosen when possible if therapy is necessary.

The placenta transfers nutrients and oxygen from the mother to the fetus and facilitates waste removal from the fetus. However, the placenta also has a number of metabolic functions, among them the synthesis of hormones, peptides, and steroids that are vital for a successful pregnancy. The placenta also presents a barrier to drug distribution from maternal blood into the fetus. Transporter proteins (e.g., P-glycoprotein [P-gp]) on both the maternal and fetal side influence drug movement; placental phase I and II drug-metabolizing enzymes also have been identified throughout gestation in the human placenta. Thus far, CYP1A1, 2E1, 3A4, 3A5, 3A7, and 4B1 and uridine diphosphate glucuronosyltransferases have been detected in the term human placenta. However, these barriers to drug movement from the mother to fetus presented by the placenta are not impenetrable. Extrapolation of data among species regarding maternal to fetal transfer of compounds is complicated by differences in placentation.[59] Humans and rats have the least number of layers. However, the endotheliochorial placentation of carnivores differs from hemochorial placentation of humans only by the presence of maternal endothelium, and it is likely that this single fenestrated layer does not present a significantly greater barrier.[60] The idea of absolute placental selectivity has been replaced with the realization that any drug administered to a pregnant animal might prudently be anticipated to cross the placenta, regardless of the degree of intimacy between fetal and placental membranes.[56,57,61] The route of administration is also likely to determine the amount of placental transfer: Routes that result in higher plasma peak concentrations (i.e., intravenously, as an intravenous infusion, and in multiple doses) are likely to expose the fetus to higher drug concentrations. Further, a "depot phenomenon" described in the human placenta reflects the accumulation of selected lipid-soluble xenobiotics in the placenta, with the placenta possibly serving as a storage site.[61]

The primary mechanism of drug movement is passive diffusion, with the amount of transfer dependent on physiochemical properties; less commonly, active transporters and facilitated diffusion contribute to drug movement.[61] Although many factors determine the rate and extent of drug transfer across the placenta, the lipid solubility of the drug and a steep maternal–fetal drug concentration gradient are probably the most important.[57] In general, nonionized compounds with high lipid solubility cross rapidly, whereas drugs with little lipid solubility cross slowly. Impermeability of the placenta to polar compounds, which generally do not penetrate cell membranes, has been described as relative rather than absolute.[57] A number of drugs that are polar at physiologic pH can cross the placenta rapidly.[57] Molecular weight influences drug movement, with those below 500 Dalton more likely and those above 1000 less likely to transfer. Protein binding precludes drug movement, whereas differences in fetal and maternal blood pH increase the accumulation of weak bases in fetal blood (humans).

Fetus and Neonate

Unique differences in drug disposition predispose the near-term fetus and neonate to adverse drug reactions. The pharmacologic principles that address risk of fetal exposure to potential teratogens have been reviewed.[61,62] The drug approval process generally precludes availability of those compounds with a demonstrated risk, but premarket assessment does not necessarily occur in dogs or cats. The responses of the fetus and newborn to individual drugs, however, vary. Differences in responses reflect, in part, differences in placental kinetics of drugs. The fetus is most sensitive to adverse effects particularly in the first trimester. The risk is positively correlated with the duration of pregnancy, with the risk greater in shorter pregnancies (e.g., dogs and cats) because this period represents a longer proportion of the pregnancy.[63]

Current efforts in human neonatology are concerned with the characterization of the pharmacokinetic differences between drugs in the near-term fetus. Differences in drug disposition compared with that of both pediatric animals and adults can lead to adverse reactions in the near-term fetus receiving drugs through the placenta. The amount of fetal protein is generally less in the neonate, which is, in turn, less than that in the adult.[56,57] Thus higher concentrations of unbound and pharmacologically active drugs can be anticipated. It is not clear if increased concentrations of unbound drug will be compensated for by increased clearance, as will occur in the adult animal. Perhaps more important are anatomic peculiarities of fetal circulation. Because the fetal liver and lungs are largely bypassed, blood reaching the heart and brain contain essentially the same concentration of drugs as present in the umbilical vein. Although fetal metabolism of drugs can contribute to the ultimate elimination of drugs in the human neonate, the amount of drug-metabolizing enzymes present in near-term animals is negligible.[57]

Although drugs administered to pregnant animals may be detectable in the fetus, they may not produce clinically important effects. Examples of drugs that have been shown to reach detectable and potentially clinically important concentrations in the fetus include salicylates and other NSAIDs, anticonvulsants (phenytoin and diazepam), local anesthetics such as lidocaine, gentamicin (in some species), and narcotic analgesics. In human infants the ratio of maternal to fetal concentration of beta-lactams approximates 1.[64] Because predicting the effects of a drug crossing the placenta is difficult, drug selection for the mother should be based, in part, on anticipated safety to the near-term fetus.

Maternal

The effects of pregnancy can alter all phases of disposition in the mother. Gastrointestinal motility and gastric acid secretion decrease and may lead to decreased drug absorption. Distribution may be influenced by decreased serum albumin, and increased Vd of drugs, resulting in lower PDCs. However, drug clearance may be more rapid as cardiac output, renal blood flow, and glomerular filtration rate increase. High progesterone concentrations may induce hepatic microsomal enzymes and increase drug metabolism.[65]

Lactation

As is the fetus, the nursing animal is an inadvertent recipient of drugs administered to the mother. Most of the pertinent information in the veterinary literature is concerned with excretion of drugs in the milk of food animals; there appears to be no information regarding small animals. Studies of humans indicate that drugs diffuse into the milk from maternal circulation. Low-molecular-weight (<200), un-ionized, highly lipid-soluble drugs that are minimally protein bound diffuse into the lactating mammary gland rapidly, whereas water-soluble drugs diffuse more slowly.[66] The pK_a of a drug largely determines its concentration in milk. Animal milk tends to be acidic compared with plasma pH. Consequently, although a drug may be nonionized in the plasma and thus more likely to diffuse into milk, it may become ionized and nondiffusible once in the milk. Such "ion trapping" can concentrate drugs in milk. The ratio of drugs in milk to plasma is predictable, being greater for weak bases and weak acids whose pK_as differ from the pH of milk by 2 pH units (+2 for acids and −2 for bases).[67] Generally, the amount of drugs excreted in milk is less than 2% of the maternal dose.[66] Greater concentrations can be expected, however, if a drug is administered to the mother intravenously, as an intravenous infusion, or in multiple doses.

Not all drugs ingested with milk during nursing will be absorbed from the gastrointestinal tract of the nursing animal. For example, milk may decrease the absorption of some drugs, whereas the pharmacokinetic properties of other drugs (i.e., aminoglycosides) preclude their absorption except in the very young. Not all drugs, however, must be absorbed to cause clinically important adverse effects. For example, antimicrobials can sometimes alter the developing flora of the pediatric alimentary tract.[27,68] Thus it is prudent to refrain from administering potentially toxic drugs to the lactating bitch or queen.

Sex

Pregnancy and lactation are obvious differences between the sexes that affect the disposition of and response to drugs. However, sex differences are relevant without the influence of active reproduction. The impact of sex on drug disposition is not well characterized in human or other animal medicine. In general, female humans, compared with male humans, are characterized by reduced smooth muscle motility, greater body fat, greater content and fluctuation in plasma volume and increased organ blood flow, xenobiotic metabolism (increased

CYP3A4, others not clear), and transporter protein activity.[69,70] It should be anticipated that sex differences are likely to be complex, as has been demonstrated for CYP enzymes in cats.[71] Female cats were characterized by greater CYP2D and lower CYP3A compared with males.

Roles of Species and Breed Differences in Drug Disposition

Differences among species in the kinetics and response to drugs are profound; Riviere[72] has offered a review in animals. Few studies have compared disposition among species, and when reported, data are generally oriented toward human medicine, with the intent to identify the (laboratory) animal most predictive of human drug disposition. Presumably, species that are physiologically similar tend to have similar drug disposition patterns, and the same dosing regimen can often be used for a particular drug.[73] However, pharmacokinetic data (Vd, clearance, and mean residence time) after intravenous administration have been compared among humans, monkeys, dogs, and rats for over 100 molecules (including many drugs).[74] Correlations between chemical structures of the compounds with pharmacokinetics allowed two categories of compounds to be identified: those characterized by high clearance, for which mathematical models would allow general extrapolation of data from one species to another, and those whose characteristics yielded incorrect extrapolations. Although the authors concluded that such an approach might be useful for extrapolation, more to the point is the reality that drugs may not be extrapolatable even with the most sophisticated of mathematical models. The combination of computation analysis of the molecular characteristics of each compound with in vivo pharmacokinetic data might ultimately be helpful in identifying the most appropriate species for predicting pharmacokinetic behavior of a particular molecule in another species. Thus caution needs to continue when extrapolating information from humans to the dog, and dog to cat. Likewise, pharmacodynamic responses may be profound.

Absorption

Gastric pH profiles have been described for the dog in anticipation of extrapolation to humans.[75] Dogs are described as poor gastric acid secretors, compared with humans as good secretors, with gastric pH fluctuating in dogs from 2.7 to 8.3 (mean 6.8). The shorter gastrointestinal tract of dogs compared with that of humans, results in a transit time (111 minutes) that is 50% of that of humans, although this may be offset by taller villi and greater bile salt concentrations. Accordingly, differences in absorption might be expected between dogs and humans in the oral absorption of drugs, particularly for enteric-coated or altered-release products.[75] Different affinities for P-gps have been demonstrated among humans, nonhuman primates, and Beagle dogs.[76] In dogs absorption of some hydrophilic compounds is more similar to that in rats, whereas absorption of others is more similar to that found in humans.[77] Another retrospective comparison between dogs and humans in the oral bioavailability of 43 drugs found close to 50% to be completely absorbed in both species. For the remaining drugs, 12 were absorbed more rapidly and to a greater (15% to 200%) extent.[78] However, the extent of absorption for drugs not well absorbed correlated poorly between the two species. In general, if the drug was well absorbed in humans, it tended to be well absorbed in dogs. Both lipid- and water-soluble drugs appear to be better absorbed in dogs, the latter suggesting more paracellular transport. The rate and magnitude of drug absorption for many drugs may be similar between dogs and cats, regardless of the route of administration. However, extrapolations must be done with caution, as is exemplified with ciprofloxacin, whose oral bioavailability in the dog is 40% (compared to 80% or better in humans) but 0% to 20% (the latter more likely with multiple dosing) in cats.[79,80] Another example is prednisone. An exception also may need to be made for slow-release preparations; rates and extent of absorption do vary among species. Dye[81,82] has demonstrated not only differences in bioavailability in cats versus dogs but also differences in pharmacokinetics related to morning versus evening dosing. Because slow-release preparations used in human patients are designed to maintain therapeutic concentrations in humans, absorption kinetics of these products can be profoundly different in the dog and cat. Use of such drugs should be based on clinical studies of these preparations in dogs and cats.

Distribution

Because most determinants of xenobiotic distribution are largely affected by cardiac output, regional blood flow, and xenobiotic chemistry, distribution differences among species might be predictable through allometric scaling.[83] However, they must also take into account differences in transport proteins. Differences in drug distribution can result in important differences in drug response. Blood volume of the cat (70 mL/kg) is less than that of the dog (90 mL/kg); PDCs of drugs whose distribution is confined to the plasma compartment may therefore differ between the species. The same amount of drug (on a per-kilogram basis) is diluted less in cats because the plasma volume is smaller. Thus drug concentrations after administration of a mg/kg dose might initially be higher in cats than in dogs. Organs that are well perfused (i.e., heart, brain) may be more susceptible to toxicity. Cats are approximately the same size as the smaller dog breeds. Thus doses determined for medium-size to large-size dogs may not be appropriate for the cat because the smaller animals have a greater body surface area. In larger animals body water makes up a larger proportion of body weight, which tends to dilute the drug. A higher dose may be needed for larger animals. Because the drug half-life may be longer (owing to increased distribution), however, the dosing interval may need to be longer.

Differences in plasma protein-binding characteristics (particularly albumin) may alter the distribution of drugs that are highly protein bound. The degree to which various drugs are protein bound varies dramatically among the species, although the clinical implication is not clear. Although the elimination characteristics of many drugs have been established for cats, few studies have determined the extent of protein binding.

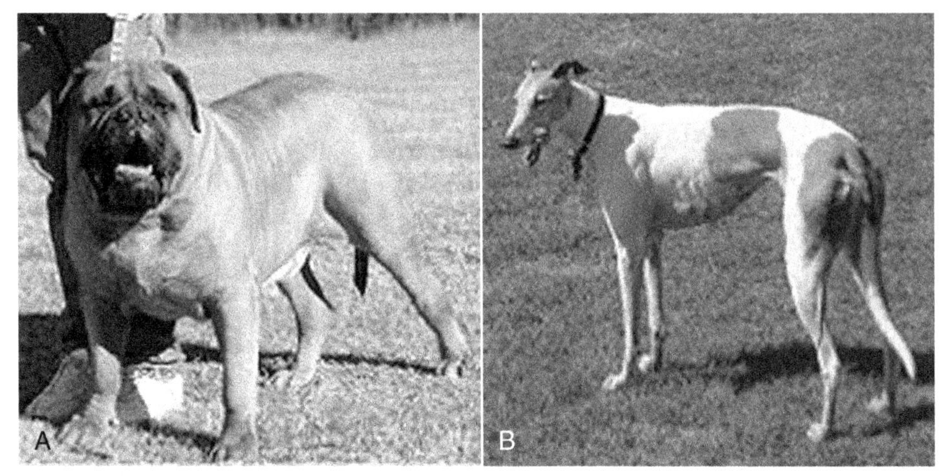

Figure 2-3 Differences in breeds may affect body composition **(A)** as well as other aspects of drug disposition. The sight hounds, represented by the Greyhound **(B)** is at risk for selected adverse drug events, in part because of a larger lean body mass compared with fat. Drugs that normally accumulate in fat may achieve higher drug concentrations in such breeds.

The interaction between disease and species should be considered when considering species differences in drug distribution. For example, the unhealthy cat does not maintain hydration as well as the dog; fluid imbalances resulting from dehydration or edema alter drug distribution. The obese cat can represent a "sink" for drugs that are lipid soluble, thus lowering PDCs potentially to submaximal levels if the dose is not appropriately increased. Weight loss in a hyperthyroid cat can have the opposite effect.

Sight hounds (e.g., Salukis, Greyhounds; Figure 2-3) offer an example of potential breed differences in drug distribution. Their lean body weight provides little fat tissue for drug distribution. As a result, they are more susceptible to overdosing with drugs that redistribute, such as thiobarbiturates.

Distribution is influenced by the multidrug transport protein P-gp. Polymorphism has been demonstrated in the Collie, yielding differences in P-gp content. Two P-gp transporting proteins are encoded by ABCB1 (previously MDR1 or PGY1) and MDR3 (also named *MDR2* and *PGY3)*; only the MDR1 gene product is thought to significantly influence drug metabolism. P-gp acts as an efflux pump by translocating drugs from the intracellular to extracellular compartments (Table 2-2) (see Chapter 3). The protein transports a large number of drugs that are chemically divergent; further, these drugs are associated with a specific CYP450 responsible for metabolism of the drugs that have been transported. Polymorphism of the MDR1 gene and P-gp have been reported in humans and are associated with altered drug disposition and thus susceptibility to adverse drug events. Interestingly, polymorphism also has been associated with an increased risk of certain illnesses (e.g., refractory seizures, Parkinson's disease, inflammatory bowel disease biliary mucoceole in dogs*). Polymorphism reflecting a mutation deletion of MDR1 that causes nonfunctional P-gp has been documented in Collie and related working-breed dogs. The incidence of the deletion is impressively high: in the U.S., in one study, 35% of Collies were homozygous and another 42% heterozygous for the mutation deletion.[84] A similarly high incidence was found in dogs in France: 20% of Collies and related breeds were found to be homozygous for the normal allele, 32% heterozygous for the deletion (carrier), and 48% homozygous for the mutant allele (affected dogs).[85] The impact of the mutation on drug safety in afflicted animals can be profound (see Chapter 3). Substrate specificity for P-pg appears to be similar among species, suggesting that human data can be used to predict which drugs might be more likely to cause adverse effects in these breeds.[86] However, protein type and amount may vary among species and breed.

*Personal communications, K. Mealey, Washington State University.

Metabolism

Human polymorphisms in CYP metabolic enzymes have been associated with therapeutic failure resulting from extremely rapid metabolism of a drug and toxic effects caused by decreased metabolism.[87] Species extrapolation among the CYP450 appears to be predictable in order of most to least: 2E1 (reasonably predictable) greater than 1A1, 1A2, and 4A (cautiously predictable) greater than 2D and 3A greater than 2A, 2B, and 2C (major caution with extrapolation).[88] Studies attempting to identify similarities between dog and human CYP activity suggest general extrapolation between the species is not prudent.[87] Although significant differences among species were not detected among rodents, rabbits, and dogs for CYP2E1, 3A2, and 4A1, comparison of animal CYP activity with human found only 2D6 to be most similar to dog.[89] Other enzymes present in dogs are CYP1A, 2C, and 2D families and subfamilies (Table 2-3).[90]

KEY POINT 2-4 The genetic basis for differences in drug transport and metabolism limits extrapolation of dosing regimens among species, and potentially, breeds. However, understanding of these polymorphisms is increasing our ability to predict increased risks associated with drug administration in some breeds.

Species differences have been documented in the handling of racemic isomers of selected drugs. Inversion (from one isomer to the other) patterns differ and are likely to result in

Table 2-2 Substrates for P-glycoprotein Transport Pump and Known Inhibitors and Inducers of Drug Transport

Substrates	Inhibitors	Inducers
Antimicrobial Drugs		
Erythromycin	Bromocriptine	Clotrimazole
Tetracycline	Carvedilol	Dexamethasone
Itraconazole	Cyclosporine	Morphine
Fluorinated quinolones (selected)	Erythromycin	Rifampin
Anticancer Drugs	Fluoxetine	Phenothiazine
Doxorubicin	Intraconazole	St. John's Wort
Vinblastine	Ketaconazole	
Vincristine	Meperidine	
Mitoxantrone	Pentazocine	
Anthelmintics	Progesterone	
Ivermectin	Quinidine	
Cardioactive Drugs	Tacrolimus	
Digoxin	Verapamil	
Quinidine		
Diltiazem		
Verapamil		
CNS-Active Drugs		
Phenothiazines		
Amitryptyline	Inhibitor of CYP3a	
Morphine	Substrate CYP3a	
Endogenous Substrates		
Bilirubin		
Steroidal Hormones		
Cortisol		
Aldosterone		
Gastrointestinal Drugs		
Cimetidine		
Loperamide		
Ondansetron		
Tacrolimus		
Immunomodulators		
Dexamethasone		
Methylprednisolone		
Cyclosporine		
Tacrolimus		
Colchicine		

CNS, Central nervous system.

Table 2-3 Cytochrome P450 Families, Their Contribution to Drug Metabolism in Humans, and Their Orthologs in Other Species

Human Isoform	% of Drugs	Canine Isoform	Feline Isoform
CYP1A1	13	CYP1A1	CYP 1A
CYP1A2		CYP1A2 (o)	
CYP2B6		CYP2B11	
CYP2E1	7	CYP2E2	CYP2E^^*
CYP2C9	18	*CYP2C1†	**CYP 2C††
CYP2D6	1.5	^CYP2D15§	CYP2D
CYP3A4	30	CYP3A12	CYP 3A
		CYP3A26	
		*polymorphism	**very low
		^ 3 variants	^^ 3 variants

*Tanaka N, Shinkyo R, Sakaki T et al: Cytochrome P450 2E polymorphism in feline liver, *Biochim Biophys Acta* 1726(2):194-205, 2005.
†Blaisdell J, Goldstein JA, Bai SA: Isolation of a new canine cytochrome P450 CDNA from the cytochrome P450 2C subfamily (CYP2C41) and evidence for polymorphic differences in its expression, *Drug Metab Dispos.* 26(3):278-283, 1998.
††Shah SS, Sanda S, Regmi NL, Sasaki K, Shimoda M. Characterization of cytochrome P450-mediated drug metabolism in cats, *J Vet Pharmacol Ther* 30(5):422-428, 2007.
§Paulson SK, Engel L, Reitz B et al: Evidence for polymorphism in the canine metabolism of the cyclooxygenase 2 inhibitor, celecoxib, *Drug Metab Dispos* 27(10):1133-1142, 1999.

different pharmacologic or toxic effects of the drugs. Induction (or presumably inhibition) of drug-metabolizing enzymes also will differentially affect the isomers.[91]

As in humans, polymorphism in drug-metabolizing enzymes has been reported in dogs[92] but is not as well described. Differences in response to anesthesia recognized in sight hounds reflect both differences in drug distribution (to lean versus fat compartments; see Chapter 1) as well as differences in metabolism. Cytochrome-mediated clearance of several anesthetic agents is less in Greyhounds compared with other (nonsight hound) dogs; documented drugs include thiopental, thiamylal, and methohexital. Clearance of propofol by Greyhounds is three times less than that by Beagles. Ketoconazole plasma concentrations were twofold higher than expected in Greyhounds in one study.[93] Further, Greyhound disposition of celecoxib, a cyclooxygenase-1 protective NSAID, indicates that breed differences may predispose this breed to adverse drug reactions. Polymorphism also has been described for CYP2C isoenzymes, again in Beagles[94] and possibly Greyhounds.[95] Polymorphism in celecoxib metabolism was attributed to CYP2D15, for which three canine variants were found.[96] In a study of 242 Beagles receiving celecoxib, approximately 50% were considered efficient metabolizers and 50% poor metabolizers, with bioavailability and maximum PDC in the latter group almost twofold higher. The impact of species differences in pharmacokinetic and pharmacodynamic considerations of enantiomers has been described.[91,97] For example, for many NSAIDs the S-isomer has a much greater affinity for cyclooxygenase-2, but the proportion of the S isomer varies among species. Further, species differ in their ability to interconvert S and R isomers.[97] For example, chiral inversion has been described for ketoprofen in cats.[98]

Other polymorphisms that have been described include thiopurine methyltransferase (TPMT), which is one of several enzymes responsible for the metabolism of the active metabolite of the prodrug azathioprine; polymorphisms resulting in

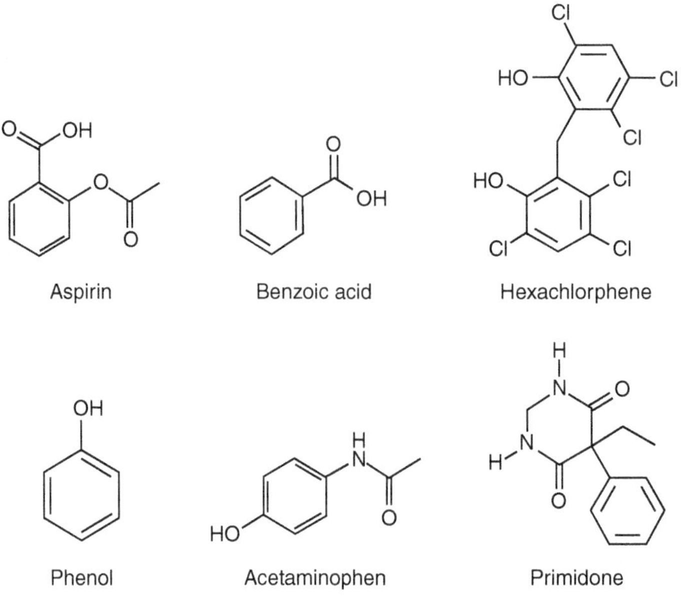

Figure 2-4 Examples of drugs (many containing phenols) whose metabolism in cats is slower owing to deficiencies in drug phase I and phase II drug-metabolizing enzymes.

deficiencies in humans have been associated with an increase in the toxic bone marrow effects of the drug. Differences in dogs have been demonstrated as well: Kidd[99] and coworkers have demonstrated that Giant Schnauzers have significantly less and Alaskan Malamutes significantly more TPMT compared with other canine breeds.

The most significant and best-characterized differences in drug disposition between the dog and cat probably result from differences in drug metabolism. Identification of phase I enzymes and their specific drug substrates is difficult, and few species differences have been described in the cat or dog. However, a recent review of CYP450 activity–based substrate metabolism in cats suggests that cats have very low activity of CYP2C, but activity of CYP2D and CYP3A approximates that of dogs or humans, depending on sex.[77] Deficiencies in demethylation and hydroxylation have been described in the cat and may be responsible for different patterns of prodrug activation (e.g., primidone; see Chapter 27) or adverse reactions to selected drugs (i.e., chloramphenicol).[100] Deficiencies in phase I demethylation and hydroxylation as well as phase II glucuronidation lead to much slower elimination of phenols and aromatic acids and amines in the cat compared with other species (Figure 2-4).[101,102] The described reaction of cats to diazepam may represent differences in the metabolites produced, as may the susceptibility of the feline liver to metabolite-induced damage.[103] Polymorphisms in drug-metabolizing enzymes have also been described in cats, which have at least three variants of CYP2E,104, although breeds were not cited.[104]

Deficiencies in phase II metabolism have long been recognized in cats. The deficiency reflects extremely low concentrations of some glucuronyl transferases. Thus many drugs excreted as glucuronide conjugates in other species are characterized by a prolonged clearance rate and half-life in the cat. Toxic levels may accumulate much more quickly in the cat, and exaggerated pharmacologic responses or toxicities occur more easily (Figure 2-4). Dosing regimens must be modified for such drugs by either decreasing the dose (especially for drugs whose dosing interval is shorter than the elimination half-life) or prolonging the dosing interval. The prototypic example is aspirin, whose half-life approximates 36 hours in cats compared with 8 hours in dogs. To prevent toxicity in the cat, aspirin is dosed every 48 to 72 hours, compared with twice daily in dogs.

Not all drugs that are conjugated with glucuronide are predisposed to toxicity in the cat. This is true for several reasons. First, the cat is deficient only in certain families of glucuronyl transferase. Cats can conjugate and excrete endogenous substrates such as bilirubin, thyroxine, and steroid hormones as well as other species. Metabolism of a variety of exogenous drugs, however, particularly phenols and aromatic acids and amines, occurs at a much slower rate in the cat than in other species.[101,102] The degrees of deficiency and potential toxicity depend on the drug substrate. For example, some phenolic compounds are sufficiently conjugated, whereas others are not. Second, glucuronide-conjugated drugs characterized by a wide safety margin are associated with few adverse reactions even if accumulation occurs. Finally, in the absence of glucuronide, drugs may be sufficiently metabolized by an alternative pathway. Some sulfates may be particularly well developed in the cat, and many drugs that are excreted as glucuronide-conjugates by the dog may be excreted as sulfated compounds by the cat. Other sulfate-conjugating systems, however, appear to be easily saturated in the cat. Unfortunately, alternate pathways of drug metabolism may also contribute to the toxicity of some drugs because they may involve phase I enzymes that catalyze the formation of toxic metabolites. Thus drugs shunted to another pathway in the cat may be very toxic to the cat but minimally toxic in other species. Deficiencies in both glucuronide and (potentially) glutathione transferase may also predispose the cat to poor scavenging systems in erythrocytes and hepatocytes, limiting the otherwise protective effects that might be realized by these systems and further contributing to toxicity. Acetaminophen is an excellent example of the potential sequelae of phase II deficiences in the cat (See Chapter 4). Because glucuronide is deficient, excessive acetaminophen is shunted to phase I enzymes, which produce toxic oxygen radicals. More metabolites are produced than can be handled, and the glutathione-scavenging system of feline erythrocytes and hepatocytes is overwhelmed, resulting in life-threatening methemoglobinemia and (potentially) hepatic necrosis. The rationale for cimetidine treatment can be understood in the context of the role of phase I metabolism, as well as that of *N*-acetylcysteine, a glutathione precursor.

Not all deficiences in metabolism occur in the cat. Although acetylation is not a common route of elimination for xenobiotics, it is an enzyme system whose deficiency in the dog is clinically relevant (e.g., procainamide). For example, the antiarrhythmic procainamide is acetylated in humans to an active metabolite. Procainamide is less potent than its acetylated metabolite and the canine dose for procainamide is considerably higher than that in humans on a mg/kg basis in order to achieve an equivalent pharmacologic response (see Chapter 14, Cardiac). A second example might be sulfonamide elimination. Sulfonamides are detoxified by *N*-acetylation in humans. In the face of deficient acetylation, shunting of the xenobiotic to an alternative pathway in dogs, with the production of the cytotoxic metabolite hydroxylamine, may be one mechanism of sulfonamide toxicity in dogs, although alternative mechanisms are likely to be responsible.[105]

Renal Excretion

In contrast to hepatic metabolism, differences in renal excretion between the dog and cat do not appear to be profoundly important to drug disposition. Glomerular filtration and active tubular secretion parallel cardiac output and thus should be predictable among species based on allometric scaling.[83] The glomerular filtration rate of cats (2.5 to 3.5 mL/min/kg) is less than that of dogs (3 to 5 mL/min/kg), suggesting that renal clearance of drugs may be faster in dogs. Although this is true of inulin, differences have not been established for most drugs. Renal disease profoundly alters the rate of drug excretion in all species. In general, serum creatinine concentrations can be used to modify the dose (decrease in proportion) or interval (prolong in proportion to abnormality). The modification should be applied only to that portion of the drug eliminated by the kidney. Note that fluid imbalances in renal disease can also alter drug distribution. Finally, differences in active transport and passive resorption—the latter influenced by differences in urinary pH—may result in differential excretion among species. However, because urine tends to be acidic in both dogs and cats, differences in the latter may not be profound.

Role of Species Differences in Target Tissues

It is difficult to predict differences in drug reaction that can be ascribed to differences in target tissues because very little is known about cats. Differences in response to selected drugs (e.g., opioids, insulin, chlorinated hydrocarbons) are known to be or are thought to be reflections of differences in tissues; however, often these differences turn out to be pharmacokinetic differences reflecting decreased or increased PDCs of active (including toxic) compounds rather than differences at the receptor level.

Feline erythrocytes (hemoglobin) appear to be more susceptible to oxidation and thus to methemoglobinemia. Drugs reported to cause methemoglobinemia in the cat include urinary antiseptics containing methylene blue[106] or azodyes, acetaminophen[101,107,108] and related compounds, benzocaine,[109] and propylthiouracil.[110] Several mechanisms have been postulated to explain the potential increased sensitivity of cats to methemoglobin formation. Lower concentrations or activities of the intracellular repair enzyme methemoglobin reductase have been postulated but not confirmed.[111,112] Faster metabolism of specific drugs to toxic metabolites that overwhelm scavenging systems has already been discussed as a likely cause for some drugs, particularly those whose elimination is shunted to alternate (toxic) pathways (i.e., acetaminophen).[107] Differences in the structure of feline hemoglobin have also been postulated. Feline hemoglobin contains up to 20 sulfhydryl groups compared with a maximum of four in other species. Sulfhydryl groups tend to be reactive and thus are susceptible to interaction with reactive parent drugs or metabolites. Thus more sulfhydryl groups would need to be maintained in a reduced state in cats.[113] Other unique considerations for the cat might include its propensity for drug-induced retinal damage; hepatic lipidosis associated with anorexia; and, potentially, an increased risk of nephrotoxicity.

Canine breed differences in response to drugs may also reflect pharmacodynamic responses. For example, brachycephalic breeds (e.g., Boxers) are more susceptible to cardiac arrhythmias (sinoatrial block) caused by acepromazine.

Miscellaneous

Differences in circadian rhythm (i.e., diurnal versus nocturnal) play a role in some differences between the dog and cat. Aminoglycosides are less likely to cause toxicity if administered during active periods. This also has been established for theophylline, for which clearance occurs more rapidly at night in the dog compared with early morning in cats. Dosing of glucocorticoids at night has been recommended for cats in order to mimic endogenous release patterns. The clinical significance of these differences has not been determined.

RECOMMENDATIONS REGARDING EXTRAPOLATION OF DOSING REGIMENS

Drug Information Sources

Extrapolation of doses of human drugs to dogs and cats and from dogs to cats should be based on a knowledge of the clinical pharmacology of the drug to be administered and on the physiologic differences of the target species. The safer the drug, the safer the extrapolation. Numerous resources are available for human drug information (e.g., *Facts and Comparisons, USP Pharmacopeia*, the package insert from the product, *Physicians' Desk Reference)*[114] to determine the safety and the determinants of disposition of a new drug. The veterinary literature and clinicians with expertise in the field, including diplomates of the American College of Veterinary Clinical Pharmacology, are additional sources.

Note that every drug that has been approved for use in humans has been studied in dogs. The studies generally have focused on *safety*, however, not efficacy. The information regarding safety (often including pertinent pharmacokinetic data, such as volume of distribution, bioavailability, and drug elimination half-life) may be obtainable through a Freedom of Information Act request, which would be processed by the Food and Drug Administration.[115]

Extrapolation of dosing regimens should be limited to relatively healthy animals, if possible, to avoid the effects of disease on drug disposition. Likewise, extrapolation to geriatric and pediatric patients is discouraged. Administration by the oral route is generally safer (although gastric irritation may be more likely). Oral administration is less preferred if the drug undergoes first-pass metabolism, however, because this can vary dramatically among animals. A 50% change in first-pass metabolism may double the pharmacologically active dose in a patient. Intravenous administration is not recommended; when it is absolutely necessary, the drug should be administered slowly (over 5 to 10 minutes or more). Drugs with long half-lives (>12 hours) should generally be avoided. If a drug is administered at an interval that is less than the drug half-life, accumulation should be anticipated and accounted for in the dosing extrapolation. Note that maximal adverse effects may not appear until accumulation is complete at steady state. Also, a drug half-life can change (as a result of disease or drug interactions). Thus a drug that initially did not accumulate (and whose dose is based primarily on volume of distribution) may begin to accumulate as disease worsens. Unless the drug can be monitored, a change in drug half-life will be missed. In such instances a dosage reduction is again indicated. On the other hand, as a patient improves, response to therapy may again change disposition, perhaps leading to therapeutic failure. The veterinarian should be prepared to treat adverse effects if they occur. If the drug half-life is long, the time necessary for abatement of the adverse reaction will also be long. In general, extrapolation of lipid-soluble drugs is discouraged because of the risk of too many species differences.

Water-Soluble Drugs

As a general rule, extrapolation of doses for drugs that are water soluble is more appropriate because these drugs are distributed to extracellular fluids (normalizing Vd) (Box 2-2); protein binding is likely to be negligible; and hepatic metabolism is minimized. Drug Vd and renal elimination may be similar among species, and the interval used for such drugs can often be extrapolated among species. The dose administered, however, probably should be reduced to compensate for differences in blood volume among animals. Increased doses are indicated for pediatric patients and for patients with edema; decreased doses are indicated for geriatric and dehydrated patients.

KEY POINT 2-5 Extrapolation of dosing regimens among species is often safer with water-soluble drugs compared with lipid-soluble drugs because disposition tends to be much simpler.

Lipid-Soluble Drugs

Lipid-soluble drugs tend to be distributed to total body water and beyond, leading to a greater risk of differences among species. They are more likely to be highly protein bound, leading to a risk of differences in tissue distribution and in the proportion of pharmacologically active drug. In contrast to water-soluble drugs, lipid-soluble drugs are more likely to require hepatic metabolism (Box 2-3). In general, the clinician should anticipate a longer half-life in cats for drugs that undergo phase I metabolism in other species. Note that species differences in phase I metabolism can be very profound. If acetylation is a major phase II route of elimination, it is likely that the drug may be metabolized faster in cats than in dogs. If phase I metabolism and glucuronidation is the major route of elimination, a longer half-life should be anticipated in cats. Although glucuronidation does not necessarily indicate that elimination of the drug will be slower in cats, until an appropriate study has established the kinetics of the drug in cats, its use is discouraged. An exception

Box 2-2

General Characteristics of Water-Soluble Drugs

- Distributed to extracellular fluid
- Characterized by a volume of distribution ≤0.3 L/kg
- Minimally protein bound
- Undergo minimal to no metabolism
- Associated with fewer drug interactions
- Less likely to be allergenic
- Less likely to be hepatotoxic
- Tend to be renally excreted
- Often characterized by a short elimination half-life
- May not accumulate and thus reach steady state

Box 2-3

General Characteristics of Lipid-Soluble Drugs

- Distributed to total body water
- May be accumulated or stored
- Characterized by a volume of distribution ≥0.6 L/kg
- More likely to be significantly protein bound
- Generally metabolized before renal excretion
- More likely to interact with other drugs
- More likely to be associated with hepatotoxicity
- More likely to be allergenic
- Often characterized by a long elimination half-life
- May accumulate and thus be characterized by a time lag to steady state

might be made if the drug can be monitored or the drug is characterized by a wide therapeutic window. Altered-release preparations are not recommended because rates of absorption among the species can be dramatic. Finally, it might be necessary to refrain from administering preparations containing propylene glycol and other unknown carriers because of adverse reactions in cats.

All Drugs

Drugs with large (>2 L/kg) Vds are not recommended because accumulation or tissue binding of the drug may occur. These factors are likely to vary among species. Prodrugs, drugs for which active metabolites contribute significant activity and slow-release drugs are not appropriate because the amount of active drug is not predictable among the species. Body surface area should be used whenever possible to determine doses of toxic drugs. Drug disposition may change as the animal improves, particularly if a disease that affects drug disposition (i.e., cardiac, renal, hepatic) is being treated. Changes in dosing regimen may again be indicated. Finally, the veterinarian should be aware of the laws regulating the use of drugs labeled for use in humans.

PATHOLOGIC FACTORS

The diseased patient is more likely to react adversely to a drug. Although such reactions occasionally reflect disease-induced differences in receptor number or sensitivity, most often they reflect differences in drug disposition. The dosage regimens recommended for a pharmaceutical preparation generally are based on controlled studies in the normal, healthy animal. However, drugs are most frequently administered to the diseased patient. Pathophysiologic changes in most body systems can alter all phases of drug disposition, predisposing the patient to adverse drug reactions (Table 2-4). The sequelae of disease on drug disposition often but not always leads to increased PDCs and thus to a greater potential for adverse drug reactions. Occasionally, however, PDCs are lower than

Table 2-4 Impact of Disease on Drug Disposition

Pharmacokinetic Changes	Impact	Sequelae
Liver disease	Decreased hepatic blood flow	Increased oral bioavailability, decreased clearance of highly extracted compounds
	Decreased phase I enzymes	Decreased hepatic clearance (longer half-life)
	Decreased phase II enzymes	Decreased hepatic clearance (longer half-life)
		Decreased hepatoprotection (increased risk of hepatoxicity)
	Decreased albumin	Increased concentration of free drug (may not be cleared more rapidly in presence of liver disease)
	Ascites	Decreased distribution of water-soluble drugs, higher drug concentrations, shorter half-life
	Decreased production of phase II enzymes	Decreased cytoprotection
Renal disease	Decreased cytoprotection	Increased risk of xenobiotic-induced nephrotoxicity
	Decreased autoregulation	Increased risk of xenobiotic-induced nephrotoxicity
	Decreased body mass (dehydration)	Decreased volume of distribution (higher xenobiotic concentration, shorter half-life)
	Increased fluid retention	Increased distribution of drugs, decreased concentration, longer half-life
	Decreased renal blood flow	Decreased renal clearance (longer half-life)
	Tubular disease	Decreased concentration of drug, decreased efficacy of urinary antibiotics, decreased clearance
	Glomerular disease	Increased risk of xenobiotic-induced nephrotoxicity
		Deceased protein-binding (increased fraction of unbound xenobiotic)
		Increased clearance of unbound fraction of highly protein-bound xenobiotics
Cardiac disease	Decreased renal blood flow	See renal disease
	Decreased hepatic blood flow	See hepatic disease
	Decreased regional blood flow	Decreased organ delivery (higher concentrations delivered to brain and heart)
Gastrointestinal disease	Decreased cytoprotection	Increased risk of gastrointestinal toxicity
	Altered permeability	Altered absorption
	Altered gastrointestinal motility	Decreased rate of absorption
	Altered P-glycoprotein	Altered absorption

anticipated (e.g., increased Vd, decreased oral bioavailability), and therapeutic failure may occur. Diseases most likely to contribute to adverse drug reactions are those affecting the kidneys, liver, and heart. Less significant effects accompany gastrointestinal, pulmonary, endocrine, and metabolic disorders. Pathologic responses that generate clinical signs of disease also may be associated with changes in drug disposition. For example, following oral administration, amoxicillin area under the curve increased in dogs rendered febrile by administration of endotoxin.[116] The cause of the increase was not clear but may have reflected increased absorption caused by lipopolysaccharide reduction of gastrointestinal transit time or fever-induced increased absorption or endotoxin-induced decreased renal clearance. The sequelae of hypovolemia affects multiple aspects of drug disposition. Because blood flow to the brain and heart are maintained, drug that might have been distributed to peripheral organs is distributed to these two organs, increasing their risk of toxicity while simultaneously limiting clearance by organs of excretion. Drug distribution to peripheral organs will then increase with successful management.

Renal Disease

Drug toxicity in renal failure may result either from increased sensitivity to the drug owing to uremia-induced alterations in tissue receptors or from decreased or increased PDCs caused by disease-induced changes in pharmacokinetics. Changes induced by renal disease have been best characterized (see Table 2-4).[117-120]

Renal blood flow is often profoundly decreased in patients with renal disease. Changes in glomerular filtration and tubular secretion tend to parallel changes in renal blood flow. The effects of changes in renal blood flow (usually decreased) on drug excretion are most profound if renal extraction of the drug is high (e.g., penicillins, sulfates, glucuronide conjugates) but are less significant for drugs that are slowly extracted (e.g., aminoglycosides, diuretics, digoxin).

Glomerular filtration of drugs and other compounds is also adversely affected in renal disease independent of changes in renal blood flow. The determinants of glomerular filtration include protein binding, glomerular integrity, and the number of functional (filtering) nephrons. The molecular size of the drug is also important because drugs with a molecular weight greater than approximately 70,000 usually cannot be filtered. Drugs that are tightly protein bound (such as NSAIDs) are not filtered until they are displaced from the protein. Factors that tend to displace such drugs from protein-binding sites may increase the rate of drug excretion in renal disease and include hypoalbuminemia, competition for protein-binding sites owing to accumulation of uremic toxins, or changes in the conformation and thus binding affinity of the protein (e.g., albumin). Changes in protein binding that have been measured in renal disease include decreased binding of acidic drugs (e.g., furosemide, NSAIDs, selected penicillins and anticonvulsants) and normal or increased binding of basic drugs owing to increased concentrations of inflammatory proteins (e.g., propranolol, diazepam, prazosin). The impact of increased clearance of otherwise protein-bound drug may be offset by the increase in plasma concentration of the free drug displaced from the protein, thus increasing elimination of unbound drug.

Although changes in active tubular reabsorption that may accompany renal disease probably do not profoundly influence the rate of drug excretion, changes in active tubular secretion can be significant. Active tubular secretion occurs in the pars recta (straight segment) of the proximal tubule. A transport system exists for a variety of organic acids (e.g., penicillins, cephalosporins, NSAIDs, sulfonamides, several diuretics) as well as bases (e.g., cimetidine, procainamide, some morphine derivatives). Distal nephron active transport may also be important for some drugs (e.g., digoxin). Excretion of these drugs is most likely to be decreased in the presence of renal disease because of decreased nephron mass, decreased renal blood flow, and decreased tubular function.

In addition to these changes, renal disease can also alter drug disposition because of changes in electrolyte, acid–base, and fluid balance. Changes in electrolytes and acid–base balance may also be important in altering receptor sensitivity to drugs, such as those affecting the cardiovascular system (e.g., hyperkalemia and its effects on responses to digitalis, quinidine, and procainamide).

KEY POINT 2-6 Serum creatinine is a reasonable indicator of the impact of renal disease on renal drug clearance.

For drugs whose elimination depends on renal function and whose clearance is known to be decreased in renal disease (Box 2-4), dosing regimens can be appropriately altered to reduce the incidence of adverse reactions.[119] Either serum creatinine or creatinine clearance is generally used to estimate glomerular filtration rate; however, because of its ease of measurement, serum creatinine is most commonly used. Decreases in the renal elimination of a renally excreted drug

Box 2-4
Examples of Drugs Characterized by Changes in Drug Disposition in Patients with Renal Disease

Changes in Protein Binding (Decreased)
Furosemide
Naproxen
Phenylbutazone
Salicylate
Warfarin

Changes in Volume of Distribution (Increased)
Cefazolin
Furosemide
Naproxen

Changes in Clearance
Aminoglycosides
Beta-lactams
Digoxin
Sulfates
Furosemide

tend to parallel increases in serum creatinine, and dosing regimens can be altered by either lengthening the dosing interval or decreasing the dose by a proportional decrease in creatinine clearance or the increase in serum creatinine (Box 2-5).

The parameter of the dosing regimen that should be altered depends on the drug. Lengthening the interval results in wider swings in PDCs during a single dosing interval and thus may not be desirable for time-dependent antimicrobial therapy but would be acceptable for concentration-dependent drugs or lengthening the interval also should be avoided for anticonvulsant or cardioactive drugs that depend on maintenance of a minimum drug concentration within a specified therapeutic range. Thus decreasing the dose may be more appropriate for these drugs. For drugs with a long elimination half-life or drugs whose effects persist in the absence of detectable drug (e.g., selected antimicrobials [e.g., concentration-dependent], glucocorticoids, nonsteroidal agents), however, it may be more appropriate to prolong the interval. Aminoglycosides previously were dosed at 12-hour intervals. Because their efficacy depends on a high PDC, yet safety is based on allowing PDCs to fall below a recommended trough concentration, prolonging the interval (i.e., from 12 to 18 or 24 hours) was more appropriate than lowering the dose in patients with renal disease sufficient to alter creatinine clearance. However, aminoglycosides are currently administered at 24-hour dosing intervals, precluding the need to prolong intervals in some renal disease patients. For other drugs whose toxicity is related to peak drug concentrations, the dose might be decreased by 50%, or the interval prolonged one half-life. Few clinical studies have addressed the impact of renal disease on the clearance of drugs in dogs or cats. Experimentally induced renal disease sufficient to cause serum creatinine to increase to 145 ± 122 μmole/L in dogs caused a slight decrease in renal clearance but no clinically significant change in elimination half-life of marbofloxacin.[121]

Hepatic Disease

The efficiency of hepatic elimination is determined by hepatic clearance and the hepatic extraction ratio of the drug.[122-125] Both, in turn, depend on hepatic blood flow; the extent of drug protein binding; and intrinsic hepatic clearance, which itself consists of hepatic uptake (the rate-limiting step of hepatic clearance), intracellular transport, metabolism, and (if applicable) biliary elimination. Drugs that are eliminated by the liver can be categorized according to their rate of extraction.[126] *Flow-limited* drugs (e.g., lidocaine, propranolol, verapamil) are so rapidly extracted by the liver that their rate of elimination depends only on the rate at which it is delivered to the liver (e.g., hepatic blood flow). Such drugs are insensitive to changes in hepatic metabolism but are very sensitive to changes in hepatic blood flow. *Capacity-limited* drugs (e.g., diazepam, prednisolone, phenylbutazone, phenytoin, theophylline, cimetidine, and antipyrine) are extracted slowly by the liver, and their elimination depends on hepatic uptake and metabolism but is independent of hepatic blood flow. The elimination of such drugs is affected by changes in hepatic metabolism but not by changes in hepatic blood flow. Some drugs are intermediate, being partially dependent on hepatic blood flow and hepatic metabolism.[123,126]

Protein binding can affect the elimination of some capacity-limited drugs because only unbound drug can be extracted by the liver. Flow-limited drugs tend to be *binding insensitive* in that hepatic extraction is so fast that binding to proteins does not alter their rate of elimination. Some capacity-limited drugs are not significantly protein bound and thus are also binding insensitive (e.g., antipyrine). In contrast, some capacity-limited drugs are *binding sensitive* (e.g., theophylline, phenytoin) because their slow rate of extraction can be increased by decreasing or increasing, respectively, protein binding.[127]

The effects of hepatic disease on drug disposition are very complex, particularly for drugs that are affected by changes in hepatic blood flow, hepatic metabolism, and protein binding (Box 2-6).[123,126] Each of these parameters may be altered in various ways in patients with liver disease. Hepatic blood flow is generally reduced in chronic liver disease because of formation of portosystemic shunts and intrahepatic shunting. Drug delivery bypasses many functional hepatocytes that would otherwise clear the drug. Plasma and tissue drug concentrations are markedly higher when dosing regimens are not appropriately altered. This is particularly important for highly extracted drugs when they are administered orally. The dose of such drugs (e.g., propranolol, verapamil, prazosin, morphine derivatives) in the presence of normal hepatic blood flow is based on decreased bioavailability owing to first-pass extraction: a large percentage of the drug does not reach systemic circulation because it is removed from portal blood by the liver the first time it passes through the liver. Decreased hepatic blood flow and intrahepatic shunting of blood can markedly increase systemic bioavailability of such drugs (Figure 2-5).[128] Studies in human patients with liver disease suggest that the intrinsic metabolism of highly extracted drugs also is reduced in patients with liver disease. In human patients with liver disease, the dose of many highly extracted drugs is reduced by 50%; such an approach is probably reasonable for the veterinary patient.

The effect of liver disease on poorly extracted (capacity-limited) drugs is more difficult to predict, particularly for drugs that are highly protein bound. Generally, hepatic metabolism is reduced in patients with liver disease. Disease is generally quite profound, however, by the time changes in drug disposition become evident. The severity of disease is manifested as a decrease in serum albumin and blood urea nitrogen levels. This has been shown by studies that have measured the clearance of

Box 2-5

Dosing Regimens for Drugs Dependent on Renal Function

New dose = old dose × pt CrCl/normal CrCl or × normal Cr/pt Cr

New interval = old interval × normal CrCl/pt CrCl or × pt Cr/normal Cr

pt = patient, Cr = creatinine, and CrCl = creatinine clearance

For example, a patient has a serum creatinine level of 2.5 mg/dL (normal is 1.2), a dosing interval for a drug given every 12 hours would be prolonged to every 24 hours, or the dose of 2 mg/kg could be reduced to 1 mg/kg.

Box 2-6

Drugs Characterized by Changes in Drug Disposition in Patients with Hepatic Disease

Changes in Blood Flow; Flow-Limited Drugs
Lidocaine
Meperidine
Metoprolol
Morphine
Pentazocine
Propranolol

Changes in Metabolism; Capacity-Limited Drugs
Chloramphenicol
Cimetidine
Diazepam
Furosemide
Prednisolone
Ranitidine
Theophylline
Warfarin

Changes in Protein Binding
Lidocaine
Meperidine
Propranolol
Diazepam
Phenylbutazone
Phenytoin

(From Williams RL: Drugs and the liver: clinical applications. In Benet LZ, Massoud N, Gambertoglio JG, editors: *Pharmacokinetic basis for drug treatment,* New York, 1984, Raven Press, pp 53-75.)

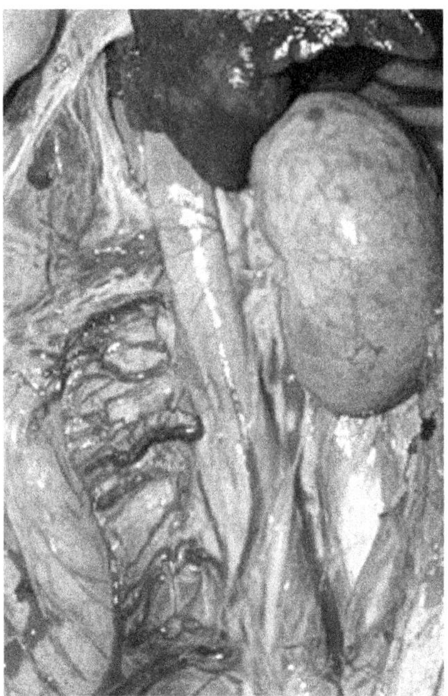

Figure 2-5 Portosystemic shunting affects drug disposition at multiple sites. Clearance of flow-limited drugs will be decreased in proportion to the fraction of blood shunted around the liver. Capacity-limited drugs may also be decreased if hepatic mass is sufficiently reduced. Accumulation of fluid in response to sodium retention may be profound, particularly in the abdomen. Albumin may be decreased, increasing the fraction of unbound drug, which may not be cleared as rapidly in the presence of disease.

antipyrine and caffeine, which are capacity-limited, binding-sensitive and binding-insensitive drugs, respectively, in dogs with experimentally induced liver disease.[129,130]

KEY POINT 2-7 If liver disease has impacted serum albumin or blood urea nitrogen, ensuring that drug metabolism is also impacted is prudent.

Because elimination of these drugs depends entirely on hepatic metabolism, their clearance might be used as a hepatic function test. Because their elimination does not necessarily correlate with the elimination of other drugs that also depend on hepatic clearance, however, they are not used to predict changes in dosing regimens for the patient with liver disease. Recommendations regarding dosing regimens for drugs not highly extracted by the liver thus are difficult to make for the patient with liver disease, in part because there is no simple test that will assess or quantitate hepatic function.[125,129-133] In general, clearance of capacity-limited drugs is probably not impaired in patients whose serum albumin and blood urea nitrogen levels are within normal limits. Common sense dictates, however, that discretion be used when administering potentially toxic drugs that depend on hepatic clearance for elimination.

Diseases of the biliary tract alter the disposition of drugs eliminated through the bile. This route of elimination is complex, however, with drugs being eliminated in feces and undergoing enterohepatic circulation. Characterizing these changes is difficult without catheterization of the biliary duct, and recommendations are very difficult to offer. Cholestasis decreases the content or activity of cytochrome P450 drug-metabolizing enzymes and thus can affect the elimination of drugs that are not secreted in bile.[134,135] In general, doses of drugs eliminated principally in the bile should be reduced, particularly if the drug is characterized by a narrow therapeutic window. Examples include selected antimicrobials (doxycycline and clindamycin), digitoxin, and naproxen.

The effects that changes in protein binding may have on hepatic drug clearance contribute to the unpredictable nature of liver disease–induced changes in drug disposition.[127,136,137] Decreased protein binding of drugs that may accompany liver disease (i.e., caused by decreased synthesis of albumin, competition for binding sites by endogenous compounds, or changes in conformation of the binding site) may increase hepatic clearance and thus compensate for reduced hepatic metabolism, although the ability of the diseased liver to compensate is not clear. Increased rather than decreased binding may occur particularly for basic drugs (e.g., lidocaine) as a result of increased production of acute-phase proteins, which may have the effect of decreasing clearance. Changes in protein binding will also affect drug distribution. Protein binding decreases the amount of drug that distributes to peripheral tissues. Drug distribution in the patient with liver disease

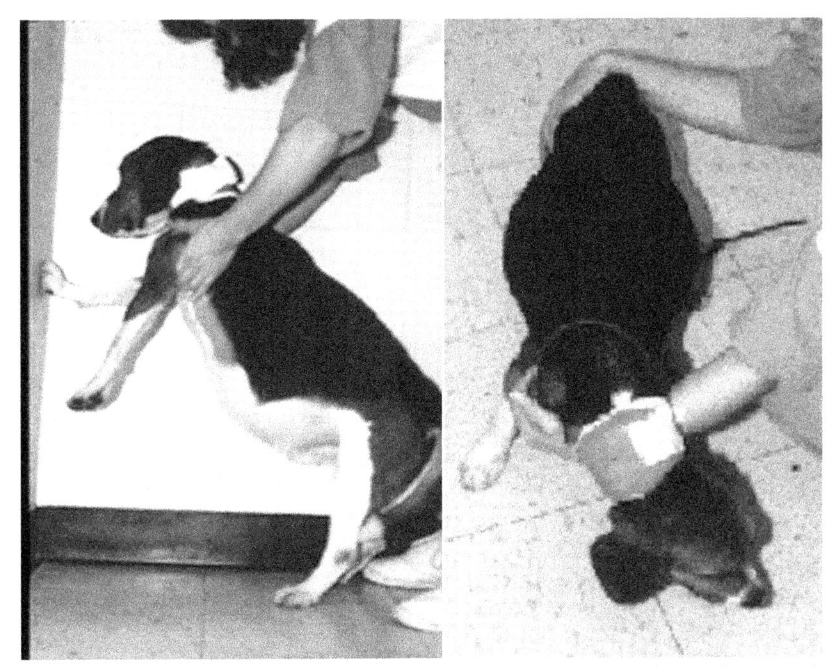

Figure 2-6 Disease can affect body composition. The ascitic compartment in an animal with liver or other disease can represent up to 30% or more of body weight. If this compartment is not one to which a drug distributes and the animal is dosed on the basis of total body weight, plasma drug concentrations may be more than 30% higher than expected. If the drug is distributed to the ascitic compartment, prolonged distribution from the compartment back to plasma may result in a longer elimination half-life.

will be further complicated by the effects of fluid, electrolyte, and acid–base imbalances, which are also likely to occur. For example, an ascitic compartment may lead to overdosing if a patient is not dosed on the basis of lean body weight and the drug does not distribute to the ascitic compartment, which may constitute up to 30% of body weight (Figure 2-6).

Cardiac Disease

Cardiac disease profoundly affects drug disposition (see Table 2-4). Primary or compensatory disturbances that lead to altered drug disposition include renal sodium and water retention, increased pulmonary and systemic venous pressures, and increased sympathetic nervous system output.[6] Sodium and water retention can cause profound changes in drug distribution owing to changes in the sizes of body compartments. In addition, increased sympathetic outflow results in redistribution of blood flow such that the heart and brain receive a higher proportion of blood and thus are exposed to more drug. Because other tissues, particularly skeletal muscle, represent a large volume to which drug is normally distributed, reduced distribution of drug to these tissues results in even higher PDCs in blood going to the heart and brain. Thus the heart and brain are more susceptible to toxicity. CNS and cardiac toxicities to lidocaine and cardiac toxicity to digoxin have been described in some patients with cardiac disease; these toxicities have been attributed to blood redistribution, which accompanies cardiac failure.

KEY POINT 2-8 Cardiac disease can affect every aspect of drug disposition. Variability may be greater as the patient responds or fails to respond to therapy.

As cardiac output decreases, reduced blood flow to the kidney and liver will have profound effects on clearance of drugs through either of these organs. Reduced blood flow reflects, in part, redistribution mediated by sympathetic output. As cardiac disease progresses, however, decreases in blood flow to both the liver and kidneys parallel decreases in cardiac output. The effects of decreased hepatic blood flow on drug elimination depend on the drug; as with liver disease, hepatic clearance of flow-limited drugs may be profoundly decreased. In the kidney, sympathetically mediated intrarenal redistribution of blood from cortical to juxtaglomerular tubules increases the likelihood of tubular reabsorption, which prolongs drug half-life.

Tissue hypoxia and decreased delivery of nutrients to the kidney and liver also contribute to decreased clearance by these organs. The metabolic capacity of the liver is reduced; thus clearance of capacity-limited drugs is impaired. Similarly, renal tubular function is impaired.

Drug absorption may be impaired in the patient with cardiac disease. This is particularly true for parenterally administered drugs. The rate of absorption is more likely to be affected than the extent of absorption; hence peak concentrations may be less, although the extent of drug absorption may not be affected. Redistribution of blood away from skeletal muscle and skin decreases the rate of drug absorption after intramuscular and subcutaneous injections. Autonomic disturbances, consisting of increased sympathetic activity and decreased autonomic tone, tissue hypoxia, and mucosal edema may decrease both the rate and the extent of gastrointestinal absorption. Decreased blood flow to the intestinal villus may decrease absorption of drugs that are normally very rapidly absorbed from the gastrointestinal tract. Finally, the effects of cardiac disease on hepatic clearance of flow-limited drugs and thus on systemic bioavailability of orally administered drugs must be considered.

Several recommendations can be made for administering drugs to the patient with cardiac disease (Box 2-7):

1. Critical drugs should be administered intravenously because absorption from all other routes is limited.
2. Drugs that are toxic (particularly to the brain and heart) should not be rapidly administered intravenously (i.e., administer over 10 to 30 minutes).
3. High drug concentrations resulting from redistribution should be compensated for by decreasing loading doses.
4. Maintenance doses of selected drugs cleared by the liver, kidney, or both should probably be lowered, although predicting which drugs and how much is difficult. Therapeutic monitoring should be used to guide alteration of dosing regimens whenever possible.

Thyroid and Other Diseases

Both hyperthyroidism and hypothyroidism can profoundly affect drug disposition, although the manner is unpredictable.[138] The effects thus far involve metabolism. In human patients with hyperthyroidism, the activities of some cytochrome P450 enzymes (e.g., hydroxylation) are increased, whereas those of others (e.g., N-demethylation) are decreased. In rats in which hyperthyroid disease had been induced, enzymes that act as cofactors were increased. Thyroidectomized animals have a general decrease in drug metabolism, although the sequelae are not always predictable. The effects of thyroid disease on drug disposition also depend on sex, with male rats having a general decrease in cytochrome P450 enzymes. The clinical sequelae of changes in drug disposition induced by thyroid disease are not well described in scientific studies, although several examples are provided in the human literature. Digoxin doses necessary to induce a clinical response are in general increased for patients with hyperthyroidism, whereas smaller doses than normal are needed for patients with hypothyroidism. Interestingly, propranolol clearance is decreased in cats with hyperthyroidism.[139]

Diseases of other body systems can also dramatically alter drug disposition. For example, gastrointestinal disease (e.g., chronic inflammatory bowel disease) alters absorption of orally administered drugs.[140] Diseases of any system may alter the response of that system to a drug. Nutrition also can alter drug-metabolizing enzymes. The effects of disease, regardless of the system, on drug absorption, distribution, metabolism, and excretion are very complex, often subtle, and very difficult to predict. Finally, as therapy becomes successful and the clinical signs of disease resolve, the sequelae of disease on drug disposition also resolve. Therapy once again may need to be adjusted as the animal responds.

Box 2-7

Examples of Drugs Characterized by Changes in Drug Disposition in Patients with Cardiac Disease

Decreased Volume of Distribution
Lidocaine
Procainamide
Quinidine
Theophylline

Decreased Clearance
Lidocaine
Prazosin
Procainamide
Quinidine
Theophylline
Digoxin*

*Clearance of digoxin is affected by other drugs used to treat cardiac disease.
(From Benowitz NL: Effects of cardiac disease on pharmacokinetics: pathophysiologic considerations. In Benet LZ, Massoud N, Gambertoglio JG, editors: *Pharmacokinetic basis for drug treatment*, New York, 1984, Raven Press, pp 89-104.)

PHARMACOLOGIC FACTORS

Drug interactions occur whenever the action of one drug is modified by the presence of another, concurrently administered drug. The incidence of interactions increases with the number of drugs included in the preparation and with the duration of treatment.[141] As such, the critical care patient may be particularly at risk; indeed, 81% of patients in a small animal intensive care unit were at risk for clinically relevant drug interactions in one study. The risk was greater in dogs with disease of the abdominal cavity and cats with cardiovascular disease.[142] Drug interactions should be expected to have a potentially profound impact on animals. In human medicine more than 50% of recent drug withdrawals in the United States have occurred because of serious drug–drug interactions, which underscores the increasing recognition of the role of interactions in adversity.[143] The author is aware of several instances of euthanasia in patients resulting from drug interactions that were not recognized until significant pathology had occurred.

The route of administration can influence the type of drug interaction. Drug interactions are not limited to interactions with active drug ingredients but may also involve interactions with additives or excipients. Interactions may occur among drugs, herbs, botanicals, and endogenous nutraceutical preparations and with foods (i.e., drug–diet interactions (Table 2-5). Interactions may also occur with containers in which the drug is stored or through which it is administered and the environment in which the drug is stored. Drug interactions can be categorized according to the phase of drug administration in which they occur: pharmaceutical, pharmacokinetic, or pharmacodynamic.

KEY POINT 2-9 The risk of drug interactions increases with the number of drugs the patient is simultaneously receiving. The negative sequealae of the interactions is likely to be greater when complicated by the presence of physiologic and pathologic factors.

Pharmaceutical Drug Interactions

Pharmaceutical drug interactions occur before the drug is absorbed and may occur before administration (Figure 2-7). Interactions can occur between two drugs or between a drug and a carrier (solvent), a receptacle (including intravenous tubing), or the environment in which it is administered (e.g., gastric environment).[144] In human medicine pharmaceutical interactions most frequently result from the addition of drugs to intravenous fluid preparations. In veterinary medicine they are most likely to occur in the critical care environment, where intravenous administration and multiple drug administration are common, or after inappropriate compounding of drugs. Drug incompatibilities can change the chemical or physical nature of a drug (Figure 2-8). Incompatible reactions can reflect degradation caused by changes in pH, binding by drugs with different charges, or other molecular interactions; changes in temperature; or exposure to ultraviolet radiation.[145] Incompatibilities may occur both with (approved) finished dosing forms or compounded preparations. A number of sources can be used to minimize the risk of drug interactions involving admixtures of drugs.[146-150]

Intravenous Preparations

A number of interactions involve drugs intended for injection (Table 2-6). Drugs that are unstable generally have a short shelf life when in solution. Reconstituted parenteral solutions should always be labeled with the new expiration date and used with strict adherence to the product label instructions after reconstitution. If directed by the label, refrigeration or freezing can prolong the shelf life. It is risky, however, to assume that cold storage will prolong the shelf life of the drug unless efficacy has been documented at the intended conditions. Freezing can increase the degradation (e.g., ampicillin), crystallization (e.g., heparin, dobutamine, furosemide), or precipitation (e.g., insulin) of drugs. Refreezing of a previously frozen and defrosted solution increases the risk of efficacy loss. Often, if specifically queried, the manufacturer of the product can provide specifit information regarding drug stability in conditions beyond those stated on the label. The proper reconstituting fluid should be used to prevent inactivation of drugs. For example, amphotericin B should be diluted only with 5% dextrose because precipitates will otherwise form; whole blood or packed red blood cells should be diluted only with 0.9% saline to prevent damage to infused cells.

Changing the pH of a solution by improperly diluting it or mixing it with another drug can be risky. The release of some insulins is pH dependent. Diluting insulin with a solution other than that provided by the manufacturer may change the pH and thus the rate of insulin release. The pH of a solution may be needed to keep the active drug dissolved or stable; changing the pH may result in precipitation or loss of stability. For example, acid-labile drugs (e.g., penicillins) can be

Table 2-5 Drug-Supplement Interactions

Drug	Supplement	Side Effect
Alprazolam	Kava	Enhanced effect
Anesthetics, sedatives	St. John's wort, valerian, kava	Increased CNS effects
Antiplatelet/anticoagulants	Garlic, ginger, ginkgo, chamomile, feverfew, bromelain, dang gui	Prolonged bleeding time
Antiviral	Garlic (allium)	Decreased effect because of CYP3A4 and P-glycoprotein induction
Cardiac stimulants	Ephedra, ginseng	Increased risk of cardiac arrhythmias
Chlorpropamide	Garlic (allium)	Hypoglycemia
CNS stimulants	Ephedra, yohimbine, guarana, ginseng, caffeine	Increased CNS stimulation
Cyclosporine	St. John's wort	Decreased effect because of CYP3A4 and P-glycoprotein induction
Digoxin	St. John's wort	Decreased effect because of P-glycoprotein induction
Diuretics	Senna, licorice	Electrolyte disturbances
Hypoglycemics	Ginseng, bilberry, dandelion, garlic, bitter melon	Hypoglycemia
Immunosuppressants	Echinacea, astragalus	Antagonizes immunosuppressive effects
Loperamide	St. John's wort	Inhibition of monoamine oxidase (enhanced effect)
Oral drugs	Senna	Decreased absorption
Propranolol	Piperine	Enhanced effect (CYP inhibition)
Selective serotonin reuptake inhibitors	St. John's wort, SAMe, silamaryn	Increased risk of side effects, serotonergic crisis
Theophylline	St. John's wort	Decreased effect because of CYP3A4 and P-glycoprotein induction
Theophylline	Piperine	Enhanced effect (CYP inhibition)
Thiazide diuretics	Ginkgo	Decreased clearance (enhanced effect)

CNS, Central nervous system; *SAMe*, S-adenosylmethionine.

destroyed in a low-pH solution. Drugs prepared as an acid salt (e.g., lidocaine hydrogen chloride) or in acidic solutions (i.e., sodium heparin) should not be combined with alkaline solutions (i.e., sodium bicarbonate).

Drugs can bind to and inactivate one another, often because of ionic attractions. Calcium in solutions causes precipitation when combined with solutions containing carbonates (e.g., sodium bicarbonate). Heparin is incompatible with several drugs, such as aminoglycoside and beta-lactam antibiotics. Thus saline rather than heparin should be used whenever possible to maintain patency of catheters through which drugs are administered. When present in sufficiently high concentrations, penicillins inactivate aminoglycosides. In fact, ticarcillin can be used therapeutically to bind gentamicin in cases of overdose. Although plasma concentrations after therapeutic dosing of either drug probably do not achieve concentrations necessary to inactivate aminoglycosides, in the critical care situation, and as a once-daily dosing regimen of aminoglycosides becomes more generally acceptable, the risk of aminoglycoside (or a fluorinated quinolone) antimicrobial inactivation by a penicillin may become greater.

Often, a pharmaceutical drug interaction involving intravenous solutions can be detected by a visual change in the appearance of the drugs. Discoloration, cloudiness, and formation of precipitate generally are indications of an interaction, and with some exceptions use of the drug should be reconsidered. Not all interactions will result in a physical change of the appearance, however. Likewise, the change in physical appearance of a drug combination does not necessarily indicate that the activity of the drug has been changed. For example, diazepam has been mixed with other preanesthetics with no observable change in drug efficacy, despite a

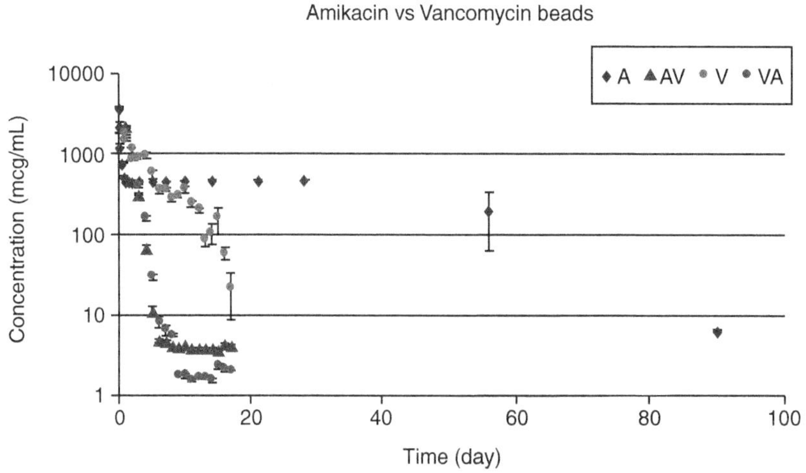

Amikacin vs Vancomycin beads

◆ A ▲ AV ● V ● VA

Concentration (mcg/mL): 10000, 1000, 100, 10, 1

Time (day): 0, 20, 40, 60, 80, 100

Figure 2-7 An example of a drug interaction is exemplified by drug efflux from calcium hydroxyapatite (plaster of Paris) beads. Individually, amikacin or vancomycin is characterized by an initial rapid release, followed by slow release from the beads over several weeks. However, when both drugs are mixed in the beads, efflux of both amikacin and vancomycin is much more rapid, being nearly complete in 1 to several days.

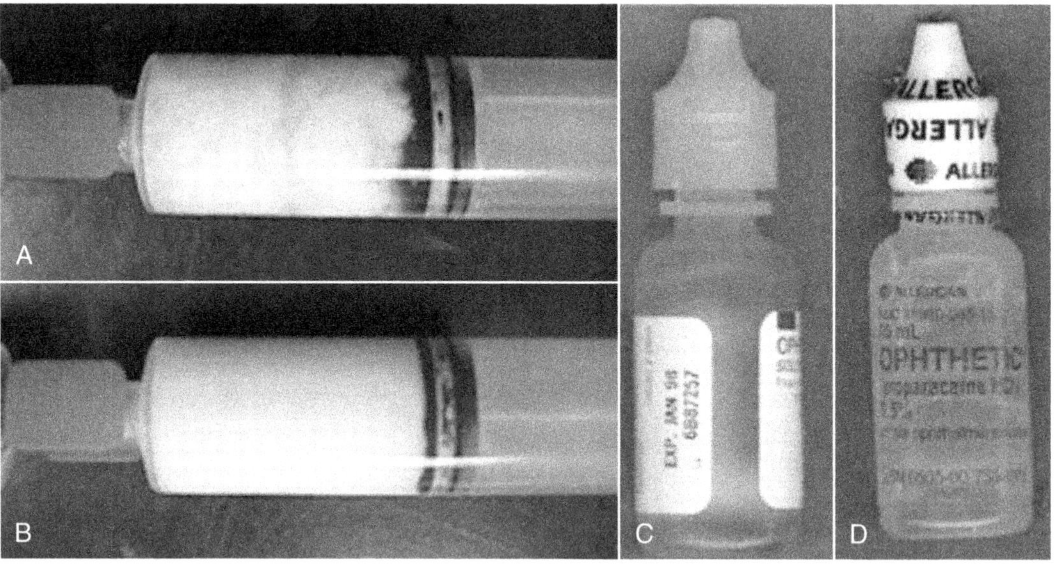

Figure 2-8 Examples of chemical changes in drugs. Transdermal gels are thermoreversible, liquefying at refrigerated temperatures **(A)** and solidifying at room temperature **(B)**. Discoloration, shown here for an ophthalmic product **(C** and **D)** and steroid.

Table **2-6** Examples of Drug Interactions in Solution

Drug or Drug Class	Incompatible Drugs	Other Risks
Amino acid solutions	Many drugs	
Aminoglycosides	Semisynthetic beta-lactams, heparin, many others; check manufacturer's label	Adsorbs to glass; use plastic for monitoring
Aminophylline	Should not be mixed with other drugs	
Amphotericin B	Use only 5% dextrose (or manufacturer suggests sterile water).	Light exposure
Ampicillin sodium	Selected diluents and drugs; check manufacturer's label	
Atropine sulfate	Bicarbonate, methicillin, promazine, warfarin, others	
Beta-lactams		
Cephalosporins	Many drugs, depending on specific antimicrobial; check manufacturer's label	Check manufacturer's recommendations regarding stability upon reconstruction.
Penicillins	As for cephalosporins; aminoglycosides	
Bicarbonate	Many drugs	
Buprenorphine	Should not be mixed with dimenhydrinate, pentobarbital	
Butorphanol	Should not be mixed with diazepam	
Blood, red blood cells	Any intravenous solution except 0.9% saline	
Calcium-containing solutions	Many drugs	
Calcium disodium EDTA	Should not be mixed with many drugs, including dextrose, metal salts	
Chloramphenicol	Many drugs	
Carbenicillin disodium	Should not be mixed with many drugs	
Cefazolin	Should not be mixed with any other drug	
Cephalothin	Should not be mixed with any other drug	
Diazepam	Cloudiness when mixed with many other drugs indicates precipitation, which will include drug; potency may be reduced.	Adsorbs to intravenous tubing and plastic containers
		Protect from light.
Digitoxin (not digoxin)	Calcium, epinephrine, vitamin B complex	
Diphenhydramine	Furosemide, methylprednisolone, pentobarbital	
Dobutamine	Alkaline solutions	Check manufacturer's label regarding discoloration.
Doxorubicin	Bicarbonate, heparin, insulin, others	Avoid prolonged contact with aluminum.
Doxycycline	Selected drugs, including lidocaine, heparin, isoproterenol, vitamin B complex	
Epinephrine	Calcium-containing solutions, ampicillin, other penicillins, pentobarbital, prochlorperazine, others	
Erythromycin	Several drugs, including selected cephalosporins, chloramphenicol, heparin, tetracyclines, and vitamin B complex	
Flunixin meglumine	Most solutions	
Furosemide	Acidic solutions cause hydrolysis; precipitates when combined with many drugs	Yellow discoloration; protect from light
Gentamicin	Many drugs, including dopamine, furosemide, heparin (see also beta-lactams, amphotericin B)	
Glycopyrrolate	Alkaline solutions	Strongly acidic solution
	Should not be diluted with saline or bicarbonate for intravenous infusion	
	Other drugs	
Heparin	Many drugs	Strongly acidic solution
		Slightly yellow discoloration is acceptable.
Hydrocortisone sodium esters	Acid pH causes hydrolysis.	Use proper dilution volume to prevent precipitation.
	Incompatible with many selected drugs	

Continued

Table 2-6 Examples of Drug Interactions in Solution—cont'd

Drug or Drug Class	Incompatible Drugs	Other Risks
Imipenem		Do not freeze.
Insulin	Check package label regarding diluents and refrigeration need and mixing lente insulin kinetics; incompatible with many drugs	Binds to intravenous tubing, selected types of glass, and plastics
Iron dextran	Oxytetracycyline, sulfonamides	
Kanamycin	See gentamicin, aminoglycosides	
Ketamine	Barbiturates, diazepam	
Lidocaine	Alkaline solutions	Loss of drug when stored in polyvinyl chloride bags (adsorption to polyvinyl chloride)
Magnesium sulfate	Many drugs, including calcium-containing drugs, sodium bicarbonate, tetracyclines, others	
Mannitol	Blood, strongly acidic, or alkaline solutions	Crystallization of high (25%) concentrations in glass containers generally can be redistributed by warming; crystallization in plastic solutions is difficult to resolve
Methylprednisolone sodium succinate	Normosol-R, Normosol-M, selected drugs	Do not dilute with a volume that is too small; precipitation may occur otherwise.
Metronidazole		Reconstituted lyophilized product is very acidic and must be buffered with bicarbonate. Ready-to-use product requires no additional handling. It is light sensitive; however, discoloration induced by light is not accompanied by loss of potency. Do not freeze.
Metoclopramide	Beta-lactams, erythromycin, sodium bicarbonate	Protect from light.
Morphine	Many drugs	
Multiple vitamin	Bicarbonate, selected cephalosporins, aminophylline, others	Decreased potency as been documented; complexes 8 hours after dilution.
Nitrofurantoin	Many drugs	
Oxyglobin	Vitamin K (see phytonadione)	Removal from foil wrap exposes hemoglobin to oxidation, with subsequent formation of methemoglobinemia (indicated by brown discoloration).
Oxytetracycline	See tetracycline	
Oxytocin	Do not mix with any other drug.	Refrigerate at <25° C; do not freeze.
Penicillin G	See also beta-lactams	Rapidly inactivates in pH <6-7 or >8
	Polyethylene glycol	
	Prochlorperazine, pentobarbital, sulfadiazine	
	Others	
Pentobarbital	Acid pH	Prepared as extremely alkaline solution
	Many drugs	
Phenobarbital	Many drugs, especially acidic solutions	
Phenylephrine	Penicillin, pentobarbital, phenobarbital, phenytoin, sodium bicarbonate	
Phenytoin	Do not mix with any other drug or intravenous solution.	
Phytonadione	Do not mix with ascorbic acid, barbiturates, phenytoin.	
Potassium chloride	Do not mix with amphotericin B.	
Pralidoxime chloride (2PAM)	Reconstitute with sterile water only; do not mix with any other drug.	

Table 2-6 Examples of Drug Interactions in Solution—cont'd

Drug or Drug Class	Incompatible Drugs	Other Risks
Procaine	Many solutions, especially alkaline	
Procainamide	Dextrose	Light yellow (but not amber) discoloration acceptable
Prochlorperazine	Many drugs; do not mix in same syringe	
Promazine	Many drugs	
Promethazine	Selected drugs	
Protein hydrolysate	Many drugs	
Propofol	Do not mix with any other drugs.	
Propranolol	Rapidly decomposes in alkaline solution	
Ringer's lactate	Alcohol in 5% dextrose, epinephrine, oxytetracycline, sodium bicarbonate, sulfadiazine	
Sodium bicarbonate	Many drugs; check package insert	
Sodium iodide	Several drugs	
Sulfonamides, sodium salts	Many drugs	
Tetracycline	Highly acidic solution may render this incompatible with many drugs.	Dark solution indicates decomposition; discoloration in multiple electrolyte solution does not indicate potency loss.
Thiopental	Many drugs	
Vancomycin	Selected drugs	
Vitamin B complex	Magnesium sulfate, erythromycin, selected others	
Warfarin	Many drugs	

cloudy discoloration. Whereas a pink discoloration of dopamine indicates inactivation, discoloration of dobutamine does not preclude efficacy if the drug is used within 24 hours. Slight yellow discoloration of procainamide is acceptable; dark discoloration indicates a loss of efficacy.

Several drugs can bind to receptacles. For example, lipid-soluble drugs (e.g., diazepam) can bind to plastic containers; insulin binds to selected glasses and to many plastics, including polyethylene and polyvinyl; aminoglycosides bind to glass. Binding to catheters and intravenous lines can be minimized by flushing each new system with a sufficient volume of solution (50 mL) before drug administration. Drugs packaged in brown bottles (e.g., diazepam, furosemide) are somewhat protected as such from ultraviolet light, and protection should be continued if they are transferred to another vial.

Oral Preparations

Oral preparations may involve drug–diet or drug–drug interactions (see Box 2-7 and Tables 2-5 and 2-6). Many drugs bind luminal contents (drug–diet interactions; Table 2-7), and oral absorption is impaired.[151] Food can alter splanchnic blood flow, gastric motility (and thus mixing and drug dissolution as well as gastric emptying), and gastric secretions. Changes in gastric secretions can alter gastric pH, which can change the percentage of ionized and thus diffusible drug. The net effect of food on drug absorption depends on the pK_a of the drug, whether the drug is labile to the effects of pH and enzymes, and the site of absorption of the drug (i.e., stomach versus intestine).[151] The sequelae may affect either the rate or extent of drug absorption. The effect of food on the rate of drug absorption is most important for drugs with a narrow therapeutic window and for drugs with a steep dose–response curve, for which a small change in PDC can cause profound differences in response to the drug. Predicting drug–diet interactions on the basis of chemical structure should be done cautiously. Whereas food will impair the oral absorption of most tetracyclines, doxycycline is minimally affected. Food reduces the absorption of ampicillin but not amoxicillin;[152] food prolongs the time to peak plasma concentrations of cefadroxil (and increases time above the minimum inhibitory concentration) but has no impact on the absorption of cephalexin.[153] Oral absorption of selected drugs is enhanced rather than decreased in the presence of food (see Table 2-2). Interactions between drugs and foods were recently well reviewed using a body-systems approach.[154]

Drug–drug interactions (see Table 2-7) in the lumen include, but are not limited to, changes in the diffusibility, dissolution rate, and particle size of orally administered drugs. Drug–drug interactions in the gastrointestinal tract can inactivate or prevent absorption of drugs. Sucralfate, cimetidine, aluminum hydroxide, and attapulgite (previously Kaopectate®) are examples of drugs that bind to and prevent the absorption of many drugs. Other drugs alter the rate of absorption by altering gastric motility (see Table 2-4; see also the discussion of pharmacokinetic interactions later in this chapter). To minimize these effects, none of these drugs should be given simultaneously with another orally administered drug.

Table 2-7 Examples of Sites of Drug–Drug Interactions

Interaction	Example Drugs
Binding to luminal contents	Tetracyclines (except doxycycline), fluorinated quinolones, antacids, sucralfate,
Absorption	
Gastric motility	Metoclopramide, anticholinergics, erythromycin
Gastric pH	Antisecretory drugs, antacids
Competition for transport proteins	See Table 2-2
Inhibition or induction of drug metabolizing enzymes	See Table 2-7
Increased splanchnic blood flow (nutrients)	
Distribution	
Competition for transport proteins in circulation	See Table 2-2
Competition for transport proteins in tissues	See Table 2-2
Altered regional blood flow	Fluid therapy, ACE inhibitors, other cardioactive drugs, phenothiazines,
Metabolism	
Competition for transport proteins	See Table 2-2
Induction of phase I enzymes (CYP 450)	See Table 2-8
Inhibition of phase I enzymes (CYP 450)	See Table 2-8
Increased phase II enzymes (glutathione)	See Table 2-8
Excretion	
Competition for transport proteins	See Box 2-8
Altered renal blood flow	Cardioactive drugs, NSAIDs, amphotericin B, aminoglycosides
Altered urinary pH	See Box 2-9

NSAIDs, Nonsteroidal antiinflammatory drugs.

Topical Preparations

Pharmaceutical interactions in topical preparations may occur between drugs or between drugs and the vehicle in which they are carried.[155,156] Both the rate and extent of drug absorption can be affected adversely. For example, macromolecular additives may bind chemically with the active drug. Methyl, ethyl, hydroxyethyl, and carboxymethyl cellulose frequently form complexes with drugs that can lead to drug precipitation. Vehicles are often selected because of their effect on drug absorption. For example, retardant vehicles (e.g., polyethylene glycol 300) interact with the drug, decreasing its absorption, whereas dimethyl sulfoxide (DMSO) is well recognized for its ability to enhance absorption of many topically applied drugs. The pluronic-lecithin vehicle of PLO gels (PLO) designed for transdermal drug delivery is thermoreversible, meaning they are semisolid at room temperature but become liquefied when refrigerated (see Figure 2-8).

The concentration of drug available for skin penetration depends on its dissolution in the vehicle. Drugs must generally dissolve in an aqueous layer of fluids that collects under the ointment base before percutaneous absorption can occur. Few drugs (and particularly water-soluble drugs) are sufficiently soluble to be dissolved in petrolatum bases; most drugs mixed in such bases are present as particles. Because few particles are located at the vehicle–skin interface, and dissolution is very slow for the particles, drugs in such preparations are likely to be ineffective. As such, lipid-soluble drugs tend to be better absorbed, particularly when prepared in lipid vehicles. Because only dissolved drug can move, the solubility of a drug in the vehicle is an important determinant of drug movement into the skin. However, a drug that has too great an affinity for the vehicle also may not be well absorbed simply because it will not leave the vehicle.[156]

Compounded Preparations

Many U.S. pharmacies now cater specifically to veterinarians and thus are prepared to address special problems in drug therapy through compounding. As important as compounding can be to the safe and effective administration of drugs to animals, compounded products present more risks of therapeutic failure than encountered with approved drugs.[157,158] Among the risks are the potential failure of the drug at the pharmaceutical phase because of interactions among the active or inactive ingredients. These risks are addressed in more depth in Chapter 4.

Pharmacokinetic Drug Interactions

Drug interactions that occur inside the body may lead to life-threatening adversities because of either therapeutic failure or increased side effects. Pharmacokinetic interactions occur when one drug alters the disposition of another drug.[159] Each stage of disposition of a drug—absorption, distribution, metabolism, or elimination—can be altered by another drug. The majority of drug interactions leading to serious adverse events in humans reflect pharmacokinetic interactions, involving either transport proteins or drug-metabolizing enzymes.[143]

Identifying the role of drug interactions in causing adverse effects is difficult; large numbers of patients generally must be studied to identify even common interactions. Predictions of drug–diet or drug–drug interactions might be facilitated by evaluation of chemistry, but caution is necessary.[154] Models that predict drug interactions are complicated by complex interactions (e.g., species, disease, and multiple drug interactions).[160] Identification of drug interactions involving dietary supplements is handicapped by the lack of a mandated surveillance mechanism; information in human medicine generally is obtained through reviews, case reports, or case series or based on open, uncontrolled studies.[161] Evidence-based information in veterinary medicine is even further limited. Several human-medicine reviews have described interactions between drugs and botanicals or herbs[161] and foods.[154] Mechanisms are often difficult to identify, in part because of broad substrate specificity. Some examples of drug–drug or drug–supplement interactions follow.

Absorption

Absorption of one drug may be hindered as a result of changes in the drug's passage through biological phases and changes in local pH; the integrity of biological membranes; regional blood flow; and, in the case of orally administered drugs, gastrointestinal motility. Each of these changes can be induced by a concurrently administered drug. Examples include the impact of an antisecretory drug on the ratio of un-ionized (diffusible) to ionized (nondiffusible) drugs. For weakly acidic drugs, a decrease in the ratio may decrease oral absorption; for weakly basic drugs, the opposite may occur. Sucralfate and cimetidine are examples of drugs that bind to and prevent the absorption of other drugs. Likewise, tetracycline and enrofloxacin are bound by divalent or trivalent cations that might be found in antacids (see Table 2-4). Finally, drugs that alter gastric motility might alter the rate of oral drug absorption. Most drugs are absorbed from the small intestine. Administration of anticholinergics decreases gastric emptying, allowing a longer time to elapse before a drug moves to the small intestine. Although extent of absorption may not be affected, peak PDCs may be lower. Metoclopramide probably has an opposite effect. In contrast to gastric motility, increasing motility of the small intestine is unlikely to alter the oral absorption of drugs because the surface area is so large that it is difficult to manipulate. However, a few drugs alter drug absorption by causing malabsorption or changing gastric blood flow (see Table 2-4). Phenytoin and phenobarbital have been associated with decreased oral absorption of vitamins.

KEY POINT 2-10 The role of drug induction and inhibition on drug transporter proteins such as P-glycoprotein is only now being delineated, but can be particularly profound for drug absorption and distribution.

Drug interactions that have an impact on absorption may also reflect altered metabolism and/or uptake in the enterocyte or liver. Drugs entering enterocytes are subject to metabolism by CYP3A, efflux mediated by P-gp, or passage into portal system and exposure to metabolic activities of the liver. Cytochrome P450 3A is the most predominant drug-metabolizing enzyme in the intestinal cell and mediates biotransformation of more than half of all drugs currently available (for humans).[162] Transporters such as the multidrug export pump P-gp, facilitate either drug absorption or efflux from the enterocyte, and drugs may act as substrates or inhibit or compete at these proteins (see Table 2-2). Both proteins (CYP 3A and P-gp) share drug substrates, and interplay between metabolic enzymes and transporters appears to confound the disposition of many orally administered drugs (Table 2-8; see also Table 2-2). Poor oral bioavailability may reflect a coordinated action of intestinal drug-metabolizing enzymes and efflux transporters. Experimentally, drug efflux by intestinal P-gp is known to prevent absorption and thus decrease the bioavailability of many CYP3A4 substrates. The interaction between P-gp and CYP3A4 at the apical intestinal membrane increases drug metabolism of those drugs that are absorbed.[163] In contrast, selected drug interactions also involve inhibition of the P-gp, resulting in increased oral bioavailability. Food–drug interactions most commonly occur in the gastrointestinal tract[154] and reflect therapeutic failure owing to reduced bioavailability of the drug. Less commonly, increased drug concentrations reflect altered appetite or gastrointestinal acidity. Those most commonly identified drug–diet (nutrient or supplement) interactions involve altered drug pharmacokinetics caused by interference with either P-gp or xenobiotic metabolizing enzymes (see the section on metabolism). Of the potential drug–nutrient interactions affecting absorption, competition among substrates for transport proteins have probably been the best described.[143,164] For example, flavenoids (found in grapefruits) are inhibitors of several P-gp substrates, which increases the risk of diet–diet or diet–drug interactions during both absorption and distribution.[164]

Distribution

Pharmacokinetic drug interactions that alter drug distribution from the central compartment to peripheral tissues usually result from competition for protein-binding sites between two or more concurrently administered drugs. Because protein binding is reversible, the drug with the highest affinity for protein (usually albumin) displaces the drug with less affinity (Box 2-8). If a highly (>80%) protein-bound drug is displaced by only a small fraction, the amount of unbound, pharmacologically active drug markedly increases, and the risk of toxicity is initially increased. Because NSAIDs are generally more than 90% protein bound, even slight displacement of the drug from its binding sites can initially result in concentrations that might increase the risk of adverse effects. Increased hepatic or renal clearance of the unbound drug tend to balance displacement of bound to unbound drug such that PDCs of free unbound drug only minimally increase (see Chapter 1).[165] However, according to its package insert, co-administration of cefovecin with other highly protein bound drugs increases the concentration of the latter. It is not clear whether increased clearance of unbound drug will be sufficient in the presence of hepatic (or renal) disease. Most drug interactions involving

Table 2-8 Members of Cytochrome P450 Superfamilies and Example Substrates, Inducers, and Inhibitors

Substrate	Inducer	Inhibitor
CYP1A2		
Acetaminophen	Insulin	Amiodarone
Amitriptyline	Omeprazole	Cimetidine
Clomipramine	Tobacco	Fluoroquinolones
Clozapine		Interferon
Imipramine		Ticlopidine
Naproxen		
Ondansetron		
Propranolol		
Theophylline		
Verapamine		
Warfarin		
Zileuton		
CYP2B6		
Cyclophosphamide	Phenobarbital	Ticlopidine
	Rifampin	
CYP2C19		
Cyclophosphamide	Carbamazepine	Cimetidine
Lansoprazole	Prednisone?	Felbamate
Omeprazole	Rifampin?	Fluoxetine
Diazepam		Indomethacin
Phenytoin		Ketoconazole
Phenobarbital		Lansoprazole
Amitriptyline		Omeprazole
Clomipramine		Paroxetine
Cyclophosphamide		Probenecid
Imipramine		Ticlopidine
Indomethacin		Topiramate
Primidone		
Progesterone		
Propranolol		
Warfarin		
CYP2C9		
NSAIDS	Rifampin	Amiodarone
Ibuprofen		Fluconazole
Diclofenac		Isoniazid
Meloxicam		Lovastatin
Naproxen		Paroxetine
Piroxicam		Phenylbutazone
Celecoxib		
Tolbutamine		Probenecid
Glipizide		Sulfamethoxazole
Losartan		Trimethoprim
Amitriptyline		Zafirlukast
Fluoxetine		
Phenytoin		
Warfarin		
CYP2D6		
Carvedilol	Dexamethasone	Amiodarone
Metaprolol	Rifampin	Celecoxib
Timolol		Chlorpromazine
Amitriptyline		Chlorpheniramine
Clomipramine		Cimetidine
Paroxetine		Clomipramine
Chlorpheniramine		Cocaine
Chlorpromazine		Doxorubicin
Codeine		Fluoxetine
Encainide		Metoclopramide
Fluoxetine		Proxetin
Flecaine		Quinidine
Lidocaine		Ranitidine
Metoclopramide		Terbinafine
Nortriptyline		
Ondansetron		
Propranolol		
Tramadol		
CYP2E1		
Enflurane	Ethanol	
Halothane	Isoniazid	
Isoflurane		
Methoxyflurane		
Sevoflurane		
Ethanol		
Theophylline		
CYP3A4,5,7		
Clarithromycin	Barbiturates	Amiodarone
Erythromycin	Carbamazepine	Cimetidine
(not azithromycin)	Glucocorticoids	Ciprofloxacin
Quinidine	Phenobarbital	Clarithromycin
Alprazolam	Phenytoin	Diltiazem
Diazepam	Rifampin	Erythromycin
Midazolam	St. John's wort	Fluconazole
Cyclosporine	Troglitazone	Itraconazole
Tacrilium	Pioglitazone	Ketoconazole
Cisapride		Norfloxacin
Chlorpheniramine		Verapamil
Amlodipine		
Diltiazem		
Felodipine		
Nifedipine		
Verapamil		
Lovastatin		
Hydrocortisone		
Progesterone		
Testosterone		

Continued

Table 2-8 Members of Cytochrome P450 Superfamilies and Example Substrates, Inducers, and Inhibitors—cont'd

Substrate	Inducer	Inhibitor	Substrate	Inducer	Inhibitor
Buspirone			Ondansetron		
Cocaine			Lidocaine		
Dapsone			Propranolol		
Codeine			Quinine		
Dextromethorphan			Terfenadine		
Finasteride			Vincristine		
Fentanyl					

NSAIDs, Nonsteroidal antiinflammatory drugs.

Box 2-8

Highly (>80%) Protein-Bound Drugs

Weak Acids (Albumin)
Nonsteroidal antiinflammatories
Coumarin derivatives
Antimicrobials
- Doxycycline
- Minocycline
- Cefovecin

Anticonvulsants
- Valproic acid
- Phenytoin
- Diazepam

Furosemide

Weak Bases (α Glycoproteins)
Several cardiac drugs
Propranolol
Lidocaine (some species)
Tricyclic antidepressants

protein binding reflect competition for albumin-binding sites because albumin is the most common binding protein, particularly for weak acids. Lipoproteins; globulins (increased with acute-phase protein increase); and, to a lesser extent, albumin bind weak bases (e.g., bupivacaine, lidocaine) (see Box 2-8).

Use of drugs that alter drug distribution to peripheral organs can alter drug delivery to the organs. For example, the use of afterload reducers may increase renal blood flow; renal clearance of drugs may also increase. Use of glucocorticoids before volume replacement in a hypovolemic patient may enhance peripheral vasoconstriction, reducing tissue distribution of other drugs. Rarely, drug interactions occur at the tissue site. For example, drugs can compete with each other at tissue-binding sites. Quinidine increases digoxin toxicity because it displaces digoxin from cardiac tissues; in contrast, hypokalemia facilitates binding of digoxin to cardiac tissue, thus enhancing digoxin cardiotoxicity.

Because P-gp is located on the cell membrane of many organs, this transporting protein can influence tissue distribution of drug. The most notable example is its presence in the blood–brain barrier, where it serves to efflux many drugs that are able to penetrate the barrier. Genetic deficiency of this protein has been associated with an increased risk of CNS toxicity in certain breeds its role in drug interactions should be anticipated (see Chapter 4 and later discussion). Drug–nutrient interactions resulting in competition for transport proteins may also affect distribution of drugs.[143,164]

Metabolism

Pharmacokinetic drug interactions frequently alter the metabolism of a concurrently administered drug (see Table 2-4).[166-170] When administering a drug metabolized by the liver, it is wise to anticipate a drug interaction if a second drug also metabolized by the liver is added to therapy. Most of the interactions result from modulation of hepatic (phase I) drug-metabolizing enzymes (see Table 2-8).

KEY POINT 2-11 Interactions at the level of drug-metabolizing enzymes are among the most dangerous, yet their predictability is complicated by the large number of enzymes, the lack of substrate specificities, and polymorphisms among animals.

Induction of drug-metabolizing enzymes should be considered as a protective mechanism that facilitates excretion of potentially toxic compounds. However, induction is a double-edged sword: although the elimination of a potentially toxic drug increases, so does potential formation of toxic or carcinogenic metabolites. Most CYP enzymes are inducible, with response to inducers varying within and among species, age, and gender. Human CYP known to be influenced by inducers include CYP 1A1/2, 2A6, 2C9, 2C19, 2E1, and 3A4 (see Table 2-8). Inducers generally act as substrates for the induced enzymes, and induction generally is dose dependent.[171] Inducers often induce more than one CYP and may significantly increase the activity of an enzyme that otherwise (constitutively) is either absent or present only in very low concentrations. Induction is accompanied by an increase in the transcription and thus intracellular concentration of the induced enzyme. Maximal induction of transcription generally requires 10 to 12 hours of exposure to a drug. Although transcription may return to baseline 18 to 24 hours (depending on dose) after the inducer is discontinued, the impact of the inducer may persist. The duration of the effect varies with the rate of enzyme degradation, which normally results in half-lives that range from 8 to 30 hours. Although not common, induction also may reflect a decrease in the rate of CYP degradation—that is, a prolongation of enzyme half-life.[172]

Barbiturates are recognized inducers of CYP; indeed, the observation that "tolerance" to hypnotics developed in dogs chronically exposed to barbiturates led to the recognition of the phenomenon of induction.[172] Phenobarbital is one of the most potent microsomal enzyme inducers known and can enhance the hepatotoxicity of other hepatotoxic drugs. Likewise, it increases the formation of and response to prodrugs and decreases the effects of itself and other drugs metabolized by the liver as clearance of these drugs is increased.[73,173,141] The CYP2B9 family, responsible for metabolism of a large number of drugs in rodents, is induced by phenobarbital. Therapeutic doses of phenobarbital have been associated with induction of CYPIA activity, as well as alpha-glycoproteins in dogs.[174] The clinical impact of this effect is demonstrated in epileptic dogs treated with phenobarbital: initial concentrations may decrease within several months of therapy despite no dose change. Interestingly, oral pentobarbital also increases the amount of CYP2C present in the intestinal tract of dogs when administered at doses consistent with that consumed by dogs fed commercial dog foods prepared from animals euthanized by pentobarbital (10 to 60 μg/gm). The impact on the metabolism of selected subtrates varies and is greatest for higher doses, but changes are also present at low doses, suggesting a potential clinical impact on therapeutic drugs.[171]

Drug interactions that reflect inhibition of drug-metabolizing enzymes may be at greater risk in causing serious adverse events. A number of inhibitors of CYP enzymes have been identified. As with inducers, the extent of inhibition is dose dependent,[172,175] with inhibitors often acting as substrates at the inhibited enzyme, and either characterized by broad enzyme interaction, being inhibitory for a number of different CYPs, or acting selectively for a single enzyme (see Table 2-8).[172] Currently, three types of drug-metabolizing enzyme inhibitors have been described: reversible, quasi-reversible, and irreversible, with reversible inhibitors being the most commonly involved in drug–drug interactions. Reversible inhibition is transient, resolving when therapy with the inhibitor is discontinued. Like induction, reversible inhibition appears to be dose dependent.[175] Reversible inhibition most commonly reflects interactions that are competitive or noncompetitive. Competitive inhibition is exemplified by a drug that blocks access to the catalytic site of the enzyme of another structurally similar drug. The drug may or may not be a substrate for the enzyme. Noncompetitive inhibition occurs when substrate binding occurs at a different site but nonetheless changes the catalytic activity of the enzyme such that it is inactivated.[172]

Generally, clearance of a concurrently administered drug metabolized by the liver is prolonged in the presence of inhibitors, increasing the potential for toxicity or for an exaggerated pharmacologic response. Additionally, prodrugs (e.g., enalapril, primidone) are less likely to be activated. Chloramphenicol, cimetidine, and imidazole antifungal drugs are examples of potent microsomal enzyme inhibitors.[73,173,141] Co-administration with potentially toxic drugs that are also metabolized by the liver should be done cautiously. Fluorinated quinolones such as enrofloxacin and marbofloxacin can increase theophylline plasma concentrations to toxic levels, presumably because of impaired hepatic clearance of theophylline.[176] Ketoconazole inhibits cytochrome P450 enzymes, including CYP3A4 in the dog.[177] However, it does not necessarily clinically affect all drugs metabolized by the liver. For example, morphine clearance was not changed in Greyhounds treated with an average of 12.7 mg/kg ketaconazole per day.[93] Although area under the curve was greater in the presence of morphine, the change was neither statistically nor clinically significant. This may reflect, however, the flow-limited nature of morphine clearance or, potentially, breed differences in drug metabolism. Other imidazoles (fluconazole and, to a lesser degree, itraconazole) also have broad enzyme inhibitory activity (see chapter 9).

Drug-induced inhibition of drug metabolism can be used for therapeutic benefit. Both cyclosporine and ketaconazole are substrates and inhibitors of both P-gp and CYP3A. As such, the combined use of the drugs may result in marked prolongation of the half-life of either drug. Ketoconazole has been used to increase blood drug concentrations of cyclosporine (owing to both inhibition of drug-metabolizing enzymes and competition with P-gp) in dogs.[178] A twofold increase in expected PDCs may occur, as indicated by a 50% dose reduction in Beagles[179] or a twofold increase in C_{max} in Greyhounds.[93] Indeed, the impact may be greater in some dogs: our laboratory has documented an elimination half-life of over 150 hours in dogs simultaneously receiving ketoconazole, yielding concentrations that exceed 4500 ng/mL. In cats, cyclosporine (4 mg/kg orally) concentrations can be expected to increase approximately twofold when administered with ketoconazole (10 mg/kg).[180] The macrolides also have broad inhibitory effects. The inhibitory effect of erythromycin may reflect inhibition of CYP3A macrolides, which appear to inhibit cyclosporine clearance. Again, in our laboratory azithromycin co-administration was associated with marked prolongation of cyclosporine half-life in a cat, leading to cyclosporine concentrations that exceeded 4500 ng/mL (therapeutic range 800-1400 ng/mL). The effect of cimetidine, another drug-metabolizing inhibitor with broad substrate specificity, is variable, ranging from no significant effect in Beagles (n=10; 15 mg/kg cimetidine every 8 hours for 8 days and 5 mg/kg once daily for cyclosporine) to 50% decrease in clearance in humans.[181] Cimetidine-induced enzyme inhibition, however, has been used to prevent metabolism of acetaminophen in humans and cats into potentially lethal toxic metabolites.[182,183] Cilastatin inhibits renal tubular drug metabolism of imipenem; the net effect may prolong the half-life of imipenem, but hepatotoxicity or renal toxicity resulting from metabolites might also be reduced (see Chapter 4). Nutrition, sex, age, and other factors can influence the way drug-metabolizing enzymes respond to drugs. Alcohol and 4-methylpyrazole competitively inhibit alcohol dehydrogenase, the drug-metabolizing enzyme that converts ethylene glycol to its lethal metabolite.

Although less common, drug clearance may also be affected by drugs that change hepatic blood flow, solely due to substrate delivery, not a limitation on metabolic rate. This interaction is significant, however, only for drugs that are characterized by extensive and rapid hepatic clearance (e.g., propanol, lidocaine) and probably is not clinically relevant.

Among the most commonly identified drug–diet (nutrient or supplement) interactions that alter drug pharmacokinetics are those reflecting drug metabolism, particularly CYP3A4.[154] Several dietary supplements are known to interact with drugs.[161] These include, but are not limited to, St. John's wort (induction of CYP3A4, particularly intestinal), echinacea (induction and inhibition of intestinal CYP), ginkgo biloba (induction of CYP219A), and grapefruit (inhibition of CYP3A4 and inhibition of P-gp).

Excretion

Pharmacokinetic drug interactions may alter urinary excretion because of changes in glomerular filtration, competition between the drug for active tubular secretion, or both (Box 2-9). Competition for carrier proteins responsible for active tubular secretion usually involves acidic drugs. Probenecid is still occasionally used to prolong the elimination of an expensive penicillin because it competes with the penicillin for a carrier protein. Renal excretion may also be affected by drugs that alter urinary pH and tubular reabsorption. Changes in urinary pH conducive to formation of a greater proportion of un-ionized drug (e.g., an acidic urinary pH and an acidic drug) encourage tubular reabsorption of a drug, thus decreasing its clearance and prolonging its elimination half-life (Box 2-10).[73,173,141] For example, overdosing of some drugs (e.g., aminoglycoside or strychnine poisoning) can be treated by hastening elimination with urinary acidifiers.

Box 2-9

Examples of Drugs That Compete for Renal Tubular Secretion

Anions (Acidic Drugs)
Penicillins
Cephalosporins
Probenecid
Sulfonamides
Aspirin
Furosemide
Nonsteroidal anti-inflammatories
Phase II metabolites (gluconic acids, glycine, and sulfate conjugates)

Cations (Basic Drugs)
Procainamide
Dopamine
Trimethoprim
Several opioid agents

Pharmacodynamic Drug Interactions

Pharmacodynamic drug interactions occur when one drug alters the chemical or physiologic response to another drug (see Table 2-6). Pharmacodynamic interactions may increase response to a drug in an additive or synergistic fashion at the same receptor (e.g., the permissive effect of glucocorticoids on alpha-adrenergic receptors; phenobarbital and clorazepate at gamma-aminobutyric receptors), at an intracellular site (e.g., epinephrine and theophylline in bronchial smooth muscle), or at different sites but with the same physiologic reaction (e.g., hypokalemia induced by cardiac glycosides and diuretics; many interactions of antimicrobials). Pharmacodynamic interactions may also decrease the response of some drugs owing to competitive antagonism at the same receptor site (e.g., atropine and anticholinesterases or atropine and metoclopramide) or antagonistic responses mediated at distant but physiologically related sites. Antagonistic pharmacodynamic interactions have been used therapeutically: oxymorphone or other mu agonistic effects are reversed with naloxone, xylazine and other chemical sedatives are reversed with tolazoline or yohimbine, and medatomidine is reversed with antipamazole.

KEY POINT 2-12 Pharmacodynamic interactions can be either detrimental or beneficial.

The most familiar pharmacodynamic interactions are probably those that act in an additive or synergistic manner to augment response to a drug. Augmentation can occur through different mechanisms of action (i.e., controlling vomiting by combining a drug active at the chemoreceptor triggering zone with a drug that acts peripherally, controlling seizures by combining phenobarbital with bromide, controlling tachycardia by combining diltiazem with digoxin or atenolol). Less commonly, augmentation may occur through similar actions at a receptor site; more often, drugs will compete with one another at the same receptor, thus resulting in antagonism. Unfortunately, often forgotten is the fact that augmentation of the desired pharmacologic response may be accompanied by augmentation of an undesirable adverse drug event (ADE). For

Box 2-10

Examples of Drugs Capable of Changing Urine pH

Urinary Acidifiers
Ascorbic acid
Methionine
Sodium acid phosphate
Ammonium chloride

Urinary Alkalinizers
Sodium bicarbonate, citrate, and acetate
Carbonic anhydrase inhibitors

example, drugs that impair renal prostaglandin synthesis (e.g., NSAIDs, angiotensin-converting enzyme inhibitors, aminoglycosides) should be used in combination cautiously because their combination increases the risk of renal failure. Likewise, ulcerogenic drugs (NSAIDs, glucocorticoids) enhance the risk of gastrointestinal ulceration when used in combination.

Pharmacodynamic interactions may decrease the response to a drug because of competitive antagonism at the same receptor site. Most commonly, these actions are desirable and are frequently the target of combined drug therapy: atropine to treat organophosphate toxicity, reversal agents for opioids and anesthetic agents. Antagonistic pharmacodynamic responses can also occur through different receptor sites or different mechanisms. The combination of a bacteriostatic antimicrobial (one that slows the growth of an organism) with a bactericidal antimicrobial (one whose efficacy depends on rapid growth) might be considered as an example. Also, the prokinetic effects of cisapride and metoclopramide are prevented by anticholinergics; calcium-containing solutions should not be combined with blood or blood components because the loss of anticoagulant effects increases the risk of microthrombi formation in the transfused blood.

Hu[161] has reviewed pharmacodynamic interactions between drugs and herbs or botanicals. These can be clinically significant, as is exemplified for selected organosulfur components of garlic, which act as anticoagulants. Increased bleeding times have been documented in patients taking garlic supplements and subsequently treated with warfarin compared with increases with warfarin alone.

REFERENCES

1. Massoud N: Pharmacokinetic considerations in geriatric patients. In Benet LZ, Massoud N, Gambertoglio JG, editors: *Pharmacokinetic basis for drug treatment*, New York, 1984, Raven Press, pp 269–282.
2. Ritschel WA: *Gerontokinetics: the pharmacokinetics of drugs in the elderly*, Caldwell, NJ, 1988, Telford Press, pp 1-16.
3. Feely J, Coakley D: Altered pharmacodynamics in the elderly, *Clin Pharm* 6:269–283, 1990.
4. Dowling P: Geriatric pharmacology, *Vet Clin North Am Small Anim Pract* 35(3):557–569, 2005.
5. National Research Council: *Nutrient requirements of dogs and cats*, Washington, DC, 2006, National Academies Press.
6. Benowitz NL: Effects of cardiac disease on pharmacokinetics: pathophysiologic considerations. In Benet LZ, Massoud N, Gambertoglio JG, editors: *Pharmacokinetic basis for drug treatment*, New York, 1984, Raven Press, pp 89–104.
7. Aucoin DP: Drug therapy in the geriatric animal: the effect of aging on drug disposition, *Vet Clin North Am Small Anim Pract* 19:41–48, 1989.
8. Morita TY, Sawada MM, A., Shimada A: Immunohistochemical and ultrastructural findings related to the blood–brain barrier in the blood vessels of the cerebral white matter in aged dogs, *J Comp Path* 133:14–22, 2005.
9. Perez-Camargo G: Cat nutrition: what is new in the old?, *Compend Cont Educ Pract Vet* 26(2A):5–14, 2004.
10. Benno Y, Nakao H, Uchida K, et al: Impact of the advances in age on the gastrointestinal microflora of beagle dogs, *J Vet Med Sci* 54:703–706, 1992.
11. Patil AR, Czarnecki-Maulden GL, Dowling KE: Effect of advances in age on fecal microflora of cats, *FASEB J* 14(4):A488, 2000.
12. Hickman MA, Bruss ML, Morris JG, et al: Dietary-protein source (soybean vs casein) and taurine status affect kinetics of the enterohepatic circulation of taurocholic acid in cats, *J Nutr* 122:1019–1028, 1992.
13. Sheaker S, Bay M: Drug disposition and hepatotoxicity in the elderly, *J Clin Gastroenterol* 18:232–237, 1994.
14. Enck RE: Pain control in the ambulatory elderly, *Geriatrics* 46:49–60, 1991.
15. Workaman BS, Ciccone V, Christophidis N: Pain management for the elderly, *Aust Fam Phys* 18:1515–1527, 1989.
16. Lawler DE, Evans RH, Larson BT, et al: Influence of lifetime food restriction on causes, time, and predictors of death in dogs, *J Am Vet Med Assoc* 226:225–231, 2005.
17. Speakman JR, van Acker A, Harper EJ: Age-related changes in the metabolism and body composition of three dog breeds and their relationship to life expectancy, *Aging Cell* 2:265–275, 2003.
18. Schultz RD: The effects of aging on the immune system, *Compend Contin Educ Pract Vet* 6(12):1096–1105, 1984.
19. Robinson EP: Anesthesia of pediatric patients, *Compend Contin Educ Pract Vet* 5(12):1004–1011, 1983.
20. Green TP, Mirkin BL: Clinical pharmacokinetics: pediatric considerations. In Benet LZ, Massoud N, Gambertoglio JG, editors: *Pharmacokinetic basis for drug treatment*, New York, 1984, Raven Press, pp 269–282.
21. Boothe DM, Tannert K: Special considerations for drug and fluid therapy in the pediatric patient, *Compend Contin Educ Pract Vet* 14:313–329, 1991.
22. Harper EJ, Turner CL: Age-related changes in apparent digestibility in growing kittens, *Reprod Nutr Dev* 40:249–260, 2000.
23. Heimann G: Enteral absorption and bioavailability in children in relation to age, *Eur J Clin Pharmacol* 18:43–50, 1980.
24. Rane A, Wilson JT: Clinical pharmacokinetics in infants and children. In Gibaldi M, Prescott L, editors: *Handbook of clinical pharmacokinetics*, New York, 1983, ADIS Health Science Press, pp 142–168.
25. Gillette DD, Filkins M: Factors affecting antibody transfer in the newborn puppy, *Am J Physiol* 210(2):419–422, 1966.
26. Morselli PL, Morselli RF, Bossi L: Clinical pharmacokinetics in newborns and infants: age-related differences and therapeutic implications. In Gibaldi M, Prescott L, editors: *Handbook of clinical pharmacokinetics*, New York, 1983, ADIS Health Science Press, pp 99–141.
27. Jones RL: Special considerations for appropriate antimicrobial therapy in neonates, *Vet Clin North Am Small Anim Pract* 17(3):577–601, 1987.
28. Shifrine M, Munn SL, Rosenblatt LS, et al: Hematologic changes to 60 days of age in clinically normal beagles, *Lab Anim* 23(6):894–898, 1973.
29. Authement JM, Wolfsheimer KJ, Catchings S, et al: Canine blood component therapy: product preparation, storage, and administration, *J Am Anim Hosp Assoc* 23:483–493, 1987.
30. Fiser DH: Intraosseous infusion, *N Engl J Med* 322(22): 1579–1581, 1990.
31. Hodge D: Intraosseous flow rates in hypovolemic "pediatric" dogs, *Ann Emerg Med* 16:305–307, 1987.
32. Sheng H-P, Huggins RA: Growth of the beagle: changes in the body fluid compartments, *Proc Soc Exp Biol Med* 139:330–335, 1972.
33. Davis LE, Westfall BA, Short CR: Biotransformation and pharmacokinetics of salicylate in newborn animals, *Am J Vet Res* 34(8):1105–1108, 1973.
34. Baggott JD: Principles of antimicrobial bioavailability and disposition. In Prescott JF, Baggot JD, Walker RD, editors: *Antimicrobial therapy in veterinary medicine*, ed 3, Ames, Iowa, 2000, Blackwell Publishing, pp 50–87.
35. Goldstein R, Lavy E, Shem-Tov M, et al: Pharmacokinetics of ampicillin administered intravenously and intraosseously to kittens, *Res Vet Sci* 59:186–187, 1995.

36. Lavy E, Goldstein R, Shem-Tov M, et al: Disposition kinetics of ampicillin administered intravenously and intraosseously to canine puppies, *J Vet Pharmacol Ther* 18:379–381, 1995.
37. Seguin MA, Papich MG, Sigle K: Pharmacokinetics of enrofloxacin in neonatal kittens, *Am J Vet Res* 65:350–356, 2004.
38. Poffenbarger EM, Ralston SL, Chandler ML, et al: Canine neonatology, Part I. Physiological differences between puppies and adults, *Compend Contin Educ Pract Vet* 12(11):1601–1609, 1990.
39. Ehrnebo M, Agurell S, Jalling B, et al: Age differences in drug binding by plasma proteins: studies on human fetuses, neonates and adults, *Eur J Clin Pharmacol* 3:189–193, 1973.
40. Horster M, Kemler BJ, Valtin H: Intracortical distribution of number and volume of glomeruli during postnatal maturation in the dog, *J Clin Invest* 50:796–800, 1971.
41. Horster M, Valtin H: Postnatal development of renal function: micropuncture and clearance studies in the dog, *J Clin Invest* 50:779–795, 1971.
42. Hellmann J, Vannucci RC, Nardis EE: Blood-brain barrier permeability to lactic acid in the newborn dog: lactate as a cerebral metabolic fuel, *Pediatr Res* 16:40–44, 1982.
43. Ginsberg G, Hattis D, Russ A, et al: Pharmacokinetic and pharmacodynamic factors that can affect sensitivity to neurotoxic sequelae in elderly individuals, *Environ Health Perspect* 113:1243–1249, 2005.
44. Hurria A, Lichtman SM: Clinical pharmacology of cancer therapies in older adults, *Br J Cancer* 98:517–522, 2008.
45. Reiche R: Drug disposition in the newborn. In Ruckesbusch P, Toutain P, Koritz D, editors: *Veterinary pharmacology and toxicology*, Westport, Conn, 1983, AVI Publishing, pp 49–55.
46. Peters EL, Farber TM, Heider A, et al: The development of drug-metabolizing enzymes in the young dog, *Fed Proc Am Soc Biol* 30:560, 1971.
47. Inman RC, Yeary RA: Sulfadimethoxine pharmacokinetics in neonatal and young dogs, *Fed Proc Am Soc Biol* 30:560, 1971.
48. Ecobichon DJ, D'Ver AS, Ehrhart W: Drug disposition and biotransformation in the developing beagle dog, *Fundam Appl Toxicol* 11:29–37, 1988.
49. Cowan RH, Jukkola AF, Arant BS: Pathophysiologic evidence of gentamicin nephrotoxicity in neonatal puppies, *Pediatr Res* 14:1204–1211, 1980.
50. Kleinman LI: Renal bicarbonate reabsorption in the newborn dog, *J Physiol* 281:487–498, 1978.
51. Bovee KC, Jezyk PF, Segal SC: Postnatal development of renal tubular amino acid reabsorption in canine pups, *Am J Vet Res* 45(4):830–832, 1984.
52. Kerner JA, Sunshine P: Parenteral alimentation, *Semin Perinatol* 3(4):417–434, 1979.
53. Otto CM, Kaufman GM, Crowe DT: Intraosseous infusion of fluids and therapeutics, *Compend Contin Educ Pract Vet* 11(4):421–431, 1989.
54. Hirschhorn N: Oral rehydration therapy for diarrhea in children: a basic primer, *Nutr Rev* 40(4):97–104, 1982.
55. Nahata MC: Sedation in pediatric patients undergoing diagnostic procedures, *Drug Intell Clin Pharm* 22(Sept):711–715, 1988.
56. Levy G: Pharmacokinetics of fetal and neonatal exposure to drugs, *Obstet Gynecol* 58(Suppl):9S–16S, 1981.
57. Welsch F: Placental transfer and fetal uptake of drugs, *J Vet Pharmacol Ther* 5:91–104, 1982.
58. Krauer B, Krauer F: Drug kinetics in pregnancy. In Gibaldi M, Prescott L, editors: *Handbook of clinical pharmacokinetics*, New York, 1991, ADIS Health Science Press, pp 1–17.
59. Carter AM: Animal models of human placentation, *Plactenta* 28(SA):S41–S47, 2007.
60. Renfree MB: Implantation and placentation. In Austin CR, Short RV, editors: *Reproduction in mammals 2. Embryonic and fetal development*, ed 2, Cambridge, 1982, Cambridge University Press, pp 26–69.
61. Syme MR, Paxton JW, Keelan JA: Drug transfer and metabolism by the human placenta, *Clin Pharmacokinet* 43(8): 487–514, 2004.
62. Farrar HC, Blumer JL: Fetal effects of maternal drug exposure, *Annu Rev Pharmacol Toxicol* 31:525–547, 1991.
63. Autio K, Rassnick KM, Bedford-Guaus SJ: Chemotherapy during pregnancy: a review of the literature, *Vet Comp Oncol* 5: 61–75, 2007.
64. Nau H: Clinical pharmacokinetics in pregnancy and perinatology. II. Penicillins, *Dev Pharmacol Ther* 10(3):174–198, 1987.
65. Papich MG, Davis LE: Drug therapy during pregnancy and in the neonate, *Vet Clin North Am Small Anim Pract* 16(3): 525–538, 1986.
66. Berlin CM: Pharmacologic considerations of drug use in the lactating mother, *Obstet Gynecol* 58(5):17S–23S, 1981.
67. Rasmussen F: Excretion of drugs by milk. In Brodie BB, Gilette JR, editors: *Handbook of experimental pharmacology, vol 28, Concepts in biochemical pharmacology, part I*, New York, 1979, Springer-Verlag, p 390.
68. Smith HW: The development of the flora of the alimentary tract in young animals, *J Pathol Bacteriol* 90:495–513, 1965.
69. Tanaka T: Gender-related differences in pharmacokinetics and their clinical significance, *J Clin Pharm Ther* 24:339–346, 1999.
70. Gandhi M, Aweeka F, Greenblatt RM, et al: Sex differences in pharmacokinetics and pharmacodynamics, *Annu Rev Pharmacol Toxicol* 44:499–523, 2004.
71. Shah SS, Sanda S, Regmi NL, et al: Characterization of cytochorme P450-mediated drug metabolism in cats, *J Vet Pharmacol Ther* 30:422–428, 2007.
72. Riviere JE: *Comparative pharmacokinetics: principles, techniques and applications*, Ames, Iowa, 2003, Blackwell Publishing.
73. Vessey DA: Hepatic metabolism of drugs and toxins. In Zakim D, Boyer T, editors: *A textbook of liver disease*, Philadelphia, 1982, Saunders, pp 197–230.
74. Jolivette LJ, Ward KW: Extrapolation of human pharmacokinetic parameters from rat, dog, and monkey data: molecular properties associated with extrapolative success or failure, *J Pharm Sci* 94:1467–1483, 2005.
75. Akimoto M, Nagahata N, Furuya A, et al: Gastric pH profiles of beagle dogs and their use as an alternative to human testing, *Eur J Pharm Biopharm* 49:99–102, 2000.
76. Xia CQ, Xiao G, Liu N, et al: Comparison of species differences of P-gps in beagle dog, rhesus monkey, and human using AtPase activity assays, *Mol Pharm* 3:78–86, 2005.
77. He Y-L, Murby S, Warhurst G, et al: Species differences in size discrimination in the paracellular pathway reflected by oral bioavailability of poly(ethylene glycol) and D-peptides, *J Pharm Sci* 87:626–633, 1998.
78. Chiou WL, Jeong HY, Chung SM, et al: Evaluation of using dog as an animal model to study the fraction of oral dose absorbed of 43 drugs in humans, *Pharm Res* 17(2):135–140, 2000.
79. Abadia AR, Aramayona JJ, Munoz MJ: Ciprofloxacin pharmacokinetics in dogs following oral administration, *J Vet Med Assoc* 42:505–511, 1995.
80. Albarellos GA, Kreil VE, Landoni MF: Pharmacokinetics of ciprofloxacin after single intravenous and repeat oral administration to cats, *J Vet Pharmacol Ther* 27:155–162, 2004.
81. Dye JA, McKiernan BC, Neft Davis CA, et al: Chronopharmacokinetics of theophylline in cats, *J Vet Pharmacol Ther* 12: 133–140, 1989.
82. Dye JA, McKiernan BC, Jones SD: Sustained-release theophylline pharmacokinetics in cats, *J Vet Pharmacol Ther* 13:278–286, 1990.
83. Riviere JE, Martin-Jimenez T, Sundlof SF, et al: Interspecies allometric analysis of the comparative pharmacokinetics of 44 drugs across veterinary and laboratory animal species, *J Vet Pharmacol Therap* 20:453–463, 1997.

84. Mealey KL, Bentjen SA, Waiting DK: Frequency of the mutant MDR1 allele associated with ivermectin sensitivity in a sample population of collies from the northwestern United States, *Am J Vet Res* 63:479–481, 2002.
85. Hugnet C, Bentjen SA, Mealey KL: Frequency of the mutant MDR1 allele associated with multidrug sensitivity in a sample of collies from France, *J Vet Pharmacol Ther* 27:227–229, 2004.
86. Martinez M, Modric S, Sharkey M, et al: The pharmacogenomics of P-glycoprotein and its role in veterinary medicine, *J Vet Pharmacol Ther* 31(4):285–300, 2008.
87. Ingelman-Sundberg M: Polymorphism of cytochrome P450 and xenobiotic toxicity, *Toxicology* 181-182:447–452, 2002.
88. Guengerich FP: Comparisons of catalytic selectivity of cytochrome P450 subfamily enzymes from different species, *Chem Biol Interact* 106:161–182, 1997.
89. Bogaards JJP, Bertrandoe M, Jacksonoe P, et al: Determining the best animal model for human cytochrome P450 activities: a comparison of mouse, rat, rabbit, dog, micropig, monkey and man, *Xenobiotica* 30:1131–1152, 2000.
90. Chauret N, Gatuhter A, Martin J, et al: In vitro comparison of cytochrome p450 mediated metabolic activities in human, dog, cat and horse, *Drug Metab Dispos* 25:1120–1126, 1997.
91. Landoli M, Soraci AL, Delatour P, et al: Enantioselective behavior of drugs used in domestic animals: a review, *J Vet Pharmacol Ther* 20:1–16, 1997.
92. Court MH, Hay-Kraus BL, Hill DW, et al: Propofol hydroxylation by dog live microsomes: assay development and dog breed differences, *Drug Metab Dispos* 27(11):1293–1299, 1999.
93. Kukanich B, Borum SL: Effects of ketoconazole on the pharmacokinetics and pharmacodynamics of morphine in healthy greyhounds, *Am J Vet Res* 69:664–669, 2008.
94. Blaisdell J, Goldstein JA, Bai SA: Isolation of a new canine cytochrome P450 CDNA from the cytochrome P4502C subfamily (CYP2C41) and evidence for polymorphic differences in its expression, *Drug Metab Dispos* 26:278–283, 1998.
95. Mealey K: Pharmacogenetics, *Vet Clin North Am Small Anim Pract Pharm* 36:961–973, 2006.
96. Paulson SK, Engel L, Reitz B, et al: Evidence for polymorphism in the canine metabolism of the cyclooxygenase 2 inhibitor, celecoxib, *Drug Metab Dispos* 27:1133–1142, 1999.
97. Lees P, Landoni MF, Giraudel J, et al: Pharmacodynamics and pharmacokinetics of nonsteroidal anti-inflammatory drugs in species of veterinary interest, *J Vet Pharmacol Ther* 27:479–490, 2004.
98. Castro E, Soraci A, Fogel F, et al: Chiral inversion of R(-) fenoprofen and ketoprofen enantiomers in cats, *J Vet Pharmacol Ther* 23:265–271, 2000.
99. Kidd LB, Salavaggione OE, Szumlanski CL, et al: Thiopurine methyltransferase activity in red blood cells of dogs, *J Vet Intern Med* 18(2):214–218, 2004.
100. Watson ADJ: Chloramphenicol toxicosis in cats, *Am J Vet Res* 89:1199–1203, 1978.
101. Welch RM, Conney AH, Burns JJ: The metabolism of acetophenetidin and N-acetyl-p-aminophenol in the cat, *Biochem Pharmacol* 15:521–532, 1966.
102. Baggott JD: *Principles of drug disposition in domestic animals: the basis of veterinary clinical pharmacology*, Philadelphia, 1977, Saunders, pp 73-112.
103. Elston TH, Rosen O, Rodar I et al: Seven cases of acute diazepam toxicity, *Proc Am Anim Hosp Assoc* Oct: 343–349, 1993.
104. Tanaka N, Shinkyo R, Sakaki T, et al: Cytochrome P450 2E polymorphism in feline liver, *Biochim Biophys Acta: General Subjects* 1726:194–205, 2005.
105. Trepanier LA: Cytochrome P450 and its role in veterinary drug interactions, *Vet Clin North Am Small Anim Pract* 36:975–985, 2006.
106. Shecter RD, Schalm CW, Kanek JJ: Heinz-body hemolytic anemia associated with the use of urinary antiseptics in the cat, *J Am Vet Med Assoc* 162:37–44, 1983.
107. Cullison RF: Acetaminophen toxicosis in small animals: clinical signs, mode of action and treatment, *Compend Contin Educ Pract Vet* 6:315–323, 1984.
108. Savides MC, Oehme FW, Leipold HW: Effect of various antidotal treatments on acetaminophen toxicosis and biotransformation in cats, *Am J Vet Res* 46:1485–1489, 1985.
109. Wilkie DA, Kirby R: Methemoglobinemia associated with dermal application of benzocaine cream in a cat, *J Am Vet Med Assoc* 192:85–86, 1988.
110. Peterson ME, Horvitz AI, Leib MS: Propylthiouracil-associated hemolytic anemia, thrombocytopenia and antinuclear antibodies in cats with hyperthyroidism, *J Am Vet Med Assoc* 184: 806–808, 1984.
111. Stolk JM, Smith RP: Species differences in methemoglobin reductase activity, *Biochem Pharmacol* 15:343–351, 1966.
112. Boothe DM: Drug therapy in cats. Mechanisms and avoidance of adverse drug reactions, *J Vet Med Assoc* 196:1297–1306, 1990.
113. Harvey JW, Kaneko JJ: Oxidation of human and animal hemoglobins with ascorbate, acetylphenylhydrazine, nitrite, and hydrogen peroxide, *Br J Haematol* 32:193–203, 1976.
114. *Physician's desk reference*, ed 64, New York, 2010, Thomas Reuters.
115. FCC Freedom of Information Act (FOIA). Accessed October 14, 2009: http://www.fcc.gov/foia/.
116. Marier JF, Beaudry F, Ducharme MP: A pharmacokinetic study of amoxycillin in febrile beagle dogs following repeated administrations of endotoxin, *J Vet Pharmacol Ther* 24:379–383, 2001.
117. Brater DC, Chennavasin P: Effects of renal disease. Altered pharmacokinetics. In Benetz LZ, Massoud N, Gambertoglio JG, editors: *Pharmacokinetic basis for drug treatment*, New York, 1985, Raven Press, pp 149–172.
118. Stern A: Drug metabolism in renal failure, *Compend Cont Educ Pract Vet* 5:913–919, 1983.
119. Riviere JE: Calculation of dosage regimens of antimicrobial drugs in animals with renal and hepatic dysfunction, *J Am Vet Med Assoc* 185(10):1094–1097, 1984.
120. Carlson GP, Kaneko JJ: Sulfanilate clearance in clinical renal disease in the dog, *J Am Vet Med Assoc* 158(7):1235–1239, 1971.
121. Lefebvre HP, Schneider M, Dupouy M: Effect of experimental renal impairment on disposition of marbofloxacin and its metabolites in the dog, *J Vet Pharmacol Ther* 1:453–461, 1998.
122. Wilkinson GR, Shand DG: A physiological approach to hepatic drug clearance, *Clin Pharmacol Ther* 18:377–390, 1975.
123. Wilkinson GR, Branch RA: Effects of hepatic disease on clinical pharmacokinetics. In Benet LZ, Massoud N, Gambertoglio JG, editors: *Pharmacokinetic basis for drug treatment*, New York, 1984, Raven Press, pp 49–70.
124. Ahmad AB, Bennet PN, Rowland M: Models of hepatic drug clearance: discrimination between the "well stirred" and "parallel-tube" models, *J Pharm Pharmacol* 35:219–224, 1983.
125. Boothe DM: Effects of hepatic disease on drug disposition. In Bonagura J, editor: *Current veterinary therapy (XII), small animal practice*, Philadelphia, 1995, Saunders, pp 758–763.
126. Williams RL: Drugs and the liver: clinical applications. In Benet LZ, Massoud N, Gambertoglio JG, editors: *Pharmacokinetic basis for drug treatment*, New York, 1984, Raven Press, pp 53–75.
127. Blaschke TF, Rubin PC: Hepatic first-pass metabolism in liver disease. In Gibaldi M, Prescott L, editors: *Handbook of clinical pharmacokinetics*, New York, 1989, ADIS Health Science Press, pp 140–149.
128. Blaschke TF: Protein binding and kinetics of drugs in liver diseases. In Gibaldi M, Prescott L, editors: *Handbook of clinical pharmacokinetics*, New York, 1989, ADIS Health Science Press, pp 126–139.
129. Boothe DM, Brown SA, Jenkins WL, et al: Disposition of indocyanine green in dogs with experimentally induced dimethylnitrosamine hepatotoxicity, *Am J Vet Res* 53:382–388, 1992.

130. Boothe DM, Jenkins WL, Brown SA, et al: Antipyrine and caffeine disposition kinetics in dogs with progressive dimethylnitrosamine-induced hepatotoxicity, *Am J Vet Res* 55:254–261, 1994.
131. Morgan DJ, Smallwood RA: Hepatic drug clearance in chronic liver disease: can we expect to find a universal, quantitative marker of hepatic function?, *Hepatology* 10:893–895, 1989.
132. Poulsen HE, Loft S: Antipyrine as a model drug to study hepatic drug-metabolizing capacity, *J Hepatol* 6(3):374–382, 1988.
133. Van Thiel DH, Hassanein T: Assessment of liver function: the current situation, *J Okla State Med Assoc* 88:11–16, 1995.
134. Rollins DE: Pharmacokinetics and drug excretion in bile. In Benet LZ, Massoud N, Gambertoglio JG, editors: *Pharmacokinetic basis for drug treatment*, New York, 1984, Raven Press, pp 249–268.
135. Kawata S, Imai Y, Inada M, et al: Selective reduction of hepatic cytochrome P450 content in patients with intrahepatic cholestasis, *Gastroenterology* 92:299–303, 1987.
136. Evans GH, Nics AS, Shand DG: The disposition of propranolol. III. Decreased half-life and volume of distribution as a result of plasma binding in man, monkey, dog and rat, *J Pharmacol Exp Ther* 186:114–122, 1973.
137. Belpaire FM, DeRick A, Dello C, et al: Alpha 1-acid glycoprotein and serum binding of drugs in healthy and diseased dogs, *J Vet Pharmacol Ther* 10(1):43–48, 1987.
138. Eichelbaum M: Drug metabolism in thyroid disease, *Clin Pharmacokinet* 1(5):339–350, 1976.
139. Jacobs G, Whittem T, Sams R, et al: Pharmacokinetics of propranolol in healthy cats during euthyroid and hyperthyroid states, *Am J Vet Res* 58(4):398–403, 1997.
140. Nimmo WS: Drugs, diseases and altered gastric emptying, *Clin Pharmacokinet* 1(3):189–203, 1976.
141. Griffin JP, D'Arcy PF: *A manual of adverse drug interactions*, ed 2, Chicago, 1979, Billing & Sons, 3–51.
142. Larson K, Gay JM, Sellon RK et al: Potential occurrence of drug interactions in small animal intensive care unit (ICU) patients, *Proceedings of the American College of Veterinary Internal Medicine*, no. 117, 2003.
143. Huang S-M, Lesko LJ: Drug-drug, drug-dietary supplement, and drug-citrus fruit and other food interactions: what have we learned?, *J Clin Pharmacol* 44:559–569, 2004.
144. Ansel HC: Ointment, creams, lotions and other dermatological preparations. In Howard C, editor: *Introduction to pharmaceutical dosage forms*, ed 2, Philadelphia, 1976, Lea & Febiger, pp 301–332.
145. Papich MG: Incompatible critical care drug combinations. In Bonagura JD, editor: *Current veterinary therapy XII, small animal practice*, Philadelphia, 1995, Saunders, pp 194–199.
146. University of the Sciences: *Remington: the science and practice of pharmacy*, ed 21, Philadelphia, 2005, Lippincott Williams & Wilkins.
147. Trissel LA: *Stability of compounded formulations*, Washington DC, 1996, American Pharmaceutical Association.
148. Trissel LA: *Handbook on injectable drugs*, ed 8, Bethesda, Md, 2000, American Society of Hospital Pharmacists.
149. *King's Guide to Parenteral Admixtures*, Napa, Calif, 1998, King Guide Publications.
150. American Society of Hospital Pharmacists: *Committee on extemporaneous formulations, Handbook on extemporaneous formulations*, Bethesda, Md, 1997, The Society, pp 1–54.
151. Toothaker RD, Welling PG: The effect of food on drug bioavailability, *Annu Rev Pharmacol Toxicol* 20:173–199, 1980.
152. Watson AD, Emslie DR, Martin IC, et al: Effect of ingesta on systemic availability of penicillins administered orally in dogs, *J Vet Pharmacol Ther* 9(2):140–149, 1986:Jun.
153. Campbell BG, Rosin E: Effect of food on absorption on cephalexin and cefadroxil in dogs, *J Vet Pharmacol Ther* 21:418–420, 1998.
154. Schmidt LE, Dalhoff K: Food-drug interactions, *Drugs* 62(10):1481–1502, 2002.
155. Idson B: Vehicle effects in percutaneous absorption, *Drug Metab Rev* 14(2):207–222, 1983.
156. Boothe DM: Topical drugs: component interactions, vehicles and the consequences of alterations, *Dermatol Rep* 6:1–8, 1987.
157. Boothe DM: Veterinary compounding in small animals: a clinical pharmacologist's perspective, *Vet Clin North Am Small Anim Pract* 36(5):1129–1173, 2006.
158. Nordenberg T: Pharmacy compounding: customizing prescription drugs, *FDA Consumer Magazine* , July 2000.
159. Pond SM: Pharmacokinetic drug interactions. In Benet LZ, Massoud N, Gambertoglio JG, editors: *Pharmacokinetic basis for drug treatment*, New York, 1984, Raven Press, pp 49–62.
160. Chien JY, Mohutsky MA, Wrighton SA: Physiological approaches to the prediction of drug-drug interactions in study populations, *Curr Drug Metab* 4:347–356, 2003.
161. Hu Z, Yang X, Ho PCL, et al: Herb-drug interactions, *Drugs* 65:1239–1282, 2005.
162. Sagir A, Schmitt M, Dilger, et al: Inhibition of cytochrome P450 3A: relevant drug interactions in gastroenterology, *Digestion* 68(1):41–48, 2003.
163. Benet LZ, Cummins CL, Wu CY: Transporter-enzyme interactions: implications for predicting drug-drug interactions from in vitro data, *Curr Drug Metab* 4:393–398, 2003.
164. Zhang S, Morris ME: Effects of the flavonoids biochanin A, morin, phloretin, and silymarinon P-glycoprotein-mediated transport, *J Pharmacol Exp Ther* 304:1258–1267, 2003.
165. Toutain PL, Bousquet-Melou A: Free drug fraction vs. free drug concentration: a matter of frequent confusion, *J Vet Pharmacol Ther* 25:460–463, 2002.
166. Hostetler KA, Wrighton SA, Molowa DT, et al: Coinduction of multiple hepatic cytochrome P-450 proteins and their mRNAs in rats treated with imidazole antimycotic agents, *Mol Pharmacol* 35:279–285, 1988.
167. Ohnhaus EE, Taras G-E, Park BK: Enzyme-inducing drug combinations and their effects on liver microsomal enzyme activity in man, *Eur J Clin Pharmacol* 24:247–250, 1983.
168. Bresnick E: The molecular biology of the induction of the hepatic mixed function oxidases. In Schenkman JB, Kupfer D, editors: *Hepatic cytochrome P-450 monooxygenase system*, New York, 1982, Pergamon Press, pp 99–156.
169. Snyder R, Remmer H: Class of hepatic microsomal mixed function oxidase inducers, *Pharmacol Ther* 7(2):203–244, 1979.
170. Schenkman JP, Kupfer D: *Hepatic cytochrome P-450 monooxygenase system*, New York, 1982, Pergamon Press, pp 99-156.
171. Kawalek JC, Howard KD, Farrell DE, et al: Effect of oral administration of low doses of pentobarbital on the induction of cytochrome P450 insoforms and cytochrome P450-mediated reactions in immature beagles, *Am J Vet Res* 64:1167–1175, 2003.
172. Hollenberg PF: Characteristics and common properties of inhibitors, inducers, and activators of CYP enzymes, *Drug Metab Rev* 34(1-2):17–35, 2002.
173. Pond SM: Pharmacokinetic drug interaction. In Benet LZ, Massoud N, Gambertoglio JG, editors: *Pharmacokinetic basis for drug treatment*, New York, 1985, Raven Press, pp 195–220.
174. Hojo T, Ohno R, Shimoda M: Enzyme and plasma protein induction by multiple oral administrations of phenobarbital at a therapeutic dosage regimen in dogs, *J Vet Pharmacol Therap* 25:121–127, 2002.
175. Levy RH, Hachad H, Yao C, et al: Relationship between extent of inhibition and inhibitor dose: literature evaluation based on the metabolism and transport drug interaction database, *Curr Drug Metab* 4(5):371–380, 2003.
176. Hirt RA, Teinfalt M, Dederichs D: The effect of orally administered marbofloxacin on the pharmacokinetics of theophylline, *J Am Vet Med Assoc* 50:246–250, 2003.

177. Kuhora M, Kuze Y: In vitro characterization of the inhibitory effect of ketaconazole on metabolic activities of CYP 450 in canine hepatic microsomes, *Am J Vet Res* 63:900–905, 2002.
178. Mouatt JG: Cyclosporin and ketoconazole interaction for treatment of perianal fistulas in the dog, *Aust Vet J* 80(4):207–211, 2002.
179. Dahlinger J, Gregory C, Bea J: Effect of ketoconazole on cyclosporine dose in healthy dogs, *Vet Surg* 27(1):64–68, 1998.
180. McAnulty JF, Lensmeyer GL: The effects of ketoconazole on the pharmacokinetics of cyclosporine A in cats, *Vet Surg* 28: 448–455, 1999.
181. D'Souza MJ, Pollock SH, Solomon HM: Cyclosporine-cimetidine interaction, *Drug Metab Dispos* 16(1):57–59, 1988.
182. Jackson JE: Cimetidine protects against acetaminophen toxicity, *Life Sci* 31:31–35, 1982.
183. Ruffalo RL, Thompson JF: Cimetidine and acetylcysteine as antidote for acetaminophen overdose, *South Med J* 75:954–958, 1982.

Pharmacogenetics

3

Katrina A. Mealey

Chapter Outline

The goal of drug therapy is to produce a specific pharmacologic effect in a patient without producing adverse effects. Unfortunately, this goal is not fully realized for every veterinary patient. If the same drug were administered to 10 patients with a particular disease, each may respond differently with respect to both drug efficacy and the likelihood of an adverse reaction. This variation in response to drug therapy can be caused by a number of patient factors, including the patient's age, health or disease status, species, gender, and breed. In many instances, however, these factors cannot fully explain the degree of interpatient variation observed. Pharmacogenetics, the study of genetic determinants of response to drug therapy, is likely the ultimate way to establish the right drug and dose for each patient, thereby optimizing efficacy and minimizing toxicity. Despite the fact that this branch of pharmacology is still in its infancy as a science, a number of important discoveries have already contributed to improved pharmacotherapy in human and veterinary patients.

Genetic variation can affect both the pharmacokinetics (i.e., drug absorption, distribution, metabolism, and excretion) and pharmacodynamics (i.e., interaction with drug transporters and receptors) of pharmaceutical agents (Figure 3-1). Currently, the greatest body of knowledge with regard to pharmacogenetics involves genetic variation in drug metabolism. Indeed, the concept of pharmacogenetics originated in the 1950s as a result of the observation in human beings that two populations of individuals existed with respect to their ability to metabolize succinylcholine, followed by the realization that this trait was inherited.[1] Approximately 1 in 3500 Caucasian subjects is homozygous for a mutation in the butyrylcholinesterase gene.[2] Because this gene is responsible for hydrolysis and inactivation of succinylcholine, patients who have the mutation experience prolonged muscle paralysis and apnea. At the time, molecular biological techniques had not yet been discovered, so the field of pharmacogenetics was initially based purely on phenotypic observations.

Modern pharmacogenetics has progressed rapidly from those initial phenotypic observations. It currently involves identifying both the phenotype and the genetic variation, or polymorphism, responsible for it. Furthermore, the pharmacogenetic traits that were first identified were monogenic—that is, they involved a polymorphism at a single gene. It is presently known that myriad genes may be involved in determining a particular drug's disposition, which increases the complexity of pharmacogenetics. Pharmacogenetics now involves systematic searches to identify functionally significant variations in DNA sequences in genes that affect drug disposition. Sequencing of the human, canine, and now feline genome should facilitate the progress of pharmacogenetics toward individualized drug therapy.

It is important to note that individualization of drug therapy encompasses two distinct, yet equally important, clinical implications. First is the ability to predict those patients at high risk for developing drug toxicity. These patients may have a polymorphism in a drug-metabolizing enzyme that results in low clearance rates for the drug. For such patients a lower drug dose or alternative drug should be administered. Second is the ability to predict those patients that are most likely to benefit from a particular drug because of appropriate receptor interactions. Patients with polymorphisms in drug receptors may be poor responders to certain pharmaceutical agents because of inappropriate drug–receptor interactions. Rather than using a trial-and-error approach to drug therapy, a veterinarian could select the drug most likely to produce the desired pharmacologic response in a particular patient, decreasing the amount of time in that the patient's disease state is poorly controlled.

Described in this chapter will be several recent discoveries in pharmacogenetics and examples of pharmacogenetically based differences in drug absorption, distribution, metabolism, excretion, and drug–receptor interactions. The role of these discoveries in clinical veterinary medicine will also be presented.

PHARMACOGENETICS OF DRUG ABSORPTION

Until recently, systemic bioavailability of orally administered drugs was considered to be a function of physicochemical characteristics of the drug and subsequent hepatic metabolism. A

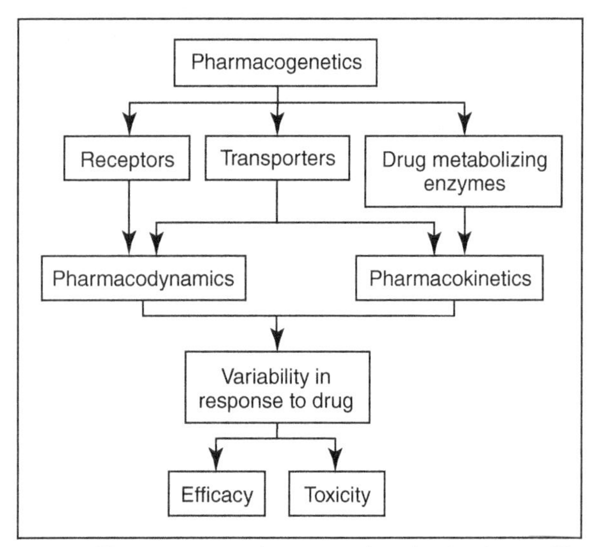

Figure 3-1 Pharmacogenetics can alter both drug efficacy and the likelihood of toxicity. Polymorphisms in drug receptors contribute to variable pharmacodynamics, and polymorphisms in drug-metabolizing enzymes contribute to variable pharmacokinetics. Interestingly, polymorphisms in drug transporters can contribute to variation in pharmacodynamics and/or pharmacokinetics, depending on the particular drug transporter involved.

number of other factors have recently been shown to affect the ability of a drug to be absorbed into the systemic circulation after oral administration. Intestinal phase I drug metabolism and active drug extrusion by efflux transporters are now considered to be among the most important determinants of oral drug bioavailability. Consequently, polymorphisms in intestinal drug-metabolizing enzymes and drug transporters should dramatically affect oral drug absorption.

In humans CYP 3A enzymes are expressed at higher levels in mature villus tip enterocytes than in hepatocytes.[3] Because intestinal villi make up such a large surface area, there is a high likelihood that absorbed drug will interact with intestinal CYP 3A enzyme, facilitating substantial first-pass metabolism. Interpatient variability in intestinal CYP 3A levels has been studied in a small sample of human patients. Elevenfold variations in CYP 3A protein content and sixfold variation in enzymatic activity were identified, suggesting that CYP 3A polymorphisms exist in the human population.[4]

Intestinal drug metabolism is thought to be important in veterinary patients also, but relatively little is known with regard to interpatient variability in enzyme activity. In dogs tissue distribution (specifically liver and duodenum) of *CYP3A12* and *CYP3A26* mRNA has been investigated by the author. Overall, expression of *CYP3A* mRNA was greater in liver than in duodenum, but the relative contributions of the two canine *CYP3A* isoforms differed. Hepatic expression of *CYP3A26* was greater than *CYP3A12* in all dogs, with *CYP3A26* making up 75.2% of the hepatic CYP3A pool. Conversely, duodenal expression of *CYP3A12* was greater than *CYP3A26* in all dogs, with *CYP3A12* composing 99.8% of the duodenal *CYP3A* pool.[5] Additionally, there was a large amount of interindividual variability among dogs. Further research is needed in this area to determine whether genetic differences account for the variation in expression of this important drug-metabolizing enzyme in hepatic and intestinal tissue among dog breeds and/or individual dogs.

Drug transporters are also known to play an important role in drug absorption. Many drug transporters have been identified in people, but the most well-characterized drug transporter is P-glycoprotein (P-gp), the product of the MDR1 (ABCB1) gene. The potential impact of transporter pharmacogenetics on drug pharmacokinetics is dramatically illustrated by P-gp. P-gp is a transmembrane protein that was first described in highly resistant tumor cell lines.[6] Tumor cells expressing P-gp were cross-resistant to various anticancer agents (anthracyclines, vinca alkaloids, taxanes, and others). P-gp has since been shown to act as an ATP-dependent pump that exports drugs from cells. P-gp is also expressed in normal mammalian tissues, where it appears to function in a protective capacity. P-gp is expressed on bile canaliculi, renal tubular epithelial cells, the placenta, brain capillary endothelial cells, and at the luminal border of intestinal epithelial cells.[7] At these locations P-gp pumps transported drugs either out of the body (into the bile, urine, or intestinal lumen) or away from protected sites (brain tissue, fetus).

KEY POINT 3-1 Intestinal and hepatic drug transporters and cytochrome P450 enzymes contribute to variability in oral drug absorption.

The significant role intestinal P-gp can play in determining oral drug bioavailability has been demonstrated in rodent studies. In *mdr*1(-/-) knockout mice, oral bioavailability of many P-gp substrate drugs (vinblastine, taxol, digoxin, loperamide, ivermectin, cyclosporine A, others) are substantially greater than in wild-type mice.[8,9] Similarly, MDR1 polymorphisms in humans have been shown to result in altered oral bioavailability of P-gp substrate drugs. Studies have shown that oral bioavailability of digoxin, a P-gp substrate, is greater in subjects with the 3435TT MDR1 genotype compared with those with the MDR1 3435CC genotype.[10] Similarly, the P-gp substrate phenytoin has been shown to have lower oral bioavailability in subjects with the MDR1 3435 CC genotype.[11]

P-gp has been fairly well characterized in dogs. Tissue distribution of P-gp in dogs is similar to that in people,[12] and it has been shown to contribute to chemotherapeutic drug resistance in vitro and in vivo.[13-15] Although its role in determining oral drug bioavailability is not well characterized, there is some evidence that P-gp is important. Bioavailability of the anticancer agent (and P-gp substrate) docetaxel was increased seventeenfold when co-administered with a P-gp inhibitor.

The MDR1 polymorphism in dogs consists of a four base-pair deletion mutation. This deletion results in a shift of the reading frame that generates several premature stop codons.[16] Because protein synthesis is terminated before even 10% of the protein product is synthesized, dogs with two mutant alleles exhibit a P-gp null phenotype, similar to mdr1 (-/-) knockout mice. Affected dogs include many herding breeds. For example, roughly 75% of Collies in the United States, France, and Australia have at least one mutant allele.[17] Other affected herding breeds, albeit affected at a lower frequency, include Old English Sheepdogs, Australian Shepherds, Shetland Sheepdogs, English Shepherd Dogs, Border Collies, German Shepherd Dogs, Silken Windhounds, McNab Shepherds, and Longhaired Whippets.[18]

One group of investigators describe a modest effect of the MDR1 deletion mutation on oral drug availability.[19] Three P-gp substrate drugs (fexofenadine, loperamide, and quinidine) were simultaneously administered to two groups of dogs, dogs homozygous for the MDR1 deletion mutation (MDR1 mut/mut) and MDR1 wild-type dogs (MDR1 WT/WT). Statistically, there were no differences in area under the curve for any drug between the two groups. Plasma concentrations of fexofenadine were significantly higher at two time points in MDR1(mut/mut) dogs than in MDR1(WT/WT) dogs.[19] The investigators suggest that P-gp limits intestinal absorption of fexofenadine, an antihistamine (H_1), in dogs.

PHARMACOGENETICS OF DRUG DISTRIBUTION

Drug distribution, the delivery of drugs from the systemic circulation to tissues, can be dramatically affected by pharmacogenetics. The drug transporter P-gp serves as an important barrier to the distribution of substrate drugs to selected tissues. For example, P-gp is a component of the blood–brain barrier, the blood–testes barrier, and the placenta. Therefore distribution of P-gp substrate drugs to these tissues is greatly enhanced in MDR1(mut/mut) dogs. MDR1(mut/mut) dogs experience adverse neurologic effects after a single dose of ivermectin (120 μg/kg). Heterozygous [MDR1(WT/mut)] or MDR1(WT/WT) dogs are not sensitive to ivermectin neurotoxicity at the 120 μg/kg dose, but MDR1(WT/mut) animals may experience neurotoxicity at ivermectin doses greater than 120 μg/kg, particularly if daily doses are administered (i.e., protocols for treatment of demodectic mange). Affected dogs also appear to have increased susceptibility to neurologic adverse effects of other avermectins, including milbemycin, selamectin (Revolution package insert), and moxidectin.[20] Interestingly, a retrospective study conducted by a national veterinary poison center reported that Collies were overrepresented in canine cases of loperamide-induced neurotoxicity.[21] Many Collies displayed signs of neurologic toxicity after administration of routinely recommended doses of the antidiarrheal agent loperamide (Imodium). Loperamide is an opioid that is generally devoid of central nervous system activity because it is excluded from the brain by P-gp.[22,23] Loperamide neurotoxicity was recently reported in a Collie that had received a routine dose (0.14 mg/kg orally).[24] The dog in this report had the MDR1(mutant/mutant) genotype. MDR1 (WT/WT) dogs do not exhibit neurologic signs after receiving even higher doses of loperamide, indicating that P-gp plays a key role in modulating distribution of substrates such as loperamide to canine brain tissue. The images in Figure 3-2 illustrate the role of P-gp in the blood–brain barrier of dogs.

KEY POINT 3-2 Dogs with the ABCB1-1Δ mutation experience greater brain penetration of drugs that are substrates for P-glycoprotein.

Less information is available regarding P-gp and the blood–brain barrier in cats. The author has received anecdotal reports of ivermectin toxicity in cats after standard doses, but whether the underlying cause is a result of altered P-gp expression or function is not currently known.

Distribution of some drugs to the testis and fetus may also be limited by P-gp. In human patients, this creates a problem for treating certain diseases. For example, the testes and brain are considered to be a sanctuary site for the human immunodeficiency virus (HIV).[25] Because HIV-1 protease inhibitors are substrates for P-gp, the virus can remain viable in these sanctuary sites, hampering effective therapy. Similarly, therapeutic concentrations of certain chemotherapeutic agents may not be achievable for testicular cancers because of active efflux by P-gp.[26] The effect of placental P-gp on distribution of drugs to the fetus is an area of active research in human medicine.[27] Understanding the role of pregnancy-associated hormones in regulating P-gp expression and function is one possible key in developing strategies to deliver drugs to the mother with minimal fetal risk.

PHARMACOGENETICS OF DRUG METABOLISM

Pharmacogenetic variation can affect both phase I and phase II metabolic enzyme activity. The pseudocholinesterase mutation serves as an example of how pharmacogenetic variation can result in dramatic differences in drug response among patients. Patients with a normal pseudocholinesterase genotype metabolize succinylcholine and recover from neuromuscular blockade rapidly, whereas those with the mutant genotype undergo sustained neuromuscular blockade that has resulted in prolonged apnea and the necessity for mechanical ventilation. A number of polymorphisms have been described in human CYP450 enzymes, many of these resulting in profound variations in clinical response. For example, CYP2D6 is a highly variable P450 pathway in humans with individuals ranging from undetectable activity (found in 6% to 10% of Caucasians) to "ultrarapid" activity (found in 3% to 10% of Europeans and 30% of one black population).[28] The ultrarapid phenotype is due to a unique gene duplication. Drugs that are substrates for CY2D6 in people include beta-receptor antagonists (propranolol, timolol, metoprolol), antiarrhythmics (quinidine, flecainide), antidepressants (amitriptyline, clomipramine, fluoxetine, imipramine), neuroleptics, and certain opioid derivatives. Depending on the patient's CYP2D6 genotype, the "typical" dose of a substrate drug may need to be decreased (poor metabolizers require ⅒ of the standard dose of nortriptyline to avoid toxicity) or increased (ultrarapid metabolizers require 5 times the standard dose to achieve therapeutic concentrations).

Relatively few polymorphisms in drug-metabolizing enzymes have been described in veterinary patients, although

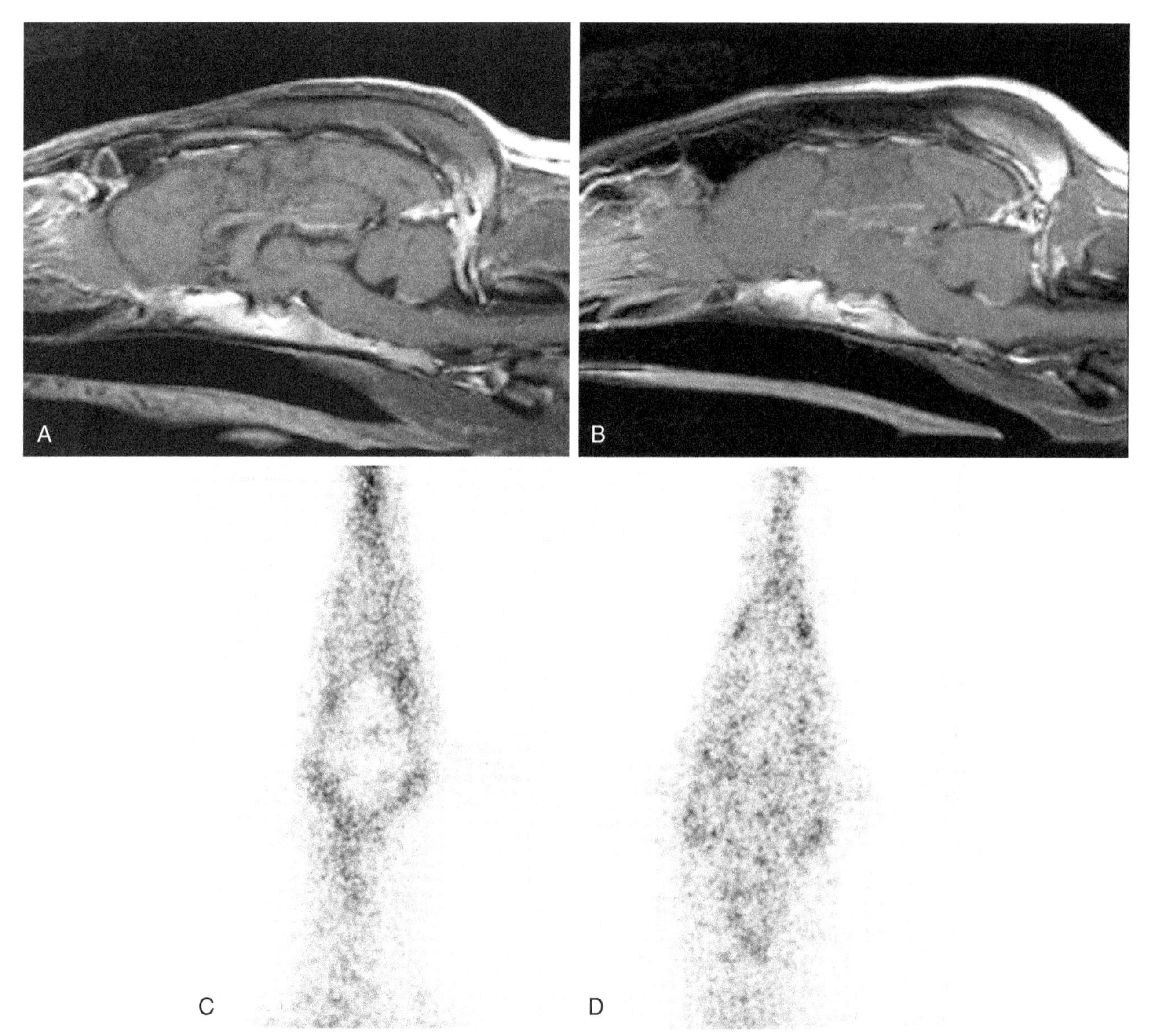

Figure 3-2 Sagittal T1-weighted post gadolinium administration magnetic resonance images displaying normal brain anatomy, tissue signal characteristics, and contrast enhancement of an MDR1 WT/WT dog **(A)** and an MDR1 mut/mut dog **(B)** showing no differences between dogs of these two genotypes. Conversely^{99m}Tc-MIBI nuclear scintigraphic neuroimaging of the brain after ^{99m}Tc-MIBI administration demonstrates the role of P-glycoprotein at the blood–brain barrier. Representative ^{99m}Tc-MIBI nuclear scintigraphic images show diminished activity in the brain compared with surrounding tissue of an MDR1 WT/WT dog **(C)** but similar activity in the brain compared with surrounding tissue of an MDR1 mut/mut dog **(D)**. (From Mealey KL, Greene S, Bagley R, et al: P-glycoprotein contributes to the blood–brain, but not blood–cerebrospinal fluid, barrier in a spontaneous canine p-glycoprotein knockout model, *Drug Metab Dispos* 36(6):1073-1079, 2008.)

this is likely to change insofar as research in this area is currently in progress. However, variation in metabolism of some drugs has been documented in dogs. CYP2B11 has been shown to have at least a fourteenfold variation in activity in mixed-breed dogs.[29] Greyhounds have been shown to have particularly low CYP2B11 activity, which results in sustained plasma concentrations of propofol, and delayed recovery compared with mixed-breed dogs.[30] The specific genetic alteration responsible for reduced CYP2B11 in Greyhounds compared with other canine breeds has not been determined. There is some evidence to suggest that CYP 2D15 may also be polymorphic in dogs. The nonsteroidal antiinflammatory drug celecoxib is metabolized to a large degree by CYP2D15. Clearance of celecoxib in Beagles is polymorphic, with about half the population being extensive metabolizers and the remainder being poor metabolizers.[31] Celecoxib has a 1.5- to 2-hour half-life in extensive metabolizers and a 5-hour half-life in poor metabolizers. One pharmacogenetic variant that has been identified in the canine CYP2D15 gene, a deletion of exon 3, results in undetectable celecoxib metabolism. The frequency and breed distribution of this polymorphism has not yet been determined. However, it is likely to have clinical significance for other drugs that are CYP2D15 substrates, including dextromethorphan, imipramine, and others.

KEY POINT 3-3 Polymorphisms in drug-metabolizing enzymes can dramatically affect drug efficacy and toxicity.

Variability in gene copy number is a phenomenon that has recently been explored in dogs.[32] Among the genes that have been demonstrated to exist in copy number variant regions in canine DNA are CYP3A12 and CYP1A. Furthermore, there appear to be breed-specific copy number variants for some dog breeds. Thus variability in gene copy number may be another source of genetic variation in drug response involving phase I enzymes.

With respect to phase II metabolic enzymes, a pan-species defect in UDP-glucuronyl transferase exists in cats. Although this is not a true example of pharmacogenetics, it serves as an example of genetic variation among species, rather than within a species, that significantly affects drug disposition. Because cats have a pseudogene, rather than a functional glucuronyltransferase gene, aceptaminophen and other drugs are not conjugated with glucuronide as they are in other species. Another pan-species phase II metabolic defect occurs in dogs. N-acetyltransferase is the enzyme responsible for metabolizing sulfonamides, procainamide, hydralazine, and other drugs. Both N-acetyltransferase genes are absent in dogs, increasing the risk for hypersensitivity reactions and adverse effect from these drugs relative to other species.[33]

A true pharmacogenetic variation exists for the thiopurine methyltrasferase (TPMT) enzyme. TPMT is a phase II enzyme that is responsible for metabolizing azathioprine and its active metabolites to their inactive forms. A ninefold range in TPMT activity exists in dogs, and activity level appears to be related to breed. Giant Schnauzers had lower TPMT activity, and Alaskan Malamutes had high TPMT activity.[34] Decreased TPMT activity has been documented to be associated with increased susceptibility to azathioprine-induced bone marrow suppression.

PHARMACOGENETICS OF DRUG EXCRETION

Drugs are eliminated from the body either unchanged or as metabolites. Renal and biliary excretion are the most important pathways of drug elimination, but excretion may occur by other routes as well. As noted previously, P-gp is expressed on renal tubular cells and biliary canalicular cells, suggesting that it may play a role in drug excretion. Concurrent administration of a P-gp–inhibitor decreases the biliary and renal clearance of doxorubicin in rats.[35] In a separate study, biliary and renal excretion of digoxin and vincristine were increased in rats after treatment with a P-gp inhibitor.[36] Further research is necessary to fully define the role of P-gp in regulating renal and biliary drug excretion in veterinary patients. However, altered biliary or renal excretion may play a role in the apparent increased sensitivity of herding breeds to chemotherapeutic drugs that are P-gp substrates. For example, MDR1(mut/mut) and MDR1(WT/mut) dogs are significantly more likely to develop hematologic toxicity, specifically neutropenia and thrombocytopenia after treatment with vincristine than ABCB1-1Δ wild-type dogs. However, these dogs tolerate cyclophosphamide at full doses.[37,38] In dogs vincristine is eliminated primarily through biliary excretion of parent drug with some urinary excretion of parent drug and metabolites.[39] The enzyme family responsible for metabolizing vincristine in dogs has not been identified. Biliary excretion of vincristine in other species is highly dependent on the P-gp–mediated drug transport.[36] The images in Figure 3-3 illustrate the role of P-gp in the biliary excretion of substrate drugs in dogs.

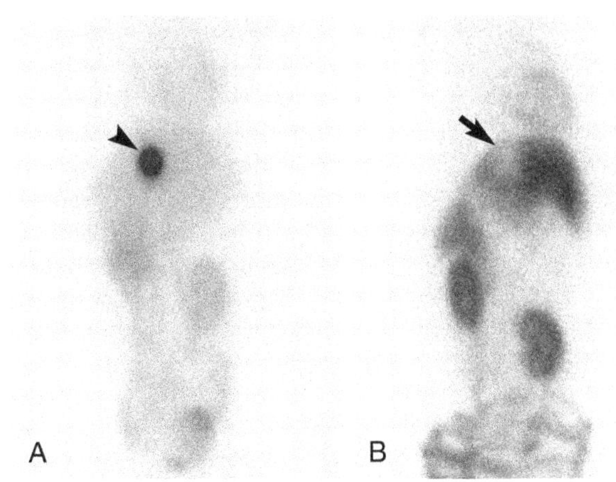

Figure 3-3 Images of the abdomen of dogs positioned in ventral recumbency on a gamma camera. Images were acquired 2 hours after intravenous injection of ^{99m}Tc-MIBI to an MDR1 WT/WT dog **(A)** and to an MDR1 mut/mut dog *(b)*. Intense uptake of ^{99m}Tc-MIBI in the gallbladder *(arrowhead)* is present in *(a)*. A void of activity in the location of the gallbladder *(arrow)* is present in **(B)**. (From Coelho JC, Tucker R, Mattoon J et al: Biliary excretion of technetium-99m-sestamibi in wild-type dogs and in dogs with intrinsic (ABCB1-1Δ mutation) and extrinsic (ketoconazole treated) P-glycoprotein deficiency, *J Vet Pharm Ther* 32:417-421, 2009.)

KEY POINT 3-4 Biliary excretion of P-glycoprotein substrate drugs is significantly decreased in dogs with the ABCB1-1Δ mutation compared with ABCB1 wild-type dogs.

PHARMACOGENETICS OF DRUG RECEPTORS

A relatively new and important area of pharmacogenetics research involves polymorphisms in genes encoding drug receptors and effector proteins. In human patients polymorphisms have been described in angiotensin-converting enzyme, beta-2 adrenergic receptors, the dopamine receptor, the estrogen receptor, and others.[40] In vitro functional studies suggest that these polymorphisms have functional significance. A polymorphism in the canine dopamine receptor D4 gene has been described, but its clinical implications are not yet understood.[41]

KEY POINT 3-5 Genetic variation in drug-metabolizing enzymes, drug transporters, and drug receptors can have a substantial impact on drug safety and efficacy.

PHARMACOGENETICS AND HYPERSENSITIVITY REACTIONS

Pharmacogenetic differences in metabolic pathways not only can affect type A adverse drug reactions (predictable; generally correlating with plasma drug concentration) but can also affect type B adverse drug reactions (idiosyncratic). Idiosyncratic toxicity to sulfonamides is similar in dogs and humans and can be characterized by fever, arthropathy, blood dyscrasias (neutropenia, thrombocytopenia, or hemolytic anemia), hepatopathy consisting of cholestasis or necrosis, skin eruptions, uveitis, or keratoconjunctivitis sicca.[42] In humans slow acetylation by NAT2 has been shown to be a risk factor for sulfonamide hypersensitivity reactions. It has been proposed that the alternative metabolic pathway in these individuals produces reactive metabolites.[43] Covalent binding of reactive metabolites of these drugs to cell macromolecules results in cytotoxicity and immune response to neoantigens. Ongoing research in one veterinary pharmacology laboratory (Department of Medical Sciences, School of Veterinary Medicine, University of Wisconsin-Madison; latrepanier@svm.vetmed.wisc.edu) is under way to characterize dogs with possible idiosyncratic sulfonamide reactions, using several methodologies, including enzyme-linked immunosorbent assay (ELISA) for antidrug antibodies, immunoblotting for antibodies directed against liver proteins, flow cytometry for drug-dependent antiplatelet antibodies, and in vitro cytotoxicity assays.

PHARMACOGENETICS IN CLINICAL PRACTICE

Scientific interest in the field of human pharmacogenetics has increased each year in parallel with the knowledge of the human genome. However, interest in this field from physicians has lagged significantly behind, presumably because relatively few significant clinical consequences can be correlated to the vast number of pharmacogenetic mutations described in the literature. There are two main reasons for this discrepancy. Up to this point, polymorphisms described in human patients either have had low allelic frequencies or the clinical relevance of a particular polymorphism was not significant. For example, a highly clinically relevant polymorphism in the human TPMT gene has been described. TMPT metabolic activity in affected patients is essentially absent, so these patients experience severe neutropenia after a "normal" dose of azathioprine. Because this TPMP polymorphism affects approximately 0.3% of the Caucasian population, pharmacogenetic testing is not routinely performed in clinical practice.[44] Conversely, the allelic frequency of a genetic polymorphism of the human MDR1 gene has been shown to be associated with lower levels of P-gp expression in the duodenum and other tissues. Although the allelic frequency of this particular MDR1 polymorphism is relatively high (>10%), it does not appear to have an important and predictable clinical impact on drug disposition. The vast majority of pharmacogenetics in human medicine is carried out for research purposes and is not performed in clinical medical practice.

In veterinary medicine, however, a commercial veterinary pharmacogenetics laboratory (Veterinary Clinical Pharmacology Laboratory, Washington State University, Pullman, WA; www.vetmed.wsu.edu/vcpl) is currently performing canine MDR1 genotyping for veterinarians, breeders, and owners in the United States. Such testing is available in Europe and Australia as well. The primary reasons that commercial pharmacogenetic testing is readily available for canine patients and not for human patients are because the MDR1 mutation in dogs has a very high allelic frequency (55% in Collies, 42% in Long-haired Whippets, and roughly 20% in Australian Shepherds), and because the polymorphism is highly predictive for serious adverse drug events, not just for ivermectin, but for chemotherapeutic drugs,[38] other antiparasitics,[45] loperamide,[24] and other drugs.[46] Box 3-1 contains a partial list of drugs that are substrates for P-gp.

KEY POINT 3-6 Pharmacogenetic testing of canine patients for the ABCB1-1Δ mutation can be used to prevent adverse drug reactions.

FUTURE DIRECTIONS

The field of pharmacogenetics, particularly in veterinary medicine, is still in its infancy. However, we have an ever-increasing arsenal of molecular tools that can be used to expand our knowledge of pharmacogenetics. Furthermore, with the recent completion of the canine and feline genome projects and the ongoing elucidation of their data, we may soon know the sequences of virtually all genes encoding drug-metabolizing enzymes, drug transporters, drug receptors, and other drug targets. With this information the traditional pharmacogenetics approach (phenotype to genotype) will likely give way to a pharmacogenomics approach (genotype to phenotype). In other words, genetic variation identified in a specific gene will be investigated to determine if it results in a variation in pharmacologic response. The convergence of these advances has the potential to individualize drug therapy for many veterinary patients.

Box 3-1

Selected P-glycoprotein Substrates

Anticancer Agents
Doxorubicin
Docetaxel*
Vincristine*
Vinblastine*
Etoposide*
Mitoxantrone
Actinomycin D

Steroid Hormones
Aldosterone
Cortisol*
Dexamethasone*
Methylprednisolone

Antimicrobial Agents
Erythromycin*
Ketoconazole*
Itraconazole
Tetracycline
Doxycycline
Levofloxacin
Sparfloxacin

Opioids
Loperamide
Morphine

Cardiac Drugs
Digoxin
Diltiazem*
Verapamil*
Talinolol

Immunosuppressants
Cyclosporine*
Tacrolimus*

Miscellaneous
Ivermectin
Amitriptyline
Terfenadine*
Ondansetron
Domperidon
Phenothiazines
Vecuronium

*Substrate of CYP 3A

(Adapted from Fromm MF: Genetically determined differences in P–glycoprotein function: implications for disease risk, *Toxicology* 181–182:299–303, 2002; Marzolini C, Paus E, Buclin T, Kim RB: Polymorphisms in human MDR1 (P–glycoprotein): recent advances and clinical relevance, *Clin Pharmacol Ther* 75:13–33, 2004; Sakaeda T, Nakamura T, Okumura K: MDR1 genotype–related pharmacokinetics and pharmacodynamics, *Biol Pharm Bull* 25:1391–1400, 2002; Sakaeda T, Nakamura T, Okumura K: Pharmacogenetics of MDR1 and its impact on the pharmacokinetics and pharmacodynamics of drugs, *Pharmacogenomics* 4:397–410, 2003; Schwab M, Eichelbaum M, Fromm MF: Genetic polymorphisms of the human MDR1 drug transporter, *Annu Rev Pharmacol Toxicol* 43:285–307, 2003.)

REFERENCES

1. Kalow W, Gunn DR: Some statistical data on atypical cholinesterase of human serum, *Ann Hum Genet* 23:239–250, 1959.
2. Kalow W: The Pennsylvania State University College of Medicine 1990 Bernard B. Brodie Lecture. Pharmacogenetics: past and future, *Life Sci* 47:1385–1397, 1990.
3. Patel J, Mitra AK: Strategies to overcome simultaneous P-glycoprotein mediated efflux and CYP3A4 mediated metabolism of drugs, *Pharmacogenomics* 2:401–415, 2001.
4. Scordo MG, Spina E: Cytochrome P450 polymorphisms and response to antipsychotic therapy, *Pharmacogenomics* 3:201–218, 2002.
5. Mealey KL, Jabbes M, Spencer E, Akey J: Differential expression of CYP3A12 and CYP3A26 in canine liver and intestine, *Xenobiotica* 38(10):1305–1312, 2008.
6. Roninson IB: The role of the MDR1 (P-glycoprotein) gene in multidrug resistance in vitro and in vivo, *Biochem Pharmacol* 43:95–102, 1992.
7. Thiebaut F, Tsuruo T, Hamada H, et al: Cellular localization of the multidrug-resistance gene product P-glycoprotein in normal human tissues, *Proc Natl Acad Sci USA* 84:7735–7738, 1987.
8. Schinkel AH, Wagenaar E, van Deemter L, et al: Absence of the mdr1a P-glycoprotein in mice affects tissue distribution and pharmacokinetics of dexamethasone, digoxin, and cyclosporin A, *J Clin Invest* 96:1698–1705, 1995.
9. Sills GJ, Kwan P, Butler E, et al: P-glycoprotein-mediated efflux of antiepileptic drugs: preliminary studies in mdr1a knockout mice, *Epilepsy Behav* 3:427–432, 2002.
10. Verstuyft C, Schwab M, Schaeffeler E, et al: Digoxin pharmacokinetics and MDR1 genetic polymorphisms, *Eur J Clin Pharmacol* 58:809–812, 2003.
11. Kerb R, Aynacioglu AS, Brockmoller J, et al: The predictive value of MDR1, CYP2C9, and CYP2C19 polymorphisms for phenytoin plasma levels, *Pharmacogenomics J* 1:204–210, 2001.
12. Ginn PE: Immunohistochemical detection of P-glycoprotein in formalin-fixed and paraffin-embedded normal and neoplastic canine tissues, *Vet Pathol* 33:533–541, 1996.
13. Mealey KL, Barhoumi R, Rogers K, Kochevar DT: Doxorubicin induced expression of P-glycoprotein in a canine osteosarcoma cell line, *Cancer Lett* 126:187–192, 1998.
14. Page RL, Hughes CS, Huyan S, et al: Modulation of P-glycoprotein-mediated doxorubicin resistance in canine cell lines, *Anticancer Res* 20:3533–3538, 2000.
15. McEntee M, Silverman JA, Rassnick K, et al: Enhanced bioavailability of oral docetaxel by co-administration of cyclosporin A in dogs and rats, *Vet Comp Oncol* 2:105–112, 2003.
16. Mealey KL, Bentjen SA, Gay JM, Cantor GH: Ivermectin sensitivity in collies is associated with a deletion mutation of the MDR1 gene, *Pharmacogenetics* 11:727–733, 2001.
17. Mealey KL, Bentjen SA, Waiting DK: Frequency of the mutant MDR1 allele associated with ivermectin sensitivity in a sample population of collies from the northwestern United States, *Am J Vet Res* 63:479–481, 2002.
18. Neff MW, Robertson KR, Wong AK, et al: Breed distribution and history of canine mdr1-1{Delta}, a pharmacogenetic mutation that marks the emergence of breeds from the collie lineage, *Proc Natl Acad Sci USA* 101:11725–11730, 2004.

19. Kitamura Y, Koto H, Matsuura S, et al: Modest effect of impaired function of P-glycoprotein on the plasma concentrations of fexofenadine, quinidine, and loperamide following oral administration in Collie dogs, *Drug Metab Dispos* 36:807–810, 2008.
20. Tranquilli WJ, Paul AJ, Todd KS: Assessment of toxicosis induced by high-dose administration of milbemycin oxime in collies, *Am J Vet Res* 52:1170–1172, 1991.
21. Hugnet C, Cadore JL, Buronfosse F, et al: Loperamide poisoning in the dog, *Vet Hum Toxicol* 38:31–33, 1996.
22. Ericsson CD, Johnson PC: Safety and efficacy of loperamide, *Am J Med* 88:10S–14S, 1990.
23. Wandel C, Kim R, Wood M, Wood A: Interaction of morphine, fentanyl, sufentanil, alfentanil, and loperamide with the efflux drug transporter P-glycoprotein, *Anesthesiology* 96:913–920, 2002.
24. Sartor LL, Bentjen SA, Trepanier L, Mealey KL: Loperamide toxicity in a collie with the MDR1 mutation associated with ivermectin sensitivity, *J Vet Intern Med* 18:117–118, 2004.
25. Choo EF, Leake B, Wandel C, et al: Pharmacological inhibition of P-glycoprotein transport enhances the distribution of HIV-1 protease inhibitors into brain and testes, *Drug Metab Dispos* 28:655–660, 2000.
26. Katagiri A, Tomita Y, Nishiyama T, Kimura M, Sato S: Immunohistochemical detection of P-glycoprotein and GSTP1-1 in testis cancer, *Br J Cancer* 68:125–129, 1993.
27. Young AM, Allen CE, Audus KL: Efflux transporters of the human placenta, *Adv Drug Deliv Rev* 55:125–132, 2003.
28. Cascorbi I: Pharmacogenetics of cytochrome P4502D6: genetic background and clinical implication, *Eur J Clin Invest* 33(Suppl 2):17–22, 2003.
29. Hay Kraus BL, Greenblatt DJ, Venkatakrishnan K: Court MH: Evidence for propofol hydroxylation by cytochrome P4502B11 in canine liver microsomes: breed and gender differences, *Xenobiotica* 30:575–588, 2000.
30. Court MH, Hay-Kraus BL, Hill DW, et al: Propofol hydroxylation by dog liver microsomes: assay development and dog breed differences, *Drug Metab Dispos* 27:1293–1299, 1999.
31. Paulson SK, Engel L, Reitz B, et al: Evidence for polymorphism in the canine metabolism of the cyclooxygenase 2 inhibitor, celecoxib, *Drug Metab Dispos* 27:1133–1142, 1999.
32. Nicholas TJ, Cheng Z, Ventura M, et al: The genomic architecture of segmental duplications and associated copy number variants in dogs, *Genome Res* 19:491–499, 2009.
33. Collins JM: Inter-species differences in drug properties, *Chem Biol Interact* 134:237–242, 2001.
34. Kidd LB, Salavaggione OE, Szumlanski CL, et al: Thiopurine methyltransferase activity in red blood cells of dogs, *J Vet Intern Med* 18:214–218, 2004.
35. Kiso S, Cai SH, Kitaichi K, et al: Inhibitory effect of erythromycin on P-glycoprotein-mediated biliary excretion of doxorubicin in rats, *Anticancer Res* 20:2827–2834, 2000.
36. Song S, Suzuki H, Kawai R, Sugiyama Y: Effect of PSC 833, a P-glycoprotein modulator, on the disposition of vincristine and digoxin in rats, *Drug Metab Dispos* 27:689–694, 1999.
37. Mealey KL, Northrup NC, Bentjen SA: Increased toxicity of P-glycoprotein-substrate chemotherapeutic agents in a dog with the MDR1 deletion mutation associated with ivermectin sensitivity, *J Am Vet Med Assoc* 223:1453–1455, 2003:1434.
38. Mealey KL, Fidel J, Gay JM, et al: ABCB1-1Delta polymorphism can predict hematologic toxicity in dogs treated with vincristine, *J Vet Intern Med* 22:996–1000, 2008.
39. El Dareer SM, White VM, Chen FP, et al: Distribution and metabolism of vincristine in mice, rats, dogs, and monkeys, *Cancer Treat Rep* 61:1269–1277, 1977.
40. Tribut O, Lessard Y, Reymann JM, et al: Pharmacogenomics, *Med Sci Monit* 8:RA152–RA163, 2002.
41. Ito H, Nara H, Inoue-Murayama M, et al: Allele frequency distribution of the canine dopamine receptor D4 gene exon III and I in 23 breeds, *J Vet Med Sci* 66:815–820, 2004.
42. Trepanier LA: Idiosyncratic toxicity associated with potentiated sulfonamides in the dog, *J Vet Pharmacol Ther* 27:129–138, 2004.
43. Spielberg SP: N-acetyltransferases: pharmacogenetics and clinical consequences of polymorphic drug metabolism, *J Pharmacokinet Biopharm* 24:509–519, 1996.
44. Becquemont L: Clinical relevance of pharmacogenetics, *Drug Metab Rev* 35:277–285, 2003.
45. Barbet J, Snook T, Gay JM, Mealey KL: ABCB1 (MDR1) genotype is associated with adverse reactions in dogs treated with milbemycin oxime for generalized demodicosis, *Vet Dermatol* 20:111–114, 2009.
46. Henik RA, Kellum HB, Bentjen SA, Mealey KL: Digoxin and mexiletine sensitivity in a Collie with the MDR1 mutation, *J Vet Intern Med* 20:415–417, 2006.

Drug-Induced Diseases

4

Dawn Merton Boothe

Chapter Outline

DEFINITIONS AND PREDISPOSING FACTORS

An adverse drug event (ADE) is any harm caused by a therapeutic or preventive (or diagnostic) intervention (Figure 4-1). The evolution of the definition in human medicine during the past decade has led to further subdivision into medication errors and adverse drug reactions (ADRs).[1] Medication errors are ADEs that result from a mistake made by the caregiver, including but not necessarily limited to administration of the wrong drug, dose, interval, or route to the wrong patient. Thus, ADEs are iatrogenic in origin. A potential subcategory of medication errors might be failure to modify a dosing regimen for recognized patient, drug, or disease factors that lead to inappropriately low or high drug concentrations at the site of action.

In contrast to medication errors, an ADR is a noxious and unintended response to a drug or other medication that occurs at a dose given with the goal of achieving the intended effect of the medication. As such, the term *ADR* implies a reaction that might cause serious harm to the patient and reflects a patient response to the inherent properties of the drug. An ADR may reflect a pharmacodynamic response or a pharmacokinetic effect. An ADR should be contrasted with the term *side effect,* which refers to an effect other than the intended effect that does not cause harm. A side effect may not be undesirable and may, in fact, be desirable or inconsequential to the health of the patient. For the purposes of this discussion, the term ADE will be used to refer to ADR with or without an iatrogenic basis. Adverse drug reactions can be further classified as either type A (type I) or type B (type II).[2-4] Type A ("augmented") adverse events generally result from drug concentrations at the site (generally estimated by plasma drug concentrations [PDCs] that either exceed the maximum or drop below the minimum therapeutic range (see Chapter 1). If the clinician is familiar with the drug and the patient, type A reactions are largely predictable and, as such, avoidable. Like type A, side effects are also generally predictable and dose dependent and for the purposes of discussion, will be included with type A adverse events in this chapter.

Generally, type A reactions are manifested as an exaggerated but normal or expected pharmacologic response to the drug (see Figure 4-1).[5] This response may be the desired response (e.g., bradycardia in a patient receiving propranolol to slow a sinus tachycardia) but also may reflect an unwanted, secondary response resulting from the drug's pharmacologic effects (e.g., bronchospasms induced by the beta-blockade effects of propranolol) (Figure 4-2). Some drugs also cause adverse events unrelated to their pharmacologic response. These reactions usually reflect damage to target cells and are referred to in this chapter as *cytotoxic adverse reactions.* Cytotoxic adverse reactions are exemplified by nephrotoxicity induced by aminoglycosides (Figure 4-3) or hepatic necrosis or methemoglobinemia induced by acetaminophen. Often, it is the metabolite of the drug rather than the drug itself that causes cytotoxicity (see Chapter 2). In such cases, drugs that induce metabolism, particularly in the liver

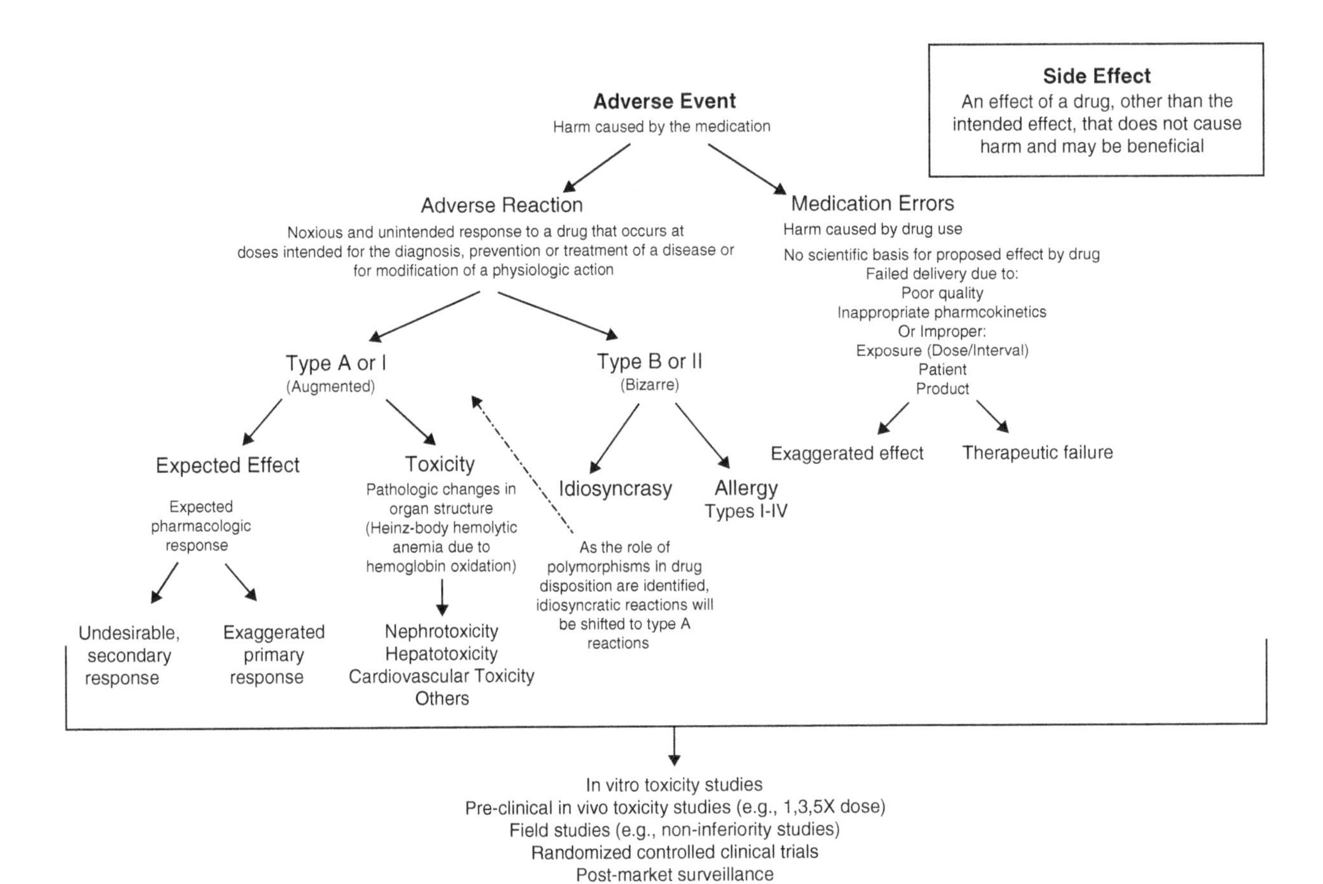

Figure 4-1 Flow chart delineating the definitions of adverse drug events (ADEs), including medication errors and adverse drug reactions (ADRs). ADEs can result in either an exaggerated response or failed response. In contrast to ADR, which implies harm to the patient, side effects do not cause harm and in some cases, may be beneficial. The risk of toxicity or ADR is assessed at several points before and during the approval process, with postmarket surveillance being perhaps the most comprehensive.

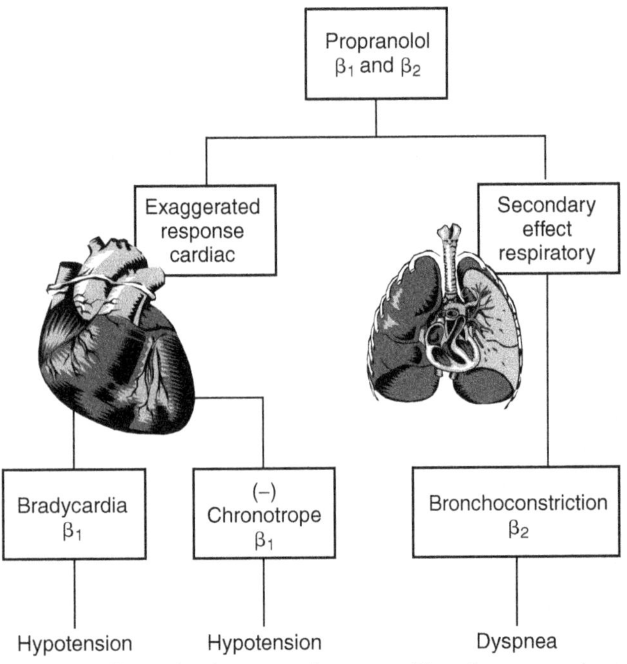

Figure 4-2 Type A drug reactions resulting from overdose. Propranolol offers an example of a type A adverse reaction that reflects both an exaggerated primary response (bradycardia, decreased contractility) and an undesirable secondary response (bronchospasm).

(e.g., phenobarbital, phenytoin; Figure 4-4), may increase the risk of toxicity, whereas drugs that decrease metabolism may reduce the risk of toxicity (e.g., cimetidine).[6-8] Cytotoxic drug reactions might be treated with drugs that scavenge radical metabolites (i.e., *N*-acetylcysteine, a glutathione precursor).

In contrast to type A events, type B ("bizarre") events are not dose or concentration dependent. As a result, these reactions are not predictable and are largely unavoidable. They occur only in a small percentage of the population receiving the drug; in human medicine they account for approximately 6% to 12% of all ADRs.[9] Generally, their incidence—indeed their existence—often is not documented until the drug is in wide use. In addition, because their cause is not well understood, treatment is generally limited to symptomatic therapy. Examples of type B adverse reactions include drug allergies or idiosyncrasies. Many of the idiosyncrasies eventually may be shown to be genetically or otherwise based (e.g., polymorphisms in transport or drug-metabolizing proteins [ivermectin toxicity of Collie-related breeds]), but the cause has yet to be identified and thus the reaction cannot be predicted. As with type A events, type B events may occur in response to the parent drug or its metabolite. This chapter will focus on allergies as type B ADRs.

This chapter discusses the mechanisms and clinical signs of the adverse events caused by selected drugs and methods by

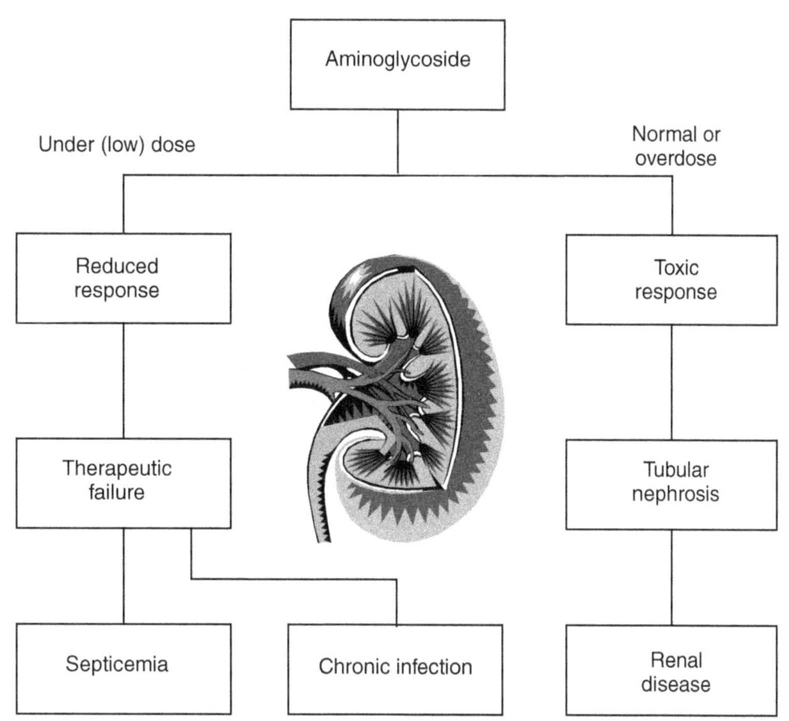

Figure 4-3 Underdose and cytotoxic response. An aminoglycoside such as gentamicin can cause two examples of a type A adverse reaction/therapeutic failure, meaning effective antimicrobial concentrations are not achieved, and a cytotoxic reaction, manifested as nephrotoxicity in response to persistent (rather than very high) plasma drug concentrations.

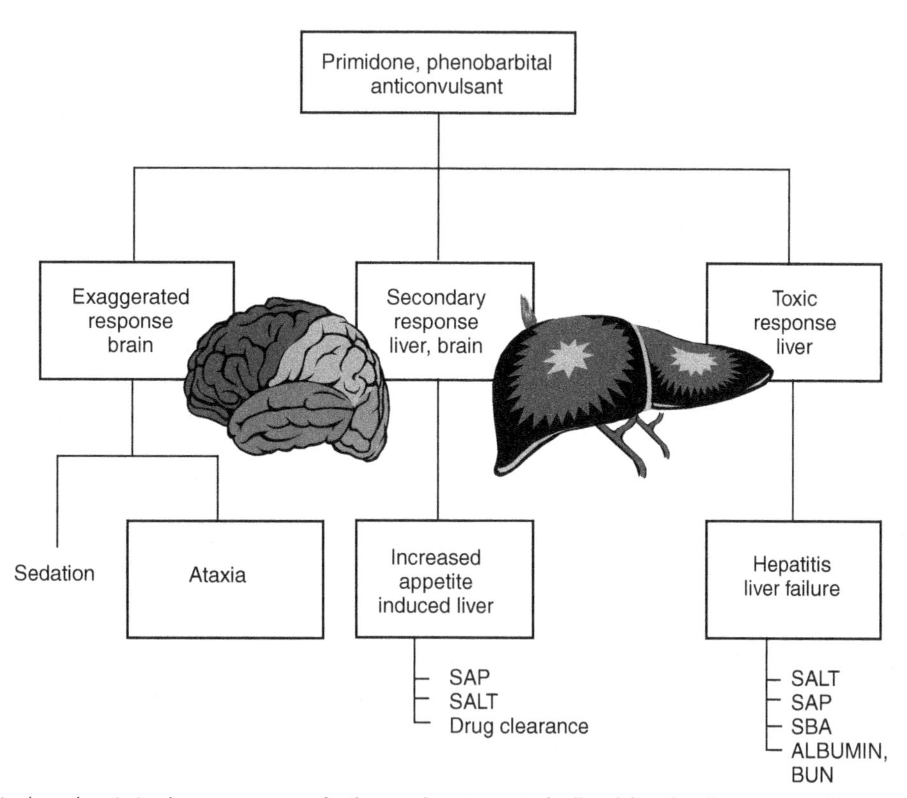

Figure 4-4 Exaggerated and cytotoxic responses. Anticonvulsants metabolized by the liver exemplify a type A adverse reaction manifested as cytotoxicity (hepatic disease). These drugs also can cause an exaggerated (but expected) response (sedation) as well as a secondary undesirable response or side effect that is not necessarily considered severe or life threatening (increased appetite, polyuria, and polydypsia). *BUN,* Blood urea nitrogen; *SALT,* serum alanine aminotransferase; *SAP,* serum alkaline phosphatase; *SBA,* serum bile acid.

which the events might be avoided or treated. Adverse events or side effects that result from the expected pharmacologic action of a drug (e.g., exaggerated pharmacologic effect) are also discussed with each drug in subsequent chapters and generally are not emphasized here. This chapter focuses more on type A than type B events because they are recognized more commonly. The list of drugs included is by no means complete but represents those drugs most commonly recognized, as well as the addition of some that are often overlooked. ADEs are also addressed in chapters that address the use of the drug.

The impact of ADEs on the monetary and health costs in human medicine were assessed in the late 1990s. The implementation of a voluntary, anonymous reporting system has facilitated medication error reporting in human medicine and thus enabled a more accurate assessment of their impact.[10] The majority (66%) of medical errors occurred during transfer of patient care within hospitals, and another 19% occurred on discharge. In a human intensive care unit (ICU) environment, 1 out of every 5 doses of medication was associated with an ADE as a result of medication errors. The veterinary profession has yet to implement a mechanism whereby ADEs due to medication errors can be assessed. Yet needs are equally applicable to veterinary medicine.[10]

Organs most susceptible to type A drug events usually are those subjected to the greatest exposure or concentration of the drug. Thus the organs with the greatest blood flow and those organs capable of drug concentration, such as the liver and kidney, are the most vulnerable to systemic drugs. Highly metabolically active organs are also more likely to manifest toxic effects for two reasons. First, such organs depend on the presence of energy, and anything that impairs acquisition of energy (including blood flow) can lead to malfunction. Second, if the metabolic activity includes metabolism of compounds, the production of potentially reactive metabolites can increase the likelihood of cytotoxicity if these metabolites interact with cellular structures. In contrast to Type A ADEs, the organs most susceptible to damage by type B reactions tend to be the organs that contain tissues that act as haptens for drug-induced allergy (e.g., skin, blood-forming units) or tissues that filter and trap immune complexes (e.g., glomerulus, joints). Organs containing a preponderance of mast cells also are more likely to manifest immune-mediated reactions (i.e., "shock organs"; see the section on allergic reactions). A summary of compounds causing predominantly type A drug reactions and, when available, their antidotes, can be found in Appendix 5. A variety of factors can influence the likelihood of adverse, and particularly toxic, reactions.[6-8] Factors that predispose a patient to the development of type A adverse events are discussed in Chapter 2.

Not all adverse reactions are clinically evident. Sometimes the reaction is not detectable unless actively sought. For example, clinical laboratory tests may detect a drug-induced hepatotoxicity (e.g., increased serum alanine transferase activity) that is otherwise clinically silent. Many drugs can directly interfere with or indirectly influence clinical laboratory tests, including endocrine function testing (discussed later).[11] Organ predisposition to drug-induced toxicity may show diurnal variations. For example, both aminoglycosides and cisplatin[12] exhibit increased renal toxicity in humans when administered in the evening as opposed to in the morning. For the aminoglycosides, safety in the morning has been attributed, in part, to the increase in glomerular filtration rate that occurs in the morning;[13] an increased sensitivity to interleukin-6–induced inflammation has been suggested for cisplatin.

PRINCIPLES OF TOXICOLOGY RELEVANT TO PHARMACOLOGY

Terminology of Toxicity and Safety Assessment

Toxicology refers to the study of poisons and their effect on living organisms.[14] A *poison* is any substance that is injurious to animals; the term is synonymous with toxic substance, toxic chemical, and toxicant. It is important to note that any drug can become a poison ("the dose makes the poison"), and the toxic response to the poison tends to correlate with the dose (or duration). *Toxic response* refers to the effects manifested by an organism in response to a toxic substance. *Toxicity* describes the quantitative amount or dose of a poison that produces a toxic response or effect. Acute toxicity generally results from a single dose or exposure or multiple doses in a 24-hour period. Most acute toxicants rapidly interfere with critical cellular processes. Subacute and subchronic toxicity occurs after 1 week to 1 month of exposure. Chronic toxicity occurs after 3 or more months of exposure.[14] These latter terms are generally applied to humans, but the relative duration of exposure applies equally to animals. Toxic chemicals can act *directly* by injuring the cells with which they come in contact or *indirectly* by injuring a group of cells that subsequently precipitate injury to others. Alternatively, toxins can act indirectly by interfering with a physiologic process on which a group of cells are vitally dependent. Toxins can act systemically (the majority), locally, or a combination of the two.[15]

An indicator of the assessment of toxicity is the LD_{50}, or the dose per unit weight of a chemical that kills 50% of animals receiving it (the median lethal dose) (Figure 4-5). The LD_{50} is both drug and species specific. The lethal dose of a drug can be compared with the dose necessary to induce the desired pharmacodynamic response (effective dose, or ED) in a targeted percent of the sample population (see Chapter 1). The ED_{50} is the dose expected to induce the response in 50% of the population; its more useful companion indicator is the EC_{50}, which describes the concentration at which 50% of individuals respond, thus removing the effects of drug absorption and distribution from consideration. Like the LD_{50}, ED_{50} and EC_{50} are generally based on single dosing and do not take into account duration of exposure. The *therapeutic index* offers a measure of the relative safety of a drug by comparing the dose producing toxicity to that causing the desired effect, or the ratio of the LD_{50} to ED_{50} (see Figure 4-5). A related term is *margin of safety* which is the ratio minimal lethal dose (LD_{01}) and the dose associated with the greatest efficacy (ED_{99}). Caution is recommended if the margin of safety (MOS) is less than 1. Alternatively, rather than measure lethality as the adverse event, the concentration necessary to cause a specific adverse event can

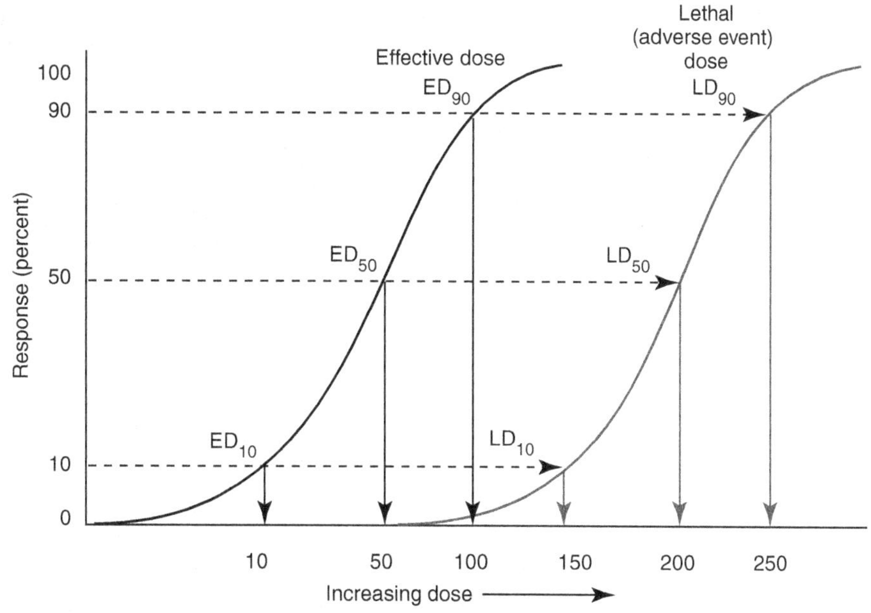

Figure 4-5 The dose necessary to cause the response in 50% of animals tested is referred to as either the *lethal dose*$_{50}$ (dose necessary to cause death; LD_{50} or 200 mg/kg) *or effective dose*$_{50}$ (dose necessary to cause targeted pharmacodynamic response; ED_{50} or 50 mg/kg), respectively. However, to induce the pharmacodynamic response of interest in the target species would require a dose of 50 mg/kg. The therapeutic index for this hypothetical drug would be the LD_{50}/ED_{50} or 200/50 = 4.

be measured and used to calculate the therapeutic index. A second set of terms by which the safety of a compound might be assessed are the *lowest observed adverse effect level* (LOAEL) and *no observed (adverse) effect level* (NOEL, or NOAEL). The LOAEL is the lowest concentration of drug associated with observed adverse effects. The NOAEL is defined as the greatest concentration of a compound that causes no detectable adverse effect. When compared with anticipated drug intake, it provides an alternative margin of safety. The absence of these effects can be used to help verify the NOAEL. The NOAEL generally is based on chronic exposure and thus may be more relevant for drugs administered at more than a single dose. NOELs and LOELs (no or lowest observed effect level, respectively) differ in that they may not indicate an adverse effect, but in fact may address a beneficial effect. All four terms are important to *risk assessment* which addresses exposure and the adverse outcomes that might be associated with exposure (see later discussion).

Other toxicologic terms relevant to drugs include *teratogen*, which is a compound that causes abnormal fetal development. It is important to note that teratogenicity is not the only form of toxicity that may occur in utero; any toxic effect that occurs in the adult is likely to occur in the developing fetus as well. *Carcinogenesis* refers to the ability of a compound, or a *carcinogen*, to cause cancer. Cancer cells are cells that have been able to avoid the sophisticated mechanisms that control normal growth, development, and division. Induction of cancer by a compound involves many variables, including duration, dose, and frequency of exposure. Generally, carcinogens take 20 years or more to induce cancer, and the cause-and-effect relationship between the compound and the cancer often is not recognized.[15,16] Although some compounds can directly interact with DNA, leading to a cancerous cell, most compounds must first be converted to a reactive metabolite to covalently bond with DNA. Damage may still be avoided if DNA repair occurs before cell division. Cellular damage increases the stimulus for division of adjacent cells, leading to a new cell type with new genotypic and phenotypic properties that can then be transformed to a malignant cell under the correct conditions. A number of compounds are recognized to be *initiating agents*, targeting molecular DNA, whereas others are considered *promoters*, acting to increase the incidence of cancer or decrease the latency period without interacting with DNA. These latter compounds must be administered repeatedly and after the initial insult. Endogenous compounds such as growth factors or hormones may act as promoters.[15]

Many compounds can induce cancer in laboratory animals when they are exposed to extremely high (supratherapeutic) doses for prolonged periods of time. Rarely do these compounds cause cancer in humans, and it is even more unlikely that they will do so in companion animals, in part because the life expectancy of companion animals generally is too short to allow emergence of cancer. Lifestyle changes that increase the risk of drug or toxicant-induced cancer in humans are likely to have the same effect in animals as well. These include but are not limited to exposure to cigarette smoke, exposure to charcoal-cooked food, chronic consumption of alcohol (unlikely in animals), and consumption of foods, many of which contain possible carcinogens.

Two mechanisms by which drugs can cause cell death are apoptosis and necrosis, each with distinct morphologic and biochemical characteristics. Apoptosis is an active process characterized by cell shrinkage, nuclear and cytoplasmic condensation, chromatin fragmentation, and phagocytosis. In contrast, necrosis is a passive process resulting in inflammation associated with cellular and organelle swelling, rupture of the plasma membrane, and spilling of cellular contents into the extracellular milieu.[17] Because apoptosis is an active process, sufficient intracellular energy must be maintained; depletion of adenosine triphosphate (ATP) may cause an apoptopic process to become a necrotic process. Not surprisingly, mitochondria appear to play a role in apoptosis. A number of toxicants cause their effects by disrupting mitochondria function and thus ATP production. However, several drugs appear to exert their toxicologic effect through induction of apoptosis (e.g., digoxin, selected chemotherapeutic agents).[17]

Genetic diversity is increasingly being identified as a cause for individual variation in response to toxins and drugs, leading to the fields of toxicogenetics and pharmacogenetics, respectively.[5,16,18] The role of polymorphic cytochrome P450s as a cause of interindividual differences in xenobiotic metabolism and drug toxicity is fairly well established. In humans polymorphism occurs less commonly in those cytochrome P450s responsible for carcinogen activation (CYP1A1 and 2, CYP1B1, CYP2E1, and CYP3A4) compared with those that are primarily responsible for drug metabolism (CYP2C9, CYP2C19, CYP2D6, and CYP3A4). Polymorphisms in drug-metabolizing enzymes have been associated with drug hypersensitivities.[6] All hepatic drug-metabolizing P450s are polymorphic with the clinically most important polymorphism in humans occurring with CYP2C9, CYP2C19, and CYP2D6.[19] Polymorphisms in cytochrome P450s of animals is now being elucidated but may play a role in adversities in certain breeds (e.g., Beagles, Greyhounds). In addition, polymorphism in P-glycoprotein (P-gp) is a well-established reason for susceptibility to adverse drug events for selected drugs in Collie-related breeds (see Chapter 2).

Postmarket Surveillance

The approval process for human-marketed drugs is designed to identify adverse reactions at several stages preclinical phase (short- and long-term animal testing): through phase III (extended clinical trials) and continuing into phase IV, which includes a mandated postmarket surveillance. However, the drug approval process for animals is not as regimented (see Figure 4-1). The requirements by the Food and Drug Administration's Center for Veterinary Medicine tend to vary with the drug undergoing approval (See Appendix 1).[20] In general, directed toxicity studies that are implemented during the approval process involve a small number (e.g., 2 to 30 but most commonly 4 of each sex) of study animals receiving the drug under conditions of exaggerated use—that is, doses (e.g.,1, 3, 5× the highest labeled dose,) and durations (e.g., 3×) of several magnitudes greater than the anticipated approved intended use. Field trials implemented during the approval process are performed in the approved species, generally as controlled (placebo or positive), randomized clinical trials, under conditions of intended use. Such studies generally involve a much larger sample population (e.g., hundreds of animals) than the directed toxicity studies. However, although toxicity studies do predict a number of adverse events that occur in the target species,[21] neither directed toxicity nor field studies are likely to involve a sample size sufficiently large to allow detection of many adverse events that occur in a very small proportion of patients (e.g., 1 in 1000 or more). Detection of such an adverse event is likely to require thousands of subjects. Further, directed studies are generally performed in a sample population of generally healthy animals unaffected by the complexities of host, drug, and disease factors associated with drug use in the target population (see Chapter 2). As such, postmarket surveillance studies and pharmacoepidemiologic studies (which focus on subgroups of target species) are particularly important to the safety assessment of approved drugs used in animal patients.[21] For the same reason, if an ADE is suspected as a result of drug therapy, the importance of reporting it (or suspicion of it) cannot be overemphasized. Note that safety assessment of human-marketed drugs are studied in dogs but with an emphasis on human rather than animal safety. Although all approved human-marketed drugs are likely to have been studied in dogs during the preclinical phase, most of this information is not generally available unless specifically requested through Freedom of Information Act mechanisms. If an ADE is suspected, it first should be reported to the manufacturer; by law, animal drug pharmaceutical companies must report adverse events reported in animals to the Food and Drug Administration (FDA). The veterinary profession, probably more so than the human-medicine community, is less likely to report adverse event perhaps because the mechanism by which the information is forwarded to the veterinary health care provider is limited in both scope and distribution. In contrast to drugs, adverse event reporting for animal dietary supplements is entirely voluntary, with no obvious mechanism for reports to be collected, assessed, or returned to the veterinary profession.

It is only through postmarket surveillance that more clinically relevant assessments of drug safety can emerge, and subtle differences in the safety of different drugs might become apparent. Assessments include hazard or risk assessment, which express the probability of harm under conditions expected with use of the drug. Hazard is the potential to cause harm—that is, the inherent toxic nature of the compound. Risk is the likelihood that harm will occur. As such, it takes into account both hazard and exposure—that is, the amount of the toxin ingested and thus dose and duration.[22] Risk–benefit analysis compares the risk associated with the use of a product and its potential benefits.[23] As such, a risk/benefit ratio addresses the acceptability of an adverse reaction by taking into account the importance, frequency, and duration of therapeutic benefit and the adverse reaction. Risk–benefit analysis generally is based on postmarket use of a product and a mechanism of surveillance that detects and assesses adverse events.[24]

Among the difficulties in assessing risk through postmarket surveillance is the attribution of the adversity to the drug. Information submitted in an ADE report is limited, and care must be taken to not assume a cause–effect relationship The FDA's Center for Veterinary Medicine has recently reviewed its ADE reporting program.[25] It defines an ADE as an undesired or lack of desired response to a drug, medical device, or (in food animals) medicated feed. As such, a distinction is not made between adverse events associated with medication errors and those associated with inherent properties of the drug. In its 2004 report, the FDA indicates that a 6-point scoring system evaluates drug reactions submitted from manufacturers, pet owners, or veterinarians. Information collected includes previous experience with the drug (i.e., historical evidence of adversities from the label information or previously submitted reports), timing of the event in relation to dosing, alternative causes, the role of overdose, and effects of dechallenge or rechallenge. Plans for improved submission include a web-based submission process.

The FDA website (http://www.fda.gov/AnimalVeterinary/SafetyHealth/ProductSafetyInformation/ucm055375.htm; accessed May 2010) can be reviewed for yearly and cumulative adverse event reports that have been reported in animals. Unfortunately, at the time of publication, the reports provide no evidence of frequency of occurrence, other than a ranking. This decision was made in part because of the inability of the FDA to standardize the number of adverse events by the number of doses administered (or units sold).

Predicting Drug Safety

Woodward[21] has demonstrated that, to some degree, studies implemented during the approval process tend to predict adversities that emerge in target species, but with marked limitations. Guengerich[26] has discussed the role of predictive toxicology based on drug chemistry in assessing clinical safety of drugs. Toxicities are likely to be predictive if the drug is characterized by a high level of intrinsic toxicity; for such drugs chemistry may often predict toxicity. Toxicity is less predictable, although still reasonably so if metabolism plays a role, but is much less predictable if the toxicity is idiosyncratic (i.e., type B or II).

IDIOSYNCRATIC REACTIONS: ALLERGIC DRUG EVENTS

The clinical manifestations of idiosyncratic ADRs vary with the type of reaction and the body system targeted. Generally, for allergies, previous exposure to the drug must occur regardless of the type of reaction, or therapy must have been sufficiently long (i.e., at 10 to 14 days for some drugs) for an allergic response to develop. However, exceptions appear to exist, as is exemplified by allergy-based reactions to sulfonamides, which may occur in as early as 5 days (see Chapter 7). Drugs generally are too small in molecular size (<1000 D) to be sufficiently antigenic. As such, drugs that induce an allergic response generally act as haptens, covalently combining with a body tissue that then also becomes antigenic. As a result, the allergic response may be directed toward the drug or tissue.[9] The hapten hypothesis is controversial because only a small percentage of persons develop a reaction, possibly because of a failure to develop tolerance. Failed tolerance may occur at one or more proposed sites. First, the role of metabolism in the formation of chemically reactive metabolites as the initial step in mediating idiosyncratic drug responses (including allergies) is increasingly supported by scientific studies. Those individuals that produce more metabolites appear to be more likely to fail to develop immune tolerance to a drug.[9] For the same reason, the dose of antigen exposure may determine the type of response. The role of CYP enzymes in idiosyncratic reactions (whether or not allergy based) is increasingly being recognized. Second, the metabolite must bind with an appropriate ligand, one with a high epitope density sufficient to induce an immune response. Third, an allergic response to a drug requires activity of an antigen-processing cell. As such, it may be more likely in the presence of inflammation, such as might be the case with a viral or bacterial infection or after stress or traumatic damage. Molecular signals that activate immune cells may also be more prevalent in the face of large concentrations of reactive metabolites because of their ability to induce oxidative stress.[9] Fourth, other factors that may determine emergence of an allergic response (i.e., failed tolerance) may include failed downregulation of regulatory factors. A balance toward protective t-helper (Th1 or 2) response may preclude emergence of an allergic response; a loss of balance may facilitate it. Accordingly, both genetic predisposition and environmental factors contribute to emergent drug allergies.[9]

KEY POINT 4-1 Drug allergies:
1. require previous exposure or treatment for 5 to 12 days.
2. generally involve metabolism to a reactive chemical, which serves as a hapten.
3. often involve binding of the hapten to a highly epitopic protein.
4. are facilitated by inflammation (e.g., infection).
5. might be manifested as types I through IV.

Type I allergic reactions (immediate or anaphylactic) are IgE mediated and result from the release of chemical mediators (e.g., histamine, serotonin, eicosanoids) from tissue mast cells or basophils. The reaction occurs within minutes after drug administration regardless of the dose administered (Figure 4-6). Clinical manifestations generally include nausea, vomiting, circulatory collapse, tachycardia, pulmonary edema, and neurologic signs. Urticaria and angioedema may also be evident. Clinical signs may be species dependent, depending on the shock organ of the species. The shock organ generally is the organ in which mast cells occur in greater numbers. In the dog the shock organs tend to be the liver and gastrointestinal tract; in the cat the shock organ generally is the lung, with fulminating pulmonary edema being a clinical manifestation.

The exact antigen that causes anaphylaxis may not be known. For example, even though anaphylaxis in microfilaremic dogs after administration of microfilaricides is well documented, the specific antigen released by the effect of the drug is not known.[27] When given to microfilaremic dogs, both dimethylcarbamazine and ivermectin can induce shock manifested as peripheral vascular collapse, dyspnea, bloody diarrhea, and other clinical signs and laboratory test results consistent with anaphylaxis.

Treatment of drug-induced anaphylaxis is directed toward prevention of the physiologic response to mediator release (i.e., epinephrine and antihistamines) and prevention of further histamine release (e.g., epinephrine and glucocorticoids;

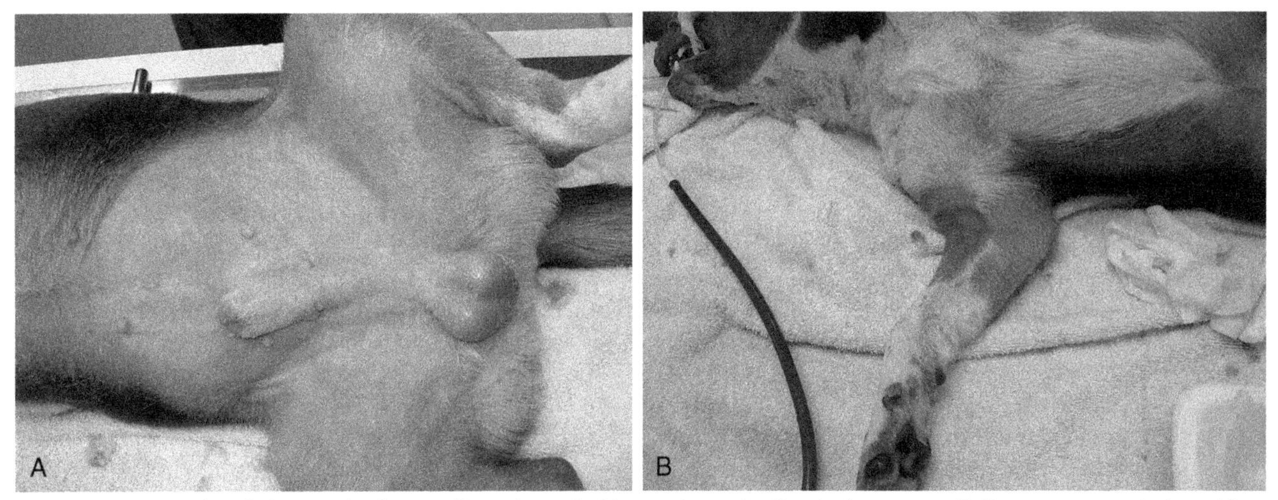

Figure 4-6 An example of dermatologic manifestation of either a type 1 allergic hypersensitivity or an anaphylactoid reaction. **A,** The former would involve antigen formation; **B,** whereas the latter would reflect a direct drug-induced histamine release from cutaneous mast cells. Skin lesions appeared 15 minutes after the puppy (undergoing an elective castration) received a preanesthetic dose of hydromorphone. (Courtesy Harry W. Boothe.)

possibly antihistamines). Ideally, antihistamines might also include the newer classes that may decrease mast cell degranulation as well as block H_1 receptors associated with histamine-mediated shock. Interestingly, and perhaps disconcertingly, glucocorticoids themselves have been associated with anaphylactic reactions (see Chapter 30).[28] Supportive therapy is also indicated. Prophylactic pretreatment in cases of anticipated anaphylaxis helps decrease the manifestations of anaphylaxis by decreasing the mast cell response. Drugs associated with type I allergic reaction in humans include penicillins, angiotensin-converting enzyme inhibitors (particularly in the first 3 weeks of therapy), nonsteroidal antiinflammatories drugs (NSAIDs), and opioids. However, the latter drugs may actually be more associated with an anaphylactic-like reaction, also referred to as an *anaphylactoid reaction.*

An anaphylactoid reaction is very similar to anaphylaxis but differs in that it is not mediated by an antigen-IgE response and thus is not allergic or immune mediated. Rather, selected drugs or compounds cause direct mast cell degranulation. Generally, these drugs are cationic (basic) and include opioids (particularly morphine [see Figure 4-6], polymyxin, radiographic contrast agents, thiacetarsamide, and amphotericin B). Hyperosmolar solutions such as mannitol can also cause direct mast cell degranulation. Adverse response to rapid intravenous administration of enrofloxacin, which is both hyperosmolar and basic, may represent an anaphlylactoid response or may simply reflect (in cats) stimulation of the chemoreceptor trigger zone. However, ciprofloxacin has been associated with an allergic response in humans,[29] and the author is aware of at least one dog treated with ciprofloxacin for which the adverse reaction met the World Health Organization category of "probable" ADR. Anaphylactoid reactions tend to be related to dose. As such, administration of a small test dose may help the clinician determine the likelihood of occurrence. Response is probably more likely with intravenous administration. In addition to the prophylactic measures for anaphylaxis, decreasing the rate of drug administration may help reduce the risk of the adverse response.

Type II reactions (cytotoxic) occur as antibody-bound blood cells become lysed and are removed from circulation. Lysis results from direct binding by either IgG or IgM. Complement may or may not be activated. Either stem cells in the bone marrow or mature circulating cells may be targeted. Targeting red blood cells, leukocytes, and platelets results in, respectively, hemolytic anemia, agranulocytosis and leukopenia, thrombocytopenia, or any combination thereof.

Type III drug reactions (immune complex disease, or serum sickness) are induced by antigen–antibody complexes involving either IgG or IgM and complement activation. Circulating antigen–antibody complexes may be filtered by and lodged in the vasculature of a number of organs, including the kidney, central nervous system (CNS), or peripheral vasculature. Clinical signs generally refer to the predominant organ affected but also include fever and lymphadenopathy. The Arthus reaction is a variation of the type III reaction and is manifested as swelling and pain at the site of drug administration. Among drug reactions in veterinary medicine, the potentiated sulfonamides are probably the most well-recognized cause of type III immune-mediated drug reaction.[30] Type IV drug reactions (delayed hypersensitivity, cell mediated) reflect cellular response at the site of the antigen. Lymphocytes and macrophages infiltrate the site and cause mediator release that perpetuates the inflammatory response.

The list of drugs that cause each type of drug-induced allergy is long and probably will remain incomplete. Although some drugs are more likely to cause a specific type of allergic reaction, any drug that causes allergy probably can cause any type of allergy, affecting any body system. Eventually, studies of structure–chemistry relationship involving metabolites and assessment of the immune system's response might allow identification of the patient at risk of developing an allergic response. Diagnosing an allergic (or any adverse) drug reaction can be very difficult and generally requires dechallenge (i.e., removal of the drug) and rechallenge. Clinical signs generally occur more promptly if the episode reflects reexposure to a previously administered allergen. The ethics of rechallenge (i.e., risk to the patient) may not justify confirmation of a presumed diagnosis. Peripheral eosinophilia and skin lesions often accompany an allergic drug response. ADRs in each of the body systems that have an allergic basis should be noted as such when possible.

Drug-induced allergy can be life threatening. Vasculitis and serum sickness are more likely to become life threatening when the kidney, liver, gastrointestinal tract, and nervous system become involved. Angioedema is life threatening if mucosal edema threatens ventilation.

Among the drugs recognized to be associated with drug allergies in dogs are the sulfonamides. Many medications contain a sulfonamide (a sulfur dioxide [SO_2] and nitrogen [N] moiety), including sulfonamide antimicrobials (derivatives of sulfanilamide in which the sulfonamide is attached to an aryl amine; e.g., sulfamethoxazole, sulfadiazine, sulfadimethoxine), "coxib" cyclooxygenase-1–sparing NSAIDs (e.g., deracoxib, firacoxib), carbonic anhydrase inhibitors (e.g., acetazolamide), diuretics (e.g., hydrochlorothiazide, chlorthalidone, furosemide), uricosurics (e.g., probenecid), drugs to treat inflammatory bowel disease (e.g., sulfasalazine), sulfonylureas (e.g., glyburide, glipizide), and selected anticonvulsants (e.g., zonisamide).[31] However, it is likely that a metabolite associated with the nitrogen moiety is responsible for the reaction, with reactions being limited to molecules containing an aryl-amine (both the sulfur and an amine moiety are attached directly to a benzene ring; sulfonylarylamine), a structure limited to sulfonamide antimicrobials. The underlying pathophysiology, clinical manifestations, and other aspects of the response have been well described[32,33] and are reviewed in Chapter 7.

ADVERSE DRUG EVENTS BY BODY SYSTEMS

Drugs causing adverse events in the various body systems are listed in tabular form in the respective sections on body systems. Discussion of the adverse reaction also can be found in the appropriate chapter. When available, treatments are offered, including tabular presentation (see Appendix 5).

Liver

The liver is vulnerable to drug-induced toxicity for several reasons (Box 4-1).[34-37] The potential for hepatotoxicity can be enhanced by dietary imbalance (high fat, low protein), presence of disease concurrent with administration of drugs that alter hepatic drug-metabolizing enzymes or hepatic blood flow,[37] and age.[38]

Drug-induced and chemical-induced liver injury have been classified into two categories.[34,35,37] Type I toxins, or intrinsic hepatotoxins, cause type A adverse events, which are predictable, dose and time dependent and occur in most, if not all, subjects exposed to appropriate doses of the substance. Any drug metabolized by the liver probably can cause some degree of type I hepatic disease simply by the production of phase I metabolites, which as a general rule tend to be toxic because of their reactivity. The longer the drug is used and the higher the dose, the more likely the ADE will occur. Type II, or idiosyncratic hepatotoxins, cause type B events, which are unpredictable and dose and time independent (consistent with Type B). Their occurrence is sporadic and not reproducible.

Drug-induced hepatotoxicity (Box 4-2) is associated with a wide range of histologic changes, from acute, reversible, and

Box 4-1
Hepatic Drug-Induced Toxicity

The liver is vulnerable to drug-induced toxicity for several reasons:

1. It receives a large portion of the cardiac output and thus is exposed to large amounts of drug.
2. The liver is a portal of entry and is exposed to the greatest concentrations of orally administered drugs.
3. The liver is the major site of metabolite formation. Thus the liver not only concentrates parent drugs but also is exposed to the greatest concentrations of their toxic metabolites.
4. The liver is a site of drug and metabolite excretion.
5. The liver is a highly metabolic organ and is susceptible to toxicities that induce hypoxia, interactions with enzymes, or loss of energy substrates.

Box 4-2
Examples of Drugs or Drug Classes Associated with Hepatotoxicity*†

Acetaminophen
Anabolic steroids
Deoxycholic acid
Diazepam (cats)
Glucocorticoids
Griseofulvin (cats)
Halothane
Isoniazid
Ketoconazole
Mebendazole
Megestrole acetate (cats)
Melarsomine
Methotrexate
Methoxyflurane
Mibolerone
Nonsteroidal antiinflammatories (including Cox-1–sparing drugs)
Oxibendazole
Phenobarbital
Phenytoin
Rifampin‡
Primidone
Sulfonamides
Thiacetarsamide

*Many other drugs that are metabolized by the liver are potentially hepatotoxic because of the production of phase I reactive metabolites.
†Microscopic lesions tend to be centrolobular in location, associated with necrosis, but otherwise nonspecific for most drugs.
‡In the author's experience, marked increase in serum alkaline phosphatase may occur but is not necessarily associated with hepatic dysfunction.

clinically benign lesions to those that cause fatal massive necrosis, chronic hepatitis, or malignancy.[34,35] Some drugs characteristically cause only a single lesion, whereas others cause multiple lesions. The lesions caused by any drug are rarely specific for that drug but can be caused by a variety of drugs or other disorders, often limiting the potential usefulness of biopsy (Figure 4-7).

Frequently, drug-induced hepatic injury is limited to select regions or zones (e.g., central, middle, or peripheral) in the lobule.[34,35] Various histologic lesions associated with drug hepatotoxicity have been described.[34,35] *Zonal necrosis* usually results from type I or predictable toxins. The production of toxic metabolites may be an important cause of zonal necrosis because drug-metabolizing enzymes predominate in zones most likely to develop necrosis. In most cases of acute injury, the process is either fatal or completely resolved. If exposure is chronic or recurring, however, the lesions may persist and progress, depending on the dose, agent, and health of the patient. *Lipid accumulation,* usually of triglycerides, may be associated with either minimal alteration of hepatic function or with both clinical and laboratory manifestations of liver dysfunction.

Nonspecific hepatitis is seldom associated with serious or progressive hepatic decompensation or failure and is fully reversible after discontinuation of the drug. *Chronic hepatitis* usually requires continued exposure and is not the result of self-perpetuation of an acute lesion. In general, prompt and complete resolution of this lesion can occur after timely discontinuation of therapy with the inciting drug. *Cirrhosis* generally requires prolonged or repeated exposure to the toxin. *Silent cirrhosis* is a term used to describe the gradual evolution of liver disease to cirrhosis without any clinical illness. Although methotrexate is among the most implicated drugs in humans, it is likely that many drugs that cause progressive liver disease do so "silently" for a long time.

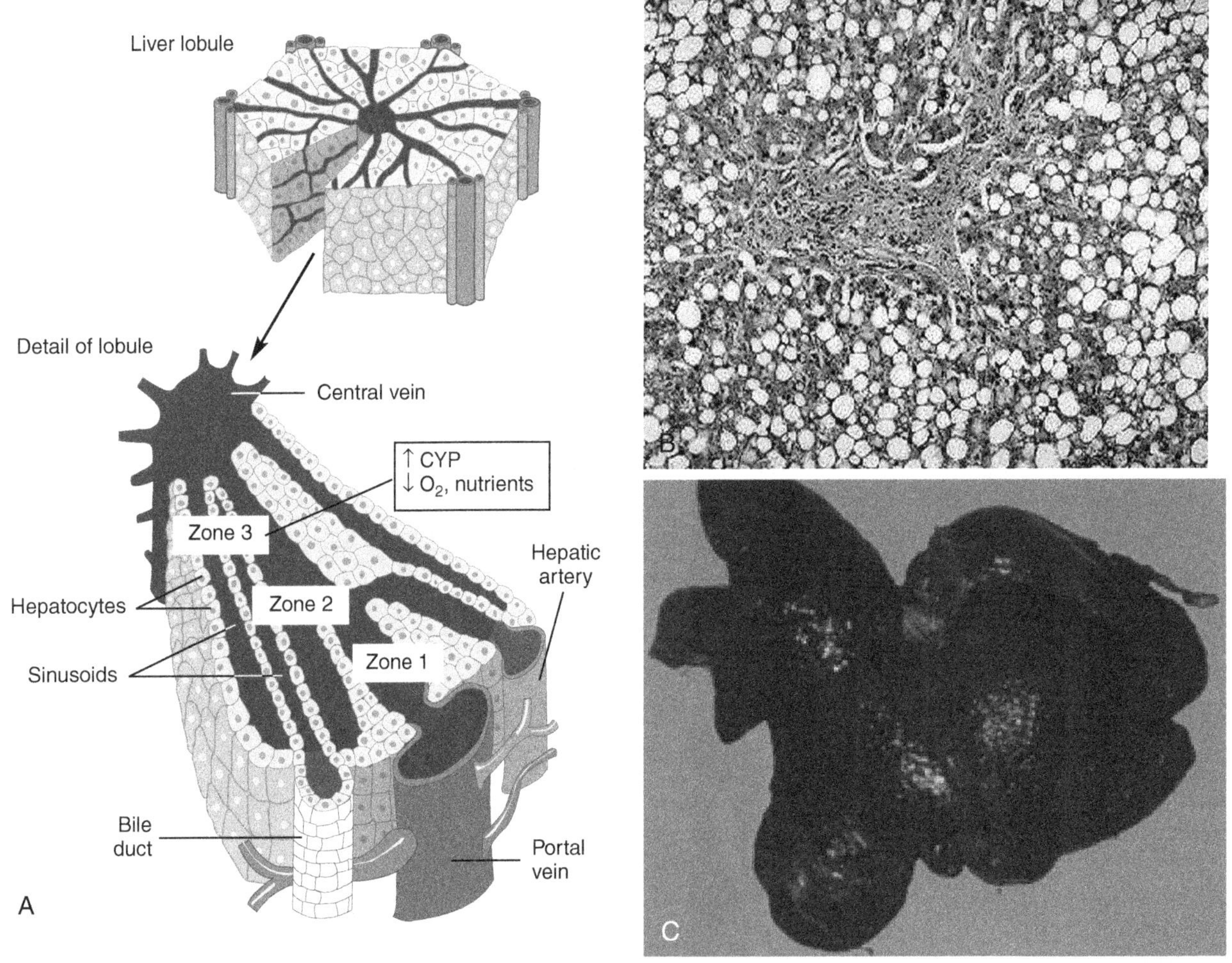

Figure 4-7 A, Drug-induced liver disease is generally nonspecific in presentation. Among the more frequent lesions are necrosis, particularly centrolobular, because hepatocytes in this region (zone 3) contain the most drug-metabolizing enzymes (i.e., production of toxic metabolites) yet receive the least oxygen. Hemorrhage and vacuolization are also common lesions. **B,** In the persistent presence of the toxin (including drug), the liver will continue to progress to irreversible changes, including the deposition of fibrous tissue as part of the cirrhotic process. **C,** A liver from a dog that died as a result of end-stage liver disease associated with phenobarbital concentrations above 50 µg/mL for 2 months. Clinical pathologic findings progressed from normal to indicative of end-stage disease within a 3-month period. (**A** from Cunningham CC, Van Horn CG: Energy availability and alcohol-related liver pathology, *Alcohol Res Health* 27(4):281-299, 2003.)

Drug-induced *cholestasis* is not well understood. Drugs can target bile ducts or canaliculi, causing primarily cholestasis without hepatocellular disease. When accompanied by an inflammatory infiltrate, systemic illness usually occurs, whereas cholestasis without inflammation is associated with no or very mild clinical signs. Recovery usually occurs after discontinuation of drug therapy.[34,35] Drugs can also affect primarily sinusoidal or endothelial cells, causing primarily *fibrosis* or *veno-occlusive disease*. Veno-occlusive disease tends to be predictable and is most commonly associated in people taking anticancer drugs. An immune basis has been recognized for some drugs causing clinical signs consistent with chronic active hepatitis.

Treatment of drug-induced liver disease is primarily supportive. Because reactive metabolites often either cause or exacerbate disease, however, use of compounds that help prevent metabolite damage to the liver should be considered. Specific examples include *N*-acetylcysteine, a precursor to intracellular glutathione; ascorbic acid, another type of oxygen radical scavenger; *S*-adenosylmethionine (SAMe), a compound that contributes to a number of methylation reactions in the body; and the herbal agent silymarin (see Chapter 19). Care must be taken to ensure that the duration of treatment exceeds the duration of activity of the toxicant, as has been demonstrated for *N*-acetylcysteine for treatment of acetaminophen toxicity.[39]

Hepatotoxic Drugs

Inhalant Anesthetics

Adverse events to inhalant anesthetics are unusual in veterinary medicine,[40,41] in part because duration of anesthetic exposure is limited. Historically, methoxyflurane administration in dogs has occasionally been associated with acute centrilobular necrosis accompanied by a mixed inflammatory infiltrate. Halothane-associated hepatic injury in the dog has not been confirmed, although a clinical case report has described acute hepatic necrosis after its use. In humans the degree and incidence of halothane-induced liver damage do not appear to correlate with the duration or number of exposures and therefore has been suggested to reflect an idiosyncratic hypersensitivity.

Mebendazole and Oxibendazole

The bendazole anthelmintics have been associated with liver pathology. Acute centrilobular hepatic necrosis and fatal fulminating hepatitis have been reported in dogs after the clinical and experimental administration of the anthelmintics mebendazole and oxibendazole.[42,43] Clinical signs were evident in as few as 2 days or as many as 10 to 14 days after administration. Although mebendazole was originally thought to be an intrinsic hepatotoxin, other studies suggest that it produces an idiosyncratic reaction.

Sulfonamides. Sulfonamide antimicrobials are associated with toxicity of multiple organs, including the liver.[30,32,33,44] Sulfonamides do not appear to differ in their likelihood of causing toxicity. In one report that supports an idiosyncratic reaction, the duration of therapy before hepatotoxicity developed ranged from 4 to 30 days, and the dose ranged from 18 to 53 mg/kg every 12 hours.[44] The mechanism of sulfonamide toxicity is discussed in more depth in Chapter 7.

Thiacetarsamide and Melarsomine. Thiacetarsamide (caparsolate) is associated with hepatic injury in humans and animals. Chronic exposures in humans are more likely to cause clinically significant hepatic disease. Hepatotoxicity is, however, a common complication of acute administration of thiacetarsamide for heartworm disease in dogs, although residual effects after therapy is completed are not expected (see Chapter 14). In normal animals melarsomine causes less hepatotoxicity and renal toxicity than thiacetarsamide.[45]

Bile Acids. Bile acids are hepatotoxic, and they contribute to the development of hepatitis in patients with cholestasis, regardless of the origin. Bile acids are also used therapeutically as choleretics. Among the bile acids present endogenously and used therapeutically, however, those that are lipid soluble (e.g., deoxycholic acid) are more hepatotoxic than those that are water soluble (e.g., ursodeoxycholic acid). Ursodeoxycholic acid rather than deoxycholic acid should be used for therapy. Bile acid therapy should be discontinued in the event of cholecystectomy.

Xylitol. The sugar alcohol xylitol is associated with life-threatening hypoglycemia and hepatic necrosis in dogs. Most cases, reported by the American Society for Prevention of Cruelty to Animals (ASPCA) Poison Control Center, reflect over ingestion of products containing xylitol as a sweetener (a small to average cookie may contain approximately 4 g xylitol). In contrast to humans, xylitol induces a ten-fold increase in insulin secretion in dogs compared to an equivalent amount of glucose. The result is a precipitous drop in serum glucose within 30 to 60 minutes after ingestion of as little as 100 mg/kg. Onset of hypoglycemia may be offset for 12 hr if xylitol-containing gum is ingested. Lethargy, ataxia, collapse, and seizures may occur. Clinical pathology may also reveal hypokalemia as potassium moves into the cell with glucose, and hypophosphatemia as a result of insulin's effects on cell permeability.[45a,b] The impact on cats is not clear. More recently, hepatic necrosis has been reported in dogs ingesting xylitol. Enzyme increases within 12 to 24 hours after ingestion of 500 mg/kg or more are followed by clinical signs and sequelae, including coagulopathies consistent with acute hepatopathy. Hyper- rather than hypophosphatemia associated with acute hepatopathy may be a poor prognostic indicator. Sorbitol does not appear to be associated with toxicity in dogs.

Kidney

Like the liver, the kidney is vulnerable to drug-induced toxicity for several reasons (Boxes 4-3 and 4-4).[46] Specific cellular or subcellular sites of nephrotoxins frequently are not known. Usually, a toxin affects more than one type of renal tissue because of the high drug concentrations to which the kidney is exposed. The glomerulus is susceptible to direct nephrotoxicity as well as to indirect toxicity such as that caused by immunologic injury.[46] Many nephrotoxins cause predominantly proximal tubular damage. This is expected in part because blood flow is greatest in the renal cortex, where

Box 4-3

Examples of Drugs Associated with Nephrotoxocity

Acyclovir
Aminoglycosides
Amphotericin B
Angiotensin-converting enzyme inhibitors
Bacitracin
Carboplatin
Cephaloridine
Cisplatin
Colistin
Cyclosporine (humans)
Foscarnet
Ganciclovir and other antiviral drugs
Iodine radiologic contrast agents (intravenous)
Methoxyflurane
Nonsteroidal antiinflammatory drugs
Polymyxin B
Sulfonamides
Tetracyclines
Thiacetarsamide
Vancomycin (in combination with other nephrotoxic drugs)

Box 4-4

Renal Drug-Induced Toxicity

The kidney is vulnerable to drug-induced toxicity for several reasons:

1. Renal blood flow accounts for 25% of cardiac output, exposing the kidneys to large amounts of blood-borne drugs.
2. Reabsorption of salt and water in the proximal tubules results in progressive concentration of drugs in the glomerular filtrate.
3. Passive drug reabsorption exposes the tubules to even greater concentrations of drug.
4. The kidney contains drug-metabolizing enzymes, thus increasing its exposure to potentially toxic metabolites.
5. The kidney is sensitive to extrarenal factors (e.g., those that induce ischemia or dehydration) that can predispose the kidney to or exacerbate drug-induced renal damage .

the proximal tubules are located. Variations in proximal tubular susceptibility to toxins may reflect different tubular functions.[46,47]

A study in human medicine focused on the use of nephrotoxic drugs in the critical care patient.[48] Reductions in renal blood flow associated with hemodynamic responses to a myriad of illnesses predisposes the ICU patient to acute renal failure which occurs in 6% of human ICU patients. Prolonged use of vasopressors increases the risk of renal hypoxia. Additionally, of note, the use of low-dose dopamine (≤3 μg/kg/min) as a nephroprotectant, particularly in patients with acute renal failure (representing at least 6% of ICU patients) was discouraged. Although renal vasodilation and urine flow increase, outcome does not improve, and the increased risk of cardiac or other adversities balances any potential nephroprotection.[48] NSAIDs were cited as a particular risk in ICU patients; newer drugs that target COX-2 do not appear to offer an advantage in regard to nephrotoxicity. Nephrotoxicity induced by NSAIDs in the critical care environment occurs rapidly and is manifested as a rapid increase in serum creatinine. If an NSAID must be used in the ICU patient, one with a short half-life is recommended, and use of other nephroactive drugs (those that alter renal blood flow) are discouraged.[48] The ICU patient also is at increased risk for aminoglycoside toxicity, with urine enzymes the earliest indicator. Clinical evidence of nephrotoxicity occurs within 5 to 10 days of therapy; once-daily (or less frequent) therapy reduces the risk. Likewise, amphotericin B often is associated with acute renal dysfunction. Sodium-containing fluids and lipid-based products are recommended in the patient at risk. The use of nacetylcysteine to protect the kidney should be considered for selected drugs.

Nephrotoxic Drugs

Most nephrotoxic drugs are discussed in relevant chapters. *Methoxyflurane* causes a dose-dependent, high-output nephrotoxicity in humans. Toxicity appears to be the result of oxalate metabolites and inorganic fluoride. Oxalate metabolites crystallize in and obstruct the tubules, whereas inorganic fluoride produces tubular necrosis.[42] Veterinary reports of methoxyflurane-induced nephrotoxicity are rare, probably because veterinary patients are at a reduced risk of developing nephrotoxicity because exposure (surgery) times are much shorter than in humans.[49]

Trivalent *arsenicals* such as thiacetarsamide denature proteins by binding to sulfhydryl groups. The glomerulus is often the first site of arsenical-induced nephrotoxicity, but proximal tubule damage predominates, probably because of the large number of enzymes that are denatured in this region.[46] Initial proteinuria is followed by tubular necrosis and degeneration.

Gastrointestinal

Stomatitis may progress to ulcerations with several drugs, particularly antineoplastic agents. Those most likely to cause stomatitis are listed in Table 4-1. A number of drugs are sufficiently caustic that ulcerations occur if the drug remains in contact with the mucosa (see Table 4-1). A number of drugs, including doxycycline and other drugs administered orally as a tablet have been associated with local mucosal damage and subsequent esophageal strictures in cats (see Chapter 19).

Although not an ADE, several drugs can cause tooth discoloration. Among the most recognized are tetracyclines, which chelate to calcium of either dentin or enamel, resulting in a yellow to brown discoloration. Oxytetracycline causes the least discoloration. The effect occurs during tooth development and is one reason that tetracyclines should not be administered to pregnant animals. The time that must lapse postpartum is not clear in animals. (It is up to 8 years of age in children.) Minocycline can cause discoloration despite animal age, probably as a result of chelation of iron resulting in insoluble complexes. Oral iron solutions can cause transient superficial discoloration of teeth, which can be removed. Other compounds associated with tooth discoloration in humans include isoproterenol, ciprofloxacin (a greenish-yellow discoloration when used in

Table 4-1 Examples of Drugs Associated with Gastrointestinal Toxicity

Ulceration/Erosions	Xerostomia		Gingival Hyperplasia	Taste disturbance	Miscellaneous	
Antineoplastic drugs	Anticholinergic-like drugs	Omeprazole (gastric)	Omeprazole (gastric)	ACE inhibitors	Angioedema	Drugs associated with allergic response (many)
Those More Likely to Cause Stomatitis		Phenytoin (gingival)	Phenytoin (gingival)	Diuretics		
Melphan	Sodium channel blockers (gingival)	Sodium channel blockers (gingival)	Griseofulvin	Griseofulvin	Microflora disruption	Many antimicrobials, especially with biliary elimination
Thiotepa	Calcium channel blockers (gingival, especially nifedipine)	Calcium channel blockers (gingival, especially nifedipine)	Metronidazole	Metronidazole		
Doxyrubicin		Antiparkinson's drugs	Carbenicillin	Carbenicillin		Drugs associated with achlorhydria
Epirubicin	Diuretics		Chlorhexidine	Chlorhexidine	Nausea/vomiting	Direct stimulation of chemoreceptor-triggering zone
Idarubicin	Bronchodilators (systemic)		Calcium channel blockers (diltiazem)	Calcium channel blockers (diltiazem)		Cardiac glycosides
Busulfan	Beta-blockers		Gold salts	Gold salts		Opioids
Procarbazine	Muscle relaxants		Vitamin D	Vitamin D		Many others
Dactinomycin	Narcotics		Sulfasalazine	Sulfasalazine		Anticancer drugs
Mitoxantrone			Cyclosporine			Drugs that alter gastric motility
Methotrexate						Erythromycin
Fluorouracil						Doxycycline (?)
Cytarabine					Teeth discoloration	Tetracyclines
Etoposide						
NSAIDs						
Those Causing Local Erosions						
Doxycycline (esophageal; cats)						
Aspirin						
Phenylbutazone						
Indomethacin						
Silver nitrate						
Hydrogen peroxide						
Isoproterenol						
Phenols						
Acids/alkalis						
Potassium chloride						
Fluorinated quinolone (especially large animal formulation)						

ACE, Angiotensin-converting enzyme; *NSAIDs*, nonsteroidal antiinflammatory drugs.

infants), and chlorhexidine (reversible yellowish-brown stains when used as a mouth rinse for more than several days).

Xerostomia (dry mouth) has been associated with anticholinergics and drugs with anticholinergic-like effects (see Table 4-1), as well as other drugs. Taste change is more discernible in humans and is caused by a number of drugs, including several antimicrobials (see Table 4-1).

Most orally administered drugs are probably capable of causing nausea or vomiting simply as a result of irritation or stimulation of the gastrointestinal tract mucosa. Erythromycin, for example, is a prokinetic agent and, as such, may cause upset in up to 50% of animals taking the drug. A patient with disease of the gastrointestinal tract is predisposed to these side effects. Many intravenous drugs also cause nausea or vomiting, particularly if given rapidly because of stimulation of the chemoreceptor-triggering zone. A number of drugs are recognized for their tendency to stimulate this zone regardless of the route of administration. Examples include digoxin, anticancer drugs, and most opioids.

Gingival hyperplasia has been reported for several drugs, including phenytoin and (in humans) calcium or sodium channel blockers.[50] The risk of its emergence might be reduced with good dental hygiene; in dogs it responded to metronidazole therapy.[51] Gingival hyperplasia is a recognized side effect of cyclosporine administration in dogs and cats (package insert, Atopica); 31% of the dogs developed gingival hyperplasia and gingivitis, which responded to metronidazole and spiramycin.[51] However, the more common effect of drugs on the oral mucosa is erosion. A number of drugs cause direct erosion with prolonged contact, especially in the feline esophagus (Table 4-1). Any drug that is antianabolic or inhibits cellular division is potentially toxic to the gastrointestinal tract by impairing the rapid turnover of epithelial cells in the mucosa (see Table 4-1). Tetracyclines and chloramphenicol are antianabolic, although long-term administration is necessary before these drugs affect the gastrointestinal tract.

Anticancer chemotherapeutic drugs best exemplify drugs that decrease epithelial cell turnover. Among the drugs most commonly causing gastrointestinal disease in veterinary medicine are the NSAIDs. These drugs inhibit prostaglandins, which in the gastrointestinal tract mucosa serve to inhibit gastric acid secretion, stimulate bicarbonate and mucus production and epithelialization, and increase blood flow. Among the NSAIDs most likely to cause gastrointestinal tract ulceration are aspirin, which also directly irritates the gastrointestinal tract mucosa, and ibuprofen, whose therapeutic range in the dog appears to be higher than the toxic range. Selected antimicrobials alter the microflora of the gastrointestinal tract and can subsequently cause diarrhea. Achlorhydria induced by a number of drugs can lead to gastrointestinal upset by changing microflora.

Torpet[50] has reviewed oral side effects of cardiovascular drugs in humans. The list of possible lesions is impressive, as are the number of drugs associated with lesions, which suggests that the oral mucosa (at least in humans) is sensitive to the effects of many drugs. Lesions include taste disturbances (diuretics, angiotensin-converting enzyme inhibitors), xerostomia (e.g., alpha-agonists and beta or calcium channel blockers, angiotensin-converting enzyme inhibitors), gingival overgrowth (calcium and sodium channel blockers) and ulcerations, as well as a number of syndromes associated with cutaneous lesions indicative of drug allergies, including angioedema (many).

Nervous System

Because of the brain's role in integrating the body, toxic injury to one of its areas can result in manifestations from another site. Likewise, drugs that cause injury to other systems can result in CNS damage caused by metabolic changes (e.g., hypoglycemia, hypoxia). The high metabolic rate of neurons and their marked need for nutritional support render this system more susceptible than others to damage.[15] Neurons are uniquely dependent on the cell body to provide support for the dendrites and axons; the axon, which is devoid of metabolic function, depends on axonal transport for supplies to meet its metabolic needs. Drugs or chemicals that interfere with axonal transport ultimately lead to axonal atrophy.[15] The CNS is also uniquely lacking in effective regenerative capacity. Lesions of CNS damage therefore persist, leading to additive effects after subsequent exposures to a toxic compound, as well as delayed manifestations when neuronal reserve can no longer compensate for the abnormalities. Some toxicities may not occur until age-related attrition of neurons causes decompensation, thus prolonging the time between cause and effect and decreasing the likelihood that the relationship between exposure and neurotoxicity will be recognized.[15]

The blood–brain and blood-CSF barriers limit the incidence of adverse events in the CNS. Increased permeability of this barrier, however, such as might occur in pediatrics or disease, predisposes animals to CNS events. All CNS-active drugs are likely to cause CNS signs if the dose is too high. Drugs that can induce seizures in epileptic patients, and should therefore be avoided, include butyrophenones, metoclopramide, tricyclic antidepressants, and reportedly (although little literature supports this fact) glucocorticoids (Table 4-2). The impact of phenothiazines on seizure activity is less clear (see Chapter 27). A number of antimicrobials can cause seizures. The fluorinated quinolones have received some attention for their possible CNS side effects and, in particular, potentiation of seizures. The mechanism of action appears to be inhibition of gamma-aminobutyric acid–receptor interactions and may (although this has not yet been proven) be facilitated by the presence of NSAIDs.[52] High doses are therefore discouraged, particularly in predisposed patients. Several other antimicrobials are associated with CNS toxicity in people.[53] These include the beta-lactams, with imipenem and cefazolin being the most epileptogenic (see Table 4-2). Metronidazole also is associated with CNS adverse effects. Clinical signs of metronidazole toxicity in the dog include ataxia, nystagmus, and stumbling. Signs may not occur for 7 to 12 days after therapy is begun (see Chapter 7). Seizures may take up to 2 weeks to resolve; therapy is supportive. Signs may be more dramatic in the cat, including seizures and blindness. Toxicity has been reported at doses as low as 30 mg/kg every 24 hours.[54] Seizures respond

Table 4-2 Examples of Drugs Associated with Adverse Drug Reactions in the Central Nervous System

Drug	Manifestation
Beta-lactams (cefazolin)	Hyperexcitability, depression, aggression, seizures
Amitraz	Sedation, ataxia, muscle weakness
Aminoglycosides	Neuromuscular blockade
Antidepressants	Hyperexcitability, depression, aggression, seizures, ataxia
Antihistamines	Sedation, excitement
Benzyl alcohol	Hypersynthesis, ataxia, aggression, depression, coma (cat)
Beta-lactams (cefazolin and imipenem)	Lowered seizure threshold, ataxia
Bismuth	Lethargy, somnolence
Butyrophenones	Lowered seizure threshold
Enrofloxacin	Seizures, exacerbated by coadministration of NSAIDs; dizziness
Erythromycin	Seizures, others
Glucocorticoids	Lowered seizure threshold with long-term therapy
Griseofulvin	Ataxia, seizures
Hexachlorophene	Neuropathy
Ivermectin	Depression, lethargy, seizures, others
Lidocaine	Seizures
Metoclopramide	Hyperexcitability, lowered seizure threshold
Metronidazole	Ataxia, nystagmus, seizures
Milbemycin	Depression, lethargy, seizures, other
NSAIDs	Nonseptic meningitis (naproxen), exacerbation of seizures caused by fluorinated quinolones
Opioids	General CNS depression
Phenobarbital	Hyperexcitability, depression
Phenothiazines	Lowered seizure threshold
Quinolones	Seizures, other
Sulfonamides	Aseptic meningitis
Vincristine	Neuropathy
Nitrofurantoin	Peripheral neuropathies

CNS, central nervous system; *NSAIDs*, Nonsteroidal antiinflammatory drugs.

to diazepam therapy. NSAIDs are associated with CNS side effects, particularly if combined with fluoroquinolones with unsubstituted piperazinyl rings (ciprofloxacin) at position 7.[55]

The CNS toxicity of the avermectins, including ivermectin, selamectin, moxidectin, and milbemycin, results from enhancement of gamma-aminobutyric acid–receptor interactions.[56-58] The role of P-gp deficiency in avermectin CNS toxicity in Collies, Australian Shepherds,[59] and related breeds has been well established (see Chapters 2 and 3).[60] Doses as small as 100 g/kg can cause toxicity in these breeds. Toxicity will, however, also occur in any animal that is sufficiently overdosed. Clinical signs, which may not occur for 2 or 3 days, include emesis, diarrhea, salivation, fever, disorientation, ataxia, trembling, seizures, depression, coma, and blindness. Although picrotoxin or physostigmine (0.06 mg/kg, slow intravenous administration) have been recommended as an antidote, success is not well documented. Treatment with neostigmine (125 μg twice at 6-hour intervals and then daily for 2 days) along with fluid therapy was associated with success in an adult cat receiving 15 mg (16 times the recommended dose) of ivermectin but was unsuccessful in two kittens, each receiving 7.5 or 15 mg of the drug.[61] Picrotoxin is associated with toxicities (seizures), and its use is not recommended unless the patient is comatose. One report cites a dose of 1 mg/min (as a 0.1% dilution in 5% dextrose) given as an intravenous drip until clinical response was evident (8 minutes). Seizures in the patient responded to anticonvulsant therapy.[62] Supportive therapy is also indicated. Collies and related breeds with the MDR1 deletion mutation may also be at risk of reaction to other CNS-active drugs that serve as a substrate for P-gp (see Chapters 2 and 3). For example, the MDR1 deletion mutation responsible for the toxicity also has been associated with loperamide toxicity in a Collie receiving 0.14 mg/kg twice daily.[63]

Amitraz has a number of effects. It stimulates alpha-2 receptors in the CNS and alpha-1 and -2 receptors in the periphery, inhibits monoamine oxidases responsible for synaptic removal of monoamines such as dopamine and norepinephrine, and inhibits the synthesis of prostaglandin E2, although the clinical impact of this latter effect is not clear. Sequelae of β2 adrenergic stimulation includes cardiovascular effects such as bradycardia and vasodilation, leading to hypotension, although peripheral alpha stimulation may cause hypertension. CNS effects of sedation, disorientation, and ataxia may progress to coma. Decreased insulin release results in hyperglycemia. Gastrointestinal effects include gastrointestinal stasis, and therefore atropine or other anticholinergics are contraindicated. Clinical signs of amitraz toxicity may reflect the vehicle, which contains xylene and propylene oxide. Signs of acute xylene toxicosis include CNS depression, ataxia, impaired motor coordination, nystagmus, stupor, coma, and episodes of neuroirritability. Treatment is largely supportive and includes alpha antagonists such as yohimbine (0.1 to 0.2 mg/kg, administered subcutaneously), which are used to reverse alpha side effects. For life-threatening hypotension, positive inotropes should be used cautiously. Control of seizures with diazepam has been contraindicated in the veterinary literature but is supported for treatment of amitraz-induced seizures in children.[64]

Metronidazole can cause CNS derangements in dogs receiving 60 mg/kg or less; duration is dose and duration dependent. Signs may not occur for 7 to 12 days after therapy is begun (see Chapter 7). Clinical signs including ataxia and nystagmus and seizures may take up to 2 weeks to resolve; therapy is supportive.

The potential for phosphate enemas to induce life-threatening CNS derangements has been well documented, particularly in cats. Toxicity is associated with hyperphosphatemia, hypocalcemia, hypernatremia, hyperglycemia, hyperosmolality, and metabolic acidosis. Onset of clinical signs (ataxia, tetany, convulsions, weak pulse, and hypothermia) is rapid and may rapidly progress to death. Treatment is supportive, including (cautious) calcium therapy. A similar phenomenon has been reported after administration of a phosphate-containing urinary acidifier in cats.[65]

Benzoic acid (alcohol or benzoate) is a preservative commonly added to oral and parenteral drugs at concentrations of 5% or higher. Benzyl alcohol can cause CNS toxicity (characterized by hyperesthesia and depression), particularly in cats. The drug is rapidly metabolized to benzoic acid and subsequently to hippuric acid and benzyl glucuronide. Glucuronide deficiency in cats results in accumulation of benzoic acid. Pharmacists may not be aware that the glucuronide deficiency of cats predisposes them to toxicity with products containing benzoic acid.[66] Although the original dose necessary to induce toxicity in the cat was as high as 2 g/kg, clinical cases and experimental studies indicate that even a lower dose can be lethal. Diets containing benzoic acid at 0.2% to 2% (0.2 to 2 gm/dL) have caused clinical toxicities. The death of up to 30 cats in England[66] led to experimental studies that determined the maximum tolerable single dose of benzoic acid to be 450 mg/kg; accumulation with multiple doses limits the highest daily dose to 200 mg/kg.[67] For example, a product containing 5% benzoic acid contains 5 g/dL or 50 mg/mL (50 mg/g for dry weight products), limiting a single dose to 9 mL/kg, or a daily dose to 4 mL (4 g/kg). Drugs also can be prepared as benzoate salts, although toxicity is less likely because less benzoate is administered on a mg/kg basis. For example, 40% of metronidazole benzoate is benzoate. A dose of 20 mg/kg delivers 12 mg/kg of metronidazole and 8 mg/kg of benzoate. A daily dose of approximately 500 mg/kg of metronidazole benzoate would be necessary to induce benzoate toxicity in the cat, a dose that would be difficult to achieve even with exceeding the recommended dose of 16 mg/kg metronidazole benzoate twice daily.

Tricyclic and other antidepressants can cause a variety of CNS disorders by virtue of their stimulatory effect on several CNS neurotransmitters and potentially inhibitory effects at other sites. Because these transmitters often modulate the normal physiology of multiple body systems, the clinical manifestations of events to these drugs can be diverse and subtle and affect other body systems. Manifestations related to the CNS include seizures, change in behavior, and depression. Many of the side effects caused in people probably cannot be detected in animals (e.g., blurred vision, dizziness, dry mouth). These drugs have not been well studied in animals, but clinical reports suggest up to 25% of animals may show an adverse reaction to these drugs. Clinical signs include increased or decreased appetite, hyperactivity, polydipsia, diarrhea, anxiety, and fear. The disposition of the drugs in humans includes lipid solubility, hepatic metabolism, and high protein binding, all of which are conducive to drug interactions. Toxicity is enhanced when drugs are used in combination. Because the effects of these drugs take several weeks to be realized, doses may be inappropriately increased, further increasing the risk of toxicity.

Peripheral neuropathies have been associated with a number of drugs. In humans peripheral neuropathy associated with nitrofurantoin occurred at doses ranging from 1.5 to 4.5 mg/kg, with a time of onset ranging from 3 weeks to 12 months. Peripheral neuropathy was severe and irreversible in some patients. The aminoglycosides cause peripheral neuromuscular blockade by interfering with calcium-mediated acetylcholine release. This effect is potentiated in the presence of other neuromuscular blockers and anesthetics.

Special Senses

Ocular Toxicity

Ocular ADRs can reflect local or systemic administration.[68] Very occasionally, systemic side effects may result from topical administration of ocular drugs.[68] Identification of adverse events affecting the eye (Table 4-3) generally depend on postmarketing surveillance systems or case reports; in some cases (e.g., fluoroquinolones in cats), follow-up toxicity studies may document the causal relationship between drug and adversity.[69] Adverse events to drugs manifested in the eye will most likely reflect systemic administration, with the retina being the most common site of reaction. Among the more commonly reported adverse events affecting the eye is acute retinal degeneration associated with exposure of the retina to a light source in patients receiving phototoxic drugs.[70] A number of drugs used to treat cardiac disease have been associated with a variety of ocular lesions, including changes (increased or decreased) in intraocular pressure.[71]

Among the most notable ADEs manifested as ocular toxicity in animals is retinal degeneration in cats after administration of fluorinated quinolones. Although fluoroquinolones do not appear to cause a similar reaction in humans, reversible (corneal epithelial damage) and irreversible macular changes occur with administration of antirheumatic quinolones, chloroquine, and hydrochloroquine.[72] Clinical signs of retinal degeneration associated with fluoroquinolone damage in cats include partial, temporary, or total blindness, with damage generally recognized to be irreversible. Although the incidence is rare, toxicity does appear to be predictable and is associated with a higher incidence in special populations, including geriatric cats and feline patients with renal disease. The mechanism of toxicity appears to reflect a deficiency of an efflux transport protein in the feline retina.* Fluorinated quinolones are structurally similar to compounds known to cause ocular toxicosis associated with accumulation in lysosomes of retinal pigment cells; additionally, fluoroquinolones have a predilection for pigmented cells of the eye. The fluoroquinolones also have been associated with phototoxicity. The combination of fluoroquinolone with ultraviolet radiation produces both a time- and concentration-dependent ocular toxicity, with a methyl group at position 8 of the quinolone ring reducing the risk.[73] Reducing exposure to sunlight (dosing at night or keeping cats indoors) might be prudent for cats receiving fluoroquinolones, particularly if in a high-risk group.[25,69] Drugs associated with fluoroquinolone retinal degeneration are discussed in more depth in Chapter 7.

*Personal communication, K. Mealey, Washington State University.

Table 4-3 Examples of Drugs Associated with Adverse Drug Reactions Involving the Eye

Drug or Drug Class	Example Drugs	Lesion
Cardiac drugs	Hydralazine	Ocular involvement of systemic lupus erythematosus
	Beta blockers	Photophobia
		Reduced tear production
		Edema, conjunctivitis
	Digoxin	Yellow vision
		Amblyopia
Aurothioglucose		Gold deposits leading to vision deficits
		Keratopathy
		Cranial neuropathy
		Retinopathy
		Conjunctivitis
Methotrexate		Retinopathy
		Visual disturbances
		Optic neuropathy
Chlorpromazine		Blurred vision
		Cataract
		Pupillary dysfunction
		Retinopathy
		Corneal epithelial damage
		Accommodation dysfunction
NSAIDS	Ibuprofen	Blurred vision
	Naproxen	Photophobia
	Piroxicam	Retinopathy
Prednisone		Cataracts
		Glaucoma (open angle)
		Proptosis
		Exophthalmia
Interferon		Ischemic retinopathy
Ethambutol		Changes in visual acuity
Isoniazid		Conjunctivitis
		Scleral icterus
		Subconjunctival hemorrhage
		(Coagulopathy)
Sulfonamides		Keratitis sicca
Tetracyclines	Minocycline	Visual disturbances
	Tetracycline	Scleral pigmentation
	Doxycycline	
Quinolones	Hydroxychloroquine	Multiple: corneal deposits, retinal toxicity,
	Chloroquine	
Fluoroquinolones	Enrofloxacin	Acute retinal degeneration
(in order of risk; cats)	Orbifloxacin	
	Marbofloxacin	
	Ciprofloxacin	
Bisphosphonates	Pamidronate, all others	Episcleritis, nerve palsy, ptosis, neuritis
Sildenafil (phosphodiesterase 6 inhibitor)	Changes in color and light perception	
	Blurred vision	
	ERG changes	
	Photophobia	
	Conjunctival hyperplasia	
Topiramate	Acute narrow-angle glaucoma	
	Uveitis	
	Mydriasis	
Phenylephrine*	Topical 10%	Systemic hypertension, may be lethal (use 2.5% instead)
Beta blockers*	Timolol	Aggravation of bronchospasm, congestive heart failure, bradyarrhythmias, sinus arrest
Carbonic anhydrase inhibitors*		Sulfonamide-based allergic reactions
Prostaglandins analogs*	Travoprost	CNS side effects (malaise, etc.)
Anticholinergics*	Cyclopentolate 2% Tropicamide	Atropine-like (dry mouth, CNS effects)
Glucocorticoids*	Dexamethasone 0.1% Prednisolone acetate 1%	Adrenal gland suppression
Chloramphenicol*		Aplastic anemia (theoretical)

ERG, Electroretinography; CNS central nervous system.
**Indicates a systemic effect from topical drug.* This section of the table is from Gray C: Systemic toxicity with topical ophthalmic medications in children, *Paediatr Perinat Drug Ther* 7(1): 23-27, 2006.

Table 4-4 Examples of Drugs Associated with Adverse Drug Reactions Involving the Ear*

Class	Drug
Aminoglycoside antimicrobials	Streptomycin
	Amikacin
	Gentamicin
	Netilmicin
	Kanamycin
	Tobramycin
Other antimicrobials	Polymixin
	Erythromycin
	Colistin
	Chloramphenicol
	Minocycline
	Vancomycin
Antiseptics	Ethanol
	Benzalkonium chloride
	Chlorhexidine
	Iodine
	Iodophors
Diuretics	Furosemide
Cancer chemotherapeutic agents	Cisplatin
Nonsteroidal antiinflammatories	Salicylates, acetaminophen, naproxen, others
Others	Propylene glycol
	Detergents

*Most drugs administered topically in the ear may be associated with ototoxicity in the presence of a perforated ear drum.

Ototoxicity

Ototoxic drugs can damage both the auditory and the vestibular apparatus (Table 4-4).[74,75] Auditory toxicity is often unrecognized, particularly in the older patient, unless complete deafness occurs. Vestibular ototoxicity might be detected as nystagmus or head tilt. Other clinical signs (e.g., tinnitus) are likely to occur in humans, but these side effects largely go unrecognized in animals. Ototoxic drugs generally are associated with loss of hair cells in the organ of Corti, although the biochemical mechanism is seldom known. Ototoxicity can be either reversible or irreversible and is more likely in the presence of a perforated ear drum if drugs are applied topically.

Aminoglycosides are well known for their ototoxic potential. Aminoglycoside-induced ototoxicity generally is irreversible. In contrast to renal tissues, aminoglycosides are not actively accumulated in perilymph, and drug concentrations generally are less in perilymph than in serum. However, because the half-life of the drug is much longer in the perilymph than in serum, surpassing that in serum by days to weeks, exposure of cells to the drug is longer. Proposed biochemical mechanisms of ototoxicity caused by aminoglycosides include impaired glucose metabolism or inhibition of polyphosphoinositide turnover. Although allowing serum drug concentrations to become undetectable does not necessarily prevent ototoxicity, low trough concentrations as should occur with once daily therapy are none-the-less the best means of preventing ototoxicity. Ototoxicity is enhanced by the presence of loop-acting diuretics such as furosemide. The potential for ototoxicity varies among the aminoglycosides. Dihydrostreptomycin was designed as an alternative to streptomycin, which was vestibulotoxic,[76] but dihydrostrptomycin also proved to be significantly cochleotoxic and was subsequently withdrawn. Streptomycin and gentamicin are more likely to cause vestibular toxicity, whereas neomycin, kanamycin, tobramycin, and amikacin sulfate are more likely to cause auditory damage. Among these, amikacin is least cochleotoxic; neomycin is so cochleotoxic (and nephrotoxic) that it cannot be used systemically. Netilmicin, the newest of the aminoglycosides, may cause the least ototoxicity. Auditory damage induced by aminoglycosides is initially characterized by the damage to outer cochlear hair cells, with progressive damage targeting inner hair cells. Initial loss impacts high-frequency hearing.[76,77] Topical application of 0.1 mL of 3% gentamicin solution to the tympanic bulla was toxic to sensory receptors of the cochlea and the vestibular apparatus in cats.[78] Fluorinated quinolones also may cause ototoxicity when given topically.

Other drugs that cause irreversible ototoxicity include the antineoplastics vincristine and vinblastine. The antineoplastic cisplatin also causes irreversible ototoxicity morphologically similar to that caused by aminoglycosides after accumulation of multiple doses, with the effect being both dose and duration independent.[77] Toxicity occurs in the hair cells of the organ of Corti and causes predominantly auditory damage. Cisplatin-induced ototoxicity can be unilateral (and hence not always recognized) or bilateral. Occasionally, ototoxic effects are transient. Chloramphenicol also has been associated with ototoxicity in the cat when applied topically with Gelfoam soaked in a concentration of 400 mg/mL.[79] Vestibular toxicity caused by chloramphenicol has been documented in humans.

Vehicles and cleansing agents also may be associated with ototoxicity. Propylene glycol is a common vehicle of topical preparations. Its use is associated with granulation and ossification of the auditory bulla and morphologic changes in the organ of Corti. Some disinfectants (e.g., 0.5% chlorhexidine in 70% alcohol) or carrier agents (e.g., propylene glycol) can cause ototoxicity. These drugs cause both vestibular and auditory side effects. Whereas chlorhexidine can cause almost complete destruction of the vestibular and auditory apparatus (in animal models), 70% alcohol does not appear to cause any ototoxicity. Quaternary ammonium disinfectants (e.g., 0.1% benzethonium or benzalkonium chloride) are among the most ototoxic compounds studied. Iodophors also cause ototoxicity, but damage will not be as profound as with quaternary ammonium compounds. Although the mechanism is not known and the extent of ototoxicity is not clear, ceruminolytic agents should not be applied topically in the presence of a perforated ear drum if the label indicates.

Reversible ototoxic ADEs are unusual. Loop-acting diuretics are among the few ototoxic drugs that cause damage that is largely reversible; however, hearing defects may be permanent. Toxicity is limited to the auditory system and reflects morphologic changes in the stria vascularis of the cochlea. The mechanism of ototoxicity is not clear but may reflect acute electrolyte disturbances in the cochlear endolymph, similar to that producing diuresis.[77] Furosemide is the least ototoxic of the loop diuretics; presumably, its combination with aminoglycosides (or other ototoxic drugs) would increase the risk of ototoxicity. Several antiseptics produce irreversible ototoxicity, presumably as a result of cell membrane damage similar to that induced in bacteria.

Aspirin, and potentially other NSAIDs, can cause transient hearing loss in humans. Clinical signs generally resolve in 48 to 72 hours. Several possible sites of damage have been recognized, including a vascular basis (i.e., loss of vasoactive prostaglandins) or impaired neurotransmission. Other drugs known to cause ototoxicity include local anesthetics (0.5% lidocaine can cause cochlear damage), tricyclic antidepressants, and, very rarely, beta-blockers. Although not ototoxic by itself, dimethyl sulfoxide should be used cautiously because of its ability to carry other drugs into the inner ear when used as a vehicle.

Integument

The skin is the organ that most commonly manifests ADEs in humans.[80] Although the reactions are generally mild, they can become life threatening. The type of lesion varies and includes almost any type of lesion described for the skin. Lesions include wheal and flare reactions, erythema, blisters, lichenoid lesions, purpura, changes in pigmentation, necrosis, pustular lesions, and changes in hair growth. The most common reactions are erythematous macular or papular rashes that resolve in several days even if untreated. These manifestations may also, however, be a precursor to a severe manifestation and thus should be observed closely. As with many organs, because the skin contains drug-metabolizing enzymes, reactions can be due to either the parent compound or its metabolites (or both).

KEY POINT 4-2 The skin may be the organ most commonly associated with adverse reactions.

Drug-induced skin events may be a manifestation of an allergic response or an autoimmune disease mediated by the skin. Both type A and type B events occur in the skin. Of the type B events, all types of allergic events (i.e., types I through IV) can involve the skin. Type IV allergic events are best exemplified by contact dermatitis. "Late" events include allergic vasculitis, purpura pigmentosa, and erythema multiforme. A distinct form of allergic (phototoxic) events has been reported in humans and animals, involving the interaction of a drug (or its metabolite) with ultraviolet radiation; the lesion often manifests in light-exposed skin (discussed later). Fixed drug eruptions are not well understood. In humans they are characterized by erythema, often with a central blister, and may occur because regulation of adhesion molecules in the epithelium is disrupted. Drugs are capable of causing autoimmune reactions in the skin, including lupus erythematosus, pemphigus, and pemphigoid skin lesions. Life-threatening drug-induced events that occur in the skin of people include the Stevens–Johnson syndrome (SJS), toxic epidermal necrolysis (TEN), hypersensitivity syndrome, serum sickness, vasculitis, and angioedema.

Lesions of SJS and TEN may be difficult to differentiate; SJS may be a milder form of TEN. Both resemble scalded skin and reflect a cell-mediated cytotoxic reaction against keratinocytes (Figure 4-8). The diseases are characterized by blistering and extensive detachment of the epidermis. The lesions are irregular in shape and are distinguished from erythema multiforme, another drug reaction of the skin, by the irregular shapes and absence of a well-defined border and edematous ring. Both TEN and SJS tend to affect the trunk, whereas erythema multiforme has an affinity for extremities. Mucous membranes are frequently involved, and patients are generally febrile, particularly with TEN. The presence of neutropenia is interpreted as a poor prognosis in human patients suffering from TEN. Treatment of TEN includes a management protocol similar to that for extensive burns; infection with *Staphylococcus aureus* (which by itself can cause a "scalded skin" lesion) is likely to complicate therapy. Drug events are the primary causes of SJS and TEN; erythema multiforme is caused by selected microorganisms, as well as by drugs. Drugs associated with TEN and SJS in humans include sulfonamides, anticonvulsants, allopurinol, oxicams, and (less frequently) other NSAIDs.

The term *hypersensitivity syndrome* has been used in the past to refer to any skin ADR. As such, however, it encompasses a wide variety of skin lesions, each treated differently. More recently, the term has been used in human medicine for a syndrome characterized by mucocutaneous eruptions, fever, lymphadenopathy, hepatitis, and eosinophilia. Arthritis or nephritis may also develop. As with SJS and TEN, sulfonamides and anticonvulsants are the most common causes of drug hypersensitivity.

Vasculitis occurs as a result of necrosis and inflammation in blood vessel walls, most commonly in the lower extremities, after antibody interaction with blood vessel walls. Drugs are the primary cause of vasculitis in humans. Penicillins, sulfonamides, thiazide diuretics, phenytoin, and propylthiouracil are the most common interaction-related drugs. Serum

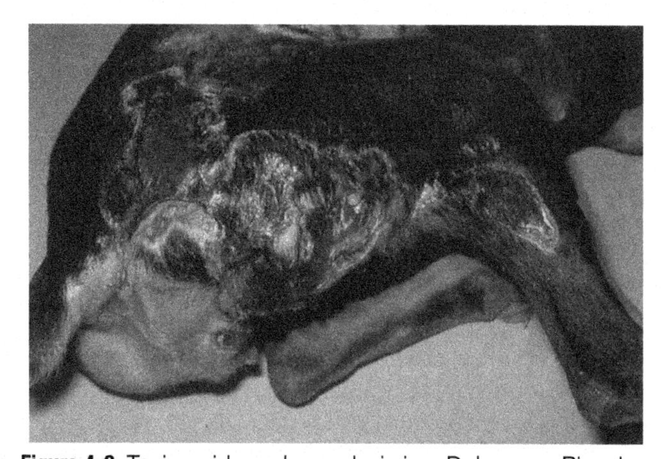

Figure 4-8 Toxic epidermal necrolysis in a Doberman Pinscher treated with chloramphenicol. Although the lesion is several weeks old, damage was evident within several days of intramuscular treatment.

sickness–like lesions in the skin also can appear as vasculitis. Lesions result from immune complex deposition in small vessels followed by complement activation and white blood cell infiltration. Lesions appear first as erythema and then progress to more severe eruption. Patients are usually febrile. Drugs that cause serum sickness manifested as dermatologic lesions in humans include selected cephalosporins, minocycline, penicillins, and propranolol.

Dermatologic manifestations of type I hypersensitivities occur at mucocutaneous junctions (including the mucous membranes of the eyes, mouth, nose, lips, or tongue) or present as pruritus, flushing, erythema, and urticaria. Of these, angioedema is the most life threatening because of the risk of upper airway obstruction. Treatment includes epinephrine (for acute respiratory distress), antihistamines, and glucocorticoids.

Skin eruptions have been attributed to a number of drugs in small animals (Table 4-5). Type I skin lesions accompany many cancer chemotherapeutic agents and gold-containing antiarthritic agents. Prednisone and phenytoin can cause alopecia. Most skin reactions reflect type B adverse drug events, however, and as such are largely unpredictable. Alopecia has been reported after oral administration of hetacillin (cat), prednisone (dog), parenteral gold therapy (dog), and phenytoin (dog and cat). Eczematous dermatitis has resulted from oral administration of sulfa drugs (dogs and cats), griseofulvin, diethylcarbamazine, and fluorocytosine. Topical neomycin–triamcinolone preparations and coal tar shampoos can produce generalized eczematous reactions. Generalized exfoliation has resulted from oral administration of quinidine, topical administration of lime sulfur dips, and the use of flea collars. Fixed drug eruptions have resulted from the oral administration of ampicillin and the intravenous administration of sodium thiacetarsamide. Pemphigus vulgaris–like reactions have followed thiabendazole oral therapy, and similar lesions have been reported with gold therapy. Erythematous dermatitis has been reported after the parenteral administration of a phenothiazine derivative. Pruritus has been reported after oral diethylcarbamazine, gold, and bromide (anticonvulsant) therapy. Purpura and lesions typical of TEN have occurred after oral administration of chloramphenicol (see Figure 4-8). Intravenous vitamin K and oral tetracyclines have caused urticaria and angioedema in the dog. Drug eruptions have also been associated with the systemic administration of levamisole. Human recombinant products such as erythropoietin have caused skin or mucocutaneous lesions typical of allergic drug events in dogs.

Hormonal therapy is often associated with predictable skin lesions, including bilaterally symmetric alopecia and hyperpigmentation (discussed later in reference to the endocrine system). The effects of glucocorticoids on the skin have been well documented and are often manifested as part of the cushingoid presentation of animals receiving therapy. Cyclosporine has been associated with changes in hair coat.[81]

Benzoic acid used as a preservative in topical preparations may cause cutaneous erythema, possibly caused by induction of inflammatory prostaglandins.[82] Ciprofloxacin was associated in a human patient with the development of erythema multiforme, which histologically was consistent with dermatitis herpetiformis.[29] Lesions developed on day 6 of therapy and responded to glucocorticoid therapy.

Photosensitization represents a novel mechanism of toxicity to selected drugs whose treatment occurs during exposure to electromagnetic radiation. Photosensitization occurs if a drug (or biological substrate) is characterized by an abnormally high reactivity to ultraviolet (UV) radiation (artificial or natural). Photosensitization requires the presence of *photosensitizers,* which induce changes in the drug after the appropriate radiation is absorbed (Box 4-5). Structural requirements of the photosensitizer to induce phototoxicity reflect its ability to absorb radiation wavelengths characterized by effective skin penetration (above 310 nm). As such, the photochemical decomposition to stable photoproducts, free radicals, and/or singlet oxygen is facilitated. The probable

Table 4-5 Examples of Drugs Associated with Adverse Dermatologic Manifestations

Drug	Manifestation
Ampicillin	Fixed drug eruption
Anticancer drugs	Alopecia
Bromide	Pruritus
Coal tar shampoos	Generalized eczema
Chloramphenicol	Purpura, TEN
Diethylcarbamazine	Eczematous dermatitis, pruritus
Erythropoietin, human recombinant	Skin or mucocutaneous lesions
Flea collars	Generalized exfoliation
5-Fluorocytosine	Eczematous dermatitis
Glucocorticoids	Alopecia, hyperpigmentation
Gold-containing drugs	Alopecia (dog), pruritus, pemphigus vulgaris–like reaction
Griseofulvin	Eczematous dermatitis
Hetacillin	Alopecia (cat)
Levamisole	Drug eruptions
Lime sulfur dips	Generalized exfoliation
Neomycin (topical)	Generalized eczema
Phenothiazine derivatives	Erythematous dermatitis
Phenytoin	Alopecia
Prednisone	Alopecia (dog)
Quinidine	Generalized exfoliation
Recombinant products, nontarget species	General skin or mucocutaneous lesions
Sulfonamides	Eczematous dermatitis
Tetracyclines (oral)	Urticaria, angioedema
Thiabendazole	Pemphigus vulgaris–like reaction
Thiacetarsamide	Fixed drug eruption
Vitamin K (intravenous)	Urticaria, angioedema
Cyclosporine	Altered hair coat
Many	Other cutaneous manifestations of allergies

TEN, Toxic epidermal necrolysis

Box 4-5

Examples of Drugs Associated with Known or Potential* Cases of Photosensitization

Acetazolamide	Isotretinoin
Alprazolam	Ketoprofen
*Amantadine	Levofloxacin
Amiloride	*Meclofenamic acid
Amitriptyline	Methotrexate
*Azathioprine	Minocycline
*Azithromycin	Nabumetone
*Benzocaine	Nalidixic acid
Captopril	Naproxen
Carprofen	Nifedipine
Chlortetracycline	Nortriptyline
Chlorothiazide	Ofloxacin
Ciprofloxacin	*Omeprazole
Clofazimine	Orbifloxacin
Clofibrate	*Osalazine
Clomipramine	Oxytetracycline
*Cyproheptadine	Paroxetine
Dacarbazine	Pentobarbital
*Danazol	*Phenobarbital
Dantrolene	Phenothiazine
Dapsone	Phenylbutazone
Diclofenac	Phenytoin
Diltiazem	Piroxicam
Doxepin	*Procaine
Doxycycline	Prochlorperazine
Enalapril	Promazine
Etretinate	Promethazine
Felbamate	*Pyridoxine
Flecainide	*Pyrimethamine
Fluoroquinolone antimicrobials	Quinidine
Fluorouracil	Silver sulfadiazine
Fluoxetine	Sulfamethoxazole
Furosemide	Sulfasalazine
Glipizide	Tetracycline
Glyburide	Tretinoin
Griseofulvin	Thiazine
Haloperidol	Tolbutamide
Hydralazine	Triamterene
Hydrochlorothiazide	Triflupromazine
Imipramine	Trimethoprim
Interferon beta	Valproic acid
Isoniazid	Vinblastine

role of fluoroquinolone antimicrobials as photosensitizers was discussed previously. Photosensitizers can be found in the cellular content of foods (e.g., flavins and porphyrins), plants or their juices, industrial chemicals (dyes, coal tar, derivatives of chlorinated hydrocarbons), and drugs. Exogenous photosensitizers may enter the body through a variety of routes, including ingestion, inhalation, injection, or direct contact with the skin or mucosa.[83] Biological targets subject to photosensitization include cell membranes, cytoplasmic organelles, and the nucleus. Photosensitization may be used therapeutically if it can be directed to targeted tissues or if UV radiation can be applied to selected sites (e.g., cancer therapy). Clinical signs vary with the photosensitizer and the amount of radiation absorbed. Signs range from mild cutaneous reactions (e.g., erythema, pruritus, urticaria and rash) to severe reactions including (in humans) genetic mutations and melanoma. Clinical signs generally occur immediately after exposure to the UV radiation. Variation may also reflect the skin type, as well as physiologic factors such as age and gender (human medicine). Photosensitivity is generally dose dependent but may not happen with the initial drug administration but rather with subsequent administration. The reaction is then referred to as a *photoallergy,* reflecting binding of the photosensitizer to a skin protein. Occasionally, the response may be delayed and may occur even in the absence of the photosensitizing substrate.

Endocrine System

The impact of xylitol on insulin secretion was discussed with its hepatotoxicity. Mechanisms of drug interference with the thyroid and adrenal axes have been documented in human patients (Table 4-6). Each axis presents several targets for drug interference. Mechanisms that decrease hormone concentrations include suppression of hormone release at each level (i.e., hypothalamus, pituitary, or target organ), often because hormone synthesis is decreased, or altered by peripheral metabolism of the hormone (e.g., thyroid hormones).[84] The latter effect is often the result of induction of hepatic drug-metabolizing enzymes. Potent inducers of hepatic drug-metabolizing enzymes include phenobarbital, phenytoin, and rifampin. Whether patients show clinical manifestations of hormone deficiency after induction of metabolizing enzymes remains to be documented. Less commonly, hormone concentrations are physiologically increased by drugs. Again, changes in hepatic metabolism are a common cause. Potent inhibitors of hepatic drug metabolism include cimetidine, chloramphenicol, and ketoconazole.

Drugs can also increase hormone concentrations by competing with and displacing the hormone from carrying proteins. The protein from which hormones are most likely to be displaced is albumin, a nonspecific carrier of many weakly acidic drugs (e.g., NSAIDs). Competition for albumin-binding sites may be less important for those hormones carried by specific carrier proteins, although competition for such binding sites has been documented. In some cases a drug may influence blood hormone concentrations simultaneously at several physiologic sites, complicating interpretation (e.g., the effects of phenytoin on thyroid hormone concentrations). Because animals differ physiologically, extrapolation between species regarding the effect of a drug must be done cautiously. Caution is also advised when extrapolating results of studies in normal animals to the animal suffering from a disease of the endocrine system. For example, propranolol decreases thyroid hormone concentrations in hyperthyroid humans but not in euthyroid dogs.[85]

In some instances the drug effect on a hormone is well known and is used either diagnostically (e.g., dexamethasone-induced decrease in cortisone or xylazine-induced growth hormone secretion)[86] or therapeutically (propranolol

Table 4-6 Drug-Induced Physiologic Changes in the Adrenocortical and Thryoid Axes*

Drug	Comment
Cortisol	
Increased	
Anticonvulsants	
Corticotropin	Diagnostic intent
Cortisone	For at least 24 hours
Estrogen	Increases binding globulin concentrations
Fluocinolone	After topical administration
Hydrocortisone	For at least 24 hours
Insulin	Marked effect with insulin-induced hypoglycemia
Lithium	
Metoclopramide	After intravenous dosing
Opiates	Within 1 hour of intravenous dosing with selected drugs
OPPPD (mitotane)†	Therapeutic intent
Prostaglandin F_2	Slight effect
Vasopressin	Mild increase
Decreased	
Barbiturates	Preoperative use
Beclomethasone	After inhalant administration
Clonidine	In growth hormone–deficient children
Danazol	Displacement from binding and increased free drug
Deoxycorticosterone	After topical administration
Dexamethasone†	Diagnostic intent
Ephedrine	Accelerated clearance caused by increased hepatic blood flow and enzyme activity
Etomidate	Direct suppression of adrenal function
Fluocinolone	After topical administration
Thyroxine	
Increased	
Dessicated thyroid	
Estrogens	Increased binding capacity of globulin for up to 1 month
Fluorouracil	Increased binding capacity
Glucocorticoids	Inhibition of conversion
Halothane	Increased release from liver
Insulin	Increased release from liver
Levothyroxine	Suppression of endogenous hormone; exogenous measured
Lithium	Report of one patient suffering from presumed drug-induced thyrotoxicosis
Phenytoin	
Propranolol	Blockage of iodothyronine deiodination in hyperthyroid and euthyroid patients
Prostaglandins	Direct effect
Tamoxifen	
Thyroid	
Thyrotropin	
Thyroid-releasing hormone (TRH)	
Decreased	
Aminosalicylic acid	Prolonged administration may cause hypothyroidism
Anabolic steroids	Decreased binding to globulins
Androgens	Decreased binding to globulins up to 1 month per administration
Anticonvulsants	
Asparaginase	
Aspirin	Displaces T_4 from binding sites to prealbumin
Barbiturates	Competition for binding to prealbumin
Bromocriptine	In hypothyroidism (response to TRH unchanged)
Carbamazepine	Induction of hepatic enzymes; increased extrathyroidal metabolism
Chlorpromazine	Increased metabolism by liver
Cholestyramine	Decreased intestinal absorption
Glucocorticoids	Up to 1 week after therapy
Diazepam	Competition for transport proteins
Furosemide	Displacement from binding sites and enhanced clearance
Growth hormone	Inhibition of thyroid-stimulating hormone (TSH) response to TRH (?)
Heparin	Modified binding to transport proteins (?) Decreased synthesis (therapeutic)
Iodides†	
Lithium	Reduced thyroidal iodine updake, iodination of tyrosine, release of T_4, hepatic metabolism of T_4 to T_3
Methimazole †	Therapeutic intent
Mitotane	Competes with T_4 for binding globulin
Penicillin	Competes for binding globulin
Phenobarbital	Induction of hepatic enzymes
Phenylbutazone	Impaired synthesis, competition for binding to albumin
Phenytoin	Displacement from binding proteins; induction of hepatic enzymes
Potassium iodide	
Propylthiouracil	Inhibits synthesis (iodination of tyrosine), therapeutic intent
Ranitidine	Slight reduction
Salicylate	Competition for transport proteins
Somatostatin	Inhibition of TSH release (?)
Stanozolol	
Sulfonamides†	
Terbutaline	Mild decrease
Triiodothyronine	

*Table reflects serum or plasma values only and is based on information reported by Young (1990).[11]

†Reported in the veterinary literature.

Table 4-6 Drug-Induced Physiologic Changes in the Adrenocortical and Thryoid Axes*—Cont'd

Drug	Comment	Drug	Comment
Triiodothyronine (Thyronine)		Anticonvulsants	
Increased		Asparaginase	
Estrogens	Increased binding capacity to transport proteins	Aspirin	
Fluorouracil	Increased binding capacity to transport proteins	Carbamazepine	Increased extrathyroidal metabolism
Heparin	Interference with binding to protein	Cimetidine	Reduced response to TRH
Insulin	45 minutes after injection; release from liver	Furosemide	
Phenytoin		Glucocorticoids	Inhibition of conversion
Prostaglandins		Iodides	Inhibition of conversion
Tamoxifen		Lithium	See under Thyroxine
Terbutaline		Phenytoin	See under Thyroxine
TRH	Percentage of free T_3 unchanged	Potassium iodide	
L-Thyroxine		Propranolol	Membrane stabilization (see under Thyroxine)
Triiodothyronine		Propylthiouracil	
Decreased		Salicylate	See under Thyroxine
Androgens	Decreased binding capacity (diminution of transport proteins)	Somatostatin	See under Thyroxine
		Stanozolol	See under Thyroxine
		Sulfonamides†	

TRH, Thyroid-releasing hormone.

or propylthiouracil-induced inhibition of thyroxine [T_4]). More commonly, the effect is undesirable. Several examples of undesired, drug-induced physiologic changes in endocrine function have been documented in small animal patients. The example most documented in small animals are the effects of drugs, and particularly glucocorticoids, on the hypothalamic–pituitary–adrenal axis. Interference with this axis can become clinically detrimental. Suppression of the adrenal axis by glucocorticoids is most marked after administration of depot (repositol) forms (e.g., those containing acetate esters).[87] Interference has also, however, been documented after administration of a single dose of prednisolone or triamcinolone; multiple doses of methylprednisolone;[87] topical administration of triamcinolone;[88] and ophthalmic administration of prednisone.[89] The impact of other steroids, including dexamethasone and betamethasone, are discussed in Chapter 17.

Glucocorticoids are not the only drugs that interfere with the hypothalamic–pituitary-adrenal axis. The imidazole antifungal drug ketoconazole inhibits the cytochrome P450 enzymes responsible for the synthesis of both sex and adrenal steroids.[90] Suppression of testosterone and cortisol has been documented in dogs after oral administration of 10 mg/kg ketoconazole once daily.[91] Hormone concentrations are lowered by day 1 and remain low at day 5. Progesterone concentrations increase as testosterone concentrations decrease. The magnitude of testosterone inhibition by ketoconazole apparently resolves, with testosterone concentrations being less predictable 1 month after therapy was started. The inhibitory effect of ketoconazole on testosterone and adrenal steroids has been used therapeutically in the treatment of prostatic cancer and benign prostatic hypertrophy and hyperadrenocorticism, respectively. The newer imidazole antifungal drugs do not appear to inhibit steroid synthesis as effectively as ketoconazole.

Drug interference with evaluation of the thyroid axis is also important because of the prevalence of thyroid dysfunction in small animals. Several drugs, targeting various sites, interfere with thyroid function testing (see Table 4-6).[92] Thyroid-stimulating hormone (TSH) response to thyroid-releasing hormone (TRH) is altered by a number of drugs that modulate neurotransmitter (e.g., serotonin, dopamine) concentrations in the brain. Glucocorticoid suppression of TSH response to TRH has been well documented. Higher doses appear to suppress hypophyseal inhibition of TSH, whereas low doses interfere with the hypothalamic response.[92] Note, however, that interference of the thyroid axis by glucocorticoids does not preclude simultaneous testing of the thyroid and adrenal axes in healthy dogs.[93,94] Antithyroid drugs such as propylthiouracil and methimazole are used therapeutically to block thyroid hormone synthesis; their mechanism occurs, at least in part, at the level of transcription.[95]

The effects of iodide- and iodine-containing products (including radiographic contrast agents) on thyroid hormone concentrations are well recognized and used therapeutically. Through hypothalamic regulation, iodines cause a rapid increase in TSH response to TRH as T_4 and triiodothyronine (T_3) concentrations decrease. Sulfonamides can have a profound effect on thyroid function.[96] Among the potential mechanisms, direct interference with the conversion of inorganic iodide to diiodotyrosine and thyroxine was demonstrated as early as 1943.[97] Decreased concentrations of peripheral hormones are associated with follicular cell hypertrophy and hyperplasia and with decreased colloid formation. Changes are profound in as early as 21 days yet resolve within 3 weeks after therapy is discontinued. These effects occur at high doses that might be used for difficult-to-treat, yet presumably susceptible, higher bacterial or protozoal infections (>60 mg/kg per day but may also occur at lower doses). The effects of sulfonamide NSAIDs and the anticonvulsant zonisamide on thyroid gland function are discussed in Chapters 29 and 27, respectively.

The effects of non-sulfonamide anticonvulsant drugs, especially phenobarbital and phenytoin, on thyroid hormone disposition are less appreciated. Several sites of interference have been identified for anticonvulsant drugs (see Chapter 27).

Hematologic

As with any drug-induced disorder, the lack of universally standardized definitions of what constitutes an adverse reaction complicates recognition of hematologic disorders induced by drugs. The criteria for drug-induced hematologic disorders have been described for humans and are based on cell count, assessment of time to onset after drug exposure and time to resolution of signs after the drug has been discontinued, and the course of the reaction.[98] Drug-induced hematologic dyscrasias may reflect a bone marrow response or an effect on peripheral tissues, including blood components (Table 4-7). Bone marrow suppression can result in pancytopenia or affect only a single cell line (i.e., anemia, leukopenia, or thrombocytopenia).[99] Both direct bone marrow suppression and toxicity to mature circulating cells may occur.

Bone marrow and peripheral cells are susceptible to both drugs and their metabolites; reactions may have an immunologic or nonimmunologic basis. Although drug allergies are a well-recognized cause of damage to stem cells of the bone marrow, many drugs are directly toxic. Discerning an immunologic basis can be difficult, however, if the antibodies involved have not been identified. Drugs most commonly associated with nonimmune-mediated bone marrow suppression include most cancer chemotherapeutic agents because of their predictable effects on DNA and cell division. Other drugs associated with nonimmune-mediated bone marrow dyscrasias include phenylbutazone, estrogen derivatives, and chloramphenicol.

Phenobarbital has caused leukopenia and other hematologic disorders when used to treat epilepsy; white cell counts normalize once the drug is discontinued. Whether or not this is an immune-mediated reaction is not clear, but its lack of dose dependency suggests a Type B reaction (See Chapter 27).

Drugs that affect blood components and the manifestations of anemia include all NSAIDs but particularly aspirin (reflecting inhibition of platelet activity), anticoagulants such as warfarin derivatives, and heparin (these generally reflect a relative overdose). Red blood cell malfunction may occur as a result of methemoglobinemia in cats (Figures 4-9 and 4-10). Although acetaminophen clearly causes hepatotoxicity, the feline red blood cell is more sensitive to the presence of radical metabolites compared with the feline liver. Several reasons have been suggested for an apparent increased sensitivity of feline red blood cells to methemoglobin formation: feline hemoglobin may be more sensitive to oxidation; feline erythrocytes may contain lower concentrations of intracellular glutathione; the proportion of subtypes of hemoglobin may differ; and, finally, feline hemoglobin may contain more sulfhydryl groups, which are reactive, than that of other species. Drugs associated with methemoglobinemia in cats include urinary antiseptics containing methylene blue or azodyes, acetaminophen and related compounds, benzocaine, DL-methionine, propylthiouracil, and methimazole.

Table 4-7 Examples of Drugs Associated with Hematologic Disturbances

Drug	Manifestation
Acetaminophen	Methemoglobinemia (especially in cats)
Anticancer drugs	Bone marrow suppression*
Azo dye (urinary antiseptics)	Methemoglobinemia (cats)
Benzocaine (and related drugs)	Methemoglobinemia (cats)
Chloramphenicol	Bone marrow suppression*
Cimetidine	Thrombocytopenia
Coumarin derivatives	Coagulation dysfunction
Erythropoietin (human recombinant)	Anemia
Estrogens	Bone marrow suppression*
Griseofulvin	Bone marrow suppression*
Heparin	Thrombocytopenia, platelet dysfunction, coagulation dysfunction
Methimazole	Methemoglobinemia
Methylene blue	Methemoglobinemia (cats)
NSAIDs	Platelet dysfunction
Phenobarbital	Neutropenia
Phenylbutazone	Bone marrow suppression*
Propylthiouracil	Methemoglobinemia
Ranitidine	Anemia

NSAIDS, Nonsteroidal antiinflammatory drugs.
*Bone marrow suppression might be manifested as anemia, leukopenia, thrombocytopenia, or any combination thereof.

Ivermectin was associated with a prolonged prothrombin time and hematomas in humans after a single oral dose, presumably because of a drug-induced vitamin K deficiency.[100]

Human recombinant erythropoietin and granulopoietin have been used to treat anemias associated with chronic renal disease and leukopenia induced by disease (e.g., parvovirus) or drugs (e.g., anticancer drugs) in dogs and cats. Unfortunately, these proteins are foreign, and antibodies may develop after 10 to 14 days, destroying not only the exogenous drug but also endogenous factors.

Drug-induced hematologic disorders have been described in the human critical care patient.[101] Among the challenges

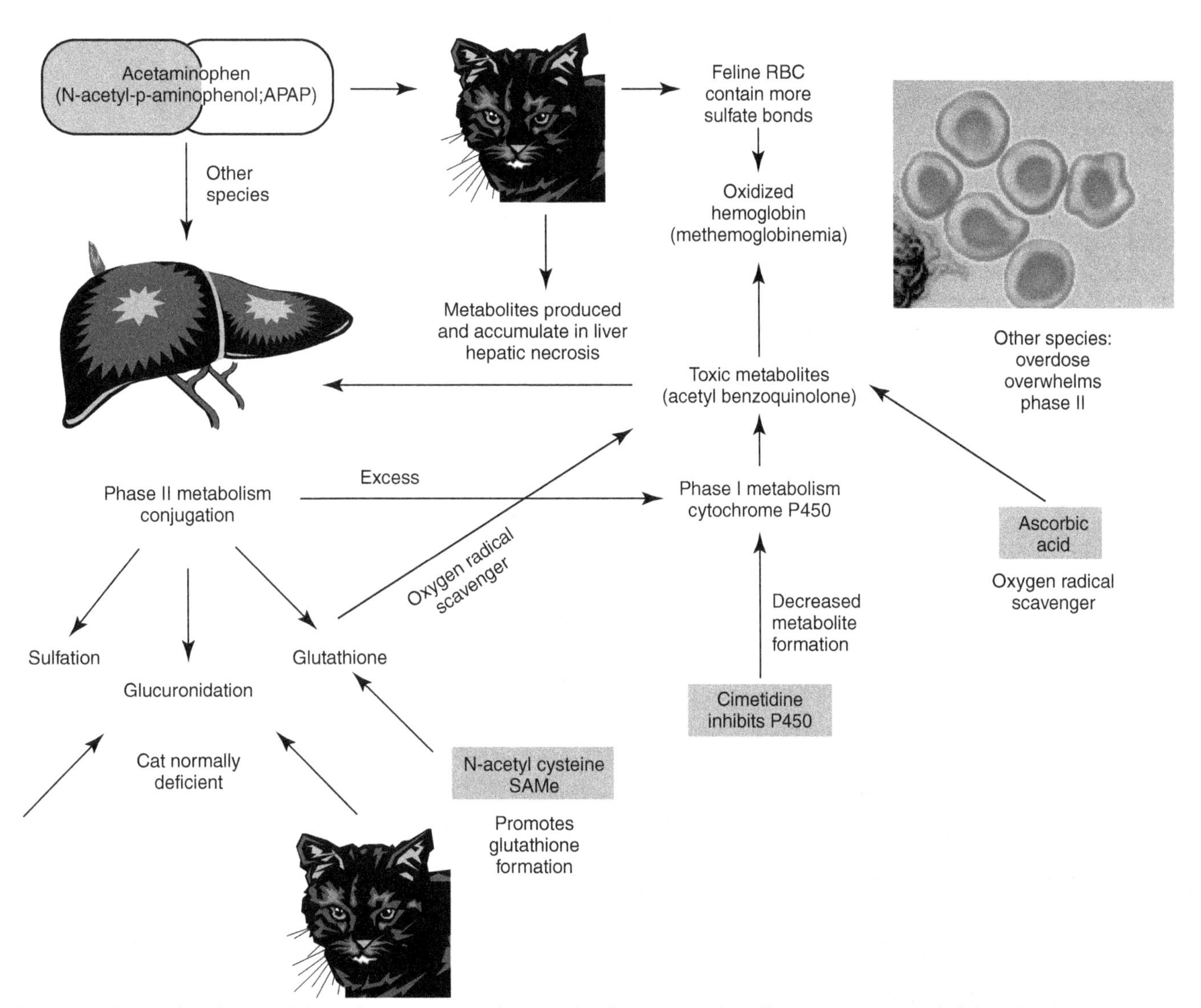

Figure 4-9 Acetaminophen toxicity reflects a cytotoxic type A adverse reaction. Because cats are deficient in glucuronidation, phase II metabolism is easily overwhelmed, and drug is shunted more aggressively back into phase I metabolism. The same process occurs in dogs after an overdose. The products of phase I metabolism are reactive and cause destruction of tissues (liver and red blood cells). Glutathione, an important phase II oxygen-radical scavenger, prevents damage but is easily depleted in cats. Supplementation in the form of *N*-acetylcysteine can decrease damage. Cimetidine is useful because it decreases phase I metabolism and thus the formation of phase I metabolites.

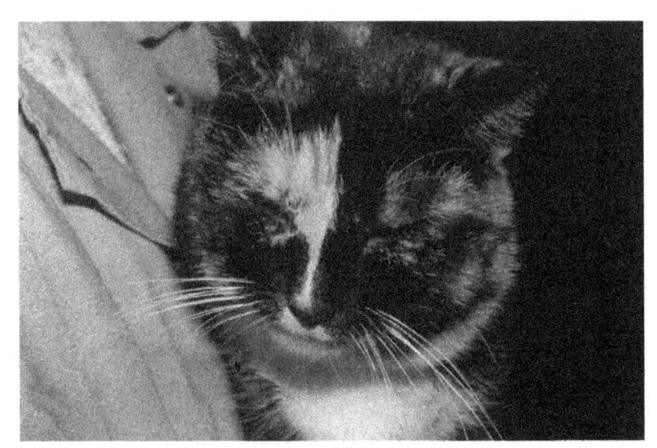

Figure 4-10 Facial edema in a cat with acetaminophen toxicosis. The mucous membranes of this cat were cyanotic.

in the ICU setting is identifying the drug as the cause, and, in the patient receiving polypharmacy, which drug. It is not clear whether ICU patients are at any greater risk to develop these dyscrasias, but certainly they are at greater risk to react adversely should they occur. Bone marrow under production is manifested as pancytopenia if the pluripotential cell is targeted or monocytopenia if a single hematopoietic cell is targeted. Neutropenia can be manifested within hours (7 to 10), thrombocytopenia in days, and anemia generally in weeks unless exacerbated by hemolysis. Bone marrow aplasia has been associated with chloramphenicol, felbamate, sulfonamides, and NSAIDs. If the effect is direct, clinical signs may resolve once the drug is discontinued, unless the effect is irreversible (e.g., selected chloramphenical reactions in humans). If indirect, immunosuppressive doses of immunomodulators may be indicated. Myelodysplasia as a prelude to acute myelogenous leukemia is associated with high doses or long durations of alkylating or topoisomerase-inhibiting anticancer drugs. Macrocytosis has been associated with drugs that negatively affect metabolic compounds needed for DNA synthesis. Examples include cobalamine, whose absorption is inhibited by neomycin, proton pump blockers, and bifuanide hypoglycemic agents, or folate, whose metabolism is inhibited by methotrexate, phenytoin, and trimethoprim. Drugs that alter the nucleotide pool may cause megablastosis (e.g., hydroxyurea, methotrexate, azathioprine, purine nucleoside analogs). Enzyme deficiencies (thiopurine methytransferase) and drug-induced erythropoietin deficiencies (e.g., cisplatin) also have been reported. Cytopenias resulting from direct effects on cells have been reported. Examples include penicillin-induced thrombocytopenia. Heparin-induced thrombocytopenia reflects binding to PF4 immunoglobulin and subsequent activation of platelets; the risk is lower with low-molecular-weight heparins. Thrombotic microangiopathies (thrombotic thrombocytopenia purpura) has been associated with the antiplatelet agents clopidogrel or ticlopidine and anticancer drugs (mitomycin-C).[101]

Respiratory System

Although compounds toxic to the lungs occasionally arrive by hematogenous routes, most pulmonary toxicities result from direct exposure of the respiratory tract through the nasopharyngeal or oropharyngeal airways and subsequently the tracheobronchial tract and alveoli.[15] Gaseous and particulate toxicants are most common. The airways may also serve as a means of systemic exposure if the toxicant is effectively and rapidly absorbed by the respiratory mucosa. Particulate matter that impacts the airways (generally 5 to 10 μm in size for the tracheobronchial tree and less than 5 μm in size for alveoli) can become trapped in the airways.

The mucociliary apparatus may remove entrapped particulate matter before a toxic response occurs. Some chemicals, however, cause direct injury to upper airways (e.g., chlorine, ammonia, water-soluble gases, and chromium). Compounds depositing in the alveoli can be removed only by blood flow (if the compound is absorbed), biotransformation by Clara cells or type II alveolar cells (which contain cytochrome P450 enzymes), or macrophages.

Pulmonary edema, manifested as an acute respiratory distress syndrome, is caused by severe exposure of the alveoli (in humans) to acute toxicants such as phosgene, chlorine, xylene, and nitrogen oxides. Because the lung is the shock organ in cats, type I allergic reactions may manifest as primarily acute respiratory difficulties. Biotransformation in the lung, as in other tissues, may be a source of a toxic compound as an innocuous chemical is converted into a toxic one (e.g., paraquat, a herbicide metabolized by type II alveolar cells). Macrophage clearance may reflect phagocytosis; macrophage death is accompanied by the release of inflammatory mediators that can damage surrounding cells and contribute to the toxic effects of a drug. Compounds that cause pulmonary injury in humans as a consequence of the inflammatory response include asbestos, beryllium, coal dust, silica, and tungsten.[15]

AVOIDING ADVERSE DRUG EVENTS

Recommendations for avoiding specific toxicities have been given or are described in specific chapters for some of the described drugs. Appendix 5 offers antidotes for many drugs. The incidence of ADEs in general, and ADRs in particular, may be reduced by several proactive actions (Box 4-6), with client education playing an important role. Type B reactions are difficult to avoid because they are unpredictable. An awareness of potential toxicities will make them less likely. Frequent patient monitoring during therapy is the best means of reducing type B adverse reactions.

REPORTING ADVERSE DRUG EVENTS

Reporting ADEs is complicated by the difficulty in identifying them. In human medicine, methods have been defined whereby the causal relationship between a suspected reaction and a suspected drug can be assessed. None is universally accepted, but each includes some or all of the following criteria: the time between the administration of the drug and the onset of the reaction or the cessation of the drug and resolution of clinical signs; the course of the reaction, which may vary if the drug is continued or interrupted; the role of the drug and underlying disease being treated as a cause of the reaction; response to readministration of the drug; results of

Box 4-6

Actions to Take to Reduce the Risk of Adverse Drug Events

1. Obtain a definitive diagnosis before treatment, including previous treatment with drugs known to be associated with type B adverse drug events.
2. Use proper drugs according to recommended protocols.
3. Use alternative (less toxic) drugs when available.
4. Thoroughly evaluate the patient before and during treatment (e.g., physical examination and clinical pathology), with an emphasis on target organs of toxicity. This includes implementation of relevant testing that might identify a genetic predisposition to adversity.
5. Modify dosing regimens when appropriate.
6. Evaluate the responses to therapy and discontinue therapy if therapeutic effects are not evident.
7. Frequently monitor the patient for remission of clinical signs and discontinue therapy as early as possible.
8. Minimize multiple drug therapy and use of drugs known to cause drug interactions. This includes avoiding, when possible, drugs metabolized by the liver or other organs.
9. Alternate administration times for patients receiving multiple drug therapy, thus reducing the potential for drug interactions.
10. Educate the client regarding potential toxicity of a drug and the clinical signs associated with its use.
11. Report adverse events.

laboratory tests; and the history of previous administration of the drug.[98]

Reporting of ADEs to the Center for Veterinary Medicine (CVM) of the FDA has markedly increased from 4000 in 1997 to nearly 25,000 a year in the past several years. The increase probably reflects, in part, the increased visibility of the CVM reporting program that accompanied improvements in the collection, analysis, and reporting of the adverse events.[25,102] Several avenues are available for reporting an ADE. The animal pharmaceutical company can be directly informed by calling the Medical Affairs officer; by law, these ADEs must be reported to the CVM. The sequelae of reporting an animal adverse event to a human drug is not clear, but mandatory reporting is probably unlikely. In such situations the second route should be pursued: the CVM. The CVM provides directions for reporting ADEs. The form (FORM FDA 1932a, "Veterinary Adverse Experience, Lack of Effectiveness or Product Defect Report") can be downloaded or printed from http://www.fda.gov/cvm/adereporting.htm or by writing to the following address: ADE Reporting System, Center for Veterinary Medicine, U.S. Food & Drug Administration, 7500 Standish Place, Rockville, MD 20855-2773. Reports also can be reported by telephone (1-888-FDA-VETS). On receipt of an ADE by the CVM, a six-part scoring system is used to evaluate each reaction. The system takes into account previous experience with the drug, alternative causes, timing of the event in the context of dosing, overdosing, and response to drug removal or rechallenge if available.[25] Recently, the CVM's approach to assessing a potential ADE insofar as it's likelihood to lead to label changes or market withdrawals has come under fire; methods of analysis may undergo reassessment, which will, it is to be hoped, further refine the assessment process and improve accuracy. Results of the ADE reporting program and analysis by the CVM can be reviewed for each drug at the previously cited website. A third alternative to ADE reporting may be the Animal Poison Control Center (APCC) affiliated with the Animal Society for Prevention of Cruelty to Animals (ASPCA) (www.aspcsaapcc.org). The latter organization should be contacted by telephone (888-426-4435) if immediate support is desired for identification and treatment of a potential ADE that may prove life threatening to the animal. Support is likely to entail a $50 consultation fee. Adverse events to animal biologics (vaccines, bacterins, and diagnostic kits) are not handled by the FDA but instead by the U.S. Department of Agriculture (800-752-6255), whereas adverse events to pesticides (topically applied external parasiticides) should be reported to the U.S. Environmental Protection Agency (800-858-PEST). Links to these agencies are available at the FDA website.

ADVERSE EVENTS TO HERBS AND BOTANICALS

Herbal or botanical products, more so than "dietary supplements" of animal origin, may be unsafe for several reasons. Adverse events are more likely when products are used in excess. Five broad classes of active chemicals exist in plants: volatile oils (e.g., catnip, garlic, citrus), fixed oils, resins, alkaloids, and glycosides. Of these, fixed oils, often used as emollients, demulcents, and bases for other agents, are among the least toxic. Resins can be strong gastrointestinal irritants. Alkaloids are among the most pharmacologically active plant chemicals and include a wide range of potentially harmful products. The risk of adverse effects to herbs is increased by the presence of many active ingredients in the same plant (see the discussion of drug interactions in Chapter 2). Indeed, herbalists often used unpurified plant extracts because of the possibility that different chemicals might interact synergistically. The amount of active ingredients may vary dramatically with the portion of the plant (i.e., leaf, flower, stem, root, seed) administered, thus influencing safety. Whereas one portion of the plant might be safe, another portion might not be. Herbalists often administer the whole plant in the belief that, in contrast to the purified extract, toxicity is reduced by a buffering effect of the whole herb. During growth of the plant, environmental contaminants may become unintended residues during the manufacturing process. Microorganisms, including bacteria, fungi, and molds, can either directly contaminate the product or produce contaminating toxins. Bacterial contamination is more likely with root products as opposed to flower or leaf products. Heavy metals such as lead, cadmium, or mercury increasingly are contaminating plants exposed to environmental pollutants. Further, unless the herbal products are grown organically, insecticides and pesticides may contaminate them. Factors during production and storage, such as storage length and conditions, can alter herbal potency and quality. Finally, herbal products might be supplemented with active ingredients (often referred to by the herbal or botanical name or simply not labeled) such as ephedrine, caffeine, or fenfluramine (the latter ingredient being one of the two ingredients in the notorious Fen-phen dietary supplements).

KEY POINT 4-3 The risk of an adverse drug effect with dietary supplements is increased by unsupervised client use; the lack of mandated premarket approval or premarket assessment of quality, safety, and efficacy; the inherent properties of herbal products; and the lack of an effective postmarket surveillance program.

The lack of quality control in labeling of herbals, botanicals, or other novel ingredients (e.g., "nutraceuticals") may contribute to the advent of adverse effects with these products.[103] Many herbal products are not labeled with the concentration per dosing unit of the ingredient of interest. Those that do may contain more or less than the labeled dose, presenting a risk of overdosing or underdosing. Manufacturers may improperly identify plants. Even if properly identified, the consumer may have difficulty in identifying a product as potentially dangerous because an herbal name often is used in place of the more easily recognized chemical name (e.g., guarana for caffeine or ma huang for ephedrine). Further, an herbal agent may be referred to by many different names. The FDA has become more proactive in directing manufacturers to list generic drug names instead of or in addition to herbal names. Proposed sources of quality assurance data for animal dietary supplements include the manufacturer of the product; the Association of American Feed Control Officials; the National Animal Supplement Council; laboratories such as Consumer Lab (www.consumerlab.com); the United States Pharmacopeia (USP) dietary supplement verification program (http://www.usp.org/USPVerified/dietarySupplements); the American Herbal Pharmacopeia (http://www.herbal-ahp.org), which offers the Botanical Safety Handbook and Herbs of Commerce; and Consumer Laboratories, a for-profit organization that provides quality assessment for a fee. However, much of its work is also independent, supported by income generated through its website. For approximately $30 per year, this site provides results of quality testing for a variety of products. Although most of the products are marketed for humans, several veterinary products recently have been evaluated for quality.

A number of other herbs have been associated with adverse effects (Table 4-8). This list is far from inclusive, in part because an effective adverse event reporting system is lacking in either human or veterinary medicine. Although infrequently reported, adverse events have occurred in veterinary patients receiving novel ingredients. The ASPCA APCC published a report of adverse reactions in 47 dogs that ingested a popular weight loss dietary supplement containing guarana (caffeine) and ma huang (ephedrine); 17% of the dogs died after the appearance of clinical signs associated with central and cardioactive compounds.

Although mechanisms for reporting adverse events in human or veterinary medicine toward herbal or botanical products currently are limited, effective mechanisms are evolving. Among the FDA's postmarket responsibilities toward (human) dietary supplements is the monitoring of product safety. Note, however, that the FDA may remove a potentially dangerous supplement only when and if the product presents an "imminent hazard to public health or safety." The burden of proof is on the FDA, not (as with drugs) on the manufacturer. The FDA recently implemented the Adverse Events Reporting System (AERS) to be used as a monitoring tool for dietary supplements as well as other medicinal products. Adverse events also can be reported for human products through the FDA's MedWatch program. Some recent FDA actions taken to address the safety of dietary supplements can be reviewed at www.consumerlab.com, at the FDA's Medwatch program, or the FDA's Center for Drug Evaluation and Research (CDER). Unfortunately, the current FDA sites for reporting adverse events to dietary supplements do not pertain to veterinary products. Reporting to the APCC may continue to be the most effective means of reporting adverse reactions of animals to medicinal agents, particularly those for which a designated watchdog does not exist (e.g., unapproved products), in part because of the APCC's ability to analyze and quickly report important trends.

Table 4-8 Examples of Therapeutic Herbs or Botanicals Associated with Adversities*

Herb	Adversity
Ginkgo biloba	Bleeding, altered platelet function
St. John's wort	Gastrointestinal disturbances, allergic reactions, fatigue, dizziness, confusion, dry mouth, photosensitivity
	Serotonin syndrome (when combined with other similarly acting drugs)
Ephedra (ma huang)	Hypertension, insomnia, arrhythmia, nervousness, tremor, headache, seizure, cerebrovascular event, myocardial infarction, kidney stones
Kava	Sedation, oral and lingual dyskinesia, torticollis, oculogyric crisis, exacerbation of Parkinson's disease, painful twisting movements of the trunk, rash
Aconitine	Cardiotoxic
Garlic	Altered platelet function
Ginger	Altered platelet function, tachycardia and/or hypertension
Ginseng	Altered platelet function
Feverfew	Altered platelet function
Echinacea	Hepatotoxicity
Valerian	Hepatotoxicity
Goldenseal root	Electrolyte disturbance
Licorice	Electrolyte disturbance
S-adenosylmethionine	Serotonin syndrome (when administered in combination with other similarly acting drugs)

*Many herbs or botanicals are associated with adversities. The use of various herbal names for each product may preclude detection of adversity. The lack of an effective adverse event reporting system hinders detection and reporting of adversities involving herbs.

ADVERSE EVENTS TO COMPOUNDED PREPARATIONS

Quality compounding is critically important to the safe and effective administration of drugs to animals, particularly the very small and very large. The role of compounding in small animal medicine was recently reviewed.[104] Compounding of animal drugs is specifically legalized by the Animal Medicinal Drug Use Clarification Act (AMDUCA; 21 C.F.R Section 530) (See Appendix 5). However, compounding must be implemented in accordance with the relevant provisions of extralabel drug use. According to the FDA, legal sources of drugs to be compounded are limited to FDA-approved finished forms of either animal or human drugs; the FDA makes no distinction as to which (animal versus human) is the preferred source for companion animal compounding. Because no other source is legalized, all other sources are considered by the FDA to be illegal, including bulk substances (e.g., pure powder) or non–FDA-approved finished drug products obtained outside of the United States. However, formulation of selected compounded prepartions is likely to be easier, yielding a better product, if prepared from pure active ingredient (i.e., bulk). The risk of supporting compounding from bulk includes the temptation to manufacture, rather than compound. Compounding, particularly for products that mimic a commercially available drug, serves as a major disincentive for manufacturers of animal drugs to pursue the approval process. Further, whereas approved animal or human drugs have undergone rigorous, scientific testing to ensure drug safety and efficacy for the patient, compounded products have not. Although pharmacists are directed to compound from written protocols and maintain written records of compounding activities, pharmacists are not currently required to ensure accuracy in product preparation, including product stability. Although a reputable pharmacy may randomly check accuracy of selected drugs, this act currently is voluntary and will be limited to selected drugs and aliquots. Although guidelines exist for establishing expiration dates of compounded products, dates are not necessarily based on scientific data. The United States Pharmacopeia has published a Pharmacist's Pharmacopeia. Further, the Pharmaceutical Compounding Accreditation Board (PCAB) has recently implemented a robust accreditation program. Adherence to its guidelines will minimize the risk of adverse reactions associated with compounded products (see www.pcab.org).

KEY POINT 4-4 The risk of an adverse drug effect with compounded products is increased by the existence of regulatory oversight and can be minimized by prescribing only through pharmacies accredited by PCAB.

The risks associated with failed delivery (too much or too little) of a compounded product are added to risks associated with the approved finished dosing form of a drug. Adverse events associated with compounded products should be reported to either the (veterinary) pharmaceutical manufacturer or the FDA; if reported to a veterinary manufacturer, the manufacturer is required by law to forward the report to the FDA, although whether this is true for a modified finished dosing form is not clear. Adverse events associated with compounded products may occur at the pharmaceutical phase (during preparation) or, largely because of failed absorption, at the pharmacokinetic phase. The more sophisticated the preparation, the more likely it is that adverse events will occur because of diminished or excessive drug delivery.

Ingredient Errors

Compounding from bulk substances is easier than from approved finished dosing forms because excipients or other materials do not interfere with product preparations. Further, excipients in the finished dosing form will not interfere with dissolution of the drug in the vehicle. However, the use of an approved finished dosing form of a drug for compounding offers a major advantage to use of a bulk substance in that the approved drug has passed stringent tests of analysis regarding drug purity and potency and the absence of contaminants. As such, products formed from bulk substances are associated with greater risks compared with products compounded from approved drugs. In contrast, for bulk substances the burden of purity and accuracy lies with the pharmacist, and there is no mechanism to ensure that this burden has been met. All products, active ingredient or excipients (fillers, preservatives, etc.), domestic or foreign, should either meet USP or equivalent standards or be purchased after FDA inspection. Drugs that are still under U.S. patents are often obtained in this manner. Bulk substances will be accompanied by a credible certificate of analysis. The need for validation of ingredient sources (including all active and inactive substances) is paramount as inexpensive bulk substances increasingly are being acquired from uninspected foreign (particularly Asian) sources.

The active drug in a compounded product might also be substituted for an alternative drug; the substituted drug may not have the same pharmacokinetic or pharmacodynamic characteristics (discussed in more detail in the next section). Veterinarians should indicate on prescriptions that unapproved substitutions are not acceptable for compounded products.

Mathematical Errors

Mathematical errors are probably the most common and potentially the most lethal reason for pharmaceutical compounding errors. Compounding is vulnerable to mathematical mistakes because of its very nature (prescription driven, small volumes) and because much of the equipment and technology that facilitate accuracy and precision of finished dosing forms are not (or should not be) used during compounding. In addition to the source of the ingredient being potentially problematic, pharmacists may substitute drugs without acquiring clinician permission. Mathematical errors may also reflect substitution of the active ingredient. For example, the active drug content may differ, as is demonstrated by metronidazole. The recipe for metronidazole benzoate should contain 1.6 mg for each 1 mg of metronidazole hydrochloride (or the dose must be similarly increased). Bromide offers another example: 1 g of the sodium bromide contains more bromide (774 mg) than the potassium salt (692 mg).

Preparation and Storage Errors

Chemical reactions (oxidation, reduction, hydrolysis) are facilitated by changes in humidity, light, pH, presence of oxidizing trace metals, and increasing environmental temperature. Excipients may enhance instability as a result of changes in pH or the presence of disintegrating agents. Degradation products (drugs or excipients) can cause adverse events. Excipients that are critical to the finished dosing form increase the risk of instability in product compounded from an approved source. Whereas approved products undergo intensive scrutiny with regard to stability and potency, compounded products do not; recipes for compounded preparations rarely are associated with studies that ensure stability or delineate conditions for storage.

Simple syrups (which tend to be acidic), preservatives, combination drugs, or other ingredients can alter drug pH and thus ionization (diffusibility) or stability. The more drugs mixed together in a single preparation, the greater the risk of chemical drug interactions. For example, weak acids and weak bases are likely to chemically inactivate one another.

Interactions may occur among the drugs or excipients. As an example, only 54% of a fluorinated quinolone (orbifloxacin) was found to be present when prepared in Lixotinic as a vehicle compared with simpler syrups.

Particle Size

Compounding from approved drugs (legal) is more difficult than from bulk drugs (illegal) because excipients are more likely to result in undissolved macroscopic or microscopic precipitates that indicate undissolved and thus nondiffusible ineffective drug. Sedimentation of undissolved particles may result in caking at the bottom of the drug receptacle; difficulty in shaking or rapid sedimentation (common) after shaking can result in erratic and unpredictable doses. Crushing of any oral tablet may result in unequal particle sizes in the preparation, which in turn will yield different surface areas and different rates of absorption. Fine crushing of the product such that it is no longer a suspension increases the concentration of soluble excipient; chemicals, including those added to the finished dosing form to facilitate degradation, can cause drug instability. Crushing an oral tablet for preparation in a syrup may also lead to unequal distribution of dissolved drug in the finished preparation, and mixing the drug such that it is equally distributed throughout the preparation may not be possible. Repackaging oral tablets or capsules into smaller dosing units may also affect drug efficacy. Diluents such as starch and dextrose might impede oral absorption. Preparation of an oral formulation from an injectable solution to enhance accuracy of dosing is more likely to be inappropriate if the drug salt is different between the preparations. If the injectable product is presented in powder form, the drug is likely to be unstable in liquids and may be destroyed when added to liquid (oral solutions). The addition of flavoring agents to oral products may increase drug instability because of changes in pH or the increased risk of microbial growth (e.g., as with syrups).

Because selected commercial oral preparations have been formulated to alter (slow or facilitate) drug delivery, reformulation of such products is discouraged. Compounding altered release products from bulk substances requires sophisticated techniques not generally available through pharmacists. Enteric-coated or spansule products should not be crushed. Although spansule products might be reformulated without crushing, the amount of drug in each spansule is not necessarily predictable, and random distribution of drug content is likely to yield erratic dosing. Cyclosporine is a complex molecule characterized by poor oral bioavailability; oral absorption requires bile acids or special formulation as a microemulsion product. As such, it is an example of a drug for which compounding should be approached cautiously and be supported by therapeutic drug monitoring. In the author's drug-monitoring laboratory, cyclosporine blood concentrations were not detectable (two different samples, 2 weeks apart) in one cat receiving a product compounded from an approved microemulsion human product. In keeping with recommendations that the unadulterated animal-approved version be used at the same dose, concentrations expected at the administered dose were detected within 1 week of the change in drug product.

Injectable Products

Administration of injectable products is inherently associated with a higher level of risk compared with administration of topical or oral products because of more rapid drug delivery, risks associated with administration of suspensions rather than solutions, potential impact of impurities (including endotoxin), and need for sterility. Actions taken to ensure sterility and removal of impurities may cause drug degradation. Endotoxin (which is essentially ubiquitous in the environment) is difficult to remove. Without testing, its absence is impossible to document, yet its presence can be lethal. The USP has generated guidelines, and state laws generally delineate regulations specifically for the compounding of injectable products. Veterinarians should be reluctant to prescribe compounded injections, and when doing so, they must be confident that the compounding pharmacist follows these criteria.

Topical Products

Although administration of topical products generally is associated with fewer risks compared with administration of systemic products (the exception is ophthalmic products, which also should be sterile), compounding the proper product can be challenging. The USP has promulgated guidelines for the compounding of topical ingredients, including guidelines designed to ensure drug dissolution and drug movement from the vehicle into the skin. For example, solid ingredients should be reduced to the smallest reasonable particle size, and the active ingredient should then be added to other substances necessary to dissolve the drug so that a uniform liquid or solid dispersion is achieved. Uniformity of dispersion should be demonstrated by spreading a thin film of the finished formulation on a flat transparent surface. Visual examination of a compounded product should be implemented to identify obvious problems with dissolution and so on. Care must be taken to ensure that ingredients are not caustic, irritating, or allergenic. Vehicle selection can be quite difficult: undissolved drug cannot pass into the skin; drug that has too great an affinity for the vehicle will remain in the vehicle. Transdermal gels are examples of products in which particular care must be exercised.

Few published reports exist that delineate adverse events resulting from inappropriate compounding. Despite indications of frequent problems with compounded products, the FDA receives few reports regarding adverse events related to compounded products. This reflects, in part, the lack of mandated reporting of adverse events. However, it also reflects the difficulty in recognizing therapeutic failure resulting from failed delivery. The latter is likely to be detected only if the information is sought and the drug or response to the drug can be easily monitored. Numerous studies have focused on accuracy in labeling of compounded products, particularly in equine medicine. Products found to be mislabeled include omeprazole, ivermectin (both pirated drugs), ketoprofen (one product contained only 50% of the labeled content, whereas 12 of 13 contained close to 100%), amikacin (the percentage of labeled content ranged from 59% to 140%; none was within 10%), and boldenone (all within 15% of labeled content, but two of five contained up to 5% of impurities).

DRUG EFFECTS ON CLINICAL LABORATORY TESTS

A drug-induced disease is often first suspected on the basis of an abnormality in a diagnostic test that cannot be easily attributed to a disease process. Many drugs cause changes in diagnostic tests but are not associated with disease. Confirming the cause-and-effect relationship between drug and abnormalities can be very difficult unless the drug can be discontinued and then readministered.

Drugs interfere with diagnostic tests either directly, at the level of the analytical procedure (in vitro), or by induction of a physiologic change in the patient (in vivo). Of the two levels of interference, it is likely that analytical interferences will occur regardless of the species from which the sample was collected. Thus interferences affecting analytical procedures are better documented in veterinary medicine because they generally can be extrapolated from human analytical testing. Mechanisms of in vitro interference vary. Drugs that interfere with endocrine testing are described as adverse drug events of the endocrine system.

If analytical (in vitro) interference by a drug is suspected, the laboratory should be contacted and questioned. This is particularly important if the patient is receiving drugs structurally similar to the drug being tested. Cross-reactivity between the drug and the test can falsely increase test values. For example, therapeutic corticosteroids cross-react with endogenous corticosteroid hormones, although the percentage of cross-reactivity varies with the assay and the drug. Some drugs cause cytotoxicity (e.g., aminoglycoside-induced nephrotoxicity); some stimulate changes without toxicity (e.g., glucocorticoid-induced alkaline phosphatase); and others interfere with hormones. Drugs can interfere with diagnostic tests in many other ways. The American Association of Clinical Pathologists publishes a handbook that summarizes changes in clinical pathology that might be drug induced. Access to this text or its information may be possible by contacting the appropriate diagnostic laboratory.

Few studies focus on the impact of drugs on clinical laboratory tests. Examples include the impact of bromide (when used as an anticonvulsant) on chloride concentrations when flame ionization is used: the two cannot be distinguished when this method is used, and bromide, being present in much higher concentrations, will artifactually increase chloride. The impact of selected antimicrobials on urine glucose also has been documented in the dog. At 22 mg/kg, cephalexin caused false-positive glucose in 50% of dogs at 6 hours and 33% of dogs at 24 hours when using selected commercially available glucose strips (Chemstrips, Boeringer Ingelheim). A tablet test (Clinitest, Miles Inc.) indicated false-positive results in 100% of dogs (n=6) at 6 and 24 hours after administration of cephalexin at 22 mg/kg; 50% of dogs receiving enrofloxacin at 5 mg/kg and 100% receiving 10 mg/kg also yielded false-positive results.[105] Enrofloxacin also caused false negatives at concentrations as low as 20 μg/mL in urine spiked with dextrose at 0.5% and above.

REFERENCES

1. Nebeker JR, Barach P, Samore MH: Clarifying adverse drug events: a clinician's guide to terminology, documentation, and reporting, *Ann Intern Med* 140:795–801, 2004.
2. Lawson DH, Richard RME: *Clinical pharmacy and hospital drug management*, London, 1982, Chapman & Hall, pp 211-237.
3. Griffin JP, D'Arcy PF: *A manual of adverse drug interactions*, ed 2, Chicago, 1979, Billing & Sons, 3–51.
4. Pirmohamed M, Breckenridge AM, Kitteringham NR, et al: Adverse drug reactions, *Br Med J*:25, 316:1295–1298, 1998.
5. Meyer UA, Gut J: Genomics and the prediction of xenobiotic toxicity, *Toxicology* 181-182:463–466, 2002.
6. Ariens EJ, Simonis AM, Offermeier J: *Introduction to general toxicology*, New York, 1976, Academic Press, pp 79-125.
7. Mitchell JR, Smith CV, Lauferburg BH, et al: Reactive metabolites and the pathophysiology of acute lethal cell injury. In Mitchell JR, Homing MG, editors: *Drug metabolism and drug toxicity*, New York, 1984, Raven Press, pp 301–318.
8. Klassen DC: Principles of toxicology. In Klassen CD, Amour MO, Doull J, editors: *Toxicology: the basic science of poisons*, ed 3, New York, 1985, Macmillan, pp 11–20.
9. Ju C, Uetrecht JP: Mechanism of idiosyncratic drug reactions: reactive metabolites formation, protein binding and the regulation of the immune system, *Curr Drug Metab* 3:367–377, 2002.
10. Schwarz M, Wiskiel R: Medication reconciliation: developing and implementing a program, *Crit Care Nurs Clin North Am* 18:502–507, 2006.
11. Young DS: *Effects of drugs on clinical laboratory tests*, ed 3, Washington, DC, 1990, American Association for Clinical Chemistry.
12. To H, Kikuchi A, Tsuruoka S, et al: Time-dependent nephrotoxicity associated with daily administration of cisplatin in mice, *J Pharm Pharmacol* 52(12):1499–1504, 2000.
13. Bleyzac N, Allard-Latour B, Laffont A, et al: Diurnal changes in the pharmacokinetic behavior of amikacin, *Ther Drug Monit* 22(3):307–312, 2000.
14. Osweiler GD: General toxicological principles. In Peterson ME, Talcott PA, editors: *Small animal toxicology*, ed 2, St Louis, 2006, Saunders.
15. Sipes IG, Dart RC: Principles of toxicology. In Wecker L, editor: *Human pharmacology: molecular to clinical*, ed 5, Philadelphia, 2009, Mosby.
16. Guengerich FP: Cytochrome P450 and chemical toxicology, *Chem Res Toxicol* 21:70–83, 2008.
17. Roberston JD, Orrenius S: Role of mitochondria in toxic cell death, *Toxicology* 181-182:491–496, 2002.
18. Ingelman-Sundberg M: Polymorphism of cytochrome P450 and xenobiotic toxicity, *Toxicology*:181-182:447–452, 2002.
19. Martinez M, Modric S, Sharkey M, et al: The pharmacogenomics of P-glycoprotein and its role in veterinary medicine, *J Vet Pharmacol Ther* 31(4):285–300, 2008.
20. Food and Drug Administration: *Information and requirements for review and approval of new animal drug applications (NADAs)*. Accessed October 14, 2009. at www.fda.gov/AnimalVeterinary/DevelopmentApprovalProcess/NewAnimalDrugApplications/default.htm.
21. Woodward KN: Veterinary pharmacovigilance. Part 6. Predictability of adverse reactions in animals from laboratory toxicology studies, *J Vet Pharmacol Ther* 28:213–231, 2005.
22. Institute of Medicine: *Perspectives, methods, and data challenges, workshop summary, nutritional risk assessment*, Washington, DC, 2007, National Academies Press.
23. Colbert BL, Biron P: *Pharmacovigellence from A to Z: adverse drug event surveillance*, Malden, Miss, 2002, Blackwell Science.

24. Hughes DA, Bayoumi AM, Pirmohamed M: Current assessment of risk-benefit by regulators: Is it time to introduce decision analyses?, *Clin Pharmacol Ther* 82:123–127, 2007.
25. Hampshire VA, Doddy FM, Post LO: Adverse drug event reports at the United States Food and Drug Administration Center for Veterinary Medicine, *J Am Vet Med Assoc* 225:533–536, 2004.
26. Guengerich FP, MacDonald JS: Applying mechanisms of chemical toxicity to predict drug safety, *Chem Res Toxicol* 20:344–369, 2007.
27. Kitoh K, Watoh K, Chaga K, et al: Clinical, hematological and biochemical findings in dogs after induction of shock by injection of heartworm extract, *Am J Vet Res* 55:1535–1540, 1994.
28. Nakamura H, Matsuse H, Obase Y, et al: Clinical evaluation of anaphylactic reactions to intravenous corticosteroids in adult asthmatics, *Respiration* 69:309–313, 2002.
29. Landor M, Lashinsky A, Waxman J: Quinolone allergy?, *Ann Allergy Asthma Immunol* 77:273–276, 1996.
30. Cribb A: Adverse reactions to sulphonamide and sulphonamide-trimethoprim antimicrobials: clinical syndromes and pathogenesis, *Adverse Drug React Toxicol Rev* 15:9–50, 1996.
31. Tilles SA: Practical issues in the management of hypersensitivity reactions: sulfonamides, *South Med J* 94(8):817–824, 2001.
32. Trepanier LA, Danhof R, Toll J, et al: Clinical findings of 40 dogs with hypersensitivity associated with administration of potentiated sulfonamides, *J Vet Intern Med* 17:647–652, 2003.
33. Trepanier LA: Idiosyncratic toxicity associated with potentiated sulfonamides in the dog, *J Vet Pharmacol Ther* 27:129–138, 2004.
34. Ockner RK: Drug-induced liver disease. In Zakim D, Boyer TD, editors: *Hepatology: a textbook of liver disease*, Philadelphia, 1982, Saunders, pp 691–722.
35. Plaa GL: Toxic responses of the liver. In Klassen CD, Amour MO, Doull J, editors: *Toxicology: the basic science of poisons*, ed 3, New York, 1985, Macmillan, pp 286–309.
36. Lee WM: Review article: drug-induced hepatotoxicity, *Aliment Pharmacol Ther* 7:4775–4785, 1993.
37. Bunch SE: Hepatotoxicity associated with pharmacologic agents in dogs and cats, *Vet Clin North Am Small Anim Pract* 23(3):659–670, 1993.
38. Schenkers B: Drug disposition and hepatotoxicity in the elderly, *J Clin Gastroenterol* 18:232–237, 1994.
39. Smith SW, Howland MA, Hoffman RS, et al: Acetaminophen overdose with altered acetaminophen pharmacokinetics and hepatotoxicity associated with premature cessation of intravenous N-acetylcystein therapy, *Ann Pharmacother* 42(9): 1333–1339, 2008.
40. Ndiritu CA, Weigel JW: Hepatorenal injury in a dog associated with methoxyflurane, *Vet Med Small Anim Clin* 72:545–550, 1977.
41. Grant PS, Meuten DJ, Pecquet-Croad ME: Hepatic necrosis associated with the use of halothane in the dog, *J Am Vet Med Assoc* 184:478–480, 1984.
42. Polzin DJ, Stowe CM, O'Leary TP, et al: Acute hepatic necrosis associated with the administration of mebendazole to dogs, *J Am Vet Med Assoc* 179:1013–1016, 1981.
43. Van Cavteren H, Marsboom R, Vanderberghe J, et al: Safety studies evaluating the effect of mebendazole on liver function in dogs, *J Am Vet Med Assoc* 183:93–98, 1983.
44. Twedt DC, Diehl KJ, Lappin MR, et al: Association of hepatic necrosis with trimethoprim sulfonamide administration in 4 dogs, *J Vet Intern Med* 11:20–23, 1997.
45. Raynaud JP: Thiacetarsamide (adulticide) versus melarsomine (RM 340) developed as macrofilaricide (adulticide and larvicide) to cure canine heartworm infection in dogs, *Ann Rech Vet* 23:1–25, 1992.

45a. Dunayer EK: New findings on the effects of xylitol ingestion in dogs, *Vet Med* :791–797, 2006.

45b. Dunayer EK: Gwaltney-Brant SM: Acute hepatic failure and coagulopathy associated with xylitol ingestion in eight dogs, *J Am Vet Med Assoc* 229:1113–1117, 2006.

46. Perazella MA: Drug-induced nephropathy: an update, *Expert Opin Drug Saf* 4(4):689–706, 2005.
47. Engelhardt JA, Brown SA: Drug-related nephropathies. Part II: Commonly used drugs, *Compend Contin Educ Pract Vet* 9: 281–288, 1987.
48. Taber SS, Mueller BA: Drug-associated renal dysfunction, *Crit Care Clin* 22:357–374, 2006.
49. Pedersoli WM: Serum fluoride concentration, renal and hepatic function test results in dogs with methoxyflurane anesthesia, *Am J Vet Res* 38:949–953, 1977.
50. Torpet LA, Kragelund C, Treibel J, et al: Oral adversed drug reactions to cardiovascular drugs, *Crit Rev Oral Biol Med* 15(1):28–46, 2004.
51. Mouatt JG: Cyclosporin and ketoconazole interaction for treatment of perianal fistulas in the dog, *Aust Vet J* 80(4):207–211, 2002.
52. Halliwell RF, Davey PG, Labert JJ: The effects of quinolones and NSAIDS upon GABA-evoked currents recorded from rat dorsal root ganglion neurons, *J Antimicrob Chemother* 27:209–218, 1991.
53. Thomas RJ: Neurotoxicity of antibacterial therapy, *South Med J* 87(9):869–874, 1994.
54. Simpson S: Treatment of metronidazole toxicity, *Standards of care: emergency and critical care medicine* 5:11, 2003.
55. Fillastre J, Leroy A, Borsa-Lebas F, et al: Effects of ketoprofen (NSAID) on the pharmacokinetics of pefloxacin and ofloxacin in healthy volunteers, *Drugs Exp Clin Res* 18:487–492, 1992.
56. Neer TM: Drug-induced neurologic disorders, *Proc Am Coll Vet Intern Med* 9:261–269, 1991.
57. Pullium JR, Seward RL, Henry RT, et al: Investigating ivermectin toxicity in collie dogs, *Vet Med* 80:33–40, 1985.
58. Tranquili WJ, Paul AJ, Todd KS: Assessment of toxicosis induced by high dose administration of milbemycin in collies, *Am J Vet Res* 52:1170–1172, 1991.
59. Mealey K, Pharmacogenetic,*Vet Clin North Am Small Anim Pract Pharm* 36:961–973, 2006.
60. Mealey KL, Bentjen SA, Waiting DK: Frequency of the mutant MDR1 allele associated with ivermectin sensitivity in a sample population of collies from the northwestern United States, *Am J Vet Res* 63:479–481, 2002.
61. Muhammad G, Abdul J, Khan MZ, et al: Use of neostigmine in massive ivermectin toxicity in cats, *Vet Hum Toxicol* 46(1): 28–29, 2004.
62. Sevine F: Letters: picrotoxin, the antidote to ivermectin in dogs?, *Vet Rec* 116:195–196, 1985.
63. Sartor LL, Bentjen SA, Trepanier L, et al: Loperamide toxicity in a collie with MDR1 mutation associated with ivermectin sensitivity in Collies, *J Vet Intern Med* 18:117–118, 2004.
64. Yilmaz HL, Yildizdas DR: Amitraz poisoning, an emerging preventive strategies epidemiology, clinical features, management, and preventive strategies, *Arch Dis Child* 88:130–134, 2003.
65. Fulton RB, Fruechte LK: Poisoning induced by administration of a phosphate-containing urinary acidifier in a cat, *J Am Vet Med Assoc* 198:883–995, 1991.
66. Davidson G: To benzoate or not to benzoate: cats are the question, *Int J Pharm Comp* 5:89–90, 2001.
67. Bedford PGC, Clarke MA: Suspected benzoic acid poisoning in the cat, *Vet Rec* 188:599–601, 1971.
68. Fraunfelder FW: Ocular adverse drug reactions, *Expert Opin Drug Saf* 2(4):411–420, 2003.
69. Wiebe V, Hamilton P: Fluoroqinolone-induced retinal degeneration in cats, *J Am Vet Med Assoc* 221:1568–1571, 2002.
70. Mauget-Faysse M, Quaranta M: Incidental retinal phototoxicity associated with ingestion of photosensitizing, *Arch Clin Exp Ophthalmol* 239(7):501–508, 2001.

71. Patel M: Ocular side effects of systemic drugs, *Optometry* 28: 33–36, 2002.
72. Buckley R, Graham E, Jones S, et al: *Oculartoxicity and hydroxychloriquine: guidelines for screening 2009 (replacing the Royal College of Ophthalmologists Guidelines, 2004)* , April 2004. http://www.library.nhs.uk/guidelinesfinder/ViewResource.aspx?resID=36837.
73. Marutani K, Matsumoto M, Otabe Y, et al: Reduced phototoxicity of a fluoroquinolone antibacterial agen with a methoxy group at the 8 position in mice irradiated with long-wave length UV light, *Antimicrob Agents Chemother* 37:2217–2222, 1993.
74. Huang MY, Schacht J: Drug-induced ototoxicity: pathogenesis and prevention, *Med Toxicol Adverse Drug Exp* 4:452–467, 1989.
75. Griffin JP: Drug-induced ototoxicity, *Br J Audiol* 22:195–210, 1988.
76. Matz G, Rybak L, Roland PS, et al: Ototoxicity of ototopical antibiotic drops in humans, *Otolaryngol Head Neck Surg* 130:S79–S82, 2004.
77. Humes HD: Insights into ototoxicity. Analogies to nephrotoxicity, *Clin Pharmacokinet* 38(4):367–375, 2000.
78. Webster JC, Carroll R, Benitez IT, et al: Ototoxicity of topical gentamicin in the cat, *J Infect Dis* 124:S138–S144, 1971.
79. Roland PS, Tybak L, Hannley M, et al: Animal ototoxicity of topical antibiotics and the relevance to clinical treatment of human subjects, *Otolaryngol Head Neck Surg* 130:S57–S78, 2004.
80. Wokenstein P, Revus J: Drug-induced severe skin reactions. Incidence, management and prevention, *Drug Saf* 13:56–68, 1995.
81. Mouatt JG: Cyclosporin and ketoconazole interaction for treatment of perianal fistulas in the dog, *Aust Vet J* 80(4):207–811, 2002.
82. Downard CD, Roberts LJ II, Morrow JD: Topical benzoic acid induces the increased biosynthesis of prostaglandin D2 in human skin in vivo, *Clin Pharmacol Ther* 57(4):441–445, 1995.
83. Quintero B, Miranda MA: Mechanisms of photosensitization induced by drugs: A general survey, *Ars Pharmaceutica* 41(1):27–46, 2000.
84. Boothe DM: Effects of drugs on endocrine testing. In Bonagura J, Kirk RW, editors: *Current veterinary therapy (XII), small animal practice*, Philadelphia, 1995, Saunders, pp 339–346.
85. Center SA, Mitchell J, Nachreiner RF, et al: Effects of propranolol on thyroid function in the dog, *J Am Anim Hosp Assoc* 17:813–822, 1981.
86. Kemppainen RJ, Sartin JL: Effects of single intravenous doses of dexamethasone on baseline plasma cortisol concentrations and responses to synthetic ACTH in healthy dogs, *Am J Vet Res* 45:742–746, 1984.
87. Spencer KB, Thompson FN, Clekis T, et al: Adrenal gland function in dogs given methylprednisolone, *Am J Vet Res* 41(9):1503–1506, 1980.
88. Roberts SM, Lavach JD, Macy DW, et al: Effect of ophthalmic prednisolone acetate on the canine adrenal gland and hepatic function, *Am J Vet Res* 45:1711–1713, 1984.
89. Zenoble RD, Kemppainen RJ: Adrenocortical suppression by topically applied corticosteroids in healthy dogs, *J Am Vet Med Assoc* 191:685–688, 1987.
90. Hostettler KA, Wrighton SA, Molowa DT, et al: Coinduction of multiple hepatic cytochrome P-450 proteins and their mRNAs in rats treated with imidazole antimycotic agents, *Mol Pharmacol* 35:279–285, 1988.
91. Willard MD, Nachreiner R, McDonald R, et al: Hormonal and clinical pathologic changes with long-term ketoconazole therapy in the dog and cat, *Proc Am Coll Vet Intern Med* 6:13.25–13.27, 1986.
92. Wenzel KW: Pharmacological interference with in vitro tests of thyroid function, *Metabolism* 30:717–732, 1981.
93. Moriello KA, Halliwell REW, Oakes M: Determination of thyroxine, triiodothyronine, and cortisol changes during simultaneous adrenal and thyroid function tests in healthy dogs, *Am J Vet Res* 48:456, 1987.
94. Reimers TJ, Concannon PW, Cowan RG: Changes in serum thyroxine and cortisol in dogs after simultaneous injection of TSH and ACTH, *J Am Anim Hosp Assoc* 18:923–925, 1982.
95. Moriyama K, Tagami T, Usui T, et al: Antithyroid drugs inhibit thyroid hormone receptor-mediated transcription, *J Clin Endocrinol Metab* 92(3):1066–1072, 2007.
96. Campbell K, Chambers MD, Davis CA, et al: Effects of trimethoprim/sulfamethoxazole on thyroid physiology in dogs, *Proc Am Coll Vet Dermatol* 11:15–16, 1995.
97. Franklin AL, Chaikoff TI: The effect of sulfonamides on the conversion in vitro of inorganic iodide thyroxine and diiodotyrosine by thyroid tissue with radioactive iodine as indicator, *J Biol Chem* 152:295–301, 1943:Accessed Dec. 18, 2009, at http://www.jbc.org/content/152/2/295.full.pdf.
98. Benichou C, Celigny PS: Standardization of definitions and criteriaforcausalityassessmentofadversedrugevents.Drug-induced blood cytopenias: report of an International Consensus Meeting, *Nouv Rev Fr Hematol* 33:257–262, 1991.
99. Stroncek DF: Drug induced immune neutropenia, *Transfus Med Rev* VII:268–274, 1993.
100. Homeida MM, Bagi IS, Ghalib HW: Prolongation of prothrombin time with ivermectin, *Lancet* 1:1346–1347, 1998.
101. Vandendries ER, Drews RE: Durg-associated disease: hematologic dysfunction, *Crit Care Clin* 22:347–355, 2006.
102. Keller WC, Bataller N, Oeller DS: Processing and evaluation of adverse drug experience reports at the Food and Drug Administration Center for Veterinary Medicine, *J Am Vet Med Assoc* 213:208–211, 1998.
103. Committee on Examining the Safety of Dietary Supplements for Horses: *Dogs, and Cats; National Research Council: Safety of dietarysupplementsforhorses,dogs,andcats*,Washington,DC,2008, National Academies Press.
104. Boothe DM: Veterinary compounding in small animals: a clinical pharmacologist's perspective, *Vet Clin North Am Small Anim Pract* 36:1129–1173, 2006.
105. Rees CA, Boothe DM: Evaluation of the effect of cephalexin and enrofloxacin on clinical laboratory measurements of urine glucose in dogs, *J Am Vet Med Assoc* 224:1455–1458, 2004.

5 Therapeutic Drug Monitoring

Dawn Merton Boothe

Chapter Outline

Therapeutic drug monitoring (TDM) is a tool for guiding the design of an effective and safe regimen for drug therapy in the individual patient. Monitoring can be used to confirm a plasma drug concentration (PDC) that is above or below the therapeutic range, thus minimizing the time that elapses before corrective measures can be implemented for the patient.[1-3] Knowledge of the principles of drug disposition (see Chapter 1) and the factors that determine these principles in the individual patient (see Chapter 2) facilitate an understanding of the use of and need for TDM.

Fixed dosing regimens are designed to generate PDCs within a therapeutic range—that is, achieve the desired effect without producing toxicity. Dosing regimens are based on the patient's clinical response to the drug. Therapeutic success is most likely to occur if doses are based on scientific studies performed in the target species intended to receive the drug for the intended reason. Marked interindividual variability has, however, been confirmed for many drugs[4,5] owing to physiologic (e.g., species, breed, age,[6] gender), pathologic (e.g., renal, hepatic, cardiac diseases)[7-10] or pharmacologic (i.e., drug interaction)[5,7,11,12] effects. Prudent clinicians modify dosing regimens when possible to compensate for the impact of some of these factors on drug disposition. However, the combined effects of these factors are often unpredictable. A trial-and-error approach to dose modification may be successful but is most appropriate when response to the drug can be easily measured. Examples include "to effect" drugs such as gas inhalants and ultrashort thiobarbiturate anesthetics, rapidly acting anticonvulsants such as diazepam, and lidocaine for the treatment of ventricular arrhythmias. The trial-and-error approach also might be reasonable for illnesses that are not serious or do not require immediate resolution and for drugs characterized by large therapeutic windows, that are generally safe at high doses, However, trial-and-error modification can be inefficient and potentially dangerous when the drug response cannot be easily measured, the drug is characterized by a narrow margin of safety, or the patient's life is threatened.

DRUGS AND INDICATIONS

TDM is not indicated for all drugs; rather, it is indicated when patient health is at risk (Box 5-1). Not all drugs can be monitored by TDM; certain criteria must be met (Box 5-2).[13] Patient response to the drug must correlate with PDC. Drugs whose metabolites are active (e.g., diazepam) or for which one of two enantiomers compose a large proportion of the desired pharmacologic response generally cannot be monitored effectively by measuring the parent drug.[14] Rather, all active metabolites, the parent drug, or both or the pharmacologically active enantiomer should be measured. The drug must be measurable at concentrations within the targeted therapeutic range in a relatively small sample size, and analytic methods must be available to detect the drug rapidly, precisely and accurately in the target species.[15] Methods must be specific for the drug of interest and able to differentiate it from other compounds. Prior to choosing a laboratory for monitoring purposes, the laboratory also should be queried regarding quality-control procedures to ensure that they are followed and assays used in animals have been validated for that species. Ideally, the laboratory will participate in some type of external validation program. Attention should be given to how the sample collected from the patient is handled. The cost of the analytic method must be reasonable. Drugs that meet these criteria and for which TDM has proved useful in veterinary medicine include, but are not limited to, selected anticonvulsants (phenobarbital, bromide, selected benzodiazepines zonisamide and levetiracetum), antimicrobials (e.g., aminoglycosides-gentamicin, and amikacin); cardioactive drugs (digoxin, procainamide, lidocaine, and quinidine); theophylline, and cyclosporine (Table 5-1).

Monitoring may be most effective if either or both minimum (C_{min}) and maximum (C_{max}) ranges have been established for the drug in the species and for the disease being treated.[4] However, the importance of the therapeutic range should not be overestimated. Although not "normals," therapeutic ranges of drugs also are population statistics, based on

Box 5-1

Drugs for Which TDM Is Most Useful

1. Serious toxicity (e.g., phenobarbital, cardiac drugs)
2. A poorly defined or difficult to detect clinical end point (e.g., anticonvulsants, behavior modifying drugs, immunomodulators)
3. A steep dose–response curve for which a small increase in dose can result in a marked increase in desired or undesired response (e.g., theophylline, phenobarbital for cats)
4. A narrow therapeutic range (e.g., most cardiac drugs)
5. Nonlinear pharmacokinetics that may lead to rapid accumulation of drugs to toxic concentrations (e.g., phenytoin or, in cats, phenobarbital)
6. Combination drug use that may lead to undesirable adverse effects caused by drug interactions (e.g., enrofloxacin-induced theophylline toxicity or chloramphenicol-induced or clorazepate-induced phenobarbital toxicity)
7. Drugs for which therapeutic failure may lead to patient harm (e.g., anticonvulsants, cardiac drugs, antimicrobials)
8. A target therapeutic range (C_{max} and /or C_{min}) has been validated in the target species with the target drug

the PDC at which most patients (e.g., 95%) with the targeted disease might be expected to respond. However, although the therapeutic range offers a reasonable target for most animals, exactly *where* in the range the individual patient will respond is not known. It is this patient-specific concentration that is identified through monitoring—that is, monitoring establishes the therapeutic range for the individual patient. As such, it is indicated to establish the baseline response in a patient that has adequately responded to therapy. Note that some animals will respond at concentrations below or above an established therapeutic range. However, dosing regimens need not necessarily be increased or decreased, respectively, for those patients unless the patient is put at risk for subtherapeutic failure or toxicity, respectively.

Therapeutic ranges do offer a target for drug therapy and are ideally based on well-controlled clinical trials in the target species. However, most recommended therapeutic ranges in animals have been extrapolated from those determined in humans. Although these ranges have proven useful, none-the-less, studies confirming the applicability of these ranges to animals are warranted. Determination of these ranges can be facilitated if adequate patient information accompanies a patient sample submitted for monitoring (see Box 5-1). Procainamide is an example of a drug for which recommended therapeutic ranges might differ between dogs and humans because of pharmacokinetic differences. Dogs do not produce the acetylated active metabolite as efficiently as humans; therefore procainamide concentrations should be higher in dogs than in humans. Primidone (rarely used currently) is an example in cats: its efficacy in dogs depends on conversion to phenobarbital, which does not happen to a significant degree in cats. Bromide offers another example of pharmacodynamic differences: whereas concentrations above 1.5 mg/mL might be considered toxic in people, they are in the low- to mid-therapeutic range in epileptic dogs. The therapeutic range for a drug also varies with the therapeutic intent (e.g., cyclosporine and perianal fistulas versus immunosuppression).

Box 5-2

When to Implement Monitoring

(1) **"Start-up": (a) Maintenance dose.** Monitoring at baseline in a responding animal to establish the therapeutic range for the patient. **(b) Loading dose maintenance dose combination (including a "mini" loading dose):** a sample should be collected after a loading dose has distributed (the day after loading bromide or within 2 hr after loading with phenobarbital) and at one half-life into the maintenance dose. If the two samples do not match, the maintenance dose should be proportionately adjusted. A steady state sample should be collected once steady state has been reached.

(2) **"Check up":** Rechecks: to proactively ensure that effective concentrations are maintained and safe concentrations are not exceeded. The frequency varies with the seriousness of therapeutic failure or the risk of toxicity. Intervals of 6 to 12 months are generally recommended for the well-controlled patient and 3 to 6 months for the poorly controlled patient. For immunomodulators, 3- to 6-month intervals for life-threatening disease.

(3) **"What's up": (a) Establish a cause for therapeutic failure or to confirm toxicity.** For patients that have not responded well to a new drug or a new dose, despite doses at the mid-to-high end of the recommended dosing range; or in previously well-controlled patients that fail therapy or develop signs of adversity. **(b) Respond to changes in patient factors:** progression or improvement of cardiac, renal, or hepatic disease; changes in clearance and, to a lesser degree, volume of distribution may change elimination half-life and thus peak or trough concentrations. **(c) Detect drug-drug or drug-diet interactions.** Changes in diet or addition of drug that may interact: baseline concentrations should be reestablished before and after a change if there is a risk that the change in diet or drug therapies may alter the disposition of the drug of interest. For example, bromide should be measured before and at steady state after the administration of a new diet; phenobarbital should be monitored before and after beginning chloramphenicol or an imidazole antifungal, cyclosporine should be monitored before and after ketaconazole (or any imidazole) or azithromycin therapy is implemented, etc.

As with clinical pathology reference ranges, the range for a specific laboratory also may vary with the methodology, and specifically whether or not metabolites are detected by the methods. As such, the laboratory should be specifically queried regarding its therapeutic range for a particular assay. Assays that are based on antibodies (e.g., enzyme-linked immunosorbent assay [ELISA], radioimmunoassay [RIA], polarized immunofluorescence [PIFA]) may detect both the parent compound and those metabolites most chemically similar to it. Monoclonal antibody–based immunoassays are less likely to detect metabolites than polyclonal antibody-based assays but nonetheless, may not be able to discriminate among very subtle changes in drug chemistry induced by metabolism. Therapeutic ranges for antibody-based assays

Table 5-1 Selected Therapeutic Drug Monitoring Data for Drugs Monitored in Small Animals*

Drug	Therapeutic Range*	Half-Life	Time to Steady State	Peak	Trough	Comments
Amikacin	2-25 μg/mL	1-2 hr	NR	0.75-1 hr	2 HL (3-6 hr)	Collect in or transfer to plastic; concentrations are likely to be nondetectable at true trough. Collect trough at 4 to 6 hr after peak for kinetics.
Amitryptyline	250-750 nmol/L (human)					
Aspirin	50-100 μg/mL	8 hr (D) 38 hr (C)	NR 8 days	2-4 hr	BND	
Benzodiazepines	100-200 ng/mL	<8 hr	NR		BND	
Bromide (sodium or potassium)	1-3.5 mg/mL	14-21 days	2-3 days		BND	Bromide will interfere with many assays that measure chloride, causing false increases.
Carbamezepine	16-51 μmol/L					Human data; includes epoxide metabolite, which contributes to efficacy. Relevance to animals questionable.
Carvedilol	Trough above 100 ng/mL	0.3 to 4.3 (D)	NR	2 hr	BND	Concentrations may be nondetectable at trough in some patients. A peak and trough might be initially collected to determine half-life and collection times for subsequent sampling.
Clomipramine	800-1600 mmol/L					Human data; relevance to animals questionable.
Cyclosporine (CsA)	Immunosuppression: 2 hr peak: 800-1400 ng/mL Immunosuppression: 12 hr trough: 400-600 ng/mL Inflammatory allergic disease: 12 hr Trough: 250 ng/mL Perianal fistula: 12 hr trough: 100-600 ng/mL	3-8 hr	NR	2 hr	BND (12 hr)	For atopy (and all other diseases), monitoring might be implemented once patient has responded to determine the range for that patient. Monitoring of peak and trough is particularly important in the presence of drugs that decrease or increase CsA metabolism or absorption.
Digoxin	0.8-2 ng/mL	36 hr (see comments)	7 days	Toxicity : 2 (glass only)	Efficacy: BND	Glass only. Do not use red rubber stopper. Marked variability in kinetics induced by disease and drug therapy indicates the need for both peak and trough concentrations such that a half-life can be calculated for this toxic drug.
Fluoxetine	350-3000 nmol/L					Human data; relevance to animals questionable.
Gabapentin	14 to 50 μmol/L					Human data; relevance to animals questionable. This is not an established range in humans but a range in which response appears to be reasonable.
Gentamicin	0.5-1.5 μg/mL 5-8 μg/mL	0.9-1.3 hr	NR	0.75-1 hr (plastic only)	2 half-lives (3-6 hr)	Collect in or transfer to plastic; concentrations are likely to be nondetectable at true trough. Collect trough at 4 to 6 hr after peak for kinetics.

Levetiracetam	5.5-20 ng/mL	2-3.6 hr (regular release product)	NR	2 hr	BND	Peak and trough recommended initially to determine patient half-life; if single samples thereafter, trough concentration should target therapeutic range. Peak concentration may need to be four-fold to eight-fold higher than trough.
Methotrexate	Less than 1 μmol/L					
Phenobarbital	14-45 μg/mL	32-75 hr	14-16 days	4-5 hr	BND	Peak and trough recommended only in difficult-to-control patients so that short half-life might be detected. Trough recommended as single sample.
Phenytoin	40 to 80 μmol/L					Inactive cross-reacting metabolite may accumulate with renal disease and cause false increase.
Primidone	Based on phenobarbital	32-75 hr	14-16 days	4-5 hr	BND	See information on phenobarbital.
Procainamide	25-50 μg/mL	2.9 hr	NR	2-4 hr	BND	
Sirolimus	5-15 ng/mL					Human data; relevance to animals questionable. This is not an established range in humans but a range in which response appears to be reasonable.
Theophylline	10-20 μg/mL	5.7 hr 7.9 hr	 NR	2 hr 2 hr	BND BND	
Thyroxine (T_4)	1-3.5 μg/dL (12.9-45 nmol/L) (D) 1-4 μg/dL (12.9-51.5 nmol/L) (C)	12-15 hr (D)	NR	4-6 hr	BND	
Free Thyroxine (fT_4)	1-3.5 ng/dL (12.9-45 pmol/L) (D) 1-4 ng/dL (12.9-51.5 pmol/L) (C)	5-6 hr (D)	NR	4-6 hr	BND	
Thyronine (T_3)	0.5-1.8 ng/mL (D) 0.4-1.6 ng/mL (C)	5-6 hr	NR			
Zonisamide	10-40 μg/mL	16-65 hr	3-10 days	2 hr (D)	BND	Peak and trough recommended initially to determine patient half-life; if single samples thereafter, trough concentration should target therapeutic range.

BND, just before next dose; *NR*, not relevant; *HL*, Half-life (elimination or disappearance); *D*, *dog*; *C*, cat

*See also Chapter 27, Anticonvulsants. Serum separator tubes, in general, should not be used for therapeutic drug monitoring samples. Some human therapeutic ranges have not been applied to animals.

generally are higher than those that detect only the parent compound. Which assay is preferred depends on the activity of the metabolites: if the metabolite is active, immunoassays may more accurately predict response compared with assays based on parent compound only. Cyclosporine, benzodiazepines, procainamide, behavior modifying drugs, and beta blockers are examples of drugs that might have active metabolites.

KEY POINT 5-1 A therapeutic range, is not a "normal," but like a "normal" is a population statistic. Monitoring should be used to determine the patient's therapeutic range, which may be below or above the population therapeutic range.

The cost of monitoring will vary among drugs, depending in part on the methods used. An advantage of high-performance liquid chromatography (HPLC) assays is their specificity for the target compound, and discrimination between parent compound and metabolites. However, assays based on HPLC tend to be more expensive because the methods are tedious, generally requiring very lengthy assay time, greater instrument and personnel dedication, and more sophisticated technology compared to that required for automated assays. Automated assays tend to more predictable, with quality assurance easier to achieve.

IMPLEMENTATION

Number and Timing of Samples: One Versus Two, Peak Versus Trough

Samples for monitoring generally are collected at peak (C_{max}, highest PDC during a dosing interval), trough (C_{min}, lowest, generally just before the next dose), or midway during the dosing interval. The type of sample and the number of samples collected depend on the goal of monitoring and the amount of drug that is eliminated during a dosing interval—that is, the elimination half-life of the drug.

For drugs with a long half-life compared to the dosing interval, because drug concentrations will not fluctuate significantly during the interval, variability in drug concentrations may reflect instrument variability, rather than drug disposition. For such drugs (e.g., bromide and, in most patients, phenobarbital or zonisamide), the timing of sample collection probably is not important and a single sample collected at any time is sufficient. However, a trough sample just before the next dose is almost always the lowest concentration that will occur with each dose, and as such is generally recommended if a minimum concentration must be maintained (e.g., anticonvulsants). In general, response to therapy and TDM should not be performed unless maintenance dosing has been sufficiently long for PDC to reach "steady state" (3 to 5 drug half-lives). An exception includes situations in which a loading dose has been administered (see below). If a loading dose is not given, the drug will accumulate (see Chapter 1) as steady state is reached (Figure 5-1). The time to steady state varies among drugs and for some drugs is quite variable among animals (see Table 5-1).

For drugs with very-long half-lives, the clinician may want to proactively assess the likelihood that the dose will result in targeted drug concentrations at steady state. Concentrations achieved after one half-life of dosing can be doubled to predict steady state concentrations. If predicted deviates substantially from target, the dose can be modified at that time, with a confirmatory check at steady state.

In contrast to drugs with a long half-life compared to the dosing interval, if the drug elimination half-life is sufficiently smaller than the interval such that peak and trough concentrations fluctuate by 25% or more, both timing and number of samples should be based on the intent of monitoring. For example, if toxicity is a concern, a single concentration might be sufficient and a peak concentration (generally 2 hr post oral dosing) is preferred. In contrast, if efficacy throughout a dosing interval is the priority, a single sample might be sufficient, but a trough sample might be preferred. The least helpful sample is one collected mid-interval. However, caution is indicated with either a single peak or a trough because in both situations the information provided with a single sample does not reflect the state of drug concentrations for the duration of the dosing interval. For drugs with short half-lives, while each dose is likely to reach or exceed peak concentrations that approximate the maximum recommended range, each trough concentration that occurs just before the next dose is likely to reach or drop below the minimum therapeutic range. If trough concentrations for such a drug are determined to be nontherapeutic and a decision is made to increase the dose, while trough concentration may exceed the target minimum as intended, peak concentrations may also become toxic. If peak concentrations are toxic and a decision is made to lower the dose, although peak concentrations may drop below the toxic range as intended, trough concentrations may then become subtherapeutic. An added advantage to collection of both peak and trough concentrations is that the elimination half-life of the drug can then be determined, providing a basis for determining the most appropriate dosing interval.

One reason that either a peak or trough might be selected is the recommended therapeutic range is based on either a peak or a trough sample. However, such recommendations generally assume the recommended dosing interval also is being followed. This is exemplified by cyclosporine, for which the recommendations for efficacy for immune suppression (extrapolated from humans) are based on the assumption of a 12-hour dosing interval and a sample collected at either a 2-hour peak or a 12-hour trough.

For some drugs, the elimination half-life changes across time in the patient. The decision to collect both a peak and trough for such drugs may depend on the elimination half-life, which in turn, can be documented as short only by collecting both a peak and a trough sample. This is exemplified by phenobarbital, for which the elimination half-life may initially be longer than the dosing interval (i.e., more than 48 hours) but after induction (i.e., several months into therapy) may be much shorter (i.e., less than 12 hours) in the same patient (Case Study 5-1). Digoxin provides a good example of the risk associated with collecting only a single sample when assessing

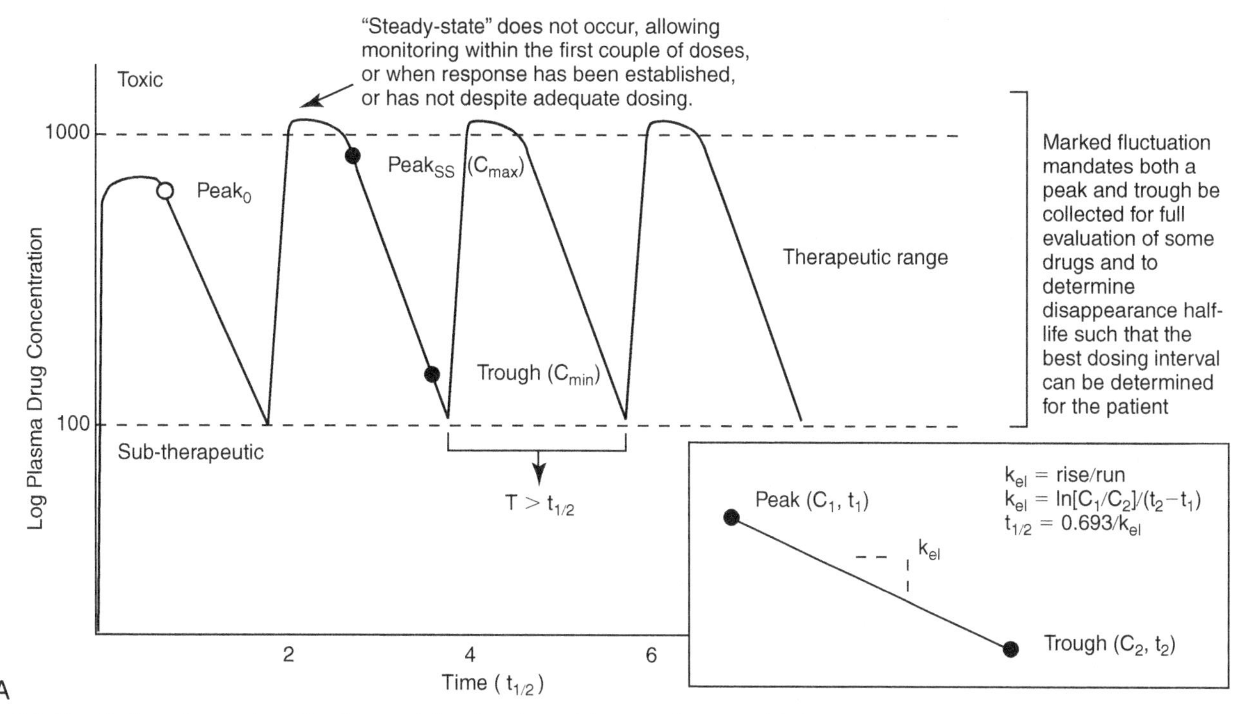

Figure 5-1 The timing of sample collection and the duration of therapy that should elapse before monitoring is implemented varies with the relationship between dosing interval and half-life of the drug. **(A)** Drug concentrations across time for a drug dosed at an interval that approximates its elimination half-life. For such drugs, concentrations fluctuate by 50% during a dosing interval, and drug concentrations at steady state will accumulate twofold compared to the first dose. Response to therapy and thus therapeutic monitoring are likely to occur within the first three to five doses. Both peak and trough samples should be collected to characterize the degree of fluctuation in drug concentrations during the dosing interval, thereby ensuring both that toxic concentrations do not occur as the drug peaks and that subtherapeutic concentrations do not occur just before the next dose. Peak and trough samples allow calculation of the elimination half-life *(inset)* and thus a more accurate determination of a proper dosing interval.

efficacy. Digoxin is characterized by a half-life that ranges from less than 12 hours, thus allowing concentrations to become subtherapeutic during a 12-hr dosing interval, to more than 36 hours (particularly in patients with renal disease), which is likely to lead to drug accumulation (Case Study 5-2). The half-life can change again if the patient responds to therapy for cardiac failure. If toxicity is suspected, a single sample collected at the time that clinical signs of toxicity appear can confirm toxicity. Neither toxicity nor efficacy can be confirmed throughout the dosing interval, however, unless two samples (peak and trough) are collected (Case Study 5-3).

If a kinetic profile of a patient is the reason for TDM, at least two samples must be collected to establish a PDC-versus-time relationship (Case Study 5-5). For such drugs, the samples preferably are collected at the peak and trough times. Regardless of the route of drug administration, with two data points, elimination (disappearance) half-life can be calculated. However, a more comprehensive kinetic profile can be built from the same two data points for a patient receiving an intravenous dose: volume of distribution (Vd) and clearance can then be estimated in addition to drug elimination half-life.

Loading doses warrant a special note. Loading is implemented with the goal of achieving steady state concentrations immediately. The advantage is to avoid the delay that otherwise will occur as steady state is gradually reached. The disadvantage is that the body will not have time to accommodate to side effects. As such, loading should be limited to situations in which failed response might be life-threatening. Although the design of the loading dose may be successful in achieving target steady state concentrations (see calculations below), the patient is not yet at steady state and will not be until the same dosing regimen has been implemented for 3 to 5 half-lives. Thus, as the patient transitions from the loading to the maintenance dose, the time to steady state begins again. If the maintenance dose fails to maintain what the loading dose achieved, then drug concentrations will gradually decline or increase until steady state is achieved (Figure 5-1, *B*). Because the majority of the change will occur in the first half-life of maintenance dosing, clinical signs of failure or toxicity may be more likely to occur during this initial half-life. Proactive monitoring after the loading dose has been absorbed and again at the first half-life will allow the clinician to assess the effectiveness of the maintenance dose. However, both samples must be collected for the assessment. Collecting a sample one half-life after the loading dose without a postload sample is minimally informative. For example, when using a loading dose for bromide, TDM should be performed three times. The first time to monitor is after oral absorption of the last of the loading doses to establish what the loading dose accomplished (i.e., day 6). The second time is at one drug half-life later

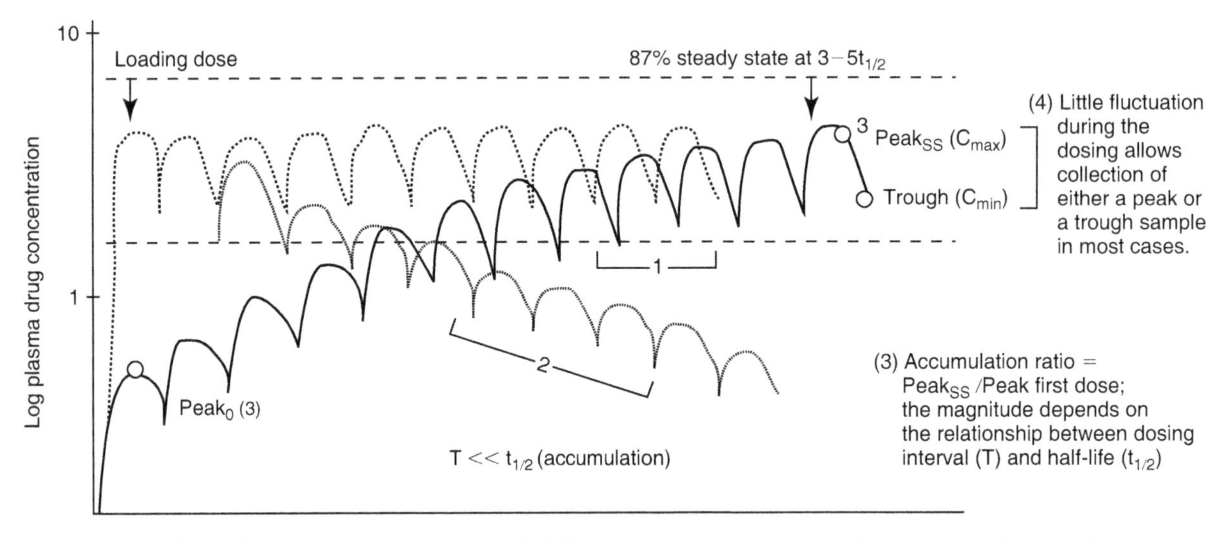

Figure 5-1, Cont'd (B) For drugs whose elimination half-life is much longer than the dosing interval, the drug will accumulate across time, with maximum accumulation occurring only at three to five drug elimination half-lives. Steady state will be achieved only at this time. The time to steady state starts over each time the dosing regimen is changed, including transitioning from a loading dose to a maintenance dose (coarse dotted lines). The maintenance dose is designed to maintain what the loading dose achieved (fine dotted line). However, if over or under dosed, drug concentrations will gradually change (decline demonstrated with fine dotted lines), until a new steady state is reached. Therapeutic failure may occur. C_1, C_2 = concentration of samples 1 and 2, respectively; k_{el} = elimination rate constant; $peak_0$ = peak following first dose; $peak_{ss}$ = peak at steady state; T = interval; $t_{1/2}$ = drug elimination half-life; t_1, t_2 = time samples 1 and 2 were collected, respectively.

(e.g., at 21 days for bromide) to ensure that the maintenance dose is able to maintain concentrations achieved by loading. Collection of this second sample at the one drug half-life point is recommended because most of the change in drug concentrations that will occur if the maintenance dose is not correct will occur during the first half-life. If the second sample (collected at one drug half-life) does not approximate the first (collected immediately after the loading doses), the maintenance dose can be modified at this time rather than wait for steady state, with the risk of therapeutic failure or toxicity. The third time to monitor bromide when using a loading dose is at steady state (e.g., 3 months) to establish a new baseline.

KEY POINT 5-2 The maintenance dose that follows the loading dose must maintain what has been achieved with the loading dose. Monitoring of drugs dosed as a load should occur shortly after the loading dose is given and then one half-life into the maintenance dose. If the two concentrations do not match, the maintenance dose should be modified.

The timing of sample collection also must take into account the pharmacodynamic response of some drugs. For example, many antimicrobials (e.g., aminoglycosides) are characterized by a half-life that is less than 2 hours (e.g., amikacin in dogs) but are given at much longer dosing intervals (e.g., 24 hours). The peak sample is important for determination of efficacy of this concentration-dependent drug. Because 12 half-lives will have elapsed before the next dose, less than 2% of the original dose will remain in the body at true trough concentrations, and concentrations are not likely to be detectable at true trough (i.e., 24 hrs after dosing). Although the absence of detectable drug may be sufficient information if safety is the reason for monitoring an aminoglycoside, kinetics (e.g., half-life) cannot be determined. Therefore collection of both a 2-hour peak and and a sample two to four elimination half-lives later will allow calculation of a half-life and extrapolation of concentrations at trough (Case Study 5-5). Cyclosporine is another example: if administered every 24 to 48 hours, because its half-life in normal dogs approximates 4 to 5 hours, little drug will be detected at 24 to 48 hours.

Specific timing of peak PDC collection is more difficult to determine accurately than that of trough concentrations. Peak PDC should be determined after drug absorption and distribution are complete (see Chapter 1). Route of drug administration can influence the time at which peak PDCs occur, which varies among drugs. For orally administered drugs, absorption is slower (1 to 2 hours), and distribution is often complete by the time peak PDCs have been achieved. The absorption rate can, however, vary widely due to factors such

CASE STUDY 5-1 THERAPEUTIC FAILURE DUE TO PHENOBARBITAL INDUCTION OF DRUG METABOLIZING ENZYMES

Signalment
3.5-year-old male Labrador Retriever

Chief Complaint
Seizures

Pertinent History
A diagnosis of epilepsy was made 6 months before presentation. Patient was suffering from severe cluster seizures. There was an initial response to phenobarbital, but seizures occurred again 6 months into therapy.

Drug of Interest
Phenobarbital

Concern
Efficacy

Other Drugs
None

Dosing Regimen
4.1 mg/kg every 12 hours, administered orally

Duration of Current Regimen
Six months. Phenobarbital concentrations at 3 months (baseline) were 35 μg/mL (peak) and 31 μg/mL (trough). Elimination half-life at that time was 40 hours.

Patient Response
Seizure control initially improved, and there was no evidence of grogginess. The patient suffered a series of cluster seizures this weekend. The referring veterinarian was interested in adding an alternative anticonvulsant (e.g., bromide).

Drug Concentration
18 μg/mL; time: 5 hours
15 μg/mL; time: 12 hours

Drug Elimination Half-Life
27 hours

Predicted Peak
NA

Predicted Trough
NA

Recommendation
Increase phenobarbital dose to 7.5 mg/kg every 12 hours (4.5 mg/kg × 30 μg/mL per 18 μg/mL), targeting a peak concentration of 30 μg/mL. Retest at new steady state (which will take only 3 to 5.5 days in this patient).

Comments
Phenobarbital concentrations decreased in this patient by nearly 50% without a decrease in dose. The elimination half-life decreased by 50%. The decrease most likely reflects induction of drug-metabolizing enzymes by phenobarbital, resulting in increased clearance and decreased drug concentrations. Induction occurs in most animals and should be anticipated by using a sufficiently high starting dose (2 mg/kg) for phenobarbital and measuring drug concentrations at steady state (approximately 2 weeks after therapy is begun) and then again at 3 months.

Follow-Up
The dose was increased to 6.5 mg/kg. Drug concentrations 1 month later were 33 mg/mL (peak) and 29 mg/mL (trough). The patient has been seizure-free for 6 months. The high phenobarbital dose and the short half-life indicate that induction, and thus metabolism, may be marked in this patient. It is possible that increased production of metabolites places this patient at risk for phenobarbital-associated hepatic disease. Accordingly, the addition of a second anticonvulsant that will allow a decrease in phenobarbital dose might be appropriate.

as product preparation, the effect of food, and patient variability. Obviously, a drug prepared as an elixir will be absorbed more rapidly than the same drug prepared as a capsule or tablet. Because food can slow the absorption of many drugs, fasting is generally indicated (if safe) before TDM. Generally, peak PDCs occur 1 to 2 hours after oral administration. Some drugs are simply absorbed more slowly than others (e.g., phenobarbital), and the time of peak PDC sample collection is longer (e.g., 2 to 5 hours for phenobarbital). For drugs administered intravenously, distribution, but not absorption is a concern. For delayed-release drugs, a sample at any time may be acceptable. For some intramuscular and subcutaneous administrations, absorption occurs rapidly (i.e., 30 to 60 minutes), but, again, drug distribution may take longer. Thus peak PDCs generally are measured 1 to 2 hours after parenteral drug administration (see Table 5-1).

Other Considerations

Sample requirements vary not only in the blood component (e.g., serum, plasma, whole blood, urine, etc) but also in the volume and sampling handling. Constituents in plasma differ substantially among species, and these constituents can interfere with the methodology of some assays. Removal of these constituents varies with the methodology, with the sample size generally being larger for assays that require more clean-up (e.g., HPLC vs. antibody-based assays). Laboratories chosen for monitoring should be queried before sample submission to ensure that the proper submission procedures are followed.

CASE STUDY 5-2 DIGOXIN-INDUCED TOXICITY; LONG ELIMINATION HALF-LIFE

Signalment
6-year-old male Dachshund cross

Chief Complaint
Congestive heart failure; renal failure

Pertinent History
The patient has been receiving digoxin therapy for 6 months. Within the last 3 months, renal disease has become decompensated. The day before presentation, the patient vomited and became ataxic and disoriented. Patient blood urea nitrogen is 82 mg/dL, and creatinine is 1.57 mg/dL.

Drug of Interest
Digoxin

Concern
Safety

Other Drugs
Enalapril, furosemide, thyroxine

Dosing Regimen
0.005 mg/kg every 12 hours, administered orally

Duration of Current Regimen
90 days

Drug Concentration
2.40 ng/mL; time: 2 hours
2.47 ng/mL; time: 12 hours

Drug Elimination Half-Life
>52 hours

Predicted Peak
NA

Predicted Trough
NA

Recommendation
Concentrations are at the upper end of the therapeutic range and are not necessarily consistent with toxicity, but a decrease in dose by about 20%, targeting 2.0 ng/mL, would be prudent. Clinical signs of uremia cannot be distinguished from clinical signs of digoxin toxicity. Prolonging the interval to at least 24 hours also would be appropriate. Collecting a peak and 24-hour trough concentration would be indicated to determine the proper dosing interval.

Comments
The prolonged half-life for digoxin in this patient presumably reflects decompensated renal disease. Note that both a peak and a trough sample were helpful in establishing the prolonged drug elimination half-life. Without both samples, the duration of the half-life and the magnitude of decreased clearance could not have been appreciated (see Case Study 5-4). Should the patient respond to therapy for its renal disease and digoxin elimination improve, monitoring is again indicated to establish a new dosing regimen because drug half-life is likely to decrease.

Follow-Up
NA

CASE STUDY 5-3 DIGOXIN THERAPY; RESPONSE AND SHORT HALF-LIFE

Signalment
8-year-old female Hound cross

Chief Complaint
Congestive heart failure resulting from mitral insufficiency

Pertinent History
The patient has been receiving digoxin therapy for 8 days. Patient has responded to therapy and is showing no evidence of toxicity.

Drug of Interest
Digoxin

Concern
Baseline check

Other Drugs
Enalapril, furosemide, a nonsteroidal antiinflammatory, and chlorpheniramine

Dosing Regimen
0.008 mg/kg every 12 hours, administered orally

Duration of Current Regimen
8 days

Drug Concentration
2.88 ng/mL; time: 1.25 hours
1.42 ng/mL; time: 9 hours

Drug Elimination Half-Life
8 hours

Continued

CASE STUDY 5-3 DIGOXIN THERAPY; RESPONSE AND SHORT HALF-LIFE—cont'd

Volume of distribution
NA

Predicted Peak
NA

Predicted Trough
NA

Recommendation
Concentrations are above the upper end of the therapeutic range, but with no evidence of toxicity, the dose should not necessarily be changed. With a 12-hour half-life, the dosing interval should not be prolonged (and could be reduced to an 8-hour dosing interval with the same total daily dose). Leave dosing regimen as is, or decrease dose by 10%.

Comments
Compare the drug half-life in this patient with the reported normal (24 hours) and with that in Case Study 5-2. Had a single sample been collected halfway through the dosing interval, concentrations would have been in the lower end of the therapeutic range, and the dose may have been inappropriately increased. The half-life in this patient indicates that the dosing interval should not be longer than 12 hours. Should a 24-hour dosing interval be used, trough drug concentrations would approximate 0.35 ng/mL.

Follow-Up
NA

CASE STUDY 5-4 THEOPHYLLINE–ENROFLOXACIN DRUG INTERACTION

Signalment
6-year-old male neutered Collie

Chief Complaint
Hyperactivity. Allergic rhinitis has been present for 2 months. There is radiographic evidence of lung lobe consolidation, and clinical signs are compatible with pneumonia that developed 1 week before presentation.

Pertinent History
Theophylline therapy begun 3 days before presentation. The patient began exhibiting signs of hyperactivity and restlessness 24 hours before presentation.

Drug of Interest
Theophylline

Concern
Toxicity

Other Drugs
Enrofloxacin 2.5 mg/kg every 12 hours orally (begun at the same time as theophylline); prednisolone 1 mg/kg every 48 hours

Dosing Regimen
21 mg/kg every 12 hours (slow-release product), administered orally

Duration of Current Regimen
3 days

Patient Response
Restlessness, pacing, irritability

Drug Concentration
47 µg/mL; time:12 hours
31 µg/mL; time: 24 hours

Drug Elimination Half-Life
19 hours

Volume of distribution
NA

Predicted Peak
Approximately 65 µg/mL

Predicted Trough
NA

Recommendation
Decrease the dose by half, or decrease the dose by 25% and prolong the dosing interval by 12 to 24 hours. Retest at the new steady state (in 3 days) and at discontinuation of enrofloxacin.

Follow-Up
After monitoring, the dosing interval was prolonged to 24 hours, and the dose was decreased by 50% from 20 to 10 mg/kg. A recheck revealed a peak and trough concentration of 12.3 µg/mL and 10.3 µg/mL at 2 and 22 hours, respectively. Near subtherapeutic concentrations indicated that either the dose might be increased or the interval decreased to 12 hours.

Comments
The fluorinated quinolones can increase concentrations of theophylline when the two drugs are given simultaneously. The mechanism is presumed to be due to impaired drug metabolism by enrofloxacin with subsequent decreased theophylline clearance. This drug interaction is well established for ciprofloxacin in humans and also has been documented for enrofloxacin. The drug elimination half-life of theophylline in this patient while receiving enrofloxacin was 19 hours, which is twice that expected in dogs.

CASE STUDY 5-5 AMINOGLYCOSIDE AND INTENSIVE FLUID THERAPY

Signalment
2-year-old male intact Staffordshire Bull Terrier

Chief Complaint
Peritonitis and bacteremia secondary to prostatic abscess

Pertinent History
Surgical correction of prostatic abscess; drug samples collected 24 hours postoperatively

Drug of Interest
Gentamicin

Concern
Efficacy and safety

Other Drugs
Antiemetics (metoclopramide); intensive fluid therapy (balanced crystalloid)

Dosing Regimen
4 mg/kg every 24 hours, administered intravenously

Duration of Current Regimen
24 hours

Patient Response
Febrile, nonresponsive

Drug Concentration
5.34 μg/mL; time: 2 hours
0.73 μg/mL; time: 9 hours

Drug Elimination Half-Life
2.4 hours

Volume of distribution:
0.45 L/kg

Predicted Peak
10 μg/mL

Predicted Trough
Nondetectable

Recommendation
A peak concentration of 10 μg/mL is sufficient for anticipated efficacy toward a microbe susceptible to gentamicin at 1 μg.mL or less. Double the dose to target 20 μg/mL (assuming a minimal inhibitory concentration of 1 to 2 μg/mL), and maintain current 24-hour dosing interval.

Follow-Up
The patient's condition remained critical for 2 more postoperative days but then began to improve progressively. The patient was discharged 10 days postoperatively.

Comments
Actual peak gentamicin concentration was lower than expected (expected: 10 μg/mL), presumably because of intensive fluid therapy. The reported volume of distribution for gentamicin in dogs is 0.25 L/kg, but it was 0.45 L/kg in this patient. Gentamicin is distributed to extracellular fluid, which was probably increased in this patient by fluid therapy. A nearly doubled distribution volume resulted in a near halving of peak concentrations. The drug elimination half-life in this patient is 2.4 hours, which is normal. Doubling of the dose will add only one drug half-life to the time that target trough concentrations (<1 μg/mL) will be reached, which currently occurs by 9 hours in this patient. Even if the drug elimination half-life were to double (to 5 hours), sufficient time will elapse during a 24-hour dosing interval to allow drug concentrations to reach the targeted 1 μg/mL. Note that the trough sample was not collected in this patient just before the next dose (i.e., at 24 hours). The drug would not have been detectable at that time; hence trough concentrations were collected after two predicted drug half-lives had elapsed.

Some drugs may require refrigeration or freezing. Sample size may vary for each drug or even for the same drug depending on the method the laboratory uses. Drugs can interact with the containers in which they are collected or mailed. In general, serum separator tubes should not be used to collect or mail samples containing drug. Drugs can bind to the silicone gel, which decreases concentrations measured in blood. Aminoglycosides can bind to glass; samples should be collected and submitted in plastic tubes. The effects of hemolysis and hyperlipidemia on drug assays vary. In general, it is wise to avoid either in sample collection. Although sample handling is often the same for each drug, the laboratory to which the sample will be submitted should be contacted before the sample is sent for TDM analysis. Details regarding timing of sample, collection, storage apparatus (i.e., tubes and anticoagulants), mailing instructions (including conditions), and cost should be known before collection.

INTERPRETATION

Information Needed for Therapeutic Drug Monitoring

For best results, a sample submitted for monitoring should be accompanied by all relevant information that the clinical pharmacologist needs to evaluate the relationship among dose, concentration, and response in the context of physiologic, pharmacologic, and pathologic factors that might alter this relationship (Box 5-3).

Box 5-3

Maximizing the Interpretation of Therapeutic Drug Monitoring

First and foremost, involve a clinical pharmacologist in the interpretation of problematic cases.

The minimum information necessary for interpretation of therapeutic drug monitoring (TDM) by a clinical pharmacologist includes the following:

1. The total daily dose of drug, presented as mg/kg for each dose. Total units (capsules, tablets, or mL) are useless if not provided in the context of mg/kg.
2. Time interval of drug administration. This is particularly important for drugs with short half-lives (e.g., aminoglycosides). If half-life is to be determined, the timing of sample collection in relation to dose must be given for both the peak and trough sample.
3. The time that the sample was collected in relationship to the dose. For example, a concentration that puts levetiracetam in the high therapeutic range means much more if that concentration was measured at 12 hours versus 2 hours.
4. The reason for TDM should be given (e.g., has the patient failed therapy, or is the patient exhibiting signs of toxicity?).
5. The disease being treated with the drug (i.e., the therapeutic range for cyclosporine varies with the syndrome being treated).
6. Patient status at the time of sample collection and/or submission.
7. Pathologic factors that might affect drug disposition. This includes the extent of disease (that is, how abnormal is the serum creatinine in a patient with renal disease, or how low is the albumin in the patient with liver disease?).
8. Concurrently administered drugs may alter drug disposition patterns and thus contribute to individual differences in drug disposition. Frequency, dose, amount, and the actual times of all drugs given to the patient must be known in order to recognize or predict potential drug interactions. For example, cyclosporine administered with azithromycin may result in concentrations that are disproportionate to the dose.
9. For selected concurrently administered drugs that can be monitored, current concentrations should be provided. For example, recommendations for a seizing patient receiving bromide at a dose that has achieved concentrations in the midtherapeutic range may differ if the phenobarbital the patient is currently receiving is in the subtherapeutic range.
10. Physiologic characteristics such as patient species, breed, and age are often important to the interpretation of the plasma drug concentration because known or predictable differences may induce drug disposition and because there may be known differences in pharmacodynamic responses. For example, cats, Greyhounds, and working (Collie-related and other) breeds are all at risk to develop toxicity with selected drugs.

Concentrations must be evaluated in the context of the clinical patient, the mechanism of drug action and the therapeutic intent of monitoring or drug administration. The history of the patient also may be important information. For example, a subtherapeutic range in a controlled seizure patient may not require manipulation if the seizure history of the patient is not severe, but higher concentrations might be prudent if historically, the patient suffers cluster seizures. The absence of seizures in a dog with subtherapeutic concentrations also is not justification for discontinuing the drug. At the other end of the range, some animals may respond only if concentrations are higher than the recommended maximum concentration. Drug concentrations need not necessarily be reduced if there is no concern regarding toxicity or unacceptable side effects, even if the maximum therapeutic range has been surpassed (e.g., bromide).

Dose Modification with Kinetic Calculations

Most dose modifications do not require kinetic calculations (discussed in more detail later). Target calculations include elimination half-life on which the proper dosing interval and time to steady state can be based, and, for a drug given intravenously, Vd or clearance. The minimum number of data points needed to develop a pharmacokinetic profile in a patient is two. Generally, for TDM these two samples consist of the peak and trough (see Figure 5-1, *A*) collected during a single dosing interval at steady state. Alternatively, for the sake of convenience, a trough sample can be collected just before a dose and the peak sample collected 2 to 5 hours (when appropriate for the drug) after dosing. This protocol assumes that the drug is handled the same way by the body during each dosing regimen and that the dose is the same. Although this may be true, conditions such as diurnal variation can alter drug disposition between dosing intervals. Oftentimes, the dose is not the same for both morning and evening.

Regardless of when the samples are collected (assuming that they are collected after absorption and distribution are complete), when the points are plotted on semilogarithmic paper, the slope between the two points reflects k_{el} (or, if non-IV administration, $k_{disappearance}$) (see Figure 5-1, *A*), which is used to determine drug half-life in the patient (see Chapter 1). Half-life can be either calculated or estimated from the PDC-versus-time curve drawn on semilogarithmic paper. The two points are connected, and the resultant line is extrapolated to both the x and y axes. For estimation, the time that must elapse between any two concentrations on the line where one concentration is twice the second is the half-life (see Figure 5-1, *A*). The half-life also can be calculated from k_{el} (the slope, or rise [C_1-C_2] over the run [$\tilde{t}_2$-t_1]). Because concentration is logarithmic, the equation becomes half-life = ln [C_1-/C_2] / [t_2-t_1]). Thus, although it is not necessary to actually plot the line to determine elimination half-life, the time that each dose was given and each sample was drawn must be known for its calculation (see Figures 5-1 and 5-2). Half-life determines the maximum time that can elapse between doses in the patient before PDCs fall below the recommended minimum effective concentration during the dosing interval (T_{max}) (see Figures 5-1, *A* and 5-2).

The Vd of drugs administered intravenously can be calculated from the peak PDC and dose (see Figure 5-2 and Case Study 5-5). If the drug is 100% bioavailable after oral, subcutaneous, or intramuscular administration, Vd can also be estimated

Elimination rate constant:	$k_{cl} = \ln (C_1/C_2)/(t_2 - t_1)$
Drug elimination half-life:	$t_{1/2} = 0.693/k_{el}$
Maximum time that can lapse between doses:	$T_{max} = \ln (C_{max}/C_{min})/k_{el}$
Amount of drug to be administered during a dosing interval:	$D_{M,max} = (V_d/F) \times (C_{max} - C_{min})$
Dose per unit time:	$D_{M,max}/T_{max}$
Dose each interval:	$\frac{D_{M,max} \times \text{Interval}}{T_{max}}$
Loading dose where Css = concentration at steady state:	$D_L = (V_d/F) \times C_{ss,max}$
Accumulation ratio: (relationship between C first dose and C at steady state):	$1/(1-[1/2]^Z)$ or $1/1-e^{T/t}{}_{1/2}$
New (proportional) dose increase:	New dose = $\frac{\text{Current dose} \times \text{new target concetration}}{\text{current concentration}}$

C_{max} = maximum PDC (peak)

C_{min} = minimum PDC (trough)

$C_{ss,max}$ = maximum (target) PDC at steady-state (ss; ed, mg/ml)

Vd = apparent volume of distribution (L/kg)

F = bioavailability (100% if IV)

Z = $T/t_{1/2}$ (Interval/half-life)

Figure 5-2 The data necessary for calculating dosing regimens can be obtained from therapeutic drug monitoring and, if necessary, from values reported in the literature, as modified (e.g., Vd) for the patient. C_1, C_2 = concentration of samples 1 and 2, respectively; C_{max} = maximum PDC (peak); C_{min} = minimum PDC (trough); $C_{ss,\ max}$ = maximum (target) PDC at steady state (mg/mL); F = bioavailability (100% if intravenous); ln = interval; K_{el} = elimination rate constant; PDC = plasma drug concentration; t_1, t_2 = time samples 1 and 2 were collected, respectively; Vd = volume of distribution (L/kg); Z = $T/t_{1/2}$ (interval [T]/half-life [$t_{1/2}$]). For patient calculation of Vd and Cl, the drug must be given IV.

from these data, assuming the drug also would be 100% bioavailable in the patient. For orally administered drugs for which the bioavailability is not known, a population bioavailability and Vd measured in normal animals must be used if new dosing regimens are to be calculated rather than proportionately adjusted. Like bioavailability, however, individual patient Vd may not be accurately estimated by population Vd. Changes in patient Vd compared with those in normal animals can be somewhat accommodated if information regarding patient factors that influence Vd, such as obesity, edema, ascites, dehydration, and serum protein concentrations, are known (see Chapters 1 and 2).

The Vd is used to calculate the amount of drug that must be administered to achieve C_{max}, the target (generally maximum) effective drug concentration (loading dose [D_L]), and the amount of drug necessary to replace drug eliminated during the dosing interval (maintenance dose, D_M) (see Figure 5-2). Once D_M and T_{max} have been established, dosing regimens can be appropriately altered to ensure that PDCs fall within a recommended therapeutic range (see Figure 5-2). For drugs with short half-lives, both a peak and a trough drug sample should be collected post dose modification to ensure that a minimum effective concentration (C_{min}) is achieved and concentrations above the maximum (C_{max}) are avoided during the designed dosing interval.

Dose Modification Without Kinetics (Proportional Adjustment)

Not all modifications in dosing regimens require pharmacokinetic calculations. If a patient has drug concentrations outside the therapeutic range, the dose should be modified to change the drug concentrations into the therapeutic range by a proportional adjustment. Generally, a dose can be proportionately modified using one of the following equations:

New dose = Old dose × Targeted PDC/ Observed patient PDC or for drugs that accumulate

New interval = Old interval × Observed PDC/ Targeted PDC

In general, targeting a 25% to 50% change is reasonable, if time allows a gradual adjustment. Because TDM identifies the therapeutic range specific for the patient, some patients will respond at the low end of the population range, some will not respond until the maximum is reached, and a smaller percentage of the population will respond at concentrations outside the recommended range.

If a patient has not responded, even for patients within the therapeutic range, drug concentrations can be gradually increased (in a stair-step fashion) until either the patient responds or the maximum end of the range is reached and the risk of adverse effects becomes too great. The direction can be reversed if drug concentrations are too high to establish a minimum effective dose. The decision as to whether to change the dose or the interval depends on the drug itself, its therapeutic index, and the need to maintain PDCs within the therapeutic range throughout a dosing interval. However, for drugs with a short half life, shortening the interval may be less expensive than increasing the dose.

Even TDM is used to ensure that the PDC stays within a targeted concentration (that is, the patient's therapeutic range) during a dosing interval, a patient may react adversely (including the failure to respond therapeutically). Disease, age, and other factors may play a role in the minimum or maximum effective concentration appropriate for each patient (see Case Studies 5-2, 5-3, and 5-5). Therefore it is imperative that PDCs be interpreted in conjunction with the desired therapeutic end point (i.e., complete eradication of seizures versus a decrease in the severity and frequency) as well as the clinical status of the patient. This is particularly important for tests for which there is great overlap between normal and abnormal ranges (e.g., digoxin, thyroid hormones).

Phenobarbital

Generally, a single trough sample should be sufficient for TDM. However, if induction of drug-metabolizing enzymes has occurred, the elimination half-life may be sufficiently short to allow excessive fluctuation in PDC during the dosing interval. This short half-life can be detected only if both peak and trough samples are measured. In a phenobarbital-naïve dog, or when phenobarbital doses are changed, baseline samples should be determined at steady state, 9 to 14 days after beginning therapy. A recheck trough sample 1 to 3 months later would be prudent to detect induction. Many of our patients respond to phenobarbital at concentrations below the minimum therapeutic range of 15 μg/mL, which suggests that a lower therapeutic range may be indicated in dogs.

Bromide

Because the elimination half-life of bromide is so long, manipulating the dose before steady state is reached may be necessary for some patients. Collection of a sample at one half-life after the start of therapy (i.e., 2-4 weeks) can be performed to proactively assess the dose; doubling the 3 weeks concentration should approximate the steady state concentration. Baseline should be established at 2.5 to 3 months. If the patient is loaded, a sample should be collected the day after loading is complete, and then at one half-life. The former sample is indicated to determine what the loading dose achieved and the latter to ensure that the maintenance dose is maintaining what the loading dose has achieved; the two samples should be within 15% of each other. If not, the maintenance dose can be adjusted proportionately. Note that a 3-week sample in a patient that received a loading dose is minimally useful without the postload monitoring sample for comparison: concentrations may increase or decrease, depending on the accuracy of the maintenance dose. In all patients, regardless of the method of dosing, a final sample should be collected at steady state to establish baseline. Finally, bromide should also be checked before and after any change in diet or medication that impacts chloride excretion has occurred.

Zonisamide

The half-life of zonisamide is generally longer than 24 hours; therefore, concentrations should not fluctuate sufficiently during a 12-hour dosing interval to routinely justify a peak and trough sample. Because toxicity is not likely to be as great a concern as therapeutic failure, a trough sample is recommended for routine monitoring. In problematic patients a peak and a trough may be justified to rule out a short half-life as a contributing cause of difficult control. Currently, zonisamide is among the drugs for which the maximum therapeutic range, which has been established in humans, can be exceeded with minimal adverse effects in dogs.

Levetiracetam

The half-life of levetiracetam (standard release) can be as short as 1 to 2 hours. However, the half-life also can be longer than 8 to 10 hours; longer half-lives should be anticipated if the slow release preparation is used. Because the duration of the half-life is not known, peak and trough samples are recommended at the beginning of therapy to determine the half-life in patients. Control is much more likely to be accomplished with an 8-hour dosing interval in a patient with a longer half-life. Once the half-life is established, a trough sample is recommended if only single samples are to be collected. A midsample concentration has little to offer, particularly given that drug concentrations may drop 50% or more from mid-interval concentrations. Thus it is prudent to identify the lowest concentration possible during the interval. The recommended therapeutic range should be targeted by trough, rather than peak, concentration. Note that in a drug with a very short half-life (e.g., 2 hours), peak concentrations in a patient may be as much as 8 times as high as trough concentrations. Levetiracetam is sufficiently safe that a high peak concentration is likely to be tolerated. Because drug concentrations do not accumulate with drugs administered at an interval substantially longer than the half-life, steady state does not occur. Therefore levetiracetam (or another drug with a short half-life) might be monitored in the first 3 to 5 days of therapy. Waiting one seizure interval to ensure that seizures are adequately controlled is reasonable. The approach for monitoring levetiracetam can be followed with other anticonvulsants associated with a short half-life compared to the dosing interval (e.g., gabapentin), unless the drug is potentially toxic. In such situations, monitoring peak and trough concentrations routinely may be prudent.

Digoxin

Although a mid-interval sample traditionally has been recommended for digoxin, unless the half-life is known to be long, a mid-interval sample provides incomplete information regarding either toxicity or efficacy. For patients in which the half-life is less than 24 hours, both a peak (2-3 hour) and trough (before next dose) sample should be collected for this drug, particularly if a 24-hour dosing interval is used. The elimination half-life is often short, particularly in animals responding to afterload reduction, and the narrow therapeutic window (which differs approximately twofold) mandates the need to know the behavior of this drug throughout the dosing interval. For example, if the half-life is 12 hr, it is likely that concentrations will be either above or below the therapeutic range (1-2 ng/mL). A single peak sample can be collected if only toxicity is the concern; a single trough sample is indicated if the question to be answered by monitoring is whether concentrations are above the minimum therapeutic range throughout the dosing interval.

Theophylline

Single trough samples may be sufficient for slow-release products such as theophylline in cats if efficacy is the concern; a peak sample would be indicated if toxicity is the concern. Both peak and trough samples should be collected in dogs receiving

CASE STUDY 5-6 PHENOBARBITAL–CHLORAMPHENICOL DRUG INTERACTION

Signalment
3.5-year-old male German Shepherd Dog

Chief Complaint
Acute onset of depression, anorexia, and lethargy. Concern: Bromism.

Pertinent History
A diagnosis of epilepsy was made 1 year before presentation. The patient was suffering from severe cluster seizures. The response to phenobarbital was initially acceptable, but seizures worsened and potassium bromide was added 6 months into therapy (see monitoring below). The dose was re-adjusted 3 months later (3 months before presentation). Although the patient has stopped seizuring, the patient was treated for a cough 1 week before presentation. Lower respiratory infection was diagnosed and antimicrobial therapy begun. Phenobarbital but not bromide was measured at that time (32 μg/mL). Three days later, the patient presented for the chief complaint. Physical examination reveals the patient to be moribund, but vital signs are otherwise normal. Clinical laboratory tests are normal. The referring veterinarian is concerned that the bromide dose is responsible for clinical signs.

Drug of Interest
Bromide (25 mg/kg bid for 3 months)

Concern
Toxicity

Other Drugs
Phenobarbital 4 mg/kg every 12 hours, administered orally (at current dose for 2 weeks; last phenobarbital collected was at steady state with the current dosing regimen); chloramphenicol 25 mg/kg every 8 hours for 3 days

Dosing Regimen
A 450 mg/kg loading dose measured 6 months before presentation was 0.9 mg/mL. The maintenance dose was 10 mg/kg every 12 hours. Although concentrations were not measured, this maintenance dose would predictably result in steady state concentrations of 0.75 mg/mL. Two months after the loading dose, a dose increase to 25 mg/kg every 12 hours was implemented. Concentrations were not subsequently measured at steady state.

Duration of Current Regimen
Bromide, 6 months; phenobarbital 1 year; chloramphenicol, 50 mg/kg tid, 4 days

Patient Response
Seizure control was improved. Patient was not groggy until recent episode.

Drug Concentration
2.10 μg/mL; time: 12 hours

Drug Elimination Half-Life
NA

Volume of distribution:
NA

Predicted Peak
NA

Predicted Trough
NA

Recommendation
Although bromide concentrations are in midtherapeutic range, they are not sufficiently increased to cause the profound nature of the clinical signs. The concentrations are comparable to the dose. Phenobarbital concentrations were measured: peak concentration was 50 μg/mL; trough concentration was 46 μg/mL. Phenobarbital elimination half-life was 58 hours. This increase occurred in a week time period.

Comments
This patient was presented for presumed bromide toxicity. The bromide concentrations were not, however, consistent with the profound depression the patient was exhibiting. Phenobarbital concentrations were checked to identify a possible contribution to lethargy in a sample of blood collected just before the onset of chloramphenicol therapy. Phenobarbital concentrations had increased in this patient by 40% to 50%, despite no dose change; it is likely that concentrations would continue to increase as a new steady state was reached. The increase was presumed to be due to chloramphenicol therapy. Chloramphenicol is a potent inhibitor of drug-metabolizing enzymes, resulting in decreased phenobarbital clearance. Drug elimination half-life had not been previously determined for phenobarbital in this patient, so a change in half-life could not be documented.

Follow-Up
Chloramphenicol therapy was discontinued. Phenobarbital therapy was discontinued for one drug elimination half-life and then restarted at the same dose. Within 48 hours, the patient was normal.

slow-release preparations. For regular preparations, both samples should be collected.

Cyclosporine

Monitoring cyclosporine is complex and is addressed in depth in Chapter 31. The elimination half-life of cyclosporine in normal dogs or cats is 4 to 8 hours, and, as such, both a peak and trough might be indicated. Recommendations may also depend on therapeutic intent (i.e., immunosuppression, treatment of chronic allergic diseases such as atopy, perianal fistulas or asthma, etc). Recommendations as drawn from humans are based on either a peak or trough concentration, although a peak concentration correlates more closely to area under the curve during a dosing interval when targeting graft-versus-host rejection. Certainly, peak target concentrations are easier to achieve than trough target concentrations in patients with a short half-life. Monitoring also is complicated by the presence of drugs which might prolong the elimination half-life due to inhibition of drug metabolizing enzymes or enhance absorption through competition with P-glycoprotein; ketaconazole and azithromycin are examples of drugs that appear to do both. For such patients, both peak (2 hours) and trough (before next dose) samples are indicated to calculate half-life. This is particularly important to determine the time to steady state, a state which will occur only in those situations where the half-life of cyclosporine is markedly prolonged. For such situations the time to steady state may be very long, and final monitoring should not take place until steady state is reached. The time to steady state can be determined only by collection of a peak and a trough sample.

Antimicrobials

Because both the aminoglycosides and fluorinated quinolones are concentration-dependent drugs, peak concentrations are of critical interest. However, determination of true peak concentration requires that two samples be collected: a peak and a second sample approximately two half-lives later. The peak sample should be collected after drug distribution has occurred, or approximately 45 to 60 minutes after dosing. A true trough sample (i.e., just before the next dose) should not be collected because it is likely that concentrations will be undetectable for both fluorinated quinolones and aminoglyclosides (given once daily with half-lives less than 3 hours). An exception might exist for determining aminoglycosides' toxicity: documentation of trough concentrations below the minimum requires a sample just before the next dose.

SUMMARY

TDM can aid clinicians in the titration of drug doses to the individual patient, thus helping prevent adverse reactions that are a direct consequence of patient variability in drug disposition. In addition, TDM ensures that optimal drug concentrations are established promptly and that therapeutic drug concentrations are maintained, which spares patients a protracted period of ineffective drug therapy.

REFERENCES

1. Wilson RC: Therapeutic drug monitoring, *Auburn Vet* 42(3): 20–22, 1987.
2. Neff-Davis CA: Therapeutic drug monitoring in veterinary medicine, *Vet Clin North Am Small Anim Pract* 18(6):1287–1307, 1988.
3. Pippenger CF, Massoud N: Therapeutic drug monitoring. In Benet LZ, et al: *Pharmacokinetic basis for drug therapy*, New York, 1984, Raven Press, pp 367–393.
4. Arnsdorf MF: Cardiac excitability and antiarrhythmic drugs: a different perspective, *J Clin Pharmacol* 29:395–404, 1989.
5. Ravis WR, Nachreimer RF, Pedersoli WM, et al: Pharmacokinetics of phenobarbital in dogs after multiple oral administration, *Am J Vet Res* 45:1283–1286, 1984.
6. Cowan RH, Jukkola AF, Arant BS: Pathophysiologic evidence of gentamicin nephrotoxicity in neonatal puppies, *Pediatr Res* 14(11):1204–1211, 1980.
7. Atkins CE, Snyder PS, Keene BW, et al: Effects of compensated heart failure on digoxin pharmacokinetics in cats, *J Am Vet Med Assoc* 195(7):945–950, 1989.
8. Frazier DL, Riviere JE: Gentamicin dosing strategies for dogs with subclinical renal dysfunction, *Antimicrob Agents Chemother* 31(12):1929–1934, 1987.
9. Frazier DL, Aucoin DP, Riviere JE: Gentamicin pharmacokinetics and nephrotoxicity in naturally acquired and experimentally induced disease in dogs, *J Am Vet Med Assoc* 192(1):57–63, 1988.
10. Dunbar M, Pyle RL, Boring JG, et al: Treatment of canine blastomycosis with ketoconazole, *J Am Vet Med Assoc* 182(2): 156–157, 1983.
11. Ravis WR, Pedersoli WM, Turco JD: Pharmacokinetics and interactions of digoxin with phenobarbital in dogs, *Am J Vet Res* 48(8):1244–1249, 1987.
12. DeRick A, Balpaire F: Digoxin-quinidine interaction in the dog, *J Vet Pharmacol Ther* 4:215–218, 1981.
13. Abbott Laboratories: Therapeutic drug monitoring, clinical guide, diagnostic division, Dallas, 1984.
14. Drayer DE: Review problems in therapeutic drug monitoring: the dilemma of enantiomeric drugs in man, *Ther Drug Monit* 10:1–7, 1988.
15. Price CP: Analytical techniques for therapeutic drug monitoring, *Clin Biochem* 17:52–56, 1984.
16. Gal P: Therapeutic drug monitoring in neonates: problems and issues, *Drug Intell Clin Pharm* 22:317–323, 1988.

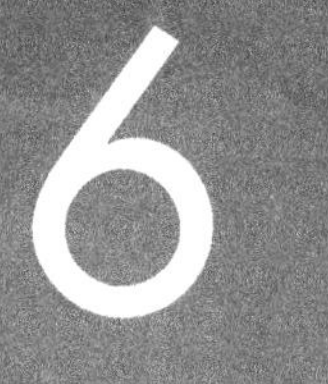

6 Principles of Antimicrobial Therapy*

Dawn Merton Boothe

Chapter Outline

JUDICIOUS ANTIMICROBIAL USE

"Even experienced practitioners may not realize that giving a patient antibiotics affects not just that patient, but also their environment, and all the other people that come into contact with that environment." Dancer's[1] statement, intended as a warning to practitioners of human medicine, emphasizes the importance of judicious antimicrobial therapy. It is understood that the goal of antimicrobial therapy is successful treatment of infection. However, the less judicious the approach taken to achieve that goal, the more likely a path to future failure is paved. The goal of antimicrobial therapy must be further modified to include avoidance of resistance, a goal that is not necessarily accomplished with successful resolution of infection. Although it might be tempting to consider that human and veterinary medicine are differentially affected by antimicrobial resistance, in reality both are inexorably linked, and what affects one will affect the other. As early as 1998, the National Foundation for Infectious Diseases estimated the cost of antibiotic-resistant bacteria to be as high as $4.5 billion annually and that they are responsible for more than 19,000 (human) deaths per year.[2] The impact is evident globally, nationally, in the community setting, in the hospital environment, and within the hospital, particularly with regard to at-risk patients (e.g., critical care).[3] Any antimicrobial used to treat a patient ultimately must be excreted into the environment; the impact of this is just now being addressed scientifically.

Empirical antimicrobial selection may become an approach of the past. As medical communities struggle to assess impact,

*The author would like to acknowledge the input regarding culture and susceptibility testing and interpretation and infection control provided by Terri Hathcock, MS, Diagnostic Veterinary Microbiologist, Auburn University.

causes, and means of avoidance, inappropriate antimicrobial use clearly is a consistent contributing factor to antimicrobial resistance. Inappropriate use includes both excessive and unnecessary use, as well as inappropriate dosing regimens. In the United States alone, approximately 350 million pounds of antibiotics are consumed annually in human medicine.[2] The numbers in veterinary medicine are less clear, but 20 million pounds were consumed by food animals during the same period.[2,4] Approximately 40% of human consumption of antimicrobials is considered unnecessary.[2] That we do not have a similar statistic regarding therapeutic antimicrobial use in veterinary patients reflects, perhaps, a somewhat cavalier attitude regarding antimicrobial stewardship both on the part of the manufacturers and the users. The veterinary profession has been intensely scrutinized by the medical community regarding its use of antimicrobial products in animals. This sometimes scientific and frequently emotional focus began with use in food animals but is shifting to companion animals.[5] Guardabassie[6] has described the role of the family pet as a reservoir of potentially resistant zoonotic organisms. Resistant strains of *Staphyloccocus intermedius, Campylobacter, Salmonella,* and *Escherichia coli* were cited as possible zoonotic concerns. At least 1% of annual salmonellosis cases in humans are assumed to be associated with companion animals.[6] Approximately 6% of *Campylobacter jejuni* infections in humans (children) are transmitted from pets.[6,7] Methicillin-resistant *Staphyloccoccus aureus* (MRSA) has been isolated in family members and pets in the same household[8-10]; methicillin-resistant *Staphylococcus intermedius** (MRSIG) has been reported in human patients[11]; and, perhaps disconcertingly, MRSA of animal origin (not previously identified in humans) has been identified in animals, albeit food animals (pigs).[12] In dogs *E. coli* strains are phylogenetically similar to pathogenic strains causing infection in humans; more than 15% of canine fecal deposits in the environment contain *E. coli* strains related to virulent human strains.[6] The concern regarding *E. coli* relates, in part, to its ability to develop resistance in the presence of antibiotic concentrations considered therapeutic.[13,14] Extraintestinal pathogenic *E. coli* (ExPEC, the "other" bad *E. coli*) appears to easily colonize the gastrointestinal tract, potentially displacing commensals and eventually emerging as infectious organisms in other body tissues, particularly in the urinary tract.[15] Further, *E. coli* is able to share mechanisms of resistance with other enteric pathogenic coliforms such as *Salmonella.*[13] Evidence exists for the transfer of resistance between *E. coli* and *Salmonella* and subsequent transfer of these organisms between animals (pet and farm animals) and humans[16]

KEY POINT 6-1 Antimicrobial use by veterinarians affects the global medical community; the veterinary hospital, the patient; and, as is increasingly being recognized, the pet owner.

**Staphylococcis intermedius* is likely to be renamed *Staphylococcus pseudintermedius*. Until official, the term *Staphylococcus intermedius* group (SIG) will be used to refer to this organism.

The pernicious advent of resistance over decades of antimicrobial use reveals that, despite their safety to the patient, antimicrobials are not innocuous drugs.[17] As in human medicine, antibiotic stewardship (i.e., judicious antimicrobial use) should become the focus for reducing resistance in veterinary medicine.[18] Prudent veterinarians and veterinary practices will implement decision-making processes (antimicrobial use paradigms) that minimize the temptation to use antimicrobials as alternative therapies. Designing a dosing regimen on the basis of cost and convenience, rather than on pharmacodynamics and pharmacokinetics, must become a paradigm of the past. Antimicrobial stewardship begins by recognizing the problems and issues and successfully implementing procedures that reasonably minimize the impact of antimicrobial use in the patient while not forfeiting the likelihood of therapeutic success. It is with this appproach this chapter emphasizes the rational basis for decision making in the selection of the proper antimicrobials.

DEFINITIONS AND GOALS

The terms *antibiotic, antibacterial,* and *antimicrobial* are often used interchangeably, despite their different meanings. *Antibiotics* are natural chemicals (e.g., penicillin) produced by organisms intended to suppress other organisms (generally, but not exclusively, bacteria), whereas *antimicrobial* refers to any compound, whether natural, synthetic, or a combination thereof, that suppresses microbial growth. *Antibacterials* target bacteria, antifungals target fungi, and so forth. The term *microbes* usually refers to bacterial organisms but also includes fungal and other (nonviral) organisms. Bacteria can be further categorized on the basis of their Gram-staining characteristics and their morphology (Box 6-1). This classification is helpful when matching bug to drug. In addition to staining characteristics, bacteria can be defined as **aerobic**—that is, those that generate energy (ATP) by aerobic respiration of oxygen. Some aerobes have minimal capacity to generate energy in the absence of oxygen and can be referred to as **obligate aerobes**. Although *Pseudomonas aeruginosa* might be classified as an obligate aerobe, it has the capacity to function, as with many other aerobes, as a **facultative anaerobe**. Facultative anaerobes prefer an oxygen-rich environment but are quite capable of switching to fermentation in the absence of oxygen. An example environment in which *P. aeruginosa* is able to survive in reduced oxygen environments (in humans) is cystic fibrosis. Other examples of facultative anaerobes include the families Enterobacteriaceae (e.g., *E. coli, Klebsiella pneumoniae, Proteus mirabilis*), Vibrionaceae (e.g., *Vibrio, Aeromonas*), and Pasteurellaceae (*Pasteurella, Haemophilus*). In contrast, **obligate anaerobes** cannot tolerate the presence of oxygen more than a few seconds. Examples include members of the family Bacteroides. *Clostridia* sp. is an example of an anaerobic organism whose oxygen toleration ranges from moderately tolerant (e.g., *Clostridia tetani*) to highly tolerant (e.g. *Clostridia perfringens*). **Microaerophilic** bacteria lie somewhere between aerobic and obligate anaerobes, in that they require low concentrations of oxygen to survive. Examples include

Box 6-1

Bergey's Classification of Medically Relevant Bacteria

Spirochetes
Spirochaetales
- Borrelia (Microaerophilic)
- Spirochaeta
- Treponema

Leptospiraceae
- Leptospira

Aerobic/Microaerophilic, Motile, Helical/Vibrioid Gram-Negative Bacteria
Campylobacter
Helicobacter

Gram-Negative Aerobic Rods and Cocci
Pseudomonadaceae
- Pseudomonas
- Xanthomonas

Legionellaceae
- Legionella

Neisseriaceae
- Acinetobacter
- Moraxella
- Neisseria

Other Genera
- Acidiphilium
- Acidomonas
- Alcaligenes
- Bordetella
- Brucella
- Flavobacterium
- Francisella

Facultatively Anaerobic Gram-Negative Rods
Enterobacteriaceae
- Citrobacter
- Edwardsiella
- Enterobacter
- Escherichia
- Klebsiella
- Kluyvera
- Morganella
- Proteus
- Providencia
- Salmonella
- Serratia
- Shigella
- Yersinia

Vibrionaceae
- Aeromonas
- Vibrio

Pasturellaceae
- Actinobacillus
- Haemophilus
- Mannheimia
- Pasteurella

Gram-Negative Anaerobic, Straight, Curved, and Helical Rods
Bacteroidaceae (Obligate anaerobes)
- Bacteroides
- Porphyromonas
- Prevotella
- Fusobacteriaceae

Anaerobic Gram-Negative Cocci
Veillonellaceae
- Acidaminococcus
- Megasphaera
- Syntrophococcus
- Veillonella

Rickettsias and Chlamydias
Rickettsiales
- Coxiella
- Rickettsia
- Rickettsiella
- Rochalimaea
- Wolbachia

Bartonellaceae
- Bartonella
- Grahamella

Anaplasmataceae
- Ehrlichia
- Neorickettsia
- Anaplasma
- Eperythrozoon
- Haemobartonella

Chlamydiales
- Chlamydiaceae
- Chlamydia

Mycoplasmas
Mycoplasmataceae
- Mycoplasma
- Ureaplasma

Spiroplasmataceae
- Spiroplasma

Gram-Positive Cocci
Aerobic, Catalase-Positive Genera
- Micrococcus
- Staphylococcus (also recognized as facultative anaerobe)

Aerotolerant, Catalase-Negative Genera
- Enterococcus
- Streptococcus (Pyogenic Hemolytic Streptococci, Oral Streptococci, Enterococci, Lactic Acid Streptococci, Anaerobic Streptococci)

Anaerobic, Catalase-Negative Genera
- Peptococcus
- Peptostreptococcus

Box 6-1

Bergey's Classification of Medically Relevant Bacteria—cont'd

Endospore-Forming Gram-Positive Rods and Cocci
Bacillus
Clostridium

Regular, Nonsporing Gram-Positive Rods
Erysipelothrix
Kurthia
Lactobacillus
Listeria
Renibacterium

Irregular, Nonsporing Gram-Positive Rods
Actinomyces
Bifidobacterium
Corynebacterium
Propionibacterium

Mycobacteria
Mycobacteriaceae
Mycobacterium

Nocardioforms
Nocardia
Nocardioides
Rhodococcus
Saccharopolyspora

(From Krieg NR, Staley JT, Hedlund B et al: *Bergey's manual of systematic bacteriology,* ed 2, Volume 4: The *Bacteroidetes, Spirochaetes, Tenericutes* (*Mollicutes*), *Acidobacteria, Fibrobacteres, Fusobacteria, Dictyoglomi, Gemmatimonadetes, Lentisphaerae, Verrucomicrobia, Chlamydiae,* and *Planctomycetes,* New York, 2010, Springer.)

Helicobacter and *Borrelia* spp.[19] When collecting a culture sample for such organisms, extreme care must be taken to prevent its exposure to oxygen. **Aerotolerant** organisms are not affected by either the presence or the absence of oxygen.

KEY POINT 6-2 Antibiotics are natural antimicrobials secreted by one microorganism to inhibit another. A microbe that secretes antibiotics also carries the genes for resistance to that antibiotic.

The term **organism** refers to either the genus or the genus and species of a microrganism. Examples include *E. coli, Staphylococcus pseudintermiedius group* (SIG), *Enterococcus faecalis,* and *Bacteroides fragilis.* For each of these organisms, multiple **strains** exist. An **isolate** refers to one **colony-forming unit** (CFU) of the resident population of that organism. This might be from any site, such as a lake, a feedlot, a surgical table, or the sample collection site of a patient. The cultured isolate is only one among what are likely to be thousands or hundreds of thousands of CFUs that make up the resident population, or **inoculum,** of the organism in the patient. Whether the inoculum in the patient represents a true infection rather than normal flora is based, in part, on the size of the inoculum—that is, how many CFUs of that organism are present in the animal.

KEY POINT 6-3 An infection is defined by the size of the inoculum, which varies with the tissue and method of culture collection.

The goal of antimicrobial therapy is to achieve sufficient concentrations of an appropriate drug at the site of infection such that the infecting organism is killed, while simultaneously avoiding side effects of the drug in the patient. In today's age of emerging resistance, the goal must be modified to include the avoidance of antimicrobial resistance. Therapeutic decisions concerning antimicrobial therapy for the infected patient are among the most challenging (Figure 6-1). Unlike most other drug therapies, antimicrobial therapy must take into account microbe, drug, and patient factors (i.e., the chemotherapeutic triangle), many of which confound successful therapy to the point of causing failure (Figure 6-2). Antimicrobial therapy is most likely to be successful when the target (and thus spectrum of antimicrobial activity) is known such that pharmacodynamics (PD) of the infecting organism can be integrated with the pharmacokinetics (PK) of the drug in the patient.

IDENTIFYING THE NEED FOR ANTIMICROBIAL THERAPY

The first decision to be made regarding antimicrobial therapy is determining the need to treat (see Figure 6-1). The decision includes confirming, to the extent possible, the existence of infection; identification of the cause of the infection bacteria (or fungal, etc), the need for treatment of the infection; and, if treatment is deemed necessary, whether antimicrobials should be part of the therapy. This first decision is probably given the least consideration yet may be the most important if resistance is to be avoided. It also may be the most difficult to make. The presence of infections frequently cannot be confirmed for a variety of reasons, such as the lack of (infection-) specific clinical signs, location in an inaccessible site, and costs associated with accurate diagnosis. Infection is supported, but not necessarily confirmed, by clinical signs or laboratory tests indicating fever, inflammation, and organ dysfunction or structural changes detected by imaging techniques such as radiology, ultrasound, and magnetic resonance imaging. Culture may support, but does not necessarily confirm, infection. Newer detection methods based on molecular diagnostic techniques (e.g., polymerase chain reaction) may ultimately prove to be important tools in the rapid bedside diagnosis of infectious diseases, including multidrug-resistant bacteria.[20] However, simply documenting the presence of these microbes may not be a sufficient indication of cause and effect. These methods may not discriminate infection (reproducing, pathogenic organisms) and colonization (the presence, growth, and multiplication of the organism without observable clinical symptoms or immune reaction), or pathogens from normal microflora. An exception can be made if cytology reveals organisms phagocytized by white blood cells, but the absence of phagocytosis does not eliminate infection.

KEY POINT 6-4 The first and most critical decision to be made regarding antimicrobial therapy is determining the need to treat. This includes confirming, as much as possible, the existence of infection; deciding if it must be treated; and, if so, whether antimicrobials should be part of the therapy.

Identifying the presence of infection is important in avoiding indiscriminate antimicrobial use. Increased risk of toxicity, cost, and inconvenience are obvious reasons that antimicrobial drugs should not be used indiscriminately. Less obvious reasons are an increased risk of superinfection and the potential emergence of resistant microbes. These latter reasons reflect, in part, the impact of antimicrobial therapy on normal flora.

Internal structures and organs (e.g., bone, heart, kidneys, the lower respiratory tract) are normally sterile. Sterility may be maintained, in part, by secretions, which constantly clean or clear the site. In addition to bulk flow, secretions may

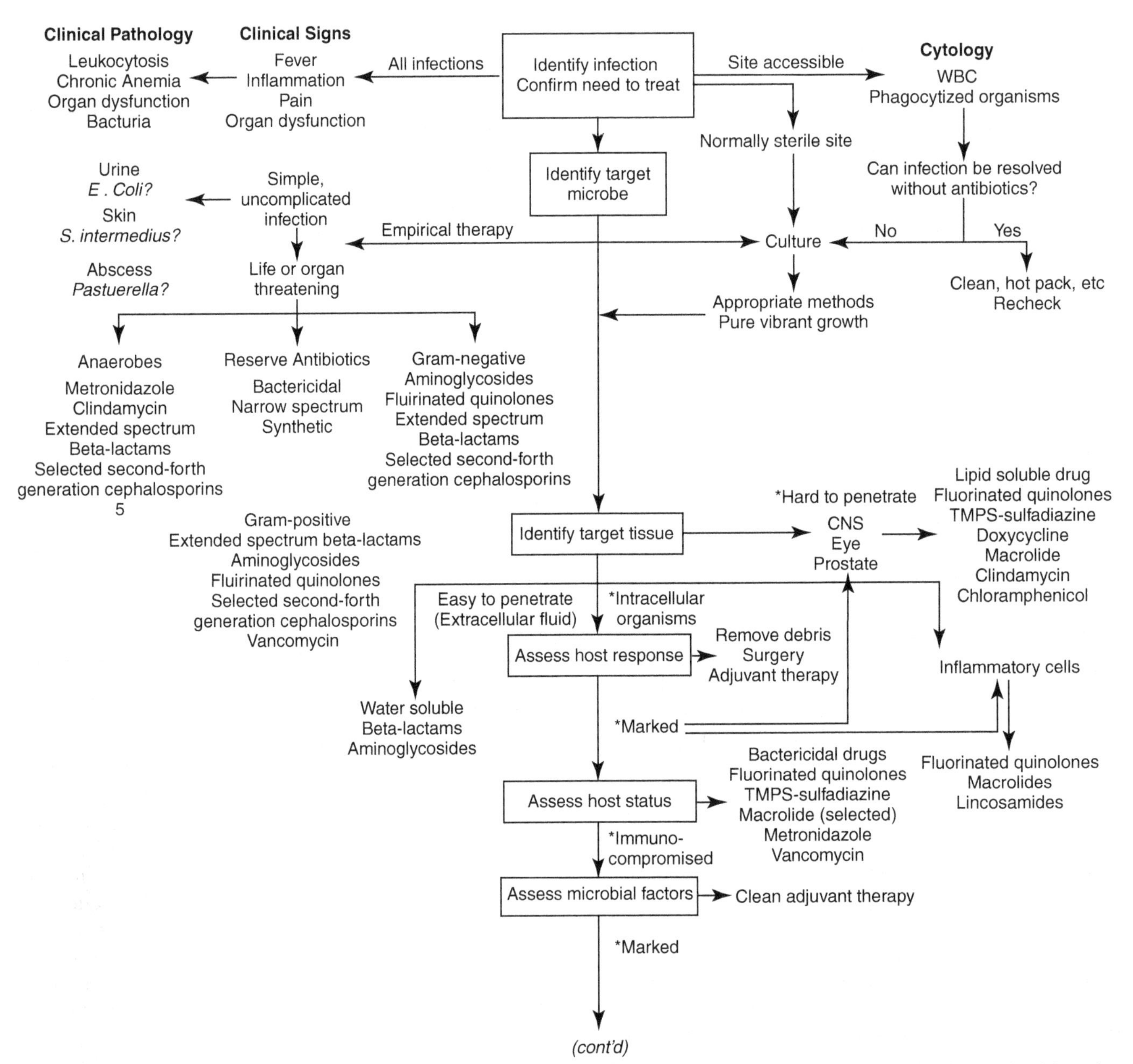

Figure 6-1 Therapeutic decision making for judicious antimicrobial therapy requires multiple steps. Antimicrobials should not be used indiscriminately; whenever possible, the most narrow-spectrum drug that targets the infecting organism should be used. Achieving adequate drug concentrations at the site of infection is critical to successful therapy. Dosing regimens should be modified for the patient; modifications should include changes in the dose and/or interval as is relevant. The asterisk at the *Design Dosing Regimen step refer to those indications previously encountered that should also lead to either a shortened interval or an increased dose, depending on whether the drug is concentration versus time dependent.

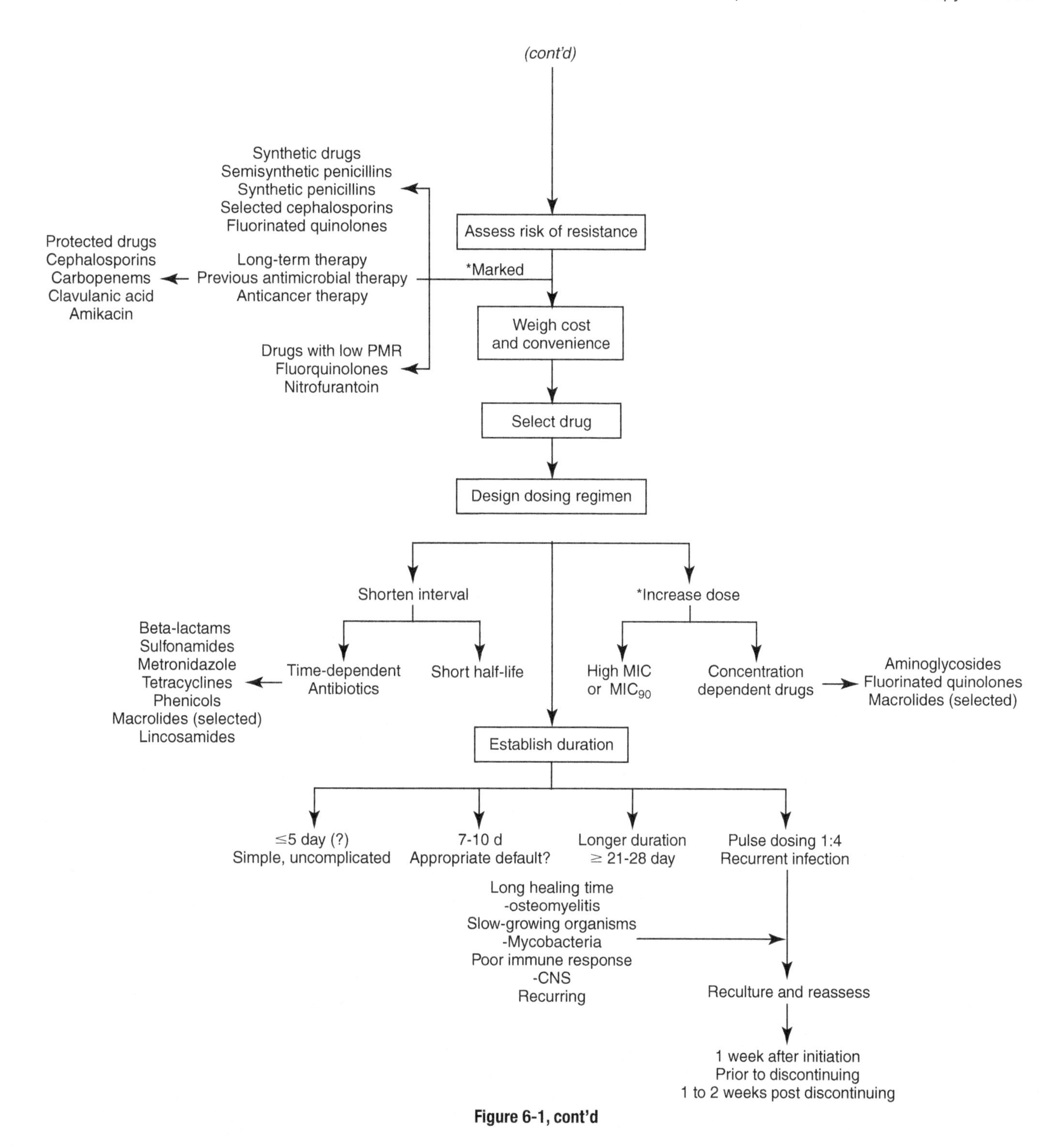

Figure 6-1, cont'd

contribute to sterility by the presence of endogenous antimicrobial compounds (e.g., tears, saliva, respiratory tract secretions, gastrointestinal acidity). However, in contrast, external (skin and conjunctiva of the eye) and internal (linings of the respiratory, digestive, and urogenital systems) surfaces are characterized by normal microflora. Normal flora may be further defined according to their contribution to host health or well-being. Most normal flora are **commensals** that appear to neither harm nor help the host. Some commensals, however, are also **opportunistic** in that they may become pathogenic, particularly if host health is impaired. A **pathogen** is a microbe that is associated with and capable of causing host damage.[21] Pathogens often reflect the normal flora of infected sites, with *E. coli, P. aeruginosa, K. pneumoniae,* and *S. aureus* being common examples of opportunistic normal flora that can become pathogenic (Table 6-1). **Mutualistic** organisms help maintain microbial balance through host–microbe interactions. They provide beneficial effects such as producing acids that lower pH and blocking colonization by more dangerous microbes. Antibiotics secreted by mutualistic organisms help maintain the composition of aerobic and anaerobic commensal bacteria, resulting in a population that is most appropriate for host

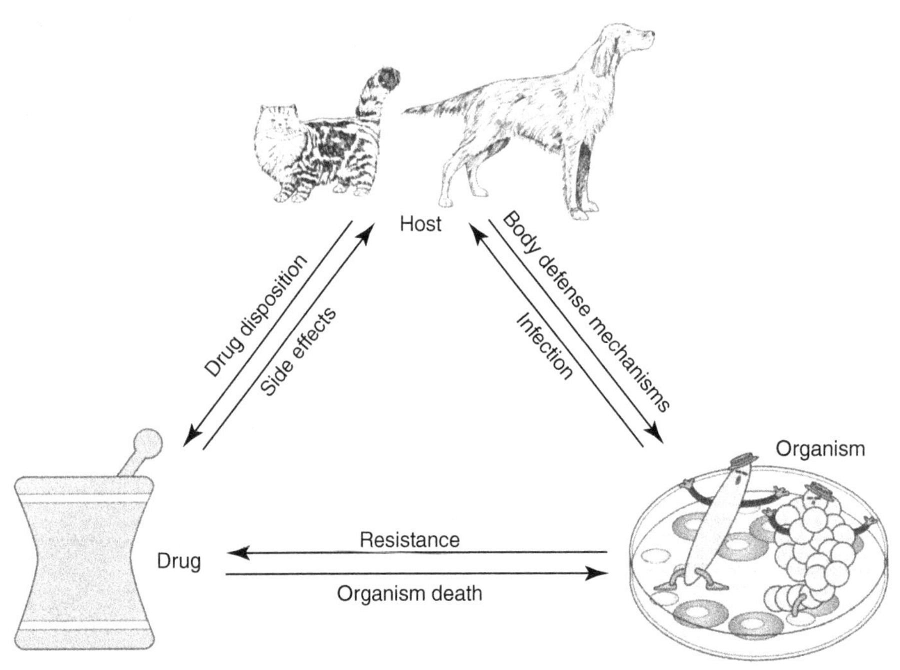

Figure 6-2 In contrast to other drug therapies, antimicrobial therapy involves not only the host and drug but also the microbe. Interactions among the three profoundly complicate successful antimicrobial therapy.

health and preventing colonization by pathogenic organisms. Opportunistic organisms may not originate from normal microflora but rather may be acquired from the environment (e.g., *Aspergillosis*, fungal organisms). **Nosocomial** organisms cause infections as a result of medical treatment, usually in a hospital or clinic setting. As such, a nosocomial infection is defined as one that arises 48 hours after hospital admission. Disruption of the environment, such as might occur with the use of antimicrobials that alter the anaerobic population, will also disrupt the balance of normal microflora, increasing the risk of infection (see the section on antimicrobial resistance). Not only will death of normal flora leave a void that can be filled in with more hardy and potentially pathogenic microbes, but the constant exposure of the microbes to antibiotics leads to ongoing development of mechanisms such that the microbes resist environmental drugs. Therefore the organisms are primed for resistance. Narrowing the spectrum of the chosen antimicrobial will help limit, although probably not prevent, the development of resistance.

KEY POINT 6-5 Discriminating among commensal versus pathogenic organisms is difficult and often cannot be determined simply by culture.

IDENTIFYING THE TARGET ORGANISM

Empirical Antimicrobial Therapy

After it has been determined that infection does exist and warrants medical management with antimicrobial drugs, identification of the target is the second critical decision to be made. Antimicrobial selection is probably most often made empirically—that is, on the basis of assumptions regarding the infecting organism and its susceptibility to drugs. These assumptions are based on historic data that identify organisms most commonly associated with infections of various body systems (see Table 6-1).[22] However, older data may not have discriminated between commensals and pathogens — indeed even today such discrimination often is not possible — which complicates the accuracy of prediction. More problematic, as resistance has emerged, the risk of incorrectly identifying the susceptibility pattern of an infecting microbe has increased. Thus the clinician should carefully balance the risk of therapeutic failure, including recurrence of infection with a resistant microbe, with the cost associated with more accurate diagnostic procedures.

The utility of Gram staining in the selection of an antimicrobial should not be overlooked as a means to narrow the spectrum of the chosen antimicrobial. Gram stain characteristics differ on account of differences in the layers penetrated by the Gram (purple) stain. The cell wall is many layers thicker in gram-positive organisms than in gram-negative ones thus rendering them more susceptible to some drugs that target the cell wall; further, the gram-positive isolates do not have an external lipopolysaccharide (LPS) covering that is present in gram-negative organisms (Figure 6-3). Whereas the LPS layer is the source of endotoxin responsible for the morbidity and mortality associated with many gram-negative infections, just as this external covering precludes stain movement into the cell wall, it also serves as a barrier to drug movement into the organism (see Figure 6-3).[23] Movement, particularly of water-soluble drugs, is generally restricted to outer membrane proteins that span the breadth of the covering (porins); however, changes in porin size and efflux pumps are mechanisms by which gram-negative organisms overcome drug movement through porins.

Table 6-1 Normal Flora and Clinically Significant Infections by Organ System (Dogs and Cats)

Organ or Site	Organism	Comment
Blood		
	Staphylococcus intermedius (D: 25%-35%)*, †, ‡ *Streptococcus* spp. (D: 18%-21%)† *Enterobacter cloacae* (D: 3%-8%, C: 7%)† *Escherichia coli* (D: 35%-45%*; D: 18%-71% & C: 14%)† *Klebsiella pneumoniae* (D: 25%-35%*: C: 14%)† *Proteus* (D: 14%)† *Pseudomonas aeruginosa* (D: 10%-20%) *Salmonella* (D: 11%-13%; C: 29%)† Obligate anaerobes (D: 10%-20%)	
Endocarditis†	*Staphylococcus intermedius* (D: 6%-33%) *Streptococcus* spp. (D: 12%-26%) *Escherichia coli* (D: 6%-30%) *Erysipelothrix rhusiopathiae* (D: 19%) *Corynebacterium* spp. (D: 19%)	
Respiratory		
Upper	*Staphylococcus intermedius* (D: 30%-35%)§, ‖, ¶	Have been isolated from nasal swabs, tonsillar and pharyngeal swabs, or tracheal and lung swabs
	Streptococcus spp. (15%-27%)§, ‖, ¶ *Corynebacterium* spp, §, ‖, ¶ *Escherichia coli*§ (15%-29%)§, ‖ *Klebsiella pneumoniae* (D: 10%-15%) ‖, ¶ *Moraxella*§, ¶ *Neisseria*§, ‖ *Pasteurella multocida* (D: 15%-34%; C: >50%)§, ‖ *Proteus* (C: <10%)§, ‖ *Pseudomonas*§ (6%-34%)§, ‖ *Bacteroides* ‖ *Clostridium* spp. § *Fusobacterium* ‖	
Rhinitis, sinusitis	*Escherichia coli* *Pasteurella multocida* *Proteus* *Pseudomonas* spp.	
Tracheobronchitis*	*Bordetella*	
Lower		
	Staphylococcus intermedius (D: 10%-15%)	Normal bronchi and lungs sterile distal to first bronchial division
	Escherichia coli (D: 30%-40%; C: 15%-20%) *Bordetella* (D: 10%-15%) *Enterococcus* *Klebsiella pneumoniae* (D: 15%-20%; C: <10%) *Pasteurella multocida* (C: >50%) *Pseudomonas* *Proteus mirabilis* (D: <10%)	
Pleuritis	*Actinomyces, Bacteroides, Corynebacterium, Fusobacterium, Nocardia, Pasteurella, Staphylococcus, Streptococcus*	
Gastrointestinal		
Oral cavity	Beta-hemolytic *Streptococcus*	Isolates from healthy dogs§
	Staphylococcus epidermidis§ *Acinetobacter*§ *Escherichia coli*§ *Moraxella*§ *Neisseria*§ *Pasteurella*§ *Proteus*§ *Pseudomonas*§ Obligate anaerobes (80%-90%)	

Continued

Table 6-1 Normal Flora and Clinically Significant Infections by Organ System (Dogs and Cats)—cont'd		
Organ or Site	**Organism**	**Comment**
Small intestine	*Escherichia coli, Klebsiella,*¶	Enteropathogenic bacteria in the stomach or small intestine associated with enterotoxin¶ or mucosal invasion
Enterobacteriaceae§	*Campylobacter fetus*¶ *Moraxella* *Neisseria* *Proteus* spp. *Pseudomonas* spp. *Salmonella typhimurium*§, ¶ *Shigella*§ *Vibrio cholerae*¶ *Vibrio parahaemolyticus*§ *Yersinia enterocolitica*¶ *Clostridium perfringens* (type A) ¶ *Bacillus*§, ¶	
Large intestine	*Enterobacteriaceae**	*Normal microflora; anaerobic make up 90% of microflora
Enterobacteriaceae§	Anaerobes	
Peritonitis		
Hepatobiliary		
	Enterobacteriaceae *Escherichia coli* *Enterobacter* *Klebsiella*	
Genital		
	Staphylococcus intermedius (D: 15%-25%)§ *Acinetobacter*§ *Escherichia coli* (30%-35%)§ *Klebsiella*§ *Moraxella,*§ *Haemophilus*§ *Pasteurella multocida (10%-25%)*§ *Proteus sp.*§ *Pseudomonas aeruginosa (<10%)* Obligate anaerobes (C: 10%-25%) *Mycoplasma* spp.§ *Ureaplasma* spp.§	Normal microflora of distal urethra and prepuce§
	Staphylococcus intermedius (D: 15%-25%)§ *Staphylococcus epidermidis*§ *Streptococcus canis, S. faecalis, S. viridans, S. zooepidemicus*§ *Corynebacterium*§ *Acinetobacter*§ *Citrobacter*§ *Enterobacter*§ *Enterococcus*§ *Escherichia coli (30%-35%)*§ *Haemophilus*§ *Klebsiella*§ *Micrococcus*§ *Moraxella,*§ *Neisseria*§ *Pasteurella multocida (15%-25%)* *Proteus*§ *Pseudomonas aeruginosa (<10%)*§ Obligate anaerobes (C: 10%-25%) Mycoplasma§ Ureaplasma§	Normal microflora of canine vagina§

Table 6-1 Normal Flora and Clinically Significant Infections by Organ System (Dogs and Cats)—cont'd

Organ or Site	Organism	Comment
Urinary Tract		
	Staphylococcus intermedius (D: <10%) *Enterococcus faecalis* (D: <10%) *Escherichia coli* (40%-50%) *Klebsiella pneumoniae* (10%-15%) *Pasteurella multocida* (C: 10%-15%) *Proteus mirabilis* (10%-15%) *Pseudomonas aeruginosa* (C: <10%)	
Central Nervous System		
	Brucella *Pasteurella*	
Ocular		
Conjunctiva	*Staphylococcus intermedius*,§, ¶ *S. albus*¶	Cultured from the conjunctival sac of clinically normal dogs or cats§¶
	Beta-hemolytic *Streptococcus* (C: 15%-25%)§, ¶ *Corynebacterium*§, ¶ *Escherichia coli*¶ *Moraxella*§ *Neisseria*§ *Pasteurella multocida* (C: 10%-20%) *Pseudomonas*§ Proteus *Bacillus*§, ¶ *Chlamydia psittaci* (C: 50%-75%) *Mycoplasma*¶	
Eye	*Leptospira* *Brucella canis* *Clostridium tetani* *Mycobacterium bovis*	
Otitis externa	*Staphylococcus intermedius* (D: 25%-30%) *Escherichia coli* (D: 10%-20%) *Proteus mirabilis* (D: 20%-25%) *Pseudomonas aeruginosa* (D: 15%-25%)	
Skin	*Staphylococcus intermedius* (D: 60%-70%) *Escherichia coli* (20%-30%) *Pasteurella multocida* (C: >50%) *Proteus mirabilis* (<10%) *Pseudomonas aeruginosa* (D: <10%)	
Wounds, abscesses	*Staphylococcus intermedius* (D: 25%-50%) *Escherichia coli* (D: 20%-30%; C: 10%-20%) *Pasteurella multocida* (C: 30%-40%) *Proteus mirabilis* (D: 10%-20%; C: <10%) *Pseudomonas aeruginosa* (D: 10%-20%) Obligate anaerobes (25%-35%)	
Musculoskeletal		
Osteomyelitis	*Staphylococcus intermedius* (D: 40%-50%) *Staphylococcus aureus* *Escherichia coli* (D: 10%-20%) *Enterococcus faecalis* (D: 10%-20%) *Proteus mirabilis* (10%-20%)	

*Numbers in parentheses refer to probable percentages of infections in this tissue that are caused by the organism, as cited by Aucoin (1993). Unless noted otherwise, the percentages refer to both dogs and cats (D = dog; C = cat). Note that the probable percentage is likely to vary geographically and may be biased toward patients referred to a specialty service.
†Numbers in parentheses refer to probable percentages of infection in this tissue that are caused by the organism, as cited by Greene (1990).
‡Number in parenthesis reflects the range of percent cited by both Aucoin (1993) and Greene (1990).
§¶ For each tissue, the symbol is defined in the *Comment* column.
**Organisms that are cultured from clinically healthy animals may be difficult to distinguish from those that cause infection.

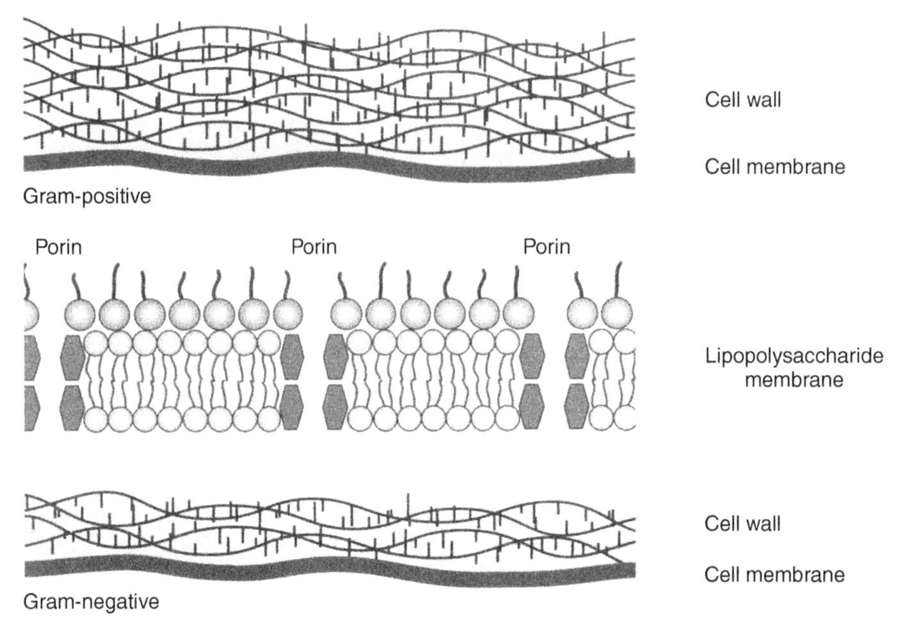

Figure 6-3 The gram-positive cell wall is thicker than the gram-negative cell wall, but the gram-negative cell wall is protected by an outer membrane including a layer of lipopolysaccharides. Endotoxin, derived from the lipopolysaccharides, contributes to the mortality and morbidity of gram-negative infections. The membrane also presents a challenge to drug movement. Although lipid-soluble drugs can diffuse through the membrane, movement of water-soluble drugs must occur through channels in outer membrane proteins called *porins,* which form aqueous channels that filter unwanted molecules. These porins are also associated with efflux pump proteins (the latter are also present in gram-positive organisms). Reduction in porin size or increased efflux pump activity are important mechanisms by which gram-negative organisms develop multidrug resistance.

In addition to Gram staining, determining the source of infection may help identify the microbe because some organisms are more likely than others to infect certain body systems. For example, genitourinary tracts are often infected with gram-negative aerobes, whereas abdominal infections generally are caused by gram-negative aerobes initially, followed by anaerobes after several days (see Table 6-1).[24,25] Skin is most commonly infected with *Staphylococcus pseudintermedius* (to be referred to as *S. intermedius* group, or SIG), abscesses with anaerobes and *Pasteurella* spp., and the urinary tract with *E. coli.* Indeed, *E. coli* is one of the more common pathogens, infecting many tissues. One study of 674 *E. coli* isolates collected from dogs found the vast majority (n=424) associated with urinary tract infections (UTIs) (n=424); however, 61 were also collected from skin, respiratory tract (52), ear (43), female (42) and male (25) reproductive tracts, and other organ systems (23). However, although *E. coli* may indeed be the most common isolate associated with UTIs, it does not necessarily represent the majority of UTIs. In a study by the author, only 50% of UTIs were caused by *E. coli,* with the remaining 50% caused by *Staphylococcus* spp., *Enterococcus* spp., *Proteus,* and others. For critical patients, organisms generally represent the normal flora of the alimentary canal or a nosocomial organism.[26] Granulocytopenic or otherwise immunoincompetent patients also are more likely to be infected by aerobic gram-negative organisms.

Even if the organism is correctly identified, the greater risk of failure associated with empirical treatment lies in the inability to correctly predict susceptibility patterns. This is not a new concern: As early as 1996, a study of critical-care patients revealed that empirical selection of antimicrobials was incorrect, on the basis of cultures collected before antimicrobials were started, in nearly 45% of patients.[27] Further, isolates of four organisms collected between 1998 and 2000 (*P. aeuriginosa, P. mirabilis, E. coli, Staphylococcus* spp.) widely considered to be susceptible to enrofloxacin (which had been approved for approximately 10 years) were characterized by a higher than expected incidence of resistance (28% for *E. coli*).[28] More recently, a high level of resistance was ascribed to drugs used empirically to treat otitis interna[29] and pyothorax.[30] Finally, our laboratory has demonstrated that more than 40% to 60% of *E. coli* associated with UTIs in dogs are characterized by resistance to first- and second-choice drugs (amoxicillin/clavulanic acid, cephalexin, potentiated sulfonamides, and enrofloxacin).[31] These differences may be regional but the absence of a robust surveillance program for dogs and cats limits empirical antimicrobial selection. These studies suggest culture and susceptibility (C&S) testing will become increasingly important.

Culture and Susceptibility Testing

C&S data can be a powerful guide for judicious antimicrobial use. However, C&S testing is only one of several tools that should support antimicrobial therapy. Among the advantages of culture is facilitation of input from a veterinary diagnostic microbiologist. As such, it has multiple roles in antimicrobial therapy: identifying the potential pathogen, providing a list of potentially effective drugs, offering guidance regarding the most effective drug, and serving as a basis for design of a dosing regimen of that drug through integration of pharmacokinetics (PK) and pharmacodynamics (PD).[32]

KEY POINT 6-6 The more at risk a patient is for resistance to be present or emerge, the more important culture and susceptibility testing becomes in the support of drug selection and design of the dosing regimen.

To date, not all infections require C&S testing to be effectively treated. Indeed, basing treatment on C&S does not guarantee therapeutic success. However, C&S can be particularly prudent for at-risk patients. It is particularly important for patients that have been treated with antimicrobials in the past several months. Testing is important to critical patients; although empirical therapy will begin before its receipt, culture of blood, urine, respiratory secretions (collected by bronchoscopy) and other pertinent body fluids (i.e., pleural, peritoneal, or cerebrospinal fluid [CSF]) should be carefully sampled before antimicrobial therapy is begun. Testing is also critical if infection by nosocomial organisms is of concern because their complex resistance patterns often require more expensive and potentially toxic drugs.[33]

Among the disadvantages of C&S testing is the time that often elapses between sample collection and receipt of results. Ideally, antimicrobial therapy will be withheld until the information is received and the accuracy of empirical choices is confirmed. The more a patient is at risk for developing resistance, the more important it may be to withhold therapy until results are received. However, treatment generally cannot be withheld. Still, if the data indicate that an incorrect choice may have been made regarding empirical antimicrobial selection, the data may no longer accurately reflect either the current infecting population or the susceptibility pattern. The clinician has several options, given that scenario (see Figure 6-1). If the patient has responded to therapy, the most prudent approach may be to stay the course, or perhaps add a second (nonantagonistic) drug to which the isolate is susceptible. If the patient has not responded sufficiently to therapy, therapy might be changed in light of the new data. However, the more prudent approach might be to reculture and wait until the new data arrive before changing course.

As with any tool, C&S data can be detrimental if misused. Contributing to improper use are the many pitfalls of testing, which begin with sampling, continue through the testing procedures and interpretation of results, and end with the design of the dosing regimen.

Culture data are only as good as the sampling methods of collection; the importance of proper culture techniques cannot be overemphasized (Box 6-2). For skin wounds the surface always contains commensals; normal flora, regardless of the site of collection, will cause background noise that must be filtered out. Swabs are often not ideal for sampling for a variety of reasons,[34] the most compelling of which is that only 3 out of 100 CFUs will actually make it to the culture stage. For anaerobes in particular, air between the fibers inhibits growth. Despite the greater level of difficulty in sample acquisition, tissue is the preferred sample. This might be an aspirate of fluids or macerated tissues (the laboratory may prefer to perform the macerating). Cleansing before sample collection is indicated, particularly for contaminated sites. For the same reason, cystocentesis is the most acceptable sample for interpretation of bacteriuria; catheterized sample often contain microbes colonizing the catheter and associated biofilm. The properly collected obligate anaerobic sample is particularly difficult to achieve and the absence of anaerobes may simply reflect improper techniques. An anerobic infection should be suspected if clinical signs are supportive (e.g., foul smell, adjacent to mucosal membranes or gas). Note that facultative anaerobes may be cultured and tested as susceptible under aerobic conditions but fail to respond to therapy as expected if the infection in the patient occurs under anaerobic conditions.

Even a properly collected culture may not confirm infection or identify the infecting pathogenic microbe. Cytology coupled with Gram staining should be considered when possible, with phagocytosis of the organism indicative of pathogenicity. Pathogenicity reflects virulence, which is often misconstrued as resistance. The chances of proper identification of the cultured isolate pathogen are greatest if vibrant growth is obtained in an otherwise sterile environment. However, for tissues characterized by a normal flora, culture may not be able to discriminate colonization and infection by normal opportunistic organisms that have become pathogenic. Most normal flora comprises commensals that are opportunistic, i.e., able to cause disease without the support of virulence factors. A population shift from colonization to infection by such organisms is more likely to occur in at-risk patients, such as the critical-care patient, or at sites for which local immunity is compromised. Infection generally reflects normal flora, such as *E. coli*, *P. aeruginosa*, *K. pneumoniae*, and *S. pseudintermedius*., although opportunistic organisms also may be acquired from the environment.

The culture may give some indication as to the quality of the sample based on evidence of contamination. If C&S data indicate contamination, the site should be resampled (tissue collection rather than swab) after proper cleansing. For example, selected organisms, such as *Bacillus* sp. and *Corynebacterium* spp. are common contaminants, and their presence in wounds may be indicative of contamination and thus, potentially, a poorly representative sample. The location of culture may also be important in identifying the organism as a contaminant. For example, whereas beta-hemolytic *Streptococcus* sp. (e.g, *S. canis)* collected from a wound may be important, it is a likely contaminant if cultured from the ear. *Streptococcus* sp. pathogenicity (i.e., the likelihood of infection) can be associated with its ability to hemolyze hemoglobin, with alpha designation (hemoglobin is simply reduced) being the least and beta (red blood cells disrupted) potentially the most hemolytic and pathogenic designation. Gamma hemolysis is actually the absence of hemolysis and is demonstrated by *Enterococcus* spp. (previously a subset of *Streptococcus* spp.). However, alpha-hemolytic also can be pathogenic under the right circumstances, such as in the patient that has undergone

Box 6-2
Techniques in Culture Sampling

Commonalities Regardless of Site*

Site preparation: Don sterile gloves. Clean wound. Do not culture purulent or necrotic debris. Thoroughly cleanse wound by removing excessive debris, flushing with saline, and blotting with sterile gauze. Change to sterile gloves before collection.

Tissue aspiration: Clean intact skin with antiseptic (e.g., 70% alcohol and 10% povidone–iodine). Allow to air dry (do not fan). Expel air from an appropriate-size syringe to which is attached a 22-Ga needle. Insert needle into intact skin at the deepest portion of the lesion. Aspirate approximately 0.5 mL fluid. Needle can be moved back and forth at different angles in skin. Remove needle with hemostat. Discard needle and recap syringe with blood-gas cap, or, particularly if anaerobes are suspected, transfer fluid to transport vial.

Swab techniques: Swab techniques are acceptable only for eye, ear, and uterus cultures. Note that only 3 of 100 colony-forming units collected in a swab are likely to be successfully cultured. Use a swab in appropriate carrier medium. The swab should be moistened with sterile, preservative-free solution if wound is not moist. Sample should be collected without touching the edge of the wound or skin. Rotate swab over 1-cm area of open wound for 4 seconds. Place swab aseptically in transport sleeve, making sure tip comes into contact with liquid transport medium (break ampule if present). One swab should be collected for each sample type (i.e., aerobic, anaerobic, and a third if cytology is of interest).

Skin or Wound Biopsy

Swab is strongly discouraged; aspirate is acceptable, but macerated tissue is preferred: Clean intact skin with antiseptic and allow to air dry (do not fan). Collect biopsy aseptically. Place in transport tube containing liquid medium. Clinical microbiology laboratory will macerate.

Bone

Place in transport system. Moisten with sterile physiologic saline as necessary.

Drain Tube Site

Treat as a contaminated wound. Care must be taken not to culture the biofilm associated with the foreign body. The drain tube should be removed, the site surgically cleaned and flushed, and the area cultured. Ideally, tissue will be collected at the presumed site of infection.

Respiratory Tract

Bronchoscopy specimens include bronchoalveolar lavage, bronchial washing, bronchial brushing, and transbronchial biopsy specimens. The bronchoscope should be passed transorally in nonintubated patients or through the endotracheal tube in intubated patients. Bronchial wash or bronchoalveolar lavage specimens should be obtained before brushing or biopsy to minimize blood in the recovered fluid.

- For lavage, sterile nonbacteriostatic 0.85% NaCl should be injected from a syringe through a biopsy channel of the bronchoscope. Recovered fluid should be placed in the transport vial.
- Bronchial brush specimens should be collected through a telescoping double catheter plugged with polyethylene glycol at the distal end (to prevent contamination of the bronchial brush) through the biopsy channel of the bronchoscope. The sample should be transported in a sterile container with a small amount of sterile nonbacteriostatic 0.85% NaCl.
- Lung aspirations should be placed in transport vial for laboratory submission.
- Pharyngeal samples are not acceptable.
- Nasal samples are of limited value. Culture requests should be limited to pathogen-specific samples, e.g., *Bordetella bronchiseptica.*

Urine

Samples should be collected by cystocentesis only. Catheterized samples generally are not preferred; if there is no alternative, collect from a fresh catheter, or (less ideal) discard the initial 5 to 10 mL of urine before collecting sample. Catheter tips or urine from a collection bag are not acceptable. Sample can be submitted in a red-top serum collection tube. Samples should be kept cold by submitting on ice and ensuring that samples are received by the laboratory within 24 hours of submission. Consider a urine paddle collection system supplied by some commerical diagnostic laboratories.

Blood Culture

Liquid medium is indicated. Volume is critical to maximize recovery. Bacteremia may consist of less than one colony-forming unit per mL of whole blood. Prepare the collection site using aseptic methods, and for blood cultures, note that at least three collections at three time points are indicated. Collection during a fever spike is recommended. For blood, the volume should be 1 part blood to 10 parts broth.

Cerebrospinal Fluid or Joint Fluids

Use blood culture bottle, and add entire sample asceptically to broth.

Other Body Fluids

See discussion of tissue aspiration.

Ocular

In general, instill 1 or 2 drops of topical anesthetic. Organisms are more readily detected in scrapings than from a swab.

- For conjunctival scrapings, scrape the lower tarsal conjunctiva with a sterilized spatula and place material directly into medium. Alternatively, use a calcium alginate swab or a cotton-tipped applicator to swab the inferior tarsal conjunctiva (inside surface of eyelid) and the fornix of the eye.
- Consider collecting a conjunctival sample first, which might help you assess the possibility of contamination. Using short, firm strokes in one direction, scrape multiple areas of ulceration and suppuration with a sterilized spatula. The eyelid should remain open, and care should be taken to avoid eyelashes. Multiple scrapings are recommended because the depth and extent of viable organisms may vary. Inoculate each scraping directly to appropriate medium.

Box 6-2

Techniques in Culture Sampling—cont'd

- Intraocular fluid should be collected using needle aspiration. Aspirate should be used to directly inoculate appropriate medium, with immediate transport to the laboratory in an anaerobic transport system.

Gastrointestinal Tract

Fecal specimens are submitted primarily for the detection of *Campylobacter, Shigella,* and *Salmonella* spp.; *Clostridium difficile;* and, in certain cases, to detect *Yersinia, Vibrio,* and *Aeromonas* spp. and enterohemorrhagic *Escherichia coli.* Care should be taken to ensure that the sample is not contaminated with urine. Fecal white blood cells should be ordered on liquid stools to indicate degree of inflammation. Stool specimens should be mixed with transport medium to maintain viability of pathogens that may be present. Sample should be collected digitally wearing a sterile glove or using a sterile fecal loop.

*The laboratory to which the sample will be submitted should be consulted before collection to ensure that its recommendations are followed. These general guidelines are offered in the absence of specific guidance.

invasive procedures such as intubation (e.g., *S. pneumonia* in humans). *Enterococcus* also has expressed beta hemolysis.The laboratory may choose not to implement susceptibility testing for those isolates considered nonpathogenic, with the interpretation of pathogenicity by the microbiologist depending on the host circumstances, including sampling site. Such decision making can only be improved with effective communication between clinician and microbiologist.

The number of organisms may be helpful in identifying the cause and effect of microbial presence and infection. Isolation of multiple organisms from a site that is easily contaminated by normal flora may represent floral colonization rather than a polymicrobial infection.[24] In contrast, pure growth generally indicates infection and the potential need for therapy. For example, *Pasteurella* as one of several organisms collected from a nasal swab may not be relevant, but if cultured as a pure isolate, it is probably indicative of infection. A related indicator of infection is the intensity of growth. For countable tissues, the number of CFUs per mL of tissue should be considered when assessing whether the inoculum represents an infection (see previous discussion of inoculum size). Vibrant growth of a single organism generally is indicative of infection by a pathogen, even in an environment that is easily contaminated. If multiple organisms are cultured and the culture was improperly collected, cleansing of the site (if possible) and reculture may facilitate correct identification of the pathogen. If the culture was a properly collected sample, those isolates characterized by lighter growth might be deemphasized in favor of organisms with significant growth. Controlling the heavier growth may facilitate the patient's capacity to eradicate the less dense population. For example, *E. coli,* SIG, or alpha-hemolytic *Streptococcus* are rapid growers, and if present together, the organisms with the greater growth might be targeted. However, *P. aeruginosa* is an example of a slow grower that is easily overwhelmed by other organisms. The impact on different growth rates exemplifies the importance of post-collection sample handing (e.g., the need to refrigerate). The presence of slow-growing organisms in a properly collected sample generally indicates the need for treatment. Specialized procedures may be necessary to identify growth in tissues normally sterile (e.g., blood culture, cerebrospinal fluid, or well-collected bronchial alveolar lavage). Thus as few as two colonies of *Pseudomonas* sp. cultured from a properly collected bronchial alveolar lavage might be considered significant, whereas the need for antimicrobial therapy might be reconsidered if growth is less than 10^5 CFUs from a site that is easily contaminated (e.g., wounds, clean-catch or catheterized urine). Patient health also should be considered: whereas, up to 10^3 CFU/mL of urine collected by cystocentesis may not be significant in normal dogs, it may be indicative of infection in a patient that is not concentrating urine (e.g., because of renal disease, diuretic or fluid therapy).

Although the susceptibility patterns of an isolate may offer clues as to pathogenicity of the cultured isolate, care must also be taken with this approach. Contaminants are often characterized by patterns of susceptibility rather than resistance. However, such an isolate may yet be a pathogen, particularly in a patient with no previous history of antimicrobial exposure. Complex patterns of resistance may suggest the isolate is an infecting pathogen rather than a colonizing commensal. This is exemplified by nosocomial organisms associated with medical treatments (arising within 48 hours of hospital admission). However, *Stenotrophomona* and *Serratia* are common contaminants of antiseptics or disinfectants that are characterized by complex patterns of resistance. Multidrug resistance (discussed later) must also be considered in the context of the inherent susceptibility of the organism, being relevant only if expressed toward drugs to which the organism should be susceptible. For example, *P. aeruginosa* may be tested toward drugs to which it is inherently resistant, yielding results that appear to suggest the isolates as multidrug resistant. However, multidrug resistance should not be considered unless expressed toward ticarcillin, carbapenems, or aminoglycosides.

The clinical microbiologist can be a powerful ally in determining the significance of isolates yielded from a sample culture. The microbiologist that is trained in veterinary medicine will be of most benefit in providing guidance regarding the relevance of the isolated microbe. However, the contributions of the clinical microbiologist will be markedly curtailed if an insufficient history of the patient from which the sample was collected is provided.

Interpreting Culture and Susceptibility Test Results

The in vitro data generated by C&S testing eventually must be applied to in vivo patient conditions. Testing methods themselves may influence results such that the data are misinterpreted. The complex nature of C&S procedures mandates standardization and a well-documented quality control program. The Committee on Laboratory Standards Institute (CLSI; previously the National Committee for Clinical Laboratory Standards [NCCLS])[35-39] validates method protocols, guidelines, and interpretive standards for C&S and molecular testing; one of its subcommittees promulgate veterinary-specific standards.[37,38] These standards and guidelines, which are applicable throughout the nation, and are often used internationally, reflect careful and exhaustive review of PD (microbial response to drug) and PK (host handling of drug) data. Because microbial populations are dynamic, standards and guidelines addressing their culture and susceptibility are likewise dynamic. Intermittent re-examination results in new guidelines and adjusted criteria, as is appropriate for changing microbial trends. CLSI publishes its findings so that clinical microbiological laboratories can access and implement the standards. An important caveat to C&S testing is that manufacturers supplying materials to the laboratory may not implement recommended changes in their materials in a timely fashion. Further, some veterinary diagnostic micribiological laboratories do not necessarily adhere to these standards but rather generate their own guidelines. Yet only CLSI standards undergo national peer review assessment and discussion among unbiased experts representing government, industry, academia, and clinical practice.

CLSI has generated guidelines for a variety of C&S testing methods. The PD information varies with the susceptibility procedures, with disk diffusion (Figure 6-4) and broth dilution (Figure 6-5) offering excellent examples of contrasts in advantages.[40] It is the latter that provides the minimum inhibitory concentrations (MICs) necessary for comparison among drugs and design of dosing regimens. The data generated from culture and susceptibility testing represents the PD portion of PK–PD integration in that it indicates what is needed to target the microbe.

KEY POINT 6-7 The veterinary clinical microbiologist is a powerful ally in the interpretation of culture and susceptibility testing data.

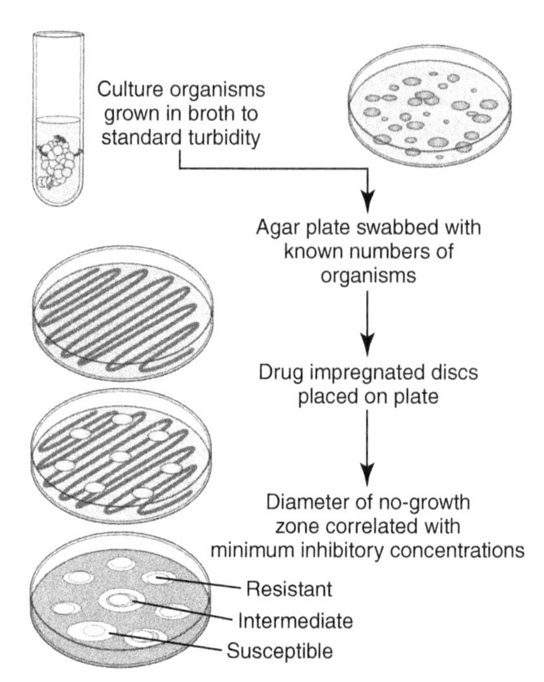

Figure 6-4 The disk diffusion method of culture and susceptibility testing. Drug diffusion from the disk results in concentrations that are higher close to the disk and gradually decrease as the diameter of the zone surrounding the disk increases. Resistant organisms can grow close to the disk despite high drug concentrations in the agar, whereas susceptible organisms will be inhibited at a standard distance from the disk. Concentrations in the agar correlate with the minimum inhibitory concentration (MIC) of the drug.

Disk Diffusion Versus Broth Dilution Techniques

Both methods of susceptibility testing require rapid growth of organisms and therefore may not be available for all organisms. Broth dilution data are particularly dependent on rapid growth, and for some organisms disk diffusion may be the only available means of obtaining data. The disk diffusion method (e.g., Kirby–Bauer) involves disks that contain a known amount of the drug of interest. The agar is streaked with a standardized inoculum of the isolated organism, and the disks are placed in standardized positions on the inoculated gel. Drug diffuses from the disk into the agar at a known rate (see Figure 6-4),[40] such that, at a standard time, the concentration in the agar correlates with the minimum inhibitory concentration (MIC) of the drug as would be determined by the broth dilution procedures (the most common method serving as a gold-standard to other methods). At the prescribed time (i.e., as specified by CLSI[35-37]), a zone of no microbial growth (in mm) is measured around the disk. Because the concentration of the drug decreases with the distance (zone) diameter from the disk, the larger the zone, the lower the concentration of drug necessary to inhibit the growth of the organism and the more likely effective drug concentrations will be achieved at the site of the infection. A susceptible ("S") designation is given if the zone is sufficiently large. Growth up to the designated zone indicates that the concentration of drug necessary to inhibit the organism is too high to achieve in the patient, leading to a resistant ("R") designation. Intermediate ("I") designation is provided for some drugs. Zone sizes necessary for an organism to be considered susceptible as opposed to resistant to a specific drug are variable and are very sensitive to disruptions in protocols, which underscores the importance of following standards. An advantage to the disk diffusion method is that multiple drugs might be simultaneously tested on one plate. This is in contrast to the more tedious and costly, yet more informative, broth dilution methods. Because disk

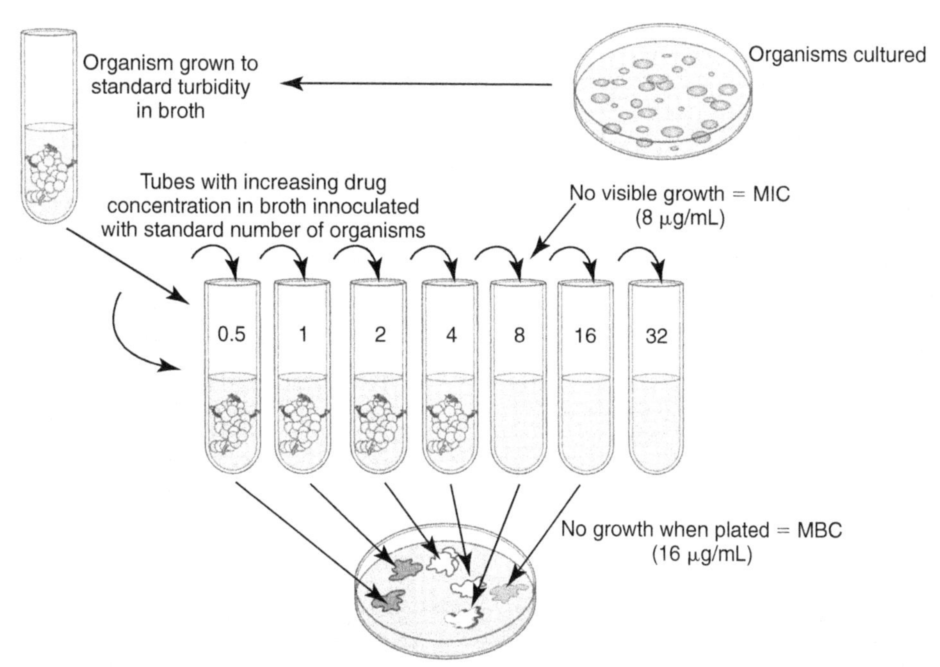

Figure 6-5 The broth dilution method of susceptibility testing provides a drug concentration to be targeted in the patient. Tubes containing serially increasing concentrations of drug are inoculated with a standard amount of the bacterial organism. At the proper time, tubes are observed for evidence of growth. The first tube (i.e., the one with the lowest concentration) that shows no evidence of growth contains the minimum inhibitory concentration (MIC) of the drug. The MIC can be used to evaluate relative drug efficacy and development of resistance and to calculate dosing regimens. This method is also one means by which the minimum bactericidal concentration (MBC) of a drug is determined. If the tubes exhibiting no growth are then used to inoculate solid agar, those tubes that yield no bacterial growth contained sufficient drug to kill, rather than simply inhibit, bacteria. The test tube that contains the lowest concentration of drug that yields no growth contains the MBC. If the MBC approximates the MIC, then the drug can be considered bactericidal.

diffusion results are reported as S, I, or R, it is described as semiquantitative.

In contrast to the disk diffusion method, the broth dilution method provides quantitative data regarding the amount of drug necessary to inhibit microbial growth (see Figure 6-5).[41] For each drug of interest, tubes of liquid media are spiked with concentrations of the drug of interest, with the highest concentration generally being that just below the CLSI threshold of susceptibility (resistant MIC breakpoint). Subsequent test tubes containing serially diluted (by half) concentrations of the drug. As such, MICs are generally reported out as logarithmic fractions or multiples of 1 μg/mL (i.e., from lowest to highest 0.0312, 0.0615, 0.125, 0.25, 0.5, 1, 2, 4, 8, 16, 32, 64, 128, 256, 512; see Figure 6-5). Each drug to be tested must involve multiple test tubes or wells. The low and high range of concentrations tested for each drug will vary depending on concentrations achieved in tissues (including blood) when administered at recommended dosing regimens to the target species. For example, the ranges tested for ticarcillin would be expected to be much higher than the concentrations tested for enrofloxacin because the maximum concentration achieved in serum after administration of a recommended dose will be much higher for ticarcillin than for enrofloxacin (see Chapter 9). Occasionally, the MIC for some drugs deviates from the aforementioned tested concentrations; generally, these are drugs marketed as combinations (e.g., trimethoprim/sulfonamide combination). PD data generated for package inserts or scientific reports also may incorporate dilutions other than those delineated by CLSI. It is important to remember that CLSI guidelines are intended only to support clinical microbiological laboratories that provide direct support for patient care.

The tubes that contain broth (standardized type and amount) of the appropriate dilutions of the drug of interest must be inoculated with a standard number of the isolated bacterial organism during the logarithmic phase of growth. Microbial growth continues under standardized conditions for the standardized period (as set by CLSI[35-37]). At the end of the incubation period, each tube is observed for evidence of growth. Evidence of growth is determined visually or using computer systems that allow miniaturized automation (see Figure 6-5 and Figure 6-6) The tube with the lowest concentration of drug that exhibits no detectable growth contains the MIC (in μg/mL), or the minimum amount of antimicrobial necessary to (in vitro) inhibit the growth of the organism cultured from the patient.[23,41] Because of the complexities of the procedures, laboratories that provide clinical C&S testing may find MIC results on the same isolate that vary, even if CLSI guidelines and interpretive standards are followed. Generally, variations within 1 broth dilution are not considered significant. Laboratories ensure that quality standards of testing are met by performing drug MIC determination for control isolates (i.e., obtained from American Testing Cell Culture: e.g, *E. coli* ATCC 25922, *Staphylococcus intermedius* ATCC 45222).[41]

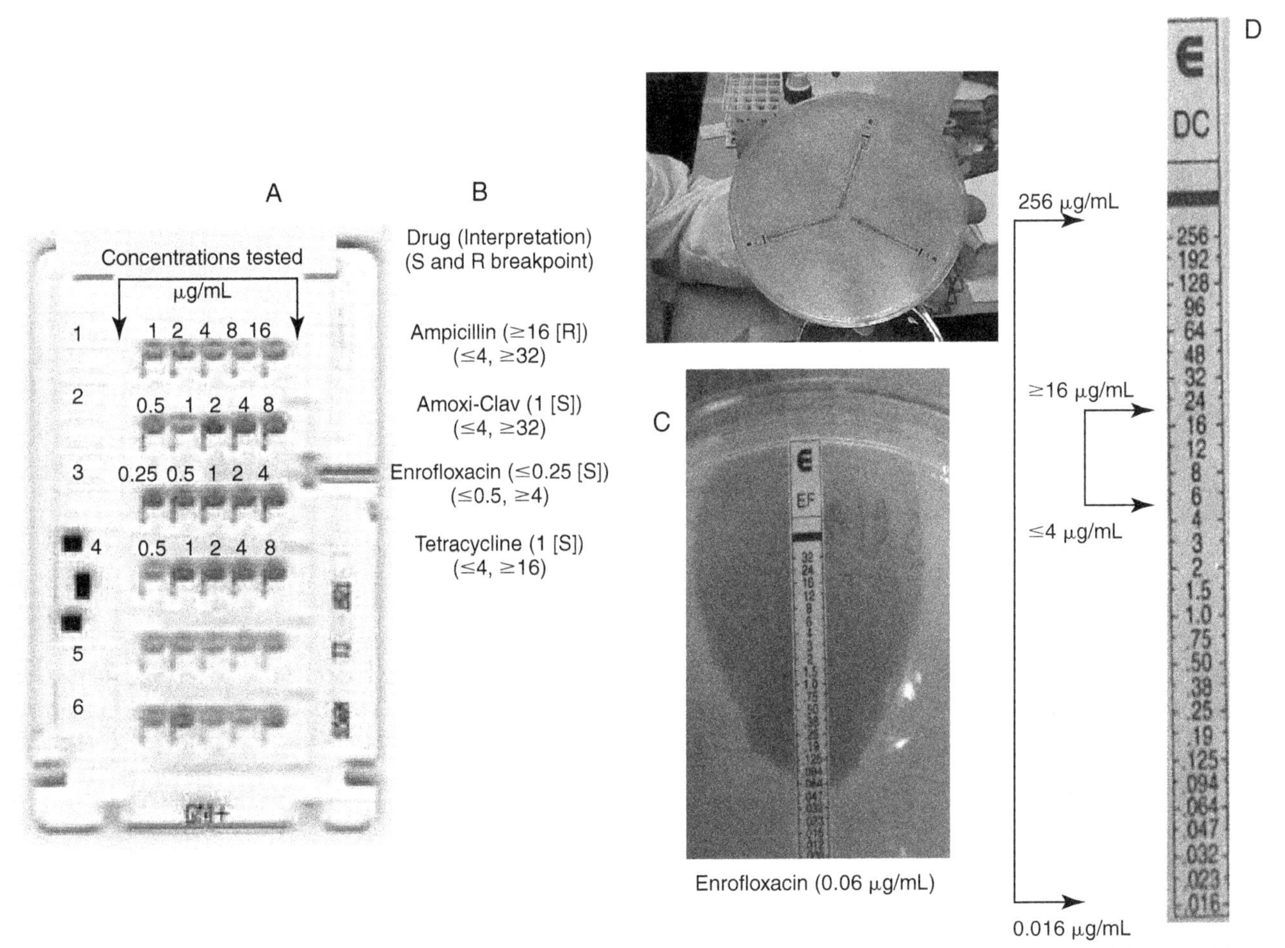

Figure 6-6 A, A commercially available antibiogram card and an E-test (C-D) with interpretation. The commercially available antibiogram card is a miniaturized broth dilution procedure that generates minimum inhibitory concentration (MIC) using a microwell design. Generally, one card is made for gram-negative isolates and another for gram-positive isolates. The size of the card limits testing of the number of drugs and the range of concentrations, with concentrations approximating the susceptible and resistant breakpoints (indicated under each drug). Some cards test only the susceptible and resistant breakpoints. Growth is indicated by a color change (all wells had growth in row 1, indicating resistance to ampicillin, but no wells had growth in row 3, indicating susceptibility to enrofloxacin). The ranges tested (above the wells) and interpretations (to the right of each drug) are provided for four of the drugs tested on the card. None of the isolates tested intermediate. A limitation of the cards is ability to indicate *how* susceptible an isolate is. This limitation is largely overcome with the E-test system **(C;** strip is enrofloxacin). Each strip releases the drug into the medium at logarithmic rates. Growth in susceptible isolates follows a tear-shaped pattern, with the point of the tear indicating the MIC. Advantages of the E-test include a very broad range of test concentrations (over16,00-fold) indicated by outer bracket (see Table 6-3), exceeding both the susceptible and resistant breakpoints (indicated by inner bracket) by several magnitudes, thus allowing assessment of how susceptible or resistant the isolate might be to the drug of interest. The MIC of this isolate is 0.06 µg/mL; for comparison, the lowest concentration that would be tested on the antibiogram. The E-test suggests that this isolate is moderately susceptible to doxycycline. The differences in the MIC between the microwell dilution and the E-test may reflect subtle differences in methodology but also the lipophilic nature of doxycline (better penetrability), thus highlighting a caveat of susceptibility testing: model drugs do not always represent the drug of interest well. Another advantage of the E-test is the smaller increments of change, and thus greater precision provided compared with tube dilution procedures. A more precise dosing regimen can thus be designed. For example, with standard tube dilution, concentrations increased from 8 to 16, whereas with E-testing, concentrations increased from 8 to 12 to 16 µg/mL. Finally, the individual nature of the test strips allows a "pick and choose" approach to individualizing drug therapy. This also, however, is a disadvantage in that costs are higher when multiple drugs are tested.

Research publications that address bacterial PD likewise should demonstrate adherence to CLSI guidelines, including quality-control procedures.

Broth dilution reports provide both the MIC (a concentration, reported in µg/mL) and (assuming CLSI procedures are followed), the CLSI interpretation of S, I, or R for that MIC. The basis of the interpretation (S, I, or R) for broth dilution procedures is addressed later in this chapter. The MIC for selected drugs may be accompanied by a "≤" or "≥". Using Figure 6-7 as an example, *Pseudomonas* have an MIC for

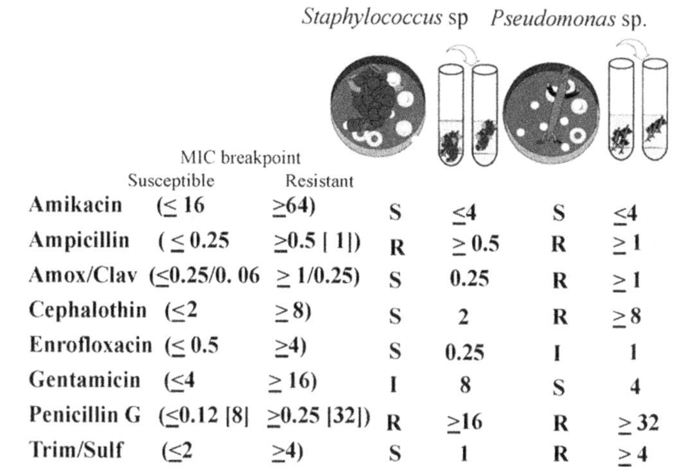

	MIC breakpoint Susceptible	Resistant	*Staphylococcus* sp		*Pseudomonas* sp.	
Amikacin	(≤ 16	≥64)	S	≤4	S	≤4
Ampicillin	(≤ 0.25	≥0.5 [1])	R	≥ 0.5	R	≥ 1
Amox/Clav	(≤0.25/0. 06	≥ 1/0.25)	S	0.25	R	≥ 1
Cephalothin	(≤2	≥ 8)	S	2	R	≥ 8
Enrofloxacin	(≤ 0.5	≥4)	S	0.25	I	1
Gentamicin	(≤4	≥ 16)	I	8	S	4
Penicillin G	(≤0.12 [8]	≥0.25 [32])	R	≥16	R	≥ 32
Trim/Sulf	(≤2	≥4)	S	1	R	≥ 4

Figure 6-7 An example of a C&S report for broth dilution. The breakpoints have been added in parantheses this report; for ampicillin and penicillin, a second breakpoint in [brackets] is for the gram-negative organisms (see text and Table 6.2). The relative in vitro efficacy of antibiotics to which an organism is susceptible can be evaluated by comparing the minimum inhibitory concentration (MIC) of the organism. For *Staphylococcus,* the resistant MIC breakpoint to MIC ratio is 64/4, whereas that for gentamicin is 16/4 or two tube dilutions from the breakpoint. Although the isolate is considered susceptible to both drugs, amikacin presumably would be more effective (although neither generally should be used alone to treat *Staphylococcus*). Differences greater than one tube dilution should be considered significant. For the beta-lactams, effective treatment of *Staphylococcus* with cephalothin (the model drug for cephalexin) may be more easily achieved (ratio of 8/2) compared to amoxicillin clavulanic acid (ratio of 0.25/0.25). However, as time-dependent drugs, elimination half-life of both drugs would need to be considered. All values (concentrations) are in μg per mL. *S* = susceptible; *R* = resistant; *I* = intermediate.

amikacin of ≤4 μg/mL. The ≤ indicates the absence of growth in the lowest concentration of amikacin tested by this laboratory (8 μg/mL); this lowest concentration may be different among laboratories that use different systems. However, often the lowest dilution tested is at or just below the lower threshold of susceptibility (the susceptible MIC breakpoint; see later definition) set by CLSI. Testing at concentrations at or very close to the susceptible breakpoint of a drug is a major disadvantage of current susceptibility testing methods: either isolate may be very susceptible to amikacin such that their actual MIC may be several tube dilutions below the lowest concentration tested (see below). As such, the closest approximation to the actual MIC for either isolate will be the concentration below the lowest dilution tested by the laboratory (i.e., ≤4 μg/mL or <8 μg/ml both indicate the same result). The isolate will be accompanied by an "S" designation, indicating susceptibility because the MIC is at or below the susceptible breakpoint determined by CLSI (Table 6-2). At the other end of the testing range, an MIC accompanied by ≥ indicates that growth was present in the highest concentration tested by the laboratory. Generally, for most automated procedures, the highest concentration tested is 1 tube dilution below the upper threshold of susceptibility (the resistant MIC breakpoint) set by CLSI for each drug (Table 6-2). For example, for cephalothin (the model drug for cephalexin in this example), the upper threshold of susceptibility (the resistant MIC breakpoint) set by CLSI is 8 μg/mL. Thus for *Pseudomonas,* growth was present in the well containing 4 μg/mL, indicating that the actual MIC is equal to or higher than 8 μg/mL (≥16 μg/mL or >8 μg/mL both indicate the same result). However, again the testing range limitations of the current procedures emerges in that level of resistance of the isolate cannot be assessed. The isolate may be characterized by low-level resistance, although this is unlikely for *P. aeruginosa* and first-generation cephalosporins (indeed, testing of *P. aerugniosa* toward cephalothin is not appropriate). However, unless the range tested extends beyond the resistant breakpoint, all that is known is that the isolate is resistant, and the MIC will be accompanied by an R designation.

KEY POINT 6-8 Culture and susceptibility testing ideally is performed following the guidelines of the Clinical Laboratory Standards Institute (CLSI).

Among the pitfalls of C&S testing are the stepwise dilutions and the range of concentrations tested for each drug. The twofold dilutions at which MIC are tested affect the design of dosing regimens at the higher MIC. Precision in the design of dose would be facilitated if MICs could be determined between the tube dilutions. For example, the dose to target 64 μg/mL would be substantially cheaper and potentially safer than that necessary to target 128 μg/mL. The limited range of concentrations tested for each drug negatively affects the ability to identify the drug to which the isolate is most susceptible (see Figure 6-6).[41] Ideally, concentrations tested by broth dilution procedures should span the range of drug concentrations that characterize the range of MICs established in a sample population of isolates of the organisms, with the highest concentration being at least one dilution above the highest drug concentration acheived in target biological fluids.[41] However, automated systems test in a very narrow range. As previously noted, because the lowest concentrations are at or just below the lower limit of susceptibility, isolates that are very susceptible to the drug of interest cannot be indentified (see Table 6-2). Therefore standard antibiograms are more indicative of resistance rather than susceptibility.

A third testing system approved by the Food and Drug Administration (FDA) offers advantages to the standard commercial broth dilution card. The "E test" (Epsilon test) combines the simplicity of disk diffusion with the informative nature of broth dilution, but goes beyond standard broth dilution procedures. (see Figure 6-6). In general, MICs generated by the E-test correlate well with MICs generated from broth dilution procedures.[42] A disadvantage of the E-test is that the length of the test strip limits the number of drugs that can be tested on a large plate (three strips for a large plate, one for a small plate), which contributes to the cost of the testing.

Table 6-2 Interpretive Standards for Disk Diffusion Equivalent Minimum Inhibitory Concentration Breakpoints for Selected Antimicrobials

Drug	Breakpoint µg/mL Susceptible[1]	Breakpoint MIC (µg/mL) Resistant[1]
Amikacin	≤16	≥64
Amoxicillin with clavulanic acid*	≤ 0.25/0.12/≤8/2*	≥ 1/0.5
Ampicillin[4]*	≤0.25[2,9] ≤0.25[3]	≥0.5 ≥ 1
Azithromycin	≤4	≥8
Carbenicillin	≤16	≥64
Cefazolin[7]	≤8	≥32
Cefotaxime	≤8	≥64
Cefoxitin	≤8	≥32
Cefpodoxime	≤2	≥8
Ceftazidime	≤8	≥32
Ceftiofur[10]*	≤2	≥8
Ceftizoxime	≤8	≥32
Ceftriaxone	≤ 8	≥64
Cefuroxime	≤4	≥32
Cephalexin*	≤ 2	≥8
Cephalothin[7]	≤2	≥8
Chloramphenicol	≤ 8 ≤ 8[9]	≥32 ≥16
Ciprofloxacin[16] (see also enrofloxacin)	≤1	≥4
Clarithromycin	≤1 ≤8	≥8 ≥32
Clindamycin[8]*	≤0.5	≥4
Difloxacin*	≤0.5	≥4
Doxycyline	≤4	≥16
Enrofloxacin*	≤0.5	≥4
Erythromycin	≤0.5 ≤0.25[9]	≥8 ≥1
Florfenicol[10]*	≤2	≥8
Gentamicin*	≤4	≥16
Imipenem/ cilastin	≤4	≥16
Kanamycin	≤16	≥64
Levofloxacin	≤2	≥8[9]
Linezolid	≤4[2] ≤4[15]	 ≥ 8
Lincomycin	≤0.5	≥4
Marbofloxacin	≤1	≥4
Meropenem	≤4	≥16
Metronidazole	≤8	≥32
Nitrofurantoin	≤32	≥128
Orbifloxacin*	≤1	≥8
Oxacillin[6]	≤2	≥4
Penicillin G	≤8[3] ≤0.12[2]	≥16 ≥0.25
Piperacillin	≤16[2] ≤64[5]	≥128 ≥128
Rifampin	≤1	≥4
Sulfadiazine	≤2	≥4
Tetracycline[14]	≤4 ≤2[9]	≥16 ≥8
Ticarcillin	≤64[5] ≤16[4]	≥128 ≥128
Ticarcillin with clavulanic acid	≤64/2[5] ≤16/2[3]	≥128/2 ≥128/2
Trimethoprim/ Sulfamethoxazole[11]	≤2/38[13] ≤0.5/9.5[9]	≥4/76 ≥4/76
Vancomycin	≤4[15] ≤1[9] ≤4	≥32 ≥32

MIC, Minimum inhibitory concentration.
*Old breakpoints replaced by Clinical Laboratory Standards Institute (CLSI) for amoxicillin–clavulanic acid for all organisms were, for *Staphylococcus* ≤4/2 = S, and ≥ 8/4 = R and for non-staphylococci, ≤8/2,=S and ≥ 32/16 = R. The provision of a separate breakpoint of ≤8 µg/mL for UTI is new.
[1]Clinical Laboratory Standards replaced by CLSI for cephalexin were ≤ 8 = S, and ≥ 32 = R. The new breakpoints were becoming official at the time of publication. Institute Interpretive standards that are based on animal pathogens are designated by an asterisk.
[2]When testing *Staphyloccocus* organisms
[3]When testing gram-negative enteric organisms
[4]Ampicillin is used to test amoxicillin
[5]When testing *Pseudomonas* organisms
[6]Oxacillin is used to treat methicillin, cloxacillin
[7]Cephalothin is used to test all first-generation cephalosporins. Does not represent cefazolin, which should be tested separately if a gram-negative organism.
[8]Clindamycin is used to test lincomycin, which is less susceptible to *Staphylococcus.*
[9]When testing *Streptococcus (S. pneumoniae* for levofloxacin)
[10]When testing pathogens associated with food animal respiratory disease
[11]Trimethoprim–sulfamethoxazole is used to test trimethoprim–sulfadiazine and ormetoprim–sulfadimethoxine
[12]For urinary tract infections
[13]For soft tissue infections
[14]Used to test chlortetracycline, oxytetracycline, minocycline, doxycycline
[15]When testing Enterococcus organisms
[16]A human criteria deemed relevant to dogs and cats. Note reduced oral bioavailability (mean of 40%) in dogs and negligible (0%-20%) in cats.

Table 6-3 Examples of Minimum Inhibitory Concentration Ranges Covered by the E-test

Drug Class	Antimicrobial Drug	CLSI Breakpoints (S, R)	MIC range (μg/mL) of E-test
Penicillins	Ampicillin	≤8, ≥32	0.5-256
	Amoxicillin–clavulanic acid	≤8/4, ≥32/16	0.25-512
Cephalosporins	Cefpodoxime	≤2, ≥8	0.12-128
Fluoroquinolones	Enrofloxacin	≤0.5, ≥4	0.06-128
Tetracyclines	Doxycycline	≤4, ≥16	0.25-512
Aminoglycosides	Gentamicin	≤4, ≥8	0.12-256
Potentiated sulfa	Trimethoprim–sulfamethoxazole	≤2, ≥8	0.06-128

CLSI, Clinical Laboratory Standards Institute; *MIC,* minimum inhibitory concentration; *R,* resistant; *S,* susceptible.

However, because the drugs can be chosen for each patient, the method lends itself well to expanded susceptibility testing in the presence of a multidrug-resistant isolate. Although E tests are tedious and expensive, the wider range of concentrations tested (up to 1600-fold differences; Table 6-3) includes MICs well below the lower and higher thresholds of susceptibility, thus allowing identification of very susceptible isolates. Further, isolates with low-level resistance might be identified, potentially justifying the use of the drug, albeit at a higher dose or in combination with another drug.

KEY POINT 6-9 The E-test, but not current broth dilution procedures, allows identification of very susceptible isolates and isolates with low-level resistance.

Because of the inherent risks of inaccuracy associated with any C&S testing procedure, results yielded from procedures that are not based on CLSI standards should be interpreted with caution. Aspects subject to variability include pH; cation content and osmolality of the media; inoculum size; media volume; temperature and duration of incubation; humidity; and, for broth dilution, the method of observing growth.[41] Accordingly, in practice, culture methods should be considered less than ideal unless CLSI protocols are followed. Further, preliminary data, quick "snap" tests, or other methods intended to generate rapid results must be interpreted cautiously; the role of the organisms in causing infection and the susceptibility of the organisms (unless identified as a multidrug-resistant microbe) may require full C&S testing. Whereas the FDA is responsible for approval of diagnostic tests for human medicine, such a pathway is not required for veterinary diagnostic tests.

Population Pharmacodynamic Statistics

Agar Gel Versus Broth Dilution Pharmacodynamics

A nonquantitative but helpful summary of PD data is an antibiogram that indicates the proportion of isolates that are susceptible (or resistant) to the drug of interest (Figure 6-8). Although it does not provide information regarding the level of susceptibility, it can provide direction regarding empirical drug selection by indicating the likelihood that an organism is susceptible to the drug of choice. The antibiogram might be generated for each practice on the basis of cumulative data summarized on an annual basis.

Population statistics generated from MICs can provide even more useful information. They are particularly helpful if MIC data is not available for an isolate infecting a patient. Population MIC statistics can be generated from a sample population of the same organism; ideally, at least 100 isolates will be collected from different patients. Pertinent PD (MIC) statistics that describe the population distribution include the range (lowest and highest MICs recorded for any isolate representing the organism), mode (the most frequently reported MIC), median (the middle MIC, the 50th percentile or MIC_{50}), and the MIC_{90} (or the 90th percentile MIC; the MIC at which 90% of the organisms are inhibited (see Figures 6-9 to 6-11) . The two-fold dilution nature of MIC determination mandates that the geometric mean (converted to account for the non-continous nature of MIC) be reported rather than arithmetic mean. If an MIC is not available for an organism infecting a patient, the MIC_{90} (or even more ideally, the MIC_{100}) of a drug for an organism is the preferred surrogate indicator of "what is needed" by the author. For example, if *S. pseudintermedius* is a known or suspected cause of pyoderma in a patient and the drug to be chosen empirically is cephalexin, the MIC_{90} of *S. intermedius* for cephelexin[43] can be used as an indicator of "what is needed"—that is, the PD target for therapy in the patient. PD information can be found on many package inserts scientific literature[43,44] or textbooks (veterinary for animal drugs, human if not), and other resources (see Table 6-4 and Chapter 7). However, the dynamic nature of microbes in response to the presence of antimicrobials may render some population data obsolete even within several years of collection. In addition to the species, a number of host factors are likely to affect the sample population statistics and its applicability to the patient. Among the more important factors is previous exposure to antimicrobials, which is likely to be associated with higher MICs compared with MICs of isolates collected from antimicrobial-naïve animals (i.e., not pathogens). Ideally, separate statistics might be promulgated for isolates collected from animals not previously exposed to antimicrobials.

KEY POINT 6-10 Recent population pharmacodynamic data such as the MIC_{90} can serve as a reasonable surrogate for patient data.

Klebsiella	No. of Isolates	Amikacin	Amoxicillin/CA	Ampicillin	Cefazolin	Cefoxitin	Ceftiofur	Cephalothin[b]	Chloramphenicol	Clindamycin	Enrofloxacin	Erythromycin	Gentamicin	Marbofloxacin	Orbifloxacin	Oxacillin	Penicillin	Tetracycline	Ticarcillin	Ticarcillin/CA	Trimethoprim/Sulfa
Enterococcus faecalis	30		97	97					83		40	28 (29)		40 (15)	10		93	63			
E. faecium	13		15	13					100		0	15		0 (11)	0		15	23			
Escherichia coli	120	98	63	48	69	65	76 (103)	46	81		63		83	65	62 (119)			68	52	64	67 (119)
Klebsiella pneumoniae	30	80	70	0	70	70	63	70	80		77		77	77	73			73	0	70	77
Proteus mirabilis	32	100	97	94	94	97	100	94	94		97		91	100	91				94	100	81
Pseudomonas aeruginosa	61	100							0		64		97	76 (50)	25				97	98	
Staphylococcus aureus	8	100	50	13	50	50	29 (7)	50	100	50	75	50	88	75	75	50	13	88			88
S. intermedius	102	92	66	17	64	64	60 (89)	64	97	43 (101)	55	43	87	63	60 (99)	72	18	42			60 (101)
S. schleifen ss coagulans	20	95	65	45	65	65	59 (17)	65	100	95 (19)	30	100	70	50	40	65	50	95			100
S. pseudintermedius	4	75	50	0	50	50	33 (3)	50	100	50	75	50	75	75	75	50	0	50			75

Figure 6-8 A cumulative antibiogram generated for the target species can be helpful in identifying drugs to which acquired resistance has emerged. The data will be specific to the facility (i.e., hospital). The number in each cell refers to the number of tested isolates designated as susceptible to the drug. When present, the number in parentheses in each cell refers to the number of isolates tested for that drug; otherwise, the number of isolates tested is indicated in the second left-hand column. Note that the data indicate that one species in a genera may not be well represented by another species in the same genera, particularly for *Enterococcus* and *Staphylococcus* genera.

Comparing PD data of a drug reveals differential susceptibility among organisms toward each drug. For example, using the antimicrobial package insert, comparison of MIC_{90} among different organisms reveals that *P. aeruginosa* tends to be susceptible (if at all) only at high concentrations compared with the more susceptible *Pasteurella multocida* (see Figure 6-11). The MIC_{90} of *P. aeruginosa* more often than not approaches or surpasses the upper threshold of susceptibility for most drugs. Thus achieving effective antimicrobial concentrations is more likely to be difficult in the patient infected with *P. aeruginosa* compared with one infected with *Pasteurella*. A review of the antimicrobial package insert reveals other differential susceptibilities.

The distribution of the MICs of organisms for drugs can help identify emerging resistance. For example, the distribution of *E. coli* for several drugs (see Figure 6-10) is bimodal, representing two different populations. The majority of isolates in the first population are characterized by an MIC well below the susceptible threshold of susceptibility (i.e., susceptible MIC breakpoint). This data demonstrates that even isolates considered susceptible are characterized by MIC that are close to the susceptible breakpoint. Further, a substantial portion of the population is higher than the upper threshold of susceptibility—that is, the MIC_{90} exceeds the resistant MIC breakpoint. It is very possible that the second population, characterized by higher MICs, probably represents isolates previously exposed to antimicrobials; as such, culture would be prudent for those animals previously exposed to antimicrobials. Finally, detecting increasing MICs determined from sequential cultures of the same organisms in a patient with recurrent infections might indicate emerging resistance, likewise, comparison of the MIC_{90} of a sample population of an organism across time can reveal emerging resistance.

The Minimum Inhibitory Concentration: Determining Susceptibility Versus Resistance

Susceptibility data based on broth dilution procedures that are reported for a patient will include the MIC, as well as a susceptible, intermediate, or resistant (SIR) interpretation.

KEY POINT 6-11 Simplistically, the MIC is the pharmacodynamic target of antimicrobial therapy, indicating the minimum concentration to be achieved at the site of infection. However, it is only a starting point.

The clinical microbiology laboratory provides the interpretation on the basis of CLSI interpretive criteria. The criteria for broth dilution procedures are presented as thresholds or breakpoint MICs (MIC_{BP}) whose values will also be in terms of the concentrations tested for each drug (i.e., multiples or

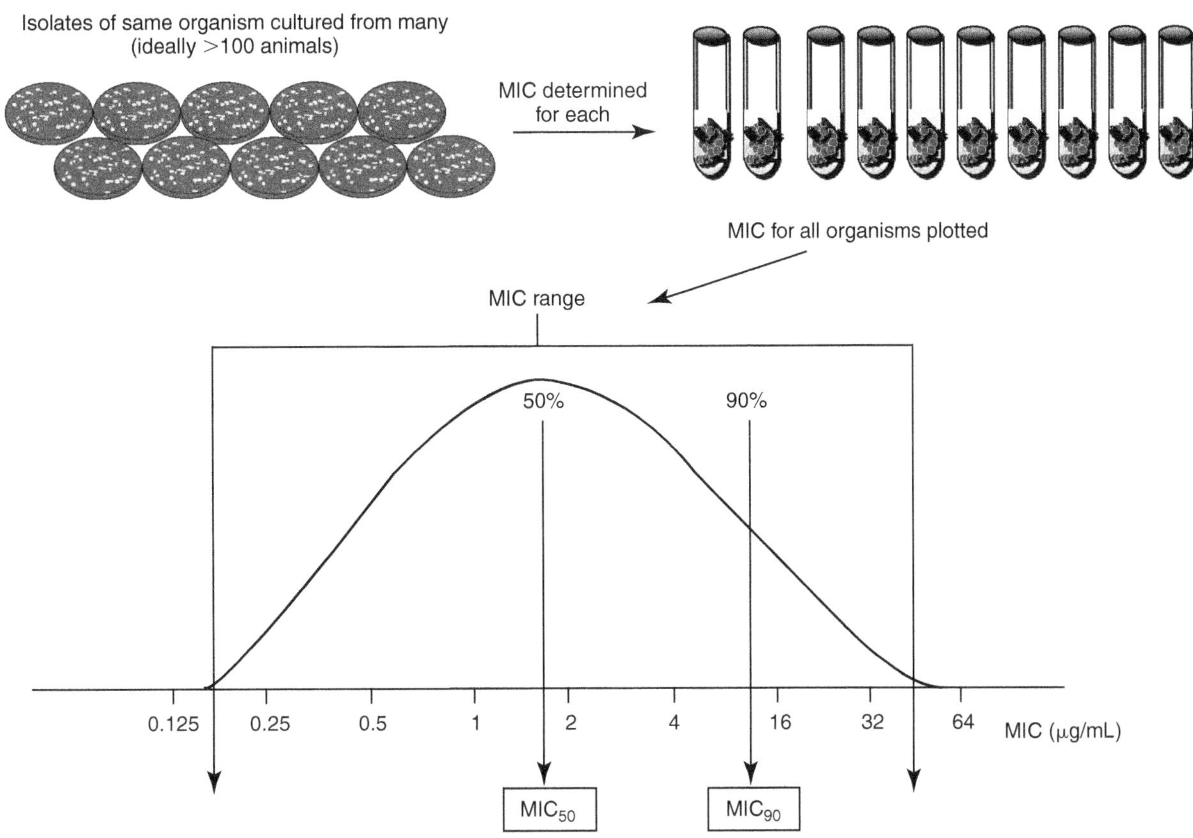

Figure 6-9 Population pharmacodynamic data. Each sample collected from a different animal (same species) yields an isolate of the organism of interest. Ideally, at least 100 representative isolates will be tested. The minimum inhibitory concentration (MIC) of each isolate is determined, and all are plotted in a distribution curve. The range represents the lowest and highest MIC determined for the isolate; the mode would be the most frequent MIC reported and the median represents the middle MIC or the 50th percentile (which, for normally distributed data, also represents the MIC) The MIC_{90} is the 90th percentile MIC. A representative package insert demonstrating the presentation of population pharmacodynamic data can be found in Figure 6-11.

fractions of 1 μg/mL) (see Table 6-2). Two breakpoints are provided for each drug. An isolate inhibited at a concentration at or below the lower threshold or susceptible MIC breakpoint will be designated "S," whereas an isolate that is able to grow after in vitro exposure to a drug concentration that equals the upper threshold or the resistant MIC breakpoint will be designated "R." The susceptible breakpoint is at least one broth dilution below the resistant breakpoint for all drugs; for some drugs the susceptible breakpoint is 2 or more broth dilutions below the resistant breakpoint, allowing for an intermediate, or "I," designation (see Figure 6-6). For example, for enrofloxacin, the susceptible and resistant MIC_{BP} are ≤0.5 and ≥4 μg/mL, respectively. Thus an isolate whose growth (under in vitro conditions specified by CLSI) is inhibited with as little as 0.5 μg/mL or less will be designated as "S." On the other hand, if growth is present in the well that contains 2 μg/mL, then 4 μg/mL (the next broth dilution) or more will be necessary to inhibit the growth of the isolate, and the isolate will be designated as "R," or resistant to enrofloxacin. An additional broth dilution occurs between 0.5 and 2 μg/mL. Isolates that are inhibited by enrofloxacin at 1 μg/mL will be designated as intermediate, or "I." An isolate with an "I" designation has developed some level of resistance, and such isolates should be treated with that drug only cautiously, at higher doses, or in combination with a complementary antimicrobial drug. The more prudent approach would be to consider "I" isolates as "R" for that drug. Use might also be considered in circumstances in which the drug accumulates in active (i.e., unbound) form at the site of infection such that concentrations exceed that achieved in plasma. Examples might include urine (produced by the normally functioning kidney) or accumulation in phagocytic white blood cells (selected drugs). Note, however, that such concentrations may yet be insufficient.

KEY POINT 6-12 Interpretive criteria for susceptibility testing by CLSI is dynamic, changing across time as microbes acquire resistance. However, once generated, the data is applicable for all laboratories in the United States.

CLSI determines the thresholds of susceptibilities—that is, the lower (susceptible) and upper (resistant) breakpoint MIC_{BP} for each drug after exhaustive evaluation of both PK data in the target species and PD data for the drug of interest toward the microbes of interest. For animal drugs approved

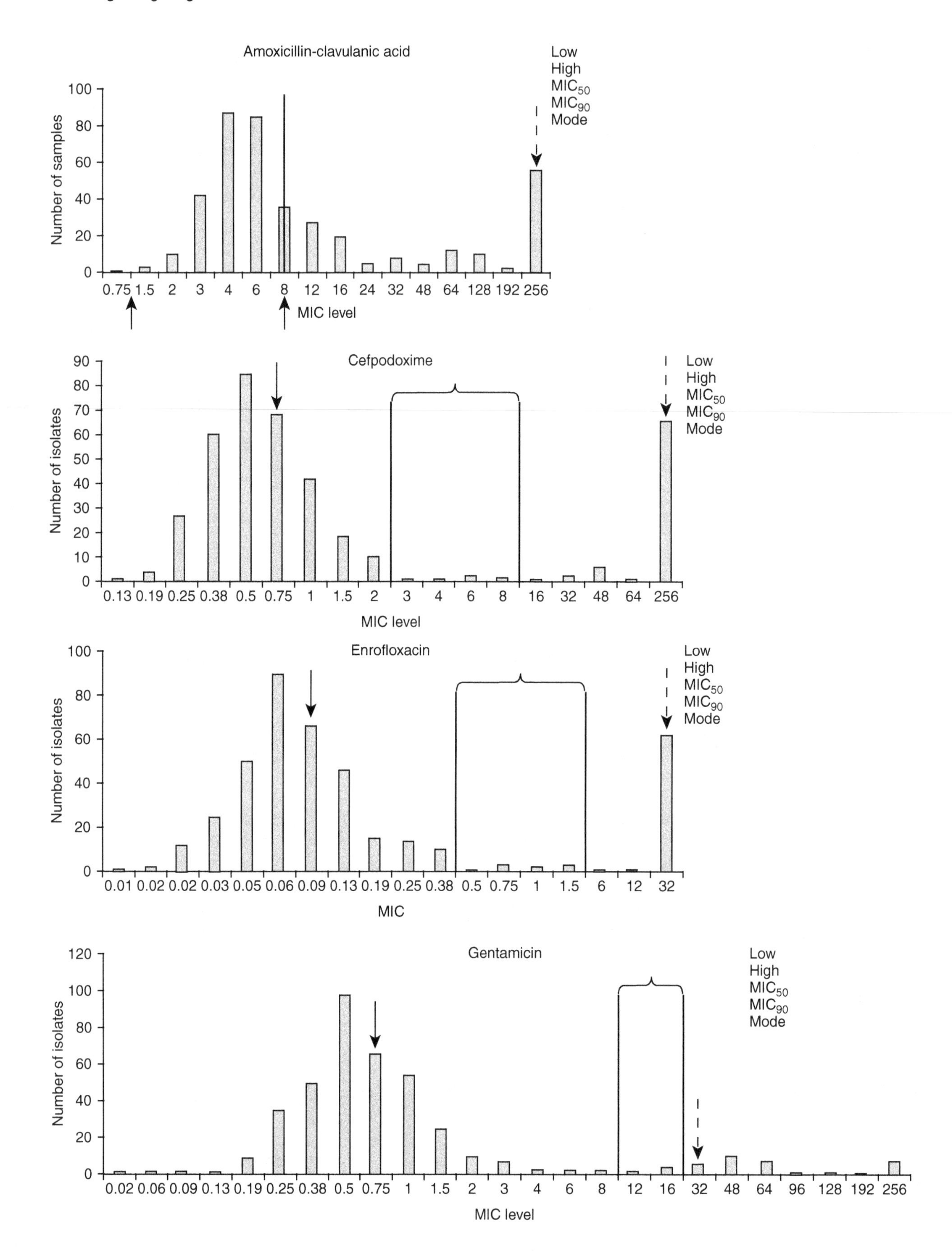
Amoxicillin-clavulanic acid
Low
High
MIC50
MIC90
Mode
Number of samples
100
80
60
40
20
0
0.75 1.5 2 3 4 6 8 12 16 24 32 48 64 128 192 256
MIC level
Cefpodoxime
Number of isolates
90
80
70
60
50
40
30
20
10
0
0.13 0.19 0.25 0.38 0.5 0.75 1 1.5 2 3 4 6 8 16 32 48 64 256
MIC level
Enrofloxacin
Number of isolates
100
80
60
40
20
0
0.01 0.02 0.02 0.03 0.05 0.06 0.09 0.13 0.19 0.25 0.38 0.5 0.75 1 1.5 6 12 32
MIC
Gentamicin
Number of isolates
120
100
80
60
40
20
0
0.02 0.06 0.09 0.13 0.19 0.25 0.38 0.5 0.75 1 1.5 2 3 4 6 8 12 16 32 48 64 96 128 192 256
MIC level

Figure 6-10 Population distributions of canine and feline *Escherichia coli* pathogens' minimum inhibitory concentration (MIC) based on E-testing for two time-dependent drugs (amoxicillin–clavulanic acid, and cefpodoxime, *upper plots)* and two concentration-dependent drugs (enrofloxacin, and gentamicin, *lower plots).* The susceptible *(left)* and resistant *(right)* breakpoints, as identifed by Committee on Laboratory Standards Institute, are indicated in brackets and lines except for amoxicillin. CLSI's new breakpoints are indicated by arrows (≤8 μg/mL for the susceptible breakpoint for isolates collected from the urinary the resistant breakpoint for other isolates; indicated by arrows below x axis). The distribution is bimodal for all drugs except gentamicin, as is indicated by a second distribution of isolates with an MIC well above the resistant breakpoint. This second population of isolates will cause the MIC_{90} *(dashed arrow)* to exceed the breakpoint. The range is represented by the lowest and highest MIC recorded (either may be limited by the range tested), the median is the 50th percentile (or MIC_{50}) *(solid arrow)* the MIC_{90} is the 90th percentile, and the mode is the most common MIC reported for that isolate and drug. Because an E-test was used, the MIC tested are not limited to two-fold dilutions. Because these isolates are pathogens that have been cultured from dogs or cats with spontaneous disease, they may represent isolates already exposed to antimicrobials which may explain the bimodal distribution (i.e., these isolates may have undergone stepwise mutations). The population distribution of drug-naïve only isolates is likely to be somewhat lower.

Fluoroquinolone A

Parameter *For oral use in dogs and cats only*	**Dose**		
	Dog Mean ± SD* (2.5mg/lb) n=6	**Dog Mean ± SD* (5.5mg/lb) n=6**	**Cat Mean ± SD* (5.5mg/lb) n=7**
Time of maximum concentration, T_{max}(h)	1.5±0.3	1.8±0.3	1.2±0.6
Maximum concentration, C_{max}, (μg/mL)	2.0±0.2	4.2±0.5	4.8±0.7
AUC0-inf (μg•h/mL)	31.2±1.6	64±8	70±6
Terminal plasma elimination half-life, $t_{1/2}$(h)	10.7±1.6	10.9±0.6	12.7±1.1

Organism	Number of Isolates	MIC_{50}	MIC_{90}	MIC Range
Staphylococcus intermedius	135	0.25	0.25	0.125–2
Escherichia coli	61	0.03	0.06	0.015–2
Proteus mirabilis	35	0.06	0.125	0.03–0.25
Beta-hemolytic Streptococcus, (not Group A or Group B)	25	1	2	0.5–16
Streptococcus, Group D enterococcus	16	1	4	0.008–4
Pasteurella multocida	13	0.015	0.06	≤0.008–0.5
Staphylococcus aureus	12	0.25	0.25	0.25–0.5
Enterococcus faecalis	11	2	2	0–4
Klebsiella pneumoniae	11	0.06	0.06	0.01–0.06
Pseudomonas spp.	9	**	**	0.06–1
Pseudomonas aeruginosa	7	**	**	0.25–1

Table: MIC Values* (μg/mL) of FQA against pathogens isolated from skin, soft tissue and urinary tract infections in dogs enrolled in clinical studies conducted during 1994-1996.

Fluoroquinolone B

Bacteria Name	Number of Isolates	MIC_{50}	MIC_{90}	MIC Range
Enterobacter spp.	9	0.11	3.66	≤0.05–3.66
Escherichia coli	28	≤0.05	0.11	≤0.05–7.3
Klebsiella spp.	8	0.11	0.11	0.11–0.23
Pasteurella spp.	8	≤0.05	≤0.05	≤0.05
Proteus spp.	15	0.92	1.83	0.11–1.83
Pseudomonas spp.	5	0.11	0.92	≤0.05–0.92
Staphylococcus spp.	193	0.23	0.46	≤0.05–1.83
Streptococcus spp.	56	1.83	3.66	0.11–7.3

Table: MIC values* (μg/mL) of FQB for bacterial pathogens isolated from skin and soft tissue infections and urinary tract infections in dogs enrolled in clinical studies conducted during 1991–1993.

Pharmacokinetic Measure	Mean Value
Peak plasma concentration (C_{MAX})	1.8 μg/mL
Time to reach C_{max} (T_{MAX})	2.8 hours
Elimination half-life ($T_{1/2}$)	9.3 hours
Area under the plasma curve (AUC0–∞)	14.5 μg•hr/mL
Total body clearance/F^a (CL/F)	375 mL/kg/hr
Steady state volume of distribution/F^b	3.8 L/kg
Volume of distribution (area)/F^c	4.7 L/kg

Table: Plasma pharmacokinetics following administration of FQB tablets (5 mg/kg body weight) to dogs (n=20).

Figure 6-11 Package insert information two fluoroquinolones, FQA (top) and FQB (bottom). Comparison of MIC_{90} among isolates for FQA suggests that *Pasteurella* sp. should be more easily treated compared with *Escherichia coli* for both drugs. Integration of pharmacokinetic data (C_{max} for these concentration-dependent drugs) and pharmacodynamic data (MIC_{90}) can be used to identify which drug is best used to treat each microbe and which dose might be used to treat the microbe. For example, for FQA at the low dose of 2.5 mg/kg, when treating *E. coli* (and no patient-specific MIC is available), the C_{max} is 2 μg/mL and the MIC_{90} is 0.06 μg/mL, resulting in a C_{max}/MIC_{90} ratio of 25. For *Proteus,* the ratio is 2/0.125, or 16. For concentration-dependent drugs, the target ratio is ≥10, suggesting the low dose may be effective for both, but the large dose might be considered for *Proteus* if the patient is considered at risk. The number of isolates of *P. aeruginosa* is not sufficient to represent the population. If the process is repeated for FQB with a C_{max} of 1.8 μg/mL at the low dose, the MIC_{90} for *E. coli is* 0.11 μg/mL, resulting in a ratio of 16. For *Proteus,* the MIC_{90} is 1.8 μg/mL, resulting in a ratio of only 1. Although the dose might be sufficient for *E. coli,* the target ratio could not be reached even at the higher dose for *Proteus*. Note that the number of organisms on which the data are based for each organism often does not reach the ideal target of 100. The smaller the sample size, the more caution is indicated when extrapolating this data to the general population. (From Pfizer, Package Insert and Fort Dodge, Package Insert)

Table 6-4 Integration of Population Pharmacodynamic (PD) and Pharmacokinetic (PK) Data and Its Role in the Design of Dosing Regimens

Time-Dependent Drugs (T > MIC 50%)				Current Dosing				Calculated Dosing	
Drug	Organism	MIC_{90}* (µg/mL)	Route	Interval (hr)	Dose (mg/kg)	C_{max} (µg/mL)	Half-life (hr)	Half-lives T > MIC	Interval (hr)
Amoxi-clav	*St. pseud*	≤ 0.5	PO	12	12.5	5.5	1	3.46	3.46
	St. aureus	4						0.46	0.46
	E. coli	32						NR	NR
Cephalexin	*St. pseud*	2	PO	12	22	20	1.3	3.32	4.32
	St. aureus	8						1.32	1.72
	E. coli	32						0.32	0.42
Cefovecin	*St. pseud*	0.25	SC	168	8	4.2	133	4.07	541.48
	St. aureus	2				(unbound)		1.07	142.39
	E. coli	1						2.07	275.42
Cefpodoxime	*St. pseud*	0.5	PO	24	5	8.2	5.6	4.04	22.60
	St. aureus	NA						NA	
	E. coli	0.5						4.04	22.60
Meropenem	*St. pseud*	NA	SC	12	20	26	0.75	NA	
	St. aureus	0.25						6.7	5
	E. coli	0.5						8.8	7
	P. aerug	2						3.7	3

Concentration-Dependent Drugs (Cmax/MIC >10-12)			Current Dosing				
Drug	Organism	MIC_{90} (µg/mL)	Route	Interval (hr)	Dose (mg/kg)	C_{max} (µg/mL)	C_{max}/MIC
Enrofloxacin	*St. pseud*	0.25	PO	24	20	7.1	28
	St. aureus	64				(plus cipro)	0.11
	E. coli	64					0.11
	P. aerug	0.5					14
Marbofloxacin	*St. pseud*	1	PO	24	5.5	4.2	4.20
	St. aureus	64					0.07
	E. coli	64					0.07
	P. aerug	0.5					8.40
Orbifloxacin	*St. pseud*	2	PO	24	2.5	2.3	1.15
	St. aureus	64					0.04
	E. coli	64					0.04
	P. aerug	16					0.14
Ciprofloxacin	*St. pseud*	0.125	PO	24	20	2.8	22
	St. aureus	0.25					11
	E. coli	64					0.04
	P. aerug	2					1.40
Gentamicin	*St. pseud*		IM	24	3	27	NR
	St. aureus	1					27
	E. coli (7)	2					13.50
	P. aerug	4					6.8
Amikacin	*St. pseud*		SC	24	10	14	NR
	St. aureus						NR
	E. coli	8					1.75
	P. aerug	8					1.75

NA, Not available; *NR*, not reached at cited dosing regimen.

in the last several decades (only since then have MIC become standard testing procedures), it is likely that some of the data were collected by the drug manufacturer during the approval process. However, both PK and PD data may be drawn from peer-reviewed literature or other sources, particularly for drugs not approved for use in the target species, or for drugs whose susceptibility thresholds are being re-evaluated by CLSI.

Three criteria must be met for CLSI to establish an MIC_{BP} for each drug. The primary and initial consideration is the population distributions, with a focus on both the statistics as well as the type (i.e., modal or bimodal; see Figure 6-10). Obvious patterns of low versus high MICs can be used to identify susceptible "cutoffs" or breakpoints. Statistics will be compared among different strains of the same species being tested. Note that some organisms may be much more susceptible to the drug of interest—that is, they have MIC_{50} and MIC_{90} that are much lower compared with other organisms (e.g., *pasteurella* and *pseudomonas*). However, CLSI generally provides only one set of criteria for all susceptible isolates.

The second consideration upon which criteria are based is, the clinical pharmacology of the drug, ideally in the target species. Among the more important PK parameters evaluated by CLSI are the peak and trough plasma drug concentrations (C_{max} and C_{min}), area under the curve (AUC) for a 24-hour dosing period, and the drug elimination half-life (see later discussion of PD indices) (Figure 6-12).[41,45-51] Volume of distribution; protein binding; and, when available, tissue (including urine) concentrations are also considered. Presumably, the MIC of an isolate considered susceptible should be below the peak plasma or tissue drug concentrations or C_{max} of a given drug when administered at a recommended dose. Indeed, selected resistant breakpoints correlate with C_{max}, as is demonstrated for amikacin when administered to dogs at 22 mg/kg. The C_{max} of 65 µg/mL (see Chapter 7) is similar to the resistant breakpoint for amikacin. However, for some breakpoints, the correlation does not exist, as is exemplified by amoxicillin/clavulanic. The C_{max} of the labeled dose of 13.5 mg/kg, administered orally, will generate a C_{max} of approximately 4 to 6 µg/mL of amoxicillin in dogs, yet the resistant breakpoint for nonstaphylococcal organisms has been ≥32 µg/mL, well beyond the concentrations that can be achieved in plasma at any reasonable dose. (In response to this disparity, CLSI has recently re-examined and readjusted the breakpoint for amoxicillin-clavulanic acid as is discussed below; see Table 6-2).Another limitation of setting breakpoints based on peak plasma drug concentrations is their lack of precision: breakpoints are limited to concentrations used for susceptibility testing and thus will be reported using twofold dilutions. As such, a resistant breakpoint concentration may be considerably higher or lower than the actual concentration achieved at the recommended dose. As such, the actual MIC reported for an infecting isolate should be compared to C_{max} reported in a sample population of the target species is an ideal default when selecting drugs (and the dosing regimen; see later discussion). The original veterinary fluoroquinolones were approved with "flexible labels" (multiple doses); for those drugs, the susceptible and resistant breakpoints reflect the C_{max} resulting from the lowest and highest labeled doses of the drug.

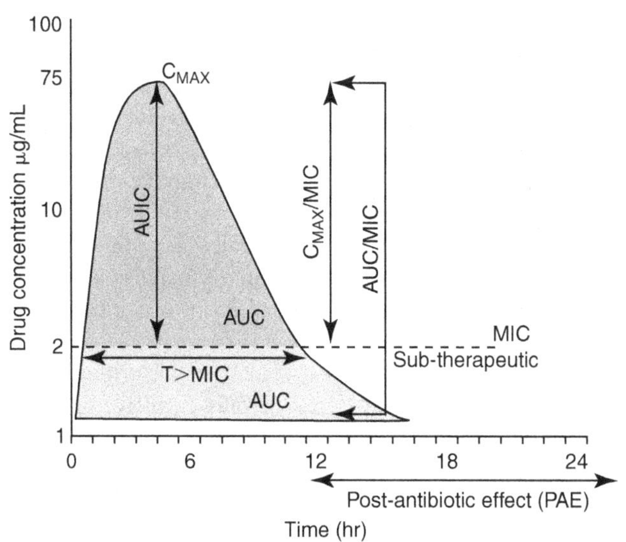

Figure 6-12 Pharmacodynamic indices (PDI) resulting from integration of pharmacokinetic (PK) data (from sample population of target or closely related surrogate species), represented here by C_{max} (µg/mL; target of 10 to 12) or area under the curve (AUC) (µg*hr/mL; target of 100-125), and microbial or pharmacodynamic (PD) data, represented here by minimum inhibitory concentration (MIC). Note that the PDI are based on (Mouton 2005 [47] and Amsterdam 2005[41]). Note that activity should be based on free (unbound) drug. The pertinent PK parameters for this hypothetical drug and infecting microbe would be as follows: C_{max} of 75 µg/mL, half-life of approximately 2 hours and AUC of 159 µg*hr/mL. The PD parameter, or MIC of the infecting organism, is 2 µg/mL. The PDI for this drug and microbe combination would be as follows: C_{max}/MIC = 37.5 (surpasses target for a concentration-dependent drug); AUC/MIC = 80 (insufficient for a gram-negative organism if a fluorinated quinolone but potentially sufficient for a gram-positive organism); and T > MIC = 8 hours, which would allow a 12, 16, or 24- (32 hr is not a reasonable interval) hour dosing interval for a time-dependent drug if the target T > MIC were 75%, 50%, or 25%, respectively. The AUIC (area under the inhibitory curve) is the integrated area of the curve above the MIC. Although somewhat similar to AUC/MIC, its use among investigators has caused confusion, leading experts in the field to focus on AUC/MIC as the area-based PDI of choice.

The third criteria that must be met as CLSI determines thresholds of susceptibility is one of clinical relevance. The MIC_{BP} must be clinically relevant—that is, the microorganisms defined as susceptible should respond clinically to the drug, and in vitro data must correlate adequately with in vivo findings.[46,51] The MIC_{BP} values established by CLSI for each drug are generally not included in the susceptibility reports. However, having this information would be helpful because the MIC of the infecting organism might then be compared with the MIC_{BP} of the drug, allowing an assessment of "level" of susceptibility of the isolate to the drug of interest (discussed in more detail later). Breakpoints set by CLSI are based on isolates collected from across the country and accordingly are relevant for any clinical microbiology laboratory that uses CLSI protocols. As such, CLSI breakpoints generally can be obtained by any microbiology laboratory that uses CLSI criteria for its testing procedures (the preferred choice). Interpretive standards generally also are delineated on package inserts (including sources such as *Physicians' Desk Reference* for human-marketed drugs or similar veterinary compendiums).

In order to simplify the use of interpretive criteria, when possible, CLSI breakpoints are generally inclusive to organisms whose spectrum is included in the drug, regardless of the site of infection. However, notable exceptions occur for both organisms and tissues. Organism exceptions generally are those either very susceptible to the drug or for organisms that easily develop in vivo resistance. For example, lower or more stringent penicillin breakpoints have been promulgated for *Staphylococcus* spp. because their beta-lactamases are particularly destructive toward penicillins compared to cephalosporins. Because destructive activity decreases the amount of drug at the site, a second set of lower breakpoints are provided. A higher breakpoint has been established for other susceptible isolates (e.g., gram-negative organisms; see Table 6-2). In contrast to *Staphylococcus, P. aeruginosa* is particularly susceptible to ticarcillin; accordingly, while another coliform is considered resistant if it is inhibited at 16 μg/mL *P. aeruginosa* is still considered susceptible even if, in vitro, it grows in the presence of 64 μg/mL (see Table 6-2). Another consideration regarding inclusivity is the generation of tissue specific breakpoints. Interpretive criteria are based on plasma drug concentrations. However, renally excreted drugs achieve much higher concentrations in urine compared to plasma. New interpretive criteria for ampicillin and amoxicillin–clavulanic acid includes a separate breakpoint that is tissue dependent: a higher breakpoint (≤8 μg/mL) has been set for *E. coli*-associated urinary tract infections, compared to much lower breakpoints for other tissues. However, caution is recommended when selecting a drug for treatment of a UTI when the "S" designation for a urinary isolate is based on breakpoints that differ from plasma (see Chapter 8) as it assumes, among other considerations, that infection occurs only in the bladder, that urine is concentrated by the patient, and the duration of exposure fulfills the needs of a time-dependent drug (see later discussion). Just as resistance can be detected in an infecting organism collected from a patient, across time, statistics may also indicate resistance (i.e., the MIC and MIC statistics [mode, median, MIC_{50}, and MIC_{90}]). Because CLSI reviews new data intermittently, their criteria for interpretive standards should result in new MIC_{BP}, and laboratories will implement these changes. The sequelae of increasing MICs in certain populations should result in an increasing number of isolates designated as "R" for drugs to which the organisms traditionally have been considered susceptible. An example is amoxicillin–clavulanic acid, whose susceptible breakpoint was recently decreased by CLSI (see Table 6-2).

Integration of Pharmacokinetics and Pharmacodynamics: How Much Is Needed Versus How Much is Achieved?

The information provided on the C&S report can be used effectively beyond the simple identification of "S" drugs. The MIC is an indicator of what is needed to target the organism and thus provides the PD information for the infecting isolate. Often, an organism will be designated as susceptible to several drugs. One advantage to the broth dilution method compared with the disk diffusion method of C&S is the ability of the former to rank the drugs according to relative efficacy based on MIC. However, the relative efficacy of antimicrobials designated as "S" against a specific pathogen should not be determined by directly comparing MICs among different drugs, even drugs in the same class. The MIC varies among the drugs for a number of reasons beyond susceptibility. These include, but are not limited to, differences in molecular weight (one drug is simply heavier than another), the ability of the drug to penetrate the organism, the number of molecules necessary to "neutralize" the target, and differences in the mechanisms of action. Further, each drug achieves different concentrations in the patient as a result of differences in disposition. Thus antimicrobials differ in potency and MIC.[47] Rather than direct comparison to an isolate MIC for one drug to an MIC for another drug, one should also consider the concentration of drug that will be achieved in the patient when the drug is administered at the recommended dose (i.e., what is achieved; C_{max}). A less than ideal method of standardizing MIC is to compare how far the MIC of the drug of interest is from the resistant breakpoint (i.e., ratio of resistant MIC breakpoint of the drug to MIC of the organism). This is less ideal, as was previously discussed, because the resistant breakpoint does not always equate with the C_{max}.

KEY POINT 6-13 The closer the MIC (or MIC_{90}) of an organism is to the C_{max}, the greater the risk of therapeutic failure and the more important the need to modify the dosing regimen for the patient.

The limitations in using MIC breakpoint as an indicator of what will be achieved in the patient reflect the serial concentration used for susceptibility testing. If a drug achieves a C_{max} of 24 μg/mL at the recommended dose, this concentration falls between 16 and 32 μg/mL serial dilutions. A susceptible breakpoint of 16 μg/mL might underestimate while a resistant breakpoint of 32 μg/mL would over overestimate what will be achieved at the recommended dose. Thus, a more relevant choice among the susceptible drugs might be based on comparing what is needed to what is achieved—in plasma (e.g., the C_{max}) when the drug is administered at the recommended dose. The ratio of C_{max} to MIC, however, requires that PK information be available for the drug of interest, ideally in the species of interest. This information often is available on package inserts for animal-approved drugs but must be collected from the literature for other drugs (see Chapter 7). The United States Pharmacopiea antimicrobial monographs published by the Journal of Veterinary Pharmacology and Therapeutics (2007) offers a compilation of PK information for a variety of antimicrobials and animal species. The integration of PD and PK is the first step in selecting a drug. However, this step is preliminary in that it does not take into account other factors that affect tissue concentrations, including host and microbial factors.

The relationship between the MIC of the infecting organism (what is needed) and the C_{max} also should be used as a basis for designing a dosing regimen.[48-50] The closer the MIC (or MIC_{90}) to the C_{max} (or the MIC_{BP}), the higher the dose and for time-dependent drugs, the shorter the interval that is indicated. For a more specific design of a dose, the MIC can serve as the targeted drug concentration (see Enhancing Antimicrobial Efficacy). If MIC data is not available from the isolate collected in the patient, population PD [MIC_{90}] data might be used as a surrogate PD indicator of how much is needed; (see Figure 6-11).

Caveats to Culture and Susceptibility Interpretation

Despite the usefulness of C&S testing, the information nonetheless reflects in vitro testing that must be applied to in vivo situations.[40,41] Results can be misleading or misinterpreted, despite ideal sampling and C&S techniques. Some of the pitfalls reflect the limitations presented by practicalities in testing (e.g., economics, technology), whereas others reflect limitations of applying in vitro data to an in vivo system. Examples include the following:

1. The limitations presented in the number of drugs and range of concentrations tested were previously addressed. The hazards of interpreting an "S" designation without knowing *how* close the MIC is to the susceptible breakpoint may facilitate emerging resistance for those isolates whose MICs are approaching the breakpoint of the drug or the C_{max} of the drug given at the recommended dose. For example, an isolate whose MIC for enrofloxacin is 0.5 μg/mL is likely to already have undergone the first step toward resistance, compared to an isolate whose MIC is 0.06 μg/mL.

> **KEY POINT 6-14** Culture and susceptibility testing is an in vitro procedure and as such, cannot accurately mimic the conditions to which the data is applied—that is, the infected patient.

2. CLSI does not provide interpretive standards for all drugs; as such, these drugs do not appear on C&S testing, and MIC_{BP} are not available. This may be a decision on the part of the manufacturer of the drug not to pursue CLSI validation, the lack of adequate data for CLSI to determine criteria, or failure of the data to correlate with patient response. For such drugs population PD and PK data as reported in the literature, for example, may be the only reasonable approach to assess antimicrobial efficacy (see later discussion).
3. For some drug classes, CLSI has established criteria for a model drug that serves to reflect patterns of susceptibility for other members in the same class. In some instances cross-susceptibility and resistance justify this approach (e.g., fluorinated quinolones might represent all veterinary fluorinated quinolones, ampicillin accurately predicts amoxicillin, and sulfamethoxazole/trimethoprim appears to predict other potentiated sulfonamides). However, exceptions to the relevance of model drugs to other members in the class occur. For example, ampicillin-sulbactam serves as a model for amoxicillin–clavulanic acid, but several diagnostic microbiologists find the latter to overestimate the efficacy of the latter. Generally, CLSI has indicated the exceptions in its interpretive guidelines (many are summarized in Table 6-2), and the veterinary diagnostic laboratory should indicate these exceptions in the C&S report. For example, cephalothin (which is no longer available) represents first-generation cephalosporins, yet cefazolin generally is less effective against *S. aureus* and more effective against *E. coli*. The spectrum of third- and fourth-generation cephalosporins is markedly disparate, and thus the class cannot be well represented by a model drug. Among the newer aminoglycosides, gentamicin is generally more effective than tobramycin against *Serratia* spp. and more effective than amikacin against *Staphylococcus,* whereas tobramycin and amikacin are more effective than gentamicin against *P. aeruginosa*.
4. Limitations in extrapolations of susceptibility data are not restricted to spectrum but also may reflect a mismatch between in vitro and in vivo response. For example, despite in vitro evidence of susceptibility, aminoglycosides should not be used to treat *Enterococcus* spp. or as sole agent to treat *Staphylococcus* spp. Potentiated sulfonamides are not considered by CLSI to be clinically effective toward enterococci, despite in vitro susceptibility. However, recent reports in the literature challenge this assessment, supporting the importance of continued surveillance of the data by CLSI. Generally, laboratories will not test drugs against organisms for which clinical efficacy has not been demonstrated. (see Figure 6-8). This is most obviously exemplified by gram-negative versus gram-positive susceptibility panels, with the drugs tested against the isolate being grouped according to anticipated efficacy for the type of organism (e.g., gram-negative isolates will not be tested against clindamycin or erythromycin; gram-positive isolates generally are not be tested against ticarcillin, which was developed for gram-negative infections; anaerobes will not be tested against aminoglycosides; methicillin-resistant *Staphylococcus* should not be tested against any beta-lactam, and *Pseuodmonas* generally is not tested against a variety of drugs to which it is consistently resistant). A more recently recognized limitation of susceptibility testing is detection of acquired resistance that is rapidly induced by the presence of the drug. This might be best exemplified by gram-negative organisms that produce extended-spectrum beta-lactamases (ESBLs). These enzymes destroy selected third- and fourth-generation cephalosporins but are induced at the site of infection by the presence of the drug.[52] Therefore ESBLs generally are not expressed by the

isolate culture in vitro. Their detection may require additional testing of the isolate in the presence of cefpodoxime and ceftazidime alone or in combination with clavulanic acid, which is not susceptible to ESBL. A fourfold or greater reduction in cephalosporin MIC when it is combined with clavulanic acid versus when present as the sole drug has been interpreted as indicative of the presence of ESBL. At the time of publication, the criteria and need for special testing of ESBL was under scrutiny. Newer ESBLs are constantly emerging as resistance evolves. For example, an ESBL produced by *K. pneumoniae*, which targets carbapenems, was recently identified, thus highlighting the need for rapid incorporation of appropriate testing procedures into microbiology testing labs.[53]

5. For any C&S method, generally only the parent drug is included in the interpretive standards, yet an active metabolite may contribute markedly to activity. For some drugs (e.g., ceftiofur), interpretive criteria include the metabolite, but for others, activity of the metabolite is not addressed. For example, most animals metabolize enrofloxacin to its de-ethylated metabolite, ciprofloxacin. Because the drugs act in an additive fashion, up to 40% to 50% of the C_{max} or area under the plasma bioactivity curve for enrofloxacin may be represented by ciprofloxacin, as has been demonstrated in dogs (see Chapter 7).[54] Consequently, efficacy of enrofloxacin may be underestimated by C&S methods, particularly because ciprofloxacin tends to be more potent than enrofloxacin toward gram-negative coliforms. PK of antimicrobial drugs characterized by activity of both parent and metabolite must be based on either bioassays, or analytic techniques that include the activity contributed by metabolites
6. As organisms are exposed to microbes, MICs increase across time. CLSI reevaluates and adjusts interpretive criteria to address these changes when possible. However, new criteria depend on the generation of new data. Current antimicrobial resistance surveillance systems focus on human medicine and thus largely address food animals (e.g., National Antimicrobial Resistance Monitoring System). Thus the lack of new data needed by CLSI to promulgate new guidelines may prevent timely reassessment. Clearly, a coordinated surveillance system for monitoring antimicrobial resistance of companion animal pathogens is needed. Additionally, the relevance of population PD data provided on labels and through scientific literature will decline with the passage of time, and caution might be taken when basing the use of a drug on population data that are more than a decade old.
7. Ideally, as MICs change, drug dosing regimens also should change. However, modification of dosing regimens cited on labels of approved drugs requires reapproval by the FDA, and manufacturers are not likely to pursue modification because of the cost associated with reapproval. Data necessary for dose modification may not be available for CLSI review. Thus modification of dosing regimens is likely to depend not only on generation of PD data but also on PK data by independent sponsors. Without CLSI direction, manufacturers of commercial antibiogram materials are unlikely to adjust the range of concentrations. Laboratories and manufacturers of C&S materials also have been slow to incorporate the new standards into their interpretations.
8. Ideally, both PK and PD data on which CLSI bases MIC_{BP} should be collected from and promulgated for the target species to be treated. However, much of this data simply does not exist for the target species. For drugs approved for use in animals, assuming the manufacturer supplied the data, CLSI interpretive standards often do exist and are published separately[38] from those established for human medicine.[39] However, some of these standards published in veterinary interpretive criteria are actually human standards that CLSI has deemed relevant to animals (see Table 6-2). For other human drugs, human interpretive standards are used but have not been evaluated for relevancy in animals. Although the standards may be equivalent among species for some drugs, for others, PK data and possibly PD data may be substantially different among species. Data should be interpreted cautiously for such drugs. Drugs that are water soluble ($Vd \leq 0.3$ L/kg) may be most applicable among species (see Chapter 1), whereas added caution is indicated for lipid-soluble drugs ($Vd \geq 0.6$ L/kg). Amikacin offers an example of a water-soluble drug for which interpretive standards might be similar between animals and humans. Ciprofloxacin offers an example of the need for caution. Although oral bioavailability of ciprofloxacin is 80% to 100% in humans, oral bioavailability averages 40% to 60% in dogs (information courtesy of Bayer Animal Health) and is 0% to 20% in cats (see Chapter 7). Accordingly, C_{max} will be about 40% to 60% lower at equivalent doses in dogs. Drugs with variable (particularly low) oral bioavailability, a large Vd (≥ 0.6 L/kg), and clearance by the liver are less likely to behave similarly among species than are drugs characterized by close to 100% oral bioavailability, a Vd indicative of extracellular distribution and renal clearance. As such, greater caution should be taken when extrapolating human interpretive criteria to animals for lipid-soluble versus water-soluble drugs.
9. The greatest caveat to the use of C&S data as a basis for drug selection and design of the dosing regimen is the disparity between the controlled environment of the in vitro test system and the dynamic in vivo environment of the host. Once the list of susceptible drugs has been narrowed down, host, drug, and microbial factors must be considered when making the final selection, as well as the design of the dose.

DRUG FACTORS THAT AFFECT ANTIMICROBIAL EFFICACY

The conditions of C&S testing cannot mimic conditions of in vivo drug behavior. Most notably, drug concentrations in the host are not static, as occurs in the in vitro system, but are dynamic, with duration of exposure dependent on elimination half-life. The importance of the PK of the drug will be addressed with discussion of concentration- and time-dependent drugs. In addition to the static exposure to drugs, in vitro systems currently do not take into account binding of drug to circulating proteins (e.g., doxycycline, cefovecin). Because only unbound drug is free to enter the microbe, and protein is not present in culture media, MICs generated from C&S should be compared with unbound, not total C_{max}. Finally, the in vitro system cannot take into account a variety of host (e.g., immunoglobulins, cytokines, secretory proteins, etc) or microbial (e.g., biofilm or other virulence factors) activities oriented toward defense.

Bactericidal Versus Bacteriostatic Antimicrobials

The MIC is a drug concentration that inhibits but does not necessarily kill the target microbe. The MIC is a reasonable clinical outcome target because the success of antimicrobial therapy usually depends on host defenses that sequester and ultimately kill the microbial population after its inhibition by the drug. Antibacterials are frequently classified according to their ability to kill (bactericidal) rather than inhibit (bacteriostatic) microbial growth. Whereas bacteriostatic activity is indicated by the MIC, bactericidal activity of a drug is indicated by its minimum bactericidal concentration (MBC). However, this classification is based on in vitro methods. The MBC can be determined in several ways. For example, those tests tubes in which no visible sign of growth was observed following the broth dilution procedures can be reinoculated on nutrient-rich agar plates (see Figure 6-5). Those test tubes that yield no growth contained concentrations that killed, rather than inhibited, the microbe. Thus the test tube with the lowest concentration that yielded no growth contained the MBC of the drug. All antimicrobial drugs are characterized by an MBC; however, those drugs whose MBC approximates the MIC (e.g., within one broth dilution) might also be considered bactericidal. The MBC is most appropriately determined based on killing curves, which measure the number of surviving bacteria after exposure to fixed concentrations of drug; the concentrations are based on those achieved in serum at defined time intervals.[41] For organisms noted as "S" to bacteridical drugs, achieving sufficient drug at the site to kill, rather than simply inhibit, the infecting pathogen is possible. For bacteriostatic drugs achieving the concentration necessary to kill the organisms without causing harm to the patient is much more difficult.[23,41] Exceptions might occur for drugs that are accumulated (in an unbound state) at the site of infection (e.g., urine or phagocytic white blood cells); in selected instances bactericidal concentrations of a bacteriostatic drug can be achieved.

KEY POINT 6-15 Bactericidal and bacteriostatic activities are defined according to vitro conditions, which may not necessarily translate to the patient.

Categorization of static versus cidal activity of a drug can be associated with its mechanism of action (Table 6-5). In general, drugs that target cell walls (beta-lactams, glycopeptides), cell membranes (polymixin B, colistin), or DNA (fluorinated quinolones) tend to act bactericidal in vitro. Ribosomal inhibitors that target more than one subunit (i.e., 30s and 50s; or 70s) also tend to be bactericidal. In contrast, drugs that target a single ribosomal subunit (tetracyclines, macrolides, lincosamides) or metabolic pathway (sulfonamides) tend to act bacteriostatic. Combinations of two bacteristatic antimicrobials that act in an additive or synergistic fashion may also result in bactericidal effects (e.g., a sulfonamide combined with a potentiating dipyrimidine). However, the distinction between

Table 6-5 Bactericidal Versus Bacteriostatic Drugs

	Target	Drug or Class	Drug
Bacteriostatic	Ribosomes		
		Tetracylines	
		Phenicols	
		Macrolides*	
		Lincosamides*	
	Metabolic pathway		
		Sulfonamides	
		Trimethoprim	
		Ormetoprim	
Bactericidal			
	Cell wall inhibitors		
		Beta-lactams	
			Penicillins
			Cephalosporins
		Vancomycin	
	Cell membrane		
		Polymyxin	
		Colistin	
	DNA		
		Fluorinated quinolones	
		Metronidazole	
	Ribosomes		
		Aminoglycosides	
		Macrolides*	
		Lincosamides*	
	RNA		
		Rifampin	
	Metabolic pathway		
		Trimethoprim–sulfonamides	
		Ormetoprim–sulfonamides	

*Accumulation in white blood cells may allow achievement of bactericidal concentrations.

bactericidal and bacteriostatic effects of a drug depends on the concentration; a bactericidal drug can be rendered nonbactericidal if concentrations sufficient to kill the organism are not reached at the site of infection the site of infection, or under conditions that slow the growth of the target organism (e.g., hypoxic environment or if used in combination with drugs that antagonize bactericidal actions). In such instances, the bactericidal drug will act in a bacteriostatic fashion. On the other hand, drugs classified as bacteriostatic may act bactericidal if high enough concentrations can be achieved, as might occur if the drug is accumulated in an unbound form (e.g., WBC or other tissues).

Because host defenses must be effective to kill those organisms whose growth is merely inhibited, achieving bactericidal concentrations of an antimicrobial drug are paramount to therapeutic success in immunocompromised hosts (e.g., viral infections, granulopoietic patients, use of immunohibiting drugs) or immunocompromised sites (septicemia, meningitis, valvular endocarditis, and osteomyelitis).[23,26]

Integration of Pharmacokinetics and Pharmacodyamics: Pharmacodynamic Indices

Although the MIC of a (presumed) infecting organism offers a target concentration for antimicrobial therapy, simply achieving the MIC of the organism in plasma may not be sufficient to ensure efficacy. Among the relationships that affect efficacy is the PK/PD relationship—that is, the dynamic relationship between the drug concentration to which the organism is exposed throughout the dosing interval (PK) and the response of the infecting organism to the drug, as estimated, for example, by the MIC (PD).[55-57] This relationship is affected by many host and microbial factors. Definitions of terms used to describe the integration of PK and PD (PD indices or PDI) are varied, depending on the author. For the purposes of this text, definitions will be drawn from Mouton.[47] It is important to note that many of the terms are based on parameters determined through in vitro testing. Therefore host and microbial factors still need to be considered. Further, most PDI are based on a 24-hr-dosing interval, thus modifications in dosing regimens should be based on a 24-hr period (Figure 6-12). The relevance of PDI to drugs with half-lives longer than 24 hr (e.g., azithromycin, cefovecin) is not clear.

Postantibiotic Exposure

Antimicrobials may continue to exert an effect even though the drug is no longer present at concentrations that exceed the MIC. The term *postantibiotic exposure* has been promoted to refer to the combined definitions that have emerged experimentally. Among the terms is the *postantibiotic effect (PAE),* which has both an in vitro and an in vivo definition.[47] The PAE is exhibited by drugs, and is defined in vitro as the period of suppression of bacterial growth after a short exposure of the organism to the antimicrobial.[47] The PAE for a drug, is determined in vitro by exposing a standard inoculum to it, removing the drug and determining the time that elapses (in hours) before the culture CFUs increase by tenfold. In vivo, the PAE is the time it takes for the number of CFUs to increase tenfold in treated animals after concentrations drop below the MIC at the tissue site.[47] Clinically, the PAE indicates the ability of a drug to inhibit bacterial growth after the drug is no longer present or is below the MIC of the infecting microbe.[49,58-60] As such, it also takes into account an effect a drug might have at subinhibitory concentrations. The impact of the PAE on antimicrobial efficacy can be profound, particularly for concentration-dependent drugs. It is the PAE that allows some drugs to be administered at long intervals despite short half-lives.[41,50, 52,59,61,62] The PAE may be absent for some organisms or some patients (e.g., some immunocompromised patients).[49] The duration of PAEs varies with each drug and each organism and the relationship between PDC and MIC (Table 6-6).[63] In general, concentration-dependent drugs appear to exhibit longer PAEs, with the duration of the PAE being proportional to the magnitude of the peak PDC (i.e., longer with higher PDC).[64] However, for each drug, and within drug classes, the PAE is markedly variable, depending on the organism.[65] Whereas beta-lactams exhibit a substantial PAE toward selected streptococci (i.e., thus making treatment less time dependent for streptococci), their PAE toward gram-negative organisms is minimal.[66] Applying information regarding the PAE to clinical patients is complicated by variable results (reflecting marked variability in methods) among investigators. The PAE is enhanced by combination antimicrobial therapy.[67-69] The duration of the PAE should be included in estimates of doses or dosing intervals. Some antimicrobials also have been associated with a postantibiotic sub-MIC effect (PASE) that may further prolong the dosing interval[70,71]; further, a postantibiotic leukocyte enhancement effect (PALE) has been described for some antimicrobials. These are incorporated in in vivo estimates of PAE. However, clinical relevance of measurements of PAE, PASE, and PALE based on in vitro observations is not clear.[66,72] These studies do point out the reasons that some antimicrobials are effective at long intervals and indicate the need for a better understanding of the relationship of PDC, MIC, and PAE in the clinical patient.

KEY POINT 6-16 The postantibiotic effect is particularly important to the efficacy of concentration-dependent drugs.

Time- Versus Concentration-Dependent Drugs

The relationship among efficacy, MIC, and the magnitude and time course of PDC can be categorized, in vitro, as either *concentration-dependent* (sometimes referred to as *dose-dependent)* or *time-dependent* (sometimes referred to as *concentration-independent)* (see Figure 6-13; and Table 6-4).[41] A third classification has emerged with characteristics from each of these classes. (e.g., as shown by fluoroquinolones). Although studies that categorize drugs are largely in vitro, the categorizations generally are supported by in vivo studies that include animal models and human clinical trials.[57] Concentration-dependent drugs, best represented by the fluoroquinolones and aminoglycosides, are characterized by efficacy that is best predicted by the magnitude of PDC (C_{max}) compared to

Table 6-6 The Duration of the Postantibiotic Effect Demonstrated by Selected Drugs Toward Selected Organisms[63,65,66]

Organism	Drug	PAE/hr	Concentration Dependent*	Time Dependent
Bacillus anthracis†	Fluoroquinolones	4-5	Aminoglycosides	Beta-lactams
	Macrolides	1-2	Fluoroquinolones	Glycopeptides
	Beta-lactams	1-2	Metronidazole	Macrolides*
	Vancomycin	1-2	Azithromycin	Linezolide*
	Rifampin	4-5	Ketolides	Tetracyclines*
Pseuodmonas aeruginosa‡	Gentamicin	4-5		Tigecycline*
	Imipenem§	Good		Clindamycin*
Staphylococcus aureus‡	Macrolides	3-4		
	Aminoglycosides	5-10		
Escherichia coli‡	Ciprofloxacin	1-2		
	Amikacin	1-2		
	Beta-lactams	0.5		
Klebsiella pneumoniae‡	Ciprofloxacin	1-2		
	Amikacin	1-2		
	Beta-lactams	0.5		
§Streptococci	Beta-lactams	Good¶		
Gram negative	Beta-lactams§	Minimal		

PAE, Postantibiotic effect.
*PAE depending on organism; efficacy enhanced by higher concentration
†Athamna 2004 [63]
‡Wang 2001[65]
§O'Reilly 2005[66]
¶Allows once-daily dosing despite short drug half-lives for aminopenicillin

the MIC of the infecting organism (see Figures 6-11 to 6-13)[73-79] For such drugs the magnitude of C_{max}/MIC (or C_{max}/MIC_{90}) generally should be 10 to 12; for more difficult infections (e.g., *P. aeruginosa,* or infections caused by multiple organisms), the higher index should be targeted.[57] The time that PDC is above the MIC—that is, the duration of exposure, (T > MIC or T > MIC_{90})—is not as important as is the C_{max}/MIC; in fact, efficacy may be enhanced (e.g., for the aminoglycosides) by a drug-free period (i.e., a long interval between doses; see Figure 6-13).[61,73,74,80-82] This may reflect, in part, the phenomenon of adaptive resistance.[83] *Adaptive resistance* refers to a reversible refractoriness to the bactericidal effects of an antibacterial agent. This phenomenon has been documented particularly for gram-negative organisms and the aminoglycosides, but it appears to occur with the quinolones as well. The resistance appears to reflect a protective phenotypic alteration in the bacteria, such as reversible downregulation of aminoglycoside active transport. Adaptive resistance occurs rapidly (within 1 to 2 hours) of antimicrobial therapy; duration reflects the elimination half-life of the drug. In humans adaptive resistance to aminoglycosides may last for up to 16 hours after a single dose of aminoglycoside, with partial return of bacterial susceptibility at 24 hours and complete recovery at approximately 40 hours.[83]

For concentration-dependent drugs, a dose that is too low is particularly detrimental. In a mouse model of *E. coli* peritonitis, the antibacterial efficacy of ciprofloxacin, but not

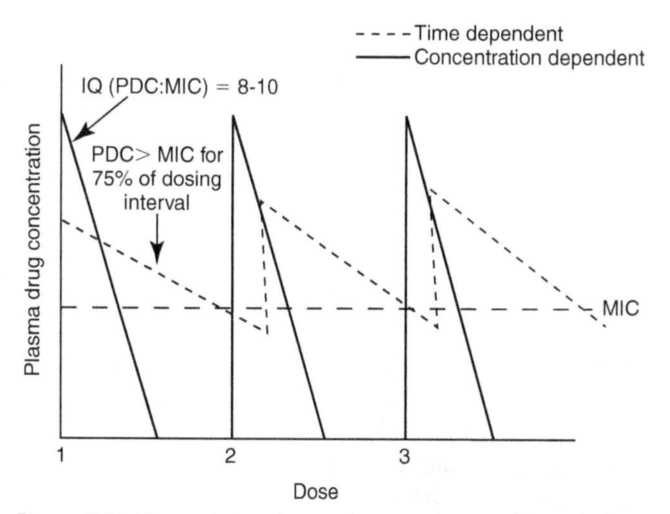

Figure 6-13 The relationship between plasma (tissue) drug concentration, and the minimum inhibitory concentration (MIC) of the organism may determine drug efficacy. The efficacy of concentration-dependent drugs (e.g., aminoglycosides; fluorinated quinolones; and, in some cases, azithromycin or other azalides) depends on a high C_{max} to MIC ratio. Doses might be increased to ensure sufficiently high plasma drug concentrations to achieve the target ratio. In contrast, for time-dependent drugs, such as beta-lactams, sulfonamides, and nonaminoglycoside ribosomal inhibitors, efficacy is maximized by ensuring that plasma drug concentration remains above the MIC for most (50% to 75%) of the dosing interval.

imipenem (or meropenem), was improved by doubling the dose. For some concentration-dependent drugs, efficacy may be both dose- and time-dependent, with the best predictor of efficacy being AUC/MIC. For example, efficacy of fluorinated quinolones can be predicted by both a C_{max}/MIC (target 10 to 12) or AUC/MIC (target 100 to 125) (see Figure 6-13).[41,84-86] The AUC/MIC may be particularly predictive for fluoroquinolones when treating gram-positive isolates; adding a second full dose may be prudent for some infections. Otherwise, concentration-dependent drugs generally can be administered at longer intervals (e.g., once a day).

In contrast to concentration-dependent drugs, efficacy of time-dependent drugs (e.g., beta-lactams) is best predicted by the time that PDC remains above the MIC. For such drugs PDC should be 2 to 4 times the MIC of the infecting microbe and should be maintained above the MIC (T > MIC) throughout a significant portion of the dosing interval (see Figures 6-12 and 6-13). However, the recommended duration of T > MIC varies from a low of 25% for carbapenems to 50% to 70% for extended-spectrum penicillins to potentially 100% for penicillin and aminopenicillins (an exception being treatment of streptococci).[56,57,61,74,87,88] With time-dependent drugs, increasing the dose may be necessary to ensure that PDCs are above (ideally severalfold) the MIC.[57] Maintaining T > MIC may be problematic for drugs with a short half-life unless the isolate is extremely susceptible (e.g., most beta-hemolytic streptococci for penicillins). Given that drug concentrations decrease by 50% every drug half-life, a C_{max}/MIC of 2 will result in a PDC that will reach the MIC in 1 half-life. The duration of the dosing interval then depends on the desired target duration (i.e., 25% to 100%) of T > MIC. If T > MIC is 100%, then the dosing interval would be 1 half-live. If T > MIC is 50%, the dosing interval would be 2 half-lives, and if T > MIC is 25%, the dosing interval could be as long as 4 half-lives. For each additional half-life to be added to the duration that T > MIC, concentrations, and thus dose, must be doubled again (i.e., quadrupuled if T > MIC = 2 half-lives, increased eightfold if T > MIC=3 half-lives, and so on). Table 6-4 demonstrates the impact of C_{max}:MIC and half-life on time-dependent drugs. Although efficacy of time-dependent drugs requires T > MIC for a sufficient time, efficacy might be enhanced by increasing the dose for drugs with a sufficiently long half-life, shortening the interval for drugs with a short half-life, or both. Constant-rate infusion,[89] or slow-release products,[90] might be ideal for time-dependent drugs with short half-lives. Drugs characterized by longer elimination half-lives might be preferred (e.g., cefovecin[43,44]). Efficacy also should be enhanced for time-dependent drugs that persist to accumulate in the unbound state in selected tissues (i.e., macrolides, clindamycin,[91] or drugs that accumulate in phagocytes.) The downside to using antimicrobial drugs with a very long half-life is that the time to steady-state concentrations and thus peak effects might be prolonged. Moreover, a "hit hard, get out quick" approach to therapy is difficult to implement with such antimicrobials.

The relationship between PDC, MIC, and time- versus concentration-dependency might be explained, in part, by the mechanism of antimicrobial action. Efficacy of the aminoglycosides or fluorinated quinolones depends on drug binding to the target (ribosome and topoisomerase or DNA gyrase, respectively); once sufficient binding occurs, protein synthesis or DNA activity, respectively, is prevented and does not re-initiate. However, beta-lactams substitute as a substrate for cell wall synthesis, and, as long as the organism is growing, it is synthesizing cell wall. Thus, the drug needs to be present as long as the organism is growing. The glycopeptides (e.g., vancomycin), which also target the cell wall, are also time-dependent drugs.

KEY POINT 6-17 Efficacy of concentration-dependent drugs can be enhanced by increasing the dose such that peak concentrations are 10 to 12 times the MIC of the infecting microbe (C_{max}/MIC ≥12).

Increasingly, CLSI is using PDI as the basis for determination of breakpoint MIC. However, not surprisingly, the optimal relationship between PDC and MIC that determines efficacy of a drug is not so simple and varies with organisms and drugs. The optimal relationship between PDC and MIC and the parameter that best predicts antimicrobial efficacy (e.g., peak PDC; the ratio of area under the drug concentration versus time curve to the organism's MIC; duration of PDC above MIC) have not been established definitively for all antimicrobials.[52,61,84,85] However, for drugs characterized by inhibition (bacteriostatic drugs), T > MIC may best predict efficacy. For some fluoroquinolones, and particularly for gram-positive organisms, efficacy is best predicted by the ratio of AUC (which is influenced by both dose and interval) to MIC rather than simply the C_{max}/MIC. The optimal AUC/MIC also varies with the organism, ranging from as low as 30 to 40 for *S. pneumoniae* and levofloxacin to greater than 350 for *P. aeruginosa* and ciprofloxacin. The area under the inhibitory curve (AUIC) reflects the integrated AUC above the MIC during the dosing interval. This parameter is similar to but varies from AUC/MIC in that it is the AUC that is above the MIC (in contrast, AUC/MIC involves the complete area). The AUIC should exceed 125 for fluorinated quinolones to achieve bacterial killing; an AUIC that exceeds 250 results in rapid killing.[57] Thus for treatment of some infections with concentration-dependent drugs, the dosing regimen might be designed to maximize both the C_{max}/MIC and the AUC/MIC. Some drugs (e.g., macrolides) are characterized by time-dependency for some organisms but concentration-dependency for others.

Table 6-4 offers examples of PDIs that are achieved using current recommended dosing regimens for selected drugs and selected PD data from selected pathogens that cause infection in dogs. The PD data are based on MIC_{90} obtained from package inserts of drugs approved in dogs or literature that provided PD data specific for canine pathogens that was more recent than package insert data. For some drugs PD was not available for canine pathogens, so PD from human pathogens was used. Doses were chosen from Table 7-1 and generally reflected the highest dose for which PK was available. When possible, nonintravenous routes were chosen because C_{max} from intravenous data may not represent C_{max} following distribution. Table 6-6 is intended to demonstrate how PDI might be used to assess a dosing regimen. It is not unusual to find that the target C_{max}/MIC (>10) often is not reached for concentration-dependent drugs) or T > MIC (50% for most) for time-dependent drugs. One could argue that the MIC_{90} is an unreasonable PD target; indeed, for some isolates it may be. The preferred PD statistic would be the MIC from the isolate infecting the patient; it can be substituted in this table for the MIC_{90}. Likewise, the 95th lower confidence interval is preferred to the mean C_{max} or half-life for the PK component of PDI. For concentration-dependent drugs, doses can be increased (whenever safety permits) to achieve the target C_{max}/MIC; for time-dependent drugs, both the dose (increase) and interval (shorten) might be modified. Alternatively, or perhaps in addition to, combination therapy might be considered. Note that the PDIs are based on plasma drug concentrations (PDCs). For some drugs, PDC underestimates concentrations in extracellular fluid. However, for others, PDC frequently overestimates by 25% to 50% or more extracellular fluid drug concentrations. Doses may need to be increased by 25% to 50% to adjust for this difference. As important as PK/PD integration is to the design of the dosing regimen, its application to the clinical patient will be facilitated by an understanding of the microbial and host factors that influence response to the drug.

KEY POINT 6-18 Efficacy of a time-dependent drug can be enhanced by ensuring that concentrations at the site of infection are above the MIC (T > MIC) for most of the dosing interval.

MICROBIAL FACTORS THAT AFFECT ANTIMICROBIAL EFFICACY

Among the most obvious ways that microbes can affect antimicrobial efficacy is the advent of resistance. However, microbes can negatively affect antimicrobials through mechanisms that do not influence MIC. These effects are not as obvious to detect as resistance but nonetheless can profoundly affect therapeutic success.

Inoculum Size

The larger the bacterial inoculum at the target site, the greater the concentration (number of molecules) of antimicrobial necessary to kill the organism. Further, more CFUs are more likely to produce greater amounts of enzymes or other materials that can destroy the drug. The "inoculum effect" of ESBL resistance describes the increasing MIC of the organisms toward cephalosporins at a larger (10^7) compared with smaller (10^5) inoculum.[92] In addition, the larger the inoculum, the greater the risk that spontaneous mutation will contribute to resistance or virulence. Note that resistance and virulence do not necessarily co-exist. In general, emerging resistance appears to be associated with *decreased* rather than increased virulence, although increasingly studies are identifying exceptions. For example, community-acquired infections may be associated with increased virulence, but less resistance. For example, although hospital-acquired infections tend to be caused by nonvirulent organisms, community-acquired infections reflect virulent organisms that can infect even the overtly healthy patient. Concern regarding MRSA reflects, in part, its apparent acquisition of virulence factors that have facilitated its transition from a hospital to community-acquired infection.

Virulence Factors

The degree of pathogenicity of bacteria (virulence) will affect antimicrobial efficacy indirectly by facilitating infection. The ability of microbes to cause disease reflects the size of the inocululm, the effectiveness of host defense mechanisms, and the intrinsic pathogenicity of the microbes resulting from the presence of virulence factors. Like biochemical mechanisms of resistance, virulence factors generally involve proteins encoded by DNA of chromosomal or shared (e.g., plasmids, transduction) origin. Contributing to the negative impact of virulence factors is host response to their effects. Virulence factors facilitate adhesion to host cell surfaces, colonization (e.g., urease of *Helicobacter pylori,* which protects it from gastric acidity), invasion (facilitated by disruption of host cell membranes or stimulation of endocytosis), immunosuppression (e.g., antibody-binding proteins), or bacterial toxins that cause local, distant, or both (e.g., endotoxin) host damage. Pathogen attachment to host cells is a crucial early step in mucosal infections and is facilitated in epithelial tissues by bacterial adherence. Adherence is a specific two-phase process involving bacterial virulence factors called *adhesins* and complementary receptors of the host epithelial cells.[93,94] Adhesins are generally found on the surface of microbes, (e.g., bacterial fimbriae) and along with other virulence factors facilitating infection, may be targets for alternative (to antimicrobial) therapy. Species differences exist among the types of receptors in the host epithelial cells. The predominant receptor type in humans is glycolipid in nature, and its presence varies with blood cell types, implying individual variation in susceptibility to bacterial adherence in several body systems. Bacterial adherence is discussed with regard to specific body systems in Chapter 8.

Another virulence factors that facilitate infection are *invasins.* Invasins are enzymes that damage physical barriers presented by tissue matrices or cell membranes, facilitating rapid bacterial spread. Examples include clostridial hyaluronidase, which is able to destroy connective tissue, and lecithinases and phospholipases of clostridial and gram-positive organisms. Bacteria have developed siderophores, which are specialized virulence factors that mediate the release or scavenging of iron critical for microbial virulence. Bacteria also have developed specialized transport systems that secrete toxic materials into the extracellular matrix. It is not clear whether the efflux proteins that transport toxins are related to those that transport drugs (see the discussion of resistance). Bacteria also facilitate invasion through materials (e.g., proteins, "slime") that prevent phagocytosis or, if the microbe is phagocytized, preclude intracellular killing. Examples include lytic enzymes of gram-positive cocci or exotoxin A produced by *P. aeruginosa*. Toxins include both endotoxins (discussed in depth later) and exotoxins. Bacterial exotoxins are among the most potent toxins known, acting on either the cell surface (e.g., *E. coli* hemolysins, "superantigens" of *S. aureus* or *Streptococcus pyogenes*); membrane; or, once the membrane is penetrated, intracellular targets (e.g., A/B toxins).

KEY POINT 6-19 *Virulence* refers to the ability of the microbe to cause infection. However, a virulent organism often is not resistant.

Biofilm

Among the most effective and probably least appreciated protective microbial factors is biofilm. Bacteria exist in either a planktonic (free floating) or sessile (attached) state; while it is the former state that characterizes C&S testing, but it is the latter state that enables persistence of the resident population, as well as the formation of biofilm.[95-97] *Biofilm* is defined as a biopolymer, matrix-enclosed bacterial population in which bacteria adhere either to one another or to a surface.[95] The outer layer of the biofilm may lose water such that it is hardened, thus providing better protection from the environment, including exposure to antimicrobials. The inner sactum of the biofilm is largely aqueous, composed of glycocalyx or slime (e.g., *Staphylococcus* spp.). In addition to passive diffusion, aqueous pores permeate the structure, allowing movement of nutrients and metabolic debris. Biofilm populations containing normal microflora in the skin or mucous membranes (e.g., urinary bladder) are lost with shedding of the skin (or bladder) surface or by the excretion of mucus; new cells and mucus are rapidly colonized by biofilm-forming bacteria. Microbes released from the surface may colonize new surfaces and subsequently produce new biofilms and new (e.g., persistent or recurring) infections. Bacterial communication during biofilm formation is sophisticated, involving quorum-sensing systems that ultimately may be targets of microbial therapy.[96] Biofilm may facilitate and protect growth of normal or pathogenic flora on foreign surfaces and can facilitate subsequent translocation of microbes to otherwise sterile tissues. Persistent, chronic bacterial infections may reflect biofilm-producing bacteria; persistent inflammation associated with immune complexes contributes to clinical signs. Dental plaque is a prototypic example of the impact that biofilm might have on preventing antimicrobial penetration. Cystic fibrosis associated with *Pseudomonas* is a disease in which biofilm contributes to mortality. Pathogens associated with biofilm in veterinary medicine include, but are by no means limited to, *Acinetobacter, Actinobacillus, Klebsiella, P. aeruginosa,* and *Staphylococcus (aureus and pseudintermedius)*.[95] Glycocalyx may contribute to protective mechanisms of other organisms as well (e.g., sulfur granules and Nocardia; Figure 6-14). Not all pathogens associated with biofilm cause infection (e.g., urinary catheters). However, because they ultimately may be

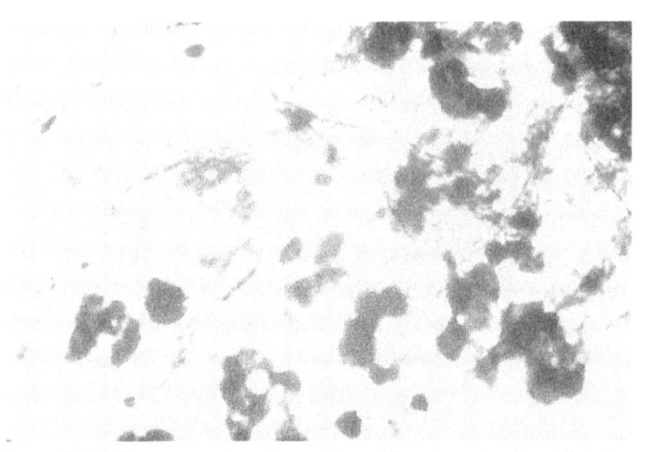

Figure 6-14 An example of combined host and microbial factors that negatively impacts therapy, *Nocardia* causes a marked inflammatory response by the host. Additionally, the organism causes secretion of calcium that combines with its biofilm, resulting in the formation of "sulfur" granules that protect the organisms from drug penetrations.

the source of infection, clinical resolution may not be possible until the biofilm is destroyed. Yet, its nature is difficult to predict based on the planktonic growth of individuals in cultures compared to the consortium that occurs in vivo.[97] Catheters (urinary or intravascular), orthopedic fixation devices, and materials used in wound management are examples of surfaces on which biofilm might develop.

KEY POINT 6-20 Biofilm can form on many foreign or natural surfaces and may profoundly decrease the likelihood of successful antimicrobial therapy.

Antimicrobial Resistance

The role of resistance in therapeutic failure of antimicrobials is well established.[23,98] The use of antimicrobials increasingly is associated with emergence of resistance. For each class of antimicrobial drugs approved for use in human medicine, resistance generally has emerged within 1 to 2 decades of use. Clinically relevant resistance toward sulfonamides, the first class of antimicrobials approved in the United States (1930s) was documented by the 1940s. Penicillins, tetracyclines, streptomycin (aminoglycoside), and erythromycin (macrolides) were all approved within a 10-year span, with resistance documented within 5 years for methicillin versus approximately 10 years for streptomycin. Resistance to nalidixic acid, the progenitor of fluoroquinolones (approved in 1950), took 3 decades to emerge, perhaps convincing manufacturers that resistance to fluoroquinolones would emerge very slowly. However, resistance to norfloxacin, the first fluoroquinolone approved in the United States, took less than 3 years to emerge, despite the fact that the lack of plasmid-mediated resistance was among the attributes of this class. Resistance to extended-spectrum cephalosporins emerged within 4 years of approval and to amoxicillin–clavulanic acid, within 5 years. Resistance to vancomycin, specifically developed to treat MRSA, emerged in its second decade of use.

KEY POINT 6-21 Antimicrobial resistance increasingly will prevent the successful empirical selection of antimicrobial drugs.

Inherent Versus Acquired Resistance

Antimicrobial resistance might be inherent to the microorganisms or acquired, either through chromosomal mutations or transfer of genetic information.[99] Generally, spectrums of antimicrobials (listed on package inserts and elsewhere) reflect inherent resistance patterns rather than acquired resistance patterns. Examples include limited efficacy of aminoglycosides toward anaerobic organisms because the drugs must be actively transported into the cell (oxygen dependent) or the resistance of gram-positive organisms, which lack an outer cell membrane, to polymyxin B, which targets the same. Acquired resistance, on the other hand, generally renders a previously susceptible organism resistant. As such, it is not necessarily predictable and can occur during the course of therapy (leading to changes in a C&S pattern). More problematically, it is often shared among microbes.

Shared resistance among bacteria reflects the ability of bacteria to incorporate extrachromosomal DNA carrying the information for resistance from other organisms. Extrachromosomal DNA (including plasmids and bacteriophages) encode for resistance to multiple drugs and can be transmitted vertically (to progeny) or horizontally, across species and genera. Transposons are individual or clusters of resistance genes bound by integrons, which move resistance genes back and forth between chromosomes to plasmids. Consequently, bacterial resistance is extremely mobile and can spread rapidly.[101] Among the mechanisms by which genetic resistance information is shared is (sexual) conjugation. Conjugation occurs particularly in gram-negative organisms and may be accompanied by genetic material that confers bacterial pathogenicity as well as altered metabolic functions. However, *Enterococcus* spp. and selected other gram-positive bacteria also transfer resistance to glycopeptides through conjugative transposons.[101] Transduction, which requires a specific receptor, involves transfer of information by a bacterial virus (bacteriophage) and is implemented especially by *Staphylococcus* spp. Resistance, including methicillin resistance, can be transferred between coagulase-negative and -positive *Staphylococcus*.[1] Transformation involves transfer of naked DNA from one lysed bacterium to another; this mechanism of transfer tends to be limited (in humans) to pneumococcal meningitis.

Although present for eons, acquired antimicrobial resistance increasingly is becoming problematic. The impact of antimicrobial resistance can be extensive. In some human intensive care units, selected isolates are characterized by a resistance prevalence of 86%. The impact of resistance on the patient includes increased morbidity, mortality, and increased hospital costs.[107] Patterns of resistance have emerged in veterinary medicine, although differences appear to occur in the ability of organisms to develop resistance to an antimicrobial, varying with species and strain. Many organisms remain predictably susceptible to selected drugs (e.g., *Brucella, Chlamydia*), whereas others are becoming problematic (e.g., *P. multocida*). Several organisms traditionally have developed resistance that can rapidly impair efficacy of new antimicrobials (e.g., *E. coli, K. pneumoniae, Salmonella, S. aureus, S. pneumoniae*). In general, these organisms have developed multidrug resistance (MDR). MDR is now considered the normal response to antimicrobials for gram-positive cocci pneumococci, enterococci, and staphylococci.[102] Among these, *Staphylococcus* spp. is considered most problematic: it is intrinsically virulent, is able to adapt to many different environmental conditions, increasingly is associated with resistance to other classes of antimicrobials, and tends to be associated with life-threatening infections.[102,103] In a veterinary teaching hospital the percentage of patients with *S. intermedius* susceptible to cephalexin and amoxicillin–clavulanic acid decreased from a high of 96% in 2005 to < 60% in 2007, a trend that appears to be emerging in other veterinary hospitals.[110]

KEY POINT 6-22 Acquired resistance can occur during the course of antimicrobial therapy.

E. coli is among the organisms that have developed multi-drug resistance.[104,105] Fluoroquinolone-resistant *E. coli* emerged as early as 1998, little over a decade after the approval of enrofloxacin for dogs or cats.[28] Multidrug-resistant *E. coli* has emerged as a cause of nosocomial infections in dogs[108] and UTIs in canine critical care patients.[104,109] The presentation is similar to the that in human critical care patients, with risk factors such as sex (males), hospital stay, and previous antimicrobial therapy being similar for both.

Factors Contributing to the Emergence of Resistance

Development of antimicrobial resistance is facilitated by several factors[111]; among the most important is exposure to antimicrobials. In the individual patient, single-dose ciprofloxacin prophylaxis increased the prevalence of ciprofloxacin-resistant fecal *E. coli* from 3% to 12% in humans.[112] Ciprofloxacin treatment for prostatitis resulted in posttreatment fecal colonization with quinolone-resistant *E. coli* that was genetically distinct from the infection-causing strains after treatment in 50% of the patients.[113] Our laboratory has demonstrated that standard doses of either amoxicillin or enrofloxacin given orally will cause close to 100% of fecal *E. coli* to become resistant to the treatment drug within 3 to 9 days of therapy; for enrofloxacin the isolates generally are multidrug resistant. As with MRSA or MRSI (*S. intermedius*), the advent of resistance by *E. coli* and other gram-negative organisms has been associated with increased cephalosporin use.[1]

The gastrointestinal flora offers a natural environment that exemplifies the impact of antimicrobials on selection pressure. The normal flora of the gastrointestinal tract is extremely diverse, with anaerobes predominating. Among the aerobes, *E. coli* are the major gram-negative and *Enterococcus* the major gram-positive organisms.[101] Environmental microbes maintain an ecologic niche through suppression of the competition by either consumption of nutrients or secretion of antibiotics. Therefore commensal organisms are constantly being exposed to antibiotics, and are "primed" to develop resistance.[101] However, the microbes producing the antibiotic, as well as surrounding normal flora, are resistant to the antibiotic. Thus genes for resistance develop along with genes directing antibiotic production.

Rapid microbial turnover in the gastrointestinal tract supports the development of resistance by ensuring active DNA replication and thus mutation potential (see previous discussion). Chromosomal (DNA) mutations (10^{-14} to 10^{-10} per cell division) are DNA mistakes that have been missed by bacterial repair mechanisms. These mistakes occur spontaneously and randomly, regardless of whether the antibiotic is present. If the mutation that confers resistance to an antimicrobial occurs in the presence of the antimicrobial when it is administered to the patient, the surviving mutant, reflecting its single-step mutation, confers a low level of resistance (see the discussion of mutant prevention concentration). The MIC of the organism is likely to increase. Further microbial turnover and continued therapy can lead to multistep mutations and rapid emergence of high-level resistance characterized by increasingly higher MIC. Stepwise mutations can lead to specific resistance such as that demonstrated toward fluorinated quinolones (stepwise mutation in the DNA gyrase gene). Nonspecific mechanisms of resistance, including that shared among organisms, are more likely to result in MDR. Microflora of the gastrointestinal tract can serve as a reservoir of resistance genes; a single drug, via integrons, plasmids, and transposons, facilitates the rapid transfer of MDR among organisms. The gastrointestinal environment exemplifies a pattern whereby resistance can emerge as a result of a combination of selection pressure and mutation. Clinically, similar mechanisms of emerging resistance are likely to occur at sites of infection.

Mutant Prevention Concentration

Drlica and coworkers[114] have hypothesized the *mutant selection window,* (see Figure 6-15) comprised of a lower threshold represented by the culture MIC of the infecting organism and an upper threshold or boundary, the MPC. Should a dose be designed such that drug concentrations fall within this window (i.e., between the MIC and MPC) at the site of infection, the mutant isolate is likely to emerge as a resistant colony. The practical application of the hypothesis explains the observed behavior of mycobacterium organisms toward fluoroquinolones (FQs). Increasing concentrations of the FQs inhibits the nonresistant (wild-type) organisms and colony numbers rapidly decrease. But this period of decline is followed by a plateau period of minimal or no growth. During this plateau phase, remaining resistant isolates recover and start to multiply again. The resistance of this emerging, second population presumably reflect a single-step (chromosomal or plasmid-mediated) mutation that resulted in an increase in the MIC to low-level resistance (e.g., MIC is close to the breakpoint). However, when these first-step mutants are exposed to even higher drug concentrations, a second rapid decline in numbers occurs, this time reflecting inhibition of the mutated, resistant organisms. Again, once sufficient bacteria recover, a second plateau occurs as the first-step mutants mutate. This stepwise or multistep mutation confers high level resistance (MIC exceeds the breakpoint several fold) that can be overcome only by very high concentrations of the FQ. The mutant selection window, which is to be avoided with initial therapy, describes drug concentrations on either side of the initial plateau for the single-step mutants. The lower boundary is defined by those drug concentrations sufficiently high to remove the majority of the wild-type competitors (MIC), whereas the higher boundary (the MPC) is defined by the concentrations necessary to inhibit the least susceptible (most resistant) isolates (the single-step mutants).[115] Above this concentration, a second mutation step (which is very rare) would be required for a population of resistant organisms to develop; the risk of this happening is reduced by preventing microbial turnover (i.e., killing all isolates).

KEY POINT 6-23 The mutant prevention concentration (MPC) is the highest MIC of any of the colony-forming units causing infection in the patient. Failure to achieve this concentration may allow resistant microbes to emerge, particularly in the at-risk patient.

On the basis of this observation, Drlica and coworkers contend that MIC-based strategies used to design dosing regimens readily select for resistant mutants.[115] Their contention is based on the observation that only one resistant mutation is needed for bacteria to grow in the presence of an antimicrobial and that infections generally contain an adequate number of CFUs for several first-step resistant mutants to be present prior to treatment. They coined the term MPC as an in vitro measure of preferred antimicrobial concentration target. If the MPC (rather than the MIC) is achieved at the site of infection, the risk of resistance is minimized because isolates that exceed the MPC concentration must have undergone a second concurrent resistance mutation step prior to therapy. As such, the MPC, not the MIC, would be the concentration targeted at the site of infection in the patient. Indeed, simply achieving the reported MIC of the infecting microbe at the site of infection is probably the approach that is most likely to yield clinically resistant organisms. Accordingly, consideration should be given to assuring that "dead bugs don't mutate." If the least susceptible of the isolates is inhibited with the dosing regimen, then the recovering population should not be resistant.

Drlica[115] has demonstrated that MPCs do not correlate to MICs. In vitro, the MPC would be defined in vitro as the (lowest) drug concentration (in the media) that yields no recovered organisms when over 10^{10} CFUs (mimicking bacterial load in the patient) are plated. Currently, determining the MPC is costly, requiring multiple testing steps and large numbers of cells; for example, standard culture procedures are based on 10^6 CFUs, whereas determination of the MPC requires at least $10^{8\text{-}10}$ CFUs. However, an MPC-based strategy to dosing clinically makes sense and should be an effective means of blocking the growth of first-step resistant mutants. Such a strategy

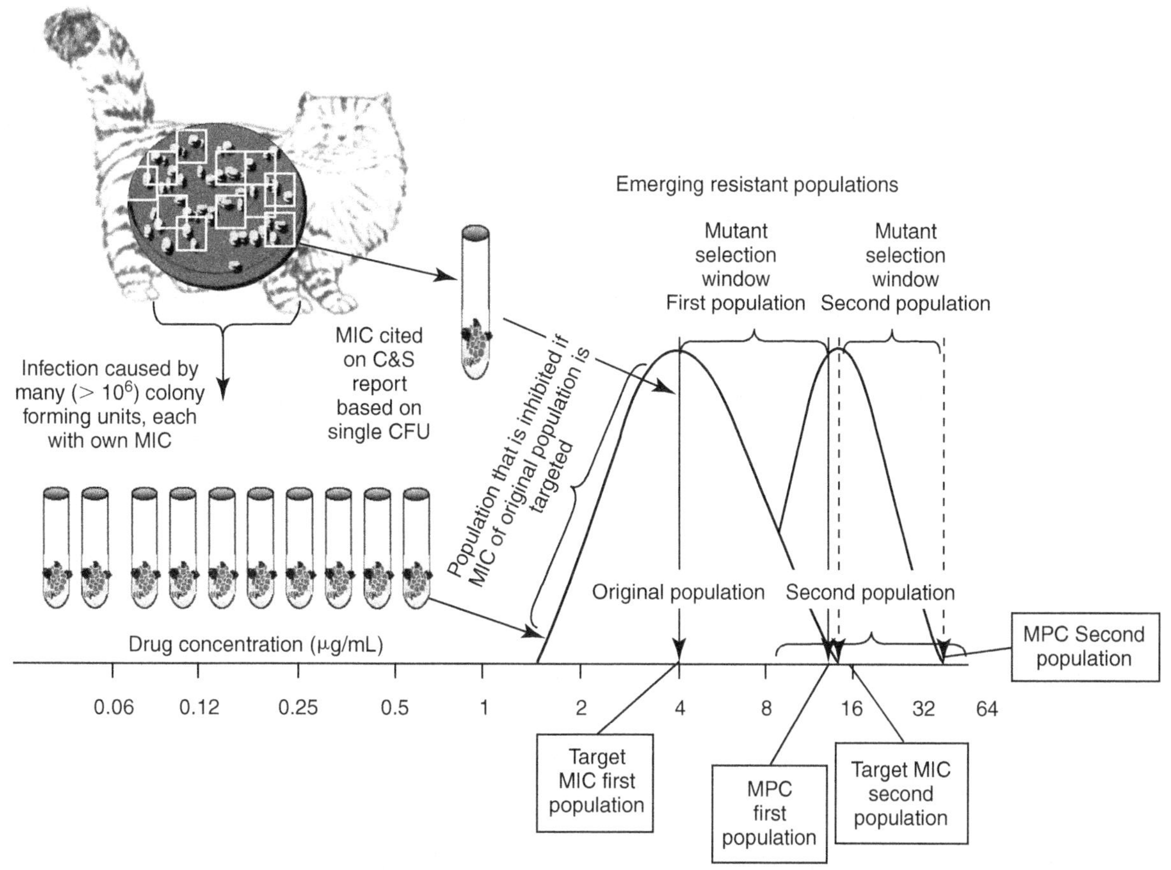

Figure 6-15 Stepwise mutation can emerge as a result of selection pressure induced by antimicrobial therapy that targets the minimum inhibitory concentration (MIC) of the infecting microbe. The mutant prevention concentration (MPC) is the concentration of drug that is necessary to inhibit first-step mutants, or the MIC of the least susceptible isolate in a resident population of pathogens. As the resident population or inoculum of wild (nonresistant) pathogen isolates reaches $10^{8\text{-}10}$ colony-forming units (CFUs), some isolates will spontaneously mutate such that resistance emerges to the drug of interest. However, when cultured, the MIC reported for the population is likely to represent the mode (the most commonly reported MIC), which in a normally distributed population, is also the MIC_{50} for the population. In contrast, the MIC of the first-step mutant will be the high end of the population MIC range. This is the concentration that should be targeted to inhibit the entire population—that is, the MPC. If the dosing regimen is designed to target the the mutant selection window, that is, the MIC of the wild population rather than the MPC (the MIC of the first-step mutant)—treatment with the drug will inhibit all isolates at or below the MIC. The void in isolates will allow the remaining, more resistant first-step mutants to recover, particularly in patients not sufficiently healthy to suppress recovering microbes. As this new population expands, a second distribution curve emerges. If recultured, the MIC of the second first-step mutant population will be higher than the wild population. If the population reaches a sufficient size (e.g., 10^8 CFUs), a second, spontaneous mutation is likely to occur, resulting in a new, higher MPC. Targeting the MPC is particularly important when using drugs for which resistance emerges in response to mutations.

would force wild-type cells to acquire two resistance mutations for growth, an event that is rare. Experimental in vitro data[114] have confirmed that MPC levels of an FQ do indeed inhibit strains that harbor first-step *gyrA* mutations (the mechanism of microbial resistance to FQ).[116] Application of the MPC is most appropriate for drugs and organisms that develop resistance by chromosomally mediated point mutations (e.g., the fluorquinolones).[117] However, the spirit of targeting the MPC might be assumed even for other drugs, in order to minimize the impact of selection pressure on emergent resistant populations. The mutant selection window can be narrowed if more than two bacterial sites are targeted, such as might occur with combination antimicrobial therapy, or with drugs that simultaneously target more than one site (e.g., the FQs).[114]

Biochemical Mechanisms of Resistance

Bacteria often respond to the presence of the antimicrobial by altering their physiology such that resistance occurs, often to multiple drugs. Microbes develop antimicrobial resistance by two primary mechanisms: modification of the target site or altered intracellular drug concentration. Methods by which intracellular drug concentration can be decreased include changes in porin sizes for gram-negative organisms (e.g., most drugs; see Figure 6-3). Porins are transmembrane proteins (e.g., OmpF) that form an aqueous channel that allows passive movement of large hydrophilic molecules. Porins are one of the few means by which drugs can gain access to intracellular targets. A change in porin size (i.e., by the addition of side chains that filter out drugs) or number increases antimicrobial resistance, as is demonstrated by the loss of the OprD protein that imparts resistance to imepenem by *Pseudomonas* spp. Closely associated with the porin proteins are efflux proteins that pump drug out of the organism; the pumps often are associated with porin proteins (e.g., FQs and tetracyclines). Most of these pumps are fueled by energy associated with proton exchange, the most notable in gram negative organisms being of the RND (resistance nodulation division) family. The best characterized in this family is the Acr-AB/TolC system, which is a complex bacterial stress response system that allows bacteria to pump out toxic molecules.[101] These and other pump systems are often characterized by a wide range of substrate specificities and, along with porins, are a common mechanism whereby an isolate can express multidrug resistance. In contrast, a number of microbes generate enzymes that destroy antimicrobials (e.g., aminoglycoside acetylases, beta-lactamases that destroy penicillins or cephalosporins, transferases that destroy chloramphenicol); in such instances resistance conferred by these mechanisms is generally limited to a single drug or drug class. Enzymatic inactivation is more likely for natural drugs to which microbes have previously been exposed (and thus presented with a greater opportunity to develop enzymes). In contrast, enzymes are less likely to destroy synthetic drugs.[118] However, plasmid-mediated enzymatic destruction of FQs has recently been described, once again highlighting the resourcefulness of bacteria.[119] Changes in target structure are another major mechanism of resistance. Example targets that have been modified include, but are not limited to, cell wall proteins (e.g., penicillin-binding proteins [PBs], particularly for MRSA [PB2] or *Enterococcus* [PB5]), or binding sites (i.e., on ribosomes, as for aminoglycosides, or DNA gyrase for FQs).[120,121] Organisms often are characterized by more than one mechanism of resistance. Multiple mechanisms are well documented for some organisms against selected beta-lactams and have been described against FQs (e.g., altered DNA gyrase and increased efflux pumps) and others. Resistance can be induced, as is exemplified by beta-lactamase formation in *Staphylococcus* spp. which greatly increases in the presence of a beta-lactam antibiotic, or for fluoroquinolone, for which efflux pump activity is markedly upregulated. Discussion of specific mechanisms of resistance will be addressed with the appropriate drugs (see Chapter 7).

Avoiding Antimicrobial Resistance

Among the approaches to reducing resistance are pharmacologic manipulations and changes in antimicrobial use practices. Pharmaceutical manufacturers have been able to manipulate antimicrobial drugs in a variety of ways such that resistance is minimized, and these options can be selected in an attempt to minimize resistance. For example, bacterial resistance has been decreased by synthesizing smaller molecules that can penetrate smaller porins (e.g., the extended-spectrum penicillins ticarcillin and piperacillin); synthesizing larger molecules that force the microbe to develop more than one point mutation (e.g., later-generation FQs), "protecting" the antimicrobial from enzymatic destruction (e.g., with clavulanic acid, which diverts the beta-lactamase from the penicillin); modifying the compound so that it is more difficult to destroy (e.g., amikacin, which is a larger and more difficult to reach molecule than gentamicin and carbapenems, later generation cephalosporins); and developing lipid-soluble compounds that are more able to achieve effective concentrations at the site of infection (e.g., doxycycline compared with other tetracyclines). Increasingly, drug design–based tactics will be implemented to minimize emergent resistance. Increasingly the role of the practitioner is equally important. A three "D"s approach might reduce the risk of emergent resistance: **De-escalate** antimicrobial use, **design** a treatment regimen that minimizes resistance (dead bugs don't mutate), and **decontaminate** the environment through proper hygiene. These approaches are exemplified by strategies implemented by intensive care units to reduce antimicrobial resistance that often involve a multitiered approach (Box 6-3). Actions include the following:

Box 6-3

Reducing Transmission of Resistant Microbes (Decontamination)

Treating infected patients in order of least-at-risk to most-at-risk
Dedicated diagnostic or handling equipment
Proper bandaging of infected sites
Dedicated bandage areas
Protection during animal handling (disposable gloves, masks, gowns, eyewear)
Decreased contact with body fluids
Dedicated disposal for contaminated materials
Proper hand washing between patients
Easy access to hand sanitizers (alchohol based)
Strict asepsis during surgery
Dedicated cleaning materials
Clean in order of cleanest to dirtiest
Proper disinfection of the following:

- Exposed or at-risk rooms
- Tables, doors, counter surfaces, floors, and so on
- Equipment (stethoscopes, keyboards, pens, and so on)
- Isolate carriers (not always necessary)

KEY POINT 6-24 The goal of antimicrobial therapy is twofold: resolving clinical signs associated with infection and avoiding emergent resistance. The two goals are not mutually inclusive.

1. **De-escalate.** De-escalation begins with not using an antimicrobial when an alternate therapy (including no therapy) is more or perhaps equally effective. Enacting primary prevention by decreasing length of hospital stay, decreasing use of invasive devices, and implementing newer approaches (e.g., selective digestive decontamination and vaccine development).[107] De-escalation also includes setting limits on the duration of antimicrobial therapy (see later discussion) and rotating the use of antimicrobial drugs on a regular schedule.[107,125] De-escalation might also refer to changing from a

higher to a lower tier category of drugs (following a "hit hard, get out quick") in a critical patient.

2. **Design:** Improving appropriate antimicrobial use through proper dosing regimens includes selection of the most appropriate drug for the bug while narrowing the spectrum. This approach also should be applied to empirical antimicrobial therapy. Design of the dosing regimen should take into account the appropriate PDI for concentration or time-dependent drugs, and when possible, targeting the MPC. More controversial approaches to design include techniques implemented in hospitals include adhering to prescribed formularies or requiring prior approval for using certain antibiotics.
3. **Decontaminate:** Approaches intended to reduce bacterial exposure are among the most important to avoiding resistance. These include improving infection control through selective decontamination procedures, prevention of horizontal transmission through proper hand-washing technique, and use of gloves and gown, or prevention by reducing exposure to bandages or other contaminated materials by identifying proper work areas and disposal sites. Other approaches include, provision of soap alternatives, easy access to disinfectants (which should complement, not replace, hand washing) and improvement of the workload and facilities for health care workers.

Improved information systems technology also plays a role. Each proposed or implemented strategy has theoretical benefits and limitations, but good data on their efficacy in controlling antimicrobial resistance are limited.[107,125] However, it is clear that decreased antimicrobial use is associated with a decrease in the advent of resistance.

Risk factors for emerging resistance in the hospital or community setting include but are not limited to increased antimicrobial use, host factors such as severity of illness and length of stay, and lack of adherence to infection control practices.[107] Consequently, among the de-escalation efforts implemented in human hospital and community environments is restricted antimicrobial use. In humans the increasing presence of drug-resistant bacterial infections among hospitalized patients is linked to the greater numbers of patients receiving inappropriate antimicrobial treatment.[123] A recent on-line report found that in human medicine, antimicrobials were often prescribed despite infection being an infrequent cause of the illness (i.e., pharyngitis). Further, the chosen antimicrobial often was inappropriate for those bacteria potentially causing infection in the treated body system.[124] Accordingly, reducing inappropriate antimicrobial use has become a priority in human medicine.

Among the more rational paradigms for antibacterial de-escalation, is an approach to empirical antimicrobial use in the hospital setting for patients with serious bacterial infections.[123] Such antimicrobial de-escalation attempts to balance the need to provide appropriate initial antibacterial treatment while limiting the emergence of antimicrobial resistance. The goal of de-escalation in this setting is to prescribe an initial antimicrobial regimen that will cover the most likely bacterial pathogens associated with infection while minimizing the risk of emerging antimicrobial resistance.[123] The three-pronged approach includes narrowing the antimicrobial regimen through culture, assessing isolate susceptibility for dose determination, and choosing the shortest course of therapy clinically acceptable. Judicious antimicrobial use combined with restricted use of ceftazidime led to a decreased antimicrobial resistance to beta-lactams, in general, in a human teaching hospital environment.[126] Note that this strategy does not exclude the use of "big gun" antimicrobials. The approach of withholding use of high-impact drugs (e.g., meropenem or vancomycin) in patients whose need for effective therapy is critical to avoid emerging resistance that might limit drug use in later patients may not be rational or in the best interest of the patient. A more appropriate approach is to use the drug correctly. However, routine use of less powerful drugs is appropriate but only if these alternatives are just as effective. Regardless of the choice, once the decision is made to use an antimicrobial, attention must be paid to dosing regimens that minimize the advent of resistance by ensuring that infecting microbes are eradicated.

Another strategy to decrease the impact of antimicrobial use on resistance is a decreased duration of therapy (see the discussion of enhancing antimicrobial efficacy). One study in human critical care patients found that reducing the duration of antimicrobial therapy from 14 days to 10 days decreased the emergence of resistance.[127] Increasingly, clinical trials will focus on demonstrating efficacy of shorter (i.e., < 5 to 7 days) treatment regimens.

Rapid detection of the correct microbe and the presence of resistance would facilitate the proper design of a therapeutic regimen. Genetic changes (e.g., mutations) that result in resistance lend themselves to molecular detection. However, molecular tests are often limited to those mutations characterized by few polymorphisms (e.g., MRSA, potentially MRSIG, and *Enterococcus* sp.). Generally, these tests require culture conditions that are often designed to facilitate expression of the resistant gene and are based on amplification techniques. Yet, as with culture, although they are able to determine phenotypic expression, they do not necessarily document the isolate as the cause of infection. Further, they generally do not detect low levels of resistance that increase the MIC but do not render the microbe as "resistant" by susceptibility testing.[122] Topical therapy should be considered when possible. Therapeutic drug monitoring may be helpful for some drugs (e.g., aminoglycosides). With at-risk patients in whom emergent mutants may not be sufficiently suppressed. Drugs inherently more resistant to bacterial inactivation should be selected (e.g., amikacin rather than gentamicin). Combination antimicrobial therapy (e.g., beta-lactamase–protected antimicrobial combinations; combination of beta-lactams with aminoglycosides) also reduces the incidence of resistance; for example, the use of an FQ reduced the advent of resistance to cephalosporins in one study.[33] Care should be taken in selecting a drug simply because of cost. Cost should be a factor only after other considerations have been taken into account. The cost of an excellent antimicrobial can be easily surpassed by the selection and use of several less expensive, but also less effective, antimicrobials.

HOST FACTORS THAT AFFECT ANTIMICROBIAL EFFICACY

Careful consideration must be given to host factors that can reduce concentrations of active drug at the site of infection.[23,75,128] The impact of host factors on antimicrobial efficacy is often underestimated; such effects can be profound.

Among such host factors is distribution of the drug to the site of the infection (drug distribution is discussed under drug factors). Thus far, discussions on antimicrobial efficacy have been focused on achieving the MIC of the infecting isolate in the patient plasma. However, infections generally are not in plasma, and patients are not generally normal. The relationship between the MIC of the infecting organisms and drug concentrations achieved at the site of infection (both magnitude and duration) is so complex that predicting efficacy is difficult. Ultimately, mathematical models that integrate the major determinants of efficacy (bactericidal activity, relationship between PDC and MIC, duration of postantibiotic effect, and susceptibility versus resistance) may prove most predictive.[129] The determinants of this relationship and the influence of drug, microbial, and host factors on efficacy warrant further discussion.

The MIC_{BP} of a drug is based on plasma C_{max}, yet infections generally occur in tissues rather than plasma. More specifically, the site of infection generally is interstitial fluid. However, detection of drug in tissues is difficult, leading to PDC as the surrogate marker of tissue concentrations. In instances in which PDCs overestimate extracellular fluid, care must be taken to adjust doses. For such drugs C&S testing may overestimate efficacy of the drug (see the section on drug distribution). On the other hand, for some tissues, drug concentrations at the site may far exceed PDC (see below). Inflammation may profoundly alter drug efficacy (Table 6-7).[23,128] Acute inflammation may initially increase drug delivery and drug concentration to the site of infection because of increased blood flow, increased capillary permeability, and increased protein release at the site (the latter effect increases the concentration of total, but not necessarily active, drug). However, chronic inflammation may do the opposite. Purulent exudate presents an acidic, hyperosmolar, and hypoxic environment that impairs the efficacy of many antimicrobials (Figure 6-16). Hemoglobin and degradative products of inflammation can bind antimicrobials.[130] Selected drugs, including aminoglycosides (and probably highly protein-bound drugs) are bound to and thus inactivated by proteinaceous debris that accumulates with inflammation. Some antimicrobials can inhibit neutrophil function. Accumulation of cellular debris associated with the inflammatory process can present a barrier to passive antimicrobial distribution. The deposition of fibrous tissue at the infected site further impairs drug penetrance and distribution (Figure 6-17).

KEY POINT 6-25 Although the host inflammatory response initially may facilitate therapeutic success, it can ultimately profoundly decrease the likelihood of success.

Table 6-7 Negative Effects of the Microenvironment on Antimicrobial Efficacy

Environmental Factor	Effect
Acidic pH	Penicillins inactivated at pH < 6.0
	Aminoglycosides and enrofloxacin more effective in alkaline pH
Hypertonicity/ hyperosmolarity	Impaired efficacy of beta-lactam antibiotics
Pus	Acidic pH
	Hypertonic
	Hyperosmolar
	Protein binding of selected drugs
	Binding to sediment (aminoglycosides)
Low O_2 tension	Aminoglycosides inactive
	Growth of organisms slowed → decreased efficacy of bactericidal drugs
	Impaired phagocytic activity of leukocytes
Large inoculum	Greater concentration of antimicrobial inactivating enzymes
	Greater concentration of drug molecules required
Leukocytes	Impaired chemotaxis, phagocytosis, metabolism

Local pH becomes more acidic as degradative products such as lysosomes, nucleic acids, and other intracellular constituents from white blood cells accumulate. The efficacy of many antimicrobials can subsequently be impaired. In humans a pH level ranging from 5.5 to 6.8 can adversely affect both host defenses and antimicrobial activity. White blood cell oxidative bursts and phagocytosis are diminished in the presence of a low pH level. Some antimicrobials are inactive at a low pH level. Erythromycin loses all of its activity when pH is below 7. Similar effects have been reported for beta-lactam antibiotics. Although beta-lactam antibiotics are weak acids and therefore less ionized in an acidic environment, they are generally less effective at a pH 6. The activities of cefoxitin, piperacillin, and imipenem (or meropenem) are significantly less at pH 6 than at pH 6.5 with piperacillin being least affected. The activity of clindamycin is similarly decreased. In addition, the accumulation of some drugs in white blood cells that might otherwise facilitate efficacy is impaired in an acidic environment. Changes in pH also lead to changes in the concentration of un-ionized and thus active drug. Weak bases such as aminoglycosides and FQs are predominantly ionized in an acidic environment and are less effective than in a less acidic environment, in part because of impaired diffusibility.

Low tissue oxygen tension, which can accompany pus, reduces white blood cell phagocytic and killing activity; slows the growth of organisms, making them less susceptible to many drugs; and specifically prevents the efficacy

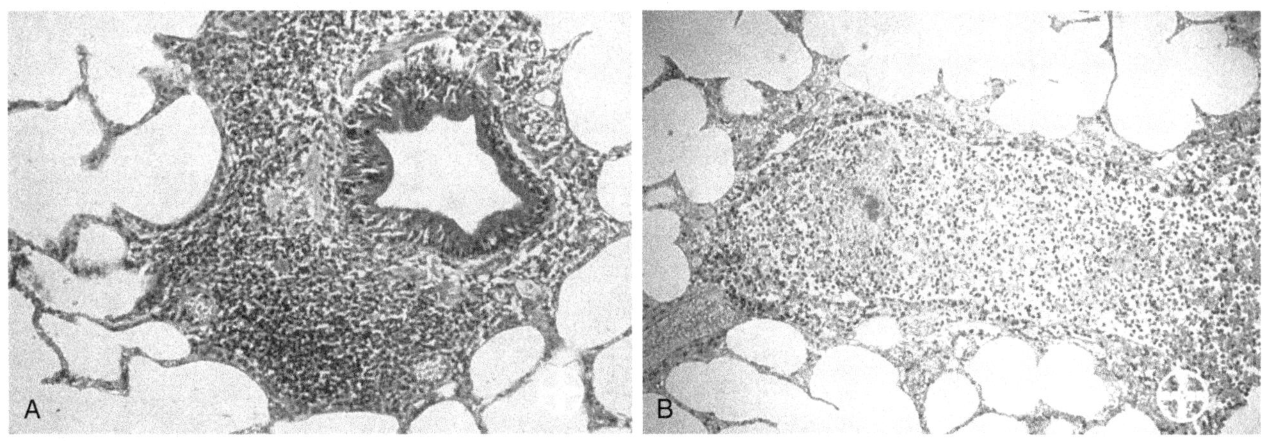

Figure 6-16 The inflammatory response to bacteria is intended to support the host in overcoming an infection. However, the response can become a confounding factor. For example, the inflammation of pneumonia of bronchitis dilutes the drug, presents a barrier to passive diffusion, and may bind and thus inactivate the drug. Local pH and thus drug ionization may impair drug action, and generation of a decreased oxygen tension further decreases drug efficacy. (Photo courtesy Bayer Animal Health.)

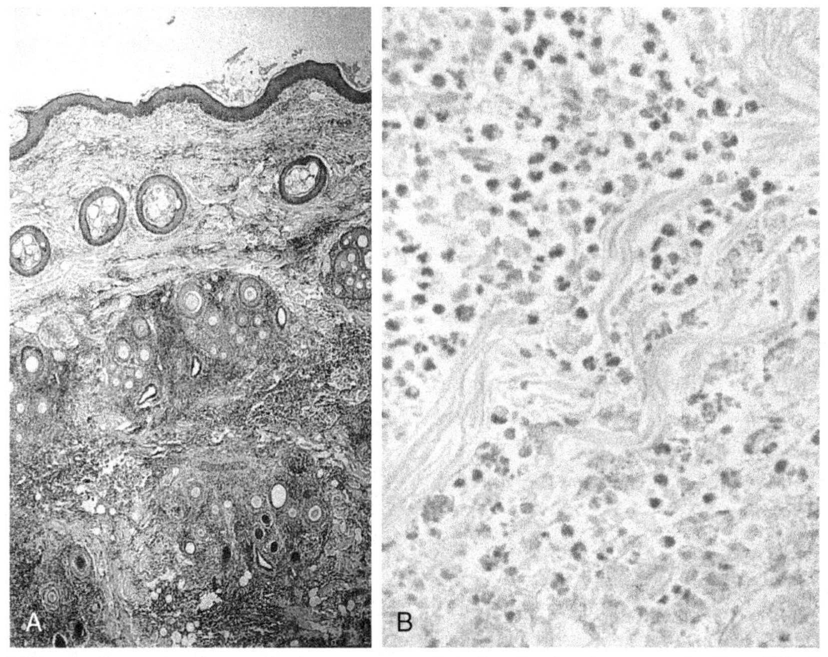

Figure 6-17 Deposition of fibrous tissue in deep pyoderma presents a barrier to drug penetration. (Photo courtesy Bayer Animal Health.)

of aminoglyosides, which depend on active transport into bacterial organisms. The aerobic component (i.e., facultative anaerobes) of a mixed infection may also be resistant to aminoglycoside therapy because the oxidative transport systems of such organisms (e.g., *E. coli)* may shut down in an anaerobic environment. Drugs that target cell walls, and beta-lactams in particular, are less effective in a hyperosmolar environment, which might occur as inflammatory debris accumulates and osmotic destruction of organisms is reduced.

Host response to infection and its impact on antimicrobial therapy may vary with the organ system infected. For example, in respiratory tract infections, mucus produced by the host can directly interfere with antimicrobial therapy. Aminoglycoside efficacy may be decreased by chelation with magnesium and calcium in the mucus. Antimicrobials may bind to glycoproteins, and mucus may present a barrier to passive diffusion. In addition, some antimicrobials may alter the function of the mucociliary apparatus, either by increasing mucous viscosity or by decreasing ciliary activity (e.g., tetracyclines).

Changes in the health of the host can lead to changes in drug disposition that can result in lower than anticipated PDCs (see Chapter 2).[50] The volume to which a drug is distributed can be affected by the fluid compartments, which vary with age, species, and hydration status. Distribution to target organs can be affected profoundly by cardiovascular

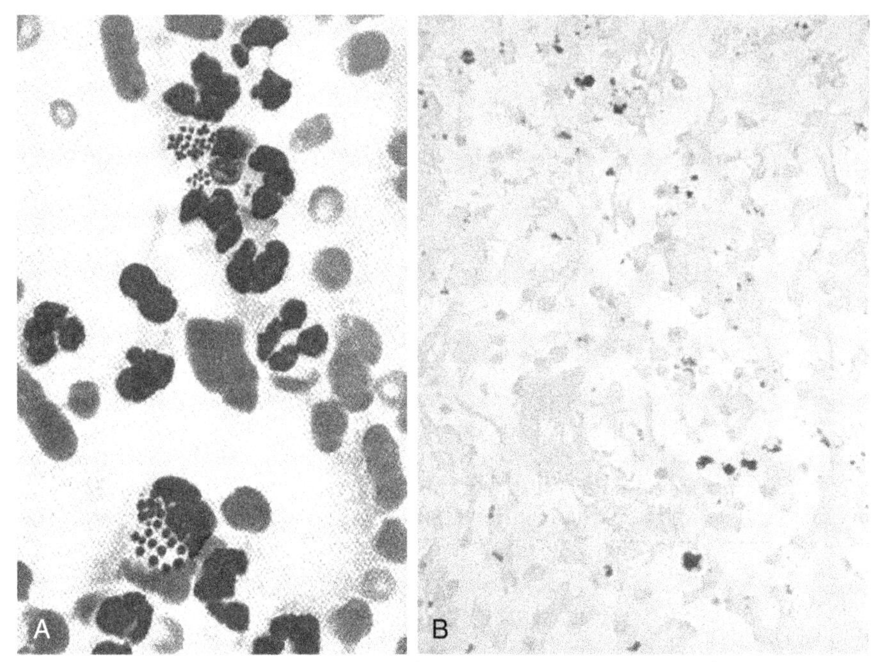

Figure 6-18 The intracellular location of organisms presents a barrier to drug penetration. Some organisms are obligate intracellular organisms, whereas others, such as *Staphyloccocus* spp., demonstrated cytologically **(A)** and by special stain of infected skin **(B),** may survive phagocytosis, serving to reinfect tissue once the phagocytic white blood cell has died.

responses, particularly in the shock patient. Elimination of the drug must be considered when selecting antimicrobials for the critical patient. Changes in glomerular filtration cause parallel changes in renal excretion of drugs. Serum creatinine concentrations should be used to modify doses or intervals of potentially toxic drugs that are excreted renally (see Chapter 2).[131] Likewise, severe changes in hepatic function may indicate selection of an antimicrobial drug not dependent on hepatic function for activation or excretion.

Host Factors That Facilitate Drug Efficacy

Host factors may also facilitate antimicrobial efficacy. Among the most important host factors are local and systemic defenses ranging from compounds that directly target microbes to healthy tissues that provide mechanical barriers and a competent immune system. The role of host defenses are beyond the scope of this chapter but cannot be underemphasized.

Other host factors that facilitate therapy include the accumulation of the drug in active form at the site of infection, which may facilitate antimicrobial efficacy and decrease the risk of resistance. Obvious examples include drugs that undergo renal or biliary excretion. For such drugs urine or bile concentrations (respectively) may exceed PDC thirtyfold to several hundredfold (see the discussion of treatment of urinary tract infections, Chapter 8). Another site of drug concentration is the phagocytic leukocyte (WBC), both in peripheral circulation and at the site of inflammation. Active concentrations of some antimicrobials (e.g., macrolides, lincosamides, and FQs) may increase concentrations 20 to 100 or more times the PDC.[28,132-137] Phagocytic accumulation may facilitate treatment of intracellular infections (e.g., *Brucella* spp., cell wall–deficient organisms, intracellular parasites, and facultative intracellular organisms such as *Staphylococcus* spp.). Thus drugs that achieve only bacteriostatic concentrations in plasma may become bactericidal inside the cell, particularly against organisms that locate and survive inside cells (Figure 6-18). Additionally, accumulated drug released by dying phagocytes at the site of infection may increase concentrations to which the infecting microbe is exposed. Accumulation of drug inside WBC has been assumed as an explanation of the disconnect of azithromycin efficacy in pulmonary infections despite low PDCs.[91] Note, however, that drug accumulation does not necessarily enhance drug efficacy. Often, the accumulated drug is sequestered into subcellular organelles, where it cannot reach the organism. In addition, the drug may become otherwise inactivated once inside the cell. The different mechanisms of action of these drugs may not occur in an anaerobic environment, and concentrations by the WBCs might be impaired in an anaerobic environment. The FQs are an example of a class of drugs whose uptake by WBCs is facilitated in an acidic environment; these drugs are distributed throughout the cytosol, where they remain active. The drug will leave the WBCs and enter a drug-free environment and thus may facilitate drug concentrations at the site of infection. Phagocytic WBCs with accumulated enrofloxacin delivered drug to inflamed tissue cages in dogs, demonstrating that accumulation may increase therapeutic response.[137] Drugs that do not accumulate in WBCs include the beta-lactams, aminoglycosides, and metronidazole. Drugs that are moderately accumulated in WBCs include chloramphenicol (onefold to fivefold) and selected sulfonamides (threefold to fivefold).[138]

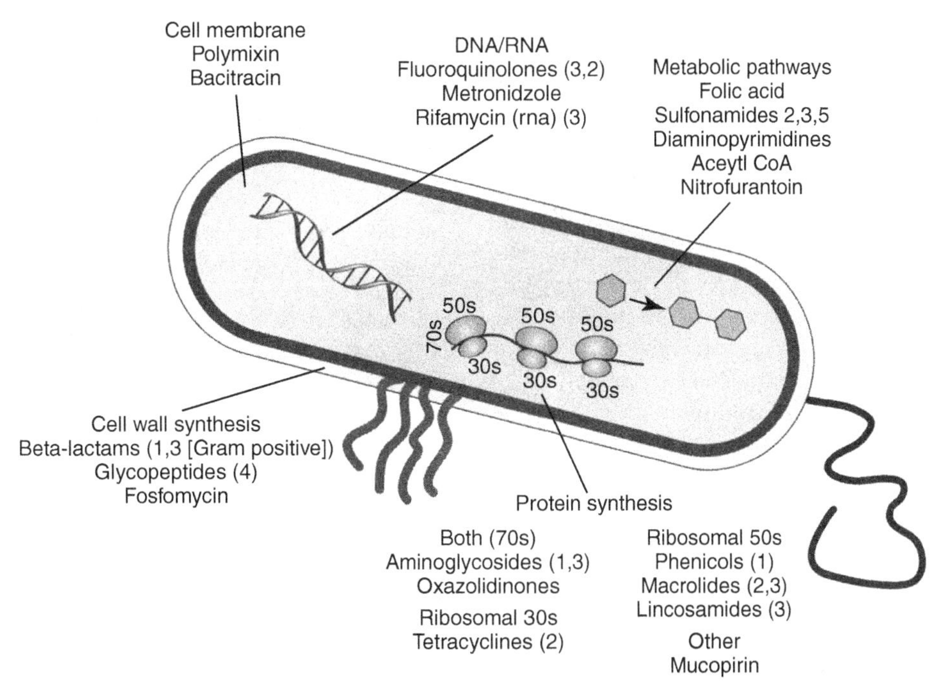

Figure 6-19 Targets of antimicrobial actions for the different classes of antimicrobial drugs. The number in parentheses refers to the major mechanism(s) of acquired resistance (other mechanisms also exist; see Chapter 7): 1 = enzymatic destruction (e.g., beta-lactamases for beta-lactams, acetylases for phenicols); 2 = increased efflux pump activity (may be associated with altered porin influx in gram-negative isolates); 3 = altered targeted site (e.g., mutations in DNA gyrase for fluoroquinolones or penicillin-binding proteins for gram-positive isolates); 4 = interfering protein and 5 = increased production of targeted metabolite. Decreased porin size is a common mechanism of resistance associated with increased efflux pump activity for many gram-negative isolates.

Another potential facilitating host factor is infection at a site that is topically accessible. In such situations several 1000-fold concentrations of the MIC may be reached with topical administration. The rationale for collecting C&S data for such infections might be controversial, but identification of the organism and some indication of susceptibility is prudent, particularly if initial therapy fails.

DRUG FACTORS THAT AFFECT ANTIMICROBIAL EFFICACY

Mechanisms of Drug Action

Knowledge of the mechanism of action (see Figure 6-19) of a particular antimicrobial is important for several reasons:

1. The mechanism of action of a drug determines whether the antimicrobial can act in a bactericidal or bacteriostatic manner (assuming proper concentrations are achieved at the tissue site; see previous discussion). Drugs that are capable of bactericidal effects at therapeutic doses are listed in Table 6-7.
2. The mechanism of action may determine whether or not the drug is concentration-dependent or time-dependent, which will impact the design of the dosing regimen.
3. The therapeutic efficacy of some antimicrobials can be impaired by host factors that alter the mechanism of action of the drug. Knowledge of the mechanism of action will facilitate anticipation of therapeutic failure.
4. The mechanism of antimicrobial action often reflects the mechanism of resistance. Identifying mechanisms by which resistance might be avoided or minimized requires an appreciation of these mechanisms of action.
5. Understanding or anticipating selected host toxicities associated with antimcirobials can be improved by understanding their mechanism of action.
6. Understanding antimicrobial mechanisms of action provides a basis for the selection of antimicrobials to be used in combination. Such drugs should be selected on the basis of mechanisms of action that complement rather than antagonize one another (see Combination Antimicrobial Therapy section).

The cell wall is an important target for several antimicrobials, protecting the hypertonic intracellular environment of the organism from the hypotonic extracellular environment.[23] A variety of proteins located in the cell wall (penicillin-bound proteins) are important in the formation of the cell wall during division of growth of the organisms. These proteins are the target of several antimicrobial agents. Destruction of the peptidoglycan layer, which provides support to the cell wall, increases the permeability of the cell wall to the hypotonic environment, resulting in osmotic lysis of the cell. Intracellular structures are also major targets for various antimicrobial agents. Binding of ribosomes, the site of protein synthesis in the cell, can either inhibit protein formation or result in the formation of faulty proteins that eventually prove detrimental to the organism. The nuclear material of microbes is another target: Interference with cellular DNA inhibits cellular division, as well as initial cellular functions. Generally, impaired DNA synthesis results in cell death. Other intracellular targets include selected metabolic pathways such as folic acid synthesis, which, when interfered with, prevents formation of materials vital to the microorganism.

Drug Disposition

Absorption

Care must be taken when selecting the antimicrobial that the disposition of the drug meets the needs of the patient (see earlier discussion of host factors). The availability of drug preparations determines drug selection in many instances because not all drugs are available for administration by all routes. To maximize plasma and thus tissue drug concentrations, intravenous administration is the preferred route for critically ill patients or difficult-to-penetrate tissues, with intramuscular and subcutaneous administration being second and third choices, respectively. Oral administration of antimicrobials, however, is preferred for long-term use, for nonhospitalized patients, and when drug therapy is targeting the gastrointestinal tract.

Note that although a drug may be 100% bioavailable after oral administration (i.e., the drug is completely absorbed), the rate of absorption may be sufficiently slow that the peak effect is minimized (although the duration of drug in circulation may be prolonged). Efficacy may be impaired, particularly for organisms with a high MIC or for concentration-dependent drugs. Slow-release preparations, either orally or parenterally administered, should be used cautiously because prolonged absorption (controlled rate of release) may be so slow that therapeutic concentrations are not achieved. The risk of resistance may be increased in such situations. Although slow-release products might improve compliance for time-dependent drugs, their use may also preclude shorter duration therapy. Topical administration is the sole route for drugs that are too toxic to the host to administer systemically. Care must be taken, however, with drugs applied to skin whose surface has been damaged. Sufficient drug absorption may occur to render the patient at risk of developing toxicity. Drugs applied to the ear canal may be ototoxic, particularly in the presence of a perforated tympanic membrane.

Distribution

Once in circulation, the antimicrobial must distribute well to target tissues (i.e., the site of infection). The principles determining drug distribution to and from tissues are discussed in Chapter 1, and movement of each antimicrobial is discussed in Chapter 7. Whereas sinusoidal capillaries, found primarily in the adrenal cortex, pituitary gland, liver, and spleen, present essentially no barrier to drug movement. Fenestrated capillaries such as those located in kidneys and endocrine glands contain pores (50 to 80 nm in size) that facilitate movement between plasma and interstitium. Because the ratio of capillary surface area to interstitial fluid volume is so large, unbound drug movement from plasma into the interstitium occurs very rapidly in these tissues.[139,140] Continuous capillaries, such as those found in the brain, CSF, testes, and prostate, present a barrier of endothelial cells with tight junctions.[139] Muscle, lungs, and adipose tissue also contain continuous capillaries.[139-141] Therapeutic antimicrobial failure in a number of body systems in humans has been associated with failed drug penetration, including soft tissue infections, osteomyelitis, prostatitis, otitis, endocarditis, ocular infections, peridontitis, and sinusitis.[141]

KEY POINT 6-26 Interstitial fluid concentrations often parallel plasma concentrations for tissue with fenestrated capillaries. The same is not likely to be true for other tissues or in the presence of host or microbial factors that impair effective drug movement.

Models for detection of drugs in tissues focus, appropriately so, on interstitial (extracellular) concentrations.[141,142] Methods that measure concentrations in tissue homogenates (including both intracellular and extracellular fluid) do not accurately represent interstitial concentrations. Extracellular fluids can be collected by a variety of methods, although a major limitation is the volume of fluid that can be collected. Detection of drug in fluids is often based on methods that require at least 1 mL or more of fluid. Of these models, those that are based on ultrafiltration techniques appear to be most accurate representations of extracellular fluid in the normal animal.[143] Tissue cages that contain an inflammagen are reasonable methods to study the impact of inflammation on drug distribution.[137] Determination of drug in tissues protected by specialized barriers is difficult, generally requiring anesthesia.[144] If concentrations are compared with plasma, data must be based on the entire time versus concentration curve (i.e., AUC, C_{max}) rather than single-point comparisons because drug does not distribute immediately into tissues. Care must also be taken to address the impact of protein binding, as can be demonstrated for cefovecin, a drug that is 90% to 99% bound to serum protein. Total serum concentrations are markedly higher than that in extraceullar fluid because the latter contains less protein.[46]

Doses for drugs generally should be higher when treating infections in tissues with continuous capillaries, particularly for water-soluble drugs. Comparison of MIC data with tissue drug concentrations may be useful when designing dosing regimens for such tissues.

Examples of different distribution patterns might be predicted somewhat based on Vd (Box 6-4; see also the section on antimicrobial drugs in Chapter 7). Although the Vd of a drug does not indicate to which tissues drug is distributed, it can be used to approximate likelihood of tissue penetration in that a lipid-soluble drug is more likely than a water-soluble drug to move beyond extracellular fluid. Urine and the central nervous system (CNS) offer two divergent examples of tissue penetration. Urine is easy to target by drugs that are renally eliminated. Other components of the urinary tract, such as the kidney and particularly the prostate, can, however, be more difficult to penetrate. Antimicrobial therapy of the CNS is very difficult, although success may be facilitated by inflammation, which enhances drug penetration. However, once

Box 6-4

Tissue Distribution Pattern of Selected Drugs

Drugs Distributed to Extracellular Fluid ($V_d \leq 0.34$ L/kg)
Beta-lactams
Aminoglycosides

Drugs Distributed to Total Body Water ($V_d \geq 0.6$ L/kg)
Chloramphenicol
Clindamycin
Doxycycline/minocycline
Erythromycin
Fluorinated quinolones
Sulfonamides/trimethoprim

Drugs Concentrated in Urine
Beta-lactams
Aminoglycosides
Fluorinated quinolones
Sulfonamides/potentiated sulfonamides
Vancomycin

Drugs Concentrated in Bile
Clindamycin
Doxycycline/minocycline
Macrolides (erythromycin)
Rifampin

Drug Penetration of the Blood–Brain Barrier
Drugs that readily enter the cerebrospinal fluid (CSF)
Chloramphenicol
Doxycycline/minocycline (unbound)
Fluorinated quinolones (for some organisms)
Metronidazole
Rifampin
Sulfonamides/trimethoprim
Drugs that enter the CSF in the presence of inflammation
Penicillins
Selected cephalosporins (e.g., cefotaxime, ceftriaxone, ceftazidime)
Fluorinated quinolones
Vancomycin
Drugs that do not enter the CSF
Aminoglycosides
Carbenicillin
Cephalothin
Cefazolin
Cefotetan
Clindamycin
Erythromycin
Tetracycline

Drugs that Accumulate in White Blood Cells
Clindamycin
Erythromycin (macrolides)
Fluorinated quinolones
Rifampin

inflammation resolves, drug distribution may again decrease. The blood–brain or CSF barrier represents a particularly challenging site because it not only prevents movement of antimicrobials into the CNS but also actively transports out or destroys some antimicrobials (i.e., penicillins and selected cephalosporins) (see Box 6-4). Care must be taken even with tissues normally characterized by excellent blood flow. For example, distribution of beta-lactams, aminoglycosides, and selected sulfonamides into bronchial secretions is generally <30% of that in plasma (see Chapter 8).[130,145,146]

Lipid-soluble antimicrobials should be used for infections that are more difficult to treat, including those associated with tissue reaction or those caused by intracellular organisms, and when the site of infection presents a distribution barrier. Tissue distribution of aminoglycosides and most beta-lactam antimicrobials is limited to extracellular fluid; in contrast, many other antimicrobials (e.g., FQs, macrolides, and trimethoprim/sulfonamide combinations) are distributed well to all body tissues, including the prostate gland and eye. Enrofloxacin approximates or surpasses unity with plasma in many tissues.[144] Imipenem (or meropenem), trimethoprim/sulfonamide, and FQs can achieve bactericidal concentrations for some infections in the CNS (particularly organisms with a low MIC); chloramphenicol will achieve bacteriostatic concentrations.[147] Accumulation of antimicrobials in WBCs facilitates treatment of intracellular infections.[132–137]

Protein binding of a drug to plasma proteins may affect antimicrobial efficacy both in the patient and in vitro as data supporting drug selection and dose design are generated. Only unbound drug is pharmacologically active (see impact on cefovecin).[45] In vivo, bound drug is retained in the vasculature; once in the interstitial fluids or inside the cell, the drug may again be bound and inactivated. In vivo C&S testing and determination of MIC occur in the absence of protein. Further, PK on which MIC_{BP} is based (C_{max} being a major consideration) frequently is based on total drug, rather than the fraction of unbound. For a drug insignificantly protein bound, this disconnect is generally not significant. However, as the fraction of bound drug increases, C&S testing may markedly overestimate efficacy by the proportion of drug that is bound (i.e., a drug that is 50% protein-bound will actually yield an "active" C_{max} that is 50% of the total). Clearance and Vd may be underestimated. Attempts should be made to base therapeutic decisions on unbound drug.[130,148]

Drug movement into bacteria must also be considered. The roles of drug pK_a and the environmental pH of a target tissue on drug efficacy have already been addressed. Ionization may impair drug movement through the LPS for drugs that passively move through this layer.

Drug Elimination

The route through which the drug is eliminated is an important consideration for two reasons. First, if the site of infection is also a route of elimination for that drug, higher drug concentrations can be expected at the site. Second, if the drug is toxic to an organ of elimination, use of the drug should be avoided if the organ is already diseased. Also, if the drug is toxic to any tissue, the drug should be used cautiously in the presence of disease of the organ of elimination or dosing regimens should be appropriately modified.

Nonantimicrobial Effects of Antimicrobials

A number of antimicrobials influence various aspects of the immune system. The phagocytosis of drugs (e.g., macrolides, lincosamides, and FQs) was previously discussed.[23,132-134,138] In addition to accumulation in WBCs, antimicrobials can influence WBC function. However, the effect can be variable. The negative effect of antimicrobials on phagocytic function has been well established, although the clinical relevance of this effect is less clear.[149] Functions that are targeted include chemotaxis (increased, decreased, or unchanged by clindamycin, erythromycin, chloramphenicol, and lincomycin and decreased or unchanged by gentamicin), phagocytosis (increased by erythromycin and chloramphenicol and decreased by tobramycin and polymyxin B), oxidative burst (increased by clindamycin, cefotaxime, and quinolones and decreased by cefotaxime, trimethoprim/sulfonamides, chloramphenicol, and erythromycin), bacterial killing (increased by cefotaxime and decreased by sulfonamides and aminoglycosides), and cytokine production or activity (interleukin 1 [IL-1] increased by cefotaxime and cefaclor and IL-10 by erythromycin; IL-1 and tumor necrosis factor decreased by cefoxitin, erythromycin, and ciprofloxacin).[138] Apoptosis of neutrophils may be accelerated.[150]

The clinical relevance of these potentially beneficial effects on phagocyte function is not clear, but relevance is supported by some studies. For example, long-term use of azithromycin appears to improve lung function in children with cystic fibrosis and is increasingly being included in its therapeutic regimen; the disease appears to progress more rapidly if azithromycin is not added to therapy. This effect of macrolides appears to target inflammation, because the effect occurs at concentrations below the MIC of the infecting organisms. Potential mechanisms include a reduction in IL-1β, IL-8, and neutrophils in bronchoalveolar lavage fluid.[151,152] In addition to the antiinflammatory effects, macrolides appear to decrease *Pseudomonas* virulence by reducing the number of pili, thus altering adherence to tracheal epithelium, altering membrane proteins, and decreasing alginate formation.[153,154]

KEY POINT 6-27 Selected antimicrobials facilitate therapeutic success through immunomodulation or their ability to decrease virulence of the infecting microbe.

Antimicrobial Effects of Nonantimicrobial Drugs

Antimicrobial effects have been described for a number of nonantimicrobial drugs at plasma concentrations achieved when the drug is used for noninfective indications. For example, a number of phenothiazines, including those with antihistaminergic effects, are antibacterial. Because these effects occur both in vitro and in vivo, the effects cannot be attributed simply to immunomodulation. Chlorpromazine is antimycotic at concentrations much higher than can be achieved safely in plasma, but its accumulation over a hundredfold in macrophages containing phagocytized pathogens facilitates effective therapy at recommended doses.[155] The less psychotically active thioridazine enhances the antimycotic activities of rifampin and streptomycin; between 2 and 3 months of use has been promoted as adjuvant therapy. Trifluoperazine and prochlorperazine inhibit *S. aureus* at concentrations of 10 to 50 μg/mL and selected other microbes (*Shigella, Vibrio*) at the same or higher concentrations and have demonstrated inhibitory effects in an animal model.[156,157] Selected cardioactive drugs, including oxyfedrine and dobutamine, exhibit antimicrobial effects, again toward selected microbes.[158] Amlodipine has broad antibacterial efficacy at concentrations as low as 5 to 10 μg/mL, with *S. aureus* being the most susceptible and gram-negative organisms (*E. coli, Klebsiella,* and *Pseudomonas*) requiring higher concentrations.[159] Other drugs with demonstrated antimicrobial effects include the antispasmodic drug dicyclomine[160] and selected nonsteroidal antiinflammatories.[161] Among the dietary supplements with recognized antibacterial effects are the flavones. Flavone dietary supplements exhibited antibacterial activity to a variety of microbes in a mouse infection model.[162,163] Chitosans have demonstrated efficacy toward a number of bacterial organisms, particularly gram-negative isolates at concentrations as low as 0.05 μg/mL.[164] Several antifungal drugs have antibacterial properties, which are addressed in Chapter 9.

Adverse Drug Events and Antimicrobials

Actions that minimize host toxicity enhance therapeutic success. However, host cells are eukaryotic, whereas the bacteria are prokaryotic. As such, targets of antibacterial therapy are sufficiently different from mammalian cells that, as a class, antibacterials (but not antifungals) tend to be safe. For example, beta-lactam antibiotics are among the safest antimicrobials because they target cell walls, a structure not present in mammalian cells. Often, even if cellular structures are present in both microbe and host, differences in the structure will result in different antimicrobial binding properties. For example, sulfonamides and FQs tend to be safe because the antimicrobials have a much greater affinity for the bacterial target enzymes than the mammalian enzymes. As with other drugs, the incidence of predictable (type A) drug reactions to most antimicrobial therapy correlates with maximum or peak PDC. However, aminoglycoside-induced nephrotoxicity and ototoxicity are an exception; toxicity tends to be related to duration of exposure and is more likely if minimum or trough PDCs are above a maximum level.[76,165,166] Occasionally, toxicity of antimicrobials does reflect their mechanism of action, if the microbial target occurs in mammalian cells and is structurally similar (see Chapter 7). For example, colistin and polymyxin target both microbial and host cell membranes. Administration of either drug is associated with a high incidence of nephrotoxicity (probably because drug is concentrated in renal tubular cells), and subsequently their use generally is limited to the topical route of administration. Drugs that inhibit protein synthesis by binding to ribosomes (e.g., tetracyclines, chloramphenicol) may cause (limited) antianabolic effects in the host at sufficiently high doses. For most antimicrobial drugs, host toxicity may occur through mechanisms unrelated to its mechanism of action, but as a result of targeting structures in host cells. Aminoglycosides cause nephrotoxicity and ototoxicity, not because of their ribosomal inhibition (their antibacterial mechanism of action) but because they actively accumulate in renal tubular (or otic hair) cells (as they do in bacterial organisms) and in lysosomes causing lysosomal disruption. Topical application is more likely to cause ototoxicity with aminoglycoside and other drugs (see Chapters 4 and 7). FQs cause retinal degeneration in cats, through mechanisms yet to be defined. Tilmicosin causes (potentially lethal) beta-adrenergic stimulation; the caustic nature of doxycycline can cause esophageal erosion in cats. Allergies are a less common adverse reaction caused by antimicrobials. Some drugs cause anaphylactoid reactions as a result of direct mast cell degranulation. True allergic reactions should be differentiated from anaphylactoid reactions (more common with intravenous administration of FQs). The latter may occur with the first dose and may be dose dependent. Anaphylactoid reactions can be minimized by administration of a small first dose before therapy. In contrast, drug-induced allergies generally require previous administration or a duration of therapy sufficient to allow antibody formation to the drug, which acts as a hapten (generally 10 to 14 days). Few drug allergies have been documented in animals. Among the most notorious are reactions to the potentiated sulfonamides.

KEY POINT 6-28 Because antimicrobial targets are prokaryotic and hosts are eukaryotic, adverse events seldom reflect the mechanism of antimicrobial activity.

Among the adverse reactions associated with antimicrobial use are those associated with drug interactions. Those most clinicaly relevant involve drug metabolizing enzymes. Examples of drugs that inhibit the metabolism of other drugs are the macrolides; chloramphenicol; and for selected drugs, the fluoroquinolones. In contrast, rifampin is an inducer. Increasingly, drugs that alter drug metabolizing enzymes are emerging as drugs that compete for or alter drug transport proteins (e.g., P-glycoprotein). Drug interactions involving antimicrobials are discussed with each class (see Chapter 8).

Adverse reactions to antimicrobials may reflect their antimicrobial success. Many orally administered drugs cause disruption of normal gastrointestinal microflora (see previous discussions). For example, the author has detected emergence of *Clostridium perfringens* in dogs treated with fosfomycin. *Streptococcus* spp. are generally associated with opportunistic infections. However, infections caused by members of this genus (*S. pyogenes* in humans and *Streptococcus canis* in animals) are associated with streptococcal toxic shock syndrome (STSS) and necrotizing fasciitis (NF).[167] These syndromes appear to reflect the presence of lysogenic bacteriophage-encoded superantigen genes encoded in the bacterial organisms.[167] The superantigen genes are powerful inducers of T-cell proliferation; the presence of the superantigens then causes release of host cytokines in quantities that may be sufficient to cause lethal effects. In one study a bacteriophage-encoded streptococcal superantigen gene was identified in the majority of *S. canis* isolates. Induction of these genes can lead to bacterial lysis and subsequent release of proinflammatory and other destructive cytokines. Indeed, use of the FQs has been associated with STSS and NF in dogs (see Chapter 7).[168]

Release of endotoxin is another example of seeming therapeutic success potentially leading to therapeutic failure (Figure 6-20). However, the clinical relevance of endotoxin release may be species dependent. Endotoxin release is a side effect of antimicrobials that occurs with therapeutic success, and it may influence antimicrobial selection for the patient infected with a large number of gram-negative organisms.[84] Endotoxins cause further release of cytokines and other mediators of septic shock (see Chapter 8). Most of these effects are mediated by the inner lipid A component of the LPS molecule that becomes exposed after antimicrobial therapy. In human patients suffering from endotoxic shock, outcome of antimicrobial therapy has been related to plasma endotoxin levels. A number of antimicrobials cause release of endotoxin from gram-negative organisms. Attempts have been made to correlate the amount of endotoxin released to the class of antimicrobial and specifically to its mechanism of action.

Continued bacterial growth or rapid cell lysis and death have been suggested as important criteria for endotoxin release after antimicrobial therapy. In contrast, the rate of bacterial killing and antimicrobial efficacy do not appear to be related to the rate and amount of endotoxin release. The amount of endotoxin release varies among the antimicrobial classes and even within the classes. Release can be related to mechanism of action. Among the drugs traditionally used to treat septicemia, aminoglycosides have been associated with the least and beta-lactams with the greatest endotoxin release (with imipenem or meropenem causing the least amount of endotoxin release among the beta-lactams).[169] The different amounts of endotoxin released by beta-lactams may reflect different affinities of the drugs for different penicillin-binding proteins. In vitro studies indicate that those beta-lactam antibiotics that specifically bind penicillin-binding protein (PBP)-3 are associated with endotoxin release, whereas those that bind PBP-2 cause little to no endotoxin release.[170] The difference may reflect the fact that PBP-3 appears to form a complex with PBP-1, 4, and 7;[171] binding of PBP-3 might thus affect a larger component of cell wall synthesis compared to binding of another PBP. The release of endotoxin by quinolones varies depending on the study. However, in a study of mouse *E. coli* peritonitis, imipenem (or meropenem) and ciprofloxacin caused less endotoxin release than did cefotaxime.[84] Selected third-generation cephalosporins also appear to be associated with less endotoxin release: In a study of septicemic patients with acute pyelonephritis, the amount of endotoxin released did not differ among cefuroxime, ciprofloxacin, or netilmicin and each was deemed safe in the septicemic patient.[172]

KEY POINT 6-29 As a class, aminoglycosides are associated with the least and beta-lactams (excluding carbapenems and selected later generation cephalosporins) the most endotoxic release.

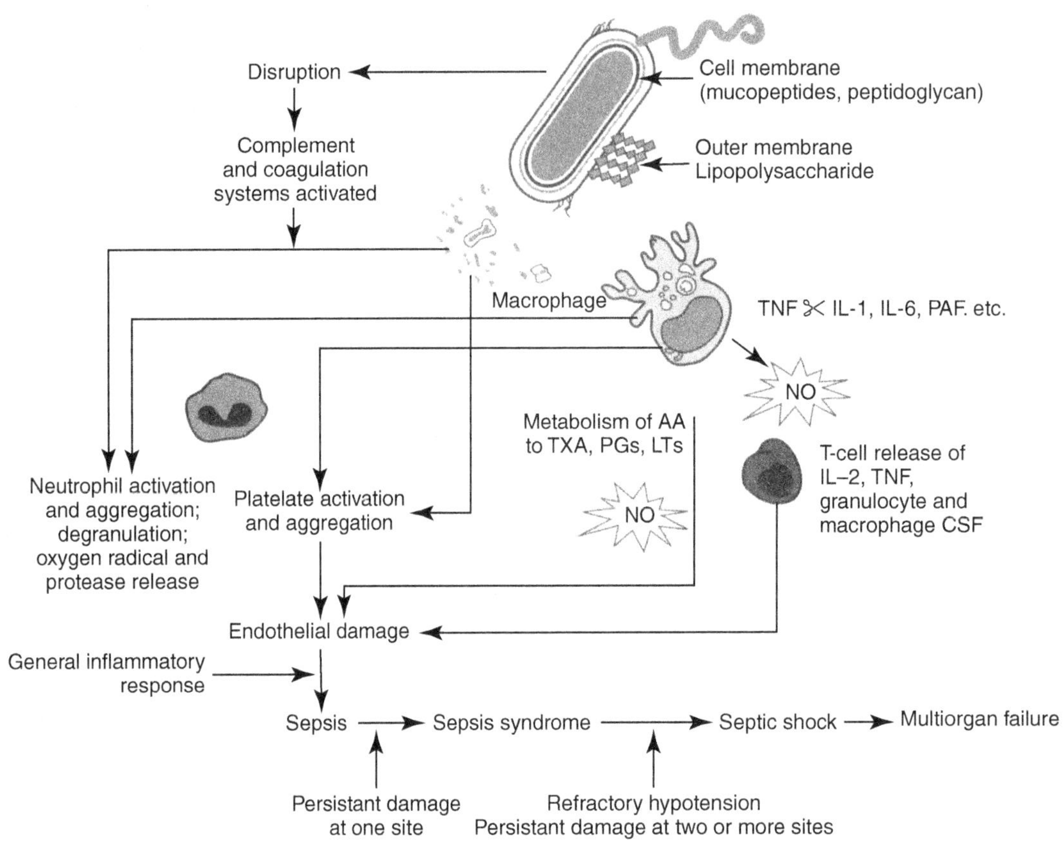

Figure 6-20 Among the adverse reactions of antimicrobial therapy is release of bacterial toxins. The risk of damage to the host is greater with a large inoculum. In this example, rapid death of gram-negative organisms can result in rapid release of endotoxin. Drugs whose mechanism results in osmotic lysis (e.g., penicillins) are more likely to be associated with sufficient endotoxin release to cause harm to the patient.

The release of endotoxin may also be dose (concentration) dependent. For example, endotoxin release is greater at half the recommended dose of ciprofloxacin (3 mg/kg versus 7 mg/kg ciprofloxacin) according to the previously described model.[84] Actions that might minimize the sequelae of endotoxin release after antimicrobial therapy have not been established. Presumably, administering a dose more slowly may decrease the rate of endotoxin release. Binding and subsequent inactivation of endotoxin by antimicrobials have been documented, particularly for cationic antimicrobials (e.g., quinolones, aminoglycosides, and polymyxin).[84,173]

ENHANCING ANTIMICROBIAL EFFICACY

Selecting the Route

Drugs may be selected on the basis of their route of administration. Not all drugs are available for parenteral or oral administration. Parenteral, and particularly intravenous, administration is indicated for life-threatening infections or whenever tissue concentrations must be maximized. Parenteral drugs are also indicated for the vomiting animal. Oral drugs are indicated for long-term use, outpatient therapy, and treatment of gastrointestinal tract illness. Topical therapy may be selected to enhance drug delivery while minimizing toxicity. Topical therapy with lipid-soluble drugs might, however, best be limited to situations in which systemic therapy of the same drug is implemented, thus preventing development of subtherapeutic drug concentrations in tissues other than the site of topical application, as might occur if topical administration alone is implemented.

Designing the Dosing Regimen

Antimicrobial therapy must be implemented in a timely fashion. An effective dose of antimicrobials administered at the first appearance of a clinical infection has a much greater therapeutic effect than therapy initiated a week later; in critical care patients, hours can mean the difference between patient recovery or death. Dosing recommendations printed on the label generally might be followed for recently approved drugs; however, exceptions occur, particularly for older drugs as we learn more about optimizing antimicrobial therapy and identify changing patterns of susceptibility. In general, to maximize efficacy, doses should be increased particularly for serious or chronic infections, tissues that are difficult to penetrate, or infections associated with detrimental changes at the site of infection. Product labels may not reflect new findings regarding antimicrobial efficacy because pharmaceutical companies may choose not to incur the costs associated with gaining approval for a new label that reflects the new dosing regimen. Dose modification beyond that on the label should be based on C&S data, current literature, and clinical signs of the patient. Adverse reactions also should be considered. Although antimicrobials are safe as a class, several are associated with dose- or duration-dependent adversities, and client counseling with informed consent is indicated when off-label dosing presents potential harm to the patient.

The approach taken to determine a dosing regimen for a patient depends on the information that is available—that is, how much is needed (PD) and how much is achieved (PK) (Table 6-4). In each instance it is assumed that patient factors are well known.

A target C_{max} can be calculated from MIC data that have been adjusted for time or concentration dependency. The dose of a drug administered intravenously is calculated as dose = target concentration * V_d For orally administered drugs, the V_d must be corrected for bioavailability (F): dose = target concentration * V_d/F (see Chapter 1). For antimicrobials the target concentration, or "what is needed," is the MIC of the infecting microbe or a reasonable surrogate, such as the $MIC_{90,}$ modified as needed to account for host, drug, or microbial factors For a concentration-dependent drug, the MIC or MIC_{90} must be multiplied tenfold to achieve the targeted PDI C_{max}/MIC ≥10. Thus for amikacin, a concentration-dependent drug, the targeted PDI for a patient infected with an *E. coli* with an MIC of 4 μg/mL is 40 μg/mL. If infection is in extracellular tissue and concentrations that are lower than in plasma are anticipated, the target C_{max} plasma may need to be multiplied by 2 or more to achieve the target in tissues. Thus the target becomes 80 μg/mL.

For amikacin the reported V_d in dogs is 0.23 L/kg. Assume an infection is in the lungs, where drug concentrations reach 50% of PDC. The dose of amikacin to target a microbe causing infection in the lungs then would be 4 μg/mL (mg/L) * 10 * 2* 0.23* L/kg or 18.4 mg/kg. If the drug is given by a route other than intravenous, the dose must be modified further for bioavailability. For example, if amikacin is generally about 70% bioavailable (F=0.7) following subcutaneous administration, the subcutaneous dose for *E. coli* would be (4 μg/mL (mg/L) * 10 * 2* 0.23* L/kg)/0.7 = 27 mg/kg. As the MIC for this *E. coli* and amikacin was quite low, next consider the same approach for a *P. aeruginosa* with an MIC of 16 μg/mL. If the infection is in the upper respiratory tract (e.g., sinus of a cat), distribution will probably be <30% of that in plasma (multiply dose by 3). The calculated dose would be 16 mg/L * 10 * 3.3*0.23 L/kg or 121 mg/kg. This is well beyond the recommended dose, and although it might be safe given once daily in a normal patient (drug concentrations would reach the target trough of 2 μg/mL by 6 to12 hours after dosing), the risk of adversity may outweigh the benefits of treatment with this dose. Combination therapy is indicated for this patient.

The design of a dosing regimen for a time-dependent antimicrobial is more complicated. For a time-dependent drug, the magnitude of C_{max} depends on how many half-lives are to elapse between doses. The ratio of C_{max}/MIC is important for determining the number of half-lives that can elapse before PDC = MIC. A good start is to multiply the MIC fourfold (C_{max}/MIC = 4) to allow a duration of two half-lives for T > MIC (each doubling of the ratio or dose provides another half-life of T > MIC). The duration of the dosing interval then depends on the desired duration of T > MIC. For T > MIC = 50%, the duration of the dosing interval is twice the number of half-lives that T > MIC; in this case, (C_{max}/MIC = 4), the dosing interval will be 4 half-lives. Although this sounds adequate, in reality, it may not be for drugs with a short half-life. For example, if the drug of interest is amoxicillin (half-life = 1 to 1.5 hr), the duration of the interval is 4 to 6 hrs, assuming all drug in plasma makes it to the site of infection. Thus, the ratio of C_{max}/MIC may need to be higher for drugs with a short half-life if a convenient dosing interval is desired. Alternatively, a drug with a longer half-life can be chosen. Using cefpodoxime as an example, based on package insert data, the MIC_{90} of *S. intermedius* is 0.5 μg/mL. Peak concentrations at 10 mg/kg approximate 15 μg/mL, yielding a ratio C_{max}/MIC of 30. The time that elapses before C_{max} and MIC reach unity is just under 5 half-lives (30 to 15 to 7.5 to 3.5 to 1.75 to 0.75. With a half-life of 4.5 hours, T > MIC duration approximates 24 hours. Theoretically, if the target is T > MIC = 50%, a dosing interval of 48 hours might be possible. However, the PDI upon which time and concentration dependency are based are limited to a 24 hr period, thus a 24-hr-dosing interval is prudent. This is particularly true if the drug is targeting tough-to-penetrate tissues or inflammatory debris: the concentration might then be reduced to 10 μg/mL, yielding a C_{max}/MIC of 10, or a duration of 2 half-lives, or 9 hours, for T > MIC. In this situation, a 24-hour dosing interval might be more appropriate; a 12-hour dosing interval might be prudent. Further, these calculations are based on a target of T > MIC of 50%. Although this target is often recommended, T > MIC of 75% to 100% might be better to minimize the risk of resistance, particularly in a patient at risk. Therapeutic drug monitoring can be used to establish or confirm a dose or interval for a drug for the individual patient and is ideally the basis of dose modification for critical patients. Unfortunately, few drugs (primarily the aminoglycosides and vancomycin) can be rapidly and accurately measured at a reasonable cost. The risks associated with these drugs, including the potential cost of using them at ineffective doses, however, may justify the cost.

Duration of Therapy

Among the most difficult decisions regarding antimicrobial therapy is the duration of administration. Generally, the duration of therapy should be 2 to 3 days beyond resolution of clinical signs. Indeed, if the dosing regimen is designed according to the saying "dead bugs don't mutate," then clinical signs of resolution should emerge rapidly. This is true, however, only if the clinical signs are discreet and able to respond rapidly. Such is not likely to be true in the absence of fever, or when radiographic resolution of inflammation or healing of inflamed skin are benchmarks. Not surprisingly, clinicians often adhere to the "longer is better" approach. However, emerging data in human medicine suggest a more pro-active approach to therapy duration reduction is prudent. Animal models have demonstrated that therapy beyond 5 days increases the intensity

Table 6-8 Examples of Synergistic Drug Combinations

Drug One	Drug Two	Organisms
Dicloxacillin	Ampicillin, penicillin, cephalothins	*Escherichia coli, Klebsiella, Pseudomonas aeruginosa*
β-Lactam: cephalothin, ampicillin, piperacillin, cefotaxime, cefamandole	Aminoglycoside: gentamicin, amikacin	*Escherichia coli, Pseudomonas, aeruginosa,* enterococci, others
Chloramphenicol	Ampicillin	*Salmonella typhimurium, Staphylococcus aureus* (effect is bacteriostatic in nature)
Penicillin	Gentamicin	*Bacteroides melaninogenicus*
Imipenem	Vancomycin	*Staphylococcus aureus*
β-Lactam, vancomycin	Aminoglycoside	*Staphylococcus aureus*
Trimethoprim/sulfonamide	Imipenem, amikacin	*Nocardia asteroides* (effect is bacteriostatic)
Imipenem	Trimethoprim/sulfonamide, cefotaxime	*Nocardia asteroides* (effect is bacteriostatic)
Ethambutol	Rifampin, aminoglycosides, ciprofloxacin (enrofloxacin), clarithromycin	*Mycobacterium avium* (effect is bacteriostatic)

From Wiedemann B, Atkinson BA: Susceptibility to antibiotics: species incidence and trends. In Lorian V, editor: *Antibiotics in laboratory medicine*, Baltimore, 1996, Williams & Wilkins, pp. 900-1168.

of drug therapy necessary to prevent emergent resistance.[174] In human medicine a number of clinical studies have investigated the impact that reduced duration of therapy might have on efficacy and resistance. In general, the longer-is-better approach is not appropriate.[175] Five days of therapy has been suggested as the upper limit in selected populations, including intrabdominal infections,[175,176] community-acquired pneumonia,[177] and other respiratory tract infections,[178] and 3 days for pneumonia characterized by a low likelihood of becoming nosocomial.[179] These studies demonstrate the increasing focus on the role of duration of therapy in the advent of resistance. However, their extrapolation to companion animals is not clear, in part because compliance differences might affect results. Exceptions for which duration of therapy might be longer include infection of sites characterized by poor local immunity (or the immunocompromised patient), tissues in which healing is prolonged, or in the presence of foreign bodies that facilitate antimicrobial growth. Exceptions also may apply to slow growing organisms.

KEY POINT 6-30 For uncomplicated infections the duration of therapy should be 5 to 7 days or less.

Combination Antimicrobial Therapy

Combination therapy can be used to achieve a broad antimicrobial spectrum for empirical therapy, treat a polymicrobial infection involving organisms not susceptible to the same drugs, reduce the likelihood of antimicrobial resistance, and reduce the risk of adverse drug reactions by minimizing doses of potentially toxic antimicrobials.[23,24,26,137] Rational combination antimicrobial therapy may be the single most effective action taken to enhance antimicrobial efficacy for the chronic or serious infection. Primary reasons to avoid combination therapy include increases in risk of suprainfection, risk of toxicity (if both drugs are potentially toxic), high cost, and inconvenience to the patient.[24]

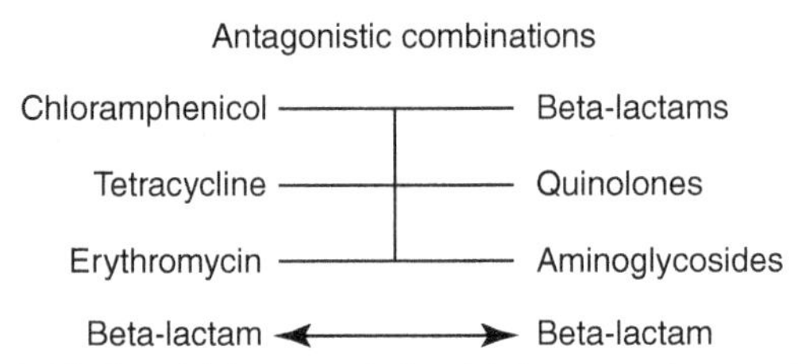

Figure 6-21 Combining antimicrobials can have different sequelae. Antagonistic antimicrobial combinations most commonly result when a drug that inhibits bacterial growth is combined with a drug whose action depends on rapid cell growth. Drugs that act at the same site may be antagonistic, additive, or synergistic (e.g., beta-lactams, depending which penicillin binding protein is targeted).

Synergism and Antagonism

Antimicrobials to be used in combination therapy should be selected rationally and based on target organisms as well as on mechanism of action (Table 6-8). Combinations might result in antagonistic, additive, or synergistic antimicrobial effects (Figure 6-21).[180] Generally, these effects are defined by in in vitro systems; clinical relevance is more difficult to establish. Also, the combined effects of two or more antimicrobials are likely to differ with the organism. Avoidance of *antagonism* is particularly important for patients with inadequate host defenses.[23,24,26,180] In general, bacteriostatic drugs that inhibit ribosomes and thus microbial growth (e.g., chloramphenicol, tetracyclines, erythromycin) should not be combined with drugs whose mechanism of action depends on protein synthesis such as growth of the organism (e.g., beta-lactams) or formation of a target protein. The bactericidal activity and continued degradation or destruction of the microbial target of beta-lactams and FQs depend on continued synthesis of bacterial proteins. Antagonistic effects have been well documented between beta-lactam antibiotics and inhibitors of ribosomal activity. The degree of antagonism between FQs and growth inhibitors is controversial; antagonism has been reported with the use of ciprofloxacin and chloramphenicol,[180] but impaired efficacy was not detected in other studies.[181] Antagonism between chloramphenicol and gentamicin has also been documented.[180] Occasionally, the combination of a bacteriostatic ribosomal inhibitor and a drug whose efficacy depends on rapid growth might enhance efficacy, even though the "-cidal" drug will act only in a "static" fashion. For example, chloramphenicol enhances the efficacy of ampicillin toward *Salmonella typhimurium* and *Staphylcoccus* spp., presumably because it inhibits the production of beta-lactamases by the organisms that might otherwise destroy ampicllin.

KEY POINT 6-31 The appropriate combination of two drugs characterized by resistance may render the microbe susceptible.

Chemical antagonism is also possible between two or more antimicrobials (see Chapter 2).[181,182] Aminoglycosides and quinolones are chemically inactivated by penicillins at sufficient concentrations. Ticarcillin has been used therapeutically to reduce the risk of toxicity in a patient overdosed with an aminoglycoside.[183] Chemical antagonism is unlikely in most clinical uses of these drugs. The risk of antagonism is increased, however, with simultaneous intravenous use of high doses of both ticarcillin and aminoglycosides, such as might occur if aminoglycosides are administered once daily. Potential chemical interactions between other antimicrobials should be identified before combination therapy. Certainly, antimicrobials should not be mixed in the same syringe or intravenous line unless a lack of antagonism has been confirmed.[182]

Drugs that have the same mechanism of action may act in an additive or synergistic fashion. For example, chloramphenicol and clindamycin bind the same 50S ribosomal subunit and will antagonize each other. Because tetracyclines bind to the 30S ribosomal subunit, combination with antimicrobials that target the 50S subunit might be considered (e.g., the phenicols, macrolides, and lincosamides) if there is scientific support. One study indicates an in vitro synergistic effect of the combined use of doxycycline and azithromycin against *P. aeruginosa*.[183a]

Additive effects probably occur when active metabolites are produced from an active parent compound, such as metabolism of enrofloxacin to ciprofloxacin.[184] Antagonistic effects might occur, however, if the drugs compete for a limited number of target sites (e.g., chloramphenicol and erythromycin). In contrast, synergistic actions might occur if the antimicrobial targets are subtly different. For example, a combination of different beta-lactams generally results in additive antimicrobial activity. If the two antimicrobials target different PBPs, however, their combined effect may actually be synergistic ("double beta-lactam therapy").[185,186] In contrast, combinations of other beta-lactam antibiotics (including combining selected cephalosporins) are antagonistic.[186] The different sequelae of combined beta-lactam therapy might be caused by the PBPs targeted by each drug.

Synergism between antimicrobials can occur if the two antimicrobials kill bacteria through independent mechanisms or through sequential pathways toward the same target.[180,187] The combination of trimethoprim and a sulfonamide exemplifies synergism resulting from sequential actions in the same metabolic pathway (see discussion of potentiated sulfonamides) (see Chapter 7). Clavulanic acid "draws" the beta-lactamase activity of the microorganism away, allowing the protective beta-lactam to impair cell wall synthesis. Synergism between beta-lactams and aminoglycosides exemplifies synergism resulting from killing by independent pathways. Synergism is expected because their mechanisms of action complement one another, but efficacy is enhanced further because aminoglycoside movement into the bacteria is enhanced by increased cell wall permeability induced by the beta-lactam (Figure 6-22).[180,188] Indeed, aminoglycoside activity against enterococci is adequate only when used synergistically with a cell wall–active antimicrobial, such as beta-lactams and vancomycin. Synergism also has been demonstrated against some strains of Enterobacteriaceae; *P. aeruginosa*; staphylococci, including MRSA; and other microorganisms. However, these organisms are not always inhibited by the combination of aminoglycoside and cell wall–active compounds. Indeed, antagonism has been described between aminoglycosides and beta-lactams against an MRSA, presumably because of induction of an aminoglycoside-modifying enzyme. Enhanced movement in a bacteria may occur with other drugs (e.g., potentiated sulfonamides, FQs) when combined with beta-lactams (see Figure 6-22). Rifampin is another drug for which combined use enchances antimicrobial efficacy of a number of drugs.

Combination therapy is a powerful tool for enhancing efficacy (Figure 6-23) as well as preventing resistance. Occasionally, the combination of drugs, which by themselves would not be expected to have efficacy against organisms not included in their spectrum, may exhibit efficacy against the organisms. For example, azithromycin and clarithromycin may exhibit synergistic effects with several other drugs against *P. aeruginosa*. When studied in patients with cystic fibrosis, the most active combinations demonstrating synergy were azithromycin combined with sulfadiazine/trimethoprim or doxycycline. Azithromycin occasionally demonstrated synergism against *P. aeruginosa* when combined with timentin, piperacillin/tazobactam, ceftazidime, meropenem, imipenem, ciprofloxacin, travofloxacin, chloramphenicol, and tobramycin.[189] In the treatment of *S. aureus*, clindamycin inhibits early rapid killing of amikacin but acts synergistically with it at 24 to 48 hours.[190]

Polymicrobial Infections

Combination antimicrobial therapy may be selected because of the presence of a polymicrobial infection (Figure 6-24).[23,24,77,191] Aminoglycosides or FQs are often combined with beta-lactams, metronidazole, or clindamycin to target both aerobic gram-positive and gram-negative infections or infections caused by both aerobes and anaerobes. The combined use of selected antimicrobials may result in therapy effective against a given microbe when either drug alone was ineffective.

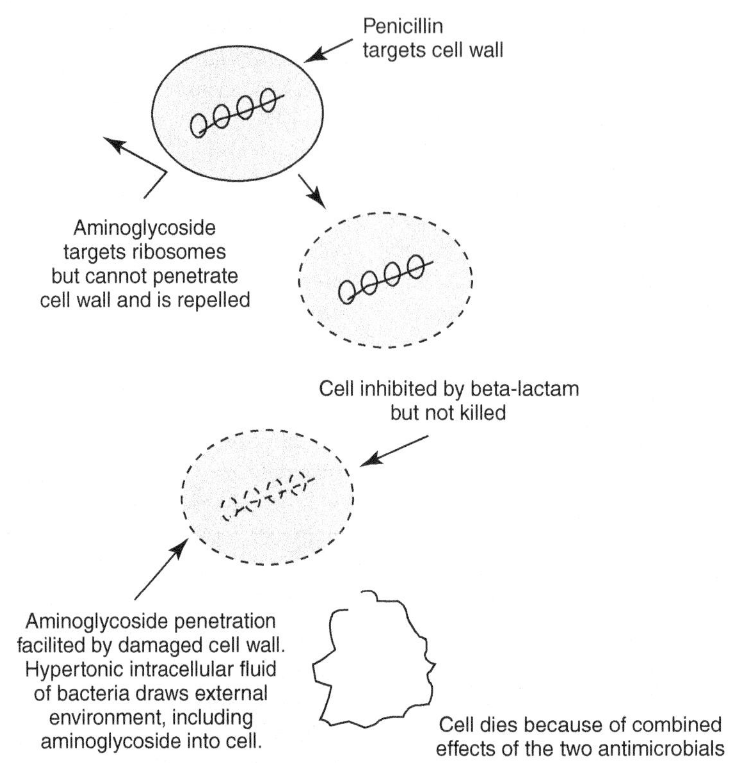

Figure 6-22 The combination of any number of drugs with a beta-lactam may result in synergistic antimicrobial effects. The prototypic example is a beta-lactam combined with an aminoglycoside, a class of water-soluble drugs whose movement through the cell to target ribosomes is limited. Changes in the cell wall permeability associated with the beta-lactam exposes the hypertonic (compared with the host) intracellular cytoplasm to the isotonic host, resulting in the influx of solutes into the organism. Intracellular access is thus facilitated for drugs also in the environment. Together, the two drugs are now more likely to kill the microbe. Such synergism has been documented in vitro between beta-lactams and a number of drugs, particularly those classified as bactericidal.

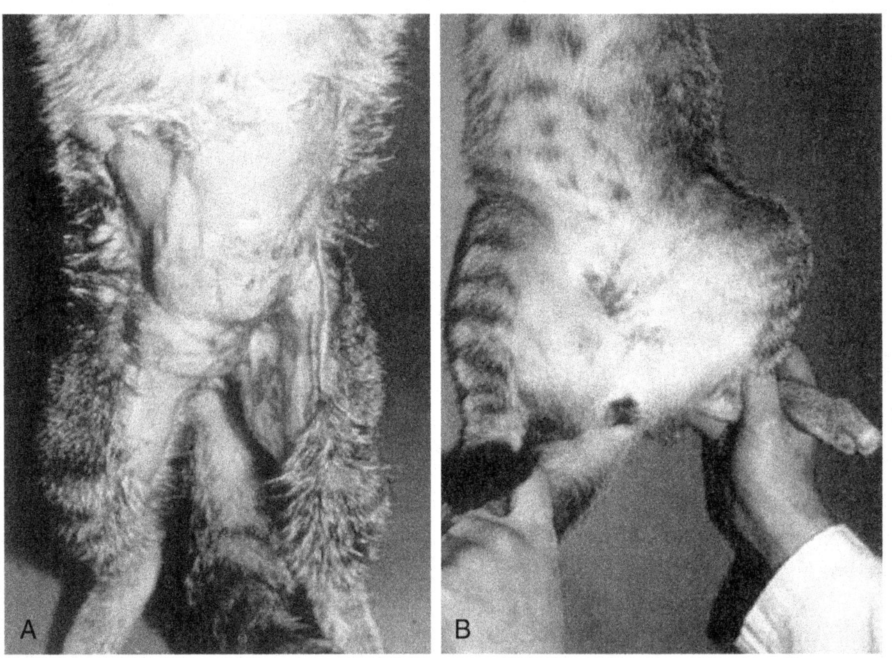

Figure 6-23 Atypical mycobacterium in a cat is associated with marked inflammation, including deposition of fibrous tissue deposition. This cat was successfully treated with a combination of sulfadiazine/trimethoprim and enrofloxacin after 3 months of therapy.

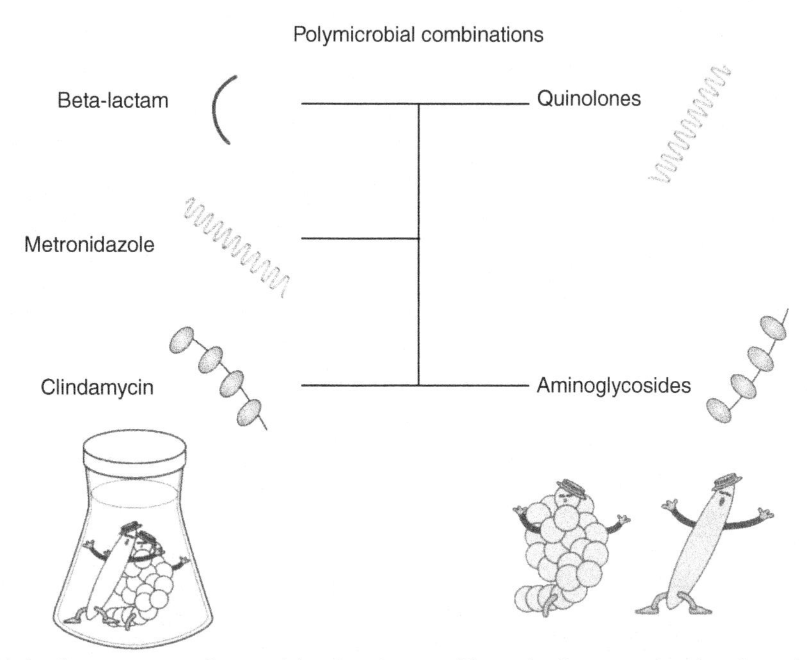

Figure 6-24 Polymicrobial infections may require combination therapy. The quinolones and aminoglycosides offer excellent aerobic gram-negative coverage; the beta-lactams (especially penicillins), metronidazole, and clindamycin offer excellent gram-positive and anaerobic coverage.

ANTIMICROBIAL PROPHYLAXIS

The prophylactic use of antimicrobials should be distinguished from treatment. The presence of infection or anticipated infection after bacterial contamination (e.g., an open fracture, contamination of abdominal contents with intestinal fluid) indicates the need for treatment rather than prophylaxis. If antimicrobial prophylaxis is to be implemented in anticipation of an invasive procedure (e.g., surgery), the following should serve as a basis for selection: The antimicrobial should target the most likely pathogenic organism, adequate concentrations of drug should be at the site of invasion before potential contamination, the antimicrobial should either have a long elimination half-life or be redosed during lengthy procedures, the least toxic drug should be selected, and the duration of therapy should be as short as possible.[23,26]

Prophylactic antimicrobials should not be used indiscriminately in the immunocompromised animal. The granulocytopenic patient is particularly predisposed to the development of suprainfection. Suprainfection occurs in 10% to 20% of human granulocytopenic patients receiving empirical broad-spectrum antimicrobials. Prolonging therapy increases the chance that suprainfection will occur.[26] Prophylactic suppression of gastrointestinal flora is recommended in human patients who are profoundly granulocytopenic for more than 2 weeks. Traditional use of nonabsorbable antimicrobials effective against aerobic gram-negative organisms (e.g., neomycin) and drugs that target anaerobic organisms (e.g., metronidazole) are being replaced by use of trimethoprim/sulfonamide combinations or FQs.[26] Trimethoprim/sulfonamide combinations are more palatable and less expensive, yet they are equally effective in preventing infections when compared with more expensive drugs in human critically ill patients. FQs allow persistence of anaerobic organisms in the gastrointestinal tract, thus reducing overgrowth of resistant gram-negative organisms and preventing rapid repopulation and overgrowth of aerobic gram-negative organisms as the antimicrobial is discontinued.

Other indications for medical prophylaxis include dentistry and prevention of recurrent, chronic infections (e.g., urinary tract, skin). The use of antimicrobials prophylactically for these conditions is discussed separately in the corresponding chapter.

SURGICAL PROPHYLAXIS*

Antimicrobial prophylaxis is defined as the administration of an antimicrobial agent in the absence of infection. The aim of antimicrobial prophylaxis is to reduce the number of viable bacteria present in the surgical wound to a level that normal host defenses can handle, thus preventing infection. Contaminating bacteria can enter the surgical wound from exogenous sources or the patient's endogenous flora. Exogenous sources include surgical equipment, the surgery room, and surgical personnel. Duration of the surgical procedure plays a role in the incidence of wound infections, especially for procedures that last longer than 90 minutes.

Endogenous bacterial sources probably play a greater role in postoperative infections than exogenous sources. Endogenous sources include skin and mucosal surfaces that are transected during surgery. Hematogenous spread of bacteria may result from overt or occult septic foci or dental manipulations.

**Harry W. Boothe*

Such sources should be either eliminated before surgery by appropriate therapeutic antimicrobial agents or avoided by not combining dental manipulations with surgery of body cavities (abdominal or thoracic) or orthopedic procedures.

Antimicrobial prophylaxis is not a substitute for good surgical practices, which include aseptic technique and gentle tissue handling. Considerations in the use of antimicrobial prophylaxis are the type of surgery, potential pathogens encountered, host competence, and pharmacologic and antibacterial properties of the antimicrobial agent.

Type of Surgery

Surgical wounds are classified as clean, clean-contaminated, contaminated, or dirty. Clean wounds are made under aseptic conditions, are closed primarily, and are not drained. Prophylactic antimicrobial therapy is not warranted for most clean procedures because bacterial contamination is minor, and the patient's competence helps prevent wound infection. Possible indications for the use of antimicrobials in clean surgical procedures are when the consequences of infection would be catastrophic (e.g., total joint replacement) or when surgical implants are used.

Clean-contaminated wounds include those made in the gastrointestinal, genitourinary, or respiratory tract without significant intraoperative spillage. Also, clean procedures in which a break in sterile procedure occurred are considered clean-contaminated. Clean-contaminated wounds may benefit from prophylactic antimicrobial therapy, and consideration of the following factors seems appropriate when contemplating the use of perioperative antimicrobial therapy: number of resident bacteria encountered, amount of spillage expected, and impact of disease condition on bacterial colonization. Resident bacterial numbers vary depending on the site of the tract incised and the nature of disease. In the normal gastrointestinal tract, resident bacteria are numerous in the oropharyngeal cavity, distal ileum, and colon. Numbers are normally much lower in the distal esophagus, stomach, and most of the small intestine. The normal genitourinary tract above the distal urethra has low bacterial populations. The normal trachea and bronchi also have relatively sparse flora. Although amount of spillage cannot always be predicted preoperatively, prophylactic antimicrobials are probably indicated if the risk of intraoperative spillage seems high. Diseases, in general, tend to modify both bacterial numbers (usually increased numbers) and populations (usually more virulent forms).

Contaminated wounds include those in which there is acute, nonpurulent inflammation or those in which gross contamination from a hollow viscus occurs. Antimicrobial prophylaxis is generally warranted when surgery is performed on contaminated wounds. Also, the presence of extensive tissue damage or accumulation of blood within wounds may warrant prophylactic drug administration, because bacterial colonization is usually promoted.

Dirty or infected wounds benefit from irrigation with antiseptics. Chlorhexidine (0.05%) is an effective wound disinfectant for infected wounds. Use of antimicrobials (systemically, topically, or both) is generally indicated before surgery to treat an infected or dirty wound. Such use is more appropriately termed *therapeutic antimicrobial therapy*.

Potential Pathogens Encountered

The most frequently encountered pathogenic bacterial contaminants of surgical wounds are *Staphylococcus* spp. and *E. coli*. The most common skin bacteria are *Staphylococcus* spp., although many other organisms may be present as transient, topical flora. The oropharynx has a mixed population of gram-positive organisms (especially *Staphylococcus* spp., *Streptococcus* spp., and *Actinomyces pyogenes*), gram-negative organisms (*Proteus, Pasteurella, Pseudomonas,* and *E. coli*), and anaerobic organisms. The stomach and small intestine have very few organisms normally present, whereas the distal ileum and large intestine have large numbers of gram-negative (especially *E. coli* and *Klebsiella, Pseudomonas,* and *Salmonella* spp.) and anaerobic organisms. Potential pathogens encountered in the genitourinary tract include both gram-positive and gram-negative organisms (especially *Staphylococcus* and *Streptococcus* spp., *E. coli,* and *Proteus* and *Pseudomonas* spp.). Pathogens of the respiratory tract (especially lower respiratory tract) include both gram-positive organisms (*Staphylococcus* spp., *Streptococcus* spp., and *A. pyogenes*) and gram-negative organisms (*Pseudomonas* spp., *E. coli,* and *Klebsiella, Pasteurella,* and *Enterobacter* spp.).

Host Competence

Host resistance may be compromised systemically or locally. Patients with systemic immunodeficiency often have chronic, recurrent, or partially responsive infections. Prophylactic antimicrobial therapy is probably indicated for such patients regardless of the surgical procedure to be performed. Secondary immunodeficiencies have been associated with a variety of diseases, including hepatic or renal failure, hyperadrenocorticism, diabetes mellitus, and neoplasia. Other factors that may affect systemic host competence include advanced age, severe malnutrition, obesity, immunosuppressive drugs, and splenectomy.

Local factors of importance in the maintenance of host competence include tissue perfusion and tissue trauma. The competence of local defense mechanisms may be affected adversely by obstruction, neoplasia, ulceration, and hemorrhage. For example, the bacterial flora of a stagnant loop of jejunum caused by intestinal obstruction resembles that of the normal distal ileum (i.e., large numbers of resident bacteria). For the purposes of selecting perioperative antimicrobials, the clinician should accurately assess host competence before the surgical procedure.

Pharmacologic and Antibacterial Properties

The primary goal to be achieved by administration of prophylactic antimicrobial agents is to produce adequate concentrations of antimicrobial at the surgical incision site at the time of wound contamination. Also important is the concept that the major risk of contamination is at the time of surgery until a fibrin seal develops between wound edges (approximately 3 to 5 hours postoperatively). Factors of importance in the use of perioperative antimicrobials are absorption (timing and route of administration), distribution, and elimination characteristics. Absorption issues are of least concern with intravenously administered antimicrobials. For most antimicrobials distribution is relatively rapid and complete within 30 to 60 minutes after intravenous administration. The concentration of drug achieved in the tissue correlates with the concentration of free drug in the serum. Highly protein-bound drugs (i.e., little free drug in the serum) achieve lower tissue concentrations than do weakly bound agents (e.g., cefazolin, gentamicin, and ampicillin). Other factors such as lipid solubility, pH, and local environment may also influence tissue penetration of the drug. Elimination of most antimicrobials is principally by way of the kidneys. The rate of elimination determines the dosing interval that is selected. More rapidly eliminated drugs require more frequent administration. Cefazolin, for example, should be administered at 2-hour intervals during the surgical procedure to maintain adequate tissue and serum levels.

The following prophylactic antimicrobial regimen seems appropriate: an intravenous dose of drug given 30 to 60 minutes before incision (i.e., at anesthetic induction) and another dose given at the completion of the procedure. If the surgical procedure lasts longer than 3 hours, an additional intraoperative dose of antimicrobial should be given approximately 2 to 3 hours after the initial dose. There is no rationale for continuing antibiotic administration longer than 24 hours after surgery in the absence of documented infection. If infection is documented, therapeutic antimicrobial therapy is initiated.

The selected drug should be bactericidal for the pathogens that are most likely to contaminate the surgical site. First-generation cephalosporins (e.g., cefazolin) are generally as effective as and less expensive than second- and third-generation cephalosporins. Surgery of the lower gastrointestinal tract may require a more elaborate schedule of prophylactic drug administration, partly because of the presence of anaerobic organisms. A second-generation cephalosporin (e.g., cefoxitin) or an aminoglycoside/anaerobic combination (e.g., amikacin and clindamycin or gentamicin and amoxicillin) should be administered systemically. The use of oral antimicrobials for prophylaxis may not be prudent, in part, because peak concentrations are likely to be less than with intravenous administration, even if bioavailability is close to 100% (and many are not).

Inappropriate perioperative antimicrobial use has been shown to increase the incidence of complications. Examples of inappropriate perioperative antimicrobial use include use of antimicrobials for clean surgical procedures, initiation of prophylactic antimicrobials postoperatively, and continuation of antimicrobial administration for longer than 24 hours. Each of these actions risks the occurrence of one or more of the following complications: reduced efficacy, suprainfection, selection of resistant bacterial pathogens, greater client cost, and a potential for higher incidence of drug-associated complications.

Although surgical prophylaxis has been integrated into the perioperative surgical plans for veterinary patients, surprising little information supports its use. In one controlled study of dogs (n = 329) and cats (n = 544) undergoing clean and clean-contaminated surgical procedures, the postoperative infection rate did not differ in placebo (9.4%) compared with the cephalexin-pretreated group (8.9%).[192] In another study investigating the impact of flushing in dogs undergoing total ear canal ablation, organisms were characterized by a higher incidence of antimicrobial resistance to cefazolin,[29] suggesting that cefazolin may not be a rational choice in all presurgical candidates.

REFERENCES

1. Dancer SJ: The problem with cephalosporins, *J Antimicro Chemother* 48:463–478, 2001.
2. Harrison PF, Lederberg J: *Antimicrobial resistance: issues and options, Forum on Emerging Infections Workshop Report, Institute of Medicine*, Washington DC, 1998, National Academy Press.
3. Evans HL, Lefrak SN, Lyman J, et al: Cost of gram-negative resistance, *Crit Care Med* 35(1):89–95, 2007.
4. Divita D: Adding up antimicrobial use, *J Am Vet Med Assoc* 219:1071–1076, 2001.
5. O'Rourke K: Small animal veterinarians may come under scrutiny for antimicrobial use, *J Am Vet Med Assoc* 221:760–761, 2002.
6. Guardabassi L, Schwarz S, Lloyd DH: Pet animals as reservoirs of antimicrobial-resistant bacteria, *J Antimicro Chem* 54: 321–332, 2004.
7. Damborg P, Olsen KE, Moller NE, et al: Occurrence of campylobacter jejuni in pets living with human patients infected with *C. jejuni*, *J Clin Microbiol* 42(3):1363–1364, 2004.
8. Gortel K, Campbell KL, Kakoma I, et al: Methicillin resistance among staphylococci isolated from dogs, *Am J Vet Res* 60(12):1526–1530, 1999.
9. Kania SA, Williamson NL, Frank LA: Methicillin resistance of staphyloccci isolated from the skin of dogs with pyoderma, *J Am Vet Med Assoc* 65:1285–1268, 2004.
10. Strommenger B, Kehrenberg C, Kettlitz C, et al: Molecular characterization of methicillin-resistant *Staphylococcus aureus* strains from pet animals and their relationship to human isolates, *J Antimicrob Chemother* 57:461–465, 2006.
11. Pottumarthy S, Schapiro JM, Prentice JL, et al: Clinical isolates of *Staphylococcus intermedius* masquerading as methicillin-resistant *Staphylococcus aureus*, *J Clin Microbiol* 42(12): 5881–5884, 2004.
12. van Loo I, Huijsdens X, Tiemersma E, et al: Emergence of methicillin-resistant staphylococcus aureus of animal origin in humans, *Emerg Infect Dis* 13(12):1834–1839, 2007.
13. Johnson JR, Clabots C, Kuskowski MA: Multiple-host sharing, long-term persistence, and virulence of *Escherichia coli* clones from human and animal household members, *J Clin Microbiol* 46(12):4078–4082, 2008.
14. Miller K, O'Neill AJ, Chopra I: *Escherichia coli* mutators present an enhanced risk for emergence of antibiotic resistance during urinary tract infections, *Antimicrob Agents Chemother* 48:23–29, 2004.
15. Russo TA, Johnson JR: Medical and economic impact of extraintestinal infections due to *Escherichia coli*: an overlooked epidemic, *Microbes Infect* 5:449–456, 2003.
16. Marsik FJ, Parisi JT, Blenden DC: Transmissible drug resistance of *Escherichia coli* and *Salmonella* from humans, animals, and their rural environments, *J Infect Dis* 132(3):296–302, 1975.
17. Davies J: Microbes have the last word. A drastic re-evaluation of antimicrobial treatment is needed to overcome the threat of antibiotic-resistant bacteria, *EMBO Rep* 8(7):616–621, 2007.
18. Owens RC, Fraser GL, Stogsdill P: Antimicrobial stewardship programs as a means to optimize antimicrobial use, *Pharmacotherapy* 24(7):896–908, 2004.

19. Schlegel HG, Jannasch HW: Prokaryotes and their habitats. In Dworkin M, editor: *The prokaryotes: a handbook on the biology of bacteria*, ed 3, vol 1, Philadelphia, 2006, Springer, pp 137–184.
20. van Hal SJ, Stark D, Lockwood B, et al: Methicillin-resistant *Staphylococcus aureus* (MRSA) detection: comparison of two molecular methods (IDI-MRSA PCR assay and geno type MRSA direct PCR assay) with three selective MRSA agars (MRSA ID, MRSA *Select*, and CHROMagar MRSA) for use with infection-control swabs, *J Clin Microbiol* 45(8):2486–2490, 2007.
21. Casadevall A, Pirofski L: What is a pathogen? *Ann Med* 34:2–4, 2002.
22. Yoshikawa TT: Empiric antimicrobial therapy. In Ristuccia AM, Cunha BA, editors: *Antimicrobial therapy*, New York, 1984, Raven Press, pp 125–135.
23. Chambers HF: General principles of antimicrobial therapy. In Brunton LL, Lazo JS, Parker KL, editors: *Goodman & Gilman's the pharmacological basis of therapeutics*, ed 11, New York, 2006, McGraw-Hill.
24. Kapusnik J, Miller RT, Sande MA: Antibacterial therapy in critical care. In Schoemaker WC, Ayers S, Grenvik A, et al, editors: *Textbook of critical care*, ed 2, Philadelphia, 1989, Saunders, pp 780–801.
25. Greene CE: *Infectious diseases of the dog and cat*, ed 3, St Louis, 2006, Saunders.
26. Githaiga A, Ndirangu M, Peterson DL: Infections in the immunocompromised patient. In Fink M, editor: *Textbook of critical care*, ed 5, Philadelphia, 2005, Saunders.
27. Hardie EM: Sepsis versus septic shock. In Murtaugh RJ, Kaplan PM, editors: *Veterinary emergency and critical care medicine*, St Louis, 1992, Mosby.
28. Boothe DM: *The accumulation of pradofloxacin in phagocytes. Abstract*, Berlin, 2006, 1st International Verafloxacin Symposium, 18.
29. Hettlich BF, Boothe HW, Simpson RB, et al: Effect of tympanic cavity evacuation and flushing on microbial isolates during total ear canal ablation with lateral bulla osteotomy in dogs, *J Am Vet Med Assoc* 227:748–755, 2005.
30. Boothe HW, Howe LM, Boothe DM, Reynolds LA, Carpenter M: Evaluation of outcomes in dogs treated for pyothorax: 46 cases (1983-2001), *J Am Vet Med Assoc* 236(6):657–663, 2010:Mar 15.
31. Shaheen BW, Boothe DM, Oyarzabal OA, Smaha T: Antimicrobial resistance profiles and clonal relatedness of canine and feline *Escherichia coli* pathogens expressing multidrug resistance in the United States, *J Vet Intern Med* 24(2):323–330, 2010:Mar-Apr.
32. Turnidge JD, Bell JM: Antimicrobial susceptibility on solid media. In Lorian V, editor: *Antibiotics in laboratory medicine*, Baltimore, 2005, Williams & Wilkins, pp 8–60.
33. Schwaber M, Cosgrove SE, Gold H: Fluoroquinolones protective against cephalosporin resistance in gram negative nosocomial pathogens, *Emerg Infec Dis* 10(1):94–99, 2004.
34. Ford A: Swab story—getting the most from wound cultures, *CAP Today*, 2009. Accessed November 12, 2009, at http://www.thepathologycenter.org/Swab%20Story.pdf.
35. Eliopoulos GM, Ambrose PG, Bradford PA, et al: *M23-A3 Development of in vitro susceptibility testing criteria and quality control parameters, Approved Guideline*, ed 3, Wayne, Penn, 2008, Clinical and Laboratory Standards Institute.
36. Cockerill FR, Wikler MA, Rex JG, et al: *M100-S19 Performance standards for antimicrobial susceptibility testing; Nineteenth Informational Supplement*, ed 3, Wayne, Penn, 2009, Clinical Laboratory Standards Institute.
37. Watts JL, Apley M, Bade DJ, et al: *M37-A3 Development of in vitro susceptibility testing criteria and quality control parameters for veterinary antimicrobial agents; Approved Guideline*, ed 3, Wayne, Penn, 2008, Clinical Laboratory Standards Institute.
38. Watts JL, Shryock TR, Apley M, et al: *M31-A2 Performance standards for antimicrobial disk and dilution susceptibility tests for bacteria isolated from animals, Approved Standard*, ed 3, Wayne, Penn, 2008, Clinical Laboratory Standards Institute.
39. Arbeit RD, Arbique JC, Beall B, et al: *MM11-A Molecular methods for bacterial strain typing, Approved Guidelines*, Wayne, Penn, 2007, Clinical Laboratory Standards Institute.
40. Turnidge JD, Bell JM: Antimicrobial susceptibility on solid media. In Lorian V, editor: *Antibiotics in laboratory medicine*, Baltimore, 2005, Williams & Wilkins, pp 8–60.
41. Amsterdam D: Susceptibility testing of antimicrobials in liquid media. In Lorian V, editor: *Antibiotics in laboratory medicine*, Baltimore, 2005, Williams & Wilkins, pp 61–142.
42. Tenover FC, Williams PP, Stocker S, et al: Accuracy of six antimicrobial susceptibility methods for testing linezolid against staphylococci and enterococci, *J Clin Microbiol* 45(9): 2917–2922, 2007.
43. Stegemann MR, Passmore CA, Sherington J, et al: Antimicrobial activity and spectrum of cefovecin, a new extended-spectrum cephalosporin, against pathogens collected from dogs and cats in Europe and North America, *Antimicrob Agents Chemother* 50(7):2286–2292, 2006.
44. Stegemann MR, Sherington J, Blanchflower S: Pharmacokinetics and pharmacodynamics of cefovecin in dogs, *J Vet Pharmacol Ther* 29:501–511, 2006.
45. Mouton JW, Dudley MN, Cars O, et al: Standardization of pharmacokinetic/pharmacodynamic (PK/PD) terminology for anti-infective drugs: an update, *J Antimicrob Chemother* 55(5):601–607, 2005.
46. Wiedemann B, Atkinson BA: Susceptibility to antibiotics: species incidence and trends. In Lorian V, editor: *Antibiotics in laboratory medicine*, Baltimore, 1996, Williams & Wilkins, pp 900–1168.
47. Levison ME, Bush LM: Pharmacodynamics of antimicrobial agents. Bactericidal and postantibiotic effects, *Infect Dis Clin North Am* 3:415–422, 1989.
48. Thompson WL: Optimization of drug doses in critically ill patients. In Schoemaker WC, Ayers S, Grenvik A, et al: *Textbook of critical care*, ed 2, Philadelphia, 1989, Saunders, pp 1181–1210.
49. Brown SA: Minimum inhibitory concentrations and postantimicrobial effects as factors in dosage of antimicrobial drugs, *J Am Vet Med Assoc* 191:871–872, 1987.
50. Schentag JJ, Nix DE, Adelman MH: Mathematical examination of dual individualization principles (I): Relationships between AUC above MIC and area under the inhibitory curve for cefmenoxime, ciprofloxacin and tobramycin, *Ann Pharmacother* 25:1050–1057, 1991.
51. Wikler MA: The breakpoint. In Lorian V, editor: *Antibiotics in laboratory medicine*, Baltimore, 1996, Williams & Wilkins, pp 1–8.
52. Pitout JD, Laupland KB: Extended-spectrum beta-lactamase-producing Enterobacteriaceae: an emerging public-health concern, *Lancet Infect Dis* 8:159–166, 2008.
53. Tolun V, Küçükbasmaci O, Törümküney-Akbulut D, et al: Relationship between ciprofloxacin resistance and extended-spectrum beta-lactamase production in *Escherichia coli* and *Klebsiella pneumoniae* strains, *Clin Microbiol Infect* 10:72–75, 2004.
54. Boothe DM, Boeckh A, Boothe HW, et al: Plasma concentrations of enrofloxacin and its active metabolite ciprofloxacin in dogs following single oral administration of enrofloxacin at 7.5, 10, or 20 mg/kg, *Vet Ther* 3(4):409–419, 2002.
55. Corvaisier S, Mairie PH, Bouvierd MY, et al: Comparisons between antimicrobial pharmacodynamic indices and bacterial killing as described by using the Zhi model, *Antimicrob Agents Chemother* 42:1731–173, 1998.

56. Nicolau DP: Predicting antibacterial response from pharmacodynamic and pharmacokinetic profiles, *Infection* 29(2):11–15, 2001.
57. McKinnon PS, Davis SL: Pharmacokinetic and pharmacodynamic issues in the treatment of bacterial infectious diseases, *Eur J Clin Microbiol Infect Dis* 23:271–288, 2004.
58. Craig WA, Vogelman B: The postantibiotic effect, *Ann Intern Med* 106:900–902, 1987.
59. Craig WA, Gudmundsson S: Postantibiotic effect. In Lorian V, editor: *Antibiotics in laboratory medicine*, Baltimore, 1996, Williams & Wilkins, pp 296–330.
60. Spivey JM: Clinical frontiers: the postantibiotic effect, *Clin Pharm* 11:865–875, 1992.
61. Schentag JJ: Correlation of pharmacokinetic parameters to efficacy of antibiotics: relationships between serum concentrations, MIC values, and bacterial eradication in patients with gram-negative pneumonia, *Scand J Infect Dis* 74: 218–234, 1991.
62. Vogelman B, Gudmundsson S, Leggett J, et al: Correlation of antimicrobial pharmacokinetic parameters with therapeutic efficacy in an animal model, *J Infect Dis* 158:831–847, 1988.
63. Athamna A, Athamna M, Medlej B, et al: In vitro post-antibiotic effect of fluoroquinolones, macrolides, beta-lactams, tetracyclines, vancomycin, clindamycin, linezolid, chloramphenicol, quinupristin/dalfopristin and rifampicin on Bacillus anthracis, *J Antimicrob Chemother* 53(4):609–615, 2004.
64. Hostacka A: Serum sensitivity and cell surface hydrophobicity of *Klebsiella pneumoniae* treated with gentamicin, tobramycin and amikacin, *J Basic Microbiol* 38(5-6):383–388, 1998.
65. Wang MG, Zhang YY, Zhu DM, et al: Postantibiotic effects of eleven antimicrobials on five bacteria, *Acta Pharmacologica Sinica* 22(9):804–808, 2001.
66. O'Reilly T, Andes DA, Ostergarrd N, et al: Evaluation of antimicrobials in experimental animal infections. In Lorian V, editor: *Antibiotics in laboratory medicine*, Baltimore, 2005, Williams & Wilkins, pp 654–718.
67. Mayer I, Nagy E: Post-antibiotic and synergic effects of fluoroquinolones and ceftazidime in combination against *Pseudomonas* strains, *Acta Biologica Hungarica* 33(5):937–947, 1994.
68. Sood P, Mandal A, Mishra B: Postantibiotic effect of a combination of antimicrobial agents on *Pseudomonas aeruginosa, Chemotherapy* 46(3):173–176, 2000.
69. Majtan V, Majtanova L: Postantibiotic effect of some antibiotics on the metabolism of *Pseudomonas aeruginosa*, *J Basic Microbiol* 38(3):221–227, 1998.
70. Zhanel GL, Karlowsky JA, Hoban DJ, et al: Antimicrobial activity of subinhibitory concentrations of aminoglycosides against *Pseudomonas aeruginosa* as determined by the killing-curve method and the postantibiotic effect, *Chemotherapy* 37(2): 114–121, 1991.
71. Jacobs MR, Bajaksouzian S, Appelbaum PC: Telithromycin post-antibiotic and post-antibiotic sub-MIC effects for 10 gram-positive cocci, *J Antimicrob Chemother* 52(5):809–812, 2003.
72. Levin S, Karakusis PH: Clinical significance of antibiotic blood levels. In Ristuccia AM, Cuhna BA, editors: *Antimicrobial therapy*, New York, 1984, Raven Press, pp 113–124.
73. John JF: What price success? The continuing saga of the toxic: therapeutic ratio in the use of aminoglycoside antibiotics, *J Infect Dis* 158:1–6, 1988.
74. Carbon C: Single-dose antibiotic therapy: what has the past taught us? *J Clin Pharmacol* 32:686–691, 1992.
75. Korzeniowski OM: Effects of antibiotics on the mammalian immune system, *Infect Dis Clin North Am* 3:469–477, 1989.
76. Maller R, Ahrne H, Holmen C, Lausen I, et al: Once- versus twice-daily amikacin regimen: efficacy and safety in systemic gram-negative infections, *J Antimicrob Chemother* 31:939–948, 1993.
77. Nördstrom L, Ringberg H, Cronberg S, et al: Does administration of an aminoglycoside in a single daily dose affect its efficacy and toxicity? *J Antimicrob Chemother* 25:159–173, 1990.
78. Powell SH, et al: Once-daily vs. continuous aminoglycoside dosing: efficacy and toxicity in animal and clinical studies of gentamicin, netilmicin, and tobramycin, *J Infect Dis* 147:918–932, 1983.
79. Blaser J: Efficacy of once- and thrice-daily dosing of aminoglycosides in in-vitro models of infection, *J Antimicrob Chemother* 27(Suppl C):21–28, 1991.
80. Vanhaeverbeek M, Siska G, Douchamps J, et al: Comparison of the efficacy and safety of amikacin once or twice-a-day in the treatment of severe gram-negative infections in the elderly, *Int J Clin Pharmacol Ther* 31:153–156, 1993.
81. Moore RD, Lietman PS, Smith CR: Clinical response to aminoglycoside therapy: importance of the ratio of peak concentration to minimal inhibitory concentration, *J Infect Dis* 155:93–99, 1987.
82. Karlowsky JA, Zhanel GG, Davidson RJ: Postantibiotic effect in *Pseudomonas aeruginosa* following single and multiple aminoglycoside exposures in vitro, *J Antimicrobial Chemother* 33(5):937–947, 1994.
83. Barclay ML, Begg EJ: Aminoglycoside adaptive resistance: importance for effective dosage regimens, *Drugs* 61(6): 713–721, 2001.
84. Nitsche D, Schulze C, Oesser S, et al: Impact of effects of different types of antimicrobial agents on plasma endotoxin activity in gram-negative bacterial infections, *Arch Surg* 131(2): 192–199, 1996.
85. Wetzstein HG: The in vitro postantibiotic effect of enrofloxacin, *Proc 18th World Buiatrics Congress,* Bologna, Italy, 18:615–618, 1994.
86. Marchbanks CR, McKiel JR, Gilbert DH, et al: Dose ranging and fractionation of intravenous ciprofloxacin agianst *Pseudomonas aeruginosa* and *Staphylococcus aureus* in an in vitro model of infection, *Antimicrob Agents Chemother* 37:1756–1763, 1993.
87. Slavik RS, Jewesson PJ: Selecting antibacterials for outpatient parenteral antimicrobial therapy: pharmacokinetic-pharmacodynamic considerations, *Clin Pharmacokinet* 42(9):793–817, 2003.
88. Preston SL: The importance of appropriate antimicrobial dosing: pharmacokinetic and pharmacodynamic considerations, *Ann Pharmacother* 38(Suppl 9):S14–S18, Jun 29, 2004:Epub.
89. MacGowan AP, Bowker KE: Continuous infusion of beta-lactam antibiotics, *Clin Pharmacokinet* 35(5):391–402, 1998.
90. Hoffman A, Danenberg HD, Katzhendler I, et al: Pharmacodynamic and pharmacokinetic rationales for the development of an oral controlled-release amoxicillin dosage form, *J Control Release* 54(1):29–37, 1998.
91. Bishai W: *Comparative effectiveness of different macrolides: clarithromycin, azithromycin, and erythromycin, Johns Hopkins Division of Infectious Diseases Antibiotic Guide*, Baltimore, 2003, Johns Hopkins, http://hopkins-abxguide.org/ (last accessed June 2010).
92. Helfand MS, Bonomo RA: β-Lactamases: a survey of protein diversity, *Curr Drug Targets Infect Disord* 3:9–23, 2003.
93. Sobel JD, Kaye D: Urinary tract infections. In Mandell GL, editor: *Mandell, Douglas, and Bennett's principles and practice of infectious diseases*, ed 7, Philadelphia, 2010, Churchhill Livingstone.
94. Coutee L, Alonso S, Reveneau N, et al: Role of adhesin release for mucosal colonization by a bacterial pathogen, *J Exp Med* 197(6):735–742, 2003.
95. Clutterbuck AL, Woods EJ, Knottenbelt DC, et al: Biofilms and their relevance to veterinary medicine, *Vet Microbiol* 121:1–17, 2007.
96. Hentzer M, Eberl L, Nielsen J, Givskov M: Quorum sensing: a novel target for the treatment of biofilm infections, *BioDrugs* 17(4):241–250, 2003.

97. Marsh PD: Dental plaque: biological significance of a biofilm and community life-style, *J Clin Periodontol* 32(Suppl 6):7–15, 2005.
98. Tomasz A: Multiple antibiotic resistant pathogenic bacteria, *N Engl J Med* 330:1247–1251, 1994.
99. Rice LB: Genetic and biochemical mechanisms of bacterial resistance to antimicrobial agents. In Lorian V, editor: *Antibiotics in laboratory medicine*, Baltimore, 2005, Williams & Wilkins, pp 441–508.
100. Fluit AC, Schmitz FJ: Resistance integrons and super integrons, *Clin Microbiol Infect* 10:272–288, 2004.
101. Kariuki S, Hart CA: Global aspects of antimicrobial-resistant enteric bacteria, *Curr Opin Infect Dis* 14:479–586, 2001.
102. Lowy FD: Antimicrobial resistance: the example of *Staphylococcus aureus, J Clin Invest* 111:1265–1273, 2003.
103. Ruscher C, Lübke-Becker A, Wleklinski CG, et al: Prevalence of methicillin-resistant staphylococcus pseudintermedius isolated from clinical samples of companion animals and equidaes, *Vet Microbiol* 136(1-2):197–201, 2009:Apr 14.
104. Cooke CL, Singer RS, Jang SS, et al: Enroflxoacin resistance in *Eschericia coli* isolated from dogs with urinary tract infections, *J Am Vet Med Assoc* 220:190–192, 2002.
105. Boothe DM, Boeckh A, Simpson RB, et al: Comparison of pharmacodynamic and pharmacokinetic indices of efficacy for 5 fluoroquinolones toward pathogens of dogs and cats, *J Vet Intern Med* 20:1297–1306, 2006.
106. Boothe DM, Boeckh A, Boothe HW: Evaluation of the distribution of enrofloxacin by circulating leukocytes to sites of inflammation in dogs, *Am J Vet Res* 70(1):16–22, 2009.
107. Hall CS, Ost DE: Effectiveness of programs to decrease antimicrobial resistance in the intensive care unit, *Semin Respir Infect* 18(2):112–121, 2003.
108. Sanchez S, McCrackin Stevenson MA, Hudson CR, et al: Characterization of multlidrug resistant *Escherichia coli* isolates associated with nosocomial infection in dogs, *J Clin Microbiol* 40(10):3586–3595, 2002.
109. Seguin MA, Vaden SL, Altier C, et al: Persistent urinary tract infections and reinfections in 100 dogs (1989-1999), *J Vet Intern Med* 17:622–631, 2003.
110. Sasaki T, Kikuchi K, Tanaka Y, et al: Methicillin-resistant *Staphylococcus pseudintermedius* in a veterinary teaching hospital, *J Clin Microbiol* 45(4):1118–1125, 2007.
111. Lautenbach E: Understanding studies of resistant organisms. Focus on epidemiologic methods. In Owens RC, Lautenbach EL, editors: *Antimicrobial resistance, problem pathogens and clinical countermeasures*, New York, 2008, Informa Healthcare, pp 61–74.
112. Hooton T: Fluoroquinolones and resistance in the treatment of uncomplicated urinary tract infection, *Int J Antimicrob Agents* 22:S65–S72, 2003.
113. Wagenlehner F, Stower-Hoffmann J, Schneider-Brachert W, et al: Influence of a prophylactic single dose of ciprofloxacin on the level of resistance of *Escherichia coli* to fluoroquinolones in urology, *Int J Antimicrob Agents* 15:207–211, 2000.
114. Drlica K: The mutant selection window and antimicrobial resistance, *J Antimicrob Chem* 52:11–17, 2003.
115. Drlica K, Zhao X, Blondeau JM, et al: Low correlation between MIC and mutant prevention concentration, *Antimicrob Agents Chemother* 50(1):403–404, 2006.
116. Ginsburg AS, Grosset JH, Bishai WR: Fluoroquinolones, tuberculosis and resistance, *Lancet Infect Dis* 3:432–442, 2003.
117. Smith HJ, Nichol KA, Hoban DJ, et al: Stretching the mutant prevention concentration (MPC) beyond its limits, *J Antimicrob Chemother* 51:1323–1325, 2003.
118. Schmitz FJ, Higgins PG, Mayer S: Activity of quinolones against gram-positive cocci: mechanisms of drug action and bacterial resistance, *Eur J Clin Microbiol Infect Dis* 21: 647–659, 2002.
119. Robicsek A, Strahilevitz J, Jacoby GA, et al: Fluoroquinolone-modifying enzyme: a new adaptation of a common aminoglycoside acetyltransferase, *Nat Med* 12:83–88, 2006.
120. Zhao X, Xu C, Domagala J, et al: DNA topoisomerase targets of the fluoroquinolones: a strategy for avoiding bacterial resistance, *Microbiology* 94:13991–13996, 1997.
121. Cohen SP, McMurray LM, Hooper DC, et al: Cross resistance to fluoroquinolones in multiple antibiotic resistant *Escherichia coli* selected by tetracycline or chloramphenicol: decreased drug accumulation associated with membrane changes in addition to OmpF reduction, *Antimicrob Agents Chemother* 33:1318–1325, 1989.
122. Leven M: Molecular methods for the detection of antibacterial resistance genes. In Lorian V, editor: *Antibiotics in laboratory medicine*, Baltimore, 2005, Williams & Wilkins, pp 509–531.
123. Kollef M: Broad-spectrum antimicrobials and the treatment of serious bacterial infections: getting it right up front, *Clin Infect Dis* 47(Suppl 1):S3–S13, 2008.
124. Vega CP: Efforts to reduce unnecessary antibiotic prescribing: are they worth it? A best evidence review, *Fam Med* 2009, http://www.medscape.com/viewarticle/585456:accessed June 2010.
125. Rice LB: Controlling antibiotic resistance in the ICU: different bacteria, different strategies, *Cleve Clin J Med* 70(9):793–800, 2003.
126. Regal RE, DePestel DD, VandenBussche HL: The effect of an antimicrobial restriction program on *Pseudomonas aeruginosa* resistance to beta-lactams in a large teaching hospital, *Pharmacotherapy* 23(5):618–624, 2003.
127. Marra AR, de Almelda SM, Correa L, et al: The effect of limiting antimicrobial therapy duration on antimicrobial resistance in the critical care setting, *Am J Infect Control* Nov 3, 2008.
128. Brumbaugh G: Antimicrobial susceptibility and therapy: concepts and controversies, Parts I and II, *Proc Am Coll Vet Intern Med* 8:525–532, 1990.
129. Li RC, Zhu ZY: The integration of four major determinants of antibiotic action: bactericidal activity, postantibiotic effect, susceptibility, and pharmacokinetics, *J Chemother* 14(6):579–583, 2002.
130. Bergan T: Pharmacokinetics of tissue penetration of antibiotics, *Rev Infect Dis* 3:45–66, 1981.
131. Lesar TS, Zaske DE: Modifying dosage regimens in renal and hepatic failure. In Ristuccia AM, Cuhna BA, editors: *Antimicrobial therapy*, New York, 1984, Raven Press, pp 95–111.
132. Easmon CSF, Crane JP: Uptake of ciprofloxacin by macrophages, *J Clin Pathol* 38:442–444, 1985.
133. Tulkens PM: Accumulation and subcellular distribution of antibiotics in macrophages in relation to activity against intracellular bacteria. In Fass RJ, editor: *Ciprofloxacin in pulmonology*, San Francisco, 1990, W. Zuckschwerdt Verlag, pp 12–20.
134. Hawkins EH, Boothe DEM, Aucoin D, et al: Accumulation of enrofloxacin and its metabolite, ciprofloxacin, in alveolar macrophages and extracellular lung fluid of dogs, *J Vet Pharmacol Ther* 21:18–23, 1998.
135. Boeckh A, Boothe DM, Wilkie S, et al: Time course of enrofloxacin and its active metabolite in peripheral leukocytes of dogs, *Vet Ther* 2:334–344, 2001.
136. Boothe HW, Jones SA, Wilkie WS, et al: Evaluation of the concentration of marbofloxacin in alveolar macrophages and pulmonary epithelial lining fluid after administration in dogs, *Am J Vet Res* 66(10):1770–1774, 2005.
137. Boothe DM, Boeckh A, Boothe HW: Evaluation of the distribution of enrofloxacin by circulating leukocytes to sites of inflammation in dogs, *Am J Vet Res* 70(1):16–22, 2009.
138. Labro MT: Interference of antibacterial agents with phagocyte functions: immunomodulation or "Immuno-Fairy Tales"? *Clin Micro Review* 40:625–650, 2000.

139. Ryan DM: Pharmacokinetics of antibiotics in natural and experimental superficial compartments in animals and humans, *J Antimicrob Chemother* 31(Suppl D):1–16, 1993.
140. Barza M: Tissue directed antibiotic therapy: antibiotic dynamics in cells and tissues, *Clin Infect Dis* 19:910–915, 1994.
141. Müller M, dela Peña A, Derendorf H: Issues in pharmacokinetics and pharmacodynamics of anti-infective agents: distribution in tissue, *Antimicrob Agents Chemother* 48(5):1441–1453, 2004.
142. Bamberger DM, Foxworth JW, Bridewell DL, et al: Extravascular antimicrobial distribution and the respective blood and urine concentrations in humans. In Lorian V, editor: *Antibiotics in laboratory medicine*, Baltimore, 2005, Williams & Wilkins, pp 719–848.
143. Brunner M, Derendorf H, Müller M: Microdialysis for in vivo pharmacokinetic/pharmacodynamic characterization of anti-infective drugs, *Curr Opin Pharmacol* 5(5):495–499, 2005.
144. Boothe DM, Boeckh A, Boothe HW, et al: Tissue concentrations of enrofloxacin and ciprofloxacin in anesthetized dogs following single intravenous administration, *Vet Ther* 2: 120–128, 2001.
145. Braga PC: Antibiotic penetrability into bronchial mucus: pharmacokinetic and clinical considerations, *Curr Ther Res* 49(2):300–327, 1989.
146. Bergogne-Bérézin E: Pharmacokinetics of antibiotics in respiratory secretions. In Pennington JE, editor: *Respiratory infections: diagnosis and management*, ed 2, New York, 1988, Raven Press, pp 608–631.
147. LeFrock JL, Prince RA, Richards ML: Penetration of antimicrobials into the cerebrospinal fluid and brain. In Ristuccia AM, Cuhna BA, editors: *Antimicrobial therapy*, New York, 1984, Raven Press, pp 397–413.
148. Craig WA, Ebert SC: Protein binding and its significance in antibacterial therapy, *Infect Dis Clin North Am* 3:407–414, 1989.
149. Labro MT: Antibacterial agents—phagocytes: new concepts for old in immunomodulation, *Int J Antimicrob Agents* 10(1): 11–21, 1998.
150. Shinkai M, Henke MO, Rubin BK: Macrolide antibiotics as immunomodulatory medications: proposed mechanisms of action, *Pharmacol Ther* 117(3):393–405, 2008.
151. Kourlas H: Anti-inflammatory properties of macrolide antibiotics, *J Pharm Pract* 19(5):326–329, 2006.
152. Amsden GW: Anti-inflammatory effects of macrolides—an underappreciated benefit in the treatment of community-acquired respiratory tract infections and chronic inflammatory pulmonary conditions? *J Antimicrob Chemother* 55:10–21, 2005.
153. Baumann U, Fischer JJ, Gudowius P, et al: A Buccal adherence of *Pseudomonas aeruginosa* in patients with cystic fibrosis under long-term therapy with azithromycin, *Infection* 29(1): 7–11, 2001.
154. Steinkamp G, Schmitt-Grohe S, Döring G, et al: Once-weekly azithromycin in cystic fibrosis with chronic *Pseudomonas aeruginosa* infection, *Respir Med* 102(11):1643–1653, 2008.
155. Amaral L, Kristiansen JE, Viveiros M, et al: Activity of phenothiazines against antibiotic-resistant *Mycobacterium tuberculosis*: a review supporting further studies that may elucidate the potential use of thioridazine as anti-tuberculosis therapy, *Antimicrob Chemother* 47(5):505–511, 2001.
156. Mazumder R, Ganguly K, Dastidar SG, et al: Trifluoperazine: a broad spectrum bactericide especially active on staphylococci and vibrios, *Int J Antimicrob Agents* 18(4):403–406, 2001.
157. Mazumder R, Chaudhuri SR, Mazumder A: Antimicrobial potentiality of a phenothiazine group of antipsychotic drug-prochlorperazine, *Indian J Exp Biol* 40(7):828–830, 2002.
158. Mazumdar K, Ganguly K, Kumar KA, et al: Antimicrobial potentiality of a new non-antibiotic: the cardiovascular drug oxyfedrine hydrochloride, *Microbiol Res* 158(3):259–264, 2003.
159. Kumar KA, Ganguly K, Mazumdar K, et al: Amlodipine: a cardiovascular drug with powerful antimicrobial property, *Acta Microbiol Pol* 52(3):285–292, 2003.
160. Karak P, Kumar KA, Mazumdar K, et al: Antibacterial potential of an antispasmodic drug dicyclomine hydrochloride, *Indian J Med Res* 118:192–196, 2003.
161. Annadurai S, Basu S, Ray S, et al: Antibacterial activity of the antiinflammatory agent diclofenac sodium, *Indian J Exp Biol* 36(1):86–90, 1998:1998.
162. Dastidar SG, Mahapatra SK, Ganguly K, et al: Antimicrobial activity of prenylflavanones, *In Vivo* 15(6):519–522, 2001.
163. Dastidar SG, Manna A, Kumar KA, et al: Studies on the antibacterial potentiality of isoflavones, *Int J Antimicrob Agents* 23(1):99–102, 2004.
164. No HK, Park NY, Lee SH, et al: Antibacterial activity of chitosans and chitosan oligomers with different molecular weights, *Int J Food Microbiol* 74(1-2):65–72, 2002.
165. Bennett WM, Plamp CE, Gilbert DN, et al: The influence of dosage regimen on experimental gentamicin nephrotoxicity: dissociation of peak serum levels from renal failure, *J Infect Dis* 140:576–580, 1979.
166. Reiner NE, Bloxham DD, Thompson WL: Nephrotoxicity of gentamicinandtobramycingivenoncedailyorcontinuouslyindogs, *J Antimicrob Chemother* 4(Suppl A):85–101, 1978.
167. Ingrey KT, Ren J, Prescott JF: A fluoroquinolone induces a novel mitogen-encoding bacteriophage in *Streptococcus canis*, *Infect Immun* 71(6):3028–3033, 2003.
168. Miller CW, Prescott JF, Mathews KA, et al: Streptococcal toxic shock syndrome in dogs, *J Am Vet Med Assoc* 209:1421–1426, 1996.
169. Trautmann M, Zick R, Rukavina T, et al: Antibiotic-induced release of endotoxin: in-vitro comparison of meropenem and other antibiotics, *J Antimicrob Chemother* 41(2):163–169, 1998.
170. Holzenheimer R: The significance of endotoxin release in experimental and clinical sepsis in surgical patients—evidence for antibiotic-induced endotoxin release? *Infection* 26(2): 77–84, 1998.
171. Bramhill D: Bacterial cell division, *Annu Rev Cell Dev Biol* 13:395–424, 1997.
172. Giamarellos-Bourboulis EJ, Perdios J, Gargalianos P, et al: Antimicrobial-induced endotoxaemia in patients with sepsis in the field of acute pyelonephritis, *J Postgrad Med* 49(2):118–122, 2003.
173. Aoki H, Kodama M, Tani T, et al: Treatment of sepsis by extracorporal elimination of endotoxin using polymyxin B-immobilized fiber, *Am J Surg* 167:412–417, 1994.
174. Tam VH, Louie A, Fritsche TR, et al: Impact of drug-exposure intensity and duration of therapy on the emergence of *Staphylococcus aureus* resistance to a quinolone antimicrobial, *J Infect Dis* 195:1818–1827, 2007.
175. Hedrick TL, Evans HL, Smith RL, et al: Can we define the ideal duration of antibiotic therapy? *Surg Infect (Larchmt)* 7(5): 419–432, 2006.
176. Hedrick TL, Sawyer RG: Duration of antimicrobial therapy for intra-abdominal infections, *Infect Med* 21(10):506–510, 2004.
177. Kolditz M, Halank M, Höffken G: Short-course antimicrobial therapy for community-acquired penumonia, *Treat Respir Med* 4(4):231–239, 2005.
178. Goff DA: Short-duration therapy for respiratory tract infections, *Ann Pharmacother* 38(9):S19–S23, 2004.
179. Dugan HA, MacLaren R, Jung R: Duration of antimicrobial therapy for nosocomial pneumonia: possible strategies for minimizing antimicrobial use in intensive care units, *J Clin Pharm Ther* 28(2):123–129, 2003.
180. Eliopoulos GM, Moellering RC: Antimicrobial combinations. In Lorian V, editor: *Antibiotics in laboratory medicine*, Baltimore, 1996, Williams & Wilkins, pp 330–396.
181. Zeiler HJ, Voight WH: Efficacy of ciprofloxacin in stationary-phase bacteria in vivo, *Am J Med* 82(5):87–90, 1987.

182. King Guide to Parenteral Admixtures, 2009. Accessed December 16, 2009, at http://www.kingguide.com.
183. Olin BR: *Drug facts and comparisons*, New York, 1992, Lippincott, p. 346.
183a. Saiman L, Chen Y, Yunhua G, et al: Synergistic activities of macrolide antibiotics against *Pseudomonas aeruginosa, Burkholderia cepacia, Stenotrophomonas maltophilia,* and *Alcaligenes xylosoxidans* isolated from patients with cystic fibrosis, *Antimicrob Agents Chemother* 46:1105–1107, 2002.
184. Kung K, Riond JL, Wanner M: Pharmacokinetics of enrofloxacin and its metabolite ciprofloxacin after intravenous and oral administration of enrofloxacin in dogs, *J Vet Pharmacol Ther* 16:462–468, 1993.
185. Hopefl AW: Overview of synergy with reference to double β-lactam combinations, *Ann Pharmacother* 25:972–977, 1991.
186. Pedler SJ, Bint AJ: Combinations of β-lactam antibiotics, *Br Med J* 288:1022–1023, 1984.
187. Richards RM, Xing DK: Investigation of synergism between combinations of ciprofloxacin, polymyxin, sulphadiazine and p-aminobenzoic acid, *J Pharm Pharmacol* 45:171–175, 1993.
188. Katou K, Nakamura A, Kato T, et al: Combined effects of panipenem and aminoglycosides on methicillin-resistant *Staphylococcus aureus* and *Pseudomonas aeruginosa* in vitro, *Chemotherapy* 51(6):387–391, 2005.
189. Saiman L, Liu Z, Chen Y: Synergistic activity of macrolide antibiotics paired with conventional antimicrobial agents against multiple antibiotic resistant *Pseudomonas aeruginosa* isolated from cytic fibrosis patients, *Antimicrob Agents Chemother* 46(4):1105–1107, 2002.
190. Watanakunakorn C, Glotzbecker C: Effects of combinations of clindamycin with gentamicin, tobramycin, and amikacin against *Staphylococcus aureus, J Antimicrob Chemother* 6:785–791, 1980.
191. Boothe DM: Anaerobic infections in small animals, *Probl Vet Med* 2:330–347, 1990.
192. Daude-Lagrave A, Carozzo C, Fayolle P, et al: Infection rates in surgical procedures: a comparison of cefalexin vs. a placebo, *Vet Comp Orthop Traumatol* 14(3):146–150, 2001.

7

Antimicrobial Drugs

Dawn Merton Boothe

Chapter Outline

The principles that guide proper antimicrobial selection are discussed in Chapter 6. This chapter focuses on the individual drugs or drug classes and their use to successfully treat bacterial infections. This includes not only resolution of clinical signs but avoidance of resistance. Characteristics discussed for each drug class include structure–activity releationship; the mechanism of antimicrobial action, including whether the drug is time- or concentration- dependent (Table 7-1); the spectrum of antimicrobial activity (Table 7-2), including pharmacodynamics (minimum inhibitory concentrations [MIC] (Tables 7-3 and 7-4) for selected organisms; mechanisms of antimicrobial resistance; clinically relevant aspects of the drug; the disposition of the drug in the patient (as it relates to both safety and efficacy); adverse drug effects; and drug interactions. The breakpoint MICs (the concentration at which an infecting isolate is considered susceptible or resistant to a drug of interest) are delineated in Chapter 6, Table 6-2). Pharmacokinetics were drawn from individual manuscripts, and the Antimicrobial's Monograph issue of the *Journal of Veterinary Pharmacology and Therapeutics*.[2] In addition, Albarellos[1] also has provided a review of disposition of selected antimicrobials; these have been included, when appropriate, in Table 7-1. Tissue distribution of antimicrobials is addressed when available; Table 7-5 provides information regarding the relative proportion of tissue versus serum concentrations of drugs, with a focus on body fluids and phagocytic cells. As a reminder (see Chapter 6), drug concentrations measured in tissue homogenates are minimally relevant to concentrations to which microbes are exposed. Data collected by ultrafiltration probes is preferred. However, interstitial fluid is not free of factors that might preclude drug activity (i.e., proteins or ionization; see discussion of cefovecin in cats); as such, dosing errors should be on the side that increase concentrations in tissues. Therapeutic indications are offered when relevant. The dissociation constant of a drug (pKa) and selected information regarding the chemical characteristics of selected drugs or preparation stability are provided for selected drugs in Table 7-6. Doses are indicated in Table 7-7; however, doses ideally should be designed on the basis of intergration of pharmacokinetic (PK) and pharmacodynamic (PD) data (see Chapter 6). Treatment of specific infection is addressed by system in Chapter 8.

Chapter 6 addressed the importance of integrating PK and PD MIC data when designing a dosing regimen. The PK parameters on which integration is most commonly based are the maximum drug concentration (for both time-dependent and concentration-dependent drugs) and elimination half-life. The latter is particularly important for time-dependent drugs but will also increase area under the curve (AUC), which predicts the efficacy of selected concentration-dependent drugs (e.g., fluoroquinolones; see Table 7-1). Among the sources of PK data to be consulted beyond this chapter are the Antimicrobial Monographs published by the United States Pharmacopiea[2] in conjunction with the Journal of Veterinary Pharmacology and Therapeutics. The PD data on which integration is based ideally is the MIC of the isolate cultured from the site of infection in the patient. If not available, the high range of the MIC or the MIC_{90} might be a reasonable population statistic surrogate indicator of "what is needed" (see Tables 7-3 and 7-4). When available, PD information for

Table 7-1 Pharmacokinetic Data for Selected Antimicrobials

Drug	Vd (L/kg)	Half-Life (hr)	Dose (mg/kg)[1]/C_{max} (μg/mL)
Amikacin (CD, I)	0.23 (D) 0.18-0.38§ 17 (C)[102]	1 [D]‡ 1.3±0.3 (C, IV)[102] 1.9±0.2 (C, IM, SC)[102]	20 (IV)/65 10 (IM, D)/14 10 (SC, D)/14‡ 10 (SC, Greyhounds)/27 F =0.9[207] 10 (IV, Greyhounds)/49[103] 10 (IV, Beagles/35)[103] 5 (IV,C)/22 (extrapolated)[102] 5 (IM, C)/17[102] 5 (SC, C)/22[102] 10 (IM, C)/38.5‡ 10 (SC, C)/39.6‡ 20 (IM, C)/65.6‡ 20 (SC, C)/67.9‡
Amoxicillin (TD, I)[67]	0.2 (D)	1 1.5†	20 (IV)/13 12.5 (PO)/5-6 (5.5) 11 (SC, D)/7 10 (SC, C)/7 40 (PO)/23†
Amoxicillin with clavulanic acid (TD, I)[26]	0.2	1-1.5 1.5 amoxicillin† 0.71 clavulanic acid	20 (IV)/13 5 (PO)/4.5-6 11 (SC, D)/7 15 (SC, C)/10 16.7 (PO, D)/11.4 amoxicillin† 4.3 (PO, D)/2.06 clavulanic acid†
Ampicillin (TD, I)	0.2-0.4 [D] 0.12‡-0.22 [C]	0.5-1.5 0.8-1.1 (Nelis, 1992) 0.2 (D)‡ 1.25 (C)‡	20 (IV)/50 12 (SC)/14 6.6 (SC)/7 30 (PO)/10 10 (PO)/3 14-16(PO)/3.4-5.5 (Nelis, 1992)
Azithromycin (TD, S)	12 (Vd_{ss}, D)[269] 23 (Vd_{ss}, C)	29 (IV), 35 (PO) (D)[269] 35 (C)[270]	24 (IV, D)/6.8 (F=0.97)[269] 24 (PO, D)/4.2[269] 5 (PO, C)/0.97±0.65 (F=0.58)[270]
Carbenicillin (TD, I)	0.19	0.25	
Cefaclor (TD, I)		2 [D]‡	25 (PO, D)/24.5 44 (PO, D)/20
Cefamandole (TD,I)			10.7 (IV, D)/9.4
Cefazolin (TD, I) (first)	0.3-0.7	0.75-1.4	15 (IV)/45 30 (IV)/90 15 (SC)/25 30 (SC)/50
Cefepime (TD, I)	0.14	1	14 (IV, D)/77 (extrapolated)[28]
Cefixime (TD, I) (third)	0.22 (Vd_{ss}) 8-18% f_{ub}	7-8 (D)‡	5 (PO, D)/2‡ 5 (PO, 6 days [D])/4.8‡
Cefodroxil (TD, I)[62] (first)		1.7 without food; 4 with food†	11 (PO, D)/10.5 22 (PO, D)/16.3-18.6‡ 44 (PO, D)/21 30 (PO, D) 35† 22 (PO, C)/17.4‡
Cefotaxime (TD, I) (third)	0.48 [D] 0.4 [D] (Vd_{ss}) 0.18‡ [C]	0.75-0.8 (D)‡ 1 (C)‡	50 (IV, IM, D)/41 50 (IM, D)/47‡ 50 (SC, D)/30‡ 10 (IV,D)/35* 10 (IM, C)/36‡ 50 (IM, C) 47‡ 50 (SC,C)/30‡

Table 7-1 Pharmacokinetic Data for Selected Antimicrobials—cont'd

Drug	Vd (L/kg)	Half-Life (hr)	Dose (mg/kg)[1]/C_{max} (μg/mL)
Cefotetan (TD, I) (third)	0.25	0.9 1.1 (D)‡	20 (IV, D)/43
Cefovecin (TD, I)	0.13 [D]	5.5 days (D) 6.9 days (C)	8 (SC, D)/121 (bound)[20] 8 (SC, C)/141 (bound)[20] 8 (SC, D)/4.2 (predicted unbound) (PI)[20] 8 (SC, C)/8.5 (predicted unbound) (PI)[20]
Cefoxitin (TD, I) (second)	0.32 [D]‡	0.7-1.3 (D)‡	60 (IV)/20 30 (IV)/10 30 (SC)/20 10 (SC)/15
Cefpodoxime (TD, I)	0.15 [D]	5.6 (PO, D) 4.7 (IV, D)	10 (PO, D)/16 (see text) 5 (PO, D) 8.2
Ceftazidime (TD, I) (third)	0.13-0.22	0.82	20 (IV)/49 30 (SC)/42.2 4.4 mg/kg, then 4.1 mg/kg/hr(CRI)/22.5
Ceftiofur (TD, I) (third)[71] (based on bioactivity)†		5-7 (D)‡	(Bioactivity) 0.22 (SC, D)/1.7‡ 2.2 (SC, D)/8.9‡ 4.4 (SC,D)/27‡
Ceftizoxime (TD, I) (third)	0.26	1	20 (IV, D)/50
Ceftriaxone (TD, I) (third)[68]†	0.24 0.27†	0.85 0.9 (IV)† 1.3 (IM)† 1.7 (SC)†	20 (IV)/45 50 (IM)/115 50 (SC)/69 F (IM, SC, D)=1.0
Cefuroxime (TD, I)			60 (IM, D)/79
Cephalexin (TD, I)(first)[60,67] (based on bioactivity)†	0.23	1.4-2.5* 1.3 (D)‡ 1.8 (D[61] increases to 2.6 at night) 4.7[59a]	20 (IV, D)/41 20 (IV, D)/24 20 (PO)/20.3 F (PO, IM, D) = 0.6 22 (PO)/20 25 (PO, D)/18.8±2.8[6] 40 (PO,D)/35† 30 (PO)/28 15 (PO, C)/11-29‡ 25 (PO, C)/15‡ 20 (SC, C)/54‡ 20 (IM, C)/61.8‡ 10-15 (PO, D)/18.6 10 (SC, D)/24.9‡ 10 (IM, D)/31.9‡
Cephalothin (first) (TD, I)[62]	0.43	0.7-0.85 1.7 without food, 2.8 with†	10 (IM)/9.3 20 (IV)/35 40 (IV)/45 20 (SC)/22 40 (SC)/30 30 (PO,D)/45 without food, 28 with food†
Cephapirin (TD, I) (first)	0.32	0.5	30 (IV)/26.9
Cephradine (TD, I)			50 (PO)/39
Chloramphenicol (TD, S)	0.85-1.77 [D]‡ 2.36 [C]‡	1.2 [D]‡ 2.7± 0.7[254] 3,3 (SC) (C)[255] 6.9 (IV) (C)[255]	33 (PO, D)/8/5 33 (SC,D)/15 50 (PO, D)/20±4 (large dogs)[252] 50 (PO, D)/27±7 (small dogs)[252] 20 (IV, C)/19.5±1.5[255] 20 (IM, C)/18.6±2.6[255] 20 (SC, C)/14.8±2.9[255] 20 (PO,C)/9.8±2.6[255] 50 total (PO, C) 8 to 25 (range)[254]

Continued

Table 7-1 Pharmacokinetic Data for Selected Antimicrobials—cont'd

Drug	Vd (L/kg)	Half-Life (hr)	Dose (mg/kg)¹/C_{max} (μg/mL)
Ciprofloxacin (CD, I) (see also enrofloxacin)	3 (D)‡ 3.85 (C)†	2.2 (D at 2.5-10 mg/kg)‡ 4.9 (D at 10 mg/kg)‡ 5.3 (D at 20 mg/kg)‡ 8.9 (D at 40 mg/kg)‡ 4.53 (C)†	10 (IV, C)/2.53 (extrapolated from terminal component)[195] 10 (PO, D)/1.4‡ 20 (PO, D)/2.8‡ 40 (PO, D)/6.6 23 (PO, D × 7day)/5.68 10 (PO, C)/0.89‖ (F = 0.3±0.1)
Clarithromycin (TD, S)	1.4 (Vd_{ss}, D)‡	3.9 (D)‡	10 (PO, D)/3.3 (F=0.7)‡
Clindamycin[261,261]	0.86 ± 0.35 (D)†	2 (IV)† 7.1 (IM)† 5 (SC)† 16.4±15.4 (C; capsule)[261] 7.5±1.7 (C; solution)[261]	11 (PO, D)/5 5.5 (PO, D)/2 10 (IV, D)/18.8 extrapolated, 7.5 postdistribution† 10 (IM, D)/7.5 (F = 1.15)† 10 (SC, D)/4.4 (F= 3.10)† 15 (PO, C)/11 11 (PO, C)/9 11(PO, C, capsule)/7.4±1.7[261] 11(PO, C, solution)/6.6±2.2
Cloxacillin (TD, I)	0.2	0.5	
Dicloxacillin (TD, I)	0.2	0.7	
Difloxacin (CD, I)		9.3 [D]‡ 6.9±0.5 (Heinen, 2002) 8.5± 0.54 (Frazier)	5 (PO, D)/1.1-1.8 10 (PO, D)/2.3 5 (PO × 5 d, D)/1.8[190] 5 (PO × 3 d)/1.79 ± 0.11[115]
Doxycyline (TD, S)	0.93 (Vd_{ss}‡)- 1.5 (D) (f_{ub} = 9%) 0.65±0.09L/kg (D) [57] 0.34 (Vd_{ss}, C)‡	7-10 (D)‡ 4.56±0.57 (D)[57] 4.6 (C)‡	5 (PO, D)/5 1.1, 0.1 (IV & CRI; D)/1.4 unbound[57] 2.5 (PO, D)/3 5 (PO, C)/6 2.5 (PO, C)/3 5 (PO, D)/3.5[158]; (see also Chapter 8)
Enrofloxacin (CD, I)	2.6 3.7-7 (D, Vd_{ss})‡ 4 (C, Vd_{ss})	0.92 (2.5)[7] 2.02 (5)[7] 2.4/3.9 (at 5 mg/kg,D)† 4.1 (5 mg/kg, D) (Heinen, 2002) 2.6/6.3 (7.5mg/kg, D) [83§] 2.9/7.4 (10 mg/kg, D)[83§] 4.1/11.7 (20 mg/kg, D) [83§] 6.7/6.1 (at 5 mg/kg, C)†	2.5 (PO, D)/1 5 (PO, D)/1.6-2 5 (PO, D for 5 d)/1.4± 0.07[190] 5 (PO, D, for 3 d/1.75±0.16 (Ciprofloxacin: 0.4)[179] 5.5 (PO, D for 7 d)/2.45‡ 5.8 (PO, D for 7 d)/1.43(Cip: 0.36)‡§ 7.5 (PO, D)/1.6 (Cip: 1)[83] 10 (PO,D)/1.7 (Cip: 1.2)[83] 11 (PO, D for 7 d)/4.56‡ 20 (PO, D)/4.2 (Cip: 1.9)[83] 2.5 (PO, C)/1.3 5 (PO, C)/2.5
Erythromycin (TD, S)	2.7 (Vd_{ss}, D)‡ 4.8±0.9	1-1.5 1.7 (D)‡ 1.35± 0.4 (IV);[267] 2.92±0.8 (estolate tablet)[267] 2.56±1.77 (ethylsuccinate suspension)[267]	10 (IV, D, lactobionate)/6.4±1.38[267] 25 (PO, D, estolate tablet)/0.3±0.17[267] 10 (IV, D)/29 (C_o)[269] 10 (PO, D)/4.9[269] 20 (PO, D, ethylsuccinate suspension)/0.17± 0.09 [269] 20 (PO)/3.5
Florfenicol (TD, S)	0.6 (C) 1.45±0.8 (D)[250]	9.2 (IM, D) 1.2 (IV, D)[250] 4 (IV, C) 5.6 (IM, C) 7.8 (PO, C)	20 (IV, D)/6.5 (at 1 hr; extrapolated from)[250] 20 (PO, D)/6.4[250] 20 (IM, D)/1.64) 22 (IM, C)/20 22 (PO, C)/27

Table 7-1 Pharmacokinetic Data for Selected Antimicrobials—cont'd

Drug	Vd (L/kg)	Half-Life (hr)	Dose (mg/kg)[1]/C_{max} (μg/mL)
Fosfomycin disodium phosphate (TD, I)	0.70 ± 0.15 (D) (Vd_{ss}) (Guiterrez, 2008)	See text	See text
Gentamicin (CD, I)	0.35±0.04 [D][97] 0.18 (Vd_{ss}[D])‡ 0.14-0.2 [C]	0.87-1.36 (D) 1.1[D]‡ 1.25±0.3 (C, IV)[101] 1.27±0.26 (C, IM)[101] 1.14±0.11 (C, SC)[101]	4 (IV)/27 8 (IV)/44 3 (IV, D)/24 (extrapolated Co,)[98] 3 (IV, D)/14 (extrapolated from B)[98] 10 (IV, D)/28 3 (IM, SC, D)/10.5[98] 4.4 (IM, D)/7.5 2.2 (IV, D)/6 10 (IV, C)/28 2 (IM, C)/4 3 (SC, C)/15-17‡ 5 (IV, C)/35 (extrapolated from B)[101] 5 (IM, C)/21.6[101] 5 (SC, C)/23.5[101]
Imipenem/cilastin (TD, I)	0.32 (D)	0.83-0.92 (IM) 1.5 (SC)	30 (IV)/180 10 (IV)/65[56] 5 (IM)/13.2 (D) F (IM, D) = 1.5 5 (SC)/8.8 (D)
Kanamycin (CD, I)	0.23-0.28	0.75-1 0.77-1 (D)‡	7.5 (IM, D)/25.8‡ 10 (IM, D)27.6±7.5‡ 15 (IM, D)/37.8‡ 25 (IM, D)/55.6‡ 39 (IM, D)/84.5‡
Levofloxacin (CD, I) (see also Ofloxacin)	1.75±0.42 (C)	8.4± 3.5 = 9.3 ± 1.6 (C)	10 (IV, C)/5.6± 1.4 (extrapolated from terminal curve) 10 (PO, C)/4.7± 0.9[200] (F=0.86±0,44)
Linezolid (TD, I)	0.63 (D)	3.6 (D)	25 (IV, D)/63 10 (IV, D)/23 25 (PO, D)/26 (F=0.96)
Lincomycin (TD, S)			22 (PO)/1.2 15 (PO)/1
Marbofloxacin (CD, I)	1.2-1.37 (D)†	9.1-14.7 PO, (D)‡ † 9.0± 2 [D] (Heinen, 2002) 11.0± 0.94 (Frazier, 2000) 11.5 (at 1 mg/kg, SC, D) 13.4 (at 4 mg/kg, SC, D) 12.7 (C)‡	2 (IV, D)/2.5 (extrapolated)[188] 1 (PO, D)/0.83‡ 2 (PO, D)/1.38‡ 2 (PO, D × 8 [D])/1.4[190] 4 (PO, D)/2.9‡ 5.5 (PO, D)/4.2±0.5 1 (SC, D)/0.78 2 (SC, D)/1.52 4 (SC, D)/3 5 (PO, D)/1.41±0.07† 6.2 (PO, C)/4.8
Meropenem (TD, I)	0.37 0.34	0.67 0.73	20 (IV)/60 (extrapolated) and 24 in ICF 20 (SC)/26 (plasma) and 11 ICF [57]
Metronidazole (CD>TD, I>S)	0.95 (D)‡ 100	4.3 4.5(D)‡	44 (IV)/60 44 (PO, D)/42
Minocycline (TD, S)	2 (D)	7-7.3 (D)	
Nitrofurantoin (S)			For urinary tract infection only
Ofloxacin (CD, I) (racemic mixture of R and S levofloxacin)		4.6 (D)	20 (PO, D)/14.2± 3.4

Continued

Table 7-1 Pharmacokinetic Data for Selected Antimicrobials—cont'd

Drug	Vd (L/kg)	Half-Life (hr)	Dose (mg/kg)[1]/C_{max} (μg/mL)
Orbifloxacin (CD, I)		4.5 = 5.2 (C)[‡] 5.4 = 5.6 (D)[‡] 7.1 ± 0.42 (D) (Heinen, 2002)	2.5 (PO, C)/2[‡] 2.5 (PO, D)/1.4-2.3[‡] 2.5 (PO, D)/1.4 ± 0.07
Oxacillin (TD, I)	0.3 (D)		40 (PO)/4.0 30 (PO)/3.0
Oxytetracycline (TD, S)	2 (D)[‡]	6 (D)[‡]	
Penicillin G (TD, I)	0.16	0.5 (D)	20,000 U/kg (IV)/30 22,000 U/kg (SC)/14
Piperacillin (TD, I)			50 (IV)/250 25 (IV)/125
Rifampin (CD, I)		8 (D)[‡]	10 (PO, D)/40[‡]
Sulfadimethoxine (TD, S)[ǀ]		13.1 (D)[‡] 10.2 (C)[‡]	55 (PO, D)/67[‡]
Sulfadiazine (TD, S)[ǀ]	1.02	9.8	
Sulfamethazine (TD, S)[ǀ]	0.5-0.6 (D)	16-17 (D)	
Tetracycline (TD, S)		1.6-2 (D)[‡] 2.5 (C)[‡]	20 (PO, D)/9 13.75 (PO, D)/7
Ticarcillin (TD, I)	0.34 (D)	1-1.25	100 (IV)/200 40 (IV)/80
Ticarcillin (TD, I) with clavulanic acid[55]		1-1.25 (ticarcillin) 0.40 (clavulanic acid)	100 (IV)/200 40 (IV)/80 F (IM, D) = 0.91 ticarcillin F (IM, D) = 0.65 clavulanic acid
Trimethoprim (TD)	1.49 (D)	2.5 (D)	
Tylosin (TD, S)	1.7(D)[‡]	0.9 (D)	10 (IM, D)/1.5[‡]
Vancomycin (TD, I)		4-6	15 mg/kgq6 hr/40 peak 5 trough μg/mL

Vd, Volume of distribution; *C*, cat;, *I*, bactericidal *D*, dog; *IV*, intravenous; *IM*, intramuscular; *SC*, subcutaneous; *T*, time dependent; *PO*, by mouth; *T*, bactericidal; Vd_{ss}, volume of distribution at steady state; *S*, bacteriostatic; *F*, bioavailability f_{ub}, fraction unbound *PI*, Package Insert, constant-rate infusion; *ICF*, intracellular fluid.

*CD or TD = Concentration or time dependency (see Chapter 6). 1 C_{max} refers to the maximum serum concentration obtained at the dose given by the route in parenthesis. Data refer to both cat and dog unless indicated otherwise (D=dog; C=cat). A new dose can be determined by proportionally changing the dose based on the desired change in C_{max}. For example, a 20 mg/kg IV dose of amikacin resulted in C_{max} of 40 μg/mL. If a patient is given 10 mg/kg IV amikacin, the resulting C_{max} should approximate about 20 μg/mL. The data should be used in conjunction with a minimum inhibitory concentration (see Chapter 6, Table 6-2).

†Source as indicated by drug name.

‡USP Veterinary Pharmaceutical Information Monographs—Antibiotics, *J Vet Pharmacol Ther* 26(Suppl 2), 2003.

§Half-life or C_{max} of ciprofloxacin (μg/mL) is that achieved from metabolism of enrofloxacin when enrofloxacin is administered at the indicated dose. The drugs should work in an additive or synergistic fashion.

¶90% protein binding in dog, 99% in cats; amount reported is peak concentration in transudate.

ǀStatic if sole agent, bactericidal if the sulfonamide is combined with a diaminopyrimidine (trimethoprim, ormetoprim)

canine and feline pathogens (e.g., see Table 7-3) is offered for selected drugs; in addition, relevant information from the human-medicine literature is provided (see Table 7-4). Care should be taken when extrapolating information regarding human pathogens to dogs and cats, although a growing amount of evidence suggests that relative susceptibility of isolates is similar for many drugs (indeed, isolates are likely to be shared), and the data are likely to include both patients that have previously received and not been exposed to antimicrobials. For time-dependent drugs, the relevant PD index (PDI) to be targeted is T > MIC, with a target of at least 50% to 75% of the dosing interval necessary to enhance efficacy, and longer to avoid resistance. An exception can be made for the carbapenems, for which T > MIC of 25% of the dosing interval is sufficient. For concentration-dependent drugs, the relevant PDI is a C_{max}/MIC ≥10.[3] This ratio should be reached at the site of infection. Alternatively, the AUC/MIC should target 125 to 250. Although as low as 30 has been supported for selected gram-positive drugs, this is particularly true for *Streptotoccus pneumoniae*, which is an organism that is particularly problematic in humans. This low AUC/MIC may not be relevant to other gram-positive organisms, including other streptococci. Because availability of AUC data is limited, this chapter will focus on C_{max}/MIC as the target for concentration-dependent drugs. For PDI for both time- and concentration-dependent drugs, doses should be modified as indicated by drug, host, and microbial factors.

The discussion of antimicrobial drugs is based on their classification by mechanism of action (Figure 7-1; see Table 7-1). The mechanism of action of each drug determines drug

Table 7-2 Spectrum of Antimicrobial Activity

Class	Drugs	MOA	G+	Stph	G-	Pse	An	My	Act	Noc	AM
Beta-lactams											
Penicillins											
Natural	Penicillin	Cell wall	3+	2+	1	N	3-4+	0	Y		
Semisynthetic	Dicloxacillin	Cell wall	4+	4+		N	N	0			
	Ampicllin	Cell wall	3+	2-3+	2-3+	N	3-4+	0	Y	Y	
	Amoxicillin	Cell wall	3+	2-3+	3+	N	3-4+	0	Y	Y	
	Amoxicillin–clavulanate	Cell wall	3+	3-4+	3+	N	3-4+	0	Y	Y	
	Ticarcillin	Cell wall	3-4+	4+	3-4+	Y	3-4+	0	Y	Y	
	Ticarcillin–clavulanate	Cell wall	3-4+	4+	4+	Y	3-4+	0	Y	Y	
Carbapenem	Meropenem	Cell wall	4+	4+	4+	Y	3-4+	0	Y	Y	
Monobactam	Aztreonam	Cell wall	N	N	4+	Y	N	0			
Cephalosporins‡											
First generation	Cephalexin	Cell wall	3+	3-4+	1-2+	N	1-2+	0	0		
	Cefazolin	Cell wall	3+	2-3+	2-3+	N	1-2+	0	0		
Second generation	Cefoxitin	Cell wall	2-3+	3-4+	3-4+	N	4+	0	0		
Third generation	Cefotaxime	Cell wall	3+	1-4+	1-4+	Y	3-4+	0			
	Ceftiofur	Cell wall	3+	2+	2-3+	N	2+	0			
	Cefpodoxime	Cell wall	3+	3-4+	3+	N	2-3+	0			
	Cefovecin	Cell wall	3+	3-4+	3+	N	2-3+	0			
Aminoglycosides	Gentamicin	Ribosomes 30&50	1+	4+§	4+	3-4+	0	Y	N/Y*	Y	Y
	Amikacin	Ribosomes 30 & 50	1+	3-4+§	4+	4+	0	Y		Y	
Fluorinated quinolones	Enrofloxacin†	Topoisomerases	1-2+	3-4+	3-4+	Y(C&S)	1+	Y	0	0	Y
	Pradofloxacin	Topoisomerases	3-4+	3-4+	3-4+	Y	3+	Y	0	0	Y
Sulfonamides	Sulfadiazine	Folic Acid synthetase	2-3+	2-3+	2+	N	2-3+	N	Y	Y	0
Pyramethamine	Trimethoprim	Folic acid reductase				N					
Tetracyclines	Doxycycline	Ribosomes 30s	2-3+	2-3+	2-3+	N	2-3+	Y	C&S		Y
Phenicols	Chorampheni-col‡	Ribosomes 50s	2-3+	2-3+	2-3+	N	2-3+	Y			
Macrolides	Erythromycin	Ribosomes 50s	3+	3-4+	1-2+	N	2-3+	Y	Y		Y
	Azithromycin	Ribosomes 50s	3+	2-4+	2+	N	2-3+	Y	Y		Y
Lincosamides	Clindamycin	Ribosomes 50s	4+	3-4+	1+	N	3-4+	Y	Y		
Nitroimidazoles*	Metronidazole	DNA-RNA	N	N	N	N	4+		C&S		Y
Oxazolidinones	Linezolid	Ribosomes 50s-70s	4+	4+	N	N	3+	Y	Y	Y	Y
Rifamycin§	Rifampin	RNA	3+	3+	N	N	Y	Y	N		Y
Glycopeptide	Vancomycin	Cell wall	4+	4+	N	N	Y	N	N		

MOA, mechanism of action; *G+*, gram-positive; *G-*, gram-negative; *Stph*, Staphylococcus; *Pse*, Pseudomonas; *An*, Anaerobes, *My*, Mycoplasma, *Act*, Actinomyces, Noc Nocadia; *AM*, atypical mycobacterium; *Y*, yes; *N*, no; *C&S*, culture and susceptibility testing. 0, No efficacy; 1, poor; 2, fair; 3, good; 4, excellent.
*Spectrum reflects inherent susceptibility and does not include acquired resistance.
†See text for specific differences, but in general enrofloxacin represents marbofloxacin, orbifloxacin, and difloxacin.
‡Generally ineffective toward enterococci.
§Generally not as sole therapy.

Table 7-3 Susceptibility Data for Feline and Canine *Escherichia coli* Pathogens (n = 595)

Drug	Resistant$_{BP}$	Mode	MIC$_{50}$	MIC$_{90}$	Range
Amoxi-clavulanate	≥32/16	4	4	32	0.5-2048
Ampicillin	≥32	2	4	512	0.25-512
Ticarcillin-clavulanate	≥128	2	2	64	2-2058
Meropenem	≥16	0.25	0.25	0.5	0.25
Cefotaxime	≥64	1	1	16	1-2048
Cefoxitin	≥32	4	4	32	0.5-2048
Cefpodoxime	≥8	0.5	0.5	256	0.12-512
Ceftazidime	≥32	0.5	0.5	16	0.25-512
Cephalothin	≥32	8	16	2048	1-2048
Gentamicin	≥16	1	1	8	1
Enrofloxacin	≥4	0.06	0.06	32	0.03-512
Ciprofloaxcin	(≥4)	0.03	0.03	32	0.3-128
TMPS	≥4/c	0.06	0.06	2	0.06
Azithromycin	≥8	8	8	64	1-512
CHPC	≥32	8	8	32	2-2048
Doxycycline	≥16	1	2	32	0.25-1024

BP, Breakpoint; *MIC,* minimum inhibitory concentration;CHPC: chloramphenicol; *TMPS,* trimethoprim-sulfonamide combination. All MIC are in µg/mL. Data is likely to include isolates from dogs or cats exposed to antimicrobials
*475 isolates are from the urinary tract. Data was generated by the author and includes isolates from animals exposed to antimicrobials.

Table 7-4 Susceptibility Data for Selected Drugs and Selected Human Pathogens Associated with Skin and Soft Tissue Infections[106]

		Enterobacter spp.		*E. coli*		*K. pneumoniae*		*P. aeruginosa*		*S. aureus*	
Drug	Resistant MIC$_{BP}$	MIC$_{50}$	MIC$_{90}$	MIC$_{50}$	MIC$_{90}$	MIC$_{50}$	MIC$_{90}$	MIC$_{50}$	MIC$_{90}$	MIC$_{50}$	MIC$_{90}$
Ciprofloxacin	≥4	≤0.25	0.5	≤0.25	>2	≤0.25	2	≤0.25	>2	≤0.25	>2
Levofloxacin	≥8	≤0.03	0.5	≤0.03	4	0.06	2	0.5	>4	0.25	>4
Doxycycline*/ Tetracycline	≥16	≤4	>8	≤4	>8					≤0.5	1
Amikacin	≥64	<1	2	2	4	1	2	2	4		
Gentamicin	≥16	≤1	≤1	≤1	2	≤1	4	2	>8	≤1	≤1
TMPS	≥4/76	≤0.5	1			0.05	1			≤0.5	≤0.5
Nitrofurantoin	≥128	≤32	64	≤32	≤32	≤32	64				
Clindamycin	≥16	>16	>16							0.12	>8
Erythromycin	≥16									0.5	>8
Linzeolid	≥8*			≤2	16					2	2
Rifampin	≥4									≤0.25	≤0.25
Vancomycin	≥32									1	1

MIC, Minimum inhibitory concentration; *BP,* breakpoint, *TMPS,* trimethoprime-sulfonamide. All MIC are in µg/mL. Data is likely to include isolates from dogs or cats exposed to antimicrobials.
*When testing *Enterococcus* spp.

efficacy (i.e., bactericidal versus bacteriostatic) and mechanisms of resistance[4]; influences time- versus concentration-dependence and duration of postantibioitic effect; and, for some drugs, affects safety. Mechanisms of action also influence the selection of combination antimicrobial therapy. For drugs that are approved for use in humans but not animals and for which information regarding use in dogs and cats is not available, PK information in humans will be summarized.

DRUGS THAT TARGET THE CELL WALL

Beta-Lactam Antimicrobials

The broad spectrum, low toxicity, and reasonable cost of beta-lactam antibiotics contribute to their frequent use for treatment of infections. In addition, their effects on cell wall synthesis result in their frequent selection for combination antimicrobial therapy. The beta-lactam antibiotics include the

Table 7-5 Serum Concentration of Drugs Achieved in (Human) Tissues*[292]

		ICF	Joint Fluid	Ascites	Pleural Fluid	Bronchial Secretions	Sinus Secretions	Middle Ear	CSF	Aqueous Humor	PMN or AM
Aminoglycosides	Amikacin	17	111 (4-7)	58 (5)	40, 21 (7.5)	21			35	0.5-4.5	
	Gentamicin	31	80	90 (0.5)	57	<8			2.5	22.5	21-73
Penicillins	Amoxicillin	40,76		83		4-23		24-50	10		
	Ampicillin	13	62	100		5	3	6-50	3.4		6
	Penicillin	17	93	39	67-88			35	8	2.5	37
	Ticarcillin	23,40,88		14		1					
	Piperacillin	35		55		4			29	4.5	<10
	Carbenicillin	22				1					
Carbapenems	Imipenem			85		20			8.5	8.5	33
	Meropenem	87 (4-12)				20-47			21	29	
Monobactam	Aztreonam	90		43	79	21			6.7	2.5	
First-generation cephalosporins	Cephalexin		66		30		10			2.5	55
	Cefodroxyl	70	98		114					42.5	
	Cefazolin	11	32 (0.5)		30	2			0	<2	<10
Cephamycins	Cefoxitin	45		117	31	11-16			52	7.5	
Oxyimino-cephalosporins	Ceftazidime	13,35		45	21	11			23.5	4.5-12.5	
	Cefotaxime	13,35	116	120 (6)	24	2		123	18-51	2.5	56
	Cefpodoxime				67 (6)						
Fluoroquinolones	Ciprofloxacin	80			26-126	26-89			25(1), 18-146 (8)	8.5-17.5	600-700
	Levofloxacin					188					1850
	Ofloxacin	49		69 (24), 93 (8)		60			42-72	14	815
Macrolides	Erythromycin base	46 (4-6)									1700-4600
	Erythromycin	6				25					
	Azithromycin	130				1692				9.3	900-70,000
Lincosamides	Clindamycin	9		44 (1-5)	92						1200
Tetracyclines	Doxycycline	47			36	17	57	42	14-22	10.5-13.5	
	Tetracycline					30	79-100			9.5-11.5	74
Sulfonamides	Sulfadiazine	50					20	57			
	Sulfamethoxazole	37						27	40		
	Trimethoprim	55					133	119			44-600
Rifampin		20 (6-9)		23 (4)	40				4		70-800
Fosfomycin		53			22					25.5	
Vancomycin			81	52	41-111				0	10.5	122
Linezolid			87			414					
Metronidazole								70	43	38.5	85-103
Chloramphenicol											964
Blisters, disks, threads											

ICF, Intracellular fluid; *CSF*, cerebrospinal fluid; *PMN*, polymorphic neutrophils. With noted exceptions (difference cited in parentheses), timing 1 to 2 hours. All concentrations are in μg/mL.

Table 7-6 Selected Chemical Characteristics of Antimicrobial Drugs

Drug	MW	Acid/Base	pKa	Predicted PC*
Amikacin	585	Base	8.1	0.0006
Amoxicillin	365	Acid	2.8, 7.2	0.0026
Clavulanate		Acid		0.069
Ampicilllin	349	Acid	2.7, 7.3	7.58
Azithromycin	749	Base	8.74	1071
Cefaclor	385	Acid		
Cefadroxil	381	Acid		
Cefazolin	454	Acid		0.81
Cefpodoxime	557	Acid		1.12
Cefotaxime	455	Acid	3.35	
Cefovecin		Acid		
Cefoxitin	427	Acid	2.2	1.65
Ceftiofur	523	Acid		
Cephalexin	347	Acid	5.3, 7.3	
Cephapirin		Acid	2.15, 5.44	
Ciprofloxacin	331	Amphoteric	6.1, 8.6	0.27
Clindamycin	425	Base	7.7	57
Doxycycline	462	Amphoteric	3.4, 7.7, 9.7	0.91
Enrofloxacin	360	Amphoteric	6.0, 8.8	3.54 (actual)
Erythromycin	733	Base	8.8	234
Gentamicin	470	Base	8.2	0.02
Imipenem	317	Acid	3.2, 9.9	0.64
Kanamycin	484		7.2	
Levofloxacin	361			0.95
Linezolid	337			
Marbofloxacin	362	Amphoteric	6.2, 8.6	0.08
Meropenem	383			0.83
Metronidazole	171			0.69
Orbifloxacin		Amphoteric		
Penicillin	334	Acid	2.7	60
Piperacillin	517			4.67
Rifampin	822	Zwitterion	1.7, 7.9	229
Sulfadiazine	250	Acid	6.4	1.54
Sulfadimethoxine	310		6.2	
Tetracycline	444		8.3, 10.2	0.40
Ticarcillin	384			9.7
Trimethoprim	290	Base	7.6	18
Tylosin	916		7.1	
Vancomycin	1449	Amphoteric	7.8, 8.9 (Basic)	13
			2.2, 9.6, 10.4, 12 (acid)	

MW, Molecular weight; *pKa,* dissociation constant *PC,* octanyl–water partition coefficient. Note that the PC is dependent on ambient pH.

cephalosporins, penicillins (including combination penicillin/beta-lactamase inhibitors), carbepenems, and monobactams (see Table 7-1).

Structure–Activity Relationship

Beta-lactam antibiotics contain a four-member beta-lactam ring as the active site. A second member ring establishes the drug as either a cephalosporin—one carbon larger—or a penicillin (Figure 7-2).[5-9] Chemically, the beta-lactams are classified as weak acids (see Table 7-6). They include natural, and semisynthetic drugs (see Table 7-2). Penicillin is a natural drug derived from the molds of the genus *Penicillium.* Penicillin serves as a base for the semisynthetic aminopenicillins (ampicillin, amoxicillin), the extended-spectrum penicillins (carbenicillin, ticarcillin, piperacillin), the carpabenems (imipenem, meropenem), and the monobactams (aztreonam).

Table 7-7 Dosing Regimens of Selected Antimicrobials*

Drug	Dose	Route of Administration	Frequency (hr)
Amikacin	15-22 mg/kg	IM, IV, SC	24 (consider monitoring)
Amoxicillin	20-30 mg/kg	IM, IV, PO, SC	6-12
Amoxicillin–clavulanic acid	10-30 mg/kg	PO	6-12
	62.5 mg/cat	PO	6-12
Ampicillin	20-60 mg/kg	PO	6-8
	10-50 mg/kg	IV	6-8
Ampicillin sulbactam	10-50 mg/kg	IM, IV	6-8
Ampicillin trihydrate	10-50 mg/kg	IM, SC	6-8
Amprolium	100 mg/dog	PO (on food or in water)	24 × 7-10 days
Azrithromycin	5-10 mg/kg (D)	PO	12-24
	5-15 mg/kg (C)	PO	12-48
	15 mg/kg loading dose	PO	
Aztreonam	12-25 mg/kg	IM, IV	8-12
Baquiloprim-sulphadimethoxine or sulphadimidine	30 mg/kg	PO	24 × 2 days then q 48 × 10-21 days
Carbenicillin	15-110 mg/kg	IM, IV, SC	6-8
Carbenicillin indanyl sodium	10-55 mg/kg	PO	8
Cefaclor	4-20 mg/kg	PO (in a fasted animal)	8
Cefadroxil	20-35 mg/kg	PO	8-12
Cefamandole	6-40 mg/kg	IM, IV	6-8
Cefazolin sodium	10-25 mg/kg	IM, IV, SC	4-8
	10-22 mg/kg	IV	1-2 times during surgery
Cefepime	50 mg/kg	IM, IV	8
Cefixime hydrochloride	5-12.5 mg/kg	PO	12-24
Cefmetazole sodium	20 mg/kg	IV	6-12
Cefoperazone sodium	22 mg/kg	IV, IM	6-12
Cefotaxime sodium	20-80 mg/kg (D)	IM, IV, SC	4-12
Cefotetan disodium	30 mg/kg	IV, SC	8
Cefovecin	8 mg/kg	SC	2-14 days based on organism MIC
Cefoxitin sodium	15-30 mg/kg (D)	IM, IV, SC	6-8
	6-40 mg/kg (D)	IM, IV	6-8
Cefpodoxime proxetil	5-10 mg/kg	PO	12-24
Ceftazidime	15-30 mg/kg	IM, IV, SC	6-12
Ceftiofur	2.2-4.4 mg/kg	SC	12-24
Ceftizoxime	25-50 mg/kg	IM, IV	8-12
Ceftriaxone	15-50 mg/kg	IM, IV	12
	25 mg/kg	IM, IV	1-2 times during surgery
Cefuroxime axetil or sodium	10-30 mg/kg	IV, PO (with food)	8-12
Cephalexin	20-60 mg/kg	PO	6-12
Cephaloridine	10 mg/kg	IM, SC	8-12
Cephalothin	10-44 mg/kg	IM, IV, SC	4-8
Cephamandole	6-40 mg/kg	IM, IV	6-8
Cephapirin	10-30 mg/kg	IM, IV, SC	4-8
Cephradine	10-40 mg/kg	IM, IV, PO	6-8
Chloramphenicol palmitate	25-50 mg/kg (D)	PO	8
	50 mg/cat	PO	12
Chloramphenicol sodium succinate	25-50 mg/kg (D)	IV, SC, IM	6-8
	50 mg/cat	IV, SC, IM	12
Chlortetracycline	25 mg/kg	PO	6-8
Ciprofloxacin	10-50 mg/kg (D)	PO	12-24
	5-20 mg/kg (D,C)	IV	12-24

Continued

Table **7-7** Dosing Regimens of Selected Antimicrobials*—cont'd

Drug	Dose	Route of Administration	Frequency (hr)
Clarithromycin	2.5-10 mg/kg (D)	PO	12-24
	62.5 mg/cat	PO	12 with clofazimine
	7.5 mg/kg (C)	PO	12 with metronidazole and amoxicillin
	5-10 mg/kg	PO	12 with rifampin and enrofloxacin
Clindamycin	5-20	PO	12-24
	25-50	PO	24 (for toxoplasmosis)
Clofazimine	4-8	PO	24
Cloxacillin	20-40 mg/kg	IM, IV, PO	4-8
Dapson	1.1	PO	8-12
Dicloxacillin	30-50 mg/kg	PO	6-8
Difloxacin	5-10 mg/kg	PO	24
Dihydrostreptomycin	20-30 mg/kg	IM, SC	24
Doxycyline	5-10 mg/kg	IV, PO	12-24
Enrofloxacin	5-20 mg/kg (D)	IM, IV, PO, SC	12-24
	5 mg/kg (C)	IM, IV, PO, SC	24
Erythromycin	10-22 mg/kg (D), maximum of 40 mg/kg	PO	8-12
	10-22 mg/kg (C)	IV, PO	8
	3-5 mg/kg (C)	IM	8
Ethambutol	15-25 mg/kg	PO	24-72
Fosfomycin	40-80 mg/kg	PO	12
Florfenicol	100-200 mg	IM, PO, SC	8 (D), 12 (C)
	25-50 mg/kg	PO, SC	8
	20 mg/kg (D)	IM, PO	6
	22 mg/kg (C)	IM, PO	12
Gentamicin	6-8 mg/kg	IV, IM, SC	24
	4-8 mg/kg (D), apply light coating	Topical	24
Hetacillin	20-44 mg/kg	PO on an empty stomach	8-12
Imipenem–cilastin	5-10 mg/kg	IM (using IM preparation), IV (slow), SC	6-8
Isoniazid	10 mg/kg (D)	PO	24
Kanamycin	10-20 mg/kg	IM, IV, SC	24
Levofloxacin	(Obtain MIC first)10 mg/kg	IV, PO	24
Lincomycin	22-33 mg/kg	IM, IV, PO	12-24
Linezolid	10-20 mg/kg	IV, PO	12-24
Marbofloxacin	2.5-5.5 mg/kg	PO	24
Meropenem	12-40 mg/kg	IV, SC	8
Methanamine mandelate	16.5 mg/kg (D only?)	PO	24 (safety not established in cats)
Methicillin	20 mg/kg	IM, IV	6
Minocycline	12.5- 25 mg/kg (D)	PO	12
	5-12.5 mg/kg (D)	IV	12
Neomycin	7-10.5 mg/kg	IM, IV, SC	24, highly nephrotoxic
	10-20 mg/kg (dilute in water)	Per rectum	6
	10-20 mg/kg	PO	12
Novobiocin	10 mg/kg	PO	8
Ofloxacin	20mg/kg	PO	24
Orbifloxacin	2.5-7.5 mg/kg	PO	24
Oxacillin	22-40 mg/kg	IM, IV, PO	6-8

Table 7-7 Dosing Regimens of Selected Antimicrobials*—cont'd

Drug	Dose	Route of Administration	Frequency (hr)
Oxytetracycline	55-82.5 mg/kg	PO	8
	7-12 mg/kg	IM, IV	12
Penicillin G, benzathine	50,000/kg	IM	2 days
Penicillin G, phenoxymethyl potassium	20-30 mg/kg	PO	6-8
Penicillin G, procaine	20,000-100,000 U/kg	IM, SC	12-24
Penicillin V potassium	10 mg/kg	PO	8
Piperacillin sodium	25-50 mg/kg	IM, IV	8-12
Piperacillin–tazobactam	3400-4500 g (D)	IV	6-8
Rifampin (in combination)	10-20 mg/kg	PO	8-12 (D), 24 (C), combined with a second antimicrobial?
Roxithromycin	15 mg/kg	PO	24
Spectinomycin	5-12 mg/kg	IM	12
Spiramycin	12.5-23.4 mg/kg	PO	24 × 5-10 days
Streptomycin	20-40 mg/kg	IM	24
Sulfadiazine	Initial dose: 220 mg/kg	PO	Once as loading dose (nocardiosis)
	Followed by: 50-110 mg/kg	PO	12 (nocardiosis)
	Loading: 50-100 mg/kg	PO	Once as loading dose (toxoplasmosis)
	Maintenance 7.5-25 mg/kg	PO	12 (toxoplasmosis)
	50 mg/kg	IV, PO	12
Sulfadiazine/trimethoprim	30 mg/kg (C)	PO,SC	12
	30 mg/kg (D)	IV, PO, SC	8-12
Sulfadimethoxine	25-100 mg/kg	IM, IV, PO	12-24
	Loading dose: 55 mg/kg	PO	Once as loading dose
Sulfadimethoxine/ormetoprim	27 mg/kg (D)	PO	24 × 14 days
	Loading dose: 55 mg/kg (D)	PO	Once as loading dose
	Followed by: 27.5 mg/kg (D)	PO	24 for a maximum of 21 days
Sulfaguanidine	100-200 mg/kg	PO	8 × 5 days
Sulfamethazine/sulfamerazine	Loading dose: 100 mg/kg	PO	Once as loading dose
	Followed by: 50 mg/kg	PO	12
Sulfamethoxazole	Loading dose: 100 mg/kg	PO	Once as loading dose
	Followed by: 50 mg/kg	PO	12
Sulfamethoxazole/trimethoprim	15 mg/kg	PO	12
Sulfasalazine	10-50 mg/kg (D), maximim of 3 g	PO	8-12, taper by 50% when response occurs
	10 mg/kg (D)	PO	8 until remission then taper to lowest effective dose
	250 mg (C)	PO	8 × 3 treatments then q24hr
	10-20 mg/kg (C)	PO	8-12 for 10 days then 24 hr
Sulfisoxazole	50 mg/kg	PO	8
Teicoplanin	3-12 mg/kg (D)	IM, IV	24
Tetracycline hydrochloride	10-33 mg/kg	PO	8-12
	7 mg/kg	IM, IV	8-12
	10-22 mg/kg (D)	PO	8-12
Ticarcillin or ticarcillin–clavulanic acid	40-110 mg/kg	IM, IV	4-8
	Initial dose: 15-25 mg/kg	IV (over 15 min)	Once
	Followed by: 7.5-15 mg/kg	IV CRI	—
Vancomycin	10-20 mg/kg (D)	PO	6 (For GI infections only)
	15 mg/kg	IV (over 30 min)	6

IM, Intramuscular; *IV,* intravenous; *SC,* subcutaneous; *D,* dog; *C,* cat.; *PO,* by mouth; *CRI,* constant-rate infusion.
*Dosing regimens ideally are based on the minimum inhibitory concentration of the infecting microbe and the appropriate PDI (e.g., C_{max}: MIC>10 for concentration-dependent drugs and T >MIC of 25 to 100% depending on the drug

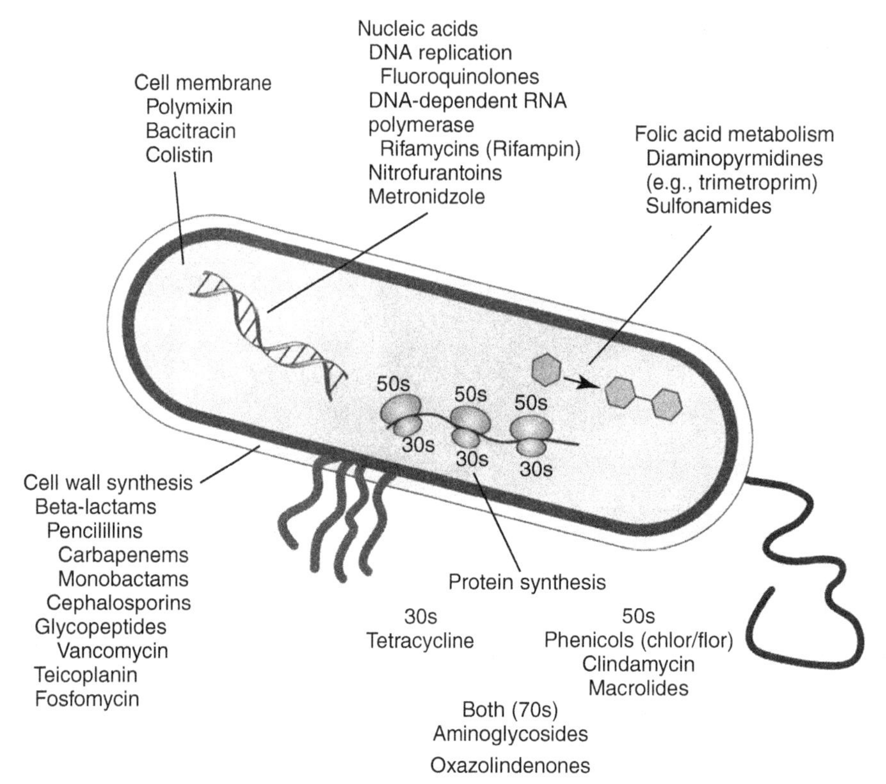

Figure 7-1 Drug mechanisms of action determine drug efficacy, bactericidal or bacteriostatic effects, mechanisms of bacterial resistance, and appropriateness of combination therapy. Occasionally, the mechanism of drug action predicts the mechanism of host toxicity.

Penicillin G is the basis for the definition of the international unit (IU) of penicillin, which is equivalent to 0.6 mg of the international pure crystalline sodium penicillin (1.6 IU/mg). The conversion of USP units varies with the salt, with 1 mg of penicillin G equivelant to the following units: sodium (1500-1750); potassium (1440-1680), and procaine (900-1050).As a group the natural penicillins are unstable and subject to hydrolysis at the beta-lactam ring. Degradation can occur when combined with other solutions. Degradation also occurs for most penicillins exposed to gastric acidity, precluding oral absorption.[9]

The cephalosporins are derived from a chemical produced by the fungus *Cephalosporium acremonium*. The six-member ring of the cephalosporins renders them more stable; this increased stability also causes them to be less susceptible to resistance. More than 22 cephalosporins are approved for use in the United States, including the cephamycins (e.g., cefoxitin, cefotetan) and oxyimino-cephalosporins (e.g., ceftazidime, cefotoxime, ceftiofur, cefpodoxime, cefovecin) (see Figure 7-2). The cephalosporins have been variably categorized, with the original "generation" designation being the most widely accepted (Table 7-8).[8,10,11] The designations began as an indicator of chronologic approval but have evolved such that each indicates relative resistance to beta-lactamase destruction; the first generation is most and the later generations least susceptible to destruction.[10] The advent of extended-spectrum beta-lactamases renders the classification less clear in that these beta-lactams specifically target later-generation drugs. Spectrum and pharmacologic properties of drugs within the generations vary, particularly in the third or later generations. Reclassifying the cephalosporins into groups according to the route of administration, and spectrum has been proposed (see Table 7-8).

Mechanism of Action

The mechanism of action of beta-lactams reflects interference with bacterial cell wall synthesis (Figure 7-3). The bacterial cell wall comprises several layers of a peptidoglycan matrix. The peptidoglycan strands are composed of five repeating disaccharide units of *N*-acetylglucosamine and *N*-acetylmuramate; these units are formed by the bacteria in stages. A pentapeptide, which ends with a D-Ala-D-Ala terminus, is attached to each of the repeating units of these disaccharides. The units are joined to form a chain or peptidoglycan strand. The resulting chains are then cross-linked to provide cell wall rigidity. Cross-linking between the D-Ala-D-Ala terminals is catalyzed by transpeptidase enzymes, one of several types of proteins that bind penicillin (referred to as *penicillin-binding proteins [PBPs]*) located in the cell wall (see Figure 7-3).[12] The bacterial substrate for the transpeptidase enzyme is the pentapeptide of the peptidoglycan and, specifically, the terminal amino acids D-Ala-D-Ala. The beta-lactam ring is the functional (active) group of all drugs in this class. It is structurally similar to the D-Ala-D-Ala terminus of the pentapeptide,

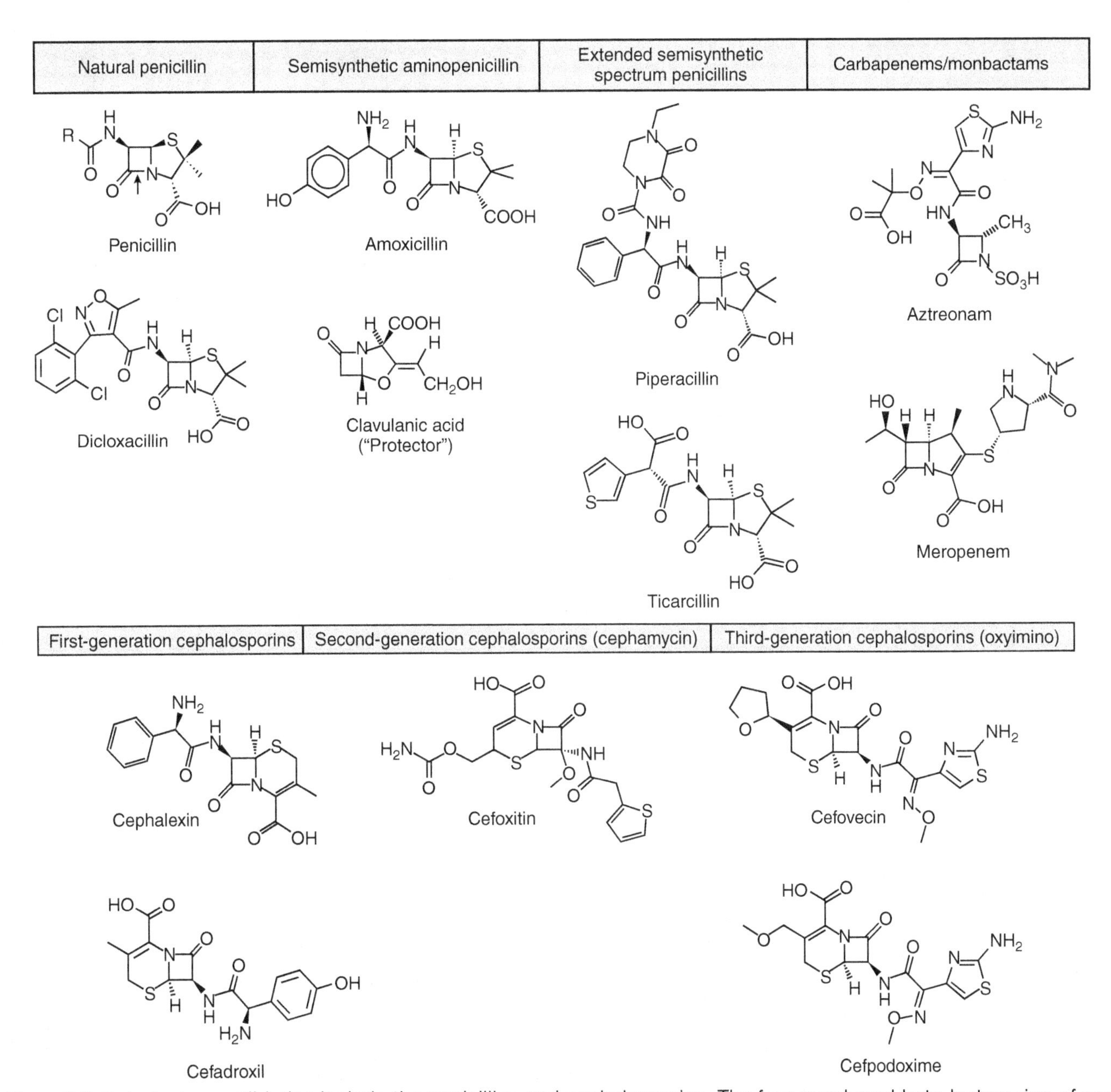

Figure 7-2 Beta-lactam antibiotics include the penicillins and cephalosporins. The four membered beta-lactam ring of each drug mimics the substrate of the transpeptidase enzyme (a penicillin-binding protein), and specifically the terminal portion of p-D-Ala-Asp-D-Ala (boxed inset). This ring structure also is the target of beta-lactamase enzyme destruction. Penicillins have an adjacent five-member ring, cephalosporins a seven-member ring. The addition of larger structures to the basic ring structure may help reduce emerging resistance by beta-lactamase rings but will not avoid methicillin resistance.

acting as a substrate and subsequently inhibiting the D-D transpeptidase enzyme (see Figure 7-3). In an actively growing cell, as peptidoglycan precursors increase in response to inhibition of synthesis, autolysins, particularly in gram-positive organisms, contribute to cell wall degradation. Degradation coupled with impaired cell wall synthesis causes the bacterial cell wall to lose rigidity. The cell becomes permeable to the surrounding environment, which, although isotonic to the host, is hypotonic to the organism. Influx of surrounding fluid into the hypertonic bacterial cell results in cytolysis, or osmotic lysis, particularly in gram-negative organisms. Cell wall instability induces the secretion of autolysins, particularly in gram-positive organisms. Because organisms continually break down and rebuild cell walls, the efficacy of the beta-lactam antibiotic ideally is constantly present and, as such, this class of drugs is considered time-dependent (see Chapter 6). However, the duration that the plasma drug concentration (PDC) should be above the MIC varies with the drug, with the desired duration being 50% to 75% of the dosing interval for most drugs. However, T > MIC may be as little as 25% to 50%

Table 7-8 Cephalosporin Grouping Based on Generation, Route, and Spectrum

Group	Drug	Generation	Route	Resistance to Beta-Lactamases	Potency (Dose)	Spectrum
1	Cefazolin Cephalothin	First	Parenteral	Staphylococcal, not enterobacterial	Moderate	High activity against gram +
2	Cefadroxil Cephalexin Cephradine	First	Oral	Staphylococcal, some enterobacterial	Moderate	High activity against gram + Some gram –
3	Cefoxitin Cefotetan Cefuroxime Cefamandole	Second	Parenteral	Many	Moderate	High activity against gram– and anaerobes
4	Ceftiofur, Cefotaxime Ceftriaxone	Third	Parenteral	Many	High	Gram –, Some gram +
5	Cefpodoxime Cefixime	Third	Oral	Many	High	High activity against gram –, some gram +
6	Ceftazidime Cefoperazone	Third	Parenteral	Many	High	High activity against gram–including *Pseudomonas* gram+
7	Cefepime Cefpirome	Fourth	Parenteral	Many	High	High activity against gram–

+, Positive; –, negative.

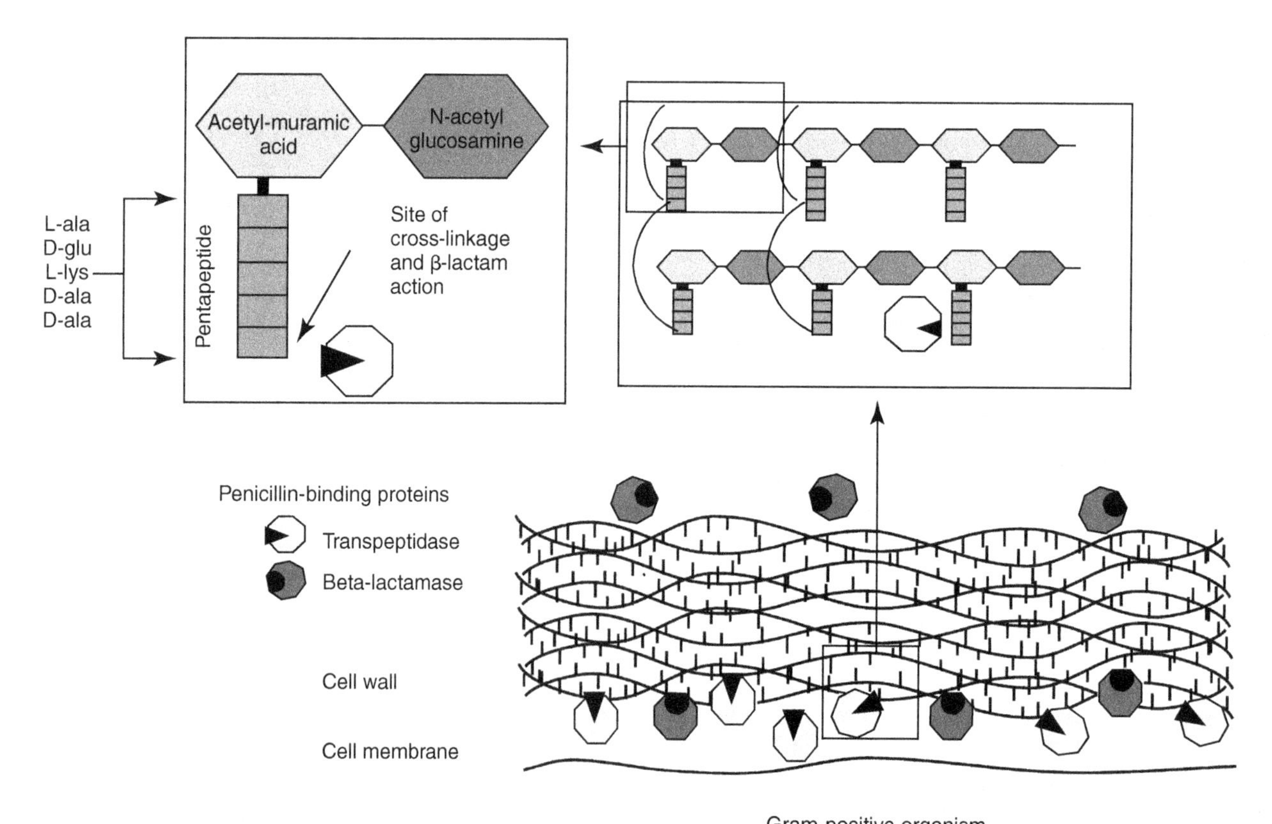

Figure 7-3 The antibacterial mechanism of action of the beta-lactams. The pentapeptide containing the D-Ala-D-Ala terminus (the structure mimicked and thus inhibited by beta-lactam antibiotics) provides the cross-linking of the strands of the cell wall, which are critical to rigidity. Two types of penicillin-binding proteins (PB) are located in the cell wall of bacteria. Transpeptidase enzymes are responsible for catalyzing the cross-bridging between the pentapeptides thus providing rigidity; changes in the structure of these proteins confers resistance to methicillin (PB-2) or other drugs. Beta-lactamase penicillin-binding proteins destroy susceptible beta-lactam antibiotics.

for carbapenems because they are characterized by more rapid bacterial killing.[13] A longer T > MIC is indicated to decrease the risk of resistance.

Although all PBPs are able to covalently bind beta-lactam antibiotics, the numbers bound and subsequent activity vary among organisms. Up to nine PBPs are encoded by the genome of *Escherichia coli;* each PBP generally has subgroups. The diversity of PBPs is responsible, in part, for differences in the spectrum of activity of the beta-lactams. High-molecular-weight PBPs (1, 2, and 3) are essential for microbial growth and survival in *Staphylocccocus* spp., whereas only PBPs 1 and 2 are critical for *Streptococcus* spp.; as such, these PBPs are the critical targets of antimicrobial therapy in these organisms.[14] In *E. coli* PBP-2 is essential for cell elongation and PBP-3 for cell division. Because PB-3 appears to complex with PBP-1, -4, and -7 as well as with other proteins,[12] effective antimicrobial binding to PBP-3 might have a greater impact than binding to other PBPs in *E. coli.* The PBP targeted is known for some drugs (e.g, cefpodoxime targets PBP-1a and 1b and PBP-3 (see package insert).

KEY POINT 7-1 The mechanism of action of the beta-lactams necessitates the presence of the drug throughout most of the dosing interval.

Although beta-lactams are very effective antimicrobials, their unique mechanism of action increases the risk of therapeutic failure in certain conditions, independent of bacterial resistance. Efficacy, particularly toward gram-negatives, is reduced in a hypertonic environment (e.g., the renal intersitium of the normally functioning kidney, an abcess) because osmotic lysis may not occur. Slow growth impairs autolysin activity, which may result in the loss of the bactericidal effect of the beta-lactam antibiotic. Examples might include the combined use of a beta-lactam with a drug that slows growth of the organisms (i.e., a ribosomal inhibitor [see Figure 7-1]), or in a hypoxic environment (e.g., abscess).

Spectrum of Activity

The spectrum of activity of beta-lactam antibiotics varies (see Table 7-2). PD data are available for both the dog and cat for limited drugs (Table 7-9), with selected information provided on human pathogens associated with skin or soft tissue infections (Table 7-10). Penicillin G, a natural antibiotic, is effective against selected gram-positive cocci and both gram-negative and gram-positive anaerobes, but it is beta-lactamase sensitive.[5] Selected enterococci are not susceptible to penicillin, and most staphylococci produce beta-lactamases. The gram-negative spectrum of penicillin G is limited but includes *Pasteurella multocida.* Penicillin V is an orally bioavailable natural penicillin, but its antimicrobial efficacy is reduced.[9] Beta-lactamase–resistant isoxazolyl-derivative penicillins include dicloxacillin, cloxacillin, methicillin, and oxacillin. These drugs are effective against gram-positive organisms, including *Staphylococcus* spp., and gram-negative and anaerobic organisms.

The spectrum of the beta-lactams was expanded with the production of the semisynthetic aminopenicillins. Amoxicillin and ampicillin (aminopenicillins) are considered broad-spectrum drugs; however, this classification has largely been muted by acquired resistance unless combined with clavulanic acid or sulbactam. They target PBP-1a. The anaerobic and gram-positive spectrum of penicillin G is maintained (although the aminopenicillins are slightly less efficacious against anaerobes). The aminopenicillins are generally effective against enterococci, although *Enterococcus faecium* often expresses resistance. In addition, many gram-negative organisms are added to the spectrum, including *E. coli, Pasteurella,* some *Proteus* species, *Klebsiella,* and selected others (e.g., *Salmonella, Shigella*). *Serratia, Enterobacter,* and *Pseudomonas* are not, however, included in the spectrum of the aminopenicillins. The spectrum of ampicillin is generally similar to that of amoxicillin, and it serves as the model drug for amoxicillin on culture and susceptibility (C&S) testing whereas amoxicillin–clavulanic acid indicates data for ampicillin–sulbactam. However, the potency of ampicillin generally is less than that of amoxicillin against enterococci and *Salmonella* but greater against *Shigella* and *Enterobacter.* The aminopenicillins are less effective compared with the penicillins against *Bacteroides fragilis,* although efficacy remains good to excellent.[9] Like penicillin, the aminopenicillins are beta-lactamase sensitive. Combination with a beta-lactamase protector (e.g., clavulanic acid or sulbactam) improves efficacy and thus broadens the spectrum against susceptible organisms that have acquired resistance through beta-lactamase production. This includes *Staphylococcus, E. coli, Klebsiella* spp., and some *Proteus* spp.[15] *Pseudomonas* spp. and other gram-negative organisms remain resistant.[7,9] Further modifications led to the extended-spectrum penicillins characterized by a markedly enhanced spectrum, particularly against gram-negative organisms, including *Pseudomonas aeruginosa, Serratia, Proteus* spp., some *Klebsiella* spp. *Shigella* spp., and *Enterobacter* spp. Examples include the carboxypenicillins carbenicillin and ticarcillin, with ticarcillin having two to four times higher activity toward *Pseudomonas* spp. than carbenicillin, and the ampicillin-derived ureidopenicillin piperacillin, which has the highest antipseudomonal activity.[5,7,16,17] The extended-spectrum penicillins are effective against anaerobic organisms, although they may be less effective than the natural penicillins. They maintain, however, good to excellent activity against *B. fragilis.*[9] The extended-spectrum penicillins are beta-lactamase sensitive; however, a ticarcillin/clavulanic acid combination product is available.

The carbapenems (imipenem and meropenem) and monobactams (aztreonam) represent the most recent members of the beta-lactam penicillins.[18] Imipenem targets PBP-1a, -1b, and -2, with its efficacy based on binding to PBP-2 and -1b. It is prepared in combination with cilastatin, which inhibits renal tubular degradation (metabolism by dehydropeptidase-1) of imipenem. As a result, drug half-life may be prolonged (although the clinical relevance of this effect in animals is questionable), and the formation of potentially nephrotoxic metabolites is reduced. Imipenem and meropenem have the broadest

Table 7-9 Susceptibility Data for Selected Beta-Lactams and Selected Feline and Canine Pathogens

		Amoxi-Clav	Cefadroxyl	Cefovecin	Cefpodoxime	Cephalexin
Acinetobacter	Mode		>32	16		>64
	MIC$_{50}$	16/8	>32	16		>64
	MIC$_{90}$	32/16	>32	32		>64
	Range	2/1-64/32	16->32	8-32		32->64
	n	16	16	16		16
	Species	D, C	D, C	D, C		D, C
	Source	1	1	1		1
	CLSI	Y	Y	Y		Y
Bacteroides spp.	Mode	≤0.5/0.25	0.5	0.25		≤0.5
	MIC$_{50}$	≤0.5/0.25	0.5	0.25		1
	MIC$_{90}$	≤0.5/0.25	16	2		16
	Range	≤0.5/0.25-8/4	≤0.25->32	≤0.06-8		≤0.5-64
	n	32	32	32		32
	Species	D, C	D, C	D,C		D, C
	CLSI	Y	Y	Y		Y
Bordetella bronchiseptica	Mode					
	MIC$_{50}$	2				
	MIC$_{90}$	4				
Clostridum spp.	Mode	≤0.5/0.25	2	0.25		≤0.5
	MIC$_{50}$	≤0.5/0.25	2	0.5		2
	MIC$_{90}$	≤0.5/0.25	16	16		16
	Range	≤0.5/0.25-1/0.5	≤0.25->32	≤0.06->32		≤0.5->64
	n	15	15	15		15
	Species	D, C	D, C	D, C		D, C
	CLSI	Y	Y	Y		Y
Coagulase-negative *Staphylococcus* spp.	Mode	≤0.5/0.25	1	0.12		1
	MIC$_{50}$	≤0.5/0.25	1	0.12		1
	MIC$_{90}$	≤0.5/0.25	4	2		4
	Range	≤0.5/0.25-1/0.5	≤0.25-8	≤0.06-8		≤0.5-16
	n	89	89	89		89
	Species	D, C	D, C	D, C		D, C
	CLSI	Y	Y	Y		Y
Coagulase-positive *Staphylococcus* spp.	Mode	≤0.5/0.25	1	0.25		1
	MIC$_{50}$	≤0.5/0.25	1	0.25		1
	MIC$_{90}$	≤0.5/0.25	2	0.5		2
	Range	≤0.5/0.25-16/8	0.5->32	0.12->32		≤0.5->64
	n	24	24	24		24
	Species	D, C	D, C	D, C		D, C
	CLSI	Y	Y	Y		Y
Corynebacterium spp.	Mode	≤0.5/0.25		1		≤0.5
	MIC$_{50}$	≤0.5/0.25	2	1		2
	MIC$_{90}$	2/1	32	4		64
	Range	≤0.5/0.25-4/2	≤0.25->32	0.25->32		≤0.5->64
	n	11	11	11		11
	Species	D, C	D, C	D, C		D, C
	CLSI	Y	Y	Y		Y

Table 7-9 Susceptibility Data for Selected Beta-Lactams and Selected Feline and Canine Pathogens—cont'd

		Amoxi-Clav	Cefadroxyl	Cefovecin	Cefpodoxime	Cephalexin
Enterobacter spp.	Mode	4/2	8	1		8
	MIC_{50}	4/2	16	1		8
	MIC_{90}	64/32	>32	32		>64
	Range	1/0.5->64/32	8->32	0.12->32		4->64
	n	39	39	39		39
	Species	D, C	D, C	D, C		D, C
	CLSI	Y	Y	Y		Y
Enterobacter cloacae	Mode	64/32	>32	2		>64
	MIC_{50}	64/32	>32	1		>64
	MIC_{90}	64/32	>32	2		>64
	Range	2/1->64/32	8->32	0.5-8		4->64
	n	20	20	20		20
	Species	D, C	D, C	D, C		D, C
	CLSI	Y	Y	Y		Y
Enterococcus spp.	Mode	1/0.5	>32	>32		>64
	MIC_{50}	1/0.5	>32	>32		>64
	MIC_{90}	1/0.5	>32	>32		>64
	Range	≤0.5/0.25-32/16	≤0.25->32	≤0.06->32		≤0.5->64
	n	45	45	45		45
	Species	D, C	D, C	D, C		D, C
	CLSI	Y	Y	Y		Y
Enterococcus faecium	Mode					
	MIC_{50}	0.5				
	MIC_{90}	1				
	CLSI					
Escherichia coli	Mode	4/2	8	0.5		8
	MIC_{50}	4/2	8	0.5	0.25	8
	MIC_{90}	8/4	16	1	0.5	16
	Range	1/0.5-64/32	4->32	0.12->32	0.12->32	2->64
	n	223	223	223	41	223
	Species	D, C	D, C	D, C	D	D, C
	CLSI	Y	Y	Y	Y	Y
Fusobacterium spp.	Mode	≤0.5/0.25	≤0.25	≤0.06		≤0.5
	MIC_{50}	≤0.5/0.25	≤0.25	≤0.06		≤0.5
	MIC_{90}	≤0.5/0.25	0.5	≤0.06		≤0.5
	Range	≤0.5/0.25-2/1	≤0.25-8	≤0.06-1		≤0.5-4
	n	66	66	66		66
	Species	D, C	D, C	D, C		D, C
	CLSI	Y	Y	Y		Y
Klebsiella pneumoniae	Mode	2/1	8	0.5		4
	MIC_{50}	2/1	8	0.5		4
	MIC_{90}	16/8	16	1		4
	Range	2/1-64/32	8->32	0.25-2		4-64
	n	16	16	16		16
	Species	D, C	D, C	D, C		D, C
	CLSI	Y	Y	Y		Y

Continued

Table 7-9 Susceptibility Data for Selected Beta-Lactams and Selected Feline and Canine Pathogens—cont'd

		Amoxi-Clav	Cefadroxyl	Cefovecin	Cefpodoxime	Cephalexin
Klebsiella spp.	Mode	2/1	8	0.5		4
	MIC$_{50}$	2/1	8	0.5		4
	MIC$_{90}$	2/1	8	1		4
	Range	1/0.5-4/2	8-16	0.25-1		2-4
	n	11	11	11		11
	Species	D, C	D, C	D, C		D, C
	CLSI	Y	Y	Y		Y
Pasteurella multocida	Mode	≤0.5/0.25	4	≤0.06		2
	MIC$_{50}$	≤0.5/0.25	4	≤0.06	≤0.03	2
	MIC$_{90}$	≤0.5/0.25	4	≤0.06	≤0.03	2
	Range	≤0.5/0.25-2/1	1-16	≤0.06-0.12	≤0.03-0.12	≤0.5-8
	n	188	188	188	32	188
	Species	D, C	D, C	D, C	D	D, C
	CLSI	Y	Y	Y	Y	Y
Peptostreptococcus spp.	Mode	≤0.5/0.25	16	0.5		16
	MIC$_{50}$	≤0.5/0.25	8	0.5		8
	MIC$_{90}$	≤0.5/0.25	32	1		16
	Range	≤0.5/0.25-2/1	≤0.25->32	0.12-2		≤0.5->64
	n	21	21	21		21
	Species	D, C	D, C	D, C		D, C
	CLSI	Y	Y	Y		Y
Porphyromonas spp.	Mode	≤0.5/0.25	≤0.25	≤0.06		≤0.5
	MIC$_{50}$	≤0.5/0.25	≤0.25	≤0.06		≤0.5
	MIC$_{90}$	≤0.5/0.25	1	≤0.06		≤0.5
	Range	≤0.5/0.25	≤0.25-1	≤0.06		≤0.5-2
	n	29	29	29		29
	Species	D,C	D,C	D,C		D, C
	CLSI	Y	Y	Y		Y
Prevotella spp.	Mode	≤0.5/0.25	≤0.25	≤0.06		≤0.5
	MIC$_{50}$	≤0.5/0.25	4	0.25		≤0.5
	MIC$_{90}$	≤0.5/0.25	32	4		64
	Range	≤0.5/0.25-1/0.5	≤0.25-32	≤0.06-8		≤0.5->64
	n	11	11	11		11
	Species	D, C	D, C	D, C		D, C
	CLSI	Y	Y	Y		Y
Proteus mirabilis	Mode	1/0.5	16	0.25		8
	MIC$_{50}$	1/0.5	16	0.25	≤0.03	8
	MIC$_{90}$	1/0.5	16	0.5	0.06	16
	Range	≤0.5/0.25-8/4	8->32	0.12-0.5	≤0.03-0.06	8-32
	n	110	110	110	14	110
	Species	D, C	D, C	D, C	D	D, C
	CLSI	Y	Y	Y	Y	Y
Proteus spp.	Mode	1/0.5	16	0.25		16
	MIC$_{50}$	1/0.5	16	0.25		16
	MIC$_{90}$	2/1	16	0.25		16
	Range	≤0.5/0.25-8/4	2->32	0.12-8		4/64
	n	71	71	71		71
	Species	D, C	D, C	D, C		D, C
	Source	1	1	1		1
	CLSI	Y	Y	Y		Y

Table 7-9 Susceptibility Data for Selected Beta-Lactams and Selected Feline and Canine Pathogens—cont'd

		Amoxi-Clav	Cefadroxyl	Cefovecin	Cefpodoxime	Cephalexin
Staphylocccocus aureus	Mode	≤0.5/0.25	2	1		2
	MIC_{50}	1/0.5	2	1	2	2
	MIC_{90}	4/2	8	2	2	8
	Range	≤0.5/0.25-16/8	1->32	0.5->32	0.12-2	1->64
	n	36	36	36	19	36
	Species	D, C	D, C	D, C	D	D, C
	Source	1	1	1	P	1
	CLSI	Y	Y	Y	Y	Y
Staphylocccous intermedius	Mode	≤0.5/0.25	1	0.12		1
	MIC_{50}	≤0.5/0.25	1	0.12	0.12	1
	MIC_{90}	≤0.5/0.25	2	0.25	0.5	2
	Range	≤0.5/0.25-16/8	0.5->32	≤0.06->32	0.12->32	≤0.5-64
	n	231	231	231	118	231
	Species	D, C	D, C	D, C	D	D, C
	Source	1	1	1	P	1
	CLSI	Y	Y	Y	Y	Y
Streptococcus spp.	Mode	≤0.5/0.25	≤0.25	≤0.06		≤0.5
	MIC_{50}	≤0.5/0.25	≤0.25	≤0.06		≤0.5
	MIC_{90}	≤0.5/0.25	2	0.5		4
	Range	≤0.5/0.25-1/0.5	≤0.25-8	≤0.06-0.5		≤0.5-16
	n	27	27	27		27
	Species	D, C	D, C	D, C		D, C
	Source	1	1	1		1
	CLSI	Y	Y	Y		Y
Streptococcus, beta-hemolytic	Mode	≤0.5/0.25	≤0.25	≤0.06		≤0.5
	MIC_{50}	≤0.5/0.25	≤0.25	≤0.06		≤0.5
	MIC_{90}	≤0.5/0.25	≤0.25	≤0.06		≤0.5
	Range	≤0.5/0.25	≤0.25-1	≤0.06-8		≤0.5-2
	n	22	22	22		22
	Species	D, C	D, C	D, C		D, C
	CLSI	Y	Y	Y		Y
Streptococcus canis	Mode	≤0.5/0.25	≤0.25	≤0.06		≤0.5
	MIC_{50}	≤0.5/0.25	≤0.25	≤0.06		≤0.5
	MIC_{90}	≤0.5/0.25	≤0.25	≤0.06		≤0.5
	Range	≤0.5/0.25	≤0.25-8	≤0.06-≤0.06		≤0.5-8
	n	66	66	66		66
	Species	D, C	D, C	D, C		D, C
	CLSI	Y	Y	Y		Y

Amoxi-Clav, Amoxicillin–clavulanic acid; *MIC,* minimum inhibitory concentration; *CLSI,* Clinical and Laboratory Standards Institute; *D,* dog; *C,* cat; y, yes. All data (except cefpodoxime) is from Stegamenn et al [20]; data for cepfodoxime is from the package insert. All MIC are in μg/mL. Data is from dogs and cats considered to be antimicrobial free[20].

antimicrobial spectrums available against bacterial organisms with cell walls, including *Pseudomonas* spp. Imipenem and meropenem are relatively resistant to beta-lactamase destruction. However, an extended beta-lactamase enzyme has recently been reported, particularly in *Klebsiella pneumoniae,*emerging as a nosocomial pathogen.[19] An advantage of the carbopenems has been their very low MICs (0.05 to 2 μg/mL) for most susceptible organisms. Meropenem is generally similar to imipenem for empirical treatment of serious infections.

Aztreonam is a monobactam (see Figure 7-2), with a high affinity for PBP-3 and lesser affinity for PBP-1a. It is particularly effective against gram-negative aerobes, including *Pseudomonas* spp. but is ineffective against gram-positive organisms and anaerobes.

Table 7-10 Susceptibility Data for Selected Human Pathogens Associated with Skin and Soft Tissue Infections[160]

Organism	Drug	Penicillin	Ampicillin	Imipenem	Meropenem	Piperacillin	Cefazolin	Cefoxitin	Ceftazidime
Enterobacter spp.	MIC_{50}		>16	0.25	≤0.06	4(4)		>32	0.25
	MIC_{90}		>16	0.5	0.12	128(64)		>32	>16
Escherichia coli	MIC50		4	0.12	≤0.06	2(1)	≤2	4	≤0.12
	MIC_{90}		>16	0.25	≤0.06	>128(4)	16	16	0.5
Klebsiella pneuomoniae	MIC_{50}		>16	0.12	≤0.06	8(2)	≤2	2	≤0.12
	MIC_{90}		>16	0.25	≤0.06	>128(16)	≥16	16	2
Proteus	MIC_{50}								2
	MIC_{90}								16
	MIC_{50}			1	1	8 (8)			
Pseudomonas aeruginosa	MIC_{90}			8	8	128 (>64)			
	MIC_{50}	8	16	≤0.06			≤2		8
Staphylococcus aureus	MIC_{90}	>32	>16	4			>16		>16

MIC, Minimum inhibitory concentration.
Parantheses refer to the combination of piperacillin with tazobactam.

The spectrum of the cephalosporins is more diverse than that of the penicillins and is not as easily categorized. Although generalizations regarding the spectrum of activity of each successive generation might be made, variability in efficacy among the drugs within and certainly among generations may result in therapeutic failure if attention is not paid to differences.[9] Thus either the package insert or C&S data should be consulted before selecting a cephalosporin, particularly beyond the first generation. In general, cephalosporins are ineffective against enterococci. With each successive generation, the cephalosporins become increasingly more resistant to beta-lactamase destruction, and all generations are generally more resistant as a class than are the penicillins. As such, they are often chosen as empirical first-choice treatment of *Staphylococcus* spp. Cephalothin (no longer commercially available) has been the drug designated by the Clinical Laboratory Standards Institute (CLSI; previously National Committee for Clinical Laboratory Standards [NCCLS]) as the model indicator for susceptibility for the first-generation cephalosporins. However, it does not represent the class equally. The aerobic spectrum of the first-generation cephalosporins is similar to that of the aminopenicillins,[9] although efficacy is more similar to amoxicillin–clavulanic acid combinations. First-generation cephalosporins such as cefazolin, cephalothin, and cephalexin are active (although not equally so) against gram-positive and gram-negative organisms such as *E. coli, K. pneumoniae*, and *Proteus mirabilis*. Among the first-generation drugs, cefazolin has better efficacy than cephalexin against gram-negative organisms (e.g., *E. coli*) but poorer efficacy against *Staphylococcus* spp.[5,9] Efficacy of cephalexin against *E. coli* is fair to poor. The anaerobic spectrum of the first-generation cephalosporins is fair but less than that of the aminopenicillins.

The second-generation cephalosporins, cefamandole, cefaclor, cefoxitin, and others, are characterized by enhanced activity toward *Enterobacter* spp., some *Proteus* spp., *E. coli*, and *Klebsiella* spp.[5] Cefoxitin has an excellent anaerobic spectrum, particularly against *Bacteroides* spp.,[5,8] although it is less effective than first-generation drugs against gram-positive organisms. Third- (cefotaxime, ceftazidime, cefpodoxime, cefoperazone, cefovecin, and the oxa-beta lactam moxalactam) and fourth-generation (cefepime; not approved in the United States) cephalosporins are generally reserved for serious gram-positive or gram-negative infections (e.g., *P. aeruginosa, Enterobacter* spp., and *Serratia* spp.). However, although the efficacy of most of the second-plus generation cephalosporins against *E. coli* tends to be good to excellent, efficacy against *P. aeruginosa*[9] is variable, and cross-efficacy among members of these generations to any organism should not be assumed. For example, cefoperazone and ceftazidime are among the most effective drugs against *P. aeruginosa,* although efficacy is less than that of the newer extended-spectrum penicillins. Cefpodoxime and cefovecin are generally effective against *E. coli* but not effective against *Pseudomonas* spp. Selected third-generation cephalosporins (e.g., cefotaxime) are effective against anaerobic organisms, whereas others (e.g., ceftazidime, ceftriaxone, and cefpodoxime) are not. Ceftiofur is a third-generation cephalosporin approved for use for canine urinary tract infections. The antimicrobial spectrum of ceftiofur includes gram-positive (*Streptococcus* spp. and *Corynebacterium* spp.), gram-negative (*Pasteurella, E. coli*, and *Salmonella* spp. but not *Pseudomonas* spp.), and anaerobic organisms. Ceftiofur is effective against many staphylococcal organisms; however, selection against *Staphylococcus* spp. should be based on C&S data.[9] The first-generation drug cefazolin has been inappropriately promoted as a generic version of ceftiofur.[19a]

The spectrum of the third-generation drugs cefpodoxime and cefovecin (the former approved in dogs and cats, the latter approved in dogs but used in cats) includes *Staphylococcus* spp.; cefovecin is also approved for use in the treatment of *Streptococcus* spp. Both drugs are effective against a variety of gram-negative organisms, including *E. coli* and *Klebsiella,* but are not generally effective toward *Pseudomonas* spp. Stegemann[20] has provided PD statistics for a large number of organisms for cefovecin, as well as selected other beta-lactams, some of which are provided in Table 7-9.

KEY POINT 7-2 The spectrum of the penicillins becomes broader as the class "extends," whereas the spectrum of the later-generation cephalosporins varies with the drug.

Resistance

Bacteria develop resistance to beta-lactams through four major mechanisms: altered or different PBPs such that antibiotic binding does not occur (e.g., staphylococcal organisms and penicillins; enterococcal organisms and cephalosporins); efflux through specific pumps; loss of or changes in porins (especially *P. aeruginosa*); and inactivation by beta-lactamases. Inactivation by beta-lactamases is most common. *Staphylococcus* resistance to penicillin appeared as early as 1942; by the late 1960s, more than 80% of medically relevant isolates were resistant to penicillin as a result of beta-lactamase production. Today more than 90% of isolates (human) produce penicillinase.[21] The approval of "protected" drugs (i.e., improved the efficacy of selected penicillins), but along with the cephalsoporins, is likely to have contributed to the emergence of altered PBP. This most notorious mechanism of resistance has yielded methicillin-resistant *Staphylococcus aureus* (MRSA) and vancomycin-resistant enterococci (VRE).

Beta-lactamases. Beta-lactamases are structurally and mechanistically similar to PBPs; indeed, certain PBPs are capable of beta-lactamase activity. Destruction of the beta-lactam (amide) ring reflects its hydrolysis (see Figure 7-2).[22] Currently, more than 400 distinct beta-lactamase enzymes are produced by gram-negative, gram-positive, and anaerobic organisms.[23,24] Selected examples are listed in Table 7-11. Altlhough clearly a major mechanism of resistance in gram-positive organisms, beta-lactamase production is also the major mechanism by which gram-negative organisms develop resistance.[22] Beta-lactamase production occurs as a result of either chromosomal mutations, particularly in gram-positive organisms, or plasmid-mediated resistance in both gram-positive and gram-negative organisms. Beta-lactamases are either constitutive, already present in the cell wall (particularly in gram-negative organisms), or induced by the presence of the antimicrobial drug (in both gram-negative and gram-positive organisms).[25] Gram-negative bacteria have the added advantage of secreting beta-lactamases into the periplasmic space such that they are strategically placed before the antibiotic can penetrate the cell wall.[9] The beta-lactams are variably susceptible to destruction by beta–lactamases; microbes vary in which enzyme they produce and whether the enzyme is constitutive or inducible (see Table 7-11).

Two major types of beta-lactamases exist: serine-based enzymes and the metallo-beta lactamases. The latter contain a zinc atom that activates water as the destructive site (see Table 7-11).[22] Several schemes have been proposed to classify beta-lactamases.The most common scheme is based on the molecular structure (Amber Classification); however, classification according to the target substrate (Bush–Jacoby Classification) may be easier to follow (see Table 7-11). According to the Amber system, Class B enzymes contain the metallo-beta lactamases, but the other three classes are serine-based enzymes. These include classes A (TEM, SHV), C (ampC, targeting cephamycins [cefotetan, cefoxitin]), and D (OXA; targeting protected drugs, such as dicloxacillin, but also protectors such as clavulanic acid). The most prevalent beta-lactamases are class A penicillinases and cephalosporinases, including clinically relevant TEM-1 and 2 or SHV-1 enzymes found in *E. coli* and *K. pneumoniae,* and PC-1 enzymes produced by *S. aureus.*[22]

KEY POINT 7-3 Microbes have been able to adapt to each pharmaceutical manipulation intended to decrease beta-lactamase activity.

TEM-1 and SHV-1 confer high-level resistance to penicillins and first generation cephalosporines but generally do not target the extended-spectrum (selected second- and third- or fourth-generation) cephalosporins or carbapenems. As such, the cephalosporins (cephalosporin C) are generally less impacted by beta-lactamases, particularly those produced by *Staphylococcus* species.[10] However, only a few cephalosporins are stable against anaerobic beta-lactamases. Selected semi-synthetic beta-lactams also are less impacted by beta-lactamases, including most third-generation cephalosporins and imipenem. The semisynthetic dicloxacillin (and oxacillin) is beta-lactamase resistant, with the exception of class D (group 2d). The combination of beta-lactam antibiotics with drugs that inhibit beta-lactamase activity (e.g., clavulanic acid, sulbactam, and tazobactam) increases the potency of the beta-lactam antibiotic, (but not the spectrum) toward susceptible organisms (see Tables 7-2, 7-9 and 7-10). Clavulanic acid irreversibly binds to some but not all beta-lactamases (see Table 7-11).[26] Combinations of beta-lactams with beta-lactamase inhibitors are particularly useful against mixed infections and have shown efficacy against selected multiresistant pathogens such as *Acinetobacter* spp. Aztreonam is generally resistant to beta-lactamase destruction but is susceptible to extended-spectrum beta-lactamases (ESBLs). The presence and diversity of beta-lactamases in canine and feline staphylococcal organisms has been described. As in other species, production is encoded by the *blaZ* gene, with all four classes of enzymes (A to D) represented genes for classes A, C, and D being plasmid mediated and class B chromosomally mediated.[27]

Microbes have adapted to each pharmaceutical manipulation intended to combat emergent resistance resulting from beta-lactamase destruction. Third-generation cephalosporins such as cefotaxime and ceftazidime initially were considered

Table 7-11 Classification of Beta-Lactamases, the Enzymes, and Drugs Targeted[5,37]

Group	Type	Subgroup	Class*	Enzyme Type	CA	Example Enzymes	Producing Organism	Target Drugs
1	Ser		C	Cephalosporinases	R	AmpC	1-6	6-8 > 1,5
						CMY-2		
2	Ser		A,D			TEM, SHV		
		a	A	Penicillinases				
		b	A	Penicillinases		TEM-1	1, 2	1
						SHV-1	2, 1	1
						PC-1	7	
				Cephalosporinases				
		be	A	Extended cephalosporinases		TEM, SHV variants		2, 5
						SHV variants		
		br	A	Inhibitor resistant	R	TEM, SHV variants	1,2,3, others	5
		c	A	Carbenicillinase		PSE, CARB	4, vibrio	1 (carbenicillin)
		d	D	Oxacillinase	R	ARI (OXA)	2,4, 10	4,5
				Carbapenemases				
		e	A	Cephalosporinase	Sus	CTX-M	1, others	
						PER		
		f	A	Carbapenemases		NCA	2, others	1,2,3,6
						IMI		
						KPC		
						GES		
						SME		
3	Met (ZN)		B	Metalloenzymes	R	IMP	4, 5, 8, 9	1, 3, 5, 8
						VIM		
						SIM		
						GIM		
4	Ser		NA	Penicillinase	R			

Keys	Example producers		Target drugs	Example drug
1	*E. coli*	1	Penicillins (e.g., Amp, Amox, Pip)	
2	*Klebsiella*	2	Oxyimino monobactams	Aztreonam
3	*Proteus*	3	Carbapenems	
4	*Pseudomonas*	4	Oxazolylpenicillins	Oxacillin
5	*Enterobacter*			Cloxacillin
6	*Serratia*			Dicloxacillin
7	*Staphylococcus*	5	Inhibitors	Clavulanic acid
8	*Bacillus*			Sulbactam
9	*Bacteroides*			Tazobactam
10	*Acinetobacter*	6	First-generation cephalosporins	
		7	Oxyimino-cephalosporins (1)	Ceftrixozime
				Cefotaxime Ceftriaxone Ceftazidime Cefpodoxime Cefovecin
		8	Cephamycins (7alphamethoxy)	Cefoxitin Cefotetan

**Amber Classification System. See text for abbreviations for enzyme types.*

indestructible by beta-lactamases.[25] However, high-level use has been accompanied by induction and selection for ESBLs in multiple-resistant coliforms,[28] particularly in those organisms that produce TEM and SHV enzymes. The genes encoding ESBLs are carried by large plasmids and are able to confer information between bacterial species and strains. The ESBLs are most commonly found in *Klebsiella* spp. (incidence in North America, 4.4%), *E. coli* (3.3% to 4.7%), or *P. mirabilis* (3.1-9.5%), but they also have been detected in other members of the family Enterobacteriaceae and in *P. aeruginosa* isolates.[29-32] The resistant gene codes for mutations in one or more amino acid (serine) substitutions in class A enzymes (TEM or SHV). The resultant change in configuration allows the enzyme to gain access to the drug despite the large oxyimino side chain of these newer-generation drugs.[24] Drugs amenable to destruction by ESBL include third-generation cefotaxime, ceftazidime and ceftriaxone, cefpodoxime, and (presumably) cefovecin.[22,33] Selected fourth-generation drugs are also susceptible, including cefepime (no longer marketed in the United States).[28] Cephamycins (e.g., second-generation cephalosporins cefoxitin, cefotetan) do not appear to be destroyed (although they are destroyed by ampC). Monobactams (i.e., aztreonam) are destroyed. Carbapenems are generally not destroyed by ESBL, nor are beta-lactamase protectors such as clavulanic acid. The use of beta-lactamase protectors appears to reduce the clinical emergence of ESBLs and may reduce the emergence of other resistant pathogens such as *Clostridium difficile* and vancomycin-resistant enterococci.[34] However, the effect (e.g., of the beta-lactamase in the presence of ESBLs) is not always predictable. Decreasesd cephalosporin usage also reduces the advent of ESBLs.

Resistance to ESBLs often is incorporated in plasmids simultaneously conferring resistance to aminoglycosides and sulfonamides.[22] Further, ESBL resistance may be associated with non–plasmid-mediated resistance mechanisms such as occurs for quinolones.[22] An "inoculum effect" of ESBLs has been described for some drugs and may explain discrepancies among studies: the MIC of the organisms toward cephalosporins increases with a larger (10^7) compared with smaller (10^5) inoculum. Because susceptibility may depend on the size of the inoculum at the site of infection,[22] ESBLs may not be detected on routine C&S testing.[31] Lack of detection of ESBLs may also reflect different levels of activity against the different cephalosporins.

Detection of ESBLs has been based on double disk diffusion techniques. The susceptible cephalosporin (e.g., cefpodoxime, ceftazidime) is incubated with the isolate as the sole drug and in the presence of a beta-lactamase inhibitor; a substantial reduction in the MIC (e.g., fourfold to eightfold) with the combination drugs compared with the cephalosporin by itself indicates an ESBL.[35,36] Not all clinical microbiology laboratories have incorporated tests for ESBLs in routine testing procedures.[22] The presence of an ESBL should be suspected with organisms resistant to or with high MIC to cefotaxime but susceptible to beta-lactam/beta-lactamase combinations.[22] The detection of an isolate with ESBL in a patient with a serious gram-negative bacillary infection should lead to the use of a carbapenem. However, a novel carbapenemase also has been described following isolation in *Serratia* spp., *K. pneumoniae* and *Enterobacter cloacae*.[19,22,37] Alternatively, combination of the cephalosporin with clavulanic acid should be considered.

KEY POINT 7-4 Extended-spectrum beta-lactamases target later-generation cephalosporins but may be missed with susceptibility testing unless special tests are performed.

Altered pencillin-binding proteins. The advent of MRSA and multidrug-resistant *Enterococcus* spp. also has been associated with cephalosporins although it is likely that beta-lactamase inhibitors contributed to its emergence.[25] The approval of the cephalosporins in the 1980s was followed by the first MRSA epidemics in the mid-1980s in the United Kingdom; the use of second- and third-generation cephalosporins also was associated with an outbreak of MRSA in Japan.[25] In humans, mortality associated with *S. aureus* bacteremia is 20% to 40%; MRSA has become a leading cause of nosocomial infections in human medicine. The term MRSA was coined in the early 1960s, when these penicillinase-resistant drugs were relatively new, and refers to resistance expressed *in vitro* to methicillin.[21] Although this discussion will focus on MRSA, increasingly, methicillin resistance is being recognized in other species and much of this information is relevant to all methicillin resistant staphylococci (MRS). Over the 30 to 40 years since MRSA was identified, MRSA infections have led to increased mortality and morbidity. The sequelae of MRSA are worse than those associated with beta-lactamase resistance because no alternative therapy remains that is predictably effective.[21] In contrast to resistance resulting from penicillinase production which is generally considered low level, infection with MRSA is considered high-level resistance. Further, MRSA isolates are essentially multidrug resistant, that is, expressing resistance to classes other than beta-lactams.

MRSA and methicillin-resistant *Staphylococcus pseudintermedius* (MRSIG)[38] are indicated by the presence of the *mecA* gene. This gene encodes a mutation in penicillin-binding protein 2a, thus reducing its affinity for the beta-lactam ring, rendering the organism resistant to all beta-lactams. The *mecA* gene is carried on the staphylococcal chromosomal cassette (SCC); currently five SCC*mec* have been described.[39] Protectors such as clavulanic acid are also unable to bind and thus are ineffective.[21] Detection of MRSA or MRSIG (or methicillin-resistance in other staphylococci [MRS]) on C&S testing generally is based on resistance to oxacillin, which is more stable than methicillin in disks used for testing. However, variability in testing methods can profoundly alter results; therefore, cefoxitin might be a more appropriate indicator of multidrug resistance in these organisms.[40] Alternative procedures such as polymerase chain reaction or latex agglutination have been used to detect the gene responsible for the formation of penicillin-binding protein 2a (mecA) of MRSA, and other techniques such as pulsed-field gel electrophoresis or multilocus sequence typing identify the specific strain of MRSA (e.g., USA100 or USA300). It is likely that this area of diagnostics will be refined in the next decade and will be applied to other MRS.

KEY POINT 7-5 Changes in the penicillin-binding protein (PBP2) by *Staphylococcus* spp. renders the microbe resistant to all beta-lactams.

Antimicrobials are associated with induction, selection, and propagation of MRSA. The wide use of cephalosporins, in particular, may have contributed significantly to the advent of MRSA. MRSA in human patients has evolved from a hospital-acquired (HA-MRSA; nosocomial) infection (usually USA100) that occurs most commonly in patients whose immune systems are compromised by a community-acquired infection (CA-MRSA), in which otherwise healthy persons are infected, usually in the skin or soft tissue. Crowded conditions, shared items, and poor hygiene increase the risk of CA-MRSA. It is CA-MRSA strain USA300 that appears to be most commonly associated with increased colonization in dogs and cats. In contrast, it is HA-MRSA (USA-100) that is most commonly associated with infections in dogs and cats.[40a] According to the Center for Disease Control, the incidence of MRSA doubled in human medicine between 1999 and 2006. The impact of MRSA (or other MRS) in veterinary medicine is increasingly problematic, not only because of its impact on the patient but also because of public health considerations. The *mec* gene has been detected in MRSA organisms infecting dogs,[40–42] and MRSA has been associated with infection in dogs.[43] However, MRSA also has been found in up to 4% of healthy dogs, with identification complicated by the need for multiple sampling sites (nasal and rectal or perineal). Risk factors for the presence of MRSA in pets or working dogs (e.g., detection and aid dogs) include contact with human hospitals (particularly if patients fed the dogs treats or were licked by the dogs) and children.[42] Infections have been isolated to family members and pets in the same household, but this is likely to reflect original transmission from humans to the pet.[40–42,44] It is likely that colonization is transient in animals. However, healthy pets have been demonstrated to be potential reservoirs for transmission of MRSA to healthy handlers and a potential health risk to immunocompromised patients (humans and presumably other animals in the household). According to the American Veterinary Medical Association, colonization by MRSA is suggested to be an occupational risk for veterinarians, although the frequency of infection associated with MRSA in veterinarians compared with other health professionals has not been documented.

MRSIG[45] has a prevalence of 0.58% to 2% in healthy dogs and up to 4% in healthy cats,[42,46] with the *mec* gene present in each canine MRSIG isolate in one study.[47] Human colonization with MRSIG is unusual.[42] However, MRSIG has been reported as a cause of infection in human patients,[42] and transmission from pets with pyoderma to humans has been confirmed.[48,49] Although the true public health significance of MRSA and MRSIG (or other multidrug-resistant organisms) in pets is not clear, the fear of infection may be as important as true risk, necessitating proper hygiene and other proactive measures such that human or animal health (including unnecessary euthanasia) is not risked.

The American Veterinary Medical Association offers a website that includes a discussion of MRSA zoonoses, including sources of guidelines that might decrease the risk presented to susceptible humans.[49a] Among the more important actions that can be taken is establishment of infection control policies and guidelines in each veterinary practice. In general, common sense approaches should prevail (e.g., minimizing intimate contact, maintaining good personal and environmental hygiene practices; see the three D's approach described in Chapter 6). This includes cleansing of hands of handlers and the paws (or body) of animals that might be exposed to MRSA, including those visiting human health care facilities. Immunocompromised patients are at most risk for MRSA infection acquired from an animal. In such cases the carrier or infected animal should be removed from the environment until successfully treated for MRSA. For dogs with skin infections, cultures are indicated to detect MRSA, particularly in animals for which infection does not resolve. Successful resolution of colonized or infected animals may require both topical (for skin infections) and systemic therapy. Evidence of successful treatment might be based on skin swabs of the ear, nose, and perianal region. Care must be taken to ensure that the laboratory providing culture procedures is well-versed in the diagnosis of MRSA, including speciation of coagulase-positive organisms.

KEY POINT 7-6 Methicillin-resistant *Staphylococcus aureus* likely originated with a human, whereas Methicillin-resistant *Staphylococcus pseudintermedius* likely originated from a dog or cat.

The multidrug resistance associated with MRSA is now evolving toward other (non–beta-lactam) antimicrobials. This reflects, in part, other resistance genes in the gene cassette carrying the *mec* gene.[42] Drugs that are affected include fluorinated quinolones and aminoglycosides. Although newer fluorinated quinolones (e.g., levfloxacin) appear to be more effective than older drugs in vitro, particularly to *Staphylococcus,* whether this translates to better clinical efficacy is unclear.[21] Glycopeptides such as vancomycin are the initial drugs used to treat MRSA in humans, although increasingly vancomycin-resistant *Staphylococcus aureus* (VRSA) infections have emerged. Linezolid and rifampin are alternative drug choices.

Multidrug resistant *Enterococcus* spp. also is an emerging issue; its emergence also appears to be correlated to use of cephalosporins. *Enterococcus faecalis* more so than *Enterococcus faecalis* is likely to develop resistance, and speciating *Enterococcus* spp. susceptibility testing might be prudent. Resistance reflects a change in penicillin-binding protein (PB-V), and the risk is increased when drugs effective against *Enterococcus* spp. are used.

Pharmacokinetics

The beta-lactams are weak acids, which favor oral absorption. Many of the beta-lactam antibiotics, however, are destroyed by the acidity of the gastrointestinal tract and thus cannot be given orally. Penicillin exceptions include penicillin V, dicloxacillin, the aminopenicillins (ampicillin and amoxicillin, including combinations with clavulanic acid), and carbenicillin (indanyl form only; effective concentrations can be achieved only in urine). Lack of stability also may affect the shelf-life of reconstituted products; expiration dates should be adhered to as indicated for the reconstituted product. Orally bioavailable cephalosporins include cephalexin, cefadroxil, and cefpodoxime (third or fourth generation). The oral bioavailability of the cephalosporins also varies among drugs and species.[5,9]

Many beta-lactams are available as intravenous or parenteral preparations. Absorption from parenteral sites tends to be rapid and complete, with the exception of products that are specifically formulated to allow slow release (e.g., esterified penicillins). Although drug concentrations may persist in circulation longer than non–slow-release preparations (an appealing aspect for time-dependent antimicrobials), older dosing regimens were designed for efficacy against organisms considerably more susceptible to drugs at the time of approval compared with current microorganisms. Thus consideration should be taken to design the dose of these products to compensate for any increase in MIC that may have emerged since the approval of the labeled dose. Selected beta-lactams are highly bound to plasma proteins. Although binding limits distribution into tissues, it also contributes to a long disappearance half-life. Cefpodoxime and, to a greater degree, cefovecin are example of beta-lactams whose long half-life reflects slow release from intravascular protein.[20]

KEY POINT 7-7 As water-soluble drugs, all beta-lactams distribute to extracellular fluid, do not penetrate sanctuary tissues well, and are renally excreted.

Distribution of beta-lactams is limited to extracellular fluid (volume of distribution [Vd or Vd_{ss}] of unbound drug generally ≤0.3 L/kg), but, barring a marked host inflammatory response, adequate concentrations of unbound drug can usually be achieved in the interstitial fluid (the site of most infections) in many tissues (see Table 7-5).[5,9] Penicillins and cephalosporins are thus widely distributed throughout most extracellular body fluids, including kidneys, lungs, joints, bone, soft tissues, and bile[5,8,11] Interstitial fluid concentrations in normal tissues generally can be predicted by, but are not necessarily equivalent to, the concentration of (unbound) drug in plasma. Comparisons of AUC frequently reveal interstitial fluids to be 30% or less than that in plasma. Among the first-generation cephalosporins, cefodroxil appears to have the better tissue-to-PDC ratio in humans (see Table 7-5). Neither penicillins nor cephalosporins traverse sanctuaries well, including mammary, prostatic, or blood–brain barriers. Imipenem, but generally not antipseudomonal penicillins such as ticarcillin and piperacillin, can reach effective concentrations in the brain. However, first- and second-generation cephalosporins should not be used for central nervous system (CNS) infections because many are destroyed by local enzymes or transported out of the CNS. Beta-lactams in general achieve 25% or less in bronchial secretions compared with PDCs (see Table 7-5).[50-52] Inflammation increases the penetration of many beta-lactams. For example, cefuroxime, cefotaxime, ceftriaxone, and ceftazidime can reach therapeutic concentrations when the cerebral spinal fluid (CSF) is inflamed.[9] Acute inflammation may also increase beta-lactam penetration of abscesses and pleural, peritoneal, and synovial fluids because of changes in vascular permeability. However, those drugs characterized by high binding to plasma protein will likewise be bound to inflammatory proteins. As response to therapy decreases, resolution of inflammation may decrease distribution. Further, if inflammation does not resolve but progresses, efficacy of beta-lactams is likely to decrease as a result of poor penetrabiltity of lipid tissue. The beta-lactams do not significantly accumulate in phagocytic cells (see Table 7-5). Beta-lactams are concentrated in the urine, enhancing efficacy for cystitis; the clinician must not assume that the high concentration will be achevied in other tissues that also are infected (e.g, nephritis or other urinary tract sites, and even high urinary concentrations may be ineffective in the presence of biofilm (see Chapter 8).

The small Vd that characterizes the unbound beta-lactams contributes to their relatively short half-lives, which often are less than 1 to 4 hours (see Table 7-1). Slow release of highly-protein bound drugs will prolong presence in the plasma. Because beta-lactams in general do not exhibit a long postantibiotic effect, dosing intervals for such drugs may be inconvenient; for critical patients, administering the drug as a constant-rate infusion may be appropriate. The attributes of constant-rate infusion for critical human patients receiving beta-lactams with short half-lives are well recognized and have been demonstrated in animal models.[3] The advantages may reflect better steady-state concentrations of drugs in peripheral tissues. Exceptions occur for selected drugs that have a longer half-life, drugs characterized by metabolism to active metabolites, or slowly absorbed or released preparations. The former includes cefpodoxime (4- to 5-hour half-life and 80% to 90% protein bound) and cefovecin (approximate 4- to 5-day half-life and 90% to 99% bound to serum proteins in dogs or cats). Penicillins designed for slow release include slow-release esters (e.g., procaine or benzathine penicillins) or highly protein-bound drugs that may be slowly released from plasma to tissue (e.g., cefovecin). For the latter, generally either absorption or distribution, rather than elimination, half-life is prolonged, resulting in a "flip-flop" model (see Chapter 1). The beta-lactam antibiotics are eliminated, in general, by active tubular secretion in the renal tubules. Clavulanic acid, which is a beta-lactam antibiotic, albeit with poor efficacy by itself, is excreted primarily in the urine of dogs.[53] With the exception of hetacillin (no longer available), hepatic metabolism does not play a role in the elimination of the penicillins. Some cephalosporins are eliminated in the urine after deacetylation by the liver, often generate no active metabolites. Examples include cephalothin, cephapirin, cefotaxime, and ceftiofur. Imipenem is degraded to inactive metabolites in the kidney. Reabsorption from the urine is facilitated by an acid urinary pH. Deacetylation of ceftiofur results in an active metabolite; dosing regimens and C&S testing are based on ceftiofur bioactivity.[54] Ceftriaxone and cefoperazone are eliminated in the bile in humans and appear to be at least partially eliminated in the bile in dogs.[9]

Disposition of selected beta-lactam antibiotics

Penicillins. Preparations of penicillin G intended for intramuscular use (e.g., procaine and benzathine) may be prepared as esters, which hydrolyze at variable rates and thus prolong absorption. Procaine penicillin is absorbed for at least 24 hours and benzathine penicillin for approximately 120 hours in some species.[9]

For the aminopenicillins the oral bioavailability of amoxicillin is greater than that of ampicillin and, unlike ampicillin, is not impaired by the presence of food.[5] Clavulanic acid appears to be about 30% to 65% orally bioavailable.[15,53,55] The absorption of both amoxicillin and clavulanic acid appears to occur through a saturable process. As with humans, a maximum rate may be reached in dogs at 10 mg/kg and 5 mg/kg, respectively. As the oral dose of amoxicillin reaches 25 mg/kg and clavulanic acid 6.25 mg/kg, amoxicillin may interfere with oral absorption of clavulanic acid. Thus ratios that favor clavulanic acid might be preferred to ensure sufficient absorption.[26] Other disposition paramenters of the aminopenicillins are summarized in Table 7-1. The disposition of amoxicillin is such that care should be taken to ensure that underdosing does not occur. This is likely to require administration beyond the label dose (12.5 mg/kg, alone or as clavulanic acid). For treatment of *S. pseudintermedius,* Stegemann[20] has reported an MIC_{90} of <0.5 μg/mL for amoxicillin-clavulanic acid (see Table 7-9). The MIC_{50} and MIC_{90} for amoxicillin-clavulanic acid and *E. coli* are 2 and 8 μg/mL, respectively. Integration of PK-PD for these organisms indicates that an alternative drug to amoxicillin with or without clavulanic acid might be considered; an exception might occur with UTI because higher drug concentrations will be achieved in the target tissue (urine). However, precaution is also suggested with this approach (see Chapter 8). Note that CLSI has recently re-set breakpoint MIC's such that many isolates considered susceptible before this change will now be considered resistant.

KEY POINT 7-8 The low C_{max} achieved for amoxicillin at the labeled dose coupled with its short half-life markedly increase the likelihood of therapeutic failure even for "susceptible" isolates.

Carbepenems. Both imipenem and meropenem have been studied in dogs.[56,57] Imipenem is minimally protein bound in dogs.[56] Peak concentrations (see Table 7-1) occur at 30 minutes for intramuscular and 50 minutes for subcutaneous administration. Extrapolated PDCs after intravenous administration appear to approximate 40 mg/L. The volume of distribution of 0.32 L/kg indicates distribution to extracellular fluid; clearance (CL) is 0.26 L/hr/kg. The elimination half-life varies almost twofold with the route (see Table 7-1). Bioavailability is high after intramuscular or subcutaneous administration.[56] In dogs given 5 mg/kg subcutaneously, targeting a 12-hour interval and a T ≥ MIC_ (25%) (acceptable for carbapenems), the highest MIC that might be treated is 2 μg/mL. The dose should be increased (approximately 30%) to adjust for ≤70% drug movement from plasma into normal interstitial fluid, particularly if the drug is given subcutaneously.

Meropenem has been studied in dogs after single dose[58] and constant-rate infusion.[57] As with imipenem, it is minimally (12%) protein bound in dogs. Clearance is 5.6 to 6.5 mL/min/kg. After a dose of 20 mg/kg, mean meropenem (μg/mL) in interstitial fluid (using ultrafiltration techniques) was 24 ± 8 μg/mL. After subcutaneous administration, C_{max} (μg/mL) in plasma and interstitial fluid, respectively, were 25 and 11 (ratio = 0.44), and AUCs were 63 and 43 μg * hr/mL, (ratio 0.68) respectively. The better ratio for AUC reflects a longer mean residence time in intracellular fluid (ICF) compared with plasma (2, 4, and 0.9 hours, respectively). Although interstitial fluid concentrations correlated very well with PDC, the doses based on plasma C_{max} values might be increased at least 40% when basing dosing on PDC to compensate for differential distribution to extracellular sites of infection. The AUC in interstitial fluid after 20 mg/kg administered intravenously or subcutaneously was 73 μg * hr/mL, and 43 μg * hr/mL, respectively, indicating that intravenous administration might be preferred to subcutaneous administration from a cost standpoint. Note that the time to maximum concentration in interstitial fluid after subcutaneous administration was 3.7 hours (2 hours for intravenous administration), indicating a potential delay in response in the acute situation.[58] Based on plasma C_{max} after 20 mg/kg administered subcutaneously in dogs, a 12-hour dosing interval, and T > MIC of 25%, the highest MIC that might be treated is 4 μg/mL. If concentrations are used to design the dosing regimen, the highest MIC that could be treated would be 1 μg/mL. Anuric renal failure in humans prolongs the half-life of meropenem fourfold.[59]

First-generation cephalosporins. Papich et al. described the tissue distribution of cephalexin.[59a] The ratio of cephalexin C_{max} or AUC in plasma versus interstitial fluid were approximately 50% and 57%, respectively. The eliminaton half-life of cephalexin appears to be somewhat route dependent, being almost twice as long as after oral administration (150 minutes) compared with intramuscular or intravenous administration (80 minutes; see Table 7-1). However, Papich et al. reported a much longer half-life of 4.7 + 1 hours in dogs after oral administration of 25 mg/kg.[59a] Plasma clearance is 2.5 mL/min/kg.[60] Bioavailability approximates 60% after either oral or intramuscular administration.[60] Oral bioavailability in dogs is affected by the time of day of administration, with C_{max} 22% lower in the evening; however, this is more than offset (as a time-dependent drug) by a prolongation of half-life by 50%.[61] The oral bioavailability of cephalexin also is affected by pretreatment with metaclopramide, which increases C_{max} and AUC, respectively, by 17% and 25%.[61] Based on the original half-life reported for cephalexin, targeting T > MIC (50%), the maximum MIC that can be treated using an oral dose of 20 mg/kg is 1 μg/mL. This is equivalent to the MIC_{50} but less than the MIC_{90} (2 μg/mL) reported for *S. intermedius* and cephalexin in dogs.[20] A dose of 40 mg/kg is needed for twice-daily dosing, or the interval should be reduced to every 8 hours. Doses would need to be further increased to compensate for differential distribution to tissues or other host or microbial factors. However, if the half-life of 5 hours is used, then twice-daily dosing of cephalexin will result in drug concentration in both plasma and interstitial fluid above the MIC_{90} for *S. intermedius*[20] for 12 hours or more.[59a] Note that the MIC_{50} and MIC_{90}, respectively, for *E. coli* and cephalexin are 8 and 16,[20] indicating that this drug should not be used to treat infections associated with *E. coli*, including urinary tract infections.

Cephalothin (no longer available in the United States, although it remains the model drug for first-generation cephalosporins at the time of publication) has been studied in dogs after oral administration at 30 mg/kg. Food affects its absorption: C_{max} of 45 μg/mL is reduced to 28 μg/mL with food at a T_{max} of 1.7 and 2.8 hours, respectively. Elimination half-life is 1.8 and 2.6 hours without and with food, respectively.[62]

Cefadroxil achieves a C_{max} of 35 μg/mL at a T_{max} of 20 minutes after an oral dose of 30 mg/kg. Food minimally affects rate or extent of absorption according to one study, but it does increase half-life from 1.7 to 4 hours.

Cefazolin has been studied in two separate groups of canine patients undergoing elective orthopedic procedures. In one study[63] clinical canine patients (n = 15) undergoing total hip replacement were administered 22 mg/kg intravenously over 2 minutes at the time of surgical positioning; animals were dosed 2 more times.[64] The distribution of the central compartment (Vc; before distribution) was 0.083 ± 0.008 L/kg. The distribution half-life approximated 5 minutes, and the elimination half-life approximated 45 minutes. Tissues from the coxofemoral joint capsule, acetabulum, and femoral cancellous bone were collected from each patient as the site was approached surgically; serum samples were collected at the same general time for each patient. Peak serum concentrations after the first dose were 178 ± μg/mL; tissue (homogenate) concentrations and mean time of collection were as follows: joint capsule, 58 + 5.7 μg/mL at 20 min, acetabulum 157 + 23 at 52 minutes and bone cancellous 227 + 29 at 68 minutes. Peak serum concentrations approximated 178 μg/mL (before distribution) and 119 μg/mL (after distribution). Based on simulations, ideal dosing was suggested to be either 22 mg/kg every 2 hours or 8 mg/kg every hour, to ensure drug concentrations remained above the MIC of *Staphylococcus* spp. (reported at 2 μg/mL).

Second- and third-generation cephalosporins. Cefuroxime is a second-generation cephalosporin approved for use in humans. Oral administration is in the form of the axetil ester; as a prodrug, desterification occurs before oral absorption. It has been studied both orally and parenterally in Beagles (n=6) as part of a toxicity study.[64a] Intravenous doses up to 500 mg/kg every 24 hours were well tolerated for 1 week. Jung[65] compared cefuroxime in serum to that in cortical tissues in dogs. At approximately 1.25 hours, after 10 and 20 mg/kg administered intravenously, serum concentrations were 12.5 and 28.7 μg/mL, respectively. The elimination half-life was 2.9 hours. Spurling[66] reported limited PDCs after oral administration in Beagles. Concentrations (μg/mL) after oral administration of the axetil form at 100 or 400 mg/kg were approximately 28.7 ± 5, and 77 ± 17, respectively.[66,67]

KEY POINT 7-9 The longer half-life of cefpodoxime renders it preferable to cephalothin for treatment of susceptible infections as long as a sufficiently high dose is used.

After a dose of 50 mg/kg ceftriaxone (third generation) was given to apparently healthy dogs, clearance was 3.61 ± 0.8 mL/kg/hr; T_{max} occurred at 30 minutes compared with 90 minutes after subcutaneous administration. Pain occurred at the injection site after both intramuscular and subcutaneous administration, whereas intravenous administration was not associated with any adversity.[68]

Based on studies in dogs after an intravenous dose of 14 mg/kg, cefepime was distributed to a volume of 0.14 l/kg, suggesting that the drug might be protein bound. However, both the elimination half-life and MRT were short at 60 minutes. Clearance was 0.13 ± 0.04 l/kg/hr. The dose necessary to maintain the breakpoint MIC of 8 μg/mL for at least two-thirds of the dosing interval (above 2 μg/mL for the entire interval) (for humans) in dogs was recommended by the author to be 40 mg/kg every 6 hours.[28]

Ceftazidime is a third-generation drug characterized by an elimination half-life of 0.8 hours in dogs. After subcutaneous injection, T_{max} occurs at 1 hour after administration of 30 mg/kg. When given an initial dose of 4.4 mg/kg followed by a constant-rate infusion of 4.1 mg/kg/hr for 36 hours, C_{max} at steady state is 22.2 μg/mL. Total body clearance is 0.19 L/kg/hr.[69] The MIC_{90} for clinical isolates (n = 101) of *P. aeruginosa* was ≤ 4 μg/mL.[69] Using 4μg/mL as the basis for a subcutaneous dose of 30 mg/kg, only 3 half-lives can elapse for T = MIC, indicating a 6-hour dosing interval might be appropriate for *Pseudomonas* spp. Ceftazidime has been studied in cats (n = 5) after intravenous and intramuscular (30 mg/kg) administration.[70] After intravenous administration, the Vd was 18 ± 0.04 L/kg; protein binding was not described. Plasma clearance was 0.19 ± 0.08 L/hr/kg, and elimination half-life was 0.77 ± 0.06 hour. After intramuscular administration, bioavailability was 82.47 ± 4.37%, resulting in a C_{max} of 89.42 ± 12.15 μg/mL, at a T_{max} of approximately 30 minutes. The authors indicated that for an 8- to 12-hour dosing interval, T > MIC would range from 35% to 52% of the dosing interval for intravenous and 48% to 72% for intramuscular administration for isolates with an MIC ≤ 4 μg/mL.

Ceftiofur is a third-generation drug approved for use in dogs for treatment of urinary tract infections. It has been studied at 0.22, 2.2, and 4.4 mg/kg administered subcutaneously in dogs (n = 9).[71] PDCs increase proportionately (see Table 7-1). It has a relatively long half-life compared with other cephalosporins, reflecting, in part, its active metabolite. Accordingly, a longer dosing interval is likely to be more reasonable for ceftiofur compared with the first-generation drugs. When administered subcutaneously, peak PDCs (C_{max}) were 1.66 ± 0.2, 8.91 ± 6.42, and 27 ± 1 μg/mL at 0.22, 2.2, and 4.4 mg/kg, respectively.[71] At the C_{max} of approximately 9 μg/mL at a dose of 2.2 mg/kg, targeting T > MIC of 50%, the highest MIC that can be treated at 12-hour intervals is 4 μg/mL. At 4.4 mg/kg administered subcutaneously, the C_{max} disproportionately increases to 29 μg/mL, and the highest MIC that could be treated using the same targets is 16 μg/mL, which actually exceeds the MIC_{BP} (≥8 μg/mL). Urine concentrations were also reported for ceftiofur bioactivity in the dog. At 24 hours, urine concentrations at 2.2 and 4.4 mg/kg were 8.1 and 29.6 μg/mL, respectively. These concentrations surpassed the the MIC_{90} for *E. coli* (4.0 μg/mL) and *P. mirabilis* (1.0 μg/mL).[71]

Cefpodoxime is a relatively new third-generation cephalosporin to be approved in dogs for treatment of canine pyoderma. Orally, it is administered as a prodrug, cefpodoxime proxetil, which is desterified in the gastrointestinal tract such that it is absorbed as cefpodoxime. According to the package insert and technical mongraphs, oral bioavailability in dogs is 63% and food does not impair absorption. At 10 mg/kg administered orally, C_{max} is variable at 16.4 ± 11 μg/mL, suggesting that dosing should err on the high side for higher MIC; T_{max} occurs at 2 to 3 hours. Plasma clearance is 23 mL/hr/kg. Cefpodoxime is excreted largely in the urine with more than 75% excreted as the parent drug. The elimination half-life of 5.6 hours (MRT 9 hours) is longer than that of many beta-lactams; therefore a longer dosing interval is possible (i.e., 12 to 24 hours, depending on the dose and MIC of the infecting microbe). PDCs after 10 mg/kg appear to approximate 1 μg/mL at the end of a 24-hour dosing interval. Thus PDC will stay above the MIC_{90} for *E. coli* (0.5), and for *S. pseudintermedius* (0.5) well beyond the targeted T>MIC of 50% to 75%. (assuming MIC does not change dramatically overtime). However, at 5 mg/kg administered orally in dogs, the highest MIC that can be treated with a 12-hour dosing interval is 4 μg/mL, and with a 24-hour dosing interval, 2 μg/mL, both of which are still above the MIC_{90} of the approved pathogens. Cefpodoxime is well tolerated in dogs at doses as high as 400 mg/kg/day for 6 months.

Tissue kinetics of cefpodoxime compared with cephalexin have been described in dogs.[59a] The free and thus diffusible fraction of drug in plasma ranged from 9% to 34%. Maximum drug concentrations after administration of 8.5 mg/kg (single dose) in dogs (n = 6) was (extrapolated from plot) approximately 10 μg/mL free drug (33±7 μg/mL total) in plasma compared with 4.3 +1.9 in interstitial fluid, suggesting less than 50% of the drug in plasma reaches interstitial tissues. Unbound AUC in plasma was not provided, but the disappearance half-life of cefpodoxime from interstitial fluid was twice as long as that from plasma (10 + 3 hours versus 5.6 + 0.9 hours, respectively). The reason for this difference is not clear, although factors that influence diffusibility from tissue into serum might also influence antibacterial activity potentially precluding drug efficacy. Nonetheless, on the basis of these data, interstitial concentrations of cefpodoxime exceeded the MIC_{90} of *S. intermedius* and *E. coli* as reported on the package insert for 24 hours.[59a] This is in contrast to cephalexin, which is <20% bound to plasma proteins and for which interstitial concentrations exceeded the MIC_{90} for *S. pseudintermedius* (as reported by Stegemann[20]) for 12 hours but did not achieve the MIC_{90} for *E. coli*.

Cefovecin (third-generation) is the newest cephalosporin to be approved in dogs at the time of this publication. Its PD and PK have been very well described including either concentrations or bioactivity in interstitial fluid in dogs or cats in part because its disposition is complicated by extensive binding to plasma proteins.[20,72,73] Accordingly, care must be taken when designing dosing regimens to base decisions on unbound, rather than total, drug. Based on protein-binding studies (microdialysis) at cefovecin concentrations ranging from 10 to 300 μg/mL in dog plasma, 96% to 98% is bound at concentrations below 100 μg/mL, with the fraction increasing to 72% at 200 μg/mL and 56% at 300 μg/mL. Avid protein-binding results in a slow release and a long elimination half-life of 136 or 133 hours when given intravenously or subcutaneously, respectively. Protein-binding also affects T_{max}, which does not occur until 6 hours (based on total drug), and the apparent Vd (0.12 L/kg), which is higher than total blood volume but considerably lower than extraceullar fluid volume. C_{max} of unbound, active drug approximates about 5 μg/mL. Predicted unbound concentrations suggest that T > MIC_{90} of, *S. pseudintermedius* (0.25 μg/mL) occurs at approximately day 12 after dosing 8 mg/kg subcutaneously; however, this is reduced to day 8 on the basis of the lowest unbound concentration predicted by the 95% confidence interval of 1 μg/mL, which is the more prudent statistic to follow (see package insert). For organisms with MIC ≥ 2 μg/mL (see Table 7-9) (e.g., *S. aureus*, not an approved indication), T > MIC of mean (predicted) unbound drug at approximately 1 to 2 days; however, if based on the lowest (95% confidence interval) predicted unbound concentrations, 2 μg/mL would not be reached in plasma. In contrast, the MIC_{90} of *Streptococcus canis* (an approved indication) is much lower (< 0.06 μg/mL); thus T > MIC exceeds 14 days even when based on the lowest predicted unbound concentration in plasma. The same is true for *Pasteurella*, the approved indication in cats; the targeted T > MIC_{90} is not reached until 12 days after treatment.

KEY POINT 7-10 The high fraction of cefovecin binding to plasma proteins prolongs its half-life, but less than 10% of total drug is active.

Studies of unbound cefovecin in tissue have been published using tissue cage models in dogs.[72] The studies demonstrate that unbound cefovecin effectively moves from plasma into tissues, as indicated by antibacterial activity against *S. pseudintermedius* across time). After 8 mg/kg administered subcutaneously in dogs, cefovecin (total) C_{max} (total, μg/mL) was 116, 32, and 40 in plasma, transudate, and exudate, respectively, with elimination half-life from transudate similar to that in plasma (147 hours and 136 hours, respectively). Antibacterial activity was detectable in transudate at 4 hours; however, T_{max} of cefovecin antibacterial activity did not occur until approximately 2 days. Interestingly, antibacterial activity in transudate actually exceeded antibacterial activity in plasma at all time points after 8 hours and far exceeded it from day 5 forward. Peak antibacterial effects for *S. pseudintermedius* persisted in transudate until day 10 after injection, with log 2 reduction in CFUs still present at day 18; activity was gone by day 21.

Urine concentrations of cefovecin have been reported in dogs after subcutaneous administration of 8 mg/kg. Peak urine (presumably unbound) concentrations of 66 μg/mL were achieved at 54 hours and approximated 2.9 μg/mL at 18 days.

These data support the use of cefovecin for treatment of susceptible isolates causing urinary tract infections. Cefovecin also is approved for use in cats. Compared with the dog, cevovecin at 8 mg/kg reaches a higher total plasma C_{max}; however, it is 99% or more bound to plasma proteins in the cat. Although mean predicted unbound concentrations approximate 10 μg/mL, the predicted variability is great, yielding as little as 0.2 if based on the lower 95% confidence interval (see package insert). The elimination half-life in cats is slightly longer at 166 hours (compared with 136 hours in dogs). The T_{max} for plasma is only 2 hours in cats (compared with 6 hours in dog). Peak concentrations of cefovecin in transudate (occurring at 1 day) were approximately 65 μg/mL (compared with approximately 30 μg/mL in dogs). However, 99% of the drug in transudate also was bound, despite the assumption that transudate is protein free. Antibacterial studies were not performed in the transudate of cats and it is not clear what impact, binding has on transudate bioactivity. The concentration of free drug in transudate in cats approximated or exceeded the MIC_{90} ($T > MIC_{90}$) *P. multocida* (0.012 μg/mL; the approved target organism in cats) for 10 days.

The percentage of a radiolabeled dose of cefovecin recovered in urine of dogs (approximately 28%) was only slightly higher than that in feces (24%), indicating that the impact of cefovecin on normal gastrointestinal microbiota may not necessarily be less than that of orally administered drugs. Although urine contamination of feces may have occurred during the collection process, a second peak in PDCs occurs in cats, indicating that enteroheptic circulation may occur.

KEY POINT 7-11 Indiscriminate use of cefovecin must be avoided such that emergence of methicillin-resistant *Staphylococcus aureus* or methicillin-resistant *Staphylococcus intermedius* will not be facilitated.

Stegemann[20] has reported the PD activity of many anaerobic and aerobic gram-positive and gram-negative (potentially) pathogenic organisms collected from dogs and cats in the United States and Europe. Isolates were tested toward cefovecin, amoxicillin–clavulanic acid, cephalexin, and cefodroxil. The number of isolates in general for each organism exceeded 25, although exceptions exist (e.g, *Klebsiella*, coryneforms). *Acinetobacter* and *Enterococcus* spp. ($n \geq 25$) were characaterized by an MIC_{50} of 16 or higher, well above the C_{max} of unbound drug; cefovecin should not be used to treat infections caused by these organisms. For the remaining isolates, integration of PD data with PK data (see Table 7-6) reveals that $T > MIC$ for cefovecin that is superior to the other three drugs studied.

Several considerations should be made when selecting cefovecin as empirical choice for treatment of (presumed) susceptible infections in the dog or cat. First, recognizing the historical relationship between cephalosporins and MRSA might lead to judicious, if not limited, use. Second, not all organisms are equally susceptible to cefovecin. Caution is recommended when using cefovecin for treatment of organisms whose $MIC_{90} \geq 2$ μg/mL. Third, if the decision is made to redose cefovecin, doing so probably should be considered at 2 to 4 days rather than 7 to 14 days for those organisms whose MIC is equal to or greater than 2 μg/mL. The need for redosing might be limited to those patients at risk for persistent and thus resistant infections. A final consideration for cefovecin therapy is the time that must lapse to detectable (4 to 8 hours in plasma or transudate) and peak (2 to 3 days) antibacterial activity of cefovecin in interstitial fluid.[72] Cefovecin may not be a wise choice if rapid antibacterial efficacy is needed. This includes the surgical patient. Because of its long time to onset and persistence, cefovecin should not be used for surgical prophylaxis. Fourth, increasingly in human medicine, the duration of antimicrobial therapy is being shortened (e.g., to 5 days or less) for treatment of uncomplicated infections such that emergent resistance might be minimized (see Chapter 6); with cefovecin, "hit hard, get out quick" is not possible.

Drug interactions. The potential synergistic and antagonistic effects of beta-lactams with other antimicrobials was discussed in Chapter 6. Synergisim resulting from enhanced antimicrobial uptake associated with altered cell wall permeability has been demonstrated for a number of antimicrobials. Antagonism should be anticipated with drugs whose impact slows organism growth (i.e., single subunit ribosomal inhibitors); efficacy of beta-lactams may be reduced to bacteriostatic rather than bactericidal effects. An exception may occur for chloramphenicol and selected Enterobacteriaceae (see the discussion of chloramphenicol). As weak acids, the beta-lactams may chemically interact with and inactivate weak bases (see the discussion of aminoglycosides). Inactivation occurs at high concentrations, as might occur with mixing of medications, or potentially, in urine. High protein binding of beta-lactams may result in drug intractions with other highly protein-bound drugs because of competition for protein-binding sites, as is exemplified for cefovecin. Drugs for which higher concentrations have been demonstrated when combined with cefovecin and include carprofen, furosemide, doxycycline, and ketoconazole (PI). It should be anticipated that concurrent use of cefovecin with other highly protein-bound drugs will result in increased free drug concentrations. Beta-lactams will compete for active tubular secretion proteins in the proximal tubule with other organic acids (e.g., penicillins, cephalosporins, nonsteroidal antiinflammatory drugs, sulfonamides, diuretics). The prototypic example drug is probenecid, the combination of which with penicillins was used therapeutically to prolong elimination before implementation of mass production technology. According to the package insert accompanying probenecid, combined use with penicillin results in a twofold to fourfold increase in penicillin drug concentrations.

Adverse Effects

Mammalian cells lack a cell wall; therefore, the beta-lactam antibiotics are very safe. Diarrhea is a common side effect that may reflect altered intestinal microbial flora. Experimentally, co-oral administration with a recombinant beta-lactamase minimally altered fecal microflora but did not negatively influence PDCs.[73a] Increasing the ratio of amoxicillin to clavulanic acid reduces gastrointestinal upset in humans (but may decrease the absorption of clavulanic acid; see previous discussion), but ratios less than 4:1 can only be accomplished using human-approved drugs, whose equivalent bioavailability has not been established in dogs and cats. The role of probiotics in preventing diarrhea has yet to be established but warrants consideration. Hypersensitivity is an infrequent reaction and occurs less often with cephalosporins. Penicilloic acid (results from breakdown of the beta-lactam ring) is the more likely mediator of hypersensitivity reactions; it is generated from the activity of several beta-lactamase or other enzymes from various sources. Thrombocytopenia has been reported to occur with some members of this class. With the exception of the carbapenems and selected later-generation cephalosporins, the beta-lactams may cause endotoxin release (see Chapter 6), which may prove detrimental to the patient, although relevance to dogs and cats is not clear.[74] Penicillins, including imipenem, antagonize gamma-aminobutyric acid type A receptors and may thus lower the seizure threshold.[75] The risk may be greater in patients with renal disease.[76] Cephalexin can cause false glucosuria.[77]

Therapeutic Use

The broad spectrum and wide safety margin of the beta-lactam antibiotics lead to their common use. Caution is recommended, however, when they are used to treat complicated infections without the benefit of C&S data. For many drugs, because of the short half-life, C_{max} achieved at recommended doses often is not sufficient to allow a convenient dosing interval. Exceptions occur for those cephalosporins with a long half-life or carpabenems for which T > MIC of 25% is acceptable. Resistance develops to beta-lactams relatively rapidly, and the drugs are not characterized by an excellent distribution pattern, with interstitial fluid concentrations of active drug often being 50% to 30% or less of plasma concentrations, depending on the tissue and the drug. Caution should be taken with third- and fourth-generation cephalosporins despite indications of susceptibility on culture data because of inducible ESBLs that require special testing, especially in the presence of a high infecting inoculum. The spectrum of natural penicillins is relatively narrow, particularly when considered in the context of resistance that has emerged through decades of use. Resistance to aminopenicillins also limits their use as empirical drugs of choice. Exceptions might include anaerobic infections. Because the extended penicillins are susceptible to beta-lactamase destruction, combination with a beta-lactamase protector (e.g., ticarcillin and clavulanic acid) or use of imipenem—which is inherently more resistant to beta-lactamase destruction—should be considered. Imipenem or meropenem should be considered before other beta-lactams for treatment of infections associated with endotoxemia because either drug is associated with the least endotoxin release. Constant-rate infusion should be considered for those penicillins with a short half-life to maintain effective concentrations in the critical patient; alternatively, and preferably, carbapenems should be considered in lieu of penicillins. Use of beta-lactamase–protected products should be considered even in uncomplicated infections. Indiscriminate use of beta-lactams, and particularly cephalosporins, should be avoided to minimize the advent of MRSIG.

The first-generation cephalosporins have been excellent first-choice antimicrobials for many infections, including urinary, skin, and respiratory tract infections. Their relative resistance to beta-lactamases produced by *Staphylococcus* spp. leads to their frequent empirical selection for infections in which *Staphylococcus* spp. are assumed to be involved. However, their empirical use increasingly is being limited, particularly at dosing regimens currently recommended. Their efficacy against *Staphylococcus* spp. as well as against many gram-negative organisms leads to their selection for surgical prophylaxis. Cefovecin should not be included in this category because of its long time to antibacterial effect and time to maximum effect and the persistence of drug concentrations well beyond the immediate postoperative period. Of the second-generation cephalosporins, cefoxitin, which is not impacted by ESBL, might be more safely considered for empirical therapy requiring a broad-spectrum antimicrobial and for anaerobic infections. With the exception of *P. aeruginosa*, cefoxitin is effective against most other organisms. The use of other second-generation and the third-generation cephalosporins is best based on C&S data because the spectra of these drugs are so variable. Caution should accompany use of second- through fourth-generation cephalosporins when based on in vitro data that may not reflect the production of ESBLs. Note also that the (over) use of cephalosporins has been associated with the emergence of multidrug-resistant microorganisms, including MRSA, *Enterococcus* spp., and *P. aeruginosa*.[25]

Beta-lactams should be the first drugs considered for combination antimicrobial therapy (if used at appropriate dosing regimens). Their unique mechanism of action facilitates movement of other drugs into bacteria, which should facilitate efficacy of other antimicrobials. The risk of resistance should also be reduced as antimicrobial movement into the cell is improved. Beta-lactams are combined with drugs effective against gram-negative organisms when broad-spectrum therapy is needed, as in the case of life-threatening infections for which the causative organisms are not known, polymicrobial infections involving anaerobes and aerobes, or gram-positive and gram-negative organisms.

Vancomycin

Vancomycin has had an important role in the treatment of human patients infected with methicillin-resistant staphylococci (see Chapter 6), but the advent of penicillinase-resistant beta-lactams and the incidence of adverse reactions have curtailed its use. Vancomycin is a large glycopeptide with three components, each of which may be responsible for its antimicrobial action on bacterial cell walls (Figure 7-4).[78] The D-Ala-D-Alanine precursor of the pentapeptide fits into a pocket formed by the large molecule, sterically interfering with further cell wall elongation. The spectrum of activity of vancomycin is limited to *Staphylococcus* and *Streptococcus* spp. and anaerobes (see Table 7-4). Selected *Enterococcus, Clostridium*, and *Corynebacterium* spp. are also generally susceptible. With the exception of enterococcal organisms, the effects of vancomycin are generally bactericidal, although they act slowly. As with other cell wall–active antimicrobials, vancomycin exhibits time-dependent killing effects, with efficacy also related to AUC. Resistance has been impeded by the high specificity of the drug. Multiple mutations are required to change the enzymes currently targeted by vancomycin. Resistance that has developed by *E. faecalis* has resulted from synthesis of a new protein that interferes with vancomycin. More recently, vancomycin-resistant staphylococci have emerged. A strain of vancomycin-intermediate *S. aureus* (VISA) has been described, the mechanism of which includes thickening of the cell wall, coupled with "clogging" of the cell wall by vancomycin itself. [79]

Although vancomycin is available as an oral preparation, this preparation is intended for topical (gastrointestinal) administration, most commonly indicated for pseudomembranous colitis caused by *C. difficile*. Systemic effects require intravenous administration. Vancomycin is distributed to most body tissues. The exception is the CNS, unless the meninges are inflamed; even then only 30% or less will penetrate. It is renally eliminated; drug concentrations may become toxic if doses are not modified for the patient with renal disease. The risk of nephrotoxicity is increased dramatically if the drug is given in combination with another nephrotoxic drug. Hypersensitivity in human patients warrants slow (60-minute) intravenous infusion of drug diluted in fluid. Ototoxicity has been reported in humans when concentrations reach 60 to 100 μg/mL.[80] Its use for veterinary patients should be limited to treatment of organisms resistant to other drugs as based on C&S data.

Teicoplanin

Teicoplanin is a mixture of several molecules (teicoplanins A_2 1-5). The molecules compose a fused glycopeptide core ring structure (teicoplanin) to which are attached two carbohydrates (differing from those in vancomycin), mannose and n-acetylglycosamine, and an acyl (fatty acid). It is the latter structure that confers better lipid solubility compared with vancomyin. Its mechanism of action and impact on bacterial killing and spectrum is similar to those of vancomycin. Its use has largely been replaced by vancomycin or daptomycin.

Fosfomycin

Fosfomycin is a phosphonic acid that contains a carbon–phosphorous bond (see Figure 7-12). It is a natural antibiotic produced by *Streptomyces fradiae*. Its in vitro spectrum is broad, and it expresses potential efficacy against isolates expressing multidrug resistance, including *E. coli* and gram-positive organisms. As a phosphoenolpyruvate analog, fosfomycin irreversibly inhibits phosphoenol pyruvate transferase, an enzyme that catalyzes the first step of cell wall peptidoglycan synthesis of microbial cell walls.[81] As a cell wall inhibitor, fosfomycin is bactericidal when present at the site of infection at therapeutic concentrations. Its

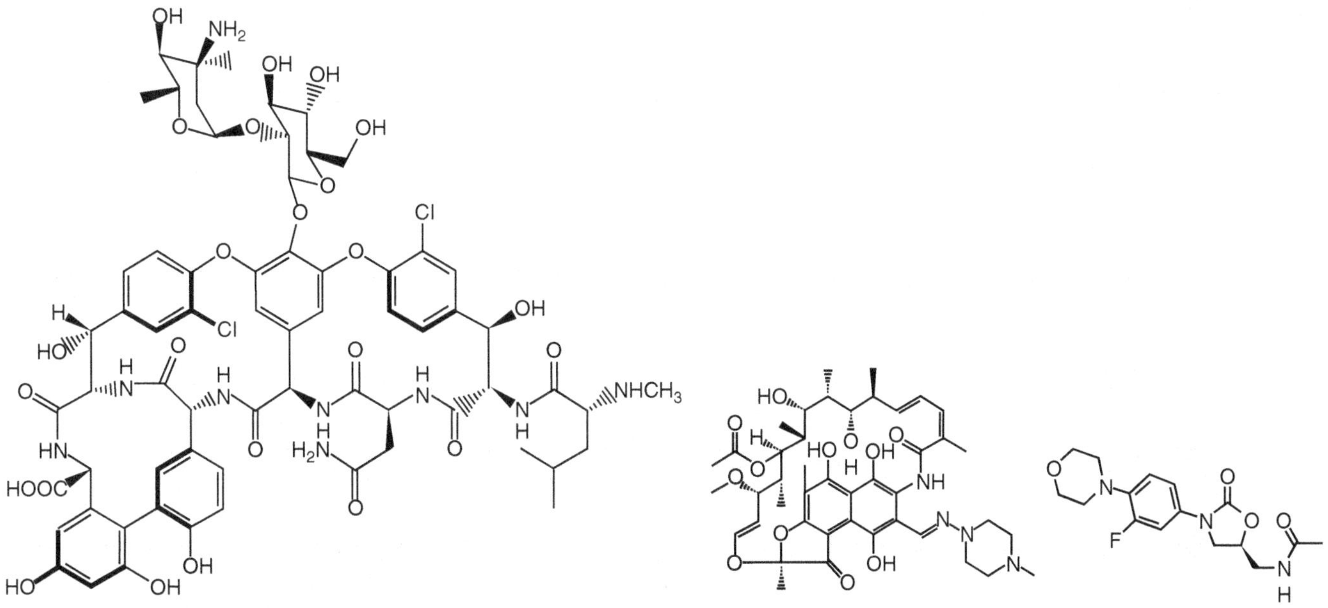

Vancomycin Rifampin Linezolid

Figure 7-4 The chemical structure of selected drugs which target resistant gram-positive microbes.

irreversible nature contributes to a concentration-dependent effect. Fosfomycin exhibits in vitro activity against a broad range of gram-positive and gram-negative aerobic microorganisms associated with uncomplicated urinary tract infections. The MIC breakpoints reported for humans are 64 (S), 28 Intermediate (I), and 256 (R). Although its mechanism of action is similar to that of the beta-lactams, fosfomycin is not susceptible to destruction by any class of beta-lactamases. Rather, resistance to fosfomycin, which is unusual, reflects the FosX or FosA enzyme, which hydrolyzes the drug in a manner similar to that of glutathione S-transferases. The gene for this protein is chromosomally mediated. Thus when resistance does occur, it is usually only toward fosfomycin (single drug resistance) with cross-resistance not occurring between fosfomycin and other classes of antimicrobial agents. Therefore resistance is not associated with multidrug resistance.[81] Further, compared with susceptible strains, fosfomycin-resistant mutants are impaired, exhibiting poorer growth rates and reduced adherence to uroepithelial cells. Fosfomycin appears to reduce bacterial adherence to uroepithelial cells, and decreased adherence is facilitated by *N*-acetylcystein[82] and urinary catheters.[83] Studies in humans have demonstrated that fosfomycin distributes well to soft tissues, reaching therapeutic breakpoints.[84] Other attributes of fosfomycin that support its use for treatment of *E. coli* urinary tract infections include renal excretion, synergistic interaction with several other classes of antimicrobials,[86] and preparation as a 3-g sachet (granules), which is mixed with water to orally deliver approximately 40 mg/kg (in humans).

The disposition of fosfomycin disodium (pure substrate) has been described in dogs (n = 8)[88] after intravenous, intramuscular, subcutaneous, and oral administration at both 40 and 80 mg/kg day for 3 days. Plasma protein binding was negligible; drug concentrations increased in a dose-dependent manner and did not change during the study period, including across each 3-day treatment period. At 40 mg/kg, peak PDCs (μg/mL) were as follows: 51.8 ± 3.4 (extrapolated peak PDC; Co, intravenous) and 5.4 ± 0.04 (oral); and at 80 mg/kg, 113 ± 12 (Co, intravenous) and 10.8 ± 0.5 (oral). Oral bioavailability (F) was 30%. Clearance was 14.9 ± 1.26 mL/kg/hr, elimination half-life was 1.3 ± 0.06 hours, and mean residence time was 1.62 ± 0.4 and 5.2 ± 0.7 (oral).

The PD and PK of fosfomycin have also been studied by the author. The distribution MIC for fosfomycin for clinical *E. coli* isolates, regardless of the presence of multidrug resistance, appears to be well below the susceptible breakpoint (≤ 64 μg/mL) for fosfomycin. In more than 100 clinical isolates collected from dogs and cats, the MIC range was 0.25 to 4 μg/mL; the MIC_{50} and MIC_{90} were, respectively, 1 and 1.5 μg/mL. Fosfomycin tromethamine was administered as a single oral dose of 80 mg/kg. After oral administration, C_{max}, elimination half-life and mean residence time were 66 ± 21 (μg/mL), 2.5 ± 1.09 hours and 5.1 ± 1.7, hours, respectively. Drug was detected at concentrations exceeding the MIC_{90} of fosfomycin for multidrug-resistant *E. coli* (1.5 μg/mL) until 7 (2.5 μg/mL) and 12 hours (9 μg/mL) after intravenous and oral administration, respectively. Drug was present in urine at concentrations above 10 μcg/mL at 24 hr post dosing. Gastrointestinal upset manifesting as mild to moderate diarrhea was observed in 4 of the 12 dogs. Food decreased oral bioavailability: without food, 109 ± 31% (95% confidence interal CI: 84%-135%) and with food, 66 ± 16% (95% CI: 52%-79%). Gender had no impact on oral bioavailability. Kill studies in our laboratory indicate that for treatment of *E. coli*, the drug is not concentration dependent, as is suggested by other studies that indicate both time- and concentration-dependent effects.[88,89] Further studies are warranted to establish efficacy for treatment of multidrug-resistant–associated urinary tract infections.

Although fosfomycin is appealing for treatment of urinary tract infections and potentially other infections caused by multidrug-resistant isolates, differences in bioavailability (oral) among different fosfomycin salts necessitates that PK be the basis, particularly of oral dosing regimens in the dog. Its efficacy appears to be both time and concentration dependent; if the latter, this should facilitate efficacy despite the short-half-life of the drug.[88] The drug appears to interact in an additive to synergistic fashion with a number of other antimicrobials.

DRUGS THAT TARGET RIBOSOMES (BACTERICIDAL)

Aminoglycosides

Despite their potential nephrotoxicity, aminoglycosides remain the cornerstone of aerobic gram-negative therapy in many complicated or serious infections. Minor differences in the chemical structures of these drugs lead to differences in efficacy and toxicity. Clinically useful aminoglycosides include neomycin, gentamicin, amikacin, netilimicin, streptomycin (or dihydrostreptomycin), and tobramycin.

Structure–Activity Relationship

Aminoglycoside compounds are composed of an amino sugar linked through glycosidic bonds to an aminocyclitol.[5,90] They vary in the amino sugar and the specific number and location of the amine groups (Figure 7-5). The different name endings indicate the microbe of origin for the natural antibiotic: The suffix "icin" (e.g., gentamicin) originates from *Micromonospora* sp., whereas the "mycin" suffix (e.g., tobramycin) derives from *Streptomyces*. Amikacin is a semisynthetic derivative of kanamycin, and netilmicin, a semisynthetic derivative of sisomicin. Tobramycin is most similar to gentamicin in both spectrum and toxicity. The aminoglycosides are polycationic, depending on the number of amine groups. Kanamycin and gentamicin have two amino sugars, whereas neomycin has three amino sugars. The amine group of gentamicins is variably methylated, yielding three different gentamicins. Streptomycin has a different aminocyclitol sugar compared with the other drugs, whereas spectinomycin is an aminocyclitol that does not contain any amino sugars.

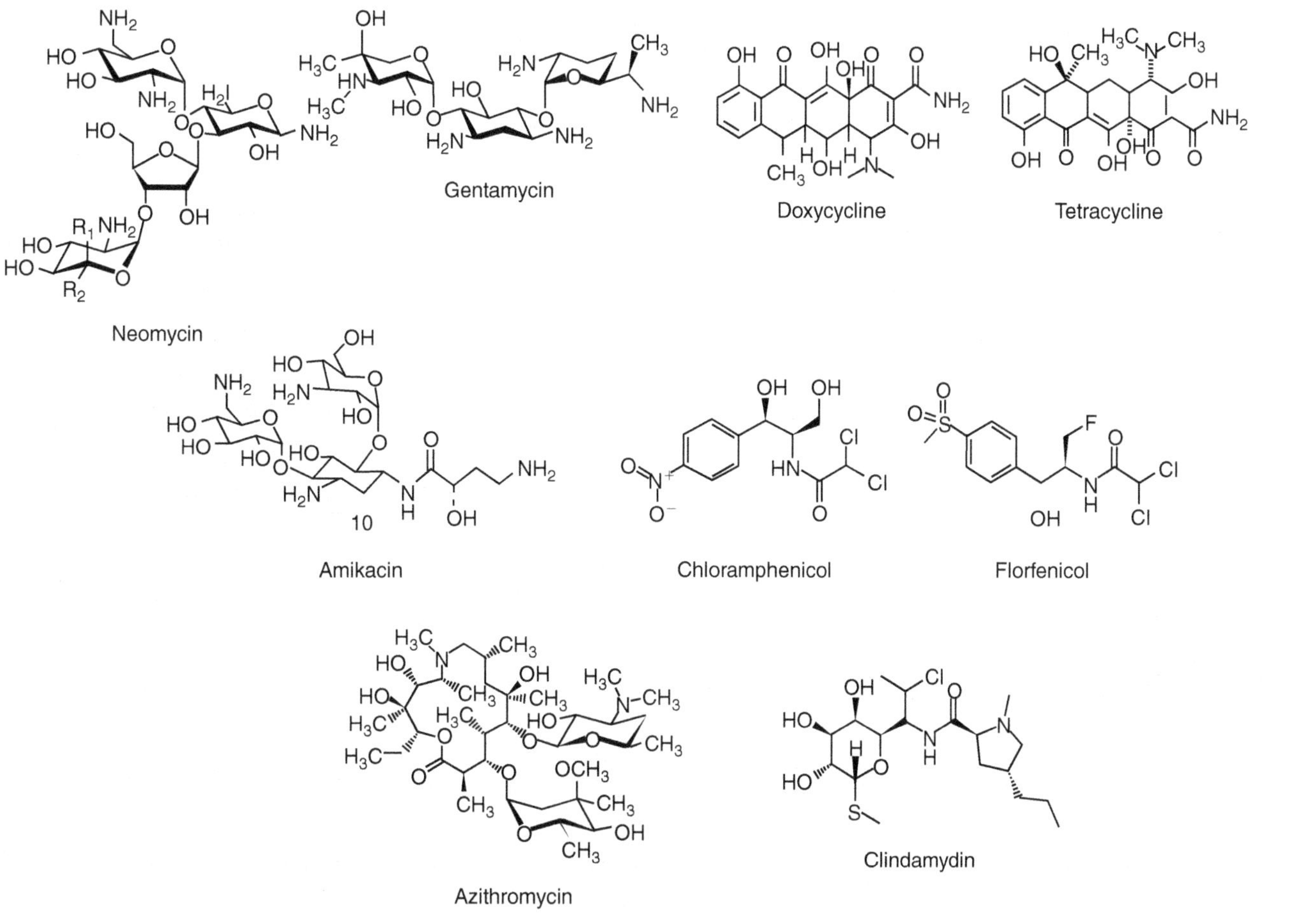

Neomycin Gentamycin Doxycycline Tetracycline Amikacin Chloramphenicol Florfenicol Azithromycin Clindamydin

Figure 7-5 Chemical structures of ribosomal inhibitors.

Mechanism of Action

Aminoglycosides target bacterial ribosomes (Figure 7-6). The drugs enter gram-negative organisms initially through porins in the lipopolysaccharide layer. Subsequent penetration of aerobic bacteria at the level of the cell membrane appears to occur in three binding stages: the negatively charged moieties of phospholipids are first ionically attracted and bound by the positive moieties of the drug, followed by the lipopolysaccharides and finally membrane proteins. Energy-dependent uptake follows binding to lipopolysaccharides. An acidic environment external to the cell membrane has been associated with increased transport, perhaps because of an increase in the membrane potential differential. However, a lower pH more commonly has been associated with increased membrane resistance; the disparity may reflect the different molecules of each aminoglycoside. An alkaline environment consistently appears to facilitate transport as does movement of cations out of the cell membrane. Uptake depends on a membrane-bound respiratory protein that is lacking in anaerobic organisms, leading to inherent resistance. The system also is deficient in facultative anaerobes such as *Enterococcus* spp. Active transport depends on a high oxygen tension in the environment rendering obligate anaerobes inherently resistant, and facultative anaerobes resistant in an anaerobic environment.[91] Cations such as calcium and magnesium in the lipopolysaccharide covering and cell membrane repel the aminoglycosides, impairing transport into bacterial cells (and renal tubular cells). Removal of calcium (e.g., through use of chelating agents such as ethylenediaminetetraacetic acid [EDTA]) or a decrease in serum calcium (i.e., hypocalcemia) facilitates aminoglycoside movement into the cell.[5,90] Hyperosmolarity and decreased pH also decrease drug movement into the cell.[80]

KEY POINT 7-12 Effiacy of aminoglycosides is dependent on active transport. Accordingly, efficacy is markedly reduced to absent in an anaerobic environment, and anaerobes are not susceptible.

Once inside the cell, aminoglycosides bind to ribosomes (see Figure 7-6). Although their mechanism of action is not completely understood, aminoglycoside antimicrobials bind to the 30S ribosomal subunit, which, as the initiator of protein synthesis, plays a crucial role in providing high-fidelity translation of genetic material.[92] Binding is so effective that polyribosome formation is prevented, and protein synthesis is impaired because of altered synthesis and misreading. Thus, in contrast to most bacteriostatic drugs, which bind to 50S ribosomes, the aminoglycosides are more likely to achieve bactericidal concentrations safely in animals. Although only a small amount of aminoglycoside appears to penetrate the cell membrane, the initial impact on ribosomes is sufficient

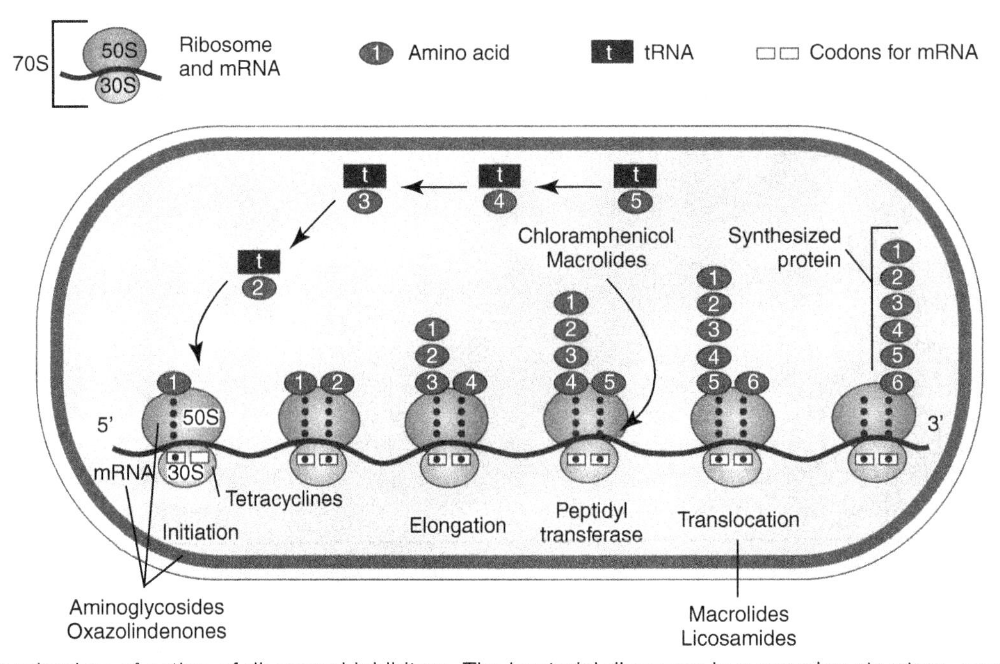

Figure 7-6 The mechanism of action of ribosomal inhibitors. The bacterial ribosome is a complex structure, composed of three RNA molecules (peptidyl and aminoacyl tRNAs and mRNA) and more than 50 proteins. The ribosome is formed as two subunits, 30S (including a 16S portion) and 50S (including a 5S portion; S referring to sedimentation rate), which join when protein synthesis is initiated and separate when completed. The process of initiation begins by the formation of a functional ribosome. The 30S subunit complexes with mRNA (which codes tRNA synthesis) and forms an initiation complex consisting of tRNA, the first amino acid (methionine), and three initiation factors (IF 1-3), one of which is an energy source, GTP. The initiation complex joins the 50S subunit, forming the (mature) 70S ribosome; it is the mature 70S ribosome that initiates protein synthesis. The mature ribosome is composed of an "A" or amino acid site (30S), the "P" or peptidyl site (50S), which contains a peptidyl transferase center; and an E or exit site adjacent to the P site. The aminoacyl tRNA carrying the amino acid binds to the A site, which then complexes to an elongation factor. Release of energy by GTP causes a conformational change or contracting motion, and the the peptide forming at the P site joins the amino acid at the A site. A nucleophilic attack initiated by the aminoacyl tRNA results in bonding of the amino acid to the growing peptide (transpeptidation); the growing peptide is then translocated to the P site. The elongation step is repeated until protein synthesis is completed.[278] The aminoglycosides inhibit ribosomal initiation (as the 30S subunit becomes activated to 70S); binding is irreversible, contributing to a bactericidal effect. Tetracyclines bind to the 16S portion of the 30S subunit of ribosomes, preventing the translocation of the amino acid from transfer RNA (tRNA) to the codon of messenger RNA (mRNA). Chloramphenicol and erythromycin prevent the transfer of peptides by binding to the 50S subunit. Erythromycin and clindamycin prevent translocation of the peptide. Drugs that act at the same site should not be used in combination.

to alter cell membrane proteins and permeability such that additional drug is able to penetrate the cell. Irreversible saturation of the ribosomes results in cell death and accounts for the concentration-dependent killing effects of the drugs; the irreversible nature of binding contributes to bactericidal effects.[92] Aminoglycosides are rapidly bactericidal, with efficacy and the postantibiotic effect of aminoglycosides correlating to peak concentrations, which ideally should be at least 10 times the MIC of the target organism.[93-97] Drugs that target the 50S ribosomal unit (e.g., chloramphenhicol, linezolid) may interfere with intracellular movement and thus rapid killing effects of aminoglycosides.[94] Because toxicity of aminoglycosides is correlated with trough concentrations (later discussed as adverse effects of aminoglycosides), treatment is implemented with once-daily therapy at high doses. This approach is both clinically[85,97,98] and experimentally[95,96,99] equal to or more efficacious and safer than the traditional frequency of administration (i.e., two to three times daily). The appropriateness of this dosing method may vary with the organism and the immunocompetence of the patient.

KEY POINT 7-13 The aminoglyosides exhibit a clinically important concentration-dependent postantibiotic effect.

Spectrum of Activity

The spectrum of activity of aminoglycosides (see Tables 7-2 through 7-4, 7-9 and 7-10) includes most aerobic gram-negative bacteria, particularly *E. coli, K. pneumoniae, P. aeruginosa, Proteus* spp. and *Serratia* spp.[5,16,80,91,101] Newer aminoglycosides such as gentamicin, tobramycin, amikacin, and netilmicin have a wider spectrum compared with older compounds such as streptomycin and kanamycin. These drugs are also effective against selective aerobic gram-positive organisms, most notably *Staphylococcus* spp. However, they generally should not be used as sole agents against gram-positive organisms. Synergism against gram-positive isolates has been demonstrated when combined with penicillins or vancomycin.[80] Aminoglycoside activity against *Enterococci* spp. is adequate only when used synergistically with a cell wall–active antibiotic, such as beta-lactams or vancomycin.[92] Among the aminoglyocsides, based on clinical isolates in humans, netilimicin has the lowest

MIC_{90} toward *Enterococcus* spp. and, along with tobramycin, *Staphylococcus* spp. Of the aminoglycosides most commonly used in dogs and cats, gentamicin has a much lower MIC_{90} than amikacin toward *Staphylococcus* spp., even accounting for differences in breakpoint MICs. Gentamicin is preferred to amikacin for treatment of *Staphylococcus* infections, based on a rabbit model of endocarditis.[101] Further, a recent comparison of activity of 1000 isolates also found gentamicin to be more effective than amikacin toward *Staphylococcus* spp.[102] In this same report, the authors noted that gentamicin also had lower MIC toward many enterobacteriacea but that amikacin achieved higher serum concentrations (and has a higher breakpoint MIC), thus negating this benefit.[102] Gentamicin and tobramycin have a very similar spectrum toward gram-negative aerobes. They and amikacin are effective against *P. aeruginosa*, *Proteus* spp. and *Serratia* spp. Gentamicin is the least effective of the three against *P. aeruginosa* but most effective against *Serratia marcescens*.[92] Amikacin generally is most effective against *P. aeruginosa*. With the exception of *Pseudomonas* species (usually an obligate aerobe, although exceptions have been reported), these organisms are facultative anaerobes and, if cultured aerobically from an anaerobic environment, may fail to respond to aminoglycoside therapy in the patient. The aminoglycosides are also effective against *Nocardia* and selected atypical mycobacterial organisms.

KEY POINT 7-14 In general, gentamicin may be more efficacious toward *Staphylococus,* spp. whereas amikacin may be more efficacious toward *Pseudomonas* spp.

Resistance

Besides the inherent resistance of anaerobic organisms (owing to decreased active transport), resistance to aminoglycosides is acquired as a result of decreased cell entry; altered porin size in the gram-negative organism is less important.[90] Resistance also includes altered ribosomal structure (uncommon except for *Enterococcus* spp.) and, more commonly, destruction by microbial enzymes inside the cell. Resistance to gentamicin involving altered ribosomal structure by *Enterococcus* spp. generally affects all aminoglycosides, as well as penicillins and vancomycin. An exception is streptomycin, which is destroyed by a different enzyme and may remain effective toward *Enterococcus*.[90]

Enzymatic destruction is the most important mechanism of acquired resistance in clinical isolates, in part because it is acquired through conjugative plasmids. Resistance reflects enzyme modification of the amino or hydroxyl groups of the drugs. The modified drug can no longer bind to ribosomes. Impact on efficacy varies among the different aminoglycosides. For example, target sites of destruction by the enzymes are harder to reach with amikacin. Consequently, amikacin is less vulnerable to resistance than are other aminoglycosides and is frequently effective toward otherwise multidrug-resistant isolates.[5,80,90] At least three different enzyme classes exist, classified by phenotypes as to phosphotransferases, acetyltransferases, and nucleotidyltransferases. Among the aminoglycosides used clinically in veterinary medicine, gentamicin and kanamycin more commonly act as substrates for phosphotransferases and acetyltransferases, wheraeas amikacin and tobramycin are more common substrates for the nucleotidyltransferases. Of the three enzymes, the phosphotransferases are more likely to be associated with high-level resistance.

Resistance to aminoglycosides by *Staphylococcus* spp. reflects chromosomal mutations in transmembrane potentials and thus drug uptake. Mutational resistance caused by changes in ribosome binding sites has been identified primarily against streptomycin, the use of which is limited. However, whereas the four gram-negative organisms most commonly causing (blood) infection in humans (*Pseudomonas, Klebsiella, E. coli,* and *Enterobacter*) remain susceptible (>95%) to the greatest number of aminoglycosides, up to 40% of *S. aureus* organisms are resistant to gentamicin. Current investigations are attempting to identify the mechanism by which enzymatic destruction of aminoglycosides might be inhibited, much the same as beta-lactamases have been used to prevent beta-lactam destruction.[92] Low-level resistance caused by multidrug efflux mechanisms has been identified in *P. aeruginosa, Burkholderia* sp. (previously *Pseudomonas), Acinetobacter,* spp. and *E. coli*.[92]

KEY POINT 7-15 Enzymatic destruction of aminoglycosides is increasingly limiting efficacy, particularly for gentamicin toward *Staphylococus* spp.

Adaptive resistance has been described for the aminoglycosides (see Chapter 6). In humans up to 40 hours may need to elapse between doses for full bacterial susceptibility to commence.[103] This phenomenon supports the once-daily use of the aminoglycosides.

Pharmacokinetics

The aminoglycosides are polar, water-soluble weak bases, and as such they are poorly absorbed from the gastrointestinal tract. An exception might occur in very young animals that are still absorbing colostrum or in the presence of inflammatory gastrointestinal disease.[90,91] Kanamycin, which is structurally very similar to amikacin, behaves similarly to amikacin.[91] Aminoglycosides are administered topically (including aerosolization and incorporation in beads) or parenterally but can be used orally for local bacterial cleansing of the gastrointestinal tract. However, absorption from body cavities may be sufficiently rapid to cause neuromuscular blockade.[90] Absorption will also occur when applied topically to large wounds with subcutaneous exposure; absorption may be sufficient to cause toxicity.[104]

Although aminoglycosides are distributed to extracellular fluids, their penetration into many tissues is considered poor (see Table 7-5). However, therapeutic concentrations can be attained in synovia and in pleural and peritoneal fluid, particularly if membranes are inflamed. Penetration of bronchial secretions is generally better than that of many beta-lactam antibiotics. However, therapeutic concentrations generally are not attained in CSF, ocular fluids, bile, milk, and prostatic secretions. Further, killing of intracellular (e.g., *Enterobacter* spp.) spp.) organisms may be limited.[94a] Intrathecal administration has been indicated for CNS infections, but the advent of third- and fourth-generation cephalsoporins and carbapenems has preempted this need.[90] Aminoglycosides are actively accumulated by renal tubular cells, but this may be of more relevance to toxicity rather than efficacy. In addition to anaerobic environments, the efficacy of aminoglycosides is reduced in an acidic environment such as might occur in the urine, ascitic fluid, and abscesses.

KEY POINT 7-16 As water-soluble weak bases, aminoglycosides are not orally absorbed, do not penetrate tissues well, and are excreted in proportion to the glomerular filtration rate.

Drug elimination half-life of the aminoglycosides is generally less than 2 to 4 hours (see Table 7-1). The aminoglycosides are eliminated by glomerular filtration, which is a relatively inefficient process. Drug accumulates in acidic urine, and alkaline urine pH facilitates reabsorption. Urine concentrations have been described for selected aminoglycosides in dogs.[105] Dosing of gentamicin (6.6 mg/kg), tobramycin (3 mg/kg), and amikacin (15 mg/kg) subcutaneously in divided doses at 8-hour intervals (not recommended) for five consecutive doses and kanamycin at 11 mg/kg at 12-hour intervals (also not recommended) for 4 doses generated mean interval urine concentrations (μg/mL) of 107 ± 33 for gentamicin: 66 ± 39 for tobramycin, 342 ± 153 for amikacin, and 473 ± 306 for kanamycin.[105]

The disposition of aminoglycosides varies somewhat among animals, primarily because of differences in glomerular filtration rates. Elimination is slower in larger animals because glomerular filtration rate decreases with body size; this may be offset by differences in Vd. Dosing based on metabolic rate normalizes the rate of elimination and might be considered in patients predisposed to aminoglycoside nephrotoxicity, although estimates of glomerular filtration rate based on extracellular fluid volume may be more accurate.[106]

A number of investigators have described the disposition of aminoglycosides in dogs or cats (Table 7-1). Gentamicin has been studied in dogs by multiple investigators. Riviere[107] described the disposition in 5-month-old Beagles (n = 11). Clearance was 4.1 ± 0.6 mL/min*kg and Vd (area) was 0.4 ± 0.04L/kg. Elimination half-life was 61 ± 8 minutes. Wilson[108] studied gentamicin (3 mg/kg) in dogs (n = 6) after intravenous, intramuscular, and subcutaneous administration. After intravenous administration, clearance was 2.29 ± 0.48 mL/min*kg and Vdss was 0.172 ± 0.025. Bioavailability approximated 95% for both intramuscular and subcutaneous routes, yielding a C_{max} of approximately 10 μg/mL for either route, with time to peak concentration for intramuscular administration being 27 minutes compared with 43 minutes for subcutaneous administration. The elimination half-life was 54 ± 15 minutes. Albarellos[204] studied gentamicin after intramuscular administration of 6 mg/kg for 5 days. After day 1, assuming 100% bioavailability, clearance was 1.24 ± 0.6 mL/min*kg (1.10 ± 0.4 by day 5), and Vd (area) was 0.084 L/kg (0.1 ± 0.05 day 5). Mean residence time was 1.48 ± 0.54 hour (1.77 ± 0.48 by day 5; significantly prolonged) and half-life ranged from 0.55 to 1.46 hours. For IV administration, the Vd_{ss} after intravenous administration was 0.23±0.04 L/kg and clearance was 2.64 ± 0.24 mL/min*kg.

Jernigan and coworkers[100] have described the disposition of several aminoglycosides in cats (see Table 7-1). After intravenous administration of gentamicin (3 mg/kg) in cats (n = 6), Vd_{ss} was 0.12 ± 0.02 l/kg and clearance was 1.1 ± 0.25 mL/kg*min. Bioavailability after subcutaneous administration was 83 ± 14.8%. Gentamicin was also studied in cats (n = 6) after intravenous, intramuscular, and subcutaneous administration of 5 mg/kg.[110] After intravenous administration, Vdss was 0.14 ± 0.02 L/kg and clearance was 1.38 ± 0.35 mL/min*kg; mean residence time was 1.8 ± 43 hour. Bioavailability after intramuscular and subcutaneous administration was 67.8 and 76.2%, respectively. Tobramycin was studied in six cats after 5 mg/kg.[111] After intravenous administration, Vd_{ss} was 0.19 ± 0.03 l/kg and clearance was 2.21 ± 0.6 mL/min*kg; mean residence time was 90 ± 16 minutes. Bioavailability after intramuscular and subcutaneous administration was 103% and 99% respectively; bioavailability was also measured at greater than 150% for both routes in one set of studies, perhaps indicating decreased clearance owing to nephrotoxicity. Finally, amikacin (5 mg/kg) was studied in cats (n = 6) after intravenous, intramuscular, and subcutaneous administration.[112] After intravenous administration, Vdss was 0.17 ± 0.02 L/kg, and clearance was 1.46 ± 0.26 mL/min*kg; mean residence time was 118 ± 14 minutes. Bioavailability after intramuscular and subcutaneous administration was 95 ± 20% and 12.3 ± 33%, respectively.

Disposition of the aminoglycosides appears to vary among breeds. Kukanich[113] has compared the PK of amikacin (10 mg/kg, administered intravenously) in Greyhounds and Beagles (n = 6 each). The volume of distribution (L/kg) was smaller (0.18 versus 0.23), but clearance was less (2.1 versus 3.3 mL*kg/min) in Greyhounds, thus elimination half-life did not differ (0.8 and 0.9 hour for Greyhounds and Beagles, respectively). The bioavailability of amikacin in Greyhounds after subcutaneous administration was approximately 90%. Although extrapolated time 0 PDC was reported for both species after intravenous administration (86 and 70 μg/mL, respectively, for Greyhounds and Beagles), this is not an appropriate target on which to base C_{max}/MIC (i.e, the C_{max} should be measured after distribution has occurred). However, compartmental analysis yielded concentrations extrapolated from the terminal curve (presumably reflecting postdistributional concentration; see Table 7-1). On the basis of these data and a target C_{max}/MIC of 8 (rather than 10), the respective subcutaneous doses (mg/kg) of amikacin recommended by the authors to target an MIC of 2, 4, and 8 μg/mL, respectively, were for the Greyhound 6, 12, and 24 and for the Beagle, 11.5, 22, and 40.

The influence of endotoxemia on gentamicin disposition has been described in cats.[114,115] Elimination half-life was shorter (77 ± 13 minutes before and 65 ± 14 after), but this change is not likely to be significant, in part because neither Vd_{ss} nor clearance was significantly different.

The disposition of aminoglycosides also differs among ages. PDCs are less in the neonate and pediatric patient because greater total body water and extracellular fluid compartments increase the Vd of the drugs from 0.25 to 0.35 L/kg (see Table 7-1). Renal clearance of aminoglycosides is less. Thus for young animals the dose of aminoglycosides should be increased; although elimination half-life may be longer, the current use of a 24-hour interval should preclude the need to lengthen it further in the pediatric patient. Disposition is also altered by disease. Dehydration and obesity increase PDCs, which may be of benefit for these concentration-dependent drugs. Intensive fluid therapy or other syndromes associated with accumulation of fluid at a site to which aminoglycosides distribute and endotoxemia decrease plasma aminoglycoside concentrations.[91] Ascites also will increase the Vd and half-life of aminoglyocosides.[116] Aminoglycosides may accumulate and cause nephrotoxicity in the fetus and should not be used during pregnancy.[90] Elimination is impaired in the patient with renal disease; dosing regimens are usually modified by lengthening the interval on the basis of serum creatinine concentration (see the section on therapeutic use).

Adverse Effects

The aminoglycosides induce a glomerular and (principally) tubular nephrotoxicity; however, because of the regenerative capacity of the proximal tubule, toxicity is largely reversible unless allowed to progress to an irreversible state (i.e., destruction of basement membrane). Toxicity results from active uptake into the renal tubular cell and disruption of cellular lysosomes (Figure 7-7). Impaired cellular respiration and synthesis of protective vasodilatory renal prostaglandins by the aminoglycoside may be important in the development of nephrotoxicity.

KEY POINT 7-17 Aminoglycoside nephrotoxicity can be minimized if kidneys are allowed a drug-free period such that drug that has been actively accumulated in the kidney can be eliminated.

Reversible renal impairment occurs in up to 25% to 55% of human patients receiving aminoglycosides for more than 3 days, although the better-designed studies indicate a rate of 10% to 20%.[90,117] In humans aminoglycoside-induced nephrotoxicity is defined as an increase in serum creatinine concentration of 0.5 mg/dL in patients for which baseline concentration is < 3 mg/dL, or an increase in 1 mg/dL if the baseline is at or above 3 mg/dL.[117]

The exact mechanism of aminoglycoside-induced nephrotoxicity is not known. Toxicity begins as the anionic phospholipids of the renal tubular cell membranes attract and bind the cationically charged drugs. The relative nephrotoxicity of the different aminoglycosides reflects differences in their renal

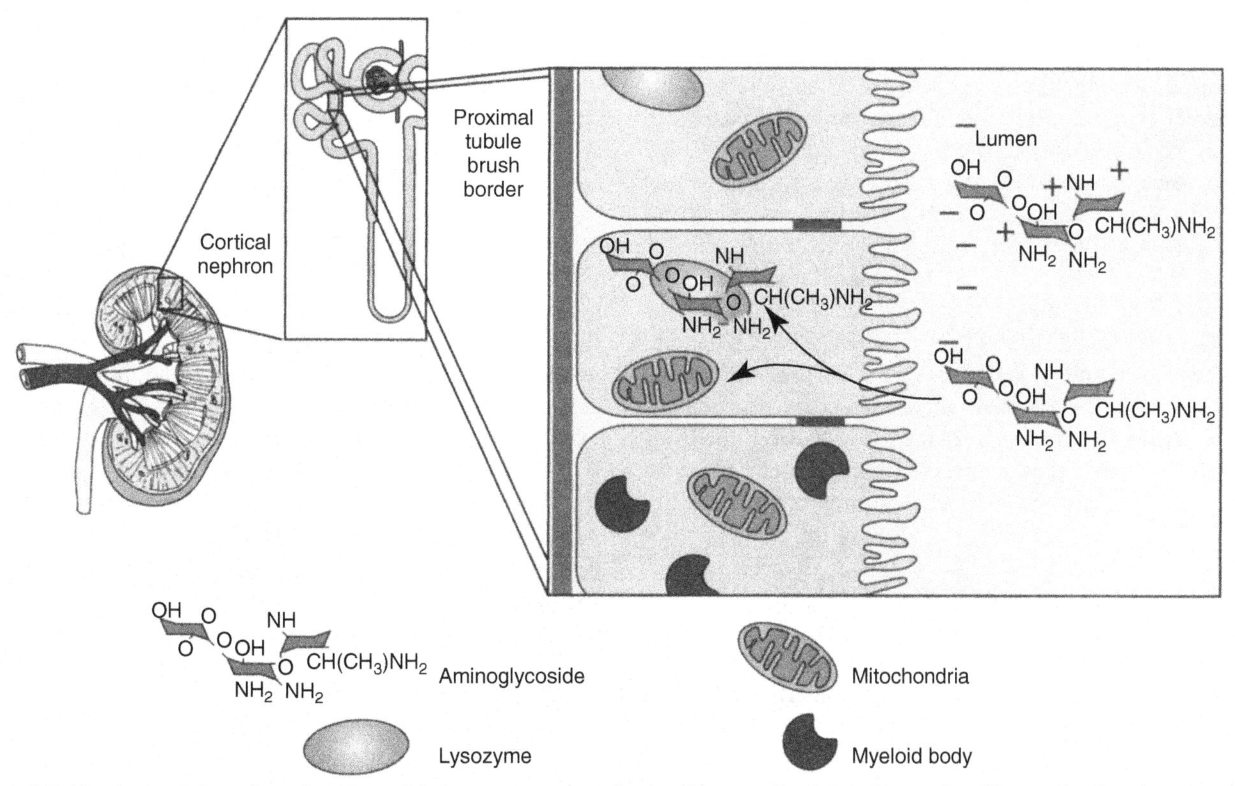

Figure 7-7 Nephrotoxicity of aminoglycosides occurs primarily in the proximal tubular cells. The cationic charge of the drugs is attracted to the anionic charge of the phospholipids in the cell membrane. The drug is actively accumulated in the cell by pinocytosis. Inside the cell the drugs accumulate in lysozymes, causing lysosomal disruption and release of myeloid bodies. Intracellular movement into lysozymes also limits intracellular efficacy. Mitochondrial function is also impaired. The effects of prostaglandin on renal blood flow may contribute to the toxicity of aminoglycosides. A number of factors increase or decrease the risk of toxicity (see text).

accumulation.[90] Nephrotoxicity may be related to the number of positively charged amino groups on the drugs; hence, neomycin is expected to be among the most nephrotoxic of the drugs.[5] An acidic local pH may enhance uptake by ionizing the aminoglycoside and thus increase the risk of toxicity. Of the clinically used aminoglycosides, neomycin is the most nephrotoxic and dihydrostreptomycin, the least. The nephrotoxicities of the other aminoglycosides are between these two extremes. Several studies have compared tobramycin and gentamicin (the latter is more concentrated), but controlled clinical trials in humans have failed to find a clinical difference in the nephrotoxicity potential between the two.[90] Studies comparing the nephrotoxic potential of amikacin with other aminolgycosides (but not gentamicin) also have been inconclusive.[90] A number of drugs increase the risk of nephrotoxicity (see the section on drug interactions).

The attraction of aminoglycoside cations to the renal tubular cell membrane can be competitively inhibited by divalent (e.g., magnesium or calcium) cations (e.g., ethylenediaminetetraacetic acid [EDTA]) or decreased in an alkaline urine (unionizing amine groups). Hypocalcemia or hypomagnesemia may increase the risk of aminoglycoside toxicity; in contrast, dietary calcium loading may protect against toxicity. Uptake of aminoglycosides also may be related to the amount of phosphatidylinositol in the cell membrane; the amount is disproportionately higher in renal cortex and cochlear tissues.[91]

Once the renal tubular cells are entered, aminoglycosides are then actively accumulated in the cell by pinocytosis; intracellular accumulation may result in concentrations greater than fiftyfold of that in plasma. Inside renal tubular cells, probably in part because of ion trapping, aminoglycosides are sequestered in lysosomes, which subsequently appear morphologically as myeloid bodies. The drugs are slowly eliminated in the urine as myeloid bodies, which contain drug, RNA, and DNA after the tubular cell dies.

The cause of tubular cell death induced by aminoglycosides remains unclear, although a number of cellular functions (in addition to lysosomal damage) are impaired; examples include phospholipases, sphingomyelinases, and ATPases. Mitochondrial respiration is decreased, impairing energy resources of the cell. Again, this may reflect interaction between the drug and mitochondrial cell membrane. Proximal tubular permeability may be impaired both directly as drugs interact with the cell membrane and indirectly as a result of impaired Na^+,K^+-ATPase activity. Aminoglycosides also alter glomerular function, perhaps by reducing the number and size of glomerular endothelial cells.[91] Finally, phospholipases important for renal prostaglandin synthesis are among the enzymes impaired by aminoglycosides. The initial decrease in glomerular filtration that accompanies aminoglycoside therapy may reflect the inability of the kidney to vasodilate in response to vasoconstrictor actions such as that signaled by angiotensin II.[91] This may reflect altered prostaglandin synthesis. As glomerular filtration declines, so may clearance of the aminoglycoside, thus increasing the risk of toxicity.[90]

The half-life of renal cortical aminoglycosides is approximately 100 hours. This and the fact that a critical aminoglycoside concentration must be reached before nephrotoxicity emerges generally preclude renal cortical nephrotoxicity before the first 3 days of therapy (Box 7-1).[117] No study has demonstrated a threshold of dosing or interval that ensures or predicts toxicity. Studies that have focused on aminoglycoside toxicity in dogs and cats have used dosing interval that ranges from 12 hours to constant intravenous infusion. Studies regarding aminoglycoside nephrotoxicity in cats have focused on doses of 35 mg/kg or more at intervals of 12 hours or less.[91] A bimodal course of aminoglycoside-induced nephrotoxicity has been described in the dog, with an initial subclinical phase characterized by a concentrating defect and an azotemic phase; different disease states might be predictable based on changes in pharmacokinetics.[108] Under experimental conditions, gentamicin at 4 mg/kg every 12 hours in dogs changes urine osmolarity within 7 days and an increase in serum creatinine by 17 days. Urinary prostaglandin E activity decreases before azotemia, which may be responsible for the state of nephrogenic diabetes insipidus. Whereas a single dose of 15 mg/kg gentamicin was associated with subclinical and morphologic changes in the kidney of young Beagles,[119] higher doses of 30 mg/kg administered at 8-hour intervals in dogs result in increases in urine gamma-glutamyltransferase within 2 days and serum creatinine within 9 to 12 days. Interestingly, a study that describes the disposition of gentamicins C1, C1a, and C2 in dogs found clearance of C1 to be twice as fast and Vd to be twice as high as for the other two gentamicins.[120] The investigators found that the renal binding of C1 is likely to be greater, suggesting that it is more likely to be nephrotoxic compared with C1a and C2.

Box 7-1

Minimization of Aminoglycoside Nephrotoxicity

1. Use once-daily therapy when appropriate.
2. Ensure adequate hydration status.If any doubt, or in a patient at risk, treat with sodium isotonic.
3. Maximize peak plasma drug concentration to ensure that C_{max}/MIC >10 and trough plasma drug concentration is < 2 μg/mL.
4. Monitor peak and trough concentration aminoglycoside concentration such that half-life and clearance can be followed.
5. Monitor urinary renal enzyme (γGT) to creatinine ratios, urine sediment, and serum creatinine.
6. Use the least nephrotoxic aminoglycoside (possible amikacin versus gentamicin).
7. Use the most effective aminoglycoside for the target organism (e.g., gentamicin for *Staphyloccocus*, amikacin for *Pseudomonas*).
8. Use combination antimicrobial therapy, particularly with synergistic antibiotics and always for gram-positive organisms
9. Avoid use of other nephrotoxic or nephroactive drugs, including antiprostaglandins, ACE inhibitors, and furosemide.
10. Administer during periods of activity (e.g., early morning in dogs, possibly evening in cats).
11. Treat with *N*-acetylcysteine.

Gentamicin (3 mg/kg) administered intravenously every 8 hours for 5 days to cats (n = 6) was not associated with changes in serum or histologic indicators of renal or vestibular dysfunction.[121] Endotoxemia appears to cause more gentamicin renal medullary accumulation in cats but does not appear to be associated with increased renal pathology.[115] Tobramycin was associated with increased serum creatinine and/or BUN in 9 of 12 cats dosed twice with tobramycin despite washout periods,[111] suggesting that it may be more nephrotoxic than other aminoglycosides, at least in cats.

No indicator of renal damage induced by the aminoglycosides is sufficiently sensitive to prevent damage; indeed, damage will continue beyond detection with current methods. Changes in urine osmolality or sodium fractional clearance typical of the initial subclinical phase may detect a concentrating defect. However, this should be preceded by a release of renal tubular enzymes such as gamma-glutamyltransferase into urine. Measurement of the enzyme has been used experimentally to measure aminoglycoside toxicity. The enzymes increase within several days after damage has begun. However, 24-hour sample collection for these procedures is impractical. Measurement of the urine creatinine to gamma-glutamyltransferase ratio in spot samples of urine have proved useful in experimental models of aminoglycoside toxicity.[123] Ratios may not, however, change until several days after toxicity has begun.[91] A change in aminoglycoside clearance may be the most sensitive indicator of aminoglycoside toxicity (see Chapter 5.[81,114,115] In humans serum creatitine may increase up to 1 week after therapy is discontinued, indicating the potential for continued damage once the drug is discontinued,[117] presumably because accumulated drug remains in the tubules. Accordingly, nephrotoxicity is best avoided (see Box 7-1 and the section on therapeutic use).

The presence of renal disease is not a contraindication for aminoglycoside use, although it certainly raises the risk. Normograms have been designed in human medicine to reduce the risk of further damage (see the section on therapeutic use). The risk of nephrotoxicity is greater if any condition of the patient depends on renal prostaglandin formation, such as hypotension, shock, endotoxemia, renal or cardiac disease, or with concurrent drug therapy that impairs prostaglandin synthesis, such as nonsteroidal antiinflammatory drugs.[5,126] Metabolic acidosis (or an acidic urine pH) also predisposes the patient to aminoglycoside nephrotoxicity because drugs are ionized and attracted to the anionic changes of cell membranes.[127] Consequently, if the source of infection is in the urinary tract, maintaining an alkaline pH will enhance the efficacy of the aminoglycosides by facilitating their diffusion back into infected tissue (and bacteria), while decreasing renal tubular cell uptake of aminoglycosides, presumably because of decreased ionization of the drugs. Aminoglycoside toxicity was demonstrated to be temporal in rats,[128] being worse when rats were resting and least when active. Accordingly, dosing in the morning may be prudent for dogs; dosing at night might be considered for cats. Some patients (e.g., pediatric dogs <14 days of age, patients with diabetes mellitus or hypothyroidism) are protected against aminoglycoside- (gentamicin)-induced nephrotoxicity because renal accumulation in the cortical tissues is limited.[130,131] Symptomatic hypomagnesemia, hypocalcemia, and hypokalemia associated with inappropriate urinary excretion of potassium despite low serum concentrations has been reported in humans after gentamicin therapy.[132] The magnitude correlated with the total cumulative dose of gentamicin. Risk factors included older age and long duration of therapy.[123] Note that hypomagnesemia and hypocalcemia may increase the risk of aminoglycoside toxicity by increasing the ease with which drugs enter the renal tubular cell.

KEY POINT 7-18 The presence of renal disease is not a contraindication for aminoglycoside use, although it certainly raises the risk of adverse effects.

Studies have attempted to identify therapies that might treat or prevent aminoglycoside-induced nephrotoxicity. The role of prostaglandin analogs (e.g., misoprostol) in the prevention or treatment of aminoglycoside toxicity has not yet been established. Melatonin administered simultaneously to rats receiving gentamicin was associated with reduced nephrotoxicity.[124] Rate receiving L-Carnitine (40 to 200 mg/kg/day, injected) beginning 4 days before receiving doses of gentamicin ranging from 50 to 80 mg/kg had less nephroxicity (based on serum creatinine and histology) compared with untreated rats. Renal gentamicin concentrations were not different, suggesting that decreased aminoglycoside uptake by the renal tubular cell was not the mechanism of prevention. Proposed mechanisms were promotion of fatty-acid oxidation, increased mitochondrial ATP, and decreased formation of oxygen radicals.[135] Again, in rats, *N*–acetylcystein (10 mg/kg intraperitoneally [IP]) protected against gentamicin (100 mg/kg subcutaneously/day × 5 days) induced nephrotoxicity.[136] This treatment apparently also has also been demonstrated to be otoprotective in human patients undergoing hemodialysis that are treated with gentamicin.[137] A federally funded human clinical trial is currently underway to validate the beneficial effects of *N*–acetylcysteine in patients with or at risk to develop aminoglycoside nephrotoxicity.

Aminoglycosides can cause an irreversible ototoxicity, although this is not likely to occur at therapeutic doses as long as trough concentrations are lower than 2 to 5 μg/mL (lower should be targeted for gentamicin, higher for amikacin). However, a single dose of tobramycin was associated with ototoxicy in humans.[80] Like nephrotoxicity, ototoxicity reflects active uptake of the drug by hair cells of the cochlea. Both auditory and vestibular toxicity may occur. As with nephrotoxicity, the ototoxic potential of each drug varies. The drugs typically should not be given to a patient with a perforated eardrum. Aminoglycosides can cause neuromuscular blockade owing to impaired calcium release at myoneural junctions. The risk appears to be dose dependent and is greater with intravenous administration, in the presence of hypocalcemia, or when combined with other agents active at the myoneural junction (e.g., anesthetics, skeletal muscle relaxants). Neuromuscular blockade can be reversed by cholinesterase inhibitors and (cautiously) calcium.

Drug Interactions

The risk of aminoglycoside ototoxicity and nephrotoxicity is increased when aminoglycosides are used in combination with one another or with nonsteroidal antiinflammatory drugs, diuretics (particularly loop-acting), angiotensin-converting enzyme inhibitors, amphotericin B, and other nephrotoxic (or nephroactive) or ototoxic drugs. The risk of neuromuscular blockade is increased with the combination of aminoglycosides and intravenous calcium, calcium channel blockers, and gas anesthetics and other neuromuscular blocking agents, including atacurium. Edrophonium will reverse the latter, whereas calcium supplementation can reverse any neuromuscular blockade.[2]

As weak bases, the aminoglycosides may chemically inactivate weak acids; inactivation has been documented in vitro[138] and in vivo[139] between tobramycin and extended-spectrum penicillins but not carbapenems.[140] Tobramycin appears more amenable to inactivation than does amikacin.[139] In vivo inactivation is more likely to occur in patients with renal disease for which PDC may be higher than in normal patients. Chemical inactivation might also occur in urine as higher concentrations are achieved. In general, the aminoglycoside is inactivated rather than the penicillin simply because the penicillin is present at much higher concentrations compared with the aminoglycoside.

Synergism between aminoglycosides and cell wall–active antimicrobials has been documented against *Enterococcus* spp. as well as some strains of Enterobacteriaceae, *P. aeruginosa*, staphylococci (including MRSA), and other microorganisms. However, these organisms are not always inhibited by the combination of aminoglycoside and cell wall–active compounds. Indeed, antagonism has been described between aminoglycosides and beta-lactams against a MRSA, presumably owing to induction of an aminoglycoside-modifying enzyme.[92]

Therapeutic Use

Despite their ability to cause nephrotoxicity, the aminoglycosides remain the most effective drugs for the treatment of serious gram-negative infections. They are also effective (combination therapy recommended), against *Staphylococcus, Nocardia, Mycoplasma*, and selected *Mycobacteria* spp. Caution is recommended in their use for infections in tissues that are difficult to penetrate and infections that may be located in an anaerobic environment. Combination therapy and topical therapy (in concert with systemic therapy) should be considered whenever possible for serious or complicated infections or in the presence of intracellular infections. Aminoglycoside-impregnated calcium hydroxyapatite or methyl methacrylate beads and methyl methacrylate cement have been used with apparent success in orthopedic procedures (see Chapter 6).[140a] Aminoglycosides cannot be given orally with the intent of systemic effects, and their use might be limited to hospitalized patients. However, once-daily therapy increases the convenience and safety of outpatient aminoglycoside therapy.

The pharmacologic rationale for once-daily (also called extended-interval) dosing of aminoglycosides includes their concentration-dependent bacterial killing, minimization of the adaptive resistance, the presence of a postantibiotic effect, and avoidance of renal cortical drug accumulation (i.e., providing a drug-free period to facilitate excretion) such that trough concentrations reach a low target.[117] As early as 1984,[141] a fixed-dose, prolonged interval was known to be safer than a reduced dose and fixed interval in regard to nephrotoxicity in dogs. Recent studies in dogs, humans, and experimental models have supported a 24-hour dosing interval (administering the total daily dose once a day) for aminoglycoside therapy. The once-daily dose of an aminoglycoside necessary to impair renal function has not been determined, in part because different drugs are studied at different doses and intervals. Because clinical patients are likely to be characterized by changes that predispose to toxicity, studies in normal animals may not be relevant. Once-daily administration of gentamicin was concluded to be safe for 5 days in dogs at a single daily dose of 6 mg/kg.[108] Maximum concentration (C_{max} (μg/mL), was 9.2 at a T_{max} of 0.48 hours. Mean trough gentamicin serum concentrations were 0.1 μg/mL. Although deemed safe, serum creatinine and urea nitrogen were increased and specific urine gravity decreased in one dog and granular casts were evident in two dogs.

Many clinical trials have been performed in humans to assess the safety and efficacy of once-versus multiple-daily dosing of aminoglycosides. Differences in objectives, patients, methodologies, and conclusions have led to confusion. Several meta-analyses have been performed in humans that focuses on clinical efficacy and either nephrotoxicity or ototoxicity in patients treated with aminoglycosides once versus multiple times daily. The number of trials included in each meta-analysis ranged from 21 to 26; the number of persons studied by each meta-analysis was 2100 to more than 3000. Barza's group[142] found that once-daily administration of aminoglycosides in patients without preexisting renal failure was as effective as multiple-daily dosing and was associated with a lower risk of nephrotoxicity and no greater risk of ototoxicity. Further, once-daily dosing was more convenient and less costly. A second (22 studies)[143] and third meta-analysis (26 studies)[144] found the rates of efficacy and toxicitity were similar and convenience and reduced cost justified the once-daily approach. Another study found that gentamicin (once or multiple times daily) and ticarcillin-clavulanic acid, either alone or combined with gentamicin, was associated with the same efficacy and nephrotoxicity renal function was better preserved with either once-daily gentamicin combined with ticarcillin–clavulanic acid or ticarcillin–clavulanic acid alone.[145] However, in humans, experts continue to advise that extended-interval aminoglycoside dosing not be used in patients with endocarditis, mycobacterial infections, or burns. Further, a simple once-daily approach to aminoglycoside therapy should not be used if the patient's creatinine clearance is less than 20 mL/min or in patients in hemodialysis because of marked alteration of PK in these patients. Rather, monitoring should be the basis of dosing in these patients.[146] Further, for obese patients (actual body weight > 20% above ideal body weight [IBW]), the dose should be reduced using the following formula that adjusts weight: obese dosing weight = IBW + 0.4 (actual weight – IBW).[147] A number of normograms have been developed for use in humans to support the design of aminoglycoside dosing regimens that will be effective yet safe in patients with renal disease. Generally, the normograms are based on creatinine clearance and other patient factors. However, in general, the normograms underestimate the dose necessary to achieve a therapeutic maximum drug concentration. Methods using probabilistic or deterministic methods are currently being investigated.[148] However, therapeutic drug monitoring continues to be the preferred method to allow calculation of individual patient PK.[117,146] Indeed, a meta-anlysis that compared once-daily multiple-dosing therapy and dosing based on PK found that basing doses on individual PK was the safest approach to dosing with aminoglycosides.[117] AUC based on two time points has enhanced prediction of dosing regimens for aminoglycosides in children with cystic fibrosis.[149] However, the distribution phase of aminoglycosides is sufficiently slow that the first sample probably should be collected no earlier than 1 hour after dosing is complete. Monitoring peak (no earlier than 1 hour, to ensure complete distribution) and detectable trough concentrations (no later than 2 to 3 half-lives after the peak to ensure concentrations are still detectable) will allow estimation of half-life, and (if given intravenously) Vd and clearance (see Chapter 5). Pretreatment and posttreatment comparisons may be useful in the early detection of significant changes in renal function, which will also help guide safe therapy. The clinical pharmacologist offering recommendations will be able to determine these parameters regardless of the actual timing (i.e., 1 versus 1.5 hours for peak, 4 versus 8 hours for trough); however, accuracy in reporting the time that samples were collected is critical for proper recommendations when the samples are collected for determination of half-life.

Maintaining hydration is probably the single most important means by which the risk of aminoglycoside-induced nephrotoxicity can be minimized. Ototoxicity also can be minimized by hydration and avoidance of topical administration, particularly in the presence of a perforated tympanum. Although gentamicin is the most economical aminoglycoside, amikacin should be considered for serious infections because of its improved resistance to antimicrobial destruction and better efficacy against some organisms, including *P. aeruginosa*. The aminoglycosides are often used in combination with other antimicrobials that have a less comprehensive gram-negative spectrum. As with imipenem, the aminoglycosides cause minimal endotoxin release in patients suffering from gram-negative infections associated with a large inoculum.[74]

DRUGS THAT TARGET NUCLEIC ACIDS

Fluorinated Quinolones

The fluorinated quinolones (FQs) are among the most recent classes of antimicrobials to be developed for treatment of bacterial infections. These synthetic drugs are minimally toxic yet have been effective in the treatment of many aerobic gram-negative organisms and selected gram-positive organisms. The desire to expand their spectrum of activity and the advent of resistance has led to innovated structural changes.

Structure–Activity Relationship

A review of the development of FQs is worthwhile, not only to facilitate understanding of their actions but also to provide insight regarding the advantages of so-called designer drugs. Two decades elapsed between the development of nalidixic acid, the progenitor of the FQs, and norfloxacin, the first of the FQs to be approved for use. Among the FQs currently used for treatment of susceptible infections in dogs and cats, ciprofloxacin was first approved for use in humans in 1986, with its veterinary counterpart, enrofloxacin, rapidly following in 1991. Extensive use of these drugs has exposed the need for improvements and newer clinical indications; pharmaceutical companies have been attentive to addressing these needs.

Nalidixic acid is the progenitor of the FQs (Figure 7-8). Synthetic manipulations, including but not limited to the addition of a fluorine atom, have broadened the antibacterial spectrum; enhanced tissue penetrability; reduced (some) side effects (perhaps while contributing to others); and, most recently, decreased the risk of resistance. Currently marketed FQs generally consist of a quinolone ring nucleus, the target of most initial structural manipulations (Figure 7-9), or a napthyridone ring structure, which replaces the nitrogen at carbon 8 on the quinolone structure (enoxacin, tosufloxacin, trovafloxacin, and gemifloxacin). The quinolone nucleus contains a carboxylic acid group at position 3 and an exocyclic oxygen at position 4 (hence the term "4-quinolones"); these are the active DNA gyrase binding sites, and thus these sites generally are not chemically manipulated. The structures yield two pKas for most FQs, rendering them amphoteric; they can act as weak bases, weak acids, or neutral compounds. For example, the carboxylic acid of enrofloxacin has a pKa of 6 and the amine group a pKa of 8.8. The side chain attached to the nitrogen at position 1 affects potency. The ethyl group at this position on nalidixic acid and the first of the clinically used FQs, norfloxacin, was replaced with a bulkier group (e.g., the cyclopropyl group of ciprofloxacin), which enhanced both gram-negative and -positive spectra. Substitution at position 5 also improved the gram-positive spectrum; however, it was the addition of a fluorine atom at position 6 that profoundly enhanced the gram-positive spectrum. The addition of a piperazyl ring, containing a heterocyclic nitrogen, at position 7 also was a critical improvement. This addition improved bacterial penetration (potency) and added *P. aeruginosa* to the gram-negative spectrum. The combination of the fluorine atom with a piperanyl ring produced the "breakthrough" class of FQs used today; norfloxacin was the first of these FQs to be approved in the United States.

Chemical manipulations continue to improve the FQs in terms of spectrum, potency, and avoidance of resistance. Substitutions on the piperazyl (e.g., ofloxacin, its L isomer, levofloxacin, and sparfloxacin) enhance the gram-positive penetration, whereas substitutions at position 8 enhance anaerobic activity (e.g., sparfloxacin, pradofloxacin, moxifloxacin). Substitutions at these sites with halogens such as chlorine or fluorine (e.g., 8-chloroquinolones or 8-fluoroquinolones [sparfloxacin]) result in ultraviolet unstable compounds (particularly the chloro substitution), which can cause phototoxicity. In contrast, substitution of a methoxy-group at the 8 position

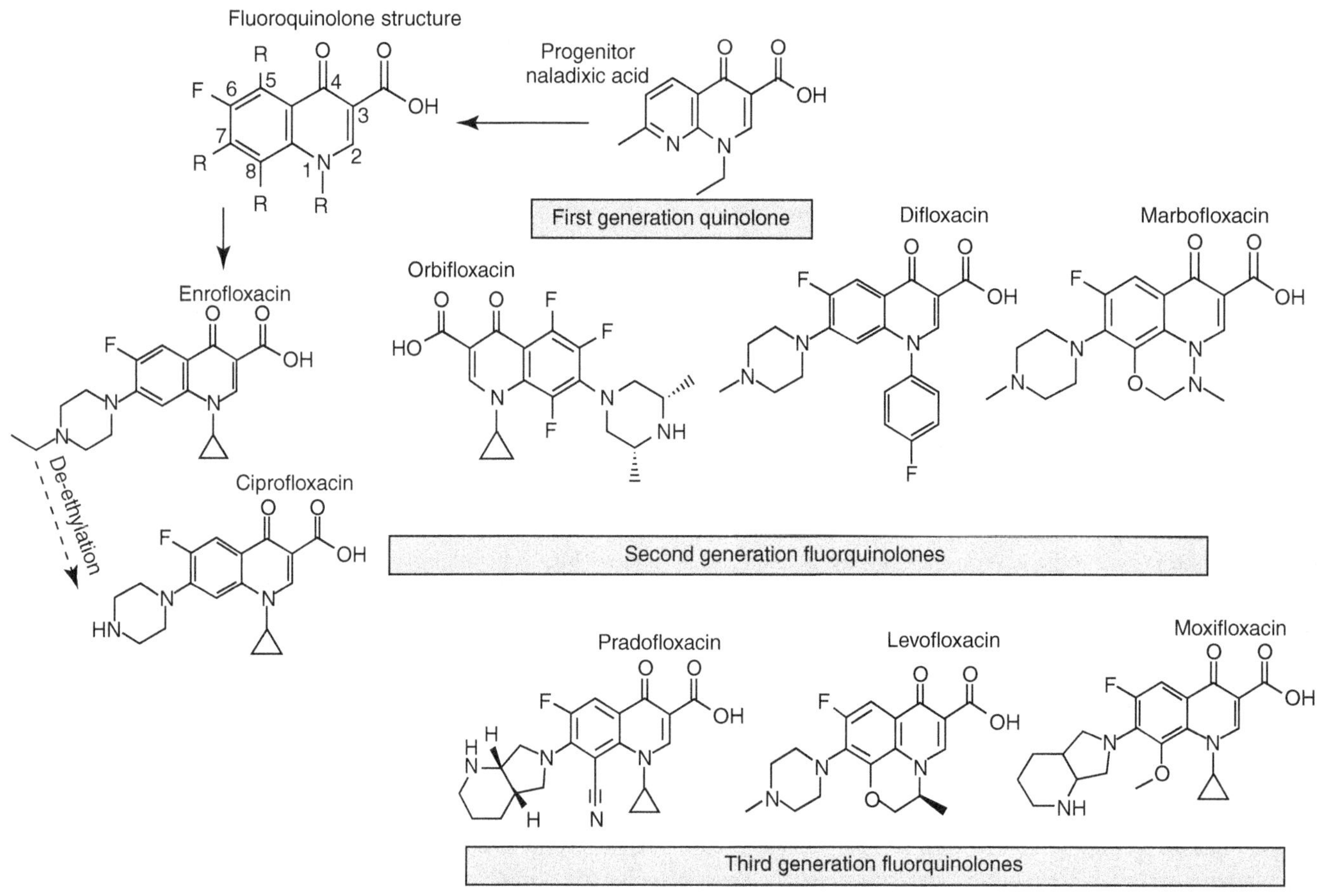

Figure 7-8 Various substitutions of the core chemical structure of the fluorinated quinolones have improved their spectrum, efficacy, and tissue penetration. The efficacy of the fluorinated quinolones depends on the ketone group at position 4 and on the carboxylic acid at position 3 (necessary for inhibition of DNA gyrase). The combination of the fluorine at position 6 (which markedly expanded the gram-positive spectrum) and the substitution of a piperyl ring at position (which enhanced efficacy towards *Pseudomonas aeruginosa* as well as increased tissue penetrability) represented a "breakthrough" for the fluorinated quinolones (e.g., enrofloxacin and its active metabolite, ciprofloxacin). Substitutions at position 8 increase the anaerobic spectrum (e.g., pradofloxacin). The addition of larger side chains may impair microbial resistance mechanisms.

(e.g., moxifloxacin, gatifloxacin) confers good anaerobic activity but without risk of phototoxicity. Recent improvements (in human medicine) focus on increasing the efficacy of FQs toward pneumococci and MRSA, as well as other gram-positive cocci, Enterobacteriaceae, *Pseudomonas*, and anaerobes, and methods by which resistance might be minimized.

KEY POINT 7-19 Chemical manipulations of fluorinated quinolones improve potency, broaden the spectrum, and decrease resistance.

Four drugs are currently approved for oral use in small animals in the United States: enrofloxacin (the first approved, for both dogs and cats, also approved for injectable [SC] use in dogs), followed rapidly by orbifloxacin (dogs and cats), difloxacin (dogs), and marbofloxacin (dogs and cats) (see Figure 7-8). Pradofloxacin may be undergoing consideration for approval for use in dogs in the United States. Variations in the chemical structures of these drugs may result in subtle differences in potency, efficacy, and tissue distribution. Human-marketed FQs, particularly ciprofloxacin and increasingly levofloxacin, continue to be prescribed by veterinarians. Care should be taken to ensure that differences in disposition between humans and dogs or cats are considered when using these drugs. In their guidance to industry, the FQs have been indicated by the Food and Drug Administration (FDA) as "drugs of interest"; as such, veterinary use of these or newer FQs approved for use in humans is likely to draw scrutiny by allied health professions, including regulatory agencies. Note that use of drugs intended for human use (including cheaper generic drugs) instead of veterinary drugs solely because the former are less expensive is likely to be a disincentive for veterinary manufacturers with regard to future approvals of drugs for animals. Further, Animal Medical Drug Use Clarification Act stipulates that the conditions underwhich extra-label drug use is allowed include the lack of availability of a veterinary approved drug that meets the patient's needs. Extra precautions should be taken when prescribing human-medicine drugs to ensure judicious use.

Because enrofloxacin was the first of the veterinary FQs to be approved for use in dogs and cats, it often is the gold standard on which subsequent drug approvals are based and

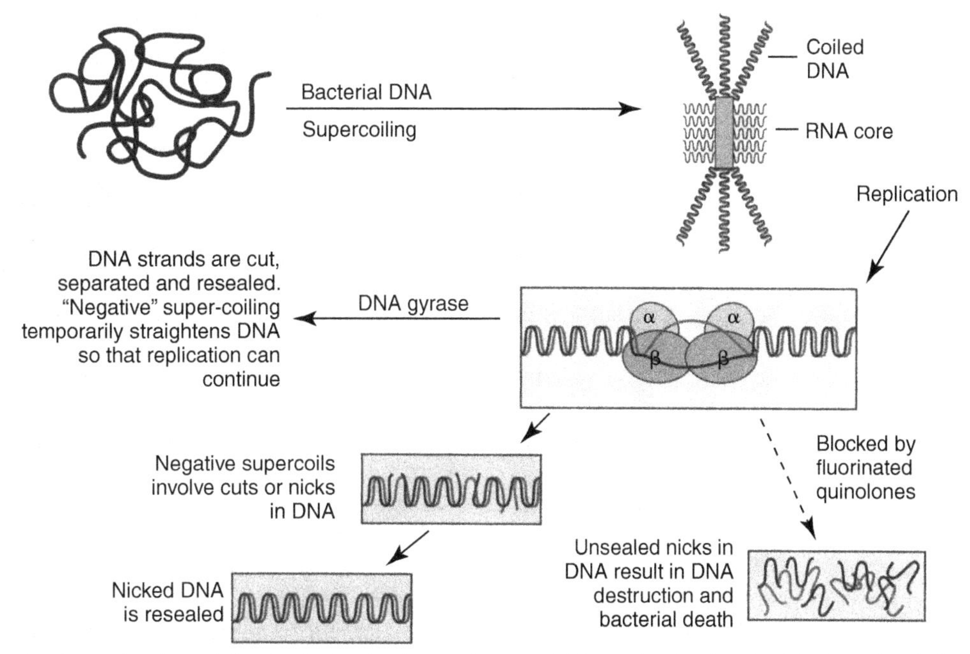

Figure 7-9 The mechanism of action of fluorinated quinolones. During DNA synthesis, the double strands of circular bacterial DNA are in a tightly (negatively) coiled state (negative referring to the direction of the coils). The DNA strands are "unzipped" to allow either messenger RNA or a new DNA strand to be synthesized. The unzipping induces stress and the subsequent formation of positive supercoils, that ultimately must be removed. DNA gyrase, a topoisomerase, directs double-stranded breaks in the DNA. After DNA synthesis, the daughter chromosomes are unlinked by topoisomerase IV. Both DNA gyrase and topoisomerase IV are essential to bacteria and either or both are targeted by the fluorinated quinolones. Drugs that target both enzymes may require multiple mutations for resistance to emerge.

upon which clinical trials evaluating FQ efficacy are based. Because it is structurally similar to ciprofloxacin and because it is metabolized (up to 50% of the AUC of bioactivity) to ciprofloxacin in many species, much of the PD information in the human literature regarding efficacy for ciprofloxacin is applicable to enrofloxacin. However, exceptions occur, particularly with regard to PK considerations. Further, some differences exist in regard to pharmacodynamics between ciprofloxacin and enrofloxacin. Although marbofloxacin has been approved for a shorter period in the United States compared with enrofloxacin, it has been used since 1994 in Europe, and a considerable amount of information is available regarding this drug. In contrast, less information is available for orbifloxacin and particularly difloxacin.

Mechanism of Action

The FQs currently are the only veterinary-approved antimicrobials that directly inhibit DNA synthesis. Bacterial DNA, is circular and can be up to 1.3 mm long, necessitating a negatively supercoiled state surrounding the RNA core (see Figure 7-9).[150,151] During DNA synthesis, the double strands of DNA must be uncoiled or "unzipped" to allow either messenger RNA to interpret or a new DNA strand to be synthesized. The unzipping of the double strands induces positive supercoiling, which leads to undue stress in the individual strands. Accordingly, DNA gyrase (topoisomerase II), directs double-stranded breaks in the DNA, thus inducing a negative supercoil configuration, balancing the positive supercoils. Once DNA polymerase passes through a break in the strand, the break is repaired. Topoisomerase IV separates the daughter DNA molecules produced by DNA replication.[152] Both DNA gyrase and topoisomerase IV are essential to bacteria replication; both are targeted by FQs either individually or sequentially, depending on the drug and organism.[151]

Bacterial topoisomerases are ATPase-dependent enzymes. Each exists as a tetramer consisting of two A and two B subunits. For DNA gyrase, the subunits are encoded by the genes *gyrA* (2517 bp) and *gyrB* (2060 bp), respectively, and for topoisomerase *parC* and *parA*, respectively. The primary enzyme responsible for activity varies with the organism and influences the target of the FQ. DNA gyrase is the primary target in *E. coli,* other gram-negative organisms, and *Mycobacterium tuberculosis,* whereas topoisomerase IV is the primary target of *S. aureus* and (probably) other gram-positive organisms.[151,153] The efficacy of the FQs against various microbes can be explained, in part, by the presence or absence of the target enzymes, as well as drug preference for different enzymes (which in turn can be related to chemical structure [see above]). For example, unlike most other bacteria, *M. tuberculosis* lacks topoisomerase IV and might be less susceptible than other microbes that have both targets. Ciprofloxacin prefers topoisomerase IV, whereas moxifloxacin prefers DNA gyrase. Accordingly, bactericidal activity of moxifloxacin might be (and clinically appears to be) better compared with ciprofloxacin against *M. tuberculosis.* Efficacy of FQs is related to the number of molecules that interfere with the target topoisomerase; interference is irreversible, resulting in concentration-dependent effects.

KEY POINT 7-20 Differences in efficacy of the fluorinated quinolones reflects, in part, the preferred topoisomerase targeted by the drug.

The MICs of the FQ for susceptible organisms tend to be low compared with most other antimicrobial drugs. DNA gyrase actions are inhibited at concentrations of 0.1 to 10 μg/mL. The precise mechanisms by which FQs kill are not fully understood, but strand breakage, autolysis associated with SOS DNA repair systems, and blockade of replication by the gyrase FQ complex may cause bacterial inhibition without bacterial killing.[154] However, the concentration of FQs necessary to inhibit the growth of organisms (MIC) is very close to that necessary to kill the organism (MBC). Although mammal DNA replication also depends on a topoisomerase, its function is somewhat different. More important, affinity of host topoisomerases is less than 0.001 of that of bacterial DNA gyrase. Thus the unique mechanism of action of the FQs renders rapid bactericidal activity with minimal effects on the host. The time to effect for FQs is very short (30 minutes); their rapidity of action often is the reason for preference of these drugs compared with other equally but more slowly effective antimicrobials (e.g., amoxicillin–clavulanic acid combinations for the treatment of selected pyodermas). Interestingly, cellular factors such as intracellular magnesium concentration, salt, and ATP may influence the affinity of FQs for their target enzymes; the clinical implications of this observation are not clear.[151]

KEY POINT 7-21 The irreversible interaction between drug and topoisomerase results in a concentration-dependent effect for the fluorinated quinolone.

The efficacy of the FQs occurs, in part, because of a long postantibiotic effect, which also is concentration dependent. Depending on the organisms, drug, and concentration, the postantibiotic effects can approximate 5 to 8 hours.[155-159] The efficacy of the FQs appears to correlate more closely with peak concentrations (i.e., concentration dependent) than with duration of PDC above the MIC.[160,161] Consequently, efficacy is more likely when C_{max}/MIC exceeds 10 or more. However, duration of time that PDCs are above the MIC (AUC/MIC) also is an effective predictor of efficacy, and may be better than C_{max}/MIC for selected organisms.[162] Analysis of multiple studies focusing on the best predictor of successful bacterial killing indicated that the area under the inhibitory curve (AUIC), an index that is similar to AUC/MIC (see Chapter 6) was the best predictor of efficacy. If AUIC is greater than 100 but less than 250, bacterial killing is slow (evident by day 7 of therapy), whereas an AUIC greater than 250 produced rapid killing, with eradication occurring within 24 hours. The effect occurred for both gram-negative and gram-positive organisms.[153] These data suggest that the most effective use of the FQs is to administer at a dose that will achieve rapid killing. A comparison of C_{max}/MIC or AUC/MIC may be helpful in comparing relative efficacy among the FQs used to treat feline or canine pathogens[164] (see Table 7-12).

Spectrum of Activity

The (human-medicine) FQs have been categorized into 3 to 4 generations based on their spectrum of activity (see Figure 7-8).[165] Athough not often used, the classification is helpful for perspective on the development of the FQs. The spectrum of nalidixic acid, the first-generation drug, is narrow. However, it was improved through pharmaceutical manipulation, yielding the second-generation drugs. This generation is exemplified by the human-marketed drug ciprofloxacin and the current veterinary FQs approved for use in dogs and cats. Their spectrum includes a broad gram-negative and less broad gram-positive spectrum. Third-generation drugs include levofloxacin, the L-isomer of ofloxacin, sparfloxacin, gatifloxacin, and moxifloxacin. This generation is characterized by enhanced potency, improved spectrum (which includes anaerobes), and reduced resistance. The fourth-generation drugs are characterized by the broadest spectrum and are exemplified by trovafloxacin. Each generation has been designed such that drug molecules target specific molecules of the target enzymes, thus increasing efficacy, and for some reducing the emergence of resistance.

The second-generation veterinary FQs have been referred to as broad in spectrum, but this term is appropriate only when referring to the gram-negative spectrum; the term *broad* is more appropriate for third-generation drugs, for which their currently is no veterinary approved example in the United States. The gram-positive spectrum is more selective, and anaerobes, in general, are not susceptible. However, other microbes are targeted, including cell wall–deficient microbes and mycobacterium. Organisms particularly susceptible to FQs include *Pasteurella* (among the lowest MICs), *E. coli, Klebsiella* spp. *E. cloacae, P. mirabilis, Citrobacter freundii*, and *S. marcescens*. *Pseudomonas* spp. also is included in the spectrum but generally is characterized by the highest MICs, with efficacy toward *Pseudomonas* spp. varying with the individual drugs (Table 7-12; see also Tables 7-3 and 7-4).[154] Among the drugs used in dogs or cats, ciprofloxacin, enrofloxacin, and marbofloxacin tend to have the lowest MICs. Ciprofloxacin is most potent toward gram-negative isolates, particularly for *E. coli* and *P. aeruginosa*.[164,166] The gram-positive spectrum includes *Staphylococcus* spp. and some *Corynebacterium*. The FQs have exhibited variable efficacy against *Streptococcus* species and *E. faecalis*.[156,167] Other susceptible organisms generally include *Campylobacter, Salmonella, Shigella*, and *Yersinia*. Efficacy of the FQs toward leptospirosis is supported by limited studies. Some rickettsial organisms may be susceptible; in vitro data and limited in vivo data indicate potential efficacy against organisms causing ehrlichiosis and Rocky Mountain spotted fever.[168]

KEY POINT 7-22 The second-generation fluorinated quinolones have a broad gram-negative spectrum and a more limited gram-positive spectrum and are generally not effective toward anaerobes.

Integration of PK and PD of the FQs reveals some differences in predicted efficacy among the FQs used in cats and dogs toward organisms within the spectrum (see Table 7-12).

Table 7-12 Pharmacodynamic Data for Selected Fluoroquinolones and Selected Feline and Canine Pathogens[164, 180]

	Enrofloxacin			Orbifloxacin			Difloxacin			Marbofloxacin			Pradofloxacin			Ciprofloxacin		
Organism	**n**	**MIC$_{50}$**	**MIC$_{90}$**	**n**	**MIC$_{50}$**	**MIC$_{90}$**	**n**	**MIC$_{50}$**	**MIC$_{90}$**	**n**	**MIC$_{50}$**	**MIC$_{90}$**	**n**	**MIC$_{50}$**	**MIC$_{90}$**	**n**	**MIC$_{50}$**	**MIC$_{90}$**
Bordetella	25/54	0.25	0.5	54	0.5	2	54	2	4	54	0.25	0.5	54	0.12	0.25			
Enterococcus	40/41	1	1	41	4	4	41	2	4	41	2	2	94	0.12	0.25			
Escherichia coli	61	0.0625	≥64	28/155	0.12	0.39/0.25	61	0.0625	≥64	61/45	0.06/≥64		155	≤0.015	0.03			
Klebsiella	32/58	0.06	0.12/0.06	58	0.12	0.25	8/58	0.25	0.11/5	11/58	0.03	0.06	58	0.06	0.06	51	0.0625	
Mycoplasma	32/70	0.12	0.5/0.25	70	0.25	0.5	70	0.25	0.5	70	0.12	0.5	70	0.03	0.06			
Pasteurella	32	≤0.03	0.03	32	≤0.06	≤0.06	32	≤0.06	<0.05	32	≤0.03	0.06	≤0.03	≤0.015	≤0.015			
Proteus mirabilis	88/28	0.125	0.25/1	15	1	8	28	0.0625	0.5	35/18	0.125	0.125/1	93	0.125	0.25	28	0.0625	0.5
Pseudomonas aeruginosa	94/58	1/0.5	>2/8	94/34	4	>8/16	94/58	2/0.125	>4/2	94/38	1/0.5	1/4	94	1	>2	58	0.125	2
Staphylococcus intermedius	119/200	0.12	0.25/0.12	51/15	0.5	0.39/0.5	19	0.25	0.25/2	135/200	0.25	0.25	200	0.06	0.06	19	0.125	0.125
Salmonella	15	≤0.03	0.25	14	0.12	0.12	14	0.25	0.25	14	0.25	0.25	14	0.06	0.12			
Staphylococcus	120/16	0.5	≥64	8	1	ND	193/16	ND/ 0.25	0.46/32	14	0.5	0.25/64		0.06	0.12	16	0.25	32
Streptococcus	33/20	05/0.25	1	33/10	1/0.25	2/≥64	33/20	0.5/ 0.125	1	33/13	0.5	1/4	33	0.12	0.12	20	0.125	1
		MIC	**MPC**		**MIC**	**MPC**		**MIC**	**MPC**		**MIC**	**MPC**		**MIC**	**MPC**		**MIC**	**MPC**
E.coli ATCC8739*		0.03-0.06	0.3-0.35		0.25	1-1.25		0.125- 0.5	1.5-1.6		0.03	0.25-0.3		0.014-0.03	0.2-0.25		0.015- 0.03	0.1-0.15
S. aureus ATCC 6538		0.06-0.125	0.5-0.61		0.5	8-9		0.125	16-18		0.15-0.5	3-3.5		0.03-0.06	0.5-0.6		0.25-0.5	5
Staphylococcus intermedius ATCC 29663		0.06-0.125	1		ND	ND		ND	ND		0.05	ND		0.03	0.15		0.125	ND

MIC, Minimum inhibitory concentration; *MPC*, mutant prevention concentration.

Based on PK reported either in the literature or on the package insert, two PDIs were determined: the C_{max}/MIC (target 10) or AUC/MIC (target 125). The PDIs were compared among drugs for the susceptible isolates of each organism at the lowest and highest labeled dose for each drug. In general, at the low dose the only organism for which the target PDIs were reached for all drugs was *E. coli*. For all other organisms, even at the high dose, targets were reached consistently only for ciprofloxacin, enrofloxacin, and marbofloxacin.[154] The authors concluded that the highest dose of the FQ is generally recommended when possible and that enrofloxacin, marbofloxacin, and ciprofloxacin performed in vitro better than difloxacin and marbofloxacin.

Levofloxacin is a human-marketed third-generation FQ that increasingly is being used in dogs and cats. It is twice as potent against gram-positive isolates (topoisomerase IV) and equally potent against gram-negative isolates (DNA gyrase) compared with ciprofloxacin, although more recent data suggest that this is not consistent (see Table 7-4).[169] For example, the $MIC_{50/90}$ (µg/mL) for human organisms isolated from skin or soft tissue infections are as follows: *S. aureus* (0.25, > 4), *E. coli* (≤0.03, 4), or *P. aeruginosa* (0.5, >4).[170] The potential efficacy of levofloxacin cannot be assessed for dogs because PK have not been established and neither C_{max} nor AUC is available. Kinetics have been reported for levofloxacin in the cat, but at 10 mg/kg, the C_{max} does not reach the MIC_{90} for *Staphylococcus* or *Pseudomonas* spp. The C_{max}/MIC_{90} is only 1 (rather than the target ≥10) for *E. coli*. The target ≥10 would be reached based on the MIC_{50} for *Staphylococcus* spp. and *E. coli* but not for *Pseudomonas* spp. The safety of levofloxacin in cats at doses that will be necessary to reach the target PDI has not been established. These data suggest that PK and PD studies are needed in the dog before levofloxacin is used and that the organisms against which levofloxacin is used in cats at the dose of 10 mg/kg should be characterized by an MIC of 0.5 µg/mL or less. Once-daily administration was demonstrated to be more effective against *Staphyloccus* spp., including an MRSA isolate, compared with twice-daily dosing.[169]

Anaerobic organisms have been considered generally resistant to the FQs. However, the spectrum of the newer drugs, particularly those substituted at position 8, has been expanded to include anaerobes. Levofloxacin, sparfloxacin, grepafloxacin, and pradofloxacin each has greater activity against anaerobes compared with older drugs. This includes the *B. fragilis* group, as well as *Clostridium, Peptostreptococcus, Prevotella,* and *Fusobacterium* spp.[171]

The FQs are effective against mycobaterial organisms. However, using *M. tuberculosis* as an example, the MIC (µg/mL) for the newer FQs are lower compared with the second-generation drugs: 1 µg/mL for levofloxacin, 0.1 to 0.5 for sparfloxacin, 0.2 to 0.25 for gatifloxacin, and 0.12 to 0.5 for moxifloxacin, compared with 0.5 to 4 for ciprofloxacin.[154] Of the FQs, gatifloxacin and moxifloxacin have been demonstrated to exceed the mutant potential concentration (MPC; see Chapter 8) for *M. tuberculosis*. Like other organisms, and despite their slow growth, the activity of FQs against *Mycobacterium* spp. is concentration dependent. However, tubercular organisms are able to enter a dormant, persistant, and antimicrobial-resistant phase, necessitating long-term therapy.

Each of the veterinary FQs has been approved with a "flexible" dosing regimen, indicating low to high doses, with the choice depending on the MIC of the infecting organism. However, as previously discussed, increasing evidence suggests that the highest concentration should be targeted whenever possible. The concept of the MPC emerged in the context of emerging FQ resistance in mycobacteria. Targeting simply the MIC is likely to select for stepwise mutants (see Chapter 6).[162] Flexibility also occurs for the interval: for enrofloxacin and orbifloxacin, the label allows once- or twice-daily dosing, whereas for marbofloxacin and difloxacin, the dose is limited to once a day. Because FQs are concentration dependent, administration of the total daily dose as a once-daily dose is generally preferred, as has been demonstrated for ciprofloxacin[173] and levofloxacin.[169] *P. aeruginosa* is an example of an organism whose tendency toward resistance suggests the higher, once-daily dose.[174] Because efficacy of an FQ is based on AUC/MIC as well as C_{max}/MIC, a second dose (not half the dose twice) might be considered, particularly for selected organisms (e.g., *S. aureus*).

KEY POINT 7-23 Failure to achieve the mutant prevention concentration (MPC) may allow emergence of multistep mutants.

The amphoteric nature of the FQs complicates the impact of pH on efficacy. For example, difloxacin was shown to be most potent (based on MIC differences) at a pH of 7.1 compared with 5.9 or 7.9, with a fourfold increase in the MIC at the alkaline pH occurring for *E. coli, K. pneumoniae, P. mirabilis,* and *S. intermedius*.[159]

Resistance

A major advantage of the FQs promoted during marketing, was the lack of clinically relevant plasmid-mediated quinolone resistance. Rather, the major mechanism of resistance reflects genetic mutations in the target topoisomerase enzymes (e.g., DNA gyrase [topoisomerase II] and topoisomerase IV). However, several observations dampen the importance of the predominance of mutational, rather than plasmid-mediated, resistance. First, history has demonstrated that resistance of any antimicrobial (plasmid or otherwise) may take several decades of intense antimicrobial use, suggesting that, as with other antimicrobials, the use of FQs ultimately was to be limited by resistance. Secondly, resistance to norfloxacin emerged as little as 3 years after its approval, regardless of the mechanism. This rapid development of resistance foretold a similar problem with other second-generation FQs. Thus, as the medical community enters the third decade of ciprofloxacin use in human medicine and the second decade of FQ use in veterinary medicine, increasing resistance, albeit not necessarily plasmid mediated, has emerged and is limiting the widespread effective use of these drugs in both human and veterinary medicine. Finally, plasmid-mediated resistance has appeared and plays a role in horizontal transmission of FQ resistance.[165] The development of FQ resistance by human bacterial organisms has influenced the decision to ban extralabel use of FQs in food animals or use as food additives (i.e., growth promotants). Clinically, the increasing pattern of resistance for veterinary FQs and ciprofloxacin has emerged toward several organisms, including *S. aureus, P. aeruginosa, E. coli,* and other gram-negative organisms (see Chapter 6). In chronic otitis of dogs, 14% of *S. pseudintermedius* cultured from the middle ear and more than 65% of *Pseudomonas* spp. cultured from the external and middle ear were resistant to enrofloxacin.[175] A prospective study of more than 300 organisms submitted to commercial laboratories found nearly 30% of *E. coli* resistant to all veterinary FQs, as well as ciprofloxacin.The MIC_{90} for *Pseudomonas* surpassed the CLSI MIC breakpoint for all drugs except ciprofloxacin, and for *E. coli* and *Staphylococcus* spp. (not including *S. intermedius)* exceeding it for all drugs by fourfold to eightfold.[154] A subsequent prospective study of more than 350 *E. coli* isolates (collected from all body tissues, with the vast majority associated with urinary tract infections) found that 30% demonstrated an MIC_{90} greater than 32 μg/mL (MIC breakpoint ≥ 4 μg/mL), with regional geographical differences demonstrated.[166] Resistance to FQs is associated with FQ use; in humans a single dose of ciprofloxacin lead to FQ-resistant microorganisms.[167] That FQ resistance can be associated with FQ use in dogs was demonstrated by Debavalya et al.:[178] Close to 100% of fecal *E. coli* developed high level resistance to FQs (associated with multi-drug resistance) within 3 to 9 days of therapy of enrofloxacin in dogs (5 mg/kg every 24 hours).

Susceptibility data from laboratories that test both ciprofloxacin and enrofloxacin may report susceptibility to ciprofloxacin but resistance to enrofloxacin. Interpretive standards on culture reports for ciprofloxacin are based on human data and may not take into account differences in oral bioavailability, just as standards for enrofloxacin do not include bioactivity contributed by ciprofloxacin. Although ciprofloxacin is more potent toward *E. coli* and *Pseudomonas aeruginosa* compared to enrofloxacin, the difference is usually within 1 tube dilution. A prospective study compared the proportion of resistance and the relative susceptibility (efficacy) among ciprofloxacin, difloxacin, enrofloxacin (alone or with ciprofloxacin), marbofloxacin, and orbifloxacin FQs toward six organisms collected from canine and feline patients.[154] The proportion of resistant isolates, which was based on CLSI interpretive criteria, did not differ among drugs, suggesting that expression of resistance by an isolate to one (second-generation) FQ might be prudently interpreted as resistance to all, despite the not uncommon finding of susceptibility to ciprofloxacin and resistance to another FQ (e.g., enrofloxacin).

Three major mechanisms of FQ resistance have been identified,[55,167] with the most studied being changes in the structure of the target topoisomerase enzymes. However, mutations, which impart resistance within the FQ class of drugs, are often accompanied by decreased expression of porin membranes and increased activity of efflux pumps, which imparts multidrug resistance.[155,169] Thus far, resistance to FQs acquired through changes in DNA gyrase has been documented clinically only after chromosomal point mutations; at least 10 different mutations have been identified so far. Resistance is stepwise, with the first step occurring primarily through mutations that reduce FQ affinity for the preferred topoisomerase target, which varies with the organism. Gram-negative bacteria tend to more commonly target DNA gyrase; changes occur more often in the *GyrA* subunit compared with *GyrB*.[141] The primary target of gram-positive organisms tends to be changes in topoisomerase IV, targeting *parC* and *parE* followed by changes in DNA gyrase. Recent evidence suggests that the drug (and its primary target) select for the mechanism of resistance.[141] High-level resistance generally reflects a second step mutation that leads to additional changes in the amino acid sequence of either (the alternate) topoisomerase target, thus further decreasing affinity, or the generation of efflux pump mechanisms. The MIC of the organisms progressively increases with each step. The role of reduced porin membranes and efflux pumps in FQ resistance was more recently discovered. Gram-negative isolates are associated with both mechanisms of reduced drug accumulation (i.e., porins and pumps), as well as decreased lipids in the lipopolysaccharide covering, impeding drug transport; gram-positive isolates *(S. aureus)* have been associated with increased drug efflux.[145,147,167] The efflux pumps affect multiple drugs, contributing to multidrug resistance, including resistance to drugs structurally unrelated to FQs.[167,169, 169a] These include tetracyclines, phenicols, and macrolides. Beta-lactams may also be involved; resistance to antiseptics and disinfectants may occur. Expression of the pump is chromosomally mediated. For example, mutations in the *mar* operon may induce the *acrAB* proteins of a stress-induced efflux pump, resulting in high-level resistance, even for isolates with no or single mutations in topoisomerase.[155] Plasmid-mediated quinolone resistance (PMQR), associated with the *qnr* gene, has recently been identified in clinical bacterial isolates, generally associated with class I integrons. However, while initially rare, in 2003, several strains of *E. coli* and *Klebsiella* spp. were found to transmit *qnr* resistance, and isolates have since been identified in the United States. The author has reported a high incidence of PMQR in clinical canine and feline *E. coli* isolates.[165a] Resistance mediated by PMQR and *qnr* tends to be low level and thus may be difficult to detect on C&S testing. Mechanisms include production of a protein that prevents quinolone binding to the target, and enzymatic destruction of the drug. Its impact appears to be related to its ability to increase the incidence of spontaneous mutations and facilitation of altered porin or efflux protein activity. Despite its low level, PMQR resistance associated with *qnr* appears to affect other drug classes, including cephalosporins (including second- and third-generation), aminoglycosides, and potentiated sulfonamides.

The emergence of stepwise resistance is generally indicated by an increase in the MIC of the organism toward the drug. In human medicine, isolates characterized by an MIC greater than 0.125 μg/mL for ciprofloxacin are treated as "reduced susceptibility," indicating that a first step toward mutation (or resistance) has occurred, whereas isolates greater than 2 µg/mL are considered to have "high-level" resistance.[165] These reports are likely, in part, to be the basis of "susceptible" MIC breakpoint promulgated by CLSI. However, it is important to note that despite a susceptible designation for some isolates, reduced susceptibility is an indication that resistance has begun and use of a FQ should be done cautiously and judiciously. Actions such as using a second dose or using the drug in combination with a second, synergistic drug should be strongly considered. Current clinical microbiology laboratories often do not perform susceptibility testing at concentrations below 0.125 to 0.25 µg/mL for FQs, thus precluding the identification of isolates that are characterized by reduced susceptibility. Thus it is important to note that reduced susceptibility to an FQ of intererest may characterize a "susceptible" isolate, and use of FQs should be done judiciously.

The term *MPC* was coined after substantial evidence emerged that resistance to FQs reflects multistep or stepwise selection of mutants when the FQ is used therapeutically at a dose that targets the MIC of a cultured infecting microble (see Chapter 6).[172] At drug concentrations below the MPC, first step mutants will continue to grow in the absence of effective host response, and may replace the wild-type (nonmutant) population.[180] Consequently, the MPC, rather than the MIC, ideally is targeted with drug therapy. Predicting the MPC on the basis of MIC is not possible; the relationship between the two appears to be larger for gram-positive than gram-negative isolates, and varies among the FQs (see Table 7-12).[180] Among the veterinary FQs, using quality assurance isolates, the ratio of MPC to MIC seems to be similar for gram-negative isolates, being less than 10, and the MPC might be reasonably targeted with doses that are within recommendations based on a C_{max}/MIC ratio of 10. However, Pasquali[181] demonstrated that the MPC/MIC for *E. coli* was fourfold to sixteenfold higher for enrofloxacin compared with ciprofloxacin. In this study the authors found that targeting the MPC for *P. aeruginosa* was not effective, postulating that the reason reflects efflux pump activity rather than point mutation (the basis of the MPC theory) as the major mechanism of resistance. Enrofloxacin and pradofloxacin have the lowest MPC/MIC ratio for gram-positive isolates; concentrations necessary to target the MPC for gram-positive isolates may be achievable with these drugs but may not be achievable at recommended doses, particularly for difloxacin and orbifloxacin. Use of the highest dose of any FQ is recommended because of the risk of resistance. If reduced susceptibility is suspected (e.g., MIC > 0.25 µg/mL), then the addition of a second dose or use as part of combination therapy might be prudent. Combination therapy has been described as a mechanism to reduce emergent resistance to FQs. For example, in an in vitro model, rifampin prevented emergence of resistance to ciprofloxacin.[169] The addition of a FQ decreased the advent of resistance to cephalosporins in another study.[182]

Newer drugs, including gemifloxacin, trovafloxacin, gatifloxacin, and pradofloxacin, may target both DNA gyrase and topoisomerase IV. Thus for these drugs, multistep resistance may be necessary to neutralize their antibacterial effects. Newer FQs appear to avoid resistance because their stereochemistry interferes with altered porin sizes and efflux mechanism. For example, for pradofloxacin the cyclopropyl ring at N1 provides bacterial killing, but the diazabicyclononyl moiety at C7 appears to physically block porins.[154] Wetzstein[180] compared the MPCs for older and newer FQs. That resistance may be more likely with older compared with newer drugs was suggested by an in vitro study,[169] in which resistance could be induced for ciprofloxacin but not levofloxacin. However, surveillance studies in humans infected with *Streptoccocus* spp. as well as other isolates, report variable findings, including lower, similar, or higher rates of resistance for levofloxacin, compared with ciprofloxacin.[169,183,184] Because resistance is likely to emerge even to the newer FQs, use based on C&S testing and design of a dosing regimen that targets the MPC as much as possible is prudent.

FQ resistance by *Mycobacterium* spp. occurs primarily as part of multidrug-resistant tuberculosis, which develops when an FQ is used as the only active agent in a failing multidrug regimen.[154] Thus combination with traditional antitubercular drugs (isoniazid, rifampin) enhances antimicrobial efficacy.[154]

Pharmacokinetics

The PK of the veterinary FQs are largely comparable among the drugs, particularly if structurally similar, although individual differences may become important for some infections. Maximum drug concentrations of the FQs do not always increase linearly with dose (see Table 7-1) This may reflect, for some drugs, variability in peak concentrations measured among different investigators, including different analytical methods. In particular, attention must be paid to the method of drug detection, with those based on bioactivity (i.e., bioassay) frequently yielding higher concentrations if an active metabolite is present (e.g., enrofloxacin and ciprofloxacin).

KEY POINT 7-24 The fluorinated quinolones are characterized by good to excellent tissue distribution because of their lipid solubility and accumulation in phagocytic white blood cells.

The only injectable preparation approved for dogs is for enrofloxacin, although an injectable preparation is available for human FQs, including ciprofloxacin. All remaining veterinary FQs approved in dogs or cats are available for oral administration. Enrofloxacin is available as a topical combination preparation. Marbofloxacin, enrofloxacin, difloxacin, and orbifloxacin are characterized by close to 100% oral bioavailability in young adult animals. A number of factors, however, influence absorption of FQs in general, and several drugs specifically. Magnesium and aluminum decrease oral absorption, and food may also, which may be undesirable for concentration-dependent drugs. The oral bioavailiabity of FQs may not be predictable, with extrapolation among species not recommended. For example, norfloxacin is characterized by 60% or less oral bioavailability in dog, and ciprofloxacin, generally less than 60%. Extrapolation of levofloxacin between humans and cats appears to be more appropriate than that of

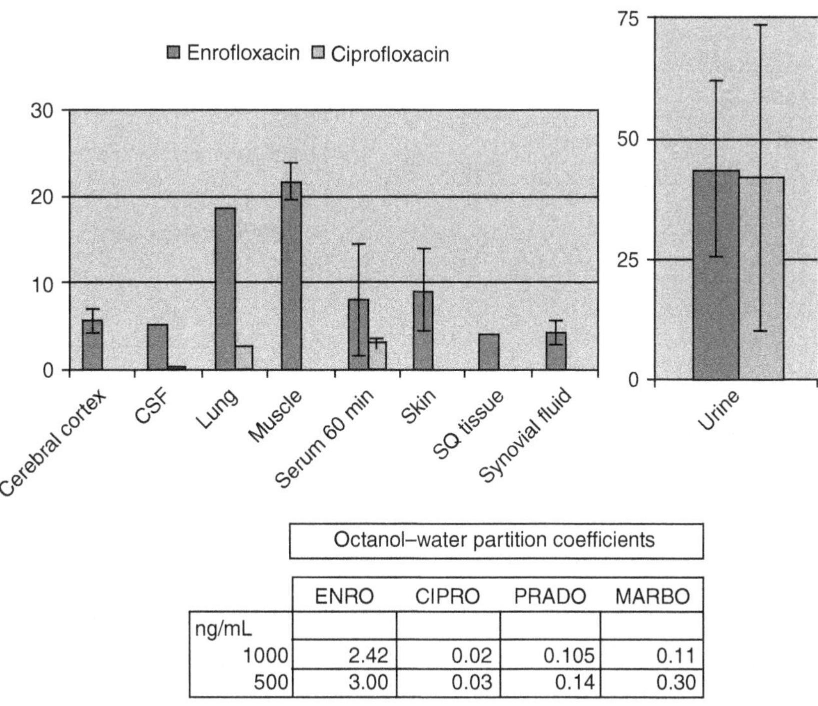

Octanol–water partition coefficients	ENRO	CIPRO	PRADO	MARBO
ng/mL				
1000	2.42	0.02	0.105	0.11
500	3.00	0.03	0.14	0.30

Figure 7-10 Selected tissue homogenate concentrations of enrofloxacin 2 hours after intravenous administration of 20 mg/kg. Concentrations in fluids are most relevant to bacterial exposure. Ciprofloxacin concentrations reflect metabolism of enrofloxacin to ciprofloxacin. Octanol–water partition coefficients suggest that enrofloxacin would distribute best into fluids at physiologic pH.

ciprofloxacin. Oral absorption also may be impaired in neonates, as has been demonstrated for enrofloxacin.[185]

As a class, the FQs are well distributed to most body tissues (see Table 7-5). Protein binding of enrofloxacin, ciprofloxacin, and marbofloxacin in dogs is 34 ± 2%, 18.5 ± 2%, and 21 ± 6%, respectively.[176] Although the Vd of the drugs ranges from a low of 1.12 (marbofloxacin) to a high of 3.2 (difloxacin), the clinical relevance of these differences is not likely to be a sufficient cause to select one over another. The respective PCs for selected FQs have been variably reported, with enrofloxacin characterized by the highest lipophilicity of the three: 2.4, 0.02, and 0.11;[187] and 3.54, 0.07, and 0.08, for enrofloxacin, ciprofloxacin, and marbofloxacin, respectively (Figure 7-10).[176] However, as with Vd, predicting tissue distribution based on PC is difficult. This reflects, in part, the common use of homogenate data for solid tissues. Homogenate data include both interstitial fluid and ICF. As such, drugs that penetrate cell membranes and accumulate in cells, not necessarily in active form, may be characterized by higher concentrations compared with drugs that distribute to interstitial fluid only. Intracellular trapping of drugs may limit access to microbes in interstitial fluid, although movement from the cell back into interstitial fluid may prolong the presence of drug in interstitial fluid by slow release from the cell. The relevance of the data is then influenced by the location of the infection (i.e., intracellular versus extracellular) and host (e.g., inflammation) or microbial (e.g., biofilm) factors that might affect efficacy. Fluid tissue concentrations (based on homogenate data) are generally greater in organs of elimination compared with plasma for all FQs. Solid tissue concentrations are often higher (e.g., if drug is trapped in the cells), particularly for the liver and kidney (organs of elimination) but also spleen and lung (perhaps reflecting phagocytic cell accumulation), prostate (perhaps reflecting ion trapping), and muscle[161,188] Homogenate tissue data are available on the package inserts of several of the veterinary approved FQs. Interestingly, the concentration of difloxacin in cortical bone (but not bone marrow), exceeds that in plasma by threefold, but did not change across a 24-hour period. This might suggest that FQs (or difloxacin) bind to bone, which may preclude activity. Frazier and coworkers[189] compared the disposition and homogenate tissue concentrations of difloxacin (5 mg/kg), enrofloxacin (5 mg/kg; ciprofloxacin also measured), and marbofloxacin (2.75 mg/kg) after multiple dosing (5 days) in the same dogs using a randomized crossover design (21 day washout period); drugs were detected using HPLC. Their studies demonstrate that the FQs accumulate in tissues with multiple dosing. Concentrations increased in the skin to reach a 4-day peak that exceeded the 1-day concentration by at least threefold. The concentrations in skin (μg/mL) at 1 and 4 days were, respectively, as follows: marbofloxacin (1.87 and 4.9), enrofloxacin (1.38 and 5.99), ciprofloxacin (0.2 and 0.5 for a total bioactivity of 1.59 and 6.9), and difloxacin (1 and 3.8). Urine concentrations also were higher at day 4 compared to day 1, with the magnitude varying for each drug. The concentrations in urine (μg/mL) were at 24 and 98 hours, respectively: marbofloxacin (14 and 50), enrofloxacin (0.14 and 1.83) plus ciprofloxacin (5.61 and 33.3 for a total bioactivity of 5.9 and 39), and difloxacin (0.56 and 1.8).

Homgenate data has been reported for enrofloxacin in anesthestized dogs (n = 4) receiving 20 mg/kg of enroflxoacin IV dogs.[188] The 1- and 2-hour serum concentrations

Table 7-13 Concentrations and Tissue to Serum Ratio for Enrofloxacin and Ciprofloxacin*

Tissue	Enrofloxacin (μg/mL)	Ratio	Ciprofloxacin (μg/mL)	Ratio
Cerebrospinal fluid	785.8	0.5	59	0.3
Joint fluid	650	0.5	170	0.7
Urine	2827	2.0	21806	94
Aqueous humor	226	0.2	64	0.3
Bile	136182	95.0	50008	216
Serum	1433	1.0	230.85	1.0

*3 hours after 4 days of oral and 1 day of intravenous 5 mg/kg enrofloxacin.

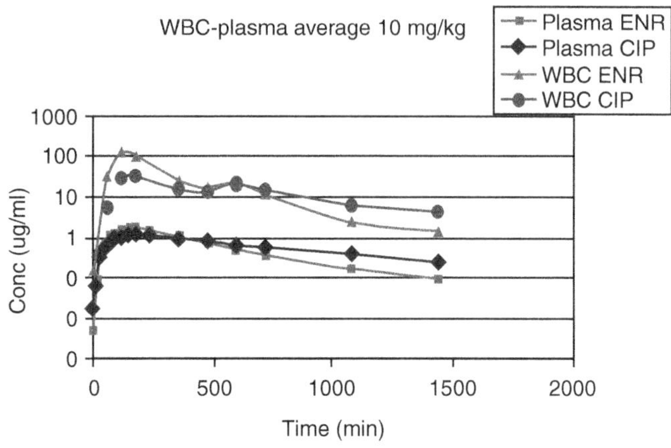

Figure 7-11 Enrofloxacin is metabolized by de-ethylation to ciprofloxacin. The two compounds will act in an additive fashion. The dotted line in the top graph indicates the predicted amount of bioactivity resulting from both enrofloxacin and its active metabolite, ciprofloxacin, after administration of 10 mg/kg. The longer half-life of ciprofloxacin can contribute to a longer duration. The graph demonstrates the accumulation of both enrofloxacin and ciprofloxacin in white blood cells (top two plots).

were 8.2 and 6.4 μg/mL (ciprofloxacin 3.1 and 2.8 μg/mL), respectively. Homogenate tissue to plasma ratios at 2 hours from lowest to highest were, in order, tracheal cartilage (0.2), aqueous humor (0.3), synovial fluid and subcutaneous tissue (0.4), peritonenal fluid and CSF (0.5), and brain (0.6).[178] For fluids located in sanctuaries, at 1 hour aqueous humor (n = 2) achieved 2.5 μg/mL enrofloxacin and 0.5 μg/mL ciprofloxacin; peak CSF concentration of 5.3 μg/mL occurred at 2 hours (one dog). For aqueous humor a second study documented, 0.23 μg/mL of enrofloxacin and 0.064 μg/mL of ciprofloxacin 3 hours after 4 days of oral and 1 day of intravenous dosing at 5 mg/kg.[180] The ratio of tissue to plasma concentrations were similar for ciprofloxacin and enrofloxacin (see Table 7-13). Another study documented that marbofloxacin (2 mg/kg, administered intravenously) achieves 0.41 μg/mL in aqueous humor at 3.5 hours in dogs.[191] Other ratios of plasma to tissue enrofloxacin after 20 mg/kg administered intravenously[192] included ligament (0.6), ear cartilage (0.7), and bone marrow (0.8). Concentrations in the prostate were 2.5-fold higher and urine 4.5-fold higher than in plasma (urine concentration of 45 μg/mL). Interstitial fluid concentrations of enrofloxacin (and formed ciprofloxacin) and marbofloxacin have also been measured using ultrafiltration. After 10 mg/kg enrofloxacin administered intravenously, the ratio of C_{max} in interstitial fluid (2.41 μg/mL) compared with plasma (5.54 μg/mL) was 0.47; the ratio for AUC, however, was 1.3, indicating that the drug appears to stay longer in interstitial fluid compared with plasma.[177] A second study[176] determined plasma to interstitial fluid ratios after 5 mg/kg, administered orally, for marbofloxacin (approximating the highest labeled dose) and enrofloxacin (the lowest once-daily dose). Plasma to interstitial fluid C_{max} ratio was 0.75 for marbofloxacin and 0.7 for enrofloxacin plus ciprofloxacin and for AUC was 1.11, for marbofloxacin and 1.3 for enrofloxacin and ciprofloxacin. The higher AUC for marbofloxacin reflected in part the higher C_{max} but also a longer elimination half-life (8.5 hours) compared with enrofloxacin (3 hours). All FQs that have been studied thus far (enrofloxacin, marbofloxacin, pradofloxacin, and ciprofloxacin) accumulate in phagocytic WBCs; concentrations may be up to 140-fold higher compared with plasma (see Table 7-5).[164,193-196] Drug in phagocytes will be distributed to sites of inflammation, thus increasing concentrations at the site of infection.[196] Impact on intracellular killing is controversial. Whereas some studies have demonstrated that FQs retain intracellular killing effects compared with macrolides,[197] another in vitro study demonstrated reduced intracellular killing ability for a variety of FQs.[184]

KEY POINT 7-25 The bioactivity of enrofloxacin can be doubled by formation of its more potent metabolite, ciprofloxacin.

The organ of elimination varies among the FQs. Difloxacin is eliminated almost exclusively by hepatic metabolism to inactive metabolites. Orbifloxacin is 40% eliminated unchanged in the urine. Marbofloxacin (clearance of 1.6 L/min) is largely excreted into the urine. However, up to 15% is metabolized in the liver to inactive metabolites,[198] with the proportion changing in the presence of renal disease.[198] Enrofloxacin also is eliminated in the urine as the unchanged drug, although approximately 25% of the drug is metabolized to ciprofloxacin, which subsequently achieves concentrations severalfold higher than enrofloxacin (Figure 7-11; see also Figure 7-8 and Table 7-13). Therapeutic concentrations of ciprofloxacin can be achieved in other tissues after administration of enrofloxacin, depending on the target organism.[161,193,199] The parent and metabolite should act in an additive fashion.[160] Because ciprofloxacin is characterized by a longer half-life than enrofloxacin in dogs (see Table 7-1), as a metabolite, ciprofloxacin can double the AUC of enrofloxacin bioactivity (see Table 7-1 and Figure 7-11).[193] Longer elimination half-lives also characterize difloxacin and marbofloxacin compared with orbifloxacin and enrofloxacin, contributing to higher AUC for these drugs (see Table 7-1). Elimination half-lives are somewhat dose dependent,[193] at least for enrofloxacin and ciprofloxacin (see Table 7-1). Alkaline urine increases the passive reabsorption of FQs from the renal tubules and may also prolong the elimination half-life. The longer half-lives should increase efficacy by increasing the likelihood that the drug will achieve the target AUC/MIC. Heinen[200] compared PDIs among the FQs after oral administration, using a bioassay that detects both parent compound and active metabolites (see Table 7-1). Based on MIC_{90} determined for *E. coli* and *Staphyloccoccus* spp. (from isolates before 1999), for no drug was the targeted AUC/MIC achieved for *Staphylococcus* spp. and only enrofloxacin achieved the C_{max}/MIC for *Staphylococcus* spp. Enrofloxacin (5 mg/kg) had the highest C_{max}/MIC toward *E. coli,* followed by marbofloxacin (2 mg/kg) and orbifloxacin (2.5 mg/kg); difloxacin (5 mg/kg) did not reach the targeted C_{max}/MIC or AUC/MIC for either organism. A similar pattern of efficacy was found among the veterinary FQs by Boothe using isolate MIC and reported C_{max},[164] with enrofloxacin plus ciprofloxacin > ciprofloxacin > marbofloxacin > orbifloxacin > difloxacin being the general pattern of magnitude in PDI. However, the higher dose was generally needed to reach desired targets for PK/PD indices; isolates had been collected from 1998 to 2000 suggesting the likelihood of achieving targeted PDI with current isolates is less likely.

The disposition of enrofloxacin in neonatal kittens differs from that in adults, appearing to be age dependent even in the pediatric patient.[185] Administration of 5 mg/kg to 2- to 8-week-old kittens[185] revealed a shorter half-life at all ages but a Vd_{ss} that was less at 2 to 4 weeks and greater at 6 to 8 weeks compared with that of adults. Accordingly, C_{max} was lower in the 6- to 8-week-old kittens. Enrofloxacin was generally poorly bioavailable at all ages.

Pradofloxacin. Pradofloxacin is a newer-generation FQ that may be undergoing approval in animals in the United States and the European Union. Structurally, it is characterized by a cyclopropyl ring at N1 (see Figure 7-8) that increases bacterial killing. A diazabicyclononyl moiety at C7 appears to physically block drug efflux through porins and targets both topoisomerases such that mutation must be multistep.[154] Its spectrum includes *P. aeruginosa*. However, many anaerobes also will be effectively targeted. At 3 mg/kg orally for 5 days in dogs, C_{max} was 1.7 ± 0.9 μg/mL and 6.2 ± 2.3 μg/mL in dogs (n = 6); half-life was 10 ± 7 hr at 3 mg/kg and 5.9 ± 1.5 hr at 12 mg/kg.[190] The long half-life results in an AUC/MIC that is favorable compared with the other FQs. Pradofloxacin also has been studied in anesthetized dogs. It appears to be well distributed among the tissues.[190] Aqueous humor concentrations achieved 0.32 μg/mL after 5 days of administration (4 oral followed by 1 IV) at 5 mg/kg of pradofloxacin.

Ciprofloxacin. Although ciprofloxacin has been studied in dogs following intravenous and oral[202] administration (Table 7.1), the studies used different animals, and limited information is available on its oral bioavailability in dogs. However, reports provided by the manufacturer indicate that ciprofloxacin is only 33% to 40% bioavailable in dogs[203] compared with nearly 80% to 100% in humans. Oral absorption of ciprofloxacin in dogs involves a dose-dependent nonlinear component that may affect its oral absorption.[202] Oral and bioavailability of ciprofloxacin in cats (using pure powder in gelatin capsules) appears to be less than that in dogs, being 20% ± 11% following single dosing and 33% ± 12% after multiple dosing.[205] Oral absorption was characterized by marked interanimal variability, suggesting that oral absorption may be minimal in some cats.[205] This suggests that oral ciprofloxacin should be avoided in cats, and oral dosing in both cats and dogs should err on the side of higher doses to compensate for unpredictable oral bioavailability. More than several human-marketed generic preparations of oral ciprofloxacin are now available at a greatly reduced cost compared with oral enrofloxacin. However, whereas bioequivalence of a generic product must be proved to the pioneer product, this proof is generated only in the species in which the drug is approved. That the PK behavior of an orally administered generic drug will behave the same way in a nonapproved species should not be assumed.

The disposition of ciprofloxacin has been described in cats after intravenous administration of 10 mg/kg (see Table 7-1). In cats Vd_{ss} of ciprofloxacin is 3.85 ± 1.34 L/k, and plasma clearance is 0.64 ± 0.28 L/hr/kg, which exceeds the normal feline glomerular filtration rate (0.15-0.25 L/h/kg), suggesting that active tubular secretion occurs.[206] AUCs after intravenous and oral administration are 17 ± 5 and 3 ± 1.2 μg*hr/mL, respectively, in cats. Drug accumulation was not significant after seven oral administrations.[205] Ciprofloxacin is metabolized into active (in humans) and inactive metabolites (N-oxide [the primary metabolite in dogs] and N-desmethyl). However, high concentrations of unchanged drug are achieved in urine, as is demonstrated after administration of enrofloxacin (see Figure 7-10).

Levofloxacin. Levofloxacin is the optical S-isomer of the racemic drug substance ofloxacin (see Figure 7-8). Compared with older FQs, its spectrum includes mycoplasma and gram-negative organisms, but the spectrum is broader toward gram-positive organisms and includes anaerobes.[207] Ofloxacin is marketed as the levo isomer (i.e., levofloxacin) rather than the racemic mixture because the L-isomer is much more active against bacterial pathogens than the R-isomer. In humans levofloxacin is well absorbed orally, is distributed to a volume of 1.1 L/kg, and is renally excreted. Concentrations in the CSF approximate 16% of that in plasma, suggesting that the drug may not be well distributed into sanctuaries. Excretion is correlated with creatinine clearance, and half-life is prolonged with renal disease, requiring dose adjustments in patients with significant renal dysfunction.[208]

Because of its spectrum and improved antibacterial activity compared with veterinary FQs, levofloxacin has been used anecdotally in dogs but does not appear to have been studied in dogs. However, ofloxacin (but not its isomers) has been studied after oral administration in young and mature Beagles.[209] Peak concentrations (measured by HPLC) at 20 mg/kg were 14.2 ± 0.4 μg/mL. The dispositions of the L-and D-isomer are likely to differ, precluding prediction of the proportion of the C_{max} represented by levofloxacin. However, even if 100% of the drug is the L-isomer, concentrations are still well below the MIC_{90} of levofloxacin. The disposition of levofloxacin has been well described in cats on the basis of a bioassay after intravenous and oral administration,[210] and it does not appear to be substantially different from that in humans. In cats the drug is well, albeit slowly, absorbed orally (T_{max} 1.6 hours), with bioavailability at 87%. The drug is rapidly distributed, reaching a Vd_{ss} of 1.75 L/kg; clearance is 0.14 L*hr/kg, and mean residence time is 13 hours (see Table 7-1). The C_{max} following oral administration was 4.7 μg/mL, indicating that the drug should be used in cats only for organisms with an MIC of 0.5 μg/mL or less.

Drug Interactions

The FQs inhibit selected hepatic drug-metabolizing enzymes and are known to prolong the elimination of selected drugs. Theophylline toxicity has been documented in humans and dogs (see Chapter 2) simultaneously receiving theophylline and ciprofloxacin or enrofloxacin.[211] Marbofloxacin also impairs the elimination of theophylline in dogs, but the effect is dose dependent, being absent at 2 mg/kg. However, at 5 mg/kg, theophylline clearance is decreased by 26% (compared with 50% reduction by enrofloxacin at 5 mg/kg IV once a day for 5 days), resulting in a change in theophylline half-life from 3.6 to 5.4 hours and a change in C_{max} from 32 (no marbofloxacin) to 44 μg/mL (5 mg/kg marbofloxacin).[212] Ciprofloxacin has been associated with increased cyclosporine concentrations, prolonged anticoagulant effects of warfarin, and enhanced hypoglycemic effects of oral hypoglycemics and insulin. Presumably, enrofloxacin and other FQs might have similar effects. Because of chelation by magnesium, calcium, and other cations, drugs such as antacids, sucralfate, and multiple vitamins should not be administered orally at the same time as a FQ. Because FQs competitively inhibit gamma-aminobutyric acid receptor binding, drugs that act similarly (e.g., selected nonsteroidal antiinflammatory drugs) when used in combination may increase the risk of seizural or other CNS activity. Enrofloxacin has been associated with false glucosuria.[77]

KEY POINT 7-26 Fluorinated quinolones can impair the metabolism of selected drugs.

The use of FQs in combination with other antimicrobials may result in synergistic activity (e.g., aminoglycosides for gram-negative organisms; beta-lactams for gram-positive or gram-negative organisms) (see Chapter 6) or antagonistic (e.g., ribosomal inhibitors).

Adverse Effects

Adverse reactions to the FQs do not reflect interaction with mammalian topoisomerases. Most adverse reactions are predictable and can be prevented with proper administration. Gastrointestinal upset manifested by vomiting, nausea, and possibly diarrhea may occur after any route of administration but particularly oral administration. The intramuscular administration of enrofloxacin frequently causes pain on injection. Nausea and vomiting have been reported when the intramuscular solution is given intravenously and may reflect mast cell degranulation and histamine release. The intramuscular solution also is very alkaline (pH 10). Diluting the drug in saline and administering it over a 30-minute period may reduce nausea and clinical signs consistent with an anaphylactoid response. FQs have been associated with allergic reactions; however, the lack of previous exposure in some (human) patients (and in the author's experience with ciprofloxacin) suggests an anaphylactoid rather than anaphylactic reaction.[213]Acute cardiovascular toxicity (hypotension, decreased left ventricular function) has been described for levofloxacin (Freedom of Information [FOI]) after an intravenous bolus (≥6 mg/kg) or intravenous infusion (≥20 mg/kg, but not ≤10 mg/kg). Increased circulating histamine concentrations accompanied the high-dose intravenous infusion, indicating a potential anaphylactoid reaction at 10, 15, 30, and 60 mg/kg intravenous bolus. Death occurred in dogs in association with neurologic and cardiac signs at 200 mg/kg, administered intravenously. Enrofloxacin also is available as a more concentrated solution (100 mg/mL) approved for use in cattle. However, it is prepared an an arganine-based vehicle, which is painful on injection and will cause perivascular inflammation if given parenterally by any route other than intravenous. Ulcers may occur if the large animal prepration is given orally.

Cartilage deformities and ligament and tendon repair. The FQs are associated with cartilage damage in dogs (and other species) (see package inserts). Enrofloxacin's original package insert cited clinical signs indicative of cartilage damage in Beagle puppies within 3 days of treatment at 12.5 mg/kg. Lesions have been documented in dogs treated with other FQs. For levofloxacin, arthropathies occurred in juvenile dogs at ≥10 mg/kg/day for 7 days (FOI). Lesions in adult dogs require much higher concentrations, as was demonstrated for levofloxacin: the no-observed-effect level was 3 mg/kg/day in normal 7- to 8-month-old dogs compared with 30 mg/kg/day in normal 18-month-old dogs. The arthropathic potential of ofloxacin (the racemic mixture of levo and the R-isomer of ofloxacin) also has been studied in dogs.[209] At 20 mg/kg for 8 days, eight out of eight 3-month-old animals developed histologic lesions, whereas only two developed clinical signs; the associated serum ofloxacin concentration was 14 μg/mL. The mechanism of cartilage damage is not known, although the most likely mechanism appears to be chelation of magnesium ions leading to dysfunction of integrins. These cell membrane proteins regulate a variety of cellular functions, including chondrocyte adherence to extracellular matrix and proteoglycan synthesis.[215] Magnesium-deficient diets in juvenile rats led to cartilage damage similar to that caused by FQs.[216] Indeed, magnesium supplementation may reverse the effects of FQs on canine chondrocytes.[217] Dogs may be among the most sensitive and the most likely to exhibit clinical lameness caused by FQ-induced cartilage damage.[204] Note that cartilage lesions as a result of FQs might be considered when FQs are used in any situation that involves growing or repairing cartilage, such as septic or immune-mediated arthritis and potentially osteoarthritis. Lesions have also been reported in other species, including humans.[218] Use of chondroprotectants (i.e., polysulfated glycosaminoglycans) might be considered if FQ therapy must be instituted in growing dogs or other situations involving cartilage growth or repair.

The FQs appear to negatively affect healing in damaged ligaments.[219] Connective tissue proteins decreased by up to 73% in dogs treated with as little as 30 to 200 mg/kg ciprofloxacin orally. Lesions were similar to those produced in magnesium-deficient dogs, suggesting that FQs induce tendon or ligament damage by antagonizing magnesium effects in the affected tissues.

The impact of FQs on bone repair also may be of concern. Based on experimental fracture healing in rats receiving placebo, cefazolin, or ciprofloxacin (50 mg/kg every 12 hours subcutaneously for any of the aforementioned drugs), fracture callus healing appeared to be impaired by FQs.[218] In vivo studies in dogs of the effects of ciprofloxacin at 30 to 200 mg/kg/day orally (equivalent to approximately 15 to 65 mg/kg bioavailable drug) in dogs on either a normal or magnesium-deficient diet found a number of proteins were decreased in both groups at all doses, including collagen, elastin, and fibronectin.[219] Of these effects, the authors concluded that magnesium deficiency increases the risk of impaired healing in the presence of FQs.

Seizures and other central nervous system disorders. Seizures and other CNS disorders have been precipitated in human and veterinary patients[220] and animal models receiving FQs;[221] predisposing factors include a preepileptic state, high doses, and concurrent use of nonsteroidal antiinflammatory drugs.[220] Newer drugs may be more likely to cause CNS side effects.[222] FQs (and imipenem) inhibit GABA release, leading to hyperexcitability;[76] inhibition of N-methyl-D-aspartate or adenosine may also be involved.[143] FQs also lower seizure threshold and impede neuromuscular transmission. Peripheral neuropathies are a recognized side effect of FQs in humans.[13,223] Clinical signs in humans have been described as severe, involving multiple organs. Onset is described as rapid (within 24 hours of onset of therapy; 84% afflicted within 1 week) and long term in duration, with symptoms lasting more than 3 months in 71% of afflicted patients and more than 1 year in 58%. The majority of cases involved levofloxacin (64%), despite ciprofloxacin (21%) being the most commonly prescribed drug. The most frequent complaints included both sensory (tingling, burning, or numbness) and motor (musculoskletal, cardiovascular, skin, gastrointestinal [cramping]) abnormalities; symptoms were described as severe in 80% of the patients.

Dose-dependent retinal degeneration. Dose-dependent retinal degeneration has been associated with use of FQs in cats. The incidence of ocular toxicity is very rare, occurring in 1 of 125,000 cats receiving enrofloxacin. The incidence at high doses is sufficiently low that toxicity was not detected in preapproval toxicity studies. During preapproval in cats, 25 mg/kg/day for 30 days and 125 mg/kg for 5 days were not associated with detectable toxicity. It is not clear whether ocular toxic-specific outcomes were addressed. Doses in clinical reports[224] in which ocular toxicity occurred (retrospective study) ranged from 4.6 to 54 mg/kg/day, with duration of dosing ranging fom 4 to 120 days. Clinical signs began with mydriasis, rapidly followed by acute blindness. Age may be a factor, with cats younger than 9 years seemingly requiring a higher (>20 mg/kg) dose. Diseases associated with changes in disposition that might result in high plasma enrofloxacin concentrations (e.g., renal disease, heart disease) may also increase the risk. Intravenous administration may increase the risk, further supporting the concentration dependence of toxicity.

Experimental studies by Bayer Animal Health in young, apparently healthy cats at 5, 20, and 50 mg/kg/day for 21 days found electroretinography changes in one of six cats at 20 mg/kg and severe changes in six of six cats within 1 week at 50 mg/kg. Manufacturers of other veterinary FQs have likewise performed follow-up ocular toxicity studies. Marbofloxacin was not associated with lesions in young cats treated with up to 27 mg/kg/day for 6 weeks or 55 mg/kg/day for 14 days. Orbifloxacin was not associated with lesions at 15 mg/kg/day orally for 30 days, but changes occurred at 45 and 75 mg/kg.[225]

KEY POINT 7-27 Among the fluorinated quinolones currently approved for use in cats in the United States, marbofloxacin appears to be the least likely to cause retinal degeneration in cats.

The mechanism of ocular toxicity appears to reflect a mutation in four amino acids of an efflux protein in the blood-retina barrier, rendering it ineffective. Effective protein activity is absent in all cats. (personal communication, Dr. Katrina Mealey, Washington State University). The FQs are structurally similar to compounds known to cause accumulation in lysosomes of retinal pigment cells and subsequent ocular toxicity. Additionally, FQs have a predilection for pigmented cells of the eye. The FQs also have been associated with phototoxicity. The combination of FQs with ultraviolet radiation produces both a time- and concentration-dependent ocular toxicity, with a methyl group at position 8 of the quinolone ring reducing the risk.[226] Reducing exposure to sunlight (dosing at night, or keeping cats indoors) might be prudent for cats receiving FQs.

Induction of bacteriophage supergenes. Induction of bacteriophage supergenes has been associated with the use of FQs, and in dog bacterial isolates, specifically enrofloxacin. Shortly after approval of enrofloxacin in Canada, seven canine cases of streptococcal toxic shock syndrome (STSS) and/or necrotizing fasciitis (NF) were reported; four of the dogs had been treated with enrofloxacin in the early stages of infection. Treatment was not only ineffective, but the syndrome appeared to be worsened by the antimicrobial therapy.[227] Further investigation has provided some insight into the possible relationships between STSS and NF and bacteriophage supergenes in *S. canis*. Using polymerase chain reaction analysis, 22 of 23 *S. canis* isolates in one study exhibited a bacteriophage-encoded streptococcal superantigen gene. Under culture conditions, induction of the bacteriophage by enrofloxacin at therapeutic concentrations resulted in a 58-fold enhancement of expression of the gene.[228] Apparently, the FQ stimulates autoingestion of a repressor protein that otherwise would prevent the bacteriophage from becoming lytic. FQs apparently also can induce bacteriophage lysis and enhanced Shiga toxin production in *E. coli*. For example, ciprofloxacin-treated mice experimentally colonized by Shiga-toxigenic *E. coli* died while their untreated colonized cohorts did not; increased Shiga toxin was demonstrated in their feces. However, induction requires ideal conditions, being dependent in part on stage and rate of growth and ideal drug concentration; conditions favoring bacteriophage induction in clinical patients have not yet been described.

Therapeutic Use

The FQs originated from nalidixic acid, itself a by product of chloroquine.[150] Nalidixic acid is characterized by a narrow spectrum, and its use was limited to treatment of urinary tract infections. Modifications of chemical structures increasingly have improved the drugs, yielding drugs that have among the broadest of antibacterial spectrums. However, caution should be exercised with selected drugs because efficacy toward specific organisms (e.g., *Pseudomonas*, spp. anaerobes) varies. The FQs also are characterized as a class among those with the greatest tissue and antimicrobial distribution patterns. However, differences in tissue distribution (e.g., enrofloxacin versus ciprofloxacin, bone distribution of difloxacin) does indicate prudence when comparing FQ use. The rapid bactericidal effect of FQs is of clinical benefit in life-threatening situations or immune-suppressed patients; concentration dependence allows once-daily dosing that improves owner compliance. Intracellular accumulation of these drugs supports use for recurrent infections caused by intracellular organisms or at sites characterized by marked inflammation. Plasmid-mediated resistance has been slow to develop, although increasingly resistance, particularly that associated with multidrug resistance, is limiting FQ use. Oral bioavailability allows prolonged administration on an outpatient basis. However, bioavailability of the different drugs varies among the species, and good oral bioavailability should not be assumed. Rather, extrapolation of oral doses should be based on scientific studies. The unique mechanism of action of these drugs renders them appealing for combination antimicrobial therapy.

However appealing these numerous attributes of the FQs, common use of these drugs is discouraged. Widespread use—and abuse—of these drugs in the past 2 decades has proved that antimicrobial resistance can and will occur. Resistance, when it does occur, is often associated with multidrug resistance affecting chemically unrelated drugs. The emergence of of MDR with newer FQs needs to be assessed. Confirmation of the need for the drug and attention to MPCs (see Chapter 6) in the design of the dosing regimen should be two hurdles that are consciously addressed each time these drugs are considered. The metabolism of enrofloxacin to ciprofloxacin and the reduced oral bioavailability of ciprofloxacin in dogs and cats coupled with the importance of ciprofloxacin as a human-medicine drug call for extra caution to be taken. Once the decision is made to use an FQ, strict adherence to the principles of antimicrobial therapy, with a special focus on proper dosing regimens, is paramount to protecting this class of antimicrobial drugs, which is so critical to the medical community.

Rifamycins

Rifamycins are macrocylic antibiotics produced by *Amycolatopsis mediterranei*. Several semisynthetic derivatives) of natural rifamycins (rifamycin SV, Rifampin, rifampicin, rifamiderifamide) have been used as extended-spectrum antibiotics.[150] Rifampin is among them. A large molecule (MW 823; see Figure 7-4) as with all rifamycins, it inhibits the B subunit of DNA-dependent RNA polymerase, suppressing RNA synthesis. Because mammalian RNA polymerase does not bind to rifamycins, its inhibition requires much higher concentrations. Rifampin can achieve bactericidal concentrations in some tissues. Effects are concentration-dependent for mycobacterium but unclear for other organisms. However, resistance develops very rapidly, markedly curtailing its use, and in general, rifampin should be used only in combination with other effective antimicrobials. Resistance may develop in as little as 2 days when it is used as the sole antimicrobial; rifampin is used experimentally to study mutation frequencies in some organisms. The use of rifampin as sole agent for treating pyoderma is addressed in Chapter 8. Resistance generally reflects a single mutation that changes the affinity of the target enzyme for the drug. Resistance (and efficacy) can be decreased with combination therapy with a number of drugs, including erythromycin, most beta-lactam antibiotics, chloramphenicol, doxycycline, and selected aminoglycosides. Rifampin has shown some efficacy against fungal microorganisms.

Spectrum

The spectrum of activity of rifampin includes primarily gram-positive (especially *Staphylococcus* spp.) organisms (see Table 7-4). However, it also is effective against *Mycobacterium*, *Neisseria*, and *Chlamydia* spp. and has been used to treat *Clostridium* and *Bacteroides* species. Rifampin has limited activity against gram-negative organisms (including *Brucella*). Resistant gram-negative organisms include *E. coli*, *Enterobacter* spp. *K. pneumoniae*, *Proteus* spp. *Salmonella* spp., and *P. aeruginosa*. However, an Internet search reveals a number of papers that indicate efficacy toward *P. aeruginosa* when combined with a number of other drugs. Highly susceptible gram-positive organisms are considered to have an MIC of 0.25 μg/mL or less; MICs are often less than 0.1 μg/mL. In contrast, the MIC of gram-negative organisms is generally 8 to 32 μg/mL; the higher MICs reflect limited penetration of gram-negative organisms. A dose of 10 mg/kg in the dog achieves a C_{max} of 40 μg/mL (see Table 7-1); accordingly, its use for gram-negative isolates (and ideally, all isolates) should be based on C&S testing.

KEY POINT 7-28 Rapid resistance to rifampin limits its use to combination therapy only.

Pharmacokinetics

Rifampin may be administered intramuscularly, intravenously, or orally with systemic effects. Oral absorption of rifampin is incomplete in humans (~40%) with peak plasma concentrations occurring in 2 to 4 hours. Concurrent feeding may reduce or delay absorption. Because it is a substrate for P-glycoprotein,[229] oral absorption may be much higher in dogs exhibiting P-glycoprotein deficiency. Approximately 75% to 80% of rifampin is bound to plasma proteins. Rifampin is very lipid soluble, distributing well to most body tissues. It concentrates in white blood cells and is characterized by immunmodulation.[230] Because rifamycins penetrate tissues and cells to a substantial degree, they are particularly effective against intracellular organisms. Rifampin is rapidly eliminated after acetylation to a metabolite (desacetyl rifampin) that is equal in efficacy to the parent compound. Whether the dog is a deficient acetylator of rifampin is unclear. Both the parent and metabolite are excreted in the bile (supporting its use for cholangitis in humans); the parent compound and metabolite undergo enterohepatic circulation. The elimination half-life of rifampin is dose dependent, being about 8 hours in dogs.

Adverse Effects

Rifampin is usually well tolerated and produces few side effects. However, gastrointestinal disturbances and abnormalities in liver function (icterus) have been reported in humans and may lead to discontinuation of therapy. Hypersensitivity reactions can also result from rifampin administration, and renal failure is a possible consequence when intermittent dosage schedules are followed. Partial, reversible immunosuppression of lymphocytes occurs. Urine, feces, saliva, sputum, sweat, and tears are often colored red-orange by rifampin and its metabolites; urine may stain. Plasma will also be orange and may be misinterpreted as hemoglobinemia. CNS depression after intravenous administration and temporary inappetence may occur. Interestingly, intermittent administration (less than twice weekly) increases the risk of side effects in humans, resulting in a flulike syndrome that is associated with clinical signs indicative of a drug reaction (eosinophilia, thrombocytopenia, hemolytic anemia [note potential for orange discoloration of plasma] and renal disease).[150] In a limited number of dogs, marked increases in serum alkaline phosphatase have been observed by the author. No other liver enzyme or function tests were affected, and dogs did not become clinically ill. The increase may reflect induction of the enzymes (much the same as glucocorticoids or phenobarbital), but monitoring of hepatic function may be prudent in at-risk dogs receiving rifampin.

Drug Interactions

Rifampin is a broad, potent inducer of microsomal enzymes, including CYP1A2, 2C9, 2C19, and 3A4;[150] as such, it will shorten the elimination half-life of a number of drugs and may increase the risk of toxicity associated with drug metabolism.[229] Therapeutic failure may occur for other drugs metabolized by the liver if modifications in dosing regimens are not made. Rifampin PDCs will decrease after multiple dosing because of induction, with plasma elimination half-life of rifampin progressively shortening by approximately 40% during the first 2 weeks of treatment in humans. Other affected drugs include the imidazoles, cyclosporine, digoxin, and several sodium channel– and beta receptor–blocking cardiac antiarrhythmics. Endogenous substrates of hepatic metabolism also may be affected; several steroids will be more rapidly catabolized.[150] Withdrawal syndromes have been reported in humans receiving opioid analgesics.[150] Because rifampin is a substrate for P-glycoprotein, dogs with the MDR-1 (ABC) deletion will have an increased risk of adverse reactions; the risk is increased if rifampin is used in combination with other drugs that interact with this protein. Finally, rifampin also has decreased biliary secretion of some compounds, notably contrast imaging media.[150] Rifampin has been used in combination with a number of drugs to enhance efficacy (and reduce resistance; see the section on resistance) for treatment of MRSA, VRE, and *Mycobacterium* spp. and others. Use in combination with doxycycline has been recommended for canine brucellosis, although clinical efficacy has not been demonstrated.[2]

KEY POINT 7-29 Rifampin is a potent inducer of drug-metabolizing enzymes.

Two other rifamycins are approved for use in humans. Rifabutin is a derivative of rifampin that is characterized by less induction of drug-metabolizing enzymes. Used for the treatment of *Mycobacterium* spp., it is characterized by unique side effects, including polymyalgia, anterior uveitis, and others. Rifapentine is used to treat tuberculosis associated with human immunodeficiency virus infections in humans. Its longer half-life allows once-weekly dosing, and its impact on drug-metabolizing enzymes has been described as intermediate.[150] Rifaximin is a semisynthetic derivative of rifamycin that is not orally absorbed. It is indicated for treatment of enteric pathogens, including *Campylobacter, C. difficile, E. coli, Helicobacter pylori,* and *Salmonella* and *Shigella*.[231] A potential advantage of rifaximin is an apparent minimal long-term effect on the gastrointestinal flora: both *E. coli* and *Enterococcus* spp. were minimally affected after 3 to 14 days of therapy. Resistance to rifaximin seems to emerge only slowly, compared with systemic use of rifampin.[231] Indications in humans have been a variety of (nonbloody) diarrheas, including small bowel overgrowth, intestinal gas, and inflammatory bowel disease.

Metronidazole

Metronidazole is deriviative of the antibiotic azomycin (2 nitro-imidazole) secreted by a streptomycete (Figure 7-12).[232] A number of other nitroimidazoles were developed from azomycin.[232] Among the other closely related imadazoles used outside the United States are tinidazole, and benznidazole, the latter being used to treat acute Chagas disease. Metronidazole impairs microbial RNA and DNA synthesis but must first undergo nitrous reduction in the organism. As such, metronidazole is a prodrug, with efficacy depending on the

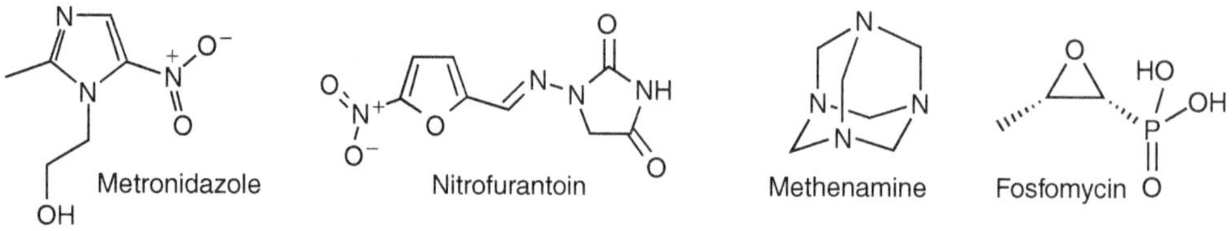

Figure 7-12 Chemical structure of miscellaneous antimicrobials.

nitrous group and a low redox potential that can be achieved only in an anaerobic environment.[233] Only organisms that live in a low-oxygen environment have developed anaerobic energy or electron-generating pathways (e.g., ferredoxins) capable of generating single electrons. Transfer of the electron to the nitrous group of metronidazole results in a highly reactive nitro radical ion. Although DNA is the primary target, other macromolecular structures may be targeted. Metronidazole will be regenerated on death of the microbe, thus facilitating its efficacy. Efficacy appears to be predominantly bactericidal, although actions may be bacteriostatic toward some organisms (e.g., *Eubacterium* spp.). Metronidazole acts as a concentration-dependent drug against trichomoniasis, and, although this is not always clear, it also appears to be concentration dependent when treating other microbes. However, time dependence has also been ascribed[234] (e.g., *Clostridium* and its efficacy appear to be similar if administered once or twice daily).[235]

KEY POINT 7-30 Metronidazole is effective only against anaerobic bacteria.

Spectrum

Metronidazole is rapidly bactericidal against all gram-negative (e.g., *B. fragilis*) and most gram-positive (e.g., *Clostridium* spp.) anaerobic bacilli, generally at MIC equal to or less than 8 μg/mL. Microaerophilic microbes such as *Helicobacter* and *Campylobacter* spp. are susceptible. Metronidazole is effective toward a number of protozoa, with efficacy dependent on the nitro group at position 5 and enhanced with substitutions at the 2 position.[236] Susceptible infections include trichomoniasis (MIC of 0.05 μg/mL if anaerobic conditions), amebiasis, and giardiasis (1 to 50 μg/mL).

Resistance

Aerobes and facultative anaerobic bacteria lack electron transport systems necessary to generate single electrons and thus are resistant to metronidazole. Further, in higher oxygen environments, oxygen will compete for the electrons generated by anaerobic organisms, thus decreasing efficacy of metronidazole. Higher doses are necessary if the infection occurs in an environment of 1% or more oxygen.[232] Interestingly, protozoa may develop resistance ot metronidazole in patients with impaired oxygen-radical scavenging abilities.[232] Microbes also acquire resistance by decreasing proteins that generate the electrons (e.g., ferredoxin). The mechanism of bacterial resistance is not totally clear, but increased production of interfering enzymes is likely. Resistance by *Helicobacter* spp. can be rapid.

Pharmacokinetics

Metronidazole is well distributed to all body tissues and can penetrate the blood–brain barrier. It is minimally protein bound (in humans). Elimination is dose dependent and occurs primarily by hepatic metabolism. At least one metabolite has 50% of the activity of the parent compound toward trichomonads. Intestinal microbes can produce a small amount of the reduced (active) metabolites. Peak concentrations in dogs after 44 mg/kg reached 42 μg/mL. Vd is 0.95 ± 0.1 L/kg, and clearance is 2.5 ± 0.54 mL/kg/min.[237] Oral bioavailability is variable, ranging from 59% to 100%. Elimination half-life in one study was 4.5 ± 9 hours (see Table 7-1). Metronidazole disposition has been described in the cat after single intraveous (5 mg/kg) administration as the salt-free product and then at 20 mg/kg orally of the benzoate salt (12.4 mg/kg active drug).[238] Extrapolated plasma concentration after intravenous administration at time 0 averaged 7.8 ± 2 μg/mL; Vd was 0.7 ± 0.3 L/kg, and plasma clearance was 91 mL/kg/hr. Elimination half-life and mean residence time were 5.3 ± 0.7 and 7.6 ± 1 hours, respectively. The benzoate salt was fairly well absorbed but was characterized by clinically significant variability, with a bioavailability of 65% ± 27% (range 28% to 80%). The C_{max} also varied, with a mean of 8.8 + 5.4, reflecting a range of 4.9 to 17.8 μg/mL; T_{max} also varied from 1 to 8 hours (mean 3.6 ± 2.9 hours). Elimination half-life and mean residence time after oral administration were 5.2 ± 0.5 and 8.7 ± 1.3 hours, respectively.

Adverse Effects

Metronidazole may discolor urine (red-brown).[232] More problematic adverse reactions include gastrointestinal upset (including hepatotoxicity when given at high doses) and CNS adversities, including seizures.[237,239] The risk of neurotoxicity is increased with intravenous administration; as such, oral administration is the preferred route whenever possible. The caustic nature of the intravenous solution also necessitates slow intravenous administration. The mechanism of neurotoxicity is not known, but in mice degenerative lesions have been demonstrated in the Purkinje cells, vestibular tracts, and several nuclei associated with equilibrium and fine motor control. These areas are also the site of the majority of gamma-aminobutyric acid–minergic receptors. In humans, characteristic lesions seen on magnetic resonance imaging indicate that the cerebellum may be most sensitive to damage; because interstitial edema was evident, with axonal swelling was suggested as a cause.[240]

In dogs, seizures are indicative of toxicity. One study in dogs (n = 21) induced seizures at doses of 60 to 110 mg/kg for a total of 10 to 110 days.[241] The most common clinical signs were vertical nystagmus, ataxia, inability to walk (≥50% each), and paraparesis (30%); less frequent neurologic signs included tetraparesis, hypermetria, tremors, head tilt, torticollis, and opisthotonus. Treatment with diazepam proved effective based on a shorter response time (resolution of debilitating clinical signs; 13 hours versus 4.5 days) as well as recovery time (return to normalcy; 11 versus 36 hours). The dose of diazepam was approximately 0.5 mg/kg, administered intravenously followed by oral administration every 8 hours for 3 days. Neurologic reaction to metronidazole has also been reported in cats (n = 2). The dose and duration associated with clinical signs were 111 mg/kg body for 9 weeks followed by 222 mg/kg/day for 2 days in one cat and 58 mg/kg for 6 months in the second.[242] Clinical signs in cats included ataxia, altered mentation, and progression to seizures. Neurologic signs resolved within days of discontinuation of the drug and supportive therapy. Histologic lesions have also been described in another 14-year-old cat that developed fatal presumed metronidaozle toxicity after treatment for inflammatory bowel disease at 73 to 147 mg/kg/day. Among the neurologic clinical signs was acute tetraparesis; lesions included diffuse, multifocal areas of necrosis throughout the brainstem.[243]

Metronidazole as either the free form or when administered as the benazoate salt was genotoxic (disruptive of lymphocytic DNA) but not cytotoxic to feline polymorphonuclear cells. Genotoxicity resolved within 7 days after the drug was discontinued.

Preparations

Metronidazole is available as either a hydrochloride (used in the approved product) salt (oral or intravenous) or, in pure drug substrate form (i.e., for compounding), the benzoate salt. It can be administered as a loading dose infused over 30 to 60 minutes in fluids, followed by an intravenous drip. It also can be given intermittently as an 8- to 12-hour maintenance dose as long as the infusion takes place slowly. For intravenous administration the dose should be neutralized with sodium bicarbonate and mixed with lactated Ringer's solution, saline, bacteriostatic water, or 5% dextrose in water (see package insert). Because intravenous administration of metronidazole is complicated, oral administration is preferred whenever possible.

The benzoate salt of metronidazole, which is not commercially available, is less bitter tasting and more tolerable than the commercially available hydrochloride salt. The oral disposition of the benzoate salt was previously described.[238] However, the benzoate moiety is larger than the hydrochloride moiety, representing 38% of the drug product. As such, when dosed on total drug weight, the dose of metronidazole benzoate should be 1.6 times the dose of metronidazole hydrochloride.[244] Further, the benzoate must be removed by desterification before its absorption; it is not clear if oral administration of the benzoate form will be as effective against gastrointestinal microbes compared with a nonbenzoate form.

Metronidazole (not studied as a salt) has been demonstrated to be stable in solutions when stored at 40° C for 90 days.[245] However, it reacts with the aluminum of needles or other canulas. Metronidazole is subject to drug interactions associated with inhibition (e.g., cimetidine) or induction (e.g., phenobarbital, prednisone, rifampin) of drug-metabolizing enzymes.

Metronidazole is available as a topical gel, which provides wound odor control. Although it can be prepared as a transdermal PLO gel, studies by the author demonstrated minimal absorption when applied to the pinna of the ear for 3 weeks at 15 mg/kg.

Metronidazole is a drug of choice for treating infections caused by obligate anaerobes, particularly those associated with gastrointestinal flora. Increasingly, it is used in lieu of oral vancomycin to treat *C. difficile*. Frequently, it is cited as a treatment for inflammatory bowel diseases in animals or humans (particularly Crohn's disease). Its efficacy may reflect, in part, immunomodulatory properties (see Chapter 19) or its ability to target those microbes most likely to produce inflammatory mediators.

DRUGS THAT TARGET FOLIC ACID

Inhibitors of Folic Acid Synthesis:/Sulfonamide/Trimethoprim or Ormetoprim Combinations

The sulfonamides are the oldest group of antibiotics used therapeutically. All sulfonamides that are currently used were derived from the first clinically relevant sulfonamide, sulfanilamide, itself a derivative of the azo dye prontosil. The discovery of its efficacy in vivo but not in vitro indicated that metabolism by the host was necessary for efficacy and contributed to the understanding of the role of drug metabolism in bioactivation. Once the metabolite was identified as the active drug, a number of manufacturers produced hundreds of different sulfonomide antimicrobial preparations. The FDA had not yet been empowered by Congress to evaluate drug safety, resulting in the lack of safety limitations. Among the vehicles in which drugs were prepared was a product containing ethylene glycol. The subsequent death of more than 100 persons, including children, ingesting the product contributed to congressional approval of the Food Drug and Cosmetic Act of 1938. It was this act that empowered the FDA to evaluate drugs for safety before marketing.

The sulfonamides were the first group of commercially available antimicrobials used systemically.[246] Their use was somewhat curtailed by the advent of the penicillins, only to increase again in the 1970s with their combination with the diaminopyridine trimethoprim. Not surprisingly, long-term use of these drugs has contributed to the development of resistance that has limited their clinical use.[246] However, a decline in their use, in part because of concerns regarding drug allergies, probably has contributed to a decline in resistance. Sulfonamides generally are used in combination with diaminopyrimidines for treatment of bacterial infections, with use of sulfonamides as sole agents generally limited to treatment of coccidiosis.

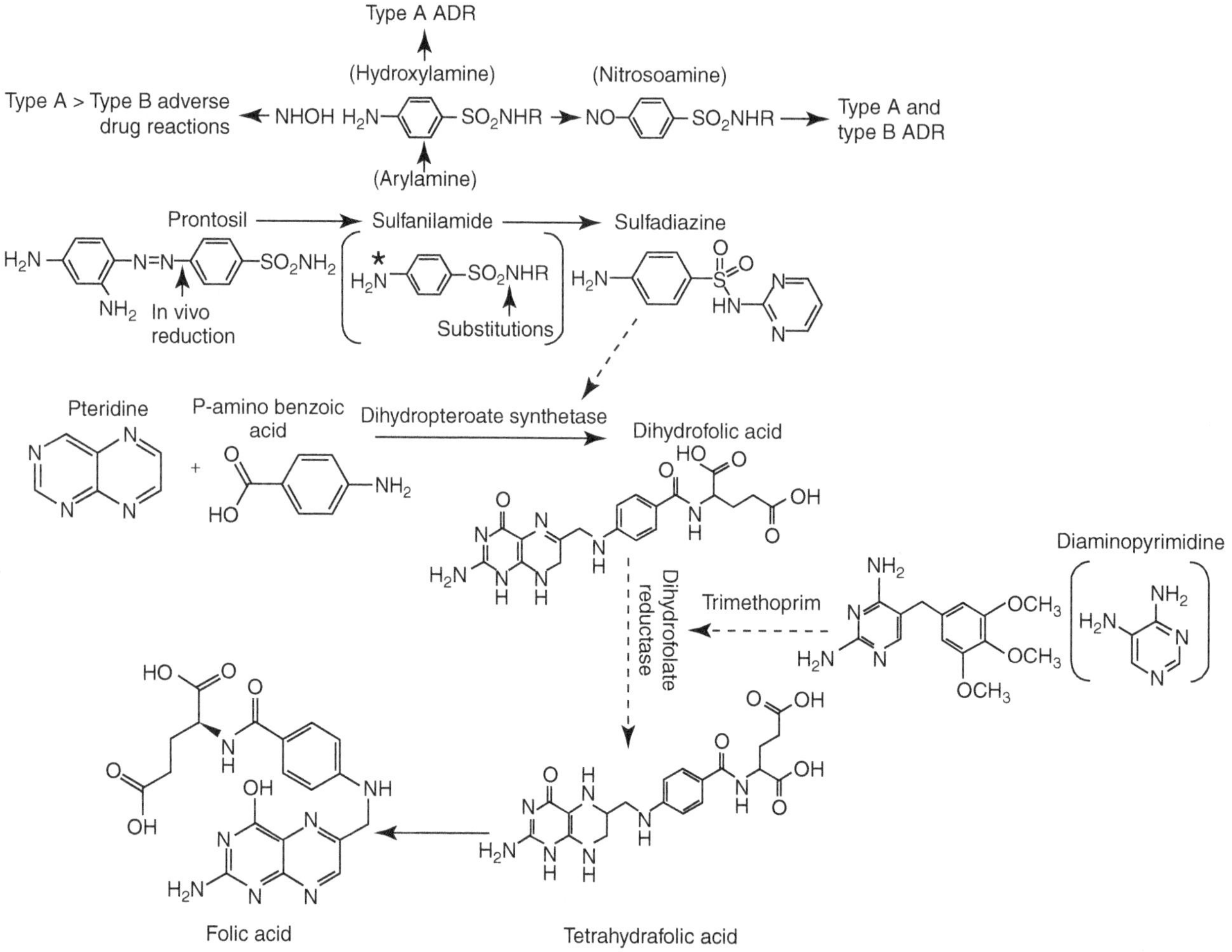

Figure 7-13 `The mechanism of action of the sulfonamides and the diaminopyrimidines. By itself, either type of drug is bacteriostatic, but the two-point sequential inhibition of folic acid synthesis results in bactericidal effects. The progenitor of the sulfonamides is sulfanilamide *(inset)*. As such, all are arylamines. Metabolism of the arylamine to a hydroxyalamine and nitroso compound contributes to the toxicities, including drug allergies, associated with sulfonamides.

Structure Chemistry Relationship

As derivatives of sulfanilamide, all sulfonamides have the same nucleus. Functional groups have been added to produce compounds with varying physical, chemical, pharmacologic, and antibacterial properties, but the active amine is in position 4 and any substitutions at this position must be freed in vivo (Figure 7-13). Although amphoteric, sulfonamides generally behave as weak organic acids and are much more soluble in an alkaline than in an acidic environment. Those of therapeutic interest have pK_a values between 4.8 and 8.6. Water-soluble sodium or disodium salts are used for parenteral administration. Such solutions are highly alkaline, somewhat unstable, and readily precipitate out with the addition of polyionic electrolytes. In a mixture of sulfonamides (e.g., the sulfapyrimidine group), each component drug exhibits its own solubility; therefore, a combination of sulfonamides is more water soluble than a single drug at the same total concentration. This is the basis of triple sulfonamide mixtures used clinically (primarily in large animals). The N-4 acetylated sulfonamides, except for the sulfapyrimidine group (sulfadiazine), are less water soluble than their nonacetylated forms. Highly insoluble sulfonamides are retained in the lumen of the gastrointestinal tract for prolonged periods and are known as "gut-active" sulfonamides. Most sulfonamides used clinically for treatment of bacterial infections are "potentiated." The "potentiator" of sulfonamides is a diaminopyrimadine; examples include trimethoprim, ormetoprim, and pyrimethamine (the latter being the preferred drug for toxoplasmosis) (see Figure 7-13).

Mechanism of Action

Folic acid is an essential bacterial substrate necessary for protein and nucleic acid metabolism. Bacterial synthesis of folic acid is accomplished in several sequential steps (see Figure 7-13). The sulfonamides are structurally similar to PABA and act as competitive substrates (antimetabolites) for the synthetase enzyme. Among the many sulfonamides used clinically are sulfadiazine, sulfamethoxazole, sulfachlorpyridazine, sulfadimethoxine, and sulfasalazine; sulfisoxazole is the model drug upon which C&S testing is based.

Because folate metabolism is required for many cellular functions, bacterial growth is inhibited; consequently, the antibacterial effects of sulfonamides as sole agents are bacteriostatic. The diaminopyrimidines trimethoprim and ormetoprim also impair folic acid synthesis but at a different point in the metabolic pathway. They prevent the conversion of dihydrofolate to tetrahydrofolate by inhibiting the reductase enzyme. By themselves, these drugs also are bacteriostatic. It is the combination of a sulfonamide antimicrobial with a diaminopyrimidine antimicrobial ("potentiated") that results in subsequent two-point inhibition of bacterial folic acid synthesis and thus bactericidal rather than bacteriostatic activity (see Figure 7-13).[5,246] Mammalian cells are not affected by these drugs because they are dependent on dietary sources of folic acid; in contrast, microbes cannot use external sources of the substrates. Further, the affinity of bacterial enzymes for the drugs is much higher than the mammalian enzymes. The competitive nature of the mechanism of killing activity of potentiated sulfonamides leads to a time-dependent effect. High inoculums may require higher doses for efficacy.

KEY POINT 7-31 The combination of the sulfanomide and the diaminopyrimidine results in bactericidal effects.

Spectrum of Activity

The spectrum of activity of sulfonamides is considered broad, but efficacy is variable because of acquired resistance. However, a decline in their use during the last decades (due to concerns regarding allergies) appears to be associated with an increased in susceptibility for a number of organisms. The spectrum of combined products includes gram-positive, gram-negative, and anaerobic organisms. The sulfonamides exhibit good to moderate activity against *E. coli; Enterobacter* spp.; *Klebsiella* spp.; *Proteus* spp.; *Pasteurella* spp.; and anaerobic organisms such as *Actinomyces, Bacteroides, Fusobacterium* spp., and selected clostridia.[247-249] The spectrum of these drugs does not include *Serratia* spp., *P. aeruginosa, Rickettsia*, or *Mycoplasma* spp. The sulfonamides exhibit good efficacy against *Brucella* spp., *Actinomyces* spp., and selected protozoal organisms such as *Pneumocystis carinii* and *Cryptosporidium* spp. Some *Chlamydia* spp. are susceptible to sulfonamides, whereas others are not. The difference appears to be based on whether the organism can obtain folic acid from the host.[249a] *Mycoplasma* organisms are not susceptible to sulfonamides. By itself, trimethoprim has a potency that is twentyfold to 200-fold less than that of sulfonamides.[246] Potentiated sulfonamides are generally useful for uncomplicated infections of many body systems.

Resistance

Inherent resistance to sulfonamides reflects, in part, the ability of the microbe to make use of host folic acid. Resistance to the sulfonamides and to trimethoprim or ormetoprim occurs relatively rapidly. Chromosomal resistance results in impaired drug penetration, reduced affinity of the enzyme for the substrate, or increased bacterial production of PABA. Plasmid-mediated resistance occurs rapidly because of altered drug penetration and decreased affinity of the enzyme for the substrate. Resistance to one sulfonamide generally results in resistance to all sulfonamides.[246] The increasing emergence of resistance has sharply curtailed the use of these drugs. The role of trimethoprim/sulfonamide combinations for the critically ill patient or for chronic infections should be based on C&S information because of the incidence of resistance.

Pharmacokinetics

The sulfonamides are generally rapidly and completely absorbed after oral administration, although there are exceptions (see the discussion of structure and chemistry). Trimethoprim and ormetoprim are well absorbed after oral administration. Sulfasalazine is poorly absorbed as an intact molecule and is used primarily for gastrointestinal diseases. After oral administration sulfasalazine is partially absorbed in the small intestine. It undergoes enterohepatic circulation and ultimately is eliminated in the urine. Most of the drug (70%) is metabolized by colonic bacteria to its component parts: sulfapyridine and 5-aminosalicylic acid. Sulfapyridine is rapidly absorbed and subsequently eliminated in urine. The 5-aminosalicylic acid may provide the major therapeutic benefit for chronic inflammatory bowel disease.[246]

Solutions intended for parenteral administration must be buffered to prevent pain and irritation caused by the alkalinity of the compounds. Topical administration is not recommended because of the effects of these drugs on wound healing. An exception is made for silver sulfadiazine and mafenide, which are used primarily for burn patients in human.[246] Sulfadiazine is combined with silver in a topical otic preparation approved for use in dogs. Protein binding of the sulfonamides varies from 15% to 99%. Examples include sulfadiazine at 30% to 50% bound, sulfadiamethoxine, at greater than 75%, and sulfasalazine up to 99% bound. Protein binding contributes to a relatively long half-life, allowing for convenient dosing intervals.

KEY POINT 7-32 The disposition of the sulfonamides, which are time dependent, is markedly variable among members of this drug class.

The tissue penetrability of the sulfonamides varies. All are distributed at least to extracellular fluid. Sulfamethoxazole (the model drug for susceptibility testing) is limited to interstitial fluid, whereas sulfadiazine is distributed to total body water.[246] Sulfadiazine penetrates most body tissues extremely well, including the prostate.[250] The penetration of these drugs varies with the sulfonamide component. Prostatic penetration is facilitated by a high pK_a. Sulfadiazine (pK_a 6.4) is among the best distributed sulfonamides but only achieved 11% of serum concentration in the prostate of dogs in one study (the original reference for this study could not be found). Drugs with a more basic pK_a may appear to better penetrate the prostate, although this may reflect ion trapping in prostatic fluids. Sulfadiazine can attain therapeutic concentrations in CSF, particularly if given intravenously, and is the preferred sulfonamide for CNS infections.[246] Trimethoprim achieves tissue concentrations four times higher than that in plasma. The combination of a sulfonamide with a diaminopyramidine at a ratio of

1:5 trimethoprim/sulfonamide results in a bactericidal effect and a tissue distribution ratio of 1:20 in most tissues.[5] This ratio, however, is described in humans, and information in dogs or for sulfadimethoxine and ormetoprim does not appear to be available.

Sulfonamides that undergo hepatic metabolism are generally acetylated. All sulfonamide antimicrobials are arylamines. The dog lacks some genes that encode for N-acetyltransferases responsible for metabolism of arylamines.[251] Thus metabolism in the dog may involve other pathways, facilitating the formation of potentially nitroso metabolites that are responsible for allergic or other idiosyncratic reactions (see the section on adverse reactions) (see Figure 7-13).[252] Drugs are renally excreted as either the parent compound or the conjugated metabolite by either glomerular filtration or active tubular secretion. Both passive reabsorption and enterohepatic circulation can prolong the elimination half-life of selected sulfonamides.[246] Acetylated metabolites of sulfonamides are often less soluble than the parent compounds, which increases the risk of renal damage should drug precipitate and form crystals. However, this is unlikely in dogs because of deficient acetylation. The risk is reduced in other species because of the use of combination products, which reduces the total amount of dose needed for efficacy. The elimination half-lives of the drugs vary with the sulfonamide component and among the species. The duration at which sulfonamides remain in the body leads to classification as short-acting (12 hours or less: sulfacetamide, sulfathiazole, and sulfisoxazole), intermediate-acting (12 to 24 hours: sulfadimethoxine, sulfisoxazole, sulfamethoxazole, sulfapyridine, sulfamethazine, and sulfadiazine), and long-acting (longer than 24 hours).[246] In the dog, according to the package insert, sulfadimethoxine concentrations are 39 μg/mL 24 hours after dosing. Peak ormetoprim at 2 hours was 1.09 μg/mL in dogs but was 0.09 μg/mL at 24 hours, indicating a half-life of about 6 hours. It is not clear whether the differences in half-life between sulfadimethoxine and ormetoprim "match" in terms of ideal proportion throughout the labeled 24-hour dosing interval.

Adverse Effects

Reactions to sulfonamide antimicrobials reflect the greatest proportion of antimicrobial adversities in the dog.[252] The adversities to sulfonamide antimicrobials but not other sulfonamides (e.g., nonsteroidal antiinflammatories, zonisamide, furosemide) probably reflect the basic structure of the sulfanilamide molecule, which is an arylamine, in which the amine group is directly attached to the benzene ring (see Figure 7-13). The susceptibility of dogs to sulfonamide toxicity may reflect the species' deficiency in acetylation and specifically N-acetylation. The proposed mechanism of toxicity reflects shunting of the sulfanilamide arylamine to an oxidative phase I pathway (see Figure 7-13). Oxidation of the arylamines yields hydroxylamine, a metabolite that can be cytotoxic at high concentrations; the metabolite also is somewhat allergenic. Hydroxylamine can be further metabolized (often spontaneously) to a nitroso compound, which is somewhat cytotoxic but is more immunogenic than the hydroxyarylamine. The potential role of the arylamine as a cause of sulfonamide toxicity is supported by the lack of apparent toxicity by other sulfonamide drugs used in dogs, which, lacking a primary arylamine, are not converted to hydroxylamine. The likelihood of adversity may be related to the type of metabolites formed and the rate of acetylation. As such, the likelihood of toxicity occurring may vary among the sulfonamide antimicrobials. The mechanism of hypersensitivity may reflect haptenization of the metabolite and a subsequent T-cell response, although other mechanisms (e.g., humoral response or cytotoxicity) may contribute.[252] Deficiencies in glutathione, ascorbic acid, or other radical scavengers may increase the risk of either type A or B reactions; the role of supplementation in preventing or treating adversities apparently has not been addressed scientifically but may be prudent. Controversy exists as to whether the parent sulfonamide might be immunogenic.[252] The "potentiator" may also be responsible for some reactions; for example, trimethoprim has been associated with skin eruptions or hepatopathy in humans; further, use of sulfadiazine as the sole coccidiostat in dogs has not been associated with drug allergies.

KEY POINT 7-33 Adversity to the sulfonamides probably reflects their metabolism to toxic or allergenic metabolites.

Type A (I) Adverse drug reactions. With the exception of thyroid-gland suppression, sulfonamides, and sulfadiazine in particular, appear to be free of type A or I adverse drug reactions at doses higher than those used therapeutically. For example, suppression of the thyroid gland was the only adverse effect evident in dogs treated with sulfadiazine at 300 mg/kg a day for 20 days. Any sulfonamide, including antimicrobial drugs, may profoundly alter thyroid physiology at high doses (25 mg/kg twice daily). The sulfonamide is a reversible substrate inhibitor of thyroid peroxidase, preventing the iodination and coupling of tyrosine residues necessary for formation of thryoxine and thyronine.[253] Whereas labled doses of sulfadiazine and trimethoprim do not appear to cause thyroid suppression at least for 4 weeks, clinical hypothyroidism has occurred in one dog treated with trimethoprim sulfadiazine at 48 mg/kg/day for 10 weeks. Experimentally induced suppression of thyroid hormone (T_4) synthesis occurred in 57% of dogs treated for pyoderma at 60 mg/kg/day for 6 weeks. Decreased thyroid hormone synthesis generally will be clinically relevant by 3 weeks of therapy but may take 6 to 8 weeks or longer and will return to normal within 3 weeks after therapy is discontinued.

Aplastic anemia has been reported in dogs receiving 30 to 60 mg/kg of sulfadiazine a day,[252] although the role of allergy versus folic acid deficiency was not documented. Because mammalian cells can use dietary folic acid, supplementation might be considered, particularly for patients that develop anemia (normocytic rather than megaloblastic)[252] consistent with folic acid deficiency while receiving a sulfonamide. Cats appear to be more sensitive to the effects of trimethoprim/sulfonamide combinations. Doses of 300 mg/kg per day for 10 to 30 days orally resulted in lethargy, anorexia, anemia, leukopenia, and increased blood urea nitrogen. Before the advent of triple and potentiated sulfonamide preparations, crystalluria was a common type I side effect, with subsequent renal damage. Nonetheless, with high doses of any sulfonamide product, prudence dictates that the hydration status of the animal be normal, particulary if urinary pH is acidic.

Type B (II) Adverse drug reactions. Although the sulfonamides are generally safe drugs, the advent of hypersensitivity drug reactions (immunologic) has limited their use. Immune-mediated diseases of the skin, kidney, liver, and eye are not dose dependent.

Sulfonamide antimicrobial toxicity in animals has been reviewed.[252,254] The incidence of systemic sulfonamide toxicity in dogs has been reported as 0.25%. In a study of dogs (n = 40), inclusion criteria included clinical signs consistent with a drug allergy and treatment with a sulfonamide antimicrobial for at least 5 days.[254] The breeds most often represented were Golden Retrievers, Miniature Schnauzers, German Shepherd Dogs, Labrador Retrievers, and Samoyeds, with Miniature Schnauzers and Samoyeds being overrepresented. The lack of representation by Doberman Pinschers was suggested to reflect decreased treatment of this breed with sulfonamides. Ages ranged from 6 months to 14 years (mean 5.7 ± 3.2), and neutered female dogs were overrepresented (60%). Three sulfonamides were represented, with 64% of afflicted dogs receiving sulfamethoxazole, 23% sulfadimethoxine, and 13% sulfadiazine; either trimethoprim or ormetoprim also were administered. No information was available regarding the proportion of sulfonamides prescribed to dogs. The frequency of each drug being administered was not determined. Doses ranged from 23 to 81 mg/kg/day, and time of onset ranged from 5 to 36 (mean 12) days. The most common clinical signs and the proportion of animals afflicted were fever (55%), thrombocytopenia (54%), hepatopathy (28%), neutropenia (27%), keratitis sicca (25%), and hemolysis (22%). Facial palsy was an unusual clinical sign. Other clinical signs included arthropathy, uveitis, skin and mucosal lesions, proteinuria, facial palsy, hypothyroidism, pancreatitis, facial edema, and pneumonitis. Dogs with hepatopathy or thrombocytopenia had a significantly lower recovery rates.[254] Dogs with hepatopathy also tended to have received the highest doses, suggesting that a toxic metabolite might be responsible and the adversity might be, in part, type A rather than type B (i.e., dose dependent and thus predictable). The fact that some animals developed adversities in as little as 5 days might also support a type A or idiosyncratic type B reaction, rather than allergy. Large breeds, with Doberman Pinschers overrepresented, appear to be at greater risk for developing arthropathy (as reviewed by Trepanier).[252]

Keratoconjunctivitis sicca is a more common side effect of sulfonamides in dogs, occurring in as many as 15% of animals receiving sulfonamides.[254] It has been reported in dogs after treatment with sulfasalazine, sulfadiazine, and sulfamethoxazole. The reaction may reflect direct cytotoxicity to the lacrimal gland rather than an allergic reaction, but nonetheless, time of onset may be months to years after therapy is initiated. Female dogs may be at greater risk. Resolution of clinical signs is more likely if the inciting drug is discontinued early; otherwise, normal function may not recur once the drug is discontinued. Prognosis is more favorable for younger dogs receiving the drug for a short period of time.

Drug Interactions

The sulfonamides have been associated with a number of drug interactions in humans.[2] Inhibition of elimination with subsequent prolonged or increased effects have been reported for oral hypoglycemic agents, dapsone when combined with trimethoprim, folate antagonists (increased risk of megaloblastic anemia), methanamine (increased risk of crystalluria), procainamide (decreased metabolism when combined with trimethoprim), and warfarin (increased anticoagulant activity with trimethoprim). In contrast, increased elimination has been reported for cyclosporine when combined with either sulfonamides or trimethoprim.[2]

Therapeutic Use

Because of the advent of resistance, the use of sulfonamides is limited to uncomplicated infections of most body systems. The concentration in urine supports the use of potentiated sulfonamides for urinary tract infections. Trimethoprim/sulfonamide combinations are indicated for treatment of infections caused by susceptible bacteria in difficult-to-penetrate tissues such as the prostate and CNS.[246] These drugs are among the drugs of choice for treating *Nocardia* and *Actinomyces* spp. Synergistic effects have been cited toward these organisms when used in combination with beta-lactam antibiotics.

DRUGS THAT TARGET RIBOSOMES (BACTERIOSTATIC)

Tetracyclines

Tetracyclines historically have been widely used, but development of resistance has largely curtailed empirical use in the last decade. However, the decline in use appears to have led to a decrease in resistance, and susceptibility increasingly is demonstrated through C&S data, potentially leading once again to more common use of these drugs.

Structure–Activity Relationship

Three naturally occurring tetracyclines are obtained from *Streptomyces*: chlortetracycline (the prototypic drug but no longer available in human-medicine preparations), oxytetracycline, and demethylchlortetracycline (see Figure 7-5). Several tetracyclines have been derived semisynthetically (tetracycline from chlortetracycline, rolitetracycline, methacycline, minocycline, doxycycline, lymecycline, and others). Elimination half-lives permit a further classification into short-acting (tetracycline, oxytetracycline, chlortetracycline), intermediate-acting (demethylchlortetracycline and methacycline), and long-acting (doxycycline and minocycline) formulations. All of the tetracycline derivatives are crystalline, yellowish, amphoteric substances that, in aqueous solution, form salts with both acids and bases. They characteristically fluoresce when exposed to ultraviolet light. The most common salt form is the hydrochloride, except for doxycycline, which also is available as doxycycline hyclate. The tetracyclines are stable as dry powders but not in aqueous solution, particularly at higher pH ranges (7-8.5). Preparations for parenteral administration must be carefully formulated, often in propylene glycol or polyvinyl pyrrolidone with additional dispersing agents, to provide stable solutions. Tetracyclines form poorly soluble chelates with bivalent and trivalent cations, particularly calcium, magnesium, aluminum, and iron. Doxycycline and minocycline exhibit the greatest liposolubility and better penetration of bacteria.

Mechanism of Action

Tetracyclines bind bacterial ribosomes and impair protein synthesis (see Figure 7-6). Bacterial ribosomal activity was described in the section on aminoglycosides. The tetracyclines bind to the 16S portion of the 30S ribosomal subunits, preventing access of the amino-acyl tRNA to the acceptor site on the mRNA ribosome complex[80] (see Figure 7-6). Because tRNA binding is prevented, amino acids cannot be added to the peptide chain, and protein synthesis is impaired. Tetracyclines are bacteriostatic in action and should not be used in the immunocompromised patient, whether disease or drug induced (i.e., glucocorticoids or anticancer drugs). Their effects are described with other bacteriostatic ribosomal inhibitors as time dependent but are probably related to AUC. The tetracyclines also inhibit matrix metalloproteinases, an action separate from their antibacterial properties.

Spectrum of Activity

Tetracyclines enter cells either through porins or active transport pumps.[80] They are considered broad spectrum (see Table 7-2), being effective against gram-positive, gram–negative, anaerobic organisms, as well as cell wall–deficient and rickettsial organisms and others. Their spectrum includes gram-negative organisms, particularly *Pasteurella* spp., and often *E. coli, Klebsiella,* and *Salmonella* spp. *P. aeruginosa* is generally not included; although susceptibility may be indicated on C&S data, caution should be exercised when selecting tetracyclines. They generally are intrinsically more effective against gram-positive organisms (see Tables 7-3 and 7-4). As such, *Staphylococcus* and *Streptococcus* spp. generally are included in the spectrum. However, the broad general use of these drugs has led to resistance by many organisms and use against gram-positive organisms should be based on C&S testing. The spectrum of action also includes *Chlamydia, Mycoplasma, Rickettsia*, and *Hemobartonella* organisms. Spirochetes (*Borrelia, Leptospirosis* spp. also are generally susceptible, and several mycobacterial organisms are susceptible. Tetracyclines target *Brucella* spp.) although in human medicine generally they are combined with rifampin or gentamicin. Tetracyclines generally are effective toward actinomycosis and are generally considered more effective than chloramphenicol.[80]

Tigecycline is a glycylcycline, a class of drugs that are synthetic analogs of the tetracyclines. Specifically, it is a glycolamide derivative of minocycline. The spectrum of this class is similar to that of the tetracyclines; however, they often remain effective against strains that have developed resistance to tetracyclines through increased efflux transport mechanisms.[80]

Resistance

Resistance to tetracyclines is plasmid mediated and inducible.[80] Most resistance to tetracyclines results from either decreased influx or increased transport of the drug out of the microbial cell. Other mechanisms include altered binding site (which may reflect a mutation) and enzymatic destruction. Cross-resistance does not necessarily occur and depends on the mechanism. Drugs that minimize the impact of efflux pumps have been developed, including the glycylcyclines.[255] These drugs also have a higher binding affinity than tetracyclines.

Pharmacokinetics

The oral absorption of tetracyclines is variable, with chlortetracycline being the least bioavailable, oxytetracycline more so, and doxycycline the most lipid soluble of the tetracyclines, being 100% bioavailable. Absorption is decreased in the presence of divalent and trivalent cations such as those present in milk products or antacids; exceptions occur for doxycycline and minocycline. Tetracyclines, particularly doxycycline, are widely distributed to most body tissues, and theoretically, inflammation need not be present for distribution into the brain[80] (see Table 7-5). Drugs will distribute through the placenta into the fetus and into milk. Doxycycline is able to penetrate cell membranes and thus gain access to intracellular organisms. Doxycycline is 99% protein bound, which prolongs its elimination half-life; note that concentrations in body fluids (see Table 7-5) are likely to reflect unbound drug, whereas that in plasma may reflect bound drug, decreasing ratios. Tetracyclines, with the exception of lipophilic tetracyclines such as minocycline and doxycycline, do not penetrate the CSF. The latter drugs are thus preferred because of better tissue penetrability for treatment of infections caused by susceptible bacteria in difficult-to-penetrate tissues, reaching 30% to 40% of plasma concentrations. Minocycline is characterized by a larger Vd in people than is doxycycline, suggesting the potential of better tissue penetrability, but may also be more bound to bone or other tissues containing cations. Tetracyclines accumulate in reticuloendothelial cells.[80] Tetracyclines are incorporated into forming bone and the enamel and dentin of teeth and cause discoloration of teeth upon eruption. The age at which this occurs in dogs and cats is not clear.

KEY POINT 7-34 Among the tetracyclines, doxycycline and minoclycline stand out for their lipid solubility and biliary excretion.

Doxycycline (PC 0.68 and pKa 3.09)[57] was studied in the dog in both plasma and interstitial fluid (using ultrafiltration) after intravenous and constant-rate influsion (to allow establishment of steady-state concentrations). The drug is 91% bound to plasma proteins in dogs, resulting in a total AUC difference sixfold higher in plasma compared with interstitial fluid. Further, the interstitial fluid C_{max} (of unbound drug) was only 0.14 μg/mL at steady-state conditions; in contrast, PDCs extrapolated from the terminal component of the elimination curve was 1.6 μg/mL. The concentration of interstitial fluid drug was equivalent to the concentration of unbound drug in plasma.[57] Vd of unbound drug was 0.65 ± 0.08 L/kg; clearance was 1.66 ± 2.21 mL*kg/min.

With the exception of doxycycline and minocycline, the tetracyclines are eliminated by both renal (approximately 60%) and biliary (40%) excretion. Presumably, minocycline is eliminated essentially in the bile, whereas the route of elimination of doxycycline is less obvious. In humans it is eliminated by both renal (41%) and biliary (59%) mechanisms. In dogs intestinal elimination of the unchanged drug appears to be the predominant route, with only about 16% of a given dose being excreted unchanged in the urine. Tetracyclines undergo enterohepatic circulation. Toxic concentrations may accumulate in patients with renal disease. Differences that justify use of minocycline instead of doxycycline are difficult to ascertain. Adverse reactions to minocycline may, however, be more likely.

The tetracyclines are available as intravenous, parenteral, and ocular preparations. Tetracyclines should not be given intramuscularly because of local tissue damage and irritation. For the same reason, tetracyclines are not indicated for topical treatment other than the eye.

Adverse Effects

Tetracyclines cause several adverse effects in small animals. Toxicity may be worsened in patients with renal disease because of decreased elimination. Gastrointestinal upset follows direct irritation of the gastrointestinal mucosa after oral administration; administration of doxycycline with food will reduce gastrointestinal side effects. Rarely, hepatotoxicity may occur. Rapid intravenous administration may result in collapse. Although the likelihood of this occurring in small animals is not clear, prudence dictates slow administration of a diluted solution (i.e., 1:10) when tetracyclines are administered intravenously. Although the mechanism is not certain, calcium binding may be important. Intravenous administration of tetracycline has caused anaphylactic shock in dogs. Diluting fluids should not contain calcium or other cations to which tetracylines might chelate. Hypersensitivity has also been reported in a dog after intramuscular administration of tetracycline. Minocycline may be more likely to cause allergic drug reactions in drugs. Lesions characterized by erythema of the skin and mucous membranes occurred in dogs after administration of most doses of minocycline. Anemia may also occur (10 mg/kg, administered intravenously). Brown to gray discoloration of teeth may occur because of chelation of tetracyclines in calcium deposits of dentin and, to a lesser degree, enamel. Tetracycline and oxytetracycline cause a yellow discoloration, whereas chlortetracycline produces a gray-brown discoloration; of all the tetracyclines, oxytetracycline causes the least tooth discoloration. Because chelation might occur in forming dentin as well as enamel, tetracyclines should be avoided from 3 weeks' gestation to at least 1 month after birth. Among the lipid-soluble tetracyclines, doxycycline may be less likely to cause discoloration. In humans minocycline may stain teeth regardless of tooth development because of chelation with iron; the drug probably has not been used sufficiently in animals to determine whether a similar effect will occur. Other side effects caused by tetracyclines include drug fever (in cats), an antianabolic effect, and a Fanconi-like syndrome in the kidneys, with the latter more likely with expired or degraded tetracyclines.[255]

Doxycycline has been associated with esophageal erosions in cats (and humans).[80] In a study of 30 cats, no orally administered tablets had passed in 30 seconds; only 40% had entered in 5 minutes. In contrast, 90% of tablets passed within 30 seconds when followed with 6 mL of water, with 100% passage at 90 seconds. For capsules only 17% had passed by 30 seconds, but 93% had passed by 60 seconds.[256] The impact of esophageal damage is not unique to doxycline; other drugs are ulcerogenic because of local effects. Indeed, the cat has been used as a model to assess the ulcerogenic potential of orally administered drugs.[257] For doxycycline, the risk may be decreased with use of the monohydrate salt. In the event that erosions do occur, among the treatments to consider would be pentoxifylline.[258]

KEY POINT 7-35 Doxycycline is only one of many drugs that might cause esophagitis in the cat.

Drug Interactions

Because of chelation with cations (magnesium, calcium, aluminum, and so on), tetracyclines should not be simultaneously administered with cation-containing drugs (e.g., antacids, sucralfate, buffered aspirin, calcium-containing supplements, fluids). Cholestyramine may also bind to tetracyclines. Tetracyclines, with the exception of doxycycline, should not be administered with food.

Because tetracyclines bind to the 30s ribosomal subunit, combination with antimicrobials that target the 50s subunit might be considered (e.g., the phenicols, macrolides, and lincosamides) with scientific support. One study indicates an in vitro synergistic effect of the combined use of doxycycline and azithtromycin against *P. aeruginosa*.[259]

Therapeutic Use

The therapeutic indications for tetracyclines are many but have decreased in recent years because of the advent of resistance. Treatment of microbial infections is best based on C&S data. Doxycycline is the preferred tetracycline because of its ability to move intracellularly compared to other tetracyclines. Doxycycline generally is indicated among first-choice therapies for obligate intracellular organisms, including ehrlichiosis, Rocky Mountain spotted fever, chlamydiosis, mycoplasmosis, and hemobartenellosis. Doxycycline also has been used to treat canine brucellosis. Other potential indications include leptospirosis and Lyme disease.

Phenicols

Chloramphenicol has been widely used in the past, but the development of resistance and human toxicity to chloramphenicol have severely curtailed its use and commercial availability. Florfenicol is a commercially available thiamphenicol derivative approved for treatment of bovine respiratory diseases complex. A sulfonyl group replaces the aromatic ring nitro group that is otherwise associated with chloramphenicol's irreversible bone marrow suppression in humans (see Figure 7-5). As chloramphenicol increasingly is difficult to obtain commercially, florfenicol may find a niche for use in small animals, particularly cats, in which the disposition is more predictable than with dogs.

Mechanism of Action

Like tetracyclines, chloramphenicol and florfenicol bind bacterial ribosomes and impair protein synthesis (see Figure 7-6). However, binding occurs at the 50s subunit with inhibition of peptidyl transferase. Actions are bacteriostatic in action, and these drugs should not be used in immunocompromised patients. As with other bacteriostatic ribosomal inhibitors, the effects of chloramphenicol and florfenicol should be considered time dependent. As with tetracyclines, although host ribosomes do not bind as effectively as do bacterial ribosomes, some host ribosomal activity will be impaired. Binding sites for chloramphenicol are close to those for clindamycin, which it competitively inhibits.[80] Chloramphenicol also inhibits mitochondrial protein synthesis in mammalian cells, with erythropoietic cells particularly sensitive.

Spectrum of Activity

Chloramphenicol is considered broad spectrum (see Table 7-1), being effective against gram-positive, gram-negative, and anaerobic organisms. *P. aeruginosa* is generally not included. The spectrum of action also includes *Chlamydia, Mycoplasma, Rickettsia*, and *Hemobartonella* organisms. As previously noted, tetracyclines are considered more effective than chloramphenicol for the latter organisms, but chloramphenicol tends to be more clinically effective for other organisms. The spectrum of activity of florfenicol is similar to chloramphenicol; although the anaerobic spectrum has not been described, it is assumed to be similar. The MIC for florfenicol of small animals generally reflects 1.0 to 8.0 μg/mL.

Resistance

Resistance to chloramphenicol is caused by destruction (acetylation) of the drug by microbial enzymes. The fluorine ring of florfenicol may impair bacterial acetylation, and thus florfenicol is more resistant to bacterial deactivation;[260] selected organisms resistant to chloramphenicol may be susceptible to florfenicol.[2]

Pharmacokinetics

Chloramphenicol is very well absorbed after oral administration in its crystalline form. Many of the originally-approved preparations are no longer available in the United States. The liquid form is less well absorbed, so much so that the palmitate form should not be used for cats because of variability in oral absorption. The chloramphenicol succinate ester is the water-soluble form intended for injection (see Table 7-1). The succinate must be hydrolyzed by plasma, hepatic, pulmonary, or renal esterases before activity. Chloramphenicol palmitate is a suspension for oral administration. Its ester is hydrolyzed by small intestinal lipases; the freed chloramphenicol is then orally absorbed. The freed chloramphenicol is among the most lipid soluble of the clinically used drugs and achieves moderate to high concentrations in most body tissues, including the CSF. It is, however, unlikely to achieve bactericidal concentrations in most tissues, including the CNS. Most of the drug is eliminated by hepatic metabolism. Glucuronidation is a major route of elimination of chloramphenicol. Cats eliminate chloramphenicol more slowly because of deficiencies in both phase I and phase II metabolism. Greater concentrations may occur in cat urine than in dog urine as a result.[261] Pediatric patients also may not eliminate chloramphenicol as efficiently as young adult dogs.

KEY POINT 7-36 Although chloramphenicol is bacteriostatic, its excellent tissue distribution and relatively long half-life render it potential appealing choice in immunocompromised patients.

Chloramphenicol was studied after single oral dose as the commercially available Chloromycetin (50 mg/kg) in dogs.[262] Although pharmacokinetics were not reported, the C_{max} (μg/mL) at T_{max} were, respectively, for Greyhounds with feeding, 21.6 ± 4.8 at 1.5 hours, or without feeding, 18.6 ± 6.7 at 3 hours; large dogs (22-26 kg), 20.0 ± 4.8 at 1.5 hours; and small dogs (11.4 to 15.5 kg), 27.5 ± 7.0 at 3 hours. Peak concentrations were notably higher in small dogs than large dogs. Half-life in Greyhounds was 3.2 hours in fasted dogs versus 1.9 hours in fed dogs; the elimination half-life (based on noncompartmental anaylsis of published data) in large dogs was 2.3 hours compared with 3.4 hours in small dogs. Average half-life among all groups was 2.7 ± 0.7 hours; mean residence time was 4.6 ± 0.67 hours. Neither oral bioavailability nor clearance was determined.

During approval for use in humans, chloramphenicol was studied in dogs.[263] Chloramphenicol was measured on the basis of an analytic procedure that detected chloramphenicol and its metabolites; therefore the relevance of the data must be considered. Homogenate tissue concentrations were described after subcutaneous administration of 35 mg/kg for 2 dogs: at 1.5 and 3 hours, plasma concentrations were 21 and 13, respectively, yielding an elimination half-life of 2.9 hours. Concentrations in the brain and CSF at the same time were 15 and 8 μg/mL (brain) and 7 and 9 μg/mL (CSF), yielding a 3-hour plasma:tissue ratio of 0.7. A second study measured chloramphenicol using a bioassay. However, only a single dog was studied after oral administration of 150 mg/kg of the crystalline powder form. The C_{max} was 45 μg/mL at 4 hours and approximately 15 μg/mL at 8 hours, yielding a disappearance half-life of 2.5 hours. This should extrapolate to a C_{max} of approximately 14 μg/mL when 50 mg/kg is administered. Although 54% of the drug was eliminated in the urine, only 6.3% of the drug in the urine was pharmacologically active. Intravenous administration of 50 mg/kg yielded an initial plasma concentration of approximately 39 μg/mL and a concentration of approximately 5 μg/mL at 8 hours, yielding a half-life of about 1.5 hours.[263]

Chloramphenicol has been studied in cats (n = 5). Oral administration of the crystalline powder in capsules yielded C_{max} (μg/mL) of 43 to 62 at 40 mg/kg, 25 to 42 at 20 mg/kg tid, and 8 to 25 at 50 mg bid.[264] Cats were also dosed with succinate intravenously, intramuscularly, subcutaneously, or orally (crystalline powder in capsules).[265] Concentrations at 30 minutes (T_{max} for each route except oral) were, respectively (μg/mL) 19.5 ± 1.5 (intravenous), 18.6 ± 2.6 (intramuscular), 14.8 ± 2.9 (subcutaneous) and 9.8 ± 2.61 (oral) after administration of 20 mg/kg (n = 5). The mean half-life of all three routes was 4.4 ± 1.38; range was 3.3 hours for subcutaneous and 6.9 hours for intravenous. AUC for each route was similar (lowest at 55 ± 7 μg*hr/mL for intravenous, highest at 67 ± 9 for subcutaneous). Finally, the bioavailability of the palmitate salt suspension is poor in cats, particularly in the fasted state.[266] Peak concentrations of the crystalline form following 100 mg/cat was 25 ± 5 (fasted) or 31 ± 3 (fed) versus 6.5 ± 1.3 (fasted) and 16 ± 3 (fed) for the succinate form.

Florfenicol has been studied in dogs and cats.[260,267] In dogs, although predictable PDCs (1.64 μg/mL) are achieved at 20 mg/kg after intramuscular administration, concentrations are unpredictable after subcutaneous administration. The drug appears to follow a "flip-flop" model, with the elimination half-life in dogs following intramuscular administration much longer (9 hours) compared with intravenous administration (<1 hour). A second study determined the oral bioavailability and described in more detail the PK of florfenicol (based on HPLC) in dogs (n = 6) after intravenous and oral administration (20 mg/kg).[267] Florenicol clearance was 1.03 ± 0.49 l*kg/hr, and the Vd_{ss} 1.45 ± 0.82 L/kg.The elimination half life is 1.11 + 0.94 hour after intravenous and 1.24 ± 0.64 after oral administration. Oral bioavailability was 95 ± 11%, with C_{max} reaching 6.18 μg/mL at a T_{max} of 0.94 hour. Florfenicol amine is a major metabolite of florfenicol, with a longer half-life in dogs (2.26 hours), but it has only 1/90 the activity of the parent compound, and its contribution to microbiological activity is considered negligible. Dogs showed no evidence of side effects after either intravenous or oral administration. The disposition of florfenicol by the intramuscular route appears to be more predicatable in cats than dogs, with C_{max} (22 mg/kg) reaching 20 μg/mL after IM administration and 27 μg/mL after oral administration (see Table 7-1).[267] Oral administration was based on a solution of 100 mg/mL. The elimination half-life was 8 hours in cats after oral administration, supporting a 12-hour dosing interval. The distribution volume in cats is supportive of a lipid-soluble drug. Adverse reactions were not noted in the six cats studied.

Adverse Effects

A major toxic concern with chloramphenicol for humans is both reversible dose-dependent and irreversible dose-independent (rare) bone marrow suppression. Reversible bone marrow suppression can also occur in animals. Dose-dependent bone marrow effects may reflect suppression of bone marrow precursor cells after mitochondrial damage. Irreversible bone marrow suppression may reflect reduction of the NO_2 group to a toxic metabolite that causes stem cell damage. Irreversible suppression should be avoided with florfenicol, which lacks the NO_2 group. Although cats appear more sensitive to chloramphenicol-induced reversible bone marrow suppression than do dogs, toxicosis appears rapidly reversible once the drug is discontinued. Toxicity to chloramphenicol occurs in cats after 7 days of therapy at 50 mg/kg, administered intramuscularly. The drug can, however, be used for 7 to 10 days safely in cats after oral administration of the crystalline form (capsules) at the rate of 50 mg/cat.[265,266] The antianabolic effects of chloramphenicol may result in impaired protein synthesis in the patient; however, despite earlier concerns, impaired immune response to vaccines does not appear to occur.

KEY POINT 7-37 Irreversible bone marrow suppression has resulted in limited availability of chloramphenicol products.

Drug Interactions

Because they compete for the same ribosomal binding site, chloramphenicol should not be used in combination with macrolides. Because they target two different ribosomal sites, the combination of chloramphenicol with tetracyclines is appealing. Interestingly, the combined use of chloramphenicol with penicillins has been demonstrated to enhance penicillin (bacteriostatic) activity in Enterobacteraceae that are otherwise resistant to penicillins because of beta-lactamase production. Chloramphenicol inhibits product of beta-lactamases in these organisms.[267a] Chloramphenicol is a potent inhibitor of drug-metabolizing enzymes and inhibits the hepatic metabolism of other drugs, potentially causing toxicity should drug concentrations increase. Prolonged sleeping times have been documented after administration of pentobarbital to dogs and cats also receiving chloramphenicol;[268] chloramphenicol has markedly prolonged phenytoin half-life[269] and phenobarbital half-life (see Chapter 2) in dogs. Phenobarbital-induced sedation and ataxia have occurred in as few as 3 days of chloramphenicol therapy. Chloramphenicol decreases the rate of elimination of digoxin.[270]

KEY POINT 7-38 Chloramphenicol is a potent inhibitor of drug-metabolizing enzymes.

Therapeutic Use

Chloramphenicol has been commercially available as a palmitate (oral) salt and a sodium succinate injectable preparation. Florfenicol is commercially available only as solution intended for (intramuscular) injection, which has been studied in dogs and cats.

Lincosamides: Lincomycin and Clindamycin

The lincosamides, including lincomycin and its congener, clindamycin, are large glycosidic antimicrobials that contain an amino side chain (see Figure 7-5). They are often used in humans as penicillin substitutes to minimize the risk of penicillin hypersensitivity. The lincosamides inhibit the 50s subunit of the bacterial ribosomes but at a site distinct from that bound by the macrolides or chloramphenicol (see Figure 7-6). Peptidyl transferase is subsequently inhibited. Efficacy is reduced when the lincosamides are used concurrently with macrolides. The ribosomal action of the lincosamides results in a bacteriostatic action against susceptible organisms at recommended doses. Clindamycin is generally bacteriostatic but can be bactericidal at concentrations that can be achieved in some tissues. As with other bacteriostatic drugs, the lincosamides are classified as time dependent, implying that plasma or tissue drug concentrations should exceed the MIC of the infecting organism for the majority of the dosing interval; efficacy also may be related to the AUC/MIC.

The spectrum of the lincosamides varies with the drug. Clindamycin is more effective against susceptible bacteria compared with lincomycin and also has greater activity toward anaerobes. The spectrum of clindamycin includes aerobic gram-positive cocci, including *Staphylococcus* and *Streptococcus* spp. as well as *Nocardia* spp. and anaerobic organisms including *B. fragilis, Fusobacterium* spp., *Clostridium perfringens, Peptostreptococcus,* and *Actinomyces* spp. Clindamycin also is effective against cell wall–deficient organisms such as *Mycoplasma* spp. Plasmid-mediated resistance reflects changes in the ribosomes and appears to be increasing against *Staphylococcus* spp. and *Bacteroides* spp. Resistance to one lincosamide generally results in resistance to others. Occasionally, resistance to macrolides may confer resistance to clindamycin if the mechanism reflects methylation of the ribosome.[80] Clindamycin is not a substrate for the macrolide efflux pump.

Because of its anaerobic and gram-positive spectrum, clindamycin often is chosen as one component of combination antimicrobial therapy. This combination also has been used to target *P. aeruginosa*; although generally ineffective as a sole agent, clindamycin may alter adherence of the microbe to epithelial cells, facilitating killing by the alternative drug.

Pharmacokinetics

Only oral preparations of clindamycin are approved in the dog and cat; an injectable preparation is approved for use in humans. Both clindamycin and lincomycin are bioavailable after oral administration, although clindamycin is more so. Food does not impair the absorption of clindamycin but does appear to impair absorption of lincomycin. Clindamycin is available as the hydrochloride, palmitate, or phosphate salts. The palmitate form is an oral prodrug, with the ester being rapidly hydrolyzed to yield free drug. The phosphate form is intended for parenteral administration, including subcutaneous, intramuscular (although it is painful), and intravenous routes. In the cat administration of 5.5 and 11 mg/kg orally generates serum concentrations above the MIC of most *S. pseudintermedius* organisms and previously *S. aureus,* but it is likely that resistance has resulted in less favorable PDI. Higher doses (11 to 20 mg/kg) will generate concentrations above the MIC of most susceptible anaerobes (see Table 7-1). In dogs oral administration of 11 mg/kg every 12 hours has been sufficient for treatment of most *Staphylococcus* spp. infections, but current MIC_{90} for clindamycin and susceptible *Staphyloccocus* spp. have not been reported. As a time-dependent drug, decreasing the interval to 8 to 6 hours may increase efficacy. Clindamycin is highly (>90%) protein bound. Distribution of the lincosamides includes most body tissues, with excellent concentrations being achieved in the skin and bones. However, it does not substantially penetrate the brain or CSF, although it can achieve concentrations effective for toxoplasmosis.[80] Its Vd in both dogs and cats approximates 1.5 L/kg. Clindamycin has been cited for its efficacy in the treatment of chronic gingivitis or periodontal disease. Unlike many other drugs with a favorable spectrum, it is able to penetrate the biofilm that protects the causative organisms. Accumulation of clindamycin in white blood cells up to fortyfold or more may increase the probability of reaching bactericidal concentrations at some sites of infection. The lincosamides are eliminated primarily by biliary excretion.

After administration of 10 mg/kg intravenously, intramuscularly, and subcutaneously in dogs, in addition to C_{max} and elimination half-life (see Table 7-1), the following were achieved: T_{max} occurred at 73 ± 16 min (intramuscular) or 47 ± 20 min (subcutaneous) and CL (mL/min/kg) 6.1 ± 1.1. The elimination half-life may vary with the route (see Table 7-2), as does mean residence time at 143 ± 34, (intravenous), 700 ± 246 (intramuscular), or 364 ± 147 (subcutaneous) minutes. Bioavailability was 115% after intramuscular and 310% after subcutaneous administration. The long half-life coupled with the highest C_{max} suggests that the subcutaneous route of administration is the preferred parenteral route for clindamycin.[272] The reason for the very high bioavailability after subcutaneous administration is not clear, although enterohepatic circulation is anticipated to increase bioavailability regardless of route of administration.

Clindamycin disposition has been reported in cats after oral administration of either a capsule or aqueous solution (see Table 7-1). [271] Peak PDCs are equivalent for both preparations, but a longer half-life for the capsule may contribute to a (not statistically significant) greater AUC for the capsule (42.6 ± 12.2) compared with the solution (35 ± 9.2). The lack of statistical difference may reflect the marked variability in half-life mean residence time for both preparations, which was approximately 6.5 hours.

Adverse Reactions, Drug Interactions, and Indications

Pseudomembranous colitis is a reported side effect in humans caused by overgrowth of *C. difficile*. The negative impact on the intestinal microbiota may persist for more than 2 weeks.[80] Because of similar mechanisms of action, this drug should not be combined with chloramphenicol or erythromycin. It has been combined with aminoglycoside treatment of polymicrobial infections involving gram-negative and anaerobic organisms. The use of clindamycin as combination antimicrobial therapy was addressed in the preceding section. Because of its ability to impair pili formation and thus adherance to tracheal epithelium, clindamycin has been associated with treatment of cystic fibrsosis associated with *P. aeruginosa* in humans, generally in association with antipseudomonadal antimicrobials.[273] However, the macrolides are more generally accepted for this use. The use of clindamycin as part of combination chemotherapy targeting protozoal disease (toxoplasmosis) is addressed in Chapter 12).

Macrolides and Azalides

Structure–Activity Relationship

The macrolides are named for their chemical structure, composed of a very large lactone (MW >750 to >1000) ring attached to a number of sugars.[274] They include the azalides, which contain a nitrogen in the ring structure (see Figure 7-13). No macrolide derivative is approved for use in dogs or cats at the time of this publication. Human-medicine drugs include the14-member rings erythromycin and clarithromycin and the 15-member ring azithromycin (an azalide semisynthetic derivative of erythromycin), spiramycin, and dirithromycin (a prodrug converted to the active erythromycylamine). The methyl group that distinguishes clarithromycin from erythromycin and the additional methyl group on azithromycin increases acid stability and enhances tissue distribution. Telithromycin is a ketolide macrolide (discussed later). Tylosin, a drug approved for use in food animals, is used to treat intestinal disorders, largely in dogs. Of the human drugs, erythromycin (first-generation), azithromycin, and to a lesser extent, clarithromycin (second-generation) are used in dogs and cats.[274] Tilmicosin is approved for use in selected food animals, but toxicity precludes its use in the injectable form in dogs and cats; information is not available regarding safety of other preparations. The second-generation macrolides differ from erythromycin only by the addition of a methyl group substitution. However, this simple change improves acid stability and tissue penetration. Further, because the methyl group enhances interaction with bacterial ribosomes, the spectrum also is improved.[274]

KEY POINT 7-39 Efficacy of the very lipid-soluble macrolides and clindamycin is facilitated further by accumulation in phagocytic white blood cells.

Mechanism of Action

Macrolides inhibit bacterial ribosomal action by binding to the 50s subunit of susceptible organisms (see Figure 7-6), and impairing the translocation step of protein synthesis. The azalides macrolides bind the ribosome at two sites.[275] Although macrolides are classified as bacteriostatic in vitro, they are bactericidal against very susceptible organisms. Further, selected drugs (e.g., azithromycin) accumulate in selected tissues at bactericidal concentrations. All macrolides generally accumulate in phagocytic white blood cells, which may facilitate distribution to the site of infection. Efficacy is enhanced in an alkaline pH, probably because of increased diffusion of the nonionized drug into organisms; as such, intracellular activity may be decreased in phagocytic cells. The antibacterial effects of the macrolides vary with the drug and are time dependent for erythromycin; antibacterial effects for azithromycin and clarithromycin are time dependent for some organisms and concentration dependent for others.

Spectrum of Activity

Like the lincosamides, the macrolides are often used in humans as penicillin substitutes to minimize the risk of penicillin hypersensitivity. Organisms are considered susceptible to the macrolides at an MIC below 2 μg/mL. For the first-generation drugs, gram-positive organisms accumulate erythromycin at concentrations that exceed that of gram-negative organisms by a hundredfold. As such, erythromycin is most effective against gram-positive organisms. *Streptococcus* spp. are susceptible at a range of 0.015 to 1 μg/mL, although resistance is increasing. Many *Staphyloccocus* organisms have remained susceptible to erythromycin, but MIC ranges of 0.12 to > 128 μg/mL for *S. aureus* indicate an increasing trend of resistance. Among the staphyloccoci, *S. pseudintermedius* remains the most susceptible. *P. multocida, Bordetella pertussis,* and *Mycoplasma* spp. are among the organisms susceptible to erythromycin. However, use should be based on C&S testing. Erythromycin generally is effective against anaerobic organisms, with the exception of *Bacterioides* spp. Macrolides are generally effective against *Campylobacter* spp.

The azolides were designed to overcome barriers presented to penetration of gram-negative organisms. Thus the spectrum of azithromycin and clarithromycin increases, particularly in terms of gram-negative bacteria, although efficacy toward selected gram-positive microbes may decrease, requiring higher MIC.[275] The actions of the azolides are bactericidal for *Streptococcus pyogenes* and *S. pneumoniae* but bacteriostatic toward staphylococci and most aerobic gram-negative organisms. Clarithromycin is effective at lower concentrations than erythromycin against *Streptococcus* and *Staphyloccus* spp. but is similar to erythromycin in efficacy against other organisms. Azithromycin has less activity against gram-positive organisms compared with erythromycin and greater activity against selected gram-negative organisms and *Mycoplasma* spp.[80] Although the spectrum of the macrolides generally includes *Actinomyces* spp., efficacy is generally less for *Nocardia* spp. Clarithromycin and azithromycin are effective against the *Mycobacterium avium* complex, *Mycobacterium leprae,* and *Toxoplasma gondii.* Compared to erythromycin, azithromycin and clarithromycin have enhanced activity against selected protozoa (e.g., *T. gondii, Cryptosporidium* spp.).

Controversy surrounds the classification of macrolides as either concentration or time dependent. The macrolides do exhibit a postantibiotic effect, with that of clarithromycin and azithromycin being longer than that of erythromycin. Azithromycin appears to be bacteriostatic against *Staphylococcus* or *Streptococcus* spp.; in vitro killing did not increase in a dose-dependent manner, suggesting that the drug is a time-dependent antimicrobial.[276]

Resistance

Acquired mechanisms of resistance to macrolides include pump-driven drug efflux from the cell (particularly in staphylococci, group A streptococci, and *S. pneumoniae*) and altered ribosomal targets (methylase enyzme; MLSB phenotype) that also confer resistance to lincosamides, which bind at the same ribosomal site. Efflux pumps contribute to resistance in *E. coli* as well.[179] Chromosomal mutations in *Bacillus subtilis, Campylobacter* spp., and gram-positive cocci alter the ribosomal binding site. Resistance of *S. aureus* to erythromycin generally is indicative of resistance to azithromycin and clarithromycin as well. The Enterobacteriaceae produce an esterase that hydrolyses the drug.

Pharmacokinetics

The macrolides and azolides are largely water insoluble and are unstable in the acidic gastric environment.[274] However, each of the macrolides is available as an oral preparation. Erythromycin also is available as a topical and ophthalmic preparation. Erythromycin base preparations generally are coated to prevent gastric degradation. Oral absorption of enteric-coated or delayed-release products designed for humans may be unpredicatable in animals.[2] Oral salts include the estolate and ethylsuccinate salts, which must be de-esterified after oral absorption, and the stearate (octadecanoate) and phosphate salts. The former (and possibly the latter) dissociate in the duodenum to be absorbed as the free base. The disposition of selected erythromycin salts has been described in dogs.[277]

After oral administration, the erythromycin base is incompletely but adequately absorbed. Food may increase acidity and thus delay absorption. Esters (stearate, estolate, ethylsuccinate) improve stability and absorption but do not appear to increase PDCs. Among the salts, estolate appears to be best absorbed orally and minimally affected by food. For the azolides, clarithromycin is characterized by greater acid stability compared with erythromycin. Clarithromycin is more rapidly absorbed (in humans), but food delays absorption and first-pass metabolism (to an active metabolite) further reduces oral bioavailability of the parent compound to 50%. Azithromycin also is absorbed rapidly, but, again, food decreases bioavailability to 43% (in humans). Erythromycin is approximately 75% protein bound; binding is as high as 96% (in humans) for the estolate salt. Protein binding for clarithromycin is concentration dependent and ranges from 40% to 70%. Despite their large moleculer size, macrolides are sufficiently lipid soluble that they diffuse through membranes, albeit slowly. With a Vd of 2 L/kg in dogs, erythromycin will reach effective concentrations in all tissues except the brain and CSF. In general, the macrolides act as weak bases and, as such, trapped in an acidic environment, including acidic intracellular organelles. Consequently, tissue concentrations will exceed plasma in many tissues. Although accumulation occurs in selected tissues (e.g., bile, bronchial secretions, phagocytic white blood cells), concentrations reach only 50% of plasma in the prostate and aqueous humor and less than 15% in the CSF. Concentrations in the middle ear will approximate 50% of those in plasma. Clarithromycin and its active metabolite are well distributed, achieving higher concentrations than erythromycin in both the middle ear and CNS. Among the macrolides, azithromycin distributes the most extensively, with a Vd that exceeds (in humans) 30 L/kg. Fibroblasts act as a reservoir, with transfer to phagocytic cells. Whereas erythromycin and azithyromycin are eliminated principally in the bile, clarithromycin is extensively metabolized to an active (14 hydroxy derivative) metabolite. Excretion is primarily by biliary secretion into the feces; enterohepatic circulation of active drug might be anticipated. Urine excretion is not significant (3% to 5%), with concentrations in urine being low (approximately 50% of plasma); an exception is clarithromycin, for which the active metabolite might achieve high concentrations in urine. The elimination half-life for azithromycin has been reported at 1 to 1.5 hours in dogs[279, 280] and cats.

The disposition of erythromycin as the estolate tablet and ethylsuccinate suspension and tablet has recently been described in dogs.[277] Intravenous administration revealed a Vd of 4.8 L/kg (see Table 7-1) and a clearance of 2.64 ± 0.84 L/hr/kg. Oral absorption of all three products was poor: the ethylsuccinate tablets did not yield predictably detectable concentrations, whereas, based on mean AUC adjusted for differences in dose, the bioavailability of the estolate tablet was only 11% (T_{max} 1.7 hr) and the ethylsuccinate suspension only 3% (T_{max}, 0.7 hr). Absorption of the suspension, in particular, was described by the authors as erratic. Peak concentrations did not reach MIC_{90} for susceptible *Staphylococcus* spp. of 0.5 μg/mL (reported by the authors) for any of the oral preparations. The apparent efficacy of erythromycin, despite poor absorption, may reflect accumulation of drug in tissues such that higher concentrations are achieved at the site of infection.[277] All dogs vomited after dosing, regardless of route of administration, with vomiting apparent 5 to 10 minutes after intravenous administration, approximately 45 minutes after oral succinate preparations, and 1 to 2 hours after the estolate tablet administration.

Limited information is available for the second-generation macrolides in animals. Azithromycin and clarithromycin absorption is influenced by uptake transporters in the intestinal epithelium. Whereas efflux transporters, such as P-glycoprotein, decrease absorption, others (organic anion-transporting proteins) facilitate uptake.[278] Azithromycin has been studied in cats and dogs (see Table 7-1).[279, 280] Bioavailability in the dog is greater than 97%. Serum protein binding is less than 25%.

Clearance is 6.0 mL*min/kg. In dogs 67% of the drug is eliminated in the bile and 33% in the urine.[279] The majority of the drug (75%) is eliminated unchanged. The remaining portion is metabolized by cytochrome P450s into a number of metabolites, which, with one exception, are inactive. Tissue concentrations (based on homogenate) at 24 hours after 20 mg/kg orally were over 101, 20, and 39 μg/mL, respectively, for liver, kidney, and lungs. After 5 days of dosing, 23 μg/mL was achieved 24 hours after the last dose in the eye but only 1.2 μg/mL in the brain (at 30 mg/kg for 5 days). In cats the maximum drug concentration (C_{max}) of 0.97 ± 0.65 μg/mL occurs at T_{max} of 0.85 ± 0.72 hr. Plasma concentrations (μg/mL) range from approximately 8 at 1 hour to 0.1 at 12 hours after intravenous administration of 5 mg/kg and approximately 1 μg/mL to 0.1 μg/mL during the same times after oral administration of 5 mg/kg. Although the elimination half-life is long, concentrations in plasma are below 0.1 μg/mL after 12 hours. However, concentrations of azithromycin approximate 0.75 to 1 μg/mL in the femur, skin, and muscle versus 10 μg/mL in tissues characterized by reticuloendothelial cells (liver, spleen, and to a lesser degree lung) and the kidney with concentrations persisting for 72 hours or more. Because tissue concentrations were based on homogenate, it is not clear how much drug is available to interstitial fluid. Clearance is 0.64 ± 0.24 L*hr/kg. Oral bioavailability is 52 ± 22%. The elimination half-life is 35 (range 29 to 51 hours).[280] The Clinical Laboratory and Standards Institute susceptible breakpoint for azithromycin (human pathogens) is 4 μg/mL. Because concentrations decline to less than 0.1 μg/mL by 12 hours, daily dosing should be considered in both cats and dogs; because time to steady state will approximate 3 to 5 days, a 15 mg/kg loading dose should be considered followed by once-daily dosing at a minimum of 5 mg/kg. Although cats do metabolize azithromycin, the unchanged drug is the predominant form in tissues. Biliary excretion is a major route of clearance in the cat.[280] Kinetics of clarithromycin become zero order (saturated) at higher doses. The large Vd of the macrolides contributes to their long elimination half-life. The half-life in cats exceeds 72 hours in some tissues.[280] In contrast to azithromycin, urinary concentrations of clarithromycin can be signifcant: up to 40% of the parent drug or its metabolite are eliminated in the urine. The mean half-life in plasma is 35 hours but varies in tissues from a low of 13 hours (fat) to a high of 72 hours (cardiac muscle).

Adverse Effects

Side effects of the macrolides are limited. With injectable products, pain may occur with intramuscular injection and thrombophlebitis with intravenous injection. Reversible cholestatic hepatitis accompanied by jaundice has been reported in humans 10 to 20 days into erythromycin therapy, especially with the estolate preparation.

Gastrointestinal upset is the most common adverse effect of the macrolides. Up to 50% of animals treated with erythromycin may exhibit vomiting. Erythromicin is motilin-like in action and characterized by marked prokinetic effects on gastrointestinal motility. This effect is dose dependent in humans and may occur more commonly in younger animals. Abdominal cramping, epigastric pain, and increased gastric emptying resulting from increased gastric motility also may occur. However, because contraction is not coordinated, efficacy as a prokinetic is limited. Gastric emptying may decrease gastric maceration of ingested food, although the impact on digestion is not likely to be significant. Azithromycin and clarithromycin do not appear to have the same gastrointestinal side effects of erythromycin. In humans allergic reactions occur rarely and are manifested as fever or skin eruptions, which resolve once therapy is discontinued. Cholestatic hepatitis is an infrequent side effect in humans.

Drug Interactions

Antacids decrease the rate (and thus peak) but not extent of absorption of azithromycin, whereas food decreases the extent by close to 50%. The macrolides may inhibit cytochrome P450 enzymes, and CYP 3A4 in particular, impairing the metabolism of other drugs.[280a] Among the macrolides, erythromycin followed by clarithromycin is most likely to be involved in significant drug interactions, although all three drugs inhibit drug-metabolizing enzymes. The effects of drugs metabolized by the liver, including selected anticonvulsants, cardiac drugs, and theophylline, are likely to increase. Drugs affected in humans include glucocorticoids, digoxin, theophylline, and warfarin. The macrolide antimicrobials (clarithromycin, roxithromycin) also increase the risk of digoxin toxicity, although this effect may be more reflective of competitive interactions with P-glycoprotein transport proteins.[281] Azithromycin is a substrate; others may be as well.[282] Among the P-glycoprotein interactions with azithromycin in cats is cyclosporine; peak cyclosporine concentrations exceeded 4500 ng/mL in a cat receiving 5 mg/kg while being treated with azithromycin.

Because they are ribosomal inhibitors, care must be taken not to combine the macrolides with drugs whose efficacy requires rapid bacterial growth, unless scientific support exists, or "-cidal" concentrations of the macrolide are achieved at the target site for both drugs. For example, synergistic effects have been documented against *B. fragilis* when erythromycin is combined with cefamandole and against *Nocardia asteroides* when combined with ampicillin. The use of erythromycin in combination with other antimicrobials is limited in small animals. Erythromycin has been used in combination with rifampin to treat *Rhodococcus equi* in horses; a similar application has not been identified in dogs or cats. Synergistic antimicrobial actions also have been reported against *P. aeruginosa* for either azithromycin or clarithromycin when combined with sulfadiazine/trimethoprim or doxycycline. In humans azithromycin has been combined with antipseudomonadal drugs, particularly for treatment of cystic fibrosis–associated *P. aeruginosa* infections. This may reflect an apparent immunomodulatory effect of azithromycin or its ability to inhibit adherence of pseudomonad organisms to respiratory epithelium. Less commonly, synergism has been demonstrated for azithromycin when combined with ticarcillin/clavulanic acid, piperacillin/tazobactam, ceftazidime, meropenem, imipenem, ciprofloxacin, travofloxacin, chloramphenicol, or tobramycin.[259]

Although not included in their spectrum, the macrolides, like clindamycin, impair the ability of *P. aeruginosa* to adhere to tracheal epithelium, the first step in respiratory tract infection. The effect occurs at least at subinhibitory concentrations and reflects decreased ability to form pili.[273] Decreased adherence to human mucins also has been demonstrated for azithromycin.[283] Other proposed effects of azithromycin include decreased alginate formation and decreased biofilm. Azithromycin has been demonstrated to impede, but not prevent, biofilm formation by *Pseudomonas* spp.[284] These attributes have led to its long-term use for treatment of cystic fibrosis in humans, generally in association with some level of antipseudomonadal antimicrobials. Antiinflammatory effects have also been attributed to azithromycin's apparent long-term efficacy for treatment of cystic fibrosis.[285,286]

Tylosin

Tylosin is a classified as a macrolide, but it is structurally somewhat different from erythromycin, leading to differences in its mechanism and spectrum. Like erythromycin, it targets the 50s ribosomal subunit, but with different sequelae. It is stable in the gastric environment and does not require enteric coating for oral administration. Like erythromycin, tylosin is distributed well to most body tissues and is eliminated by hepatic metabolism and biliary excretion. Approved for use in the United States for treatment of swine dysentery and other large animal syndromes, tylosin also has been used in small animals to treat infections of the gastrointestinal tract (associated with chronic inflammatory bowel disease) and bacterial pyodermas. Its spectrum is not clear but includes selected gram-positive and gram-negative organisms.

Ketolides

Like the azolides, the ketolides are semisynthetic modifications of erythromycin designed to minimize barriers to penetration in gram-negative organisms.[275] Telithromycin is the first ketolide approved for clinical use in humans; the drug was developed specifically for treatment of upper and lower respiratory tract infections caused by organisms resistant to the macrolides.[287] Like the macrolides and azalides, the ketolides are well distributed into tissues, with concentrations being maintained in humans sufficiently long to allow a 24-dosing interval. Thus far, the ketolides have not been used or studied in veterinary medicine, perhaps because azithromycin currently meets the needs of infections that might otherwise be treated with ketolides.

MISCELLANEOUS ANTIMICROBIALS

Oxazolidinones

Oxazolidinones are a new group of synthetic antimicrobials effective against gram-positive bacteria, including methicillin- and vancomycin-resistant staphylococci, vancomycin-resistant enterococci, penicillin-resistant pneumococci, and anaerobes.[288] Linezolid is the first of this class of drugs to be approved for use in the United States (see Figure 7-4). Oxazolidinones inhibit the initiation of protein synthesis by binding at the P site of 50S ribosomal subunit; it also binds to the 70S subunit. Oxazolidinones compete with chloramphenicol and lincomycin for binding of the 50S subunit, which indicates that they have close binding sites, even though oxazolidinones do not inhibit peptidyl transferase as do chloramphenicol and lincomycin. Oxazolidinones may inhibit formation of the ribosomal initiation complex, similar to aminoglycosides. The mechanism is sufficiently different from other 50S binders that resistance to other protein synthesis inhibitors does not cross over to the oxazolidinones. Efficacy against *Staphylococcus* spp. is characterized by an MIC_{90} between 1 and 4 μg/mL in humans; methicillin resistance does not appear to affect susceptibility. Linezolid also is effective against enterococci; even intermediate isolates appear to be susceptible at 1 μg/mL.[288] Streptococci also are susceptible. Anaerobic activity is comparable to clindamycin.[289] Linezolid is effective toward atypical mycobacterium[290] and both *Actinomyces* and *Nocardia* sp. Activity toward *S. pneumoniae* is generally bactericidal but bacteriostatic against staphylococci and enterococci. [291, 292] Antibacterial effects appear to be time dependent, with efficacy related to AUC/MIC. Resistance thus far is rare.

Disposition includes good oral absorption and good tissue penetration. Linezolid accumulates in bone, lung, vegetations, hematoma, and CSF. Concentrations in sanctuaries are lower than those in plasma.[293] Linezolid has been approved by the FDA for treatment in humans of complicated skin infections or nosocomial pneumonia caused by MRSA, concurrent bacteremia associated with either vancomycin-resistant *E. faecium* or CA pneumonia caused by penicillin-resistant *S. pneumoniae*.[288] It has become the drug of choice for treatment of resistant gram-positive infections. The oxazolidinones have been minimally used in dogs and cats, and their use is discouraged unless warranted on the basis of C&S testing and until kinetic studies are available in the target species (e.g., cats).

Linezolid PK has been described in the dog after oral and intravenous administration (see Table 7-1).[293] Oral absorption is rapid and complete, allowing intravenous and oral dosing to be the same. The drug is minimally protein bound. Clearance is 2.0 ± 0.3 mL*min/kg. The drug appears to undergo limited metabolism to inactive metabolites that are extensively enterohepatic recycled. Renal excretion occurs for parent compounds and metabolites. In humans renal disease causes accumulation of metabolites that may contribute to adverse effects.[294]

Linezolide appears to be well tolerated in humans. Myelosuppression has occurred in humans. Additionally, it is an inhibitor of monoamine oxidases, and care should be taken in patients also receiving serotonergic or adrenergic drugs or dietary supplements. Peripheral neuropathies have been associated with long-term use. Drug interactions involving cytochrome P450 do not appear to occur. Linezolide inhibits mitochondrial protein synthesis, causing hyperlactatemia in humans.[294] Linezolid may decrease intracellular movement of aminoglycosides, affecting rapid killing. [94] Based on in vitro killing curve studies, linezolid efficacy against MRSA was enhanced most by rifampin, compared with vancomycin or gentamicin; indeed, efficacy of the latter was reduced by linezolid, with activity antagonistic toward gentamicin.

MISCELLANEOUS ANTIBIOTICS

Daptomycin. Daptomycin is a lipopeptide derived from *Streptomyces* that was discovered several decades ago but has been reconsidered for treatment of vancomycin-resistant gram-positive organisms. Its spectrum includes gram-positive and anaerobic microbes. However, its mechanism involves binding to the cell membrane, and although bactericidal, daptomycin is associated with an increased risk of toxicity. It acts in a concentration-dependent fashion.[80] Vancomycin-resistant drugs require higher concentrations. Daptomycin is minimally orally bioavailable, requiring intravenous administration for systemic effects. It cannot be given intramuscularly because of direct toxicity. It is not involved in any clinically relevant drug interactions. Although largely renally excreted, it is approximately 92% bound to plasma proteins in humans. The result is a longer half-life that allows once-daily dosing in humans. Daptomycin causes skeletal muscle damage in dogs at doses that exceed 10 mg/kg and peripheral neuropoathies at higher doses.[80] Dispostion has been described for Beagles after once- and twice-daily dosing.[295] When given at 5, 25, or 75 mg/kg intravenously, peak serum concentrations were 58, 165, and 540 μg/mL, respectively (total drug); concentrations extrapolated from the terminal component of the curve approximated

30, 100, and 300 μg/mL, respectively. The elimination half-life appeared to be between 2 and 3 hours, which may indicate that the drug is not as highly protein bound in dogs compared with people. All doses caused skeletal muscle damage, as indicated by serum creatine phosphokinase; damage, however, was worse with 8-hour administration of 25 mg/kg than with once-daily administration of 75 mg/kg.[295]

Fusidic Acid. Fusidic acid is a steroidlike antimicrobial that interferes with ribosomal translocation (peptidyl tRNA). Efficacy is limited to gram-positive bacteria. It is bactericidal at high concentrations against both coagulase-positive and coagulase-negative staphylococci. It is available as oral, intravenous, topical, and ocular preparations. In humans it is characterized by 90% oral bioavailability. Adverse reactions include granulocytopenia, rash, and hepatotoxicity; thrombophlebitis; and venospasm, which may accompany intravenous infusion. Resistance develops rapidly when used as a sole agent. Drugs with which it has been combined include the aminoglycosides, quinolones, rifampin, and vancomycin. However, combination therapy has not precluded development of MRSA.

Topical Antimicrobials

The advantage of topical antimicrobials is achievement of very high concentrations at the site of infection and avoidance of side effects that otherwise might occur with systemic therapy.

Bacitracin

Bacitracin is a complex polypeptide isolated from *B. subtilis*. It inhibits peptidoglycan synthesis in bacteria by interfering with the enzyme responsible for movement of cell components through the membrane. Its spectrum of activity includes gram-positive and very few gram-negative organisms. Systemic use causes nephrotoxicity, and use is limited to topical administration. The drug is not absorbed after oral administration and can be used to treat gastrointestinal infections caused by susceptible organisms.[5,297]

Polymyxins

Polymyxins are a group of large acetylated decapeptides produced by *Bacillus* spp. At least six compounds have been identified, of which only two, polymyxin (polymyxin B) and colistin (polymyxin E), are used clinically. Polymyxins are cationic detergents that interact and interfere with the phospholipid of the bacterial cell membrane, resulting in increased permeability. The polymyxins are thus bactericidal. However, a number of compounds can interfere with their activity, including divalent cations, purulent exudate, fatty acids, and quaternary ammonium compounds. The spectrum of activity of the polymyxins includes most gram-negative organisms, including *P. aeruginosa*. Two exceptions include *Proteus* spp. and most *Serratia* spp. The drugs are weak bases (pK_a 8 to 9) and are not orally bioavailable. As such, they have been used to "sterilize" the gastrointestinal tract.

Elimination is principally by way of the kidneys, which are also the primary sites of toxicity. Glomerular and tubular epithelial damage has limited their usefulness. Other side effects include respiratory paralysis (after rapid intravenous administration), CNS dysfunction, fever, and anorexia. Use of the polymyxins is primarily limited to topical administration. However, pemphigus vulgaris has been reported in association with topical use for otitis externa in the dog.[296] Polymyxin protects against gram-negative endotoxemia by binding to the anionic lipid component of the lipopolysaccharide at concentrations much lower than those associated with toxicity. Relevance to treatment in dogs or cats is not established.

Novobiocin

Novobiocin is derived from coumarin and is effective against both gram-positive and gram-negative organisms. The drug is particularly efficacious against *Staphylococcus* spp. Its mechanism of action is not certain but involves both cell membrane and cell wall synthesis. Novobiocin causes a number of toxic effects when used systemically, including bone marrow suppression, nausea, vomiting, and diarrhea. Its use is limited to topical application.[5,297]

Mupirocin

Mupirocin (pseudomonic acid) is a naturally occurring fermentation product of *Pseudomonas fluorescens*. It is available as a cream or ointment, and its use has been largely limited to topical application. Although it acts to inhibit protein synthesis, its mechanism is novel in that it prevents incorporation of isoleucine into proteins by binding to isoleucyl transfer-RNA synthetase.[297] Its unique mechanism precludes cross-resistance with other antibacterials. Resistance is unusual, low level, and generally overcome by higher concentrations. The spectrum of mupirocin includes aerobic gram-positive cocci (high efficacy toward *S. aureus*, *S. epidermidis*, and beta-hemolytic streptococci) and selected gram-negative cocci. An advantage to mucopirin is that it minimally affects normal flora. Its indications in human medicine include prophylaxis in ulcers, operative wounds, and burns and treatment of skin infections. In humans mupirocin has proved efficacious as an oral antibiotic. In addition, mupirocin has proven useful in the management of secondary pyodermas or superinfection of chronic dermatoses. Mupirocin is generally not associated with side effects; local burning, stinging, itching, or pain has been reported in about 1% of human patients.[297]

Silver Sulfadiazine

Silver sulfadiazine (see the discussion of sulfonamides) is approved for use in humans in a polypropylene glycol vehicle and in a water-soluble gel. It is approved for use in dogs combined with enrofloxacin as an otic preparation. The synergistic coupling of the silver with sulfadiazine results in efficacy against *P. aeruginosa* as well as a broad range of gram-positive and other gram-negative organisms. The silver component interferes with the cell wall. Silver sulfadiazine has been approved for use in the treatment of human burn patients, but other antimicrobials have proved more efficacious (e.g., iodophors; combinations of povidone iodine with neomycin, polymyxin, and bacitracin [Neosporin]; and silver sulfadiazine–cerium nitrate cream). However, the low toxicity, low hypersensitivity, and low level of resistance warrants its continued use in veterinary patients.[297]

Urinary Antiomicrobials

Nitrofurans. The nitrofurans are synthetic compounds whose antimicrobial activity occurs through the 5-nitrofuran group (see Figure 7-12).[5,297] Nitrofurantoin and furazolidone are examples. They are weak acids. These drugs block oxidative reactions necessary for formation of bacterial acetyl coenzyme A. They are bacteriostatic in action. The spectrum of activity of nitrofurantoin includes a number of gram-positive or gram-negative organisms, but its use should be based on C and S testing. The spectrum also includes selected protozoa. Nitrofurans are orally bioavailable but require an acidic environment to cross cell membranes. Use is limited to urinary tract infections, and ideally those associated with an acidic pH. Because 50% of nitrofurantoin is eliminated in urine in an active form, the drug is appropriate for treatment of urinary tract infections. Its use is, however, limited by gastrointestinal and systemic toxicity. Systemic toxicities in humans include peripheral neuropathy at therapeutic doses. The time to onset ranges from 3 weeks to over 12 months (median: 2 to 3 months). Although not common, peripheral neuropathy can be both severe and irreversible. Old age and renal disease increased the risk of toxicity.[271] Albeit rare, pulmonary pneumonitis and fibrosis have been associated with long-term (6 months or more) use in humans and may be insidious in onset. The use of nitrofurantoin is limited to infections of the urinary tract that are not susceptible to other drugs. However, a current advantage to this drug is limited resistance among those organisms considered susceptible, including *E. coli* and selected other organisms.

Methenamine. Methenamine (hexamine; hexamethylenetetramine is the name for commercial uses) is a chemical that releases formaldehyde and ammonia on hydrolysis (see Figure 7-12). It is usually sold as the hippurate salt. The degree of hydrolysis, and thus antibacterial efficacy, is pH dependent, requiring an acidic pH. The drug is bactericidal in an acid environment and bacteriostatic in a more alkaline environment. Therefore it is less effective in the presence of urease-producing bacteria that alkalinize the urine. Its spectrum of activity includes both gram-positive and gram-negative organisms. Methenamine is orally bioavailable and reaches high concentrations in urine.[220] The chemical is used primarily to treat urinary tract infections in dogs. Generally, it is used in combination with urinary acidifiers to enhance antibacterial actions. Its safety in cats could not be verified.

REFERENCES

1. Albarellos GA, Landoni MF: Current concepts on the use of antimicrobials in cats, *Vet J* 180(3) (Jun): 304–316, 2009.
2. United States Pharmacopeia (USP) Antibiotic Monographs, *J Vet Pharmacol Ther* 26(Suppl 2), 2003.
3. Mattoes HM, Kim M-K Kuti JL, et al: Clinical advantage of continuous infusion β-lactams, *Serious Hospital Infections* 13(3): 1–8, 2001.
4. Rice LB: Genetic and biochemical mechanisms of bacterial resistance to antimicrobial agents. In Lorian V, editor: *Antibiotics in laboratory medicine*, Baltimore, 2005, Williams & Wilkins, pp 441–508.
5. Neu HC: Principles of antimicrobial use. In Brody TM, Larner J, Minneman KP, et al, editors: *Human pharmacology: molecular to clinical*, St Louis, 1994, Mosby, pp 616–701.
6. Kapusnik J, Miller RT, Sande MA: Antibacterial therapy in critical care. In Schoemaker WC, Ayers S, Grenvik A, et al, editors: *Textbook of critical care*, ed 2, Philadelphia, 1989, Saunders, pp 780–801.
7. Bush LM, Calmon J, Johnson C: Newer penicillins and lactamase inhibitors, *Infect Dis Clin North Am* 3:571–594, 1989.
8. Donowitz GR: Third generation cephalosporins, *Infect Dis Clin North Am* 3:595–612, 1989.
9. Vaden S, Riviere J: Penicillins. In Adams R, editor: *Veterinary pharmacology and therapeutics*, ed 8, Ames, Iowa, 2001, Iowa State University Press, pp 818–827.
10. Williams JD, Naber KG, Bryskier A, et al: Classification of oral cephalosporins. A matter for debate, *Inter J Antimicro Agents* 17:443–450, 2001.
11. Caprile KA: The cephalosporin antimicrobial agents: a comprehensive review, *J Vet Pharmacol Ther* 11:1–32, 1988.
12. Bramhill D: Bacterial cell division, *Annu Rev Cell Dev Biol* 13:395–424, 1997.
13. Anonymous: Antimicrobial treatment guidelines for acute bacterial rhinosinusitis, *Arch Otolaryngol Head Neck Surg* 130:S1–S45, 2004.
14. Chambers H: Penicillin-binding protein - mediated resistance in pneumococci and staphylococci, *J Infect Dis* 179(Suppl 2): S353–S359, 1999.
15. Bywater RJ, Palmer GH, Buswell JF, et al: Clavulanate-potentiated amoxycillin: activity in vitro and bioavailability in the dog, *Vet Rec* 116(2):33–36, 1985.
16. Brown SA: Treatment of gram-negative infections, *Vet Clin North Am* 18:1141–1166, 1988.
17. Papich M: Treatment of gram-positive bacterial infections, *Vet Clin North Am* 18:1267–1286, 1988.
18. Sobel JD: Imipenem and aztreonam, *Infect Dis Clin North Am* 3:613–624, 1989.
19. Yigit H, Queenan AM, Anderson GJ, et al: Novel carbapenem-hydrolyzing β-lactamase, KPC-1, from a carbapenem-resistant strain of *Klebsiella pneumoniae*, *Antimicrob Agents Chemother* 45(4):1151–1161, 2001.

19a. Human Drug Product Not Equivalent to Veterinary Ceftiofur; CVM Update, July 1997. Accessed June 2010, at http://www.fda.gov/AnimalVeterinary/NewsEvents/CVMUpdates/ucm127855.

20. Stegemann MR, Passmore CA, Sherington J, et al: Antimicrobial activity and spectrum of cefovecin, a new extended-spectrum cephalosporin, against pathogens collected from dogs and cats in Europe and North American, *Antimicrob Agents Chemother* 50(7):2286–2292, 2006.
21. Lowy FD: Antimicrobial resistance: the example of *Staphylococcus aureus*, *J Clin Invest* 111:1265–1273, 2003.
22. Helfand MS, Bonomo RA: β-Lactamases: a survey of protein diversity, *Curr Drug Targets Infect Disord* 3:9–23, 2003.
23. Li XZ, Mehrotra M, Ghimire S, et al: Beta-lactam resistance and beta-lactamases in bacteria of animal origin, *Vet Microbiol 15* 121(3-4):197–214, 2007.
24. Rodriguez-Banõ J, Navarro MD, Romero L, et al: Clinical and molecular epidemiology of extended-spectrum β-lactamase-producing *Escherichia coli* as a cause of nosocomial infection or colonization: implications for control, *Clin Infect Dis* 42:37–45, 2006.
25. Dancer SJ: The problem with cephalosporins, *J Antimicro Chemother* 48:463–478, 2001.
26. Vree TB, Dammers E, van Duuren E: Variable absorption of clavulanic acid after an oral dose of 25 mg/kg of Clavubactin and Synulox in healthy dogs, *J Vet Pharmacol Therap* 26:165–171, 2003.

27. Malik S, Christensen H, Peng H, et al: Presence and diversity of the β-lactamase gene in cat and dog staphylococci, *Vet Microbiol* 123:162–168, 2007.
28. Chaudhary U, Aggarwal R: Extended spectrum -lactamases (ESBL): an emerging threat to clinical therapeutics, *Indian J Med Microbiol* 22(2):75–80, 2004.
29. Jacoby GA, Medeiros AA, O'Brien TF, et al: Broad-spectrum, transmissible beta-lactamases, *N Engl J Med* 319:723–724, 1988.
30. Jacoby GA, Medeiros AA: More extended-spectrum beta-lactamases, *Antimicrob Agents Chemother* 35:1697–1704, 1991.
31. Jacoby GA: Extended-spectrum beta-lactamases and other enzymes providing resistance to oxyimino-beta-lactams, *Infect Dis Clin North Am* 11:875–887, 1997.
32. Decre D, Gachot B, Lucet JC, et al: Clinical and bacteriologic spectrum of extended-spectrum beta-lactamase-producing strains of *Klebsiella pneumoniae* in a medical intensive care unit, *Clin Infect Dis* 27:834–844, 1998.
33. Sturenburg E, Mack D: Extended-spectrum beta-lactamases: implications for the clinical microbiology laboratory, therapy, and infection control, *J Infect Dis* 47:273–295, 2003.
34. Lee N, Yuen KY, Kumana CR: Clinical role of beta-lactam/beta-lactamase inhibitor combinations, *Drugs* 63(14):1511–1524, 2003.
35. Antonio O, Weigel LM, Rasheed K, et al: Mechanisms of decreased susceptibility to cefpodoxime in, *Escherichia coli, Antimicrob Agents Chemother* 46(12):3829–3836, 2002.
36. Tenover FC, Raney PM, Williams PP: Confirmation methods for *Escherichia coli* with isolates the flqA locus and genetic evidence that Topoisomerase IV is the primary target and DNA gyrase is the secondary target. The Fluoroquinolone Toxicity Research Foundation, Collected during Project ICARE, *J Clin Microbiol* 41:3142–3146, 2003.
37. Queenan AM, Bush K: Carbapenemases: the versatile β-lactamases, *Clin Microbiol Rev* 20(3):440–458, 2007.
38. Devriese LA, Hermans K, Baele M, et al: *Staphylococcus pseudintermedius* versus *Staphylococcus intermedius, Vet Microbiol* 133(1-2):206–207, 2009.
39. Leonard FC, Markey BK: Methicillin-resistant *Staphylococcus aureus* in animals: a review, *Vet J* 75:27–36, 2008.
40. Kania SA, Williamson NL, Frank LA: Methicillin resistance of staphyloccci isolated from the skin of dogs with pyoderma, *J Am Vet Med Assoc* 65:1268–1285, 2004.
40a. Faires MC, Tater KC, Weese JS: An investigation of methicillin-resistant *Staphylococcus aureus* colonization in people and pets in the same household with an infected person or infected pet, *J Am Vet Med Assoc* 235(5):540–543, 2009.
41. Gortel K, Campbell KL, Kakoma I, et al: Methicillin resistance among staphylococci isolated from dogs, *Am J Vet Res* 60(12):1526–1530, 1999.
42. Weese JS, van Duijkeren E: Methicillin-resistant *Staphylococcus aureus* and *Staphylococcus pseudintermedius* in veterinary medicine, *Vet Microbiol* Jan 27: 140(3-4):418–429, 2010.
43. Walther B, Wieler LH, Friedrich AW, et al: Methicillin-resistant *Staphylococcus aureus* (MRSA) isolated from small and exotic animals at a university hospital during routine microbiological examinations, *Vet Microbiol* Feb 5: 127(1-2):171–178, 2008.
44. Strommenger B, Kehrenberg C, Kettlitz C, et al: Molecular characterization of methicillin-resistant *Staphylococcus aureus* strains from pet animals and their relationship to human isolates, *J Antimicrob Chemother* 57:461–465, 2006.
45. Devriese LA, Hermans K, Baele M, et al: *Staphylococcus pseudintermedius* versus *Staphylococcus intermedius, Vet Microbiol* 133(1-2):206–207, 2009.
46. Ruscher C, Lubke-Becker A, Wleklinski C-G, et al: Prevalence of methicillin-resistant *Staphylococcus pseudintermedius* isolated from clinical samples of companion animals and equidaes, *Vet Microbiol* Apr 14: 136(1-2):197–201, 2009.
47. El Zubeir IEM, Kanbar T, Alber J, et al: Phenotypic and genotypic characteristics of methicillin/oxacillin-resistant *Staphylococcus intermedius* isolated from clinical specimens during routine veterinary microbiological examinations, *Vet Microbiol* 121:170–176, 2007.
48. Pottumarthy S, Schapiro JM, Prentice JL, et al: Clinical isolates of *Staphylococcus intermedius* masquerading as methicillin-resistant *Staphylococcus aureus, J Clin Microbiol* 42(12):5881–5884, 2004.
49. Guardabassi L, Loeber ME, Jacobson A: Transmission of multiple antimicrobial-resistant *Staphylococcus intermedius* between dogs affected by deep pyoderma and their owners, *Vet Microbiol* 98:23–27, 2004.
49a. Methicillin-resistant *Staphylococcus Aureus*. Accessed January 1, 2010, at http://www.avma.org/reference/backgrounders/mrsa_bgnd.asp
50. Braga PC: Antibiotic penetrability into bronchial mucus: pharmacokinetic and clinical considerations, *Curr Ther Res* 49(2):300–327, 1989.
51. Bergogne-Bérézin E: Pharmacokinetics of antibiotics in respiratory secretions. In Pennington JE, editor: *Respiratory infections: diagnosis and management*, ed 2, New York, 1988, Raven Press, pp 608–631.
52. Bergan T: Pharmacokientics of tissue penetration of antibiotics, *Rev Infect Dis* 3:45–66, 1981.
53. Bolton GC, Allen GD, Filer CW: Absorption, metabolism and excretion studies on clavulanic acid in the rat and dog, *Xenobiotica* 14(6):483–490, 1984.
54. Brown SA: Pfizer Animal Health, personal communication.
55. Garg RC, Keefe TJ, Vig MM: Serum levels and pharmacokinetics of ticarcillin and clavulanic acid in dog following parenteral administration of Timentin, *J Vet Pharmacol Ther* 10(4):324–330, 1987.
56. Barker CW, Zhang W, Sanchez S, et al: Pharmacokinetics of imipenem in dogs, *Am J Vet Res* 64:694–699, 2003.
57. Bidgood TL, Papich MG: Comparison of plasma and interstitial fluid concentrations of doxycycline and meropenem following constant rate intravenous infusion in dogs, *Am J Vet Res* 64:1040–1046, 2003.
58. Bidgood T, Papich MG: Plasma pharmacokinetics and tissue fluid concentrations of meropenem after intravenous and subcutaneous administration in dogs, *Am J Vet Res* 63:1622–1628, 2002.
59. Krueger WA, Neeser G, Schuster H, et al: Correlation of meropenem plasma levels with pharmacodynamic requirements in critically ill patients receiving continuous veno-venous hemofiltration, *Chemotherapy* 49(6):280–286, 2003.
59a. Papich MG, Davis JL, Floerchinger AM, et al: Cefpodoxime and cephalexin plasma pharmacokinetics, protein binding, and tissue distribution after oral administration to dogs. Accepted, *Am J Vet Res*, 2010 in press.
60. Carli S, Anfossi P, Villa R, et al: Absorption kinetics and bioavailability of cephalexin in the dog after oral and intramuscular administration, *J Vet Pharmacol Ther* 22:308–313, 1999.
61. Prados AP, Ambros L, Montoya L, et al: Chronopharmacological study of cephalexin in dogs, *Chronobiol Int* 24(1):161–170, 2007.
62. Campbell BG, Rosin E: Effect of food on absorption of cefadroxil and cephalothin in dogs, *J Vet Pharmacol Ther* 21:418–420, 1998.
63. Richardson DC, Aucoin DP, DeYoung DJ, et al: Pharmacokinetic disposition of cefazolin in serum and tissue during canine total hip replacement, *Vet Surg* 21(1):1–4, 1992.
64. Marcellin-Little DJ, Papich MG, Richardson DC, et al: Pharmacokinetic model for cefazolin distribution during total hip arthroplasty in dogs, *Am J Vet Res* 57(5):720–723, 1996.
64a. WHO Food Additives Series: 49 Toxicological evaluation of certain veterinary drug residues in food. Accessed June 2010, at http://www.inchem.org/documents/jecfa/jecmono/v49je04.htm).

65. Jung H-H, Mischkowsky T: Measurements of cefuroxime concentration in bone in dogs and man, *Arch Orthop Trauma Surg* 94:25–28, 1979.
66. Spurling NW, Harcourt RA, Hyde JJ: An evaluation of the safety of cefuroxime axetil during six months oral administration to beagle dogs, *J Toxicol Sci* 11:237–277, 1986.
67. Sakamoto H, Hirose T, Mine Y: Pharmacokinetics of FK027 in rats and dogs, *J Antibot* 38(4):496–504, 1985.
68. Rebuelto M, Albarellos G, Ambros L: Pharmacokinetics of Ceftriaxone administered by the intravenous, intramuscular or subcutaneous routes to dogs, *Vet Pharm Therap* 25:73–76, 2002.
69. Moore KW, Trepanier LA, Lautzenhiser SJ, et al: Pharmaocinetics of ceftazidime in dogs following subcutanoeus administration and continuous infusion and the association with in vitro susceptibility of *Pseudomonas aeruginosa*, *Am J Vet Res* 61:1204–1208, 2000.
70. Albarellos GA, Ambros LA, Landoni MF: Pharmacokinetics of ceftazidime after intravenous and intramuscular administration to domestic cats, *Veterinary Journal* 178:238–243, 2008.
71. Brown SA, Arnold TS, Hamlow PJ, et al: Plasma and urine disposition and dose proportionality of ceftiofur and metabolites in dogs after subcutaneous administration of ceftiofur sodium, *J Vet Pharmacol Ther* 18(5):363–369, 1995.
72. Stegemann MR, Sherington J, Blanchflower S: Pharmacokinetics and pharmacodynamics of cefovecin in dogs, *J Vet Pharmacol Therap* 29:501–511, 2006.
73. Stegemann MR, Sherington J, Coati N, et al: Pharmacokinetics of cefovecin in cats, *J Vet Pharmacol Therap* 29:513–524, 2006.
73a. Harmoinen J, Mentula S, Heikkilä M, et al: Orally administered targeted recombinant beta-lactamase prevents ampicillin-induced selective pressure on the gut microbiota: a novel approach to reducing antimicrobial resistance, *Antimicrob Agents Chemother* 48:75–79, 2004.
74. Trautmann M, Zick R, Rukavina T, et al: Antibiotic-induced release of endotoxin: in-vitro comparison of meropenem and other antibiotics, *J Antimicrob Chemother* 41(2):163–169, 1998.
75. Kumar GAV, Kothari VM, Kirsihman A, et al: Benzathine penicillin, metronidazole and benzyl penicillin in the treatment of tetanus: a randomized, controlled trial, *Ann Trop Med Parasitol* 98:59–63, 2004.
76. Semel JD, Allen N: Seizures in patients simultaneously receiving theophylline and imipenem or ciprofloxacin or metronidazole, *South Med J* 84:465–468, 1991.
77. Rees CA, Boothe DM: Evaluation of the effect of cephalexin and enrofloxacin on clinical laboratory measurements of urine glucose in dogs, *J Am Vet Med Assoc* 224(9):1455–1458, 2004.
78. Ingerman MJ, Santoro J: Vancomycin: a new old agent, *Infect Dis Clin North Am* 3:641–652, 1989.
79. Walsh TR, Howe RA: The prevalence and mechanisms of vancomycin resistance in *Staphylococcus aureus*, *Annu Rev Microbiol* 56:657–675, 2002.
80. Chambers HF: Protein synthesis inhibitors and miscellaneous antibacterial agents. In Brunton LL, Lazo JS, Parker KL, editors: *Goodman & Gilman's the pharmacological basis of therapeutics*, ed 11. Accessed January 2009, at http://www.accessmedicine.com/content.aspx?aID=949328.
81. Fillgrove KL, Pakhomova S, Schaab MR, et al: Structure and mechanism of the genomically encoded fosfomycin resistance protein, FosX, from *Listeria monocytogenes*, *Biochemistry* 46:8110–8120, 2007.
82. Marchese A, Bozzolasco M, Gualco L, et al: Effect of fosfomycin alone and in combination with N-acetylcysteine on *E. coli* biofilms, *Int J Antimicrob Agents* 22(Suppl 2):95–100, 2003.
83. Marchese A, Gualco L, Debbia EA, et al: In vitro activity of fosfomycin against gram-negative urinary pathogens and the biological cost of fosfomycin resistance, *Int J Antimicrob Agents* 22(Suppl 2):53–59, 2003.
84. Sauermann R, Marsik C, Steiner I, et al: Immunomodulatory effects of fosfomycin in experimental human endotoxemia, *Antimicrob Agents Chemother* 51(5):1879–1881, 2007.
85. Olay T, Vicente MV, Rodríguez A: Efficacy of fosfomycin + vancomycin or gentamicin in experimental endocarditis due to methicillin-resistant *Staphylococcus aureus* (MRSA), *J Chemother* 1(4 Suppl):391–392, 1989.
86. Schito GC: Why fosfomycin trometamol as first line therapy for uncomplicated UTI? *Int J Antimicrob Agents* 22(Suppl 2):79–83, 2003.
87. Sack K, Schulz E, Marre R, et al: Fosfomycin protects against tubulotoxicity induced by Cis-diaminedichloroplatin and cyclosporin A in the rat, *J Mol Med* 65(11):525–527, 1987.
88. Gutierrez OL, Ocampo CL, Aguilera JR, et al: Pharmacokinetics of disodium-fosfomycin in mongrel dogs, *Res Vet Sci* 85:156–161, 2008.
89. Kawaguchi K, Hasunuma R, Kikuchi S, et al: Time- and dose-dependent effect of fosfomycin on suppression of infection-induced endotoxin shock in mice, *Biol Pharm Bull* 25(12):1658–1661, 2002.
90. Riviere J, Spoo W: Aminoglycosides. In Adams R, editor: *Veterinary pharmacology and therapeutics*, ed 8, Ames, Iowa, 2001, Iowa State University Press, pp 828–840.
91. Bamberger DM, Foxworth JW, Bridwell DL, et al: Extravascular antimicrobial distribution and the respective blood and urine concentrations in humans. In Lorian V, editor: *Antibiotics in laboratory medicine*, Baltimore, 2005, Williams & Wilkins, pp 799–809.
92. Vakulenko SB, Mobashery S: Versatility of aminoglycosides and prospects for their future, *Clin Microbiol Rev* 16:430–450, 2003.
93. Maller R, et al: Once- versus twice-daily amikacin regimen: efficacy and safety in systemic gram-negative infections, *J Antimicrob Chemother* 31:939–948, 1993.
94. Jacqueline C, Caillon J, Le Mabecque V, et al: In vitro activity of linezolid alone and in combination with gentamicin, vancomycin or rifampicin against methicillin-resistant *Staphylococcus* aureus by time-kill curve methods, *J Antimicrob Chemother* 51(4):857–864, 2003.
95. Powell SH, Thompson WL, Luthe MA, et al: Once-daily vs. continuous aminoglycoside dosing: efficacy and toxicity in animal and clinical studies of gentamicin, netilmicin, and tobramycin, *J Infect Dis* 147:918–932, 1983.
96. Blaser J: Efficacy of once- and thrice-daily dosing of aminoglycosides in in vitro models of infection, *J Antimicrob Chemother* 27(Suppl C):21–28, 1991.
97. Reiner NE, Bloxham DD, Thompson WL: Nephrotoxicity of gentamicin and tobramycin given once daily or continuously in dogs, *J Antimicrob Chemother* 4(Suppl A):85–101, 1978.
98. Vanhaeverbeek M, Siska G, Douchamps J, et al: Comparison of the efficacy and safety of amikacin once or twice a day in the treatment of severe gram-negative infections in the elderly, *Int J Clin Pharmacol Ther* 31:153–156, 1993.
99. Blaser J, Stone BB, Zinner SH: Efficacy of intermittent versus continuous administration of netilmicin in a two-compartment in vitro model, *Antimicrob Agents Chemother* 27:343–349, 1985.
100. Roudebush P, Fales WH: Antibacterial susceptibility of gentamicin resistant organisms recovered from small companion animals, *J Am Anim Hosp Assoc* 18:649–652, 1982.
101. Asseray N, Caillon J, Roux N, et al: Different aminoglycoside-resistant phenotypes in a rabbit *Staphylococcus aureus* endocarditis infection model, *Antimicrob Agents Chemother* 46(5):1591–1593, 2002.
102. Forgan-Smith WR, McSweeney RJ: Gentamicin and amikacin—an in vitro comparison using 1000 clinical isolates, *Intern Med J* 8:383–386, 2008.
103. Barclay ML, Begg EJ: Aminoglycoside adaptive resistance: importance for effective dosage regimens, *Drugs* 61(6):713–721, 2001.

104. Mealey KL, Boothe DM: Nephrotoxicosis associated with topical administration of gentamicin in a cat, *J Am Vet Med Asso* 204:1919–1921, 1994.

104a. Kihlström E, Andåker L: Inability of gentamicin and fosfomycin to eliminate intracellular Enterobacteriaceae, *J Antimicrob Chemother* 15(6):723–728, 1985.

105. Ling GV, Conzelman GM Jr, Franti CE, et al: Urine concentrations of gentamicin, tobramycin, amikacin, and kanamycin after subcutaneous administration to healthy adult dogs, *Am J Vet Res* 42(10):1792–1794, 1981.

106. Peters AM: The kinetic basis of glomerular filtration rate measurement and new concepts of indexation to body size, *Eur J Nucl Med Mol Imaging* 31(1):137–149, 2004.

107. Riviere JE, Coppoc GL: Pharmacokinetics of gentamicin in the juvenile dog, *Am J Vet Res* 42(9):1621–1623, 1981.

108. Wilson RC, Duran SH, Horton CR Jr: Bioavailability of gentamicin in dogs after intramuscular or subcutaneous injections, *Am J Vet Res* 50(10):1748–1750, 1989.

109. Baggot JD, Ling GV, Chatfield RC: Clinical pharmacokinetics of amikacin in dogs, *Am J Vet Res* 46(8):1793–1796, 1985.

110. Wright LC, Horton CR Jr, Jernigan AD, et al: Pharmacokinetics of gentamicin after intravenous and subcutaneous injection in obese cats, *J Vet Pharmacol Ther* 14(1):96–100, 1991.

111. Jernigan AD, Hatch RC, Wilson RC: Pharmacokinetics of tobramycin in cats, *Am J Vet Res* 49(5):608–612, 1988.

112. Jernigan AD, Wilson RC, Hatch RC: Pharmacokinetics of amikacin in cats, *Am J Vet Res* 49(3):355–358, 1988.

113. Kukanich B, Coetzee JF: Comparative pharmacokinetics of amikacin in Greyhound and Beagle dogs, *J Vet Pharmacol Ther* 31:102–107, 2007.

114. Jernigan AD, Hatch RC, Wilson RC, et al: Pharmacokinetics of gentamicin in cats given Escherichia coli endotoxin, *Am J Vet Res* 49(5):603–607, 1988.

115. Jernigan AD, Hatch RC, Wilson RC, et al: Pathologic changes and tissue gentamicin concentrations after intravenous gentamicin administration in clinically normal and endotoxemic cats, *Am J Vet Res* 49(5):613–617, 1988.

116. Kim H-S, Sohn I-J, Min DI: Pharmacokinetics of amikacin and effect of ascites in Korean patients, *Am J Health-Syst Pharm* 59:1855–1857, 2002.

117. Kim M-J, Bertino JS Jr, Erb TA, et al: Application of bayes theorem to aminoglycoside-associated nephrotoxicity: comparison of extended-interval dosing, individualized pharmacokinetic monitoring, and multiple-daily dosing, *J Clin Pharmacol* 44:696–707, 2004.

118. Shy-Modjeska JS, Riviere JE, Rawlings JO: Application of biplot methods to the multivariate analysis of toxicological and pharmacokinetic data, *Toxicol Appl Pharmacol* 72(1):91–101, 1984.

119. Riviere JE, Hinsman EJ, Coppoc GL, et al: Morphological and functional aspects of experimental gentamicin nephrotoxicity in young beagles and foals, *Vet Res Commun* 7(1):211–213, 1983.

120. Isoherranen N, Lavy E, Soback S: Pharmacokinetics of gentamicin C_1, C_{1a}, and C_2 in beagles after a single intravenous dose, *Antimicrob Agents Chemother* 44(6):1443–1447, 2000.

121. Jernigan AD, Hatch RC, Brown J, et al: Pharmacokinetic and pathological evaluation of gentamicin in cats given a small intravenous dose repeatedly for five days, *Can J Vet Res* 52(2):177–180, 1988.

122. Jernigan AD, Wilson RC, Hatch RC, et al: Pharmacokinetics of gentamicin after intravenous, intramuscular, and subcutaneous administration in cats, *Am J Vet Res* Jan: 49(1):32–35, 1988.

123. Grauer GF, Greco DS, Behrend EN, et al: Estimation of quantitative enzymuria in dogs with gentamicin induced nephrotoxicosis using urine enzyme/creatinine ratios from spot urine samples, *J Vet Intern Med* 9(5):324–327, 1995.

124. Brown SA, Garry FB: Comparison of serum and renal gentamicin concentrations with fractional urinary excretion tests as indicators of nephrotoxicity, *J Vet Pharmacol Ther* 11:330–337, 1988.

125. Frazier DL, Aucoin DP, Riviere JE: Gentamicin pharmacokinetics and nephrotoxicity in naturally acquired and experimentally induced disease in dogs, *J Am Vet Med Assoc* 192:57–63, 1988.

126. Boothe DM: Adverse renal effects of selected drugs, Veterinary previews, Purina Publication for Veterinarians, *Veterinary Learning Systems* 2:10–13, 1995.

127. Hsu CH, Kurtz TW, Easterling RE, et al: Potentiation of gentamicin nephrotoxicity by metabolic acidosis, *Proc Soc Exp Biol Med* 146:894–897, 1974.

128. Julien N, Karzazi M, Labrecque G, et al: Temporal modulation of nephrotoxicity, feeding, and drinking in gentamicin-treated rats, *Physiol Behav* 68(4):533–541, 2000.

129. Prins JM, Weverling GJ, van Ketel RJ, et al: Circadian variations in serum levels and the renal toxicity of aminoglycosides in patients, *Clin Pharmacol Ther* 62:106–111, 1997.

130. Cowan RH, Jukkola AF, Arant BS: Pathophysiologic evidence of gentamicin nephrotoxicity in neonatal puppies, *Pediatr Res* 14:1204–1211, 1980.

131. Brown SA, Nelson RW, Moncrieff CS: Gentamicin pharmacokinetics in diabetic dogs, *J Vet Pharmacol Ther* 14:90–95, 1991.

132. Chambers HF: Aminoglycosides. In Brunton LL, Lazo JS, Parker KL, editors: *Goodman & Gilman's the pharmacological basis of therapeutics*, ed 11, New York, 2006, McGraw Hill.

133. Kes P, Reiner Z: Symptomatic hypomagnesemia associated with gentamicin therapy, *Magnes Trace Elem* 9(1):54–60, 1990.

134. Ozbek E, Turkoz Y, Sahna E, et al: Melatonin administration prevents the nephrotoxicity induced by gentamicin, *Br Med J (Intl Ed)* 85(6):742–746, 2000.

135. Kopple JD, Ding H, Letoha A, et al: L-carnitine ameliorates gentamicin-induced renal injury in rats, *Nephrol Dial Transplant* 17:2122–2131, 2002.

136. Mazzon E, Britti D, de Sarro A, et al: Effect of N-acetylcysteine on gentamicin-mediated nephropathy in rats, *Eur J Pharmacol* 424(1):75–83, 2001.

137. Feldman L, Efrati S, Eviatar E, et al: Gentamicin-induced ototoxicity in hemodialysis patients is ameliorated by N-acetylcysteine, *Kidney Int* 72(3):359–363, 2007.

138. Konishi H, Goto M, Nakamoto Y, et al: Tobramycin inactivation by carbenicillin, ticarcillin and piperacillin, *Antimicrob Agents Chemother* 23:654–657, 1983.

139. Uber WE, Brundage RC, White RL, et al: In vivo inactivation of tobramycin by piperacillin, *Ann Pharmacother* 25:357–359, 1991.

140. Ariano RE, Kassume DA, Meatherall RC, et al: Lack of in vitro inactivation of tobramycin by imipenem/cilastin, *Ann Pharmacother* 26:1075–1077, 1992.

140a. Atilla A, Boothe HW, Tollett M, Duran S, Campos Diaz H, Boothe DM: In vitro elution of amikacin and vancomycin from impregnated plaster of Paris beads. Accepted for publication, *Vet Surg* 39: 715–721, 2010.

141. Riviere JE, Carver MP, Coppoc GL, et al: Pharmacokinetics and comparative nephrotoxicity of fixed-dose versus fixed-interval reduction of gentamicin dosage in subtotal nephrectomized dogs, *Toxicol Appl Pharmacol* 75(3):496–509, 1984.

142. Barza M, Loannidis JPA, Cappelleri JC, et al: Single or multiple daily doses of aminoglycosides: a meta-analysis, *Br Med J* 312:338–345, 1996.

143. Bailey TC, Little JR, Littenberg B, et al: A meta-analysis of extended-interval dosing versus multiple daily dosing of aminoglycosides, *Clin Infect Dis* 24(5):786–795, 1997.

144. Ali MZ, Goetz MB: A meta-analysis of the relative efficacy and toxicity of single daily dosing versus multiple daily dosing of aminoglycosides, *Clin Infect Dis* 24(5):796–809, 1997.

145. Gilbert DN, Lee BL, Dworkin RJ, et al: A randomized comparison of the safety and efficacy of once-daily gentamicin or thrice-daily gentamicin in combination with ticarcillin-clavulanate, *Am J Med* 105(3):182–191, 1998.
146. Wallace AW, Jones M, Bertino JS: Evaluation of four once-daily aminoglycoside dosing nomograms, *Pharmacotherapy* 22(9):1077–1083, 2002.
147. Woeltje KF, Ritchie DJ: Antimicrobials. In Carey CF, Lee HH, Woeltje KF, editors: *The Washington manual of medical therapeutics*, ed 29, Philadelphia, 1998, Lippincott-Raven, pp 250–251.
148. Rougier F, Claude D, Maurin M, et al: Aminoglycoside nephrotoxicity, *Curr Drug Targets Infec Disord* 4:153–162, 2004.
149. Kingsley P, Coulthard D G, Peckham SP, Conway et al: Therapeutic drug monitoring of once daily tobramycin in cystic fibrosis—caution with trough concentrations. Accessed April 2007, at http//www.cysticfibrosismedicine.com 6(2):125–130, 2001.
150. Neu HC: The quinolones, *Infect Dis Clin North Am* 3:625–640, 1989.
151. Schmitz FJ, Higgins PG, Mayer S: Activity of quinolones against gram-positive cocci: mechanisms of drug action and bacterial resistance, *Eur J Clin Microbiol Infect Dis* 21:647–659, 2002.
152. Petri WA Jr: Chemotherapy of tuberculosis, Mycobacterium avium complex disease, and leprosy. In Brunton LL, Lazo JS, Parker KL, editors: *Goodman & Gilman's the pharmacological basis of therapeutics*, ed 11, New York, 2006, McGraw-Hill.
153. Ng EY, Truckis M, Hooper DC: Quinolone resistance mutations in topoisomerase IV: Relationship to target of fluoroquinolones in *Staphylococcus aureus*, *Antimicrob Agents Chemother* 40:1881–1888, 1996.
154. Ginsburg AS, Grosset JH, Bishai WR: Fluoroquinolones, tuberculosis and resistance, *The Lancet Infect Dis* 3:432–442, 2003.
155. Power EGM, Bellido JLM, Phillips I: Detection of ciprofloxacin resistance in gram-negative bacteria due to alterations in gyrA, *J Antimicrob Chemother* 29:9–17, 1992.
156. Prescott JF, Yielding KM: In vitro susceptibility of selected veterinary bacterial pathogens to ciprofloxacin, enrofloxacin and norfloxacin, *Can J Vet Res* 54:195–197, 1990.
157. Witte W, Grimm H: Occurrence of quinolone resistance in *Staphylococcus aureus* from nosocomial infection, *Epidemiol Infect* 109:413–421, 1992.
158. Wetzstein HG, Schmeer N: Bactericidal activity of enrofloxacin against *Escherichia coli* growing under strictly anaerobic conditions, *Proceedings of the 95th General Meeting, American Society of Microbiologists,* Washington, DC, A-37, 1995.
159. van de Hoven R, Wagenaar JA, Walker RD: In vitro activity of difloxacin against canine bacterial isolates, *J Vet Diagn Invest* 12:218–233, 2000.
160. Wetzstein HG: The in vitro postantibiotic effect of enrofloxacin, *Proc 18th World Buiatrics Congress*, Bologna, Italy 18:615–618, 1994.
161. Walker RD, Stein GE, Hauptman JG, et al: Pharmacokinetic evaluation of enrofloxacin administered orally to healthy dogs, *Am J Vet Res* 53:2315–2319, 1992.
162. McKinnon PS, Davis SL: Pharmacokinetic and pharmacodynamic issues in the treatment of bacterial infectious diseases, *Eur J Clin Microbiol Infect Dis* 23:271–288, 2004.
163. Schentag JJ, Meagher AK, Forrest A: Fluoroquinolone AUIC break points and the link to bacterial killing rates. Part 1: In vitro and animal models, *Ann Pharmacother* 37(9):1287–1298, 2003.
164. Boothe DM, Boeckh A, Slimpson RB, et al: Comparison of pharmacodynamic and pharmacokinetic indices of efficacy for 5 fluoroquinolones toward pathogens of dogs and cats, *J Vet Intern Med* 20(6):1297–13306, 2006.
165a. Shaheen BS, Nayak R, Boothe DM: Identification of novel mutations and high incidence of plasmid mediated quinolone resistance determinants among extended-spectrum cephalosporins in *Escherichia coli* isolates from companion animals in the United States, *Presented at the American Society of Microbiology Conference Antimicrobial Resistance in Zoonotic Bacteria and Foodborne Pathogens*, Toronto, June 8-11, 2010.
165. Hopkins KL, Davies RH, Threlfall EJ: Mechanisms of quinolone resistance in *Escherichia coli* and *Salmonella*: recent developments, *Int J Antimicrob Agents* 25:358–373, 2005.
166. Riddle C, Lemons CL, Papich MG, et al: Evaluation of ciprofloxcin as a representative veterinary fluoroquinolone in susceptibility testing, *J Clin Microbiol* 38(4):1636–1637, 2000.
167. Pfaller MA, Jones RN: Trends in ciprofloxacin nonsusceptibility and levofloxacin resistance among *Streptococcus pneumoniae* isolates in North America, *J Clin Microbiol* 39(7):2748–2750, 2001.
168. Breitschwerdt EB, Papich MG, Hegarty BC, et al: Efficacy of doxycycline, azithromycin, or trovafloxacin for treatment of experimental rocky mountain spotted fever in dogs, *Antimicrob Agents Chemother* 43(4):813–821, 1999.
169. Kang SL, Rybak MJ, McGrath BJ, et al: Pharmacodynamics of levofloxacin, ofloxacin, and ciprofloxacin, alone and in combination with rifampin, against methicillin-susceptible and -resistant *Staphylococcus aureus* in an in vitro infection model, *Antimicrob Agents Chemother* 38(12):2702–2709, 1994.
170. Fritsche TR, Sader HS, Jones RN: Epidemiology of antimicrobial resistance: species prevalence, susceptiblity profiles and resistance trends. In Lorian V, editor: *Antibiotics in laboratory medicine*, Baltimore, 2005, Williams & Wilkins, pp 815–850.
171. Hecht DW, Wexler HM: In vitro susceptibility of anaerobes to quinolones in the United States, *Clin Infect Dis* 23:S2–S8, 1996.
172. Drlica K, Zhao X, Blondeau JM, et al: Low correlation between MIC and mutant prevention concentration, *Antimicrob Agents Chemother* 50(1):403–404, 2006.
173. Sánchez Navarro MD, Sayalero Marinero ML, Sánchez Navarro A: Pharmacokinetic/pharmacodynamic modelling of ciprofloxacin 250 mg/12 h versus 500 mg/24 h for urinary infections, *J Antimicrob Chemother* 50:67–72, 2002.
174. Marchbanks CR, McKiel JR, Gilbert DH, et al: Dose ranging and fractionation of intravenous ciprofloxacin against *Pseudomonas aeruginosa* and *Staphylococcus aureus* in an in vitro model of infection, *Antimicrob Agents Chemother* 37:1756–1763, 1993.
175. Cole LK, Kwochka K, Kowalski J, et al: Microbial flora and antimicrobial susceptibility patterns of isolated pathogens from the horizontal ear canal and middle ear in dogs with otitis media, *J Amer Anim Hosp Assoc* 212:534–538, 1998.
176. Boothe DM, Smaha T, Carpenter M, et al: Emerging resistance in canine and feline *Escherchia coli* pathogens: a pilot surveillance study, Submitted to *J Vet Int Med*, March 2009.
177. Hooper DC: Emerging mechanisms of fluoroquinolone resistance *Emerg Infect Dis* 7(2), 2001. Accessed November 12, 2009 at www.cdc.gov/ncidod/eid/vol7no2/hooper.htm.
178. Debavalya N, Boothe DM, Hathcock T: Multi-drug resistance in fecal *Escherichia coli* following routine enrofloxacin but not amoxicillin therapy in dogs, *Am Coll Vet Int Med (Proceedings)*, 2008.
179. Shaheen BS, Boothe DM, Oyarzabal O, et al: The contribution of gyrA mutation and efflux pumps to fluoroquinolone and multi-drug resistance in canine and feline pathogenic *Escherichia coli* isolates from the US. In print, *Am J Vet Res*, 2010.
179a. Shaheen BW, Boothe DM, Oyarzabal OA, et al: Antimicrobial resistance profiles and clonal relatedness of canine and feline Escherichia coli pathogens expressing multidrug resistance in the United States, *J Vet Intern Med* Mar-Apr: 24(2):323–330, 2010.
180. Wetzstein HG: Comparative mutant prevention concentrations of pradofloxacin and other veterinary fluoroquinolones indicate differing potentials in preventing selection of resistance, *Antimicrob Agents Chemother* 49(10):4166–4173, 2005.

181. Pasquali F, Manfreda G: Mutant prevention concentration of ciprofloxacin and enrofloxacin against *Echerichia coli, Salmonella Typhimurium* and, *Pseudomonas aeruginosa, Vet Microbiol* 119:304–310, 2007.
182. Schwaber M, Cosgrove SE, Gold H: Fluoroquinolones protective against cephalosporin resistance in gram negative nosocomial pathogens, *Emerging Infectious Diseases* 10(1):94–99, 2004.
183. Karlowsky JA: Susceptibilities to levofloxacin in *Streptococcus pneumoniae, Haemophilus influenzae*, and *Moraxella catarrhalis* clinical isolates from children: results from 2000-2001 and 2001-2002 TRUST studies in the United States, *Antimicrob Agents Chemother* 47(6):1790–1797, 2003.
184. Seral C, Barcia-Macay M, Mingeot-Leclercq P, et al: Comparative activity of quinolones (ciprofloxacin, levofloxacin, moxifloxacin and garenoxacin) against extracellular and intracellular infection by *Listeria monocytogenes* and *Staphylococcus aureus* in J774 macrophages, *J Antimicrob Chemother* 55:511–517, 2005.
185. Seguin A, Papich MG, Siegle KJ, et al: Pharmacokientics of enrofloxacin in neonatal kittens, *Am J Vet Res* 65:350–356, 2004.
186. Bidgood TL, Papich MG: Plasma and interstitial fluid pharmacokinetics of enrofloxacin, its metabolite ciprofloxacin, and marbofloxacin after oral administration and a constant rate intravenous infusion in dogs, *J Vet Pharmacol Therap* 28:329–341, 2005.
187. Isaccs A, Boothe DM, Axlund T: Comparative distribution of fluorquinolons in the brain and cerebral spinal fluid of dogs, 2010 (In preparation)
188. Boothe DM, Boeckh A, Boothe HW, et al: Tissue concentrations of enrofloxacin and ciprofloxacin in anesthetized dogs following single intravenous administration, *Vet Ther* 2:120–128, 2001.
189. Frazier DL, Thompson L, Trettien A, et al: Comparison of fluoroquinolone pharmacokinetic parameters after treatment with marbofloxacin, enrofloxacin, and difloxacin in dogs, *J Vet Pharmacol Therap* 23:293–302, 2000.
190. Boothe DM, Boothe HW, Doornink M: Pharmacokinetic and pharmacodynamic indices of pradofloxacin efficacy in canine serum, and subcutaneous interstitial fluid, Presented as a final report to Bayer Animal Health, Berlin, Germany, 2006.
191. Regnier A, Concordet D, Schneider M, et al: Population pharmacokientics of marbofloxacin in aqueous humor after intravenous administration in dogs, *Am J Vet Res* 64:899–993, 2003.
192. Boothe DM, Boeckh A, Boothe HW, et al: Tissue concentrations of enrofloxacin and ciprofloxacin in anesthetized dogs following single intravenous administration, *Vet Ther* 2:120–128, 2001.
193. Boeckh A, Boothe DM, Wilkie S, et al: Time course of enrofloxacin and its active metabolite in peripheral leukocytes of dogs, *Vet Ther* 2:334–344, 2001.
194. Hawkins EC, Boothe DM, Guinn A, et al: Concentration of enrofloxacin and its active metabolite in alveolar macrophages and pulmonary epithelial lining fluid of dogs, *J Vet Pharmacol Ther*: Feb: 21(1):18–23, 1998.
195. Boothe HW, Jones SA, Wilkie WS, et al: Evaluation of the concentration of marbofloxacin in alveolar macrophages and pulmonary epithelial lining fluid after administration in dogs, *Am J Vet Res* 66:1770–1774, 2005.
196. Boothe DM, Boeckh A, Boothe HW: Evaluation of the distribution of enrofloxacin by circulating leukocytes to sites of inflammation in dogs, *Am J Vet Res* Jan: 70(1):16–22, 2009.
197. Carbon C: Clinical relevance of intracellular and extracellular concentrations of macrolides, *Infection* 23:S10–S14, 1995.
198. Lefebvre HP, Schneider M, Dupouy V, et al: Effects of experimental renal impairment on disposition of marbofloxacin and its metabolites in the dog, *J Vet Pharmcol Ther* 21:453–461, 1998.
199. Boothe DM, Boeckh A, Boothe HW, et al: Plasma concentrations of enrofloxacin and its active metabolite ciprofloxacin in dogs following single oral administration of enrofloxacin at 7.5, 10, or 20 mg/kg, *Vet Ther* 3(4):409–419, 2002.
200. Heinen E: Comparative serum pharmacokinetics of the fluoroquinolones enrofloxacin, difloxacin, marbofloxacin, and orbifloxacin in dogs after single oral administration, *J Vet Pharmacol Therap* 25:1–5, 2002.
201. Abadıá AR, Aramayona JJ, Munõz MJ, et al: Disposition of ciprofloxacin following intravenous administration in dogs, *J Vet Pharmacol The* 17:384–388, 1994.
202. Abadıá AR, Aramayona JJ, Munõz MJ, et al: Ciprofloxacin pharmacokinetics in dogs following oral administration, *J Vet Med* 42:505–511, 1995.
203. Dalhoff A, Bergan T: Pharmacokinetics of fluoroquinolones in experimental animals. In Kuhlman J, Dalhoff A, Zeiler HJ, editors: *Quinolone antibacterials*, Berlin, 1998, Springer Verlag, pp 188–189.
204. Albarellos G, Montoya L, Ambros L, et al: Multiple once-daily dose pharmacokinetics and renal safety of gentamicin in dogs, *J Vet Pharmacol Therap* 27:21–25, 2004.
205. Albarellos GA, Kreil VE, Landoni MF: Pharmacokinetics of ciprofloxacin after single intravenous and repeat oral administration to cats, *J Vet Pharmacol Therap* 27:155–162, 2004.
206. Miyamoto K: Use of plasma clearance of iohexol for estimating glomerular filtration rate in cats, *Am J Vet Res* 62(4):572–575, 2001.
207. Marchetti F, Viale P: Current and future perspectives for levofloxacin in severe *Pseudomonas aeruginosa* infections, *J Chemother* 15(4):315–322, 2003.
208. Fish DN, Chow AT: The clinical pharmacokinetics of levofloxacin, *Clin Pharmacokinet* 32(2):101–119, 1997.
209. Yoshida K, Yabe K, Nishida S, et al: Pharmacokinetic disposition and arthropathic potential of oral ofloxacin in dogs, *J Vet Pharmacol Therap* 21:128–132, 1998.
210. Albarellos GA, Ambros LA, Landoni MF: Pharmacokinetics of levofloxacin after single intravenous and repeat oral administration to cats, *J Vet Pharmacol Therap* 28:363–369, 2005.
211. Intorre L, Mengozzi G, Maccheroni M, et al: Enrofloxacin-theophylline interaction: influence of enrofloxacin on theophylline steady state pharmacokinetics in the beagle dog, *J Vet Pharmacol Ther* 18:352–356, 1995.
212. Hirt RA, Teinfalt M, Dederichs D: The effect of orally administered marbofloxacin on the pharmacokinetics of theophylline, *J Vet Med Assoc* 50:246–250, 2003.
213. Landor M, Iashinsky A, Waxman J: Quinolone allergy? *Ann Allergy Asthma Immunol* 77:273–276, 1996.
214. Davenport CM, Boston RC, Richards DW: Enrofloxacin and magnesium deficiency on matrix metabolism in equie articular cartilage, *Am M Vet Res* 62:160–166, 2001.
215. Ergerbacher M, Edinger J, Tschulenk W: Effects of enrofloxcin and ciprofloxacin hydrochloride on canine and equine chondrocytes in culture, *Am J Vet Res* 63:704–708, 2001.
216. Stahlmann R, Forster C, Shakiboei M, et al: Magnesium deficiency induces joint cartilage lesions in juvenile rats which are identical to quinolone-induced arthopathy, *Antimicrob Agents Chemother* 39:2013–2018, 1995.
217. Ergerbacher M, Wolfesberger B, Gabler C: In vitro evidence for effects of magnesium supplementation on quinolone-treated horse and dog chondrocytes, *Vet Pathol* 38(2):143–148, 2001.
218. Huddleston PM, Hanssen AD, Rouse MS et al: *Ciprofloxacin inhibition of experimental fracture-healing*, The Fluoroquinolone Toxicity Research Foundation, 2003.
219. Shakibaei M, de Souza P, van Sickle D: Biochemical changes in achilles tendon from juvenile dogs after treatment with ciprofloxacin or feeding a magnesium-deficient diet, *Arch Toxicol* 75(6):369–374, 2001.

220. Halliwell RF, Davey PG, Lambert JJ: The effects of quinolones and NSAIDS upon GABA-evoked currents recorded from rat dorsal root ganglion neurons, *J Antimicrob Chemother* 27:209-218, 1991.
221. De Sarro A, Cecchetti V, Fravolini V, et al: Effects of novel 6-desfluoroquinolones and classic quinolones on Pentylene-tetrazole-induced seizures in mice, *Antimicrob Agents Chemother* 43(7):1729-1736, 1999.
222. Lode H: Potential interactions of the extended-spectrum fluoroquinolones with the CNS, *Drug Safety* 21:123-135, 1999.
223. Cohn JS: Peripheral neuropathy associated with fluoroquinolones, *Ann Pharmacother* 34(1), 2001.
224. Gelatt KN, Van der Woerdt A, Ketring KL, et al: Enrofloxacin associated retinal degeneration in cats, *Vet Ophthalmol* 4:99-106, 2001.
225. Wiebe V, Hamilton P: Fluoroqinolone-induced retinal degeneration in cats, *Am Vet Med Assoc* 221:1508-1571, 2002.
226. Marutani K, Matsumoto M, Otabe Y, et al: Reduced phototoxicity of a fluoroquinolone antibacterial agen with a methoxy group at the 8 position in mice irradiated with long-wave length UV light, *Antimicrob Agents Chemother* 37:2217-2222, 1993.
227. Miller CW, Prescott JR, Mathews KA, et al: Streptococcal toxic shock syndrome in dogs, *J Am Vet Med Assoc* 209:1421-1426, 1996.
228. Ingrey KT, Ren J, Prescott JF: A fluoroquinolone induces a novel mitogen-encoding bacteriophage in, *Streptococcus canis, Infect Immun* 71(6):3028-3033, 2003.
229. Baciewicz AM, Chrisman CR, Finch CK, et al: Update on rifampin and rifabutin drug interactions, *Am J Med Sci* 335(2):126-136, 2008.
230. Ziglam HM, Daniels I, Finch RG: Immunomodulating activity of rifampicin, *J Chemother* 16(4):357-361, 2004.
231. Adachi JA, DuPont HL: Rifaximin: a novel nonabsorbed rifamycin for gastrointestinal disorders, *Clin Infect Dis* 42:541-547, 2006.
232. Phillips MA, Stanley SL Jr: Chemotherapy of protozoal infections: amebiasis, giardiasis, trichomoniasis, trypanosomiasis, leishmaniasis, and other protozoal infections. In Brunton LL, Lazo JS, Parker KL, editors: *Goodman & Gilman's the pharmacological basis of therapeutics*, ed 11, New York, 2006, McGraw-Hill.
233. Muller M: Mode of action of metronidazole on anaerobic bacteria and protozoa, *Surgery* 93:165-171, 1983.
234. Levett PN: Time-dependent killing effect of *Clostridium difficile* by metronidazole and vancomycin, *J Antimicrob Chemother* 27:55-62, 1991.
235. Karjagin J, Pähkla R, Karki T, et al: Distribution of metronidazole in muscle tissue of patients with septic shock and its efficacy against, *Bacteroides fragilis in vitro, J Antimicrob Chemother* 55:341-346, 2005.
236. Nix DE, Tyrrell R, Muller M: Pharmacodynamics of metronidazole determined by a time-kill assay for Trichomonas vaginalis, *Antimicrob Agents Chemother* 39(8):1848-1852, 1995.
237. Neff-Davis CA, Davis LE, Gillette EL: Metronidazole: a method for its determination in biological fluids and its disposition kinetics in the dog, *J Vet Pharmacol Ther* 4(2):121-127, 1981.
238. Sekis I, Ramstead K, Rishniw M, et al: Single-dose pharmacokinetics and genotoxicity of metronidazole in cats, *J Feline Med Surg* 11:60-68, 2009.
239. Fitch R, Moore M, Roen D: A warning to clinicians: metronidazole neurotoxicity in a dog, *Probl Vet Neurol* 2:307-309, 1991.
240. Heaney CJ, Campeau NG, Lindell EP: MR imaging and diffusion-weighted imaging changes in metronidazole (Flagyl)-induced cerebellar toxicity, *Am J Neuroradiol* 24:1615-1617, 2003.
241. Evans J, Levesque D, Knowles K: Diazepam as a treatment for metronidazole toxicosis: a retrospective study of 21 dogs, *J Vet Intern Med* 17:304-310, 2003.
242. Caylor KB, Cassimatis MK: Metronidazole neurotoxicosis in two cats, *J Am Anim Hosp Assoc* 37(3):258-262, 2001.
243. Olson EJ, Morales SC, McVey AS, et al: Putative metronidazole neurotoxicosis in a cat, *Vet Pathol* 42:665-669, 2005.
244. Davidson G: To benzoate or not to benzoate: cats are the question, *Int J Pharm Compound* 5:89-90, 2001.
245. Wu Y, Fassihi R: Stability of metronidazole, tetracycline HCl and famotidine alone and in combination, *Int J Pharm* 290: 1-13, 2005.
246. Petri WA Jr: : Sulfonamides, trimethoprim-sulfamethoxazole, quinolones, and agents for urinary tract infections. In Brunton LL, Lazo JS, Parker KL, editors: *Goodman & Gilman's the pharmacological basis of therapeutics*, ed 11, New York, 2006, McGraw-Hill.
247. Hirsch DC, Biberstein EL, Jang SS: Obligate anaerobes in clinical veterinary practice, *J Clin Microbiol* 10:188-191, 1979.
248. Hirsch DC, Indiveri MC, Jang SS, et al: Changes in prevalence and susceptibility of obligate anaerobes in clinical veterinary practice, *J Am Vet Med Assoc* 186(10):1086-1089, 1985.
249. Indiveri MC, Hirsch DW: Susceptibility of obligate anaerobes to trimethoprim-sulfamethoxazole, *J Am Vet Med Assoc* 188:46-48, 1986.

249a. Kuo CC, Wang S, Grayston JT: Antimicrobial activity of several antibiotics and a sulfonamide against *Chlamydia trachomatis* organisms in cell culture, *Antimicrob Agents Chemother* 12(1):80-83, 1977.

250. Sharer WC, Fair WR: The pharmacokinetics of antibiotic diffusion in chronic bacterial prostatitis, *Prostate* 3(2):139-148, 1982.
251. Trepanier LA, Ray K, Winand NJ, et al: Cytosolic arylamine N-acetyltransferase (NAT) deficiency in the dog and other canids due to an absence of NAT genes, *Biochem Pharmacol* 54(1):73-80, 1997.
252. Trepanier LA: Idiosyncratic toxicity associated with potential sulfonamides in the dog, *J Vet Pharmacol Therap* 27:129-138, 2004.
253. Hall IA, Campbell K, Chambers MD, et al: Effect of trimethoprim-sulfamethoxazole on thyroid function in dogs with pyoderma, *J Am Vet Med Assoc* 202:1959-1962, 1993.
254. Trepanier LA, Danhof R, Toll J, et al: Clinical findings in 40 dogs with hypersensitivity associated with administration of potentiated sulfonamides, *J Vet Intern Med* 17:647-652, 2003.
255. Chopra I: New developments in tetracycline antibiotics: glycylcyclines and tetracycline efflux pump inhibitors, *Drug Resist Updat* 5:119-125, 2002.
256. Westfall DS, Twedt DC, Steyn PF, et al: Evaluation of esophageal transit of tablets and capsules in 30 cats, *J Vet Intern Med* 15(5):467-470, 2008.
257. Carlborg B, Densert O: Esophageal lesions caused by orally administered drugs. An experimental study in the cat, *Eur Surg Res* 12(4):270-282, 1980.
258. Apaydin BB, Paksoy M, Art T, et al: Influence of pentoxifylline and interferon-alpha on prevention of stricture due to corrosive esophagitis, *Eur Surg Res* 33:225-231, 2001.
259. Saiman L, Liu Z, Chen Y: Synergistic activity of macrolide antibioitics paired with conventional antimicrobial agents against multiply antibiotic resistant P aeruginosa isolated from CF patients, *Antimicrob Agents Chemother* 46(4):1105-1107, 2002.
260. Park B-K, Lim J-H, Kim M-S, et al: Pharmacokinetics of florfenicol and its metabolite, florfenicol amine, in dogs, *Res Vet Sci* 84:85-89, 2008.
261. Papich MG, Riviere J: Chloramphenicol. In Adams R, editor: *Veterinary pharmacology and therapeutics*, ed 8, Ames, Iowa, 2001, Iowa State University Press, pp 868-897.

262. Watson ADJ: Chloramphenicol in the dog: observations of plasma levels following oral administration, *Res Vet Sci* 16:147–151, 1974.
263. Glazko AJ, Wolf LM, Dill WA, et al: Biochemical studies on chloramphenicol (chloromycetin), *J Pharm Exp Ther* 96:445–449, 1949.
264. Watson AD: Chloramphenicol 2. Clinical pharmacology in dogs and cats, *Aust Vet J* 68(1):2–5, 1991.
265. Watson ADJ: Plasma chloramphenicol concentrations in cats after parenteral administration of chloramphenicol sodium succinate, *J Vet Pharamcol Therap* 2:123–127, 1979.
266. Watson ADJ: Effect of ingesta on systemic availability of chloramphenicol from two oral preparations in cats, *J Vet Pharmacol Therap* 2:117–121, 1979.
267. Papich MG: Florfenicol pharmacokinetics in dogs and cats (Abstract No. 235), 17th Annual Veterinary Medical Forum, American College of Veterinary Internal Medicine, Chicago, IL, June 10-13, 1999.

267a. Michel J, Bornstein H, Luboshitzky R, et al: Mechanisms of chlorampenicol-cephalordine synergism on Enterobacteiaeae, *Antimicrob Agents Chemother* 7(6):845–849, 1975.

268. Adams HR, Dixit BN: Prolongation of pentobarbital by chloramphenicol in dogs and cats, *J Am Vet Med Assoc* 156(7):902–905, 1970.
269. Sanders JE, Yeary RA, Fenner WR, et al: Interaction of phenytoin with chloramphenicol or pentobarbital in the dog, *J Am Vet Med Assoc* 175(2):177–180, 1979.
270. Turco JD: Pharmacokinetics and interactions of digoxin with phenobarbital in dogs, *Am J Vet Res* 48(8):1244–1249, 1987.
271. Boothe DM, Brown SA, Fate GD, et al: Plasma disposition of clindamycin microbiologic activity in cats after single oral doses of clindamycin hydrochloride as either capsules or aqueous solution, *J Vet Pharmacol Ther* 19:491–494, 1996.
272. Lavy E, Ziv G, Shem-Tove M, et al: Pharmacokinetics of clindamycin HCl administered intravenously, intramuscularly, and subcutaneously to dogs, *J Vet Pharmacol Therap* 22:261–265, 1999.
273. Yamasaki T, Ichimiya T, Hirai K, et al: Effect of antimicrobial agents on the piliation of *Pseudomonas aeruginosa* and adherence to mouse tracheal epithelium, *J Chemother* 9:32–37, 1997.
274. Asaka T, Manaka A, Sugiyama H: Recent developments in macrolide antimicrobial research, *Curr Top Med Chem* 3:961–989, 2003.
275. Schlunzen F, Harms JM: Structural basis for the antibiotic activity of ketolides and azalides, *Structure* 11:329–338, 2003.
276. Dorfman MS, Wagner RS, Jamison T, et al: The pharmacodynamic properties of azithromycin in a kinetics-of-kill model and implications for bacterial conjunctivitis treatment, *Adv Ther* 25(3):208–217, 2008.
277. Albarellos GA, Kreil VE, Ambros LA, et al: Pharmacokinetics of erythromycin after the administration of intravenous and various oral dosage forms to dogs, *J Vet Pharmacol Ther* 31(6):496–500, 2008.
278. Garver E, Hugger ED, Shearn SP, et al: Involvement of intestinal uptake transporters in the absorption of azithromycin and clarithromycin in the rat, *Drug Metab Dispos* 36:2492–2498, 2008.
279. Shepard RM, Falkner FC: Pharmacokinetics of azithromycin in rats and dogs, *J Antimicrob Chemother* 25(Suppl A):49–60, 1990.
280. Hunter RP, Lynch MJ, Ericson JF: Pharmacokinetics, oral bioavailability and tissue distribution of azithromycin in cats, *J Vet Pharmacol Ther* 18(1):38–46, 1995.

280a. Haddad A, Davis M, Lagman R: The pharmacological importance of cytochrome CYP3A4 in the palliation of symptoms: review and recommendations for avoiding adverse drug interactions, *Support Care Cancer* 15(3):251–257, 2007.

281. Bizjak ED, Mauro VF: Digoxin-macrolide drug interaction, *Ann Pharmacother* 31(9):1077–1079, 1997.
282. Sugie M, Asakura E, Zhao YL, et al: Possible involvement of the drug transporters P glycoprotein and multidrug resistance-associated protein Mrp2 in disposition of azithromycin, *Antimicrob Agents Chemother* 48(3):809–814, 2004.
283. Carfartan G, Gerardin P, Turck D, et al: Effect of subinhibitory concentrations of azithromycin on adherence of *Pseudomonas aeruginosa* to bronchial mucins collected from cystic fibrosis patients, *J Antimicrob Chemother* 53:686–688, 2004.
284. Gillis RJ, Iglewski BH: Azithromycin retards *Pseudomonas aeruginosa* biofilm formation, *J Clin Microbiol* 42(12):5842–5845, 2004.
285. Kourlas H: Anti-inflammatory properties of macrolide antibiotics, *J Pharm Pract* 19(5):326–329, 2006.
286. Amsden GW: Anti-inflammatory effects of macrolides—an underappreciatedbenefitinthetreatmentofcommunity-acquired respiratorytractinfectionsandchronicinflammatorypulmonaryconditions? *J Antimicrob Chemother* 55:10–21, 2005.
287. Lorenz J: Telithromycin: the first ketolide antibacterial for the treatmentofcommunityacquiredrespiratoryinfections, *IntJClin Pract* 57:519–529, 2003.
288. Bozdogan B, Applebaum PC: Oxazolidinones: activity, mode of action, and mechanism of resistance, *Int J Antimicrob Agents* 23:113–119, 2004.
289. Yagi BH, Zurenko GE: An in vitro time-kill assessment of linezolid and anaerobic bacteria, *Anaerobe* 9(1):1–3, 2003.
290. Ntziora F, Falagas ME: Linezolid for the treatment of patients with mycobacterial infections: a systematic review, *Int J Tuberc Lung Dis* 11(6):606–611, 2007.
291. Brown-Elliott BA, Ward SC, et al: In vitro activities of linezolid against multiple *Nocardia* species, *Antimicrob Agents Chemother* 45(4):1295–1297, 2001.
292. Smith AJ, Hall V, Thakker B, et al: Antimicrobial susceptibility testing of *Actinomyces* species with 12 antimicrobial agents, *J Antimicrob Chemother* 56(2):407–409, 2005.
293. Slatter JG, Adams LA, Bush EC, et al: Pharmacokinetics, toxicokinetics, distribution, metabolism and excretion of linezolid in mouse, rat and dog, *Xenobiotica* 32(10):907–924, 2002.
294. Garrabou G, Soriano A, Lopez S, et al: Reversible inhibition of mitochondrial protein synthesis during linezolid-related hyperlactatemia, *Antimicrob Agents Chemother* 51(3):962–967, 2007.
295. Oleson FB Jr, Berman CL, Kirkpatrick JB, et al: Once-daily dosing in dogs optimizes daptomycin safety, *Antimicrob Agents Chemother* 44(11):2948–2953, 2000.
296. Rybníček J, Hill PB: Suspected polymyxin B-induced pemphigus vulgaris in a dog, *Vet Dermatol* 18(3):165–170, 2007.
297. Spann CT, Turtrone WD, Weinberg JM: Topical antibacterial agents for wound care: a primer, *Dermatol Surg* 29:620–626, 2003.

8 Treatment of Bacterial Infections

Dawn Merton Boothe

Chapter Outline

This chapter focuses on the treatment of bacterial infections on a systems basis. In addition, selected organisms are discussed because of their unique nature and the difficulties encountered when treating such infections. In general, the ease with which microbes appear to become resistant requires dosing regimens that are based on scientific studies demonstrating both efficacy toward the microbe and pharmacokinetics in the target species; if the latter is not available, extrapolated doses should be promulgated by persons with expertise (e.g., a veterinary clinical pharmacologist). Because of limited evidence-based information in veterinary medicine, data from the human-medicine literature may serve as a basis for recommendations. Information supporting the judicious use of antimicrobial drugs is found in Chapters 6 and 7. This includes but is not limited to data referring to drug concentrations achieved in the plasma at recommended doses (see Table 7-7), and other pharmacokinetic data (see Table 7-1) and tissue-to-drug ratios of antimicrobial drugs (see Table 7-5). In addition, population pharmacodynamic data are available that indicate the concentration of drug necessary to inhibit the microbes (minimum inhibitory concentration [MIC]) for selected drugs: See Table 7-3 *(Escherichia coli)*, Table 7-4 (human data for selected microbes for which veterinary information could not be consistently found), Tables 7-9, and 7-10 (data for beta-lactams), and Table 7-12 (fluoroquinolones). Selected pharmodynamic data are also provided in this chapter for infections associated with specific body systems. This includes an example of regional cumulative antimicrobial susceptibility antibiograms that might help guide empirical therapy, which is increasingly discouraged as resistance emerges (Figure 8-1). The clinician is encouraged to consider the approach to individualized antimicrobial therapy presented in Chapter 6. This includes Figure 6-1, which is an algorithm for antimicrobial therapy that is intended to minimize the risk of antimicrobial resistance, particularly in the at-risk patient. Algorithms have also been offered for infections of selected body systems. Preventing resistance is among the more important considerations that must be made by veterinarians using antimicrobials. (Box 8-1). A three "Ds" approach includes "detergent" (address hygiene at multiple levels), "de-escalating" drug use, and "design" dosing optimal regimens. Hygiene, which goes beyond simple hand washing, also is a critical component of preventing emerging resistance. Resistance is also minimized by de-escalating drug use. This includes simply decreasing the number of antimicrobial drugs prescribed and dispensed. However, de-escalating also entails moving to a lower tier of drug classes (i.e., one that is less broad in its actions and less "effective" toward microbes that tend to develop multidrug resistance). Although it is critical to use the best drug possible such that the infecting population is killed, once this is accomplished, de-escalation to a less-important lower tier class of drugs should be possible. First-tier drugs might include both narrow and broader spectrum beta-lactams (amoxicillin with without clavulanic acid), clindamycin, tetracyclines, and potentiated sulfonamides. Second-tier drugs might include those drugs characterized by spectra purposefully extended to target organisms not generally susceptible to first-tier drugs. Newer drugs such as third-generation cephalosporins, extended-spectrum penicillins, and fluoroquinolones might be included in this category. Therapy should be based on culture and susceptibility testing data, whenever possible, and population pharmacodynamic statistics if patient MIC data are not available. Third-tier drugs include those that tend to be reserved for treatment of microbes associated with either inherent or acquired resistance. Their use should be based on culture and susceptibility testing data and should be de-escalated to a lower-tier drug as soon as possible. Examples might include drugs that target multidrug-resistant gram-negative (aminoglycosides, carbapenems) and gram-positive (glycopeptides, linezolids) organisms. The American College of Veterinary Internal Medicine[1] and the International Society of Companion Animal Infectious Disease (publications pending) have promulgated guidelines intended to minimize emerging resistance.

KEY POINT 8-1 A three-pronged approach is indicated for preventing antimicrobial resistance: escalating hygiene, de-escalating antimicrobial drug use, and optimizing dosing regimens such that the infecting inoculum is eradicated, not simply inhibited.

INFECTIONS OF THE CENTRAL NERVOUS SYSTEM AND SPECIAL SENSES

Meningitis

Meningitis serves here as the prototypic infection of the central nervous system (CNS).

Physiology and Pathophysiology

Infections of the CNS are uniquely problematic for three reasons: cellular components reflect functional specialization, a major portion of the CNS is sequestered from the rest of the body by physiologic barriers, and tissues of the CNS are closely confined within rigid skeletal structures such that swelling cannot occur without subsequent and potentially lethal damage. Cellular specialization is of diagnostic benefit in the identification and localization of infections of the CNS because clinical signs are often referred to a specific region of the brain.

The course of CNS infection is affected by the relationship of the brain and spinal cord to the vasculature, meninges, and skeletal structure. The brain is suspended in cerebrospinal fluid (CSF) and is surrounded by the meninges (pia mater and arachnoid [together forming the leptomeninges] and the dura mater). Infections of the leptomeninges tend to involve their entire surface that surrounds the brain and spinal cord. In contrast, infections of the dura mater tend to be limited and sharply circumscribed. With persistent infection of the meninges, increased intracranial pressure results from extensive cerebral edema and hydrocephalus. Infections of the spinal cord meninges are less limited and often extend longitudinally the length of the cord.[1]

About 85% of CSF is produced by the choroid plexus of the lateral, third, and fourth ventricles. The CSF flows into the subarachnoid space, circulates around the brain and spinal cord by bulk flow, and is reabsorbed through the arachnoid. The CSF is totally recirculated in 3 to 4 hours. The choroid plexus is physiologically similar to renal tubules, even containing similar secretory mechanisms. Indeed, specialized transport systems allow the movement of organic acids (including many beta-lactams) against a concentration gradient out of the CSF. In cases of infections involving the ventricles, because of the flow pattern of CSF, intrathecal administration of drugs does not result in predictable drug concentrations in the ventricles. Rather, drug must be directly instilled into the ventricles. Infections of the CNS can impair CSF reabsorption across the arachnoid villi, resulting in hydrocephalus.[1]

Capillaries of the brain and spinal cord (with the exception of the choroid plexus) differ from other capillaries. First, the vascular endothelium is characterized by tight junctions rather than intracellular clefts. Second, they are surrounded by the foot processes of astrocytes (see Figure 29-1). Both form a barrier to passive diffusion of drugs and their compounds. Only compounds that are actively transported or are of sufficient lipid solubility can pass out of the capillaries into the brain. The barrier affects the movement of antimicrobials. In addition, impaired movement of immunoglobulins, complement, and other mediators of the immune response affects antimicrobial selection in that bacteriostatic drugs are much less desirable.[1,2]

Cumulative Antimicrobial Susceptibility Report
Canine Isolates from 1/ 1/ 07 to 1/ 1/ 10

	No. of Isolates	Amikacin	Amoxicillin/CA	Ampicillin	Cefazolin	Cefpodoxime	Ceftiofur	Cephalothin[b]	Chloramphenicol	Clindamycin	Enrofloxacin	Erythromycin	Gentamicin	Marbofloxacin	Oxacillin	Penicillin	Rifampin	Tetracycline	Ticarcillin	Ticarcillin/CA	Trimethoprim/Sulfa
Enterococcus faecalis	128		98	96					84		52	17 (127)		54 (110)		96	54	46 (116)			
Enterococcus faecium	52		31	27					96		6	12		13 (46)		27	54	25 (48)			
Escherichia coli	486	98	68	53	71	70	75 (444)	57 (442)	85		69		85	71				69 (439)	55	68	73
Klebsiella pneumoniae	100	67	60	0	58	61	57 (87)	58 (93)	70		63		64	64				59 (93)	0	61	71
Proteus mirabilis	136	99	95	91	90	96	98 (117)	91 (129)	90		95		92	98				0 (129)	94	100	90
Pseudomonas aeruginosa	250	98							6 (246)		56		89	80 (223)					94	96	
Staphylococcus aureus	30	97	37	17	37	33	21 (28)	37	100	37	50	37	90	50	37	20	93	87			93
Staphylococcus intermedius[b]	480	94	77	20	76	69	72 (411)	78 (441)	98	49 (477)	63	49	90	67	78	18	98 (476)	53 (430)			65
Group G beta streptococci	20	45	100	100	100	65	100 (12)	100 (19)	70	95	60	0	65	65		100	100	47 (19)			100

Feline Isolates from 1/ 1/ 07 to 1/ 1/ 10

	No. of Isolates	Amikacin	Amoxicillin/CA	Ampicillin	Cefazolin	Cefoxitin	Cephalothin[b]	Chloramphenicol	Clindamycin	Enrofloxacin	Erythromycin	Gentamicin	Marbofloxacin	Oxacillin	Penicillin	Rifampin	Tetracycline	Ticarcillin	Ticarcillin/CA	Trimethoprim/Sulfa
Enterococcus faecalis	14		100	100				93		43	14		36 (11)		100	64	29			
Enterococcus faecium	7		57	43				100		14	0		14		29	14	57			
Escherichia coli	59	100	81	44	86	85	70 (53)	93		81		86	81				70 (53)	47	81	81
Pseudomonas aeruginosa	9	100						0		44		100	100					89	89	
Staphylococcus intermedius[c]	12	92	58	17	58	58	58	100	25	33	25	92	33	64	17	100	33			33
Staphylococcus aureus	9	100	78	11	78	78	78	100	33	67	33	100	89	78	11	100	100			100

Continued

Figure 8-1 Cumulative antimicrobial susceptibility reports for canine *(top)* and feline *(bottom)* organisms isolated from samples collected during the years 2007 to 2010 at a veterinary teaching hospital. The data are geographically restricted to Alabama and are from a teaching hospital that has a wide referral base. Accordingly, the data may not be relevant to other areas of the United States nor to patients with first time infections. No attempt has been made to separate data according to history, including previous antimicrobial exposure. Ideally, each practice would generate a cumulative report at frequent intervals (e.g., yearly or every other year). The report might serve as a basis for empirical selection of antimicrobials. However, the number of isolates must be sufficient to represent the population; ideally, at least 100 isolates of each organism should be sampled. Drugs that are not included in the antibiogram for each organism generally are not included because the use of the drug for that organism is inappropriate. Each cell indicates the percentage of the tested isolates that were considered susceptible to the drug on the basis of Clinical and Laboratory Standards Institute (CLSI) guidelines promulgated in 2008. The *first row* lists the drugs to which susceptibility was determined for the organisms. The *far left column* names the genus and species of the organisms isolated and for which susceptibility was determined. The *second from the left column* indicates the total number of isolates tested. For some drugs not all isolates were tested; in such instances the total number of isolates tested is indicated in parentheses in that cell. New CLSI interpretive criteria for selected drugs (approved in 2010), including amoxicillin–clavulanic acid cephalexin and its model drug, cephalothin, are likely to result in a marked decrease in the percentage of susceptible isolates. Cephalothin continues to act as a class drug, representing first-generation cephalosporins (see Chapter 6 for a discussion of limitations of model drugs; e.g., cephalexin should not be used to treat *E. coli,* as a general rule). *Staphylococcus intermedius* represents what is currently referred to as *S. intermedius* group. (Data provided by Terri Hathcock, MS, Diagnostic Veterinary Microbiologist, Infection Control Officer, College of Veterinary Medicine, Auburn University.)

Box 8-1

Treatment of Multidrug-Resistant Microorganisms

1. Avoid emergent resistance.
   - A. Address hygiene both in the hospital and at home. Clean bedding. Reduce exposure to environment or family members that might carry resistant organisms.
   - B. Base drug on culture and susceptibility data. Wait for data if possible. If not, base empirical therapy on local cumulative antimicrobial susceptibility data (see Figure 8-1).
   - C. De-escalate antimicrobial use. Avoid using antimicrobials when possible. De-escalate to lower-tier drug as soon as possible. Decrease duration of therapy.
   - D. Use drug with a spectrum that is as narrow as possible, minimizing selection pressure.
   - E. Optimize dosing regimens (see 4) such that all infecting colony-forming units (including colony-forming units with mutant prevention concentration) are killed (not inhibited), especially in at-risk patients.
   - F. Consult experts (e.g., specialists, including clinical pharmacologists, veterinary diagnostic microbiologists).
2. Treat underlying cause of recurrent infections.
3. Implement adjuvant therapies.
4. Base design of dosing regimen on culture data, including minimum inhibitory concentrations.
   - A. Pharmacodynamic indices should surpass that recommended for efficacy; for example, concentration-dependent drugs, C_{max}/MIC >12, AUC/MIC > 250 (AUC/MPC ≥ 22); time-dependent drugs T > MIC more than 75%.
   - B. Intravenous dosing should be considered to ensure that the highest concentrations of drug will be obtained. If the site can be topically reached, topical administration should accompany systemic therapy.
5. Use drug combinations known to produce either additive or synergistic effects. Use full dose of both drugs. De-escalate as soon as possible.
6. Gram positive:
   - A. Methicillin-resistant *Staphylococcus,* spp., non–Vanconmycin-resistant *Enterococcus* spp.
     - i. Rifampin combined with any other drug to which the organism is susceptible
     - ii. Vancomycin (not Vancomycin-resistant *Enterococcus*). Vancomycin must be given intravenously for systemic therapy (oral drug is for gastrointestinal therapy only).
     - iii. Linezolid
     - iv. Aminoglycosides should not be used as sole agents for treatment of multidrug-resistant gram-positive infections. In general, gentamicin is more efficacious against-*Staphylococcus* spp. than amikacin.
     - v. Choramphenicol is a bacteriostatic drug; care must be taken to ensure that killing effects are achieved.
     - vi. Potential alternatives include fusidic acid or fosfomycin (evidence needed).
     - vii. Some evidence exists that the combination of vancomycin with a carbapenem may enhance efficacy.
   - B. For vancomycin-resistant *Enterococcus* spp., use beta-lactams with known susceptibility.
7. Gram-negative:
   - A. Combination therapy is based on culture and susceptibility testing data.
   - B. The laboratory should test specifically for presence of extended-spectrum beta-lactamases, particularly for third-generation cephalosporins. Testing may be indicated for carbapenem targeting extended-spectrum beta-lactamases in *Klebsiella pneumoniae.* Otherwise, the presence of AMP-C indicates the use of carbapenems.
   - C. The most effective drug or drug combination should be used initially, with de-escalation to a lower-tier drug when possible (i.e., within 5 days).
8. *Clostridium difficile*
   - A. Discontinue antimicrobial therapy that may be contributing to overpopulation.
   - B. If therapy is indicated, treat with metronidazole; alternative is oral vancomycin.

Vascular damage associated with infection can affect the course of infection. Hypertrophy of the endothelium (as might occur with persistent bacterial infection) or infection of the endothelial cells (as occurs with Rocky Mountain spotted fever, for example) can cause thrombosis or embolization to arteries or veins. Loss of capillary integrity contributes to cerebral edema and movement of microorganisms into the brain. At the same time, capillary permeability facilitates movement of antimicrobials that normally cannot cross the cerebral or meningeal capillaries into the site of infection.[1,2]

The inflammatory response of the CNS also differs from that in other body tissues. The response tends to be less intense and is characterized by infiltration of microglial cells and proliferation of astrocytes. Abscessation is slower and involves gliosis rather than fibrosis. Host response to infection in the CNS involves antibody, cell-mediated immunity, and complement-mediated immunity. Normally excluded from the CNS, antibody in the CNS indicates damage to the blood–brain barrier or synthesis of immunoglobulin from cells that have been able to penetrate the brain parenchyma. Antibody protection is important in bacterial meningeal infections and may determine the outcome. Cell-mediated immunity, on the other hand, is the predominant host response to fungal or intracellular parasites. Infections by selected organisms, such as *Mycoplasma* spp., may lead to a host response to both the infecting organism and host proteins (e.g., myelin). Despite the role of the immune system in bacterial infections of the CNS, host defenses remain inadequate for control of the infection. Indeed, the relative lack of opsonization, complement, and immunoglobulins may allow bacterial survival in the subarachnoid space.[1,2]

Bacterial products can contribute to the development of cerebral edema. Release of cytokines and tumor necrosis factor is mediated by materials such as endotoxin of gram-negative organisms and teichoic acid produced by *Staphylococcus aureus*. Whereas changes in capillary permeability may increase antimicrobial movement across the blood–brain barrier, antimicrobial therapy may initially worsen cerebral edema, as bacterial death causes release of more mediators of inflammation. Inflammation, hemorrhage, hydrocephalus, and edema may cause displacement of the brain or spinal cord. Herniation may be a life-threatening sequela.[1] The potential release of endotoxin may be an important consideration in the initial selection of an antimicrobial; drugs that minimize endotoxin release yet still penetrate the blood–brain barrier include meropenem and the fluoroquinolones.

Antimicrobial Selection

Successful antimicrobial therapy of CNS infections is facilitated by use of a bactericidal drug and maximization of plasma drug concentrations such that bactericidal concentrations are achieved in the CNS. The CNS is relatively immunoincompetent, thus increasing the concentration of drug necessary for effective therapy. Studies in animal models have shown that the rapid bactericidal killing in the CSF requires drug concentrations that exceed the minimum bactericidal concentration (not MIC) by tenfold to twentyfold.[2] To maximize drug concentrations at the site of infection, drugs that can be given intravenously are preferred to oral preparations. Antimicrobials to treat the CNS are often selected empirically because of difficulties encountered when collecting culture and susceptibility data. Most infections reach the CNS by a hematogenous route. Organisms most likely cultured from or infecting the CNS are delineated in Table 6-1; however, the lack of predictability of the infecting organism mandates the need for a properly collected culture sample. After the most likely infecting organism and drugs effective against the organism have been selected, antibiotics should be selected next on the basis of movement into the CNS. Drug penetration of the blood–brain barrier is particularly challenging because the barrier not only prevents movement of antimicrobials into the CNS but also actively transports out or destroys some antimicrobials (i.e., selected beta-lactams) (see Table 7-5).

KEY POINT 8-2 Doses of antimicrobials, particularly those that are water soluble, may have to be increased tenfold or more to achieve effective concentrations in the brain.

To enter the CNS, antimicrobials must penetrate the epithelium of either the choroid plexus or the cerebral endothelium; both are characterized by tight junctions. Antimicrobials generally are not metabolized in the CNS; concentrations thus reflect a balance between penetration and elimination via the blood–brain or blood–CSF barrier.[3] Passive diffusion is the major mechanism of drug movement. Drugs that are more likely to penetrate the barrier are characterized by high lipid solubility, small molecular weight, and low protein binding.[2] Whereas lipid-soluble drugs enter the CNS through transcellular pathways, water-soluble drugs must move through paracellular pathways and thus depend on the opening of tight junctions. Several transport mechanisms facilitate influx (as well as efflux; see below and Chapter 27) of selected drugs (e.g., penicillins, ceftriaxone), but this accounts for only a low concentration of drug movement. Antimicrobial movement into the CNS thus is generally slow, with peak concentrations often not occurring until several hours after drug administration. Methods intended to increase permeability of and thus antimicrobial movement into the CSF (e.g., hyperosmotic solutions, receptor-specific antibodies, inflammatory mediators) have not been well evaluated.[3] Once selected drugs successfully penetrate the CNS, drug efflux may decrease intracellular concentrations. Penicillins (but not ceftriaxone, carbapenems, nor ampicillin) are actively transported from the CNS; active transport can be inhibited by probenicid.[4] Interestingly, the action of this pump is inhibited by meningeal inflammation. Therefore inflammation will increase inward movement of several antimicrobial, including many beta-lactams and vancomycin. However, as treatment is effective, increased influx declines such that within 5 days of therapy, penicillin CSF half-life and drug concentrations in humans markedly decrease. This is in contrast to drugs with a low affinity for active transport system; for such drugs concentrations tend to remain clinically relevant throughout CNS infection. Active transport mechanisms do not appear to affect CSF concentrations of fluoroquinolones or aminoglycosides.[3]

Antimicrobial therapy also is likely to be affected by the presence of purulent material. As in all body systems, the microenvironment can negatively affect antibacterial therapy. In the presence of meningitis, lactate accumulates in the CSF, causing the pH to decrease. Antibacterial activity of weakly basic antimicrobials may decrease, particularly for the aminoglycosides and potentially for the fluoroquinolones.[2] The dynamics of CSF are altered by disease and drugs. At best, CSF production is unaltered, although several studies have demonstrated decreased CSF production. Glucocorticoids may further decrease CSF production; however, rather than prolonging the half-life of the drug in the CNS, glucocorticoids appear to decrease or not change CSF antimicrobial concentrations.[5]

Drug movement into the CNS was summarized in Box 6-4 and Table 7-5. Because of the impact of normal physiology and drugs, dosing regimens designed for treatment of CNS infection tend to differ from traditional therapy, in that doses often are much higher. The risk of toxicity that might accompany such increases must be weighed against the need to penetrate the CNS in concentrations sufficient to cause bactericidal effects (see Table 7-5). In general, selected beta-lactams (meropenem more than imipenem; cefoxitin, ceftazidime and cefotaxim), trimethoprim/sulfonamide, fluorinated quinolones, rifampin, and metronidazole can achieve bactericidal concentrations for some infections in the CNS; chloramphenicol and doxycycline or minocycline achieve bacteriostatic concentrations.[6] Amikacin may achieve effective concentrations as well. Drugs that should be avoided or whose doses should be further markedly increased for treatment of CNS infections because of poor penetration include many beta-lactams, including carbenicillin, cephalothin, cefazolin, cefotetan; and clindamycin, erythromycin, and tetracycline. Drugs recommended for treatment of meningitis in humans are increased by at least 50% to 100% or more when safety is not an issue, with intervals being reduced for time-dependent drugs, to ensure that adequate concentrations reach the CNS. For other drugs, doses for treatment of CNS infections are increased several-fold compared with other infections. For example, beta-lactam doses in particular are increased as follows: penicillin normally dosed at 1 million U is increased 1 to 4 million U to 24 million U/person; aztreonam is increased threefold, and several third-generation cephalosporins (cefotaxime, ceftazidime, ceftriaxone) are increased sevenfold to twentyfold. Aminoglycoside doses are either not increased or increased twofold (e.g., amikacin). Doxycycline is increased twofold, and sulfonamides are increased fourfold to fivefold. Because of local immunoincompetence, duration of therapy for patients with infections of the CNS should be at least 10 to 14 days and up to 21 days.[2] The need for 4 to 6 weeks of therapy, as has been suggested in dogs, is not clear; it may not be necessary.[7] Intrathecal administration of antimicrobials that might be systemically toxic at concentrations necessary to be effective in the CNS might be a reasonable alternative. However, this method has not been well studied, particularly in animal patients. Further, because distribution of intrathecally administered drug into the CSF is uneven, drug concentrations may not be adequate at some sites.

Adjuvant therapy. Because of the harm associated with inflammation in a closed system, antiinflammatories should be considered when treating CNS infections (e.g., meningitis). Corticosteroid therapy may be indicated during initial stages of treatment of meningitis to minimize the effects of inflammation and loss of capillary integrity.[2,7] Experimentally, methylprednisolone decreases leukocyte accumulation, CSF outflow resistance, and brain water content in animals with bacterial meningitis.[2] Dexamethasone also reverses the development of brain edema and, compared with methylprednisolone, has the added advantage of decreasing CSF pressure and lactate. Note that these studies did not include comparisons with antimicrobial therapy. Nonetheless, glucocorticoid therapy may be beneficial early during the course of therapy; indeed, treatment before antibacterial therapy may minimize the effects of mediators of inflammation released by dying bacteria.[2] A study of infants with bacterial meningitis treated with ceftriaxone and either a placebo or dexamethasone found the duration of infection and degree of inflammation in the latter group to be shorter and less, respectively, although mortality or long-term neurologic sequelae did not differ between the two groups.[8] In an analysis of five clinical trials in adult humans with bacterial meningitis, the incidence of side effects was the same in the group treated with glucocorticoids (dexamethasone), but both mortality and persistence of clinical signs were improved in the group treated with steroids, leading the authors to conclude that a single dose is justified if given at the beginning of antimicrobial therapy.[9,10] Dexamethasone can be used (0.1 to 0.15 mg/kg every 6 hours up to 4 days), particularly in the presence of cerebral edema.[2]

KEY POINT 8-3 A well timed but limited duration of treatment with glucocorticoids may be indicated in the patient with bacterial meningitis to prevent organ-threatening inflammation.

Treatment of cerebral edema should also include mannitol. If intensive monitoring is available, high-dose barbiturate therapy might be useful for these patients. Barbiturates decrease cerebral metabolic demands and cerebral blood flow and provide protection against oxygen radicals.

Adverse reactions. Because of altered permeability of the blood–brain barrier, the infected CNS is more likely than the normal CNS to respond adversely to antimicrobials. Seizures are the most likely manifestation. The antimicrobial most likely to cause seizures include selected beta-lactams (see Chapters 6 and 7), most notably imipenem (but not meropenem), metronidazole, and fluoroquinolones, particularly in patients also receiving nonsteroidal antiinflammatories. In general, seizures that develop as a result of drug therapy should be treated as with any acute seizural manifestation, with diazepam the preferred anticonvulsant of choice.

Ocular Infections

The principles of ocular therapy are discussed in Chapter 27.

Microbial Targets

Whitley[11] has provided a review of isolates cultured from ocular tissues of clinically normal dogs and dogs with ocular disease (Table 8-1). The most common organism associated

Table 8-1 Microbial Flora Associated with Infections at Selected Tissue Sites

Site		Percent (%)*
Eye[11]	*Staphylococcus* spp. (coagulase –)	0-11
	Staphylococcus spp. (coagulase +)	16-42
	Streptococcus spp. (beta hem)	17-22
	Streptococcus spp. (alpha hem)	2-9
	Streptococcus canis	16.5
	Corynebacterium spp.	3.5
	Enterococcus spp.	0-5.6
	Escherichia coli	4-17
	Proteus spp.	0-2.6
	Proprionobacterium	0-2.6
	Pseudomonas aeruginosas	0-9.5
Wound[92]	*No growth*	16
(n = 213)	**Gram-positive**	53
	Staphylococcus spp. (coagulase–)	5
	Staphylococcus intermedius	12
	Oral and other *Streptococcus* spp.	6
	Streptococcus canis	7
	Bacillus spp.†	6
	Actinomyces spp.	3
	Corynebacterium spp.	2
	Gram-negative	47
	Pasteurella multocida	15
	Pasteurella canis	5
	Other *Pasteurellaceae*	2
	Enterobacteraceae	7
	Vibrionaceae	4
	Non-glucose fermenters	16
Urine[105]	*Escherichia coli*	45
(n = 8354)	*Staphylococcus* spp. total	12
	Proteus mirabilis	6-12
	Klebsiella pneumoniae	7-12
	Enterococcus spp.†	6-9
	Enterococcus faecalis	(2-4)
	Enterococcus faecium	(1-3)
	Streptococcus spp.	5
	Pseudomonas aeuruginosa	3
	Mycoplasma spp.	2-3
	Enterobacter spp.	2-3

*Proportions are approximate.
†Considered a contaminant.

with bacterial conjunctivitis in dogs is *Staphylococcus* spp. (*aureus* [68% of infections] or *epidermidis* [27% of infections]). A variety of other organisms, including *Corynebacterium* spp. and gram-negative rods, make up the remaining infections. Most of the infecting organisms are considered normal ocular flora.[11] Bacterial infection complicating keratoconjunctivitis sicca generally is caused by *Staphylococcus* spp. (32% to 69% of dogs) and *Streptococcus* spp. (9% to 25%); *Pseudomonas* spp. (5% to 18% of infections) is the most common gram-negative isolate. In cats *Mycoplasma felis* and *gatea* are the more common isolates associated with conjunctivitis; however, they also are commonly isolated in normal cats, calling into question the role of the organism in disease. *Chlamydia (Chlamydophila felis)*[12] may be a concurrent pathogen, although both it and *Mycoplasma* spp. may reflect infection secondary to primary feline herpesvirus infection.

Like conjunctival infections, corneal infections (including ulceration) are most commonly caused by *Staphylococcus* spp., followed by *Streptococcus* spp. (together making up approximately 65% of infections). Other causes include *Corynebacterium* spp. and gram-negative rods (including *Pseudomonas* spp.).

Drug Preparations

Characteristics of topical ophthalmic antibacterial drugs to consider are the spectrum, and their lipid versus water solubility, with lipid solubility being more important if tissue penetration is of importance. Because of the ability to administer high concentrations of antimicrobials with topical administration, traditional classification of bacteriostatic versus bactericidal (fungal or viral -static or -cidal) may not be relevant to antiinfective drugs, and susceptibility data might underestimate topical efficacy. Ophthalmic drugs indicated for treatment of ocular infections are available as single or multiple antimicrobial agents (Table 8-2a and Table 8-2b). Generally, either gram-negative or gram-positive organisms are targeted using individual agents; mixed infections can be targeted with combination products or drugs characterized by a broad spectrum. Whereas few drugs are approved for use in animals, multiple human products are commercially available. Others can be compounded, which might include "fortification" of commercial products. However, the nuances of ocular preparations mandate that extreme caution be taken when formulating or modifying a product intended for topical ocular therapy (see Chapter 23).[11]

KEY POINT 8-4 Whereas high concentrations of drugs might be achieved with topical ophthalmic drug administration, lipid solubility remains important if deeper tissues are to be penetrated with systemic antimicrobials.

Drugs that target gram-negative organisms include the water-soluble, weakly basic aminoglycosides. At the high concentrations achieved topically, they are generally also effective against *Staphylococcus* spp. and include tobramycin (0.3%; drug of choice for treatment of *Pseudomonas* spp.), gentamicin (available with the glucocorticoid betamethasone), and neomycin (less effective toward *Pseudomonas* spp. and generally available only in combination with other antimicrobials). Polymyxin B, whose systemic use is precluded by nephrotoxicity, is a water-soluble drug, characterized by limited intraocular distribution. The fluoroquinolones also target gram-negative organisms, including *Pseuodmonas* spp. as well as *Staphyloccoccus* spp. In contrast to the aminoglycosides, the fluoroquinolones are lipid soluble. Drugs include ciprofloxacin, and ofloxacin and its L-isomer, levofloxacin. Systemic fluoroquinolones have been associated with retinal degeneration in cats (see Chapter 7). The adversity reflects accumulation due to a missing transport pump in the blood-retinal barrier (personal communication,

Table **8-2a** Selected Topical Preparations for Treating Ophthalmic Infections

Drug	Effect	Target	Solubility	Trade Name	Manufacturer
Gentamicin 0.3%, solution, ointment	Antibacterial	Gram-negative	Water	*Gentocin (V)*	Schering–Plough
Polymyxin B 1 mg/mL	Antibacterial	Gram-negative	Water	*Terramycin (V)*	Pfizer
Tobramycin 0.3%	Antibacterial	Gram-negative	Water	*Tobrex*	Alcon
Tobramycin 0.3%/loteprednol etabonate 0.5%	Antibacterial, antiinflammatory	Gram-negative	Water	*Zylet*	Bausch & Lomb
Tobramycin 0.3% dexamethasone 0.1% suspension	Antibacterial, antiinflammatory	Gram-negative	Water	*Tobradex*	Alcon
Ciprofloxacin 0.3% solution and ointment	Antibacterial	Gram-negative>gram-positive	Lipid	*Ciloxan*	Alcon
Neomycin 0.35%/polymyxin B, 10,000 IU/mL/ Hydrocortisone 1%	Antibacterial, antiinflammatory	Gram-negative>gram-positive	Water	*Cortisporin*	King
Neomycin 0.35%/ dexamethasone 0.1%	Antibacterial, antiinflammatory	Gram-negative>gram-positive	Water	*Neodecadron*	Merck
Neomycin 0.35%/polymyxin B 10,000 IU/mL/dexamethasone 1%	Antibacterial, antiinflammatory	Gram-negative>gram-positive	Water	*Maxitrol*	Mertik
Norfloxacin 0.3% solution	Antibacterial	Gram-negative>gram-positive	Lipid	*Chibroxin*	Merck
Ofloxacin 0.3% solution	Antibacterial	Gram-negative>gram-positive	Lipid	*Ocuflox*	Allergan
Bacitracin ointment 500 U/g	Antibacterial	Gram-positive	Water	*AK-Tracin*	***
Erythromycin 0.5% ointment	Antibacterial	Gram-positive	Lipid	***	***
Levofloxacin 0.5% solution	Antibacterial	Mixed	Lipid	*Quizin*	Santen
Morifloxacin 0.5%	Antibacterial	Mixed	Lipid	*Vigamox*	Alcon
Polymyxin/bacitracin/zinc	Antibacterial	Mixed	Water	*Polytracin, Polysporin*	***
Polymyxin B/bacitracin/ neomycin	Antibacterial	Mixed	***	*Neosporin, Polymycin*	***
Sulfacetamide 10% solution, ointment	Antibacterial	Mixed	Lipid	*Bleph-10*	Allergan
Chloramphenicol 0.5% solution, 1% ointment	Antibacterial	Mixed, *Mycoplasma, Chlamydia*	Water	*Chloroptic (0.5%)*	Allergan
Tetracycline 1%	Antibacterial	Mixed, *Mycoplasma, Chlamydia*	***	*Achromycin*	Storz/Lederle
Natamycin suspension 5%	Antifungal	Antifungal	***	*Natacyn*	Alcon
Trifluridine 1%	Antiviral	Antiviral	***	*Viroptic*	Monarch
Valganciclovir HCl	Antiviral	Antiviral	***	*Valcyte*	Roche
Vidarabine 3% ointment	Antiviral	Antiviral	***	***	***
Idoxuridine 0.1% solution	Antiviral	Antiviral	***	*Compounded*	***

Katrina Mealey, Washington State University). It is not clear if the adversity may occur with topical use, but prudence suggests that safety not be assumed.[13] Drugs that target gram-positive organisms include the lipid-soluble erythromycin (0.5%; bacteriostatic), whose efficacy is limited by resistance, and the water-soluble bacitracin, which, like polymyxin B, is most known for its nephrotoxicity associated with systemic therapy. An example of a triple-antibiotic combination is one containing neomycin, polymyxin B, and bacitracin (see Table 8-2a). Broad-spectrum topical antimicrobials include chloramphenicol (prohibited for use in food animals), tetracyclines (drugs of choice for ocular *Mycoplasma* or *Chlamydia*), and the sulfonamides. Each is lipid soluble. Whitley[11] has described a preparation of vancomycin (3.1%) and cefazolin (3.3%) compounded from injectable products., although the combination might be improved by replacing cefazolin with a drug with a broader gram-negative spectrum.

Topical antifungal are limited and include the polyene natamycin. Its spectrum includes all fungal agents except dermatophytes. The imidazoles must be compounded from intravenous solutions (i.e., miconazole, fluconazole, and

Table 8-2b Subconjunctival Doses of Drugs Also Used Systemically

Drug	Dose (mg)	Target
Bacitracin	5000-10,000 U	Gram-positive
Clindamycin	15 to 50	Gram-positive
Erythromycin	100	Gram-positive
Amikacin	25-100	Gram-negative
Gentamicin	10 to 20	Gram-negative
Polymyxin B	100000 U	Gram-negative
Streptomycin	40-100	Gram-negative
Neomycin	100-500	Gram-negative >positive
Penicillin	500,000-1,000,000U	Gram-positive >gram-negative
Ampicillin	50-150	Mixed
Carbenicillin	100-250	Mixed
Cefazolin	50-100	Mixed
Ceftazidime	100	Mixed
Ticarcillin	1000	Mixed
Chloramphenicol	40-100	Mixed

itraconazole). Their spectrum includes opportunistic, dimorphic fungi and dermatophytes.

Treatment of Selected Infections

Use of systemic antimicrobials for treatment of ocular infections is complicated by poor drug penetration. Therefore topical therapy is indicated for external ocular infections, and subconjunctival administration is recommended for serious corneal or anterior chamber infections. For bacterial endophthalmitis, intravitreal antimicrobial therapy is indicated, although extreme caution is indicated for this route.[13] Treatment of intraocular infections can be supported with systemic therapy of lipid-soluble drugs that can achieve bactericidal concentrations. In addition to antibacterials, collagenase inhibitors such as *N*-acetylcysteine, sodium citrate, bacitracin, and tetracycline compounds have been recommended for treatment of corneal infections.

Treatment with tetracycline is indicated for control of *Mycoplasma* and *Chlamydia* spp. Cats may develop hypersensitivity manifested as acute conjunctivitis with topical treatment.[14] Oral therapy with tetracycline (5 mg/kg bid) stops shedding within 6 days. Azithromycin starting at 7 to 10 mg/kg qd for 2 weeks, followed by 5 mg/kg qd for 1 week, followed by 5 mg/kg qod for 14 days has been advocated, although the need for the complicated dosing regimen or the long duration is not clear. The presence of sneezing may indicate infection with feline calicivirus (FCV), for which supportive therapy is indicated. Conjunctivitis, often accompanied by ulcerative keratitis, can be a manifestation of feline herpesvirus (FHV-1), In addition to supportive therapy, topical preparations are available for its treatment (see also Chapter 10).[15] Antivirals include vidarabine, trifluridine, and idoxuridine (the latter must be compounded). These are generally virustatic, requiring frequent application (every 1 to 2 hours is preferred, but every 4 to 6 hours is acceptable).

Systemic treatment of experimentally induced *Chlamydia psittaci* with 19 days of amoxicillin–clavulanic acid (12.5 to 25 mg/kg bid) has been compared with doxycycline (10 to 15 mg/kg qd; positive control) in 5-month-old cats (n = 24; 8 per group) using a randomized, placebo-controlled, blinded design.[15a] Outcome was based on clinical scoring, including respiratory signs or corneal changes; other clinical signs were not described. Both treatments were associated with rapid clinical improvement and reduced chlamydial isolation, with amoxicillin–clavulanic acid being associated with less isolation. However, five of eight of the cats treated with amoxicillin–clavulanic acid, but no doxycycline-treated cats, became positive 3 weeks after treatment. These cats became negative again with 4 weeks of retreatment with amoxicillin–clavulanic acid and remained negative 6 months later.

Systemic therapy was described in cats experimentally infected with *C. felis*. Once the organisms was detected, cats were treated with azithromycin (10 mg/kg qd for 3 days followed by twice weekly) (n = 9; two untreated negative controls, two doxycycline-treated positive controls [10-15 mg/kg qd]).[16] At the end of the 21-day treatment period, untreated control cats were also treated. Despite an initial response to treatment (negative isolation to day 14), infection was eradicated in only one of five cats treated with azithromycin compared with both cats receiving doxycycline. However, it is not clear if the dosing regimen for azithromycin resulted in effective drug concentrations.

Otic Infections

Otitis Externa

Pathophysiology. Inflammation of the ear canal and the proximal pinna affects up to 20% of dogs, whereas fewer (up to 6% of) cats are affected.[17] A number of causes can be identified in otitis externa, and their resolution is paramount to successful therapy. Possible causes include foreign bodies, allergies, parasites (e.g., mites, chiggers), skin disorders of a keratinous or sebaceous origin, and autoimmune disorders. Structural characteristics of the ear also can predispose the animal to otitis externa, including pendulous ears, higher number of ceruminous glands, the vertical and horizontal paths of the canal, hair in the ear canal, stenotic ear canals, or neoplasm. Environmental factors also can contribute to the difficulty in treating otitis externa, including external conditions that perpetuate excessive moisture (e.g., humidity, bathing) or heat or irritants (e.g., irritating medicaments or shampoos). The presence of yeast or bacteria that are part of the normal flora perpetuates the inflammatory process, and, with time, the inflammatory process itself will cause proliferative changes that complicate therapy. One of the more important predisposing factors to otitis externa is inappropriate treatment, including undertreatment and overtreatment.[17] Ultimately, in some animals surgical treatment will be indicated (Figure 8-2).

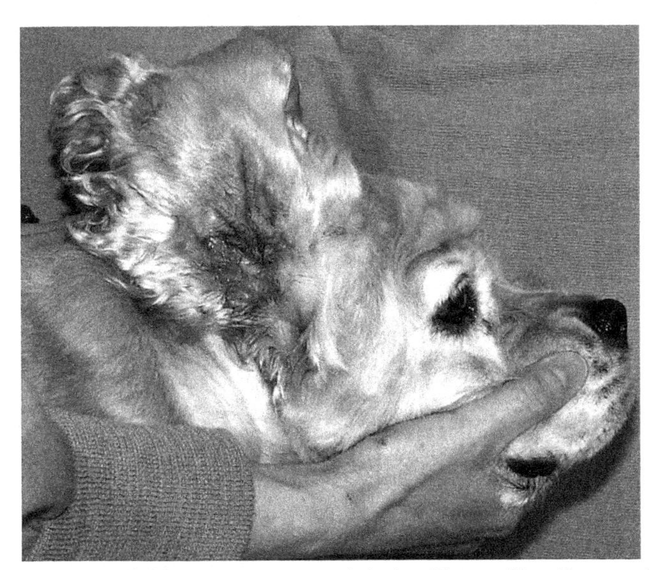

Figure 8-2 Otitis externa associated with proliferation and inflammation may fail to respond to topical and systemic antimicrobial therapy despite intensive cleaning. (Photo courtesy Harry W. Boothe, Jr, DVM, MS, DACVS, Auburn, AL.)

Microbial Targets. Bacterial organisms found in normal ears include *S. epidermidis* and *Staphylococcus intermedius (Staphylococcus pseudintermedius*; see Chapter 6) and *Micrococcus* spp. Coliforms are found less commonly. Infection usually can be distinguished from colonization by the presence of large numbers of organisms, particularly if the culture is pure. Infection also is indicated by the presence of inflammation and phagocytized bacteria. Inflammation reflects, in part, the breakdown of fatty materials by organisms into irritating by-products. *S. intermedius* is the most common organism (30% to 50%) associated with otitis externa, followed by *Pseudomonas aeruginosa, Proteus* spp., *Streptococcus* spp., *E. coli,* and *Corynebacterium* spp. The infecting organism also appears to be time dependent in that acute otitis is generally associated with *Staphylococcus,* whereas chronic otitis more commonly involves *Pseudomonas* spp. This may refelect, however response to chronic antimicrobial therapy.

Petersen[18] reported on the frequency and susceptibility of *S. intermedius* and *P. aeruginosa* in canine ear samples (n = 553) submitted to a state diagnostic laboratory between 1992 and 1997. Sampling methods varied. *S. intermedius* was isolated from 50% of ear samples but was the sole isolate in only 32% of the samples positive for *S. intermedius. P. aeruginosa* was isolated from 28% of ear cultures and was the sole isolate in 33% of *P. aeruginosa* samples.

The susceptibility of both *S. intermedius* and *P. aeruginosa* isolated from canine skin and ears appears to be changing across time (Table 8-3). A number of investigators have described their susceptibility. A review of the data suggests that the incidence of methicillin resistance is increasing, with a decrease in susceptibility of *Staphylococcus* spp. in general emerging in isolates collected during the period between 2003 to 2006. Morris[19] focused on the susceptibility of methicillin-resistant isolates, including both coagulase-positive (*S. aureus,* and *S. intermedius*), as well as *Staphylococcus schleiferi* (including both coagulase-negative and positive subspecies; see also the discussion of *Pyoderma).* Of the total number of resistant isolates found in skin or ear, 28% of the methicillin-resistant *S. aureus* (MRSA), 40% of the methicillin-resistant *S. intermedius* (MRSI), and 33% of the methicillin-resistant *Staphylococcus schleiferi* (MRSS; presumed to be coagulase-positive subspecies *schleiferi*) were in the skin, and 5% MRSA, 26% MRSI, and 47% MRSS were located in the ear. Rubin[20] described the susceptibility of 106 canine *P. aeurginosa* isolates cultured from soft tissue infections, including otitis externa and interna (see Table 8-3). No information was available regarding previous antimicrobial therapy in these animals. The limited amount of data precludes assessment across time; however, *Pseudomonas* is an organism recognized for its inherent resistance to multiple drugs, with an increasing tendency of resistance toward drugs to which it is normally considered susceptible (e.g., fluoroquinolones).

The combined data, particularly from *Staphylococcus* spp. isolates, demonstrate the limited susceptibility of these organisms to drugs most often used systemically or topically to treat organisms infecting the skin or ear. Culture and susceptibility data might increasingly become the basis for drug selection and dose design. Although the applicability of culture and susceptibility testing to the topical treatment of otitis externa may be controversial, the incidence of resistance is sufficient to justify culturing even in the earliest stages of infection, particularly in those patients at risk for recurrence, such that emergent resistance can be detected. Susceptibility testing is clearly recommended if gram-negative organisms are expected or in the face of severe or chronic otitis, failed antimicrobial therapy, and the presence of inflammatory cells. Testing is also recommended if systemic therapy is anticipated. Care should be taken to appropriately prepare and collect cultures from infected ears. Frustratingly, the accuracy of susceptibility testing may be questioned simply because of differences in laboratories. Schick[21] compared the results of cultures simultaneously submitted from dogs with otitis. Swabs were rubbed together to ensure similar samplings. Labs agreed regarding the presence of *Pseudomonas* spp. only 83% of the time. Susceptibility of the isolates to amikacin varied in 13 of 16 samples, for gentamicin 10 of 16, and for enrofloxacin 9 of 16.

In cats *Pasteurella multocida* joins *Staphylococcus* and *Streptococcus* spp. as a commonly infecting organism; the coliforms and *Pseudomonas* spp. are less common causes. *Malassezia pachydermatis* is an opportunistic yeast that occurs in up to 49% of normal dogs and 23% of normal cats. The numbers increase in dogs with otitis, however, being present in 80% or more of dogs. Although it is likely that *Malassezia* spp. contributes to otitis externa, its role is not clear. Nonetheless, therapy should target this organism as well.

Antimicrobial and Adjuvant Options. The public health implications of treating methicillin-resistant *Staphylococcus* spp. in dogs or cats are addressed in the discussion of *Pyoderma.* Because successful treatment of otitis externa is critically dependent on proper cleaning, it is difficult to separate antimicrobial therapy from adjuvant therapy. The goals of

Table 8-3 Percent Susceptibility of Canine *Staphylococcus* spp. and *Pseudomonas aeurginosa* Isolates

ORGANISM	*S. INTERMEDIUS*				MRSA[19]	MRSI[19]	MRSS[19]	*P. AEURUGINOSA*				
Collection Site	**Skin[18†]**	**Ear[18†]**	**Multiple*†‡**		**Multiple‡**	**Multiple‡**	**Multiple‡**	**Skin[18]**	**Ear[18]**	**Multiple***		**Ear[20]**
Years	1992-1997[18]	1992-1997	2003-2005	2006-2007	2003-2004	2003-2004	2003-2004	1992-1997	1992-1997	2003-2005	2006-2007	2003-2006
Sample size (n)	497	553	196	102	39	57	49	42	311	98	61	106
Drugs												
Amikacin			100	92				100		95	100	96
Amoxicillin-clavulanic			96	66				0	0			1
Ampicillin	28	48	20	17								0
Cefazolin				64								0
Cefotaxime												74
Cefpodoxime												0
Ceftazidime												94
Ceftiofur												3
Cephalothin	99	99	96	64				0	0			0
Chloramphenicol			99	97	90	95	100			0	0	1
Ciprofloxacin	99	99	82					95	88	76		84
Clindamycin	78	88	79	43	28	32	86					
Difloxacin												57
Enrofloxacin			77	55	10	55	35			18	64	69
Levofloxacin												84
Marbofloxacin					10	57	29				76	73
Orbifloxacin											25	48
Erythromycin	79	90	77	43	15	35	88					
Gentamicin	97	98	97	87	92	81	88	100		93	97	93
Impenem												99
Meropenem												99
Oxacillin	99	99		72								
Penicillin	28	49	23	18								
Piperacillin								100	99	100		
Piperacillin/tazobactam												95
Tetracycline	55	74	65	42	64	82	86		0	0		2
Ticarcillin								98	82	90	97	
TMPS	71*	82	76	66	97	68	100	0		0	0	43

MR: Methicillin-resistant *SA: Staphylococcus aureus; SI: Staphylococcus pseudintermedius;SS: Staphylococcus* strains; *TMPS*, trimethoprim–sulfonamide.
*Unpublished data by author representing hospital population.
†Includes both resistant and susceptible isolates.
‡Most isolates are from skin or ear.

therapy for otitis externa are to identify and resolve the primary factors, reduce inflammation, and control or eradicate infection. Sedation or anesthesia may be necessary for proper cleansing. Cleansing should remove irritating oils, waxes, and other debris that might serve as a nidus of infection by providing a microenvironment favorable to the growth of microorganisms. Ear cleaning should be less aggressive in the presence of severely swollen or proliferative canals; in such patients initial therapy might begin with antiinflammatory doses of glucocorticoids and antimicrobials, both systemically and topically.

KEY POINT 8-5 The goals of therapy for otitis externa are to identify and resolve the primary factors, reduce inflammation, and control or eradicate infection. Repetitive sedation or anesthesia may be necessary for proper cleansing.

Ceruminolytics contain various surface active agents or emulsifiers (dioctyl sodium sulfosuccinate, carbamide peroxide, squalene, propylene glycol, glycerin, oil) that dissolve wax accumulation and associated debris. They should be used as an initial flush. Less messy water-soluble agents (dioctyl sodium sulfosuccinate, propylene glycol) are often preferred.[22] Carbamide peroxide, a common ingredient of human preparations that is seldom found in veterinary preparations, releases nascent oxygen, causing a bubbling action that softens and removes debris. Combination products may contain drying agents such as isopropyl alcohol, silicone dioxide, and alpha hydroxy acids (lactic, malic, or salicylic acid). In addition to their drying effects, these materials may also have mild antimicrobial effects.[22]

Flushing solutions facilitate removal of debris. Although water and saline are the safest, some products contain germicidal ingredients. Chlorhexidine can be diluted to a 0.05% solution and used topically. Although ototoxicity should lead to cautious use in the presence of a perforated eardrum, one study failed to provide evidence of damage after 21 days of therapy in dogs with experimentally traumatized membranes; the power of the study to detect a significant difference is not stated.[22] Povidone–iodine at 0.1% to 1% can provide bactericidal activity in flushing solutions, although it can cause contact irritation. Because of ototoxicity, solutions with less than 0.5% iodine are preferred if the eardrum is ruptured. Iodine might also be administered as a polyhydroxidine complex (Xenodine). Because it contains 0.5% of titratable iodine, it is less irritating and provides a longer duration of activity. Efficacy against *Pseudomonas* spp. has been established with this product. It must be used in an aqueous environment and therefore should be used within 2 hours after cleaning to maximize its effects.[22] Acetic acid is a relatively inexpensive agent, available as white or brown vinegar in a 5% solution. Antimicrobial effects occur because of direct damage as well as acidification of the local environment. The acidic pH may also facilitate removal of necrotic debris. *Pseudomonas* spp. succumbs to a 2% solution within 1 minute of contact,[22] whereas a 5% solution is effective against *Staphylococcus* spp. *Streptococcus* spp., *E. coli,* and *Proteus* spp. The preparation is irritating at 2% to 5% concentrations, however, and inhibition of wound healing and ototoxicity may occur at concentrations of 2.5%. Dilutions of 1:1, 1:2, or 1:3 in water daily or every other day have been recommended.

Topical antimicrobial treatment of otitis externa is generally indicated regardless of whether systemic therapy is implemented. Topical products intended specifically for treatment of otitis externa (Tables 8-4 and 8-5) generally contain various drugs intended to target bacteria, yeast, and inflammation. Vehicles are designed to maximize drug solubility (only dissolved drug will passively diffuse) but must also allow drug movement from the vehicle into tissues. Antibacterial agents often include products that are associated with severe systemic toxicity when given orally or parenterally; topical administration generally is not associated with systemic adversities.

On the basis of a MEDLINE search and review of the literature in human medicine, the ototopic use of antimicrobials does not appear to be associated with an increased risk of antimicrobial resistance.[23] However, the relevance to canine or feline ear, for which the pathophysiology is substantially different, is not clear. Ototoxicity is, however, likely for many antimicrobial drugs when administered in the ear canal, especially in the presence of a perforated tympanic membrane (see later discussion).

KEY POINT 8-6 Topical treatment of otitis externa is generally indicated regardless of whether systemic therapy is implemented.

Topical antimicrobials generally are selected on the basis of cytology and potentially Gram staining. A number of products are commercially available (see Table 8-4). For selected drugs, ophthalmic (directly or diluted) or injectable (diluted) products may also be used. Vehicles used in topical products represent a balance between drug solubility and drug delivery.It may be necessary for vehicles to be pH balanced to maximize solubility. Demulcents (polyethylene or propylene glycol or glycerin) act to suspend non–water-soluble drugs; the glycol agents may irritate an already irritated ear. DMSO is included in some otic preparations as a vehicle, although it also has significant antiinflammatory effects. The agent is very hygroscopic and as such is an effective carrier agent for other drugs included in an otic preparation. In addition, DMSO provides mild antibacterial and antifungal actions as well as antiinflammatory and antifibroplastic effects. Other vehicles used to administer drugs useful for otic disorders include solutions, lotions, ointments, and other oil-based products. Occlusive oils may be undesirable for exudative lesions. Ointments and oil-based products can, however, be used in cases of chronic otitis externa that are dry. Generally, topical preparations should be applied twice daily. A number of home remedies have been recommended for treatment of otitis externa (see Table 8-5). Caution is recommended when making new preparations or modifying old preparations. A number of drug interactions between drugs and their vehicles can inhibit the efficacy of any of the drugs. In addition, drugs must be dissolved to be effective, and the addition of solid drugs (i.e., as powders or crushed tablets) to ointment vehicles (e.g., petrolatum jelly) is likely to yield an occlusive but minimally effective agent. Some acceptable modifications of commercially available products are noted in Table 8-5.

Table 8-4 Examples of Commercially Available Topical Products Used for Treatment of Otitis Externa

	ACTIVE INGREDIENT			
Product	**Antibacterial**	**Antifungal**	**Antiinflammatory**	**Vehicle/Other Ingredients**
Baytril Otic	Enrofloxacin 0.5%	Silver sulfadiazine 1%	—	Benzyl alcohol
Coly-Mycin*†	Colistin 0.3% Neomycin		Hydrocortisone 1%	Polysorbate 80, acetic acid, sodium acetate
Derma 4‡	Neomycin 0.25%	Nystatin	Triamcinolone acetonide 0.1%	Polyethylene, mineral oil, gel (ointment)
Forte-Topical‡	Neomycin 0.25% Polymyxin Procaine penicillin G		Hydrocortisone acetate 0.2% Hydrocortisone sodium succinate 0.125%	Suspension
Gentocin otic	Gentamicin 0.3%		Betamethasone valerate 0.1%	Hydroxycellulose, glacial acetic acid, water, ethanol, alcohol, glycerin, propylene glycol
Liquichlor‡	Chloramphenicol		Prednisolone 0.17%	Mineral oil, petrolatum (ointment), squalane, tetracaine 0.42%
Neo-Predef‡	Neomycin 0.35%		Isoflupredone acetate 0.1%	Anhydrous lanolin, petrolatum, mineral oil (ointment)
Otic solution*	Polymyxin B Neomycin		Hydrocortisone 1%	
Otomax†	Gentamicin 0.3%	Clotrimazole	Betamethasone valerate 0.1%	Ointment
Panolog‡	Neomycin	Nystatin	Triamcinolone acetonide 0.1%	Polyethylene, mineral oil, gel (ointment)
Postatex	Orbafloxacin	Posaconazole	Mometasone	—
Tobrex ophthalmic*	Tobramycin 0.3%			
Tresaderm‡	Neomycin 0.32%	Thiabendazole	Dexamethasone 0.1%	Glycerin, propylene glycol, water, alcohol

*Human preparation.
†Second-line product.
‡First-line product.

Table 8-5 Homemade Otic Products or Modifications of Commercially Available Otic Products

Drugs	**Antimicrobial**	**Antiinflammatory**	**Modification**
Baytril	Enrofloxacin 22.7 mg/mL	None	Dilute 1:1 up to 1:25 in water, 5% DMSO, saline, Synotic
Novalsan solution	Chlorhexidine diacetate 2%	None	Dilute 1:1 in water
Silvadene	Silver sulfadiazine 0.5%	None	Mix 1:1 with water
Synotic	Enrofloxacin* 22.7 mg/mL	Fluocinolone acetonide	Replace 1 mL of Synotic solution with 1 mL of injectable preparation
Tris-EDTA	Tris-EDTA	None	6.05 mg EDTA, 12 g tromethamine (Trizma base), 1 L distilled water. pH must be adjusted to 8 with hydrochloric acid.† Autoclave
Xenodine	Polyhydroxidine 1%	None	Dilute 1:5 with water

DMSO, Dimethyl sulfoxide.
*Represents a modification.
†Addition of 0.3 g Gentocin/L has been recommended; see text for precautions.

Note that modification of a product may alter the stability, and a shelf-life of 1 week or less might be prudent unless data exist to support a longer beyond-use date. Several in-practice compounded preparations have been described elsewhere.[24]

Examples of antibacterials used in otic preparations to target gram-negative organisms include the aminoglycosides gentamicin (0.3%), tobramycin (0.3%), and neomycin (0.33%) and the cell membrane–active agents colistin (0.3%) and polymyxin B (5000 IU/mL). Topical aminoglycosides also target *Staphylococcus* spp. whereas systemically, amikacin is more effective toward *Pseudomonas* spp., and gentamicin is more effective toward *Staphylococcus* spp., systemic use of an aminoglycoside as sole therapy for treatment of *Staphylococcus* spp. is discouraged. An otic preparation for amikacin can be compounded from the commercially available injectable product by adding 30 to 50 mg/mL to sterile saline or Tris-EDTA. Because aminoglycosides are more effective in an alkaline environment, they should be used either before or 1 or more hours after acidifying agents. Silver sulfadiazine (0.5%) is an ointment approved for humans to prevent or treat infection in burn patients. Its spectrum also includes *Pseudomonas* spp. However, the product, as approved in humans, may cause skin irritation. Silver sulfadiazine (1%) is available in commercial products combined with enrofloxacin (0.5%) or as a micronized powder (e.g., www.spectrumrx.com) that can be reconstituted in sterile water to a 0.5% to 1% solution (5 and 10 mg/mL, respectively). An otic preparation containing orbafloxacin and posaconazole as an antifungal drug with mometasone as an antiinflammatory has recently been approved for dogs (Table 8-4). A number of other antimicrobials have been administered topically, including the narrow-spectrum fusidic acid for treatment of *Staphylococcus* spp., antipseudomonadals such as colistin or polymyxin B (10,000 U/mL of Neosporin GU,[24] fluoroquinolones (discussed later), and ticarcillin (which also targets *Staphylococcus* spp.). Ciprofloxacin and ofloxacin are available as human otic preparations. Ciprofloxacin is generally more potent than enrofloxacin against *Pseudomonas* spp.

Trothmethamineethylenediamine-tetraacetate (EDTA, Tris-EDTA, or commercial Triz/EDTA) is a topically applied compound that chelates cations, thus rendering the cell wall and membrane of both gram-positive and gram-negative organisms more permeable to antimicrobials. Penetration of antibacterials subsequently is facilitated. Treatment should be timed such that microorganisms are exposed to Tris-EDTA before peak concentrations of antimicrobials reach the site of infection. Direct addition of antibiotics such as gentamicin to the buffer solution may be less desirable than pretreatment with Tris-EDTA, followed later by antimicrobials (to allow time for chelation of cations). Because cations are also removed from the lipopolysaccharide covering, EDTA may be particularly effective for treatment of gram-negative organisms. Aminoglycosides in particular are facilitated because cations that otherwise would repel positively charged drugs such as aminoglycosides are removed. Synergisim has been demonstrated with Tris-EDTA and aminoglycosides (amikacin and neomycin) against *S. intermedius, Proteus mirabilis, P. aeruginosa,* and *E. coli.* Combination solutions appear to be stable for at least 3 months.[25]

KEY POINT 8-7 Pretreatment of an infected site with *tris*-EDTA has the potential to enhance efficacy of many antimicrobials against many bacteria.

However Tris-EDTA synergisim also has been demonstrated, albeit in vitro, for other drugs. These include fluoroquinolones and amoxicillin. Tris-EDTA also appeared to have a synergistic effect with 0.15% chlorhexidine digluconate in an open, unblinded clinical trial in dogs (n = 11) with chronic otitis externa associated with both gram-negative and gram-positive infections. Enrofloxacin was also used in these dogs.[26]

A common otic preparation compounded by veterinarians for treatment of otitis externa combines 12 mL of 100 mg/mL enrofloxacin in 8 oz (240 mL) of T8 (alcohol combined with the spermicide nonoxynol-9), 4-8 mg of dexamethasone phosphate, and 1 to 2 mL of DMSO, yielding a final product of 0.5% enrofloxacin and 0.0016 to 0.0032% dexamethasone. Because T8 can be irritating, Tris-EDTA might be substituted, although the advantages of pretreatment with Tris-EDTA will be lost.

Topically applied antifungal otic agents generally target *M. pachydermatis* and include the imidazoles clotrimazole (1%), miconazole (1%), and the benzimidazole thiabendazole (1%) and the polyene macrolides nystatin and amphotericin B. Among these, those containing thiabendazole might be considered first line.[17,22] Ketoconazole is available as a topical preparation that can be reformulated into solutions that can be used topically.[24] The allylamine, terbinafine, is also effective against *Malassezia* spp. and is available as a 1% solution.

Antiinflammatories often are included in topical otic solutions. Examples include DMSO (60%) and glucocorticoids. Among the glucocorticoids used topically, the order of potency (which should not be confused with efficacy) is fluocinolone > betamethasone or dexamethasone > isoflupredone > triamcinolone > prednisolone (prednisone should not be administered topically) > hydrocortisone. Note that sufficient drug may be absorbed with topical therapy that the hypothalamic–pituitary–adrenal axis will be affected.[27]

Several clinical trials have addressed the topical treatment of otitis externa. A preparation containing marbofloxacin (0.3%), clotrimazole (1%), and dexamethasone (0.09%) (10 gtt/ear/day) was prospectively compared with one containing polymyxin B (5.5 IU/mL), miconazole (2.3%), and prednisolone acetate (0.5%) (5 gtt/ear/bid) in dogs (n = 140; ages 4 months to 16 years) with clinical signs indicative of acute or subacute otitis externa.[28] Treatments were randomized. Exclusion criteria included treatment within the previous 10 days with topical or systemic antimicrobials (including antifungals), nonsteroidal antiinflammatories, glucocorticoids (previous 14 days), or a long-acting steroidal anti-inflammatory drugs (previous 60 days). The presence of concurrent auricular disease, including ear parasites, foreign bodies, and neoplasia or hyperplasia were also a basis for exclusion. Pregnant or nursing dogs were excluded. Culture (swab) revealed disease was associated with *Staphylococcus* spp. (39.5%; 82% *S. intermedius*), *Pseudomonas* spp. (12.9%; *P. aeruginosa* predominant), *Enterobacteraceae* spp. (17%; *Proteus*, spp. *E. coli*), and *Malassezia* spp. (58%). *Streptococcus* spp. and other gram-positive isolates represented another 11.4%, whereas 10.5% were infected with other gram-negatives; 8.6% of ears were cultured as no growth. Susceptibility testing indicated that 85% of isolates were susceptible to marbofloxacin. Interestingly, 43.5% were susceptible to polymyxin B, a drug generally considered ineffective against *Staphylococcus* spp. and other gram-positive as well as selective gram-negative organisms (e.g., *Proteus* spp.). Ears were scored for severity of otitis (0-3, with 3 most severe) and cultured (in addition to baseline) before, in the event of failure, or 2 weeks into therapy if the cause was *Pseudomonas* spp. Approximately 75% of yeast were susceptible to both antifungals studied. Owners and investigators were blinded to the treatment groups. Ears were cleaned according to a predefined schedule, based on the underlying classification scheme (erythematous [EO] or suppurative [SO]) approximately 2 to 3 times per week (with physiologic saline on days 0, 2, 4 (EO) or days 1 and 6 (SO).

Response was assessed on days 7 and 14, with treatment continued to day 14 if indicated on day 7 assessment. The preparations were found to be equivalent with regard to success (58% for the marbofloxacin preparation compared to 41% for the polymyxin-based preparation; failure to identify this difference as significant may have reflected the sample size), but the marbofloxacin preparation was considerd superior in terms of control of pain, pus, appearance, and odor on day 14. The differential response apparently was not statistically significant, although better efficacy would be expected for marbofloxacin based on the limited spectrum of polymyxin B.

Systemic therapy is indicated for severe infections but should be coupled with topical therapy and should be based on culture and susceptibility testing. Doses should be designed with the site of infection in mind; distribution is likely to be limited to the site, particularly with marked inflammation. Water-soluble drugs might be administered topically, and lipid-soluble drugs systemically. No data support selection of the same versus different but complementary antimicrobials when both topical and systemic therapy are used. The advantage of using the same antimicrobial topically as administered systemically is increased likelihood of effective drug concentrations at the site of infection. The advantages of combination therapy have been discussed previously (see Chapter 6) and are particularly appealing for the treatment of chronic, minimally responsive otitis externa. Oral antifungals such as ketoconazole or itraconazole may be indicated for control of infection caused by *Malassezia* spp. (see Chapter 9). Glucocorticoids may be necessary for rapid control of inflammation regardless of the cause or duration of infection. General principles of glucocorticoid therapy should be followed (see Chapter 30).

Treatment of Specific Causes of Otitis Externa

Acute otitis externa. Although ultimately the normal ear is clean and dry, severe swelling or proliferation indicates less aggressive therapy initially and the potential need for glucocorticoid therapy (topical or systemic). Once swelling is decreased, cleaning will be more effective. If the tympanic membrane is intact, initial cleaning begins with an application of a ceruminolytic, which can then be rinsed with water, or an antimicrobial solution such as chlorhexidine, povidone, polyhydroxidine iodine, or acetic acid. If the tympanic membrane is ruptured, only water or saline should be used for cleansing because many of the cleansing agents are ototoxic. Cleansing can be accomplished at home, although initial cleaning might be more thorough if performed under general anesthesia, particularly in intractable patients. For ears in which a large amount of debris has accumulated, removal of material may require alligator forceps through an otoscope and flushing with either an open-ended Tomcat catheter or a 3.5 to 5 French feeding tube and syringe or an in-house vacuum system. Hair that might obstruct drainage of the ear canal or facilitate collection of debris should be removed.

Because otitis externa tends to be associated with similar pathogens, regardless of the underlying cause, topical medication applied after cleaning generally contains an antimicrobial, antifungal, and glucocorticoid. Glucocorticoids decrease not only swelling and proliferation but also apocrine and sebaceous secretions. Note that topical administration does not preclude suppression of the hypothalamic–pituitary–adrenal axis, and the long-term use of these products is discouraged. In the event of moderate to marked swelling of the ear canal and pinna, short-term use of systemic glucocorticoids may be indicated. Note that care should be taken not to use glucocorticoids in combination with nonsteroidal antiinflammatories (including treatment intended for control of osteoarthritis). To minimize the risk of antimicrobial resistance, products that contain commonly used first-line antimicrobial and antifungals directed toward *Malassezia* spp. might be chosen for acute (nonrecurring) otitis externa. Culture and susceptibility data are the best basis for selection of the most appropriate second-line antimicrobial. In the event of moderate swelling of the ear canal and pinna, topical antimicrobial therapy probably should be accompanied by systemic therapy. Therapy for acute otitis externa should be followed through rechecks at 10- to 14-day intervals. Resolution generally requires 2 to 4 weeks.

Chronic otitis. Resolution of chronic or recurring otitis includes treatment of specific diseases of the ear that allow perpetuation of infection or inflammation. Culture and susceptibility data collected during cleansing of the ears under general anesthesia should be the basis of antimicrobial selection, particularly systemic. Thorough visual examination accompanied by cytologic examination can help identify other underlying causes. Antiinflammatories (e.g., oral prednisolone at 0.5 mg/kg every 12 hours, tapered when indicated) are indicated in the presence of marked inflammation and when proliferation precludes effective examination. Topical therapy with intense cleansing should be implemented; several months of topical therapy may be indicated. Systemic therapy should accompany topical therapy if deeper infection is suspected (i.e., marked proliferation or ulceration).[23]

Bacterial otitis. The need for antimicrobial therapy for bacterial otitis externa should be based on cytologic evidence of inflammatory debris and intracellular organisms supports bacterial infection. A first-line product containing neomycin or chloramphenicol might be appropriate. Severe inflammation may indicate the need for a lipid soluble systemic antimicrobial therapy. Among the more commonly selected systemic antimicrobials are amoxicillin–clavulanic acid, a fluorinated quinolone, or a first-generation cephalosporin.[22] Failure to respond to first-line medicaments may indicate the need for culture. Some authors recommend discontinuing antimicrobial therapy for 3 to 5 days before culture; however, while a false negative might be ignored, a false positive is a clear indicator that therapy may fail. Otic preparations containing gentamicin or tobramycin might represent the second line of medicaments for infections resistant to neomycin or chloramphenicol.

Otitis caused by *Pseudomonas* spp. can be among the more frustrating problems to treat and often is the incentive behind the formation of homemade otic products. Flushing with an acetic acid–based solution is indicated. Commercially available otic products have been modified by the addition of drugs effective against *P. aeruginosa* (amikacin, enrofloxacin, polymyxin B, or colistin sulfate) or the addition of antiinflammatory drugs. Several alternatives can be considered for refractory cases. Enrofloxacin has been added to commercially available otic solutions, but it (or ciprofloxacin or marbofloxacin) also may be the oral antimicrobial of choice. Note that ciprofloxacin is more potent against *Pseudomonas* spp. and may be preferred topically; oral enrofloxacin will result in ciprofloxacin exposure, as well as enrofloxacin. The maximum end of the fluoroquinolone dosing regimen should be considered when treating a refractory case of *Pseudomonas*-induced otitis externa (i.e., 20 mg/kg once daily for enrofloxacin, 30 to 40 mg/kg orally for ciprofloxacin in dogs). Other products to be used in resistant cases include silver sulfadiazine, xenodine, and chlorhexidine (1.5%).

Malassezia pachydermatis. *Malassezia pachydermatis* is an opportunistic organism that, in large numbers, causes proliferatory changes in the ear. Its presence may contribute to bacterial otitis, and thus its control may be important in the treatment of otitis. Because control of inflammation may be paramount to controlling infection by *Malassezia,* spp. glucocorticoids such as those provided in otic preparations may be indicated. Ketoconazole appears to be among the most efficacious antifungal drugs, followed by miconazole, nystatin, clotrimazole, and amphotericin B.[22] Thiabendazole (the active antifungal in Tresaderm), however, may be sufficiently effective, allowing other antifungals to be reserved for resistant cases. Routinely used cleaning and drying solutions should be used on a daily to alternate-day basis to facilitate control.

Ear mites generally occur in young animals, and their presence is determined by direct examination. Carbaryl and pyrethrin-based products should be used for at least a 3-week cycle to ensure killing of adults and immature mites. Products containing thiabendazole should be selected because the product probably kills all stages of mites, including eggs. Polyhydroxidine iodine may also be effective when administered once weekly for 4 weeks. *Otodectes* can be treated with ivermectin given orally once a week for 4 weeks or subcutaneously every 10 to 14 days. With severe infestations ivermectin should be combined with other topical miticides. Because other portions of the body may harbor mites that infest the ear, affected animals should be dipped.

Seborrheic otitis or ceruminous otitis usually accompanies endocrinopathies. Secondary bacterial and *Malassezia* spp. infections are not uncommon with this disorder. The first-line medications should be effective for management of most cases, but longer-term management may require a combination of cleansing, drying, and glucocorticoid products applied once to thrice weekly. Cocker Spaniels and other breeds occasionally develop what appears to be a local hypersensitivity to cerumen, resulting in a progressively inflammatory, proliferative disease that ultimately may result in calcification of auricular cartilages. Control of inflammation initially may require oral glucocorticoids accompanied by topical application of a potent (e.g., dexamethasone or fluocinolone) glucocorticoid. Topical antimicrobials (antibacterial and antifungal) probably are also indicated; systemic antimicrobial therapy may also be necessary. The ears should be frequently flushed with cleansing and drying agents. For some animals long-term, low-dose glucocorticoid therapy may be necessary.

Swimmer's ear generally occurs because frequent swimming encourages low-grade inflammation and subsequent maceration. Ears should be kept clean and dry. Topical antiinflammatory therapy and, in some cases, topical antimicrobial therapy may be necessary. Products should be used on the day of swimming and for several days after.

Otitis Media

Otitis media associated with infection of the middle ear generally results from extension of otitis externa through a perforated eardrum.[17,29] A perforated eardrum may be hard to detect and must be distinguished from a "false" eardrum. Indications that infection of the external ear has extended into the middle ear include persistence of otitis externa, pain, swelling or narrowing of the ear canal, and evidence of neurologic involvement such as facial palsy (ptosis or paralysis of the lip or ear) or vestibular abnormalities. Less commonly, infection may follow extension from the pharynx by way of the auditory tube or hematogenous spread. Radiographs and surgical exploration may be necessary for both diagnosis and treatment. Debris should be cytologically examined for evidence of predisposing conditions. Fungal infections (e.g., aspergillosis, infection caused by *Malassezia*) spp., foreign bodies such as grass awns, neoplasia, inflammatory polyps, and tumors, including cholesteatoma, are among the more common causes of otitis externa. Calcification of auricular cartilage may also predispose subjects to the development of infection. Breeds apparently predisposed to otitis media include Cocker Spaniels and German Shepherd Dogs.

Medical management of otitis media is often unsuccessful unless accompanied by surgical management, particularly if inflammation is severe and chronic or if the ear canal is stenotic. Surgical intervention may be the most cost-effective means of management and should provide the most accurate diagnosis. Treatment includes removal of debris and topical application of an antimicrobial with or without an antifungal preparation until the infection appears resolved. After debris is cleaned from the external canal, myringotomy (under general anesthesia) may be necessary to clean debris, collect a sample for culture and cytologic examination, and relieve pain associated with the infection. Intraoperative infusion of the bulla may be an effective means of providing higher concentrations of an antimicrobial,[29] but duration of exposure is not clear and residual effects should not be anticipated. However, flushing the bulla is an effective means of reducing the microbial flora.[30] In a retrospective study of 34 dogs afflicted with otitis media, the most likely causative organisms were *Enterococcus* and *Streptococcus* spp., *Pseudomonas* spp., *Proteus* spp., and *E. coli*.[30] The varied population among animals limits empirical prediction of either the organism or, as was demonstrated in the study, susceptibility. Disconcertingly, empirical antimicrobial selection was inappropriate on the basis of culture and susceptiblitity data in nearly 60% of the patients. This probably reflects, in part, previous antimicrobial therapy.[30] This study also demonstrated that the preflushing and postflushing cultures often did not match, and postflushing culture was recommended.

Systemic antibacterial therapy should begin in conjunction with topical therapy; current recommendations are to continue therapy for at least 4 to 6 weeks. For fungal infections (e.g., one caused by *Malassezia* spp.), oral therapy with an imidazole antifungal (e.g., thiabendazole, ketoconazole, itraconazole) should be implemented. For severe inflammation glucocorticoids may be given topically or, if indicated, systemically for the first 1 to 3 weeks of treatment. Topical glucocorticoid therapy can be continued if inflammation persists after resolution of infection. When used as a vehicle, DMSO may also impart antiinflammatory effects. Daily flushes of 5% acetic acid in water (1:1 to 1:3) may further control symptoms. Therapy must be continued until the tympanic membrane is repaired (generally 21 to 35 days). Control of the inflammatory process may be necessary before tympanic healing is complete. Should the tympanum not heal, debris may once again accumulate, and the ear must be flushed again.

Topical therapy of otitis media is complicated by the risk of ototoxicity, which is complicated by inflammation.[29] Although response to inflammation may decrease the risk of ototoxins reaching the inner ear, assessing the degree of protection is difficult. Ototoxins can affect either the vestibular apparatus or the cochlea; subtle changes in response to ototoxins may be difficult to detect. Either the active ingredient or the vehicle of a topical preparation may be ototoxic. Among the known ototoxins that might be used to treat the ear topically are chlorhexidine, fluoroquinolones, aminoglycosides, polymyxins, eruthromycin, detergents, and alcohols.[32] The lack of data regarding the ototoxic potential of a given product does not necessarily mean that the product is safe. In general, direct application of any antimicrobial to the external ear in the presence of a perforated eardrum is discouraged.

Otitis interna

Otitis interna or labyrinthitis resulting from infection of the inner ear also occurs as a result of extension from otitis externa and media (see discussion of otitis externa), movement of organisms through the auditory tube, or hematogenous spread. Foreign bodies, tumors (including cholesteatoma), or other occlusive or inflammatory objects may predispose the subject to infection.[31] Clinical signs vary with the extent of vestibular dysfunction, which in turn reflects the extent of infection and accompanying inflammation. Continuation of infection into the meninges is more likely in cats than in dogs.

Cultures that reflect infecting organisms might be obtained by sampling the middle ear; alternatively, myringotomy may be necessary. Both topical and systemic antimicrobial therapy should be implemented. Because yeast is often present, topical therapy should include antifungal drugs (e.g., nystatin). A number of antimicrobials can be used for treatment of otitis interna, although distribution is likely to be limited for many (see Table 7-5). A lipid-soluble drug is preferred, and combination therapy should be considered to minimize the risk of resistance. Examples include the fluoroquinolones and chloramphenicol; the latter, however, is not likely to reach killing concentrations at the site of infection. Ototoxicity of antimicrobial drugs must be considered.[32]

INFECTIONS OF THE SKIN

Pyoderma

Pathophysiology

Pyoderma is defined as a bacterial infection in skin associated with pus. Both the normal organ (skin) and the diseased local environment (pus) present barriers to drug movement and therefore efficacy.[33] As such, pyoderma is a complex disease that may be difficult to treat effectively. The location of the infection in the skin, and particularly the depth (surface infection to cellulitis), confounds therapy.[34,35] Consequently, one of the goals of therapy for pyoderma is to prevent the progression of clinical signs. Whereas a surface infection (e.g., intertrigo) is generally amenable to topical antimicrobial therapy, superficial skin structures (e.g., impetigo, superficial folliculitis) may be less responsive; however, even these infections may yet respond to proper topical therapy in lieu of systemic therapy. Certainly, as infection becomes more deep-seated, systemic antimicrobial therapy becomes more important (Figure 8-3, *A*).[33-35] Lesions of deep pyoderma begin in the distal portion of the hair follicle, often extend below the follicle, and may be accompanied by furunculosis and a granulomatous response. As the disease worsens, antimicrobial penetration becomes more limited, and successful therapy is more difficult to achieve, requiring higher doses and, for time-dependent drugs, shorter intervals .[33-35] Cellulitis is the most severe manifestation of pyoderma and involves infection of the dermis and adjacent subcutaneous tissues. Although uncommon, infection at this depth can become life threatening if sepsis develops.

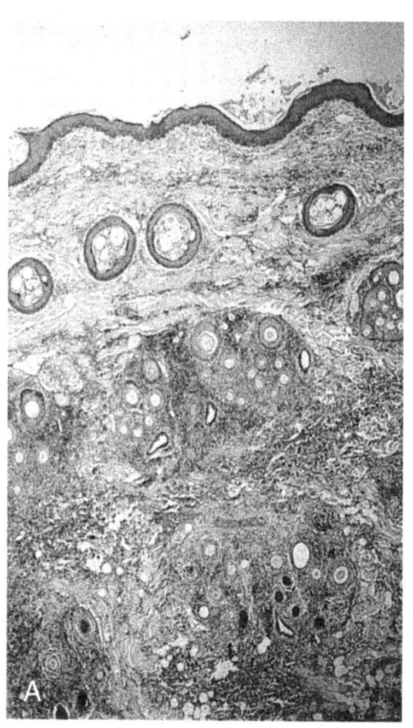

Figure 8-3 A, Histologic section of deep pyoderma. Scarring and accumulation of inflammatory debris present both mechanical and functional barriers to drug penetration.

Continued

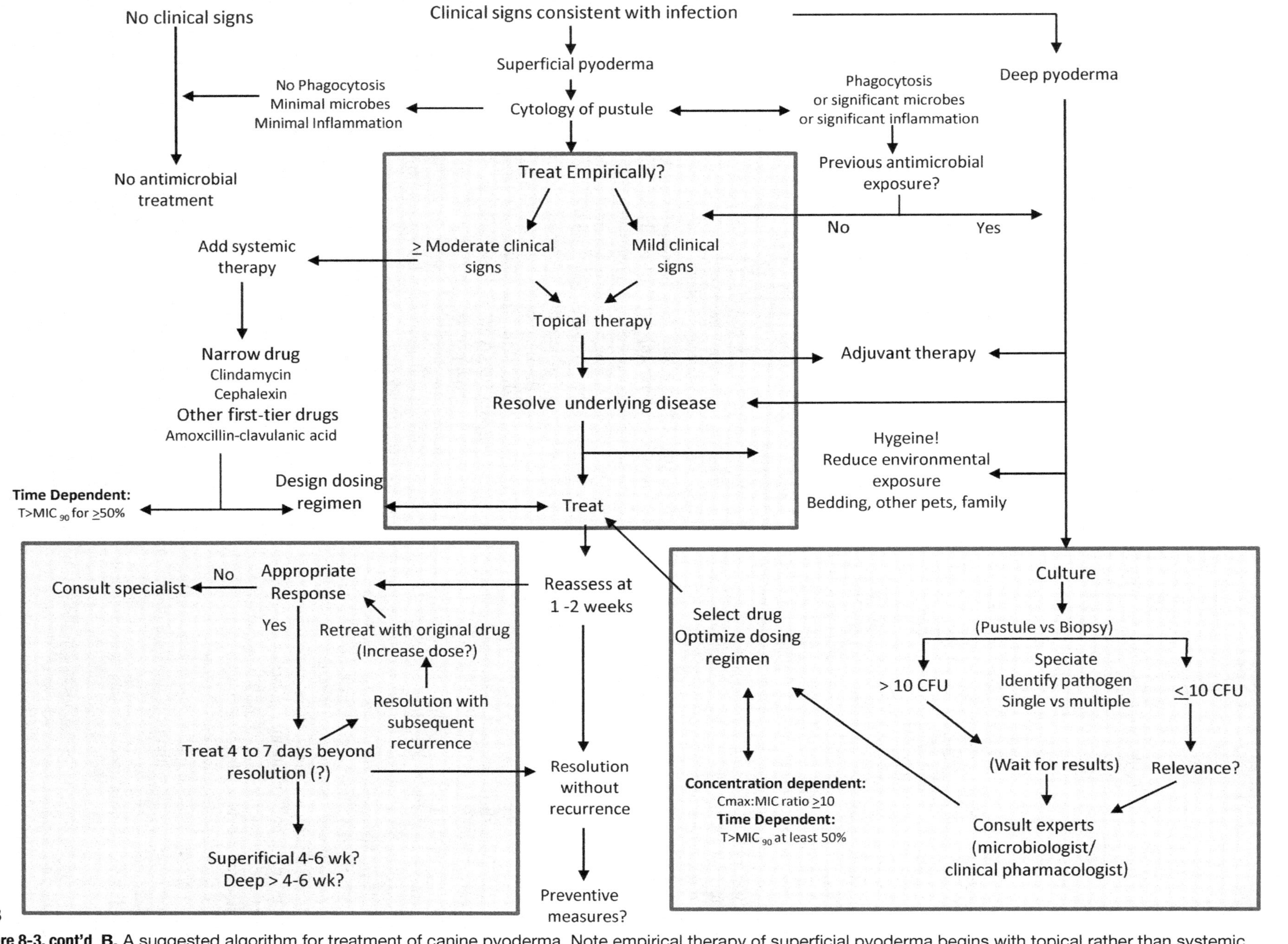

Figure 8-3, cont'd B, A suggested algorithm for treatment of canine pyoderma. Note empirical therapy of superficial pyoderma begins with topical rather than systemic therapy *(center)*; treatment of deep pyoderma begins with culture and susceptibility testing *(lower right)*. Once the decision is made to use systemic therapy, narrow spectrum, first-tier drugs should be chosen first *(upper left)*. Topical therapy is a part of all therapies. Removal of underlying disease may be paramount to therapeutic success. Dosing regimens should be designed to minimize the advent of resistance; if successful, subsequent recurrences may continue to respond to first-tier drugs. Initial therapy should be reassessed within 7 to 10 days; failure to respond at this time should lead to alternate therapies, which may involve reculture and consultation with specialist. In responders, evidence regarding the duration of therapy is not clear and until such data exist, current recommendations focus on 4 to 6 weeks. (*A*, Photograph courtesy Bayer Animal Health.)

KEY POINT 8-8 Focusing on topical therapy as the sole method of delivery of antmicrobial therapy should minimize the need for systemic antimicrobial therapy, which might contribute to resistance.

Not all pyodermas are difficult to treat; indeed, most will respond to initial therapy. Therapy with superficial pyodermas should begin with topical therapy only (see Figure 8-3, *B*) However, some patients that initially respond to antimicrobial therapy experience recrudescence after therapy is discontinued. The most likely cause for recrudescence is failure or inability to control underlying skin diseases that predispose the skin to persistent or recurrent infections. Examples include ectoparasitism, seborrhea (cornification disorders), allergies (atopic dermatitis, flea or food allergies), and endocrinopathies (hyperadrenocorticism or hypothyroidism).[33-35] Anatomic abnormalities such as skin folds (intertrigo) also predispose the patient to bacterial infection.[33-35] Failure or inability to correct these underlying factors increases the risk of therapeutic failure, and emergent resistance if multiple courses of antimicrobials are implemented. In addition to the physiologic barriers presented by the normal animal, a number of other factors complicate treatment of pyoderma. These include the effects of the infecting microbe; mechanical, functional, and structural sequelae of progressive disease; and limitations of the drugs themselves. Although the sequelae of these interacting factors are difficult to predict in the individual patient, their impact can be minimized by decision making that is based on these interactions.

The surface of the skin normally presents several barriers to bacterial invasion and colonization. Cells of the stratum corneum desquamate from the surface of the skin and hair follicles, and the lipid-rich environment between the cells impedes bacterial movement.[34,35] Epithelial proliferation follows injury to the skin, decreasing the likelihood of bacterial invasion. Sebum and sweat contain antibacterial chemicals such as inorganic salts[34,35] and lipids.[36] Finally, resident microflora may be important by helping to keep invading microflora in check. Differences in the incidence and ease of treatment of pyoderma in dogs versus cats and other species may reflect anatomic and physiologic differences in their skin.[34,35] Canine skin may be predisposed to pyoderma because the stratum corneum is thin and compact and contains less lipid material. Therefore canine stratum corneum may present a less efficient barrier to bacterial invasion compared with that of other species. Canine hair follicles lack a lipid–squamous "plug," which may facilitate bacterial penetration into the hair follicle.[34,35,37] Finally, the pH of canine skin is higher than that of other species, perhaps providing an environment more conducive to bacterial proliferation.[34,35]

Skin also has a well-developed immune response, composed of proteins, immunoglobulins located in the basement membrane, cells of the immune system located in the dermis and epidermis, and regional lymphoid tissue.[34,35] However, materials released from microbes facilitate invasion, impair cellular phagocytosis, and damage host tissues. Under normal circumstances components of bacteria that penetrate the skin stimulate a humoral response (immunoglobulins G and M), which in turn activates effector mechanisms leading to an acute inflammatory response.[34,35] Soluble mediators released by organisms (e.g., hemolysin, epidermolytic toxin, leukocidin) may damage host tissues or alter host response.[34,35] *Staphylococcus* spp. in particular plays a role in perpetuating the inflammatory response. Cutaneous mast cells triggered by antistaphylococcal immunoglobulin E may increase epidermal permeability and facilitate bacteria or bacterial antigen penetration in patients with allergic skin disease.[34-36] Most staphylococci associated with canine pyoderma produce "slime," a material that facilitates bacterial adhesion to cells. Staphylococcal organisms contain protein A, which impairs antibody response, activates complement, and causes chemotaxis.[38] Some staphylococcal organisms release superantigens (enterotoxin), which may cause interleukin release and an inappropriately large T-lymphocyte response in the skin.[34-36,39] Finally, selected *Staphylococcus* spp. suppress or prevent intracellular killing once phagocytized by leukocytes.[40] Viability of the organisms will be maintained inside the phagocyte, allowing not only survival but perhaps also continued replication inside the cell. Subsequent release of the organism on the death of the phagocyte allows reinfection, leading to persistent or recurrent infections.

The phagocytic white blood cells (initially neutrophils) that respond to inflammatory mediators use a number of oxidative (e.g., myeloperoxidase) and nonoxidative (e.g., bactericidal permeability-increasing protein) mechanisms to kill phagocytized invading bacteria.[41] Unfortunately, host responses to bacterial invasion may become deleterious and can negatively affect therapy. The inflammatory response to infection may facilitate bacterial penetration, is responsible for clinical signs associated with the disease, and may preclude antimicrobial penetration of the skin. The severe and persistent inflammatory response leads to pruritus, and self-trauma further aggravates bacterial penetration. The disease may develop an autoimmune component.[34,35] These long-term changes, in conjunction with inflammatory disease, predispose the patient to recurrent pyoderma.

As bacterial skin disease progresses, pathologic changes become barriers to drug distribution at the site of infection, and dosing regimens should be modified accordingly. The barriers vary with the site of infection, ranging from very superficial structures (epidermal and hair follicle) to deep structures below the hair follicle. Hair follicles may rupture, leading to furunculosis. Granulomatous changes and keratinaceous debris may act as foreign bodies, perpetuating the inflammatory response.[34,35] These deeper structures may become isolated by fibrous tissue as disease progresses unchecked. Foci of organisms located in these isolated beds of scar tissue are a likely cause of recurrent infections with deep pyoderma (see Figure 8-3, *A*), as can intracellular survival of phagocytized organisms (see Figures 6-17 and 6-18).[34,35]

KEY POINT 8-9 As bacterial skin disease progresses, pathologic barriers impede drug distribution to the infecting organism. Dosing regimens should be modified accordingly.

Microbial Flora

The microflora of the skin is composed of both resident and transient organisms. Resident organisms in the skin of dogs include *Micrococcus* spp. beta-hemolytic streptococci, aerobic diphtheroids, *Propionibacterium acnes,* and *Staphylococcus* spp. *Pseudomonas, Proteus,* and *Corynebacterium* organisms have also been cultured from normal dogs. Among the resident organisms cultured from the skin of normal dogs, only *S. intermedius* is a likely initial cause of pyoderma. *S. intermedius* has recently been reclassified to *Staphylococcus pseudintermedius*; however, the original terminology will be used throughout this text until the newer terminology has been accepted and is in general use. *S. aureus* and other *Staphylococcus* spp. are much rarer causes of superficial pyodermas in dogs.[34,35,37] *S. intermedius* is involved in approximately 90% of canine pyodermas.[33-35] The resident status of *S. intermedius* in the skin is debatable. Although cultured frequently from either the skin or hair of normal dogs, *S. intermedius* may simply be a contaminant or a transient organism, acting as a "nomad," proliferating only when environmental circumstances are supportive of growth.[42] The microflora of dogs with pyoderma differs from the microflora of the skin in normal dogs. Even skin not clinically affected by pyoderma is characterized by increased staphylococcal colonization.[34,35] Eventually, *Staphylococcus* spp. become the predominant organism in the skin. It can change the local environment, allowing proliferation of other organisms. Thus, even when disease has progressed to the point that gram-negative infections (e.g., *E. coli, Proteus* spp., and *Pseudomonas* spp.)[34,35] are involved (generally deep pyodermas), *S. intermedius* is likely to be involved. In fact, if *S. intermedius* is not cultured from the skin lesion, the laboratory or culture technique may be questioned.[33] When pyoderma is treated, concomitant infection with *S. intermedius* should be assumed, and control of infection by *S. intermedius* in such cases should facilitate treatment of other organisms, including gram-negative bacteria.

Several studies have addressed microbes causing skin infections, including prevelance of methicillin-resistant *Staphylococcus* spp. (MRS) in dogs and cats. Among the caveats to the studies will be differences in methodology, particularly as it pertains to sample collection. Ideally, samples are based on tissue samples following adequate cleansing; more often than not, however, samples are collected by swabs. Diagnostic aids can be useful to discriminate infection from colonization in the skin. Gram staining and cytology are particularly helpful. The presence of rods indicates a mixed infection (with gram-negative organisms); intracellular organisms indicate phagocytosis and thus infection rather than colonization. Cytology may help stage or identify the cause of disease: Mononuclear infiltrations indicate deep, chronic infections; large numbers of *Staphylococcus* spp. in pustules may indicate hyperadrenocorticism.[34,35]

Petersen and coworkers[18] reported on the frequency and susceptibility of *S. intermedius* and *P. aeruginosa* in samples collected between 1992 and 1997 from canine skin and ears (n = 497) and submitted to a state diagnostic laboratory (see Table 8-3). The method of sample collection was not provided but reflects methods used by practitioners. *S. intermedius* was isolated from 89% of skin samples and was the only isolate cultured from 47% of samples. *P. aeruginosa* was isolated from 7.5% of skin samples, with the frequency of collection from the skin increasing during the 6-year period of the study. Of the isolates yielding *P. aeruginosa*, it was the only isolate in 33% of samples. Although *Staphylococcus* isolates were susceptible to drugs generally chosen empirically as first-choice treatment for pyoderma, as in the author's institution, MRS appears to have begun increasing in the early 2000s. This is indicated by the difference in isolates collected from 2003 to 2005, versus 2006 and 2007 (Table 8-3). These data demonstrate that initially the proportion of susceptible isolates collected from skin,and other tissues was nearly 100% for drugs traditionally selected empirically, only to decrease to nearly 65% susceptible during this period. These data underscore the limitations that appear to be emerging regarding empirical selection of antimicrobials even for those conditions traditionally considered safe, such as pyoderma. They also underscore the importance of appropriate dosing regimens to minimize the advent of resistance.

KEY POINT 8-10 Methicillin-resistant *Staphylococcus* increasingly is being identified in association with pyoderma.

The public health significance of treating MRS is addressed in greater depth in Chapter 7. The role of previous antimicrobial therapy facilitating multidrug-resistant *Staphylococcus* spp. has been well established (see Chapter 6). A report from Sweden demonstrated that *S. intermedius* isolates from dogs with recurring pyoderma were more likely to be characterized by resistance than isolates of first-time infections.[43] Approval and subsequent use of betalactamase inhibitors and cephalosporins are particularly well associated with MRSA and MRSI. Overproduction of beta-lactamases coupled with changes in penicllin-binding proteins contribute to oxacillin/methicillin-resistant *Staphylococcus* spp., whether *aureus* (MRSA) or *intermedius* (MRSI).

KEY POINT 8-11 The role of previous antimicrobial therapy facilitating emergence of multidrug resistant *Staphylococcus* has been well established.

Abraham[44] prospectively studied the frequency of *Staphylococcus* spp. as a cause of infection in cats. No cat had received antimicrobials within the previous 7 days. The prevalance of coagulase-negative isolates was higher than coagulase-positive isolates in all cats, and the proportion of each was similar in healthy cats compared to cats with inflammatory skin disease (ISD). For healthy cats (n = 50); 21 were coagulase-positive isolates (n = 17/50, or 34% of all healthy cats) and 49 were coagulase-negative (n = 49/50 cats or (98% of all cats). This compares to ISD cats (n = 48) of which 25 were coagulase-positive isolates (n = 24/48 or 50% of cats) compared to 46 coagulase-negative isolates (n = 46/48 or 96% of cats). Of the coagulase-positive isolates, approximately 50% were *S. aureus* and *S. intermedius*, respectively, in both groups. Specifically, in healthy cats 10 and 11 of 21 coagulase-positive (48% and 52%) isolates were *S. aureus* and *S. intermedius*, respectively.

From the ISD cats, 14 and 11 of 25 (56% and 44%) were *S. aureus* and *S. intermedius,* respectively. The proportions of staphylococci infections differ between dogs and cats.[45] In a separate study by the same group, 74% of healthy dogs (n = 37/50) were positive for growth compared with 88% of dogs with ISD (n = 52/59).[45] The total number of isolates (from different body regions) cultured was greater in ISD dogs compared with healthy dogs. For both healthy and ISD groups, coagulase-positive isolates far outweighed coagulase-negative isolates, and *S. intermedius* outnumbered *S. aureus.* For coagulase-positive isolates in the 52 ISD dogs, the frequency of isolation of *S. aureus, intermedius,* and *schleiferi* subsp. *coagulans* (SSc) (all coagulase positive isolates) was, respectively, 10, 134, and 6 isolates each, compared with 8, 69, and 0 isolates, each respectively, in the 37 healthy dogs (2 coagulase-negative isolates). In the healthy dogs, 9 isolates of coagulase-negative *S. schleiferi* subsp. *schleiferi* [SSs] were identified, indicating the possible importance of subspeciated *S. schleiferi.* Methicillin resistance occurred in both coagulase-positive (MRSA, MRSI, MRSSc) and -negative (MRSSs) isolates and was more frequent for MRSI and in ISD (n = 4 MRSI, n = 1 MRSA, MRSC = 1, MRSS = 1) compared with healthy (MRSI = 1, MRSA = 0, MRSC = 1, MRSS = 0) dogs.

Other staphylococci are being recognized for their increasing role in canine pyoderma. *S. schleiferi* has recently been recognized for its increasing role, particularly in recurrent infections;[45,47,48] it was the second most common *Staphylococcus* organism cultured in one study. The increasing recognition of this organism is important because multiple antimicrobial resistances can occur with *S. schleiferi,* [45,49] whereas the incidence of multiple drug resistance (meaning resistance that includes drug classes other than beta-lactams) by *S. intermedius* remains low (see the discussion of antimicrobial resistance below). Concern might heighten if laboratories cannot or do not distinguish between *S. schleiferi* and *S. intermedius,* much as *S. intermedius* was confused with S. *aureus* in the 1970s. Further *S. schleiferi* exists as either coagulase-negative (*schleiferi* subspecies), which generally indicates contaminants, or coagulase-positive (*coagulans* subspecies), which has a greater clinical significance. The increasing prevalence of *S. aureus* infections coupled with the emergence of *S. schleiferi* warrants more caution and vigilance in the prevention of zoonosis.[50]

The role of *P. aeruginosa* as the sole infectious organism in canine pyoderma (n = 20) was retrospectively studied in 66 dogs with mixed or pure infections associated with pyoderma.[46] As with Petersen,[18] the incidence of *Pseudomonas* as the sole agent of pyoderma was observed to be increasing. Seven of the dogs presenting with deep pyoderma had not been previously presented for skin disease; these dogs responded well to 3 to 4 weeks of fluoroquinolone therapy. The remaining 13 dogs had a protracted history of skin disease that had been treated with antimicrobials, immunomodulatory drugs, or both. Of these dogs, 11 had been previously treated with antimicrobials effective against *Staphylococcus* spp. Antimicrobials to which isolates should potentially have been susceptible but were resistant included enrofloxacin (40%; half of these dogs had previously been treated with a fluoroquinolone), ticarcillin (36%), ciprofloxacin (25%), and gentamicin or amikacin and norfloxacin (5%). Interestingly, all isolates were susceptible to marbofloxacin, a questionable finding based on likely cross-resistance among fluoroquinolones. Doses of drugs used to treat the infection ranged from 6 to 13 mg/kg for enrofloxacin qd, or 5 to 12 mg/kg bid; norfloxacin at 18 to 23 mg/kg qd, marbofloxacin at 3 to 5 mg/kg qd, and cephalexin 20 to 25 mg/kg bid. All but two dogs responded after treatment for 3 to 12 weeks (mean 4.8 weeks). However, a potentially important observation that some dogs responded to cephalexin was interpreted to potentially imply that *Pseudomonas* was only a secondary pathogen in some of the dogs.

Considerations in Drug Selection

For most antimicrobials used to treat canine pyoderma, adverse events or side effects become less important to the selection and other considerations can take precedence. Exceptions might occur for erythromycin; up to 50% of animals should be expected to develop gastrointestinal upset when treated with erythromycin.[51] Gastrointestinal side effects in particular are likely to increase if higher doses of antimicrobials are used. Immune-mediated side effects caused by potentiated sulfonamides may limit their long-term use.[52] Sulfonamides are also able to decrease thyroid hormone synthesis at high doses that might otherwise be indicated to effectively treat pyoderma.

Drug Movement to the Site of Infection

Distribution of antimicrobials applied topically is limited by the presence of the stratum corneum, although distribution of topically applied drugs should be be enhanced in the presence of inflammation. Accumulation of inflammatory debris, however, also impedes drug movement after either topical or systemic administration. Shampooing not only removes inflammatory debris but also softens the stratum corneum, thus facilitating movement of topically applied antimicrobials to deeper tissues. Distribution of systemically administered antimicrobials to the skin is somewhat limited even with normal conditions. Despite the skin being the largest organ of the body, blood flow to the skin represents only 9% of the cardiac output. Drug distribution to the skin takes longer than to tissues with greater blood flow. Although skin is well perfused, blood supply to the epidermis consists of capillaries that lie under the epidermis, and drugs must passively diffuse to the epidermis and, with folliculitis, through the hair follicle. The plexi of arteries and veins that supply the skin include arteriovenous anastomoses that allow blood to bypass capillary beds. Blood supply to the skin can be altered easily in disease, particularly in the extremities and deep dermis.

Many antimicrobials used to treat pyoderma are lipid soluble, although the degree varies with each drug. Drugs that are characterized by a favorable distribution pattern to the skin include the fluoroquinolones, the sulfonamides (including those potentiated), the macrolides (erythromycin), the lincosamides (clindamycin and lincomycin), and chloramphenicol.[53] The distribution of water-soluble drugs (beta-lactams, aminoglycosides) to interstitial fluid of skin should be anticipated to be less than that of plasma, particularly in the presence of physical barriers presented by fibrosis. Note that the poorer distribution of beta-lactams coupled with their time dependence indicates that those drugs with longer elimination half-lives are preferred. The presence of marked inflammatory cells may be taken advantage of with use of antimicrobials that accumulate in white blood cells (e.g., fluoroquinolones, clindamycin, macrolides, rifampin); higher intracellular concentrations may also facilitate intracellular killing of microorganisms that may survive phagocytosis.

Antimicrobial Resistance

Antimicrobial resistance may affect antimicrobial therapy of pyoderma or other infections associated with staphylococci. Resistance to penicillins by *S. aureus* or *S. intermedius* generally reflects an increase in chromosomally mediated beta-lactamase production.[49] However, use of beta-lactamase protectors (e.g., beta-lactams coupled with clavulanic acid or sulbactam) or beta-lactamase–resistant drugs (e.g., cephalosporins) has led to adaptation by *Staphylocccus* spp. through mutations in the penicillin-binding proteins (PBP-2) encoded by the *mecA* gene, located on the staphylococcal chromosomal cassette (SCC_{mec}). The expression of this gene prevents efficacy of any beta-lactam antibiotic.

S. aureus has developed an increasing pattern of resistance against many antimicrobials (discussed in depth in Chapter 6). Indeed, the proportion of *S. aureus* susceptible to drugs generally chosen to treat pyodermas is consistently less than that of *S. intermedius*. In contrast, *S. intermedius* has not appeared to be as adaptable; antimicrobial resistance in *S. intermedius* has been slow to emerge, and the impact of previous antimicrobial use on the susceptibility pattern of the microbe to other drugs has been controversial.[34,35] However, although *S. intermedius* is a species distinct from *S. aureus*, transmission between these organisms of plasmids responsible for multiple antimicrobial resistance may be a factor that appears to be contributing to antimicrobial failure in canine pyoderma.[34,35] In humans antimicrobial resistance is a rapidly emerging concern in dermatology.[54] In patients with skin wounds, *S. aureus* (44% methicillin resistant) and *P. aeruginosa* were the most common bacteria isolated. The incidence of MRSA increased from 26% in 1992 to 75% in 2001. Resistance was not limited to *Staphylocccus* spp.; *P. aeruginosa* resistance to quinolones increased in deep wounds from 19% in 1992 to 56% in 2001, and in superficial wounds from 0 to 18% by 2001. Although these statistics have been generated from human medicine, their changing pattern mimics what is occuring in veterinary medicine. Several studies have demonstrated the advent of MRS in veterinary patients (see previous discussion).

The frequency of methicillin resistance in coagulase-positive and -negative *Staphylococcus* spp. in dogs with and without skin disease was previously cited.[45] As early as 1998, in a retrospective study of 131 *S. intermedius* strains isolated from apparently healthy dogs and another 187 *S. intermedius* strains isolated from dog pyodermas, the proportion of multidrug-resistant (three or more drug classes) strains increased from 10.8% in 1986 to 1987 to 28% in 1995 to 1996.[55] In dogs with pyoderma, 26% of the isolates in one study were associated with multidrug resistance, including resistance to methicillin, albeit in only 2 of 57 cases. However, although not revealed in the phenotype, close to 50% of the organisms studied carried the gene (*mec*A) responsible for formation of PBP2a, the penicillin-binding protein that confers resistance to methicillin. *S. schleiferi* was the second most common *Staphylococcus* organism cultured; most were resistant to methicillin (coagulase-negative versus positive subspeciation not provided). [49] That previous antimicrobial therapy may have been associated with *Staphyloccoccus* antimicrobial resistance was supported by the more common isolation of *S. schleiferi* in dogs currently receiving antimicrobials (10 of 12) compared with dogs that were not (5 of 28).[47] A multiclinic prospective study that compared susceptibility in organisms isolated from samples from first-time and recurrent cases of canine pyoderma (n = 394 *Staphylococci*) found that resistance to macrolides, lincosamides, fusidic acid, tetracycline, and streptomycin was significantly greater in recurrent cases (45%) compared with the first-time cases (20%). Identification of *S. schleiferi* was not addressed. Resistance was not detected in penicillinase-stable beta-lactams.[43]

More recently, Morris[19] retrospectively determined the proportion of *Staphyloccoccus* isolates expressing methicillin resistance in dogs and cats. Samples were collected from a variety of tissues; the method varied with the clinician; isolates were processed at a veterinary teaching hospital according to Clinical and Laboratory Standards Institute (CLSI) guidelines. Isolates included *S. aureus* (n = 139; resistant isolates = MRSA), *S. intermedius* (n = 463; MRSI), and *S schleiferi* (n = 148; MRSSs vs MRSSc not distinguished). The frequency of resistance for each *Staphylococcus* spp. was as follows: MRSA 35% (more commonly associated with deep infections), MRSS and MRSSc, together, 40% (more commonly associated with superficial infections), and MRSI, 17%. The higher percentage of resistance in this hospital population probably reflects the referral nature of the patients and the likelihood that patients had previously received antimicrobials. The frequency of MRSA was the same in both dogs and cats, whereas MRSI and MRSS were higher in dogs compared with cats. Of the resistant isolates, 28% of MRSA, 40% of MRSI, and 33% of MRSS were in the skin, and 5% of MRSA, 26% of MRSI, and 47% of MRSS were located in the ear. Among the organisms, MRSS remained most susceptible to all drugs save the fluoroquinolones, but susceptibility to the fluoroquinolones was ≤35% (see Table 8-3). Although chloramphenicol was the most consistently effective drug, its use as the sole agent should be questioned.

A study of healthy cats (n = 50) and cats with ISD (n = 48) found that four healthy cats and one ISD cat harbored a coagulase-positive MRS.[44] In healthy dogs (n = 50), zero of six *S. aureus* isolates were MRSA, whereas one *S. intermedius* (n = 34) isolate was MRSI. In dogs with ISD (n = 48), one of six *S. aureus* isolates were MRSA, whereas 4 of 52 *S. intermedius* isolates were MRSI.[45]

Note that not all multidrug-resistant *Staphylococcus* organisms are methicillin resistant. Disconcertingly, MRS is expanding to include drug classes other than beta-lactams.[56] Fluoroquinolone resistance may be associated with MRSA (ciprofloxacin and levofloxacin) and also has been associated with emergent MRSA,[57] although it is not clear if the resistant isolates emerge once other microbes are inhibited by drugs, or if fluoroquinolones facilitate infection by increasing adherence of MRSA at the site of infection. On the other hand, multidrug resistance not in association with methicillin resistance (e.g., to clindamycin, chloramphenicol, doxycycline) also has emerged. Finally, resistance to vancomycin occurs with acquisition of the vanA resistance gene, usually from enterococci, which also prevents the drug from binding to the target peptidoglycan. Resistance to linezolid also has been documented.

The prudent clinician will take a proactive approach to prevent the development of antimicrobial resistance among organisms that cause canine pyoderma. Previous antimicrobial use should be considered in the selection of an antimicrobial without the benefit of culture and susceptibility data. Susceptibility data should be considered as a basis for selection of antimicrobials for patients with a history of recent antimicrobial use. Persistent infections imply therapy has failed; recurrent infections may have previously been successfully treated, but underlying disease or other factors that as yet are not identified or cannot be corrected, have facilitated return. Certainly, previously used drugs that failed should be avoided if the infection is considered persistent rather than recurrent, with selection best based on susceptibility testing for both. Perhaps more so than gram-positive isolates, resistance more likely may be encountered in gram-negative organisms associated with deep pyoderma,[34,35] and culture and susceptibility data become increasingly important for antimicrobial selection with these infections. Resistance is more likely to develop with long-term therapy (as must occur for deep pyoderma) and conditions that are likely to result in subtherapeutic concentrations at the site of infection (e.g., beta-lactam antibiotics, particularly those with short half-lives compared with the dosing interval). Repetitive cultures that yield increasing MICs for the same drug may indicate development of resistance, and alternative drugs or combination antimicrobial therapy should be considered in such cases.[53]

Antimicrobial Selection

The number of antimicrobials recommended for initial therapy of pyoderma increases with the number of papers published regarding therapy. Clinician preferences vary, appropriately so, with experience. Although clinicians might not agree on their first-choice antimicrobial, there is little disagreement regarding the target organism. Initial therapy should be topical. If a decision is made that systemic drugs are indicated, therapy should begin with an orally bioavailable drug effective against *S. intermedius*. Ideally, the dosing interval should be 12 hours or longer to facilitate owner compliance; as such, time-dependent drugs with half-lives of less than 4 hours (e.g., amoxicillin, and potentially cephalexin) should be avoided in clients unwilling to dose every 8 hours. Subsequent considerations regarding drug selection vary with the severity of the disease. The more severe the disease, the greater the care that must be taken with antimicrobial selection. Tissue penetration should be increasingly predictable as the infection deepens. Detection and avoidance of resistance become increasingly important as the duration of therapy and the risk of subtherapeutic drug concentrations at the site of infection increase. With few exceptions, adverse effects are not a common cause of therapeutic failure and, as such, may not have a major impact on antimicrobial selection. Cost often has a major impact on selection. Clients may be reminded, however, that they might as well spend their money on an appropriate drug and dosing regimen rather than on prolonged therapy with an inappropriate drug or dosing regimen.

A number of drugs are indicated for initial therapy of pyoderma. Among the most frequent first-choice drugs for first time infections are beta-lactam antibiotics that tend to be resistant to *Staphylococcus* beta-lactamases. Cephalexin has been the treatment of choice for many clinicians. It and cefadroxil were among the earliest studied.[58] As time-dependent drugs, based on integration of maximum drug concentrations and MIC_{50} or MIC_{90}, high doses and frequent intervals may be indicated (Tables 8-6 and 8-7). The approval of cefpodoxime, a third-generation cephalosporin, has been a potentially important addition to the armamentarium of drug therapy for treatment of canine pyoderma. Attributes include an MIC_{90} for *S. intermedius* of 0.5 μg/mL and plasma drug concentrations that remain above this MIC for longer than 24 hours, with a dose of 10 mg/kg (but not 5 mg/kg if the 95th percentile of animals is targeted). The large structure of cefpodoxime appears to render it less susceptible to the development of resistance due to production of cephalosporinases. Another recently approved drug that will facilitate compliance is cefovecin. Based on plasma concentrations of unbound drug or interstitial concentrations,[59] concentrations will remain above the MIC_{90} of *S. intermedius,* as reported on the package insert for at least 13 (plasma) to 18 days (interstitial fluid); the duration, however, will be much less if the 95th percentile is used. The advantages of this drug mandate its judicious use such that emergent methicillin resistance is minimized.

Amoxicillin–clavulanic acid also is chosen as an initial drug for treatment of canine pyoderma. Its efficacy is similar to the first-generation drugs cephalexin and cefadroxil, although cephalexin is probably the most cost effective. Amoxicillin–clavulanic acid may be less likely than either first-generation cephalosporin to induce resistant bacteria at subinhibitory concentrations.[34,35] However, its short half-life and low C_{max} at recommended dose compared with the MIC_{50} or MIC_{90} for *S. intermedius* mandate an unacceptably short dosing interval if the targeted pharmacodynamic indices are to be achieved. The interpretive standards for amoxicillin have recently been updated by CLSI, causing many isolates previously considered susceptible now to be classified as resistant. Alternatively, beta-lactamase–resistant beta-lactams such as oxacillin and dicloxacillin might be used for initial or long-term therapy, although the cost may preclude their selection until initial therapy fails. Data regarding the current state of susceptibility of *Staphylococcus* spp. to these drugs is not available. A disadvantage of the beta-lactams is their failure to accumulate in phagocytic white blood cells. Further, distribution into tissues characterized by marked inflammation and fibrosis may be limited.

Table 8-6 Pharmacokinetic and Pharmacodynamic Indices for Treatment of Canine *Staphylococcus pseudintermedius**

Time-Dependent	Source†	Dose	C_{max}	MIC_{50}	Half-Life	C_{max}/MIC_{50}	T> MIC	Interval (h)+	MIC_{90}	C_{max}/MIC_{90}	$T>MIC_{90}$
Amoxicillin–clavulanic acid (1)	59	24	12	4	1.25	3.0	1.878	3.2813	32	0.375	None
Cefadroxyl	59	30	30	8	1.7	3.8	3.4	5.95	16	1.875	None
Cefovecin*	59	8 (SC)	4.2	0.5	130	8.4	390	682	1	4.200	390
Cefpodoxime	PI, 131	5	8.2	0.5	5	16.4	20	35	256	0.032	None
Cephalexin	59	30	28	16	3	1.8	2	4	512	0.055	None
Doxycycline		5	6	2	8	3.0			32	0.188	None
Concentration‡ Dependent											
Ciprofloxacin	131	20	2.8	0.03	NA	93	NA	NA	32	0.088	NA
Difloxacin	PI, 131	10	2.3	0.25	NA	9.2	NA	NA	32	0.072	NA
Enrofloxacin†	131	20	6	0.06	NA	100.0	NA	NA	32	0.188	NA
Marbofloxacin	PI, 131	5.5	4.2	0.25	NA	16.8	NA	NA			NA
Orbifloxacin	PI, 131	2.5	2	0.125	NA	16.0	NA	NA	32	0.063	NA

MIC, Minimum inhibitory concentration; *TMPS,* trimethoprim–sulfonamide; *SC,* subcutaneous; *NA,* not applicable; *PI,* package insert.
C_{max} = Peak plasma drug concentration when administered at the cited dose. Data collected from literature or package inserts (also see Table 7-1).
MIC = Refers to either the MIC_{50} or MIC_{90} (50th or 90th percentile, respectively) reported for *S. intermedius* in the cited reference.
C_{max}/MIC = Calculated by dividing C_{max} by MIC; for concentration-dependent drugs, a ratio of >12 was chosen to minimize resistance.
T>MIC = Calculated by dividing C_{max} by MIC; for each doubling, plasma drug concentration is above the MIC (T>MIC) for one half-life.
Interval = Based on avoiding resistance; that is, a T>MIC for 75% of the dosing interval. Calculated by multiplying T>MIC by 1.75. A target interval is reached if considered sufficiently convenient to facilitate compliance.
Dose is in mg/kg, half-life is in hours; target C_{max}/MIC_{50} or C_{max}/MIC_{90} (preferred) is ≥10 and for most drugs, T >MIC is 50% of dosing interval.
*Unbound drug
†Reference number
‡With ciprofloxacin
§See Table 7-1

KEY POINT 8-12 A beta-lactam with a longer half-life should be selected for treatment of pyoderma; doses may need to be increased to adjust for reduced tissue distribution.

Chloramphenicol may also be an effective first-choice antimicrobial, although concerns for human exposure and its bacteriostatic nature to the drug may preclude its use. Decreased use of this drug because of toxicity concerns has probably contributed to its consistent efficacy against *Staphylococcus* spp., including methicillin resistance. If chloramphenicol is chosen, care must be taken to use it at appropriate dosing intervals. MIC_{90} data for *S. intermedius* was not available, but doses can be designed around MIC (generally 8 µg/mL in our hospital) from the patient's data when available. Its use as sole agent for treatment of methicillin resistance should be avoided if possible because of its bacteriostatic nature. In our hospital, it has proven largely ineffective for treatment of MRS or multidrug resistant organisms. Combination with rifampin might be considered.

For infections that do not respond to initial therapy and become increasingly complicated, a drug that targets both *S. intermedius* and gram-negative organisms might be selected. Because bactericidal concentrations at the site of infection are desirable,[37] a drug that is likely to distribute to and through the inflammatory site is desirable. The use of beta-lactams should be de-emphasized for infections associated with marked inflammatory debris or scarring because these drugs do not penetrate these barriers well.[53]

Appropriate drugs should be based on susceptibility testing. Lipid-soluble drugs include the fluoroquinolones and potentiated sulfonamides (i.e., trimethoprim– or ormetoprim–sulfonamide combinations), erythromycin, azithromycin, and lincomycin or clindamycin; of these, only the potentiated sulfonamide and fluoroquinolones are classified as bactericidal. Each of these classes, except the potentiated sulfonamides, also accumulate in phagocytic WBC. Increasingly common reports of immune-mediated diseases such as keratitis sicca or impaired thyroid hormone secretion may decrease the use of potentiated sulfonamides, particularly at high doses and for long-term therapy. An advantage might, however, be once- to twice-daily therapy (sulfadimethoxine/ormetoprim), which has proved effective for some authors.[34,35] A cautious reminder, however: efficacy based on resolution of clinical signs does not preclude emerging resistance.

The fluoroquinolones, such as enrofloxacin and marbofloxacin, are the drugs of choice for complicated infections. They are characterized by rapid bactericidal activity, and their spectrum includes both *S. intermedius* and gram-negative organisms.[34,35,37] These drugs distribute very well to the skin.[60] Inflammatory debris and fibrous tissue should be traversed well with little impact on antimicrobial efficacy.[60] Efficacy of the fluoroquinolones is maintained despite slow growth of organisms or low oxygen tension.[61] All fluoroquinolones that have been studied accumulate in white blood cells,[40,62–66] thus increasing drug at the site of inflammation.[67] Fluoroquionlones are able to penetrate the lipopolysaccharide covering of gram-negative organisms. Their spectrum includes *Pseudomonas* spp., although increasing resistance to this organism and to *S. aureus* is reported. In one study of 383 isolates, the MIC for enrofloxacin against *S. intermedius* from 1995 to 1999 ranged from 0.063 to 64 mg/mL; the MIC_{50} and MIC_{90} were 0.125 and 0.25 mg/mL, respectively. Two resistant strains were found, but only among isolates collected in 1999. However, the authors concluded that the emergence of resistant mutants following 10 in vitro passages suggests that inappropriate use might favor the development of resistant strains in vivo. Like enrofloxacin, the MICs of marbofloxacin for *S. intermedius* are low, ranging from 0.125 to 2 μg/mL; MIC_{50} and MIC_{90} are both 0.25 μg/mL (according to the package insert). The fluoroquinolones are concentration-dependent drugs; doses should achieve a target C_{max}:MIC of greater than 8 to 10. Both enrofloxacin (with its active metabolite ciprofloxacin) and marbofloxacin achieve nearly 2 μg/mL in plasma at 5 mg/kg, yielding an inhibitory quotient of about 8. Tissue concentrations are likely to be even higher. Following administration of 5 mg/kg of enrofloxacin daily for 3 days, concentrations reached 1.9 and 4.2 μg/mL in the biopsied skin of animals with superficial and deep pyoderma, respectively, compared with 1.5 μg/mL in plasma and normal skin[68]; ciprofloxacin was not measured in either tissue. However, these studies are based on homogenate data, and relevancy to clinical response is not clear.

Despite favorable skin distribution of fluoroquinolones, use of high doses are recommended when possible. In one study, based on *Staphylococcus* organisms isolated from dogs with spontaneous disease (antimicrobial history unknown), a target C_{max}:MIC_{90} ≥10 might be achievable based on the highest dose and the MIC_{50} for four of five fluoroquinolones used clinically in dogs (the exception being difloxacin), with ratios greatest for enrofloxacin and ciprofloxacin. However, no drug was able to achive the target when using the MIC_{90} (Table 8-6).[131] However, if the isolate is known to be susceptible to fluoroquinolones, the ratio of C_{max}: MIC_{90} can be achieved for ciprofloxacin, enrofloxacin, or marbofloxacin using the MIC_{90} at the high dose.[131] These findings were supported by a study that found the MICs of orbifloxacin for *S. intermedius* isolates to be higher compared with enrofloxacin or marbofloxacin. In a study of 254 isolates (69 skin and 171 ear), the MICs for orbifloxacin ranged from 0.016 to 8 mg/mL; MIC_{50} and MIC_{90} were 0.5 and 1 μg/mL, respectively. Peak concentrations at 2.5 mg/kg achieve 2 μg/mL, yielding an inhibitory quotient at 2. Data are not available for 5 and 7.5 mg/kg. However, extrapolating doses for 7.5 mg/kg from 2.5 mg/kg, a ratio of 6 might be anticipated. Orbifloxacin exhibited a concentration-dependent, bactericidal effect against *S. aureus* reference strain, but a time-dependent bactericidal effect against *S. intermedius*.[69] Tissue concentrations for comparison with MIC data are not available for orbafloxacin.

Newer third-generation fluorquinolones may have the advantage of potentially being effective toward isolates resistant to second-generation drugs. This susceptibility should not be assumed but should be based on culture data and doses (using known pharmacokinetic data) designed around MIC.

Like the fluoroquinolones, clindamycin and the macrolides (including the azalide azithromycin) accumulate in white blood cells, distribute well to skin, and target *Staphyloccoccus* spp.; however, neither is characterized by a gram-negative spectrum. Although these drugs are bacteriostatic in action, bactericidal concentrations may be achieved in some tissues, including phagocytic WBC. (see Chapter 7). These may be reasonable choices for treatment of canine pyoderma. Note, however, that azithromycin will not reach steady-state concentrations for 4 to 7 days after therapy is begun; accordingly, a loading dose (twice the maintenance dose) should be given the first 2 days. In an uncontrolled study of superficial pyoderma in dogs (n = 21), clindamycin at 11 mg/kg every 24 hours for 14 to 42 days (depending on response) yielded a clinical score of excellent in 71% of animals within 14 days of initiating therapy. However, the authors noted that clinical response should be evaluated at 14 and 28 days because resistance developed. Cultures should be considered to detect resistance.[70] Azithromycin (10 mg/kg daily) was effective in 90% of dogs with either superficial or deep bacterial pyoderma in an uncontrolled clinical trial.[71] Interestingly, rifampin as sole therapy may be effective for treatment of *S. pseudintermedius* (but not *S. aureus*), although clinical trials supporting this approach are indicated. Accumulation in phagocytic cells may facilitate its efficacy.

The use of aminoglycosides for treatment of complicated pyoderma should be limited to life-threatening conditions associated with sepsis (e.g., cellulitis) or to organisms with known (i.e., based on susceptibility data) resistance to enrofloxacin. The aminoglycosides are generally effective against *Staphylococcus* spp. (particularly gentamicin) and gram-negative organisms including *Pseudomonas* (particularly amikacin). However, aminoglycosides generally should not be used as sole agents to treat *Staphyloccoccus* spp. unless evidence supports such use under the intended conditions. Combination with rifampin should be considered. For gram-negative organisms, resistance is less likely to develop against amikacin than against gentamicin, particularly for *Pseudomonas* spp. The aminoglycosides do not distribute well through inflammatory debris and fibrous tissue, are not effective against facultative aerobes (i.e., in the presence of reduced oxygen tension), and are not accumulated in white blood cells.[40] Therefore care must be taken to ensure that an adequate dose is given. Once-daily administration is encouraged, and combination antimicrobial therapy with a beta-lactam effective against the target organism should be strongly considered.

As sole therapy, rifampin is generally discouraged in part because resistance develops rapidly (indeed, resistance to rifampin is used experimentally to detect mutation frequencies). However, in an open, uncontrolled clinical trial in dogs (n = 20; all but 2 were superficial pyoderma), 40% were *S. pseudintermedius* positive.[71a] Treatment with rifampin at 5 mg/kg once daily for 10 days was clinically successful in 90% of dogs; the two dogs that failed therapy had deep pyoderma. Recurrence did not occur for at least 1 month in responders.

Table 8-7 Susceptibility Data for Selected Canine Gram-Positive Pathogens[76,131]

	Drug	Amoxicillin-Clavulanic Acid	Cefadroxyl	Cephalexin	Cefovecin	Cefpodoxime
	MIC_{BP} (sus)	≤0.25 (≤8/2:urine)		≤2		≤2
	MIC_{BP} (res)	≥1		≥8		≥8
Organism	**(Dose) (mg/kg)/**	**(13.5)**	**(11)**	**(25)**	**(8[SC])**	**(10)**
	C_{max} (μg/mL)	**6**	**10.5**	**19**	**4.2**	**16**
Coagulase-negative *Staphylococcus* spp.	Mode	≤0.5/0.25	1	1	0.12	
	MIC_{50}	≤0.5/0.25	1	1	0.12	
	MIC_{90}	≤0.5/0.25	4	4	2	
	Range	≤0.5/0.25-1/0.5	≤0.25-8	≤0.5-16	≤0.06-8	
	n	89	89	89	89	
	Species	D, C	D, C	D, C	D, C	
	Source	76	76	76	76	
	CLSI	Y	Y	Y	Y	
Coagulase-positive *Staphylococcus* spp.	Mode	≤0.5/0.25	1	1	0.25	
	MIC_{50}	≤0.5/0.25	1	1	0.25	
	MIC_{90}	≤0.5/0.25	2	2	0.5	
	Range	≤0.5/0.25-16/8	0.5->32	≤0.5->64	0.12->32	
	n	24	24	24	24	
	Species	D, C	D, C	D, C	D, C	
	Source	76	76	76	76	
	CLSI	Y	Y	Y	Y	
***Enterococcus* spp.**	Mode	1/0.5	>32	>64	>32	
	MIC_{50}	1/0.5	>32	>64	>32	
	MIC_{90}	1/0.5	>32	>64	>32	
	Range	≤0.5/0.25-32/16	≤0.25->32	≤0.5->64	≤0.06->32	
	n	45	45	45	45	
	Species	D, C	D, C	D, C	D, C	
	Source	76	76	76	76	
	CLSI	Y	Y	Y	Y	
Staphylococcus aureus	Mode	≤0.5/0.25	2	2	1	
	MIC_{50}	1/0.5	2	2	1	2
	MIC_{90}	4/2	8	8	2	2
	Range	≤0.5/0.25-16/8	1->32	1->64	0.5->32	0.12-2
	n	36	36	36	36	19
	Species	D, C	D, C	D, C	D, C	D
	Source	76	76	76	76	
	CLSI	Y	Y	Y	Y	Y
Staphylococcus intermedius	Mode	≤0.5/0.25	1	1	0.12	
	MIC_{50}	≤0.5/0.25	1	1	0.12	0.12
	MIC_{90}	≤0.5/0.25	2	2	0.25	0.5
	Range	≤0.5/0.25-16/8	0.5->32	≤0.5-64	≤0.06->32	0.12->32
	n	231	231	231	231	118
	Species	D, C	D, C	D, C	D, C	D
	Source	76	76	76	76	
	CLSI	Y	Y	Y	Y	Y
***Streptococcus* spp.**	Mode	≤0.5/0.25	≤0.25	≤0.5	≤0.06	
	MIC_{50}	≤0.5/0.25	≤0.25	≤0.5	≤0.06	
	MIC_{90}	≤0.5/0.25	2	4	0.5	
	Range	≤0.5/0.25-1/0.5	≤0.25-8	≤0.5-16	≤0.06-0.5	
	n	27	27	27	27	
	Species	D, C	D, C	D, C	D, C	
	Source	76	76	76	76	
	CLSI	Y	Y	Y	Y	

Continued

Table 8-7 Susceptibility Data for Selected Canine Gram-Positive Pathogens[76,131]—cont'd

	Drug	Amoxicillin-Clavulanic Acid	Cefadroxyl	Cephalexin	Cefovecin	Cefpodoxime
***Streptococcus,* β-hemolytic**	Mode	≤0.5/0.25	≤0.25	≤0.5	≤0.06	
	MIC_{50}	≤0.5/0.25	≤0.25	≤0.5	≤0.06	
	MIC_{90}	≤0.5/0.25	≤0.25	≤0.5	≤0.06	
	Range	≤0.5/0.25	≤0.25-1	≤0.5-2	≤0.06-8	
	n	22	22	22	22	
	Species	D, C	D, C	D, C	D, C	
	Source	76	76	76	76	
	CLSI	Y	Y	Y	Y	
Streptococcus canis	Mode	≤0.5/0.25	≤0.25	≤0.5	≤0.06	
	MIC_{50}	≤0.5/0.25	≤0.25	≤0.5	≤0.06	
	MIC_{90}	≤0.5/0.25	≤0.25	≤0.5	≤0.06	
	Range	≤0.5/0.25	≤0.25-8	≤0.5-8	≤0.06-≤0.06	
	n	66	66	66	66	
	Species	D, C	D, C	D, C	D, C	
	Source	76	76	76	76	
	CLSI	Y	Y	Y	Y	
Staphylococcus intermedius		**Ciprofloxacin**	**Difloxacin**	**Enrofloxacin**	**Marbofloxacin**	**Orbifloxacin**
	Mode	0.16	0.5	0.19	0.31	0.87
	MIC50	0.125	0.25	0.25	0.25	0.5
	MIC90	0.125	2	0.25	1	2
	Range					
	n	19	19	19	16	15
	Species	D, C	D, C	D, C	D, C	D, C
	Source	131	131	131	131	131
	CLSI	Y	Y	Y	Y	Y

MIC, Minimum inhibitory concentration; *BP,* breakpoint as established by CLSI; *SC,* subcutaneous; *D,* dog; *C,* cat; *CLSI,*: A yes (Y) indicates that data was collected following the guidelines of the Clinical and Laboratory Standards Institute; Source = reference.

Designing a Dosing Regimen

Perhaps an often overlooked reason that bacterial pyoderma is difficult to resolve in dogs is use of an inappropriate dosing regimen of an otherwise appropriate drug. Although the importance of culture and susceptibility testing for chronic, recurrent, and deep pyoderma cannot be denied, it is critical to realize that in vitro conditions do not and cannot mimic the microenvironment of the host. They also do not reflect the ability of the drug to reach the site of infection, including inside white blood cells, nor do they take into account active metabolites. The effects of underlying skin disease including changes in the patient's immune status (local or systemic) also cannot be taken into account by the in vitro system. Thus it is critical that both the dose and interval of a dosing regimen be designed such that drug concentrations are maximized at the site of infection.

In general, the dose of an antimicrobial should be as great as possible when treating complicated pyoderma to ensure effective concentrations at the site of infection. Twice the recommended dose has been suggested by some authors, and this is a reasonable starting point, but it is likely to be insufficient for some drugs in some patients, particularly if the drug is time dependent and characterized by a short half-life.[34,35] Doses up to fourfold higher than recommended may be necessary for organisms whose MIC for the drug is close to breakpoint or in the presence of factors that will decrease the movement or efficacy of antimicrobial at the site of infection. Higher doses are critical for concentration-dependent drugs (see Table 8-6). The greater the inflammatory response at the site (and particularly fibrosis) and the deeper the infection, the more important the need for increasing the dose. If necessary, selection of an antimicrobial might be made with an emphasis on safety so that doses can be increased with minimal risk of side effects. High tissue concentrations in relation to the MIC of the infecting organism are particularly important to the antimicrobial efficacy of selected drugs, most notably the aminoglycosides and the fluoroquinolones. For concentration-dependent drugs (aminoglycosides and fluoroquinolones), antimicrobial efficacy is enhanced in the presence of a high C_{max}:MIC ratio in part because of an enhanced postantibiotic effect. In addition, both aminoglycoside efficacy and safety are facilitated by a moderately long drug-free period during a dosing interval. Thus for aminoglycosides once-daily administration of the total daily recommended dose should be considered for pyoderma. With the fluoroquinolones, the dose should likewise be modified to maximize plasma (and thus tissue) drug concentration; this is particularly important for organisms whose MIC approaches the breakpoint for enrofloxacin (4 μg/mL). Once-daily dosing with enrofloxacin at a high dose (15 to 20 mg/kg) is recommended. However, because efficacy of fluoroquinolones also is based on area under the curve (see Chapter 6), the addition of a second dose may also enhance efficacy for complicated pyoderma.

For time-dependent antimicrobials, the interval of drug administration must be considered. These include the beta-lactams and bacteriostatic antimicrobials. For these drugs the duration that the drug concentration at the site is above the MIC is more important to antimicrobial efficacy. Thus for beta-lactams, antimicrobial efficacy is likely to be facilitated more by a shorter dosing interval than by increasing the dose. For example, to improve the efficacy of amoxicillin–clavulanic acid or cephalexin, the dose should be increased such that 2 to 4 times the MIC is reached and then an 8-hour dosing interval should be used in lieu of 12-hour intervals when treating cases at risk for development of resistance. Unfortunately, owner compliance is less likely with this regimen and may be a reason for considering an alternative class of drugs for treatment of complicated pyodermas. The long half-life of cefpodoxime supports its use at 10 mg/kg at 24-hour dosing intervals for many susceptible organisms. Cefovecin is particularly appealing; it should be effective with a single dose, particularly if the underlying cause of the disease can be identified and corrected. If healing is critical to resolution of infection (to be differentiated from resolution of clinical signs), a second dose may be indicated.

Duration of Therapy

An insufficient duration of therapy is another common cause of therapeutic failure in the treatment of pyoderma with an otherwise appropriate antimicrobial. However, clinical trials are indicated to establish if the issue may also be a less-than-ideal dose (i.e., a dose that fails to achieve the highest MIC of the infecting colony) that would allow a shorter duration. Recommendations have varied with authors, although the consensus is that the duration of therapy for pyoderma increases with the severity of infection.[34,35] Historically, therapy has extended 7 to 21 days (depending on the severity of infection) after surface healing has occurred. However, whether this is based on resolution of infection versus resolution of clinical signs has not been established. Superficial infections should resolve within 3 to 4 weeks of antimicrobial therapy if the patient is immunologically normal. Recommendations for deep pyoderma or the presence of immune compromise have suggested at least 4 to 6 weeks of therapy. Treatment for 12 weeks or longer is not unusual. Evaluation by the clinician at 7 days and then at 14-day intervals may be prudent, and reculture might be considered to reconfirm infection and should be implemented to detect resistance. Clinical evaluation should continue for several more weeks after therapy has been discontinued to ensure resolution.

Several authors have suggested alternative dosing regimens for antimicrobials for patients whose disease will not resolve. Examples include dosing once daily, every other day, or pulse dosing. Pulse dosing involves administration of a drug using full dosing regimens either 2 days a week or every other week. With the every-other-week approach, if recurrence is prevented, the duration of the "off" week can be gradually increased. Intervals of greater than 3 weeks are, however, likely to result in recrudescence.[34,35] Conceivably, the risk of resistance should be increased if infecting microorganisms are exposed to intermittent concentrations of drugs. Clinically, however, this does not appear to happen, although clinical trials that focus on emerging resistance (rather than resolution of infection) are lacking. It is possible that the impact of prolonged antimicrobial therapy on normal skin microflora might be minimized by pulse dosing, particularly if dosing occurs at levels high enough to target those colony-forming units (CFUs) with the highest MIC whose survival otherwise would facilitate emergence of a resistant population. If pulse dosing is to be implemented, a drug with a narrow spectrum (i.e., oxacillin, clindamycin, erythromycin) should be used to minimally affect the normal flora; further, high doses should be used to ensure efficacy against targeted organisms. Compliance may be an issue with pulse dosing, and care must be taken to ensure that drug therapy is maintained. Pulse dosing with cephalexin on the weekend (15 mg/kg every 12 hours) decreased the number of relapses compared with placebo (n = 13) after 1 year of therapy for prevention of relapse of idiopathic superficial or deep pyodermas in dogs (n = 28). The time to relapse also was greater in the treatment group (6.6 months) compared with the placebo group (2.5 months). Dogs were assigned to either group after clinical resolution was acheived following cephalexin at 15 mg/kg twice daily until 2 weeks beyond clinical cure. Dogs did not receive other systemic antibacterial drugs or any antiinflammatory.

Other Clinical Trials

Efficacy for treatment of pyoderma exists for both enrofloxacin[72,73] and marbofloxacin.[74] In an open (uncontrolled) study of dogs with superficial pyoderma (n = 66) caused predominantly by *S. intermedius*, marbofloxacin was effective in 86% and improved in another 8% after 21 to 28 days of therapy.[74] In another study 81% of dogs with recurrent superficial or deep pyoderma (n = 228) associated primarily with *S. intermedius* receiving marbofloxacin (2 mg/kg) for 3 to 16 weeks were classified as having responded at 1 week after cessation of therapy; at 1 month 70% of the dogs were still classified as responders, whereas 11% were classified as having relapsed.[75]

The efficacy of azithromycin for treatment of canine pyoderma (n = 26; 8 superficial and 18 deep) was studied prospectively using open uncontrolled design and was reported as an abstract.[71] Underlying disease was accepted and diagnosis was based on cytologic examination. The duration of azithromycin (10 mg/kg qd) varied with the deepness of the lesions ranging from 5 to 10 days. Eighty-eight percent of dogs recovered, with dogs that had superficial lesions requiring 5 to 7 days and dogs that had deep lesions requiring 7 to 10 days. Side effects occurred in only 24% of dogs, these included intense salivation, anorexia, and vomiting. One dog required antiemetic therapy (metaclopramide).

Stegemann and others[76] reported the efficacy of cefovecin for treatment of canine pyoderma and skin wounds. Dogs (n = 354) were from the United Kingdom and were evaluated in three studies, each using a randomized parallel design such that dogs received either amoxicillin–clavulanic acid (12.5 mg/kg bid for 2 weeks; n = 112) as positive control or cefovecin (8 mg/kg, administered subcutaneously; n = 242). The blinding method varied for each study, with a double-dummy design (each dog received placebo) implemented in one of the studies (Study B). Exclusion criteria included antimicrobial use within the past 14 days, short-acting glucocorticoids in the previous 10 days, or long-acting corticosteroids for 30 days. Up to 0.5 mg/kg/day of methylprednisolone or prednisone was allowed to control intense pruritis. Concurrent otitis was treated topically. Parasitic and fungal diseases were ruled out, and bacteria were confirmed by culture (sampling technique not delineated). Animals were evaluated 28 days after the final treatment. The most common organism cultured was *S. intermedius* (data are included in Table 8-7) (n = 223), with the MIC_{50} and MIC_{90} being 0.12 and 0.25 μg/mL, respectively. The next most common isolate was *E. coli* (MIC_{50} and MIC_{90} of 0.1 and 1 μg/mL, respectively). The number of treatments did not differ between groups and depended on clinical response, with nearly 50% of animals with superficial pyoderma in both groups responding after a single 14-day course of therapy; for animals with deep pyoderma, the numbers approximated 30% for both groups. For animals with deep pyoderma, 89% of animals enrolled in two of the studies had responded by the end of the third course of treatment (42) days, which is consistent with the recommendation to treat deep pyoderma for 4 to 6 weeks. Cefovecin was considered numerically more effective in treatment of superficial pyoderma. Criteria for success varied with the study and ranged from total absence of clinical signs to mild clinical signs. The study targeted a "noninferiority" classification of cefovecin, demonstrating that it was not worse than the positive control. Clinical success with cefovecin averaged 97% (study A & C) and 87% (study B) for all indications, compared with 92.5% and 80%, respectively, for amoxicillin–clavulanic acid. For cefovecin the lowest proportion of responders was for deep pyoderma (n = 13), at 77% for the double-dummy study versus 96% for the other two studies; only one animal with deep pyoderma was treated with amoxicillin–clavulanic acid. The incidence of side effects was similar in both groups, except for vomiting, which occurred more commonly in the group receiving amoxicillin–clavulanic acid.

KEY POINT 8-13 The long half-life of cefovecin will facilitate appropriate dosing. However, the impact of persistent drug concentrations must be monitored, and indiscriminate use of this potentially important drug must be avoided.

The efficacy of pradofloxacin (n = 56, 3 mg/kg by mouth qd) was compared with that of amoxicillin–clavulanic acid (positive control; n = 51, 12.5 mg/kg by mouth bid) for the treatment of deep pyoderma in dogs (n = 56) using a multicenter, randomized blinded controlled clinical trial.[77] Treatment continued until 2 weeks past remission, for a maxium treatment period of 9 weeks; final assessment took place 2 weeks later. Exclusion criteria included antiinfective or antiinflammtory drugs in the previous 14 days. Inclusion criteria required a positive culture (swabs; two attempts made before exclusion); positive cultures were found in only 71% (n = 92) of the 130 dogs studied. Bacteria isolated were predominantly *Staphylococcus* spp. (n = 115), with other organisms including but not limited to *Enterococcous* spp. (n = 5), *Pseudomonas* spp. (2), and *E. coli* (2). For the pradofloxacin group, 86% achieved clinical remission and recurrence did not occur during the 2 week posttreatment period. For the amoxicillin–clavulanic acid group, 73% (n = 37) achieved clinical remission; for the remaining dogs, 3 improved, 5 did not respond, and 6 had recurrence of clinical signs within 2 weeks of remission.

Topical Therapy

Topical antimicrobial therapy may be the only method of antimicrobial administration needed to treat selected surface and superficial pyodermas. Antiseptic bathing (e.g., benzoyl peroxide, chlorhexidine, ethyl lactate, iodine, or triclosan) should be considered as initial sole therapy in uncomplicated pyodermas. Topical antimicrobials also might be considered, particularly for localized infections. Mupirocin might be considered for treatment of localized dermatologic problems, including interdigital abcesses, pressure point pyodermas, and secondary pyodermas associated with lick dermatitis. Early use of mupirocin, in particular, may be beneficial in limiting the recurrence of pyodermas. The efficacy of mupirocin 2% ointment (bid for 3 weeks) was reported as good to excellent in an open, uncontrolled design for treatment of chin acne in cats (n = 25). Therapy had to be discontinued in one cat because of a contact allergy.[78]

Topical antimicrobial therapy should also be considered an adjuvant for superficial and deep pyodermas. Shampoos remove debris that might impede drug movement or affect drug efficacy. In addition, the combined effect of a topical and systemic antimicrobial may result in additive or synergistic antibacterial effects in the patient with pyoderma. Although irritating with long-term use, products that contain benzoyl peroxide tend to be the most efficacious in controlling bacterial growth and removing accumulated debris on the skin.[79] Products containing chlorhexidine, sulfur, triclosan, and ethyl lactate are also acceptable. Shampoos should be used twice weekly.[34,35]

KEY POINT 8-14 The combined effect of a topical and systemic antimicrobial may result in additive or synergistic antibacterial effects in the patient with pyoderma.

A human clinical trial examined the effect of terbinafine cream (1%) compared with gentamicin (0.1%) using a contralateral design in patients with pyoderma associated with *S. aureus*.[80] After treatment, *S. aureus* could not be isolated in any patient treated with gentamicin and in only three patients treated with terbinafine; a negative control was not reported. Both groups markedly improved during the treatment period and treatments did not differ significantly. The authors concluded that terbinafine might be beneficial for treatment of *S. aureus*, particularly that associated with fungal infections. Checkerboard MIC studies have demonstrated that the combined effect of benzoyl peroxide and terbinafine is greater than that of either drug alone against *Candida* spp., *S. aureus,* and *Pseudomonas* spp., resulting in additive or synergistic effects against all three isolates.[81]

Adjuvant Therapy

The importance of adjuvant therapy should not be overlooked in the treatment of pyoderma.[34,35] Adjuvant therapy may target the underlying skin disease or support antimicrobial therapy. Antihistamines (see Chapter 29) and 3-omega fatty acids should be considered when appropriate in conjunction with antimicrobial therapy to control the inflammatory response associated with infection or the underlying disease. Antimicrobial efficacy will be complicated by coadministration of drugs that alter the immune response. Most notably, glucocorticoids should not be used in patients with pyoderma. Although these drugs effectively ameliorate the inflammatory response and are useful in cases of pruritus leading to self-trauma, they also may facilitate the spread of bacterial infection.[34,35] Other adjuvant therapies to consider include immunomodulatory therapy and topical antimicrobial therapy. Although immunomodulatory therapy (levamisole and cimetidine) may prove beneficial, there is often a bimodal effect with these drugs: if the proper dose is not given, immunosuppression rather than enhancement of the immune system may occur.[34,35]

Adjvant therapy may include immunomodulators. In a pilot study human recombinant interferon alpha-2b (1000 IU/day by mouth) was only minimally effective compared with placebo in dogs with idiopathic recurrent superficial pyoderma.[82] Analgesic therapy also should be considered, particularly in animals that are experiencing pain. To prevent immunosuppression, nonsteroidal antiinflammatories should be considered. Indeed, meloxicam proved better than a placebo in control of pain associated with pyotraumatic dermatitis or folliculitis.[83] Tepoxalin might be worthwhile because it targets both prostaglandins and leukotrienes, the latter implicated in perpetuation of chronic inflammatory allergic diseases such as atopy (see Chapter 31). It is reasonable to consider the use of nonsteroidals, and tepoxalin in particular for treatment of pruritis associated with pyoderma. In a report from the Czech Republic, dogs (n = 18) with recurrent pyoderma received either cephalexin or cephalexin and an immunomodulator (characterized by natural killer cell activity, lymphocyte proliferation, and enhanced macrophage activity). The study did not appear to be randomized or blinded; further, dogs had previously received glucocorticoids. The authors reported that dogs receiving the immunomodulator had a better cure rate and a shorter time to cure.[84]

Juvenile Cellulitis (Puppy Strangles)

Juvenile cellulitis is probably more appropriately addressed as an immune-mediated disease, but its potential microbial-based pathophysiology as well as its presentation warrant inclusion under bacterial infections. Juvenile cellulitis is an unusual but often painful nonpruritic inflammatory condition afflicting puppies generally from 4 weeks to 4 months of age.[85,86] Clinical signs of inflammation generally involve the face or head. Its presentation may begin as a mild inflammation (e.g., redness and edema at tips of ears) but may rapidly become severe. Lymphadenopathly of nodes draining the inflamed areas (e.g., submandibular) has led to the misnomer "puppy strangles"; prescapular and other lymph nodes may become involved. Lesions range from (granulomatous) inflammation to pustules, ulcers, or erosions; fistulae may develop. Pustular otitis externa may be present. Less commonly, other areas of the body may be involved, including the abdomen, thorax, feet, vulva, prepuce, or anus. The extent of lesions may result in systemic illness; leukocytosis caused by neutrophilia and anemia typical of chronic disease may be present. Occasionally, other body systems will be involved (e.g., sterile suppurative arthritis)[87]. Cytologic examination reveals sterile pyogranulomatous inflammation; cultures generally are negative. Histopathology generally reveals granulomas and pyogranulomas consisting of clusters of large epithelioid macrophages. The cause of juvenile cellulitis is unknown, but the syndrome responds well to immunosuppressive doses (prednisolone at 2 mg/kg/day for up to 3 weeks), indicating a potential immune dysfunction. Hypersensitivity to (previously eradicated) microorganisms has been proposed. Therapy should be early and aggressive to prevent scarring. Antimicrobials are indicated only if supported by diagnostics. Although an etiologic agent has not been identified, a streptococcal-based reaction is suspected. Ideally, a lipid-soluble drug effective against *Streptococcus* spp. would be indicated to penetrate inflamed tissues. Fluoroquinolones are not recommended, not only because of questionable efficacy toward *Streptococcus* spp. but also because of age-related effects on cartilage as well as the potential induction of bacteriophage toxolysins carried by *Streptococcus* spp. (see Chapter 7). Assuming that there is a need for antimicrobial therapy targeting *Streptococcus* spp. high doses and frequent intervals of penicillin beta-lactams (amoxicillin–clavulinic acid) are indicated. Supportive therapy (e.g., cleaning of wounds, use of astringents) are indicated as needed. Analgesic therapy should be considered.

Wounds

The use of systemic antimicrobials for treatment of wounds is controversial, particularly in human medicine, for which diabetic and decubitus ulcers present a profound problem. Although the pathophysiology of these wounds may differ from that of the most common wounds treated in veterinary medicine, the principal approach should be similar. Disruption of skin or other tissue exposes the wound to infection, dehydration associated with fluid loss occurs, immunity is compromised, and scarring occurs. In contrast to the noninfected surgical wound that heals by primary intention, all open skin wounds, including those healing by secondary intention,[88] will be colonized with microbial organisms. This does not, however, indicate infection or the need for antimicrobial therapy. Host factors largely will determine if growth of the microbial population will be limited to colonization, with healing proceeding normally. Chronic wounds in particular are predisposed to infection because extensive synthesis of new, primarily granulation, tissue must occur. Scar tissue, which contains no epidermal appendages, is more extensive. As such, multiple aspects of the skin immune system are absent. Chronic wounds are further complicated by the presence of fibronectin, an adhesive glycoprotein that, while intended to serve as a matrix adhesive, also binds bacteria. Neutrophil and macrophage influx is critical to keeping bacteria in check.

KEY POINT 8-15 All open skin wounds, including those healing by secondary intention,will be colonized with microbial organisms. This does not, however, indicate infection or the need for antimicrobial therapy.

Colonizing microbes generally do not penetrate to deeper tissues, whereas infecting microbes will; accordingly, swabs are undesirable culture methods. Whether colonization progresses to infection depends on the number of organisms per gram of tissue (thus tissue samples rather than swabs are critically important to proper culture) and the ability of the patient to mount an effective immune reponse. Infection generally requires greater than 100,000 CFU/g tissues in a wound. An exception occurs for beta-hemolytic *Streptococcus*, which is particularly virulent in humans. Successful wound healing depends on an organism load below 100,000 CFU/gm. Studies generally demonstrate that in contrast to acute wounds, systemically administered drugs generally do not reach deeper tissues where infection occurs. This reflects not only the changes associated with healing but also the formation of biofilm (see Chapter 6). The impact of biofilm on healing of chronic wounds can be profound. Infections involving biofilm are resistant to host immune responses and more resistant to antimicrobials and topical antibacterials. The moist environment generally associated with chronic wounds facilitates biofilm, as does fibroinnectin.

KEY POINT 8-16 The impact of biofilm on healing of chronic wounds can be profound, leading to resistance to host immune responses and resistance to both systemic and topical antimicrobials.

In human medicine the consensus is that wound care should be optimal. Wound care should prevent microbial growth, which will inevitably occur on the surface of the wound, from progressing from colonization to infection. Accordingly, cleansing, débridement, nutritional support, and actions that enhance oxygenation, including increased perfusion, are paramount to success. A variety of wound-assessment tools have been developed in human medicine.[88] Wound care should be thoroughly reviewed before implementing systemic antimicrobial therapy. Topical antimicrobials are considered the key to successful management of wounds and are indicated if there is a risk that colonization will progress to infection. In humans *wound contamination* is treated simply with irrigation and cleansing with sterile water or saline. Likewise, *wound colonization* is treated with irrigation and cleansing of wounds, removal of necrotic tissue and foreign bodies, and nanocrystalline silver dressings. *Critical colonization* may require systemic antimicrobials but should be accompanied by medicated bandages and the topical application of slow-release antimicrobials (e.g., topical silver and cadexomer iodines). *Wound infection* is an indication that systemic antimicrobials should be added to topical therapy. Both systemic and topical medications are particularly critical in the face of poor wound perfusion.

KEY POINT 8-17 Topical antimicrobials are considered the key to the successful management of wounds and are indicated if there is a risk that colonization will progress to infection.

The most common topical antimcirobials used for wound management in humans are mupirocin, neomycin, bacitracin, polymyxin, erythromyicn, gentamicin, and silver sulfadiazine. Other topical antimicrobials to consider include fusidic acid and metronidazole. Their use for wound management was reviewed by Spann et al.[89] In addition to these traditional drugs, newer antimicrobials are under development. These include protegrin-1, an antimicrobial peptide that occurs naturally in a number of mammalian tissues, including neutrophils. These are particularly effective against gram-positive organism, including MRSA and vancomycin-resistant *Enterococcus* spp. Other topically applied antimicrobials are under investigation (see Box 8-1).

The use of antiseptics on wounds is controversial, in part because of their impact on wound healing. This impact appears to be concentration dependent.[90] Topical antiseptics include sodium chloride, (preferred) chlorhexidine, and povidone-iodine. The Food and Drug Administration has approved povidone-iodine for short-term treatment of superficial and acute wounds, indicating that its impact on wound healing is neither positive nor negative. A potential reason for using antiseptics, rather than antimicrobials, on wounds, is to prevent antimicrobial resistance. However, care should be taken not to use antiseptics and disinfectants indiscriminately. Resistance has developed toward most antiseptics or disinfectants for many microbes, with the mechanisms similar to those for which antimicrobial resistance has emerged. For example, a number of organisms, including *Pseudomonas* spp., have become resistant to quarternary ammonium compounds, *Klebsiella* and *E. coli* have expressed resistance to chlorine, and peroxides are among the compounds toward which the most resistance has emerged.[91]

KEY POINT 8-18 Resistance that has developed toward most antiseptics or disinfectants by many microbes occurs by way of mechanisms similar to those that result in antimicrobial drug resistance.

Occlusive or vapor-permeable dressings may reduce the risk of bacterial contamination. Note that for all levels of infection, appropriate cleansing, including débridement, is key to the success of antimicrobial therapy, whether topical or systemic.

Dog or cat bite wounds may be deep, penetrating wounds. As such, the risk for infection may be greater compared with more superficial skin wounds. However, particularly with cat bite wounds that are open and in which the risk of cellulitis is minimal, antimicrobial therapy may not be indicated (Figure 8-4). Hot-packing is an important component of therapy.

The microbiology of canine bite wounds was recently reviewed prospectively.[92] Wounds were clipped and cleansed with 70% alcohol. Culture samples were collected before cytologic samples, using swabs, which may limit accuracy and preclude colony counts. Swabs were inserted deep within puncture wounds or deep pockets. Both aerobic and anaerobic cultures were collected from dogs (n = 50) in which wounds were inflicted within the previous 72 hours. A total of 104 wounds were studied, with 21 assessed cytologically as infected and 83 noninfected. However, based on growth, 75% were positive. Sixty-six of the 83 noninfected (cytologically) wounds yielded positive growth, for a total of 213 isolates. Aerobic isolates were equally represented by gram-negative and gram-positive organisms (see Table 8-1). Anaerobic organisms were cultured in 17 of 50 wounds; 17 yielded anaerobic organisms. The most common anaerobic organisms (obligate) were *Prevotella melaninogenica* (59%) followed by *Clostridium* and *Peptostreptococcus* spp.

Cat bite wounds have also been studied (Australia).[93] *P. multocida* historically is recognized to be a causative agent on the basis of wounds in humans. However, as in the dog, a range of aerobic and anaerobic organisms are associated with feline bite wounds. In humans the sequelae of cat bites result in infection with a variety of aerobes, including *Staphylococcus* spp., *Streptococcus* spp., including alpha-hemolytic; *Moraxella* spp., Enterobacteriaceae spp., *Weeksella zoohelcum;* and *Capnocytophaga*. Anaerobic organisms include a number of *Fusobacterium* spp., *Bacteroides* spp., *Porphyromonas* spp., *Prevotella* spp., *Peptostreptococcus* spp., and *Propionobacterium* spp. Bite wounds as they develop in cats include *Pasteurella* spp. (the most common facultative anaerobe), *Bacteroides* spp. (including *Prevotella, Porphyromonas;* 29%), *Fusobacterium* spp. (19%), *Peptostreptococcus* spp. (13%), and *Actinomyces* spp. Closed abscesses in cats contain an average of three isolates, although as many as eight have been identified. Isolates have been confirmed to be of oral origin. Accordingly, the role of *Porphyromonas,* and particularly *Porphyromonas gingivalis,* is increasingly recognized for its importance.

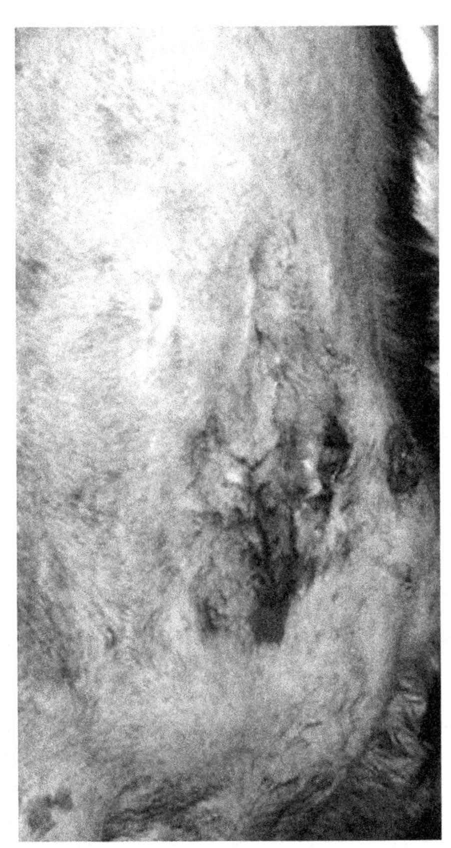

Figure 8-4 Feline abscesses are an example of an infection that may not require treatment with antimicrobials, particularly if the abscess is open and draining well. Treatment is indicated if associated with a risk of cellulitis.

Miscellaneous Infections

Dapsone is an antimicrobial that inhibits para-aminobenzoic acid metabolism to folic acid. Selected mycobacterial strains, most notably *Mycobacteria leprae* or *Mycobacteria lepraemurium,* are exquisitively sensitive to its effects. In addition, the drug appears to be capable of some form of immunomodulation and may prove beneficial in deep skin infections associated with a pyogranulomatous response for which no organism has been identified. Because of difficulty associated with identifying infectious organisms such as *Nocardia* spp. and atypical mycobacterial organisms, however, use of dapsone should be reserved until a susceptible organism has been identified or other causes of inflammatory skin disease have been ruled out. The drug has not been studied in animals, and in humans, it is characterized by marked differences in disposition. Hemolytic episodes have been reported in humans; however, generally these individuals are suffering from metabolic defects of red blood cells. Dapsone also is used to treat bites caused by brown recluse spiders in humans. When Dapsone is administered within 48 hours of the bite, tissue necrosis is markedly decreased and wound healing is subsequently faster.

INFECTIONS OF THE MUSCULOSKELETAL SYSTEM

Osteomyelitis

Because bacterial myositis is rare unless it accompanies infection of the surrounding soft tissues, this discussion is limited to bacterial infections affecting the skeletal structures.

Pathophysiology

Similar to models described in humans,[94] infections of the bone occur by a hematogenous route, secondary to a contiguous focus or direct inoculation through surgery or trauma.[95] The metaphyses of long bones are the most common sites of hematogenous infection.[94] Blood flow becomes slow and turbulent in this region, and capillaries lack phagocytic cells. Acute infection causes local cellulitis resulting in leukocyte accumulation, increased bone pressure, decreased pH, and reduced oxygen tension. Contiguous infections generally result from direct inoculation of the bone because of trauma, extension from surrounding soft tissues, or contamination associated with surgery. Vertebral osteomyelitis most commonly reflects a hematogenous source of infection, usually from an artery. Because each artery supplies two adjacent vertebrae, the infection usually involves two vertebrae. Secondary osteomyelitis is further classified on the basis of the presence or absence of vascular insufficiency.

Both hematogenous and secondary osteomyelitis can be classified as acute or chronic. Acute osteomyelitis is a suppurative infection accompanied by edema, vascular congestion, and small vessel thrombosis. Vascular supply to the site of infection becomes compromised as the infection extends into the soft tissue. Both medullary and periosteal blood supplies can become compromised, resulting in necrotic, ischemic, and ultimately dead bone forming a sequestrum. Bacteria located in this tissue become isolated, with acute osteomyelitis progressing to chronic osteomyelitis. Chronic osteomyelitis is characterized by local bone loss, a nidus of infected dead bone or scar tissue, an area of ischemic soft tissue, persistent drainage, and sinus tracts. The clinical course can be refractory. The risk of infection continues even in apparently cured osteomyelitis because of this nidus of infection. Indeed, the term *arrested* is often used instead of the term *cured* when referring to successful therapy in human patients. The presence of foreign bodies facilitates sustained infection through formation of biofilm (see Chapter 6), promotion of virulence factors (e.g., adherence receptors), and their negative impact on local immune function.[95] Successful treatment of osteomyelitis is less likely in the presence of necrotic surrounding soft tissue, foreign bodies, bone instability, nonunion, or septic joints. Consequently, surgical removal of the nidus of infection and foreign bodies often must accompany antimicrobial therapy.

KEY POINT 8-19 Successful treatment of osteomyelitis is less likely in the presence of necrotic soft tissue, foreign bodies, bone instability, nonunion, or septic joints.

In addition to the classes of osteomyelitis based on route of infection, a more clinically relevant classification system (Ciemy-Mader) developed in humans[94] yields 12 distinct stages based on patient status, anatomic considerations, cause of infection, treatment factors, and prognosis. The advantages of this approach is that stages delineate factors that complicate therapy. Four stages are described on the basis of anatomic considerations, with each stage characterized by additional complications.

Stage 1 (medullary) occurs early; the primary site of infection is endosteal or may include infected intramedullary pins. Therapy may simply include antimicrobials but may also include surgical débridement or removal of the surgical foreign body. Stage 2 (superficial) osteomyelitis occurs as a result of extension of infection from soft tissue. As such, a secondary contiguous focus exists; this focus requires surgical débridement in conjunction with antimicrobial therapy. Stage 3 (localized) osteomyelitis is characterized by full-thickness infection of the cortices with sequestration that requires surgical removal. Stage 4 (diffuse) osteomyelitis involves the full diameter of the infected bone and may cross a joint. Bone instability occurs as a result of either infection or surgical treatment. Therapy includes débridement, management of dead space, and stabilization. Each of these four stages can be further categorized on the basis of the status of the host: A (normal), B (local or systemic compromise), or C (treatment of the infection is more life threatening than the osteomyelitis). Local compromise includes chronic lymphedema, venous stasis, compromise of major vessels, arteritis, and extensive scarring fibrosis. Systemic compromise includes malnutrition, evidence of metabolic disease (e.g., renal or liver disease, diabetes mellitus), malignancy, age extremes, or immunosuppression. These stages are dynamic, being affected by therapy, progression of disease, and host status.

Microbial Targets

Hematogenous osteomyelitis is usually caused by a single pathogenic organism, with *Staphylococcus* spp. (50% to 70%) predominating and *S. intermedius* most common. Vertebral osteomyleitis also is most commonly caused by *Staphylococcus* spp. Common sites of infection in humans that lead to vertebral osteomyelitis are the genitourinary tract, skin and soft tissue, respiratory tract, mouth, endocardium, and intravenous lines.[94] Multiple pathogenic organisms are usually involved with contiguous infections, and as in hematogenous infections, *Staphylococcus* spp. is one of the most common organisms isolated. Gram-negative and anaerobic organisms are also commonly involved.[94] The most common gram-negative are *E. coli, Klebsiella, Pasteurella, Serratia,* and *Proteus* spp. The most common anaerobes are *Bacteroides, Fusobacterium,* (including *F. necrophorum*), *Clostridium* spp., and others. The risks of therapeutic failure associated with osteomyelitis outweigh the risks associated with culture and susceptibility testing; accordingly, drug selection and the design of the dosing regimen should be culture based. Care must be taken with sample collection to ensure that proper techniques are followed.

Antimicrobial Therapy

Clinical trials have provided only limited direction in the successful treatment of osteomyelitis, being handicapped by variations in duration (acute versus chronic), organisms studied, the model of osteomyelitis used, mode of infection (in nonspontaneous models), presence of foreign material, previous surgical procedures, and previous antimicrobial therapy. Among the critical host factors of concern when treating osteomyelitis is drug distribution to the site. Distribution may be limited because of changes in blood flow, presence of inflammation, and poor local immunity. Note that some drugs distribute to the bone only to bind to calcium or other cations (e.g., tetracyclines, potentially fluoroquinolones) (Table 8-8). As with other sites of infection, drug penetration in osteomyelitis is determined by the molecular weight and the lipid solubility of the drug. Protein-bound drugs do not distribute to the site of infection. The mechanisms of capillary transport in osteomyelitic bone are similar to those in normal bone,

Table 8-8 Concentrations of Selected Antimicrobials in Bone Experimentally Infected with *Staphylococcus aureus*

Drug	Dose	CONCENTRATIONS (μg/m) Serum	Bone	Bone to Serum Ratio	Breakpoint MIC
Beta-lactams					
Nafcillin	40 mg/kg	21.9	2.1	0.095	≤2 to ≥4
Moxalactam	40 mg/kg	65.2	6.2	0.095	≤8 to ≥64
	5 mg/kg	45.6	3.2	0.07	≤8 to ≥32
Cefazolin	15 mg/kg	67.2	2.6	0.04	≤8 to ≥32
Cephalothin	40 mg/kg	34.8	1.3	0.04	≤8 to ≥32
Aminoglycosides					
Tobramycin	5 mg/kg	14.3	1.3	0.09	≤4 to ≥16
Others					
Clindamycin	70 mg/kg	12.1	11.9	0.98	≤0.5 to ≥4
Vancomycin	2-3g (28.5-43 mg/kg)	35	5.3*	0.15	≥14

MIC, Minimum inhibitory concentration.
*Monitoring recommended.
Adapted from Mader JT, Calhoun J: Osteomyelitis. In Mandell G, Bennett JE, Dolin R, editors: *Principles and practice of infectious diseases,* ed 4, New York, 1995, Churchill Livingstone, pp. 1039-1050.

although permeability ratios to the site of the drugs differ. A blood-bone barrier does not appear to exist. However, the impact of the intramedullary infection on blood distribution may limit drug delivery. The impact of biofilm on successful therapy also may be profound, particularly in the presence of foreign bodies.

Determining the extent of drug distribution to potential sites of infection in bone is difficult. Distribution studies often are based on cannulation of nutrient artery and the ipsilateral femoral vein. Detection of drug in bone is limited by recovery of the drug, which tends to be low because tissue is lost during the extraction procedure. Volume of distribution studies generally have shown that concentrations of biologically active drug in the interstitial fluid space of normal cortical bone are equivalent to that in the serum, regardless of the lipophilicity of the drug. The characteristics of cefazolin have resulted in its use for surgical prophylaxis in patients undergoing orthopedic surgical procedures.[96] Cefazolin readily traverses capillaries of both normal and osteomyelitic bone, and the pathophysiology of osteomyelitis enhances penetration. Although the volume of spaces (plasma and interstitial) increases in osteomyelitis by 330% and 941%, respectively, the distribution of cefazolin increases proportionately. Cefazolin is not as highly protein bound in dogs as it is in humans (35% versus 80%); accordingly, effective concentrations of pharmacologically active drug should be expected in normal bone tissues of dogs.[96] However, other drugs appear to penetrate infected bone better than cefazolin. The prophylactic use of antimicrobials increasingly is not considered necessary (see Chapter 6). Although the long half-life of cefovecin might support its indication for treatment of osteomylitis caused by susceptible bacteria, it is not indicated for prophylaxis. Not only will maximum concentrations take up to 8 to 24 hours to achieve (with efficacy depending on the MIC_{90} of the target microbe), but therapy cannot be discontinued after surgery (the elimination half-life causes drug to persist for 1 to 2 weeks), as is indicated for prophylaxis.

In experimental rabbit models of osteomyelitis caused by *S. aureus,* drugs characterized by the best bone-to-serum ratio were, in order, clindamycin, vancomycin, moxalactam (a beta-lactam antibiotic), tobramycin, cefazolin, and cephalothin (see Table 8-8).[94]

Because of the potential difficulty in achieving high concentrations at the osteomyelitic site, a number of methods of local drug delivery might be considered, particularly for infections associated with multidrug-resistant organisms. Advantages include high local concentrations for a longer period of time and avoidance of systemic exposure to antimicrobials that might otherwise be toxic. Among those methods most considered are antimicrobial-impregnated beads. Two forms of beads have been used. Beads made of polymethyl methacrylate (PMMA) are nonbiodegradable; their use in horses has been reviewed, and much of the information is applicable to dogs and cats.[97] A number of commercially available PMMA cements are available; additionally, compounding pharmacies are beginning to offer antimicrobial-impregnated beads. Mixing drug in PMMA results in an exothermic reaction, causing tissue damage and the potential release of toxins; bone-healing and phagocytic function may be impaired. Antimicrobials are added in powder form but must be heat stable. More recently, calcium-based (e.g., sulfate, plaster of paris) antimicrobial-impregnated beads have been studied. In contrast to the PMMA, these beads are biodegradable and their formation is not exothermic. However, beads should be sterilized using non–heat-based methods. The advantages of calcium sulfate includes osteoconductivity, potentially facilitating bone healing; the biodegradable nature often precludes the need for retrieval surgery. Even more recently, biodegradable matrices are being studied.

KEY POINT 8-20 Local drug delivery may be a viable adjuvant for treatment of problematic osteomyelitis, particularly if infection involves a multidrug-resistant organism.

Regardless of the matrix type, antimicrobial release or elution tends to be bimodal, with an initial rapid release (12 to 48 hours) followed by a slower release over weeks or months. For PMMA, elution rates (based on in vitro studies) vary with antimicrobial concentration, pore and bead size, and permeability of the cement (which, in turn, can be affected by the amount and type of antimicrobial). The form (e.g., liquid versus powder form) of the antimicrobial will also influence elution. Host factors influencing elution rates include surface area available for bead exposure, blood flow, and fluid content. In general, concentrations in the first stage of elution surrounding the area can be anticipated to exceed the MIC_{90} of most susceptible organisms by more than a hundredfold, increasing the likelihood of a quick kill. Concentrations during the second phase of elution will be much lower but may still surpass the MIC_{90} of infecting microbes by several to a hundredfold. Sayegh[97] indicates that encapsulation of the beads during healing results in therapeutic concentrations being achieved up to 2 to 3 mm surrounding the beads.

Atilla and others[98] have demonstrated that the combination of drugs in beads alters their elution rate, causing it to be more rapid. Atlhough concentrations are initially higher, the duration of effective concentration may be shorter. The authors also demonstrated that, interestingly, the elution rate may change even if drugs are not mixed in the same bead but are in different beads. Antimicrobial-impregnated beads can be used to treat bone, synovial structures, and other soft tissues; use of PMMA in joints is discouraged, however, because it tends to be irritating. Indications include refractory infections, particularly osteomyelitis, and prophylaxis after surgery of contaminated wounds.

A disadvantage of beads, particulary PMMA-based beads, is the foreign nature. Further, the PMMA can inhibit phagocytic function. Heat-damaged tissue may facilitate infection. Host response to the cement may also facilitate infection by *S. aureus*, and microorganisms can secrete materials that protect against host defense mechanisms. As such, they may be associated with risk of infection, as has been described in a series of human patients (n = 20). Cultures of gentamicin-loaded beads removed 2 weeks after implantation from prosthesis-related infections revealed 90% to be infected. Of the 28 isolates, nearly 70% were gentamicin-resistant.[99] Interestingly, 12 of the 18 infected patients were considered infection free before removal of the infected beads. Most common isolates were *P. aeruginosa* and *S. aureus*. In contrast, the prosthetic devices in the area of the beads tended to not be infected.

The use of tobramycin antimicrobial-impregnated calcium sulfate beads in a series of dogs (n = 6) was recently reported.[100] The beads are commercially available, approved for use as bone filler. Sites included forelimb and hindlimbs. Infecting organisms included *S. intermedius*, *S. aureus*, and *P. aeruginosa*. The number of beads implanted ranged from four to nine; one dog that received a total hip replacement received 24 beads. Beads generally lost their radio-opacity by 4 weeks and were no longer visible radiographically by 6 to 8 weeks. Clinical signs associated with infection resolved in all but one dog.

A case report described the successful use of a commercially available gentamicin-impregnated collagen sponge (CollaRx) in the treatment of septic arthtritis associated with MRSA in a dog.[12] Other matrices are under investigation, with a focus on those that slow release or are biodegradable. However, a commonality of most of the studies addressing drug elution from foreign matrices is of questionable applicability to the patient. This includes studies that expose representative pathogens (e.g., *Staphylococcus* spp.) to eluent containing the antimicrobial. The accuracy of concenterations measured *in vitro* from eluent representing matrices incubated in buffer as predictors of interstial concentrations in a surgical patient receiving these drug delivery devices is debatable. As such, studies are needed based on concentrations measured *in vivo* using ultrafiltration probes that collect interstitial fluid.

Medical management of chronic osteomyelitis in humans has not been well supported by well-designed controlled clinical trials; the knowledge base in veterinary medicine is even more limited. Variability in risk factors, pathophysiology of infection, and etiologic agents and failure to identify the organism preclude the generation of consensus regarding recommendations in humans. Further, outcome measures of therapeutic success are not always identified or clear. A large trial using expensive therapies for extended periods of time is prohibitively expensive and is complicated by the ability of pathogens to cause low-grade symptoms or lie dormant for many years, requiring long-term follow-up.[95] It is not surprising, therefore, that recommendations have been based on historical observations, experimental models, and nonrandomized trials.[95] Retrospective studies have been helpful but generally are more representative of complicated cases.[101]

Although drug distribution to healthy bone is adequate, the detrimental effects of osteomyelitis minimize drug distribution to the site of infection. As such, culture-based drug selection and dosing regimen design is likely to be paramount to therapeutic success. Parenteral antimicrobial therapy should begin with drugs targeting the most likely organisms; drug therapy can be changed if indicated on the basis of susceptibility data. Duration of therapy for osteomyelitis is generally recommended for 4 to 6 weeks, in part because tissue revascularization after débridement requires at least 3 to 4 weeks.[95] However, as with other therapies, the evidence for duration of therapy is limited by the lack of clinical trials. The need for longer term therapy might be anticipated for chronic osteomyelitis.

The first 2 weeks of therapy should be by parenteral administration (data from the start of therapy or after surgical débridement). For acute hematogenous osteomyelitis, the causative agent must be properly identified. Mismanagement with inappropriate antimicrobial can lead to extension of the infection, necrosis, and the formation of sequestra, as well as emergence of resistance. If the patient has not responded to specific antimicrobial therapy (i.e., based on culture) within

48 hours, surgical intervention is indicated for human patients. Bone biopsy specimens are necessary for culture for human patients[94] unless the patient also has positive blood cultures. Because of its excellent distribution characteristics, oral quinolone therapy may be an acceptable alternative for gram-negative and *Staphylococcus* spp. infections. Note, however, that the activity of the second-generation fluoroquinolones against anaerobes and other gram-positive organisms (e.g., *Streptococcus* spp., some *Corynebacterium* spp.) is less predictable, whereas third-generation fluoroquinolones have a broader spectrum. In addition, although bone concentrations of difloxacin are high (see package insert), concentrations do not decline over time, suggesting that the drug is bound and thus inactive. Whether this is true for other fluoroquinolones is not clear. Clindamycin, metronidazole, or amoxicillin–clavulanic acid can be used in combination with the quinolones to provide gram-positive and anaerobic coverage. Intravenous therapy generally is recommended, in part because antimicrobials most commonly associated with clinical success (e.g., cefazolin and vancomycin) are characterized by poor oral bioavailability. However, because of the potential risks and inconvenience, alternative therapies, such as oral antimicrobial therapy, have been considered. The potential efficacy of oral therapy is more reasonable with the availability of several drugs that are safe and highly bioavailable after oral administration. Several oral antimicrobial agents have undergone evaluation for the treatment of acute and chronic osteomyelitis in human medicine. Oral antimicrobials are considered for treatment of acute osteomylitis in children and chronic infection caused by atypical gram-positive and selected gram-negative organisms. Choices include the fluoroquinolones, clindamycin, and linezolid, the latter being reserved for MRS or potentially enterococci.[95] Retained foreign material or prosthetic devices complicate oral management of osteomyelitis, and therapy is more likely to fail with oral rather than intravenous therapy.[95] Despite these drawbacks, a number of studies have supported oral therapy for chronic osteomyelitis. In general, oral therapy with ciprofloxacin as sole agent compares favorably to parenteral therapy with single or combination antimicrobials. However, resistance in gram-positive organisms appears to develop rapidly. Rifampin used in combination with other antimicrobials appears to be effective for treatment of staphylococcal orthopedic implant-related infections. Thus whereas intravenous antimicrobials for 2 weeks followed by long-term oral (ciprofloxacin) therapy appears to be effective, longer-term therapy (3 to 6 months or more) with a combination of ciprofloxacin and rifampin was associated with a 100% cure rate compared with a 58% cure rate for ciprofloxacin only.[95] A meta-analysis study of 22 trials involving 927 human patients with orthopedic devices associated with *S. aureus*–induced osteomyelitis offers some insight into antimicrobial therapy. Disconcertingly, most of the studies were characterized as poor in quality, impaired by inappropriate methods and statistical analysis. However, a trend of improvement was detected for the combination of rifampicin–ciprofloxacin compared with ciprofloxacin alone. Use of ticarcillin for bone infections associated with *Pseudomonas* spp. was described as favorable. Therapeutic success with oral fluoroquinolones did not differ from success with intravenous beta-lactams. Comparison of locally placed PMMA gentamicin bead chains compared with parenteral antimicrobials could not be evaluated well because all patients received systemic therapy.[102]

Chronic contiguous osteomyelitis may be particularly difficult to resolve. Assessment of vascular integrity by cutaneous oxygen tension can be useful for determining the extent of damaged tissue to be removed.[94] Hyperbaric oxygen therapy may facilitate healing in tissues characterized by low oxygen tension. Dead space can be managed short term with antimicrobial-impregnated acrylic beads; the beads are generally replaced with a cancellous bone graft after 2 to 4 weeks. Hyperbaric oxygen is an important adjunct therapy for human patients with osteomyelitis. It serves to restore intramedullary oxygen tension and thus facilitates phagocytic killing. Furthermore, it supports collagen production, angiogenesis, and wound healing.[94]

Infections associated with prosthetic devices involving cement are particularly problematic to resolve. Infections generally occur at the bone–cement interface. Infectious pathogens are numerous and, in humans, often include microorganisms considered to be contaminants of cultures (e.g., corynebacteria, propionibacteria, and *Bacillus* spp.). PMMA cement may predispose the site to infection, as previously discussed. Infection can be treated with removal of the prosthetic device and 6 weeks of antimicrobial therapy followed by reimplantation or surgical removal and débridement with immediate reimplantation accompanied by polymethyl methacrylate cement inpregnated with an antimicrobial (an aminoglycoside). When the prosthesis cannot be removed, lifelong antimicrobial therapy has been implemented for human patients, assuming that the microorganism is sufficiently susceptible to oral antimicrobial therapy and the patient can tolerate the therapy.

Septic Arthritis

Pathophysiology

Septic arthritis most commonly reflects hematogenous inoculation. Patients with osteoarthritis or immune-mediated arthritis, trauma, or intraarticular inflammation are predisposed to infections in the inflamed joint. Trauma may predispose to infection because of a loss of vascular integrity. Synovial tissue is very vascular, and the lack of a basement membrane facilitates bacterial penetration. Bacteria can contribute to the process of inflammation through production of tissue-damaging mediators such as proteases. *S. aureus* is among the organisms most commonly causing infection in humans, in part because of its ability to bind to bone sialoprotein, a glycoprotein of joints.[103] It is able to contribute to destruction of cartilage because of the production of chondrocyte proteases. Infection often affects a single joint and usually is limited to the joint. Exceptions are made in the presence of predisposing factors that affect multiple joints (e.g., immune-mediated arthritis). Drug distribution into inflamed synovium occurs more rapidly and results in higher concentrations than in uninflamed joints.

Clinical signs associated with septic arthritis include fever, limited joint motion, and swelling of peripheral joints associated with joint tenderness. Synovial fluid analysis discriminates between septic and nonseptic causes of arthritis. In general, septic arthritis more commonly is associated with increased polymorphonuclear leukocytes. The presence of immunomodulating drugs (e.g., glucocorticoids) may blunt leukocyte infiltration. In human patients the presence of bacteria can be detected in approximately 33% of cases by cytologic examination of a smear of synovial fluid. Cytologic examination should include Gram stains. Synovial fluid should be cultured; for human patients blood culturing also is recommended.[103] False-negative cultures may not, however, rule out bacterial arthritis; in human patients with documented infection, synovial fluid cultures were negative 10% of the time. Radiographic examination may help rule in arthritis.

Microbial Targets

The most common causes of septic arthritis reported in animals are bacterial in origin. The potential for viral causes should not be ignored. In human patients two syndromes of arthritis are described: acute and chronic, nonarticular. The syndromes are caused by different types of organisms, with mycobacterial or fungal infections of the joint largely responsible for the chronic form. According to surgical texts, organisms most commonly associated with septic joints include *Staphylococcus* spp., *Streptococcus* spp., *E. coli,* and *Pasteurella* spp.

Antimicrobial Therapy

In human patients septic arthritis is treated aggressively. Empirical therapy is begun after culture collection using an intravenously administered antimicrobial effective against *S. aureus.* Examples include cefuroxime, cefotaxime, and ceftriaxone; the role of extended-spectrum beta-lactamases and therapeutic success has not been addressed, and the prudent clinician might consider combining therapy with a drug that is not vulnerable to these destructive enzymes. The use of fluoroquinolones for treatment of infections associated with joints or ligaments should be done cautiously. Their impact on healing cartilage may be similar to that of cartilage in growing animals, and evidence has emerged that demonstrates their negative impact on ligaments. Use of chondroprotective disease-modifying agents (including both glucosamine and chondroitin sulfates) should be considered in any patient with joint disease receiving any fluorinated quinolone. Note that fluoroquinolones have been associated with impaired healing in tendons[103a]; the impact on other skeletal tissues is not clear. The use of an antimicrobial-impregnated collagen sponge was addressed previously.

KEY POINT 8-21 The use of a fluoroquinolone for treatment of infections associated with joints or ligaments requires caution.

Duration of therapy for treatment of septic arthritis in humans generally is at least 3 weeks, although these recommendations are based on older retrospective studies.[101] Shorter treatment periods are being promoted, particularly in children. Similarly, a recent trend is oral treatment after a brief period of intravenous therapy. Response to antimicrobial therapy is based, in humans, on repetitive analysis of synovial fluid collected by joint aspiration. Persistence of infusion beyond 7 days is interpreted as the need for surgical drainage. Use of appropriate antimicrobials early in the course of arthritis will minimize damage to the joint.[103]

Adjuvant Therapy

Because septic arthritis can be accompanied by the loss of collagen and erosion of articular surfaces, therapy with disease-modifying agents should strongly be considered. Injectable products such as polysulfated glycosaminoglycans (Adequan), pentosan polysulfate, and hyaluronic acid (the latter perhaps in combination with either of the former) are more apt to act more rapidly than oral products. Oral disease-modifying agents such as chondroitin sulfates, keratan sulfates, and glucosamines (e.g., Cosequin) also should be strongly considered until the joint is healed.

URINARY TRACT INFECTIONS (UTIs)

UTIs include but are not limited to pyelonephritis, ureteritis, cystitis, urethritis, and prostatitis. Infection occasionally is restricted to urine (bacteriuria).[104] Identification of the site of a UTI may be difficult, as might be discrimination of the infection as primary or secondary. However, because infection in any region of the urinary tract can be accompanied by or result in infection throughout the tract, terminology inclusive of all sites (i.e., UTI) often is preferred to terms limited to a single site of infection (e.g., upper or lower UTI). However, the site of infection has implications because of potential differences in ease of treatment, including drug distribution. The incidence of UTIs in dogs is higher (estimated at 14%) than that in cats (1% to 3%).[104] However, it is not clear whether this takes into account occult infections (see later discussion).

Microbial Targets

Because the urinary tract is a site for which bacterial contamination is common, the size of the inoculum should be considered when identifying target pathogens and the need for treatment. This need increases in the face of emerging antimicrobial resistance. Generally, the urinary tract is sterile above the urethra. *Bacteriuria* simply refers to the presence of bacteria in the urine. Infection of the urinary tract begins with bacterial adherence to uroepithelial cells of the urinary mucosal surface. The number of CFUs indicative of infection is higher than that for tissues for which contamination is unlikely and is influenced by both the method of sample collection and the gender. In his retrospective evaluating risk factors associated with UTI in dogs (n = 8354) from 1969 to 1995, Ling et al.[105] defined clinically important bacteriuria when samples were collected by catheterization as ≥100,000 CFUs/mL in female dogs and ≥10,000 CFUs/mL in males, whereas ≥100,000 CFUs were considered significant in either gender if collected midstream. In an uncontaminated cystocentesis, any growth was considered significant. Other investigators (e.g., Seguin[106])

Table 8-9 Pharmacokinetic and Pharmacodynamic Indices for Treatment of Canine and Feline *Escherichia coli* Associated with Urinary Tract Infections

Drug	Resistant BP (μg/mL)	Mode (μg/mL)	MIC_{50} (μg/mL)	MIC_{90} (μg/mL)	Range	Dose (mg/kg)	C_{max} (μg/mL)	Half-Life	C_{max}: $MIC_{50}^{\dagger}$	T>MIC (hr)
Amoxicillin-clavuanic acid	≤ 1 is susceptible	4	4	32	0.5-2048	13.5	6	1.25	NA	1
Ampicillin	0.5-1	2	4	512	0.25-512	30	10	1	NA	2
Meropenem	16	0.25	0.25	0.5	0.25	20 (SC)	26	0.75	NA	4.5
Cefotaxime	64	1	1	16	1-2048	50 (IM)	47	0.75	NA	6
Cefoxitin	32	4	4	32	0.5-2048	30 (SC)	10	1	NA	2
Cefpodoxime	8	0.5	0.5	256	0.12-512	10	16	5	NA	20
Ceftazidime	32	0.5	0.5	16	0.25-512	30 (SC)	42	1	NA	6
Cephalothin (cephalexin)	8	8	16	2048	1-2048	25	19	1	NA	1
Gentamicin	16	1	1	8	1	4.4	7.5	NA	7.5	NA
Enrofloxacin	4	0.06	0.06	32	0.03-512	20	6	NA	100	NA
Ciprofloxacin	4	0.03	0.03	32	0.3-128	20	2.8	NA	93	NA
Azithromycin	8	8	8	64	1-512	24‡	4	35	NA	0
CHPC	32	8	8	32	2-2048	50	20	3	NA	6
Doxycycline	16	1	2	32	0.25-1024	5	5	5	NA	5

BP, Breakpoint, *MIC,* minimum inhibitory concentration; *NA,* not applicable; *SC,* subcutaneous; *IM,* intramuscular; *TMPS,* trimethoprim–sulfadoxine; *CHPC,* chloramphenicol.
*475 isolates are from the urinary tract. Personal data of author (in press).
†Data based on MIC_{50}, but MIC_{90} preferred. However, this data includes dogs previously exposed to antimicrobials. MIC_{90} is likely to be lower if only antimicrobial-naïve dogs are considered (see Table 8-11). The MIC_{90} of susceptible isolates is likely to be lower (see Table 8-11).
‡This dose is approximately twofold higher than recommended.
§Doses are those delineated in Table 7-1.
C_{max}/MIC (target ≥10) and T >MIC (target generally 50% of dosing interval) are likely to be higher and longer, respectively, for renally excreted drugs if infection is limited to the bladder, biofilm is minimal, and renal concentration is normal.

have considered growth significant in cystocentesis samples only if CFUs are greater than 1000. This seems to be a reasonable basis for criteria when considering treatment of UTI, as long as the criteria are considered in the context of the circumstances surrounding the infection, including the presence of clinical signs. The presence of three or more different organisms was considered by Ling et al.[105] as indicative of contamination regardless of the method of collection and indicated the need to resample and reculture.

Historically, *E. coli* has been recognized as the predominant cause of UTIs in both dogs and cats (Table 8-9).[107,108] *Staphylococcus* spp. and other gram-positive organisms historically have accounted for 25% of UTIs in dogs. Other cited causative agents in the dog include *Proteus, Klebsiella, Enterobacter,* and *Pseudomonas* spp.[110] *Proteus* and *Staphylococcus* spp. cause urinary alkalinization and as such often are associated with struvite formation in dogs. In the cat, organisms other than *E. coli* that cause UTIs have included *Proteus, Klebsiella, Pasteurella, Enterobacter, Pseudomonas,* and *Corynebacterium* spp.[108] *Mycoplasma* spp. also should be considered as a less common cause of UTIs.[111]

KEY POINT 8-22 The need to treat a urinary tract infection should be carefully critiqued. Resolution of the cause of the infection is critical to therapeutic success, including avoidance of resistance.

Enterococcus spp. increasingly is competing with *E. coli* as the predominant organism associated with UTI. Ling and coworkers[105] found that most UTIs were caused by a single agent, with *E. coli* the organism most commonly isolated (45%; see Table 8-1). The number of animals exhibiting signs associated with UTI was not indicated in the study nor was identification of the UTI as a first occurrence or a recurrence. Although UTIs occurred more frequently in female dogs, the frequency of specific organisms causing UTIs was generally similar between genders, with the exception of *Proteus* and *Enterococcus* spp., which were cultured more freqently from females (10.5% and 9.6%, respectively) compared with males (5% and 5% to 6%, respectively). Multiple organism infections were more likely to be found in females than in males. Age did not appear to be an important predictive factor of the most likely pathogen. The majority of infections were associated with ≥100,000 CFUs/mL, whereas approximately 20% of infections, regardless of the number of infecting organisms or the gender of the dog, were characterized by ≤1000 CFUs/mL.

A retrospective study of UTI in dogs admitted to a veterinary teaching hospital and subsequently diagnosed with UTI (n = 240)[112] found that *E. coli* was the causative organism in 50% of the cases. Although the majority of the remaining organisms were gram-negative coliforms (e.g., *Proteus, Klebsiella* spp.) selected gram-positive organisms *(Staphylococcus* and *Enterococcus* spp. being the majority) also were cultured.

The causative agents associated with recurrent UTI (defined later) appears to be similar in that *E. coli* is most common. However, the causative agents in the remainder may differ. Seguin[106] retrospectively examined recurrent UTIs in dogs (n = 441 isolates from 373 positive cultures). *E. coli* (47%) was the most commonly isolated, followed by *Enterococcus* spp. (21%). Other organisms included *Proteus* (7.7%), *Klebsiella* (5.9%), *Staphyloccoccus* (5.2%), and *Pseudomonas* spp. (4.1%). Mixed infections occurred in 17% of the cultures. In a prospective study of dogs receiving glucocorticoids (n = 127), the most common organism isolated was *E. coli* followed by *Enterococcus* spp. A retrospective study in cats (n = 141) with diabetes mellitus[113] also identified *E. coli* as the most common organism. However, a study of 123 specimens collected from asymptomatic cats found *Enterococcus faecalis* to be the most commonly isolated organism (43%), with *E. coli* the second most common (32%).[114] There does not appear to be any information regarding the causative agent associated with infection in different regions of the urinary tract.

Limited information is available regarding the susceptibility of organisms causing UTI. Attention to this issue in clinical studies generally addresses patterns of susceptibility but not the level; however, the latter becomes important to the detection of emerging resistance in those isolates considered susceptible based on CLSI criteria. Boothe and coworkers[115] (see Table 7-3) have described the proportion of *E. coli* isolates susceptible to traditional first-choice antimicrobials, with regional differences apparent. Decreasing susceptibility is likely to limit empirical predictability of those drugs that remain effective. These data underscore the importance of susceptibility methods that allow discernment of different levels of susceptibility. The data also underscore the importance of designing dosing regimens that maximize doses or (for time-dependent drugs) intervals such that resistance might be minimized (see Chapter 6).

In a retrospective study of UTI in dogs receiving glucocorticoids,[116] organism susceptibility was recorded (n = 32): trimethorpim–sulfonamide (97%), amoxicillin–clavulanic acid (76%), tetracycline (70%), ampicillin (61%), and cephalexin (52%). Interestingly, only 7% were susceptible to enrofloxacin, but only 6 dogs were receiving enrofloxacin.

Pathophysiology

The clinical signs of UTI vary with the site of infection. As with other body systems, the inflammatory response largely is responsible for the clinical signs of UTI. Bacteriuria can be asymptomatic, detected on urinalysis but causing no clinical signs.[109] Acute cystitis can cause dysuria but rarely causes signs of systemic inflammation. Acute pyelonephritis, however, is often associated with signs of systemic inflammation, including fever. As in any body system, evidence of inflammation is not necessarily evidence of infection and the need for antimicrobial therapy. Likewise, absence of inflammation does not rule out bacterial infection.

Possible sources of UTI include ascension from the urethra and hematogenous and lymphatic factors. Ascending infection is by far the most common route of infection, although the kidney is predisposed to develop infection associated with blood-borne organisms. In both humans and dogs the origin of bacteria infecting the urinary tract is generally fecal, with the frequency of infection by a particular strain depending on the virulence of the organism. Pathogens generally travel along the urethra to the bladder. Anatomic deformity and turbulent urine flow may facilitate antegrade movement of organisms toward the bladder. Female patients are more predisposed to ascending infection because of the shorter length of the tract and increased risk of contamination. Once in the bladder, infection can continue to ascend the ureter to the kidney, particularly if vesicoureteral reflux is present.

Because *E. coli* is consistently the most common organism associated with UTI, a focus on its pathophysiology is warranted. *E. coli* can be identified based on the presence of selected antigens that serve as a basis for serotyping: O, or somatic (more than 140 serotypes); K, or capsular (which may be associated with more virulence factors); and H, or flagella (necessary for ascending infection and renal invasion). *E. coli* is also represented by a number of pathogenic strains based on the presence of specific virulence factors that facilitate infection. Strains are broadly categorized as intestinal or extraintestinal; the latter group generally is recognized to originate from intestinal strains that subsequently acquire virulence factors that facilitate extra-intestinal survival. Among the extraintestinal strains are uropathogenic *E. coli* (UPEC) represented by many different serotypes.[109] Initial infection by UPEC depends on adherence to uroepithelial cells (e.g., pili or fimbriae). Type 1 pili are among the most important virulence factors facilitating invasion, adherence, and persistence of *E. coli* infections; similar factors are associated with infection by *Proteus* spp. and *Klebsiella* spp.[117b] Toxins are released; examples include hemolysin, causing uroepithelial cell death (thus providing nutrients for UPEC) and cytotoxic necrotizing factor, which stimulates apoptosis and inflammatory cell chemotaxis. Other virulence factors act to scavenge environmental iron necessary for extra-intestinal survival of the bacteria (e.g., enterobactin, which itself is inactivated by lipocalin 2, a bacteriostatic factor secreted by host leukocytes); others impair the hosts' defensive ability to scavenge iron. Factors also facilitate uroepithelial cell penetration by *E. coli;* rapid intra-epithelial proliferation of microbes is accompanied by biofilm formation. Exfoliation of surface uroepithelial cells that occurs with urination is an important host protective mechanism but may facilitate recurrence as infected uroepithelial cells are exposed from the deeper layers. Inflammatory cells respond to cell destruction.

Much of the understanding associated with UPEC pathogenesis comes from contrasting it to a UPEC strain that is associated with much less pathogenicity, causing asymptomatic bacturia (ASB; strain 83792). This strain has been used prophylactically to infect the bladder of humans afflicted with UTI associated with more pathogenic UPEC; this unique approach to treatment is currently undergoing clinical trials.[117c]

Understanding the role of virulence factors in UTI is a prelude to identifying therapies and alternative antimicrobials. Among the factors targeted are adherence factors, in part because of their critically important role in initial infection. *E. coli* contains adhesins that bind to the glycolipid receptors. Mannose-containing receptors are present on most Enterobacteriaceae. On entry into the lower urinary tract *E. coli* organisms associated with canine UTI appear to adhere primarily through these mannose-sensitive adhesins, initiating colonization. In contrast, mannose-resistant fimbriae and other adhesins appear to be critical for colonization of the renal structures. Binding between receptor and adhesin changes the receptor-bearing cell. The severity of a UTI may be correlated with the degree of adherence to uroepithelial cells. Organisms causing acute pyelonephritis in human patients are characterized by higher adherence compared with organisms causing asymptomatic bacteria.[117] The interaction between microbe and receptors may offer a target for treatment. Treatment with mannose or similar molecules has been proposed to block the receptors, thus reducing adherence.[117] However, while this may decrease infection in the bladder, some of the most pathogenic *E. coli* do not recognize mannose (e.g, UPEC associated with renal infection). Further, interaction between the pathogen and the mannose receptor may be important in the initiation of host defense. Cranberry juice extract contains proanthocyanidins that appear to block uroepithelial cell adherance (Type pili) receptors, presumably precluding bacterial adherence. Several antimicrobials interfere with bacterial expression of fimbrial adhesins and thus may prevent bacterial attachment and colonization. Examples include penicillin, ampicillin, amoxicillin, and streptomycin. Once-daily administration of antimicrobials at reduced (one half to as little as one eighth) doses also may be able to prevent UTIs because of interference with fimbrial expression or formation.[119] The role of fosfomycin for this indication requires further development. Among the adherence factors, biofilm has a profound influence on UTI, particularly persistent or recurrent UTI caused by *E. coli*.[117a,b] Although bioifilm clearly contributes to infections associated with urinary catheters, its role in chronic UTI is less appreciated. Biofilm physically and functionally contributes to antimicrobial resistance. A crystalline-based biofilm produced in association with urease production (and urinary alkalinization) appears to contribute to, and indeed, be necessary for the formation of struvite crystals. Use of compounds such as iodoacetamide (IDA) and *N* -ethyl maleimide (NEM) that inhibit enzymes necessary for the formation of the biofilm matrix of these crystials is an area of investigation.

Predisposing Factors

A number of microbial factors increase the risk of UTI.[104] Siqueira and coworkers[118] have described virulence factors associated with *E. coli* isolated from dogs with UTI (n = 51) and pyometra (n = 52) and feces of healthy dogs (n = 55). These include but are not limited to other microbial antigens, production of toxins such as hemolysin or urease, and the mucoid polysaccharide capsules (e.g., *Pseudomona* spp.). Urease producers (*Staphylococcus, Proteus,* or *Mycoplasma* spp.) increase the risk of struvite urolithiasis, predominantly in dogs.

Other host factors increase the risk of UTI. Anatomic predispositions to infection include perineal urethrostomy (particularly in cats). Bacterial infection is rarely the initial cause of disease of the lower urinary tract in cats, but development of infection is a common sequela.[108] The role of viruses in feline lower urinary tract disease has been reviewed.[120] Viruses that have been isolated from the urinary tract of cats with spontaneous disease include feline calicivirus, bovine herpesvirus 4, and feline syncytium-forming virus.[121] Other potential uropathogens include mycoplasmas and ureaplasmas.[111,121] Risk factors have been described in cats with diabetes mellitus, with infection present in 18 of 141 cats.[113] Hyperthyroidism also is a risk factor. Immunosuppressive therapy is a risk factor, as has been demonstrated prospectively in dogs, (n = 127) receiving glucocorticoids (prednisolone or methylprednisolone): 18% were positive (compared with a matched control set of dogs not receiving glucocorticoids) on at least one culture.[116]

Recurrent UTIs reflect either persistence or relapse of the infection or reinfections.[106,109] Persistent or relapsing infections reflect therapeutic failure, whereas reinfection reflects a new bacterial species or strain following a period of urine sterility (i.e., negative urine culture). *Superinfection* refers to infection with a different organism that emerges during treatment of the original organism. Discriminating among persistence, relapse, or reinfection is difficult. Drazenovich and coworkers[122] used pulsed-field gel electrophoresis (PGFE) to pulsotype *E. coli* isolates associated with persistent UTI in dogs in an attempt to discriminate between recurrence and reinfection. Interestingly, of the *E. coli* in their study (n = 12 dogs, 47 isolates), only two dogs had the same PFGE genetic pattern (pulsotype); further, few virulence factors were identified among infecting isolates. Frietag and coworkers[123] studied whether antimicrobial susceptibility profiles could predict a recurrent infection as persistent or relapsing, versus reinfection, with pulsotypes as the determining factor. Susceptibility was effective only 58% of the time in predicting the pattern of recurrence. However, the study group included only five cats (17 isolates); the interval between diagnosis ranged from 6 weeks to 2.5 years. Of the 17 isolates, 9 unique isolates were identified, with no more than 2 from each cat, but susceptibility patterns differed within and between clones. Because PGFE is based largely on chromosomal DNA (i.e., does not include plasmid DNA) and detects the presence of the gene but not its expression, pulsotypes may not be the most appropriate standard on which to base recurrence patterns.

Causes of recurrent UTI (defined as 2 or more in a 6-month period) were retrospectively studied in dogs (n = 100).[106] The median age was 7.7 years. Persistence (defined as same organism and same susceptibility pattern; 42%) and reinfection (different isolate; 50%) were equally responsible for recurrence. Superinfections were identified in 2% of dogs; it is not clear how many animals were cultured while on antimicrobial therapy; the proportion may be higher if superinfections are prospectively sought. Dogs younger than 3 years of age were at greater risk, whereas dogs older than 10 years were associated with a decreased risk of recurrence. This may reflect, in younger dogs, anatomic or other underlying causes being more important to recurrence. Females were at greater risk than males, and sporting dogs, nonsporting dogs, and hounds were at risk compared with other breeds. *E. coli* (56%) and *Enterococcus* spp. (21%) were the most common organisms. Multiple isolates were present in 18% of infections. An underlying cause (or causes) was found in 71 of the dogs; correction occurred in approximately 25 of these. Disorders include abnormal micturition, anatomic defects, altered urothelium (i.e., tumors or uroliths), altered urine composition (hypoadrenocorticism or diabetes mellitus), and impaired immunity (e.g., chemotherapy, hyperadrenocorticism). Dogs treated without removing the underlying cause of disease were more likely to be considered poorly controlled (74.5%), with duration of a disease-free period being less than 8 weeks. Correction of underlying disease or therapy intended to prevent reinfection (i.e., low-dose, long-term antimicrobials) was associated with better control. Over 29% of the infections were associated with multidrug resistant microbes, with abnormal micturition more commonly associated with resistant organisms. Interestingly, 87% of the dogs in which relapse occurred were initially presented for a problem other than UTI, and 50% of the dogs studied were asymptomatic for UTI. Sediments in 15% of the dogs were not indicative of infection, and these isolates in particular tended to be resistant. The authors concluded that culture and susceptibility testing may be indicated in the presence of a predisposing disorder.

The need for preemptively culturing urine in animals predisposed to infection was supported by the prospective findings of Torres and others[116] and Bailiff and others[113] Torres and others[116] studied UTI in dogs (n = 127) receiving glucocorticoids; 18% were positive (compared with a matched control set of dogs not receiving glucocorticoids) on at least one culture, although no dog had clinical signs of UTI. However, pyuria or bacturia predicted positive culture 90% and 95% of the time, respectively. The most common organism isolated was *E. coli*, followed by *Enterococcus* spp. Superinfection was present in 6 of 52 dogs whose urine was cultured while receiving glucocorticoids; each dog was receiving cephalexin (22 mg/kg bid by mouth), and the cultured isolate was resistant to cephlexin. Bailiff et al.[113] retrospectively studied 141 cats with diabetes mellitus. Of these, 13% also had UTI, with *E. coli* the most common organism. Risk factors were female and low body weight; no treatment-related risk factors were identified, including level of diabetic control, or glucosuria.

KEY POINT 8-23 Culture and susceptibility testing should be strongly considered as the basis of therapy in any urinary tract infection that is not occurring for the first time.

Occult UTIs are not limited only to animals with underlying disease; it is possible that "asymptomatic bacteria" is a more appropriate term. Occult UTI appears to occur more commonly than previously thought in cats.[114] In a study of 123 specimens collected from asymptomatic cats, 38% were positive. Positive cultures were more prevalent in older female cats. In contrast to most studies, *E. faecalis* was the most commonly isolated organism (43%), with *E. coli* the second most common (32%).

Other factors may contribute to recurrence or reinfection. Urinary tract catheterization contributes to an increased risk of UTI in an experimental model of male feline cystitis.[124] Catheterization is a common cause of ascension of bacteria from the urethra to the bladder. In human patients one catheterization results in infection in 1% of patients, and infection develops in most, if not all, patients within 3 to 4 days of placement of an indwelling, open-drainage catheter system.[109] A study of infection in cats after perineal urethrostomy found that while the surgical procedure does not predispose the cat to recurrent bacterial UTI, surgical alteration of the urethral surface coupled with underlying uropathy may increase the risk and thus prevalence of ascending infection.[125] Catheters should be used only in cats for which obstruction is likely if catheterization is not performed.[126] Urinary calculi will contribute to canine and feline lower UTIs. One study reports growth of bacteria in urine or calculi of 41% of cats with urinary calculi.[127] *Staphylococcus* spp. were responsible for most (45%) of these infections. Pyometra may serve as a source of reinfecting organisms,[128] as might tumors (e.g., transmissible venereal tumors).[129]

Resistant Urinary Tract Infection

Resistant microbes, and particularly *E. coli*, are increasingly common causes of UTI (Figure 8-5; see also Table 7-3). In a prospective study of *E. coli* isolates, the majority of which were associated with UTI in dogs (n = 240) at a teaching hospital, Boothe and coworkers[115] found the rate of resistance of *E. coli* to common first-choice antimicrobials limited empirical selection of an appropriate antimicrobial at that hospital (Figure 8-5). The percentage of organisms resistant to first-choice drugs exceeded 50% for ampicillin (e.g., amoxicillin) and was 40% or more for drugs considered relatively invulnerable resistant to beta-lactam resistance (i.e., amoxicillin–clavulanic acid and cephalothin). Moreover, 40% of the *E. coli* organisms also were resistant to trimethoprim–sulfamethoxazole. Disconcertingly, 40% of organisms were resistant to fluoroquinolones, the first choice for complicated infections, and 50% were resistant to extended-spectrum penicillins (carbenicillin, piperacillin, and ticarcillin). Indeed, the only drugs to which *E. coli* was predictably susceptible were nitrofurantoin and the aminoglycosides, particularly amikacin. Third-generation cephalosporins ceftiofur and particularly ceftazidime also exhibited susceptibility, although extended-spectrum beta-lactamases (see Chapter 7) were not tested. Several factors were associated with UTI resistance in these organisms, with antimicrobial therapy within the past 5 days and duration of hospital stay being the most important. The incidence of resistance in this retrospective study is in contrast to earlier reports of UTI resistance. For example, in a 2001 study, *E. coli* isolates (the majority being UTI) cultured from dogs were susceptible to norfloxacin (90%), enrofloxacin (87.5%), gentamicin (90.7%), and amikacin (85.9%).[130] The proportion of *E. coli* classified as resistant to amoxicillin or amoxicillin–clavulanic acid is likely to increase in the next few years because CLSI has lowered the breakpoints for these two drugs (along with cephalexin). Other investigators have reported *E. coli* resistance, particularly to fluoroquinolone.

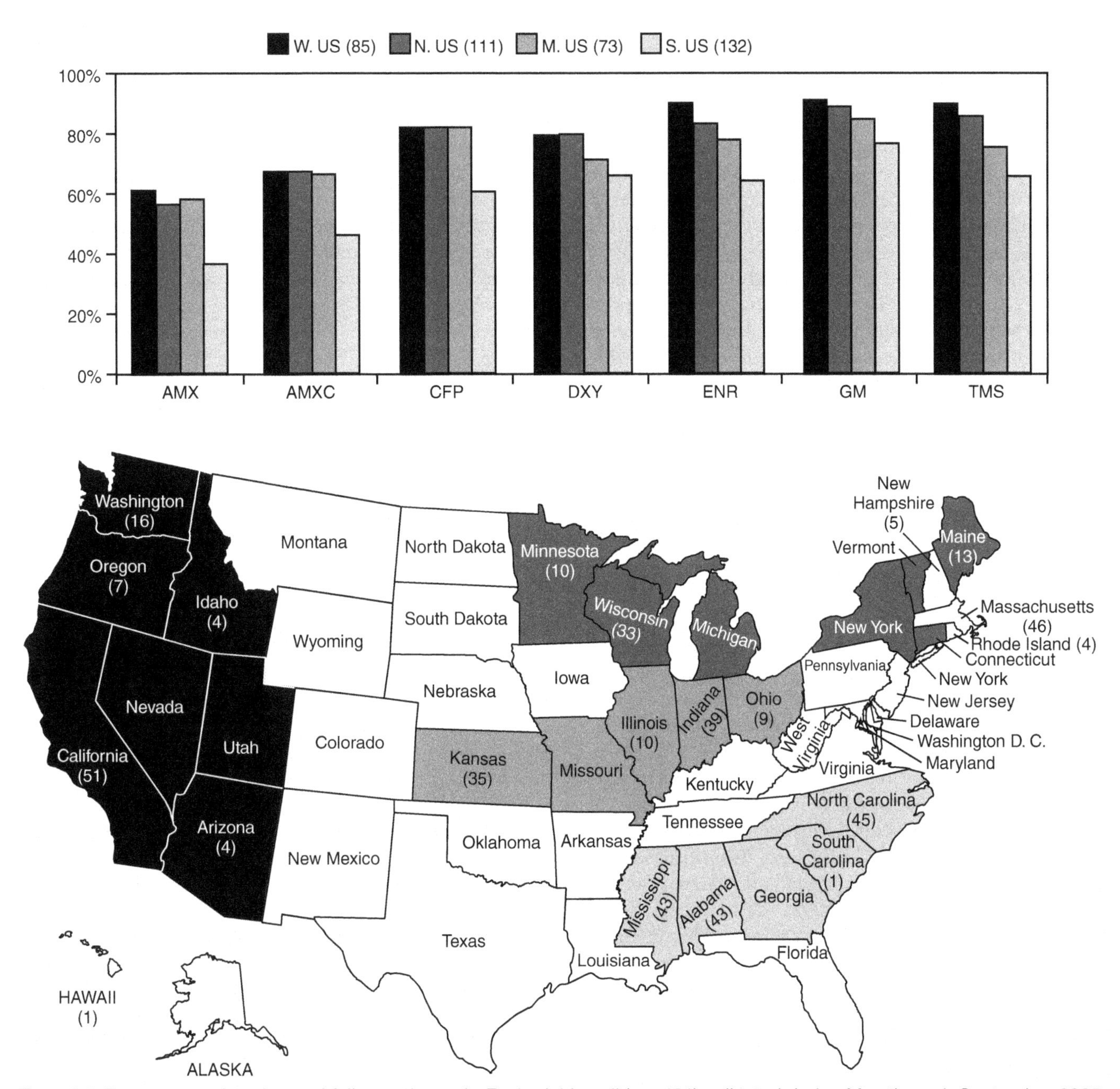

Figure 8-5 Percentage of canine and feline pathogenic *Escherichia coli* (n = 401) collected during May through September 2005 susceptible to selected antimicrobials. Resistance differed by regions (regions delineated in map), with the south characterized by the lowest level of susceptibility for each drug. *AMX,* Amoxicillin; *AMXC,* amoxicillin–clavulanic acid; *CFP,* cefpodoxime; *DXY,* doxycycline; *ENR,* enrofloxacin; *GM,* gentamicin; *TMS,* trimethoprim sulfonamide.

In a study by the author of *E. coli* organisms (n = 50)—most of which were isolated from the urine—the MIC_{90} for the fluroquinolones was greater than 64 μg/mL, suggesting high-level multistep resistance.[131] Multidrug-resistant *E. coli* has emerged as a cause of nosocomial infections in dogs[132] and UTI in canine critical care patients.[106,133] Data generated by the author suggest that resistance to fluoroquinolones is multidrug in nature, reflecting not only mutations in topoisomerases but also induction of efflux pumps.[134] *E. coli* is not the only organism associated with UTI to which resistance has emerged in clinical cases. *Enterococcus* resistance in particular has emerged, probably reflecting its presence as the major gram-positive aerobe in the gastrointestinal tract, although its role as a uropathogen is not clear.

Although in vitro resistance may not necessarily predict in vivo failure, evidence in human medicine suggests otherwise. As in dogs, *E. coli,* is the most prevalent uropathogen in humans. However, antimicrobial resistance to first-choice drugs, trimethoprim–sulfonamethoxazole (TMP-SMX) and ampicillin, often exceeds 30% in humans. In women with UTI caused by *E. coli* characterized by in vitro resistance to TMP-SMX and subsequently treated with the combination drug, approximately 50% were bacteriologic failures and another 40% clinical failures.[135] Previous antimicrobial therapy profoundly affected the likelihood of resistance, with the risk greater if the antimicrobial of interest has been used. Again, in women the most important independent risk factors for TMP-SMX resistance in nonhospitalized cases was use of the antimicrobial within the past 3 months. Those who had taken any antimicrobial were more than twice as likely to be infected with a resistant isolate; use of TMP-SMX within the past 2 weeks was associated with a sixteenfold greater risk of infection with a resistant isolate.[135] Interestingly, trimethoprim by itself results in cure rates that are similar to combination with sulfamethoxazole; because it is associated with fewer side effects, it is the preferred drug for treatment of uncomplicated UTI by some.[135]

Urinary catheterization is not only a recognized risk factor for UTI but also for antimicrobial resistance. Catheterization has resulted in bacteriuria in previous bacteria-free urine and has been associated with changes in urine microflora, as well as increased resistance.[136] Although aseptic techniques will reduce the risk of infection, infection is not prevented. The risk of persistent UTI in cats with experimentally induced cystitis was increased with catheter placement, despite the use of a closed system of urine drainage.[110] The risk of infection can be correlated with duration of catheter placement, with the risk being reduced in patients catheterized for less than 3 days.[137] Previous antimicrobial therapy is likely to contribute to the risk: resistance in dogs catheterized more than 5 days was strongly associated with the advent of resistant microrganisms.[115] Catheter type influences the risk of infection, probably because of its impact on biofilm formation (see Chapter 6) and bacterial swarming.[138] However, isolation of organisms within microcosms associated with biofilm and subsequently isolated from urine collected from the catheter—or from the catheter tip itself—does not necessarily indicate infection[137]; The incidence of resistance in *E. coli* collected from catheters tips is greater than that collected by cystocentesis[112] If infection is present, the causative organism should be identified based on cystocentesis, or urine collected from the passage of a fresh, sterile catheter. However, catheterization should be kept to a minimum. Intermittent catheterization in spinal patients offers unique challenges. In humans, risk of resistance was related to frequency of catheterization (three times was associated with a greater risk than six times per day) and bladder overfilling (overfilling increased risk); previous indwelling catheterization also increased the risk. Trauma to the urethera during catheterization in itself did not increase the risk of infection, but the development of "false passages" or strictures resulting from repeat trauma did. Hydrophilic catheters appeared to reduce the risk of infection. Antimicrobials should be used judiciously in spinal patients. Whereas symptomatic infections are treated, asymptomatic bacteriuria is not necessarily treated; not surprisingly, long-term prophylactic antimicrobial therapy is associated with an increased risk of infection. As such, antimicrobials therapy tends to be limited to treatment of symptomatic infections or prophylaxis during initial (short-term) catheterization.[139] The efficacy of antimicrobial infusion at the end of catheterization is not clear, with studies generating conflicting results. However, in contrast to multiple systemic dosing, single local infusion of high concentrations of drug is less likely to lead to resistance and potentially might do less harm than systemic therapy. Local intravesicular infusion of an antimicrobial might be considered of inducing minimal risk to resistance.

Difficulties encountered in the successful treatment of UTI, and particularly multidrug-resistant UTI, mandate that approaches be taken to prevent resistance, which includes preventing infection. Because previous use of antimicrobials consistently is a major predictor of emerging resistance, the question of the need to treat should be the first consideration for all infections. If reasonable alternatives exist to antimicrobial drug therapy, they might be considered first or in addition to antimicrobial therapy.

Prevention of Urinary Tract Infection

A number of host factors prevent or limit bacterial infection in the bladder.[109] Among the host factors important in preventing infection are normal micturition, normal anatomic barriers, systemic immunocompetence, mucosal defense barriers, and the inherent antibacterial properties of urine. Recurring infections are most likely to reflect failed host defenses, whether originating spontaneously or iatrogenically (e.g., immunosuppressive drugs).[106] Support of factors can be targeted with adjuvant therapies instead of antimicrobial treatment, when possible, or to facilitate antimicrobial therapy, particularly in the patient at risk for recurrent infections.

The decision to treat or not treat an infection might take into account the size of the inoculum (i.e., CFU/mL of urine) but should also take into account host factors (e.g., clinical signs, history, ability to control underlying cause, contributing factors, previous response to therapy). The location of infection may play a major role in determining the need for therapy. Whereas asymptomatic bacteriuria will often resolve or become self-limiting if left untreated, bacterial pyelonephritis is likely to progress.[104,117] Virulence testing or serotyping eventually may be helpful in the decision to treat or not treat. The normal flora of the vulva and prepuce may be an important host defense mechanism against infecting microorganisms of the urinary tract. Normal flora may prevent colonization by pathogenic organisms or disrupt metabolism of pathogens. Secretory antibodies may coat infecting organisms, preventing adherence, and reduced antibody production may promote infection. Mucus may have other antibacterial effects. In the bladder, mucosal secretion of surface mucopolysaccharides is important to host defense by preventing attachment of bacteria. Destruction of this layer facilitates infection. Treatment with sulfonated glycosaminoglycans intraluminally may coat the uroepithelium and thus provide a barrier to bacterial adherence. Administration of carbenoxolone (a licorice derivative) stimulates secretion of mucosal polysaccharide and (in rabbits and humans) increases the clearance of *E. coli* infection. In the bladder, the composition of urine can affect bacterial growth. Urine concentration (unless extreme) is not likely to affect bacteria (bacteria are generally hypertonic compared with their environment), but high concentrations of urea or other compounds or low pH may impair bacterial growth. The addition of prostatic fluid inhibits bacterial growth. Exceptions include selected *Staphylococcus* and *Proteus* spp., which are relatively resistant to the antibacterial effects of urea.[109] Tamm–Horsfall protein secreted by the cells of the ascending loop of Henle binds to *E. coli* by way of mannose-containing side chains and, as such, probably acts as a urinary bacterial defense mechanism. Other factors that help prevent or reduce bacterial infection include frequent urination, a small residual urine volume in the bladder, and rapid urination.

KEY POINT 8-24 The use of adjuvant therapies, particularly in the prevention of urinary tract infections, should be considered carefully, particularly with regard to clinical evidence of efficacy.

Therapy

The Need for Drug Therapy

The presence of bacteriuria is not necessarily an indication of the need for antimicrobial therapy (Figure 8-6). Antimicrobial therapy should be used only when reasonable evidence of infection exists. Bacterial UTI occurs much less frequently in cats than in dogs, and even the presence of clinical signs indicative of cystitis should not be interpreted as a need for antimicrobial drug therapy.

In humans, to prevent resistance, treatment generally is not indicated in asymptomatic bacteriuria except under certain conditions in which the patient is at risk, such as during pregnancy or invasive surgical procedures.[140] Likewise, for veterinary patients the risk of emerging resistance must be weighed against the risk of failing to treat. If the patient is one for which aminoglycoside therapy is inadvisable, the need for treatment should be even more closely examined. With *Enterococcus* bacteriuria, treatment should not be implemented unless the need is clear. Clearly, if the decision is made to treat a UTI, therapy must be aggressive, designed to kill invading pathogens as well as emerging mutants as rapidly as possible. Nonantimicrobial alternatives should be considered in lieu of or in addition to antimicrobial therapy.

The Sequelae of Drug Therapy

The traditional goal of drug therapy for UTI is to eliminate bacteriuria in animals exhibiting clinical signs and urinalyses consistent with UTI. However, four sequelae of antimicrobial therapy may occur.[104,109] *Cure* can be defined as negative urine cultures during and after (usually 1 to 2 weeks) antimicrobial therapy. Quantitative bacterial counts should decrease within 48 hours after initiation of an appropriate antimicrobial. Cure does not rule out the possibility of reinfection. UTIs may reflect first-time or recurrent infections. *Chronic UTI* is often used to refer to persistence of infection. The previously defined terms *recurrence, persistence,* and *relapse* often are used interchangeably when referring to UTIs. *Persistence,* or recurrence, can refer to presence of significant or low numbers of bacteria after 48 hours of therapy. If the numbers are significant, antimicrobial resistance or insufficient drug concentrations (e.g., improper dose, poor oral absorption, poor renal elimination) should be suspected. If numbers are very low, a continuous source of bacteria in the urinary tract (e.g., urinary calculi, prostate, kidney) or contamination from the lower urinary tract might be suspected.[109] In such cases, cultures can identify persistent organisms after therapy has been discontinued. An appropriate approach would be classification of recurrent or persistent infections into three categories. *Relapse* occurs when the same organism causes infection 1 to 2 weeks after therapy has been discontinued. Relapse generally occurs within 1 to 2 weeks of cessation of therapy and may reflect either a very deep-seated infection or an abnormality of the urinary tract (e.g., structural, renal, or prostatic infection). The presence of a different organism is considered *reinfection* (i.e., a new infection). A new infection also can occur by the same organism located outside of the urinary tract. Generally, reinfection occurs more than 1 to 2 weeks after cessation of therapy. *Superinfection* may also occur and reflects infection with an additional organism during the course of antimicrobial treatment.[104] Evidence of persistent or relapsing infection or superinfection should lead to more aggressive therapy and to the use of bactericidal rather than static drugs. Among the common causes of complications associated with UTI, antimicrobial resistance, unidentified underlying disease, and inappropriate dosing regimen should be considered.

Identification of the Target

In all but simple UTI, culture is indicated. Culture is recommended in patients whose history includes exposure to antimicrobial therapy within the last 3 months; exposure may include any household member, including other pets. The more complicated the infection or the greater the patient is at risk for resistance to emerge, the more important it is to base therapy on susceptibility data. In human patients diagnosis of UTI in asymptomatic patients is. based on at least two clean-catch midstream urine collections. The same organism should be present in significant (see previous discussion) amounts in both cultures. A single culture is sufficient in the presence of symptoms. Urinary cultures should be the basis of antimicrobial selection in complicated infections (e.g., reinfection or relapse, history of antimicrobial use in the past 4 to 6 weeks)[104] or if the infection represents a risk to the patient's health. Infection after recent urinary catheterization also should lead to culture collection. Increasingly, culturing at the outset, even in simple, first-time infections, may become prudent.

Quantitative urine culture (i.e., colony counts) should be implemented to facilitate discrimination of harmless bacterial contaminations (e.g., from the urethra) from pathogenic organisms (see previous discussion). Bacterial counts of more than 10^5 CFU are clearly indicative of infection regardless of the method of collection, whereas counts between 10^3 and 10^5 organisms are considered suspect if not collected by cystocentesis or if collected from female dogs. Counts of less than 1000 CFU should lead to a second culture and, in the absence of clinical signs or mitigating circumstances, consideration of alternative therapies. Methods have been described for

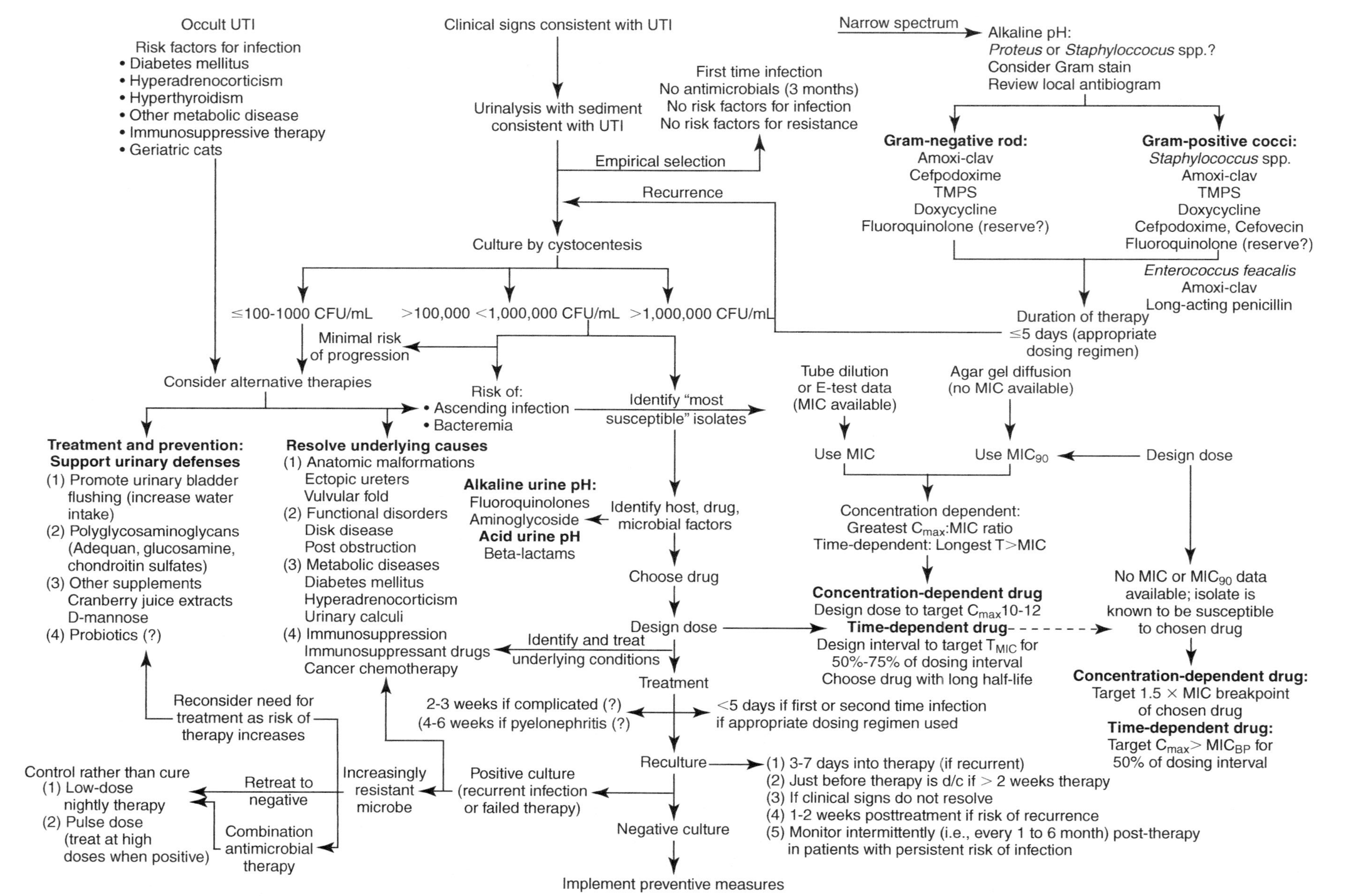

Figure 8-6 Suggested algorithm for treatment of urinary tract infections in dogs or cats. Treatment should be begun with assessing the need to treat with antimicrobial drugs (*upper left*) versus alternative therapies. Empirical treatment (*upper right*) should be pursued only for uncomplicated infections, including animals not recently exposed to antimicrobials (this may include any household member or pet). Culture and susceptibility data (*lower right*) should be used to both select drug and design the dose; in its absence, population pharmacodynamic data (MIC_{90}) can be used if the identity of the infecting microbe is known. Treament of recurring infections (*lower left*) requires a series of reassessments, including recultures. With continued recurrence, the need for continued therapy should be balanced with the risk of therapy to the patient; prophylactic therapy might be considered to prevent recurrence once the urine has been cleared of infection (*far lower left*).

culture procedures performed in practice.[104] In addition to the method of collection, consideration must be given to sample handling. Samples should be kept refrigerated if the time from collection to processing by the lab is anticipated to exceed 12 hours, unless an appropriate amount of preservative is added. A viable alternative for submission of urine samples that will be in transit longer than 12 hours is collection and subsequent submission using a "paddle" apparatus (e.g., UriCult®).

Antimicrobial Selection

Presumably, a drug that is renally excreted should be selected for treatment of UTIs. Urinary concentrations of such drugs often surpass serum concentrations (up to 300-fold), which is particularly helpful for concentration-dependent drugs (Table 8-10). Susceptibility data do not take these higher concentrations into account, but this may be appropriate. Several caveats must be recognized when basing antimicrobial selection on renal elimination and anticipation of high urine drug concentrations:

KEY POINT 8-25 The design of the dosing regimen for treatment of a urinary tract infection should be based on plasma, not urine, drug concentrations.

1. Drug is not likely to be concentrated in some situations. Examples include but are not limited to fluid therapy, diuretic use, renal disease, and other diseases (e.g., hyperadrenocorticism).
2. Drugs characterized by a short elimination half-life may be limited in efficacy if they are time dependent in action. However, plasma elimination half-life may not accurately reflect contact time of drug in the urine if the drug is excreted renally. Contact can be enhanced by drug administration immediately after micturition or before an anticipated micturition-free period (e.g., at night).
3. Intraepithelial growth and biofilm may preclude drug efficacy even if concentrations are high in urine.
4. If the UTI is associated with infection in the blood (or in the presence of bacteremia), kidney, or prostate, then antimicrobial selection should be based on anticipated plasma (or tissue) drug concentrations and serum breakpoint MICs. A similar approach should be taken for recurrent infections or complicated infections.

A prudent approach for treatment of UTI is choice of a renally excreted drug but dosing based on drug concentrations achieved in plasma. Data from a few prospective studies, including animal model studies and human patient–based clinical trials, generally demonstrate that breakpoints based on plasma drug concentrations rather than urine appear to moderately predict outcomes associated with treatment of UTI.[45] For example, maximum efficacy of aminopenicillins in treating UTI in human clinical trials is achieved when plasma drug concentrations are maintained above the MIC for 30 hours or more.[271] Accordingly, CLSI interpretive criteria for infections in other tissues are relevant to UTI. Drugs that are not eliminated in urine might be characterized by lower concentrations in urine compared with tissues but still can be beneficial for

Table 8-10 Mean Urine Concentrations for Antimicrobials Used to Treat Urinary Tract Infections in Dogs

Drug	Dose	Route	Freq*	Mean Urine Drug Concentration (μg/mL)
Penicillins				
Penicillin G	37,000 U/kg	PO	8	295 ± 210
Penicillin	500 (7 mg/kg)	PO		100
Amoxicillin	11 mg/kg	PO	8	202 ± 93
Ampicillin	500 mg (7 mg/kg)	PO		500
Indanyl carbenicillin	26 mg/kg	PO	8	309 ± 55
	382 mg	PO		1000
	500 mg	PO		300
Cephalosporins				
Cefaclor	500 mg	PO		900
Cefadroxil	500 mg	PO		1800
Cephalexin	500 mg	PO		1000
Cephradine	500 mg	PO		1000
Aminoglycosides				
Gentamicin	2 mg/kg	SC	8	107 ± 33
Amikacin	5 mg/kg	SC	8	342 ± 143
Tobramycin	2.2 mg/kg	SC	8	66 + 39
Fluorinated quinolones				
Enrofloxacin	5 mg/kg	PO	12	40 ± 10
Other				
Sulfisoxazole	1000 mg	PO		100
Trimethoprim	100 mg	PO		30-160
Trimethoprim–sulfadiazine	13 mg/kg	PO	12	55 ± 19
	4.4 mg/kg	PO	8	100
Nitrofurantoin	100 mg	PO		100
	1000 mg	PO	8	200
Nalidixic acid	18 mg/kg	PO		138 ± 65
Tetracycline	500 mg (7 mg/kg)	PO	8	300 123 ± 40
Chloramphenicol	33 mg/kg	PO		30
Erythromycin	500 mg	PO		
Fosfomycin	80 mg/kg	PO	12-24	

PO, By mouth; *SC*, subcutaneously.
*Frequency.
†Assumes normal renal function.
Modified from Barsanti[107]

UTI if dosing regimens are appropriate. Some drugs used to treat UTIs (e.g., indanyl–carbenicillin, nitrofurantoin) are recognized not to achieve effective concentrations in other tissues, and therefore use in areas other than the urinary bladder should be done cautiously.

As resistance to *E. coli* and other uropathogens increases, empirical therapy for UTI increasingly will be limited (Table 8-9). Caution is recommended because of the recent recognition of the growing incidence of antimicrobial resistance. Among the organisms frequently causing UTIs in dogs and cats, *E. coli, Proteus* spp., *P. aeruginosa,* and *Enterobacter* spp. are among the organisms that vary widely in their susceptibility pattern and for which empirical therapy is more risky (Table 8-11; see also Tables 7-3 and 7-9). Empirical therapy, if it is to be pursued, is indicated only for *uncomplicated infection*—that is, those patients in which no underlying structural, neurologic, or functional abnormality can be identified.[104] The absence of previous antimicrobial therapy should also be interpreted as uncomplicated. Once relapse occurs (see later discussion), an infection should no longer be considered uncomplicated.

Attention should be paid to the pH of the urine compared with the pK_a of the chosen drug. In the presence of an alkaline pH, weakly basic antimicrobials might be considered (aminoglycosides, and fluoroquinolones, with the latter being amphoteric but more effective in an alkaline urine). Because urease producers may alkalinize the urine, drugs targeting such organisms (e.g., *Proteus, Staphyloccocus,* and some *Klebsiella* spp.) should be selected. In the presence of an acidic urinary pH (perhaps caused by *E. coli*), weakly acid drugs (e.g., penicillins, cephalosporins, potentiated sulfonamides) might be better empirical selections. However, if the drug is highly concentrated in the urine, even a predominantly ionized drug (e.g., a weak base in an acidic environment), may be sufficiently un-ionized to ensure effective concentrations.

Infections uncomplicated by previous antimicrobial therapy or in regions for which resistance has minimally emerged may respond to empiric therapy. *E. coli* or *Enterobacter* spp. traditionally have been considered responsive to trimethoprim–sulfadiazine, third-generation cephalosporins (cefpodoxime, cefovecin), or amoxicillin–clavulanic acid combinations. Among these, penicillins may be preferred because of their effects of fimbriae. Approximately 60% of *E. coli* are resistant to cephalexin. *Klebsiella, Proteus,* and *Staphylococcus* spp. are likely to respond to a first- or third-generation cephalosporin or to amoxicillin–clavulanic acid. Amoxicillin or ampicillin (preferably combined with a beta-lactamase protector) should be effective if a decision is made to treat *Enterococcus* spp. (see Tables 7-9, 8-3, and 8-6). However, for Enterobacteriaceae in particular, integration of pharmacokinetics and pharmacodynamics raise concerns regarding efficacy for drugs with short elimination half-lives, particularly if infection involves tissue other than the urinary bladder. In the absence of an MIC, the more stringent MIC_{90} (see Tables 8-9 and 8-11) and C_{max} from package inserts or the literature (see Table 7-1) can be used to design dosing regimens. The highest end of the dosing regimen is indicated, particulary for at-risk patients. For selected concentration-dependent drugs, C_{max}:MIC should exceed 10 to 12, and for time-dependent drugs, T>MIC should be at least 50% if not more of the dosing interval (generally, initial target concentrations should exceed the MIC by at least two to four fold (see Table 8-9). For time-dependent drugs, those with longer half-lives might be preferred (e.g., cefovecin and cefpodoxime). Although the package insert for cefovecin indicates that MIC_{90} concentrations for *E. coli* (1 μg/mL) are not achieved after a recommended dose of 8 mg/kg subcutaneously, predicted unbound plasma drug concentrations will be maintained at or above this concentration for 3 days. Cefovecin is approved for treatment of canine *E. coli* UTI in Canada at 8 mg/kg. Note that neither cefovecin nor cefpodoxime are effective against *Enterococcus* spp., indicating that the Gram-staining characteristics of the infecting organism might facilitate proper antimicrobial choice for empirical treatment of a UTI in dogs or cats. Because resistance in *E. coli* toward fluoroquinolones with rare exception is associated with MDR, their use for treatment of UTI should be considered second tier and ideally, be based on culture and susceptibility testing. Care should be taken using the fluoroquinolones for *Enterococcus* spp., for which efficacy can be variable. Boothe et al demonsrated that for *E. coli,* when using the MIC_{90} for fluoroquinolones, the C_{max}:MIC_{90} failed to reach ≥10—as is suggested for concentration-dependent drugs—even with the highest dose for each drug. (see Tables 7-12 and 8-9 for additional MIC data).[131] However, for isolates that are known to be susceptible to ciprofloxacin, enrofloxacin, and marbofloxacin reached the target C_{max}:MIC_{90} at the high (but not low) dose. Even with susceptibility data that provide MIC, because the tested concentrations are close to the breakpoint MICs, isolates considered susceptible to fluoroquinolones may have already developed low-level resistance, increasing the risk of emergent resistance in at-risk patients.[142] Certainly an "I" to any one fluoroquinolone should be interpreted as emerging resistance to others. Isolates with MIC approaching the breakpoint should be treated with alternative drugs, combination drugs, or "added doses" (e.g., high dose, twice daily). Marbofloxacin is preferred for cats at risk for retinal adversities, particularly if dosing twice daily. Although ciprofloxacin is more potent against gram-negative isolates, dosing should be increased to compensate for differences in oral bioavailability and oral dosing should not be used in cats. Fluoroquinolones are also effective against *Mycoplasma* and *Ureaplasma* spp.

A summary of treatment of UTI in humans might offer some guidance for empirical therapy in dogs or cats. In women with risk factors for infection with resistant bacteria, or in the setting of a high prevalence of TMP/SMX resistance, a fluoroquinolone or nitrofurantoin is recommended for empirical treatment. The goal of treatment is eradication of infection using shorter courses of therapy (i.e., 3 days) with once-daily dosing of a selected drug or a single dose of a particularly efficacious antimicrobial.[141] The role of nitrofurantoin is increasing for treatment of UTI in women, particularly in the presence of increasing antimicrobial resistance to other urinary antimicrobials. Resistance among uropathogens to nitrofurantoin generally is consistently at a low level despite its use for 5 decades. An advantage to nitrofurantoin is its minimal effect on the normal gut flora. Consequently, selection pressure for antimicrobial resistance is reduced compared with other antimicrobials.[135] Further, nitrofurantoin does not share cross-resistance with more commonly prescribed antimicrobials, and its use is justified from a public health perspective as a fluoroquinolone-sparing agent. For

Table 8-11 Susceptibility Data (μg/mL) for Drugs for Gram-Negative Pathogens Collected from Antimicrobial-Free Dogs and Cats*

	Drug	Amoxicillin–Clavulanic acid	Cefadroxyl	Cephalexin	Cefovecin	Cefpodoxime
	MIC_{BP} (sus)	≤0.25 ≤8/2 (urine)		≤2		≤2
	MIC_{BP} (res)	> 1		≥ 8		≥ 8
Escherichia coli	Mode	4/2	8	8	0.5	
	MIC_{50}	4/2	8	8	0.5	0.25
	MIC_{90}	8/4	16	16	1	0.5
	Range	1/0.5-64/32	4->32	2->64	0.12->32	0.12->32
	n	223	223	223	223	41
	Species	D, C	D, C	D, C	D, C	D
	Source	76	76	76	76	P
	CLSI	Y	Y	Y	Y	Y
Klebsiella pneumoniae	Mode	2/1	8	4	0.5	
	MIC_{50}	2/1	8	4	0.5	
	MIC_{90}	16/8	16	4	1	
	Range	2/1-64/32	8->32	4-64	0.25-2	
	n	16	16	16	16	
	Species	D, C	D, C	D, C	D, C	
	Source	76	76	76	76	
	CLSI	Y	Y	Y	Y	
Pasteurella multocida	Mode	≤0.5/0.25	4	2	≤0.06	
	MIC_{50}	≤0.5/0.25	4	2	≤0.06	≤0.03
	MIC_{90}	≤0.5/0.25	4	2	≤0.06	≤0.03
	Range	≤0.5/0.25-2/1	1-16	≤0.5-8	≤0.06-0.12	≤0.03-0.12
	n	188	188	188	188	32
	Species	D, C	D, C	D, C	D, C	D
	Source	76	76	76	76	P
	CLSI	Y	Y	Y	Y	Y
Proteus mirabilis	Mode	1/0.5	16	8	0.25	
	MIC_{50}	1/0.5	16	8	0.25	≤0.03
	MIC_{90}	1/0.5	16	16	0.5	0.06
	Range	≤0.5/0.25-8/4	8->32	8-32	0.12-0.5	≤0.03-0.06
	n	110	110	110	110	14
	Species	D, C	D, C	D, C	D, C	D
	Source	76	76	76	76	P
	CLSI	Y	Y	Y	Y	Y

	Drug	Ceftazidime	Cefotaxime	Imipenem	Meropenem	Piperacillin/tazobactam
	MIC_{BP} (sus)	≤8	≤8	≤4	≤4	≤16
	MIC_{BP} (res)	≥32	≥64	≥16	≥64	≥128
Pseudomonas spp.	MIC_{50}	2	32	1	1	1
	MIC_{90}	8	>64	4	2	2
	Range	0.25-128	0.25-64	0.15-16	1-8	4-64
	n	106	106	106	106	106
	Species	D	D	D	D	D
	Source	20	20	20	20	20
	CLSI	Y	Y	Y	Y	Y

	Drug	Ciprofloxacin	Difloxacin	Enrofloxacin	Marbofloxacin	Orbifloxacin
	MIC_{BP} (sus)	≤1	≤0.5	≤0.5	≤1	≤1
	MIC_{BP} (res)	≥4	≥4	≥4	≥4	≥8
Escherichia coli	Mode	0.35	0.69	0.4	0.67	0.66
	MIC_{50}	0.0625	0.25	0.0625	0.25	0.125

Continued

Table 8-11 Susceptibility Data (µg/mL) for Drugs for Gram-Negative Pathogens Collected from Antimicrobial-Free Dogs and Cats*—cont'd

	Drug	Ciprofloxacin	Difloxacin	Enrofloxacin	Marbofloxacin	Orbifloxacin
Escherichia coli	MIC_{90}	≥64	≥64	≥64	≥64	≥64
	Range					
	n	61	61	61	45	45
	Species	D, C	D, C	D, C	D, C	D, C
	Source	131	131	131	131	131
	CLSI	Y	Y	Y	Y	Y
Proteus spp.	Mode	0.08	0.64	0.17	0.21	0.72
	MIC_{50}	0.065	1	0.125	0.125	1
	MIC_{90}	0.5	4	1	1	8
	n	28	28	28	18	15
	Species	D, C	D, C	D, C	D, C	D, C
	Source	131	131	131	131	131
	CLSI	Y	Y	Y	Y	Y
Pseudomonas spp.	Mean	0.25	0.93	0.45	0.69	1.3
	MIC_{50}	0.125	1	0.5	0.5	1
	MIC_{90}	1	16	8	8	16
	n	58	58	58	38	34
	Species	D, C	D, C	D, C	D, C	D, C
	Source	131	131	131	131	131
	CLSI	Y	Y	Y	Y	Y
Pseudomonas spp.	MIC_{50}	0.25	2	1	0.25	8
	MIC_{90}	8	≥32	32	16	>32
	Range	0.015-32	0.015-32	0.015-32	0.015-32	0.015-32
	n	106	106	106	106	106
	Species	D	D	D	D	D
	Source	20	20	20	20	20
	CLSI	Y	Y	Y	Y	Y

MIC, Minimum inhibitory concentration; *BP*, breakpoint, *SC*, subcutaneous; Y indicates that data were collected following guidelines of Clinical Laboratory and Standards Institute (CLSI). *D*, dog; *C*, cat; *Y*, yes; *P*, package insert.
*Pharmacokinetic data from Table 7-1.
†Based on cephalothin.

example, single-dose ciprofloxacin prophylaxis increased the prevalence of ciprofloxacin-resistant fecal *E. coli* from 3% to 12%.[135] After treatment with ciprofloxacin for prostatitis, 50% resulted in post-treatment fecal colonization with quinolone-resistant *E. coli* genetically distinct from the prostatic infection. Indeed, in humans, although flouroquinolones are effective as short-course therapy for acute cystitis, widespread empirical use is discouraged because of potential promotion of resistance.[140] An exception is made for acute (nonobstructive) pyelonephritis but only if culture results direct continuing therapy.

Beta-lactams and fosfomycin are also considered second-line (to TMP-SMX) agents for empirical treatment of cystitis in humans. Fosfomycin may be a reasonable first choice for treatment of UTI in dogs if data support its use for treatment of canine UTI. Advantages to fosfomycin tromethamine justify consideration of its use in dogs. Despite many years of use in humans, it is characterized by an extremely low incidence of resistance. Indeed, canine and feline isolates expressing MDR maintain susceptibility to fosfomycin.[135a] Further, pharmacokinetics in dogs support its use for treatment of UTI. Its role for treatment of UTI in dogs is emerging; a prudent approach might be as a second- or third-tier drug because of its importance in human medicine. In general, drugs metabolized by the liver (chloramphenicol) or excreted in the bile (macrolides, clindamycin) do not achieve high concentrations in the urine and should generally be avoided for treatment of UTI. Doxycycline might be appropriate if susceptibility data is available, although concentrations achieved in urine might be bacteriostatic.

Duration of Therapy

The "test for cure"[104] (or perhaps, more appropriately, "response") can be based on a second culture 3 to 5 days into therapy. Cure should be anticipated only if the organism count is less than 100 per mL of urine. Urine culture a second time just before discontinuation of therapy has been recommended,[104] particularly if antimicrobial prophylaxis is to be implemented. The duration for successful treatment of uncomplicated lower UTIs might be as short as 3 to 5 days, particularly if doses are designed to target all infecting isolates, including those with the highest MICs.[104] Such an approach is more likely to be successful if high doses and appropriate intervals are chosen. Treatment may need to be extended, however, if infection occurs anywhere other than the uroepithelium. Traditionally, a 10- to 14-day therapeutic regimen has been recommended for the first episode of therapy; the evidence for this recommendation is limited and clinical trials demonstrating appropriate duration of therapy are needed. Shorter-term antimicrobial therapy (a single high dose) has proved effective for female human patients with a lower UTI. Drugs that have been used successfully in humans for short-term dosing include trimethoprim–sulfonamide combinations, aminoglycosides, selected cephalosporins, and fluoroquinolones. Both single-dose and 3-day antimicrobial treatment regimens have been studied with dogs receiving amikacin and a trimethoprim–sulfonamide combination. Therapy was not uniformly successful, suggesting that caution should be used with this treatment regimen.[143] However, these studies were implemented before understanding the importance of reaching targeted PDI (i.e., C_{max}:MIC > 10-12 and T>MIC for more than 50% of the dosing interval). Factors that should preclude single-dose antimicrobial therapy for a lower UTI include recurrence, historical poor response to single-dose therapy, underlying predisposing factors to a UTI (including structural abnormalities or metabolic disorders, such as diabetes mellitus, and hyperadrenocorticism), and either pyelonephritis or symptoms of a UTI that have occurred for more than 7 days.

For infections that reflect a relapse, the duration of therapy should be at least 2 weeks; however, for human patients suffering from a relapse, a higher cure rate occurred with a 6-week course of therapy. For animals a duration of 4 to 6 weeks is recommended.[104] The duration also might be based on the cause of the relapse and whether the underlying cause is curable and treated. Because relapse is likely to occur shortly after antimicrobial therapy is discontinued, cultures should be collected again 7 to 10 days after cessation of therapy to detect the recurrence. In general, regardless of the sequence of UTI, doses should always maximize efficacy and avoidance of resistance. A new antimicrobial should be selected if infection occurs more than 10 days after cessation of therapy;[104] as more time elapses between cessation of therapy and the presence of bacteriuria, the more likely it is that reinfection is the cause of recurrence.

In the event of relapse after 6 weeks of therapy, 6 months of therapy or more may be necessary. A 3- to 6-month duration of therapy may be indicated for animals. However, clinical trials are lacking to document these recommendations as well. Greater care must be taken, in the selection of antimicrobials for longer-term therapy, with special consideration to toxicity. Drugs that are used for long-term therapy in human patients include amoxicillin, cephalexin, trimethoprim–sulfonamide combination, or a fluorinated quinolone. Cultures should be repeated monthly, and as long as significant bacteria are not present, the drug need not be changed. Should relapse occur after a drug is discontinued, the same drug or a new drug should be administered for a longer course of therapy. Long-term therapy may be particularly important for animals in which renal parenchymal damage is a risk. As with first-time infection, and perhaps more so, the need for treatment must be balanced with the disadvantages of treatment (or the risks of not treating should be balanced with the benefits of treating).

Clinical Trials

Despite the frequency of UTI in dogs and cats, the number of clinical trials examining therapy are limited. Pradofloxacin (n = 27 dogs; 5 mg/kg) has been compared with doxycycline (n = 23; 5 mg/kg load, followed by 2.5 mg/kg bid for 2 doses, then 2.5 mg qd) and amoxicillin–clavulanic acid (n = 28; 62.5 mg/kg bid for 10 days) in cats with clinical signs of UTI.[144] Cats were not randomly assigned; assignment to treatment group was based on susceptibility; if more than one drug was designated susceptible, animals were assigned to keep groups balanced. All cats receiving pradofloxacin responded, with 13% and 10%, respectively, of the doxycycline and amoxicillin--clavulanic acid groups remaining infected after treatment. However, the proportion of responders was not different among treatment groups, probably reflecting small sample size.

Efficacy of cefovecin (8 mg/kg, administered subcutaneously) was compared with that of cephalexin for treatment of canine (n = 129) UTI.[145] Efficacy was based on elimination of the pretreatment uropathogen. Exclusion criteria included local or systemic antimicrobials within the previous 14 days, or short- (7 days) or long-acting (30 days) glucocorticoids. The study was implemented as a multicenter, blinded, randomized study, with cephalexin (15 mg/kg, administered orally bid) serving as the positive control. Animals were treated for 14 days. The most common uropathogen was *E. coli* (60%), followed by *P. mirabilis* (12%) and *S. intermedius* (12%). As would be expected on the basis of the cephalexin MIC_{90} of *E. coli*, the overall cure rate for animals infected with *E. coli* was 79% in the cefovecin group compared with 36% for cephalexin. Bacteria were eliminated in 59% of cefovecin-treated dogs compared with 35% of cephalexin-treated dogs. Of the infecting isolates, 90.5% of *E. coli* infections were eradicated compared with 53% of *E. coli* infections for cephalexin. Of infections caused by *S. intermedius*, 6 of 6 were eliminated by cefovecin, compared with 7 of 10 for cephalexin; for *Proteus mirabilus*, 9 of 9 were eliminated by cefovecin, compared with 5 of 7 for cephalexin. Interestingly, although 319 dogs with clinical signs of UTI were evaluated for inclusion, only 137 (43%) actually were bacteriuric.

Prophylaxis

Long-term prophylaxis can be implemented for patients at risk for recurrence. Prophylaxis (by definition) can occur only after the infection has been eradicated. The use of low doses of antimicrobials in the presence of bacteriuria is likely to lead to the generation of resistant organisms and is contraindicated. Thus prophylactic antimicrobial therapy of UTIs is indicated for reinfection but not relapse (the latter suggests that the organism was never completely eradicated). The antimicrobial chosen for long-term prophylaxis should be both safe and inexpensive. Trimethoprim–sulfonamide combinations (monitor for immune-mediated reactions), nitrofurantoin, and fluoroquinolones are examples. However, neurologic side effects with nitrofurantoin may preclude its use, particularly long term. Fosfomycin might also fill this role. The dose for prophylaxis is generally reduced to 30% to 50% of the full dose.[104] Subtherapeutic concentrations of drugs often are sufficiently inhibitory to prevent infection of the uroepithelium. The drug should be administered at night to maximize contact of the drug with the urinary tract. Intermittent urine cultures (monthly) are indicated to detect breakthrough infections in animals receiving long-term antimicrobial prophylaxis. Negative cultures for 6 to 9 months or more may indicate that prophylaxis is no longer necessary.

Adjuvant Therapy

Diuresis has been advocated in the treatment of UTIs in humans. Advantages include rapid dilution of bacteria, removal of infected urine, and subsequent rapid reduction of bacterial counts. In patients with pyelonephritis, an added advantage may be enhanced host defenses: medullary hypertonicity inhibits leukocyte migration, and high ammonia concentration inactivates complement. In the presence of vesicoureteral reflux, however, diuresis may increase the risk of acute urinary retention.

Use of drugs to modify urinary pH may facilitate the antibacterial effects of urine. The presence of ionizable organic acids (hippuric and gamma-hydroxybutyric acid) in an acidic pH may enhance the antibacterial activity of the urine. Antibacterial activity may be increased by ingestion of cranberry juice (if urinary pH is acidic), which contains precursors of hippuric acid. Cranberry juice extract also should be considered because of its potential ability to block adherence receptors. Methenamine, available as a hippuric acid or mandelate salt, releases formaldehyde at a urinary pH of 5.5 or less, which also can increase antibacterial activity of urine.

Local urinary analgesics, such as phenazopyridine, rarely are indicated for the management of UTIs. Dysuria is most likely to respond to appropriate antimicrobial therapy. These drugs cause methemoglobinemia and are contraindicated in cats.

Drugs or nutraceutical products that enhance polysulfated glycosaminoglycan synthesis (e.g., Adequan, pentosan polysulfate, glucosamine, chondroitin sulfate) might be considered for patients with complicated UTI. Such products may cover or help repair the uroepithelium, thus decreasing bacterial adherence. Gunn-Moore and Shenoy[146] prospectively studied the effects of 60 days oral n-acetyl glucosamine in cats (n = 40) with feline idiopathic cystitis using a randomized, double-blinded, placebo controlled study. Response was based on owner assessment. Both groups improved significantly, with 26 of 40 cats suffering recurrences. Although the power of the study was large, the size of the placebo response limited the ability to detect a significant difference between treatment groups. Improvement in both groups was potentially attributed to owners, most of whom changed the cats to moist rather than dry diets. The quality of the glucosamine was not addressed. Wallius and Tidholm[147] studied the effects of polysulfated glycosaminoglycans (PGAGs) in cats (n = 19) with clinical signs indicative of cystitis but culture negative. Cats were randomly assigned to receive either saline placebo or 3 mg/kg PGAGs on days 1, 2, 5, and 10. Assessment was based on owner perceptions of improvement. A treatment effect could not be detected because clinical signs resolved in essentially all cats (save one from each group). As with the previous study, the authors of this study could not conclude that PGAGs were not beneficial for treatment of inflammation, including that associated with UTI. Treatment with mannose or similar molecules may block mannose receptors, thus reducing adherence.[119]

The use of probiotics in the treatment of UTIs in human patients was reviewed by Lenoir-Wijnkoop.[148] In general, *Lactobacillus* spp. are most commonly recommended for treatment of UTI. However, selected species are likely to emerge as more effective than others and microbiota may need to originate from the target species. The use of probiotics in the treatment of renal oxalate stones in human patients was also reviewed by Lenoir-Wijnkoop and coworkers.[148] The absence of *Oxalobacter formigenes* from fecal microbiota increases the risk of kidney stones. Although no study has demonstrated an association between probiotic therapy and decreased renal stones, both animal and human studies have documented that *O. formigenes* can become established in the gastrointestinal tract, and establishment reduces urinary oxalate concentrations.

Pyelonephritis

Treatment of pyelonephritis may require hospitalization with intravenous fluid administration. Oral antimicrobial therapy is acceptable for mild to moderate cases as long as oral therapy is tolerated well. Because renal dysfunction can be life threatening, antimicrobial selection should ultimately be based on culture and susceptibility data. Therapy can be initiated empirically; however, resistance among *E. coli* organisms should lead to selections with known susceptibility. Combination therapy should be considered. Urine is not likely to be concentrated, thus added attention must be paid to ensure that effective concentrations reach the target tissue. Pyelonephritis can be associated with bacteremia, particularly gram-negative bacteremia. Clinical signs indicative of severe, life-threatening infection should lead to parenteral antimicrobial therapy with predictably effective drugs (e.g., aminoglycosides, fluoroquinolones, extended-spectrum beta-lactams, and third-generation cephalosporins known to not be extended-spectrum beta-lactam producers). Combination therapy also should be strongly considered. The high concentration of antimicrobial that facilitates treatment of the lower urinary tract (bladder and lower) may not occur in pyelonephritis; thus close attention must be paid to using sufficiently high doses and frequent dosing. Drugs whose efficacy is dependent on a hypotonic environment (compared with the target organism), such as beta-lactams, fosfomycin, or vancomycin, may be less effective in the face of medullary hypertonicity, although this may be less than normal in the face of pyelonephritis. Nonetheless, if drug combinations are used, at least one of the two drugs should not target cell walls. As with infection lower in the tract, bacterial numbers should decrease dramatically within the first 48 hours of treatment. For uncomplicated pyelonephritis, 14 days of therapy may be sufficient of treatment. Cultures should be repeated as previously indicated during and within 1 to 2 weeks of discontinuation of therapy. Complications such as abscessation may require surgical intervention and longer-term therapy.

KEY POINT 8-26 *E. coli* resistance to fluoroquinolones, when it does emerge, is generally characterized by multidrug resistance.

KEY POINT 8-27 Treatment of pyelonephritis should be approached as a potentially life-threatening disease requiring aggressive but appropriate antimicrobial therapy.

Prostatitis

Pathophysiology

Bacterial prostatitis can present as either an acute or chronic infection. One does not necessarily precede or follow the other. Among the causes of prostatic infection, ascending infection and urine reflux appear to be most likely. Acute prostatitis often is accompanied by fever, pain, and symptoms typical of a UTI. Palpation of the prostate reveals tenderness, swelling, and (potentially) a fluctuant surface (Figure 8-7). Care should be taken when palpating the prostate so that the risk of bacteremia is minimized. Chronic bacterial prostatitis most commonly is caused by gram-negative coliforms, with *E. coli* being most common, followed by *Klebsiella* spp., *Enterobacter* spp., *P. mirabilis,* and *S. aureus.*

Antimicrobial Selection and Use

Antimicrobial penetration into the noninflamed canine prostate is limited. Drugs that are basic and lipid soluble appear to diffuse through tissues best, including macrolides (e.g., erythromycin and presumably azithromycin and clarithromycin), fluoroquinolones, and trimethoprim–sulfonamide combinations. The intense inflammatory response that accompanies acute prostatitis facilitates antimicrobial movement into the prostate,[109] although high doses should be used to ensure adequate concentrations at the site of infection. Parenteral antimicrobials based on culture (prostatic fluid or urine) should be used in the presence of life-threatening infection; otherwise, oral therapy is acceptable. Duration of therapy should be at least 4 weeks to minimize the risk of progression to chronic prostatitis. Prostatic abscessation generally requires surgical intervention. Chronic prostatitis in human patients is difficult to cure unless infected tissue is surgically excised. Chronic prostatitis generally results in relapse. Therapy, when successful, generally requires 1 to 2 months of therapy. Antimicrobials that penetrate the noninflamed prostate (e.g., fluoroquinolones, trimethoprim–sulfonamide combinations, or macrolides) should be selected.[109]

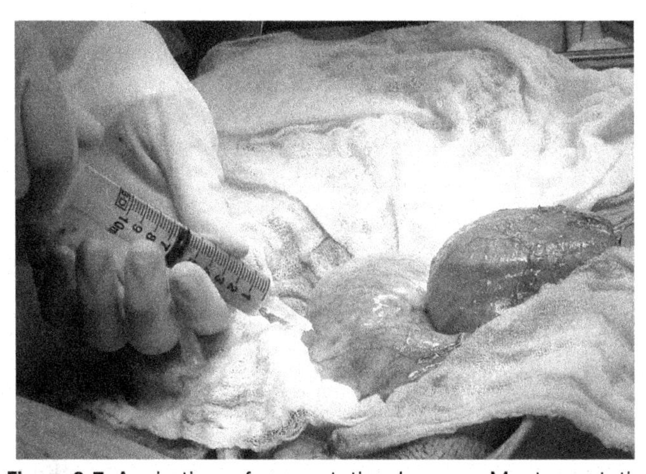

Figure 8-7 Aspiration of a prostatic abscess. Most prostatic abscesses require surgical removal. Abscessation carries the risk of peritonitis and bacteremia. Fluid should be submitted for culture and susceptibility testing. (Photo courtesy Harry W. Boothe, DVM, MS, DACVS, Auburn, AL.)

Adjuvant therapy for the treatment of prostatitis includes stool softeners and, if indicated, analgesics. Neutering should be considered.

INFECTIONS OF THE UTERUS

Endometritis

Endometritis is associated with sanguineous or purulent vaginal discharge in either the pregnant bitch (if the cervix is open) or nonpregnant bitch.[149] As with many organ systems, organisms causing uterine infections tend to be members of the normal flora of the reproductive tract. Organisms most commonly associated with uterine infections include *Streptococcus* spp., *E. coli, Salmonella, Campylobacter, Mycoplasma,* and *Chlamydia* spp.[149] Bacterial infections of the uterus resulting in endometritis can be responsible for infertility, abortion, stillbirths, and fetal death. Treatment of endometritis differs in the presence of pregnancy (live fetuses) in part because of potential injury to developing fetuses. Regardless of the antimicrobial, any type of placentation is sufficiently intimate to allow movement of drug administered to the dam or queen to cross the placenta and enter the fetus. In general, however, the fetus can excrete water-soluble drugs more easily than lipid-soluble drugs because water-soluble drugs can be eliminated in the allantoic fluid. In contrast, drug-metabolizing enzymes of the fetal liver are immature and essentially nonfunctional. Although metabolizing activity increases as the term of pregnancy ends, activity remains sufficiently weak that drug elimination is probably ineffectual. Thus lipid-soluble drugs tend to remain in the fetus. When possible, drugs that are water soluble should be selected for treatment of infections in the pregnant bitch.

The beta-lactams are preferred with amoxicillin combined with clavulanic acid or a cephalosporin as first choice, assuming the target organism is included in the spectrum. Care should be taken to avoid cephalexin if an *E. coli* is suspected. Culture and susceptibility data should be the basis for antimicrobial selection for treatment of endometritis, even if antimicrobials are begun before results are received. Should susceptibility data indicate beta-lactams as resistant, aminoglycosides can be used. Pediatric (and presumably fetal) canine kidneys are protected from aminoglycoside damage because the cortical regions do not fully develop until several weeks postpartum. Fluoroquinolones also appear to be safe for the developing fetus (e.g, enrofloxacin at 15 mg/kg), although the risk of cartilage damage even in the developing fetus might lead to an alternative class of drugs. Response to antimicrobial therapy is indicated by resolution of vaginal discharge, which should occur within several days of beginning therapy. Therapy should continue for 2 to 3 weeks.[149] In the case of fetal death, prostaglandin therapy may be indicated to evacuate the uterus. Evidence of septicemia indicates more dramatic and aggressive therapy (see the section on bacteremia).

Pyometra

Although bacterial infection is secondary to the cystic changes associated with pyometra, the infection is the primary cause of illness and death. Organisms most commonly associated with pyometra include *E. coli* (the majority of infections), hemolytic *Streptococcus, Staphylococcus, Klebsiella, Pasteurella, Pseudomonas, Proteus,* and *Moraxella* spp.[150] Wadas and coworkers[128] demonstrated that *E. coli* associated with pyometra in dogs was derived from fecal flora and was also identical to those simultaneously cultured from the urine. Hagman and Kühn[151] confirmed that *E. coli* was from the normal flora and was the same as that cultured from the urinary bladder. Host and microbial factors (see Chapter 6) play a large role in the pathogenesis of pyometra and response to drug therapy. In addition to the obvious impact of inflammatory and other debris on antimicrobial efficacy, the local immune response of the uterus is impaired.[150] Complications such as bacterial peritonitis and endotoxin contribute to mortality. Endotoxin concentrations generally are increased before implementation of drug therapy, further complicating antimicrobial selection.[150]

Surgical removal of the infected uterus is the treatment of choice; however, antimicrobial therapy should be implemented regardless of whether ovariohysterectomy is performed. Prostaglandin therapy may be implemented in selected cases (see Chapter 23).

Culture and susceptibility data should be collected before empirical therapy with a bactericidal drug that includes *E. coli* in its spectrum is begun. Although a beta-lactam antibiotic is generally an excellent first choice, concern with rapid cell death and release of lethal quantities of endotoxin should lead to (1) selection of a carbapenem (meropenem or imipenem), the beta-lactam associated with the least endotoxin release; (2) combination therapy with a non–beta-lactam antimicrobial (e.g., an aminoglycoside or fluorinated quinolone) that is administered before (1 to 2 hours) the beta-lactam; or (3) slow administration of the beta-lactam, perhaps over the course of 1 hour. Therapy for pyometra should include supportive measures such as fluid rehydration and, if indicated, therapy for endotoxic shock. Glucocorticoid therapy is discouraged unless the patient is characterized as adrenocortico-deficient (see Chapter 30).

RESPIRATORY TRACT INFECTIONS

Principles of Antimicrobial Treatment

A major barrier to passive drug movement from the blood to the site of infection in the respiratory tract is the bronchial–alveolar–blood barrier.[152,153] Whereas drugs of a molecular weight up to 1000 can move easily through the open junctions of the capillaries, drugs must passively diffuse through the tight junctions of the alveolar epithelial cells.[152] Movement of drugs into bronchial secretions occurs primarily by passive diffusion and is more likely to occur for drugs with favorable physiochemical characteristics such as high lipophilicity and low molecular weight (<450). Few drugs achieve concentrations in respiratory tissues equal to concentrations in the plasma.[154] Thus achieving simply the MIC in the plasma against an organism infecting the respiratory tract is likely to result in therapeutic failure.[154-156] Rather, the targeted plasma drug concentration must be sufficiently great to ensure that the MIC will be reached at the site of infection. The relationship between plasma and bronchial drug concentrations can be described by the partition ratio,[152,153] which is the area under the plasma drug concentration versus time curve in plasma divided by the same in bronchial secretions. Such a relationship would compare not only peak concentrations but also the time that drug stays in tissues, which generally is longer than in plasma. Collection of sequential bronchial secretion samples necessary for kinetic analysis is, however, difficult, and such information currently is not available for many drugs. A more practical relationship is the ratio of bronchial drug concentration to plasma drug concentration. This ratio has been established for a number of antimicrobial drugs and is often available in package inserts and textbooks. The ratio can serve as a basis for antimicrobial selection and dose manipulation.[152,153] Ratios can be further manipulated to take into account phagocytic accumulation of antimicrobials.[154]

Among the antimicrobial classes, the penicillin antibiotics are characterized by one of the lowest plasma to bronchial tissue drug concentrations (mean of 9%), although variation exists among the individual drugs (see Table 7-5). For example, amoxicillin reaches four to five times higher concentrations in bronchial secretions than ampicillin when given at the same dose, although this is probably due to higher plasma concentrations.[152,153] As little as 1% of some beta-lactams and no more than 23% of plasma amoxicillin, however, reaches bronchial secretions. An exception can be made for meropenem, which appears to reach approximately 50% of plasma concentrations (see Table 7-5). The cephalosporins may be distributed slightly, albeit probably not clinically, better than the penicillins (mean of 15%), again with variation among the individual members. For example, cephalexin achieves only 15% of plasma concentrations, whereas cefoxitin and cefotaxime reach 25% of plasma concentrations. Selected third-generation cephalosporins may reach even higher concentrations.[152,153]

KEY POINT 8-28 Among the antimicrobial classes, the penicillin antibiotics are characterized by one of the lowest (often less than 10%) plasma to bronchial tissue drug concentrations.

Of the aminoglycosides, amikacin distributes into bronchial secretions somewhat better than most beta-lactams, generally reaching 20% to 30% of plasma concentrations. Clindamycin achieves 61% of plasma concentrations. Tetracyclines, and particularly doxycycline (38%) and minocycline, can reach 30% to 60% of plasma concentrations after a single dose. Macrolides such as erythromycin generally distribute well into bronchial secretions (41% to 43%), although newer drugs such as azithromycin (which can accumulate up to 200-fold in pulmonary tissues) distribute much better than erythromycin.[152,153] The fluoroquinolones reach 70% or more of plasma concentrations; they also accumulate over fiftyfold to a 100-fold in alveolar macrophages. The potentiated sulfonamides have variable distribution. Whereas trimethoprim reaches 100% of serum concentrations in bronchial fluid, the sulfonamide component may achieve much lower concentrations. For example, sulfamethoxazole achieves only 18% of serum concentrations. Metronidazole, useful for anaerobic infections, achieves 100% of plasma concentrations in respiratory secretions.[152,153] For drugs with a long elimination half-life (e.g., doxycycline, the azalides), the ratios of bronchial concentrations to plasma concentration may increase with repetitive dosing as drugs accumulate.[152,153]

Inflammation generally increases concentrations of selected antibacterials (e.g., beta-lactams and aminoglycosides) in bronchial secretions because of local vasodilation and vascular permeability. Excessive inflammation can, however, preclude antimicrobial distribution (Figure 8-8).[152,153] In such instances, a drug that accumulates in white blood cells should be considered. Mucus produced in response to a bacterial infection in the respiratory tract can also interfere with antimicrobial therapy.[152,153] Aminoglycoside efficacy may be decreased by chelation with magnesium and calcium in the mucus. Antimicrobials may bind to glycoproteins, and mucus may present a barrier to passive diffusion. In addition, some antimicrobials may alter function of the mucociliary apparatus, either by increasing mucous viscosity or decreasing ciliary activity (e.g., tetracyclines). Because of these negative effects, drugs that decrease mucous viscosity (e.g., expectorants or bromhexine, a drug available outside of the United States) or are mucolytic (e.g., acetylcysteine) may facilitate antimicrobial therapy.[152,153] Cysteine-containing drugs may facilitate penetration of antimicrobials.[157] *N*-acetylcysteine may be given by any route and reach effective concentrations in the lung. In addition to its mucolytic effects, the drug imparts some anti-inflammatory effects (oxygen radical scavenging) and appears to help bacterial penetration of the mucopolysaccharide capsule of gram-negative bacteria. The use of *N*-acetylcysteine is addressed in Chapter 20.

Increasingly, the nonantimicrobial benefits of selected antimicrobial drugs are being realized. The effects of long-term azithromycin use on lung function and progression of cystic fibrosis is discussed later in this chapter. The azolides have demonstrated synergistic effects against *P. aeruginosa* with a number of antimicrobials (see the discussion of bacterial rhinitis and sinusitis).

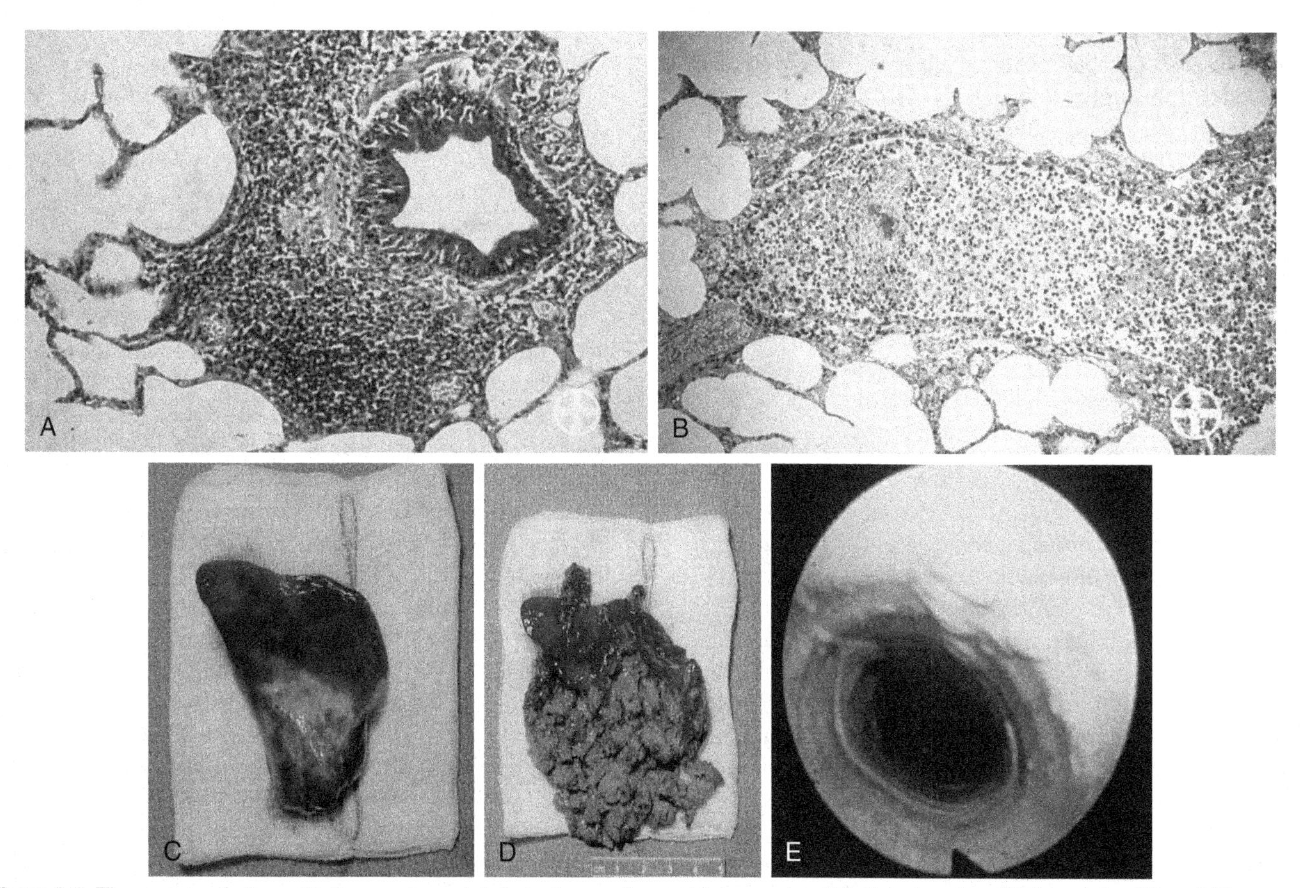

Figure 8-8 The accumulation of inflammatory debris in the peribronchiolar region **(A)**, the alveolus **(B)**, lung lobe **(C** and **D)**, or trachea **(E)** is likely to impair drug distribution to the site of infection and may hinder the activity of the drug that is able to penetrate the debris. (Courtesy Bayer Animal Health.)

Bacterial Rhinitis and Sinusitis in Cats

Pathophysiology

The pathophysiology of bacterial rhinitis and sinusitis has not been confirmed in cats, but the role of viral disease in chronic infection increasingly is evident (see the section on microbial targets). Acute manifestations of rhinitis are likely to reflect viral infections; causative agents include FHV-1 (generally identified as the causative agent in the majority of cases), FCV, and *Chlamydia* spp.

Viruses can cause profound local changes in the respiratory epithelium of upper airways. In humans rhinoviral adherence to the epithelium upregulates production of biogenic amines, tumor necrosis factor (TNF), and other cytokines, as well as leukotrienes.[158] At the same time, viruses suppress local immune response. The negative impact of viral infections on local (and potentially systemic) immune mechanisms, particularly if coupled with lysis of nasal turbinates, as can occur in cats, likely predisposes the nares and sinuses to secondary bacterial infection. As the syndrome progresses, the role of viral organisms is likely to become less important. The loss or reduction of mucociliary tract function probably has a profound impact on the pathophysiology of respiratory tract infections in dogs and cats (see Chapter 20). Impaired removal of inflammatory and bacterial debris or bacterial biofilm allows accumulation and retention of material that not only is responsible for clinical signs (e.g., sneezing) but also contributes to infection by promoting an environment conducive to microbial growth. Successful therapy is confounded by (presumed) limited drug distribution to the nares and sinuses, particularly in the face of chronic inflammatory debris. Bacterial adherence to epithelial cells might also profoundly affect therapeutic success. Initial clinical response may be followed by recrudescence of clinical signs and failed response to repeated antimicrobial therapy.

KEY POINT 8-29 Although the initial role of viruses in the pathophysiology of upper respiratory disease is clear, the role of bacteria in perpetuating the syndrome is not clear despite multiple studies that have demonstrated a microbial presence.

Complicating the treatment of chronic sinusitis is the inability to discriminate commensal organisms from pathogens (see Chapter 6). Culture of nasal flushes may be a better means to assess infection than rhinoscopy-guided biopsy.[159] Cytology may be important in distinguishing a bacterial infection from sinusitis that is primarily chronic allergic inflammatory in origin and more likely to respond to immunomodulatory therapy (see Chapter 20). Properly identifying an infectious cause helps prevent the indiscriminate use of antimicrobials, which may contribute to the emergence of resistant bacterial infection.

Microbial Targets

Several studies have addressed the microbes associated with upper respiratory disease in cats, with varied results. Variability reflects, in part, variation in study methods and often failure to discriminate commensals from infection. A common void is lack of data in control animals. Johnson and coworkers[160] have studied the organisms associated with rhinosinusitis in affected (10) cats, comparing the flora to normal cats (7). Aerobic bacteria were present in 5 of 7 normal and 9 of 10 affected cats; *Mycoplasma* spp. was present in only 2 of 10 diseased cats. Potential pathogens were cultured more frequently from diseased cats, but it was not clear if their growth reflected infection as opposed to colonization of previously diseased tissue. FHV-1 was detected using polymerase chain reaction (PCR) in 4 of 7 normal cats and 3 of 10 diseased cats. *Bordetella bronchiseptica* was cultured in 1 cat with disease that had been vaccinated with the same strain. In the review Johnson and coworkers[160] also indicated that a previous study (by the same investigators) found that swab culture of 15 of 21 cats with rhinitis yielded *Pseudomonas* spp. (53%) and *E. coli* (40%). Both *Pasteurella* (4 of 11) and *Pseudomonas* spp. (7 of 11) also have been cultured from the frontal sinuses of affected cats.

Bannasch and Foley[161] evaluated pathogens in animal shelter cats that were either normal (n = 259) or afflicted with clinically mild to severe upper respiratory infection (n = 314). The proportion of all isolates identified for all cats were FCV (54.7%), FHV-1 (28%), *Mycoplasma* spp. (14.4%), *B. bronchiseptica* (9.5%), and *C. felis* (2.8%). Unfortunately, the incidence of pathogens in controlled versus affected cats was not described, limiting interpretation of the role of pathogens in disease. More recently, Spindel and coworkers[162] cultured cats with feline rhinitis before a clinical trial. Organisms most frequently cultured or detected based on PCR from nasal swabs included FHV-1 (75%), *Mycoplasma* spp. (75%), and *Bordetella* spp. (47.5%). Additionally, *Staphyoloccoccus* and *Streptococcus* were recovered in 12.5% and 10% of cases, respectively. Hartmann and colleagues[163] prospectively studied cats (n = 39) presented to a veterinary teaching hospital with clinical signs of upper respiratory disease or conjunctivitis. Cats were tested for FCV, FHV-1, *C. felis,* and *Mycoplasma* spp.; 37 of 39 cats had at least one organism present. Both *C. felis* and *Mycoplasma* spp. were each present in approximately 50% of cats, with both present in 28% of cats and neither in approximately 5%. The role of other microorganisms was not addressed. Finally, Veir and coworkers[164] described bacterial and viral pathogens isolated from nasal and pharyngeal swabs in affected (acute rhinitis) cats (n = 52). However, the impact of the findings on the relevance to clinical signs was limited by the lack of studies in control cats. Cultures in affected cats included an anterior nares swab (using a urethral swab after mucus was removed) and pharyngeal swabs from the oropharyngeal area. Infectious organisms were also detected using PCR for FHV-1, FCV, *Mycoplasma,* and *Chlamydia* spp. Eleven different organisms were cultured from nasal swabs, with the most common being *Mycoplasma* (48%) and *Pasteurella* spp. (32%). Thirteen different organisms were cultured from the pharyngeal swab, with the most common being *Pasteurella* (73%), *Mycoplasma* (52%), and *Moraxella* spp. (21%); *Flavobacterium* spp. was cultured from 17% of animals. Pharyngeal and nasal swabs matched in only 12% of the animals. *Bordetella* sp. was present only in nasal swabs (n = 3; 5%). FHV-1 was detected in 69% of the nasal swabs despite being PCR positive in 82% of cases. The authors considered *B. bronchiseptica, C. felis*, FCV, and FHV-1 as the primary pathogens, although detection of FHV-1 did not always indicate infection. Nine afflicted cats were negative for primary organisms in nasal culture but positive in pharyngeal culture. Agreement between nasal and pharyngeal data was considered moderate for FHV-1 and *Mycoplasma* PCR; substantial for FHV-1 isolation, *Mycoplasma* culture, and FCV; and perfect for *C. felis*. Collection of nasal swab data was described as difficult, time consuming, and uncomfortable for the subjects. The authors concluded that information yielded from aerobic culture of either nasal discharge or pharynx of cats is not sufficiently useful to justify collection; accordingly, empirical therapy was suggested by the authors. Previous studies had revealed that 80% of aerobic (non-*Mycoplasma* spp.) isolates were susceptibile to amoxicillin–clavulanic acid, cephalosporins, chloramphenicol, enrofloxacin, and tetracylines.

Based on these studies, although consensus has not been reached, the most likely initiating pathogens associated with rhinitis are FHV-1 and FCV. If bacteria are involved in the initiation, *Mycoplasma* spp., *B. bronchiseptica,* and *C. felis* are the primary bacterial causes.[162] Previous antimicrobial history might be important for discerning the role of gram-negative organisms, particularly in sinusitis.

Antimicrobial Drugs and Treatment

Care must be taken to ensure proper antimicrobial selection and dosing regimen in to minimize the advent of resistance in upper respiratory tract infections. Indiscriminate therapy must be avoided. As infection becomes chronic, persistent antimicrobial therapy is likely to encourage development of resistant organisms through antimicrobial selection pressure. Although the normal lung may be well perfused, marked inflammatory debris will affect the ability of the drug to reach the site in effective concentrations (see Figure 8-8). Drug distribution to normal bronchial or sinus secretions is limited; inflammatory debris may pose an even greater risk of poor delivery. Even drug concentrations that achieve the MIC of the infecting organisms may contribute to antimicrobial failure. As weaker organisms die (e.g., *P. multocida)*, persistent environmental changes coupled with the continued presence of antimicrobials will select the more hardy organisms (e.g., *B. bronchiseptica)*. Eventually, organisms largely resistant to most clinically relevant bacteria (e.g., *P. aeruginosa)* emerge. In part because of the concern of emerging resistance and the desire to avoid the indiscriminate use of antimicrobials, fever in humans with acute rhinitis is not to be interpreted as secondary bacterial infection, nor is a change in the color of the discharge. Secondary bacterial infection is considered in cases for which acute clinical signs persist for 10 days or more or worsens after 5 to 7 days. Treatment is implemented for 10 to 14 days.[158]

Curing chronic rhinitis or sinusitis in cats may be an unreasonable expectation, particularly if damage to nasal turbinates precludes adequate mucociliary tract function or other local immune protections. Control of clinical signs, particularly during flare-ups, may be a more reasonable expectation. Little information exists regarding the role of bacteria in persistence of infection, but human patients with cystic fibrosis are frequently infected with *P. aeruginosa,* so much so that its appearance is generally associated with a downward spiral in clinical response. Consequently, much research has focused on infection by this organism, some of which may apply to cats with chonic sinusitis or rhinitis. The propensity of infection of cystic fibrosis patients with *P. aeruginosa* may reflect, in part, adherence of the organism to epithelial cells as well as generation of biofilm.[165] Isolates causing infection appear to be different from isolates infecting other tissues. Biofilm may be induced by the presence of hypoxia and appears to be associated with resistant organisms; low oxygen tension also may cause emergence of the more resistant, nonmucoid pseudomonad organisms. Hypermutability of the organism has been associated with antimicrobial-induced selection pressure.[165] "Late" infection with *Burkholderia* sp. and aspergillosis has been recognized.

Although chronic sinusitis or rhinitis is generally not life threatening in cats, a therapeutic approach similar to that for cystic fibrosis might be reasonable. Thus focusing on removal of organized bacterial debris is an important component of therapy.[166] Two rules of antimicrobial therapy recommended in patients with cystic fibrosis may apply to chronic sinusitis or rhinitis: (1) Antimicrobial selection should be based on periodic isolation and identification of pathogens and their susceptibility, and (2) indiscriminate use should be avoided. Rather, a rational, clinical endpoint should be considered in the context of duration of therapy.[165] Even with appropriate culture techniques, identifying the infecting organism may be difficult. For example, nonmucoid *Pseudomonas* spp., which tends to cause early infections in humans with cystic fibrosis, is slow growing and harder to culture, making MIC determination more difficult.

KEY POINT 8-30 Effective therapy of URI in cats may depend more on adjuvant therapy that alters the environment rather than repetitive antimicrobial therapy. Antimicrobial therapy might be approached with the goal of control, rather than cure, with dosing regimens designed to ensure eradication of infection with each therapeutic interlude.

When the decision to use antimicrobials is made, their use should be aggressive, designed to achieve effective concentrations—sufficient to kill even the potential mutants. Lipid-soluble drugs and drugs that concentrate in phagocytic cells should be considered; as infection progresses, combination (double to triple) therapy should be implemented. Pulse dosing at intervals sufficiently long to allow the microflora to normalize as much as possible is a reasonable approach. Early antipseudomonadal therapy designed to eradicate infection is recommended in humans with cystic fibrosis to prevent infection by resistant pseudomonads. Long-term azithromycin appears to improve lung function and slow the progression of the disease in humans with cystic fibrosis and increasingly is included in the therapeutic regimen.[167,168] The effects of azithromycin may be immunomodulatory insofar as they occur at concentrations below the MIC of the infecting organisms. Proposed mechanisms have included, among others, a reduction in inteleukins (IL)-1β, IL-8, and neutrophils in bronchoalveolar lavage fluid; reduction in immune complexes directed toward the biofilm produced by mucoid *P. aeruginosa;* and impaired adherence of *P. aeruginosa* to the epithelium.[169] Azithromycin and clarithromycin also have exhibited in vitro synergistic effects against both mucoid and nonmucoid *P. aeruginosa*. The most active combinations demonstrating synergy in patients with cystic fibrosis were azithromycin–sulfadiazine–trimethoprim and azithromycin–doxycycline. Azithromycin occasionally demonstrated synergism when combined with extended-spectrum beta-lactam antibiotics (meropenem, imipenem, and others), ciprofloxacin, chloramphenicol, and tobramycin.[170] Azithromycin has a long half-life in lung tissues of cats (see Chapter 7) and is a reasonable choice for combination, but not sole, therapy of cats with sinusitis infected with *Pseudomonas* spp. Care should be taken in using antistaphylococcal drugs (unless specifically indicated on the basis of culture and susceptibility data) because of the potential advent of MRS.[165] When used, doses should be modified to ensure concentrations that well exceed the MIC of the infecting organisms for most of the dosing interval.

Several clinical trials have examined the efficacy of selected antimicrobials. The efficacy of amoxicillin (22 mg/kg by mouth bid, tablet form) was compared with that of azithromycin (15 mg/kg by mouth; n = 10) in shelter cats (n = 31) suspected to have bacterial rhinitis (on the basis of nasal discharge). Treatments were randomized, but blinding was not addressed; negative controls were not included.[171] Animals had been cultured before initiation of antimicrobial therapy.[164] Response was based on clinical signs assessed before and every 3 days until infection resolved. Failures in one group were subsequently crossed over to the alternative drug for an additional 9 days. For azithromycin, 3 of 10 cats (30%) initially responded, whereas 6 were switched to amoxicillin. For amoxicillin 8 of 21 (38%) responded, whereas 13 were switched to azithromycin. In the second treatment period, 5 of 10 (50%) responded to amoxicillin, and 3 of 6 (50%) responded to azithromycin. No differences were detected in clinical outcome or scores at cross-over; the limitation may be sample size. At the time of the report, the cost of amoxicillin treatment (drug alone) was approximately 35% of that for azithromycin, but the inconvenience of twice-daily dosing was not included in the cost assessment. However, some limitations of this study complicate interpretation. No loading dose was given for azithromycin; therefore azithromycin was not quite at steady state at the 9-day crossover time, and treatment did not occur while drug concentrations were at steady state. For the same reason, because a washout was not implemented to accommodate for the long half-life of azithromycin, those cats switched from azithromycin to amoxicillin were likely to have significant azithromycin concentrations during at least 6 days of the second treatment period.

Pradofloxacin (5 mg/kg [n = 13] or 10 mg/kg [n = 12] qd) also has been compared with amoxicillin (22 mg/kg every 12 hr; n = 15) for treatment of feline rhinitis in shelter cats (n = 40) using a randomized design (blinding not addressed; no control included); cats that failed the first therapy (7 days' duration) were treated with the alternative therapy.[162] Organisms most frequently cultured or detected based on PCR from nasal swabs included FHV-1 (75%), *Mycoplasma* (75%), and *Bordetella* spp. (47.5%). Additionally, *Staphyloccoccus* and *Streptococcus* were recovered in 12.5% and 10% of cases, respectively. Response rates were 67% for amoxicillin and 85% and 92%, respectively, for 5 and 10 mg/kg pradofloxacin. Differences were not statistically significant, but this may reflect the small number of animals: All except one cat that failed initial therapy responded to the second therapy. Because cats that were infected with *Mycoplasma* spp. responded after treatment with amoxicillin (n = 3), *Mycoplasma* spp. may not have been associated with infection.

Although the contribution of *Chlamydia* spp. to upper respiratory infection (URI) is less clear, several studies have examined reponse to therapy. Experimentally induced *C. felis* was not eradicated, but clinical signs resolved in cats receiving 10 to 15 mg/kg azithromycin for 3 days, followed by twice-weekly for 3 weeks. In contrast to azithromycin, infection was eradicated at 5 to 10 mg/kg doxycycline for 3 to 4 weeks.[16] Differences in the pathogenicity among strains may complicate application of the experimental infections to spontaneous disease; however, studies suggest that azithromycin may not offer sufficient advantages to doxycycline for treatment of chlamydiosis in cats.[16] Hartmann and coworkers[163] prospectively studied cats (n = 39) presented to a veterinary teaching hospital with clinical signs of upper respiratory disease or conjunctivitis. Cats were tested for FCV, FHV-1, *C. felis* and *Mycoplasma;* 37 of 39 cats had at least one organism present with the breakdown as follows: FCV (72%), *C. felis* (59%), *Mycoplasma* spp. (46 to 64%), FHV (28%) and the combination of *C. felis* and *Mycoplasma* spp. (28%) or FHV-FCV (13%); 10% had all four organisms present. The study was placebo controlled and double blinded; all cats were randomly assigned to receive either doxycycline (5 mg/kg bid by mouth) or pradofloxacin (5 mg/kg qd) for 42 days. Cats in both groups responded within 1 week of therapy, including those cats with viral, but not microbial, infection. *Mycoplasma* spp. was eliminated in all cats; *C. felis* was eliminated in all doxycycline-treated cats (n = 22) but remained in 4 of the 17 pradofloxacin-treated cats.

Inhalant therapy coupled with systemic therapy prolongs duration of eradication (mean of 8 months extended to 12 months) of *Pseudomonas* spp. infections in human patients with cystic fibrosis. However, the depth of penetration of sinuses in cats with inhaled therapy is questionable. Nevertheless, inhalant therapy should be helpful if coupled with appropriate systemic therapy. The ability to achieve high aminoglycoside concentrations in the presence of mucoid material is important because of the negative effects such debris has on aminoglycoside therapy; inhalation of aminoglycosides (28 days on, 28 days off) has been successful as sole therapy in humans with cystic fibrosis. The use of topical (e.g., ophthalmic solution) aminoglycoside therapy often implemented by clinicians dealing with chronic sinusitis in cats might provide therapeutic benefits similar to inhalant therapy; however, inhalant therapy also should be considered. Aerosolization of polypeptides such as polymyxin–colistin whose systemic use is precluded by systemic toxicity also has been used in human patients to treat *Pseudomonas* infections. Aerosolized doses of 500,000 to 1 million IU of colistin twice daily (potency of 30,000 IU/mL) have been used for several months.[165] Aerosolization of beta-lactams might also be considered.

Facilitating removal of bacterial and host debris, although important, may be difficult. Use of drugs intended to "dry" secretions (i.e., decongestants, antihistamines) generally are not prudent unless serous secretions (e.g., those associated with acute viral infection) are prolific. Methods of assisted mechanical clearance used in human patients are not likely to be effective in the upper airway disease of cats. Recombinant human DNase digests polymeric extracellular DNA and reduces the viscosity of pulmonary secretions; as such, it has become the cornerstone of mucolytic therapy in patients with cystic fibrosis. The drug is delivered by inhalation and is generally used as maintenance rather than limited to acute exacerbations. Cost may preclude its use in cats. Inhaled hypertonic saline has also increased fluidity of secretions; pretreatment with adrenergic agonists may be prudent to minimize the risk of irritant bronchoconstriction. The use of *N*-acetylcysteine as a mucolytic is described in Chapter 20.

The efficacy of once daily L-lysine (250 mg if less than 5 months or 500 mg if greater than 5 months of age) was studied for its impact on emergent URI in animal shelter cats (n = 144 treated and 147 nontreated cats). No difference was found in the subsequent incidence of URI that emerged between the two treatment groups.[172]

Bacterial Tracheobronchitis

Pathophysiology

Infectious tracheobronchitis is a contagious disease in dogs. Although it is generally mild and self-limiting, it can become serious, particularly if multiple bacteria become involved. Likelihood of infection reflects, in part, variability among strains. Host ciliated epithelial cell receptors are recognized by fimbrial and nonfimbrial filamentous (hemagglutinin and pertactin) adhesions. Upon colonization, exotoxins (adenylate cyclase-hemolysin, dermonecrotic toxin, and tracheal cytotoxin) and endotoxin impair the host response (e.g., phagocytosis, humoral and cell-mediated response) and cause local damage. Recent evidence suggests the organism may not be limited to an extracellular location but may survive intracellularly under some conditions.[173] The mucosal defense generally is able to clear most organisms within 3 days of infection. *Bordetella* spp. will, however, persist for up to 14 weeks after infection.[174,175] Active attachment to cilia and ciliostasis induced by *Bordetella* spp. appear to be important reasons for bacterial persistence. Whereas the disease generally is self-limiting to 7 to 10 days' duration, systemic signs indicative of pneumonia dictate the need for antimicrobial therapy.

KEY POINT 8-31 Canine tracheobronchitis generally is a self-limiting disease, with antimicrobial therapy generally not indicated unless infection persists beyond 7 to 10 days.

Microbial Targets

B. bronchiseptica remains the primary bacterial pathogen associated with infectious tracheobronchitis in dogs and appears to be the only agent that has induced classic kennel cough either experimentally or spontaneously. However, other viral organisms (e.g., canine parainfluenza virus and canine adenovirus type-2) may initiate or complicate the syndrome and *Mycoplasma* spp. may worsen it.[173] Chalker and colleagues[176] reviewed the role of pathogens and specifically mycoplasmas in canine respiratory disease. Dogs were from two groups: a rehoming kennel with a history of endemic canine infectious respiratory disease (n = 210; samples collected from nonvaccinated dogs with variable clinical signs during 1999 to 2002) and a training center (n = 153; dogs vaccinated regularly, with only sporadic outbreaks). At least 12 different *Mycoplasma* spp. were cultured from both groups of animals, with isolates obtained from tonsillar, tracheal, and bronchial lavage samples. Isolates were speciated on the basis of PCR. Differences in the two groups were limited to the lower respiratory tract *(Mycoplasma cynos)*; its presence was associated with an increased severity of disease. Previous studies by the same group in the same rehoming facility based on bronchial alveolar lavage (n = 209) indicated that canine respiratory coronavirus predominated in dogs with mild disease, *B. bronchiseptica* in dogs with moderate disease, and *Streptococcus equi* subsp. *zooepidemicus* in dogs with severe disease, with the bacterial load being greater in dogs with more severe disease.[177] *Pasteurella* spp. may also be involved (as reviewed by Chalker et al.[177])

Therapy should be based on culture and susceptibility data because organisms other than *Bordetella* spp. frequently complicate infection. It is likely that *Mycoplasma* spp. also play a role in infectious tracheobronchitis in dogs, and drug selection should include this organism. Despite the presence of other organisms, once the need for antimicrobial therapy is identified, therapy should include a drug with known efficacy against *B. bronchiseptica* (see later discussion). Culture of *B. bronchiseptica* does not necessarily indicate infection; the significance of growth depends on the number of colonies and sample location. Whereas isolation from the trachea is significant, isolation from the nares or pharynx is likely to be significant only if growth is moderate to heavy.[178] First-choice antimicrobials generally include the tetracyclines, chloramphenicol, and the macrolides (including erythromycin, clarithromycin, and azithromycin). Fluoroquinolones should be based on culture and susceptibility support. Glucocorticoids should not be used in the presence of bacteriostatic drugs; alternative mechanisms to control cough (e.g., narcotic antitussives) should be considered. Prophylaxis might be considered in animals exposed to *B. bronchispetica*; treatment, however, is not always indicated because the disease tends to be self-limiting.

Because of the location of the organism and the difficulty of drug penetration into bronchial secretions, aerosolization of selected antimicrobials (aminoglycosides, polymyxin B) should be considered as an adjunct to systemic antimicrobial therapy for kennel cough. Systemic therapy should include a drug that penetrates bronchial secretions well. Drugs with known in vitro efficacy against both *B. bronchiseptica* and

Mycoplasma spp. include the fluoroquinolones, doxycycline or minocycline, chloramphenicol, and the macrolides. Among these, only the fluoroquinolones typically are associated with bactericidal concentrations. Accumulation of the macrolides in lung tissue may, however, result in bactericidal concentrations of these otherwise bacteriostatic drugs. Vaccination should be used to immunize dogs against the primary pathogens of infectious tracheobronchitis.

Bacterial Pneumonia

Bacterial pneumonia is much more common in dogs than in cats.

Microbial Targets

Although *B. bronchiseptica* and *S. zooepidemicus* are among the bacterial organisms commonly associated with pneumonia, many other organisms can cause infection, including *E. coli, Pasteurella, Klebsiella, Staphylococcus,* and *Pseudomonas* spp.[175] The potential for *Mycoplasma* spp. and anaerobic organisms (particularly in the presence of abscessation) as a cause of infection should not be ignored. Generally, the respiratory tract is sterile below the larynx. *Mycoplasma* spp. were associated with pneumonia in cats on the basis of isolation in large numbers and pure growth. Clinical signs resolved on treatment with doxycycline or ciprofloxacin, potentially supporting their role.[179] Foster and coworkers[180] also retrospectively reviewed the microbiology associated with lower respiratory tract infection in cats (n = 21; Australia); isolates were collected by bronchoalveolar lavage between 1995 and 2000. Organisms were identified as pathogens on the basis of purity of growth, absence of oral contaminants, and a review of supportive clinical signs and diagnostic indicators (e.g., radiographs). *Mycoplasma* spp. was the sole pathogen in 11 of 19. Other infecting organisms included a combination of *Mycoplasma* spp. with *P. multocida,* or *B. bronchiseptica. Pasteurella* spp. was a cause of infection with other microbes in two other animals. Other infectious organisms include toxoplasmosis, cryptococcosis, mycobacterium, and miscellaneous bacteria. Other studies reporting on the bacteria associated with airways of healthy cats have identified *Pasteurella* spp., *Pseudomonas* spp., *Staphylococcus* spp., *Streptococcus* spp., *E. coli,* and *Micrococcus* spp. Those organisms most commonly reported as the causes of pneumonia in cats included *P. multocida, E. coli, K. pneumoniae, B. bronchiseptica, Streptococcus canis, Mycobacterium* spp., and Eugonic Fermenter-4.

Antimicrobial and Adjuvant Therapy

Cytology and culture collected by tracheal wash, bronchoscopy, bronchoalveolar lavage, or lung aspiration should serve as the basis for treatment. Cultures of the pharyngeal area should not be the basis of antimicrobial selection for infections of the respiratory tract. The more severe the infection, the more important lipid solubility becomes to drug selection and the greater the need to choose a drug that accumulates in inflammatory cells. Doses should be sufficiently high to establish bactericidal concentrations of drug at the site of infection. Among the antimicrobials, fluoroquinolones such as enrofloxacin should be considered because of their spectrum and lipid solubility. In addition, accumulation by alveolar macrophages might enhance drug distribution at the site of inflammation.[63,65-67] Accumulation has been documented for enrofloxacin, marbofloxacin, and pradofloxacin. Combination therapy should be considered to not only broaden the spectrum of antimicrobials but also to enhance efficacy. Aerosolization should be considered in addition to (never instead of) systemic antimicrobial therapy, particularly in severe cases. Aerosolization may be particularly important for infections associated with *B. bronchiseptica.*

Mobilization of respiratory secretions may be important to resolution of infection. In addition to physical techniques such as coupage, mucolytic and mucokinetic agents should be administered. Bronchodilators may also facilitate movement of respiratory secretions as well as facilitate airway movement. Their use is controversial, with some authors suggesting that their antiinflammatory effects may be detrimental. As such, control of inflammation in a nonimmunosuppressive manner may be of benefit. Therefore theophylline should be considered because of its antiinflammatory effects. Theophyllilne can cause ventilation perfusion mismatching, and oxygen therapy should be available to patients when this drug is administered in moderate to severe cases. Alternatively, β_2-selective bronchodilators such as terbutaline may be indicated; they may also facilitate ciliary activity by decreasing viscosity of airway secretions. Combination therapies also should be considered (e.g., theophylline, terbutaline) to facilitate bronchodilation. *N*-acetylcysteine (200 to 500 mg orally or intravenously bid) should be considered for adjuvant therapy in infections associated with marked inflammatory debris. Intravenous administration (e.g., Mucomyst®) is preferred in patients whose clinical signs are indicative of serious or life-threatening inflammation. The drug will facilitate antimicrobial penetration through mucoid debris present at the site of infection but also through the lipopolysaccharide membrane of gram-negative organisms. Treatment might continue until resolution of radiographic signs indicative of pneumonia, which may require up to 6 weeks. The use of non–immune-suppressing antiinflammatories should be considered in the presence of fulminating inflammation. Among the bronchodilators that might be used, theophylline is the most effective antiinflammatory. Pentoxyfylline also might be considered (see Chapter 20). Drugs that decrease bronchial secretions, including diuretics, should be avoided. Further, dehydrated patients should be rehydrated to facilitate the functions of the mucociliary tract.

Pyothorax

Pathophysiology

Pyothorax, otherwise known as *empyema,* refers to the accumulation of white blood cells in the pleural space.[181] Organisms reach the pleural space by direct introduction (most commonly by way of a foreign body), hematogenous or lymphatic spread, or extension from an adjacent structure.[182,183] In cats, parapneumonic spread currently appears to be the most common route of infection. The physiologic forces that keep the pleural space essentially free of fluid are overcome

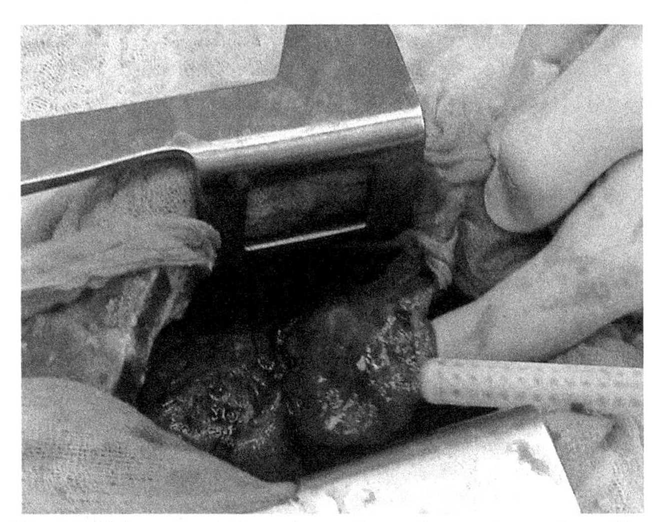

Figure 8-9 Intraoperative view of pyothorax in a dog. The inflammatory response can be profound, requiring analgesic therapy. Intrathoracic lavage with fluids containing heparin may increase the chance of long-term survival. (Photo courtesy of Harry W. Boothe, DVM, MS, DACVS, Auburn, AL.)

by inflammation, resulting in an increase in regional blood flow, capillary hypertension, increased capillary permeability, and increased oncotic draw (by inflammatory proteins) of fluid into the pleural space (Figure 8-9). Lymphatic drainage becomes progressively more important as oncotic draw into capillaries is lost, but accumulation of inflammatory debris and fibrosis ultimately preclude lymphatic drainage of the pleural space. Gram stain of fluids collected by thoracentesis can be a rapid method of diagnosing the bacterial cause of infection. The incidence of anaerobic organisms as either sole agents (particularly in cats) or in combination with other bacteria is high. Thus samples submitted for culture should include both aerobic and appropriately collected anaerobic specimens. The presence of a foul smell (reflecting the production of organic matter by-products) is supportive of infection by anaerobic organisms.

Microbial Targets

In cats anaerobes predominate as the causative organisms of pyothorax. Organisms include Bacteroideaceae (*Bacteroides, Porphyromonas,* and *Prevotella* spp.), *Fusobacterium, Actinomyces, Nocardia, Peptostreptococcus, Clostridium, Propionibacterium, Pasteurella,* and *Mycoplasma* spp. Barrs and Betty[182] recently reviewed feline pyothorax and observed that infecting flora is similar to oropharyngeal flora. Aspiration of oral flora was suggested as the most likely mechanism of infection in 15 of 18 cats in one study.[183] Causative organisms in the dog include but are not necessarily limited to *Fusobacterium, Actinomyces, Nocardia, Corynebacterium, Streptococcus, Bacteroides, Pasteurella, E. coli, Klebsiella,* and *Peptostreptococcus.*[181] The most common aerobic organisms isolated in dogs in a retrospective study were *P. multocida* (37%), followed by *E. coli* (26%); anaerobic organisms included *Fusobacterium* (13%) and *Bacteroides* spp. (10%). *Actinomyces* organisms were collected in 26% of the patients.[184] In a more recent retrospective study of pyothorax in dogs Boothe and coworkers[185] found *E. coli* to be the most common infecting organism.

Both cytology and culture and susceptibility data should be an important component of antimicrobial selection for treatment of pyothorax. A retrospective study[185] revealed that empirical therapy resulted in inappropriate antimicrobial selection in 35% of the patients. Further, some dogs with cytologic evidence of infection yielded no growth on culture, whereas other dogs had no cytologic evidence of bacteria despite growth on culture. Multiple organisms should be suspected in all cases of pyothorax even if only a single culture is identified; infections were mixed in 46% of patients, with 65% of the organisms being gram negative, 17% gram positive, and 17% to 43% anaerobic.[185] Because such a high percentage of infections may involve anaerobic organisms, antimicrobial selection might most appropriately include drugs effective against anaerobes.

KEY POINT 8-32 Both cytology and culture and susceptibility data should be an an important component of antimicrobial selection for treatment of pyothorax.

Fungal organisms also should be considered as a cause of pyothorax.

Antimicrobial and Adjuvant Therapy

For both dogs and cats, nonsurvivors usually die or are euthanized within the first several days of hospitalization.[182,183,185] Removal of inflammatory debris is a critical component of effective antimicrobial therapy for the patient with pyothorax. Drainage by thoracentesis alone is not likely to be effective; indeed, up to an 80% mortality rate can be expected with this approach. Progression to a chronic stage can be expected in many patients in whom drainage has been inadequate, increasing both mortality and cost compared with patients in whom drainage was adequate. Thus therapy should include chest tube drainage (potentially by continuous water seal suction at 20 cm).

Adequate hydration will be important to offset the risk of hypotension induced by continuous removal of pleural effusion. Effective removal of debris not only will remove mediators associated with morbidity but also will facilitate antimicrobial distribution. Response to antimicrobial therapy should be based on repeated cytology and Gram stains. Clinical signs and cytologic findings should improve once chest tube drainage is in place. Bacteria generally are undetectable 2 to 3 days after therapy is begun; however, serial cultures should be used to confirm the absence of growth. Antimicrobial selection should be based on culture and susceptibility data. Unfortunately, growth often does not occur despite cytologic evidence of bacteria. An anaerobic environment should be assumed even if aerobes are cultured because many of these organisms are able to survive and grow in an anaerobic environment.

Bilateral chest tube placement may be necessary in some patients, whereas surgical intervention may be critical to many. In a retrospective study of pyothorax in dogs, medical management was successful (based on absence of disease for 1 year) in only 25% of dogs, as opposed to 78% that were surgically managed.[184] Boothe and coworkers[185] retrospectively compared drainage, chest tube–based drainage and lavage, and surgical intervention followed with chest tube placement in dogs (n = 46) with pyothorax. There was no difference in either short-term or long-term survival. In cats antimicrobial therapy coupled with needle thoracentesis is associated with a 50% to 80% mortality rate, indicating that chest tube placement with intermittent thoracic lavage is preferred.[183] Lavage not only facilitates exudate drainage but also dilutes inflammatory debris and the inoculum, which should facilitate antimicrobial penetration. Lavage may also cause débridement of pleura and breakdown of adhesions. Recommended lavage fluids include warmed 0.9% NaCl or lactated Ringers solution at a rate of 10 to 30 mL/kg with each lavage. Up to 25% of lavage fluid may not be recovered. Hypokalemia is a potential complication; it may be necessary to add potassium to lavage fluid. Use of intrapleural fibrinolytics in an attempt to reduce adhesions is generally discouraged. However, Boothe and colleagues[185] demonstrated that lavage with physiologic saline containing heparin (10 IU/mL) was positively associated with long-term survival in dogs with pyothorax. The addition of antimicrobial therapy to lavage fluid probably offers no added benefit and may be a detriment if it irritates the pleura.

Antimicrobials initially should be administered intravenously to ensure that the highest concentration reaches the site of infection. Once response is achieved, oral therapy can be implemented. Combination antimicrobial therapy should be considered for the treatment of pyothorax, in part because of the frequent mixed nature of infection. In particular, antimicrobials that are not effective in an anaerobic environment (e.g., aminoglycosides) should not be used as sole agents in the treatment of pyothorax. A penicillin should be considered with initial therapy because the spectrum includes anaerobic organisms and synergistic interactions that occur with a number of antimicrobials. However, limited susceptibility to aminopenicillins (ampicillin, amoxicillin) may indicate the need for extended-spectrum beta-lactams.[115] Because many of the organisms (including anaerobes) associated with pyothorax produce beta-lactamases, protected drugs or drugs inherently resistant to beta-lactamases should be selected, although increasingly these drugs are also limited in susceptiblity. The use of cephalosporins for the treatment of pyothorax is generally not recommended because their efficacy against anaerobes is less than that of penicillins unless the anaerobic spectrum of the drug is confirmed (e.g., cefoxitin) or combination therapy is implemented. The aminoglycosides (particularly amikacin) are among the drugs to which *Nocardia* spp. is very susceptible and should be considered in combination with a beta-lactam for treatment of this organism. The advantages of fluoroquinolones include lipid solubility, general potency, and accumulation in phagocytic white blood cells, which will not only facilitate intracellular killing but also increase movement of drug to sites of inflammation. The newer-generation fluoroquinolones, including the cyanofluoroquninolone pradofloxacin, have an enhanced spectrum against anaerobic organisms compared with their earlier counterparts.

For initial therapy, particularly in serious cases, the author prefers a combination of parenteral (intravenous) meropenem, particularly in serious cases, and amikacin. If ampicillin is used, it should be protected with sulbactam and should be given at a high dose at least every 4 hours. The most appropriate dose and interval should be based on the MIC of the infecting organism when possible. Amikacin should be given once daily. Therapy should be continued for 3 to 5 days or until improvement is evident (e.g., 7 to 10 days). At that time, assuming improvement is evident, oral therapy can be implemented. The author prefers high doses of amoxicillin–clavulanic acid (25 to 30 mg/kg every 8 hours) and a sulfadiazine/trimethoprim combination (30 to 45 mg/kg twice daily) based on both drugs. Alternatively, metronidazole or clindamycin and a second or third-generation fluoroquinolone as sole therapy may be reasonable choices. Synergistic actions against *Nocardia* spp. have been documented (in vitro) with a number of antimicrobial combinations, including amikacin and sulfadiazine–trimethoprim.[186] Other drugs that have shown efficacy against *Nocardia* or *Actinomyces* spp. and are characterized by adequate distribution to the pleural space include clindamycin, minocycline, and doxycycline.[186] Precaution is advised, however, when using these bacteriostatic drugs in combination with a bactericidal drug.

Involvement of anaerobic organisms and presence of devitalized tissues is likely to mandate an extended period of antimicrobial therapy, with 4 to 6 weeks being a reasonable target.

INFECTIONS OF THE GASTROINTESTINAL TRACT

Oral Cavity

Pathophysiology

Dental diseases are associated with both the accumulation of dental plaque and the emergence of pathogenic organisms. The type of microbe appears to be more important in the initiation of disease, where the microbial load is more important for persistence (i.e., chronicity) of disease[187] The impact of periodontal disease on general health warrants a proactive approach to management. Effective prevention can be realized with effective control of the microbes located in subgingival or supragingival plaque. Mechanical débridement is important to treatment, with antimicrobial therapy indicated with probing depths that exceed 5 mm.[187] Therapy should target those microorganisms capable of destroying periodontal connective tissues. Specifically, therapy should target the eradication of organisms such as *Porphyromonas gingivalis* and *Prevotella intermedia*: their absence is a predictor of resolution of disease.

Microbial Targets

The aerobic and anaerobic flora from gingival pockets of 49 dogs with severe gingivitis and periodontitis were cultured. The susceptibility of each isolate to four antimicrobial agents currently approved for veterinary use in the United States (amoxicillin–clavulanic acid; clindamycin; cefadroxil; and enrofloxacin) was determined. In a study of organisms cultured from canine gingivitis and periodontitis, the combination of amoxicillin–clavulanic acid had the highest susceptibility against aerobes (94%) and anaerobes (100%) compared with clindamycin, cefadroxil, and enrofloxacin. Enrofloxacin had the highest in vitro susceptibility activity against aerobic gram negatives.[188] Similar findings were reported in cats (n = 40): susceptibility against all isolates was greatest with amoxicillin–clavulanic acid (92%). Anaerobes were equally (99%) susceptible to amoxicillin–clavulanic acid and clindamycin, whereas susceptibility to aerobes was greatest to enrofloxacin (90%).[189]

Antimicrobial and Alternative Treatments

Use of culture and susceptibility data as a basis for antimicrobial selection in the mouth is complicated by normal polymicrobial anaerobic growth. Culture of a relatively pure growth may indicate the organism as the cause of infection. Representative cultures should be obtained from infections in deeper, isolated tissues (e.g., abscessation or osteomyelitis). Care should be taken in collection of the anaerobes; these organisms can be exquisitely sensitive to oxygen. Because infections are likely to involve anaerobic organisms, drugs that target anaerobes and distribute well to the mucosa and (if indicated) bone should be selected. Examples include clindamycin; the aminopenicillins, including amoxicillin–clavulanic acid combinations; and metronidazole. Among these drugs, clindamycin has proved the most effective in penetrating the glycocalyx and other material serving as a barrier to antimicrobial penetration in the presence of plaque. Metronidazole–fluoroquinolone combinations (e.g., ciprofloxacin [humans] or enrofloxacin) have been shown to act synergistically in the treatment of periodontitis. Pradofloxacin was demonstrated to be effective against subgingival bacteria associated with periodontal disease in dogs.[187] Anaerobic organisms, including *Bacteroides* species, produce beta-lactamases, and therefore, clavulanic acid combinations should be considered for more complicated or serious infections. The role of gram-negative organisms in causing infections should not be ignored even in the presence of abscessation.

Prophylactic antimicrobial use has been commonplace for dental procedures but not warranted for healthy animals. Decreasing the microbial load is probably a more appropriate goal than is proplyaxis. The duration of antimicrobial therapy before the procedure depends on the intent of prophylaxis. Protection of the patient predisposed to endocarditis during the procedure is particularly important. A single dose of antimicrobials timed such that peak plasma concentrations occur as the dental procedure is begun may be sufficient for most animals. For an orally administered drug, the time of administration should approximate the time to peak tissue concentrations, which is generally 1 to 2 hours after administration. For intravenously administered drugs, drug concentrations will not be highest at the tissue site until distribution has occurred, generally 30 to 60 minutes after administration. If the intent of prophylactic therapy is to decrease the bacterial load of the oral cavity before the procedure, then the drug should be administered several days before the procedure. Because the oral cavity contains a large population of normal organisms, prophylaxis for surgical procedures involving the oral cavity often has been extended to 1 week or longer before or after the procedure. A novel drug delivery system has recently been designed for treatment of periodontal disease in dogs. Doxycycline, characterized by a broad antimicrobial spectrum, is prepared in a vehicle that is injected into the periodontal pocket after dentistry. The moist environment causes the vehicle to gel, resulting in a slow-release drug delivery system. In clinical trials associated with Food and Drug Administration approval, animals receiving the drug after dental work improved more rapidly than animals treated with a placebo. The cleaning procedure itself, however, appeared to be the more important means of improving the health of the local environment.

Antiseptic agents can prove beneficial in home care dentistry.[190] Chlorhexidine is considered one of the most efficacious products and is indicated for patients with periodontal disease. It is available in several 12% preparations: an oral acetate rinse (Nolvadent, Fort Dodge); a more palatable gluconate solution (CHX Oral Cleansing Solution, VR_x Products), or a gluconate gel. In addition to having an immediate bactericidal effect, chlorhexidine adsorbs to the tooth pellicle, which serves as a reservoir, allowing continuous release of chlorhexidine. Chlorhexidine has caused toxicity when applied as a disinfectant in catteries after grooming by the cats. Although there are no reports of chlorhexidine toxicity when used for periodontal disease in cats, research focused primarily on Beagles suggests that caution should be exercised when this product is used for cats. Fluoride-containing products also should be used cautiously because dogs appear to be more susceptible than other species to acute toxicosis.

Esophagus and Stomach

Primary infections of the upper gastrointestinal tract are unusual. Thus treatment of infections generally includes resolution of the underlying cause.[191]

Megaesophagus

Regardless of the cause of megaesophagus, aspiration pneumonia is a serious, potentially life-threatening complication. The continuous use of antimicrobials for prevention of pneumonia in cases of unresolvable megaesophagus is controversial and probably not indicated unless continuous bacterial infection has been documented. The inflammatory response of aspiration pneumonia is likely to be induced by chemicals (including hydrochloric acid) or foreign bodies. Accordingly, drugs that control the inflammatory response with minimal immune suppression should be used in a timely fashion (see Chapter 20). The treatment of pneumonia was discussed earlier.

KEY POINT 8-33 The continuous use of antimicrobials for prevention of pneumonia in cases of unresolvable megaesophagus is controversial and probably not indicated unless continuous bacterial infection has been documented.

Stomach

Vomiting originates from many central and peripheral causes, including acute gastritis. Acute gastritis, in turn, has many causes and is most likely to respond when the underlying cause is resolved, which generally occurs in 1 to 5 days. Bacteria are an unlikely cause of vomiting, and antimicrobial therapy rarely is indicated. Therapy is supportive, including fluids and appropriate additives (e.g., potassium if vomiting is profuse) and antiemetics.

The normal flora of the stomach of dogs consists of large spiral bacteria, including *Helicobacter* species.[192] Spiral bacterial and a nonpathogenic chlamydial organism occur in the feline stomach. The role of spiral organisms (most notably *Helicobacter* spp.) in gastrointestinal diseases in dogs and cats is currently being investigated, but it is likely that these organisms will become the target of drug therapy in the medical management of several diseases. Numbers of bacteria in the gastrointestinal tract gradually increase distally to the ileocecal valve.[193] Numbers of bacteria abnormally increase when normal bowel defenses are impaired. Several mechanisms exist to protect the normal gastrointestinal tract from infection. Among the most important are gastric and bile acids, which limit the concentration of bacteria. In humans more than 99.9% of ingested coliform bacteria are killed at a pH of less than 4 within 30 minutes. In contrast, no reduction of bacteria occurs in the stomach in the presence of achlorhydria.[194] Among the reasons that *Helicobacter pylori* has been recognized for its pathogenicity in the cause of human gastrointestinal disorders is its ability to alter the gastrointestinal pH and thus increase host susceptibility to other infections.[194] Treatment for *Helicobacter* is discussed in Chapter 18.

Drugs that contribute to bacterial overgrowth include antisecretory drugs and antacids. Mucus and mucosal tissue integrity provide physical barriers and help clear bacteria from the upper and small intestine.[194]

Small and Large Intestines

Normal Control Mechanisms

Intestinal motility. Intestinal motility has several roles in the prevention of gastrointestinal bacterial infection. Gastrointestinal motility and diarrhea help remove offending pathogens from the gastrointestinal tract, not unlike the cough reflex does in the respiratory tract. Bowel stasis increases the risk of bacterial overgrowth in the small intestine and contributes to the risk of inflammatory bowel disease. Antimotility drugs (e.g., opioids) increase the risk of overgrowth;[194] in contrast, the use of prokinetic drugs may be beneficial if decreased motility is a factor in the development of diarrhea. Obstruction or stasis of intestinal or bile flow and decreased mucosal blood flow contribute to bacterial infections in the intestinal tract.[193]

Normal microflora. Microflora is established at 2 to 3 weeks of life. The population remains stable under normal conditions but does vary among species. The high-meat diet of carnivores supports a predominant population of streptococci and *Clostridium perfringens* and suppresses *Lactobacillus*.[193] Anaerobes comprise the majority of intestinal microflora, outnumbering aerobic organisms by tenfold to 1000-fold;[193] in humans 99.9% of enteric microbes are anaerobic. Aerobic gram-negative coliforms in humans include *E. coli, Klebsiella, Proteus,* and enterococci.[194] The normal microflora is important to the control of infecting microorganisms in the gastrointestinal tract. Normal floral bacteria compete for available nutrients, maintain redox potentials, and produce antibacterial compounds that prevent colonization by infecting organisms. Normal flora also have a number of physiologic functions. Microflora produce volatile fatty acids and vitamins as well as metabolize bile acids and some drugs. Indigenous (anaerobic) microbes attach to the intestinal epithelial surface and act synergistically with host immune mechanisms to interfere with experimental *Salmonella* infections.[194] Gram-negative aerobes such as *Proteus* spp., *Enterobacter* spp., and *E. coli* act in concert with host immune mechanisms to prevent infection with *Vibrio* species. Gram stains of fecal smears might be used to help identify a loss of balance in the normal microflora of dogs or cats. In meat eaters, normally 75% of the flora is represented by gram-negative organisms and 25% gram-positive. A loss of gram-positive or an increase (that might include *Clostridium*) may be supportive of an imbalance.

In the presence of diarrhea, anaerobic numbers decline because the organisms require stasis and a low oxygen potential. In the presence of antimicrobials, the loss of normal microflora in humans can shift the balance of bacteria to gram-negative aerobes and replacement of anaerobes with organisms such as *Pseudomonas* spp., *Klebsiella* spp., anaerobes such as *Clostridium* spp., and yeast *(Candida)*.[194] Diarrhea associated with antimicrobial use has long been associated with disruption in the balance of normal microflora, in part because of the loss of toxic products produced by normal microflora. The number of organisms (e.g., *Salmonella*) needed to cause infection is markedly reduced after administration of a single dose of selected antimicrobials (e.g., for *Salmonella* spp., streptomycin). Resistance to infection can be restored with a return of the normal enteric flora (in humans, especially *Bacteroides* spp.). Outbreaks of gastrointestinal infections in humans, particularly with *Salmonella* spp., can be associated with antimicrobial exposure.[194]

Host immunity. Host intestinal immunity plays an important role in the prevention of gastrointestinal infection. The intestine is normally in a state of physiologic inflammation because of the presence of neutrophils, macrophages, plasma cells, and lymphocytes. The loss of neutrophils and their phagocytic capability results in an increased susceptibility to gram-negative (rod) infections originating in the gastrointestinal tract.[194] Secretory IgA is resistant to intraluminal degradation and as such provides an important source of local immune protection. The intestinal antibodies are directed toward a variety of bacterial antigens, including endotoxin, capsular material, and exotoxins. In addition, they may have bactericidal, opsonic, or neutralizing effects on bacteria.[194] In the nursing animal, several compounds produced by the mother are important. In humans breast milk contains lactoferrin, lysosome, phagocytic activity, oligosaccharide fractions, and other materials that afford protection to the newborn.

Factors facilitating infection. A number of microbial factors facilitate gastrointestinal infection. Factors that determine bacterial virulence and pathogenicity are well represented by *E. coli* and include production of enterotoxins, the capacity to invade, induction of hemorrhagic colitis, and expression of adherence and enteroaggregation.[194] Production of enterotoxins (defined as having a direct effect on intestinal mucosa such that fluid secretion increases) by organisms such as *Staphylococcus* spp., *C. perfringens, Bacteroides* spp., and *E. coli)* can result in disruption of fluid fluxes across the intestinal mucosa. The organisms producing enterotoxins generally are part of the normal microflora but, in the presence of predisposing factors (e.g., garbage enteritis, bacterial stasis, bacterial overgrowth), proliferate in the small intestine. Noninvasive organisms can induce diarrhea by actions of exotoxins that stimulate adenyl cyclase and subsequently sodium, chloride, and water secretion into the intestinal lumen. Cytotoxins produced by several pathogens cause mucosal destruction and a subsequent inflammatory response.[193,194] Some organisms *(Salmonella,* particularly in the ileum, and *Shigella* spp.) are capable of causing mucosal invasion, resulting in hemorrhagic feces. Enterohemorrhagic *E. coli* produces cytotoxins, and the enterotoxin produced by *C. perfringens* also causes cytotoxicity. The pathogenesis of *Campylobacter jejuni* and *H. pylori* infections also has been attributed to cytotoxins.[194]

Adherence factors contribute to the ability of organisms to colonize the intestinal epithelium and cause infection. Adherence antigens generally are fimbrial in nature but are distinct from those responsible for urinary adherence. A number of distinctly different adhesions have been described for enteric microorganisms. Invasiveness, as represented by *Shigella* spp. and selected strains of *E. coli,* results in the destruction of epithelial cells and superficial inflammation. The degree of invasiveness depends on the protein to which the organism is bound and may also depend on the production of cytotoxic exotoxins.[194] Newer antimicrobial agents may target the adherence of toxins, acting to prevent their synthesis or antagonizing their effects and thus blocking the ability of the microbe to infect. Drugs also may minimize the actions of enterotoxins. Other virulence factors that facilitate infection in the gastrointestinal tract include motility, chemotaxis, and production of mucinase.[194] The ability of *H. pylori* to alter gastric acidity has already been mentioned.

Treatment of bacterial diarrhea. The role of bacteria in causing diarrhea and the treatment of these causative organisms are also discussed in Chapter 19. The role of translocation of bacteria is addressed in Chapter 26. Several diarrheal syndromes have been described in small animals.[193] Neonatal colibacillosis occurs in dogs and cats. Puppies are generally only 1 week old, but diarrhea can persist in older puppies. Factors contributing to infection with *E. coli* include immunologic incompetency (including failure of passive transfer), immaturity of intestinal epithelial cells (nonselectively permeable) for the first 2 to 3 days of life, and exposure to *E. coli* in colostrum. The syndrome of bacterial overgrowth is a cause of chronic or recurrent diarrhea; German Shepherd Dogs appear to be predisposed. Increased numbers (more than 10^5/mL) of *E. coli* and enterococci (considered normal flora) and selected anaerobes (e.g., *Clostridium* spp.) are found in duodenal secretions of affected dogs. Underlying factors are not well described but include motility disorders, hypochlorhydria, and deficiency of secretory antibody (IgA). Animals generally respond to antimicrobial therapy.

Adjuvant therapy. The importance of fluid therapy for patients with diarrhea induced by bacterial infections should not be overlooked. The composition of electrolyte losses in severe diarrhea is similar to that of serum, and both intravenous and oral rehydration therapy should reflect this composition. Absorption of oral solutions depends on the intact intestinal mucosa. Sodium and glucose should be present in equimolar concentrations; amino acids (e.g., glycine) might be added in veterinary preparations to facilitate electrolyte absorption.[193] In humans an oral recipe is recommended to contain 3.5 g NaCl, 2.5 g $NaHCO_3$, 1.5 g KCl, and 20 g glucose (dextrose) per liter of boiled water.[194]

INFECTIONS ASSOCIATED WITH BACTEREMIA

Bacteremia is defined as the presence of live bacteria in the bloodstream. Bacteremia does not necessarily lead to sepsis (the systemic inflammatory response to infection) unless microbial growth overwhelms host defenses.

Infective Bacterial Endocarditis

Causative organisms of infectious endocarditis (IE) are not limited to bacteria but include *Chlamydia* spp., *Mycoplasma* spp., fungi, and viruses. Because more is known about bacteremia caused by bacteria, it serves as the basis of discussion here. Regardless of the type of infecting organisms, the events that allow development of IE are probably the same. IE includes infection and colonization of the endocardial and adjacent surfaces of the cardiac valves, their supportive structures, and the wall of the heart. The incidence in dogs and cats appears to be low (0.06% to 6.6% based on necropsy findings).[195]

The incubation period of IE, that is, the time that elapses between the bacteremic event and the onset of clinical symptoms, may be up to 2 weeks. Historically, IE has been classified in humans on the basis of the progression of untreated disease. Acute disease is characterized by a fulminant course of events, characterized by high fever, evidence of systemic involvement, leukocytosis, and death generally within a couple of days (taking as long as several weeks). Subacute (death in 6 to 12 weeks) and chronic (duration longer than 12 weeks) IE are characterized by a slower course with low-grade fever and vague clinical signs.[195]

Pathophysiology

Microbial factors. Several independent events lead to the development of IE.[196] The endothelial surface of the valve first must be altered (e.g., by blood turbulence induced by valvular insufficiency) such that bacteria can adhere to and colonize it. Initially, the damaged surface induces the deposition of platelets and fibrin, forming a nonbacterial thrombotic endocarditis. Organisms with the ability to adhere to platelets or fibrin have the advantage of inducing disease with smaller inoculums. Bacterial adhesion to the thrombus forming on the damaged valvular surface is critical to the initial stages of IE. The thrombus provides a protective environment for bacterial growth in that phagocytic and other host defenses are impaired below the surface.[196] This thrombus provides a surface for bacterial adherence and colonization. Organisms particularly capable of adherence include *S. aureus, S. epidermidis,* and *P. aeruginosa.* Colonization is followed rapidly by the formation of a protective sheath of fibrin and platelets, which facilitates bacterial multiplication and vegetative growth. Transient bacteremia such as might occur during dental, gastrointestinal, or urogenital procedures can lead to colonization of a thrombus that has formed on a previously damaged valve. Infecting organisms tend to be nonpathogenic organisms associated with the mucosal surface (e.g., *P. acnes, Actinomyces* spp., *S. epidermidis*) or organisms that are resistant to complement-mediated bactericidal activity (e.g., *E. coli, P. aeruginosa, Serratia marcescens*). Within genera of bacteria, differences in the ability of strains to cause infection also might be related to their lack of encapsulation (thus allowing adherence). Dextran, a complex polysaccharide produced by some organisms (e.g., *Streptococcus*) spp., is an example of an extracellular molecule that may facilitate bacterial adhesion to the valvular surface. Some organisms are able to directly bind to endothelial surfaces; indeed, endothelial cells may ingest some organisms (e.g., *S. auerus*) as the initial event. Some organisms are potent stimulators of platelet aggregation (e.g., *Staphylococcus* and *Streptococcus* species), thus facilitating growth of the vegetative lesion as well as formation of thrombi in systemic circulation.[196]

Host factors. Host defenses can both impair and facilitate the formation of the vegetative lesion. Although humoral antibodies should decrease the number of circulating bacteria, they also may facilitate bacterial invasion by stimulating agglutination. Constant antigenic challenge results in the formation of circulating antibodies. Rheumatoid factors (anti-IgG IgM antibodies) develop in 50% of human patients within 6 weeks of developing IE. Antinuclear antibodies also are formed. Circulating immune complexes are more likely with long illnesses. Although antibodies may provide some protection, they also may contribute to the development of glomerulonephritis, musculoskeletal abnormalities, and low-grade fever. Interestingly, platelets provide the host with some defenses during the course of IE. Low-molecular-weight cationic proteins (thrombodefensins, or platelet microbicidal protein [PMP]) are released after exposure of the platelet to thrombin. These appear to damage the bacterial cell membrane or wall and may act synergistically with select antimicrobials to cause bactericidal effects. Organisms resistant to PMP may be more likely to contribute to the pathophysiology of IE.[196]

Complications of infectious endocarditis. Complications of IE that may require medical management develop in several organs. In humans myocardial abscesses are found in 20% of cases autopsied, generally as a result of acute staphylococcal endocarditis. Embolism is common, most commonly occurring in the splenic, renal, coronary, or cerebral circulation. The kidney is often afflicted in patients with IE because of septic embolization (with or without abscessation), infarction, or glomerulonephritis. Cerebral emboli occur in 33% of human cases of IE, leading to arteritis, abscessation, and infarction. Splenic abscesses, although potentially common, may not be clinically evident. Petechiae may indicate arteritis of the vascular supply of the skin or immune complex deposition.[196]

Antimicrobial therapy. Despite the low incidence of therapeutic success, venous blood culture is probably the most important diagnostic tool for IE. Multiple blood cultures (at least three are recommended in the first 24 hours for human patients) are more likely to yield a positive result. Bacterial counts in blood are generally low, and growth can be slow. Cultures should be held 3 weeks. Newer technologies may include methods that detect bacterial cell constituents.

Empirical therapy should begin after cultures have been collected. In human patients *Staphylococcus* and *Streptococcus* spp. are among the most common causes of IE. In dogs, *S. aureus, E. coli,* and beta-hemolytic streptococci are the most commonly isolated.[195] Antimicrobial selection should be broadly based, however, targeting gram-negative as well as gram-positive organisms. Anaerobic organisms also should be included in the spectrum. The same approach is indicated for culture-negative IE. Drug distribution is less of a concern for IE, thus minimizing the need for lipid-soluble drugs. An exception must be made if bacterial embolization of organs (e.g., spleen, brain, or kidneys) has occurred or if the original source of infection remains a potential source of continuing infection. Antimicrobials should be based on efficacy in the presence of potential immune suppression. Bactericidal concentrations should be achieved in blood or tissues, indicating intravenous therapy. Consideration should be given to release of endotoxin. Combination therapy should be considered not only to enhance the spectrum of a single antimicrobial but also to enhance efficacy. Beta-lactams should be considered because of their broad spectrum as well as their ability to increase antimicrobial delivery into bacteria. Imipenem or meropenem stand out among the beta-lactams for their minimal release of endotoxin. Likewise, the fluoroquinolones and the aminoglycosides cause minimal release of endotoxin.

KEY POINT 8-34 Empirical antimicrobial selection for infective endocarditis should be broadly based, but properly collected cultures should be attempted first.

Peritonitis and Other Intraabdominal Infections

Pathophysiology

Infection of the abdomen includes infections of the peritoneal space, retroperitoneal space, and the viscera, including the liver, pancreas, spleen, and kidney.[197] In veterinary medicine peritonitis is most commonly secondary to an intraabdominal infection. Bacteremia is a common finding in infections associated with aerobic organisms but less common if infection involves anaerobes. Bacteria can gain access to the peritoneal cavity directly by way of transmural migration, through the (damaged) intestinal wall, or through other intraabdominal abscesses. In patients with liver disease, organisms that might otherwise be removed from portal circulation can gain access to the peritoneum through lymph or blood. Fever, abdominal pain, nausea, vomiting, and diarrhea are common clinical signs associated with peritonitis. Analysis of peritoneal fluid collected by paracentesis should provide the basis of diagnosis and the need for surgical intervention. Surgical correction is indicated for both diagnostic and therapeutic intervention. Peritoneal fluid can also provide a basis for initial antimicrobial therapy as well as culture and susceptibility data.

The causative organisms of peritonitis are likely to vary with the source; each organ is characterized by its own natural flora. Gastric flora is variable, depending on the state of hydrochloric acid secretion, but can include flora from the oral cavity. The flora of the small intestine is also variable, but in the presence of disease (including achlorhydria), the number of organisms also increases. Large bowel organisms can be present in small bowel obstructions, stasis, and so forth. *E. coli,* enterococci, and anaerobes (e.g., *Bacteroides, Fusobacterium, Peptostreptococcus* spp.) are among the likely causative organisms. The primary flora of the large bowel are anaerobic.

Penetration of organisms into the peritoneal cavity generally is insufficient for the development of peritonitis. Chemical damage such as that associated with bile peritonitis may cause necrosis that increases the severity of peritonitis. The presence of free hemoglobin in the peritoneal cavity contributes to peritoneal infection, perhaps by providing iron required for bacterial metabolism. Intraperitoneal fluid and fibrin increase the inflammatory response to microbial organisms. Fibrin may serve to trap organisms, yet allow abscess formation. In addition, it causes abdominal organisms to adhere to one another. Bacteria produce a number of substances that contribute to the pathophysiology of peritonitis. Endotoxin concentrations increase rapidly in the presence of peritonitis; aerobic organisms possess more endotoxin with greater biologic activity than anaerobic organisms. Anaerobic organisms, however, produce collagenases and proteolytic and other enzymes. In addition, anaerobes may be more resistant to granulocyte killing mechanisms.[197]

The mixture of organisms may contribute to the pathophysiology of infection and may increase (synergistically) the pathogenicity of infection. On the other hand, facultative organisms may facilitate the growth of anaerobic organisms by reducing the oxygen tension of the environment. Each bacterial component may contribute differently to the peritoneal infection. Early peritonitis may be characterized predominantly by infection with gram-negative aerobes; later peritonitis reflects abscessation by obligate anaerobes. Either stage can be lethal.

Antimicrobial and Adjuvant Therapy

Antimicrobials should be used to control or prevent bacteremia, to limit infection locally, and to prevent an inflammatory response to infection. The presence of inflammation indicates a need for surgical intervention, including drainage of the abdomen. Therapy should begin immediately after cultures are collected, but antimicrobials should be modified on the basis of data received after therapy has begun.

Infections are generally polymicrobial. Data generated from human patients are likely to be applicable to small animals.[197] Antimicrobial therapy should target a mixed infection, with organisms most likely derived from the gastrointestinal tract. *E. coli, Klebsiella, Enterobacter,* and *Proteus,* spp. are among the more common aerobic (but facultative anaerobic) organisms. In human patients infection that develops during hospitalization most commonly involves highly resistant strains of aerobic gram-negative organisms: *Acinetobacter* spp., *Serratia* spp., and *P. aeruginosa.*[197] *Bacteroides, Clostridium, Fusobacterium, Peptococcus,* and *Peptostreptococcus* spp. are among the most common obligate anaerobic organisms. Antimicrobial therapy should include anaerobic organisms because they often are involved even when not present on culture. Several factors impair culture of anaerobic organisms. Cultures require longer time for growth and susceptibility testing. In addition, susceptibility data often have not been standardized for anaerobic organisms.

Data from human patients indicate that survival of subjects with peritonitis is decreased if initial therapy is inappropriate, even if "adequate" therapy is ultimately implemented.[197] Thus initial antimicrobial therapy is very important. Combinations of two or more antimicrobials are generally selected for treatment of peritonitis; however, care must be taken to avoid antagonistic combinations (see Chapter 6). Attention should be given to the potential release of endotoxin. Antimicrobials need not be effective against all organisms. Eradication of the most virulent organisms may remove the synergistic effect of multiple organisms, thus allowing host defenses to destroy organisms not affected by antibiotics. Clindamycin is particularly appealing because of its efficacy against approximately 95% of anaerobic organisms and has been effective as the sole agent in infections caused by mixed infections with anaerobic Enterobacteriaceae. In addition, it is effective against *Staphylococcus* spp. Metronidazole is also a good choice because of its efficacy against anaerobes. In addition, it may have efficacy against *E. coli* in mixed aerobic–anaerobic infections. Beta-lactams, and particularly penicillins, remain excellent choices for treatment of abdominal infections. The penicillins are preferred because of their efficacy against anaerobes compared with cephalosporins. Beta-lactamase protectors provide enhanced efficacy against both aerobes and selected anaerobes. The carbapenems have among the broadest efficacy of the antimicrobials currently available; that of ticarcillin is also broad, especially when combined with clavulanic acid. Aminoglycosides are indicated for resistant aerobic gram-negative and selected positive organisms and provide synergistic activity when combined with beta-lactams. They are not, however, efficacious against anaerobic organisms and have limited efficacy against facultative anaerobes when in an anaerobic environment. Likewise, care must be taken in the selection of a first-generation cephalosporin. Cefoxitin, a second-generation drug, includes many gram-negative organisms and *Bacteroides fragilis* in its spectrum. The synergism expressed between fluoroquinolones and metronidazole in treatment of peridontitis may reasonably be expressed in treatment of peritonitis as well, which suggests that this combination is appealing.

KEY POINT 8-35 Survival of peritonitis is decreased by inappropriate initial antimicrobial use, even in patients in which appropriate therapy ultimately is implemented.

Intravenous administration is recommended to maximize drug delivery to the gastrointestinal tract, which may be poorly perfused. Once gastrointestinal function is normal, oral administration can be reinstituted. Irrigation of the peritoneal area and the peritoneum is recommended. Although bactericidal activities of the host (specifically opsonins) may be diluted by irrigation, dilution of microbes and fibrin is of greater advantage. Addition of heparin will further reduce fibrin deposition and the risk of adhesions or pockets of microbial growth. Although povidone–iodine can decrease the incidence of intraabdominal infection when used as an irrigant, it also may impair host defenses. More important, cytotoxicity and proinflammatory effects can worsen inflammation associated with peritonitis, hence it is to be avoided. Intraperitoneal administration of antimicrobials does not appear to offer distinct advantages over intravenous administration. An exception is made with peritoneal dialysis as adjuvant therapy; antimicrobials should be added to the peritoneal lavage to maintain antibiotic concentrations in the peritoneal fluid.

Prophylactic therapy includes use of preoperative cleansing with diet, as well as cathartics and enemas to reduce the total fecal and bacterial mass. Oral antimicrobials should be used to cleanse the gastrointestinal tract. Gastrointestinal flora are susceptible to oral neomycin (aerobic gram-negative organisms) and metronidazole (anaerobes). Intravenous antimicrobials should also be used preoperatively for patients for which the surgical procedure is accompanied by a high risk of contamination.

Peritoneal dialysis as a method of treating peritonitis should be accompanied by antimicrobial use. Contamination from organisms inhabiting the skin (e.g., *Staphylococcus* spp.) is the most common source of infection in patients receiving peritoneal dialysis as a means of controlling renal failure.

Sepsis and Septic Shock Syndrome

Definitions

Sepsis is defined by clinical evidence of a systemic response to an infection (e.g., tachycardia, fever, or hypothermia), with severe sepsis associated with hypotension or organ failure.[198,199] Sepsis syndrome is characterized by altered perfusion of organs (e.g., respiratory or renal dysfunction), whereas septic shock is sepsis syndrome accompanied by hypotension that is not responsive to fluid therapy but is responsive to pharmacologic intervention. Refractory shock, on the other hand, is septic shock that (in humans) lasts longer than 1 hour and does not respond to conventional pharmacologic therapy. The systemic inflammatory response syndrome can result from sepsis but may also indicate a response to any number of systemic mediators of inflammation. Multiorgan response and potential failure is involved. Note that none of these definitions is based on the presence of bacterial (or other microbial) infection; rather, each is based on clinical signs. Presumably, at some time during the course of infection, bacteremia (positive blood cultures) and endotoxemia (presence of endotoxin in the blood) have been evident if a diagnosis is made. Regardless, because the syndrome can be a progressive, fatal clinical situation, management is intensive and meticulous (see Box 8-2).

Shortfalls of human studies regarding treatment of sepsis include inappropriate models and limited outcome measures, particularly mortality, which precludes identification of benefits of therapies. Although information can be drawn from the human literature, the relevance of findings to dogs or cats is often not clear. In a review of the state of sepsis in veterinary patients, Otto[200] calls for the refinement of consensus guidelines for staging and treatment of sepsis in veterinary patients, as has been promulgated in humans[199] (Box 8-2). In her editorial, she reports that respondents to a survey (approximately 100 small animal practices) reported an incidence of sepsis in 1% to 5% of feline patients, with a 10% to 25% survival rate, and 6% to 10% of dogs, with a 25% to 50% survival rate. A 50% survival rate has been cited for dogs (as reviewed by Hopper and Bateman[201]). Survival differs with the cause of sepsis, being 97% for pyometra compared with 40% for peritonitis. Although this section will attempt to address therapy of sepsis, such a review should not be substituted for a comprehensive review of the current state of sepsis management in veterinary patients, which is likely to be a dynamic approach evolving over the next decade.

Although ultimately, novel therapies may target specific mediators of disease (e.g., biomarkers), currently treatment is limited to supportive care.[200] Application of human treatments to dogs or cats will require validation through studies, particularly for polypeptide therapies, which may be antigenic in animals.[200]

Pathophysiology

Systemic disease caused by gram-negative bacteria is the most common cause of the sepsis syndrome. Bacterial translocation of indigenous bacteria from the gastrointestinal tract to extraintestinal sites is the most likely source of the bacteria. The lipid moiety of the lipopolysaccharide (LPS) covering of gram-negative organisms is the most common virulence factor. It is LPS that triggers the host response to bacterial invasion, including both humoral and cellular aspects. Although the host response may be successful in killing the microbes, the negative sequelae increase host mortality. Cytokines and, in particular, TNF and interleukin-1 (IL-1; the classic endogenous pyrogen) are produced by macrophages and monocytes within minutes of contact with LPS (Figure 8-10). Each is capable of inducing fever and inflammation. TNF in particular has been implicated as the most potent mediator of the pathophysiology of sepsis. TNF alone, however, probably is not sufficient to be lethal; yet, when present with other released mediators and, in particular, interferon-γ, the effects of TNF become more lethal. The majority of lethal effects caused by TNF can be attributed to its effects on tissue metabolism, cardiac function, and vascular tone. Nitric oxide (endothelial-derived relaxing factor) is being delineated as an important

Box 8-2

Management of Severe Sepsis[199]

1. Early (first 6 hours) goal-directed resuscitation for septic-induced shock is based on fluid therapy: goals for successful therapy are based on central venous pressure, mean arterial pressure, urine output, and central venous or mixed venous–oxygen saturation. Insufficient response indicates the need for treatment with packed cells or dobutamine infusion (or both).
2. Diagnosis should be based on cultures collected before initation of antimicrobial therapy if collection does not significantly delay treatment.
   a. Cultures include two blood cultures (one percutaneously and the other through any catheter in place 48 hours or longer) and a quantitative culture from other obviously or potentially infected sites. If cultures in the vascular device and blood yield the same organism, the catheter might be considered the source of infection.
   b. Imaging diagnostic tools should be used in an attempt to identify the source of infection.
3. Intravenous antimicrobial therapy with a sufficiently broad-spectrum drug should be empirically initiated within 1 hour of diagnosis of sepsis.
   a. Decisions to cure infections should take precedence over decisions that minimize superinfection.
   b. Empirical selection should include one or more drugs that target all likely pathogens and adequately penetrate the presumed infected tissue.
   c. Recently used antimicrobials should be avoided.
   d. Antimicrobial therapy should take into account local resistance patterns (e.g., the possibility of methicillin-resistant *Staphylococcus* infections).
   e. Restriction of antimicrobials as a strategy to reduce the development of antimicrobial resistance or to reduce cost is not an appropriate initial strategy in this patient population.
   f. Monitoring can be helpful if information is provided in a timely fashion.
   g. Experienced clinicians (pharmacists and pharmacologists) should be consulted to ensure that doses maximize efficacy and minimize toxicity.
   h. The antimicrobial regimen should be assessed daily to maximize efficacy, prevent resistance, reduce toxicity, and minimize cost.
   i. Combination therapy is recommended for certain infections (e.g., *Pseudomonas* spp.) or neutropenic patients with severe sepsis.
   j. De-escalation of antimicrobial therapy should be implemented as soon as possible, based on susceptibility data, including limitation of combination therapy to 3 to 5 days.
   k. Anatomic infections requiring control at the source must be identified early and treated appropriately, using the least invasive but most effective intervention.
4. Fluid therapy: natural/artificial colloids and/or crystalloids:
   a. Evidence does not support one over the other.
   b. Fluid challenges should be implemented to assess patient response to fluids, which should be based on CVP and should be continued as long as hemodynamic improvement continues.
   c. Fluid rates should be substantially decreased if indicators of cardiac filling increase without evidence of hemodynamic improvement.
5. Vasporessors (e.g., norepinephrine):
   a. Perfusion should be maintained in the face of life-threatening hypotension even if hypotension has not been resolved.
   b. Response is based on mean arterial pressure as measured by an arterial catheter.
   c. Norepinephrine or dopamine are preferred initial choices with epinephrine indicated in norepinephrine non-responders.
6. Inotropic support:
   a. Dobutamine should be administered in the face of myocardial dysfunction, as based on increased cardiac filling pressures and low cardiac output.
   b. Combined vasopressor/inotrope (norepinephrine, dopamine) is indicated if cardiac output is not measured.
7. Glucocorticoids:
   a. Intravenous hydrocortisone (targeting relative adrenal insufficiency) is given if blood pressure responds poorly to fluid resuscitation of vasopressor therapy.
   b. Dexamethasone should be avoided because of the potential for suppression of the hypothalamic–pituitary–adrenal axis.
   c. An ACTH stimulation test is not used to identify those patients for which glucocorticoid therapy is indicated.
   d. Oral fludrocortisone is administered if the steroid used has no mineralocorticoid activity.
   e. Steroid therapy is discontinued when vasopressor therapy is no longer needed.
8. (Recombinant Human Activated Protein C) is indicated in patients assessed at high risk for death, if no contraindication exists. This therapy is not currently recommended in animals because of the risk of allergic response).
9. Blood products:
   a. Red blood cells are recommended after hypoperfusion has resolved to maintain hemoglobins above 6 g/dL.
   b. Platelets are recommended when counts are below 5000 mm^3 and can be considered when counts are between 5000 and 30,000 mm^3.
   c. Erythropoeitin is not indicated unless for reasons other than sepsis.
   d. Fresh frozen plasma should not be used to correct clotting abnormalities, and antithrombin should not be administered for treatment of severe sepsis or shock.

mediator of the lethal effects of TNF. The inducible nitric oxide synthase is the likely cause of hypotension associated with septic shock.[198]

Humoral mediators contribute to the systemic response to LPS. The coagulation pathway can be directly initiated by either LPS or TNF and other cytokines (most commonly through the extrinsic pathway). The fibrinolytic pathway also can be activated. Disseminated intravascular coagulopathy is not an uncommon sequela of septic shock. Complement activation and platelet-activating factor contribute to the response. The relationship between the mediators of septic shock is intricate and yet to be defined. These relationships, however, lead to the

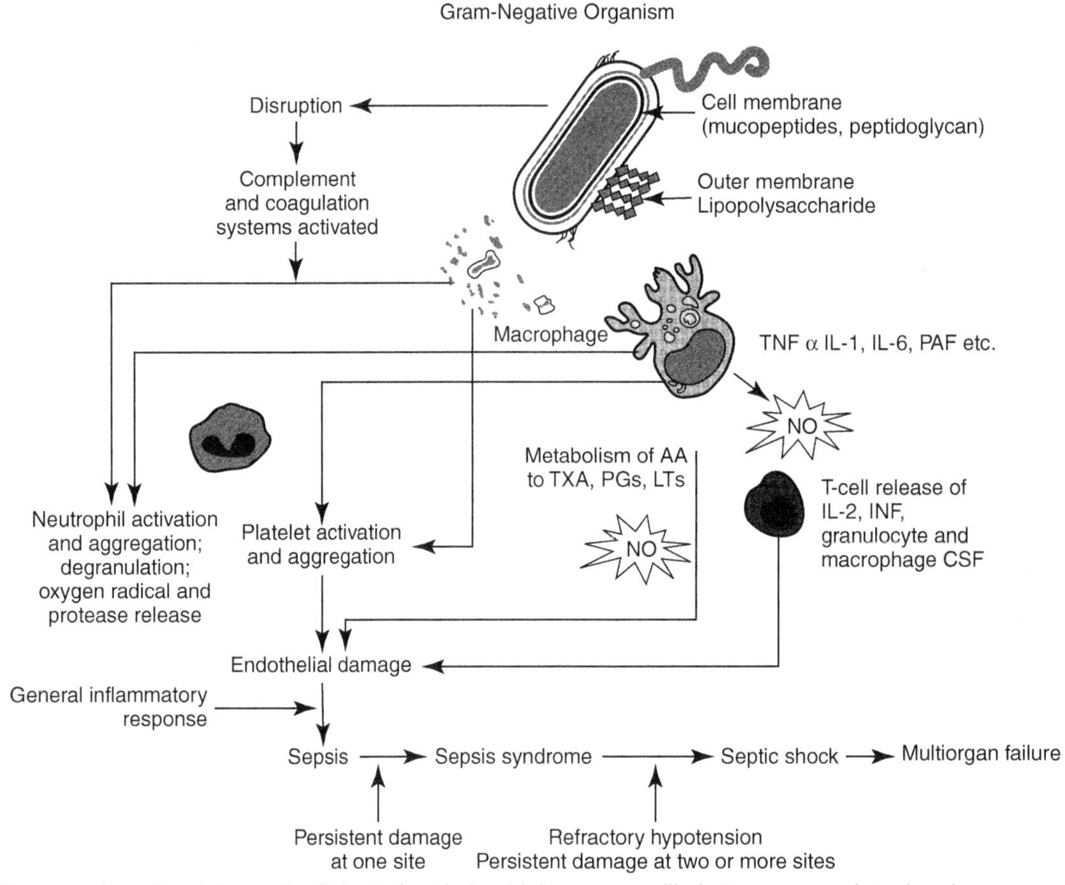

Figure 8-10 The sequelae of endotoxemia. Selected antimicrobials are more likely to cause endotoxin release, most notably the beta-lactams (with imipenem being an exception). The aminoglycosides cause little endotoxin release. *AA,* Amino acids; *CSF,* colony stimulating factor; *IL,* interleukin; *INF,* interferon; *LTs,* leukotrienes; *PAFs,* platelet-activating factor; *PGs,* peptidoglycans; *TNF*-α, tumor necrosis factor-α; *TXA,* thromboxane synthase A.

progressive nature of the syndrome, as well as the difficulty in pharmacologically manipulating response.

Splanchnic ischemia and specifically intestinal mucosal ischemia may play a major role in bacterial translocation. Selected drugs may increase the risk owing to detrimental effects on the mucosa, including glucocorticoids, nonsteroidal antiinflammatories, and vasopressors. Drugs that target anaerobic bacteria may facilitate the growth of gram-negative organisms; their growth might be supported by antisecretory drugs that alter gastric pH and enteral nutrition. However, adequate nutrition is important to maintenance of the mucosal barrier. The most important means to prevent bacterial translocation is to protect the gastrointestinal barrier through maintenance of gastrointestinal perfusion, avoidance of increased gastric pH, and selective bacterial decontamination.

Studies that document the microbes associated with sepsis in animals are limited. Greiner and coworkers[202] (in Germany) retrospectively described the microbes associated with sepsis in cats (n = 292) during the period of 1994 to 2005. Only 23% of the cats had positive cultures. Of the microbes cultured, the distribution of gram-positive and -negative organisms was equal. For gram-negative (43%), 31% of the total isolates were Enterobacteriaceae (16% *E. coli,* 8% *Enterobacter* spp., and 4% *Salmonella* spp.). The breakdown for gram-positive isolates (45% of total) was as follows: *Staphylocccous* coagulase negative (11%), *Streptococcus* spp. (11%), and miscellaneous gram-positive (14%). Obligate anaerobes represented another 12%. Overall susceptibility for all aerobic or facultative anaerobic organisms was highest for enrofloxacin (76%), followed by chloramphenicol (69%), gentamicin (67%), and cephalexin or amoxicillin–clavulanic acid (64%). For the remaining drugs, less than 50% of isolates were susceptible (doxycycline, trimethoprim sulfonamide, ampicillin).

Antibacterial Therapy

Successful antimicrobial therapy of sepsis will be enhanced by anticipation (i.e., looking for clinical signs), early diagnosis, aggressive yet appropriate antimicrobial therapy, and intensive supportive therapy. Identifying and correcting the cause of sepsis (e.g., loss of gastrointestinal mucosal integrity, granulocytopenia, foreign bodies) is an underlying focus of management. Although antimicrobial therapy is the cornerstone of therapy, it can also contribute to the pathophysiology.

In human critical care environments, an apparent increase in the incidence of sepsis is attributed to an increase in the severity of illnesses, the complicated nature of care, including invasive procedures and immunosuppressive drugs, as well as the longer survivial of patients with chronic illnesses. The high morality rate of sepsis (35% to 50%) reflects, in part, unacceptable delays in appropriate treatment. This partially reflects the difficulty in identifying sepsis. One of the most important predictors of outome in human patients with severe sepsis is prompt and appropriate antimicrobial therapy. Appropriate therapy includes use of drugs that target the infecting microbe within 1 hour of the recognition of sepsis. A major risk factor for mortality is failure to initiate antimicrobial therapy with a drug to which the causative agent is susceptible within 24 hours of receipt of susceptibility results. Disconcertingly, even subsequent correction of previously inappropriate therapy may not reduce the risk of death. Septic patients are predisposed to infection with resistant microbes (Box 8-3). Initial antimicrobial selection must cover a wide range of organisms, including resistant isolates, which makes adequate coverage difficult to achieve. Yet initial adequate antimicrobial therapy is the most important determinant of outcome. A meta-analysis[203] in humans focused on mortality as an outcome indicator of appropriate versus inappropriate therapy in patients with severe sepsis (septic patients). *Appropriate* was defined as treatment with at least one antimicrobial to which all causative microorganisms (based on blood cultures) were susceptible within 24 hours of identification of the organism; *inappropriate* was defined as administration of an antimicrobial agent to which at least one of the infecting microorganisms was resistant or the lack of an antimicrobial to which the organisms were considered susceptible within 24 hours of microbial isolation. Of the 904 patients studied, 23% received inappropriate therapy. After adjusting for confounding factors, the overall 28-day mortality was greater in the inappropriate group (28%) compared with the appropriate group (39%).

In addition to the most appropriate drugs, adequate coverage also includes proper modification of dosing regimens for the critical septic patient. Increased volume of distribution, decreased protein, and altered blood flow to organs of clearance complicate design of dosing regimens.[158] The highest doses of antimicrobials are recommended in human critical care patients; intervals of time-dependent drugs should be designed to avoid resistance.[204] Decreased doses or longer intervals should not necessarily be implemented in critical patients with altered renal function unless the risk of toxicity is imminent. Monitoring should be considered.

The approach to antimicrobial therapy in the critical care patient should be to "hit early, hit hard, and get out fast."[204]

Box 8-3

Risk Factors for Colonization with Resistant Microbes

- Hospital stay longer than 5 days
- Previous hospital stay longer than 2 days within past 90 days
- Antimicrobials, especially broad-spectrum, within the past 90 days
- Antimicrobial resistance in the environment
- Poor underlying condition
- Immunocompromised (including use of immunosuppressive drugs) or neutropenic patient
- Invasive procedures/hardware

Accordingly, therapy should be initiated early with a broad-spectrum antimicrobial that targets all potential pathogens, including resistant organisms, at doses designed to kill. Therapy should then be de-escalated to a narrow spectrum as soon as possible, generally on the basis of culture and susceptibility testing. Because human critical care patients often succumb to illnesses that do not necessarily occur in veterinary patients (i.e., pneumonia, particularly that associated with ventilatory support caused by *Streptococcus pneumoniae)*, initial treatment should not necessarily reflect empirical therapy in humans. However, resistance patterns are potentially similar. A number of risk factors have been identified for colonization with resistant organisms (see Box 8-3). Patients that fall into these categories warrant consideration as candidates for second- or third-tier choices. The initial therapy in these patients should be based on resistance data promulgated for dogs or cats in the treatment facility. Accordingly, surveillance programs that monitor patterns of resistance must be promoted in the interest of increased patient survivial and judicious antimicrobial use. Concerns in humans are the same for veterinary patients. These concerns include MRS and, increasingly, resistant gram-negative infections. Up to 40% of *E. coli* infections in humans are resistant to ampicillin; a similar pattern has been reported in veterinary medicine. The advent of extended-spectrum beta-lactamases is decreasing efficacy of third-generation cephalosporins. Increasing resistance to fluoroquinolones (10% in human medicine, more in veterinary medicine) is limiting their use as well. Accordingly, carbapenems are considered more often.

KEY POINT 8-36 The approach to antimicrobial therapy in the critical care patient should be to "hit early, hit hard, and get out fast." Initial therapy should target any potential infecting organism (including nosocomials) with de-escalation to less potent drugs as therapy progresses.

Allthough evidence is lacking that confirms combination antimicrobial therapy improves the chances of a favorable outcome in human medicine, the consensus is that combination therapy is reasonable, and is indicated for treatment of selected organisms (e.g., *Pseudomonas* spp.). Combination therapy may be the reason that patient response to antimicrobials has improved (in human medicine) during the last several decades. Combination therapy should be considered not only to increase efficacy (particularly if the antimicrobials act synergistically) but also to reduce the advent of resistance. For bacteremia, antimicrobial combinations should be chosen that provide a broad spectrum, enhance (synergistic) efficacy against gram-negative organisms, and minimize resistance. In the presence of sepsis, selected drugs should also minimize endotoxin release. Organisms particularly adept at developing resistance include *Pseudomonas, Serratia,* and *Enterobacter* spp. Combination therapy is particularly important in neutropenic patients. Monotherapy, generally with a carbapenem, a fluoroquinolone (e.g., enrofloxacin), or a third-generation cephalosporin (e.g., ceftazidime), may be effective if the cause is a highly susceptible gram-negative organism. However, the prudent clinician will use a combination of drugs likely to be effective against the suspected organism. Combination therapy (discussed in Chapter 6) may be important to decrease the risk of resistance as well as enhance efficacy against the infecting microbe. For example, aminoglycosides should never be used alone because of their poor penetrability. The combination of an animoglycoside with a beta-lactam with either cefazolin or ampicillin–sulbactam might be indicated for treatment of bacterial translocation associated with parvovirus; because puppies are likely to be drug naïve, *E. coli* resistance is likely to be minimal for these drugs. In contrast, the combination of aminoglycosides with carbapenems may be indicated in the patient with a previous history of antimicrobial therapy. Treatment regimens should be changed if indicated by culture and susceptibility data. Design of dosing regimens is discussed in Chapter 6; monitoring as a tool to ensure adequate drug concentrations is particularly important for the septic patient.

Antimicrobial de-escalation, which is important to minimize the advent of resistance, is a two-pronged approach. Narrowing the spectrum as soon as possible is important in minimizing selection pressure.[204] Further, decreasing the duration of therapy increasingly is being associated with an improved outcome in human medicine.[204] Using hospital-acquired pneumonia as an example, studies in humans have demonstrated a reduced proportion of relapses in shorter-duration (5 to 8 days) treatment groups, with response to therapy as an indicator of the need for therapy. In contrast, infections associated with *S. aureus* bacteremia may require longer durations of therapy because of the potential to cause septic emboli. Catheter-related bacteremia in immunocompromised animals is an example of a condition for which duration of therapy might be 14 days. Therapy for neutropenic patients might continue as long as neutropenia persists. Therapy for infections of areas with poor blood supply may need to be longer; examples include valvular disease (4 to 6 weeks) or necrotic tissue (e.g., osteomyelitis; up to 8 weeks).

Adjuvant Therapy

Drugs that target inflammatory mediators associated with sepsis are also discussed in Chapters 31 and 32. Cardiovascular support can be provided in the form of volume replacement and positive inotropes/pressors. Fluid therapy should be intensive, with the goal of reestablishing normal perfusion. A number of colloids and some crystalloids are available. Drugs intended to maintain or increase blood pressure should be used cautiously. Certainly, adrenergic agents such as dopamine, dobutamine, norepinephrine, and isoproterenol should be administered only in the presence of adequate volume replacement and in conjunction with intensive monitoring of central venous pressure and, ideally, pulmonary wedge pressure. Fluid therapy likely will need to be more intensive in the presence of pressor agents, dobutamine in particular. Vasoconstrictive drugs should be avoided. Thus, although dopamine at low doses (5 μg/kg per minute) may be preferred in the presence of impaired renal perfusion, dobutamine may be preferred otherwise. Of the two, dobutamine (5 to 10 μg/kg) is more likely to increase oxygen delivery and consumption in tissues.[205]

Hopper and Bateman[201] reviewed the hemostatic dysfunctions associated with sepsis, with a focus on the integration of hemostatic and inflammatory signals. The inflammatory mediators associated with multiple organ dysfunction syndrome systemically activate coagulation, causing intravascular fibrin formation typical of disseminated intravascular coagulation. The primary means by which inflammation associated with sepsis mediates coagulation is through mediator-induced expression of the procoagulant tissue factor (Factor III). Example mediators include endotoxin, TNF-α lipoprotein, and growth factor. Increased coagulation, in turn, contributes to inflammation, which can increase patient morbidity or mortality associated with sepsis. Endogenous tissue factor pathway inhibitor (TFPI) blockade may decrease mortality. Heparin, including low-molecular-weight heparin, increases the release of TFPIs from endothelial cells, platelets, and that stored with lipoproteins. Despite its role in the pathophysiology, clinical trials in humans receiving recombinant TFPIs have failed to demonstrate a difference in 28-day mortality rates. Antithrombin (AT, previously antithrombin III) binds to and inhibits thrombin and Factor Xa, as well as a number of other factors. High- (but not low-) molecular-weight (LMW) heparin and other glycosaminoglycans of sufficient length bind to and sterically hinder AT, potentiating its anticoagulant activity. Thus, while both unfractionated and low-molecular-weight heparin inactivate Factor Xa, only low-molecular-weight heparin (LMH) targets AT. The latter's longer half-life allows its intermittent subcutaneous use in place of constant-rate infusions of unfractionated heparins. However, in addition to its anticoagulant effects, AT has substantial antiinflammatory effects; these effects require AT binding to endothelial cells, an action that is prevented by binding to heparin. Its antiinflammatory effect has led to studies examining potential efficacy of AT therapy for patients with sepsis. Despite its potential antiinflammatory effects, evidence demonstrating the beneficial effects of AT with clinical trials of humans with sepsis is lacking. The Surviving Sepsis Campaign Guidelines currently do not support treatment with AT. Protein C (PC) is a vitamin K–dependent protein that directly inactivates or enhances the inactivation of a number of coagulation factors, including Factors Va and VIII. It also has direct antiinflammatory actions. Activation of PC is accomplished by thrombomodulin (TM) located in endothelial cells; activation is enhanced 1000-fold if thrombomodulin is bound to thrombin. Therefore thrombin, which is one of the most procoagulant substances in the body, contributes to the primary anticoagulant pathway. Receptors on the surface of the cell bind to PC such that it concentrates at sites of TM–thrombin complexes. Clinical trials have demonstrated that human septic patients are deficient in PC (possibly because of increased destruction, increased consumption, decreased formation possibly related to vitamin K deficiency), and this deficiency affects survival. Although the same has been demonstrated in dogs, an impact on outcome was not demonstrated. Administration of recombinant PC has been associated with improved positive outcomes in human patients. However, species specificity necessitates a fifteenfold to twentyfold higher dose of the human recombinant product when administered to dogs. Further, it is rapidly eliminated. However, antigenicity precludes readministration.

Correction or prevention of impaired tissue perfusion (i.e., with fluid replacement or pressor agents) helps prevent decreased microcirculation. Additional preventive measures might be implemented in the presence of normal platelet counts and coagulation times. Synthetic colloids (which themselves can prolong bleeding times), or the combination of crystalloids and low-dose heparin, are indicated to maintain microcirculatory flow. Evidence of disseminated intravascular coagulation (prolonged coagulation times and low platelet counts) indicates the need for replacement of coagulation factors. Heparin therapy should be implemented with caution in the presence of disseminated intravascular coagulation to minimize the risk of bleeding. Certainly, heparin therapy is indicated in the presence of pulmonary thromboembolism.

The advent of oliguria or anuria indicates the need for diuretic therapy. Opiate antagonists have been shown to reverse the course of septic shock in selected studies. Because patients with prolonged hypotension were particularly responsive, it is likely that the drugs (e.g., naloxone) provide a transient vasopressor effect. Naloxone, however, appears to have no clinically relevant effect in patients in septic shock.

The intravenous administration of polyclonal immunoglobulin increasingly is emerging as a therapy associated with an increase in survival. The use of IgM, in particular is associated with decreased morality.[206,207]

The role of drugs intended to ameliorate the signs of sepsis syndrome is controversial. Glucocorticoids, nonsteroidal antiinflammatories, and lazeroids (an investigational category of drugs; see Chapters 29 and 30) are variably effective to noneffective, depending on the study. The most important variabilities that appear to affect response to these drugs are dose and timing of administration. For glucocorticoids, most studies in human patients afflicted with sepsis have failed to show a significant benefit to survival; some patients dosed with glucocorticoids were more likely to develop suprainfections. Yet experimental studies have shown that, when provided sufficiently early (within 4 hours of sepsis), "shock" doses of glucocorticoids may ameliorate release of the more important mediators of septic shock. Similarly, nonsteroidals (and, in particular, flunixin meglumine) may decrease the release of or response to a number of mediators of septic shock.[208] Again, however, timing of administration is critical: Benefits are most likely to be realized when administration occurs within several hours of the onset of sepsis. Unfortunately for veterinary patients, clinical signs of sepsis are usually not identified until the critical period of antiinflammatory administration has passed.

Among the indications for glucocorticoids in septic patients is replacement therapy in the face of relative adrenocorticotrophic deficiency (see Chapter 30). A recent clinical trial in humans explored the impact of hydrocortisone therapy on 28-day survival rates and found no difference between groups. Although responders responded more rapidly if treated with hydrocortisone, the incidence of superinfection and subsequent recurrence of septic shock increased.[209] Nonetheless, the current criteria for use of glucocorticoids, as delineated in the Surviving Sepsis Campaign Guidelines, are based on hypotension responsiveness to fluid and vasopressor therapy.

The advent of recombinant technologies has led to the development of granulocyte colony-stimulating factors. These drugs are likely to prove useful for selected patients (most notably granulocytopenic patients). Treatment protocols have not, however, been well established. Therapy with antiserum has enjoyed a resurgence of interest in human medicine. Administration of serum from patients that have recovered from shock induced by *Pseudomonas* spp. or patients "immunized" with mutant strains of *E. coli* has increased the survival of patients suffering from profound shock. Monoclonal antibodies that bind endotoxin, TNF, and other mediators of shock have been or are being studied. Pentoxifylline is a methylxanthine derivative that is accompanied by properties not present in other methylxanthines. Among those potentially beneficial in sepsis is the ability to scavenge oxygen radicals and alter the rheologic properties of blood, thus facilitating microcirculation.[270]

A number of adjuvant therapies have been studied for their ability to ameliorate clinical signs associated with sepsis. The use of low doses of an antimicrobial that binds endotoxin (e.g., polymyxin B; PMB) yet is otherwise nephrotoxic has not been well studied in either dogs and cats. A very early study reported that lipopolysacharides (LPS) modified with PMB was less lethal in dogs compared to PMB alone.[272] A placebo-controlled clinical trial in naturally occurring parvovirus-associated endotoxic dogs (n = 30) compared PMB and ampicillin to ampicillin alone.[273] Treatment with PMB (12,500 IU/kg, IM, every 12 hr for 5 days) administered with ampicillin (10 mg/kg IM, every 12 hr) was associated with greater hemodynamic improvement and lower serum TNFα concentrations compared with dogs receiving ampicillin alone (other supportive therapy in both groups included fluid therapy, colloidal solutions, metoclopramide, ranitidine and sucralfate). Serum urea nitrogen and creatinine actually were higher numerically in the control group. In cats, the effect of PMB was studied both ex vivo and in vivo, the latter using a randomized, blinded, placebo-controlled experimental model of low dose endotoxin infusion in cats (n = 12).[274] Ex vivo, TNFα release was less in whole blood cultures. In vitro, response to endotoxin was significantly less in cats receiving PMB (1 mg/kg over 30 minutes, 30 minutes after LPS administration) compared with cats receiving only LPS. The authors interpreted this response as supportive for clinical trials addressing the clinical use of PMB in cats with sepsis.

A polyvalent equine origin antiserum against LPS endotoxin has been used in small animals (SEPTI-serum, Immvac, Inc., Columbia MO 75201); 4.4 mL/kg diluted 1:1 with intravenous crystalloid fluids was administered slowly over 30 to 60 minutes.[275] The product should be administered before treatment with antimicrobials that might cause the release of endotoxin. Retreatment, if necessary, is recommended 5 to 7 days after the first treatment. The equine origin may result in anaphylaxis; patients should be monitored closely.

Use of sucralfate rather than antisecretory drugs is indicated if the patient is at risk for gastrointestinal ulceration in the face of possible bacterial translocation. Prevention of reperfusion injury is likely to be important, although pharmacologic interventions have not yet been well defined. Selective (e.g., gram-negative [polymyxin B, neomycin] and fungal organisms [amphotericin B]) decontamination of the gastrointestinal flora coupled with endotoxin binders (e.g., kaolin pectate, activated charcoal) might be considered. Use of dilute chlorhexidine or betadine enemas has been anectodally helpful in puppies with parvovirus.

Prophylaxis remains an important tool for the prevention of sepsis. Among the more important tools in the critical care environment is meticulous adherence to cleanliness policies in the environment to minimize nosocomial infections.[210] Prophylactic antimicrobials are discussed later.

ANAEROBIC INFECTIONS

Anaerobes differ from other bacteria in that they do not require the presence of molecular oxygen for metabolic activity and growth but instead depend on fermentative processes. Strict anaerobes cannot tolerate the presence of oxygen, and few are clinically significant. Growth of *obligate* anaerobes depends on an environment characterized by reduced oxygen tension and low oxidation-reduction (redox) potential. Most clinically significant anaerobic organisms are obligate and include the genera *Fusobacterium, Bacteroides, Clostridium,* (selected species), *Peptostreptococcus* (enteric *Streptococcus*), and *Peptococcus* spp. Although *oxygen-tolerant* anaerobes cannot utilize oxygen, they can grow in its presence. Oxygen-tolerant organisms include *Clostridium perfringens* and *Propionibacterium* spp. Finally, *facultative* anaerobes are characterized by flexible oxygen requirements and can grow in the presence or absence of oxygen. Facultative anaerobes, which are clinically important in small animals, include *Staphylococcus* spp. and the enteric gram-negative bacilli such as *E. coli* and *Klebsiella* and *Pasteurella* spp.[211,212] Like aerobic organisms, anaerobic organisms are also classified by their gram-staining characteristics. Gram-positive cocci include *Peptococcus* and *Peptostreptococcus.* Gram-positive rods include those that form spores (*Clostridium* spp.) and those that do not (*Actinomyces* and *Propionibacterium* spp.). Gram–negative anaerobic rods include *Bacteroides* and *Fusobacterium* spp.

Results of studies investigating the incidence of anaerobic organisms as causative agents of infections in veterinary medicine have been relatively consistent. The most frequently isolated organisms in one study[213] were *Bacteroides, Peptostreptococcus, Fusobacterium,* and *Porphyromonas* spp. These organisms represented 70% of the isolates. Other previously reported clinically significant isolates include *Clostridium, Propionibacterium, Actinomyces,* and *Peptococcus* spp.[212] Some older studies suggest that *Clostridium* spp. are more commonly isolated, but this finding may reflect inappropriate culturing techniques or regional differences in prevalence of selected genera.

Pathogenesis

Anaerobic infections are endogenous in origin because the causative organisms are most commonly members of the normal bacterial flora that occur in surrounding uninfected tissues. The normal bacterial flora of the body are predominantly anaerobic. Anaerobic organisms are particularly prevalent on mucous membrane surfaces, as exemplified by an anaerobic to aerobic ratio of 1000:1 in the large intestine (colon) and 10:1 in the oral cavity.[193] Anaerobic organisms, and particularly *Bacteroides* spp., are also prevalent in the female reproductive tract (vagina). Infections by anaerobic organisms usually require a break in the normal skin or mucosal defense barriers, thus allowing penetration and contamination, or a break in the host's immune defenses. Thus certain areas of the body are more predisposed to the development of anaerobic infections. The most common sites of anaerobic infections reported in small animals are the oropharynx, skin (including bite wounds), respiratory tract, abdomen, reproductive tract, musculoskeletal system, and CNS. Anaerobic organisms are also causes of bacteremia.

Anaerobic bacteria, particularly gram-negative rods, are often considered serious pathogens because they are capable of producing toxins and enzymes, which enhance their pathogenicity. Both *Bacteroides* (especially *B. fragilis*) and *Fusobacterium* spp. produce potent toxins that not only cause tissue necrosis but also enhance the spread of infection. *Bacteroides* spp. may also produce collagenase. Clostridial organisms also produce a variety of toxic compounds that, in addition to tissue necrosis, may cause hemolysis, disseminated intravascular coagulation, and renal failure.[211] Several organisms produce compounds that destroy leukocytes, thus debilitating a component of the host's immune system.[211]

Diagnosis of anaerobic infections is often difficult. *Bacteroides* and *Fusobacterium* spp. are often difficult to visualize in Gram stains when in the presence of exudates and tissue debris. Gram-positive organisms may appear as gram-negative, or they may assume usual morphology in older exudates or after antibacterial therapy.[211] Improper culturing techniques are probably the most common cause for failure to isolate all infective organisms.[211,214]

Anaerobic infections should be suspected when an infection is characterized by one or more of the following: close proximity to a mucous membrane; a putrid, foul-smelling exudate; necrotic or gangrenous tissue; gas; a blackish discoloration of tissues (which may fluoresce under ultraviolet light if caused by *Bacteroides melaninogenicus*); sulfur granules (indicating infection caused by a variety of different organisms, including *Actinomyces* spp.)[185] a subacute onset of inflammation; and leukocytosis associated with a high fever.[211,215] Anaerobic infections also should be suspected when cultures are negative despite observation of organisms with a Gram stain and in cases of endocarditis associated with negative blood cultures. Closed-space infections such as pyothorax; pyometra; and brain, lung, or intraabdominal abscesses are frequently caused by anaerobic infections. Other infections commonly caused by anaerobes include aspiration pneumonia, peritonitis associated with bowel contamination, chronic osteomyelitis associated with open fractures, bite wounds, penetrating foreign bodies, and solid tumors with a necrotic center.

Factors Affecting Selection of Antimicrobials

Factors that contribute to therapeutic (antimicrobial) failure for anaerobic infections include improper culturing techniques, mixed infections, and inactivation of the antimicrobial. Culture information important for the proper management of anaerobic infections. Failure to isolate anaerobic organisms caused by improper culturing techniques should be suspected whenever routine aerobic cultures of purulent exudate yield no growth.

Most clinically significant anaerobes are obligate and thus cannot survive exposure to oxygen for more than a few seconds. In addition, facultative bacteria generally grow faster than anaerobic organisms and thus may overgrow and mask anaerobic organisms, particularly if specimen culturing is delayed.[211] The best specimens for anaerobic culture are aspirates or tissue biopsy specimens (1 cm^2) rather than swabs.[216,217] Suitable aspirates include those of infected body fluids (i.e., peritoneal, pericardial, pleural), aspirates of pus (from abscesses, deep wounds, or pyometra), tracheal or percutaneous lung aspirates, surgical tissue specimens (including samples from deep infections, bone biopsy material, and sequestra), and blood.[216,217] All air or gas bubbles should be removed from both the needle and syringe immediately after sample collection.[215] Urine; swabs for the oropharynx, upper airway, external airway, and external reproductive tract; sputum or nasal exudates; and bronchoscopy brushings or aspirates (unless obtained with a double-lumen sleeve) are generally considered inappropriate. Culture samples should be placed in culture vials.[215] Specialized transport receptacles should be devoid of oxygen and contain anaerobic media that will also allow isolation of aerobic organisms. Specimens collected in plastic syringes should also be placed in transport tubes because oxygen can slowly permeate through the syringe. Specimens generally should be kept at room temperature until transported.

Many anaerobic infections are caused by more than one organism. Both anaerobic–anaerobic and anaerobic–aerobic mixed infections have been reported in small animals. A mean of 1.7 to 1.9 anaerobic organisms were isolated per specimen in several studies. Samples usually also contained facultative anaerobes.[214,218] According to one study, 80% of infections with obligate anaerobes simultaneously contained facultative anaerobic or aerobic organisms, with members of the family Enterobacteriaceae being the most common organisms isolated.[213] These include *E. coli,* followed by *Pasteurella* spp. and *S. intermedius.* Mixed bacterial infections are often more virulent than infections caused by single organisms.[211] Because synergistic mechanisms develop between facultative and anaerobic organisms, infection by multiple organisms may promote the overgrowth of commensal anaerobes such as *Actinomyces* spp.[208,212,219] *Bacteroides* spp. can inhibit phagocytic activity of surrounding white blood cells when present in mixed infections. Commensal bacteria may act as symbiotes by producing growth factors required by pathogenic anaerobic organisms. Facultative organisms may also provide a more favorable environment for anaerobes by removing oxygen and adding reducing substances.[212] The number of microorganisms located within an abscess may also have an effect on drug efficacy because antimicrobial inactivation is more likely.

The environmental conditions surrounding an anaerobic infection can be detrimental to the activity of antimicrobial drugs. These effects, discussed in Chapter 6, are very likely to be marked in some anaerobic infections. The inflammatory exudate that usually accompanies anaerobic infections can have profound effects on drug efficacy. Cellular membranes, breakdown products of phagocytic cells, and inflamed tissues are all capable of binding to and reducing the effective concentration of pharmacologically active antimicrobial drugs.[155] Host tissues may also produce local enzymes that destroy antimicrobials.[155]

The anaerobic environment that characterizes anaerobic infections can also profoundly alter the efficacy of antimicrobials. The *oxidation-reduction potential* (referred to as EH), which measures the anaerobiosis associated with an abscess, is estimated to be approximately −400 mV in human abscesses, which is indicative of an environment free of oxygen. The lack of oxygen has profound effects on two activities important to the success of antimicrobial therapy. The first is its effect on white blood cells. To kill selective organisms, white blood cells must be able to initiate oxidative bursts, an activity that is very difficult to accomplish in the anaerobic environment.[220,221] In addition, white blood cell chemotaxis in response to bacterial factors is reduced in anaerobic environments.[215] The second detrimental effect of an anaerobic environment relates to the mechanism of transport or action of the drugs. The efficacy of aminoglycosides and the combination of trimethoprim–sulfamethoxazole are particularly affected. Aminoglycosides require active transport into cells by mechanisms dependent on oxygen. In addition, the mechanism of action of these antimicrobials depends, in part, on cellular respiration processes that utilize oxygen. The lack of oxygen renders these antimicrobials ineffective; all anaerobic organisms are thus resistant to aminoglycosides. The aerobic component of a mixed infection may also be resistant to aminoglycoside therapy because the oxidative transport systems of such organisms (e.g., *E. coli*) may shut down in an anaerobic environment.

The development of resistance by anaerobic organisms to selected antimicrobials is an important cause of therapeutic failure. As with other bacteria, plasmid-mediated, transferable drug resistance and the inability of drugs to penetrate bacterial cells are important mechanisms by which anaerobic organisms develop resistance to antimicrobials.[215] Several studies have concentrated on the development of resistance to beta-lactam antibiotics. Anaerobic organisms, and particularly *B. fragilis,* develop resistance to these drugs primarily by blocking all penetration by the drug or by producing beta-lactamase enzymes that inactivate the drug. *B. fragilis* is particularly adept at developing resistance because of the production of beta-lactamases (penicillinases or cephalosporinases), enzymes that cleave the beta-lactam ring, thus effectively destroying antimicrobial activity. Most strains of *B. fragilis* produce a chromosomally mediated beta-lactamase, which inactivates many cephalosporins, particularly first-generation drugs. In addition to this cephalosporinase, many strains of *B. fragilis* can acquire novel beta-lactamases that are characterized by greater impact on the penicillins than the cephalosporins. One study found that some strains of *B. fragilis* could produce beta-lactamases that are capable of inactivating cefoxitin and imipenem, two drugs that historically have been effective for the treatment of anaerobic infections.[221] Several of these strains are, however, capable of producing massive quantities of the cephalosporinase. Although this enzyme does not have much specific activity against cefoxitin, the drug is inactivated because of the vast quantities produced. Cefoxitin resistance of this nature can be transferred to other strains of *Bacteroides* spp. A study that investigated the emerging resistance patterns of *B. fragilis* to various antimicrobial agents over a 3-year period found that resistance to cefoxitin, originally the most active drug against this species, doubled in 2 years.[221]

Bacteroides spp. also possess a sophisticated system of resistance. In the aforementioned 3-year study, resistance to clindamycin did not increase, and no organisms were resistant to metronidazole or chloramphenicol. Although tetracyclines were the drug of choice for infections caused by *B. fragilis* in the early 1950s, almost 66% of the organisms were resistant to the drug. Variation in anaerobic (e.g., *B. fragilis*) resistance patterns have been described for different geographic regions. In addition, various patterns have been described according to the site of tissue or sample collection. One study found that organisms isolated from the blood were more resistant to piperacillin, cefoxitin, and clindamycin than were the same isolates obtained from the abdominal cavity. Experimental studies have shown that resistance genes can be naturally transferred from *B. fragilis* to *E. coli*. This finding may have profound implications for the treatment of mixed anaerobic–aerobic infections, particularly those originating from colonic bacteria. One study[213] has documented a 29% incidence of resistance of *Bacteroides* spp. to ampicillin; in contrast, 100% were susceptible to amoxicillin, clavulanic acid, and chloramphenicol, and most were susceptible to metronidazole. Only 83% were susceptible to clindamycin.

Clostridium difficile has been associated with hospital outbreaks of illness in hospital environments (based on the author's personal experience).[222] Its ability to form spores to minimize exposure to oxygen renders it resistant to most environmental disinfectants, with the exception of chlorine bleach. Animals receiving anticancer or antibacterial chemotherapeutic agents are at a risk of developing infection when exposed to environmental clostridial spores. Treatment in such situations generally is accomplished with metronidazole until clinical signs resolved; feces should be negative for enzyme-linked immunosorbent assay (ELISA) toxin (1 to 15 days).

Antimicrobial Drugs

The successful treatment of an anaerobic infection depends on altering the local environment in a manner designed to reduce bacterial proliferation and checking the spread of infection into adjacent tissues. The first goal is achieved by surgical débridement of dead tissue. At the time of surgery, pockets of pus should be drained, trapped gas released, and any obstructions to drainage eliminated. Surgery should also improve circulation to the site of infection, which will improve oxygenation of tissues. Local spread of infection is managed by administration of an antimicrobial. Although the number of antimicrobials that can be used to treat anaerobic infections is limited, there are several that are effective and safe. Resistance does not yet seem to have impaired empirical selection of anaerobes (Table 8-12), although caution is still indicated in patients that previously received antimicrobials or those at risk for therapeutic failure for other reasons.

Beta-Lactam Antibiotics

Penicillin G, a natural antibiotic, is the prototype penicillin. The anaerobic susceptibility of the semisynthetic aminopenicillins ampicillin and amoxicillin is similar to that of penicillin G. In contrast to penicillin G, they are effective after oral administration. Penicillins are the drug of choice for clostridial infections and for *Peptostreptococcus* spp. They are generally effective against *Fusobacterium* and *Actinomyces* spp. Although the penicillins are effective against many *Bacteroides* spp., several species, including *B. melaninogenicus* and *B. fragilis*, both of which are clinically important, are uniformly resistant to most penicillins,[211] with the exception of piperacillin.[220] A 33% rate of resistance by *Bacteroides* spp. to penicillin G has been reported in veterinary patients. A large percentage of these strains was also resistant to ampicillin and cephalothin.[214] Jang and colleagues[213] reported that 29% of *Bacteroides* isolates in veterinary medicine are resistant to ampicillin. The efficacy of penicillin (and cephalosporin) antibiotics against *B. fragilis* can be improved by combining the antibiotic with clavulanic acid or sulbactam. Indeed, Jang and colleagues[213] reported all *Bacteroides* isolates to be susceptible to amoxicillin–clavulanic acid. Both of these drugs have a greater affinity for beta-lactamases than do the beta-lactam antibiotics and preferentially bind to and inactivate the bacterial enzyme. The efficacy of amoxicillin against *B. fragilis* is greatly enhanced when combined with clavulanic acid.[223] The addition of clavulanic acid also enhances the efficacy of amoxicillin against several gram-negative enteric organisms, which may be important factors in the pathogenesis of mixed infections. Jang and coworkers[213] found 100% of clostridial organisms to be susceptible to ampicillin, compared with 80% of isolates that were susceptible to clindamycin.

The cephalosporins are very similar to the penicillins in pharmacokinetic characteristics but as a class are less efficacious against anaerobes. First-generation cephalosporins (e.g., cephalothin, cefazolin, and cefadroxil) may be effective against many anaerobic organisms, with the exception of *B. fragilis*; use should be based on susceptibility testing. The second-generation cephalosporin cefoxitin is, however, one of the most effective antibiotics against anaerobic infections, including *B. fragilis*, although resistance is increasing, as was previously noted. As a second-generation cephalosporin, cefoxitin is also effective against many gram-negative enteric organisms, which enhances its utility for the treatment of mixed infections. Many *Clostridium* spp. are resistant to most

Table 8-12 Susceptibility Data for Selected Anaerobic Pathogens Collected from Antimicrobial-Free Dogs and Cats[76]

	Drug	Amox-Clav	Cefadroxil	Cefovecin	Cephalexin
	MIC_{BP} (sus)	≤0.25			≤2
	MIC_{BP} (res)	> 1			≥ 8
Bacteroides spp.	Mode	≤0.5/0.25	0.5	0.25	≤0.5
	MIC_{50}	≤0.5/0.25	0.5	0.25	1
	MIC_{90}	≤0.5/0.25	16	2	16
	Range	≤0.5/0.25-8/4	≤0.25->32	≤0.06-8	≤0.5-64
	n	32	32	32	32
	Species	D, C	D, C	D, C	D, C
	Source	76	76	76	76
	CLSI	Y	Y	Y	Y
	Mode	≤0.5/0.25	2	0.25	≤0.5
Clostridum spp.	MIC_{50}	≤0.5/0.25	2	0.5	2
	MIC_{90}	≤0.5/0.25	16	16	16
	Range	≤0.5/0.25-1/0.5	≤0.25->32	≤0.06->32	≤0.5->64
	n	15	15	15	15
	Species	D, C	D, C	D, C	D, C
	Source	76	76	76	76
	CLSI	Y	Y	Y	Y
	Mode	≤0.5/0.25	≤0.25	≤0.06	≤0.5
Fusobacterium spp.	MIC_{50}	≤0.5/0.25	≤0.25	≤0.06	≤0.5
	MIC_{90}	≤0.5/0.25	0.5	≤0.06	≤0.5
	Range	≤0.5/0.25-2/1	≤0.25-8	≤0.06-1	≤0.5-4
	n	66	66	66	66
	Species	D, C	D, C	D, C	D, C
	Source	76	76	76	76
	CLSI	Y	Y	Y	Y
	Mode	≤0.5/0.25	16	0.5	16
Peptostreptococcus spp.	MIC_{50}	≤0.5/0.25	8	0.5	8
	MIC_{90}	≤0.5/0.25	32	1	16
	Range	≤0.5/0.25-2/1	≤0.25->32	0.12-2	≤0.5->64
	n	21	21	21	21
	Species	D, C	D, C	D, C	D, C
	Source	76	76	76	76
	CLSI	Y	Y	Y	Y
	Mode	≤0.5/0.25	≤0.25	≤0.06	≤0.5
Porphyromonas spp.	MIC_{50}	≤0.5/0.25	≤0.25	≤0.06	≤0.5
	MIC_{90}	≤0.5/0.25	1	≤0.06	≤0.5
	Range	≤0.5/0.25	≤0.25-1	≤0.06	≤0.5-2
	n	29	29	29	29
	Species	D, C	D, C	D, C	D, C
	Source	1	1	1	1
	CLSI	Y	Y	Y	Y
	Mode	≤0.5/0.25	≤0.25	≤0.06	≤0.5
Prevotella spp.	MIC_{50}	≤0.5/0.25	4	0.25	≤0.5
	MIC_{90}	≤0.5/0.25	32	4	64
	Range	≤0.5/0.25-1/0.5	≤0.25-32	≤0.06-8	≤0.5->64
	n	11	11	11	11
	Species	D, C	D, C	D, C	D, C
	Source	76	76	76	76
	CLSI	Y	Y	Y	Y

MIC, Minimum inhibitory concentration; *BP,* breakpoint, *SC,* subcutaneous; A Y indicates that data were collected following the guidelines of Clinical Laboratory Standards Institute (*CLSI*). *D,* dog; *C,* cat; *Y,* yes.
*Pharmacokinetic data from Table 7-1

cephalosporins; thus alternative antimicrobials should be considered for infections caused by these organisms. Currently, piperacillin and cefoxitin remain the most active beta-lactam antibiotics for the treatment of human anaerobic infections. Because of the variable nature of susceptibility patterns and the unique mechanisms and characteristics of beta-lactams exhibited by anaerobic bacteria, however, culture and susceptibility monitoring of these pathogens in crucial. The carbapenems are the newest class of beta-lactam antibiotics and are among the the most effective beta-lactam antibiotics against anaerobic infections.

Other Antimicrobials

Chloramphenicol is one of the most effective antimicrobial drugs against all strains of anaerobic bacteria, including penicillin-resistant *B. fragilis*.[213] Its utility, however, is decreased by its bacteriostatic nature as well as by its tendency to cause adverse reactions, particularly in the cat, and concerns regarding human exposure. Clindamycin is a lincosamide antimicrobial whose mechanism of action is similar to that of chloramphenicol. Like chloramphenicol, it is bacteriostatic against anaerobic organisms. Clindamycin is more efficacious for the treatment of anaerobic infections than its parent drug, lincomycin. Clindamycin is also concentrated in white blood cells at the site of infection, which is considered to be an important factor in the efficacy of this drug. This is an active energy process, however, which may not occur in the oxygen-deficient environments that characterize anaerobic infections. The spectrum of activity of clindamycin includes anaerobic organisms. It is generally very effective against most strains (83% cited by Jang et al.[213]) of *B. fragilis*, including those resistant to penicillin, and is very effective against veterinary isolates of *Clostridium*. Clindamycin is not, however, effective against *C. difficile*, and its use may be associated with pseudomembranitis or other gastrointestinal disorders related to microbial overgrowth. Although fluoroquinolones are generally not considered sufficiently broad in spectrum to include anaerobes, newer-third generation drugs may be very effective. An example is pradofloxacin, whose efficacy includes anaerobes associated with gingival disease in dogs and cats.[267]

SELECTED ANAEROBIC INFECTIONS

Clostridum difficile

C. difficile is reaching epidemic proportions in human patients. Antimicrobial exposure results in suppression of normal flora and is a major risk factor with clindamycin, penicillins, and cephalosporins. A more recent study in humans found fluoroquinolones to be the primary risk factors for the emergence of a clonal-based outbreak in a hospital.[224] Transmission is fecal to oral through contaminated environment and hands of health care personnel in human patients (as with MRSA), and a new strain with increased virulence has emerged. Outbreaks have increased in the hospital setting, although community-acquired infections are increasing in Europe.[225] Outbreaks have been reported in veterinary hospitals as well.[222] Clinical signs range from mild diarrhea to pseudomembranous colitis and toxic (and potentially fatal) megacolon. Toxin binds to intestinal cells and disrupts tight junctions, leading to inflammation and watery diarrhea, the hallmark of infection. Toxins are downregulated by the *tcdC* gene; deletions of this gene leads to clinical signs. A binary toxin also has been described, although its role in human disease is not well defined. A seasonal pattern has been described for selected human hospitals.[226] Epidemiologic description in humans is complicated by diagnosis based on the presence of toxin rather than organism culture. Resistance to newer 8-methoxy fluoroquinolones used to treat the organism (e.g., gatifloxacin and moxifloxicin) has already emerged.[227]

C. difficile may massively increase its exotoxin production in the gastrointestinal tract in the presence of subinhibitory plasma clindamycin concentrations because of increased bacterial synthesis of exotoxin.[228] The use of metronidazole, a popular antigiardial drug, for the treatment of anaerobic infections in dogs and cats has markedly increased. The drug is consistently effective against most anaerobes, including *B. fragilis* as well as most other strains of *Bacteroides*. Metronidazole is also effective for treatment of human cases of *C. difficile*. It is generally not effective against *Actinomyces* or *Propionibacterium*. Its mode of action probably results from disruption of bacterial DNA after bacterial metabolism to toxic metabolites. The low oxidation-reduction potential of the anaerobic environment is conducive to bacterial formation of toxic metabolites.

Vancomycin is the drug of choice for humans for the treatment of antibiotic-associated colitis caused by *C. difficile*. Its mechanism of action results from inhibition of bacterial cell wall synthesis. Thus its actions are primarily bactericidal. Its spectrum includes *Clostridium*, gram-positive bacilli (*Bacillus*, *Actinomyces*), and *Propionibacterium*.

The sulfonamides can be effective against many anaerobic organisms. Caution should be taken, however, because of the patterns of resistance that have been noted for veterinary anaerobic isolates. For serious or difficult anaerobic infections, sulfonamide use should be based on susceptibility data.

Clostridum tetani

Tetanus is caused by the neurotoxin tetanospasmin produced by vegetative *Clostridum tetani*, a motile, gram-positive spore-forming anaerobe.[229] Spores contaminating an anaerobic site (e.g., in the presence of a foreign body or tissue necrosis) vegetate. The toxin, tetanospasmin, enters axons of local motor neurons, and by retrograde movement reaches the axonal body in the spinal cord. Eventually the toxin reaches the brain, where it acts to cleave the protein responsible for fusion of the gamma-aminobutyric acid–containing synaptic vesicle with the neuronal cell membrane.[230] As such, it inhibits the release of inhibitory neurotransmitters gamma-aminobutyric acid as well as glycine, resulting in presynaptic blockade for selected synapses of the spinal cord (predominant site) and brain. Dogs and cats are considered fairly resistant to tetanus and therefore are not generally vaccinated; indeed, vaccination is not protective in humans, necessitating revaccination with exposure.[231] Clinical signs generally occur within 5 to 10 days of wound acquisition, although delays of up to 3 weeks have been reported.[231] Wounds closer to the head are associated with more rapid onset of generalized tetanus. Relative resistance of carnivores to the toxin may result in signs localized to the wound area, manifested as stiffness that usually spreads to the opposite limb or beyond. Generalized tetanus is associated with a guarded prognosis and is characterized as extreme muscle rigidity, manifested as a stiff gait, difficulty in standing or lying down, and hyperthermia. Intracranial signs accompany localized tetanus, resulting in hypertonic facial muscles (e.g., trismus or lockjaw) and reflex muscle spasms. Animals have difficulty with prehension or swallowing solid food. Dysuria, urine retention, constipation, and gas distention are not unusual. Autonomic clinical signs may not appear until several days after rigidity has occurred. Signs include ptyalism, tachycardia, tachypnea, and hypertension.[231] Death, when it occurs, usually results from respiratory compromise.[229] Untreated cases can prove fatal, although natural resistance often limits the disease to localized or mild cases.

Treatment focuses on antimicrobial therapy in an attempt to decrease formation of neurotoxin and neutralization with antitoxin of any toxin not yet bound to nerve tissue. The intravenous route is preferred to the intramuscular or subcutaneous routes (the latter may require 48 to 72 hours for therapeutic concentrations to be reached). Antitoxin (100 to 1000 U/kg, <20,000 U total) should be administered every 5 to 10 minutes; the dose should be decreased for larger dogs. Pretreatment of anaphylaxis is appropriate; administration of a test dose (0.1 to 0.2 mL) subcutaneously or intradermally may help identify those at risk (formation of a wheal at the site). Localized injection at the wound site (1000 U) may be helpful; likewise, intrathecal (I–10 U) injection has been shown experimentally to reduce morbidity and mortality rates in dogs, probably because of better access to neurotoxin bound to nervous tissue. In humans 500 U is injected proximal to the wound. Recovery is slow and progressive, even when antitoxin is administered. Recovery at sites were tetanospasmin is bound requires formation of new receptors, which takes approximately 3 weeks.[231]

Local and systemic antibiotic therapy should be used to eradicate vegetative clostridial organisms, thus reducing the amount of toxin released. Metronidazole is superior to penicillin G and tetracyclines. Penicillins inhibit type A gamma-aminobutyric receptors, which is the target of tetanus toxin. Studies comparing the time to recovery and mortality of penicillin with those of metronidazole for treatment of tetanus in humans are controversial, with studies ranging from improved outcome for metronidazole to no differences between treatments.[230] The studies are complicated by differences in the form of penicillin studied, limiting conclusions. However, because of the possible impact of penicillin, metronidazole might be preferred; at the very least, procaine penicillin probably should be avoided because it may exacerbate CNS symptoms.[230]

Animals should be removed from stimulating environments. Supportive therapy for tetanus includes control of autonomic signs, reflex spasms, or convulsions. Anticholinergics may be indicated to treat bradyarrhythmias. Phenothiazines (chlorpromazine preferred) combined with barbiturates (pentobarbital or phenobarbital) have been recommended as the preferred treatment.[229] Caution with the use of phenothiazines is recommended for patients with seizures; phenothiazines lower seizure threshold and can worsen seizures associated with other disorders. However, use for treatment of muscle rigidity may preclude concerns regarding seizures. Further, a retrospective study of acepromazine use in dogs experiencing seizures found no increase in seizure activity associated with acepromazine. However, acepromazine may be sufficiently different from other phenothiazines to warrant caution in extrapolating information to phenothiazines as a class.[232] Phenobarbital should be administered as a loading dose (12 mg/kg to achieve the lower end of the recommended range for epilepsy). Glycopyrrolate should be administered to control bradycardia that may occur with the combined use of these drugs. Benzodiazepines (e.g., diazepam) may be useful for controlling spasms and hyperexcitability; methocarbamol is a less effective centrally acting skeletal muscle relaxant. Methocarbamol, dantrolene (a peripherally acting skeletal muscle relaxant), or gamma-aminobutyric acid antagonist may be useful, including in combination, for the control of spasticity. Tetanus-induced respiratory compromise requires intubation and respiratory support, which may require sedation, paralytic agents, or both. Linnenbrink[231] discussed the limited use of supraphysiologic concentrations (2 to 4 mmol/L) of magnesium for control of autonomic dysfunction in human patients. Magnesium decreased rigidity and imparted a dose-sparing effect on sedatives. Hypocalcemia occured but generally did not need correcting. The loss of tendon reflexes was monitored as an indication of toxicity. Successful management of tetanus in two dogs has been reported.[233] Therapy included a combination of general anesthetics (pentobarbital, propofol), anticonvulsants (diazepam, including by constant-rate infusion, phenobarbital), and muscle relaxants (diazepam, methocarbamol), including phenothiazine sedatives (for muscle rigidity). Supportive therapy was intensive and crucial to therapeutic success, with full recovery requiring several weeks.

Clostridium botulinum

Botulism in dogs is almost exclusively caused by type C *Clostridium botulinum* organisms that release the neurotoxin in a vegetative state.[110] Although released in the inert form, cleavage by tissue or bacterial proteinases generates the dichain metalloproteinase neurotoxin, which is similar to tetanus toxin. Generally, clinical signs result from ingestion of the preformed toxin, in part because adult animals generally are resistant to colonization by the organism, although antimicrobial therapy can facilitate colonization. The toxin is absorbed by intestinal lymphatics as with nutrient proteins; toxin complexed with other proteins appears to protect the toxin from intestinal degradation. At the nerve terminal, the toxin prevents the presynaptic release of acetylcholine by irreversibly binding. The toxin is characterized by a very high affinity for the presynaptic membrane receptors, making it one of the most potent toxins. At this point the toxin is susceptible to inactivation by antitoxin. However, once receptor-mediated endocytosis has moved the toxin into the cell, antitoxin activation can no longer occur. Of the two chains, the L chain is more likely to inhibit acetylcholine release. Clinical sequelae, evident within hours but delayed for up to 6 days, include paralysis and degeneration of the affected synapse with subsequent lower motor neuron and parasympathetic dysfunction. Death generally does not occur unless paralysis extends to the respiratory tract. Recovery follows formation of new terminal axons and neuromuscular junctions with cranial nerve, neck, and forelimb functions generally returning to normal first.

Therapy focuses on supportive care; spontaneous recovery generally will occur in all animals if respiratory function is not affected. Antitoxin is ineffective if nerve endings have been penetrated, which generally occurs rapidly; however, treatment may be beneficial if oral absorption of the toxin is ongoing. Type C antitoxin (10,000 to 15,000 U, intravenously or intramuscularly) should be administered twice, with each dose 4 hours apart. The antitoxin remains in the system for 40 days, mitigating the need for follow-up therapy. Penicillin or metronidazole can be administered to reduce the intestinal growth of *C. botulinim*, although the efficacy of this practice is questionable and may be contraindicated if organism death is thought to increase toxin release. Neuromuscular potentiators (aminopyridine, diaminopyridine, guanidine hydrochloride) have not proved effective.

Clostridium perfringens

C. perfringens capable of producing an enterotoxin can cause severe diarrhea.[234] Binding of the toxin to intestinal epithelial cells increases permeability, causing fluid and ion secretion, cell death, and sloughing of the intestinal mucosa. Sporulation leading to enterointoxication can occur after antimicrobial therapy, increased intestinal pH, dietary alteration, and immunosuppression; it also is associated with viral enteritis. Enterotoxemia can cause rapid death. Very occasionally, clinical signs may occur after ingestion of contaminated meat or as a result of nosocomial infections. Therapy includes antimicrobials and intensive fluid therapy. Antimicrobials that are variably effective include metronidazole, ampicillin, amoxicillin–clavulanic acid, tylosin, clindamycin, and tetracyclines.

MISCELLANEOUS INFECTIONS

L-Form Bacterial Infection

L-form bacteria either have a deficient cell wall or lack one altogether. Their role in causing infections in animals is not well understood. A number of organisms are capable of becoming cell wall deficient, including *Staphylococcus* and *Streptococcus* species. Information regarding the causes of an organism assuming this structural state are not clear, nor is the role of L-forms in the cause of disease. Presumably, the infection starts in the skin and progresses as multiple abscesses form and then dehisce. Bacteremia can lead to polyarthritis. Because of their cell wall–deficient state, microorganisms are difficult to detect by light microscopy but can be visualized inside phagocytes by electron microscopy. Drugs whose antibacterial effects do not target the cell wall are indicated. Tetracyclines have been the drug of choice.[235]

Hemobartonellosis (Hemotropic Mycoplasmosis)

The causative agent of feline infectious anemia was recently reclassified as *Mycoplasma* on the basis of RNA sequence analysis, leading to a change in terminology to hemotrophic mycoplasmosis. Mycoplasma are gram-negative organisms that lack a cell wall. At least two variants have been identified in the cat, with the large form, Ohio strain *(Mycoplasma haemofelis)* being more pathogenic compared with the small form, California strain *(Candidatus Mycoplasma haemominutum)*; the latter apparently has not been associated with disease.[236] *Mycoplasma haemocanis* has been associated with anemia in splenectomized dogs, although the distinction between *M. haemofelis* and *M. haemocanis* is not clear.

Experimentally, inoculation is followed by a period of 2 to 34 days before clinical signs and anemia associated with parasitemia appear; this second period persists from 18 to 30 days. Mortality rates are highest during this phase, with hematocrit levels returning to near normal in surviving cats. Recovered cats remain carriers for years and may experience recrudescence of clinical signs. Anemia reflects predominantly extravasular rather than intravascular hemolysis. Inclusions and other changes in the surface of the red blood cell result in osmotic fragility, reduced deformability, and subsequent removal from the bloodstream by the spleen. Afflicted animals may have lowered resistance to concurrent infections; an association with feline leukemia virus (but apparently not feline immunodeficiency virus) may worsen the pathopyhysiology of either syndrome.[236]

Doxycycline is the treatment of choice (5 mg/kg orally every 24 hours for 21 days) but will not necessarily eradicate the infection. Care should be taken to either administer a liquid preparation or follow capsules with a liquid wash to prevent esophageal damage. Experimentally, azithromycin was ineffective at 15 mg/kg orally twice daily for 7 days for treating large-form mycoplasma in cats.[237] Cats remained PCR positive and anemic after treatment. In contrast to azithromycin, fluoroquinolones may be effective for treatment. Dowers[238] prospectively compared 2 weeks of treatment with enrofloxacin at a low (5 mg/kg po qd) and high dose (10 mg/kg po qd) to doxycycline (5 mg/kg po bid) in cats (n = 16, 4 per group, including a no treatment group) experimentally infected with large form *H. felis*. All treatment cats responded. The high dose enrofloxacin group had fewer days of anemia compared to the other groups; 1 doxycycline and 2 high-dose enrofloxacin cats cleared of organisms based on PCR and remained disease free for at least 6 months. Ishak et al.[268] studied the efficacy of marbofloxacin (2.75 mg/kg daily for 2 weeks beginning 16 days after infection) for treatment of experimentally induced *M. haemofelis* infection in cats (n = 12; including 6 untreated control). Marbofloxacin was associated with more rapid hematologic response. However, PCR-based detection of organisms (viral numbers not quantified) did not differ from that of the nontreated group, indicating that infection was not consistently eradicated. Nonetheless, the authors concluded that marbofloxacin was a reasonable treatment option. Tasker et al.[269] also studied the efficacy of marbofloxacin (2 mg/kg orally daily for 4 weeks) for treatment of *M. haemofelis* in experimentally infected cats with or without chronic feline immunodeficiency virus (n = 6/group, 3 cats from each group treated). Organism counts were reduced and animals improved, but animals were not cleared.

Dowers et al.[239] also compared the efficacy of pradofloxacin at a low (5 mg/kg orally qd) and high dose (10 mg/kg orally qd) to doxycycline (5 mg/kg orally bid) in cats (n = 23) experimentally infected with *M. haemofelis*. Therapy was initiated when cats became positive on PCR and continued for 6 weeks. However, cats that became PCR negative by day 42 (the last day of treatment) were also treated with methylprednisolone sodium acetate (20 mg/kg intramuscularly) in an attempt to cause recrudescence after immunosuppresion. The number of days of anemia did not differ among treatment groups; all were less than the control group. Organism copy numbers were significantly lower in the low-dose group compared with the doxycycline group for 4 of the 5 posttreatment weeks. Four of 6 cats in the high-dose and 2 of 6 cats in the low-dose pradofloxacin group tested negative (cPCR) on day 42 of treatment and were immunosuppressed. None of the doxycycline cats yielded negative PCR results. Immunosuppression yielded transiently positive results in 5 of the cats; 1 cat became persistently negative. By day 28 of glucocorticoid therapy, however, 4 of the 6 transiently positive cats (3 low doses and 1 high dose) became negative. These studies consistently indicated that, under experimental conditions, fluoroquinolones may play a role in the treatment and possible clearing of *M. haemofelis* and are reasonable alternatives when doxycycline fails or cannot be used. Lappin[240] prospectively evaluated the efficacy of imidocarb (5 mg/kg intramuscularly; repeated in 2 weeks) for treatment of experimentally induced (11 cats) chronic haemobartonellosis. Both the large form (*M. haemofelis;* n = 4; 3 treated, 1 control), and small form (*M. hemominutum*; n = 3, 2 treated, 1 control) were studied. Three cats were infected with both organisms. Side effects were limited to irritation at the injection site. Both control cats remained PCR positive throughout the study. One cat inoculated with both forms and one cat inoculated with *M. haemofelis* became persistently negative at weeks 4 and 6 after treatment (the remaining cats became negative at week 2 but positive at weeks 4 and 6) and were subsequently treated with methylprednioslone. One cat died as a result of undetermined causes, and the second became PCR positive. Imidocarb does not appear to be a reasonable alternative for clearing chronically infected cats.

KEY POINT 8-37 Doxycycline remains the drug of choice for treatment and eradication of feline mycoplasma, with high-dose fluoroquinolones a potential treatment alternative.

The concurrent use of immunosuppressive doses of glucocorticoids is controversial. Glucocorticoids may increase the number of microogranisms in the blood and may exacerbate accompanying concurrent infections.[236]

Bartonellosis and Coxiella

Bartonella is an aerobic, gram-negative, intracellular organism, probably transmitted by ticks. It targets cells of the immune system, living in endothelial and red cells. The organism is associated with a reduction in CD8+ cells and the expression of adhesion molecules. The association with *Bartonella* and IE has been described.[241] All seropositive dogs were also seropositive for *Anaplasma phagocytophilum*. Its association with valvular disease in people results in a poor prognosis. Treatment should be at least 2 weeks in duration. Potentially effective drugs include doxycycline.

Brucellosis

Pathogenesis

An infectious disease, brucellosis draws attention because of its insidious nature, difficulty to treat, and zoonotic potential. *Brucella canis,* the causative agent of brucellosis in dogs, is a small gram-negative coccobacillus. Among *Brucella, B. canis* stands out in morphology, biochemistry, and immunology. Among its differences compared with other organisms is its zoonotic potential: The disease can be transmitted only between members of Canidae. Cats are only transiently infected after experimental infection. Dogs are susceptible to infection with *Brucella abortus* but do not appear to be important to the spread of infection. Infection by *Brucella* involves penetration of mucous membranes after contact with contaminated fluids from an infected urogenital tract or an aborted fetus. Phagocytized organisms are transported to lymphatic and genital tissues, where multiplication occurs. Leukocyte-associated bacteremia can persist for years. Organisms can be intermittently shed from infected animals (during estrus, breeding, or abortion).[242]

Although antibodies are generated against *Brucella* species, as with most intracellular organisms, cell-mediated immunity is the primary mechanism of host defense. Cell-mediated immunity can provide protection against reinfection, although persistent infection may be necessary to provide persistent protection. Immune response to inflamed infected tissues (e.g., spermatozoa) contributes to infertility. Immunosuppressive drugs appear to increase the risk of infection but may not alter the course of the disease in dogs already infected. Spontaneous recovery can occur but may take up to 5 years. During this period infection might be associated with bacteremia. As with other blood-borne organisms, *Brucella* may localize in tissues other than the urogenital tract. Discospondylitis; anterior uveitis; and, less commonly, glomerulopathy or meningoencephalitis may result. Diagnosis is based on agglutination tests, agar-gel immunodiffusion, or ELISA.[242] Therapy with antibiotics does alter the progression of the disease.

Antimicrobial and Adjuvant Therapy

A number of antimicrobial drugs are effective in vitro against *Brucella* but may not be able to eradicate infection. Antimicrobial therapy can relieve symptoms, shorten the duration of illness, and reduce the likelihood of complications yet not eradicate the organism.[243] Success will be enhanced by a combination of effective drugs at high doses for at least 4 weeks. Drugs should be able to penetrate cell membranes; accumulation in phagocytic cells should further facilitate success. Among effective antimicrobials, lipid-soluble tetracyclines (minocycline and doxycycline) are particularly efficacious when used at a high dose and in combination with an aminoglycoside. The World Health Organization has also recommended doxycycline in combination with rifampin, although doxycycline with streptomycin was found to be more effective in the treatment of discospondylitis.[243] Fluoroquinolones should also be effective when combined with aminoglycosides,[243] although clinical trials documenting efficacy in dogs have not been reported. An added advantage of these drugs is intracellular accumulation. Fluoroquinolones may not, however, be effective as sole agents against brucellosis. Human patients intolerant of tetracyclines also responded well to combinations of trimethoprim–sulfonamides and aminoglycosides. Antimicrobial therapy should not be discontinued too early; sequential titers can be used to assess response to therapy.

Infected dogs should be neutered as soon as possible. Glucocorticoids or other immunosuppressive therapy may be indicated for treatment of infections associated with life-threatening or organ-threatening inflammation (e.g., CNS). Currently, prevention is best implemented through good hygiene practices, neutering of infected animals, and vaccination of cattle.

Leptospirosis

The genus *Leptospira* belongs to the family Treponemataceae, which contains all spirochetes, including *Borrelia* species. Leptospirosis is primarily a disease of wild and domestic animals; humans are infected only occasionally.[244] However, it is a reemerging disease for reasons that are not yet known.[245]

Pathogenesis

Leptospirosis generally causes an acute generalized infection or interstitial nephritis. Leptospires are motile spirochetes; *Leptospira interrogans* tends to be the pathogenic organism in animals. At least three antigenically distinct serovars cause disease in dogs; infection in cats is rare.[234] Infection occurs through the mucosa or abraded skin and can occur between animals or in animals that come in contact with the contaminated environment. Once the mucosa is penetrated, the organism multiplies rapidly in the bloodstream. Inflammation causes parenchymal damage, particularly in the liver and kidney. Persistence in renal tubular cells leads to colonization of the kidney.[244] Chronic active hepatitis can be a sequela of infection in dogs.

Leptospirosis can present as a peracute infection manifested by shock and death. Less acute presentation involves fever, anorexia, vomiting, and dehydration. Clinical laboratory tests may reveal thrombocytopenia, electrolyte alterations, and liver damage. Diagnosis is based on serologic testing (paired serum titers). Leptospires are very difficult to recover, with urine analysis by dark field microscopy providing the best chance of discovery.

Antimicrobial Therapy

Treatment focuses on eradication of the causative organism and supportive therapy. Acute renal failure may require intensive management. Antibiotics should inhibit the multiplication of the organism as well as eradicate it. Response manifested as a decrease in fever should be apparent within several hours of administration.[234] Drugs shown to be effective in vitro include most penicillins, third-generation cephalosporins, and tetracyclines but not first- and second-generation cephalosporins. Not all penicillins appear to be able to eradicate the organisms, but high doses of penicillin G, ampicillin, and amoxicillin are among the more effective choices in clearing the urine.[244,245] Procaine penicillin G (40,000 units/kg intramuscularly or subcutaneously every 24 hours or a divided dose given every 12 hours) is the antibiotic of choice for leptospiremia. It may be necessary to decrease the dose if the animal is in renal failure (e.g., dividing the dose by the serum creatinine), although the real risk of side effects in the presence of renal disease is not clear. Penicillin clears infection with leptospirosis if continued for a sufficient period of time. An injectable form of penicillin should be used for 14 days or until azotemia resolves; an oral form (amoxicillin [22 mg/kg every 8 hours]) can then be initiated. Intravenous ampicillin or amoxicillin (22 mg/kg every 6 to 8 hours) have also been used successfully during initial therapy. Doxycycline can also be used for initial therapy and to clear leptospiremia.[234,245] Initial penicillin therapy of 2 weeks' duration can also be followed by doxycycline (5 mg/kg twice daily) for 6 to 8 weeks to achieve elimination of the carrier state.

KEY POINT 8-38 Procaine penicillin is the antibiotic of choice for leptospiremia and may clear the infection if administered for a sufficient length of time.

In human patients doxycycline appears to be beneficial for the prevention of infection even after exposure, whereas the penicillins do not appear to prevent infection after exposure (despite their ability to eradicate infection).[244] Clearing tissues may be more difficult than clearing urine; doxycycline for 2 weeks appears to be the most frequently recommended for clearing the carrier state in dogs.[245] Fluoroquinolones (ciprofloxacin and enrofloxacin) also appear to be effective against leptospires, although clinical studies supporting their use are lacking. Hamsters experimentally infected with *L. interrogans* responded to ciprofloxacin.[246] In vitro studies of five serovars of *Leptospira* indicated efficacy on the basis of MICs (0.05 to 0.20 μg/mL), although the effect was bacteriostatic; bactericidal concentrations were tenfold to a hundredfold higher.[247] Orbifloxacin has proved ineffective.[234] Experimentally, the macrolides also appear effective.[234] Protection is best implemented by prevention of exposure and elimination of reservoirs.

Most dogs presenting with leptospirosis have developed renal disease.[245] Thus supportive therapy should focus on treatment of acute renal failure and its associated signs (i.e., uremic gastritis, hypertension). Leptospirosis may be the most widespread zoonotic disease in the world, and vaccination is important to prevention. Gloves should be worn when handling carrier animals.

Lyme Borreliosis

Like *Leptospira* species, *Borrelia* species belong to the family Treponemataceae. *Borrelia* are motile spirochetes that have an outer slimelike layer. They are rapidly killed by desiccation and ultraviolet lights. *Borrelia* infect both humans and animals; up to 15 *Borrelia* species cause disease. The Centers for Disease Control and Prevention has designated Lyme disease as the most common vector-borne infection in the United States. However, the disease may be overdiagnosed in humans.[248]

Ixodes species are the primary insect vectors of the spirochete *Borrelia burgdorferi*. Lyme borreliosis afflicts primarily humans and dogs, although cats can be infected experimentally. Organisms are able to adhere to many different types of mammalian cells as well as avoid elimination by phagocytic cells.[248] The immune response appears to be initially suppressed during infection, apparently allowing the organisms to spread. The disease is multisystemic, with nonspecific clinical signs such as relapsing fever (during which borreliae are present in blood), anorexia, lethargy, and lymphadenopathy. Polyarthritis might result in episodic lameness; clinical signs often do not develop until several months after infection.[248,249] Heart block, which occurs in humans,[248] has been reported in one infected dog. Clinical laboratory changes are also variable, depending on the site of localization of the infection. Diagnosis is facilitated by serum titers, although interpretation is complicated by interlaboratory variability and overlap between titers indicative of clinical versus subclinical infection. Resolution of natural disease in humans appears to be dependent on class II major histocompatibility complex genes.

According to the the 16th Consensus Conference on Anti-infective Therapy,[250] the goal for treatment of borreliosis is eradication of infection (not negative serology) such that progression to chronic disease might be prevented. Treatment should be implemented for 14 to 21 days. Based on in vitro testing, antimicrobials effective against *B. burgdorferi* include, in order of most to least effective, ceftriaxone, erythromycin, amoxicillin, cefuroxime, doxycycline, tetracycline, and penicillin G.[249] In human medicine the first line of oral therapy for the primary phase of illness is amoxicillin or doxycycline, with cefuroxime–axetil implemented as second line. Azithromycin is indicated if first or second line cannot be administered. Treatment for the subsequent phases include ceftriaxone (intravenous or intramuscular) or penicillin (intravenous), doxycycline, and amoxicillin (orally) for 21 to 28 days. Antimicrobial therapy based on clinical response includes, in order of preference, tetracyclines (doxycycline is the drug of choice), high doses of ampicillin or amoxicillin, and erythromycin and its derivatives.[248] Third-generation cephalosporins (e.g., ceftriaxone) are also generally effective. One study in humans found similar clinical cure rates for ceftriaxone (85%) compared with doxycycline (88%).[251] No information appears to be available regarding the efficacy of cefpodoxime; however, initial studies by the manufacturer may have indicated a lack of in vitro susceptibility.[251a] Accordingly, the use of either cefpodoxime or cefovecin should be based on susceptibility data. The organisms appear to be resistant to ciprofloxacin (and presumably enrofloxacin and other veterinary fluoroquinolones) and to the aminoglycosides. Oral therapy is sufficient except in cases of neurologic signs; intravenous therapy should be instituted in such cases. *B. burgdorferi* is a potent inducer (in vitro) of TNF-alpha and interleukin-1β. Antimicrobial therapy in humans is occasionally characterized by a Jarisch–Herxheimer reaction, which may reflect release of spirochetal endotoxin and subsequent septic shock syndrome.[248] Supportive therapy includes nonsteroidal antiinflammatories as needed for joint lameness. Disease-modifying chondroprotective agents should be strongly considered. Care should be taken when combining nonsteroidals with doxycycline or minocycline because of the competition for protein-binding sites and the potential for adverse reactions to the nonsteroidal drug. Glucocorticoids should be limited to treatment of acute spirochetemia; recrudescence of spirochetemia will be facilitated with their use. Prevention focuses on eradication of the vector.

Higher Bacteria: Nocardiosis and Actinomycosis

Pathogenesis

Nocardiosis is generally presented as a localized infection. The organism is an acid-fast, aerobic, soil-borne actinomycete, usually introduced through the respiratory tract. Traumatic penetration may result in a localized skin infection.[252,253] *Actinomyces* are commensal anaerobic organisms found in the oral cavities of animals. Infection commonly follows penetrating wounds, such as inhalation of grass awns. *Actinomyces* are distinctive in their configuration, presenting as filamentous growth with true branching.

The taxonomy of *Nocardia* is currently evolving, but *Nocardia asteroides* is among the more commonly identified pathogens. Culture is made difficult sometimes by the slow growth that characterizes this organism when present in mixed cultures from clinical material. Rapidly growing bacteria often obscure the smaller *Nocardia* colonies. Colony characteristics may take up to 2 to 4 weeks to be noticed. Gram staining may help identify the organisms earlier, although smears may also be negative. *Nocardia,* but not *Actinomyces,* stains acid fast, although acid-fast staining in *Nocardia* is also variable. *Nocardia* appears as beaded, branching filaments when Gram stained but will not stain with hematoxylin and eosin preparations or in periodic acid-Schiff stains for fungi (see Figure 6-14)).[252] In human patients, positive cultures and smears occur in only one third of the cases. Pus from a fistula or abscess will facilitate identification. *Nocardia* and *Actinomyces* also stain gram positive, but again staining is irregular.[254]

Nocardiosis is an opportunistic infection. In humans a number of underlying diseases, most of which are accompanied by an altered immune system, predispose the patient to nocardiosis. Infections occur because the organism is able to evade bacterial protective mechanisms of the host. Immune T cells and neutrophils are important to eradication of *Nocardia. Nocardia* may be resistant to oxidative bursts of neutrophils. Filamentous log-phase cells of *Nocardia* are more virulent and toxic to macrophages than are the coccoid stationary-phase organisms, which can be easily phagocytized.

Nocardia produces suppurative necrosis and abscess formation. In humans *Nocardia* in skin seldom causes a marked fibrotic response; rather, granulation tissue will be loose, with bands of fibrous tissue surrounding the lesions. Confluent abscesses form with little to no encapsulation. Extension to the pleura or chest wall may result in empyema, subcutaneous abscesses, or sinus tracts. Occasionally, bony involvement may occur. Calcium-containing "sulfur granules" present a barrier to bacterial penetration and may indicate reversion of the organism *(Actinomyces)* to an L-form.

Antimicrobial and Adjuvant Therapy

A number of antimicrobials are effective against both *Actinomyces* and *Nocardia.* An anaerobic environment and hence infection with *Actinomyces* should be assumed unless proved otherwise, thus leading to more conservative antimicrobial selection. Penicillins (penicillin G, amoxicillin) are generally preferred, although resistance and L–form organisms can preclude their efficacy.[254] Clavulanic acid can reduce the risk of resistance. The formation of protective calcium granules by certain strains of *Actinomyces* limits antibiotic penetration into the organisms. The formation of these granules is stimulated by the presence of penicillin antibiotics. Trimethoprim–sulfonamide combinations are also very effective, although high doses are recommended. Combinations of penicillins with trimethoprim–sulfonamide result in synergistic actions against *Nocardia* and *Actinomyces*[186] (high doses and frequent intervals). Clindamycin and erythromycin are also effective, particularly against L-forms.[254] The aminoglycosides are highly effective against *Nocardia* and *Actinomyces,* and synergistic activity has been documented against this organism with combinations. Minocycline (and presumably doxycycline) also is effective, although use of this bacteriostatic drug may preclude combinations with other antimicrobials.

Treatment for both *Nocardia* and *Actinomyces* should occur for at least 6 weeks, with high doses at frequent intervals (see the discussion of respiratory tract infections in this chapter). Treatment should continue beyond resolution of clinical signs. Adjuvant therapy should include drainage and lavage of empyema and, when indicated, chest tube drainage or surgical débridement. Lavage should continue for several days until cytologic examination of aspirated fluid indicates resolution of infection and fluid accumulation decreases (5 to 10 days; see previous discussion of empyema). The author has often recommended initial hospitalization and intravenous therapy with amikacin and amoxicillin–clavulanic acid or, for serious, life-threatening infections, a carbapenem followed 10 to 14 days later with very high (45 to 60 mg/kg twice daily; note the risk of thyroid gland suppression at this dose) oral sulfadiazine, with trimethoprim replacing the aminoglycoside and high, frequent doses of amoxicillin-clavulanic acid replacing the carbapenem. The amoxicillin–clavulanic acid combination should be continued with the sulfonamide for 4 to 6 weeks or more. The beta-lactam should be administered at 6- to 8-hour intervals.

Mycobacteria

Mycobacteria are composed of a number of aerobic, acid-fast bacteria. They vary markedly in host affinity and ability to cause disease. Disease is frequently accompanied by granulomatous inflammation because of their ability to survive phagocytosis. The acid-fast nature of these microorganisms reflects the large amount of lipid material in the cell wall. Constituents of the cell wall stimulate the granulomatous response. The organisms are more resistant than most organisms to environmental changes (e.g., pH, heat) and are more resistant to disinfection. Some organisms (most notably *Mycobacterium avium*) can survive in the environment for several years. They are, however, very susceptible to 5% phenol or 5% household bleach. Generally, organisms causing disease are characterized by one of three forms.[235] *Tuberculosis* generally is internal in location. Infecting organisms include *Mycobacterium tuberculosis* (more common in dogs) and *Mycobacterium bovis* (more common in cats). *Leprosy* is characterized by localized cutaneous nodules; *Mycobacterium lepraemurium* is probably the most common infecting organism (in cats). *Atypical mycobacteria* generally presents as a spreading subcutaneous inflammatory disease (Figure 8-11); among the several organisms causing this complex is *M. avium.* Dogs and cats are most commonly infected by owners with disease or exposure to infected farm animals.

Tuberculosis

Dogs and cats are more susceptible to infection by tuberculous mycobacteria than by atypical mycobacteria. Infection generally occurs through the respiratory or alimentary tract. Local multiplication at the site of infection results in a granulomatous response at the primary complex (site of deposition) and local lymph nodes. Particularly in cats, however, a granulomatous response may develop only in surrounding lymph nodes. For tuberculosis respiratory infections are more common in dogs; intestinal infections are more common in cats. Infection can be followed by elimination of the organisms in animals with a sufficient immune response. The more common sequelae are location within phagocytic cells, intracellular multiplication, and granuloma formation as the body attempts to eradicate the organism. Organisms that outpace the host immune system can cause disseminated disease. Immunity is incurred by the cell-mediated response, but factors that facilitate an adequate response in the host are not known. Diagnosis can be facilitated with intradermal skin testing in dogs with the highest concentration of antigen used in humans. Cats do not react strongly to intradermal testing. Diagnosis can be facilitated by the presence of acid-fast organisms in tissue biopsy material.

Antimicrobial therapy is complicated by the fastidious nature of the organism. Drug penetration into the organism is likely to be more difficult than for other organisms; intracellular survival further complicates efficacy of drugs reaching the site of infection. Treatment should generally include combination therapy for at least 6 to 9 months. A combination of isoniazid (10 to 20 mg/kg orally once daily) plus rifampin (10 to 20 mg/kg orally every 12 to 24 hours) plus ethambutol (15 mg/kg orally every 24 hours) is the most effective therapy (in humans), although isoniazid-resistant organisms have become increasingly difficult to treat. More rapid remission is likely with intravenous administration. The isoniazid can also be administered prophylactically (6 to 12 months) in cases of exposure. The fluoroquinolones are also effective against

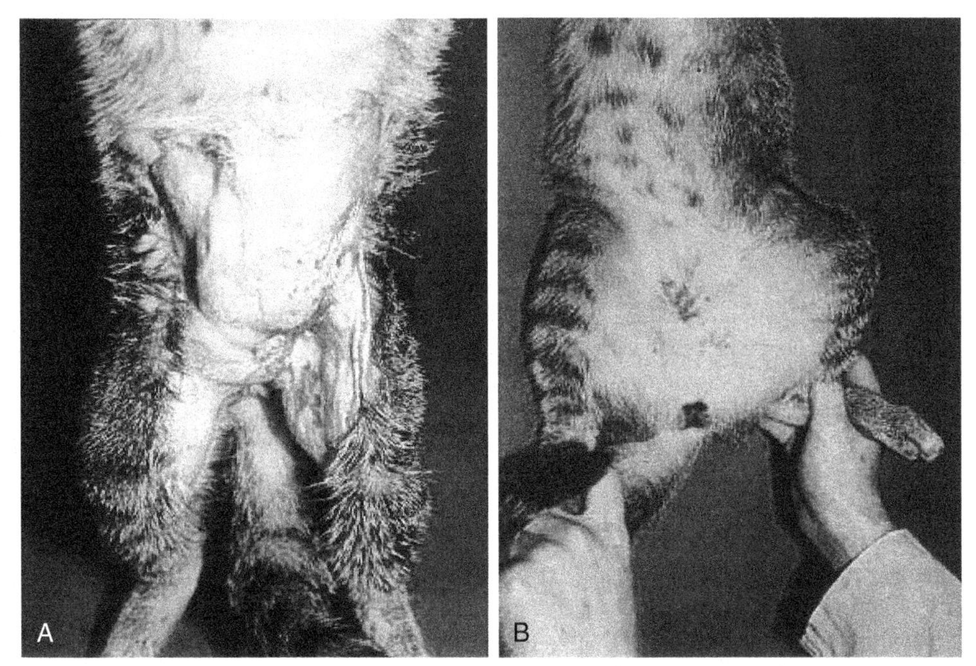

Figure 8-11 Atypical mycobacterium in a cat before *(A)* and 3 months after *(B)* treatment with a combination of enrofloxacin and sulfadiazine–tribrissen. Note the granulomatous tissue and multiple fistulous tracts. (Photographs courtesy Katrina Mealey, DVM, PhD, DACVIM, DACVCP, Washington State University, Pullman, WA.)

selected species of mycobacteria. *M. avium* (see later discussion of atypical mycobacteria) is an exception, although it does also respond to other drugs used to treat atypical mycobacteria. Infected animals remain a health hazard because they serve as temporary sources of dissemination in the environment.

Leprosy

Feline leprosy is caused by *M. lepraemurium,* also the causative organism of rat leprosy. The infection causes rapidly growing, soft, fleshy nodules in the skin and subcutaneous tissues, usually on the head or extremities. Infected cats are generally healthy, and the lesions are not painful. Feline leprosy may comprise two different clinical syndromes, one tending to occur in young cats and caused typically by *M. lepraemurium* and another in old cats caused by a single novel mycobacterial species.

Diagnosis is generally based on the presence of granulomatous inflammation and acid-fast organisms in biopsy specimens or impression smears; PCR may also be available. Treatment includes surgical removal and antimicrobial therapy. Drugs include dapsone (1 mg/kg [dogs] orally every 8 hours or 50 mg [cats] orally every 12 hours) for 2 weeks or clofazimine (8 mg/kg orally every 24 hours for 6 weeks and then twice weekly thereafter). Rifampin may also be useful. Cats with feline leprosy caused by a slow-growing mycobacterium responded well to a combination of two or three antibiotics:[255] rifampicin (10 to 15 mg/kg once a day), clofazimine (25 to 50 mg once daily or 50 mg every other day) or clarithromycin (62.5 mg per cat every 12 hours).

Atypical Mycobacteria

Both slow-growing organisms *(M. avium)* and rapid-growing organisms (e.g., *Mycobacterium fortuitum, Mycobacterium chelonei)* cause disease in dogs and cats, although the rapid-growing organisms are more common. These organisms are ubiquitous in natural environments (especially wet soils) and generally are not pathogenic. Infection is generally acquired after trauma to the skin; the location of entrance into the body determines the presentation of the disease. Penetration into subcutaneous tissue appears to promote pathogenicity. Generally, infection presents as a localized but spreading infection characterized by granulomatous inflammation and acid-fast organisms. Multiple fistulous draining tracts are evident, usually in the caudal abdominal, inguinal, or lumbar subcutaneous tissues (see Figure 8-11). Cats are usually clinically healthy even if cutaneous involvement is extensive. Less commonly, fever, anorexia, and weight loss occur. Hypercalcemia as a result of the release of parathormone-like hormone from macrophages associated with the inflammatory response may occur,[275] and has, in the author's experience, occurred in a cat infected with atypical mycobacteria. Diagnosis of atypical mycobacterium is difficult in part because organisms are not abundant. Tissue biopsy specimens should be taken from the subcutaneous tissues because organisms are more likely to be located in the panniculus. Nocardiosis should be considered as a differential. Bacterial culture provides the definitive diagnosis.

Therapy focuses on antimicrobial drugs. Antitubercular drugs are generally ineffective against atypical mycobacterial species. Quinolones, aminoglycosides (particularly amikacin), and doxycycline (or minocycline) are effective and can be used in combination if more aggressive therapy is desired. Other combinations include clofazimine, rifampin and the azolides, azithromycin, or clarithromycin. Other drugs that might be beneficial include trimethoprim–sulfonamide combinations and clofazimine. High doses are recommended to maximize drug delivery into the granulomatous tissue. Surgical debulking may be indicated for large granulomatous masses. Care should be taken not to discontinue drugs too early. At least 4 to 6 weeks of therapy should be anticipated.

Horne and Kunkel[256] retrospectively reported on 10 cases of rapidly growing mycobacterium in cats (n = 10); 6 of 10 yielded *M. fortuitum* on culture, 2 of 10 *Mycobacterium abcessus,* and 1 of 10 *Mycobacterium goodii.* Five of the cases resolved. Susceptibility patterns for the drugs were as follows ("I" considered resistant): amiikacin (9 of 10), kanamycin (3 of 10), gentamicin (7 of 10), cefoxitin (6 of 10), imipenem (8 of 10), doxycycline (4 of 10), minocycline (7 of 10), ciprofloxacin (7 of 10), moxifloxacin (7 of 8), clarithromycin (5 of 10), azithromycin (5 of 10), trimethoprim sulfamethoxazole (6 of 8), linezolid (2 of 8), and amoxicillin–clavulanic acid (3 of 10). Organisms were resistant to ceftriaxone, cefepime, cefotaxin, and erythromycin. The drugs used to treat all cases varied but included marbofloxacin, clarithromycin, minocycline or doxycycline, cefodroxil, and a potentiated sulfonamide. The drug most commonly associated with resolution appeared to be clarithromycin. The duration of treatment ranged from 3 to 21 months (median 7 months).

Melioidosis and Tularemia

Melioidosis is caused by *Burkholderia (Pseudomonas) pseudomallei,* a bipolar, aerobic, gram-negative motile bacillus occurring predominantly in Southeast Asia, northern Australia, and the South Pacific. It is characterized by fever, myalgia, dermal abscesses, and epididymitis.[257] Effective antimicrobials include tetracyclines, chloramphenicol, trimethoprim–sulfonamide combinations, amoxicillin–clavulanic acid, and novobiocin–tetracycline. High doses of parenteral ceftazidime for 2 weeks has proved most effective; imipenem–cilastin may also be effective.

Tularemia, caused by *Francisella tularensis,* is a tick-transmitted disease of both dogs and cats.[258] Infection begins with localized lymphadenopathy followed by bacteremia and multiple organ involvement. Clinical signs vary and include fever, mucopurulent nasal or ocular discharge, abscess at the site of inoculation (or associated with lymphadenopathy), myalgia, shivering, and signs indicative of septicemia. Preferred antimicrobial therapy in human patients includes the aminoglycosides. Chloramphenicol or tetracyclines may be associated with relapses. The fluoroquinolones also may be effective.

RICKETTSIAL AND ANAPLASMID DISEASES

Rickettsial and *anaplasmid* organisms are fastidious, obligate intracellular parasites that appear as pleomorphic coccobacilli. They multiply by binary fission, contain both DNA and RNA, and are capable of synthetic and energy-producing reactions. Their life cycle involves insect reservoirs (primarily ticks) and mammals.[259] The rickettsial organisms have undergone reclassification such that two families exist: *Anaplasmataceae* and *Rickettsiaceae*. *Ehrlichia* has recently been reclassified from the family Rickettsiaceae to the family Anaplasmataceae; other animal pathogens in this family include *Anaplasma* and *Neorickettsia.* Reclassification has resulted in renaming *Ehrlichia platys* as *Anaplasma platys, Ehrlichia risticii* as *Neorickettsia risticii,* and *Cowdria* sp. as *Ehrlichia* sp. The family Rickettsiaceae is limited to Rickettsia. *Coxiella burnetii,* the causative agent of Q fever, is not included in either group and stands out additionally because of its robust nature outside of host cells and presentation of disease.[259]

Although advances in recent years have increased our knowledge regarding the physiology of these organisms and the pathophysiology of the disease, much information is still missing. The pathogenesis of the other rickettsial organisms reflects vasculitis caused by proliferation of the organisms in endothelial cells. Diagnosis is generally based on serologic testing. Serologic evidence of disease generally does not, however, occur until several weeks after clinical signs have developed.

Ehrlichiosis

Pathophysiology

Diseases caused by *Ehrlichia* can be varied in presentation and often mimic other diseases, making diagnosis difficult.[236] Disease can present in an acute, clinical, or subclinical phase. The acute phase lasts 2 to 4 weeks, during which the organisms replicate in the mononuclear phagocytic cells of the liver, spleen, and lymph nodes. Infected cells travel to the lung, kidney, and meninges, where endothelial inflammation can occur. Nonspecific clinical signs during this phase include fever, anorexia, weight loss, ocular and nasal discharge, and edema. Additional clinical signs depend on the severity of infection in each organ and include dyspnea, neurologic abnormalities, and lymphadenopathy. Platelet consumption, sequestration, and destruction contribute to thrombocytopenia, which often characterizes this phase. Leukopenia and anemia become more likely as the disease progresses. The subclinical phase occurs at 6 to 9 weeks and is characterized by pancytopenia. An adequate immune response should eradicate the disease, but immunoincompetence leads to chronic infection. Clinical signs in chronic disease vary with the severity of infection and can range from asymptomatic to severe. Bleeding tendencies, anemia, chronic weight loss, and debilitation are nonspecific clinical signs. Abdominal tenderness, ophthalmic complications (anterior uveitis, retinal detachment), and neurologic abnormalities may be present. Secondary infections (bacterial and, less commonly, fungal) may reflect immune suppression. Diagnosis is based on clinical laboratory changes and serologic diagnosis using indirect fluorescent antibody. Treatment is oriented toward eradication of the infecting organism and supportive therapy based on clinical signs. Therapy in chronic stages may also require targeting opportunistic infections in the immunosuppressed animal.

Causative Organisms

Disease caused by canine ehrlichiosis generally targets blood-forming units. Ehrlichiosis is caused by *E. canis,* the brown dog tick, and *Rhipicephalus sanguineus* serves as the primary insect vector. Other infections carried by this vector *(Babesia canis* and *Hepatozoon canis)* can simultaneously infect the host. *E. canis* is a pleomorphic organism that circulates in peripheral monocytes. Infection is transmitted through the saliva of the tick into the bloodstream of the host. Transmission has also occurred between hosts (patients) through blood transfusions. Although the dog is the primary target of *E. canis*, infections in cats is suspected but has not yet been documented.[260] Other *Ehrlichia* organisms infecting animals include *Ehrlichia chaffeensis* in dogs (mononuclear cells), *Ehrlichia ewingii* (granulocytes, dogs), *Anaplasma phagocyophila* (formerly *Ehrlichia equi*, probably responsible for a significant number of granulocytic ehrlichiosis in dogs in northeastern and upper Midwestern states and California[260]), *Anaplasma platys* (previously *Ehrlichia platys*; platelets in dogs) and *N. risticcia* (formerly *Ehrlichia risticcia*), which can cause infection in monocytic and granulocytic cells of dogs or cats (or horses).

Antimicrobial and Supportive Therapy

Doxycycline or minocycline are the treatment of choice (10 mg/kg orally every 24 hours for 4 weeks) for ehrlichiosis.[260] Although fluoroquinolones (e.g., enrofloxacin) appear to be effective for the treatment of *Rickettsia rickettsii* at a dose of 3 mg/kg orally twice daily, based on experimental infection, they do not appear to be effective at 10 mg/kg orally twice daily for the treatment of ehrlichiosis.[261] The effects of combination therapy with doxycycline and enrofloxacin on antimicrobial efficacy against ehrlichiosis have not been established, but the combination might be considered for patients that do not respond to doxycycline. Chloramphenicol is also effective against ehrlichiosis but is less ideal clinically than tetracyclines and enrofloxacin; its use might be limited to puppies if tetracyclines are not acceptable because of brown discoloration of teeth. However, doxycycline is less likely to cause discoloration (see Chapter 7). Imidocarb diproprionate is as effective as doxycycline (5 mg/kg intramuscularly followed by a second injection 2 weeks later), but care must be taken to minimize the side effects of this drug. It recently has been approved in the United States. It should be used to treat patients that have not responded to doxycycline or enrofloxacin. Because chloramphenicol targets a different ribosomal target site than doxycycline, combination therapy with the two drugs might be considered but should be based on clinical trials,

Imidocarb (6.6 mg/kg intramuscularly, two injections, 2 weeks apart) was ineffective in clearing *Ehrlichia* in dogs (n = 10 treated and n = 5 untreated controls) experimentally infected.[262] However, twice-daily administration of doxycycline at 5 mg/kg orally bid for 4 weeks cleared five of the imidocarb-treated dogs; two control dogs spontaneously cleared as well.[263]

Supportive therapy for ehrlichiosis includes fluid and electrolyte therapy; blood or blood component transfusions; hematinics (vitamins, iron if bleeding has been extensive); and, less commonly, drugs that stimulate erythropoiesis. Anabolic steroids should be used cautiously in the presence of liver involvement. Short-term glucocorticoids may be indicated in severe cases to minimize immune-mediated destruction of platelets or immune-mediated arthropathies, vasculitis, or meningitis. Serologic titers generated by ehrlichiosis are not protective, and reinfection may occur. Platelet counts may decrease despite rapid clinical improvement in response to doxycycline. Serum antibodies may not be useful because they remain elevated for months after therapy. Monitoring PCR may be the best method of evaluating therapeutic success; because it cannot differentiate dead from live organisms, a strong positive the week after completing doxycycline suggests persistent infection.[260]

Long-term prophylaxis might be considered in endemic areas or kennels and consists of tetracycline (3 to 6 mg/kg once daily orally) or reposital tetracycline (200 mg intramuscularly twice weekly). Davoust and coworkers[264] reported a prophylactic program based on French military dogs (614; average weight 29 kg) returning after 4 months of stay in an area highly endemic for ehrlichiosis. The study was coupled with detection of plasma doxycycline concentrations (n = 124 dogs) and its association with chemoprevention. Dogs were treated with doxycycline (100 mg [approximately 3 mg/kg] by mouth qd). In 10 of these dogs, the time course of doxycycline was determined. Peak doxycycline (approximately 5 hours) in these dogs ranged from about 1 to 1.7 μg/mL; half-life approximated 9 hours. The drug was assayed by high-performance liquid chromatography; the peak concentrations were based on total drug. At 24 hours, concentrations ranged from 0.26 to 0.4 μg/mL. Spot checks on 114 dogs in the field yielded concentrations that were above 2 μg/mL. Of the 614 dogs, 4% (n = 24) were seropositive; concentrations were not determined in these dogs. They were asymptomatic. Based on a previous report that demonstrated an MIC of equal to or less than 0.03 μg/mL for ehrlichia and doxycycline, the authors concluded that the chemoprevention program was appropriate.

Rocky Mountain Spotted Fever

Causative Organism

The causative agent of Rocky Mountain spotted fever is *R. rickettsii*. It is transmitted primarily by *Dermacentor* species, with the American dog tick being the principal vector in the eastern United States and the wood tick the principal vector in the western United States. Transmission of disease requires tick attachment to the host for at least 5 hours and up to 20 hours; thus the disease might be prevented by routine checks of the animal's body.[265] The incidence of infection in dogs caused by this organism only now is being appreciated. Unrecognized and untreated illness can lead to death, although the severity of clinical signs depends, in part, on the degree and location of the initial vascular damage induced by the organisms. Diagnosis is complicated by cross-reactivity to several nonpathogenic members of *Rickettsia* and should be based on both acute and convalescent serum titers or direct immunofluorescence in skin biopsy material.[265]

Pathophysiology

Organisms are transmitted through the saliva of the tick into the bloodstream, where they replicate in endothelial cells of small blood vessels and capillaries. Damaged endothelial cells become inflamed. Vessels become permeable, causing extravasation of fluid into perivascular spaces. Depending on the severity of infection, clinical signs may indicate edema, hemorrhage, hypotension, or shock. Infection in vessels of the CNS may lead to neurologic signs and a more rapid deterioration of clinical signs.

Other clinical signs vary and may require medical management, depending on which organs are infected: Cardiac abnormalities may include conduction abnormalities or other life-threatening arrhythmias; the respiratory system may be characterized by clinical signs reflecting pulmonary edema, which is minimally responsive to diuretic therapy; ocular abnormalities range from subconjunctival inflammation to retinal detachment; and, in severe cases, acute renal failure occurs as a result of decreased renal perfusion. Severe inflammation causing vascular obstruction can lead to gangrene of peripheral limbs, ears, lips, scrotum, or mammary glands. Other less specific clinical abnormalities include fever, anorexia, depression, muscle pain, polyarthritis, and weight loss.[265] In addition to increases in liver enzymes and serum bilirubin, clinical laboratory tests may reveal the need to treat thrombocytopenia; severe acute infection may also cause leukopenia and anemia. Hypoproteinemia, azotemia, hyponatremia, and hypocalcemia may also be present. Treatment is focused on both eradication of the organisms and supportive therapy of derangements in the infected body system.

Antimicrobial and Supportive Therapy

Tetracyclines remain the treatment of choice for rickettsial infections. Although tetracycline may be sufficient, drugs characterized by better lipophilicity (e.g., doxycycline, minocycline) may be more advantageous. Chloramphenicol is also effective, but less so than tetracyclines. Fluoroquinolones are also effective experimentally,[265] although clinical efficacy has not been established. Combinations of both doxycycline and enrofloxacin may be additive to synergistic, but the effects of this antimicrobial combination on rickettsial organisms has not been established. Clinical response should be rapid except in cases with severe vascular sequelae (i.e., neurologic or renal damage). Supportive therapy should target abnormalities previously described. These include electrolyte abnormalities and replacement of colloid (protein). Vascular permeability, however, will complicate volume replacement (with either crystalloids or colloids) and, if too intensive, may contribute to peripheral (including pulmonary) edema.

Breitschwerdt et al.[266] reported the efficacy of azithromycin (3 mg/kg by mouth qd) and trovofloxacin (5 mg/kg by mouth bid) compared with doxycycline (5 mg/kg by mouth bid) in dogs (n = 16; 4- to 5-month-old beagles; four per group, including untreated control) experimentally infected with *R. rickettsii*. Treatment duration was for 7 days (starting day 5 post infection), except for azithromycin, which was used for only 3 days. Drug concentrations were measured after the last treatment, with peak concentrations (μg/mL) evident at 1 hour: 0.15 (azithromycin), 3.5 (doxycycline), and 1 (trovafloxacin). Whereas all three antimicrobials caused rapid improvement in a number of outcome measures, ocular lesions were rare with doxycycline or trovafloxacin but present in all azithromycin-treated dogs. Based on PCR, DNA was present though day 21 after infection, although organisms were not isolated. The authors concluded that fluoroquinolones might be a reasonable alternative to doxycycline. Although azithromycin was discouraged as a first-line treatment by the authors, the half-life of the drug was not known at the time of the study, leading to the shorter duration of therapy. As such, azithromycin (which has a 29-hour half-life in dogs) would not have yet reached steady state at the time that it was discontinued. Further, a dose used was lower than that currently recommended; as such, azithromycin might be reconsidered through controlled studies.

Other Rickettsial-Like Diseases

Canine cyclic thrombocytopenia is caused by *E. platys,* an organism that replicates in platelets. Cyclic thrombocytopenia occurs at 10- to 14-day intervals. Both platelet numbers (as low as 20,000) and aggregation are impaired. Treatment should be with tetracyclines as described for *E. canis. Neorickettsia helminthoeca* is one of the causative agents of salmon poisoning disease, which is transmitted after ingestion of fish containing the trematode vector. Like other rickettsial diseases, it is treated with tetracyclines. Hemobartonellosis is caused by a hemotrophic organism that causes acute or chronic anemia in dogs or cats. Damaged red blood cells are removed by the host's immune system. The host is not able to resolve infection without treatment. Tetracyclines are the drug of choice. Supportive therapy may include glucocorticoids at immunosuppressive doses. Metronidazole (40 mg/kg orally once daily for 3 weeks) has been used to treat resistant infections.[265]

REFERENCES

1. Morley PS, Apley MD, Besser TE, et al: American College of Veterinary Internal Medicine: Antimicrobial drug use in veterinary medicine, *J Vet Intern Med* 19(4):617–629, 2005.
2. Tunkel AR, Scheld MW: Acute meningitis. In Mandell GL, editor: *Mandell, Douglas, and Bennett's principles and practice of infectious diseases*, ed 7, New York, 2010, Churchill Livingstone.
3. Lutsar I, McCracken GH, Friedland IR: Antibiotic pharmacodynamics in cerebrospinal fluid, *Clin Infect Dis* 27:1117–1119, 1998.
4. Nau R, et al: Pharmacokinetic optimization of the treatment of bacterial central nervous system infections, *Clin Pharmacokinet* 35:223–246, 1998.
5. Lutsar I, McCracken GH Jr, Friedland IR: Antibiotic pharmacodynamics in cerebrospinal fluid, *Clin Infect Dis* 27(5):1117–1127, 1998.
6. LeFrock JL, Prince RA, Richards ML: Penetration of antimicrobials into the cerebrospinal fluid and brain. In Ristuccia AM, Cuhna BA, editors: *Antimicrobial therapy*, New York, 1984, Raven Press, pp 397–413.
7. O'Brien DP, Axlund TW: Brain disease. In Ettinger SJ, Feldman EC, editors: *Textbook of veterinary internal medicine*, ed 6, St Louis, 2005, Saunders.
8. Shembesh NM, Elbargathy SM, Kashbur IM, et al: Dexamethasone as an adjunctive treatment of bacterial meningitis, *Indian J Pediatr* 64(4):517–522, 1997.
9. van de Beek D, de Gans J, McIntyre P, et al: Steroids in adults with acute bacterial meningitis: a systematic review, *Lancet Infect Dis* 4:139–143, 2004.
10. Tunkel AR, Hartman BJ, Kaplan SL, et al: Practice guidelines for the management of bacterial meningitis, *Clin Infect Dis* 39(9):1267–1284, 2004.
11. Whitley RD: Canine and feline primary ocular bacterial infections, *Vet Clin North Am* 30:1151–1167, 2000.

12. Owen MR, Moores AP, Cox RJ: Management of MRSA septic arthritis in a dog using a gentamicin-impregnated collagen sponge, *J Small Anim Prac* 45:609–612, 2004.
13. Kern TJ: Antibacterial agents for ocular therapeutictics, *Vet Clin North Am Small Anim Pract* 34:655–668, 2004.
14. Ramsey D: Feline *Chlamydia* and calicivirus infections, *Vet Clin North Am Small Anim Pract* 30(5):1015–1028, 2001.
15. Stiles J: Feline herpes virus, *Vet Clin North Am Small Anim Pract* 30(5):1001–1014, 2001.

15a. Sturgess CP, Gruffydd-Jones TJ, Harbour DA, et al: Controlled study of the efficacy of clavulanic acid-potentiated amoxycillin in the treatment of *Chlamydia psittaci* in cats, *Vet Rec* 149(3):73–6, 2001.

16. Owen WMF, Sturgess CP, Harbour DA, et al: Efficacy of azithromycin for the treatment of chlamydophilosis, *J Feline Med Sur* 5:302–311, 2003.
17. Radlinsky MG, Mason DE: Diseases of the ear. In Ettinger SJ, Feldman EC, editors: *Textbook of veterinary internal medicine*, ed 6, St Louis, 2005, Saunders.
18. Petersen AD, Walker RD, Bowman MM, et al: Frequency of isolation and antimicrobial susceptibility patterns of *Staphylococcus intermedius* and *Pseudomonas aeruginosa* isolates from canine skin and ear samples over a 6-year period (1992-1997), *J Am Anim Hosp Assoc* 38:407–413, 2002.
19. Morris DO, Rook KA, Shofer FS, et al: Screening of *Staphylococcus aureus, Staphylococcus intermedius*, and *Staphylococcus schleiferi* isolates obtained from small companion animals for antimicrobial resistance: a retrospective review of 749 isolates (2003-04), *European Society of Veterinary Dermatology (ESVD)* 17:332–337, 2006.
20. Rubin J, Walker RD, Blickenstaff K, et al: Antimicrobial resistance and genetic characterization of fluoroquinolone resistance of *Pseudomonas aeruginosa* isolated from canine infections, *Vet Microbiol* 131(1-2):164–172, 2008.
21. Schick AE, Angus JC, Coyner KS: Variability of laboratory identification and antibiotic susceptibility reporting of *Pseudomonas* spp. isolates from dogs with chronic otitis externa, *Vet Dermatol* (Apr) 18(2):120–126, 2007.
22. Royschuk RAW: Management of otitis externa, *Vet Clin North Am Small Anim Pract* 26:921–951, 1994.
23. Weber PC, Roland PS, Hannley M, et al: The development of antibiotic resistant organisms with the use of ototopical medications, *Otolaryngol Head Neck Surg* 130:S89–S94, 2004.
24. Morris DO: Medical therapy of otitis externa and otitis media, *Vet Clin North Am Small Anim Pract* 34:541–555, 2004.
25. Sparks TA, Kemp DT, Wooley RE, et al: Antimicrobial effect of combinations of EDTA-Tris and amikacin or neomycin on the microorganisms associated with otitis externa in dogs, *Vet Res Commun* 18(4):241–249, 1994.
26. Ghibaudo G, Cornegliani L, Martina P: Evaluation of the in vivo effects of Tris-EDTA and chlorhexidine digluconate 0.15% solution in chronic bacterial otitis externa: 11 cases, *Vet Dermatol* 15, 65-65:2004.
27. Walsh P, Aeling JL, Huff L, et al: Hypothalamic-pituitary-adrenal axis suppression by superpotent topical steroids, *J Am Acad Dermatol* 28:618–622, 1993.
28. Rougier S, Borell D, Pheulpin S, et al: A comparative study of two antimicrobial/anti-inflammatory formulations in the treatment of canine otitis externa, *Vet Dermatol* 16(5):299–307, 2005.
29. Gogghelf LN: Diagnosis and treatment of otitis media in dogs and cats, *Vet Clin Small Anim Prac* 34:469–488, 2004.
30. Hettlich BF, Boothe HW, Simpson RB, et al: Effect of tympanic cavity evacuation and flushing on microbial isolates during total ear canal ablation with lateral bulla osteotomy in dogs, *J Am Vet Med Assoc* 227:748–755, 2005.
31. Dyer Inzana K: Peripheral nerve disorders. In Ettinger SJ, Feldman EC, editors: *Textbook of veterinary internal medicine*, ed 6, St Louis, 2005, Saunders.
32. Pickrell JA, Oehme FW, Cash WC: Ototoxicity in dogs and cats, *Semin Vet Med Surg Small Anim* 8:42–49, 1993.
33. Ihrke PJ: Bacterial infections of the skin. In Greene C, editor: *Infectious diseases of the dog and cat*, Philadelphia, 1990, Saunders, pp 72–79.
34. Ihrke PJ: *Bacterial skin disease in the dog: a guide to canine pyoderma*, Trenton, New Jersey, 1996, Bayer Corporation, Veterinary Learning Systems.
35. Ihrke PJ: Deep pyoderma. In Ihrke PJ, editor: *Bacterial skin disease in the dog: a guide to canine pyoderma*, Trenton, New Jersey, 1996, Bayer Corporation, Veterinary Learning Systems, pp 35–44.
36. White PD: *Understanding and treating skin inflammation*, Trenton, New Jersey, 1996, Bayer Corporation, Veterinary Learning Systems, *Proc North Am Vet Conf Int Symp*, pp 5–12.
37. Lloyd D: *Treating staphylococcal skin disease in the dog*, Trenton, New Jersey, 1996, Bayer Corporation, Veterinary Learning Systems, *Proc North Am Vet Conf Int Symp*, pp 13–20.
38. Cox HU, Schmeer N, Newman SS: Protein A in *Staphylococcus intermedius* isolates from dogs and cats, *Am J Vet Res* 47:1881–1884, 1986.
39. Morales CA, Schultz KT, DeBoer DJ: Antistaphylococcal antibodies in dogs with recurrent staphylococcal pyoderma, *Vet Immunol Immunopathol* 42:137–147, 1994.
40. Tulkens PM: Accumulation and subcellular distribution of antibiotics in macrophages in relation to activity against intracellular bacteria. In Fass RJ, editor: *Ciprofloxacin in pulmonology*, San Francisco, 1990, W Zuckschwerdt Verlag, pp 12–20.
41. Aucoin DP: Intracellular-intraphagocytic dynamics of fluoroquinolone antibiotics: a comparative review, *Compend Contin Educ Pract Vet* 18(2) (Suppl):9–13, 1996.
42. DeBoer DJ: Immunomodulatory effects of staphylococcal antigen and antigen-antibody complexes on canine mononuclear and polymorphonuclear leukocytes, *Am J Vet Res* 55:1690–1696, 1994.
43. Holm BR, Petersson U, Morner A: Antimicrobial resistance in staphylococci from canine pyoderma: a prospective, *Vet Rec* 151:600–605, 2002.
44. Abraham JL, Morris DO, Griffeth GC, et al: Surveillance of healthy cats and cats with inflammatory skin disease for colonization of the skin by methicillin-resistant coagulase-positive staphylococci and *Staphylococcus schleiferi* ssp. schleiferi, *European Society of Veterinary Dermatology (ESVD)* 18:252–259, 2007.
45. Griffeth GC, Morris DO, Abraham JL, et al: Screening for skin carriage of methicillin-resistant coagulase-positive staphylococci and *Staphylococcus schleiferi* in dogs with healthy and inflamed skin, *European Society of Veterinary Dermatology (ESVD)* 19:142–149, 2008.
46. Hillier A, Alcorn JR, Cole LK: Pyoderma caused by Pseudomonas aeruginosa infection in dogs: 20 cases, *European Society of Veterinary Dermatology (ESVD)* 17:432–439, 2006.
47. Frank LA, Kania SA, Hnilica KA, et al: Isolation of *Staphylococcus schleiferi* from dogs with pyoderma, *J Am Vet Med Assoc* 222:451–454, 2003.
48. Bes M, Guerin-Faublee V, Freney J, et al: Isolation of *Staphylococcus schleiferi* subspecies coagulans from two cases of canine pyoderma, *Vet Rec* 150:487–488, 2002.
49. Kania SA, Williamson NL, Frank LA: Methicillin resistance of staphyloccci isolated from the skin of dogs with pyoderma, *J Am Vet Med Assoc* 65:1268–1285, 2004.
50. Hnilica K: Staphylococcal pyoderma, an emerging problem, *Compend Contin Educ Pract Vet* 26:560–568, 2004.
51. Kunkle GA, Sundlof S, Deisling K: Adverse side effects of oral antibacterial therapy in dogs and cats: an epidemiologic study of pet owners' observations, *J Am Anim Hosp Assoc* 31:46–55, 1995.

52. Cribb AE, Lee BL, Trepanier L, et al: Adverse reactions to sulphonamide and sulphonamide-trimethoprim antimicrobials: clinical syndromes and pathogenesis, *Adverse Drug React Toxicol Rev* 15:9–50, 1996.
53. Neu HC: Principles of antimicrobial use. In Wecker L, editor: *Brody's human pharmacology: molecular to clinical*, Philadelphia, 2009, Mosby.
54. Valencia IC, Kirsner RS, Kerdel FA: Microbiologic evaluation of skin wounds: alarming trend toward antibiotic resistance in an inpatient dermatology service during a 10-year period, *J Am Acad Dermatol* 50:845–849, 2004.
55. Pellerin JL, Bourdeau P, Sebbag H, et al: Epidemiosurveillance of antimicrobial compound resistance of Staphylococcus intermedius in clinical isolates from canine pyodermas, *Comp Immunol Microbiol Infect Dis* 21:115–133, 1998.
56. Popovich K, Hota B, Rice T: Phenotypic prediction rule for community-associated methicillin-resistant, *Staphylococcus aureus, J Clin Microbiol* 45(7):2293–2295, 2007.
57. Weber SG, Gold HS, Hoper DC, et al: Fluoroquinolones and the risk for methicillin-resistant *Staphylococcus aureus* in hospitalized patients, *Emerg Infect Dis* 9(11):1415–1422, 2003.
58. Kung K, Riond JL, Wanner M: Pharmacokinetics of enrofloxacin and its metabolite ciprofloxacin after intravenous and oral administration of enrofloxacin in dogs, *J Vet Pharmacol Ther* 16:462–468, 1993.
59. Stegemann MR, Sherington J, Blanchflower S: Pharmacokinetics and pharmacodynamics of cefovecin in dogs, *J Vet Pharmacol Therap* 29:501–511, 2006.
60. Vancutsem PM, Babish JC, Schwark WS: The fluoroquinolone antimicrobials: structure, antimicrobial activity, pharmacokinetics, clinical use in domestic animals and toxicity, *Cornell Vet* 80:173–186, 1990.
61. Wetzstein HG: The in vitro postantibiotic effect of enrofloxacin, Bologna, Italy, *Proc 18th World Buiatrics Congress* 18:615–618, 1994.
62. Caprile KA: The cephalosporin antimicrobial agents: a comprehensive review, *J Vet Pharmacol Ther* 11:1–32, 1988.
63. Hawkins E, Boothe DM, Guinn A, et al: Accumulation of enrofloxacin and its active metabolite, ciprofloxacin, in canine alveolar macrophages, *J A Vet Pharmcol Ther* 21:18–23, 1998.
64. Boeckh A, Boothe DM, Wilkie S, et al: Time course of enrofloxacin and its active metabolite in peripheral leukocytes of dogs, *Vet Ther* 2:334–344, 2001.
65. Boothe HW, Jones SA, Wilkie WS, et al: Evaluation of the concentration of marbofloxacin in alveolar macrophages and pulmonary epithelial lining fluid after administration in dogs, *Am J Vet Res* 66:1770–1774, 2005.
66. Boothe DM: *The accumulation of pradofloxacin in phagocytes*, Berlin, 2006, Abstract, 1st International Verafloxs Symposium, 18.
67. Boothe DM, Boeckh A, Boothe HW: Evaluation of the distribution of enrofloxacin by circulating leukocytes to sites of inflammation in dogs, *Am J Vet Res* 70(1):16–22, 2009.
68. Stegemann M, Heukamp U, Scheer M, et al: Kinetics of antibacterial activity after administration of enrofloxacin in dog serum and skin: in vitro susceptibility of field isolates, *Suppl Compend Contin Educ Pract Vet* 18(2):30–34, 1996.
69. Ganiere JP, Medaille C, Etore F: In vitro antimicrobial activity of orbifloxacin against *Staphylococcus intermedius* isolates from canine skin and ear infections, *Res Vet Sci* 77:67–71, 2004.
70. Bloom PB, Rosser EJ: Efficacy of once-daily clindamycin hydrochloride in the treatment of superficial bacterial pyoderma in dogs, *J Am Anim Hosp Assoc* 37:537–542, 2001.
71. Ramadinha RR, Ribeiro SS, Peixoto PV, et al: *Evaluation of the efficiency of azithromycin (azitromicina) for treating bacterial pyodermas in dogs*, 2002, World Small Animal Veterinary Association Congress.
71a. Senturk S, Ozel E, Sen A: Clinical efficacy of rifampicin for treatment of canine pyoderma, *Acta Vet Brno* 74:117–122, 2005.
72. Miller WH: *The use of enrofloxacin in canine and feline pyodermas and otitis in dogs*, 1992, Proceedings 1st Int Symposium on Baytril, p 33-39.
73. Paradis M, Lemay S, Scott DW, et al: Efficacy of enrofloxacin in the treatment of canine pyoderma, *Vet Dermatol* 1:123–127, 1990.
74. Paradis M, Abbey L, Baker B, et al: Evaluation of the clinical efficacy of marbofloxacin (Zeniquin) tablets for the treatment of canine pyoderma: an open clinical trial, *Vet Dermatol* 12:163–169, 2001.
75. Horspool LJ, Van Laar P, Van Den Bos R, et al: Treatment of canine pyoderma with ibafloxacin and marbofloxacin fluoroquinolones with different pharmacokinetic profiles, *J Vet Pharmacol Therap* 27:147–153, 2004.
76. Stegemann MR, Coati N, Passmore CA, et al: Clinical efficacy and safety of cefovecin in the treatment of canine pyoderma and wound infections, *J Small Anim Pract* 48:378–386, 2007.
77. Mueller RS, Stephan B: Pradofloxacin in the treatment of canine deep pyoderma: a multicentred, blinded, randomized parallel trial, *European Society of Veterinary Dermatology (ESVD)* 18:144–151, 2007.
78. White SD, Bordeau PB, Blumstein P, et al: Feline acne and results of treatment with mupirocin in an open clinical trial: 25 cases (1994-1996), *Vet Dermatol* 8:157–164, 1997.
79. Kwochka KW, Kowalski JJ: Prophylactic efficacy of four antibacterial shampoos against *Staphylococcus intermedius* in dogs, *J Am Vet Med Assoc* 52:115–118, 1991.
80. Nolting S, Bräutigam M: Clinical relevance of the antibacterial activity of terbinafine: a contralateral comparison between 1% terbinafine cream and 0.1% gentamicin sulphate cream in pyoderma, *Br J Dermatol* 126:56–60, 2006.
81. Burkhart CG, Burkhart CN, Isham N: Synergistic antimicrobial activity by combining an allylamine with benzoyl peroxide with expanded coverage against yeast and bacterial species, *Br J Dermatol* 154:341–344, 2006.
82. Thompson LA, Grieshaber TL, Glickman L, et al: Human recombinant interferon alpha-2b for management of idiopathic recurrent superficial pyoderma in dogs: a pilot study, *Vet Ther* 5:75–81, 2004.
83. Viking HO, Frendin J: Analgesic effect of meloxicam in canine acute dermatitis—a pilot study, *Acta Vet Scand* 43:247–252, 2002.
84. Špruček F, Svoboda M, Toman M, et al: Therapy of canine deep pyoderma with cephalexins and immunomodulators, *Acta Vet Brno* 76:469–474, 2007.
85. White SD, Rosychuk RAW, Stewart U, et al: Juvenile cellulitis in dogs: 15 cases (1979–1988), *J Am Vet Med Assoc* 195: 1609–1611, 1989.
86. Scott DW, Miller WT, Griffin CE: *Small animal dermatology*, ed 6, Toronto, 2001, Saunders, pp 1163–1167.
87. Hutchings SM: Juvenile cellulitis in a puppy, *Can Vet J* 44(5):418–419, 2003.
88. Wysocki AB: Evaluating and managing open skin wounds: colonization versus infection, *AACN Clinical Issues: Advanced Practice in Acute and Critical Care* 13(3):382–397, 2002.
89. Spann CT, Tutrone WD, Weinberg JM, et al: Topical antibacterial agents for wound care: a primer, *Dermatol Surg* 29(6):620–626, 2003.
90. Drosou A, Falabella A, Kirsner RS: Antiseptics on wounds: an area of controversy, *Wounds,* May 10, 2003. Accessed November 12, 2009, at www.woundsresearch.com/article/1585.
91. Aiello AE, Larson E: Antibacterial cleaning and hygiene products as an emerging risk factor for antibiotic resistance in the community, *Lancet Infect Dis* 3:501–506, 2003.

92. Meyers B, Schoeman JP, Goddard A, et al: The bacteriology and antimicrobial susceptibility of infected and non-infected dog bite wounds: fifty cases, *Vet Microbiol* 127:360–368, 2008.
93. Love DN, Malik R, Norris JM: Bacteriological warfare amongst cats: what have we learned about cat bite infections? *Vet Microbiol* 74(3):179–193, 2000.
94. Mader JT, Calhoun J: Osteomyelitis. In Mandell GL, editor: *Mandell, Douglas, and Bennett's principles and practice of infectious diseases*, ed 7, New York, 2010, Churchill Livingstone.
95. Shuford JA, Steckelberg JM: Role of oral antimicrobial therapy in the management of osteomyelitis, *Curr Opin Infect Dis* 16:515–519, 2003.
96. Cunha BA, Crossling HR, Pasternak HS, et al: Penetration of cephalosporins into bone, *Infection* 12:80–84, 1984.
97. Sayegh AI: Polymethylmethacrylate beads for treating orthopedic infections, *Compend Contin Educ Pract Vet* 25(10):789–795, 2003.
98. Atilla A, Boothe HW, Tollett M, et al: In vitro elution of amikacin and vancomycin from impregnated plaster of paris beads, *Vet Surg* 39(6):715–721, 2010.
99. Neut D, van de Belt H, Stokroos I, et al: Biomaterial-associated infection of gentamicin-loaded PMMA beads in orthopaedic revision surgery, *J Antimicrob Chemother* 47:885–891, 2001.
100. Ham K, Griffon D, Seddighi M, et al: Clinical application of tobramycin-impregnated calcium sulfate beads in six dogs (2002-2004), *J Am Anim Hosp Assoc* 44:320–326, 2008.
101. Vinod MB, Matussek J, Curtis N, et al: Duration of antibiotics in children with osteomyelitis and septic arthritis, *J Paediatr Child Health* 38:363–367, 2002.
102. Stengel D, Bauwens K, Sehouli J, et al: Systematic review and meta-analysis of antibiotic therapy for bone and joint infections, *Lancet Infectious Diseases* 1:175–188, 2001.
103. Smith JW, Piercy EA: Bone and joint infections. In Mandell GL, Bennett JE, Dolin R, editors: *Principles and practice of infectious diseases*, New York, 1995, Churchill Livingstone, pp 1032–1038.
103a. Haddow LJ, Chandra Sekhar M, Hajela V, et al: Spontaneous Achilles tendon rupture in patients treated with levofloxacin, *J Antimicrob Chemother* 51(3):747–748, 2003.
104. Bartges JW: Urinary tract infections. In Ettinger SJ, Feldman EC, editors: *Textbook of veterinary internal medicine*, ed 6, St Louis, 2005, Saunders.
105. Ling GV, Norris CR, Franti CE, et al: Interrelations of organism prevalence, specimen collection method, and host age, sex, and breed among 8,354 canine urinary tract infections (1969-1995), *J Vet Intern Med* 15:341–347, 2001.
106. Seguin MA, Vaden SL, Altier C, et al: Persistent urinary tract infections and reinfections in 100 dogs (1989-1999), *J Vet Intern Med* 17:622–631, 2003.
107. Barsanti JA: Genitourinary infections. In Greene C, editor: *Infectious diseases of the dog and cat*, ed 3, St Louis, 2006, Saunders.
108. Lees GE: Bacterial urinary tract infections, *Vet Clin North Am Small Anim Pract* 26:297–316, 1996.
109. Sobel JD, Kaye D: Urinary tract infections. In Mandell GL, editor: *Mandell, Douglas, and Bennett's principles and practice of infectious diseases*, ed 5, Philadelphia, 2010, Churchill Livingstone.
110. Barsanti JA: Botulism. In Greene CE, editor: *Infectious diseases of the dog and cat*, ed 3, St Louis, 2006, Saunders.
111. Senior DF, Brown MB: The role of Mycoplasma species and Ureaplasma species in feline lower urinary tract disease, *Vet Clin North Am Small Anim Pract* 26:305–308, 1996.
112. Boothe D, Smaha T: Escherichia coli *antimicrobial resistance in small animals: the scope of the problem*, Louisville, KY, June 2006, Presented at the American College of Veterinary Internal Medicine, J Vet Intern Med, 2006.
113. Bailiff NL, Nelson RW, Feldman EC, et al: Frequency and risk factors for urinary tract infection in cats with diabetes mellitus, *J Vet Intern Med* 20:850–855, 2006.
114. Litster A, Moss S, Platell J, et al: Occult bacterial lower urinary tract infections in cats: urinalysis and culture findings, *Vet Microbiol* 136:130–134, 2009.
115. Boothe DM, Smaha T, Carpenter M et al: Emerging resistance in canine and feline Escherichia coli pathogens: a pilot surveillance study, Submitted to J Vet Int Med March 2009.
116. Torres SMF, Diaz SF, Nogueira SA, et al: Frequency of urinary tract infection among dogs with pruritic disorders receiving long-term glucocorticoid treatment, *J Am Vet Med Assoc* 227:243–349, 2005.
117. Senior DF, deMan P, Svanborg C: Serotype, hemolysin production and adherence characteristics of strains of Escherichia coli causing urinary tract infection in dogs, *Am J Vet Res* 53:494–498, 1992.
117a. Hatt JK, Rather PN: Role of bacterial biofilms in urinary tract infections, *Curr Top Microbiol Immunol* 322:163–192, 2008.
117b. Soto SM, Smithson A, Martinez JA, et al: Biofilm formation in uropathogenic Escherichia coli strains: relationship with prostatitis, urovirulence factors and antimicrobial resistance, *J Urol* 177(1):365–368, 2007.
117c. Roos V, Ulett GC, Schembri MA, et al: The asymptomatic bacteriuria Escherichia coli strain 83972 outcompetes uropathogenic E. coli strains in human urine, *Infect Immun* 74(1):615–624, 2006.
118. Siqueira AK, Ribeiro MG, Leite DS, et al: Virulence factors in Escherichia coli strains isolated from urinary tract infection and pyometra cases and from feces of healthy dogs, *Res Vet Sci* 86:206–210, 2009.
119. Soto SM, Smithson A, Martinez JA, et al: Biofilm formation in uropathogenic Escherichia coli strains: relationship with prostatitis, urovirulence factors and antimicrobial resistance, *J Urol* 177(1):365–368, 2007.
120. Kruger JM, Osborne CA, Vetna PJ, et al: Viral infections of the feline urinary tract, *Vet Clin North Am Small Anim Pract* 26:281–296, 1996.
121. Kruger JM, Osborne CA: The role of uropathogens in feline lower urinary tract disease. Clinical implications, *Vet Clin North Am Small Anim Pract* 23:101–123, 1993.
122. Drazenovich N, Ling GV, Foley J: Molecular investigation of Escherichia coli strains associated with apparently persistent urinary tract infection in dogs, *J Vet Intern Med* 18:301–306, 2004.
123. Freitag T, Squires RA, Schmid J, et al: Antibiotic sensitivity profiles do not reliably distinguish relapsing of persisting infections from reinfections in cats with chronic renal failure and multiple diagnoses of Escherichia coli urinary tract infection, *J Vet Intern Med* 20:245–249, 2006.
124. Barsanti JA, Shotts EB, Crowell WA, et al: Effect of therapy on susceptibility to urinary tract infection in male cats with indwelling urethral catheters, *J Vet Intern Med* 6:64–70, 1993.
125. Griffin DW, Gregory CR: Prevalence of bacterial urinary tract infection after perineal urethrostomy in cats, *J Am Vet Med Assoc* 100:681–684, 1992.
126. Lees GF: Use and misuse of indwelling urethral catheters, *Vet Clin North Am Small Anim Pract* 26:499–505, 1996b.
127. Ling GV, Granti CE, Ruby AL, et al: Epizootiologic evaluation and quantitative analysis of urinary calculi from 150 cats, *J Am Vet Med Assoc* 196:1459–1462, 1990.
128. Wadas B, Kuhn I, Lagerstedt AS, et al: Biochemical phenotypes of Escherichia coli in dogs: comparison of isolates isolated from bitches suffering from pyometra and urinary tract infection with isolates from faeces of healthy dogs, *Vet Microbiol* 52:293–300, 1996.
129. Batamuz EK, Kristensen F: Urinary tract infection: the role of canine transmissible venereal tumor, *J Small Anim Pract* 37:276–279, 1996.

130. Oluoch AO, Kim CH, Weisiger RM, et al: Nonenteric Escherichia coli isolates from dogs: 674 cases (1990-1998), *J Am Vet Med Assoc* 218(5):732, 2001.
131. Boothe DM, Boeckh A, Simpson RB, et al: Comparison of pharmacodynamic and pharmacokinetic indices of efficacy for 5 fluoroquinolones toward pathogens of dogs and cats, *J Vet Intern Med* 20:1297-1306, 2006.
132. Sanchez S, McCrackin Stevenson MA, Hudson CR, et al: Characterization of multidrug resistant Eschericia coli isolates associated with nosocomial infection in dogs, *J Clin Microbiol* 3586-3595, 2002.
133. Cooke CL, Singer RS, Jang SS, et al: Enrofloxacin resistance in Eschericia coli isolated from dogs with urinary tract infections, *J Am Vet Med Assoc* 220:190-192, 2002.
134. Shaheen BW, Boothe DM, Wang C: The contribution of gyrA mutation and efflux pumps to fluoroquinolone resistance and the emergence of multi-drug resistance, in canine and feline clinical E. coli isolates from US, Accepted, *Am J Vet Res*, 2010.
135. Hooton T: Fluoroquinolones and resistance in the treatment of uncomplicated urinary tract infection, *Int J Antimicrob Agents* 22:S65-S72, 2003.
135a. Hubka P, Boothe DM: Susceptibility of multidrug resistant canine and feline Escherichia coli isolates to fosfomycin, Submitted to *Vet Microbiol*, May 2010.
136. Barsanti JA, Blue J, Edmunds J: Urinary tract infection due to indwelling bladder catheters in dogs and cats, *J Am Vet Med Assoc* 187:384-388, 1985.
137. Smarick SD, Haskins SC, Aldrich J: Incidence of catheter associated urinary tract infections among dogs in a small animal intensive care unit, *J Am Vet Med Assoc* 224:1936-1940, 2004.
138. Godfrey H, Fraczyk L: Preventing and managing catheter-associated urinary tract infections, *Br J Community Nurs* 10(5):205-206, 208-212:2005.
139. Wyndaele JJ: Complications of intermittent catheterization: their prevention and treatment, *Spinal Cord* 40:536-541, 2002.
140. Nicolle L: Best pharmacological practice: urinary tract infections, *Expert Opin Pharmacother* 4(5):693-704, 2003.
141. Schito GC: Why fosfomycin trometamol as first line therapy for uncomplicated UTI? *Int J Antimicrob* 22:S79-S83, 2003.
142. Baquero F: Low-level antibacterial resistance: a gateway to clinical resistance, *Drug Resist Updat* 4:93-105, 2001.
143. Rogers KS, Lees GE, Simpson RB: Effects of single-dose and three-day trimethoprim-sulfadiazine and amikacin treatment of induced Escherichia coli urinary tract infections in dogs, *Am J Vet Res* 49:345-349, 1988.
144. Litster A, Moss S, Honnery M, et al: Clinical efficacy and palatability of pradofloxacin 2.5% oral suspension for the treatment of bacterial lower urinary tract infections in cats, *J Vet Intern Med* 21:990-993, 2007.
145. Passmore CA, Sherington J, Stegeman MR: Efficacy and safety of cefovecin (Convenia™) for the treatment of urinary tract infections in dogs, *J Small Anim Prac* 48:139-144, 2007.
146. Gunn-Moore DA, Shenoy CM: Oral glucosamine and the management of feline idiopathic cystitis, *J Feline Med Surg* 6: 219-225, 2004.
147. Wallius BM, Tidholm AE: Use of pentosan polysulphate in cats with idiopathic, non-obstructive lower urinary tract disease: a double-blind, randomised, placebo-controled trial, *J Feline Med Surg* 11(6):409-412, 2009.
148. Lenoir-Wijnkoop I, Sanders ME, Cabana MD, et al: Probiotic and prebiotic influence beyond the intestinal tract, *Nutr Rev* 65(11):469-489, 2007.
149. Linde-Forsberg C: Abnormalities in pregnancy, parturition and periparturient period. In Ettinger SJ, Feldman EC, editors: *Textbook of veterinary internal medicine*, ed 6, St Louis, 2005, Saunders.
150. Root Kustritz MV: Cystic endometrial hyperplasia and pyometra. In Ettinger SJ, Feldman EC, editors: *Textbook of veterinary internal medicine*, ed 6, St Louis, 2005, Saunders.
151. Hagman R, Kühn I: Escherichia coli strains isolated from the uterus and urinary bladder of bitches suffering from pyometra: comparison by restriction enzyme digestion and pulsed-field gel electrophoresis, *Vet Microbiol* 84:143-153, 2002.
152. Bergogne-Bérézin E: Pharmacokinetics of antibiotics in respiratory secretions. In Pennington JE, editor: *Respiratory infections: diagnosis and management*, ed 2, New York, 1988, Raven Press, pp 608-631.
153. Braga PC: Antibiotic penetrability into bronchial mucus: pharmacokinetic and clinical considerations, *Curr Ther Res Clin Exp* 49(2):300-327, 1989.
154. Chiu LM, Amsden GW: Intrapulmonary pharmacokinetics of antibacterial agents: implications for therapeutics, *Am J Respir Med* 1:201-209, 2002.
155. Levin S, Karakusis PH: Clinical significance of antibiotic blood levels. In Ristuccia AM, Cunha BA, editors: *Antimicrobial therapy*, New York, 1984, Raven Press, pp 113-123.
156. Bergan T: Pharmacokinetics of tissue penetration of antibiotics, *Rev Infect Dis* 3:45-66, 1981.
157. Braga PC, Scaglione F, Scarpazza G, et al: Comparison between penetration of amoxicillin combined with carbocysteine and amoxicillin alone in pathological bronchial secretions and pulmonary tissue, *Int J Clin Pharmacol Res* 5(5):331-340, 1985.
158. Anonymous: Antimicrobial treatment guidelines for acute bacterial rhinosinusitis, *Arch Otolaryngol Head Neck Surg* 130: 1S-45S, 2004.
159. Berryessa NA, Johnson LR, Kasten RW, et al: Microbial culture of blood samples and serologic testing for bartonellosis in cats with chronic rhinosinusitis, *J Am Vet Med Assoc* 233(7):1084-1089, 2008.
160. Johnson LR, Foley JE, De Cock HEV, et al: Assessment of infectious organisms associated with chronic rhinosinusitis in cats, *J Am Vet Med Assoc* 227(4):579-585, 2005.
161. Bannasch MJ, Foley JE: Epidemiologic evaluation of multiple respiratory pathogens in cats in animal shelters, *J Feline Med Surg* 7:109-119, 2005.
162. Spindel ME, Veir JK, Radecki SV, et al: Evaluation of pradofloxacin for the treatment of feline rhinitis, *J Feline Med Surg* 10:472-479, 2008.
163. Hartmann AD, Helps CR, Lappin MR, et al: Efficacy of pradofloxacin in cats with feline upper respiratory tract disease due to *Chlamydophila felis* or *Mycoplasma* infections, *J Vet Intern Med* 22:44-52, 2008.
164. Veir JK, Ruch-Gallie R, Spindel ME, et al: Prevalence of selected infectious organisms and comparison of two anatomic sampling sites in shelter cats with upper respiratory tract disease, *J Feline Med Surg* 10:551-557, 2008.
165. Gibson RL, Burn JL, Ramse BW: Pathophysiology and management of pulmonary infections in cystic fibrosis, *Am J Respir Crit Care Med* 168:918-951, 2003.
166. Chernish RN, Aaron SD: Approach to resistant gram-negative bacterial pulmonary infections in patients with cystic fibrosis, *Curr Opin Pulm Med* 9(6):509-515, 2003.
167. Baumann U, Fischer JJ, Gudowius P, et al: A buccal adherence of *Pseudomonas aeruginosa* in patients with cystic fibrosis under long-term therapy with azithromycin, *Infection* 29(1):7-11, 2001.
168. Steinkamp G, Schmitt-Grohe S, Coring G, et al: Once-weekly azithromycin in cystic fibrosis with chronic *Pseudodomonas aeruginosa* infection, *Respir Med* 102(11):1643, 2008.
169. Carfartan G, Gerardin P, Turck D, et al: Effect of subinhibitory concentrations of azithromycin on adherence of *Pseudomonas aeruginosa* to bronchial mucins collected from cystic fibrosis patients, *J Antimicrob Chemother* 53(4):686-688, 2004.

170. Nguyen D, Emond MJ, Mayer-Hamblett N, et al: Clinical response to azithromycin in cystic fibrosis correlates with in vitro effects on *Pseudomonas aeruginosa* phenotypes, *Pediatr Pulmonol* 42(6):533–541, 2007.
171. Ruch-Gallie RA, Veir JK, Spindel ME, et al: Efficacy of amoxycillin and azithromycin for the empirical treatment of shelter cats with suspected bacterial upper respiratory infections, *J Feline Med Surg* 10:542–550, 2008.
172. Rees TM, Lubinski JL: Oral supplementation with L-lysine did not prevent upper respiratory infection in a shelter population of cats, *J Feline Med Surg* 10:510–513, 2008.
173. Keil DJ, Fenwich B: Canine respiratory bordetellosis: keeping up with an evolving pathogen. In Carmichael L, editor: *Recent advances in canine infectious diseases*, Ithaca, 2000, International Veterinary Information Service, A0104.0100 Canine respiratory bordetellosis: keeping up with an evolving pathogen (Last Updated: 13–Jan–2000).
174. Ford RB: Canine infectious tracheobronchitis. In Greene C, editor: *Infectious diseases of the dog and cat*, ed 3, St. Louis, 2006, Saunders.
175. Hawkins EH: Diseases of the lower respiratory system. In Ettinger SJ, Feldman EC, editors: *Textbook of veterinary internal medicine*, ed 4, Philadelphia, 1995, Saunders, pp 767–811.
176. Chalker VJ, Owen WMA, Paterson C, et al: Mycoplasmas associated with canine infectious respiratory disease, *Microbiology* 150:3491–3497, 2004.
177. Chalker VJ, Brooks HW, Brownlie J: The association of *Streptococcus equi* subsp. *zooepidemicus* with canine infectious respiratory disease, *Vet Microbiol* 95:149–156, 2003.
178. Keil D: Canine respiratory bordatellosis: keeping up with an evolving pathogen. In Carmichael L, editor: *Recent advances in canine infectious diseases*, Ithaca, 2000, International Veterinary Information Service, A0104.0100.
179. Finegold SM: Anaerobic bacteria: general concepts. In Mandell GL, Bennett JE, Dolin R, editors: *Principles and practice of infectious diseases*, New York, 1995, Churchill Livingstone, pp 2156–2172.
180. Foster SF, Martin P, Allan GS, et al: Lower respiratory tract infections in cats: 21 cases (1995-2000), *J Feline Med Surg* 6:167–180, 2004.
181. Bauer T, Woodfield JA: Mediastinal, pleural and extrapleural diseases. In Ettinger SJ, Feldman E, editors: *Textbook of veterinary internal medicine*, ed 4, Philadelphia, 1995, Saunders, pp 812–842.
182. Barrs VR, Betty JA: Feline pyothorax: new insights into an old problem: part 1. antiopathogenesis and diagnostic investigation, *The Veterinary Journal* 179:163–170, 2009.
183. Barrs VR, Betty JA: Feline pyothorax: new insights into an old problem: part 2. treatment recommendations and prophylaxis, *The Veterinary Journal* 179:171–178, 2009.
184. Rooney MB, Monnett E: Medical and surgical treatment of pyothorax in dogs: 26 cases (1991-2001), *J Am Vet Med Assoc* 221:86–92, 2002.
185. Boothe HW, Boothe DM, et al: Pyothorax in dogs: a retrospective study of organisms and antimicrobials, *J Am Vet Med Assoc* 15:236(6):657–663, 2010.
186. Eliopoulos GM, Moellering RC: Antimicrobial combinations. In Lorian V, editor: *Antibiotics in laboratory medicine*, Baltimore, 1996, Williams & Wilkins, pp 330–396.
187. Stephan B, Greife HA, Pridmore A, et al: Activity of pradofloxacin against *Porphyromonas* and *Prevotella* spp. implicated in periodontal disease in dogs: susceptibility test data from a European multicenter study, *Antimicrob Agents Chemother* 52(6):2149–2155, 1097–1123:2008.
188. Harvey CE, Thornsberry C, Miller BR: Antimicrobial susceptibility of subgingival bacterial flora in dogs with gingivitis, *J Vet Dent* 12:151–155, 1995.
189. Harvey CE: Antimicrobial susceptibility of subgingival bacterial flora in cats with gingivitis, *J Vet Dent* 12:157–160, 1995.
190. West-Hyde L, Floyd M: Dentistry. In Ettinger SJ, Feldman EC, editors: *Textbook of veterinary internal medicine*, ed 4, Philadelphia, 1995, Saunders, pp 1097–1123.
191. Jergens AE: Diseases of the esophagus. In Ettinger SJ, Feldman EC, editors: *Textbook of veterinary internal medicine*, ed 6, St Louis, 2005, Saunders.
192. Simpson KW: Disease of the stomach. In Ettinger SJ, Feldman EC, editors: *Textbook of veterinary internal medicine*, ed 6, St Louis, 2005, Saunders.
193. Greene CE: Gastrointestinal and intra-abdominal infections. In Greene C, editor: *Infectious diseases of the dog and cat*, ed 3, St Louis, 2006, Saunders.
194. Guerrant RL: Principles and syndromes of enteric infection. In Mandell GL, editor: *Mandell, Douglas, and Bennett's Principles and practice of infectious diseases*, ed 7, New York, 2010, Churchill Livingstone.
195. Haggstrom J, Kvart C, Pedersen HD: Acquired valvular heart disease. In Ettinger SJ, Feldman EC, editors: *Textbook of veterinary internal medicine*, ed 6, St Louis, 2005, Saunders.
196. Sheld WM, Sande MA: Endocarditis and intravascular infections. In Mandell GL, editor: *Mandell, Douglas, and Bennett's principles and practice of infectious diseases*, ed 7, New York, 2010, Churchill Livingstone.
197. Levison ME, Bush LM: Peritonitis and other intra-abdominal infections. In Mandell GL, editor: *Mandell, Douglas, and Bennett's principles and practice of infectious diseases*, ed 7, New York, 2010, Churchill Livingstone.
198. Young LS: Sepsis syndrome. In Mandell GL, Bennett JE, Dolin R, editors: *Principles and practice of infectious diseases*, New York, 1995, Churchill Livingstone, pp 690–705.
199. Dellinger RP, Levy MM, Carlet JM, et al: Surviving sepsis campaign: international guidelines for management of severe sepsis and septic shock: 2008, *Crit Care Med* 36(1):296–327, 2008.
200. Otto CM: Sepsis in veterinary patients: what do we know and where can we go? *J Vet Emerg Crit Care* 17(4):329–332, 2007.
201. Hopper K, Bateman S: An updated view of hemostasis: mechanisms of hemostatic dysfunction associated with sepsis, *J Vet Emerg Crit Care* 15(2):83–91, 2005.
202. Greiner M, Wolf G, Hartmann K: Bacteraemia in 66 cats and antimicrobial susceptibility of the isolates (1995-2004), *J Feline Med Surg* 9(5):404–410, 2007.
203. Harbarth S, Garbino J, Pugin J, et al: Inappropriate initial antimicrobial therapy and its effect on survival in a clinical trial of immunomodulating therapy for severe sepsis, *Am J Med* 115:529–535, 2003.
204. Glynn CM, Azadian B: Empire antimicrobial therapy for severe sepsis in the intensive care unit: in early, hit hard, out early, *Curr Anaesth Crit Care* 16:221–230, 2005.
205. Hardie EM: Sepsis versus septic shock. In Murtaugh RJ, Kaplan PM, editors: *Veterinary emergency and critical care medicine*, Philadelphia, 1992, Mosby.
206. Kreymann KG, de Heer G, Nierhaus A, et al: Use of polyclonal immunoglobulins as adjunctive therapy for sepsis or septic shock, *Crit Care Med* 35(12):2677–2685, 2007.
207. Laupland KB, Kirkpatrick AW, Delaney A: Polyclonal intravenous immunoglobulin for the treatment of severe sepsis and septic shock in critically ill adults: a systematic review and meta-analysis, *Crit Care Med* 35(12):2686–2692, 2007.
208. Hardie EM, Kolata RJ, Rawlings CA: Canine septic peritonitis: treatment with flunixin meglumine, *Circ Shock* 11:159–173, 1983.
209. Sprung CL, Annane D, Keh D, et al: Hydrocortisone therapy for patients with septic shock, *N Eng J Med* 358(2):111–124, 2008.

210. Ogeer-Gyles JO, Mathews KA, Sears W, et al: Development of antimicrobial drug resistance in rectal *Escherichia coli* from dogs hospitalized in an intensive care unit, *J Am Vet Med Assoc* 229:694–699, 2006.
211. Dow SW, Jones RL, Adney WS: Anaerobic bacterial infections and response to treatment in dogs and cats: 36 cases (1983–1985), *J Am Vet Med Assoc* 189:930–934, 1986.
212. Dow SW, Jones RL: Anaerobic infections. Part I. Pathogenesis and clinical significance, *Compend Contin Educ Pract Vet* 9(7):711–719, 1987.
213. Jang SS, Breher JE, Dabaco LA, et al: Organisms isolated from dogs and cats with anaerobic infections and susceptibility to selected antimicrobial agents, *J Am Vet Med Assoc* 210:1610–1614, 1997.
214. Hirsch DC, Indiveri MC, Jang SS, et al: Changes in prevalence and susceptibility of obligate anaerobes in clinical veterinary practice, *J Am Vet Med Assoc* 186:1086–1089, 1985.
215. Giamarellou H: Anaerobic infection therapy, *Int J Antimicrob Agents* 16(3):341–346, 2003.
216. Dow SW, Curtis CR, Jones RI, et al: Results of blood culture from critically ill dogs and cats: 100 cases (1985–1987), *J Am Vet Med Assoc* 195:113–117, 1989.
217. Dow SW, Jones RL, Royschuk RA: Bacteriologic specimens: selection, collection, and transport for optimum results, *Compend Contin Educ Pract Vet* 11(6):686–701, 1989.
218. Hirsch DC, Biberstein EL, Jang SS: Obligate anaerobes in clinical veterinary practice, *J Clin Microbiol* 210:188–191, 1979.
219. Brook I: Pathogenesis and management of polymicrobial infections due to aerobic and anaerobic bacterial, *Med Res Rev* 15:73–82, 1995.
220. Tally FP: Factors affecting the choice of antibiotic in mixed infections, *J Antimicrob Chemother* 22(Suppl A):87–100, 1988.
221. Tally FP, Cuchural GJ: Antibiotic resistance in anaerobic bacteria, *J Antimicrob Chemother* 22(Suppl A):63–71, 1988.
222. Weese JS, Armstrong J: Outbreak of *Clostridium difficile*-associated disease in a small animal veterinary teaching hospital, *J Vet Intern Med* 17:813–816, 2003.
223. Indiveri MC, Hirsch DC: Clavulanic acid–potentiated activity of amoxicillin against, *Bacteroides fragilis, Am J Vet Res* 46:2207–2209, 1985.
224. Loo VG, Poirier L, Miller MA, et al: A predominantly clonal multi-institutional outbreak of *Clostridium difficile*-associated diarrhea with high morbidity and mortality, *N Engl J Med* 353(23):2442–2449, 2005.
225. Efron PA, Mazuski JE: *Clostridium difficile* colitis, *Surg Clin North Am* 89(2):483–500, 2009.
226. Nguyen GC, Kaplan GG, Harris ML, et al: A national survey of the prevalence and impact of *Clostridium difficile* infection among hospitalized inflammatory bowel disease patients, *Am J Gastroenterol* 103(6):1443–1450, 2008.
227. McDonald LC, Killgore GE, Thompson A, et al: An epidemic, toxin gene-variant strain of *Clostridium difficile, N Engl J Med* 353(23):2433–2441, 2005.
228. Gerber M, Walch C, Löffler B, et al: Effect of sub-MIC concentrations of metronidazole, vancomycin, clindamycin and linezolid on toxin gene transcription and production in Clostridium difficile, *J Med Microbiol* 57(Pt 6):776–783, 2008.
229. Greene CE: Tetanus. In Greene CE, editor: *Infectious diseases of the dog and cat*, ed 3, St Louis, 2006, Saunders.
230. Kumar GAV, Kothari VM, Kirsihman A, et al: Benzathine penicillin, metronidazole and benzyl penicillin in the treatment of tetanus: a randomized, controlled trial, *Ann Trop Med Parasitol* 98:59–63, 2004.
231. Linnenbrink T, McMichael M: Tetanus: pathophysiolgy, clinical signs, diagnosis, and update on new treatment modalities, *J Vet Emerg Crit Care* 16(3):199–207, 2006.
232. Tobias KM, Marioni-Henry K, Wagner R: A retrospective study on the use of acepromazine maleate in dogs with seizures, *J Am Anim Hosp Assoc* 42:283–289, 2006.
233. Low RM, Lambert RJ, Pesillo SA: Successful management of severe generalized tetanus in two dogs, *J Vet Emerg Crit Care* 16(2):120–127, 2006.
234. Greene CE, Sykes JE, Brown CA, Hartmann K: Leptospirosis. In Greene CE, editor: *Infectious diseases of the dog and cat*, ed 3, St Louis, 2006, Saunders.
235. Greene CE: Bacterial diseases. In Ettinger SJ, Feldman EC, editors: *Textbook of veterinary internal medicine*, ed 4, Philadelphia, 1995, Saunders, pp 367–376.
236. Sykes JE: Feline hemotrophic mycoplasmosis (feline hemobartonellosis), *Vet Clin Small Anim* 33:773–789, 2004.
237. Westfall DS, Jensen WA, Reagan WJ, et al: Inoculation of two genotypes of Haemobartonella felis (California and Ohio variants) to induce infection in cats and the response to treatment with azithromycin, *Am J Vet Res* 62:687–691, 2001.
238. Dowers KL, Olver C, Radecki SV, et al: Use of enrofloxacin for treatment of large-form *Haemobartonella felis* in experimentally infected cats, *J Am Vet Med Assoc* 221:250–253, 2002.
239. Dowers KL, Tasker S, Radecki SV, et al: Use of pradofloxacin to treat experimentally induced *Mycoplasma haemofelis* infection in cats, *Am J Vet Res* 70:105–111, 2009.
240. Lappin MR: Effects of imidocarb diproprionate in cats with chronic haemobartonellosis, *Vet Ther* 3(4):144–149, 2002.
241. MacDonald KA, Chomel BB, Kittleson MD, et al: A prospective study of canine infective endocarditis in northern California (1999-2001): emergence of *Bartonella* as a prevalent etiologic agent, *J Vet Intern Med* 18:56–64, 2004.
242. Greene CE, Carmichael LE: Canine brucellosis. In Greene CE, editor: *Infectious diseases of the dog and cat*, ed 3, St Louis, 2006, Saunders.
243. Young EJ: Brucella species. In Mandell GL, editor: *Mandell, Douglas, and Bennett's principles and practice of infectious diseases*, ed 7, New York, 2010, Churchill Livingstone.
244. Farrar BM: Leptospira species. In Mandell GL, editor: *Mandell, Douglas, and Bennett's principles and practice of infectious diseases*, ed 7, New York, 2010, Churchill Livingstone.
245. Langston CE, Heuter KJ: Leptospirosis: A re-emerging zoonotic disease, *Vet Clin North Am Small Anim Pract* 33:791–807, 2004.
246. Shalit I, Barnea A, Shahar A: Efficacy of ciprofloxacin against *Leptospira interrogans* serogroup icterohaemorrhagiae, *Antimicrob Agents Chemother* 33:788–789, 1989.
247. Takashima I, Ngoma M, Hashimoto N: Antimicrobial effect of a new carboxyquinolone drug, Q-35, on five serogroups of *Leptospira interrogans, Antimicrob Agents Chemother* 37:901–902, 1993.
248. Steere AC: Borrelia burgdorferi (Lyme disease, Lyme borreliosis). In Mandell GL, editor: *Mandell, Douglas, and Bennett's principles and practice of infectious diseases*, ed 7, New York, 2010, Churchill Livingstone.
249. Greene CE, Staubinger RK: Borreliosis. In Greene CE, editor: *Infectious diseases of the dog and cat*, ed 3, St Louis, 2006, Saunders.
250. 16th Consensus Conference on Anti-infective Therapy: Lyme borreliosis: diagnosis treatment and prevention, Institut Pasteur, Centre d'Information Scientifique, Paris, France, December 2006. Accessed November 12, 2009 at www.infectiologie.com/site/medias/english/Lyme_shortext-2006.pdf.
251. Dattwyler RJ, Luft BJ, Kunkel MJ, et al: Ceftriaxone compared with doxycycline for the treatment of acute disseminated Lyme disease, *New Engl J Med* 337:289–295, 1997.
252. Lerner PI: Nocardia species. In Mandell GL, editor: *Mandell, Douglas, and Bennett's principles and practice of infectious diseases*, ed 7, New York, 2010, Churchill Livingstone.
253. Russo TA: Agents of actinomycosis. In Mandell GL, editor: *Mandell, Douglas, and Bennett's principles and practice of infectious diseases*, ed 7, New York, 2010, Churchill Livingstone.
254. Edwards DF: Actinomycosis and nocardiosis. In Greene CE, editor: *Infectious diseases of the dog and cat*, ed 3, St Louis, 2006, Saunders.

255. Malik R, Hughes MS, James G, et al: Feline leprosy: two different clinical syndromes, *J Feline Med Surg* 4(1):43–59, 2002.
256. Horne KS, Kunkle GA: Clinical outcome of cutaneous rapidly growing mycobacterial infections in cats in the southeastern United States: a review of 10 cases (1996-2006), *J Feline Med Surg* 11(8):627–632, 2009.
257. O'Brien CR, Greene CE, Greene RT: Miscellaneous bacterial infections. In Greene CE, editor: *Infectious diseases of the dog and cat*, ed 3, St Louis, 2006, Saunders.
258. Greene CE, DeBay BM: Tularemia. In Greene CE, editor: *Infectious diseases of the dog and cat*, ed 3, St Louis, 2006, Saunders.
259. Saah AJ: Introduction to rickettsiosis, ehrlichisoses, and anaphlasmosis. In Mandell GL, editor: *Mandell, Douglas, and Bennett's principles and practice of infectious diseases*, ed 7, New York, 2010, Churchill Livingstone.
260. Cohn LA: Ehrlichiosis and related infections, *Vet Clin North Am Small Anim Pract* 33(4):863–884, 2003.
261. Neer TM, Eddlestone SM, Gaunt SD, et al: Efficacy of enrofloxacin for the treatment of experimentally induced *Ehrlichia canis* infection, *J Vet Intern Med* 13:501–504, 1999.
262. Eddlestone SM, Neer TM, Gaunt SD, et al: Failure of imidocarb dipropionate to clear experimentally induced *Ehrlichia canis* infection in dogs, *J Vet Intern Med* 20(4):840–844, 2006.
263. Eddlestone SM, Diniz PP, Neer TM, et al: Doxycycline clearance of experimentally induced chronic *Ehrlichia canis* infection in dogs, *J Vet Intern Med* 21(6):1237–1242, 2007.
264. Davoust B, Keundjian A, Rous V, et al: Validation of chemoprevention of canine monocytic ehrlichiosis with doxycycline, *Vet Microbiol* 107:279–283, 2005.
265. Breitschwerdt EB: Obligate intracellular bacterial pathogens. In Ettinger SJ, Feldman EC, editors: *Textbook of veterinary internal medicine*, ed 6, St Louis, 2005, Saunders.
266. Breitschwerdt EB, Papich MG, Hegarty BC, et al: Efficacy of doxycycline, azithromycin, or trovafloxacin for treatment of experimental rocky mountain spotted fever in dogs, *Antimicrob Agents Chemother* 43(4):813–821, 1999.
267. Silley P, Stephan B, Greife HA, et al: Comparative activity of pradofloxacin against anaerobic bacteria isolated from dogs and cats, *J Antimicrob Chemother* 60(5):999–1003, 2007.
268. Ishak AM, Dowers KL, Cavanaugh MT, et al: Marbofloxacin for the treatment of experimentally-induced *Mycoplasma haemofelis* infection in cats, *J Vet Intern Med* 22:288–292, 2008.
269. Tasker S, Caney SM, Day MJ, et al: Effect of chronic FIV infection, and efficacy of marbofloxacin treatment, on *Mycoplasma haemofelis* infection, *Vet Microbiol* 117(2-4):169–179, 2006.
270. Quezado ZM, Hoffman WD, Banks SM, et al: Increasing doses of pentoxifylline as a continuous infusion in canine septic shock, *J Pharmacol Exp Ther* 288(1):107–113, 1999.
271. Turnidge J, Paterson DL: Setting and revising antibacterial susceptibility breakpoints, *Clin Microbiol Rev* 20(3):391–408, 2007.
272. From AH, Fong JS, Good RA: Polymyxin B sulfate modification of bacterial endotoxin: effects on the development of endotoxin shock in dogs, *Infect Immun* 23(3):660–664, 1979.
273. Sentürk S: Evaluation of the anti-endotoxic effects of polymyxin-E (colistin) in dogs with naturally occurred endotoxic shock, *J Vet Pharmacol Ther* 28(1):57–63, 2005.
274. Sharp CR, DeClue AE, Haak CE, et al: Evaluation of the anti-endotoxineffectsofpolymyxinBinafelinemodelofendotoxemia, *J Feline Med Surg* 12(4):278–285, 2010.
275. Macintir D: Treatment of severe parvoviral enteritis, Proceedings Central Veterinary Conference, 2008. http://veterinary calendar.dvm360.com/avhc/article/articleDetail.jsp?id=567275 &sk=&date=&pageID=3. (Accessed July 12, 2010.)
276. Kallas M, Green F, Hewison M, et al: Rare causes of calcitriol-mediated hypercalcemia: a case report and literature review, *J Clin Endocrinol Metab* 95: 3111–3117, 2010.

9 Treatment of Fungal Infections

Dawn Merton Boothe

Chapter Outline

Currently, only nine antifungal drugs, representing five classes, are approved for use in the United States.

FUNGAL PHYSIOLOGY

The pathogenic fungi affecting humans and animals are eukaryotes, generally existing as either filamentous molds (hyphal forms) or intracellular yeasts (Table 9-1).[1] Dimorphic fungi grow in the host as a yeastlike form but as molds in vitro at room temperature. Some fungi (e.g., *Coccidioides immitis, Histoplasma,* and *Rhinosporidium* species) grow inside host cells, dividing into spores until released from the cell as it ruptures. The fungal cell wall is a target for several of the antifungal drugs (Figure 9-1). It is rigid and contains chitin, a structural component, and polysaccharides. These generally preclude Gram staining and serve as a barrier to drug penetration. The cell membrane is complex and, unlike bacteria but as with higher eukaryotes, contains sterols.[2] Ergosterol is the primary sterol component of fungal cell membranes, regulating both permeability and membrane-bound enzymes. Because it also is a major component of organelle membranes, it also influences mitochondrial respiration and oxidative phosphorylation.[3] The rate of chitin synthesis is influenced by ergosterol content, being inhibited at high concentrations and stimulated at low concentrations. Fungal content of ergosterol influences drug efficacy and the potential risk of resistance for some drugs. Microtubular structures found in all eukaryotic cells support the cellular cytoskeleton and mitotic spindle; they support not only cell division but also cellular integrity. Organelle position and movement are supported by microtubules. The tubules in turn are comprised of tubulin, a heterodimer containing α and β subunits. Because microtubules are constantly being assembled and dissembled, impaired microtubular synthesis alters integral cellular function.

Table 9-1 Classification of Selected Fungi of Medical Importance

Level	Name	Disease or Infecting Organism
Kingdom	**Fungi**	
Subkingdom	Amastigomycotera	
Phylum	Zygomycota	
Class	Zygomycetes	
Order	Mucorales	
Family	Mucoraceae	
Genus	*Absidia*	*Absidia (Zygomycosis, mucormycosis)*
	Mucor	*Mucor (Zygomycosis, mucormycosis)*
	Rhizopus	*Rhizopus (Zygomycosis, mucormycosis)*
Family	*Several others*	
Order	Entomophthorales	
Family	Basidiobolaceae	
Genus	*Basidiobolus*	*Basidiobolus* sp.
Subkingdom	Eumycotera	
Phylum	Ascomyta	
Subphylum	Saccharomycotina	
Order	Saccharomycetales	
Family	Saccharomycetaceae	Budding yeasts
Genus	*Saccharomyces*	Budding yeasts
Genus	*Debaryomyces*	*Candida**
	Khyveromyces	*Candida**
	Lodderomyces	*Candida**
	Pichia	*Candida**
Subphylum	Pneumocystiodiomycetes	
Order	Pneumocystidiales	
Family	Pneumocystideaceae	
Genus	*Pneumocystis jirovecii*	Pneumocystis pneumonia
Subphylum	Euascomycotina	
Order	Eurotiales	
Family	Eurotiaceae	
Genus	*Eurotium, Emericella*	*Aspergillus**
Genus	*Talaromyces*	*Penicillium**
Order	Onygenales	
Family	Gymnoascaceae/ Ajellomycetaceae	
Genus	*Ajellomyces*	*Blastomyces dermatitidis**
		*Histoplasma capsulatum**
		*Paracoccidioides braziliensis**
Family	Gymnoascaceae/ Arthrodermataceae	
Genus	*Arthroderma*	*Microsporum*
		Trichophyton
		Epidermophyton
Class	Pyrenomycetes/ Sordariomycetes	
Order	Ophiostomatales	
Family	Ophiostomataceae	
Genus	*Ophiostoma*	*Sporothrix schenckii**
Order	Hypocreales	
Family	Many	*Fusarium*
Order	Clavicipitales	
Family	Clavicipitaceae	
Genus	Ergot alkaloids	St. Anthony's fire
Phylum	Basidiomycota	
Subphylum	Holobasidiomycont Basidiomycot	
Class	Phragmobasidiomycetes/ Tremellomycetes	
Order	Trichosporonales	*Trichosporon asahii**
Order	Filobasidiales	
Family	Filobasidiaceae	
Genus	*Filobasidiella*	*Cryptococcus neoformans**
Phylum	**Fungi Imperfecti/ Deuteromycota**	
Form–Class	Blastomycetes	
Form–Order	Cryptococcales	
Form–Family	Cryptococcaceae	
Genus	*Candida*	*Candida*
Genus	*Cryptococcus*	*Cryptococcus*
Genus	*Malassezia*	*Malassezia*
Genus	*Pityrosporum*	*Pityrosporum*
Genus	*Rhodotorula*	*Rhodotorula*
Genus	*Trichosporon*	*Trichosporon*
Form–Class	Hyphomycetes	
Form–Order	Moniliales	
Form–Family	Moniliaceae	
Genus	*Aspergillus*	*Aspergillus*
Genus	*Blastomyces*	*Blastomyces*
Genus	*Coccidioides*	*Coccidioides*
Genus	*Epidermophyton*	*Epidermophyton*
Genus	*Geotrichum*	*Geotrichum*
Genus	*Hostoplasma*	*Hostoplasma*
Genus	*Microsporum*	*Microsporum*
Genus	*Paracoccidioides*	*Paracoccidioides*
Genus	*Penicillium*	*Penicillium*
Genus	*Sporothrix*	*Sporothrix*
Genus	*Trichophyton*	*Trichophyton*
Genus	Others	
Form–Family	Dematiaceae	*Alternaria*
Genus	*Alternaria*	*Bipolaris*
Genus	*Bipolaris*	*Cladophialophora*
Genus	*Cladophialophora*	*Curvularia*
Genus	*Curvularia*	*Helminthosporium*

*Teleomorphic form or sexually producing state.
(From Reference Guide to the Classification of Fungi and Fungal-like Protists, with Emphasis on the Genera with Medical Importance (circa 2007), accessed December 17, 2009, at http://www.sbs.utexas.edu/mycology/bio329/pdf_files/sp2007/refguidefungal_sp2007.pdf.)

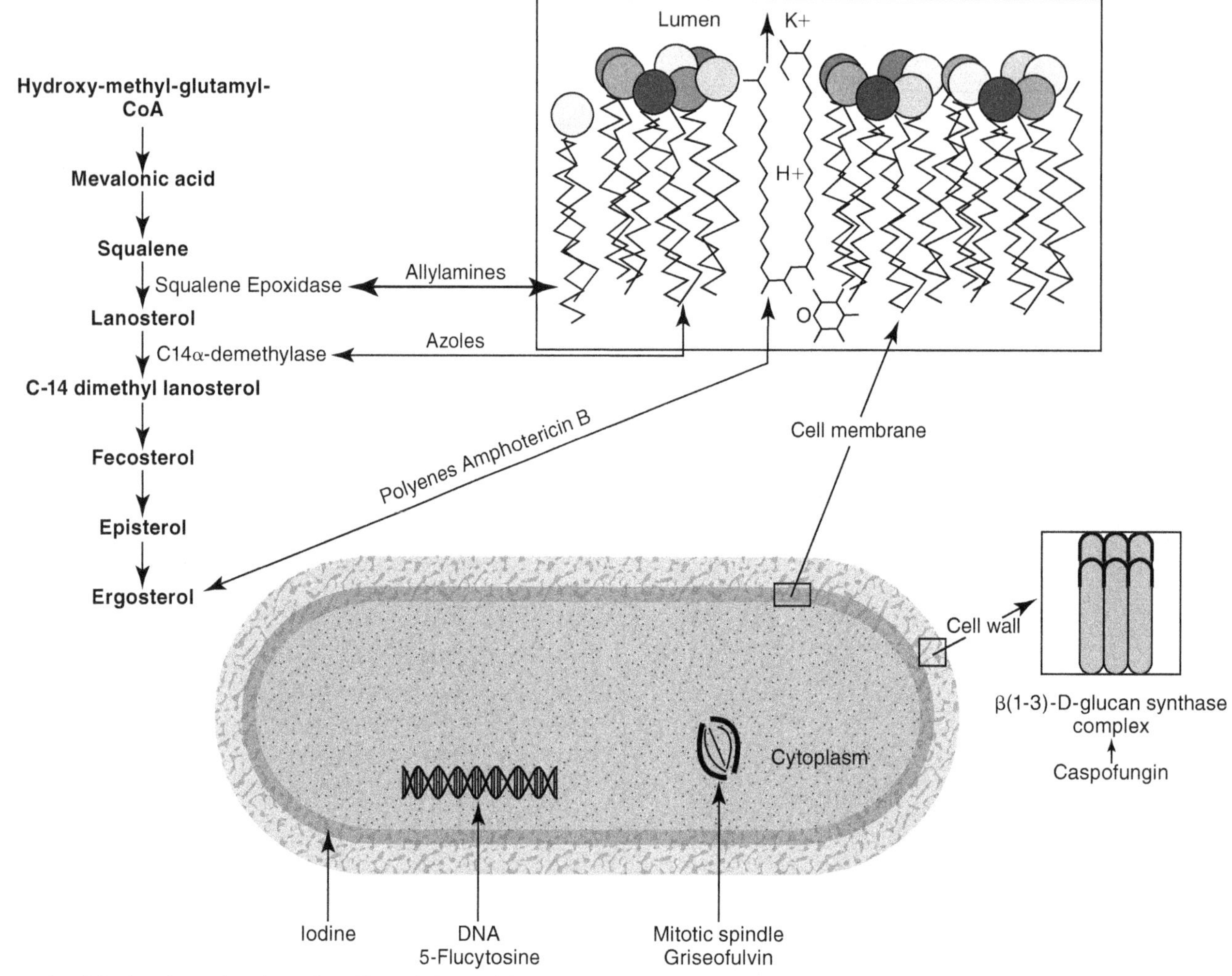

Figure 9-1 Mechanism of action of antifungal drugs. Most clinically relevant antifungals target cell wall ergosterol through different mechanisms. Amphotericin B binds to it, creating channels in the cell membrane. Azoles impair ergosterol synthesis by targeting C-14 α-demethylase while allylamines (e.g., terbinafine) inhibit squalene epoxidase. Drugs or drug classes that do not target ergosterol include 5-flucytosine, which impairs DNA synthesis upon its intracellular conversion to 5-fluouracil; griseofulvin, which impairs formation of the mitotic spindle; and caspofungin, an echinocandin that targets β-D-glucan synthesis in the fungal cell wall. Iodine may precipitate cellular proteins.

PATHOPHYSIOLOGY OF INFECTION

Fungal infections differ from bacterial infections in several respects, and pathogenic fungi have developed several characteristics that complicate antimicrobial therapy.[4] Some of the differences in the eukaryotic structure of fungal organisms compared with the prokaryotic structures of bacteria were delineated in the preceding section. Other differences exist. For example, *Cryptococcus* and occasionally *Sporothrix schenkii* produce an external coating or slime layer that encapsulates the cells and causes them to adhere and clump together.[2] Whereas many fungal organisms produce exotoxins in vivo, there is no conclusive evidence that fungi produce endotoxins. Fungal organisms are characterized by a low invasiveness and virulence. In fact, most animals will overcome a fungal infection. Factors that predispose the patient to infection include necrotic tissue, a moist environment, and immunosuppression. Innate immunity generally rapidly identifies and destroys fungal organisms that present pathogen-associated molecular patterns recognized by specific receptors on host cells. Pattern recognition receptors include the lectinlike receptor dectin-1, which binds beta-glucan in the fungal cell wall, and the Toll-like receptors. Binding by neutrophils and macrophages results in a cascade of intracellular events that cause rapid clearance in tissues of exposure. Organisms that are able to penetrate these tissues initiate an immune response. Immunity to fungal organisms appears to be T-cell mediated, with tumor necrosis factor-alpha (TNF-α) being a major signaling cytokine, although all but dermatophytes also stimulate antibody production.[5] In response, fungal organisms impair an effective immune response through a number of mechanisms. A number of molecules scavenge oxygen radicals generated by inflammatory cells (melanin, mannitol, catalase). The cell wall of *Histoplasma capsulatum* contains β-glucan, which covers and hides α-glucan, preventing recognition by phagocytic cells. Further, it is able to survive intracellular locations in phagocytic cells by a number of mechanisms. Phenotype switching prevents receptor recognition by host cells.[5] Gliotoxin is an immunosuppressive mycotoxin, produced particularly well by *Aspergillus fumigatus*.[5]

KEY POINT 9-1 The slow-growing nature of fungal infections requires long-term therapy. However, antifungal drugs are inherently more toxic than antibacterial drugs because fungal targets are often similar to mammalian targets.

Although an adequate immune response and recruitment of appropriate inflammatory cells to the site of infection is critical to resolution of fungal infections, progression to uncontrolled, pyogranulomatous inflammation is often deleterious. Proper early cellular recruitment may determine the difference between success and failure. The positive effects of some antifungals may include their immunomodulatory capabilities. These beneficial effects, which are largely based on in vitro studies, with an occasional murine mouse model verification, have been reviewed by Ben-Ami and colleagues.[5] Amphotericin B, the azoles, and the echinocandins have been studied most. Among the effects is downregulation of inflammatory cytokine genes. The use of antiinflammatories should be considered in critical situation. The use of glucocorticoids is addressed in the section on the treatment of fungal infections, but other antiinflammatories that minimally affect lymphocytic-mediated immunity (e.g., nonsteroidal antiinflammatories, leukotriene receptor antagonists) should be considered as long as attention is paid to potential negative drug interactions involving imidazoles in particular. Manipulation of the immune response in combination with antifungal drugs is a more recent area of focus that is likely to affect treatment of fungal disorders.

Fungal infections can be primarily superficial and irritating (e.g., dermatophytosis) or systemic and life threatening (e.g., dimorphic fungal infections including blastomycosis, cryptococcosis, histoplasmosis, and coccidioidomycosis). Fungal organisms may exhibit an affinity for certain tissues, such as the dermatophytes for keratin and *H. capsulatum* for macrophages. Animals may develop a hypersensitivity to the infecting organism (as is often seen in dermatophyte infections), which can result in a pathologic response to the infection as well as facilitate dissemination. The role of proteolytic enzymes in infections caused by dermatophytes is being investigated. On the other hand, the lack of hypersensitivity may also indicate a poorer prognosis for recovery.[2]

Information regarding antifungal drug use in animals is limited. Human literature often focuses on candidiasis, an infection that is much less common in dogs and cats; as such, relevance of information must be considered. The risk factors for fungal infection have been recently reviewed.[7] Using candidiasis as an example, broad-spectrum antimicrobials or immunosuppressive drugs (glucocorticoids, chemotherapy) play a major role. Malnutrition, malignancy, age extremes, and neutropenia also predispose to candidiasis. Similar risk factors occur for aspergillosis, although increased organ transplantation and its accompanying immunosuppression probably has contributed to not only the increased incidence of infection but also the emergence of newer species. Likewise, the increased invasiveness of life-extending procedures coupled with increased survival is contributing to an increased incidence of infection. Improved diagnostic techniques are allowing identification of previously unknown organisms; for example, other filamentous organisms that are emerging in human medicine include the *Zygometes (Mucor, Rhizopus, Rhizomucor, Absidia,* and *Cunninghamella), Fusarium, Paecilomyces,* and *Scedosporium.*

Several factors can lead to therapeutic failure or relapse after antifungal therapy.[4] Most antifungals are fungistatic in action, with clearance of infection largely dependent on host response.[6] In humans relapsing infections are not uncommon for selected *Trichophyton* species and for invasive mycoses in immunocompromised patients. In the latter group, aspergillosis infections are particularly problematic. As with bacteria, the pattern of fungal disease is constantly changing. The advent of acquired immunodeficiency syndrome in human patients has been important in the development of new strains of resistant organisms, and there remains a continuing need for development of new antifungal agents. However, this represents only one of many factors that increase the risk of fungal infection. In some instances, therapeutic failure reflects poor penetration of drug into infected tissues (particularly the central nervous system and bone) or into those organisms that are encapsulated.

Several organisms, particularly the superficial pathogens and systemic opportunistic organisms, have a primary resistance to antifungal drugs, contributing to therapeutic failure. Like antibacterial resistance, antifungal resistance can be intrinsic (primary) or acquired (secondary). A third type of resistance, referred to as *clinical resistance,* involves the progression or relapse that occurs despite laboratory-documented susceptibility to the treatment drug.[8] Primary resistance occurs with amphotericin B to filamentous fungi and dermatophytes. The risk factors for acquired resistance have not been well identified. Because resistance is an increasingly emerging problem, dosing regimens should maximize antifungal plasma concentrations. However, much more so than antibacterial drugs, antifungal drugs present a risk of toxicity causing the design of dosing regimens to be much more restrictive compared to antibacterial therapy.

Toxicity of antifungals is a common cause of therapeutic failure. Because both the antifungal target organism and the host cells are eukaryotic, the cellular targets of fungal organisms are substantially different from those of bacterial organisms. As a result, antibacterials generally are ineffective against fungal organisms, and, in contrast to most antibacterials, antifungals are often toxic or associated with undesirable side effects in the host. The incidence of side effects has limited the number of effective yet safe antifungal drugs available. Some strategies for reducing toxicity have allowed dose escalation, increasing the likelihood of efficacy and decreasing the risk of resistance. Their use (e.g., liposomal amphotericin B products) are particularly important in the immunosuppressed patient. A potentially important strategy for avoidance of resistance is combination therapy.[8,9] Combination therapy, if correctly designed, should also enhance efficacy and reduce toxicity through more rapid response to therapy. Dose reduction may be possible. Finally, a common reason for therapeutic failure is discontinuing therapy after resolution of clinical signs but before eradication of infection. Therefore antifungal therapy should extend well beyond clinical cure.

As with antibacterials, efficacy is influenced by the relationship between plasma or tissue concentrations, minimum inhibitory concentration (MIC) of the infecting microbe and antifungal. Studies for antifungal organisms generally begin with killing curves followed by animal models; however, as with antibacterials, their relevance also must be supported by pharmacokinetic studies that determine drug concentrations at the site of infection coupled with pharmacodynamic studies that determine susceptibility in terms of end points of efficacy.[10]

Compared with bacterial testing, antifungal culture and susceptibility testing have not been well developed as a tool for the treatment of fungal infections. As with antibacterial testing, antifungal testing is principally identification of resistant microbes rather than a description of the level of susceptibility.[8] In vitro susceptibility testing of antifungal agents is highly dependent on test conditions, and interlaboratory results vary markedly. Interpretation of culture and susceptibility data may be limited by a lack of standardized testing methods for some drugs and organisms. As with bacteria, the MIC for a fungal organism is the concentration of the antifungal drug that inhibits the growth of the fungus under standardized conditions (Table 9-2). The minimum lethal concentration is the concentration that kills the organisms.[1] Correlation between MIC and clinical response is poor, and assessment of antifungal agents appears to be best accomplished through efficacy studies in animal models. Fortunately, the need for fungal culture and susceptibility testing may not be as critical for fungal organisms as it is for bacterial organisms because, with the exception of 5-flucytosine, fungal development of resistance to antimicrobial therapy is not common.[11] Resistance is more likely with a rapidly growing organism exposed to high concentrations of an antifungal for a long period of time.[1] However, resistance does occur, and as with antibacterials, use of previous antifungal drugs appears to increase the risk of resistance. This has been demonstrated for *Candida,* the MICs of which tend to be higher in human patients previously treated with antifungals than in drug-naïve patients. Mechanisms of resistance of fungal organisms are similar to those of bacterial organisms (e.g., failure to accumulate in cells, altered target structures, formation of alternative pathways).[12] The advent of newer antifungal agents and resistance among fungal organisms is, however, likely to cause in vitro testing of antifungals to become more important to therapeutic success.

KEY POINT 9-2 Resistance by fungal organisms is not as common as in bacterial organisms, but it is more likely in those that are rapidly growing.

One author notes that never before have so many new antifungals been under development, ranging from entirely new compounds with new targets to modifications of existing drugs (e.g., cyclodextrin–itraconazole and polyethylene glycol–amphotericin B).[13] Newer concepts being explored include combinations of antifungals with one another or with nonantibiotic compounds. Newer therapies may focus on immunomodulation[14] with a balance between recruitment (cytokines, chemokines, lymphokines, and growth factors) and antiinflammatory effects. The need for new therapies is timely, as the epidemiologic behavior of fungal organisms, at least as they occur in human medicine, increasingly is shifting toward opportunistic organisms for which traditional antifungals often are characterized by limited efficacy.[7]

ANTIFUNGAL DRUGS

The primary agents used to treat fungal infections are the natural antibiotics; the polyene macrolides (amphotericin B as the prototype); the synthetic agents, including the azoles (ketoconazole as the prototype); and the newer allylamine antifungals (Figure 9-2). Flucytosine has a less important role in the treatment of dimorphic fungal diseases, particularly in animals. The natural antibiotic griseofulvin belongs to no group but has an important place in the armamentarium against dermatophytosis. As recently as 1988, the treatment of systemic fungal infections in humans emphasized the use of amphotericin B, ketoconazole, and flucytosine. In the decade that followed, further development of the azole derivatives has led to a new age in the treatment of systemic fungal diseases. Currently, antifungal therapy is most effective when based on an understanding of the therapeutic ratio of the drug in the infection being treated. For amphotericin B, this ratio tends to be small because of its toxicity. The newer azole derivatives have proved to provide much of the efficacy of amphotericin B without its toxicity. Doses for selected antifungal drugs are found in Table 9-3.

POLYENE MACROLIDE ANTIBIOTICS: AMPHOTERICIN B

Structure–Activity Relationship

Examples of polyene (i.e., multiple double-bond; see Figure 9-1) antifungal drugs include amphotericin B, nystatin, and pimaricin. Each antibiotic is produced by a different species of *Streptomyces* (family Actinomyces). Amphotericin B was developed in the 1960s and was so successful in fulfilling the need for a broad-spectrum antifungal that further advancement of antifungal therapy was largely ignored. These drugs are very large molecules, consisting of a macrolide containing a large lactone ring. The polyene contains three to eight double bonds, which represent the lipophilic portion of the molecule. The number of double bonds categorizes the polyenes into trienes, tetraenes (natamycin [paramycin]), and pentanes; amphotericin B and candicidin are heptanes, whereas nystatin is classified as a pseudo-heptane/tetraene.[3] A hydroxylated hydrocarbon backbone represents the hydrophilic portion of the molecule. These compounds are insoluble in water and are unstable, and they will rapidly decompose if exposed to sunlight.

Table 9-2 Minimum Inhibitory Concentrations for Selected Antifungal Drugs

	Amphotericin B		Ketoconazole	Itraconazole		Fluconazole	Voriconazole	Clotrimazole	5-Flucytosine	Griseofulvin
Range (MIC_{50}, MIC_{90})	Bossche*	Mallie Li	Bossche	Bossche	Li	Bossche	Li	Bossche	Bossche	Bossche
Alternaria alternata			0.063-0.25							
Aspergillus flavus	12.5–>25	0.38-0.32 (3,16)	0.5–>10	0.063-0.13	0.047-3 (0.5, 1)	NA	0.125-0.5 (0.19,0.38)	0.5-2	10–>100	—
Aspergillus fumigatus	0.14–>25	0.012-3 (0.25, 1)	0.12–>25	0.001-10	0.023-32 (0.75,2)	NA	0.023-3 (0.19, 0.25)	0.1-10	0.5–>100	—
Aspergillus niger	0.12 -> 25	0.016-0.38 (0.125,0.25)			0.19-32 (1.5, 4)		0.032-0.5 (0.19-0.38)	1-100	0.5-10	
Blastomyces dermatitidis	0.05–0.78	<0.03-1 (<0.06, 0.05)	0.005–>2	0.063-0.13	≤0.03-16 (≤ 0.03, 0.25)	NA	≤0.03- >16 (≤0.03, 0.25)	0.13-3.13	0.06–>100	—
Candida albicans	0.04–>4	0.002-2 (0.064, 0.19)	0.01–>100	0.063-128	0.003-32 (0.094, 0.5)	0.125–>80	0.002-32 (0.008, 0.04)	0.01-50	0.016-100	>100
Coccidioides immitus	0.15-96 >	0.25-2 (0.5, 1)		0.05-0.64	0.125-1 (0.5, 1)	NA	≤0.03-5 (0.125, 0.5)	0.1-3.4	>97	—
Cryptococcus neoformans	0.04-2.8		0.063-32	0.001-0.5	0.63 (MIC_{90})	NA		0.02-4	0.1–>100	—
Histoplasma capsulatum	0.0007–>100	<0.03-2 (0.25, 1)	0.063-3.12	0.063-0.0	≤0.03-0.5 (≤0.03, 0.06)	NA	≤0.03-2 (0.25, 1)	0.1-1	NA	—
Malassezia furfur	0.3–>2.5		0.01-0.4	0.001-1		NA		0.2-12.5	>100	—
Microsporum canis	1.8-100>		0.5-16	0.063-0.25		NA		0.03–2	NA	0.1–>18
Microsporum gypseum	2.3–>100		0.002-0.004	NA		0.1-2		NA	0.5-3.13	
Sporothrix schenckii	0.4–>100		0.25–>64	0.001-4	0.4 (MIC_{90})	NA		0.5-10	1.6-3.12	—
Trichophyton mentagrophytes	5.6–>100		0.001–>64			NA		0.01-20	NA	0.1–>30
Trichophyton sp.	5.42 -> 100		0.1-12.5	0.03-0.25		1-64		0.015-2	NA	0.1–>30

MIC, Minimum inhibitory concentration.

*Data from Bossche HV: Itraconazole: a selective inhibitor of the cytochrome P-450 dependent ergosterol biosynthesis. In *Recent trends in the discovery, development, and evaluation of antifungal agents,* Proceedings of an International Telesymposium, Barcelona, Spain, JR Prouse Science, pp. 207–222, 1987; Mallie M, Bastide JM, Blancard A et al: In vitro susceptibility testing of *Candida* and *Aspergillus* spp. to voriconazole and other antifungal agents using Etest®: results of a French multicentre study, *Int J Antimicrob Agents* 25:321–328, 2005; Li RK, Ciblak MA, Nordoff N et al: In vitro activities of voriconazole, itraconazole, and amphotericin B against *Blastomyces dermatitidis, Coccidioides immitis,* and *Histoplasma capsulatum, Antimicrob Agents Chemother* 44(6):1734–1736, 2000.

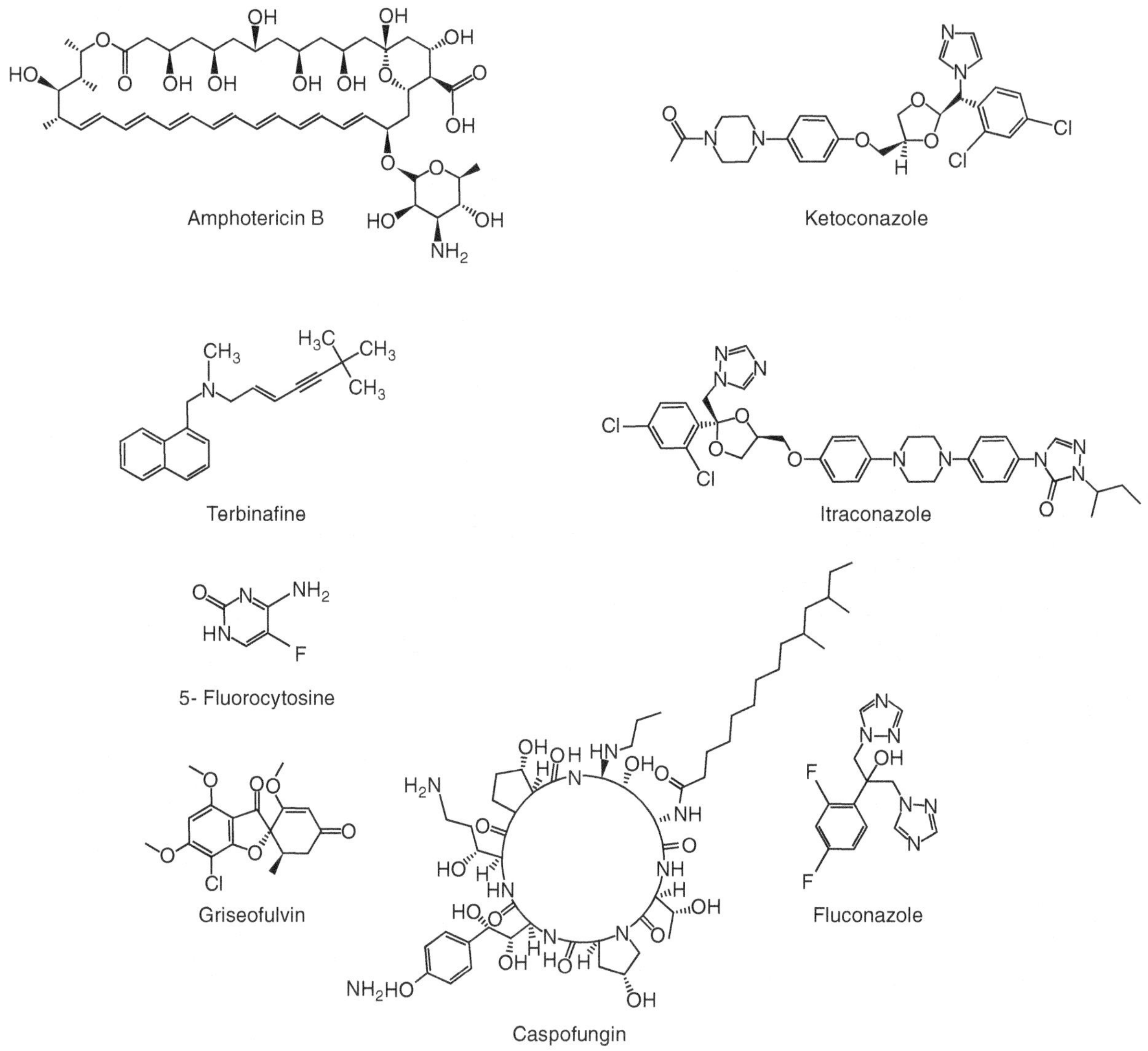

Amphotericin B

Ketoconazole

Terbinafine

Itraconazole

5- Fluorocytosine

Griseofulvin

Caspofungin

Fluconazole

Figure 9-2 Chemical structures of selected antifungal drugs.

Mechanism of Action

Polyene macrolides bind with the sterol portion of the phospholipids that make up the fungal cell membrane. Amphotericin has a much higher affinity for *ergosterol,* the major sterol component of fungal cell membranes, than for cholesterol, the major sterol in mammalian cell membranes (Figure 9-3).[1] The interaction of the drug and the sterol results in the formation of channels or pores in the cell membrane (Figure 9-4). The result is an increase in cell permeability and disruption in proton gradient flow; loss of membrane fluidity may alter H+-ATPase activity.[3] Altered K^+/H^+ exchange results in the loss of K^+ and Mg^{2+} from the cell. Cellular metabolism is disrupted; internal acidification of the fungal cell and the loss of important organic molecules from the cell result in irreversible cell damage. The efficacy of some of the drugs can be related to their ability to bind to ergosterol. However, the polyenes also are associated with the formation of lethal reactive oxygen molecules. Polyenes also are defined according to the concentration of drug necessary to cause erythrocyte hemolysis,

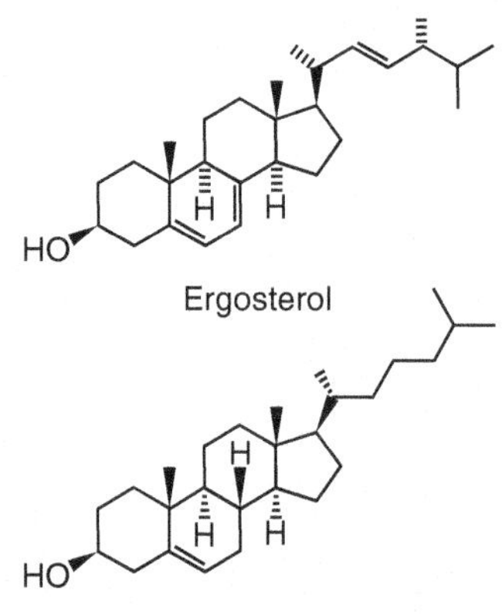

Figure 9-3 Cholesterol, the major sterol of mammalian cells, is structurally similar to ergosterol, the major sterol of fungal cell walls. Binding of amphotericin B to cholesterol results in complicated pharmacokinetics as well as host toxicity.

Table **9-3** Dosing Recommendations for Antifungal Drugs (1)

Drug		Indication	Dose	Route	Interval (hr)
Amphotericin A (1,2)	(Fungizone [AmBD])	Test dose	0.25-0.5 mg/kg	IV	Once
		General mycoses	0.15-1 mg/kg in 30 mL 5% D/W	Rapid IV infusion (over 5 minutes through a butterfly catheter after flushing catheter with 10 mL 5% dextrose)	48 or 3 × per week to a cumulative dose of 4-12 mg/kg (D) or 4-6 mg/kg (C)
			0.15-1 mg/kg in 200-500 mL 5% D/W via peripheral venous catheter	IV (over 4-6 hrs)	48 or 3 × per week to a cumulative dose of 4-12 mg/kg (D) or 4-6 mg/kg (C)
		Blastomycosis	Initial dose: 0.5 mg/kg (D)	IV	48 or 3 × per week to a cummulative dose of 4-10 mg with ketaconazole
			Followed by: 0.15-0.25 mg/kg (D)	IV	1 × per month with ketaconazole
		Cryptococcosis	0.5-0.8 mg/kg	SC	48 or 2-3 × per week. Dilute to <20 mg/mL in 5% dextrose
			0.15-0.4 mg/kg (C)	IV	48 or 2-3 × per week for 3-4 weeks. Total cumulative dose of 4-6 mg/kg with flucytosine
		Histoplasmosis	Initial dose: 0.5 mg/kg (D)	IV	3 × per week to a cumulative dose of 4-6 mg with ketaconazole
			Followed by: 0.15-0.25 mg/kg	IV	1 × per month with ketaconazole
			0.25 mg/kg (C)	IV	48 × 4-8 weeks with ketaconazole
			0.15-0.5 mg/kg (C)	IV	1 × per month with ketaconazole
		Gastroinestinal pythiosis	1-2 mg/kg (D)	IV	48 or 3 × per week to a cumulative dose of 12-24 mg/kg
		Resistant filamentous fungi	2-2.5 mg/kg	IV	48 or 3 × per week to a cumulative dose of 15-30 mg/kg
		Leishmaniosis	0.5-0.8 mg/kg	IV	48 to a cumulative dose of 8-16 mg/kg
		Pulmonary fungal disease	Systemic dose diluted in 5% D/W	Aerosol (nebulization)	Use the chosen systemic dose, prepared as 5 mg/mL in 5% dextrose
		CNS fungal disease	0.2-0.5 mg	Intrathecal	48 or 2-3 × per week. Dilute in 5 mL cerebrospinal fluid or 10% dextrose
		Fungal cystitis	50 μg/mL prepared in 5% D/W	Urinary bladder infusion	24; repeat once if necessary.
Amphotericin B, colloidal dispersion (ABCD) (1,2)	(Amphotec) (Amphocel)*	Test dose	0.25-0.5 mg/kg	IV	Once
		General mycoses	1-2.5 mg/kg	IV	48 or 3 × per week to a cumulative dose of 15-30 mg/kg
Amphotericin B, lipid complex (ABLC) solution (1,2)	(Albecet)	Test dose	0.25-0.5 mg/kg	IV	Once
		General mycoses	1-2.5 mg/kg	IV	48 or 3 × per week to a cumulative dose of 12-30 mg/kg
		Blastomycosis, severe	1-2 mg/kg (D)	IV	3 × per week to a cummulative dose of 12-24 mg/kg
		Cryptococcosis	1 mg/kg (C)	IV	48 or 3 × per week to cumulative dose of 12 mg/kg

Table 9-3 Dosing Recommendations for Antifungal Drugs (1)—cont'd

Drug		Indication	Dose	Route	Interval (hr)
Amphotericin B, liposomal (AmBD) (1,2)	Ambisome (B LamB)	Test dose	0.25-0.5 mg/kg	IV	Once
		General mycoses	1-4 mg/kg (D)	IV	48 or 3 × per week to a cumulative dose of 12-30 mg/kg
		Leishmaniosis	3-4 mg/kg (D)	IV	48 or 3 × per week to a cumulative dose of 12-30 mg/kg
			250-300 mg/(D)	PO (on food)	24 × 7-12 days
			60-100 mg (C)	PO	24 × 5 days
			300-400 (C)	PO (on food)	24 × 5 days
		Coccidiosis prophylaxis	28.8 mg/L water	PO (in water)	24 × 14 days
			1.25 g of 20% powder	PO (on food)	24 × 14 days
		Coccidiosis treatment	150 mg/kg	PO	24 × 14 days with sulfadimethoxine
Captan powder 50%		Dermatomycoses	30 mL/1 L of water (2 tbsp/gal of water)	Topical. Do not rinse	2-3 × per week
Chlorhexidine diacetate		Fungal skin infection	1 mL of 2% solution to 9 mL water	Topical	PRN
Clotrimazole		Dermatophytosis	Apply to lesions	Topical	12 until culture is negative
		Antifungal	60 mL of 1 g/dL in polyethylene glycol	Topical (intranasal)	Over 1 hr (under general anesthesia); repeat in 3-4 weeks PRN
Enilconazole		Nasal aspergillosis	5% solution	Topical (instill into nasal sinus)	12 × 7-10 days
			10-20 mg/kg (10% solution diluted 50:50 with water)	Topical (instill into nasal sinus)	12 × 10-14 days
		Dermatophytes	Dilute to 0.2% solution	Wash affected area???	72-96 × 4 treatments
Fluconazole (3)		Blastomycosis	5 mg/kg	PO	12
		Cryptococcosis	2.5-10 mg/kg	PO (with food)	12-24
			150-200 mg/C	PO	24 or divide dose and administer q8h
Flucytosine (combination therapy)		Cryptococcus	125-250 mg/C	PO	Divide dose and administer q6-8h. Do not use as sole therapy
			150-175 mg/kg	PO	Divide dose and administer q6-8
			25-50 mg/kg	PO	6
		Urinary candidiasis	50-75 mg/kg Maximum of 100 mg/kg	PO	8. Alkalinize urine to > 7.4
Griseofulvin (microsize) (3)		Dermatophytosis	10-30 mg/kg	PO (with fatty meal)	24 or divide dose and administer q8-12h
			50 mg/kg	PO (with fatty meal)	24 or divide dose and administer q8-12h
			80-130 mg/kg	PO (with fatty meal)	24 or divide dose and administer q8-12h
Griseofulvin (ultramicrosize) (3)			5-10 mg/kg	PO	24
			20-50 mg/kg	PO	24

Table 9-3 Dosing Recommendations for Antifungal Drugs (1)—cont'd

Drug	Indication	Dose	Route	Interval (hr)
Iodide, potassium	Sporotrichosis, pythiosis	0.4 mL/kg (D)	PO	24
		30-100 mg/C	PO	24 or divide dose and administer q 8-12h x 10-14 days
Itraconazole(4)	Systemic mycoses or generalized dermatomycosis	5-10 mg/kg	PO	12-24
Ketoconazole(4)	Systemic and cutaneous mycoses, protothecosis, aspergillosis	10-20 mg/kg (D)	PO	12-24
	Systemic and cutaneous mycoses, protothecosis, aspergillosis	10 mg/kg (C)	PO	12-24
	Sporotrichosis	5-10 mg/kg (C)	PO	12-24
	Sporotrichosis	15 mg/kg (D)	PO	12
	Candidiasis	10 mg/kg	PO	8
	Aspergillosis	10 mg/kg	PO	24
	CNS mycoses	15-20 mg/kg	PO	12
	Malassezia canis	10 mg/kg (D) or		24 × 30 days
	Malassezia canis	5 mg/kg (D)	PO	12
	Dermatophytosis	10 mg/kg	PO	24
	Coccidiodomycosis	10-30 mg/kg (D)	PO	24 × 3-6 months or divide dose and administer q 12 × 3-6 months
	Blastomycosis	10 mg/kg (20 mg/kg if ocular or central nervous system)	PO	12 × 2-3 months
	Histoplasmosis	10 mg/kg	PO	12-24 × 3 months
	Cryptococcosis	10 mg/kg	PO	24 (in combination with another antifungal)
Lufenuron	Coccidiodomycosis (adjuvant)	50-100 mg/kg (D)	PO	24
		15 mg/kg	PO	24
	Dermatophytosis	50-100 mg/kg	PO	Two treatments 2 weeks apart, then monthly
		80-100 mg/kg (C)	PO	Two treatments 2 weeks apart, then monthly
	Systemic mycoses	5 mg/kg (D), 15 mg/kg (C)		Two treatments 2 weeks apart then monthly
Miconazole	Dermatophytosis	Apply topically as directed	Topical	12-24
	Ocular fungal infections	Apply topically as directed	Topical	4-12 times per day
Natamycin	Ocular fungal infections	Several drops	Topical	3-8
Povidone–iodine		Apply light coating	Topical	12-24
Sodium hypochlorite (bleach)	Rinse	1:20 (0.5%) in water	Topical spray	Every 5-7 days

Continued

Table 9-3 Dosing Recommendations for Antifungal Drugs (1)—cont'd

Drug	Indication	Dose	Route	Interval (hr)
Terbinafine	Dermatophytosis	30-40 mg/kg (D)	PO	24
Voriconazole(5)	Aspergillosis, susceptible fungal infections	3-6 mg/kg (D)	PO	12-24; use higher dose once daily. Dose has not been verified

C, cat; *CNS*, central nervous system; *D*, dog; *D/W*, dextrose in water; *IV*, Intravenous; *PO*, by mouth; *PRN*, as needed; *SC*, subcutaneous.

1. Minimum of treatment time reflects infectious agent. See text for renal-saving tactics. For nondermatophytes a minimum of 2 months, generally 4 to 6 months, extends to 8 to 10 months for cryptococcosis and beyond for coccidiodomycosis, and always should be 1 to 2 months beyond resolution of clinical signs. Doses collected from *Greene's Infectious Diseases of the Dog and Cat* (2006 and other resources)
2. Precede with 0.1 to 0.25 mg test dose diluted in 10 mL in dextrose. Dilute calculated dose in 10 to 60 mL (rapid) or 250 to 1000 ml (slow infusion) 5% dextrose. See text for rapid versus slow infusion techniques. Administration may be subcutaneous, although concentrations greater than 20 mg/mL are locally irritating. Total cumulative dose varies with target organism from 4 to10 mg/kg in dogs (8-12 mg/kg if coccidioidomycosis) or 4-8 mg/kg in cats. Higher daily and cumulative doses are generally indicated for lipid-complexed amphotericin (see text). See text for more specific guidance for each organism and combination therapy protocols. Use at 30-day intervals for prevention of relapse (scientific basis for this approach is lacking).
3. Duration for dermatophytosis 4-6 weeks; may be longer with long-haired breeds
4. Lower dose is given bid, higher once daily.
5. Induction in dog may result in decreased drug concentrations. Monitoring would be ideal if available.

*Amphocel (Amphocil) is no longer available in the US.

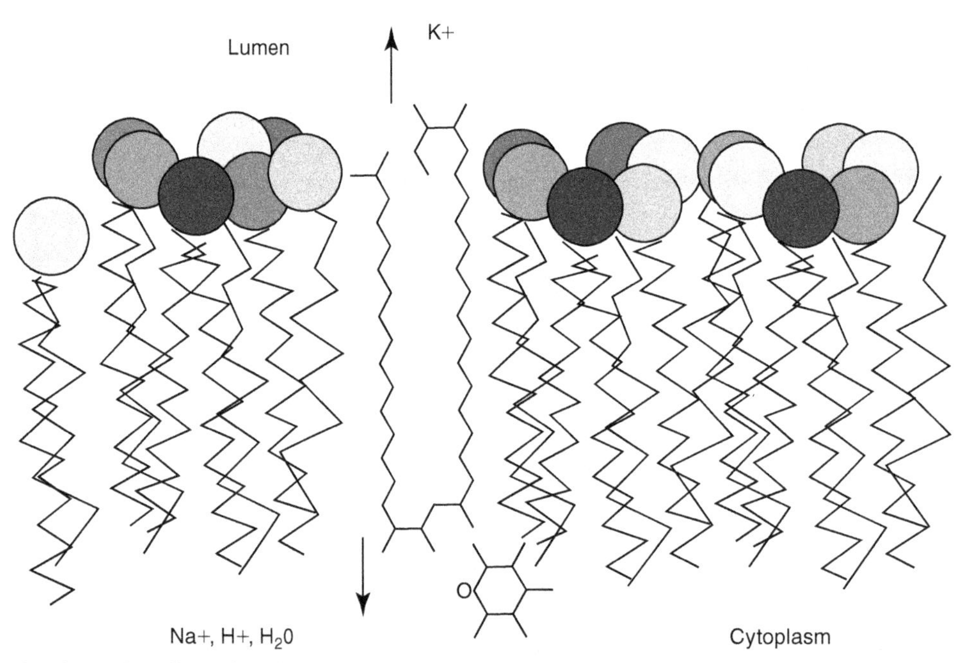

Figure 9-4 The mechanism of antifungal action and nephrotoxicity of amphotericin B reflect binding of the drug to ergosterol, the major sterol in fungal cell walls. Binding results in cell membrane permeability and the loss of critical micronutrients and electrolytes.

presumably because of cholesterol binding. Pimaricin causes lysis at low concentrations, limiting use to topical application, whereas amphotericin B and nystatin cause lysis at much higher concentrations.[3]

Amphotericin is fungistatic but can be fungicidal at high concentrations. At high concentrations the drug directly disrupts the fungal cell membrane. As with some other select antifungal drugs, amphotericin appears to have some immunomodulating characteristics. Both humoral and cell-mediated immunity may be enhanced, thus increasing the host's ability to overcome infection. Amphotericin B activates macrophages and stimulates TNF-α and interleukin-1 (IL-1), both of which facilitate macrophage killing by way of nitric oxide–dependent pathways.[5,14]

Spectrum of Activity and Pharmacodynamics

Despite the advent of the azole antifungal drugs, amphotericin B remains the most effective agent against most of the major fungal pathogens. The indications for amphotericin therapy include most systemic fungal diseases, including those caused by the dimorphic fungi (histoplasmosis, blastomycosis, cryptococcosis, and coccidioidomycosis) and disseminated sporotrichosis, phycomycosis, aspergillosis, and candidiasis. Amphotericin B has greater activity against some organisms (e.g., *Candida* and *Aspergillus* species and coccidioidal meningitis) than the newer azoles and particularly fluconazole. Amphotericin B is not effective against dermatophytes. Amphotericin MICs appear to correlate well with efficacy in animal models and human patients.[10] The MICs of

Table 9-4 Pharmacokinetic Data for Liposomal Amphotericin B Preparation in the Dog[22]

	Dose mg/kg	Day	*C_{max} µg/mL	AUC µg hr/mL	Vdss L/kg	CL mL hr/kg	HL hr
Liposomal	0.25	1	0.21±0.9	1.7±0.4	1.67±1.4	112±43	4.6±2.0
(Ambisome)		30	1.55±0.55	5.0±1.3	0.2±0.6	47±16	2.5±0.8
	1	1	1.5	9.5±4.0	0.96±0.81	79±44	8.3±4.5
		30	12	109±40	0.08±0.02	8.7±4	5.5±1.7
	4	1	20	143±34	0.3±0.09	26±8	8.4±2.2
		30	95	1452±423	0.04±0.03	1.8±1	16.0±4.7

AUC, Area under the curve; *CL*, clearance; *HL*, half-life; *VDss*, volume of distribution at steady state.
*Numbers without standard deviation were extrapolated from plots.

amphotericin B toward selected fungal microbes are listed in Table 9-4.[15,16] Although these are based on humans, they represent a reasonable target for isolates infecting animals as well. In addition to the MIC, the minimum fungicidal concentration (MFC) has been reported for selected organisms infecting humans (or animals).[15] The MFC_{50} and MFC_{90}; µg/mL) are, respectively, *Blastomyces dermatitidis* (0.125, 0.5); *H. capsulatum* (0.5, 2), and *C. immitis* (4, 16). In killing-curve studies, amphotericin B consistently exhibits concentration-dependent killing. However, killing is variable among organisms, being fungicidal toward *Candida* sp. but not toward many yeasts and other organisms. As a concentration-dependent drug, amphotericin B may exhibit a long post-antifungal effect (PAFE), which, like the postantibiotic effect of concentration antimicrobials, varies in duration with the organism and the relationship of the MIC to the plasma drug concentration (PDC).[10] However, it can prolong the dosing interval of the drug. A PAFE of only 0.5 hours occurs at approximately 2 hours exposure at drug concentrations that reflect 0.5 times the MIC, but this duration is prolonged to approximately 10 hours at 32 times the MIC for *Candida* and *Cryptococcus neoformans;* the PAFE for the latter may exceed 12 hours.[10]

KEY POINT 9-3 Despite the advent of the azole antifungal drugs, amphotericin B remains the most effective agent against most of the major fungal pathogens.

Sufficient data exist to integrate Ambisome pharmocokinetics and pharmacodynamics toward selected microbes that infect the dog (Table 9-4; see also Table 9-2). Two targets are considered: the MFC and a 12-hour PAFE (targeting PDCs that equal the MIC_{90} of the infecting microbe by 32). Based on the C_{max} of dogs for Ambisome measured at day 1 and day 30 of dosing, the MFC of *B. dermatitidis* and *H. capsulatum* will be achieved on the first day of dosing at 1 mg/kg. Assuming the PAFE as described in animal models would be exhibited by dimorphic fungal organisms infecting dogs, based on MIC_{90} for *B. dermatitidis* of 0.05 µg/mL (see Table 9-2), a target of 1.6 µg/mL (32 times the MIC) is indicated to achieve a 10 to 12-hour PAFE. Again, the target will be reached in dogs on day 1 with a 1 mg/kg dose of Ambisome; the 12-hour PAFE could be added to the time the PDCs are above the MIC (which in turn, is based on half-life). For *H. capsulatum*, the MIC_{90} is 1 µg/mL; accordingly, a target of 32 µg/mL (for at least 2 hours) might be indicated to achieve a 10 to 12-hour PAFE. Assuming linear kinetics, reaching the target on day 1 will require a dose of approximately 4 mg/kg, which is likely not to be tolerated (an exception may occur for lipid-based products). However, the target is likely to be approached with 30 days of dosing at 2.5 mg/kg. *C. immitis* is less susceptible to the killing effects of amphotericin B; the MFC_{90} (11 µg/mL) is likely to be reached on day 1 of dosing at 2.5 mg/kg, but 30 days of dosing will be required to reach the MFC_{90} or the 12-hour PAFE. These calculations were based on the MIC_{90} of the respective organisms; if the MIC of the infecting microbe is known, then a lower dose might be reasonable.

Resistance

The incidence of resistance to amphotericin B is low and has been documented primarily for *Candida.* The development of resistance may be related to changes in the number of sterol components in the fungal cell wall, with low ergosterol content associated with resistance.[3] *Pythium insidiosum*, classified as a pseudofungus, (the cause of what was previously and inappropriate referred to as fungal phycomycosis), as with other oomycetes, is largely devoid of cell membrane sterol. As such, they are inherently resistant to polyenes.[1] However, other mechanisms of resistance also exist, probably reflecting multiple mechanisms. Some organisms are able to resist concentrations that exceed 2 µg/mL. The azole derivatives may contribute to amphotericin B resistance by preventing the formation of ergosterol, the target of amphotericin B.[1]

Amphotericin appears to act synergistically with the following: 5-flucytosine against cryptococcosis, tetracyclines against coccidioidomycosis, and imidazoles (discussed later) for a variety of fungal disorders. The use of synergistic combinations may enhance efficacy while reducing the potential of toxicity.

Preparations

Because amphotericin is unstable, it is prepared with desoxycholate as a lyophilized cake form (amphotericin B; previously Fungizone®; AmBD). Supplies were limited at the time of publication,[8] perhaps reflecting declining use in human medicine in favor of newer lipid-based formulations.

Desoxycholate—also referred to as deoxycholate, a bile salt—is added to aid solubilization of the lyophilized cake form of the drug, which, when reconstituted, is in a colloidal suspension. Reconstitution should be with sterile water only; the solution will remain stable for 1 week if refrigerated. Storage should include protection from light, although protection during therapy is probably not necessary; potency is unaffected after light exposure of up to 24 hours. Labeled directions indicate that dilution should occur only with 5% dextrose to prevent drug precipitation and inactivation; Trissel's *Handbook on Injectable Drugs* (http://online.statref.com/titles/titleinfopage.aspx?titleid=141) indicates that normal saline is incompatible with amphotericin B, leading to a 43% drop in drug concentrations within 2 hours. Although the drug has been mixed by veterinarians with 0.45% NaCl and 2.5% dextrose with no apparent change, the basis for this observation is unclear, and the prudent clinician would avoid the combination and provide sodium loading (see the section on therapeutic use) through a different catheter. In general, amphotericin B should not be mixed with other drugs; although known to be compatible with some, it is incompatible with many others. The drug should be administered only intravenously, with exceptions for localized treatment in selected body tissues or fluids (e.g., aqueous humor, cerebrospinal fluid [CSF]). For small animals, which do not require a complete vial, the reconstituted drug can be divided into smaller aliquots and frozen.

Amphotericin also has been complexed to lipid mixtures in an attempt to reduce nephrotoxicity. Reticuloendothelial cells phagocytize the lipid component, facilitating directed delivery to the site of fungal infection. Drug uptake by the hepatic and splenic macrophages, bone marrow, and inflammatory tissues is thus enhanced. For liposomal products, some studies have shown that amphotericin B is selectively transferred from liposomes to fungal but not host cell membranes. Prolonged antifungal activity (compared with nonliposomal preparations) has been documented for these preparations. Each product is injectable and differs in the lipid makeup as well as the ratio of lipid to amphotericin B. Lipid-based products include a lipid complex (ABLC; Abelcet) suspension that forms a tightly packed ribbonlike structure and is the largest of the lipid-based products (250 nm); a colloidal dispersion of cholesterol sulfate, which forms 122 nm disks (Amphotec or Amphocil [ABCD]); and a single-layered liposomal product, Ambisome (LAmB; see Table 9-4), which is the simplest and smallest (60 to 70 nm) of the molecules.[17,18] The differences among these products have recently been reviewed.[19] Amphotericin B also has been administered with a lipid vehicle (intralipid; AMB-IL) rather than 5% dextrose. Although nephrotoxocity appears to be reduced in some patients, it does not appear to be decreased in the patients at most risk for toxicity, and therefore liposomal lipid-based products should be considered.[18a] Administration of AMB-IL also is not recommended because of mixed product is unstable. The differences among the lipid-based or lipid-containing products and their clinical use in humans have recently been reviewed.[19]

Amphotericin is also available as a topical preparation (Fungizone), including cream, lotion, and ointment forms.

Pharmacokinetics

Amphotericin is not water soluble and thus is not bioavailable after oral administration. It is more than 90% bound to circulating serum lipoproteins (including cholesterol). Penetration into the pleura, peritoneum, inflamed tissues, CSF, and aqueous humor may result in a drug concentration two thirds of that in the plasma. The metabolism and excretion of amphotericin is not well characterized and is complex, being complicated by binding to cholesterol, which is structurally similar to ergosterol (see Figure 9-3). Biliary elimination may be the primary method of excretion (in humans only 3% of the drug is eliminated in the urine); however, concentrations are detectable in both bile and urine for up to 7 weeks in human patients.

The pharmacokinetics of the various amphotericin B preparations, including those complexed to lipids, vary markedly in humans; interpretation of kinetics is complicated by the lack of discrimination between free amphotericin B and that complexed to the various carriers. Because of its small size, Ambisome is characterized by the slowest uptake, and the highest PDCs. In humans, peak PDCs (μg/mL) vary with the dose (indicated in mg/kg), reflecting differences in volume of distribution that vary on account of tissue uptake: AmBD, 2.9 μg/mL at 1 mg/kg); Albecet (ABLC), 1.7 μg/mL at 5 mg/kg); Amphotec (ABCD), 3.1 μg/mL at 5 mg/kg; and Ambisome (LAmB), 83 μg/mL at 5 mg/kg. For LAmB, concentrations appear to be both dose and time dependent in dogs (Table 9-4). An advantage of the liposomal product is that it accumulates at sites of infection and targets the fungal cell wall, with release of amphotericin into the cell.[19] For ABLC (and LAmB), tissue or fungal phospholipases appear to release amphotericin B at the site of infection. However, the colloidal form of amphotericin B (Amphocil), which is taken up by reticuloendothelial cells, was demonstrated in humans to accumulate in lung tissues to a greater concentration than Ambisome, suggesting that it might be preferable for respiratory infections.[20] This finding requires further support by animal model or clinical studies. That LAmB may be preferred for central nervous system (CNS) infections is supported by the study and review of Ibrahim and coworkers,[21] who address the potential inability of ABLC to penetrate the brain in mice or rabbit models. Comparing dosing ranges, LAmB was effective without nephrotoxicity at 5 to 20 mg/kg in animal models of disease, with highest tolerated doses being 30 to 50 mg/kg (as reviewed by Adler).[19] Although ABLC was efficacious at doses ranging from 5 to 15 mg/kg, nephrotoxicity and decreased efficacy occurred at 15 mg/kg compared to 5 mg/kg. (as reviewed by Adler).[19]

The pharmacokinetics of Ambisone (LAmB) have been described in Beagles (n = 10 per group) as part of a toxicity study in humans and compared historically to AmBD (see Table 9-4).[22] Dogs received 0.25 to 16 mg/kg/day as an intravenous infusion over 5 minutes, with PDCs determined on days 1, 14, and 30. Dogs receiving 8 and 16 mg/kg daily did not finish the treatment period because of severe weight loss (n = 17/20); this same pattern of weight loss was also described in dogs receiving AmBD at 0.75 mg/kg every other day (as reviewed by Bekersky and coworkers[22]). However, dogs tolerated 4 mg/kg Ambisone daily with peak concentrations at this dose were markedly variable, ranging from 18 μg/mL at day 1 to 94 μg/mL at day 30. Concentrations of Ambisone were a hundredfold higher than other formulations: A dose of 0.6 to 0.75 of AmBD resulted in peak amphotericin concentrations of 1.25 to 4.4 μg/mL after multiple dosing. This compares to a peak concentration of 54 ± 16 μg/mL at 4 mg/kg daily. Ambisome kinetics were nonlinear, with clearance and distribution decreasing as dose increased, potentially reflecting saturation of distribution and clearance processes. For example, although dose only increased 64-fold in the study, area under the curve (AUC) on day 1 at 0.25 mg/kg was 2.6 μg*hr/mL (compared) to 2592 μg hr/mL at 16 mg/kg, representing a 2500-fold increase. Multiple dosing also resulted in accumulation at each dose, with 30-day to 1 day AUC ratios being 2.5 and 10 at low (0.25 mg/kg) and intermediate (4 and 8 mg/kg) doses, respectively. (see Table 9-4). Kinetics are likely to be equally complex in other dogs and cats, and lack of predictability may limit use.

Toxicities and Side Effects

Nephrotoxicity is the major side effect associated with the use of amphotericin B. Renal function becomes impaired in more than 80% of patients receiving amphotericin,[4,23,24] with serum creatinine at least doubling in 40% to 60% in human.[23] Although largely reversible, renal toxicity depends on total cumulative dose and duration of therapy. In human patients chronic renal disease occurs in close to 50% of patients receiving more than approximately 60 mg/kg total dose compared with only 17% who receive less than 57 mg/kg. The proportion decreases to 8% in those receiving less than 14 mg/kg total dose.[23] Although renal function usually returns to normal before completion of therapy, some residual damage often persists after discontinuation of the drug. Two mechanisms are important in renal toxicity. Intense arterial vasoconstriction occurs within 15 minutes of administration and lasts 4 to 6 hours. The mechanism is unknown but can lead to acute tubular nephrosis secondary to ischemia. Nerve degeneration, angiotensin II receptor blockage, adrenergic blockade, and potent vasodilators do not prevent renal vasoconstrictive effects. Amphotericin B may activate formation of vasoconstrictive (thromboxane) arachidonic acid metabolites, which suggests that direct vasoconstriction may be responsible. Amphotericin B can increase calcium fluxes. Histologic lesions are most profound in regions vulnerable to hypoxia or areas rich in oxygen.[23]

KEY POINT 9-4 Liposomal-based amphotericin is among the safest with regard to nephrotoxicity.

Distal renal tubular toxic effects result from binding of membrane cholesterol in the tubular cell membrane (see Figure 9-4). Altered electrolyte fluxes result in acidification abnormalities (metabolic acidosis), hypokalemia, and concentrating defects (polyuria, polydipsia). Renal tubular acidosis is common, dose related, and generally reversible (although resolution may take several months) and generally precedes significant decreases in glomerular filtration rate (GFR). Potassium and magnesium wasting in humans can lead to substantial deficits.[23] Magnesium deficits appear at 2 weeks and are maximal at 4 weeks. Both potassium and magnesium should be monitored; electrolyte abnormalities may persist for several weeks after therapy is discontinued. Rarely, hyperkalemia has been reported in association with rapid infusion as potassium shifts from the intracellular compartments. The risk is greater in patients with renal failure. Concentration defects occur in essentially all human patients, are not related to azotemia, and may persist for months. Urine specific gravity may not be an effective measure by which to assess renal damage.

Ampohtericin B toxicity has been documented in dogs. Ceylan and colleagues[24] described the nephrotoxicity of AmBD in dogs (n = 18; cross-bred) receiving 0.5 mg/kg in 25 mL 5% dextrose in water as a 4- to 5-minute intravenous bolus; 1 mg/kg in 50 mL as a 4- to 5-minute bolus, or 2 mg/kg in 1000 mL over 4 to 5 hours. Dogs were treated for 12 days. Side effects (vomiting, diarrhea, anorexia, fever, tachycardia, and phlebitis) were evident in all dogs by day 3 but were worse in dogs receiving 1 mg/kg and least in dogs receiving 2 mg/kg. Indicators of renal damage (blood urea nitrogen, creatinine) were increased in all groups by day 5 but were highest in the 1 mg/kg group. Serum calcium was significantly decreased compared with baseline in the 1 mg/kg and 2 mg/kg groups. Hematologic indicators of anemia were evident in the 1 mg/kg group. Among the indicators of nephrotoxicity studied was urine γ-GGT, which was significantly higher than baseline in all groups by day 5 of therapy but did not differ among groups or times during treatment. On the basis of this study, the authors suggested that infusion over a 4- to 5-hour period (or fluid support) decreases the risk of aminoglycoside toxicity. However, no study has determined the long-term effects of any method of administration of amphotericin B on renal failure in dogs or cats.

In their pharmacokinetic study of LAmB (Ambisome) in Beagles at doses ranging from 0.25 to 16 mg/kg daily for 30 days, Bekersky and coworkers[22] reported that no dogs died as a result of the drug; however, dose-dependent tubular nephrosis was present at 1 mg/kg, and 70% and 100% of dogs in the 8 and 16 mg/kg treatment group, respectively, were euthanized before the end of the study because of 25% or more body weight loss. Vomiting and diarrhea were evident in all groups, including a liposomal (i.e., without amphotericin B) control, but were worse in the 4, 8, and 16 mg/kg treatment groups. Azotemia was not present in the 1 mg/kg group. Azotemia was described as moderate and clinically significant toward the end of the 30-day treatment period in the 4 mg/kg group, with creatinine increasing from a baseline of 0.7.1 ± to 2.3 ± 0.4 mg/dl by study end. Serum potassium was not clinically affected. The authors concluded that dogs tolerated up to 4 mg/kg well, despite peak amphotericin B concentrations ranging from 18 to 94 μg/mL.

Acute anaphylactic-type reactions such as vomiting, fever, and chills can occur with the use of amphotericin B and have been reported with lipid complex preparations as well.[25] Up to 30% of dogs receiving AmBD develop fever.[26] The frequent incidence of these reactions often leads to pretreatment for anaphylaxis (one-time use of a short-acting glucocorticoid does not enhance the toxicity of amphotericin B; see the discussion of "cocktail" in the following section).

Other side effects associated with amphotericin B include nausea and anorexia, thrombophlebitis, cardiac arrhythmias and related toxicities, hepatic dysfunction, and CNS signs (if given intrathecally) (see discussion on therapeutic use). Several side effects can be prevented by proper treatment (see following discussion of therapeutic use).

Drug Interactions

Amphotericin B interacts in an additive to synergistic fashion with a number of antifungal agents (see the discussion of combination therapy), although this effect seems to be most consistent with flucytosine. Although synergistic effects should be expected with azoles, this combination may be antagonistic if azole therapy is begun first.

In general, drugs that are renally active are not recommended for patients also receiving amphotericin B. In humans cyclosporine and tacrolimus (calcineurin inhibitors) will enhance nephrotoxicity. However, these immunomodulators tend to be safer, as far as nephrotoxicity is concerned, in both dogs and cats, and the combination may not be as dangerous. The nephrotoxicity of amphotericin also may be enhanced with catabolic drugs such as glucocorticosteroids, antineoplastic drugs, antiprostaglandins (glucocorticoids and nonsteroidal antiinflammatory drugs), and other nephrotoxic antibiotics. One study demonstrated that diuretic therapy during, but not just before, amphotericin B therapy increased the risk of nephrotoxicity more than twelvefold (as reviewed by Bagnis and Deray[23]). Although diuretics have been used for a "protective" effect, the potential benefits are limited to mannitol, and even it may be associated with electrolyte disturbances. Combination with digoxin may enhance nephrotoxicity and hypokalemia. Declining renal function in association with amphotericin B therapy may affect clearance of co-administered drugs. Because it is renally excreted, 5-flucytosine toxicity may be enhanced if renal function declines with amphotericin B.

Therapeutic Use

Most of the advice and studies addressing the recommended method of administration of amphotericin B are based on the non-lipid preparation (AmBD).

Multiple strategies may help reduce toxicities or side effects to amphotericin B. The first focuses on prevention of an anaphylactoid reaction by pretreatment (to prevent vomiting, fever, chills, and anaphylaxis) with antihistamines (diphenhydramine 0.5 mg/kg, administered intravenously) and short-acting glucocorticosteroids (e.g., hydrocortisone sodium succinate, 0.5 mg/kg, administered intravenously). Because the reaction appears to be associated with direct mast cell degranulation (because of the cationic nature of amphotericin B), pretreatment with a small test dose (0.1 mg/kg for cats or 0.25 mg/kg for dogs diluted in 10 mL infused over 15 minutes) may help identify animals that are likely to have an adverse reaction during infusion. Whereas lipid products may be characterized by less nephrotoxicity, they are more likely than nonlipid products to cause vomiting, nausea, and phlebitis.[38] As such, pretesting is indicated with their use as well.

In addition to dilution protocols (see discussion under Toxicity), strategies are intended to minimize amphotericin-B induced nephrotoxicity. Although what constitutes amphotericin B nephrotoxicity may vary, an increase in creatinine of as little as 25% may be considered significant in some patients.[18] Azotemia precedes tubular dysfunction in humans, allowing for early detection (i.e., before irreversible damage). Urine sediment initially should be monitored for evidence of nephrotoxicity. Serum chemistries tend to be less sensitive indicators of nephrotoxicity. Urine γ-gt has been used to assess lipid-based amphotericin B toxicity. The drug should be temporarily discontinued (24 to 48 hours) if the blood urea nitrogen level becomes abnormal.[27]

KEY POINT 9-5 Nephrotoxicity caused by amphotericin B might be minimized by several approaches, including pretreatment with sodium-containing fluids.

First and foremost, pretreatment with sodium-containing fluids is particularly important for preventing renal toxicity, including that associated with renal arterial vasoconstriction; posttherapy treatment might also be prudent. Secondly, amphotericin B can be administered with a "cocktail" intended to protect the kidney. Administration of the dose diluted in 5% dextrose is accompanied by mannitol (0.5 mg/kg) to maintain glomerular filtration rate and sodium bicarbonate (1 to 2 mg/kg) to prevent cellular acidification defects. The mannitol and sodium bicarbonate should not be added directly to the amphotericin B solution but given through another catheter in order to avoid precipitation of amphotericin B. The ability of cocktails to prevent nephrotoxicity is controversial. The treatment is based on one small study in dogs[31] for which mannitol was demonstrated to protect the kidney. However, a subsequent study (using isolated perfused rat kidneys) found mannitol to impart a protective effect, presumably by reducing renal tubular edema by virtues of its osmotic effect.[32] Binding of cellular cholesterol prevented toxicity, supporting the presumed mechanism of direct cytotoxicty. This study also demonstrated a synergistic toxic effect of amphotericin B in the presence of hypoxia. Only one clinical trial, in humans, has addressed renoprotection by mannitol, and it failed to identify an effect. However, this clinical trial, although randomized, involved only 11 patients and is probably not conclusive (as reviewed by Bagnis and Deray[18,23]) Although such cocktails generally are not harmful as long as the solutions are not mixed with amphotericin B, mannitol has been associated with electrolyte abnormalities in the human-medicine literature.[23] Deray[18] indicates that mannitol decreases renal medullary blood flow and PO_2. As such, the use of mannitol remains controversial. A relatively recent study describes the nephroprotective effects of *N*-acetylcysteine (10 mg/kg daily) in a rat model of amphotericin-induced nephrotoxicity;[33] administration began 1 day before amphotericin was started. As previously described, amphotericin should not be mixed with solutions containing electrolytes, acidic solutions, or preservatives because these materials may cause drug precipitation. The rate at which amphotericin B is administered may also reduce the incidence of nephrotoxicity.

The third strategy by which amphotericin B toxicity might be reduced is administration with lipids or as a specialized delivery system (in lipids). Conventional amphotericin B is not recommended in humans in the presence of renal insufficiency, hypokalemia, hypomagnesemia, tubular acidoses, or polyuria.[18] Lipid preparations are designed to deliver more drug selectively to the site of infection,[34] thus allowing higher doses (see the section on preparations). The liposomal products tend to be very expensive. In contrast to liposomes, fat emulsions are easy to prepare and administer and tend to be more cost effective. These products appear to be equal in efficacy to nonliposomal products but safer with regard to nephrotoxicity. However, the use of intralipid as the vehicle (AmB-IL) is associated with other difficulties that limit its use (see previous discussion).

The safety of liposomal or lipid-based products may allow delivery of higher doses without an increased risk of nephrotoxicity, with the incidence of nephrotoxicity reduced by 8% to 28%, depending on the preparation.[18,23] Although several studies are available that address the safety of these products individually, and LAmB (Ambisome) in particular,[35] none appears to have compared all three products. However, in general, the liposomal product LAmB (Ambisome) is recognized to be the safest with regard to nephrotoxicity. Ambisome achieves the highest concentrations in humans compared with other amphotericin preparations but is well tolerated renally.[17,19] In general, efficacy of LAmB is equal to or exceeds that of AmBD and is consistently better tolerated. Survival rates in humans for the product ranges from 99% to 100% (visceral leishmaniasis; three studies, n ≅ 400), 37% to 78% (aspergillosis; five studies, n ≅ 400), 84% to 93% for cryptococcosis (two studies, n ≅ 280), 98% for histoplasmosis (one study, n = 55), and 20% to 69% for zygomycosis (three studies, n ≅ 130).[35] That LAmB may be preferred for CNS infections is supported by the study and review of Ibrahim and coworkers,[21] who found LAmB generally superior to ABLC in treating CNS infections, as indicated by response and decrease in fungal load. Abelcet (ABLC) and LamB were generally characterized as having the lowest incidence of all side effects (fever, chills, nausea, dyspnea, hypertension, hypotension, tachycardia, and nephrotoxicity) with the exception of hypokalemia (42% with LamB). Ambisome was associated with abnormal hepatic function tests in approximately 20% of human patients.[17] Abelcet causes fewer infusion-related side effects in humans, and therefore a test dose is not necessarily indicated, whereas Amphotec is more likely to cause infusion side effects and should be given as a short infusion only.

One study reports the efficacy and safety of a liposomal product when used at higher than recommended cumulative doses for treatment of canine blastomycosis.[36] In another study, although the products were equally efficacious, the degree of nephrotoxicity between a fat emulsion and standard amphotericin B was no different.[37] Amphotericin B also has been administered with a lipid vehicle (intralipid) rather than 5% dextrose. Although nephrotoxocity appears to be reduced in some patients, it does not appear to be decreased in the patients at most risk for toxicity, and therefore liposomal lipid-based products should be considered.[18] Further studies documenting the efficacy and safety of liposomal or fat emulsion products containing amphotericin B are needed.

A fourth strategy that can be used to minimize adverse events associated with amphotericin B is administration using alternative routes. Localized mycotic infections have been treated with localized administration of amphotericin, which may reduce the incidence of nephrotoxicity. Subconjunctival, intravitreal, intrathecal, intranasal (human aspergillosis: 5 mg/mL in water administered as aerosol), and intraperitoneal routes have been reported. Oral administration has been used for treatment of gastrointestinal candidiasis and presumably might be used for other gastrointestinal fungal disorders.[29] Both LamB and ABLC have been demonstrated to have enhanced efficacy when administered as an aerosol for pulmonary infections (as reviewed by Adler).[19] Amphotericin B (AmBD) can be mixed in sterile water to 200 mg/kg and infused into the bladder for fungal cystitis. For fungal infections of the CNS, the drug can be given (0.2 to 0.5 mg in either 5 mL of CSF or 10% dextrose) intrathecally (under general anesthesia) two to three times per week.[27]

Combination antifungal therapy is a fifth stategy that is strongly encouraged to enhance efficacy and thus decrease the duration of antifungal exposure to the host. For example, as reviewed by Adler,[19] efficacy of LamB is enhanced when combined with micafungin (zygomycosis, aspergillosis) and voriconazole (aspergillosis).

Although a sixth strategy whereby amphotericin B toxicity can reduced includes variation in doses, frequency of administration, concomitant therapy, and duration of therapy, no protocol has proven to be superior to others. Some literature supports rapid intravenous administration (bolus) in less debilitated dogs; slow intravenous administration might be more prudent in cats. A dose (0.25 to 0.5 mg/kg) can be diluted in 300 to 1000 mL of 5% dextrose and administered in an indwelling catheter over 2 to 6 hours, or it can be diluted in as little as 10 to 60 mL (30 recommended) and given over 2 to 10 minutes through a butterfly catheter[27] (flush catheter after infusion). The slow infusion method has the added advantage of additional fluids, which may reduce the incidence of nephrotoxicity,[28] especially in debilitated animals. The advantages of dilution and slow infusion is preferred and was previously discussed (see Toxicity). It is recommended that the small bolus be preceded or followed up with supplemental fluid, preferably normal saline. One report of an uncontrolled clinical trial describes the successful and apparently safer administration of amphotericin B after twice- or thrice-weekly subcutaneous administration (0.5 to 0.8 mg/kg diluted in 400 to 500 mL of fluid such that amphotericin B is less than 20 mg/L) for several months for treatment of cryptococcosis in dogs and cats.[30] However, only five successful cases were described, and further confirmation should be expected before this route is routinely embraced.

The sequence of repetitive treatments is also controversial. Some authors recommend alternate-day therapy, whereas others recommend daily therapy at a smaller dose. Doses also vary. Daily doses range from 0.15 to 0.5 mg/kg every other day (e.g., on Monday, Wednesday, Friday) until a cumulative dose of 4 to 12 mg/kg (depending on the organism or if therapy is combined with another antifungal) AmBD has been reached. Starting at a low dose (0.15 to 0.25 mg/kg) and gradually increasing the dose until the desired daily dose has been reached may reduce the severity of side effects. For particularly resistant infections, a dose of 1 mg/kg has been used on an alternate-day basis.

Other Polyenes

The spectrums of piramicin (natamycin) and nystatin are similar to that of amphotericin B. Pirimacin is used primarily to treat fungal keratitis, although efficacy toward *Aspergillus* may be questionable.[3] Aerosolization of piramycin for treatment of susceptible fungal disorders also should be considered. The toxicity of nystatin precludes parenteral administration, although a liposomal product is being formulated. Currently, use of nystatin is limited to superficial and mucosal mycoses.

AZOLE DERIVATIVES

Structure–Activity Relationship

The azole derivatives (imidazoles and triazoles) include a large number of predominantly synthetic drugs. These drugs consist of a five-member ring with other aromatic rings attached by a carbon nitrogen bond. Imidazoles contain two nitrogen atoms and include clotrimazole, econazole, enilconazole, miconazole, and ketoconazole. Triazoles contain three nitrogen atoms and include fluconazole, itraconazole, and voriconazole (see Figure 9-1).[4,39-41] Among the newer azoles are posaconazole and voriconazole. Voriconazole, a synthetic deriviative of fluconazole, is the first of the second-generation triazole compounds to be approved by the Food and Drug Administration. Voriconazole contains a fluorine molecule and a methyl group, which greatly enhances its spectrum compared with that of fluconazole.[42] Other triazoles have been patented. Most compounds generally are not available as solutions because they tend to be insoluble in water (an exception is fluconazole). They are, however, soluble in organic solvents such as propylene glycol.

Mechanism of Action

The azoles target fungal sterol ergosterol. However, in contrast to amphotericin B, the imidazole derivatives do not bind to ergosterol but rather block its synthesis. The azoles inhibit fungal cytochrome P450 enzymes with sterol14α-demethylase as the primary fungal target; however, other synthesizing enzymes also are targeted.[3] Decreased cell membrane ergosterol alters cell membrane function but also is accompanied by an increase in 14-methylsterols, compounds that are potentially toxic. Cell membrane function fluidity decreases as cell permeability increases, resulting in a fungistatic effect (fluconazole and ketoconazole). At higher concentrations, selected drugs (miconazole, econazole, clotrimazole) also interfere with cell membrane fluidity and physiochemical intracellular processes (e.g., secretory vesicles, mitochondrial respiration), resulting in fungicidal effects. Efficacy of selected agents against gram-positive organisms may reflect this latter effect.[3] Chitin synthesis increases in concert with decreased ergosterol synthesis, but its irregular distribution contributes to altered cell wall function. Because azoles also generate and detoxify intracellular hydrogen peroxide, selected drugs also express antibacterial, antiprotozoal, and anthelmintic activities. The imidazoles are also characterized by immunomodulatory effects, which may facilitate effective therapy.[5] Because their mechanism of action depends on cell wall synthesis, the onset of action of the imidazoles may result in a lag time to therapeutic efficacy. In addition, a long elimination half-life of some members of this class (e.g., itraconazole) results in a lag time as steady-state concentrations are achieved.

KEY POINT 9-6 The mechanism of action of the azoles will result in a lag time to efficacy, which may be prolonged further because of the time that must elapse before steady state concentrations are reached.

Spectrum of Activity and Pharmacodynamics

Although the imidazole derivatives are more selective in their cellular activity than amphotericin B (i.e., impairing the synthesis of rather than binding to ergosterol), their spectrum of activity is broad and includes the dermatophytes ("ringworm": *Microsporum* and *Trichophyton* species), yeasts, dimorphic fungi (blastomycosis, histoplasmosis, cryptococcosis, coccidioidomycosis), *Eumycetes, Actinomyces,* and some *Phycomycetes.*[1,4,11,27,40,43] The efficacy against these organisms varies. Studies comparing the efficacies of the azoles in animals are limited at the time of this publication, although several are pending in the human-medicine literature.

KEY POINT 9-7 Although not as efficacious as amphotericin B, the spectrum of the imidazoles is the broadest of the clinically used antifungal drugs.

In vitro MIC data regarding the relative susceptibility of selected organisms to itraconazole emphasize the variable susceptibility of fungal organisms to these drugs. Table 9-2 provides MIC_{90} data for selected organisms and itraconazole. For dermatophytes, the MIC_{90} for *Microsporum* species is 250 μg/mL versus for *Trichophyton* species 4 μg/mL. For other *Eumycetes,* MIC_{90} concentrations range from 0.130 μg/mL to more than 128 μg/mL.[11,44] Fluconazole generally is considered to be fungistatic in action. This has been demonstrated for *Candida* sp. and *C. neoformans.*[10] However, more recent data suggest that fungicidal activity may occur toward *Candida*. Like fluconazole, itraconazole more consistently exerts a time-dependent, fungistatic effect toward most organisms. The MFC_{50} and MFC_{90} (μg/mL) have been reported for *B. dermatitidis* (0.125, 3, respectively), *H. capsulatum* (2, 16), and *C. immitis* (>16 for both).[15] However, it may exert fungicidal effects towards *Aspergillus*. The long half-lives of the imidazoles will facilitate convenience of dosing despite their time-dependent killing effects. Efficacy of itraconazole will be enhanced by the formation of its active metabolite, hydroxyl-itraconazole, which may surpass the parent.[45] As with other azoles, the spectrum of the third-generation imidazoles, posaconazole (similar in structure to itraconazole) and voriconazole (similar in structure to fluconazole), includes a variety of infecting fungal organisms. Their spectrums are very similar.[10] Posaconazole has been demonstrated to be more potent than fluconazole toward *Candida* and should be effective against the dimorphic fungal organisms,[46] although little information is available regarding its use. As with other azoles, voriconazole is fungistatic toward yeasts, exhibiting time-dependent killing, but for some filamentous organisms may be -cidal. Its spectrum includes *Candida* sp., with MIC generally being 1 to 2 log lower than fluconazole; however, MICs are higher for fluconazole-resistant strains than for nonresistant strains. Voriconazole also is effective against *C. neoformans, Trichosporon beigelii,* and *Saccharomyces cerevisiae*. Additionally, it is very effective against *Aspergillus* sp., including some strains resistant to amphotericin B; indeed, it is approved for the treatment of *Aspergillosis* in humans. Time-killing studies with *Aspergillus* demonstrate that, in general, amphotericin B is more efficacious but itraconazole less efficacious than voriconazole. Activity against *B. dermatitidis, C. immitis,* and *H. capsulatum* appears to be "reasonable" but "less" toward *S. schenckii*. Li[15] compared the MICs of amphotericin B, itraconazole, and voriconazole and found voriconazole to be more active in vitro than amphotericin B for the mold forms of *H. capsulatum, B. dermatitidis,* and *C. immitis,* with activity being fungicidal (MFC_{50}, MFC_{90}, respectively) toward *B. dermatitidis* (0.125, 4) and some *H. capsulatum* (8, ≥ 32) (see Table 9-2). Fungicidal activity toward *C. immitis* is difficult to achieve (>32 for the MFC_{50}). Activity *Aspergillus* also is fungicidal (MFC not provided) toward several dematiaceous molds.[15] Many dematiaceous and hyaline molds resistant to amphotericin B (e.g., *Scedosporium, Fusarium, Paecilomyces, Alternaria)* are susceptible to voriconazole. However, zygomycetes are not susceptible.[42] Cutaneous infections by *Leishmania* species are clinically susceptible to ketoconazole.[47] Clotrimazole and miconazole are common drugs used topically for treatment of dermatophytosis (e.g., Conofite) or yeast (e.g., otic preparations such as Otomax). Both drugs, as well as other imidazoles (e.g,) appear to exhibit efficacy against gram-positive organisms including staphylococci and anaerobes.

Resistance

Resistance to the azoles has been sporadic, generally occurring in immunocompromised patients receiving long-term therapy. Failed drug accumulation in the cell is a major mechanism of resistance (e.g., *Candida* sp., *C. neoformans, Aspergillus flavus,* and *A. fumigatus*), caused by either decreased influx or formation of efflux proteins. Two major efflux transport proteins have been identified, particularly for *Candida* sp. toward fluconazole: the multidrug-resistant protein, major facilitator superfamily (MFS; a proton-motive-force–based mechanism; e.g., CaMDR1) and the ATP-binding cassette (e.g., CDR1 and 2). Resistance to azoles also may reflect altered interaction between the drug and targeted fungal CYP 450 enzyme; fluconazole appears more susceptible than itraconazole to mutations that alter drug-receptor fit. Gene amplification leading to enhanced synthesis of the target protein also has been identified as a mechanism of resistance to azole derivatives. Finally, fungal organisms may circumvent the synthetic pathway inhibited by azoles or compensate for altered enzyme activity; for example, inhibition of ergosterol may result in the accumulation of 14-methylated sterols that are less toxic than other compounds.[3] Resistance to fluconazole appears to be increasing. Widespread use of fluconazole for treatment of *Candida* has been associated with increased resistance of the drug for selected species. Whereas many molds (e.g., *A. fumigatus*) are inherently resistant to fluconazole,[3] resistance of *Aspergillus* isolates to itraconazole is rare. Combinations with nonantagonistic antifungal agents might be considered for treatment of infections by organisms associated with antifungal resistance.

Pharmacokinetics

Only selected pharmacokinetic information is available for the imidazoles in dogs or cats (Table 9-5).Oral absorption of the imidazole derivatives varies with the drug and among animals. For many drugs oral preparations are not available. For example, enilconazole (imazalil) is not orally bioavailable. For other imidazoles the rate of absorption varies from 1 to 4 hours. Oral absorption often depends on gastric pH, product preparation, and the presence of other drugs.[48] Absorption of itraconazole and ketoconazole is enhanced by gastric acidity; these drugs should be administered with food.[49] Alkalinizing drugs administered orally will decrease their absorption. Cyclodextrins are used to form complexes with the drugs, thus rendering the liphophilic drug soluble in solution, making oral solutions available for some drugs (e.g., Sporonix solution). In general, oral bioavailability should be anticipated to be better for these solutions than for capsules. Peak PDCs of itraconazole occur between 1 to 5 hours in cats and dogs. Bioavailability of capsules is approximately 20% in dogs and may be as little as 10% in cats, compared with close to 50% for the solution in cats and dogs.[50,51] Decreased bioavailability may be responsible for therapeutic failure associated with low PDCs in some animals (cats and dogs). Unpredictable oral administration of itraconazole prepared as a capsule limits its usefulness in humans; the solution, on the other hand, generates more predictable concentrations.[17] Care should be taken with compounded preparations; oral absorption generally is not verified for these products, and adequate oral bioavailability should not be assumed. Fluconazole is characterized by the best oral bioavailability among the imidazoles, being completely absorbed in cats;[52] however, its efficacy, compared with that of itraconazole, is limited.

KEY POINT 9-8 Absorption of itraconazole and ketoconazole is enhanced by gastric acidity; these drugs should be administered with food.

Table 9-5 Pharmacokinetic Data for Selected Imidazoles in the Dog

Drug	Dose (PO, Once) mg/kg	C_{max} µg/mL*	AUC (infinity) µg hr/mL	Half-Life hr	Oral Bioavailability %
Itraconazole[52]	5	3.55 ± 2.81		51	20 capsule
	10	13.5 ± 8.5			
Voriconazole[55]	3	6.5*	32 (IV); 89(PO)†	6.3	138
	3 (30 days)	1.69± 0.83†	18 (IV);52		
	6 (30 days)	4.54±2.22			
	12 (30 days)	10.34 ± 5.1			
Posaconazole[56]	10	3-3.5+	43-57	7	65-72 (cyclodextrin)
	10	0.2 (± 22%) at 7.6 hr	7.5	15	37-48 (methylcellulose)
	10 (fed)	0.7 (± 28%) at 8 hr	27		
	40 (fed)	2.1 (±31%) at 9 hr	105		

AUC, area under the curve; *D*, dog; *IV*, intravenous; *PO*, By mouth.
*50% protein bound.
†The lower C_{max} and AUC after 30 days of dosing reflects autoinduction.
Vehicle dependent+

Distribution to tissues also varies among the imidazoles. Ketoconazole is up to 99% protein bound; the highest tissue levels occur in the liver, lung, and kidney (and cerumen). Itraconazole is also very highly protein bound in humans.[4] There is minimal penetration of the CSF by ketoconazole, although fluconazole penetrates the CSF well, with serum to CSF PDCs ranging from 0.58 to 0.89 µg/mL. The volume of distribution of ketoconazole is only 0.87 L/kg in dogs compared with 17 L/kg 5 L/kg for itraconazole in dogs[51] and cats, respectively.[50] The volume of distribution of fluconazole is 1.14 L/kg in cats, with high concentrations occurring in the CSF and aqueous humor.[52] The difference in distribution volume reflects, in part, distribution and accumulation to fat.[51] Drug concentrations of itraconazole in the skin may exceed that in plasma by threefold to tenfold, with drug detectable 2 to 4 weeks after therapy is discontinued.[51] Although distribution of itraconazole to the CSF appears to be limited, therapeutic concentrations appear to be achieved in patients suffering from cryptococcal meningitis. Among the azole derivatives, fluconazole has the best tissue distribution pattern and can achieve effective concentrations in CSF.

KEY POINT 9-9 Among the imidazoles, fluconazole is characterized by the best oral bioavailability and distribution into the central nervous system.

With the exception of fluconazole, the azole derivatives are eliminated by extensive oxidative (cytochrome P450) metabolism with excretion as inactive metabolites into the bile and urine. However, metabolism of itraconazole generates an active hydroxylated metabolite, whose AUC may exceed that of the parent compound.[53] Metabolism may be dose dependent; elimination rate constants are lower and half-lives are longer at higher doses and with longer therapy. In contrast to the other imidazoles, fluconazole is eliminated principally (70%) in the urine. The half-life of the imidazoles varies, with that of ketoconazole being relatively short (1.4 hours in dogs). Fluconazole and itraconazole have longer half-lives, ranging from 22 to 32 hours in humans. The half-life of fluconazole in cats is 25 hours.[52] The half-life of itraconazole in dogs is 51 hours (itraconazole)[52] versus 40 to 70 hours in cats (itraconazole);[50] The longer drug elimination half-life must be taken into account because it results in a longer time to steady-state concentration and maximum therapeutic effect. However, it also allows the flexibility of once-daily (10 mg/kg) rather than twice-daily (5 mg/kg) dosing.

The disposition of voriconazole is complicated. Its disposition has been reported in dogs as part of a preclinical study (see Table 9-5).[55] Beagles (n = 4) received multiple doses (8) of 6 mg/kg orally or 3 mg/kg intravenously using a crossover design; disposition was studied on day 1 and day 30 for each route. The AUC after single and multiple dosing (µg*h/mL) after the intravenous dose was 32 and 18, respectively, and after the oral dose 89 and 52, respectively, suggesting autoinduction. Other relevant parameters after single oral dosing were as follows: C_{max}, 6.5 µg/mL at T_{max} of 3 hours and apparent bioavailability of 138%. The drug was 51% protein bound, indicating a concentration of approximately 3.25 µg/mL of active drug. For a safety study, Beagles (n = 6) also received oral doses of 3, 6, or 12 mg/kg for 1 month. The apparent volume of distribution was 1.3 L/kg and clearance was 24 mL/min/kg, resulting in a calculated half-life of 6.3 hours. The C_{max} increased in a slightly disproportionate dose-dependent manner, being 1.69 ± 0.83 µg/mL at 3 mg/kg and 10.3 ± 5.1 µg/mL at 12 mg/kg 30 days after oral dosing. However, cytochrome P450 increased in a dose-related manner, resulting in a 1.7-fold increase in relative liver weight at the highest compared with the lowest dose. Autoinduction in dogs, which does not occur in humans, resulted in an increased clearance after multiple dosing, with these effects dissipating approximately 1 month after the drug was discontinued. For example, the mean C_{max} after a single oral dose of 3 mg/kg in dogs was 6.5 µg/mL but only 1.7 after 30 days dosing at the same dose. Although 55% to 87% of the drug ultimately was eliminated in the urine in dogs, only 5% was as the parent drug, indicating extensive hepatic metabolism. A major pathway of metabolism was generation of the N-oxide and hydroxylation metabolites as well as glucuronidation. The dose of voriconazole recommended for dogs can be based on pharmacokinetic–pharmacodynamic integration. The MIC_{90} of most infecting microbes for which data are available will be achieved after 30 days at 3 mg/kg, even accounting for 50% protein binding in dogs. An exception occurs, however, for *H. capsulatum*, for which a higher dose is indicated. With a half-life of 6 hours, based on time-dependent killing, at least twice the MIC of the infecting microbe should be targeted to allow for a 12-hour dosing interval. In humans dosing regimens are designed to reach 3 to 6 μg/mL in the plasma; accordingly, a dose of 3 to 6 mg/kg twice daily is recommended. However, the half-life in humans is long (6 to 24 hours, depending on the dose), and steady-state concentration requires 5 to 6 days of dosing. As such, a loading dose consisting of a double daily dose is recommended for the first day of therapy. This is not necessary in dogs: the shorter half-life precludes accumulation to a steady state. However, the shorter half-life will necessitate twice-daily dosing. Because of autoinduction in dogs, dosing regimens should not be extrapolated for cats from dogs without the support of pharmacokinetic studies.

Voriconazole is cleared primarily by hepatic metabolism to inactive metabolites by CYP 2C19 (the primary isoenzyme), 2C9, and 3A4 being involved. Selected humans are considered "poor metabolizers" of the drug because of variation in CYP 2C19. In humans the dose is halved in the presence of mild to moderate liver disease. The relevance of this to dogs, which autoinduce, is not known.

Very limited pharmacokinetic information is available for dogs receiving posaconazole (see Table 9-5).[56] It was studied in two different vehicles (cyclodextrin or methylcellulose) during preclinical investigations. Absorption from the cyclodextrin vehicle was better, resulting in a higher C_{max}, greater AUC, and better oral bioavailability. Although the half-life following intravenous administration was approximately 8 hours, the effective half-life is 15 hours after oral administration, probably reflecting slow absorption, as is indicated by a T_{max} of 8 to 9 hours. Food enhanced absorption, increasing C_{max} and AUC fourfold. Although C_{max} increased more than two fold with multiple dosing, AUC was the same, indicating accumulation is not likely to be a clinical concern.

Preparations

Ketoconazole, itraconazole, and fluconazole are available for oral administration. Solutions are available for some products. Although their safety has not been documented for animals, fluconaozle (Diflucan) is available as an intravenous preparation that appears to be safe in cats when administered as a slow intravenous drip at 5 mg/kg. The solubility of imidazoles is poor and potentially toxic; solubilizing agents may cause adverse reactions. Cats also appear to tolerate a slow intravenous drip of itraconazole (5 mg/kg) with no adverse effects, although neither product is commercially available. Ketoconazole also is available in a topical preparation and a shampoo. Clotrimazole and miconazole are recommended only for localized dermatophyte or yeast infections susceptible to topical treatment. Clotrimazole has been used topically to treat nasal aspergillosis. Enilconazole is a topically effective azole that has been used to treat nasal aspergillosis but is available in the United States only as a 13.8% poultry dip. It is available in Canada as a 10% solution approved for use in dogs and horses. The poultry dip has been used topically in the United States at a dilution of 1:50 in water in dogs and cats with no apparent adverse effects. Terconazole is a new, topically active triazole that apparently has not yet been used for animals. However, an otic preparation containing posaconazole (with orbifloxacin and an anti-inflammatory) has recently been approved for dogs.

Drug Interactions

The azoles may interact synergistically with a number of antifungal agents. Synergism with polymyxin B is benefited in otic prepraitions.[3] Ketoconazole and, presumably, other azole antifungals have synergistic antifungal activities with 5–flucytosine against *Candida* and *Cryptococcus* and with amphotericin against a variety of organisms. However, timing of amphotericin B and azole therapy is important. Azoles impair ergosterol synthesis, and therefore their use before amphotericin B may decrease its efficacy which is dependent on active cell wall synthesis. Amphotericin B should begin either simultaneously with (azoles are characterized by a lag time to effect) or before azole administration. Enhanced efficacy has also been demonstrated for terbenifine and topical therapy (see Therapeutic Use).

Because the efficacy of the azoles depends on interaction with P450 (an oxidative enzyme responsible for drug metabolism), drug interactions at the level of drug or steroid metabolism should be anticipated in the patient. The azoles are both inhibitors and inducers of CYP isoenzymes; the extent to which an azole inhibits metabolism often depends on its relative affinity for host compared to fungal CYP 450.[3,57] All of the clinically relevant imidazoles inhibit some CYP. These include: CYP3A4 (ketoconazole, itraconazole, fluconazole, voriconazole; (ketoconzole has a higher affinity than itraconazole); 2C19 and 2C9 (ketoconazole, fluconazole, voriconazole); 2D6 (ketoconazole); 2C8 (ketoconazole and voriconazole); and 1A2 and 2E1 (ketoconazole). However, as has been demonstrated in dogs, voriconazole is an autoinducer and species differences in CYP interactions may be profound. When present, inhibition can be clinically relevant. It can be beneficial (e.g., the combination of ketoconazole with cyclosporine in an attempt to prolong cyclosporine clearance in order to decrease the daily cost of this drug (see Chapter 31).[58] In the author's laboratory, the effect of ketoconaozle on cyclosporine concentrations appears to be quite variable, ranging from no effect to a dramatic increase. Kukanich and Borum[59] found that ketoconazole (approximately 13 mg/kg for 5 days) did not appear to affect the intravenous disposition of morphine in Greyhounds.

However, more commonly, inhibition is associated with adverse reactions. The author is aware of two cases of marked increases in phenobarbital concentrations (to over 85 μg/mL) in epileptic dogs receiving fluconazole or itraconazole, respectively, for treatment of Malassezia; one of the dogs was euthanized resulting from (assumed) liver disease. More recently, a dog receiving deracoxib and also developed a perforated duodenal ulcer receiving ketaconazole for a skin yeast infection.

Itraconazole appears to cause autoinhibition; changes in the elimination half-life of intractonaozle have been documented in cats receiving long-term therapy (>6 weeks).[50] In humans, the risk of drug interactions involving voriconazole is high, perhaps more so than with the other azoles. Their magnitude and impact in dogs and cats needs to be clarified. Clinically relevant drug interactions have been documented for a number of drugs administered in concert with voriconazole; avoidance of other drugs administered by the liver would be prudent.[42]

KEY POINT 9-10 All imidazoles appear to impact drug-metabolizing enzymes, with inhibition being most common and clinically relevant.

Not all drug interactions involve inhibition of CYP. Clotrimazole is a potent inducer of CYP3A and miconazole of CYP 1A and 2E; even ketoconazole is an inducer of CYP 2, although it is less potent than clotrimazole (see Chapter 2 for drugs metabolized by CYP isozymes). As previously discussed, voriconazole is an inducer of CYP in dogs. Ketoconazole interferes with sex hormones and corticosteroids by displacing them from globulins and perhaps by interfering with their synthesis. Ketoconazole inhibits lanosterol14-demethylase (cholesterol synthesis; CYP51) and two hydroxylase enzymes responsible for steroid metabolism as well as a key enzyme involved in testosterone synthesis. As a result of its effects on steroid synthesis, ketoconazole has been used to treat hyperadrenocorticism and to impair testosterone synthesis in patients with prostatic hypertrophy or prostatic cancer. Ketoconazole has caused lightening of the hair coat of some dogs.[60] Willard and coworkers[60] reported depressed basal cortisol and testosterone concentrations and ACTH response by cortisol at 30 mg/kg/day. A rebound response was seen after ketoconazole was discontinued. Serum progesterone concentrations were also decreased. Aldosterone was not decreased. Cats receiving 30 mg/kg/day for 30 days developed dry hair coat and weight loss but no changes in testosterone or progesterone concentrations.[61]

Finally, not all clinically relevant drug interactions involving imidazoles reflect effects on cytochrome P450. The imidazoles in general are substrates for P-glycoprotein, and ketoconazole is a known inhibitor.[62] Accordingly, other drugs that serve as substrates for P–glycoprotein are likely to be absorbed to a greater extent. Thus ketoconazole can affect (increase) cyclosporine A concentrations following oral administration without affecting cyclosporine elimination half-life as has been documented in the author's laboratory.

Toxicities and Side Effects

In general, the imidazoles are not characterized by the complex toxicities that are associated with amphotericin B. Because the azoles interfere with synthesis of ergosterol rather than binding the sterol, the host toxicities typical of those induced by amphotericin do not occur.[63] Gastrointestinal toxicities are the most common and are not severe.[4,40,27,54,64] Nausea and vomiting can usually be prevented by administration of the drug with food. Hepatotoxicity with ketoconazole has been reported in humans. Mayer and colleagues[65] retrospectively reported adverse effects of ketoconazole in dogs. Medical records in Australia (n = 296), Germany (n = 35), and the United States (n = 301) were reviewed, and adverse events were reported in 92 (14.6%). Doses ranged from 2.6 to 33.4 mg/kg, with an average daily dose of 11.2 mg/kg. The frequency of adverse events was as follows: vomiting (7.1%), anorexia (4.9%), diarrhea (1.1%), and lethargy (1.9%). Uncommon side effects included pruritis (0.6%) and ataxia, polyuria, and polydipsia; causal relationships were difficult to establish for the uncommon reactions.

Side effects to itraconazole are limited to gastrointestinal symptoms (nausea and vomiting), which may be related in part to the vehicle if associated with the oral solution (a cyclodextrin carrier).[3] One case of cutaneous drug eruption typical of erythema multiforme caused by itraconazole has been reported in a dog;[67] idiopathic vasculitis has also been reported.[54] Fluconazole is associated with very few side effects; hematologic disorders may occur particularly in profoundly ill patients; otherwise, side effects appear to be limited to gastroinestinal and cutaneous reactions.

Isolated cases of hepatotoxicity have been reported with itraconazole and fluconazole. A retrospective study of dogs with blastomycosis found 5% to 10% of dogs treated with itraconaxole (5 to 10 mg/kg bid) developed hepatotoxicity with the effect dose dependent.[119] A dose dependency has been documented in one case with fluconazole. Patients with impaired liver function may be predisposed to worsening hepatic function induced by the azole antifungal drugs. The occurrence of liver disease in animals treated with itraconazole is controversial. Cats receiving 5 and 10 mg/kg twice daily showed no adverse effects (including weight loss) after receiving itraconazole for 6 weeks.[50] However, one study of enilconazole applied as a 0.2% solution once every 3 days to Persian cats in a cattery indicated potential gastrointestinal signs in the cats, including salivation, anorexia, increased liver enzymes, and emesis and muscle weakness.[66] Nausea, vomiting, skin rash, thrombocytopenia, and hypokalemia have also been reported with fluconazole therapy. The author dealt with acute hepatopathy in a cat treated topically with a commercial over the counter preparation of clotrimazole; the owner treated a large cutaneous wound topically several times a day. The hepatopathy resolved within several days of discontinuing therapy.

Voriconazole is associated with a number of side effects. Interestingly, voriconazole (but no other azole) causes vision disturbances in humans. Disturbances are characterized by loss of color discrimination, blurred vision, bright spots, wavy lines, and photophobia; up to 30% of human patients are afflicted, although the drug rarely is discontinued because of this effect. Visual hallucinations are reported in 5% of human patients. Experimentally, voriconazole produced dose-dependent changes in the electroretinogram of dogs at plasma levels comparable to those in humans.[68] Skin rashes also commonly occur; although most are mild, occasional severe reactions (e.g., Stevens–Johnson syndrome) occur. Clinical signs resolve when the drug is discontinued. As with other azoles, voriconazole is associated with increased hepatic leakage enzymes as well as serum alanine phosphatase; increased liver weight occurred experimentally in dogs after 1 month of dosing at 3 mg/kg.[68] Hepatotoxicity should be assumed to be dose and duration dependent. Although most changes are asymptomatic, severe hepatopathy has been reported in humans receiving voriconazole, with effects apparently dose dependent. Hepatic function might be measured before and 2 weeks into therapy and then every 2 to 4 weeks. The use of *N*-acetylcysteine, *S*–adenosylmethionine, or other hepatoprotectants might be considered. Again, because dogs appear to autoinduce, the impact of voriconazole on the liver is not clear. Other gastrointestinal side effects include nausea, vomiting, diarrhea, and abdominal pain.[42] Although voriconazole is not nephrotoxic, nor is it eliminated in the urine, the carrier of the intravenous preparation may accumulate in patients with impaired renal function, and therefore the intravenous preparation should not be used in these patients.[42]

Therapeutic Use

In general, itraconazole and fluconazole are more efficacious against many organisms than ketoconazole; however, the spectrum of fluconazole is limited compared with that of itraconazole. Ketoconazole has been used effectively for dermatophyte infections; mucocutaneous candidiasis; and many systemic mycoses in both dogs and cats. Ketoconazole has been reported to be effective in the treatment of dermatophytosis,[70,71] blastomycosis,[72] histoplasmosis,[73] coccidioidomycosis,[74] and cryptococcosis.[75] Ketoconazole probably should not be used alone for treatment of canine blastomycosis; recommendations are to use amphotericin in addition to ketoconazole. Higher doses also are indicated for systemic cryptococcosis and coccidioidomycosis. Ketoconazole also has proved effective for treatment of *Malassezia* dermatitis, and candidiasis. It is available as a topical shampoo that can be useful for treatment of dermatophytosis or *Malassezia.* Ketoconazole has little efficacy (43%) against *Aspergillosis* species, fluconazole more efficacy (although some isolates, including *A. fumigatus,* are inherently resistant), and itraconazole most efficacy (60% to 70%). Fluconazole has been used successfully to treat ketoconazole-resistant strains of *Candida.* Equal efficacies of itraconazole and fluconazole have been shown for cryptococcal meningitis, despite relatively poor penetration of the CSF by itraconazole. Both are equally effective in *Candida*-induced pyelonephritis. Comparison of ketoconazole and fluconazole reveals fluconazole to be more active against coccidioidal meningitis.

Among the imidazoles, itraconazole and fluconazole are being used more consistently than the others for systemic treatment of susceptible fungal infections. For itraconazole[76] conditions successfully treated include blastomycosis[54] (including ocular[77]), histoplasmosis,[78] cryptococcosis (including meningitis),[79-81] sporotrichosis,[82] aspergillosis,[83] dermatophytosis,[64] dermatophytic pseudomycetomas,[84,85] phaeohyphomycosis,[86] and cutaneous *Alternaria.*[87] Efficacy against *Aspergillosis* is better than that clinically recognized for any other agent (not including newer drugs), and although resistance is rare, treatment failure rates of up to 50% have been reported for itraconazole. In animals administration of itraconazole at a rate of 5 mg/kg twice daily is efficacious in the treatment of blastomycosis and histoplasmosis. After administration of 10 mg/kg, the C_{max} for itraconazole in dogs was 13.5 ± 8.5 µg/mL versus 3.55 ± 2.81 µg/mL at 5 mg/kg. Although the MIC_{90} of most infecting fungal organisms will be achieved at 5 mg/kg, at the higher 10 mg/kg dose, the MFC for itraconazole will be achieved for *B. dermatitidis,* almost reached for *H. capsulatum,* but not reached for *C. immitus.* However, the incidence of adverse effects may be greater at this higher dose.[54] Concentrations will be higher at steady state. The efficacy of itraconazole against coccidioidomycosis is equivocal, requiring long-term therapy. Relapse of disease appears to be common. Despite the larger MIC for dermatophytes compared to other susceptible fungal organisms, itraconazole at 1.5 to 3 mg/kg every 24 hours was effective in 8 of 15 cats in one uncontrolled clinical trial for treatment of dermatophytosis.[64] Fluconazole is only modestly effective toward sporotrichosis; itraconazole should be considered first-line therapy.[69]

KEY POINT 9-11 In general, itraconazole and fluconazole are more efficacious against many organisms than ketoconazole; however, the spectrum of fluconazole is limited compared with that of itraconazole.

Itraconazole has been used to treat canine blastomycosis (5 mg/kg/day); sporotrichosis (7.5 mg/kg/day); and, in conjunction with surgery, nasal aspergillosis (10 mg/kg/day). In cats it has proved effective for treatment of cryptococcosis and histoplasmosis. The dermatologic pharmacokinetics of itraconazole support pulse therapy, which has been used in human medicine for treatment of selective dermatologic fungal disorders. Treatment occurs for 2 consecutive weeks of daily administration each month for 3 consecutive months.[88] One report of itraconazole used to treat dermatophytosis noted similar success with this technique.[64]

There are few reports regarding the efficacy of fluconazole for treatment of fungal infections in animals; infections that have been treated include blastomycosis,[89] cryptococcosis,[74] and nasal aspergillosis.[90] Efficacy has, however, been demonstrated toward a variety of fungal disorders in humans. Pulse dosing (once weekly) of fluconazole also has been described for treatment of skin infections in people.

Enilconazole has excellent in vitro activity against a number of organisms, but its topical use is limited to dermatophytes and nasal aspergillosis. Miconazole also is limited to topical use; combination with polymyxin B yields synergistic activity.

Newer azoles are likely to prove even more efficacious than fluconazole and itraconazole for the treatment of aspergillosis and coccidioidomycosis. Voriconazole is approved for treatment of selected infections, but in particular aspergillosis. The maintenance dose in humans is approximately 2 to 5 mg/kg twice daily. In human patients who have not responded adequately to traditional therapy for treatment of aspergillosis, 38% had a partial to complete response to voriconazole used as salvage therapy. In a study of invasive aspergillosis in humans, 53% of patients receiving voriconaozle responded (partial to complete) within 12 weeks compared with only 32% of patients receiving amphotericin B; survival rates were 71% and 58%, for each drug, respectively.[42] Because of superior clinical response, safety, and survival, treatment of immuncompromised human patients with voriconazole was demonstrated to be economically superior to treatment with amphotericin B.[91] For *Pseudallescheria/Scedosporium*, major pathogens in human immunocompromised hosts normally resistant to amphotericin B and *Fusarium* sp., response rate was 30% to 63% and 50%, respectively, for the two species. Despite excellent in vitro efficacy against *C. neoformans* and good CNS penetration, voriconazole is not recommended for treatment of *Cryptococcosis*, in part because of its failure in human patients. The same may be true for blastomycosis, histoplasmosis, and coccidiodomycosis. Although effective in animal models, successful therapy with voriconazole for these organisms has not been demonstrated in humans. A salvage approach might be considered for these organisms.[42]

A single case report describes the successful treatment with posoconazole of a fungal disorder caused by *Mucor* (Zygomycetes class; Mucorales order) species on the nose of a 15-year-old cat.[91a] After poor response to fluconazole, the cat was treated at 5 mg/kg daily for 3 months, with initial response evident in 2 weeks and continued response for the remainder of the 3-month treatment period.

Terbinafine was shown to enhance efficacy when combined with itraconaozle or fluconazole when treating candidiasis characterized by low susceptibility to the azoles.[92] Indeed, combination with benzoyl peroxide topically enhanced treatment of candidiasis associated with *Pseudomonas* and *Staphylococcus aureus* infections in humans.[93]

BENZIMIDAZOLES

Benzimidazoles (e.g., thiabendazole) may be better known for their anthelmintic activity, but many also are characterized by a broad range of antifungal activity at relatively low doses. Benzimidazoles bind to β-tubulin of the microtubule. Not only is mitosis blocked, but selected organelles also are displaced, such as mitochondria in hyphal tips, which alters linear growth. Unfortunately, resistance generally caused by point mutations in the β-tubulin genes, limits the antifungal activity of the drugs. The spectrum of thiabendazole is limited to the dermatophytes (toward which activity can be -cidal) and, to a lesser degree, *A. fumigatus*, penicillinosis, and some *Fusarium* species. Thiabendazole also is effective against *Pneumocystis carinii*. Its use as an antifungal is largely limited to topical therapy (e.g., otitis externa).

ECHINOCANDINS

The echinocandins are the first new antifungal drugs to be developed in the last 15 years.[94] Originally elucidated from different fungal organisms, including *Aspergillus*, they are synthetically modified lipoproteins derived from fermentation broth of a number of organisms.[95] Included in the chemicals identified thus far are aculeacin A, echinocandin B, pneumocandin B, enfumafungin, and papulacandins. These chemicals inhibit the synthesis of β-D-glucan (the major glucan in the cell wall of *Aspergillus*), disrupting the fungal cell wall (see Figure 9-1). Their novel mechanism of action results in rapid fungicidal effects for some organisms with minimal side effects.[96] Caspofungin (see Figure 9-2) is the first of the drugs to undergo approval in the United States. Its spectrum of activity is limited but does include *Candida* sp. and *Aspergillus* sp.; the drug is approved to treat the latter. Other drugs include micafungin and anidulafungin, both approved to treat candidiasis.

The large molecular weight of the echinocandins and poor oral absorption limit use to intravenous administration. Drug does not distribute well into the urine or CNS. Concentrations in the lungs approximate those in the plasma. The compounds undergo phase I metabolism to inactive metabolites. Despite its metabolism by the liver,[97] capsofungin does not serve as a substrate for major CYP 450. However, selected drugs will alter capsofungin, disposition, including cyclosporine (which increases it). In humans caspofungin acetate is characterized by an elimination half-life of 9 to 10 hours but is administered once daily. Capsofungin is involved in few drug interactions. Side effects are unusual but include phlebitis, fever, nausea, skin rash, and abnormal liver function. Despite low CNS concentrations, human cases of cerebral aspergillosis have responded to caspofungin treatment. The ability to kill *Aspergillus* is controversial; generation of cell wall–deficient colonies in vitro may be associated with organism viability. The optimal dose has not yet been established in humans; generally a loading dose of 70 mg is followed up by doses of 50 to 70 mg daily. A ceiling dose of 1 mg/kg has been suggested, but doses of micafungin as high as 300 mg daily (up to 8 mg/kg daily) was not associated with toxicity in humans.[94] Efficacy has been demonstrated against fluconazole-resistant strains of *Candida*. However, *Cryptococcus* is resistant. Although *Fusarium* is resistant, *Scedosporium* is moderately susceptible and *Saccharomyces* is susceptible.

FLUCYTOSINE

Structure–Activity Relationship

5-Flucytosine (FLU; 5-fluorocytosine) was originally developed as an anticancer drug much the same as its sister anticancer drug, 5-fluorouracil. It is a water-soluble powder.

Mechanism of Action

As an antimetabolite, FLU interferes with DNA synthesis after its conversion to 5–fluorouracil, a substitution compound that prevents synthesis in the fungal cell.[4,40] The compound enters the cell by way of cytosine permease, which also takes up adenine, guanine, hypoxanthine, and cytosine.[3] The enzyme responsible for conversion of FLU to 5–fluorouracil is a cytosine deaminase, an enzyme whose absence in mammalian cells renders FLU relatively specific for fungal cells. The effect of FLU depends on subsequent metabolism: if converted by pyrimidine processing enzymes to a uridine monophosphate derivative, inhibition of thymidylate synthase and DNA synthesis yields -cidal effects. Alternatively, it can be converted by way of a pyrimidine salvage pathway resulting in metabolism to a uridine-5'-triphosphate derivative. Subsequent incorporation into RNA results in impaired protein synthesis and fungistatic effects *(Candida, Cryptococcosis)*. Many organisms are intrinsically resistant to FLU because they either lack the permease enzyme or have a defective deaminase enzyme. Resistance also develops relatively rapidly, particularly for aspergillosis followed by cryptococcosis and candidiasis (especially *Candida krusei*).[3] Secondary resistance usually reflects a decrease in an enzyme responsible for formation of uridine monophosphate. Use in combination with another antifungal agent reduces the development of resistance.

Spectrum of Activity

The spectrum of activity of FLU is limited and includes cryptococcosis, candidiasis and some cladosporiosis, aspergillosis, chromomycosis, and sporotrichosis. It has been the treatment of choice for cryptococcosis in humans.[4,40] Combination therapy is usually indicated (e.g., amphotericin, ketoconazole). When FLU is used alone, resistance develops rapidly. Synergism occurs with amphotericin B and probably with ketoconazole (or other imidazoles).

Pharmacokinetics

Oral absorption of FLU is rapid and close to complete. Peak plasma concentrations occur in 1 to 2 hours. Distribution is large, to total body water. Protein binding is minimal, and CSF concentrations reach up to 90% of plasma concentrations. Penetration of aqueous humor and joints is good. The half-life of FLU is 3 to 6 hours. Most of the drug is excreted into the urine unchanged. Renal clearance is similar to that of creatinine and thus may be significantly decreased if renal dysfunction is present. Doses will probably need to be modified for patients with renal disease.

Preparations

Flucytosine is available as an oral preparation.

Side Effects

Because FLU interferes with DNA synthesis, body systems composed of rapidly dividing cells are adversely affected. Bone marrow depression is manifested as anemia, leukopenia, and thrombocytopenia (pancytopenia). This toxicity may be serious and is more common in patients with renal disease. Gastrointestinal toxicity is manifested as nausea, vomiting, and diarrhea, but it is not usually serious. Reversible, erythemic, alopecic dermatitis has been reported in dogs.

GRISEOFULVIN

Structure–Activity Relationship

Griseofulvin (see Figure 9-1) is produced from a *Penicillium* species bacterium. The drug is insoluble in water.

Mechanism of Action

Griseofulvin enters fungi through an energy-dependent transport system. Griseofulvin inhibits fungal mitosis by binding to the microtubules that form the mitotic spindle. The formation of microtubules from tubulin is inhibited. Formation of cytoplasmic microtubules responsible for transport of endogenous compounds also is inhibited. Other drugs, such as colchicine and vincristine, which also bind to and inhibit the microtubule, do so at a site that is different from that of griseofulvin. Griseofulvin also probably inhibits nucleic acid and fungal wall synthesis. It is not certain if griseofulvin is fungistatic or fungicidal. Resistance probably reflects decreased drug uptake.

Spectrum of Activity

The spectrum of activity of griseofulvin reflects the presence of an energy-dependent transport system in the fungal organism. Those with prolonged energy-dependent transport systems are susceptible, whereas those with independent systems of short duration are not. Efficacy is limited to dermatophytes: *Microsporum, Trichophyton,* and *Epidermophyton*. Because of its distribution into keratin, griseofulvin remains the drug of choice for fungal infections of the nails.

Pharmacokinetics

Oral absorption varies because of water insolubility and depends on particle size and preparation. Absorption is increased in the presence of fat. The rates of dissolution and disaggregation alter the bioavailability of different products. Bioavailability of the ultramicrosize is at least 50% greater than that of the microsize. Although griseofulvin penetrates the stratum corneum, it does not achieve effective concentrations topically. Griseofulvin is widely distributed to most tissues, but it is deposited and concentrated in keratin precursor cells. Thus it is incorporated in new keratin of skin, nails, and hair and (in humans) is secreted in perspiration. Although new keratin formed during treatment with griseofulvin is resistant to fungus, griseofulvin does not destroy fungi that infect the outer layers of the skin. New hair, skin, or nail growth accompanied by shedding of older growth is necessary before the fungus is affected; new growth is the first to be free of disease. Thus skin infections require 4 to 6 weeks of therapy, whereas toenails may require up to a year of therapy. Long hair breeds probably should be treated for a longer period of time compared to short hair breeds.

KEY POINT 9-12 Treatment with griseofulvin must be sufficiently long for new growth to replace infected growth.

Hepatic metabolism of griseofulvin by dealkylation is significant; metabolites are not active. The half-life reportedly is 24 hours in the dog. Half of the drug is excreted as metabolites in the urine. The rest is excreted through the bile unchanged in the feces.

Preparations

Griseofulvin is available for oral use as either a microsize (particle size 10 μm) or ultramicrosize (particle size 2.7 μm; e.g., Fulvicin, Gris-PEG) tablets. The drug should be administered with a fatty meal, particularly if the microsize preparation is used. Duration of therapy is *at least* 4 to 6 weeks (new hair growth must occur) and possibly longer. The drug should be administered at least once a day despite initial reports that recommend one weekly administration.

Side Effects and Drug Interactions

Side effects to griseofulvin are not uncommon. Nausea, vomiting, and diarrhea can be minimized by administration of the dose in divided increments with a meal. Hepatotoxicity may occur, and use in liver disease should be avoided. Idiosyncratic toxicity has been reported in the cat, manifested as gastrointestinal upset, neurologic disease, and bone marrow suppression.[98] The reaction appears to be both dose and duration independent. Signs may not be reversible, depending on the severity. Cats with feline immunodeficiency disorders may be more likely to develop neutropenia.[99] Certain feline breeds (e.g., Persian, Siamese, Abyssinian) may be more commonly affected.[98] At very high doses, the drug is teratogenic and carcinogenic in animals. The drug should not be given during the first two trimesters of pregnancy. Use with a shampoo (miconazole or chlorhexidine) enhances efficacy.

Griseofulvin is a potent inducer of microsomal enzymes. The clinical sequelae of this drug interaction are not well known, although increased metabolism of other drugs should be anticipated.

ALLYLAMINES AND THIOCARBAMATES

The allylamines (e.g., terbinafine, naftifine) and the much older thiocarbamates (e.g., tolnaftate) competitively inhibit squalene epoxidase, blocking conversion of squalene to lanosterol, leading to squaline accumulation and ergosterol depletion in the cell membrane. Terbinafine has a much higher affinity for fungal compared with mammalian squaline epoxidase. Aviod uptake of terbinafine into body fat and epidermis enhances and potentially limits its efficacy to dermatophytes and superficial pathogens of the skin. Antifungal effects are -cidal in these organisms; it has proved more efficacious than griseofulvin for both acute and chronic dermatophyte infections in humans. Efficacy has also been demonstrated against *S. schenckii* and *Aspergillus* (*A. flavus* more so than *A. fumigatus*). Although it is not clear if effective tissue concentrations are acheived, in vitro activity toward *B. dermatitidis, C. immitis,* and *H. capsulatum* has also been described as excellent. Some strains of *Crypotococus* sp. also are susceptible. In vitro activity also has been demonstrated toward *Rhizopus, Alternaria, Phialophora, Chrysosporium,* and *Exophiala* spp.[3,100] Fungistatic efficacy has been demonstrated against yeasts,[101] with activity being poor toward *Candida.*[3] Increasingly, terbinafine has enhanced the efficacy of other antifungal drugs when used in combination for treatment of a variety of fungal disorders and pythiosis.[100b] Terbinafine expresses some antibacterial activity; for example, when combined with benzoyl peroxide, its topical spectrum (in human) is expanded to include *Pseudomonas* and *Staphylococcus.*[100b] In contrast to terbinafine, tolnaftate is limited to treatment of dermatophytes. Resistance to the allylamines is rare, but the drugs potentially can be affected by multidrug resistance efflux mechanisms.[3]

Terbinafine, available in oral and topical preparations, is well absorbed (80% in humans) after oral administration, although fat facilitates absorption. High concentrations occur in the stratum corneum, sebum, and hair. The drug is metabolized by the liver in humans; the elimination half-life is sufficiently long to allow once-daily administration, with steady state not occurring for 10 to 14 days in humans.[3,102] An abstract reporting pharmacokinetics in cats suggested that a dose of 20 to 40 mg/kg once daily provided sufficient concentration of drug in the skin. The drug was well tolerated at this dose.[103] Side effects of terbinafine after oral administration are limited to gastrointestinal and skin symptoms; hepatobillary dysfunction is a rare adverse event.[3] Because inhibition of ergosterol synthesis occurs at a step before cytochrome P450 involvement, the allylamines do not affect steroid synthesis as do the imidazoles.

KEY POINT 9-13 Although the distribution of terbinafine supports its efficacy to treat dermatophytes, it may also enhance the efficacy of other antifungal drugs toward other organisms.

IODIDES

The mechanism of antifungal action of the iodides is not known. Iodide is rapidly and completely absorbed orally. Distribution is to the extracellular fluid. Thyroid uptake will concentrate the drug up to 50 times that in plasma. Iodide is available as a 20% Na and K^+ salt oral or intravenous preparation. Both salts have been used successfully to treat canine and feline cutaneous or lymphocutaneous forms of sporotrichosis, and, as such, it remains the drug of choice.[104,105] Oral Na^+ preparations are usually used. Iodide toxicity is more common in cats and is manifested as sweating; tachycardia; dry, scaly coat; diarrhea; and polyuria/polydipsia. Cardiomyopathy has been reported in cats. Treatment causing clinical signs of iodinism should be discontinued for 1 week and then reinstituted at a lower dose. Iodine has also been reported to be effective for various other fungal diseases, particularly as a topical ointment for localized skin infections. Topical iodine preparations continue to be available and might be used to treat fungal rhinitis (discussed later).

LUFENURON

Lufenuron is a chitin synthetase inhibitor used for the control of fleas in dogs and cats. Its use for the treatment of dermatophytes is controversial. A retrospective study of dogs and cats found that dogs treated with once-daily administration of 50 to 60 mg/kg responded (based on skin scraping) within 21 days. Cats received doses that ranged from 50 to 266 mg/kg, with response in 8 to 12 days. However, clinical trials have not been able to accomplish what the retrospective study implied. A study describing efficacy at a single dose of about 80 mg/kg every 2 weeks until culture cure was followed by clinical trials that failed to eradicate or prevent infection at 140 mg/kg. When combined with weekly enilconazole shampoos, 60 mg/kg every 30 days caused clinical response in most cats in a cattery after several weeks of therapy; however, not all animals became culture negative, and relapse occurred.[3] Several abstract reports have failed to demonstrate efficacy, despite differences in duration or dose. This includes studies using established animal models for which itraconazole is effective.[106] Moriello and colleagues[107] could not demonstrate a protective effect of lufenuron (30 or 122 mg/kg monthly for 2 months) when used before experimental infection of juvenile cats with *Microsporum canis*. Studies based on combination rather than sole therapy may provide more information.

KEY POINT 9-14 Several abstract reports have failed to demonstrate efficacy of lufenuron in the treatment of fungal infections, despite differences in duration or dose.

COMBINATION THERAPY

Combination antifungal therapy has been reviewed in human medicine,[108] including the molecular basis.[9] Indications include patients at risk (immunocompromised). Few clinical studies provide conclusive evidence for or against combination therapy.[108] In vitro studies examining combination therapy often used different methods, limiting the ability to determine a consensus. Among the difficulties with clinical studies is the more common use of combinations in patients with greater severity of disease, thus biasing results. Not surprisingly, sample size is often too small to demonstrate significant differences. In vitro data for *C. neoformans* exposed to ampohtericin B, when combined with imidazoles, indicates, in order of minimal to most synergistic effect, fluconazole = itraconazole < posaconazole.[9] The combination of flucytosine with itraconazole indicated the most synergistic activity toward *C. neoformans.* In contrast, for candidiasis, the order of least to most synergistic activity when imidazoles are combined with terbinafine was fluconazole < posaconazole < itraconazole < voriconazole.[9] In animal (mice) models, the addition of fluconazole offered no benefit to amphotericin B for treatment of cryptococcosis. Flucytosine potentiated the effect of fluconazole but not posaconazole for treatment of *C. neoformans*. The most effective combination was amphotericin with flucytosine; the addition of fluconazole to this combination reduced the fungal burden even more. The efficacy of voriconazole toward aspergillosis was enhanced by caspofungin.

The combination of antifungals with other drugs not traditionally considered antifungal may offer enhanced clinical response. For example, combination therapy with antibacterials that target DNA may enhance efficacy. Examples include the fluroquinolones and the rifamycins.[9] Rifampin has shown some efficacy against fungal microorganisms *(H. capsulatum, Aspergillus* sp., and *B. dermatitidis)* when combined with amphotericin B. Amphotericin B apparently facilitates movement of rifampin through the fungal cell wall into the organism, where RNA polymerase then can be accessed. A beneficial effect has been demonstrated in vivo (but not in vitro) for trovafloxacin combined with fluconazole or amphotericin G. In vitro efficacy has been demonstrated for the latter. The combination of traditional antifungal agents with terbinafine or chitin synthesis inhibitors (e.g., caspofungin) may also prove to be effective combinations for treatment of selected infections (e.g., coccidioidomycosis, aspergillosis, and others).

Among the drug combinations currently being actively researched are antifungal agents with immunomodulators. Included are cytokines such as granulocyte or macrophage colony-stimulating factors or interferon γ-1b. In contrast, the impact of calcineurin antagonists (e.g., tacrolimus and cyclosporine) is one of exacerbation, at least for cryptococcal meningitis.

THERAPEUTIC USE OF ANTIFUNGAL AGENTS

Dermatologic Fungal Infections: Dermatophytosis

A number of fungal organisms inhabit the hair coats of dogs and cats. *Alternaria, Cladosporium,* and yeasts may be associated with dermatitis. Dermatophytes can be isolated from normal animals or can be a cause of infection. Dermatophyte infections generally are self-limiting, with ability to mount an inflammatory response being an important determinant of infection control. Accordingly, drugs such as glucocorticoids, which mute the inflammatory response, predispose a patient to dermatophyte infection; dermatophytosis infection is 3 times more prevalent in cats infected with feline immunodeficiency virus than in noninfected cats.[66] The route of drug administration (topical versus systemic therapy) depends on the extent of infection, with the exception of *Trichophyton* infections, which should be treated systemically.

Topical therapy is indicated for all patients with dermatophytosis and may be the sole therapy for local, nondiffuse lesions. Hair coat preparation before medication should include clipping and bathing to remove hair and crusts. Several medicaments are available as shampoo, ointment, or cream formulations for topical therapy (see Table 9-5). Active ingredients include povidone–iodine, chlorhexidine, and imidazole. Other active ingredients that can be applied topically include captan, lime sulfur, and sodium hypochlorite. Short-term topical glucocorticoid therapy might be considered to control acute inflammation when present. Topical administration of enilconazole emulsion has been useful for treatment of feline dermatophytosis.

Moriello[66,107] retrospectively evaluated in vitro and in vivo studies of treatments for dermatophytosis in dogs and cats. Topical treatments consistently found to be effective when administered once or twice weekly were lime sulfur (1:16), 0.2% enilconazole rinse (twice weekly; response in as early as 5 weeks), and a combined 2% miconazole–chlorhexidine shampoo. Captan, chlorhexidine (as sole agent), and povidine–iodine were generally ineffective.

Response to systemic therapy is likely to be more rapid if combined with topical therapy.[66] Systemic therapy should probably be preceded with a total body clip. Griseofulvin is the treatment of choice for long-term systemic antifungal therapy of dermatophytosis,[109] although expense mandates that a diagnosis of dermatophytosis be confirmed. Care should be taken that the proper dose and duration of therapy are followed; treatment probably should be longer for longer-haired animals. Cure was reported in 63 to 70 days in one study with a mean of 41 days at 50 mg/kg in another study (as reviewed by Moriello).[66] For infections that do not respond to griseofulvin, an imidazole can be used. Ketoconazole has been used successfully, particularly when dosed at 10 mg/kg daily for 20 days. Itraconazole has, however, proved more efficacious for treatment of dermatophytes in human patients and has proved efficacious experimentally in cats infected with *M. canis*.[110] Itraconazole was effective at 10 mg/kg once daily for 56 days or for 28 days followed by a week-on week-off pulse dosing for 56 to 70 days.[111] Interestingly, low-dose itraconazole (1.5 to 3 mg/kg) in 15-day cycles required a shorter time period at 1 to 3 cycles or 15 to 45 days. However, only 8 of 15 cats were successfully treated in this study, and two of these cats required a second cycle. Using an open clinical trial, a protocol using itraconazole (10 mg/kg once daily) and lime sulphur rinses (cat coat saturated with rinse at 8 ounces per gallon of water) every 7 days for 21 days was associated with successful treatment of dermatophytosis in shelter cats.[111a] Cure was longer with higher fungal load (18.4+ 9.5 days) compared to smaller loads (14.5+5.7 days). Cats tolerated the rinses well. Efficacy of lufenuron was not substantiated in controlled studies. Terbinafine has demonstrated efficacy toward dermatophytosis in dogs and cats, although higher doses (>30 to 40 mg/kg) generally are required to achieve a mycologic cure. Time to cure in dogs varied from 21 to more than 126 days and from 28 to 84 days in dogs. A lower dose (10 to 30 mg/kg) may also be effective in both dogs and cats, although treatment should be expected to be approximately 60 to 90 days.[107] Use of terbinafine at 30 mg/kg for 2 weeks resulted in a cure of 11 of 12 cats with *M. canis,* and at 8.25 mg/kg daily, it eradicated spores from asymptomatic carrier cats (as reviewed by Bossche[3]). The use of systemic terbenafine at either a low (10 to 20 mg/kg) or high (30 to 40 mg/kg) dose once daily was compared with placebo treatment in cats (n = 9 per group) ranging between 1.5 and 4.5 months of age that were experimentally infected with *M. canis.* Cats were treated for 120 days. Response in the low-dose treatment group did not differ from that of the control group but did in the high-dose group; the number of cats cured per group was not provided. PDCs did not differ between the two dose groups, but concentrations in the hair were significantly higher with the higher dose.[112] Drug accumulated with multiple dosing, with concentrations at 3 months higher than at 2 months, suggesting peak effects may take up to 3 months (or more). Median concentrations in plasma at 9 and 120 days were 1.4 mg/L and 4.1 mg/L respectively, in the low-dose cats compared with 1.7 and 5.5 mg/L respectively, in the high-dose cats. Median concentrations in the hair at 9 and 120 days were 1 mg/L and 1.2 mg/L, respectively, in the low-dose cats compared with 1.9 and 3.6 mg/L respectively, in the high-dose cats. The highest concentration achieved in the hair in any one cat was 7.92 μg/mL; this compares with humans receiving only 6 mg/kg, for which concentrations reach 2.40 to 55 μg/g.

Additional topical therapies for treatment of dermatophytosis or other dermatologic fungal disorders are also addressed in Chapter 22. Environmental cleansing may be important to treatment of dermatophytosis. This might be accomplished with either 2% chlorhexidine or 0.5% sodium hypochlorite.

Yeast or Yeastlike Infections

Malassezia

Malassezia (Pityrosporum) is a commensal organism that inhabits the skin, ear canal, anal sacs, vagina, and rectum of dogs. It is now recognized to be the causative agent of either localized or generalized pruritic inflammatory skin disease in dogs. The pathogenesis of the infection is controversial and appears to involve hypersensitivity to the organism. Postulated predisposing factors include allergic disease such as atopic dermatitis, diseases of cornification, chronic inflammatory skin disease, and previous therapy with antibiotics or glucocorticoids.

Therapy for *Malassezia* is directed toward removing predisposing factors and killing the causative agent.[113] Antimicrobial therapy ideally should include both systemic and topical drugs. Ketoconazole and itraconazole are the systemic drugs of choice and should be given for at least 30 days. Topical therapy may be sufficient in some cases. Antifungal shampoos containing chlorhexidine, miconazole, or ketoconazole should be given at least twice weekly for a minimum of 6 weeks. Shampoos that resolve any exudate (e.g., benzoyl peroxide) may facilitate topical penetration of the antifungal drug. An acetic acid rinse (white vinegar and water at a ratio of 1:1) used twice weekly as a degreasing agent after shampooing may also prove beneficial as well as inexpensive. Application of eniloconazole emulsion may also be beneficial. The emulsion can be applied with a sponge or by whole-body immersion; the diluted product appears to remain stable for 4 to 6 weeks when protected against light, although use of a fresh dilution is recommended for each treatment.

Cole and coworkers[114] studied in vitro the addition of 0.1% ketaconaozle to an ear rinse containing EDTA tromethamine and benzyl alcohol (T8 Solution) for treatment of canine otitis associated with *Malassezia*. The low concentration was sufficient to inhibit fungal growth. By itself, EDTA and thromethamine had no effect. Ahman and coworkers[115] studied pulse dosing of itraconazole (5 mg/kg orally qd, 7 days on, 7 days off, 7 days on) for treatment of *Malassezia pachydermatitis* associated with greasy seborrheic dermatitis in Devon Rex cats (n = 6). Assessment was not blinding; control cats were not studied. Clinical signs associated with seborrhea resolved in all cats, with dramatic improvement recorded in the second week, supporting the role of *Malassezia* in the disease.

Negre and coworkers[116] systematically reviewed the literature (before 2007) with regard to the treatment of skin disorders associated with *Malassezia*. Clinical trials in peer-reviewed veterinary literature were considered if they focused on treatment of *Malessezia* associated with dermatitis and involved more than five dogs. Studies were assessed for quality based on methods intended to select subjects that adequately represented the target population and minimized bias. Trials were classified by size of the study groups. Outcome measure assessment had to include both clinical evidence of response as well as the extent of reduction in fungal colony counts. Only

8 of 35 studies met the full criteria and another 6 met all but the mycologic requirement. Eleven studies were evaluated for evidence of efficacy for azole derivatives. Based on their review, 2% miconazole with 2% chlorhexidene was the only topical product for which good evidence existed. Fair evidence existed for either ketoconazole at 10 mg/kg daily or itraconazole at 5 mg/kg daily for 3 weeks.

Candidiasis

In the yeast phase, candidiasis normally occurs in the gastrointestinal, respiratory, or urogenital mucosa. The organism is acquired at birth and occurs at mucocutaneous junctions in the skin and in several organs inside the body. Factors that alter normal microflora (e.g., prolonged, high-dose, broad-spectrum antimicrobial therapy) predispose to the development of candidiasis. Cell-mediated immunity is important in the control of disease, and prolonged immunosuppression increases the risk of further spread. Generally, microcirculation of the organs filters organisms, leading to embolization.

Topical infection can be treated with topical antifungal products, including polyene macrolides, imidazoles, and gentian violet (1:10,000). Systemic therapy can be treated with amphotericin B, 5-flucytosine (combined with another antifungal drug), or the imidazoles.

Systemic Fungal Diseases

Therapeutic success with antifungal drugs can be enhanced by long-term therapy, generally one to several months beyond the resolution of clinical signs; avoidance of immunosuppressive drugs; and use of combination therapy, particularly for infections that are difficult to penetrate or are life or organ threatening.

Blastomycosis

Blastomyces organisms become established in the lungs and then disseminate throughout the body. The presence of clinical signs in dogs is indicative of disseminated disease and the need for aggressive therapy. Preferred sites of infection in dogs are the skin, eyes, bones, lymph nodes, subcutaneous tissues, nasal passages, and brain. These tissues are difficult to penetrate with most antifungal drugs, thus increasing the likelihood of therapeutic failure. Immunosuppression is common in dogs with blastomycosis, further hindering therapeutic success. The use of radioimmunoassay tests based on the major surface protein W1-1 is predictive of active infection, confirming absence of infection 100% of the time.[117] The authors concluded that the test is more accurate than those based on the A antigen and thus may be more relevant to assessing response to therapy. When the titer is used, concentrations are high initially but decline during therapy, persisting for months.[117]

Amphotericin B has been the treatment of choice for blastomycosis.[118] Although high doses are more effective, the risk of nephrotoxicity may necessitate a less aggressive approach; lipid-based products should be considered particularly in patients at risk. The total cumulative dose for amphotericin B (AmBD) generally is 4 to 6 mg/kg for dogs and 4 mg/kg in cats; a higher dose should be anticipated for lipid-based products. A maintenance dose of 0.15 to 0.25 mg/kg intravenously once monthly after the cumulative dose was reached was recommended in the early 1980s, but the scientific basis of this approach is questionable. Doses range from 0.15 to 0.5 mg/kg thrice weekly in dogs and cats, depending on renal function. Severe cases or intolerance to amphotericin B might be treated with a lipid complexed drug (see Table 9-3). Renal-sparing measures should be taken for patients with preexisting renal disease. Despite aggressive therapy, a relapse rate of 17% has been reported in dogs.[26] Combination therapy of amphotericin B with an imidazole should be considered whenever possible and is particularly important for infections in tissues that are difficult to penetrate, such as the brain and eye. However, because of mechanisms of action, it is important to begin the two drugs simultaneously. Of the imidazoles, ketoconazole has been used alone to treat blastomycosis in humans, but it is less successful for animals as a sole agent. Ketoconazole can be used at 10 to 10 mg/kg/day (up to 30 mg/kg/day for difficult-to-penetrate tissues [e.g., eye, CNS]) when combined with amphotericin B. Because imidazoles are characterized by variation in drug disposition among animals, efficacy might be enhanced by increasing the dose. Although sequential use of amphotericin B followed by ketoconazole has been recommended, the two apparently can be used in combination immediately with little to no increased risk of toxicity. The rapid effects of amphotericin B are critical for life-threatening or organ-threatening infections. Itraconazole or possibly fluconazole are more likely to be effective than ketoconazole for the treatment of blastomycosis. Although itraconazole is more likely to be effective as sole therapy,[119] combination therapy with amphotericin B is still recommended. Therapy should continue for at least 60 days or 1 month beyond resolution of disease indicators, whichever is longer. In their retrospective study of dogs with pulmonary blastomycosis, Crews[119a] found 79 dogs survived, 38 died, and 8 were euthanized. Most dogs were treated with itraconazole alone (n = 89) with does in 14 of these dogs less than recommended. No information was provided regarding survival rates among the different treatments, including 20 dogs treated with a combination of amphotericin B and an imidazole. No significant effect could be demonstrated in dogs loaded for 5 days (dose not given) with itraconazole.

With proper therapy up to 80% of dogs with blastomycosis can be effectively treated.[54] The severity of pulmonary involvement appears to be a prognostic factor for both initial survival and the likelihood of relapse. Therapy may result in an initial worsening of respiratory disease, presumably because of an inflammatory response to dying organisms. A short course of short-acting glucocorticoids might be considered concurrently as therapy is initiated.[120] Of the remaining 20% of animals that survive initial therapy, some may die within the first 2 weeks of therapy. Relapse can occur in up to 20% of infected animals within the first 6 months after therapy, but relapse after 1 year is rare.

Histoplasmosis

Host macrophages phagocytize the yeast phase of *Histoplasma*, and the organism then undergoes replication. The intracellular location is a mitigating factor in the hematogenous and lymphatic dissemination of the organisms from the lungs to other tissues. In most patients cell-mediated immunity brings the infection under control. The gastrointestinal tract may also be a primary site of infection, although dissemination from the lungs appears to be more likely.[121] Although pulmonary infection may be self-limiting, therapy is indicated to prevent dissemination of infection.

Ketoconazole has been the drug of choice for mild pulmonary histoplasmosis.[121] One study, however, reported that only itraconazole (5 mg/kg orally twice daily for 60 to 130 days; because the half-life is sufficiently long in cats, 10 mg/kg once a day for the same duration might be used) was effective against histoplasmosis in cats after ketoconazole had failed,[78] and consequently, it is the preferred treatment. Fluconazole might be considered if the CNS is involved. For more severe pulmonary infection or gastrointestinal infection, therapy should be more aggressive and include itraconazole combination therapy with amphotericin B (0.15 to 0.5 mg/kg intravenously 3 times a week, increasing to up to 1 mg/kg every other day to a total cumulative dose of 7 to 8.5 mg/kg). Both of the latter drugs are much more effective (up to a hundredfold) than ketoconazole against histoplasmosis. The prognosis for patients with pulmonary histoplasmosis is fair to good but guarded when the disease has disseminated. Acute respiratory distress might warrant a course of antiinflammatories. In a retrospective study of airway obstruction associated with chronic histoplasmosis in dogs,[122] resolution of respiratory clinical signs occurred in less than 1 week in those dogs treated with glucocorticoids alone compared with a mean of 2.6 weeks if combined with an antifungal and 9 weeks if receiving an antifungal only. The use of glucocorticoids was not associated with development of active or disseminated histoplasmosis. Treatment should continue for at least 60 days or 1 month beyond resolution of disease indicators, whichever is longer.

Cryptococcosis

Cryptococcus organisms infect the upper respiratory tract or the alveoli, potentially causing granulomas at both sites. Once established in the respiratory system, they can disseminate to other tissues. Infection of the CNS by either dissemination or direct extension is common. Cutaneous and ocular lesions are common in cats.

Cell-mediated immunity is critical to the host's ability to overcome a cryptococcal infection Cryptococcal organisms have several features that affect their virulence. The capsule inhibits plasma cell function, phagocytosis, and leukocyte activity. Fever is uncommon (25% of dogs), particularly in cats. Immunosuppression is essentially necessary for cryptococcosis to develop in humans. Underlying diseases are, however, not often identified in cats or dogs with cryptococcosis. A risk factor for therapeutic failure in cats, which are generally more commonly infected with *Cryptococcus* than are dogs, is co-infection with immunosuppressive viruses.[123] The impact of the use of glucocorticoids in patients with severe *Cryptococcus* infection is not clear. Using a murine model of CNS and pulmonary cryptococcosis treated with fluconazole (5 or 15 mg/kg every 8 hours), investigators found that whereas dexamethasone (0.15 mg/kg every 8 hours intraperitoneally) for 3 days, 30 minutes before fluconazole) administration did not have a deleterious effect on successful therapy with fluconazole, response was much better with early (1 day) as opposed to later (8 days) into infection. Because pharmacokinetics confirmed that fluconazole concentrations in the plasma and tissue remained above the MIC at both time points and did not change across time, the authors concluded that the number of fungal organisms influenced outcome. Although dexamethasone was not associated with beneficial or deleterious effects, the authors did not address whether sufficient animals had been studied to detect a difference;[124] however, their study does support the early rather than later use of glucocorticoids.

Amphotericin B has been the treatment of choice for cryptococcosis.[79,80,85] Doses should start at 0.5 to 0.8 mg/kg 2 to 3 times a week (0.25 to 0.5 mg/kg in cats); the drug can be given subcutaneously once diluted as long as the concentration does not exceed 20 mg/mL. A total cumulative dose at the higher end is recommended for cryptococcosis (4 to 8 mg/kg in one source, but up to 9 to 12 mg/kg in another for cats), reflecting longer duration of therapy. Initial therapy with a low dose and a subsequent increase in dose has been suggested for cats. Combination with 5-flucytosine or the imidazoles is likely to improve therapeutic success and is indicated for CNS infections because amphotericin B cannot sufficiently penetrate the blood–brain barrier. Ketoconazole has been used successfully to treat cryptococcosis. Itraconazole (10 mg/kg orally once daily), however, and fluconazole are more effective than ketoconazole against cryptococcosis. Cats appear to tolerate itraconazole better than ketoconazole.[79] Both drugs, but especially fluconazole, are characterized by better tissue penetrability and can be used to treat CNS infection. One study with cats reported that 16 of 28 were cured of cryptococcosis after treatment with itraconazole (100 mg orally once daily) for a mean of 4 to 16 months,[81] with duration dependent on resolution of disease indicators. Combination with either flucytosine (50 mg/kg every 6 hours) or terbinafine should also be considered.[100] Response to therapy can be correlated to a decline in antigen titer.[125] The prognosis for recovery is favorable if the CNS is not involved.

Coccidioidomycosis

Coccidioidomycosis begins as an alveolar infection that spreads to peribronchiolar tissues and the lung surface. Cell-mediated immunity is important in overcoming the infection. In immunodepressed animals or in animals with massive exposure, pulmonary infection becomes extensive, and the infection disseminates first to mediastinal and tracheobronchial lymph nodes and then to other tissues. Organs that are subsequently infected include, in order of likelihood, bone, joints, visceral organs, the heart and pericardium, testicles, eyes, and brain.

Coccidiodomycosis is the most difficult of the dimorphic fungal infections to treat, and antifungal therapy is particularly long.[126] The duration varies with both the site of infection and the drug and can be for the life of the animal in some cases of disseminated disease. Whereas respiratory infections may spontaneously resolve, untreated disseminated infections will result in death. Ketoconazole has been the drug of choice for treatment in the past and is associated with a 60% cure, with CNS or orthopedic involvement being associated with worse prognosis. Ketoconazole therapy should extend at least 1 year beyond resolution of clinical signs. However, itraconazole is more effective and should be considered; the duration is likely to be the same. Amphotericin B is also effective for the treatment of coccidioidomycosis; encapsulated or otherwise modified formulations should be considered such that therapy can continue for a longer period of time. A lower maintenance dose of either ketoconazole or amphotericin B has been recommended once clinical signs are in remission, although this approach (i.e., using lower doses) should be used very cautiously. Therapy with itraconazole may occur for a shorter time, although this has not been well established in animals. Fluconazole is indicated for CNS infections. Combination therapy (i.e., amphotericin B with an imidazole) should be strongly considered for treatment of coccidioidomycosis. Deterioration of clinical signs and a rising complement fixation test are both indications for combination therapy with amphotericin B. In general, duration of therapy should be at least 8 to 12 months; relapse is common, particularly in cats.[127]

Paracoccidioidomycosis

Paracoccidiodomycosis, caused by *Paracoccidioides brasiliensis,* is a severe infection of the lungs and other body systems associated with granulamatous response in humans. Although rare in animals, one case was reported in South America in a Doberman Pinscher that presented with cervical lymphadenopathy.[128]

Aspergillosis

Aspergillosis can occur as either the localized form, involving cavities of the ears, nose, or sinuses; or the disseminated form, occurring primarily in the lung of immunocompromised animals. Both systemic and topical therapy should be implemented with either form of the disease. Systemic therapy should consist of an imidazole; among the drugs itraconazole is the most efficacious against aspergillosis. Itraconazole was effective in treatment of aspergillosis or penicillinosis in two cats, although hepatotoxicity developed in a third; topical treatment with clotrimazole resulted in cure for this animal.[129] Itraconazole therapy for 10 weeks cured one dog infected with systemic and subsequent respiratory infection with *Aspergillus niger.*[130] Topical therapy has included amphotericin B; thiabendazole; and enilconazole, a topical imidazole available in Europe but not the United States. Enilconazole might be the most effective treatment when directly infused into the nasal passages through fenestrated tubes.[131] The 10% solution is diluted 1:1 with water and administered through surgically placed nasal tubes within 2 to 3 minutes. The solution emulsifies within several minutes of mixing; nasal tubes must be flushed after treatment. The total daily dose of 20 mg/kg is administered in two divided doses daily. Topical clotrimazole might be considered instead of enilconazole. One study reported response of refractory fungal rhinitis to surgical débridement combined with a povodine–iodine (see Chapter 11 for definition) wound dressing changed every 2 to 3 days; treatment continued until granulation tissue was present.[132]

Steinbach and coworkers[133] retrospectively examined the impact of combination or sequential antifungal therapy on invasive aspergillosis in humans or in experimental animals and found interactions ranging from synergy to antagonism. Amphotericin B combined with 5-fluorocytosine was the most commonly used combination (49%), with others including amphotericin B with itraconazole (16%) or rifampin (11%). Combination therapy was associated with improvement in 63% of patients, generally with amphotericin B combined with either 5-fluorocytosine or rifampin. However, combination of rifampin with the azoles was discouraged because induction by the former was apt to decrease concentrations of the latter, potentially below that considered effective. Combinations of amphotericin B with itraconazole were considered indifferent. In retrospective studies of animal model reports, amphotericin B plus 5-fluorocytosine, rifampin, or itraconazole was described as indifferent, whereas amphotericin B with micafungin was described as a positive interaction. Sequential therapy also was associated with benefits: Improvement was noted with amphotericin B or itraconazole followed by voriconazole but not with itraconazole followed by amphotericin B.[133] Indeed, azoles followed by amphotericin B (rather than opposite sequence) were found to be antagonistic, as might be expected based on the mechanism of action of the two drug classes. The use of capsofungin alone or with other antifungal drugs may provide alternative therapies for treatment of aspergillosis; terbinafine might also be considered in combination.

The use of voriconazole in animals for treatment of aspergillosis is very appealing but has not yet been described. The potential side effects of voriconazole and its complex pharmacokinetics suggest that use should be based on scientific studies that establish dosing regimens necessary to achieve MICs demonstrated for targeted fungal organisms, as well as studies that establish safety after several weeks of therapy at that dose.

Subcutaneous Mycoses

Sporotrichosis

Sporotrichosis occurs in three clinical forms: cutaneous, cutaneolymphatic, and disseminated. Disseminated disease generally involves most internal organs. The treatment of choice for both dogs and cats is supersaturated potassium iodide (SSKI).[134] Itraconazole at 5 to 7.5 mg/kg every 12 to 24 hours has been recommended.[126] Cats are more sensitive than dogs to the side effects of SSKI. Treatment should continue for at least 30 days beyond clinical remission. Immunosuppressive drugs should be avoided, if possible, for the duration of the animal's life; recurrence in clinically cured animals has been reported after immunosuppressive doses of glucocorticoids. Imidazoles (e.g., ketaconazole or itraconazole) should be used to treat animals that cannot tolerate or do not respond to SSKI. Other antifungals (e.g., terbinafine) might be combined with iodine.

Rhinosporidiosis

Rhinosporidium rarely causes disseminated disease in animals and is essentially limited to the nasal tissues. Surgical excision is the treatment of choice.[135] For recurrences dapsone may be useful. Alternatively, ketoconazole or itraconazole may be successful.

Pythiosis

Originally referred to as *phycomycosis*, pythiosis, a granulomatous disease, is caused by a number of taxonomically diverse nonseptated hyphal *Oomycetes*. The cell wall of *Oomycetes* differs from that of true fungi. Most notably is the limited amount of sterols in the fungal cell wall; hence antifungal agents are often ineffective against infections caused by these organisms. No antifungal agent has proved efficacious against this organism. However, two cases of gastrointestinal pythiosis were treated postoperatively (and apparently successfully) with a combination of itraconazole (10 mg/kg daily) or combined with terbinafine (7.5 mg/kg qd).[136] Up to 20 mg/kg itraconazole daily has been recommended.[126] Brown[137] described the MIC of *Pythium insidiosum* and *Lagenidium* sp toward a number of antifungal agents and found that the relative efficacy to be azoles (limited) < terbinafine and caspofungin (minimal to moderate inhibition) < mefenoaxam (profound efficacy). The latter drug is a fungicide used in agriculture and is approved by the Environmental Protection Agency. Its mechanism is inhibition of RNA polymerase.

REFERENCES

1. McGinnis MR, Rinaldi MG: Antifungal drugs: mechanisms of action, drug resistance, susceptibility testing, and assays of activity in biological fluids. In Lorian V, editor: *Antibiotics in laboratory medicine*, ed 4, Baltimore, 1996, Williams & Wilkins, pp 176–211.
2. Carter GR, Chengappa MM: *Essentials of veterinary bacteriology and mycology*, ed 4, Philadelphia, 1991, Lea & Febiger.
3. Bossche VH, Engelen M, Rochette F: Antifungal agents of use in animal health—chemical, biochemical and pharmacological aspects, *J Vet Pharmacol Therap* 26:5–29, 2003.
4. Bennett JE: Antimicrobial agents: antifungal agents. In Brunton LL, Lazo JS, Parker KL, editors: *Goodman & Gilman's the pharmacological basis of therapeutics*, ed 11, New York, 2006, McGraw-Hill.
5. Ben-Ami R, Lewis RE, Kontoyiannis DP: Immunocompromised hosts: immunopharmacology of antifungal drugs, *Clin Infect Dis* 47:226–235, 2008.
6. Marichal P: Mechanisms of resistance to azole antifungal compounds, *Current Opinion in Anti-Infective Investigational Drugs* 1:318–333, 1999.
7. Richardson M, Lass-Flörl C: Changing epidemiology of systemic fungal infections, *Clin Microbiol Infect* 14(Suppl 4):5–24, 2008.
8. Kontoyiannis DP, Lewis RE: Antifungal drug resistance of pathogenic fungi, *Lancet* 359:1135–1144, 2002.
9. Lupetti A, Nibbering PH, Campa M, et al: Molecular targeted treatments for fungal infections: the role of drug combinations, *Trends Mol Med* 9(6):269–276, 2003.
10. Groll AH, Piscitelli SC, Walsh TJ: Antifungal pharmacodynamics: concentration-effect relationships in vitro and in vivo, *Pharmacotherapy* 21(8s):133s–148s, 2001.
11. Grant SM, Clissold SP: Itraconazole. A review of its pharmacodynamic and pharmacokinetic properties and therapeutic use in superficial and systemic mycoses, *Drugs* 3:310–344, 1989.
12. Ghannoum MA, Rice LB: Antifungal agents: Mode of action, mechanisms of resistance, and correlation of these mechanisms with bacterial resistance, *Clin Microbiol Rev* 12:501–517, 1999.
13. Steinbach WJ, Stevens DA, Denning DW, et al: Advances against Aspergillosis, *Clin Infect Dis* 37(Suppl 3):S155–S156, 2003.
14. Committee on New Directions in the Study of Antimicrobial Therapeutics: New Classes of Antimicrobials, Committee on New Directions in the Study of Antimicrobial Therapeutics: Immunomodulation, National Research Council. Promising Approaches to the Development of Immunomodulation for the Treatment of Infectious Diseases: Report of a Workshop. In: *Treating Infectious Diseases in a Microbial World: Report of Two Workshops on Novel Antimicrobial Therapeutics*. National Academies Press. Accessed July 10, 2010 at http://books.nap.edu/openbook.php?record_id=11471&page=37.
15. Li RK, Ciblak MA, Nordoff N, et al: In vitro activities of voriconazole, itraconazole, and amphotericin B against *Blastomyces dermatitidis*, *Coccidioides immitis*, and *Histoplasma capsulatum*, *Antimicrob Agents Chemother* 44(6):1734–1736, 2000.
16. Mallie M, Bastide JM, Blancard A, et al: In vitro susceptibility testing of *Candida* and *Aspergillus* spp. to voriconazole and other antifungal agents using Etest®: results of a French multicentre study, *Int J Antimicrob Agents* 25:321–328, 2005.
17. Quilitz R: The use of lipid formulations of amphotericin B in cancer patients, Cancer Control: Journal of the Moffitt Cancer Center, September/October 1998. http://www.moffitt.org/moffittapps/ccj/v5n5/toc. Accessed on November 18, 2009.
18. Deray G: Amphotericin B nephrotoxicity, *J Antimicrobol Chemother* 49(Suppl S1):37–41, 2002.

18a. Adler-Moore JP, Proffit RT: Amphotericin B lipid preparations: what are the differences? *Clin Microbiol Infect* 14(Suppl 4):25–36, 2008.

19. Ranchère JY, Latour JF, Fuhrmann C, et al: Amphotericin B intralipid formulation: stability and particle size, *J Antimicrob Chemother* 37(6):1165–1169, 1996.
20. Vogelsinger H, Weller S, Djanani A, et al: Amphotericin B tissue distribution in autopsy material after treatment with liposomal amphotericin B and amphotericin B colloidal dispersion, *J Antimicrob Chemother* 57:1153–1160, 2006.
21. Ibrahim AS, Gebremariam T, Husseiny MI, et al: Comparison of lipid amphotericin B preparations in treating murine zygomycosis, *Antimicrob Agents Chemother* 52(4):1573–1576, 2008.
22. Bekersky I, Boswell GW, Hiles R: Safety and toxicokinetics of intravenous liposomal amphotericin B (AmBisome®) in beagle dogs, *Pharm Res* 16(11):1694–1701, 1999.
23. Bagnis CI, Deray G: Amphotericin B nephrotoxicity, *Saudi J Kidney Dis Transplant* 13(4):481–491, 2002.
24. Ceylan E, Akkan HA, Tutuncu M, et al: Nephrotoxic effect of amphotericin B administered in different doses and infusion model in dogs, *Acta Vet Brno* 72:229–234, 2003.
25. Schneider P, Klein RM, Dietze L, et al: Anaphylactic reaction to liposomal amphotericin (AmBisome®), *Br J Haematol* 102:1108, 1998.
26. Legendre AM, Selcer BA, Edwards DF, et al: Treatment of canine blastomycosis with amphotericin B and ketoconazole, *J Am Vet Med Assoc* 184(10):1249–1254, 1984.
27. Greene CE: Antifungal chemotherapy. In Green CE, editor: *Infectious disease of the dog and cat*, ed 3, St Louis, 2006, Saunders.
28. Rubin SI, Krawiec DR, Gelberg H, et al: Nephrotoxicity of amphotericin B in dogs: a comparison of two methods of administration, *Can J Vet Res* 53:23–28, 1989.
29. Stevens DA: Oral amphotericin B as an antifungal agent, *J Mycol Med* 6(S II):1–2, 1996.
30. Malik R, Craig AJ, Wigney DI, et al: Combination chemotherapy of canine and feline cryptococcosis using subcutaneously administered amphotericin B, *Aust Vet J* 73:124–128, 1996.
31. Olivero JJ, Loazno-Mendez J, Ghafary EM, et al: Mitigation of amphotericin B nephrotoxocity by mannitol, *Br J Med* 1:550–551, 1975.
32. Zager RA, Bredl CR, Schimpf BA: Direct amphotericin B-mediated tubular toxicity: assessments of selected cytoprotective agents, *Kidney Int* 41:1588–1594, 1992.

33. Feldman L, Efrati S, Daishy V, et al: N-acetylcysteine ameliorates amphotericin-induced nephropathy in rats, *Nephron Physiol* 99:23–27, 2005.
34. Leenders ACAP, de Marie S: The use of lipid formulations of amphotericin B for systemic fungal infections, *Leukemia* 10:1570–1575, 1996.
35. Lanternier F, Lortholary O: Liposomal amphotericin B: what is its role in 2008? *Clin Microbiol Infect* 14(Suppl 4):71–83, 2008.
36. Krawiec DR, McKiernan BC, Twardock RA, et al: Use of an amphotericin B lipid complex for treatment of blastomycosis in dogs, *J Am Vet Med Assoc* 209:2073–2075, 1996.
37. Randal SR, Adams LG, Whate MR, et al: Nephrotoxicity of amphotericin B administered to dogs in a fat emulsion versus five percent dextrose solution, *Am J Vet Res* 57:1054–1058, 1996.
38. Greene CE: *Infectious disease of the dog and cat*, ed 3, St Louis, 2006, Saunders.
39. Cleary JD, Taylor JW, Chapman SW: New drug developments. Itraconazole in antifungal therapy, *Ann Pharmacother* 26:502–509, 1992.
40. Benson JM, Nahata MC: Clinical use of systemic antifungal agents, *Clin Pharm* 7:424–438, 1988.
41. Pasko MT, Piscitelli SC, Slooten V, et al: Fluconazole: a new triazole antifungal agent, *DICP Ann Pharmacother* 24:860–867, 1990.
42. Johnson LB, Kauffman CA: Voriconazole: A new triazole antifungal agent, *Clin Infect Dis* 36:630–637, 2003.
43. van Custum J, van Gerven F, Janssen PAJ: The in vitro and in vivo antifungal activity of itraconazole. In *Recent trends in the discovery, development, and evaluation of antifungal agents, Proceedings of an International Telesymposium*, Barcelona, Spain, 1987, JR Prouse Science, pp 177–192.
44. Borgers M: Changes in fungal ultrastructure after itraconazole treatment. In *Recent trends in the discovery, development, and evaluation of antifungal agents, Proceedings of an International Telesymposium*, Barcelona, Spain, 1987, JR Prouse Science, pp 193–206.
45. Abdel-Rahman SM, Jacobs RF, Massarella J, et al: Single-dose pharmacokinetics of intravenous itraconazole and hydroxypropyl-beta-cyclodextrin in infants, children, and adolescents, *Antimicrob Agents Chemother* 51(8):2668–2673, 2007.
46. Carrillo-Munoz AJ, Quindos G, Rusega M, et al: Antifungal activity of posaconazole compared with fluconazole and amphotericin B against yeasts from oropharyngeal candidiasis and other infections, *J Antimicrob Chemother* 55:317–319, 2005.
47. Hart DT, Lauwers WJ, Willemens G, et al: Perturbation of sterol biosynthesis by itraconazole and ketoconazole in Leishmania mexicana infected macrophages, *Mol Biochem Parasitol* 33:123–134, 1989.
48. Hardin TC, Graybill JR, Techick R, et al: Pharmacokinetics of itraconazole following oral administration to normal volunteers, *Antimicrob Agents Chemother* 9:1310–1313, 1988.
49. Van Peer A, Woestenbourghs R, Heykants J, et al: The effects of food and dose on the oral systemic availability of itraconazole in healthy subjects, *Eur J Clin Pharmacol* 36:423–426, 1989.
50. Boothe DM, Herring I, Calvin J, et al: Itraconazole disposition following single oral and intravenous and multiple oral dosing in healthy cats, *Am J Vet Res* 58:872–877, 1997.
51. Heykants J, Michiels M, Meuldermans W, et al: The pharmacokinetics of itraconazole in animals and man. An overview. In *Recent trends in the discovery, development, and evaluation of antifungal agents, Proceedings of an International Telesymposium*, Barcelona, Spain, 1987, JR Prouse Science, pp 223–250.
52. Vaden SL, Heit MC, Hawkins EC, et al: Fluconazole in cats: pharmacokinetics following intravenous and oral administration and penetration into cerebrospinal fluid, aqueous humor and pulmonary epithelial lining fluid, *J Vet Pharmacol Ther* 20:181–186, 1997.
53. Groll AH, Piscitelli SC, Walsh TJ: Antifungal pharmacodynamics: concentration-effect relationships in vitro and in vivo, *Pharmacotherapy* 21(8 Pt 2):133S–148S, 2001.
54. Legendre AM, Rohrback R, Toal RL, et al: Treatment of blastomycosis with itraconazole in 112 dogs, *J Vet Intern Med* 10:365–371, 1996.
55. Roffey SJ, Cole S, Comby P, et al: The disposition of voriconazole in mouse, rat, rabbit, guinea pig, dog and human, *Drug Metab Dispos* 31(6):731–741, 2003.
56. Nomeir AA, Kumari P, Hilbert MJ, et al: Pharmacokinetics of SCH 56592, a new azole broad-spectrum antifungal agent, in mice, rats, rabbits, dogs, and cynomolgus monkeys, *Antimicrob Agents Chemother* 44(3):727–731, 2000.
57. De Coster R, Beerens D, Haelterman C, et al: Effects of itraconazole on the pituitary-testicular-adrenal axis: an overview of preclinical and clinical studies. In *Recent trends in the discovery, development, and evaluation of antifungal agents, Proceedings of an International Telesymposium*, Barcelona, Spain, 1987, JR Prouse Science, pp 251-262.
58. Bossche HV: Itraconazole: a selective inhibitor of the cytochrome P-450 dependent ergosterol biosynthesis. In *Recent trends in the discovery, development, and evaluation of antifungal agents, Proceedings of an International Telesymposium*, Barcelona, Spain, 1987, JR Prouse Science, pp 207–222.
59. Kukanich B, Borum SL: Effects of ketoconazole on the pharmacokinetics and pharmacodynamics of morphine in healthy greyhounds, *Am J Vet Res* 69:664–669, 2008.
60. Willard MD, Nachreiner R, MacDonald R, et al: Ketoconazole-induced changes in selected canine hormone concentrations, *Am J Vet Res* 47:2504–2509, 1986a.
61. Willard MD, Nachreiner RF, Howard VC, et al: Effect of long term administration of ketoconazole in cats, *Am J Vet Res* 47:2510–2513, 1986b.
62. Kim RB: Drugs as p-glycoprotein substrates, inhibitors, and inducers, *Drug Metab Rev* 34(1&2):47–54, 2002.
63. van Cauteren H, Coussement W, Vandenberghe J, et al: The toxicological properties of itraconazole. In *Recent trends in the discovery, development, and evaluation of antifungal agents, Proceedings of an International Telesymposium*, Barcelona, Spain, 1987, JR Prouse Science, pp 262-271.
64. Manciati F, Pedonses F, Zulline C: Efficacy of oral administration of itraconazole to cats with dermatophytosis caused by, *Microsporum canis, J Am Vet Med Assoc* 213:993–995, 1998.
65. Mayer UK, Glos K, Schmid M, et al: Adverse effects of ketoconazole in dogs—a retrospective study, *Vet Dermatol* 9:199–208, 2008.
66. Moriello KA: Treatment of dermatophytosis in dogs and cats: review of published studies, *Vet Dermatol* 15:99–107, 2004.
67. Plotnick AN, Boshoven EW, Prsychuk RA: Primary cutaneous coccidioidomycosis and subsequent drug eruption to intraconazole in a dog, *J Am Anim Hosp Assoc* 33:129–143, 1997.
68. Background document for the Antiviral Drug Products Advisory Committee meeting: *Voriconazole, Food and Drug Administration Center for Drug Evaluation and Research, Division of Special Pathogen and Immunologic Drug Products*, 2001, Pfizer Global Research & Development NDAs, pp 21–266 and 21-267.
69. Castro LGM, Belda W Jr, Cuce LC, et al: Successful treatment of sporotrichosis with oral fluconazole: a report of three cases, *Br J Dermatol* 128(3):352–356, 1993.
70. Medleau L, Chalmers SA: Ketoconazole for treatment of dermatophytosis in cats, *J Am Vet Med Assoc* 100:77–78, 1992.
71. Mundell AC: New therapeutic agents in veterinary dermatology, *Vet Clin North Am Small Anim Pract* 20:1541–1556, 1990.
72. Dunbar M, Pyle LR, Boring JG, et al: Treatment of canine blastomycosis with ketoconazole, *J Am Vet Med Assoc* 182:156–157, 1983.
73. Noxon JO, Diglio K, Schmidt DA: Disseminated histoplasmosis in a cat: successful treatment with ketoconazole, *J Am Vet Med Assoc* 181:817–819, 1982.

74. Malik R, Wigney DI, Muir DB, et al: Cryptococcosis in cats: clinical and mycological assessment of 29 cases and evaluation of treatment using orally administered fluconazole, *J Med Vet Mycol* 30:133–144, 1992.
75. Noxon JO, Monroe We, Chinn DR: Ketoconazole therapy in canine and feline cryptococcosis, *J Am Anim Hosp Assoc* 22:179–183, 1986.
76. Tucker RM, Williams PL, Arathoon EG, et al: Treatment of mycoses with itraconazole, *Ann NY Acad Sci* 544:451–470, 1988.
77. Finn MJ, Stiles J, Krohne SG: Visual outcome in a group of dogs with ocular blastomycosis treated with systemic antifungals and systemic corticosteroids, *Vet Ophthalmol* 10(5):299–303, 2007.
78. Hodges RD, Legendre AM, Adams LG, et al: Itraconazole for the treatment of histoplasmosis in cats, *J Vet Intern Med* 8:409–413, 1994.
79. Medleau L, Green CE, Rakich PM: Evaluation of ketoconazole and itraconazole for treatment of disseminated cryptococcosis in cats, *Am J Vet Res* 51:1454–1548, 1990.
80. Malik R, Krockenberger M, O'Brien CR, et al: Cryptococcosis. In Greene CE, editor: *Infectious diseases of the dog and cat*, ed 3, St Louis, 2006, Saunders.
81. Medleau L, Jacobs GJ, Marks MA: Itraconazole for the treatment of cryptococcosis in cats, *J Vet Intern Med* 9:39–42, 1995.
82. Peaston A, Sporotrichosis: *J Vet Intern Med* 7:44–45, 1993.
83. Legendre AM: Antimycotic drug therapy. In Bonagura JD, Kirk RW, editors: *Current veterinary therapy XII*, Philadelphia, 1995, Saunders, pp 327–331.
84. DeBoer DJ, Moriello KM, Cairns R: Clinical update on feline dermatophytosis—part II, *Compend Contin Educ Pract Vet* 17:1471–1480, 1995.
85. Medleau L, Rakich PM: Microsporum canis pseudomycetomas in a cat, *J Am Anim Hosp Assoc* 30:573–576, 1994.
86. Michaud AJ: Phaeohyphomycotic rhinitis due to *Exophiala jeanselmei* in a domestic cat, *Feline Pract* 21:19–21, 1993.
87. Simons EG: Phaeohyphomycosis in a cat caused by *Alternaria infectoria*, *Mycoses* 36:451–454, 1993.
88. Guptal AK, Sibbald GR, Lynde CW, et al: Onychomycosis in children: prevalence and treatment strategies, *J Am Acad Dermatol* 36:395–402, 1997.
89. Hill B, Moriello KA, Shaw SE: A review of systemic antifungal agents, *Vet Dermatol* 6:59–66, 1995.
90. Sharp NH, Harvey CE, Obrien JA: Treatment of canine nasal aspergillosis/penicillinosis with fluconazole, *J Small Anim Pract* 32:513–516, 1991.
91. Wenzel R, Del Favero A, Killber C, et al: Economic evaluation of voriconazole compared with conventional amphotericin B for the primary treatment of aspergillosis in immunocompromised patients, *J Antimicrob Chemother* 55:352–361, 2005.
91a. Wray JD, Sparkes AH, Johnson EM: Infection of the subcutis of the nose in a cat caused by *Mucor* species: successful treatment using posaconazole, *J Fel Med Surg* 10:523–527, 2008.
92. Barchiesi F, de Francesco LF, Scalise G: In vitro activities of terbinafine in combination with fluconazole and itraconazole against isolates of *Candida albicans* with reduced susceptibility to azoles, *Antimicrob Agents Chemother* 41(8):1812–1814, 1997.
93. Burkhart CG, Burkhart CN, Isham N: Synergistic antimicrobial activity by combining an allylamine with benzoyl peroxide with expanded coverage against yeast and bacterial species, *Br J Dermatol* 154:341–344, 2006.
94. Denning DW: Echinocandins: a new class of antifungal, *J Antimicrob Chemother* 49:889–991, 2002.
95. Renslo AR: The echinocandins: total and semi-synthetic approaches in antifungal drug discovery, *Anti-Infective Agents in Medicinal Chemistry* 6:201–212, 2007.
96. Denning DW: Echinocandin antifungal drugs, *Lancet* 362(9390):1142–1151, 2003.
97. Anhthu H: Caspofungin acetate: an antifungal agent, *Am J Health-Syst Pharm* 58(13):1206–1214, 2001.
98. Helton KA, Nesbitt GH, Caciolo OL: Griseofulvin toxicities in cats: literature review and report of seven cases, *J Am Anim Hosp Assoc* 22:453–458, 1986.
99. Sheltin GH, Grant CK, Linenberg ML, et al: Severe neutropenia associated with griseofulvin therapy in cats with feline immunodeficiency virus infection, *J Vet Intern Med* 4:317–319, 1990.
100. Ryder NS: Activity of terbinafine against serious fungal infections, *Mycoses* 42(Suppl 2):115–119, 1999.
100a. Burkhart CG, Burkhart CN, Isham N: Synergistic antimicrobial activity by combining an allylamine with benzoyl peroxide with expanded coverage against yeast and bacterial species, *Br J Dermatol* 154(2):341–344, 2006.
100b. Cavalheiro AS, Maboni G, de Azevedo MI, et al: In vitro activity of terbinafine combined with caspofungin and azoles against, *Pythium insidiosum*, *Antimicrob Agents Chemother* 53(5):2136–2138, 2009.
101. Balfour JA, Faulds D: Terbinafine: a review of its pharmacodynamic and pharmacokinetic properties and therapeutic potential in superficial mycosis, *Drugs* 43:259–284, 1992.
102. Feargemann J, Zehender H, Jones T, et al: Terbinafine levels in serum, stratum corneum, dermis-epidermis (without stratum corneum), hair, sebum, and eccrine sweat during and after 250 mg terbinafine orally once per day in man, *J Invest Dermatol* 24:523–528, 1990.
103. Sparks AH: Terbinafine in cats: a pharmacokinetic study, Edinburgh, Scotland, 1996, *Proc Third World Cong Vet Dermatol*.
104. Werner AH, Werner BE: Feline sporotrichosis, *Compend Contin Educ Pract Vet* 15:1189–1198, 1993.
105. Moriello KA, Granks P, Delany-Lewis D, et al: Cutaneous-lymphatic and nasal sporotrichosis in a dog, *J Am Anim Hosp* 24:621–626, 1988.
106. Ben-Ziony A: Use of lufenuron for treating fungal infections of dogs and cats: 297 cases (1997-1999), *J Am Vet Assoc* 217:1510–1513, 2000.
107. Moriello KA, Deboer DJ, Schenker R, et al: Efficacy of pre-treatment with lufenuron for the prevention of *Microsporum canin* infection in a feline direct topical challenge model, *Vet Dermatol* 15:357–362, 2004.
108. Ostrosky-Zeichner L: Combination antifungal therapy: a critical review of the evidence, *Clin Microbiol Infect* 14(Suppl 4):65–70, 2008.
109. DeBoer DJ, Moriello KA: Cutaneous fungal infections: dermatophytosis. In Greene CE, editor: *Infectious diseases of the dog and cat*, ed 3, St Louis, 2006, Saunders.
110. Moriello KA, DeBoer DJ: Efficacy of griseofulvin and itraconazole in the treatment of experimentally induced dermatophytosis in cats, *J Am Vet Med Assoc* 207(4):439–443, 1995.
111. Colombo S, Cornegliani L, Vercelli A: Efficacy of Itraconazole as a combined continuous/pulse therapy in feline dermatophytosis: preliminary results in nine cases, *Vet Dermatol* 12(6):347–350, 2001.
111a. Newbury S, Moriello K, Verbrugge M, et al: Use of lime sulphur and itraconazole to treat shelter cats naturally infected with *Microsporum canis* in an annex facility: an open field trial, *Vet Derm* 18:324–331, 2007.
112. Kotnik T, Kozuh Erzen N, Kuzner J: Drobnic-Kosorok M: Terbinafine hydrochloride treatment of Microsporim canis experimentally induced ringworm in cats, *Vet Microbiol* 83:161–168, 2001.
113. Ihrke PJ: Malassezia dermatitis and hypersensitivity. In *Antimicrobial therapy: applications in dermatology, Proceedings from an International Symposium, the North American Veterinary Conference*, Orlando, Florida, January, 1996, pp 45–48.
114. Cole LK, Luu DH, Rajala-Schultz PJ, et al: In vitro activity of an ear rinse containing tromethamine, EDTA, benzyl alcohol and 0.1% ketoconazole on *Malassezia* organisms from dogs with otitis externa, *Vet Dermatol* 18(2):115–119, 2007.

115. Åhman S, Perrins N, Bond R: Treatment of *Malassezia pachydermatis*-associated seborrhoeic dermatitis in Devon Rex cats with itraconazole—a pilot study, *Vet Dermatol* 8:171–174, 2007.
116. Negre A, Bensignor E, Guillot J: Evidence-based veterinary dermatology: a systematic review of interventions for *Malassezia* dermatitis in dogs, *Vet Dermatol* 0:1–12, 2008.
117. Klein BS, Squires RA, Lloyd JK, et al: Canine antibody response to *Blastomyces dermatitidis* WI-1 antigen, *Am J Vet Res* 61(5):554–558, 2000.
118. Legendre AM, Selcer BA, Edwards DF, Stevens R: Treatment of canine blastomycosis with amphotericin B and ketoconazole, *J Am Vet Med Assoc* 184(10):1249–1254, 1984.
119. Areceneaux KA, Taboada J, Hosgood G: Blastomycosis in dogs: 115 cases (1980–1995), *J Am Vet Med Assoc* 213:658–664, 1998.
119a. Crews LJ, Feeney DA, Jesse DR, et al: Utility of diagnostic tests for and medical treatment of pulmonary blastomycosis in dogs: 125 cases (1989-2006), *J Am Vet Med Assoc* 232:222–227, 2008.
120. Legendre AM: Antimycotic Drug therapy. In Bonagura J, editor: *Kirk's current veterinary therapy small animal pract XIII*, Philadelphia, 2000, Saunders, pp 327–334.
121. Greene CE: Histoplasmosis. In Greene CE, editor: *Infectious diseases of the dog and cat*, ed 3, St Louis, 2006, Saunders.
122. Schulman RL, McKiernan RC, Schaeffer DJ, et al: Use of corticosteroids for treating dogs with airway obstruction secondary to hilar lymphadenopathy caused by chronic histoplasmosis: 16 cases (1979-1997), *J Am Vet Med Assoc* 214:1345–1348, 1999.
123. Jacobs GJ, Medleau L, Calvert C, et al: Cryptococcal infection in cats: factors influencing treatment outcome, and results of sequential serum antigen titers in 35 cats, *J Vet Intern Med* 11(1):1-4, 1997.
124. Lortholary O, Nicolas M, Soreda S, et al: Fluconazole, with or without dexamethasone for experimental cryptococcosis: impact of treatment timing, *J Antimicrob Chemother* 43:817–824, 1999.
125. Flatland B, Greene RT, Lappin MR: Clinical and serological evaluation of cats with cryptococcosis, *J Am Vet Med Assoc* 209:1110, 1996.
126. Greene R: Coccidioidomycosis and paracoccidioidomycosis. In Greene CE, editor: *Infectious diseases of the dog and cat*, ed 3, St Louis, 2006, Saunders.
127. Greene RT, Troy GC: Coccidioidomycosis in 48 cats: a retrospective study (1984–1993), *J Vet Intern Med* 9:86–91, 1995.
128. Ricci G, Mota FT, Wakamatsu A, et al: Canine paracoccidioidomycosis, *Med Mycol* 42(4):379–383, 2004.
129. Tomsa K, Gluas TM: Zimmer fungal rhinitis and sinusitis in three cats, *J Am Vet Med Assoc* 222(10):1380–1384, 2003.
130. Kim SH, Yong HC, Yoon JH, et al: Aspergillus niger pulmonary infection in a dog, *J Vet Med Sci* 65:1139–1140, 2003.
131. Kuehn NF: Nasal aspergillosis. In Bonagura JD, Twedt DC, editors: *Current veterinary therapy XIV*, St Louis, 2009, Saunders.
132. Moore AH: Use of topical povidone-iodine dressings in the management of mycotic rhinitis in three dogs, *J Small Anim Pract* 44(7):326–329, 2003.
133. Steinbach WJ, Stevens DA, Denning DW, et al: Combination and sequential antifungal therapy for invasive Aspergillosis: review of published in vitro and in vivo interactions and 6281 clinical cases from 1966 to 2001, *Clin Infect Dis* 37(Suppl 3):S188–S224, 2003.
134. Rosser EJ, Dunstan RW: Sporotrichosis. In Greene CE, editor: *Infectious diseases of the dog and cat*, ed 3, St. Louis, 2006, Saunders.
135. Castellano MC, Breitschwerdt EB: Rhinosporidiosis. In Greene CE, editor: *Infectious diseases of the dog and cat*, ed 3, St Louis, 2006, Saunders.
136. Rakich PM, Grooter AM, Tang K-N: Gastrointestinal pythiosis in two cats, *J Vet Diagn Invest* 17:262–269, 2005.
137. Brown TA, Grooters AM, Hosgood GL: In vitro susceptibility of *Pythium insidiosum* and a *Lagenidium* sp to itraconazole, posaconazole, voriconazole, terbinafine, caspofungin, and mefenoxam, *Am J Vet Res* 69(11):1463–1468, 2008.

10 Antiviral Therapy

Dawn Merton Boothe

Chapter Outline

Approximately 80 families and 4000 species of viruses are known to date, and more than 60% of illnesses afflicted humans in developed countries are caused by viruses. However, the development of drugs intended to prevent and treat viral diseases has been frustratingly protracted. Despite the long and intensive search for effective antiviral drugs, very few compounds have clinical applications. Currently, at least 23 antiviral drugs have been approved for use in human medicine; none is approved for use in animals. Unfortunately, unlike the situation with many other anti-infectious drugs, applications for human antiviral drugs in veterinary patients often have been limited because the etiologic agents of viral diseases vary so widely. In recent years, however, given the similarities between feline and human immunodeficiency viruses[1] and potentially other viruses, information regarding pathophysiology and drugs with potential efficacy are increasingly applicable to veterinary use. Further, trends have developed toward development of drugs that are broadly effective against viral diseases. The development of species-specific recombinant proteins (e.g., interferons [IFNs]) has increased our knowledge base and promises to improve the therapeutic armamentarium for viral disease afflicting dogs and cats. Although these drugs are discussed in greater depth in other chapters, their support of treatment for antiviral diseases will be addressed here.

For a number of reasons, the development of effective antiviral drugs is more difficult than development of other anti-infectious agents. Drugs that target the viral processes must penetrate host cells to be effective, potentially limiting their distribution. Because the mechanisms by which viruses replicate must involve the host genome, drugs that are effective against viruses also are likely to have a negative effect on the host, with most antiviral drugs subsequently being characterized by a narrow therapeutic window. Clinical signs during the stages of infection when viruses might be most conducive to pharmacologic therapy often being mild to absent, and the need for antiviral therapy is not recognized until antiviral response is unlikely. Therapy is further complicated by viral latency, the ability of the virus to incorporate its genome into the host genome such that clinical infection becomes evident again without re-exposure to the organism. Selection of the most appropriate antiviral drugs is handicapped by the lack of broad-spectrum antivirals and the lack of rapid tests to identify the infecting virus. Newer polymerase chain reaction tests have at least helped in the more rapid diagnosis of some viral disease (e.g., parvovirus in dogs).

KEY POINT 10-1 The development of effective antiviral drugs is limited by the latent nature of disease, inherent host toxicity to viral drugs, and rapid emergence of viral resistance. Differences in viral diseases limits application of human antiviral drugs to dogs or cats.

In vitro susceptibility testing of viruses requires sophisticated and expensive techniques such as cell cultures. In vitro inhibitory testing procedures have not been standardized, and results vary with the assay system, cell type, and viral inoculum. Additionally, results may not correlate with therapeutic efficacy of antiviral drugs.[2] The lack of correlation between in vitro testing and clinical efficacy reflects, in part, the requirement of some antiviral drugs for activation (i.e., metabolism of a prodrug, generally by the host).[2] Not only is the spectrum of antiviral drugs narrow, but additionally, a drug often targets a specific viral protein (usually a polymerase or transcriptase enzyme) involved in viral nucleic acid synthesis.[2] The limited mechanism of action tends to facilitate the development of antiviral resistance, which can occur rapidly, often reflecting substitution of only a single, although critical, amino acid in the target protein. Drugs that simply inhibit single steps in the viral replication cycle are virustatic. Consequently, viral replication is only temporarily halted, although in human medicine, chronic drug therapy may suppress reactivation of the disease caused by the virus and thus prevent clinical signs of disease. Because drugs often inhibit only active replication, viral growth often resumes once therapy is discontinued.

Antiviral drugs often cannot eliminate nonreplicating or latent viruses, and effective antiviral therapy generally also depends on an adequate host immune response. Consequently, those antiviral drugs that enhance the immune system of the host may be more likely to eradicate infection, as might combinations of antiviral and immune-enhancing drugs. Conversely, it is the overexpression of the immune response and the subsequent immune (e.g., feline immunodeficiency virus [FIV] and feline leukemia virus [FeLV]) or inflammatory response (e.g., feline infectious peritonitis [FIP]) that causes continued pathophysiology. The complex cascade of the immune system with dual pathways that balance a response renders pharmacologic management of just the right amount of immunomodulation in the right direction difficult in the face of viral diseases.

Prions *(protein infectious virion)* are infectious agents composed entirely of propagated misfolded protein that is resistant to endogenous straightening. The term *prion* refers to the unidentified unit of infection. The method of propogation is not clear but appears to involve abnormal refolding of protein such that aggregates of tightly packed beta sheets accumulate to form amyloid. Accumulation occurs only in neural tissues and is uncontrollable and invariably lethal. Among the diseases affecting dogs or cats that are thought to be associated with prions is feline spongiform encephalopathy. Because these agents are not treatable, they will not be considered further in this chapter.

VIRAL REPLICATION

Viruses are composed of a core genome consisting of either double-stranded or single-stranded DNA or RNA surrounded by a protein shell known as a *capsid.* Some viruses are further surrounded by a lipoprotein membrane or envelope. Both the capsid and lipoprotein membrane may be antigenic. Viruses cannot replicate independently and must usurp the host's metabolic machinery to replicate. Therefore viruses are obligate intracellular parasites. The host's pathways of energy generation, protein synthesis, and DNA or RNA replication provide the virus with the means of viral replication. For some viruses, replication is initiated by viral enzymes.[2] DNA viruses include poxvirus, herpesvirus, adenovirus, hepadnavirus, and papillomavirus. RNA viruses include rubella virus, rhabdovirus (rabies), picornavirus, arenaviruses, arboviruses, orthomyxovirus, and paramyxovirus (canine distemper) (Table 10-1).

Cells respond to viral infection in three ways: infection may have no impact on the cell or its function, cellular death may occur (which may preclude subsequent infection), or the cell may be transformed such that host control of cell growth is lost to viral activities. Viral replication occurs in five or six sequential steps (Figure 10-1): cell entry, including host cell attachment, generally through specific receptors, followed by host cell penetration; disassembly or uncoating resulting in release of viral genome; transcription of viral genome (or viral messenger RNA), which is dependent on virus-specified enzyme; translation of regulatory (early) or structural (late) viral proteins; post-translation modifications (including proteolytic cleavage, myristoylation, glycosylation); assembly of virion components; and release of the virus, generally by budding or cell lysis.[2] For DNA viruses, viral DNA is transcribed to host mRNA by host cell mRNA polymerase (or, for poxvirus, viral RNA polymerase). Replication of RNA viruses requires virion enzymes to synthesize mRNA. Double stranded RNA (dsRNA) viruses contain RNA molecules that are transcribed into proteins. Two groups of single stranded RNA (ssRNA) viruses exist. The RNA genome of positive-sense ssRNA viruses is directly translated as mRNA by the host. In contrast, the RNA genome of negative sense ssRNA viruses must first be translated to mRNA by viral RNA-dependent RNA polymerase; host ribosomes subsequently translate to the protein.

Retrovirues are unique viruses that contain a single strand of RNA that must first be translated, via reverse transcriptase, to a DNA copy of the viral RNA template. The DNA is then incorporated into the host genome (as a provirus), duplicated, and subsequently transcribed into genomic RNA and mRNA for translation into viral proteins.[2]

A number of host mechanisms protect against viral infection. However, the host response not only may fail to protect but also may perpetuate the disease. Antibodies will be generated in response to viral infection, but these do little to overcome the initial infection. Rather, in part because viral activity is generally intracellular and thus inaccessible to antibodies, antibodies generally protect against subsequent infection. Unfortunately, the presence of circulating antibodies can contribute to the disease process of some infections (e.g., FIP). Cell-mediated immunity (CMI) plays a critical role in overcoming and preventing viral infection. However, viruses that can avoid an effective CMI response may cause latent or, if the cell does not result in the loss of normal cellular housekeeping activities, persistent infections. Mechanisms by which this can be accomplished included downregulation of major histocompatibility complex production such that the infected cell is not recognized by T cells; cells are generated that are not detectable by the host immune system; and infection is limited to cells located in an immunoprivileged site, such as the brain. Viruses that are particularly adept at causing persistent, chronic infections include paramyxoviruses, selected herpesviruses, and retroviruses.

KEY POINT 10-2 Host response often cannot effectively eradicate infection, even in the presence of drugs, but often contributes to the diseases process.

In addition to the directed immune response, the host will mount a number of nonspecific protective mechanisms. These include increased body temperature, activity of natural killer cells and phagocytes, and hormones. The role of IFN increasingly is being revealed as a target of pharmacotherapy. Viral infection begins with interaction between the virus and its specific host cell receptor. It is this interaction that initiates the host activation of multiple signal transduction cascades that mount a host defense. Ultimately, these mechanisms cause the nucleus to activate diverse immunoregulatory genes and proteins that cause the intracellular environment to be antagonistic toward viral replication.[3] Phosphorylations activate several

Table 10-1 Classification of Viruses by Genome Type

Genomic Type		Family (Viridae)	Genus (Virus)	Disease
DNA				
	ssDNA	Reoviridae		
		Parvoviridae	Parvovirus	Canine parvovirus, feline panleukopenia (distemper)
	dsDNA	Adenoviridae	Adenovirus	Canine infectious hepatitis, blue eye (CAV1), respiratory disease (CAV2)
		Herpesviridae	Herpesvirus	Canine herpes (CHV, reproductive), feline herpes (FHV-1; rhinotracheitis)
		Papillomaviridae		Canine papillomas
		Parvoviridae		
		Poxviridae		
RNA	dsRNA	Reoviridae	Rotavirus	
	(+)ssRNA	Coronaviridae	Coronavirus, feline coronavirus (FoCV)	Canine corona virus (gastrointestinal), feline infectious peritonitis
		Caliciviridae	Vesivirus	Feline calicivirus (respiratory)
		Flaviviridae	West Nile virus	
		Hepeviridae	Hepatitis virus E	
		Picornaviridae	Enterovirus	Polio, bovine, and porcine enterovirus
			Rhinovirus	
			Hepatitis virus A	
			Erbovirus	Equine rhinitis virus B
			Aphthovirus	Foot and mouth disease
	(-)ssRNA	Filoviridae	Ebola, Marburg	
		Paramyxoviridae	Parainfluenza virus	Kennel cough (dog)
			Mumps virus	Mumps
			Morbillivirus	Measles, canine distemper
			Newcastle virus	Newcastle disease
		Rhabdoviridae	Rabies virus	Rabies
		Orthomyxoviridae	Influenza A (including canine), B, C virus	Canine influenza (respiratory)
	ssRNA	Retroviridae*	Lentivirus (HIV, FIV)	Human, feline AIDS
			Gammaretrovirus	Feline infectious leukemia

*Many virus members contain oncogenes.
ds, Double strand; *ss*, single strand.

families of transcription factors. Among the antiviral genes regulated are those encoding interferon (IFN), including α-1 and -β regulators. Several viral cell receptor–initiated events have been identified for their ability to induce activation that ultimately involves IFN. For example, chemokine receptor binding to human immunodeficiency virus (HIV) envelope or glycoproteins, and poxvirus and measles virus binding to T and B cell membrane–bound glycoprotein each initiate such events. The 2–5A pathway is an example of an endogenous antiviral protective system that induces IFN through dependent RNase and 2'-5' oligoadenylate synthetase (OAS). Viral infection stimulates OAS, which ultimately leads to destruction of both viral and cellular rRNA. Subsequent cell death is similar in appearance to that caused by apoptosis. Viral replication is subsequently prevented.[4] Activation of IFN-based and other defense mechanisms also can occur through nonreceptor–mediated mechanisms.[3] Not surprisingly, viruses have developed several mechanisms that evade IFN-mediated cell responses. An example includes production of soluble IFN receptors that preclude interaction with normal receptors (e.g., poxviruses and herpesviruses) that would otherwise activate the cascades, downregulation of IFN synthesis (adenovirus), and blocking of phosphorlyations.[3]

The pathophysiology of infection, including molecular mechanisms, has recently been described for FeLV[5] and FIV,[1] including the role of selected cytokines in the immune response.[6]

ANTIVIRAL DRUGS

Few antiviral drugs have been studied in animals (Tables 10-2, 10-3), and widespread clinical use of antiviral drugs is not common in veterinary medicine. Only a selection of the

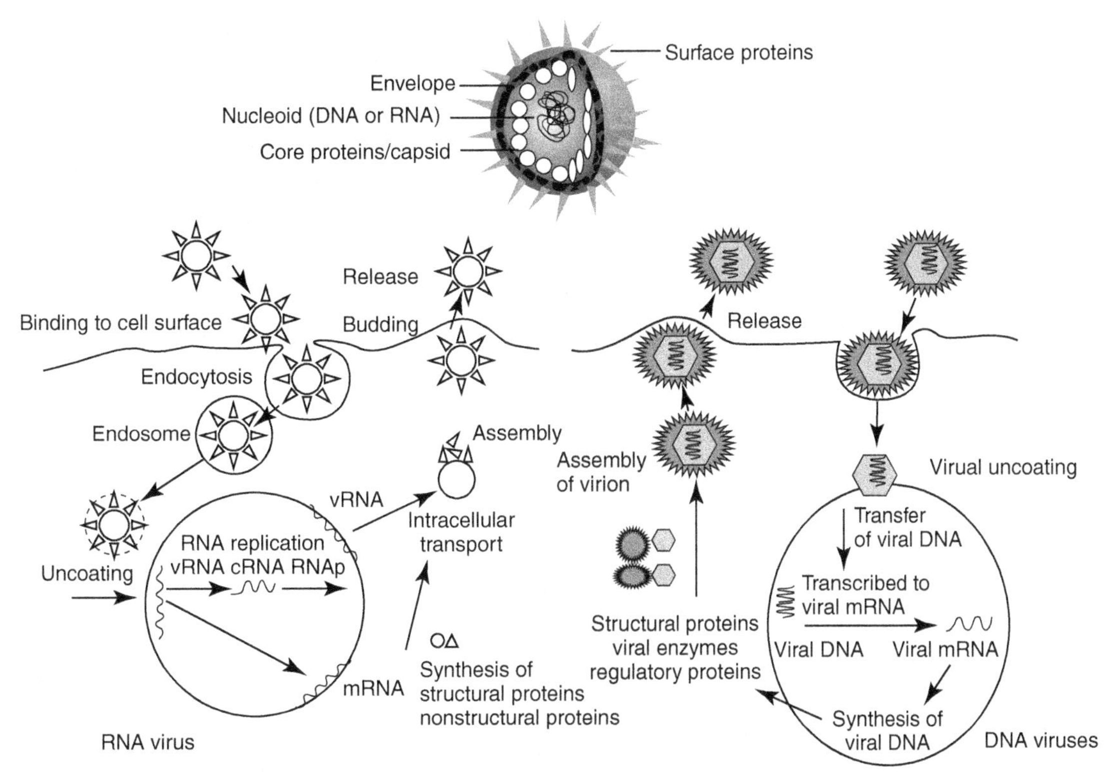

Figure 10-1 Replication of a representative RNA virus and DNA virus. Targets of antiviral drugs are presented before or during infection (including cell penetration), inside the cell (including viral replication, assembly and release), and during dissemination of progeny. The latter also includes preventing immunosuppression or the overzealous host response. *cRNA,* Replication intermediate; *mRNA,* messenger RNA; *RNAp*, RNA polymerase; *vRNA,* viral RNA.

more promising agents and their purported attributes are briefly discussed; alternatively, when pharmacokinetic information is available, because such information is so limited, it also is provided even if the drug is not an accepted therapy for canine or feline viruses.

Antiviral drugs are most practically categorized by the major viruses targeted by the drug, which tends to limit direct applicability to animal diseases. Although data specific to veterinary use are increasing, much information regarding antiviral drugs continues to reflect extrapolation from the human-medicine literature. This is particularly true for pharmacokinetics, and unless stated otherwise, such information is human in origin. Yet the disposition of antiviral drugs tends to be complex, often requiring prodrug activation, protein binding, and hepatic clearance, all of which tend to vary among species. The drugs are often characterized by a narrow therapeutic window. As such, extrapolation of dosing regimens should be done cautiously. Immune-modulating drugs in particular are not well understood, and mechanisms of action have not yet been fully elucidated. Very few human antiviral drugs have been studied or reported to be used for treatment of viral disorders in dogs or cats and the evidence provided by the few clinical trials performed in animals often is characterized by limitations in study design. Consequently, the inclusion in this chapter of information regarding antiviral drugs should not be interpreted as justification for use but rather treated as a springboard for additional studies. Two categories of drugs have been and are currently being pursued for the pharmacologic treatment of viral diseases. *Antiviral chemicals* directly interfere with the virus, whereas *biologic response modifiers* stimulate the host's immune system, thereby increasing the host's ability to overcome viral invasion. The latter are discussed in greater depth elsewhere in this book.

Targets of Antiviral Therapy

Potential targets in the viral life cycle that might be pharmacologically inhibited are expressed during extracellular stages of viral infection (i.e., penetration), intracellular stages (i.e., replication, assembly, and viral release), and dissemination. Those expressed during extracellular stages include specific enzymes whose release is required for skin and mucosal barrier penetration by some viruses, specific cell receptors required for penetration by other viruses, and specific precursor "fusion" proteins that must be activated before cell penetration by some viruses. Antivirals that diminish penetration of host cells by the virus are more viral specific and thus not as inherently toxic as those that prevent viral replication by interfering with viral nucleic acid, DNA, and protein synthesis. Because cell penetration is enhanced by viral-induced immunosuppression, pharmacologic immunomodulation may also help prevent viral penetration.[7] Thus these drugs are inherently more useful during the early stages of infection, which are often missed because of the lack of clinical signs. Classes of antivirals that target cell entry include soluble receptor decoys and antireceptor antibodies. Uncoating of the virus can be targeted by ion channel blockers, capsid stabilizers, and fusion protein inhibitors.[2]

Table 10-2 Antiviral Drugs with Potential Application in Dogs or Cats

Class	Drug	Mechanism	Viral Target	Veterinary Indications	Comments
Pyrimidine nucleoside	Idoxurine	Incorporated into DNA as thymidine analogue	Herpesvirus	Herpetic keratitis	Neoplasia and infertility limits to topical
	Trifluridine	Incorporated into DNA as thymidine analogue	Herpes simplex virus Cytomegalovirus Adenoviruses	Herpetic keratitis	Topical
	Sorivudine	DNA: thymidine analogue (thymidine Kinase)	Varicella-zoster virus		
Purine nucleoside	Vidarabine	Host phosphorylation; analogue of adenosine; competitive inhibition DNA polymerase; ribonucleoside reductase, other RNA activities	DNA viruses: herpesvirus Poxvirus Rhabdoviruns Hepadnavirus Selected RNA tumor viruses	Herpetic keratitis	Toxicity limits IV administration to life-threatening situations.
	Acyclovir Valacyclovir (prodrug)	Acyclovir: Synthetic analogue of guanosine; viral activation (thymidine kinase) and host phosphorylation: inhibition of DNA polymerase	DNA viruses Herpes virus	Feline rhinovirus? Veterinary use limited by differences in viral thymidine kinase	Topical, oral, parenteral (acyclovir). Oral (valacyclovir). Acyclovir associated with renal disease in dogs
	Penciclovir Famiciclovir (prodrug)	Guanine nucleoside, targeting thymidine kinase (herpes) or phosphotransferase (cytomegalovirus)	DNA viruses Herpesvirus Cytomegalovirus	Feline herpes virus	Less potent than acyclovir but accumulated in cell
	Ganciclovir	Guanine nucleoside			
	Ribavirin	Multiple enzymes inhibited, capping and polypeptide synthesis	DNA and RNA viruses (broad spectrum) Herpesvirus Orthomyxovirus Poxvirus Picornavirus Rhabdovirus Rotavirus Retrovirus	Feline calicivirus (limited efficacy against rhinovirus)	Oral, Aerosol Lesions worsened in cats with calici
Antiretroviral	Zidovudine (AZT)	Thymidine analogue; inhibition of RNA dependent DNA polymerase (reverse transcriptase)	Retroviruses		Relatively safe in cats; studied alone and in combination with lamivudine
	Lamivudine		Retroviruses HIV, FIV	FIV	Relatively safe in cats; studied in combination with AZT
	Didanosine	Purine nucleoside	HIV, FIV (including AZT resistant strains)		
Miscellaneous	Foscarnet Amantadine Rimantadine	DNA polymerase Interference with viral attachment, penetration or intracellular releases; viral mRNA transcription, assembly	Herpes Influenza A Influenza C Sendai virus Pseudorabies	Rhinovirus (prophylaxis); FeLV?	Oral, intranasal, subcutaneous, aerosol
	Oseltamivir (prodrug)	Neuraminidase inhibitor	Influenza A Influenza B		
	Suramin	Inhibition of reverse transcriptase		FeLV?	
	Inosiplex	Suppression of viral mRNA; induce T-cell differentiation			

Table **10-3** Doses of Selected Antiviral Drugs

Drug	Indication	Dose	Route	Interval (hr)
Famciclovir	See text			
Foscarnet sodium		20-30 mg/kg (D)	IV, PO	8
Idoxuridine 0.1% solution	Ocular herpes virus infection	1 drop in each eye (C)	Topical (ophthalmic)	4-8
Idoxuridine 0.5% ointment		Apply to local lesion	Topical	4-8
Interferon alpha-2 (human recombinant)	Non-neoplastic feline leukemia virus–FeLV-associated disease (low dose)	15-30 IU/cat	IM, PO, SC	24h × 7 days on and off cycles
		0.5-5 IU/kg (C)	PO, SC	24h × 7 days on and off cycles
	FeLV appetite stimulation	1 IU/cat	PO	24h × 7 days on and off cycles
	Feline infectious peritonitis (nonexudative)	30 IU/cat (C)	PO	24h × 7 days on and off cycles
	Feline infectious peritonitis (exudative)	2000 IU/Cat	IM	24
	Ocular herpes	10 IU	PO	24
		25-50 IU/mL saline	Topical (both eyes)	4-6
	Indolent ulcers	60-100 IU	PO, SC	24
Interferon bovine beta	Non-neoplastic FeLV-associated disease (high dose)	10,000-1,000,000 IU/kg	PO, SC	24h × 7 days on and off cycles
	Feline infectious peritonitis (exudative)	20,000 IU/C	IM	24h × 14-21 days
	Acute feline herpesvirus in kittens	10,000 IU/kg	SC	24h × 21 days
Interferon, feline recombinant	Immunostimulation	1 million IU/kg	SC	48h; reduce to 7 d when responding
Lactoferrin	Feline immunodeficiency virus stomatitis	40 mg/kg (C)	Topical	24
Lysine	Immunostimulation	500 mg/cat	PO	24h or divide dose and administer q 12h for life
Oseltamivir	Susceptible virus infections	2 mg/kg (D)	PO	12h × 10 days
Propionibacterium acnes	Immunostimulation	<7 kg: 0.1-0.2 mg/dog	IV	4 × per week in first week, 2 × per week at 3- to 4-day intervals, followed by 1 × per week until clinical signs abate or stabilize. Maintenance dose once per month.
Propionibacterium acnes	Feline retrovirus infection	15 μg/kg	IV	Biweekly for 2-3 weeks
Ribavirin	Susceptible virus infections	11 mg/kg	IM, IV, PO	24h × 7 days
Trifluridine ophthalmic solution	Ocular herpesvirus infection	1-2 drops of a 0.1% solution	Topical	3-8
Vidarabine	Ocular herpesvirus infection	Apply 0.3 cm (0.125 inches)	Topical	4-8
Zidovudine	Susceptible virus infections	5-25 mg/kg (C)	PO, SC	8-12

C, cat; *D*, Dog; *IM*, intramuscular; *IV*, intravenous; *PO*, by mouth; *SC*, subcutaneous.

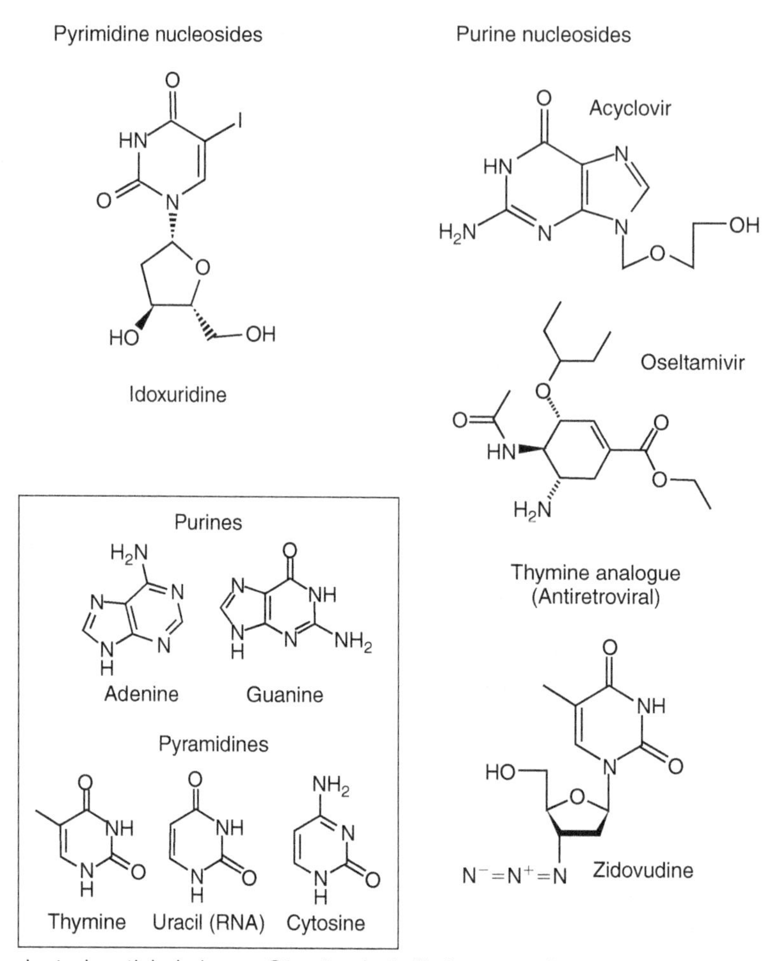

Figure 10-2 Structures of selected antiviral drugs. Structural similarity to purine or pyrimidine bases of host RNA or DNA *(box)* results in limited host safety.

Currently, targets expressed during intracellular stages of viral infection are the most common sites of pharmacologic intervention. Drugs include antivirals as well as a number of other classes of drugs (e.g., immunomodulators). Viral replication depends on macromolecular synthesis (by the host) of viral genome and on genome replication, transcription, and translation. Classes of drugs that inhibit transcription include inhibitors of viral DNA or RNA polymerase, reverse transcriptase, helicase, primase, or integrase. Natural substances capable of inhibiting viral transcription and translation (e.g., IFN) are much more potent than synthetic compounds. Viral replication is targeted by antisense oligonucleotides and ribozymes. Many antiviral drugs are nucleoside or nucleotide analogs, whose chemical structures allow prevention of viral replication by blocking nucleic acid metabolism (Figure 10-2; see also Figure 10-1). However, viral replication is so closely connected to vital functions of the host cell that agents capable of inhibiting viral replication usually injure host cells as well. Although such drugs are more likely to be broad in their antiviral spectrum, most also are potential teratogens, mutagens, and (particularly in humans) carcinogens. Further, they are associated with a variety of other host toxicities, with bone marrow suppression a not uncommon occurrence.[7]

Fewer agents have been developed that block viral translation. Classes of drugs that inhibit viral translation include IFNs, antisense oligonucleotides, and ribozymes. In addition, regulatory proteins might be inhibited. Another category of intracellular targets are specific enzymes, such as RNA or DNA polymerase, or reverse transcriptase of retroviruses, whose expression is required for the maintenance of the viral life cycle. Antiviral agents designed to block expression of these enzymes may have increased selectivity for viruses compared with the host, although their antiviral spectrum frequently is limited. Finally, assembly of synthesized viral macromolecules and release of the assembled virus may be pharmacologically inhibited. For example, IFN-induced inhibition of RNA tumor viruses occurs at assembly, although the mechanism is unknown.[7]

Posttranslational modifications such as proteolytic cleavage may be targeted by some drug classes (e.g., protease inhibitors). IFNs and drugs that inhibit specific proteins target viral assembly. Finally, antiviral antibodies and cytotoxic lymphocytes target the release of viruses from the host cell.

The final stage of viral infection that might be targeted pharmacologically is release of the new viral progeny from the infected host cell. Viruses can leave cells by causing cellular lysis or budding. With lysis, virus leaves in a sudden burst that kills the host cell. With budding, interaction between the virus and cell receptor induces changes that allow fusion of viral and cellular membranes, thus allowing the progeny to gradually leave the infected cell by budding. An example target for drugs during viral release is the neuraminidase in influenza viruses, a virulence factor that cleaves the sialic acid (neuraminic acid) residues from the glycan portion of cell receptors recognized by viral hemagglutinin.[8]

Viral infection may be also be pharmacologically inhibited during dissemination, which for some viruses appears to depend primarily on virally-induced host immunosuppression. Thus dissemination is another stage in which modulation of the immune system may help the host overcome viral infection.[7] Biological response modifiers emerge with a role in modification of host response, whether it be inhibition of viral-induced immunosuppression or inhibition of an overzealous host response. The biological response modifier most commonly studied for its effect on viral infections and showing the most promise in efficacy has been IFN.

Antiviral-Induced Nephrotoxicity

Among the toxicities caused by antiviral drug is nephrotoxicity. The risk of antiviral drug–induced nephrotoxicity has increased as drugs have become more effective and novel in their action and as combination drug therapy has been implemented in response to increasing viral resistance.[9] Acute tubular necrosis has been associated with a number of antiviral drugs (e.g., foscarnet, acyclovir, IFN, and cidofovir). However, variable renal lesions have been ascribed to a number of drugs, reflecting three major mechanisms: transporter defects, apoptosis, and mitochondrial injury. Glomerular disease resulting in proteinuria and, occasionally, the nephrotic syndrome has been mediated by either immune-mediated complexes (IFN) or crystal deposit (foscarnet). Crystalline deposits in the renal tubule (e.g., acyclovir, ganciclovir, and indinavir) can cause intrarenal obstruction. Isolated tubular defects may occur; examples include a Fanconi-like syndrome (cidofovir, tenofovir), distal tubular acidosis (e.g., acyclic nucleotide phosphonates, foscarnet), and nephrogenic diabetes insipidus (NDI: foscarnet).[9] A major contributor to toxicity is intratubular cell drug accumulation mediated by ion-transport systems. For example, nephrotoxicity associated with cidofovir and adefovir appears to be facilitated by transport mediated by a transport protein.[10] Limited use of antiviral drugs in veterinary medicine probably precludes effective evaluation of the advent of nephrotoxicity in animals with viral infections subsequently treated with antiviral drugs. However, among the clinical signs of toxicosis to accidentally ingested acyclovir in dogs were signs consistent with acute renal failure.[11]

Antiherpesvirus Drugs

Pyrimidine Nucleosides

A variety of pyrimidine nucleosides (both halogenated and nonhalogenated) effectively inhibit the replication of herpes simplex viruses with limited host cell toxicity. The exact mechanism of action of these compounds appears to reflect substitution of pyrimidine for thymidine, causing defective DNA molecules.

Idoxuridine. Idoxuridine (5-iodo-2-deoxyuridine, IDU; Stoxil) was the first of the nucleoside analogues to prove useful in the treatment of viral diseases. Idoxuridine resembles and is substituted for thymidine. After phosphorylation, it is incorporated into both viral and host cell DNA. Altered DNA is susceptible to breakage, resulting in faulty transcription and altered viral proteins. The spectrum of antiviral activity is limited to DNA viruses, particularly members of the herpesvirus group. Resistance to IDU develops rapidly.[2] The ability of IDU to cause neoplastic changes, genetic mutation, and infertility limits its use to topical, primarily ophthalmic, infections. IDU is available as an ophthalmic ointment or solution. It is currently approved for use in the treatment of herpes keratitis in humans and has proved useful for the treatment of feline herpetic keratitis. One drop of a 0.1% solution is usually applied to the affected eye every hour; the 0.5% ointment can be applied every 2 hours.[12,13] Topical application of IDU to the conjunctiva has been associated with irritation, pain, pruritus, inflammation, and edema of the conjunctiva and punctate areas on the cornea. Resistance of viruses to the drug develops readily both in vitro and in clinical cases.

Trifluridine. Trifluridine (triflurothymidine; TFT; Viroptic) is a halogenated (fluorinated) pyrimidine that is similar and often considered superior to IDU. TFT monophosphate irreversibly inhibits thymidylate synthetase, and TFT triphosphate competitively inhibits DNA polymerase incorporation of thymidine into DNA. Like IDU, it is preferentially incorporated into both viral and host DNA, and late virus-specific DNA transcription is inhibited.[2] Trifluridine has in vitro inhibitory effects against herpes simplex virus (types 1 and 2), cytomegalovirus, and selected adenoviruses. Clinical resistance to TFT has been reported. As with IDU, the primary therapeutic indication for TFT is herpetic keratitis. TFT is prepared as a 0.1% ophthalmic solution and is usually applied 6 to 8 times per day. Trifluridine is frequently preferred to IDU for the treatment of human and feline herpetic keratitis in order to prevent toxicities associated with IDU.[12,13] Adverse reactions include discomfort on application and palpebral edema.[2]

Sorivudine. Sorivudine is a pyrimidine nucleoside analog characterized by potency that results in a relative selectivity for varicella-zoster virus (VZV). The drug is initially phosphorylated by viral thymidine kinase and then metabolized to diphosphate by viral thymidylate kinase. As such, sorivudine triphosphate is a competitive inhibitor of viral DNA replication. Unlike acyclovir, however, sorivudine is not incorporated into viral DNA. Inhibitory concentrations of sorivudine are 1000-fold lower for VZV than are those of acyclovir. Cellular uptake in cells infected with herpesvirus is fortyfold greater than in uninfected cells. Clinical resistance has not yet been detected.[2]

Sorivudine (in humans) is well absorbed after oral administration and is characterized by 98% protein binding. The elimination half-life is 5 to 7 hours, although half-life increases with age. Elimination appears to be urinary, with minimal hepatic metabolism. Side effects are primarily gastrointestinal (nausea, vomiting, and diarrhea). Hepatic enzymes may increase. Long-term administration has caused hepatic neoplasms in rodents. Sorivudine (probably its metabolite) appears to negatively interact with 5-fluorouracil by inhibiting the enzyme responsible for fluorouracil metabolism.[2] Sorivudine is available in both oral and intravenous preparations but only as investigational drugs.

Purine Nucleosides

Certain purine nucleosides have proved to be effective antivirals and are used as systemic agents. Several of these antiviral drugs deserve special mention.

Vidarabine. Vidarabine (Vira-A) was initially investigated for its efficacy as a cancer chemotherapeutic drug. An analog of adenine, vidarabine is phosphorylated by host enzymes and competitively inhibits viral DNA polymerase. It is substituted for adenine into DNA, thus inhibiting viral DNA polymerase. Mammalian DNA is also inhibited, although to a lesser extent. Ribonucleoside reductase, RNA polyadenylation, and transmethylation reactions also are inhibited.[2] Vidarabine selectively inhibits DNA viruses, particularly herpesviruses. It is also effective against poxviruses, rhabdoviruses, hepadnaviruses, and selected RNA tumor viruses.[2] Until recently, the drug was prepared as an injectable suspension. It is poorly water soluble, however, and must be dissolved in large volumes of fluid before intravenous use. A 3% ophthalmic ointment continues to be available. On intravenous administration, vidarabine is deaminated to hypoxanthine arabinoside which has 10% of the potency of the parent compound, but reaches concentrations that exceed the parent compound by fifteenfold after constant intravenous infusion. The drug is eliminated renally but predominantly as the hypoxanthine metabolite. The elimination half-life of the metabolite is approximately 3.5 hours. Adverse reactions are more likely with intravenous administration and include gastrointestinal upset (vomiting, diarrhea) and central nervous system (CNS) derangements (hallucinations, ataxia, tremors, and painful peripheral neuropathies with long-term use). In addition, vidarabine is probably mutagenic and carcinogenic. Phlebitis, hypokalemia, rash, elevated transaminases, and pancytopenia as well as inappropriate concentrations of antidiuretic hormone have been reported in humans. Systemic use in humans is reserved for life-threatening infections (e.g., herpes encephalitis). Although vidarabine is preferred over IDU for topical therapy of herpetic keratitis, the advent of acyclovir has reduced its use. Vidarabine can be useful for patients that have developed resistance to acyclovir or in combination with acyclovir for life-threatening infections.[2] Literature regarding its use in the cat is limited, but topical administration of the 3% ointment appears to be well tolerated in cats.[12,13]

Acyclovir and Valacyclovir. Acyclovir is an acyclic synthetic purine nucleoside analog that substitutes for guanosine in DNA synthesis. Valacyclovir is an L-valyl ester prodrug of acyclovir. Efficacy of acyclovir depends on activation of the drug to its monophosphate derivative by viral thymidine kinase. Subsequent phosphorylation to the diphosphate and then triphosphate form is mediated selectively by cells infected with herpesvirus. The formation of acyclovir-GTP results in the inhibition of viral DNA polymerase and incorporation of acyclovir-GTP into viral DNA, which terminates viral DNA synthesis. The drug has a greater affinity for viral (versus host) thymidine synthetase. Antiviral activity of acyclovir is limited essentially to herpesviruses. The in vitro activity of acyclovir is 100 times that of vidarabine and 10 times that of IDU. Viral resistance to acyclovir results from mutation to strains that are characterized by a reduction in viral thymidine kinase (the most common mechanism), altered substrate specificity, or altered viral DNA polymerase.[2]

Acyclovir is available in topical, oral (capsule), and parenteral (powder to be reconstituted) preparations. The bioavailability of the oral preparations (in humans) is poor (10% to 30%) and decreases with increasing doses.[2] In contrast, valacyclovir, which is rapidly and completely converted to acyclovir, increases bioavailability of acyclovir to 50% (in humans). Acyclovir distributes to all body fluids, including cerebrospinal fluid. It is eliminated primarily unchanged by glomerular filtration and tubular secretion and accumulates in patients with renal failure. The elimination half-life in adults with normal renal function is 1.5 to 6 hours; this can increase to 20 hours in anuric patients.

Toxicity of acyclovir, regardless of the preparation, is limited. Oral administration (of both acyclovir and valacyclovir) is associated with gastrointestinal upset. Intravenous administration may cause renal insufficiency and (rarely) CNS side effects. Cats experimentally infected with feline herpesvirus type 1 (FHV-1) that received 60 mg/kg daily of valacyclovir orally became ill within 6 to 9 days of therapy, necessitating termination of the study in 12 days. White blood cell counts declined, yet no difference was found in viral pathology in treated versus untreated cats, leading the authors to assess valacylovir as an unlikely option for treatment of FHV-1.[14] Renal dysfunction is reversible and may reflect concentration in urine to the point that crystallization occurs[2] (see previous discussion). Rapid infusion, dehydration, and inappropriate urine flow increase the risk of renal damage. Phlebitis also may accompany intravenous administration. A retrospective review (January 1995 through March 2000) of acyclovir toxicoses in dogs (n = 105) following accidental ingestion reported by The American Society for Prevention of Cruelty to Animals National Animal Poison Control Center found clinical signs developing in 6 of 10 dogs within 3 hours of ingestion of doses ranging from 40 to 2195 mg/kg. [11] The most common clinical signs were vomiting, diarrhea, anorexia, and lethargy, with polyuria and polydipsia reported in only 1 dog. Treatment included standard decontamination procedures, (i.e., induction of emesis, administration of activated charcoal), diuresis, and supportive care.

Veterinary use of acyclovir may be limited, probably because of differences among infecting viruses in viral thymidine kinase for acyclovir. In addition, antiviral resistance is increasing. Acyclovir is unable to eliminate latent infections. It is available as an ophthalmic ointment, a topical ointment and cream, an intravenous preparation, and various oral formulations.

KEY POINT 10-3 Veterinary use of acyclovir may be limited, probably because of differences in viral thymidine kinase for acyclovir.

Penciclovir and Famciclovir. Like acyclovir, penciclovir is an acyclic guanine nucleoside. Its spectrum of activity (herpes simplex virus and VZV) is also similar to that of acyclovir. Penciclovir (up to 77% bioavailable) is formed from its prodrug famciclovir. Penciclovir is a hundredfold less potent than acyclovir but is accumulated to higher concentrations than is acyclovir in infected cells.[2] Plasma elimination half-life in humans is approximately 2 hours, and elimination is renal. Although, like acyclovir, the drug is well tolerated orally, chronic administration appears to be tumorigenic, causing testicular toxicity in animals.

The pharmacokinetics and safety of penciclovir resulting from oral administration of famciclovir have been reported in cats (n = 8) at 62.5 mg (half of a 125-mg tablet; 9 to 18 mg/kg) orally after single and multiple dosing (every 8 or 12 hours; 4 cats per group) for 3 days.[15] The maximum drug (C_{max}; ng/mL) concentration following a single dose was 330 ± 120, and the elimination (disappearance) half-life was 3.1 ± 0.9 hr. Using a multiple-dosing, 12-hour dosing regimen, the C_{max} of penciclovir (ng/mL) did not change significantly from single dosing (multiple 12-hour dosing C_{max} [ng/mL] of 330 ± 180 at a T_{max} of 5 hours) but did with 8-hour dosing (multiple 8-hour dosing C_{max} of 680 ± 290) μg/mL. This increase is practically expected with a 3-hour half-life in the face of an 8-hour dosing interval (accumulation ratio of 1.4), but altered clearance cannot be ruled out without intravenous pharmacokinetic studies. The half-life did not change with multiple dosing, although the duration of dosing may not have been enough to allow emergence of drug interactions and the sample size may not have been sufficient to detect a difference. Dose normalization of C_{max} and area under the curve (AUC; 24 hours) yielded no significant differences between the two dosing intervals; again, limitations in sample size may have precluded detection of differences. Adverse effects may have included decreases in packed cell volume (by 27%) and total protein (by 10%). However, these changes may have reflected frequent blood draws during the study. White blood cell counts increased (neutrophils and monocytes) by 54% after the last dose. Although the cats tolerated dosing well, the target concentration suggested for treatment of FHV-1 is 3500 ng/m (based on the review of Thomasy et al.[15]), which was approximately tenfold higher than the C_{max} achieved in this study. Further studies must verify the safety of the drug at doses necessary to achieve this concentration.

Ganciclovir. Ganciclovir is structurally similar to acyclovir, with the addition of a hydroxymethyl group on the acyclic side chain. Its spectrum includes herpesvirus, with particular efficacy against cytomegalovirus; effective concentrations are tenfold to a hundredfold lower than the concentrations effective against other herpesviruses.[2]

Unfortunately, similar concentrations are inhibitory to bone marrow progenitor cells. As with other guanine nucleosides, ganciclovir inhibits viral DNA synthesis after monophosphorylation mediated by viral thymidine kinase (herpes) or phosphotransferase (cytomegalovirus). Diphosphates and triphosphates of ganciclovir are formed by cellular enzymes. The triphosphate competitively inhibits deoxyguanosine triphosphate incorporation into both viral and host DNA, with preferential inhibition of viral over host DNA polymerase. Intracellular concentrations (which exceed acyclovir concentrations by at least tenfold) decline much more slowly than those of acyclovir, resulting in a cellular elimination half-life of approximately 24 hours. Hence the drug is given once daily in humans.[2] Resistance most commonly reflects point mutations or deletions in viral DNA, resulting in reduced formation of viral phosphotransferase.

Ganciclovir is poorly bioavailable in humans (9%, with food). More than 90% of the absorbed drug is eliminated renally, with an (plasma as opposed to cell) elimination half-life of 2 hours. Elimination half-life increases proportionately with creatinine clearance. The primary adverse effect is myelosuppression, with neutropenia occurring in up to 40% and thrombocytopenia in 5% to 20% of patients. Myelosuppression more commonly occurs with intravenous administration and is generally reversible by 1 week after discontinuation of therapy, but it can be persistent and fatal. Treatment with granulocyte colony-stimulating factor may minimize neutropenia.[2] The risk of myelosuppression is increased when ganciclovir is combined with other cytotoxic drugs. Side effects in the CNS also are frequent, occurring in up to 15% of human patients. Clinical signs include convulsions and coma. Other adverse effects include infusion-related phlebitis, azotemia, anemia, fever, hepatic dysfunction, nausea, vomiting, and eosinophilia. Therapeutic use of ganciclovir includes cytomegalovirus retinitis, particularly in humans with acquired immune-deficiency syndrome–induced immunodeficiency. Ganciclovir is also used for treatment of any infection or prevention of infection (particularly in transplant recipients) associated with cytomegalovirus.

Ribavirin. Ribavirin (1-β-D-ribofuranosyl-1,2,4-triazole-3-carboxamide; Virazole) is a purine nucleoside analog that is activated by viral phosphorylation and subsequently prevents the formation of mRNA and translation of viral genome.[12,13] The action of ribavirin involves specific inhibition of virus-associated enzymes, inhibition of the capping of viral mRNA, and inhibition of viral polypeptide synthesis. Thus it is effective against both DNA and RNA viruses and is a broad-spectrum antiviral drug. Susceptible viruses include adenoviruses, herpesviruses, orthomyxoviruses, poxviruses, picornaviruses, rhabdoviruses, rotaviruses, and retroviruses. Viral resistance to ribavirin is rare. Ribavirin is well absorbed in humans, widely distributed in the body, and eliminated by both renal and biliary routes as both parent drug and metabolites; it has a plasma half-life of 24 hours in humans. It does not have a wide margin of safety in domestic animals. Toxicity is manifested by anorexia, weight loss, bone marrow depression, anemia, and gastrointestinal disturbances. It has been successfully administered by topical, parenteral, oral, and aerosol routes. Ribavirin is administered as an aerosol to human patients afflicted with respiratory viral infections, thus avoiding the hematopoietic toxicities associated with systemic use of the drug. In the cat, in vitro investigations revealed marked antiviral activity against a strain of calicivirus but little efficacy for rhinotracheitis.[12,13] However, Povey[16] studied the oral administration of 25 mg/kg every 8 hours for 10 days in cats that had been experimentally infected with calicivirus. Pathologic lesions in infected cats worsened, primarily because of severe thrombocytopenia that presumably was drug induced. Cats also developed liver disease, although clinical signs resolved 1 week after the drug was discontinued.

Miscellaneous Antiherpes Drugs

Foscarnet

Foscarnet (phosphonoformic acid) is an inorganic trisodium salt that interferes directly with herpes viral DNA polymerase. The drug may also be effective in treating retroviral infections owing to similar interference with reverse transcriptase. Direct actions preclude the need for intracellular activation. Foscarnet has a hundredfold greater affinity for viral as opposed to host DNA polymerase-α.[2] Point mutations in DNA polymerase are responsible for resistance. Foscarnet is poorly bioavailable after oral administration. The drug is concentrated in bones, resulting in complicated plasma elimination. Elimination (in humans) is bimodal with an initial 4- to 8-hour elimination half-life followed by a 3- to 4-day half-life. It is eliminated primarily by the kidneys, with clearance decreasing proportionately with creatine clearance.

Major side effects in human patients include nephrotoxicity and hypocalcemia, which can become symptomatic. Serum creatinine increases in up to 50% of patients but decreases after therapy is stopped. Acute tubular necrosis, crystalluria, and interstitial nephritis have occurred. Sodium loading before therapy may decrease the risk of renal toxicity. Because foscarnet is highly ionized at physiologic pH, metabolic abnormalities are common in human patients. Calcium and phosphorus may decrease or increase. Decreases in ionized calcium may be sufficient to cause clinical signs consistent with tetany. Other CNS side effects reported in human patients (up to 25%) include tremors, irritability, seizures, and hallucinations. Fever, nausea, vomiting, anemia, leukopenia, and hepatic dysfunction also have been reported. Indications in human patients include cytomegalovirus retinitis and herpes infections that are resistant to acyclovir. The disposition of foscarnet and its precursor, thiophosphonoformate (TPFA), have been studied in normal cats. Whereas foscarnet was only 8% bioavailable, TPFA was 44%; however, only 14% of the drug is converted to foscarnet.[16a] The half-life of foscarnet was approximately 3 hrs with clearance of 1.88 ml/min/kg, being similar to renal clearance. Foscarnet has been shown to be effective prophylactically in the treatment of feline rhinotracheitis. Its efficacy against retroviruses warrants further investigation for the treatment of FeLV. Currently, foscarnet is given to immunocompromised human patients and is being studied in the cat for treatment of retroviral infections.

Antiretroviral Drugs

Zidovudine

All clinically used (human-approved) antiretroviral agents are 2′,3′- dideoxynucleoside analogs. Zidovudine (AZT; Retrovir) is a thymidine analog. Within the virus-infected cell, the 3′-azido group substitutes for the 3'-hydroxy group of thymidine. The azido group is then converted to a triphosphate form, which is used by retroviral reverse transcriptase and incorporated into DNA transcript.[12,17] The 3' substitution prevents DNA chain elongation and insertion of viral DNA into the host cell's genome, preventing viral replication. Thus the shared mechanism of action of these drugs is inhibition of RNA-dependent DNA polymerase (reverse transcriptase). This enzyme is responsible for conversion of the viral RNA genome into double-stranded DNA before it is integrated into the cell genome. Because these actions occur early in replication, the drugs tend to be effective for acute infections but relatively ineffective for chronically infected cells.[2] Cellular α-DNA polymerases are inhibited only at concentrations a hundredfold greater than those necessary to inhibit reverse transcriptase, thus rendering this drug relatively safe to host cells. Cellular γ-DNA polymerase, however, is inhibited at lower concentrations. Zidovudine is effective against a variety of retroviruses at low concentrations (<0.001 to 0.04 μg/mL. The intracellular elimination time of AZT is 3 to 4 hours.[2]

In human patients AZT is rapidly absorbed, with a bioavailability of 60% to 70%. Food impairs absorption. Concentrations in the cerebrospinal fluid are approximately 50% of those in plasma. The plasma elimination half-life is 1 to 1.5 hours. In human patients AZT undergoes first-pass metabolism.

Among the toxicities caused by AZT is myeloid suppression. The concentration necessary to suppress (human) myeloid cells is higher than that associated with antiviral activity, but nonetheless is still relatively low at 0.3 to 0.6 μg/mL.[2] Although metabolites appear to be void of antiviral toxicity, at least one may contribute to myeloid toxicity. Granulocytopenia and anemia are the major adverse effects of AZT in human patients. The risk of toxicity increases in human patients with low ($CD4^+$) lymphocyte counts, high doses, and prolonged therapy. Idovudinzidovudine may cause Heinz body anemia in cats,[21] suggesting that complete blood counts should be performed on cats receiving AZT. Granulocyte colony-stimulating factor is indicated for management of granulocytopenia. CNS side effects are more likely as therapy is begun. Other side effects reported in humans include myopathy (characterized by weakness and pain), neurotoxicities, hepatitis (uncommon), and esophageal ulceration. Resolution of myopathy occurs slowly after drug therapy is discontinued. The risk of myelosuppression is increased by drugs that inhibit glucuronidation or renal excretion. Therapeutic indications for AZT in humans include treatment of HIV infections. Treatment with AZT prolongs survival, decreases the incidence of opportunistic infections, increases measures of immune function, and decreases HIV antigens and RNA. Zidovudine has been combined with didanosine or zalcitabine for more sustained $CD4^+$ lymphocyte response.

The disposition of AZT has been studied in cats. It is rapidly absorbed in cats after intragastric or oral administration. Administration of a single dose of 25 mg/kg in normal cats by either route generates maximum serum concentrations of 28 ± 7 and 29 ± 15 μg/mL, respectively. Bioavailability for the intragastric route is 70 ± 24%, and for the oral route 95 ± 23%. The elimination half-life is approximately 1.5 hours and volume of distribution 0.82 L/kg. Drug concentrations were above the effective concentration 50 (EC_{50}) of 0.19 μg/mL for FIV for at least 24 hours after either intravenous or oral administration.[18] The drug appears safe at this dose despite drug concentrations being well above that associated with myeloid suppression of human cells. Side effects in cats at 25 mg/kg (administered intravenously) were limited to transient restlessness, mild anxiety, and hemolysis.[18]

KEY POINT 10-4 The disposition and safety of AZT support its use in cats.

Lamivudine

Lamivudine is among the more potent drugs against human immunodeficiency virus (HIV) and also has been studied in cats. As with AZT, it is rapidly absorbed in cats after intragastric or oral administration. Administration of a single dose of 25 mg/kg in normal cats by either route generates maximum serum concentrations of 50 ± 38.5 and 40 ± 40 μg/mL, respectively, with bioavailability for the intragastric route being 88 ± 45%, and for the oral route 80 ± 52%. The elimination half-life is approximately 2 hours and volume of distribution is 0.6 L/kg. The effective concentration 50 (EC_{50}) for lamivudine ranges from 0.8.7 (mutant) to 11 μg/mL (wild type) for FIV and is present for at least 24 hours after either intravenous or oral administration.[19] As with AZT, lamivudine appears safe in cats at 25 mg/kg with similar side effects.[19]

The disposition of the combination of AZT (5 mg/kg) and lamivudine (3 mg/kg) has also been studied in normal and FIV-infected cats after single and multiple (7-day) dosing.[20] Median AZT concentrations (ng/mL) were (median followed by range) 3.67 (2.67 to 4.66) at first dose and 3.65 (3.54 to 3.76) at steady state for AZT and 2.86 (2.62 to 3.08) at first dose and 3.89 (3.27 to 3.08) ng/mL (31.7 to 102.4 ng/mL) at steady state. These concentrations were comparable to those achieved in humans, although direct comparisons are precluded by different doses. Volume of distribution, clearance, and half-life were similar with combined therapy to that reported for individual therapy by Zhang and coworkers.[18,19]

Didanosine

Didanosine is a purine nucleoside effective against HIV, including strains that have developed resistance to AZT. Although it is tenfold to a hundredfold less potent than AZT, it is more active in quiescent cells and in nondividing (human) monocytes and macrophages. It also is not toxic for hematopoietic precursor cells or lymphocytes at clinically relevant concentrations. It is metabolized inside the cell to its active derivative (ddATP), which competitively inhibits virus preferentially to host reverse transcriptase. Oral bioavailability of didanosine is about 40% in humans. Because it is very acid labile, food decreases absorption by 50% or more. Didanosine is available as both tablets and powder, with the tablet being 20% to 25% more bioavailable than the powder. Only about 20% of drug in plasma distributes to the cerebrospinal fluid. Up to 60% of the drug is excreted unchanged through the kidneys, with a plasma elimination half-life of up to 1.5 hours. Intracellular metabolism may be responsible for some plasma elimination. Side effects include painful peripheral neuropathy and pancreatitis. High doses increase the risk for both. A history of pancreatitis predisposes the patient to this side effect. Up to 70% of human patients develop pancreatitis, although hyperamylasemia will occur in up to 20%. Other adverse effects include diarrhea; rashes; CNS signs, including insomnia and seizures; optic neuritis; and, rarely, hepatic failure or cardiac dysfunction. Animal studies also have found gastrointestinal, bone marrow, hepatic, and renal dysfunction. Didanosine (33 mg/kg orally per day for 6 weeks) was used to develop a model of antiretroviral peripheral neuropathy in normal and infected SPF kittens.[21a] Didanosine is approved for treatment of advanced HIV infections in human patients intolerant of or resistant to AZT. Stavudine, a thymidine nucleoside, and zalcitabine, a cytosine nucleoside, are alternatives to AZT therapy for human patients.[2]

Miscellaneous Antiviral Drugs

Amantadine

Amantadine and its derivative rimantadine are synthetic antiviral agents that appear to act on an early step of viral replication after attachment of virus to cell receptors. Interference of release of infectious viral nucleic acid into the host cell through the transmembrane domain of the viral M2 protein is proposed. The effect seems to lead to inhibition or delay of the uncoating process that precedes primary transcription. Amantadine may also interfere with the early stages of viral mRNA transcription. Amantadine also prevents virus assembly during virus replication. Viruses affected at usual concentrations include different strains of influenza A and C (but not B) virus, Sendai virus, and pseudorabies virus. It is almost completely absorbed from the gastrointestinal tract, and about 90% of a dose administered orally is excreted unchanged in the urine over several days (according to data for humans). The main clinical use has been to prevent infection with various strains of influenza A viruses. In humans, however, it also has been found to produce some therapeutic benefit if taken within 48 hours after the onset of illness. Amantadine and its derivatives may be given by the oral, intranasal, subcutaneous, intraperitoneal, or aerosol routes. It produces few side effects, most of which are CNS related; stimulation of the CNS is evident at very high doses. Acute toxicity generally reflects its anticholinergic effects and includes cardiac, respiratory, renal, or CNS toxicity.

Oseltamivir

Oseltamivir is prepared as an ester prodrug. On release by esterases in the gastrointestinal tract, the carboxylate form acts as a selective inhibitor of influenza A and B viral neuraminidases by inducing a conformation change at the enzymatic active site. The viruses cannot leave the infected cell and therefore aggregate at the cell surface and are unable to spread. Concentrations achieved in humans after oral administration of a therapeutic dose is 0.35 μg/mL of the carboxylate form. In humans the half-life is approximately 6 to 10 hours. It is excreted by renal tubular excretion; probenecid prolongs the half-life by twofold. The drug has not yet been studied in dogs or cats despite its anecdotal use for treatment of parvovirus in dogs.

Suramin

Suramin is a polysulfonate hexasodium salt capable of inhibiting reverse transcriptase; it has been studied for use in treating FeLV (discussed later).

Inosiplex

Inosiplex (Isoprinosine) is a compound formed from inosine and the para-acetamidobenzoate salt of 1-dimethylamino-2-propanol. Inosiplex can inhibit cytopathic effects of several viruses in culture. In vivo experiments, however, suggest that optimal activity of inosiplex occurs with therapeutic administration after viral infection and requires an adequate host immune response. The mechanism of antiviral activity appears to involve specific suppression of viral mRNA. Inosiplex does not appear to be as efficacious as several antimetabolite antiviral compounds. Inosiplex can also induce T-cell differentiation similar to that induced by thymic hormones, apparently by augmenting RNA synthesis. Thus inosiplex may be more useful as an immunopotentiator in immunodeficient patients (see earlier discussion of biologic response modifiers).[12,17,22]

Interferon and Its Inducers

Interferons (IFNs) are addressed in greater depth in Chapter 3. They are a group of multiple-gene inducible cellular glycoproteins that interact with cells and render them resistant to infection by a wide variety of RNA-containing and DNA-containing viruses. In addition, IFNs have numerous other effects on target cells, including a reduction in the rate of cell proliferation and alterations in the structure and function of the cell surface, the distribution of cytoskeletal elements, and the expression of several differentiated cellular functions. Interferons induce the synthesis of new proteins that are responsible for the activation of cellular endonucleases that degrade viral mRNA. Human IFNs are classified as α, β, or γ, depending on their physical stability, immunologic neutralization properties, host range, and homology in amino acid sequence. Viral infections generally are associated with the expression of IFN α and β genes. Those used in clinical trials have been produced by induction of synthesis by human white blood cells; fibroblasts; lymphoblasts; and, more recently, recombinant DNA techniques in bacteria. Numerous modes of antiviral action have been proposed. In addition to their ability to establish an antiviral state in host cells, they also appear to modulate the immune system of the host.

Interferons inhibit the replication of a wide variety of viruses. Among the RNA-containing viruses, the togaviruses, rhabdoviruses, orthomyxoviruses, paramyxoviruses, reoviruses, and several strains of picornaviruses and oncornaviruses are sensitive to inhibition by IFNs. Among the DNA-containing viruses, the poxviruses and several strains of herpes simplex types 1 and 2 viruses, as well as cytomegalovirus, are inhibited by IFNs. Adenoviruses are generally resistant. There are extreme variations in sensitivity to IFNs among different types and even strains of virus. In addition, the responses in different model and test systems can be extraordinarily variable. Interferons appear not to be as useful in the therapy of viral infections as was hoped initially. Interferons are usually administered parenterally but recently also have been used orally with some success. Although rare at recommended dosages, side effects may occur at higher levels.

To date, at least five feline IFN-alpha (feIFN) subtypes have been encoded,[23] each of which (1, 2, 3, 5, and 6), when expressed in a Chinese hamster ovary cell line, has exhibited antiviral activity against vesicular stomatitis virus– and feline calicivirus–infected cells.[24]A recombinant feline IFN omega (rFeIFN-ω) is an insect- (silkworm-) generated (rather than microbial-based) product (Virbagen Omega) that is licensed by the U.S. Department of Agriculture for the treatment of retrovirus infections in cats.

Several substances induce IFN and have been tested for the prevention and treatment of viral infections and for treatment of neoplastic diseases. Although effective in some model systems, IFN inducers have not yet been found to be clinically useful because of their toxicity. High-molecular-weight inducers include polyriboinosinic acid/polyribocytidylic acid or poly(I)/poly(C); low-molecular-weight inducers include tilorone, aminobromophenylpyrimidinone, and aminoiodophenylpyrimidinone.

Miscellaneous Alternatives or Adjuncts to Antiviral Drugs

Lymphocyte T-Cell Immune modulator is an immune-regulating single polypeptide extracted and purified from bovine-derived stromal cells (ProLab manufacturers). The product package insert indicates that lymphocyte counts rapidly increased in cats (n = 23) with FIV or FeLV after treatment (1 mL) at 0, 7, and 14 days followed by monthly doses. Clinical scores became significantly better after the third dose. Red blood cell counts also increased in severely anemic cats. A clinical trial was not available for review, and no information was provided regarding control animals. As a biologic, the product has not been considered for approval by the Food and Drug Administration but had received conditional licensing by the United States Department of Agriculture as of November 2009.[24a]

Several drug classes continue to be investigated mainly because of their in vitro antiviral activities. Their potential clinical usefulness remains obscure in most instances. Included among these agents are thiosemicarbazones, guanidine, benzimidazoles, arildone, phosphonoacetic acid, rifamycins and other antibiotics, and several natural products.

Lysine is an essential amino acid. Herpes simplex viral proteins are rich in L–arginine, and in vitro tissue culture studies suggest that viral replication is enhanced in the presence of a high L-arginine to L-lysine ratio. In contrast, when the ratio is low (i.e., lysine > arginine), viral replication and the cytopathogenicity of herpes simplex virus have been found to be inhibited. The effects of lysine may reflect antagonism of arginine-growth promoting effects, although the site of interaction is not known. Replacement of viral arginine with lysine-yielding nonfunctional proteins also has been proposed.

Mycophenolic acid (MPA) is a non-nucleoside noncompetitive, reversible inhibitor of eukaryotic inosine monophosphate dehydrogenase. Inhibition of lymphocyte proliferation has led to its use to treat host versus graft rejection in human transplant recipients. Because microbial RNA and/or DNA synthesis also is inhibited, MPA has the potential for inhibiting infecting parasites and microbes, the latter including viruses. Mycophenolic acid appears to impair viral replication of a variety of viruses, including Sindbis virus, HIV herpesvirus, hepatitis B virus, orthopoxviruses, dengue virus, West Nile virus, and double-stranded RNA avian reoviruses.[25] It also appears to potentiate the inhibitory effects of cyclic guanosine analogs (e.g., acyclovir, penciclovir, and ganciclovir) against herpesviruses, the nucleoside analogs against HIV. However, its use as a broad-spectrum antiviral agent against positive- and negative-stranded RNA viruses has not been established.[25]

TREATMENT OF SELECTED VIRAL INFECTIONS

Treatment of viral diseases in small animals is nonspecific and seldom includes antiviral drugs. Therapy tends to be supportive, focusing on fluid and electrolyte supplementation, prevention or treatment of secondary bacterial infection, and treatments that support the function and structure of the organ targeted by the infection. By far, the most important approach to management of viral diseases in dogs and cats is prevention and, in particular, an effective vaccination program. In addition, isolation of infected animals and cleansing of environments contaminated with potentially infecting viruses are important ways to limit the spread of viral infections.

Treatment of Selected Canine Viral Infections

Canine Parvoviral Enteritis

Parvoviral enteritis, caused by canine parvovirus-2 (CPV-2), is among the most common and fatal viral infections afflicting dogs, including most members of the family Canidae. Infection by this highly contagious virus generally reflects contact with infected feces. Animals, humans, and objects can serve as vectors. After exposure viral replication begins in the lymphoid tissue of the gastrointestinal tract, from where it disseminates to the intestinal crypts of the small intestine. The virus localizes in the epithelium of the tongue, oral and esophageal mucosa, small intestine, and lymphoid tissue. Because CPV-2 infects the germinal cells of the intestinal crypt, cell turnover is impaired and villi shorten. Mitotically active myeloid cells and lymphoid cells are also targeted, leading to neutropenia and lymphopenia. Complications of intestinal damage include bacteremia, endotoxemia, and disseminated intravascular coagulation (DIC). Infections are most severe in puppies younger than 12 weeks of age because of their immature immune system. Clinical signs include vomiting (which can be severe), diarrhea, and anorexia. Animals may be febrile. Clinical pathology may reveal leukopenia. Myocarditis can develop in patients infected in utero or less than 8 weeks of age. Diagnosis is based on clinical signs, leukopenia (generally proportional to the severity of illness), and enzyme-linked immunoassay (ELISA) antigen testing.

The clinical efficacy of rfeIFN-omega has been evaluated for the treatment of dogs with experimental and spontaneous parvoviral enteritis. Martin and coworkers[26] treated experimentally infected Beagle puppies with rFeIFN-omega (2.5 MU/kg) for 3 consecutive days and reported 1 of 5 deaths compared with 5 of 5 in untreated controls. De Mari and coworkers[27] studied spontaneous disease using a multicentric, double-blind, placebo-controlled study. Clinical signs of the IFN-treated (2.5 million units/kg/day for 3 consecutive days) animals (n = 43) improved significantly during the 10-day study period compared with those of control animals (n = 49). Only 3 deaths occurred in the IFN group compared with 14 deaths in the placebo group, resulting in a 4.4 reduction in mortality. This increased to a 6.4–fold reduction in mortality in unvaccinated dogs.

Oseltamivir has been used to treat parvovirus, although this use is not based on a randomized clinical trial. One (abstract form) study reports a decrease in mortality of parvovirus by 75% to 100% (2 mg/kg orally every 12 hours); cost will be approximately $0.25/kg. However, neuraminidase does not appear to be a virulence factor for parvovirus, including the release of viruses from the cell. In contrast, bacterial neuraminidases are also produced by a large number of respiratory mucosal pathogens and are necessary for biofilm formation by *Pseudomonas aeruginosa*. Use of viral neuraminidase inhibitors prevents biofilm formation by microbial organisms. Accordingly, the use of oseltamivir for its *nonviral* indications warrants further consideration for its potential impact on intestinal bacterial translocation; well-designed clinical trials are needed to demonstrate efficacy.

KEY POINT 10-5 Efficacy of oseltamivir for treatment of parvovirus, if it is scientifically demonstrated, may reflect its impact on bacterial translocation rather than viral inhibition.

Symptomatic therapy for canine parvoviral enteritis focuses on restoration of fluids and electrolytes and on prevention or treatment of bacteremia or endotoxemia. Fluid therapy is the single most important treatment and should be aggressive and continued as long as the patient is vomiting or diarrhea is present. Among the antiemetics, metoclopramide originally was among the most successful, with ondansetron considered for animals that fail to respond. Maropitant may be the better choice. Treatment of diarrhea is generally not indicated. The use of narcotic motility modifiers (e.g., loperamide, diphenoxylate) has been recommended if necessary,[28] but their use may prolong the presence of undesirable toxins in the gastrointestinal lumen. Thus their use is discouraged. Antimicrobial therapy should focus on both gram-negative coliforms and anaerobic organisms. In general, an injectable beta-lactam combined with an aminoglycoside has proved efficacious. Fluid therapy, once-daily dosing, and the immature nature of pediatric canine kidneys provide protection against aminoglycoside-induced renal disease. Fluorinated quinolones should not be used if possible because of the risk of cartilage damage. Ceftiofur has been used because of its potential for intravenous administration and its efficacy against *Escherichia coli*, one of the major contributors to secondary bacterial complications of parvovirus. Note, however, that efficacy and safety at doses necessary to control the systemic bacterial complications of parvovirus have not been documented. In addition, efficacy against anaerobic organisms of the gastrointestinal tract has not been studied. Cefazolin should be equally effective as ceftiofur against *E. coli* associated with translocation, although more frequent administration may be necessary and efficacy against anaerobes may be less.

Parvoviruses are extremely stable, being resistant to environmental conditions and many chemical disinfectants. Canine parvovirus is susceptible to sodium hypochlorite (1 part household bleach to 1:32 parts water). Exposure to diluted bleach must be long in duration.

Canine Distemper

Canine distemper[29] spreads by aerosolization to the epithelium of the upper respiratory tract. Multiplication in tissue macrophages leads to spread to lymphatics; tonsils; bronchial lymph nodes; and ultimately to lymphatic tissues of the gastrointestinal tract, liver, and other organs. Additional spread generally is hematogenous. Leukopenia characterized by lymphopenia develops as the virus proliferates in lymphoid tissues. Animals with adequate immunity are able to clear infection within 8 to 9 days. In dogs with an insufficient immune response, the virus spreads to other tissues, including the skin and other organs. Persistent viral infection of the CNS appears to develop in dogs that are not able to generate circulating IgG antibodies to the viral envelope. Immune complex deposition in the CNS may facilitate viral infection. Lesions and their sequelae in the CNS vary with the age and immunocompetence of the dog, the pathogenicity of the virus, and the duration (acute versus chronic) of infection. Acute encephalitis is more likely in young or immunosuppressed dogs and reflects direct viral damage. Demyelinating polioencephalomalacia is characterized by minimal inflammation. Continued infection in the CNS leads to progressive increases in the immune response, ultimately contributing to continued and widespread damage. Chronic infection is associated with increased concentrations of antimyelin antibodies, activation of macrophages, and release of reactive oxygen radicals. Despite resolution of inflammation in surviving animals, canine distemper virus can persist in infected brain tissues.

Clinical signs vary with the extent of infection and include general listlessness; fever; upper respiratory tract infection (similar to kennel cough); keratoconjunctivitis sicca; serous to mucopurulent discharge; and vomiting and diarrhea, often associated with tenesmus. Animals may become severely dehydrated. Neurologic signs generally develop after recovery (generally at 1 to 3 weeks but potentially up to several months) and tend to be progressive. Mature animals can abruptly develop neurologic signs despite prior vaccination and no previous evidence of disease. Clinical signs of CNS involvement vary with the area of the CNS affected and with the magnitude of damage and include hyperesthesia, cervical rigidity, seizures, cerebellar signs, paraparesis or tetraparesis, and myoclonus. Diagnosis is based on immunologic testing of IgM (ELISA). Measurements of IgG in both serum and cerebrospinal fluid may be useful for detecting chronic CNS infections. Immunocytology may also be helpful in the diagnosis of canine distemper, although the need for special equipment renders this aid less practical.

The most appropriate approach for limiting morbidity and mortality associated with canine distemper is proper vaccination.[29] Treatment continues to be largely supportive and focuses on prevention or treatment of bronchopneumonia (usually caused by *Bordetella bronchiseptica*), fluid and electrolyte support with supplementation of B vitamins as needed, and treatment of neurologic signs. Progression of neurologic signs may provide justification for treatment of cerebral edema (e.g., single administration of dexamethasone).[29] Seizures should be treated with anticonvulsant medications (diazepam for immediate control, phenobarbital or bromide for long-term control). Myoclonus is not treatable. Chronic inflammatory forms of distemper (including optic neuritis, encephalitis) may require long-term glucocorticoid therapy. Glucocorticoids that are more effective in their ability to control oxygen radicals (e.g., methylprednisolone) may offer an advantage, although this has not been clinically addressed with controlled studies. Therapy with ascorbic acid intravenously has not been proved to be clinically useful but nonetheless has been recommended.[29] Infections associated with measles in children apparently have responded favorably to two treatments with vitamin A (200,000 IU or 60 mg) if given within 5 days of the onset of clinical signs.[29] Canine distemper virus is extremely susceptible to common disinfectants.

Infectious Canine Hepatitis

Infectious canine hepatitis[30] initially localizes in the tonsils and spreads to regional lymph nodes and then to the bloodstream. The virus rapidly disseminates to all tissues, with hepatic parenchymal cells and vascular endothelial cells serving as the primary targets. Cytotoxic effects of the virus cause injury to the liver, kidney, and eye. In immunocompetent animals, infection is cleared within 7 days. Acute hepatic necrosis tends to develop in immunoincompetent animals. Although acute necrosis is the most common cause of death in animals surviving the initial phases of infection, it also can be self-limiting. Animals that respond with a partial neutralizing antibody tend to develop chronic active hepatitis, which can progress to fibrosis. Although renal lesions may develop with acute infection, progression to chronic renal disease apparently does not occur. Animals, however, remain prone to pyelonephritis. Ocular location of the virus occurs in about 20% of animals and can cause severe anterior uveitis and corneal edema. Ocular lesions tend to be self-limiting unless complications develop. DIC is a frequent acute complication of infectious canine hepatitis, probably triggered by widespread endothelial damage and activation of the clotting cascade. Decreased hepatic function and inability to clear products of degradation and to synthesize clotting factors contribute to DIC. Clinical signs in the acute stages of infectious canine hepatitis include enlargement of lymphoreticular tissues, fever, coughing, abdominal tenderness associated with hepatomegaly, and hemorrhagic diathesis.

Less commonly, icterus and CNS signs may develop. Ocular lesions may be associated with blepharospasm, photophobia, cloudiness of the cornea, and ocular discharge. Diagnosis is based on clinical laboratory changes consistent with damage caused by infectious canine hepatitis and serologic testing.

Therapy is supportive and should continue until the liver has adequately healed from acute damage. Among the alternative therapies that might be considered is lactoferrin. Inhibition of growth has been demonstrated toward a number of viruses by the iron-binding protein lactoferrin. This endogenous compound is found in mucosal membranes, milk, and other tissues where it imparts other antimicrobial effects. Among the viruses targeted is canine herpesvirus, as has been demonstrated using in vitro techniques (canine kidney cells). The effects targeted viral replication and were independent of the iron-binding effects of the drug.[31] Impaired interaction between the virus and cell receptors leading to altered viral–host cell attachment was a suggested mechanism.

Therapy focuses on fluid and electrolyte support, treatment as indicated for DIC (including both replacement therapy and anticoagulant therapy), and treatment for hepatic encephalopathy as needed in acute stages. Hypertonic glucose (0.5 mL/kg of a 50% solution given intravenously over 5 minutes) may be helpful in the presence of hypoglycemia. Polyinosinic–polycytidylic acid, an IFN inducer, has been used experimentally but is not a practical therapy. Persistence of chronic liver disease should be treated appropriately.

Infectious canine hepatitis is very resistant to many chemical disinfectants, including chloroform, ether, acid, and formalin. Chemical disinfectants that appear to be useful include iodine, phenol, and sodium hydroxide. The application of steam (5 minutes at 50° to 60° F) may be a reasonable method of disinfection for instruments.

Canine Infectious Tracheobronchitis (Kennel Cough)

The most common causative organisms of kennel cough are canine parainfluenza virus, a single-stranded RNA virus, and *B. bronchiseptica*.[32] Other viruses and bacterial infections are also associated with the syndrome. Bacterial causes of tracheobronchitis are discussed in Chapter 8. Viral transmission occurs primarily by aerosol or, for some viruses, oronasal contact. The lack of viral replication in macrophages limits infection of the virus to the upper respiratory tract, although it is the viral-induced damage to the respiratory epithelium that allows secondary bacterial infection. *B. bronchiseptica* preferentially attaches to the respiratory epithelium, replicates on respiratory cilia, and releases potent toxins that impair phagocytosis and cause ciliostasis, allowing infection by opportunistic organisms. The most common clinical signs associated with canine infectious tracheobronchitis (ITB) is paroxysmal nonproductive coughing, often associated with retching. Edema of the vocal folds is responsible for the characteristic honking sound of the cough. History includes exposure to other dogs, often at a boarding facility. Diagnosis is based on history and clinical signs. Culture of the upper airways (by bronchoscopy or transtracheal wash) can support diagnosis of a bacterial component. Rising antibody titers may be helpful in identifying a specific viral etiology. Therapy focuses on control of cough and, in cases complicated by persistent bacterial infection, (as evidenced by mucopurulent discharge that emerges after viral phase) antimicrobials. Glucocorticoids may be helpful for controlling cough but do not appear to shorten the clinical outcome. Antitussive therapy should include both peripheral bronchodilators and centrally active drugs. Narcotic derivatives are more likely than non-narcotics to control cough associated with ITB. Aerosol therapy may be helpful in cases associated with marked accumulation of respiratory secretions or pneumonia. Mucolytics, such as *N*-acetylcysteine, may be very irritating to the respiratory tract and can be given orally or parenterally.

Parainfluenza virus is susceptible to sodium hypochlorite, chlorhexidine, and benzalkonium solution. Control of outbreaks in a kennel may require isolation of the entire facility for up to 2 weeks. Vaccines are available; intranasal vaccination may lead to clinical signs typical of ITB.

Canine Papillovirus

Papillovirus is a largely self-limiting infection. However, antiviral therapy might be considered in nonresponders or in the interest of improving the comfort of animals. One uncontrolled clinical trial reported response of infection with nonspecific immunomodulation. Dogs (n = 16) presenting with papillomas in the oral mucosae and palate were treated with 2 mg *Propionibacterium acnes* intramuscularly once per week. Response was realized in 2 weeks, with resolution of lesions occurring within 5 weeks in younger animals. However, in older animals response required treatment 3 times per week, with regression of lesions beginning at week 3 and completed by week 6. No significant side effects of therapy were reported, leading the authors to conclude that *P. acnes* would be a reasonable alternative for treatment of canine papillomas that have not naturally regressed.[33] Other anecdotal treatments have included IFN-alpha-2a, 1-3 million IU/dog, orally 3 times per week.

Yagci and coworkers[34] prospectively studied the positive effects of azithromycin (10 mg/kg once daily for 10 days) for treatment of canine oral (n = 12) or cutaneous (n = 5) papillomatosis using a double-blinded controlled design. Dogs were assigned to treatment groups based on entry into the study; 10 dogs (7 oral and 3 cutaneous) received treatment, whereas 7 did not. Cutaneous lesions on 1 dog in the placebo group spontaneously resolved at day 41. However, skin lesions in the 10 dogs with cutaneous lesions in the treatment group resolved in 10 to 15 days (although not stated in the report, it is assumed that all dogs with oral lesions also had skin lesions). The number of animals with oral lesions that responded was not provided. Recurrence of lesions was not evident during the 8-month follow-up period of the study.

Treatment of Selected Feline Viral Infections

Feline Panleukopenia

Feline panleukopenia[35] is caused by parvovirus transmitted by direct contact between cats or between cats and vehicles acting as vectors. As with other parvoviruses, cells that are rapidly dividing are particularly susceptible to infection, including bone marrow, lymphoid tissue, and intestinal mucosal crypt cells. In utero infection can cause a number of reproductive disorders in the pregnant cat, ranging from loss of fetuses if infection occurs early in the pregnancy to birth of affected kittens. Injuries in kittens occur in the CNS, particularly the cerebellum, optic nerve, and retina. Panleukopenia causes acute signs, including fever; depression; anorexia; and, less frequently, vomiting. Dehydration can be extreme. Other potential clinical signs include ulceration, bloody diarrhea and icterus, and signs indicative of DIC. Queens infected during pregnancy may be diagnosed with infertility, and dead fetuses may mummify. Kittens affected in utero present with classic signs of cerebellar hypoplasia.

Diagnosis generally is based on a complete blood count. Therapy is symptomatic and focuses on fluid and electrolyte replacement (with vitamin B) and maintenance, antiemetics (generally metaclopramide), and broad-spectrum antimicrobials to control secondary infection. The use of antivirals has not been established. Diazepam or other appetite stimulants can be attempted in anorectic cats that are not vomiting. Blood transfusions may be indicated in the presence of severe anemia.

*Feline Infectious Peritonitis (FIP)**

The treatment of FIP has recently been reviewed.[36] Although caused by a coronavirus, the pathophysiology of infection is complex, in part because a variety of coronaviruses are capable of infecting cats. Further, cat susceptibility to infection and subsequent development of FIP vary unpredictably.[37] The underlying relationship between FIP virus and non-FIP feline corona virus (FeCoV) cannot yet be discriminated based on current serology methods alone. The role of polymerase chain reaction based assays has to be defined; the ABCD Guidelines for FIA indicates that it cannot diagnose FIP in that positive results have been obtained in healthy carriers and negative results may occur in cats with FIP. Rivalta's test—based on high protein content, inflammatory mediators, and fibrinogen present in fluids of the effusive form—is characterized by a high predictive value.[37a] Among the feline corona viruses are strains whose pathogenicity and virulence vary from minimal, with replication limited to the gastrointestinal epithelium, to the virulent strains causing (FIP). Variability in virulence exists even within strains causing FIP. Cats infected with non-FIP corona virus are at risk to develop FIP as some strains appear to rapidly mutate to the virulent form. Virulence may be related to the ability of the virus to infect and replicate within macrophages. The "S" protein on the viral envelope appears to be responsible for viral attachment, membrane fusion, and virus-neutralizing antibody production. Infection and subsequent reinfection among carrier cats (e.g., in catteries or multiple-cat households) probably facilitates mutation. Cats do not develop FIP unless preexisting corona antibodies exist. Antibodies to the virus facilitate monocytes and macrophage infection (antibody-dependent enhancement), leading to dissemination. Cats that develop antibodies before mounting an effective cell-mediated response to FeCoV appear to develop the effusive form of FIP on reinfection; a partial cell-mediated response may result in the noneffusive form of the disease.

Clinical signs of FIP reflect immune-complex deposition (Arthus-type reaction) in smaller vessels. Clinical signs of FIP vary with the site of virus and immune complex deposition and generally reflect either an effusive or noneffusive form. Immune complexes that form in response to the virus or the specific viral antigen include both antiviral antibodies and complement. Activation of complement leads to the release of vasoactive amines, endothelial retraction, and increased epithelial permeability, which in turn allows exudation of the protein-rich exudate typical of FIP. If vascular permeability is the predominant effect, the effusive form develops. Less severe permeability with subsequent recruitment of inflammatory cells appears to lead to the pyogranulomatous inflammation characteristic of the noneffusive form. Neutrophil accumulation and subsequent release of lysozymes cause vascular necrosis. Systemic involvement may reflect spread of viral-infected macrophages and subsequent complement activation or deposition of immune complexes from circulation into tissues. Pyogranulomata develop, the magnitude of which reflects the size, number, and amount of antibody and antigens. Regions of high blood pressure and turbulence appear to be more common sites of deposition. Effusive FIP causes ascites with or without pleural effusions. Noneffusive FIP tends to be vague in presentation and includes fever, weight loss, anorexia, and depression. Ocular lesions are common, characterized by iritis, hypopyon, and hyphema. Pyogranulomata may be present in the vitreous or the retina. Neurologic signs are not uncommon and include ataxia, nystagmus, and seizures. Meningitis may lead to tremors, hyperesthesia, behavioral changes, or cranial nerve defects. Hydrocephalus also may develop.

Investigations into treatment of FIP have focused on both antiviral therapy (particularly IFN) as well as control of the immune response. A number of drugs have been studied for potential efficacy against FIP, some with little hope of being clinically applicable. For example, in one in vitro study, the rank of CD_{50}: ED_{50} (the ratio of a cytotoxic to effective dose) of drugs toward FIP was pyrazofuin > 6-azauridine > 3-deazaguanosine > hygromycin B > fusidic acid > dipyridamole. Compounds with no effect were caffeic acid, carbodine, 3-deazauridine, 5-fluoroorotic acid, 5-fluorouracil, D(+)glucosamine, indomethacin, D-penicillamine, rhodamine, and taurine.[38] More recent in vitro studies have demonstrated the potential efficacy of ribavirin or adenine arabinoside, but neither acyclovir nor AZT.

A variety of studies (as reviewed by Hartmann and others[36]) have focused on minimizing the immune and thus inflammatory response. However, studies have been characterized by a number of limitations, including failure to accurately diagnose FIP and limited sample size. Glucocorticoids with or without

*The European Advisory Board and Cat Diseases (ABCD) has published guidelines for the viral disease of major feline or human public health significance. Each guideline provides an excellent review of the pathophysiology of the disease and an evidence-based approach to the diagnosis, prevention, and treatment of the diseases (Table 10-4). Although the availability of diagnostic and treatment aids will vary among countries, the principles and applications are relevant to all.

cyclosphosphamide have been associated with variable success in uncontrolled studies. Despite in vitro studies, ribavirin has not been proven effective and appears to be too toxic at doses that are necessary to achieve effective concentrations. Case reports have described variable success with thromboxane synthetase inhibitors, melphalan, chlorambucil, tylosin (for its immunomodulatory effects), promodulin, human IFN, *P. acnes* and the "paraimmunity" inducer Baypamum have all been reported either as single cases or in clinical trials. No clear effective treatment has emerged.

According to the ABCD, low dose human IFN- α is contraindicated and SC high dose was ineffective in cats with FIP. Most recently, efficacy of feline recombinant-omega IFN has been studied. A series of 12 cases of spontaneous FIP treated with a combination of glucocorticoids and recombinant feline-omega IFN (10^6 IU/kg administered subcutaneously every 48 hours until clinical improvement followed by once weekly); complete remission (over 2 years) was reported in 4 cats and partial remission (2 to 5 months) in another 4. However, all survivors were older cats (older than 5 years), with the effusive form of the disease.[39] Hartmann and coworkers Ritz and coworkers[399] failed to find a treatment effect compared to placebo for rF-INFω in cats (n = 37) whose FIP was confirmed histologically and immunohistochemically (ability to detect a significant difference may have been limited by sample size). Effusive disease was also treated with dexamethasone or prednisolone. rF-INFω was administered at 10^6 IU/kg subcutaneously daily for 8 days and then weekly thereafter. Despite ongoing and historical studies, effective treatment of FIP remains elusive. Anecdotal reports suggest efficacy of pentoxifylline for the effusive form of FIP. Supportive therapy includes fluids as necessary, antimicrobials, ascorbic acid, vitamin B, and vitamin A.

Options for treatment of ocular FIP (Table 10-4) include topical and oral glucocorticoids (prednisolone or dexamathasone) or a combination thereof. As a primary T-cell, rather than B-cell inhibitor, cyclosporine is not recommended. As with systemic disease, anecdotal reports suggest efficacy of pentoxifylline. Intracameral tissue plasminogen activase has been anecdotally suggested if fibrin does not resolve.

Preventive efforts toward FIP infection are also complicated by the futility of identifying and removing carriers: serologic testing will identify only previous exposure to coronavirus, which will be true for the majority of cats. Vaccines thus far have proved ineffective because antibodies sensitize to rather than protect from the disease. Strains and route of inoculation will influence outcome of vaccination. Because animals will have been exposed by the time diagnosis is made, isolation is not necessary. However, environmental cleansing should be relatively easy. Although FeCoV is relatively stable in the environment, it is easily destroyed by most common detergents and disinfectants, including diluted (1:32) sodium hypochlorite solution.

Feline Respiratory Disease

Feline rhinovirus (FRV) and calicivirus (FCV) are the major viral causes of respiratory disease in the cat,[40] but a number of bacterial organisms contribute to the pathogenesis, including *B. bronchiseptica, Mycoplasma* spp., and *Chlamydia psittaci.* Other viral organisms (e.g., reovirus, poxvirus) also may contribute. Rhinovirus is a herpesvirus. Natural routes for both viral infections are by way of the nasal, oral, and conjunctival mucosae. Viral replication of rhinovirus occurs primarily in the nasal mucosal epithelium and, for calicivirus, throughout the respiratory epithelium. Growth of rhinovirus tends to be restricted to areas of lower body temperature; thus lesions tend to be limited to the nasal mucosa and the pharynx. Lesions reflect necrosis and result in the typical clinical signs of marked sneezing, pyrexia, depression, and anorexia; cats may salivate. Conjunctivitis with chemosis and hyperemia are common, with mucopurulent discharge of the nares and eyelids developing. Oral ulceration is rare. Several syndromes have been described, including the classical acute rhinosinusitis and corneal disease; an atypical disease that may be accompanied by a systemic response (including fading kitten syndrome), and chronic rhinosinusitis disease. For the latter, damage to nasal turbinates can be extensive and permanent, leaving the infected cats susceptible to lifelong chronic upper respiratory tract infections (e.g., rhinitis, sinusitis) and conjunctivitis. Rhinosinusitis may also reflect a chronic allergic inflammatory response.[40b] Calicivirus infection has variable clinical signs because it is more likely to affect the lungs. Oral lesions (tip of the tongue, mouth, and nose) are the most predominant sign, reflecting epithelial necrosis; fever and mild respiratory and conjunctival signs also occur. Feline calicivirus also has been associated with chronic gingivitis and stomatitis. Sneezing and ocular and nasal discharge are not as common as with rhinovirus. Pulmonary lesions begin with alveolitis. Lameness also may occasionally develop. An often lethal, highly virulent form of FVC resulting in systemic disease has been reported, with the disease more severe in adults compared to kittens.[40a] The syndrome is associated with a systemic inflammatory response syndrome. Diagnosis using molecular-based assays should be made only cautiously for FVC as the presence of virus and clinical signs are poorly correlated.

Similarities between human and feline herpesvirus infection justifies the potential application of human antiherpetic drugs to treatment of feline infections. Accordingly, information regarding their use for treatment of feline respiratory infections is increasing. For example, using infected feline kidney cells, the inhibitory concentration (50%) was determined for a number of antiviral drugs toward FHV-1. In vitro efficacy of IDU and that of ganciclovir were approximately equivalent and approximately twice that of cidofovir and penciclovir. Foscarnet appeared to be comparatively ineffective.[41] Also using in vitro techniques, cidofovir decreases cytopathic effects and viral load FHV-1 of feline corneal epithelia at concentrations of 0.05 and 0.02 mg/mL. However, cytotoxic effects also were evident in cultured cells.[42] Van der Meulen and coworkers[43] reported on the in vitro efficacy of six antiviral drugs [acyclovir, ganciclovir, cidofovir, foscarnet, adefovir, and 9-(2-phosphonylmethoxyethyl)-2, 6-diaminopurine (PMEDAP)], using an in vitro plaque reduction assay (embryo-derived feline kidney cells). Of the six drugs, ganciclovir, PMEDAP, and cidofovir were most effective in reducing

Table **10-4** Summary of the European Advisory Board on Cat Disease Guidelines for Feline Viral Diseases*[37a, 40a, 40b, 69a, 73, 74]

Disease	Cause	Diagnosis	Vaccine	Prevention	Treatment
FVC	Calicivirus	PCR?	Two injections, at 9 and 12 weeks (4 weeks acceptable with repeat every 2 weeks until 12 weeks of age); third at 16 weeks in high risk situations; 52 weeks; then yearly (high risk) or every 3 yr booster queen before mating.	Sodium hypochlorite (5% bleach; 1:32). Individual cages for non-household member cats.	**Antivirals:** None **Immunomodulators:** rFINFω (IV) Stomatitis: Immunosuppressants (glucocorticoids, others [IV]), human or rfIFNω (IV), including intralesional Highly virulent strain: glucocorticoids, IFN (III) **Supportive therapy**: Stomatitis: Stomatitis: cleaning-extraction, antimicrobials Highly virulent: fluid therapy, antimicrobials
Rhinotracheitis	Feline herpes virus (alpha)	PCR; positive may indicate low level shedding or viral latency	All kittens: at 9 weeks and 12 weeks. Unvaccinated adults: two vaccinations, 2 to 4 weeks apart. Booster: annual for high risk; if > 3 yr between boosters, two vaccinations 2-4 weeks apart. Otherwise booster every 3 yr.		**Antivirals (III):** Trifluridine topically every hr × 24 then every 4 hr Idoxuridine topically every 2 to 4 hr Ganciclovir topically Acyclovir topically and oral L-lysine 250 mg bid to 400 mg once daily **Immunomdulators (III):** rfIFNω: 1 MU/kg every 24 to 48 hr 50,000-100,000 U PO every 24 hr 10 MU/19 ml 0.9% NaCl: 2 gtt OU 5×/day for 10 days **Supportive (fluids etc):** Appetite stimulants (feeding tube if necessary) Antimicrobials Mucolytics, including nebulization with saline
Panleukopenia	Feline parvovirus	Latex agglutination based tests; PCR	All kittens: Start at 4 weeks with inactivated product (if exposed), or 6 to 9 weeks otherwise. Repeat every 3 to 4 weeks until 12 weeks (if started at 4 weeks) or 16 weeks. Booster at 1 yr and then 3 yrs or more. Adult cats: one vaccination; booster at 1 yr. Booster queens before breeding; kittens may require extra vaccination at 16 to 20 weeks. Avoid modified live in pregnant queens.	Isolate from susceptible kittens. Passive immunization of exposed young kittens, unvaccinated adults. Virus extremely stable; cleanse with sodium hypochlorite, formaldehyde (gas for room disinfection), sodium hydroxide or peracetic acid.	**Antivirals:** None **Immunomodulators:** Immune serum rFINFω (IV) **Supportive:** Fluids, antimicrobials (including anaerobic spectrum) Enteral or parenteral nutrition (IV?) Antiemetics Plasma or whole blood if hypoproteinemic

Table **10-4** Summary of the European Advisory Board on Cat Disease Guidelines for Feline Viral Diseases*[37a, 40a, 40b, 69a, 73, 74]—cont'd

Disease	Cause	Diagnosis	Vaccine	Prevention	Treatment
Infectious peritonitis	Feline corona virus group 1	Clinical signs Rivalta's test Others?		Isolation of cats not necessary. Clean as with standard disinfectants. Wait 2 months after seropositive cats removed before introduction of new cat.	**Antivirals:** none **Immunodulators:** rFINFω (IV) Immunosuppression: Prednisolone or Dexamethasone (III) Pentoxyfylline (IV) Cyclophosphamide (with glucocorticoids) (IV) Thromboxane synthetase inhibitors (ozagrel) (III)
Immunodeficiency virus	Retrovirus (lentivirus)	ELISA; Western blot for inconclusive results	Routine vaccination of FIV-positive cats controversial; inactivated vaccines recommended.	Neuter cats (to avoid fight-induced transmission). Shelters: segregate FIV+ cats.	**Antivirals:** AZT (5-10 mg/kg stomatitis: III); (do not use if anemic) **Immunomodulators** rf-IFNω(?) rh-IFNα (III) Stomatitis: Glucocorticoids others Neutropenia: Filgastrim (III) Anemia: rh-erythropoietin (IV; 100 IU/kg SC every 48 hr rh-insulin-like growth factor (III)
Leukemia	Gamma retrovirus	ELISA; PCR for inconclusive results	Generally recommended at 8-9 and 12 weeks; booster annually and then at 2 to 3 yr intervals in cats older than 3 to 4 yr. Note: response to other vaccines may be insufficient. Do not vaccinate sick FeLV + Cats. Vaccinate healthy FeLV and FIV + Cats.	Neuter cats (to avoid fight-induced transmission). Hospital and shelters: segregate FIV+ cats Test and remove multicat households. Shelters: euthanize sick cats; house-positive cats individually.	**Antivirals:** AZT (I) **Immunomodulators:** rf-IFNω (I) Avoid immunosuppressants unless cancer or stomatitis Neutropenia: Filgastrim
H5N1 (swine flu)	Influenza type A	Clinical signs	NA	Strict isolation; standard medical disinfectants.	Supportive; contact regulatory authorities

*The number (I-IV) by each treatment is the evidence number suggested by ABCD Guidelines for that disease where I = the highest level of evidence reflecting well designed randomized, controlled clinical trials in the target species; II = well-designed controlled studies in target species with spontaneous disease but an experimental setting; III = nonrandomized clinical trials, case series, uncontrolled studies with dramatic results; and IV = expert opinion, case reports, nontarget species studies or pathophysiologic justification.

plaque numbers and thus were cited as potentially viable candidates for treatment. In another in vitro study penciclovir was found to be much more potent (concentration by which plaques were reduced by 50% of 1.6 μg/mL) against FHV than acyclovir (24 μg/mL) and trifluorothymidine (5.7 μg/mL).[44]

Although in vitro studies are useful for identifying potential drugs, clinical trials are necessary to support their use. However, well-controlled clinical trials are limited. Stiles[45] retrospectively described the use of a variety of drugs for treatment of FHV-1 in cats (n = 17). Drugs included IDU (n = 7), vidarabine (n = 4), and trifluridine (n = 3) as well as recombinant human alpha-IFN (PO, n = 3) in conjunction with topical administration of antiviral agents. Williams followed up on his 2004 *in vitro* study[46] with a clinical trial involving cats (n = 30) with clinical signs associated with and demonstrated to be positive for FHV-1. Acyclovir ointment (0.5%) was applied 5 times daily; cats had been previously treated (for 21 days) with topical chlortetracycline three times daily for treatment of Chlamydia. No placebo or other control groups were studied. Cats that were FHV-1 positive did not respond to the 21 days of chlortetracycline therapy, but did respond to acyclovir in a median of 12 days of treatment. Cats that were treated only 3 times a day with acyclovir (due to poor owner compliance) did not respond initially, but did respond when the frequency of treatment was increased. Based on these studies and anecdotal reports, ocular herpetic infections can be treated topically with, in order of efficacy, trifluridine (1%) or idoxuridine (0.1%), vidarabine (3%), and acyclovir (3%). Each must be applied at 4-hour intervals for 1 week beyond the resolution of clinical signs.[47] Preference as to idoxuridine or trifulridine as first choice may depend on cost and tolerance (irritation).

Anecdotal reports suggest the potential efficacy of other drugs. For example, famciclovir (31 mg or ¼ of a 125-mg tablet orally twice daily for 10 days) has been used for acute flare-ups in cats not exhibiting systemic signs of illness associated with upper respiratory tract infections. In their review, Caney and coworkers[48] report that FHV-1 might be treated with topical use of trifluorothymidine (trifluridine; most potent; hourly the first 24 hours, then hourly during the waking hours, to every 4 hours as soon as re-epithelialization has occurred), IDU (every 2 to 4 hours for the first 24 hours, then 4 to 6 times daily until 1 week beyond clinical resolution of signs) and vidarabine. It is best if treatment is started early, but the duration of therapy should be limited to 2 to 3 weeks because of the risk of epithelial toxicity. Oral administration of AZT also should begin early, although it is a hundredfold less potent against FHV than it is toward human herpes simplex.

Other drugs might be considered for treatment of feline viral respiratory infections, although evidence for use is limited. Among those most commonly cited is lysine. Using a placebo-controlled design, L-lysine administration (400 mg in food once daily) was associated with a decrease in the incidence of conjunctivitis in cats with experimentally induced viral respiratory diseases.[49] Animals were infected 5 months before the study such that infections were latent. Viral expression was induced by either the stress of rehousing or administration of glucocorticoids. The drug caused a delay in onset of clinical signs (average delay of 7 days) and a decrease in episodes of viral shedding 5 months but only in rehoused cats and not glucocorticoid-treated cats. The 400-mg dose yielded a maximum plasma concentration of about 450 nmol/mL after single dosing (two cats; time not noted) and approximately 300 nmol/mL at 3 hours after 30 days of therapy.[49] Stiles and colleagues[50] also studied the impact of lysine (500 mg orally twice daily) beginning 6 hours before experimental infection of cats (n = 4; an additional 4 cats received placebo). Because arginine is an essential amino acid, both arginine and lysine were analyzed in plasma. Lysine did not affect arginine concentrations, supporting its safe use in cats. Despite the small number of animals, clinical scores differed between the two treatment groups between days 5 and 15 after infection; however, the scores of the two groups were similar during the final week of the 21-day study, as resolution of clinical signs caused the scores to return to baseline (preinfection).This study provides some evidence of support; failure to maintain a significant difference at 21 days may reflect sample size. However, the efficacy of once-daily L–lysine (250 mg if less than 5 months or 500 mg if greater than 5 months) also was studied for its impact on emergent upper respiratory infection in animal shelter cats (n = 144 treated and 147 nontreated cats). No difference was found in the subsequent incidence of upper respiratory infection that emerged between the two treatment groups.[51]

KEY POINT 10-6 A consensus cannot yet be determined from clinical trials that address the efficacy of lysine for treatment of upper respiratory infections in cats.

Interferon also has been studied. Human recombinant drug has been used at 5 to 25 U per day orally, whereas rFeIFN-ω is recommended at 2 drops of 500,000U/mL saline topically 5 times a day. Sandmeyer and coworkers[52] studied the in vitro effect of rFeIFN-ω n cultured corneal epithelial cells infected with FHV-1. Concentrations of 100,000 IU/mL significantly reduced virus-induced pathology without causing cytotoxicity. Siebeck and coworkers[53] also studied in vitro the impact of recombinant human IFN α-2b and rFeIFN-ω in FHV-1 using feline kidney cells. Both plaque number and size were reduced by 100,000 U/mL of both recombinant IFNs; neither product at any concentration (up to 500,000 U/mL) caused cytotoxicity. The feline product was more effective but only at higher concentrations. Ohe and coworkers[53a] demonstrated in vitro sensitivity to recombinant feline IFN (the IFN type was not provided but the product is produced in Japan) by 5 strains of FCV causing breakthrough disease in vaccinated cats. No well-controlled study has identified drugs useful for treatment of feline calicivirus.

Supportive therapy for respiratory disease associated with viral infections must also be directed toward the secondary bacterial infection associated with the syndrome. This includes both removing debris that might support bacterial growth at the site of infection and controlling bacterial infection and inflammation. Antimicrobial therapy is best based on an appropriately collected culture, which may be difficult. Empirical selection should target the most likely infecting organisms (e.g., fluorinated quinolones, doxycycline, azithromycin). Note that ineffectual antibacterial therapy is likely to contribute to infection by *P. aeruginosa*. Alternating antimicrobial therapy may reduce the development of resistance; higher doses should be used not only because penetrability is likely to be impaired but also because minimizing the advent of resistance is important. Combination therapy should be considered with acute flare-ups associated with bacteria (see Chapter 8). Because oral medication may be difficult to administer, injections and medications that can be given once daily may be preferred. Nasal decongestants may be helpful during the acute phases, but note that α–adrenergic decongestants may contribute to nasal mucosal necrosis owing to impaired blood flow. Antihistaminergic products are probably preferable; among them are newer drugs that may have better efficacy than older antihistamines if they preclude mast cell degranulation (Zyrtec [cetirizine], 2.5 mg/cat daily). However, their use should be discontinued in the presence of purulent secretions. At this point, liquefaction of secretions may be paramount to success; a dysfunctional mucociliary apparatus may contribute to infection by providing an optimal environment for microbial growth. Mucolytic drugs and mucokinetics may facilitate movement of accumulated respiratory secretions. *N*-acetylcysteine can be given by injection (125 mg), although oral administration (⅛ tsp sprinkled on food) might be helpful despite significant first-pass metabolism of the compound.

Aerosolization or local installation of saline also may be helpful if lesions tend to predominate in upper airways.

The impact of glucocorticoids on viral-induced feline respiratory infections is not well studied. In general, immune suppression is discouraged because of the risk of recrudescence of latent infections. However, in one study, administration of methylprednisolone (5 mg/kg intramuscularly) did not statistically increase shedding of FHV in experimentally infected cats compared with pretreatment shedding, although the power of the study to detect a significant difference was low.[49]

Feline Viral Neoplasia: Feline Leukemia Virus

FeLV is caused by an oncornavirus subfamily of retroviruses. Its pathophysiology has been well reviewed.[5] Viral replication depends on the presence of reverse transcriptase (RNA-dependent DNA polymerase). The enzyme makes a provirus (a copy of DNA) that is subsequently inserted into the host genome. The binding site of FeLV is the major envelope glycoprotein (gp70); antibodies to this envelope provide protective immunity. Malignant cells also contain the feline oncornavirus cell membrane antigen (FOCMA); high levels of FOCMA antibodies render the cat resistant to viral-induced leukemia or lymphoma. FeLV is contagious, with transmission occurring by way of the saliva after close contact between cats. Iatrogenic transmission can occur through contaminated blood or instruments that penetrate (e.g., needles). Initial infection is characterized by malaise and lymphadenopathy. Cats that mount an adequate immune response recover. FeLV spreads hematogenously to the bone marrow in cats that do not mount an immune response. Cats can become latently infected, with the virus residing undetected (by ELISA, fluorescent antibody testing, or viral culture) in the bone marrow.

Cats infected with FeLV die as a result of viral-induced neoplasia (lymphoma or leukemia), suppression of the bone marrow (anemia), or infections caused by FeLV-induced immunosuppression. Bone marrow suppression occurs because FeLV can block differentiation of erythroid progenitors. Other mechanisms may also be involved. Platelet and leukocyte abnormalities also may occur, and a panleukopenia-like syndrome induced by FeLV has been described. Immunosuppression reflects disruption of T-cell function, ultimately affecting both cellular and humoral immunity. Immune complex disease has been described and can be induced experimentally with antibodies to gp70. Glomerulonephritis may be a sequela. Other disorders include those of the reproductive tract (infertility, abortions, endometritis), lymphadenopathy (most severe in submandibular lymph nodes), osteochondromas, and olfactory neuroblastomas. Diagnosis of FeLV is based on fluorescent antibody testing and ELISA. The indications and advantages for each are described elsewhere.[54]

Treatment of FeLV-related diseases varies with the syndrome resulting from the infection and, for most syndromes, is discussed in other chapters. Lymphoma is generally fatal in 1 to 2 months if not treated. Prognosis for complete remission is relatively good for the otherwise healthy cat.[54] Treatment focuses on combinations of chemotherapeutic drugs and, for selected cancers (e.g., nasal lymphoma), radiation therapy. Single-agent glucocorticoids are relatively ineffective and are palliative only. The most commonly used combination of chemotherapeutic agents is cyclophosphamide, vincristine, and prednisone. Other drugs that might be added to this regimen, depending on the cell type and response, include doxorubicin and, less commonly, L-asparaginase, cytosine arabinoside, and methotrexate. Antiemetics may be necessary, as might appetite stimulants (cyproheptadine, diazepam, megestrol acetate).

Treatment of the cancer component of viral diseases is addressed in Chapter 33. Bone marrow suppressive disease has been treated with repetitive blood transfusions. Prednisolone may increase the life span of erythrocytes if immune-mediated destruction is contributing to anemia, but glucocorticoids also will contribute to immune suppression. Human recombinant (and, when available, canine recombinant) growth factors may be useful for increasing bone marrow production of precursor cells despite the fact that most animals with anemia have high endogenous concentrations. Response to human recombinant erythropoietin (100 U/kg, subcutaneously 3 times weekly) requires about 3 to 4 weeks. This product should be reviewed before its use. Likewise, recombinant granulocyte colony-stimulating factor may be of benefit in the treatment of leukopenias. Development of antibodies to both of these products may limit their use beyond several weeks.

No antiviral drug has been shown to clear a FeLV viremic cat. Drugs that target reverse transcriptase, such as AZT, offer the most promise for effective therapy. Zidovudine suppresses viral replication but will not eliminate the virus. Experimentally, the drug can prevent viremia when administered (60 mg/kg per day divided every 8 hours) within 96 hours of infection. Zidovudine (30 mg/kg per day) inhibited antigenemia in kittens and prolonged survival time from 35 to 102 weeks. Myelosuppression, however, occurred in 33% of the treated cats.

In another study AZT (10 to 20 mg/kg twice daily for 42 days) prevented retroviral infection in cats if administered immediately after virus exposure. Replication also may have been reduced when it was administered to previously infected animals.[55] Serum-neutralizing antibodies developed in some of the infected cats, and the cats became resistant to subsequent viral challenge. However, progression of disease was not altered in cats if treatment was withheld until day 28 after infection, although the level of viremia was much lower than in untreated cats. Zidovudine appeared to be nontoxic in uninfected cats, although 3 of 12 infected kittens became anorectic and icteric and were vomiting after 40 days of treatment. Zidovudine may be beneficial in reducing FeLV-associated diseases; one study reported improved health status and a reduction of oral lesions in cats with FeLV-associated stomatitis.

In their review of antiviral therapy in cats, Caney and coworkers[48] acknowledge the controversy regarding the efficacy of AZT for treatment of FIV and FeLV but report that positive cats with gingivitis or neurologic disorders have responded clinically to either oral or subcutaneous administration, with reversible anemia being the major side effect. Kociba and coworkers[56] studied the effect of leukocyte-derived human IFN-α on FeLV-associated erythroid aplasia but found no beneficial effects. Other drugs have been studied for potential efficacy against FeLV. Phosphomethoxyethyl adenine (PMEA), another reverse transcriptase inhibitor, also has been studied in cats. Cats with stomatitis associated with FeLV responded better to PMEA (AZT was also given at 5 mg/kg every 12 hours), but adverse reactions to the drug are likely to limit its use. The combination of AZT with IFN (1.6×10^6 U/kg, SC, sid) or IFN by itself may reduce antigenemia, but antibody development may reverse the effect. Cogan[55] evaluated the efficacy and safety of suramin (10 to 20 mg/kg) in two FeLV-infected cats. Although toxic signs were limited to vomiting and anorexia (both resolving between treatments), viremia in both peripheral blood cells and serum did not resolve. Serum viral infectivity transiently decreased during treatment but was significantly higher 14 days after treatment was discontinued. Previous in vitro studies by the same author revealed a 90% inhibition of infectivity at drug concentrations of 100 mg/mL. Immunomodulating therapies also have been studied or reported after empiric use in cats with FeLV-related diseases. Immunomodulators may provide the most effective means of treating or controlling FeLV-related diseases.

KEY POINT 10-7 Although the efficacy of AZT for treatment of FIV and FeLV is controversial, gingivitis or neurologic disorders associated with disease may respond clinically.

A clinical case of feline epitheliotrophic T-cell lymphoma with paraneoplastic eosinophilia that failed initial therapy responded when rhINFa2b was added. Response was based on clinical, hematogenous, and sonographic evaluation. Relapse coincided with detection of antibodies directed toward the IFN.[58]

Other immunomodulatory drugs have been studied for treatment of FeLV. Antibodies that target gp70 have proved useful experimentally only when given within 3 weeks of the initial infection. Immunostimulants including IFN-α, staphylococcal protein A (10 μg/kg twice weekly for 10 weeks, then monthly), *P. acnes* (0.5 mL intravenously twice weekly for 2 weeks, then weekly), acemannan (2 mg/kg twice weekly), and evening primrose (550 mg daily) have been used with variable success, but no well-designed study has proved efficacy. Staphylococcal protein A has reversed viremia in a few cats, but only a small number of cats have been studied. Ultimately, combinations of therapies (e.g., antiviral drugs combined with immune modulators) may prove most beneficial. For example, response to *Staphylococcals* protein A (intraperitoneal) and IFN (oral) or the combination thereof was studied in a clinical trial of 36 cats with spontaneous FeLV infection (animals with tumors were excluded). No differences were found in clinical scores, clinical pathology, or survival time, although the authors reported that owners reported improved health more often in those cats treated with *Staphylococcals* protein A, leading the authors to recommend this form of immunomodulation in conjunction with supportive care.[59]

Adoptive immunotherapy using autologous lymph node cells that have been activated and expanded ex vivo using interleukin-2 (IL-2) in short-term cultures resulted in clinical improvement within 2 to 4 weeks and lasting at least 13 months in 9 of 18 cats with FeLV; 4 of the 18 cats became antigen free.[60]

Feline Immunodeficiency Virus

Pathophysiology of infection. FIV, like HIV, is caused by a lentivirus.[21] The pathophysiology of infection with FIV has been reviewed.[1,6] FIV continues to serve as a model for the study of human lentiviruses, and information regarding transmission, pathogenesis, host response, and immune dysfunction antiviral strategies is often shared among the two syndromes.[61] As with FeLV, transmission of FIV among cats occurs by way of saliva or blood, presumably through bite wounds. Transmission also can occur in utero or through milk ingested by nursing infants. Whereas CD4 receptors on T-cells serve as receptors for HIV, CD4 is not the receptor for FIV. One group of investigators has identified CD134 (OX40) as a primary receptor.[62] However, CD4 cells decrease early in infection, and therefore FIV causes progressive disruption of normal immune function. Viral replication begins in lymphoid tissues and salivary glands and spreads to mononuclear cells and nonlymphoid organs. Clinical signs may occur during the initial phases of viremia. The cause of the decrease is not known, but the result is an inversion of the normal CD4/CD8 ratio in infected cats. CD8 cells may increase, contributing to the inversion. Formation of immunoglobulins (dysregulation may lead to hypergammaglobulinemia in some cases) and cytokines also is disrupted. Several phases of infection have been described after infection with FIV: an acute phase, followed by a clinically asymptomatic phase that varies in duration, and a terminal phase. Other phases have been described by other investigators.

As with HIV, clinical signs of FIV are highly variable, reflecting different tissues and the role of secondary pathogens. Secondary bacterial infections reflect opportunistic microflora. Infections by fungal (e.g., *Cryptococcus*) and protozoal (e.g., *Toxoplasma*) organisms also should be anticipated. Abnormal neurologic signs are not uncommon and may reflect an inflammatory response to altered astrocyte metabolism. Changes in behavior are most commonly reported, followed by seizures, paresis, motor abnormalities, and disrupted sleep patterns. Direct damage is the most common cause of neurologic signs, although secondary infection by *Toxoplasma* or *Cryptococcus* spp. should be considered. Abnormalities in renal function and wasting disease also may reflect either abnormal function or an inflammatory response in the respective organs. Ocular diseases include anterior uveitis (caused by either FIV or opportunistic secondary organisms), glaucoma, vitreal changes, retinal degeneration, and retinal hemorrhage. Respiratory disease generally reflects secondary infection. Neoplasia is a common reason for presentation. A number of tumor types have been reported in FIV-infected cats, including lymphomas (usually B cell) and leukemias. Diagnosis is based on clinical signs and serologic testing.

Treatment. Therapy of FIV has largely focused on supportive care. Antiviral therapy thus far has been unrewarding, but newer information may provide potentially effective choices. Both AZT and PMEA have been studied; although neither drug thus far has prevented infection, onset to detectable viremia and immunologic changes can be prolonged. A trend toward normalization of inverted CD4:CD8 ratios and clinical evidence of improvement in diseases such as stomatitis have occurred. Of the two drugs, AZT is most likely to improve the quality of life of a cat infected with FIV. In general, improvements in the cat's general condition, immune status, and quality of life can be expected, along with a longer life span. Benefits of immunomodulators in cats with FIV are not clear, and assessment of scientific studies is clouded by the additional use of antimicrobials and other drugs. Immunostimulation should be avoided, however, because of the association of enhanced immune response with enhanced production of FIV experimentally.

In human patients with AIDs, highly active antiretroviral therapy has essentially revolutionized therapy, often rendering the lethal disease into a chronic but often manageable disease. The combination therapy is designed to suppress viral replication while preserving and potentially repairing the host immune response. Combination therapy generally includes two antiretroviral drugs such as AZT or lamivudine, which target early viral replication, with an HIV-1 protease inhibitor that targets later stages of replication. Other antiretroviral drugs approved for use in humans include ddi (didanosine), ddc (zalcitabine), D4T (stavudine), 3TC (lamivudine), and most recently Ziagen (abacavir). The first protease inhibitor approved in the United States was saquinavir (late 1995); others approved since then include ritonavir, indinavir, nelfinavir, and amprenavir. This approach has proved to be effective in decreasing viral loads and improving the CD4:CD8 ratio in human patients with AIDS; mortality and morbidity of HIV infection have subsequently been reduced. However, treatment paradigms have shifted from "hit hard and early" to delaying aggressive therapy until clinical signs have progressed. Whether a similar approach should be considered for treatment of FIV is not clear, although the indications and criteria for decision making have been reviewed.[63] Unfortunately, although FIV, like HIV, is susceptible to nucleoside analogs, it may not be susceptible to currently prescribed HIV-1 protease inhibitors, although this may change for newer protease inhibitors.[20]

FIV is susceptible in vitro to a number of nucleoside analogs, including AZT, zalcitabine, didanosine, and lamivudine in vitro at concentrations similar to those necessary to inhibit HIV-1. However, identifying the proper dose will be important; for example, subinhibitory concentrations of AZT increased the (in vitro) mutation frequency of FIV in a dose-dependent manner.[64]

As with patients with HIV, feline patients infected with FIV and subsequently treated with AZT show delayed onset of viremia, reduced plasma virus loads, and clinical improvement. Zivudine has been successfully used at 5 to 15 mg/kg orally every 12 hours to treat FIV-induced neurologic manifestations and 5 mg/kg subcutaneously every 12 hours to treat stomatitis, conjunctivitis, and alopecia; it improved the CD4:CD8 ratio. Quality and quantity of life also improved.[18] However, Hayes and coworkers[65] studied the effect of AZT in kittens, focusing on pathophysiology of the disease at the thymus. The loss of thymic function in kittens infected with FIV appears to reflect an inflammatory process that continues even if viral burden is significantly reduced. In 8-week-old kittens experimentally infected with FIV, zidovudine monotherapy reduced viral load in peripheral blood lymphocytes, plasma, and thymus, compared with saline-controlled kittens. However, an impact on neither thymus lesions nor CD4 could be detected, and neither thymic involution nor CD4 cell decline were prevented.[65]

According to Jordan and coworkers,[20] combination therapy with AZT and lamivudine demonstrated some clinical benefit in infected cats receiving experimental bone marrow transplants, although specifics were not provided. Using in vitro methods, AZT or lamivudine alone or in combination were somewhat effective in FIV-infected peripheral blood mononuclear cells, with the combination resulting in an additive or synergistic effect.[66] Follow-up in vivo studies were performed in specific pathogen-free cats receiving the combination before infection, at the same time as infection, or 2 weeks after infections. Doses were high (50 to 75 mg/kg every 12 hours). The authors found that the combination was helpful in preventing (five of six cats) but not treating infection. Both infection and antibody seroconversion were delayed in all treatment groups. However, adverse drug reactions (anemia and neutropenia) occurred at either treatment dose, although these resolved when the dose was dropped to 10 mg/kg twice daily.

Interferon. Using in vitro techniques, viral replication was decreased in feline cell lines infected with FIV and subsequently treated rFeINF-ω, but not rFeIFN-γ. A similar effect was found with simultaneous infection and treatment of peripheral mononuclear blood cells: replication was decreased with both rhIFN-α2 and rFeINF–ω, but not rFeIFN-γ. Pretreating 3 days before infection did not improve efficacy of rFeIFN-γ.[67] The effect of subcutaneous administration of rFeIFN-v (1 million U/kg per day) for 5 consecutive days on day 0, 14, 60 was studied in 81 cats experimentally infected with FeLV or FeLV/FIV (based on ELISA) using a multicentric double-blinded placebo controlled design.[68] All cats were exhibiting clinical signs associated with infection, but the study did not include cats with malignancy. The treatment group receiving IFN therapy was associated with less mortality, improvement in hematologic indicators, and improved clinical scores compared with placebo-treated cats.[68] However, in another study, although well tolerated, rf-IFN α did not significantly alter CD4:CD8 ratios or proviral load in cats with experimentally induced chronic FIV infection after treatment at either a high dose at 10^6 U/kg per day subcutaneously for 5 days or a lower dose of 10^4 U/cat orally per day for 6 weeks.[48]

Pedretti and coworkers[57] reported on the administration of a low dose (10 IU/kg) of natural human IFN-α (a combination of at least 9 different α subtypes) in naturally infected cats (n = 24; six placebo-treated cats). The product was diluted in phosphate-buffered saline, fortified with bovine albumin, filtered, and administered over the gums. The product was administered using a 7-days-on, 7-days-off cycle for 6 months; after 2 months of no therapy, another round was instituted. Treatment was considered easy by practitioners and was well tolerated with no overt side effects in cats. All treated cats survived the treatment period except for one cat that was seriously ill at study start; in contrast, only one placebo-treated cat survived the initial 6-month treatment period. Fever and lymphadenopathy resolved in the treatment group by day 10 of therapy but persisted throughout the study in the placebo group. However, viremic counts (excluding two cats with outlying high counts) did not change among groups. Survivability of CD4 cells was better in treated cats, although CD8 counts slowly increased such that the balance between CD4 and CD8 cats was not maintained. White cell counts declined in placebo cats. The placebo group, but not the treatment group, was characterized by progressive liver disease and failure. The authors indicated that the favorable response probably reflected the downregulation of inflammatory cytokines realized only with low (1 to 10 IU/kg) doses and the loss of this control such that proinflammatory responses occur with higher doses.

In a study of 40 naturally infected FIV cats treated with AMD3100 (a bicyclam chemokine receptor inhibitor; 0.5 mg/kg every 12 hours, administered subcutaneously), PMEA (10 mg/kg twice a week), or a combination of the two drugs for 6 weeks, stomatitis improved with either PMEA or the combination therapy. Further, the provirus load decreased in the AMD3100group compared with other groups.[69, 69a] However, treatment in either PMEA group was accompanied by decreased red blood cell, hemoglobin, and hematocrit counts; serum magnesium was decreased in the AMD3100 group. The authors concluded that the combination therapy was less effective than the use of the bicyclam alone. Guidelines of the ABCD recommend its use for treatment of FIV.

Bleomycin inhibits HIV viral replication apparent through oxygen-radical generation that also characterizes its anticancer effects. The use of bleomycin in combination with highly active antiretroviral therapy, particularly in those situations in which resistance has developed, has been recommended;[70] efficacy in cats infected with FIV has not yet been reported.

The efficacy of two acyclic phosphonyl adenine nucleosides, (fluoro, or FPMPA and methoxyethyl; PMEA) ameliorated clinical symptoms of FIV. Response included the incidence and severity of stomatitis, immunologic parameters such as relative and absolute CD4+ lymphocyte counts, and virologic parameters, including proviral DNA levels in peripheral blood mononuclear cells. However, of the two FPMPA was not associated with hematologic side effects, even at 2.5-fold higher dose, compared with PMEA.[71]

Because of its efficacy in mice, 16alpha-bromo-epiandrosterone (epiBr), a synthetic derivative of the natural hormone dehydroepiandrosterone (DHEA), also has been evaluated for efficacy against experimentally induced FIV infection in cats.[72] Two treatment regimens were studied: 5 consecutive days for weeks 0, 4, 8, and 16, or treatment 1 week before infection and continuing for 4 weeks after infection. All animals were studied for 20 weeks. For both groups, compared with control animals, CD4: CD8 T-cell ratio and total CD4 cell counts were less and CD8 cells higher from weeks 2 through 20 after infection. Although virus load was initially higher in treated cats, viremia subsequently declined to less than that of controls, and treated cats had higher FIV–p24 antibody responses.[72]

REFERENCES

1. Elder JH, Sundstrom M, de Rozieres S, et al: Molecular mechanisms of FIV infection, *Vet Immunol Immunopathol* 123:3–13, 2008.
2. Hayden FG: Antiviral agents (non-retroviral). In Hardmen J, Limbird L, editors: *Goodman & Gilman's the pharmacologic basis of therapeutics*, ed 10, New York, 2001, McGraw-Hill, pp 1313–1347.
3. Grandvaux N, tenOever BR, Servant MJ, et al: The interferon antiviral response: from viral invasion to evasion, *Curr Opin Infect Dis* 15:259–267, 2002.
4. Castelli J, Hassel BA, Wood KA, et al: A study of the interferon antiviral mechanism: apoptosis activation by the 2–5A system, *J Exp Med* 186(6):967–972, 1997.
5. Levy LS: Advances in understanding molecular determinants in FeLV pathology, *Vet Immunol Immunopathol* 123:14–22, 2008.
6. Willett BJ, Hosie MJ: Chemokine receptors and co-stimulatory molecules: unravelling feline immunodeficiency virus infection, *Vet Immunol Immunopathol* 123:56–64, 2008.
7. Carrasco L: The replication of animal viruses. In Shugar D, editor: *Viral chemotherapy*, vol I, New York, 1984, Pergamon, pp 111–148.
8. Hayden FG: Antiviral agents (nonretroviral). In Brunton LL, Lazo JS, Parker KL, editors: *Goodman & Gilman's the pharmacological basis of therapeutics*, ed 11, New York, 2006, McGraw-Hill.
9. Izzedine H, Launay-Vacher V, Deray G: Antiviral drug–induced nephrotoxicity, *Am J Kidney Dis* 45:804–817, 2005.
10. Chilar T, Lin DC, Pritchard JB, et al: The antiviral nucleotide analogs cidofovir and adefovir are novel substrates for human and rat renal organic anion transporter 1, *Mol Pharmacol* 56:570–580, 1999.
11. Richardson JA: Accidental ingestion of acyclovir in dogs: 105 reports, *Vet Hum Toxicol* 42(6):370–371, 2000.
12. Dolin R: Antiviral chemotherapy and chemoprophylaxis, *Science* 227:1296–1303, 1987.
13. Gustafson DP: Antiviral therapy, *Vet Clin North Am Small Anim Pract* 16:1181–1189, 1986.
14. Nasisse MP, Dorman DC, Jamison KC, et al: Effects of valacyclovir in cats infected with feline herpesvirus 1, *Am J Vet Res* 58:1141–1144, 1997.
15. Thomasy SM, Maggs DJ, Moulin NK, et al: Pharmacokinetics and safety of penciclovir following oral administration of favciclovir to cats, *Am J Vet Res* 68:1252–1258, 2007.
16. Povey RC: Effect of orally administered ribavirin on experimental FCV infection in cats, *Am J Vet Res* 39:1337–1341, 1978.

16a. Straw JA, Loo TL, de Vera CC, et al: Pharmacokinetics of potential anti-AIDS agents thiofoscarnet and foscarnet in the cat, *J Acquir Immune Defic Syndr* 5(9):936–942, 1992.

17. De Clercq E: New selective antiviral agents active against the AIDS virus, *Trends Pharm Sci* 8:339–345, 1987.
18. Zhang W, Maudin JK, Schmidt C, et al: Pharmacokinetics of zidovudine in cats, *Am J Vet Res* 66:835–840, 2004.
19. Zhang W, Maudin JK, Schmidt CW, et al: Pharmacokinetics of lamivudine in cats, *Am J Vet Res* 66:841–846, 2004.
20. Jordan HL, Pereira AS, Cohen MS, et al: Domestic cat model for predicting human nucleoside analogue pharmacokinetics in blood and seminal plasma, *Antimicrob Agents Chemother* 45(7):2173–2176, 2001.
21. Sellon RK, Hartmann K: Feline immunodeficiency virus infection. In Greene CE, editor: *Infectious diseases of the dog and cat*, ed 3, St Louis, 2006, Saunders.

21a. Zhu Y, Antony JM, Martinez JA, Glerum, et al: Didanosine causes sensory neuropathy in an HIV/AIDS animal model: impaired mitochondrial and neurotrophic factor gene expression, *Brain* 130(Pt 8):2011–2023, 2007.

22. Tavares L, Roneker C, Johnston K, et al: 3'-Azido-3'-deoxythymidine in feline leukemia virus-infected cats: a model for therapy and prophylaxis of AIDS, *Can Res* 47:3190–3194, 1987.

23. Wonderling R, Powell T, Baldwin S, et al: Cloning, expression, purification and biological activity of five feline IFN-alpha subtypes, *Vet Immunol Immunopathol* 89:13–27, 2002.
24. Baldwin SL, Powell TD, Sellins KS, et al: The biological effects of five feline IFN-alpha subtypes, *Vet Immunol Immunopathol* 99(3-4):153–167, 2004.
24a. Gingerich DA: Lymphocyte T-cell immunomodulator (LTCI): Review of the immunopharmacology of a new veterinary biologic, *Int J Vet Res* 6(2):61–68, 2008.
25. Robertson CM, Hermann LL, Coombs KM: Mycophenolic acid inhibits avian reovirus replication, *Antiviral Res* 64:55–61, 2004.
26. Martin V, Najbar W, Gueguen S, et al: Treatment of canine parvoviral enteritis with interferon-omega in a placebo-controlled challenge trial, *Vet Microbiol* 89(2–3):115–127, 2002.
27. de Mari K, Maynard L, Eun HM, et al: Treatment of canine parvoviral enteritis with interferon-omega in a placebo-controlled field trial, *Vet Rec* 152(4):105–108, 2003.
28. McCaw DL, Hoskins JD: Canine viral enteritis. In Greene CE, editor: *Infectious diseases of the dog and cat*, ed 3, St Louis, 2006, Saunders, pp 63–73.
29. Greene CE, Appel MJ: Canine distemper. In Greene CE, editor: *Infectious diseases of the dog and cat*, ed 3, St Louis, 2006, Saunders, pp 25–41.
30. Greene CE: Infectious canine hepatitis and canine acidophil cell hepatitis. In Greene CE, editor: *Infectious diseases of the dog and cat*, ed 3, St Louis, 2006, Saunders, pp 41–47.
31. Tanaka T, Nakatani S, Xuan X: Antiviral activity of lactoferrin against canine herpes virus, *Antiviral Res* 60:193–199, 2003.
32. Ford RB: Canine infectious tracheobronchitis. In Greene CE, editor: *Infectious diseases of the dog and cat*, ed 3, St Louis, 2006, Saunders, pp 54–61.
33. Megid J, Júnior JGD, Nardi G: Efficacy of canine papillomatosis treatment using *propionibacterium acnes (P. acnes)*. Paper presented at the *International Symposium on Predictive Oncology and Intervention Strategies*, February 7-10, Nice, France, 2004, in poster session 995 (Immunotherapy).
34. Yagci BB, Ural K, Öcal N, et al: Azithromycin therapy of papillomatosis in dogs: a prospective, randomized, double-blinded, placebo-controlled clinical trial, *Vet Dermatol* 19:194–198, 2008.
35. Greene CE, Addie DD: Feline parvovirus infections. In Greene CE, editor: *Infectious diseases of the dog and cat*, ed 3, St Louis, 2006, Saunders, pp 78–88.
36. Hartman K, Ritz S: Treatment of cats with feline infectious peritonitis, *Vet Immunol Immunopathol* 123:172–175, 2008.
37. Addie DD, Jarrett O: Feline coronavirus infection. In Greene CE, editor: *Infectious diseases of the dog and cat*, ed 3, St Louis, 2006, Saunders, pp 88–102.
37a. Truyen U, Addie D, Belák S, et al: Feline panleukopenia. ABCD guidelines on prevention and management, *J Feline Med Surg* 11(7):538–546, 2009.
38. Barlough JE, Shacklett BL: Antiviral studies of feline infectious peritonitis virus in vitro, *Vet Rec* 135(8):177–179, 1994.
39. Ishida T, Shibanai A, Tanaka S, et al: Use of recombinant feline interferon and glucocorticoid in the treatment of feline infectious peritonitis, *J Feline Med Surg* 6(2):107–109, 2004.
39a. Ritz S, Egberink H, Hartmann K: Effect of feline interferon-omega on the survival time and quality of life of cats with feline infectious peritonitis, *J Vet Intern Med* 21(6):1193–1197, 2007.
40. Gaskell RM, Dawson S, Radford A: Feline respiratory disease. In Greene CE, editor: *Infectious diseases of the dog and cat*, ed 3, St Louis, 2006, Saunders, pp 145–154.
40a. Radford AD, Addie D, Belák S, et al: Feline calicivirus infection. ABCD guidelines on prevention and management, *J Feline Med Surg* 11(7):556–564, 2009.
40b. Thiry E, Addie D, Belák S: Feline herpesvirus infection. ABCD guidelines on prevention and management, *J Feline Med Surg* Jul; 11(7):547–555, 2009.
41. Maggs DJ, Clarke HE: In vitro efficacy of ganciclovir, cidofovir, penciclovir, foscarnet, idoxuridine, and acyclovir against feline herpesvirus type-1, *Am J Vet Res* 65(4):399–403, 2004.
42. Sandmeyer LS, Keller CB, Bienzle D: Effects of cidofovir on cell death and replication of feline herpesvirus-1 in cultured feline corneal epithelial cells, *Am J Vet Res* 66(2):217–222, 2005.
43. van der Meulen K, Garre B, Croubels S, et al: In vitro comparison of antiviral drugs against feline herpesvirus 1, *BMC Vet Res* 2:13, 2006.
44. Williams DL, Fitzmaurice T, Lay L, et al: Efficacy of antiviral agents in feline herpetic keratitis: results of an in vitro study, *Curr Eye Res* 29(2-3):215–218, 2004.
45. Stiles J: Treatment of cats with ocular disease attributable to herpesvirus infection: 17 cases (1983-1993), *J Am Vet Med Assoc* 207(5):599–603, 1995.
46. Williams DL, Robinson JC, Lay E, et al: Efficacy of topical aciclovir for the treatment of feline herpetic keratitis: results of a prospective clinical trial and data from *in vitro* investigations, *Vet Rec* 157:254–257, 2005.
47. Stiles J: Ocular infections. In Green CE, editor: *Infectious diseases of the dog and cat*, ed 3, St Louis, 2006, Saunders, pp 974–991.
48. Caney SMA, Helps CR, Finerty S, et al: Treatment of asymptomatic chronically FIV-infected barrier-maintained cats with recombinant feline interferon omega, *J Vet Int Med* 17:423, 2003.
49. Maggs DJ, Nasisse MP, Kass PH: Efficacy of oral supplementation with L-lysine in cats latently infected with feline herpesvirus, *Am J Vet Res* 64:37–42, 2003.
50. Stiles J, Townsend WM, Rogers QR, Krohne SG: Effect of oral administration of L-lysine on conjunctivitis caused by feline herpesvirus in cats, *Am J Vet Res* 63:99–103, 2002.
51. Rees TM, Lubinski JL: Oral supplementation with L-lysine did not prevent upper respiratory infection in a shelter population of cats, *J Feline Med Surg* 10:510–513, 2008.
52. Sandmeyer LS, Keller CB, Bienzle D: Effects of interferon-α on cytopathic changes and titers for feline herpesvirus-1 in primary cultures of feline corneal epithelial cells, *Am J Vet Res* 66: 210–216, 2005.
53. Siebeck N, Hurley DJ, Garcia M, et al: Effects of human recombinant alpha-2b interferon and feline recombinant omega interferon on in vitro replication of feline herpesvirus-1, *Am J Vet Res* 67:1406–1411, 2006.
53a. Ohe K, Takahashi T, Hara D, et al: Sensitivity of FCV to recombinant feline interferon (rFeIFN), *Vet Res Commun* 32(2):167–174, 2008.
54. Hartmann K: Feline leukemia virus infection. In Greene CE, editor: *Infectious diseases of the dog and cat*, ed 3, St Louis, 2006, Saunders, pp 105–131.
55. Cogan DC: Effect of suramin on serum viral replication in feline leukemia virus-infected pet cats, *Am J Vet Res* 47:2230–2232, 1986.
56. Kociba GJ, Garg RC, Khan KNM, et al: Effects of orally administered interferon-α on the pathogenesis of feline leukaemia virus-induced erythroid aplasia, *Comp Haematol Inter* 5(2):79–83, 1995.
57. Pedretti E, Passeri B, Amadori M, et al: Low dose interferon-α treatment for feline immunodeficiency virus infection, *Vet Immunol Immunopathol* 109:245–254, 2006.
58. Cave TA, Gault EA, Argyle DJ: Feline epitheliotrophic T-cell lymphoma with paraneoplastic eosinophilia–immunochemotherapy with vinblastine and human recombinant interferon alpha2b, *Vet Comp Oncol* 2(2):91–97, 2004.
59. Macaw DL, Boon D, Jargons AE, et al: Immunomodulation therapy for feline leukemia virus infection, *J Am Anim Hosp Assoc* 37(4):356–363, 2001.
60. Blakeslee J, Noll G, Richard O: Autologous lymph node lymphocytes, *J Acquir Immune Defic Syndr Hum Retrovirol* 18(1):1–6, 1998.

61. Giannecchini S, Di Fenze A, D'Ursi AM, et al: Antiviral activity and conformational features of an octapeptide derived from the membrane-proximal ectodomain of the feline immunodeficiency virus transmembrane glycoprotein, *J Virology* 77(6):3724–3733, 2003.
62. Shimojima M, Miyazawa T, Ikeda Y, et al: Use of CD134 as a primary receptor by the feline immunodeficiency virus, *Science* 20; 303(5661):1192–1195, 2004.
63. Louie M, Markowitz M: Goals and milestones during treatment of HIV-1 infection with antiretroviral therapy: a pathogenesis-based perspective, *Antiviral Res* 55:15–25, 2002.
64. LaCasse RA, Remington KM, North TW: The mutation frequency of feline immunodeficiency virus enhanced by 3'-Azido-3'-deoxythymidine, *J Acquir Immune Defic Syndr Hum Retrovirol* 12(1):26–32, 1996.
65. Hayes KA, Phipps AJ, Francke S, et al: Antiviral therapy reduces viral burden but does not prevent thymic involution in young cats infected with feline, *Immunodefic Virus Antimicrob Agents Chemother* 44(9):2399–2405, 2000.
66. Arai M, Earl DD, Yamamoto JK: Is AZT/3TC therapy effective against FIV infection or immunopathogenesis? *Vet Immunol Immunopathol* 85(3-4):189–204, 2002.
67. Tanabe T: Feline immunodeficiency virus lacks sensitivity to the antiviral activity of feline IFN-γ, *J Interferon Cytokine Res* 21(12):1039–1046, 2001.
68. de Mari K, Maynard L, Sanquer A, et al: Therapeutic effects of recombinant feline interferon-v on feline leukemia virus (FeLV)-infected and FeLV/feline immunodeficiency virus (FIV)-coinfected symptomatic, *J Vet Intern Med* 18:477–482, 2004.
69. Stengel C, Klein D, Egerbink H: Placebo-controlled double blind treatment study in naturally feline immunodeficiency virus infected cats using the chemokin receptor inhibitor 1,1-Bis 1,4,8,11-tetra-azacylotetradekan (AMD3100), *J Vet Int Med* 17:381, 2003.
69a. Gfuffydd-Jones T, Hartmann K, Hosie MJ, et al: Feline leukaemia. ABCD guidelines on prevention and management, *J Feline Med Surg* 11(7):565–574, 2009.
70. Georgiou N, van der Bruggen T, Oudshoorn M, et al: Mechanism of inhibition of the human immunodeficiency virus type 1 by the oxygen radical generating agent bleomycin, *Antiviral Res* 63:97–106, 2004.
71. Artmann K, Kuffer M, Balzarini J: Efficacy of the acyclic nucleoside phosphonates(S) -9- (3-fluoro-2- phosphonylmethoxypropyl)adenine(FPMPA)and-(2-phosphonylmethoxyethyl)adenine (PMEA) against feline immunodeficiency virus, *J Acquir Immune Defic Syndr Hum Retrovirol* 17(2):120–128, 1998.
72. Pedersen NC, North TW, Rigg R, et al: 10-16alpha-Bromo-epiandrosterone therapy modulates experimental feline immunodeficiency virus viremia: initial enhancement leading to long-term suppression, *Vet Immunol Immunopathol* 94(3-4):133–148, 2003.
73. Hosie MJ, Addie D, Belák S, et al: Feline immunodeficiency. ABCD guidelines on prevention and management, *J Feline Med Surg* 11(7):575–584, 2009.
74. Thiry E, Addie D, Belák S, et al: H5N1 avian influenza in cats. ABCD guidelines on prevention and management, *J Feline Med Surg* 11(7):615–618, 2009.

Disinfectants, Antiseptics, and Related Biocides

11

Harry W. Boothe

Chapter Outline

Disinfectants, antiseptics, and biocides are expected to play an even more important role in the future in controlling microbes in both the veterinary patient and hospital.[1] When used properly, disinfectants, antiseptics, and biocides contribute to both the prevention and the treatment of disease. Despite the fact that there are as many as 300 biocidal products available, about 14 of these are in more than 90% of the registered products in the United States.[2] The veterinary clinician need be familiar with relatively few biocidal products to make an informed decision regarding their selection and use.

DEFINITIONS

Definitions of appropriate terms, characteristics of disinfectants and antiseptics by chemical type, factors affecting disinfection and antisepsis, and disinfection and antiseptic practices germane to veterinary practice are reviewed in this chapter (Box 11-1). It is hoped that through greater understanding of the properties of disinfectants and antiseptics, veterinary clinicians will use them appropriately.

The distinction between disinfectants and antiseptics is not always clear (Table 11-1). Antiseptics are usually the weakest and least toxic of the surface antimicrobials.[3] Antiseptics may be used on intact skin or mucous membranes before a surgical procedure or in the treatment of open wounds. Regardless of their use, antiseptics should exert a sustained effect against microorganisms without causing tissue damage.[4] Although some specific biocides may be used as both disinfectants and antiseptics (e.g., alcohols and iodines), it is not generally recommended that an antiseptic be used for the purpose of disinfection, and vice versa.

KEY POINT 11-1 Use of an antiseptic for the purpose of disinfection, and vice versa, is generally *not* recommended.

CHARACTERISTICS OF DISINFECTANTS AND ANTISEPTICS BY CHEMICAL TYPE

The characteristics of the following 10 types of disinfectants, antiseptics, and biocides are presented: alcohols, aldehyde compounds (formaldehyde and glutaraldehyde), chlorhexidine, chlorine and chlorine compounds, ethylenediaminetetraacetate (EDTA), ethylene oxide, iodine and iodine compounds, peroxygen compounds (including hydrogen peroxide), phenols (including bisphenols and halophenols), and quaternary ammonium compounds. Mechanism of action (presumed or established), classification as to level of biocidal activity, commonly available preparations, efficacy, and uses are presented for each chemical type (Figure 11-1).

Alcohols

Alcohols possess the following features desirable for a disinfectant: bactericidal action against vegetative forms, relative inexpensivness, ease of availability, and relative nontoxicity when used topically.[5] Alcohols are used alone or in combination with phenols, chlorhexidine, iodines, and quaternary ammonium compounds.[6] Alcohols appear to exhibit their antimicrobial effect by denaturing proteins. Lysis of some microorganisms may occur, although the bacteriostatic action of alcohols is due to the inhibition of cell metabolites. Some water is required for alcohols to be most effective. Alcohols are considered to have intermediate-level biocidal activity. Two forms of alcohol are used most commonly: ethyl alcohol and isopropyl alcohol. Ethyl alcohol has enhanced virucidal properties and reduced toxicity compared with isopropyl alcohol, which has slightly greater bactericidal action.

When used alone, alcohols are more effective antiseptics than disinfectants. Alcohols are not good cleaning agents and are not recommended in the presence of physical dirt.[7]

Box 11-1

Disinfection and Antisepsis Definitions

Sterilization: The act or process, physical or chemical, that destroys or eliminates all forms of life, especially microorganisms.

Disinfection: The killing of pathogenic agents by chemical or physical means directly applied. Disinfection processes differ from sterilization procedures, primarily in their lack of sporicidal activity.

Disinfectant: An agent, usually chemical, that frees from infection by destroying disease-producing or other harmful microorganisms. This term generally refers to substances applied to inanimate objects.

High-level disinfectant: An agent that has effectiveness against bacterial endospores under the proper conditions. High-level disinfectants are to be used on critical items (items that, if contaminated, impart a substantial risk of infection to the patient).

Intermediate-level disinfectant: An agent that inactivates the tubercle bacillus but does not necessarily kill bacterial spores. These disinfectants may be used on semicritical items, which carry an intermediate risk of inducing infection in the patient.

Low-level disinfectant: An agent that rapidly kills vegetative forms of bacteria and fungi but cannot be relied on within a practical period of time to destroy bacterial endospores, tubercle bacillus, or small nonlipid viruses. These disinfectants are indicated only for use on noncritical items that carry relatively little risk of inducing infection in the patient.

Antiseptic: A substance that prevents or arrests the growth or action of microorganisms on living tissue either by inhibiting their activity or by destroying them.

Biocide: A chemical or physical agent, usually broad spectrum, that inactivates microorganisms.

(From Block SS: *Disinfection, sterilization, and preservation*, ed 5, Philadelphia, 2001, Lippincott Williams & Wilkins; and Greene CE: *Infectious diseases of the dog and cat*, ed 3, St Louis, 2006, Saunders)

Table 11-1 Categorization of Biocides: Disinfectants, Antiseptics, or Both

Biocides Most Appropriately Used as Disinfectants	Biocides Most Appropriately Used as Antiseptics	Biocides Effective as Both Disinfectants and Antiseptics
Aldehyde compounds (formaldehyde and glutaraldehyde)	Chlorhexidine	Alcohols
Chlorine and chlorine compounds	Dilute sodium hypochlorite solution (Dakin's solution)	Chloroxylenols
Ethylene oxide	EDTA	Iodines
Hydrogen peroxide	Iodophors	
Phenols		
Quaternary ammonium compounds		

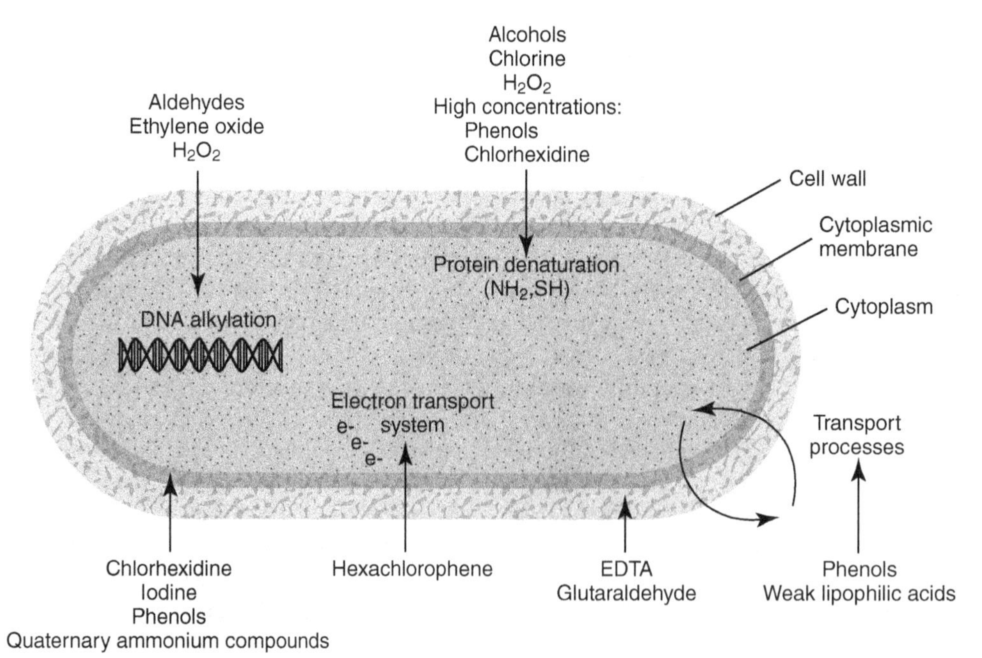

Figure 11-1 Diagram showing targets within the microbe for selected disinfectants, antiseptics, and biocides.

Alcohols are widely used for both hard-surface disinfections and skin antisepsis.[8] In appropriate concentrations, alcohols provide the most rapid and greatest reduction in microbial counts on intact skin. Alcohols should not be used in open wounds. Alcohols should be allowed to evaporate thoroughly from the skin to be fully effective and to decrease irritation.[7] Because of their inability to destroy bacterial spores, alcohols are not recommended for disinfection of surgical instruments.

Aldehyde Compounds (Formaldehyde and Glutaraldehyde)

Formaldehyde (3% to 8% solutions) exhibits intermediate-level to high-level disinfection. It is sporicidal, with its mechanism of action being the ability to combine with protein, RNA, and DNA in the spore.[9] Formaldehyde does not penetrate well, and its fumes are irritating.[6] It is used infrequently as a disinfectant in veterinary hospitals.

Glutaraldehyde (1,5-pentanedial) has been used as a chemosterilizing agent for approximately 40 years.[10,11] It displays potent bactericidal, fungicidal, virucidal, mycobactericidal, and sporicidal activity.[11-13] Glutaraldehyde acts on proteins by denaturation and on nucleic acids by alkylation.[14] It is classified as an intermediate-level to high-level biocide.

Factors that influence the activity of glutaraldehyde include time of contact, temperature, concentration, pH, and the presence of soiling material.[12] Glutaraldehyde shows a very marked, temperature-dependent activity.[12] The pH affects the stability and biocidal activity of glutaraldehyde. Glutaraldehyde is more stable at acid pH, but it is more active at alkaline pH (around 8 to 8.5). As pH increases, the number of reactive sites to which glutaraldehyde binds is increased, thus enhancing its lethal effect.[12] At alkaline pH, glutaraldehyde penetrates more extensively into the spore, where it fixes the cortex.[11] The negative effect of organic matter is more apparent when lower concentrations of glutaraldehyde are used. Alkaline glutaraldehyde (2%) takes longer to be effective in the presence of organic matter.[6] Glutaraldehyde has a dual role against bacterial biofilms (a characteristic of some bacteria that makes them more resistant to disinfection): an ability to penetrate the biofilm and inhibit microbial cells protected by the film and an acceleration of the detachment rate of bacteria from the biofilm.[12]

Disinfectants containing 2% glutaraldehyde are considered high-level disinfectants, with recommended contact times of 10 to 30 minutes. Exposure times of 6 to 10 hours frequently result in sterilization. Glutaraldehyde is used widely as a disinfectant for heat-labile equipment (e.g., endoscopes). Glutaraldehyde disinfectants are not as noxious, irritating to the skin, or corrosive as formaldehyde; however, precautions should be taken with their use. Gloves, safety goggles, and proper ventilation are recommended to minimize risks to those disinfecting the equipment, and glutaraldehyde-disinfected equipment should be thoroughly rinsed with sterile water before use to reduce risk to the patient.[11] Stabilized glutaraldehyde solutions are safe and effective preoperative skin antiseptics for elective clean-contaminated surgical procedures in dogs.[15]

KEY POINT 11-2 Under proper conditions, 2% glutaraldehyde is considered a high-level disinfectant.

Chlorhexidine

Chlorhexidine is a cationic bisbiguanide, not related to hexachlorophene, that was first synthesized in 1950.[16] It is available as a solution and as a scrubbing agent. Chlorhexidine solution is used principally as a topical antiseptic on skin wounds and mucous membranes, but it is also used as a pharmaceutical preservative. Chlorhexidine scrub is used to preoperatively prepare the surgeon and patient. Chlorhexidine exhibits a broad spectrum of antibacterial activity, strong binding to the skin, ability to adsorb to negatively charged surfaces in the mouth (e.g., tooth and oral mucosa), persistence, low toxicity, and a minimal negative effect on activity by blood or other organic material.[7] Chlorhexidine has its major antibacterial action by interference with the function of cellular membranes, with the primary site of action being the cytoplasmic membrane.[8,13,14,16,17] Rupture of the cytoplasmic membrane of the microbe occurs without lysis of the cell wall. Chlorhexidine has low-level to intermediate-level biocidal activity.

Chlorhexidine has a very rapid bactericidal effect as well as persistence of action.[14] It has limited fungicidal and virucidal properties.[6] Chlorhexidine is more effective against gram-positive than gram-negative bacteria and exhibits a bacteriostatic effect against some bacteria.[6,7] Acquired resistance to chlorhexidine has been observed, notably in staphylococci.[8,18] The optimum range of pH for activity of chlorhexidine is 5.5 to 7. Chlorhexidine is incompatible with anionic detergents and inorganic anionic compounds;[6] thus standing soap lather should be removed by rinsing before chlorhexidine solution is applied to the skin. Chlorhexidine forms a precipitate when diluted with electrolyte solutions, but this precipitate does not affect antimicrobial activity.[19]

Chlorhexidine is available as an alcoholic solution (scrub) that is used in the preoperative skin preparation of the surgeon and patient and as an aqueous solution. Two preparations that are used commonly in veterinary hospitals are chlorhexidine gluconate (scrub) and chlorhexidine diacetate or gluconate (solution). There are few reports of adverse reactions with chlorhexidine. Chlorhexidine scrub should be used only on intact skin, never in wounds. Negligible absorption from the alimentary tract occurs, and the incidences of skin irritation and hypersensitivity are low. Chlorhexidine is ototoxic when placed in the middle ear cavity, and its use on the brain or meninges is contraindicated. In general, chlorhexidine solution (0.05%) is an effective and well-tolerated wound antiseptic in veterinary patients.[19,20]

KEY POINT 11-3 Chlorhexidine solution (0.05%) is generally an effective and well-tolerated wound antiseptic.

Chlorine and Chlorine Compounds

Chlorine disinfectants are readily available, inexpensive, have a broad antimicrobial spectrum, and present minimal environmental hazards.[3] Mechanism of action appears to be through oxidation of peptide links and denaturation of proteins.[14] Intracellular accumulation results in inhibition of essential enzyme systems.[13] Chlorine compounds are classified as intermediate-level disinfectants. Two factors that affect the biocidal activity of chlorine are pH and the presence of organic material. The greatest influence on the antimicrobial activity of chlorine in solution appears to be pH. With decreasing pH there is increasing biocidal activity. This increased activity at lower pH is due to a higher concentration of undissociated hypochlorous acid, which has a greater bactericidal action than the dissociated form. Organic matter consumes available chlorine and reduces its antibacterial efficacy.[21] This negative effect is particularly evident in solutions with low levels of chlorine. Small additions of iodine or bromine to chlorine solutions greatly enhance their bactericidal activity.[21]

Sodium hypochlorite appears to be the chlorine compound most frequently used as a disinfectant in veterinary hospitals. It is an effective virucidal agent.[22] Sodium hypochlorite was first introduced as an antiseptic in 1915 as Dakin's solution (0.4% available chlorine).[23] Although still used as a wound antiseptic, sodium hypochlorite is used more frequently as a disinfectant in veterinary hospitals as a 0.16% solution (1:32 dilution of 5.25% stock solution) of liquid bleach.

EDTA

EDTA, especially in combination with Tris buffer ([hydroxymethyl]aminomethane), has been shown to have antibacterial properties, particularly against certain gram-negative bacteria. Tris-EDTA acts by increasing cell wall and membrane permeability through chelation of divalent cations and by slowing degradation of ribosomes.[13,24,25] The clinical use of Tris-EDTA has been limited largely to four major pathogens: *Pseudomonas aeruginosa, Proteus vulgaris, Escherichia coli,* and *Staphylococcus aureus.*[24] Tris-EDTA decreases the minimal inhibitory concentration for these bacteria when selected antimicrobials are added in vitro.[26] It also potentiates the antimicrobials effects of chlorhexidine diacetate in lavage solutions.[27]

Tris-EDTA solution is inexpensive and readily available. It has been used as an irrigant in combination with antimicrobials in the treatment of otitis externa, bacterial rhinitis, and multiple fistulae in dogs.[24] Formulations of other biocidal agents (e.g., chloroxylenol) may contain EDTA. Such preparations have enhanced efficacy against *P. aeruginosa* organisms.[28]

Ethylene Oxide

Recognition of the biocidal activity of ethylene oxide did not take place until more than 60 years after its discovery in the 1850s. Ethylene oxide was patented in the United States in 1936 for use as a gas-phase biocide.[10] It is a high-level disinfectant when used under proper conditions. Variables that are critical to the action of ethylene oxide include prehumidification, temperature, and concentration. Ethylene oxide sterilization is used for heat-labile equipment. Ethylene oxide is an alkylating agent that exhibits its bactericidal and sporicidal activities because of its reaction with nucleic acids.[8,29] It may be combined with either carbon dioxide or fluorocarbons. Because of its toxicity, mutagenicity, carcinogenicity, and capacity to irritate eyes and mucous membranes, ethylene oxide sterilization for heat-labile equipment is being challenged by other, safer techniques, such as plasma sterilization (see later discussion of peroxygen compounds).

Iodine and Iodine Compounds

The first reference to the use of iodine for wounds was made in 1839.[10,30] Iodine is an excellent, prompt, effective biocide with a broad range of action. Of the seven different forms of iodine that are present in pure aqueous iodine solutions, only two play a role in the disinfection processes: molecular iodine (I_2) and hypoiodic acid (HOI). Molecular iodine has superior sporicidal and cysticidal properties compared with HOI. Iodine acts by decreasing the oxygen requirements of aerobic microorganisms.[14] Iodine also interacts preferentially with thiol groups in proteins of the cytoplasmic membrane.[14,30,31] Although bacterial resistance to iodine seems to be uncommon, bacterial resistance to povidone–iodine has been reported.[18] Iodine has comparatively low reactivity with proteins, except blood, and pH has little effect on antimicrobial efficacy. Blood reduces the efficacy of iodine by converting it into nonbactericidal iodide.

KEY POINT 11-4 Use of iodophor in body cavities is *not* recommended.

Two main groups of iodine preparations are used clinically: preparations releasing free iodine and those containing complex-bound iodine. Preparations that release free iodine have intermediate-level biocidal activity. Preparations that release free iodine include *iodine topical solution,* an aqueous solution containing 2% iodine and 2.4% sodium iodide; *strong iodine solution (Lugol's solution),* an aqueous solution containing 5% iodine and 10% potassium iodide; *iodine tincture,* containing 2% iodine and 2.4% sodium iodide in aqueous ethanol (1:1); and *strong iodine tincture,* containing 7% iodine and 5% potassium iodide in 95% ethanol. Iodine tincture preparations are both more efficacious and more toxic than aqueous solutions, including iodophors.

Preparations containing complex-bound iodine have low-level to intermediate-level activity. Iodophors are the most commonly used preparations that contain complex-bound iodine. The iodine in iodophors is bound to a carrier of high molecular weight (e.g., polyvinylpyrrolidone). Such carriers tend to increase the solubility of iodine; provide a sustained-release reservoir; reduce the equilibrium concentration of free molecular iodine; improve the wetting properties of the iodine; and aid in penetration of iodine in organic soil, including fat.[30]

The best known iodophor is povidone–iodine. Povidone–iodine compounds have a pH of about 5. The bactericidal properties of iodophors depend on the liberation of free iodine.[32] The amount of free iodine in iodophor preparations depends on concentration, being greatest in a 0.07% solution of povidone–iodine.[33] Dilutions of iodophors demonstrate more rapid bactericidal action than a full-strength povidone–iodine solution.[34] Although in vitro studies have shown povidone–iodine to be highly effective against selective bacteria, including methicillin-resistant *S. aureus,*[35] in vivo studies provide conflicting data regarding efficacy.[23] LeVeen et al.[32] conclude that on the basis of clinical and experimental evidence, free iodine is not liberated from povidone–iodine in therapeutic concentrations. Clinical studies indicate that povidone–iodine is suitable as an antiseptic on intact skin.[32]

Iodine-containing preparations, particularly iodophors, are used frequently as antiseptics. Iodophors are available in a variety of forms, including 10% solution, 2% cleansing solution (scrub), and 2% aerosol spray. Presurgical skin disinfection of surgeon and patient, disinfection of mucous membranes, and wound disinfection are the most common uses of iodophors. Povidone–iodine also has been reviewed favorably as an oral antiseptic.[36] Cutaneous absorption of iodine, particularly in traumatized skin, can lead to increased serum iodine levels. Systemic iodine toxicity is also possible when iodophors are used to treat large, open wounds.[23] Also, iodophors produce adverse effects when placed in the peritoneal cavity; hence their use in the peritoneal cavity is not recommended.[32]

Peroxygen Compounds

Hydrogen peroxide has historical and current application as a disinfectant and antiseptic. As a 3% solution, hydrogen peroxide has limited bactericidal effectiveness and is usually classified as an intermediate-level biocide.[23] It is an oxidizing agent and acts by denaturing proteins and lipids of microorganisms.[14,29] Hydrogen peroxide (3%) provides an effervescent cleansing action; however, because of its cytotoxicity, hydrogen peroxide is inappropriate as an antiseptic.[23,37] As a 58% solution, however, and in the presence of an electromagnetic field, hydrogen peroxide becomes a gas plasma. As a gas plasma, hydrogen peroxide destroys microorganisms and is classified as a high-level disinfectant. Hydrogen peroxide (58% solution) is sporicidal by virtue of its effect on the outer spore layers and the spore core.[38] Because the process temperature associated with plasma sterilization does not exceed 50° C, plasma sterilization is particularly well suited to heat-labile materials that cannot be steam sterilized.[39] Because of its relative safety, plasma sterilization is emerging as an alternative to ethylene oxide gas in the sterilization of heat-labile articles. Other peroxygen compounds, such as peracetic acid and ozone, have limited use in veterinary medicine.

Phenols

Carbolic acid, a phenol, is the oldest example of an antiseptic compound.[40] Phenols have a wide spectrum of activity against bacteria, viruses, and fungi, but they have minimal sporicidal activity.[6] They act on the cytoplasmic membrane, producing leakage and disrupting membrane transport.[13] Phenols are classified as low-level to intermediate-level biocides. While used sparingly in veterinary medicine, phenolic biocides are still widely used throughout the world.[41] Two classes of phenol derivatives that have potential interest are the bisphenols (e.g., triclosan and hexachlorophene) and halophenols (chloroxylenol).[8]

Triclosan, a broad-spectrum antimicrobial agent, is used as a topical antiseptic and is frequently formulated with EDTA.[8,42] Hexachlorophene, a chlorinated phenol derivative, was used as a presurgical antiseptic primarily by surgeons, but its toxicity has limited its use.[43] Chloroxylenol has been used extensively as a preservative, disinfectant, and topical antiseptic.[28]

Quaternary Ammonium Compounds

Introduced in 1916, quaternary ammonium compounds are surface-active cations that exhibit low-level biocidal activity.[10] They bind irreversibly to the phospholipids and proteins of the cytoplasmic membrane of microbes, impairing permeability.[13,14] Quaternary ammonium compounds are much more effective in preventing the growth of bacteria than in killing them, and they are far more effective against gram-positive than gram-negative bacteria.[6] Quaternary ammonium compounds possess a narrow margin of safety and can fail when exposed to resistant microorganisms.[43]

Quaternary ammonium compounds with a carbon chain length of 14 demonstrate the highest level of bactericidal activity.[44] They were used initially as an adjunct to surgery, such as in presurgical patient preparation, but this use has been curtailed, in part because of the observation that skin bacteria survive beneath the layer of applied quaternary ammonium compound. Additionally, quaternary ammonium compounds tend to be inactivated by lipids in organic matter, and their activity is adversely affected by soap, hard water, and gauze.[43] Quaternary ammonium compounds are currently used primarily for environmental disinfection of floors, walls, and equipment surfaces. Benzalkonium chloride is used as a topical antifungal agent for horses at a concentration of 0.15%.

FACTORS AFFECTING DISINFECTION AND ANTISEPSIS

A successful disinfection plan requires initial consideration of microbial susceptibility and environmental conditions.[45] Factors of importance when selecting a chemical biocide include the degree of microbial killing required; the nature and composition of the surface item or device to be treated; amount of organic matter present; number and resistance of microorganisms present; presence of microbial biofilms; and cost, safety, and ease of use of the available agents.[2] Critical items, which, if contaminated, impart a substantial risk of infection, must be sterilized. Noncritical items, which touch only the intact skin of the patient during routine use, can be disinfected. The greater the risk of infection associated with the use of a device, the more complete must be the degree of microbial killing on that device. The nature and composition of the device or surface to be treated affects the ease with which that device may be disinfected. Smooth, nonporous, and cleanable surfaces (e.g., table surfaces) are easiest to disinfect, whereas crevices, joints, and pores (e.g., surgical clamps) constitute barriers to the penetration of liquid biocides.[2]

The amount of organic material present has a major impact on the efficacy of most disinfectants. Physical cleaning before disinfection is often the most important step in the disinfection process.[2] Endoscopes and accessories are particularly challenging to clean properly. Organic material has an especially profound effect on the biocidal efficacy of chlorine and iodine-based disinfectants and quaternary ammonium compounds.[2]

Negative effects of organic material are particularly profound with weak concentrations and with low-level disinfectants.

The number and resistance of microorganisms present can influence biocidal efficacy. In general, the higher the level of microbial contamination, the longer must be the exposure to the chemical biocide before the entire microbial population is killed.[2] Microorganisms vary widely in their resistance to chemical biocides, with bacterial spores being most resistant, then protozoal cysts, coccidial oocysts, tubercle bacilli, small nonlipid viruses, fungi, vegetative bacteria, and medium-size lipid viruses.[37] Differences in resistance exhibited by various vegetative bacteria are relatively minor, with staphylococci and enterococci being the more resistant gram-positive bacteria and *Pseudomonas, Proteus, Klebsiella, Enterobacter,* and *Serratia* spp. showing greater resistance than other gram-negative bacteria.[2,8] The resistance of some bacteria, such as *Pseudomonas* and *Serratia* spp., may relate in part to the production of a glycocalyx-based biofilm.[8,43,46]

Some bacteria (e.g., *Klebsiella pneumoniae, Serratia* and *Pseudomonas* spp.) produce biofilms.[43,47,48] Biofilms are collections of bacteria in a community that form in an exopolysaccharide extracellular matrix.[48] They surround bacteria and make them more resistant to disinfection. Biofilms may be encountered in medical implants, such as catheters, sutures, and orthopedic prostheses, and seem to present a barrier to penetration by disinfectants and antiseptics.[8,25,43,46,48] Biofilms serve as nidi of contamination as well as sources of bacterial products, such as toxins.[48] The reduced accessibility of the bacteria included in the biofilm appears to be the major factor in resistance development.[47] Resistance depends on the nature of the disinfectant, with greater resistance reported with selected quaternary ammonium compounds (e.g., benzalkonium chloride) and less resistance with oxidizing agents (e.g., sodium hypochlorite and hydrogen peroxide) and phenolic derivatives.[47] Intrinsic and acquired resistances to disinfectants have been observed, notably *Staphylococci, Pseudomonas,* and *Enterobacter* spp.[3,8,18,46] Potential for acquired bacterial resistance is rated very low, low, and moderate for alcohols, triclosan, and chlorhexidine, respectively.[42] Although concerns about the use of chlorhexidine, triclosan (a bisphenol), and quaternary ammonium compounds and possible bacterial resistance to them and to antimicrobials have been raised,[49] antimicrobial-resistant pathogens (e.g., methicillin-resistant *S. aureus*) did not demonstrate resistance to biocides at the currently used contact times and concentrations.[34]

Cost may be a factor in selection of disinfectants and antiseptics. One of the major impacts on cost of a disinfection procedure is the dilution of biocide used. Although overdilution of a biocide will reduce its net cost, overdilution may also significantly reduce its biocidal potency. The manufacturer's recommendations should be followed when diluting a biocide. Selection of biocides should be based primarily on efficacy and safety, not cost. Ease of use of a biocide can affect disinfection practices. Those agents with wider safety margins are likely to be easier to use. Other causes of disinfection failure include poor disinfectant penetration or coverage, insufficient contact time, and inadequate temperature and humidity while the disinfectant is being applied.[3,46]

DISINFECTION AND ANTISEPTIC PRACTICES

Veterinary Hospital Disinfection

Types of disinfection practices in a veterinary hospital include immersion disinfection; disinfection of surfaces, including cabinets, tables (examination, treatment, and surgery), kennels, lights, and chairs; and environmental disinfection.[40] Agents that have been used for immersion disinfection include 2% alkaline glutaraldehyde, isopropyl alcohol (thermometers), chlorhexidine diacetate, and quaternary ammonium compounds. Of these agents, only 2% alkaline glutaraldehyde is reliable. Because the disinfection of surgical instruments by immersion lacks the safety of heat-pressure sterilization, immersion disinfection is not recommended for instruments to be used during aseptic surgery.

Surface disinfection in a veterinary hospital can be particularly important in minimizing spread of disease. Thorough cleaning of the surface before disinfection is a critical step. Other factors that improve the efficacy of surface disinfection include adequately covering the surface with the disinfectant and maintaining contact for a sufficient time. Agents that are used as surface disinfectants include sodium hypochlorite and quaternary ammonium compounds. Sodium hypochlorite is used as a 0.16% solution (1:32 dilution of 5.25% solution) of liquid bleach to disinfect kennels and tables. Such a solution has been shown to be effective in neutralizing parvovirus.[50] Quaternary ammonium compounds are surfactants that have both cleansing and disinfecting properties. Despite their cleansing properties, quaternary ammonium compounds have reduced biocidal efficacy in the presence of organic material; hence cleaning of surfaces before their use is indicated. Quaternary ammonium compounds have been recommended for the routine disinfection of environmental surfaces.[43] Effective environmental disinfection of large-animal holding facilities using a peroxygen compound (4% peroxymonosulfate) has been described.[51]

Surgical Antisepsis

Surgical antisepsis is the application of antimicrobial chemicals to skin, mucosa, and wounds to reduce the risk of infection.[52] Surgical antisepsis most commonly involves the removal or reduction of normal flora by the topical application of antimicrobial substances to the intact skin before a surgical procedure. Distinguishing between antiseptic use on intact skin and that on mucous membranes or in wounds is important. Different formulations and concentrations of antiseptics are indicated depending on their use. Preparations containing alcohol or detergents (scrubs) are to be used only on intact skin. The concentration of antiseptic used in wounds is less, in general, than that of preparations applied to intact skin.

Surgical Preparation of the Skin

The purpose of a surgical hand scrub or alcohol-based hand rub is to remove transient flora and reduce resident flora for the duration of surgery in case of glove tears.[7,53] Regardless of the biocidal agent used, the technique of hand washing is important. The primary problem with hand hygiene is not a paucity of good products but rather the laxity of practice.[7] Nails should be short, and artificial nails and nail polish are discouraged.[7] Debris should be removed from under the fingernails with a nail cleaner after the hands and forearms have been washed thoroughly. The subungual area has higher microbial counts, and contamination of the hands can increase when gloves create a warm, moist environment.[7,40] Duration of washing is important both for mechanical action and to allow antimicrobial products sufficient contact time to achieve the desired effect.[7] Although the American College of Surgeons suggests that a surgical scrub of 120 seconds, including brushing of the nail and fingertip areas, is adequate,[7] longer scrubs may be performed by veterinary surgeons.

Selection of an appropriate biocidal agent for surgical hand scrubbing should be made in three stages: One should determine what characteristics are desired, review and evaluate the evidence of safety and efficacy in reducing microbial counts, and consider the personnel acceptance of the product and the costs.[7] Antiseptic treatment of the skin should not be toxic, should not cause skin reactions, and should not interfere with the normal protective function of the skin.[52] Antiseptic agents used to prepare the skin of the surgeon or patient include alcohols, chlorhexidine, iodophors, and chloroxylenols.

Alcohols, in appropriate concentrations (60% to 90%), provide the most rapid and greatest reduction in microbial counts on skin.[7,52] Alcohols are not good cleansing agents, and they are not recommended in the presence of physical dirt. They should be allowed to evaporate thoroughly from the skin to be fully effective and to decrease irritation.[7] Immersion of the surgeon's hands and arms in alcohol has been shown to be an effective technique.[7] Waterless, alcohol-based hand rinse products (rubs) effectively reduce microbial counts on skin.[54] Hand rubs have been shown to be effective within application times of 90 to 180 seconds.[53] Alcohol is also used on the intact skin of the veterinary patient before surgery as a defatting agent.[55]

Chlorhexidine gluconate has both rapid and persistent antibacterial activity when used as a presurgical scrub. Its persistence is probably the best of any agent currently available for hand washing.[7] The activity of chlorhexidine is not significantly affected by blood or other organic material.[7] The incidence of skin irritation to chlorhexidine scrub seems low. Chlorhexidine scrub may be the ideal agent for surgical preparation of the skin.[33] Both 2% and 4% formulations in a detergent base are readily available.

Iodophors, particularly povidone–iodine, are used frequently in the presurgical preparation of surgeons and veterinary patients. The antimicrobial effects of iodophors are similar to those of iodine. Recommended levels of free iodine for antiseptics are 1 to 2 mg/L.[7] Povidone–iodine scrub has been found to be equally effective as chlorhexidine gluconate scrub in reducing the number of bacteria on canine skin for up to 1 hour after application.[56] Iodophors are rapidly neutralized in the presence of organic materials such as blood.[7] They have a propensity toward skin irritation, and cutaneous absorption can cause thyroid dysfunction. Iodophors are available as a surgical scrub (2%) and as a solution (10% and 2%).

Chloroxylenols and bisphenols are synthetic phenol derivatives that have been used sparingly as a presurgical scrub of surgeons and veterinary patients. They are less effective than either chlorhexidine or iodophors in reducing skin flora, but chloroxylenols may have a lower incidence of skin irritation than iodophors.[7] Their activity is only minimally affected by organic matter.[7] Formulations used as a presurgical scrub include 3% chloroxylenol, 1.5% parachlorometaxylenol, and 1% to 2% triclosan.[7,42]

Surgical Preparation of Mucous Membranes

Antisepsis of mucous membranes, particularly the oral mucosa, presents particular problems. The bacterial colonization of the oral cavity is very high, and the efficacy of oral antiseptics is affected by dilution effects as well as inactivation due to salivary proteins.[36] Also, an increase in antiseptic concentration is limited by local irritation and a high absorption rate with the risk of systemic intoxication.[36] Only a few solutions are useful as oral antiseptics: povidone–iodine, chlorhexidine, and hexetidine.[36] Povidone–iodine solution has been shown to reduce inflammation and the progression of periodontal disease as well as bacteremia after dental extractions.[36]

Chlorhexidine solution is an effective agent for the prevention and treatment of oral disease.[16] Its effectiveness stems from its ability to adsorb to negatively charged surfaces in the mouth, such as the tooth and mucosa. Hexetidine is used as a 0.1% solution for local infections and oral hygiene. It has been shown to have similar antimicrobial efficacy against common buccal organisms as 0.2% chlorhexidine.[57]

Wound Antisepsis

When topically treating a contaminated wound with an antiseptic solution, the clinician should choose an appropriate type and concentration of antiseptic that has both antibacterial properties and minimal negative effects on wound healing. Antiseptics that appear to fulfill these criteria include chlorhexidine solution, povidone–iodine solution, and sodium hypochlorite solution (Dakin's solution). Chlorhexidine diacetate solution (0.05%) has a wide spectrum of antimicrobial activity as well as minimal deleterious effects on wound healing.[58] Its sustained residual activity seems to be an advantage in wound therapy. Dilution of the stock solution with sterile water, 0.9% sodium chloride, or lactated Ringer's solution does not adversely affect its antibacterial activity.[19]

Povidone–iodine solution appears to be most effective and least tissue toxic in concentrations of 0.1% to 1%.[33] Povidone–iodine concentrations greater than 0.5% are cytotoxic to the canine fibroblast in vitro.[33] Povidone–iodine should be used judiciously on large wounds because of the potential for systemic absorption of iodine.

A dilute Dakin's solution (0.005% sodium hypochlorite) has been shown to be both bactericidal and not damaging to fibroblasts.[58] Dakin's solution has been used as an effective irrigant for human wounds since World War I, and its use has persisted to the present. In vivo studies on the efficacy of Dakin's solution in canine wounds are not available.[33]

REFERENCES

1. King LJ: History and future perspectives of the use of disinfectants in animal health, *Rev Sci Tech* 14:41–46, 1995.
2. Favero MS, Bond WW: Chemical disinfection of medical and surgical materials. In Block SS, editor: *Disinfection, sterilization, and preservation*, ed 5, Philadelphia, 2001, Lippincott Williams & Wilkins, p 881.
3. Kahrs RF: General disinfection guidelines, *Rev Sci Tech* 14: 105–122, 1995.
4. Brown CD, Zitelli JA: A review of topical agents for wounds and methods of wounding—guidelines for wound management, *J Dermatol Surg Oncol* 19:732–737, 1993.
5. Ali Y, Dolan MJ, Fendler EJ, et al: Alcohols. In Block SS, editor: *Disinfection, sterilization, and preservation*, ed 5, Philadelphia, 2001, Lipipncott Williams & Wilkins, p 229.
6. Jeffrey DJ: Chemicals used as disinfectants: active ingredients and enhancing additives, *Rev Sci Tech* 14:57–74, 1995.
7. Larson EL: APIC guideline for handwashing and hand antisepsis in health care settings, *Am J Infect Control* 23:251–269, 1995.
8. McDonnell G, Russell AD: Antiseptics and disinfectants: Activity, action, and resistance, *Clin Microbiol Rev* 12:147–179, 1999.
9. Rossmoore HW: Nitrogen compounds. In Block SS, editor: *Disinfection, sterilization, and preservation*, ed 5, Philadelphia, 2001, Lippincott Williams & Wilkins, p 383.
10. Hugo WB: A brief history of heat, chemical and radiation preservation and disinfection, *Int Biodeterioration Biodegrad* 36:197–217, 1995.
11. Scott EM, Gorman SP: Glutaraldehyde. In Block SS, editor: *Disinfection, sterilization, and preservation*, ed 5, Philadelphia, 2001, Lippincott Williams & Wilkins, p 361.
12. Russell AD: Glutaraldehyde: current status and uses, *Infect Control Hosp Epidemiol* 15:724–733, 1994.
13. Denyer SP, Stewart GSAB: Mechanisms of action of disinfectants, *Int Biodeterioration Biodegrad* 41:261–268, 1998.
14. Maris P: Modes of action of disinfectants, *Rev Sci Tech* 14:47–55, 1995.
15. Lambrechts NE, Hurter K, Picard JA, et al: A prospective comparison between stabilized glutaraldehyde and chlorhexidine gluconate for preoperative skin antisepsis in dogs, *Vet Surg* 33:636–643, 2004.
16. Denton GW: Chlorhexidine. In Block SS, editor: *Disinfection, sterilization, and preservation*, ed 5, Philadelphia, 2001, Lippincott Williams & Wilkins, p 321.
17. Barrett-Bee K, Newboult L, Edwards S: The membrane destabilising action of the antibacterial agent chlorhexidine, *FEMS Microbiol Lett* 119:249–254, 1994.
18. Chapman JS: Characterizing bacterial resistance to preservatives and disinfectants, *Int Biodeterioration Biodegrad* 41:241–245, 1998.
19. Lozier S, Pope E, Berg J: Effects of four preparations of 0.05% chlorhexidine diacetate on wound healing in dogs, *Vet Surg* 21:107–112, 1992.
20. Amber EI, Henderson RA, Swaim SF, et al: A comparison of antimicrobial efficacy and tissue reaction of four antiseptics on canine wounds, *Vet Surg* 12:63–68, 1983.
21. Dychdala GR: Chlorine and chlorine compounds. In Block SS, editor: *Disinfection, sterilization, and preservation*, ed 5, Philadelphia, 2001, Lippincott Williams & Wilkins, p 135.
22. Kennedy MA, Mellon VS, Caldwell G, et al: Virucidal efficacy of the newer quaternary ammonium compounds, *J Am Anim Hosp Assoc* 31:254–258, 1995.
23. Doughty D: A rational approach to the use of topical antiseptics, *J Wound Ostomy Continence Nurs* 21:224–231, 1994.
24. Ashworth CD, Nelson DR: Antimicrobial potentiation of irrigation solutions containing Tris-(hydroxymethyl) aminomethane-EDTA, *J Am Vet Med Assoc* 197:1513–1514, 1990.
25. Russell AD: Biocide use and antibiotic resistance: the relevance of laboratory findings to clinical and environmental situations, *Lancet Infect Dis* 3:794–803, 2003.
26. Wooley RE, Jones MS: Action of EDTA-Tris and antimicrobial agent combinations on selected pathogenic bacteria, *Vet Microbiol* 8:271–280, 1983.
27. Klohnen A, Wilson DG, Hendrickson DA, et al: Effects of potentiated chlorhexidine on bacteria and tarsocrural joints in ponies, *Am J Vet Res* 57:756–761, 1996.
28. Stubbs WP, Bellah JR, Vermaas-Hekman D, et al: Chlorhexidine gluconate versus chloroxylenol for preoperative skin preparation in dogs, *Vet Surg* 25:487–494, 1996.
29. Joslyn LJ: Gaseous chemical sterilization. In Block SS, editor: *Disinfection, sterilization, and preservation*, ed 5, Philadelphia, 2001, Lippincott Williams & Wilkins, p 337.
30. Gottardi W: Iodine and iodine compounds. In Block SS, editor: *Disinfection, sterilization, and preservation*, ed 5, Philadelphia, 2001, Lippincott Williams & Wilkins, p 159.
31. Russell AD: Similarities and differences in the responses of microorganisms to biocides, *J Antimicrob Chemother* 52:750–763, 2003.
32. LeVeen HH, LeVeen RF, LeVeen EG: The mythology of povidone–iodine and the development of self-sterilizing plastics, *Surg Gynecol Obstet* 176:183–190, 1993.
33. Lemarié RJ, Hosgood G: Antiseptics and disinfectants in small animal practice, *Compend Contin Educ Pract Vet* 17:1339–1351, 1995.
34. Weber DJ, Rutala WA, Sickbert-Bennett EE: Outbreaks associated with contaminated antiseptics and disinfectants, *Antimicrob Agents Chemother* 51:4217–4224, 2007.
35. Goldenheim PD: *In vitro* efficacy of povidone–iodine solution and cream against methicillin-resistant *Staphylococcus aureus*, Postgrad Med J 69:S62–S65, 1993.
36. Rahn R: Review presentation on povidone-iodine antisepsis in the oral cavity, *Postgrad Med J* 69:S4–S9, 1993.
37. Greene CE: Environmental factors in infectious disease. In Greene CE, editor: *Infectious diseases of the dog and cat*, ed 3, St Louis, 2006, Saunders, p 991.
38. Block SS: Peroxygen compounds. In Block SS, editor: *Disinfection, sterilization, and preservation*, ed 5, Philadelphia, 2001, Lippincott Williams & Wilkins, p 185.
39. Jacobs PT, Lin S: Sterilization processes utilizing low-temperature plasma. In Block SS, editor: *Disinfection, sterilization, and preservation*, ed 5, Philadelphia, 2001, Lippincott Williams & Wilkins, p 747.
40. Heit MC, Riviere JE: Antiseptics and disinfectants. In Adams HR, editor: *Veterinary pharmacology and therapeutics*, ed 8, Ames, Iowa, 2001, Iowa State University Press, p 783.
41. Goddard PA, McCue KA: Phenolic compounds. In Block SS, editor: *Disinfection, sterilization, and preservation*, ed 5, Philadelphia, 2001, Lippincott Williams & Wilkins, p 255.
42. Kampf G, Kramer A: Epidemiologic background of hand hygiene and evaluation of the most important agents for scrubs and rubs, *Clin Microbiol Rev* 17:863–893, 2004.
43. Terleckyj B, Elsinger EC, Axler DA: Antiseptics and disinfectants—current issues, *J Am Podiatr Med Assoc* 85:439–445, 1995.
44. Merianos JJ: Surface-active agents. In Block SS, editor: *Disinfection, sterilization, and preservation*, ed 5, Philadelphia, 2001, Lippincott Williams & Wilkins, p 283.
45. Grow AG: Writing guidelines to require disinfection, *Rev Sci Tech* 14:469–477, 1995.
46. Russell AD: Mechanisms of bacterial resistance to biocides, *Int Biodeterioration Biodegrad* 36:247–265, 1995.
47. Ntsama-Essomba C, Bouttier S, Ramaldes M, et al: Resistance of *Escherichia coli* growing as biofilms to disinfectants, *Vet Res* 28:353–363, 1997.

48. Morck DW, Olson ME, Ceri H: Microbial biofilms: prevention, control, and removal. In Block SS, editor: *Disinfection, sterilization, and preservation*, ed 5, Philadelphia, 2001, Lippincott Williams & Wilkins, p 675.
49. Russell AD: Bacterial adaptation and resistance to antiseptics, disinfectants and preservatives is not a new phenomenon, *J Hosp Infect* 57:97–104, 2004.
50. McGavin D: Inactivation of canine parvovirus by disinfectants and heat, *J Small Anim Pract* 28:523–535, 1987.
51. Patterson G, Morley PS, Blehm KD, et al: Efficacy of directed misting application of a peroxygen disinfectant for environmental decontamination of a veterinary hospital, *J Am Vet Med Assoc* 227:597–602, 2005.
52. Crabtree TD, Pelletier SJ, Pruett TL: Surgical antisepsis. In Block SS, editor: *Disinfection, sterilization, and preservation*, ed 5, Philadelphia, 2001, Lippincott Williams & Wilkins, p 919.
53. Suchomel M, Gnant G, Weinlich M, et al: Surgical hand disinfection using alcohol: the effects of alcohol type, mode and duration of application, *J Hosp Infect* 71:228–233, 2009.
54. Larson EL, Aiello AE, Heilman JM, et al: Comparison of different regimens for surgical hand preparation, *AORN J* 73:412–420, 2001.
55. Shmon C: Assessment and preparation of the surgical patient and the operating team. In Slatter D, editor: *Textbook of small animal surgery*, ed 3, Philadelphia, 2003, Saunders, p 162.
56. Osuna DJ, DeYoung DJ, Walker RL: Comparison of three skin preparation techniques in the dog. Part I: Experimental trial, *Vet Surg* 19:14–19, 1990.
57. Ashley KC: The antimicrobial properties of two commonly used antiseptic mouthwashes—corsodyl and oraldene, *J Appl Bacteriol* 56:221–225, 1984.
58. Swaim SF, Lee AH: Topical wound medications: a review, *J Am Vet Med Assoc* 190:1588–1593, 1987.

12 Drugs for the Treatment of Protozoal Infections

Randy C. Lynn and Dawn Merton Boothe

Chapter Outline

Protozoal infections can provide diagnostic as well as therapeutic challenges for the small animal clinician. The situations can range from the simple treatment of a young kitten with coccidiosis to the more robust challenges of chronic giardiasis in a breeding kennel. Although several of the protozoa are well characterized and relatively easy to treat, others are poorly understood and have no specific agents available for therapy. Three types of infections caused by major pathogens are presented here: common enteric coccidia, toxoplasmosis, and giardia. The pathogens are known to affect dogs and cats, and two are significant zoonotic agents.

This chapter does not include the protozoa that appear only sporadically in the veterinary literature (*Balantidium, Pentatrichomonas, Entamoeba, Hammondia, Besnoitia,* and *Sarcocystis* spp.). These organisms are not adequately documented as pathogens of dogs and cats and thus require no therapy. Also excluded are selected protozoal pathogens that are partially characterized but have no effective treatment available. Textbooks of parasitology or infectious disease should be consulted for a complete discussion of these sporadic, spurious, or untreatable pathogens.[1,2]

Therapy of protozoal infections, which are often zoonotic, must include use of therapeutic agents along with supportive therapy and proper hygiene and husbandry to clean up the environment and prevent spread to other animals and people. No therapeutic agent, no matter how safe or effective, can be expected to treat these diseases without supportive therapy and hygiene. Table 12-1 lists the therapeutic agents discussed in the text. These drugs are discussed below as well as in specific chapters.

COMMON ENTERIC COCCIDIOSIS

Biology

The most common protozoa in small animal veterinary medicine are the coccidians, which cause a condition termed *coccidiosis.* Coccidia are very host specific. Dogs and cats are infected with several species in the genus *Isospora.* Diagnosis is readily made by conventional fecal floatation techniques using concentrated sugar or salt solutions. Careful identification of coccidia oocysts may reveal the presence of spurious coccidia from other genera, especially *Eimeria* spp., which commonly parasitize food animals, thus indicating coprophagy. Nevertheless, coccidia are ubiquitous in young dogs and cats and commonly cause disease, especially in those with suboptimal nutrition, immune status, or stress.

Coccidia are obligate intracellular parasites that depend on dispersion of fecal oocysts for transmission. This fact alone illustrates the importance of hygiene. There are four species that infect dogs (*Isospora canis, Isospora ohioensis, Isospora burrowsi,* and *Isospora neorivolta*) and two that infect cats (*Isospora felis* and *Isospora rivolta*). Although direct ingestion of the oocyst is the primary means of infection, rodents can serve as paratenic hosts if they ingest the oocyst and then are eaten by the definitive host.

Coccidia have life cycles that are more complex than other infectious agents (Figure 12-1). Each life cycle includes both sexual and asexual phases. This is important to remember because the therapeutic agents used to treat and control coccidia are primarily effective against the asexual stage of the life cycle.

KEY POINT 12-1 Hygiene must be addressed for effective resolution of coccidian infections.

Table 12-1 Dosing Regimens for Selected Antiprotozoal Drugs

Drug	Indication	Species	Dose (mg/kg)	Interval (hr)	Route	Duration (days)	Comments
Albendazole	Giardiasis	Dog	25	12	PO	2	
Allopurinol	Leishmaniasis	Dog	20	24	PO		
		Dog	15	24	PO		With meglumine antimoniate
Aminosidine	Leishmaniasis	Dog	5	12	IM	3-4 weeks	
Amphotericin B	Leishmaniasis	Dog	0.8-2.5	24	IV		
Amphotericin B, Liposomal	Leishmaniasis	Dog	3 To total of 15	24	IV		
Amprolium	Coccidiosis	Cat	60-100	24	PO	7	
		Dog	300-400	24	PO	5	
			1.5 tsp/gal in water		PO	10	
Atavaquone	Babesiosis	Dog	13	8	PO	10	With azithromycin
Azithromycin	Cryptosporidiosis	Cat	7-15	12	PO	5-7	
		Dog	5-10	12	PO	5-7	
Clindamycin	Hepatozoonosis	Dog	10	8	PO	14	With sulfadiazine-trimethoprim and clindamycin
	Neosporosis	Dog	7.5-15	8	PO	28-56	
			15-22	12	PO	28-56	
Decoquinate	Hepatozoonosis	Dog	10-20	12	PO	2 years	
Diminazene	Babesiosis	Dog	3.5	Once	IM		With imidocarb
	Cytauzoonosis	Cat	2	Once	SC	Repeat in 2-4 weeks	
Febendazole	Giardiasis	Dog	50	24	PO	3	
Furazolidone	Coccidiosis	Cat	8-20	12-24	PO	5	
		Dog	8-20	12-24	PO	5	
	Giardiasis	Cat	4	12	PO	7-10	
Imidocarb proprionate	Babesiosis	Dog	5-6.6		IM	Repeat in 2 weeks	
		Dog	7.5	Once	IM		With diminazene
	Cytauzoonosis	Cat	5	Once	SC	Repeat in 2 weeks	
Meglumine antimoniate	Leishmaniasis	Dog	100	24	SC	3-4 weeks	
Metronidazole	Giardiasis	Cat	10-25	12	PO	5-7	
		Dog	10-25	12	PO	5-7	
			50	24	PO	3	
Paramycin	Cryptosporidiosis	Cat	125-165	12	PO	5	
		Dog	125-166	12	PO	5	
Pentamidine	Babesiosis	Dog	16.5	24	IM	48	
	Leishmaniasis	Dog	4	Twice weekly	IM	3 to 4 weeks	
Phenamidine	Babesiosis	Dog	15	24	IM	48	
Ponazuril	Toxoplasmosis, neosporosis	Dog	10-20	24	PO	10-14*	
	Coccidiosis	Dog	20	Once weekly	PO	Repeat in 1 week*	
Pyramethamine	Hepatazoonosis	Dog	0.25	12	PO	14	With sulfadiazine–trimethoprim and clindamydin
	Neosporosis	Dog	1	24	PO		With sulfonamide at 15-30 mg/kg

Continued

Table 12-1 Dosing Regimens for Selected Antiprotozoal Drugs—cont'd

Drug	Indication	Species	Dose (mg/kg)	Interval (hr)	Route	Duration (days)	Comments
Quinacrine	Coccidiosis	Cat	10	24	PO	5	
	Giardiasis	Cat	9	24	PO	6	
		Dog	6.6	24	PO	5	
Rinidazole	Trichomoniasis	Cat	10-50	12-24‡	PO	14	
Sulfadiazine-trimethoprim	Hepatazoonosis	Dog	15	12	PO	14	With pyrimethamine and sulfadiazone-trimethoprim
	Neosporosis	Dog	15-20	24	PO	28-56	
			10-15	8	PO	28-56	
Sulfadimethoxine	Coccidioisis	Cat	50-60	24	PO	5-20	
		Dog	50-61	24	PO	5-21	
Sulfadimethoxine-amprolium	Coccidiosis	Dog	25/150	24	PO	14	
Sulfadimethoxine-trimethoprim	Coccidiosis	Dog	55/11	24	PO	7-23	
Sulfaguanidine	Coccidioisis	Cat	150-200	24	PO	6	
			100-200	8	PO	5	
		Dog	150-200	24	PO	6	
			100-200	8	PO	5	
Tinidazole	Trichomoniasis	Cat	15				Not reported
Trypan blue	Babesiosis	Dog	10§	Once	IV		
Tylosin	Cryptosporidiosis (to reduce diarrhea)	Dog	11	12	PO	28	

*Based on experimental infection in mice.
†Anectdotal.
‡Clinical signs recur at lower dose; safety at higher dose not established.
§Use a 1% solution.

The oocyst is passed in the feces, and, after suitable exposure to air, heat, and moisture, the oocyst sporulates. This process may take only a few hours or a few days, depending on the species of coccidia and on the environmental conditions. During sporulation each oocyst develops into two sporocysts that contain four sporozoites each; thus each oocyst contains a total of eight infective sporozoites.

After ingestion the sporozoites are liberated from the oocyst and invade the enterocytes that line the small intestine. Once inside the enterocytes, the sporozoites turn into trophozoites, which undergo asexual fission (properly termed *schizogony* or *merogony)* to produce many daughter schizonts. After 4 days the enterocyte ruptures and releases the multiple schizonts (or meronts). This schizont stage is the place in the life cycle where therapeutic agents have a chance to break the life cycle. Because the schizonts are released from the cell only every 4 days, the therapeutic agent should be present in the gut for several multiples of this period, usually 14 to 21 days. The daughter schizonts are capable of infecting new enterocytes and repeating the cycle of fission into many daughters and rupture of the subsequent enterocytes. The number of asexual cycles has been determined for each species of coccidia; the small animal pathogens typically have two or three asexual cycles before entering the sexual stage of the life cycle.

The schizont, produced by the last cycle of asexual fission, enters another enterocyte and develops into either a male or a female gametocyte. The female gametocyte enlarges and forms a singular large cellular structure within the enterocyte. The male gametocyte undergoes fission to produce many small biflagellate male sex cells. The enterocytes rupture, and the motile male sex cells fertilize the female gametocytes, which mature to a zygote and then pass out in the feces in the form of an oocyst. The fresh oocysts are exposed to the external environment, where they sporulate and infect new hosts.

The repeated intracellular invasion of enterocytes and subsequent rupture can produce substantial pathology to the gut, especially if the infected host is young, weak, malnourished, or stressed. Normal animals, in otherwise good health, usually experience coccidial infection followed by an effective immune response that limits and eliminates the infection without therapeutic intervention. Most clinicians prefer to intervene when coccidia are identified in a fecal floatation. Therapy is usually successful in eliminating the coccidial oocysts, although it is not known how many of these animals

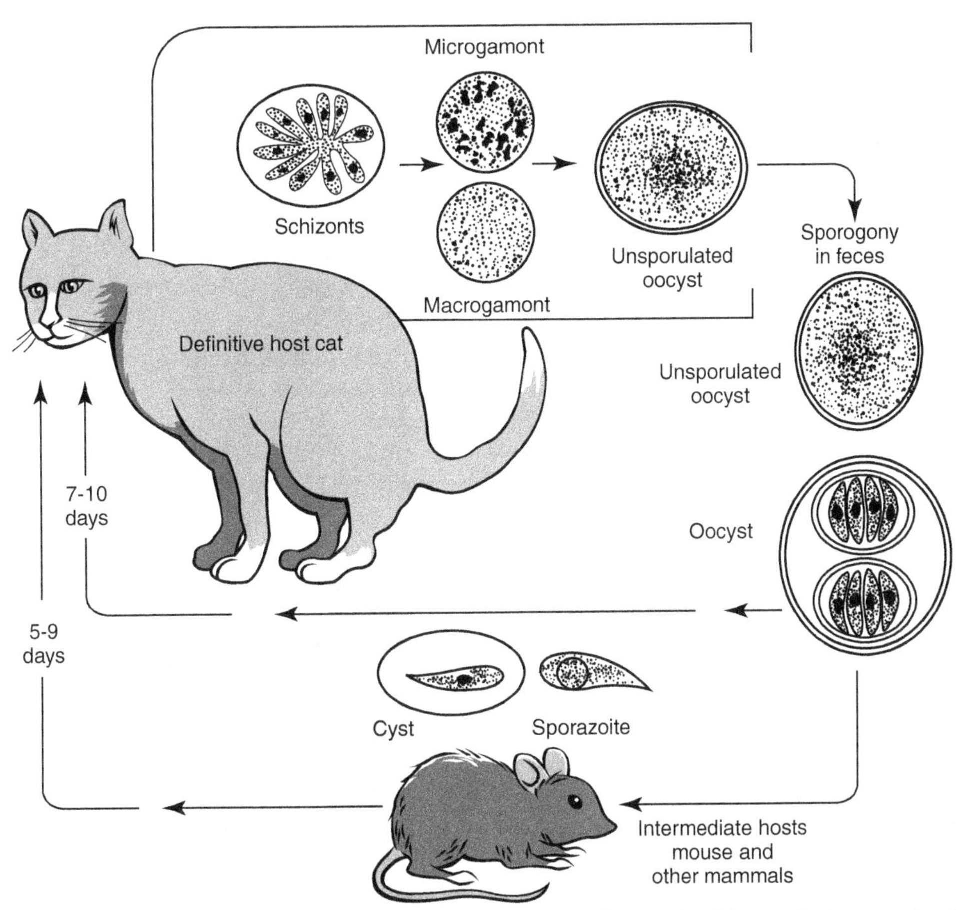

Figure 12-1 Life cycle of *Isospora felis,* which is typical of the *Isospora* spp. The mode of transmission may be direct, via ingestion of sporulated oocysts from the environment, or indirect, via ingestion of cysts in prey animals. Sexual and asexual reproduction of the parasite occurs in the intestines of the definitive host (in this case, a cat), and unsporulated oocysts are shed in the feces of definitive hosts. (From Dubey JP, Greene CE: Enteric coccidiosis. In Greene CE, editor: *Infectious diseases of the dog and cat,* ed 2, Philadelphia, 1998, Saunders, p. 511.)

would have spontaneously cleared the infection without intervention.

Treatment

Sulfas and Potentiated Sulfas

Use of sulfonamides is the treatment of choice for small animal coccidia as well as a number of other protozoal organisms. Unfortunately there is a paucity of research information to support their efficacy. Two pivotal studies on sulfamethoxine and sulfaguanidine against coccidia support their utility; however, these two agents are no longer available in the United States.[3,4] Clinicians have empirically substituted more readily available sulfonamides and enjoyed apparent clinical success.[5] Currently there is one simple sulfa and three potentiated sulfas that are commonly used in the United States: sulfadimethoxine (Albon), sulfadimethoxine with ormetoprim (Primor), sulfadiazine with trimethoprim (Di-Trim, Tribrissen), and sulfamethoxazole with trimethoprim (Bactrim, Septra).

KEY POINT 12-2 Use of sulfonamides is the treatment of choice for small animal coccidians.

Sulfonamide Chemistry and Mechanism of Action

The sulfonamides are discussed in more depth in Chapter 7. Each is a structural analog of para-aminobenzoic acid that competitively inhibits the dihydropterate synthetase step in the synthesis of folic acid, which is required for synthesis of RNA and DNA. Inhibition by sulfas impairs protein synthesis, metabolism, and growth of the pathogen. A vast array of sulfa agents have been created and described; all but a few have been lost in the sands of time. The important differences among these agents involve their solubility, duration of action, and activity against key pathogens. Fortunately, the three sulfas included in this discussion demonstrate acceptable performance in all three categories; solubility is adequate, they are given once or twice daily, and they have a reasonably broad spectrum of action. The sulfa drugs are primarily effective against the schizont stages of coccidian; thus prolonged treatment may be required for the drug to effectively block the life cycle.

Potentiator Chemistry and Mechanism of Action

The diaminopyrimidine potentiators (trimethoprim and ormetoprim) act in concert with sulfonamides by blocking the next step (dihydrofolate reductase) in folic acid synthesis. Chemically the diaminopyrimidines are related to pyrimethamine, which has antimalarial properties. The agents are highly selective inhibitors of dihydrofolate reductase. This sequential blockade produces significant potentiation of activity. It is a classic case of drug potentiation.

Drug Disposition

The sulfonamides are weak acids that are well absorbed from the gastrointestinal tract and are widely distributed in the body. Sulfadimethoxine and sulfamethoxazole have high serum protein binding, which provides decreased body clearance and long half-lives. They undergo metabolic alteration in the liver and subsequent renal clearance. Trimethoprim and ormetoprim are also well absorbed from the gut, widely distributed, and then hydroxylated and excreted through the urinary tract.

Toxicity and Adverse Effects

The long history of sulfa use in veterinary medicine has resulted in a wide array of toxic and idiosyncratic reactions in animals. Historically, the most common and most avoidable reactions result from crystallization in the urinary tract with secondary crystalluria, hematuria, and urinary obstruction. Recent reviews in human medicine indicate that the improved solubility of the modern preparations has decreased the risk of crystalluria; nevertheless, it is still prudent to ensure adequate water intake and proper hydration during sulfa therapy.[6] The human-medicine literature also suggests that the sulfonamides may be directly nephrotoxic.[6] Hematopoietic disorders (thrombocytopenia and leukopenia) have also been reported as a result of sulfa therapy. Sulfaquinoxaline especially has been associated with hypothrombinemia, hemorrhage, and death in puppies receiving therapy for coccidia.[7]

Idiosyncratic reactions in animals and people often include immune-mediated phenomena such as hypersensitivity reactions, drug fever, urticaria, nonseptic polyarthritis, focal retinitis, and hepatitis. Fortunately, these reactions occur at very low rates when the drugs are used at recommended dose rates and for less than 2 weeks.

Preparations

There are four sulfa products that are currently available for use in small animal medicine: sulfadimethoxine, sulfadimethoxine with ormetoprim, sulfadiazine with trimethoprim, and sulfamethoxazole with trimethoprim. Each is available in a variety of formulations.

Sulfadimethoxine

Sulfadimethoxine is a rapidly absorbed, long-acting sulfonamide. It is not acetylated in the dog and is excreted unchanged in the urine. It is approved for treatment of coccidiosis in dogs and cats. It has a wide margin of safety; dogs given multiple oral doses of 160 mg/kg by mouth daily for 13 weeks showed no signs of toxicity.[8]

It is important that all treated animals receive adequate water intake to prevent dehydration and crystalluria, as well as proper nutrition, during therapy for coccidiosis. Therapy is available as a 40% injection (Albon); in 125-, 250-, and 500-mg tablets (Albon); as a pleasant-tasting 5% suspension (Albon); and as a 12.5% oral solution (Albon, Di-Methox). The approved therapy is an initial dose of 55 mg/kg, orally or by subcutaneous or intravenous injection, for the first day and subsequent doses of 27.5 mg/kg orally once daily for 12 to 21 days. It seems reasonable that, because coccidia are enteric pathogens, the oral route would be most effective.

Sulfadimethoxine with Ormetoprim

Sulfadimethoxine with ormetoprim is the most recently approved potentiated sulfonamide. It constitutes a rational combination that potentiates the action of both drugs by blocking two sequential steps in the synthesis of folic acid. Ormetoprim is a diaminopyrimidine potentiator with very low mammalian toxicity. The available tablets contain 100/20, 200/40, 500/100, or 1000/200 mg sulfadimethoxine/mg ormetoprim, respectively (Primor). The tablets are designated by the total weight of active ingredient in each tablet; thus Primor 120 contains 100 mg of sulfadimethoxine and 20 mg of ormetoprim. The approved starting dose is 55 mg/kg orally on the first day of treatment and then 27.5 mg/kg orally once per day for 14 to 21 days. Treatment should not extend beyond 21 days.[8]

It is interesting to note that the only recent controlled study of coccidiosis therapy for dogs was conducted with this drug combination. In that study, 32.5 mg/kg or 66 mg/kg was given continuously in the food for 23 days, subsequent to experimental oocyst infection. The higher dose of 66 mg/kg provided better results and did not produce any adverse reactions.[9]

Sulfadiazine or Sulfamethoxazole with Trimethoprim

Sulfadiazine with trimethoprim is the potentiated sulfa with the most years of actual use in veterinary medicine. For many years it was the only potentiated sulfa approved for use in animals. Trimethoprim is a diaminopyrimidine potentiator with very low mammalian toxicity. The available tablets contain 25/5, 100/20, 400/80, or 800/160 mg sulfadiazine/mg trimethoprim, respectively (Tribrissen, Di-Trim). The tablets are designated by the total weight of active ingredient in each tablet; thus Tribrissen 30 contains 25 mg sulfadiazine and 5 mg trimethoprim. The approved dose is 30 mg/kg orally or 26.4 mg/kg by subcutaneous injection daily for up to 14 days. The preferred dose for bacterial infections in dogs and cats is 30 mg/kg once or twice daily and may be indicated for severe coccidial infections. The manufacturer recommends that animals with marked hepatic parenchymal damage, blood dyscrasias, or previous sulfonamide sensitivity should not be given this product.[8,10]

Sulfamethoxazole with trimethoprim is a readily available product approved for use in people (Bactrim, Septra); it is not currently approved for use in animals. Because of its similarity to veterinary potentiated sulfonamides and because low-cost generics are available, it is widely used in veterinary medicine. There is some controversy regarding the appropriate dosing regimen for this human-labeled product in animals, but many clinicians gain acceptable clinical results using the same dose as sulfadiazine.

Sulfamethoxazole with trimethoprim is available in a fixed combination of 5:1 sulfamethoxazole to trimethoprim as tablets and pediatric suspension. The available single-strength tablets contain 400/80 mg and double-strength tablets contain 800/160 mg trimethoprim, respectively (Bactrim, Septra). The pediatric oral suspension contains 40 mg sulfamethoxazole and 8 mg trimethoprim per milliliter. The dose for bacterial infections and coccidiosis in dogs and cats is 30 mg/kg once daily for 10 days[10] and may be indicated in severe coccidial infections.

Amprolium

Amprolium (Amprol, Corid) is an antiprotozoal drug that is a structural analog of thiamine. It is freely soluble in water, methanol, and ethanol. The close structural similarity between amprolium and thiamine allows amprolium to compete with thiamine for absorption into the parasite. It is most effective against the first-generation schizont stage and thus is more effective for prevention than treatment.

At very high doses, amprolium may produce thiamine deficiency in the host. Thiamine deficiency can be treated by adding thiamine to the diet, although excessive thiamine supplementation may decrease the efficacy against the pathogen. In dogs adverse reactions are apparently rare and may consist of neurologic abnormalities, depression, anorexia, and diarrhea.[10]

Amprolium is approved for use in the drinking water or feed of poultry and cattle for the prevention and treatment of coccidia. Treatment for dogs and cats requires adapting the approved formulations to small animal use. The target dose for treatment of dogs is 100 to 200 mg/kg by mouth daily in food or water.[10] Dogs may be treated by mixing 30 mL (2 Tbs) of 9.6% amprolium solution to 1 U.S. gallon (3.8 L) of drinking water and offering it as the sole source of drinking water.[11] Alternatively, 1.25 g of 20% amprolium powder can be mixed with daily ration sufficient for four puppies.[12] Amprolium should be provided in either the food or the water but not in both for a period of 7 days. It may be given as a treatment for coccidia or as a preventive measure for 7 days before puppies are shipped or to bitches just before whelping.

Cats may be treated at a dose of 60 to 100 mg/kg by mouth once daily for 7 days, which may be accomplished by direct oral administration.[13] Placement of medication in food or water may be more unreliable for cats than for dogs owing to the finicky eating habits of many cats.

Furazolidone

Although the nitrofurans (nitrofurazone and furazolidone) have been reported in the literature as being effective in the treatment of coccidiosis and were once widely available for oral treatment of food animals, they have been systematically eliminated from the veterinary marketplace in the United States because of concerns regarding carcinogenicity. Furazolidone apparently inhibits numerous microbial enzyme systems, especially those related to carbohydrate metabolism, but the actual mechanism of action remains to be determined.[14] Furazolidone is still available in a dosage form that is approved for human use (Furoxone). Potential toxicity includes gastrointestinal disturbance, peripheral neuritis, decreased spermatogenesis, and weight gain.[15] Dogs and cats can be treated with 8 to 20 mg/kg orally, 1 to 2 times daily, for 5 days.[10,13] The product is available in 2 formulations approved for use in people (Furoxone): 100-mg tablets and an oral liquid containing 3.34 mg/mL.

Quinacrine

Quinacrine has demonstrated useful activity in the treatment of coccidiosis. Efficacy is variable, as is the relationship between plasma and tissue concentrations. Commercial production in the United States. (Atabrine) was discontinued in 1993.

TOXOPLASMOSIS

Biology

Toxoplasmosis is caused by *Toxoplasma gondii,* an obligate intracellular coccidian parasite. The parasite and the disease occur worldwide and have serious zoonotic impact. The domestic cat and other cats serve as the definitive hosts of this parasite. All other warm-blooded animals serve as intermediate hosts. In the United States, infection rates range from 0% to 100% in cats, 30% in dogs, and 30% to 60% in people. Although infection and seroconversion are common, clinical disease and diagnosis are rare.[16]

Enteroepithelial Life Cycle

The enteroepithelial life cycle of *T. gondii* in cats is similar to the life cycle of the common enteric coccidia (Figure 12-2). *Toxoplasma* oocysts are ingested from the environment; alternatively, tissue cysts may be ingested by carnivorism. Once ingested, bradyzooites are released that penetrate the epithelial cells and begin a cycle of asexual reproduction. The sexual stage of the cycle proceeds when the zooites differentiate into microgametes and macrogametes. The macrogametes are fertilized by the microgamete, and the resulting union produces an oocyst that is shed in the feces to begin the cycle again. It is believed that the enteroepithelial life cycle and the resulting oocysts occur only in cats; therefore only cats shed infective oocysts.

Extraintestinal Life Cycle

The extraintestinal life cycle occurs in all warm-blooded animals, including cats. This cycle begins when oocysts or infected tissues are ingested. The bradyzoites or sporozoites penetrate intestinal cells and undergo asexual reproduction and then break out of the gastrointestinal tract to infect virtually all other tissues, including the brain, striated muscle, and liver. After entering these extraintestinal tissues, they penetrate the cell and multiply until the cell is destroyed. The tachyzoites are released to infect other cells, and the cycle repeats. Eventually, the tachyzoites form tissue cysts that remain viable and infective for the life of the animal. These tissue cysts are infective to all warm-blooded animals and infect all animals who ingest the infected tissues. It is the ubiquitous tissue migration and replication across innumerable species that makes the pathogen so insidious and dangerous.

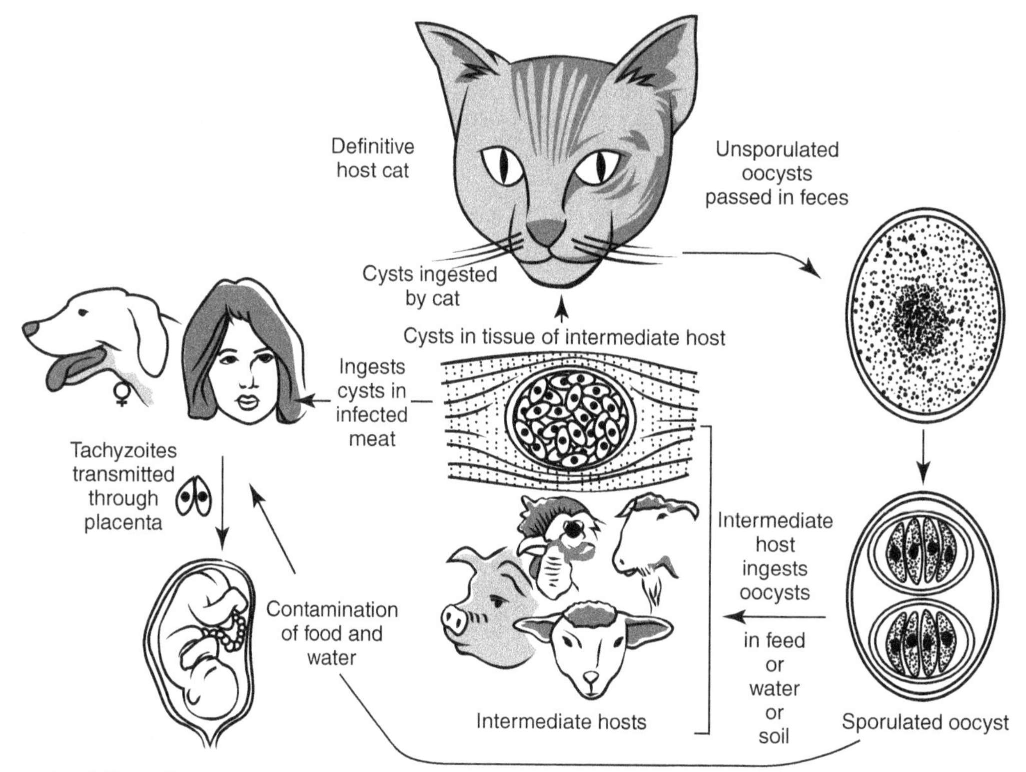

Figure 12-2 Life cycle of *Toxoplasma gondii.* (From Dubey JP, Lappin MR: Toxoplasmosis and neosporosis. In Greene CE, editor: *Infectious diseases of the dog and cat,* ed 2, Philadelphia, 1998, Saunders, p. 494.)

Congenital Transmission

If the host is infected during pregnancy, then the tachyzoites move across the placenta to infect the developing fetus. Infection during the first half of the pregnancy leads to more severe disease in the fetus. Women infected during pregnancy risk congenital malformation, mental retardation, and death of the unborn fetus. Women should be cautioned to avoid exposure to cat feces and to refrain from consuming undercooked meat during pregnancy.

Clinical Signs

Clinical signs in cats are most severe in prenatally infected kittens. Such kittens may be stillborn or die before weaning. Clinical signs relate to pathology in the liver, lungs, and central nervous system. Adult cats typically demonstrate anorexia, lethargy, dyspnea, weight loss, icterus, vomiting, diarrhea, stiff gait, shifting leg lameness, or neurologic deficits. Ocular lesions may include uveitis in the anterior and posterior chambers, iritis, iridocyclitis, and detached retina. In severe cases respiratory or central nervous system involvement may cause death.[17]

Infected dogs may show clinical signs related to respiratory, neuromuscular, or gastrointestinal pathology. Generalized toxoplasmosis is characterized by fever, tonsillitis, dyspnea, diarrhea, and vomiting.[17] More devastating clinical signs may be seen in dogs with neurologic or muscular involvement. Seizures, neurologic deficits, tremors, ataxia, paresis, or paralysis may be seen in these animals. Ocular lesions in dogs are infrequently reported.[17]

Diagnosis

Antemortem diagnosis of toxoplasmosis is a significant diagnostic challenge primarily because of the usual lack of clinical signs in infected animals. Fecal floatation for infected cats may reveal small oocysts that are indistinguishable from other coccidia. It is also important to realize that infected cats shed oocysts for only 1 to 2 weeks after their first exposure, thereafter forming a protective immunity that prevents further shedding of oocysts. Many other tools have been applied to the diagnosis of toxoplasmosis, including clinical chemistry, which may reveal elevated liver enzymes; cytology, which may detect tachyzoites; radiology, which could suggest inflammation of target organs; serology, which would reveal a past infection; and parasite isolation. Unfortunately, no simple, specific, and timely diagnostic tool is available to detect an active case of toxoplasmosis.

Treatment

Treatment of toxoplasmosis may have several goals: to prevent shedding of oocysts from infected cats, to prevent transmission of toxoplasmosis by ingestion of infected tissues, to prevent tachyzoite replication in nonfeline host tissues, and to prevent prenatal infections. In some cases the goal may be to alleviate clinical signs of an active infection.

Clindamycin

Clindamycin is currently considered the drug of choice for treating toxoplasmosis. Structurally, clindamycin is a congener of lincomycin. Clindamycin is well absorbed (90%)

after oral administration and is widely distributed in most tissues, except the central nervous system. It readily crosses the placenta and is extensively bound to plasma proteins. The drug is metabolized in the liver and excreted primarily in the urine and bile.[18] Gastrointestinal upset is sometimes reported in animals receiving clindamycin. Severe, even fatal, pseudomembranous enterocolitis has been reported in people, caused by overgrowth of *Clostridium difficile.*

KEY POINT 12-3 Clindamycin is currently considered the drug of choice for treating toxoplasmosis.

Treatment of systemic *Toxoplasma* infection in dogs can be accomplished with oral or intramuscular clindamycin at 10 to 20 mg/kg twice daily for 2 weeks.[17,19] Cats can be treated for systemic infections with oral or parenteral clindamycin at 10 to 12.5 mg/kg twice daily for 2 to 4 weeks; this antimicrobial is also useful to control shedding of oocysts.[20] The drug should be given with caution to cats with pulmonic toxoplasmosis; parenteral administration to experimentally infected cats resulted in several deaths.[10]

Clindamycin is available in two veterinary formulations (Antirobe): capsules containing 25, 75, or 150 mg and an oral solution containing 25 mg/mL. Similar clindamycin formulations are available for use in humans (Cleocin): 75- and 150-mg oral capsules, an oral pediatric suspension (15 mg/mL), and an injectable solution containing 150 mg/mL.

Sulfa Plus Pyrimethamine

The more time-tested therapeutic regimen for toxoplasmosis is a combination of sulfonamide and pyrimethamine. The sulfonamides were discussed previously. Pyrimethamine is structurally and pharmacologically similar to the folic acid antagonist trimethoprim. Pyrimethamine is primarily used in veterinary medicine to treat toxoplasmosis and equine protozoal myelitis, or "equine toxoplasmosis." Little pharmacokinetic data are available for pyrimethamine use in dogs and cats, but in humans it is well absorbed after oral administration. It is well distributed to the kidneys, liver, spleen, and lungs. The metabolic pathway is unclear, but pyrimethamine metabolites may be found in the urine.

Pyrimethamine can cause anorexia, malaise, vomiting, depression, and myelosuppression. Concomitant oral administration of folinic acid or brewer's yeast may help alleviate some of these clinical signs. Because toxicity may develop rapidly in cats, they should have frequent hematologic monitoring. It is a teratogen in rats but is sometimes used by pregnant women.[10]

Dogs and cats are treated for systemic *Toxoplasma* infections at a dose of 30 mg/kg sulfa and 0.25 to 0.5 mg/kg pyrimethamine orally twice daily for 2 weeks. Cats may be treated to control shedding of oocysts at a dose of 100 mg/kg sulfa and 2 mg/kg pyrimethamine orally once daily for 1 to 2 weeks.[17]

Pyrimethamine alone is available in 25-mg tablets (Daraprim) and in combination tablets containing 25 mg pyrimethamine and 500 mg sulfadoxine (Fansidar). These dosage forms are likely to be difficult for most cat owners to administer.

Monensin

Monensin is an ionophore coccidiostat that is fed to poultry and cattle to enhance feed efficiency. It forms ionic complexes that move across biological membranes. The net effect is disturbance of mitochondrial function, which inhibits growth of the pathogen. It is not well absorbed from the gastrointestinal tract, and thus oral administration provides effective concentrations only in the gastrointestinal tract. It can be toxic if high doses are given. Shedding of *Toxoplasma* oocysts may be controlled in cats by mixing monensin in the feed at 0.2% on a dry matter basis and feeding for 1 to 2 weeks.[17] Monensin is available in several feed-additive formulations designed for incorporation into a finished feed. Formulating such feeds for cats is beyond the capabilities of most cat owners.

Toxoplasmosis is the most common infection of the central nervous system in human patients with acquired immunedeficiency syndrome, resulting in a number of studies in human patients regarding efficacy. Standard regimens include combinations of pyrimethamine with either sulfadiazine or clindamycin, although side effects limit use. A potentially less toxic combination includes atovaquone suspension (approximately 20 mg/kg every 12 hours) and either pyrimethamine (1 mg/kg once daily after a loading dose of approximately 3 mg/kg) or sulfadiazine (20 mg/kg every 6 hours). In one study up to 82% of patients receiving atovaquone as part of combination therapy responded therapeutically, with 28% discontinuing therapy as a result of gastrointestinal adverse events (including taste of atovaquone). The combination of atovaquone and pyrimethamine was recommended as the first-choice combination, with sulfadiazine substituting for pyrimethamine in patients unable to tolerate the former.[21]

GIARDIA

Biology

Giardia (Giardia duodenalis = Giardia lamblia) are protozoan parasites that are motile by means of flagella. They exist extracellularly in the lumen of the gastrointestinal tract. They are ubiquitous pathogens that can inhabit and cause disease in most mammals and are well-known pathogens in dogs, cats, and people. Recent surveys show that 36% of puppies in the United States are infected with *Giardia*.[22] Despite this prevalence, the condition in pet animals remains underdiagnosed on account of inappropriate fecal examination techniques. It is a pathogen with zoonotic potential, insofar as *Giardia* frequently causes disease in people, but there is some uncertainty as to whether the same species and strains infect people and pets. More extensive information about this issue can be found elsewhere.[1,23-26]

The life cycle of *Giardia* is direct and simple (Figure 12-3). The cyst of the *Giardia* is passed in the feces. It is nonmotile and protected by a distinct wall. Although very susceptible to drying, the cysts can survive for weeks or months in cool water. Infections are often traced back to contaminated drinking water. Once ingested, the cysts break open and trophozoites are released into the small intestine. The trophozoites are flattened on one side with a ventral sucking disk that attaches

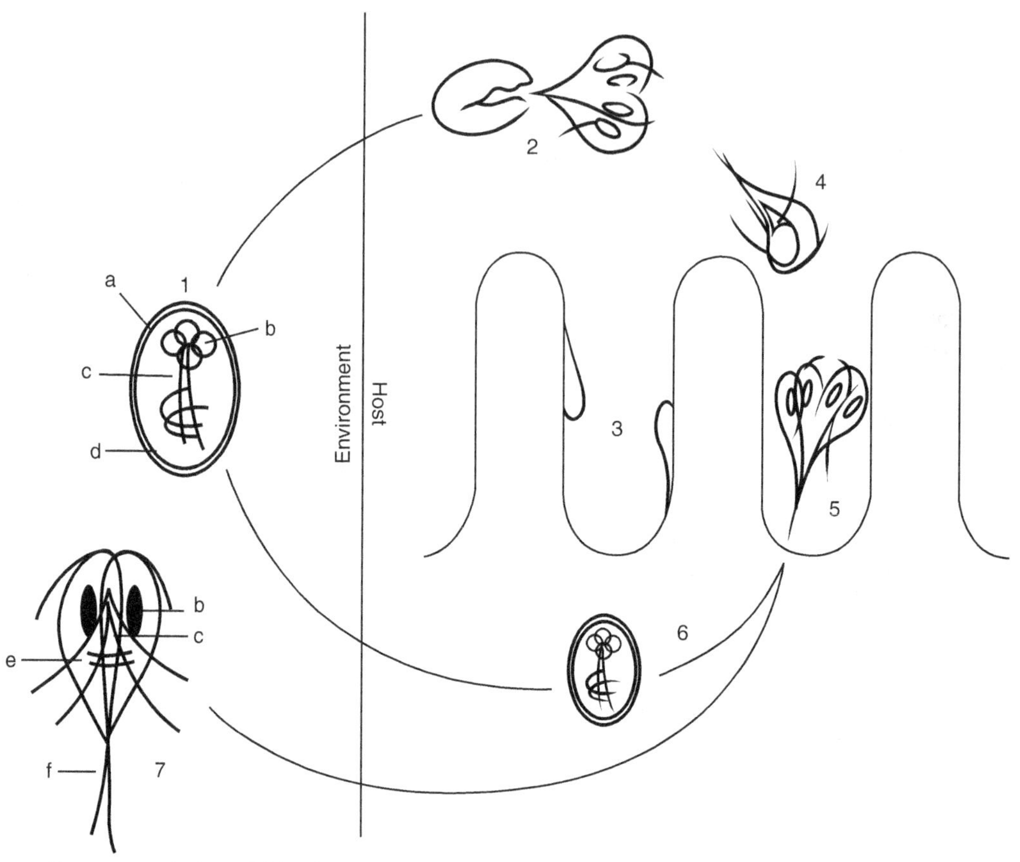

Figure 12-3 Schematic representation of *Giardia* life cycle and structural features of *Giardia* cysts and trophozoites visible by light microscopy. Infection begins when a cyst *(1)* is ingested by the host. Excystation *(2)* in the upper small intestine results in the release of an incompletely divided pair of trophozoites. Trophozoites attach to villous epithelial surfaces *(3)* or swim freely *(4)* in the lumen of the small intestine, where asexual division of trophozoites *(5)* also takes place. Encystment *(6)* of trophozoites, probably in the lower ileum or in the colon, results in the passage of infective cysts in the feces. Trophozoites *(7)* may also be passed into the environment, but they die quickly. Key to organelles: *a,* cyst wall; *b,* nuclei; *c,* axonemes; *d,* adhesive-disk fragments; *e,* median bodies; and *f,* flagella. (From Kirkpatrick CE: Giardiasis. *Vet Clin North Am Small Anim Pract* 17: 1377, 1987.)

to the brush border surface of the villous epithelium. The trophozoites obtain their nutrients by way of the host cell membrane. The flagella provide locomotion from one attachment site to another. The trophozoites reproduce by binary fission. After several divisions the trophozoites encyst and are shed in the feces; they are immediately infective.

Conventional fecal floatation techniques make identification of the parasite difficult because concentrated salt floatation media distort the trophozoites. Preferred methods of diagnosis include microscopic examination of saline smears, which readily show the motile trophozoites. Alternatively, a zinc sulfate centrifugal method may be used to concentrate the giardial cysts and improve sensitivity.[1] Improved techniques for evaluation of duodenal aspirates and fecal enzyme-linked immunosorbent assay (ELISA) testing have recently become available.

Treatment

Albendazole

Albendazole is a broad-spectrum benzimidazole commonly used for treatment of nematode and trematode infections in large animals. Early evidence suggested that albendazole is 100% effective in treating giardiasis in dogs.[27] The dose given in that study was 25 mg/kg orally twice a day for four doses. Albendazole is available in an oral suspension (Valbazen) containing 113.6 mg/mL.

Albendazole, like other benzimidazoles, is well absorbed (about 50% bioavailable) and converted in the liver to its active metabolites, albendazole sulfoxide and albendazole sulfone. These active metabolites are thought to bind to tubulin molecules, which prohibits the formation of microtubules and disrupts cell division. There is also evidence that benzimidazoles can inhibit fumarate reductase, which blocks mitochondrial function, thus depriving the parasite of energy and resulting in death. The parent drug and its metabolites are excreted primarily in the urine.

Albendazole has been shown to be teratogenic, thus limiting its use in pregnant animals. Dogs treated with 50 mg/kg twice daily may develop anorexia, and cats treated with 100 mg/kg per day for 14 to 21 days showed weight loss, neutropenia, and mental dullness.[10] More recently, the drug was shown to be toxic to dogs and cats in clinical use.[28,29] Reported toxicities include myelosuppression (anemia, leukopenia, and thrombocytopenia), abortion, teratogenicity, anorexia, depression, ataxia, vomiting, and diarrhea. Veterinarians are advised to use due caution with this product in dogs.

Fenbendazole

Fenbendazole is currently approved by the U.S. Food and Drug Administration (FDA) for removal of gastrointestinal helminthes in dogs. Recently, it has shown excellent activity against *Giardia*.[28,30,31] The approved dose and the effective dose against *Giardia* is 50 mg/kg orally once daily for 3 days. Treatment of giardiasis is not an approved use for this product.

The drug is well tolerated and has a good safety profile. The only reported adverse effects are vomiting and diarrhea. This time-tested anthelmintic should enjoy more widespread use in the treatment of *Giardia* in dogs. Fenbendazole (50 mg/kg orally once daily for 5 days) was variably effective in treating cats concurrently infected with *Giardia* and *Cryptosporidium parvum*.[32] Although the number of oocysts decreased the first week after treatment (compared with controls), no difference was detected the second week (the power of the study was not addressed). Only 50% (4 of 8) of cats treated with fenbendazole were negative 3 weeks after treatment.

Furazolidone

There is a report of successful treatment of giardiasis in cats with furazolidone.[33] As noted previously, furazolidone was once widely available for oral treatment of food animals. Presently, the nitrofurans have been systematically eliminated from the veterinary marketplace in the United States because of concerns regarding carcinogenicity. Furazolidone is still available in a dosage form that is approved for human use (Furoxone). Toxicity includes gastrointestinal disturbance, peripheral neuritis, decreased spermatogenesis, and weight gain.[15] Cats can be treated with a dose of 4 mg/kg twice daily for 7 to 10 days.[26,34] The product is available in two formulations approved for use by people (Furoxone): 100-mg tablets and an oral liquid containing 3.33 mg/mL.

Metronidazole

The nitroimidazoles represent a very useful class of drugs that have broad-spectrum activity against trichomonads, amebas, *Giardia*, as well as anaerobic cocci and *Bacillus* spp. The prototypical nitroimidazole is metronidazole, which has become the drug of choice for treatment of *Giardia*. Other drugs in the class (ipronidazole, tinidazole, nimorazole, ornidazole, and benznidazole) have been used to control *Giardia*, although none of these is currently available in the United States. None of the nitroimidazole drugs is approved for use in animals. The FDA strongly warns against their use in food-producing animals because this class of drug has been shown to produce tumors in laboratory rodents.

KEY POINT 12-4 Metronidazole has become the drug of choice for treatment of *Giardia*.

Metronidazole (Flagyl) is well absorbed from the gastrointestinal tract. It has very low protein binding and is well distributed in the body. After entering the target cell, it interacts with the protozoal DNA, where it causes a loss of helical structure and strand breakage.[12] The liver extensively metabolizes the drug, and in humans hepatic transformation is responsible for 50% of the elimination. Patients receiving cimetidine or phenobarbital may require adjustment in the dosage because of drug interaction. Metronidazole toxicity may be seen with high doses. Neurologic toxicity includes ataxia, nystagmus, seizures, tremors, and weakness.[12,35] Numerous studies have demonstrated that metronidazole is an effective treatment for giardiasis,[36-40] although efficacy is rarely 100%. Dogs may be treated orally with 12.5 to 32.5 mg/kg twice daily; therapy should be continued for 8 days. Cats may be treated orally with 17.4 mg/kg once daily for 8 days.[12] The commercially available product (Flagyl) is formulated in 250- and 500-mg tablets. Parenteral formulations are also available, but their usefulness is questionable insofar as the giardial trophozoites remain in the lumen of the gastrointestinal tract. Efficacy of metronidazole benzoate (25 mg/kg orally twice daily) for treatment of giardia was studied prospectively in experimentally infecting cats that had been vaccinated for giardiasis (n = 16) and cats that had not been vaccinated (n = 16). All cats had been shedding giardia for 3 months and were confirmed positive 1 week before treatment. All cats were negative by the 15-day posttreatment period.

Quinacrine

Quinacrine has also been shown to be useful in treating giardiasis in dogs and cats.[40] Unfortunately, commercial production of the product (Atabrine) was discontinued in 1993.

MISCELLANEOUS DRUGS AND PROTOZOAL INFECTIONS

Drugs

Folate Antagonists

Folate antagonists used to treat protozoal disease are categorized as type 1 or type 2. Type 1 antagonists include the sulfonamides and sulfones, which mimic para-aminobenzoic acid, thus targeting dihydropteroate synthase. Type 2 antifolates include the diaminopyrimidines, such as pyrimethamine, biguanidines, the triazine metabolites (discussed later), and quinazolines. These drugs target dihydrofolate reductase, preventing the formation of tetrahydrofolate, a cofactor necessary for the biosynthesis of thymidylate, purine nucleotides, and selected amino acids.[41] Type 1 folate antagonists are discussed in greater depth in Chapter 7. Pyrimethamine is characterized by an 80- to 90-hour half-life in humans. Although not a first-line antimalarial drug, it, along with a sulfonamide (sulfadiazine), is the first choice for treatment of toxoplasmosis. Other drugs with which it is given include clindamycin and the macrolides; the drug also has been administered with dapsone, but this may increase the risk of agranulocytosis. The drug is relatively well tolerated in humans.

Dapsone also is a folate antagonist, (similar to para-aminobenzoic acid, it should be considered a type 1 folate antagonist) shown to be useful against *Pneumocystis carinii*.[42]

Synergy has been demonstrated toward some organisms when dapsone is combined with pyrimethamine and trimethoprim; efficacy was greater compared with sulfonamide combinations toward selected organisms.

Atovaquone

Atovaquone is a hydroxymapthoquinone used for the treatment and prevention of selected protozoal disease in humans, including malaria. It is available as either the sole drug, or in combination with proguanil. Proguanil is a biguanide prodrug that must be converted to the triazine metabolite, cycloguanil. The combined drug minimizes the risk of resistance. Synergy also has been demonstrated with the combination toward some organisms. The mechanism of action of atovaquone includes, but probably is not limited to, impaired mitochondrial function in the protozoal organism, probably at the level of electron transport. Dihydroorotate dehydrogenase has been the suggested mitochondrial enzyme targeted by atovaquone.[41] Resistance to atovaquone, reflecting single point mutations, occurs rapidly when atovaqone is used alone.[41] The pharmacokinetics have been cited as a contributing factor to resistance: slow uptake and high lipophilicity may result in prolonged exposure of the protozoa to subtheraeputic concentrations.

Triazines

Toltrazuril is a triazine coccidiostat used in poultry; ponazuril is the major metabolite. Toltrazuril targets the mitochondrial respiratory chain of the susceptible protozoal organism; at higher concentrations, it also blocks pyrimidine formation.[43] Ponazuril has been shown to be active against *Sarcocystis neurona* both in vitro and in vivo and has been approved for use in horses to treat protozoal encephalitis caused by *Sarocystis.* Efficacy also has been demonstrated in vivo against *Neospora caninum.*[44] In vitro studies with toxoplasmosis indicates that ponazuril interferes with tachyzoite division. Disease regressed in mice treated with 100 mg/kg of toltrazuril and ponazuril, but recrudescence occurred with the ponazuril-treated mice but not those treated with toltrazuril.[43] At 10 or 20 mg/kg, ponazuril treatment 1 day before or 3 days after infection followed by 10 days of therapy completely protected mice against acute toxoplasmosis. Treatment with 20 mg/kg but not 10 mg/kg once before and daily for 6 days after infection, followed by 10 days of therapy, also protected against fatal toxoplasmosis.[45]

Using a murine model of neosporosis, either toltrazuril or ponazuril administered at 20 mg/kg in drinking water completely prevented the formation of cerebral lesions and decreased polymerase chain reaction (PCR) detection by 90%.[46] Ponazuril is being used at 20 mg/kg once weekly for 2 weeks for coccidia in dogs (see other doses).

Other Nitroimidazoles

Tinidazole and ronidazole are newer nitromidazoles that have been used with variable success for treatment of protozoal disease. Of the two, the kinetics have been described for tinadazole in dogs and cats after single intravenous (15 mg/kg) and oral doses (15 mg/kg or 30 mg/kg). Oral bioavailability was described as completed, with peak plasma concentrations after oral administration of 15 mg/kg being 17.8 and 22.5 μg/mL in dogs and cats, respectively, and after 30 mg/kg, 37.9 μg/mL in dogs, and 33.6 μg/mL in cats. The apparent volume of distribution in dogs and cats was 0.67 and 0.54 L/kg, respectively. The elimination half-life in dogs was 4.4 hours, compared with 8.4 hours in cats, suggesting 8- to 12-hour dosing intervals in both species. However, plasma drug concentrations were above the minimum inhibitory concentration of tinidazole-susceptible bacteria for 24 hours in cats and 12 hours in dogs after a single oral dose of 15 mg/kg. No adverse events were reported.

Other Nitrofurans

Numerous nitrofurans have been studied for efficacy against protozoal organisms. Among them, nifurtimox demonstrated significant efficacy against Chagas disease. Although nifurtimox is available in the United States, access can be gained only through the Centers for Disease Control and Prevention (CDC), presumably to allow tracking of human cases of Chagas infections. Trypanocidal effects reflect partial reduction and formation of reactive oxygen radicals; the organisms have low concentrations of glutathione and thus have a limited capacity to scavenge the oxygen radicals. However, like the organisms, host toxicity also reflects oxygen radical formation. The ability of *N*-acetylcysteine to protect the host apparently has not been studied. Although absorbed well after oral administration, metabolism is sufficiently rapid that concentrations of the parent compound remain low; efficacy of the metabolites is not known. Side effects include gastric upset and weight loss.

Quinolones

The quinolone-containing drugs are classified as two types: Type 1 drugs include the 4-aminoquinolones such as chlorquinolone, whereas the type 2 drugs include the aryl-amino alcohols such as quinine and quinidine. Their use has been principally for the treatment of malaria in humans, but they occasionally are used to treat other parasites. Quinine is the primary alkaloid of cinchona, the bark of a South American tree, and has been used medicinally since the early 1600s. The drug is still derived primarily from natural sources. Quinidine differs from quinine only by the orientation of an alcohol group, resulting in greater potency and toxicity. Chloroquine is characterized by less toxicity and greater efficacy compared with quinine.[47] However, widespread resistance to chloroquinine has markedly reduced its use. The mechanism of action of these drugs is not well known, with a number being proposed. These include inhibition of protein sythnthesis, inhibition of FV lipase or aspartic proteinases and inhibition of DNA or RNA synthesis.[41] Quinine and similar drugs increase the refractory period of muscle, antagonizing the action of physostigmine on skeletal muscle.[47] Respiratory distress and dysphagia occur in humans with myasthenia gravis. Quinine is well absorbed after oral administration. The drug is extensively metabolized and is characterized by an elimination half-life of about 11 hours, but this can increase (owing to decreased clearance) to close to 20 hours with repetitive dosing.[47] Side effects also include hypoglycelmia (which can be life-threatening), hypotension, and central nervous system side effects.

Diaminidines

The diaminidines include diminazene aceturate and pentamidine isethionate (approved in the United States to treat *Pneumocystis* pneumonia), and a carbanilide member, imidocarb diproprionate. The latter is approved for use in the United States to treat canine babesiosis. The mechanism of action of these drugs is not clear and may vary for the individual parasite. Proposed mechanisms include cationic interactions with DNA or nucleotides or interference with polyamine uptake or function. Efficacy within a genus of protozoa may vary with the species. Efficacy of pentamide is particularly good against *Pneumocystis*, hence its importance in human medicine. As a class, the diamidines are fungicidal toward some organisms, although their usefulness was largely replaced by amphotericin B.[47]

In humans pentamidine has a half-life of about 6 hours but is very slowly eliminated in the urine. The drug is extensively accumulated in tissues, which may explain its apparently prophylactic efficacy against for some organisms. Side effects can be life threatening and may reflect anticholinergic- or histaminergic-like responses (perhaps reflecting mast cell degranulation and histamine release). Clinical signs include tachycardia, dyspnea, vomiting, and (in humans) fainting or dizziness. Sterile abscesses have been reported in humans after intramuscular injection. Pancreatitis and either hyperglycemia or hypoglycemia (the latter potentially life-threatening) also have been reported.[47]

Sodium Stibogluconate

Sodium stibolugonate (SSG) is a pentavalent antimonial compound used for the treatment of leishmaniasis. As with several other antiprotoazoal drugs, SSG is available only through the CDC. Its mechanism of action is not known, but bioenergetics, including glycolysis and fatty acid metabolism and generation of ATP and GTP of amastigotes is impaired. The drugs may be prodrugs with generation of Sb^{3+} being the toxic compound. The preservative chlorocresol may contribute to the activity of the compound. The drug is eliminated in humans in two phases: a short 2-hour phase followed by a longer 30- to 75-hour phase. Accumulation of the drug in macrophages may facilitate efficacy. Resistance is limiting efficacy of the drugs for treatment of leishmaniasis; increasingly higher doses are required. Currently, when given (20 mg in humans) daily for 10 days, the drug yields an 85% to 90% cure rate.[47] The drug is relatively well tolerated, with pain at the injection site, chemical pancreatitis (high incidence), hepatitis, bone marrow suppression, myalgia, and malaise being reported side effects in humans.[47]

Miscellaneous Protozoal Infections

Leishmaniasis

Leishmaniasis is caused by protozoa of the Trypanosomatidae family. In mammals the organisms reside in macrophages as amastigotes. Two major forms occur. The cutaneous form is caused by a number of species, including *Leishmania major, Leishmania tropica,* and *Leishmania mexicana.* The visceral form is caused by *Leishmania* of the *donovani* complex. The dog is the major reservoir for human visceral leishmaniasis in Mediterranean countries.[48] Whereas the cutaneous form has been reported in the United States and other countries, the visceral form has largely been limited to Asia and the Middle East, with afflicted dogs generally having traveled to endemic countries.[49] Recently, the visceral form has been described in a kennel of Foxhounds in Oklahoma; additional multiple dog outbreaks have since been reported.

Two reviews have addressed treatment of leishmaniasis.[50,51] The latter is a systemic review of the literature. The goal of treatment ranges from resolution of clinical signs to eradication of organisms. Because experimental infections are difficult to establish, clinical trials tend to focus on spontaneous disease. Therapeutic response is based on decreased *Leishmania*-specific antibody concentrations and return of parasite-specific cell mediated immunity.[50] Improvement persists unless organisms have not been cleared.

A number of studies have focused on the role of altered immune response in refractory infections caused by intracellular protozoal infections.[48] Resistance to leishmaniasis may reflect Th-1–mediated immunity. Among the cytokines important for an effective Th-1 response, IL-1 is among the most potent inducers. Depending on the immune response, infection in dogs can cause manifestations that range from asymptomatic subclinical disease to complete manifestation.[52] In one study dogs experimentally infected with *Leishmania infantum* failed to express IL-4 compared with control dogs. Further, in infected but asymptomatic dogs, although both Th-1 and Th-2 cytokines were produced, cell-mediated immunity reflected preferential expression of Th-1 cytokines.[52] IL-12 augmented interferon-gamma production by peripheral blood mononuclear cells in dogs either experimentally or naturally infected with canine visceral leishmaniasis, suggesting that IL-12 may be a feasible cytokine therapy in infected dogs refractory to therapy.[48]

Treatment with antiprotozoal drugs traditionally has included pentavalent antimony compounds, including SSG (obtainable through the CDC) and meglumine antimoniate. Baneth and Shaw[50] reviewed the efficacy of antimony for treatment and cure of leishmaniasis in dogs. Cure rate is considered low, although clinical signs often improve. Use has been limited more recently by the emergence of *L. infantum,* which is resistant to therapy.

KEY POINT 12-5 Successful therapy of leishmaniasis ultimately may require appropriate immunomodulation.

The use of a liposomal antimony preparation for treatment of leishmaniasis was studied in experimentally infected Beagles (n = 6). Dogs first received an intravenous injection of a commercial product (Glucantime; Rhône-Mérieux, France; 9.9 μg/kg antimony), and 1 week later the same dose of antimony was given as a liposomal preparation intravenously for 2 days, then subcutaneously for 8 days. The cycle was repeated

10 days later. The disposition of antimony was characterized for both antimony preparations. Regarding the disposition, for the liposomal and nonliposomal preparations, the results were, respectively: C_{max} at steady state (μg/mL) 51, 114; volume of distribution at steady state (L/kg), 0.4 ± 0.16 and 0.2 ± 0.06; clearance (l*hr/kg) 0.009 ± 0.005 and 0.17 ± 0.05; area under the curve (μg/hr/mL) 1494 ± 1038 and 61.2 ± 14; and elimination half-life*hr) 33.1 ± 13.8 and 6.1 ± 0.7. Response to therapy was addressed only in terms of total protein and gamma globulin concentrations treatment and at long-term follow-up. These increased 3 months after treatment with the free form of antimony but not the liposomal form.[53]

Allopurinol is metabolized by *Leishmania* to an inactive analog of inosine, which is then incorporated into the RNA of the parasite, causing faulty protein translation. It can be used alone or in combination with other drugs. Although clinical signs are likely to improve, clinical cure is unlikely. Survival (78% for more than 4 years in one study) is more likely if renal insufficiency is not present when therapy is begun; the proportion of survivors is similar to that in dogs treated with antimony. Among the clinical sequelae of leishmaniasis is progressive renal disease. The efficacy of allopurinol (10 mg/kg twice daily for 6 months) in slowing the progression of renal disease associated with proteinuria was prospectively studied in dogs (n = 12; 5 no treatment controls) without proteinuria or renal insufficiency, asymptomatic dogs with proteinuria (n = 10; 5 no treatment controls), and symptomatic (azotemic) dogs (n = 8) with proteinuria and renal insufficiency.[54] Compared with untreated controls, proteinuria was decreased in dogs that already had proteinuria and the progression slowed of tubular but not glomerular disease in all asymptomatic dogs. Finally, azotemia resolved in the symptomatic dogs. Cure of visceral leishmaniasis with the combined use of fluconazole and allopurinol for 4 months has also been reported.[55]

A number of other drugs have been studied for their potential efficacy. Among the drugs used to treat leishmaniasis is the antifungal agent, amphotericin B (see Chapter 9). Baneth and Shaw[50] reviewed use of amphotericin B for treatment of leishmaniasis. In general, efficacy is limited by emerging renal disease after total cumulative doses ranging from 8 to 26 mg/kg. This study reported that 27 of 28 naturally infected dogs that responded to amphotericin B (out of a total of 30 infected dogs) remained in clinical remission for 12 months after treatment of 0.5 to 0.8 mg/kg intravenously 2 to 3 times a week for a total cumulative dose of 15 mg/kg (as reviewed by Baneth and Shaw[50]). In another study 100% of 16 dogs diagnosed with leishmaniaisis were clinically cured (no organisms in the bone marrow and 87% negative on PCR) at the end of 4 to 5 weeks of amphotericin B prepared as the desoxycholate salt in soybean oil (0.8 to 2.5 mg/kg). However, 6 dogs (including 2 dogs that never became negative) subsequently became PCR positive for infection at some point in the posttreatment follow-up. Of these 6 dogs, 3 became clinically ill again. The authors concluded that a single negative PCR result should not be interpreted as clinical cure.[56] Oliva and coworkers[57] reported the failure of liposomal amphotericin B (3 to 3.3 mg/kg for 3 to 5 treatments) to cure dogs (n = 13) with cutaneous leishmaniasis. Although animals responded clinically very rapidly, recrudescence of clinical signs returned 4 months later and lymph node aspirates remained positive. Of 17 dogs treated with amphotericin B prepared in a lipid, 14 were treated successfully, as indicated by negative bone marrow PCR results at 1 to 3 months after therapy; however, the timing of recheck may have been inappropriately short.

Pentamidine (4 mg/kg intramuscularly every 3 days for 8 treatments) has also been used successfully in resolving clinical signs in a small number of dogs naturally (n = 3) or experimentally (n = 5) infected with *L. infantum*. Two of the experimental animals were cured. Other drugs that have been used with variable efficacy include metronidazole, itraconazole, ketoconazole, and terbinafine.

Noli and Auxilia[51] systematically reviewed the literature for evidence of effective therapy for treatment of *L. infantum*. Clinical trials that addressed prevention or treatment (n = 47) were reviewed from 1980 to 2004. Good evidence was found to support the use of meglumine antimony (at least 100 mg/kg for 3 to 4 weeks). Fair evidence existed for pentamidine (4 mg/kg twice weekly) and aminosidine (5 mg/kg twice daily) for 3 to 4 weeks. Aminosidine is an aminoglycoside antimicrobial whose efficacy is similar to that of antimony, but its use is limited by emergent nephrotoxicity. Insufficient evidence existed for allopurinol alone, amphotericin B, ketoconazole, enrofloxaxcin, metronidazole, or combinations thereof.

Trypanosomosis

Trypanosomiasis is caused by protozoa of the genus *Trypanosoma* spp. Two major diseases occur: that associated with *T. brucei* in subsahara Africa and that associated with *T. cruzi*, occurring largely in Latin America. Infection with *T. bruceia* is transmitted by the tsetse fly and occurs either in small vessels or connective tissue. The disease is of major regional economic importance, impacting food producing and companion animals as well as humans. Resistance has emerged toward the three primary chemotherapeutic agents, with underdosing and delay in treatment being major mitigating factors.[51a] Treatment of experimentally induced *T. brucei brucei* in dogs has been studied. The use of diaminazene aceturate (7 mg/kg) as a single dose, or pentamidine esethionate (4 mg/kg, IM, at either every other day for 6 treatments [Group 2] or at 3, 2, 14, 16 days [Group 3]), was studied in dogs (n = 4 per group and 3 untreated controls) 14 days after experimental infection with *T. brucei brucei*. All dogs were parasitemic by day 7 of infection. By day 7 posttreatment, parasitemia had cleared in all dogs but not the control animals (these died by day 28 postinfection). However, one dog in the diaminazene group relapsed at day 42 (dog died at day 70); the remaining dogs remained free of parasites through the 77 day study period. Two dogs treated with pentamidine (group 3) also died, without evidence of parasitemia. Serum liver enzymes increased more significantly in the diaminazine group. The authors concluded that pentamidine at 4 mg/kg every other day for 2 weeks was a reasonable choice for treatment of trypanosomosis in dogs. Chagas disease is caused by *T. cruzi* which is transmitted by the kissing (reduviid) bug. Infection occurs after rubbing feces from the bug into the bitewound made by the bug; infection also can be acquired by eating the bug. The acute stage occurs within weeks after initial infection and is followed by a latent and then chronic stage. The chronic stage in humans impacts the nervous (neuritis and other neuropathies), digestive (e.g., megaesophagus or megacolon; reflecting in part neurologic damage) and cardiovascular systems (cardiomyopathy). Cardiovascular disease in dogs is generally associated with right-sided cardiac dysfunction, and its sequelae, including arrhythmias, pleural effusion, ascites, and hepatomegaly. Treatment focuses on parasiticides and supportive care. Intracellular amastigotes destroy intramural neurons; inflammation, fibrosis, and cell death result in organ damage and clinical signs. Antiparasiticides include azoles (benznidazole) or nitros (nifurtimox). The latter may be associated with gastrointestinal signs, peripheral neuropathy, and hemolytica anemia.

Cryptosporidiosis

Cryptosporidiosis is a ubiquitous protozoal disease spread by the fecal–oral route and associated with immunosuppressive diseases in dogs or cats. *C. parvum* is the strain that most commonly infects mammals. Clinical manifestations reflect malabsorption or secretory diarrhea through unknown mechanisms. Signs are similar to those associated with giardiasis, although mucus is more common with infections by the latter. The syndrome may be self-limiting. Like giardia, cryptosporidiosis is a zoonotic concern. In humans nutritional approaches (including probiotics, low-fat diets, high-fiber diets, simple carbohydrates) to treatment are generally effective, with antimicrobial therapy reserved for nonresponders. Antiprotozoal therapy has largely been ineffective. Tylosin (11 mg/kg by mouth twice daily for 28 days) may help reduce diarrhea. Clindamycin was ineffective in single cases for treatment of cryptosporidiosis in cats. The aminoglycoside paramycin may be effective following oral (not parenteral) administration. When paramycin is used in cats (150 mg/kg every 12 to 24 hours orally for 5 days), fecal oocysts were cleared from infected cats,[58] but when it was used to treat feline trichomoniasis, 25% of the cats developed acute renal failure. Azithromycin has been used with some success in the treatment of cattle and might be considered as an alternative therapy in dogs or cats. Nitazoxanide, approved for use in humans to treat *Giardia*, is a derivative of nitrothiazole found to be effective against a wide range of parasites and bacteria. The use of this drug in dogs and cats has not yet been reported.

Fenbendazole (50 mg/kg orally once daily for 5 days) was variably effective in treating cats concurrently infected with *Giardia* and *C. parvum*.[32] Although the number of oocysts decreased the first week after treatment compared with controls, no difference was detected the second week (the power of the study was not addressed). Only 50% (four of eight) of cats treated with fenbendazole were negative 3 weeks after treatment.

Trichomoniasis

Tritrichomonas foetus, the cause of trichomoniasis in cattle, is an emerging protozoal enteric pathogen of domestic cats. Infection occurs in the lumen of the colon, where inflammatory colitis and explosive, chronic, foul-smelling diarrhea result.[59] The disease may be prevalent in high-density cat populations such as catteries or show environments and therefore may be more prevalent in purebred cats. A number of treatments have been tried without consistent therapeutic success, including metronidazole, fenbendazole, albendazole, pyrantel pamoate, sulfadimethoxine, trimethoprim–sulfadiazine, furazolidone, tylosin, enrofloxacin, amoxicillin, clindamycin, paromomycin, and erythromycin.[59]

Trichomonads generate pyruvate through glycolysis and reductive fermentation. The latter pathway is targeted by 5-nitroimidazole antibiotics such as metronidazole. Reduction of the nitroimidazoles in hydrogenosomes generates anion radicals, which accumulate to toxic concentrations in the protozoal cell. Metronidazole as sole therapy generally has been ineffective against *T. foetus* infection in cats: Transient improvement is generally followed by recrudescence of clinical signs.[60] Gookin and coworkers[60] found that, based on in vitro comparison of metronidazole, ronidazole, and tinidazole, ronidazole was the most potent toward *T. foetus* isolated from a cat with spontaneous disease. Ronidazole was then prospectively studied for its efficacy in a cat naturally infected, and 10 specific pathogen-free (SPF) kittens experimentally infected with *T. foetus.* Ronidazole at 30 to 50 mg/kg every 12 hours for 14 days resolved clinical signs and cured (based on PCR results) all 11 cats. Relapses occurred at 10 mg/kg. Kather and coworkers[61] reported in vitro susceptibility for *T. foetus* collected from four Bengal cats with spontaneous disease. Omeprazole and paromomycin were ineffective, and metronidazole, ronidazole, and furazolidone were equally effective at 0.625 to 2.5 μg/mL. However, ronidazole was characterized by greater lethality.

In SPF kittens experimentally infected with *T. foetus,* ronidazole (10 mg/kg every 12 hours for 2 weeks) initially was effective but relapse occurred in 5 of 5 cats 2 to 20 weeks after treatment. However, at 30 to 50 mg/kg, 10 of 10 cats remained negative for 21 to 30 weeks after treatment. Likewise, treatment with 10 mg/kg ronidazole for 2 weeks resolved clinical signs of infection in a spontaneously diseased cat, with clinical signs returning at 85 days.[60]

Cytauxzoonosis

Cytauxzoonosis is a generally fatal tick-borne protozoal disease that afflicts cats. The bobcat appears to be the reservoir host. Cytauxzoon has an erythrocytic phase, which morphologically cannot be distinguished from babesiosis, as well as a tissue phase. Schizonts develop in monocytes, which then marginate into the vascular endothelium, often occluding the vessel. Schizonts then develop into merozoites, which, on release into the blood and tissue, invade other cells, including erythrocytes. Clinical signs rapidly progress, with the course of the disease generally being less than 1 week. Clinical signs generally include pale mucous membranes, dehydration, dyspnea, icterus, anorexia, and severe lethargy. Treatment with either diminazene aceturate (2 mg/kg subcutaneously, repeated in 2 to 4 weeks) or imidocarb dipropionate (5 mg/kg, subcutaneously, repeated in 2 weeks) should be considered.[62]

In one report, 6 of 7 cats diagnosed with cytauxzoonosis responded to 2 intramuscular injections (2 to 4 weeks apart) of either diminazene aceturate or imidocarb dipropionate (2 mg/kg). However, the seventh cat died after the first injection of diminazine.[63] Drugs generally shown to be ineffective include paravaquone (20 or 30 mg/kg intramuscularly daily), buparaquone (5 or 10 mg/kg intramuscularly daily), sodium thiacetarsamide, and tetracyclines.[62,64]

Babesiosis

Babesiosis is a tick-borne hematozoan disease afflicting dogs and cats. Dogs are known to host *Babesia canis* (large and more important form) and *Babesia gibsoni* (small form), both of which cause hemolytic anemia, whereas cats are infected with *Babesia felis,* among others. However, other body systems may also be involved. In dogs the disease can present as hyperacute, acute, chronic, and subclinical. Greyhounds appear to have a higher prevalence compared with other breeds of dogs. Treatment with imidocarb dipropionate (approved by the FDA for this use) is generally successful. A number of protocols for treatment have been described. Imidocarb at 7.5 mg/kg can be followed with diminazene (3.5 mg/kg) or given in two doses (5 to 6.6 mg/kg 14 days apart). Imidocarb is the preferred drug with concurrent infection with *Erhlichia.* A single dose of imidocarb should be protective. Phenamidine (15 mg/kg once a day, for two doses), pentamidine (16.5 mg/kg, two doses 24 hours apart), or trypan blue (10 mg/kg of a 1% solution intravenously, once) also have been suggested for severe infections when the anticholinergic properties of the diamidine derivatives are a concern. Clindamycin at 25 to 50 mg/kg daily for 7 to 10 days also may be useful. For cats the antimalarial drug primaquine, (0.5 mg/kg orally or intramuscularly) has been recommended. However, because the lethal dose is 1 mg/kg, extreme caution should accompany use of this drug in cats. Another drug that may be useful is atovaquone.

The mechanism of action of atovaquone against other protozoa is believed to involve the inhibition of cytochrome *b* and electron transport. The antiprotozoal drug atovaquone has proved effective for treatment of at least two *Babesia* species, *Babesia microti* and *Babesia divergens,* when combined with azithromycin.[65] The combined use of atovaquone (13 mg/kg orally every 8 hours) and azithromycin (10 mg/kg orally once daily) was successful in the treatment of babesiosis in dogs.[65] Of 11 dogs remaining infected with *B. gibsoni* (Asian genotype) despite therapy with either imidocarb. diproprionate alone (dose: 6 to 6.6 mg/kg intramuscularly) for two doses 1 to 2 weeks apart, diminazene aceturate (3.5 mg/kg intramuscularly) for two doses 2 weeks apart, or a combination of the two, 8 became PCR negative compared to 11 of 11 controls that remained positive. [65]

Evidence (PCR) of infection was absent in 80% of treated dogs, whereas it was present in all dogs in a placebo group of similar size. No adverse events were reported in treated animals. Treatment was limited to animals that did not require hospitalization, indicating a need to study acutely ill animals. However, the lack of any other known effective therapy warrants consideration of this combination for treatment in acutely ill animals as well. Of the two preparations (atovaquone or atovaquone combined with proguanil) currently available in the United States, the single product is probably less likely to cause gastrointesintal side effects.[65]

Hepatozoonosis

Hepatozoonosis is a tick-transmitted hemosporazoon disease infecting dogs. The organism is similar to *Babesia.* The clinical syndrome is characterized by a stiff gait and myalgia, inactivity, and weight loss and profound leukocytosis (mature neutrophilia: 70,000 to 200,000 cells/μL). Periosteal proliferation and increased alkaline phosphatase may be present. Severe hyperesthesia may be manifested as stiffness. Analgesic therapy, probably with nonsteroidal antiinflammatory drugs, is indicated. Tepoxalin (Zubrin) might be considered for its ability to target leukotrienes (prevalent in white blood cells) as well as prostaglandins. Definitive diagnosis appears to have been facilitated using an ELISA-based test. Treatment with triple combination therapy (TCP) may resolve clinical signs and has dramatically improved the prognosis in dogs. Therapy includes trimethoprime sulfadiazine (15 mg/kg orally, twice daily), clindamycin (10 mg/kg orally, three times daily), and pyrimethamine (0.25 mg/kg orally, once daily), each administered for at least 14 days. Efficacy with imidocarb dipropionate (5 mg/kg subcutaneously, given once) alone or combined (at 6 mg/kg subcutaneously, every 14 days) with tetracycline (22 mg/kg orally, thrice daily) for 14 days) is less effective. Treatment with the coccidiostat toltrazuril (5 to 10 mg/kg subcutaneously or orally, once daily for 3 to 5 days, or 5 mg/kg orally, twice daily for 4 days) may resolve clinical signs, but the risk of relapse may be great. Decoquinate (10 to 20 mg/kg orally, twice daily; continuous therapy) may be indicated to prevent relapses after TCP.

Neospora Caninum

N. caninum is a *Toxoplasma gondii*-like protozoan for which canids are the only known definitive host. The life cycle involves cysts containing bradyzoites in the intermediate host and rapidly dividing tachyzoites in multiple tissues of the definitive host. The intestinal phase in the definitive host is similar to that of coccidiosis and leads to passage of nonsporulated oocysts in feces. Clinical disease, which is most severe in puppies, presents as hind limb paresis that rapidly progresses to rear limb paralysis and occasionally rigid hyperextension of limbs. Other signs include dysphagia, jaw muscle paralysis, muscle atrophy, and heart failure. Neosporosis in adult dogs generally includes neurologic disease but also may manifest as encephalomyelitis, polymyositis, myocarditis, or dermatitis. Puppies can be infected transplacentally. A canine kidney cell model, recombinant canine interferon alpha (IFN-alpha), beta (IFN-beta), and gamma (IFN-gamma) inhibited the growth of *N. caninum* tachyzoites. However, the effect was associated with the suppression of the host cell viability.[66] Treatment is similar to that for toxoplasmosis.

Protothecosis

Prototheca are achlorophyllous algae, related to green algae and ubiquitous in the environment. Their importance as a cause of infection in immunocompromised infections is increasing in human medicine.[67] Infections are either subcutaneous to cutaneous, synovial or systemic. Infection is generally preceded by skin or wound infections. Therapy with amphotericin B requires high concentrations, which may include local as well as systemic therapy. Duration of treatment in humans ranges from several days to months. Tetracyclines (doxycycline) may act synergistically. Imidazoles and flucytosine have been used systemically successfully, and a number of local therapies have been successful (gentian violet, polymyxin B, clotrimazole, neomycin, hydrogen peroxide, and potassium iodide). Protothecosis in cats usually is cutaneous, whereas dogs may present with a variety of clinical manifestations. The most common presenting sign in dogs is protracted hemorrhagic diarrhea, with the colon the most common site.[68] Treatment in dogs has included amphotericin B rectally in an enema form (3% cream), itraconazole, and ketoconazole.

SUMMARY

Therapy of protozoal infections in small animals may range from simple to complex therapeutic dilemmas. The best treatment of each case must be determined by considering the life cycle of the pathogen, the general physical condition of each animal, and the animal's environment. Therapy must include adequate attention to supportive therapy to control clinical signs and support normal body function. Therapy also should include adequate hygiene to limit reinfection and disease transmission. The selection and administration of the specific antiprotozoal agent are only parts of the overall therapeutic picture.

REFERENCES

1. Bowman DD: *Georgis' parasitology for veterinarians*, ed 9, St Louis, 2009, Saunders.
2. Greene CE: *Infectious diseases of the dog and cat*, ed 3, St Louis, 2006, Saunders, pp 667–807.
3. Boch J, Gobel E, Heine J, et al: *Isospora*-infektionen bei hund und katze, *Berl Munch Tierarztl Wochenschr* 94:384–391, 1981.
4. Correa WM, Correa CNM, Langoni H, et al: Canine isosporosis, *Canine Pract* 10(1):44–46, 1983.
5. Dubey JP: Intestinal protozoa infections, *Vet Clin North Am Small Anim Pract* 23(1):37–55, 1993.
6. Cribb AE, Lee BL, Trepanier LA, et al: Adverse reactions to sulphonamide and sulphonamide–trimethoprim antimicrobials: clinical syndromes and pathogenesis, *Adverse Drug React Toxicol Rev* 15(1):9–50, 1996.
7. Patterson JM, Grenn HH: Hemorrhage and death in dogs following the administration of sulfaquinoxaline, *Can Vet J* 16(9):265–268, 1975.
8. Entriken TL, editor: *Veterinary pharmaceuticals and biologicals* [VPB] 1999/2000, ed 11, Lenexa, Kan, 1998, Veterinary Medicine Publishing.
9. Dunbar MR, Foreyt WJ: Prevention of coccidiosis in domestic dogs and captive coyotes (*Canis latrans*) with sulfadimethoxine-ormetoprim combination, *Am J Vet Res* 46(9):1899–1902, 1985.
10. Plumb DC: *Veterinary drug handbook*, ed 3, Ames, Iowa, 1999, Iowa State University Press.
11. Smart J: Amprolium for canine coccidiosis, *Mod Vet Pract* 52:41, 1971.
12. United States Pharmacopeial Convention (USP): *USP drug information update,* Rockville, MD, 1998, pp. 1289-1586.
13. Dubey JP, Greene CE: Enteric coccidiosis. In Greene CE, editor: *Infectious diseases of the dog and cat*, ed 3, St Louis, 2006, Saunders, pp 775–784.
14. Fraser CM, editor: *The Merck veterinary manual*, ed 7, Rahway, NJ, 1991, Merck & Co.
15. Brander GC, Pugh DM, Bywater RJ, et al: *Veterinary applied pharmacology and therapeutics*, ed 5, Philadelphia, 1991, Baillière Tindall.
16. Lappin MR: Protozoal and miscellaneous infections. In Ettinger SJ, Feldman EC, editors: *Textbook of veterinary internal medicine*, ed 6, St Louis, 2005, Saunders, pp 438–646.
17. Dubey JP, Lappin MR: Toxoplasmosis and neosporosis. In Greene CE, editor: *Infectious diseases of the dog and cat*, ed 3, St Louis, 2006, Saunders, pp 754–755.
18. Hardman JG, Limbird LE, Gilman AG, et al: *Goodman & Gilman's the pharmacological basis of therapeutics*, ed 9, New York, 1996, McGraw-Hill.
19. Greene CE, Cook JR, Mahaffey EA: Clindamycin for treatment of *Toxoplasma* polymyositis in a dog, *J Am Vet Med Assoc* 187(6):631–634, 1985.
20. Lappin MR, Greene CE, Winston S, et al: Clinical feline toxoplasmosis, *J Vet Intern Med* 3:139–143, 1989.
21. Chirgwin K, Hafner R, Leport C, et al: Randomized phase II trial of atovaquone with pyrimethamine or sulfadiazine for treatment of toxoplasmic encephalitis in patients with acquired immunodeficiency syndrome: ACTG 237/ANRS 039 study, *Clin Infect Dis* 34:1243–1250, 2002.
22. Hahn NE, Glaser CA, Hird DW, et al: Prevalence of *Giardia* in the feces of pups, *J Am Vet Med Assoc* 192:1128–1129, 1988.
23. Barlough JE: Canine giardiasis: a review, *J Small Anim Pract* 20:613–623, 1979.
24. Kirkpatrick CE: Feline giardiasis: a review, *J Small Anim Pract* 27:69–80, 1986.
25. Zajac AM: Giardiasis, *Compendium* 14(5):604–611, 1992.
26. Barr SC, Greene CE, Gookin JL: Enteric protozoal infections. In Greene CE, editor: *Infectious diseases of the dog and cat*, ed 3, St Louis, 2006, Saunders, pp 736–750.
27. Barr SC, Bowman DD, Heller RL, et al: Efficacy of albendazole against giardiasis in dogs, *Am J Vet Res* 54(6):926–928, 1993.
28. Meyer EK: Adverse events associated with albendazole and other products used for treatment of giardiasis in dogs, *J Am Vet Med Assoc* 213(1):44–46, 1998.
29. Stokol T, Randolph JF, Nachbar S, et al: Development of bone marrow toxicosis after albendazole administration in a dog and cat, *J Am Vet Med Assoc* 210:1753–1756, 1997.
30. Barr SC, Bowman DD, Heller RL: Efficacy of fenbendazole against giardiasis in dogs, *Am J Vet Res* 55:988–990, 1994.
31. Zajac AM, LaBranche TP, Donoghue AR, et al: Efficacy of fenbendazole in the treatment of experimental *Giardia* infection in dogs, *Am J Vet Res* 59:61–63, 1998.
32. Keith CL, Radecki SV, Lappin MR: Evaluation of fenbendazole for treatment of *Giardia* infection in cats concurrently infected with *Cryptosporidium parvum*, *Am J Vet Res* 64:1027–1029, 2003.
33. Kirkpatrick CE: Giardiasis in a cattery, *J Am Vet Med Assoc* 187(2):161–162, 1985.
34. Sherding RG, Johnson SE: Diseases of the intestines. In Birchard SJ, Sherding RG, editors: *Saunders manual of small animal practice*, ed 3, St Louis, 2006, Saunders, pp 702–738.
35. Dow SC, LeCouteur RA, Poss ML, et al: Central nervous system toxicosis associated with metronidazole treatment of dogs: five cases (1984-1987), *J Am Vet Med Assoc* 195(3):365–368, 1989.
36. Boreham PFL, Phillips RE, Shepherd RW: The sensitivity of *Giardia intestinalis* to drugs in vitro, *J Antimicrob Chemother* 14:449–461, 1984.
37. Kirkpatrick CE, Farrell JP: Feline giardiasis: observations on natural and induced infections, *Am J Vet Res* 45(10):2182–2188, 1984.
38. Zimmer JF: Treatment of feline giardiasis with metronidazole, *Cornell Vet* 77:383–388, 1987.

39. Watson ADJ: Giardiasis and colitis in a dog, *Aust Vet J* 56: 444–447, 1980.
40. Zimmer JF, Burrington DB: Comparison of four protocols for the treatment of canine giardiasis, *J Am Anim Hosp Assoc* 22:168–172, 1986.
41. Olliaro P: Mode of action and mechanisms of resistance for antimalarial drugs, *Pharmacol Ther* 89(2):207–219, 2001.
42. Hughes WT: Use of dapsone in the prevention and treatment of *Pneumocystis carinii* pneumonia: a review, *Clin Infect Dis* 27:191–204, 1998.
43. Darius AK, Melhorn H, Heydorn AO: Effects of toltrazuril and ponazuril on *Hammondia heydorni* (syn. *Neospora caninum*) infections in mice, *Parasitol Res* 92:520–522, 2004.
44. Mitchell SM, Zajac AM, Davis WL, et al: Mode of action of ponazuril against Toxoplasma gondii tachyzoites in cell culture, *J Eukaryot Microbiol* 50:689–690, 2003.
45. Mitchell SM, Zajac AM, Davis WL, et al: Efficacy of ponazuril in vitro and in preventing and treating *Toxoplasma gondii* infections in mice, *J Parasitology* 90(3):639–642, 2004.
46. Gottstein B, Eperon S, Dai WJ, et al: Efficacy of toltrazuril and ponazuril against experimental *Neospora caninum* infection in mice, *Parasitol Res* 87(1):43–48, 2001.
47. Tracy JW, Webster LT: Drugs used in the chemotherapy of protozoal infections: amebiasis, giardiasis, trichomoniasis, trypanosmiasis, leshmaniasis and other protozoal infections. In Hardman JG, Limberd E, editors: *Goodman & Gilman's the pharmacologic basis of therapeutics*, ed 11, New York, 2006, McGraw-Hill.
48. Strauss-Ayali D, Baneth G, Shor S, et al: Interleukin-12 augments a Th1-type immune response manifested as lymphocyte proliferation and interferon gamma production in Leishmania infantum-infected dogs, *Int J Parasitol* 35(1):63–73, 2005.
49. Schantz PM, Steurer FJ, Duprey ZH, et al: Autochthonous visceral leishmaniasis in dogs in North America, *J Am Vet Med Assoc* 226(8):1316–1322, 2005.
50. Baneth G, Shaw SE: Chemotherapy of canine leishmaniosis, *Vet Parasitol* 106:315–324, 2002.
51. Noli C, Auxilia ST: Treatment of canine old world visceral leishmaniasis: a systematic review, *Vet Dermatol* 16:213–232, 2005.
51a. Apka PO, Ezeokonkwo RC, Eze CA, et al: Comparative efficacy assessment of pentamidine isethionate and diminazene aceturate in the chemotherapy of, *Trypanosoma brucei brucei* infection in dogs, *Vet Parasitol* 151:139–149, 2008.
52. Chamizo C, Moreno J, Alvar J: Semi-quantitative analysis of cytokine expression in asymptomatic canine leishmaniasis, *Vet Immunol Immunopathol* 103(1-2):67–75, 2005.
53. Valladares JE, Riera C, Gonzalez-Ensenyat P, et al: Long term improvement in the treatment of canine leishmaniosis using an antimony liposomal formulation, *Vet Parasitol* 97:15–21, 2001.
54. Plevraki K, Koutinas AF, Kaldrymidou H, et al: Effects of allopurinol treatment on the progression of chronic nephritis in Canine Leishmaniosis (*Leishmania infantum*), *J Vet Intern Med* 20:228–233, 2006.
55. Colakoglu M, Fidan Yaylali G, et al: Successful treatment of visceral leishmaniasis with fluconazole and allopurinol in a patient with renal failure, *Scand J Infect Dis* 38(3):208–210, 2006.
56. Cortadellas O: Initial and long term efficacy of a lipid emulsion of amphtericin B desoxcycholate in the management of canine leishmaniasis, *J Vet Intern Med* 17:808–812, 2003.
57. Oliva G, Gradoni L, Ciaramella P, et al: Activity of liposomal amphotericin B (AmBisome) in dogs naturally infected with Leishmania infantum, *J Antimicrob Chemother* 36:1013–1019, 1995.
58. Barr SC, Jamrosz GF, Hornbuckle WE, et al: Use of paromomycin for treatment of cryptosporidiosis in a cat, *J Am Vet Med Assoc* 205:1742, 1994.
59. Gookin JL, Levy MG: *Trichomoniasis in cats: recognition and resilience*, Denver, 2001, Proc 19th ACVIM 755.
60. Gookin JL, Copple CN, Papich MG, et al: Efficacy of Ronidazole for treatment of feline Tritrichomonas foetus infection, *J Vet Int Med* 20:536–543, 2006.
61. Kather EJ, Marks SL, Kass PH: Determination of the in vitro susceptibility of feline Tritrichomonas foetus to 5 antimicrobial agents, *J Vet Intern Med* 21:966–970, 2007.
62. Lobetti: 2002. Cytauxzoonosis. World Small Animal Veterinary Association, Mexico City, 2003. Accessed July 20, 2010 at http://www.vin.com/proceedings/Proceedings.plx?CID=WSAVA2002&PID=2593.
63. Greene CE, Latimer K, Hopper E, et al: Administration of diminazene aceturate or imidocarb dipropionate for treatment of cytauxzoonosis in cats, *J Am Vet Med Assoc* 215(4):497–500, 1999, :Aug 15.
64. Bondy PJ, Cohn LA, Kerl ME: Feline cytauxzoonosis, *Compend Contin Educ Pract Vet* 27(1):69–75, 2005.
65. Birkenheuer AJ, Levy MG, Breitschwerdt EB: Efficacy of combined atovaquone and azithromycin for therapy of chronic *Babesia gibsoni* (Asian genotype) infections in dogs, *J Vet Intern Med* 18(4):494–498, 2004.
66. Nishikawa Y, Iwata A, Nagasawa H, et al: Comparison of the growthinhibitoryeffectsofcanineIFN-alpha,-betaand-gammaon canine cells infected with *Neospora caninum* tachyzoites, *J Vet Med Sci* 63(4):445–448, 2001.
67. Thiele D, Bergmann A: Protothecosis in human medicine, *Int J Hyg Environ Health* 204:297–302, 2002.
68. Strunck E, Billups L, Avgeris S: Canine protothecosis, *Compend Contin Educ Pract Vet* 26:96–102, 2004.

Drugs for the Treatment of Helminth Infections: Anthelmintics

13

Tad B. Coles and Randy C. Lynn

Chapter Outline

Practicing veterinarians commonly use drugs to treat and prevent helminth infections in small animals. The life cycle and biology of the most important parasites are well understood by graduate veterinarians and are not discussed here; however, current textbooks of parasitology may be consulted for review.[1-4] Gastrointestinal parasites are among the most common infectious agents that veterinarians in small animal practice face. A landmark parasite prevalence study evaluated more than 6000 canine fecal specimens from all 50 states and the District of Columbia.[5] The results indicate that parasites are common in American dogs. Nationwide, 36% of the samples tested were positive for roundworm *(Toxocara canis)*, hookworm *(Ancylostoma caninum)*, or whipworm *(Trichuris vulpis)*. Even more surprising, 52% of the samples from the southeastern United States were positive for at least one nematode. In a recent study of the results of heartworm and fecal testing in the western United States, the importance of annual testing and routine use of preventives was highlighted.[6] Clinics in 11 states were surveyed, and local dogs with no history of travel were diagnosed with heartworms in every state but Idaho and Wyoming. The prevalence of intestinal parasites in companion animals in Ontario and Quebec, Canada, during the winter was recently evaluated.[7] The fact that 30% of feline and 39% of canine fecal samples were positive for gastrointestinal parasites prompted the authors to recommend that all veterinarians follow the Companion Animal Parasite Council (CAPC) guidelines[8] regarding use of year-round broad-spectrum deworming protocols. Another reason for following CAPC guidelines, in this instance regarding routine heartworm testing and prophylaxis, is concern about animals moving from heartworm-endemic areas to those with limited heartworm exposure. These concerns were realized when Hurricane Katrina resulted in thousands of dogs and cats being shipped from Louisiana, where heartworm prevalence is quite high, to shelters across the United States.[9]

KEY POINT 13-1 Helminth infections are common in pets.

KEY POINT 13-2 Testing, treatment, and prevention of helminth infections in pets have profound zoonotic implications.

Although these parasites are important to the health of dogs, several are also important zoonotic pathogens. Ascarid larvae migrate through human tissues, causing a variety of signs correlated to the location of the migration. These are primarily *Toxocara* species ascarids, but the raccoon ascarid, *Baylisascaris procyonis,* is being increasingly implicated as a cause of human disease in the United States.[10] The Centers for Disease Control and Prevention (CDC) have published *Guidelines for Veterinarians: Prevention of Zoonotic Transmission of Ascarids and Hookworms of Dogs and Cats,* which is an excellent resource and is available online as a PDF download.[11]

KEY POINT 13-3 The raccoon ascarid is an emerging zoonotic threat.

Worldwide, helminth infections are a major animal and human health concern,[12] with hookworms infecting large numbers of people worldwide, especially those of low economic status.[13] More than 30% of the human population, in vast areas of South America and Asia, is infected with hookworms. More than half of the population is infected with hookworms in many southern areas of the African continent. Experts estimate that a billion people, more than a fifth of the planet's human inhabitants, harbor hookworms.[14] One study showed that nearly all dogs in a remote community of northeastern India were infested with one or more zoonotic gastrointestinal parasites.[15] This study demonstrated that dogs played a major zoonotic role both in transmitting parasites that use dogs as their definitive and paratenic host and in mechanically transmitting and spreading the dissemination range of an array of human-specific parasites. A recent feline study in metropolitan Rio de Janeiro revealed an 89.6% prevalence of overall gastrointestinal helminth parasites in cats.[16]

KEY POINT 13-4 The practicing veterinarian who judiciously uses anthelmintics is in a unique position to have a dramatic impact on the health of pets and people.

Through the prudent use of anthelmintics in companion animals, the practicing veterinarian is in a unique position to positively affect not only the patient's health but also public health.

ANTHELMINTICS

In this chapter anthelmintics that are approved by the U.S. Food and Drug Administration (FDA) and commercially available in the United States are grouped together by class according to their generic names. The literature on antiparasitic drugs is enormous. In the interest of both economy and readability, only a few references are listed for each drug. These will guide the veterinarian who needs more specific information about the subject. Table 13-1 provides a general overview of anthelmintic drug spectrum against the common canine and feline helminths.

Since the last edition of this text was published, there have been considerable changes, most notably the more widespread use of ivermectin and the emergence of other macrocyclic lactones. New information on avermectin toxicity is covered in the ivermectin section. Drug manufacturers have discontinued production of many tried-and-true anthelmintics such as dichlorvos (Task Capsules) and diethylcarbamazine citrate (Filaribits). In addition, some drugs, such as N-butyl chloride, have simply been superseded. For simplicity's sake, discontinued products and drugs that are not widely available do not appear in the current edition; however, an earlier edition of this text can certainly be consulted for information about them. The latest information about diethylcarbamazine citrate can be obtained from the American Heartworm Society 2005 guidelines for the diagnosis, prevention, and management of heartworm infection in dogs.[17] This organization produced similar guidelines for cats in 2007[18] and updated the guidelines for dogs in 2010.[18a]

New anthelmintic products are continuously researched and frequently launched. The Compendium of Veterinary Products provides a comprehensive list of commercially available products approved by the FDA.[19] An exhaustive review of the pharmacology, mechanism of action, pharmacokinetics, and efficacy of anthelmintics is beyond the scope of this chapter. There are excellent texts available for those interested in more exhaustive information on anthelmintics.[20-22] Pharmacologic activity against nonhelminths, such as flukes, fleas, and ticks, by some anthelmintics and anthelmintic drug combinations may be mentioned, but such activity is not the focus of this chapter.

Macrolides

Macrolides, which include both avermectins and milbemycins, have revolutionized the control of parasites in both humans and animals. Ivermectin is the best known agent in this class. The dual activity of some macrolides, such as ivermectin and selamectin, against endoparasites, such as helminths, and ectoparasites, such as fleas, gave rise to the term *endectocide*. These products are similar in that they are large complex macrocyclic structures produced by soil microorganisms in the *Streptomyces* genus. They are generally regarded as the most effective and least toxic parasiticides yet developed. Commercially, they have crushed the competition. Many conventional drugs that were direct competitors of this class were retired from common use and eventually discontinued by the manufacturer.

KEY POINT 13-5 Macrolides are large complex macrocyclic products of soil microorganisms. This class includes the most effective, least toxic parasiticides.

Macrolides are excreted in the feces as active drug. Drugs in this class, especially the avermectins, are toxic to dung-feeding insects, but not birds, plants, and earthworms. Elimination of coprophagous insects appears to delay processing of nutrients, but the overall environmental impact of this finding is unclear.[23]

Although originally believed to act by disturbing gamma-aminobutyric acid (GABA)–mediated neurotransmission, it now appears that they act with high affinity to a nematode-specific glutamate-gated chloride channel.[24,25] Macrolides trigger chloride ion influx, which hyperpolarizes the parasite neuron and prevents initiation or propagation of normal action potentials. The selectivity of macrolides is due to different glutamate function in invertebrates compared with that of vertebrates. Glutamate acts as an inhibitory neurotransmitter in invertebrates and an excitatory neurotransmitter in mammals.[2] The net effect is paralysis and death of the target parasite.

Despite their beneficial activities, macrocyclic lactones have several flaws. They are ineffective against cestodes and trematodes, and they are sometimes expensive. That said, the U.S. patent on ivermectin has now expired, allowing generic competitors to enter the market and reduce the cost of ivermectin treatment, but to date the cost savings have not been realized on products for dogs and cats to the same degree as those for horses and food animals. Although macrolides are generally regarded as the most effective and least toxic parasiticides yet developed, toxicity may occur with overdosage, especially in Collies, many of which are unusually sensitive to macrolide endectocides. An excellent summarized overview of the pharmacology, indications, dosing, precautions, and side effects of commercially available macrocyclic lactones is available online as a PDF download from the United States Pharmacopeial Convention, Inc.[23]

KEY POINT 13-6 Macrolides are ineffective against trematodes and cestodes.

Table 13-1 Anthelmintic Medications

	DRUG ACTIVITY AGAINST COMMON CANINE & FELINE HELMINTHS								
	TAPEWORMS						HEARTWORM		
Drug	*Dipylidium*	*Taenia*	*Echinococcus*	Roundworm	Hookworm	Whipworm	Preventative	Microfilaricide	Adulticide
Macrolidex									
Ivermectin(Iver)				CF	CF		CF	C	C*F*
Milbemycin(Milb)				CF	CF	C	CF	C	
Moxidectin(Mox)					C		C	C	
Selamectin				CF	F		CF		
Benzimidazoles									
Albendazole									
Febantel(Feb)				CF	CF	C			
Fenbendazole		C		CF	CF	C			
Tetrahydropyrimidines									
Pyrantel(Pyr)				CF	CF				
Piperazines									
Piperazine				CF					
Isoquinolones									
Praziquantel(Praz)	CF	CF	C						
Epsiprantel	CF	CF							
Arsenicals									
Melarsomine									C
Miscellaneous									
Dichlorophen	CF	CF							
Combinations									
Emodepside+Praz	F	F		F	F				
Pyr+Praz	CF	CF		CF	CF				
Pyr+Praz+Feb	C	C	C	C	C	C			
Iver+Pyr				C	C		C		
Iver+Pyr+Praz	C	C		C	C		C		
Milb+Lufenuron				C	C	C	C	C	
Imidicloprid+Mox				CF	CF	C	CF		

C = Canine, F = Feline. Some activities listed are not approved and may require higher than approved doses.
*when used in combination with doxycycline - use with caution and only in special circumstances after consulting references.

Ivermectin

Ivermectin was the first commercially available macrolide, released for use in animals in 1981.[24] The avermectins were isolated from the fermentation broth of *Streptomyces avermitilis*. The discovery of its anthelmintic activity was made after administration of the actinomycetic broth to mice infected with the nematode *Nematospiroides dubius*. Ivermectin is effective against many nematodes and arthropods. In particular, ivermectin is very effective against immature *Dirofilaria immitis*.

KEY POINT 13-7 Ivermectin, the first macrolide used commercially, revolutionized the control of parasites in humans and other animals.

Administration of ivermectin to pregnant rats, mice, and rabbits produced teratism only at or near doses that were maternally toxic. There was no teratogenesis in cattle, sheep, and dogs when ivermectin was administered to pregnant animals at four times the recommended dose. Although toxicity for aquatic animals is high, the binding of ivermectin in soil reduces its concentration to levels that have minimal effect on the environment, as previously discussed. The acute oral LD_{50} in mice varied from 11.6 to 87.2 mg/kg; and the LD_{50} for rats was 42.8 to 52.8 mg/kg. In a 14-week study with rats, the "no-effect" level was 0.4 mg/kg.

Ivermectin is well absorbed (95%) after oral administration and well distributed to most tissues except the central nervous system. It is largely eliminated unchanged in the feces and is metabolized to a small degree in the liver by oxidation. In dogs the terminal half-life is approximately 48 hours. No teratism was observed in fetuses when pregnant bitches received repeated oral doses of ivermectin of 0.5 mg/kg. A single oral dose of 2 mg/kg and repeated oral doses of 0.5 mg/kg per day for 14 weeks were well tolerated by dogs.[26]

Avermectin Toxicity. It is important not to administer avermectins concurrently with drugs that could increase avermectin blood–brain barrier penetration, such as ketoconazole, itraconazole, cyclosporine, and calcium-channel blockers.[27] Selamectin toxicity information is addressed in detail later, in the selamectin section. According to a popular veterinary pharmaceutical clinical text, signs of ivermectin toxicity in dogs, in order of frequency, are ataxia, blindness, mydriasis, tremors, and vomiting.[28] Other signs include dehydration, depression, diarrhea, hyperthermia, bradycardia, sinus arrhythmia, coma, seizures, and death.[26,29,30] A recent retrospective study of ivermectin toxicosis cases evaluated at a poison control center revealed clinical signs in the following order of frequency: ataxia, lethargy, tremors, mydriasis, and blindness.[30a]

The apparent LD_{50} for Beagles is 80 mg/kg.[26] The primary clinicopathologic sign in dogs is decreased serum iron values.[22] A common reference used by clinical veterinarians states that death could occur with doses above 40 mg/kg, tremors at 5 mg/kg, and mydriasis at 2.5 mg/kg and that signs of toxicity rarely occur at doses below 1 mg/kg.[28] But a recent retrospective poison control center study revealed that clinical signs may develop between 0.2 to 2.5 mg/kg.[30a] A wide variety of signs were noted, including more severe signs like coma and seizure, at doses below 1 mg/kg. In fact, death was noted in dogs that received 1 to 2.5 mg/kg doses of ivermectin.

A common presenting history is that of a dog that was in close proximity to horses during deworming and later started showing signs of disease. Dogs that develop clinical signs within 4 to 6 hours of ivermectin ingestion typically develop severe clinical signs, whereas dogs with signs developing 10 to 12 hours after exposure tend to have much milder clinical signs.[29] It is not uncommon for dogs with ivermectin toxicity to have seizures. When seizures are severe and uncontrolled for a considerable period of time, hemolytic anemia and muscle damage may occur. Some severe cases present with seizures and miosis, which warrants a poor prognosis. It is possible that severe seizures and miosis on presentation may be associated with severe brain damage.[31]

Clinical signs of ivermectin toxicity in cats, in order of frequency, are ataxia, mydriasis, tremors, hyperesthesia, and hypothermia.[28] Dogs are about 10 times as likely as cats to have ivermectin toxicity.[28]

Some Collies are unusually sensitive to the toxic effects of ivermectin, although it is safe for all breeds at the approved dose of 0.006 mg/kg (6 mcg/kg). Early studies indicated that some genetic lines of Collies developed severe adverse reactions when ivermectin was given at a dose of 100 to 200 mcg/kg (16 to 32 times the label dose), producing mydriasis, ataxia, tremors, drooling, paresis, recumbency, excitability, stupor, and coma. At that time Australian Shepherds, Border Collies, Shetland Sheepdogs, and Old English Sheepdogs were also reported to be sensitive to ivermectin. The lethal dose for some Collies was reported to be 1/200th that of Beagles.[32]

After Collies were also found to be more sensitive to loperamide,[33] the canine multidrug resistance (MDR1) gene was identified and found to be mutated in ivermectin-sensitive Collies.[34] MDR1 codes for a glycoprotein that is an integral part of the blood–brain barrier. There are many excellent sources of information about the MDR1 gene mutation and mechanisms of ivermectin toxicity associated with increased GABA activity.[29,30,35] The mutant MDR1 allele was found in 35% of the 40 Collies that were tested in one study, about the same percentage of Collies that are sensitive to ivermectin.[36] A survey of DNA from 4000 purebred dogs revealed that the MDR1 mutation was present in seven breeds of Collie lineage and two sighthound breeds, although the mutation was not identified in all breeds known to have ivermectin sensitivity.[37]

It was found that the potential for ivermectin sensitivity could be estimated by genotypic or polymerase chain reaction (PCR)–based testing for the MDR1 mutation.[38] In this study the mutant MDR1 allele was found in Australian Shepherds, Miniature Australian Shepherds, English Shepherds, German Shepherd Dogs (white), Longhaired Whippets, McNab Shepherds, Old English Sheepdogs, Shetland Sheepdogs, Silken Windhounds, and Longhaired Whippet.[23,37] Sensitivity to ivermectin was also noted in Australian Cattle Dogs, Bearded Collies, and Border Collies, but the mutant MDR1 allele was not found in these breeds.[37] More recently, the relationship with P-glycoprotein, the product of the ABCB1 (formerly MDR1) gene, was studied in depth by looking for the ABCB1-1Δ allele in a DNA study of 5368 dogs.[39] The ABCB1-1Δ allele was found in Collies, Longhaired Whippets, Standard and Miniature Australian Shepherds, Shetland Sheepdogs, Old English Sheepdogs, Border Collies, Silken Windhounds, and German Shepherd Dogs.

The fact is, until a particular dog is tested, its susceptibility to ivermectin toxicity is unknown. Washington State University, College of Veterinary Medicine, Veterinary Clinical Pharmacology Lab, provides genetic testing to determine the presence of the MDR1 mutant gene. Table 13-2 was adapted from information available at the aforementioned institution's website.[40] The general practitioner can also use this table when presented with a dog that has had a known exposure to ivermectin to determine prognosis and the appropriate level of treatment. As noted previously, a common finding when taking history on ivermectin and moxidectin exposure cases is that the dog was present while the owner was deworming a horse. It is not unusual for horses to spit out a small amount of dewormer, which is ingested by the dog. If the amount ingested can be quantified, then this table can help the veterinarian estimate prognosis and determine how aggressive to get with treatment. Obviously, the risk of a severe toxicity is much greater with a Collie than with another breed.

Another presentation to consider is dogs with the habit of eating horse feces. Dogs that are not ivermectin sensitive are probably not at risk, but an ivermectin-sensitive dog that eats the feces of a horse that has been treated with ivermectin within the last few days may have a severe, even fatal reaction. Ivermectin reaches maximum fecal concentration 2 to 3 days after the horse is treated.[41] By 4 days posttreatment, 90% of the drug has been excreted in the feces. Owners of ivermectin-sensitive coprophagic dogs should treat feces from ivermectin-treated horses as toxic waste and dispose of it in a manner that will prevent the dog from eating it.

Regarding treatment of ivermectin toxicity, although there is some evidence that intravenous administration of physostigmine may be of some benefit for dogs[42] and neostigmine may help treat cats[43] suffering from severe ivermectin intoxication, adverse events associated with these treatments typically outweigh benefit, thus the mainstay of care given by most veterinarians is supportive and symptomatic.[26] Inducing emesis, giving activated charcoal, providing fluid therapy, supplying parenteral alimentation, and maintaining respiratory support and normal body temperature are essential. This supportive care may be needed for an extended period of time because the half-life of ivermectin is 2 days and the half-life of moxidectin is 19 days.[30]

There is no antidote for ivermectin and moxidectin toxicity, but veterinarians should consider lipid rescue, a promising therapy adapted from human medicine. Dr. Guy Weinberg initially described the use of an intravenous lipid emulsion (Intralipid) to treat local anesthetic toxicity (bupivacaine) in humans. He coined the term "lipid rescue." One of the studies to support human use of lipid rescue was an experiment on dogs that were overdosed with bupivacaine and rescued from certain toxicity with intravenous lipid emulsion.[44] Dr. Weinberg established a noncommercial website (www.lipidrescue.com) to disseminate information and foster discussion of cases. Since then, lipid rescue has been used to treat nonbupivacaine toxicities in other species. Although support is certainly anecdotal, in 2008 a veterinary online contributor to the lipid rescue website described an ivermectin-overdosed dog that had clinical signs of toxicity and recovered nicely after activated charcoal, supportive care, and an intravenous lipid emulsion were administered. More recently, a case report of a puppy with moxidectin toxicosis was published describing the use of an intravenous lipid emulsion given as a bolus of 2 mL/kg, followed by 4 mL/kg/hr for 4 hours beginning 10 hours after exposure and repeated at 0.5 mL/kg/min for 30 minutes beginning 25.5 hours after exposure.[45] The 16-week-old dog presented with acute onset seizures, paralysis, and coma soon after exposure to moxidectin. Diazepam, glycopyrrolate, and intravenous fluids were given along with respiratory ventilation and other supportive care. The puppy improved dramatically within 30 minutes of the second dose of Intralipid. Although ideal dosages have not been established, the typical recommendation is for bolus administration of 1.5 mL/kg of intravenous lipid emulsion, followed by 0.25 mL/kg/min for 30 to 60 minutes.[46] Other brands of intravenous lipid emulsion, such as Liposyn, can also be considered. It is best to have the product available ahead of time rather than try to acquire it in the midst of an emergency. Dr. Weinberg's lipid rescue website (mentioned previously) describes preparation of a kit to have on hand.

Dogs. Ivermectin (Heartgard) tablets are administered orally at a dose level of 0.006 mg/kg (6 mcg/kg) at monthly intervals to prevent the establishment of the *D. immitis*. The initial dose should be given within 1 month of the first exposure to mosquitoes and throughout the period of the year when mosquitoes are active. The last treatment must be given

Table 13-2 Breeds Affected by MDR-1 Mutation

Breed	Approximate Frequency
Collie	70%
Longhaired Whippet	65%
Australian Shepherd	50%
Australian Shepherd, Mini	50%
Silken Windhound	30%
McNab Shepherd	30%
Shetland Sheepdog	15%
English Shepherd	15%
German Shepherd Dog	10%
Herding Breed Cross	10%
Mixed Breed	5%
Old English Sheepdog	5%
Border Collie	< 5%

(Data from Washington State University, College of Veterinary Medicine, Veterinary Clinical Pharmacology Lab. (2010). Affected breeds Retrieved Jan 26, 2010, from http://www.vetmed.wsu.edu/depts-VCPL/breeds.aspx.)

to dogs within 1 month after the last exposure to mosquitoes. Ivermectin alone has minimal activity against the adult heartworm in the short term. It is active on the third- and fourth-stage larvae and the circulating microfilariae. A single oral dose of ivermectin administered within 2 months of infection prevents the establishment of adult worms in the heart. A single oral dose of 0.05 mg/kg is adequate to clear the circulating microfilariae when given to dogs 4 weeks after the administration of an adulticide, although ivermectin is not approved as a microfilaricide.[47] Review of the original reference is suggested for more complete information. When ivermectin (0.006 mg/kg) is given to heartworm-positive dogs over several months, the circulating microfilariae are eliminated, resulting in an occult infection. Thus dogs receiving monthly ivermectin should be tested annually with an occult heartworm test.[17,48,49]

Knight provides an excellent review of heartworm testing and suggested chemoprophylaxis timing for various regions in the United States.[50] The American Heartworm Society guidelines for diagnosis, prevention, and management of heartworm infection in dogs should also be consulted.[17] Although there is no FDA-approved microfilaricide, macrocyclic lactones are the safest and most effective microfilaricidal drugs available for use in heartworm-positive dogs.[17] Compared with ivermectin, milbemycin is a more potent microfilaricide and causes quicker clearance of microfilariae.[17]

Short-term use of ivermectin alone has minimal effect on adult heartworms, but when given continuously over a prolonged period, for 1 to 2 years, or when combined with doxycycline, it may have some utility for treating dogs with adult heartworm infection. The older the adult heartworms are when first exposed to ivermectin, the longer it takes them to die; because they continue to cause damage during this time, long-term ivermectin therapy generally is not a substitute for melarsomine (Immiticide) therapy.[17] In addition, a mild hypersensitivity reaction has been observed in dogs with circulating microfilariae that are treated with ivermectin. Many products that contain ivermectin have precautions suggesting removal of adult heartworms and microfilariae before initiating ivermectin heartworm prophylaxis.

Regarding the combination of ivermectin and doxycycline as a heartworm adulticide; it has been found that *Wolbachia* spp. bacteria are filarial species endosymbionts—that is, their presence is necessary for filial worm survival—and that eliminating this bacteria from heartworm-positive dogs and cats will decrease host antigenic response.[51,52] In fact, one study of heartworm-positive dogs comparing groups that were treated with three drugs (i.e., melarsomine, doxycycline, and ivermectin), two drugs (i.e., doxycycline and ivermectin), doxycycline alone, ivermectin alone, and melarsomine alone, led the authors to conclude that the combination of doxycycline and ivermectin was synergistic and could eliminate adult heartworms with less potential for severe thromboembolism than melarsomine alone.[52] This is discussed in greater depth in the melarsomine section.

Ivermectin given as a single subcutaneous injection or orally administered at 0.2 mg/kg demonstrated high efficacy against the immature and adult *T. canis, A. caninum, Ancylostoma braziliense, Uncinaria stenocephala, Strongyloides stercoralis, Capillaria* spp., and *Filaroides hirthi*.[53] At that dose its activity against *Toxascaris leonina* and *T. vulpis* is erratic.[23] When treating respiratory nematode parasites a higher dose, 0.4 mg/kg by subcutaneous injection or orally every 2 weeks for 2 to 3 doses has been recommended recently for *Oslerus (Filaroides) osleri, F. hirthi, Aelurostrongylus abstrusus,* and *Capillaria aerophila* infections.[54]

Several combination products containing ivermectin are available. A combination product (Heartgard Plus) containing ivermectin and pyrantel pamoate is available. See the discussion of combination products for more information.

Cats. Ivermectin is FDA approved as a monthly heartworm preventive in cats (Heartgard Chewable for Cats). The approved monthly oral dose of 0.024 mg/kg is effective in preventing the development of *D. immitis* and hookworms *(A. braziliense* and *Ancylostoma tubaeforme)*.[55-57] Feline roundworm *(Toxocara cati)* infections have been controlled with 0.2 to 0.3 mg/kg of ivermectin and lungworm *(A. abstrusus)* infections with 0.4 mg/kg of ivermectin.[58-60] *Capillaria* species are rarely implicated in feline cystitis, and infestations are thought to be self-limiting usually, but in one case a single dose of ivermectin 0.2 mg/kg, administered subcutaneously, was successfully used to treat the condition in a cat.[61]

Milbemycin Oxime

Milbemycin oxime was the second macrocyclic lactone approved by the FDA. It is a fermentation product of *Streptomyces hygroscopicus aureolacrimosis*. It has structural similarities to ivermectin and is believed to work by a similar mechanism of action and have similar pharmacokinetic properties with regard to absorption, metabolism, and excretion. Although an LD_{50} was never determined for dogs, single oral doses of 200 mg/kg were tolerated in laboratory Beagles. Collie dogs tolerated single oral doses of 10 mg/kg without toxicity.

KEY POINT 13-8 Milbemycin, the second macrolide used commercially, is similar to ivermectin.

Dogs. Milbemycin oxime tablets (Interceptor) are formulated to deliver a minimum dose of 0.5 mg/kg of body weight. When given every 30 days it is effective in preventing heartworms *(D. immitis)*.[62-64] It also kills *A. caninum, T. canis,* and *T. vulpis*.[65-68,23] One study indicates that milbemycin may help control raccoon roundworm *(B. procyonis)* infections in dogs and thus decrease the zoonotic potential of a parasite that can have devastating effects in humans, including death.[69]

KEY POINT 13-9 Milbemycin is safe for nursing and pregnant animals.

Milbemycin oxime has been extensively tested with regard to safety. It is nontoxic to Collies at up to 20 times the recommended dose and is safe when given to pregnant and nursing animals.[70,71] Milbemycin oxime, like ivermectin, is known to kill heartworm microfilariae and inhibit the release of new microfilariae. Thus all dogs receiving routine monthly heartworm prophylaxis with milbemycin should be tested with adult antigen tests.[72-74,49,17]

KEY POINT 13-10 Use of milbemycin may help control the raccoon roundworm, which has human health implications.

Cats. Milbemycin oxime (Interceptor) is approved for use in cats. The product is effective in preventing in heartworm *(D. immitis)* at a monthly dose of 0.5 mg/kg[75] and removing roundworms *(T. cati)* and hookworms *(A. tubaeforme)* at a monthly dose of 1.5 mg/kg.[76,23]

Moxidectin

Moxidectin was the third macrolide to enter the parasite market. It is a chemically altered product of *Streptomyces aureolacrimosus noncyanogenus* and has a similar range of activity and safety margin as ivermectin and milbemycin oxime. Moxidectin is currently approved in the United States for injectable use as a heartworm (*D. immitis*) preventive and hookworm (*A. caninum* and *U. stenocephala*) treatment in dogs (ProHeart 6) and for topical use in combination with imidacloprid to prevent heartworms, treat fleas, and control and treat ear mites and intestinal parasites in dogs and cats (Advantage Multi). The combination product is reviewed later in this chapter. The oral use of moxidectin in dogs is covered in the previous edition of this text. Moxidectin toxicity was discussed previously in the Avermectin Toxicity section.

KEY POINT 13-11 Moxidectin, the third macrolide used commercially, is also similar to ivermectin and milbemycin.

KEY POINT 13-12 Moxidectin is available as a sustained-release injectable heartworm preventive and hookworm treatment.

KEY POINT 13-13 Moxidectin combined with imidacloprid is available as a topical heartworm preventive and flea treatment that controls ear mites and internal parasites.

Dog. Moxidectin injection (ProHeart 6) was launched in the United States in 2001 with an indication to prevent heartworms and treat hookworms in dogs. The label for the sustained-release injectable product instructed that it was to be given no more often than once every 6 months. The FDA had concerns about safety as a result of adverse event reports that it received, and the manufacturer voluntarily recalled the product from the U.S market in 2004 to address those safety concerns.[77] During that time the product remained on the market in Australia, Japan, and parts of Europe. In 2008 the product was reintroduced to the U.S. market with a new label under a postmarketing surveillance initiative based on human drug programs and known as a Risk Minimization Action Plan (RiskMAP), which includes veterinarian training and use of a pet-owner consent form. This is the first veterinary drug to be marketed under RiskMAP, a strengthened risk minimization and restricted distribution program.[78] The new label advises not to administer the drug to sick, debilitated, or underweight dogs or those with a history of weight loss and states that the product should be used with caution in dogs with preexisting allergic disease, including food allergy, atopy, and flea allergy dermatitis. The label also warns not to administer moxidectin injection within 1 month of vaccinations.[79]

Injectable moxidectin is indicated for use in dogs 6 months of age and older for the prevention of heartworm disease. It should be given at 0.17 mg/kg by subcutaneous injection within 1 month of the dog's first exposure to mosquitoes or within 1 month of the dog's last dose of monthly heartworm preventive. The sustained-release injection provides a 6-month window of protection from heartworms.[79] However, it does not clear microfilariae or remove adult heartworms.[23] A challenge study comparing efficacy and adverse reactions among four groups of dogs given placebo or moxidectin at 0.06, 0.17, or 0.5mg/kg and inoculated with 50 *D. immitis* third-stage larvae 180 days later revealed 100% efficacy at the label dose (0.17 mg/kg).[80] However, one of eight dogs given the lower dose (0.06 mg/kg) was infected. The authors speculated that the failure of protection was a result of individual pharmacokinetic variation because the moxidectin serum concentration in the unprotected dog was at the limit of quantitation (lowest detectable quantity) 8 days after treatment and undetectable thereafter compared with others in that group that had detectable concentrations until at least day 14 and for as long as 55 days for most of the other dogs.[80] Both the frequency and size of injection-site granulomas correlated positively with the moxidectin dose.[80]

Moxidectin sustained-release injection is also indicated for the treatment of hookworms *A. caninum* and *U. stenocephala*; although it will eliminate larval and adult stages of those parasites, reinfection may occur in less than 6 months, making its use less than ideal when attempting to control recurrent hookworm disease.

Selamectin

Prepared by semisynthetic modification of doramectin,[81] selamectin (Revolution) is the latest macrolide to enter the U.S. marketplace. This product is unique among other macrolides used in small animals in that it is formulated for convenient topical administration. It is simply "spotted" onto the skin of the pet. It was the first macrocyclic lactone approved for use in dogs and cats to provide activity against both internal and external parasites. However, the discussion here focuses on the activity of selamectin against internal parasites.

KEY POINT 13-14 Selamectin is the latest macrolide to be used commercially in the United States.

KEY POINT 13-15 Selamectin is unique among macrolides in its topical formulation and extreme broad spectrum against internal and external parasites.

It is produced as a fermentation product of *S. avermitilis*, which is then chemically modified.[82] The pharmacokinetics after topical administration has been studied extensively. The topical bioavailability varies greatly among species. In dogs the bioavailability is only 4%, but it is much greater in cats (74%). The terminal half-life was much longer in both species after topical administration than after intravenous administration, suggesting sustained release from an extravascular depot. The half-life after topical administration was 11 days for dogs and 8 days for cats.[23] The product is absorbed in sufficient quantities and persists for sufficient time to control the target parasites. The approved topical dose is a minimum of 6 mg/kg for dogs and cats.

Selamectin is approved for the prevention of heartworm *(D. immitis)* in both dogs and cats when applied topically every month.[8] Extensive studies proved that the drug's efficacy against heartworms remained[84,85] even when bathing followed application. The bathing study demonstrated that after topical application efficacy is not likely to be decreased by inadvertent swimming or exposure to rainstorms. The drug is not effective in clearing microfilariae. In cats selamectin is also effective in removing hookworm *(A. tubaeforme)* and roundworm *(T. cati)*. This effect is undoubtedly due to the greater topical bioavailability observed in cats.[82] Selamectin is effective against roundworms in dogs[23] and lungworms *(A. abstrusus)* in cats,[86] but these are not label-approved indications. The drug has labeled indications in dogs for activity against ear mites, sarcoptic mange mites, and ticks and in cats for activity against ear mites, but these indications are not the focus of this chapter.

KEY POINT 13-16 Selamectin has much greater bioavailability after topical administration on cats compared with dogs.

The safety of selamectin has been established in both dogs and cats and even for use in puppies and kittens over 6 weeks of age. It is also safe to use in ivermectin-sensitive Collies and in breeding dogs and cats.[84] Selamectin did not cause any abnormalities when applied topically to ivermectin-sensitive Collies at 40 mg/kg.[22] However, avermectin-sensitive Collies given a topical overdose of 10 times the label dose had hypersalivation.[28] Clinical signs of dogs reported to the ASPCA Animal Poison Control Center are, in order of frequency, hypersalivation, agitation, diarrhea, facial edema, and hyperactivity.[28] In cats the signs in decreasing frequency are vomiting, anorexia, hyperesthesia, hyperthermia, and mydriasis.[28] If cats are exposed orally to selamectin they invariably have hypersalivation and sometimes vomit, but topical overdoses at 10 times the label dose in cats did not cause any abnormality.[28] Although the insert recommends that dogs should be tested for existing heartworm infections before selamectin administration, it also notes that hypersensitivity reactions were not observed when heartworm-infected dogs were treated with selamectin at 3 times the label dose.[87] Clinical studies have confirmed the wide safety margin demonstrated in the laboratory studies.

Benzimidazoles

The benzimidazoles represent a large family of broad-spectrum agents that have been in widespread use for many years in a vast array of animal species. Several excellent review articles[88-90] discuss the history, mode of action, and spectrum of activity of this useful class of anthelmintics.

Thiabendazole, the first benzimidazole discovered, represented a major step forward when it became available in the early 1960s.[91] At the time of its introduction, thiabendazole was a true broad-spectrum product that was very safe to the host animal. Since that time, parasite resistance to the benzimidazoles has been discovered in several species.

KEY POINT 13-17 Introduced to the market in the early 1960s, thiabendazole was the first benzimidazole used commercially and was a major advancement in anthelmintics. It is not commercially available as an anthelmintic for small animals.

Considerable effort has been devoted to determining benzimidazole mechanism of action. Conventional wisdom holds that benzimidazoles bind to tubulin molecules, which inhibit the formation of microtubules and disrupt cell division.[92,93] It has a much higher affinity for nematode tubulin versus mammalian tubulin, thus providing selective activity against parasites. Evidence also indicates that the benzimidazoles can inhibit fumarate reductase, which blocks mitochondrial function and kills the parasite by depriving it of energy.

The benzimidazoles are poorly soluble and thus are generally given by mouth. They are more effective in horses and ruminants because of their slow transit through the cecum and rumen. Proper use in small animals requires that the benzimidazoles be given for a minimum of 3 days in a row. The dose is usually more effective when divided into two doses per day, thus prolonging the contact time with the parasite.

KEY POINT 13-18 Benzimidazoles are not very soluble.

Because both albendazole and oxfendazole were found to be teratogenic, their use is limited to nonpregnant animals. For simplicity, febantel, a nonbenzimidazole drug that is metabolized to a benzimidazole, thus sharing efficacy and mechanism of action, is included in this section with the other benzimidazoles.

Albendazole

Albendazole is the newest benzimidazole. It has potent broad-spectrum anthelmintic activity, but is not approved for use in dogs and cats. Albendazole has demonstrated a broad spectrum of anthelmintic activity against gastrointestinal nematodes; lung nematodes, including inhibited larval forms; cestodes; and lung and liver trematodes in farm animals, companion animals, and humans. Albendazole (Albenza or Zentel) is used overseas to treat humans with intestinal helminth infections, hydatid disease, or cysticercosis. It is commonly used for treatment of nematode and trematode infections in large animals (Valbazen).

KEY POINT 13-19 Albendazole is the latest benzimidazole to be used commercially, but it is not approved for use in dogs or cats.

Albendazole, like other benzimidazoles, is well absorbed (about 50% bioavailable) and converted in the liver to the active metabolites albendazole sulfoxide and albendazole sulfone. These active metabolites are thought to bind to tubulin and inhibit fumarate reductase. The parent drug and its metabolites are excreted primarily in the urine.

Because albendazole was shown to be teratogenic, its use is limited to nonpregnant animals. Dogs treated with 50 mg/kg twice daily may develop anorexia. Cats may exhibit lethargy, depression, and anorexia when treated.[28] When cats were given 100 mg/kg/day for 14 to 21 days, they displayed weight loss, neutropenia, and mental dullness.[28] When used clinically, albendazole may be associated with significant toxicity, including myelosuppression (leukopenia, anemia, and thrombocytopenia), abortion, teratism, anorexia, depression, ataxia, vomiting, and diarrhea.[94,95] Recent evidence suggests that it may cause aplastic anemia in dogs and cats.[28] Veterinarians are advised to use due caution with this product.

Albendazole is available as an oral suspension (Valbazen) containing 113.6 mg/mL. Dogs can be treated for lungworms *(F. hirthi)* at a dose of 25 to 50 mg/kg twice daily for 5 days, with the treatment repeated in 2 to 3 weeks, and for bladder worms *(Capillaria plica)* at a dose of 50 mg/kg twice daily for 10 to 14 days.[28] Both dogs and cats can be treated for the lung fluke *(Paragonimus kellicotti)* at a dose of 25 mg/kg twice daily for 14 days or 50 mg/kg orally once daily for 21 days.[28] Although albendazole is effective against these uncommon parasites, ivermectin and praziquantel are more convenient therapies and likely to be just as effective.

Febantel

Febantel is a prodrug that is metabolized to fenbendazole and oxfendazole, which are undoubtedly the active parasiticides.[90] The oral acute toxic dose in mice, rats, and dogs is more than 10 g/kg (10,000 mg/kg). At oral doses above 150 mg/kg per day for 6 days, transient salivation, diarrhea, vomiting, and anorexia may be seen in dogs and cats. Febantel is not available in a single-entity formulation but only in combination with praziquantel and pyrantel, which are discussed in the section on combination products.

Fenbendazole

Fenbendazole (Panacur) is a commercially successful benzimidazole that is widely used in dogs. The oral LD_{50} for rats and mice is more than 10 g/kg (10,000 mg/kg).[28] Fenbendazole does not have embryotoxic or teratogenic effects in rats, sheep, or cattle. In the rabbit fenbendazole was fetotoxic but not teratogenic, and no carcinogenesis was observed in lifetime studies of rats and mice. In a 6-month toxicity study in dogs, no effect was observed at 4 mg/kg or less.

KEY POINT 13-20 Febantel is metabolized to fenbendazole and oxfendazole, which are probably the active molecules.

KEY POINT 13-21 Fenbendazole is used in a wide variety of species, including dogs, cats, livestock, horses, and zoo animals.

Fenbendazole is a broad-spectrum anthelmintic with activity against a wide variety of nematodes and cestodes in dogs, cats, cattle, sheep, goats, horses, and many zoo animals. Absorbed fenbendazole is metabolized to at least two active metabolites, oxfendazole sulfoxide and oxfendazole sulfone. It undergoes enterohepatic cycling in ruminants, which prolongs effective blood levels.[96] In the United States fenbendazole is approved for control of helminth parasites of horses, cattle, and dogs.

KEY POINT 13-22 Fenbendazole has a broad spectrum of activity against many nematodes and cestodes.

Dogs. Fenbendazole is approved only for use in dogs 6 weeks of age and older. Fenbendazole granules (Panacur) are mixed in the feed at a dose level of 50 mg/kg and given to dogs for 3 consecutive days for the removal of *T. canis, T. leonina, A. caninum, U. stenocephala, T. vulpis,* and *Taenia pisiformis.*[97] It has shown excellent activity against *Giardia* spp. in dogs at the approved dose.[95,98] At longer-than-approved duration of therapy (i.e., 50 mg/kg daily for 10 to 14 days), it has been used to treat the lung fluke, *P. kellicotti,* in dogs.[28] Fenbendazole is relatively safe, and there are no known contraindications to its use in dogs.

Cats. Fenbendazole is not currently approved for use in cats. When given at a dose of 50 mg/kg for 5 days, it is effective against ascarids, hookworms, *Strongyloides,* and *Taenia* spp. tapeworms.[28] Treatment of *A. abstrusus, P. kellicotti,* and *C. aerophila* may require 14 days of therapy.[28]

Tetrahydropyrimidines

The tetrahydropyrimidines include the numerous salts of pyrantel, morantel, and the investigational compound oxantel, which is available outside the United States. They all act as nicotinic agonists, which disturb the neuromuscular system, causing contraction and subsequent tonic paralysis.[99-102] In vitro experiments indicate that pyrantel is 100 times more powerful than acetylcholine. It seems that the nicotinic acetylcholine receptors of invertebrate parasites are essential for neurologic function but differ in physiology and distribution in mammals.[103] In ruminants these products are rapidly metabolized to inactive metabolites; therefore higher doses are required to treat ruminants compared with monogastric animals.[20]

KEY POINT 13-23 Tetrahydropyrimidines are nicotinic agonists. They cause contraction and subsequent tonic paralysis of parasites.

KEY POINT 13-24 Pyrantel is 100 times more powerful than acetylcholine.

Pyrantel

Pyrantel was introduced in the United States as a broad-spectrum anthelmintic for sheep in 1966[22] and is now available under a wide variety of trade names in the form of tablet, paste, oral suspension, and medicated feed.[104] The tartrate salt of pyrantel is a white powder, soluble in water, that is used in horses and swine. Pyrantel tartrate is well absorbed after oral administration in the rat, dog, and pig. Plasma levels peak within 3 to 6 hours.[22] Pyrantel tartrate is rapidly metabolized and in dogs is primarily eliminated by way of the urinary tract, but pyrantel pamoate is poorly absorbed from the gastrointestinal tract and is primarily eliminated through the feces with less than 15% excretion through the urinary tract.[104]

KEY POINT 13-25 Pyrantel pamoate is poorly absorbed, which contributes to its safety in young animals.

The pamoate salt of pyrantel is a yellow powder, insoluble in water. It is available as a ready-to-use suspension and as tablets for dogs and horses. The fact that pyrantel pamoate is poorly absorbed from the intestine adds to its safety in very young or weak animals. Pyrantel salts are stable in solid form but photodegrade when dissolved or suspended in water, resulting in reduction of potency.

Dogs. Pyrantel pamoate is available as a tablet, chewable tablet, and palatable suspension (Nemex and many other trade names) and is indicated for the removal of *T. canis, T. leonina, A. caninum,* and *U. stenocephala* from dogs and puppies.[105-108] The drug has also been used to treat *Physaloptera* stomach worms in dogs, although such use is not approved.[104,109] Pyrantel may have some effect on tapeworms as well, but other drugs are commonly used to treat tapeworm infections in small animals. The recommended dose of 5 mg/kg of pyrantel pamoate suspension is administered orally or mixed with a small amount of feed.[104] For animals weighing 2.25 kg or less, the dose is increased to 10 mg/kg. Tablets may be administered directly or placed in a small portion of food. Pyrantel pamoate is safe for nursing and weanling pups, pregnant bitches, males used for breeding, and dogs infected with *D. immitis.* The oral LD_{50} is greater than 690 mg/kg in dogs.[22] In chronic toxicity studies dogs had no adverse effects when given 20 mg/kg daily for 3 months but did have ill effects at 50 mg/kg or above daily.[22] Pyrantel pamoate is compatible with organophosphates and other antiparasitic and antimicrobial agents.

Cats. Pyrantel pamoate products used in dogs are not labeled for cats but are considered very safe and effective against some common feline parasites, the ones that are similar to those afflicting dogs and are listed as indications on the canine label. The oral dose range of 5 to 20 mg/kg is reportedly efficacious against ascarids, hookworms, and *Physaloptera* spp., with the dose repeated in 2 to 3 weeks in some cases.[22,27,28,104] Pyrantel pamoate is labeled for cats as a combination product with praziquantel (Drontal), which is described later, in the combination product section.

Cyclic Depsipeptides

The cyclodepsipeptide PF1022A, isolated from *Mycelia sterilia,* was found to have low toxicity and strong anthelmintic properties when tested against *Ascaridia galli* in chickens, making it one of the most promising deworming prospects to emerge since the discovery of avermectins and milbemycin.

Emodepside

Emodepside is the first cyclic depsipeptide to be approved for use against animal parasites in the United States. It is a semisynthetic derivative of PF1022A, mentioned previously. The product binds to a presynaptic latrophilin receptor in parasitic nematodes, which results in flaccid paralysis and death.[110] It has low to moderate acute toxicity in mammalian species. The oral LD_{50} in rats is greater than 500 mg/kg and is more than 2000 mg/kg when applied to the skin. Studies in rats and rabbits suggest that emodepside may interfere with fetal development.[111] Women who are pregnant or may become pregnant should avoid direct contact with emodepside and wear disposable gloves if product handling is necessary. Emodepside is only available commercially as a combination product, combined with praziquantel, and as such is discussed in detail later, in the section on broad-spectrum combinations.

KEY POINT 13-26 Emodepside is the first cyclic depsipeptide approved in the United States.

KEY POINT 13-27 Pregnant women should use care if they must handle this drug.

Piperazines

Piperazine was used to treat human gout in the early 1900s because it acts as an excellent uric acid solvent. Its anthelmintic activity was discovered in the 1950s.[22] Since then, a wide variety of piperazine salts have been derived. The various salts of piperazine (adipate, hydrochloride, sulfate, monohydrate, citrate, and dihydrochloride) are used as anthelmintics in swine, poultry, horses, dogs, and cats. Piperazine is quite safe to use in these species but has a narrow spectrum of action, limited primarily to roundworms.[93,27] Anthelmintic activity depends on the salt freeing its piperazine base in the gastrointestinal tract. The amount of piperazine (base) in each salt varies widely. The citrate salt contains 35% piperazine; adipate salts, 37%; phosphate salts, 42%; and dihydrochloride salts, 50% piperazine base.[96]

Piperazine paralyzes worms by blocking the action of acetylcholine and GABA at the neuromuscular junctions, and the worms are eliminated by intestinal peristalsis.[20,112] It acts by hyperpolarizing nerve membranes at the neuromuscular junction, leading to flaccid paralysis of the parasite.[22] Piperazine is also one of the active ingredients in a number of combination anthelmintic products. Piperazine should not be used in combination with pyrantel pamoate because the modes of action are antagonistic.

KEY POINT 13-28 Piperazine paralyzes worms by blocking acetylcholine and GABA, and the worms are eliminated by intestinal peristalsis; thus it may not work well in the face of gastrointestinal hypomotility.

Piperazine is rapidly absorbed from the gastrointestinal tract and rapidly cleared by urinary excretion. Elimination is virtually complete within 24 hours.[96] It may not be effective in animals with intestinal hypomotility because the paralyzed worms may recover from the drug effect before they are passed in the stool. Piperazine should be used with caution in animals with hepatic or renal dysfunction. Occasional adverse reactions observed in dogs include ataxia, diarrhea, and vomiting.

Piperazine is available as tablets, solution, and soluble powder under many proprietary names (Pipatabs, Puppy Paste, Happy Jack KittyKat Paste, Tasty Paste). It is practically nontoxic. The oral LD_{50} for rats is 4.9 g/kg and for mice is 11.4 g/kg. Treatment for intoxication is symptomatic and supportive. Piperazine can be administered to animals of all ages.

Dogs and Cats

Piperazine is usually administered orally at 45 to 65 mg of base per kilogram,[96] although higher doses (100 to 250 mg/kg) have been reported in the literature.[107,113-115] Piperazine is effective against adult roundworms *T. canis, T. cati,* and *T. leonina.*

Isoquinolones

The cesticidal isoquinolones are represented by two closely related drugs: praziquantel and epsiprantel. This cesticidal class is the safest and most effective yet approved in the United States. They attack the parasite neuromuscular junction and the tegument. These drugs cause increased cell membrane permeability to calcium and resulting loss of intracellular calcium. This effect produces an instantaneous contraction and paralysis of the parasite.[116] The second effect is a devastating vacuolization and destruction of the protective tegument.[92,117] The combined effects of paralysis and tegmental destruction provide excellent activity against cestodes.

KEY POINT 13-29 Isoquinolones are the safest and most effective cesticidal drugs approved in the United States.

Praziquantel

Praziquantel was the first cesticidal isoquinolone approved in the United States. It has marked anthelmintic activity against a wide range of adult and larval cestodes and trematodes of the genus *Schistosoma*. Oral administration results in nearly complete absorption and rapid distribution throughout the body and across the blood–brain barrier. Although 80% of the drug is eliminated in the urine, the main site of inactivation is the liver, with only trace amounts of the unchanged drug excreted primarily in the urine.[22,91] Praziquantel has high oral bioavailability, high protein binding, and a marked first-pass effect. The oral half-life in dogs is reported to be 30 to 90 minutes[22] to 3 hours.[28]

KEY POINT 13-30 Praziquantel, the first approved cesticidal isoquinolone in the United States, has marked anthelmintic activity against cestodes and trematodes.

Praziquantel is a very safe anthelmintic. Rats tolerated daily administration of up to 1000 mg/kg for 4 weeks, and dogs tolerated up to 180 mg/kg per day for 13 weeks. Vomiting is typically observed at high dosage rates. Injected doses of 200 mg/kg were lethal in cats.[28] Praziquantel did not induce embryotoxicity, teratogenesis, mutagenesis, or carcinogenesis, nor did it affect the reproductive performance of test animals. Occasional adverse experiences in clinical use include pain on injection, anorexia, diarrhea, salivation, vomiting, sleepiness, staggering, and weakness. Overdoses have been reported to cause diarrhea, depression, incoordination, tremors, salivation, and vomiting.

KEY POINT 13-31 Praziquantel has a wide margin of safety.

Dogs and cats. Praziquantel (AmTech, Droncit) is administered orally or injected subcutaneously at 2.5 to 7.5 mg/kg for the removal of *Dipylidium caninum, Taenia taeniaeformis, T. pisiformis, T. hydatigena, T. ovis, Mesocestoides corti, Echinococcus granulosus, Echinococcus multilocularis, Spirometra* spp., *Diphyllobothrium latum, D. erinacei,* and *Joyeuxiella pasquali.*[118-124,96] The product insert has extensive information about using this drug to help control *E. multilocularis,* including the life cycle of the parasite, difficulty of diagnosis, and other public health considerations.[125] Praziquantel injection is not intended for use in puppies or kittens younger than 4 weeks of age. Several combination products contain praziquantel; see the section on combination products for more information.

Epsiprantel

Epsiprantel (Cestex) was the second cesticidal isoquinolone to be approved in the United States. Unlike its cousin praziquantel, epsiprantel is poorly absorbed after oral administration. Less than 0.1% is recovered from the urine; there are no known metabolites.[28] It is eliminated in the feces unchanged.[22] Because of the low bioavailability, systemic toxicity and teratogenic effects are very unlikely, but the safety of epsiprantel in pregnant dogs and cats has not been proved. In acute toxicity studies in mice and rats, the oral minimum lethal dose of epsiprantel was shown to be more than 5000 mg/kg. Doses as high as 36 times the label dose were well tolerated in dogs and caused vomiting in some kittens.[28] Cats given the drug at 40 times the label dose for 4 days had minimal signs. Dogs given 90 times the label dose for 14 days had no significant adverse events.[126]

KEY POINT 13-32 Like praziquantel, epsiprantel, the second cesticidal isoquinolone approved in the United States, has a wide margin of safety, but unlike praziquantel, it is poorly absorbed orally.

Epsiprantel treatment as an oral film-coated tablet, at 2.75 mg/kg for cats or 5.5 mg/kg for dogs, effectively removes *D. caninum, T. taeniaeformis, T. pisiformis,* and *T. hydatigena* after a single dose.[127,128] Evidence suggests that the drug is effective against *E. granulosa* and *E.multilocularis*, but the data are insufficient to recommend a dosage that will completely clear the infection from those treated.[129] Epsiprantel was given concurrently with diethylcarbamazine (in dogs), antiinflammatory drugs, insecticides, and nematocides with no incompatibilities observed.[126] It should not be used in puppies and kittens younger than 7 weeks of age.

Arsenicals

Heavy metals like arsenic and antimony are well represented in the history of anthelmintics. To date, safer and more effective drugs for the most common parasites have largely replaced arsenicals. Their use is now limited to removal of adult *D. immitis*. Thiacetarsemide (Caparsolate) is no longer available commercially in the United States[130] and thus will not be covered in this chapter. The therapeutic effect of arsenicals depends on a reaction between the arsenic salt and sulfhydryl-containing enzymes.[131] Inactivation of parasite enzyme systems causes death. Because arsenic is widely known as a toxin in man and animal, caution is required when using these products.

KEY POINT 13-33 Arsenicals typically have a narrow margin of safety.

Melarsomine

Although contraindicated in cats, melarsomine dihydrochloride (Immiticide), the only arsenical anthelmintic commercially available in the U.S. veterinary market, has 92% to 98% efficacy against adult *D. immitis* in dogs.[132-136] The arsenic content of the product is less than that of thiacetarsemide, making melarsomine less toxic to the patient. Melarsomine is labeled to be administered intramuscularly at a dose of 2.5 mg/kg for two injections given 24 hours apart to dogs at low risk of thromboembolic complications.[17] Dogs that have moderate risk of thromboembolism may be treated with an alternative three-injection regimen of a single injection followed by a rest period of 1 to 2 months, after which two standard injections are given.[17] This later three-injection regimen is reportedly less hazardous for the patient and more efficacious and therefore is the preferred regimen recommended by the American Heartworm Society, regardless of the stage of disease (unless melarsomine is otherwise contraindicated).[17, 18a] Melarsomine is contraindicated in dogs with severe heartworm disease associated with caval syndrome.[28] Injections should only be made deep into the lumbar epaxial muscles along L3 to L5. Peak blood level is achieved in about 11 minutes after injection, and the half-life is 3 hours.[28]

KEY POINT 13-34 Melarsomine is the only commercially available arsenical anthelmintic.

About one third of dogs treated will have injection site reactions, most of which resolve within a week, but firm nodules at the injection site can persist indefinitely.[28] Additional adverse reactions include elevated hepatic enzymes, coughing, gagging, depression, lethargy, anorexia, fever, pulmonary congestion, and vomiting.[27] This drug exemplifies the problem of parasite removal by poisoning the patient just enough to kill the parasite, hopefully without damaging the patient too much. It has a narrow therapeutic range. The toxic dose is only 2.5 to 3 times the recommended dose and can result in panting, pulmonary inflammation, salivation, vomiting, edema, and death. Safety has not been determined in breeding, pregnant, or lactating dogs. That said, clinical studies indicate that the treatment is well tolerated even in dogs that have clinical signs of heartworm disease.[135,137,138]

As previously mentioned in the ivermectin section of this chapter, the American Heartworm Society guidelines for diagnosis, prevention, and management of heartworm infection in dogs should be consulted before treating a heartworm-infected dog with melarsomine.[18a] Treatment with a macrocytic lactone before administration of melarsomine should be considered along with other methods to reduce the potential for melarsomine adverse reactions. For example, as previously mentioned in the ivermectin section, one study of heartworm-positive dogs comparing groups that were treated with three drugs (i.e., melarsomine, doxycycline and ivermectin), two drugs (i.e., doxycycline and ivermectin), doxycycline alone, ivermectin alone, or melarsomine alone led the authors to conclude that the combination of doxycycline and ivermectin was synergistic.[52] All dogs treated with ivermectin plus doxycycline (with or without melarsomine) were free of microfilariae in 9 weeks. This may be related to the elimination of *Wolbachia* sp. bacteria, which are filarial endosymbionts. The authors found that the administration of doxycycline plus ivermectin for several months before (or without) melarsomine resulted in elimination of adult heartworms with less severe thromboembolism than did treatment with melarsomine alone.[52]

KEY POINT 13-35 The prudent practitioner will consult American Heartworm Society guidelines before using melarsomine.

Miscellaneous

Dichlorophen

Dichlorophen (Happy Jack Tapeworm Tablets) is a chlorinated analog of diphenylmethane. It has low toxicity for mammals. The oral LD_{50} is 2690 mg/kg for rats, and the acute oral LD_{50} in dogs is 1000 mg/kg. Dichlorophen has bacteriostatic, fungicidal, and cesticidal properties. It causes electron transport–linked phosphorylation to uncouple in the parasite mitochondria and is relatively safe in the host because of low gastrointestinal absorption.[91] Dichlorophen may be given orally as an "aid in the removal" of *D. caninum* and *T. pisiformis* tapeworms from dogs.[139] The drug may be administered orally in tablet or capsule form at 220 mg/kg after an overnight fast. The tapeworms are killed, digested, and eliminated in an unrecognizable form. Animals occasionally vomit or develop diarrhea after treatment with dichlorophen.

KEY POINT 13-36 Dichlorophen is not absorbed well from the gastrointestinal tract, which improves its safety profile.

KEY POINT 13-37 Dichlorophen aids in the removal of tapeworms from dogs.

BROAD-SPECTRUM COMBINATIONS

The veterinary practitioner is always looking for anthelmintic products that cover an ever-increasing spectrum of parasites. Broad-spectrum products provide two important advantages. First, they obviate dosing with several different products at once when a patient has a mixed parasite infection, making administration easier. Second, they provide peace of mind that a treated animal will be cleared of possibly undiagnosed parasites. For instance, a puppy from the animal shelter will be better served by use of a product that is effective in removing both roundworms and hookworms than a product that is effective against only roundworms. There are two ways to increase the spectrum of anthelmintics: either by tackling the arduous task of discovering a single broad-spectrum chemical or by combining several compatible active ingredients to build the desired spectrum of activity.

KEY POINT 13-38 Broad-spectrum anthelmintic combinations make treating mixed parasitic infections easier and may treat common undiagnosed parasites; therefore they are associated with increased veterinary and owner confidence.

Combination anthelmintic products are briefly reviewed in this section, but not combinations that are formulated to treat or prevent fleas or other nonhelminth parasites. In many cases combination-product formulation and dosing regimens are different from those of the single-entity drug ingredients. The toxicity and mechanism of action of the individual ingredients are covered earlier in this chapter.

Emodepside Plus Praziquantel

This product is formulated for use in cats (Profender) as a topical spot-on that contains 1.98% emodepside and 7.94% praziquantel. The prefilled applicators deliver a minimum dose of 3 mg/kg emodepside and 12 mg/kg praziquantel when applied to the skin. The active ingredients are readily absorbed through the skin, enter systemic circulation, and act on target parasites in the gastrointestinal tract. It is labeled for use in cats and kittens that are at least 8 weeks of age and is considered safe to use in heartworm-positive cats.[111] The product is safe and effective in removing roundworms, *T. cati* (adults and fourth-stage larvae); hookworms, *A. tubaeforme* (adults, immature adults, and fourth-stage larvae); and tapeworms, *D. caninum* and *T. taeniaeformis*.[140-142] The topical emodepside–praziquantel product was very effective and safe when used in a large-scale clinical study comparing it with topical selamectin–oral epsiprantel.[143]

Pyrantel Plus Praziquantel

Two-way combination products containing pyrantel and praziquantel are approved for use in the United States in both dogs (Virbantel) and in cats (Drontal).

Dogs

The canine product is formulated to deliver 5 mg of praziquantel and 5 mg of pyrantel pamoate per kilogram. A single dose is given to dogs to remove tapeworms *(D. caninum* and *T. pisiformis)*, hookworms *(A. caninum, A. braziliense,* and *U. stenocephala)*, and roundworms *(T. canis* and *T. leonina)*.

Cats

The feline product is formulated to deliver at least 5 mg of praziquantel and 20 mg of pyrantel pamoate per kilogram. A single dose is given to cats and kittens to remove tapeworms *(D. caninum* and *T. taeniaeformis)*, hookworms *(A. tubaeforme)*, and roundworms *(T. cati)*. The product is 98% effective and well tolerated. Cats maintained in conditions of heavy or constant parasite exposure should be reevaluated in 2 to 4 weeks. This combination product should not be used in kittens weighing less than 1.5 pounds or those younger than 4 weeks of age.

Pyrantel Plus Praziquantel Plus Febantel

A three-way combination of pyrantel, praziquantel, and febantel (Drontal Plus) is available in the United States and many other parts of the world. This product is formulated to deliver at least 25 mg febantel, 5 mg praziquantel, and 5 mg pyrantel pamoate per kilogram. A single dose is given to dogs to remove tapeworms *(D. caninum, T. pisiformis, E. granulosus, E. multilocularis)*, hookworms *(A. caninum, U. stenocephala)*, roundworms *(T. canis, T. leonina)*, and whipworms *(Trichuris vulpis)*.[144,145] It is interesting to note that a single dose of this combination is effective against nematodes, especially whipworms, but that febantel alone requires three daily doses to effectively remove nematodes. This combination of ingredients may be synergistic. This product should not be used in pregnant dogs, dogs weighing less than 2 pounds, or puppies younger than 3 weeks of age.

Ivermectin Plus Pyrantel

Ivermectin combined with pyrantel pamoate is available in flavored chunks or tablets (Heartgard-30 Plus, Iverhart Plus, Tri-Heart Plus) for dogs. Pyrantel pamoate is added to provide action against gastrointestinal parasites because the heartworm-preventive dose of ivermectin, which is safe for Collies, is not effective against these important parasites. The product is formulated to deliver a target dose of 0.006 mg (6 mcg) of ivermectin and 5 mg of pyrantel pamoate per kilogram of body weight. Given orally to dogs every 30 days, it treats and controls roundworms *(T. canis, T. leonina)* and hookworms

(*A. caninum, A. braziliense,* and *U. stenocephala*) and prevents heartworms (*D. immitis*).[146] At a minimum, the product should be given at monthly intervals during the heartworm season. Adult heartworms do not produce detectable levels of microfilariae when exposed to ivermectin, so an antigen test should be used to reveal the presence of adult heartworms.[17] Safety tests have revealed that the ivermectin–pyrantel combination is well tolerated.[147] This medication should not be given to dogs younger than 6 weeks of age. (See the ivermectin section of this chapter for a discussion of administration of ivermectin to dogs harboring adult heartworms, a procedure that carries some risk and is not a labeled indication for use.)

Ivermectin Plus Pyrantel Plus Praziquantel

Ivermectin combined with pyrantel pamoate and praziquantel is available in flavored tablets (Iverhart Max) for dogs. Adding praziquantel to the two-way combination product previously mentioned extends the parasite spectrum to include tapeworms. This product is formulated to deliver a target dose of 0.006 mg (6 mcg) of ivermectin, 5 mg of pyrantel pamoate, and 5 mg of praziquantel per kilogram. Given orally to dogs every 30 days, it treats and controls roundworms (*T. canis, T. leonina*), hookworms (*A. caninum, A. braziliense,* and *U. stenocephala*), and tapeworms (*D. caninum, T. pisiformis*) and prevents heartworms (*D. immitis*). At a minimum, the product should be given at monthly intervals during the heartworm season. Adult heartworms do not produce detectable levels of microfilariae when exposed to ivermectin, so an antigen test should be used to reveal the presence of adult heartworms.[17] This medication should not be given to dogs younger than 8 weeks of age or those with existing heartworm infections. (See the ivermectin section of this chapter for a discussion of administration of ivermectin to dogs harboring adult heartworms, a procedure that carries some risk and is not a labeled indication for use.)

Milbemycin Oxime Plus Lufenuron

A two-way combination of milbemycin oxime and lufenuron (Sentinel) is approved for use in dogs. It is formulated to deliver a minimum dose of 0.5 mg of milbemycin oxime and 10 mg of lufenuron per kilogram of body weight. When given every 30 days, it is effective in preventing heartworms (*D. immitis*). The product also kills hookworms (*A. caninum*), removes and controls roundworms (*T. canis* and *T. leonina*) and whipworms (*T. vulpis*), and controls fleas. This medication should not be used in puppies younger than 4 weeks of age or those that weigh less than 2 pounds. This product is approved for concurrent administration with nitenpyram (Capstar) for quick knockdown of existing flea populations.

Imidacloprid Plus Moxidectin

A new combination product (Advantage Multi) contains imidacloprid for external parasites and moxidectin for internal parasites. The canine product provides a minimum of 10 mg/kg of imidacloprid and 2.5 mg/kg moxidectin, whereas the feline product provides the same dose of imidacloprid and 1 mg/kg moxidectin. It is important not to use the canine product on cats because cats are more sensitive to moxidectin than dogs.

Dogs

The canine product is approved for the prevention of heartworms (*D. immitis*), for the treatment and control of adult and larval hookworms (*A. caninum, U. stenocephala*), adult and larval roundworms (*T. canis, T. leonina*), and whipworms (*T. vulpis*).[148] The canine product has not been tested in dogs that weigh less than 1.36 kg (3 lb) or are younger than 7 weeks of age. Nor has it been tested in breeding, pregnant, or lactating dogs. Dogs should be tested for the presence of heartworm before administration. The canine product is not effective against adult heartworm or for clearing microfilariae. It was well tolerated at 5 times the label dose. Oral ingestion of the product by dogs may cause serious reactions, including depression, salivation, dilated pupils, incoordination, panting, and generalized tremors. Thus it is important to prevent dogs from licking the product from the application site.

Cats

The feline product is approved for the prevention of heartworm, *D. immitis;* for the treatment and control of adult and larval hookworm, *A. tubaeforme;* and adult and larval roundworm, *T. cati.* It should not be used on cats that weigh less than 0.9 kg (2 lb) or on cats younger than 9 weeks of age. This product was well tolerated when given at 5 times the label dose in 9-week-old kittens. Cats dosed with a single dose at 10 times the label dose exhibited mild transient hypersalivation. Oral ingestion of the product may cause hypersalivation, tremors, vomiting, and decreased appetite.

This combination is also effective in treating fleas in dogs and cats and ear mites in cats.

REFERENCES

1. Foreyt WJ: *Veterinary parasitology reference manual,* ed 5, Ames, Iowa, 2001, Blackwell.
2. Mehlhorn H, editor: *Encyclopedic reference of parasitology: diseases, treatment, therapy,* ed 2, New York, 2001, Springer-Verlag.
3. Taylor MA, Coop RL, Wall RL: *Veterinary parasitology,* ed 3, Ames Iowa, 2007, Blackwell.
4. Bowman DD: *Georgi's parasitology for veterinarians,* ed 9, Philadelphia, 2008, Saunders.
5. Blagburn BL, Lindsay DS, Vaughan JL, et al: Prevalence of canine parasites based on fecal floatation, *Compend Cont Educ Pract Vet* 18(5):483–523, 1996.
6. Bowman DD: Spread of companion animal vector-borne parasitic disease in the US and Europe: Concerns relative to travel, national disasters, shelter-source animals and wildlife. 2nd Canine Vector-Borne Disease (CVBD) Symposium, *Mazara del Vallo, Sicily,* Italy, 2007.
7. Blagburn BL, Schenker R, Gagne F, et al: Prevalence of intestinal parasites in companion animals in Ontario and Quebec, Canada, during the winter months, *Vet Ther* 9(3):169–175, 2008.
8. Companion Animal Parasite Council. Accessed February 19, 2010, at http://www.capcvet.org/.
9. Bowman DD, Torre CJ, Mannella C: Survey of 11 western states for heartworm (Dirofilaria immitis) infection, heartworm diagnostic and prevention protocols, and fecal examination protocols for gastrointestinal parasites, *Vet Ther* 8(4):293–304, 2007.
10. Murray WJ, Kazacos KR: Raccoon roundworm encephalitis, *Clin Infect Dis* 39(10):1484–1492, 2004.

11. Centers for Disease Control (CDC): Guidelines for veterinarians: prevention of zoonotic transmission of ascarids and hookworms of dogs and cats. Accessed February 19, 2010, at http://www.cdc.gov/ncidod/dpd/parasites/ascaris/prevention.pdf.
12. Urbani C, Albonico M: Anthelminthic drug safety and drug administration in the control of soil-transmitted helminthiasis in community campaigns, *Acta Trop* 86(2-3):215–221, 2003.
13. Hotez PJ, Bethony J, Bottazzi ME, et al: Hookworm: "The Great Infection of Mankind," *PLoS Med* 2(3):e67, 2005.
14. Hotez PJ, Pritchard DI: Hookworm infection, *Sci Am* 272(6):68–75, 1995.
15. Traub RJ, Robertson ID, Irwin P, et al: The role of dogs in transmission of gastrointestinal parasites in a remote tea-growing community in northeastern India, *Am J Trop Med Hyg* 67(5):539–545, 2002.
16. Labarthe N, Serrao ML, Ferreira AM, et al: A survey of gastrointestinal helminths in cats of the metropolitan region of Rio de Janeiro, Brazil, *Vet Parasitol* 123(1-2):133–139, 2004.
17. American Heartworm Society 2005 Guidelines for the diagnosis, prevention and management of heartworm (Dirofilaria immitis) infection in dogs, American Heartworm Society. Accessed January 25, 2009, at http://www.heartwormsociety.org/article_48.html.
18. American Heartworm Society 2007 Guidelines for the diagnosis, prevention and management of heartworm (Dirofilaria immitis) infection in cats, American Heartworm Society. Accessed January 26, 2009, at http://www.heartwormsociety.org/article_47.html.
18a. American Heartworm Society 2010 Guidelines for the diagnosis, prevention and management of heartworm (Dirofilaria immitis) infection in dogs, American Heartworm Society. Accessed July 18, 2010, at http://www.heartwormsociety.org/veterinary-resources/canine-guidelines.html.
19. North American Compendiums: *Compendium of veterinary products*, ed 10, Port Huron, Mich, 2007, North American Compendiums.
20. Campbell WC, Rew RS, editors: *Chemotherapy of parasitic diseases*, New York, 1985, Plenum Press.
21. Vanden Bossche H, Thienpoint D, Janssens PG, editors: *Chemotherapy of gastrointestinal helminths*, New York, 1985, Springer-Verlag.
22. Riviere JE, Papich MG, editors: *Veterinary pharmacology and therapeutics*, ed 9, Ames, Iowa, 2009, Wiley-Blackwell.
23. United States Pharmacopeia: Macrocyclic lactones (veterinary-systemic). The United States Pharmacopeial Convention, Inc. Accessed Jan 26, 2009, at http://www.usp.org/pdf/EN/veterinary/macrocyclicLactones.pdf.
24. Shoop WL, Mrozik H, Fisher MH: Structure and activity of avermectins and milbemycins in animal health, *Vet Parasitol* 59(2):139–156, 1995.
25. Wolstenholme AJ, Rogers AT: Glutamate-gated chloride channels and the mode of action of the avermectin/milbemycin anthelmintics, *Parasitology* 131(Suppl):S85–S95, 2005.
26. Paul A, Tranquilli W: Ivermectin. In Kirk RW, editor: *Current veterinary therapy X*, ed 10, Philadelphia, 1989, Saunders, pp 140–142.
27. Papich MG: *Saunders handbook of veterinary drugs*, ed 2, Philadelphia, 2007, Saunders.
28. Plumb DC: *Plumb's veterinary drug handbook*, Ames, Iowa, 2008, Blackwell.
29. Dorman DC: Neurotoxic drugs in dogs and cats. In Bonagura JD, editor: *Kirk's current veterinary therapy XII*, Philadelphia, 1995, Saunders, pp 1140–1145.
30. Rumbeiha WK: Parasiticide toxicosis: avermectins. In Bonagura JD, editor: *Kirk's current veterinary therapy XIV*, St Louis, 2009, Saunders, pp 125–127.
30a. Merola V, Khan S, Gwaltney-Brant S: Ivermectin toxicosis in dogs: a retrospective study, *J Am Anim Hosp Assoc* 45(3):106–111, 2009.
31. Gwaltney-Brant S: ASPCA Animal Poison Control Center—veterinary toxicologist, *Personal Communication*, January 26, 2010.
32. Pulliam JD, Seward RL, Henry RT, et al: Investigating ivermectin toxicity in Collies, *Vet Med* :33–40, 1985:(June).
33. Hugnet C, Cadore JL, Buronfosse F, et al: Loperamide poisoning in the dog, *Vet Hum Toxicol* 38(1):31–33, 1996.
34. Mealey KL, Bentjen SA, Gay JM, et al: Ivermectin sensitivity in collies is associated with a deletion mutation of the mdr1 gene, *Pharmacogenetics* 11(8):727–733, 2001.
35. Mealey KL: Therapeutic implications of the MDR-1 gene, *J Vet Pharmacol Ther* 27(5):257–264, 2004.
36. Mealey KL, Bentjen SA, Waiting DK: Frequency of the mutant MDR1 allele associated with ivermectin sensitivity in a sample population of collies from the northwestern United States, *Am J Vet Res* 63(4):479–481, 2002.
37. Neff MW, Robertson KR, Wong AK, et al: Breed distribution and history of canine mdr1-1Delta, a pharmacogenetic mutation that marks the emergence of breeds from the collie lineage, *Proc Natl Acad Sci U S A* 101(32):11725–11730, 2004.
38. Geyer J, Doring B, Godoy JR, et al: Development of a PCR-based diagnostic test detecting a nt230(del4) MDR1 mutation in dogs: verification in a moxidectin-sensitive Australian Shepherd, *J Vet Pharmacol Ther* 28(1):95–99, 2005.
39. Mealey KL, Meurs KM: Breed distribution of the ABCB1-1Delta (multidrug sensitivity) polymorphism among dogs undergoing ABCB1 genotyping, *J Am Vet Med Assoc* 233(6): 921–924, 2008.
40. Washington State University, College of Veterinary Medicine, Veterinary Clinical Pharmacology Lab: (2010). Affected breeds. Accessed January 26, 2010, at http://www.vetmed.wsu.edu/depts-VCPL/breeds.aspx.
41. Perez R, Cabezas I, Sutra JF, et al: Faecal excretion profile of moxidectin and ivermectin after oral administration in horses, *Vet J* 161(1):85–92, 2001.
42. Tranquilli WJ, Paul AJ, Seward RL, et al: Response to the physostigmine administration in collie dogs exhibiting ivermectin toxicosis, *J Vet Pharmacol Ther* 10:96–100, 1987.
43. Muhammad G, Abdul J, Khan MZ, et al: Use of neostigmine in massive ivermectin toxicity in cats, *Vet Hum Toxicol* 46(1):28–29, 2004.
44. Weinberg G, Ripper R, Feinstein DL, et al: Lipid emulsion infusion rescues dogs from bupivacaine-induced cardiac toxicity, *Reg Anesth Pain Med* 28(3):198–202, 2003.
45. Crandell DE, Weinberg GL: Moxidectin toxicosis in a puppy successfully treated with intravenous lipids, *J Vet Emerg Crit Care (San Antonio)* 19(2):181–186, 2009.
46. Weinberg G: Lipid rescue resuscitation from local anaesthetic cardiac toxicity, *Toxicol Rev* 25(3):139–145, 2006.
47. Hribernik TN: Canine and feline heartworm disease. In Kirk RW, editor: *Current veterinary therapy*, Philadelphia, 1989, Saunders, X, pp 263–270.
48. Bowman DD, Johnson RB, Ulrich ME, et al: Effects of long-term administration of ivermectin or milbemycin oxime on circulating microfilariae and parasite antigenemia in dogs with patent heartworm infections. *Proceedings of the Heartworm Symposium Austin*, Tex, 1992, American Heartworm Society.
49. Lok JB, Knight DH: Macrolide effects on reproductive function in male and female heartworms. *Proceedings of the Heartworm Symposium Auburn*, 1995, Ala, American Heartworm Society.
50. Knight DH: CVT update: heartworm testing and prevention in dogs. In Bonagura JD, editor: *Kirk's current veterinary therapy: XIII*, Philadelphia, 2000, Saunders, pp 777–782.
51. Bazzocchi C, Ceciliani F, McCall JW, et al: Antigenic role of the endosymbionts of filarial nematodes: IgG response against the Wolbachia surface protein in cats infected with Dirofilaria immitis, *Proc Biol Sci* 267(1461):2511–2516, 2000.

52. McCall JW, Genchi C, Kramer L, et al: Heartworm and Wolbachia: therapeutic implications, *Vet Parasitol* 158(3):204–214, 2008.
53. Bowman DD: *Georgi's parasitology for veterinarians*, ed 7, Philadelphia, 1999, Saunders.
54. Sherding RG: Respiratory parasites. In Bonagura JD, Twedt DC, editors: *Kirk's current veterinary therapy XIV*, St Louis, 2009, pp 666-671.
55. Nolan TJ, Niamatali S, Bhopale V, et al: Efficacy of a chewable formulation of ivermectin against a mixed infection of *Ancylostoma braziliense* and *Ancylostoma tubaeforme* in cats, *Am J Vet Res* 53(8):1411–1413, 1992.
56. Knight DH: Guidelines for diagnosis and management of heartworm (Dirofilaria immitus) infection. In Bonagura JD, editor: *Kirk's current veterinary therapy: XII*, Philadelphia, 1995, Saunders, pp 879–887.
57. Merial LTD: Heartgard® chewables for cats [package insert], 2006.
58. Blagburn BL, Hendrix CM, Lindsay DS, et al: Anthelmintic efficacy of ivermectin in naturally parasitized cats, *Am J Vet Res* 48(4):670–672, 1987.
59. Kirkpatrick CE, Megella C: Use of ivermectin in treatment of *Aelurostrongylus abstrusus* and *Toxocara cati* infections in a cat, *J Am Vet Med Assoc* 190(10):1309–1310, 1987.
60. Hawkins EC: Diseases of the lower respiratory system. In Ettinger SJ, Feldman EC, editors: *Textbook of veterinary internal medicine,* ed 4, Philadelphia, 1995, pp 767–811.
61. Bedard C, Desnoyers M, Lavallee MC, et al: Capillaria in the bladder of an adult cat, *Can Vet J* 43(12):973–974, 2002.
62. Bater AK: Efficacy of oral milbemycin against naturally acquired heartworm infection in dogs. *Proceedings of the Heartworm Symposium* 1989 Charleston, SC, 1989, American Heartworm Society.
63. Bradley RE: Dose titration and efficacy of milbemycin oxime for prophylaxis against *Dirofilaria immitis* infection in dogs. *Proceedings of the Heartworm Symposium* 1989 Charleston, SC, 1989, American Heartworm Society.
64. Grieve RB, Frank GR, Stewart VA, et al: Chemoprophylactic effects of milbemycin oxime against larvae of Dirofilaria immitis during prepatent development, *Am J Vet Res* 52(12):2040–2042, 1991.
65. Bowman DD, Parsons JJ, Grieve RB, et al: Effects of milbemycin on adult *Toxocara canis* in dogs with experimentally induced infection, *Am J Vet Res* 49(11):1986–1989, 1988.
66. Bowman DD, Johnson RC, Hepler DI: Effects of milbemycin oxime on adult hookworms in dogs with naturally acquired infections, *Am J Vet Res* 51(3):487–490, 1990.
67. Bowman DD, Lin DS, Johnson RC, et al: Effects of milbemycin oxime on adult *Ancylostoma caninum* and *Uncinaria stenocephala* in dogs with experimentally induced infections, *Am J Vet Res* 52(1):64–67, 1991.
68. Blagburn BL, Hendrix CM, Lindsay DS, et al: Efficacy of milbemycin oxime against naturally acquired or experimentally induced *Ancylostoma* spp. and *Trichuris vulpis* infections in dogs, *Am J Vet Res* 53(4):513–516, 1992.
69. Bowman DD, Ulrich MA, Gregory DE, et al: Treatment of Baylisascaris procyonis infections in dogs with milbemycin oxime, *Vet Parasitol* 129(3-4):285–290, 2005.
70. Blagburn BL, Hendrix CM, Lindsay DS, et al: Milbemycin: Efficacy and toxicity in beagle and collie dogs. *Proceedings of the Heartworm Symposium* 1989 Charleston, SC, 1989, American Heartworm Society.
71. Sasaki Y, Kitagawa H, Murase S, et al: Susceptibility of rough-coated collies to milbemycin oxime, *Nippon Juigaku Zasshi* 52(6):1269–1271, 1990.
72. Blagburn BL, Hendrix CM, Lindsay DS, et al: Post-adulticide milbemycin oxime microfilaricidal activity in dogs naturally infected with *Dirofilaria immitis*. *Proceedings of the Heartworm Symposium* 1992 Austin, Tex, 1992, American Heartworm Society.
73. Bowman DD: Anthelmintics for dogs and cats effective against nematodes and cestodes, *Compend Cont Educ Pract Vet* 14(5):597–599, 1992.
74. Lok JB, Knight DH, LaPaugh DA, et al: Kinetics of microfilaremia suppression in *Dirofilaria immitis*-infected dogs during and after a prophylactic regimen of milbemycin oxime. *Proceedings of the Heartworm Symposium* 1992 Austin, Tex, 1992, American Heartworm Society.
75. Stewart VA, Hepler DI, Grieve RB: Efficacy of milbemycin oxime in chemoprophylaxis of dirofilariasis in cats, *Am J Vet Res* 53(12):2274–2277, 1992.
76. Blagburn BL, Hendrix CM, Vaughan JL, et al: Efficacy of milbemycin oxime against *Ancylostoma tubaeforme* in experimentally infected cats. 37th Annual meeting of the American Association of Veterinarian Parasitologists. Boston, Mass, 1992.
77. Glickman LT, Glickman NW, Moore GE, et al: Safety profile of moxidectin (Proheart 6) and two oral heartworm preventives in dogs, *Intern J Appl Res Vet Med* 3(2):49–61, 2005.
78. Food and Drug Administration, Center for Veterinary Medicine: ProHeart® 6 (moxidectin) Questions and Answers, June 5, 2008. Accessed January 29, 2009, at http://www.fda.gov/cvm/Proheart6FAQ.htm.
79. Anonymous: ProHeart 6 client information and product label. Fort Dodge Animal Health, 2008. Accessed January 29, 2009, at http://www.proheart6.com/.
80. Lok JB, Knight DH, Wang GT, et al: Activity of an injectable, sustained-release formulation of moxidectin administered prophylactically to mixed-breed dogs to prevent infection with Dirofilaria immitis, *Am J Vet Res* 62(11):1721–1726, 2001.
81. Bishop BF, Bruce CI, Evans NA, et al: Selamectin: a novel broad-spectrum endectocide for dogs and cats, *Vet Parasitol* 91:163–176, 2000.
82. Thomas CA: Revolution: a unique endectocide providing comprehensive conveient protection, *Compend Cont Educ Pract Vet* 21(Suppl 9):2–25, 1999.
83. McTier TL, McCall JW, Jernigan AD, et al: *UK-124,114, a novel avermectin for the prevention of heartworms in dogs and cats*, Tampa, Fla, American Heartworm Symposium, American Heartworm Society, Batavia, Ill, 1998.
84. Thomas CA: Revolution safety profile, *Compend Cont Educ Pract Vet* 21(Suppl 9):26–31, 1999.
85. Boy MG, Six RH, Thomas CA, et al: Efficacy and safety of selamectin against fleas and heartworms in dogs and cats presented as veterinary patients in North America, *Vet Parasitol* 91(3-4):233–250, 2000.
86. Fisher MA, Shanks DJ: A review of the off-label use of selamectin (Stronghold/Revolution) in dogs and cats, *Acta Vet Scand* 50:46, 2008.
87. Pfizer Animal Health. Revolution (selamectin) package insert. Accessed January 29, 2009, at http://www.revolution4dogs.com/PAHimages/compliance_pdfs/US_EN_RV_compliance.pdf.
88. Campbell WC: Benzimidazoles; veterinary uses, *Parasitology Today* 6(4):130–133, 1990.
89. Lacey E: Mode of action of benzimadzoles, *Parasitology Today* 6(4):112–115, 1990.
90. McKellar QA, Scott EW: The benzimidazole anthelmintics: a review, *J Vet Pharmacol Ther* 13:223–247, 1990.
91. Adams HR, editor: *Veterinary pharmacology and therapeutics*, ed 7, Ames, Iowa, 1995, Iowa State University Press.
92. Frayha GJ, Smyth JD, Gobert JG, et al: The mechanisms of action of antiprotozoal and anthelmintic drugs in man, *Gen Pharmacol* 28(2):273–299, 1997.
93. Reinemeyer CE, Courtney CH: Antinematodal drugs. In Adams HR, editor: *Veterinary pharmacology and therapeutics*, ed 8, Ames, Iowa, 2001, Iowa State University Press, pp 947–979.
94. Stokol T, Randolph JF, Nachbar S, et al: Development of bone marrow toxicosis after albendazol administration in a dog and cat, *J Am Vet Med Assoc* 210:1753–1756, 1997.

95. Meyer EK: Adverse events associated with albendazole and other products used for treatment of giardiasis, *J Am Vet Med Assoc* 213(1):44–46, 1998.
96. United States Pharmacopeia: *USP Drug Information Update (September, pp 1289-1586)*, Rockville, MD, 1998, United States Pharmacopeial Convention.
97. Intervet/Schering-Plough Animal Health. Panacur C Canine Dewormer Product Insert. Accessed January 30, 2009, at http://www.compasnac.com/intervet.htm.
98. Barr S: Enteric protozoal infections. In Greene C, editor: *Infectious diseases of the dog and cat*, St Louis, 2006, Saunders, pp 736–750.
99. Aubry ML, Cowell P, Davey MJ, et al: Aspects of the pharmacology of a new anthelmintic: pyrantel, *Br J Pharmacol* 38:332–344, 1970.
100. Eyre P: Some pharmacodynamic effects of the nematodes: methypyrdine, tetramisole and pyrantel, *J Pharm Pharmacol* 22:26–36, 1970.
101. Martin RJ: Neuromuscular transmission in nematode parasites and antinematodal drug action, *Pharmacol Ther* 58(1):13–50, 1993.
102. Martin RJ: Modes of action of anthelmintic drugs, *Vet J* 154(1):11–34, 1997.
103. Londershausen M: Approaches to new parasiticides, *Pestic Sci* 48(4):269–292, 1996.
104. United States Pharmacopeia (2005). Tetrahydropyrimidines (veterinary—oral-local). The United States Pharmacopeial Convention, Inc. Accessed January 26, 2009, at http://www.usp.org/pdf/EN/veterinary/tetrahydropyrimidines.pdf.
105. Linquist WD: Drug evaluation of pyrantel pamoate against *Ancylostoma, Toxocara*, and *Toxascaris* in eleven dogs, *Am J Vet Res* 36(9):1387–1389 & 1695, 1975.
106. Klein JB, Bradley RE, Conway DP: Anthelmintic efficacy of pyrantel pamoate against the roundworm, *Toxocara canis*, and the hookworm, *Ancylostoma caninum*, in dogs, *Vet Med Small Anim Clin* 73:1011–1013, 1978.
107. Jacobs DE: Control of *Toxocara canis* in puppies: a comparison of screening techiques and evaluation of a dosing programme, *J Vet Pharmacol Ther* 10:23–29, 1987.
108. Clark JA: Physaloptera stomach worms associated with chronic vomition in a dog in Western Canada, *Can Vet J* 31(12):840, 1990.
109. Clark JN, Daurio CP, Barth DW, et al: Evaluation of a beef-based chewable formulation of pyrantel against induced and natural infections of hookworms and ascarids in dogs, *Vet Parasitol* 40:127–133, 1991.
110. Harder A, Holden-Dye L, Walker R, et al: Mechanisms of action of emodepside, *Parasitol Res* 97(Suppl 1):S1–S10, 2005.
111. Bayer Healthcare: Profender (emodepside/praziquantel) Topical Solution Product Insert, Bayer Healthcare, 2007. Accessed January 31, 2009, at http://www.bayerdvm.com/resources/docs/Profender-Label.pdf.
112. Roberson EL: Chemotherapy of parasitic diseases. In Booth NE, McDonald LE, editors: *Veterinary pharmacology and therapeutics*, ed 6, Ames, Iowa, 1988, Iowa State University Press, pp 882–927.
113. English PB, Sprent JFA: The large roundworms of dogs and cats: effectiveness of piperazine salts against immature *Toxocara canis* in prenatally infected puppies, *Austr Vet J* 41:50–53, 1965.
114. Sharp ML, Sepesi JP, Collins JA: A comparative critical assay on canine anthelmintics, *Vet Med Small Anim Clin* 68:131–132, 1973.
115. Jacobs DE: Anthelmintics for dogs and cats, *Int J Parasitol* 17(2):511–518, 1987.
116. Andrews P, Thomas H, Pohlke R, et al: Praziquantel, *Med Res Rev* 3(2):147–200, 1983.
117. Arundel JH, Bossche Hvd, Thienpoint D, et al: *Chemotherapy of gastrointestinal helminths*, New York, 1985, Springer-Verlag.
118. Gemmell MA, Johnstone PD, Oudemans G: The effect of praziquantel on *Echinococcus granulosus, Taenia hydatigena* and *Taenia ovis* infections in dogs, *Res Vet Sci* 23:121–123, 1977.
119. Andersen FL, Conder GA, Marsland WP: Efficacy of injectable and tablet formulations of praziquantel against mature *Echinococcus granulosus*, *Am J Vet Res* 39(11):1861–1862, 1978.
120. Thakur SA, Prezioso U, Marchevsky N: Efficacy of droncit against *Echinococcus granulosus* infection in dogs, *Am J Vet Res* 39(5):859–860, 1978.
121. Thomas H, Gonnert R: The efficacy of praziquantel against cestodes in cats, dogs, and sheep, *Res Vet Sci* 24:20–25, 1978.
122. Andersen FL, Conder GA, Marsland WP: Efficacy of injectable and tablet formulations of praziquantel against immature *Echinococcus granulosus*, *Am J Vet Res* 40(5):700–701, 1979.
123. Gemmell MA, Johnstone PD, Oudemans G: The effect of route of administration on the efficacy of praziquantel against *Echinococcus granulosus* infections in dogs, *Res Vet Sci* 29:131–132, 1980.
124. Kruckenberg SM, Meyer AD, Eastman WR: Preliminary studies on the effect of praziquantel against tapeworms in dogs and cats, *Vet Med Small Anim Clin* 76:689–697, 1981.
125. Bayer Healthcare. Droncit (praziquantel) injectable cestocide for dogs and cats. Accessed January 30, 2009, at https://www.bayerdvm.com/Products/droncit/droncit-labels.cfm.
126. Pfizer Animal Health: Cestex (epsiprantel) veterinary tablets, 2000. Accessed January 30, 2009, from http://www.pfizerah.com/PAHimages/compliance_pdfs/US_EN_CE_compliance.pdf.
127. Corwin RM, Green SP, Keefe TJ: Dose titration and confirmation tests for determination of cestocidal efficacy of epsiprantel in dogs, *Am J Vet Res* 50(7):1076–1077, 1989.
128. Manger BR, Brewer MD: Epsiprantel, a new tapeworm remedy, preliminary efficacy studies in dogs and cats, *Br Vet J* 145:384–388, 1989.
129. United States Pharmacopeia: Epsiprantel veterinary—oral-local, 2008, The United States Pharmacopeial Convention, Inc., Accessed Jan 26, 2009, at http://www.usp.org/pdf/EN/veterinary/epsiprantel.pdf.
130. Plumb DC: *Veterinary drug handbook*, ed 5, Stockholm, Wisconsin, 2005, PharmaVet.
131. Gilman AG, Rall TW, Nies AS, et al: *Goodman and Gilman's the pharmacological basis of therapeutics*, ed 8, New York, 1990, Pergamon Press.
132. Dzimianski MT, McCall JW, McTier TL, et al: Preliminary results of the efficacy of RM 340 administered seasonally to heartworm antigen and microfilaria positive dogs living outdoors in a heartworm endemic area. *Proceedings of the Heartworm Symposium* 1992 Austin, Tex, 1992, American Heartworm Society.
133. Keister DM, Dzimianski MT, McTier TL, et al: Dose selection and confirmation of RM 340, a new filaricide for the treatment of dogs with immature and mature Dirofilaria immitis. *Proceedings of the Heartworm Symposium* 1992 Austin, Tex, 1992, American Heartworm Society.
134. Keister DM, Tanner PA, Meo NJ: Immiticide: review of discovery, development and utility. *Proceedings of the Heartworm Symposium* 1995, Auburn, Ala, 1995.
135. Miller MW, Keister DM, Tanner PA, et al: Clinical efficacy and safety trial of melarsomine dihydrochloride (RM340) and thiacetarsemide in dogs with moderate (Class 2) heartworm disease. *Proceedings of the Heartworm Symposium* 1995, Auburn, Ala, 1995.
136. Rawlings CA, McCall JW: Melarsomine: a new heartworm adulticide, *Compend Cont Educ Pract Vet* 18(4):373–379, 1996.
137. Vezzoni A, Genchi C, Raynaud JP: Adulticide efficacy of RM 340 in dogs with mild and severe natural infections. *Proceedings of the Heartworm Symposium* 1992, Austin, Tex, 1992, American Heartworm Society.
138. Case JL, Tanner PA, Keister DM, et al: A clinical field trial of melarsomine dihydrochloride (RM340) in dogs with severe (Class 3) heartworm disease. *Proceedings of the Heartworm Symposium* 1995, Auburn, Ala, 1995.

139. Reinemeyer CR, Courtney CH: Anticestodal and antitrematodal drugs. In Adams HR, editor: *Veterinary pharmacology and therapeutics*, ed 8, Ames, Iowa, 2001, Iowa State University Press, pp 980–991.
140. Altreuther G, Borgsteede FH, Buch J, et al: Efficacy of a topically administered combination of emodepside and praziquantel against mature and immature *Ancylostoma tubaeforme* in domestic cats, *Parasitol Res* 97(Suppl 1):S51–S57, 2005.
141. Charles SD, Altreuther G, Reinemeyer CR, et al: Evaluation of the efficacy of emodepside+praziquantel topical solution against cestode (*Dipylidium caninum, Taenia taeniaeformis*, and *Echinococcus multilocularis*) infections in cats, *Parasitol Res* 97(Suppl 1):S33–S40, 2005.
142. Reinemeyer CR, Buch J, Charles SD, et al: Evaluation of the efficacy of emodepside plus praziquantel topical solution against ascarid infections (*Toxocara cati* or *Toxascaris leonina*) in cats, *Parasitol Res* 97(Suppl 1):S41–S50, 2005.
143. Altreuther G, Buch J, Charles SD, et al: Field evaluation of the efficacy and safety of emodepside/praziquantel spot-on solution against naturally acquired nematode and cestode infections in domestic cats, *Parasitol Res* 97(Suppl 1):S58–S64, 2005.
144. Bowman DD, Arthur RG: Laboratory evaluation of Drontal plus (febantel/praziquantel/pyrantel) tablets for dogs. *Proceedings of the American Association of Veterinary Parasitology*, Minneapolis, Minn, 1993.
145. Cruthers LR, Slone RL, Arthur RG: Efficacy of Drontal plus (praziquantel/pyrantel/febantel) tablets for removal of *Ancylostoma caninum, Uncinaria stenocephala* and *Toxascaris leonina. Proceedings of the American Association of Veterinary Parasitology,* Minneapolis, Minn, 1993.
146. Clark JN, Daurio CP, Plue RE, et al: Efficacy of ivermectin and pyrantel pamoate combined in a chewable formulation against heartworm, hookworm, and ascarid infections in dogs, *Am J Vet Res* 53(4):517–520, 1992.
147. Clark JN, Pulliam JD, Daurio CP: Safety study of a beef-based chewable tablet formulation of ivermectin and pyrantel pamoate in growing dogs, pups and breeding adult dogs, *Am J Vet Res* 53(4):608–612, 1992.
148. Arther RG, Atkins C, Ciszewski DK, et al: Safety of imidacloprid plus moxidectin topical solution applied to cats heavily infected with adult heartworms (Dirofilaria immitis), *Parasitol Res* 97(Suppl 1):S70–S75, 2005.

Therapy of Cardiovascular Diseases

14

Dawn Merton Boothe

Chapter Outline

CARDIOVASCULAR PHYSIOLOGY AS IT PERTAINS TO CARDIOVASCULAR DRUGS

Membrane Ion Movements and the Action Potential

Predicting the nuances of pharmacodynamic responses to cardiac drugs depends, in part, on understanding the electrophysiology of myocardial cells. Selected mechanisms of ion movement into the cell are demonstrated in Figure 14-1. The action potential duration (APD) of myocardial cells is long compared with that of nerves, reflecting the well-orchestrated coordination of multiple ion channels and associated transport proteins.[1] The magnitude and direction of the ion flow, and thus current, depends on both transmembrane voltage and ion concentration gradients. Two types of myocardial cells will be discussed: those capable of automaticity (i.e., spontaneous

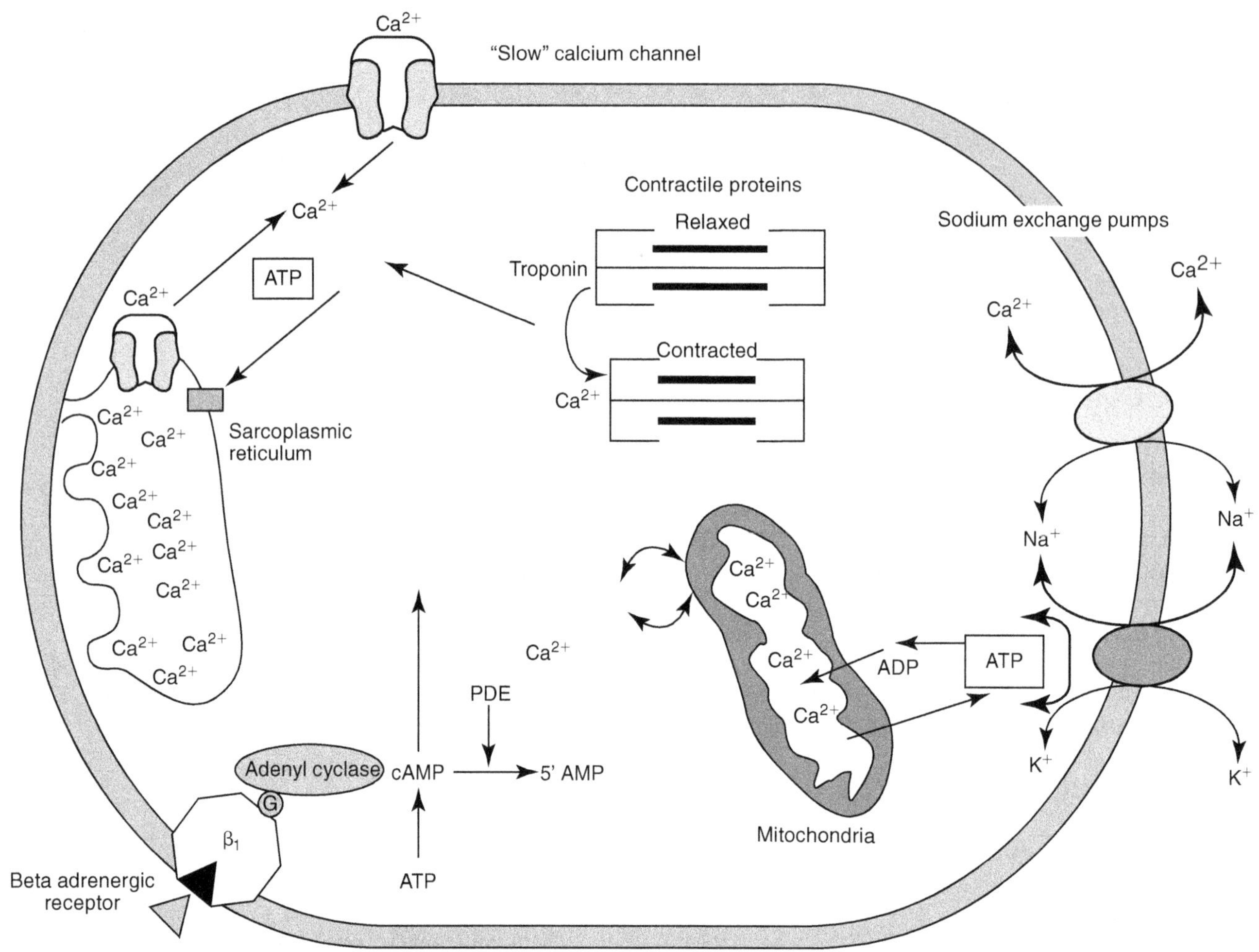

Figure 14-1 Calcium can enter the myocardial cell through several mechanisms, including the slow calcium channel, the sodium–calcium exchange ATPase pump, and beta 1 adrenergic receptor stimulation. Increased intracellular concentrations of calcium lead to the release of sarcolemmal calcium. Calcium leads to the interaction between actin and myosin, causing myocardial contractility. Sequestration of calcium in the sarcoplasmic reticulum causes myocardial relaxation. Sodium and potassium channels are not shown in this diagram. *ATP,* Adenosine triphosphate; *cAMP,* cyclic adenosine monophosphate; *PDE,* phosphodiesterase.

depolarization), exemplified by cells that normally serve as pacemakers (e.g., sinoatrial [SA] node) and those cells not normally capable of automaticity (e.g., atrial and ventricular myocardial cells). Although overlap exists, the electrophysiology of each differs from one another (Figure 14-2).

Nondepolarizing cells

In nondepolarizing cells, the resting membrane potential (RMP) of -80 to -90 (inside compared with outside) reflects the relative distribution of sodium, potassium, and chloride across the cell membrane. The external and internal concentration of sodium approximates 145 and 15 mmol/L, respectively (ratio of 9.7), whereas that of potassium approximates 4 (range 3 to 6) and 145 mmol/L respectively (ratio of 0.027). Chloride ions contribute to the RMP only by virtue of their influence on cellular electrical responses to incoming signals. At rest the distribution of ions is not at equilibrium but is in a dynamic state, constantly subject to internal and external influences. The major driving force for the negative RMP is ion movements through channels (molecular pores) that span the myocardial cell membrane. These channels generally exist in either an open (conducting) or closed (resting) state, with a third state of "inactivation" reflecting a period in which the nonconducting channel cannot be activated. The state of channels targeted by cardiac drugs markedly influences their impact on the action potential. Drugs with greater affinity for inactivated channels generally are more influential than those that target other states.

KEY POINT 14-1 Differences in response of pacemaker versus nonpacemaker cells to cardioactive drugs reflects, in part, differences in membrane electrophysiology and ion flow.

Movement of ions through the channels follows both concentration and electrical (i.e., electrochemical) gradients. Ion flow is also influenced by energy-dependent pumps that actively and selectively direct ion movement against the electrochemical gradients. A "leak current" allows a constant, albeit smaller, ion flux. At rest the status of all channels influencing the membrane potential is static, save for a specific ("inward rectifier") channel that is permeable only to potassium, allowing it to efflux down an electrochemical gradient. This efflux is countered by a Na+,K+-ATPase pump, which

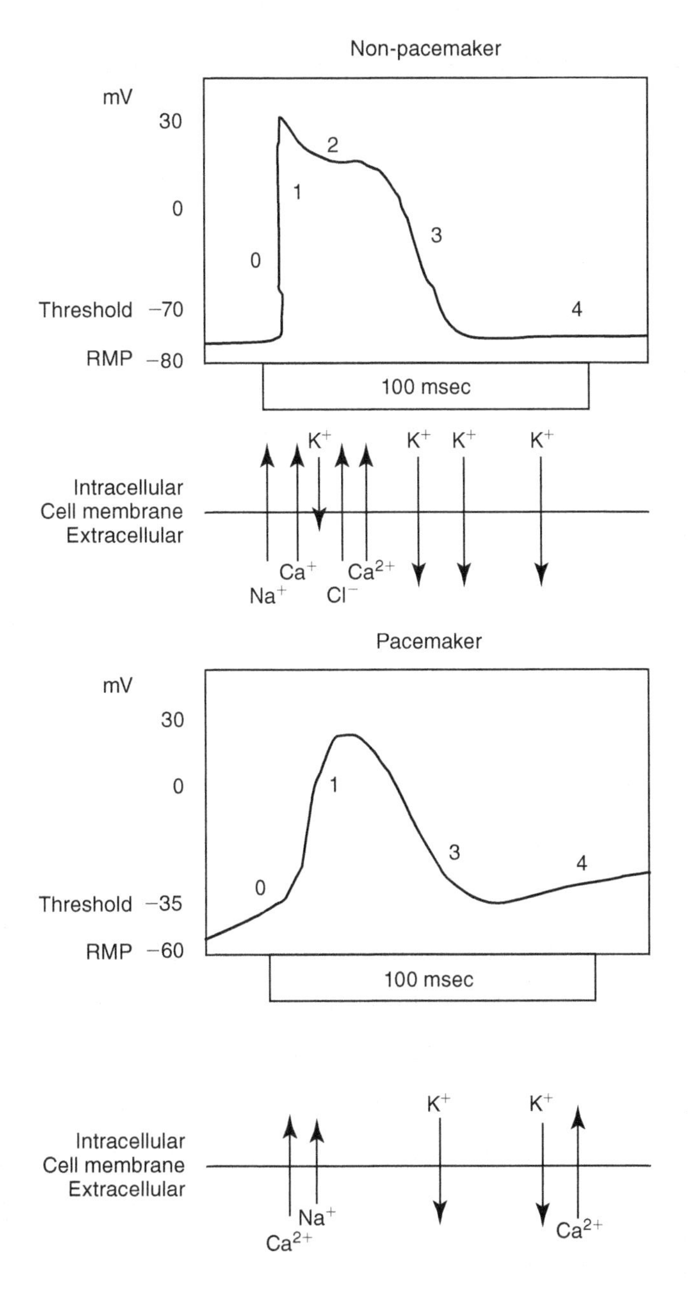

Figure 14-2 The action potential (AP) occurs in four phases. The ions responsible for and the configuration of each phase differ between cells capable of automaticity (i.e., pacemaker) and non-pacemaker (i.e., nondepoloarizing) cells. Phase 0 occurs when the resting membrane potential (RMP) reaches threshold, resulting in the generation of the AP. The rapid upswing in the membrane potential reflects sodium (non-pacemaker) and, to a lesser degree, calcium influx. In cells capable of automaticity *(bottom),* calcium is the primary ion moving inward during phase 0. This calcium influx stimulates release of calcium from the sarcoplasmic reticulum. The small influx of calcium in non-depolarizing cells is important to intracellular calcium fluxes. Phase 1 represents the early phase of repolarization. An influx of chloride and decreased efflux of potassium lead to reestablishment of the membrane potential. During phase 2 electrogenic movement of calcium through "slow" channels prolongs repolarization, causing a plateau phase. With phase 3, the membrane potential reaches the diastolic resting level. In cells capable of automaticity, this phase is characterized by a gradual depolarization, probably because of calcium influx, until threshold is reached. The heart rate is determined by the slope of phase 4; tissues with the steepest phase 4 slope will serve as the cardiac pacemaker.

exchanges 3Na+ for 2K+, thus maintaining the intracellular concentration necessary for the gradient. Accordingly, potassium has the greatest influence on the RMP, and very slight changes in extracellular potassium can influence potassium flux, the RMP, and the cardiac cell cycle.

KEY POINT 14-2 Potassium has the greatest influence on the resting membrane potential. As such, even slight changes in extracellular potassium can influence potassium flux, the resting membrane potential, and the cardiac cell cycle.

Myocardial sodium channels are the primary gatekeepers of the action potential in nonpacemaker cells (see Figure 14-1). They are voltage gated and closed at rest. Membrane depolarization in nonpacemaker cells (see Figure 14-2) increases selective permeability in sodium channels. The concentration gradient causes an initial sodium influx, stimulating more voltage-gated sodium channels to open, thus perpetuating a self-regenerating action potential (phase 0, depolarization). Sodium channels inactivate when depolarization is complete and must go through a resting (recovery) period before they can be reactivated. Membrane permeability reestablishes itself largely in response to potassium ion efflux, and the membrane potential begins to decline back toward the RMP (phase 1, early repolarization). As the membrane potential continues to repolarize (phase 3), the ability of sodium channels to reactivate increases, until the RMP is once again reached (phase 4). Because sodium influx and sodium channel recovery is rapid, sodium channels are referred to as "fast," in contrast to "slow" calcium channels, which take longer to recover. Drugs with greater affinity for inactivated sodium channels generally are more able to affect the refractory period and the APD compared with those that target either resting or open channels. Sodium influx during phase 0 depolarization influences other ion channels and their ion movements.

Among the ions most influenced by sodium flux in nonpacemaker cells are potassium channels, of which multiple types, exist, varying in tissue and intracellular location, and control (Table 14-1). Inward rectifier potassium channels are among the channels that determine the RMP. Depolarization causes conformational changes in transient potassium channels, which rapidly inactivate, and delayed rectifier potassium channels, which include both slow and rapid inactivators (each voltage gated). Efflux of potassium through these channels causes the membrane to begin to repolarize. Initially, the outward potassium current is balanced by an inward depolarizing current of calcium through L-type channels, causing the plateau, or phase 2, of repolarization in nonpacemaker (but not pacemaker) cells. Increased activity of delayed rectifier channels increases potassium efflux, which, when coupled with closing calcium channels, results in late repolarization (phase 3; see Figure 14-2). Slower delayed rectifier potassium

Table 14-1 Potassium Channels Active in the Cardiovascular System

Channel	Designation	Regulation	Role
1. Tandem (or two) pore domain	*K_{2p} 1-7,9-12,13,15-18 **KCNK	Oxygen, pH, mechanical stretch, G proteins	Leak K^+ Establish RMP
2. Inward rectifier	K_{ir} 1-7 or IRK; KCNJ	ATP (K_{ir} 6); G-proteins	Inward K flow (some "weak" channels allow efflux) Establish RMP
3. Calcium activated	K_ca BK (also Maxi-K or slo1; K_ca-1 KCNMA) SK (K_ca 2-4; KCNN, KCNT) IK; K_ca-5, KCNU	Calcium; or other signals (sodium, chloride) (BK also responds to voltage; SK responds to sodium)	BK: large ion flow SK: small ion flow
4. Voltage gated	K_va	Transmembrane potential	Contribute to AP repolarization; limits frequency of AP
Delayed rectifier	K_va 1,2,3,7,10		Repolarization
Outward rectifying	K_va 10 (KCNH)		
Inward rectifying	K_va 11 (KCNH)		
Transient			
A-Type	K_va 1,3,4 (KCNA, KCNC, KCND)		Repolarization (efflux)
Slowly activating	K_va12 (KCNH)		

channels remain open to ensure net outward potassium efflux such that the membrane potential becomes more negative, causing rapid delayed rectifier and inwardly rectifying potassium channels to open. The delayed rectifier K^+ channels close when the membrane potential is restored to about -80 to -85 mV, but the inwardly rectifying potassium channels remain open throughout phase 4, thus maintaining the RMP. Because potassium channels generally remain open as long as the membrane is not at its resting potential (i.e., is in some state of depolarization), potassium channels also influence the duration of the action potential. Thus the influence of potassium channels in nondepolarizing cells includes the RMP and the rate of repolarization. In pacemaker cells (discussed in greater depth later in this chapter), potassium channels influence the RMP, the rate of repolarization, and the initial rate of phase 4. Consequently, potassium and drugs that target potassium channels potentially influence all cardiac (e.g., depolarizing and nondepolarizing) tissues.

KEY POINT 14-3 Inward flux of sodium is the primary ion responsible for phase 0 of nondepolarizing cells, whereas calcium influx is the primary ion in pacemaker cells.

Calcium also plays a major role in both nondepolarizing and depolarizing myocardial cells. The extracellular to intracellular calcium ratio of myocardial cells approximates 10, generating a calcium ion flow down both a concentration and electrical gradient. In contrast to the vasculature, in which channel movement is predominantly receptor mediated, calcium flux in the myocardium is predominantly voltage dependent. At least three types of voltage-gated calcium channels exist in the cardiovascular system, with differences reflecting conductance and sensitivity to voltage: T, N, and L types.[2] The N-type (neuronal) calcium channels are located predominantly in neural tissues and markedly differ in responsiveness compared with L and T calcium channels. The best characterized of the calcium channels are of the L-type (long-lasting, large), and they are the predominant influencing channel during the states of the cardiac action in which the membrane potential is positive. Despite being voltage gated, calcium L-channels contain receptors (similar to those in the vasculature) that influence calcium channel flow and are subject to drug-induced blockade. In contrast to L-type channels, T-type (transient, tiny) channels are more active at negative potentials and are the predominant channel of influence at rest. As such, whereas L- channels are activated at high voltages, T-channels are activated at low voltages.

In nonpacemaker cells, in response to sodium influx, extracellular calcium enters the cell through L-type channels as repolarization begins. The influx is sufficient to stimulate release of intracellular calcium from the sarcoplasmic reticulum and other Ca^{2+} stores (e.g., mitochondria). This (initial sodium and subsequent) calcium ion flow links the action potential to excitation–contraction coupling in nondepolarizing cells.[3] The duration of contraction is determined by the rate of intracellular calcium removal from actin and myosin sites in the cytosol by either resequestration into the sarcolemma (or other stores) or efflux from the cell. Efflux is accomplished by at least two pumps, both of which exchange sodium for calcium. The $Na^+/Ca2^+$ ATP-ase pump exchanges 1 Na^+ for 3 Ca^{2+} but has only a minor influence on phase 2 of repolarization. The plateau of phase 2 repolarization in nondepolarizing cells is primarily influenced (sustained) by a balance between inward movement of calcium through L-type channels and outward movement of K^+ through the slow delayed rectifier potassium channels.[4]

As with sodium channels, calcium channels exist in resting (closed, but responsive), open, or inactivated (unresponsive) states, and recovery must occur before the resting (responsive) state is achieved. Because both current movement and recovery of calcium channels are slower compared with those of sodium channels, the term *slow channels* is used to refer to ion movement through calcium channels. Hormones, neurotransmitters, and inorganic ions influence calcium channels. As with sodium channels, those drugs with a greater affinity for inactivated calcium channels are more effective.

Pacemaker Cells

Ion flow in cells capable of automaticity inherently is different from that of nondepolarizing cells to allow for spontaneity. Spontaneous depolarization occurs in response to ion fluxes across the cell membrane. The spontaneity of pacemaker cells reflects several electrophysiologic differences between pacemaker and nonpacemaker cells. In contrast to nonpacemaker cells, pacemaker cells have only a few sodium channels. They tend to be in an inactivated state, rendering the cell less responsive to sodium-induced depolarization. However, sodium can influence depolarization, albeit slightly, because more sodium channels are open in the resting state for pacemaker fibers compared with nonpacemaker cells, allowing sodium ions to continually flow down the concentration gradient into the cell. As a result, the maximum RMP of pacemaker cells is only about -60 mV. Second, calcium channels, rather than sodium channels, are responsible for phase 0 of the action potential in pacemaker cells. Third, depolarization is slow, beginning with calcium influx through T-channels until L-channels are activated to initiate phase 0 (depolarization). Fourth, phase 2 is not apparent in pacemaker cells. Fifth, as with nonpacemaker tissues, repolarization in pacemaker cells is initiated by potassium efflux. However, in contrast to nonpacemaker cells, repolarization continues beyond the RMP (-60 mV), resulting in a hyperpolarized (phase 4) membrane. As such, phase 4 in pacemaker cells is a "prepotential," consisting of an initial reduction in potassium efflux, followed by opening of transient T calcium channels. Calcium influx decreases the membrane potential, causing it to become increasingly positive until the firing level (approximately -40 mV) is reached and L-channels are opened.

Automaticity

The rate (slope) of phase 4 in pacemaker cells is influenced by a number of factors. The slope determines the rate at which the action potential threshold of pacemaker cells is reached. Thus the slope of phase 4 determines the rate of spontaneous depolarization, and the cells that set the pace of the heart, the pacemaker cells, are those tissues with the steepest slope. Under normal circumstances, because it is characterized with the steepest slope, the SA node sets the pace. It is followed by conducting tissues, the Purkinje fibers, and, finally, myocardial tissue. As the default pacemaker, the SA node is innervated by both sympathetic and parasympathetic fibers. Vagal activation associated with acetylcholine (ACh) decreases the slope of phase 4 and thus SA nodal pacemaker rate; these actions reflect increased potassium conductance (efflux) and decreased slow inward Ca^{2+} and Na^{+} movement. Vagal activity also causes the cell to become hyperpolarized, increasing the time needed to reach threshold. However, in atrial fibers, vagal tone facilitates K^{+} channel-mediated repolarization, thus shortening the APD. Finally, vagal tone inhibits sympathetic activity, but the heart rate will increase only if sympathetic outflow (norepinephrine under normal conditions and epinephrine with pathologic conditions) is sufficient. Sympathetic tone, in turn, inhibits vagal tone. Changes in the serum concentration of ions, particularly potassium, also influence SA pacemaker activity. Hyperkalemia increases K^{+} conductance and thus efflux, resulting in bradycardia, whereas hypokalemia increases the rate of phase 4 depolarization (causing tachycardia), presumably by decreasing potassium conductance during phase 4. The slope of phase 4 can change in diseased myocardial tissue (e.g., hypoxia, acidosis, conditions that alter membrane permeability), and the generation of faster impulses may allow these tissues to take over as pacemakers.

KEY POINT 14-4 The cell with the steepest slope of phase 4 sets the heart rate. Although the sinoatrial node is the normal pacemaker, nonpacemaker cells can emerge as pacemakers if cell permeability is altered by disease, hypoxia, trauma or drugs.

Conduction Velocity

The interrelationship between phase 4 and phase 0 of the action potential (the rate of depolarization) determines the conduction velocity—that is, the speed of impulse propagation through pacemaker and nonpacemaker cardiac fibers. Conduction depends on the magnitude of the depolarizing current and the geometric (physical) relationship between myocardial cells. Conduction velocity is directly proportional to the rate and magnitude of phase 0 depolarization. Thus factors that slow the rate or magnitude of sodium (for nondepolarizing cells) or calcium (for pacemaker cells) flow during phase 0 also influence conduction velocity. Conduction velocity, in turn, influences the ability of the impulse to depolarize surrounding cardiac fibers. The faster and the greater the magnitude of depolarization, the more likely the impulse will depolarize surrounding cardiac fibers. For nonpacemaker cells, sodium is the major determinant of conduction velocity by virtue of its impact on the rate and extent of phase 0 upswing. However, calcium conductance during phase 0, albeit slight, also is able to influence phase 0 of nondepolarizing cells. For pacemaker cells, calcium is the major determinant of conduction velocity, with sodium an influencing factor.

Refractory Periods

Myocardial cells are neither excitable nor responsive to additional stimuli during the early and intermediate phases of the action potential cycle. Further, they are only partially responsive if stimulated before complete repolarization has occurred—that is, as the RMP returns to normal. Refractory periods (RPs) describe the period of time (or proportion of the APD) in which cells are nonresponsive. During the absolute refractory period (ARP), cells are totally nonresponsive. In contrast, cells may be partially (effective; ERP) or relatively (RRP) refractory to stimuli, with the state dependent on the number of open (i.e., recovered from inactivation) sodium channels. The ARP occurs when sodium channels are closed. Tissues will not respond to any stimuli, no matter how strong. The ERP is the shortest interval that can occur before a premature impulse can propagate a response.[5] It includes the ARP plus a shorter period following the ARP that reflects the opening of some sodium channels but not enough to transmit an impulse. The RRP follows the ERP and represents a state in which a sufficient number of sodium channels are open such that a very strong stimulus might be propagated. The refractory periods are protective in that they limit the rate at which myocardial tissues can respond to impulses, thus ensuring sufficient time for cardiac filling and ejection to occur before the next contraction occurs. Proper direction of impulse propagation is also facilitated. Because sodium channels during these periods are refractory to reopening, unilateral (one direction only) conduction is ensured along a myocardial fiber, precluding the premature regeneration of an action potential and inappropriate coordination between excitation–contraction coupling. Loss of unilateral conduction is a contributing factor to re-entrant or circus rhythms.

Afterload and Preload

Both *afterload* and *preload* are variably defined depending on the source. Each is determined by the law of Laplace ($T = PR/2$, where T is wall tension, P is chamber or vessel pressure, and R is chamber or vessel radius). *Preload* occurs just before (end-diastolic) and afterload just after contraction. Preload is often referred to as the end-diastolic filling pressure, or the end-diastolic volume. Preload reflects the combined factors that influence passive (i.e., relaxed) ventricular wall stress at the end of diastole. Among the most important factors is the volume of blood that fills the ventricles. Increased filling volume enlarges the ventricular chamber, causing either tension or pressure or both to increase. A greater force is necessary for contraction to overcome the tension. Preload pressure occurs in the heart, is highest at the end of filling, or the end of diastole, and is virtually the same in the ventricle and its atria. Other measures of preload have included end-diastolic fiber length or stretch. *Afterload* is presented outside the heart (aorta) and is the pressure against which the heart must pump to effectively empty the ventricular chamber. At the point that ejection begins (beginning of systole), the aortic valves open and aortic pressure = peripheral resistance = arterial pressure = ventricular pressure. Afterload is also referred to as myocardial wall tension, or the force that must be generated by the heart for myocardial fiber shortening (contraction) to occur such that blood is ejected from the ventricle. Among the most important factors influencing afterload is peripheral resistance.

KEY POINT 14-5 The primary determinant of preload, or ventricular filling, is blood volume. The primary determinant of afterload is peripheral (arterial) resistance.

Myocardial Contractility

Contraction of both cardiac and smooth muscle depends on Ca^{2+}. The inotropic state of the muscle reflects the relationship between resting fiber length and peak isometric tension. The myocardium develops force for contraction and thus the strength to pump blood by forming cross-bridges between actin and (tropo) myosin myofilaments in cardiac muscle. The amount of force that the muscle can generate depends on the number of cross-bridges that form when myosin engages actin. Energy in the form of adenosine triphosphate (ATP) causes a sliding motion between the proteins of the myofilaments and cardiac muscle to shorten and develop force. The interaction between proteins in the myofilament is regulated by troponin, which is found at regular intervals on the tropomyosin fibers. Troponin is formed from three subunit proteins: T binds to tropomysin, I inhibits the actin-binding site on tropomyosin, and C binds to calcium.[4] Calcium binding of troponin C forces a conformational change in the troponin complex, causing troponin I to move away from tropomyosin, thus allowing cross-bridging between actin and myosin. The force that develops as actin and myosin interact depends on both the affinity and amount of calcium binding to troponin. The amount is regulated by the concentration of intracellular calcium. It is only as intracellular calcium is removed that troponin I moves back into position; thus contraction will continue until all intracellular calcium is removed.

Multiple mechanisms influence myocardial intracellular (cytosolic) calcium (see Figure 14-1). Extracellular calcium can enter through two sources: movement through (slow) electrogenic or voltage-gated calcium L channels embedded in T-tubules, which ensures that calcium is delivered in close proximity to the sacroplasmic reticulum, and movement though Na^{+}-Ca^{2+} ATP channels, which is dependent on cell membrane ATPase.[3,6] Cytosolic calcium flow is modulated primarily by β-adrenergic receptors; increased cyclic adenosine monophosphate (cAMP) activates protein kinase, which in turn increases calcium movement through the L-channels.[4] Opening of slow calcium channels in response to depolarization causes intracellular calcium to rise rapidly, stimulating subsequent release from intracellular storage sites (sarcoplasmic reticulum and, to a lesser degree, mitochondria). The contracted myocardial muscle relaxes as intracellular calcium concentration falls as a result of resequestration into the sarcoplasmic reticulum and efflux from the cell, both of which are energy (ATP) dependent. Disorders of lusitropy (i.e., disorders of diastolic relaxation) occur if intracellular calcium does not decrease. The velocity and extent of cardiac muscular contraction are regulated by sarcomere length.[4] Length (stretch) reflects preload, or the transmural filling pressure. An optimal stretch maximizes the relationship between actin and myosin filaments, allowing more Ca^{2+}-activated cross-bridges and more forceful contractions. In the normal cat and dog, the upper limit of filling pressure in the left ventricle stretches the sarcomere to the length that generates peak tension during contraction. With sustained systolic overloading of the heart, however, the ideal sarcomere stretch is exceeded, cross-bridging decreases and myocardial contractility declines. Abnormalities of the excitation–contraction coupling mechanism contribute to the pathogenesis of cardiomyopathies and chronic hemodynamic overloading.

KEY POINT 14-6 Both cardiac contraction—mediated by intracellular release of calcium—and cardiac relaxation–mediated by reuptake of intracellular calcium—increase myocardial energy and thus oxygen demands.

The most important factor regulating myocardial contractility is stimulation of cardiac sympathetic nerves; cAMP serves as the secondary messenger, altering intracellular calcium flux and myocardial contractility. Myocardial cAMP is produced by adenylyl cyclase, which in turn is regulated by either stimulation or inhibition of adenine or guanine nucleotide proteins. Many cell surface receptors interact with proteins that regulate adenylyl cyclase. An increase in intracellular cAMP causes phosphorylation of proteins that increase calcium influx through the "slow" calcium channels, and the release, reaccumulation, and storage of calcium in the sarcoplasmic reticulum. Cyclic AMP is degraded by several phosphodiesterases (PDEs) isoenzymes, each of which has been associated with specific pharmacodynamic actions. At least 11 isoforms have been named. Inhibition of these enzymes causes the same effect as an increase in either adenylyl or guanylyl cyclase and thus cAMP or cGMP, respectively (see Figure 14-1). The pharmacodynamic response varies with tissue site: PDE II is located in smooth muscle of the urinary bladder detrusor muscle; PDE III in the heart, systemic vascular smooth muscle, and platelets (cAMP); PDE IV in bronchial smooth muscle and pulmonary circulation (cAMP); PDE V in the smooth muscle of the corpus cavernosum, visceral smooth muscle, skeletal muscle, platelets, kidney, lung, cerebellum, and pancreas (cGMP); and PDE VI in the retina (responsible for transduction).

KEY POINT 14-7 The most important factor regulating myocardial contractility is stimulation of cardiac sympathetic nerves.

Adrenergic Receptors

The adrenergic nervous system has a major physiologic role in modulating normal myocardial inotropic and chronotropic states and the time-variable tension that develops as ventricles contract. Both the myocardium and peripheral vasculature are innervated with sympathetic nerve terminals. Under normal conditions norepinephrine released from nerve endings in the heart acts as the primary regulator. Circulating catecholamines released from the adrenal gland play a less important role in normal conditions, but their influence increases as myocardial failure progresses. Molecular cloning techniques have identified nine subclasses of receptors: alpha (α) 1 (three subclasses); α 2 (three subclasses); and β 1, 2, and 3.[7] Adrenergic receptors are linked to different G protein–coupled receptors, which differentially influence secondary messenger systems (sometimes the same one). Beta receptors are linked to adenylyl cyclase through Gs proteins. Beta agonists regulate cell processes by increasing cAMP, thus influencing downstream effects through cAMP-dependent protein kinases (see the discussion of smooth muscle). In contrast, α receptors are linked to Gi proteins, which oppose the actions of Gs proteins, thus decreasing cAMP.

KEY POINT 14-8 Norepinephrine from local nerve endings is the primary regulator of the heart under normal circumstances, but circulating catecholamines (e.g., epinephrine) predominate with myocardial failure.

In the normal heart, stimulation of the sympathoadrenal system is the primary method by which the heart adjusts to transient changes in workload. The myocardium possesses predominantly β receptors whereas vascular smooth muscle is rich in α receptors. Both β receptors and α receptors are subdivided into two types. Beta-1 receptors predominate in the myocardium, increasing inotropy (strength of contraction) and chronotropy (rate of impulse generation) (see Figure 14-1). Myocardial effects of adrenergic receptors are achieved through increased magnitude of the calcium current, slowed channel inactivation, and increased magnitude of K^+ and Cl^- repolarizing currents. Pacemaker current and thus sinus rate increase.[5] Beta-2 receptors (and recently described β-3 receptors) are also located in the heart, but their function is not clear. Disease affects the state of receptors. Continued stimulation of adrenergic receptors, such as that which accompanies diseases states (e.g., congestive heart failure) or long-term adrenergic therapy, results in a dampening or desensitization of response to receptor stimulation. Desensitization reflects internalization and destruction of cell surface receptors. For example, β-1 receptors decrease up to 75% (β-2 receptors are spared) in human patients with congestive heart failure, leading to a compensatory increase in sympathetic signal outflow, which likely contributes to the pathophysiology (see the discussion of myocardial remodeling).[7] The function of myocardial β-3 receptors is not clear, but they may provide feedback inhibition of contractility; an imbalance in myocardial disease may contribute to the pathophysiology of myocardial disease.[8]

In vascular smooth muscle, α-2 receptors mediate vasodilation (Figure 14-3). Most α activity in the cardiovascular system is mediated by way of α-1 receptors. Effects include contraction of vascular (and nonvascular) smooth muscle. A-2 receptors inhibit neurotransmitter release but also mediate vascular contraction (as do α-1 receptors). Subtypes 1 and 2 of either α or β receptors can be selectively pharmacologically stimulated (agonists) or inhibited (antagonists) to manage cardiovascular disease.

Smooth Muscle of the Vasculature

Myocardial oxygen demand is directly related to heart rate, myocardial wall tension, and the inotropic state of the myocardium.[3,9] Myocardial wall tension is determined by the size (diameter) of the ventricle and intraventricular pressure. Thus tension is affected by preload (end-diastolic volume and stretch) and afterload (aortic blood pressure). Drugs that decrease systemic arterial pressure through dilation of arterioles decrease left ventricular afterload. Following the path of least resistance, a larger volume of blood will be ejected from the ventricular chamber into systemic circulation, thus

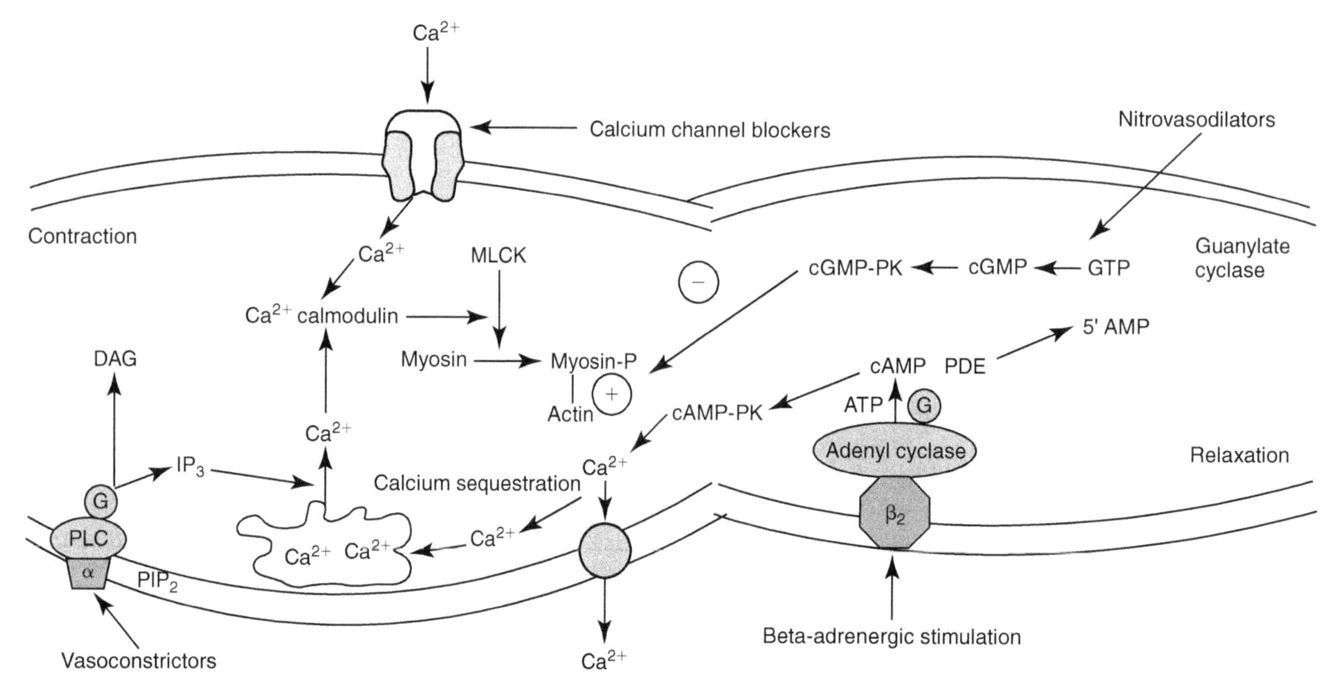

Figure 14–3 Contraction of vascular smooth muscle (vasoconstriction) reflects an influx of calcium, although mechanisms may differ from those in the myocardial cell. Calcium influx occurs through receptor-mediated channels or, less commonly, voltage-gated channels. Intracellular calcium combines with calmodulin. Myosin light-chain kinase (MLCK) is activated, and myosin light chain is phosphorylated (Myosin-P), promoting the interaction between myosin and actin. Cyclic adenosine monophosphate (cAMP) appears to stimulate sequestration and efflux of intracellular calcium and through cAMP protein kinase (cAMP-PK) decreases MLCK, causing vascular smooth muscle to relax (an action opposite to that in the myocardial muscle cell). Cyclic guanosine monophosphate (cGMP) also causes relaxation, probably through nitric oxide–mediated mechanisms. Intracellular calcium also can be released from the sarcoplasmic reticulum after hydrolysis of membrane phosphatidylinositol (PIP_2) and subsequent formation of the secondary messenger inositol triphosphate (IP_3). *ATP,* Adenosine triphosphate; *DAG,* diacylglycerol; *GTP,* guanosine triphosphate; *PDE,* phosphodiesterase; *PLC,* phospholipase C.

diverting blood from the pulmonary vasculature. Left ventricular filling (preload) and thus myocardial wall size and tension will decrease, as will myocardial oxygen demand. An advantage of preload or afterload is that the decrease in cardiac work occurs without affecting myocardial contraction.

KEY POINT 14-9 A number of mediators act to cause arterial constriction and thus increase peripheral resistance.

The excitation–contraction coupling in vascular smooth muscle depends on calcium influx, which enters the cell through either voltage-sensitive (electrogenic) signals associated with depolarization or, more commonly, through receptor-operated Ca^{2+} channels. Intracellular calcium also is released from the sarcoplasmic reticulum in response to membrane phosphatidylinositol hydrolysis and formation of the secondary messenger inositol triphosphate.[2] Intracellular calcium interacts with calmodulin, activating myosin light-chain kinase (MLCK) to phosphorylate myosin light chain. Cross-bridging between myosin and actin causes smooth muscle to contract. Cyclic AMP decreases both MLCK and intracellular calcium, causing relaxation of vascular smooth muscle. As with cAMP, the secondary intracellular messenger cGMP causes vascular smooth muscle relaxation, although the mechanism is different (see Figures 14-1 and 14-3). Endothelium-derived relaxing factor (EDRF; chemically related to nitric oxide) and endothelium-derived constricting factor (EDCF) are among the vasoactive substances released by the endothelial cell that control the hemodynamics of the cardiovascular system. Intracellular response to EDRF (or nitric oxide) is probably signaled by cGMP. Other mediators of vascular smooth muscle response include, but are not limited to, prostacyclin, histamine, and acetylcholine. Mediators released from the endothelial cell generally act locally on vascular smooth muscle (Figure 14-4); an exception might include mediators released from the pulmonary vasculature, which may be sufficient to modulate a systemic response.

Systolic and diastolic pressures are, respectively, the upper and lower limits of the oscillations around mean arterial pressure. The mean arterial pressure is the arterial pressure over time and is defined as the diastolic pressure plus one third of the pulse pressure. Arterial blood pressure is the product of cardiac output (determined by stroke volume and heart rate) and total peripheral resistance. Total peripheral resistance is the sum of resistance in all vascular beds. It is also affeccted by aortic impedance (resistance to flow) and diastolic arterial pressure, which in turn is determined by the sympathetic nervous system, the renin–angiotensin–aldosterone system and arginine vasopressin system, vascular (extracellular fluid) volume, and aldosterone or other volume active hormones.[43]

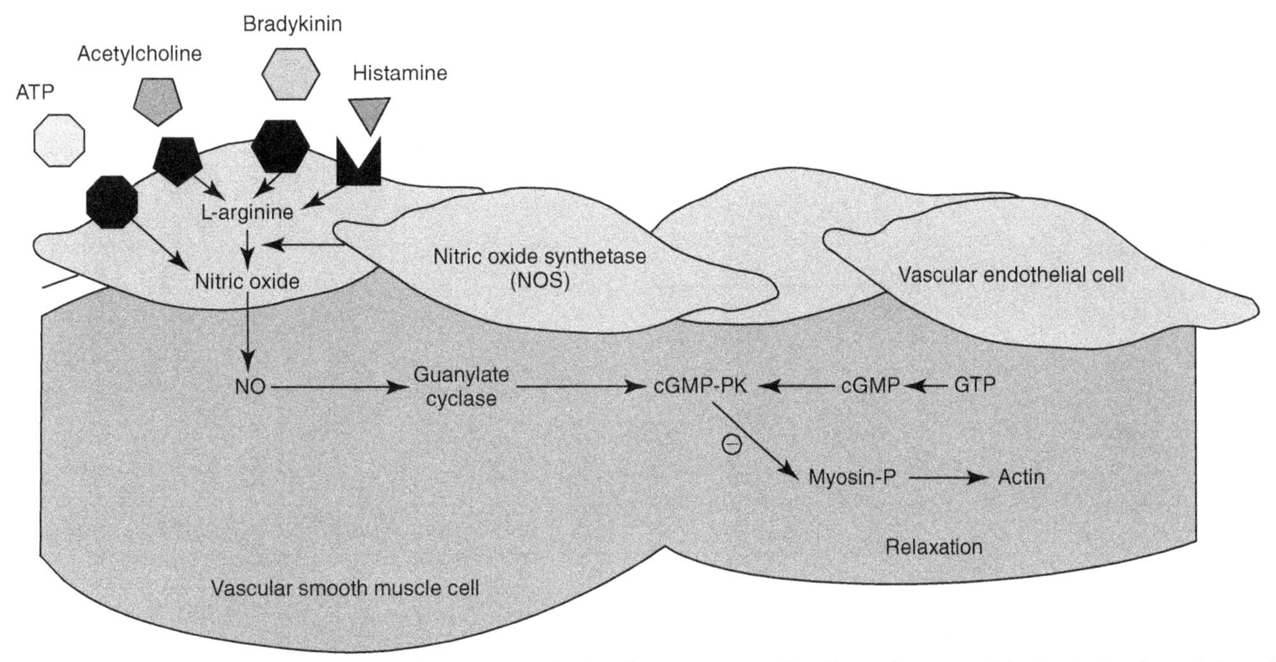

Figure 14-4 Vasoactive mediators responsible for vasodilation (e.g., prostacyclin, histamine, acetylcholine) stimulate nitric oxide synthetase to convert L-arginine to nitric oxide (NO) in the endothelial cells. Nitric oxide enters the smooth muscle cell and stimulates guanylate cyclase such that cyclic guanosine monophosphate (cGMP) is released. *ATP,* Adenosine triphosphate; *cGMP-PK,* cGMP-dependent protein kinase; *GTP,* guanosine triphosphate; *Myosin-P,* phosphorylated myosin.

The Renin–Angiotensin–Aldosterone System

The renin–angiotensin–aldosterone system (RAAS) plays an important role in regulating blood volume, arterial pressure, and cardiac and vascular function (Figure 14-5).[10] An additional but critically important role in cardiac repair and remodeling has recently emerged. RAAS regulation of arterial pressure is accomplished through constriction of resistance vessels, mediated by several mechanisms. Included are direct stimulation of AGII receptors and indirect stimulation through facilitation of norepinephrine. Vasopressin also is a potent mediator of peripheral vasoconstriction by way of V-1 receptors. Its increase reflects either increased release from sympathetic nerve terminal endings or decreased reuptake.[11]

Other neurohumoral–endocrine mediators of RAAS are produced by a number of organs, resulting in both local and systemic responses. Contributing organs include the kidney, brain, heart, vasculature, adipose tissue, gonads, placenta, and pancreas. In the kidney, renin is produced in the juxtaglomerular cells, and angiotensinogen in the proximal tubular cells. The majority of the effects of RAAS reflect its most potent mediator, angiotensin II (AGII), which in turn is dependent on renin. Renal renin release is stimulated by hypotension, decreased sodium delivery to the distal tubules, or direct stimulation of β-1 adrenergic receptors. Renin catalyzes proteolytic cleavage of circulating angiotensinogen to the decapeptide, angiotensin I. Angiotensin I is then converted to AGII by angiotensin-converting enzyme (ACE), located in vascular endothelium with the majority of systemic release coming from the lungs. AGII is further degraded by angiotensinoginases located in red blood cells AG III and IV.

ACE is a kinase II metallopeptidase enzyme bound to the membrane of a variety of cells, but particularly endothelium, epithelium, neuroepithelium, and brain cells.[12] Organs respond to both systemic and local renin, with local response influenced by local concentrations of ACE and angiotensin receptors. Concentrations of ACE differ among tissues, with that in the renal tubular brush border the greatest (300- and 10-fold higher than the left ventricle and lung, respectively). Thus, although the kidney is the most important site of renin release, it also is a target of the RAAS, responding to both systemic and urinary renin. Renal AGII concentrations exceed circulating AGII more than 1000-fold, causing renal vasoconstriction and sodium retention. Degradation of AGII yields angiotensin III (AgIII), which has 40% of the pressor and 100% of the aldosterone effects of AGII.

Through AGII, RAAS modulates responses to low sodium intake and provides for long-term control of renal function, body fluid volumes, and arterial pressure. In the healthy canine kidney, response to AGII results in increase in both preglomerular and postglomerular vascular resistance, although the predominant effect is on the efferent rather than afferent arteriole. Renal blood flow consequently decreases, but glomerular capillary pressure increases.[12] AGII regulates body fluid content by directly stimulating thirst centers in the brain; adrenal release of aldosterone, which mediates increased renal sodium and fluid retention; and posterior pituitary release of vasopressin (antidiuretic hormone, ADH), a component of the arginine vasopressin system (AVP). Vasopressin increases renal fluid retention through V2 receptors in renal tubular cells. In addition to its vascular effects, AGII released from endothelial cells also facilitates cardiac hypertrophy and vascular

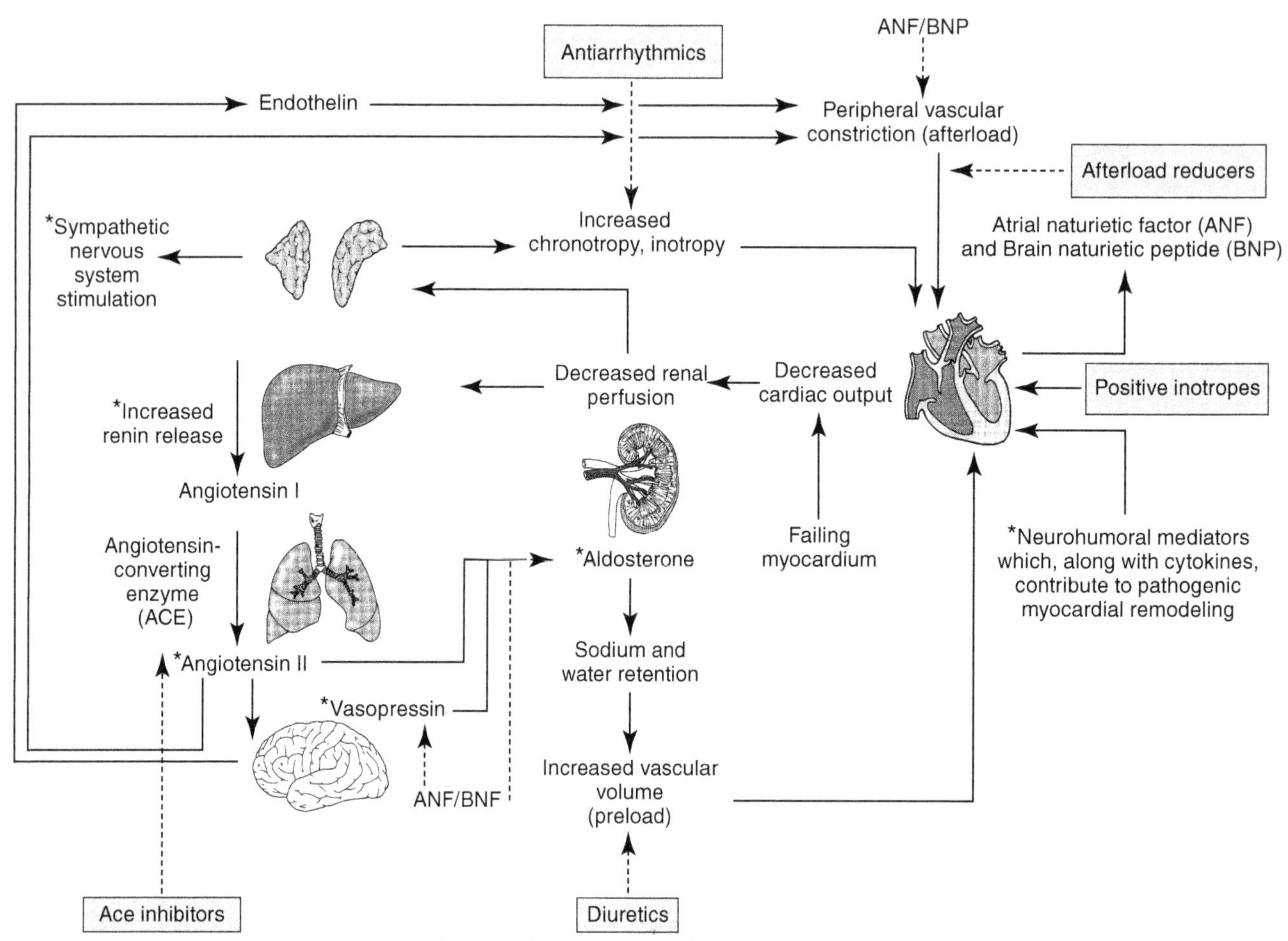

Figure 14-5 Neuroendocrine responses to decreased peripheral perfusion associated with the failing left ventricle may initially result in increased contractility, increased cardiac output, and increased tissue perfusion. Systems activated include the sympathetic adrenergic system, the renin–angiotensin–aldosterone system, and the arginine vasopressin system. Compensatory mechanisms, however, lead to increased afterload (adrenergic stimulation, angiotensin release) and increased preload (aldosterone, release of vasopressin), both of which may detrimentally increase the workload on the failing heart. Mediators signaling these responses contribute to myocardial remodeling (indicated by asterisk*), leading to progressive myocardial failure. Therapeutic approaches that target these mediators (shaded boxes) are intended to not only alter the negative sequlae of increase preload, afterload and cardiac response, but also remodeling. *ACE,* Angiotensin-converting enzyme; *dashed line,* inhibited.

hypertrophy. Notably, production of inflammatory cytokines is increased from both normal and abnormal (damaged) myocardial tissue, contributing to the negative sequelae of cardiac remodeling.[13] AGII is prothrombotic and may induce cardiac muscle hypertrophy.

KEY POINT 14-10 The effect of the renin–angiotensin–aldosterone system is complex. It comprises both systemic as well as local systems, multiple receptors and mediators, and complex receptor–mediator interactions.

KEY POINT 14-11 Ultimately, the negative sequelae of compensation contribute to the progression of myocardial disease and failure

Renal vascular response to AGII is mediated by AGII receptors (ARs), a transmembrane G-coupled protein receptor consisting of several subtypes that vary in location, numbers, affinity for AGII, and secondary messenger systems. The most well known of the subtypes, AR-1, preferentially binds AGII and AGIII, mediating the classic angiotensin RAAS responses on blood pressure and water and electrolyte balance. Included are water, sodium intake, renal sodium retention, secretion of vasopressin and aldosterone, and cell growth/proliferation. In addition to AR-1, AR-2 receptors also bind AII and AIII.[14-16] However, AR-2 receptor density is greatest in the brain, including areas involved with fluid and electrolyte regulation and balance, arterial pressure, cognition, behavior, and locomotion. Concentrations of AR-2 also are high in steroid-producing glands, including the adrenal glands and ovaries.[16] Because of the central location of AR-2, AGII and AGIII can modulate many body functions and responses. Expression of AR-2 is particularly high during fetal development, but it persists in the adult brain, supporting a role in neuronal function. In the brain, AR-2 appears to oppose the traditional RAAS effects of AR-1 on drinking behavior and vasopressin secretion. Other effects mediated by AR-2 receptors are regulation of cell proliferation, apoptosis, and cellular differentiation.[16] Again, AR-2 appears to attenuate AR-1 mediated apoptosis, pressor, and chronotropic effects. Like AR-1 receptors, several secondary systems appear to signal AR-2 effects, including the mitogen-activated protein kinase (MAPK) and nitric oxide/cGMP pathways.[16]

Regulation of RAAS effects through angiotensin receptors is complex, possibly involving feedback inhibition pathways, responses that vary with duration of exposure, and systems that may oppose one another. Likewise, pharmacologic management of heart disease through manipulation of AR receptors may be complex.[15] Disease is likely to contribute to variability in response to AGII and its modulating drugs. For example, in the failing heart the expression of AR-1 decreases, whereas that of AR-2 does not change or increases. Both receptors are associated with effects that initially, in moderation, might benefit the patient, but with progression become detrimental. Not surprisingly, a link has been described between AR and β-adrenergic receptors. Both AR-1 and β receptors interact with G proteins, with AR-1 through activation of phospholipase C and β-receptors through activation of adenylyl cyclase. Diamerization of the two receptors has been described in vitro and occurs in vivo.[17] This integration will further complicate pharmacologic manipulation.

Among the mediators stimulated by AGII are vascular endothelial production of nitric oxide and endothelin (ET-1), both of which contribute to regulation of renin release. Nitric oxide appears to oppose, whereas endothelin appears to reinforce, the vascular effects of AGII. Endothelins are peptide vasoconstrictors released from endothelial cells; three have thus far been identified: ETs 1 through 3. Endothelins exert their effects through a number of endothelin receptors (ET) including ET-A, associated with vasoconstriction and vascular smooth muscle proliferation, and ET-B, which promotes both constriction and dilation, clearance of endothelin, and production of endothelial cell prostacyclin and nitric oxide. Endothelin receptor antagonists have facilitated understanding of the role of endothelins in vascular regulation and ultimately may offer a mechanism of pharmacologic manipulation. Endothelin is the most potent vasoconstrictor known. In addition to direct vascular effects, endothelin modulates plasma concentrations of both atrial natriuretic factor (ANF), arginine vasopressin (AVP), and aldosterone. Additionally, endothelin contributes to vascular remodeling.

Mechanisms other than ACE modulate formation of AGII. Opposing effects of ACE are regulated in part by AR, but other body systems also modulate the influence of ACE. For example, ACE also inhibits breakdown of bradykinin. Bradykinin consequently increases, resulting in vasodilation and naturiesis.[18] The vasodilatory effects of bradykinin are mediated in the vascular endothelium through arachidonic acid derivatives, nitric oxide, and endothelium-derived hyperpolarizing factor in the vascular endothelium. The mechanism of natriuresis is not clear.[12] Bradykinin also has beneficial effects on cardiac remodeling, which helps oppose the negative sequelae of AGII.

The Role of Nitric Oxide

For decades, researchers have attempted to identify a factor released from endothelial cells, referred to as *EDRF*, which is responsible for mediating a number of stimuli causing vasodilation. Ultimately, nitric oxide (NO) was recognized to be the smallest and most basic mediator of vascular response.[19] Released as a gas (and thus often mistaken for nitrous oxide [N_2O], or "laughing gas"), it is synthesized in response to NO synthetase (NOS) enzymes from L-arginine and oxygen or by sequential reduction of inorganic nitrate (see Figure 14-4). However, as a free radical, NO is very reactive and unstable and interacts with oxygen on exposure to air to form the pollutant nitrogen dioxide (NO_2). Two major classes and three isoforms of NOS have been identified.[19-21] Constitutive NOS (cNOS or NOS-1) is continuously produced and includes two isoforms synthesized either by vascular endothelial cells (eNOS) or neurons (nNOS). Constitutive NOS, which is calcium dependent, tends to mediate cell responses through cellular receptors. Responses of cNOS include that mediated by vascular mediators such as acetylcholine, norepinephrine, histamine, and substance P. Not surprisingly, response is rapid. Inducible NOS (iNOS or NOS-2) is produced as needed by inflammatory cells (e.g., macrophages, neutrophils, and Kuppfer cells), generally after exposure to cytokines (e.g., tumor necrosis factor or interleukins) or bacterial lipopolysaccharides. Production of NO from iNOS requires new protein synthesis and is characterized by a delay of several (2 to 4) hours.

Regardless of origin, NO causes its effect by diffusing across cellular membranes to intracellular targets. Cytosolic cGMP is the major intracellular messenger (see Figure 14-4) causing physiologic response to NO. Responses include dilation of blood vessels, inhibition of thrombogenesis, cytotoxic responses, and neuronal signaling. However, because NO contains an unpaired electron in its outer orbit, it is a free radical. As such, it can contribute to the formation of other radicals while simultaneously scavenging oxygen radicals. The half-life of NO is so short that studies involving NO generally are based on its oxidation end products nitrates and nitrites.[20] However, despite its very short half-life, NO has many important and complex actions in the body. Under basal conditions, peripheral vasoconstriction is locally relieved by intermittent cNOS-induced NO in response to sheer stress and endothelial cell receptor stimulation. Inflammation and immune signals also induce NO release by way of iNOS. NO inhibits platelet aggregation and adhesion, contributing to antithrombogenic mechanisms in the vascular endothelium. NO may ameliorate the detrimental effects of norepinephrine on the growth of cardiac myocytes and fibroblasts, suggesting that increased NO bioavailability may prevent or reverse remodeling in patients that have experienced heart failure.[22] Modulation of inflammation varies, however, with cell type and the source of NO production (i.e., iNOS versus cNOS). Although targeting NO production through drug therapy may appear to be a reasonable approach to the treatment of a variety of cardiovascular disorders, the complex nature of its release and the events leading to its release currently preclude predictable and safe modulation. It is likely, however, that selective modulation of NO ultimately will provide a therapeutic approach to many disorders.

PATHOPHYSIOLOGY OF CARDIAC DISEASE AS IT RELATES TO DRUG THERAPY: CONGESTIVE HEART FAILURE

Neural–Humoral–Endocrine Compensatory Mechanisms in the Myocardium and Vasculature

Congestive heart failure (CHF) refers to the inability of the heart to deliver blood necessary to meet the metabolic demands of body tissues. Backward failure is the most common form, reflecting increased end diastolic pressure and atrial pressures. Venous and capillary pressures increase to the point that fluid transudates into interstitial tissues, resulting in the clinical manifestations that result from heart failure, including (left sided) pulmonary and circulatory edema or (right-sided) ascites. Patients generally are hypervolemic and thus are referred to as "wet." Less commonly, forward failure reflects decreased cardiac output and poor periperhal perfusion ("cold") resulting in exercise intolerance or cool extremities. Backward failure ultimately may lead to forward failure.

Mechanisms that compensate for loss of contractility or abnormal loading on the heart initially maintain cardiac output in the normal range either at rest or with limited exercise. Clinical signs of disease may not be evident (preclinical stage). However, the negative sequelae of compensation ultimately contribute to the progression of myocardial disease and failure. Decompensation occurs when cardiac output is no longer sufficient to support circulation despite compensatory mechanisms

Regardless of the cause of cardiac failure, decreased blood pressure and compromised organ perfusion initiate complex interactive compensatory responses of the neural, hormonal, and endocrine systems.[11,23] Neuroendocrine changes reflect "fight or flight" stimuli, affecting blood pressure and fluid volume (see Figure 14-5). Baroreceptors and the vasomotor center interact with the sympathetic and parasympathetic systems to increase heart rate, myocardial contractility, and blood pressure and to activate the RAAS. Although cardiac output may increase, the responses contribute to fluid accumulation and myocardial remodeling, which ultimately lead to irreversible myocardial failure.

The kidney directs responses designed to increase arterial blood volume in response to poor renal perfusion accompanying the failing heart. Renal compensatory mechanisms are mediated by RAAS in the juxtaglomerular apparatus. Renal glomerular arterioles are exquisitely sensitive to catecholamines; their reflex vasoconstriction exacerbates diversion of blood flow from the glomerulus. However, renal arteriolar underperfusion coupled with adrenergic stimulation causes the release of renin in pressure-volume–sensitive receptors of the afferent arterioles. In response to decreased renal plasma flow and glomerular filtration rate (GFR), the filtration fraction increases, normalizing renal excretory function. Proximal tubular function is maintained (and possibly enhanced) such that a greater percentage of sodium and water is reabsorbed from the filtrate. Decreased sodium in the filtrate causes further renin release. Fluid retention initiated by these changes increases ventricular filling. Actin and myosin interaction are optimized with myocardial cell stretching (sarcomere length–active tension relationship or Frank–Starling phenomenon), leading to improved contractility. Stroke volume and cardiac output increase, as does cardiac work. Effective restoration of blood volume and ventricular filling will improve renal perfusion but at a new equilibrium characterized by increased ventricular filling pressures and intravascular and interstitial fluid volumes.

Myocardial disease is accompanied by changes in concentrations of components of the RAAS. For example, AGII increases twofold to threefold in the left ventricle and kidneys and tenfold in plasma. Because AGII is produced by mechanisms other than ACE (e.g., chymase), the impact of ACE inhibitors on resolution of increased AGII is variable among tissues. Inhibitors of ACE may vary in their relative impact on efferent or afferent arterioles; the impact may also vary within renal zones.

Other systems influenced by RAAS also change in the diseased heart. ANF and atrial natriuretic peptide (ANP, or atriopeptin) production by atrial myocytes is stimulated by atrial stretch in the heart and a number of other signals (adrenergic stimulation, AGII, endothelin, increased sodium) associated with congestive heart failure. Brain natriuretic factor, although originally identified in brain tissue, is secreted by ventricular myocytes and interacts with ANF receptors, causing similar effects. The effects of ANF are mediated by at least three receptors (NPRA1-3 or A-C), two (NPRA 1 and 2) of which are linked to cGMP and the third to G-protein. ANF inhibits AVP activated by RAAS. Renal response to ANF includes dilation of the afferent glomerular arteriole, renal sodium wasting, and decreased renin secretion; aldosterone secretion from the adrenal gland also decreases. Vascular smooth muscle is relaxed. As such, normally, ANF induces natriuresis, diuresis, and vasodilation, inhibits renin and aldosterone secretion, and appears to attenuate vasoconstriction. . Interestingly, ANF also influences adipose tissue, causing, among other things, release of amino acids. Although plasma concentrations of ANF are increased in heart failure, response is blunted for reasons that are not clear. Diagnostically, detection of ANF has been used to differentially diagnose acute dyspnea. e.g., that associated with pulmonary edema.

Circulating ET-1 increases in both plasma and the left ventricle in response to a number of signals, including norepinephrine, AVP, and interleukin-1. Increases parallel the progression of myocardial injury and correlate with increased pulmonary arterial pressures. ET-1 may play a role in the pathophysiology of pulmonary hypertension of heart failure in humans.[24]

Heart failure not only is the result of dysfunction of the RAAS but also reflects several abnormalities of the second major compensatory system, the adrenergic nervous system.[17,25,26] Indeed, the two systems appear to influence each other, affecting both the heart and peripheral vasculature. Loss of myocardial contractile support is partially compensated for by increases in plasma catecholamines released from the adrenal gland; autonomic imbalance occurs as the parasympathetic system fails to "check" adrenergic response. This may reflect the reduced sensitivity of baroreceptors.[26] The failing heart becomes increasingly dependent on circulating, rather than local catecholamines. In the failing heart, maximum contractile and heart rate response are decreased for several reasons. In the later stages of failure, myocardial response to sympathetic nerve stimulation is blunted as a result of decreased synthesis, storage, and release of myocardial norepinephrine. Beta-1 receptors decrease and inhibitory guanine nucleotide–binding proteins (G_i) increase.[27] Sustained adrenergic signaling associated with myocardial injury causes downregulation of β-1 receptors and uncoupling of both β-1 and β-2 receptors from G proteins. Because β receptors are diamerized with AR, AR-1 decreases in concert with β receptors.[17]

KEY POINT 14-12 Heart failure is the result of integrated altered functions of the renin–angiotensin–aldosterone system; the adrenergic nervous system; and their integrated influences on afterload, preload, heart rate, and myocardial remodeling.

As the heart fails, α-adrenergic–mediated vasoconstriction in response to circulating catecholamines causes regional peripheral vasoconstriction, ensuring preservation of arterial blood pressure. Differential vasoconstriction among the vascular beds causes blood flow to be redistributed to organs with the highest metabolic requirements (i.e., brain, heart, and active skeletal muscles). Accordingly, renal blood flow is restricted, resulting in activation of the RAAS. Autoregulation of intrarenal blood flow (e.g., efferent renal arteriolar constriction) helps maintain glomerular filtration despite systemic redistribution. Venoconstriction and fluid retention increase preload, providing some compensation for decreased cardiac output.

Although the goal of compensatory mechanisms is to increase cardiac output, eventually the secondary sequelae prove detrimental and both diastolic and systolic cardiac dysfunctions emerge. In the peripheral vasculature, vasoconstriction mediated by AGII, circulating catecholamines, AVP, and ET-1 results in persistent and significant increased systemic vascular resistance. Mechanical vascular stiffness, reflecting intramural sodium and water content, worsens resistance. The vasculature, particularly in skeletal muscle, can no longer autoregulate. Increased resistance tends to raise (maintain) blood pressure and organ perfusion, but at a cost: the marked increase in cardiac afterload causes a proportionate decrease in stroke volume. The heart must work harder, using more oxygen to affect the same cardiac output. Because stroke volume is less, the end-diastolic volume (preload) in the heart is greater, increasing myocardial wall tension. Myocardial diastolic relaxation, necessary for myocardial perfusion, is impaired. Increasing myocardial oxygen and energy needs cannot be met as myocardial perfusion decreases. Thus increased peripheral resistance represents a vicious cycle as it worsens the failing heart. Abnormal relaxation during diastole also has been associated with direct changes in the myocardial cell. These include abnormal sarcoplasmic reticulum regulation of intracellular Ca^{2+} and decreased density of Ca^{2+}-ATPase.[27] Drugs that increase cAMP thus may influence either contractility (inotropy) or diastolic relaxation (lusitropy).

Negative Sequelae of Myocardial Remodeling

In the last decade, as more data regarding the role of RAAS and related systems in the progression of myocardial failure have emerged, therapies have been designed to minimize the negative sequelae of compensatory mechanisms. Accordingly, the traditional goals of therapy have been to lower venous pressure (diuretics), decrease afterload on the failing heart (vasodilators), decrease heart rate (e.g., β blockers, calcium channel blockers [CCBs], or digoxin), and increase myocardial contractility (positive inotropes).[28] However, the traditional view of CHF as a hemodynamic syndrome characterized by fluid retention, high venous pressure, and low cardiac output has been modified over the last decade. This change reflects a response to a number of unanticipated findings in reviews of clinical trials testing traditional therapies targeting neurohumoral responses in humans. Notably, clinical trials failed to demonstrate long-term survival with traditional therapies. Further, drugs that initially caused a favorable response often shortened, rather than lengthened, survival time. For example, vasodilators such as α-adrenergic blockers, short-acting L-type CCBs, inoxidil, prostacyclin, and phosphodiesterase inhibitors failed to prolong survival despite effective afterload reduction. Inotropic agents increased contractility by increasing cAMP but shortened long-term survival as cardiac energy needs and arrhythmias increased. Increased calcium flux associated with their use may also have contributed to diastolic dysfunction.[28] In concert with these findings, selected drugs that initially worsened clinical signs (e.g., β-adrenergic drugs) were associated with improved long-term survival. Finally, several classes of drugs were associated with improved survival through mechanisms other than that expected on the basis of their known pharmacologic effects. For example, selected diuretics (e.g., spironolactone) and drugs active in the RAAS, including ACE inhibitors and angiotensin II–receptor blockers, appeared to slow myocardial deterioration and remodeling.[28-30]

The findings of the clinical trials reoriented investigators to the potential impact of disease and drug therapies on myocardial deterioration, progressive remodeling, and maladaptive hypertrophy. For example, worsening of disease despite effective afterload reduction appears to have reflected, in part, increased release of neurohumoral mediators (norepinephrine, AGII, and endothelin), stimulating further proliferation and remodeling. Inhibition of inappropriate mediators through drugs such as β blockers may decrease maladaptive myocardial proliferation, and progressive dilation of the heart was proposed as a mechanism.[28] The impact of remodeling and its prevention on the progression of CHF is now a well-recognized target of therapy. The extent of progressive remodeling is associated with clinical outcome, and the key to improved survival for CHF that has emerged as a result of these findings is the blunting of the progressive deterioration, remodeling, and proliferation associated with disease.[28]

Remodeling reflects a number of cellular and biochemical activities that lead to myocardial hypertrophy, fibrosis, altered excitation–contraction coupling, apoptosis, altered cellular metabolism, and discordant electrophysiologic responses. The negative sequelae of remodeling include altered ventricular myocardial wall and chamber dimensions and altered geometry. Although myocyte hypertrophy does not appear to be associated with negative sequelae in the failing heart,[31] the responses also include maladaptive proliferation and chronic dilation, leading to eccentric hypertrophy. Myocardial cell life span is shortened, initiating a vicious cycle of myocardial cell death, increased load on surviving myocytes, and compensatory proliferation. Consequently, myocardial cell death and remodeling and dilation increase. Elongation of cardiac myocytes increases cardiac chamber size but also increases individual myocyte tension, further stimulating hypertrophy.[24] Several mediators recognized for their neurohumoral compensatory responses contribute to cardiac remodeling, offering a target of therapy. In particular, AG II contributes to several aspects of cardiac remodeling through AG II type 1 (AT1) receptors.[32] Fibroblast gene expression increases, leading to increased density and proliferation, and myocyte hypertrophy.[31] Aldosterone activates several genes responsible for synthesis of myocardial extracellular matrix.[33] The myocardium appears to include a local RAAS regulated in part by AG II that supports cardiac fibrosis; the more severe the failure, the more aldosterone is activated, with local activation occurring independently of systemic effects.[34] Underlying proliferation and remodeling is inflammation; both are associated with increased gene expressions of proinflammatory cytokines.[35] Inflammatory cytokines, NO, and reactive oxygen species act as negative inotropes, contributing to cardiac remodeling.[35] NO also impairs mechanical myocardial function by increasing intracellular cGMP, reducing calcium current and desensitizing myofilaments. NO has both negative inotropic and chronotropic effects on the heart and has been associated with myocardial necrosis.[24] Free radicals also decrease calcium sensitivity and calcium accumulation in the sarcoplasmic reticulum.[36] Calcium sensitization is further reduced by pathologic conditions such as acidosis or hypoxia. These changes determine the long-term prognosis in patients with heart failure.[28] In the heart damaged by myocardial infarction, proinflammatory cytokines (e.g., tumor necrosis factor [TNF]-α, IL-1b, and others) stimulate cardiac fibroblasts to alter the extracellular matrix (ECM), primarily through AGII and AR-1 receptors. Plasma TNF-α has been positively correlated with the severity of CHF in humans and is increased in dogs and cats with heart failure.[24] Eventually, damaged and normal tissue is replaced with scar tissue that maintains structural integrity but limits chamber size. Remodeling involves production of structural proteins, including fibronectin, collagens (Col) I and III, tissue inhibitors of matrix metalloproteinases (TMPs) and "secondary" growth factors. Apoptosis may contribute to progressive left ventricular dysfunction, as is supported by increased plasma apoptosis–signaling surface receptors that trigger programmed cell death in patients with heart failure.[24] Angiotensin receptor density also increases in area macrophages.[37]

KEY POINT 14-13 Several mediators recognized for their neurohumoral compensatory responses contribute to cardiac remodeling, with angiotensin and its subsequent influences playing a major role.

As the understanding of the pathophysiology of CHF has advanced, the tools with which disease and response to therapy can be monitored also will advance. Preferred biomarkers have been circulating molecules associated with neurohumoral responses to the failing heart, such as endothelin, natriuretic peptides, AGII, and endothelin or markers of myocardial damage (e.g., creatine kinase isoenzymes and troponins). Increased cardiac troponin (I or T) has emerged as the preferred gold-standard marker for acute events involving the myocardium, whereas increased B-type natriuretic peptide may be preferred for identification of cardiac diseases as a cause of dyspnea. Boswood[38] has addressed the status of biomarkers in feline and canine cardiac disease.

Management should attempt to correct maladaptive responses in cardiovascular function and inflammatory and proliferative responses (Tables 14-2 and 14-3). Functional changes reflect short-term hemodynamic neurohumoral responses initiated by the endocrine system that are intended to improve cardiac performance, vascular tone, and salt and water excretion. As such, traditional approaches to treatment of congestive heart failure have included drugs that decrease preload (e.g., diuretics), afterload (e.g, ACE inhibitors), and heart rate (e.g., beta-blockers). However, drugs that slow the progression of myocardial disease by virtue of their effects on myocardial inflammation, remodeling, necrosis, or apoptosis represent the newest group of drugs used to treat the failing heart. Selected drugs (including those in current use) that improve hemodynamic effects by blocking neurohumoral stimuli may prove most beneficial because of their simultaneous inhibition of proliferative stimuli. Accordingly, attempts should be made to select those drugs in each category with demonstrable muting of myocardial remodeling.

VASODILATOR THERAPY

Vasodilator drugs can be categorized according to the type of vessels that they dilate: arterioles (i.e., resistance vessels: arterial dilators), veins (i.e., capacitance vessels: venodilators), or both. All three types of vasodilators can be useful in the patient with CHF. Arterial vasodilators target resistance vessels, relieving vasoconstriction that accompanies CHF or primary hypertension. Normally, vasoconstriction maintains systemic pressure in the normal range of 100 to 110 mm Hg. However, the critical organs (i.e., the brain, kidneys, and

Table 14-2 Timing of Cardioactive Drug Use

Stage	Drug or Drug Class	Target Effect	Asymptomatic	SYMPTOMATIC				
				Mild	Moderate	Severe		
						No arrhythmias	Arrhythmias	
							Ventricular	Atrial
II B_2	ACE Inhibitor	Peripheral vasoconstriction (Increased afterload)	+	+	+	+	+	+
		Remodeling						
II B_2	Beta blocker	Remodeling	+	+	+	+	+	+
III B_2 C	Spironolactone	Edema (volume overload)		+	+	+	+	+
		Remodeling						
III B_2 D	Furosemide	Edema (volume overload)			+	+	+	+
III B_2 D	Beta blockers	Supraventricular tachycardias Ventricular tachycardias			+*		+	
III B_2 D	Digoxin	Supraventricular tachycardias						+
	Pimobendan	Decreased contractility (systolic failure)				+	+	+
		Increased afterload, preload						
IV D	Hydralazine	Peripheral vasoconstriction (increased afterload)			+	+	+	+
IV D	Amlodipine	Peripheral vasoconstriction (increased afterload)				+	+	+
IV	Amiodarone	Arrhythmias					+	+
		Diastolic failure						
IV D_1	Nitroprusside	Peripheral vasoconstriction and volume overload				+	+	+
IV	Dobutamine	Decreased contractility						+

*Consensus could not be reached regarding the early use of beta-blockers for myocardial protection.
+= indicated for use. The New York Heart Association and International Small Animal Cardiac Health council provides a functional classification of CHF: Class I (asymptomatic); II (clinical signs with strenuous exercise); III (clinical signs with routine daily activities or mild exercise), and IV (severe clinical signs at rest). The American College of Veterinary Internal Medicine has promulgated a complementing classification system for CVMI based on structural changes: Stage A (high risk but no identifiable disorder), B (structural disease without clinical signs, subclassified as 1 [no radiographic or echocardiographic changes] and 2 [significant regurgitation with evidence of left-sided heart enlargement], C (structural disease with current or historical clinical signs), and D (end-stage disease refractory to standard therapies).

heart) are effectively perfused at pressures 20 to 30 mm Hg less than normal. This "reserve" allows arterial dilating agents to decrease systemic blood pressure and cardiac afterload without compromising critical organ blood flow. As peripheral resistance decreases, in the patient with CHF, stroke volume increases. In the presence of mitral insufficiency, the regurgitant fraction that enters the pulmonary circulation and reenters the heart is reduced. Finally, with reduction in volume overload, the end-diastolic volume of the left ventricle is reduced, wall tension is reduced, and myocardial perfusion increases. Venodilators increase the volume of the capacitance vessels, also reducing preload to the right, and subsequently left, ventricle. Preload reducers may also relieve some pulmonary vascular congestion. Potential negative inotropic effects of peripherally acting drugs tend to be masked by baroreceptor-mediated increase in sympathetic tone[2] in the normal animal.

KEY POINT 14-14 More than any class of drugs, cardioactive drugs are associated with adverse effects, and their use should be implemented only if they are well understood and proper monitoring tools are available.

Arterial Vasodilators

In the 1980s the role of increased resistance in cardiac failure became a focus of therapy. Drugs that decrease peripheral resistance do so by dilating arterial or resistance vessels. The inclusion of peripheral vasodilators in the armament of treatment for CHF, particularly in its early stages, has proved useful in reducing the dependency on digitalis for long-term treatment. However, their efficacy as venodilators increasingly is being challenged. Those drugs whose mechanisms also contribute to the inhibition of neurohumoral endocrine compensatory responses are more likely to address both the

Text continued on p.491.

Table 14-3 Doses of Selected Cardiovascular Drugs

Drug	Indication	Dose	Route	Interval (hr)
Acepromazine	Arterial thromboembolism	0.15-0.3 mg/kg	SC	8-12
Amiodarone	Antiarrhythmic	Initial dose: 10-25 mg/kg	PO	12 × 7 days
		Followed by: 5-7.5 mg/kg	PO	12 × 14 days
		Thereafter: 7.5 mg/kg	PO	24
	Doberman cardiomyopathy	Initial dose: 10 mg/kg	PO	12 × 7 days
		Thereafter: 8 mg/kg	PO	24
Amlodipine besylate	Systemic hypertension	0.625 mg/cat. Increase to 1.25 mg/cat if needed	PO	24
		0.125-0.25 mg/kg (C)	PO	24
		0.1 mg/kg (D)	PO	12 initially, then slowly increase (weekly) to:
		0.2-0.4 mg/kg (D)	PO	24
Amrinone	Positive inotrope support	1-2 mg/kg (D). Maximum of 100 mg	PO	12
		0.1 mg/kg/min (D)	IV (over 5 min)	To effect
Aprindine		1-2 mg/kg (D). Maximum of 100 mg	PO	12
		0.1 mg/kg/min (D)	IV (over 5 min)	To effect
Aspirin	Antithrombotic therapy	5-10 mg/kg (D)	PO	12-48
		6-25 mg/kg (C)	PO	2 × per week
		80 mg/cat	PO	48
	Hypertrophic cardiomyopathy	160 mg/cat	PO	2 × per week
	Postadulticide heartworm	5-10 mg/kg (D)	PO	24
	Disseminated intravascular coagulation	7.5-15 mg/kg	PO	24-48 × 10 days. Use lower dose if other anticoagulants are concurrently administered
Atenolol	Beta blockade	6.25-50 mg (D)	PO	12
		0.25-1 mg/kg (D)	PO	12-24
		2-3 mg/kg (C)	PO	12-24
		5-12.5 mg/cat	PO	24
	Hypertension	2 mg/kg	PO	24
Atropine	Sinus bradycardia	0.022-0.044 mg/kg	IM, IV, SC	To effect
		0.04 mg/kg	PO	6-8
	Atropine response test	0.044 mg/kg	IV	Once
Benazepril	Afterload reduction or hypertension	0.25-1 mg/kg	PO	24
	Renal disease	0.5-1 mg/kg (C)	PO	24
		0.25-0.5 mg/kg (D)	PO	24
Bretylium tosylate	Refractory ventricular arrhythmias	5-10 mg over 8 min	1-2 mg/min	Every 1-2 as needed to control arrhythmias
Calcium chloride (contains 0.273 mg elemental calcium)	Ventricular asystole	0.1-0.3 mL/kg of a 10% solution (100 mg/mL $CaCL_2$)	IV (slowly)	To effect
	Hypocalcemia	0.068-0.13 mEq (0.05-0.1 mL/kg of a 10% solution)	IV (slowly)	To effect
Calcium gluconate (contains 0.093 mg elemental calcium)	Ventricular asystole	0.5-1.5 mL/kg of a 10% solution (100 mg/mL $CaCL_2$)	IV (slowly)	To effect
Captopril	Vasodilator, Congestive heart failure	0.25-2 mg/kg (D)	PO	8-12
		2-3 mg/cat	PO	8
		3-6.25 mg/cat	PO	12
	Hypertension	0.5-2.0 mg/kg (D)	PO	8-12

Table 14-3 Doses of Selected Cardiovascular Drugs—cont'd

Drug	Indication	Dose	Route	Interval (hr)
Carvedilol	Cardiac beta blockade	0.5-0.9 mg/kg; start at 0.1 mg/kg and increase in 0.25 mg/kg increments	PO	12 to effect
Clopidogrel	Antiplatelet	1-2 mg/kg (D)	PO	24
		Load: 10 mg/kg (D)	PO	For acute effect
		18.75-75 mg/cat	PO	12
Coenzyme Q	Dilated cardiomyopathy	30-90 mg/dog	PO	12
Dalteparin	Thromboembolic disease	100-150 IU/kg (D)	SC	8
Deferoxamine mesylate	Cardiac arrest	5-15 mg/kg	IM, IV, SC	2 × 2 doses. then 8 × 3 doses
	Cardiac arrest	10 mg/kg	IM, IV	2 × 2 doses. then 8 × 3 doses
Dexrazoxane	Iron chelation for doxorubicin-induced cardiotoxicity	25 mg/kg (ratio of 10-20:1 dexrazoxane-doxorubicin)	IV	
Dicoumarol	Anticoagulant	Initial dose: 5 mg/kg	PO	Once
	Anticoagulant	Maintenance dose: 1.3-2.6 mg/kg	PO	24
Diethylcarbamazine	Heartworm prophylaxis	6.6 mg/kg (D)	PO	24
Digitoxin	Heart failure, supraventricular tachyarrhythmias	0.03-0.1 mg/kg/day (D)	PO	Divide dose and administer every 8-12
		0.005-0.015 mg/kg (C)	PO	24; monitor
		0.22 mg/m^2 (D)	PO (tablet)	12; monitor
		0.18 mg/m^2 (D)	PO (elixir)	12; monitor
Digoxin	Congestive heart failure	0.005-0.02 mg/kg (D)	PO (tablet)	12; monitor
		0.22 mg/m^2 (D)	PO (tablet)	12; monitor
	Supraventricular tachyarrhythmias	0.0025-0.004 mg/kg (C)	PO (tablet)	12; monitor
		0.18 mg/m^2	IV, PO	If intravenous, give 25%-50% of dose every 1 hr; if orally, 12 hr
	Dilated cardiomyopathy	0.005-0.008 mg/kg (D)	PO (elixir)	12; monitor
		0.003-0.004 mg/kg (C)	PO (elixir)	12; monitor
		0.0055-0.011 mg/kg (D)	IV (Cardoxin)	Give 25%-50% of dose every 1 hr
		2-3 kg: 0.0312 mg (C)	PO (Cardoxin)	48; monitor
		4-5 kg: 0.0312 mg (C)	PO (Cardoxin)	24-48; monitor
		>6 kg: 0.0312 mg (C)	PO (Cardoxin)	12; monitor
Diltiazem	Hypertension, hypertrophic cardiomyopathy, supraventricular tachyarrhythmias	0.125-0.35 mg/kg	IV (slowly)	Every 15 minutes as needed to a total dose of 0.75 mg/kg
	Acute atrial tachycardia	0.05-0.15 mg/kg	IV (slowly)	Every 5 minutes as needed to a total dose of 0.1-0.3 mg/kg
		0.25 mg/kg	IV (slowly)	Every 15 minutes as needed to a total dose of 0.75 mg/kg
		0.5-2 mg/kg	PO	8
		1.75-2.5 mg/kg (C)	PO	8
	Hypertrophic cardiomyopathy	7.5 mg (C)	PO	8-12

Continued

Table **14-3** Doses of Selected Cardiovascular Drugs—cont'd

Drug	Indication	Dose	Route	Interval (hr)
Diltiazem, extended release (XR and cardiazem CD)	See diltiazem	1/2 of 60 mg tablet or 10 mg/kg (C) cardiazem	PO	24
		30 mg (C) extended release	PO	24
Disopyramide PO_4		Ventricular dysrhythmias	6-22 mg/kg (D)	PO
Dobutamine	Inotropic agent	5-20 µg/kg (D)	IV CRI	
		2.5-15 µg/kg (C)	IV CRI (caution)	
Dopamine hydrochloride	Inotropic agent	2-25 µg/kg. Up to 50 µg/kg if severe hypotension or shock	IV CRI	
	Renal vasodilator: (acute renal failure)	2-5 µg/kg (low dose) in 5% D/W	IV CRI	
	Acute heart failure	2-10 µg/kg (40 mg in 500 mL)	IV CRI	
Enalapril	Hypertension, heart failure, valvular insufficiency	0.2-1 mg/kg (D) 1-2.5 mg/cat	PO	12-24
	Progressive renal disease	0.25-0.5 mg/kg (C)	PO	12-24
		1.25 mg/kg (C)	SC	6
		5 mg/kg (C)	PO	24
Epinephrine		Use 1:10,000 (0.1 mg/mL) of 1 m/mL (1:1000)	Dilute 1 mL of 1 mg/mL (1:1000) in 10 mL saline to make 1:10000	
	Cardiac arrest	0.2 mL/kg (0.05-0.5 mg or 0.5-5 mL)	IV, IT	As needed every 5-15 min
		10-20 µg/kg	IV	As needed every 5-15 min
		200 µg/kg	IV	As needed every 5-15 min
		0.8-2 mg/kg	IT	As needed every 5-15 min
	Anaphylaxis	0.1- 0.2 mL/kg (0.01-0.02 mg/kg)	IM, IV, SC	As needed every 5-15 min
		2.5-5 µg/kg	IV	As needed every 5-15 min
		50 µg/kg	IT	As needed every 5-15 min
Esmolol	Selective β [1] blockade, ventricular arrhythmias	0.05-0.1 mg/kg (D)	IV (slow bolus)	Every 5 min to a total cumulative dose of 0.5 mg/kg
		Loading dose: 200-500 µg/kg	IV (slow bolus)	Once
		Maintenance dose: 25-200 µg/kg	IV CRI	
Furosemide	Diuresis with acute renal failure	5-20 mg/kg	IM, IV, PO	8-12 or as needed. Adjust to lowest dose possible
	Hypertension	1-2 mg/kg. Maximum of 8 mg/kg for acute renal failure	PO	12
	Hypercalcemia	1-2 mg/kg	IM, IV, PO, SC	8-12
		0.1-1 mg/kg	IV CRI	
Gemfibrozil	Hyperlipidemia	7.5 mg/kg	PO	12
Glycopyrrolate	Sinus bradycardia, SA block, AV block	0.005-0.010 mg/kg	IM, IV	As needed
		0.01-0.02 mg/kg	SC	8-12
Heparin	Lipoprotein lipase provocative test	100 IU/kg	IV	Test lipids before and 15 min after heparin

Table **14-3** Doses of Selected Cardiovascular Drugs—cont'd

Drug	Indication	Dose	Route	Interval (hr)
Hydralazine	Vasodilator, heart failure	Initial dose: 0.5 mg/kg	PO	Once
		Then titrate up to 1-3 mg/kg (D)	PO	12
		0.5-0.8 mg/kg (C)	PO	12
	Hypertension	0.5-2.0 mg/kg (D)	PO	8-12
		2.5 mg/cat	PO	12
	Acute arterial thromboembolism	0.5-2 mg/kg (D)	IM, PO	12
		2.5 mg/cat. Maximum of 10 mg/cat	PO	12
Hydrochlorothiazide	Antihypertensive agent	0.5-2 mg/kg	PO	12-24
	Diuretic	2-4 mg/kg (D)	PO	24
Inamrinone	Low-output heart failure	Loading dose: 1-3 mg/kg	IV (over 2-3 min)	Once
		Followed by: 30-100 μg/kg	IV CRI	
Insulin, Regular	Hyperkalemia	0.25-0.5 IU/kg (D)	IV	Once. Follow with 50% dextrose
Isopropamide iodide	Sinus bradycardia, SA or AV block	0.2-0.4 mg/kg	PO	8-12
Isoproterenol	Bradycardia, AV block, cardiac arrest	0.04-0.08 μg/kg	IV CRI	
		0.4 mg in 250 mL 5% D/W	IV (slowly)	To effect
Isosorbide dinitrate	Vasodilator	2.5-5 mg/animal	PO	12
Isosorbide mononitrate	Vasodilator	5 mg/dog	PO	12
Ivermectin	Heartworm preventive	6 μg/kg (D)	PO	Monthly
	Microfilaricide	50-200 μg/kg	PO	Once every 2 weeks following adulticide administration
Levamisole	Microfilaricide	10-11 mg/kg (D)	PO	24 × 6-12 days
Lidocaine	Ventricular arrhythmias	Initial dose: 2-4 mg/kg (D)	IV (slow bolus)	Administer at 10-15 min increments to a maximum of 8 mg/kg
		Followed by: 25-80 μg/kg (D)	IV CRI	
		Initial dose: 100 to 400 μg/kg	IV (slowly)	Once
		Followed by: 250 to 750 μg/kg	IV (slowly)	To effect
		15-50 μg/kg	IV CRI	
Lisinopril	Afterload reduction (vasodilator)	0.25-0.50 mg/kg. Maximum of 1 mg/kg	PO	24
Lufenuron/milbemycin	Heartworm preventive	1 tablet per appropriate-size dog	PO	Monthly
Melarsomine dihydrochloride	Dirofilariasis	2.5 mg/kg (D)	IM (deep lumbar)	24 × 2 days, repeat in 4 months
Metaraminol	Vascular support during shock	0.01-0.1 mg/kg	IV (slowly)	To effect
Methoxamine hydrochloride	Vasopressor: cardiac arrest, shock	100-800 μg/kg (D)	IV (slowly)	As needed
		200-250 μg/kg	IM	To effect
		40-80 μg/kg	IV	To effect
Metoprolol	Atrial fibrillation, hypertrophic cardiomyopathy	5-50 mg/dog	PO	8
	Beta blockade	0.5-1 mg/kg (D)	PO	8
		2-15 mg/cat	PO	8
		12.5-25 mg/cat	PO	12
Mexiletine hydrochloride	Ventricular arrhythmias	4-10 mg/kg (D)	PO	8-12. Use cautiously
		5-8 mg/kg (D)	PO	8-12. Use cautiously
	Doberman cardiomyopathy	5-8 mg/kg	PO	8 until dog responds to amiodarone

Continued

Table **14-3** Doses of Selected Cardiovascular Drugs—cont'd

Drug	Indication	Dose	Route	Interval (hr)
Milbemycin oxime	Heartworm, hookworm, roundworm, whipworm prophylaxis	0.5-0.99 mg/kg	PO	Monthly
	Heartworm preventive	2 mg/kg (C)	PO	Monthly
Milrinone	Low-output heart failure	0.5-1 mg/kg (D)	PO	12
Moxidectin	Heartworm preventive	3 μg/kg (D)	PO	Monthly
	Heartworm preventive	0.17 mg/kg	SC	6 months
Nadolol	Beta blockade	0.25-0.5 mg/kg	PO	12
Nicotinamide	Vacor toxicosis	Initial dose: 500-1000 mg	IM	Once
	Hyperlipidemia	Initial dose: 1.5 mg/kg	PO	12
Nicotinamide		Gradually increase to: 12.5 mg/kg	PO	12
		50 to 100 mg/cat	PO	24
	See nicotinamide (also known as vitamin B_3)			Niacin can be dosed as nicotinamide with fewer side effects
Nifedipine	Arterial vasodilator, calcium antagonist	1 mg/kg (D)	PO	12-24
Nitroglycerin 2% ointment	Dilated cardiomyopathy	5-30 mm (D)	Topical	4-12
	Heart failure	0.6-5.1 cm (0.25-2 inches)/dog	Topical	6-8
		1.3 cm (0.5 inch)/2.2 kg (D)	Topical	12
		0.3-0.6 cm (0.125-0.25 inches)/cat	Topical	4-6
		4-12 mg/dog. Maximum of 15 mg	Topical	6-8
		2-4 mg (1/4 inch) (C)	Topical	12
		2.5-10 mg	Transdermal	12 on, 12 off
Nitroprusside	Vasodilator for acute congestive heart failure	0.5 μg/kg (C)	IV CRI	Use 50 μg/mL dilution (1.26 mL to 60 mL 5% dextrose)
		1-2 μg/kg (D). Maximum of 10 μg/kg	IV CRI	Use 50 μg/mL dilution (1.26 mL to 60 mL 5% dextrose)
Norepinephrine bitartrate	Cardiovascular disorders	0.05-0.3 μg/kg	IV	
Norepinephrine bitartrate	Vasopressor	2-4 mg/500 mL (4-8 μg/ml)	IV	Infuse to effect
Phenoxybenzamine hydrochloride	Acute hypertension from pheochromocytoma	0.2-1.5 mg/kg (D)	PO	12
		0.5 mg/kg (C)	PO	12
		2.5 mg. Increase in 2.5-mg increments to a maximum of 10 mg	PO	12
	Endotoxemia	0.25-0.5 mg/kg (D)	PO	6-8
		2.5-10 mg/cat	PO	24
		0.25 mg/kg (C)	PO	8
		5-15 mg (D)	PO	24
		2.5-30 mg (D)	PO	8
		0.5 mg/kg (C)	PO	24
		0.25 mg/kg (C)	PO	8
Phentolamine	Hypertension from pheochromocytoma	0.02-0.1 mg/kg (D)	IV	To effect
	Vasodilator	0.15 mg/kg	IV (slowly)	As needed
		0.1 mg/kg (D)	IV	15 min, to effect
		1 mg/kg (D)	IM, SC	15 min, to effect
		1-3 μg/kg	IV CRI	

Table **14-3** Doses of Selected Cardiovascular Drugs—cont'd

Drug	Indication	Dose	Route	Interval (hr)
Phenytoin	Ventricular arrhythmias	2-4 mg/kg (D). Maximum of 10 mg/kg	IV	Increase by 2 mg/kg increments to effect
	Ventricular arrhythmias	10 mg/kg (D)	IV	8
	Ventricular arrhythmias	30-50 mg/kg (D)	PO	8
	Ventricular arrhythmias	20 mg/kg (C)	PO	7 days
Pimobendan	Dilated cardiomyopathy	0.1-0.3 mg/kg (D)	PO	12
Prazosin	Arterial vasodilation, functional urethral obstruction	1 mg/15 kg (D)	PO	8-12
Procainamide	Ventricular arrhythmias	25-50 μg/kg/min (D)	IV CRI	500-1000 mg in 500 mL 5% D/W, to effect
		Initial dose: 6-8 mg/kg (D). Maximum of 15 mg/kg	IV (over 5 min)	Once
		Followed by: 25-40 μg/kg (D)	IV CRI	
		6-20 mg/kg (D)	IM	4-6
		8-23 mg/kg (D)	PO	6-8; monitor
		6.6-22 mg/kg	PO	4 or up to every 8 if sustained-release formulation; monitor
		62.5 mg/cat	PO	6; monitor
		Initial dose: 1-2 mg/kg (C)	IV	Once
		Followed by: 10-20 μg/kg (C)	IV CRI	
		3-8 mg/kg (C)	IM, PO	6-8; monitor
		20 mg/kg (D)	PO (sustained-release formulation)	8; monitor
Propantheline bromide	Sinus bradycardia	0.25-1 mg/kg (D)	PO	8
		7-30 mg/dog	PO	8
		0.8-1.6 mg/kg (C)	PO	8
		7.5 mg/cat	PO	8
Propranolol	Ventricular hypertrophy, aortic stenosis	0.125-0.25 mg/kg (D)	PO	12
		0.2-1 mg/kg (D)	PO	8
		0.4-1.2 mg/kg (C)	PO	8-12
	Ventricular arrhythmias	0.02-0.06 mg/kg	IV (over 2-3 min)	8 or to effect
		0.44-1.1 mg/kg (D)	PO	8
		Initial dose: 0.25-0.5 mg/cat	IV (slowly)	Once
		Followed by: 2.5-5 mg/cat	PO	8
	Hypertrophic cardiomyopathy, valvular insufficiency	0.3-1 mg/kg (D). Maximum of 120 mg/day	PO	8
		≤5 kg: 2.5 mg/cat	PO	8-12
		>5 kg: 5 mg/cat	PO	8-12
	Hypertension	2.5-10 mg/dog	PO	8-12
		2.5-5 mg/cat	PO	8-12
	Tachyarrhythmias from endocrinopathies	0.15-0.5 mg/kg (D)	PO	8
		0.3-1 mg/kg (D)	IV	8-12 or to effect
		2.5-5 mg (C)	PO	8-12
Propylthiouracil (PTU)	Hyperthyroidism	10 mg/kg (C)	PO	8
		50 mg/cat	PO	8-12
		11 mg/kg	PO	12
		150 mg/dog	PO	24
Quinidine	Cardiac arrhythmias	4-8 mg/kg (C)	IM	8
		10-20 mg/kg (C)	PO	6-8

Continued

Table **14-3** Doses of Selected Cardiovascular Drugs—cont'd

Drug	Indication	Dose	Route	Interval (hr)
Quinidine gluconate	Cardiac arrhythmias	6-20 mg/kg (D)	IM, IV (slow), PO	6-12. 1 mg quinidine base = 1.65 mg quinidine gluconate
	Ventricular tachycardia	6.6-22 mg/kg	IM	2-4 (or every 8-12 if sustained-release formulation)
		6-20 mg/kg (D)	PO	6-8
	Conversion of rapid supraventricular tachycardia	6-11 mg/kg	IM	6
Quinidine sulfate	Cardiac arrhythmias	6-22 mg/kg (D)	PO	6 or every 8 if extended capsules. 1 mg quinidine base = 1.2 mg quinidine sulfate
	Ventricular tachycardia	6-22 mg/kg	PO	2 until arrhythmia controlled, then every 6-8 hr
Selamectin	Parasiticide	6 mg/kg	Topical	Monthly heartworm preventive
Sildenafil	Pulmonary hypertension	0.25-3 mg/kg	PO	12
Sotalol	Ventricular arrhythmias	1-3 mg/kg 10 mg/cat	PO	12
		20 mg/kg (D)	PO	12
Spironolactone	Ascites	1-2 mg/kg (D). Maximum of 4 mg/kg	PO	12
	Diuretic, heart failure	2-4 mg/kg	PO	24
		1-2 mg/kg (D)	PO	12
	Primary hyperaldosteronism, hepatic insufficiency	1 mg/kg (C)	PO	12
		12.5 mg (C)	PO	24
Spironolactone/ hydrochlor-othiazide	Diuretic, antihypertensive agent	2 mg/kg	PO	12-24
Taurine	Dilated cardiomyopathy	500 mg/dog	PO	12
		250-500 mg/cat	PO	12
Terbutaline	Bradyarrhythmias	2.5-5 mg/dog	PO, SC	8
		0.625 mg/cat	PO	8
Tocainide	Ventricular arrhythmias	17-25 mg/kg (large D)	PO	8
		30 mg/kg (small D)	PO	8
Vasopressin, aqueous	Non-responsive shock	1.2U/kg	Intratracheal	
Verapamil hydrochloride	Supraventricular arrhythmias	Initial dose: 0.05-0.15 mg/kg (D) or 1 mg/kg if normal myocardial function	IV (bolus)	Once
		Followed by: 2-10 μg/kg/min	IV CRI	To effect
		50 μg/kg (D)	IV (slowly)	Repeat at 5-minute intervals until total dose is 150-200 μg/kg
		25 μg/kg (C)	IV (slowly)	Repeat at 5-minute intervals until total dose is 150-200 μg/kg
		0.11-0.33 mg/kg	IV (slowly)	Repeat at 5-minute intervals until total dose is 150-200 μg/kg

Table 14-3 Doses of Selected Cardiovascular Drugs—cont'd

Drug	Indication	Dose	Route	Interval (hr)
Verapamil hydrochloride		1-3 mg/kg (D)	PO	6-8
		10-15 mg/kg	PO	Divide dose and administer every 8-12
		1.1-2.9 mg/kg (C)	PO	8
	Hypertension, conversion of rapid supraventricular tachycardia	1.1-4.4 mg/kg	PO	8-12

SC, Subcutaneous; *PO*, by mouth; *C*, cat; *D*, dog; *IV*, intravenous; *IM*, intramuscular; *CRI*, constant-rate infusion; *D/W*, dextrose in water. *IT*, intratracheal; *SA*, sinoatrial; *AV*, atrioventricular.

hemodynamic and proliferative alterations that accompany the progressively failing heart compared with those drugs whose actions decrease only resistance. For the latter group, although initially beneficial, their use may contribute to a worsening of disease, particularly if the degree of afterload reduction stimulates a hemodynamic response that counters decreased resistance. Thus care should be taken in the timing of therapy and its implementation.

KEY POINT 14-15 Because drugs that decrease peripheral resistance can cause hypotension and reflex tachycardia, care must be taken to avoid overzealous therapy and worsening of the neurohumoral compensatory responses initiated by cardiac failure.

Hydralazine

Hydralazine is a pure arterial vasodilator whose mechanism is not completely understood. Arteriolar smooth muscle is directly relaxed, perhaps by inhibiting calcium fluxes into the cell.[9] Conversion to NO and increased cGMP also have been suggested.[39] The decrease in peripheral vascular resistance caused by hydralazine is associated with an increase in cardiac performance.[40] Coronary and venous vasculature is not affected. Hydralazine lowers mean arterial pressure, total systemic resistance, and left ventricular filling pressures, causing an overall increase in cardiac performance in dogs with left ventricular failure.[40] In addition to its vasodilatory effects, hydralazine has been associated with a number of other effects that might benefit the patient with CHF. A positive inotropic effect has been described, perhaps reflecting stimulation of cAMP through β-receptors.[41] Hydralazine acts as an antioxidant by inhibiting membrane-bound enzymes that form free radicals, including super oxide.[42] More recently, hydralazine inhibition of prolyl hydroxylase domain (PHD) enzymes has been described, ultimately leading to an increase in vascular endothelial growth factor [VEGF], which has a number of positive effects. Endothelial cell growth is associated with angiogenesis, coronary vessel density, and improved myocardial perfusion;[39] VEFG also is antiapoptotic and cardioprotective in animal models.

Hydralazine binds to smooth muscle, resulting in a biological half-life that is longer than its plasma half-life. The drug is well absorbed after oral administration in both dogs and humans. However, in humans it is subject to first-pass metabolism with elimination by acetylation. The extent of first-pass metabolism in the dog, which is deficient in acetylation, is not described. Peak effects occur in the dog at 3 to 5 hours.[3] The incidence of adverse reactions may be significant. Hydralazine frequently causes increased heart rate; this effect may prove to be detrimental to the patient with CHF because of increased myocardial oxygen demands. β-blocker therapy (or, historically, in the case of myocardial failure, digitalis therapy) may be indicated to slow the heart rate. Hypotension may occur but is largely prevented by proper dose titration.[3] If sufficient, hypotension may activate the RAAS.[43] In humans, hydralazine has been associated with a variety of immune-mediated reactions, including a well-described drug-induced lupuslike syndrome.[9] A previous indication for hydralazine include afterload reduction in patients with moderately early to late signs of CHF. Hydralazine should be administered in small increments until an effective dose is reached. The advent of the ACE inhibitors has largely replaced the use of hydralazine, which currently is limited to animals that cannot tolerate or respond to ACE inhibitor therapy. In a canine model of chronic left ventricular dysfunction, however, hydralazine combined with nitrate therapy can cause a more marked increase in stroke volume compared with ACE inhibitors alone.[44] As the beneficial effects of hydralazine on the failing heart are realized, its use may increase.

Calcium Channel Blockers

Structure–Activity Relationship

Five types of calcium channels have been identified, with the L, N, and T subtypes the best characterized (the other two being P/Q and R subtypes). Each comprises a major subunit, α1, which is the major pore-forming unit of the channel, and associated subunits α2, β, γ and δ, which modulate α1. Calcium channels can be broadly blocked by large divalent (cadmium and manganese). Currently, 10 CCB cations have been approved for use in human medicine, all targeting the α-1 subunit.[45] Three categories target L-channel blockers, each targeting different domains of the α1 subunit: phenylalkylamines, represented by verapamil; benzothiazepines, represented by diltiazem (Figure 14-6); and the dihydropyridines, represented by nifedipine (including amlodipine, felodipine, nicardipine, and others). A newer category of CCBs, represented

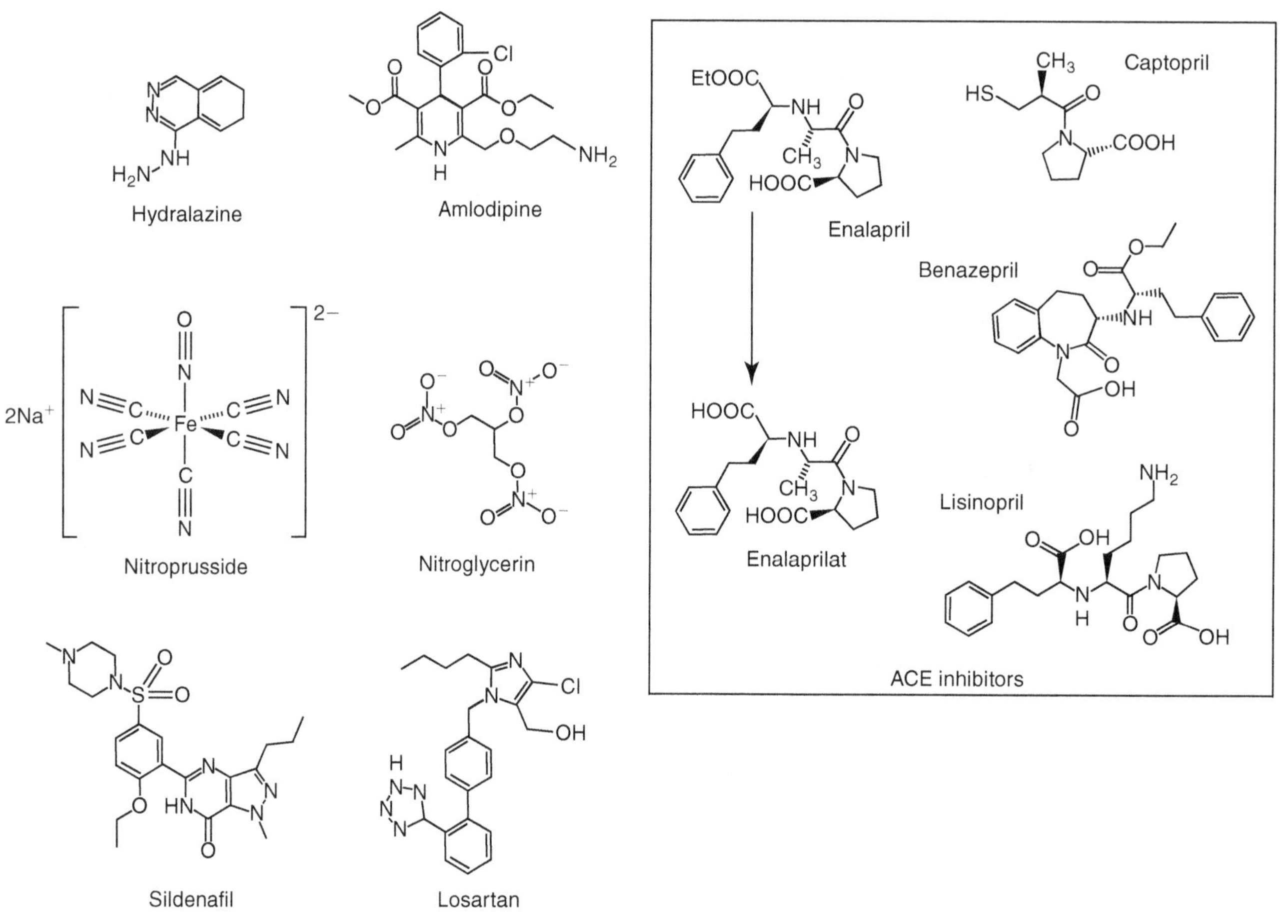

Figure 14-6 Structures of selected vasoactive drugs. *Inset:* Many of the angiotensin–converting enzyme inhibitors (ACE inhibitors) are prodrugs that must be metabolized to the active "prat" form.

by mibefradil, selectively block T-type channels.[45] The drugs vary among classes in pharmacodynamic effects and adverse events.

Pharmacodynamic Effects

Although calcium channel (or entry) blockers are also referred to as *calcium antagonists,* they do not directly antagonize calcium. Rather, they inhibit the entry of calcium into the cell or inhibit its mobilization from intracellular stores. CCBs inhibit the voltage-dependent channels in vascular smooth muscle at significantly lower concentrations than that necessary to interfere with the release of intracellular calcium or receptor-operated channels.[2] The pharmacodynamic effects of the CCBs reflect differences in potency at the various tissue receptors (i.e., either cardiac or vascular).

The effects of calcium entering cells by way of L-type channels is better documented than that entering T-type channels. Most clinically used CCBs block exclusively L-type channels, which are the most effective in the vasculature. Vasodilator effects of CCBs are primarily arterial, with little to no venodilator effects. Coronary vasodilation is significant but variable among drugs. The order of vasodilator potency of prototypical drugs from each class is nifedipine > verapamil > diltiazem. This may be balanced by differences in oral bioavailability; as such, the magnitude of the hemodynamic effects of the calcium channel antagonists also reflects the route of administration. Bioavailability is reduced (in humans) as a result of first-pass metabolism for nifedipine > verapamil > diltiazem. The impact of bioavailability on therapy can be complex. For example, whereas oral bioavailability of diltiazem is only 50%, chronic therapy is facilitated by decreased metabolism, which increase bioavailability. Diltiazem (discussed in greater depth as a class IV antiarrhythmic) is metabolized by acetylation, a phase II conjugation system; however, deficiencies in clearance in the dog have not been described.

All three prototypic drugs are available as oral preparations. Both verapamil and diltiazem are available as an intravenous solution for the rapid treatment of supraventricular arrhythmias. Hypotension, bradycardia, and tachycardia (generally reflex) are the predominant clinical indicators. In patients with poor myocardial reserve, exacerbation of CHF may result in peripheral or pulmonary edema. Further clinical pharmacology and side effects may be addressed for specific drugs under the appropriate category.

Amlodipine is a congener of nifedipine. Nifedipine causes vasodilation at concentrations that have little effect on the heart. Like nifedipine, amlodipine affects predominantly smooth rather than cardiac muscle and decreases total peripheral resistance. However, even at doses causing vascular effects, amlodipine has little effect on sinus node function and cardiac conduction. Thus a major advantage to amlodipine compared with other CCBs is that it may not cause reflex cardiac stimulation.

Vasodilator effects of selected CCBs may reflect modulation of NO. For example, amlodipine, but neither nifedipine nor diltiazem, experimentally causes NO release from canine coronary microvessels.[46] The clinical relevance of this finding is not yet clear but may imply that such CCBs are particularly effective for treatment of heart failure. Calcium channel blockade appears to have no effect on thrombus formation.[47,48] The effect of amlodipine on myocardial contractility is not clear, but most evidence to date does not support a clinically relevant positive inotropic effect.

At physiologic pH, with a pKa of 8.6, amlodipine is largely ionized, which contributes to a gradual association with the calcium channel receptor. Onset of action is thus a gradual event if therapy is begun with a loading dose. Among its peripheral vasodilatory effects, amlodipine prevents coronary vasospasm in response to a number of vasoconstrictive stimuli. Amlodipine has a protective effect against myocardial injury in an animal model of heart failure; the mechanism may be inhibition of NO induction mediated, in turn, by cytokines. Amlodipine inhibits ouabain-induced production of IL-1a, IL-1b, and IL-6, an action that appears to be calcium dependent in mononuclear cells.[35]

Clinical Pharmacology

In humans, amlodipine disposition is markedly variable. Peak concentrations following single oral administration do not occur for 6 to 12 hours; bioavailability ranges from 64% to 90% and is not affected by food. Protein binding is approximately 95% in human hypertensive patients. The elimination half-life is long. Approximately 90% of the drug is metabolized to inactive products. Based on limited information, the disposition of amlodipine in dogs appears similar to that in humans. Oral bioavailability in dogs is 88%; at least 50% of the drug is cleared by nonrenal mechanisms, and renal clearance includes that of both parent compound and its metabolites. The elimination half-life of amlodipine in dogs is 30 hours; little of the drug is excreted unchanged in the kidneys.[49] As with many cardiovascular drugs, amlodipine contains a chiral carbon. In humans each contributes to approximately 50% of the total area under the curve (the balance leaning toward S), but only the S enantiomer is pharmacologically active. The S-isomer is characterized by a longer half-life (49.6 hours) in humans compared with the R-isomer (35 hours); the long half-life allows once-daily dosing.[50] Enantiomer information is not available for dogs. Steady-state concentrations are not achieved for 5 to 10 days. Although administration of a loading dose may decrease the time to reach steady state, delayed response also reflects drug-receptor binding kinetics. Despite its use in cats, no pharmacokinetic data could be found for amlodipine in cats.

KEY POINT 14-16 The delay in efficacy of amlodipine in cats may be only partially overcome by starting therapy with a loading dose.

Drug Interactions and Side Effects

As a class, CCBs are involved in a number of drug interactions. Drugs that generally inhibit drug-metabolizing enzymes (e.g., cimetidine, chloramphenicol) will prolong the elimination and thus the cardiovascular effects of several CCBs. Selected CCBs can, in turn, prolong the elimination of drugs (e.g., cyclosporine, theophylline, and digoxin). The effects vary with the drug and are more likely with diltiazem and verapamil, but are largely absent for amlodipine. Side effects of CCBs vary with the primary pharmacodynamic effect. The major toxicities associated with CCBs are excessive vasodilation, which may activate the RAAS; negative inotropy; and depression of sinus nodal rate and atrioventricular conduction (negative chronotropy). These latter effects may be of therapeutic benefit (see the discussion of antiarrhythmics). Overzealous therapy associated with activation of the RAAS has been demonstrated in normal dogs receiving 0.57 mg/kg orally twice daily for 6 days.[53] A number of oral adverse drug events have been attributed to cardiovascular drugs.[51] Among them is gingival hyperplasia, particularly by nifidipine and its congeners, including amlodipine.[52] Amlodipine has been associated with gingival hyperplasia in dogs; the risk may be worsened in animals receiving other drugs associated with this adverse drug event (ADE)(e.g., cyclosporine).

Clinical Use

Amlodipine, a congener of nifedipine, is often the drug of choice for treatment of feline hypertension.[54] Because its actions are independent of the renin–angiotensin–converting enzyme system, the renal afferent (rather than efferent) artiole is preferentially dilated with amlodipine. Although renal perfusion and glomerular filtration are preserved in renal stressor states such as hypotension, increased glomerular perfusion may activate the RAAS, which may worsen renal disease in the impaired kidney. Accordingly, amlodipine should not be used as the sole afterload reducer in animals with myocardial failure associated with neural humoral compensatory mechanisms. As such, the use of amlodipine in dogs tends to be limited to hypertension associated with minimal compensatory mechanism. Mathur and coworkers[55] have demonstrated an antihypertensive effect of amlodipine (0.25 mg/kg orally daily) in cats with surgically induced hypertension associated with renal insufficiency.

Other indications for amlodipine therapy include afterload reduction in dogs whose myocardial failure has not responded or for those that have developed an intolerance to enalapril and diuretics. In human patients a synergistic effect occurs when amlodipine or another peripherally acting CCB is combined with ACE inhibitors. The complementary actions of CCBs and ACE inhibitors may facilitate control of systemic hypertension while minimizing detrimental renal effects. In humans the co-administration of amlodipine and ACE inhibition at low doses has been suggested to provide superior renoprotective benefits compared with those of either drug alone.[56] When combined with other therapies, a lower dose may be indicated (see Table 14-3). To guide therapy, clinicians should monitor patients with a targeted pressure of less than 150 mm Hg. Response should occur in 24 to 48 hours.

The use of amlodipine in veterinary cardiology has been reviewed.[57] Using an open, uncontrolled study, Jepson and coworkers[58] prospectively studied for 7 years (1998-2004) the efficacy of amlodipine (0.625 mg/cat/day) in hypertensive cats (n=141; median 15 years of age), with systolic blood pressure (SBP) 195 mm Hg; (184 and 214 mm Hg, 25th and 75th quartile, respectively). The dose of amlodipine was increased to 1.25 mg/cat if SBP remained above 160 mmHg. Phosphate-restricted diets were offered for azotemic cats, with aluminum hydroxide initiated if hyperphosphatemia became uncontrolled. Predictors of duration of survival in cats that did not survive to study end (n=89) were limited to urine protein: creatinine ratios (UPC), with the decline significant.

Helms[59] studied transdermal absorption of amlodipine (0.625 mg once daily) using a nonrandomized (oral dosing occurred first), nonblinded design in client-owned cats (n=6) with systolic hypertension (SBP ≥180 to 220 mm Hg depending on underlying cause). Oral doses were titrated up until SBP < 180 mm Hg was achieved; the final dose was maintained for 7 days, and blood was collected at that point. Cats were then crossed over to transdermal amlodipine at the same oral dose established for each cat. Blood pressure was recorded at 3 and 7 days, and plasma amlodipine was determined 12 hours after the last dose at 7 days for both treatment groups. After oral dosing SBP decreased a median of 73.5 mm Hg below baseline; after 7 days of transdermal dosing, SBP remained 52 mm Hg below baseline. The relative decrease was greater after oral compared with transdermal administration. Plasma amlodipine concentrations ranged from 5.7 to 18.7 ng/mL after oral administration compared with 1.4 to 4.5 ng/mL after transdermal administration. The lack of a crossover design may be a limitation of the study because a time effect could not be considered. This may be particularly important for a drug with a half-life that is likely to exceed 30 hours (the canine half-life) in cats (resulting in time to steady state of 3 to 6 days) coupled with further delay related to drug receptor interactions. This could result in a substantial hold-over effect from the first treatment simply as a result of drug concentrations. Further, a cumulative effect for the sequential treatment groups would not be identified. Post transdermal SBP was not compared with post oral SBP, so it is not clear if the decline was significant.

Although diltiazem is not recognized for vasodilatory actions, it apparently can improve GFR and enhance urine production in dogs with leptospirosis. The presumed mechanism is renal arterial vasodilation and subsequent reversal of renovasoconstriction. Mathews and Monteith[60] retrospectively studied the impact of diltiazem on acute renal failure in dogs (n = 11; seven dogs received standard care) associated with leptospirosis. Diltiazem was administered intravenously at 0.1 to 0.5 mg/kg slowly, followed by 1 to 5 μg/kg/min within 60 hours of admission and was continued until serum creatinine stabilized. Compared with standard therapy, renal recovery defined by reduction in serum creatinine occurred almost twice as fast in the diltiazem-treated group compared with the standard group, without a change in systemic blood pressure.

For cats with hyperthyroidism, the degree of hypertension associated with hyperthyroidism generally is mild, unless accompanied by renal insufficiency. Because hyperthyroidism-induced hypertension associated with hyperthyroidism alone is due to high-adrenergic output (causing increased cardiac inotropy and rate), β blockers are preferred to calcium channel blockers for control of hypertension. However, the addition of amlodipine may be indicated in hyperthyroid hypertensive cats that also exhibit renal insufficiency.

Angiotensin-Converting Enzyme Inhibitors

Structure–Activity Relationship

ACE inhibitors are carboxyalkyl dipeptide or tripeptide drugs whose chemistry yields three classes of drugs (see Figure 14-6): the sulfhydryl-containing drugs, which are structurally related to captopril; dicarboxyl-containing drugs related to enalapril (including lisinopril, benazepril, ramipril, and quinapril); and phosphorous-containing drugs related to fosinopril.[18] At least nine drugs have been approved in the United States for use in humans. Those approved for veterinary use are in the dicarboxyl group, including enalapril (United States), and ramipril and imidapril (Canada and Europe). With exception of lisinopril, each is a prodrug, being metabolized, at least in part, by CYP 3A4, to their respective active form (enalaprilat, benazeprilat, ramiprilat, and imidaprilat, respectively). Although differences exist in potency for ACE, all appear clinically equal in the inhibition of RAAS, and no compelling reason exists to select one ACE inhibitor over another based on pharmacodynamic response.[18]

Pharmacodynamic Effects

The primary effect of ACE inhibition is prevention of the conversion of AGI, which is relatively inactive, to the active AGII. However, ACE inhibitors also inhibit bradykinin inactivation. Because bradykinin stimulates prostaglandin synthesis, pharmacodynamic actions of ACE inhibitors may reflect bradykinin or prostaglandin activity.[18] However, of the two actions ACE inhibition is a more sensitive and measurable indicator of the complex dose–response relationship that characterizes the primary actions of ACE inhibitors (see the section on clinical pharmacology).[61] Actions of ACE inhibition target the neurohumoral and renal compensatory responses associated with myocardial failure. The detrimental sequelae of neurohumoral compensatory effects involving the RAAS have been previously reviewed. Specific inhibition of ACE decreases circulating levels of AGII and aldosterone. Effects include vasodilation (arterial), decreased systemic blood pressure, increased cardiac output, and reduced heart rate. Aldosterone secretion is reduced (but not obliterated), and natriuresis (loss of sodium in urine) occurs. Mild venodilation reduces some preload. ACE inhibitors also target a variety of mediators associated with myocardial remodeling. In the normal feline kidney, ACE inhibitors mildly increase Na^+ and Cl^- urinary excretion and may increase K^+ excretion. The ACE inhibitors have a positive inotropic effect on the heart but do not increase heart rate. The mechanism is unclear, but with enalapril it is associated with increased cardiac vasoactive intestinal peptide in rats.[62]

Primary cardiac effects increase their importance in the management of cardiac disease accompanied by CHF. Inhibition of ACE also increases circulating concentrations of the endogenous stem cell regulator Ac SDKP (*N*-acetyl-seryl-aspartyl-lysyl-proline), which may contribute a cardioprotective effect.[18]

KEY POINT 14-17 Because angiotensin and its downstream signals contribute so much to progressive myocardial failure, ACE inhibitors offer much more than simply afterload reduction in the patient with congestive heart failure.

Clinical Pharmacology

Pharmacokinetic–Pharmacodynamic Relationship. The use of ACE inhibitors has been reviewed in dogs and cats.[12,61,63] The exact relationship among ACE inhibitors, ACE inhibition, impaired AGII production, pharmacodynamic responses (blood pressure and cardiovascular), and pharmacokinetics is complex.[61] Most ACE inhibitors used in animals (e.g., enalapril and benazepril) are prodrugs, which are more easily absorbed than the active metabolite. Those that are not prodrugs include captopril and lisinopril.[64] In addition to passive oral absorption, prodrugs are actively transported in the jejunum by peptide carrier-mediated transport (PEPT). Substrate specificity has been described for the different transport proteins.[61] The importance of transport on drug absorption is not clear. Food does not appear to affect absorption. Parent compound oral bioavailability is low (20% to 40% in dogs); only a fraction of the low bioavailability appears to reflect first-pass metabolism by hepatic carboxyl esterases to active metabolites. Maximum drug concentrations occur approximately 30 minutes after administration in the dog. A small amount of drug not metabolized on first pass will be metabolized by esterases located in tissues.[61]

Tissue distribution and subsequent action of ACE inhibitors is among the most complex of drugs, being influenced by lipophilicity; systemic and local binding; receptor numbers and affinity; and, for prodrugs, presence of local metabolizing enzymes. Protein binding and its profound impact on pharmacokinetic–pharmacodynamic relationships are described later in this chapter. Lipophilicity determines distribution, particularly of the prodrug, into sanctuaries such as the brain, where local esterases produce the active compound. Accordingly, lipophilic prodrugs such as fosinopril are more likely to affect the central nervous system compared with less lipophilic drugs such as enalapril.[61] Elimination of ACE inhibitors (i.e., active metabolite) is largely renal. However, the magnitude excreted renally varies with the drug.[61] In dogs enalaprilat is largely (85% to 95%) eliminated by renal clearance, whereas benazeprilat and ramiprilat are cleared through both the kidney (45%) and bile. Fosinopril is also cleared (in humans) by liver and kidneys.

Protein binding of ACE contributes to complex pharmacokinetic–pharmacodynamic responses.[61] Binding to proteins is both nonspecific, to albumin, yielding an inactive state, or specific, to ACE (located in circulation or tissue vascular endothelium), resulting in an active complex. Nonspecific binding is nonsaturable, whereas specific binding is saturable, with the latter resulting in nonlinear pharmacokinetics. Based on modeling, circulating ACE represents approximately 5%, 10%, and 30% of the total ACE pool in dogs, cats, and humans, respectively, with the balance represented by tissue ACE. Endothelial ACE occurs in many tissues but predominates in the lungs. Tissue endothelial ACE acts locally (paracrine) but also is released such that it can act systemically (hormonally). Bound, endothelial ACE is regularly cleaved to yield circulating ACE, which, is in turn, bound to circulating plasma proteins (in an inactive form) to ensure a steady supply of either ACE or its inhibitors. Endothelial ACE is accessible to ACE inhibitors in the extracellular space, facilitating an immediate response to ACE inhibitors. However, because the drug is bound to ACE, the (active) ACE inhibitor will not be detected (analytically). If drug is detectable, then all available tissue binding sites are saturated. Thus a decline in response that reflects a decline in drug concentrations occurs only after tissue sites are not saturated, which occurs only at drug concentrations that are not detectable. As such, the saturable nature of binding to ACE by the ACE inhibitor results in a nonlinear dose–response curve (detectable concentrations do not correlate well to response). Thus, in contrast to most drugs for which the terminal component of the plasma-concentration versus time is a reasonable guide to duration of effect, for ACE inhibitors the terminal curve reflects what is generally considered distribution for other drugs. The true terminal curve for ACE inhibitors reflects slower elimination at very low, but largely non-detectable concentrations. The slower elimination occurs as receptors become unsaturated, and free drug is eliminated; as such, it must take into account both elimination from the body and the relationship between drug and receptors—that is association–dissociation interactions. Consequently, the true terminal elimination phase of ACE inhibitors is physiologically (rather than pharmacokinetically) based, being influenced by receptor numbers (total binding capacity), the affinity between drug (metabolite) and receptor, and the amount of drug available for binding.[61]

Because bound, nondetectable drug is active drug, the pharmacodynamic (biologic) half-life of the ACE inhibitor might be anticipated to be much longer than the (detectable) plasma elimination half-life. Indeed, the complex pharmacokinetic–pharmacodynamic relationship of ACE inhibitors affects the design of a dosing regimen, particularly when adjusting doses for disease. This complexity reflects several characteristics. First, for most drugs, response correlates with the time course of drug concentrations. However, for ACE inhibitors response correlates better with tissue concentrations that are not detectable. Second, saturation of tissue receptors is characterized by a lag time. Therefore the slope of the true terminal phase of the plasma elimination curve is very flat, and maximum response may not be realized for several days.[61] Third, once saturation occurs, further increases in dose are not likely to cause an increase in response. However, a very low dose (e.g., 0.03 mg/kg) might not be prudent because saturation will take longer and the maximal response may occur more slowly than with higher doses (e.g., 0.125 mg/kg). Simulation studies examining the pharmacokinetic–pharmacodynamic relationship of benzeprilat and ACE inhibition predict ACE inhibitor doses higher than 0.125 mg/kg every 24 hours will increase ACE inhibition very little,[65] a finding supported by a study of ramilprat in cats.[66] King and coworkers[67] also demonstrated that increasing doses of 0.25, 0.5, and 2 mg/kg were well tolerated in cats but did not result in a comparable increase in ACE inhibition.

KEY POINT 14-18 The complex relationship between drug and tissue receptors includes a persistent effect in the absence of detectable drug and a saturable dose–response relationship.

For ACE inhibitors, neither circulating nor tissue concentrations significantly differ after 8 days of therapy. Consequently, the pharmacodynamic response tends to exceed the time course of the metabolite by several orders of magnitude based on measured elimination half-life of the metabolite. For example, the elimination half-life of enaliprat in dogs approximates 61 minutes, compared with a predicted pharmacodynamic half-life of 17 to 19 hours.[61] For benazeprilat ACE inhibitory activity approximates 100% after multiple dosing at 0.25 mg/kg once daily and persists throughout each 24-hour dosing interval,[68] despite the fact that the plasma elimination half-life of benazepril is 1.4 hours in dogs (39 ± 6 min for benazilprilat). This is consistent with the predicted pharmacokinetic–pharmacodynamic half-life of 17 to 19 hours.[61,65] In cats receiving benazeprilat, plasma ACE was inhibited at 0.25 mg/kg, with 90% of activity persisting at 24 hours after a single dose.[65] The modeled terminal elimination half-life of the active metabolite is approximately 28 hours compared with a measured half-life of approximately 60 minutes. Finally, in Beagles ramipril and ramiprilat elimination half-lives are 0.5 and 0.75 hours, respectively,[69] with the pharmacokinetic–pharmacodynamic half-life predicted to be approximately 23 hours.[61] In cats benazeprilat is excreted predominantly (about 85%) through the bile. Plasma half-life is approximately 1 hour, but the pharmacokinetic–pharmacodynamic half-life is characterized by an elimination half-life of 28 hours following single oral dosing.[61]

Contributing to the complex pharmacokinetic–pharmacodynamic relationship will be variability among normal animals resulting from differences in disposition, in receptor number and affinity. Further, concentrations accumulate with multiple dosing up to 50% in dogs.[68,70] It is likely, however, if these differences in plasma disposition will translate to differences in pharmacodynamic response. Indeed, the pharmacokinetic–pharmacodynamic relationship between ACE and ACE inhibition is likely to mitigate differences in response among animals that reflect altered clearance because of disease, unless the disease also affects drug-receptor interaction. For example, a decrease in renal function that prolongs the half-life of an ACE inhibitor twofold is not likely to translate into a duration of effect that is twice as long. As such, benazepril (cleared predominantly by the liver) offers no advantage to enalapril (renally cleared) in the renal-compromised patient. The complex nature between pharmacokinetics and pharmacodynamics must be taken into account in studies that attempt to describe changes in response associated with disease, age, gender, drug interactions, and so forth. Such studies must address not only changes in pharmacokinetics but also the ways in which these changes influence (if at all) the physiologic response. Additionally, such studies must also address the impact of those factors on the interaction between drug and receptor (i.e., ACE), including the impact on the amount of ACE and its affinity for the drug. Finally, none of the discussion thus far has addressed the response of the body to inhibition of ACE. Because mechanisms other than ACE exist for formation of AGII, response to ACE inhibitors may decline within 24 hours after a maximum response has been realized despite maintenance of drug-receptor interactions.[61]

Dose modification in the diseased patient. Response to ACE inhibitors can be influenced by several factors. Sodium depletion in the dog shifts the ACE inhibitory mechanism of action from decreased renal AGII to enhanced kinin activity. Decreased circulating ACE associated with ACE inhibitors may correct after several days to weeks, a phenomenon referred to as *angiotensin escape*. Plasma renin activity may increase as negative feedback is lost. This effect may vary with the drug but is higher in hypertensive than in normotensive dogs.[12] However, response to therapy (perhaps muted) may continue because of inhibition at the tissue level or alternative mechanisms of action. Variability in ACE inhibitory response also may reflect genotype differences in plasma and tissue ACE concentration or receptors. Genetic polymorphism appears to influence response in humans; ACE gene polymorphism has been demonstrated in dogs.[12]

The impact of liver disease on formation of active drug has not been determined for all prodrug ACE inhibitors. However, severe liver disease does not appear to impact metabolism of benazepril to benazeprilat in dogs.[71] Dose modification in response to renal disease–induced altered drug disposition for drugs cleared by the kidney is complicated by the apparent lack of correlation of response to active drug concentration in plasma or vascular tissue.[12,61] The impact of renal failure on ACE inhibitory pharmacokinetics (drug disposition) and pharmacodynamics (drug–receptor–response interaction) has been summarized by Lefebvre and Toutain.[12] The impact on overall ACE inhibition reflects not only changes in drug concentration associated with altered clearance of drug from plasma but also distribution to tissue endothelial ACE and binding kinetics to ACE. Based on mathematical modeling in dogs with experimentally induced renal disease (GFR decreased by 50%), enapirilat clearance may decrease up to 45%, with changes in the area under the curve markedly varying from 30% to 40%. These changes are offset somewhat by decreased binding (decreased potency), such that enaliprilat inhibitory activity increased by about 65% in the first 24 hours. In contrast, neither benazeprilate nor ramiprilat response appears to be affected by renal disease in dogs.[72] Dose adjustment for benazepril is not necessary in cats with renal insufficiency.[73]

In the cat the impact of increasing the dose of ACE inhibitors may vary with the intent (e.g., hypertension versus progressive renal disease). For example, feline hypertension in patients with low or undetectable plasma renin activity and aldosterone responded poorly to enalapril at 0.25 mg/kg once daily, but the response (decreased ACE activity) doubled when a second dose was added.[74] In contrast, although benazepril was associated with a decrease in blood pressure and an increase in GFR in a surgical model of renal insufficiency, increasing the dose of benazepril (from 0.25 up to 2 mg/kg daily for 6.5 months) did not result in a proportional improvement in response in cats with chronic renal failure.[12,75] Indeed, overzealous increase in dosing may put patients at risk for initiation of neurohumoral responses that may contribute to renal dysfunction. These studies highlight the complex nature of dose–response relationship of ACE inhibitors and underscore the need for monitoring response when changing doses regardless of species or disease state.

KEY POINT 14-19 Overzealous therapy with angiotensin-converting enzyme inhibitors may activate or potentiate the very neurohumoral endocrine responses targeted with therapy.

Ramipril and ramilprilat kinetics have been studied in both dogs[72] and cats.[66] In Beagles (n=10) the elimination half-life of free drug is 11.5 ± 6.0 minutes; this increased to 14.9 ± 7.2 minutes when renal impairment was surgically induced.[72] After renal impairment, GFR was decreased by 58%. Although clearance of the free fraction of drug and metabolite was reduced, no pharmacodynamic changes occurred in renally impaired dogs, leading the authors to conclude that dose adjustment was not necessary in renal disease. In cats ramipril and its active metabolite ramiliprat have been reported after single and multiple oral dosing (0.125 to 1 mg/kg daily).[66] Peak concentrations of ramiprilat occur in 1.5 hours, and the mean elimination half-life ranged from approximately 20 to 30 hours, depending on the route. Steady-state concentrations of metabolite were present after 2 days of dosing, and food did not affect oral absorption. Although a dose-dependent effect on ACE activity was present with single dosing, after multiple dosing the maximum inhibition of ACE was the same for all doses. Detectable drug was still present 72 hours after the last dose. Inhibition was still present 24 hours after the last dose. Based on their study, the authors concluded that the elimination of the active metabolite would not be altered in patients with renal disease; a dose of 0.125 mg/kg daily was suggested as a basis for further studies.

Adverse Events

Potential adverse drug events associated with ACE inhibitors have been reviewed[12] and are largely limited, in dogs and cats, to the sequalae of hypotension (previously discussed) and to nephropathies induced by pharmacodynamic response to the drugs. In general, the risk is more likely in patients also receiving diuretics or in the face of impaired renal function. However, acute hypotension is a risk as therapy is begun, particularly in renin-dependent (sodium-depleted) patients. Clinical signs indicative of hypotension may include fatigue and apathy. Increased dietary salt or decreased diuretic therapy may be indicated initially as ACE inhibitor therapy is begun. Acute renal failure may occur as a result of altered renal perfusion. The RAAS, and particularly AGII, is the principal autoregulatory mechanism that maintains renal perfusion in the presence of low arterial pressures. In the kidney, angiotensin regulates both renal blood flow and GFR by modulating constriction of the postglomerular efferent arteriole in the presence of reduced GFR. In addition, tubular sodium is reabsorbed, and renin release is inhibited. Inhibition of ACE and AGII precludes constriction of the postglomerular efferent arteriole (Figure 14-7).[76] As ACE inhibitor therapy is begun, total peripheral vascular resistance, renal vasoconstriction, and renal perfusion pressure decrease. Net glomerular filtration decreases in concert with decreased glomerular hydrostatic pressure. Decreased glomerular filtration after ACE inhibitor therapy is more likely to occur in the presence of excessive vasodilation, moderate to severe volume depletion, or minimal myocardial reserve. In patients with mild to moderate cardiac dysfunction, renal filtration generally is maintained despite initiation of ACE inhibitor therapy as long as afterload is decreased such that cardiac output (and thus GFR) can increase. As heart failure progresses, the risk of acute renal decompensation increases because reflex efferent arteriolar tone becomes increasingly important to the maintenance of glomerular filtration in these patients. All ACE inhibitors are equally likely to have a negative impact on renal function in patients at risk. This includes benazepril, for which clearance depends on liver metabolism.

KEY POINT 14-20 Renal adverse events associated with angiotensin-converting enzyme inhibitors are more likely if renal autoregulation is impaired by drug or disease.

Initial acute ACE inhibitor treatment of at-risk patients can decrease both creatinine clearance and GFR. Assuming that renal damage is not irreversible, however, chronic treatment generally causes GFR to return to baseline levels. An initial increase in serum urea nitrogen and creatinine associated with initiation of therapy may actually indicate a positive renal response; in human patients an increase from baseline of up to 30% in serum creatinine is acceptable as long as the GFR remains above the minimum of 20 mL/min. However, GFR is not routinely measured in animals and an "acceptable" increase in GFR has not been established. Accordingly, an increase in either serum urea nitrogen or creatinine concentrations may indicate the need to decrease or temporarily discontinue therapy in dogs and cats. Although deterioration of renal function associated with ACE inhibitor therapy is generally reversible if therapy is discontinued, damage may become irreversible if decreased GFR persists. Therapy is contraindicated with preexisting hypotension, hypovolemia, hyponatremia, and acute renal failure. ACE inhibition may potentiate hypotensive episodes in surgical patients. However, withdrawal of therapy to prevent hypotension should be reconsidered in patients receiving ACE inhibitors for treatment of hypertension. Should it occur, hypotension can respond to fluid therapy, and as such, ACE inhibition probably should be continued up to the surgical procedure. Sodium depletion can

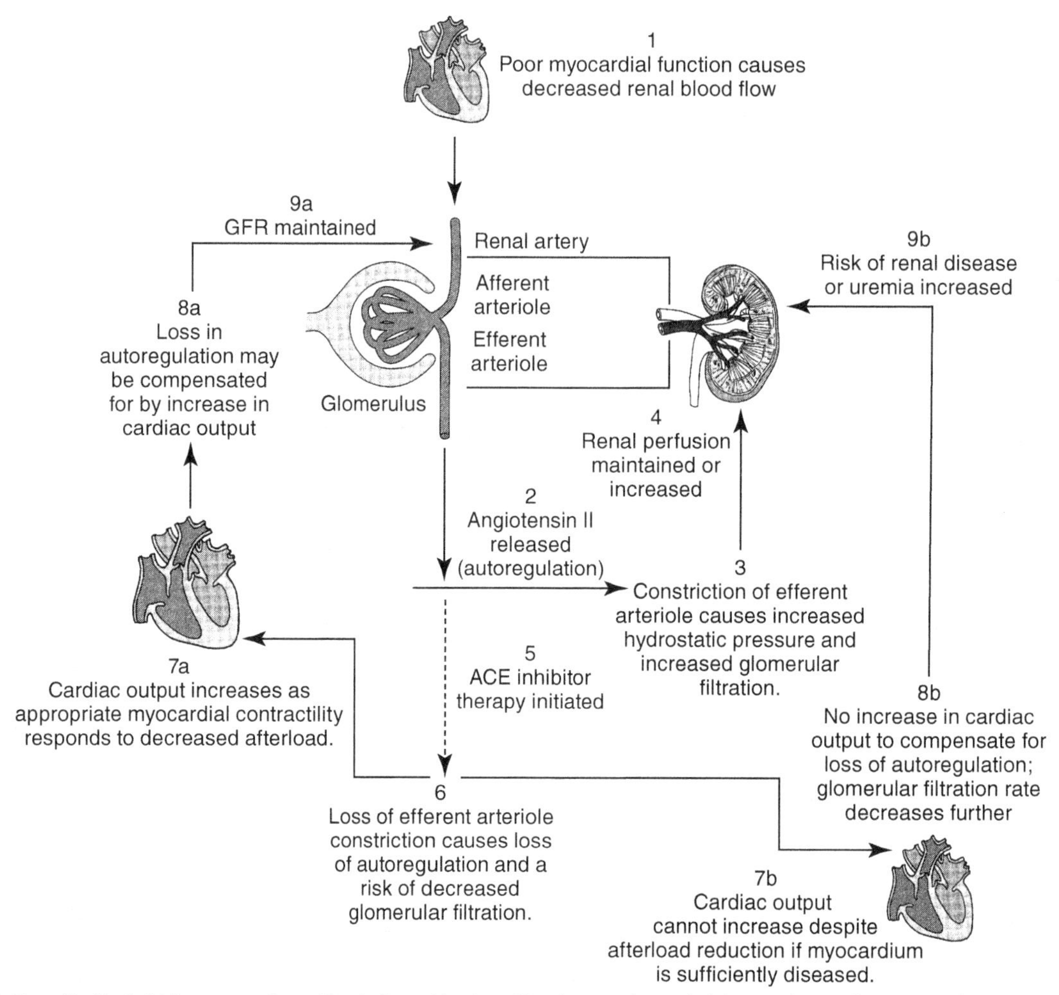

Figure 14-7 Despite their kidney-sparing effects in patients with glomerulonephritis, angiotensin-converting enzyme (ACE) inhibitors may contribute to renal disease in patients whose renal blood flow is threatened. In such patients maintenance of glomerular filtration may depend on increased efferent arteriolar tone (vasoconstriction). Use of ACE inhibitors reduces this tone. In patients whose cardiac function is sufficient (including those that respond to decreased afterload), increased cardiac output can compensate for decreased efferent arteriolar tone, thus maintaining glomerular filtration rate. In patients that are sodium depleted or have severe myocardial dysfunction, glomerular filtration rate may decline. *Dashed line,* inhibited.

activate the RAAS in normal dogs and cats. Experimentally, the use of ACE inhibitors and the subsequent loss of renal autoregulation in the presence of sodium restriction is accompanied by a decrease in renal blood flow, GFR, and filtration fraction. Accordingly, the use of ACE inhibitors in the presence of a low-sodium diet should be accompanied by frequent monitoring of renal function, particularly in patients predisposed to renal dysfunction.

The BENCH (BENazepril in Canine Heart Disease) study group reported the long-term tolerability of benazepril in dogs with CHF.[77] Although the authors found plasma creatinine concentrations to be lower in the benazepril group than in the placebo group, a significant difference could not be demonstrated. However, serum creatinine levels tended to be higher than normal more often in the placebo group, leading the investigators to suggest that improved renal function was associated with benazepril. No abnormalities in electrolytes were associated with benazepril.

Although aldosterone production is impaired in the presence of ACE inhibitor therapy, hyperkalemia is unlikely even in the presence of high-potassium diets, unless the patient is otherwise predisposed to potassium retention. Potassium monitoring might be indicated in the presence of dietary sodium restriction[78] or when combined with potassium-sparing diuretics such as spironolactone. Because the impact of aldosterone on sodium retention and potassium excretion is muted, the combination of ACE inhibitors with potassium-wasting diuretics decreases the risk of hypokalemia.[78] The impact of ACE inhibitor therapy on erythropoiesis associated with renal disease is unclear, but studies suggest renal erythropoietin production probably will not normalize in response to ACE inhibitor therapy. As such, supplementation may be indicated.

The ACE inhibitors reportedly cause a dry cough in up to 20% of human, particularly female, patients. Onset ranges from 1 to 26 weeks of therapy, with clinical signs resolving within the first week of discontinuing therapy. The mechanism may reflect accumulation of pulmonary bradykinin or prostaglandins; interestingly, treatment with aspirin has reduced cough, suggesting a possible role for prostaglandins.[18]

Despite their ability to decrease proteinuria (discussed at more length later in this chapter), ACE inhibitors have been associated with the advent of proteinuria in human patients. Therapy need not be discontinued if it develops. Therapy also has been associated with skin rashes and angioedema. The latter is not dose related and generally occurs soon after dosing, within the first week of therapy.[18] Neutropenia, glycosuria, and hepatotoxicity are rare side effects reported in humans.

The ACE inhibitors should not be used in pregnant animals. In human women therapy in the first trimester appears to be safe but results in multiple fetopathologies (potentially related to fetal hypotension) when administered in the second and third trimester.

Drug Interactions

Lefebvre and Toutain[12] reviewed the literature addressing clinically relevant adverse reactions that might reflect interactions between ACE inhibitors and simultaneously administered drugs. Because AGII and aldosterone synthesis can occur in the absence of ACE, drugs that contribute to hypotension, sodium loss, or alteration of renal autoregulation should be avoided or used cautiously in patients receiving ACE inhibitors. The risks of combining ACE inhibitors and diuretics on renal dysfunction have been documented in humans and dogs. AGII and aldosterone may increase, despite the administration of furosemide in patients receiving ACE inhibitors. Further, the diuretic effect can decrease proportionately with GFR when combined with ACE inhibitors. However, the combined use of ACE inhibitors and sodium-wasting diuretics, and specifically furosemide, decreases the risk of hypokalemia.[78] The impact of combined use of nonsteroidal antiinflammatory drugs (NSAIDs) and ACE inhibitors is less clear. Although presumably, NSAIDs that minimize cyclooxygenase-(COX-) 1 inhibition are less likely to be associated with nephropathy, in human patients the risk is equivalent when either traditional or newer NSAIDs are used. A number of studies have investigated the sequelae of combined NSAID and ACE inhibitor therapy in normal dogs and dogs with experimentally induced decreased renal function. In general, no significant detrimental impact on renal function has been reported. However, this should not be interpreted as proof of no effect, and the combined use should be avoided or undertaken cautiously, with additional attention to monitoring of renal function. Note that NSAIDs may attenuate antihypertensive actions of ACE inhibitors, although the impact may be less with those drugs that target principally COX-2. ACE inhibitors may increase the risk of nephrotoxocitiy induced by other agents, including contrast dye.[79]

The combination of ACE inhibitors with angiotensin receptor blockers (ARBs) might be considered for a beneficial therapeutic effect. However, a meta-analysis that studied the combined use of ACE inhibitors and ARBs found the addition of an ARB to ACE inhibitor therapy was not associated with a reduced mortality rate compared with ACE inhibitor treatment alone. The addition of an ARB did not affect exercise capacity, functional capacity, and quality of life. Of the outcome measures studied, only the rate of hospitalization was reduced with the combination of therapy.[80]

Beta blockers normalize β-receptor signaling and antagonize cytotoxic effects of circulating catecholamines, which increased with heart failure.[80] Additionally, β blockers may also directly block AGII-mediated pathways. As such, β blocker therapy combined with ARBs and ACE inhibitors theoretically might completely remove the effects of angiotensin in cardiac patients. However, results of clinical trials regarding use of the combination in humans are controversial. A meta-analysis found that, compared with ACE inhibitors alone, the combination did not improve survival rates, although hospital stays did shorten.[80] Further, subgroup analysis suggested that the addition of ARBs is redundant and combined use of ARBs with ACE inhibitors and β blockers potentially puts the patient at an increased risk of adverse drug events. A subsequent study using the ARB candesartan demonstrated that when it was combined with β blockers in patients also taking ACE inhibitors, it does tend to increase the risk of adverse events.[81]

Hypotension has been reported with the combined use of the β blocker atenolol, the ACE inhibitor quinapril, and an overdose of the selective serotonin reuptake inhibitor fluvoxamine, treatment with aminophylline was successful.[82]

Other reported drug interactions include decreased drug absorption when combined with antacids, although the clinical relevance of this finding in light of the relationship between plasma drug concentrations and responses is questionable.

Clinical Use in Canine Patients with Myocardial Disease

The role of ACE inhibitors in general for treatment of CHF associated with myocardial failure in dogs has been well established, with use emerging as part of cornerstone therapy. However, the timing of administration in the progression of diseases remains to be fully defined. The most extensively studied of the ACE inhibitors is enalapril, although captopril, benazepril, and lisinopril have also been studied. More recently, ramipril is being studied in dogs and cats. Captopril, the efficacy of which was demonstrated in an experimental model of canine mitral regurgitation (see BENCH study group)[83] was the first generally accepted ACE inhibitor to be used in dogs and cats. Captopril can induce positive hemodynamic effects within 1 hour of therapy, although the effects are short lived (4 hours).[84] Its short half-life led to dosing at 8-hour intervals. Subsequently, the safety and efficacy of quinipril were demonstrated when administered once daily (0.5 mg/kg) compared with captopril (0.5 mg/kg every 8 hours or 24 hours, respectively) in dogs (n=92) with CHF.[85]

Enalapril administered at 12-hour dosing intervals was also demonstrated to be of benefit in dogs with experimentally induced heart failure. The first placebo-controlled study demonstrating efficacy of ACE inhibitors in dogs with spontaneous myocardial disease (dilated cardiomyopathy [DCM] or mitral regurgitation) was the Cooperative Veterinary Enalapril (COVE) Study.[86] This multicenter study involving 211 dogs demonstrated that enalapril therapy (for 28 days) was associated with improved longevity and quality of life.[86] The IMPROVE[87] study group reported in the same issue that enalapril (0.5 mg/kg twice daily) was associated with lower heart rate and mean systemic and pulmonary arterial pressures in dogs (35 with DCM, 22 with mitral regurgitation) compared with dogs in the placebo group. Dogs continued to receive traditional therapies (i.e., digoxin or diuretic). Ettinger and coworkers[88] subsequently established the beneficial effects of enalapril for dogs (n=110; 15 locations throughout the United States) with either DCM or other chronic acquired heart disease (primarily mitral insufficiency). Although the study was not well controlled for stage of disease or differences in conventional therapy, results supported the importance of ACE inhibition in improving the quality of life and, particularly in dogs with DCM, prolonging life. The mean time to treatment failure (including treatment with traditional cardiovascular drugs) increased from 77 days in the placebo group to 156 days in the enalapril-treated group. Although more dogs died suddenly in the enalapril treatment group, all but one had preexisting ventricular arrhythmias for which they were receiving antiarrhythmic therapy. The BENCH study group[83] focused on long-term survival afforded by the addition of benazepril to dogs (n=162) with class (International Small Animal Cardiac Health Council [ISACHC]) II or III heart failure associated with chronic valvular disease (n=125) or DCM (n=37). This prospective, randomized, placebo-controlled, double-blinded European study was multicenter (n=16) and multicountry (n=4). It studied benazepril (0.25 mg/kg once daily) as either sole therapy or as an add-to traditional therapy for up to 34 months. Mean survival significantly improved from 158 days in the placebo group to 428 days in the treatment group. Survival rates at 1 year were 20% and 49%, respectively, for the two groups. High-risk dogs had not been removed from the study group, suggesting that survival would improve in less severely afflicted animals. The risk of progression to a worsening class of heart failure was also reduced, whereas quality of life measures were improved in the benazepril group. Benefits could also be demonstrated in subgroup analysis for those dogs with cardiovascular disease, but not the smaller sample of dogs afflicted with DCM. Adverse events to benazepril were slightly less (not statistically so) than to placebo.

KEY POINT 14-21 Evidence of clinical efficacy of angiotensin-converting enzyme inhibitors is provided among clinical trials based on improved quality of life, improved survival, and objective measures of cardiac function.

Pouchelon and coworkers[89] retrospectively addressed the efficacy of benazpril in dogs with Class II and III CHF (n=141). Dog were classified as untreated if they did not receive benazepril before the appearance of clinical signs of CHF; these dogs served as controls. For the treated dogs, the mean dose was 0.3 ± 0.13 mg/kg. Median survival times were greater (3.3 years) in the treatment group (n=34) compared with untreated dogs (1.9 years, n=59 dogs) for all breeds except Cavalier King Charles Spaniels.

Controversy still exists regarding when ACE inhibitor therapy should be initiated in the patient with CHF, if and when it is the preferred vasodilator, and its position in the sequence of drugs. For humans, ACE inhibitors are indicated for any patient with left ventricular systolic dysfunction even in the absence of clinical signs of overt cardiac failure.[64] Studies in humans suggest that inhibition of ACE in patients with systolic dysfunction can prevent or delay the progression of heart failure, decrease the incidence of sudden death, and improve the quality of life.[64] Although treatment plans have been offered for enalapril, based on severity of disease,[88] the importance that ACE inhibitors may have in attenuating myocardial remodeling and the need for early intervention may supersede treatment plans based on severity.

KEY POINT 14-22 The timing of initiation of angiotensin-converting enzyme inhibitor therapy in relation to other drugs remains controversial.

To minimize negative sequelae of afterload reduction, particularly that leading to activation of the RAAS, treatment with enalapril or other ACE inhibitors might be initiated at a lower dose[90] (see Table 14-3) with increased increments at weekly intervals until clinical signs indicate improvement or further increases cannot be tolerated. Renal function should be monitored weekly for the first month of therapy in patients predisposed to adverse renal effects.

The role of ACE inhibitors in cats with hypertrophic cardiomyopathy (HCM) is not clear. However, using an experimental feline banding model of pressure-overload left ventricular hypertrophy, 4 weeks of enalapril (0.5 mg/kg orally once daily) was associated with less intraventricular septum and free-wall diastolic thickness as well as decreased arterial (systolic and mean) pressure compared with placebo. Renal function and other physiologic parameters did not differ between placebo and treatment groups.[91]

ANGIOTENSIN-CONVERTING ENZYME INHIBITORS AND TREATMENT OF PROGRESSIVE RENAL DISEASE

The use of ACE inhibitors for the treatment and attenuation of progressive renal disease in humans and animals has been well reviewed.[12] The evidence of efficacy is not clear, but therapy is generally accepted as beneficial. It is likely that a combination of therapies will be most beneficial.[92] ACE inhibitors have repeatedly been demonstrated to provide superior renoprotective effects in patients with renal disease compared with other vasoactive drugs.[93] The potential application of ACE inhibitors for this indication emerged as early as 1985, following a demonstrable beneficial effect on proteinuria and accompanying renal damage in a rat model of renal failure. Potential application to a variety of human renal diseases was demonstrated over the next decades, with use in animals lagging not far behind. A meta-analysis[94] of clinical trials in humans with hypertension found a small benefit, probably reflecting reduction in blood pressure.

This study was met with controversy, indicating that the role of ACE inhibitors in progressive renal disease has yet to be clearly defined. Benefits demonstrated in dogs and cats have resulted in the approval of benazepril in Europe and Australia for treatment of chronic progressive renal diseases in animals.

ACE inhibitors have three potential positive effects in the patient with renal disease: control of systemic and glomerular capillary hypertension, delayed progression of glomerulosclerosis and tubulointerstitial disease, and decreased proteinuria.[12] In humans control of the progression of renal disease depends on control of systemic hypertension but this is not necessarily the mechanism whereby ACE inhibitors impart renoprotection. Systemic hypertension may accompany chronic renal disease in 50% to 93% of dogs and cats, and a similar dependency might be expected in animals. Hyperperfusion and hypertension accompanying renal diseases initially enhances the filtration capacity of remaining nephrons. However, this compensation for nephron loss occurs at a cost. AGII-mediated hypertension leads to distention of the glomerular capillary and mechanical strain on the glomerular mesangial cell. Podocyte coverage becomes inadequate, changing the size exclusion of the glomerulus such that permeability is increased. The exposed mesangial cells stimulate extracellular matrix proliferation and release of proinflammatory cytokines. Inflammatory and other proteins are increasingly filtered through the damaged glomerulus. The protein is toxic to tubular epithelials cells and stimulates further cytokine release. Included is transforming growth factor-β, which stimulates excessive renal deposition of extracellular matrix in both the glomerulus and tubulointerstitium. Persistent inflammation mediated by AGII leads to glomerular and tubulointerstitial fibrosis, a characteristic of end-state renal disease.[12]

In humans and experimental models, ACE inhibitors have demonstrated renoprotection in selected states of nephrotoxicosis associated with renal vascular hypertension. Examples include experimentally induced cyclosporine nephrotoxicity,[95] in which ACE inhibitors decrease renal vascular resistance, increase GFR, and promote diuresis in experimentally induced doxorubicin nephprotoxicity.[96] Beneficial effects of ACE inhibitors include decreased deposition of extracellular matrix. The effects of ACE inhibitors have been demonstrated in humans to be greater if therapy is begun early in a variety of renal diseases, with polycystic renal disease being the sole disease thus far that has not responded to therapy.[12]

KEY POINT 14-23 Efficacy of angiotensin-converting enzyme inhibitor therapy for progressive renal disease in dogs or cats depends on use early in disease.

In dogs a variety of studies have attempted to demonstrate renoprotective effects of ACE inhibitors. Studies in dogs have predominantly involved enalapril, whereas benazepril has been the drug of choice for cats for reasons that are not clear other than approval status of the drugs in the country of origin of each study. Results varied with the disease, the model (including experimental versus spontaneous nephropathies), and doses studied (enalapril at 0.5 mg/kg every 24 hours to 2 mg/kg every 12 hours). Outcome measures generally include objective measures such as azotemia, renal plasma flow, GFR, survival rates, weight gain or loss, and histopathology or more subjective measures such as appetite. In a canine experimental model, differences were limited to fewer histologic lesions after 6 months of treatment (1 mg/kg every 12 hours for 2 weeks followed by 0.5 mg/kg every 12 hours) compared with untreated controls. A controlled study in X-linked hereditary nephritis in Samoyeds demonstrated increased survival time in treated dogs (enalapril at 2 mg/kg every 12 hours from 4 weeks of age); therapy was begun before proteinuria could be detected. In the treatment group increased serum creatinine was delayed in onset and progression was slowed, although the magnitude of azotemia did not change. The life span of afflicted dogs increased 36%,[97] an outcome measure that must be considered in the context of studies that found up to 53% increased survival time in dogs receiving a modified diet.[98] In a third study, a difference in serum creatinine level could not be detected in untreated dogs versus enalapril-treated (0.5 mg/kg every 12 to 24 hours) dogs with spontaneous idiopathic renal disease. However, this lack of a difference probably reflected the small number of animals studied because serum creatitine levels had not increased more than 0.2 mg/dL in 13 of 16 treated dogs compared with 1 of 14 untreated dogs by the end of the 6-month study period.[99]

In cats benazepril has proved effective for treatment of hypertension associated with experimental feline renal disease[75] and cats with HCM.[100,100a] Cats with experimentally induced chronic renal failure responded to benazepril (0.5 to 2 mg/kg once daily), although serum creatinine levels did not differ from those of the control group.[75] In cats with polycystic renal disease, enalapril-treated (0.5 mg/kg once daily) cats had less azotemia compared with untreated cats, although GFR did not differ.[101] Although the potential efficacy of ACE inhibition for treatment of progressive renal disease may be less clear in cats than in dogs, sufficient evidence exists to warrant its consideration as early in the disease as possible.

ANGIOTENSIN-CONVERTING ENZYME INHIBITORS AND TREATMENT OF PROTEINURIA

Among the specific renal indications of ACE inhibitors is proteinuria. Proteinuria appears to be correlated with renal disease, so much so that it is a marker of the progression of disease. Decreased proteinuria can be correlated with improved renal function, perhaps by preventing the inflammatory effects of protein in the tubule. Proteinuria is a demonstrated risk factor for the progression of chronic renal failure in cats.[102]

In humans, ACE inhibitors are considered superior to other vasoactive drugs in decreasing proteinuria, although the mechanism still is not understood and may depend on the cause of proteinuria. Use as part of combination therapy is likely to be the key.[103] The mechanism may reflect maintenance of podocyte function in the face of glomerular hypertension; ACE inhibitors decrease podocyte hypertrophy. Reduced filtration pressure has been demonstrated in cats with experimental chronic renal disease.[102] Whether control of systemic hypertension is sufficient to control podocyte function has yet to be demonstrated; additional direct effects on podocytes or mesangial cells may occur. Regardless of the mechanism, renal function improves in concert with reduction of proteinuria in human patients. Reduction of proteinuria appears to be dose dependent, occurs rapidly, and remains drug dependent in that proteinuria will recur once the drug is discontinued.

Response of canine proteinuria to ACE inhibitors is variable, but again this may reflect limitations in study design. Finco and coworkers[104] were not able to demonstrate a renoprotective effect caused by decreased proteinuria in experimental renal disease in dogs.[104] However, in another experimental model of renal failure, the urine protein to creatinine ratio was lowered in dogs receiving enalapril (0.5 mg/kg every 12 hours) for 6 months.[105] In a prospective, blinded study of dogs with spontaneous glomerulonephritis, enalapril (0.5 mg/kg) twice daily (but not once daily) reduced the urinary protein to creatinine ratio to less than 50% of baseline, although response required 1 to 3 months. The ratio decreased by 4.2 in treated dogs, compared with a 1.9 increase in placebo-treated dogs.[99] In cats benazepril also has proved effective for treatment of proteinuria associated with spontaneous renal diseases.[106]

Mizutani and coworkers[107] prospectively studied the effect of benazepril (0.5 to 1 mg/kg) in cats (n=61) with chronic renal disease using a randomized, placebo, double-blinded parallel design. Cats were studied for up to 6 months. The urine protein to creatinine ratio was reduced in benazapril-treated cats; further, fewer cats progressed to stage 4 renal disease in the treatment group compared with the placebo group. Using a randomized, double-blinded parallel design, King and coworkers[102] also prospectively studied the impact of benazepril (0.5-1 mg/kg daily) in cats (n=192; 96 treatment and placebo control each) with chronic renal disease (creatinine ≥ 2 mg/dL; urine specific gravity ≤ 1.025). Cats were treated for up to 1119 days. Proteinuria was significantly reduced based on the urine protein to creatinine ratio. Response was present at the first posttreatment sampling time (7 days) and was greatest in those with the highest ratios, although response was significant also in cats with low ratios ($p \leq 0.02$). Survival time (which was inversely related to initial urine protein to creatinine ratio in the placebo group) did not differ between placebo and treatment groups (637 ± 480 for benazepril; 520 ± 323 placebo), although variability was marked for both treatment groups, limiting the power to detect a significant difference. Quality of life also did not differ between groups, although appetite improved more in treated cats with initial urine protein to creatinine ratio of 1 or higher. Therapy was well tolerated. Adverse events did not differ between treatment groups; creatinine concentrations did not differ between the groups, including as therapy began.

Angiotensin II Receptor Antagonists

The development of losartan, the first approved AGII receptor antagonist (ARA), represents a concerted pharmaceutical development endeavor to design a drug based on the core structure of the pharmacologic target. Currently, seven ARA drugs have been approved in the United States. Although each is devoid of agonistic activity, only very minor molecular changes can render the drugs as potent agonists.[18] Generally, ARA receptors have a 10,000-fold greater affinity for AR-1 compared with AR-2 receptors. Potency varies among drugs, with candesartan being most and losartan being least potent for AR-1 blockade. However, losartan is metabolized to an active, more potent compound. Blockade of AR-1 is competitive, but inhibition of AGII response is described as insurmountable, perhaps because of the slow release of drug from the receptor.[18] Regardless of the mechanism, maximal response to AGII is attenuated; blockade is effective despite increased concentrations of AGII or missed doses. Blockade generally attenuates most biologic effects of AGII. This includes peripheral vasoconstriction, pressor response (rapid and slow), the release of vasopressin, adrenal catecholamines or aldosterone, the advent of thirst, altered renal function, cellular hypertrophy, and hyperplasia.[18]

In humans oral bioavailability of the various ARA products is generally less than 50%, and protein binding is greater than 90%. Hepatic metabolism varies among the drugs: candesartan and olmesartan are prodrugs, losartan (14%) is metabolized (CYP2C9 and 3A4) to a metabolite more potent than the parent compound, and several others are metabolized to inactive metabolites. The half-life is variable among drugs, ranging from 2.5 hours for losartan (6-9 hours for its active metabolite) to 24 hours for telmisartan. Losartan is excreted both renally and by hepatic metabolism, with liver, but not renal, disease affecting disposition. Losartan is a competitive antagonist of thromboxane A2 and impairs platelet aggregations.[18]

The pharmacokinetics of ARAs have not been well established in dogs and cats. Several studies in dogs reflect preclinical studies for human products. Limited pharmacokinetic and pharmacodynamic data of losartan potassium were reported in dogs after oral administration of 5 to 20 mg/kg.[107a] Oral bioavailability ranged from 22% to 33%. The elimination half-life approximated 2 to 2.5 hours after oral administration but only 40 minutes after intravenous administration. The volume of distribution of 0.3 L/kg suggested limited tissue distribution; the drug is very highly (>95%) bound to plasma proteins. Clearance approximated hepatic blood flow; the proportion of drug converted to the active metabolite was not measured. Maximum drug concentration was dose dependent, with a low of 0.8 ± 4 μg/mL at 5 mg/kg to 2.9±1.6 at 20 mg/kg. Pharmacodynamically, an unbound plasma drug concentration of 3 ng/mL (total drug of 96 ng/mL) was determined to the 50th percentile concentration needed to block a pressor response. This concentration was almost achieved at the lowest oral dose of 5 mg/kg, suggesting a dose between 5 and 10 mg/kg. Irbesartan has been studied in dogs alone or in combination with hydrochlorthiazide.[107b] Dogs were treated with 30 mg/kg once daily for 8 days. Maximum drug concentrations at day 8 were 4.3±1.0 μg/mL, with an elimination half-life of 21±3.7 hours. Although pharmacodynamic response did not relate well with plasma drug concentrations, the effective concentration (EC_{50}) associated with decreasing systemic or diastolic blood pressure was 3.3 ± 0.4 μg/mL, potentially supporting a dose of 30 mg/kg once daily. A lag time to efficacy of several days would be expected.

Indications for ARA treatment in humans include hypertension, diabetic nephropathy, stroke prophylaxis, and heart failure in patients intolerant to ACE inhibition. It is not clear whether antagonism of AGII receptors is more efficacious than therapy with ACE inhibitors. Compared with ACE inhibitors, ARAs differ in their impact on the RAAS in several aspects. Because non-ACE alternative pathways exist for generation of AGII, ACE inhibitors cannot completely attenuate its effects. In contrast, ARAs will effectively block all AGII effects. However, AGII receptors can still be activated. Because ARAs will result in a several-fold increase in renin, AGII concentrations will increase. Finally, inhibition of ACE also results in the inhibition of other pathways; this effect will not occur with ARAs, resulting in persistence of substrates (e.g., bradykinin, Ac-SDKP). Losartan has proved comparable in efficacy to enalapril, but efficacy compared with captopril was variable among studies. In human medicine, ACE inhibitors remain the first-line drugs of choice, with ARAs reserved for nonresponders. The combined use of ACE inhibitors and ARAs is controversial and requires further study.[18] The ARAs have also been used alone or in combination with ACE inhibitors or amlodipine to treat proteinuria.

Arterial and Venous Dilators

Organic Nitrates

Organic nitrates activate cGMP, which ultimately decreases actin and myosin interaction, leading to relaxation of vascular smooth muscle and arterial and venous dilation (see Figure 14-4). At low concentrations venodilation predominates, and net systemic vascular resistance is usually not affected. Coronary vessels are directly dilated. Pharmacologic effects occur rapidly. First-pass metabolism precludes oral administration of nitrates; therapeutic routes include intravenous, sublingual, and topical (transdermal ointment).

Nitroglycerin is a member of the organic nitrate group. Although all vascular smooth muscle might be relaxed, the dose of nitroglycerin administered causes predominantly venous dilation and preload reduction. Pulmonary and systemic congestion and myocardial workload are reduced.[108] Nitroglycerin is available for intravenous and sublingual use and as an ointment. The 2% ointment form has been the most commonly used preparation in veterinary medicine. It can be applied to the hairless portion of an animal's skin (abdomen or ear). Gloves should be used by the caregiver to avoid percutaneous absorption of drug. The clinical indication for use is limited to acute (emergency) treatment of CHF.

Sodium Nitroprusside

Nitroprusside (see Figure 14-6)[9] contains cyanide, which oxidizes intracellular sulfhydryl groups to produce methemoglobin; NO is simultaneously released. Activation of cGMP causes vasodilation (see Figure 14-3). The NO system that activates nitroglycerin is different from that activating nitroprusside, accounting for differences in vascular beds targeted by each drug.[9] Both arterioles and venules are dilated by nitroprusside; systemic and pulmonary vasculatures are targeted. Nitroprusside is one of the most potent vasodilators available. The advantages of nitroprusside over other vasodilator drugs include its potency, its effect in both preload and afterload reduction, immediate hemodynamic effects, extremely short half-life, and low cost. Nitroprusside must be administered by constant intravenous (IV) infusion using an infusion pump; the potential for hypotension necessitates close monitoring. Free cyanide released during intracellular metabolism is cleared in part by transulfation of thiosulfate yielding thiocyanate, which itself is potentially toxic. Overdosing of nitroprusside may yield excessive cyanide, causing severe lactic acidosis; the risk is increased in patients with liver disease or those receiving diuretics (decreased thiosulfate stores). Co-administration of sodium thiosulfate may be indicated in at-risk patients. Clearance of the toxic end product, thiocyanate, may be decreased in patients with renal disease, particularly if infusion continues beyond 24 to 48 hours. Monitoring of thiocyanate should be considered in at-risk patients; concentrations should not exceed 0.1 mg/mL.[9] Feline hemoglobin may be predisposed to oxidation and methemoglobin formation. The primary indication of sodium nitroprusside is treatment of severe (catastrophic) CHF. Nitroprusside is administered as a constant-rate infusion using a dedicated line and an infusion pump (1-10 μg/kg/min, starting at 1 μg/kg/min in dogs and 0.5 μg/kg/min in cats; increasing 0.5-1 μg/kg/min every 5 minutes to maintain systolic pressure at 90-1000 mm Hg). Nitroprusside is inherently unstable and will decompose under alkaline conditions and with exposure to light.

Prazosin

Prazosin is an α-adrenergic receptor blocker. However, it also is a venous dilator (perhaps owing to inhibition of cAMP) and thus might be considered as both a preload and an afterload reducer. Despite significant first-pass metabolism in humans, prazosin is effective after oral administration. Prazosin is an effective antihypertensive agent. However, tolerance develops rapidly. It is more effective when used in combination with other drugs. Clinical use of prazosin is limited because hydralazine affords a much better reduction in peripheral resistance and increase in cardiac output.

Phosphodiesterase Inhibitors

Several selective inhibitors of phosphodiesterase (PDE) V have been approved for treatment of penile erectile dysfunction in humans. These include sildenafil (Viagra), tadalafil (Cialis), and vardenafil (Levitra). In contrast to most other PDE inhibitors, PDE V inhibits breakdown of cGMP. Subsequent release of NO in nerve terminals of endothelial cells causes smooth muscle relaxation and increased blood flow. PDE V is located in corpus cavernosum smooth muscle, vascular and visceral smooth muscle, skeletal muscle, platelets, kidney, lung, cerebellum, and pancreas. Potency of tadalafil with PDE V is more than 9000-fold compared with that of other PDE isoforms except for PDE VI (retina) and PDE XI (in skeletal muscle), for which potency is 700- or 14-fold greater, respectively, indicating a relative selectivity for PDE V. Disposition of tadalafil in humans is characterized by oral absorption that is not impaired by food (bioavailability not reported on package insert), greater than 90% binding to plasma proteins, and a volume of distribution approximating 1 L/kg. In humans tadalafil is metabolized by CYP 3A4 to inactive catechols. In humans the elimination half-life is 17 hours. Drug interactions caused by inhibition or induction of CYP 3A4 may result in clinically relevant adverse drug events. For example, the dosing interval is prolonged from 12 hours to 72 hours in humans concomitantly receiving imidazole antifungals or other inhibitors of CYP 3A4. Despite hepatic metabolism, renal insufficiency may increase area under the curve and C_{max} twofold to fourfold, whereas moderate hepatic disease does not appear to affect disposition. Although systemic hypotension is not a common side effect of tadalafil, PDE V inhibitors in general potentiate nitrate-induced hypotension and co-administration is contraindicated. Care is indicated when combined with α-blocker therapy. Visual disturbances in humans reflect temporary impairment of color vision, reflecting inhibition of PDE VI in the retina. The PDE V inhibitors have been used with variable success to treat pulmonary hypertension in dogs.

KEY POINT 14-24 Selectivity of phosphodiesterase inhibitors reflects specificity for different enzymes and the presence of specific enzymes in different tissues.

ANTIARRHYTHMIC DRUGS

Cardiac Arrhythmias

Underlying molecular causes of arrhythmias have been reviewed in humans.[1] Arrhythmias result from a combination of factors, including genetic predisposition, external stressors and subsequent myocardial remodeling, as well as iatrogenic contributions. Ischemia, electrolyte imbalances, activation of the RAAS and other systems, and pharmacologic therapy are among the triggers for arrhythmias.[1] Inherited causes of arrhythmias are rare, but generally pathophysiology is straightforward, particularly if associated with mutations in ion channel genes. In contrast, arrhythmias associated with acquired heart disease are complex. Structural and electrical remodeling, hemodynamic changes, and neuroendocrine signals each influence ion channel function, intracellular calcium response, and intercellular communication and matrix composition.

Regardless of the source, all cardiac arrhythmias arise from two primary abnormalities: impulse initiation, which includes spontaneous automaticity and triggered activity, and impulse propagation—that is, conduction (generally manifested as reentrant arrhythmias). Impulse initiation establishes heart rate and is determined primarily by the rate of diastolic depolarization—that is, the slope of phase 4. In the normal heart the slope (heart rate) is autonomically controlled, being decreased by acetylcholine released from parasympathetic nerves and increased by norepinephrine released from the adrenal cortex. Stroke volume decrementally decreases as heart rate increases; accordingly, cardiac output may ultimately decrease with faster rates. The slope of phase 4 can be affected by a number of abnormal conditions. Enhanced automaticity occurs when the rate of spontaneous diastolic depolarization increases sufficiently to allow emergence of pathologically slowed or increased rates (e.g., sinus tachycardia). Ectopic foci (pacemakers that normally are latent) may emerge and may cause tachycardia if the frequency exceeds that of the sinoatrial node. Arrhythmias of initiation may also be triggered by an abnormal depolarization (phase 0), resulting in secondary upstrokes in the action potential. Two types of triggered arrhythmias occur. Delayed after-depolarization (DAD) occurs after a normal action potential and is followed by an overload of intracellular calcium. Examples include arrhythmias associated with myocardial failure, myocardial ischemia, adrenergic stress, and digoxin toxicity. Early after-depolarization (EAD) upstrokes occur during phase 3 repolarization and follow abnormally long cardiac action potentials. They generally result from abnormal inward sodium or calcium channel currents or exchange pumps and are associated with very slow heart rates or low extracellular K^+ or in association with drugs that cause prolonged action potential duration.

KEY POINT 14-25 Arrhythmias reflect altered impulse initiation (automaticity) or impulse propagation (conduction).

Drugs that decrease automaticity do so through several mechanisms. Some decrease the rate (slope) of phase 4 spontaneous depolarization, suppressing the ectopic focus such that the sinoatrial node is allowed to resume its dominance. Automaticity might also be reduced by lengthening the time needed to attain threshold potential by increasing either the excitation threshold (more positive; e.g., Na^+ or Ca^{2+} channel blockers) or the diastolic membrane potential (i.e., hyperpolarization, or more negative). Finally, spontaneous discharge might be reduced by prolonging the action potential duration, such as might occur with prolonged effective or absolute refractory periods.[5] Triggered automaticity can be impaired by inhibiting the development of after-depolarizations or interfering with inward sodium or calcium channels. Shortening (rather than prolongation) of the action potential duration will inhibit EADs. Although the mechanism is not well known, magnesium will also inhibit EADs.[5]

KEY POINT 14-26 Automaticy can be reduced by prolonging the effective refractory period or increasing the time it takes for the membrane potential to reach threshold (phase 4).

Arrhythmias associated with conduction abnormalities are exemplified by reentrant arrhythmias. Reentrant arrhythmias may be either anatomic or functional. Functional reentrant arrhythmias are exemplified by pathologies such as ischemia that markedly slow conduction. Anatomic arrhythmias involve two or more pathways that travel to the same region of the heart but differ in electrophysiology (e.g., refractory period or conduction speed). Emergence of reentrant arrhythmias reflects the unique histologic make up of myocardial muscle. The geometric connection of myocardial cells to one another facilitates rapid movement of impulses throughout the myocardium such that the heart acts as a single large cell (Figure 14-8). One region might receive signals from several different pathways. Coordination of impulse conduction ensures that myocardial fibers are excited in a sequence that maximizes pump efficiency. Normally, retransmission of an impulse received in a specific region from an alternative (i.e., second) direction is prevented because either the signals arrive simultaneously, thus canceling one another, or the fiber remains refractory from the first impulse and cannot respond to the second. However, if the refractory period is abnormally short, or conduction of the reentering, alternative impulse is markedly slowed, the fiber will no longer be refractory from the first impulse. The impulse can be reinitiated and travels in the opposite direction, until it returns to the region again, generating a (circus) reentrant arrhythmia (see Figure 14-8). Altered membrane channel and ion movements with injured cardiac tissue channels slow movement through fast Na^+ channels (phase 0) and slow Ca^{2+} channels. Conduction is accordingly slowed, potentially generating reentrant arrhythmias.

Clinically relevant antiarrhythmics act to prevent reentrant arrhythmias by blocking specific ion channels or by targeting autonomic function, thus altering initiation, or conduction or action potential duration (thus refractory periods)

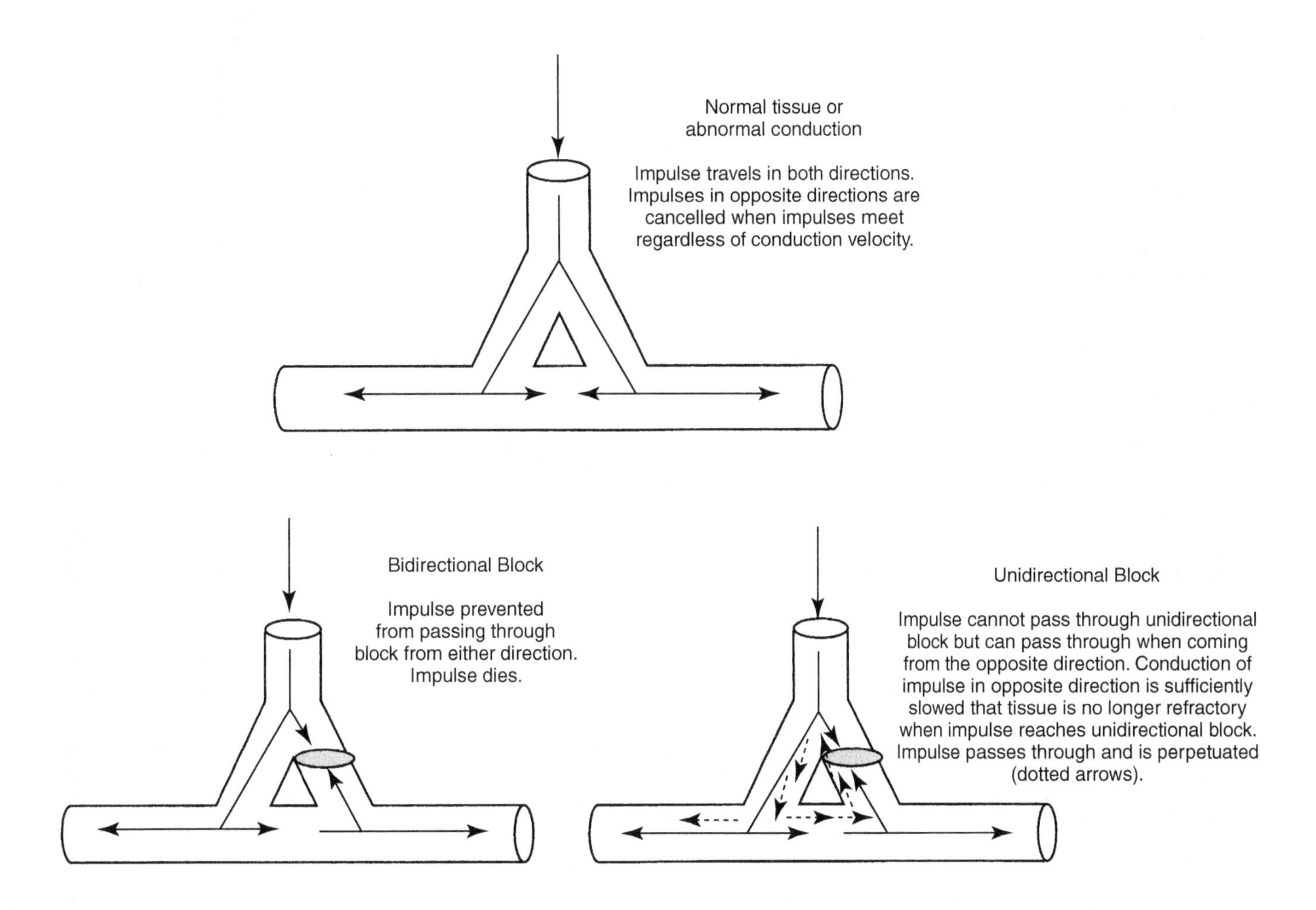

Figure 14-8 In the normal myocardium, electrical impulses travel down one or more paths of a bifurcated myocardial cell. Bifurcations allow coordination of contractions in all directions such that myocardial emptying is efficient and complete. Several mechanisms exist to ensure that impulses travel only in the proper direction. Those impulses that travel in opposite directions will be canceled by one another, precluding their transmission in the wrong direction. In the presence of a unidirectional block (i.e., resulting from damaged myocardium), transmission of one of the impulses will be prevented. However, although the impulse that normally would be canceled is now able to pass through the damaged tissue in the other direction, it will meet tissue that remains refractory from the first impulse. Consequently, it will not be transmitted any further. However, if conduction of the second unimpeded impulse is slowed, the myocardium will no longer be refractory when the impulse passes through the unidirectional block. Therefore the myocardium is receptive to the electrical impulse of this misdirected impulse, and the signal will be transmitted. Because of the combined effects of the unidirectional block and slowed conduction, the impulse may be perpetuated, resulting in a circus or reentrant arrhythmia. Drugs can reduce the arrhythmia by causing a bidirectional block, which prevents the second impulse from traveling through the damaged site, or by increasing the rate of conduction of the second impulse such that it reaches myocardial tissue while it is still in its refractory state from the first impulse.

of cardiac fibers. Initiation and thus automaticity can be suppressed through blockade of ion channels or drugs that facilitate adenosine or acetylcholine (thus increasing the maximum diastolic or resting potential) or antagonize adrenergic receptors (thus decreasing the slope of phase 4). Acceleration of conduction or prolongation of the ERP or APD causes the second impulse to reach tissue still refractory from the first impulse. Examples include Ca^{2+} channel blockers, β-adrenergic receptor antagonists, and digitalis glycosides. Slowed conduction caused by these drugs may increase the risk of functional reentrant arrhythmias. However, because reentrant arrhythmias respond best to drugs that prolong the refractory period, such drugs nonetheless remain effective for treatment of reentrant arrhythmias if the effective refractory period is prolonged. Examples of drugs that prolong ERP or APD might include drugs that delay recovery of sodium channels (particularly those that target inactivated channels) or potassium channel blockade (the delayed rectifier channels is particularly amenable to drug blockade), or drugs that prolong the APD. However, potassium channel blockade is also particularly conducive to causing arrhythmias, perhaps in part because of the importance of potassium channels in multiple phases of the action potential cycle.

KEY POINT 14-27 Reentrant arrhythmias can be decreased by increasing the rate of conduction or prolonging the effective refractory period.

In general, the complex action of antiarrhythmic drugs renders antiarrhythmic therapy generally inefficient and risky. All antiarrhythmic drugs are proarrhythmogenic. A major contributing factor to both inefficiency and risk is lack of knowledge regarding the particular electrophysiologic mechanism that underlies each arrhythmia or the drug. For example, the number of potassium channels, their differences in location, control, and role in the action potential complicate understanding, let alone predicting the impact of potassium channel blockade on cardiac function or rhythm. Increasingly, the arrhythmogenicity of drugs is likely to be understood as the differences in potassium channel impact by these drugs are understood. For example, blockade of delayed rectifier potassium current (I_{k5}) in the presence of high (β) adrenergic output predictably causes torsades de pointes in dogs.[110a]

Differences in clinical actions of antiarrhythmic drugs reflect in part different affinities of ion channel–blocking drugs for target receptors on the ion channel proteins, with some drugs targeting specific receptor subtypes. Affinity may change with conformation of the protein channel. As such, affinities are often state dependent (i.e., occurring only in the open, conducting state; in the closed, resting state; or during the inactivated, recovering state). Further, cardiac drugs often target more than one channel, and changes induced by a drug in one current generally influences the other currents. Direct and indirect (through the autonomic system) effects on cardiac contractility contribute to adverse effects.[5] Finally, most antiarrhythmic drug target channels in both normal and abnormal tissues. Electrolyte abnormalities and hypokalemia in particular often predispose arrhythmogenicity and may increase adverse effects to antiarrhythmics.[109,110] Indeed, a randomized human clinical trial that focused on the use of antiarrhythmic drugs for prevention of sudden death found that sudden death actually increased, primarily because of the proarrhythmic effects of drugs that target ion channels.[111] Accordingly, antiarrhythmics should be considered dangerous,[109,111] and their use should be pursued, whenever possible, under the guidance of clinicians with appropriate expertise (i.e., cardiologists).

Antiarrhythmic cardiac drugs fall into four main classes according to their dominant electrophysiologic effect on myocardial cells[5,112] (Figure 14-9). Although this classification serves to couple electrophysiologic actions with antiarrhythmic effects, increasing emergence of the complex mechanisms of actions of these drugs complicates the classification, and care should be taken not to assume that drugs within classes behave the same way; indeed, most drugs have multiple effects that cross into multiple classes.

KEY POINT 14-28 All antiarrhythmics are proarrhythmic, and their use should be initiated cautiously and only if proper monitoring tools are available.

Class I Antiarrhythmic Drugs

Class I agents comprise the standard membrane-stabilizing drugs such as lidocaine, quinidine, and procainamide. These agents work by selectively blocking the fast Na^+ channels and depressing phase 0 of the action potential through the direct membrane-stabilizing or "local anesthetic" effect. Accordingly, class I drugs increase the threshold of excitability and decrease the rate of spontaneous phase 4 depolarization, thus reducing the emergence of ectopic foci (decreased automaticity). Although decreased phase 0 depolarization also decreases conduction velocity (thus prolonging conduction and increasing the risk of re-entrant arrhythmias), effects on automaticity and generation of ectopic foci appear to predominate over effects on conduction velocity. Some class I drugs also prolong action potential duration, especially the effective refractory period, and as such are particularly useful in treating reentrant arrhythmias.[113] Class I agents can be further subdivided according to their effects on the refractory period and the rate of repolarization. Class 1A are intermediate blockers, including quinidine and procainamide. Class 1 B are rapid blockers, including lidocaine and mexiletine. Class 1C blockers are characterized by slow blocking kinetics and include flecainide, propafenone, and moricizine.

The risk of proarrhythmogenicity of antiarrhythmics is increased in dogs and cats by virtue of the dearth of scientifically based data supporting their use. However, regarding the data that do exist, when comparisons are made between dogs and humans, the concentrations at which antiarrhythmic effects of class I drugs are realized generally are similar. However, marked differences in pharmacokinetics exist; indeed, an exception to the generalization occurs for procainamide because of differences in its metabolism between dogs and humans.[114]

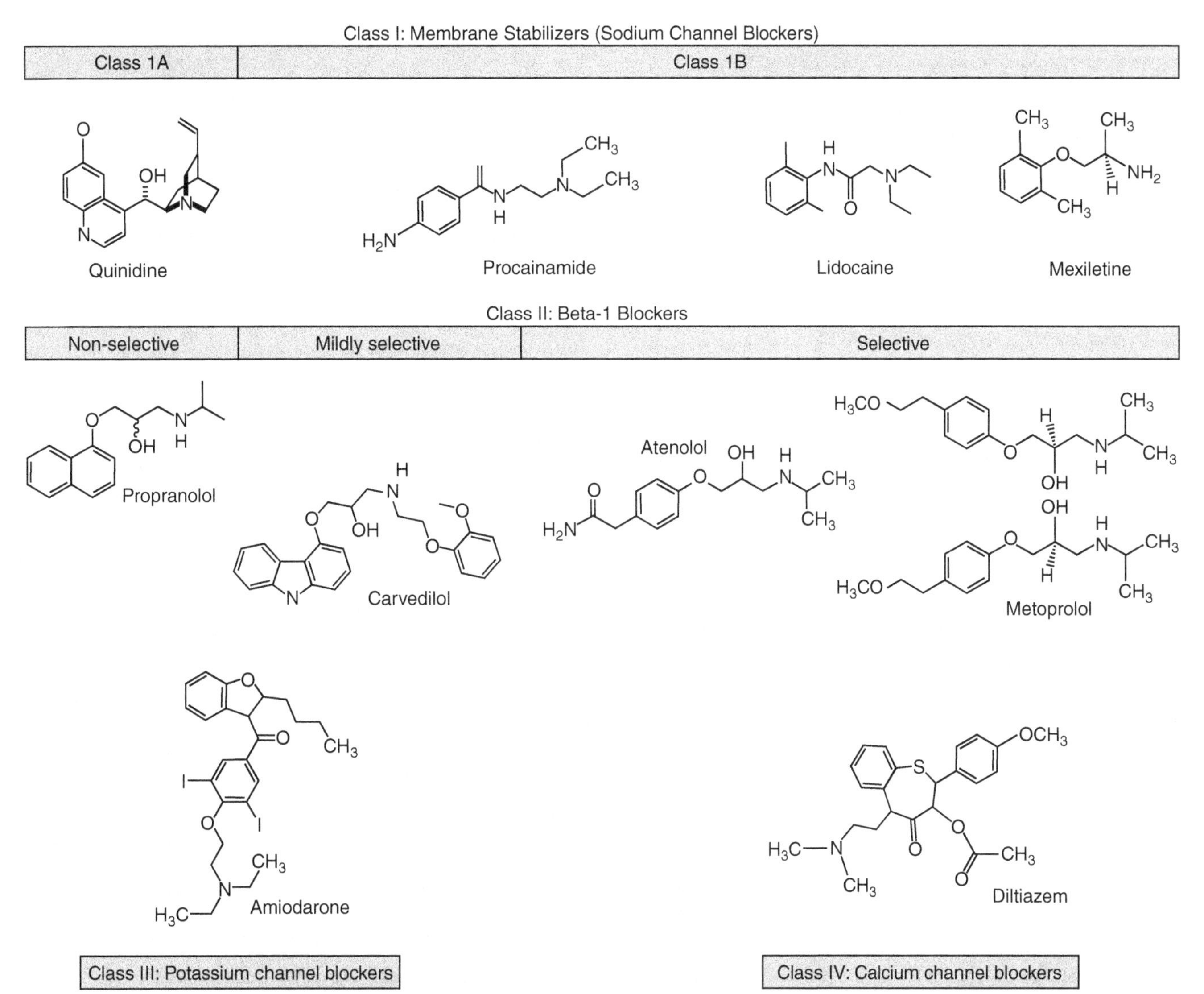

Figure 14-9 Structures of selected antiarrhythmic drugs. The drugs are classified by their mechanism of action, although much overlap occurs, particularly with potassium channel effects. Metoprolol exemplifies the chiral carbon present on most β blockers (some have two). Rotation of the four groups around the carbon yields enantiomers (stereoisomers that are non-superimpos-ablemirror images). Although similar in structure, the enantiomers are likely to be different in both pharmacokinetic and pharmacodynamic properties. Most products are sold as racemic mixtures of both isomers, although only one may be active. The body is likely to handle the isomers differently. Class 1C drugs are not shown.

KEY POINT 14-29 Although antiarrythmics are classified according to the major ion targeted, newer data indicate that this scheme is simplistic and much overlap occurs among the classes.

Class IA Drugs

Class 1 A drugs increase the threshold for excitability and decrease automaticity, reduce the rate of phase 0 depolarization and thus slow conduction, prolong both the effective refractory period and the action potential duration, and delay repolarization. A shared arrythmogenic effect of sodium channel blockers with atrial flutter reflects slowed conduction. Subsequent slowing of atrial flutter may allow more signals to be transmitted through the atrioventricular node, causing the heart rate to increase.

Quinidine

Quinidine, derived from the bark of the cinchona plant, is a diastereomer of the antimalarial drug quinine. Quindine affects most types of cardiac muscles.[5,112] Its efficacy against supraventricular and ventricular arrhythmias facilitates its classification as a broad-spectrum antiarrhythmic. Quinidine has both direct and indirect effects. For direct effects, quinidine blocks open Na^+ channels, increasing the threshold for excitability and decreasing automaticity, thus suppressing ectopic pacemakers. Blockade of multiple K^+ currents prolongs action potentials, particularly at slow heart rates. Electrophysiologically, quinidine increases the QRS complex; the QT interval may also be prolonged, causing *torsades de pointes* at therapeutic or subtherapeutic concentrations in some patients.[5] Because it also prolongs the effective refractory period, especially in the atria, quinidine is particularly useful for treatment of reentrant arrhythmias such as atrial fibrillation.[112, 113,2,115] In the atria quinidine also has an indirect effect through antivagal ("atropine-like") actions, contributing to undesirable side effects, and specifically, tachycardia.

KEY POINT 14-30 Blockade of sodium channels might be expected to affect nondepolarizing cells more than depolarizing cells.

KEY POINT 14-31 The anticholinergic effects of quinidine – which initially result in an increased heart rate –contribute to its efficacy in the treatment of atrial fibrillation.

Although given intravenously (which markedly increases the risk of cardiotoxicity) and intramuscularly, quinidine is most practically administered orally. Intramuscular injection is painful. Quninidine has been prepared as different salts to manipulate (prolong) oral absorption. Quinidine sulfate is absorbed rapidly after oral administration,[5,112] whereas the gluconate form is absorbed more slowly. Despite marked (90%) binding to α glycoproteins, quinidine distributes rapidly to most tissues, resulting in a large volume of distribution. In states of high stress, it may be necessary to increase doses of quinidine to overcome increased binding associated with increased inflammatory and other α glycoproteins, although this may be an issue more commonly encountered in humans with myocardial infarction. Quinidine binds to tissue, including cardiac proteins. Hepatic metabolism is mediated by CYP3A and is extensive, with excretion of parent compound or metabolites in the urine. Variability in metabolism is marked among patients and can be influenced by other drugs, necessitating individualized therapy. The duration of action of quinidine may be shortened or lengthened by drugs that target CYP3A4. The half-life is about 6 hours, but the dosing interval may be prolonged with slow-release preparations.

Quindine disposition has been studied in Beagle dogs (n=4). An intravenous dose of 1 mg/kg distributed to a volume of 1.17 ± 0.40 L/kg and was cleared at a rate of 5.90 ± 0.40 mL/min/kg, yielding an elimination half-life of 3.46 ± 1.44 h and mean residence time (MRT) of 3.34 ± 1.25 h. After oral administration of the sulfate salt (100 mg orally), C_{max} was 2162 ± 598 ng/mL and oral bioavailability was 73%.[116]

Quindine can cause or be affected by drug interactions, particularly by drugs that affect CYP 2D6 and 3A. It is a potent inhibitor of CYP 2D6, prolonging the elimination of selected drugs or preventing the formation of active drug (e.g., morphine from codeine).[5] Its clearance is affected by other drugs that impair (e.g., cimetidine, verapamil) or induce (e.g., phenobarbital, phenytoin, rifampin) CYP 2D6. Clearance of quinidine was decreased in normal Beagles (n=4) by 50% after treatment with the CYP3A substrate inhibitor ketoconazole. The elimination half-life (hr) increased from 3.46 ± 1.44 to 6.78 ± 1.98; C_{max} increased from 2162 ± 598 to 3295 ± 636 ng/mL.[116] Quindine clearance also is prolonged by drugs that alkalinize the urine (e.g., carbonic anhydrase inhibitors, thiazide diuretics). Quindine decreases digoxin clearance and may compete with it for P-glycoprotein–mediated efflux. Competition at cardiac binding sites also may displace digoxin, further increasing plasma digoxin concentrations, which may exacerbate digoxin-induced cardiac arrhythmias.[117]

Quinidine is associated with cardiotoxicity-induced arrhythmias such as atrioventricular blockade or ventricular arrhythmias. Sudden death caused by syncope has been reported. The atropine-like (antivagal) effects of quinidine probably account for some potentially serious side effects. Loss of vagal tone, important to the control of conduction in the atrioventricular node, may increase impulse conduction to the ventricles, resulting in *paradoxical acceleration,* an undesirable increase in heart rate in the patient with supraventricular tachycardias (including atrial fibrillation). This loss of vagal tone also impacts drugs whose cardiac effect is based on enhanced vagal tone. In humans, digitalization prior to therapy is indicated. Quinidine is also an α-adrenergic blocking agent and can cause vasodilation and potential hypotension. Gastrointestinal symptoms (e.g., nausea, vomiting, diarrhea) may occur, particularly with the sulfate form.

As a broad-spectrum drug, quinidine may be effective for acute or chronic management of supraventricular and ventricular arrhythmias. However, its efficacy particularly targets atrial arrhythmias. Quinidine is contraindicated in the presence of complete A-V heart block. Daily doses range from 5 to 15 mg/kg; therapeutic concentrations are 2 to 6 μg/mL. The drug can be given intravenously, but only with extreme caution.

Procainamide

Procainamide differs from the local anesthetic procaine only by replacement of an ester with an amide (see Figure 14-9). Like quinidine, procainamide blocks open Na^+ channels and outward K^+ channels. Thus it decreases automaticity, increases refractory periods, and slows conduction as well as prolongs the action potential duration. Its *N*-acetyl metabolite (in which the dog is deficient) is active and accounts for a major proportion of activity in humans. Although the metabolite does not block Na^+ channels, it does prolong the action potential duration (a K^+-blocking effect).[5] The metabolite is equal in efficacy but less potent than the parent compound in the control of ventricular arrhythmias.[118] The effects of procainamide on automaticity, excitability, responsiveness, and conduction are similar to those produced by quinidine. Indirect effects (those affecting the autonomic nervous system) are significantly weaker, with no α-adrenergic blockade or paradoxical acceleration.[5]

KEY POINT 14-32 Because the acetyl metabolite of procainamide targets potassium channels, decreased efficacy can be anticipated in dogs compared to humans.

Procainamide is rapidly and almost completely absorbed after oral administration, although the rate varies with the preparation. Peak concentrations occur within 45 to 75 minutes with a capsule but take longer with tablets. Bioavailability in the dog approximates 85%.[119] Only about 20% of the drug is protein bound to glycoproteins in humans.[5] Distribution occurs to most tissues except the brain,[5] yielding a large (1.44 L/kg in dogs) volume of distribution.[119] Procainamide is extensively biotransformed by the liver to metabolites. In humans, *N*-acetylprocainamide is a major active metabolite, contributing significantly to antiarrhythmic effects. In dogs acetylation is deficient and therapeutic concentrations reflect principally the parent drug whereas for humans, it reflects both parent and metabolite. In dogs the mean concentration necessary to control arrhythmias in ouabain (a cardiac glycoside)-intoxicated dogs was 33.8 μg/mL, with a range of 25 to 48.5 μg/mL.[120] This compares with a therapeutic range of concentration of 5 to 30 μg/mL for the combined parent and metabolite in humans. The elimination half-life of procainamide in the normal dog is 2.5 to 2.8 hours.

The fluoroquinolones decrease clearance of procainamide or its *N*-acetyl metabolite in humans. The extent and target (parent versus metabolite) varies with the fluoroquionlone drug. In humans ciprofloxacin decreases clearance of both by nearly 20%; competition appears to be occurring for renal tubular transport proteins.[121] Toxicities of procainamide include cardiotoxicity, similar to that induced by quinidine; hypotension with rapid intravenous administration (bolus); and gastrointestinal signs (anorexia, nausea, vomiting, diarrhea). Cardiac toxicity is indicated by a 50% widening of the QRS complex or by bradyarrhythmias or tachyarrhythmias.

Procainamide is available as oral capsules, tablets, and sustained-release tablets. Intravenous preparations are available for acute or unstable situations. Intravenous infusion is a reasonable approach for the treatment of the acute patient and may be preferred to rapid bolus, which may be associated with hypotension. Procainamide also can be administered intramuscularly (15 to 20 mg every 2 hours [dog] or 8 to 16 mg every 3 to 6 hours [cat]). An advantage to procainamide over other antiarrhythmics is ease of converting from an intravenous to an oral preparation. The transition is best accomplished by stopping an infusion, and, at one elimination half-life, administering the first oral dose (125 to 500 mg every 6 to 8 hours, for a total of 33 mg/kg per day).

Procainamide is a broad-spectrum antiarrhythmic drug. In general, its effectiveness as a ventricular antiarrhythmic drug parallels or exceeds that of quinidine, and it is useful for patients who have failed quinidine therapy. Arrhythmias for which procainamide have proved useful include ventricular[122] and, to a lesser degree, supraventricular types. Procainamide can suppress digitalis-induced toxicity but fatalities may occur.

Disopyramide

The pharmacologic effects and spectrum of disopyramide are similar to those of procainamide and quinidine. Although it is effective in controlling supraventricular arrhythmias, its primary use is for ventricular tachyarrhythmias. Disopyramide has been studied in the dog.[123] It is quickly absorbed after oral administration, but it undergoes rapid metabolism and clearance. Its half-life is less than 2 hours in the dog, necessitating multiple daily administrations. Like quinidine, disopyramide has potent antivagal effects and can therefore increase the ventricular rate dramatically in patients with supraventricular tachycardias. More important, disopyramide also has a negative inotropic effect on the heart and can be lethal for patients with preexisting myocardial disease. Clinical indications for disopyramide are probably limited by its potential adverse affects on the heart.[124]

Class IB Drugs

Class IB drugs include agents such as lidocaine and its congeners and phenytoin. Lidocaine (see Figure 14-9), widely used as a local anesthetic, is the prototypic class IB drug. Increasingly, it is being used for a variety of conditions (discussed later). Lidocaine preferentially binds to open (phase 0) and inactivated (phases 1 through 3) channels. Therefore cardiac tissues with long action potential duration or tissues that are rapidly firing (because more time is spent in the inactivated state), such as ischemic tissues, are more affected by lidocaine. Because atrial tissues have a very short action potential compared with ventricles, lidocaine preferentially targets arrhythmias in the abnormal Purkinje system and ventricles. In contrast, it minimally affects the sinoatrial node, atria, or atrioventricular node, although it has been used to successfully treat supraventricular arrhythmias in a limited number of dogs.[125] Additionally, abnormal ventricular tissues are preferentially affected compared to normal myocardial tissues. Lidocaine also minimally affects the autonomic system.

Lidocaine suppresses automaticity, increases the threshold, and hyperpolarizes (increases the resting membrane potential) of Purkinje fibers. Increased conduction velocity may facilitate inhibition of reentrant arrhythmias. The action potential duration is either unaffected or shortened. Lidocaine efficacy is dependent on potassium; hypokalemia will minimize its efficacy.

KEY POINT 14-33 Lidocaine targets inactive sodium channels, which are more prevalent in diseased, rapidly beating tissues, thus minimizing binding to normal or atrial myocardial tissues.

Lidocaine is well absorbed orally, but it is subject to first-pass metabolism, with only one third of the drug reaching systemic circulation. Rectal bioavailability ranges from 32% to 56%, depending on the preparation.[126] Peak concentrations in dogs after intravenous administration of 6 mg/kg approximate 10 μg/mL, declining to 0.1 μg/mL by 3 hours, with the elimination half-life approximating 50 minutes.[127] After intramuscular administration, absorption is complete, with peak concentrations at the same dose approximating 1.8 μg/mL at 30 minutes. Distribution is rapid to a volume of approximately 1.4 L/kg.[127,128] About 70% of the drug is bound to protein (glycoprotein). Lidocaine is cleared by hepatic metabolism to active and inactive metabolites. Clearance in female dogs (n=4; dose of 2 mg/kg infused over 5 minutes) was 27.5 ± 6.0 mL/min/kg. As a flow-limited drug, systemic clearance of lidocaine should decrease in proportion with hepatic blood flow. Portosystemic shunting will increase oral bioavailability; experimentally induced portosystemic shunting in dogs increases it from 15% to 80%.[129] Lidocaine is prepared for intravenous administration. Lidocaine can be administered intravenously as a rapid bolus or as a continuous intravenous infusion. It can also be given intramuscularly in emergency situations. Topical creams, salves, or gels and patches are intended for local anesthetic use only and will not provide antiarrhythmic efficacy.

As an antiarrhythmic, lidocaine is indicated for emergency treatment of ventricular arrhythmias. Pharmacologic effects occur rapidly. Lidocaine has several undesirable effects. Although lidocaine may decrease the risk of acute death associated with ventricular fibrillation, one study demonstrated decreased hospital survival, mitigating its routine use. The primary toxicity in the dog occurs in the central nervous system, with symptoms that range from drowsiness or agitation to muscle twitching and convulsions at higher plasma concentrations. Therapeutic and toxic lidocaine concentrations have been established experimentally. In an study of canine myocardial infarction, inhibition of electrically stimulated ventricular tachycardia responded to mean concentrations of 3.5 μg/mL (1 mg/kg intravenously followed by 80 μg/kg/min).[130] Wilcke and coworkers[131] compared effective and toxic concentrations in six dogs. Minimum effective concentrations for experimentally induced ouabain toxicity (outcome measure was eradication of ventricular tachycardia) ranged from 3.8 to 7.65 μg/mL (mean 6.25 μg/mL). The time necessary to eradicate the arrhythmia ranged from 0.3 to 1 hour after infusion of 1480 mg/hr. However, neurologic manifestations of toxicity appeared at 6.3 to 10.4 μg/mL (mean 8.21 μg/mL) (tonic extension) and became more exaggerated (cortical seizures) at 7.3 to 11.2 μg/mL (mean 9.58 μg/mL). Other neurologic manifestations of lidocaine toxicity include anxiety, sedation, and disorientation. The risk of toxicity with intravenous administration is greater in the cat compared with the dog; however, the cat s prone to cardiac toxicity. Cardiac suppression will occur at higher doses; exacerbation of heart failure has been reported in human patients with poor left ventricular function.[5] Lidocaine can worsen first-degree or second-degree atrioventricular block and is contraindicated for patients with third-degree heart block because of suppression of ventricular automaticity. A large intravenous bolus may cause sinus arrest; cats are more prone to this adversity.

Drug interactions involving lidocaine are limited. Care should be taken when mixing lidocaine solution with other drugs to avoid pharmaceutic direct drug-drug interactions. Selected drug interactions reflect competition with other basic drugs for binding sites on glycoproteins, although their clinical relevance is not clear. Lidocaine increases hepatic blood flow: a 12-hour infusion of 76 μg/kg/min increased hepatic arterial blood flow 1.6- to 9.2-fold.[128] Despite its flow-limited behavior, lidocaine appears to decrease its own clearance, with the impact being demonstrable following longer infusions compared with bolus administration.[128,132] Changes were more profound in one study following a 24-hour compared with a 90-minute infusion period.[132] Another study found that multiple administration of lidocaine (once daily) was associated with a decrease in hepatic intrinsic clearance from 1224 ± 859 to 285 ± 104 mL/min/kg.[128] Lidocaine metabolism is inhibited by a number of drugs, including midazolam and thiamylal.[133]

Tocainide (no longer marketed in the United States) and mexiletine are class IB antiarrhythmic drugs that are similar in chemistry and mechanism of action to lidocaine but modified to reduce first-pass metabolism, thus allowing oral administration. For example, tocainide is 100% orally bioavailable. Using a model of canine myocardial infarction, tocainide prolonged conduction intervals and the effective refractory period by 26% to 31% in damaged tissue compared with 6% to 8% in the noninfarcted zone.[134] Tocainamide has been used for long-term management of ventricular arrhythmias, particularly those that respond to lidocaine or fail to respond to procainamide. Arrhythmias that are refractory to lidocaine are not likely to respond to tocainide. Tocainide is prepared as a racemic mixture. Both the R and S enantiomers appear to have greater antiarrhythmic activity alone compared with the racemic mixture, whereas the racemic mixture appears more toxic than either enantiomer alone. Consequently, safety and efficacy might be improved if single enantiomer preparations become available.[135] Tocainaide may be more likely than lidocaine to cause CNS and gastrointestinal adverse reactions. Bone marrow dyscrasias and pulmonary fibrosis have limited use of tocainide. Blood dyscrasias have occurred in dogs.[110] Contraindications to lidocaine should be followed for tocainide.

After intravenous administration of tocainide, spontaneous premature ventricular complexes were reduced in dogs with experimentally induced myocardial infarction.[136] In Doberman Pinschers (n=23) with cardiomyopathy, tocainide at 15 to 25 mg/kg every 8 hours reduced the number of ventricular premature complexes short term by at least 70% in 80% of treated dogs; ventricular tachycardia was corrected in 90% of affected dogs. Serum concentrations at 2 hours and 8 hours were 6.2 to 19.1 mg/L and 2.3 to 11.1 mg/L, respectively. Long-term control was more difficult in animals whose left ventricular shortening fraction was less than 17%. Although efficacious, tocainide therapy may be limited by side effects. Anorexia and gastrointestinal disturbances occurred in 35% of dogs, with peak concentrations being higher in afflicted dogs (14 μg/mL) compared with dogs not exhibiting toxicity (11 μg/mL). Serious adverse effects occurred in 58% of dogs treated longer than 4 consecutive months and included progressive corneal endothelial dystrophy; renal dysfunction occurred in 25% of the dogs.[137]

Mexiletine, like tocainide, is a structural analog of lidocaine, indicated for oral management of life-threatening ventricular arrhythmias. Like lidocaine, it decreases the the APD more than the ERP such that the ratio of ERP/APD increases (package insert). Normal cardiac tissue is minimally impacted. In humans and dogs, mexiletine is characterized by high oral bioavailability, low first pass metabolism, 50-60% bound to plasma protein, and a volume of distribution of 5-7 liters/kg. Clearance in humans is primarily hepatic via CYP2D6 metabolism (hence, major differences in metabolizer phenotypes may occur), with some CYP1A2; metabolites are largely inactive. extensive metabolizer phenotypes. In dogs, most of the drug may be renally excreted, although its plasma elimination half-life approximates 10-12 hours; liver disease may prolong clearance. Mexiletine exists as a racemic mixture; in humans, the S isomer is characterized by a higher area under the curve (mean R/S ration = 0.8). [137a] In dogs, mexiletine has demonstrated stereoselective effects, with *R*-(-)-mexiletine being more potent in the prevention of ventricular tachycardia than S-(+)- mexiletine. [137b]

In human clinical trials involving mexiletine, approximately 40% of study participants withdrew from studies because of adverse effects; this rate was similar to treatment groups receiving quinidine or procainamide. Rarely, mexiletine has been associated with liver disease, warranting monitoring in patients with abnormal tests indicative of liver disease. Although mexiletine does not cause heart block in normal animals, it occasionally exacerbates pre-existing conduction disturbances; its use is contraindicated in the presence of 2nd or 3rd degree heart block. Mexiletine is arrhythmogenic: sustained ventricular arrhythmias worsened in approximately 10% of human patients receiving mexiletine. Minimum therapeutic plasma concentrations appear to approximate 0.5 mcg/ml in humans (range 0.05 to 2 mcg/ml). Dosing intervals are designed to minimize fluctuation.

Studies of mexiletine in dogs are largely experimental in nature, supporting use in humans. Experimentally, including studies using canine models, it suppresses induced ventricular arrhythmias. Mexiletine (5 mg/kg) (or esmolol at 1.25 mg/kg or verapamil at 0.4 mg/kg) was limited in its success in preventing torsades de pointes in a canine model involving blockade of delayed rectifying current and β-adrenergic stimulation. [110a] However, mexiletine (4.5 mg/kg load followed by 1.5 mg/kg/hr infusion) was able to partially prevent the proarrhythmic effects of β-adrenergic A-V blockade (sotalol 4.5 mg/kg load followed by 1.5 mg/kg/hr infusion) in diuretic (furosemide and hydrochlorthiazide)-induced hyopkalemic dogs. Mexiletine prevented sotalol-associated torsades de pointes that was electrically induced in the dogs. [110b] Pharmacodynamic effects of melixetine were determined in three canine models of arrhythmias. The minimum effective plasma concentrations (μg/ml) of mexiletine necessary to suppress arrhythmias were 1.8 ± 0.6 when induced by digitalis, 3.7+0.9 for adrenaline, and 2.2 ± 0.4 for coronary ligation μg/mL.[110c] The plasma elimination half-life in dogs is 3 to 4 hr. Mexiletine may be more effective when used in combination with other drugs. For example, it was more effective at in preventing experimentally induced ventricular arrhythmias in dog myocardium when combined with quinidine. [110d]

Like tocainide, mexiletine is more likely than lidocaine to cause central nervous system and gastrointestinal toxicity. Mexiletine induces seizures in dogs at 25 mg/kg; vomiting occurs at 15 to 30 mg/kg. However, the drug was well tolerated at 15 mg/kg for 13 weeks in normal dogs. [138b] Contraindications to lidocaine should be followed for mexiletine.

Phenytoin is an anticonvulsant with a limited spectrum of cardiac antiarrhythmic activity. Its mechanism and impact are similar to those of lidocaine. Its primary use in veterinary medicine has historically been management of digitalis-induced arrhythmias; phenytoin will shorten atrioventricular nodal and Purkinje refractory period in digitalized patients.

Class IC Drugs

Class IC drugs cause effects similar to those of the class IB drugs except that they do not prolong the refractory period. Examples include encainide, flecainide, lorcainide, and propafenone. Conduction velocity is depressed. In addition to sodium channel blockade, flecainide also blocks (in vitro) delayed rectifier potassium channels and calcium channels. Action potential duration is shortened in Purkinje cells (as a result of blockade of late-opening sodium channels) but prolonged in ventricular tissues (because of potassium channel blockade). In contrast to most class 1B drugs, flecainamide affects atrial tissues, prolonging the action potentials proportionately with rates, rendering it effective for atrial arrhythmias. However, it affects normal as well as abnormal tissues. Flecainide studies in dogs have been largely experimental. In one study concentrations of 610 ± 111 ng/mL increased the electrically induced defibrillation threshold in dogs.[138] The arrhythmogenicity of flecainamide can be lethal. Reentrant ventricular tachycardia may emerge when treating atrial arrhythmias, heart block may occur in conduction disturbances, and congestive heart failure can be exacerbated if ventricular performance is poor.[5]

Propafenone is a Na^+ channel blocker that is similar to flecainide, including K^+ channel blockade. It is prepared as a racemic mixture with the S-(+) isomer also exhibiting β-adrenergic antagonism in some (human) patients at concentrations at or above 1 μg/mL. Its efficacy is greater with atrial than with ventricular arrhythmias. It is eliminated through CYP2D6 metabolism as well as renal excretion, generally undergoing first-pass metabolism to an equipotent active metabolite. At least one other metabolite is active. Metabolism can be saturated with only small dose increases, resulting in disproportionately high plasma drug concentrations. Inhibitors of CYPD26 will contribute to high drug concentrations. It is available in slow-release preparations. Dosing is modified in human patients with liver disease.

Class II Antiarrhythmic Drugs

Class II antiarrhythmic drugs are β-adrenergic receptor blocking agents. Although discussed here because they affect cardiac arrhythmias, β-blockers have a number of potentially positive effects, particularly on the failing heart. Abbott[26] has reviewed β blockade in the management of systolic dysfunction. β-adrenergic stimulation causes the following effects, which are antagonized by β blockers: decreased magnitude and inactivation of calcium current, increased magnitude of potassium and chloride repolarizing currents, increased pacemaker activity, and increased DAD- and EAD-mediated arrhythmias.[5,9] Adrenergic signals stimulate atrial chronotropic β receptors more so than ventricular receptors. As such, β-blocking drugs (propranolol, alprenolol, and metoprolol) are most effective in slowing atrial compared with ventricular rates and are more effective during states of adrenergic stress.[139] Beta blockers decrease pacemaker current and thus sinus rate.[5] Because β blockers increase atrioventricular nodal conduction and prolong atrioventricular nodal refractoriness, they are useful for reentrant arrhythmias associated with the atrioventricula node.[5] In acutely ischemic myocardial tissue, β blockers increase the energy necessary to fibrillate the heart and thus may decrease mortality (in humans) if used in the first couple of weeks after myocardial infarct.[5]

A number of clinical trials have revealed the efficacy of β-blockade in the treatment of heart failure, reflecting a major effect on remodeling associated with the failing heart.[140] The effects of β blockade in chronic heart failure have been described as protective. Effects considered protective include decreased heart rate, decreased energy consumption, and antifibrillatory effects. Prevention of adrenergic overactivation decreases myocardial cell necrosis. Beta blockers that induce an upregulation of β receptors improve contractility. These benefits tend to outweigh negative inotropic effects that might lead to deterioration of hemodynamics and decompensation, although care must be taken in patients experiencing acute failure. The success of the "paradoxical intervention" may not be obvious until 2 to 3 months after initiation of additional β blocker therapy.

KEY POINT 14-34 In addition to slowing the heart rate—particularly in the presence of high sympathetic tone—β blockers also provide cardioprotection and slowing of progressive myocardial failure.

Drug therapy with β blockers presents pharmacokinetic and pharmacodynamic challenges generally not encountered by many other drugs. Among the challenges are the potential sequelae of interactions between drugs and receptors. Pharmacodynamically, chronic exposure of receptors to agonists or antagonists may cause receptors to be internalized and destroyed, resulting in decreased response or desensitization. Desensitization of β receptors may accompany long-term β blockade therapy. However, initiation of therapy at low doses may attenuate desensitization, an approach that is recommended in human patients with CHF.[7] Patients are monitored closely for acute adversities, and the dose is gradually increased only as low doses are tolerated. Low-dose metoprolol therapy simultaneously reduces vascular resistance and avoids reflex tachycardia, an advantage previously recognized only for carvedilol.[141] Use of low doses may also decrease the rebound effect that has been documented in humans once β blockade is discontinued. Rebound is associated with worsening heart failure and arrhythmias. Down-titration (decreasing the dose as the drug is discontinued over a 2-week period) reduces the rebound effects.[142] Use of β blockers in states of excessive adrenergic stimulation may allow unopposed α-adrenergic stimulation–mediated hypertension. Beta-blockers should be tapered rather than suddenly decreased to avoid the negative sequelae of receptor up regulation.

Beta blockers are not equal in efficacy. Protective effects of carvedilol and metoprolol were compared in progressive CHF in humans.[143] Carvedilol performed better in preventing cardiovascular-related illness in a clinical trial (COMET) involving human patients with heart failure associated with ischemia or idiopathic cardiomyopathy (see later discussion). Pharmacokinetically, distribution into the central nervous system—which may be important for maximal response—varies with lipophilicity, with effects of water-soluble drugs (atenolol, nadolol) potentially muted compared with those of more lipophilic drugs (e.g., metoprolol). Distribution is complicated by binding to both albumin and α-glycoproteins, the latter a protein whose concentration increases with inflammation; this may be more relevant to acute myocardial infarction. Binding decreases concentration of active drug; however, because clearance of flow-limited drugs generally is not affected by protein binding, a compensatory increase in drug clearance should not be anticipated and the risk of drug interactions at the level of protein binding increases. Lipophilic β-adrenergic drugs generally are characterized by hepatic clearance that is flow-limited (exceptions are the water-soluble atenolol and nadolol, which are predominantly renally excreted). For flow-limited drugs, the rate of substrate delivery (hepatic blood flow) determines clearance. As such, oral administration is characterized by significant (if not total) hepatic extraction and first-pass metabolism. Beta blockers interact with P-glycoprotein, with carvedilol being an example; its impact is sufficient to warrant its therapeutic use for inhibition of drug transport, which otherwise would result in multidrug resistance. [143a] The impact of disease and its successful treatment may impact response. Progressive cardiac disease or improvement thereof might profoundly alter clearance; disposition will be markedly altered in patients with liver disease associated with portosystemic shunting. Pharmacokinetics are further complicated by production of metabolites that are variably active. For example, for carvedilol, M4 and M5 are equipotent to the parent drug; M14 appears to be responsible for greater antioxidant effects compared with the parent. The hydroxymetabolite of metoprolol has 20% of the parent compound in dogs.[144]

Finally, most β-adrenergic blockers contain at least one chiral carbon, and thus are present as two isomers, each differing both kinetically and dynamically from the other.[141] The stereometric character of β-blockers markedly complicates their use. Complicating interpretation, the isomers can be described according to their spatial orientation (S versus R) or the direction in which they rotate light (+ or −); the two are not necessarily related. Blockade of β-1 receptors is achieved predominantly by the S isomer for most drugs. An exception occurs for sotalol, for which the R isomer exhibits more β blocker activity. In the dog the (−) isomer (based on rotation of polarized light; not related to R or S terminology is almost twofold more potent than the (+) isomer of metoprolol.[145] In contrast, non–β-1-blockade effects (e.g., blockade of α receptors, antiarrhythmic activity) generally are not stereoselective. All β blockers are marketed as a racemic mixture; exceptions include imolol (marketed as the S isomer), labetolol (which contains two chiral carbons), and nadolol (which contains three chiral carbons); all these are marketed as a mixture of four isomers. Absorption of β blockers does not appear to be stereoselective, although timolol may be stereoselectively metabolized by intestinal epithelial cells.[141] Binding to proteins may be steroselective, with selectivity varying with the binding protein. Distribution to tissues does not appear to be stereoselective beyond that determined by differences in protein binding. However, β blockers appear to be stored at terminal nerve endings in a stereoselective manner, with preferential storage of the (−) isomer, particularly for water-soluble drugs such as atenolol. Metabolism of β blockers is very complicated. Each isomer may be stereoselectively metabolized to active metabolites, which maintain the chiral carbon; as such, metabolites may be stereoselectively active or further metabolized. For metoprolol and carvedilol (but not significantly for other lipid-soluble drugs), metabolism is stereoselective, resulting in stereoselective plasma drug concentrations. In humans concentrations of the (+) carvedilol isomer (the less active isomer) are approximately twice that of the (−) isomer with regard to C_{max} and area under the curve; for metoprolol the concentrations of the isomers are almost equivalent, with the (−) isomer up to 30% higher than the (+) isomer. Renal clearance of water-soluble drugs (atenolol, nadolol) does not appear to be stereoselective. Drug interactions also may be stereoselective. In humans CCBs (verapamil and diltiazem) decrease first-pass metabolism. However, the inhibition is stereoselective for verapamil (but not diltiazem) toward the (+) R-isomer of propranolol. Cimetidine and quinidine also have exhibited stereoselective inhibition of β blockers. Finally, genetic polymorphism has been demonstrated for enzymes responsible for CYP-mediated drug metabolism in humans (and should be anticipated in dogs), although differences do not appear to be stereoselective.[141]

KEY POINT 14-35 Like many cardioactive drugs, enantiomers and active metabolites contribute to variability in disposition among patients.

Nonselective B Blockers

Propranolol is the prototype β blocker. It is a competitive, nonselective β blocker of both β-1 and β-2 receptors. Like all β blockers, propranolol is most effective in the presence of elevated sympathetic tone. Its negative chronotropic effect is less likely in conditions not associated with elevated levels of catecholamines (e.g., less effective if associated with hypokalemia, fever, some heart diseases). It will slow ventricular rates in patients suffering from supraventricular arrhythmias, including those induced by digitalis toxicity, but is rarely able to convert a supraventricular arrhythmia to a normal sinus rhythm. As a β-1 blocker, propranolol is also a negative inotrope. This pharmacologic effect might be detrimental in the patient with small cardiac reserve (e.g., the patient with decompensated CHF) during acute treatment. Propranolol has been studied in euthryoid and hyperthyroid cats.[146] Changes in disposition induced by hyperthyroidism suggest that a lower dose is indicated for oral administration because of increased bioavailability. Clinical indications of propranolol (β blockers) as an antiarrhythmic include reduction of ventricular rate in cases of supraventricular tachycardias, hypertrophic and other forms of obstructive heart disease, and hyperthyroidism. The effects of propranolol are dose, time, duration and route dependent; although oral administration may be associated with decreased bioavailability of the parent drug, formation of a more effective metabolite may cause better response with oral administration.[146b]

The toxic effects of propranolol are the result of nonselective β blockade and include bradyarrhythmias, hypotension, heart failure, bronchospasm, and hypoglycemia, particularly in diabetics. In an intact experimental canine model, insulin (4 IU/min intravenously with glucose) was shown to be superior to epinephrine for treatment of acute propranolol toxicity.[147]

Nadolol (5 to 10 mg orally every 6 to 12 hours [cat]; 40 to 60 mg orally every 6 to 12 hours [dog]) also is a nonspecific β blocker that is renally excreted. Side effects and contraindications typical of propranolol occur for nadolol.[110] Sotalol is another non-specific β-blocker that also prolongs the APD and ERP of atrial and ventricular fibers (Class III).

Selective Beta Blockers

Metoprolol is a relatively selective, lipophilic β-1 blocker. It is marketed as a racemic mixture, although the (−) isomer provides the predominant β blockade effect. The clinical pharmacology of metoprolol exemplifies the complexities associated with therapeutic use. Metoprolol undergoes hepatic clearance to several metabolites, of which the α-hydroxyl metabolite, the product of metabolism steroselective for the S(−) isomer is active. However, the proportion of this metabolite formed from the parent compound may not be clinically significant. O-Demethylation and N-dealkylation appear to be the major metabolites formed in dogs.[148]

The β-blocking effect of α-hydroxymetoprolol has been compared with that of metoprolol after intravenous administration in the dog. The dose–response relationship was linear for both compounds, but the metabolite required 10 times the plasma concentration of the metoprolol (5 times the dose) for therapeutic equivalence. The volume of distribution for the metabolite was 2 liters/kg compared with 3.5 liters/kg for metoprolol, whereas clearance was 3.5 mL/kg/min for the metabolite compared with 20 mL/kg/min for metoprolol. The net effect of these differences resulted in an elimination half-life for the α-hydroxy metabolite of 7 hours compared with 2 hours for the parent compound. Approximately 5% of an intravenous dose of metoprolol was metabolized to the active metabolite.[144] In Beagles (n=4, 8 years old, all female) receiving 1.37 mg/kg metoprolol orally, the area under the curve (0-48 hours; μg/mL/hr) was 2 for α-hydroxymetoprolol, compared with 4.39 for metoprolol acid and 1.89 for metoprolol. Peak plasma concentrations (estimated from concentration versus time curve) of metoprolol and its metabolites were 400 ng/mL at 0.5 hour for metoprolol, compared with 100 ng/mL at 3 hours for α-hydroxymetoprolol. An intravenous dose of 2 mg/kg resulted in a decrease in heart rate in normal dogs by 35% at a concentration of 379 ± 24 ng/mL; the concentration of the α-hydroxyl metabolite was approximately 38 ng/mL. A similar intravenous dose of the metabolite (2 mg/kg) resulted in a 25% reduction in heart rate. These studies suggest that the active metabolite of metoprolol may not play a major role in cardiac response, although the impact on other effects (i.e., antiarrhythmic, cardioprotective) is not clear.

Stereoselective pharmacodynamic effects of metoprolol also have been described in dogs. The concentration (μg/mL) necessary to achieve 50% of the inhibitory effect for each isomer were as follows: for V_{max} 250 ± 80 (R) versus 70 ± 30 (S), dP/dtmax: 450 ± 210 (R) versus 70 ± 40 (S) and heart rate, 520 ± 210 (R) versus 82 ± 27 (S). As such, the (S) isomer was more potent than the (R) isomer at a ratio of 3.7, 6.8, and 6.3 for V_{max}, dp/dt_{max}, and heart rate, respectively.[145] Stereoselectivity has also been reported for the disposition of metoprolol in anesthetized dogs, (although applicability to awake dogs is not clear). The peak times to maximum inhibitory effect of either metoprolol isomer occurred at 90 to 120 minutes-Because the isomers were not given intravenously, volume of distribution(Vd) and CLs could not be corrected for bioavailability (F); however, differences occurred in Vd/F, CLs/F, and area under the curve between the isomers;.[145] Another investigator[149] documented that hepatic clearance of metoprolol in dogs is slightly selective for the (S) isomer.

Metoprolol is prepared as an oral tartrate (Lopressor®), and slow-release succinate salt (Toprol XI®); the latter allows once-daily dosing in humans. The slow-release preparation does not appear to have been studied in dogs or cats. Indications of the slow-release preparation in humans include hypertension as well as treatment of stable CHF.

Verapamil (3 mg/kg) inhibited clearance of metoprolol in dogs approximately 50% to 70%. The effect is profound after oral administration, abolishing first-pass metabolism, with inhibition selective toward O-demethylation of the (S) isomer.[149]

A large multicenter clinical trial studied the use of metoprolol for treatment of acquired heart disease and particularly DCM compared with a placebo in dog.[149a] The drug did not appear to decrease mortality rates but did improve ventricular function as well as quality of life.

Carvedilol represents one of the more recently (third) generation of β blockers associated with potential antiarrhythmic, antihypertensive, and antiremodeling effects.[150-152] Carvedilol is specifically approved to reduce cardiovascular mortality in human patients. Although it is characterized by β_1 and β_2 as well as α-adrenergic blockade, it is relatively (mildly) β_1-selective in human patients. Vascular endothelium contains β1 and β2 receptors as well as α-1 receptors, each targeted by carvedilol. As such, it decreases total peripheral resistance and preload without compromise of cardiac output or causing reflex tachycardia. This advantage however, might be minimized by low-dose therapy of other (i.e., not carvedilol) β blockers.[153]Advantages compared with traditional selective β blockers such as metoprolol include reduced mortality in human patients with left ventricular failure, perhaps resulting from a more complete antagonism of sympathetic activation.[140,142,154,155] Carvedilol benefits do not reflect a reduction in heart rate as much as improvement in left ventricular function. Additional advantages may include antioxidant and antiproliferative properties and inhibition of apoptosis in the heart.[150-152,156] Finally, carvedilol may inhibit the synthesis of endothelin in coronary arteries.[157] Carvedilol appears to protect against doxorubicin-induced cardiomyopathy.[158] In a rabbit model of ischemia, carvedilol provided superior cardioprotection, probably because of antioxidant and antineutrophil effects.[159] Similar effects were reported in a human patient receiving doxorubicin.[160]

KEY POINT 14-36 An advantage of carvedilol compared with other selective β blockers is α-adrenergic blockade, which may decrease afterload.

Carvedilol has been relatively well studied in dogs, It is well absorbed and undergoes extensive hepatic metabolism, including glucuronidation and subsequent biliary excretion.[161] The kinetics and selected pharmacodynamics have been studied in anesthetized[162] and awake[163,164] dogs. In anesthetized dogs the elimination half-life was 54 minutes (compared with 2.4 hours in humans), and the volume of distribution was 2 L/kg. When studied at doses ranging from 10 μg to 630 μg/kg, heart rate did not decrease, although reports in awake dogs indicate otherwise. Pulmonary and systemic pressures decreased in treated animals but increased in control animals, consistent with the β blockade effect of the drug. The authors recommend an optimal plasma drug concentration of 100 ng/mL, achieved after intravenous infusion of 150 to 310 μg/mL. Disposition was characterized by marked variability. The median peak concentration (extrapolated) of carvedilol after intravenous administration of 1.75 μg/mL was 476 ng/mL (range 203 to 1920 ng/mL), elimination half-life ($t_{1/2}$) was 282 minutes (range 19 to 1021 minutes), and MRT was 360 minutes (range 19 to 819 minutes). Volume of distribution at steady state was 2 L/kg (range 0.7 to 4.3 L/kg). After oral administration of 1.5 mg/kg, the median peak concentration was 24 μg/mL (range 9 to 173 μg/mL), time to maximum concentration was 90 minutes (range 60 to 180 minutes), $t_{1/2}$ was 82 minutes (range 64 to 138 minutes), and MRT was 182 minutes (range 112 to 254 minutes). Median bioavailability after oral administration of carvedilol was 2.1% (range 0.4% to 54%). However, the bioavailability of active metabolites (M4 and M5, which are equipotent to parent drug in humans) was not determined, and it is not clear whether these metabolites are produced in dogs. On the basis of these data, monitoring should be considered to adjust dose. The half-life of 3 hours suggests 8-hour dosing. However, pharmacodynamic studies were also performed.[164] Normal dogs were studied at baseline and after multiple-dose (>5 days) oral administration of carvedilol (1.5 mg/kg of body weight orally every 12 hours). Dogs were challenged with isoproterenol. Carvedilol had no effect on heart rate or blood pressure in six of eight dogs at baseline or study end, but heart rate reduced after multiple dosing in two of eight dogs. Carvedilol attenuated isoproterenol-induced changes in heart rate by 54% to 76% through 12 hours and by 30% at 24 hours. The effects of isoproterenol on blood pressure was attenuated by 80% to 100% through 12 hours. Based on normal dogs, an oral dose of 1.5 mg/kg was recommended every 12 hours. The magnitude of β-blockade response correlated strongly to peak plasma carvedilol concentration, suggesting that therapeutic drug monitoring may be clinically useful. Carvedilol also has been compared to bisopropol (see later discussion).

The efficacy of carvedilol and metoprolol for the treatment of chronic heart failure has been compared in humans. The efficacy of these drugs has also been compared with that of standard therapy in humans.[154,165] No difference could be demonstrated in most outcome measures between carvedilol versus metoprolol treatment, although blood pressures were lower in carvedilol compared with metoprolol patients. Patients receiving either carvedilol or metoprolol significantly improved compared with those receiving standard therapy.[154] More recently, the results of the COMET study, which compared carvedilol with metoprolol, have been reported. The COMET study was a randomized, double-blind, parallel comparison of carvedilol at approximately 0.3 mg/kg twice a day and metoprolol tartrate at approximately 0.7 mg/kg twice a day. Patients (n=3000) were studied for 58 weeks and had stable chronic heart failure, New York Heart Association (NYHA) functional class II to IV, with left ventricular dysfunction. Patients continued ACE inhibition and diuretics. Patients were randomly assigned to receive either carvedilol or metoprolol and followed for 58 months. Endpoints were cardiovascular events (which may be less relevant in dogs or cats), and the proportion of such events in each group (584 for carvedilol versus 667 for metoprolol), although statistically significant, may not be as clinically relevant.

In a study of myocardial perfusion in dogs receiving either carvedilol (2 mg/kg) or metoprolol (4 mg/kg) orally, carvedilol was associated with greater increase in myocardial perfusion and decrease in blood pressure, whereas metoprolol was associated with greater decrease in heart rate.[166] Carvedilol appears to be an inhibitor of P-glycoprotein, at least as was demonstrated in vitro in cancer cells: the LD_{50} of doxorubicin in breast cancer cells increased by twentyfold (200 to 10 ng/mL)[167] despite doxorubicin cardioprotection.[160]

Oyama and coworkers[168]prospectively failed to find a significant impact of carvedilol (0.3 mg/kg twice daily) in dogs with DCM (n=16; n=7 placebo) using a placebo-controlled, double-blinded randomized design. Endpoints for which significant differences were not documented included changes in ventricular function, activation of neurohumoral compensatory responses, or owner-perceived quality of life. However, animal death reduced sample size and the power of the study to detect a significant difference was not reported. Marcondes-Santos and coworkers[169] found some beneficial effect of carvedilol when added to traditional therapy (digoxin, benazepril, codeine) in dogs (n=13) with chronic mitral valvular disease; 12 control dogs with disease did not receive carvedilol. Dogs were studied using a prospective blinded parallel study. A tendency for improvement occurred for quality of life and a reduction in SBP, and improved disease classification during the 3-month study period.

Atenolol (see Figure 14-9) is a selective β_2 blocker. In humans its use is associated with greater mortality compared to non-atenolol β blockers. The difference presumably reflects a risk of ventricular fibrillation that is greater with atenolol compared to others. Compared to most other clinically used selective β blockers, atenolol is much less lipid soluble and thus less likely to penetrate the central nervous system; increased mortality may be related to the lack of centrally mediated vagal tone, which would otherwise counteract the risk of fibrillation.[170] The implications of this difference among β blockers is not clear for dogs or cats. Little information is available regarding active metabolites or stereoisomers.

Atenolol is 90% bioavailable after oral administration in normal adult cats.[171] Elimination half-life in normal adult cats is 3.44 ± 0.5 and 3.65 ± 0.39 hours after intravenous and oral administration, respectively. A dose of 3 mg/kg orally generates a peak plasma concentration of 0.48 ± 0.16 μg/mL and will block cardioresponsiveness to isoproterenol for 12, but not 24, hours, suggesting a 12-hour dosing interval. Using a prospective, randomized, crossover, blinded study, atenolol (6.25 mg every 12 hours) was studied in healthy cats as either an oral or transdermal preparation.[172] Peak (2-hour) and trough (12-hour) concentrations were measured after 1 week of administration.Therapeutic concentrations (250 ng/mL) were reached in six of seven cats (579 ± 212 ng/mL) 2 hours after oral administration, but in only two of seven cats (177 ± 123 ng/mL) following transdermal administration. Trough plasma atenolol concentrations were 258 ± 142 ng/mL following oral administration and 62.4 ± 17 ng/mL following transdermal administration. The authors concluded Monitoring might be considered in animals that must receive atenolol transdermally. Atenolol is indicated for cats with HCM associated with outflow obstruction and respiratory distress. Henik and coworkers[173] reported the efficacy of atenolol (1 to 2 mg/kg PO every 12 hours) for control of hypertension in hyperthyroid cats (n=20). Although heart rate was decreased, SPB was not well controlled, indicating the need for an additional vasodilator. Crandell and Ware[174] described the successful use of atenolol for treatment of cardiac toxicity associated with phenylpropanolamine overdose in a dog.

KEY POINT 14-37 Transdermal delivery of atenolol in cats is not predictable and should be implemented only if monitoring is available.

Esmolol is a β_1-selective blocker (S enantiomer) characterized by a very (ultra) short half-life owing to metabolism by erythrocyte esterases. Methanol is a metabolite of esmolol in humans, but its formation does not appear to be clinically relevant. Duration of effect is about 10 minutes; therefore its effects will rapidly dissipate once the drug is discontinued.[5] It is administered intravenously and has proved useful in dogs for acute ventricular arrhythmias associated with inhalation anesthesia and surgical removal of hyperactive thyroid glands.[110] In anesthetized dogs receiving a constant-rate infusion, steady-state concentrations occurred in 10 minutes, with duration of β blockade paralleling drug concentrations.[175] Peak β blockade occurred within 15 seconds after loading with a 500 μg/kg constant-rate infusion and at 30 to 45 seconds after switching to a maintenance dose of 12.5, 25, or 50 μg/kg/min. Duration of β blockade was less than 15 minutes once drug was discontinued. Esmolol has been proved to be effective for treatment of cats with HCM and left ventricular outflow tract obstruction.[176]

Bisoprolol is among the β-1 selective blockers that have prolonged the life span of humans with cardiac disease. Among its distinguishing characteristics is less lipophilicity than other drugs; consequently, the parent drug is eliminated by both hepatic metabolism and renal excretion (approximately 50% each) in dogs.[177] Bisoprolol is less lipophilic than other β blockers, including carvedilol; the implication is not clear, but pharmacodynamic data for bisoprolol apparently are not yet available in dogs. However, Beddies and coworkers[177] compared the pharmacokinetics of carvedilol and bisoprolol (1 mg/kg either drug) after both intravenous and oral administration in 12 Beagles using a parallel nonrandomized study design (six dogs per group; oral drug was followed by intravenous drug). Intravenous administration of bisoprolol resulted in a C_{max} (presumed to be extrapolated) of 408 ± 75 (presumed to be ng/mL) with a 3.9 ± 0.3 hour half-life. Volume of distribution was 2.4 ± 0.6 L/Kg, and clearance 0.42 ± 0.08 L/h/kg). After oral administration of bisoprolol, the C_{max} was 322 ± 261 at 1.1 ± 0.7 hr. Oral bioavailability of bisoprolol was 91.4% compared with 14.3% for carvedilol. For carvedilol, after intravenous administration, C_{max} (presumed to be extrapolated) for carvedilol was 788 ± 348 (presumed to be ng/mL) and half-life 1 ± 0.2 hour. Volume of distribution was 2.9 ± 0.6, and clearance 2.1 ± 0.5 L/hr/kg. After oral administration the C_{max} of carvediolol was 51 ± 42 at 1.1 ± 07 hours.

Class III Antiarrhythmic Drugs

Class III drugs prolong the cardiac action potential and refractory period by selective potassium channel blockade. As such, they have no effect on the fast Na^+ conductance and prolong APD without slowing conduction velocity. They generally do not cause β-blockade; sotalol is an example exception. There are two members of this class: bretylium and amiodarone. Bretylium is used as an antifibrillatory drug in humans. It accumulates in sympathetic nerve terminals, where it blocks norepinephrine release, but only after an initial release of stored neurotransmitter. Bretylium is minimally effective in dogs, in part because it affects primarily the Purkinje fibers and ventricles, limiting its spectrum of activity. It is not used clinically in veterinary medicine but is used in human medicine for ventricular arrhythmias. It reportedly can cause defibrillation in cases of ventricular fibrillation in humans and has been investigated for similar effects in dogs.[178] Because it causes the release of norepinephrine from adrenergic neurons, it may be associated with untenable, undesirable side effects.

Amiodarone is a structural analog of thyroid hormone; its mechanism may involve interaction with nuclear thyroid hormone receptors.[5] It blocks activated sodium channels, calcium channels, and multiple potassium channels. Conduction velocity is slowed, the action potential duration is prolonged, and repolarization is delayed. Further, it noncompetitively blocks adrenergic receptors. It also inhibits cell-to-cell coupling, which may be important to its effects in diseased tissues. It is a powerful antiarrhythmic drug useful for both atrial and ventricular arrhythmias.[179] In the normal canine heart, however, amiodarone causes negative inotropic effects.[180] It also causes both α-blocking and nonselective β-blocking effects. Proarrhythmogenic effects are more likely in the presence of hypokalemia. Amiodarone is metabolized via CYP 3A4 to an active metabolite in dogs. Amiodarone, however, shows only moderate efficacy for the treatment of arrhythmias (supraventricular or ventricular) in dogs and cats,[110] although it was more effective than bretylium in preventing sustained ventricular tachycardia or fibrillation in a canine model of reperfusion arrhythmia.[178] Therapeutic concentrations of 0.5 to 2 μg/mL (1 to 2.5 μg/mL)[181] have been recommended.[5] Because it is very lipophilic, with lipid to plasma ratios may be as high as 300:1, amiodarone accumulates in cells (myocardial concentrations exceed plasma by 15 fold), and is slowly released, resulting in a lag time to onset and long duration of maximum effect. Generally, a loading dose is administered for several weeks, followed by a maintenance dose. Adverse effects tend to persist as the drug is eliminated over a period of weeks to months; one half- the peak effect is reached only after 21 days following drug discontinuation. Lipophilicity also limits oral absorption (bioavailability in humans is 30%). Adverse effects require long-term therapy, with the most serious being pulmonary fibrosis, which can be rapidly fatal. Other side effects include corneal deposits, hepatic dysfunction, neurologic dysfunctions (up to 40% in humans), including peripheral neuropathy, muscular weakness, and altered thyroid function (hyperthyroidism and hypothyroidism). Photosensitivity and blue discoloration of the skin have been reported. Amiodarone is associated with drug interactions.

Saunders and coworkers[182] retrospectively studied the effect of amiodarone (median loading and following maintenance doses of 16.5 and 9 mg/kg/day) for treatment of atrial fibrillation in dogs (n=17). A variety of cardiac diseases were studied. Cardioconversion to normal sinus rhythm occurred in six dogs, and heart rate was decreased by at least 20% in 13 dogs. The drug was discontinued in five dogs because of adversities, including bradycardia and increased liver enzymes. Kraus and coworkers[181] retrospectively studied amiodarone toxicity in Doberman Pinschers (n=22) with occult DCM. All dogs were simultaneously receiving either tocainamide or mexiletine; some dogs also were receiving other antiarrhythmics. All dogs had been dosed with a loading dose (9.0-12.1 mg/kg) followed by a maintenance dose (range 4.3 to 6.3 mg/kg). Serum amiodarone concentrations ranged within and between animals, in part because of dose changes, but roughly ranged from 1.5 to 3.7 μg/mL at doses that ranged from 200 to 400 mg/kg once (for higher concentrations) to (for lower concentrations) twice daily. Adverse events that emerged during loading or maintenance included anorexia and vomiting associated with increased liver enzymes in up to 45% of dogs. Dogs often responded to temporary discontinuation of the drug, but persistent hepatic involvement necessitated discontinuation of therapy for some dogs.

Hepatopathy associated with amiodarone therapy has been reported in a series of 4 cases (3 of which were Doberman Pinchers).[182a] Doses ranged from 8 to 10 mg/kg per day with duration as short as 6 weeks and as long as 8 months. Patients were receiving other drugs, including melixetine. Concentrations of amiodarone approximated 1.7 mcg/ml at the time of toxicity. Hepatopathy included increased serum liver enzymes in all dogs, and hyperbilirubinerma in 2 of the dogs. No risk factors were identified other than left ventricular dysfunction. Because the drug had been used by the authors in only 10 dogs, the incidence of hepatopathy was described as 40% in this small population of dogs. Hepatopathy resolved in 3 cases after amiodarone was discontinued despite continuation of other cardiac drugs (including melixetine); one dog died suddently.

Sotalol is a class III potassium blocking antiarrhythmic drug with nonselective β-blocking properties. Studies in dogs appear to be limited to experimental studies supporting its use in humans. For example, sotalol disposition was described in dogs (n=3). Oral absorption was rapid and oral bioavaiability 75 to 90%; elimination half-life was 4.5 ± 1 h.[177a] the volume of distribution is larger (by 4 fold) than total body water. [177b] Excretion appears to be renal. Plasma concentrations necessary to achieve 50% and 100% of β-blockade after isoproterenol administration were 1-2 and 2.3 to 3.4 μg/ml, respectively.[177b] In an early canine model, the relative efficacy of β-blockade following isoproterenol stimulation was l-propranolol > propranolol >>sotalol >bunolol. [146b] Sotalol is largely cleared in dogs by renal excretion; volume of distribution ranges from 1.1 to 1.6 L/kg. The half-life is shorter in dogs at 4 to 5 hrs compared to 7 to 18 hrs in humans. Experimentally, sotalol has been used to induce torsades de pointes in hyokalemic dogs (2.5 meg/L).

Class IV Antiarrhythmic Drugs

Class IV antiarrhythmic drugs are the CCBs. Those blockers particularly effective on the vasculature are discussed with the vasodilator drugs. Diltiazem and verapamil have been used in both dogs and cats for their effects on heart rate. Both drugs are also, however, characterized by negative inotropic effects, with verapamil being a more effective but less safe negative inotrope.

Because calcium entry into myocardial cells is regulated primarily by slow channels, the CCBs also affect the heart. Specialized tissues capable of automaticity and atrioventricular conduction tissues are particularly affected by CCBs. The differences in pharmacologic effects induced by these drugs often reflect their impact on recovery of slow calcium channel.[2] CCBs that do not alter the rate of recovery (e.g., nifedipine and its congener amlodipine) will have little effect on conducting tissues. Drugs that do delay recovery of the channels can also delay conduction. For example, verapamil and diltiazem decrease the rate of recovery of calcium channels and thus not only decrease the magnitude of the cardiac action potential but also slow conduction through the atrioventricular node. The faster that atrioventricular nodal stimulation occurs, the more effective the atrioventricular nodal blockade is. Both drugs are useful for supraventricular arrhythmias. However, verapamil also has been shown to be useful in the treatment of experimentally induced ventricular tachycardias in dogs.[183] Because of their effect on slow calcium channels, CCBs also decrease myocardial contractility.[2] Verapamil also appears to provide cardioprotective effects in dogs with acute Chagas disease, which is characterized by destruction of sympathetic nerve terminals and alterations of β-receptor density.[184] A proposed mechanism is increased adrenergic adenylyl cyclase activity.

KEY POINT 14-38 Calcium channel blockers active in the heart target cells normally capable of automaticity and thus are more useful for supraventricular arrhythmias.

Hypotension, bradycardia, and tachycardia (generally reflex) are the predominant clinical indicators of CCB overdose. In patients with poor myocardial reserve, exacerbation of CHF may result in peripheral or pulmonary edema

Diltiazem

Diltiazem (see Figure 14-9) is the most commonly used CCB in veterinary medicine, in part because it has been studied in both dogs and cats. It exerts its greatest effects in the sinoatrial and atrioventricular nodes, tissues in which slow Ca^{2+} influx is largely responsible for phase 0 depolarization. Diltiazem slows sinus rate and atrioventricular conduction. The ventricular rate is reduced in patients with atrial fibrillation or flutter, but primary ventricular arrhythmias are generally unresponsive to diltiazem. Myocardial oxygen demand decreases in response to the effects of diltiazem. Cardiac side effects include hypotension, bradycardia, and various degrees of heart block. In human patients a therapeutic range of 50 to 300 ng/mL has been identified and can be used as a target for clinical response in animals.

The magnitude of the hemodynamic affects of the CCB reflects the route of administration. Bioavailability is reduced as a result of first-pass metabolism for nifedipine > verapamil > diltiazem, with bioavailability of diltiazem only 50% after oral administration. However, the extent of metabolism decreases with chronic administration, facilitating chronic oral therapy. Diltiazem is metabolized by acetylation, which is deficient in the dog but not in the cat; the impact of acetylation deficiencies in the dog on diltiazem disposition has not been studied.

In an attempt to identify a product that allows convenient (once to twice daily) dosing intervals, the disposition of several diltiazem products has been studied in cats. Comparison of intravenous, standard, and slow-release (CD) diltiazem preparations reveals a disappearance half-life of 120 minutes for the intravenous and oral preparations, but 460 minutes (7 hours) for the CD preparation. The bioavailabilities of the oral preparations are 71% (standard) and 36% (CD). The higher bioavailability of the standard preparation for cats compared with humans (30%) may reflect less first-pass metabolism, despite the fact that cats are efficient acetylators. Peak plasma concentrations for the standard preparation occurred at 45 minutes; peak steady-state concentrations of CD should occur at 1 to 2 days. Diltiazem is approximately 55% to 65% bound to serum proteins in cats. Maximum prolongation of the PR interval is less than 20% for either preparation, occurring at approximately 18 hours, when plasma diltiazem concentrations are between 50 and 100 ng/mL. The pharmacodynamic effects have not been studied in cats with HCM. However, on the basis of the pharmacokinetic data, the standard diltiazem product is administered at 1 mg/kg every 8 hours, but the CD product (prepared in gelatin as either 60-mg or 90-mg capsules) can be administered at 10 mg/kg every 24 hours. An extended-release diltiazem (Dilacor XR) also was studied in cats (n=13; 10 normal and 3 with HCM) after oral administration of either 30 or 60 mg (9.3 to 14.8 mg/kg, obtained as 60-mg tablets in 120-mg capsules; tablets were halved [with difficulty] to yield 30 mg fractions). Peak serum concentrations following 60 mg (8 cats; concentrations not measured until 6 hours) were markedly variable, ranging from approximately 71 to 1500 ng/mL (mean 787 ± 488 ng/mL); by 24 hours, concentrations were 196 ± 232 (range 5 to 920) ng/mL. At 30 mg (5 cats), peak concentrations were 448 ± 370 (20 to 800) at 6 hours and 43 ± 24 (20 to 88 ng/mL) at 24 hours. Variability in absorption indicates that monitoring, if available, would be a useful tool for targeting effective concentrations.[185] The recommended dose is one half of one of the pellets given once or twice daily.

Diltiazem appears to be relatively safe in cats. A retrospective study of client-owned cats (n=25) with HCM treated with 60 mg diltiazem once daily, reported side effects evident at 60 mg per cat included lethargy, gastrointestinal disturbances (vomiting, diarrhea), and weight loss (36%). Clinical signs appeared in 1 to 7 days.[185] Diltiazem has been studied in cats after single-dose transdermal administration. Therapeutic concentrations (50 to 200 ng/mL) were not acheived in any cat (n = 6).[185a] Administration as a transdermal gel is not recommended until multiple dosing has been documented to predictably achieve therapeutic concentrations.

Diltiazem has been studied in dogs.[186,187] The PR interval is prolonged approximately 20% at plasma concentrations of 60 ng/mL. In dogs suffering from atrial fibrillation or CHF, diltiazem (0.5 to 1 mg/kg every 8 hours) can be used for its negative chronotropic effects to reduce heart rate in the presence of sustained supraventricular arrhythmias. Diltiazem can be used either alone or in combination with digoxin. Because of its negative inotropic effects, however, it must be used cautiously in patients with myocardial failure, and digitalization may be indicated before diltiazem therapy is begun. The drug can be used intravenously (0.2 to 0.4 mg/kg, followed by infusion of 4 to 8 μg/kg per minute), although extreme caution is recommended.

A single case of diltiazem toxicity has been reported in a dog that accidentally ingested between 95 and 109 mg/kg of a slow-release product.[188] Clinical signs included cardiac arrhythmias, bradycardia, hypotension, mental depression, and gastrointestinal upset. The patient was treated with a temporary pacemaker. Costello and Syring[189] reviewed the toxicity associated with CCBs in general. Therapeutic strategies discussed for treatment included calcium as the initial therapy to increase availability to cells. Response should be monitored by electrocardiogram and heart rate. Glucagon may improve or reverse bradycardia and hypotension through unclear mechanisms that increase cAMP. Experimental doses used in dogs were 0.2 to 0.25 mg/kg bolus followed by 150 μg/kg/min constant-rate infusion. Because calcium blockade may cause hypoinsulinemia (and hyperglycemia) at the level of insulin release from pancreatic β cells, insulin and dextrose may be indicated (4 U/min in 20% dextrose and potassium supplementation as needed), as is a pacemaker. Finally, drugs that act as direct agonists at calcium channels may be beneficial, although no drug is clinically available or described with this effect. Among the drugs studied is 4-aminopyridine.

Verapamil

Verapamil is similar to diltiazem in its actions. It undergoes first-pass metabolism after oral administration in humans. Although it is available in both intravenous and oral preparations, caution is recommended with intravenous use. It has been studied for the treatment of acute supraventricular tachycardia in the dog at a dose of 0.05 to 0.15 mg/kg up to 0.2 to 5 mg/kg.[110,190] Supraventricular arrhythmias that do not respond to class IA drugs often respond to oral verapamil therapy.[110] Among the CCBs used in small animals, verapamil is associated with the greatest negative inotropic effects and as such should be used cautiously in animals with ventricular myocardial dysfunction. Further, verapamil may be associated with more drug interactions than diltiazem.

Miscellaneous Antiarrhythmic Drugs

Digoxin, a cardiac glycoside traditionally recognized as a positive inotrope used to improve cardiac muscle contractility in the failing heart, is also a negative chronotrope as a result of both its direct (inhibition of Na^+,K^+-ATPase pump) and indirect (cholinergic-like) effects. In fact, its most common use in the treatment of canine CHF is probably as a negative chronotrope rather than a positive inotrope. Vagomimetic effects inhibit atrioventricular nodal calcium currents and activate acetylcholine-mediated atrial potassium channels. Cardiac glycosides increase the slope of phase 4, particularly in the presence of low extracellular potassium. Indirectly, glycosides hyperpolarize the RMP and shorten atrial action potential durations but increase atrioventricular nodal refractory periods, thus enhancing activity against atrial reentrant arrhythmias.[6] Although digoxin is less effective in slowing the heart rate in the presence of high catecholamine output compared with nonadrenergic stress conditions, only moderate decreases in heart rate are necessary to improve cardiac function. Use of digoxin as a negative chronotrope is discussed in greater depth along with its positive inotropic effects.

Dofetilide is a pure delayed rectifier K^+ channel blocker. As such, it has no extracardiac adverse events. Its efficacy is in the maintenance of normal sinus rhythm in the patient with atrial fibrillation. It is renally excreted, with dose modification necessary with renal disease. The drug is available only through limited distribution. Ibutilide also is a pure delayed rectifier K^+ channel blocker whose use is limited to intravenous administration because of extensive first-pass metabolism. It is metabolized by the liver, with a duration in humans ranging from 2 to 12 hours. Among the more common side effects is torsades de pointes.

Moricizine is a phenothiazine analog that blocks Na^+ channels. It has been used to chronically treat ventricular arrhythmias but has been associated with increased mortality when used acutely to treat myocardial infection. Characterized by first-pass metabolism, its long duration of action in humans (many hours) probably reflects active metabolites.

Atropine is considered an antiarrhythmic by virtue of its blockade of vagally mediated cardiac slowing in some bradyarrhythmias. It is useful, however, only for short-term management. Longer-acting orally administered anticholinergics (e.g., propantheline) are indicated only rarely for bradyarrhythmias, with pacemaker placement being the preferred treatment.

Adenosine is an endogenous nucleoside. It must be administered as a rapid intravenous bolus. Adenosine can acutely block reentrant supraventricular arrhythmias and (rare) ventricular tachycardia associated with DAD events. Transient asystole is a not-uncommon adverse event that lasts less than 5 seconds because of rapid intracranial domination. Atrial fibrillation and bronchospasm are rare events. The effects of adenosine are ameliorated by methylxanthine derivatives.

Magnesium is an antiarrhythmic indicated in patients with torsades de pointes, probably by inhibition of ion flow responsible for EAD. When given intravenously, it has also been used for treating arrhythmias associated with digoxin toxicity. Chronic oral magnesium therapy has not been demonstrated to decrease arrhythmias.

POSITIVE INOTROPES

A positive inotrope increases and a negative inotrope decreases myocardial contractility. Although intuitively, the use of a drug that increases cardiac contractility is reasonable in the patient with a failing myocardium, proof of clinical efficacy of positive inotropes has largely been lacking, and their use is controversial.[191] The advent of newer positive inotropes, such as pimobendan (an inodilator), may provide more clear direction.

Positive inotropic agents increase cardiac force by mechanisms involving increased intracellular Ca^{2+}-concentration. Most mechanisms increase the quantity of calcium available for binding, which in turn augments contractile protein interaction in the myocardial cell (see Figure 14-1). Mechanisms include increasing cAMP production by stimulating adenylyl cyclase; sensitizing myocardial cells (proteins) to calcium, decreasing cAMP degradation by inhibiting PDEs; altering the Na^+,Ca^{2+}-ATPase exchange pump; and, finally, directly stimulating the proteins in the cell membrane that control calcium channels (see Figure 14-1). However, increased intracellular calcium is also associated with adverse effects. It increases the risk of calcium overload in myocardial cells, which will decrease lusitropy (diastolic relaxation). Additional negative sequaelae include apoptosis, necrosis, and the development of tachycardia and arrhythmia. Further, the increase in contractility increases energy/ATP and oxygen consumption.[192]

KEY POINT 14-39 Inherent in the increased contractility associated with many positive inotropes is increased myocardial oxygen demand.

Digitalis and Other Cardiac Glycosides

Digitalis was used as a cardiac drug as early as the 1200s,[3,6,193] with its beneficial effects in the failing heart recognized by 1785. That its efficacy reflected increased myocardial contractility was described in 1958. In addition to improved hemodynamics, digoxin slows atrioventricular conduction and thus heart rate, a critical benefit in patients with atrial fibrillation. The popularity of digoxin reflected, in part, its use for treatment of tachycardia associated with rheumatic heart disease, a common cardiac malady of the mid twentieth century. Cardiac glycosides currently are used to increase circulation in patients with CHF and to slow the ventricular rate in the presence of supraventricular tachycardia (e.g., atrial fibrillation and flutter), with the latter negative chronotropic effect probably of more benefit. The therapeutic margin of the cardiac glycosides is narrow, but to date they have not been effectively replaced with an alternative safer drug. This is apt to change in the next decade with safer and more effective drugs that are in various stages of development (e.g., selective PDE inhibitors and calcium sensitizers) being identified and developed.

Structure–Activity Relationship

Digitalis refers to both digoxin and digitoxin. Digitalis is obtained from the dried leaf of the foxglove plant *(Digitalis purpurea).* The active component of cardiac glycosides is an aglycone, which is released from attached sugars by hydrolysis (Figure 14-10).[3,6] Cardiac glycosides contain a steroidal nucleus containing a lactone ring (at C17) and one or more glycosidic residues (C3). Although the term *digitalis* has been used interchangeably with the term *cardiac glycosides,* current use is largely limited to digoxin in humans.

Mechanism of Action and Pharmacodynamic Responses

Cardiac glycosides are potent but reversible inhibitors of the α subunit of cell membrane–bound Na^+,K^+-activated adenosine triphosphate (Na^+,K^+-ATPase) "pump" (see Figures 14-1 and 14-11). The enzymatic activity is impaired, leading to like impairment of active transport, or exchange of sodium for potassium and a gradual increase in intracellular sodium. Cardiac fibers (both cell membrane and sarcoplasmic membrane) possess a second ATPase pump that exchanges Na^+ for Ca^{2+}; this pump is one of two ATP-ase pumps that extrude intracellular calcium after contraction (the second being a Ca^{2+}-ATPase pump). As sodium increases in the cell in response to glycoside inhibition of the Na^+,K^+-ATPase pump, exchange of Na^+ for Ca^{2+} is augmented, increasing calcium influx. Only a small increase in intracellular calcium occurs, but it is sufficient to cause a marked increased in Ca^{2+} release from the sarcoplasmic reticulum during systole (see Figures 14-1 and 14-2). Myocardial contractility improves, resulting in an increase in left ventricular function in both the normal and failing myocardium.[6] In humans the increased contractility occurs at serum concentrations of 1.4 ng/mL.[6]

At 1 to 2 ng/mL, digoxin also indirectly increases efferent vagal (cholinergic) tone and decreases sympathetic nervous activity. Increased vagal tone is associated with inhibiting Ca^{2+}

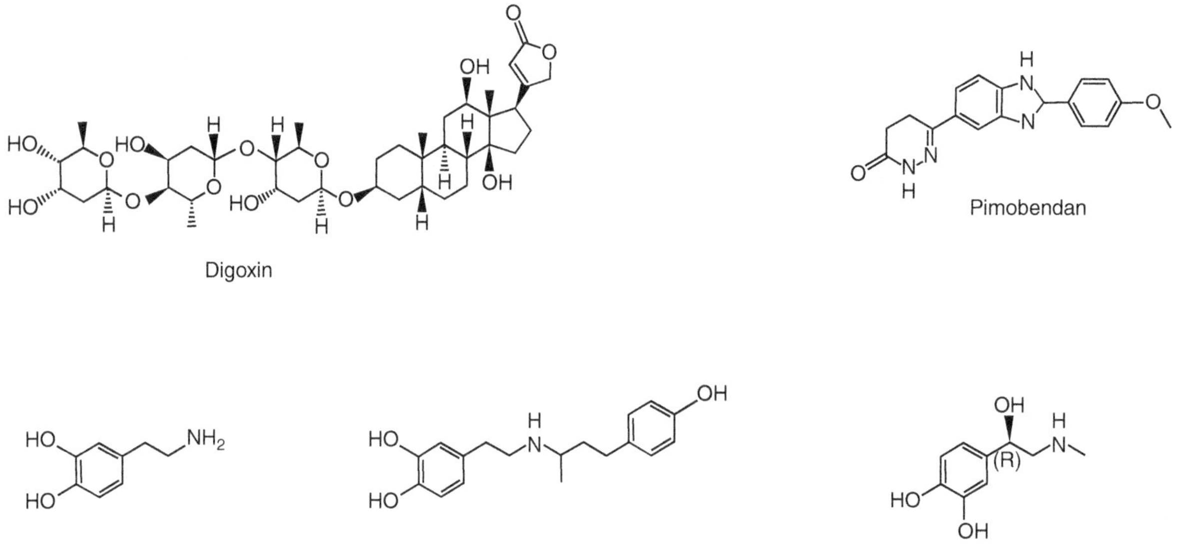

Digoxin

Pimobendan

Dopamine

Dobutamine

Epinephrine

Figure 14-10 Chemical structure of selected drugs with positive inotropic effects.

currents; decreasing automaticity; increasing the diastolic RMP; increasing the ERP, and decreasing conduction velocity, particularly in atrial and atrioventricular nodal tissues. Paradoxically, in nonconducting atrial fibers, acetylcholine-mediated potassium currents are increased, which shortens atrial action potentials. Therefore digoxin may contribute to or cause atrial tachycardias, including reentrant arrhythmias such as atrial fibrillation. The risk is greater in the diseased heart. However, although more impulses are transmitted to the AV node by fluttering or fibrillating atrial tissues, the vagal effects of digitalis decrease the number of atrial impulses that are transmitted by the atrioventricular node to the ventricles. Consequently, digoxin is indicated for slowing of ventricular rates in patients with supraventricular tachycardias such as atrial fibrillation. Electrocardiographically, digoxin prolongs the PR interval and depresses the ST segment (the latter mechanism is not understood).[6]

KEY POINT 14-40 The direct effects of digoxin alter potassium, calcium and sodium flux across the myocardial cell membrane. The indirect effects increase vagal tone. Therefore digoxin is associated with a variety of cardiac arrhythmias .

In addition to increased vagal tone, the indirect effects of digoxin on heart rate also reflect decreased sympathetic nervous system activity.[6] Digoxin decreases neurohumoral activation associated with heart failure.[6] Inhibition of the sodium pump in neuronal cells, particularly in the baroreceptor, results in stimulation of parasympathetic and inhibition of sympathetic nerves. Digoxin appears to directly alter carotid baroreflex responsiveness to changes in carotid sinus pressure in animals with heart failure.[6] Digoxin is less effective as a negative chronotrope for tachycardias associated with marked sympathetic drive such as occurs with CHF. However, even minor reductions in heart rate may markedly improve

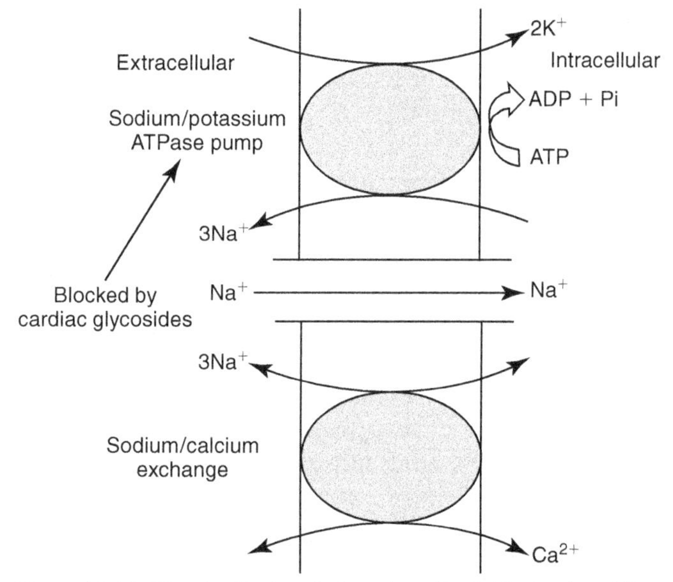

Figure 14-11 Direct effects of digoxin reflect blockade of the sodium/potassium ATPase pump. The resulting increase in intracellular sodium initiates the sodium/calcium ATPase pump. Increased intracellular calcium is sufficient to stimulate intracellular release of calcium, increasing contractility. Myocardial arrhythmias caused by digoxin reflect, in part, disruption in cell membrane fluxes of sodium, potassium, and calcium. *ADP,* Adenosine diphosphate; *ATP,* adenosine triphosphate.

myocardial function. Heart rate will be slowed, particularly in patients with a rapid heart rate, with effects generally occurring at serum digoxin concentrations of 1.3 ng/mL.[6] Digitalis has only minor indirect effects in ventricular tissue.

The effects of cardiac glycosides on myocardial oxygen demand depend on the net effect on cardiac function. Mechanistically, energy utilization shifts from one ATPase pump to another, which might minimize the increase in oxygen needs.

In normal hearts oxygen demand increases proportionately with increased contraction.[3] If ventricular volume decreases and systolic wall stress declines, however, as would be expected in an animal with myocardial failure, improved cardiac function and subsequent decreased fiber length will compensate for the increased oxygen demand caused by improved contractility.[3,191]

KEY POINT 14-41 The efficacy of digoxin probably reflects its negative chronotropic effects more than its positive inotropic effects.

Cardiac glycosides can cause peripheral arterial and venous vasoconstriction, but these effects are more likely in the normal animal.[6] Pulmonary vasoconstriction is induced by all cardiac glycosides except digoxin. Effects in the vasculature are more common after intravenous administration and occur in less than 15 minutes; indeed, with oral administration vasodilation predominates. Thus oral digitalization with digoxin will minimize the risk of adverse effects caused by cardiac glycoside–induced vasoconstriction.[191]

Detrimental effects on myocardial remodeling are a potentially important deterrent to cardiac glycoside therapy. Ouabain (a largely experimental cardiac glycoside) induces mRNA and subsequent production of IL-1b, IL-6, and TNF-α in human peripheral blood mononuclear cells. In an experimental model of myocardial failure, high doses of digoxin increased myocardial necrosis, cellular infiltration, intracardiac IL-1b, TNF-α, and mortality. However, no death occurred among control animals treated with 10 mg/kg.[35]

Clinical Pharmacology

Digoxin and digitoxin are the two most widely used cardiac glycoside preparations. The disposition of both drugs have been studied in dogs[194-197] and is variable among animals and preparations. Oral bioavailability of digoxin varies from 40% to 90%, depending on the preparation. Up to 90% of the alcohol (i.e., elixir) is absorbed, with peak concentrations occurring in 45 to 60 minutes.[3] Variation in bioavailability of tablets is affected by differences in dissolution between products. Absorption is retarded by food. Compared with digoxin, oral absorption of the more lipid-soluble glycoside, digitoxin, is much more complete and thus predictable. Interestingly, in humans *Eubacterium lentum,* a normal microbial inhabitant, metabolizes digoxin to inactive metabolites in a small percentage of the population, leading to unexpected decreased bioavailability. Both digoxin and digitoxin are distributed slowly, in part because of a large volume of distribution that includes most body tissues but also reflects concentration in cardiac tissues. Although the volume of distribution of digoxin is large, it is distributed primarily to cardiac and skeletal muscle, indicating that dosing should be based on lean body weight.[6] Only 25% of digoxin is protein bound, whereas most of digitoxin (90%) is protein bound. Accordingly, response to digoxin should be faster and the dose of digitoxin should be higher (to compensate for high protein binding). Digoxin is primarily eliminated unchanged in the kidneys. The half-life varies from 21 to 60 hours,[3] with a working average of 1.7 days. Half-life is variable in the same animal, ranging from 46 to 154 hours in one study.[3] Elimination half-life is strongly influenced by renal function. Because variability increases as renal function changes with the progression of cardiac disease or response to therapy, monitoring of both a peak and a trough is strongly recommended. For example, our laboratory has demonstrated an elimination half-life for digoxin to be as short as 9 hours in animals concurrently receiving an ACE inhibitor and diuretic therapy but longer than 48 hours in animals with presumed renal dysfunction.

KEY POINT 14-42 The half-life of digoxin is markedly variable, and monitoring of both peak and trough samples may be prudent, particularly in patients that have responded to therapy.

In contrast to digoxin, digitoxin is metabolized by the liver to digoxin and other metabolites. Its metabolism is affected by factors that alter the microsomal system but generally not hepatic disease. Despite binding to serum proteins and hepatic metabolism, a half-life of 8 to 12 hours in dogs (parent compound) is shorter than that of digoxin, which may necessitate more frequent dosing. Digitoxin undergoes a small enterohepatic cycle.

Population kinetic analysis has been used to describe the disposition of digoxin in a population (n=161; 32 studied prospectively) of dogs with naturally occurring heart disease.[198] Covariable data collected included serum creatitine and potassium, body weight and body surface area, and formulation of digoxin administered. Dosing regimens (dose, intervals), formulation of digoxin, type and state of cardiac disease, and adjuvant medications and method of monitoring (time of sample collection, analytic technique) varied among animals. The rate of oral absorption was markedly variable. The slowest absorbers (n=19) were prospectively studied and as such had been admitted 2 hours before dosing, compared with the remaining 142 cases, in which dosing occurred at home. Based on the reported rate constant, the absorption half-life in the slow absorbers approximated 6.1 hours compared with 1 hour for the fast absorbers. The type of formulation (Lanoxin tablets versus elixir) did not statistically influence the absorption rate constant. These data suggest that the stress of admission may profoundly affect the rate of absorption and perhaps the peak plasma drug concentration of digoxin, indicating that patients ideally be dosed at home before monitoring. Elimination rate constants (and thus half-life) were not reported. Potassium was negatively correlated to volume of distribution corrected for oral bioavailability (Vd/F), potentially reflecting displacement of digoxin from its tissue binding sites (Na^+/K^+ ATPase) by potassium, resulting in a smaller volume of distribution. Creatinine was a poor predictor of changes in digoxin clearance even when corrected for bioavailability (Cl/F).

Preparations and Dosing Information

Digoxin is available for intravenous or oral administration. Intravenous administration results in pharmacologic effects in 5 to 30 minutes, with a maximal effect in 2 hours. Intravenous administration might (very cautiously) substitute for oral dosing in animals intolerant to the latter. Digoxin should not be given intramuscularly because it is erratically absorbed and causes pain and tissue necrosis. Oral administration results in pharmacologic effects in 1 to 2 hours, although peak effects will not occur until steady state is reached. Digoxin elixir is more orally bioavailable, and it may be necessary to decrease doses by 15%. If deemed necessary, oral digitalization is best accomplished with digoxin tablets. In the absence of a loading dose, steady-state concentrations can be achieved within 48 hours of oral dosing in most patients. If necessary, a prudent intravenous loading dose is administration of the oral daily maintenance dose over a 12-hour period.[191] Doses should be calculated on lean body weight; toxicosis is likely to be minimized if dosing is based on body surface area (0.44 mg/m^2). Daily doses should be divided if warranted on the basis of drug elimination half-life (as calculated from therapeutic drug monitoring) to minimize fluctuation in plasma drug concentrations.

KEY POINT 14-43 The therapeutic window of digoxin is narrow, but the risk of adversities might be minimized if attention is paid to the risk factors presented by disease- and drug-related factors.

Drug Interactions

The concurrent administration of quinidine increases plasma concentrations of digoxin; the mechanism may reflect displacement from tissue binding sites, although this mechanism is controversial.[117,199] Quinidine also appears to decrease renal digoxin clearance by decreasing renal blood flow.[200] Verapamil also increases concentrations of digoxin.[191] Interactions between digitalis and diuretics have been reported and stem primarily from the effects on potassium (hypokalemia). Diuretics do not seem to alter the disposition of digoxin.[201] Phenobarbital has been reported to increase (rather than decrease) digoxin concentrations; the clinical relevance of this report is not clear.[201,202] Administration of β-adrenergic agonists increases the likelihood of arrhythmias. Amphotericin B may also cause hypokalemia and thus potentiate digitalis intoxication.

Clinical Efficacy

Inotropic response to digoxin is greatest in the initially depressed state of the failing heart. Stroke volume increases as ventricular emptying improves, with a reduction in end-diastolic volume.[191] This positive effect is less likely if intrinsic compensatory mechanisms are maintaining cardiac output. The inotropic response to digoxin occurs before evidence of electrophysiologic changes. As a positive inotrope, withdrawal of digoxin in human patients with mild to moderate CHF and a normal sinus rhythm resulted in a significant (compared to placebo) worsening of clinical signs. In patients with severe CHF, fewer patients receiving digoxin died or were hospitalized as a result of CHF during the study period. Retrospectively, digoxin effects were best when concentrations were below 1 ng/mL. However, it is not clear if this effect is due to decreased heart rate or a positive inotropic effect: clinically, animals may have the greatest improvement immediately before accumulated glycoside toxicosis.[191] Digoxin may also decrease myocardial remodeling: ouabain increased mediators associated with ventricular remodeling after myocardial infarction.[35] Digoxin modulates neurohumoral and autonomic states.[35] Currently, in humans digoxin therapy generally is reserved for patients with heart failure accompanied by atrial fibrillation or for patients with a sinus rhythm but who have not yet sufficiently responded to ACE inhibitors and adrenergic receptor antagonists.

Proof of efficacy of digoxin in the treatment of CHF in dogs has been difficult to establish, in part because of poorly designed clinical trials.[191] Studies are complicated by failure to control variables and, most notably, adjunct therapy. Subclinical measures based on hemodynamic response often have not been included, making it more difficult to identify efficacy. Different levels of disease also influence outcome; response to digoxin may be less obvious in the terminal stages of congestive cardiomyopathy (shortening fraction of 20%).[191] Clinical trials based on survival analysis similarly have been fraught with poor methodologies. Controversy also exists regarding the relative efficacy of digoxin versus digitoxin in the treatment of CHF in dogs.[191] Early studies with dogs receiving either drug revealed greater clinical improvement in dogs with CHF treated with digoxin (85%) than digitoxin (55%) but a greater risk of toxicity (based on electrophysiologic changes in the PR interval.[203,204] It is likely, however, that digitoxin was underdosed in these studies.[191] Current consensus among cardiologists is that digoxin is the preferred drug on the basis of both pharmacodynamics and pharmacokinetics.

Knight[191] offered a description of the canine patient most likely to respond to digoxin therapy. Such a patient is asymptomatic, with CHF characterized primarily by systolic ventricular dysfunction accompanied by supraventricular tachycardia, including sinus tachycardia, atrial flutter, and fibrillation. Chronic mitral regurgitation is included in the indications, although timing of the use of digoxin as treatment in this syndrome may be less clear unless myocardial failure is evident. Digoxin is not indicated for the compensated patient that is asymptomatic (including normal sinus rhythm; plus or minus diuretics). Aggressive treatment may be necessary to control heart rate. Whereas vagally mediated effects occur at subtoxic concentrations (50% of the toxic dose), the direct effects on atrioventricular nodal conduction occur only at full digitalization—that is, as toxic concentrations are approached.[191] Such concentrations may be more necessary in patients with atrial flutter or fibrillation for which response might be dependent on atrioventricular nodal effects. The negative chronotropic effects are decreased in the presence of concurrent sympathetic stimulation, which is more likely as the severity and chronicity of heart failure increases. Thus sinus tachycardia is most likely to normalize if cardiac function improves sufficiently to minimize sympathetic stimulation. β-adrenergic blockers or CCBs may be useful adjunct therapies if heart rate remains unacceptably high in patients receiving digoxin.[191]

Controversy exists regarding whether digoxin should precede, accompany, or follow vasodilator therapy and, more specifically, ACE inhibitor therapy. Preference generally favors the latter. Digoxin is, however, indicated for symptomatic patients that cannot tolerate ACE inhibitors and for patients that presented with moderate to severe clinical manifestations of decompensation, particularly if the patient is no longer responsive to diuretic or vasodilator therapy.[191]

Monitoring

Monitoring recommendations for digoxin are extrapolated from human medicine. The traditional recommended therapeutic range of 0.8 to 2.0 ng/mL is intended to prevent toxic concentrations but not necessarily identify efficacy. Maximal contractile activity in humans generally occurs at concentrations between 0.5 and 1.5 ng/mL.[205] Neurohormonal benefits may occur at concentrations of 0.5 to 1 ng/mL.[6] Although inotropic effects will continue to increase as drug concentrations increase, peak effects are likely to be limited by toxicity. Because the risk of death increases at higher concentrations associated with maximal contractility, concentrations below 1 ng/mL are recommended for humans.

Therapeutic concentrations of digitoxin and digoxin differ. For digitoxin recommended concentrations are 1.4 to 2.6 ng/mL.[3] The recommended range for digoxin is likely to vary with the laboratory but generally is 1 to 2 ng/mL or 1.5 to 2.5 ng/mL.[195] Because the time needed for C_{max} to decline to C_{min} is one half-life, the dosing interval should not exceed patient half-life. The targeted concentration for either cardiac glycoside in the individual animal should be based on clinical signs, including response to therapy. Traditionally, single samples (generally mid trough) have been collected at mid interval for monitoring. However, based on 2 hr peak and 12 hr trough samples, the author has documented a shortening of digoxin half-life in a patient treated with ACE inhibitors (presumably due to increased glomerular filtration rate and thus renal digoxin clearance) or other therapy. In such patients plasma drug concentrations can fluctuate twofold during a dosing interval, causing the patient to become both toxic or subtherapeutic. For such patients design of a dosing regimen might best be based on both peak and trough concentrations (at 2 and 11.5 hours after oral administration at home). If only a single sample is possible, selection of the time of collection depends on the intent of monitoring. If toxicity is of concern, a peak sample should be collected 1 to 2 hours after administration at home; if efficacy is of concern, then a trough sample should be collected just before the next dose. However, neither situation will provide guidance regarding drug concentrations throughout the dosing interval.

Toxicity and Side Effects

Digitalis intoxication is not uncommon, although improper use plays a large role in the incidence of adversity. In addition, signs of toxicity are more easily recognized than are signs of efficacy, contributing to the perceived narrow therapeutic margin. It is likely that with proper use the risk–benefit ratio is not as narrow as perceived. Serious toxic effects of digitalis are due to altered electrical activity, which reflects changes in intracellular calcium, sodium, and potassium changes and thus the electric potential formed across the cell membrane. Digitalis causes an increase in automaticity and ectopic beats. As concentrations surpass 2 ng/mL, the risk of sinus bradycardia or arrest, prolongation of atrioventricular conduction, heart block, or increased sympathetic nervous activity with increased automaticity increases. The negative chronotropic effects of digitalis can be ameliorated with atropine.

KEY POINT 14-44 The risk of hypokalemia, which increases the risk of digoxin toxicity, is increased in the anorectic patient receiving potassium-wasting diuretics. Potassium supplementation may be indicated.

Digoxin binds preferentially to the phosphorylated form of Na^+,K^+-ATPase, whose concentration is decreased by extracellular potassium. Thus hypokalemia increases digoxin toxicity by facilitating binding to the target protein.[6] Increased intracellular calcium also contributes to the arrhythmogenicity of digoxin.[6] The increased calcium causes the cytoplasmic membrane to become unstable immediately after repolarization and cell membrane permeability to Na^+, Ca^{2+}, and K^+ increases. Ion flow of Na^+ and Ca^{2+} follows the concentration gradient, tending to hypopolarize the membrane (i.e., it moves toward 0 mV); flow of potassium is less important because concentration and electrochemical gradients for potassium tend to balance one another. Dysrhythmias tend to worsen as calcium increases as the risk of after-depolarization–mediated automaticity increases.[5]

Because the mechanism of arrhythmogenicity for digoxin is the same as the mechanism of efficacy (positive inotropic and negative chronotropic effects), it is not surprising that cardiac glycosides are characterized by a narrow safety margin. Any cardiac antiarrhythmia may be induced by digitalis. An electrocardiogram should be useful in diagnosing digitalis toxicity if compared with an electrocardiogram obtained before drug administration. Changes in sodium, calcium, or potassium increase the risk of arrhythmias associated with automaticity. In the atrium digoxin shortens the action potential, predisposing it to atrial fibrillation.[5] The negative chronotropic effects of digoxin also can directly slow sinus nodal activity, leading to heart blockade. Arrhythmias include sinus bradycardia; disturbances of atrial rhythm; atrioventricular conduction, including complete atrioventricular block (third-degree heart block); and disturbances of ventricular rhythm, especially premature beats. Ventricular tachycardia and flutter may also occur. The likelihood and severity of toxicity are related to the severity of cardiac disease. Toxic effects with digitalis are frequent and can be lethal if allowed to persist. Dogs with severe cardiomegaly and CHF are probably at greater risk of developing ectopic ventricular arrhythmias. Other factors predisposing to digoxin toxicity include but are not limited to hypokalemia, hypercalcemia, hypomagnesemia, hypothyroidism, acid–base imbalances, and abnormal renal function.[6] Combination therapy with selected drugs also predisposes the patient to toxicity. The cat is more sensitive to digoxin than the dog.

Digoxin also causes noncardiac toxicities as a result of impaired Na^+-K^+ pump activity on neuronal and secretory organs. Frequently, the earliest indications of digoxin toxicity are gastrointestinal adversities including anorexia; nausea; vomiting; and, less frequently, diarrhea. Vomiting also results from direct stimulation of the chemoreceptor trigger zone. Neurologic effects include malaise and drowsiness.

The most frequent cause of digoxin toxicity is probably overdosing, which includes failure to individualize dosing regimens. The potential for toxicity is increased with hypokalemia because binding to the Na^+-ATPase pump is facilitated. This may occur, for example, if the patient is also receiving diuretic therapy that causes potassium loss (furosemide, thiazides, and other "nonsparing" diuretics). Digitalis toxicity can be diagnosed and the risk minimized by plasma drug concentration monitoring. Therapeutic concentrations of digitoxin and digoxin differ. For digitoxin concentrations greater than 3.4 ng/mL are considered toxic.[3] For digoxin the risk of toxicosis is greater if concentrations exceed 2 to 2.5 ng/mL.[195] Because of overlap between toxicity and efficacy, concentrations should be considered in the context of clinical signs.

The treatment of cardiac glycoside intoxication includes (1) discontinuation of digitalis therapy for at least one drug elimination half-life; (2) discontinuation of potassium-depleting diuretics; and (3) administration (as needed) of phenytoin, which blocks atrioventricular nodal effects of digitalis (bradyarrhythmias), lidocaine (for ventricular arrhythmias)[206] (1-3 mg/kg intravenously), and oral potassium supplementation (e.g., potassium chloride), but only if hypokalemia exists.[3] Atropine may be useful to treat sinus bradycardia and second- or third-degree heart block induced by cholinergic augmentation. Procainamide also has been shown experimentally to be useful for treatment of digoxin-induced ventricular arrhythmias in the canine heart when plasma drug concentrations approximate 8 to 12 ng/mL.[207,208] Cholestyramine can be used as a binding agent to decrease absorption from the gastrointestinal tract (including drug undergoing enterohepatic circulation).

The large volume of distribution of digoxin prevents the use of techniques for increasing clearance as an approach to decreasing the risk of toxicity in the case of overdose. Purified ovine antibody fractions (Fab) to digoxin (DIGIBIND® or DIGIFAB®) have proved to be an effective antidote to life threatening digoxin toxicity (e.g, ventricular arrhythmias) following massive overdose in humans. Although they have been successfully used by the author to treat an accidental overdose of digoxin, their cost is likely to be prohibitive. The drug costs $700-800 per vial; an adequate dose may result in a cost of thousands of dollars. Dosing is complicated, being based on the total amount of digoxin in the body. This can be estimated on the basis of the amount ingested and the average bioavailability or on serum digoxin concentrations and the average volume of distribution.[6] Toxicity can recur once the Fab has been eliminated 1 to 2 days after therapy, particularly in patients with impaired renal function.

Clinical Use

The recent approval of pimobendan for use in dogs should result in a decline in the use of cardiac glycosides as positive inotropes. Clinical uses of digitalis have included restoration of adequate circulation in patients with CHF and reduction of the ventricular rate as a treatment of atrial fibrillation or flutter. Both syndromes require long-term treatment. If there is no urgency in treatment, the drug can be administered orally. Maximal effect is achieved in four half-lives. Digoxin is the cardiac glycoside drug of choice except for the patient with renal disease; digitoxin should then be administered. Calculation of digoxin doses should be based on lean body weight, and dosages should be reduced in the obese patient or in the presence of ascites. Electrolyte disorders should be corrected before dosage.

Calcium Sensitizers

A disadvantage of drugs that increase intracellular calcium are the deleterious effects of intracellular Ca^{2+} overload, including cardiac arrhythmias, and cell injury that could ultimately lead to myocardial cell death.[209] Additionally, positive inotropic effects generally are associated with increased myocardial oxygen consumption. Calcium sensitizers are positive inotropic drugs that increase cardiac contractility by direct effects on cardiac myofilaments or the cross-bridge interaction, without altering intracellular Ca^{2+}-concentration.[192] Calcium sensitizers target "downstream" calcium sites, particularly the cardiac excitation–contraction coupling process. Examples of targeted sites include Ca^{2+} binding to troponin C, thin filament regulatory sites and/or directly on the cross-bridge cycling. Because efficacy is not dependent on an increase in intracellular calcium, they do not induce the negative sequelae generally associated with increased intracellular calcium (arrhythmias, cell injury, and death) or does energy activation increase. Further, calcium sensitizers can potentially reverse myocardial contraction dysfunction that accompanies pathologic conditions such as acidosis. Three classes of calcium sensitizers have been described according to the type of interaction between calcium and cellular sites. Class I sensitizers target the interaction between troponin C and calcium, thus increasing the calcium sensitivity of troponin C (e.g., pimobendan and levosimendan). Class II sensitizers directly interact with the thin filaments, facilitating actin–myosin interaction such as might occur if the troponin C/Ca^{2+}-complex is stabilized without altering the Ca^{2+}-affinity of troponin C. Class III sensitizers directly interfere with activation steps of the cross-bridge-cycle.[192] Although their efficacy is not certain, Ca^{2+} sensitizers are clinically more effective than the agents that are purely downstream regulators of calcium.[209]

Disadvantages of calcium-sensitizing agents may include the prolongation of myocardial relaxation and possible exacerbation of impaired diastolic function (decreased lusitropy). The risk is greatest if calcium sensitivity of myofilaments increases at low (diastolic) calcium concentrations. The risk is reduced by drugs that increase myofilament calcium sensitivity only during high-calcium conditions (i.e., systole), thus enhancing systole without changing diastolic function.

Current calcium-sensitizing drugs generally are characterized by marked inhibition of PDE.[36] For example, the impact of levosimendan and pimobendan on lusitropy ranges from no impact to improvement.[192] The ideal calcium sensitizer would not inhibit PDE.

Phosphodiesterase Inhibitors

Selective PDE inhibition has yielded therapeutic options for treatment of cardiovascular disorders. At least five PDE isoenzymes have been described; affinity for cyclic nucleotides may account for differences in activity. For example, the affinity of PDE III (located in the heart and systemic smooth muscle vasculature) for cAMP is greater than that for cGMP, whereas PDE V (limited in location to the retina, corpus cavernosum, and cerebral and pulmonary vasculature) has a greater affinity for cGMP.[210] PDE inhibitors, including amrinone, pimobendan, and vesnarinone, prevent the breakdown of cAMP, increasing intracellular cAMP concentration. In myocardial cells, PDE inhibition results in an increase in myocardial contractility. PDE inhibitors also inhibit nitrite accumulation, with pimobendan being the most and amrinone the least potent inhibitor.[35]

Methylxanthine Derivatives

Methylxanthine derivatives have been classified as PDE inhibitors, but the mechanism of action is controversial. Their positive inotropic effects may actually reflect altered calcium fluxes or other mechanisms. Of the methylxanthines, theophylline is the most cardiopotent. The positive inotropic effects of these drugs are complex because they have a variety of pharmacologic actions. In addition to their cardiac effects, these drugs have significant central nervous system, renal, and smooth muscle effects. Thus their use for cardiac disease is limited.

Fatal toxicities can and often do occur during chronic oral or rapid intravenous administration of methylxanthines, probably as a result of cardiac effects. Tachycardia and central nervous system signs (restlessness, hyperexcitability, sensory disturbances) can be correlated with increased plasma concentrations. Plasma monitoring may be used to control toxicity. Local gastrointestinal irritation and nausea, vomiting, and diarrhea may occur with oral administration. These can be prevented by administration of the drugs with food. Therapeutic uses for the methylxanthines in cardiac disease are limited. In veterinary medicine theophylline has been used to treat CHF. Currently, these drugs should be used only in cardiac patients with respiratory disease.

Bipyridines

Bipyridines are nonglycosidic, noncatecholamine positive inotropes that have cardiac effects similar to catecholamines. The mechanism of action of these drugs is probably inhibition of PDE and increased intracellular cAMP concentrations. However, unlike catecholamines, myocardial oxygen consumption does not increase and may actually decrease in patients with CHF. Differences in potency and toxicity when compared with theophylline may reflect selective PDE isoenzyme inhibition for each group of drugs. The bipyridines inhibit PDE III only, whereas theophylline may be a nonselective inhibitor of PDE. Amrinone was the first of this class of drugs to be used therapeutically, but side effects limited its use. Milrinone is more potent than amrinone (20 to 30 times) yet characterized by a toxic to therapeutic ratio of 100 in normal dogs. Milrinone is a selective PDE III inhibitor. It lowers pulmonary vascular resistance in patients with CHF and pulmonary hypertension. Peripheral vasodilation is another major therapeutic benefit of PDE III inhibitors. Milrinone increases renin secretion, presumably by increasing cAMP in juxtaglomerular cells.[211] Side effects at higher doses limit long term use. Intravenous milrinone lowers pulmonary vascular resistance in human patients with CHF and pulmonary hypertension.[210]

Intravenous or oral administration of milrinone results in marked positive inotropic effects in patients with CHF. Effects are dose dependent. Contractility increases up to 100% at plasma concentrations of 200 mm/L after infusion of 10 µg/kg per minute in anesthetized dogs versus only 60% in patients receiving digitalis. An oral dose of 1 mg/kg increases contractility by 90% and decreases blood pressure by 10%. As with the cardiac glycosides, animals with very poor myocardial function may not be able to respond to the bipyridines. In contrast to cardiac glycosides, heart rate increases 40%. As with drug disposition, individual animal response to milrinone appears to be quite variable.[212] Pilot studies indicate an elimination half-life of about 1.4 hours for milrinone in dogs, although this is likely to be quite variable.[212] Oral bioavailability approximates 92%. Milrinone does not appear to be as effective a positive inotrope for people as it is for dogs. In clinical trials in dogs with CHF, approximately 80% of animals reportedly respond to milrinone.[213] Survival data were not reported for dogs. Milrinone appears to be substantially safer than digoxin when given at an oral dose of 0.5 to 1 mg/kg twice daily. However, exacerbations of arrhythmias may occur in some animals. Ruptured chordae tendineae (4%) and sudden death (13%) were other complications reported in clinical trials with dogs with CHF.

Pimobendan and levosimendan

Pimobendan is a benzimidazole–pyridazinone derivative that acts as a specific type III PDE inhibitor, causing positive inotropy. However, its efficacy may reflect actions as a calcium sensitizer. Pimobendan enhances calcium–troponin C interaction. Pimobendan increases sensitivity at low concentrations, increasing the risk of diastolic dysfunction resulting from decreased lusitropy (relaxation). However, neither pimobendan nor its congener, levosimendan, affect or improve myocardial lusitropy. In addition to its positive inotropic effects, pimobendan prolongs the action potential duration by enhancing calcium current through L-type calcium channels in the sarcolemma. However, prolonged action potential duration may increase the risk of QT syndrome. In contrast to the other Ca^{2+}-sensitizers, both pimobendan and levosimendan cause vasodilation of both the arterial and venous vessels, reflecting activation of the Ca^{2+}-dependent K^+-channels (and ATP-sensitive K^+-channels for levosimendan); As such, pimobendan is referred to as an *inodilator*. Additionally, pimobendan is associated with a reduction of proinflammatory cytokines that initiate or perpetuate myocardial remodeling associated with progressive CHF.[35] As such, pimobendan appears to provide some level of cardioprotection. Finally, pimobendan also exerts antithrombotic effects. [192,209] In contrast to pimobendan, an advantage of levosimendan is that it appears to sensitize to calcium without influencing PDIII activity unless higher concentrations are achieved. As such, levosimendan may be the perfect "designer" drug for treatment of systolic dysfunction in patient with CHF. Treatment with levosimendan improved hemodynamics and patient survival in one study, although the study groups were too small to allow mortality assessment. Improvement occurred even in patients treated with beta-adrenoceptor blockers, which currently are associated with the best evidence of improved hemodynamics and survival in patients with chronic heart failure.[209]

KEY POINT 14-45 The potential efficacy of the inodilator pimobendan reflects not only its positive inotropic effects but also calcium sensitization, vasodilation, and cardioprotection.

Pimobendan is prepared as a mixture of stereoisomers. In humans, although the pharmacokinetics of the enantiomers is the same, the l-isomer is 1.5 times more potent in increasing strength of contraction than the d-isomer. In humans both enantiomers accumulate in red blood cells, with the respective (+)- and (−)-pimobendan ratio (red blood cell: plasma) being 5.8 and 8.4. Similar data could not be found in dogs. Food may slow or impair oral absorption. Oral bioavailability is 60 to 65%, In normal dogs, peak plasma drug concentration (C_{max}) for the parent and metabolite following administration of 0.2 mg/kg orally was 3.09 ± 0.76 ng/mL and 3.66 ± 1.21 ng/mL, respectively. Pimobendan is highly (>90%) protein bound in dogs. The apparent volume of distribution at steady state (presumably of unbound drug) is 2.6 L/kg. In dogs pimobendan is demethylated to an active metabolite (UDCG-212) that contributes substantially to its pharmacodynamic effects. The metabolite is a more potent inhibitor of PDIII; however, its mechanism of calcium sensitization may be different from that of the parent compound. Metabolism appears to occur primarily by CYP1A2 (in humans), although its contribution to metabolism is variable, ranging from 18 to 76%; CYP3A4 accounts for less than 10% of elimination. The active metabolite is then excreted by sulfation or glucuronidation and eliminated through feces. Elimination half-life of pimobendan and its metabolite in dogs are 0.5 and 2 hours, respectively (which is similar to both isomers in humans).

A delay occurs between peak pimobendan concentration and peak left ventricular contractility response; further, response persists beyond elimination of drug. In both dogs and humans, effects are still evident at 8 hours, despite a short half-life in either species. In humans pharmacodynamic effects include increased ejection fraction, mean shortening velocity, cardiac index, and stroke volume index (each increased 50% to 60%). Left ventricular end-systolic dimension, SBP, and diastolic blood pressure are decreased 8% to 11% in humans. However, although pimobendan improves morbidity and the physical exercise capacity of human heart failure patients, decreased mortality has not yet been demonstrated.

Pimobendan has been used extensively in dogs with acquired cardiac disease including mitral valve insufficieny and dilated cardiomyopathy; its use should be considered in dogs with systolic dysfunction associated with primary myocardial disease or chronic volume loading. The labeled dose of pimobendan in dogs is 0.5 mg/kg administered every 12 hours and given at least 1 hour before food. Dosing is usually started at the low end of the dose range. Pimobendan can be combined with a variety of cardiac drugs, including diuretics, ACE inhibitors, or digoxin. However, the positive inotropic effects may be reduced when given in conjunction with calcium channel antagonists or β-adrenergic antagonists.

Pimobendan has been compared to levosimendan and milrinone in anesthetized dogs.[213a] All three drugs increased myocardial contractility, venous and arteriolar vasodilation, left ventricular -arterial coupling and mechanical efficiency; levosimendan increased myocardial efficiency. The clinical use of pimobendan in dogs has been reviewed.[214-216a]

In normal dogs pimobendan moderately reduced systemic and pulmonary vascular resistance, markedly reduced left ventricular end-diastolic pressure, and moderately increased heart rate and cardiac output. Myocardial blood flow also is increased. A lusitropic effect also has been demonstrated in the left ventricle of normal dogs.[54] Efficacy in diseased dogs may be superior to that in humans. Summaries of the field (clinical) trial (n=355 dogs) supporting approval of pimobendan found efficacy to be equivalent to that of enalapril in dogs with grades II to IV CHF associated with either valvular disease or DCM. Dogs also received diuretics and, as needed, digoxin for supraventricular arrhythmias. Side effects were similar in both groups.

Kanno and coworkers[219] described the effects of pimobendan (0.25 mg/kg twice daily) on cardiac, hemodynamic, and neurohumoral factors in dogs with mild mitral regurgitation. Dogs were treated for 4 weeks. Pimobendan was associated with a decrease in SBP and the degree of regurgitation, an increase in renal blood flow and glomerular filtration rate, decreased norepinephrine concentrations, and improved heart size. Using a randomized, placebo controlled, double-blinded study in dogs (10 English Cocker Spaniels, 10 Doberman Pinschers) with DCM, when added to standard therapies (i.e., furosemide, enalapril, digoxin), pimobendan (0.3 to 0.6 mg/kg/day) was demonstrated to improve heart failure class, and to prolong survival in Doberman Pinschers (mean of 329 days compared with 50 in placebo group).[216] O'Grady and coworkers[220] also found that the addition of pimobendan (0.25 mg/kg PO every 12 hr) to standard diuretic (furosemide) and afterload reduction (benazepril) therapy was associated with a longer time (130.5 days) to treatment failure in Doberman Pinschers with DCM and CHF compared with the placebo group (63 ± 14 days).

Pimobendan also has proven useful for treatment of degenerative mitral valvular disease. The QUEST study[221] compared the impact of pimobendan (n=124) versus benazepril (n=128) on mortality in dogs from Europe, Canada, and Australia afflicted with myxomatous mitral valve disease. Of the dogs reaching an endpoint associated with decline the median time was 267 days for pimobendan compared to 140 for benazepril. Pimobendan (0.2 to 0.3 mg/kg twice daily) did not have a sustained positive effect on echocardiographic values of asymptomatic dogs (some were receiving ACE inhibitors) (n=24) with mitral valve disease using a randomized, blinded design. An initial increase in systolic function at 30 days did not persist to study end (6 months). However, a major limitation of the study was the sample size.[222]

KEY POINT 14-46 Pimobendan can be safely combined with other traditional drug therapies for congestive heart failure.

Other studies have compared pimobendan to ACE inhibitor therapy in an attempt to identify the most effective approach. Using a prospective, randomized, single-blinded parallel design, the clinical efficacy and safety of pimobendan was compared in a 6-month study to ramipril in client-owned dogs (n=43) with mild to moderate heart failure associated with mitral valve disease. Treatment was well tolerated in both groups; pimobendan-treated dogs were only 25% as likely to have an adverse outcome related to heart failure (odds ratio 4.09, 95% confidence interval 1.03 to 16.3, P=0.046). However, despite randomization, dogs receiving ramipril began with a higher overall score, suggesting this group had more severe disease.[217] The efficacy of pimobendan (n=41) was also compared to benazepril as a positive control (n=35) in dogs with atrioventricular disease using a parallel, randomized, blinded multicenter clinical trial (VetSCOPE). Animals were assessed at 56 days, and long-term survival was determined.[218] Scores in dogs receiving pimobendan improved compared with those of animals not receiving pimobendan; further, long-term survival was greater at 415 days compared with 128 for dogs not receiving pimobendan.

Timing of pimobendan administration in the progression of myocardial disease may be important. Discontinuation of pimobendan improved mitral regurgitation in two dogs[57] led to a double blinded parallel clinical trial comparing the effect of either pimobendan or benazepril in dogs (Beagles; n=12; 6 per group) with asymptomatic, naturally occurring mitral valvular disease.[223] Increased systolic function associated with a longer regurgitant jet characterized by a greater velocity was detected in the pimobendan group within 15 days of initiation of therapy. Histologic mitral valvular lesions were worse (moderate to severe) in three dogs at the end of the 512-day treatment period in the pimobendan group compared with the benazepril group (mild to slight in six dogs).

Evidence exists that pimobendan can be combined with standard cardiovascular drugs with no apparent adverse effects, as has been suggested by clinical trials assessing efficacy. In addition, Fusellier and coworkers[224] failed to detect significant differences in adversities when pimobendan was combined with meloxicam in 10 Beagles using a randomized, crossover design. However, dogs were studied 4 times (placebo, meloxicam, pimobendan, and the combination), and the power to detect a significant difference was not addressed, indicating that an adverse reaction cannot be ruled out.

Pimobendan has been associated with histologic damage to the endocardium, myocardium and valves, particularly at high intravenous disease. [224a] A randomized, blinded, controlled clinical trail in Beagles (n=12) with mitral valvular disease comparing the impact of 512 days of therapy with either benazepril and pimobendan found that pimobendan was associated with an increase in the maximum area and peak velocity of the regurgitant jet turbulence. Further, acute focal hemorrhages, endothelial papillary hyperplasia, and infiltration of chordae tendinae with glycosaminoglycans occurred in the pimobendan-treated dogs. These studies support avoiding pimobendan use unless indicated.

Beta-Adrenergic Agonists

The β-adrenergic agonists include the catecholamines (norepinephrine, epinephrine, isoproterenol, dopamine, and dobutamine). Catecholamines increase contractility through β-adrenoceptor–mediated accumulation of cyclic AMP and subsequent phosphorylation of regulatory proteins, by protein kinase A (PKA). Proteins targeted include L-type Ca^{2+} channels, phospholamban (regulates the calcium pump), ryanodine receptors (a class of intracellular calcium channels), TnI and myosin-binding protein C (see Figure 14-1). These drugs are the most potent myocardial stimulants, each causing increased contractility. However, depending on the drug, potent peripheral vasomotor responses may limit their use clinically as positive inotropes but may also justify their use as pressor agents.

Dopamine

Dopamine is an endogenous catecholamine (norepinephrine) precursor with selective β_1 activity. It is widely used as a cardiac stimulant. Because it stimulates the release of norepinephrine, however, it has α-receptor-, β_2-receptor-, and dopaminergic-receptor–mediated actions as well. Its inotropic effects are due to β_1-receptor stimulation in the heart. At low doses (4 μg/kg per minute) in dogs, dopamine increases stroke volume and cardiac output and stimulates renal dopaminergic receptors, causing increased renal blood flow and diuresis. This is useful during situations of systemic vasoconstriction (e.g., shock), during which it is important to maintain renal blood flow. At high doses, however, it causes α-adrenergic stimulation and vasoconstriction. This may potentially reduce renal blood flow. Vasoconstriction can be reversed with alpha-adrenergic blocking drugs (e.g, phenothiazines). Dopamine appears to increase systolic pressure without significantly affecting diastolic pressure.

Dopamine is not effectively absorbed orally. It is rapidly metabolized by the body by monoamine oxidize and catechol O-methyl transferase (COMT) and has a half-life of less than 2 minutes. Dopamine is most commonly marketed as a solution that is further diluted with saline or dextrose. The drug is administered intravenously. Because the pharmacologic effects of dopamine are short lived, it is usually administered by constant infusion, and rate of administration can be used to control the intensity of effects.

KEY POINT 14-47 Beta agonists markedly increase myocardial oxygen demand and thus are arrythmogenic.

Cardiac arrhythmias may occur following dopamine therapy due to α-adrenergic activity. Dopamine should not be used in the hypovolemic patient (in part because of the potential for enhanced vasoconstriction in response to α-adrenergic activity). Tissue sloughing may occur in the event of perivascular leakage. Indications include cardiogenic, or endotoxic, shock and oliguria. Dopamine has been compared to norepinephrine as a pressor agent in humans; although statistical difference in 28 day mortality could not be demonstrated between the two groups, dopamine was associated with more life-threatening arrhythmias.[223a] Dopamine can be diluted in a variety of fluids; an exception is fluids containing sodium bicarbonate or other alkaline infusions that will inactivate the drug. It will remain stable for at least 24 h after dilution.

Dopamine receptors are present in the cat, with D1 receptors identified in the feline renal cortex. The concentration appears to be lower than that in rats, dogs, and humans. The status of dopamine receptors in the feline renal vasculature is not clear. However, fenoldopam, a dopamine agonist, exhibits 300-fold greater affinity than dopamine for feline dopamine receptors, suggesting that failure of feline renal response to dopamine reflects a lack of dopamine receptors.[225] This suggestion is supported by the observation that low-dose dopamine can provide effective diuresis in the dog but not the cat, yet higher doses of dopamine do increase diuresis and natriuresis in the cat.[225,226] Fenaldopam is used for treatment of emergency hypertension and to stimulate systemic vasodilation, natriuresis, and diuresis in human patients with renal disease.[227] Dopamine is likewise indicated in veterinary patients to induce diuresis in dogs with oliguric renal failure, in dogs and cats as a pressor agent in the presence of hypotension, and to provide inotropic support in the failing congestive heart.

Dobutamine

Dobutamine is a synthetic drug that is similar to dopamine but with the addition of a large bulky molecule that reduces non-β_1 effects. Dobutamine is a more effective inotrope than dopamine and is not associated with increased cardiac rates at lower doses. Therapeutic and pharmacologic ranges, respectively, are 0.1-10 μM; 10-100 μM.[228] Dobutamine appears to increase cardiac contractility with less cardiac oxygen consumption than other catecholamines. Dobutamine does not dilate the renal vascular bed as does dopamine, although in a canine model of endotoxic shock it increased urine output and mesenteric blood flow at 5 and 10 μg/kg per minute, probably resulting from cardiac effects.[229] Because of its greater selective effect on contractility as opposed to increasing heart rate, it is preferred to dopamine as a positive inotrope for treatment of CHF that is severe and eminently life threatening. Its arrhythmogenicity is less than that of epinephrine and is not likely to occur (in normal dogs or dogs with ventricular ectopic beats) until therapeutic doses have been exceeded.

Dobutamine is not effective orally and has a plasma half-life of approximately 2 minutes because of metabolism by COMT. It is therefore usually administered by constant-rate intravenous infusion. The drug is metabolized in the liver to inactive glucuronide conjugates. Like dopamine, dobutamine is prepared as a solution to be diluted with dextrose or variety of fluids, but is inactivated by alkaline solutions such as those containing sodium bicarbonate. It is stable for only 6 hours after dilution. The major indication for dobutamine is short-term therapy for refractory CHF. It is the preferred drug (e.g., compared with digoxin) because its short half-life reduces the potential for toxicity and the inotropic effects of dobutamine are greater. Treatment beyond 48 hours is discouraged, in part because of the development of tolerance. In people, however, a residual effect occurs for up to several months. Dobutamine and volume replacement are indicated for treatment of hemorrhagic shock.[230] Likewise, in dogs with septic shock, dobutamine (5 to 10 μg/kg per minute) increases mesenteric blood flow and urine output when administered in conjunction with fluid therapy.[229]

The dose generally recommended is 2.5 to 20 μg/kg/min in dogs and 0.5-5 μg/kg/min in cats, starting with an initial dose of 2.5 to 5 μg/kg/min and increasing 1-2 μg/kg/min every 5 to 30 minutes. Improvement should occur within 30 minutes. The most common side effect is ventricular arrhythmias, which are less likely to occur if doses of 15 μg/kg per minute are not exceeded. Arrhythmias should not be treated with β-adrenergic blockers; rather, the dose should be decreased until arrhythmias resolve. Animals with very severe CHF and very poor myocardial function may not be able to respond to dobutamine because of little contractile reserve. Tachyphylaxis may occur within 72 hours of continuous treatment owing to downregulation of β1 - receptors.

Epinephrine

Epinephrine is one of the most potent vasopressor drugs known. It causes an immediate rise in blood pressure as a result of (1) direct myocardial stimulation and a positive inotropic effect, (2) an increased heart rate or positive chronotropic effect, and (3) vasoconstriction in many vascular beds. As with the other catecholamines, its cardiac effects are due to direct interaction with β_1-receptors and cells of the pacemaker and conducting tissues. Cardiac systole is shorter and more powerful. Because the formation of cAMP requires ATP, however, epinephrine causes the greatest increase in the rate of energy usage and myocardial oxygen demand. This increase in oxygen need may be detrimental to the failing heart. Increased work and myocardial oxygen consumption result in *reduced* cardiac efficiency.

Epinephrine is rapidly metabolized in the gastrointestinal tract and does not reach therapeutic plasma concentrations after oral administration. Absorption is more rapid after intramuscular versus subcutaneous administration because of local vasoconstriction. Epinephrine is rapidly metabolized by the body. The liver plays an important but not essential role in the metabolism of epinephrine. Two enzymes catalyze its degradation: COMT and monoamine oxidase.

Epinephrine is available in several forms of solution that can be used for intravenous, inhalation, and nasal administration. Because of the decreased efficiency of cardiac work, epinephrine is not used simply as a positive inotropic agent. Ventricular arrhythmias can be expected. In addition, central nervous system signs may occur. The primary indication for epinephrine in treatment of cardiac disease is acute cardiac life support (see the discussion of "crash cart" drugs) or for pressor support in patients insufficiently responsive to norepinephrine.

Isoproterenol

Isoproterenol is a nonspecific β-agonist that, like epinephrine, increases myocardial oxygen demand. Tachycardia and the potential for other arrhythmias tend to exclude its use for the cardiac patient.

Miscellaneous Agents

Miscellaneous inotropic agents include calcium when given as a slow intravenous injection or infusion. Care must be taken with the administration of calcium because it can cause cardiac rigor and standstill at high doses; attention must be given to the amount of calcium per dosing unit (e.g., ml or oral dosing form) among the different oral or injectable salts (see Table 14-3). The gluconate form is preferred to calcium chloride. Glucagon is also a positive inotropic agent.

Phenylpropanolamine is used primarily to treat urinary incontinence, but toxicity is manifested predominantly in the cardiac system. Toxicity was reported in a 5-year-old, female Labrador Retriever receiving 48 mg/kg. Clinical signs included tachypnea, tachycardia, and ataxia. Cardiac arrhythmias were characterized by multiform ventricular tachycardia, left ventricular dilation with a focal dyskinetic region in the dorsal intraventricular septum, and elevations in creatinine kinase and cardiac troponin I. Diagnostic tests were attributed to myocardial necrosis following transient infarction or directed myocardial toxicity. All abnormalities resolved within 6 months.[174]

Coenzyme Q, also called *ubiquinone,* is a natural fat-soluble compound similar to vitamin K in structure and ubiquitous in plants and animals. It acts as an antioxidant to protect cell membranes from free radical activity. Coenzyme Q plays a role in the conversion of 95% of energy needs; organs with the highest energy needs have the highest coenzyme Q concentrations. The use of the compound has been in patients with severe CHF (150 to 225 mg/day), particularly for those whose endogenous concentrations fall below 2 μg/mL. The effects of coenzyme Q on myocardial cells is controversial. In cultured myocardial cells, coenzyme Q stimulates beating activity, probably by stimulating the formation of mitochondrial ATP.[231] In humans undergoing valve replacement, coenzyme Q appeared to scavenge hydroxyl but not superoxide anions.[232] Singh and coworkers[233] demonstrated a protective effect of coenzyme Q in patients receiving the compound within 3 days after acute myocardial infarction. However, a lack of effect on ventricular function was reported in patients with CHF.[234] Coenzyme Q may block apoptosis.[235] Foods highest in coenzyme Q include beef, spinach, sardines, albacore tuna, and peanuts. Beta blockers, statin (cholesterol-lowering drugs) and other cardiovascular drugs can decrease coenzyme Q. Coenzyme Q is available as a dietary supplement, generally in capsules ranging in size from 10 to 60 mg.

Nutritional intervention with essential nutrients, including L-arginine and L-carnitine, also has been recommended as effective adjunctive therapy for prevention and control of cardiovascular disease.[236]

NEGATIVE INOTROPES

The negative inotropes most commonly used in clinical practice are those that block β-receptors (propranolol, which is nonselective, or atenolol, which selectively blocks β_1-receptors) or CCBs (diltiazem). By virtue of their mechanisms of action, drugs in either of these categories also tend to act as negative chronotropes; often this action is desirable. Both groups of drugs have been previously discussed as antiarrhythmics. These drugs are further discussed under treatment of HCM.

The primary indication for the use of negative chronotropes in veterinary medicine is feline HCM, a cardiac disease characterized by a thickened cardiac muscle; poor distensibility and compliance, and thus poor cardiac filling; and, depending on the degree of ventricular hypertrophy, obstruction to cardiac outflow. Atrial fibrillation is not uncommon in this syndrome and generally causes a tachycardia that worsens this syndrome. Thus the negative chronotropic effects of these drugs are of benefit in cats suffering from hypertrophic cardiomegaly.

TREATMENT OF SPECIFIC VASCULAR DISORDERS

Acquired Valvular Diseases

Chronic Mitral Valve Insufficiency

Pathophysiology. Chronic mitral valve insufficiency (CMVI; chronic valvular disease) results from endocardiosis of the mitral valve. It is the most common cardiovascular disorder in the dog, leading to death resulting from CHF in 7% of all dogs before the age of 10 years. The pathophysiology has been well reviewed.[237] The initiating cause is unknown. However, because the leaflets are stiff and malformed, their motion is abnormal. Because they fail to accurately oppose one another during systole, blood regurgitates into the left atrium. The abnormal motion and regurgitant fraction contribute to sheer stress on the valve leaflets. Endothelial damage may result in an imbalance in local growth factors. The progression of disease reflects a number of factors, including the volume of forward (reduced) and backward (regurgitant) flow, the size of the left atrium, and the compliance of the atria and pulmonary arterial tree. The progression of disease and the manifestations of clinical signs reflect both the underlying disease and compensatory mechanisms. The decrease in forward flow and thus cardiac output activates neural, humoral, and renal compensatory mechanisms as well as remodeling (hypertrophy and dilation) of the left atrium and ventricles.

Increased circulating blood volume and arterial resistance generally are sufficient to support cardiac output, even for a number of years. The compensatory mechanisms, including cardiac remodeling, that maintain forward flow do so, however, at the cost of worsening the regurgitant fraction. The regurgitant fraction that accompanies CMVI is determined by the degree of valvular deformity; the amount of afterload (systemic impedance) placed on the left ventricle; and, as disease progresses, the amount of dilation of the valvular annulus and misalignment of papillary muscles as the left ventricle enlarges.[90] Mitral regurgitation becomes uncompensated (symptomatic) when the leaking valves are no longer able to keep pulmonary capillary pressures from exceeding the threshold associated with pulmonary edema or maintaining forward cardiac output.[237] Decreased myocardial contractility will inevitably emerge, although progression will be slow. However, the point at which impaired contractility contributes significantly to pathophysiology and clinical signs is not clear.[237]

Clinical signs indicative of cardiac disease may reflect left atrial overfilling and decreased atrial compliance rather than myocardial dysfunction. The development of pulmonary congestion and edema reflects pressure in the left atrium, which in turn depends on volume of the left atrium and compliance in the left atrial wall. If the rate of increase of the regurgitant fraction is sufficiently slow, left atrial compliance can gradually increase, and pulmonary congestion does not develop until later in the disease. In contrast, a sudden increase in the regurgitant volume such as might occur with a ruptured chordae tendineae will cause a rapid rise in atrial and thus pulmonary capillary pressure and pulmonary edema.[90] Coughing associated with pulmonary edema may reflect edema of the bronchial walls and the accumulation of excess mucus. Left atrial enlargement can be great, with two potential sequelae. Pressure on the mainstem bronchus or the recurrent laryngeal nerve may stimulate coughing. In addition, the enlarged atria are predisposed to atrial tachycardias (premature supraventricular beats, atrial flutter, atrial fibrillation). Ventricular dilation also can predispose the development of ventricular tachycardia. Any of the arrhythmias can contribute to the progression of disease. Occasionally, the left atrial wall can rupture, leading to hemopericardium and cardiac tamponade.[90] Although not well described in dogs, remodeling as described in multiple animal models should be assumed to contribute to the progression of CHF in dogs.

Clinical signs associated with CMVI that require medical management are variable, in part because of variable progression of the disease and the different pathophysiologic sequelae, each characterized by its own set of overlapping clinical signs. Decreased forward flow may result in weakness, decreased stamina, or syncope; enlarged left atria with mainstem compression (or primary bronchomalacia[240a]) can present as coughing (which can be sufficiently paroxysmal as to cause syncope); elevated left atrial and pulmonary capillary pressures may result in respiratory distress (tachypnea, loss of sinus arrhythmia, or dyspnea), coughing (deep and resonant), wheezing, or orthopnea if increase is sufficiently slow or fulminating, pulmonary edema, ventricular fibrillation, and sudden death if rapid; or right heart failure characterized by pleural effusion and ascites.[90] Among the difficulties in recognizing the need for treatment is distinguishing clinical signs associated with mitral regurgitation and its sequelae from similar clinical signs that may be associated with a host of illnesses unrelated to myocardial disease. As noted by Haggstrom and coworkers,[237] the tendency is to overdiagnose pulmonary edema–associated CHF. The role of molecular or other markers of disease (e.g., brain natriuretic peptide [BNP] or canine-specific N-terminal brain natriuretic peptide [NT-proBNP]) in the the diagnosis of disease is being defined and may assist in the diagnosis of cardiac disease as a cause of respiratory distress.[237a] Clinical signs, coupled with sequential radiography, should help clinicians distinguish early signs of mitral regurgitation from other causes.

KEY POINT 14-48 Care must be taken not to overdiagnose pulmonary edema and prematurely implement therapy for treatment of chronic mitral valve insufficiency.

Drug Therapy. The goals of therapy for CHF associated with CMVI are to increase tissue perfusion in order to relieve symptoms such that quality of life is improved; stabilize the disease, thus reducing hospital admissions; and decrease mortality or prolong survival by either slowing the progression of or, ideally, reversing myocardial systolic or diastolic dysfunction associated with left ventricular myocardial remodeling. The severity of symptoms of CHF may vary dramatically, with acute episodes of cardiac decompensation often accompanying comorbidity.

The traditional approach to treatment of CHF has been in response to resolution of clinical signs. During the last 2 decades, therapy focused on minimizing the impact of compensatory neurohumoral endocrine mechanisms. These included volume overload and increased afterload. Targets of therapy include decreasing fluid volume with diuretics (spironolactone, furosemide) and ACE inhibitors; decreasing afterload (ACE inhibitors, arterial dilators); and minimizing cardiac arrhythmias. Arrhythmias requiring management, most commonly are supraventricular tachycardias (β blockers, CCBs, or digoxin) but occasionally include ventricular arrhythmias (e.g., procainamide, melixetine, sotalol). Because impaired myocardial contractility does not emerge until late in the progression, positive inotropes (digoxin, pimobendan) generally have been the last class of drugs to be added to the armentarium.

KEY POINT 14-49 The traditional therapeutic goals of congestive heart failure—targeting compensatory mechanisms—should be expanded to include slowed progression of myocardial damage.

However, as in humans, treatment of CHF increasing will be oriented toward preventing myocardial remodeling that occurs in response to the compensatory changes. These treatments will include new applications of traditional drugs, as well as the addition of new drugs for traditional targets and new drugs for new targets.

Various pharmacotherapies in humans have been reviewed by Lonn et al.[238] Those clearly associated with improved survival are the ACE inhibitors and β-blockers, whereas diuretics and digoxin improve clinical signs. In contrast, class I antiarrhythmics, CCBs (including class IV antiarrhythmics), and digoxin have been associated with increased mortality rates. Newer classes of drugs in use (e.g., calcium sensitizers) have not been available for a sufficient length of time for data to have been generated for review. Future classes of drugs may include drugs that target ANP, such as neutral endopeptidase inhibitors (e.g., ecadotril), or drugs that target myocardial inflammation and remodeling, including antioxidants and anticytokines.

Currently, the cornerstones of pharmacotherapy in dogs for CHF include diuretics (preload reduction), drugs that impair the renin–angiotensin–aldosterone axis, β-adrenoceptor antagonists, vasodilators (afterload reduction), and, in some cases, positive inotropic drugs. The standard of care for treatment includes, at a minimum, an afterload reducer, ACE inhibitor, a β blocker, and the addition of a diuretic as needed to treat congestion. Digoxin, an aldosterone antagonist, and an angiotensin receptor antagonist are added as indicated in selected patients (Table 14-2). Although these therapies are based on clinical trials that have demonstrated subsequent decreased mortality or morbidity with the addition of each agent, the actual proportion of patients responding to therapy has been small, indicating a need for improved medical management.[238] Because the progression of CHF in dogs appears similar to that in humans, it is reasonable to assume that pharmacodynamic effects on the slowing of progression of myocardial disease may be similar in both species. [238a-e]

Among the factors confounding treatment of CHF in dogs (or cats) is the lack of pharmacokinetic studies supporting the design of effective and safe dosing regimens. Enatiomers, active metabolites, drug interactions, and the impact of disease or its treatment on drug disposition are just some of the factors that complicate effective use of cardioactive drugs in dogs and cats. The lack of pharmacokinetic studies is consistent limitation for many human-approved drugs used in dogs or cats. Also among the difficulties associated with effective management of CHF is the point at which therapy is initiated. This is particulary problematic for the patient with mitral regurgitation which may be characterized by a long preclinical stage.[240] Preferences among clinicians may reflect experience rather than scientific studies. Several considerations may guide choices. Animals with left atrial enlargement and mainstem bronchus compression may have normal myocardial function. Reduction of systemic resistance (afterload) may allow more blood to exit the aortic valve, thus decreasing the regurgitant fraction through the mitral valve and left atrium such that coughing is resolved. The size of the left ventricle also may decrease, which may reduce the size of the mitral annulus, further reducing the regurgitant fraction. ACE inhibitors initially, followed by amlodipine and/or hydralazine, are indicated to decrease systemic vascular resistance in early phase II CHF.[237,239,240] Theophylline, hydrocodone, or butorphanol might be considered for control of cough in early phases of the disease. [237,240] In addition to their effects on afterload, in the patient with evidence of compensatory mechanisms, ACE inhibitors have the added advantage of decreasing sodium and water retention and thus blood volume, helping to reduce the regurgitant fraction. As disease progresses, ACE inhibitors may be favored over amlopdipine by virtue of their, the beneficial effects on myocardial remodeling. Although hydralazine might also support myocardial revascularization and impart cardioprotection its positive inotropic effects may not be desireable in early stages of insufficiency. However, it may be indicated in dogs coughing due to mainstem bronchi compression that do not sufficiently respond to ACE inhibitors and may be useful for reducing.[241] Care should be taken with all afterload reducers to avoid hypotension and potential activation of the RAAS.

As clinical signs progress, diuretics are indicated for reduction of sodium and water retention. Treatment of patients with pulmonary (interstitial) congestion does not differ much from treatment of atrial enlargement. Pulmonary congestion implies that atrial compliance is high, resulting in increased left atrial pressures and pulmonary capillary pressure. Afterload reduction and diuretics are indicated in that order, depending on the severity of clinical signs; positive inotropes are indicated in the presence of myocardial dysfunction. Diuretics initially may play a more active role in the presence of pulmonary edema, but a decreasing need may be evident after several weeks of therapy. Although diuretics are among the first classes of drugs used to treat the sequelae of CMVI, caution is recommended. Overuse can lead to reduced cardiac output, hypokalemia, acid–base imbalances, and activation of the RAAS and its associated negative sequelae. As such, use might be reserved for late phase II or early phase III CHF.[240] The need for diuretics might be offset by the use of ACE inhibitors; further, and once diuretic therapy is begun, ACE inhibitors may allow for a substantial (up to 50%) dose reduction.[37,240a] Spironolactone might be considered first not only because its mechanism targets aldosterone but also because it imparts cardioprotective effects.[240a,242] However, its efficacy as a diuretic is probably least, whereas fursosimide is the most effective. In the case of acute cardiogenic pulmonary edema (i.e., that which is life threatening), nitroprusside may be indicated for afterload reduction and nitroglycerin for pre-load reduction. Morphine may be helpful. Its central effects may reduce stress and anxiety and the negative sequelae of vascular responses to stress. Respirations may deepen and slow, resulting in improved ventilation. In addition, ventilation may result in pooling of blood in the splanchnic vasculature, reducing preload. The enlargement of the left atrium may be associated with supraventricular tachycardias. Ventricular rates greater than 180 beats per minute (bpm) may reduce cardiac output; therapy should target reduction to 150 to 160 bpm or less. Digoxin has been the preferred antiarrhythmic drug because of its impact not only on heart rate but also on baroreceptor function. Either diltiazem or selective β_1-blockers or metoprolol are added if response is insufficient. However, recent revelations of the impact that β-blockers have on myocardial remodeling may support their initial use for treatment of supraventricular tachycardia. Cardiac decompensation may occur in some patients if the heart rate drops below 150 bpm; animals whose heart rate depends on sympathetic activity may be particularly sensitive to β-blockade.[90]

KEY POINT 14-50 As with vasodilators, overuse of diuretics may result in activation or worsening of neurohumoral compensatory mechanisms.

Until recently, digoxin has been the only orally bioavailable positive inotrope recommended for improved contractility.[90] In the absence of afterload reducers, increased myocardial contractility actually might increase the regurgitant fraction. Thus its use should be limited to animals that have not responded to afterload reduction alone or in combination with diuretic therapy. The use of pimobendan for treatment of CMVI is increasing. Patients benefit from both positive inotropic effects of vasodilation; the American College of Veterinary Internal Medicine's "Guidelines for the diagnosis and treatment of canine chronic valvular heart disease" recommends its use for management of both actue and chronic heart failure.[242a] The use of pimobendan in canine patients with heart disease was previuosly discussed and has recently been reviewed again.[242b]

Right-sided heart failure is described as a common complication of CMVI.[90] Because the right ventricular wall is thinner than the left ventricular wall, it is more compliant and thus better able to adjust to the increased volume associated with tricuspid insufficiency. It does not, however, adjust as well to increases in pulmonary pressure. Right ventricular stroke volume can markedly decrease in the face of very small increases in pulmonary pressure, resulting in decreased delivery to the left ventricle and decreased cardiac output. The use of systemic vasodilators in the presence of pulmonary hypertension may further decrease cardiac output. Unfortunately, pulmonary hypertension often does not respond selectively to pharmacologic management (see the section on pulmonary hypertension).

Rupture of the chordae tendineae has been described as possibly the most frequently encountered complication of CMVI.[90] The sequelae of rupture appear more dependent on the type (i.e., first, second, or third order) rather than the number of those that rupture. The negative sequelae generally reflect the inability of the left atrium to accommodate to the rapid increase in left atrial pressure. Patients may present in severe respiratory distress as pulmonary capillary pressure and pulmonary (interstitial and alveolar) edema develop. Right-sided heart failure (manifested as pleural effusion or ascites) also may be present. Treatment includes aggressive diuretic therapy (furosemide at 8 mg/kg intravenously every 6 hours). Rapidly acting positive inotropes (dobutamine or dopamine) may facilitate emptying of the left ventricle and thus decrease the size of the mitral annulus. Afterload reducing agents appear to be of no benefit and may be deleterious if cardiac output decreases. Preload reducing agents are probably less beneficial with right-sided failure.

Tricuspid Valvular Insufficiency

Because a normally functioning left ventricle ensures forward movement of blood in the right ventricle, incompetence of the tricuspid valve generally does not lead to cardiac insufficiency unless accompanied by an underlying disease (e.g., pulmonary hypertension, heartworm disease, CMVI). Identification of any underlying disorder leading to tricuspid valvular insufficiency is critical to successful management of cardiac insufficiency. Loop diuretics (furosemide) or aldosterone antagonists (spironolactone) (or a combination thereof) may be indicated for management of ascites. Spironoloactone may be more effective for right-sided, compared to left-sided therapy. Digoxin may be helpful in the presence of myocardial failure, and antiarrhythmic drugs may be necessary to control tachycardia.[90] Treatment of pulmonary hypertension associated with heart failure is discussed below.

Diseases of the Myocardium

Dilated Cardiomyopathy (DCM)

Pathology. The cause of DCM in dogs is not known, although a number of causes have been proposed (e.g., viral, nutritional, toxins, hereditary). Often, secondary changes cannot be distinguished from primary changes (i.e., which is cause and which is effect). Biochemical changes similar to those accompanying DCM in humans have been identified in dogs, including decreased myocardial carnitine or myoglobin concentration, decreased β-receptor–mediated cAMP (e.g., downregulation of receptors or decreased intracellular proteins), decreased intracellular regulatory proteins (e.g., light chains), or altered calcium release from the sarcoplasmic reticulum. Among these causes, decreased carnitine has received the most attention.[243] Carnitine is responsible for the transport of fatty acids into mitochondria, where they are subjected to β-oxidation; carnitine deficiency then might be characterized by altered energy metabolism and lipid accumulation in the myocardium. Clinical trials have, however, suggested that carnitine deficiency is a secondary rather than a primary disorder of DCM. In contrast to the cat, taurine deficiency is not a common disorder accompanying DCM in dogs. Although decreased plasma concentrations of both taurine and carnitine have been reported in American Cocker Spaniels with DCM, amino acid supplementation alone does not appear to resolve the disease.[190,243] A reversible taurine-deficient DCM has been described in related Golden Retrievers (n=5). Improvement occurred within 3 to 6 months of taurine supplementation. Substantial systolic function was maintained with cardiac drugs (but not taurine) discontinued in four of five dogs.[245]

All four cardiac chambers are enlarged in dogs with DCM, although left-sided enlargement predominates in some breeds (e.g., Boxers, Doberman Pinschers).[190] The myocardial muscle generally is pale, thin (compared with chamber size), and flabby. The mitral annular ring is dilated, and papillary muscles are often atrophied. The primary physiologic dysfunction accompanying the pathologic changes is poor systolic ventricular function characterized by decreased rate of ventricular development, reduced fractional shortening, ejection fraction, and rate. Diastolic dysfunction is characterized by increased end-diastolic pressures in the ventricles, atria, and venous circulation.[190] Valvular insufficiency, cardiac arrhythmias, and compensatory neurohumoral and renal mechanisms complicate therapy.

As with CMVI, a number of clinical signs develop in DCM, depending on the severity of dysfunction and the level of compensation by neurohumoral and renal mechanisms. In contrast to CMVI, myocardial dysfunction characterizes DCM at the outset, and positive inotropic support is the mainstay of therapy. In addition, the use of afterload reducers may offset the progression of disease, potentially prolonging the life of the animal.[190] The variable clinical signs are similar among breeds, although their frequencies may vary among selected breeds. Giant breeds are more likely to present with clinical signs reflecting right-sided heart failure (ascites, weight loss, fatigue), whereas clinical signs of left-sided heart failure are more common in Boxers and Doberman Pinschers.[190] In working dogs, exercise intolerance may serve as an indicator of dysfunction relatively early in the disease compared with nonworking dogs for whom the disease might present as a rapid progression of deterioration.

Although myocardial dysfunction characterizes DCM, many dogs are diagnosed before overt heart failure occurs. Syncope or episodic weakness may be the primary clinical sign in animals in which disease is characterized by cardiac arrhythmias. Variability in the cardiac dysfunction also occurs among breeds, and recognition of these differences may direct drug therapy. For example, up to one third of Boxers diagnosed with DCM are asymptomatic, with DCM characterized by ventricular arrhythmias but normal myocardial indices.[190] Asymptomatic giant breeds may have atrial fibrillation with only mild changes in myocardial function. In contrast, disease in asymptomatic Doberman Pinschers generally is characterized by ventricular arrhythmias and marked impairment of myocardial function.[190] Whereas atrial fibrillation is a common finding in giant breeds, sudden death in otherwise asymptomatic Doberman Pinschers and Boxers is more common than in other breeds because of the advent of fatal ventricular arrhythmias.[190]

Clinical signs of DCM that may direct drug therapy include weak arterial pulses, irregular pulses with pulse deficits (indicative of ventricular or atrial arrhythmias), pulsus alternans (alternating arterial pulse in the absence of cardiac arrhythmias, indicative of severe myocardial failure), lung sounds indicative of pulmonary interstitial edema, and clinical signs associated with right-sided heart failure (previously discussed). A number of changes in clinical pathologic parameters also may modify drug selection. Of concern is evidence of renal dysfunction or, particularly in patients with right-sided failure, hepatic dysfunction, which may lead to modification of the dosing regimen of cardiac drugs or might predispose the patient to worsening renal disease (e.g., use of ACE inhibitors or diuretics). Electrocardiography and echocardiography are important tools for the selection of myocardial drugs and subsequent monitoring of efficacy in the dog with DCM. An electrocardiogram should be used to confirm the type and severity of cardiac arrhythmia. Echocardiography can be used, in concert with clinical signs and an electrocardiogram, to assess prognosis or response to drug therapy. Assessment might include the degree of chamber dilation, mitral valve configuration and closure, and systolic performance. Ejection phase indices including left ventricular fractional shortening, ejection fraction, and velocity of circumferential shortening decline with decreasing systolic function.[190]

KEY POINT 14-51 When treating dilated cardiomyopathy with drugs excreted renally, care must be taken to modify the dosing regimen as renal function declines (or improves) with cardiac function.

Drug Therapy. The best-case scenario to be expected when treating DCM has been improved quality and length of life. Therapy should be selected such that clinical signs are minimized; additionally, use of appropriate therapy may slow the progression of myocardial dysfunction. During the progression of diseases, diuretics, positive inotropes, vasodilators, ACE inhibitors, and antiarrhythmics are apt to play a role in drug management. They are used in a variety of combinations, depending on the nature and severity of clinical signs associated with the disease in the individual animal. Individualization of therapy is paramount to proper use of the drugs and thus to achieving the goals of drug management. Therapeutic drug monitoring is indicated when drugs are used for which monitoring is available (see Chapter 5).

Antiarrhythmic drugs may or may not be indicated for the patient with DCM associated with atrial or ventricular arrhythmias but without clinical signs of CHF. Despite the fact that sudden death may be a sequela of ventricular arrhythmias, no evidence exists that their control with antiarrhythmics prolongs life. Indeed, in human patients antiarrhythmic drugs may be proarrhythmic in some cases, thus increasing the risk of sudden death.[246a] The proarrhythmic effects of these drugs occur in dogs as well, although reports largely relate to experimental situations. Well-controlled clinical trials regarding the use of antiarrhythmic drugs for dogs with DCM are lacking. Among the drugs reported to cause variable levels of success in the treatment of ventricular arrhythmias are procainamide,[246] tocainide,[247] and propranolol.[246] Historically, Sisson and Thomas[247a] recommend the use of procainamide to treat frequent ventricular premature depolarizations or ventricular tachycardias in dogs with DCM. Refractory arrhythmias can be treated with the addition of propranolol or a change to quinidine, tocainide, or mexiletine.

Antiarrhythmic therapy when supplemented with conventional therapy for CHF (ACE inhibitors, furosemide, and digoxin) is associated with a longer life span in Doberman Pinschers (n=19) with DCM and sudden ventricular tachycardia: median (and range) survival from the first episode increased from 11 (3 to 38) to 197 (78 to 345) days, respectively. Treatment consisted of tocainide (n=6; 15 to 20 mg/kg every 8 hours) or mexiletine (n=7; 5 to 8 mg/kg every 8 hours), with the addition of procainamide (15 to 20 mg every 8 hours), quinidine gluconate (8 to 9 mg/kg every 8 hours), amiodarone (10 mg/kg every 12 hours for 1 to 2 weeks, followed by 5 to 10 mg/kg every 24 hours) or β-adrenergic antagonists (propranolol 0.5 mg/kg every 8 hours, or metoprolol or atenolol at 0.5 mg/kg every 12 hours).[253]

KEY POINT 14-52 Control of ventricular arrhythmias in the patient with dilated cardiomyopathy with currently available drugs is controversial and evidence thus far does not clearly support benefits.

Atrial fibrillation is among the most common atrial arrhythmias associated with DCM. Digoxin is the antiarrhythmic drug of choice not only for its negative chronotropic effect (including atrioventricular nodal impulse suppression) but also for its positive inotropic effects (discussed previously in this chapter). Although only a weak positive inotrope, digoxin remains useful because it slows heart rate and normalizes baroreceptor function.[240] However, the positive inotropic effects can be marked in some dogs with DCM.[248,249] Negative chronotropic effects likewise will benefit most patients.[250] Both pharmacologic effects act to reduce activation of the RAAS.[249] Studies in human patients with DCM have detailed the reduction of clinical manifestations, improved capacity for exercise, and slowed progression of disease induced by digoxin therapy.[189] The RADIANCE and DIG trials in humans showed that patients in heart failure denied digoxin had worsening of signs, quality of life, exercise tolerance, and hemodynamic status. Digoxin has been indicated for treatment of heart failure in dogs with supraventricular tachycardia. Use in dogs with normal myocardial function should be pursued cautiously; however, discretion must be used in treatment of these dogs because other drugs will control signs with less danger of toxicity. In general, digoxin should be instituted in late phase II in the presence of myocardial failure (to treat atrial fibrillation) and reserved for phase III (as diuretic therapy is initiated) in dogs without myocardial failure.[240] Its use as a positive inotrope has largely been replaced by pimobendan.

Should digoxin fail to control the heart rate, a CCB (e.g., diltiazem) or a β-adrenergic blocking drug (propranolol, atenolol) is indicated. Either type of drug also can be used to treat persistent sinus tachycardias. Although no study has documented increased efficacy of one class of drugs over another for dogs, β-blockade apparently has improved survival rates for human patients with cardiac failure. Although the risk of sudden detrimental effects on myocardial function and cardiovascular effects has lead to a call for caution when β-blockers are used in the patient with severe heart failure, evidence regarding improvement in human patients suggests otherwise. Selected CCBs can have a similar effect; diltiazem may be the least likely to detrimentally affect cardiac function in patients with severe disease.[190]

The role of β-blockade in dogs with DCM is controversial. The role of β-blockers for treatment of heart failure is currently being investigated (see discussion under antiarrhythmics) as a means of decreasing the progression of myocardial disease. Metoprolol and carvedilol are the most promising.[151]

KEY POINT 14-53 Digoxin may be the drug of choice for treatment of atrial fibrillation associated with myocardial failure.

ACE inhibitors are indicated for dogs with DCM and clinical signs of cardiac failure. In a clinical trial of 110 dogs in 15 locations throughout the United States, when enalapril was used in combination with other drugs indicated for treatment of DCM, the mean number of days until treatment failure increased from 56.6 (placebo) to 143 (enalapril).[88] Less clear is the indication in the absence of clinical signs. Both increased afterload and preload (sodium and water retention) may be contributing to the progression of disease without causing overt clinical signs of decompensation. The presence of an ACE inhibitor may reduce the necessary dose of other drugs used to control clinical signs (e.g., furosemide). ACE inhibitors have been the cornerstone of chronic heart failure therapy, being implemented as early as phase II. In addition to their effects on afterload reduction and reduction of electrolyte abnormalities, they may blunt pathologic remodeling such that the progression of heart failure is slowed. Both duration and quality of life may be improved with their use. When used in combination with diuretics, the diuretic dose should be reduced; The dose of the ACE inhibitor might be increased (doubled for enalapril) in patients that fail to respond; it is not clear if dose increase results in enhanced response.

Diuretics are indicated for patients with signs of congestion. For severe pulmonary edema, therapy should be aggressive (intravenous, high doses). Oral therapy is indicated for control and long-term management. Dogs should be closely monitored for the advent of dehydration, excessive preload reduction, and subsequent decreases in cardiac output or azotemia. Although not common, hypokalemia may occur. In patients that are refractory (e.g., pleural effusion or ascites) to furosemide (particularly those with right-sided heart failure in which oral absorption may be reduced), parenteral rather than oral therapy may improve response. Alternatively, butamide is more orally bioavailable than furosemide in humans and may likewise be better absorbed in dogs.[190] Alternative managements include the addition of a thiazide diuretic to furosemide therapy, a venodilator, or an ACE inhibitor.

Extreme sodium restriction activates the RAAS and may contribute to renal dysfunction; use of ACE inhibitors may compound renal dysfunction. Thus diuretic therapy (and a marked dietary sodium restriction) should not be used indiscriminately. Some clinicians suggest that diuretic therapy should be implemented only in conjunction with ACE inhibitors.[237] Combined use should allow the diuretic dose to be decreased by 50% or more in earlier phases of disease, although higher doses may be necessary to affect sufficient diuresis in later stages. Furosemide has been the cornerstone of therapy; potassium-sparing diuretics may be added for more effective therapy. However, spironolactone increasingly should be considered because of the importance of aldosterone-receptor blockade (including contributions to altered myocardial remodeling) in cardiovascular therapy.

The evidence for use of pimobendan to treat congestive heart failure associated with dilated cardiomyopathy was previously discussed whether to use it prior to the onset of clinical signs associated with heart failure is not clear; the PROTECT study currently in process aims to evaluate timing of pimobendan treatment in DCV.

Therapy also should target neurohormonal abnormalities.[240] These include ACE inhibitors (as previously described), aldosterone antagonists, β blockers (e.g., carvedilol or metoprolol), which blunt adrenergic (sympathetic) responses; neutral endopeptidase inhibitors (e.g. ecadotril), which prevents the breakdown of ANP (thus moderating activation of the RAAS; and AGII receptor blockers (e.g. losartan). Antioxidants and anticytokine therapies will increase as more information becomes available.

Both milrinone and amrinone are used short term in human patients with heart failure. The vasodilating properties of these positive inotropic drugs are beneficial. In dogs with DCM, the positive inotropic effects of milrinone improve hemodynamic function and clinical signs.[252] Long-term use of milrinone has been limited by evidence of increased mortality rates in human patients.[190] The absence of coronary arterial disease in dogs may, however, minimizes the risk associated with the use of milrinone for long-term treatment of DCM. Despite its potential benefits, milrinone is not generally used to treat DCM. The positive inotropes dobutamine, dopamine, and amrinone are recommended less frequently than in the past, except for emergency therapy (rescue) of myocardial failure (phase IV). These drugs markedly increase oxygen demand, influence ion flow and may worsen arrhythmias (including tachycardia). Dobutamine is the preferred drug; vasodilators should be used simultaneously. Miscellaneous agents such as morphine (redistribution of blood volume), epinephrine, and calcium chloride should be used for specific indications in phase IV severe heart failure or as rescue drugs for cardiopulmonary rescuscitation.[240]

Nutritional agents may also have a role in treatment of myocardial disease. Taurine has essentially eliminated DCM in cats. The role of carnitine in dogs is less clear. Support for use includes treatment of DCM in Cocker Spaniels with taurine and carnitine. Other potential nutritional therapy includes supplementation with omega fatty acids (oil of fish origin), which may improve appetite and blunt cardiac cachexia.

Pentoxifylline therapy in human patients with DCM positively correlated to improved left ventricular function.[24,252] The use of pentoxifylline as an adjunctive therapy for CHF in adult Doberman Pinschers with idiopathic DCM has been studied in a double-blinded, placebo-controlled clinical trial when added to conventional heart failure therapy (ACE inhibitor, diuretics, and digoxin).[24]

Treatment of catastrophic CHF includes use of sodium nitroprusside and dobutamine.

Feline Dilated Cardiomyopathy

The recognition that DCM in cats was largely reversible with the administration of taurine has all but eliminated DCM in cats.[244,254] Most commercial feline diets now contain sufficient taurine to prevent the syndrome. A history of unconventional foods or homemade diets will help identify the occasional cat with cardiac disease associated with taurine deficiency. The clinical presentation of DCM in cats is similar to that in dogs, although pleural effusions are more common. Systemic thromboembolism is another potential complication. Plasma taurine concentrations are often but not always low (<30 nM/mL). Systemic thromboembolism apparently can increase, and fasting can decrease, plasma taurine concentrations. Taurine supplementation largely reverses the clinical signs and electrocardiographic abnormalities associated with taurine deficiency. Most animals respond to taurine supplementation (250 to 300 mg/day orally) within 3 to 6 weeks of therapy. Mortality rates are highest, however, during the initial 2 to 3 weeks of therapy. Echocardiography is the preferred method for monitoring response to therapy because response times can markedly vary. Adjuvant therapy may be necessary until clinical response.

Diuretics (furosemide) can be used to manage pulmonary edema and pleural effusions; differences in dosing regimens for cats compared with dogs should be observed. Cats may appear to be dehydrated (based on skin turgor), but this is more likely to represent redistribution of fluids to the pleural cavity or lungs. Fluid may be necessary in the presence of azotemia associated with low-output failure and hypotension but should only be administered cautiously and slowly. Digoxin (0.0035 to 0.0055 mg orally every 12 to 24 hours) may be indicated until the response to taurine is evident. The use of pimobendan for treatment of poor myocardial contractility has not been reported in cats. Differences in response compared with that of dogs might be anticipated if cats do not metabolize pimobendan to an active metabolite. However, anecdotally, cats appear to respond to the positive inotropic effects. Emergency management of myocardial failure may require administration of dobutamine (2 to 5 μg/kg per minute); common side effects of dobutamine administration in cats include seizures and vomiting. Vasodilator therapy should be implemented. Afterload reduction might be accomplished with ACE inhibitors in the presence of compensatory neurohumoral mechanisms or amlodipine (or both). Renal function should be closely monitored, however, particularly in the patient with azotemia.

Alternative therapies include hydralazine (0.5 to 0.8 mg/kg every 12 hours) to control systemic resistance and 2% nitroglycerin topically (¼ inch topically every 8 to 12 hours) for (short-term management) preload reduction. Adjuvant therapy may be required to treat or prevent thromboembolism. Provided that a properly prepared diet is fed, most drugs and taurine supplementation generally can be discontinued within 2 to 3 months of therapy. Failure to respond, particularly in the presence of normal plasma taurine concentrations, may indicate an idiopathic DCM.

Thromboembolism

Treatment of thromboembolism is addressed in depth in Chapter 15.

Feline Aortic Thromboembolism

Feline aortic thromboembolism (FATE) is not an uncommon sequela of feline cardiomyopathy. Thrombus formation reflects the combined result of altered endocardial surface (exposed collagen, von Willebrand factor or tissue factor, hemostatic/inflammatory blood components [e.g., hypercoagulability] and blood flow). In the cat the underlying defect in blood components has not been identified, although vitamin B_{12} and arginine have been identified as deficient in one study (as reviewed by Smith and Tobias).[255] Blood flow derangements usually accompany and may be correlated with the magnitude of left atrial enlargement. Cats with any type of cardiomyopathy are at risk to develop FATE. The pathophysiology and treatment were reviewed by Smith and Tobias,[255] and use of selected antithrombotic agents for its treatment also is discussed in Chapter 15.

The goals of therapy include, in addition to rest, control of pain, improved systemic perfusion, (including prevention of further embolism), and supportive therapy as necessary. The latter should address treatment of primary cardiac disease. Newer NSAIDs preferentially target COX-2. As such, the inhibitory effects of prostacyclin will be subdued while the pro-platelet activity will not be. Accordingly, other than the use of aspirin, which is recognized for its unique antiplatelet effect, NSAIDs — particularly those known to be preferential for COX-2, — should be avoided in cats with FATE or cardiac disease in general, unless scientific studies support their use. The use of alternative antiplatelet drugs is discussed in Chapter 16. Opioids and tramadol are reasonable drugs for controlling pain. Resolution of embolism and reinstitution of perfusion are difficult. No controlled clinical trials have established appropriate therapy. Fluid therapy appropriate for the cardiac status is indicated. Scientific evidence regarding the efficacy of acepromazine (as an arterial dilator) is lacking, and the risk of contributing to hypotensive shock warrants avoidance. Smith and Tobias[255] reviewed the use of tissue type plasminogen activator (see Chapter 15). The treatment is expensive, and although reperfusion may occur, the risk of mortality associated with FATE, hyperkalemia, and other complications is 50% to 70%.

Hypertrophic Cardiomyopathy

Pathophysiology. HCM is a disease that principally affects cats but occasionally is diagnosed in dogs. It is characterized by hypertrophy of the nondilated left ventricular free wall not associated with any other disease that can cause cardiac hypertrophy. Baty[256] and Abbott[256a] have reviewed feline HCM. Several etiologies of HCM are likely in cats, including altered muscle proteins, calcium transport, catecholamine physiology, or trophic factors.[190] A familial basis probably contributes to risk.[256] Hyperthyroidism and possibly hypertension are likely causes of HCM that may require drug management. The syndrome can be symmetric or asymmetric (disproportionate hypertrophy of the intraventricular septum, left ventricular free wall, or papillary muscles). Recognition of different forms of HCM may lead to different approaches to drug therapy. Regardless of the cause or type of HCM, the primary physiologic abnormality of HCM is diastolic dysfunction with systolic anterior motion of the mitral valve and increasingly recognized component, contributing to outflow obstruction and often accompanied by mitral regurgitation.[256a] Causes of the dysfunction include increased wall thickness, impaired ventricular relaxation, and ischemic myocardial fibrosis.[190] Obstruction to systolic outflow may occur in some cats, but it is not clear if the obstruction is the cause or the effect of HCM, nor is the clinical relevance of the obstruction well described. Clinical manifestations of HCM may include manifestations of the possible sequelae of HCM, including pleural effusions and arterial thromboembolism. Diagnosis is based on echocardiography, with adjuvant diagnostics as indicated to identify the underlying cause. The role of increased circulating concentrations of cardiac troponin I (CTnI) in diagnosis and response to treatment is evolving.[256]

Treatment. Treatment for HCM should be based on physical examination and radiographic, electrocardiographic, and echocardiographic findings. The goals of drug therapy, depending on the severity of disease, include improvement in diastolic ventricular filling and treatment or prevention of pulmonary edema and thromboembolism. Drug therapy may not be indicated in asymptomatic cats. Left atrial enlargement, outflow obstruction (left ventricular), or serious cardiac arrhythmias are, however, indications for drug management.[190]

Acute pulmonary edema requires both oxygen and diuretic therapy. Diuresis generally is accomplished with furosemide. In severe cases of acute edema, nitroglycerin ointment may be indicated. Improvement in diastolic function generally has been accomplished with either β-blockade or CCBs. Both act to decrease cardiac rate and myocardial contractility. Both propranolol (a β blocker) and diltiazem (a CCB) have been studied. Propranolol, a nonselective β blocker, was the original cornerstone of therapy, although no clinical trial provides evidence of its efficacy in cats.[257] Selective β blockers are used long term to increase ventricular volume, decrease contractility, and reduce outflow tract obstruction. The most important effect of β blockade appears to be antagonism of catecholamine effects.[257] Benefits in cats include decreased heart rate and reduced severity of left ventricular outflow obstruction. In human patients myocardial perfusion also is improved. Beta blockade may have a minimal effect on systolic function if used at proper doses.[257] Note that the oral dose of propranolol should be reduced by 25% to 50% in cats with hyperthyroidism because of increased bioavailability.[146]

The choice of treatment for HCM may reflect cardiologist preference more than direction by clinical trials. Beta blockade may be preferred in the presence of left ventricular outflow obstruction. A test dose of esmolol may provide further support of a β-blocking drug.[190] A disadvantage of nonselective blockade by propranolol is potential respiratory distress secondary to bronchoconstriction that may accompany blockade of β_2-receptors of the smooth muscle of the bronchial tree. Both atenolol (atenolol [cats] 12.5 mg once daily orally, increase 50% or administer twice daily if heart rate does not slow sufficiently; treat on an individual basis), a selective β_1-receptor blocker, and diltiazem will minimize the risk of bronchospasm. β blockers also are preferred by some cardiologists if the heart rate is increased. An added advantage of atenolol is once-daily therapy, which may improve owner compliance. Controversy exists regarding preference of propranolol or other β blockers versus diltiazem. Some consideration might be given to selection of β-blockers based on penetrability of the myocardium; atenolol may be characterized by the least penetrability. The role of carvedilol in treatment of feline HCM is currently unclear.

In cats diltiazem has proved efficacious for the treatment of HCM because of its both negative inotropic and chronotropic effects. Compared with propranolol, diltiazem may have the additional benefit of directly enhancing myocardial relaxation and dilating coronary vessels.[258,259] Comparisons between propranolol and verapamil in human patients with HCM support the additional benefits of CCBs compared with β-blockade. Propranolol caused deterioration of systolic performance without improving diastolic function.

KEY POINT 14-54 The choice of diltiazem versus a β blocker for treatment of feline hypertrophic cardiomyopathy may largely be a matter of clinician preference.

Compared with verapamil, diltiazem can minimally affect the inotropic state of the heart or peripheral vasculature at doses that produce coronary vasodilation.[258,259] A controlled clinical trial in 17 cats with HCM compared responses to diltiazem, verapamil, and propranolol. Cats receiving propranolol or verapamil in general did poorly, with so few surviving that data analysis was precluded. In contrast, all cats (12) receiving diltiazem improved to the point of becoming asymptomatic with no adverse effects at 1.75 to 2.5 mg/kg orally administrated every 8 hours. Diuretic and aspirin therapies were discontinued without the development of circulatory congestion or thromboembolism. The survival rate for the diltiazem-treated cats was threefold greater than for the propranolol cats. Thickness of the left ventricular wall improved in cats after therapy with diltiazem. Mean heart rate decreased in diltiazem-treated cats; however, heart rate increased during stressful conditions. This might be interpreted as reduction in the resting rate reflects improved cardiac performance rather than depression of electrical activity in the sinoatrial node, which is a more physiologically appealing approach to control of cardiac rate. The authors found that cats receiving diltiazem did not require the addition of propranolol for control of their disease. This might suggest that propranolol (or atenolol) be reserved for cats whose heart rate exceeds 270 bpm.[258,259] Cats with HCM secondary to hyperthyroidism also appear to benefit from diltiazem therapy.

Two preparations of diltiazem (0.5 to 1.5 mg/kg orally [dog]; 1.75 to 2.45 mg/kg 2 to 3 times daily orally [cat]) are available to facilitate ease of administration. Diltiazem CD can be given at a rate of 10 mg/kg once daily orally. Diltiazem XR is prepared as a capsule that contains four 60-mg pellets (total 240-mg capsule). Cats can be dosed by removing one of the pellets and administering half of the pellet once daily. An intravenous preparation of diltiazem is also available for emergency life-threatening supraventricular tachycardias (0.2 to 0.4 mg/kg administered intravenously, followed by 0.4 mg/kg per minute). Response to therapy is manifested as clinical improvement, including resolution of pulmonary edema and reduction in heart rate.

The role of ACE inhibitors in cats with HCM is not clear. A retrospective study (as reviewed by Baty)[256] found that enalapril might improve clinical signs and reduce outflow obstruction. In a clinical study in Switzerland, left ventricular wall thickness was reduced compared with baseline in cats with HCM (n=32) receiving standard therapy (diltiazem 9 mg/kg once daily, at 6 plus-minus aspirin) with benazapril (0.33-0.75 mg/kg once daily) but did not decrease in cats receiving standard therapy alone.[100] In another study, as reviewed by Abott, outcome measures including echocardiograhic findings and diastolic function were not significantly improved by ramipril compared to placebo in Maine coon cats with HCM but without heart failure. Likewise, 4 months of spironolactone therapy did not improve echocardiograhic indicators of diastolic functioin in a similar colony of Maine coon cats. [100a] However, limitations in sample size must be considered before these negative findings are interpreted as evidence against efficacy; assuming proper precautions are taken with use, either an ACE in hibitor or spironolactone might be considered in the treatment of HCM. In her review Baty[256] also addressed a large clinical trial comparing atenolol, diltiazem (long acting), and enalapril in addition to furosemide in cats; results were not yet available at the time of publication. The use of these and other drugs known to reduce the impact of neurohumoral signals on myocardial remodeling in the treatment of hypertrophic cardiomyopathy is being defined.

In cats with HCM, only those cardiac arrhythmias that are symptomatic or life threatening should be treated with antiarrhythmic drugs. Examples include sustained or paroxysmal ventricular tachycardia.[190] Prevention of arterial thromboembolism generally should be implemented as previously discussed. The use of aspirin for prevention of thromboembolism in cats with HCM, however, remains controversial. Aspirin does impair feline platelet activity when dosed at 25 mg/kg every 3 days. Collateral circulation also may improve.[257] Yet no controlled studies provide proof of efficacy. One study reports a 75% incidence of recurrent thromboembolic disease in cats receiving aspirin therapy.[257]

A small number of cats are afflicted with intermediate or intergrade cardiomyopathies. This poorly categorized and poorly understood form of myocardial disease (often referred to as *restrictive cardiomyopathy* because of the presence of extensive endocardial fibrosis) is characterized by normal to modestly decreased systolic function, dilated atria, and normal to dilated ventricular chambers. Some cats have mild obstruction or mitral regurgitation. Diastolic dysfunction is generally more detrimental than systolic dysfunction. As with HCM, CHF, pleural effusion, pulmonary edema, and arterial thromboembolism are potential complications associated with these cardiomyopathies. Because of the variable manifestations of this form of myocardial disease, treatment likewise is variable and not clear. Furosemide is indicated for control of pulmonary edema and pleural effusions. Caution is recommended when a β-blocker or a CCB is used in the presence of decreased diastolic function. Nitroglycerin or ACE inhibitors may be indicated in some cases. Digoxin is indicated in the presence of atrial tachycardia or fibrillation associated with reduced systolic function. Supraventricular tachycardia that does not respond to digoxin may respond to propranolol, atenolol, or diltiazem.

Myocardial hypertrophy associated with hyperthyroidism reflects high volume overload, increased sympathetic tone, systemic hypertension, and the direct effect of thyroid hormones on myocardial contractile proteins. Both systolic and diastolic pressures are often elevated. Increased systemic pressures reflect in part increased vascular resistance caused by high sympathetic outflow, vascular remodeling, and potentially renal disease. A variety of cardiac arrhythmias (ranging from tachycardia to heart block) are associated with hyperthyroidism. Cardiac drugs generally are not necessary, however, if hyperthyroidism is not associated with CHF and in the absence of marked cardiomegaly. Propranolol and diltiazem are beneficial in the patient with HCM associated with hyperthyroidism; verapamil does not appear to be of benefit.[258,259] In the presence of cardiac disease, diuretics, antithyroid medications, ACE inhibitors or other vasodilators (for hypertension), and digoxin (for DCM) should be used as previously described.

Hypertension

Systemic Hypertension

Systemic hypertension occurs in both cats and dogs, although more commonly in cats, and is associated with a number of underlying causes. The most likely are hyperthyroidism (23% to 87% of afflicted cats) and chronic renal disease. The pathophysiologic cause of hypertension in renal disease is not well known but may include abnormal salt excretion, activation of the sympathetic nervous system or RAAS, altered renopressor mediators, and anemia-induced increased cardiac output.[43] Hyperthyroidism apparently causes hypertension by increasing β-receptor number and activity in the myocardium. A thyroid-hormone–specific adenylyl cyclase system mediates the cardiovascular response. Other causes of systemic hypertension include diabetes mellitus, acromegaly, and primary aldosteronism.[190] Occasionally, the recent history may include therapy with steroids (glucocorticoids, progestogens, anabolic steroids).[43] An underlying cause cannot, however, be identified for all cases of systemic hypertension.

Clinical signs of hypertension in the cat include signs related to the underlying disease or signs specific to hypertension. The most common sign specific to hypertension is blindness (83% in one study) associated with retinal detachment or hyphema. Less commonly, signs related to cerebral vascular accident (e.g., seizures, ataxia, sudden collapse) may occur. Diagnostic tests may reveal the underlying causes or associated abnormalities that may require medical management.[43] Azotemia may not be evident despite chronic renal disease as the precipitating cause. Kidneys may be small. Systolic murmurs and gallop rhythms may be auscultated, but tachycardia is not common. Mild to moderate cardiomegaly may be evident radiographically, but pleural effusion and pulmonary edema are unusual; renal disease will increase the likelihood of abnormal fluid retention. Left ventricular hypertrophy is likely but should not be confused with HCM. Ocular changes are easy to monitor and should be used to establish a baseline before implementation of therapy. Hemorrhage may be present in any chamber of the eye. Retinal hemorrhage should be interpreted as an indication of hypertension. Cats with retinal detachment have a higher pressure than cats without detachment.[43] Retinal arteries may be tortuous.

Proper measurement of blood pressure is paramount to successful management of systemic hypertension. Measurements should be taken after an animal has had proper time to acclimate to its surroundings and under conditions of minimal stress.[43] Among the indirect methods used to measure systemic blood pressure in cats, the Doppler and photoplethysmographic methods are probably preferred.[190] Care must be taken to follow proper techniques with the appropriate equipment when blood pressure is indirectly measured.[43] Several readings should be taken over several days unless contraindicated by clinical signs of hypertension. With indirect methods, normal blood pressure (mm Hg) in the unsedated cat is 118 (Doppler leg method) to 123/81.2 (mean arterial pressure 96.8)[43] and in dogs is 133/76 (Dinamap on the tail). Antihypertensive therapy is indicated if the indirect systolic pressure or diastolic pressure is greater than 170 or 100 mm Hg, respectively.[43]

KEY POINT 14-55 Effective treatment of hypertension is vitally dependent on valid measurement of blood pressure.

Returning systolic pressure to normal (i.e., 120 mm Hg) may be an unrealistic goal of therapy; targeting less than 170 mm Hg in cats is more reasonable.[43] Response to therapy should be based on appetite and body weight, ophthalmic examinations, and monitoring of blood pressure. Management of hypertension associated with renal disease should include medical management of that disorder. Additional management includes dietary manipulation (low sodium); diuretics; propranolol; and arterial vasodilators, including α-receptor antagonists, CCBs (amlodipine), hydralazine, and ACE inhibitors.[190] Dietary changes probably should be postponed until drug therapy is stabilized.

Amlodipine is generally the preferred medication for treatment of systemic feline hypertension, followed by a combination of amlodipine with either an ACE inhibitor or a β-blocker in refractory cases. Hydralazine should be reserved for cases that continue to fail to respond, in part because of the potential for activation of the RAAS.[43] For cats with severe ocular manifestations or neurologic signs, therapy must be more aggressive. Sodium nitroprusside can be given as a constant-rate infusion, but the risk of adverse reactions to this arterial and venous dilator requires administration by an infusion pump with constant monitoring. Alternatively, hydralazine coupled with furosemide can be administered, with the addition of a β-blocker (propranolol or atenolol) if response is not sufficient within 12 hours.[43]

Long-term management should be based on repetitive monitoring of blood pressure (weekly until the animal is stable at a sufficiently low pressure) and body weight, as well as the underlying disease causing hypertension. If renal disease is the underlying cause, monitoring also should include an ocular examination and serum potassium concentrations. Once control is acceptable, monitoring should take place at 3-month intervals. Multiple drug combinations are more likely to be associated with adverse effects (including sleeping, ataxia, and anorexia).

Emergency treatment of hypertension might be accomplished orally, although a loading dose may be necessary for amlodipine. Nitroprusside tends to be the preferred treatment for intravenous administration because of ease of titration. Acepromazine can be used as well, although its longer half-life precludes titration and hypotension associated with higher doses may negatively affect renal function. Sedation may be an unwanted side effect.

Use of enalapril and amlodipine has been studied in dogs with experimentally induced myocardial infarction. Although both drugs preserved left ventricular volume and function during the healing process, enalapril more effectively limited hypertrophy.[260] The role of carvedilol in the management of feline hypertension has not yet been well described.

Pulmonary Hypertension

The pulmonary vasculature is a low-resistance, low-pressure, high-capacitance system. It is influenced by right ventricular cardiac output, pulmonary venous pressure, and pulmonary vascular resistance. Pulmonary hypertension (sustained mean pulmonary arterial pressure [PAP] >30 mm Hg; normal 10 to 14 mm Hg) has been categorized by the World Health Organization, largely on the basis of underlying disease, into five categories: (pulmonary) arterial hypertension (I), (pulmonary) venous hypertension (II), chronic alveolar hypoxia (III), chronic thromboembolic disease (IV), and miscellaneous causes (V). Classes II, III, and IV are most relevant to dogs or cats. As reviewed by Johnson and coworkers[261a] in a retrospective study of pulmonary hypertension in dogs (n=53), increased venous pressure caused by myocardial disease, including PDA, represented 46% of cases, followed by alveolar hypoxia (pulmonary fibrosis, pneumonia, others; 23%), and thromboembolism (including that associated with heartworm disease; 20%), with 9% of cases associated with miscellaneous causes. Pulmonary vascular changes (in addition to thromboembolism) that influence hypertension include vasoconstriction, and proliferation of smooth muscle and endothelium.

A number of mediators influence pulmonary vascular response. Arachidonic acid metabolites balance one another by either inhibiting (e.g., prostacyclin, released from endothelial cells in response to prostacyclin synthase) or stimulating (e.g., thromboxane, mediated by thromboxane synthase) vasoconstriction, platelet aggregation, and vascular proliferation. Endothelin and serotonin cause potent vasoconstriction and pulmonary arteriolar smooth muscle proliferation and, for endothelin, potentially fibrosis. In contrast, NO and vasoactive intestinal peptides cause vasodilation and inhibit platelet activation and vascular smooth muscle proliferation. In human patients hypertension is associated with a decrease of vasodilatory mediators (e.g., prostacyclin, NO) and an increase in vasoconstrictive mediators (e.g., thromboxane, serotonin, endothelin). The role of mediators in pulmonary hypertension of dogs is not well defined, although endothelin has been demonstrated to be higher in dogs with heartworm disease compared with other diseases that might cause pulmonary hypertension. However, chronic pulmonary overcirculation is associated with pulmonary vascular remodeling in the dog characterized by pulmonary arterial hypertrophy and increased resistance that may exceed systemic pressure, resulting in right to left shunts. In contrast, pulmonary venous hypertension such as that associated with myocardial disease generally is reduced by pulmonary edema with alveolar hypoxia as a compensatory response that minimizes pulmonary perfusion to poorly ventilated airways. Chronic hypoxia also can lead to pulmonary vascular remodeling.

Treatment of pulmonary hypertension in dogs was recently reviewed.[261b] Treatment of pulmonary hypertension focuses on treatment of underlying disease. Oxygen therapy induces vasodilation and is the only therapy associated with decreased mortality in humans. Vasodilatory drug therapy is implemented if the underlying cause cannot be identified or effectively treated. Vasodilators associated with variable efficacy include hydralazine, CCBs, prostacyclin analogs (e.g., epoprostenol), endothelin receptor antagonists (e.g., bosentan) and PDE inhibitors (e.g., sildenfil). Response and justification for long-term therapy is based on the magnitude by which pulmonary arterial pressure is reduced.

KEY POINT 14-56 Vasodilators are variably effective in the treatment of pulmonary hypertension; treatment is best accomplished if the underlying cause is corrected.

PDE-V is located (in humans) in the pulmonary vasculature and the corpus cavernosum. Other locations may occur in dogs. Inhibition of PDE-V specifically results in accumulation of cGMP. Drugs that specifically targeted PDE-V include, but are not limited to, sildenafil and the longer-acting tadalafil. Sildenafil (2 mg/kg once or twice daily; range 0.5 to 3mg/kg orally every 8 to 24 hours) has been studied retrospectively in dogs (n = 13) with pulmonary hypertension PAP≥ 25 mm Hg at rest for a duration of 3 days to 5 months.[262] Underlying causes included chronic pulmonary diseases, valvular heart disease, patent ductus arteriosus, and pulmonary thromboembolism; a cause was not identified in five dogs. Ten of the dogs were receiving concurrent mediations oriented toward treating underlying disease. In six of eight dogs for which PAPW as determined before and after treatment, PAP decreased from 4 to 37 mm Hg at approximately 2 days into therapy. However, systolic pressure also decreased a median of 33 mm Hg (beginning pressure was 135/90 mm Hg). A number of clinical signs resolved among treated dogs, including cardiogenic ascites, which resolved in one of two dogs. Median survival time was increased 91 days. Complications associated with therapy were difficult to discern in part because of the number of other drugs dogs were receiving; one dog died after discharge when treated with nitroglycerin. The reported use of tadalafil in dogs is limited to a case report in a Yorkshire Terrier with idiopathic hypertension.[263] Treatment (1 mg/kg every 48 hours) resulted in a 20% reduction (105 to 80 mm Hg) in pulmonary arterial hypertension. However, systemic hypotension occurred, and the dog was euthanized 10 days after therapy began.

Pimobendan has been effective in reducing (but not significantly) the ratio of pulmonary to systemic vascular resistance in human patients with chronic emphysema[263a] However, pimobendan was associated with an actue reduction of tricuspid regurgitation flow velocity and NTproBNP in dogs with pulmonary hypertension associated with mitral insufficiency.[237b]

Hydralazine may induce preferential dilation of the pulmonary arterial tree compared with the systemic vasculature. Hydralazine decreases pulmonary vascular resistance in both normal lungs and in lungs with experimentally induced embolization.[261] Because hypoxia can worsen pulmonary arterial vasoconstriction, oxygen therapy is critical to the treatment of pulmonary hypertension associated with CMVI. Aggressive diuretic therapy is indicated to reduce pulmonary edema as well as pulmonary hypertension. Bronchodilator therapy may facilitate bronchiolar smooth muscle spasm, facilitating air movement. In humans CCBs (e.g., diltiazem, nifedipine) are effective in only 10% of patients and only at high doses. A 20% reduction in pulmonary arterial hypertension supports long-term therapy.

Prostacyclin is both a systemic and pulmonary vasodilator. When administered by continuous intravenous infusion it improves mortality and exercise tolerance in human patients with primary pulmonary hypertension. Intravenous prostacyclin also improves right-sided heart structure and function.[210] Prostacyclin analogs are characterized by half-lives longer than the endogenous compound but sufficiently short that constant infusion is necessary. Most problematic is the cost, which is likely to be prohibitively expensive. Examples include epoprostenol (intravenous) and treprostinil (subcutaneous). Two alternative route preparations are available in the U.S. Iloprost is an inhalant form that is administered 6 to 12 times daily; beraprost is an oral preparation administered every 6 hours. A low dose of a systemic PDE III inhibitor may enhance the cAMP-dependent pulmonary vasodilatory response to inhaled prostacyclin.[210] Studies do not appear to have addressed their use in dogs or cats.

Endothelin-receptor antagonists include bosentan, which targets both ET-A and -B and is approved in the United States. Cost may be prohibitive. Drugs available outside the United States include sitaxentan and ambrisentan, both ET-A antagonists. As such, vasoconstriction is minimized (ET-A blockade), but ET-B remains responsive to endothelin, thus promoting its clearance and contributing to vasodilation.

Theophylline is a nonselective PDE inhibitor. Additional benefits include fair bronchodilation, as well as some antiinflammatory control. However, is can be associated with ventilation perfusion mismatching, particularly with intravenous administration. Therefore oxygenation is important. The impact of theophylline in mismatching in patients suffering from hypertension is not known.

L-arginine, a substrate of NO synthase, anecdotally has been associated with reduction in pulmonary arterial hypertension.

Unless hyperthyroidism is accompanied by renal insufficiency, the degree of hypertension associated with hyperthyroidism generally is mild. Because hyperthyroidism-induced hypertension is due to high adrenergic output (causing increased cardiac inotropy and rate), β blockers are preferred to calcium channel blockers. However, the addition of amlodipine may be indicated in hyperthyroid hypertensive cats with renal insufficiency.

Cardiac Arrhythmias

Treatment of cardiac arrhythmias is not innocuous and should be pursued with caution. The greater the extent of myocardial disease, the greater the risk of cardiac arrhythmias, including sudden death. No clear guidelines have emerged among cardiologists regarding first-choice antiarrhythmics or which arrhythmias should be treated. However, a consensus does indicate that not all arrhythmias require treatment. Arrhythmias associated with sudden death (e.g., ventricular arrhythmias, severe bradyarrhythmias including third-degree heart block), syncope, or clinical signs reflecting myocardial failure such as weakness should be treated.

Supraventricular Arrhythmias

Supraventricular Premature Contractions. Ectopic foci that generate premature contractions in the region of the sinoatrial node, atria, atrioventricular node, or junctional tissue generally are not serious enough to cause clinical signs and, as such, require no medical therapy. If clinical signs are evident, therapy should be directed toward the underlying disease. If antiarrhythmic therapy is deemed necessary, drugs are selected for their ability to slow atrioventricular nodal conjunction (e.g., digitalis glycosides, β- blockers, or CCBs). Drugs associated with negative inotropic effects should be used cautiously if myocardial failure is associated with the supraventricular premature contractions.

Supraventricular Tachycardias

Supraventricular tachycardia includes sinus, atrial, or junctional tachycardia; atrial flutter; and atrial fibrillation. Therapy should be considered for heart rates above 220 or 260 bpm in the dog and cat, respectively. The most likely underlying cause is atrial enlargement resulting from dilation. Sinus tachycardia is the most common type of supraventricular tachycardia in dogs and is generated by increased sympathetic tone. Treatment includes digitalis glycosides (if CHF is present), the β blockers (e.g., nonselective propranolol or the preferred selective blockers atenolol, metoprolol, or carvedilol), the class III antiarrhythmic amiodarone (less ideal), or the CCBs (e.g., diltiazem). The most appropriate drug should be based on the underlying cause of the tachycardia. Atrial tachycardia may reflect an autonomic dysfunction (generally not amenable to treatment) or, less commonly, a reentrant circuit. For reentrant causes, class IA antiarrhythmics (especially quinidine), digitalis, or a β blocker is indicated. Atrioventricular nodal or junctional tachycardias can be similarly treated.

Gelzer and Kraus[264] reviewed the management of atrial fibrillation. Atrial fibrillation occurs in the presence of multiple reentering wavelets; its development is facilitated by a large atrium. The authors[264] suggest that treatment is indicated when the average heart rate from a Holter recording exceeds 150 bpm in dogs and at any heart rate in cats with atrial fibrillation. The most efficacious antiarrhythmic drugs are those that increase the wavelength (distance traveled by the depolarization impulse during the refractory period). Although this might be accomplished by either increasing the speed of conduction or increasing the refractory period, the former is not a recognized mechanism of action of antiarrhythmic drugs. Treatment may be unnecessary if the ventricular rate is less than 150 bpm in asymptomatic dogs with no evidence of cardiac disease. Treatment of atrial fibrillation should focus on slowing the ventricular response such that cardiac filling improves and myocardial oxygen demand decreases. In symptomatic dogs the atria can be targeted with class IA drugs (quinidine or, less preferred, procainamide), or conduction through the atrioventricular node can be targeted with digitalis, glycosides, CCBs, or β blockers. Although quinidine prolongs wavelength, its paradoxical acceleration (induced by anticholinergic effects) may increase the ventricular response rate, leading to worsening clinical signs. Quinidine can be used to convert atrial fibrillation to a sinus rhythm in dogs. Successful conversion is, however, generally limited to large-breed dogs with no evidence of underlying cardiac disease and is not recommended in dogs with cardiac failure.

Among the drugs, digitalis probably is the preferred treatment for atrial fibrillation despite the fact that it facilitates the arrhythmia by decreasing the impulse wavelength.[264] Although Gelzer and Kraus[264] recommend monitoring a trough sample 3 to 7 days after starting therapy, for reasons previously discussed, both a peak and trough sample might be prudent to determine half-life at baseline and in response to therapy. Decreased conduction within the atrioventricular node will decrease the ventricular rate. Additionally, positive inotropic effects may benefit the patient with myocardial failure. Previously mentioned precautions should be followed when negative chronotropes that also are negative inotropes are used; CCBs and β blockers may need to be reserved for patients that have not sufficiently responded to digoxin. According to Gelzer and Kraus,[264] a CCB is preferred in animals with a rapid ventricular rate resulting from enhanced sympathetic tone. An exception can be made for acute management, in which case digitalis is begun simultaneously with a CCB; β blockers are generally reserved for cases that do not respond to other drugs. Because of a potential protective effect on the diseased myocardium, however, β blockers might be indicated earlier and perhaps preferentially to diltiazem or other CCBs if chronic activation of the sympathetic system is contributing to cardiac failure.

KEY POINT 14-57 Digoxin is probably the preferred drug for treatment of atrial fibrillation. However, treatment in dogs may not be indicated unless the heart rate exceeds 150 bpm. Atrial fibrillation should be treated in all cats.

Emergency management of supraventricular arrhythmias is indicated in the presence of sustained arrhythmias in patients that are hemodynamically unstable. Beta blocker therapy includes propranolol (0.02-0.06 mg/kg, slow intravenous administration every 8 hours) or esmolol. Esmolol (0.05-0.1 mg/kg intravenously every 5 minutes up to 0.5 mg/kg) has a shorter half-life compared to propranolol. Failure to convert can be followed with CCB therapy with little risk of negative inotropic effects. Diltiazem (0.25 mg/kg intravenously over 2 minutes followed by 0.25 mg/kg every 15 minutes) can be implemented until conversion occurs, up to a maximum dose of 0.75 mg/kg. Verapamil also has been used (0.05 mg/kg, slow intravenous administration up to 0.15 mg/kg).

KEY POINT 14-58 Emergency management of supraventricular or ventricular arrhythmias is indicated in the presence of sustained arrhythmias in patients that are hemodynamically unstable.

Despite the traditional consensus that lidocaine is indicated only for ventricular arrhythmias, Johnson and coworkers[125] described the impact of lidocaine at a standard dose in five dogs with complex supraventricular arrhythmias. In each case normal sinus rhythm was achieved and then maintained with mexiletine.

Ventricular Arrhythmias

The importance of any ventricular arrhythmia depends on the ventricular rate, duration of the arrhythmia (tachycardia), and the severity of underlying cardiac disease. The clinical sequelae of a detrimentally rapid ventricular rate and insufficient ventricular filling include weakness, syncope, seizures, collapse, and clinical signs indicative of CHF.

Ventricular tachycardias are caused by a variety of underlying disorders, including but not limited to primary cardiac disease, metabolic disorders causing acid–base or electrolyte imbalances, infectious disorders, neoplasia, and trauma. Resolution of the underlying cause is paramount to successful therapy of ventricular tachycardias. Not all ventricular premature contractions require treatment. Generally, ventricular premature contractions that are multifocal, occur more frequently than 25 per minute, or occur in repetitive runs that result in a heart rate of 130 bpm or more should be medically managed. Those that are associated with clinical signs or those that occur in breeds at risk for sudden death (e.g., German Shepherd Dogs, Boxers) might also be treated, although this is controversial.

Ventricular arrhythmias that are considered life threatening should be managed with intravenously administered lidocaine. Generally, a slow intravenous bolus (4 to 8 mg/kg [dogs]; 0.5 to 1 mg/kg [cats]) is followed by a constant infusion (22 to 66 μg/kg per minute [dogs]; 10 to 20 μg/kg per minute [cats]). Once sufficient response has occurred, oral therapy can be phased in. Procainamide can be administered intravenously (2 to 20 mg/kg over 30 minutes followed by a constant infusion of 2 to 40 μg/kg per minute [dogs]; 1 to 2 mg/kg intravenous bolus followed by 10 to 20 μg/kg per minute infusion [cats]) or, in less critical patients, intramuscularly or orally (6.6 to 22 mg/kg every 2 to 6 hours [dogs]) in patients that do not respond to lidocaine. Quinidine also can be used (6.6 to 22 mg/kg orally, intramuscularly every 6 hours). Eradication of the ventricular arrhythmia may not be a reasonable expectation. Insufficient response should lead to confirmation of the diagnosis; evaluation of acid–base or electrolyte disturbance; and, if necessary, addition of a second class IA antiarrhythmic or β blocker (see discussion of precautions in myocardial failure). Ventricular pacing devices may be necessary for animals that continue to fail to respond to antiarrhythmic therapy.

Response (hemodynamic, antiarrhythmic, and adverse) to a single intravenous bolus dose of procainamide was demonstrated to not differ from a single intravenous dose of lidocaine in dogs with postoperative ventricular arrhythmias.[265] Neither drug was associated with undesirable hemodynamic changes. Specific information regarding the study (e.g., doses) could not be found.

Bradyarrhythmias

Bradycardia is defined as a heart rate of less than 70 bpm and usually results from sinus nodal or atrioventricular conduction disturbances. Both conduction and automaticity (decreased) disturbances cause bradycardias. In general, medical management of bradyarrhythmias is unreliable, and placement of a pacemaker device is the preferred method of management.

Sinus brachycardia usually is clinically asymptomatic, with the most common clinical sign being syncope or episodic weakness. For animals that are symptomatic, long-acting anticholinergic drugs (e.g., propantheline) might be helpful. Failure to respond will require pacemaker placement.

Atrioventricular nodal block can be first, second, or third degree, depending on the severity. With third-degree block, there is no conduction between the atria and the ventricles. The ventricular escape rhythm approximates 40 bpm. Pacemaker placement is the preferred method of treatment, but emergency cases can be treated with isoproterenol (constant-rate infusion). If the ventricular rate increases in response to atropine, an orally active long-acting (relative to atropine) anticholinergic such as propantheline might be effective. Diphenoxylate reportedly also has been useful.

Pericardial Effusion

Pathophysiology

Accumulation of fluid in the pericardial sac most commonly reflects a disorder of the pericardium but can also occur as a manifestation of myocardial failure.[190,266] Causes include but are not limited to pericarditis (septic or foreign body), neoplasia, and idiopathic hemorrhage. If accumulation is severe, cardiac tamponade may develop. Increased intrapericardial pressure and diastolic collapse of the right atrium and potentially the right ventricle can result in reduced preload to the left ventricle, decreased cardiac output, and hypotension. Systemic compensatory mechanisms may be activated in an attempt to maintain cardiac output. Chronic disease ultimately can lead to pleural effusion and (in extreme cases) pulmonary edema.

Pharmacologic Management

Because pericardial effusion often does not respond sufficiently to pharmacologic management, pericardiocentesis and surgical alternatives such as pericardiectomy or balloon dilation should be anticipated if the underlying cause cannot be rapidly resolved. In cats with feline infectious peritonitis, high doses of glucocorticoids may decrease the accumulation of pericardial fluid. Glucocorticoids also have been recommended for dogs with idiopathic hemorrhagic pericardial effusion that has not responded to pericardiocentesis.

HYPERTHERMIA

Hyperthermia requires treatment in dogs and cats when temperatures exceed 106° F. Temperatures below 106° F may be beneficial (e.g., inhibition of viral replication, stimulation of white blood cell function). In contrast, temperatures of 107° F are life threatening and may lead to permanent organ damage, alkalosis or superimposed acidosis, electrolyte derangements (hypernatremia or hyponatremia, hypokalemia, hypophosphatemia, and hypocalcemia), disseminated intravascular coagulopathy, and acute renal failure (particularly with exertional heat stroke). Hyperthermia can occur for a variety of reasons, most classified as either true fever (endogenous or exogenous pyrogens directly alter the hypothalamic thermostat) or inadequate heat dissipation (e.g., classic heat stroke or exertional heat stroke associated with excessive exercise). Pathologic hyperthermia is less common and includes malignant hyperthermia, a muscular disorder that appears to reflect drug- (e.g., halothane) induced alterations in calcium kinetics. In all cases treatment begins by removing the inciting cause. Antipyretics (e.g., dipyrone or other NSAIDs) are indicated in situations involving a reset thermostat (i.e., a true fever) but only if the body temperature is 106° F or higher. Injectable preparations are preferred. Relatively selective COX inhibitors (e.g., carprofen) may be equally or more effective than nonselective drugs because prostaglandins formed by COX-2 are responsible for mediating fever.

Phenothiazines may also be beneficial, in part by inducing peripheral vasodilation. Use of α-agonists or other drugs that induce peripheral vasoconstriction is discouraged. Treatment of hyperthermia associated with inadequate heat dissipation focuses on rapid cooling of the body, correction of electrolyte and fluid imbalances, and prevention of complications. Cold water should be avoided for cooling because it may induce vasoconstriction, decrease heat dissipation, and rebound hyperthermia.[267] Spraying the patient with cool water in the presence of fans is the preferred method of cooling. Crystalloid therapy should be aggressive; colloidal therapy may be indicated. The use of NSAIDs in treatment of hyperthermia resulting from inadequate heat dissipation should not be ruled out, in part because of the inhibitory effects timely administration of these drugs can have on multiorgan failure associated with cytokine and other mediator release. Malignant hyperthermia is less likely to respond to external cooling, although this should be implemented; bromocriptine and neuromuscular paralysis (e.g., pancuronium) may help control muscle rigidity.[267]

SHOCK

Shock reflects a state in which tissue perfusion is inadequate to meet tissue metabolic needs.[268] Tissue perfusion may be inadequate because of low or unevenly distributed blood flow.[269] Selection of the most appropriate therapy is facilitated by categorizing shock first as to the functional disturbance and second as to primary cause.

Classification Of Shock

Hypovolemic Shock

Hypovolemic shock is one of the more common causes of shock in small animals.[268] Causes include but are not limited to hemorrhage, trauma, and severe dehydration such as that which accompanies renal dysfunction, vomiting, or hypoadrenocorticism.[269] Physiologically, hypovolemic shock can present in three stages. The earliest stage is accompanied by compensatory mechanisms (e.g., increased heart rate, increased vascular resistance) designed to maintain blood pressure. As volume loss progresses, the second or middle stage is characterized by tachycardia with low systemic blood pressure and hypothermia. Capillary refill time is prolonged, and pulse pressure is poor. Blood is shunted away from less vital organs to the brain and heart, and blood clotting abnormalities may be accompanied by increased capillary permeability. Urine output decreases. If hypovolemia persists, the final stage of decompensation occurs. This stage is largely irreversible[268] and is characterized by vascular dilation and pooling of blood in peripheral tissues. Poor cardiac filling leads to insufficient cardiac and brain perfusion. Death reflects myocardial failure, cardiac arrhythmias, respiratory failure associated with pulmonary edema, and cardiopulmonary arrest.[268]

Cardiogenic Shock

Cardiogenic shock is a state of low cardiac output associated with diastolic or systolic dysfunction. The heart is unable to function as a pump, and blood delivery to organs is insufficient. Causes include myocardial failure (acquired or congenital) and cardiac arrhythmias. Iatrogenic cardiogenic shock also can be drug induced.[269] Clinically, because the underlying cause of shock is inadequate blood flow, cardiogenic shock presents similarly to hypovolemic shock, with the primary difference of increased atrial filling pressures accompanied by pulmonary edema.[269]

Distributive Shock

Distributive shock occurs when blood flow is distributed improperly to tissues. Improper distribution reflects a rapid, marked increase in peripheral vasodilation, vascular capacitance, and peripheral pooling of blood.[269] Causes generally include those associated with the release of vasoactive mediators, most notably endotoxemia (see Chapter 8) or other causes of sepsis and anaphylaxis or anaphylactoid reactions. Injured and ischemic tissues (e.g., due to hypovolemic or cardiogenic shock) also lead to the release of vasoactive and procoagulant mediators. Vascular occlusive diseases such as saddle thrombi and pulmonary thromboembolism (e.g., dirofilariasis) also cause distributive shock.[269] For example, with sepsis distributive shock might initially be "warm" in that blood flow is increased in peripheral tissues. As shock progresses and venous pooling continues, fluid is lost from the vascular space, venous return decreases, cardiac output decreases, and tissues become underperfused or "cool."

Pathophysiology

Ideally, treatment of shock should focus on early reversal based on the underlying cause. As shock progresses, the underlying pathophysiology is the same, and treatment is oriented toward prevention and reversal of inadequate tissue perfusion. Some type of damage is likely to occur in any tissue subjected to a period of hypotension (mean arterial blood pressure <50 mm Hg). These include cell ischemia, inadequate oxygen delivery, and the generation of proinflammatory/procoagulant mediators.[269]

Sequelae of cellular ischemia. Tissues suffer damage from inadequate tissue oxygenation in 5 to 10 minutes, and the damage is irreversible at 15 to 20 minutes.[269] Mitochondrial dysfunction accompanies ATP depletion, leading to anaerobic metabolism and lactic acid accumulation. Cell membrane (ATPase) pumps become disrupted, and intracellular destructive enzymes are released. Accumulation of intracellular calcium leads to the activation of enzymes that disrupt cellular homeostasis. Intracellular sodium and chloride increase, and magnesium and potassium decrease. ATP breakdown yields hypoxanthine and generation of xanthine oxidase (converted from xanthine dehydrogenase), which produces oxygen free radicals.[269] With reperfusion, hyperemia occurs once blood flow is reestablished if the period of impaired oxygenation or poor tissue perfusion is short. The duration of hyperemia is determined by the extent of mediator release (potassium, hydrogen, NO, adenosine, adrenomedullin, the latter a hypotensive peptide first discovered in pheochromocytomas). On the other hand, if blood flow is less than 20% of normal for longer than 5 minutes, reperfusion after perfusion failure leads to reoxygenation injury. Injury reflects the production of self-destructive enzymes and metabolites and derangements in blood clotting.[269] Together the consequences of reperfusion injury include uneven distribution of blood flow and focal ischemia (perhaps exacerbated by inappropriate thrombosis), swelling of capillary endothelial cells and subsequent plugging by leukocytes migrating to the area, and increased microvascular viscosity and interstitial edema.[269]

Oxygen free radicals. The generation of oxygen free radicals by mitochondria, macrophages, and neutrophils sets the stage for reperfusion injury should blood flow be reestablished after a sufficiently long period of poor perfusion, causing perhaps the most detrimental sequelae of shock.[269] Xanthine oxidase metabolizes molecular oxygen into radicals such as superoxide anion, hydrogen peroxide, and the hydroxyl radical (see Chapter 29). Enzymes that normally scavenge oxygen free radicals (e.g., superoxide dismutase, catalase, and glutathione) are overwhelmed as tissues reperfuse. Production of oxygen free radicals is exacerbated by mediators released in response to oxygen free radicals, including cytokines (including TNF), interleukins (which also induce procoagulant activity), and prostaglandins.[269]

Role of nitric oxide. NO can be either protective or detrimental in the patient with sepsis and endotoxemia. Under basal physiologic conditions, NO serves as a free oxygen radical scavenger, limiting toxicity associated with superoxide and other radicals. Inhibition of platelet aggregation and leukocyte adhesion limits ischemia–reperfusion injuries.[21] During shock large amounts of iNOS are formed; as such, NO becomes a major contributor to the pathophysiology of shock.[21,269] Peroxynitrous acid, generated from the reaction of NO with oxygen free radicals, destroys cellular macromolecules, causing mitochondrial and cell membrane dysfunction, production of prostaglandins, and programmed cell death (apoptosis). The coagulation cascade is activated, ultimately leading to disseminated intravascular coagulation. Arteriovenous shunting (possibly caused by iNOS) contributes to maldistribution of blood flow, particularly in endotoxic and other septic shock, and may be a cause of irreversibility.[269]

Thus, although the initial responses of the body to iNOS might lead to important compensatory responses, ultimately the responses may prove to be detrimental. Nevertheless, inhibition of NOS is undesirable because systemic vascular resistance is improved only at the cost of loss of blood flow to vital organs. Platelet aggregation increases, along with the risk of thrombus formation and disseminated intravascular coagulation.[269] Analogs of L-arginine, such as L-NAME (*N*-nitro-L-arginine methyl ester) competitively inhibit NO production by either cNOS or iNOS from L-arginine. Treatment of human patients in septic shock with L-NAME, however, led to pulmonary hypertension and reduced cardiac output.[270] Drugs that selectively inhibit iNOS but not cNOS may be a more appropriate focus of investigation.

Gastrointestinal barrier. The sequelae of ischemia and hypoxia in the gut have profound clinical implications for the patient undergoing shock. Potent vasoconstrictors (endothelins), cytokines, and other mediators act in concert with leukocyte migration and epithelial necrosis to increase capillary permeability, transcapillary fluid filtration, and interstitial edema. Diarrhea is a common clinical complication of resuscitation from shock and may indicate the loss of the protective mucosal barrier in the gastrointestinal tract. Bacterial translocation and endotoxin absorption result in release of massive quantities of proinflammatory mediators, predisposing the patient to septicemia and, ultimately, to the systemic inflammatory response syndrome (see Chapter 29).[269] This syndrome is characterized by multiorgan dysfunction.

The compensatory mechanisms implemented to counter the pathophysiologic sequelae (decreased tissue perfusion and oxygen delivery) of shock involve the neural, hormonal, and renal reflexes previously described for cardiovascular diseases. Vasoconstriction maintains arterial blood pressure and redistributes blood flow to vital organs (cerebral and coronary vessels). Cardiac output is increased by increasing heart rate and a fluid shift from interstitial to intravascular sites. Although compensatory mechanisms support the patient during the initial stages of shock, increased vascular resistance and myocardial oxygen demand ultimately will contribute to the demise of the patient.

Treatment

Successful therapy for shock focuses on reestablishing blood flow, blood pressure, and blood volume to normal or above normal (see Table 14-4).[269] Monitoring response to therapy can, however, be difficult. Muir[269] recommends that response to therapy and a good prognosis be based on frequent monitoring of behavior, level of consciousness, arterial blood pressure, tissue oxygenation, heart and respiratory rate and rhythm, mucous membrane color, capillary refill time, and urine output. Clinical pathology data should focus on packed cell volume, total protein, and serum lactate.

KEY POINT 14-59 Successful therapy for shock focuses on reestablishing blood flow, blood pressure, and blood volume to normal or above normal.

Treatment of shock should maximize tissue perfusion and oxygen delivery to and consumption by peripheral tissues and minimize the effects of proinflammatory and procoagulant mediators. For septic shock (discussed more extensively in Chapter 8) therapy also focuses more aggressively on prevention of endotoxin release and its effects. Regardless of the cause of shock, appropriate therapy is summarized by the acronym VIP: **V**entilation to facilitate blood oxygenation, **I**nfusion of fluids to restore blood volume, and support of the myocardial **P**ump to facilitate blood delivery (flow) to tissues.[269]

Fluid therapy. Fluid therapy should be aggressive but not overzealous. Care should be taken not to reduce packed cell volume and total protein to less than 20% and 3.5 g/dL, respectively, to minimize the risk of pulmonary or interstitial edema. Administration of hypertonic saline provides rapid but short-term (30 to 120 minutes) hemodynamic improvement in hypovolemic or endotoxic shock; duration of improvement can be extended if hypertonic saline is combined with a colloid.

Blood and blood substitutes. Treatment of hypotensive shock secondary to hemorrhage in which 25 mL/kg or more of blood is lost should include whole blood or packed red blood cells. Blood substitutes should be used when blood products are not available or for animals for which the risk of a transfusion reaction is too great.

Pressor drugs. Positive inotropic drugs are indicated to maintain arterial blood pressure and regional blood flow in patients whose myocardial function does not improve sufficiently after administration of fluids. Pressor drugs also are indicated for patients whose cardiac contractile activity is compromised. Dopamine and dobutamine have been the preferred pressor drugs; dopamine may be preferred for bradycardic animals. [229] Improved blood flow to the gastrointestinal tract will help minimize the risk of gastrointestinal mucosal damage and subsequent multiorgan failure.[229] Volume replacement must occur before either drug can be used successfully. Refractory hypotension is often associated with septic shock. Underlying mechanisms include vasopressin deficiency, activation of ATP-sensitive K^+ channels (in response to accumulation of lactate and hydrogen), and overproduction of NO (which precludes vascular smooth muscle contraction). Activation of K^+ channels causes hyperpolarization, precluding interaction of vasoconstrictors with smooth muscle receptors. Among the current therapies is treatment with vasopressin. [269a] In patients with septic or hypovolemic shock, vasopressin is released biphasically. Osmotic overstimulation may cause rapid release of endogenous vasopressin. However, only 20% of the total pool is available for rapid release. Slower release results in relative deficiency by 1 hour of sustained hypovolemic shock in humans. Whereas arterial pressure is minimally affected in healthy subjects, patients in vasodilatory shock express an exaggerated response to exogenous vasopressin therapy. Mechanisms include replacement of endogenous stores, inhibition of K^+ channels, and decreased synthesis of nitric acid. Treatment at physiologic doses (0.01-0.04 units [70-kg human adult]) has been described as the best vasopressor drug; doses of first-line vasoproessors can be reduced, thus reducing the risk of adverse effects with these drugs. The drug can be given intratracheally.[269b] Yoo[269c] described a vasopressin dose determination study in dogs with experimentally-induced hemorrhagic shock. A dose of 0.4 IU/kg was the most effective dose, providing more hemodynamic response in decompensated shock compred to 1.6 IU/kg. Treatment ideally occurs when endogenous concentrations are lowest. Other benefits of vasopressin include increase urine output; improved cerebral, coronary, and pulmonary blood flow; and increased serum cortisol. Side effects occurring at nonphysiologic doses include platelet aggregation and renal, mesenteric, pulmonary, and coronary vasoconstriction. Vasopressin should be used only with caution in patients with cardiovascular disease. The use of glucocorticoids may be indicated in patients non-responsive to pressor agents as a result of functional adrenocorticodeficiency (See Chapter 30).

Miscellaneous drugs. The use of drugs intended to minimize the damage of oxygen free radicals has not been well established in animals such that a standard protocol can be followed. The use of glucocorticoids is controversial (see Chapter 30). Their potential benefits to the endotoxic shock patient have been delineated. In general, the efficacy of these products to limit vascular response to vasoactive compounds depends on the time of administration. Efficacy is greatest when administered before or within several hours of the onset of the pathophysiologic response to shock. Although survival (several hours) has been documented after use of glucocorticoids (compared with placebo) in human and animal clinical trials, long-term survival (beyond several days) has not been documented. Use of glucocorticoids in human patients with endotoxic or septic shock has been associated with an increased risk of infection in some studies but no increased risk in others. The use of glucocorticoids in veterinary medicine remains controversial. Of the drugs to be used, methylprednisolone may be preferred in most causes of shock because of its potential ability to scavenge oxygen free radicals. Administration should be short term.

KEY POINT 14-60 The use of drugs intended to minimize the damage of oxygen free radicals has not been well established in animals.

A number of NSAIDs have been studied for their ability to block response to mediators of endotoxic shock. Indomethacin and ibuprofen have shown efficacy in human patients. Flunixin meglumine has been studied in dogs. As with glucocorticoids, however, the effects of NSAIDs must be realized within the first 2 hours of the onset of endotoxic shock (i.e., before mediators have been able to stimulate response). Prolonged therapy with NSAIDs is not advised because of toxic effects. Although gastrointestinal toxicity is the major concern in most animals, the patient suffering from endotoxic shock may be more predisposed.

Despite the lack of scientific data to support clinical response to drugs that scavenge oxygen free radicals, their use should be strongly considered, particularly if there is little risk of toxicity (See Chapter 29).

The use of antimicrobials in patients suffering from or predisposed to endotoxic or septic shock is discussed elsewhere (see Chapter 8). Patients that have suffered vascular compromise are at risk of suffering the consequences of translocation of enteric pathogens. Prophylactic therapy should be oriented toward minimization of gastric erosion or ulceration (see Chapter 19) and selective decontamination of the digestive tract (targeting gram-negative aerobic pathogens). In humans oral antimicrobials that are not absorbed are recommended: a paste containing 2% polymyxin, 2% tobramycin, and 2% amphotericin (to target fungal organisms) for the oral cavity and a solution of polymixin (100 mg), tobramycin (80 mg), and amphotericin B (500 mg) for the gastrointestinal tract (about 0.1 mL/kg every 6 hours) have been recommended.[271] However, this therapy is intended to reduce the incidence of nosocomial infections in the intensive care environment. The incidence of pneumonia, urinary tract infections, and catheter-related septicemia can be decreased. The role of selective digestive decontamination in patients subject to shock (with the exception of endotoxic shock) is less clear.

Cardiopulmonary Cerebrovascular Resuscitation

Generally, the goal of cardiopulmonary cerebrovascular resuscitation (CPCR) is to maintain or preserve neurologic function. It is beyond the scope of this chapter to discuss the causes of and recognition of the need for CPCR. Obviously, prevention is the key to success, and treatment of underlying diseases likely to cause cardiopulmonary arrest should be reviewed. Success is more likely if the cardiopulmonary arrest is associated with reversible conditions (e.g., anesthetic overdose, upper airway obstruction, hemorrhage, electrolyte imbalances). The focus of this discussion is on drugs used in CPCR. Which drugs are proper and when their use is indicated in the patient are controversial. Cardiac rather than respiratory arrest is discussed. The pharmacologic effects, side effects, and other pertinent clinical pharmacologic data for each of the drugs have been discussed elsewhere; discussion here is limited to the use of the drugs during or immediately after CPCR.

"Crash Cart" Drugs

Drugs that should be carried in a crash cart include epinephrine, atropine, magnesium chloride, naloxone, lidocaine, sodium bicarbonate, and bretylium tosylate.[272]

Epinephrine remains the mainstay of acute cardiac life support. It is intended to promote systemic vasoconstriction such that blood flow is diverted to the coronary and cerebral circulation. It is indicated for pulseless ventricular tachycardia, ventricular fibrillation, electromechanical dissociation (pulseless electrical activity), and ventricular asystole. The standard dose is 10 to 20 μg/kg (1 mg in humans) or 10 mL of a 1:10,000 solution repeated every 3 to 5 minutes. The optimal dose may be very high, ranging from 0.45 to 2 mg/kg (Table 14-4). For humans the American Heart Association has recommended a fivefold increase in the dose to 5 mg if there is no response to the initial 1 mg dose.[267]

KEY POINT 14-61 Epinephrine remains the mainstay of acute cardiac life support.

Atropine has little indication in CPCR with the exception of bradycardia, pulseless electrical activity, and ventricular asystole. The dose for electromechanical dissociation and asystole is 1 mg intravenously, repeated every 3 to 5 minutes. In humans complete vagal blockade occurs at 0.04 mg/kg (3 mg); this dose is discouraged. Likewise, a total dose below 0.5 mg can cause parasympathomimetic effects and also is discouraged.[267]

Isoproterenol is a pure, nonselective β-agonist drug. As such, it is a positive inotrope but can also cause peripheral vasodilation. It will increase myocardial oxygen demand. Currently, its use is limited to bradyarrhythmias that do not respond to atropine.[272]

Bicarbonate provides little benefit and may in fact harm patients in metabolic acidosis. Acidosis associated with cardiac arrest is best treated with ventilatory and circulatory support. Potentially harmful effects of bicarbonate include arrhythmogenic alkalemia; increased generation of CO_2; hyperosmolarity; hypokalemia; paradoxical central nervous system and myocardial intracellular acidosis; and a leftward shift in the oxyhemoglobin dissociation curve, limiting delivery of O_2 to tissues.[267] When used, bicarbonate therapy ideally should be guided by blood gas analysis (pH <7.15 to 7.2).[267] Indications or situations in which bicarbonate may prove beneficial for humans requiring CPCR include hyperkalemia; tricyclic antidepressant overdose; prolonged cardiac arrest (protracted hypoperfusion-induced acidosis); and postresuscitation, bicarbonate-responsive, and anaerobic lactic acidoses.[267] Sodium bicarbonate (1 mEq/kg intravenously) may be used after epinephrine in patients suffering from a prolonged cardiac arrest who have shown improvement in cardiovascular or cerebral recovery. It should be followed by correction of any deficit (monitored) that is greater than 5 mEq/kg. The bicarbonate-induced hypercarbia tends to be transient and generally harmless to the heart if used in conjunction with epinephrine.[272]

KEY POINT 14-62 Bicarbonate provides little benefit and may in fact harm patients in metabolic acidosis.

Calcium administration does not appear to enhance cardiac performance during CPCR. Ischemia associated with cardiac arrest causes intracellular accumulation of calcium, which can disrupt membranes and uncouple oxidative phosphorylation. Calcium can cause coronary vasospasm and will exacerbate the arrhythmic tendency of the unstable myocardium and impair relaxation.[267,272] It will also exacerbate digoxin toxicity. Calcium causes precipitation when combined with sodium bicarbonate. Calcium is not recommended except in cases of prolonged cardiac arrest or absent or ineffective pump activity. Calcium chloride (10% solution contains 100 mg/mL Ca^{2+}) is associated with the longest and most predictable increase in plasma ionized calcium.[272] In human patients 1 g of calcium chloride (approximately 15 mg/kg) is generally sufficient, although toxicity may occur at this dose. Other indications for calcium include hyperkalemia, ionized hypocalcemia, and CCB overdose.[267]

Crystalloids (including hypertonic resuscitation and balanced electrolyte solutions) are indicated if the cause of cardiac arrest is hypovolemia. Inappropriate fluid load can, however, contribute to decreased cerebral blood flow and decreased coronary blood flow.[272] The production of lactic acid will be enhanced in critically ill hyperglycemic patients, which can lead to or contribute to cell injury. Dextrose infusions are considered by the American Heart Association to be harmful to humans.[267] As such, dextrose-containing fluids should be avoided. Isotonic saline or Ringer's lactate is preferred as the resuscitation fluid.

KEY POINT 14-63 If crystalloid therapy is indicated in the shock patient, isotonic saline containing fluids free of dextrose is indicated.

Several routes of drug administration can be used to support resuscitation. Central venous catheter placement is ideal for immediate drug delivery to the heart. A sufficient bolus of a compatible isotonic fluid should follow any drug administered through peripheral tubing. Intracardiac injections probably offer no increased benefit compared with central intravenous administration. Potential complications include cardiac tamponade, coronary vessel laceration, and pneumothorax. Intracardiac bolus may destabilize the electrical properties of the heart.

Alternative routes of administration can be considered in the absence of venous access. Intratracheal administration is an effective alternative route to central intravenous administration for selected drugs during CPCR.[272] In general, the dose is doubled and the drug is administered through a catheter in 10 to 20 mL of liquid for the drugs to reach the alveoli, where they will be subsequently absorbed. Insufflation will facilitate drug absorption. Doses of all drugs administered intratracheally should be increased by twofold to 2.5-fold. The duration of action of the drugs may be longer after intratracheal administration than after intravenous administration. Drugs shown to be effective after intratracheal administration include epinephrine, lidocaine, atropine, and naloxone. There are several drugs that should not be given via intratracheal administration because of the risk of tissue damage. Examples include sodium bicarbonate (depletes surfactant), norepinephrine, and calcium chloride.[267] Drugs should not be mixed in the same syringe before intratracheal administration.

Table **14-4** Crash Cart Drugs

Drug	Indication	Dose	Comments
Amiodarone	Defibrillation	*5-10 mg/kg IV	
Atropine	Bradycardia, asystole, PEA	0.022-0.04 mg/kg IV	Repeat at 3 to 5 intervals as needed. Avoid more than 0.04 mg/kg and less than 0.5 mg total dose; exception may be PEA, which may require 0.4 mg/kg IV
Bicarbonate	Hyperkalemia, prolonged cardiac arrest	1 meq/kg IV	Therapy should be guided by blood gases and generally is reserved for resuscitative attempts lasting longer than 20 minutes. Ventilatory support critical.
Bretylium	Ventricular flutter	5-10 mg/kg IV	
Calcium chloride	Prolonged cardiac arrest with ineffective activity, severe hypocalcemia, severe hyperkalemia	15 mg/kg slow IV	Monitor electrocardiogram. 10% solution of calcium chloride contains more calcium per mL than other calcium salts
Calcium gluconate	Prolonged cardiac arrest with ineffective activity, severe hypocalcemia, severe hyperkalemia	10 mg/kg/hr in any fluid	Monitor electrocardiogram. 10% solution of calcium gluconate contains less calcium per mL than calcium chloride.
Dexamethasone	Pulseless idioventricular arrhythmia	2-4 mg/kg IV	
Dobutamine	Positive chronotrope, positive inotrope	2.5-10 μg/kg/min (D)	Any IV fluid
Dopamine hydrochloride	Positive chronotrope, positive inotrope	5-20 μg/kg/min, to effect	Any nonalkaline IV fluid
	Low dose (renal vasodilation)	1-4 μg/kg/min	
	Mid dose	5-10 μg/kg/min	
	High dose	10-20 μg/kg/min	
Epinephrine	Fine ventricular fibrillation, PEA, asystole, positive inotropic and vascular support, status asthmaticus	10-20 μg/kg (0.02 mg/kg)	Repeat at 3- to 5-minute intervals as needed. Up to 0.2 mg/kg total dose may be indicated. IV(double dose if IT)
		10 mL of 1:10,000 sol	Repeat at 3- to 5-minute intervals as needed
		0.005-1.5 μg/kg/min, to effect CRI	
Flumezanil	Diazepam reversal	0.02 mg/kg, IV	
Isoproterenol	Bradyarrhythmias		Limit to atropine nonresponders
Lidocaine	Ventricular tachycardia, flutter	Initial dose: 2-6 mg/kg	May be of more benefit post-resuscitation; use in 5% dextrose. 0.9% NaCl less preferred
		Followed by: 25-80 μg/kg	
Magnesium chloride	Ventricular tachycardia	5-10 ml of 2% solution, IV	
	Ventricular flutter	25 to 40 mg/kg, IV	IV over 5 minutes followed by CRI
Magnesium sulfate 25%	None	Up to 1 mEq/kg/day	5% dextrose, diluted to <20%
Naloxone	Narcotic reversal, PEA	0.02-0.04 mg/kg, IV	
Nitroprusside	Hypertensive crisis	1-10 μg/kg/min	5% dextrose
	Pulmonary edema	0.5-5 μg/kg/min.	Start low, and increase slowly. Monitor blood pressure
Procainamide	Ventricular tachycardia, flutter	4-8 mg/kg IV	40-60 μg/kg/min
Vasopressin	Vascular support, asystole	0.04 to 0.8 units/kg, IV	
	Post-resuscitation vascular support	0.001 units/kg/hr	
Yohimbine	Anesthetic reversal	0.1 to 0.2 mg/kg, IV	

IV, Intravenous; *PEA,* pulseless electrical activity; *IT,* intratracheal; *CRI,* constant-rate infusion.
*Chemical defibrillation (in absence of electrical defibrillation): 1 mg potassium chloride and 6 mg acetylcholine/kg, followed by 1 mL/10 kg 10% calcium chloride. Amiodarone also has been suggested at 5-10 mg/kg IV. Chemical defibrillation is rarely effective.

Intraosseous administration is another alternative to intravenous use in small animals. The bone marrow provides a large venous access; the most common sites during CPCR are either the trochanteric fossa of the femur or distal cranial femur.[272]

Specific Conditions

Cardiac asystole refers to the complete absence of electrical activity. Therapy is oriented toward stimulating any electrical activity and then modifying the activity to generate a rhythm with a pulse.[267] Epinephrine generally remains the drug of choice for cardiac arrest. Doses should be sufficient (> 0.01 mg/kg) to cause positive inotropic and peripheral vasoconstrictive effects yet low enough (<0.2 mg/kg) to avoid ventricular fibrillation. In an experimental model of cardiac arrest in dogs, declining renal function was positively correlated with the amount of epinephrine administered and the energy required for defibrillation.[273] Because of its short duration of action, epinephrine should be administered every 3 minutes. Longer-term inotropic support should be provided with a less effective pressor drug such as dopamine or dobutamine. Electrolyte imbalance should be treated with the appropriate electrolyte. Bicarbonate is useful only in the previously described indications.

Ventricular fibrillation is best converted to a normal rhythm by electrical defibrillation. Potassium chloride, bretylium, and magnesium chloride have been used to pharmacologically treat defibrillation in the dog. Among these, magnesium chloride (5 to 10 mL of a 2% solution administered intravenously) may be best. Once an organized rhythm has been established, epinephrine may be beneficial for increasing vascular tone and improving blood flow to the brain. The initial dose should be low (0.02 mg/kg) and increased tenfold (0.2 mg/kg) in nonresponsive patients. Very high doses may, however, excessively increase myocardial oxygen demand. Lidocaine may prove useful for "coarsening" fibrillation, rendering it more amenable to electroconversion. In addition, it may increase vascular tone response to epinephrine.[267] Bretylium has proved useful in some human cases of refractory ventricular fibrillation. The drug is administered immediately (1 minute) before electrical defibrillation. Refractory cases also may require correction of severe acidosis. Precaution is, however, taken to ensure that the pH is increased to no higher than 7.5 because of increased resistance to defibrillation.[267]

Ventricular tachycardia also is most amenable to electrical shock. Lidocaine is the drug of choice for control of ventricular tachycardia. Alternatives include procainamide (and, for humans, bretylium). Magnesium sulfate (25 to 40 mg/kg intravenously over 5 minutes) may be useful in refractory cases or in cases of ventricular flutter; constant-rate infusion over 4 to 8 hours is indicated if the patient responds.

Electromechanical dissociation (EMD; pulseless electrical activity) generally is fatal when caused by myocardial diseases. Treatable causes in humans include hypovolemia (e.g., acute blood loss, which should be treated with volume replacers), pericardial tamponade, and tension pneumothorax.[267] Epinephrine or atropine (0.04 to 0.08 mg/kg intravenously) may be useful when EMD is associated with hypotension or pleural or pericardial disorders. Pulseless electrical activity is likewise accompanied by a poor prognosis, although naloxone, dexamethasone sodium phosphate, and calcium have been recommended. Calcium is most likely to be of benefit with hypocalcemia or extreme hyperkalemia.[267]

Bradyarrhythmias are most amenable to nondrug therapy. The slower the rate and the wider the ventricular complex on the electrocardiogram, the more ineffective will be the cardiac contractility.[267] Atropine is most useful with narrow complex bradyarrhythmias. However, atropine should be used cautiously such that potentially lethal tachycardia might be prevented in hypoxic patients. A low dose (0.022 mg/kg) is indicated unless vagolytic arrest is present. Dopamine and epinephrine may be helpful for inotropic support. Isoproterenol is controversial because of peripheral vasodilation.

Anesthetic or narcotic overdoses should be reversed if possible. Naloxone (0.02-0.04 mg/kg intravenously) is indicated for any narcotic. Yohimbine or atipamezole (0.1 to 0.2 mg/kg intravenously) is indicated in the presence of α-2 antagonists and may be effective for other chemical restraining agent, including ketamine or barbiturates.[267a,b] Flumazenil (0.02 mg/kg intravenously) is indicated for reversal of diazepine depressant effects.

Postresuscitation monitoring and care are critical to successful CPCR. Dobutamine is preferred to dopamine by many clinicians for postresuscitation inotropic support. SBP should be maintained above 90 mm Hg. Urine formation should be maintained at 1 to 2 mL/kg per hour. Furosemide may be indicated in the face of decreasing urine output. Neurologic function should be assessed along with the need for iron chelators, CCBs, or oxygen free radical scavengers. Vasopressin (0.04 to 0.8 units/kg intravenously or 0.001 units/kg/hr) may be indicated in patients whose vasculature remains nonresponsive to epinephrine.

HYPERLIPIDEMIA

The metabolic pathway of lipid formation and metabolism is complex,[274,275] offering several targets of pharmacologic control. Although coronary artery disease associated with atherosclerotic plaques is not a disease of dogs and cats, drug therapies for the disease play role in the treatment of hyperlipidemias in animals. As such, an in-depth discussion of lipid metabolism is warranted. Lipoproteins are macromolecules consisting of lipids (cholesterols, triglycerides, phospholipids) and proteins (apolipoproteins or apoproteins; e.g., apo-A [I-V], apo-B, apo-C [II and III], and apo-E). Together, cholesterol and triglycerides comprise the major lipid particles in the body, with each having important functions. Cholesterol provides stability to cell membranes, facilitates membrane transport, and serves as a basis for the synthesis of steroids and bile acids. Triglycerides serve as a source of energy storage, being lightweight compared to glycogen. Cardiac and skeletal muscle extract triglycerides from circulating proteins and, through lipolysis, convert them to fatty acids as an energy source (Kreb's cycle for ATP production and gluconeogenesis in selected tissues) and glycerol.

Both cholesterol and triglycerides are insoluble in water, and as such they circulate as lipoproteins, with apoproteins providing structural rigidity to lipoproteins. However, the proteins also serve as ligands or cofactors in lipoprotein metabolism. Spherical lipoproteins are structured such that the most water-soluble components (apoproteins, phospholipids, and unesterified cholesterol) face outward and surround the most lipid-soluble core components (cholesterol esters, triglycerides). In addition to transport, apoproteins facilitate recognition of enzymes that remove or process the lipids within the lipoprotein. Several classes of lipoproteins have been classified according to their density, lipid content, and surface protein. These include in order of density chylomicrons (least dense at ≤ 0.95g/mL), very low-density lipoprotein (VLDL) cholesterol, intermediate-density lipoprotein (IDL) cholesterol, low-density lipoprotein (LDL) cholesterol ("bad" cholesterol), and high-density lipoprotein (HDL) cholesterol ("good cholesterol") (most dense at 1.06g/mL). Generally, total cholesterol, triglycerides, and HDL are measured directly, with VLDL and LDL estimated though calculation.

Three pathways exist for formation of lipoproteins. The exogenous pathway of lipoprotein formation begins with digestion and absorption of dietary fat. Dietary cholesterol must be esterified, a process mediated by acyl coenzyme A cholesterol acyltransferase (ACAT-2,) located in both the intestinal epithelial cell and liver. In the epithelial cell, cholesterol and triglyceride are packaged into chylomicrons. Chylomicrons contain the largest proportion of triglycerides (fat) of any of the lipoproteins, with a triglyceride to cholesterol ratio of 10:1 (i.e., more than 90% triglycerides). Therefore, although chylomicrons are very large, their fat content renders them the least dense of the lipoproteins. The high fat content of chylomicrons also provides the buoyancy necessary for their accumulation at the top of undisturbed (>12 hours) plasma. Formation of chylomicrons depends on microsomal triglyceride transfer protein (MTP), which acts to transfer the triglyceride to an apolipoprotein. The apolipoproteins will form the outside surface of chylomicrons and are synthesized in intestinal epithelial cells or are acquired from HDLs once the chylomicron is secreted into lymph. Chylomicrons enter plasma at the thoracic duct. Once in circulation, fatty acids are released from the triglycerides in chylomicrons in tissue that produce lipoprotein lipase (LPL); insulin provides a permissive effect. Its absence in humans is associated with severe hypertriglyceridemia and pancreatitis. Tissues that contain LPL are exemplified by adipose tissue and skeletal and cardiac muscles. Fatty acids released from triglycerides are either immediately used as a source of energy by surrounding tissues or stored for future energy needs in adipocytes. The chylomicron remnants that remain once triglycerides have been removed contain dietary cholesterol and they are rapidly metabolized by the liver.

The *endogenous pathway* for generation of lipoproteins reflects hepatic synthesis of VLDLs and subsequent uptake of circulating VLDLs by tissues. Triglyceride synthesis is regulated in the liver and other tissues through coenzyme A (CoA) diacylglycerol acyltransferase enzymes that catalyze the final step. Triglycerides intended for lipoprotein synthesis are transferred (along with other lipids) to the endoplasmic reticulum, where they, along with cholesterol, will combine with newly synthesized apoB-100 to form VLDLs. Transfer cannot occur without MTP, and its absence (or the absence of triglycerides) prevents formation of VLDLs and subsequent lipoproteins. Like chylomicrons, VLDLs are very large, containing a large amount of core triglyceride (ratio of triglycerides: cholesterol of 5:1). Although VLDLs contribute to plasma turbidity, they do not float with chylomicrons on the surface of undisturbed plasma. The VLDLs are synthesized in the liver endoplasmic reticulum in response to increased free fatty acids.

The VLDLs are released into circulation, taken up by tissues that produce LPL, and processed by LPL to yield fatty acids, glycerol, and a VLDL remnant or IDLs. The free fatty acids are either used as an energy source or stored in the cell as fat (Box 14-1).

The IDLs either are removed by the liver in response to LPL or are metabolized by way of hepatic triglyceride lipase to form LDLs. The LDLs are composed primarily of cholesterol esters and contain essentially no triglycerides. Because they have a longer half-life than other lipoproteins, LDLs accumulate to a higher plasma concentration compared with either VLDLs or IDLs. Hence the LDLs carry the majority of cholesterol (the "bad" cholesterol) in the body. The LDLs also are removed from circulation primarily by the liver in proportion to LDL receptor expression, with a smaller amount taken up by LDL receptors in tissues. Tissue uptake results in the release of free cholesterol, which is subsequently esterified such that it accumulates in cells. Most clearance occurs in the liver. Increased expression of LDL receptor expression is a major means by which cells regulate free cholesterol content. A number of signals increase LDL receptor expression, thereby decreasing circulating LDL, including thyroxin and estrogen, decreased consumption of saturated fats and cholesterol, and pharmacologic anticholesterol drugs (statins).

Among LDLs, densities vary, with the smaller, denser, less buoyant particles potentially more amenable to oxidation.[274] Oxidized (radical) lipoproteins damage vascular endothelium and are scavenged by a receptor mediated process in macrophages (forming foam cells). It is the inflammatory and immunologic response to oxidized LDL and at the vascular endothelium of coronary vessels that contributes to atherosclerosis and its subsequent morbidity in humans. Although it is cholesterol that is considered "bad", it appears that it is the fatty acids, not cholesterol, that are oxidized to atherogenic metabolites. As such, triglycerides, not cholesterol, are the source of atherosclerotic mediators, and thus the lipoproteins containing the largest component of triglycerides should be considered the greatest risk. What is not clear is why transport of cholesterol by HDL would decrease this risk.

HDLs facilitate the transport of cholesterol from peripheral tissues (including atherogenic plaques) to the liver. As such, HDLs contain more cholesterol (as ester) than triglyceride in their core compared with other lipoproteins and are of higher density than the other lipoproteins. This mechanism of "reverse cholesterol transport," the third pathway of lipid metabolism, is complex and not well understood.[274]

Box 14-1
Fatty Acids

Fatty acids contain variable lengths of carbons that may or may not include double bonds. Nomenclature of fatty acids involves an ending with "oic" [or simply "ic"] acid [the acid referring to the carboxylic acid that each contains] with the number of carbons followed by the number of double bonds [e.g., arachidonic acid, C 20:0, contains 20 carbons and no double bonds, whereas arachidonic acid C20:4 contains 4 double bonds]. A saturated fat contains carbons with as many hydrogens as possible, meaning it contains no double bonds or functional groups. Such fats are straight and as such, can be packed very tightly, thus allowing storage of a lot of energy in a small space. Such fats also offer no opportunity for lipid peroxidation. Unsaturated fats contain variable numbers of functional groups or, more commonly, (alkene) carbon double bonds. The more double bonds, the greater the risk of oxygen radical formation (peroxidation). The fatty acid that extends on either side of each double bond can exist in one of two configurations: *cis*, for which both ends are on the same side of the double bond, or *trans*, for which each end is on a different side. Steric hindrance presented with fatty acid ends being on the same side of the bond as in *cis* fatty acids causes the molecule to bend or kink. However, the ends of a *trans* fat are on opposite sides, do not compete for space and thus remain largely straight, such as might occur with saturated fats. Most naturally occurring unsaturated fatty acids contain only three double bonds, each in the *cis* position. The few naturally occurring *trans* fatty acids are generally found in the meat and dairy products of ruminant animals (originating from the rumen). Saturated fats and *trans* unsaturated fats tend to be solid at room temperature and are less amenable to oxidation. The term *trans* is used when referring to fats because it is the common name used to refer to all unsaturated fats. This probably reflects the fact that most fats that are consumed are unsaturated plant fats that are artificially partially hydrogenated such that a *trans* configuration is produced. Because they are more saturated, they are less conducive to oxidation (degradation) into smaller fatty acids, ketones, and aldehydes, and because they are less likely to become rancid, their shelf-life is prolonged. Presumably, fats that contain unsaturated (oxidizable) double bonds should be less safe than the fats whose carbon bonds are "saturated" with hydrogen. However, because unsaturated fats might also be considered more fluid, thus allowing flexibility in cell membranes, polyunsaturated fats have also been considered safer, although absorption of unsaturated dietary fats that are oxidized during the cooking of food may increase their atherogenecity. Despite the fact that *trans*, partially hydrogenated (unsaturated) fats are less oxidizable, the amount of *trans* fats in the diet correlates with the advent of atherosclerosis. Although the mechanism is not well understood, it may simply reflect increased total unsaturated fat content. Coronary heart disease in humans correlates with the amount of both saturated and unsaturated fat; however, saturated fats appear to be less atherogenic than disproportionate carbohydrates in the diet [the latter perhaps contributing to increased formation of saturated fat formation in the body]; fish also decreases the risk of alherosclerosis. *Trans* fats in particular seem to reduce the amount of HDL, thus increasing the risk of coronary artery disease. Thus consumption of *trans* fats is recommended to be as low as possible.

Pathophysiology of Dislipidemias

Hyperlipidemia is defined as increased concentrations of triglycerides or cholesterol. In humans hyperlipidemia results from a combination of dietary, genetic, and metabolic factors.[275] In veterinary medicine, primary idiopathic hyperlipidemia appears to be familiar in Miniature Schnauzers and Beagles but has been reported in other breeds and occasionally in cats. Secondary hyperlipiemia is associated with other disorders, such as diabetes mellitus, hyperadrenocorticism, pancreatitis, and hypothyroidism.

Treatment of Hyperlipidemia

In humans the choices for treatment of hypertriglyceridemia vary with the category, three of which are defined according to concentration (mg/dL) of triglycerides (borderline high [150-199], high [200-499], or very high [≥500]), with a focus on the risk of coronary heart disease. Pharmacotherapy targets synthesis of cholesterol and includes the statins, niacin, bile acid sequestrants, and fibric acid derivatives.

Statins. *Statins* competitively inhibit (hepatic) HMG-CoA reductase and thus block the rate-limiting step in cholesterol synthesis. At higher doses the more potent drugs (e.g., atorvastatin, simvastatin) also reduce triglycerides associated with increased VLDL. In humans statins have proved effective in reducing morbidity and mortality associated with hyperlipidemia and coronary heart disease.[275] Six products are approved for use in the United States, with lovastatin, simvastatin, and pravastatin the most commonly prescribed. Each statin is structurally similar to HMG-CoA. LDL receptor expression increases, causing LDL-C concentrations to decrease. Humans taking the highest doses of the most potent statins realize up to a 45% reduction in triglycerides. A similar reduction can be achieved with niacin and fibric acid derivatives, but fibric acid may not decrease LDL-C. The statins have a number of nonlipid-lowering cardioprotective effects, although mechanisms are not known. These include inhibition of enhanced vascular endothelial nitric oxide production, inhibition of vascular smooth muscle proliferation, facilitation of apoptosis, and stabilization of vascular atherosclerotic plaques. Platelet aggregation is decreased. Oral bioavailability is variable among drugs (30% to 85%); simvastatin and lovastatin are administered as prodrugs.[275] All undergo extensive first-pass metabolism, resulting in systemic bioavailability of 5% to 30%. Atorvastatin, lovastatin, simvastatin, and others (but not pravastatin, fluvastatin, and rosuvastatin) are metabolized by CYP 3A4, increasing the risk of drug interactions. Entry into the liver for several statins is mediated by transport proteins, which may compete with other drugs. Most metabolites have some degree of activity. Those products that make it to systemic circulation are highly bound to proteins. Elimination half-lives are generally less than 4 hours (exceptions are 20-hour atorvastatin and rosuvastatin), and effect appears to be time dependent in that lovastatin is slightly more effective when given as 40 mg twice daily, as opposed to 80 mg once daily. Elimination of parent and metabolites is largely biliary. Two potentially serious side effects of statins have been reported: hepatotoxicity and myopathy. Statins cause increased liver enzymes in 3% of human patients. However, the incidence of serious hepatotoxicity is rare (1 case per million users annually). Hepatic enzymes should be measured at baseline and repeated at 3 to 6 months, then yearly thereafter if normal. Myopathy (rhabdomyolysis; approximately 0.01% and monitored by serum creatine kinase) appears to be dose dependent and is most commonly associated with gemfibrozil. Myopathy can be associated with myoglobinuria and, rarely, death. Niacin will increase the risk (discussed later), as will macrolide antimicrobials, cyclosporine, imidazole antifungals, and inhibitors of CYP3A4. Creatine kinase might be monitored in at-risk patients (e.g., drug interactions).[275] Combined use of statins with other drugs can reduce either LDLC-C or triglycerides greater than statin use alone; current treatment of dyslipidemias (such as that which characterizes prediabetes) increasingly is based on combination therapy. Combination with bile acid sequestrants can reduce LDL-C by another 20% to 30%; the addition of niacin will reduce concentrations even further (up to 70% in humans), although the risk of myopathy increases with high statin and niacin doses. Combination with fibrates is particularly effective when treating hypertriglyceridemia.[275]

Niacin. Niacin (nicotinic acid) is a water-soluble compound that in its amide form (nicotinamide) acts as a B vitamin complex. However, only niacin lowers lipids (although nicotinamide can act as a source of niacin) and only at doses higher than that associated with B vitamin activity.[275] Triglycerides may reduce up to 45%; LDL-Cholesterol (LDL-C) decreases up to 30%, and HDL-C increases up to 40% (humans). The mechanism reflects inhibition of hormone-sensitive lipase-induced lipolysis in adipose tissue. The transport and esterification of free fatty acids to the liver is inhibited, and hepatic triglyceride synthesis is decreased. Adipocyte adenylyl cyclase may be the ultimate enzyme inhibited. Niacin may also inhibit diacylglycerol acyltransferase 2, the rate-limiting enzyme of triglyceride synthesis. Niacin also enhances LPL activity, thus promoting the clearance of chylomicrons and VLDL triglycerides. The identification of a niacin receptor may ultimately lead to development of drugs that target the receptor.[275] In humans administration of regular or crystalline niacin (2 to 6 g divided into 2 to 3 daily doses) causes maximal effects within 4 to 7 days. The high dose is necessary to ensure sufficient niacin; at lower doses most is converted to nicotinamide. The half-life of niacin is only 30 to 60 minutes in humans, necessitating at least twice-daily dosing; an extended-release preparation allows once-daily dosing. Use in humans is limited by cutaneous flushing, skin rashes, and dyspepsia. Flushing, interestingly, resolves after 1 to 2 weeks of stable dosing but will return if several doses are missed and is minimized by starting at a low dose (e.g., 100 mg twice daily in humans) that is gradually increased (weekly) to a maximum total daily dose of 2 g. Co-administration of aspirin also will reduce flushing.[275] Dyspepsia is reduced if administered with a meal. Niacin is contraindicated in patients with gastrointestinal ulceration. Hepatotoxicity is a serious but rare adverse reaction to niacin. All sustained-release niacin (over-the-counter) preparations have been associated with hepatotoxicity (including fulminating hepatic necrosis), particularly at high doses; the risk may be less with Niaspin an FDA-approved extended release coated tablet. Toxicity may take several years to develop and has occurred in human patients who tolerated crystalline niacin. Niacin increases the risk of statin-induced myopathy; the statin dose should be reduced to approximately 25% when used in combination.[275] Niacin should either be avoided or used cautiously in diabetics (types I or II); any change in insulin need should be anticipated for insulin-dependent diabetics. The risk of niacin-induced hyperglycemia might be reduced (but probably not avoided) in the diabetic patient with use of sustained-release niacin.[275]

Bile acid (resin) sequestrants. Cholestyramine and colestipol are anion-exchange resins prepared as hygroscopic powders and administered as chloride salts.[275] The highly positively charged particles bind to the negatively charged bile acids, precluding their absorption. Hepatic synthesis consequently increases, resulting in lowered cholesterol. As with statins, LDL receptors increase and LDL-C decreases. However, because statins are more effective, generally resins are used as second-line treatment. Unfortunately, resin-induced increase in bile-acid production causes an increase in hepatic triglyceride synthesis, leading to potentially marked increases in serum triglyceride concentrations, and severe hypertriglyceridemia is a contraindication for use; an exception is colesevelam, which does not appear to significantly increase triglycerides. Resins are not orally absorbed. Rarely, hyperchloremic acidosis may occur. Cholestyramine and colestipol are administered as a slurry, which is associated with gastrointestinal upset (including dyspepsia and bloating); again, the exception is colesevelam, which is administered as a soft-gel capsule. Cholesteramine and colestipol will impair the absorption of many drugs. Resins generally are administered before or with a meal. Although colesevelam is less likely to affect absorption of other drugs, it nonetheless should be administered 1 hour after or 3 to 4 hours before any other orally administered drug. Additional flavoring may facilitate administration of cholesteryamine and colestipol.[275]

Fibric acid. The ester form of ethyl chlorophenoxyisobutyric (clofibrate) was the first to be approved in the United States, but its use was not associated with a reduction in mortality associated with coronary heart disease. Gemfibrozil is a nonhalogenated phenoxypentanoic acid and as such is not halogenated fibrates. Its use has been demonstrated to reduce mortality rates in men. The mechanism by which fibric acid derivatives decrease cholesterol is not certain, but they appear to interact with and stimulate peroxisome proliferator-activated receptors. Fatty acid oxidation is stimulated, LPL synthesis and apoA-I and II expression increase, and apoC-III (an inhibitor of lipolytic processing) expression is reduced. Most fibric acids also are antithrombotic, inhibiting coagulation and enhancing fibrinolysis. Those (human) patients most likely to respond are those with dysβlipoproteinemia (type III). In human patients with mild hypertriglyceridemia, gemfibrozil may cause triglyceride to decrease up to 50% without a change in LDL-C. In contrast, with second-generation drugs (fenofibrate, bezafibrate, ciprofibrate) LDL may decrease up to 20% and up to 30% in patients with marked hypertriglyceridemia (400-1000 mg/dL). Fibric acids have been the drugs of choice for treatment of severe triglyceridemia and chylomicronemia. Fibric acid compounds usually are well tolerated. Side effects are not uncommon, occurring in 5% to 10% of human patients; however, discontinuation of the drug is generally unnecessary. Side effects reflect the gastrointestinal tract, cutaneous lesions (rash, urticaria, alopecia), increased liver enzymes, and myalgias. Myopathies may occur in patients receiving clofibrate, gemfibrozil, or fenofibrate, including up to 5% of patients receiving a combination of statins with gemfibrozil. Minor increases in liver transaminases and alkaline phosphatase have been reported. Gemfibrozil will inhibit transport-mediated hepatic uptake of statins and compete with statins for glucuronidation (an exception being fenofibrate), potentially increasing concentrations of both drugs. Effects of oral anticoagulants are potentiated, and the risk of choleliths may increase. Both renal and hepatic diseases are contraindications to fibric acid administration.

Inhibition of dietary cholesterol absorption. Ezetimibe appears to inhibit a transport protein specific to cholesterol (and plant sterol) absorption. Whereas cholesterol absorption may be markedly decreased, triglyceride absorption will not be affected; serum cholesterol concentrations may decrease up to 50%, whereas triglyceride may decrease only up to 5%. Cholesterol synthesis generally increases; hence ezetimibe is often coupled with a statin. Increased LDL receptor expression is accompanied by decreased LDL-C. Because ezetimibe is insoluble in water, it has not been studied intravenously, and bioavailability is not known. However, after intestinal epithelial glucuronidation, it is absorbed to undergo enterohepatic recirculation, with 70% excreted in the feces and about 10% in the urine. Ezetimibe has been associated with rare allergic reactions.

Dirlotapide is a selective inhibitor of MTP. MTP is required for the assembly and secretion of apolipoprotein B (apoB)-containing lipoproteins, the primary structural protein of plasma VLDLs. Consequently, MTP inhibitors block the assembly and release of lipoproteins into the blood stream. In field trials, serum lipids were decreased in obese dogs treated with dirlotapide, but changes were not clinically significant. However, depending on the pathophysiology of hypertriglyceridemia, consideration might be given to the potential for dirlotapide, particularly in combination with other therapies (e.g., gemfibrozil), for treatment.

HEARTWORM DISEASE (DIROFILARIASIS)

Physiology and Pathophysiology

Both the adult worms and the microfilariae of *Dirofilaria immitis* are responsible for the clinical signs associated with heartworm disease. Heartworms live 5 to 7 years in dogs (2 to 3 years in cats) but are most susceptible to adulticide therapy while young. Maximal microfilaria production occurs after 8 to 18 months of adult worm development, and microfilariae live about 18 to 24 months. The adults are covered with a canine antigen that provides an immunologic sanctuary, protecting the worm against immunologic rejection. However, its subsequent absence contributes to a marked inflammatory host response on worm death. The severity of heartworm disease and the onset of clinical signs reflect, in part, the number of infecting worms. Large numbers of worms are more likely to cause greater pulmonary hypertension, thromboembolism, and risk of vena cava syndrome. Experimentally, the endothelium of the pulmonary artery responds to the presence of heartworms within 3 days. Endothelial damage leads to edema associated with vascular permeability. Trophic factors released by platelets and leukocytes stimulate the multiplication of smooth muscle cells, which subsequently migrate from the interna to media, where they continue to rapidly multiply. Cells continue to divide and produce collagen.

Arteries dilate, become tortuous, and develop aneurysms. Obstructed blood flow is rerouted to regions of normal lungs. Interstitial pulmonary edema worsens. Pulmonary disease further worsens as fragments of dead worms are carried distally into the smaller pulmonary arteries. Villous proliferation is coupled with thrombi formation and a granulomatous response to the dead heartworms. Pulmonary blood flow may be totally obstructed, and the caudal pulmonary lung lobes may become consolidated. Decreased endothelium-dependent relaxation can be correlated with pulmonary arterial blood pressure in dogs with heartworms, suggesting that this may be an important factor in the development of dirofilariasis-induced pulmonary hypertension.[276,277,277a] Increased pulmonary vascular resistance can cause acute right-sided heart failure.

The clinical signs associated with heartworm disease and its treatment again depend on the number of worms present but also on the duration of infection and the host response, which can be quite variable. Coughing and dyspnea, the most common clinical signs, reflect disease of the caudal lung lobe arteries. Pulmonary edema and inflammatory response to dead heartworms are the most likely inciting causes. Dyspnea also might reflect ventilation perfusion mismatching as blood flow is diverted to patent arteries. Exercise intolerance is most likely to be associated with right ventricular hypertrophy and dilation resulting from severe arterial disease and impaired pulmonary blood flow. Mild to moderate hypoxemia worsens pulmonary hypertension. Right-sided CHF increases the magnitude of exercise intolerance and may lead to overt signs of right-sided heart failure such as ascites and an enlarged liver. Thromboembolism worsened by the inflammatory response to dead heartworms often is accompanied by hemoptysis; this was particularly true after treatment with thiacetarsamide. Blood loss resulting from vascular and airway rupture is most likely to occur after coughing in areas of severe vascular and parenchymal disease.

Occult Heartworm Disease

The incidence of occult disease can vary (from 5% to 67% of infected dogs) depending on geographic region. Occult infections may be caused by infection of one sex only

(57% to 85% of occult infections), prepatent infections (particularly in colder months), drug-induced adult worm sterility, or immune-mediated elimination of microfilariae. Immune-mediated destruction of microfilariae occurs in the presence of excessive IgG production directed toward the microfilariae. A granulomatous reaction may follow phagocytosis of antibody–microfilaria–leukocyte complexes. Up to 15% of dogs with occult heartworm disease can be expected to develop immune-mediated pneumonitis characterized by coughing and dyspnea. Radiographically, the reaction causes diffuse interstitial and alveolar infiltrates. Tracheal lavage may reveal an eosinophilic exudate, and clinical laboratory tests reveal eosinophilia, basophilia, and hypergammaglobulinemia. Other potential sequelae of immune-mediated destruction of microfilariae include CHF, vena cava syndrome, and severely enlarged pulmonary arteries.

Therapy

Current recommendations for treatment and prevention of heartworm disease as recommended by the American Heartworm Society can be reviewed at http://www.heartwormsociety.org.[277a]

Pretreatment Assessment

Pretreatment evaluation should focus on assessment of the risk of complications after adulticide therapy. In general, the risk of treatment was greater for thiacetarsemide compared to melarsomine, the currently approved canine adulticide. Diagnostic measures weigh the likelihood of success against the risk of side effects or complications. The extent and type of supportive therapy should be determined on the basis of the severity of infection before treatment. The development of thromboembolism is the complication most amenable to pretreatment assessment.

Up to 70% of dogs with severe heartworm disease may have an occult infection; as the number of adult heartworms increases, the number of microfilariae produced by each female decreases.[277] The presence of occult disease also may indicate a greater likelihood of immune-mediated microfilarial disease. Infection indicated by positive tests should be confirmed before adulticide therapy is implemented. Antigen tests that quantitate antigen indirectly provide information regarding the adult heartworm load and can be of benefit in the assessment of the severity of infection. Radiographs are an important baseline test for assessing the severity of disease, with a focus on the caudal pulmonary lung field. Right ventricular enlargement should be assessed carefully by radiographic means. Cardiac ultrasonography is the preferred method of assessing right ventricular function and the extent and impact of pulmonary hypertension. Ultrasonography also might be helpful in identifying those animals with a high worm burden.

Ideally, a minimum database consisting of a complete blood count, routine serum chemistries, and urinalysis should be collected as part of the pretreatment evaluation. Findings of hypoalbuminemia, increased liver enzyme activity, azotemia, and proteinuria should lead to more intensive assessment of renal and hepatic function. Although renal dysfunction should be interpreted as a cause for concern, evidence of hepatic dysfunction should be expected in some animals, particularly those with evidence of right-sided CHF, and is not necessarily indicative of a decision not to treat. Up to a tenfold increase in liver enzyme activity can be tolerated before treatment. Leukocytosis is indicative of an inflammatory response in the lung parenchyma. Evidence of thrombocytopenia should lead to more aggressive evaluation of thromboembolic disease, including the presence of low-grade disseminated intravascular coagulopathy. Overt signs of bleeding and abnormal coagulation parameters may be absent in patients with low-grade disseminated intravascular coagulopathy; however, thrombocytopenia should persist.

Severe Pulmonary Arterial Disease and Pretreatment Therapy

Severe pulmonary arterial disease is indicated by the tortuosity and enlargement of the pulmonary lobar arteries, which in normal animals should not exceed in diameter the width of the ninth rib. Approximately 10% of infected dogs can be expected to have severe disease. Evidence of pulmonary thromboembolism before treatment should lead to a pretreatment course of glucocorticoids (1 to 2 mg/kg per day) until clinical and radiographic indicators of thromboembolism begin to resolve (generally 3 to 7 days). Glucocorticoids should not, however, be used routinely because of their ability to increase survival of adult heartworms. Because of the role that platelets have in causing the thromboembolic (including inflammatory) response, drugs such as aspirin, which impair platelet activity, may be beneficial. However, care should be taken to avoid COX-2 preferential drugs that may increase the risk of thromboembolism.

Anticoagulants such as heparin can increase pulmonary blood flow and reduce the severity and incidence of thromboembolic disease, including associated signs such as coughing and hemoptysis. Antithrombotic therapy generally consists of aspirin (4 to 6 mg/kg per day) for 2 to 3 weeks before treatment. Aspirin therapy is continued during and 3 to 4 weeks after adulticide therapy. Attention should be paid to the development of gastrointestinal side effects with protracted aspirin use, although they are less likely to occur with the low dose used for thromboembolic disease. Aspirin should not be used in the presence of hemoptysis. Evidence of gastrointestinal side effects should lead to therapy with sucralfate and H_2-receptor blockers; misoprostol might be avoided because of the unknown impact of this prostaglandin on pulmonary blood flow in the face of pulmonary arterial disease. Low-dose heparin (50 to 70 U/kg subcutaneously every 8 hours) may further increase survivability after therapy[278] and is particularly crucial if there is evidence of disseminated intravascular coagulopathy (decreasing platelet count). For such patients heparin therapy should be continued for at least 7 days, and until the platelet count exceeds 150,000/μL, therapy can be continued for several weeks if needed.

If the severity of pulmonary arterial disease reflects a large burden of adult worms, the likelihood of fatal complications after adulticide therapy can be decreased by reducing the adult heartworm burden surgically (by way of the jugular vein), partial adulticide therapy (with melarsomine dihydrochloride), or cage confinement and antithrombotic therapy. Partial adulticide therapy (see package insert) involves injecting only the first of the two adulticide injections of drug, followed by a 30-day hiatus in patient activity. At the end of 1 month, the full treatment protocol is implemented. Because up to 50% of animals with severe pulmonary arterial disease can be expected to have signs associated with right-sided CHF, therapy with diuretics and a low-sodium diet may be indicated.

KEY POINT 14-64 To prevent fatal complications in patients with dirofilariasis, large worm burdens should be decreased before full adulticide therapy.

KEY POINT 14-65 The duration of retroprotection of macrolides varies with the drug but generally ranges from 3 to 4 months.

Pneumonitis

Glucocorticoids (prednisone 1 to 2 mg/kg per day or dexamethasone 0.2 to 0.4 mg/kg per day) are indicated to control the inflammatory response of pneumonitis. A parenteral route can be used for severely affected animals. Clinical improvement should occur within the first 24 hours, with radiographic resolution of pulmonary infiltrates associated with the pneumonitis in 3 to 5 days. Glucocorticoids should be discontinued when radiographic lesions are maximally resolved. Adulticide therapy should begin as soon as possible.

Prophylactic Therapy

Prophylaxis may be seasonal or throughout the year, depending on geographic location. Prophylaxis between May and October may be sufficient in the northern half of the country. Prophylaxis may contribute to collateral protection of unprotected dogs by decreasing the reservoir population, particularly in areas where mosquito and dog populations are low. Therapy should begin at 6 to 8 weeks of age if the season is appropriate. Once-daily administration of diethylcarbamazine (DEC) has been replaced with a macrolide antibiotic. Diethylcarbamazine (2.5 to 3 mg/kg orally once daily) affected L3 to L5 molting stage; however, efficacy may be lost with as little as three missed doses. DEC was safe when given to heartworm-negative dogs. But when administered to a dog infected with as few as 50 microfilariae/mL blood, DEC causes a severe anaphylactic-like reaction in up to 85% of animals. The reaction is characterized by depression, lethargy, vomiting, diarrhea, bradycardia, and shock, followed by death. Hepatomegaly and thrombocytopenia occur. Treatment is supportive (e.g., fluids, shock doses of glucocorticoids).

The macrolide antimicrobials are effective for the prevention of heartworm disease when given monthly, a distinct advantage to DEC therapy, particularly for owners whose compliance with daily therapy is poor. Macrolides are effective against microfiariae, third- and fourth-stage larvae, and potentially adult worms, with younger worms most susceptible to their effects. Efficacy is greatest for 1 month, but an additional month generally can be expected. Moxidectin is unique in its longer half-life of 20 days, its chemical side chains (compared with other avermectins), and its availability in slow-release microspheres. Oral choices of macrolide antibiotics include ivermectin (2-day half-life) (Heartgard; Merck; 6 to 12 μg/kg by mouth monthly at 6 weeks or older; 24 μg/kg by mouth monthly in cats), milbemycin oxime (Interceptor; Novartis; 0.5 to 1 mg/kg or 500 to 1000 μg/kg monthly by mouth) in dogs at 8 weeks or older; and moxidectin (ProHeart, Fort Dodge; 3 to 6 μg/kg by mouth monthly). Topical options include selamectin (Revolution, Pfizer; 6 to 12 mg/kg, topical in dogs 6 weeks or older), and moxidectin topical (with imidacloprid; Advantage Multi for dogs).[279] Moxidectin also is available as an injectable slow-release product (ProHeart, Fort Dodge, 170 μg/kg as microspheres subcutaneously every 6 months in dogs 6 months or older) in several countries.[280] It was voluntarily withdrawn in the United States (but not other countries) in 2004 for potential and controversial safety issues but was reintroduced in 2008. An advantage of this product is retroprotection of 4 months and full protection that extends beyond its 6-month labeled claim. Ivermectin is highly effective in preventing heartworm infections in dogs when given monthly (5.98 μg/kg). It does not control other helminthes but is available in a combination product with pyrantel, which controls hookworms and roundworms. Milbemycin controls roundworms, hookworms, and whipworms. Selamectin is effective against hookworms and roundworms, as well as fleas (adults), ear and sarcoptic mange mites, and selected ticks.

The duration of retroactive protection varies with the macrolide. Ivermectin, but not milbemycin, appears to retroactively protect against infection if given as long as 4 months after infection. Both drugs are effective at 3 months after infection. Retroactive efficacy (and partial adulticide effects of ivermectin) may warrant prophylactic therapy during the off season, particularly in light of a recent survey finding that 80% of respondents failed to give their dogs monthly heartworm preventive on the due date. Unlike DEC, the avermectins do not appear to cause adversity when given as preventives to heartworm-positive dogs. In a review, McCall[281] summarizes the "safety-net" (reachback) and adulticide effects of macrocyclic lactones. Up to 95% efficacy against adults may be realized, but treatment requires 9 to 30 months, with continuous monthly therapy resulting in better efficacy. Increased dose and shorter intervals do not appear to affect efficacy. The effect is greater on younger worms than on older worms, supporting better efficacy with earlier as opposed to later treatment. Among the drugs, efficacy in killing mature worms is ranked ivermectin > selamectin and moxidectin injectable > milbemycin.

The microfilaricidal effect of macrolides at prophylactic doses has several implications. First, adulticide therapy need not be followed by microfilaricide therapy; prophylactic therapy will lead to resolution of microfilaria. Second, microfilaria testing should precede initiation of prophylaxis therapy to prevent mistaking pretreatment infection for therapeutic failure and to minimize the risk of the sequelae of rapid microfilaria kill. Third, administration of a macrolide antibiotic

Table 14-5 Safe and Toxic Doses of Macrocyclic Lactones in ABCB1 Deficient Dogs[282]

	Labeled (Safe) Doses		Toxic Doses	
	μg/kg/month		μg/kg	
Drug	Oral	Topical	ABCB1 (-)	Wild type
Ivermectin	6		>120 PO	>2500 PO
Milbemycin	50 to 1000		12,500 PO	200,000 PO
Moxidectin	3	2500	90 PO (oral form) 1000 PO (topical form)*	>900 PO
Selemectin		6000	60,000 topical 15,000 PO	

PO, By mouth.
*As might occur with accidental ingestion.

(except moxidectin) at prophylactic doses is the most frequent cause of iatrogenic occult infections resulting from either microfilaricidal effects or sterilization of the female adult worm. Most adult infections become occult within 6 (2 to 9) months after beginning therapy. It is important that antigen testing rather than concentration tests be used as screening procedures in animals to be treated prophylactically.

The American Heartworm Society suggests that efficacy of prophylactic products should be tested at 3 months (4 for injectable 6-month product), after the start of the new product, or at the restart of lapsed prophylaxis. A negative status should be confirmed by testing before the change (i.e., change in drugs or re-initiation of lapsed prophylaxis). A positive test before the change or at 3 months indicates failure of the original drug or infection during the lapse in therapy. A negative test at 3 months should be followed by retesting at 8 to 9 months; a positive result at that time indicates that infection may have occurred before or during transition to the new drug, or failure of the new drug. A positive test after 9 months indicates failure of the new product or noncompliance.

Adverse reactions associated with macrocyclic lactones were addressed in Chapter 4. Adversities generally involve the central nervous system. Mealey[282] reviewed the impact of the *MDR1* (currently *ABCB1)* gene product P-glycoprotein on the safe use of macrocyclic lactones in dogs. Mealey[282] underscores the fact that all macrocyclic lactones are safe in all dogs, regardless of the presence of the deletion, when used at the approved preventive dose (Table 14-5). Adversities occur when used off label (e.g., treatment of mange at daily doses of 300 to 600 μg/kg). Accidental overdose is more likely with large animal preparations because of unintentional exposure[283] or intentional exposure with a miscalculated compounded product.[282] Internet-based recipes offered by lay users will contribute to increased risk of toxicity with off-label use of large animal products.[282] Known safe and toxic doses (in μg/kg) in gene-deficient dogs are provided in Table 14-5. Because the proposed mechanism of central nervous system adversities (disorientation to seizures) reflects enhanced chloride ion flow through gaba-channels, anticonvulsant drugs that do not target the GABA receptor (e.g., levetiracetam, zonisamide to a lesser degree) might be preferred over those that do (e.g., benzodiazepines, phenobarbital).

KEY POINT 14-66 P-glycoprotein deficiency leading to macrocyclic lactone toxicity in Collies and working breeds of dogs can be detected on the basis of a molecular test.

In 2004 Proheart (injectable moxidectin) was voluntarily withdrawn from the U.S. market; no other country withdrew the product. In support of its reintroduction in 2008, Fort Dodge provided to the Center for Veterinary Medicine a review of adverse events associated with its injectable product and two other unnamed oral monthly products. The data, which were collected from medical records of animals receiving the drugs or vaccines (alone or in combination), have been published.[284] In addition to the adverse events, the report offers a reasonable perspective on the difficulties associated with assessing adverse events as they currently are reported in veterinary medicine. Among the adverse events examined was association of treatment with cancers. Differences were limited to the incidence per 10,000 days at risk for mast cell tumors (0.024 for animals treated with one of the heartworm preparations, 0.043 for animals receiving vaccinations only, and 0.072 for Proheart 6 only), with no relationship demonstrated regarding the number of doses received (from 1 to 5). Allergic rates and all other safety profiles were similar among the three preventives studied. Interestingly, all heartworm preventives studied were associated with an increased incidence of allergic reactions. The apparent lack of substantial differences in adverse events for Proheart 6 compared with monthly preventives should be weighed against the risk of the sequelae of therapeutic failure as a result of poor compliance.

Adulticide Therapy

Melarsomine

Melarsomine is a trivalent arsenical that offers several advantages to the older arsenical, thiacetarsamide.[285] Because it is unstable in an aqueous solution, it is manufactured as a lyophilized powder that must be reconstituted immediately before use. Although its mechanism of action is not clear, it is equal to or better in efficacy for treatment of dirofilariasis based on controlled clinical trial in dogs with class 2 (moderate) heartworm disease. Melarsomine also is characterized by a wider therapeutic index than thiacetarsamide, although the margin is still considered low. Death associated with pulmonary inflammation can occur with as little as three times the recommended dose. However, melarsomine may be less likely than thiacetarsamide to cause pulmonary arterial vasoconstriction.[286] Melarsomine is administered deeply through an intramuscular route (2.5 mg/kg twice at 24-hour intervals) in dogs with mild to moderate disease. One half of worms, primarily males, die after the first injection; the remaining die with second treatments. According to the package insert, a 10% death rate is expected in dogs with class III disease when two doses are given initially. As such, in dogs with severe heartworm disease (see package insert for characteristics), an alternative dosing regimen consisting of one 2.5 mg/kg injection, followed 1 month later by the full regimen, is recommended. However, the alternative regimen increasingly is being implemented as the rule rather than the exception, regardless of the state of disease. The American Heartworm Society cites the alternative regimen as being not only safer but also more effective, resulting in fewer treatment failures. Reaction to the intramuscular injection can be expected in at least 30% of animals being treated and is minimized by making sure that the injection is deep. Care should be taken to ensure that the needle is appropriate for the depth of muscle, that injection is complete before needle withdrawal, and that sites of injection are alternated. Local reaction should be limited to edema and slight pain. Other side effects to mesarlomine reflect reaction to the dead heartworms or the drug (hepatotoxicity).

Clinically ill patients should be stabilized before treatment. Instead of melarsomine, macrocyclic lactones delivered at prophylactic doses may be administered with the intent to kill adult worms. The American Heartworm Society recommends treatment with a macrocyclic lactone for 6 months if immediate therapeutic intervention is not necessary. Treatment also will decrease circulating microfilariae and kill migrating larvae. Reduction in antigenic mass may reduce the risk of thromboembolism. In worms less than 4 months in development, ivermectin will also stunt immature worms and reduce female worms. Finally, administration for at least 3 months (or injection of slow-release moxidectin) will allow development of immature worms to a stage susceptible to melarsomine killing.

Efficacy varies with the drug and duration. Efficacy generally requires at least 1 year of therapy, with older worms requiring up to 2 years of therapy. When administered as prophylactic doses, ivermectin and selamectin reduce adult numbers by 56% after 16 months of therapy; abnormalities in surviving worms may decrease their life span. Precardiac larvae and young (less than 7 months) worms are most susceptible to ivermectin, with susceptibility inversely correlated with worm age. Treatment of older worms may require melarsomine to prevent continued development of disease as worms slowly die. Moxidectin (parenteral) and milbemycin are associated with rapid microfilaria killing and therefore should be used cautiously. Further, milbemycin does not appear to reduce worm counts, although it may sterilize female worms. The slow death of adults associated with macrocycline lactones may decrease the risk of thromboembolic disease; however, animals should be monitored at least every 4 to 6 months until worms are dead.

Complete killing of adult worms may not be necessary for clinical improvement. Further, clinical signs may not improve if residual worms are killed (i.e., through retreatment). Because surviving worms may not produce microfilariae, antigen testing is the most accurate method of evaluating successful therapy. Worms continue to die for up to 1 month after therapy; therefore antigen testing generally should occur at 5 to 6 months after therapy. Worms that survive adulticide therapy tend to be antigen-producing females; accordingly, the absence of antigen at 6 months indicates successful therapy. The presence of antigens at a later date (after a negative test) is indicative of reinfection rather than therapeutic failure.

Alternative Adulticides

The impact of preventives on maturing or adult heartworms was addressed under prophylaxis. Alternative adulticides do not appear to be effective. Levamisole efficacy is variable and unpredictable and generates iatrogenic occult infections. Side effects, including emesis, nervousness, ataxia, hallucinations, and seizures, are not unusual. Interestingly, tetracycline antimicrobials decrease microfilaria production and some adulticide effects in *Onchocerca* spp. owing to death of a symbiotic gut microbe (*Wolbachia* spp. of the order Rickettsiales). A surface protein on the organisms may contribute to pulmonary and renal inflammation. Tetracyclines also may cause infertility in female worms. McCall[287] reported that the combination of doxycycline (10 μg/kg) with ivermectin (6 μg/kg) for several months will eliminate heartworms. The study involved six groups of five dogs experimentally infected with adult heartworms. Groups received either placebo, ivermectin (6 μg/kg for 36 weeks), doxycycline (10 μg/kg/day for 18/36 weeks), or both drugs with or without melarsomine. All dogs treated with the combination were amicrofilaremic after week 9, and antigen test scores gradually decreased in these animals. In dogs treated with either ivermectin or doxycycline, counts decreased but some microfilariae were still present at 36 weeks. With regard to the adult worms, the percentage of reduction was 20% for ivermectin, 9% for doxycycline, and 78% for the combination. In dogs also treated with melarsomine, the percentage of reduction was 100% for melarsomine alone compared with 93% for melarsomine, ivermectin, and doxycycline. On the basis of these findings, further clinical studies are warranted to assess the use of tetracyclines (specifically doxycycline) in the treatment of heartworms.

The risk of pulmonary embolism is greater with a larger worm load and rapid kill and in dogs with moderate to severe radiographic changes. Small dogs (<15 kg) may be at greater risk. Clinical signs of embolism (fever, cough, hempotysis, right-sided heart failure) generally occur within 7 to 10 days but may occur at any time up to 4 to 6 weeks after treatment; exercise often is not restricted in afflicted animals. The most critical therapy for preventing thromboembolism is exercise restrictions for at least 1 month after therapy. Glucocorticoids have been recommended (0.5 mg/kg alternate days) for clinically affected animals; impact on efficacy of melarsomine has not been determined. Routine use of aspirin for prevention of pulmonary thromboembolism is not recommended and, according to the American Heartworm Society, may be contraindicated. Other potential reactions to dead or dying worms include exsanguination because of disseminated intravascular coagulopathy. Treatment of pulmonary thromboembolism is controversial and includes careful fluid therapy; use of heparin (75 IU/kg subcutaneously thrice daily until platelet count has normalized [5-7 days]) and aspirin (5 to 7 mg/kg/day) has been advocated by some but remains controversial. Cough suppressants should be used as indicated; antimicrobial use should be implemented only in the face of nonresponsive fever. The role of vasodilator therapy in management of pulmonary thromboembolism is controversial. Hydralazine has shown some efficacy in improved cardiac output in dogs with heart failure associated with heartworm disease. Alternative therapies recommended by Atkins and coworkers[53] include amlodipine or diltiazem.

Right-sided heart failure may accompany pulmonary thromboembolism or postcaval syndrome. Treatment may include diuretics (furosemide, spironolactone), ACE inhibitors (targeting fluid retention and myocardial remodeling), and aspirin (targeting thromboembolic disease). Digoxin has not proved effective and is not generally recommended unless treatment focuses on supraventricular arrhythmias or refractory heart failure.

Microfilaricide Therapy

Because of the microfilaricide effect of macrocyclic lactones, the need for microfilaricide therapy is increasingly considered unnecessary as a follow-up to adulticide therapy. Regardless of the drug used, microfilariae generally resolve after several months of prophylactic therapy in the treated or untreated heartworm-infested dog. No drug is approved for use as a microfilaricide in the United States. However, if rapid removal of microfilariae is warranted, the macrocyclic lactones can be used, although duration of efficacy varies. A single dose may be insufficient to clear microfilariae; subsequent doses can be administered as needed. Ivermectin (unapproved as a microfilaricide) is 90% effective after a single dose (0.05 mg/kg or 50 μg/kg orally; approximately 8 times the preventive dose) 4 weeks after adulticide therapy is complete. Large animal preparations have been diluted 1 to 9 mL with propylene glycol (Ivomec) or water (Eqvalan) and administered at a rate of 1 mL/20 kg; however, this may increase the risk of adverse reactions. Administration in the morning is recommended to allow observation for the day. Care should be taken to avoid overdosing, particularly in Collie or related breeds that might be predisposed to toxicity (discussed later). Because milbemycin is the most potent and potentially more consistently effective microfilaricide, it can be used for rapid kill (0.5 mg/kg). Alternatively, prophylactic doses of any macrolide could be reduced to a 2-week interval. Animals should be hospitalized for the first 8 hours after therapy, particularly if rapid-kill doses are administered. Rapid kill of large numbers of microfilariae 4 to 8 hours after the first dose rarely is accompanied by acute circulatory collapse. Predisposed animals include dogs weighing less than 16 kg or harboring more than 10,000 microfilariae per mL of blood, although reactions have occurred in animals with as few as 5000 microfilariae per mL of blood. Pretreatment with antihistamines and glucocortocoids should be considered in predisposed animals. Therapy includes fluid support and shock doses of short-acting glucocorticoids. Pretreatment with prednisolone may decrease adverse effects in dogs with a high microfilarial load. Clinical signs are not likely with subsequent microfilaricide treatment. Predisposed animals might also be treated with prophylactic doses of ivermectin. Moxidectin and selamectin also are microfilaricidal, although an appropriate dose has not been recommended.

Avermectin Toxicities

Adverse reactions to ivermectin and milbemycin microfilaricide therapy are more likely in Collies and Collielike dogs, including Border Collies and Old English Sheepdogs, than in the general population. Toxicity reflects a gene mutation in the p-glycoprotein efflux pump (homozygous or affected present in 35% of studied collies). Toxicity is characterized by acute ataxia, mydriasis, weakness, and seizures. Coma and death may follow. Toxicity predictably occurs at 10 times the recommended dose (50 μg/kg) for ivermectin and 5 times for milbemycin. Moxidectin and selamectin appear to be safe in collies at 10 times and 5 times, respectively, the prophylactic dose. Less common (<5%) toxicities occur in other dogs and are limited to lethargy and vomiting, which generally occur within 2 hours after drug administration. Occasionally, tachycardia, tachypnea, weakness, and pale mucous membranes accompany therapy. Treatment of toxicity includes fluid administration, glucocorticoids, and other supportive therapy. Animals with a very high microfilarial load may be more likely to have an adverse reaction to microfilaricide doses; adversity might be reduced in such animals by reduction of the dose of ivermectin by one third.

A concentration microfilarial test should be performed 3 to 4 weeks after microfilaricide treatment with ivermectin. Persistence of microfilariae after adulticide treatment (within the past year) may reflect failure of microfilaricide therapy (approximately 10% of animals) or a surviving gravid female. Microfilaricide therapy should be repeated, and, should microfilaria still persist, an adult antigen test should be repeated 60 to 90 days after adulticide. If the test is positive, the adult worms most likely are young females, and repeated adulticide therapy may not be effective. Therapy should be withheld for 1 year, but microfilaricide therapy should begin. When given at doses that are microfilaricidal, ivermectin also will prevent infection. Ivermectin can be used as a preventive in older or severely affected animals that are heartworm positive but for which adulticide therapy is not immediately or ever anticipated. Ivermectin not only will prevent further infection in these animals but also will reduce the microfilarial load, thus decreasing the risk of future adulticide complications. When a microfilaricide is administered, any animal will be protected against reinfection that may have occurred during the 1 to 2 months that elapsed between adulticide and microfilaricide therapy. Because the prophylactic doses of ivermectin can reduce microfilariae, causing an occult disease (generally within 6 months of prophylactic therapy), antigen testing rather than microfilarial concentration is the recommended method of screening for heartworm disease in animals on a monthly preventive program.

A number of other drugs are microfilaricidal, including fenthion, diethylcarbamazine, levamisole (11 mg/kg orally once daily for 7 to 10 days), and dithiazanine iodide (4.4 to 8.8 mg/kg orally once daily for 7 to 10 days); the latter drug is approved by the Food and Drug Administration for this use in dogs. The safety and efficacy of these products are not, however, predictable.[288] Treatment usually requires multiple days of therapy.

Feline Heartworm Disease

Differences exist in the pathyophysiology of heartworm infection as it occurs in the cat compared with the dog. Cats are more resistant to infection; accordingly, the rate of infection is lower[277] both in incidence and worm count (generally less than 6 and often only 2 or 3); further, the life expectancy of adult worms is shorter (2 to 3 years). Diagnostic limitations caused by low antigen load may underestimate the true prevalence of infection in cats. Despite the low worm load, the pathophysiology of the disease is similar in cats but more exaggerated, and sudden death is more frequent. Proliferation and inflammation are marked in the cat, and trophic factors from leukocytes may largely be responsible for the differences in the magnitude of response.[277] However, worm-mediated immune suppression may preclude emergence of clinical signs. The magnitude of thromboembolism apparently does not correlate with the number of infecting worms. Pulmonary infiltrates with eosinophils may develop. Paroxysmal coughing and dyspnea are the most common presenting signs, yet vomiting may be the only sign in some cats. Acute pulmonary thromboembolism is not unusual. Other clinical signs that may require pharmacologic management include tachycardia or bradycardia and neurologic disturbances (e.g., ataxia, blindness, seizures). Right-sided heart failure may occur with chronic disease, as might pleural effusions. Diagnosis of heartworm disease in the cat is more difficult than in the dog. Microfilariae usually are absent, and antigen testing tends to be less sensitive than in the dog because of the low worm burden. Even very sensitive tests, capable of detecting one female worm, may fail as a result of the frequency of unisex (male) infections in cats. Although antibody tests can detect either sex of larva or adult, they cannot discriminate active from past infection. Further, tests vary with the age of larvae. Nonselective angiography and echocardiography can be helpful in diagnosing feline heartworm diseases, although serologic testing based on adult antigens should be used to confirm the diagnosis.

Several preventives are currently approved in the United States for use in cats, including ivermectin (Heartgard for Cats: 55 µg/cat up to 2.3 kg or 5 lb; 165 µg/cat up to 7 kg or 15 lb, oral;), selamectin (Revolution for cats; 15 mg/cat if 2.3 kg or less, 45 mg for cats > 2.3 kg, topical) and moxidectin topical (with imidacloprid; Advantage Multiplex for Cats, 2.3, 4, and 8 mg topical for <2.3 kg (5 lb), 2.3 to 4.1 kg and > 4.1 kg (9 lb) cats, respectively).[289,290] The need for adulticide therapy in cats is controversial. Infection may be self-limiting in asymptomatic cats or in cats with mild pulmonary infiltrates with eosinophils. Cats may respond to low doses of glucocorticoids. Adulticide should be reserved for cats that maintain clinical signs despite glucocorticoid therapy. Cats with low worm burden are more amenable to treatment. The worm burden might be surgically reduced in cats with a larger worm number. Thiacetarsemide has been studied in uninfected cats (n=14), and all but one cat reacted adversely; 66% developed lethargy, depression, and anorexia, and at least one third vomited.[291] Three of 14 cats undergoing the treatment protocol developed clinical signs consistent with fulminating pulmonary edema typical of anaphylaxis or an anaphylactoid reaction. All three of the cats died. Nine other cats developed acute respiratory signs. A follow-up study[292] with 23 cats (17 with heartworms) found no adversity to thiacetarsamide therapy. Yet Rawlings and Calvert[277] report findings similar to those of Turner et al.[291] when treating cats with spontaneous infections. Melarsomine appears to be more toxic to cats than dogs; the American Heartworm Society notes that doses as low as 3.5 mg/kg may be toxic. Of the macrolide antimicrobials, ivermectin (24 µg/kg every 30 days for 2 years) has been demonstrated to reduce worm burden by 65% compared to untreated cats.

Cats also are at risk of developing acute pulmonary thromboembolism within the first 3 weeks of adulticide therapy. Glucocorticoids and heparin (50 to 70 U/kg subcutaneously every 8 hours) with or without aspirin therapy should be administered in the face of thromboembolism. Platelet counts should be monitored and antithrombotic therapy implemented if counts decrease below 100,000/mL. The presence of allergic pneumonitis may delay adulticide therapy. Treatment with prednisolone (1 to 2 mg/kg per day) for several days should resolve clinical signs, but clinical signs may return during adulticide therapy.

Microfilaricide therapy is largely unnecessary for cats because of the low incidence of microfilariae-positive disease. If microfilariae are present, ivermectin is an effective microfilaricide. Prophylaxis can be implemented with ivermectin (24 µg/kg), milbemycin oxime (2 mg/kg), or selamectin (6 to 12 mg/kg).

Geographic differences in infection incidence is marked, with differences reflecting weather, economic foundation, and so forth. Clinicians should be aware that disease can occur at 3 months. Heartworms secrete substances that prevent vascular responses, and stimulate (possibly protective) inflammation. Note that the disease includes several processes. These include fibrosis, scarring, and similar lesions at the microcapillary level; alveolar capillary fibrosis; lesions up to the fourth or fifth obstruction of cross-sectional area of right or left caudal lobar arteries, and reduced blood flow. Occult disease with adult worms producing microfilariae worsens the disease (eosinophilic infiltrates or pneumonitis).

REFERENCES

1. Shah M, Akar FG, Tomaselli GF: Molecular basis of arrhythmias, *Circulation* 112(16):2517–2529, 2005.
2. Michel T: Treatment of myocardial ischemia. In Brunton LL, Lazo JS, Parker KL, editors: *Goodman & Gilman's the pharmacological basis of therapeutics*, ed 11, New York, 2006, McGraw-Hill, pp 823-844.
3. Miller MW, Adams RH: Digitalis, positive inotropes and vasodilator drugs. In Riviere J, Papich M, editors: *Veterinary pharmacology and therapeutics*, ed 9 Ames, Iowa, 2009, Iowa State University Press, pp 541-574.
4. Klabunde RE: *Cardiology physiology concepts*, Philadelphia, 2005, Lippincott Williams & Wilkins.
5. Roden DM: Antiarrhythmic drugs. In Brunton LL, Lazo JS, Parker KL, editors: *Goodman & Gilman's the pharmacological basis of therapeutics*, ed 11, New York, 2006, McGraw-Hill, pp 899–932.

6. Rocco TP, Fang JC: Pharmacotherapy of congestive heart failure. In Brunton LL, Lazo JS, Parker KL, editors: *Goodman & Gilman's the pharmacological basis of therapeutics*, ed 11, New York, 2006, McGraw-Hill, pp 869-897.
7. Schwinn DA, Duke JB: New advances in receptor pharmacology, *Revista Mexicana de Anestesiologia* 27:83–87, 2004.
8. Cheng H-J, Zhang Z-S, Onishi K, et al: Up-regulation of runctional β3-adrenergic receptor in the failing canine myocardium, *Circ Res* 89:599–606, 2001.
9. Hoffman B: Therapy of hypertension. In Brunton LL, Lazo JS, Parker KL, editors: *Goodman & Gilman's the pharmacological basis of therapeutics*, ed 11, New York, 2006, McGraw-Hill, pp 845-868.
10. Jackson EK: Renin and angiotensins. In Brunton LL, Lazo JS, Parker, editors: *Goodman & Gilman's the pharmacological basis of therapeutics*, ed 11, New York, 2006, McGraw-Hill, pp 789–821.
11. Pool PE: The clinical significance of neurohormonal activiation, *Clin Ther* 19:53–67, 1997.
12. Lefebvre HP, Toutain PL: Angiotensin-converting enzyme inhibitors in the therapy of renal diseases, *J Vet Pharmacol Ther* 27(5):265–281, 2004.
13. Luft FC: Cardiac angiotensin is upregulated in the hearts of unstable angina patients, *Circ Res* 94:1530–1532, 2004.
14. Gulati K, Lall SB: Angiotensin II–receptor subtypes characterization and pathophysiological implications, *Indian J Exp Biol* 34(2):91–97, 1996.
15. Gallinat S, Busche S, Raizada MK, et al: The angiotensin II type 2 receptor: an enigma with multiple variations, *Am J Physiol Endocrinol Metab* 278(3):E357–E374, 2000.
16. Gendron L, Payet MD, Gallo-Payet N: The angiotensin type 2 receptor of angiotensin II and neuronal differentiation: from observations to mechanisms, *J Mol Endocrinol* 31(3):359–372, 2003.
17. Barki-Harrington L, Luttrell LM, Rockman HA: Dual inhibition of β-adrenergic and angiotensin II receptors by a single antagonist: a functional role for receptor–receptor interaction in vivo, *Circulation* 108(13):1611–1618, 2003.
18. Jackson EK: Renin and angiotensin. In Brunton LL, Lazo JS, Parker KL, editors: *Goodman & Gilman's the pharmacological basis of therapeutics*, ed 11, New York, 2006, McGraw-Hill.
19. Whittle BJR: Nitric oxide in physiology and pathology, *Histochem J* 27:727–737, 1995.
20. Adams HR: Physiologic, pathophysiologic and therapeutic implications for endogenous nitric oxide, *J Am Vet Med Assoc* 209:1297–1302, 1996.
21. Parratt JR: Nitric oxide in sepsis and endotoxemia, *J Antimicrob Chemother* 41:31–39, 1998.
22. Klein L, O'Connor CM, Gattis WA, et al: Pharmacologic therapy for patients with chronic heart failure and reduced systolic function: review of trials and practical considerations, *Am J Cardiol* 91:18F–40F, 2003.
23. Ruffolo RR Jr, Feuerstein GZ, Ohlstein EH: Recent observations with β-adrenoceptor blockade. Beneficial effects in hypertension and heart failure, *Am J Hypertens* 11(1Pt 2): 9S–14S, 1998.
24. Blum A, Miller H: Pathophysiological role of cytokines in congestive heart failure, *Annu Rev Med* 52:15–27, 2001.
25. White CM: Catecholamines and their blockade in congestive heart failure, *Am J Health Syst Pharm* 55(7):676–682, 1998.
26. Abbott JA: B-blockade in the management of systolic dysfunction, *Vet Clin North Am Small Anim Pract* 34(5):1157–1170, 2004.
27. Tanigawa T, Yano M, Kohno M, et al: Mechanism of preserved positive lusitropy by cAMP-dependent drugs in heart failure, *Am J Physiol Heart Circ Physiol* 278(2):H313–H320, 2000.
28. Katz AM: Heart failure: a hemodynamic disorder complicated by maladaptive proliferative responses, *J Cell Mol Med* 7:1–10, 2003.
29. Kasma S, Toyama T, Kumakura H, et al: Effect of spironolactone on cardiac sympathetic nerve activity and left ventricular remodeling in patients with dilated cardiomyopathy, *J Am College Cardio* 41:574–581, 2003.
30. Hayashi M, Tsutamoto T, Wada A, et al: Immediate administration of mineralocorticoid receptor antagonist spironolactone prevents post-infarct left ventricular remodeling associated with suppression of a marker of myocardial collagen synthesis in patients with first anterior acute myocardial infarction, *Circulation* 107:2559–2565, 2003.
31. Grobe JL, Mecca AP, Lingis M, et al: Prevention of angiotensin II-induced cardiac remodeling by angiotensin-(1–7), *Am J Physiol Heart Circ Physiol* 292:736–742, 2007.
32. Bolton K, Machado JM, Speth RC, et al: Prevention of angiotensin II-induced cardiac remodeling by angiotensin-(1–7), *Am J Physiol Heart Circ Physiol* 292:736–742, 2007.
33. Fejes-Tóth G, Náray-Frjes-Tóth A: Early aldosterone-regulated genes in cardiomyocytes: clues to cardiac remodeling, *Endocrinology* 148(4):1502–1510, 2007.
34. Zannad F, Dousset B, Alla F: Treatment of congestive heart failure. Interfering with the aldosterone-cardiac extracellular matrix relationship, *Hypertension* 38:1227–1232, 2001.
35. Matsumori A, Sasayama S: The role of inflammatory mediators in the failing heart: immunomodulation of cytokines in experimental models of heart failure, *Heart Fail Rev* 6: 129–136, 2001.
36. Dorigo P, Floreani M, Santostasi G, et al: Pharmacological characterization of a new Ca^{2+} sensitizer, *J Pharmacol Exp Ther* 295:994–1004, 2000.
37. Gurantz D, Cowling RT, Varki N, et al: IL-1β and TNF-α upregulate angiotensin II type 1 (AT1) receptors on cardiac fibroblasts and are associated with increased AT1 density in the post-MI heart, *J Mol Cell Cardiol* 38(3):505–515, 2005.
38. Boswood A: Editorial: the rise and fall of the cardiac biomarker, *J Vet Intern Med* 18:797–799, 2004.
39. Knowles HJ, Tian YM, Mole DR, et al: Novel mechanism of action for hydralazine: induction of hypoxia-inducible factor-1α, vascular endothelial growth factor, and angiogenesis by inhibition of prolyl hydroxylases, *Circ Res* 95(2):162–169, 2004:Jul 23.
40. Kittleson MD, Hamlin RL: Hydralazine pharmacodynamics in the dog, *Am J Vet Res* 44(8):1501–1505, 1983.
41. Rabinowitz B, Parmley WW, Har-Zahav Y, et al: Correlation between effects of hydralazine on force and on the cAMP system of ventricular myocardium in dogs and cats, *Cardiovasc Res* 20(3):215–220, 1986.
42. Hare JM: Nitroso-redox balance in the cardiovascular system, *N Engl J Med* 351:2112–2114, 2004.
43. Henik RA: Diagnosis and treatment of feline systemic hypertension, *Compend Contin Educ Pract Vet* 19:163–178, 1997.
44. Cohn JN: Nitrates versus angiotensin-converting enzyme inhibitemmors for congestive heart failure, *Am J Cardiol* 72(8):21C–24C, 1993:discussion, 24C-26C.
45. Michel T: Treatment of myocardial ischemia. In Brunton LL, Lazo JS, Parker KL, editors: *Goodman & Gilman's the pharmacological basis of therapeutics*, ed 11, New York, 2006, McGraw-Hill.
46. Zhang X, Hintze TH: Amlodipine releases nitric oxide from canine coronary microvessels: an unexpected mechanism of action of a calcium channel-blocking agent, *Circulation* 97(6):576–580, 1998.
47. Beaughard M, Brasset M, John G, et al: Failure of calcium channel blockade to reduce platelet-mediated cyclic flow variations in dogs with coronary stenosis and endothelial injury, *J Cardiovasc Pharmacol* 26(4):577–583, 1995.
48. Behrend EN, Grauer GF, Greco DS, et al: Comparison of the effects of diltiazem and aspirin on platelet aggregation in cats, *J Am Anim Hosp Assoc* 32:11–18, 1996.

49. Stopher DA, Beresford AP, Macrae PV, Humphrey MJ: The metabolism and pharmacokinetics of amlodipine in humans and animals, *J Cardiovasc Pharmacol* 12(Suppl 7):S55–S59, 1988.
50. Laufen H, Leitold M: Enantioselective disposition of oral amlodipine in healthy volunteers, *Chirality* 6(7):531–536, 1994.
51. Torpet LA, Kragulund C, Reibel J, et al: Oral adverse drug reactions to cardiovascular drugs, *Crit Rev Oral Biol Med* 15(1):28–46, 2004.
52. Jorgensen MG: Prevalence of amlodipine-related gingival hyperplasia, *J Periodontol* 68(7):676–678, 1997.
53. Atkins CE, Rausch WP, Gardner SY, et al: The effect of amlodipine and the combination of amlodipine and enalapril on the renin-angiotensin-aldosterone system in the dog, *J Vet Pharmacol Ther* 30(5):394–400, 2007.
54. Beaucage P, Massicotte J, Boileau JF, et al: Effects of first and second generation calcium channel blockers on diastolic function of the failing hamster heart: relationship with coronary flow changes, *J Cardiovasc Pharmacol* 42(1):142–150, 2003.
55. Mathur S, Syme H, Brown CA, et al: Effects of the calcium channel antagonist amlodipine in cats with surgicallly induced hypertensive renal insufficiency, *Am J Vet Res* 63(6):833–839, 2002.
56. Locatelli F, Del Vecchio L, Andrulli S, et al: Role of combination therapy with ACE inhibitors and calcium channel blockers in renal protection, *Kidney Int Suppl* 82:S53–S60, 2002.
57. Tissier R, Chetboul V, Moraillon R, et al: Increased mitral valve regurgitation and myocardial hypertrophy in two dogs with long-term pimobendan therapy, *Cardiovasc Toxicol* 5(1):43–51, 2005.
58. Jepson RE, Elliott J, Brodbelt D, et al: Effect of control of systolic blood pressure on survival in cats with systemic hypertension, *J Vet Intern Med* 21(3):402–409, 2007.
59. Helms SR: Treatment of feline hypertension with transdermal amlodipine: a pilot study, *J Am Anim Hosp Assoc* 43(3):149–156, 2007.
60. Mathews KA, Monteith G: Evaluation of adding diltiazem therapy to standard treatment of acute renal failure caused by leptopirosis: 18 dogs (1998-2001), *J Vet Emerg Crit Care* 17(2):149–158, 2007.
61. Toutain PL, Lefèbvre HP: Pharmacokinetics and pharmacokinetic/pharmacodynamic relationships for angiotensin-converting enzyme inhibitors, *J Vet Pharmacol Ther* 27(6):515–525, 2004.
62. Duggan KA, Ye VZ: Angiotensin-converting enzyme inhibition with enalapril increases the cardiac concentration of vasoactive intestinal peptide, *Ann NY Acad Sci* 805:713–716, 1998.
63. Lefebvre HP, Brown SA, Chetboul V, et al: Angiotensin-converting enzyme inhibitors in veterinary medicine, *Curr Pharm Des* 13(13):1347–1361, 2007.
64. Jackson EK, Garrison JC: Renin and angiotensin. In Brunton LL, Lazo JS, Parker KL, editors: *Goodman & Gilman's the pharmacological basis of therapeutics*, ed 11, New York, 2006, McGraw-Hill.
65. King JN, Maurer M, Toutain PL: Pharmacokinetic/pharmacodynamic modelling of the disposition and effect of benazepril and benazeprilat in cats, *J Vet Pharm Therap* 26:213–224, 2003.
66. Desmoulins PO, Burgaud S, Horspool LJ: Pharmacokinetics and pharmacodynamics of ramipril and ramiprilat in healthy cats, *J Vet Pharmacol Ther* 31(4):349–358, 2008.
67. King JN, Humbert-Droz E, Maurer M: Plasma angiotensin converting enzyme activity and pharmacokinetics of benazepril and benazeprilat in cats after single and repeated oral administration of benazepril HCL, *J Vet Pharmacol Ther* 22(6):360–370, 1999.
68. King JN, Mauron C, Kaiser G: Pharmacokinetics of the active metabolite of benazepril, benazeprilat, and inhibition of plasma angiotensin-converting enzyme activity after single and repeated administrations to dogs, *Am J Vet Res* 56:1620–1628, 1995.
69. Nordström M, Abrahamsson T, Ervik M, et al: Central nervous and systemic kinetics of ramipril and ramiprilat in the conscious dog, *J Pharmacol Exp Ther* 266(1):147–152, 1993.
70. King JN, Maurer M, Morrison CA, et al: Pharmacokinetics of the angiotensin-converting-enzyme inhibitor, benazepril, and its active metabolite, benazeprilat, in dog, *Xenobiotica* 27:819–829, 1997.
71. Kitagawa H, Ohba Y, Kuwahara Y, et al: An angiotensin converting enzyme inhibitor, benazepril can be transformed to an active metabolite, enazeprilat, by the liver of dogs with ascitic pulmonary heartworm disease, *J Vet Med Sci* 65(6):701–706, 2003.
72. Lefebvre HP, Jeunesse E, Laroute V, et al: Pharmacokinetic and pharmacodynamic parameters of ramipril and ramiprilat in healthy dogs and dogs with reduced glomerular filtration rate, *J Vet Intern Med* 20(3):499–507, 2006.
73. King JN, Strehlau G, Wernsing J, et al: Effect of renal insufficiency on the pharmacokinetics and pharmacodynamics of benazepril in cats, *J Vet Pharmacol Ther* 25(5):371–378, 2002.
74. Uechi M, Tanaka Y, Aramaki Y, et al: Evaluation of the renin-angiotensin system in cardiac tissues of cats with pressure-overload cardiac hypertrophy, *Am J Vet Res* 69(3):343–348, 2008.
75. Brown SA, Brown CA, Jacobs G, et al: Effects of the angiotensin converting enzyme inhibitor benazepril in cats with induced renal insufficiency, *Am J Vet Res* 62(3):375–383, 2001.
76. Malomvolgyi B, Koltai MZ, Hadhazy P, et al: Captopril produces endothelium-dependent relaxation of dog isolated renal arteries. Potential role of bradykinin, *Arch Int Pharmacodyn Ther* 330(1):39–52, 1995.
77. Pouchelon JL, King J, Martignoni L, et al: The BENCH (BENazepril in Canine Heart Disease) Study Group, Long-term tolerability of benazepril in dogs with congestive heart failure, *J Vet Cardiol* 6(1):7–13, 2004.
78. Roudebush P, Allen TA, Kuehn NF, et al: The effect of combined therapy with captopril, furosemide, and a sodium-restricted diet on serum electrolyte concentrations and renal function in normal dogs and dogs with congestive heart failure, *J Vet Intl Med* 8(5):337–342, 1994.
79. Mignat C, Unger T: ACE inhibitors. Drug interactions of clinical significance, *Drug Saf* 12(5):334–347, 1995.
80. Scow DT, Smith EG, Shaughnessy AF: Combination therapy with ACE inhibitors and angiotensin-receptor blockers in heart failure, *Am Fam Physician* 68(9):1795–1798, 2003.
81. Hennekens CH, Kowalczykowski M, Hollar D: Lack of deleterious interaction between angiotensin receptor blockers and β-blockers in the treatment of patients with heart failure, *J Cardiovasc Pharmacol Ther* 11(2):149–152, 2006.
82. Roberge RJ, Rossetti ML, Rosetti JM: Aminophylline reversal of antihypertensive agent toxicity, *Vet Hum Toxicol* 43(5):285–287, 2001.
83. Bench Study Group: The effect of benazepril on survival times and clinical signs of dogs with congestive heart failure: results of a multicenter, prospective, randomized, double-blinded, placebo-controlled, long-term clinical trial,, *J Vet Cardiol* 1:7–18, 1999.
84. Kittleson MD, Johnson LE, Pion PD, et al: The acute haemodynamic effects of captopril in dogs with heart failure, *J Vet Pharmacol Ther* 16(1):1–7, 1993.
85. Morisse B, Kersten U: Treatment of heart failure in dogs with ACE inhibitors: Comparison of quinapril and captopril, *Tier Prax* 23(5):489–496, 1995.
86. Cove Study Group: Controlled clinical evaluation of enalapril in dogs with heart failure: Results of the cooperative veterinary enalapril study group, *J Vet Intern Med* 9:243–252, 1995.
87. The IMPROVE Study Group. Acute and short-term hemodynamic, echocardiographic, and clinical effects of enalapril maleate in dogs with naturally acquired heart failure: results of the invasive multicenter prospective veterinary evaluation of enapril study, *J Vet Intern Med* 9:234–242, 1995.

88. Ettinger SJ, Benitz AM, Ericsson GF, et al: Live Study Group. Effects of enalapril maleate on survival of dogs with naturally acquired heart failure. The long-term investigation of veterinary enalapril, *J Am Vet Med Assoc* 213(11):1573–1577, 1998.
89. Pouchelon JL, Jamet N, Gouni V, et al: Effect of benazepril on survival and cardiac events in dogs with asymptomatic mitral valve disease: a retrospective study of 141 cases, *J Vet Intern Med* 22(4):905–914, 2008.
90. O'Grady MR: Acquired valvular heart disease. In Ettinger SJ, Feldman EC, editors: *Textbook of Veterinary Internal Medicine*, ed 4, Philadelphia, 1995, Saunders, pp 944–958.
91. Ishikawa Y, Uechi M, Hori Y, et al: Effects of enalapril in cats with pressure overload-induced left ventricular hypertrophy, *J Feline Med Surg* 9(1):29–35, 2007.
92. Codreanu I, Perico N, Remuzzi G: Dual blockade of the renin-angiotensin system: the ultimate treatment for renal protection? *J Am Soc Nephrol* 16(Suppl 1):S34–S38, 2005.
93. Vogt L, Navis G, de Zeeuw D: Renoprotection: a matter of blood pressure reduction or agent-characteristics? *J Am Soc Nephrol* 13(Suppl 3):S202–S207, 2002.
94. Casas JP, Chua W, Loukogeorgakis S, et al: Effect of inhibitors of the renin-angiotensin system and other antihypertensive drugs on renal outcomes: systematic review and meta-analysis, *Lancet* 366(9502):2026–2033, 2005.
95. Lassila M, Finckenberg P, Pere AK, et al: Comparison of enalapril and valsartan in cyclosporine A-induced hypertension and nephrotoxicity in spontaneously hypertensive rats on high-sodium diet, *Br J Pharmacol* 130(6):1339–1347, 2000.
96. Mansour MA, El-Kashef HA, Al-Shabanah OA: Effect of captopril on doxorubicin-induced nephrotoxicity in normal rats, *Pharmacol Res* 39(3):233–237, 1999.
97. Grodecki KM, Gains MJ, Baumal R, et al: Treatment of X-linked hereditary nephritis in Samoyed dogs with angiotensin converting enzyme (ACE) inhibitor, *J Comp Pathol* 117(3):209–225, 1997:Oct.
98. Burkholder WJ, Lees GE, LeBlanc AK, et al: Diet modulates proteinuria in heterozygous female dogs with X-linked hereditary nephropathy, *J Vet Intern Med* 18(2):165–175, 2004.
99. Grauer GF, Greco DS, Getzy DM, et al: Effects of enalapril versus placebo as a treatment for canine idiopathic glomerulonephritis, *J Vet Intern Med* 14(5):526–533, 2000.
100. Amberger CN, Glardon O, Glaus T, et al: Effects of benazepril in the treatment of feline hypertrophic cardiomyopathy Results of a prospective, open-label, multicenter clinical trial, *J Vet Cardiol* 1(1):19–26, 1999.
100a. Abbott JA: Feline Hypertrophic Cardiomyopathy: An Update, Veterinary Clinics of North America: Small Animal Practice, *Topics in Cardiology* 4(4):685–700, 2010.
101. Miller RH, Lehmkuhl LB, Smeak DD, et al: Effect of enalapril on blood pressure, renal function, and the renin-angiotensin-aldosterone system in cats with autosomal dominant polycystic kidney disease, *Am J Vet Res* 60(12):1516–1525, 1999.
102. King JN, Gunn-Moore DA, Tasker S, et al: Benazepril in renal insuficiency in cats study group. Tolerability and efficacy of benazepril in cats with chronic kidney disease, *J Vet Intern Med* 20(5):1054–1064, 2006.
103. Ruggenenti P, Schieppati A, Remuzzi G: Progression, remission, regression of chronic renal diseases, *Lancet* 357(9268): 1601–1608, 2001.
104. Finco DR, Brown SA, Brown CA, et al: Progression of chronic renal disease in the dog, *J Vet Intern Med* 13(6):516–528, 1999.
105. Brown SA, Finco DR, Brown CA, et al: Evaluation of the effects of inhibition of angiotensin converting enzyme with enalapril in dogs with induced chronic renal insufficiency, *Am J Vet Res* 64(3):321–327, 2003.
106. Watanabe T, Mishina M, Wakao, Y: Studies of the ACE inhibitor benazepril in an experimental model and in clinical cases of renal insufficiency in cats (abst), *J Vet Intern Med* 13:252, 1999.
107. Mizutani H, Koyama H, Watanabe T, et al: Evaluation of the clinical efficacy of benazepril in the treatment of chronic renal insufficiency in cats, *J Vet Intern Med* 20(5):1074–1079, 2006.
107a. Christ DD, Wong PC, Wong N, et al: Pharmacokinetics and pharmacodynamics of the angiotensin II receptor antaonist losartan potassium (DuP 753/MK 954) in the dog, *J Pharm Ext Ther* 268(3):1999–1205, 1994.
107b. Huang Xm Qiu F, Xie HT, et al: Pharmacokinetic and pharmacodynamic interaction between irbesartan and hydrochlorothiazide in renal hypertensive dogs, *J Cardiovasc Pharm* 46:863–869, 2005.
108. Spargo OM, Tait AR, Knight PR, et al: Effect of nitroglycerin-induced hypotension on canine spinal cord blood flow, *Br J Anaesth* 59:640–647, 1987.
109. Côté E, Ettinger SJ: Electrocardiography and cardiac arrhythmias. In Ettinger SJ, Feldman EC, editors: *Textbook of veterinary internal medicine*, ed 7, St Louis, 2010, Saunders, pp 1159-1187.
110. Muir WW: Antiarrhythmic drugs: treatment of cardiac arrhythmias, *Vet Clin North Am Small Anim Pract* 27(5): 957–988, 1991.
110a Gallacher DJ, Van de Water A, vand der Linde H, et al: In vivo mechanisms precipitating torsades de pointes in a canine model of drug-induced long-QT1 syndrome, *Cardiovas Res* 76: 247–256, 2007.
110b. Chézalviel-Guilbert F, Davy JM, Poirier JM, et al: Mexiletine antagonizes effects of sotalol on QT interval duration and its proarrhythmic effects in a canine model of torsade de pointes, *J Am Coll Cardiol* 26(3):787–792, 1995.
110c. Hashimoto K, Ishii M, Komori S: Antiarrhythmic plasma concentrations of mexiletine on canine ventricular arrhythmias, *J Cardiovasc Pharmacol* 6(2):213–219, 1984.
110d. Costard-Jaeckle A, Liem LB, Franz MR: Frequency-dependent effect of quinidine, mexiletine, and their combination on postrepolarization refractoriness in vivo, *J Cardiovasc Pharmacol* 14(6):810–817, 1989.
111. Katz AM: Selectivity and toxicity of antiarrhythmic drugs: molecular interactions with ion channels, *Am J Med* 104:179–195, 1998.
112. Miller MW, Adams RH: Antiarrhythmic agents. In Riviere J, Papich M, editors: *Veterinary pharmacology and therapeutics* ed 9, Ames, Iowa, 2009, Iowa State University Press, pp 575–601.
113. Anyukhovsky EP, Sosunov EA, Feinmark SJ, et al: Effects of quinidine on repolarization in canine epicardium, midmyocardium, and endocardium: II. In vivo study, *Circulation* 96(11):4019–4026, 1997.
114. Hashimoto K, Shibuta T, Satoh H, et al: Quantitative analysis of the antiarrhythmic effect of drugs on canine ventricular arrhythmias by the determination of minimum effective plasma concentrations, *Jpn Circ J* 47:92–97, 1983.
115. Sosunov EA, Anyukhovsky EP, Rosen MR: Effects of quinidine on repolarization in canine epicardium, midmyocardium, and endocardium: I. In vitro study, *Circulation* 96(11):4011–4018, 1997.
116. Kuroha M, Shirai Y, Shimoda M: Multiple oral dosing of ketoconazole influences pharmacokinetics of quinidine after intravenous and oral administration in beagle dogs, *J Vet Pharmacol Therap* 27:353–359, 2004.
117. Colvin RA, Ashavaid TF, Katz AM, et al: Amiodarone, verapamil, and quinidine do not affect equilibrium binding of digoxin, *J Cardiovasc Pharmacol* 16(4):519–522, 1990.
118. Bagwell EE, Walle T, Drayer DE, et al: Correlation of the electrophysiological and antiarrhythmic properties of the N-acetyl metabolite of procainamide with plasma and tissue drug concentrations in the dog, *J Pharmacol Exp Ther* 197(1):38–48, 1976.

119. Papich MG, Davis LE, Davis CA, et al: Pharmacokinetics of procainamide hydrochloride in dogs, *Am J Vet Res* 47(11):2351–2358, 1986.
120. Papich MG, Davis LE, Davis CA: Procainamide in the dog: antiarrhythmic plasma concentrations after intravenous administration, *J Vet Pharmacol Ther* 9(4):359–369, 1986.
121. Bauer LA, Black DJ, Lill JS, et al: Levofloxacin and ciprofloxacin decrease procainamide and N-acetylprocainamide renal clearances, *Antimicrob Agents Chemother* 49(4):1649–1651, 2005.
122. Davis J, Glassman R, Wit AL: Method for evaluating the effects of antiarrhythmic drugs on ventricular tachycardias with different electrophysiologic characteristics and different mechanisms in the infarcted canine heart, *Am J Cardiol* 49(5):1176–1184, 1982.
123. Cook CS, Gwilt PR, Kowalski K, et al: Pharmacokinetics of disopyramide in the dog. Importance of mono-N-dealkylated metabolite kinetics in assessing pharmacokinetic modeling of the parent drug, *Drug Metab Dispos* 18(1):42–49, 1990.
124. Schmidt JJ, Frederick LG, Garthwaite SM: Rapid infusions of bidisomide or disopyramide in conscious dogs: effect of myocardial infarction on acute tolerability, *J Cardiovasc Pharmacol* 20(2):236–250, 1992.
125. Johnson MS, Martin M, Smith P: Cardioversion of supraventricular tachycardia using lidocaine in five dogs, *J Vet Intern Med* 20:272–276, 2006.
126. Ritschel WA, Grummich KW, Hussain AS, et al: Rectal bioavailability of lidocaine in the dog: evaluation of first-pass elimination, *Methods Find Exp Clin Pharmacol* 9(8):497–502, 1987.
127. Wilcke JR, Davis LE, Neff-Davis CA, et al: Pharmacokinetics of lidocaine and its active metabolites in dogs, *J Vet Pharmacol Ther* 6(1):49–57, 1983.
128. Ngo LY, Tam YK, Tawfik S, et al: Effects of intravenous infusion of lidocaine on its pharmacokinetics in conscious instrumented dogs, *J Pharm Sci* 86(8):944–952, 1997.
129. Gugler R, Lain P, Azarnoff DL: Effect of portacaval shunt on the disposition of drugs with and without first-pass effect, *J Pharmacol Exp Ther* 195(3):416–423, 1975.
130. Krejcy K, Krumpl G, Todt H, et al: Lidocaine has a narrow antiarrhythmic dose range against ventricular arrhythmias induced by programmed electrical stimulation in conscious postinfarction dogs, *Naunyn Schmiedebergs Arch Pharmacol* 346(2):213–218, 1992.
131. Wilcke JR, Davis LE, Neff-Davis CA: Determination of lidocaine concentrations producing therapeutic and toxic effects in dogs, *J Vet Pharmacol Ther* 6(2):105–111, 1983.
132. LeLorier J, Grenon D, Latour Y, et al: Pharmacokinetics of lidocaine after prolonged intravenous infusions in uncomplicated myocardial infarction, *Ann Intern Med* 87(6):700–706, 1977.
133. Nagashima A, Tanaka E, Inomata S, et al: A study of the in vitro interaction between lidocaine and premedications using human liver microsomes, *J Clin Pharm Ther* 30(2):185–188, 2005.
134. Hiromasa S, Li ZY, Coto H, et al: Selective effects of tocainide in canine acute myocardial infarction, *Int J Cardiol* 27(1): 79–86, 1990.
135. Uprichard AC, Allen JD, Harron DW: Effects of tocainide enantiomers on experimental arrhythmias produced by programmed electrical stimulation, *J Cardiovasc Pharmacol* 11(2):235–241, 1988.
136. Wallace AA, Stupienski RF, Heaney LA, et al: Antiarrhythmic actions of tocainide in canine models of previous myocardial infarction, *Am Heart J* 121(5):1413–1421, 1991.
137. Calvert CA, Pickus CW, Jacobs GJ: Efficacy and toxicity of tocainide for the treatment of ventricular tachyarrhythmias in Doberman pinschers with occult cardiomyopathy, *J Vet Intern Med* 10(4):235–240, 1996.
137a. Grech-Belanger, Turgeon J, Gilbert M: Steroselective disposition of mexiletine in man, *Br J Clin Pharmac* 21:481–487, 1986.
137b. Turgeon J, Uprichard AC, Bélanger PM, et al: Resolution and electrophysiological effects of mexiletine enantiomers, *J Pharm Pharmacol* 43(9):630–635, 1991.
138. Hernandez R, Mann DE, Breckinridge S, et al: Effects of flecainide on defibrillation thresholds in the anesthetized dog, *J Am Coll Cardiol* 14(3):777–781, 1989.
138a Carlier J: Hemodynamic, electrocardiographic and toxic effects of the intravenous administration of increasing doses of mexiletine in the dog. Comparison with similar effects produced by other antiarrhythmics, *Acta Cardiol Suppl* 25:81–100, 1980.
139. Boucher M, Dubray C, Duchene-Marullaz P: Pharmacological evidence for differences in the β-adrenoreceptor populations mediating atrial and ventricular chronotropic responses in the unanaesthetized dog, *J Auton Pharmacol* 4(4):279–86, 1984.
140. Nuttall SL, Langford NJ, Kendall MJ: B-blockers in heart failure. 1. Clinical evidence, *J Clin Pharm Ther* 25:395–398, 2000.
141. Mehvar R: Sterospecific pharmacokientics and pharmacodynamics of β-adrenergic blockers in humans, *J Pharm Pharmaceutic Sci* 4(2):185–200, 2001.
142. DiLenarda A, Sabbadini G, Salvatore L, et al: Long term effects of carvedilol in idiopathic dilated cardiomyopathy with persistent left ventricular dysfunction despite chronic metoprolol, *J Am Coll Cardiol* 33:1926–1934, 1999.
143. Remme WJ, Torp-Pedersen C, Poole-Wilson PA, et al: Carvedilol protects better against vascular events than metoprolol in heart failure. Results from COMET, *J Am Coll Cardiol* 49: 963–971, 2007.
143a. Takara K, Sakaeda T, Okumura K: Carvedilol: a new candidate for reversal of MDR1/P-glycoprotein-mediated multidrug resistance, *Anticancer Drugs* 15(4):303–309, 2004.
144. Regardh CG, Ek L, Hoffmann KJ: Plasma levels and β-blocking effect of α-hydroxymetoprolol–metabolite of metoprolol in the dog, *J Pharmacokinet Biopharm* 7(5):471–479, 1979.
145. Yin XX, Zhang YD: Pharmacokinetic-pharmacodynamic modeling of metoprolol enantiomers in the dog, *Yao Hsueh Hsueh Pao-Acta Pharmaceutica Sinica* 32(6):411–415, 1997.
146. Jacobs G, Whitten T, Sams R, et al: Pharmacokinetics of propranolol in healthy cats during erythroid and hyperthyroid states, *Am J Vet Res* 58:398–403, 1997.
146a. Kaplan H, Commarato MA: Relative beta adrenergic receptor blocking activity in dogs after intravenous and intraportal vein administration: bunolol, propronolol, their leveoisolmers and sotalol, *J Pharm Exp Therp* 185(2): 395–405, 1973.
147. Kerns W, Schroeder D, Williams C, et al: Insulin improves survival in a canine model of acute β-blocker toxicity, *Ann Emerg Med* 29:748–757, 1997.
148. Fang J, Semple HA, Sog J: Determination of metoprolol, and its four metabolites in dog plasma, *J Chromatography B* 809:9–14, 2004.
149. Murthy SS, Nelson WL, Shen DD, et al: Pharmacokinetic interaction between verapamil and metoprolol in the dog. Stereochemical aspects, *Drug Metab Dispos* 19(6):1093–1100, 1991.
150. Feuerstein GZ, Ruffolo RR Jr: Carvedilol, a novel multiple action antihypertensive agent with antioxidant activity and the potential for myocardial and vascular protection, *Eur Heart J* (Suppl F 16):38–42, 1995.
151. Keating GM, Jarvis B: Carvedilol: a review of its use in chronic heart failure, *Drugs* 63(16):1697–1741, 2003.
152. Kowey PR: A review of carvedilol arrhythmia data in clinical trials, *J Cardiovasc Pharmacol Ther* 10 (Suppl 1):S59–S68, 2005.
153. Mehvar R, Brocks DR: Stereospecific pharmacokinetics and pharmacodynamics of β-adrenergic blockers in humans, *J Pharm Pharm Sci* 4(2):185–200, 2001.

154. Sanderson JE, Chan SK, Yip G, et al: β-blockade in heart failure: a comparison of carvedilol with metoprolol, *J Am Coll Cardiol* 34(5):1522–1528, 1999.
155. Kotsinas A, Gorgoulis V, Zacharatos P, et al: Antioxidant agent nimesulid and β-blocker metoprolol do not exert protective effects against rat mitochondrial DNA alterations in Adriamycin-induced cardiotoxicity, *Biochem Biophys Res Commun* 254:651–656, 1999.
156. Feuerstein G, Yue TL, Ma X, Ruffolo RR: Novel mechanisms in the treatment of heart failure: inhibition of oxygen radicals and apoptosis by carvedilol, *Prog Cardiovasc Dis* 41(1 Suppl 1):17–24, 1998.
157. Ohlstein EH, Arleth AJ, Storer B, et al: Carvedilol inhibits endothelin-1 biosynthesis in cultured human coronary artery endothelial cells, *J Mol Cell Cardiol* 30(1):167–173, 1998.
158. Kalay N, Basar E, Ozdogru I, et al: Protective effects of carvedilol against anthracycline-induced cardiomyopathy, *J Am Coll Cardiol* 48(11):2258–2262, 2006:Dec 5.
159. Feuerstein G, Liu GL, Yue TL, et al: Comparison of metoprolol and carvedilol pharmacology and cardioprotection in rabbit ischemia and reperfusion model, *Eur J Pharmacol* 351(3): 341–350, 1998.
160. Fazio S, Palmieri EA, Ferravante B, et al: Doxorubicin-induced cardiomyopathy treated with carvedilol, *Cardiol* 21(10): 777–779, 1998.
161. Schaefer WH, Pilitowski J, Hwang B, et al: Metabolism of carvedilol in dogs, rats, and mice, *Drug Metab Dispol* 26(10): 958–969, 1998.
162. Sawangkoon S, Miyamoto M, Nakayama T, et al: Acute cardiovascular effects with pharmacokinetics of carvedilol in healthy dogs, *Am J Vet Res* 61:57–60, 2000.
163. Arsenault WG, Boothe DM, Gordon SG, et al: Pharmacokinetics of carvedilol after intravenous and oral administration in conscious healthy dogs, *Am J Vet Res* 66(12):2172–2176, 2005.
164. Gordon SG, Arsenault WG, Longnecker M, et al: Pharmacodynamics of carvedilol in conscious, healthy dogs, *J Vet Intern Med* 20:297–304, 2006.
165. Kukin ML, Kalman J, Charney RH, et al: Prospective randomized comparison of effect of long-term treatment with metoprolol or carvedilol on symptoms, exercise, ejection fraction, and oxidative stress in heart failure, *Circulation* 99:2645–2651, 1999.
166. Beller KD, Diedrich F, Sponer G: The effect of carvedilol on contrast echocardiography in comparison to metoprolol in conscious dogs, *Arzneimittelforschung* 49(10):830–834, 1999.
167. Jonsson O, Behnam-Motlagh P, Persson M, et al: Increase in doxorubicin cytotoxicity by carvedilol inhibition of P-glycoprotein activity, *Biochem Pharmacol* 58(11):1801–1806, 1999.
168. Oyama MA, Sisson DD, Prosek R, et al: Carvedilol in dogs with dilated cardiomyopathy, *J Vet Intern Med* 21(6): 1272–1279, 2007.
169. Marcondes-Santos M, Tarasoutchi F, Mansur AP, et al: Effects of carvedilol treatment in dogs with chronic mitral valvular disease, *J Vet Intern Med* 21(5):996–1001, 2007.
170. Aursnes I, Osnes JB, Tvete IF, et al: Does atenolol differ from other β-adrenergic blockers? *BMC Clinical Pharmacology* 7:4 doi:10.1186/1472-6904-7-4. Accessed July 2007.
171. Quinones M, Dyer DC, Ware WA, et al: The pharmacokinetics of atenolol in normal cats,, *Am J Vet Res* 57:1050–1053, 1996.
172. MacGregor JM, Rush JE, Rozanski EA, et al: A comparison of oral versus transdermal atenolol administration in cats, *Am J Vet Res* 69(1):39–44, 2008.
173. Henik RA, Stepien RL, Wenholz LJ, et al: Efficacy of atenolol as a single antihypertensive agent in hyperthyroid cats, *J Feline Med Surg* 10(6):577–581, 2008.
174. Crandell JM, Ware WA: Cardiac toxicity from phenylpropanolamine overdose in a dog, *J Am Anim Hosp Assoc* 41(6): 413–420, 2005.
175. Quon C, Gorczynski: Pharmacodynamics and onset of action of esmolol in anesthetized dogs, *Am Soc Pharmacol Exp Ther* 237(3):912–918, 1986.
176. Bonagura J, Stepien R, Lehmkuhl L: Acute effects of esmolol on left ventricular outflow obstniction in cats with hypertrophic cardiomyopathy: a Doppler echocardiographic study, *J Vet Int Med* 5:123, 1991.
177. Beddies G, Fox PR, Papich MD, et al: Comparison of the pharmacokinetic properties of bisoprolol and carvedilol in healthy dogs, *Am J Vet Res* 69(12):1659–1663, 2008.
177a. Schnelle K, Garrett ER: Pharmacokinetics of the -adrenergic blocker sotalol in dogs, *J Pharm Sci* 62(3):362–375, 1973.
177b. Tawara K: Studies on the pharmacokinetics and effects of beta-adrenergic blocking agents, sotalol (author's transl), *Hokkaido Igaku Zasshi* 52(3):245–259, 1977.
178. Rosalion A, Snow NJ, Horrigan TP, et al: Amiodarone versus bretylium for suppression of reperfusion arrhythmias in dogs, *Ann Thorac Surg* 51(1):81–85, 1991.
179. Sicouri S, Moro S, Litovsky S, et al: Chronic amiodarone reduces transmural dispersion of repolarization in the canine heart, *J Cardiovasc Electrophysiol* 8(11):1269–1279, 1997.
180. Ware WA, Muir WW, Swanson C: Effects of amiodarone on myocardial performance in normal canine hearts and canine hearts with infarcts, *Am J Vet Res* 52(6):891–897, 1991.
181. Kraus MS, Thomason JD, Fallaw TL, et al: Toxicity in Doberman Pinschers with ventricular arrhythmias treated with amiodarone (1996-2005), *J Vet Intern Med* 23(1):1–6, 2009.
182. Saunders AB, Miller MW, Gordon SG, et al: Oral amiodarone therapy in dogs with atrial fibrillation, *J Vet Intern Med* 20(4):921–926, 2006.
182a. Jacobs G, Calvert C, Kraus M: Hepatopathy in 4 dogs treated with amiodarone, *J Vet Intern Med* 14(1):96–99, 2000.
183. De Micheli A, Medrano GA, Iturralde P, et al: Effects of verapamil in ventricular tachycardias. An experimental and clinical study, *Acta Cardiol* 52(1):1–15, 1997.
184. Chen G, Barr S, Walsh D, et al: Cardioprotective actions of verapamil on the β-adrenergic receptor complex in acute canine Chagas' disease, *J Mol Cell Cardiol* 28(5):931–941, 1996.
185. Wall M, Calvert CA, Sanderson SL, et al: Evaluation of extended-release diltiazem once daily for cats with hypertrophic cardiomyopathy, *J Am Anim Hosp Assoc* 41:98–103, 2005.
185a. Davidson G: update on transdermals for veterinary patients, *Internat J Pharmaceut Compound* 9:178-182, 2005.
186. Maskasame C, Lankford S, Bai SA: The effects of chronic oral diltiazem and cimetidine dosing on the pharmacokinetics and negative dromotropic action of intravenous and oral diltiazem in the dog, *Biopharm Drug Dispos* 1:521–537, 1992.
187. Nakamura S, Suzuki T, Sugawara Y, et al: Metabolic fate of diltiazem: Distribution, excretion, and protein binding in the rat and dog, *Arzneimittelforschung* 37:1244–1252, 1987.
188. Syring RS, Costello MF, Poppenga RH: Temporary transvenous cardiac pacing in a dog with diltiazem intoxication, *J Vet Emerg Crit Care* 18(1):75–80, 2008.
189. Costello M, Syring RS: Calcium channel blocker toxicity, *J Vet Emerg Crit Care* 18(1):54–60, 2008.
190. Meurs KM: Myocardial disease: canine. In Ettinger SJ, Feldman EC, editors: *Textbook of veterinary internal medicine*, ed 7, St Louis, 2010, Saunders, pp 1320-1328.
190a. MacDonald K: Myocardial disease:feline. In Ettinger SJ, Feldman EC, editors: *Textbook of veterinary internal medicine*, ed 7, St louis, 2010, Saunders, pp 1328-1341.
191. Knight D: Efficacy of inotropic support of the failing heart, *Vet Clin North Am Small Anim Pract* 27(5):879–904, 1991.
192. Brixius K, Hoyer HK, Schwinger RHG: Ca^{2+} -sensitisers—a promising option to treat heart failure? *Cardiovas Drug Ther* 19:423–428, 2005.

193. Hogan DF, Green HW III: Dilated cardiomyopathy. In Bonagura JD, Twedt DC, editors: *Kirk's current veterinary therapy XIV*, St Louis, 2009, Saunders, pp 792-797.
194. Breznock EM: Application of canine plasma kinetics of digoxin and digitoxin to therapeutic digitalization in the dog, *Am J Vet Res* 34:993–999, 1973.
195. De Rick A, Belpaire FM, Bogaert MG, et al: Pharmacokinetics of digoxin, *Am J Vet Res* 39:811–818, 1978.
196. Button C, Gross DR, Johnston JT, et al: Pharmacokinetics, bioavailability, and dosage regimens in dogs, *Am J Vet Res* 41:1230–1237, 1980.
197. Button C, Gross DR, Allert JA: Application of individualized diogxin dosage regimens to canine therapeutic digitalization, *Am J Vet Res* 41:1238–1242, 1980.
198. Whittem T, Hogan D, Sisson D, et al: The population pharmacokinetics of digoxin in dogs with heart disease, *J Vet Pharmacol Therap* 23:261–263, 2000.
199. Doering W: Quinidine-digoxin interaction: pharmacokinetics, underlying mechanism and clinical implications, *N Eng J Med* 301(8):400–404, 1979.
200. Koren G, Klein J, Giesbrecht E, et al: Effects of quinidine on the renal tubular and biliary transport of digoxin: in vivo and in vitro studies in the dog, *J Pharmacol Exp Ther* 247(3): 1193–1198, 1988.
201. Ravis WR, Pedersoli WM, Turco JD: Pharmacokinetics and interactions of digoxin with phenobarbital in dogs, *Am J Vet Res* 48(8):1244–1249, 1987.
202. Pedersoli WM, Ganjam VK, Nachreiner RF: Serum digoxin concentrations in dogs before, during, and after concomitant treatment with phenobarbital, *Am J Vet Res* 41(10): 1639–1642, 1980.
203. Detweiler DK: Comparative pharmacology of cardiac glycosides, *Fed Proc* 26:1119–1124, 1977.
204. Ettinger S: Therapeutic digitalization of the dog in congestive heart failure, *J Am Vet Med Assoc* 148(5):525–531, 1966.
205. Weiss M, Kang W: Inotropic effect of digoxin in humans: mechanistic pharmacokinetic pharmacodynamicmodel based on slow receptor binding, *Pharmac Res* 21(2):231–236, 2004.
206. Akiyama K, Hashimoto K: Effects of lidocaine, disopyramide and verapamil on the in vivo triggered ventricular arrhythmia in digitalized canine heart, *Jpn J Pharmacol* 53(4):419–426, 1990.
207. Endou K, Yamamoto H, Sata T: Comparison of the effects of calcium channel blockers and antiarrhythmic drugs on digitalis-induced oscillatory afterpotentials on canine Purkinje fiber, *Jpn Heart J* 28:719–735, 1987.
208. Hashimoto K, Ishii M, Komori S, et al: Canine digitalis arrhythmia as a model for detecting Na-channel blocking antiarrhythmic drugs: a comparative study using other canine arrhythmia models and the new antiarrhythmic drugs propafenone, tocainide and SUN 1165, *Heart Vessels* 1:29–35, 1985.
209. Endoh M: Mechanism of action of Ca^{2+} sensitizers—update 2001, *Cardiovasc Drugs Ther* 15(5):397–403, 2001.
210. Watanabe E, Shiga T, Matsuda N, et al: Low-dose systemic phosphodiesterase III inhibitor pimobendan combined with prostacyclin therapy in a patient with severe primary pulmonary hypertension, *Cardiovasc Drugs Ther* 17(4):375–379, 2003.
211. Chiu YJ, Hu S-H, Reid IA: Inhibition of phosphodiesterase III with milrinone increases renin secretion in human subjects, *J Pharmacol Exp Ther* 290:16–19, 1999.
212. Kittleson MD: Efficacy and safety of milrinone for treating heart failure in dogs, *Vet Clin North Am Small Anim Pract* 27(5):905–918, 1991.
213. Keister DM, Kittleson MD, Bonagura JD, et al: Milrinone. A clinical trial in 29 dogs with moderate to severe congestive heart failure, *J Vet Int Med* 4(2):79–86, 1990.
213a. Pagel PS, Hettrick DA, Warltier DC: Comparison of the effects of levosimendan, pimobendan, and milrinone on canine left ventricular-arterial coupling and mechanical efficiency, *Basic Res Cardiol* 91(4):296–307, 1996.
214. Fuentes VL: Use of pimobendan in the management of heart failure, *Vet Clin North Am Small Anim Pract* 34(5):1145–1155, 2004.
215. Gordon SG, Miller MW, Saunders AB: Pimobendan in heart failure therapy—a silver bullet? *J Am Anim Hosp Assoc* 42: 90–93, 2006.
216. Fuentes VL, Corcoran B, French A, et al: A double-blind, randomized placebo-controlled study of pimobendan in dogs with dilated cardiomyopathy, *J Vet Intern Med* 16(3):255–261, 2002.
216a. Adrian Boswood: Current use of pimobendan in canine patients with heart disease, Veterinary Clinics of North America: small animal practice, Volume 40, Issue 4, *Topics in Cardiol* 40(4):571–580, 2010.
217. Smith PJ, French AT, Van Israel N, et al: Efficacy and safety of pimobendan in canine heart failure caused by myxomatous mitral valve disease, *J Small Anim Pract* 46(3):121–130, 2005.
218. Lombard CW, Jones O, Bussadori CM: Clinical efficacy of pimobendan versus benazepril for the treatment of acquired atrioventricular valvular disease in dogs, *J Am Anim Hosp Assoc* 42:249–261, 2006.
219. Kanno N, Kuse H, Kawasaki M, et al: Effects of pimobendan for mitral valve regurgitation in dogs, *J Vet Med Sci* 69(4): 373–377, 2007.
220. O'Grady MR, Minors SL, O'Sullivan ML, et al: Effect of pimobendan on case fatality rate in Doberman Pinschers with congestive heart failure caused by dilated cardiomyopathy, *J Vet Intern Med* 22(4):897–904, 2008.
221. Haggstrom J, Boswood A, O'Grady M, et al: Effect of pimobendan or benazepril hydrochloride on survival times in dogs with congestive heart failure caused by naturally occurring myzomatous mitral valve disease: the QUEST study, *J Vet Intern Med* 22(5):1124–1135, 2008.
222. Ouellet M, Bélanger MC, Difruscia R, et al: Effect of pimobendan on echocardiographic values in dogs with asymptomatic mitral valve disease, *J Vet Intern Med* 23(2):258–263, 2009.
223. Chetboul V, Lefebvre HP, Sampedrano CC, et al: Comparative adverse cardiac effects of pimobendan and benazepril monotherapy in dogs with mild degenerative mitral valve disease: a prospective, controlled, blinded, and randomized study, *J Vet Intern Med* 21(4):742–753, 2007.
223a. De Backer D, Biston P, Devriendt J, et al: SOAP II Investigators, Comparison of dopamine and norepinephrine in the treatment of shock, *N Engl J Med* 362(9):779–789, 2010.
224. Fusellier M, Desfontis JC, Le Roux A, et al: Effect of short-term treatment with meloxicam and pimobendan on the renal function in healthy beagle dogs, *J Vet Pharmacol Ther* 31(2): 150–155, 2008.
224a. Chetboul V, Lefebvre HP, Sampedrano CC, et al: Comparative adverse cardiac effects of pimobendan and benazepril monotherapy in dogs with mild degenerative mitral valve disease: a prospective, controlled, blinded, and randomized study, *J Vet Intern Med* 21(4):742–753, 2007.
225. Flournoy WS, Wohl JS, Albrecht-Schmitt TJ, et al: Pharmacologic identification of putative D1 dopamine receptors in feline kidneys, *J Vet Pharmacol Ther* 26(4):283–290, 2003.
226. Wohl JS, Schwartz DD, Flournoy S: Renal hemodynamic and diuretic effects of low dosage dopamine in anesthetized cats, *J Vet Emerg Crit Care* 17(1):45–52, 2007.
227. Murphy MB: Dopamine: a role in the pathogenesis and treatment of hypertension, *J Hum Hypertension* 14:S47–S50, 2000.
228. Li C, Tsai CS, Cheueh SH, et al: Dobutamine inhibits monocyte chemoattractant protein-1 production and chemotaxis in human monocytes, *Anesth Analg* 97:205–209, 2003.

229. DeBacker D, Zhang H, Manikis P, et al: Regional effects of dobutamine in endotoxic shock, *J Surg Res* 65(2):93–100, 1996.
230. Luo X, Huang Y, Hayes JK, et al: Effects of dobutamine, epinephrine and norepinephrine on the hemodynamics of dogs during hemorrhagic shock, *Acta Anaesthesiol Sinica* 35(2): 610–671, 1997.
231. Kishi T, Okamoto T, Takahashi T, et al: Cardiostimulatory action of coenzyme Q homologues on cultured myocardial cells and their biochemical mechanisms, *Clin Investig* 71 (Suppl 8):S71–S75, 1993.
232. Zhou M, Zhi Q, Tang Y, et al: Effects of coenzyme Q10 on myocardial protection during cardiac valve replacement and scavenging free radical activity in vitro, *J Cardiovasc Surg* 40(3):355–361, 1999.
233. Singh RB, Wander GS, Rastogi A, et al: Randomized, double-blind placebo-controlled trial of coenzyme Q10 in patients with acute myocardial infarction, *Cardiovasc Drugs Ther* 12(4):347–353, 1999.
234. Langsjoen PH: Lack of effect of coenzyme Q on left ventricular function in patients with congestive heart failure, *J Am Coll Cardiol* 35(3):816–817, 2000.
235. Kagan T, Davis D, Lin L, Zakeri Z: Coenzyme Q10 can in some circumstances block apoptosis, and this effect is mediated through mitochondria, *Ann N Y Acad Sci* 887:31–47, 1999.
236. Kendler BS: Nutritional strategies in cardiovascular disease control: an update on vitamins and conditionally essential nutrients, *Prog Cardiovasc Nurs* 14:124–129, 1999.
237. Haggstrom J, Duelund Pedersen H, Kvart C: New insights into degenerative mitral valve disease in dogs, *Vet Clin North Am Small Anim Pract* 34(5):1209–1226, 2004.
237a. Oyama MA, Singletary GE: The use of NT-proBNP assay in the management of canine patients with heart disease, *Vet Clin North Am: Small Anim Pract* 40(4):545–558, 2010.
237b. Atkinson KJ, Fine DM, Thombs LA, et al: Evaluation of pimobendan and N-terminal probrain natriuretic peptide in the treatment o fpulmoanry hypertension secondary to degenerative mitral vlavule disase in dogs, *J Vet Intern Med* 23(6): 1190–1196, 2009.
238. Lonn E, McKelvie R: Drug treatment in heart failure, *Brit Med J* 320:1188–1192, 2006.
238a. Goussev A, Sharov VG, Shimoyama H, et al: Effects of ACE inhibition on cardiomyocyte apoptosis in dogs with heart failure, *Am J Physiol* 275(2 Pt 2):H626–31, 1998 Aug:PubMed PMID: 9683452.
238b. Zac V, Rastogi S, Mishra S, et al: Atenolol is inferior to metoprolol in improving left ventricular function and preventing ventricular remodeling in dogs with heart failure, *Cardiology* 112(4):294–302, 2009.
238c. Tanimura M, Sharov VG, Shimoyama H, et al: Effects of AT1-receptor blockade on progression of left ventricular dysfunction in dogs with heart failure, *Am J Physiol* 276(4 Pt 2):H1385–92, 1999.
238d. Mishima T, Tanimura M, Suzuki G, et al: Effects of long-term therapy with bosentan on the progression of left ventricular dysfunction and remodeling in dogs with heart failure, *J Am Coll Cardiol* 35(1):222–229, 2000.
238e. Morita H, Khanal S, Rastogi S, et al: Selective matrix metalloproteinase inhibition attenuates progression of left ventricular dysfunction and remodeling in dogs with chronic heart failure, *Am J Physiol Heart Circ Physiol* 290(6):H2522–H2527, 2006.
239. Sisson D: Evidence for or against the efficacy of afterload reducers for management of heart failure in dogs, *Vet Clin North Am Small Anim Pract* 27(5):945–956, 1991a.
240. Atkins C, Bonagura J, Ettinger S, et al: Guidelines for the dianosis and treatment of canine chronic valvular heart disease, *J vet inter Med* 23(6):1142-1150, 2009.
241. Keene BW, Bonagura JD: Management of heart failure in dogs. In Bonagura JD, Twedt DC, editors: *Kirk's current veterinary therapy XIV*, St Louis, 2009, Saunders.
242. Slight SH, Joseph J, Granjam VK, et al: Extra-renal mineralocorticoids and cardiovascular tissue, *J Mol Cell Cardiol* 31:1175–1184, 1999.
242a. Atkins C, Bonagura J, Ettinger S, et al: Guidelines for the diagnosis and treatment of canine chronic valvular hear disease, *J Vet Intern Med* 23:1142–1150, 2009.
242b. Boswood A: Current use of pimobendan in canine patients with heart disease, *Vet Clin N Amer Small Anim Pract* 40(4):571-580, 2010.
243. Keene BW: L-carnitine supplementation in the therapy of canine dilated cardiomyopathy, *Vet Clin North Am Small Anim Pract* 27(5):1005–1010, 1991.
244. Sisson DD, Knight DH, Helinski C, et al: Plasma taurine concentrations and M-mode echocardiographic measures in healthy cats and in cats with dilated cardiomyopathy, *J Vet Int Med* 5(4):232–238, 1991.
245. Bélanger MC, Ouellet M, Queney G, et al: Taurine-deficient dilated cardiomyopathy in a family of golden retrievers, *J Am Anim Hosp Assoc* 41(5):284–291, 2005.
246. Harpster NK: Boxer cardiomyopathy: a review of the long term benefits of antiarrhythmic therapy, *Vet Clin North Am Small Anim Pract* 21:989–1004, 1991.
246a. Podrid PJ: Proarrhythmia, a serious complication of antiarrhythmic drugs, *Curr Cardiol Rep* 1(4):289–296, 1999.
247. Calvert CA: Effect of medical therapy on survival of patients with dilated cardiomyopathy, *Vet Clin North Am Small Anim Pract* 21:919, 1991.
247a. Sisson DD, Thomas WP: Myocardial diseases. In Ettinger SJ, Feldman EC, editors: *Textbook of Veterinary Internal Medicine*, ed 4, Philadelphia, 1995, Saunders.
248. Kittleson MD, Eyster GE, Knowlen GG, et al: Efficacy of digoxin administration in dogs with idiopathic congestive cardiomyopathy, *J Am Vet Med Assoc* 186:162–165, 1985.
249. Ferguson DW, Berg WJ, Sanders JS, et al: Sympathoinhibitory responses to digitalis glycosides in heart failure patients: direct evidence from sympathetic neural recordings, *Circulation* 80:65, 1989.
250. Wright KN: Assessment and treatment of supraventricular tachyarrhythmias. In Bonagura JD, Twedt DC, editors: *Kirk's current veterinary therapy XIV*, St Louis, 2009, Saunders, pp 722-727.
251. Cleland JG: Progression from hypertension to heart failure: mechanisms and management, *Cardiology* 92(Suppl 1): 10–19, 1999.
252. Skudicky D, Bergemann A, Sliwa K, et al: Beneficial effects of pentoxifylline in patients with idiopathic dilated cardiomyopathy treated with angiotensin-converting enzyme inhibitors and carvedilol: results of a randomized study, *Circulation* 103(8):1083–1088, 2001.
253. Calvert CA: Influence of antiarrhythmia therapy on survival times of 19 clinically healthy Doberman Pinschers with dilated cardiomyopathy that experienced synocope, ventricular trachycardia, and sudden death (1995-1998), *J Am Anim Hosp Assoc* 40:24–28, 2004.
254. Pion PD, Kittleson MD, Thomas WP, et al: Response of cats with dilated cardiomyopathy to taurine supplementation, *J Am Vet Med Assoc* 201:275–284, 1992.
255. Smith SA, Tobias AH: Feline arterial thromboembolism: an update, *Vet Clin North Am Small Anim Pract* 34(5):1245–1271, 2004:Sep.
256. Baty CJ: Feline hypertrophic cardiomyopathy: an update, *Vet Clin North Am Small Anim Pract* 34(5):1227–1234, 2004.
256a. Abbott JA: Feline hypertrophic cardiomyopathy: An update, *Vet Clin North Am Small Anim Pract* 40(4):683-670, 2010.

257. Fox PR: Evidence for or against efficacy of β-blockers and aspirin for management of feline cardiomyopathies, *Vet Clin North Am Small Anim Pract* 27(5):1011–1022, 1991.
258. Bright JM, Golden AL, Gompf RE, et al: Evaluation of the calcium channel blocking agents diltiazem and verapamil for treatment of feline hypertrophic cardiomyopathy, *J Vet Int Med* 5:272–282, 1991.
259. Bright JM: Evidence for or against the efficacy of calcium channel blockers for management of hypertrophic cardiomyopathy in cats, *Vet Clin North Am Small Anim Pract* 27(5):1023–1034, 1991.
260. Jugdutt BI: Effects of amlodipine versus enalapril on left ventricular remodelling after reperfused anterior myocardial canine infarction, *Can J Cardiol* 13(10):945–954, 1997.
261. Lupi-Herrera E, Furuya ME, Sandoval J, et al: Effect of hydralazine on vascular mechanics in a canine lobar preparation of pulmonary embolism, *Lung* 70(5):291–309, 1992.
261a. Johnson L, Boon J, Orten C: Clinical characteristics of 53 dogs with Dopper-derived evidence of pulmonary hypertension, *J Vet Intern Med* 13(5):440-447, 1999.
261b. Kellihyan HB, Stepien RL: Pulmonary hypertension in dogs: Diagnosis and therapy, *Vet Clin North Am Small Anim Pract* 40(4):623-641, 2010
262. Bach JF, Rozanski EA, MacGregor J, et al: Retrospective evaluation of sildenafil citrate as a therapy for pulmonary hypertension in dogs, *J Vet Intern Med* 20(5):1132–1135, 2006.
263. Serres F, Nicolle AP, Tissier R, et al: Efficacy of oral tadalafil, a new long-acting phosphodiesterase-5 inhibitor, for the short-term treatment of pulmonary arterial hypertension in a dog, *J Vet Med A Physiol Pathol Clin Med* 53(3):129–133, 2006.
263a. Yamazaki Y, Matsumoto H, Takeda A, et al: Effects of pimobendan on pulmonary hypertension in patients with chronic pulmonary emphysema, *Nihon Kyobu Shikkan Gakkai Zasshi* 35(8):847–853, 1997.
264. Gelzer AR, Kraus MS: Management of atrial fibrillation, *Vet Clin North Am Small Anim Pract* 34(5):1127–1144, 2004.
264a. Dimich I, Lingham R, Narang J, et al: Esmolol prevents and suppresses arrhythmias during halothane anaesthesia in dogs, Can J Anaesth 39(9):83–86, 1992.
265. Chandler JC, Monnet E, Staatz AJ: Comparison of acute hemodynamic effects of lidocaine and procainamide for postoperative ventricular arrhythmias in dogs, *J Am Anim Hosp Assoc* 42:262–268, 2006.
266. Tobias AH: Pericardial diseases. In Ettinger SJ, Feldman EC, editors: *Textbook of veterinary internal medicine*, ed 7, St Louis, 2010, Saunders, pp 1342–1352.
267. Marini JJ, Wheeler AP: *Critical care medicine: the essentials*, Baltimore, 1997, Williams & Wilkins.
267a. Verstegen J, Fargetton X, Zanker S, et al: Antagonistic activities of atipamezole, 4-aminopyridine and yohimbine against medetomidine/ketamine-induced anaesthesia in cats, *Vet Rec* 128 (3):57–60, 1991.
267b. Hatch RC, Zahner JM, Booth NH: Meperidine-acepromazine-pentobarbital anesthesia in cats: reversal by 4-aminopyridine and yohimbine, Am J Vet Res 45 (12):2658–2662, 1984.
267c. Hatch RC, Kitzman JV, Clark JD: Reversal of pentobarbital anesthesia with 4-aminopyridine and yohimbine in cats pretreated with acepromazine and xylazine, Am J Vet Res 45 (12):2586–2590, 1984.
268. Waddell LS, Drobatz KJ, Otto CM: Corticosteroids in hypovolemic shock, *Compend Contin Educ Small Anim Pract* 20:571–588, 1998.
269. Muir WW: Shock, *Compend Contin Educ Small Anim Pract* 20:549–571, 1998.
269a. Dunser MW, Wenzel V, Mayr AJ, et al: Management of vasodilatory shock: defining the role of arginine vasopressin, *Drugs* 63:237–256, 2003.
269b. Efrati O, Barak A, Ben Abraham, et al: Hemodynamic effects of tracheal administration of vasopressin in dogs, *Resuscitation* 50(2):227–232, 2001.
269c. Yoo JH, Park C, Hahm D, et al: Determination of optimal dose of arginine vasopressin in hemorrhagic shock in dogs, *J Vet Med Sci* 69:755–758, 2007.
270. Avontuur JAM, Biewenga M, Buijk SLCE, et al: Pulmonary hypertension and reduced cardiac output during inhibition of nitric oxide synthesis in human septic shock, *Shock* 9: 451–454, 1998.
271. Marino PL: *The ICU Book*, ed 2, Philadelphia, 1997, Lippincott Williams & Wilkins.
272. Wingfield WE: Cardiopulmonary arrest and resuscitation in small animals. Part II: advanced and prolonged life support, *Emerging Sci Technol* Spring:21–31, 1996.
273. Izzat NN, Hawkins EP, Rosborough JP, et al: Renal function following cardiac arrest and resuscitation in the canine, *Resuscitation* 32(3):251–261, 1996.
274. Kingsbury KJ, Bondy G: Understanding the essentials of blood lipid metabolism, *Prog Cardiovascu Nurs* 18(1):13–18, 2003.
275. Mahley RW, Bersot TP: Drug therapy for hypercholesterolemia and dyslipidemia. In Brunton LL, Lazo JS, Parker KL, editors: *Goodman & Gilman's the pharmacological basis of therapeutics*, ed 11, New York, 2006, McGraw-Hill, pp 933–966.
276. Matsukukura Y, Washizu M, Kondo M, et al: Decreased pulmonary arterial endothelium relaxiation in heartworm infected dogs with pulmonary hypertension, *Am J Vet Res* 58:171–174, 1997.
277. Rawlings CA, Calvert CC: Heartworm disease. In Ettinger SJ, Feldman EC, editors: *Textbook of Veterinary Internal Medicine*, ed 4, Philadelphia, 1995, WB Saunders, pp 1046–1068.
277a. Atkins C: Canine heartworm disease. In Ettinger SJ, Feldman EC, editors: *Textbook of Veterinary Internal Medicine*, ed 8, St Louis, 2010, Saunders, pp 1353-1380.
278. Vezzoni A, Genchi C: Reduction of post-adulticide thromboembolism complications with low dose heparin therapy. In Otto GF, editor: *Proceedings of the Heartworm Symposium*, Washington DC, 1989, American Heartwork Society, p 73.
279. Arther RG, Bowman DD, Slone RL, et al: Imidacloprid plus moxidectin topical solution for the prevention of heartworm disease *(Dirofiloria immitis)* in dogs, *Parasitol Res* 97(Suppl 1): S76–S80, 2005.
280. Holm-Martin M, Atwell R: Evaluation of a single injection of a sustained-release formulation of moxidectin for prevention of experimental heartworm infection after 12 months in dogs, *Am J Vet Res* 65(11):1596–1599, 2004.
281. McCall JW: The safety-net story about macrocyclic lactone heartworm preventives: a review, an update, and recommendations, *Vet Parasit* 133(2-3), 2004. State of the Heartworm (AHS Symposium 2004). Proceedings of the 11th Triennial Symposium of the American Heartworm Society 2004, 24 Oct;197–206, 2005.
282. Mealey KL: Canine ABCB1 and macrocyclic lactones: heartworm prevention and pharmacogenetics, *Vet Parasitol* 158(3):215–222, 2008.
283. Snowden NJ, Helyar CV, et al: Clinical presentation and management of moxidectin toxicity in two dogs, *J Small Anim Pract* 47(10):620–624, 2006.
284. Glickman LT, Glickman NW, Moore GE, et al: Safety profile of moxidecting (ProHeart 6) and two oral heartworm preventatives in dogs, *J Appl Res Vet Med* 3(2):49–61, 2005.
285. Raynaud JP: Thiacetarsamide (adulticide) versus melarsomine (RM 340) developed as macrofilaricide (adulticide and larvicide) to cure canine heartworm infection in dogs, *Ann Rech Vet* 23:1–25, 1992.
286. Maksimowich DS, Bell TG, Williams JF, et al: Effect of arsenical drugs on in vitro vascular responses of pulmonary artery from heart worm infected dogs, *Am J Vet Res* 58:389–393, 1997.

287. McCall JW, Genchi C, Kramer L, et al: Heartworm and Wolbachia: therapeutic implications, *Vet Parasitol* 158(3): 204–214, 2008.
288. Blagburn BL: Microfilaricidal therapy: review and update, *Vet Med* 89:630–638, 1994.
289. Arther RG, Atkins C, Ciszewski DK, et al: Safety of imidacloprid plus moxidectin topical solution applied to cats heavily infected with adult heartworms *(Dirofilaria immitis)*, *Parasitol Res* 97(Suppl 1):S70–S75, 2005.
290. Arther RG, Charles S, Ciszewski DK, et al: Imidacloprid/moxidectin topical solution for the prevention of heartworm disease and the treatment and control of flea and intestinal nematodes of cats, *Vet Parasitol* 133(2-3):219–225, 2005.
291. Turner JL, et al: Thiacetarsamide in normal cats: pharmacokinetic, clinical laboratory and pathologic features. In Otto GF, editor: *Proceedings of the Heartworm Symposium*, Washington, DC, 1989, Amerian Heartworm Society, p 135.
292. Dillon AR: The effects of thiacetarsamide administration to normal cats. In Soll MD, editor: *Proceedings of the Heartworm Symposium*, Batavia, Ill, 1992, American Heartworm Society.

15 Drugs Acting on Blood or Blood-Forming Organs

Dawn Merton Boothe

Chapter Outline

DRUGS STIMULATING MEDULLARY POEISIS

Bone Marrow Regulation

The bone marrow contains nonhematopoietic (osteoblasts, of pluripotential stromal origin) and hematopoietic (osteoclasts, of macrophage/monocyte origin) stem cells as well as nonosteogenic cells such as platelets and lymphocytes. Interaction is critical to hematopoiesis, with both nonhematopoietic and nonosteogenic cells contributing to regulation of hematopoietic cells and medullary poiesis. Multiple factors control the commitment, proliferation, and differentiation of bone cell precursors. These include but are not limited to cytokines, growth factors, systemic hormones, and transcriptional regulators. Cell–cell and cell–matrix interactions maintain contact between osteoblastic cells and osteoclast marrow precursors and between the stroma and hematopoietic cells. Among the interacting signals are adhesion molecules, including but not limited to integrins, selectins, and cadherins. Osteoclastogenesis is stimulated by interleukin (IL)-1 and tumor necrosis factor (TNF). The latter is released from marrow mononuclear cell lines in response to NFκB ligand (RANKL), IL-6, IL-11, macrophage colony-stimulating factor (M-CSF) and granulocyte-macrophage colony-stimulating factor (GM-CSF) released from the stroma. Megakaryocytes appear to play a major role in the regulation of hematopoiesis through expression of a number of mediators such as RANKL, n-methyl d aspartate-type glutamate receptors, calcium-sensing receptors, osteonectin, and osteocalcin. Another example is thrombopoietin, which simultaneously regulates megakaryopoeisis and inhibits osteoclastogenesis.[1]

Red Blood Cell Formation

Hematopoiesis

Hematopoiesis occurs through differentiation of stem cells that are formed early in embryonic life. Differentiation occurs in a series of steps in which burst-forming units (BFUs) and colony-forming units (CFUs) are formed for each of the major cell lines. These undifferentiated cells continue to proliferate and differentiate under the influence of a number of cellular and humoral factors that are produced by bone marrow and peripheral tissues.

Erythropoietin (EPO) is the most important regulator of the proliferation of committed erythroid cells (see the discussion of erythropoiesis-stimulating agents [ESAs]) (Figure 15-1).[2] The kidney is the major site of EPO production, where it is released in response to anemia or hypoxia. Among the more important regulators of the myeloid series are granulocyte colony-stimulating factor (G-CSF) and granulocyte/macrophage colony-stimulating factor (GM-CSF). Several vitamins are needed for red and white blood cell formation (hematopoiesis and granulopoiesis, respectively).[2,3]

Drugs Affecting Red Blood Cell Formation

Pharmacologic therapy (Table 15-1) for anemia is oriented toward (1) providing components needed for red blood cell (RBC) production (e.g., proteins, vitamin B_{12}, and folic acid), including hemoglobin synthesis (iron and other minerals); and (2) stimulating bone marrow formation of RBCs.

KEY POINT 15-1 Blood cell formation cannot occur without adequate nutritional support, regardless of the effectiveness of drug therapy.

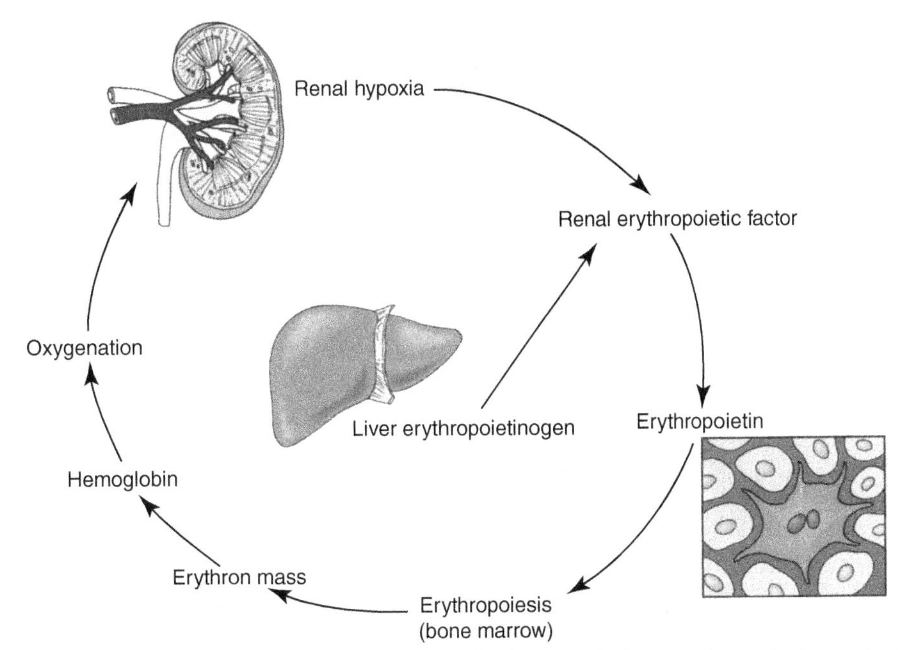

Figure 15-1 Red blood cell formation is stimulated in the kidney. Erythropoietic factor release is stimulated by hypoxia. Erythropoietin stimulates erythroid precursors and the release of reticulocytes into circulation.

Components Needed for Red Blood Cell Production

Vitamin B_{12}

Vitamin B_{12} (cyanocobalamin), the "maturation factor," is essential for DNA synthesis, and its deficiency inhibits nuclear maturation and division. Because cells that rapidly multiply are affected first, reduced RBC proliferation and a "maturation arrest" in the bone marrow are among the first indications of a vitamin B_{12} deficiency. The erythroblast cannot continue to divide, becomes very large, and is referred to as a *megaloblast* (megaloblastic anemia). The mature erythrocyte is also large and is referred to as a *macrocyte*. Although its oxygen-carrying capacity is adequate, the enlarged cell is very fragile because of its large size, and it has a reduced life span.[2,3]

Vitamin B_{12} is a porphyrin-like compound with a ring containing a centrally located cobalt.[2] It can be acquired from both the diet and microbes in the gastrointestinal tract. Most microbial production is in the large intestine, however, where B_{12} is not readily absorbed because it is dependent upon receptor mediated uptake. Dietary deficiency of B_{12} is unlikely and usually results from poor absorption (including pancreatic enzyme deficiency) from the gastrointestinal tract. Absorption of B_{12} is complicated (Figure 15-2) and depends on several factors.[2] Gastric acid and pancreatic enzymes are needed to release B_{12} from dietary and salivary binding proteins.[2] To avoid being digested, B_{12} is protected by binding to intrinsic factor (excreted by the exocrine pancreas in cats[4]) and R protein, which are secreted by the parietal cells. The bound B_{12} complex is carried to the ileum, where B_{12} is adsorbed to highly specific receptor sites on the brush border. Vitamin B_{12} enters the cell by pinocytosis and then enters the blood, where it is bound with transcobalamin, the plasma carrier. Excessive vitamin B_{12} is stored in large quantities in the liver and is slowly released as needed. Vitamin B_{12} is excreted into the bile but undergoes enterohepatic cycling. Interference with absorption by the ileum will result in continuous depletion of B_{12}. Many months of defective vitamin B_{12} absorption are necessary, however, before vitamin B_{12} deficiency occurs. The anemia resulting from B_{12} deficiency is also referred to as *pernicious anemia*. Exclusive uptake of cobalamine in the ileum as led to its detection in serum as a tool for diagnosing disease of the ileum.[4] Deficiency has been described (in cats) by increased serum methylmalonic acid (MMA) coupled with serum cobalamine at or below 100 ng/mL (the lowest detectable concentration). However, the description of clinical and biochemical signs associated with deficiency focused on the gastrointestinal tract and did not address tests indicative of anemia.

Vitamin B_{12} is available as a parenteral preparation in the pure form of cyanocobalamin or the more highly protein bound hydroxocobalamin. Hydroxocobalamin may provide more sustained effects than cyanocobalamin when given by injection.[2] Vitamin B_{12} is also available for oral administration in the pure form or in combination with other vitamins and minerals. Methylcobalamin is another congener of vitamin B_{12} and represents one of the two intracellular active forms of the vitamin (the other being deoxyadenosylcobalamin).[2] Foods high in vitamin B_{12} include selected microbial sources and animal (meat) products. There are no significant toxicities associated with therapy. Indications for B_{12} therapy are limited to situations of B_{12} malabsorption such as ileectomy, gastrectomy, malabsorption syndromes, or chronic administration of cimetidine or other antisecretory drugs because an acid environment is necessary for release of B_{12} from the diet and for intrinsic factor activity. In one study[4] response to cobalamin treatment (250 μg subcutaneously once weekly in cats (n = 19) with gastrointestinal disease was prospectively studied, with a focus on indicators

Table **15-1** Doses of Drugs Acting on Blood or Blood-Forming Units

Drug	Dose	Route	Frequency (Days)
Aspirin	0.5 mg/kg (normal dogs)	PO	12
(antithrombotic)	5-10 mg/kg (heartworm)	PO	24
Clopidogrel	1-2 mg/kg (D)	PO	24
	Load: 10 mg/kg (D)	PO	For acute effect
	18.75-75 mg/kg (cat)	PO	12
Danazol	5-10 mg/kg (dog)	PO	12
	5 mg/kg (cat)	PO	12
Desmopressin acetate	0.4 μg/kg	SC	24
nasal drop (0.01% spray)	2-4 drops	Nasal mucosa	
	0.1-0.2 mg	PO*	
Erythropoietin (rhEPO)	50-100 U/kg	SC	3/wk†
Fluoxymesterone	0.2-1 mg/kg	PO	1
Folic acid	5 mg (dog)	PO	24
	2.5 mg (cat)	PO	24
Folinic acid	1 mg/kg	PO	24
Heparin‡			
Heartworms	50-70 U/kg	SC	8
	10-100 U/kg	IV (load)§	
	5-10 U/kg	IV infusion	Every hour
Thromboembolism	100-300 U/kg	IV (load)	
	10-50 U/kg	IV infusion	
DIC, mild	5-10 U/kg	SC	8
	75-200 U/kg	SC	8
DIC, severe	300-500 U/kg	SC	8
	750-1000 U/kg	SC	8
Nandrolone decanoate	1-5 mg/kg	IM	7
Nandrolone phenylproprionate	1 mg/kg	IM	7
	25-50 mg/kg (dog)	IM	7-14
	10-20 mg/kg (cat)	IM	7-14
Oxymetholone	1 mg/kg	PO	1
Protamine‖	1-1.5 mg/1 mg heparin	IV	
Stanozolol¶	0.25-3 mg/kg	PO	1
	2-10 mg/kg	IM	7
Testosterone			
Proprionate	2.2 mg/kg	IM	7
Enanthate	4-7 mg/kg	IM	7
Vitamin B_{12}	100-200 μg (dog)	PO, SC	
	50-100 μg (cat)	PO, SC	
Vitamin K_1 (phytonadione)	1 mg/kg (liver disease)	PO	24
	0.125-1.25 mg/kg coumarin or short-acting rodenticides	IM, SC, PO	12
	5 mg/kg (loading dose) (indandione) or long-acting rodenticides	SC, PO	—
	2.5 mg/kg	SC, PO	24
Warfarin†	0.1-0.2 mg/kg (dog)	PO	24
	0.5 mg/kg (cat)	PO	24

PO, By mouth; *SC,* subcutaneous; *IV,* intravenous; *DIC,* disseminated intravascular coagulation; *IM,* intramuscular.
*Dose for the oral preparation has not been substantiated. As of this writing, the acetate preparation is no longer available in the United States.
†Monitor packed cell volume twice weekly for the first several months, and modify dose as appropriate.
‡Adjust dose by monitoring activated partial thromboplastin time to 1.5 to 2.5 times baseline.
§Or in blood products, incubated for 30 minutes before administration.
‖No more than 50 mg/10 min. Dose is reduced if time lapses between heparin overdose and protamine administration.
¶Approved for use in dogs and cats.

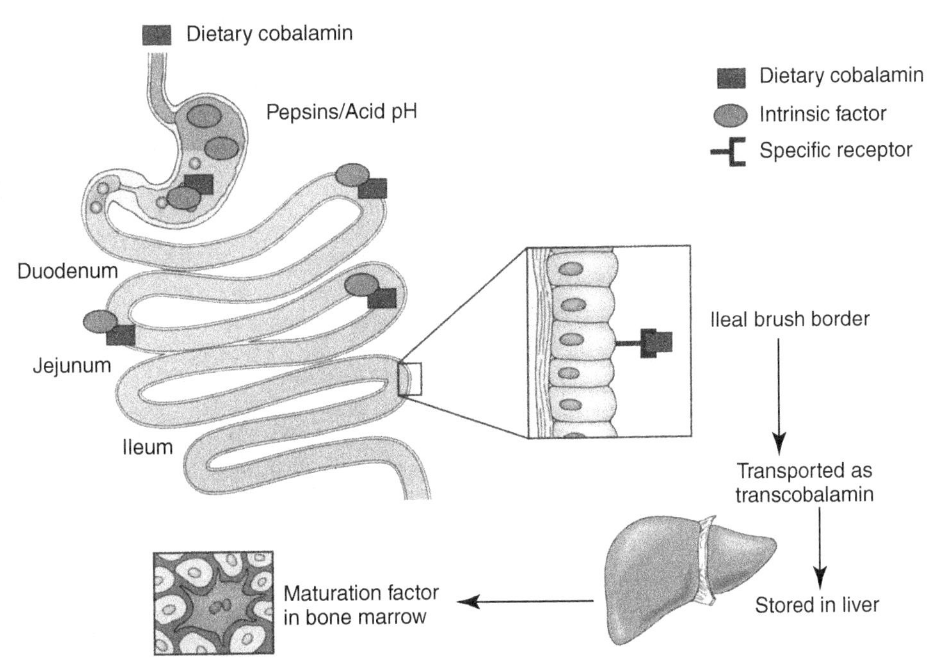

Figure 15-2 The absorption of vitamin B_{12} from the gastrointestinal tract is complicated and depends on the release of intrinsic factor and hydrochloric acid from the stomach. The drug complexes with a receptor. This complex is protected as it passes to the ileum, where it is absorbed by receptor-mediated pinocytosis.

of gastrointestinal health. Indicators of cobalamin deficiency (serum MMA, cysteine) improved and were correlated with weight gain and folic acid use, however, improvements in indices of red blood cell health were not addressed.

Folic Acid

Folic acid (pteroylglutamic acid) is a cofactor needed for DNA synthesis because it promotes the formation of a nucleotide necessary for DNA formation. Folic acid is also necessary for RNA synthesis, and it serves as a methyl donor for the formation of vitamin B_{12}.[2] Folic acid is acquired from the diet, although it can also be formed by microbes. Dietary sources include yeast, liver, kidney, and green vegetables. Folic acid is also stored in the liver but not as avidly as is vitamin B_{12}. It undergoes enterohepatic circulation but is destroyed daily by catabolic processes. Daily requirements are high, and serum levels will fall rapidly several days after dietary deficiency. Gastrointestinal absorption of folic acid is not as complex as that of vitamin B_{12}, although it requires protein digestion and the presence of dihydrofolate reductase in the small intestine. Jejunal pathology can result in folate deficiency. The degree of folic acid binding to plasma proteins is not well understood.

Folic acid is available as both a parenteral and an oral (pure or combined product) form. The minimum daily requirement in humans is 50 μg/day, but this can increase to 100 to 200 or more in patients with high cell turnover rates (e.g., hemolytic anemia).[2] In humans the most popular form of folic acid supplementation is as part of a multivitamin preparation containing 400 to 500 μg of pteroylglutamic acid. In high disease states, 1 to 2 1-mg tablets are consumed. This dose may be the source of the recommended dose for cats and dogs. Compared with commercially available products, the dose recommended for small animals seems excessive, and it is not clear that such a high dose is necessary. There are, however, no apparent significant toxicities associated with therapy.

Indications for therapy are inadequate intake as a result of the administration of several drugs (methotrexate, potentiated sulfonamide antibiotics, some anticonvulsants such as phenytoin), liver diseases, malabsorption, or other chronic debilitating diseases.. Folinic acid (leucovorin) is a formyl derivative of tetrahydrofolic acid and as such does not require the action of dihydrofolate reductase in order to act as a folate by contributing a carbon moiety. In humans, administration of folinic acid increases serum folate activity owing to 5-methyltetrahydrofolate. Folinic acid apparently serves as a substrate for inhibitors of dihydrofolate reductase such as methotrexate, or diaminopyrimidines such as trimethoprim or ormetoprim, and as such, can resolve some deficiencies associated with folic acid deficiency. However, it will not replace deficient folic acid or any of its derivatives prior to the tetrahydrofolate step in folic acid use.[2] As such, leucovorin can be used clinically to circumvent the actions of dihydrofolate reductase (e.g., methotrexate) and replace materials in the folic acid pathway beyond tetrahydrofolate, but can not prevent folic acid deficiency. Leucovoran also inhibits thymidylate synthtase and as such, facilitates anticancer efficacy of 5-fluorouracil.

Hemoglobin Synthesis: Iron

Hemoglobin consists of a heme portion and a globin portion. The heme portion is formed from a pyrrole ring, four of which combine to form a protoporphyrin compound. This in turn combines with iron to form heme. Four hemes combine with the globulin globin to form hemoglobin. Several factors are necessary for hemoglobin formation.

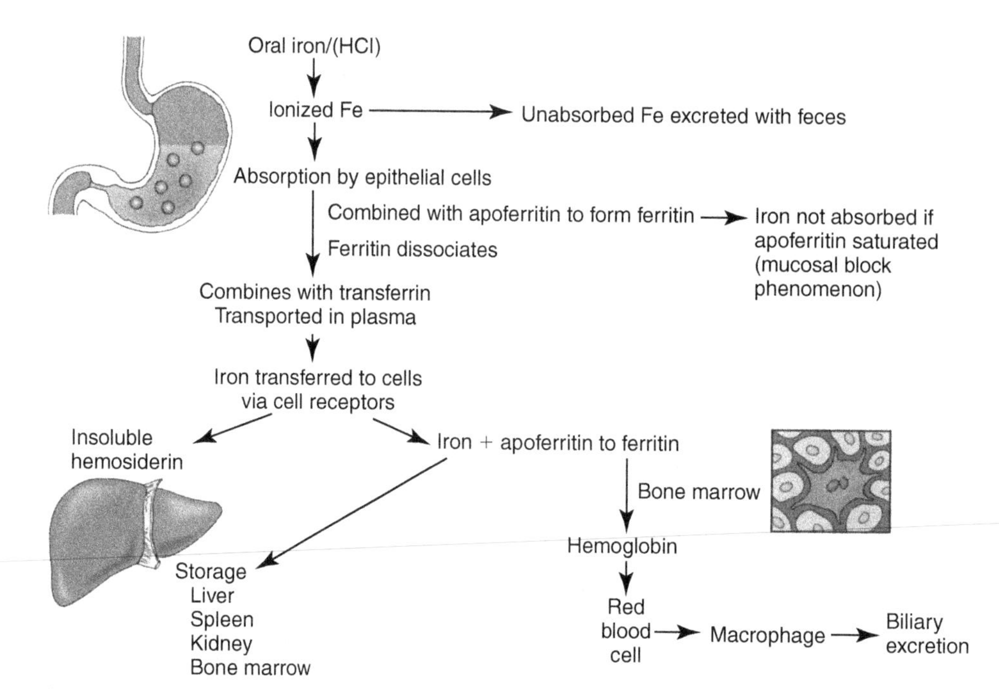

Figure 15-3 Absorption of usable iron from the gastrointestinal tract is maximized in an acidic environment. Iron combines with apoferritin in cells to form ferritin, the soluble form of iron. Iron is bound to transferrin in plasma. Saturation of apoferritin leads to saturation of transferrin. Excessive iron is stored as hemosiderin, a nonsoluble form of iron. In the presence of saturation, iron is eliminated in the gastrointestinal tract.

Iron is a component of hemoglobin, myoglobin, and other substances, such as those found in cytochrome and electron transport systems.[2,3] Approximately 65% of total body iron is present in hemoglobin, 4% as myoglobin, and 1% in cytochromes and electron transport systems. The remaining 15% to 30% is stored as either ferritin, the soluble form of iron stores, or hemosiderin, the insoluble stores. Oral absorption of iron is slow, complicated, and not well understood (Figure 15-3). It is available in the diet in either a heme form, which makes up a small percentage of the total but readily absorbed form, or in a nonheme (ferric oxide) form. The nonheme form represents the largest dietary fraction, but its absorption is profoundly affected by dietary factors. Nonheme iron must be converted to the ferrous form for absorption to occur; conversion depends on an acidic environment. Absorption of iron is increased by hydrochloric acid and decreased in situations that decrease acid production in the stomach (e.g., chronic use of antisecretory drugs).

Iron is absorbed primarily from the proximal jejunum, where it immediately combines in the enterocyte with apoferritin to form ferritin. When transferred out of the enterocyte, ferritin dissociates, and iron combines with the globulin transferrin. Iron is transported in the plasma in this form, but the binding is loose so iron can be easily transferred to tissues. Iron is transferred to cells by way of specific receptors that interact with transferrin, especially in the liver. In cells, iron again combines with apoferritin to become ferritin. Small quantities are also stored as the very insoluble hemosiderin; the quantity of this storage form increases when the total quantity of iron in the body is much more than apoferritin can accommodate. When apoferritin is saturated, transferrin cannot release iron, and it thus becomes close to 100% bound (estimated iron stores).

There is no mechanism for the excretion of iron other than by the gastrointestinal tract. Gastrointestinal tract elimination occurs by (1) exfoliation of enterocytes containing iron, (2) biliary elimination, and (3) elimination in diet of iron not absorbed. Total body iron is regulated by altering the rate of absorption. If all the apoferritin in the enterocyte is combined with iron, the amount of iron in the enterocyte is high, and absorption from the diet is slowed. Absorption is faster if iron stores are depleted. This mechanism has been referred to as the *mucosal block phenomenon*.

Preparations. Iron is available in both oral and parenteral preparations. Oral preparations are prepared as ferrous (bivalent) or ferric (trivalent) salts. Ferrous salts tend to be the treatment of choice for oral supplementation and are dosed according to their iron content.[2] Examples of bivalent ferrous salts include sulfate (20% iron), gluconate (12%), and fumarate (33%). The ferrous bivalent salts are more soluble in the gastric environment and are absorbed three times faster than the trivalent salts. The efficacy of polysaccharide oral iron products approximates that of ferrous products. Slow-release iron products have not been well studied. These products may be continued for several months; toxicities and side effects are dose related.

KEY POINT 15-2 Response of anemia to iron supplementation should be anticipated only if the cause is iron deficiency. Excessive iron therapy should be avoided because excessive iron cannot be easily excreted.

Parenteral preparations are indicated if oral preparations cannot be tolerated or are not feasible. Iron dextran administered by intramuscular injection generally is preferred. Parenteral administration results in a more rapid accumulation of iron stores, which may take months (in humans) with oral therapy. Other indications for parenteral therapy include diseases of the gastrointestinal tract that preclude iron absorption or that will exacerbate another disease (e.g., inflammatory bowel disease) or intolerance of oral supplementation.[2] Much of the iron given intramuscularly remains at the site of injection for several months. The remaining iron enters the plasma but must first be phagocytized by reticuloendothelial cells for processing. This may take several months, and evaluation of total body iron may be difficult until all of the iron is processed.[2]

In human patients iron injection is preceded by a test dose (approximately 0.5 mL). It is given only in a large muscle mass and is associated with long-term discomfort, local skin discoloration, and a perceived risk of malignant change at the site of injection. Selected iron dextran preparations also can be administered intravenously. Dosing is based on a conversion of body weight (0.66 × weight in kilograms) and on the patient's hemoglobin level compared with the desired hemoglobin level (14.8 g/dL).[2] After an initial 0.5-mL test dose, the calculated dose is given in 2-mL increments each day until completed. Side effects associated with intravenous administration include malaise, fever, arthralgias, urticaria, and generalized lymphadenopathy.[2]

Drug interactions. Several drugs, including tetracyclines and antacids, and several foods bind to and precipitate iron when given orally. Absorption is enhanced in the presence of ascorbic acid because it reduces ferric iron to its ferrous state and prevents formation of insoluble and unabsorbable iron compounds.[5]

Clinical use. Indications for iron therapy are limited to treatment or prevention of iron deficiency such as occurs with blood loss or successful therapy with anabolic steroids or recombinant EPO in a patient suffering from chronic anemia. The efficacy of "shotgun" products is questionable. As with any hematinic preparation, provision of these compounds will be ineffective if the nutritional status of the animal is poor. Shotgun preparations are products that contain a combination of hematinic agents such as vitamin B_{12}, folic acid, pyridoxine, riboflavin, nicotinic acid, pantothenic acid, thiamine, biotin, ascorbic acid, and vitamin E. The need for inclusion of all of these products is not clear. An exception might be made for ascorbic acid, which enhances oral absorption of iron, and pyridoxine, which is useful in human patients with selected anemias. One human patient with pure red cell aplasia has responded to riboflavin. Occasionally, these products might be considered dangerous because some additives may be sufficiently high to mask clinical signs of other nutrient deficiencies that ultimately may become life threatening.[2]

Bone Marrow Stimulation

Erythropoiesis-Stimulating Agents

EPO, an endogenous glycosylated protein hormone (MW 30,000 daltons), is the most important regulator of committed erythroid progenitor proliferation.[2] Extensive glycosylation is responsible for the activity of the molecule.[6] The kidney (peritubular cell) is the primary source of endogenous EPO, although the liver produces a small amount in some species. Insufficient oxygen delivery to tissues is the primary stimulus for promotion of the transcription and thus production and secretion of EPO[2] (see Figure 15-1). Hypoxia or anemia will increase synthesis by a hundredfold or more. However, renal disease, damage to the bone marrow, or deficiencies of iron or other essential vitamins can impair synthesis. Inflammatory cytokines also impair secretion (as well as iron delivery). Prostaglandins appear to increase and nonsteroidal anti-inflammatory drugs appear to decrease EPO production.

KEY POINT 15-3 Formation of antibodies to foreign erythropoietin may lead to therapeutic failure as long as 12 months after the beginning of therapy. As such, treatment should be reserved for states of erythropoietin deficiency or for those limited indications for which efficacy has been demonstrated through well-designed clinical trials. Iron deficiency might be anticipated in some animals.

Mechanism of Action

Once released from the renal cell, EPO travels to the bone marrow, where it binds to receptors on the surface of committed erythroid progenitors. The influence of EPO (including ESAs) on RBC production occurs at several steps. EPO binding initiates changes in intracellular phosphorylation.[2] Additionally, EPO stimulates proliferation and differentiation of erythroid precursors, including BFU–erythroid CFUs: erythroid, erythroblasts, and reticulocytes.[2] Recombinant human EPO also stimulates the release of reticulocytes from the bone marrow into the blood, where they subsequently mature.[7-11]

Preparations

Human EPO has been isolated and cloned and can be synthesized in large quantities with recombinant techniques using a mammalian (hamster cell line). ESAs include two recombinant EPO (rEPO) products. Epoetin is a recombinant human product (rhEPO), available in two products that differ in their glycosylated carbohydrate patterns: alpha (Epogen, Eprex) and beta (Procrit). A second ESA is darbepoetin, a recombinant hyperglycosylated analog of the human protein, often referred to as a *second-generation EPO*. Hyperglycosylation increases stability. Darbepoetin is dosed in μg/kg, whereas epoetin is dosed as units/kg for epoetin: a dose of 6.25 to 12.5 μg/kg of darbepoetin is equivalent in humans to a dose of 2500 to 5000 units/kg of rhEPO (0.0025 μg darbepoetin to 1 unit epoetin).[12] Albumin is included as a vehicle in both epoetin alpha and darbepoetin. However, because of the concern regarding potential transmission of disease carried by albumin, alternative vehicles such as polysorbate 80 have been used to formulate epoetin beta.[13] Products are intended for intravenous or subcutaneous administration. Both canine (rcEPO)[14] and feline (rfEPO)[15] recombinant products have been developed but are not yet commercially available. Canine EPO is more closely homologous to feline EPO compared with rhEPO and will be preferred in cats should rcEPO approval precede the feline product.

Disposition

The disposition of ESAs has not been well characterized in either humans or animals. Glycosylation (addition of carbohydrates) prolongs elimination compared with the endogenous proteins. In humans the elimination half-life of rh-EPO is about 6 to 9 hours after intravenous administration, with a very small volume of distribution (0.055 L/kg). As with most endocrine products, plasma half-life may not necessarily reflect biological half-life.[9,11] Glycosylation of darbepoetin is greater than that of epoetin, leading to an accordingly longer (threefold) biological half-life in humans. Dosing subsequently can be reduced to every other day (3 times weekly).[2]

Adverse Effects

Antibody formation. Use of ESAs is associated with immunogenicity, and relevant side effects should be anticipated when administering foreign protein products intended to mimic endogenous protein products.[16] Pure red cell aplasia (PRCA) is a recognized, albeit rare, sequela of rEPO in humans.[17] In 1998 a formulation was approved internationally that varied from the U.S. product by vehicle, storage, and handling. The use of the product was associated with an increased incidence of PRCA, leading to the assumption that the differences increased the immunogenicity of the product.[18] The increased frequency of disease facilitated its characterization.Clinically manifested as a rapid onset of severe anemia, refractoriness to rhEPO therapy, and a low reticulocyte count, PRCA is associated with high concentration of EPO-neutralizing antibodies, probably of IgG origin.[6,19] Diagnosis is confirmed by the presences of EPO neutralizing antibodies in circulation, absence of bone marrow red cells and normal to elevated transferrin saturation. Testing no longer appears to be available for either eryropoietin or antibodies for dogs or cats. In one study, greater than 95% of human cases afflicted with chronic renal disease received the drug subcutaneously for a mean of nine months before the onset of PRCA. Antibodies resolved in 80% of patients when the drug was discontinued but only in the presence of immunosuppressive therapy.[13,17,19] A lower incidence of PRCA was found in patients with cancer chemotherapy–related anemia, probably because anticancer therapy led to immunosuppression.[13] The incidence of PRCA has been reduced by methods intended to reduce immunogenicity. These included changes in processing that contributed to immunogenicity (such as freeze drying), changes in packaging (replacement of rubber stoppers with Teflon, removal of silicone lubricant in prefilled syringes), and a shift from subcutaneous to intravenous administration.[13] Darbepoetin may be associated with less immunogenicity compared with rhEPO, as is shown by response in one human patient to darbepoetin despite development of rhEPO-induced PRCA.[20]

Because of the foreign nature of EPO, adverse effects reported in humans also should occur with rhEPO administration in animals. Local and systemic allergic reactions include cellulitis, fever, arthralgia, and mucocutaneous ulcerations, which occurred in 12% of animals treated in a pilot study.[21-23] Signs resolve with drug withdrawal but may reappear when treatment is resumed. Because antibodies directed toward the foreign rhEPO may stimulate production of antibodies targeted toward endogenous EPO, RBCs, hematocrit, and hemoglobin may progressively decrease starting as early as 2 weeks of therapy.[21-23] Antibodies are indicated by a bone marrow myeloid-to-erythroid cell ratio of less than 8. Discontinuation of rhEPO will result in resolution of antibody formation and, to some degree, the anemia (i.e., that caused by antibodies), but drug therapy cannot be reinstituted.[22] The incidence of antibody formation is high, developing in 63% to 100% of healthy dogs receiving EPO.[24] Red cell aplasia was associated with anti-Epogen antibodies in two out of three dogs treated longer than 90 days and seven out of eight cats treated for 180 days or more. For the cats, 70% were refractory to further EPO therapy, requiring transfusion therapy until anti-epoetin antibody concentrations decreased (2 to 4 months after rhEPO was discontinued. Because both exogenous and native EPO may be impaired, aplastic anemia resulting from bone marrow failure may ultimately occur. Immunosuppressive therapy directed toward antibody formation, although apparently successful in humans, has not been addressed in veterinary medicine. Antibodies generally require 2 to 12 months after therapy is discontinued for eradication. Species specificity of rEPO should minimize the advent of anti-EPO antibodies as has been demonstrated for both the dog[24,25] and cat.[15] Randolph and coworkers[15] have demonstrated that the feline recombinant product not only does not induce antibodies but also will re-establish erythropoiesis in most cases of rhEPO-induced red cell aplasia. Unfortunately, the same does not appear to be true for the canine recombinant preparation[25] in dogs, suggesting that even species-specific origin of rEPO may be associated with antibodies.

Miscellaneous adverse effects. Other adverse effects that may require monitoring in patients receiving EPO include systemic hypertension, iron deficiency, hyperkalemia, and polycythemia.[8] Flulike symptoms occur in some human patients receiving the drug intravenously. Hypertension occurs in many human patients with renal disease as the hematocrit normalizes. Patients who begin the use of rhEPO when in a state of hypertension are likely to experience a further increase in blood pressure. The mechanism of hypertension is not known but may include increased blood viscosity or peripheral vasoconstriction. Blood pressure increases within as little as 2 weeks of therapy and tends to stabilize by month 4. Increased blood pressure has been reported in 40% to 50% of dogs or cats treated with ESAs.[26] It may be necesary to adjust drug therapy for hypertension (e.g., increase amlodipine dose).[27] Polycythemia is another likely sequela of ESAs if response to therapy is not monitored on the basis of packed cell volume (PCV).[27] Other miscellaneous adverse effects of rhEPO in dogs and cats include seizures (one in six dogs, two of eleven cats[26]), particularly in animals with moderate to severe azotemia and as a terminal clinical sign.[27] Depleted iron stores should be anticipated in patients with iron deficiency (discussed later).[22] Pain on subcutaneous injection (a route being used less frequently in humans in order to minimize PRCA) varies with products, with the alpha (e.g., Eprex) being more painful in humans than the beta (Procrit). In an animal model involving renal ablation, rhEPO actually hastened the progression of chronic renal disease. However, the clinical relevance of this finding has not been documented.

Indications and Clinical Use

The primary indication for ESAs in humans is anemia of chronic renal disease (CRD).[7,8,21,23,28] Most human patients receiving renal dialysis also receive ESAs. Indications in animals are likely to be similar to those in humans, particularly for renal disease, because clinical signs of weakness, somnolence, depression, and poor appetite associated with CRD in cats (and presumably dogs) is due to anemia. Decisions must be made regarding the product (epoetin, alpha or beta, versus darbepoetin), route (intravenous versus subcutaneous), and dosing regimen (dose and interval). Subcutaneous administration of epoetin—which can cause pain on administration—has been associated with better response in humans, although it appears to be more immunogenic. In contrast, darbepoetin appears to be equally efficacious regardless of the route.[29] Preference among the ESA products is not yet clear; evaluation of darbopoetin currently is ongoing.[30] Advantages of darbopoetin may include faster response time, particularly with front end loading, decreased dosing intervals, and decreased risk of immunogenicity. The average dose of darbepoetin used in human patients with CRD or cancer ranged from 3.5 to 5 µg/kg 1 to 3 times per week; preliminary studies indicate that administration as infrequent as once every 3 weeks may be sufficient.

Because it has been available longer, more information is available regarding rhEPO use in both humans and animals. In humans with CRD, rhEPO normalizes the hematocrit, hemoglobin concentration, and RBCs after administration of 15 to 300 U/kg rhEPO 3 times weekly. Some human patients have required 500 U/kg. A stair-step approach has been used for nonresponding CRD in human patients in that the dosage continues to be increased until the desired response is achieved.[8] When the desired response is achieved (a hematocrit of 30% to 40%), a smaller maintenance dose (25 to 100 U/kg three times a week) is given to maintain the hematocrit above 30%.[8] Normalizing the PCV in patients with underlying renal disease may be associated with a greater risk of cardiovascular side effects.[31] Because of convenience and cost, in humans the maintenance dose generally has been given subcutaneously, whereas the induction dose is often given intravenously. However, intravenous administration increasingly is being used for maintenance dosing to minimize the risk of immunogenicity (in human patients).[18] The intravenous route in humans has the added advantage of convenience in those individuals with chronic access ports (i.e., human patients undergoing dialysis), a situation that is less likely in animals.

Erythropoetin therapy is indicated in dogs or cats with a PCV of 20% to 25% or less owing to renal disease (see Table 15-1). To date, of the commercially available products, reports (whether scientific or anecdotal) of use in animals are limited to alpha EPO. Recombinant human EPO has been used in small animals with chronic anemia.[21,22,23] When administered in uremic animals with CRD, the hematocrit of most patients normalizes within 3 to 4 weeks of therapy, and the clinical well-being of patients improves. Response to therapy is indicated by reticulocytosis, and an increase in hematocrit of 0.5% to 1% each day. Hypokalemia associated with uremia in cats should also resolve, in part because of improved appetite.[22] White blood cells and platelets do not seem to be affected. Caution is indicated for patients that are hypertensive before rhEPO therapy. Informed consent should be obtained before use because of the high incidence of antibody formation. Initial treatment should begin at 100 U/kg (or, if a slower increase is acceptable, 50 to 75 U/kg) subcutaneously 3 times a week until the target hematocrit (originally 37% to 45% in dogs or 30% to 40% in cats; more recently 30% to 35% for dogs and 25% to 30% in cats) has been reached.[27] Generally, response requires approximately 4 weeks. The PCV should be measured twice weekly for the first several months of therapy. The dose is decreased to a maintenance dose of 50 to 100 U/kg and the frequency of administration to twice weekly once the target PCV has been achieved. The dose should be titrated to maintain the PCV in the mid-target range. If the PCV does not increase sufficiently, the dose of rhEPO can be increased in 25- to 50-U/kg increments. The maintenance dose will vary for each patient. A maximum dose has not been established in animals, although weekly doses of 300 to 1050 U/kg have been reported.[22]

Among the more common causes of ESA therapeutic failure in humans is iron deficiency. Iron therapy generally is begun along with rhEPO. Iron therapy is not easily monitored. In humans serum ferritin and transferrin iron saturation are the most common tests used.[32] An increasing percentage of hypochromic red blood cells and decreasing content of hemoglobin in reticulocytes may also reveal iron deficiency but will not reveal iron overload. Iron gluconate and iron sucrose are considered the safest of the intravenous iron medications.[32] However, because intravenous iron dextran therapy is more expensive and is associated with anaphylactic therapy, oral iron therapy is preferred.[2,8] Further, the body can control iron content with oral but not intravenous administration. Differences in the gastrointestinal absorption of iron may alter response to rhEPO therapy. Addition of 200 mg of oral iron, however, appears to successfully maintain adequate iron stores in human patients with CRD receiving rhEPO. Oral iron supplementation in dogs is recommended at 100 to 300 mg of ferrous sulfate daily (20- to 60-mg elemental iron) and for cats 50 to 100 mg (10 to 20 elemental).[27] Iron dextran (10 to 20 mg/kg for dogs and 50 mg total dose for cats) is recommended by intramuscular administration (deep) for animals that cannot tolerate oral supplementation. Note that oral absorption of iron may not occur until serum ferritin is below 30 to 50 ng/mL (human patients). Erythropoiesis improves, however, even in human patients whose transferrin saturation is above that diagnostic of iron deficiency (16%).[33]

Anemias other than that associated with CRD also may be associated with decreased levels of endogenous EPO in animals and thus might respond to supplementation. However, the potential application of these indications in veterinary medicine must be balanced by the lack of scientific support and the adversities that are more likely in animals compared with humans if rh-EPO is used (e.g., antibody production). These have been reviewed by Langston and coworkers[27] and others.[2,34] An enzyme-linked immunosorbent assay (ELISA) kit developed to detect canine EPO may be helpful in identifying the need for supplementation although access at the time of publication is not known.[35]

The most common nonrenal use of ESAs in humans is anticipation of autologous blood transfusion; use of rhEPO increased the number of autologous units collected, and pretreatment may decrease the need for allogenic transfusion therapy. Although the need is less clear, a similar approach should be of benefit in animals; experimentally, pretreatment with iron and rhEPO in dogs resulted in higher hematocrit levels after transfusion than those in pretreatment with iron and saline.[27] Selected (nonmyeloid) cancer anemias associated with chemotherapy may respond to EPO supplementation, including multiple myeloma and myelodysplastic diseases (the latter defined on the basis of cytopenia, dysplastic hematopoietic precursor cells and less than 30% blasts in the bone marrow).[2,27,34] Anemia associated with cancer may reflect an inadequate EPO response; in humans the ratio of measured to predicted EPO (the latter based on population studies) of less than 0.9 is interpreted as an indication of potential response. Response may be related to dose: One retrospective study of multiple myeloma in humans reported a higher overall survival in patients who received a high dose (greater than 60,000 U/week) rather than a lower routine dose.[36] The use of ESAs in human cancer patients has been reviewed,[38] and guidelines for such use have been published.[38,39]

A combination of rhEPO and immunosuppressive therapy apparently was not successful in cats with pure red cell aplasia (not associated with previous rhEPO therapy) but may have prolonged survival rates of dogs with myelofibrosis.[27] An interesting and potentially relevant application of ESA is for patients in the intensive care unit. In human patients in the intensive care unit, blood loss, including that associated with repetitive phlebotomy for diagnostic testing, can be significant. The veterinary patient—particularly the smaller one—may be similarly predisposed. Relative EPO deficiencies in these patients further predispose to anemias, as is indicated by transferrin saturations of less than 20% in the majority of patients. The use of rhEPO decreases the number of transfusions needed in these patients. The use of exogenous EPO in viral immunosuppressive diseases is tempting but controversial and might best be based on demonstration of endogenous EPO deficiency. Whereas endogenous EPO appears to be low and thus exogenous therapy is of benefit in human patients with HIV-associated anemia, EPO concentrations are increased in feline patients with feline leukemia virus.[27] However, the PCV increased after 2 weeks of rhEPO in nonanemic cats positive for feline immunodeficiency virus; antibodies did not appear with this short-course therapy. Other uses of rhEPO in dogs have been characterized by variable success. The use of rHEPO in racing animals is likely to be associated with the production of antibodies and therefore is discouraged not only for ethical and legal reasons but also for health reasons. Human growth factors (granulopoietin and EPO) were associated with bone marrow recovery in a dog with ehrlichiosis.[40] However, therapy took several months before response in peripheral counts were realized. The use of EPO in patients with pancytopenia associated with parvovirus is controversial, particularly in light of one case of fulminant infection in a human patient with immunodeficiency who was subsequently treated with rhEPO.[41] Evaluating response of drug-induced bone marrow depression to rHEPO is complicated by the impact of discontinuing the inciting drug.

Therapeutic Failure

The most likely reason for a patient not to respond to rhEPO is inappropriate therapy. If the anemia is not associated with CRD, rhEPO therapy may be ineffective if endogenous rhEPO concentrations are maximally increased. Failure in a patient with low endogenous rhEPO may occur for several reasons. The dosage may be insufficient. Failure of an anemic animal to respond to rhEPO may indicate the development of antibodies directed toward rhEPO, as previously discussed.[22] Animals that develop antibodies should recover, with antibodies potentially resolving within 3 to 4 weeks in dogs. Recovery may depend in part on the severity of renal disease, with recovery less likely in those animals with severe renal disease. In humans pure red cell aplasia as a result of antibody formation may be treated with a low dose (3.3 mg/kg) of cyclosporine.[6,42] Differences in vehicles, stabilizers, and handling were identified as possible contributors to autoantibodies in human patients with renal disease who were receiving recombinant EPO; changes in response to these problems has dramatically reduced the incidence of antibody formation.[16] Response to ESAs is likely to require iron supplementation.[22] Chronic inflammatory disease decreases response to rhEPO, as do myelophthisic diseases that replace bone marrow with fibrous tissue. Alternatively, anemia may persist because patient nutrition is not sufficient to support increased EPO.

Granulopoietin and Related Products

At least six growth factors influence granulopoiesis.[2] Formation of both granulocytes and macrophages from multipotential stem cells is stimulated by stem cell factor, a glycoprotein produced by bone marrow stromal cells; IL-1 and IL-6, inflammatory cytokines that mediate many of the systemic manifestations of acute inflammation; and IL-3. GM-CSF, along with G-CSF, is produced by a variety of tissues in response to cytokines such as IL-1, TNF, and endotoxin.[2,5] Supplementation with exogenous factors stimulates the proliferation of various cell types, with the type affected depending on the factor or combination of factors. IL-3 increases both platelets and granulocytes, and GM-CSF administered by itself stimulates granulocyte and macrophage proliferation. When given in combination with IL-3, however, GM-CSF stimulates thrombopoiesis, and when combined with EPO and IL-3, erythropoiesis is stimulated as well.[43]

As with EPO, recombinant products have been developed for therapeutic stimulation of granulopoiesis. Both recombinant canine (rcGSF) and recombinant feline (rfGSF) G-CSF have been cloned, but neither is commercially available at this time. Feline GSF has much closer homology with rcGSF than with rhGSF and thus is the preferred product. Despite their lack of availability, the factors are increasingly being studied for treatment of neutrophil disorders in dogs and cats.[5,44]

In normal dogs G-CSF (5 μg/kg per day) will increase neutrophil counts over fourfold within 24 hours, reaching a maximum of approximately 72,000/mL by 19 days, with counts returning to normal within 5 days after discontinuation of therapy.[44] In dogs afflicted with cyclic neutropenia, rcGSF (2.5 μg/kg every 12 hours) prevents neutropenia and associated clinical signs, although cycling of neutrophils is not prevented. Chemotherapy-induced neutropenia (induced by mitoxantrone) was minimized in dogs receiving rcGSF for 20 days. Studies in normal cats receiving rcCSF reveal an approximately threefold increase in neutrophil count that persists until the drug is discontinued. No adverse effects occur.[44] Cohn et al.[45] demonstrated that plasma G-CSF concentrations increased just after the onset of neutropenia in puppies (n = 8) experimentally exposed (oronasal) to parvovirus. Neutrophil counts rebounded within 2 to 3 days, and G-CSF concentrations decreased before neutropenia resolved, questioning the benefits of exogenous therapy. However, recombinant human G-CSF did correct canine cyclic hematopoiesis in one study.[46]

Other compounds have been studied for their effect on granulopoiesis. An extract of *Serratia marcescens* activates interferon- α and interferon-γ, as well as IL-1, IL-6, and GM-CSF, and induces myeloproliferation either directly or through release of other cytokines.[44]

Vincristine

Vincristine has demonstrated efficacy in the treatment of thrombocytopenia. Its mechanism is not clear, but several have been proposed. These include decreased upregulation of glycoprotein receptors on platelets, thereby reducing interaction with von Willebrand factor (vWF) and platetet aggregation, or reduction in immunglobulin G (IgG) autoantibodies that damage endothelial cells or suppress von Willebrand factor–cleaving protease activity.[47] Other mechanisms suggested in the veterinary literature have included impaired macrophage phagocytosis of platelets and effects at the bone marrow (increased megakaryocyte fragmentation and stimulation of thrombopoiesis).[48] For acute episodes of thrombocytopenia purpura in humans, vincristine treatment has been considered a salvage treatment (1.4 mg/m^2 followed by 1 mg on days 4 and 7).[49] However, its success in these patients has led to more frequent use as first-choice therapy. A retrospective study in humans found patient outcome (survival) to be better when vincristine therapy was administered initially as opposed to 3 days into treatment.[50] The authors subsequently encourage the early, initial use of vincristine as part of combination therapy, including traditional modalities. Dogs with severe immune-mediated thrombocytopenia (IMT; platelet count less than 15,000/μL) appear to be respond similarly. In a prospective study, Rozanski and coworkers[48] found that platetet counts in dogs with IMT increased more rapidly in patients that received prednisone (1.5 to 2 mg/kg/day) and vincristine (0.02 mg/kg) as opposed to prednisone alone. Further, animals refractory to prednisone alone for 7 days responded rapidly when vincristine was added to therapy. However, all dogs also were treated with doxycycline (10 mg/kg/day) for 7 days. Because IMT in dogs is characterized by increased antiplatelet antibodies on platelet surface, response to vincristine might be expected in this syndrome more than other causes of thrombocytopenia. Because vincristine is a relatively safe drug, initial therapy with vincristine should be considered in dogs with moderate to severe IMT.

TREATMENT OF DISORDERS OF HEMOSTASTIS

Anabolic or Androgenic Steroids

Chemistry

Anabolic steroids are synthetic compounds structurally related to testosterone. They have protein-anabolic activity similar to that of testosterone but ideally minimal androgenic effects (i.e., minimal masculinization) (Table 15-2).[51,52] Testosterone is the sole endogenous androgen in most mammals. Its androgenic effects and rapid elimination have led to the manufacture of synthetic compounds. Chemical manipulations that have produced clinically useful anabolic steroids include (Figure 15-4) (1) alkylation (addition of a methyl [CH_3] group) at the 17β position (e.g., methyl-testosterone, stanozolol), which impairs hepatic metabolism, thus prolonging elimination half-life; (2) esterification of the 17β hydroxyl group (e.g., Deca-Durabolin) such that absorption from parenteral sites is prolonged; and (3) modification of the steroidal ring structure. The sequelae of changes in the steroidal structure vary with the modification and include prolonged absorption or elimination.

KEY POINT 15-4 The role of anabolic steroids in the treatment of anemia is primarily chronic, nonregenerative anemias that fail to respond to erythropoietin.

Mechanism of Action

The mechanism of hematinic action of anabolic steroids on the cellular level is typical of the steroidal compounds.[52-55] Anabolic steroids enter the RBCs, where they enhance

Table 15-2 Anabolic and Androgenic Activity of Selected Steroids

Generic Name	Trade Name	Anabolic	Androgenic
Injectable		(1=low)	(5 = very high)
Testosterone cypionate, enanthate		4	3-4
Nandrolone decanoate	Deca-Durabolin	4	2-3
Stanozolol	Winstrol	2-3	1
Oral			
Oxymetholone	Anadrol	5	5
Oxandrolone	Oxydrin	2-3	1
Stanozolol	Winstrol	2-3	1

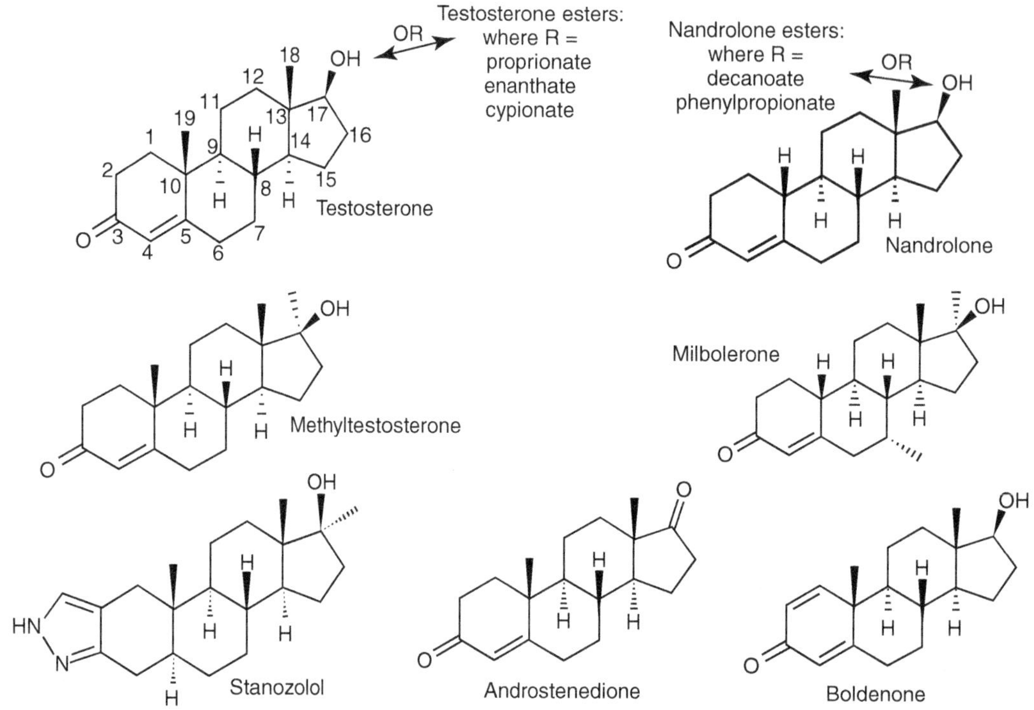

Figure 15-4 Chemical structures of several anabolic steroids. Rings and their positions are indicated for testosterone. Esters on R-groups also alter absorption characteristics. Methylation (methyltestosterone, stanozolol) increases anabolic activity as well as toxicity. Nandrolone is a nonmethylated anabolic steroid. Mibolerone has little anabolic activity, whereas the double bond at C1 and C2 contributes to marked activity with boldenone. Nonmethylated products tend to be less efficacious but less hepatotoxic.

glycolysis and the formation of steroidal 17-keto metabolites. These metabolites are delivered to tissues, including the bone marrow, where they interact with a cytosolic receptor in the appropriate cell and are transferred to the cell nucleus. In the nucleus they induce the formation of RNA and synthesis of an effector protein that brings about the pharmacologic effect.

The sequelae of steroid-induced nuclear transcription are manifold.[54,55] The proposed sequelae on RBC formation include (1) stimulation of EPO production by way of EPO-stimulating factor, (2) differentiation of stem cells into EPO-stimulating factor–sensitive cells (e.g., hemocytoblasts), and (3) direct stimulation of erythroid-progenitor cells. Anabolic steroids also increase intracellular concentrations of 2,3-bisphosphoglycerate in erythrocytes; oxygen release into tissues is subsequently increased.

Efficacy of the anabolic steroids on the RBC mass depends on the presence of supportive materials.[54,55] This includes adequate concentrations of androgen dehydrogenase in the RBC, adequate EPO concentrations, and sufficient bone marrow cellularity. Thus the effectiveness of anabolic steroids in treating anemia may be limited depending on the cause (i.e., renal disease accompanied by low EPO levels). Administration of high doses of these steroids may cause a negative feedback inhibition.

Pharmacologic Effects

The difference in the pharmacologic effects of these drugs among the various tissues and, specifically, whether an androgenic versus an anabolic effect will predominate cannot be attributed to differences in target tissue receptor structure because there appears to be only one androgen receptor type. Differences in response may be concentration dependent (e.g., reproductive tissues requiring higher concentrations than nonreproductive tissues), with drugs differing in their binding to the androgen receptor. However, mibolerone has little anabolic effect despite tight receptor binding and methylation; in contrast, boldenone, which is not methylated, has marked anabolic activity, attributed to a double bond at positions 1 and 2 (see Figure 15-4).[56]

The effect of several anabolic steroids in renal EPO was studied in the perfused canine kidney exposed to 4 hours of hypoxia.[57] Activities important to secretion of EPO included a double bond at position 4 and 5 and the absence of a methyl group at position 10 (see Figure 15-4). Alternatively, differences in response may reflect conversion of the drug by target tissues to an active metabolite that subsequently causes the pharmacologic effect.[54,55] In the presence of continued administration, anabolic steroids initiate and maintain a positive nitrogen balance, although the response is short-lived in intact males.[52,54,55] The anabolic effects of stanozolol have been studied in dogs. Based on urine excretion of urea, retention of intravenously administered radiolabeled amino acid was increased in sled dogs (n = 10) receiving stanozolol either 2 mg/dog orally twice daily (increased from a baseline of 30% to posttreatment retention of 50%), or 25 mg weekly for 4 weeks (increased from 27% to 67%). The authors[58] concluded that such an effect might be beneficial with acute or chronic conditions characterized by protein loss. Anabolic steroids antagonize glucocorticoid-induced protein catabolism by competitively inhibiting glucocorticoid binding to glucocorticoid receptors. Although anabolic steroids appear to vary in their ability to antagonize the effects of glucocorticoids, protein anabolism may be induced in patients experiencing glucocorticoid-induced protein catabolism. Anabolic steroids also reduce urinary excretion of nitrogen, sodium, potassium, chloride, and calcium.

As part of their anabolic activity, these compounds increase the circulating RBC mass (and possibly granulocytic mass). Red blood cell indices, hemoglobin, and hematocrit increase in various types of anemia. White blood cell mass may increase in cases of pancytopenia, although white blood cell response takes longer than the RBC response. Response by thrombocytes is slower and less predictable.[52,54,55]

Pharmacokinetics

The absorption and disposition of anabolic steroids depend on the type of preparation, the presence of specific receptors, and the species to which it is administered.[52,54,55] Most anabolic steroids depend on hepatic metabolism for elimination, with those metabolites that are anaologs of the parent compound accompanied by metabolic activity.[56] The risk of abuse in athletes (including the racing animal) has led to metabolic profiling of some steroids. Among the steroids, Beagle hepatic microsomal metabolism of steroids yielded hydroxylated and oxidized metabolites testosterone, methyltestosterone, mibolerone, and boldenone, with testosterone a metabolite of boldenone and androstenedione a major metabolite of testosterone (see Figure 15-4).

Preparations

Anabolic steroids have been divided into two categories depending on the presence or absence of an alkyl (CH_3) group at the 17-carbon position, although the relevance of this division is probably less important than the impact of the individual drugs (see Figure 15-4).[54,55] Oral and parenteral preparations are available, with the alkylated products being better absorbed orally. Oil-based parenteral preparations are intended for slow release. Examples of alkylated anabolic steroids include methyltestosterone, (oral), oxymetholone (oral), stanozolol (oral and parenteral), methandrostenolone, ethylestrenol, and norethandrolone (see Table 15-1). Examples of nonalkylated anabolic steroids include testosterone cypionate or enanthate, oxymetholone, and nandrolone in its decanoate form (parenteral).

Toxicity Versus Efficacy

A review of risks in human athletes includes cardiovascular adversities, increased risk of cancer, behavioral disorders, and increased risk of tendon damage.[59] Hepatotoxicity is the most common serious adverse effect associated with androgenic or anabolic steroids.[54,55] Toxicity ranges from mild increases in clinical laboratory tests to hepatocellular carcinoma (in humans). Drugs alkylated at the 17-carbon position are more likely to cause hepatotoxicity (see Figure 15-4). Although the mechanism is not known, the drugs or their metabolites may be carcinogenic or may increase the metabolism of other drugs to carcinogenic or hepatotoxic compounds. Cholestatic liver damage occurs early and can be significant but is apparently reversible if the drug is discontinued before irreversible hepatic lesions develop. It is not clear if the hepatotoxic effects that occur in humans are likely in dogs or cats.

Masculinization is a major undesirable (or desirable) side effect of anabolic steroids in humans.[52,54,55,59] Virilization can occur but is seldom objectionable in dogs or cats. In dogs and cats, anabolic steroids increase libido in males, interfere with the female reproductive cycle, and cause masculinization of fetuses if administered during pregnancy. Other undesirable consequences of anabolic steroid therapy in dogs include hyperplasia of the perineal glands and stimulation of androgen-dependent tumors, such as anal carcinomas and prostatic carcinomas. In humans edema resulting from water retention occurs.[52,54,55]

Clinical Indications

The use of anabolic steroids for treatment of renal disease and catabolic effects associated with cachexia are addressed in their respective chapters. Human recombinant EPO has largely replaced anabolic steroids in the treatment of chronic anemias, particularly those associated with renal disease. Anabolic steroids are, however, indicated for treatment of chronic, nonregenerative anemias that fail to respond to EPO; for animals that react adversely to EPO; or for hematopoietic diseases that are not typically associated with decreased concentrations of EPO.[54,55] Of human patients with aplastic anemias who have failed conventional therapy of anemia, 50% or more have responded to anabolic steroids.[54,55] Anabolic steroids have been used in conjunction with anticancer chemotherapeutic drugs to protect bone marrow production of RBCs, thus allowing longer and perhaps more toxic chemotherapy.[52,54,55] Anabolic steroids presumably help decrease the catabolic effects of cancer. Treatment several weeks before cancer chemotherapy may enhance response to anabolic steroids. Use of anabolic steroids for cancer has not been established in dogs and cats.

Hematopoietic response to anabolic therapy is variable, and the time to clinical improvement is long, frequently 3 or more months. Cellularity of the bone marrow appears to determine rate of response to anabolic steroids. Cessation of therapy may result in recurrence of the underlying diseases. Among the anabolic steroids, nandrolone decanoate has the greatest hematopoietic effect.[54,55] Leukocyte and thrombocyte counts may also increase after therapy with anabolic steroids, although these effects are slower in onset and less likely, particularly for thrombocytes. Danazol is the anabolic steroid of choice in the treatment of thrombocytopenia, especially that which is immune mediated. Beneficial effects probably include impaired clearing of IgG-labeled platelets and decreased antibody formation. Response to therapy may take several months, and relapse may occur when danazol therapy is discontinued. Anabolic steroids and, in particular, danazol, have been used with some benefit for patients with hemolytic anemia. Benefits include not only expansion of the RBC mass but also impaired complement activation and binding to RBCs. Human patients suffering from anemia caused by renal disease respond to continuous administration of anabolic steroids. RBC indices improve, as well as appetite, muscle mass, and strength.

In general, the following approaches should be used with anabolic steroids in dogs and cats (see Table 15-1). State restrictions regarding the use of these drugs should be observed. Nandrolone decanoate is the drug of choice except in cases of thrombocytopenia, for which danazol is the drug of choice. Several months of therapy may be necessary before a clinical response is observed. The dose should be decreased once the maximum therapeutic effect occurs. Relapse of disease may occur once the drug is discontinued, and hepatotoxicity is a potential contraindication for use of these drugs.

A final consideration regarding anabolic steroids is use in racing dogs. In addition to potential performance-enhancing abuse, testosterone, methyltestosterone, and mibolerone are used to prevent estrus.[56] Detection of urinary metabolites in racing animals is an ongoing field of study.[56]

Oxygen-Carrying Solutions

Oxygen-carrying solutions (often referred to as *blood substitutes)* offer the advantages of oxygen delivery to tissues similar to that of blood, without the concerns of transmission of disease. Two types of blood substitutes have been developed to both carry and deliver substantial amounts of oxygen to tissues: free hemoglobin–based oxygen-carrying solutions (HBOCs) and fluorocarbons.[60,61] Fluorocarbons are chemicals that are miscible with blood and can carry as much as 5.25 mL of oxygen per 100 mL of blood, depending on oxygen tension. Although the oxygen-carrying capacity of these compounds is not adequate for total blood replacement, their low viscosity makes them potentially useful in disorders characterized by abnormalities in microcirculation. In addition, use of these agents in nonvascular tissue (e.g., the peritoneal cavity) may enhance supplementing oxygen exchange in tissues during respiratory failure.

Of the two blood substitutes pursued for clinical use, HBOCs (e.g., oxyglobin, approved for use in dogs) have proved most useful. Free, unmodified hemoglobin (purification involves washing, lysing, ultrafiltering, and pasteurizing) is not an effective blood substitute. Free hemoglobin decreases the amount of oxygen released from tissues by reducing concentrations of 2,3-diphosphoglycerate such that the oxyhemoglobin dissociation curve shifts to the left. As a result, the Pa_{50} of oxygen in HBOCs is reduced from 28 mm HG to 10 mm Hg. In addition, the free smaller dimers of hemoglobin are more readily cleared by the kidneys, resulting in a short half-life (20 minutes), as well as an increased risk of nephrotoxicity. Smaller molecules also may be responsible for the increase in vascular (systemic and pulmonary) resistance that may accompany use of HBOCs, including Oxyglobin use. Enlarging the size of the hemoglobin molecules by cross-linking (e.g., with fumarate or dasprin [HemAssist]), polymerization techniques (e.g., using oxidized raffinose [Hemolink] or gluteraldehyde [Oxyglobin and Hemopure]) or surface conjugation reduces the negative sequelae of free smaller molecules.[62] Surface conjugation techniques have the added advantage of blocking the hemoglobin receptor site that interacts with and blocks nitric oxide, thus reducing the risk of vasoconstriction. Of the HBOC products, Oxyglobin, the first approved for use by the Food and Drug Administration, is a bovine hemoglobin–based product indicated for the treatment of canine anemia. Human hemoglobin–based products also have been developed (PolyHeme, a surface conjugated product); recombinant products are currently being studied. Intended indications for newer products extend beyond supplementation of oxygen in critically anemic patients, including sensitizing of cancer cells or scavenging of nitric oxide.[62]

Manipulation of the hemoglobin tetramer by cross-linking, polymerization, and other methods yields products with variable molecular weights: for Oxyglobin the average MW is 200 kDa (range 64-500 kDa) whereas conjugation of surface proteins (e.g., polyethylene glycol [Enzon] yields lower molecular weight products (117-125); recombinant products may be as small as 64 kDa. Among the advantages of the larger molecular weight (discussed later) is the ability of the compounds to act as colloids, increasing preload, stroke volume, and cardiac output (similar to hetastarch, plasma, and dextran-70), with the added advantage of increased oxygen delivery.[62] In general, using experimental canine models of acute hemorrhagic hypovolemia, use of a bovine HBOC either increases oxygen delivery or arterial oxygen content, although studies generally have not been able to consistently demonstrate both occurring.[62] One study concluded that treatment of acute anemia in dogs with 15 mL/kg of a bovine HBOC was able to increase oxygen content equivalent to packed RBCs.[63] In canine models of hemorrhagic hypovolemia, intestinal perfusion and oxygenation appear to be maintained; however, increased systemic vascular resistance and decreased cardiac output have also been demonstrated.

Oxyglobin (Biopure Corp., www.oxyglobin.com; availability at the time of publication is not clear) is a polymerized bovine HBOC fluid. Oxyglobin increases plasma and total hemoglobin concentrations and thus increases arterial oxygen content. Its molecular weight imparts colloidal properties similar to those of dextran 70 and hetastarch. Its polymerized nature precludes renal filtration and renal side effects of hemoglobinuria. Because the solution is free of RBC walls, antigens associated with transfusion reactions are largely absent. Likewise, the absence of plasma reduces reactions associated with isoantibodies. However, antibodies may develop to bovine hemoglobin, and caution is recommended with repeated administration 10 or more days apart. As a foreign protein, anaphylactic reactions are possible.

Oxyglobin is eliminated similarly to hemoglobin by reticuloendothelial cells. Its elimination half-life in dogs is estimated to range between 30 and 40 hours, with 90% of the drug eliminated within 5 to 7 days. Conditions for HBOCs studied in controlled canine clinical trials included immune-mediated hemolysis (n = 30), blood loss (gastrointestinal, traumatic, surgical, rodenticide intoxication; n = 25), and ineffective erythropoiesis (idiopathic, RBC aplasia, ehrlichiosis; n = 9). Relative to pretreatment, plasma hemoglobin concentration significantly increased ($P = 0.001$) and clinical signs associated with anemia (lethargy/depression, exercise intolerance, and increased heart rate) significantly improved ($P = 0.001$) after treatment with Oxyglobin. Treatment success was defined as the lack of need for additional oxygen-carrying support (i.e., blood transfusion) for 24 hours after the completion of infusion with the HBOC. Success in the treatment group was 95% compared with 32% in untreated control dogs.[64]

Side effects of HBOCs include circulatory overload and its negative sequelae (e.g., pulmonary edema, pleural effusion, increased central venous pressure, dyspnea, coughing), particularly in patients already suffering from volume overload (e.g., congestive heart failure) or in cases of accidental overdose (>10 mL/kg/hr). Hypertension is a recognized side effect of HBOC use. Smaller molecules are potentially more likely to reduce nitric oxide and subsequent increased vascular resistance.[62] Species are likely to differ in their vasoactive response. Oxyglobin caused a 30% increase in peripheral vascular resistance in isovolemic dogs; hypertension also has been induced in hypovolemic cats.[62]

Vasoconstriction may be sufficiently profound that tissue perfusion is compromised. Further, standard methods of assessing adequate volume resuscitation may be ineffective in the presence of HBOCs.[65] Oxyglobin mildly decreases PCV immediately after infusion and increases total and plasma hemoglobin concentrations for at least 24 hours. PCV and RBC counts are not accurate measures of anemia for 24 hours after administration. Overhydration should be avoided with the use of an HBOC because of its plasma-expanding properties; likewise, administration of other colloidal solutions is discouraged. Central venous pressure or clinical signs indicative of circulatory overload should be monitored during and immediately after administration of Oxyglobin, particularly in normovolemic patients or patients with cardiac disease. Cats also may be predisposed to volume overload: One retrospective study of Oxyglobin use in cats with anemia found that 29 of 72 developed volume overload compared with 37 of 72 that responded to therapy. Hypothermia appeared to increase the risk once body temperature was returned to normal.[66]

Transient changes or side effects after administration of Oxyglobin reported by Biopure Corp. include yellow-orange discoloration of the skin, sclera, and gums; red to dark green discoloration of feces; brown-black discoloration of urine; vomiting; diarrhea; and decreased skin elasticity within 48 hours of dosing. The frequency and intensity of these clinical signs are dose dependent. HBOC solutions may interfere with several laboratory tests, particularly those based on colorimetric procedures (see package insert) or hemostatic tests based on optical methods. Pulse oximetry, blood gas analysis, and related procedures generally are not affected.

Oxyglobin may be warmed to 37° C before administration. As long as it is not frozen, it will remain stable for up to 24 months. Care should be taken to avoid temperatures that are too cold in the refrigerator. Oxyglobin is intended as a one-time use only at a recommended dose of 30 mL/kg intravenously at a rate of up to 10 mL/kg/hr. Although animals may not need the full 30 mL/kg; according to the manufacturer, 10 mL/kg may be sufficient in some cases. The foil bag in which the product is contained is oxygen impermeable. Once the bag is opened, oxygen can penetrate the plastic bag, resulting in the oxidation of the hemoglobin, as evidenced by the formation of methemoglobinemia. Unlike intact RBCs, which can reduce methemoglobinemia, HBOC solutions cannot. A brown discoloration will appear when approximately 25% of the hemoglobin has been oxidized. The product also offers an excellent environment for bacterial growth, even with refrigeration. The product should be used within 4 days of opening. Retrospective studies using HBOCs have been performed in both dogs[67] and cats.[66] However, neither study was accompanied by a non–HBOC-treated group, and the retrospective nature of the study precluded implementation of methods to reduce bias. A retrospective study of immune-mediated hemolytic anemia found that all dogs treated with Oxyglobin died, but the study did not address bias introduced by selection of only those most severely afflicted animals for treatment with HBOCs.[67] Gibson and coworkers[66] retrospectively studied HBOC use in 72 cats treated for anemia, including hemolytic anemia associated with acetaminophen toxicosis. Although 37 cats improved after a mean dose of 14.6 mL/kg (4.8 mL/hr), adverse events (not necessarily associated with HBOC) occurred in 44, including pleural effusions (n = 21) and pulmonary edema (n = 8). The anemic crisis was survived by 23 cats; euthanasia or death of the remaining cats was attributed to the underlying disease rather than administration of the HBOC.[66] Oxyglobin also has been used successfully in a variety of other species.[62]

The use of Oxyglobin was reviewed retrospectively in cats (Germany) (n = 53, treated, 48 studied).[68] The drug was generally administered by a fluid pump at 5 mL/kg/hr. Bags had been stored for 24 hours or less at 4° C. Some cats were treated more than once in a 24-hour period. The bases of treatment varied but included the general condition of the patient, the current hematocrit or hemoglobin level, and underlying disease. Cats receiving blood products were excluded from the study. Domestic Shorthair represented the predominant breed (n = 37); ages ranged from 0.3 to 14 years. Indications were blood low anemia (n = 25), hemolysis (n = 13), and ineffective erythropoiesis (n = 8). Reasons for administration of Oxyglobin rather than blood included lack of availability of feline blood products (including compatible donor) or to reduce loss of previously opened (within 24 hours) product coupled with reduced availability of feline donors. All patients also received Ringer's lactate. An overall survival rate was not offered, but a survival rate was offered for each group. Hemoglobin changes ranged from −0.8 to 3.3 in the blood loss group (decreased in 5 cats) with a 24-hour survival rate of 72%. In the hemolytic group, hemoglobin changed from 0.2 to 5.2 gm/dL for a 24-hour survival rate of 84%. In the group with ineffective erythropoiesis, hemoblogin changed from −0.5 to 2.4 g/dL, with an 88% survival rate. Of the cats treated, 11 of the 48 had some type of cardiac disease; in this subgroup (which included cats from each of the preceding treatment groups), adverse reactions that might be related to treatment occurred in seven cats. These included pulmonary edema, pleural effusion, or respiratory distress; one of the cats died within 6 hours, and four died within 28 hours as a result of volume overload after receiving a range of 6.7 to 20 mL/kg in the 24-hour period.

DRUGS ACTING ON COAGULATION OR CLOTTING

Hemostastis has been reviewed[69] elsewhere. Briefly, it occurs in three steps (Figure 15-5), with the role players varying somewhat with the site or rate of flow: high shear vessels include the smaller to medium arteries, whereas low shear vessels include the larger arteries or veins. Platelet adherence occurs in the presence of damaged tissue or disrupted endothelium; platelets also will adhere to one another. Platelet adherence is mediated by laminin, collagen,or fibrinonectin in low shear vessels and adenosine diphosphate (ADP) and vWF in high shear stress vessels. Adherence is followed by platelet activation, during which granular contents of platelets are released. The contents recruit more platelets but also integrate platelet activation with the inflammatory process through release of mediators such as IL-1, platelet-activating factor, and serotonin. In high shear stress vessels, ADP and vWF are the primary mediators of activation, whereas thromboxane is the primary activator in low shear stress vessels. Thrombin will activate platelets (by way of protease-activated receptors) in any vessel. Because thrombin is not inhibited by cyclooxygenase inhibition, it is considered the strongest of the activators. Platelet adherence and subsequent activation are then followed by assembly of glycoproteins, causing aggregation. Again, the role players vary with the site, with vWF and glycoprotein Ib-IX-V mediating the response in high shear flow rates and fibrinogen in low shear flow vessels. The final common pathway to platelet aggregation is the glycopeptides IIb through IIIa receptors; this protein is the target of several investigative antithrombotic drugs in humans.[69]

Although a number of endogenous compounds play a role in platelet aggregation, a number of exogenous substances do as well (e.g., infectious organisms, complement factors). Further, endogenous factors provide balance, preventing coagulation. Among the most important antiplatelet mediators are nitric oxide and prostacyclin, both released from the

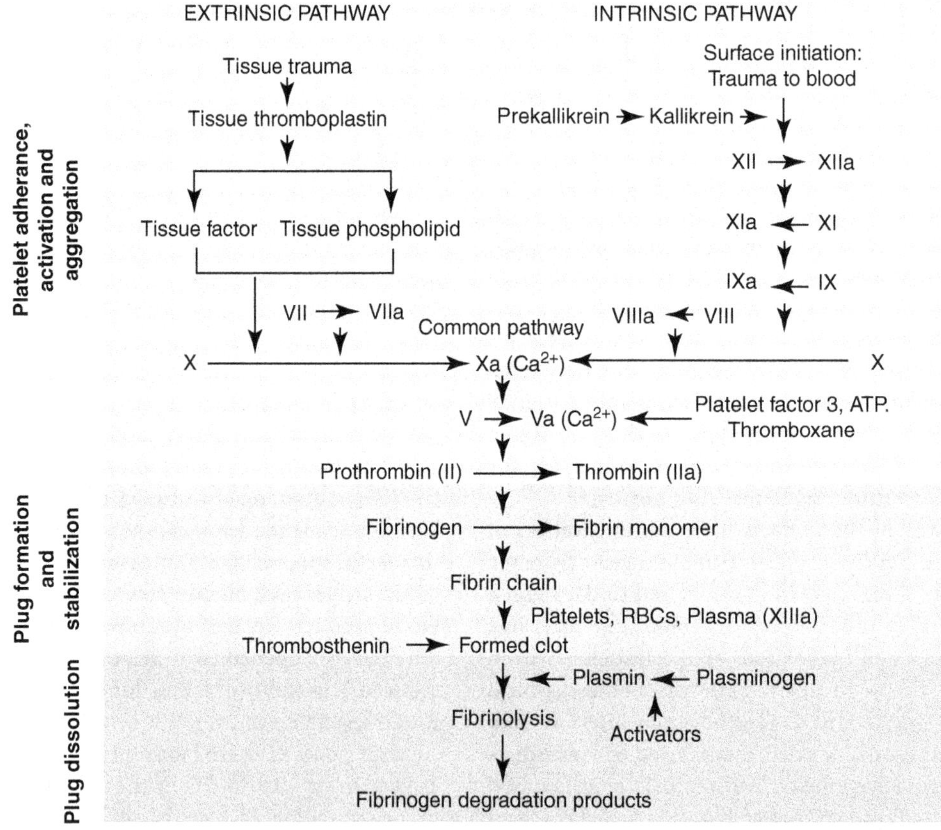

Figure 15-5 Hemostasis occurs in several phases: vascular and platelet, coagulation, and fibrinolysis. Each phase must remain in equilibrium to maintain a normal state of hemostasis. Endogenous procoagulants and anticoagulants function in each phase. The vascular and platelet phase is composed of vascular wall contraction and platelet adherence. Damage to the vessel exposes subendothelial collagen, which stimulates platelet adherence, which, in turn, depends on von Willebrand factor. Activation of the coagulation phase relies on a complex series of interdependent events. Injury results in activation of procoagulant substances in a cascade manner. Activation (designated by a lower case *a*, e.g., Xa) generally occurs as a result of proteolysis of a small molecule from the inactive factor. The major events in the coagulation cascade include formation of thromboplastin as a result of tissue trauma (designated as intrinsic if the blood is damaged and extrinsic if the vascular structures are damaged); transformation of prothrombin to thrombin; and rapid conversion of fibrinogen into fibrin. Calcium is involved as a factor at several steps. The fibrinolytic phase is initiated by the conversion of plasminogen to plasmin, which degrades fibrin.

endothelium. These two mediators appear to act synergistically to inhibit platelet adhesion, activation, and aggregation. Aggregation leads to the organized deposition of coagulation proteins with the formation of a temporary platelet plug. It ultimately should be stabilized in a cross-linked fibrin network. The final step in hemostasis is plug removal, which is accomplished through the initiation of fibrinolysis following activation of plasminogen to plasmin (see Figure 15-5). Disorders reflect not only failed hemostasis but increased risk of thrombosis as a result of a hypercoagulable state induced by disease or, less commonly, drugs.

Hemostatic Drugs

Hemostatic drugs are used to prevent or attenuate bleeding. They can be administered either topically or systemically. In general, topical agents either act as a factor in the coagulation cascade or stimulate some aspect of the coagulation cascade (see Figure 15-5).

Topical

Lyophilized concentrates of one or more clotting factors are available as topical preparations. These preparations usually provide an artificial factor or structural matrix that facilitates clotting (Figure 15-6). An intact hemostatic mechanism is necessary for their efficacy. These are absorbable products and are indicated for capillary oozing from small, superficial vessels. Examples of concentrated factors include thromboplastin (prothrombin is converted to thrombin, used locally in surgery), thrombin (converts fibrinogen to fibrin; available as powder, solution, or sponge), and fibrinogen. Examples of artificial matrices include absorbable gelatin sponge and oxidized cellulose (treated surgical gauze that promotes clotting) (see Figure 15-6).

Astringents act locally by precipitating proteins. These agents do not penetrate tissues and thus are restricted to surface cells. They can be damaging to surrounding tissues. Examples include ferric sulfate, silver nitrate (e.g., sticks; see Figure 15-6), and combinations that include tannic acid (e.g., STA).

Epinephrine and norepinephrine are hemostatic drugs only by virtue of their vasoconstrictive effects. They may be included in topical medications or injectable local anesthetics to decrease blood flow to the tissues.

Systemic

Fresh blood or blood components are hemostatic drugs only in states of (coagulation) factor deficiency. Examples include plasma (contains electrolytes, albumin, and some coagulation factors), fresh frozen plasma (plasma in which factors V and VII are stable), cryoprecipitate, and platelet-rich plasma.

Vitamin K. Vitamin K is a hemostatic drug only in instances of vitamin K deficiency. It is necessary for hepatic synthesis

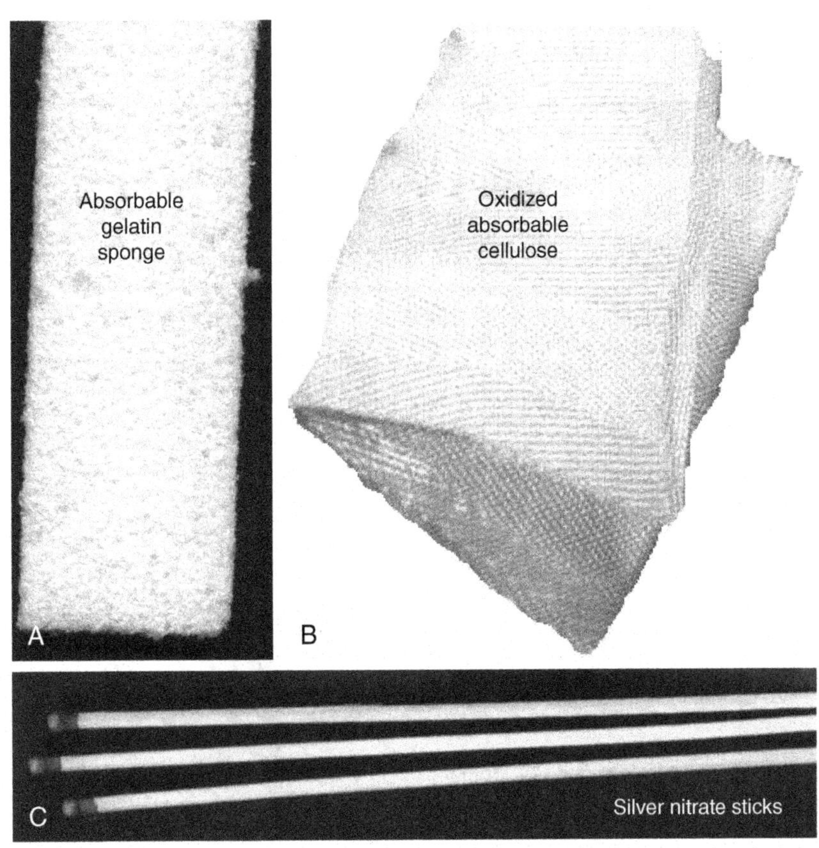

Figure 15-6 Examples of coagulants **(A)**.Oxidized cellulose (Surgicel shown here) provides a matrix for clotting **(B)**. Gelfoam also provides an artificial structural matrix that initiates the clotting process **(C)**. Products that contain silver nitrate (shown here), tannic acid, or salicylic acid precipitate proteins and cause coagulation by destroying tissue. Their use is limited to small, topical lesions.

of coagulation factors II, VII, IX, and X (Figure 15-7). Several forms of vitamin K are available for therapeutic use. Vitamin K_1 (phytonadione), the plant form, can be given parenterally and orally. It is more effective and more rapid in onset compared with other vitamin K analogs. However, anaphylactic reactions have been reported with intravenous administration, particularly with those preparations containing polysorbate 80, a known releaser of histamine in dogs. The drug can also be given intramuscularly. The effects of vitamin K_1 occur within 1 hour of administration,[3,70] although several hours are needed to resolve bleeding tendencies as coagulation proteins are replaced.

Vitamin K_2 (menaquinone) is the natural animal and microbial form of vitamin K. Vitamin K_3 (menadione) is one of several synthetic forms. It must be metabolized to the active state. Vitamin K_3 usually is absorbed too slowly to be used effectively in acute conditions, but it can be used for chronic therapy once the acute crisis has been resolved. In states of hypocoagulation, vitamin K_1 is the preferred form, administered either subcutaneously or orally (3 mg/kg subcutaneously in multiple sites followed by 1 mg/kg every 24 hours parenterally or orally).[71] Fat will enhance the oral absorption of vitamin K.

The most common use of vitamin K is treatment of rodenticide toxicity (see later discussion of anticoagulants). Duration of treatment for rodenticide poisoning will vary according to the toxicant. Toxicities from rodenticides containing coumarin or warfarin should be treated for 4 to 6 days; intoxication with diphacinone or brodifacoum requires treatment for at least 14 days.[71] For toxicity with longer-acting rodenticides (i.e., indandiones), the dose of vitamin K is often reduced for subsequent weeks:[71] 0.5 mg/kg, week 2; 0.25 mg/kg, weeks 3 and 4. Prothrombin time should be monitored for 2 days after vitamin K is discontinued to detect residual rodenticide toxicity. Screening tests should remain normal for 3 to 4 days after therapy has been discontinued.

Protamine sulfate. Protamine sulfate is a low-molecular-weight, positively charged drug that binds to heparin, forming a salt and neutralizing its anticoagulant effects. It is used as a procoagulant only in instances of heparin overdosing. Protamine should be used cautiously because it also has anticoagulant activity, probably by impairing thrombin and fibrinogen. It is difficult to dose accurately because the dose is based on the amount of heparin to be antagonized (1 to 1.5 mg protamine for each 1 mg of heparin). In addition, the dose decreases as time elapses after heparin was administered.[72] No more than 50 mg should be given in a 10-minute period.

Desmopressin. Desmopressin acetate (deamino 8-D-arginine vasopressin) is a synthetic analog of vasopressin and antidiuretic hormone that is used to treat central diabetes insipidus However, the drug also transiently increases serum concentrations of vWF in part through the release of preformed vWF from endothelial cells and macrophages as well as release of preformed Factor VIII.[73] Increased release was

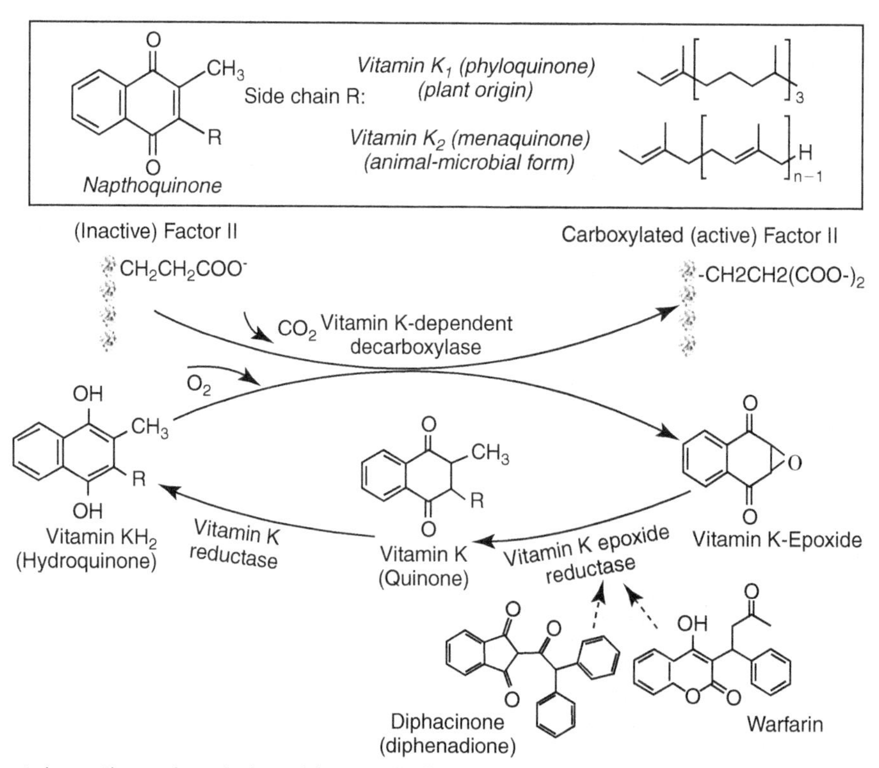

Figure 15-7 Vitamin K catalyzes the carboxylation of factors II, VII, IX, and X. As part of the reaction, the oxidized vitamin must be reduced to continue activation of coagulation factors. Coumarin derivatives block the reduction of vitamin K, rendering it incapable of activating coagulation factors. The arrow on warfarin identifies the chiral carbon that leads to S and R enantiomers. Both isomers are highly (>95%) bound to plasma proteins. Enterohepatic circulation was evident in cats 4 hours after administration.

demonstrated 1 hour after infusion in normal and afflicted dogs, although increase in afflicted dogs was greater.[74] Kraus and coworkers[75] have demonstrated that desmopressin decreases buccal mucosal bleeding time in Doberman Pinschers afflicted with vWF A similar response has been demonstrated for Greyhounds with vWF deficiency treated with 1 mg/kg desmopressin diluted in 1 mL of saline.[76] The maximum response occurs 1 to 2 hours after treatment, although it may occur after as little as 10 minutes of infusion, with effects lasting 2 hours after intravenous administration.[69] The increase is sufficient to provide improved coagulation activity in animals suffering from von Willebrand disease that undergo surgery.[71] Desmopressin is generally administered by slow intravenous infusion over 20 to 30 minutes in humans after dilution in a minimum of 100 mL of physiologic saline. However, the intranasal (human) preparation also can be given subcutaneously at 1 U/kg.[69] Rapid infusion may result in tachycardia, flushing, tremor, and abdominal discomfort. Repetitive administration results in depletion of the storage pools and loss of procoagulant effect and may increase the risk of tachyphylaxis.[71,73]

Recombinant human factor VIIa. The role of tissue factor (TF), a transmembrane glycoprotein receptor located in multiple extravascular tissues, is key to the initiation of hemostasis. It is through activation of Factor VII (FVII) bound to receptors located on TF that Factors IX and X are activated, leading to platelet activation and subsequent coagulation. A recombinant FVII product, derived from transfected baby hamster kidney cells, is chemically identical to activated FVII. The drug product was developed for treatment of human hemophiliacs (A and B) who had developed antibodies (following multiple blood transfusions) to Factors VIII or IX.[77] Theoretically, although FVIIa should effect hemostasis through a TF factor, afflicted hemophiliacs are not able to mount an effective coagulative response primarily through loss of an amplified response by FVIII and IX. However, supraphysiologic doses appear to stimulate hemostasis (thrombin formation) by way of TF-independent pathways. Although activation of Factor X is not as effectively amplified as in the normal patient, more effective platelet involvement yields a more stable fibrin clot than would be formed in Factor-deficient patients. The fibrin clot is actually denser than that in normal patients. Because rhFVII requires exposed TF and activated platelets, its effects tend to be limited locally. The drug has been used on a compassionate-use basis for treatment of hemophiliacs undergoing procedures associated with a risk of bleeding or in patients suffering from refractory bleeding. The use of rhFVII has been described in dogs, including those suffering from either A or B hemophilia. Use in homozygote von Willebrand's disease was not as successful. However, hypersensitivity reactions developed in several animals within 30 minutes of treatment, and all animals developed antibodies within 2 weeks of therapy. Nonetheless, should safety be improved, suggested potential applications of rhFVII therapy in animals, beyond treatment of factor deficiencies, have included disseminated intravascular coagulation (DIC), thrombocytopenia or thrombocytopathia, anticoagulant rodenticide toxicosis, overzealous anticoagulant therapy, high-risk surgeries, and liver and gastrointestinal diseases.[77]

Fibrinolysin inhibitors. Fibrinolysin inhibitors prevent the activity of plasmin (fibrinolysin) and therefore promote the persistence of clots (see Figure 15-5). The lysine analog aminocaproic acid is one of the few examples. Its therapeutic use is limited to treatment after an overdose of a fibrinolytic agent. It theoretically acts by substituting for lysine-binding sites, forming a complex with plasminogen, precluding its conversion to plasmin (e.g., inhibits streptokinase).[78] It was studied after intravenous administration (1750 mg of 250 mg/mL solution followed by 250 mg/mL every hour for 9 hours) in a canine (n = 4; 10-21 kg) model of urokinase and venous injury–induced thrombosis. Aminocaproic acid inhibited plasmin formation completed, compared with heparin (20,000 U intravenously every 3 hours), which inhibited it by approximately 80%.[79]

Antihemostatic Drugs

Feline aortic thromboembolism (FATE) is a useful model for the discussion of treatment of thromboembolic disease. With FATE the goals of therapy are to reduce the formation of the thrombus, prevent embolization, improve collateral blood flow, control pain, and provide supportive care. Because thrombus formation in the heart (atria) is facilitated by blood stasis associated with atrial enlargement and endothelial damage, supportive therapy may include cardiogenic support. Drugs used to limit the formation of thrombi include anticoagulants, thrombolytics, and antithrombotics.

Anticoagulants

Anticoagulants interfere either directly or indirectly with the clotting cascade (see Figure 15-5). Several in vitro anticoagulants are used for blood collection intended for transfusion therapy and should be considered as drugs. Examples include citrate phosphate dextrose, acid citrate dextrose, sodium citrate, and heparin. All except heparin (discussed later) act by effectively removing Ca^{2+} from the cascade system. In vivo anticoagulants include heparin and the vitamin K antagonists.

Heparins

Heparin is a heterogeneous mixture of sulfated (anionic) polysulfated glycosaminoglycans (PSGAG) (Figure 15-8). Glycosaminoglycans are a family of structurally diverse and distinct polyanionic complex carbohydrates. Included in this group are heparin, heparan sulfate, chondroitin 4-sulfate, chondroitin 6-sulfate, dermatan sulfate, keratin sulfate, and hyaluronic acid. Each of the glycosaminoglycans is composed of repeating polysaccharides consisting of an amino sugar (e.g., glucosamine or galactosamine) and uronic (e.g., glucuronic or iduronic) acid or a hexose (galactose; keratin sulfate only). Each is ubiquitous in location. Among them, heparan sulfate proteoglycans are diverse in location with those that are endothelial derived serving as the primary endogenous anticoagulant. They are an integral part of stromal matrices, basement membranes, and almost all cell surfaces where they provide cohesion between vessels and vascular stroma.[43] Endogenous

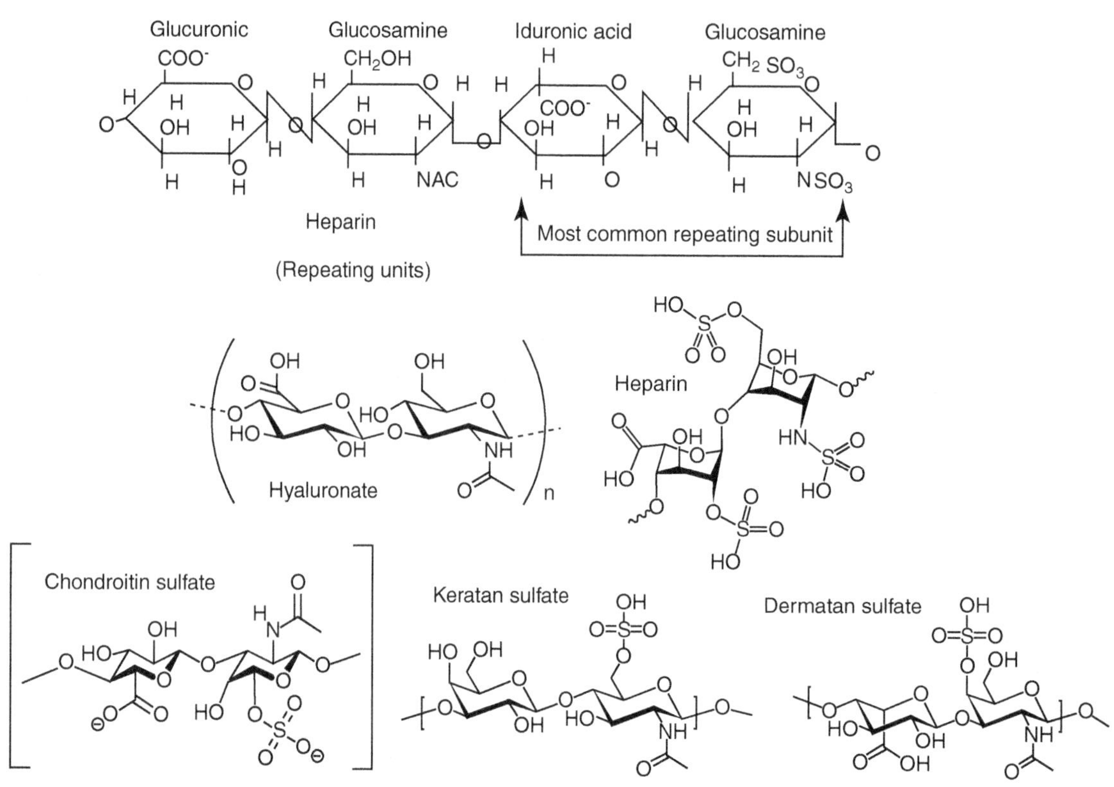

Figure 15-8 Heparin is a heterogeneous mixture of sulfated, anionic, and polysulfated glycosaminoglycans. The subunits include uronic acid, sulfonaminoglycosamine, *N*-acetylglucosamine, and a pentasaccharide sequence. Heparin is one of many polysulfated glycosaminoglycans (PGAGs) found throughout the body. Other structurally similar PGAGS include hyaluronate, heparin sulfates, chondroitin sulfates, keratan sulfates, and dermatan sulfates.

synthesis results in multiple compounds that vary in the lengths of carbohydrate chains Heparin and heparan sulfate are the most complex members of this class of compounds and are characterized by the greatest biologic diversity.[43] Proteoglycans are formed when proteins, which serve as the core for the PGAG, are posttranslationally (in the Golgi apparatus) modified with the addition of glycosaminoglycan chains. Each is sulfated to variable degrees, depending on the repeating subunits of which the disaccharide is composed.

Heparin was so named because of its initial discovery in high concentrations in the liver. It is often located attached to serine residues of core proteins (e.g., coagulation factors). Commercially available heparin is prepared from porcine intestinal mucosa and bovine lung. It is stored in mast cells, along with other PGAGs, including chondroitin and dermatan sulfate. Heparin also is stored in the body in basophils and, to a lesser extent, in vascular endothelium. Tissues with high concentrations of mast cells serve as a source of heparin. Heparin is a highly sulfated (generally 2 to 3 per subunit) glycosaminoglycan composed of alternating sequences of sulfoaminoglycosamine and uronic acid units and smaller amounts of *N*-acetylglucosamine (see Figure 15-8). Its structure also includes a unique and specific sulfated glucosamine pentasaccharide sequence that binds to antithrombin (AT) III and thus serves as the active site of the molecule. The number of active sites in a molecule of heparin is variable, but it is present in only about 30% of the molecules. In its native state, the molecular weight is quite variable, ranging from 3 to 50 kDa.

The molecular weight of commercial unfractionated heparin (UFH) generally varies from 1800 to 30,000 daltons (mean 15,000, representing about 45 monosaccharide chains).[80] However, heparin also has been prepared through filtration methods as fractionated or low-molecular-weight (LMW) heparins, which normally make up less than 5% of endogenous heparin. The LMW heparins generally are only 1000 to 10,000 daltons in size and are specifically defined as an average weight of 8000 daltons or less, with at least 60% of the product being less than 8000 daltons in size (see Figure 15-8). A variety of LMW heparins have been made, with each varying by the method of fractionation or depolymerization. The LMW heparins have much higher affinity for AT (by way of Xa) compared with UFH and thus are more potent, providing 70 units/mg of antifactor Xa and a ratio of antifactor Xa to AT activity of 1.5 or more.[80] Doses of fractionated LMW preparations are thus lower than unfractionated products (Table 15-3). Preparations of UFH also contain contaminants such as dermatan sulfate; these contaminants may be present in LMW heparin preparations but in diluted form. Intentional contamination of heparins with oversulfated chondroitin sulfates is addressed with adverse reactions. Some of these compounds also have anticoagulant activity, albeit less than heparin.[81]

Mechanism of action. Heparin interacts with many proteins, probably by electrostatic forces between the polyionic groups of the glycosaminoglycan and the cationic groups of proteins. Example proteins include proinflammatory chemokines, growth factor, extracellular matrix proteins, and leukocyte

Table 15-3 Doses of Unfractionated Heparin and Low Molecular Weight Heparin

Drug	Category	Indication	Dose	Route	Interval (h)
Dalteparin	(LMWH)	Thromboembolic disease	100-150 IU/kg (D)	SC	8
			50 mg/cat		12 (C)
			180 IU/kg (C)	SC	6
Enoxaparin	(LMWH)	Thromboembolic disease	0.8 mg/kg (D)	SC	6
			1.25 mg/kg (C)	SC	6
			5 mg/kg (C)	PO	24
Heparin	(UFH)	Arterial thromboembolism, thrombophlebitis	Initial dose: 100-200 IU/kg. Maximum of 500 IU/kg (D)	IV	Once
			Initial dose: 375 IU/kg (C)	IV	Once
			Maintenance dose: 100-300 IU/kg	SC	6-8
		Prophylaxis	Low dose: 10-50 IU/kg	SC	8-12 (Monitor APTT to 1.5 to 2 times pretreatment baseline)
		Feline thromboembolism associated with cardiomyopathy	Induction: 1000 IU/kg	IV	Once
			Maintenance: 50 IU/kg	SC	8
		During acute pancreatitis	50-100 IU/kg	SC	8-12
		Disseminated intravascular coagulation	75-100 IU/kg	IV, SC	6-8
			5000 IU/500 mL blood	IV	As needed
		Low dose	5-10 IU/kg	IV infusion	1
		Burns	100-200 IU/kg	IV, SC	8 × 1-4 treatments
		Closed chest lavage	1000 IU/L fluid at 20 mL/kg	Intrathoracic	12
		Lipoprotein lipase provocative test	100 IU/kg	IV	Test lipids before and 15 min after heparin

LMWH, Low-molecular-weight heparin; *D,* dog; *SC,* subcutaneous; *C,* cat; *PO,* by mouth; *UFH,* unfractionated heparin; *IV,* intravenous; *APTT,* activated partial thromboplastin time.

proteins. Intracellular effects reflect interaction of heparin or heparan sulfates with cell surface-binding proteins (which are not necessarily true receptors) followed by endocytotic internalization.

The most recognized sequelae of protein–heparin interaction are the anticoagulant actions of heparin.[43] However, this effect is indirect, reflecting facilitation of the actions of endogenous anticoagulant proteins. The most notable is AT, one of several endogenous serine proteinase inhibitors (serpins) whose thrombin inhibition occurs only in the presence of heparin. Long chains of heparin bind to specific lysine residues on AT. At low heparin concentrations (0.1 to 1 U/mL), AT rapidly inhibits the activity of the clotting factors IIa (thrombin), Xa, and IXa, resulting in prolongation of activated partial thromboplastin time (APTT) and thrombin time (TT); prothrombin time (PT) is only mildly affected. At high heparin concentrations (>5 U/mL), heparin interacts with heparin cofactor II (HCII), which binds only to thrombin, causing further inhibition. Binding of heparin to AT or HCII results in a stable complex (Figure 15-9). Binding induces conformational change in the anticoagulant complex such that the active sites of the inhibitor is exposed, facilitating binding to the clotting factors. As such, heparin increases the velocity, but not magnitude, of interaction between the endogenous anticoagulants and clotting factors. The rate of interaction can increase 10,000-fold

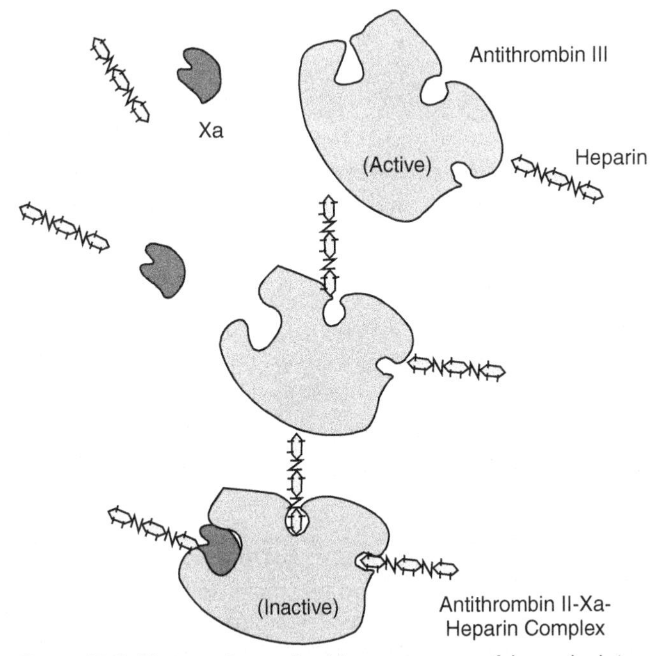

Figure 15-9 The pentasaccharide sequence of heparin interacts with the amino residues of antithrombin III, changing the conformation of antithrombin II and its ability to interact with factors IXa, XIa, XIIa, and, in particular, II and Xa. Heparin may directly interfere with factor X.

in the presence of heparin. The anticoagulant and clotting factor complex will remain intact after activity is inhibited; as such AT is a "suicide" substrate.[54] In contrast, heparin will be released to interact with other molecules. Other inhibitors, whose concentrations are less than one hundredth of that of AT are also inhibited at high concentrations; these include plasminogen activator inhibitor, protein C inhibitor, and tissue factor pathway factor inhibition of Xa. Heparin also inhibits factors IXa and to some degree Xia; the kallikrein–kinin system and, through binding to complement C1, the complement system are inhibited. Factor VIIa is minimally inhibited.

Because the specific AT-binding site of heparin is generally absent in other glycosaminglycans (limited in heparin sulfates and absent in chondroitin and dermatan sulfates), these latter compounds are characterized by minimal anticoagulant activity.

Simultaneous inhibition of both AT and thrombin requires molecules greater than 5400 MW. LMW heparins generally act through AT inhibition of Xa rather than IIa. Thus LMW heparin fractions are more potent anticoagulants (a lower concentration inhibits Xa) compared with high-molecular-weight (HMW) fractions,[81] but HMW heparins may be more effective anticoagulants because their large structure facilitates simultaneous binding of both AT and thrombin simultaneously.[72] Whereas the ratio of antiXa:IIa activity for UFH is generally 1:1, the same ratios range from 2 to 4:1 up to 9:1 for LMW heparins in humans.[82] Lower ratios might be expected for dogs because LMW heparin appears to have less effect on AT.

KEY POINT 15-5 Although fractionated low-molecular-weight heparins are more potent inhibitors of Xa, products that contain high-molecular-weight fractions may actually be more effective anticoagulants because their large structure facilitates simultaneous binding of both antithrombin and thrombin.

The effect of heparin on thrombin and Xa occurs only when the factors are not bound to platelets or fibrin; platetet factor IV blocks the interaction between heparin and AT. However, heparins have an antiplatelet effect because of a high affinity for platelet factor IV. Most heparin preparations also inhibit platelet aggregation, negating effects of platelet-derived growth factor on vascular smooth muscle and leading to their descriptor as *platelet-active anticoagulants*. vWF (platelet factor VIII) is among the factors bound and inhibited by heparin.[80] Heparins also bind to vascular endothelium, causing release of two other endogenous PGAGs and altering vascular endothelial permeability.[81]

Heparin has other effects not related to its anticoagulant activity. In human patients heparin may prove useful for prevention of atherosclerosis and for accelerated formation of collateral circulation in the presence of thrombosis (angiogenesis).[81,83] Heparin can inhibit or modulate selected targets of an allergic inflammatory response, including neutrophils and T cells. Heparins appear to decrease leukocyte adherence to vascular endothelium and facilitate leukocyte migration along a chemoattractant gradient to sites of inflammation. Derivatives of low anticoagulant activity block superoxide anion generation, probably by interacting with superoxide dismutase. Heparin appears to impair mast cell degranulation by altering intracellular calcium release through blockade of inositol 1,4,5-triphosphate receptors.[43] Heparin also appears able to influence tumor cell metastasis. Tumor cell invasion from the vasculature probably involves host degradative enzymes, including heparinases, which target both heparin and heparan sulfate. Exogenous heparin inhibits the hydrolysis of heparan sulfate. Heparins with low anticoagulant activity have reduced the metastasis of several tumor types in various experimental models.[43] Smooth muscle cell proliferation such as that which accompanies atherosclerosis and bronchial asthma also is influenced by heparin and heparan sulfate.[84] Heparin inhibits capillary endothelial growth but binds with high affinity to fibroblast growth factors and potentiates their growth-promoting effects.[54] As such, heparin facilities growth of smooth muscle of the vasculature (including pulmonary), airways, intestine, and contractile cells such as fibroblasts and renal glomerular mesangial cells. Effects can be correlated with molecular size and sulfation of heparin; heparin and other heparans may serve as reservoir for growth factors. Endogenous heparin has been implicated in diseases characterized by smooth muscle proliferation; manipulation of selected members of the heparins may ultimately prove to be a therapeutic alternative to treatment.[43] Finally, heparin liberates lipoprotein lipase and can decrease serum triglyceride concentrations, thus "clearing" lipemia.[72,54]

Drug disposition. The complex chemistry of heparin and its binding to proteins and cells leads to complex disposition. Absorption and distribution of heparin are limited by the large size and polarity. Studies characterizing heparin elimination are generally based on response to therapy (i.e., changes in the APTT). However, more recent studies in animals have detected the drug chemical in blood.[85]Absorption of heparin after oral administration or by aerosolization is negligible; as such, heparin is a parenteral anticoagulant. Subcutaneous absorption is rapid; intramuscular administration is generally contraindicated because of the risk of hemorrhage. Heparin is metabolized by heparinase in the liver and by reticuloendothelial cells. Metabolites of heparinase activity are excreted in the urine. The anticoagulant activity of the metabolites apparently has not been addressed. The elimination half-life of heparin appears to depend on molecular weight. The LMW fractions are cleared less rapidly compared with larger molecules, leading to a half-life two to three times longer than that of endogenous heparin. As such, molecules with a higher affinity for AT activity will be cleared more rapidly than those responsible for anti-Xa activity.[86] It is perhaps for this reason that UFH remains the preferred heparin in situations in which a rapid resolution of response upon discontinuation of therapy is desired (e.g., surgical patients or other patients at risk for bleeding).

The pharmacodynamics and elimination half-time of response (based on anti Xa activity) of dalteparin (Fragmin; anti-Xa activity of 2500 U/mL) have been reported in dogs

(Table 15-4). Targeted therapeutic ranges based on anti-Xa activity approximates 0.3 U/mL for UFH and 0.5 U/mL for LMW heparin.[87] Dose response indicates increasing effects with increasing dose, with response more rapid in onset and of greater magnitude with intravenous compared with subcutaneous administration. Response occurs in 2 minutes with intravenous administration, compared with 2 hours with subcutaneous administration. Peak APTT and TT at 2 hours after subcutaneous administration of 200 IU/kg were similar to that measured at 1 minute after 25 IU administered intravenously. Peak effects after intravenous administration approximated 1.75 times baseline for APTT and up to 2.5 times baseline (TT); return to baseline occurred at approximately 1 hour. The impact of subcutaneous administration on APTT and TT was muted: peak effect was no more than 1.25 times baseline for either APTT or TT at all doses. Return to baseline appeared to be dose dependent for both routes but generally was faster (1 to 4 hours, but up to 8 hours) after intravenous compared with SC administration (6 to 10 hours). The authors noted that significant anticoagulant activity lasted up to 3 hours, but even the highest subcutaneous doses failed to affect either APTT or TT to a clinically significant degree. The authors also concluded that monitoring LMW heparin administration in dogs would best be accomplished by measuring anti-FXa activity with chromogenic substrates.[88] The influence of LMW heparin on APTT and TT in dogs appears to be less than that in humans, suggesting species differences in coagulation response. However, this may reflect a shorter APTT in normal dogs compared with normal humans.

The pharmacodynamics (based on anti-Xa activity) of 5 days' treatment of dalteparin (100 IU/kg subcutaneously twice daily) or enoxaparin (1 mg/kg subcutaneously twice daily) was compared with that of UFH (250 IU/kg subcutaneously every 6 hours) in cats (n = 5) using a randomized (for the first treatment) crossover design with a 14-day washout between treatments. Peak activity for all three products occurred at approximately 2 to 4 hours, with the maximum effect of each product in anti-Xa (U/mL) approximating 0.6 (UFH), 0.45 (enoxaparin) and 0.3 (dalteparin). Concentrations reached the human therapeutic range of 0.5 to 1 U/mL anti-Xa activity in only one cat receiving dalteparin. For each drug mean activity was not detectable before the next dose (trough). These data led the investigators to conclude that higher doses than those studied are indicated,[87] Vargo and coworkers drew similar conclusions in their study of rhe effect of dalteparin (100 IU/kg SC, b.i.d, for 13 days) in healthy cats (n = 8) (based on anti-Xa activity). Activity was measurable in only 4 cats; activity present by 4 hr after a single dose (the first sampling time) and returned to baseline by 6 hr; in these cats. Prothrombin time and APTT were not significantly altered by dalteparine administration; although sample size was small, clinical values were essentially unchanged in the cats.[88a] The half-life of heparin is prolonged in renal or liver failure.[81] Bioavailability (subcutaneously) of the LMW heparins appears to be similar in humans, approximating 80% to 90%,[82] and approximates 100% in dogs.[89]

Preparations. Because heparin is a heterogeneous mixture, only about 33% of the molecules i the drug preparation inhibit coagulation, and correlation between heparin plasma concentration and anticoagulant activity is not possible. Correlation between dose and response is further complicated by differences in effects based on molecular weight. The concentration of heparin is standardized by bioassay as units of activity, with 1 unit of heparin (referred to as a *Howell unit)* being equivalent to approximately 2 μg of pure heparin, which in turn (according to the Online Medical Dictionary; http://www.online-medical-dictionary.org/) is the amount of heparin that will maintain anticoagulant activity in 1 mL of feline blood for 24 hours at 0° C.[90] Heparin is available as a sodium or lithium salt. The sodium salt is usually the preferred preparation for in vivo use. LMW heparins currently available for prevention of acute deep vein thrombosis or pulmonary thromboembolism in the United States include dalteparin, enoxaparin (also approved for extended use in prevention of deep vein thrombosis), and ardeparin. The cost for treating a cat with enoxaparin for 1 month has been estimated at $80 (US). Storage of diluted drug (20 mg/mL) and storage in either glass vial or individual tuberculin syringes for up to 4 weeks does not result in statistical

Table 15-4 Pharmacodynamic Response to Plasma Anti-factorXa (Dalteparin) in Healthy Dogs[88,89]

Dose*	Route	Max anti Xa activity	Max APTT (min) (sec)	Max TT (min)‡	Time to max (min)	Duration (hr)‡ APTT	TT	Half-life (min)
		0.1†	15.3±1.5	15.5±0.4	§			
50	SC	0.23±0.0	15.5±1.4	17.2±1.2	120	6	6	81
100	SC	0.43±0.5	16.6±0.1	18.0±1.9	120	8	8-10	123
200	SC	0.9±0.18	19.4±2.4	25.5±4.0	120-180	10	10	182
25	IV	0.43±0.1	18.2±1.3	24.8±2.5	2	1	1	50
50	IV	0.88±0.18	21.2±0.8	39.8±12.4	2	2	2-8	
100	IV	1.86±0.17	26.8±4.2	>500	2	3	4	75

APTT, activated partial thromboplastin time; *TT,* thrombin time; *SC,* subcutaneous; *IV,* intravenous.
*Dose is U anti Xa/kg.
†Reflects 0 time measurement
‡Thrombin time measured at at 3 IU/mL.
§Time to max generally was similar for anti-Xa, APTT, and TT.
||Time to return to baseline for APTT and TT, which often differed.

differences of activity. A generic LMW heparain has recently been approved.

Drug interactions and side effects. Heparin stands out as a drug that will interact with many other drugs. Heparin should not be mixed with any other drug. Hemorrhage is the major complication of heparin therapy, occurring in 18% to 22% of human patients receiving heparin.[81] Hemorrhage is less likely to occur with low dosages and constant intravenous infusion (as opposed to intermittent intravenous administration). Hypersensitivity may play a role in hematoma formation.[91] The incidence of hemorrhage can be reduced by (1) confirmation of the need for therapy; (2) use of the appropriate dose and frequency; (3) avoidance of combination therapy with other antihemostatic drugs, including aspirin and other salicylates; and (4) monitoring of the effects of therapy with clotting or coagulation tests. Use of LMW heparin should also be considered. At higher doses the APTT can be useful for assessing the likelihood of hemorrhage. Monitoring APTT is less useful when low doses of heparin are given. Heparin is contraindicated for the bleeding patient and for DIC unless replacement blood or plasma therapy is given (see later discussion of clinical indications). Excessive therapy (theoretically) might be treated with protamine sulfate, a compound that complexes with heparin. It is dosed according to the amount of heparin to be neutralized (see previous discussion of protamine). The risk of bleeding in surgical patients receiving LMW heparin has not been well assessed; however, the longer duration of action of these products may contribute to an increased risk of bleeding. In human patients undergoing cardiovascular surgery, although all antithrombotic drugs studied increased the risk of bleeding, the use of the LMW product enoxaparin was associated with the greatest amount of blood loss and need for blood transfusions.[92]

Heparin-induced thrombocytopenia has been reported in 5% to 30% of human patients receiving heparin and is more likely to occur with bovine as opposed to porcine preparations.[81,93,94] Two types (type I and type II, similar to type A and type B adverse reactions) of thrombocytopenia have been described. Several days of therapy are necessary for type I thrombocytopenia to occur; it resolves once therapy is discontinued. Type I thrombocytopenia occurs less frequently with LMW heparins. Type II thrombocytopenia occurs in fewer people, is more severe and rapidly fulminating, and is characterized by a longer time to onset (6 to 10 days). Type II thrombocytopenia may be an allergic response to the secondary and tertiary structures of heparin and has caused paradoxical thrombosis.[81]Antibody formation toward heparin bound to platelet factor IV has been demonstrated.[80] The syndrome is recognized by a greater than 50% decrease in platelets that cannot be explained by other causes and/or skin lesions at the site of injection.[80] As with type I thrombocytopenia, the incidence of type II thrombocytopenia is likely to be less with LMW heparins. However, cross-reactivity of 20% or more toward heparin antiplatelet antibodies has been reported for LMW heparins; heparanioids such as danaparoid have been suggested for human patients demonstrated to develop heparin-induced thrombocytopenia.

A small number of human patients have developed skin necrosis with both UFH and LMW heparin. Lesions are similar to those caused by toxic epidermal necrolysis and can be lethal. The cause is unknown.

In human patients receiving long-term therapy, heparin has induced osteoporosis. The mechanism is not known but does not seem to involve prostaglandin E_2. The effect is more dramatic with UFHs. LMW heparins have an osteopenic or calcium-sparing effect, although the sequelae and nature of this effect are not characterized.[81]

Liver leakage enzymes increase in up to 93% of human patients receiving heparin. The increases peak approximately 7 days into therapy and then return to normal, with no obvious detrimental clinical sequelae. Heparin also interferes with and falsely increases bile acids. When used as an in vitro anticoagulant, heparin falsely increases blood urea nitrogen, bile acids, and sodium and potassium salts. Finally, heparin can interfere with several hormones. It interferes with thyroid hormones, causing decreases in both thyronine and thyroxine. It is a predictable and potent inhibitor of aldosterone secretion in human patients, causing natriuresis and the potential for hyperkalemia, particularly in predisposed patients.[95,96] The effects of heparin on the renin–angiotensin–aldosterone system may be responsible for its antihypertensive effects.[97]

A unique side effect of heparin recently identified reflects adulteration of heparin ingredients by the addition of synthetic or animal origin oversulfated (4 sulfates per disaccharide unit) chondroitin sulfates (OSCS). Acute reactions in humans (which are potentially lethal) reflect two mechanisms: direct interaction with kallikrein and release of C3a and C5a anaphylatoxins.[98] Hypotensive patients (e.g., those undergoing renal dialysis) and patients receiving angiotensin-converting enzyme inhibitors (which inhibit degradation of bradykinin) were at risk of reacting adversely. Because LMW heparins are processed from UFHs, contamination is also possible, although contaminants will be diluted compared with unfractionated preparations. The dog, rat, and pig were studied as models for toxicologic evaluation (as reported by manufacturers Sanofi–Aventis) of contaminated heparins; however, the dog was not selected because cardiovascular toxicity did not occur after administration of doses (0.83, 2.09, 10 mg/kg) considered clinically relevant (although coagulation disorders precluded dosing higher than 10 mg/kg). Consequently, the dog probably is less sensitive to the effects of OSCS, which is consistent with the relative safe use of polysulfated aminoglycans (i.e., Adequan) in dogs compared with humans.

N-acetylcystiene (NAC) manifests some actions similar to heparin. It has been used as a renoprotectant and hepatoprotectant agent in humans undergoing surgery. Compared with placebo controls, human patients receiving 150 mg/kg NAC followed by 150 mg/kg as a 24-hour infusion had lower postoperative PTs and prolonged coagulation times (based on thromboelastometry tracings); further, platelet aggregation also was decreased. Blood loss increased in these patients, leading the investigators to warn that patients receiving NAC preoperatively had an increased risk of bleeding.[99]

Clinical indications and use. Clinical indications for heparin therapy include the prevention or treatment of venous or pulmonary embolism (e.g., nephrotic syndrome, autoimmune hemolytic anemia, hyperadrenocorticism, or heartworm disease) and atrial fibrillation with embolization (e.g., feline cardiomyopathy) and as an anticoagulant for diagnostic use and blood transfusion.

Thromboembolism. Heparin remains the drug of choice when rapid anticoagulant activity is necessary in acute thrombosis; in humans heparin is continued for 4 to 5 days to allow time to onset of oral anticoagulants. Generally, heparin is effective only on the fluid phases of thrombin-dependent proteins and is ineffective toward clot-bound factors. However, heparin not only prevents further thrombosis but also appears to facilitate resolution of the thrombus, promoting recanalization through activation of tissue plasminogen activator[81] and stimulating angiogenesis. Efficacy of therapy does not seem to be related to the anatomic location of the thrombus. Heparin and other antithrombotic agents have not been well studied in dogs and cats. Many studies that focus on pharmacokinetics and pharmacodynamics are performed in normal animals; response to drugs may be much different in the face of diseases requiring therapy. In human patients (and possibly dogs), the dose of heparin necessary to control coagulation may be greater than that in the normal patient who is not suffering from a coagulopathy.[100] For thrombosis, heparin is administered parenterally; deep subcutaneous or intrafat injection prolongs persistence of therapeutic concentrations. Large hematomas can occur with deep intramuscular injection. Heparin is also administered intravenously, either intermittently or as a constant infusion. In human patients the use of weight-based nomograms to determine initial and maintenance heparin infusion rates results in a higher percentage of patients reaching the targeted activated thromboplastin time (APTT) range earlier in the course of therapy.[101] Monitoring is particularly important to establish effective doses. Doses are variable with author, route, species, and intent. Generally, subcutaneous doses range from 150 to 250 U/kg in dogs and from 250 to 375 U/kg in cats every 8 hours. The dose of heparin in normal cats necessary to maintain therapeutic concentrations of heparin (as established in humans, 0.35 to 0.7 U/mL) in one study was 300 U/kg of heparin every 8 hours.[85]

For most causes of thromboembolism, therapy is more likely to be successful in patients if heparin is administered at a rate to cause the APTT time to be 1.5 to 2.5 times baseline or the activated clotting time (ACT) to be 1.2 to 1.5 times baseline (prolongation by 15 to 20 seconds).[80,101-103] However, monitoring APTT generally is ineffectual if low doses of heparin (or LMW heparin) are given. Rather, anti-Xa activity should be measured.[88] A baseline should be established before therapy is begun, and monitoring should occur 2 hours after a subcutaneous dose; measurements might be immediate. Alternatively, targeting anti-Xa activity of 0.35 to 0.7 IU/mL has been recommended in human patients requiring higher doses of UFH to maintain targeted APTT; less heparin was needed in one study, decreasing the risk of bleeding.[80] Replacement of AT should accompany heparin therapy when indicated (e.g., nephrotic syndrome, DIC). Gradual discontinuation of heparin therapy has been recommended to prevent a hypercoagulable state.[102,104] Long-term heparin therapy can be accomplished at home with subcutaneous injections, or warfarin therapy can be implemented (see later discussion of vitamin K antagonists).

LMW heparins (e.g., enoxaparin) have been studied in humans and to some degree in dogs and cats. Advantages when compared with HMW heparins include specificity of action, better absorption after subcutaneous injection, more predictable dose–response relationship because of improved prediction of pharmacokinetics, and prolonged elimination half-life. Reduced incidence of bleeding (in nonsurgical patients) because of more specific targeting of Xa compared with thrombin and other factors, as well as reduced thrombocytopenia, has also been suggested as an advantage of LMW heparins.[81,105] Because LMW heparin does not effectively affect thrombin, APTT and TT are minimally affected and therefore should not be used to monitor response. Rather, anti-Xa activity should be measured. According to Mischke and Grebe,[88] in humans an anti-Xa activity target of 0.3 to 0.6 U/mL at 4 hours is suggested for patients at high risk of thrombosis (the lower target intended to minimize the risk of bleeding complications; a target of 0.14 to 0.34 has been recommended for patients with acute myocardial infection already receiving thrombolytic therapy) and 0.4 to 0.9 U/mL for low-risk patients.[80,88] Whether the targets appropriate for dogs are also appropriate for cats has yet to be established. However, if the same targets are relevant, a dose of 100 U/kg of LMW heparin (dalteparin) would achieve the targeted anti-Xa activity in dogs at 2 to 4 hours (see Table 15-4)

A retrospective study of cats with FATE and treated with dalteparin found the drug, when administered at 99 U/kg either once or twice daily, to be both convenient and effective. Mean follow-up time of 172 days was associated with recurrence in 8 of 43 cats, with complications related to bleeding described as infrequent.[103] The use of LMW heparin (dalteparin, starting daily dose of 102 IU/kg subcutaneously) has been compared to warfarin (0.08 mg/kgl using PT and an international normalized ratio target of 2 to 3) for treatment of arterial thrombosis in cats.[106] Dalteparin increased mean survival time to 255 days compared with 69 days for warfarin-treated cats, although the differences were not statistically significant, probably due, in part, to small sample size. Further, 17% of the warfarin-treated cats exhibited bleeding adverse events, whereas none of the LMW heparin–treated cats did.

Supportive therapy for treatment of FATE includes the use of analgesics to control pain. The use of newer nonsteroidal antiinflammatories that are more potent for cyclooxygenase 2 (responsible for prostacycline formation) than cyclooxygenase 1 (responsible for thromboxane formation) might prudently be avoided. Their use may shift the balance toward thrombogenesis (see Chapter 29). Use of opioid analgesics, including a fentanyl patch and/or constant-rate infusion, should be considered. Acepromazine should be avoided for either treatment or prevention of thromboemblism; its vasodilatory properties are not likely to facilitate collateral circulation and hypotension-induced decreased blood flow may increase the risk of thrombus growth.[103]

For prevention of pulmonary thromboembolism, heparin can be administered at a lower dose (30 to 75 U/kg). Monitoring ACT or APTT may not be useful at these doses. Hemorrhage, however, remains a potential side effect in at-risk patients (i.e., those undergoing surgery).

A Cochrane review in human medicine found insufficient evidence to recommend use of LMW heparin instead of vitamin K antagonists.[107]

In patients suffering from severe heartworm disease, low-dose heparin given 1 to 2 weeks before treatment and 3 to 6 weeks after treatment improves survival rates compared with no treatment or with aspirin therapy.[108] In the event of thrombosis associated with adulticide therapy, heparin should be administered (50 to 70 U/kg every 8 hours) for at least 7 days (assuming the platelet count increases to above 150,000/mm^3).

LMW heparins have been recommended as treatment or prevention of thrombosis associated with immune-mediated hemolytic anemia.

Disseminated Intravascular Coagulaopathy

Heparin is used with blood and plasma for the treatment of DIC. The use of heparin for treatment of DIC remains controversial.[71] Its efficacy for DIC depends on adequate concentrations of AT (≥40% of normal). Replacement therapy with either whole fresh blood or fresh or fresh frozen plasma is indicated if AT levels are not normal or for actively bleeding patients. A loading dose is generally followed by a maintenance dose; the loading dose can be preincubated with blood or plasma in order to maximize effects on AT Maintenance dosing should be based on changes in APTT rather than on a fixed dose. This is particularly true in patients suffering from DIC because the synthesis of cofactors varies among patients with DIC. Although normal dogs respond rapidly to heparin therapy, identification of changes in APTT in DIC patients may be difficult. Neutralization of heparin with polybrene (hexadimethrine bromide)[71] can be used to distinguish changes in the APTT due to heparin from those due to DIC once a baseline APTT has been established. The recommended dose of heparin is markedly variable, ranging from a low of 75 to 100 U/kg administered subcutaneously (a dose unlikely to change APTT but likely to be sufficient to target AT) to a high of 750 to 1000 U/kg (severe disease with organ damage caused by microthrombosis) every 8 hours. An intravenous bolus of 5000 U or 80 U/kg followed by constant-rate infusion of 5 to 18 U/kg/hr also has been recommended. For a hypercoagulable state, a subcutaneous dose of 200 to 300 U/kg every 6 hours is recommended. The APTT should be monitored every 6 hours. In general, if higher doses are used, the APTT should be prolonged by 1.5-fold to twofold. Once a therapeutic response is established, the APTT and platelet count should be monitored daily. Heparin should not be abruptly discontinued in patients with DIC because of the risk of rebound hypercoagulability associated with AT deficiency. Nonanticoagulant uses of heparin are increasing in human medicine. Anecdotal reports in humans indicate that heparin can be beneficial for the treatment of asthma and allergic inflammation.

DIC has been reviewed in cats,[109] including its treatment. Of the 46 cats studied retrospectively, 43 died or were euthanized, precluding conclusions regarding the most effective therapies.

Vitamin K Antagonists (Oral Anticoagulants)

The oral anticoagulants differ primarily in their duration and magnitude of effect. Studies of their importance in veterinary medicine have focused primarily on their toxic rather than their therapeutic indications,[11] although these drugs are being used increasingly to treat thromboembolic diseases.

Chemistry. The vitamin K antagonists consist of two groups: the coumarin derivatives (dicoumarol and warfarin) and the indandione anticoagulants. Both interfere with the hepatic synthesis of vitamin K–dependent clotting factors II, VII, IX, and X and anticoagulant proteins C and S (see Figure 15-7).[95] They block the reduction of vitamin K by vitamin K epoxide after its use in factor synthesis, thus effectively reducing the concentration of vitamin K. Two points related to this mechanism are important. First, the anticoagulant activity occurs only in vivo; second, there is a delay in anticoagulant activity (and therefore therapeutic or toxic effect) for 8 to 12 hours because of the persistence of factors synthesized before administration. Factor VII has the shortest half-life and therefore is the first factor to become deficient. Antithrombotic effects occur in 4 to 6 days after therapy is begun, however, as serum concentrations of factors IX and X decrease. Serum concentrations of the anticoagulant protein C also decrease but more rapidly than clotting factors, thus possibly rendering the patient hypercoagulable. Other factors that might contribute to the hypercoagulable state increased thrombin generation as a result of the release of procoagulant platelet-derived factors, expression of tissue factor in response to damaged endothelium, and release of platelet factor IV by activated platelets with subsequent neutralization of heparin.[80] Heparin therapy might be used for the first 2 to 5 days after warfarin therapy is begun to prevent this hypercoagulable state.

Disposition. Warfarin contains a chiral carbon (see Figure 15-7) and is marketed as a racemic mixture. The S isomer is approximately 5.5 times more potent than the R isomer with regard to anticoagulant activity in all species pharmacodynamically studied.[110] The vitamin K antagonists are rapidly and completely orally absorbed. Warfarin is 75,000 times more soluble in water than is dicoumarol and is characterized by much better oral bioavailability.[72] Peak levels occur in 1 hour. There are, however, marked differences in product bioavailability, and products should be interchanged with caution. For products used as rodenticides, warfarin derivatives often have a drug half-life up to 7 days, whereas the indandione diphacinone has an elimination half-life of 30 days.[11] All coumarin derivatives are highly bound to serum albumin, limiting the distribution volume to plasma volume. Vitamin K antagonists are metabolized by the liver to inactive metabolites by the cytochrome P450 system and subsequently conjugated to glucuronide. They undergo an enterohepatic cycle.

Although response does not relate in a dose-dependent manner to plasma drug concentrations, the disposition of warfarin, including its enantiomers, has been reported in cats (n = 10) after single intravenous administration of 0.5 mg/kg and then at 0.1, 0.25, and 0.5 mg/kg (n = 4) orally of the racemic mixture.[110] The disposition of the S isomer resulted in significantly higher area under the curve compared with the R isomer, in part because of longer mean residence time and half-life, which were approximately twice as long in the S (approximately 24 hours) compared with the R (11 hours) isomers. Variability was great, with a range that varied almost threefold (11 to 38 hours) for both half-life and mean residence time for the S isomer. A dose-dependent effect was evident. Problematically, distribution of warfarin throughout the study tablets was even. Anticoagulant potency of the two isomers was not studied in cats.

Preparations. Vitamin K antagonists are prepared for therapeutic use as tablets and solutions (e.g., warfarin, dicoumarol). They are, however, more commonly used as oral rodenticides.

Drug interactions. A variety of factors can increase the activity of warfarin anticoagulants. Hypoproteinemia, antimicrobial therapy, hepatic disease, hypermetabolic states, pregnancy, and the nephrotic syndromes are some examples. Drug interactions are most significant when used therapeutically for chronic treatment. Because they are highly protein bound, they will be displaced by (or will displace) other drugs that are protein bound, and their anticoagulant effects may be increased to the point of toxicity. Examples include acetylsalicylic acid and other nonsteroidal antiinflammatory drugs. Drug interactions occur with other antihemostatic agents.

Clinical use. Clinical use of the coumarin derivatives in dogs and cats is increasing as monitoring techniques improve and doses are refined. The high incidence of recurrent thromboembolism in cats receiving aspirin has led to renewed interest in the use of warfarin for management of arterial thromboembolism. Currently, cardiologists are recommending use of warfarin even in the absence of prior thromboembolic events once adequate left atrial enlargement (left atrial to aortic ratio <2) has been confirmed by echocardiography.[111] The drug is discontinued if atrial size should normalize (ratio of <1.25).

Warfarin therapy for humans is characterized by doses that vary as much as twentyfold. Variability should be anticipated as a result of species differences in drug disposition, warfarin preparations, the target disease, and the presence of other drugs that may interact with warfarin. Accurate dosing should be based on drug-response monitoring. For long-term anticoagulant needs, or in combination with heparin (100 U/kg every 8 hours) for acute treatment of thromboembolism, warfarin can be administered at 0.1 to 0.2 mg/kg (or one fourth to one half of a 1-mg tablet in cats) orally every 24 hours.[70,111]

The PT should be measured at baseline before initiation of therapy. Heparin therapy (when also being used) may prolong the prothrombin (as well as ACT and APTT), but a baseline should still be established. Warfarin therapy should be monitored by 4 to 5 days of therapy. Beginning monitoring earlier may help detect changes more easily. Monitoring techniques should be standardized. An optimum sampling time of 2 hours has been recommended.[111] The target response to warfarin therapy varies. Recommendations have included an increase in baseline prothrombin of 1.3 to 1.6 times baseline to 1.5 to 2.5 times baseline.[111]

A standardized approach to interpreting prothrombin response has been recommended based on an international reference preparation of standardized human brain thromboplastin. The international normalized ratio (INR) is determined for the patient (INR = patient prothrombin/control PT^{ISI}), where ISI is the international sensitivity index of the thromboplastin control used to determine the prothrombin. The ISI is provided by the manufacturer of the thromboplastin control. Standardization is important because controls can vary by more than twofold. A target INR of 2 to 3 has been recommended for prevention of feline thromboembolism while minimizing the risk of bleeding. Either the dose or the interval can be manipulated to achieve the target INR (or prothrombin). Tablet size restrictions may, however, make it difficult to fine-tune warfarin therapy. The dosing interval might be prolonged to as long as 48 hours for some patients.[102] Heparin therapy can be discontinued approximately 3 days after warfarin therapy is begun; prothrombin should be expected to decrease as a result. After the patient is sent home, monitoring can be decreased to 2-week intervals.

Warfarin therapy has been combined with aspirin to treat or prevent recurrent thromboembolism or increased risk of thromboembolism. Although the combination is rational, the risk of bleeding is intensified. Not only are both platelets and coagulation factors targeted with this combination, but drug interactions between these two highly protein-bound drugs can also complicate safe therapy.

Toxicity. Toxicity manifested as hemorrhage has been the major veterinary medical concern with vitamin K antagonists. Secondary poisoning resulting from the ingestion of a rodent that has eaten treated bait is the most common cause of toxicity. Toxicity can also occur, however, by overdosing warfarin for treatment of thromboembolism. Treatment for anticoagulant rodenticide toxicity is symptomatic and specific. Specific therapy is vitamin K. Vitamin K_1 is a very effective antidote, but it must be given as long as the anticoagulant is present in the body at toxic levels. This time varies, depending on the drug, from several days to several weeks after ingestion. Vitamin K_3 (menadione) is much less expensive but is also far less effective and never should be used as the sole antidote in cases of severe coagulopathy. Treatment with vitamin K will preclude the therapeutic benefits of warfarin for up to 3 weeks.

Fibrinolytics (Thrombolytics)

Fibrinolytic agents increase the activity of plasmin (fibrinolysin), the endogenous compound that is responsible for dissolving clots.[112]

Streptokinase and Streptodornase

Streptokinase and streptodornase are synthesized by streptococcal organisms. Urokinase is prepared from cultures of human renal cells. Streptokinase, streptodornase, and urokinase are used in the treatment of wounds that do not respond to antibacterial therapy, burns, ulcers, chronic eczemas, ear hematomas, otitis externa, osteomyelitis, chronic sinusitis, or other chronic lesions. They are available as powders for local or systemic administration. Streptokinase may be useful for the treatment of feline thromboembolic disease. In an experimental model, streptokinase reduced mean thrombus weight after administration of a loading dose (90,000 IU/cat) and a constant maintenance infusion of 45,000 IU (studied for only 3 hours). Clinical use of streptokinase has not been reported.[70]

Tissue Plasminogen Activator

Tissue-type plasminogen activator (tPA) activates plasminogen bound to fibrin. Its use should be limited to cases of thrombosis (rather than prevention). Some studies have indicated a potential use for tPA for dissolution of thrombi in cats, but side effects should be minimized before general use of the drug can be accepted. Although 50% of cats with spontaneous aortic thrombosis treated with tPA (0.25 to 1 mg/kg per hour for a total dose of 1 to 10 mg/kg) had resolution of clinical signs, 70% of the cats treated died from reperfusion injury, heart failure, or other side effects.[70]

Clinical Use

Cost and lack of refined doses and selectivity have limited the use of thrombolytic drugs for treatment of (pulmonary) thromboembolism in dogs and cats.

Antithrombotics

Platelet activity is controlled by substances generated both outside and inside the platelet. Adenophosphate, prostaglandins, thromboxane, serotonin, cAMP, and GMP are generated within the platelet, where they interact with platelet receptors or with the platelet itself. Modulation of all platelet activity can be achieved by interaction with these compounds. Among platelet receptors are two P2YP type purinergic receptors that are activated by ADP and coupled with G-protein (Gq). Activation causes platelet shape to change, induces phosphatidylinositol turnover and platelet aggretation. This response is offset by a second receptor type coupled to Gi. Activation of this receptor by ADP inhibits adenylyl cyclase and decreases cAMP, resulting in muted platelet activation. Both receptors must be stimulated for platelets to activate.

The thienopyridines ticlopidine and clopidogrel are ADP antagonists with antiplatelet activity. Their inhibitory effects on P_{2Y12} G1-coupled adenosine receptors are irreversible, targeting both primary and secondary aggregation to a variety of agonists. Ticlopidine has been extensively studied in human patients with thromboembolic disease. Inhibition occurs in 2 to 5 days. The thienopyridines also inhibit the conformation change of glycoprotein IIb/IIa induced by ADP. Because binding of fibrinogen and vWF is prevented, thrombrus progression is inhibited. Because both ticlopidine and clopidrogel are prodrugs, pharmacodynamic tests must occur in vivo and pharmacokinetics must be based on the active metabolite. The enzyme responsible for metabolism has not yet been identified.[54] Maximum effects are delayed up to 8 to 11 days; a loading dose (twice maintenance) is suggested in humans. Effects persist for several days after discontinuation of therapy; this may reflect an irreversible nature of inhibition and the need for new platelets. Serious side effects are rare in humans but include neutropenia and thrombocytopenia. The drug has proved equal to aspirin in the prevention of human stroke. Ticlopidine has been studied in dogs. A dose of 62 mg/kg every 24 hours inhibits platelet aggregation in normal dogs, but higher doses may be necessary in the presence of thromboembolic disease.[3,113] It is not clear if the cat metabolizes ticlopidine to the active drug. However, ticlopidine also has been studied in cats (n = 8) at 50, 100, and 200 mg/cat once daily orally and 250 mg/cat every 12 hours for 10 days using (apparently) a nonrandomized crossover design with at least 14 days between treatments.[114] Outcome measures included oral mucosal bleeding times and platelet aggregation (blood aggregometry). Significant reduction in platelet aggregation occurred with doses at 100 mg and above, although effects were present on all three test days (3, 7, and 10) only for the 250-mg twice-daily dose. Ticlopidine was associated with dose-dependent anorexia and vomiting, which occurred shortly after dosing, causing the authors to conclude that clinical utility of ticlopidine was limited. However, cats developed tolerance to these side effects. One of the eight cats was removed from the study because of sudden death, although the death could not be attributed to the drug.

Clopidogrel is related to ticlopidine and is less likely to cause neutropenia. Also a prodrug, its onset of action also is slow, with the loading dose in humans being 4 times the maintenance dose. Clopidogrel has been studied for its effect on thrombolysis, based on the observation that platelet activation may decrease thrombolysis or facilitate rethrombosis.[115] Clopidogrel had no impact on thrombolysis in cats with experimentally induced (tPA) thrombosis after 3 days of oral therapy (75 mg), although only three cats were studied. However, a follow-up study in blood collected from cats (n = 9) found no effect.[115] The pharmacokinetic-pharmacodynamic relationship of clopidregel was described in dogs (n = 8) receiving approximately 1 mg/kg PO every 24 hr for 3 days followed by either 0.5 or 1 mg/kg every 24 hr for 3 days (n = 5).[115a] Indices of platelet inhibition (e.g, ADP-induced platelet aggregation decreased by 80 to 93% from baseline) were present by day 3 in either treatment group, with the duration of effect lasting 3 to 7 days. Peak metabolite concentration 210 + 200 ng/ml occurred 1 hour after administration; the rapid disappearance and low (below detectable) concentrations of the metabolite precluded complete pharmacokinetic description. Experimentally, clopidogrel (5 mg/kg) proved more effective than aspirin (5 mg/kg) when combined with t-PA (80 μg/kg) or heparin (200 U/kg) for prevention of experimentally induced coronary artery occlusion.[115b]

Dipyridamole is a vasodilator that inhibits cAMP phosphodiesterase and increases cAMP in the platelet. When used alone, it minimally affects platelet activity but acts synergistically with aspirin to inhibit platelet activity.[116]

Aspirin causes an irreversible and thus long-lasting negative effect on platelet activity, which is clinically manifested as prolonged bleeding time. Aspirin irreversibly inactivates prostaglandin G and H synthetase, the enzyme that catalyzes the initial conversion of arachidonic acid to thromboxane A_2. Two types of this enzyme are present: the constitutive form responsible for conversion of arachidonic acid to prostaglandin H (and ultimately thromboxane) and an inducible form that activates cells in response to growth factors during inflammation. The antiplatelet effects of aspirin result from acetylation of the constitutive form of the enzyme.[117] Platelets are not able to synthesize proteins and thus cannot regenerate the enzyme necessary for thromboxane formation. The irreversible nature of platelet inhibition allows aspirin administration to occur at 3-day or longer intervals. Reduced formation of the various eicosanoids responsible for platelet aggregation and coagulation accounts for the variety of different pharmacologic (therapeutic and toxic) responses to aspirin. Side effects of aspirin can, however, be minimized by taking advantage of the dose–response relationship between aspirin and its many pharmacologic effects.

Prospective, controlled studies that support the efficacy of aspirin as an antithrombotic either as a preventive or treatment for FATE are limited. In a retrospective study of cats with acute FATE, survival did not differ between cats receiving 5 mg (n = 12) versus ≥ 40 mg/cat (n = 34) every 72 hours.[118] An advantage of the lower dose might be inhibition of thromboxane synthetase (causing platelet aggregation) without inhibition of prostacyclin synthetase (inhibition of platelet aggregation). However, the power of the study to detect a treatment difference was not described, and failure to detect a significant difference should not be interpreted as equal efficacy between the two doses. On the other hand, the incidence of side effects was lower in the low-dose aspirin group.

One study reported that a very high dose of aspirin (650 mg/cat) in cats before initiation of thrombus formation improved collateral circulation compared with controls that did not receive aspirin,[119] suggesting that aspirin prophylaxis might help reduce recurrence and that therapy should be initiated as soon as possible in the acute event.

The antiplatelet effect of aspirin can be separated to a large degree from its other actions by administration of a low dose (0.5 mg/kg every 12 hours in a normal dog). One retrospective study of the use of an ultralow dose of aspirin (0.5 mg/kg) versus (unfractionated) heparin (75-125 U/kg every 6 to 8 hours) in 151 dogs with immune-mediated hemolytic anemia being treated with prednisolone and azathioprine found the percentage of animals surviving the hospital stay to be 84% for the aspirin group versus approximately 54% for either the heparin-treated or no-antihemostatic-drug–treated group.[120] Survival at 1 year was 67% for the aspirin-treated group versus 46% for the heparin-treated group and 34% for the no-antihemostatic-drug–treated group. The study was biased by the assignment of treatments: Coagulopathy was worse in the heparin group compared with the aspirin group. Nonetheless, the study supports the potential efficacy of aspirin at very low doses compared with no antihemostatic drug; its inclusion in the treatment regimen is made more prudent because of the potential for glucocorticoid therapy to worsen the risk of thromboemblism (see Chapter 30).

Other "low doses" suggested for aspirin include 10 mg/kg in heartworm-infested dogs and 25 mg/kg twice weekly in cats.[72,117,121] Although experimental studies reveal antiplatelet activity for aspirin, clinical response is variable.[122,123] Aspirin, however, remains a component of therapy directed toward prevention and treatment of arterial thrombosis,[2,117,124] including severe pulmonary arterial thrombosis associated with heartworm disease.[108] Coupled with cage confinement, aspirin (4 to 6 mg/kg per day) administered for 2 to 3 weeks before caparsolate therapy may improve survival after treatment.[108] Aspirin is still the most commonly used drug for prevention of arterial thrombosis in cats (25 mg/kg orally every 72 hours) despite the lack of clinical proof of efficacy.[70] Recurrence of thrombosis may, however, be as high as 75%.

Interestingly, one report in a canine model of coronary thrombosis describes a synergistic antiplatelet effect when administered with metoclopramide.[125] Aspirin was administered at 0.03 to 0.1 mg/kg intravenously and metoclopramide at 0.1 or 0.3 mg/kg intravenously. The effect of metoclopramide was attributed to either $s5HT_2$ or antagonism of $alpha_2$.

Other drugs with antiplatelet activity are available but have not been sufficiently studied in animals. These include the tirofiban and abciximab, inhibitors of glycoprotein (IIb/IIIa), a platelet surface integrin that serves as a receptor for fibrinogen and vWF. For example, abciximab is the Fab fragment of a human monoclonal antibody directed toward the receptor used to treat coronary thromboembolism. Propranolol has been found to be ineffective as an inhibitor of platelet activity.[71,126]

Homocysteine

The recognition of arterial damage in two infants with inborn errors of metabolism resulting in an increase of homocysteine led to the investigation of the possible role of homocysteine in thromboembolic disease.[127] However, homocysteine accumulation generally is accompanied by an increase of its precursor, S-adenosylhomocysteine (SAH). This demethylated product of numerous S-adenosylmethionine (SAM)-dependent transmethylation reactions may cause a potent feedback inhibition, resulting in hypomethylation of reactions critical to thrombogenic control. In homocystinuria, lowered plasma homocysteine is accompanied by lowered SAH concentrations and restored transmethylation reactions. It is not clear if increased homocysteine (or SAH) is a cause or effect (and thus a marker) of thromboembolic disorders. Because the kidneys are responsible for clearing up to 70% of homocysteine, concentrations increase in concert with creatinine in patients with renal disease, reaching increases of threefold to fivefold above baseline. Other factors that increase homocysteine include decreased folate and vitamin B concentrations and cardiovascular disease itself.

REFERENCES

1. Compston JE: Bone marrow and bone: a functional unit, *J Endocrinol* 173:387–394, 2002.
2. Kanshansky K, Kipps TJ: Hematopoietic agents: growth factors, minerals, and vitamins. In Brunton L, Lazo JS, Parker KL, editors: *Goodman and Gilma's the pharmacologic basis of therapeutics*, ed 11, New York, 2006, McGraw-Hill.

3. Adams HR: Drugs acting on blood and blood elements. In Adams HR, editor: *Veterinary pharmacology and therapeutics*, ed 7, Ames, Iowa, 1995, Iowa State University Press, pp 531–543.
4. Ruaux CG, Steiner JM, Williams DA: Early biochemical and clinical responses to cobalamin supplementation in cats with signs of gastrointestinal disease and severe hypocobalaminemia, *J Vet Intern Med* 19:155–160, 2005.
5. Weiss DJ: Leucocyte disorders and their treatment. In Kirk RW, editor: *Current veterinary therapy XI*, Philadelphia, 1995, Saunders, pp 452–456.
6. Locatelli F, Aljama P, Barany P: Erythropoiesis-stimulating agents and antibody-mediated pure red-cell aplasia: where are we now and where do we go from here? *Nephrol Dial Transplant* 19:288–293, 2004.
7. Eschbach JW, Adamson JW: Recombinant human erythropoietin: implications for nephrology, *Am J Kidney Dis* 11: 203–209, 1988.
8. Eschbach JW, Adamson JW: Guidelines for recombinant human erythropoietin therapy, *Am J Kidney Dis* 16, (Supp l): 2–8, 1989.
9. Faulds D, Sorkin EM: Epoetin (recombinant human erythropoietin); a review of its pharmacodynamic and pharmacokinetic properties, *Drugs* 38(6):863–899, 1989.
10. Schwenk MH, Halstenson CE: Recombinant human erythropoietin, *DICP* 23:528–535, 1989.
11. Schulman A, Lusk R, Lippincott CL, et al: Diphacinone-induced coagulopathy in the dog, *J Am Vet Med Assoc* 188:402–405, 1986.
12. Patton J, Reeves T, Wallace J: Effectiveness of darbepoetin alfa versus epoetin alfa in patients with chemotherapy-induced anemia treated in clinical practice, *Oncologist* 9(4):451–458, 2004.
13. Bennett CL, Luminari S, Nissenson AR: Pure red-cell aplasia and epoetin therapy, *N Engl J Med* 351(14):1403–1408, 2004.
14. MacLeod J, Tetreault J, et al: Expression and bioactivity of recombinant canine erythropoietin, *Am J Vet Res* 59(9):1144, 1998.
15. Randolph JF, Scarlett JM, Stokol T, et al: Expression, bioactivity and clinical assessment of recombinant feline erythropoietin, *Am J Vet Res* 65:1355–1366, 2004.
16. Casadevall N, Rossert J: Importance of biologic follow-ons: experience with EPO, *Best Pract Res Clin Haematol* 18(3):381–387, 2005.
17. Evens AM, Bennett CL, Luminari S: Epoetin-induced pure red-cell aplasia (PRCA): preliminary results from the research on adverse drug events and reports (RADAR) group, *Best Pract Res Clin Haematol* 18(3):481–489, 2005.
18. Schellekens H: Immunologic mechanisms of EPO-associated pure red cell aplasia, *Best Pract Res Clin Haematol* 18(3):473–480, 2005.
19. Carson KR, Evens AM, Bennett CL, et al: Clinical characteristics of erythropoietin-associated pure red cell aplasia, *Best Pract Res Clin Haematol* 18(3):467–472, 2005.
20. Asari A, Gokal R: Pure red cell aplasia secondary to Epoetin alpha responding to darbepoetin alpha in a patient on peritoneal dialysis, *J Am Soc Nephrol* 15:2204–2207, 2004.
21. Cowgill L: Application of recombinant human erythropoietin (r-Hu-EPO) in dogs and cats. In Kirk RW, editor: *Current Veterinary Therapy XI*, Philadelphia, 1992, Saunders, p 484.
22. Cowgill L: CVT update: use of recombinant human erythropoietin. In Bonagura J, editor: *Current Veterinary Therapy XII*, Philadelphia, 1995, Saunders, pp 961–966.
23. Cowgill LD, Polzin DJ, Osborne CA, et al: Results of recombinant human erythropoietin clinical trial, *Proc 12th ACVIM Forum* 12:490–492, 1994.
24. Randolph J, Stokol T, Scarlett JM, et al: Comparison of biological activity and safety of recombinant canine erythropoietin with that of recombinant human erythropoietin in clinically normal cogs, *Am J Vet Res* 60(5):636, 1999.
25. Randolph JF, Scarlett J, Stokol T, et al: Clinical efficacy and safety of recombinant canine erythropoietin in dogs with anemia of chronic renal failure and dogs with recombinant human erythropoietin-induced red cell aplasia, *J Vet Intern Med* 18: 81–91, 2004.
26. Cowgill LD, James KM, Levy JK, et al: Use of recombinant human erythropoietin for management of anemia in dogs and cats with renal failure, *J Am Vet Med Assoc* 212(4):521–528, 1998.
27. Langston CE, Reine NJ, Kittrell D: The use of erythropoietin, *Vet Clin North Am Small Anim Pract* 33(6):1245–1260, 2003.
28. Adamson JW, Eschbach JW: Treatment of the anemia of chronic renal failure with recombinant human erythropoietin, *Proc 9th ACVIM Forum* 9:603–610, 1991.
29. Cervelli M, Gray N, McDonald S, et al: Randomized cross-over comparison of intravenous and subcutaneous darbepoetin dosing efficiency in haemodialysis patients, *Nephrology* 10(2):129, 2005.
30. Glaspy J: Phase III clinical trials with darbepoetin: implications for clinicians, *Best Pract Res Clin Haematol* 18(3):407–416, 2005.
31. Besarab A, Bolton WK, Browne JK, et al: The effects of normal as compared with low hematocrit values in patients with cardiac disease who are receiving hemodialysis and epoetin, *N Engl J Med* 339:584–590, 1998.
32. Eschbach JW: Iron requirements in erythropoietin therapy, *Best Pract Res Clin Haematol* 18(2):347–361, 2005.
33. Wingard RL, Parker RA, Ismail N, et al: Efficacy of oral iron therapy in patients receiving recombinant human erythropoietin, *Am J Kidney Dis* 25:433–439, 1995.
34. Garton JO, Gertz MA, Witzig TE, et al: Epoetin alfa for the treatment of anemia of multiple myeloma, *Arch Intern Med* 155:2069–2074, 1995.
35. Giampaoli S, Facciabene A, Mennuni C: A protocol to guide development of a sensitive ELISA for canine erythropoietin, *Vet Clin Pathol* 32(4):199–201, 2003.
36. Baz R, Brand C, McGowan B, et al: High dose recombinant human erythropoietin use is associated with increased overall survival in patients with multiple myeloma, *2005 American Society of Clinical Oncology Annual Meeting*, abst 6621.
37. Bohlius JF, Langensiepen S, Engert A: Effectiveness of erythropoietin in the treatment of patients with malignancies: methods and preliminary results of a Cochrane review, *Best Pract Res Clin Haematol* 18(3):449–454, 2005.
38. Djulbegovic B: Erythropoietin use in oncology: a summary of the evidence and practice guidelines comparing efforts of the Cochrane Review group and Blue Cross/Blue Shield to set up the ASCO/ASH guidelines, *Best Pract Res Clin Haematol* 18(3):455–466, 2005.
39. Lichtin A: The ASH/ASCO clinical guidelines on the use of erythropoietin, *Best Pract Res Clin Haematol* 18(3):433–438, 2005.
40. Aroch I, Harrus S: The use of recombinant human granulocyte colony stimulating factor and recombinant human erythropoietin in the treatment of severe pancytopenia due to canine monocyte ehrlichiolsis, *Israel J Vet Med* 6, 2001.
41. Borwkoski J, Amrikachi M, Hudnall SD: Fulminant parvovirus infection following erythropoietin treatment in a patient with acquired immunodeficiency syndrome, *Arch Pathol Lab Med* 124(3):441–445, 2001.
42. Duffield JS, Mann S, Horn L, et al: Low-dose cyclosporin therapy for recombinant erythropoietin-induced pure red-cell aplasia, *Nephrol Dial Transplant* 19:479–481, 2004.
43. Tyrrell DJ, Kilfeather S, Page CP: Therapeutic uses of heparin beyond its traditional role as an anticoagulant, *Trends in Pharmaceutical Science* 16:198–204, 1995.
44. Kruth SA: Cytokines and biological response modifiers in small animal practice. In Kirk RW, editor: *Current veterinary therapy XI*, Philadelphia, 1995, Saunders, pp 452–456.

45. Cohn LA, Rewerts JM, McCaw D, et al: Plasma granulocyte colony-stimulating factor concentrations in neutropenic, parvoviral enteritis-infected puppies, *J Vet Intern Med* 13: 581–586, 1999.
46. Lothrop CD, Warrren DJ, Souza LM, et al: Correction of canine cycline hematopoiesis with recombinant human granulocyte colony stimulating factors, *Blood* 72:1324–1328, 1988.
47. Ferrara F, Annunziata M, Pollio F, et al: Vincristine as treatment for recurrent episodes of thrombotic thrombocytopenic purpura, *Ann Hematol* 81(1):7–10, 2002.
48. Rozanski EA, Callan MB, Hughes D: Comparison of platelet count recovery with use of vincristine and prednisone or prednisone alone for treatment for severe immune-mediated thrombocytopenia in dogs, *J Am Vet Med Assoc* 220(4): 477–481, 2002.
49. Chamouni P, Lenain P, Buchonnet G, et al: Difficulties in the management of an incomplete form of refractory thrombotic thrombocytopenic purpura, the usefulness of vincristine, *Transfus Sci* 23:101–106, 2000.
50. Ziman A, Mitri M, Klapper E, et al: Combination vincristine and plasma exchange as initial therapy in patients with thrombotic thrombocytopenic purpura: one institution's experience and review of the literature, *Transfusion* 45:41–49, 2005.
51. Dennis JS: Anabolic steroids: their potential in small animals, *Compend Contin Educ Pract Vet* 12:1403–1419, 1990.
52. Bagatelle CJ, Brenner WJ: Androgens in men—uses and abuses, *N Engl J Med* 334:707–714, 1996.
53. Molinari PF: Erythropoietic mechanism of androgens: a critical review and clinical implications, *Haematology* 67(3): 442–460, 1982.
54. Majerus PW, Tollefsen DM: Blood coagulation and anticoagulant, thrombolytic, and antiplatelet drugs. In Brunton L, Lazo JS, Parker KL, editors: *Goodman and Gilman's the pharmacologic basis of therapeutics*, ed 11, New York, 2006, McGraw-Hill.
55. Snyder PJ: Androgens. In Brunton L, Lazo JS, Parker KL, editors: *Goodman and Gilman's the pharmacologic basis of therapeutics*, ed 11, New York, 2006, McGraw-Hill.
56. Williams TM, Kind AJ, Hill DW: Drug metabolism: in vitro biotransformation of anabolic steroids in canines, *J Vet Pharmacol Ther* 23(2):57–66, 2000.
57. Paulo LG, Fink GD, Roh BL, et al: Effects of several androgens and steroid metabolites on erythropoietin production in the isolated perfused dog kidney, *Blood* 43:39–47, 1974.
58. Olson ME, Morck DW, Quinn KB: The effect of stanozolol on 15nitrogen retention in the dog, *Can J Vet Res* 64(4):246–248, 2000.
59. Maravelias C, Dona A, Stefanidou M, et al: Adverse effects of anabolic steroids in athletes: a constant threat, *Toxicol Lett* 158(3):167–176, 2005.
60. Lowe KC: Blood transfusion or blood substitution, *Vox Sang* 51:257–263, 1986.
61. Gould SA, Sehgal LR, Rosen AL, et al: Red cell substitutes: an update, *Ann Emerg Med* 14:798–803, 1985.
62. Day TK: Current development and use of hemoglobin-based oxygen-carrying (HBOC) solutions, *J Vet Emerg Crit Care* 13(2):77–93, 2003.
63. Kelly N, Rentko VT: Comparative cardiovascular response by Oxyglobin versus packed red blood cells in acute anemia, *J Vet Emerg Crit Care* 8(3):252, 1998.
64. Rentko VA, Wohl J, Murtaugh R, et al: Clinical trial of a hemoglobin based oxygen-carrying (HBOC) fluid in the treatment of anemia in dogs, *J Vet Intern Med* 10:177–178, 1996.
65. Driessen B, Jahr JS, Lurie F, et al: Inadequacy of low-volume resuscitation with hemoglobin-based oxygen carrier hemoglobin glutamer-200 (bovine) in canine hypovolemia, *J Vet Pharmacol Therap* 24:61–71, 2001.
66. Gibson GR, Callan MB, Hoffman V, et al: Use of a hemoglobin-based oxygen-carrying solution in cats: 72 cases (1998–2002), *J Am Vet Assoc* 221(1):96–102, 2002.
67. Grundy SA, Barton C: Influence of drug therapy on survival of dogs with immune-mediated hemolytic anemia: 88 cases (1989–1999), *J Am Vet Med Assoc* 218(4):543–548, 2001.
68. Weingart C, Kohn B: Clinical use of a haemoglobin-based oxygen carrying solution (Oxyglobin®) in cats (2002-2006), *J Feline Med Surg* 10:431–438, 2008.
69. McMichael M: Primary hemostasis, *J Vet Emerg Crit Care* 15:1–8, 2005.
70. Meurs KM: Primary myocardial disease. In Ettinger SJ, Feldman EC, editors: *Textbook of Veterinary Internal Medicine*, ed 6, St Louis, 2005, Saunders.
71. Greene RA, Thomas JS: Hemostatic disorders: coagulopathies and thrombosis. In Ettinger SJ, Feldman EC, editors: *Textbook of veterinary internal medicine*, ed 4, Philadelphia, 1995, Saunders, pp 1946–1963.
72. Adams HR, Carr AP: Hemostatic and anticoagulant drugs. In Adams HR, editor: *Veterinary pharmacology and therapeutics*, ed 7, Ames, Iowa, 1995, Iowa State University Press, pp 544–559.
73. McMichael M: Primary hemostasis, *J Vet Emer Crit Care* 15(2):1–8, 2005.
74. Johnstone IB: Desmopressin enhances the binding of plasma von Willebrand factor to collagen in plasmas from normal dogs and dogs with type I von Willebrand's disease, *Can Vet J* 40(9):645–648, 1999.
75. Kraus KH, Turrentine MA, Jergens AE: Effect of desmopressin acetate on bleeding times and plasma von Willebrand factor in Doberman pinscher dogs with von Willebrand's disease, *Vet Surg* 18(2):103–109, 1989.
76. Sato I, Parry BW: Effect of desmopressin on plasma factor VIII and von Willebrand factor concentrations in Greyhounds, *Aust Vet J* 76:809–812, 1998.
77. Kristensen AT, Edwards ML, Devey J: Potential uses of recombinant human factor VIIa in veterinary medicine, *Vet Clin North Am Small Anim Pract* 33(6):1437–1451, 2003.
78. Brockway WJ, Castellino FJ: The mechanism of the inhibition of plasmin activity by ε-aminocaproic acid, *J Biol Chem* 246(14):4641–4647, 1971.
79. Takeda Y, Parkhill TR, Nakabayashi M: Effects of heparin and ε-aminocaproic acid in dogs on plasmin-^{125} I generation in response to urokinase injections and venous injury, *J Clin Invest* 51:2678–2685, 1972.
80. Hirsh J, Warkentin TE, et al: Heparin and low-molecular-weight heparin: mechanisms of action, pharmacokinetics, dosing, monitoring, efficacy, and safety, *Chest* 119(Suppl):64S–94S, 2001.
81. Freedman MD: Pharmacodynamics, clinical indications, and adverse effects of heparin, *J Clin Pharmacol* 32:584–596, 1992.
82. Weitz JI: Low-molecular-weight heparins, *N Engl J Med* 337(10):688–698, 1997.
83. Folkman J, Shing S: Control of angiogenesis by heparin and other sulfated polysaccharides, *Adv Exp Med Biol* 313: 355–364, 1992.
84. Burden TS, Buhler FR: Regulation of smooth muscle proliferative phenotype by heparinoid-matrix interactions, *Trends in Pharmaceutical Science* 9:94–98, 1988.
85. Kellerman DL, Lewis DC, Myers NC, et al: Determination of a therapeutic heparin dosage in the cat, *Proc Am Coll Vet Intern Med* 14:748, 1996.
86. Brieger D, Dawes J: Production method affects the pharmacokinetic and ex vivo biological properties of low molecular weight heparins, *Thromb Haemost* 77(2):317–322, 1997.
87. Alwood AJ, Downend AB, Brooks MB, et al: Anticoagulant effects of low-molecular-weight heparins in healthy cats, *J Vet Intern Med* 21:378–387, 2007.
88. Mischke R, Grebe S: The correlation between plasma anti-factor Xa activity and haemostatic tests in healthy dogs, following the administration of a low molecular weight heparin, *Res Vet Sci.* 69(3):241–247, 2000.

88a. Vargo CL, Taylor SM, Carr A, et al: The effect of a low molecular weight heparin on coagulation parameters in healthy cats, *Can J Vet Res* 73(2):132–136, 2009.
89. Grebe S, Jacobs C, Kietzmann M, et al: Phamacokinetics of low-molecular-weight heparins Fragmin D in dogs, *Berl Munch Tierarztl Wochenschr* 113(3):103–107, 2000.
90. Online Medical Dictionary
91. Grodman-Gross CA, Sastri SV: Heparin-associated hematomas: possible allergic reaction, *DICP Ann Pharmacother* 21:180–183, 1987.
92. McDonald SB, Renna M, Spitznagel EL, et al: Preoperative use of enoxaparin increases the risk of postoperative bleeding and re-exploration in cardiac surgery patients, *J Cardiothorac Vasc Anesth* 19(1):4–10, 2005.
93. Greinacher A, Michels I, Schäfer M, et al: Heparin-associated thrombocytopenia in a patient treated with polysulphated chondroitin sulphate: evidence for immunological crossreactivity between heparin and polysulphated glycosaminoglycan, *Br J Haematol* 81:252–254, 1992.
94. Shumate MJ: Heparin-induced thrombocytopenia, *N Engl J Med* 333:1006, 1995.
95. Aull L, Chao H, Coy K: Heparin-induced hyperkalemia, *DICP* 24:244–246, 1990.
96. Oster JR, Singer I, Fishman LM: Heparin-induced aldosterone suppression and hyperkalemia, *Am J Med* 98:575–586, 1995.
97. Susic D, Mandal AK, Jovovic D, et al: Antihypertensive action of heparin: role of the renin-angiotensin aldosterone system and prostaglandins, *J Clin Pharmacol* 33:342–347, 1993.
98. Kishimoto TK, Viswanathan K, Ganguly T, et al: Contaminated heparin associated with adverse clinical events and activation of the contact system, *N Engl J Med* 358(23):2457–2467, 2008.
99. Niemi TT, Munsterhjelm E, Pöyhiä R, et al: The effect of N-acetylcysteine on blood coagulation and platelet function in patients undergoing open repair of abdominal aortic aneurysm, *Blood Coagul Fibrinolysis* 17(1):29–34, 2006.
100. Mungall D, Raskob G, Coleman R, et al: Pharmacokinetics and dynamics of heparin in patients with proximal vein thrombosis, *J Clin Pharmacol* 29:896–900, 1989.
101. Gunnarsson PS, Sawyer WT, Montague D, et al: Appropriate use of heparin, *Arch Intern Med* 155:526–532, 1995.
102. Hawkins EC: Diseases of the lower respiratory system. In Ettinger SJ, Feldman EC, editors: *Textbook of veterinary internal medicine*, ed 4, Philadelphia, 1995, Saunders, pp 767–811.
103. Smith SA, Tobias AH: Feline arterial thromboembolism: an update, *Vet Clin Small Anim* 34:1245–1271, 2004.
104. Lauer MA, Houghtaling PL, Peterson JG: Attenuation of rebound ischemia after discontinuation of heparin therapy by glycoprotein IIb/IIIa inhibition with eptifibatide in patients with acute coronary syndromes observations from the platelet IIb/IIIa in unstable angina: receptor suppression using integrilin therapy (PURSUIT) trial, *Circulation* 104:2772, 2001.
105. Frydman AM, Bara L, Woler M, et al: The antithrombotic activity and pharmacokinetics of enoxaparin, a low molecular weight heparin, in humans given single subcutaneous doses of 20 to 80 mg, *J Clin Pharmacol* 28:609–618, 1988.
106. DeFrancesco TC, Moore RR, Atkins CL, et al: Comparison of dalteparin and warfarin in the longterm management of feline arterial thromboembolism, *Proc ACVIM*: #281, 2005.
107. Van der Heijden JF, Hutten BA, Büller HR, et al: Vitamin K antagonists or low-molecular-weight heparin for the long term treatment of symptomatic venous thromboembolism, *Cochrane Database Syst Rev* , 2001, Issue 3, Art. No.: CD002001. doi:10.1002/14651856.CD002001, 2008.
108. Rawlings CA, Calvert CA: Heartworm disease. In Ettinger SJ, Feldman EC, editors: *Textbook of veterinary internal medicine*, ed 4, Philadelphia, 1995, Saunders, pp 1046–1068.
109. Estrin MA, Wehausen CE, Jessen CR, et al: Disseminated intravascular coagulation in cats, *J Vet Intern Med* 20: 1334–1339, 2006.
110. Smith CE, Rozanski EA, Freeman LM, et al: Use of low molecular weight heparin in cats: 57 cases (1999-2003), *J Am Vet Med Assoc* 225(8):1237–1241, 2005.
111. Harpster NK, Baty C: Warfarin therapy of the cat at risk of thromboembolism. In Bongura J, editor: *Current veterinary therapy XII*, Philadelphia, 1995, Saunders, pp 868–873.
112. Witty LA, Krichman A, Tapson VF: Thrombolytic therapy for venous thromboembolism: utilization by practicing pulmonologists, *Arch Intern Med* 154:1601–1604, 1994.
113. Boudreaux MK, Dillin AR, Ravis WR: Effects of treatment with aspirin or aspirin/dipyrimadole combination in heartworm negative, heartworm infected and embolized heartworm-infected dogs, *Am J Vet Res* 52:1992–1999, 1991.
114. Hogan DF, Ward MP: Effect of clopidogrel on tissue-plasminogen activator-induced in vitro thrombolysis of feline whole blood thrombi, *Am J Vet Res* 65:715–719, 2004.
115. Hogan DF, Andrews DA, Talbott KK, et al: Evaluation of antiplatelet effects of ticlopidine in cats, *Am J Vet Res* 65:327–332, 2004.
115a. Brainard BM, Kleine SA, Papich MG, et al: Pharmacodynamic and pharmacokinetic evaluation of clopidogrel and the carboxylic acid metabolite SR 26334 in healthy dogs, *Am J Vet Res* 71(7):822–830, 2010.
115b. Yao SK, Ober JC, Ferguson JJ, et al: Clopidogrel is more effective than aspirin in preventing coronary artery reocclusion after thrombolysis, *Trans Assoc Am Physicians* 106:110–119, 1993.
116. Boudreaux MK, Dillin AR, Sartin EA, et al: Effects of treatment with ticlopidine in heartworm negative, heartworm infected and embolized heartworm-infected dogs, *Am J Vet Res* 52:2000–2006, 1991.
117. Patrono C: Aspirin as an antiplatelet drug, *N Engl J Med* 330:1287–1294, 1994.
118. Smith SA, Tobias AH, Jacob KA, et al: Arterial thromboembolism in cats: acute crisis in 127 cases (1992–2001) and long-term management with low-dose aspirin in 24 cases, *J Vet Intern Med* 17:73–83, 2003.
119. Schaub RG, Gates KA, Roberts RE: Effect of aspirin on collateral blood flow after experimental thrombosis of the feline aorta, *Am J Vet Res* 43(9):1647–1650, 1982.
120. Weinkle TK, Center SA, Randolph JF, et al: Azathioprine and ultra-low-dose aspirin therapy for canine immune-mediated hemolytic anemia, *Proc ACVIM* , 2004.
121. Jackson ML: Platelet physiology and platelet function: inhibition by aspirin, *Compend Contin Educ Pract Vet* 9:627–638, 1987.
122. Rawlings CA, Keith JC, Lewis RE, et al: Aspirin and prednisolone modification of radiographic changes caused by adulticide treatment in dogs with heartworm infection, *J Am Vet Med Assoc* 183:131–132, 1983.
123. Rawlings CA, Keith JC, Losonsky JM, et al: Aspirin and prednisolone modification of postadulticide pulmonary arterial disease in heartworm-infected dogs: arteriographic study, *J Am Vet Med Assoc* 44:821–827, 1983.
124. Chastain CB: Aspirin: new indications for an old drug, *Compend Contin Educ Pract Vet* 9:165–170, 1987.
125. Duval N, Grosset A, O'Connor SE: Combination of aspirin and metoclopramide produces a synergistic antithrombotic effect in a canine model of coronary artery thrombosis, *Fundam Clin Pharmacol* 11:57–62, 1997.
126. Allen DG, Johnstone IB, Crane S: Effects of aspirin and propranolol alone and in combination on hemostatic determinants in the healthy cat, *Am J Vet Res* 46:660–663, 1985.
127. Brattström L, Wilcken D: Homocysteine and cardiovascular disease: cause or effect? *Am J Clin Nutr* 72:315–323, 2000.

Fluids, Electrolytes, and Acid–Base Therapy

16

Reid P. Groman and Michael D. Willard

Chapter Outline

PHYSIOLOGY

Water

Water accounts for 60% of lean body weight in adult animals, with variation between species. This percentage is affected by fat and age. Obese and older animals tend to have a smaller percentage of body weight composed of water, whereas up to 90% of body weight in neonates is water. Approximately two thirds of this water is present within cells (intracellular fluid [ICF] compartment) and one third is extracellular fluid (ECF). Of the ECF, three fourths is interstitial fluid and one fourth of the ECF volume is plasma. Thus plasma accounts for only 5% of body weight.[1,2]

Water freely diffuses through cell membranes. Consequently, all body compartments have approximately the same osmolality (290 to 310 mOsm/kg in dogs and 300 to 330 mOsm/kg in cats).[3] Osmotic force is the prime determinant of distribution of water across cell membranes (i.e., the partitioning of water between the ECF and ICF). Plasma sodium is the primary determinant of ECF osmolality. Glucose and urea make minor contributions as well, which is reflected in the following calculation:

$$\begin{aligned}\text{Plasma osmolality (mOsm / kg)} &= 2[\text{Na} + \text{K}] \\ &+ [\text{serum glucose in mg / dL} \div 18] \\ &+ [\text{BUN in mg / dL} \div 2.8]\end{aligned}$$

In the laboratory osmolality is measured by freezing point depression or vapor pressure osmometry. The measured value is often higher than the calculated value because this equation does not include all osmotically active particles present in plasma.

As can be seen from the preceding formula, sodium is principally responsible for ECF osmolality. Osmolality in the ICF is principally determined by potassium, magnesium, phosphates, and proteins. To promote water movement from one compartment to another, the osmolality of one or more compartments must change.[4] Tonicity, or effective osmolality, refers to the osmotic pressure of a solution—Osmotic pressure is the pressure required to prevent water movement across a semipermeable membrane. When the relationship between tonicity and osmolality is under consideration, it is important to distinguish between permeant and impermeant solutes. Permeant solutes (e.g., urea) move freely across cell membranes and do not induce net water movement when introduced into a solution (i.e., they are ineffective osmoles). Impermeant solutes (e.g., sodium and glucose) induce water movement when introduced into a solution and are called *effective osmoles,* because they do not readily cross cell membranes. Glucose, to the extent that it causes hyperglycemia, is an impermeant solute and does contribute to ECF osmolality. However, glucose administration usually does not cause hyperglycemia because it is rapidly taken up by cells in the presence of insulin. The implication is that tonicity is less then osmolality.

The capillary walls are freely permeable to sodium, chloride, and glucose. As a result, these substances are osmotically inactive across capillary membranes. However, plasma proteins are limited in their ability to cross capillary membranes, and plasma volume is ultimately maintained by the colloid osmotic pressure (COP), COP is the force created by macromolecules present within the vasculature that prevents water from escaping to the extravascular space. Thus, COP is essentially the pressure exerted by plasma proteins. Albumin contributes to roughly 75% of COP in healthy patients, with globulins making up the remainder. At the venous end of the capillary bed, plasma proteins exert an osmotic force in excess of the hydrostatic gradient, resulting in a net fluid flux from the interstitium into the vessels. Thus albumin is important for distribution of water between the intravascular and interstitial compartments, and plasma proteins in general play a key role in the maintenance of intravascular fluid volume.[1] This is in contrast to the osmotic equilibrium governing water distribution across the ECF and ICF compartments.

The amount of available water in the body is determined by a balance between intake and loss.[1] Water intake occurs by drinking and eating, which are controlled by thirst and hunger. Alterations in water intake can occur with neurologic disease and congenital abnormalities. Animals normally lose water through urine, feces, and expired air. To a lesser extent, evaporation from the skin surface promotes water flux across the epidermis. Obligatory urinary and fecal losses are determined by the solute load that must be excreted. Respiratory losses of water are affected by ambient temperature and humidity. Water losses may increase as a result of vomiting, diarrhea, and polyuria. Rarely, clinically relevant water losses arise through traumatized tissues or with cavitary effusions. Fever also can be responsible for increasing loss of water.[5] Fluid losses, such as those incurred by vomiting, diarrhea, and polyuria, are often classified as isotonic (i.e., small solutes are lost in proportion to their concentration in plasma), but more commonly these losses are slightly hypotonic, with sodium concentrations of 80 to 120 mg/dL. This is manifested by hypernatremia, which is commonly observed with dehydration. To maintain hydration homeostasis, urine output *may* exceed the obligatory urine output, the latter being the volume required for elimination of solutes. While the term *free water* is well recognized and accepted, this fluid resembles a hypotonic crystalloid in content, as opposed to water. Water excretion is due to modification of antidiuretic hormone (ADH) secretion. ADH is normally released from the posterior pituitary gland when osmoreceptors in the hypothalamus detect hypertonicity or when baroreceptors in the cardiovascular system sense hypovolemia. Release of ADH promotes water retention. For water to be excreted by the kidneys, there must be adequate delivery of tubular fluid to the ascending limb of the loop of Henle, and the renal collecting ducts must remain impermeable to water in the absence of ADH.[6]

Sodium

Sodium is the osmolar skeleton of the ECF. Under normal conditions the kidneys regulate its elimination, excreting as much sodium as is ingested. Renal sodium excretion is normally regulated by aldosterone, atrial natriuretic factors (ANF), and intrinsic renal mechanisms (e.g., renal blood flow [RBF], glomerular filtration rate [GFR], and glomerulotubular balance). *Glomerulotubular balance* refers to the ability of the kidney to maintain a relatively constant fractional reabsorption of sodium, despite changes in GFR. If there is expansion of the effective circulating volume (i.e., overhydration, hypervolemia), the cardiac atria distend with subsequent release of ANF. ANF and other natriuretic factors inhibit both the formation and effects of angiotensin and decrease sodium reabsorption from the renal medullary collecting ducts. Conversely, when atrial receptors detect a decrease in volume, sympathetic tone is increased and ANF release is inhibited. Further, decrements in renal perfusion and the associated decrease in delivery of sodium (and/or chloride) to the macula densa activate the renin–angiotensin–aldosterone system, promoting sodium to be reabsorbed from the renal tubules and collecting ducts.[7]

Potassium

The regulation of total body and plasma potassium concentration is important to the extent that potassium alterations may profoundly affect the resting membrane potential (RMP) of cardiac and neuromuscular cells.[8] Hypokalemia lowers the RMP, making it more difficult to achieve an action potential with subsequent contraction of a muscle. Hyperkalemia raises the RMP, which may result in an action potential of decreased amplitude or, in extreme cases, continuous depolarization of the cell membrane. Although the majority of the body's potassium is found within cells, it is the plasma concentration that corresponds with and contributes to relevant myocardial and neuromuscular abnormalities.

Potassium homeostasis can be conceptualized as having both an internal and an external balance. *External balance* refers to the total amount of potassium in the body and is determined by the balance between intake versus loss. Potassium enters the body principally through ingestion, and almost all ingested potassium is absorbed. A small amount of potassium is normally excreted in the feces, although the colon may serve as an important route for potassium excretion in disease states. Normal potassium loss occurs predominantly through the kidneys, the amount determined by ECF potassium concentration, delivery of sodium and water to the distal tubule and collecting ducts, as well as the secretion of aldosterone. Although the kidneys normally eliminate potassium efficiently, renal mechanisms cannot maintain normal plasma serum potassium concentrations when grossly excessive amounts of potassium are ingested.[9]

Internal potassium balance refers to the distribution of potassium between the ICF and ECF compartments. The Na-K ATPase enzyme pump found in cellular membranes actively transports potassium into the cell and maintains a high intracellular potassium concentration (i.e., approximately 150 mEq/L) relative to the ECF (approximately 4 mEq/L). In hyperkalemic states insulin and β2-adrenergic activity augment the transport of potassium into the cells, safely storing additional potassium until it can be eliminated.[9] The internal balance mechanisms may be thought of as a temporary measure designed to allow the kidneys and, to a lesser extent, the colon time to restore potassium balance.[8,10]

Acid–Base Balance

The body must deal with very large amounts of acid (H^+) that are generated daily by normal metabolic processes. This is important because H^+ is very reactive, and small amounts (i.e., nanoequivalents) can have detrimental effects on protein structure and function (i.e., enzymes, cell membranes, and receptors). Normal blood pH is 7.40. Many metabolic functions are exquisitely sensitive to pH, and normal function can only occur within a very narrow pH range. If, for example, a patient's pH falls to 7.20 (which represents an increase of approximately 20 nEq H^+/L), myocardial dysfunction, vasodilation, or dysrhythmias may be observed.[11,12]

Changes in $[H^+]$ are opposed by buffer systems within the body. These systems consist of a buffer pair of an acid (H^+ donator) and its conjugate base (H^+ acceptor) as follows:

$$\underset{acid}{HA} \leftrightarrow H^+ + \underset{base}{A^-}$$

Weak acids and their conjugate bases constitute the most effective buffer pairs in the body, insofar as they are minimally dissociated and readily capable of accepting or donating H^+ in the presence of changes in H^+ load. This is in contrast to strong acids, which are highly dissociated in most biological fluids.

It was noted 100 years ago that the hydration of CO_2 in the presence of carbonic anhydrase forms H_2CO_3 (carbonic acid), and carbonic acid acid will ionize into and achieve equilibrium with its conjugate base, bicarbonate (HCO_3^-), and H^+, almost instantaneously:

$$CO_2 + H_2O \xleftrightarrow{\text{carbonic anhydrase}} H_2CO_3 \longleftrightarrow HCO_3^- + H^+$$

By rearranging the variables in the preceding equation, applying laws of mass action, and recognizing that H_2CO_3 exists in almost continuous equilibrium with dissolved CO_2, the value of dissolved CO_2 was substituted, giving rise to the following equation:

$$[H^+] = K_a\left(\frac{[CO_2]}{HCO_3^-}\right)$$

Ultimately, the partial pressure of CO_2 in the blood (pCO_2) was substituted for dissolved CO_2, the concept of pH was defined (the negative logarithm of $[H^+]$), and the following equation was derived:

$$pH = pK_a + \log\left(\frac{HCO_3^-}{PCO_2xSC}\right)$$

where pKa is the logarithm of the ionization constant K_a for H_2CO_3 and SC is the solubility coefficient of CO_2 in blood (0.03).

This is the classic *Henderson–Hasselbalch equation,* fundamental to appreciating traditional acid–base chemistry and interpreting acid–base derangements. This equation shows that the pH of the ECF varies when either $[HCO_3^-]$ or pCO_2 is altered.

There are two categories of acid found in the body: nonvolatile (produced by metabolism of proteins) and volatile (derived from CO_2) produced by cellular respiration throughout the body.[11] Nonvolatile (also called *fixed)* acid (H^+) is primarily excreted by the kidneys, whereas volatile acid (CO_2) is eliminated by way of the lungs. On a daily basis, small pH changes within the body are counteracted by multiple complex and often opposing physiochemical processes that, for the sake of simplicity, are presented as (1) the actions of intracellular and extracellular buffering systems (chemical buffering), (2) modulation of ventilation (physiologic buffering), and (3) renal reclamation and elimination. There are many buffer systems throughout the body. The principle intracellular buffers are hemoglobin, phosphate, and proteins, which are capable of buffering both volatile and nonvolatile acids. The principle extracellular buffer systems are calcium carbonate and phosphate of bone, in addition to the bicarbonate-carbonic acid system, which reacts only with nonvolatile acid. Hemoglobin and albumin account for most of the nonbicarbonate buffering capacity. The HCO_3^- buffering system is capable of responding to an acute change in $[H^+]$, and the $HCO_3^-/H_2CO_3/CO_2$ equilibrium equation (see Equation 16-1) allows changes in pH to be further modulated by changes in ventilation. This "open system" greatly enhances the buffering capacity of the HCO_3^- system and is capable of buffering changes in pH within minutes of an acid or alkali load. Finally, the kidneys play a major role in maintaining pH by increasing or decreasing acid elimination in the urine. Although hours to days may be required for this system's buffering ability to reach completion, it is clinically the most reliable of all the adaptive mechanisms to normalize pH.

Acid–base physiology may be viewed as having an external and an internal balance, as described for potassium. *External balance* refers to the elimination of acid from the body, whereas internal balance allows for the body to safely sequester excessive acid until it can be excreted. The pH of the ECF is largely determined by how effectively these mechanisms function.

A perceived limitation to traditional acid–base physiology is that it is too simplistic, ascribing changes in pH to either respiratory (changes in pCO_2) or metabolic (changes in bicarbonate) causes, thereby neglecting the contribution of other variables in solution. To address this, *nontraditional* or *quantitative* approaches to acid–base chemistry and analysis are described.[13] The terms *Stewart approach* and *Fencl–Leith approach* are variants of the often confusing and misunderstood *nontraditional* approaches to acid–base analysis. The nontraditional approach subdivides metabolic causes into two independent variables, those associated with a strong ion difference (SID) ions that are totally dissociated (e.g., sodium, chloride, potassium, lactate) and A_{TOT} (ions of weak acids that are partially dissociated, e.g., phosphate and albumin). The nontraditional approach defines the pCO_2 (respiratory contribution) as an independent variable. According to the quantitative approach, changes in HCO_3 are explained by alterations in SID, A_{TOT}, and pCO_2. It has been demonstrated that if enough A_{TOT} and SID determinants are measured, an approximate pH can be calculated. The perceived strength of the quantitative approach is that it provides an estimate of the "contribution" of individual electrolyte derangements to an acid–base imbalance when pH is not measured. However, the quantitative approach is only a means of estimating the metabolic contribution to pH when it is not otherwise measured, but not the pH itself; the pH is also highly dependent on the respiratory component, the pCO_2. The traditional system utilizes an overview parameter such as bicarbonate, total CO_2, or base deficit to quantify the metabolic contribution. The Stewart approach breaks down the metabolic component into two large groups: SID and A_{TOT}; however, it does not further define the contributions. The Fencl–Leith modification is the only truly semiquantitative approach, insofar as it it breaks down the metabolic contribution into six individual components (water [marked by serum sodium], bicarbonate [marked by chloride], albumin, lactate, ketones [if measured], phosphate, and the effect of unmeasured ions). Advocates of the nontraditional approach find that it is more accurate, avoiding some of the oversimplifications associated with the traditional, albeit more familiar, Henderson–Hasselbalch equation. Both are simplifications of a complex dynamic system, and both suffer from inherent inaccuracies.[13] For practical purposes, benefits of the nontraditional approach are best appreciated when pH and a blood gas analyzer are not available to the clinician. Other advantages to this approach, when compared with traditional acid–base chemistry, are less clear and remain a topic of recurrent deliberations. Importantly the astute clinician should appreciate that all methods of acid–base analysis merely quantitate the magnitude of a disorder. Similarly, acid–base findings may provide subtle clues to pathogenetic mechanisms, but they do not characterize or define a disease or its management. Such inferences mandate evaluation of the complete history, thorough physical examination, and results of other laboratory tests. To remain consistent with concepts taught in most clinical settings, the traditional approach (Henderson–Hasselbalch) to analyzing acid–base disturbances is discussed.

The blood bicarbonate concentration is normally regulated by the kidneys. The kidneys reabsorb filtered bicarbonate and regenerate bicarbonate that has been consumed in the process of buffering acid. In this way, bicarbonate may be conceptualized as a kind of conveyer belt, combining with nonvolatile acid (i.e., H^+), thereby maintaining a stable pH in the face of an acid load. When bicarbonate combines with H^+, carbonic acid (H_2CO_3) is formed, which dissociates to form CO_2 and water. CO_2 is eliminated by ventilation (see Equation 16-1). When organic anions (e.g., lactate, pyruvate, gluconate, acetate, citrate, ketones) are metabolized, a hydrogen ion is carried along in the process. This alters the carbonic acid $H_2CO_3 \leftrightarrow H^+ + HCO_3$ equilibrium (mass action), shifting it rightward, generating new bicarbonate. Many processes in the body directly or indirectly use a chloride–bicarbonate counterporter. When chloride is excreted (e.g., into the stomach lumen), a "new" bicarbonate anion moves in the opposite direction (into the ECF). Similar counterporters exist in red blood cells, renal tubules, and small intestinal epithelial cells.

When nonvolatile acid is present in excess, it reacts with bicarbonate and other buffer systems, especially intracellular protein and phosphate.[14] The plasma bicarbonate concentration decreases as the bicarbonate combines with H^+ and forms H_2CO_3, the pH decreases, which by definition is an acidosis. More specifically, it is a metabolic acidosis because the disorder promotes the accumulation of excessive nonvolatile acid. The body will try to reestablish pH by lowering the pCO_2 (hyperventilation). This is the appropriate and anticipated compensatory response. Although less common, excessive loss of HCO_3^- (as occurs with some types of diarrhea) may cause a metabolic acidosis with a similar compensatory response.[15] When the primary derangement promotes accumulation of excess volatile acid (an increase in pCO_2), pH decreases and the acid–base disorder is described as a respiratory acidosis. Respiratory acidosis, by definition is an increase in pCO_2,. In patients with primary respiratory acidosis, the kidneys respond by increasing excretion of acid.[15]

By definition, metabolic alkalosis is an elevation in pH caused by excessive plasma bicarbonate. Alkalosis decreases pulmonary ventilation, which elevates the pCO_2 Conversely, reduction of pCO_2 produces an alkalosis, the terms hyperventilation and respiratory alkalosis often used interchangeably. In response to a primary respiratory alkalosis, renal acid excretion is reduced.[16]

The kidneys respond to respiratory acid-base disorders over several hours to days. The pulmonary response to metabolic acid-base disorders occurs in a matter of minutes. In dogs it is possible to predict the approximate degree of a compensation; anticipated compensation is less clear or predictable in cats. Compensatory mechanisms are not efficient enough to return the pH within the normal range. These defense mechanisms do not correct the acid-base disturbance but merely minimize the change in pH imposed by the disturbance. Moreover, overcompensation for a primary acid–base disorder does not occur,[11]

DISEASE-INDUCED CHANGES

Sodium

Changes in plasma sodium concentration usually reflect changes in total body water content. Hyponatremia and hypernatremia primarily cause clinical problems by promoting neuronal edema or dehydration (ICF), respectively. The severity of clinical signs is thought to correspond with the rate of change rather than with the magnitude of hyponatremia or hypernatremia. If changes in serum sodium occur slowly, the brain can usually adjust the number of osmotically active molecules to prevent cerebral fluid gain or loss. This underscores the fact that severe hyponatremia or hypernatremia should be corrected gradually rather than quickly.[17] When the serum sodium abnormality has been gradual in onset, the patient's sodium should be corrected slowly, not lowered faster than 1 mmol/L/hr or increased at a rate exceeding 0.5 mmol/L/hr.

Hypernatremia

Naturally occurring disease processes resulting in hypernatremia are usually disorders of free water loss.[7,18] Rarely, hypernatremia results from the addition of sodium (e.g., ocean water ingestion, hypertonic saline or sodium bicarbonate administration). Hypernatremia is a reflection of inadequate water relative to sodium content in the ECF. While ECF volume is determined by the total sodium content (not concentration) in the body, plasma sodium concentration is not a measurement of a patient's volume status. The thirst mechanism is so effective that hypernatremia seldom occurs in animals that have access to adequate amounts of water and are not vomiting or regurgitating. Hypernatremia often develops in hospitalized patients, and a methodical preemptive diagnostic approach, including serial evaluation of electrolytes and quantification of fluid intake and loss, permits rapid recognition of water imbalance and prevent wide variations in serum sodium. Hypernatremia should prompt consideration of the disorders listed in Box 16-1.

Hyponatremia

Because naturally occurring diseases rarely produce sodium losses in excess of water, hyponatremia in the clinical setting is almost invariably due to excess water in the ECF.

Hyponatremia may be caused by several mechanisms, and a systematic approach to cause and correction is advised. Sodium and its attendant ions account for approximately 95% of the osmotically active substances in extracellular water. While hyponatremia is commonly associated with hypoosmolality, plasma osmolality must be assessed to appropriately determine of the cause of hyponatremia (Box 16-2).[7]

Hyponatremia with concurrent normal plasma osmolality suggests laboratory error or pseudohyponatremia. Pseudohyponatremia may occur with hyperlipidemia because the lipid occupies space in the volume of serum obtained for analysis; the concentration of sodium itself is not affected. Hyponatremia with concurrent plasma hyperosmolality suggests that other osmotically active particles (e.g., glucose, mannitol) are drawing water out of the ICF and into the plasma, thus diluting the sodium that is present.[7,19] This is often called translocational hyponatremia because it is caused by translocation of sodium across cell membranes.

Hypoosmolar hyponatremia in a patient producing large volumes of dilute urine reflects impaired free water excretion (e.g., inappropriate ADH secretion).

Volume and hydration status may further suggest causes of hyponatremia. Overtly hypovolemic patients often have

Box 16-1

Causes of Hypernatremia

Normal Loss of Free Water with Inadequate Replacement
- Failure to provide water to an animal that can drink
- Inadequate fluid therapy for an animal that cannot drink
  - Unconscious animal
  - Animal that is not being fed or watered by mouth
  - Animal with an oral, pharyngeal, or esophageal disease that prevents ingestion
  - Adipsia

Excessive Loss of Free Water with Inadequate Replacement
- Diabetes insipidus
- Heat stroke
- Fever, hyperthermia
- Hypotonic fluid losses
  - Diarrhea
  - Vomiting
  - Polyuria
- Excessive intake of sodium
  - Salt poisoning
  - Administration of sodium
    - Hypertonic saline
    - Sodium bicarbonate

Box 16-2

Evaluation of the Patient with Hyponatremia

Normoosmolal Patients
- Look for artifact (i.e., pseudohyponatremia due to hyperproteinemia)

Hypoosmolal Patients
- Hypovolemic patients
  - Gastrointestinal loss of hypotonic fluid with water replacement
  - Hypoadrenocorticism
  - Salt-losing nephropathies
  - Sequestration of fluids or sodium in third spaces

Hypervolemic Patients
- Congestive heart failure
- Nephrotic syndrome
- Hepatic disease (especially cirrhosis)

Normovolemic Patients
- Primary polydipsia
- Administration of hypotonic fluids

Hyperosmolal Patients
- Hyperglycemia
- Mannitol infusion

an obvious source of fluid loss. Hyponatremia in an overhydrated patient is often observed with (but is not the cause of) cavitary effusions associated with congestive heart failure, advanced oliguric renal failure, or severe hepatic disease (usually cirrhosis). These disorders may be associated with such exuberant water retention that patients become hyponatremic in the face of total body sodium excess. Patients with congestive heart disease or cirrhosis are often described as having decreased effective circulating volume (ECV). ECV is the *volume* of arterial blood effectively perfusing tissue. ECV is a dynamic quantity and not a measurable, distinct compartment. The fluid retention seen with ineffective cardiac output is appropriate (because of release of ADH and angiotensin II), whereas the fluid retention observed with renal failure and cirrhosis is a component of the disease process itself. These patients have decreased ECV and consequent reduction in GFR and RBF; as a result, the body attempts, albeit ineffectively, to retain the fluid within the ECF.[7]

Hypoosmolar hyponatremia may be seen with chronic gastrointestinal disease. These patients may be hypernatremic early in the course of their disease, but sustained ADH release, excessive water consumption, or both may ultimately lead to hyponatremia. Diseases associated with third-space losses (e.g., pancreatitis, peritonitis) promote ADH release, and hyponatremia may be seen in affected patients. It is a common misunderstanding that hyponatremia in this setting is a result of the fluid accumulation itself. The hyponatremia, however, is due to changes in ADH, and fluid accumulation is not the proximate cause. Cutaneous fluid losses (e.g., burns) may be isonatremic with little change in plasma sodium or may be associated with hyponatremia.[7,19]

Similarly, sodium may be lost from the body as a result of hypoadrenocorticism or following administration of thiazide diuretics. Diuretics decrease the kidney's diluting capacity and increase sodium excretion. These patients may be distinguished from those with gastrointestinal loss of hypotonic fluid by evaluating the urinary sodium concentration (fractional excretion of sodium [FE Na^+]). FE Na^+ is not a test but rather a calculation based on the concentrations of sodium and creatinine in blood and urine.

Under normal circumstances, the body's response to hypovolemia and hyponatremia is to impede renal sodium losses as a means of restoring ECF. Consequently, little sodium would be found in the urine (FE Na^+ <1%). Animals in which renal losses are the cause of the hyponatremia will, however, have substantial urinary sodium concentrations (FE Na^+ >3%).[19]

Hyponatremia and hypoosmolality occur uncommonly in well-hydrated euvolemic dogs and cats. Although rare, primary polydipsia (also called *psychogenic polydipsia*) syndromes associated with inappropriate ADH release or overzealous administration of hypotonic fluids are described, and are possible causes of hyponatremia in this setting.[7]

Chloride

Most often, changes in plasma chloride concentration are clinically relevant because they affect acid-base status. In particular, hypochloremia is associated with metabolic processes that are coupled with alkalosis.[20] Similarly, hyperchloremia tends to be associated with acidosis.

Hypochloremia

The major causes of hypochloremia are increased loss caused by vomiting of gastric contents or excessive administration of loop diuretics (e.g., furosemide).[21] Chloride losses caused by gastric vomiting are usually associated with hypokalemia and metabolic alkalosis. Occasionally, a paradoxical aciduria is also seen. Physical examination and laboratory findings often corroborate a history of vomiting. Rarely, administration of large doses of sodium without corresponding administration of chloride (e.g., high doses of sodium penicillin or sodium bicarbonate) may cause hypochloremia. When a hypochloremic patient is also hyponatremic, hyperkalemic, or both, the clinician should consider hypoadrenocorticism. If, however, the clinician corrects the plasma chloride concentration to account for changes in plasma free water, for example:

$$[\text{Dogs: Corrected } Cl^- = \text{plasma Cl in mEq/L} \times (146 \text{ plasma Na in mEq/L})$$
$$\text{Cats: Corrected } Cl^- = \text{plasma Cl in mEq/L} \times (156 \text{ plasma Na in mEq/L})]$$

patients with hypoadrenocorticism may have a normal or increased corrected chloride concentration.[20] Changes in chloride are often interpreted with changes in free water, which alters sodium and chloride concentrations proportionally. This can be done by correcting the chloride concentration for changes in sodium using the preceding formulas. Primary disorders of chloride (i.e., acid–base disturbances) have abnormal corrected chloride values, whereas disorders of free water do not; determination of corrected chloride values seldom affects diagnostic or therapeutic decisions in a given patient. Its determination is only to permit the interested clinician to quantitatively assess the contribution of bicarbonate (marked by changes in chloride) to the metabolic component of an acid–base disturbance.

Hyperchloremia

Hyperchloremia is principally found in animals that are simultaneously hypernatremic as a result of the loss of free water and in patients that have received fluids containing proportionally more chloride than sodium relative to plasma values. Examples include administration of 0.9% saline, hypertonic saline, parenteral nutrition, and especially 0.9% saline supplemented with potassium chloride. Hyperchloremia may also be observed in patients that have a metabolic acidosis associated with a normal anion gap (i.e., hyperchloremic metabolic acidosis). This biochemical finding is commonly seen in animals with small bowel diarrhea caused by loss of bicarbonate-rich, chloride-poor fluid.[20] It can also be seen with regurgitation or vomiting of duodenal contents and in patients with renal tubular acidosis.

Potassium

Changes in the plasma potassium concentration are clinically important because of the effect of potassium on cellular metabolism, RMPs, and the subsequent strength of contraction when an action potential is generated.[9] Hypokalemia and hyperkalemia both cause muscular weakness and predispose to cardiac dysrhythmias. Although there is variation between patients, plasma potassium concentrations ≥ 8.0 mEq/L or ≤ 2.0 mEq/L are generally considered life threatening, although less dramatic changes can be dangerous if there are concomitant electrolyte derangements (e.g., hyponatremia, hypocalcemia, or hypercalcemia) or if the changes occur rapidly.[10] Potassium is highly labile, and changes in pH of the ECF may cause significant alterations in serum potassium, particularly in critically ill patients.

Hyperkalemia

Hyperkalemia may be artifactual (i.e., pseudohyperkalemia) or real. If hyperkalemia is real, it is either iatrogenic (increased intake or administration) or spontaneous. The major cause of spontaneous hyperkalemia is decreased urinary excretion caused by renal, urinary tract or adrenal disease (Box 16-3).[10]

Pseudohyperkalemia, an in vitro increase in potassium concentration, may be observed with marked thrombocytosis (generally ≥ 800,000/ul). Because the elevation in potassium in this setting is due to leakage from disrupted or dying cells, it is important to measure plasma or serum potassium concentrations shortly after a sample is obtained to avoid drawing erroneous conclusions about a patient's electrolyte status. Similarly, animals with white blood cell counts equal to or greater than 100,000/ul (e.g., leukemia) may rarely have pseudohyperkalemia because of transcellular leakage of potassium.[22,23] Neonates, Akitas, and English springer spaniels are known to have a high potassium content within their red blood cells and hemolysis may cause hyperkalemia [24] If there is doubt as to whether the hyperkalemia is artifactual or real, one should obtain a lithium heparin–anticoagulated blood sample and promptly harvest the plasma.[21]

The list of drugs that may cause hyperkalemia is extensive.[10] With the exception of overexuberant infusion of potassium chloride in intravenous fluids and administration of drugs that inhibit production or activity of aldosterone (e.g., enalapril, spironolactone), significant hyperkalemia caused by drug administration is rare and generally only occurs if there is underlying renal or adrenal dysfunction. Only the more common causes are provided in Box 16-3.

Decreased urinary potassium excretion may be due to severe primary renal dysfunction (e.g., typically anuric or oliguric primary renal failure), postrenal causes (e.g., uroperitoneum, uretheral obstruction) or to secondary renal dysfunction resulting from aldosterone deficiency (i.e., hypoadrenocorticism). Disorders promoting development of edema or cavitary effusions or enteritis (especially whipworm infection)[25-27] are sometimes associated with the development of mild hyperkalemia, the exact pathogenetic mechanism of which remains unclear . The clinician should rule in or rule out hypoadrenocorticism early in the diagnostic evaluation because it has an excellent prognosis if recognized and treated promptly. An adrenocorticotropic hormone (ACTH)–stimulation test is required for definitive diagnosis, although resting serum cortisol concentrations may be used to screen for its presence. Dogs with resting cortisol levels of more than 2 ug/dL rarely have hypoadrenocorticism,[28] and in such cases the submission of a post-ACTH (stimulated) cortisol sample may not be indicated.

Box 16-3

Causes of Hyperkalemia

Artifactual

Pseudohyperkalemia
Lysis of red blood cells that have high potassium concentrations (generally seen only in selected breeds and families)
Thrombocytosis
Extreme leukocytosis

Iatrogenic

Administration of potassium chloride or other potassium-containing drug
Potassium-sparing diuretics
Trimethoprim-sulfa
Propranolol
Angiotensin-converting enzyme inhibitors (e.g., enalapril)
Heparin
Massive digitalis overdose

Decreased Excretion

Acute renal failure (especially anuric or oliguric)
Hypoadrenocorticism
Third-space disorders

Miscellaneous

Gastrointestinal (e.g., whipworms)

Hypokalemia

Hypokalemia results from reductions in dietary intake or increased losses through the urinary or gastrointestinal tract. Decreased intake is unlikely to cause hypokalemia unless the diet is severely deficient or when potassium-free intravenous fluids are administered to an inappetent patient. Potassium translocation from ECF to ICF may be seen in patients receiving parenteral nutrition, insulin, sodium bicarbonate, or glucose-containing fluids.[8,9] Similarly, alkalemia may reduce serum potassium levels as extracellular potassium moves intracellularly in exchange for hydrogen ions.

Increased loss of potassium is the most important cause of hypokalemia in dogs and cats. Vomiting and diarrhea lead to gastrointestinal losses, whereas drug therapy (e.g., furosemide) and renal failure or polyuria result in renal losses. The latter is commonly observed in older cats and may be detected in the absence of azotemia. Hyperaldosteronism is an uncommon disorder of cats that may cause profound hypokalemia. If the cause of hypokalemia is unclear after routine evaluations, the clinician may calculate the fractional excretion of potassium (FE_K). Animals that are hypokalemic as a result of nonrenal causes should have normal (approximately 4% to 6%) to decreased FE_K, whereas cats with potassium-losing nephropathies usually have values above 6% to 10%.[8,29,30]

Miscellaneous Minerals

Miscellaneous minerals that occasionally are of concern to the clinician are phosphorus and magnesium. Severe hypophosphatemia capable of causing clinical signs is principally seen in ketoacidotic diabetic patients that are overtreated with insulin and occasionally in emaciated cats receiving enteral or parenteral nutrition,[31,32] although hypophosphatemia can be seen from time to time in patients with other diseases.[33] The most clinically relevant consequence of hypophosphatemia is hemolysis. Hyperphosphatemia is commonly seen in patients with renal disease but seldom requires special considerations when formulating fluid therapy. Magnesium is primarily absorbed in the jejunum and ileum, while the kidneys regulate magnesium balance. Hypomagnesemia is primarily due to renal or gastrointestinal losses.[34] Hypomagnesemia may cause cardiac dysrhythmias and neuromuscular irritability. Hypomagnesemia is increasingly recognized feature of ketoacidotic diabetes mellitus. It is also seen in dogs with severe protein-losing enteropathy.[35] Depletion of magnesium has a permissive effect on potassium exit from the ICF leading to ECF accumulation of potassium, which is subsequently lost from the body. This potassium deficiency is refractory to supplementation until the magnesium deficit is also corrected. Similarly, hypocalcemia may occur as a secondary electrolyte abnormality when there is a magnesium deficit. Hypermagnesemia is primarily associated with renal disease. Excessive provision of magnesium (e.g., in diet or intravenous fluids) is also reported.[36,37]

Acid–Base Status

Traditional evaluation of acid–base status is best accomplished by blood gas analysis, integrating information provided by the pH, pCO_2, and bicarbonate. When evaluating blood gas values, consideration is first given to pH.[11] The normal pH of blood analyzed at 37° C is 7.35-7.45. If the pH is abnormal, is the patient acidemic (pH < 7.35) or alkalemic (pH > 7.45) If it is abnormal, by definition an acid–base disorder exists. If the pH is normal, an acid–base disorder is unlikely but should not be ruled out, because there may be a mixed acid-base disturbance (i.e., more than one primary acid–base disturbance occurring concurrently) or (uncommonly) a fully compensated acid–base disturbance. These circumstances are not always readily distinguishable. The reader is referred to other references for information on mixed disorders.[38]

If the pH is abnormal, the clinician should try to determine which component (respiratory or metabolic) is the primary contributor (Table 16-1). Subsequently, evaluation for appropriate compensation of the primary disorder is undertaken. Generally, the pH will vary in the direction of the primary disorder. The other component is the secondary or compensatory component attempting to restore pH to normal. When both components vary in the same direction at the pH, both disorders are primary, i.e., a mixed disorder is present. In the dog there are guidelines for expected compensation in acid-base disorders (see Table 16-1); however, it is not possible to extrapolate these guidelines from the dog to the cat. Results of blood gas analysis are interpreted in light of anamnesis and clinical examination findings to most appropriately determine the most probable cause of the acid–base disorder.[11]

Table 16-1 Expected Findings and Compensation in Normal Dogs with Simple Acid–Base Disturbances

	pH	Primary Abnormality	Normal Compensatory Response
Metabolic acidosis	↓	↓ HCO_3	↓ P_{CO2} by 0.7 mm for each 1 mEq/L ↓ in HCO_3
Metabolic alkalosis	↑	↑ HCO_3	↑ P_{CO2} by 0.7 mm for each 1 mEq/L ↑ in HCO_3
Respiratory acidosis	↓	↑ P_{CO2}	
Acute			↑ HCO_3 by 1.5 mEq/L for each 10 mm ↑ in P_{CO2}
Chronic			↑ HCO_3 by 3.5 mEq/L for each 10 mm ↑ in P_{CO2}
Respiratory alkalosis	↑	↓ P_{CO2}	
Acute			↓ HCO_3 by 2.5 mEq/L for each 10 mm ↓ in P_{CO2}
Chronic			↓ HCO_3 by 5.5 mEq/L for each 10 mm ↓ in P_{CO2}

Metabolic Acidosis

Metabolic acidosis is probably the most widely recognized canine and feline acid–base disorder . The most common causes of metabolic acidosis in these species are listed in Box 16-4. Acidosis from accumulation of lactic acid is thought to be the most common cause of metabolic acidosis. In the setting of poor peripheral perfusion, anaerobic metabolism often predominates, with subsequent production of lactic acid.[39] The acidemia is not actually due to dissociation of the lactate; the lactate simply reflects the anaerobic metabolism that has released protons. Therefore lactic acidosis may be seen in conjunction with other disorders. Lactic acidosis is usually diagnosed by elimination of other causes of acidosis, presence of elevated anion gap, and physical examination findings suggesting ischemia or volume depletion. Blood lactate levels may be measured (i.e., hand-held monitors or standard blood gas analyzers).[20,21,40] The anion gap, although reported with other serum chemistry measurements, is actually a calculated value $[(Na + K) - (HCO_3 + Cl)]$. The electrolytes used in the formula are called measured cations (Na, K) and measured anions (HCO_3, Cl). Ions not included in the formula are called unmeasured cations and unmeasured anions.

Most dogs and cats with diarrhea do not develop a significant acidosis. Occasionally, patients with profuse diarrhea lose excessive amounts of bicarbonate in the feces and consequently develop an inorganic (hyperchloremic) metabolic acidosis. This acidosis may occur simultaneously with lactic acidosis in some patients with concomitant dehydration or hypovolemia.[20]

Renal failure causes acidosis when the kidneys cannot adequately excrete H^+, regenerate HCO_3^-, or both. Renal ammonium excretion is the principle means of eliminating protons, and this is usually adequate until renal failure becomes severe. Acidosis from renal dysfunction may have a normal anion gap

Box 16-4

Common Causes of Metabolic Acidosis

- Lactic acidosis caused by decreased perfusion
  - Dehydration
  - Poor cardiac output
- Renal failure
- Diabetic ketoacidosis
- Hypoadrenocorticism
- Addition of acid to the body
  - Ethylene glycol intoxication
  - Salicylate intoxication
  - Ammonium chloride

initially, but an increased anion gap is expected in more severely uremic patients as unmeasured anions accumulate. Hypoadrenocorticism causes an acidosis in part because aldosterone is needed for the secretion of H^+ into collecting duct fluid; thus it may be thought of as a functional renal disease (i.e., without structural nephron damage). Specific renal tubular defects (renal tubular acidosis) are uncommon in dogs and cats but should be on the list of differential diagnoses for patients with a hyperchloremic acidosis and normal anion gap.[20]

Diabetic ketoacidosis occurs when there is excessive production of ketone bodies, especially b-hydroxybutyrate, generally causing an increased anion gap acidosis.[41]

When ethylene glycol is ingested, it is metabolized by the liver to glycolic acid. This often results in severe acidemia that is refractory to standard treatments, largely because acid metabolites continue to be produced until all of the ethylene glycol is metabolized.[42] The acidosis typically occurs before there is any evidence of renal injury. History may be informative, and several quantitative colorimetric in-house test kits are available. Calcium oxalate crystalluria often precedes overt renal failure. Both monohydrate (i.e., "picket fence") and dihydrate (i.e., "Maltese cross") calcium oxalate crystals may be observed in urine sediment. Markedly increased anion and osmolol gaps are seen shortly after exposure.[43] A high anion gap acidosis may be documented within 3 hours and persists for at least 24 hours.

Metabolic Alkalosis

Clinically significant metabolic alkalosis in dogs and cats is usually due to vomiting of gastric contents, diuretic therapy, or excessive administration of bicarbonate. Other causes of alkalemia (e.g., severe hypokalemia, severe hypomagnesemia) are clinically less important.[16,20]

Vomiting of gastric contents causes loss of H^+ as well as loss of Cl^- and water. Hypovolemia and concurrent hypochloremia prevent the relative excess of bicarbonate from being eliminated in the urine, reflecting the body's priority of restoring ECF volume. To restore ECF volume, the body reclaims sodium and water from the renal tubules. To efficiently reabsorb sodium (a cation), a negatively charged ion(s) must be reabsorbed (generally Cl^- or HCO_3^-) simultaneously to maintain electroneutrality. If insufficient amounts of Cl^- are present to accompany the reclaimed sodium, bicarbonate will be reabsorbed instead, even though total body bicarbonate is in excess.[20] Similar pathogenic mechanisms may be observed when excessive furosemide administration promotes a brisk diuresis with chloride-rich urine. Both of these circumstances are considered chloride-responsive alkaloses because complete resolution can only occur if chloride-replete fluids are a component of therapy. Clinically important chloride-resistant alkalosis is uncommon in dogs and cats.[20]

Respiratory Alkalosis

Respiratory alkalosis, or primary hypocapnia, is relatively common, occurring when alveolar ventilation exceeds the amount required to eliminate the CO_2 produced by metabolism; hyperventilation from any cause (e.g., excitement, pain, fear, hypoxemia, sepsis, liver disease) causes PCO_2 to decrease and can result in an alkalosis.[44,45] The alkalosis itself, however, rarely causes detrimental effects in the patient, but this should not dissuade the clinician from seeking out the underlying cause.

Respiratory Acidosis

Respiratory acidosis, or primary hypercapnia, is occasionally diagnosed in dogs or cats with naturally occurring diseases; more commonly it is associated with sedation and anesthesia. Carbon dioxide diffuses more rapidly across the alveolar membrane than oxygen, and hypoventilation is for all practical purposes the only cause of, and therefore defines, respiratory acidosis. Primary hypoventilation may be seen in patients with upper airway obstruction, neuromuscular weakness that impairs breathing (e.g., myasthenia gravis, hypokalemia, botulism), muscular rigidity that prevents breathing (e.g., tetanus, seizures), chest wall or pleural cavity disorders (e.g., pneumothorax, pleural effusion, flail chest), and chronic obstructive pulmonary disease.[46]

Blood Gas Analysis

Blood gas analysis mandates precise technique and thus properly trained support staff.[11,21] Hand-held "point-of-care" units have made blood gas analysis feasible for many practices.[47] However, the total serum CO_2 (TCO_2) available on most chemistry panels from commercial veterinary laboratories may be used as a rough surrogate marker for HCO_3^- and as such may be used as an approximation of the metabolic contribution to acid–base derangements when HCO_3 is not measured.[21]

Although TCO_2 is less expensive and is more widely available than blood gas analyzers, relying on this measurement requires the clinician to make assumptions that may be incorrect for a given patient.[21] One must speculate whether an abnormal bicarbonate concentration is due to a primary metabolic or a respiratory derangement. Suppositions should be supported by careful evaluation of history, physical examination, and ancillary laboratory data. Major alterations in bicarbonate concentrations are often but not invariably primary events (i.e., low or high TCO_2 representing primary metabolic acid–base disorders). It is reasonable to rely on the TCO_2 provided that the apparent acid–base abnormality is consistent with what the clinician infers from the history and physical examination findings. However, compensation of primary disturbance cannot be assessed, particularly if a pH value is not available.

FLUIDS

Calculation

Fluid therapy is a complex topic and this section is not all encompassing. However, basic principles of fluid therapy are discussed. Planning fluid therapy requires consideration of maintenance needs, estimated hydration deficit, and assessment of ongoing losses.

Maintenance Fluid Needs

Maintenance fluid requirements (i.e., the amount of fluid necessary to replace insensible losses and obligatory urinary losses) vary with the animal's size, age, and occasionally diet (i.e., eating a diet containing excessive solute such as sodium increases the patient's water requirements for maintenance). Ambient temperature and humidity also affect maintenance requirements. Studies have been performed evaluating basal metabolic rate in companion animals. The optimal formula for determining the maintenance needs for dogs and cats is controversial. In general, smaller animals need more milliliters per kilogram daily than do larger animals. For most domestic species, estimates of daily water requirements range from 40 mL/kg/day (large dogs) to 60 mL/kg/day (cats and small dogs).[48,49] The daily maintenance water requirement for a healthy cat or dog weighing between 6 and 60 kg is as follows: (30 x BW[kg]) + 70. Studies using indirect calorimetry suggest that for animals weighing less than 10 kg or more than 50 kg, a more precise formula is as follows: 97 × body weight (0.655).[50] Water is present in foods and is generated as foods are metabolized. Maintenance requirements should be provided to patients not consuming sufficient quantities of water on their own.

The combination of variables (e.g., age, hydration status, perfusion, cardiac and renal function) makes it difficult to calculate exactly how much fluid an individual patient needs. In general, as long as the estimated amount of required fluids is provided and the patient is assessed frequently, clinically significant problems referable to fluid therapy are likely to be avoided. With the exception of the conditions listed in subsequent sections, providing slightly more fluid than is believed necessary is in most cases recommended insofar as it is more common to underestimate fluid needs than to overestimate them. However, patients with myocardial dysfunction, oliguric renal disease, severe anemia, severe hypoalbuminemia, or pulmonary edema can be seriously harmed by excessive fluid administration.

Deficit Fluid Needs

Fluid deficit should be estimated when patients are initially examined. Although there are guidelines for estimating degree of dehydration (Table 16-2), there are many pitfalls in this approach. Any excited or dyspneic animal that is breathing through its mouth may have dry, tacky oral mucous membranes, whereas nauseated animals may have moist membranes in the face of dehydration. Weight loss causes some degree of decreased skin turgor, while but obese animals may not have changes in skin turgor even when they are 8% to 10% dehydrated.[51]

Table 16-2 Determination of Degree of Dehydration

Manifestation	Degree (%)
Loss of skin elasticity	5
Oral mucous membranes becoming tacky	6-7
Prolonged capillary refill time	6-8
Skin tenting that persists	8-10
Eyes sunken back into orbits	10
Cool extremities, early shock	10-12

Findings of increased hematocrit and plasma proteins support the clinical suspicion of dehydration (i.e.. animals that are hemoconcentrated and hyperproteinemic are usually dehydrated). However the clinician seldom knows what these parameters were shortly before the animal became ill, and the hematocrit and total protein values by themselves are not a reliable means to assess hydration status. Many animals with chronic illness have anemia of chronic disease; dehydration may cause them to have a spuriously normal hematocrit value. Likewise, patients can be hypoproteinemic, and dehydration may cause them to have a seemingly normal serum protein concentration. There are many possible causes for a well-hydrated dog or cat to be hyperproteinemic, generally due to elevated globulin fraction (e.g., heartworm disease, ehrlichiosis, chronic dermatitis, feline infectious peritonitis). Alterations in body weight may be useful in assessing changes in hydration status because changes in body weight generally reflect changes in fluid content. When treating dehydrated patients, the clinician may interpret an increase in body weight as an encouraging sign that hydration is being restored. However, an increase in body weight in a well-hydrated patient may be an early indicator of fluid overload. Patient history should not be overlooked. Any animal that is not drinking or eating but has ongoing losses (e.g., vomiting, diarrhea, polyuria, tachypnea) is or will become dehydrated.

In general, because of the problems associated with determining the degree of dehydration, slightly overestimating the deficit is recommended unless the patient has syndromes mentioned in the discussion of maintenance fluid requirements. The dehydration deficit is determined by the following formula:

$$\text{Body weight (kg)} \times \text{estimated percentage dehydration} \times 1000 = \text{milliliters needed}$$

Deficit fluids can be administered more rapidly than maintenance fluids when patients are closely and frequently monitored. One half of the dehydration deficit can be administered as a bolus, with the remainder replaced as a constant rate infusion over 12 to 24 hours. Cats have smaller blood volumes per body weight than dogs (i.e., 50 to 60 mL/kg as opposed to 80 to 90 mL/kg in the dog) and can become fluid overloaded with smaller fluid doses than dogs. Once the estimated deficit is replaced, the animal should be re-examined, assessing for evidence of further deficits.[51]

Ongoing Losses

Ongoing losses can be divided into normal, insensible losses (e.g., from respiration, normal urine and fecal losses, skin evaporation) and those that are not normal (e.g., vomiting, diarrhea, polyuria, fever, tachypnea). In general, insensible respiratory losses involve water but not electrolytes (i.e., "free water"), whereas abnormal losses often involve electrolytes as well as water. Therefore the clinician should characterize the nature of fluid losses when choosing a fluid to administer. Careful assessment of body weight (i.e., with an accurate scale that measures ounces or tenths of a pound) remains a reliable means of monitoring for ongoing fluid balance in an individual patient. It is also important to weigh the animal after it has urinated and before it is fed. Because approximately 60% of body weight, rapid changes in body weight usually reflect changes in body water content as opposed to muscle mass or fat. One kilogram represents approximately 1000 mL of water. Frequent measurement or close estimation and matching of "ins and outs" (e.g., oral intake, parenteral fluids, urine production, vomiting, and diarrhea) can help prevent gross errors in approximation of patient requirements.

Choice of Fluid

There are several categories of fluids and additives available (Box 16-5). Crystalloid solutions (e.g., physiologic saline solution [PSS; 0.9% saline solution], 5% dextrose in water [D5W], Ringer's solution) are composed of electrolytes and nonelectrolytes that can pass freely out of the vascular space. Isotonic *replacement* crystalloids have an electrolyte composition similar to that of extracellular fluid, with a relatively high sodium and low potassium concentration. The terms *high* and *low* refer to the concentrations of sodium and potassium *relative to each other* in the fluid bag itself; it is important to note that the sodium and potassium are both essentially normal when compared with ECF and plasma. The most widely available isotonic replacement solutions are 0.9% saline, lactated Ringer's solution (LRS), Plasmalyte A (Baxter Healthcare Corp), and Normosol-R (Hospira, Inc). In true hypovolemia a very small concentration gradient exists between ECF and ICF spaces. Consequently, water shifts do not occur across the cell membrane. Intravascular crystalloid equilibrates with the interstitial space, with 20% to 25% of the infused volume remaining within the intravascular space 1 hour after infusion. Metabolism of the lactate in LRS or acetate and gluconate in Normosol-R or Plasmalyte A provides base to the body. When used for long-term therapy, there is a tendency for patients to develop mild to moderate hypokalemia. Normal ongoing losses typically have lower sodium and higher potassium than normal ECF, and therefore administering replacement solutions does not provide adequate potassium. Hypernatremia is less often encountered

Box 16-5

Selected Fluids and Fluid Additives Commonly Used in Dogs and Cats

- Crystalloids
  - Physiologic saline solution (0.9% saline, physiologic saline solution)
  - Hypertonic saline (7%)
  - Lactated Ringer's solution
  - Ringer's solution
  - 5% Dextrose in water
  - 0.45% Saline plus 2.5% dextrose
- Colloids
  - Plasma
  - Dextran-70
  - Hetastarch (hydroxyethyl starch)
- Additives
  - Potassium chloride
  - Potassium phosphate
  - 50% Dextrose
  - Sodium bicarbonate
  - Calcium chloride
  - Calcium gluconate
  - Magnesium sulfate

with use of replacement solutions for ongoing losses, unless renal sodium excretion is impaired. Thus potassium supplementation is almost always indicated, but switching to a commercially available isotonic maintenance fluid with a lower sodium concentration (e.g. Normosol-M [Hospira, Inc]) for long-term therapy after rehydration is not always necessary. Commercially available maintenance solutions (Table 16-3) are designed to fulfill the electrolyte requirements of patients with normal daily losses that are unable to maintain adequate fluid and electrolyte intake, and may be used to replenish obligate and insensible net ongoing losses. As these fluids have a relatively high potassium concentration (13 mEq/L), they should not be administered rapidly (0.5 mEq/kg/hr [suggested maximum rate of potassium administration] × 13 mEq/L = 38.5 mL/kg/hr = maximum rate of administration). Hypotonic solutions include Normosol M (Hospira), D5W, and 0.45% saline. Although the osmolality of D5W is 252 mOsm/L (which is close to being isotonic), the glucose is rapidly taken up by cells and metabolized after it is administered to the patient. Therefore administering glucose solutions is essentially equivalent to giving free water (unless hyperglycemic diuresis with subsequent dehydration results). Administration of D5W does not significantly contribute to meeting caloric needs (D5W has 170 kcal/L) and it is not intended to treat severe hypoglycemia. *Symptomatic* hypoglycemia is initially treated with bolus injection of 25% or 50% dextrose. Subsequently, adding a sufficient volume of 50% dextrose to a balanced isotonic crystalloid to produce a final dextrose concentration of 2.5% to 5% is usually sufficient for *maintaining glycemic status* on a nonemergent basis. Rapid infusion of hypotonic solutions can cause severe dilution of serum electrolytes, especially sodium. Although there are rare indications for hypotonic fluids

Table 16-3 Electrolyte Composition of Commercially Available Fluids

	Glucose (g/L)	Sodium (mEq/L)	Chlorine (mEq/L)	Potassium (mEq/L)	Calcium (mEq/L)	Magnesium (mEq/L)	Buffer (mEq/L)	Osmolality (mOsm/L)
D5W	50	0	0	0	0	0	0	252
D10W	100	0	0	0	0	0	0	505
PSS	0	154	154	0	0	0	0	308
PSS + D5W	50	154	154	0	0	0	0	560
½ PSS + D5W	50	77	77	0	0	0	0	406
½ PSS + D2.5W	25	77	77	0	0	0	0	280
Ringer's	0	147.5	156	4	4.5	0	0	310
LRS	0	130	109	4	3	0	28	272
LRS + D5W	50	130	109	4	3	0	28	524
Normosol-R	0	140	98	5	0	3	50	296
Normosol-M and 5% Dextrose	50	40	40	13	0	3	16	364

D10W, 10% dextrose in water; *D5W,* 5% dextrose in water; *D2.5W,* 2.5% dextrose in water; *PSS,* physiologic (i.e., 0.9%) saline solution; *LRS,* lactated Ringer's solution; *½ PSS,* 0.45% saline solution.
Modified from Chew DJ, DiBartola SP: *Manual of small animal nephrology and urology,* New York, 1986, Churchill Livingstone.

(e.g., recalcitrant hypernatremia or as a vehicle for delivery of specific drugs), they are seldom required in most clinical situations. Infusion of hypertonic (7.5%) saline creates a large osmotic gradient, and water is drawn from the intracellular and, to a lesser extent, interstitial compartment causing a rapid, albeit transient (<30 min), expansion of intravascular volume. Combining hypertonic saline with 6% hetastarch or dextran 70 prolongs the beneficial effects. Hypertonic solutions are reported to be safe and effective for the treatment of hypovolemic hypotension and may have a role in minimizing intracranial pressure. Their use is contraindicated with hypernatremia and dehydration, and as is true with all crystalloids, excessive volume is associated with cardiac failure. Crystalloids containing preservatives (e.g., benzyl alcohol) are not recommended because they may have adverse effects, especially in cats.[52]

Colloidal solutions (e.g., dextran 70, hetastarch 6%, Oxyglobin) are retained in the intravascular space to a greater degree than crystalloids and draw fluids from the cellular and interstitial compartments into this compartment.[51] Although both colloids and isotonic crystalloids can be used to rapidly expand intravascular volume in animals in shock, colloids are generally more effective (and effective at lower doses) than crystalloids.[53] It generally requires two to four times as much isotonic crystalloid solution to expand the ECF compartment as it does with dextran or hetastarch. Hetastarch and dextrans are primarily indicated for rapid volume expansion. Dextrans and hetastarch may also be used to maintain plasma COP in patients with severe hypoalbuminemia. Anaphylactic reactions have been reported with both hetastarch and dextrans, but they are uncommonly observed. Low-molecular-weight dextrans (i.e., dextran 40) have been reported to cause renal failure, and they are not routinely employed in clinical practice. Both hetastarch and dextrans may also cause coagulation abnormalities when administered at high doses. Clinically significant hemorrhage is rare.

Purified hemoglobin both acts as a strong colloid and increases the oxygen-carrying capacity of the blood. Stroma-free, hemoglbin-based, oxygen-carrying solutions (e.g., Oxyglobin) are used to treat anemia in a variety of species. Indications also include volume resuscitation in hypovolemic states. The greatest advantage of Oxyglobin is its ability to carry oxygen to tissues and offload oxygen more effectively than blood because it is not limited by red cell flow; it has also been shown to improve microvascular perfusion, thus improving oxygen tension in injured tissues. Human serum albumin (HSA) obtained from purified human plasma is available commercially and has been used in critically ill companion animals with pancreatitis, peritonitis, acute hepatic failure, and protein-losing enteropathy. In addition to its role in maintaining colloid osmotic pressure, albumin has many other properties that may benefit critically ill patients, including maintenance of the selective permeability of the microvascular barrier, and as a carrier of a number of substances, including bilirubin, fatty acids, hormones, and drugs. Most commercially available albumin products are prepared as 5% or 25% solutions. The chemical structure of human albumin is not identical to canine or feline albumin, and type III hypersensitivity reactions, which are sometimes severe and fatal, are reported after the administration of HSA in healthy dogs.[54] Until further studies suggest otherwise, routine use of HSA is discouraged unless all other means of restoring albumin or colloid osmotic pressure have failed. Lyophilized canine albumin has recently become available commercially. If this product is shown to have a favorable side effect profile (compared with human albumin products), it would be expected to prove useful in the management of severely ill hypoalbuminemic dogs with correspondingly low colloid osmotic pressure.

Clinicians often need to tailor a fluid for a specific patient. This is usually done by adding potassium chloride, 50% glucose, potassium phosphate, calcium gluconate, calcium chloride, magnesium sulfate, sodium bicarbonate, or a combination thereof. The specific amounts are discussed under specific disorders.

Route of Administration

Fluids may be administered orally, intravenously, subcutaneously, intraosseously, or peritoneally.[55] Whenever oral intake is inadequate or not feasible (e.g., subject refuses to drink adequate volumes, vomits, does not absorb fluids sufficiently quickly for desired effect), parenteral administration is preferred. Intravenous administration is the quickest way to replenish an underexpanded ECF and is the standard of care for acute replacement of fluid losses (e.g., due to shock) or maintaining ECF volume during anesthetic procedures. This route allows uninterrupted infusion, which is expected to be advantageous to severely ill, hemodynamically unstable animals. Venous catheter access can be difficult because of the patient's size or temperament, vascular collapse, or prior use of veins for catheters or venipuncture. Routine catheter care is mandatory to prevent infection, phlebitis, extravasation, and clotting within the catheter lumen.

Subcutaneous fluid administration is technically easier than intravenous administration and is usually adequate when the need for fluids is not severe or acute. Owners can usually be taught to administer subcutaneous fluids at home. From 50 to 200 mL may be injected per site, and several sites may be injected at one time. Poor absorption may be observed if excessive fluids are administered at one site. Although more commonly administered once daily, subcutaneous fluids may be given as frequently as every 6 hours if clinically indicated and tolerated by the patient. If fluid from the prior injections has not been absorbed, however, it is necessary to determine the reason before more fluids are administered. Severely dehydrated animals may absorb subcutaneous fluids very slowly because of poor peripheral vascular perfusion. Furthermore, administration of hypertonic or irritating solutions under the skin is discouraged, because fluids may be drawn from the central compartment or cause injury to local and adjacent tissues.[55] Subcutaneous fluids are often considered to be relatively safe in patients with heart disease, but this is an incorrect assumption and fluid overload may rapidly ensue.

Intraperitoneal administration permits the infusion of large volumes of fluids, and absorption generally occurs more quickly than with subcutaneous administration. This route is occasionally used for neonates whose veins are not readily accessible with a catheter. The clinician can administer a warmed (not hot) isotonic fluid aseptically with a 23- to 20-gauge needle or similar bore size over-the-needle catheter. Fluids given by this route may be administered over a short period (i.e., less than 5 minutes) until the abdomen becomes obviously distended (usually about 20 mL/kg). Patient discomfort and respiratory distress indicate that an excessive volume was administered into the peritoneal cavity. Aseptic technique must be used so that bacteria are not introduced. On balance, intraperitoneal administration does not offer clear advantages over intravenous, intraosseous, or subcutaneous routes, which are preferred.

Intraosseous administration[56] is accomplished by using either a specifically designed needle, a bone marrow aspiration needle, or an 18- to 20-gauge spinal or hypodermic needle. The needle is inserted into the marrow cavity of the humerus or femur; less common sites are the tibia and ilium. Fluids are then administered as for intravenous administration. Gravity drip rates of approximately 10 mL/min may be reached. Absorption occurs more quickly than with subcutaneously administered fluids, and it may be easier to obtain access to the marrow cavity in very small animals than to the jugular or cephalic vein.[55-58] In rare cases pain may be seen as a consequence of infection, administration of cold solutions, or excessive administration rate.

The administration of crystalloid solutions rectally as an enema is described, because the normal colon will avidly absorb intraluminal water. This technique is seldom used in the clinical setting for provision of fluid deficits. Moreover, intravenous administration is mandatory for volume-depleted patients, and subcutaneous fluids are so easy to administer that there is essentially no reason for rectal administration. However, it may be used in select emergencies to modify core body temperature in a severely hypothermic or hyperthermic patient.

Determining Adequacy of Fluid Therapy

Fluid requirements should be evaluated and adjusted regularly. Generally fluid therapy is not abruptly discontinued but rather is gradually tapered to maintenance, or lower than maintenance rates over 12 to 24 hours. A common mistake with long-term intravenous fluid therapy is failing to adjust fluid rates as the condition of the pet changes. Close monitoring of body weight is useful to corroborate the observed efficacy of fluid therapy. Physical examination parameters compatible with dehydration (e.g., skin turgor, dry oral mucous membranes) should improve with appropriate fluid therapy, assuming there are no intercurrent disease processes associated with weight loss or development of tachypnea. Frequent observation of respiratory rate and effort and thoracic auscultation are expected to permit early detection of pulmonary edema. Similarly, new cardiac murmurs or gallop rhythms not audible before fluid therapy was instituted often presage overt clinical signs of fluid overload.

Because urine output is affected by myriad factors, it is not possible to define what constitutes normal urine output for many patients. As a general rule, urine output should be 1 to 2 mL/kg/hr. Although urine output is seldom quantified, it should be apparent if a patient is producing reasonable volumes of urine that is not extremely concentrated. This is not reliable for patients with renal failure, and some attempt must be made to quantify urine output when oligoanuria is a concern (e.g., weighing urine-soaked diapers, catching all urine in ambulatory patients) if a urinary catheter and closed collection system is not in place. Central venous pressure (CVP) is a measure of the hydrostatic pressure within the central venous compartment that provides an assessment of intravascular blood volume and cardiac function. It is typically measured by a percutaneously placed jugular catheter, which has its tip in the cranial vena cava. The catheter can be attached to either an electric pressure transducer or a water manometer. When interpreted in concert with other diagnostic findings, CVP is most useful for guiding fluid therapy in seriously ill animals with oliguric renal disease or myocardial dysfunction.[55]

ELECTROLYTES

Considerations for Therapy

Therapy for electrolyte disorders primarily consists of supplementing electrolytes or decreasing their plasma concentrations by promoting excretion, dilution, or sequestration. The major electrolyte disturbances capable of causing clinical signs in dogs and cats, and thus requiring therapy, are hypokalemia and hyperkalemia. It is rarely necessary to address hyponatremia specifically, except with regard to some patients with hypoadrenocorticism. Hypoadrenocorticism is relatively uncommon, but volume replacement and management of hyperkalemia are usually the major goals for such patients in a crisis. Similar to hyponatremia, hypernatremia usually does not require specific treatment and often will correct itself as the underlying disease is being treated.

Hyponatremia

Hyponatremia is almost universally due to retention of free water except in patients with hypoadrenocorticism. Primary sodium loss (e.g. diarrhea) is not common. Unless the hyponatremia is severe enough to cause clinical signs, the clinician should first identify and correct the underlying disorder. Neurologic clinical manifestations (due to an osmotic shift of water into brain cells) are rarely observed with acute hyponatremia. To prevent rapid changes in the patient's sodium, the initial fluid chosen should have a sodium concentration similar to the serum sodium. It is recommended that sodium be raided no faster than 1 mEq/L/hour, although there is debate regarding the pace and degree of sodium correction. There is a risk of neurologic complications (myelinolysis), which typically occurs 3 to 4 days after aggressive correction of hyponatremia and may include weakness, ataxia, quadriparesis, and hypermetria.[59,60] Buffered isotonic crystalloids such as LRS are generally preferable to PSS for this purpose because plasma normally has approximately 145 mEq Na/L and 110 mEq Cl/L. PSS contains 154 mEq of each per liter, whereas LRS has 130 mEq Na/L and 109 mEq Cl/L. The sodium concentration in Normosol-R (140 mEq/L) is slightly greater than that of LRS. Therefore administration of PSS adds too much chloride relative to the amount of sodium, although this is seldom clinically significant. It is rare that hypertonic saline solutions are needed to replace sodium in small animals.[7,17]

Hypernatremia

Spontaneous hypernatremia is almost always due to loss of free water, and is not a reflection of total body sodium content. Sodium gain (e.g., ocean water ingestion or overzealous fluid administration) is less common. If the patient is hypovolemic, rapid administration of isotonic crystalloid (including saline) is likely to cause rapid changes in sodium and therefore is discouraged. The initial fluid for correcting volume deficits should have a sodium equal to (or slightly below) that of the patient so as not to change sodium too rapidly. Subsequently, *slow* administration of a hypotonic crystalloid (e.g., D5W, 0.45% NaCl) may be appropriate. Hypernatremia by itself is seldom associated with signs, and lowering the plasma sodium concentration too quickly is likely, be more detrimental to the patient than the actual hypernatremia. If the hypernatremia existed for more than a few hours, it is often appropriate to administer PSS, a mixture of physiological saline solution plus 5% dextrose in water, or 0.45% NaCl/2.5% dextrose. Conservative administration of either solution decreases serum tonicity slowly enough to prevent neurologic complications. To minimize the risk of neuronal overhydration, serum sodium should not be lowered at a rate exceeding 0.5 mEq/L/hr.[7,61]

Hypochloremia

Hypochloremia is principally found in patients with excessive losses caused by gastric vomiting or diuretic administration and is of clinical relevance principally because of its effects on systemic acid–base balance. Administration of PSS with or without potassium chloride is usually adequate to replace the chloride and resolve the problem.

Hyperchloremia

Hyperchloremia may be managed by administration of an alkalinizing fluid such as LRS (Cl = 98 mEq/L), Plasmalyte, or Normosol-R (Cl = 110 mEq/L). Isotonic saline (Cl = 154 mEq/L) is seldom indicated for treating hyperchloremia, even for the initial management of patients with hyponatremia caused by hypoadrenocorticism. Even in patients with true hyperchloremia (i.e., not corrected for water), hypotonic fluids should not be administered without careful assessment of sodium status.

Hypokalemia

Supplemental administration of potassium is routine in small animal medicine because hypokalemia is a common abnormality, especially in inappetent hospitalized patients receiving more than 2 to 3 days of intravenous fluids. With rare exceptions, all anorexic animals on maintenance fluids should receive potassium in excess of that contained in most replacement fluids because of obligatory losses of potassium into the urine. Animals with polyuria or other avenues of potassium loss may have even greater needs. Only pets that have or are prone to hyperkalemia should not receive potassium supplementation. It is not possible to predict with confidence exactly how much potassium a particular patient will need; therefore the patient's plasma potassium concentration should be periodically monitored when receiving supplemental potassium.

If the patient can accept oral fluids and is not vomiting, oral administration of potassium gluconate is usually an efficient means of replenishing plasma potassium.[62] There is great interpatient variability in the amount of enteral potassium needed to correct hypokalemia.[29,30,63]

Intravenous supplementation of potassium is common but mandates frequent monitoring of both the patient and the serum potassium concentration. As a general rule, potassium should not be infused at a rate exceeding 0.5 mEq/kg per hour, although if necessary, carefully monitored patients may receive greater rates without consequence. If it is necessary to administer 0.5 mEq/kg per hour or more, continuous electrocardiographic monitoring for cardiotoxic effects (i.e., bradycardia, tall T waves, small P waves, ventricular arrhythmias, ventricular fibrillation, and asystole) is recommended. Table 16-4, in addition to the other tables in this chapter, provides guidelines for determining how much potassium to add to fluids for intravenous administration. Many clinicians routinely start by adding 15 to 20 mEq K/L to maintenance fluids while periodically monitoring the animal's plasma potassium concentration.

Potassium may also be added to fluids intended for subcutaneous administration, the safe amount depending on the *total osmolality* of the solution and *not the potassium concentration* in the fluid bag. General guidelines suggest that solutions containing potassium in quantities greater than 35 mEq/L should not be given subcutaneously.[8] If the clinician experiences difficulty correcting hypokalemia despite seemingly appropriate potassium supplementation, the serum magnesium concentration should be checked.[64,65]

Hyperkalemia

Therapy for hyperkalemia depends on the severity of clinical signs and the magnitude of the hyperkalemia. The clinician should always look for the cause of hyperkalemia, because it often indicates significant renal or adrenal disease. If hyperkalemia is mild (e.g., 5.5 to 6.5 mEq/L) and is not expected to rise rapidly, it is appropriate to screen for common associated syndromes (e.g., hypoadrenocorticism, renal failure, iatrogenic potassium administration). Administration of potassium-free fluids (e.g. 0.9% NaCl) is often advised without qualification. However, isotonic replacement solutions (K ≤4 mEq/L) will similarly "dilute" a hyperkalemic patient and augment renal potassium excretion. Therapy with any balanced, buffered isotonic crystalloid may be appropriately selected for treating mild hyperkalemia, particularly insofar as many patients will be somewhat dehydrated. If the patient is also hyponatremic (i.e., hypoadrenocorticism), 0.9% saline (higher concentration of sodium compared with buffered isotonic solutions) may be administered if the clinician monitors for excessive rate of lowering of plasma sodium. If the patient has hyperkalemia of sufficient magnitude to cause cardiotoxicity (i.e., usually ≥8 mEq/L), additional therapy may be warranted (Table 16-5).[10] The routine use of sodium bicarbonate for managing hyperkalemia is generally discouraged. However, this drug may be given in an acute setting to a patient that has concurrent metabolic acidosis. Administration of dextrose and insulin decreases blood potassium concentration but can also decrease serum phosphorus concentration, which only rarely causes problems (i.e., hemolytic anemia).[66] Slow administration of 10% calcium gluconate may be administered for rapid correction of hyperkalemic cardiotoxicity. It does not lower the potassium level but transiently protects the heart until other measures (i.e., fluid administration) decrease the plasma potassium concentration.[8]

Hypophosphatemia

Optimal management of hypophosphatemia depends somewhat on whether the clinician is trying to prevent hypophosphatemia or to treat associated problems (e.g., hemolytic anemia) caused by hypophosphatemia. Severe hypophosphatemia is often seen as a complication of diabetic ketoacidosos. Other causes include hyperparathyroidism and hyperalimenation. If the patient has a dangerously low serum phosphorus concentration (e.g., 1.0 to 1.5 mg/dL) but does not yet have clinical signs, a simple rule of thumb is to provide one quarter of the maintenance potassium being given in the intravenous fluids (assuming maintenance rates are being used) as potassium phosphates and the remainder as potassium chloride.[66] The patient's serum phosphorus concentration is then monitored two to three times daily until it is out of the danger zone (i.e., serum phosphorus >2 mg/dL), at which time the phosphorus supplementation is stopped. If the animal is experiencing hemolysis, then a constant-rate infusion of 0.01 to 0.03 mmol phosphate/kg per hour may be given.[31,32,66] Greater rates of phosphorus adminstration (e.g., 0.05 to 0.1 mmol/kg per hour) are described but seldom required to treat hypophosphatemia.[31] The patient must be monitored three to four times daily, however, to ensure that the serum phosphorus concentration is increasing and that the serum calcium concentration is not decreasing. Severe, symptomatic hypocalcemia might result from excessive phosphorus administration.

Table 16-4 Approximate Amount of Potassium to Add to Fluids for Intravenous Administration

Serum Potassium (mEq/L)	mEq Potassium to Add to Fluids	Maximum Rate of Infusion (mL/kg/H)
3.5-4.0	15/L	30
3.0-3.5	28/L	16
2.5-3.0	40/L	12
2.0-2.5	60/L	8
<2.0	80/L	6

Table 16-5 Symptomatic Therapy for Hyperkalemia

Treatment	Dose
Potassium-free fluids	Physiologic saline solution or 5% dextrose
Calcium gluconate	0.5-1.0 mL 10% calcium gluconate/kg intravenously (10-15 minutes)
Dextrose and insulin	0.5 U regular insulin/kg + 2 g dextrose per unit insulin
Sodium bicarbonate	Based on blood gas analysis or 1-2 mEq/kg

Hypomagnesemia

If hypomagnesemia needs to be treated or prevented, magnesium sulfate or magnesium chloride should be administered in D5W or 0.9% NaCL. Initial dosing guidelines are 0.75 to 1 mEq/kg/day given intravenously by constant-rate infusion, although 0.15 to 0.30 mEq/kg may be given over 10 to 15 minutes for life-threatening cardiac arrhythmias.[67] Because magnesium is a divalent ion, 1 mEq is equivalent to 0.5 mmol. Magnesium should not be added to LRS, or given in the same fluid line as calcium-containing fluids or insulin.

ACID–BASE STATUS

Considerations for Therapy

In general, the clinician should always attempt to determine the underlying cause of the acid–base abnormality and correct it. If the acidemia or alkalemia is so severe that it puts the patient at significant risk, however, symptomatic therapy is needed.

Metabolic Acidosis

A blood pH below 7.20 puts a patient at risk for arrhythmia, hypotension, and myocardial dysfunction. For such patients administration of sodium bicarbonate may be considered. A patient with blood pH below 7.1 is considered to be at high risk for cardiovascular complications, and prompt bicarbonate therapy should be considered. The goal of such therapy is to raise the pH to approximately 7.20 or slightly greater, not to correct the pH so that it returns to the normal range. Sodium bicarbonate should not be given to patients with respiratory acidosis or decreased respiratory drive. If too much base is administered, a patient may become alkalemic after the cause of the acidemia (e.g., diabetic ketoacidosis, lactic acidosis) is corrected.[20]

Metabolic Alkalosis

Alkalosis is important because of the chloride abnormalities that may be associated with it. The alkalosis does not cause the hypochloremia but may potentiate it and therefore enhance the effects of high pH on the myocardium. Most dogs and cats with clinically important metabolic alkalosis have a chloride-responsive condition (e.g., vomiting gastric contents, excessive furosemide administration in anorexic animals). Correction of volume depletion and supplementation with chloride (e.g., PSS occasionally with potassium chloride supplemented) is usually adequate to correct the problem.[20]

Respiratory Acidosis and Alkalosis

Respiratory acidosis and alkalosis require therapy directed at the cause of the problem and seldom require symptomatic therapy.

Drugs Used to Correct Acid-Base Abnormalities

The main drugs used to alter blood and body pH are sodium bicarbonate and fluids containing bicarbonate precursors. In particular, LRS has often been used to treat acidosis. Under normal circumstances, hepatic metabolism of lactate causes consumption and elimination of protons (i.e., H^{++}), thus raising the pH.[20] If the lactate is not metabolized (e.g., the patient already has lactic acidosis), LRS may cause a mild dilutional acidosis similar to saline or will not affect acid–base status. Moreover, the lactate in LRS will never cause a lactic acidosis because it is a salt. Even when the lactate is not metabolized, however, expanding the ECF may improve peripheral perfusion. Similar fluids such as Normosol-R and Plasmalyte are considered to be just as effective. Sodium bicarbonate ($NaHCO_3$) can be used to correct acidemia. It works rapidly by providing base, which titrates H^+. Sodium bicarbonate is not always beneficial and is seldom required for acidotic patients. Its use is particularly controversial for patients with lactic acidosis.[68,69] When $NaHCO_3$ is added to the blood, a small percentage of it is converted to CO_2 almost immediately. Traditionally, if this CO_2 cannot be exhaled, it may exacerbate preexisting acidemia. More commonly, however, the respiratory acidosis offsets the bicarbonate-induced metabolic alkalosis, with negligible, if any, increase in pH. Clinicians should appreciate that when $NaHCO_3$ is given to patients with diabetic ketoacidosis, they may become alkalotic after the ketone bodies are metabolized (rebound phenomenon). Physiologically, most patients can deal with alkalosis better than with acidosis.

Various formulas can be used to help the clinician decide how much bicarbonate (HCO_3) to administer.[20] The following is suggested for most situations when $NaHCO_3$ is indicated:

$$\text{mEq to administer} = \text{body weight in kg} \times 0.3 \times \text{calculated } HCO_3 \text{ deficit}$$

The body weight is multiplied by 0.3 to approximate the ECF volume, which is where the HCO_3 will first be distributed. There will eventually be diffusion of HCO_3 into the cells, and additional HCO_3 may have to be administered to retain the desired effect in the ECF. For that reason some clinicians utilize a factor of 0.5 instead of 0.3.

The calculated HCO_3 deficit *to treat* is not the same as "base deficit" (a calculation provided by a blood gas analysis). To calculate the HCO_3 deficit *to treat*, the clinician must first decide what plasma concentration of HCO_3 is desired. It is appropriate to aim for a plasma concentration of approximately 14 to 15 mEq/L if the HCO_3 concentration is less than that initially. The patient's HCO_3 concentration is then subtracted from the desired HCO_3 concentration (e.g., 15 mEq/L). The resulting number is the calculated HCO_3 deficit *to treat* for this patient at this time. Once the total amount of HCO_3 to be administered is calculated, it is administered intravenously, usually over 1 to 4 hours. After several hours, this HCO_3 will distribute to the ECF and later to the ICF, and the patient should be reevaluated to determine whether more HCO_3 is needed.

$NaHCO_3$ is not a benign drug, although severe adverse effects are rare and complications can be minimized if it is used judiciously. Hypernatremia, hypervolemia, hypokalemia, ionized hypocalcemia, hypotension, nausea, and paradoxical intracellular acidosis, are possible.[70] The recognition of potential adverse effects of $NaHCO_3$ led investigators to develop other forms of base that could be administered to restore acid–base status while circumventing the problems associated with $NaHCO_3$. THAM (tris hydroxymethyl aminomethane) is sodium free and has a free amino group that buffers protons. THAM administration doesn't result in generation of CO_2. This drug never gained widespread acceptance, in part because of reported side effects including respiratory depression, hyperkalemia, and hepatotoxicity. Carbicarb (1:1 mixture of sodium bicarbonate and sodium carbonate) has been shown in animal studies of metabolic acidosis to be superior to $NaHCO_3$ in preserving or improving cardiac output and intracellular pH. However, further development of this drug was abandoned, in large part because it was not convincingly demonstrated to be superior to $NaHCO_3$. Ethylene glycol intoxication often necessitates aggressive $NaHCO_3$ therapy. Large amounts of acid are produced as ethylene glycol is metabolized to glycolic acid[20]; therefore it may be difficult to give $NaHCO_3$ in sufficient amounts to maintain a safe pH, depending on how much ethylene glycol was ingested.

SPECIAL CONSIDERATIONS

Shock

Shock is a syndrome characterized by the presence of severe clinical signs, including altered mental status, mucous membrane color, capillary refill time, heart rate, and pulse quality. Shock may be classified as hypovolemic, cardiogenic, or distributive. Obstructive shock, as described, is less commonly discussed as a distinct entity as its pathophysiology is believed to overlap with other classifications. Classification schemes, including this one, tend to be oversimplifications because relatively few global clinical parameters represent many complex dynamic processes occurring at the cellular level. Hypovolemic shock occurs when loss of blood volume causes a severe decrease in tissue perfusion and oxygenation. Causes include hemorrhage and severe dehydration. Cardiogenic shock is caused by myocardial failure with or without arrhythmias that decrease cardiac output. In obstructive shock inadequate tissue perfusion results from obstruction of blood flow within the vasculature. Obstructive shock may be seen in animals with massive pulmonary thromboembolism, pericardial effusion, or gastric dilation/volvulus. Distributive shock is characterized by nonuniform loss of peripheral vascular resistance. Resistance in specific tissue beds may be increased, decreased, or normal. Although cardiac output may be increased, the clinical picture is generally one of vasodilation. The vascular and cellular events result in the global release of inflammatory mediators, leading to the systemic inflammatory response syndrome (SIRS). Sepsis may lead to distributive shock. If there is refractory hypotension, it is further defined as septic shock. Further, patients may have distributive shock subsequent to trauma or other severe inflammatory processes in the absence of an infectious cause (e.g., pancreatitis, anaphylaxis).[71] Appropriate treatment of a patient in shock requires characterizing the shock syndrome present in a given patient.[53,72]

Hypovolemic Shock

The immediate need is to reestablish effective circulating blood volume. Appropriate resuscitation fluids are isotonic crystalloids (e.g., LRS, PSS, Normosol R) with or without the addition of colloids or hypertonic saline. If isotonic crystalloids are used alone in patients with ongoing blood loss, a decrease in vascular volume may be expected after initial resuscitation as redistribution occurs across the extracellular space. With colloids a more steady state of vascular volume expansion is expected. Hypertonic saline should be used cautiously or not at all for patients that are already hypernatremic. Colloids (e.g., dextran 70, 6% hetastarch) are sometimes used with hypertonic saline; or they may be used alone. Hetastarch is given at a dose of 5 to 20 mL/kg in dogs and 5 mL/kg in cats over 5 to 10 minutes, although doses of up to 40 mL/kg per day are described. To prevent hypervolemia, the rate of infusion of isotonic crystalloids should be decreased by 40% to 60% after colloids are started. In the face of ongoing blood loss, optimal therapy ideally should include blood products. If the patient is symptomatic for anemia and blood products are not available, Oxyglobin may be given.[53,58,72-74]

Unless there is suspicion for hypoadrenocorticism, steroids are generally not recommended. Vasopressors are not generally indicated for hypovolemic patients. In particular, clinicians should avoid α-agonists that increase blood pressure by causing vasoconstriction, unless patients are severely hypotensive and the clinician must time while other interventions are implemented.[53]

Obstructive Shock

Gastric dilation/volvulus (GDV) is the prototype disorder characterized by obstructive shock. Distention of the stomach with food and air compresses the portal vein and vena cava. This compression can occur with dilation and does not require volvulus. Fluids for resuscitation should be administered through large-bore cephalic catheters because fluid administration through saphenous catheters will be ineffective. Balanced electrolyte solutions are administered at 60 to 90 mL/kg in the initial hour of treatment. Hypertonic saline/dextran solutions can also be used initially (5 mL/kg over 5 to 10 minutes) but must be followed by isotonic crystalloids to maintain perfusion.[75] Once resuscitation is under way, the stomach is decompressed by carefully passing an orogastric tube. If passage of the tube is not possible, the stomach is trocarized. Because ischemia and reperfusion appear to be important mechanisms of injury, administration of free radical scavengers may eventually become important in the early treatment of this disorder. There is no evidence supporting the use of glucocorticoids or nonsteroidal inflammatory agents in gastric dilation/volvulus patients.

Cardiogenic Shock

Treatment of cardiogenic shock is directed toward improving myocardial contractility, reducing afterload and preload and controlling dysrhythmias. The clinician should examine the patient frequently to ensure that fluid therapy does not lead to decompensation because these patients are often volume intolerant. It is typically inadvisable to administer crystalloids in edematous cardiac patients. For the rare patient that must receive fluids (e.g., as a vehicle for drug administration), limited amounts of sodium should be given (e.g., 0.45% NaCl).[76] Maintenance rates or less are then carefully administered. CVP measurement can be particularly useful in monitoring these patients.

Distributive Shock

Distributive shock is principally seen in animals with SIRS. In SIRS release of various inflammatory mediators causes abnormal blood flow regulation with subsequent tissue hypoxia, even when there is normal to increased cardiac output (hence the term *hyperdynamic shock*). Increased vascular permeability may cause plasma volume to leak into interstitial tissues, further reducing tissue perfusion.[77-80]

It can be difficult to effectively treat some patients with SIRS. Blood volume should be maintained as for hypovolemic shock. Either isotonic or hypertonic crystalloids may be used. The clinician must also identify and eliminate the cause of the inflammation, which usually includes broad-spectrum antibiotic therapy. Pharmacologic therapies directed at specific inflammatory pathways have been investigated, but none have been found to be effective to date.[81] There is limited evidence supporting the administration of nonsteroidal antiinflammatory agents and corticosteroids, and their use is generally discouraged. A syndrome of relative adrenal insufficiency (RAI) is described in critically ill humans and animals, and patients with RAI *may* benefit from low (i.e., physiologic) doses of corticosteroids. Criteria for the diagnosis of RAI in animals and humans have been published, but at present the syndrome is not widely recognized.[82]

Hypoglycemia is relatively common in critical illness, and intravenous glucose supplementation may be needed. Most patients require fluid support, and adding hypertonic glucose to balanced isotonic fluids to create a fluid with a final glucose concentration of 5% is recommended. Although intermittent boluses of hypertonic glucose may be administered (0.5 gm/kg of 10% to 25% dextrose solution), continuous infusion of hypertonic solutions through a peripheral vein may cause thrombophlebitis. The addition of hypotonic glucose-containing fluids (e.g., D5W) at maintenance rates can usually maintain blood glucose concentrations of more than 100 mg/dL in volume-sensitive patients.

Renal Disease

Fluid therapy for patients with renal disease should first correct significant fluid, electrolyte, and acid–base abnormalities and subsequently produce a diuresis to eliminate normally excreted substances that have been retained. It is important to distinguish patients with oliguric renal disease from those with polyuric renal disease and also to determine if pets have chronic kidney disease or acute on chronic kidney injury. Severely hypoalbuminemic patients with proteinuric nephropathy present special challenges. Oliguria describes a patient that is producing less than 1 to 2 mL urine/kg per hour, although some clinicians define *oliguria* as less than 0.25 mL/kg per hour.[83] Anuria is a more severe situation indicating negligible urine production. Polyuria means that greater than normal amounts of urine being produced. Most patients with chronic kidney disease are polyuric until they are preterminal, when they may become oliguric. Patients with acute renal injury similarly may be polyuric or oliguric–anuric.

Polyuric Renal Failure

The first goal of fluid therapy for patients with polyuric renal failure is to correct dehydration (which is commonly present with decompensated renal failure) and severe electrolyte or acid–base abnormalities. If the patient is seriously ill, intravenous fluids are usually preferred to prevent delayed uptake from subcutaneous depots or vomiting of orally administered fluids. The next step is to provide sufficient fluids to match urinary losses. Occasionally, pharmacologic attempts are made to further augment renal function and urine production with diuretics (e.g., furosemide). This should not be done unless the patient is euhydrated and on intravenous fluids or is overhydrated. The use of appropriate and aggressive crystalloid therapy is generally adequate, and although this makes sense intuitively, there is limited evidence to support the use of diuretics in this setting.

As much fluid as possible should be administered without overhydrating the patient. The amount of fluid administered is slowly increased as damaged kidneys recover and adapt to the increased demand placed on them. As a general rule of thumb, therapy is begun by replacing deficits and weighing the patient. Fluids are then administered at 1.5 to 2 times the calculated maintenance rate or more, if necessary to keep up with renal losses. If the patient does not gain weight inappropriately and does not have signs of fluid overload (i.e., gallop rhythm, murmur, pulmonary crackles), the clinician can slowly increase the amount of fluids administered each day, usually by 15% to 30%. Although loop diuretics (e.g., furosemide) are sometimes also required, vigilant therapy with balanced crystalloids often produces an adequate diuresis. When fluid-induced diuresis is brisk, the rate of intravenous fluid administered is slowly decreased (e.g., 10% to 25%) each day, and the body weight is closely monitored to prevent the patient from becoming dehydrated.[84] Recording the volume of urine produced over a given time (e.g., 24 hours) is advisable. Measurement of CVP is *not* useful in this setting.

Oliguric and Anuric Renal Failure

Oligoanuric renal failure is more difficult to manage than polyuric renal failure. Oligoanuria is observed with severe acute renal injury and occasionally in preterminal chronic renal disease.[83] In the latter situation there is usually little that can be offered to help the patient besides renal replacement therapy or transplantation. In the former situation, it is important to try to quickly convert the oliguria to polyuria by replacement of the fluid deficit and then administration of furosemide, osmotic diuretics, or dopamine, although none of these drugs has been proved to benefit or alter the prognosis of anuric renal failure patients. Furosemide, administered either as a bolus or as a constant-rate infusion, is typically the first way that the clinician attempts to convert an oliguric patient to a polyuric state. Although once highly regarded, dopamine is generally of dubious value in patients with established oliguric, acute renal failure.

If furosemide therapy fails to convert an oliguric patient to a polyuric state, osmotic diuresis may be attempted by administering a bolus of mannitol (1 gm/kg intravenous bolus) followed by additional boluses or a constant-rate infusion (1 to 2 mg/kg/minute). Alternatively, 10% to 20% dextrose may be administered. The use of dextrose is favored by some clinicians because it may be metabolized if it cannot be excreted. The clinical significance of this is uncertain. However, if this is the case, the clinician should be able to detect glucose in newly formed urine, with the recognition that some patients with acute renal failure already have glucosuria as a result of proximal renal tubular damage. The body weight should be monitored closely to prevent excessive overhydration. Serum electrolytes should also be monitored. It is important that maintenance fluids be initiated immediately after infusing dextrose or mannitol to prevent renal hypoperfusion. If urine production is not increased by these measures, infusions should be discontinued before overhydration, pulmonary edema, and hypertonicity occur (i.e., before half of the total calculated volume is administered).[83]

Great care must be taken not to volume overload oliguric patients. If life-threatening overhydration occurs, all intravenous therapies are discontinued. Diuretics may be administered, but these patients may not improve without hemodialysis or hemofiltration. CVP should be monitored. CVP values consistently greater than 10 to 12 cm H_2O are *compatible with* but not diagnostic for fluid overload. CVP values between 5 and 10 cm H_2O suggest that the patient may tolerate additional fluid challenge. [85] Another technique is to measure urine output and administer fluids accordingly, using a technique sometimes called "ins and outs."[84] The patient is initially rehydrated over 6 to 8 hours. The clinician next divides the day into six 4-hour intervals. The amount of urine produced over each interval is given back to the patient over the subsequent interval.

Oligoanuric renal failure patients are predisposed to hyperkalemia and severe acidosis, Serum magnesium abnormalities are also common. If the patient is well hydrated and remains oliguric or anuric, all intravenous fluids are discontinued. Alternatively, the clinician may elect to replace only insensible losses with intravenous fluids at this time, but this has inherent risks. Body weight is assessed several times daily. Consideration of referral for hemodialysis is appropriate in persistently (i.e., duration longer than 24 hours) oliogoanuric patients.

The healing phase of acute renal failure may be accompanied by an intense diuresis that can require administration of several times the calculated daily maintenance volume. If an oliguric or anuric patient becomes polyuric, it is necessary to guard against dehydration. The rate of fluid administration must be slowly decreased when the patient is being weaned off intravenous fluids.[83] Excessive losses of potassium may occur during the healing, polyuric phase.

Urethral Obstruction

The clinical condition of dogs and cats with urethral obstruction depends on the duration and severity of the obstruction. Less commonly, bilateral ureteral obstruction will result in oligoanuria; in this situation the bladder is small or empty. When urethral obstruction is diagnosed, intravenous fluids should be instituted immediately, with the rate based on the degree of hypoperfusion and dehydration present. Hyperkalemia, if severe and associated with bradydysrhythmias, should be treated aggressively before relieving the obstruction. If acidosis is present and hyperkalemia is not associated with life-threatening signs, fluid resuscitation alone will often be sufficient to correct these values. A balanced isotonic electrolyte solution is recommended for initial therapy in most cases.[86] These patients often develop severe polyuria after the obstruction is relieved (e.g., postobstructive diuresis), the severity of which generally depends on the degree of renal tubular damage or loss of urine-concentrating ability. It is common for severely affected patients to have daily fluid needs that exceed their calculated maintenance values during this healing period.[86]

Proteinuric Nephropathies

Glomerular diseases that have progressed in duration or severity to cause hypoalbuminemia are recognized in companion animals. Some patients with severe proteinuria will have clinical and clinicopathologic features of nephrotic syndrome. By definition, nephrotic syndrome implies glomerular protein loss sufficient to cause hypoalbuminemia, in addition to edema (or ascites) and hypercholesterolemia. Although it is postulated that patients with nephrotic syndrome have more severe glomerular lesions and a less favorable prognosis than patients that do not fulfill these criteria, this is not the case for dogs.

When choosing fluid therapy, the clinician must consider both the need for diuresis and the effects of further dilution of serum albumin concentrations by aggressive administration of crystalloids in addition to effects on blood pressure.[87] The patient may already have edema, ascites, or pleural effusion resulting in part from the hypoalbuminemia. Further dilution of plasma albumin concentrations with intravenous fluids may unmask or exacerbate fluid retention. Uncommonly, cavitary effusions will be of sufficient severity to require removal by paracentesis. Judicious administration of a loop diuretic can be used at this time; the diuretic causes fluid loss from the vascular compartment that is ideally replaced by fluid from the third space. If too much fluid is removed from the vascular compartment, renal hypoxia and damage may result.[87] Removal of cavitary effusions is generally discouraged. Such withdrawal, especially if repeated, will further lower the body albumin concentration and make fluid reaccumulation more likely.

If the patient's cardiovascular status is rapidly deteriorating because of severe hypoalbuminemia or if it is necessary to perform a procedure (especially one requiring anesthesia) in a patient with marginal cardiovascular status, a synthetic colloid (e.g., hetastarch, dextrans) can ge given. Alternatively, plasma may be administered. However, synthetic colloids are more effective in maintaining osmotic pressure in the vascular space. Moreover, the amount of plasma required to replace the deficit in albumin is relatively large, and the ability of administered albumin to maintain vascular expansion is usually gone within 24 to 72 hours (as it is with artificial colloids). Plasma is indicated only for patients with clinically significant coagulopathies that require invasive procedures. Many patients with glomerular disease are hypertensive, and blood pressure must be monitored carefully lest fluid therapy cause worsening of the hypertension with subsequent retinal or central nervous system injury.

Cardiac Disease

Most animals with cardiac failure do not need parenteral fluid therapy. Animals that are eating and drinking can usually be managed by offering distilled water and using diuretics as needed. However, if the patient is severely dehydrated, is anorexic, or has concurrent renal failure or other organ failure, fluid therapy may be needed. Treatment of such animals in severe cardiac failure is similar to the treatment of those with oliguric renal failure; the clinician must be careful not to overhydrate the patient. Measurement of CVP is useful; however, pulmonary artery catheters (i.e., Swan–Ganz) provide information (e.g., pulmonary wedge pressure) that is not available from CVP catheters. It is important to note that pulmonary artery catheters are most useful for monitoring cardiovascular status but not fluid balance in critically ill patients. Fluid administration is controversial with many cardiac diseases. Because of their lower sodium content, hypotonic solutions may be more appropriate when fluids are deemed necessary because patients with heart disease are often unable to appropriately excrete sodium. However, it is not the sodium concentration of the fluid, per se, but the volume of fluid that contributes to this situation. Similarly, sodium bicarbonate administration is often discouraged because of the relatively high sodium load.[88]

Electrolyte abnormalities in patients with cardiac disease must be treated carefully. Oral potassium supplementation is best for hypokalemic animals that are not vomiting. Hypokalemic patients are more prone to digitalis toxicity and supraventricular arrhythmias.[8] Marked repeatable hyponatremia is usually an indication that cardiac disease is advanced. Cautious sodium administration is appropriate only for patients with severe, symptomatic hyponatremia (rare). Even then, only enough sodium to alleviate or prevent central nervous system signs should be administered.

Patients with simultaneous cardiac and renal failure are among the most difficult to manage. The clinician must identify the cause of the renal and cardiac diseases and treat each. If the underlying causes cannot be determined or treated, it is best to monitor CVP and "ins and outs" while giving small amounts of fluids with minimal amounts of sodium.[88] In general, fluids are administered as rapidly as possible without excessively increasing the CVP (e.g., >10 to 12 cm H_2O).

Gastrointestinal Disorders

Acute Vomiting

Acute vomiting commonly causes fluid deficits.[89] The severity of the deficit will depend on the severity and cause of the vomiting and on whether the animal will eat or drink. Although vomiting is considered an alimentary tract disorder, vomiting is often caused by extragastrointestinal disorders (e.g., renal failure, adrenal failure, hepatic failure, hypercalcemia, pancreatitis, diabetic ketoacidosis). The therapy for most animals with moderate to severe acute vomiting includes not being fed or watered until the vomiting diminishes, which means that the patient has ongoing losses (both insensible and from vomiting) and no intake. Therefore, even if such an animal is not dehydrated at the time of examination, it will usually become so shortly.

If mild dehydration is present or anticipated, subcutaneous fluids are often adequate. If the dehydration is or will probably become severe or if the animal appears to be going into shock, intravenous fluids are indicated. Until the electrolyte and acid–base status are known, 0.9% saline, Normosol-R, or LRS are generally acceptable choices. Although hypokalemia is common in animals with acute vomiting, supplemental potassium should not be administered until it is known that the patient is not hyperkalemic as a result of adrenal or renal dysfunction. One of the most common causes of severe vomiting in young animals is parvoviral enteritis, which will be discussed later with acute diarrhea.

Chronic Vomiting

Most patients with chronic vomiting (i.e., that lasting 2 weeks or longer) are not overtly dehydrated when presented to the veterinarian. The fact that the animals have had the disease for so long usually means they were able to compensate for their fluid losses. If unable to compensate, they typically would have been been brought in earlier as emergencies (e.g., in hypovolemic shock). Some of these patients will be dehydrated because of a recent worsening of their disease. Even when the animal's fluid status is acceptable, however, there may be significant electrolyte and acid–base abnormalities.

Fluid therapy must be tailored for each individual. Hypokalemia is common if the patient does not have adrenal insufficiency or severe renal failure, both of which can cause chronic vomiting. It is not possible to predict with accuracy what a given patient's acid–base status is, even when the cause of the vomiting is known. Animals with high intestinal obstruction occasionally have a hypokalemic, hypochloremic, metabolic alkalosis that is thought to reflect gastric outflow obstruction, whereas some animals with seemingly pure gastric fluid losses can have a normal pH or are acidemic. If therapy must begin before the electrolyte and acid–base status are known (i.e., the patient is severely dehydrated), then balanced isotonic solutions (e.g., Normosol-R, PSS, LRS) are usually acceptable.

Potassium supplementation is not recommended until a potassium deficit is confirmed. If renal failure and hypoadrenocorticism have been eliminated and hypokalemia is present, it is appropriate and generally safe to add 14 to 20 mEq/L of potassium chloride to crystalloid solutions and administer it at a maintenance rate.[8]

Acute Diarrhea

Many animals with acute diarrhea are not dehydrated unless the diarrhea is profuse, vomiting is present, or the patient is anorexic. Acute parvoviral enteritis is an important cause of acute diarrhea, vomiting, and anorexia. In severe cases intravenous fluid therapy is indicated regardless of the cause.[89] Treatment initially should correct hypovolemia and hydration deficits. Subsequently, when the serum potassium is determined, 20 mEq/L of potassium chloride may be added to isotonic crystalloids. If hyperkalemia is marked, up to 40 mEq/L may be added to intravenous fluids. With parvoviral enteritis, the clinician must also be concerned with hypoglycemia (discussed later), which may result from sepsis or diminished capacity for glycogenolysis and gluconeogenesis in a sick puppy.[90]

Chronic Diarrhea

Most patients that are brought to the veterinarian because of chronic diarrhea are not overtly dehydrated. The fact that the animals have had diarrhea for so long and are just now being examined suggests that they are able to compensate for their fluid losses. If they had been unable to maintain hydration during the previous 2 or more weeks, they probably would have been brought in earlier in hypovolemic crisis. A recent worsening of the disease may cause dehydration, in which case it is reasonable to start fluids (usually a balanced isotonic crystalloid supplemented with 20 mEq/L potassium chloride). Hypokalemia is the most common electrolyte problem in these patients, but acute renal failure and hypoadrenocorticism, two of the most common causes of noniatrogenic hyperkalemia, occasionally cause disease characterized predominantly by diarrhea. The acid–base status cannot be predicted, and the clinician should not administer alkalinizing or acidifying solutions until at least the TCO_2 (and ideally the blood pH) is known.

Another major concern for animals (especially dogs) with chronic diarrhea is hypoalbuminemia. Protein-losing enteropathies may produce serum albumin concentrations of less than 1.5 g/dL. Not all such dogs have ascites or edema.[89] The clinician should avoid excessively diluting the remaining albumin in severely hypoalbuminemic patients because it can cause further pooling of fluid in third spaces and depletion of effective circulating volume. If the animal needs increased oncotic pressure, synthetic or natural colloids may be administered. However, albumin that has been administered intravenously can be lost rapidly into the intestines of animals with protein-losing enteropathies. Synthetic colloids (e.g., hetastarch) are typically more effective for management of these patients, unless they are simultaneously coagulopathic.

Pancreatic Disease

Acute Pancreatitis

Acute pancreatitis is a potentially fatal disease that usually has no specific therapy, although cats can have pancreatitis caused by bacterial, viral, or protozoal infections. Affected dogs usually are anorexic and yet vomit gastrointestinal secretions, leading to severe dehydration. The primary therapies available are fluid therapy (to enhance pancreatic perfusion) and initially withholding oral intake in patients that are vomiting.[89] If an inflamed pancreas is poorly perfused, the inflammatory state may progress from a relatively mild, edematous one to a severe hemorrhage or necrotic condition with a poorer prognosis.

The most common mistakes in treating dogs with pancreatitis are thought to be premature oral feeding and inadequate administration of fluids.[91] The former concern is now being debated. Not only must the fluid deficit be replaced, but a normal effective circulating volume also must be attained so that visceral perfusion is improved. Severe abdominal inflammation may cause fluid to pool in the abdomen or peripancreatic tissues and thus be unavailable for organ perfusion. Furthermore, there may be pooling of fluid in the intestines because of poor motility and serosal peritoneal inflammation.

It is important to monitor the serum albumin concentration. If the albumin concentration drops and the patient is judged to be inadequately perfused, plasma or hetastarch may be useful.[92] Although contentious, there is some thought that administration of plasma may replenish circulating proteases, thus offering some protection against enzymes released from the diseased pancreas,[89] as well as supply antithrombin, which may be helpful in treating disseminated intravascular coagulation.

Diabetic Ketoacidosis

Animals with diabetic ketoacidosis are often, but not invariably, severely dehydrated and acidotic when first examined. Fluid administration and judicious use of insulin generally produce favorable outcomes if the patient does not have severe pancreatitis or other severe concurrent illness.[41] Most dogs and cats with severe diabetic ketoacidosis are treated initially with fluids until dehydration and electrolyte/acid–base abnormalities are at least partially corrected before beginning therapy with insulin, but this is not a universally accepted tenet of therapy. A balanced isotonic replacement solution is used. It is generally not necessary to administer $NaHCO_3$ to these patients, and clinicians are discouraged from its use unless it is determined that a profound metabolic acidosis exists after fluid deficits have been replaced. Many ketoacidotic patients will become hypokalemic once therapy is begun; therefore it is reasonable to start supplementing potassium with the initial fluids once it is determined that the patient is not hyperkalemic.[41] Hypophosphatemia is a potential problem of aggressive insulin therapy, and serum phosphate concentrations must be monitored, especially if anemia is developing. If the patient becomes severely hypophosphatemic, the intravenous fluids should be supplemented with potassium phosphate (see previous discussion on phosphorus). The patient must be monitored to prevent hypocalcemia and hyperphosphatemia.[66] Hypomagnesemia should be anticipated in ketoacidotic diabetic patients.

Hepatic Disease

The main concerns regarding administration of fluids to a patient with hepatic disease are hypoalbuminemia, hypoglycemia, fluid and salt retention, and electrolyte abnormalities. Fluids restricted in sodium (e.g., half-strength PSS plus 2.5% or 5% dextrose) should be used to help avoid fluid retention in dogs with chronic hepatic disease prone to ascites (e.g., cirrhosis). Addition of glucose to the fluids (i.e., 2.5% to 5%) guards against hypoglycemia. If hypoalbuminemia is severe, administration of colloids in addition to crystalloids should be considered. Large volumes of plasma often are required to significantly increase plasma albumin concentrations, and hypoalbuminemia is not necessarily an indication for plasma administration. Plasma is primarily administered to patients that are coagulopathic. The administration of human albumin may effectively increase serum albumin, but its use is controversial because some patients have died after using it. Hypokalemia predisposes the patient to hepatic encephalopathy; supplemental potassium chloride in the intravenous fluids prevents this occurrence. Acid–base abnormalities are difficult to predict and must be assessed in each patient. In general, the clinician should prevent alkalemia because it predisposes the patient to hepatic encephalopathy.[93]

Hypoglycemia

Hypoglycemia may be caused by various diseases (e.g., septicemia, hypoadrenocorticism, hepatic insufficiency, insulinoma, starvation of a neonate, iatrogenic overdose of insulin). Regardless of its cause, symptomatic hypoglycemia that is causing weakness, coma, or convulsion should be treated.[94] For emergencies 1 mL/kg of 50% dextrose/kg is drawn up, diluted 1:1 with PSS, and administered intravenously, slowly to effect. For a more prolonged effect, dextrose may be added to maintenance fluids. In most cases 2.5% dextrose given at maintenance rates will maintain the blood glucose concentration in a safe range (i.e., >80 mg/dL). In rare cases it may be necessary to administer 5% instead of 2.5% dextrose to achieve this goal.

Hypocalcemia

Symptomatic hypocalcemia is usually caused by puerperal tetany, hypoparathyroidism, resection of parathyroid tumors, ethylene glycol intoxication, or inappropriate administration of a hypertonic phosphate enema. Regardless of its cause, hypocalcemia causing clinical signs (i.e., tetany, convulsions) should be treated.[95] While calcium gluconate 10% and calcium chloride 10% may be obtained, calcium chloride is thought to be more potent (10% calcium gluconate has 0.46 mEq Ca/mL, whereas 10% calcium chloride has 1.36 mEq Ca/mL); therefore there is potential for overdosage and cardiotoxicity may, in addition to the phlebitis and perivascular tissue injury observed if extravastion occurs. Similar tissue injury is observed if calcium chloride is given by the subcutaneous route. Calcium gluconate is therefore selected over calcium chloride for treating hypocalcemia, except in extremely rare circumstances (i.e., hepatic disease impairing metabolism of gluconate). Approximately 0.5 to 1.5 mL of 10% calcium gluconate is administered per kilogram, or 5 to 15 mg/kg may be administered slowly to effect over 10 to 30 minutes. Such a treatment usually lasts a few hours, although some animals will need additional therapy within 1 to 3 hours. Once the crisis is over, calcium may be added to the intravenous fluids to provide constant infusion. In general, 10 mL of 10% calcium gluconate is added to 500 mL of 0.9% NaCl and administered at maintenance rates. Then the serum calcium level and clinical signs are monitored, and the amount of calcium in the intravenous fluids is increased if necessary. Alternatively, the clinician may administer 1 to 2 mL calcium gluconate/kg (diluted 1:1 in sterile PSS) subcutaneously.[96]

Hypercalcemia

Symptomatic hypercalcemia in dogs is usually due to hypercalcemia of malignancy, vitamin D intoxication, primary hyperparathyroidism, hypoadrenocorticism, granulomatous disease, or chronic renal disease causing tertiary hyperparathyroidism.[97] In the first two conditions, it is important to rapidly decrease the plasma concentration of calcium to prevent renal injury. This is ultimately best accomplished by elimination of the cause (e.g., removing or treating the malignancy causing hypercalcemia of malignancy, removing the parathyroid adenoma). While searching for the cause, however, the clinician may administer 0.9% NaCl to promote diuresis and enhance urinary calcium excretion. However, potassium concentrations must be monitored to prevent hypokalemia.[98] Furosemide promotes natriuresis and calciuresis if the patient is adequately hydrated. Administration of 1 mg prednisolone/kg daily may enhance calcium excretion and reduce bone resorption as well as intestinal calcium absorption. However, steroid administration may make it more difficult to diagnose the cause of the hypercalcemia if it is due to a lymphoid malignancy. Severe cases may be treated with salmon calcitonin, pamidronate, or clodronate. Saline diuresis and furosemide are successful in controlling hypercalcemia in the short term in most patients. Prognosis depends on the underlying disease.

SURGERY

Dehydration should be corrected before surgery and anesthesia, if possible. Even after deficits have been corrected, animals undergoing prolonged general anesthesia usually benefit from intravenous fluid support. Unless the patient has cardiac disease or is hypoproteinemic or anemic, isotonic crystalloids (e.g., PSS, LRS) are usually administered at 4 to 5 mL/kg per hour. Severe hypoproteinemia or anemia should be corrected with blood products or synthetic colloids before the patient is anesthetized.

If the clinician anticipates significant loss of blood during the procedure, he or she may need to increase the basal rate by 5 to 10 mL/kg per hour. If there is substantial blood loss or the hematocrit falls to less than 20% to 25% during the procedure, strong consideration should be given to administering red blood cells (either as packed red cells or whole blood) or administering purified hemoglobin. If one is attempting to correct for blood loss during the procedure with crystalloids, approximately three times the estimated volume of blood lost should be given.

REFERENCES

1. Rose BD, Post TW: Regulation of water and electrolyte balance. *Clinical physiology of acid-base and electrolyte disorders*, ed 5, New York, 2001, McGraw-Hill, p 239.
2. Edelman IB, Leibman J: Review: anatomy of body water and electrolytes, *Am J Med* 27:256, 1959.
3. Hardy RM, Osborne CA: Water deprivation test in the dog: maximal normal values, *J Am Vet Med Assoc* 174:479, 1979.
4. Guyton AC: Partition of the body fluids: osmotic equilibria between extracellular and intracellular fluids. In *Textbook of medical physiology*, ed 11, Philadelphia, 2006, Saunders, p 286.
5. Rose BD, Post TW: Regulation of plasma osmolality. In *Clinical physiology of acid-base and electrolyte disorders*, ed 5, New York, 2001, McGraw-Hill, p 285.
6. Sterns RH, Spital A: Disorders of water balance. In Kokko JP, Tannen RL, editors: *Fluids and electrolytes*, ed 2, Philadelphia, 1990, Saunders, p 139.
7. DiBartola SP: Disorders of sodium and water: hypernatremia and hyponatremia. In DiBartola SP, editor: *Fluid, electrolyte, and acid-base disorders in small animal practice*, ed 3, St Louis, 2006, Saunders, pp 47–79.
8. DiBartola SP: Autran de Morais HS: Disorders of potassium: hypokalemia and hyperkalemia. In DiBartola SP, editor: *Fluid, electrolyte, and acid-base disorders in small animal practice*, ed 3, St Louis, 2006, Saunders, pp 91–121.
9. Rose BD, Post TW: Potassium homeostasis. In *Clinical physiology of acid-base and electrolyte disorders*, ed 5, New York, 2001, McGraw-Hill, p 372.
10. Willard MD: Disorders of potassium homeostasis, *Vet Clin North Am* 19:241, 1989.
11. DiBartola SP: Introduction to acid-base disorders. In DiBartola SP, editor: *Fluid, electrolyte, and acid-base disorders*, ed 3, St Louis, 2006, Saunders, p 229.
12. Rose BD, Post TW: Acid-base physiology. In *Clinical physiology of acid-base and electrolyte disorders*, ed 5, New York, 2001, McGraw-Hill, p 299.
13. Autran de Morais HS: Strong ion approach to acid base disorders. In DiBartola SP, editor: *Fluid electrolyte and acid base disorders in small animal practice*, Philadelphia, 2006, Saunders, p 311.
14. Rose BD, Post TW: Regulation of acid-base balance. *Clinical physiology of acid-base and electrolyte disorders*, ed 5, New York, 2001, McGraw-Hill, p 325.
15. Rose BD, Post TW: Introduction to simple and mixed acid-base disorders. In *Clinical physiology of acid-base and electrolyte disorders*, ed 5, New York, 2001, McGraw-Hill, p 535.
16. Rose BD, Post TW: Metabolic alkalosis. In *Clinical physiology of acid-base and electrolyte disorders*, ed 5, New York, 2001, McGraw-Hill, p 551.
17. Rossi NF, Schrier RW: Hyponatremic states. In Maxwell MH, Kleeman CR, editors, et al: *Clinical disorders of fluid and electrolyte metabolism*, ed 4, New York, 1987, McGraw-Hill, p 461.
18. Hardy RM: Hypernatremia, *Vet Clin North Am* 19:231, 1989.
19. DiBartola SP: Disorders of sodium and water. In DiBartola SP, editor: *Fluid electrolyte and acid base disorders in small animal practice*, Philadelphia, 2006, Saunders, p 53.
20. DiBartola SP: Metabolic acid base disorders. In DiBartola SP, editor: *Fluid electrolyte and acid base disorders in small animal practice*, Philadelphia, 2006, Saunders, p 269.
21. DiBartola SP, Green RA, Autran de Morais HS, et al: Electrolytes and acid-base. In Willard MD, Tvedten H, editors, et al: *Small animal clinical diagnosis by laboratory methods*, ed 4, Philadelphia, 2004, Saunders, p 117.
22. Bellevue R, Dosik H, Spergel G, et al: Pseudohyperkalemia and extreme leukocytosis, *J Lab Clin Med* 85:660, 1975.
23. Reimann KA, Knowlen GG, Tvedten HW: Factitious hyperkalemia in dogs with thrombocytosis, *J Vet Intern Med* 3:47, 1989.
24. Degen M: Pseudohyperkalemia in Akitas, *J Am Vet Med Assoc* 190:541, 1987.
25. Willard MD, Fossum TW, Torrance A, et al: Hyponatremia and hyperkalemia associated with idiopathic or experimentally induced chylothorax in four dogs, *J Am Vet Med Assoc* 199:353, 1991.
26. Bissett SA, Lamb M, Ward CR: Hyponatremia and hyperkalemia associated with peritoneal effusion in four cats, *J Am Vet Med Assoc* 218:1590, 2001.
27. Graves TK, Schall WD, Refsal K, et al: Basal and ACTH-stimulated plasma aldosterone concentrations are normal or increased in dogs with *Trichuris*-associated pseudohypoadrenocorticism, *J Vet Intern Med* 8:287, 1994.
28. Lennon EM, Boyle TE, Hutchins RG: Use of basal serum or plasma cortisol concentrations to rule out a diagnosis of hypoadrenocorticoism in dogs: 123 cases (2000–2005), *J Am Vet Med Assoc* 231:413–416, 2007.
29. Dow SW, Fettman MJ, LeCouteur RA, et al: Potassium depletion in cats: renal and dietary influences, *J Am Vet Med Assoc* 191:1569, 1987.
30. Dow SW, LeCouteur RA, Fettman MJ, et al: Potassium depletion in cats: hypokalemic polymyopathy, *J Am Vet Med Assoc* 191:1563, 1987.
31. Justin RB, Hohenhaus AE: Hypophosphatemia associated with enteral alimentation in cats, *J Vet Intern Med* 9:228, 1995.
32. Adams LG, Hardy RM, Weiss DJ, et al: Hypophosphatemia and hemolytic anemia associated with diabetes mellitus and hepatic lipidosis in cats, *J Vet Intern Med* 7:266, 1993.
33. Harkin KR, Braselton WE, Tvedten H: Pseudohypophosphatemia in two dogs with immune-mediated hemolytic anemia, *J Vet Int Med* 12:178, 1998.
34. Khanna C, Lund EM, Raffe M, et al: Hypomagnesemia in 188 dogs: a hospital population-based prevalence study, *J Vet Int Med* 12:304, 1998.
35. Kimmel SE, Waddell LS, Michel KE: Hypomagnesemia and hypocalcemia associated with protein-losing enteropathy in Yorkshire terriers: five cases (1992-1998), *J Am Vet Med Assoc* 217:703, 2000.
36. Brautbar N, Massry SG: Hypomagnesemia and hypermagnesemia. In Maxwell MH, Kleeman CR, et al: *Clinical disorders of fluid and electrolyte metabolism*, ed 4, New York, 1987, McGraw-Hill, p 831.
37. Toll J, Erb H, Birnbaum N, et al: Prevalence and incidence of serum magnesium abnormalities in hospitalized cats, *J Vet Int Med* 16:217, 2002.
38. Autran de Morais HS: Mixed acid-base disorders. In DiBartola SP, editor: *Fluid electrolyte and acid base disorders in small animal practice*, ed 3, Philadelphia, 2000, Saunders, p 298.
39. Hindman BJ: Sodium bicarbonate in the treatment of subtypes of acute lactic acidosis: physiologic considerations, *Anesthesiology* 72:1064, 1990.
40. Rose BD, Post TW: Metabolic acidosis. In *Clinical physiology of acid-base and electrolyte disorders*, ed 5, New York, 2001, McGraw-Hill, p 578.
41. Nelson RW: Diabetes mellitus. In Ettinger SJ, Feldman EC, editors: *Textbook of veterinary internal medicine*, ed 7, St Louis, 2010, Saunders, pp 1782–1796.

42. Clay KL, Murphy RC: On the metabolic acidosis of ethylene glycol intoxication, *Toxicol Appl Pharmacol* 39:39, 1977.
43. Grauer GF, Thrall MA, Henre BA, et al: Early clinicopathologic findings in dogs ingesting ethylene glycol, *Am J Vet Res* 45:2299, 1984.
44. Rose BD, Post TW: Respiratory alkalosis. In *Clinical physiology of acid-base and electrolyte disorders*, ed 5, New York, 2001, McGraw-Hill, p 673.
45. Johnson RA: Autran de Morais H: Respiratory acid base disorders. In DiBartola SP, editor: *Fluid, electrolyte, and acid-base disorders*, ed 3, St Louis, 2006, Saunders, p 293.
46. Rose BD, Post TW: *Respiratory acidosis, Clinical physiology of acid-base and electrolyte disorders*, ed 5, New York, 2001, McGraw-Hill, p 647.
47. Shiroshita Y, Tanaka R, Shibazaki A, et al: Accuracy of a portable blood gas analyzer incorporating optodes for canine blood, *J Vet Int Med* 13:597, 1999.
48. Muir WW, DiBartola SP: Fluid therapy. In Kirk RW, editor: *Current veterinary therapy VIII*, Philadelphia, 1983, Saunders, p 28.
49. Bell FW, Osborne CA: Maintenance fluid therapy. In Kirk RW, editor: *Current veterinary therapy X*, Philadelphia, 1992, Saunders, p 37.
50. Rivers JPW, Burger LH: Allometry in dog nutrition. In *Nutrition of the dog and cat*, Waltham Symposium No. 7, Cambridge, 1989, Cambridge University Press, p 67.
51. DiBartola SP, Bateman S: Introduction to fluid therapy. In DiBartola SP, editor: *Fluid, electrolyte, and acid-base disorders*, ed 3, St Louis, 2006, Saunders.
52. Ryan CP: Toxicity associated with lactated Ringer's solution containing preservatives, *Fel Pract* 12:7, 1982.
53. Day TK, Bateman S: Shock syndromes. In DiBartola SP, editor: *Fluid, electrolyte, and acid-base disorders in small animal practice*, ed 3, St Louis, 2006, Saunders, pp 540–564.
54. Francis A, et al: Adverse reactions suggestive of type III hypersensitivity in six healthy dogs given human albumin, *J Am Vet Med Assoc* 239:873–879, 2007.
55. Hansen BD: Technical aspects of fluid therapy. In DiBartola SP, editor: *Fluid, electrolyte, and acid-base disorders in small animal practice*, ed 3, St. Louis, 2006, Saunders, pp 344–376.
56. Otto CM, Crowe DT: Intraosseous resuscitation techniques and applications. In Kirk RW, Bonagura JD, editors: *Current veterinary therapy XI*, Philadelphia, 1992, Saunders, p 107.
57. Fiser DH: Intraosseous infusion, *N Engl J Med* 322:1579, 1990.
58. Okrasinski EB, Krahwinkel DJ, Sanders WL: Treatment of dogs in hemorrhagic shock by intraosseous infusion of hypertonic saline and dextran, *Vet Surg* 21:20, 1992.
59. O'Brien DP, Kroll RA, Johnson GC, et al: Myelinolysis after correction of hyponatremia in two dogs, *J Vet Int Med* 8:40, 1994.
60. Brady CA, Vite CH, Drobatz KJ: Severe neurologic sequelae in a dog after treatment of hypoadrenal crisis, *J Am Vet Med Assoc* 215:222, 1999.
61. Rose BD, Post TW: Hyperosmolal states: hypernatremia. In *Clinical physiology of acid-base and electrolyte disorders*, ed 5, New York, 2001, McGraw-Hill, p 746.
62. Fournier G, Pfaff-Poulard C, Methani K: Rapid correction of hypokalaemia via the oral route, *Lancet* 2:163, 1987.
63. Dow SW, Fettman MJ, Curtis CR, et al: Hypokalemia in cats: 186 cases (1984-1987), *J Am Vet Med Assoc* 194:1604, 1989.
64. Whang R: Refractory potassium repletion: a consequence of magnesium deficiency, *Arch Intern Med* :152, 1992.
65. Bateman S: Disorders of magnesium. In DiBartola SP, editor: *Fluid, electrolyte, and acid-base disorders*, ed 3, St Louis, 2006, Saunders, p 217.
66. Willard MD, Zerbe CA, Schall WD, et al: Severe hypophosphatemia associated with diabetes mellitus, *J Am Vet Med Assoc* 190:1007, 1987.
67. Dhupa N: Magnesium therapy. In Kirk RW, Bonagura JD, editors: *Current veterinary therapy XII*, Philadelphia, 1995, Saunders, p 132.
68. Narins RG, Cohen JJ: Bicarbonate therapy for organic acidosis: the case for its continued use, *Ann Intern Med* 106:615, 1987.
69. Stacpoole PW: Lactic acidosis, *Ann Intern Med* 105:276, 1986.
70. Hartsfield SM: Sodium bicarbonate and bicarbonate precursors for treatment of metabolic acidosis, *J Am Vet Med Assoc* 179:914, 1981.
71. Brady CA, Otto CM: Systemic inflammatory response syndrome, sepsis, and multiple organ dysfunction, *Vet Clin N Am* 31:1147, 2001.
73. Schertel ER, Tobias TA: Hypertonic fluid therapy. In DiBartola SP, editor: *Fluid therapy in small animal practice*, ed 2, Philadelphia, 2000, Saunders, p 496.
74. Rudolff E, Kirby R: Colloid fluid therapy. In Bonagura JD, Twedt DC, editors: *Kirk's Current veterinary therapy XIV*, St Louis, 2009, Sanders, pp 61–67.
75. Allen DA, Schertel ER, Muir WW, et al: Hypertonic saline/dextran resuscitation of dogs with experimentally induced gastric dilatation-volvulus shock, *Am J Vet Res* 52:92, 1991.
76. Ware WA: Myocardial diseases of the dog. In Nelson RW, Couto CG, editors: *Small animal internal medicine*, ed 3, St Louis, 2003, Mosby, p 106.
77. Haskins SC: Management of septic shock, *J Am Vet Med Assoc* 200:1915, 1992.
78. Jafari HS, McCracken GH: Sepsis and septic shock: a review for clinicians, *Pediatr Infect Dis J* 11(9):739, 1992.
79. Weeren FR, Muir WW: Clinical aspects of septic shock and comprehensive approaches to treatment in dogs and cats, *J Am Vet Med Assoc* 200:1859, 1992.
80. Bone RC: Toward an epidemiology and natural history of SIRS (systemic inflammatory response syndrome), *J Am Med Assoc* 268:3452, 1992.
81. Lefering R, Neugebauer EA: Steroid controversy in sepsis and septic shock: a meta-analysis, *Crit Care Med* 23:294, 1995.
82. Burkitt JM, Haskins SC: Relative adrenal insufficiency in dogs with sepsis, *J Vet Internal Med* 21(2):226–231, 2007.
83. Cowgill LD, Elliot DA: Acute renal failure. In Ettinger SJ, Feldman EC, editors: *Textbook of veterinary internal medicine*, ed 5, Philadelphia, 2000, Saunders, p 1615.
84. Chew DJ, Gieg JA: Fluid therapy during intrinsic renal failure. In DiBartola SP, editor: *Fluid, electrolyte, and acid-base disorders in small animal practice*, ed 3, St Louis, 2006, Saunders, pp 518–540.
85. Allen DG: Special techniques. In Allen DG, editor: *Small animal medicine*, Philadelphia, 1991, JB Lippincott, 1991, p 1035.
86. Stone EA, Barsanti JA: *Urologic surgery of the dog and cat*, Philadelphia, 1992, Lea & Febiger, p 119.
87. Polzin D, Osborne CA, O'Brien T: Diseases of the kidneys and ureters. In Ettinger SJ, editor: *Textbook of veterinary internal medicine*, ed 3, Philadelphia, 1989, Saunders, p 1962.
88. Bonagura JD, Lehmkuhl LB, Autran de Morais H: Fluid and diuretic therapy in heart failure. In DiBartola SP, editor: *Fluid, electrolyte, and acid-base disorders in small animal practice*, ed 3, St Louis, 2006, Saunders, pp 490–518.
89. Simpson KW, Birnbaum N: Fluid and electrolyte disturbances in gastrointestinal and pancreatic disease. In DiBartola, editor: *Fluid electrolyte and acid-base disorders*, ed 3, St Louis, 2006, Saunders, p 429.
90. Heald RD, Jones BD, Schmidt DA: Blood gas and electrolyte concentrations in canine parvoviral enteritis, *J Am Anim Hosp Assoc* 22:745, 1986.
91. Williams DA: Exocrine pancreatic disease. In Ettinger SJ, Feldman EC, editors: *Textbook of veterinary internal medicine*, ed 5, Philadelphia, 2000, Saunders, p 1345.
92. Logan JC, Callan MB, Drew K, et al: Clinical indications for use of fresh frozen plasma in dogs: 74 dogs (October through December 1999), *J Am Vet Med Assoc* 218:1449, 2001.

93. Schenker S, Breen KJ, Hoyumpa AM: Hepatic encephalopathy: current status, *Gastroenterology* 66:121, 1974.
94. Feldman EC, Nelson RW: Beta-cell neoplasia: Insulinoma. In *Canine and feline endocrinology and reproduction*, ed 3, Philadelphia, 2004, Saunders, p 613.
95. Feldman EC, Nelson RW: Hypocalcemia and primary hypoparathyroidism. In *Canine and feline endocrinology and reproduction*, ed 3, Philadelphia, 2004, Saunders, p 716.
96. Feldman EC: Disorders of the parathyroid glands. In Ettinger SJ, Feldman EC, editors: *Textbook of veterinary internal medicine*, ed 7, St Louis, 2010, Saunders, pp 1722–1751.
97. Elliott J, Dobson JM, Dunn JK, et al: Hypercalcemia in the dog: a study of 40 cases, *J Small Anim Pract* 32:564, 1991.
98. Green T, Chew DJ: Calcium disorders. In Silverstein DC, Hopper K, editors: *Small animal critical care medicine*, St Louis, 2009, Saunders, p 56.

17 Drugs Affecting Urine Formation

Dawn Merton Boothe

Chapter Outline

RENAL PHYSIOLOGY AND DRUG THERAPY

Extracellular Fluid

The physiology of body fluids and the role of the kidney are also addressed in Chapters 16 and 18 The volume of extracellular fluid (ECF) is determined primarily by total body sodium content for two reasons: First, sodium is the major constituent of ECF; secondly, active transport mechanisms control sodium in intracellular and extracellular compartments.[1] Control of ECF involves cardiovascular, renal, and central nervous systems. Because these systems are closely integrated, one system can compensate for the failure of another system, thus ensuring that salt and water excretion remain appropriate even with changes in blood pressure. Among the compensatory mechanisms is autoregulation of renal blood flow through efferent arteriolar resistance. Because regulatory mechanisms adjust both short- and long-term sodium and water transport rates, small increases in mean arterial blood pressure can cause a marked increase in sodium excretion, ultimately changing total body sodium.[1] However, a check-and-balance system exists whereby if sodium balance becomes negative, as sodium concentration in the ECF decreases, causing thirst and water intake to decrease accordingly until ECF sodium concentration normalizes. A positive balance does the opposite, resulting in an increase in water intake. These integrated systems maintain a sodium and water excretion that equals that of intake minus any lost through nonrenal mechanisms (e.g., feces, sweat).

Renal Transport of Fluids and Electrolytes

The proximal tubules are responsible for 66% of the sodium and glomerular filtrate reabsorbed by the kidney. The primary pathway of fluid and electrolyte reabsorption in the renal tubule begins in the lumen and progresses through the cell and the interstitial fluid and into the capillary. Two water-permeable cell membranes are traversed during reabsorption. In the proximal tubule, active sodium ion reabsorption from the lumen into the cell generates an osmotic gradient in the lumen that leads to an almost simultaneous movement of water into the cell. Sodium reabsorption that begins with entry across the luminal membrane continues with movement across the basolateral membrane into the interstitial space (Figure 17-1). Basolateral movement is the energy-dependent process, fueled by a Na/K-dependent ATPase located on the basolateral membrane. The exchange rate of two K^+ for each three Na^+ entering the interstitial fluid provides an electrochemical gradient that favors passive entry of Na^+ from the lumen into the cell. The concentration gradient generated by the basolateral movement determines the rate of sodium movement from the lumen. Chloride (and to a lesser degree, other anions) follows sodium, maintaining electroneutrality of the reabsorbate and

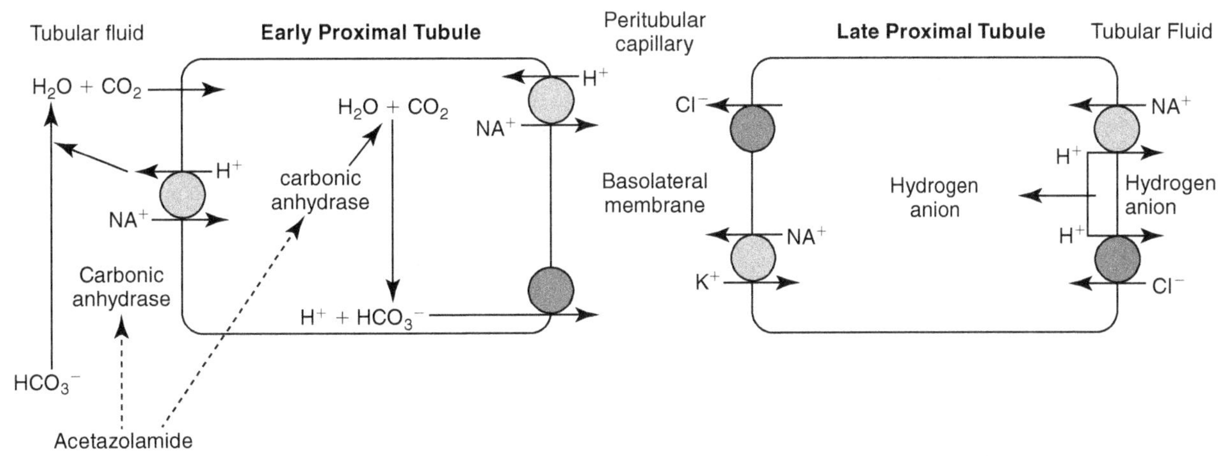

Figure 17-1 Movement of fluids and electrolytes into the proximal tubule and predominant sites of action of selected diuretics. The proximal tubule is the primary site of fluid resorption. Sodium enters the renal tubular cell by several mechanisms, including concentration-dependent passive diffusion, concentration-independent active transport, and countertransport with hydrogen. This latter mechanism yields bicarbonate and, although it occurs spontaneously, is also catalyzed by carbonic anhydrase. As sodium, chloride, and water are resorbed, the concentration of the remaining solute in the urine increases, causing an osmotic draw of fluid back into the tubule. Consequently, resorption of fluids is self-limiting to some degree. *Dashed lines* reflect inhibited actions, and *solid lines* reflect stimulation.

a slight electronegativity of the cell compared with the luminal contents. The concentration gradient also favors passive movement of potassium from the interstitium into the cell, where it is used to continue the Na-K exchange. Although movement of sodium from the lumen into the cell is passive (albeit at the cost of an active basolateral efflux), sodium reabsorption into the cell is facilitated by three additional entry mechanisms: diffusion with chloride (quantitatively the most important), co-transport with uncharged or acidic anions, and countertransport with hydrogen ions (important to acid–base regulation and the site of carbonic anhydrase action). Although transport of sodium, water, and other electrolytes raises interstitial pressure, movement into peritubular capillaries facilitates continued reabsorption. Bicarbonate processing also occurs in the proximal tubule.

Unlike the proximal tubule, cells of the descending limb of the loop of Henle do not appear to be equipped with specialized transporting systems. The cells are relatively impermeable to sodium, chloride, and potassium but are permeable to water. Water moves from the lumen into the interstitium, causing electrolyte concentrations to progressively increase in the lumen until a maximum is reached at the bend. Diuretic drugs do not appear to be active in the descending portion of the tubule. In the ascending limb of the loop, chloride is transported "uphill," achieving intracellular concentrations that are higher than predicted (based on the Nernst equation).[2] Chloride movement occurs by a Na (downhill), K^+-$2Cl^-$ (uphill) co-transport system, with Na^+, K^+-ATPase in the peritubular membrane providing the energy source. High intracellular chloride concentration facilitates chloride movement into the interstitium. The ion transports in the ascending loop of Henle are critical for proper function of the countercurrent mechanism in the renal medulla. The ascending loop of Henle tubule is not permeable to water, and fluid in the lumen becomes progressively diluted (Figure 17-2). About 25% of sodium-chloride reabsorption and 40% of potassium reabsorption occurs in the ascending loop of Henle, although only about 15% of the filtrate is reabsorbed in this region.[2] In contrast to the proximal tubules, Na^+-H^+ exchange does not appear to occur in the loop of Henle, and little if any bicarbonate is processed.

Reabsorption of water and electrolytes in the distal tubule and collecting ducts is variable. Sodium and chloride are reabsorbed against a concentration gradient. Because the early distal tubule is impermeable to water, an unfavorable concentration gradient is generated that limits the effectiveness of a sodium pump. Sodium and potassium contents in the urine are closely regulated by an aldosterone-sensitive mechanism in the distal late tubule (see Figure 17-2). Aldosterone signals the synthesis of a protein that increases the sodium and potassium permeability of the luminal membrane. As sodium moves in, potassium simultaneously moves from the interstitium into the cell. Electrogenic movement of sodium into the cell causes an electronegativity in the lumen that attracts potassium from the cell. Whether potassium is reabsorbed or excreted is determined primarily by plasma potassium, which in turn tends to depend on dietary intake.[2]

In the medullary collecting ducts, only small amounts of sodium chloride and potassium are reabsorbed. Antidiuretic hormone increases permeability of the cell membrane to water, which moves from the lumen, following the previously established medullary osmotic gradient. Less than 5% of filtered sodium is reabsorbed in the distal tubule and medullary collecting system under normal conditions.[2]

Atrial Natriuretic Hormone

Atrial natriuretic hormone (ANH), a "natriuretic factor" first described in 1984, is involved in the control of ECF. It is synthesized from a prohormone and stored as a peptide in granules in atrial myocardial cells. Concentrations increase

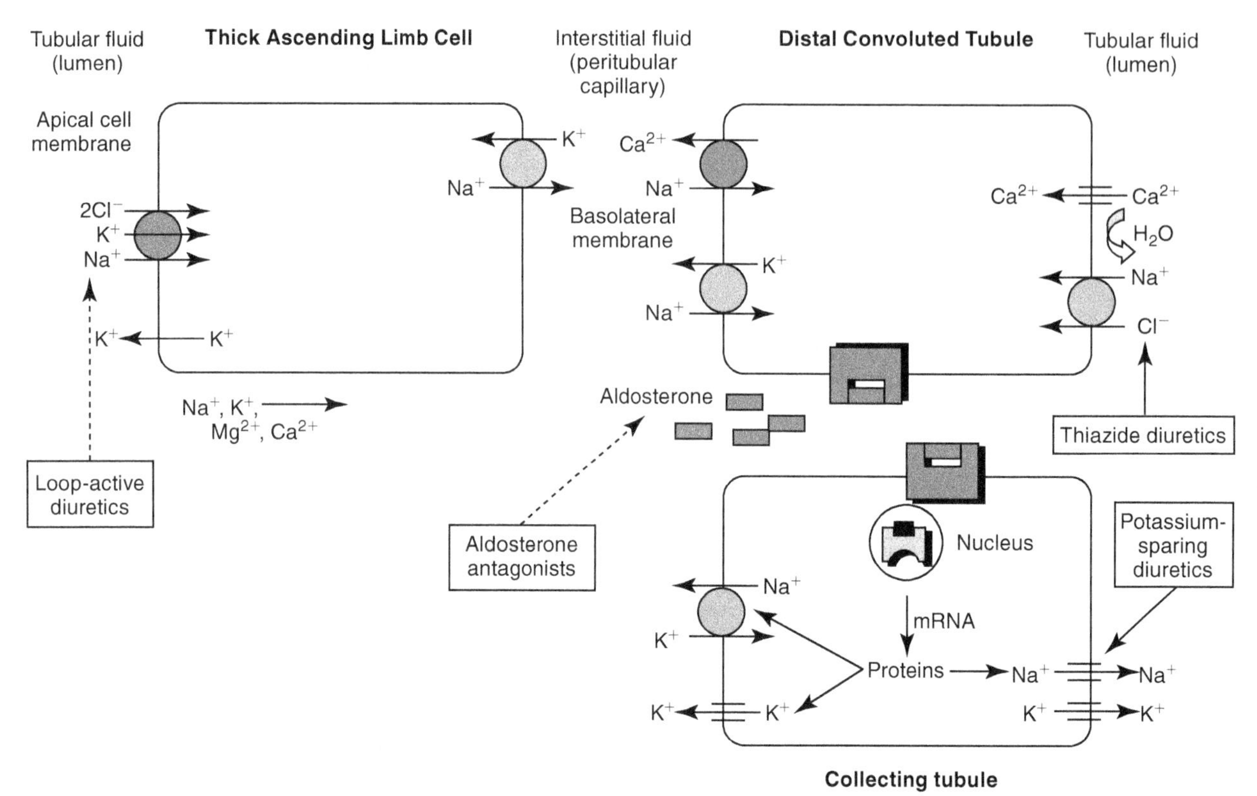

Figure 17-2 Movement of fluids and electrolytes in the thick ascending loop of Henle, the distal tubule, and the collecting ducts. Sites of action of selected diuretics also are indicated *(dashed lines* reflect inhibited actions, and *solid lines* reflect stimulation). In the ascending loop of Henle, electrolytes, but not water, are able to pass from the lumen into the cells. Up to 25% of the sodium and 40% of potassium is resorbed by way of a countertransport mechanism across a concentration gradient. In addition, chloride is actively transported into the cell. In the distal tubule, aldosterone plays a major role in fluid and electrolyte transport. Aldosterone mediates uptake of luminal sodium; sodium is exchanged for potassium, which is excreted into the lumen. Because of its location distal to most diuretics, efficacy of diurectics may be markedly decreased in high aldosterone states (e.g., congestive heart failure, liver disease). Aldosterone acts through steroid receptors. Like most steroidal compounds, the effects of aldosterone depend on nuclear transcription of effector proteins.

above baseline when either the ECF expands, blood pressure increases, or dietary salt intake increases. Renal blood flow and glomerular filtration are subsequently increased. Sodium excretion also increases, presumably by a direct tubular action. Peripheral vasodilation can result in decreased blood pressure. Effects occur rapidly but are not sustained, suggesting that ANH is a mechanism that can restore equilibrium rapidly.[2]

Reduction of ECF is beneficial in conditions associated with inappropriate fluid retention such as in certain cardiac, renal, and liver diseases. Although the cause of ECF expansion differs in each disease, the commonality is salt and water retention. Because sodium is the primary cationic constituent of ECF, sufficient renal excretion of sodium ultimately reduces ECF.

DIURETIC THERAPY

Therapeutic Use of Diuretics

Three strategies exist for movement of inappropriate fluid accumulation (edema): correction of the underlying disease (often not possible), restriction of dietary or other sodium intake, and administration of diuretics. Of these, diuretics remain the cornerstone for treatment of edema or volume overload, particularly that which is life threatening.[1] Although diuretics increase the rate of urine formation, their therapeutic indications include maintenance of urine flow; mobilization and reduction of inappropriate ECF stores, such as that manifested as edema or ascites; correction of specific ion imbalances; reduction in the rate of intraocular fluid formation; reduction of blood pressure; and reduction of pulmonary capillary wedge pressure.[2]

Targets of Diuretic Therapy

Diuretics are classified by their mechanism of action and include the loop diuretics, carbonic anhydrase inhibitors, thiazides, osmotic diuretics, and potassium-sparing diuretics (Figure 17-3, Table 17-1). Rational selection of diuretics relies on an appreciation of their mechanisms of action. With the exception of the osmotic diuretics and carbonic anhydrase inhibitors (the latter targets sodium bicarbonate), each class targets sodium or chloride reabsorption of tubular cells, effectively preventing the establishment of the normal ion gradient by renal tubular cells.[1-3] Diuretics that increase net urinary excretion of sodium chloride or sodium bicarbonate also are referred to as *natriuretic*. The efficacy and use of each class of diuretics varies with their site of action and the

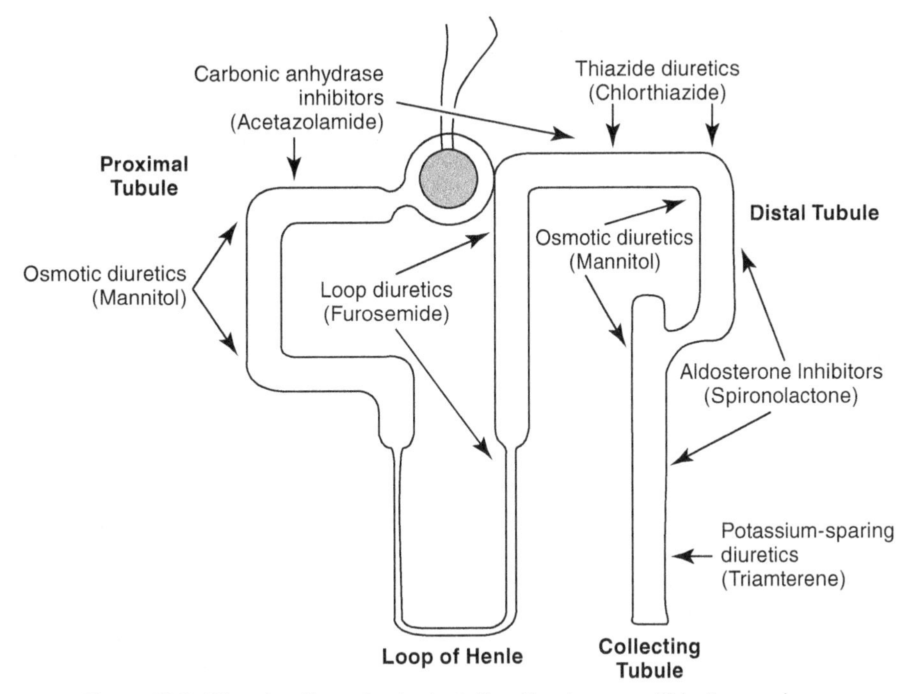

Figure 17-3 Site of action of selected diuretic classes within the nephron.

mechanism by which sodium reabsorption is inhibited. The mechanisms of sodium resorption that are targeted by diuretic therapy vary in location within the renal tubule and include electrogenic passive diffusion (proximal and late distal tubule and collecting system); exchange with hydrogen (generated by the actions of carbonic anhydrase and bicarbonate reabsorption); co-transport with glucose, organic acids, and phosphate (proximal tubule); reabsorption along with chloride reabsorption (late proximal tubule); and co-transport with chloride and potassium (by way of the thick ascending limb of the loop of Henle, which results in formation of medullary interstitial hyperosmolarity).

KEY POINT 17-1 Rational selection of a diuretic should be based on the underlying pathophysiology and the mechanism of action of the drug. Differences in patient disposition and response may require increased dosing or shorter intervals.

Principles of Diuretic Therapy Use

Several principles can guide diuretic therapy[4]: (1) The pattern of electrolyte excretion varies with the class of diuretic. (2) Maximal response to each drug class is limited by the site of action of the diuretic; as such, assuming drug delivery to the site of action has been appropriate, diuretic failure will occur to all members of the same drug class. class. (3) The combination of two (or more) diuretics with different mechanisms of action should cause additive and may cause synergistic effects.[2]

When used to reduce ECF volume, the selection of the most appropriate diuretic should be based on the cause of ECF volume retention. Diuretic selection for the patient with acute renal failure also should take into account the ability of the diuretic to reach the target tissue despite reduction in renal blood flow. The impact of the direct or indirect actions of the diuretic on systemic sequelae beyond decreased ECF volume (e.g., metabolic acidosis, hypokalemia) should be considered. Several diuretics also influence renal physiology by virtue of their effects on renal vasculature and may be preferred during states of reduced renal blood flow. Finally, several diuretics target physiologic processes that are not unique to the kidney (i.e., carbonic anhydrase inhibitors) and thus may be used therapeutically for reasons other than diuresis.

Factors Limiting Response to Diuretics

Two types of tolerance to diuretic therapy have been described in human patients. Short-term tolerance, or "braking," occurs after the first dose and probably reflects a response to protect intravascular volume. Restoration of diuretic-induced loss of volume will resolve this type of tolerance. Long-term administration of loop diuretics can cause tolerance that reflects hypertrophy of the distal nephron in response to prolonged exposure to increased solute concentration. Sodium reabsorption increases accordingly, decreasing diuresis. Because thiazides target regions of the nephron that hypertrophy, a combination of thiazides with loop-acting diuretics results in a synergistic diuretic response in some human patients.

Several other factors may negatively affect response to diuretic therapy. Most diuretics are present at physiologic pH as uncharged molecules or organic ions and reach the renal tubular cell by active tubular secretion. The degree of ionization can affect the rapidity with which drugs are transported to renal receptors. Declining renal blood flow can preclude drug delivery to the site of diuretic action. For drugs that must reach distal sites (e.g., thiazides), it may be necessary to double doses to achieve a clinical response. For each diuretic a threshold (in drug concentration) must be reached before diuresis will occur. Lack of response may reflect simply an underdose for that patient, and dose titration is indicated. With renal disease characterized by proteinuria, many diuretics will remain bound to plasma proteins present in the tubular lumen and thus will remain inactive. Administration of the diuretic with albumin appears to facilitate response to diuretics in human patients with edema associated with the nephrotic syndrome. Resistance to diuretic therapy also may reflect the presence of another drug that decreases response. For example, nonsteroidal antiinflammatory drugs (NSAIDs) can alter intrarenal prostaglandin regulatory mechanisms, and a number of drugs compete for active tubular secretion of the diuretic into the tubular lumen.

In addition to their direct tubular effects, all diuretics indirectly influence renal tubular function. Accommodation to the effects of a diuretic in a normal animal may result in the

Table 17-1 Doses of Selected Diuretic Drugs

Drug	Indication	Dose	Route	Interval (hrs)
Chlorothiazide	Diuretic	10-40 mg/kg	PO	12
	Partial antidiuretic hormone (ADH) deficiency/diabetes insipidus	20-40 mg/kg	PO	12
Chlorpropamide	Partial antidiuretic hormone (ADH) deficiency/diabetes insipidus	10-40 mg/kg (D)	PO	24
Demeclocycline	Inappropriate antidiuretic hormone (ADH) secretion	3-12 mg/kg	PO	6-12
Dopamine hydrochloride	Renal vasodilator: (acute renal failure)	2-5 μg/kg (low dose) in 5% D/W	IV CRI	
Ethacrynic acid	Diuretic, pulmonary edema	0.2-0.4 mg/kg	IM, IV	4-12
Furosemide	Diuresis with acute renal failure	5-20 mg/kg	IM, IV, PO	8-12 or as needed. Adjust to lowest dose possible
	Hypertension	1-2 mg/kg; maximum of 8 mg/kg for acute renal failure	PO	12
	Hydrocephalus, brain edema	0.5-2 mg/kg	PO	12
	Ascites from hepatic failure	1-2 mg/kg	PO, SC	12-24
	Hypercalcemia	1-2 mg/kg	IM, IV, PO, SC	8-12
		5 mg/kg	IV	As needed
		2-5 mg/kg	IV	To effect
		0.1-1 mg/kg	IV CRI	
Hydrochlororthiazide	Diuretic	2-4 mg/kg (D)	PO	24
	Antihypertensive agent	0.5-2 mg/kg	PO	12-24
	Nephrogenic diabetes insipidus	0.5-5 mg/kg	PO	12
	Hypoglycemia	2-4 mg/kg (D)	PO	12 (with diazoxide)
		2-4 mg/kg	PO	12
Mannitol 20%	Oliguric renal failure	0.25-0.5 g/kg of a 15% to 25% solution	IV (over 15-60 min)	Repeat every 4-6 hr if necessary
	Glaucoma	1-3 g/kg	IV (over 15-20 min)	Repeat every 4-8 hrs if necessary
	Central nervous system edema	1.5 g/kg	IV	Once
Spironolactone	Ascites	1-2 mg/kg (D); maximum of 4 mg/kg	PO	12
	Diuretic, heart failure	2-4 mg/kg	PO	24
		1-2 mg/kg (D)	PO	12
	Primary hyperaldosteronism, hepatic insufficiency	1 mg/kg (C)	PO	12
		12.5 mg (C)	PO	24
Spironolactone/ hydrochlorothiazide	Diuretic, antihypertensive agent	2 mg/kg	PO	12-24
Triamterene	Diuretic	1-2 mg/kg (D)	PO	12

loss of any pharmacologic effect several days after the start of diuretic therapy. Response to any diuretic will be modulated by internal homeostatic mechanisms that normally direct body fluid volumes and osmolar concentrations. For example, if a diuretic fails to cause a net sodium excretion (such as occurs with mannitol), ECF contraction will increase the concentration of electrolytes, stimulating water intake and replenishment of the lost volume.[2] Refractoriness to thiazides can develop rapidly as a result of salt-retaining mechanisms being activated. Edema (ascites) associated with liver disease may not respond to diuretic therapy because signals from the cirrhotic liver indicate a depleted rather than an exaggerated ECF.[2]

Finally, refractoriness to diuretic therapy may reflect pharmacokinetic changes. The oral bioavailability of some diuretics (e.g., furosemide) is quite variable in human patients and unpredictable in the individual patient. It may be necessary to try several doses before the most effective one is found. Some diuretics (spironolactone, amiloride) are more effective after metabolism by the liver, although this also may be species dependent. Although the elimination half-life of several diuretics is sufficiently long to allow twice-daily elimination (in human patients), several of the loop diuretics are characterized by an elimination half-life of 2 to 3 hours. For such drugs the pharmacologic effect is decreased once the drug is no longer present. Rebound reabsorption of sodium by the nephrons has been described in such cases, suggesting that constant-rate intravenous infusion may provide better response. In addition, in patients that are not responding well, small increases in diuresis in the presence of the drug potentially will be magnified to clinically significant increases if the response is continuous.

Refractoriness to diuretic therapy can be approached by cage rest (which may improve renal circulation), an increase in the dose of the diuretic, intravenous administration, the use of a more effective diuretic (such as a loop-active diuretic), or a decrease in interval such that the drug is present at the site for a longer period of time (constant infusion). For constant-rate intravenous infusion, a loading dose (full to double dose) should be given, followed by a maintenance dose given each hour. Continued refractoriness should lead to the addition of a second diuretic that works through a different yet complementary mechanism of action (e.g., thiazides with a loop-acting drug).

DIURETICS

Osmotic Diuretics

Osmotic diuretics increase the osmolality of extracellular fluid, enhancing flow of water from tissues to interstitial fluid and plasma. For a solute to act as an osmotic diuretic, it must be freely filtered at the glomerulus, not reabsorbed by the renal tubule, and be pharmacologically and metabolically inert. Mannitol (Figure 17-4) is the most commonly used osmotic diuretic; others include urea, glycerol, and isosorbide. As the concentration of an osmotic diuretic increases in the renal tubular lumen, osmotic forces overcome the movement of water with sodium into the renal tubular cell. Eventually, as water retention in the urine increases, sodium concentration decreases and passive sodium reabsorption is reduced. Sodium loss is, however, relatively small. Although mannitol appears to work throughout the renal tubule, the principal site of action appears to be the loop of Henle (see Figure 17-3).[1] Mannitol is distributed to ECF and thus extracts water

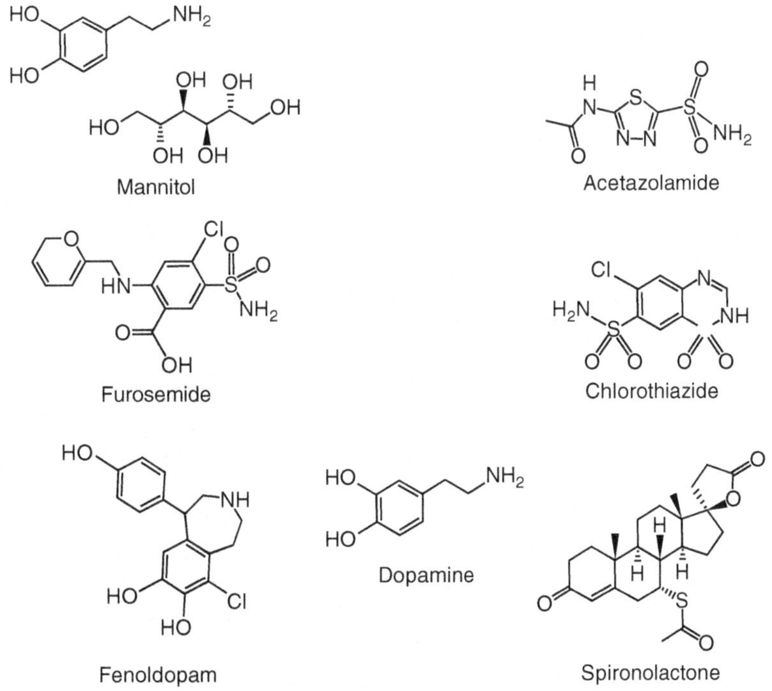

Mannitol
Acetazolamide
Furosemide
Chlorothiazide
Fenoldopam
Dopamine
Spironolactone

Figure 17-4 Chemical structures of selected diuretics.

from intracellular compartments, increasing ECF, decreasing blood viscosity, and inhibiting renin release.[1] The impact on intracellular compartments is therapeutically beneficial in patients with cerebral edema and glaucoma.[1] Renal blood flow increases, removing NaCl and urea from the renal medulla and decreasing renal medullary tonicity. Medullary tonicity also may be reduced further by a prostaglandin-mediated increase in renal medullary blood flow. Mannitol is not absorbed after oral administration. In humans it is characterized by an elimination half-life of approximately 1 hour.

KEY POINT 17-2 Osmotic diuretics will be useful for reducing intracellular edema only if they surround but do not enter the target cell.

The major adverse effect of osmotic diuretics is increased ECF, which can be detrimental in patients with pulmonary edema or cardiac failure. Hyponatremia resulting from water extraction causes headaches, nausea, and vomiting in human patients.[1] In contrast, loss of water in excess of electrolytes can cause hypernatremia and dehydration. Osmotic diuretics generally are contraindicated in anuria of severe renal disease or in patients that are not responsive to test doses. Mannitol and urea also are contraindicated for patients with active cranial bleeding. Glycerin (but not mannitol) can be metabolized, causing hyperglycemia.

Mannitol is most commonly used to treat acute renal failure resulting from an acute reduction in glomerular filtration or acute changes in renal tubular permeability. Mannitol provides protection to the tubules in that it attenuates reduction in glomerular filtration rate (GFR) associated with acute tubular nephrosis if the drug is administered before an ischemic insult.[1] Efficacy (experimentally) for treatment of nephrotoxicity, however, is documented only when administered before the toxin; clinical efficacy is even less obvious. Mannitol is particularly indicated for treatment of toxic nephrosis because the concentration of the toxin in the urine will be reduced by the osmotic draw of water by the solute. In contrast to diuretics that act on tubular segments, osmotic diuretics usually maintain their effect in the oliguric state that accompanies acute renal failure because they will continue to be filtered by the glomerulus. If the tubular cell becomes permeable, however, as may occur with certain toxins or prolonged tubular ischemia, the osmotic diuretics may lose their efficacy. Yet in patients with acute tubular nephrosis, mannitol may convert an oliguric patient to a nonoliguric state.[1]

Mannitol is distributed to ECF and thus is not effective in movement of fluids from interstitial tissues. ECF volume will initially increase and may prove detrimental to the patient with decompensated cardiac function. Plasma osmolality increases after treatment with mannitol. Cerebrospinal fluid (CSF) and aqueous humor formation subsequently decrease. Whether mannitol will cross the blood–brain barrier is unclear. However, because mannitol is distributed into interstitial fluids but does not penetrate cell membranes, intracellular edema will also be reduced. As such, mannitol is used to treat selected causes of cerebral edema associated with increased intracellular fluid volume. The use of mannitol for treatment of acute brain injury is discussed in Chapter 27. A Cochrane review failed to find conclusive evidence regarding its efficacy, although the number of eligible clinical trials for review was limited.[5] Mannitol can be used to decrease brain mass before neurosurgery. The use of mannitol to facilitate diagnosis of ureteral obstruction has been described.[6]

Carbonic Anhydrase Inhibitors

Two types of carbonic anhydrase are located in the proximal tubule, both targeted by carbonic anhydrase inhibitors: type II, located in the cytoplasm; and type IV, located in the luminal and basolateral membranes (see Figure 17-1). In the lumen, H^+ (generated from the Na^+-H^+ transporter) reacts with HCO_3^- to form H_2CO_3, which, in the presence of brush border carbonic anhydrase, rapidly decomposes to water and CO_2. The CO_2 rapidly diffuses into the tubular cell, where it reacts with water to form H_2CO_3. This reaction normally proceeds slowly but is markedly accelerated by carbonic anhydrase in the cytoplasm. Because intracellular H^+ is low (because of Na^+-H^+ co-transport), H_2CO_3 spontaneously ionizes to form H^+ and HCO_3^-. An electrochemical gradient moves $Na^+HCO_3^-$ into the interstitial space, with water following. Chloride becomes concentrated in the lumen and diffuses down its gradient into the interstitium (see Figure 17-1).[1] Carbonic anhydrase inhibitors target both the cytoplasmic and membrane-bound carbonic anhydrase, completely impairing $NaHCO_3$ reabsorption in the proximal tubule (see Figure 17-3). The collecting tubule is a secondary target. As a result, urine concentrations of bicarbonate increase, and up to 35% of the filtered load is excreted. Because hydrogen ions are not generated by the conversion of bicarbonate to CO_2 and H_2O, they are not available for exchange with sodium. Thus the amount of acid and ammonia excreted in urine also decreases. The loss of titratable acid and ammonia secretion in the collecting duct results in an increase in urinary pH to approximately 8 and the potential development of metabolic acidosis.[1] At least 65% of sodium bicarbonate is reabsorbed through carbonic anhydrase–independent mechanisms. Sodium and chloride not reabsorbed in the proximal tubule are delivered to the loop of Henle, where most of the chloride and sodium subsequently are absorbed. Up to 70% of potassium is excreted because of the increased sodium load. Bicarbonate remains in the urine, contributing to alkalinity. Ultimately, however, much of the bicarbonate that remains in the proximal tubular lumen is resorbed distally in the nephron by mechanisms that are not well understood.

Several sequelae result from the diuretic mechanism of carbonic anhydrase inhibitors. First, metabolic acidosis develops as bicarbonate is lost in the proximal tubules. Second, the filtered load of HCO_3^- decreases to the point that the uncatalyzed (spontaneous) reaction between CO_2 and water leads to HCO_3 reabsorption. This in turn decreases the response of the renal tubule to carbonic anhydrase inhibitors. Thus the diuretic effect of these drugs is self-limiting. However, in patients refractory to alternative diuretic therapy, the combination of acetazolamide with diuretics that block sodium resorption distally may result in marked naturiesis. Thus carbonic anhydrase inhibitors may be useful for combination therapy.[1] In the distal tubule, as sodium is reabsorbed, potassium excretion markedly increases. Carbonic anhydrase is located in other tissues. Aqueous humor and CSF formation are both decreased by carbonic anhydrase inhibitors. Accordingly, the major indication for their use is glaucoma. The effect in the eye is direct and is not influenced by metabolic acidosis. The effect of carbonic anhydrase inhibition in the brain is not as well understood and may result from both the direct effects and the development of metabolic acidosis. Although carbonic anhydrase also is located in the gastric mucosa, only large doses of inhibitors reduce gastric acid secretion. Carbonic anhydrase activity in red blood cells will be impaired, causing an increase in CO_2 levels in peripheral tissues and decreased levels in expired air. Carbonic anhydrase can increase delivery of solutes to the macula densa. Tubuloglomerular feedback may be triggered, increasing afferent arteriolar resistance and reducing renal blood flow and GFR.

Side effects of carbonic anhydrase inhibitors are not common. Large doses may cause drowsiness. Side effects can also result from urinary alkalinization or metabolic acidosis. Hepatic encephalopathy can be induced as renal ammonia is diverted from the urine. Precipitation of calcium phosphate may cause calculus formation. Respiratory or metabolic acidosis can be worsened. Carbonic anhydrase inhibitors are contraindicated in patients with cirrhosis or other causes of hepatic encephalopathy or conditions associated with acidosis. The impact of carbonic anhydrase inhibitors on urinary pH can reduce the rate of excretion of weak bases.[1]

Acetazolamide (Figure 17-4) is a potent, reversible inhibitor of carbonic anhydrase. Its primary indication in veterinary medicine is for the treatment of glaucoma with the intent to decrease aqueous humor formation. It is used less commonly to control CSF formation in patients with hydrocephalus or other causes of increased cerebral fluid pressure. Acetazolamide is characterized by some antiepileptic activity, although tolerance rapidly develops to this effect. Occasionally, acetazolamide might be used to alkalinize the urine. Indications might be for selected causes of crystalluria and to facilitate excretion of weakly acidic drugs, such as phenobarbital, and salicylate. Because its efficacy is self-limiting, combination with sodium bicarbonate may be indicated if persistent urinary alkalinization is desired.

Acetazolamide is orally bioavailable, with peak concentrations occurring within 2 hours after administration. The drug is eliminated by active tubular secretion with some passive reabsorption. In humans the drug is totally eliminated in 24 hours. The drug is relatively safe, although metabolic acidosis may occur (is is usually self-limiting). In patients with hepatic encephalopathy, alkaline urine may increase the amount of urinary ammonia reabsorbed because a greater proportion will be un-ionized. This may result in exacerbation of neurologic dysfunction, and this drug should not be used in patients with severe hepatic dysfunction. Acetazolamide decreases iodide uptake by the thyroid gland (perhaps similar to other sulfonamide antibiotics) and should be avoided in hypothyroid patients or patients undergoing thyroid testing. Whether the drugs can render a euthyroid patient hypothyroid is not known. Drugs that depend on urine acidity are less effective when used with acetazolamide. This includes urinary antiseptics such as methenamine, which is rarely if ever indicated in veterinary medicine; efficacy of weakly acidic antibiotics might also be impaired, whereas that of weak bases will be enhanced.

Methazolamide is among the orally administered carbonic anydrase inhibitors used to treat glaucoma in dogs. Its impact on intraocular pressure and aqueous humor flow rate was described in Beagles receiving a single dose of 25 or 50 mg (10 dogs per group; 5 control) followed by multiple twice-daily dosing for 9 days.[7] A diurnal difference in intraocular pressure was measured in all animals, being highest in the morning. At 25 and 50 mg, intraocular pressure decreased in the morning but increased in the evening compared with baseline. Compared with baseline, aqueous humor flow rate increased in both groups. Although response to 50 mg (compared with 25) was greater for both intraocular pressure and aqueous humor flow rate, the difference was not significant, perhaps reflecting a small sample size.

Thiazide Diuretics

The thiazide diuretics, represented by chlorothiazide (see Figure 17-4), were developed to enhance the potency of carbonic anhydrase inhibitors.[1] Although most do inhibit carbonic anhydrase to some degree, their efficacy as diuretics reflects their ability to directly inhibit sodium chloride co-transport in the distal tubule, perhaps by competing with chloride for binding (see Figure 17-2).[1] Newer diuretics have been developed that act at the same site as the thiazides but are not thiazides; the term *thiazide-like diuretics* is applied to these latter drugs. The primary site of action of these drugs also is the distal tubule (see Figure 17-3), a site characterized by avid binding for thiazide diuretics. Although some action has also been described in the proximal tubule, this may reflect the weak carbonic anhydrase action of these drugs. Compared with other diuretics, the thiazide diuretics are less effective in causing sodium excretion because close to 90% of reabsorption of sodium from the urine has occurred by the time passage through the distal and collecting tubules is complete. Because the tubular site of potassium secretion is distal to the site of thiazide action, potassium excretion is increased and more sodium is reabsorbed. Thiazides have variable effects on calcium excretion, with excretion *decreasing* with chronic administration. Thiazides cause magnesium excretion, and the potential advent of hypomagnesia is being recognized in humans receiving thiazides long term.[1]

The thiazides vary in their oral bioavailability, with that of chlorothiazide being the poorest (10% bioavailable in humans). The degree of protein binding varies among the drugs, and thus delivery to the kidneys via glomerular filtration may be limited. Active tubular secretion of the drugs can be antagonized by probenecid. Likewise, the elimination half-life of the drugs is also variable, with that of chlorothiazide being very short (1.5 hours in humans). For hydrochlorothiazide bioavailability (in humans) is 65%, whereas the elimination half-life is 2.5 hours. Thus the duration of diuretic effect is quite variable. The potency also is variable, with chlorothiazide 10 times more potent than hydrochlorothiazide. Thus doses also are quite variable.

The thiazide diuretics are characterized by a wide safety margin, and clinical toxicity is rare. As with the loop diuretics, most serious toxicities reflect overzealous use. Volume depletion, hypotension, hyponatremia, hypochloremia, hypomagnesemia, and hypercalcemia have been reported. Potassium depletion can be clinically significant, particularly in patients with primary or secondary hyperaldosteronism. Oral potassium supplementation is indicated for patients that become hypokalemic; this is particularly important for patients receiving digoxin because the risk of digoxin toxicity is enhanced in the hypokalemic patient. Alternatively, the thiazides can be used in combination with a potassium-sparing diuretic. Like the carbonic anhydrase inhibitors, thiazides may exacerbate neurologic dysfunctions associated with cirrhotic liver disease. Thiazides appear to diminish the effects of insulin, particularly in the hypokalemic patient, and should not be given to patients with diabetes mellitus.

Thiazides are involved in a number of drug interactions. They can diminish the effectiveness of anticoagulants, uricosuric drugs (for treatment of gout), and insulin and may increase the effects of anesthetics, digitalis glycosides, lithium, and vitamin D. Thiazides do provide additive or synergistic effects when combined with loop diuretics. Efficacy of the thiazides is decreased by NSAIDs and methenamines (because of alkalinization of urine). Hypokalemia induced by the thiazides may be worsened by amphotericin B or corticosteroids. Quinidine has reportedly caused lethal drug interactions with thiazides by causing ventricular tachycardia; however, this may reflect thiazide-induced hypokalemia.[1]

Thiazides are used primarily in the treatment of early congestive heart failure. Although they may be less effective as diuretics, thiazides, in contrast to most other diuretics, minimally affect the composition of ECF. Thiazides may directly decrease glomerular filtration, particularly after intravenous administration. Thus they should not be given to patients with compromised renal function. Thiazides decrease renal excretion of calcium and are contraindicated in patients with hypercalcemia. In contrast, bromide excretion may be facilitated, and thiazides may be useful for treatment of bromide toxicity.

Drugs That Interfere with Renal Epithelial Sodium Transport

Potassium-Sparing Diuretics

Diuretics that are not associated with kaliuresis include the aldosterone antagonists (see later discussion), triamterene, and amiloride.[1] The primary indication for the latter drugs is their ability to spare potassium wasting. Because they cause only a small amount of sodium wasting, however, they usually are combined with another diuretic. Both triamterene and amiloride impair electrogenic sodium reabsorption in the late distal tubule and the collecting systems, after much sodium reabsorption has already occurred. Because the normal electrical potential across the tubular epithelium is lost, the driving force for potassium secretion is reduced. The potassium-sparing effects of these drugs are most effective in the patient whose potassium excretion has markedly increased (i.e., by hyperaldosteronism or therapy with potassium-wasting diuretics). Like the thiazides, amiloride decreases calcium excretion into the urine. The impact of either triamterene or amiloride on renal hemodynamics is minimal.

The drugs are orally bioavailable (50% to 60% in human patients). Both triamterene and amiloride are actively secreted into the proximal tubule (the route by which they reach their site of action), although a portion of triamterene undergoes hepatic metabolism to a metabolite that is active in humans. Both liver disease and hepatic disease can increase the risk of adverse reactions to triamterene. The most serious toxicity is hyperkalemia that is more likely to occur in a patient receiving angiotensin-converting enzyme inhibitors or aldosterone inhibitors. As such, the drugs are contraindicated in patients at risk for or already have developed hyperkalemia. NSAIDs and dietary potassium intake increase the risk of hyperkalemia. As a pteridine derivative, triamterene is a weak folic acid antagonist. Folic acid deficiency leading to megaloblastic anemia has been reported in human patients with cirrhosis.[1] Triamterene also can reduce glucose tolerance. Amiloride, like triamterene, can cause gastrointestinal upset (vomiting, diarrhea). In general, these drugs are not effective diuretics unless combined with another diuretic and, usually, thiazides.

Aldosterone Antagonists

Aldosterone and mineralocorticoid agonists cause sodium and water retention in exchange for potassium and hydrogen excretion.[1] Spironolactone (see Figure 17-2) competitively antagonizes the actions of aldosterone and other mineralocorticoids by binding to the receptor such that it is not active. The site of action is limited to the late distal tubule and the collecting duct (see Figure 17-3). Aldosterone causes sodium and water retention by interacting with mineralocorticoid receptors. Interaction with specific DNA sequences results in the expression of multiple gene products called *aldosterone-induced proteins*. The proteins appear to activate or increase the expression of preexisting yet "silent" sodium channels and pumps in the cell membrane. Sodium moves into the cell from the luminal membrane, causing an electronegative lumen that is conducive to potassium excretion. As such, spironolactone (see Figure 17-4) is effective as a diuretic only in the presence of aldosterone, and efficacy will be impaired in the presence of high concentrations of aldosterone. In addition to several segments of the nephron, aldosterone receptors occur in the colon and salivary glands. Unlike the thiazides and carbonic anhydrase inhibitors, spironolactone causes calcium excretion in the urine. Spironolactone has no effect on renal hemodynamics. However, it has a variety of effects on the diseased myocardium. The recently discovered beneficial effects of spironolactone on both acute myocardial damage[8] and chronic cardiac remodeling[9] are briefly discussed in

Chapter 14 Spironolactone conceivably should be the drug of choice in high aldosterone states such as congestive heart failure or portal hypertension, but its efficacy is less than that of the loop-acting diuretics. Consequently, sole therapy with spironolactone occurs early in the respective syndrome or in combination with other diuretics. Supporting its early use in patients with congestive heart failure is the recognition that, in these patients, spironolactone promotes magnesium and potassium retention, increases uptake of myocardial norepinephrine, attenuates formation of myocardial fibrosis, and decreases mortality associated with both progressive ventricular dysfunction and malignant ventricular arrhythmias.[10,11] Indeed, its apparent positive effects of decreasing mobidity and mortality rates led to early termination of a clinical trial examining these effects in humans.[10]

KEY POINT 17-3 Because of its site of action, spironolactone might enhance the efficacy of any naturietic that acts proximal to its site of action in the distal tubule (see Figure 17-3).

Spironolactone is 60% to 70% bioavailable (in humans), is highly protein bound, and undergoes extensive first-pass metabolism and enterohepatic circulation.[1] In humans spironolactone is characterized by a short half-life (1.4 hours). Its active metabolite (canrenone, which is available outside of the United States as canrenoate, a prodrug of canrenone); however, has an elimination half-life that is much longer (16.5 hours). It is not clear what proportion of the drug is metabolized to the active metabolite in dogs and cats. Spironolactone (or other mineralocorticoid receptors) are the only diuretics that do not require access to the tubular lumen in order to cause diuresis (although the active metabolite apparently does).[1]

The most serious toxicity of spironolactone, like other potassium-sparing diuretics, is hyperkalemia, which is more likely to occur when the drug is given in combination with potassium-wasting diuretics and oral potassium supplementation. The contraindications and side effects that characterize the potassium-sparing diuretics also pertain to spironolactone. In addition, spironolactone has induced metabolic acidosis in patients with cirrhosis. Diarrhea, gastritis, gastric bleeding, and peptic ulceration have been reported in human patients receiving the drug; consequently, it is contraindicated in patients with gastric ulceration. Central nervous system adverse effects such as drowsiness, lethargy, ataxia, and confusion have been reported in human patients. Androgen side effects (e.g., gynecomastia impotence) have been reported in human patients. Finally, the ability of spironolactone to induce malignancy has been raised.[1] Aspirin (salicylates) reduce the efficacy of spironolactone by competing for active tubular secretion. Spironolactone alters the elimination of digitalis glycosides.

Spironolactone is most commonly used to control edema associated with hyperaldosteronism. It is generally, however, combined with either a thiazide or a loop-acting diuretic. Edema associated with hypertension and liver disease are among the more common indications. Spironolactone is the drug of choice for treatment of edema associated with chronic liver disease (secondary to hyperaldosteronism) in human patients.[1] Rarer indications include syndromes associated with potassium depletion.

High-Ceiling Diuretics

The efficacy of diuretics acting on the proximal tubule is limited by the marked reabsorptive capacity of the thick ascending limb of the loop of Henle. Diuretics that act beyond the loop of Henle also are limited in efficacy because only a small percentage of the filtrate reaches that area. In contrast, drugs that act at the loop of Henle tend to be very effective.[1] The term *high ceiling* refers to the peak diuretic effect of these drugs, which far surpasses that of other diuretics. The primary site of action is the thick ascending limb of the loop of Henle, where the drugs bind to and impair the luminally located $Na^+K^+2Cl^-$ co-transport mechanism (see Figure 17-2). Because of their site of action, these drugs also are referred to as *loop diuretics*.[1] Two isoforms of the $Na^+K^+Cl^-$ co-transport enzyme exist with the second isoform located in the apical membrane of the thick ascending loop. The second is located in many body tissues.[12] The efficacy of high-ceiling loop diuretics reflects the large amount of filtrate that reaches this region of the kidney and the lack of a very efficient reabsorptive region beyond the loop. Ethacrynic acid is a phenoxyacetate derivative, and furosemide is a sulfonamide derivative (see Figure 17-4). Furosemide is the member of this class used in small animal patients. Abbott and Kovacic[12] reviewed the use of furosemide in veterinary medicine.

Furosemide causes a profound increase in Na^+ and Cl^- urinary excretion. Ultimately, as ECF decreases in response to furosemide, glomerular filtration decreases and proximal tubular reabsorption of sodium is enhanced. Species differences should be expected in response to furosemide. Dogs respond across a broad therapeutic range. Cats respond in a narrower range, but with a more rapid and intense saluresis and diuresis compared with dogs.[12] Doses in cats greater than 10 mg/kg, administered intramuscularly, may be associated with lethargy and decreased appetite that may last 24 to 48 hours after dosing. In dogs the dose above which intolerance occurs is 50 mg/kg, administered intramuscularly. Blood pressure will decline in both species at these doses, with hypotension more profound in cats.[12] Morbidity at higher doses may reflect volume contraction, hypotension, electrolyte abnormalities, and activation of neurohumoral endocrine responses. At massive doses furosemide inhibits carbonic anhydrase activity in the proximal tubule, but this minimally affects diuretic actions at normal doses. Like the thiazides, the mechanism of action of furosemide is proximal to the site of Na^+ and K^+ exchange; thus potassium excretion is increased. Furosemide also markedly enhances the excretion of calcium and magnesium but does not increase calcium reabsorption in the distal tubule, as do the thiazides. Thus furosemide is indicated for treatment of hypercalcemia, although care must be taken to replace sodium and chloride losses. Because furosemide increases the excretion of acid and ammonia in the distal nephron, diuretic-induced metabolic alkalosis may develop. This can be exacerbated if ECF is rapidly mobilized such that its volume contracts. The kidney's ability to excrete a concentrated urine during hydropenia or a dilute urine during states of water diuresis is impaired by furosemide.

KEY POINT 17-4 In addition to its loop-diuretic effects, furosemide is useful for a variety of other physiologic effects, particularly in the vasculature

Furosemide will increase renal blood flow if volume depletion is avoided. The effect is, however, variable. NSAIDs attenuate the diuretic response to loop diuretics, perhaps by altering prostaglandin-mediated increases in blood flow. Loop diuretics block tubuloglomerular feedback, presumably by inhibiting transport of NaCl to the macula densa.[1] Because of this effect, they also are powerful stimulants of renin release; prostaglandin (prostacyclin) release may be involved in this response. During states of volume depletion, renin activation also may reflect stimulation of the sympathetic nervous system and of intrarenal baroreceptor mechanisms.

Loop diuretics, particularly furosemide, increase venous capacity, possibly because of prostaglandin release. Although this effect is short lived, it enhances the initial diuretic response. This effect is likely to be blunted or inhibited by NSAIDs, including newer drugs that are more potent toward COX-2 compared with COX-1. Decreased peripheral vascular resistance also has been reported.[12] The hemodynamic effects of furosemide may be of particular benefit in the patient with pulmonary edema: The capacity of veins increases, and left ventricular filling pressures subsequently decrease. Impaired electrolyte transport in other tissues generally is clinically irrelevant, with the exception of the endolymph, which may contribute to the ototoxicity characteristic of this group of diuretics. The pulmonary effects may contribute to potential efficacy in the treatment of the acute respiratory distress syndrome or acute lung injury (the latter when combined with albumin). In the dog furosemide dilates gastrointestinal vascular beds.[12]

Furosemide appears to be renoprotective in states of ischemic damage; this may reflect a reduction in oxygen consumption in response to inhibition of co-transport. However, it also has antioxidant effects and protects against free radicals at low doses (0.1 mg/kg/day in rats).[12] Nonetheless, the use of furosemide in acute renal failure has not been consistently demonstrated to reduce patient mortality rates in humans.[12]

Furosemide has a variety of actions other than vascular in the lungs. It attenuates bronchospasm in response to a number of stimuli and stimulates bronchodilation. Furosemide inhibits laryngeal irritant receptors in anesthetized dogs. Clinical signs of dyspnea may be relieved with inhaled furosemide.[12]

Interestingly, furosemide appears to have anticonvulsant properties. Its mechanism may reflect an increase in threshold and decreased seizure propagation. Intraneuronal chloride may be maintained; this may reflect interaction with potassium chloride co-transport enzymes. Interaction may impart neuroprotection. Seizure-induced cellular swelling may be reduced.[12] Furosemide may reduce production of CSF. The target enzymes are present in the choriod plexus. A 50% reduction in CSF has been reported in cats treated with 50 mg/kg intravenously. However, furosemide should not be used to reduce CSF or intracerebral pressure in the presence of or at a dose sufficient to induced hypotension.[12] Furosemide has been associated with a decrease in intracranial pressure but is more effective if it follows a dose of mannitol.[12] In contrast to thoracic lymph flow, furosemide appears to decrease ascitic transudate from selected neoplasms.

Furosemide is rapidly absorbed from the gastrointestinal tract. Bioavailability is only about 60%, however, ranging from 10% to 100% in the individual patient. Thus several different oral doses must be given before therapeutic failure can be assumed. Intravenous administration is indicated in patients for whom lack of response due to oral absorption must be avoided. Alternatively, a drug that is 100% bioavailable after oral administration (e.g., bumetanide or torsemide in human patients) should be given. Furosemide is highly protein bound, which limits delivery through the glomerulus, but it is able to reach its site of action by active tubular secretion.

The most common toxicity associated with furosemide therapy generally reflects overzealous administration, resulting in altered electrolyte and fluid balance. Depletion of body sodium can cause hypotension, reduced GFR, circulatory collapse, and thromboembolic episodes. In the patient with liver disease characterized by activation of the renin–angiotensin–aldosterone system, furosemide can induce hepatic encephalopathy. Continued Na^+ delivery results in continued exchange for H^+ and K^+, causing hypochloremic alkalosis. Hypokalemia likewise can occur, particularly in patients with insufficient dietary intake or patients receiving digoxin therapy. Hypomagnesemia and hypocalcemia are less common, albeit possible, consequences of overzealous furosemide therapy.[1] Furosemide depletes total body iodide, which may be of benefit in states of hyperiodism.[12] Because of its impact in the developing fetus, furosemide is not recommended in pregnant or lactating animals. Furosemide increases lymph flow through the thoracic duct in dogs at 8 to 10 mg/kg. Accordingly, it might be avoided in animals with pleural effusion. Ototoxicity can lead to tinnitus (in human patients), deafness, vertigo, and (described in humans) "a sense of fullness in the ears." Ototoxicity most commonly occurs with rapid intravenous administration, more with ethacrynic acid than with furosemide, and generally is reversible. Contraindications for furosemide therapy include severe Na^+ or volume depletion, hypersensitivity to sulfonamides, and anuria that has not responded to a test dose of furosemide. In human patients furosemide should not be used during pregnancy. Chronic use of furosemide may result in renal hypertophy.[12] The impact of furosemide on mucociliary transport rates is controversial, with some studies showing a detrimental effect.[12] Avoidance of furosemide in patients with inflammatory lung disease, particularly that which is associated with airway secretions, is prudent. Although it contains a sulfur moiety, furosemide does not contain an aryl amine (see Chapters 4 and 7), and patients that are allergic to sulfonamides are not likely to show a cross-reactivity to furosemide. However, cross-allergy has been reported, albeit rarely, in humans. The sulfur moiety may play a role in pancreatitis, which has been reported rarely in humans.[12] Furosemide may directly inhibit insulin secretion; however, this effect is species specific, occurring in dogs and humans but not mice.

Drug interactions involving furosemide may become clinically important. Furosemide is chemically incompatible with a number of drugs (demonstrated for diazepam, dopamine, dobutamine, metoclopramide, and morphine). As such, its use as a constant-rate infusion should be through its own line and not "piggybacked" onto lines containing other drugs. When administered as a constant-rate infusion, furosemide will likely have to be diluted. Stability has been demonstrated for at least 8 hours when diluted fivefold (to a concentration of 10 mg/mL) in either 5% dextrose, lactated Ringer's solution, 0.9% saline, or sterile water.[13] Dilution to 5 mg/mL with water or 5% dextrose is also apparently safe, but 0.9% saline or lactated Ringer's solution may result in cloudiness. Presumed precipitation with the latter probably reflects decreased solution pH.

Because it is highly protein bound (in humans), furosemide may compete with other drugs for protein-binding sites; clinically relevant interactions have been attributed to competition. For example, anticoagulant activity may be enhanced in the presence of furosemide. Other drugs known to interact with furosemide, perhaps because of competition for protein binding, include propranolol and lithium (both characterized by higher plasma drug concentrations). Competitive binding may affect thyroid function tests; initial displacement of thyroxine, causing higher free concentrations, may negatively inhibit thyroid-stimulating hormone.[12] The freed thyroxine will be cleared more rapidly and thus may not be interpreted as high. It is possible that total thyroxine will decrease; the low thyroid-stimulating hormone may be interpreted as hypothyroid.

Potential ototoxicity induced by furosemide is enhanced by aminoglycosides (synergistic) and cisplatin. The risk of cardiac arrhythmias induced by digoxin also are increased by furosemide. Both NSAIDs and probenecid block diuretic response to furosemide, the former perhaps resulting from attenuation of response to renal prostaglandins and the latter from competition for active tubular secretion. In contrast, the thiazides act synergistically with furosemide to induce diuresis. The nephrotoxic potential of other drugs (e.g., cephalosporins, aminoglycosides) is enhanced by furosemide.

Furosemide is used for a variety of indications (see Table 17-1). Treatment of hypertension is limited to animals that have not responded to other therapies. Among the most common indications is edema of a variety of causes that reflect increased hydrostatic pressure and potentially decreased oncotic draw. However, edema associated with vascular permeability generally is not an indication; fluid loss in such cases generally is at the cost of decreases in total body water.

Furosemide is the drug of choice for the management of acute pulmonary edema. Its use in the long-term management of sodium retention might be postponed until other, less effective diuretics become ineffective. Edema associated with the nephrotic syndrome appears to respond only to loop diuretics. For the patient with refractory edema, furosemide can be combined with other diuretics, preferably potassium sparing, such as the thiazides or spironolactone. Doses much higher than normal may be necessary to induce diuresis in patients with renal disease for two reasons. First, renal tubular function is abnormal, and response to furosemide may be impaired. Second, drug delivery to the site of action may be decreased. Administration as a constant-rate infusion (0.66 mg/kg load followed by 0.66 mg/kg/hr) will induce more diuresis, natriuresis, and calciuresis but less kaliuresis compared with intermittent bolus administration.[14] An advantage of constant-rate infusion is avoidance of toxic concentrations that have been associated with ototoxicy in humans. Because of its effects on iodine depletion, it may be useful in the cat with hyperthyroidism before radioiodine treatment, facilitating uptake, as has been demonstrated in humans receiving 40 mg/kg/day for 5 days. Its use as an adjunct to surgery or to control thyroid storm in hyperthyroid cats warrants consideration.

Proteinuria caused by glomerular nephritis may also reduce the efficacy of furosemide because it binds to protein in the urine. The massive doses necessary for acute renal failure may cause hepatotoxicity. Once oliguria has been definitively established, furosemide therapy should be discontinued. Because loop diuretics interfere with the kidney's ability to produce a concentrated urine, when combined with hypertonic saline, furosemide can be used to treat life-threatening hyponatremia. The use of furosemide to facilitate diagnosis of ureteral obstruction also has been described.[6]

Pressor Agents

Drugs that increase cardiac output should, by virtue of increased renal blood flow and glomerular filtration, increase urine output. Among the pressors used to support myocardial depression and hypotension is the positive inotrope dopamine (see Chapter 14). Dopamine receptors in the renal vasculature of several species induce renal vasodilation, with the effect accomplished at low doses of dopamine. Higher doses cause release of epinephrine and subsequent renal arterial vasoconstriction. Dobutamine does not have a similar effect in the renal vasculature. Consequently, dopamine may be the preferred inotropic drug in the face of hypotension that threatens renal function. However, Sigrist[15] has retrospectively reviewed the role of dopamine in acute renal failure, including meta-analyses assessment in humans. In humans many of the studies cited for use have been implemented in animal models or healthy individuals. Because mortality does not change, the incidence of side effects no longer justifies its use. The lack of consistent response in the presence of disease may reflect receptor desensitization; further, profoundly ill patients are likely to realize changes in pharmacokinetics and pharmacodynamics that increase the risk of adversity. Finally, it is not clear if increase urine production stimulated through hemodynamic changes is in fact a positive response or if urine production is an indicator of improvement. Effects in animals are more likely to be realized in animal models of acute renal failure when administered in advance of the insult.

KEY POINT 17-5 Dopamine receptor activity of the feline kidney is different from that of the canine kidney and accordingly is less responsive to dopamine.

Species differences exist in the renal response to dopamine. Although dopamine receptors are present in the feline renal cortex, their numbers are lower compared with those of other species.[16] The cat is among the species for which diuretic doses of dopamine do not cause renal arterial vasodilation, perhaps because of fewer dopamine receptors in the renal vasculature. Higher doses of dopamine do increase diuresis and natriuresis.[17]

Fenoldopam (see Figure 17-4) is a dopamine DA-1 agonist with no α or β adrenergic receptor effects used for treatment of emergency hypertension in humans. It also stimulates systemic vasodilation, natriuresis, and diuresis in human patients with renal disease.[18] Renoprotection has been described, supporting its use in acute renal failure.[19,20] In a dog exsanguination[21] or aortic clamp (n = 8 Labrador Retrievers)[19] models, fenoldopam (0.1 μg/kg/min) maintained renal blood flow before, during, and after induction of acute hypovolemia.[21] Zimmerman-Pope and coworkers[22] attempted to study the impact of fenoldopam on renal function after nephrotomy but found that the model insufficiently affected renal function. Unlike dopamine, feline kidneys respond to fenoldopam. It exhibited a 300-fold greater affinity for feline dopamine receptor, compared with dopamine, suggesting that feline vasculature contains the receptors but lacks dopamine.[17] Wohl and colleagues[23] found no effect of low-dose (3 μg/kg/min) dopamine on indices of renal diuresis (urine output, renal blood flow, sodium excretion, fractional excretion, or creatinine clearance) in anesthetized healthy cats (n = 12). Arterial blood pressure did transiently decrease. In contrast, Simmons and coworkers[20] found that feline kidneys responded to fenaldopam. Ketamine and diazepam were used to induce anesthesia for instrumentation purposes only; healthy awake cats were studied (n = 6). A 12-hour pretreatment assessment of baseline (an infusion of 2.2 mL/kg/hr of saline) was followed by fenoldopam infusion over 2 hours (0.5 μg/kg/min). Parameters were then studied for 12 hours. Fenoldopam increased urine output, sodium excretion, and fractional excretion (with comparable changes in urine specific gravity); creatinine clearance also increased after a transient decrease. The effects were delayed: GFR was increased at 6 hours after fenoldopam administration, coinciding with increases in urine output. Central venous pressure simultaneously decreased. Studies in humans thus far have not clearly demonstrated a beneficial effect of fenoldopam in patients with acute renal failure; further studies are indicated.

THE USE OF DIURETICS IN SELECTED CLINICAL CONDITIONS

Congestive Heart Failure

The intial diuretic selection for human patients with mild congestive heart failure is a thiazide; however, most patients will require a loop diuretic. In human patients the rate of oral absorption of diuretics is slowed, requiring longer to maximal response. Delivery of loop diuretics to their site of action is normal, and doses do not necessarily need to be increased unless there is evidence of renal insufficiency. Renal response to diuretic therapy may be decreased, however, requiring more exposure to drugs. Although a dose increase may be indicated, a decrease in interval may be more likely to cause a response. A thiazide diuretic should be added to therapy if dietary salt retention coupled with a loop diuretic have not been effective. Attention should be paid to ensure that hypokalemia and volume depletion do not occur with this combination. The use of spironolactone may increase as its effects on cardiac remodeling are further described.

KEY POINT 17-6 In patients with congestive heart failure, care must be taken with diuretics to avoid overzealous therapy that may stimulate neurohumoral endocrine responses.

Cirrhosis

Ascites that accompanies cirrhotic liver disease generally reflects a state of hyperaldosteronism and subsequent sodium and water retention. Therefore spironolactone is the diuretic of choice for human patients. Although the amount of diuresis can be expected to be only moderate, this is desirable because greater diuresis may negatively affect intravascular volume. In human patients repeated large-volume paracentesis minimizes the need for more potent diuretics. The active metabolites of spironolactone allow once-daily dosing, although 3 to 4 days must elapse before full pharmacologic effects are realized. Insufficient response to spironolactone indicates the need for an additional diuretic; spironolactone should be continued. For human patients a thiazide is used initially, and a loop diuretic is used in place of the thiazide only if response has been inadequate. The decreased response to a loop diuretic in a patient with cirrhosis is not understood but does not reflect decreased drug delivery. Rather, the tubular cells do not respond maximally. Although higher doses may be of benefit, decreasing the interval may be more likely to increase response.

Nephrotic Syndrome

Response to diuretics in patients with the nephrotic syndrome may be less than ideal if hypoalbuminemia is sufficient to decrease binding of the diuretic (e.g., <2 g/dL). Unbound drug will diffuse into tissues (i.e., volume of distribution will increase), removing the drug from the site of action in the renal tubule. In such patients addition of albumin to the therapeutic regimen will increase response. Binding to albumin in tubular fluid also decreases response and is more likely to occur when urine albumin concentrations exceed 4 g/dL. Dose increases (twofold to threefold) may help compensate for increased tubular binding of the diuretic. Because tubules in patients with nephrotic syndrome may not respond to drugs in general as well as those in the normal patient, decreasing the interval (such that the duration of exposure is longer) also may increase response.

DRUGS THAT ALTER RENAL CONSERVATION OF WATER: ANTIDIURETIC HORMONE

Antidiuretic hormone (ADH) is released by the posterior pituitary in response to increased plasma osmolality (as little as 2%, or 280 mOsm/kg) and depleted ECF volume. The latter might occur, for example, resulting from acute causes such as hypovolemia, sodium depletion, and hemorrhage or chronic causes such as cardiac failure, hepatic cirrhosis with ascites, hypothyroidism, and excessive use of diuretics.. Antidiuresis involves the hypothalamus, neurohypophysis, posterior pituitary, and kidney. Neurons of osmoreceptors, baroreceptors, and higher cerebral centers stimulate the hypothalamus. Calcium-mediated degranulation results in the release of ADH as well as oxytocin and other mediators. A number of chemical mediators are also associated with the release of ADH, including angiotensin II, prostaglandins, and acetylcholine. Inhibitors of release include opioids, atrial natriuretic peptide, and γ-aminobutyric acid.

The actions of ADH are receptor mediated. At least two receptors have been identified. Both receptors are located in the kidney, although the specific tissue site varies. Glomerular, vasa recta, and interstitial medullary receptors (V1) participate in the control of the GFR, medullary blood flow, and prostaglandin synthesis, respectively. The predominant effect of ADH occurs in the collecting duct and is mediated by V2 receptors. In the presence of ADH, the collecting ducts of the cortex and medulla become permeable to water, which follows the osmotic drag.

A number of therapeutic drugs can alter ADH secretion either directly or indirectly. Drugs that alter the osmolality of urine may indirectly alter the secretion of ADH. Drugs that stimulate ADH secretion include the vinca alkaloids, cyclophosphamide, tricyclic antidepressants, and isoproterenol. Inhibitors of ADH secretion include ethanol, mineralocorticoids, and glucocorticoids. The effect of mineralocorticoids results from volume depletion that accompanies sodium loss. Inhibition by glucocorticoids, on the other hand, probably results from both a central effect and cardiac effects. Drugs that inhibit prostaglandin synthesis also will facilitate the action of ADH. Lithium is an example of a drug that inhibits the effects of ADH.

DRUGS THAT ALTER URINARY pH

Urinary acidification or alkalinization depends on normal renal function. Changes in urine pH are at best modest, and the effect on systemic acid–base status is equally modest. In the face of renal deficiency, the use of acidifying salts may be harmful. Changes in urinary pH are implemented to enhance efficacy of a drug in the urine, to enhance solubility of a drug or other solute in the urine, to facilitate urinary excretion of a toxin, or to promote an unfavorable environment for microbial growth. Excretion of an acidic compound is likely to be enhanced if the pK_a of the compound is within the range of 3 to 7.5; for a basic compound a pk_a 7.5 to 10.5 is necessary.

Urinary Acidifiers

Ammonium chloride is a urinary acidifier. Ammonium ion (NH_4^+) serves as a proton donor. Ammonia (NH_3) formed by the kidney is excreted in an acid urine as the ammonium ion. In states of acidosis, renal production of ammonia is stimulated, increasing the concentration of a proton acceptor, thus buffering urinary acid by allowing secretion of protons in tubular fluid. The ammonium of orally administered ammonium chloride is converted by the liver to urea, freeing hydrogen ion, which subsequently decreases bicarbonate. Thus efficacy depends on hepatic conversion of ammonia to urea. Of the urinary acidifiers, ammonium chloride probably provides the most consistent changes in pH. The use of ammonium chloride is contraindicated in hepatic insufficiency.

Acetohydroxamic acid (5 mg/kg every 8 hr orally) is structurally similar to urea that acts as a potent and irreversible inhibitor of bacterial urease. It has been used in humans as adjuvant therapy to treat urinary tract infections associated with urease-producing bacteria (e.g, *Staphylococcus, Klebsiella, Corynebacterium urealyticum,Pseudomonas,* and *Providencia*). Approximately 15% of patients have had laboratory findings characteristic of a hemolytic anemia; accordingly, care might be particularly taken in cats.

Other urinary acidifiers include DL-methionine, ethylenediamine dihydrochloride, and sodium acid phosphate. Methemoglobinemia has been reported in cats receiving phosphate-containing urinary acidifiers.

Cysteine Urolithiasis

Cystinuria also is generally accompanied by increased urinary excretion of lysine, arginine, and ornithine in the urine. Cystine is a non-esssential amino acid composed of two cysteine amino acids joined at their sulfur atoms. It can be synthesized in the body from the essential amino acid, methionine. Cystine solubility in urine decreases as pH increases, predisposing to urolith formation. Cysteine urolithiasis represents a small proportion of uroliths in the dog (1% to 22%).[24] Cystinuria appears to decline with age in dogs with uroliths.[24] Therapies have been variable in choice and effect. Dietary management has included low methionine or sodium diets, the latter reducing the transport of cysteine into the urine in return for sodium.[24] Pharmacologic management has included conversion of cysteine to a more soluble compound with the heavy metal chelator D-penicillamine or tioproinin. However, side effects limit the successful use of D-penicillamine. The use of tioproinin has been reported in an open study of 88 dogs with cystinuria and uroliths.[24] Dogs in which uroliths had been removed were treated with 30 mg/kg, and dogs with uroliths present received 40 mg/kg orally every 12 hours. Treatment duration ranged from 1 month to 13 years (mean 2.8 years), with the median less than 1 year. Stones resolved in 63% of dogs receiving tioproinin, with the mean time to dissolution being 1.6 months. However, uroliths re-formed in 12 of the dogs (between 3 to 36 months) receiving tioproinin prophylactically at 30 mg/kg, with dissolution occurring in five of those when the dose was increased to 40 mg/kg. Side effects occurred in 12% of animals, with the most common being myopathy related to chewing or swallowing and aggression. Disconcertingly, proteinuria (n = 3) and thrombocytopenia (n = 4) also were reported. The authors emphasized the potential importance of lifelong therapy.

Because the potential for cysteine crystal formation is enhanced in an acidic urinary pH, one strategy for prevention of cysteine uroliths has been an increase in urinary pH. Urine pH should be sustained at or above 7.5 to dissolve or prevent the formation of cystine uroliths. Although sodium bicarbonate can be used to maintain an alkaline urine pH, dietary sodium may enhance cystinuria in humans. Further, alkalinization was not a successful treatment in six cysteinuric dogs also receiving tioproinin.[24] Thus potassium citrate may be the preferred urinary alkalinizer in patients with cystine uroliths.

Calcium Oxalate Urolithiasis

Close to 50% of urinary calculi in cats are calcium oxylate rather than struvite, with cats older than 7 years of age more commonly afflicted.[25] Uroliths composed of calcium are difficult to dissolve with diet or medications.[26-30] Medications that alter urine concentrations of calcium are likely to detrimentally alter normal calcium homeostasis. Thiazide diuretics decrease renal excretion of calcium by virtue of their effect on the Na-Cl transporter: decreased intracellular sodium results in increases calcium reasorption via the $Na^+/Ca2^+$ countertransporter. Volume contraction results in both sodium and calcium reabsorption. Potentiation of the effects of parathyroid hormone on tubular reabsorption of calcium may also be beneficial. Although human patients suffering from normocalcemic hypercalciuria benefit from thiazide therapy, efficacy in comparable small animal patients has not been established. Thiazides may prove useful for patients whose hypercalciuria is associated with normocalcemia but are contraindicated for hypercalcemic patients. Hypokalemia is a potential undesirable side effect of thiazide therapy and can be prevented by oral administration of potassium citrate.

Potassium citrate therapy may also benefit the patient with calcium oxalate urolithiasis. Citrates complex with calcium to form salts that are more soluble than oxalate salts. Citrate also is metabolized to bicarbonate, which may alkalinize the urine, and in dogs, may increase citrate excretion in the urine. Low concentrations of citrate occur in up to 63% of patients with calcium oxalate urolithiasis, but a similar role has not been identified in dogs or cats. Potassium citrate is available in a wax matrix, slow-release preparation. Delayed absorption results in prolonged maintenance of urine citrate concentrations. Potassium citrate is more likely to be effective in dogs with calcium oxalate urolithiasis if hypocitraturia can be documented. Dosing regimens may be guided by measuring urinary pH, which should be maintained at or above 7. Vitamin B_6 (2 to 10 mg/kg every 24 hours) and B_{12} (1 mg/kg every 24 hours) has been recommended to decrease oxalate urolithiasis although clinical trials supporting this use are controversial. Supplementation may be indicated in cases of potential vitamin B deficiency (e,g., senior cats with bowel disease). Dietary management and encouragement of fluid intake (including slightly salting the diet) also are recommended.

Anaerobic microbial oxalate degradation in the gastrointestinal tract appears to be an important mechanism by which the incidence of hyperoxaluria occurs. Deficiency of *Oxalobacter formigenes* may be associated with calcium oxalate. Supplementation of gastrointestinal flora with the organism in human volunteers was associated with a reduction in urinary oxylate excretion, which suggests that this may be an alternative therapy.[31]

Urate Urolithiasis

In addition to low-protein diets, dissolution of urate stones can be facilitated by urine alkalinization and administration of allopurinol.[26-30] Urinary pH should be maintained at 7 to 7.5 with oral sodium bicarbonate or potassium citrate. Allopurinol competitively inhibits xanthine oxidase, the enzyme that forms uric acid from xanthines. Plasma and thus urinary concentrations of uric acid are decreased. Because serum concentrations of xanthine increase with allopurinol therapy, urinary alkalinization is recommended with allopurinol therapy in human patients suffering from gout to prevent the formation of xanthine stones. Although allopurinol is recommended for treatment of Dalmatian urate urolithiasis, its use for patients with urate stones associated with portosystemic shunting should be implemented cautiously because the efficacy of allopurinol depends, in part, on hepatic metabolism. Alkalinization also is not recommended for these patients because of the potential for hepatic encephalopathy. The disposition of allopurinol has been described in Dalmations.[32] After oral administration of 10 mg/kg, peak plasma concentrations (C_{max}) was 6.43 ± 0.18 μg/mL at 3 hours, and the elimination half-life approximated 2.5 to 3 hours. A dosing regimen was not recommended by the authors because of the variability of hyperuricosuria in dogs and the lack of determination of a dose–response relationship to identify a target therapeutic concentration.

Although generally safe, allopurinol is associated with several adverse effects in humans. Included are cutaneous reactions; fever and malaise; and sequelae of drug interactions. Sequential urine urate: creatinine ratios have been advocated for monitoring response to dietary and medical management of urate urolithiasis. A controlled study in healthy dogs, however, found no relationship between random urine samples and 24-hour quantitation of uric acid excretion.[33] Thus 24-hour uric acid measurements probably provide the best means for evaluating response to therapy. Note, however, that urates are easily crystallized and may be difficult to measure in urine. Medications should be continued at least 4 weeks after radiographic evidence of stone dissolution. If dissolution is not evident by 6 to 8 weeks, it is possible that the stones are composed of materials other than urate.

REFERENCES

1. Jackson EK: Diuretics. In Hardman JG, Limbird LE, editors: *Goodman and Gilman's the pharmacological basis of therapeutics*, ed 9, New York, 2001, McGraw-Hill, pp 757–787.
2. Okusa MD: Diuretic drugs. In Wecker L, editor: *Brody's human pharmacology: molecular to clinical*, St Louis, 2010, Mosby.
3. Gross DR: Diuretics. In Adams R, editor: *Veterinary pharmacology and therapeutics*, Ames, Iowa, 1995, Iowa State University Press, pp 523–530.
4. Brater DC: Diuretic therapy, *N Engl J Med* 339(6):387–395, 1998.

5. Wakai A, Roberts I, Schierhout G: Mannitol for acute traumatic brain injury, *Cochrane Database of Systemic Reviews* , 2007:Issue 1. Art. No.: CD001049. doi: 10.1002/14651858.CD001049.pub4.
6. Choi H, Won S, Chung W, et al: Effect of intravenous mannitol upon the resistive index in complete unilateral renal obstruction in dogs, *J Vet Intern Med* 17:158–162, 2003.
7. Skorobohach BJ, Ward DA, Hendrix DV: Effects of oral administration of methazolamide on intraocular pressure and aqueous humor flow rate in clinically normal dogs, *Am J Vet Res* 64(2):183–187, 2003.
8. Hayashi M, Tsutamoto T, Wada A, et al: Immediate administration of mineralocorticoid receptor antagonist spironolactone prevents post-infarct left ventricular remodeling associated with suppression of a marker of myocardial collagen synthesis in patients with first anterior acute myocardial infarction, *Circulation* 107:2559–2565, 2003.
9. Kasma S, Toyama T, Kumakura H, et al: Effect of spironolactone on cardiac sympathetic nerve activity and left ventricular remodeling in patients with dilated cardiomyopathy, *J Am Coll Cardio* 41:574–581, 2003.
10. Soberman JE, Weber KT: Spironolactone in congestive heart failure, *Curr Hypertens Rep* 2(5):451–456, 2000.
11. Soberman J, Chafin CC, Weber KT: Aldosterone antagonists in congestive heart failure, *Curr Opin Investig Drugs* 3(7):1024–1028, 2002.
12. Abbott LM, Kovacic J: The pharmacologic spectrum of furosemide, *J Vet Emerg Crit Care* 18(1):26–39, 2008.
13. Adin DB, Hill RC, Scott KC: Short-term compatibility of furosemide with crystalloid solutions, *J Vet Intern Med* 17(5):724–726, 2003.
14. Adin DB, Taylor AW, Hill RC, et al: Intermittent bolus injecdtion versus continuous infusion of furosemine in normal adult greyhound dogs, *J Vet Intern Med* 17:632–636, 2003.
15. Sigrist NE: Use of dopamine in acute renal failure, *J Vet Emerg Crit Care* 17(2):117–126, 2007.
16. Flournoy WS, Wohl JS, Alnrecht-Schmitt TJ, et al: Pharmacological identification of putative D1 dopamine receptors in feline kidneys, *J Vet Pharmacol Therap* 26:283–290, 2003.
17. Wohl JS, Schwartz DD, Flournoy WS, et al: Renal hemodynamic and diuretic effects of low-dosage dopamine in anesthetized cats, *J Vet Emer Crit Care* 17:45–52, 2007.
18. Murphy MB: Dopamine: a role in the pathogenesis and treatment of hypertension, *J Hum Hypertens* 14:S47–S50, 2000.
19. Halpenny M, Markos F, Snow HM, et al: The effects of fenoldopam on renal blood flow and tubular function during aortic cross-clamping in anaesthetized dogs, *Eur J Anaesthesiol* 17(8):491–498, 2000.
20. Simmons JP, Wohl JS, Schwartz DD, et al: Diuretic effects of fenoldopam in healthy cats, *J Vet Emerg Crit Care* 16(2):96–103, 2006.
21. Halpenny M, Markos F, Snow HM, et al: Effects of prophylactic fenoldopam infusion on renal blood flow and renal tubular function during acute hypovolemia in anesthetized dogs, *Crit Care Med* 29(4):855–860, 2001.
22. Zimmerman-Pope N, Waldron DR, Barber DL, et al: Effect of fenoldopam on renal function after nephrotomy in normal dogs, *Vet Surg* 32(6):566–573, 2003.
23. Wohl JS, Schwartz DD, Flournoy WS, et al: Renal hymodynamic and diuretic effects of low-dosage dopamine in anesthetized cats, *J Vet Emerg Crit Care* 17(1):45–52, 2007.
24. Hoppe A, Denneberg T: Cystinuria in the dog: clinical studies during 14 years of medical treatment, *J Vet Intern Med* 15:361–367, 2001.
25. Lekcharoensuk C, Lulich JP, Osborne CA, et al: Association between patient-related factors and risk of calcium oxalate and magnesium ammonium phosphate urolithiasis in cats, *J Am Vet Med Assoc* 217:520–525, 2000.
26. Osborne CA, Hoppe A, O'Brien TO: Medical dissolution and prevention of cystine urolithiasis. In Kirk RW, Bonagura JD, editors: *Current veterinary therapy X: small animal practice*, Philadelphia, 1989, Saunders, pp 1189–1193.
27. Senior DF: Medical management of urate urolithiasis. In Kirk RW, Bonagura JD, editors: *Current veterinary therapy X: small animal practice*, Philadelphia, 1989, Saunders, pp 1178–1181.
28. Dieringer TM, Lees GE: Nephroliths: approach to therapy. In Kirk RW, Bonagura JD, editors: *Current veterinary therapy XI: small animal practice*, Philadelphia, 1992, Saunders, pp 889–891.
29. Buffington CA, Sokolowski JH: *Proceedings of the 16th Annual Waltham/OSU Symposium: Nephrology and Urology*, Vernon, Calif, 1992, Kal Kan Foods, Inc.
30. Lulich JP, Osborne CA: Canine calcium oxalate urolithiasis: risk factor management. In Kirk RW, Bonagura JD, editors: *Current veterinary therapy X: small animal practice*, Philadelphia, 1992, Saunders, pp 893–899.
31. Duncan SH, Richardson AJ, Kaul P, et al: Oxalobacter formigenes and its potential role in human health, *Appl Environ Microbiol* 68(8):3841–3847, 2002.
32. Ling GV, Case LC, Nelson H, et al: Pharmacokinetics of allopurinol in Dalmatian dogs, *J Vet Pharmacol Ther* 20(2):134–138, 1997.
33. Osborne C, Bartges JW: *Personal communication*, December 1993, University of Minnesota.

18 Treatment of Urinary Disorders

India F. Lane and Jennifer E. Stokes

Chapter Outline

MANAGEMENT OF ACUTE RENAL FAILURE

Pathophysiology

Acute renal failure results from a sudden, severe decline in renal function, which may be initiated by prerenal, renal, or postrenal causes. Although several specific renal diseases can cause acute renal decompensation, in veterinary medicine acute *intrinsic* renal failure is most commonly caused by a nephrotoxicant or an infectious or ischemic injury. The proportionately high blood flow and large capillary surface area in the kidney increase the organ's sensitivity to blood-borne toxicants. Additionally, the sophisticated transport mechanisms, intensive metabolic activity, and refined concentrating mechanisms found in renal tubules increase the likelihood of toxic injury. Glomeruli, too, are susceptible to direct destruction and immunologic injury. The most common nephrotoxicants encountered in veterinary medicine are ethylene glycol and therapeutic agents such as aminoglycosides, amphotericin B, cisplatin, radiographic contrast agents, and analgesics. Additional nephrotoxins include lilies, which are toxic in cats only, and raisins and grapes, which are toxic in dogs.[1]

Ischemic injury may result from any insult that compromises perfusion of afferent arteriolar blood flow. Hypoperfusion from shock, dehydration, or hypotension is the most common mechanism of renal ischemia. Trauma, anesthesia, cardiac output failure, and persistent vomiting or diarrhea are potential ischemic events encountered in small animals. Thrombosis, hyperviscosity, and polycythemia are additional, less common disorders that interfere with renal blood flow. Angiotensin-converting enzyme (ACE) inhibitors, widely used in the management of congestive heart failure in dogs and proteinuric disorders, inhibit production of the vasopressor angiotensin II. In the glomerulus angiotensin II blockade preferentially dilates efferent arterioles, which may lead to loss of glomerular capillary pressure and reduction in glomerular filtration (see Chapter 14). The vasodilatory effect is most prominent in diseased or poorly perfused kidneys and can lead to progressive azotemia or overt acute renal failure in treated patients.[2,3]

The administration of nonsteroidal antiinflammatory drugs (NSAIDs) may inhibit vasodilatory prostaglandin production in the kidneys. The effect of NSAIDs is minimal in healthy kidneys but can be devastating when superimposed on marginally functioning kidneys, hypovolemia, or other vasoconstrictive states (anesthesia, surgery, sepsis, heart failure, liver failure, nephrotic syndrome).[4] In these disorders renal blood flow and glomerular filtration rate become increasingly dependent on prostaglandin synthesis; administration of NSAIDs can precipitate renal ischemia and failure. Many systemic diseases increase the risk of acute renal failure by ischemic or vascular mechanisms. These disorders include pancreatitis, hepatic failure, immune-mediated hemolytic anemia, heat stroke, disseminated intravascular coagulopathy, rickettsial disease, babesiosis, and bacterial endocarditis.[5,6]

Both toxicant and ischemic insults to nephrons lead to impairment of cellular transport mechanisms, cellular swelling, and death. Cellular hypoxia and intracellular calcium overload lead to additional membrane damage and oxygen free radical formation. Vascular congestion and tubular obstruction result from cellular swelling and act as common mechanisms perpetuating renal ischemia and renal failure.[7] Therapeutic measures employed in acute renal failure attempt to support renal excretory function, attenuate cellular damage, and favor renal recovery.

General Considerations in Management

Goals of management of established acute renal failure are to (1) treat or minimize underlying disease processes; (2) correct fluid, electrolyte, and acid–base disorders; (3) initiate a diuresis; (4) manage systemic complications; and (5) establish a prognosis. The first principle in managing any disease process is to "treat the treatable." In acute renal failure "treatable" problems may include dehydration or hypovolemia, postrenal obstruction, cardiac or hepatic disease, leptospirosis, rickettsial disease, bacterial endocarditis, pyelonephritis, hypercalcemia, renal lymphoma, and hemoglobinuria. Early recognition of potential toxicant-induced renal failure allows for treatment with specific antidotes (e.g., 4-methylpyrazole or ethanol for ethylene glycol) or with nonspecific measures such as gastric lavage, fluid therapy, and cathartics. Administration of any potentially nephrotoxic agents should be stopped.

KEY POINT 18-1 Early recognition and treatment of reversible disease, appropriate fluid therapy, and maintaining urine production are the keys to medical management of acute renal failure.

Fluid Therapy

After identification of underlying disorders, the management of acute renal failure relies largely on management of fluid, electrolyte, and acid–base imbalances. Fluid deficits are estimated (estimated percentage dehydration × body weight in kilograms = liters required) and replaced rapidly, within 4 to 6 hours. Initial fluid choices include 0.9% saline or other replacement solutions. Low-sodium fluids such as 0.45% saline/2.5% dextrose or half-strength lactated Ringer's solution in 2.5% dextrose may be used for patients with cardiac insufficiency or hypernatremia. Fluids for maintenance requirements (40 to 60 mL/kg per day) and ongoing losses (polyuria, vomiting, diarrhea) should be added to the daily fluid total. In most cases rehydration fluid requirements will equal two to three times maintenance requirements; careful calculation of deficits and ongoing needs is recommended to prevent underestimation of fluid needs (Table 18-1).

Urine output should be measured during the rehydration phase to document appropriate diuresis and to calculate future fluid requirements. After adequate volume replacement, urine output should reach at least 1 to 2 mL/kg per hour. Oliguric patients, in which urine output is less than 1 mL/kg per hour, require additional treatment. If the animal is not overhydrated, mild volume expansion may be considered. Administration of an additional 3% to 5% of the animal's body weight in fluid should eliminate any remaining, undetected volume deficits and enhance renal perfusion and glomerular filtration rate (GFR).[8] If volume expansion is attempted, the patient must be carefully monitored for signs of overhydration, including inappropriate weight gain, systemic hypertension, increased bronchovesicular sounds, tachypnea, tachycardia, restlessness, chemosis, and serous nasal discharge. Note that dry mucous membranes can be a consequence of uremia and are not good indicators of hydration status in acute renal failure.[9] Appropriate volume expansion is documented by a modest increase in body weight and modest reductions in the hematocrit and plasma protein concentrations. Volume overload is a common complication of fluid therapy in oligoanuric renal failure patients. Roughly two thirds of dogs and cats referred for hemodialysis management of uremic crises are hypervolemic. Without dialytic support this complication can be difficult to reverse unless urine production increases.[9]

KEY POINT 18-2 Fluid therapy must be tailored to the individual patient, based on variable urine production and ongoing losses. If urine production is poor, significant adjustments in fluid rate and pharmacologic treatments are usually necessary.

Methods to Enhance Urine Production

If urine production remains poor after rehydration and volume expansion, pharmacologic manipulation of oliguria is warranted. Furosemide, dopamine, and osmotic diuretics have been standard options for management of oliguric and anuric renal failure despite a lack of clinical studies confirming efficacy (see Chapter 17 and for dopamine, see Chapter 14). Despite the lack of proven clinical efficacy, furosemide (2 to 3 mg/kg intravenously every 6 to 8 hours) is often chosen as an initial treatment for oliguria because it is readily available and easy to administer. A constant-rate infusion (CRI) of furosemide (1 mg/kg per hour) has also been recommended.[8,10]

As a loop diuretic, furosemide helps increase tubular flow and improve renal blood flow but does not significantly affect GFR.[7] It is also speculated that the activity of furosemide may

Table **18-1** Drugs Used in the Management of Acute Renal Failure

Agent	Actions	Dosage	Adverse Effects	Contraindications
Agents Used to Enhance Urine Production				
Furosemide	Loop diuretic ↑ RBF	2-3 mg/kg IV q 6-8h 2-6 mg/kg IV q 30-60 min 0.25-1 mg/kg/h IV CRI	Volume depletion, hypokalemia	Gentamicin, nephrotoxicity
Dopamine	↑ RBF, ↑ GFR ↑ Natriuresis	1-5 μg/kg/min IV CRI	Arrhythmias, hypertension, vomiting	
Mannitol	Osmotic diuresis ↓ Cellular edema Free radical scavenger	0.5-1.0 g/kg IV slow bolus (10%-20% solution) 1-2 mg/kg/min IV CRI (5%-10% solution)	Pulmonary edema, GI upset	Overhydration, cardiac disease
10%-20% Dextrose	Osmotic diuresis Caloric support	25-50 mL/kg IV slow infusion q8-12h	Volume expansion, hyperglycemia, hyperosmolality	
Agents Used to Treat Hyperkalemia				
Calcium gluconate (10% solution)	Cardioprotection	0.5-1.0 mL/kg IV slow bolus	Arrhythmias	
Sodium bicarbonate	Alkalinization of ECF	0.5-2 mEq/kg IV slow bolus	Hypernatremia, ↓ ionized calcium, hypokalemia	Hypocalcemia
Dextrose	↑ Insulin	0.1-0.5 g/kg IV (102 mL/kg 25% solution)	Hyperglycemia, hyperosmolality	
Insulin/dextrose	Intracellular movement of potassium	0.25-0.5 U/kg insulin with 1-2 g dextrose per unit Insulin given	Hypoglycemia	
Sodium polystyrene sulfonate	Exchange resin	0.5 g/kg PO or per rectum or 6 hrs	Nausea, constipation, gastrointestinal ulcers	
Agents Used to Treat Metabolic Acidosis				
Sodium bicarbonate	Alkalinization	See text for dosage information	Hypernatremia, hypokalemia, ↓ ionized calcium	
Agents Used to Treat Nausea/Vomiting				
Famotidine	H_2 antagonist	0.5-1 mg/kg IV q 12-24 hr		
Ranitidine	H_2 antagonist	2 mg/kg IV q 8-12 hr		Severe renal or hepatic failure (adjust dose)
Dolasetron	Serotonin recepter antagonist	0.6 mg IV q 6 hr		
Metoclopramide	Dopamine antagonist	0.2-0.4 mg/kg IV or 1-2 mg/kg q 24 hr IV CRI	CNS signs, interference with dopamine, constipation	GI obstruction, seizures
Misoprostol	Prostaglandin analog	1-5 μg/kg PO q 6-12 hr	GI upset, uterine Contraction	Pregnancy, hypertension, seizures

RBF, Renal blood flow; *IV*, intravenous; *GFR*, glomerular filtration rate; *CRI*, constant-rate infusion; *GI*, gastrointestinal; *ECF*, extracellular fluid; *CNS*, central nervous system.

protect cells of the thick ascending loop of Henle by reducing active transport at this site. Furosemide may be useful in managing overhydration and hyperkalemia and enhancing toxin elimination in acute renal failure.[9] Furosemide has been shown to exacerbate gentamicin toxicity and should be avoided in patients recently treated with aminoglycosides.[11] If urine output does not increase in 30 to 60 minutes, furosemide may be repeated at 4 to 6 mg/kg intravenously at 30- to 60-minute intervals; concurrent dopamine administration should also be considered. The efficacy of furosemide in reversing oliguria appears to be improved with the concurrent administration of dopamine.[12] Dopamine in this instance may improve delivery of furosemide to sites of activity. If diuresis is established with furosemide administration, intravenous bolus doses may be repeated every 6-8 hours or a CRI can be maintained at 0.25 to 1 mg/kg/hr.[9] In healthy Greyhounds a furosemide infusion resulted in more diuresis, natriuresis, and calciuresis and less kaliuresis than bolus doses.[13] High-dose furosemide did not increase survival rates in people with acute renal failure in a prospective, double-blinded, randomized placebo-controlled trial.[14] An influence on survival in cats and dogs has not been established. Extracellular fluid volume and potassium requirements should be carefully addressed during furosemide treatment.

Dopamine is a catecholamine (a norepinephrine precursor) that in low doses causes increases in renal blood flow. In dogs dopamine acts at specific splanchnic and renal receptors to cause efferent arteriolar vasodilation, enhancing renal blood flow and sodium excretion. Dilation of mesenteric, coronary, and intracerebral vascular beds also is expected. Effects on GFR are modest.[15] In cats dopamine appears to stimulate α-adrenergic receptors, leading to increased blood pressure and natriuresis.[16] Dopamine must be administered as a CRI, ideally with an automated fluid infusion pump. Dopamine is administered diluted in nonalkaline fluids, usually normal saline or dextrose solutions. Infusion rates of 1 to 5 μg/kg per minute are recommended. Infusion is usually started at 1 to 2 μg/kg per minute while the patient is monitored for changes in heart rate or rhythm. Tachycardia, ectopic or premature ventricular beats, nausea, vomiting, and hypertension are adverse effects, predominantly seen at higher doses. The pressor effects of dopamine are variable and can be detrimental to renal function; monitoring of urine output and degree of azotemia is imperative in individual patients. The half-life of dopamine is approximately 2 minutes; effects are withdrawn within 10 minutes after the infusion is discontinued. The drug is metabolized to inactive compounds by monoamine oxidase and catechol-O-methyltransferase in the kidney, liver, and plasma.[17] Recent prospective, randomized, double-blinded, placebo-controlled trials in humans have failed to show efficacy of low-dose dopamine in management of acute renal failure. Dopamine may also cause detrimental gastrointestinal, respiratory, endocrine, and immunologic effects.[18] Use of dopamine for management of acute renal failure has fallen out of favor, except as needed for pressor response.

Fenoldopam and other new selective dopamine subtype DA-1 receptor agonists may more effectively increase renal blood flow in dogs[8] and possibly in cats. Results of these selective dopaminergic compounds have not been reported in clinically affected patients in acute renal failure.

KEY POINT 18-3 The primary benefit of diuretic administration is to increase urine production and simplify management. Minimal, if any, benefits on glomerular filtration rate or survival are likely.

Osmotic diuretics currently represent the optimal pharmacologic option for enhancing urine flow. Osmotic agents such as mannitol enhance urine production by increasing both intravascular volume and tubular fluid flow. Mannitol is freely filtered at the glomerulus and poorly reabsorbed in renal tubules, creating an osmotic effect such that water is not reabsorbed from the tubular lumen. Osmotic agents also prevent tubular and vascular obstruction by minimizing cellular swelling. Mannitol also possesses weak renal vasodilatory and cellular free radical scavenging actions.[19] Adverse effects of mannitol infusion include volume overload and pulmonary edema, gastrointestinal upset, and central nervous system effects (usually at high doses). The drug is contraindicated for overhydrated or dehydrated patients and for patients with preexisting cardiac disease or suspected intracranial hemorrhage. Mannitol (20% to 25% solution) may be administered at a dosage of 0.5 to 1.0 g/kg intravenously as a slow bolus (over 15 to 20 minutes).[20] Another protocol entails administration of partial dosages (0.5 mg/kg each) every 15 minutes for three treatments.[21] Urine output should improve within 1 hour. A second bolus may be attempted if the agent is unsuccessful, but the potential for volume overexpansion and edema formation increases. When mannitol is beneficial, intermittent bolus injections (0.5 to 1 g/kg intravenously every 6 to 8 hours) or CRI of a 5% to 10% solution (2 to 5 mL/min) may be given up to 2 g/kg per day.[13] Lower doses given more frequently (0.25 to 0.5 g/kg intravenously every 4 hours) or a CRI of 1 to 2 mg/kg/min also have been recommended.[9] One author recommends maintaining diuresis with an infusion of mannitol diluted in lactated Ringer's solution.[8]

Hypertonic dextrose solutions have been useful as an alternative osmotic agent. Once the renal threshold for glucose transport has been exceeded, dextrose solutions create effects similar to those of mannitol on tubular flow and urine output. Solutions of 10% or 20% dextrose are formulated and administered as intermittent slow boluses of 25 to 50 mL/kg (over 1 to 2 hours) two or three times per day. The initial infusion rate may be as high as 2 to 10 mL/min in order to rapidly create hyperglycemia. The infusion rate may subsequently be dropped to 1 to 5 mL/min.[21,22] Advantages of dextrose solutions include low cost, availability, and relative safety. Dextrose solutions also provide nominal caloric supplementation. Urine glucose is easily monitored to ensure that sufficient hyperglycemia and filtration of glucose are continuing; urine volume still must be quantitated because glycosuria can occur without significant increases in urine production. Dextrose solutions may be inferior to mannitol in other respects, however, because the osmotic effects on cellular swelling and tubular obstruction will be minimized by intracellular equilibration of glucose across cell membranes, an effect that does not occur with mannitol.[8] Hypertonic glucose also lacks the vasodilatory and free radical scavenging effects of mannitol. The rapid movement of glucose intracellularly does, however, minimize the potential development of vascular overload and pulmonary edema.

For patients who become fluid overloaded and have decreased renal output, fluid removal is an essential part of management. Standard treatment in human medicine that is also available for veterinary patients includes peritoneal dialysis and hemodialysis. A promising new treatment is cross-linked polyelectrolyte sorbents. This oral solution can absorb as much as 50 times its weight in gastrointestinal water (up to a liter of fluid in a 30 kg dog) as well as urea, creatinine, and potassium, allowing an alternative to renal excretion of excessive fluid and solutes.[23]

The choice of initial treatment protocol for oliguria varies with clinician preference, experience, available technical support, and patient variables. Furosemide or dopamine (or both) historically were employed initially, but this practice must be critically assessed because dopamine may actually cause detrimental effects. Mannitol is probably, however, the preferred agent for treatment of nephrotoxic and ischemic renal failure in patients that are not overhydrated. If one protocol is ineffective, another protocol may be attempted. Polyuric renal failure generally is easier to manage and has a better prognosis than oliguric renal failure. The effects of all measures to reverse oliguria appear to diminish as the duration of oliguria is prolonged.

Management of Hyperkalemia and Metabolic Acidosis

Patients with acute renal failure may be hypokalemic, normokalemic, or hyperkalemic. Hyperkalemia is most likely observed with oliguric or anuric renal failure. Management of hyperkalemia and other electrolyte disturbances is ideally based on serum electrolyte determinations; however, an estimate of potassium status can often be made on the basis of an electrocardiogram. Administration of potassium-free fluids and initiation of a diuresis is usually sufficient to correct mild to moderate hyperkalemia. Longer-term control of mild hyperkalemia may be gained with exchange resins. Sodium polystyrene sulfonate (Kayexalate) is given as a suspension in 20% sorbitol (2 g/kg/day by mouth or by rectum in 3 to 4 divided doses). Nausea, constipation, and gastrointestinal ulceration or erosion are possible complications of this product and have limited its tolerance in veterinary patients.[9]

Peaked T waves, bradycardia, prolonged PR intervals, flattened P waves, and widened QRS complexes may be seen with moderate elevations in serum potassium. Severe hyperkalemia may result in a loss of P waves, idioventricular rhythms, atrial standstill, or ventricular fibrillation and represents a life-threatening emergency. With severe electrocardiographic changes, administration of calcium gluconate (0.5 to 1 mL/kg of a 10% solution given intravenously over 10 to 15 minutes) offers cardioprotective actions. Calcium ions counteract potassium without lowering serum potassium; other measures must be initiated to prevent subsequent cardiac toxicity.[24]

Bicarbonate administration facilitates an intracellular shift of potassium ions and is another useful initial treatment for moderate hyperkalemia. Sodium bicarbonate is administered as a slow intravenous injection of 0.5 to 2 mEq/kg.[24] Alternatively, bicarbonate deficits can be determined on the basis of serum bicarbonate, total CO_2, or base deficit measurement. The deficit is calculated by the formula: 0.3 × body weight (kg) × base deficit *or* (20 − serum bicarbonate or total CO_2 concentration). A portion of the deficit (usually one fourth or one half) is given as a slow bolus or in fluids, and the acid–base status is reassessed. An advantage of sodium bicarbonate administration is concurrent correction of coexisting metabolic acidosis. In the absence of hyperkalemia, bicarbonate administration is reserved for severe acidosis (blood pH <7.2 or total CO_2 <12 to 15 mEq/L). Overzealous bicarbonate administration may have serious detrimental results, including hypernatremia, hyperosmolality, ionized calcium deficits, reduced plasma potassium concentrations, metabolic alkalosis, and paradoxical acidosis of the cerebrospinal fluid.

An alternative method of therapy for acute hyperkalemia includes the administration of glucose (dextrose 0.1 to 0.5 g/kg as a 20% solution *or* 1 to 2 mL/kg 50% dextrose diluted to 25%).[20] Administration of glucose triggers endogenous insulin secretion; both glucose and insulin facilitate intracellular movement of potassium. Protocols utilizing insulin and glucose (0.25 to 0.5 U/kg insulin followed by 1 to 2 g glucose per unit of insulin administered) have also been recommended. Exogenous insulin administration can promote hypoglycemia; blood glucose monitoring is required.

Disorders of calcium are occasionally found in acute renal failure. Hypercalcemia may be a cause of acute renal damage. Calcium levels usually drop with fluid or diuretic administration; investigation into the etiology of hypercalcemia should proceed, however. Severe hypocalcemia is rare except in ethylene glycol intoxication. Alkalinizing therapy may further reduce ionized calcium levels, resulting in symptomatic hypocalcemia. Calcium administration may be necessary in some cases.

Maintenance Fluid Therapy

Once a diuresis has been established, and in cases of nonoliguric acute renal failure, fluid therapy should be tailored to match urine volume and other sensible and insensible losses. Insensible losses (e.g., water lost from respiration) are estimated at 13 to 22 mL/kg per day. Urine output (the most variable sensible loss in patients with renal failure) is quantitated during 6- or 8-hour intervals; the amount lost is replaced during an equivalent period. Ongoing gastrointestinal losses also are estimated and replaced. Some clinicians factor in a 3% to 5% estimate to provide for subclinical dehydration each day, regardless of physical examination findings (except for signs of overhydration). Intervals can be extended as the animal is stabilized.

Fluid composition during maintenance therapy should be tailored to the individual. Polyionic replacement solutions that provide buffering activity and electrolyte replacement (e.g., lactated Ringer's solution, Normosol-R, Plasma-Lyte 56) may be administered during the first few days of treatment, especially if gastrointestinal or electrolyte losses are great. For longer-term therapy, lower sodium solutions designed to meet maintenance fluid needs (e.g., half-strength lactated Ringer's solution or 0.45% saline in 2.5% dextrose, Normosol-M, or Plasma-Lyte 56) are preferred, insofar as most ongoing losses will consist of free water losses in polyuria.[8] Alternating administration of 5% dextrose solutions with high-sodium replacement solutions may also be effective in preventing hypernatremia in patients requiring long-term fluid therapy.[21] Potassium supplementation in excess of amounts supplied in commercial fluids is usually required during the maintenance phase of treatment; a total of 20 to 30 mEq KCl per liter of fluid administered is typically sufficient.

Other Considerations

Multiple complications may be encountered during the course of treatment of acute renal failure. Complications are usually a result of uremia and include oral ulceration, vomiting, diarrhea, malnutrition, infection, hemorrhage, anemia, hypertension, and neurologic deterioration. Most of these complications are best ameliorated by minimizing azotemia. Anorexia and vomiting are typically due to activation of the chemoreceptor trigger zone, uremic gastritis, and mucosal intestinal ulceration. Management of gastrointestinal complications of uremia is described in the later discussion of chronic renal failure. Note that metoclopramide and histamine-2 receptor blockers such as ranitidine and famotidine are renally excreted; doses should be modified for severely uremic animals. Aggressive nutritional support may be required in patients with acute renal failure undergoing long periods of treatment. A diet providing 2 to 3 g protein/kg per day and 70 to 110 kcal/kg per day is optimal for critically ill patients with renal failure. A reduced protein diet is designed to minimize uremia and acidosis associated with acute renal failure. In recovering, mildly azotemic patients, a high-protein diet may enhance renal recovery.[25]

Although often considered a hallmark of chronic disease, anemia may become severe in the course of acute renal failure because of depressed erythropoiesis and hemorrhage. Transfusion support and attention to gastrointestinal or generalized hemorrhage may be needed. Careful attention to aseptic care of intravenous catheters, urinary catheters, and wounds is important to prevent infection in patients with acute renal failure. Neurologic disturbances, including ataxia, stupor, tremors, head bobbing, and seizures, may be observed in animals with severe anemia. Neurologic symptoms may be attributed to hypocalcemia, uremic encephalopathy, cerebral edema, dialysis, or an underlying toxicant (e.g., ethylene glycol). Resolution of uremia, control of hypocalcemia, or administration of low-dose diazepam may be required for management.

Cellular Protectants

Many agents have been investigated as potential cellular protectants or stimulants of cellular regeneration in acute renal failure. Agents such as magnesium, adenosine triphosphate (ATP), thyroxine, and glycine have been considered for their potential to restore intracellular energy stores. Atrial natriuetic peptide (ANP), brain natriuetic peptide (BNP), and other similar peptides increase GFR and have renoprotective effects in ischemic renal injury. ANP has caused severe hypotension in patients with renal failure, but BNP appears to increase GFR without causing systemic hypotension.[26] Oxygen free radical scavengers and calcium channel blockers have been investigated as methods of alleviating reperfusion injury in renal epithelial cells. Growth factors may promote cellular repair and regeneration. Most of these agents remain in the experimental stages, however, and have found limited clinical application in human or veterinary medicine. Manipulation of the cell biology of acute renal failure is likely to provide therapeutic options in the future, however.[27,28]

MANAGEMENT OF CHRONIC KIDNEY DISEASE

Many varied insults can lead to progressive renal dysfunction in small animals. Infectious diseases, obstructive disorders, hypercalcemia, glomerular disease, and some neoplastic disorders may be identified and specific treatment pursued. In many cases, however, a specific etiology is not determined, and management is directed toward alleviation of clinical signs; correction of metabolic consequences; and, ideally, slowed progression of the disease process. Principles of medical management are to (1) stage the disease and pursue appropriate diagnostic strategies, (2) consider renoprotective maneuvers that may retard progression of renal damage, (3) identify and manage sequelae of renal failure (hypertension, anemia, metabolic acidosis, and gastrointestinal ulceration), (4) intervene as necessary in crises, and (5) plan and initiate appropriate monitoring and follow-up evaluations. Excellent reviews of staging criteria and management considerations are available,[29] and updated guidelines are available from the International Renal Interest Society (IRIS) at iris-kidney.org. In general, dietary and other therapeutic maneuvers should be instituted in a stepwise approach, with serial monitoring implemented to tailor management (Figure 18-1).

Pathophysiology

The clinical and pathophysiologic consequences of renal disease result from complex events set into motion as excretory, homeostatic, and other renal functions are lost. When approximately 66% of total nephron mass is lost, fluid excretion per nephron is increased to facilitate waste excretion. Solute diuresis in remaining nephrons and developing tubular dysfunction lead to polyuria and compensatory polydipsia. As nephron loss progresses to 75% or greater, excretory function is compromised and azotemia develops. With progressive reduction in GFR, excretion of phosphorus and endogenous acids is impaired, leading to hyperphosphatemia, hypocalcemia, metabolic acidosis, and secondary hyperparathyroidism. Diseased kidneys also fail to produce or regulate other important metabolic and endocrine compounds, leading to systemic hypertension, anemia, and a catabolic state. Widespread polysystemic effects of uremia are possible as well, affecting gastrointestinal mucosa, neuromuscular function, cardiopulmonary function, and immunologic function. Management strategies are designed to blunt these effects of progressive renal dysfunction (Table 18-2).

Dietary Strategies

Protein

Reduction in protein intake (compared with protein content of maintenance commercial dog foods) has been advocated for dogs and cats with renal disease. Dietary protein restriction has been advocated on the basis of the hyperfiltration theory of progressive renal disease.[30] In rats with induced renal disease, the compensatory response of remaining nephrons includes increases in single nephron blood flow, single nephron filtration rate, and elevated glomerular capillary pressure.[31] These responses are ultimately detrimental in rodent models, leading to progressive renal injury,[30] an effect that can be blunted by reduced protein diets that minimize glomerular hypertension.

Although glomerular hypertension and hypertrophy occur in dogs with experimental renal disease,[32] a significant effect of protein restriction alone on the course of renal failure in dogs or cats has not yet been demonstrated.[33-36] Reduction in protein intake is undeniably beneficial in moderately to severely affected patients by reducing the production of nitrogenous wastes and acid by-products that contribute to uremia and metabolic acidosis. In such patients (usually with blood urea nitrogen >60 to 75 mg/dL or mmol/L), moderate restriction of protein intake can be expected to reduce blood urea concentrations, alleviate metabolic acidosis, and indirectly minimize phosphorus intake.[37] Recommended dietary

Patient Monitoring Flowsheet: Chronic Renal Failure

Date				
Patient History*:				
Current medications				
Current diet				
Caloric intake				
Appetite				
Physical Examination*:				
Body weight				
Body condition				
Hydration status				
Blood pressure				
Fundic examination				
Clinical Pathology:				
Packed cell volume*				
Plasma protein*				
Serum albumin				
BUN/Urea*				
Creatinine*				
Phosphorus				
Calcium				
Sodium				
Potassium				
TCO_2 or HCO_2				
Urine-specific gravity				
Urine pH				
Urine protein				
Sediment				
Comments:				

Figure 18-1 Example of a flowsheet for monitoring the clinical and clinicopathologic features of chronic renal failure. *Minimal components of frequent serial monitoring.

protein intake for initial management is 2 to 3.5g/kg per day in dogs. This level is generally provided by diets containing high biologic value protein at approximately 13% of gross energy when fed at maintenance caloric requirements.[37] The protein requirement for dogs in renal failure is higher than the minimum protein requirements for healthy dogs; however, most commercial maintenance diets are 20% to 30% protein. In cats protein requirements are 3.5 to 4.0 g/kcal per day and may be provided by diets containing approximately 21% of gross energy as protein.[37] Products that provide high-quality protein in homemade diets include eggs, liver, cottage cheese, and lean meats.

Further reduction in protein intake should be reserved for refractory patients in which signs of uremia persist on the previously described diet. Excessive protein restriction may lead to protein malnutrition, hypoalbuminemia, and anemia. Protein or other nutrient deficiencies can inadvertently develop if adequate quantities of a moderately restricted diet are not consumed; intake of adequate energy should take precedence in dietary formulations. Protein depletion also may adversely affect renal function by contributing to alterations in renal hemodynamics and accentuating muscle catabolism, anemia, and acidosis. Animals with protein malnutrition exhibit weight loss, poor hair coats, and muscle wasting. Although reduced protein intake may improve clinical signs of renal disease, this dietary maneuver is unlikely to prevent renal disease in normal animals, dramatically slow progression of renal disease, or enhance renal function. Thus the role of reduced protein intake in animals with early renal disease is less clear. Again, moderate restriction of protein may be appropriate in these individuals, with regular monitoring for evidence of protein malnutrition and for progression of azotemia.

KEY POINT 18-4 Progressive reduction in phosphorus and protein intake is justified in chronic kidney disease in an effort to reduce nitrogenous wastes, acid by-products, and mineral deposition in the kidneys and other soft tissues.

Table 18-2 Drugs Used in the Management of Chronic Renal Failure

Agent	Action	Dosage	Adverse Effects	Contraindications
Agents Used to Treat Hyperphosphatemia/Hyperparathyroidism				
Aluminum hydroxide	Phosphorus binder	30-100 mg/kg/day PO	GI upset, constipation, aluminum toxicity	
Aluminum carbonate				
Calcium acetate	Phosphorus binder	60-90 mg/kg/day PO	Hypercalcemia	
Calcium carbonate	Phosphorus binder	90-150 mg/kg/day PO	Hypercalcemia	Hypercalcemia
Calcitriol	↑ Serum calcium ↓ PTH	2.5-3.5 mg/kg/day PO or 0.75-5.0 mg/kg/day PO, effective dose varies	Hypercalcemia	Hypercalcemia, hyperphosphatemia
Agents Used to Treat Metabolic Acidosis				
Sodium bicarbonate	Alkalinizing	8-12 mg/kg PO q 8-12 hr	Hypernatremia	Hypertension
Potassium citrate	Alkalinizing Potassium supplement	35 mg/kg PO q 8 hr		
Calcium acetate	Alkalinizing Phosphorus binder Calcium supplement	100 mg/kg/day PO	Hypernatremia	
Agents Used to Treat Systemic Hypertension				
Furosemide	Loop diuretic	2-4 mg/kg/day PO	Volume depletion	
Enalapril	ACE inhibition	0.25-0.5 mg/kg PO q 12-24 hr	Renal decompensation, GI upset	
Benazepril	ACE inhibition	0.5-1.0 mg/kg PO q 24 hr		
Diltiazem	Calcium channel blocker	0.5-1.0 mg/kg PO q 8-12 hr (D) 1.0-2.25 mg/kg PO q8-12h (C)	Hypotension Bradycardia	Avoid using with beta-blockers
Amlodipine	Calcium channel blocker	0.625-1.25 mg/kg orally q 24 hr	As for diltiazem	
Atenolol	Beta-adrenergic antagonist	2 mg/kg/day	Hypotension	
Propranolol	Beta-adrenergic antagonist	2.5-10 mg PO q 8-12 hr (D) 2.5-5 mg PO q 8-12 h (C)	Hypotension, bronchoconstriction	
Prazosin	Alpha-adrenergic antagonist	0.25-2.0 mg PO q 8-12 hr (D) 0.25-1.0 mg PO q 8-12 hr (C)	Hypotension, GI upset	
Agents Used to Treat Anemia				
Recombinant human erythropoietin	↑ Erythropoiesis	100 U/kg SC 3 times weekly; taper when target hematocrit reached	Polycythemia hypertension, seizures	Untreated iron deficiency, hypertension
Stanozolol	Anabolic steroid	1-4 mg/dog PO q 12 hr; not recommended in cats	As for nandrolone	As for nandrolone
Agents Used to Treat Anorexia, Vomiting				
Famotidine	H_2 antagonist	0.5-1 mg/kg PO or IV q 24 hr		Severe renal or hepatic failure
Ranitidine	H_2 antagonist	0.5-2.0 mg/kg PO q 12 hr		Severe renal or hepatic failure
Metoclopramide	Dopamine antagonist	0.2-0.4 mg/kg SC, IM, or PO q 8 hr	CNS signs, constipation	GI obstruction, seizures
Misoprostol	Prostaglandin analog	1-5 μg/kg PO q 6-8 hr	GI upset, uterine contraction	Pregnancy, hypertension, seizures
Sucralfate	Mucosal protectant	0.25-1.0 g PO q 6-8 hr	Constipation	
Diazepam	Benzodiazepine	0.05-0.15 mg/kg IV	Sedation	
Agents Used in the Management of Glomerular Disease				
Enalapril	ACE inhibition	0.5 mg/kg PO q12-24h	Hypotension Hypercalcemia	
Benazepril	ACE inhibition	0.5-1 mg/kg PO q24h	Decreased renal perfusion as for enalapril	

Continued

Table 18-2 Drugs Used in the Management of Chronic Renal Failure—Cont'd

Agent	Action	Dosage	Adverse Effects	Contraindications
Fish oil	Omega-3 fatty acid supplementation	Dietary supplement, see labels	Coagulopathy, Gastrointestinal irritation (high doses)	Pregnancy
Aspirin	Cyclooxygenase inhibition	0.5-5 mg/kg PO q 12 hr	Coagulopathy, Gastrointestinal ulceration	
Furosemide	Diuretic	2.2 mg/kg PO q 12-24 hr	Dehydration, Hypokalemia	Volume depletion
Colchicine	Prevent amyloid deposition	0.01-0.03 mg/kg/day PO	Gastrointestinal irritation	Severe renal or hepatic failure
DMSO	Antifibrotic (amyloidosis)	90 mg/kg SC 3 times weekly (diluted solution, see text)	Local effects, Hypotension	Dehydration

PO, By mouth; *GI*, gastrointestinal; *PTH*, parathyroid hormone; *ACE*, angiotensin-converting enzyme; *D*, dog; *C*, cat; *SC*, subcutaneous; *IV*, intravenous; *IM*, intramuscular; *CNS*, central nervous system; *DMSO*, dimethylsulfoxide.

Phosphorus

Restriction of dietary phosphorus is advocated for patients with renal failure to minimize hyperphosphatemia, secondary hyperparathyroidism, and dystrophic mineralization. Feeding to maintain a calcium × phosphorus solubility product below 60 to 70 is recommended to minimize soft tissue and renal mineralization. In experimental studies in dogs with induced renal disease, phosphorus and calcium restriction improved survival times but did not prevent renal mineralization.[38] In a prospective clinical study in cats, feeding a phosphorus- and protein-restricted diet, and administering phosphorus binders if needed, improved survival times from a mean of 383 days to 616 days.[39] Cats fed the renal diet also had reduced plasma urea and phosphorus concentrations when compared with cats fed other diets.

Although phosphorus restriction can be advocated more reliably and earlier than protein restriction, most diets formulated for renal disease are restricted in both protein and phosphorus content because meat proteins are the primary source of phosphorus in the diet. Appropriate canine diets are 0.13% to 0.28% phosphorus on a dry weight basis, providing 0.3 to 0.5 mg phosphorus/kcal, whereas feline diets are approximately 0.5% phosphorus, providing 0.9 mg phosphorus/kcal.[40] Supplemental phosphate-binding agents may be required if dietary restriction is inadequate to minimize hyperphosphatemia and normalize the calcium × phosphorus solubility product (see later discussions of dietary supplements and secondary hyperparathyroidism).

Sodium

Moderate sodium restriction is beneficial for dogs with renal disease, particularly those with systemic hypertension. Although single nephron adaptive responses are remarkably efficient for maintaining solute and water balance in renal disease, handling of large fluid and solute loads is limited, and conservation of water and solute is impaired. Sodium excretion increases with declining GFRs to maintain homeostasis; however, response to a sodium challenge may be impaired, and excess sodium intake could lead to volume expansion. Conversely, sodium cannot be maximally conserved in the presence of acute restriction in intake or volume depletion. Diets should provide 15 to 50 mg/kg per day, usually 0.1% to 0.3% on a dry matter basis.[41] Changes in sodium intake should be made gradually if possible to prevent rapid changes in fluid homeostasis and extracellular fluid volume. A recent study of the effects of dietary sodium intake on renal function in normal cats and cats with experimentally induced renal disease indicated that low sodium intake may actually contribute to hypokalemic nephropathy and progressive renal injury in cats.[42] More research must be done to determine the optimal level of sodium intake for cats with renal insufficiency or failure.

Lipids

Abnormalities of lipid metabolism in renal disease may lead to hypercholesterolemia, hypertriglyceridemia, and elevated low-density lipoprotein concentrations. High saturated fatty acid intake has been shown to accelerate glomerulosclerosis and progressive renal injury in rat models. Dietary lipid composition may be manipulated to minimize hypercholesterolemia, minimize inflammation, and protect renal hemodynamic function. In one study of dogs with induced renal failure, dogs fed a diet supplemented with omega-3 polyunsaturated fatty acids (provided by menhaden fish oil) had reduced intraglomerular pressure, reduced proteinuria, and better indices of renal function than dogs supplemented with omega-6 polyunsaturated fatty acids.[43] Supplementation of omega-3 polyunsaturated fatty acids may be expected to favor vasodilatory eicosanoid production, inhibit intrarenal platelet aggregation, and minimize systemic and glomerular hypertension. Whether any appreciable effect of dietary lipid manipulation will be seen over the long-term course of chronic renal failure remains unknown.[43,44]

Energy

Appropriate caloric intake is a frequently overlooked goal of dietary management of renal failure patients. A catabolic state may be perpetuated despite the best manipulations of dietary content if sufficient calories for body energy requirements are not ingested. Energy depletion and protein malnutrition in turn exacerbate azotemia and hamper renal compensatory or regenerative responses. Energy requirements for patients with chronic renal failure have been estimated at 60 to 110 kcal/kg per day; a reasonable starting point is 75 kcal/kg per day.[31] Frequent monitoring of body weight and body condition is imperative to ensure that appropriate weight is maintained.

As renal failure progresses, intake of appropriate calories becomes more important than the composition of the diet. Caloric supplements composed of fat and carbohydrate sources may be offered to provide additional energy. Occasionally, obese patients with renal disease are encountered. Because obesity may contribute to systemic hypertension and impair other organ system functions, weight reduction is desirable in these patients. Adjustments in weight must be gradual, however, and excessive restriction of calories and protein intake should be avoided.

Dietary Supplements

Intestinal Phosphate-Binding Agents

If dietary phosphorus reduction is ineffective in maintaining a serum phosphorus level of less than 6 mg/dL and a calcium × phosphorus solubility product less than 70, phosphorous-binding agents may be administered.[45] These agents are generally ineffective if dietary phosphorus is not restricted concurrently and are most effective when given just before or with a meal. Liquid or encapsulated preparations are preferable to tablet forms because they more readily mix with ingesta in the intestinal tract. These agents prevent absorption of ingested phophorus or phosphorus secreted in saliva, bile, or intestinal fluid. Tablet forms can be crushed and given with food. Aluminum-based products (aluminum hydroxide, aluminum carbonate) are widely available and are administered at daily dosages of 30 to 100 mg/kg divided into two or three feedings.[46] Magnesium-based products should be avoided in patients with renal failure.[45]

Calcium-based products (calcium acetate, 60 to 90 mg/kg per day; calcium carbonate, 90 to 150 mg/kg per day) are alternative phosphorus-binding agents with additional alkalinizing effects. Calcium-based products can also be used to minimize or correct hypocalcemia. Calcium acetate is recommended in normocalcemic to mildly hypercalcemic patients, insofar as calcium carbonate is more likely to lead to hypercalcemia. Calcium-based products and aluminum-based agents also may be administered concurrently for added phosphorus-binding effects.[37,45] Serum calcium and phosphorus concentrations should be monitored every 2 weeks initially, then monthly or as needed during chronic therapy. Adverse effects of phosphorus-binding agents include nausea, gastrointestinal upset, constipation, and hypophosphatemia. Toxic effects of aluminum are theoretically possible with long-term administration, including anemia, encephalopathy, and osteomalacia.[47] Aluminum toxicity appears to be unlikely in dogs and cats.

Alkalinizers

Although dietary protein restriction helps reduce acid metabolites and metabolic acidosis, alkalinization therapy may be required in animals with moderate to severe metabolic acidosis. Chronic untreated metabolic acidosis may accelerate protein catabolism and azotemia, promote renal ammoniagenesis contributing to progressive renal tissue damage, and lead to increased calcium and potassium losses. Acid–base derangements also likely contribute to the clinical manifestations of renal failure, including anorexia, vomiting, and weight loss.[48,49] Alkalinizing therapy is ideally planned on the basis of serial blood gas analyses. Serum total CO_2 (TCO_2) measurement is a reasonable guide to management in most patients. Oral alkalinization is recommended when bicarbonate or TCO_2 measurements fall below 15 to 17 mmol/L, whereas parenteral supplementation may be needed if the TCO_2 falls below 10 to 12 mmol/L.

Alkalinizing agents include potassium citrate (35 mg/kg orally every 8 hours or 0.3 to 0.5 mEq potassium/kg orally every 12 hours) and calcium carbonate or calcium acetate (100 mg/kg daily).[31,50] These agents are particularly valuable when hypokalemia (potassium citrate), hyperphosphatemia, or hypocalcemia (calcium-based agents) is a concurrent problem (discussed elsewhere). Oral sodium bicarbonate may be administered at 8 to 12 mg/kg every 8 to 12 hours (1 mEq/cat every 8 to 12 hours for cats). Household baking soda supplies approximately 4000 mg bicarbonate per teaspoon (or 12 mEq bicarbonate/g); 5- and 10-grain tablet preparations are also available. Alternatively, a 1 mEq/mL solution of bicarbonate can be prepared by adding 5 or 6 tablespoons of baking soda to 1 L of water (or one third of an 8 ounce box is added to 1 quart of water).[48] Because of the added sodium intake, sodium bicarbonate may be inadvisable in hypertensive patients, and some clinicians prefer to use alternative alkalinizing agents in all renal failure patients. It is questionable, however, whether the sodium salt in sodium bicarbonate contributes to hypertensive disease in dogs and cats.

Dosages of all alkalinizing agents may be titrated to effect. The goal of treatment is to modify bicarbonate concentrations to approximately 18 to 24 mmol/L. Overcorrection of acidosis can lead to metabolic alkalosis, hypokalemia, or ionized calcium deficits.

Potassium

Renal failure and metabolic acidosis have been identified as risk factors for hypokalemic myopathy in cats.[51,52] Increased fractional excretion of potassium is observed, although 24-hour potassium loss is variable. Hypokalemia may be exacerbated by chronic metabolic acidosis, especially in cats fed acidifying diets. Potassium depletion in turn induces acidosis and depresses GFR, intensifying renal disease and potassium loss.[52-54] From these observations it has been hypothesized that supplementation of potassium in cats with renal insufficiency may stabilize or improve renal function. A beneficial effect on renal function and overall outcome in chronic kidney disease has not yet been proven; however, potassium supplementation can increase total body potassium somewhat and appears to be well tolerated.

Most commercial renal diets have been adjusted to provide potassium beyond requirements for healthy animals, but cats with mild to moderate hypokalemia (K 3.5 to 4.5 mEq/L) will benefit from potassium supplementation at 2 to 5 mEq/day.

Low-dose supplementation (2 mEq/cat per day) may be justified in normokalemic cats to prevent potassium depletion.[52] Cats with severe hypokalemia may require intensive replacement with intravenous potassium chloride or increased supplementation (5 to 10 mEq/day). Potassium supplementation may be initiated at 1 to 6 mEq/kg per day if other dietary measures do not correct the hypokalemia.[31] Potassium concentration should be carefully monitored in cats and in dogs undergoing fluid diuresis for renal disease. Chronically, dogs with polyuric renal failure also may become hypokalemic but seem more resistant to this sequela of renal disease. Some renal failure diets may in fact oversupply potassium for canine needs.

Potassium supplements are available in powder or liquid form for long-term oral administration. Potassium gluconate powder mixed in food appears to be the most palatable and best-tolerated product; flavored potassium gluconate elixirs also are available. A relatively new flavored gel preparation also may be acceptable to cats. Potassium citrate solution or diluted potassium chloride for injection (dilute 1:1 with water) also may be given orally. Gastrointestinal ulceration, nausea, vomiting, and food aversion may develop with liquid preparations.

Summary of Dietary Recommendations

On the basis of current information, the ideal diet for small animals in mild to moderate chronic renal failure should be moderately reduced in protein, phosphorous, and sodium content; contain high-quality protein sources; be highly digestible; and provide adequate potassium, nutrient, and caloric density. In a recent study, feeding a diet appropriately modified in protein, phosphorus, lipids, and sodium was associated with stable renal function and delayed onset of uremia in dogs with moderate chronic renal failure.[55] These dogs had a better perceived quality of life, lower risk of death, and prolonged survival (>13 months) compared with dogs fed a maintenance diet. In these studies other treatments appropriate to the stage and consequences of renal failure were initiated as needed, lending support to the long-term benefits of a carefully crafted and monitored treatment regimen for chronic renal diseases. Similarly, in 45 cats with mild to moderate renal failure followed for up to 2 years, cats fed a renal diet had significantly lower all-cause mortality rates and no uremic crises or renal mortality compared to cats fed a maintenance diet. Cats fed the diet formulated for renal disease also had reduced azotemia and acidosis during the study period.[56] The composition and nutrient profiles for commercial renal diets are available in manufacturers' product information and summarized in a review by Bartges and Brown.[57]Dietary supplements or homemade diets may be required to meet the needs of individual patients.

KEY POINT 18-5 The overall effects of feeding a diet formulated for renal disease include enhanced quality and length of life.

Management of Anorexia and Vomiting

The best dietary strategy is ineffective if the patient becomes anorectic, cannot consume adequate calories for energy needs, or is vomiting and intolerant of enteral feeding. Many metabolic consequences of renal failure may affect appetite, including hydration status, severity of uremia, degree of anemia, acidosis, secondary hyperparathyroidism, gastrointestinal complications, and electrolyte imbalances. In the sick, uremic animal, correction of dehydration, acidosis, electrolyte abnormalities, and gastrointestinal complications should be accomplished before attempting to introduce a therapeutic renal diet[58] Supplementation of water-soluble vitamins and correction of anemia also may improve appetite. ACE inhibitors, some antimicrobials, and many other therapeutic agents can contribute to anorexia, and their potential benefit should be reviewed critically in intolerant patients.

In anorectic patients with chronic renal failure, a review of previous diets, dietary habits, and drug therapy is advised. As with all dietary changes, new diets should be introduced gradually, and small, more frequent meals may be preferable for many patients. Owners and nursing staff can tailor the feeding schedule and feeding environment to enhance appetite by avoiding hurried, noisy feeding or feeding in close association with painful or stressful procedures. Some animals respond to hand feeding or feeding during petting and socialization, especially in a quiet ward or outside the hospital area. Warming of food, moistening food, and ensuring easy access to food are practical methods of improving acceptance.[58] Flavoring agents can also be added, including animal fat, bouillon, clam juice, tuna broth, brewer's yeast, garlic, butter, or cottage cheese.[37] An added benefit of flavored liquids is enhanced fluid intake, although broths high in sodium and phosphorus should be avoided. Supplementation of vegetable oils, margarine, cream, or complex sugars may be used to increase caloric intake.[31] If oral ulcers that limit food intake are observed, application of xylocaine gels or cool tea flushes may be used to alleviate pain. Enteral feeding using esophagostomy or gastrostomy tubes are another option for managing chronic renal failure in dogs and cats. They allow easy administration of medications and fluids in addition to providing adequate nutrition to an anorectic or hyporexic patient.

Gastrointestinal effects of uremia include mucosal irritation from nitrogenous waste products, impaired gastrointestinal mucosal barriers, and hypergastrinemia. Central receptors for appetite and nausea also are affected by retained substances and increased parathyroid hormone (PTH) concentrations. Anorexia, vomiting, and diarrhea are common complications of advanced renal failure. In patients with chronic renal failure, sporadic vomiting, nausea, and anorexia may be alleviated by the administration of histamine blockers such as cimetidine (5 mg/kg orally, intramuscularly, or intravenously every 6 to 8 hours), famotidine (0.5 to 1 mg/kg orally every 12 to 24 hours), or ranitidine (0.5 to 2 mg/kg orally every 12 hours). Cimetidine inhibits hepatic metabolism of many drugs, including β-blockers and calcium channel blockers, and should be avoided in patients receiving these drugs. Alternately, administration of a proton pump inhibitor (omeprazole 0.7 to 1.5 mg/kg orally every 12 to 24 hours in cats or 0.5-1 mg/kg orally every 24 hours) may be effective in cases refractory to histamine blockers. The addition of sucralfate, a gastrointestinal mucosal protectant, may be useful for patients with severe gastritis or suspected gastrointestinal hemorrhage. Because sucralfate is most effective in an acidic stomach environment, other antiemetics or antacid medications should be given at least 30 minutes after administration of sucralfate when used concurrently. For refractory vomiting metoclopramide (0.2 to 0.4 mg/kg subcutaneously, intramuscularly, or orally every 8 hours) may be administered to improve gastric emptying and reduce centrally mediated nausea. Dolasetron is a serotonin receptor antagonist that has been used extensively in people to decrease nausea and vomiting associated with chemotherapy and anesthesia. Little published information is available about the efficacy and pharmacokinetics of this drug in dogs or cats, but its use in veterinary medicine is growing. It has potential use in managing nausea and vomiting in dogs and cats caused by chemotherapy; anesthesia; enteritis; and metabolic diseases, including renal failure. A dose of 0.6 mg/kg intravenously or orally every 24 hours is recommended to prevent nausea and vomiting, whereas a higher dose of 1 mg/kg intravenously or orally every 24 hours is recommended for treatment of clinical emesis and nausea. It can be used in combination with other antiemetics, including metoclopramide.[59] Ondasetron, another serotonin receptor antagonist, was shown to be about twice as effective as metoclopramide in alleviating nausea and vomiting in uremic human patients.[60] Maropitant, a novel synthetic nonpeptide neurokinin type 1 (NK1) selective receptor antagonist, prevents and treats emesis and is licensed for use in dogs. The dose of 1 mg/kg orally or subcutaneously every 24 hours for up to 5 days is recommended for dogs to manage nausea and vomiting caused by a variety of factors, whereas a higher dose is recommend for prevention of motion sickness.[61] Maropitant has not been approved for use in cats. One published study concerning its use in cats demonstrated that it is safe and effective in reducing the incidence of vomiting induced in laboratory cats by xylazine administration or motion sickness.[62]

Misoprostol, a synthetic prostaglandin analog, inhibits gastric acid and pepsin secretion and has a cytoprotective effect on gastric mucosa. The drug may be useful in renal failure–induced gastritis at a dosage of 1 to 5 μg/kg orally every 6 to 8 hours. Transient gastrointestinal upset is a possible adverse effect of misoprostol administration that may be managed by adjusting the drug dosage and giving the drug with food.[17] Anorexia or gastrointestinal complications of drug administration must be addressed quickly in patients with renal failure, however, because dehydration and renal decompensation can occur.

Pharmacologic manipulation of appetite also has been attempted in anorectic patients. In the short term, intravenous administration of low-dose diazepam (0.05 to 0.15 mg/kg intravenously) may be successful in reviving appetite or stimulating food intake. Oral administration of benzodiazepines, such as oxazepam, may result in unacceptable sedation. Oral diazepam also has been associated with behavior changes and incidences of hepatic failure in cats. The metabolism of benzodiazepines may be reduced with concurrent administration of cimetidine. Cyproheptadine, dosed at 2 to 4 mg/cat orally every 12 to 24 hours, is an additional appetite stimulant. Other agents, such as anabolic steroids, glucocorticoids, and progestins, are of questionable benefit in stimulating appetite. Glucocorticoids are not recommended for most patients with renal failure because they may promote tissue catabolism, contribute to gastrointestinal ulceration, and result in fluid and sodium retention and glomerular hyperfiltration. Mirtazapine is a noradrenergic and specific serotonergic antidepressant that has been used in dogs and cats for management of nausea and vomiting, although no published data confirm its efficacy and safety.

KEY POINT 18-6 Pharmacologic management plays an important role in ameliorating the effects of systemic hypertension and proteinuria, two key risk factors for progression of chronic kidney disease in dogs and cats.

Management of Systemic Hypertension

In animals with chronic kidney disease, the afferent arteriole dilates, which leads to increased intraglomerular pressure. The kidney is susceptible to hypertensive damage, on account of both elevated systemic arterial blood pressure and intraglomerular pressure. In dogs there is a close association between elevated intraglomerular pressure and progressive renal injury. Systemic hypertension is observed in more than 60% of dogs and cats with renal disease, particularly in animals with glomerular disorders, renal vascular disease, and renal neoplasia.[41] Multiple mechanisms may contribute to the development of hypertension in renal failure, including decreased glomerular filtration, impaired sodium and water handling, local activation of the renin–angiotensin–aldosterone system, and impaired production of renal vasodilatory substances. High systolic blood pressure (>163 mm Hg) in dogs at the time of diagnosis of chronic renal failure was associated with increased risk of developing a uremic crisis and dying, compared with dogs that had lower blood pressure.[63] Controlling hypertension may decrease the rate of progression of chronic renal failure. Clinical signs of hypertension in small animals are usually manifestations of ocular complications, including blindness, retinal hemorrhages, retinal detachment, and glaucoma, but they may include cardiac failure, neurologic signs, hemorrhage, and effusions. Overt signs are often inapparent, however, and blood pressure recordings should be routinely monitored in patients with renal disease.

Moderate restriction of sodium intake is one step in management of mild systemic hypertension. Dietary sodium content of 0.1% to 0.3% sodium by dry matter is recommended for initial management.[41,64] Most commercial "renal" diets provide appropriate sodium content, limiting sodium intake to 10 to 40 mg/kg per day. Sodium restriction should be gradual so as not to precipitate volume depletion. If necessary, additional sodium restriction may be accomplished by feeding homemade diets or diets formulated for cardiac disease.

Pharmacologic manipulation of blood pressure may be indicated in animals with moderate to severe hypertension (systolic blood pressure >180-200 mm Hg), clinical signs attributable to hypertension, or persistent hypertension despite sodium restriction. There is evidence that dogs with renal failure have great variability in blood pressure, and it may be appropriate to initiate antihypertension drugs in dogs with intermittently elevated blood pressure (>160/100 mm Hg).[46] The choice of agent must be based on the potential risks and benefits in the individual animal and the clinician's experience and preference. A variety of agents have been proposed for use in hypertension, including ACE inhibitors and calcium channel blockers, diuretics and β-blockers.

In dogs ACE inhibitors are the first choice for management of hypertension. Inhibition of angiotensin II production leads to decreased aldosterone secretion, decreased blood pressure, efferent arteriolar dilation, and reduced intraglomerular capillary pressure. In glomerular disease ACE inhibitors are helpful in controlling hypertension and minimizing proteinuria. In dogs with experimentally induced chronic renal insufficiency, enalapril was shown to decrease proteinuria and glomerular capillary pressure after 3 and 6 months of therapy, respectively. Dogs receiving enalapril had fewer glomerular and tubulointerstitial lesions than the placebo-treated group.[65]

KEY POINT 18-7 Angiotensin-converting enzyme inhibitors are the first choice antihypertensive agent for dogs. They are administered at low doses initially and titrated to achieve ideal effect without worsening azotemia or electrolyte disturbances.

Potential risks of ACE inhibitor administration include hypotension; decreased renal perfusion; hyperkalemia; gastrointestinal upset; and, rarely, myelosuppression or seizures. Excessive reductions in renal perfusion and GFR are most worrisome because they may lead to acute decompensation of renal failure. To prevent this complication, administration of ACE inhibitors is initiated at a low dosage while blood pressure, blood urea nitrogen, and creatinine concentration are measured. The drug may be slowly increased to an effective dosage. Starting dosages of enalapril and benazepril are 0.25 to 0.5 mg/kg orally per day. Benazepril is less likely to cause renal damage than enalapril and has been shown to decrease systolic blood pressure in dogs and cats. A dose of 0.5 to 1 mg/kg orally every 24 hours successfully decreased blood pressure in cats with experimentally induced renal disease, without decreasing GFR.[66] Irbesartan (5 mg/kg orally every 12 to 24 hours) is an angiotensin II–receptor blocker that will also lower blood pressure in dogs.[67] Further research is needed to determine whether all cats and dogs with chronic renal failure or renal insufficiency would benefit from ACE inhibitor therapy. This class of drugs may be renoprotective without lowering systemic blood pressure.

Calcium channel blockers such as diltiazem or amlodipine also are attractive agents for the management of hypertension in patients with renal failure. Amlodipine (0.625 to 1.25 mg/cat daily by mouth) has become the preferred agent for cats.[68] In dogs that are nonresponsive to ACE inhibitors or in which the drugs are contraindicated, amlodipine (0.05 to 0.25 mg/kg orally every 24 hours) can be administered. Calcium channel blockers reduce blood pressure by peripheral vasodilatory effects; potency varies with the preparation. Calcium channel blockers increase peripheral resistance, leading to a decrease in blood pressure, but they also dilate afferent renal arteriole, which can be detrimental. There are some concerns about possible detrimental effects of calcium channel blockers, which were associated with exacerbation of renal injury, proteinuria, or both in studies of people and diabetic dogs. Newer classes of calcium channel blockers may offer increased renoprotective effects by dilating both the efferent and afferent renal arterioles.[67] Calcium channel blockers also possess cytoprotective qualities that may be helpful in acute or chronic renal damage. Calcium channel blockers are negative inotropes and may cause hypotension, cardiac arrhythmias, and gastrointestinal upset in some patients.

KEY POINT 18-8 The calcium channel blocker amlodipine is the first-line antihypertensive agent for cats.

Diuretics are the mainstay of treatment of early volume-dependent hypertension in human patients; however, they may contribute to dehydration and potassium loss and may be inadvisable for patients with chronic renal failure. The diuretic spironolactone acts by inhibiting aldosterone. Aldosterone has hemodynamic effects that preferentially dilate the afferent arteriole, raising intraglomerular pressure; thus spironolactone and eplerenone (another aldosterone antagonist) may be useful drugs in the management of patients with renal failure.[67] Further studies are necessary.

Beta-blockers such as propranolol and atenolol are agents with negative inotropic and vasodilatory actions. Atenolol (2 mg/kg daily for cats, 0.25 to 2 mg/kg daily for dogs) may be preferred over propranolol because of its duration of action and β_1-receptor specificity. Atenolol is less likely to cause bronchoconstrictive side effects than propranolol.[64] Both diuretics and β-blocking agents appear to be minimally effective in dogs with hypertension of renal failure, although β-blockers may be effective in cats.[69] Clinical application now is limited.

Serial monitoring of blood pressure, hydration status, and renal and cardiac function is imperative for the appropriate management of hypertensive disease (reduction to approximately 150 to 170 mm Hg). Weekly blood pressure recordings should be made initially as dietary and then pharmacologic management is initiated. Biweekly or monthly recordings can be continued during maintenance treatment. Refractory hypertension may respond to combination therapy or addition of a direct vasodilator such as hydralazine. Administration of a calcium channel blocker with a β-blocking agent is not recommended because of additive negative inotropic effects. Control of hypertension in patients with renal failure may slow the progression of disease and minimize the ocular, cardiovascular, and neurologic complications that can develop with uncontrolled hypertension.

Management of Secondary Hyperparathyroidism

Hyperphosphatemia, hypocalcemia, and impaired activation of vitamin D metabolites contribute to the development of secondary hyperparathyroidism in animals with renal failure.

PTH plays an important role in regulating plasma calcium and phosphorous concentrations through effects on the gastrointestinal tract, kidney, and bone. The primary stimulus for PTH release is a drop in plasma calcium concentration; in renal failure phosphorous retention and hyperphosphatemia may lead to hypocalcemia. Additionally, and perhaps more important, impaired conversion of 25-hydroxycholecalciferol (25-hydroxyvitamin D) to the active 1,25-hydroxycholecalciferol (1,25-hydroxyvitamin D, or calcitriol) by 1-α-hydroxylase impairs gastrointestinal absorption of calcium. Calcitriol also plays an important role in the regulation of PTH by exerting an inhibitory (negative feedback) effect on PTH production and release.

The classic effect of secondary hyperparathyroidism in animals with renal failure is the development of renal osteodystrophy, usually seen as "rubber jaw," which results from excessive calcium and phosphorous removal from bone. This complication appears to be rare in dogs and cats but may develop with long-standing disease or juvenile renal disease. Secondary hyperparathyroidism has, however, been implicated as a contributor to many other manifestations of uremia in human patients, including anemia, glucose intolerance, hyperlipidemia, encephalopathies, neuropathies, cardiac damage, muscle damage, and immunologic dysfunction. Furthermore, soft tissue mineralization associated with hyperparathyroidism may contribute to the progression of renal failure.

Dietary restriction of phosphorus, administration of phosphorus-binding agents, and calcium supplementation may be sufficient to minimize secondary hyperparathyroidism in early chronic renal failure (see earlier discussions of phosphorus binders and alkalinizers). Supplementation of the active vitamin D metabolite calcitriol may be valuable in further management of hyperparathyroidism and renal failure. Calcitriol acts to enhance calcium absorption in the intestines, enhance reabsorption of calcium in the kidneys, facilitate PTH-mediated removal of calcium from bone, and directly inhibit PTH secretion.[70,71] Calcitriol supplementation should help normalize plasma calcium and phosphorous concentrations and minimize the clinical and clinicopathologic effects of secondary hyperparathyroidism.

Calcitriol supplementation has been recommended in low-dose (2.5 to 3.5 ng/kg per day)[70] and high-dose (6.6 ng/kg per day)[71] protocols. Formulations of 250- and 500-ng capsules are available; other doses may be prepared by special order from compounding pharmacies. Serum calcium concentrations should be normal, and serum phosphorus concentrations should be maintained at less than 6 mg/dL before initiation of calcitriol supplementation. Frequent monitoring of calcium and phosphorus concentrations is required during administration. The first assessment should be completed 7 to 14 days after initiation of treatment, followed by monthly rechecks. Ideally, efficacy of treatment should be assessed by PTH measurements on pooled blood samples obtained before and during the first 6 months of treatment. The major complication of calcitriol supplementation is the development of hypercalcemia. Hypercalcemia can be managed by adjusting calcium-based phosphorus-binding agents used concurrently, reducing the dosage of calcitriol, or discontinuing administration of calcitriol temporarily and reinstituting the drug at a lower dosage when calcium concentrations return to normal.[70] If phosphorus-binding agents are required to help normalize serum phosphorus, calcium acetate or aluminum-based binding agents may be preferable to calcium carbonate to minimize the propensity for hypercalcemia.

KEY POINT 18-9 When administered and monitored appropriately, calcitriol appears to improve quality and length of life in dogs with moderate-stage chronic kidney disease.

Calcitriol administration reportedly results in rapid reduction of serum PTH levels, normalization of serum calcium concentrations, and subjective improvement in the general well-being of treated dogs.[70] Some investigators advocate its use early in renal failure as a method of improving quality of life in patients with renal failure and as a method of potentially slowing progression of renal disease. However, other investigators reserve calcitriol supplementation for animals in which hyperparathyroidism has been documented.[71] Preliminary results from a double-blind randomized controlled clinical trial of calcitriol administration in dogs with spontaneous mild to moderate chronic kidney disease indicate prolonged survival and reduced mortality in dogs receiving calcitriol. PTH measurements and ionized calcium measurements were conducted frequently so that the dosage could be tailored appropriately; effective doses ranged from 0.75 to 5.0 ng/kg/day.[72] As with other medical manipulations in patients with renal failure, careful monitoring of treatment is essential, with the potential benefits and possible risks weighed for each individual patient.

Management of Anemia

Progressive, nonregenerative anemia is a common complication of chronic renal dysfunction. Moderate to severe anemia is responsible for many of the clinical signs of renal disease, including apathy, lethargy, weakness, poor appetite, and poor body condition. A number of pathophysiologic mechanisms probably contribute to the anemia observed in renal failure, including depressed erythrocyte production, shortened red blood cell life spans, concurrent chronic inflammatory disease, and blood loss caused by gastrointestinal bleeding.[73] Gastrointestinal blood loss and erythropoietin lack appear to be the most important mechanisms of anemia. Dramatic responses to erythropoietin supplementation are seen in some cases.

Recombinant human erythropoietinrh (EPO), a genetically engineered replica of human erythropoietin, became available in the late 1980s and has been used in dogs and cats with anemia of renal failure. Erythropoietin is administered at an initial dosage of 100 U/kg subcutaneously three times weekly until the hematocrit is normalized. A rapid loading phase of 150 U/kg/day for the first week has been recommended for severely anemic (<14% packed cell volume) patients.[46] Target hematocrits are 0.37 to 0.45 L/L in dogs and 0.30 to 0.40 L/L in cats. Initial monitoring includes reevaluation of packed cell volume or hematocrit measurements at 7- to 14-day intervals. In most cases rapid, progressive increases in red blood cell count, hemoglobin concentration, and hematocrit are observed, along with improvement in clinical parameters such as appetite, body condition, alertness, and activity.[74,75] Lower initial dosages (50 to 75 U/kg) may be used if a slower response is desired, in hypertensive patients, or if the drug is cost prohibitive. If a response is not observed in 3 to 4 weeks, the dosage may be increased incrementally to 125 to 150 U/kg three times weekly. If a poor response is seen, the animal should be evaluated for untreated blood loss, iron deficiency, concurrent inflammatory disease. As target hematocrits are reached, the dosage and frequency of administration are tapered, with required maintenance dosages usually at 75 to 100 U/kg every 4 to 7 days. Follow-up monitoring can then be performed at monthly intervals if a stable clinical course has been observed.

Unfortunately, resistance to rhEPO is observed in some dogs and cats after several weeks of treatment. Anti-rhEPO antibodies are formed in 25% to 50%[74] of treated patients, blocking the erythropoietin effect. A rapid decline in hematocrit, red blood cell count, and hemoglobin concentration, along with erythroid hypoplasia of the bone marrow, is observed 4 to 16 weeks after initiation of therapy. Anti-rhEPO antibodies may also interfere with remaining endogenous erythropoietin and result in life-threatening anemia or a transfusion-dependent anemia. Because of the potential development of cross-reacting antibodies, rhEPO treatment is generally reserved for dogs and cats with symptomatic severe anemia, usually when the hematocrit drops below 20% to 25% in dogs or 17% to 20% in cats. Anecdotal evidence suggests that darbepoetin, a second-generation erythropoietin analog with a longer duration of action, may be less antigenic in dogs and cats than rhEPO.

A suboptimal response to rhEPO treatment also may be attributed to depleted iron stores. Iron status, including serum iron concentration and total iron-binding capacity, should be evaluated before initiating treatment and reevaluated monthly or if apparent resistance to treatment is observed. Some authors recommend iron supplementation for all animals treated with rhEPO.[74] Ferrous sulfate is given orally at a dosage of 100 to 300 mg/day (dogs) or 50 to 100 mg/day (cats). Gastrointestinal side effects may be minimized by dividing the dose into smaller doses. Iron dextran can be given intramuscularly to ensure administration; however, anaphylaxis and iron overload are possible. Systemic and intrarenal hypertension are additional consequences of rhEPO administration that may develop as a result of the increased red cell volume and adaptive increased peripheral vascular resistance. Initiation of rhEPO treatment is contraindicated for patients with uncontrolled hypertensive disease. Other adverse effects uncommonly observed with rhEPO administration include allergic reactions, fevers, seizures, vomiting, and polycythemia.[76]

Ideally, recombinant feline and canine EPO would be used in anemic patients with chronic renal failure, but these products are not available commercially. Recombinant canine EPO (rcEPO) was shown to be effective in stimulating erythropoiesis in 19 dogs with anemia caused by chronic renal failure but had less efficacy in dogs with red cell aplasia caused by previous therapy with rhEPO.[77]

The androgenic effects of anabolic steroids also may stimulate red blood cell production in renal failure patients. Androgens increase renal and extrarenal erythropoietin secretion, stimulate erythroid precursors in the bone marrow, and may stimulate heme synthesis. Testosterone esters, nandrolone decanoate, and stanozol are readily available and inexpensive agents, but they may be controlled substances in some areas. These agents have been recommended for their nonspecific effects on appetite, strength, body condition, and general well-being, effects that are largely anecdotal. Administration of anabolic steroids may promote sodium and fluid retention and cause hepatotoxicity, so their use in animals with renal or cardiac dysfunction is not entirely innocuous. For the most part, rhEPO has replaced anabolic steroids in the management of renal failure.[46]

MANAGEMENT OF GLOMERULAR DISEASE

Pathophysiology and General Considerations

Glomerular disease is a common cause of proteinuria and progressive renal disease in dogs and is encountered occasionally in cats. In glomerulonephritis (GN) the deposition of immune complexes in glomerular capillary walls initiates a local inflammatory response, including complement activation, activation of the membrane attack complex, chemotaxis of neutrophils and macrophages, and production of oxygen free radicals. Immune complexes may form in circulation in response to numerous antigens or when antibodies react with endogenous or planted glomerular antigens in situ. GN in dogs has been associated with numerous systemic infectious and inflammatory diseases, including canine adenovirus, bacterial endocarditis, brucellosis, dirofilariasis, ehrlichiosis, borreliosis, neoplasia, pancreatitis, systemic lupus erythematosus, and other immune-mediated and chronic inflammatory disorders (including neoplastic disease). In cats feline leukemia virus, feline infectious peritonitis, polyarthritis, pancreatitis, and other immune-mediated diseases are implicated. Many of these are treatable diseases; however, a source of antigen is not identified in many cases of GN; familial and idiopathic glomerulopathies are recognized.[78]

Proteinuria is a typical sequela of glomerular damage and may be the earliest detectable laboratory abnormality. Leakage of protein across the glomerulus can lead to tubulointerstitial injury and progression of renal damage. In humans, dogs, and cats, proteinuria is linked to progression of renal disease. Two studies have shown that higher urine protein:creatinine ratios in cats are inversely related to survival in cats with chronic renal failure and proteinuria. Benazepril has been shown to decrease proteinuria in cats.[79]

In renal amyloidosis deposition of amyloid A, derived from the acute phase reactant serum amyloid A, predominates. In dogs and cats, renal amyloidosis is usually a component of reactive systemic amyloidosis triggered by chronic inflammatory disease.[80] Familial forms of systemic amyloidosis are observed in the Abyssinian cat and Chinese Shar-Pei dog. In both GN and renal amyloidosis, glomerular surface area, function, and permeability are affected, leading to proteinuria and glomerular hyperfiltration. Ultimately, the nephron becomes nonfunctional; azotemia and renal failure ensue.[81]

Other sequelae of progressive glomerular disease include systemic hypertension, hypercoagulability, hyperlipidemia, and nephrotic syndrome.[41,82] Systemic hypertension develops commonly in glomerular disease as a result of sodium retention and complex intrarenal mechanisms leading to depressed vasodilatory and enhanced vasoconstrictive responses. A hypercoagulable state is favored not only by loss of antithrombin III but also by increased concentrations of fibrinogen; factors V, VIII, and X; and enhanced platelet aggregability in glomerular disease.[82] Dogs with antithrombin III concentrations less than 70% of normal and with fibrinogen concentrations of more than 300 mg/dL are at high risk for thromboembolic events.

Goals of management of glomerular disease are (1) to identify and treat the underlying disease process if possible, (2) to minimize proteinuria, and (3) to manage the consequences of glomerular disease and renal failure as they occur. Additional information about the disease and improved management strategies can be expected if renal lesions are appropriately characterized in biopsy specimens.[78]

KEY POINT 18-10 Pharmacologic treatment should be initiated in dogs and cats with persistent proteinuria (urine protein creatinine > 2.0 or >0.5, respectively). Medical management is most effective when initiated early in the disease process (before azotemia) and when a treatable underlying disease can be identified.

Glomerulonephritis

If an underlying disease process is not found or is not reversible, adjunctive treatments are initiated. Intervention is recommended early in the disease process and should be instigated before the development of renal azotemia when possible. Once a dog or cat is diagnosed with persistent proteinuria (urine protein:creatinine ratio >2 or >0.5, respectively), medical intervention should be considered.[83]

ACE inhibitor therapy should be initiated at the time of diagnosis of GN. Enalapril (0.5 mg/kg orally every 12 to 24 hours) has been shown to decrease proteinuria, serum creatinine, and blood pressure, compared with a placebo, in dogs with idiopathic membranous and membranoproliferative GN.[84] Enalapril is used in proteinuric, normotensive dogs as well as hypertensive dogs with GN. Benazepril has not been objectively assessed for treatment of GN in dogs but may be as efficacious. Dosages should be started low and titrated to effect while renal function and blood pressure are monitored carefully because administration of ACE inhibitors can cause acute decompensation of renal function, especially if volume status is poor.

Immunosuppressive therapy is often considered to counter the immunologic components of glomerular diseases. Corticosteroids, although often potent immunosuppressive and antiinflammatory agents, have potential disadvantages in the treatment of glomerular disease. Steroids may increase glomerular permeability and worsen proteinuria. Steroid treatment may accelerate muscle catabolism, worsen azotemia, contribute to hypercoagulability and thromboembolism, exacerbate hypertension, and immunosuppress already-debilitated patients.[85] Because of these effects and the lack of convincing evidence of the efficacy of steroids in glomerular disease, steroid treatment is generally reserved for patients in which the underlying disease process is steroid responsive, such as systemic lupus erythematosus.[81] One histologic variant of glomerular disease in humans, minimal change disease, is responsive to corticosteroids; if lesions are consistent with this diagnosis in a dog, corticosteroid treatment should be more strongly considered.[78] Other cytotoxic agents such as azathioprine, cyclophosphamide, and chlorambucil may be chosen for immunosuppressive effects in cases of rapidly progressive GN. Human patients with membranous nephropathy respond best to a combination of corticosteroid and alkylating agent.[78] However, efficacy of many of these agents as single agents or in combination has not been adequately determined in dogs. Cyclosporine was not beneficial for dogs with idiopathic GN in one study.[86]

Inflammation may be modified by other means. Thromboxane synthetase inhibitors are effective in decreasing proteinuria, platelet aggregation, and thromboxane generation in experimental models of GN and can prevent histologic development of GN if administered at the time of the glomerular insult.[87] The drug may decrease proteinuria even when administered after the insult.[88] The NSAID aspirin is advocated in glomerular disease for its antithrombotic effects, but it may also influence glomerular inflammation by inhibiting platelet activation and aggregation. Low-dose aspirin administration (0.5 to 5 mg/kg every 12 hours) is designed to allow inhibition of platelet cyclooxygenase without affecting prostacyclin formation, an important vasodilatory compound and an antagonist of platelet aggregation.[89] Low-dose aspirin administration also may reduce the risk of thromboembolic complications in dogs with glomerular disease.[78]

Dietary lipid composition has been shown to affect glomerular hypertrophy, glomerular capillary pressure, and renal function in dogs with experimentally reduced renal mass (15/16 nephrectomy).[90] In humans with nephrotic syndrome, omega-3 fatty acid supplementation has been effective in reducing triglyceride concentration and platelet aggregation.[91] These effects may be important because hypercholesterolemia may contribute to progressive glomerular damage and increased proteinuria.

Dietary protein is also manipulated in glomerular disease. Although protein supplementation may appear logical in patients with urinary protein loss and hypoalbuminemia, moderate restriction of protein has been more effective in minimizing proteinuria and effective protein loss. Recommendations are similar to those for other types of chronic renal failure. Certainly, protein synthesis is affected by dietary protein intake, however, and appropriate dietary protein levels must be determined for individual patients. Sodium restriction also is implemented, as for chronic renal failure, and is particularly important in glomerular disease to prevent or minimize hypertension and edema.

Diuretics may be required for management of the edematous patient with nephrotic syndrome. Furosemide (2.2 mg/kg orally every 12 to 24 hours) is reasonably effective. Patients should be monitored for volume depletion or hypokalemia associated with furosemide administration.

A logical overall approach to the patient with GN is as follows. Baseline measurements of renal function, albumin, blood pressure, antithrombin III levels, and urinary protein loss are measured. Dietary manipulation, ACE inhibitor therapy, fatty acid supplementation and aspirin administration are initiated, and the patient is reevaluated in 1 to 2 weeks. Reductions in the urine protein:creatinine ratio, along with stable renal function, indicate good response. Ancillary treatment for renal failure or nephrotic syndrome may be initiated as needed in individual cases. Although some cases resolve with treatment of underlying disease or spontaneous remission, many cases are steadily progressive. Patients with nephrotic syndrome or established azotemia have a poor prognosis.

KEY POINT 18-11 Dietary management, angiotensin-converting enzyme inhibitor administration, fatty acid supplementation, and aspirin provide the cornerstones for management of glomerular disease. Goals of treatment include a reduction in urine protein creatinine, avoidance of complications, and stable renal function.

Renal Amyloidosis

Renal amyloidosis carries a poor prognosis, especially if renal failure and uremia are evident. Underlying inflammatory and neoplastic diseases should be identified and managed if possible; however, few interventions will affect established amyloid deposits. Dimethylsulfoxide (DMSO) has been suggested in the treatment of amyloidosis. The drug may enhance solubilization of amyloid fibrils, reduce serum amyloid A protein concentrations, and reduce associated interstitial inflammation and fibrosis. The latter effect is most likely to be beneficial in improving renal function and reducing proteinuria. Long-term management of a few dogs with DMSO injections has been described.[81,92] DMSO (90% solution) may be diluted 1:4 with sterile water and administered subcutaneously at a dosage of 90 mg/kg three times weekly.[81] Adverse effects of DMSO include nausea, a garliclike odor, and pain on injection. Oral daily dosages have been described, ranging from 250 to 300 mg/kg per day.[93,94]

Colchicine is another agent that impairs the release of serum amyloid A from hepatocytes and may prevent the production of amyloid-enhancing factor.[78] The agent is used to prevent development and progression of amyloidosis in human patients with familial Mediterranean fever. Like DMSO, the agent is unlikely to be helpful after the development of renal failure. Low doses of colchicine (0.01 to 0.03 mg/kg daily) may be considered prophylactically for Chinese Shar-Pei dogs with recurrent fevers and joint disease, which may be precursors to systemic or renal amyloid deposition.[78,81] Both colchicine and DMSO are most effective in the early phases of amyloid deposition; colchicine may reduce proteinuria as well. As with other types of glomerular disease, metabolic complications such as hypertension and hypercoagulability must be identified and addressed.

DIALYTIC THERAPY

Dialytic therapy is available to remove excess water or solutes from plasma using osmotic gradients across a semipermeable membrane. In hemodialysis the membrane is an extracorporeal synthetic membrane, whereas in peritoneal dialysis the peritoneum serves as the membrane for exchange. By these methods urea, creatinine, and other retained molecules can be eliminated in the patient with renal failure. Although peritoneal and hemodialysis techniques have been described in many animal models, their clinical application in small animal veterinary medicine has been limited by the extensive technical, equipment, and financial requirements involved.[95-102] Dialytic therapy is generally considered most appropriate as a temporary, short-term measure in reversible renal and postrenal disorders. It can, however, be an effective means of supplementing medical management in refractory end-stage chronic renal failure. It is also used to manage feline transplant recipients and cats with ureteral obstruction before surgical intervention. Intermittent hemodialysis has been successful in reducing the average urea concentration in dogs and cats with chronic renal disease and moderate azotemia.[100,101,103] Indications for dialytic therapy in acute renal failure include failure of conservative therapy; refractory oliguria or anuric, life-threatening fluid overload; or life-threatening electrolyte or acid–base disturbances. Hemodialysis also is useful in the early management of toxicoses, especially ethylene glycol intoxication, as well as adjunctive treatment of refractory leptospirosis. In chronic renal failure, dialysis is considered when uremic signs are unresponsive to therapy, usually when azotemia is advanced. The procedure requires reliable vascular access, an appropriate hemodialyzer and dialysis delivery system, and dedicated technical team.[101,103] Currently, hemodialysis is available at the University of California–Davis Companion Animal Dialysis Unit, Davis, California, and San Diego, California; and the Animal Medical Center, New York, New York. Continuous renal replacement may be available at additional specialty centers or veterinary teaching hospitals. The development of additional centers for intermittent dialysis in dogs may increase the application of the technique for improved management and prolonged survival in selected cases. Peritoneal dialysis may be initiated in the practice or referral center setting after placement of an intraabdominal dialysis catheter.[98] Straight, acute peritoneal dialysis catheters are available for emergency dialysis, whereas column disk or T-fluted catheters are preferred for long-term dialysis. Dialysate solutions of 1.5% to 4.25% dextrose are infused to create an osmotic gradient within the abdomen. Substances such as urea, creatinine, phosphorus, electrolytes, and other uremia molecules can pass through intercellular channels of the peritoneum into the dialysate for removal. A dedicated technical support team is required to manage the frequent exchanges and potential complications of the procedure. Peritonitis, hypoalbuminemia, electrolyte abnormalities, and leakage around the catheter are common complications.[99]

RENAL TRANSPLANTATION

Renal transplantation is the definitive mode of management of chronic renal diseases in human patients and has become a viable option in veterinary medicine in selected circumstances. A successful clinical renal transplantation program has been developed for cats at the Veterinary Medical Teaching Hospital, University of California, Davis,[104-106] and is now available at several veterinary referral hospitals in the United States and Canada. With transplantation of a healthy donor kidney and appropriate immunosuppressive therapy, uncomplicated cases can expect good-quality posttransplant survival times of 1 to 3 years. Of 61 cats receiving renal transplants between 1996 and 1999 at the University of Davis, approximately 60% survived 6 months after the operation, whereas the 3-year survival rate was about 40%.[107] Cats 10 to 14 years of age had a higher risk of death, especially during the 6-month postoperative period.[107] The best candidates for renal transplantation are cats in early renal failure, with less than 20% weight loss and no other disease conditions. Candidates are screened for cardiac disease, neoplasia, concurrent metabolic disease, urinary tract infection, feline leukemia virus, and feline immunodeficiency virus.

Immunosuppressive therapy with cyclosporine and prednisolone is initiated perioperatively and continued indefinitely. Treatment is monitored by frequent measurements of trough blood levels of cyclosporine. Potential complications of transplantation include anesthetic and surgical complications, obstruction of the transplanted ureter, infections caused by immunosuppression, pyelonephritis, postoperative hypertension, central nervous system disease, hypercalcemia, and acute or chronic graft rejection.[107,108] De novo malignant neoplasia was diagnosed in 9.5% of 95 feline transplant recipients 2 to 28 months after transplantation and may be associated with immunosuppressive therapy.[109]Transplantation cannot be regarded as a cure for renal disease or an option for emergency treatment of renal failure, but it can be expected to provide an improved quality of life and enhanced survival in some cats with renal failure. Details of the program, surgical procedure, and criteria for case selection are available.[105,106] Canine transplantation remains problematic, although newer immunosuppressive strategies have been developed.[110]

MANAGEMENT OF MICTURITION DISORDERS

Physiology of Micturition

The storage phase of micturition is characterized by sympathetic dominance, with sympathetic innervation to the bladder and urethra supplied by the hypogastric nerve. Activation of β-adrenergic receptors in the urinary bladder facilitates relaxation of the detrusor muscle, whereas stimulation of α-adrenergic receptors in the bladder neck and urethra facilitates smooth muscle contraction and closure of the outlet. Additional urethral resistance is supplied by the striated muscle of the external urethral sphincter. As bladder volume and pressure increase with filling, afferent information is transmitted to the central nervous system by way of the pelvic nerve and spinal afferent pathways. Voiding is initiated by voluntary control centers in the cerebral cortex and midbrain. Efferent impulses are transmitted by spinal pathways and the pelvic nerve in the parasympathetic system, initiating contraction by stimulating cholinergic receptors in the detrusor muscle of the urinary bladder. The sympathetic input to the bladder and urethra is inhibited, allowing outlet resistance to drop appropriately. After complete voiding, the system is reset for storage.[111]

Disorders of urine storage usually result in urine leakage, whereas disorders of voiding result in urine retention, incomplete voiding, or incontinence. Most disorders of micturition can be classified and managed according to the status of urinary bladder (hypocontractile or hypercontractile) and urethral (hypotonic or hypertonic) function.[112,113] Diagnosis is usually based on evaluation of historical, physical, and observational findings, although specialized urodynamic testing is required in some instances. Pharmacologic agents are valuable in the management of functional micturition disorders; manipulation of urinary bladder or urethral smooth muscle tone can aid in facilitating normal micturition. Because pharmacologic activity is directed at the end organ (postganglionic receptors in the urinary bladder or urethra), agents are applied similarly in both neurogenic and non-neurogenic disorders (Table 18-3). Practical reviews regarding the management of major micturition disorders are available.[114,115]

KEY POINT 18-12 Pharmacologic manipulation of micturition is aimed at the target end-organ receptors (in the urinary bladder or urethral muscle), so treatments are applied similarly regardless of the cause of the dysfunction.

The Hypocontractile Urinary Bladder

Problems resulting in hypocontractile urinary bladders include sacral or suprasacral neurologic lesions, acute or chronic overdistention of the urinary bladder, disorders causing general muscle weakness, or dysautonomia. Urinary bladder contraction is primarily controlled by parasympathetic (cholinergic) input. Cholinergic agents have been used to promote bladder emptying in atonic bladders, although the success of orally administered agents is unreliable.[116] Bethanechol chloride is administered at starting dosages of 1.25 to 2.5 mg (cats), 5 mg (small dogs), and 10 mg (larger dogs) every 8 to 12 hours. Full effects of the drug should be apparent within 1 to 2 days. When effective, voiding is usually observed within 2 hours. The dosage may be increased by 2.5- to 5-mg increments up to 25 mg every 8 hours in dogs and 7.5 mg every 8 hours in cats if ineffective.[113] Parenteral administration of bethanechol (2.5 to 10 mg given subcutaneously every 8 hours) may be effective in refractory dogs with bladder atony; however, the likelihood of adverse effects is increased with this route.[117,118]

Table 18-3 Pharmacologic Agents Used in the Management of Micturition Disorders

Agent	Actions	Dosages	Adverse Effects	Contraindications
Agents Used to Increase Bladder Contractility				
Bethanechol (Urecholine)	Parasympathomimetic	Dog: 5-25 mg PO three times daily Cat: 1.25-5.0 mg PO three time daily	Vomiting, cramping Ptyalism, anorexia	Urethral obstruction, GI disease, hyperthyroidism
Cisapride	Smooth muscle prokinetic			
Agents Used to Decrease Bladder Contractility				
Oxybutynin (Ditropan)	Anticholinergic, antispasmodic	Dog: 1.25-5 mg PO two to three times daily Cat: 0.5-1.25 mg PO two to three times daily	Vomiting, diarrhea, urine retention, sedation	Glaucoma, cardiac disease, GI obstruction
Propantheline (Pro-Banthine)	Anticholinergic	Dog: 7.5-15 mg PO three times daily Cat: 5-7.5 mg/cat PO three times daily or as needed	As for oxybutynin	As for oxybutynin
Dicyclomine (Bentyl)	Anticholinergic, smooth muscle relaxant	Dog: 10 mg/dog PO three times daily Cat: not determined	As for oxybutynin	As for oxybutynin
Imipramine (Tofranil)	Tricyclic antidepressant, anticholinergic and adrenergic effects	Dog: 5-15 mg PO twice daily Cat: 2.5-5 mg PO three times daily	Tremors, seizures, tachycardia, excitability	
Agents Used to Increase Urethral Resistance				
Diethylstilbestrol (DES)	Reproductive hormone (female)	Dog: 0.1-1.0 mg/dog PO daily for 5 days, followed by 0.1-1.0 mg q 5-14 days as needed	Signs of estrus, bone marrow suppression, pyometra	Immune-mediated disease, pregnancy
Stilbestrol	Reproductive hormone (female)	Dog: As for DES, *or* 0.01-0.02 daily (see text)	As for DES	As for DES
Estriol	Reproductive hormone (female)	Dog: 0.5-2 mg/dog PO q 24-48 hr	As for DES, GI upset	As for DES
Premarin (conjugated estrogen)	Reproductive hormone (female)	Dog: 0.02 mg/kg PO q 48-72 hr or as needed	As for DES	As for DES
Testosterone proprionate	Reproductive hormone (male)	Dog: 2.2 mg/kg SC or IM q 2-3 days Cat: 5-10 mg IM as needed	Aggression, prostatic disease, perianal disease	Prostate disorders
Testosterone cypionate	Reproductive hormone (male)	Dog: 2.2 mg/kg IM or 200 mg/dog IM q 30-60 days	As for testosterone propionate	Prostatic disease
Phenylpropanolamine	Alpha-agonist	Dog: 1.5 mg/kg PO two to three times daily Cat: 1.5-2.2 mg/kg PO two to three times daily	Tachycardia, hypertension, restlessness, anorexia	Cardiac disease, glaucoma, hypertensive disease
Ephedrine (Pseudoephedrine)	Alpha-agonist	Dog: 1.2 mg/kg PO two to three times daily Cat: 2-4 mg/cat PO two to three times daily	As for phenylpropanolamine	
Deslorelin	GnRH analog	Dog: 5-10 mg depot injection once or twice (see reference for details)		
Agents Used to Decrease Urethral Resistance				
Phenoxybenzamine (Dibenzyline)	Alpha-antagonist, urethral smooth muscle relaxation	Dog: 0.25 mg/kg PO twice daily Cat: 1.25-7.5 mg/cat PO once to twice daily	Hypotension, GI upset, tachycardia	Cardiac disease, glaucoma, diabetes mellitus, renal failure
Prazosin (Minipress)	Alpha-antagonist, urethral smooth muscle relaxation	Dog: 1 mg/15 kg PO three times daily Cat: 0.5 mg PO three times daily or 0.03 mg/kg IV	As for phenoxybenzamine	As for phenoxybenzamine

Table **18-3** Pharmacologic Agents Used in the Management of Micturition Disorders—Cont'd

Agent	Actions	Dosages	Adverse Effects	Contraindications
Baclofen (Lioresal)	Skeletal muscle relaxant	Dog: 5-10 mg PO three times daily Cat: Not recommended	Weakness, pruritus, GI upset	
Dantrolene (Dantrium)	Skeletal muscle relaxant	Dog: 1-5 mg PO two to three times daily Cat: 0.5-2 mg/kg PO three times daily, 1.0 mg/kg IV	Weakness, GI upset, sedation, hepatotoxicity	Cardiopulmonary disease
Diazepam (Valium)	Benzodiazepine, skeletal muscle relaxant	Dog: 2-10 mg/dog PO three times daily Cat: 1-2.5 mg/cat PO three time daily (*or* 0.5 mg/kg IV)	Sedation, polyphagia, paradoxical excitement, hepatotoxicity	Hepatic disease, pregnancy

PO, By mouth; *GI,* gastrointestinal; *SC,* subcutaneous; *IM,* intramuscular; *IV,* intravenous.

Adverse effects of cholinergic agents include muscarinic effects such as salivation, defecation, and abdominal cramping. Vomiting, diarrhea, and anorexia also are possible complications. Overdosage or parenteral administration can (rarely) result in a cholinergic crisis and death; atropine is useful as an antidote. Parasympathomimetic agents are contraindicated in the face of urinary or gastrointestinal obstruction and should be used with caution in animals with bronchial disease or ulcerative gastrointestinal disease. Bethanechol administration may increase smooth muscle tone at the bladder neck and outlet;[119] urethral resistance must be minimized with α-antagonists, striated muscle relaxants, or both before bethanechol treatment is initiated. Intermittent urinary catheterization or indwelling urinary catheterization may be necessary during early therapy to ensure a patent outlet and to maintain a small urinary bladder, facilitating recovery of smooth muscle function.

Recovery of urinary contractile function is most likely in animals with acute overdistention of urinary bladder or with reversible neurologic lesions creating detrusor atony. Alternative pharmacologic agents enhancing bladder motility are lacking; cholinesterase inhibitors, β-antagonists, dopamine antagonists, and prostaglandin treatments have been investigated in human beings but have not received much attention in veterinary patients. Increased urinary frequency and enhanced contractile indices have been observed with cisapride administration in human patients.[120,121] This prokinetic agent increases acetylcholine release at neuromuscular junctions and may ultimately be valuable in stimulating bladder smooth muscle in dogs and cats, but urinary effects remain unproved and availability is limited to veterinary compounding pharmacies.[115,122]

The Hypercontractile Urinary Bladder

Accommodation, or compliance, of the urinary bladder may be affected by congenital disorders, chronic inflammation, infiltrative masses, neurologic disorders, or idiopathic causes. In cats bladder hypercontractility (detrusor instability) has been described in feline leukemia–associated urinary incontinence.[123] Filling of the bladder is impaired, and involuntary bladder contractions occur at low bladder pressures and volumes. Clinically, disorders of bladder accommodation are manifested by urinary incontinence and pollakiuria. Management of urinary bladder storage dysfunction may include treatment of urinary tract infections, correction of neurologic disorders, or pharmacologic intervention.

KEY POINT 18-13 Urinary bladder overactivity is rare in small animals but responds well to pharmacologic treatment. Treatment of urinary tract infection and inflammation and consideration of behavioral disorders should precede trial treatment.

Agents with anticholinergic properties may be used to alleviate the signs associated with bladder contractility or reduced bladder storage function. These agents appear to be quite effective in dogs and cats with idiopathic and feline leukemia–associated urinary incontinence but may be less effective in bladders with severe inflammatory disease, neoplastic diseases, or fibrotic changes. Oxybutynin, with anticholinergic, antispasmodic, and local anesthetic actions on the urinary bladder, has been used in veterinary patients and is available in tablet form (5-mg tablets) and in a liquid syrup. In dogs dosages of approximately 0.2 mg/kg have been effective.[123] Small dogs usually respond to 0.75 to 1.25 mg oxybutynin every 8 to 12 hours, whereas larger dogs may require 2.5 to 5 mg every 8 to 12 hours. In cats a dosage of 0.5 to 1.25 every 8 to 12 hours is recommended.[124] Long-acting formulations have recently become available. Tolterodine is a competitive, pure muscarinic receptor antagonist that is the drug of choice in humans for treating destrusor instability in human beings, which results in a hyperactive or hyperreflexive bladder. It has fewer side effects than oxybutynin, which was previously the drug of first choice.[125] At this time there is not information on appropriate doses in veterinary patients.

Other agents with anticholinergic or antispasmodic activity include dicyclomine, tricyclic antidepressants, propantheline, and tolterodine. Dicyclomine is a similar, less expensive agent that has been as effective as oxybutynin in preliminary studies in dogs. Dosages of 5 to 10 mg every 8 hours are recommended in dogs.[126] Use of this drug in cats has not been reported.

The tricyclic antidepressant imipramine is another agent with anticholinergic properties. Imipramine also has mild stimulatory effects on α- and β-receptors in the bladder and urethra, which serve to further facilitate urine storage.

Recommended dosages of imipramine are 5 to 15 mg orally every 8 to 12 hours in dogs and 2.5 to 5 mg orally every 12 hours in cats.[112] Propantheline is an alternative anticholinergic agent. Recommended dosages of propantheline range from 5 to 7.5 mg as needed in cats (frequency varies from every 8 hours to every 2 or 3 days)[112,127,128] and 7.5 to 30 mg every 12 hours in dogs.[113] Starting doses of 5 mg/day in cats and 7.5 to 15 mg every 12 hours in dogs are reasonable.

Ptyalism is a common complication of anticholinergic administration in cats that can be minimized by placing the product in gelatin capsules. Other adverse effects of anticholinergic agents include drowsiness, ileus and vomiting, constipation, and urine retention. Dry mouth, dry eyes, and mydriasis have been reported in humans. Anticholinergic agents are contraindicated in animals with glaucoma. Many alternative agents have been employed for detrusor instability in people, including tolterodine, β-agonists, calcium channel blockers, and other smooth muscle relaxants. Success rates have varied, and these agents have not been investigated in veterinary medicine.

The Hypotonic Urethra

Reproductive Hormones

Poor outlet resistance (urethral incompetence) is a common disorder of middle-aged, neutered, medium- to large-breed dogs, and predisposing factors include caudal bladder position, a short urethra, poor urethral tone, neutering, breed, and obesity. German Shepherd Dogs, Doberman Pinschers, Old English Sheepdogs, Springer Spaniels, Boxers, Rottweilers, Weimaraners, and Irish Setters are overrepresented.[129] Urethral incompetence can also be attributed to congenital, inflammatory, and neurogenic disorders. Because of the prevalence of this problem in older, neutered animals, reproductive hormone supplementation has been used extensively with good results. Affected animals do not appear to be deficient in reproductive hormones; improved continence observed with reproductive hormone administration is likely due to a variety of effects on the urethra. The major action of reproductive hormones in the lower urinary tract may be sensitization and upregulation of α-adrenergic receptors in the bladder neck and urethra. Mucosal integrity, collagen content, and capillary vascularity in the urethra also are enhanced by estrogens, contributing to a more effective urethral mucosal "seal."[130]

KEY POINT 18-14 Urethral sphincter mechanism incompetence is the most common cause of urinary incontinence in dogs. Most affected dogs leak urine intermittently at rest and respond well to alpha-adrenergic agents, reproductive hormones, or a combination of the two.

Diethylstilbestrol and stilbestrol are effective and reasonably safe choices for female dogs with urethral incompetence. Diethylstilbestrol is initially administered at a total dosage of 0.1 to 1 mg (approximate 0.02 mg/kg) orally each day for 5 to 7 days, followed by a similar dosage administered every 5 to 14 days.[112] Daily estrogen treatment, using minimal dosages of stilbestrol, also has been recommended. The protocol includes starting dosages of 0.04 to 0.06 mg orally administered daily for 1 week and then reduced at weekly intervals to 0.01 mg daily. After 4 weeks the treatment is discontinued. A prolonged residual effect may be observed. If incontinence recurs, the protocol may be repeated or the drug may be administered indefinitely at 0.01 to 0.02 mg/dog daily.[131] Commercially available alternative estrogens include conjugated estrogens (Premarin, 0.02 mg/kg orally every 2 to 4 days and estriol, 0.5 to 2.0 mg/dog every 2 to 3 days). As for diethylstilbesterol, daily loading doses are advised for the first 5 to 7 days. More frequent dosing (two to three times per week) are usually necessary with these preparations.

Response to estriol was studied in a group of 129 incontinent adult spayed female dogs in an open label trial. Dogs were given 2 mg of estriol daily for 1 week, then the dose was reduced at weekly intervals to the minimal effective dose (0.5 to 2 mg/dog every 24 to 48 hours). Veterinarians reported continence in 61% and improvement in an additional 22% of the dogs; owner-reported responses were slightly less favorable.[132] Favorable experience with natural, conjugated estrogen (similar to Premarin) has been described in nine incontinent large-breed dogs followed in a prospective manner. All dogs responded well to estrogen administration; daily administration was continued until 2 weeks of continence had been achieved. In seven of nine dogs in which dose information was reported, maintenance dosages ranged from 0.625 mg to 1.25 mg per dog, administered orally every 12 to 72 hours. In the remaining two dogs, administration every 4 to 7 days was effective.[133] No hematologic effects of estrogen were observed in estrogen-treated dogs in either study.[132,133]

Significant inter-animal variation in accumulation and recirculation of the drug was noted in pharmacokinetic studies.[134] Potential adverse effects of estrogen administration include bone marrow suppression, alopecia, behavioral changes, and signs of estrus, although the risks are minimal when the drug is used properly. Periodic monitoring of complete blood counts is advised for dogs receiving long-term estrogen administration. In addition to toxic effects, estrogens frequently cause signs of estrus in cats and are not recommended in that species.[112]

Many spayed female dogs respond well to estrogen administration. A response rate of 60% to 70% can be expected.[131] A residual effect may be observed in some dogs such that the drug can be discontinued intermittently; however, most dogs require constant treatment and ultimately become refractory to the drug. Dosage and frequency adjustments can be attempted when treatment failure occurs; however, switching to or combining with an alternative agent may be more effective.

Testosterone administration may be used similarly for the treatment of urethral incompetence in male dogs and cats. The potential for adverse effects is significant; effects include aggression, other behavioral changes, prostatic disease, and aggravation of disorders such as perianal adenomas and perineal hernias. Other disadvantages of the drug include the ineffectiveness of oral preparations and its classification as a controlled drug. Testosterone proprionate may be administered parenterally at dosages of 2.2 mg/kg subcutaneously or intramuscularly (dogs) or 5 to 10 mg/cat every 2 to 3 days. Testosterone cypionate or testosterone enanate may be administered every 30 to 60 days at a similar dosage. Some dogs require higher doses; a dosage of 200 mg/dog administered intramuscularly has been effective.[135] Experiences with oral preparations (methytestosterone) for urinary incontinence have not been reported. The many disadvantages of this drug limit its application in the treatment of urinary incontinence, although it may be useful in some neutered male dogs with acquired urethral incompetence. If the product is minimally effective or frequent injections are required, alternative agents should be used.

KEY POINT 18-15 When used at appropriate dose and frequency of administration, estrogen treatment of urinary incontinence is safe in dogs and highly unlikely to cause bone marrow suppression.

α-Adrenergic Agonists

Sympathomomimetic agents (Alpha-agonists) are effective agents for the treatment of urethral incompetence. α-adrenergic agents probably enhance urethral closure through release of endogenous norepinephrine and direct stimulation of α-receptors in the bladder neck and urethra. The agents are usually well tolerated and may be used in animals of either sex. Phenylpropanolamine preparations are effective and available from veterinary suppliers. The agent is no longer found in over-the-counter decongestant preparations. Approximate dosages of 1.5 to 3 mg/kg orally every 8 to 12 hours are recommended. The best responses appear to be gained by starting at a dosage of at least 1.5 mg/kg every 8 hours and then adjusting the dosing frequency after a few weeks. Many dogs can be maintained with once- or twice-daily administration of phenylpropanolamine, especially in timed-release formulations. Ephedrine (ephedrine, pseudoephedrine) is an alternative α-agonist also available in over-the-counter preparations. However, many of these preparations are also under pharmacist control at this time and cannot be purchased in bulk amounts. Dosages are similar to phenylpropanolamine (1.2 mg/kg orally every 8 to 12 hours).[112] Dogs usually receive 12.5 to 50 mg orally two to three times daily. Efficacy of ephedrine compounds is slightly less predictable than that of phenylpropanolamine.

KEY POINT 18-16 Phenylpropanolamine remains the most reliable pharmacologic treatment for urethral incompetence in dogs. Adjustments in dose, frequency, and type of product may improve response in the small percentage of affected dogs with refractory incontinence.

In cats the administration of α-agonists is somewhat problematic. One-half of a 25-mg phenylpropanolamine tablet may be given orally every 8 to 12 hours. Some experts recommend sprinkling 1/12 of a 75-mg capsule onto food twice daily.[136] The effectiveness of α-agonists in cats is questionable, however. Only small portions of the urethra are composed predominantly of smooth muscle and expected to respond to α-agonists. Fortunately, pure urethral incompetence is rare in cats.

Adverse effects of α-agonists include anorexia, weight loss, hyperexcitability, and tachycardia. The author has observed occasional instances of gastrointestinal upset and skin eruption with phenylpropanolamine administration. Systemic hypertension is a serious theoretical complication, although it has not yet been reported with clinical use.[137,138] The drug should be avoided or used cautiously in dogs with cardiac or hypertensive disorders, including renal disease and diabetes mellitus. In human patients the drug is contraindicated in the face of prostatic hypertrophy, hyperthyroidism, and glaucoma.

Response to appropriate dosages of phenylpropanolamine are usually good. Excellent clinical responses or "cures" can be expected in 75% to 90% of dogs,[131,137,139,140] with significant improvement noted in almost all patients treated with the drug. In a large (n = 50) prospective, blinded, placebo-controlled study, Scott et al.[141] found 55% of treated dogs (phenylpropanolamine 1 mg/kg orally every 8 hours) became continent after 7 days of treatment, as opposed to 26% of placebo-treated dogs. After 28 days the percentage of continent dogs rose to 85.7% in the phenylpropanolamine group, as opposed to 33% of placebo-treated dogs.[141] In another randomized, double-blinded study, female dogs responded well to phenylpropanolamine (1.5 mg/kg every 12 hours); 21 of 24 dogs were continent and another 2 improved.[142]

Although most resources recommend administration of phenylpropanolamine two or three times daily for best effect, the dose is adjusted to the minimal amount needed to achieve continence. As with reproductive hormones, it is usually beneficial to start with the optimal dose until continence is achieved. However, a recent investigation in healthy intact Beagles challenges this assumption. Dogs were treated with phenylpropanolamine at once-, twice-, or thrice-daily intervals. Urodynamic changes (increased urethral pressure) were similar for all dosing frequencies, leading the authors to recommend once-daily treatment for incontinent dogs.[143] Desensitization of receptors was suspected with thrice-daily administration. Responses in intact Beagles may not parallel those in incontinent spayed dogs; however, reduced frequency of administration may be effective in some dogs and may prevent development of tolerance during long-term treatment.

Although over-the-counter availability of ephedrine and pseudoephedrine makes their use convenient, outcomes are slightly less favorable with these agents. With ephedrine compounds, 82.4%[144] and 74%[139] continence rates are reported. In another group of nine female dogs studied in a crossover design, improvement in continence score, maximal urethral closure pressure, and functional area of the urethral pressure profile was observed after pseudoephedrine (1.5 mg/kg every 8 hours) administration.[138]

Although most dogs exhibit excellent response to alpha agonists, refractory incontinence does occur. Patients that do not respond tend to be younger dogs with congenital urethral incompetence or dogs in which incontinence develops before or soon after ovariohysterectomy. These patients may respond to an increased therapeutic dosage; combination treatment with reproductive hormones; or other treatment modalities, such as urethral injection of collagen.

Alternative agents currently under investigation include gonadotropin-releasing hormone (GnRH) analogs and duloxetine. Reichler[145] reported their experience with luprolide, buserelin, and deslorelin, GnRH analogs that suppress the release of sex hormone. Their use in incontinence is based on the theory that chronically unsuppressed follicle-stimulating hormone (FSH) and luteinizing hormone (LH) release (due to lack of negative feedback) in ovariectomized dogs may contribute to urinary incontinence. Administration of analogs paradoxically results in reduced FSH and LH over time. In 12 of 13 dogs with refractory incontinence, the drug appeared useful, either alone or in combination with alpha agonists. Deslorelin (5 to 10 mg depot injection) became the preferred treatment in this study. In a subsequent trial, 9 of 23 incontinent dogs treated with long-acting leuprolide were continent for prolonged periods (70 to 575 days); another 10 of the dogs had partial response. These 23 dogs, however, also responded to phenylpropanolamine, with 92% overall reduction in urine leakage.[146] Urethral closure pressures did not increase in these dogs, however. The only urodynamic parameter that changed after depot leuprolide injection in spayed Beagles was cystometric threshold volume (an indicator of capacity and accommodation).[147] There were no apparent adverse effects of GnRH treatment reported in this study, but long-term use of these drugs in dogs has not been evaluated. GnRH analogs may prove to be a valuable long-acting treatment that would alleviate the need for daily or weekly medication; however, availability and cost of GnRH analogs limit their use in the United States.

Duloxetine, a serotonin and norepinephrine reuptake inhibitor, has proven useful in women with stress incontinence and may improve striated muscle resistance as well as bladder capacity.[148] Adverse effects included nausea, fatigue, insomnia, constipation, diarrhea, and headache, but these symptoms were infrequent and mild. Experience is limited in small animals at this time.

For incontinent dogs that fail to respond to appropriate pharmacologic treatment, a search for underlying urinary tract infection, neurologic abnormalities, and other causes of incontinence is indicated. For refractory female dogs, a bulking agent such as collagen can be injected into the urethral submucosa to generate increased urethral resistance. This minimally invasive, endoscopic-assisted procedure provides significant improvement for up to several years and can be repeated when effectiveness wanes.[149-151] Alternatively, surgical options, including episioplasty, colposuspension, or urethropexy, are reasonable for some dogs that fail to respond to medical management.[152,153] Many dogs undergoing urethral injections or surgical procedures require phenylpropanolamine treatment after surgery to achieve the best outcome.

The Hypertonic Urethra (Functional Urethral Obstruction)

Inappropriate urethral resistance may lead to functional urethral obstruction and urine retention. Urethral inflammation or spasm can develop after urethral obstruction with uroliths or urethral plugs. Urethral resistance also may be uncoordinated with bladder contraction as a result of neurologic disorders or idiopathic causes. Urethral resistance also may increase when bethanechol is administered for hypocontractile urinary bladders; the drug also stimulates contractions of musculature at the bladder neck. In these situations pharmacologic manipulation may be instituted to decrease smooth or striated muscle contractility in the urethra and reduce outlet resistance.

Alpha-Adrenergic Antagonists

Alpha-adrenergic antagonists are the preferred agents for decreasing urethral smooth muscle tone and are experimentally effective in reducing overall urethral resistance in dogs.[154] Their activity is less predictable in cats, in which striated muscle predominates in the urethra. Phenoxybenzamine has been a commonly used α-antagonist in both dogs and cats.[155,156] Phenoxybenzamine irreversibly inactivates α-receptors and may have a central effect on striated musculature.[157] The drug is available in 10-mg capsules and is dosed at approximately 0.25 mg/kg orally every 12 to 24 hours.[112] Total dosages usually range from 5 to 20 mg (dogs) and 2.5 to 5 mg (cats). Efficacy may be discerned by judging the quality of urine stream produced. Phenoxybenzamine is expensive and unavailable in some areas. The drug's availability may be further limited because of the discovery of its carcinogenic potential in rats[157] as well as its obsolescence relative to newer alpha antagonists used in human beings.

An alternative, and more selective, α_1-antagonist is prazosin, a drug that has been recommended in the management of heart failure and systemic hypertension in dogs. Extrapolated dosages are 1 mg per 15 kg body weight orally every 8 to 12 hours in dogs; dosages of 0.25 to 0.5 mg every 12 to 24 hours seem reasonable for cats. Because total dosages of 1.5 to 3 mg orally every 8 hours are used for functional urethral obstruction in humans, however, lower dosages may be effective in small animals. Prazosin was shown to produce superior urethral pressure reduction compared with phenoxybenzamine, although prazosin therapy was associated with a significant drop in blood pressure.[158] Additional α-blocking agents have included terazosin and doxazosin.[157,159] No reports are available regarding their use in small animals, although a starting dose of 0.125 to 0.25 mg/dog orally every 24 hours can be extrapolated from human dose recommendations.

Tamsulosin is a newer antagonist that exhibits strong selectivity for urinary α_1 receptors (α_{1A}) over vascular α_1 receptors (α_{1B}), minimizing the risk of hypotension.[160,161] Because glucuronidation is probably required for metabolism, tamsulosin cannot currently be recommended for use in cats. In experimental studies in dogs, doses of 1 to 100 μg/kg intravenously and orally have been used to evaluate the effect of tamsulosin on urethral pressure and arterial blood pressure.[160,162,163] Oral tamsulosin doses of 1 to 10 μg/kg produced dose-dependent blockade of phenylephrine-induced urethral pressure.[163] For clinical application in dogs, 10 μg/kg orally every 24 hours is recommended on the basis of anecdotal evidence.

Silodosin is another commercially available α_1 antagonist that shows even greater α_{1A} receptor selectivity in canine tissues than does tamsulosin and may prove to be a useful therapy, but veterinary clinical data and experience with silodosin are lacking at this point.[164]

Adverse effects of α-antagonists include hypotension, reflex tachycardia, and gastrointestinal irritation. Nausea can be minimized by administration of the drug with food. The drug may be dangerous to animals with cardiac disease receiving other vasodilators or diuretics and to animals with renal disease, in which drops in perfusion pressure could precipitate an acute crisis. Any evidence of weakness should prompt withdrawal of the drug or adjustment of the dosage.

Striated Muscle Relaxants

If manipulation of urethral smooth muscle does not sufficiently improve voiding, addition of a striated muscle relaxant may be considered. Striated muscle relaxants are particularly useful in dysuric patients with upper motor neuron lesions and in cats with functional urethral obstruction. In this species striated muscle predominates in the distal urethra and likely contributes most to functional obstruction. The most common muscle relaxant used for urethral resistance is the benzodiazepine diazepam. The drug serves as a short-acting muscle relaxant by centrally mediated actions, and its effect on urethral striated muscle is variable.

Diazepam (0.2 to 0.5 mg/kg orally) is recommended as a temporary agent to facilitate bladder expression or to augment weak voiding; the agent is given 15 to 30 minutes before expression.[156] Dosages for cats range from 1.25 to 2.5 mg/cat every 8 to 12 hours; sedation is common with higher dosages.[155,156] In dogs total dosages of 2 to 10 mg/dog are given.[117,118] Adverse effects of diazepam administration include sedation, weakness, and paradoxical excitement. In cats behavior changes and idiosyncratic hepatotoxicity are additional concerns. Alprazolam is a reasonable alternative if chronic administration is needed.

Dantrolene is an alternative striated muscle relaxant that has been investigated in cats. Dantrolene acts as a direct muscle relaxant by inhibiting calcium movement from the sarcoplasmic reticulum in muscle cells. The agent (1 mg/kg, administered intravenously) was effective in reducing segmental urethral pressures in healthy male cats[165] and in moderately reducing urethral pressures in a small group of recently obstructed cats.[166] The effect on urethral musculature was enhanced by the concurrent administration of prazosin.[166] Recommended oral dosages are 1 to 5 mg/kg orally every 8 hours in dogs and 0.5 to 2 mg/kg orally every 8 hours in cats.[167] Potential adverse effects include sedation, dizziness, weakness, and gastrointestinal upset; the drug is contraindicated in patients with cardiopulmonary disease. Hepatotoxicity is a worrisome adverse effect of dantrolene administration in humans, usually after long-term treatment at high dosages.[17] Although oral dantrolene has been recommended for several years, clinical reports regarding its use in small animals are lacking. Other striated muscle relaxants include baclofen, cyclobenzaprine, and botulinum toxin injections.[159] On the basis of anecdotal reports relayed to the authors, baclofen cannot be recommended because of poor tolerance of the drug in dogs and cats.

Treatment of detrusor–urethral dyssynergia has been unrewarding in reported cases.[155,168-170] In the authors' experience, dogs with dysfunctional voiding in the absence of compressive neurologic disease are often responsive to manipulation of smooth muscle resistance.[171] Pharmacologic manipulation of urethral tone in cats with dyssynergia or functional obstruction and dogs with suspected striated urethral dyssynergia is less rewarding. Recovery is also related to the degree of detrusor damage sustained by the time of diagnosis. In chronic cases circumvention of urethral resistance using intermittent urinary catheterization or urethral stents may be necessary for temporary or prolonged relief of obstruction.[159]

PHARMACOLOGIC AGENTS THAT TARGET URETERAL MOTILITY

With an increase in obstructive ureteroliths observed in small animal practice, interest in pharmacologic strategies to promote passage of ureteroliths through the urethra has increased. Fluid therapy and diuretics may be useful in increasing urine flow and hydrostatic pressure proximal to a ureterolith, but this approach must be done with caution so that affected animals, especially those with complete obstruction, are not overhydrated. Alleviating ureteral spasm can be attempted. Alpha antagonists, calcium channel blocking agents, and antiinflammatory agents can facilitate ureteral relaxation.[172] These drugs do appear to facilitate ureterolith passage in humans but have not been well studied in dogs or cats. Glucagon appears to reduce ureteral contractions in dogs and has been used in cats with ureteral obstruction. In cats, however, the drug did not appear overly efficacious and can lead to acute adverse reactions, characterized by tachypnea, dyspnea, and gastrointestinal signs.[173] Amitriptyline, a tricyclic antidepressant, reduced smooth muscle activity in human and pig ureteral segments in ex vivo studies. Further study of the effects of amitriptyline on feline ureters is warranted. Tamsulosin (see the discussion of the hypertonic urethra in this chapter) has become the agent of choice for medical management of small ureteroliths in humans.

DRUGS USED IN THE MANAGEMENT OF FELINE LOWER URINARY TRACT DISEASE

Idiopathic hematuria, dysuria, and urethral obstruction represent a common clinical problem encountered in cats. *Feline urologic syndrome, idiopathic feline lower urinary tract disease (iFLUTD), idiopathic feline cystitis,* and *feline interstitial cystitis* all are terms that have been used to describe this combination of clinical signs when urinary tract infection, urolithiasis, neoplasia, and other causes have been ruled out. Many pharmacologic agents and treatment strategies have been proposed to manage this disorder and prevent its recurrence. The apparent efficacy of any treatment for cats with idiopathic disease should be considered in light of the usual self-limiting nature of this disorder, and pharmacologic agents should be administered only after assessment of the likely benefits and possible risks of each treatment.[127,174] Recent publications suggest a relationship among stress, alterations in the feline nervous system, and the development of iFLUTD, with an increased emphasis on environmental and behavioral influences.[175-177] Moisture intake and environmental modifications appear to be the most effective treatments in cats with recurrent idiopathic disease; however, pharmacologic agents have a place in short-term symptomatic relief and in reducing discomfort and recurrence in refractory cases.

KEY POINT 18-17 Idiopathic lower urinary tract signs in cats are usually self-limiting. Pharmacologic agents are reserved for cats with refractory idiopathic cystitis, after dietary, water intake, and environmental modifications have failed to sufficiently alleviate recurrences.

HISTORICAL TREATMENT STRAGEGIES

Urinary Acidifiers

Manipulation of urine pH, usually by dietary means, has been a long-standing strategy for management of feline lower urinary tract disease (FLUTD). The strategy is most likely to be helpful in cats in which struvite crystalluria is a significant component of obstructive FLUTD and does not eliminate recurrence in all cats with idiopathic disease.[127,178] Most urologic diets are designed to promote acid to neutral urine in fed cats; additional acidification is rarely necessary or wise.

Overacidification is another possible complication of urine acidification in cats; young cats and cats with renal insufficiency are most susceptible. Long-term administration of urinary acidifiers may contribute to metabolic acidosis, hypokalemia, bone and mineral imbalances, renal failure, and calcium oxalate urolithiasis.[179-181] Heinz body anemia and methemoglobinemia have been observed in kittens treated with DL-methionine as well as in adult cats treated with high dosages.[182] Arrhythmias and central nervous system depression are serious complications of high-dose ammonium chloride administration. Both agents are contraindicated in patients with hepatic disease because the administration of an ammonium load may potentiate hepatoencephalopathy. Serial monitoring of clinical status, complete blood counts, acid–base, and electrolytes is recommended during therapy.

Urinary Antiseptics

Urinary antiseptic agents have been considered as adjunctive treatment in FLUTD because of their antiviral activity.[127] Viruses including herpesvirus, feline syncytia-forming virus, and feline calicivirus have been implicated in the etiopathogenesis of FLUTD, although a consistent cause-and-effect relationship has been difficult to establish. The agents are more commonly used for antibacterial and antifungal properties, but these are uncommon causes of urinary disease in cats. The most commonly suggested antiseptic for small animal usage is methenamine, a cyclic hydrocarbon administered in combination with either mandelic acid (methenamine mandelate) or hippuric acid (methenamine hippurate). Mandelic acid and hippuric acid serve to acidify the urine and may exhibit some additional antimicrobial activity. With sufficient contact time in acidic urine, methenamine is converted to formaldehyde, a potent antimicrobial agent. Methenamine is contraindicated for patients with renal or hepatic insufficiency, and its use may contribute to overacidification like other urinary acidifiers. Use of other antiseptics or analgesics containing methylene blue or azodyes is discouraged in cats because of the potential for development of Heinz body hemolytic anemia.

Glucocorticoids

Glucocorticoids have been recommended to alleviate urinary bladder or urethral inflammation in cats with iFLUTD. Anti-inflammatory effects of glucocorticoids on leukocyte migration, vascular permeability, and arachidonic acid metabolism would be expected to suppress the inflammatory symptomatology and hematuria associated with this disorder. Treatment is based on the assumption that persistent inflammation leads to hematuria. Although it appears that glucocorticoids do little to alter the course of typical iFLUTD,[183] some clinicians recommend glucocorticoid administration (prednisone or prednisolone 1 to 2 mg/kg every 24 hours) in cats exhibiting chronic, recurrent, or refractory idiopathic hematuria and dysuria.[184] No convincing evidence has been presented to establish that glucocorticoids alter the natural course of iFLUTD or prevent recurrence, however.

Glucocorticoid administration also presents certain risks. Refractory urinary tract infection and pyelonephritis may develop, especially when glucocorticoids are administered to cats with indwelling urinary catheters.[185] Prophylactic antimicrobial treatment does not appear to reduce the risk of catheter-induced infection. Glucocorticoids must be considered contraindicated for cats with urinary catheters in place or with evidence of bacteriuria. The catabolic effects of glucocorticoids also may be hazardous in debilitated, azotemic, or dehydrated cats.[127]

CONTEMPORARY TREATMENT STRATEGIES

Antispasmodic Agents

Agents that relax smooth or striated muscle of the urinary tract have been advocated for symptomatic relief of pollakiuria, dysuria, and stranguria in cats with FLUTD.[128,184,186] The anticholinergic agents propantheline and oxybutynin have been recommended for their antispasmodic effects on the urinary bladder. In one small controlled study, propantheline administration did not affect resolution of clinical signs at 5 days after treatment compared with placebo administration;[187] however, this agent has little direct smooth muscle relaxant properties. If antispasmodic agents are administered, cats should be monitored for urine retention; the loss of a frequent mechanical washout of urine theoretically could delay resolution of inflammation or predispose cats to urinary tract infection.

Agents acting on urethral musculature also have been recommended to facilitate urination in dysuric cats and to alleviate functional urethral obstruction in postobstructed cats. Phenoxybenzamine and prazosin are α-adrenergic antagonists that serve to inhibit urethral smooth muscle contracture. These agents may be helpful in minimizing resistance in the preprostatic and prostatic portions of the urethra in cats;[188-189] striated muscle components of the urethra are not affected. Diazepam or dantrolene may be more effective in relaxing skeletal muscle in the postprostatic urethra.[165,166,189] Phenothiazine derivatives, such as acepromazine[188] and aminopropazine, may also be effective as direct smooth and striated muscle relaxants and can be particularly useful in minimizing anxiety of acutely affected cats.

Analgesia

For acute flare-ups of lower urinary tract signs, short-term analgesic treatments may be useful to reduce the discomfort associated with bladder and urethral inflammation. Butorphanol (0.5 to 1.25 mg/cat orally every 4 to 6 hours) has been recommended;[190] longer-acting buprenorphine can be considered as well. Both agents can be given as subcutaneous injections if this is less stressful to the cat.[186] NSAIDs have also been recommended for analgesic and antiinflammatory effects. No controlled studies are available to demonstrate a response from any of these agents.

Anxiolytic Agents

A variety of other agents have been considered for treatment of nonseptic, idiopathic inflammatory cystitis (interstitial cystitis [IC]) in human patients, and many have been suggested for similar usage in cats. In some ways the disease in cats does appear to mimic IC in women, a disorder characterized by dysuria, pollakiuria, and painful urination without demonstrable cause. Pathophysiologic mechanisms identified in women with IC have been documented in affected cats,[178,191-193] including increased mast cell numbers in the urinary bladder, decreased urinary glycosaminoglycan excretion,[191] and altered urinary bladder permeability.[193]Additional investigations have focused on the influence of neurogenic mediators of inflammation in IC, in which sensory input from afferent neurons in the urinary bladder may trigger inflammatory and pain responses.[192]

A variety of anxiolytic and antidepressant agents have been investigated in IC, including antihistamines, doxepin, and amitriptyline (Elavil). Amitriptyline is a tricyclic antidepressant with multiple actions, including (1) potentiation of neurotransmitter activity in the central nervous system, (2) inhibition of histamine release, (3) potent antihistaminic properties, and (4) anticholinergic activity.[194] As an antidepressant and antianxiety agent, amitriptyline has been used in small animals for behavioral modification, elimination disorders, chronic pruritus, and self-mutilation.[195,196] The agent has shown promise for the treatment of IC in women and has been recommended for alleviation of anxiety and pain associated with iFLUTD.[192] Eleven of fifteen cats treated with amitriptyline were free of chronic iFLUTD signs for 6 months in one study, and nine were asymptomatic for 12 months or longer.[197]

Amitriptyline may be less effective for treating acute than chronic episodes of iFLUTD. Amitriptyline administration (5 mg/day orally) had no beneficial effect in treating 31 cats with acute, nonobstructive iFLUTD, and they were significantly more likely to have recurrence of hematuria and pollakiuria within 7 days of discontinuation of amitriptyline, compared with cats administered a placebo. Clinical signs usually resolved within 7 days, regardless of whether a placebo or amitriptyline was administered.[198] A second placebo-controlled study of 24 cats with iFLUTD did not show a benefit of daily amitriptyline (10 mg/cat) administered for 1 week.[199]

For cats in which amitriptyline is indicated, a starting dosage of 5 mg/cat every 24 hours is empirically recommended; the dose is adjusted to effect a mild calming behavior in the cat, which is usually achieved with dosages of 2.5 to 12.5 mg/cat per day.[192] Long-term treatment is recommended, along with elimination of environmental stresses, in cats affected by severe, recurrent idiopathic disease. Adverse effects of amitriptyline administration in human patients include anticholinergic effects (dry mouth, blurred vision, constipation), hypotension, drowsiness, and cardiac arrhythmias.[194] Sedation, vomiting, and disorientation have been reported in dogs treated with the drug,[195] whereas transient sedation has been the most common adverse effect observed in cats. Amitriptyline may also predispose to bacterial cystitis by causing urinary retention and decreased frequency of urination.[198] Clomipramine (0.5 mg/kg/day) is a good alternative anxiolytic agent that seems to be more tolerable for cats.

Behavioral-modification drugs have been used in treatment of iFLUTD, but results are only anecdotal. Fluoxetine and paroxetine, two selective serotonin reuptake inhibitors, have been used with some success to treat compulsive disorders in cats and dogs. They are dosed at 0.5 to 1 mg/kg orally every 24 hours. Although considered safe, sedation, anxiety, poor appetite, constipation, lowered seizure threshold, and difficulty in controlling diabetic patients are possible side effects. These drugs should not be used concurrently with monoamine oxidase inhibitors, selegiline, or L-tryptophan.[200] In a recent prospective clinical trial involving 12 cats, feline facial pheromone was compared with a placebo as treatment for iFLUTD. Although there was no statistical differences between the two groups, more of the pheromone-treated cats had less severe and fewer episodes of iFLUTD,[201] and further studies are warranted. Modification of environment and attention to behavioral issues must be done concurrently to minimize the neuroendocrine influences on the disease. Environmental enrichment, reduction in intercat conflict or aggression, change of feeding method, and litter box management are included in the potential modifications.[176]

Glycosaminoglycans

Pentosan polysulfate (PPS; Elmiron) is a synthetic polysaccharide that augments the protective glycosaminoglycan layer of the urinary bladder. Orally administered PPS has resulted in good long-term responses (>6 to 12 months) in some women with IC[202] and may be effective in reducing clinical episodes in cats with recurrent or chronic idiopathic disease. The currently recommended dosage for cats is 8 mg/kg orally every 12 hours.[190] Oral glucosamine has been suggested as an alternative glycosaminoglycan. In a controlled study of 40 cats treated for 6 months, there was no difference in owner assessments of each cat's health and number of days with lower urinary tract signs between glucosamine-treated cats and placebo-treated cats.[201] Cats in both groups were somewhat improved owing to the introduction of canned cat food; however, recurrences were still frequent.

INTRAVESICULAR AGENTS USED IN LOWER URINARY TRACT DISEASE

Infusion of antimicrobial and antiinflammatory agents into the urinary bladder has been attempted as a form of local therapy in dogs and cats with lower urinary tract disease. The idea of directly applying antiseptic, antiinflammatory, or analgesic agents to diseased mucosa is enticing. Even saline infusion may provide symptomatic relief of lower urinary tract symptoms. Simple urohydrodistention provides temporary relief of symptoms in some women with IC.[203] Presumably, extreme distention of the urinary bladder may stimulate and exhaust mast cell degranulation, induce urinary glycosaminoglycan production, and cause ischemic degeneration of bladder sensory nerve endings. Released inflammatory mediators also can be flushed with the infused solution. Instillation of solutions into the urinary bladder requires placement of a urinary catheter, however, and urohydrodistention requires general or regional anesthesia. Furthermore, agents instilled into the urinary bladder often are rapidly voided and may be altered with inflammation; enhanced permeability to salicylate infusion has been documented in cats with idiopathic cystitis.[193] Thus the risk of significant systemic absorption of intravesicular agents is difficult to predict.

Antifungal Agents

Primary fungal infections of the lower urinary tract are rare, and *Candida* spp. are the most common cause of funguria in dogs and cats. *Candida* spp. are normal florae of the gastrointestinal system, upper respiratory tract, and genital mucosa. Infections in dogs and cats are usually due to *Candida albicans,* although other species have been reported. Candiduria in humans occurs when predisposing factors are present, such as indwelling urinary catheters, diabetes mellitus, drug therapy (antibiotic, steroids, cancer chemotherapeutic), and lower urinary disease. In dogs and cats, these same factors are likely to be relevant. In a report of 31 cases of candiduria in dogs and cats, 35% of the patients had diabetes mellitus.[204]

Unlike management of funguria in humans, in which correction of the underlying condition often resolves the infection, treatment of all cases of funguria in dogs and cats is recommended. The drug of first choice in humans with a persistent infection is fluconazole, and this is likely true for dogs and cats. The condition should be managed as a complicated urinary tract infection, and treatment should be continued for at least 2 to 4 weeks, with resolution confirmed by negative urine culture. If the infection persists beyond 4 weeks of therapy, then antifungal susceptibility testing should be done because *Candida* organisms can develop resistance to azole drugs.[204] Previously reported doses of fluconazole are 2.5 to 5 mg/kg orally every 24 hours in dogs and 2.5 to 10 mg/kg orally every 12 hours in cats.[17] An alternative treatment to oral or injectable antifungals is intravesicular infusions of 1% clotrimazole into the urinary bladder, using a Foley catheter. A dose of 9 mL/kg infused by a urinary catheter weekly for 3 weeks was successful in treating a diabetic cat. A diabetic dog was successfully treated with 7 mL/kg injected into the bladder, with ultrasound assistance, for four treatments. This treatment may be a useful alternative to oral fluconazole, although further studies are needed to prove efficacy and safety.[204]

Dimethylsulfoxide

The free radical scavenging agent DMSO has been applied intravesicularly as a local antiinflammatory and analgesic agent. The drug and its metabolites neutralize free radical hydroxides and free radical oxygen, modulate platelet aggregation and prostaglandin metabolism, decrease fibroplasia, and provide local analgesia. In high concentrations DMSO may have antibacterial activity, but it also creates mucosal edema and hemorrhage.[205] The agent has been used in the management of interstitial and radiation-induced cystitis in human patients, cyclophosphamide-induced cystitis in dogs, and idiopathic cystitis in cats.[184,203,206] DMSO infusion may be considered for cats with chronic, refractory idiopathic disease, especially those with thickened urinary bladder walls.

The treatment regimen for cats involves instillation of 10 to 20 mL of 10% medical grade DMSO (Rimso-50) into the urinary bladder with the cat under general anesthesia. The solution is left in the urinary bladder for 10 minutes and then removed. The process can be repeated 2 weeks after the initial application if needed.[184] Up to 25 mL of 25% to 50% intravesicular DMSO is empirically recommended for dogs. In cats instillation of 45% veterinary grade DMSO for 3 days after induction of salicylate/ethanol bladder wall injury did not alter the subsequent inflammatory response or infection rate.[185] The drug also may have contributed to renal lesions observed in these cats and appeared to be locally irritating.[185] Intravascular hemolysis and hemoglobinuria may result if significant quantities of DMSO are absorbed.

Bacillus Calmette–Guérin Therapeutic

Bacillus Calmette–Guérin (BCG) Therapeutic is a bacterial product of attenuated *Mycobacterium bovis,* with muramyl dipeptide as the predominant active compound. Intravesicular BCG cell wall infusion is used as an alternative to radical surgery in human patients with carcinoma of the urinary bladder. The agent promotes a local inflammatory reaction that appears to suppress superficial cancerous lesions by incompletely understood mechanisms.[207] Effects of T cells and natural killer cells also lead to its use as an immunostimulant. The agent must be administered by way of nontraumatic urethral catheterization and handled as hazardous infectious material. Local irritation and hematuria are commonly observed after infusion; systemic adverse effects are rare but may include fever, nausea, diarrhea, anemia, leukopenia, ureteral obstruction, shock, and death. The agent is contraindicated for patients with urinary tract infections or fevers and those receiving immunosuppressive therapy. In dogs injection of intralesional BCG has been variably helpful during surgical resection of transitional cell carcinomas. Severe granulomatous reactions are possible.

Infusion of other chemotherapeutic agents (doxorubicin, thiotepa) is rarely attempted in veterinary medicine because of the advanced stage of disease usually present at diagnosis. Local infusions are not expected to penetrate beyond the submucosa, whereas most neoplasms have infiltrated the muscularis or serosa in small animals.[208]

Piroxicam

Piroxicam (Feldene), a potent NSAID, appears to have antitumor activity in some animals with urinary tract neoplasia.[209] In dogs with transitional cell carcinoma, sustained remissions are possible in selected individuals, whereas maintenance of stable disease may be obtained in many. For neoplastic disease, piroxicam is administered daily at 0.3 mg/kg/day. Piroxicam (administered daily or every other day) also has been considered for the treatment of chronic inflammatory bladder disorders. Clinical experience supports this practice; the safety and efficacy of the drug have not been critically evaluated, however.[174] Gastrointestinal ulceration is common; concurrent administration of gastrointestinal protectants is recommended.

REFERENCES

1. Mazzaferro EM, Eubig PA, Hackett TB, et al: Acute renal failure associated with raisin or grape ingestion in 4 dogs, *J Veter Emerg Crit Care* 14:203, 2004.
2. Toto RD: Renal insufficiency due to angiotensin-converting-enzyme inhibitors, *Miner Electrolyte Metab* 20:193, 1994.
3. Longhofer SL, Ericsson GF, Cifelli S, Benitz AM: Renal function in heart failure dogs receiving furosemide and enalapril maleate, *J Vet Intern Med* 7:123, 1993.
4. Murray MD, Brater DC: Renal toxicity of the nonsteroidal anti-inflammatory drugs, *Annu Rev Pharmacol Toxicol* 32:435, 1993.
5. Forrester SD, Lees GE: Renal manifestations of polysystemic diseases. In Osborne CA, Finco DR, editors: *Canine and feline nephrology and urology*, Baltimore, 1995, Williams & Wilkins, p 491.
6. Lobetti RG, Jacobson LS: Renal involvement in dogs with babesiosis, *J S Afr Vet Assoc* 72:23, 2001.
7. Lane IF, Grauer GF, Fettman MJ: Acute renal failure: Part I: Risk factors, prevention and strategies for protection, *Compend Contin Educ Pract Vet* 16:15, 1994.
8. Chew DJ: Fluid therapy during intrinsic renal failure. In Dibartola SP, editor: *Fluid therapy in small animal practice*, Philadelphia, 1992, Saunders, p 554.
9. Cowgill LD, Francey T: Acute uremia. In Ettinger SJ, Feldman E, editors: *Textbook of veterinary internal medicine*, ed 6, St Louis, 2005, Saunders.
10. MacIntyre DK, Royer N: Management of acute renal failure in critical patients: technical concerns, Lake Buena Vista, Fla, 1995, Proc 13th Am Coll Vet Intern Med Forum, p. 10.
11. Adelman RD, Spangler WL, Beasom F, et al: Furosemide enhancement of experimental gentamicin nephrotoxicity: comparison of functional and morphological changes with activities of urinary enzymes, *J Infect Dis* 140:342, 1979.
12. Lindner A, Cutler RE, Goodman WG: Synergism of dopamine plus furosemide in preventing acute renal failure in the dog, *Kidney Int* 16:158, 1979.
13. Adin DB, Taylor AW, Hill RC, et al: Intermittent bolus injection versus continuous infusion of furosemide in normal adult greyhound dogs, *J Vet Intern Med* 17:632, 2003.
14. Cantarovich F, Rangoonwala B, Lorenz H, et al: High-dose furosemide for established ARF: a prospective, randomized, double-blinded, placebo-controlled, multicenter trial, *Am J Kidney Dis* 44:402, 2004.
15. Denton MD, Chertow GM, Brady HR: "Renal-dose" dopamine for the treatment of acute renal failure: scientific rationale, experimental studies and clinical trials, *Kidney Int* 49:4, 1996.
16. Clark KL, Robertson JM, Drew GM: Do renal tubular dopamine receptors mediate dopamine-induced diuresis in the anesthetized cat? *J Cardiovasc Pharmacol* 17:267, 1991.
17. Plumb DC: *Veterinary drug handbook*, ed 5, Philadelphia, 2005, Wiley-Blackwell.
18. Debaveye YA, van den Berghe GH: Is there still a place for dopamine in the modern intensive care unit? *Anesth Analg* 98:461, 2004.
19. Burnier M, Schrier RW: Protection from acute renal failure, *Adv Exp Med Biol* 212:275, 1986.
20. Kirby R: Acute renal failure as a complication in the critically ill animal, *Vet Clin North Am Small Anim Pract* 19:1189, 1989.
21. Ross LA: Fluid therapy for acute and chronic renal failure, *Vet Clin North Am Small Anim Pract* 19:343, 1989.
22. Finco DR, Low DG: Intensive diuresis in polyuric renal failure. In Kirk RW, editor: *Current veterinary therapy VII, small animal practice*, Philadelphia, 1980, Saunders, p 1091.
23. Cowgill LD, Francey T, Strickland AD, et al: Reduction of dialysis dependency with an oral cross-linked polyelectrolyte sorbent (CLP) in ESRD (abstract), *ASAIO J* 48(2):177, 2002.
24. Kintzer PP, Peterson ME: Hypoadrenocortism. In Bonagura JD, Twedt DC, editors: *Kirk's current veterinary therapy XIV*, St Louis, 2009, Saunders.
25. White JV, Finco DR, Crowell WA, et al: Effect of dietary protein on functional, morphologic and histologic changes of the kidney during compensatory hypertrophy, *Am J Vet Res* 52:1357, 1991.
26. Venkataraman R, Kellum JA: Novel approaches to the treatment of acute renal failure, *Expert Opin Invest Drugs* 12:1353, 2003.
27. Brady HR, Brenner BM, Lieberthal W: Acute renal failure. In Brenner BM, editor: *Brenner and Rector's the kidney*, ed 5, Philadelphia, 1996, Saunders, p 1200.
28. Schrier RW, Wang W, Poole B, et al: Acute renal failure: definitions, diagnosis, pathogenesis, and therapy, *J Clin Invest* 114:5, 2004.
29. Elliott J, Watson ADJ: Chronic kidney disease: staging and management. In Bonagura JD, Twedt DC, editors: *Kirk's current veterinary therapy XIV*, St Louis, 2009, Saunders, pp 883–892.
30. Hostetter TH, Olson JI, Rennke HG, et al: Hyperfiltration in remnant nephrons: a potentially adverse response to renal ablation, *Am J Physiol* 241:F85, 1981.
31. Brown SA: Canine renal disease. In Wills JM, Simpson KW, editors: *The Waltham book of clinical nutrition of the dog and cat*, Oxford, England, 1994, Pergamon, p 313.
32. Brown SA, Finco DR, Crowell WA, et al: Single-nephron adaptations to partial renal ablation in the dog, *Am J Physiol* 258:F495, 1990.
33. Finco DR, Brown SA, Crowell WA, et al: Effects of dietary phosphorus and protein in dogs with chronic renal failure, *Am J Vet Res* 53:2264, 1992.
34. Finco DR, Brown SA, Crowell WA, et al: Effects of dietary protein intake on geriatric dogs with reduced renal mass, *Am J Vet Res* 55:867, 1994.
35. Polzin DJ, Osborne CA, O'Brien TD, et al: Effects of protein intake on progression of canine chronic renal failure, *J Vet Intern Med* 7:125, 1993.
36. Adams LG, Polzin DJ, Osborne CA, et al: Effects of dietary protein and calorie restriction in clinically normal cats and in cats with surgically induced chronic renal failure, *Am J Vet Res* 54:1653, 1993.

37. Polzin DJ, Osborne CA: Conservative medical management of chronic renal failure. In Osborne CA, Finco DR, editors: *Canine and feline nephrology and urology*, Baltimore, 1995, Williams & Wilkins, p 508.
38. Brown SA, Crowell WA, Barsanti JA, et al: Beneficial effects of dietary mineral restriction in dogs with marked reduction of functional renal mass, *J Am Soc Nephrol* 1:1169, 1991.
39. Elliott J, Rawlings JM, Markwell PJ, et al: Survival of cats with naturally occurring chronic renal failure: effect of dietary management, *J Small Anim Pract* 41:242, 2000.
40. Polzin D, Osborne C, Ross S: Chronic kidney disease. In Ettinger S, Feldman E, editors: *Textbook of Veterinary Internal Medicine*, St Louis, 2005, Elsevier.
41. Acierno MJ: Systemic hypertension in renal disease. In Bonagura JD, Twedt DC, editors: *Kirk's current veterinary therapy XIV*, St Louis, 2009, Saunders.
42. Buranakarl C, Mathur S, Brown SA: Effects of dietary sodium chloride intake on renal function and blood pressure in cats with normal and reduced renal function, *Am J Vet Res* 65:620, 2004.
43. Brown SA: Dietary fatty acid supplementation and chronic renal disease, Lake Buena Vista, Fla, 1995, Proc 13th Am Coll Vet Intern Med Forum, p. 470.
44. Bauer JE: Management of spontaneous canine renal disease by dietary polyunsaturated fatty acids, Lake Buena Vista, Fla, 1995, Proc Am Coll Vet Intern Med Forum, p. 477.
45. Chew DJ, Dibartola SP, Nagode LA, et al: Phosphorus restriction in the treatment of chronic renal failure. In Kirk RW, Bonagura JD, editors: *Current veterinary therapy XI, small animal practice*, Philadelphia, 1992, Saunders.
46. Polzin DJ, Osborne CA, Ross S: Chronic kidney disease. In Ettinger SJ, Feldman E, editors: *Textbook of veterinary internal medicine*, ed 6, St Louis, 2005, Saunders.
47. Llach F, Bover J: Renal osteodystrophy. In Brenner BM, editor: *Brenner and Rector's the kidney*, ed 5, Philadelphia, 1996, Saunders, p 2187.
48. Autran de Morais H: Dibartola SP: Acid-base disorders. In Bonagura JD, Twedt DC, editors: *Kirk's current veterinary therapy XIV*, St Louis, 2009, Saunders.
49. Giovanetti S, Cupisti A, Barsotti G: The metabolic acidosis of chronic renal failure: pathophysiology and treatment, *Contrib Nephrol* 100:48, 1992.
50. Lulich J, Osborne CA, O'Brien T, et al: Feline renal failure: questions, answers, questions, *Compend Contin Educ Pract Vet* 14:127, 1992.
51. Dow SW, Lecouteur RA, Fettman MJ, et al: Potassium depletion in cats: hypokalemic polymyopathy, *J Am Vet Med Assoc* 191:1563, 1987.
52. Dow SW, Fettman MJ: Renal disease in cats: the potassium connection. In Kirk RW, Bonagura JD, editors: *Current veterinary therapy XI, small animal practice*, Philadelphia, 1992, Saunders, p 820.
53. Dow SW, Fettman MJ, Smith KR, et al: Effect of dietary acidification and potassium depletion on acid-base balance, mineral metabolism and renal function in adult cats, *J Nutr* 120:569, 1990.
54. DiBartola SP, Buffington CA, Chew DJ, et al: Development of chronic renal disease in cats fed a commercial diet, *J Am Vet Med Assoc* 202:744, 1993.
55. Jacob F, Polzin DJ, Osborne CA, et al: Clinical evaluation of dietary modification for treatment of spontaneous chronic renal failure in dogs, *J Am Vet Med Assoc* 220:1163, 2002.
56. Ross S, Osborne C, Polzin D, et al: Clinical evaluation of effects of dietary modification in cats with spontaneous chronic renal failure (abstr.), *J Vet Intern Med* 19(3):433, 2005.
57. Bartges JW, Brown SA: Summary of dietary recommendations in urinary diseases. In Bonagura J, editor: *Kirk's current veterinary therapy XIII*, Philadelphia, 2000, Saunders, p 841.
58. Osborne CA, Lulich JP, Sanderson SL, et al: Treatment of uremic anorexia. In Bonagura JD, editor: *Kirk's current veterinary therapy XII, small animal practice*, Philadelphia, 1995, Saunders, p 966.
59. Ogilvie GK: Dolasetron: a new option for nausea and vomiting, *J Am Anim Hosp Assoc* 36:481, 2000.
60. Ljutic D, Perkovic D, Rumboldt Z, et al: Kidney, *Blood Press Rev* 25:61, 2002.
61. de la Puente-Redondo VA, Siedek EM, Benchaoui HA, et al: The anti-emetic efficacy of maropitant (Cerenia) in the treatment of ongoing emesis caused by a wide range of underlying clinical aetiologies in canine patients in Europe, *J Small Anim Pract* 48:93–98, 2007.
62. Hickman MA, Cox SR, Mahabir S, et al: Safety, pharmacokinetics and use of the novel NK-1 receptor antagonist maropitant (Cerenia) for the prevention of emesis and motion sickness in cats, *J Vet Pharmacol Ther* 31:220–229, 2008.
63. Jacob F, Polzin DJ, Osborne CA, et al: Association between initial systolic blood pressure and risk of developing a uremic crisis or of dying in dogs with chronic renal failure, *J Am Vet Med Assoc* 222:322, 2003.
64. Stepien RL, Henik RA: Systemic hypertension. In Bonagura JD, Twedt DC, editors: *Kirk's current veterinary therapy XIV*, St Louis, 2009, Saunders.
65. Brown SA, Finco DR, Brown CA, et al: Evaluation of the effects of inhibition of angiotensin converting enzyme with enalapril in dogs with induced renal insufficiency, *Am J Vet Res* 64:321, 2003.
66. Brown SA, Brown CA, Jacobs G, et al: Effects of the angiotensin converting enzyme inhibitor benazepril in cats with induced renal insufficiency, *Am J Vet Res* 62:375, 2001.
67. Brown SA: Renoprotective mechanisms of angiotensin inhibition, Minneapolis, 2004, Proc 22nd American Coll of Vet Intern Med, p. 712.
68. Henik RA, Snyder PS, Volk LM: Amlodipine bisylate therapy in cats with systemic arterial hypertension secondary to chronic renal disease (abstr.), San Francisco, 1994, Proc 12th ACVIM Forum, p. 976.
69. Ross LA: Hypertension and chronic renal failure, *Semin Vet Med Surg Small Anim* 7:221, 1992.
70. Chew DJ, Nagoda LA, Carothers MA et al: Calcitriol treatment of renal secondary hyperparathyroidism in dogs and cats, Washington, DC, 1993, Proc 11th Am Coll Vet Intern Med Forum, p. 164.
71. Polzin DJ, Ross S, Osborne CA: Calcitriol. In Bonagura JD, Twedt DC, editors: *Kirk's current veterinary therapy XIV*, St Louis, 2009, Saunders.
72. Polzin DJ, Ross S, Osborne C, et al: Clinical benefit of calcitriol in canine chronic kidney disease (abstr.), *J Vet Intern Med* 19(3):433, 2005.
73. King LG, Giger U, Diserens D, et al: Anemia of chronic renal failure in dogs, *J Vet Intern Med* 6:264, 1992.
74. Cowgill LD: Medical management of the anemia of chronic renal failure. In Osborne CA, Finco DR, editors: *Canine and feline nephrology and urology*, Baltimore, 1995, Williams & Wilkins, p 539.
75. Cowgill LD, Feldman B, Levy J, et al: Efficacy of recombinant human erythropoietin (rHuEPO) for anemia in dogs and cats with renal failure, *J Vet Intern Med* 4:126, 1990.
76. Cowgill LD: CVT Update: use of recombinant human erythropoietin. In Bonagura JD, editor: *Kirk's current veterinary therapy XII, small animal practice*, Philadelphia, 1995, Saunders, p 961.
77. Randolph JF, Scarlett J, Stokol T, et al: Clinical efficacy and safety of recombinant canine erythropoietin in dogs with anemia of chronic renal failure and dogs with recombinant human erythropoietin-induced red cell aplasia, *J Vet Intern Med* 18:81, 2004.

78. Vaden S: Glomerular diseases. In Ettinger SJ, Feldman EC, editors: *Textbook of veterinary internal medicine*, ed 6, Philadelphia, 2005, Saunders, p 1786.
79. Elliot J: Importance of proteinuria in cats with chronic renal failure, Minneapolis, 2004, Proc 22nd American Coll Vet Intern *Med*, p. 708.
80. DiBartola SP, Benson MD: Pathogenesis of reactive systemic amyloidosis, *J Vet Intern Med* 3:31, 1989.
81. Grauer GF, DiBartola SP: Glomerular diseases. In Ettinger SJ, Feldman RN, editors: *Textbook of veterinary internal medicine*, ed 4, Philadelphia, 1996, Saunders, p 1760.
82. Relford RL, Green RA: Coagulation disorders in glomerular diseases. In Kirk RW, Bonagura J, editors: *Current veterinary therapy XI, small animal practice*, Philadelphia, 1992, Saunders, p 827.
83. Lees GE, Brown SA, Grauer GF, et al: Assessment and management of proteinuria in dogs and cats, *2004 ACVIM Forum Consensus Statement (Small Animal)*, 2004.
84. Grauer GF, Greco DS, Getzy DM, et al: Effects of enalapril versus placebo as a treatment for canine idiopathic glomerulonephritis, *J Vet Intern Med* 14:526, 2000.
85. Llach F: Hypercoagulability, renal vein thrombosis, and other thrombotic complications of nephrotic syndrome, *Kidney Int* 28:429, 1985.
86. Vaden S: The effects of cyclosporin versus standard care in dogs with naturally occurring glomerulonephritis, *J Vet Intern Med* 9:259, 1995.
87. Longhofer SL, Culham CA, Frisbie DD, et al: Effects of thromboxane synthetase inhibition on immune complex glomerulonephritis, *Am J Vet Res* 52:480, 1991.
88. Grauer GF, Frisbie DD, Snyder PS, et al: Treatment of membranoproliferative glomerulonephritis and nephrotic syndrome in a dog with a thromboxane synthetase inhibitor, *J Vet Intern Med* 6:77, 1992.
89. Vaden SL, Brown CA: Glomerular disease. In Bonagura J, Twedt DC, editors: *Kirk's current therapy XIV*, St Louis, 2009, Saunders.
90. Brown SA, Brown CA, Crowell WA, et al: Dietary lipid composition alters the chronic course of canine renal disease, *J Vet Intern Med* 10:168, 1996.
91. Hall AV, Parbtani A, Clark WF, et al: Omega-3 fatty acid supplementation in primary nephrotic syndrome: effects on plasma lipids and coagulopathy, *J Am Soc Nephrol* 3:1321, 1992.
92. Spyridakis L, Brown SA, Barsanti JA, et al: Amyloidosis in a dog: treatment with dimethylsulfoxide, *J Am Vet Med Assoc* 189:690, 1986.
93. Gruys E, Sijens RJ, Biewenga WJ: Dubious effect of dimethylsulfoxide therapy on amyloid deposits and amyloidosis, *Vet Res Commun* 5:21, 1981.
94. Cowgill LD: Diseases of the kidney. In Ettinger SJ, editor: *Textbook of veterinary internal medicine*, ed 2, Philadelphia, 1983, Saunders, p 1843.
95. Carter LJ, Wingfield WE, Allen TA: Clinical experience with peritoneal dialysis in small animals, *Compend Contin Educ Pract Vet* 11:1335, 1989.
96. Crisp MS, Chew DJ, DiBartola SP, et al: Peritoneal dialysis in dogs and cats: 27 cases (1976-1987), *J Am Vet Med Assoc* 195:1262, 1989.
97. Thornhill JA, Hartman J, Boon GD, et al: Support of an anephric dog for 54 days with ambulatory peritoneal dialysis and a newly designed peritoneal catheter, *Am J Vet Res* 45:1156, 1984.
98. Ross LA, Labato MA: Peritoneal dialysis. In DiBartola SP, editor: *Fluid, electrolyte, and acid-base disorders in small animal practice*, ed 3, St Louis, 2006, Saunders.
99. Lane IF, Carter LJ, Lappin MR: Peritoneal dialysis: an update on methods and usefulness. In Kirk RW, editor: *Current veterinary therapy XI, small animal practice*, Philadelphia, 1992, Saunders, p 865.
100. Cowgill LD: Veterinary hemodialysis: state of the art/science, San Antonio, Texas, 1996, Proc 14th Am Coll Vet Intern Med Forum, p. 368.
101. Langston CE: Hemodialysis. In Bonagura J, Twedt DC, editors: *Kirk's current veterinary therapy XIV*, St Louis, 2009, Saunders.
102. Cowgill LD, Francey T: Hemodialysis. In DiBartola SP, editor: *Fluid, electrolyte, and acid-base disorders in small animal practice*, ed 3, St Louis, 2006, Saunders.
103. Langston CE, Cowgill LD, Spano J: The application of hemodialysis in uremic cats: a review of 24 cases, *J Vet Intern Med* 10:168, 1996.
104. Gregory CR, Gourley IM, Kochin EJ, et al: Renal transplantation for treatment of end-stage renal failure in cats, *J Am Vet Med Assoc* 201:285, 1992.
105. Gregory CR: Renal transplantation in cats, *Compend Contin Educ Pract Vet* 15:1325, 1993.
106. Gregory CR, Gourley IM: Organ transplantation in clinical veterinary medicine. In Slatter DH, editor: *Textbook of small animal surgery*, ed 2, Philadelphia, 1993, Saunders, p 95.
107. Adin CA, Gregory CR, Kyles AE, et al: Diagnostic predictors of complications and survival after renal transplantation in cats, *Vet Surg* 30:515, 2001.
108. Aronson LR, Drobatz KJ: Hypercalcemia following renal transplantation in a cat, *J Am Vet Med Assoc* 21:1034, 2000.
109. Wooldridge JD, Gregory CR, Mathews KG, et al: The prevalence of malignant neoplasia in feline renal-transplant recipients, *Vet Surg* 31:94, 2002.
110. Lothrop C: Simultaneous bone-marrow transplantation and renal transplantation for end-stage renal disease in dogs, 2005, Proc 23rd Annual Forum of the American College of Veterinary Internal Medicine, p. 515.
111. deGroat WC, Booth AM: Physiology of the bladder and urethra, *Ann Intern Med* 92:312–315, 1980.
112. Lane IF, Westropp JL: Urinary incontinence and micturition disorders: pharmacologic management. In Bonagura JD, Twedt DC, editors: *Current veterinary therapy XIV*, St Louis, 2009, Saunders.
113. Barsanti JA: Urinary incontinence. In Lorenz MD, Cornelius LM, editors: *Small animal medical diagnosis*, ed 2, Philadelphia, 1993, Lippincott, p 345.
114. Lane IF: Treating urinary incontinence, *Vet Med* 98:58, 2003.
115. Fischer JR, Lane IF: Treating functional urinary obstruction, *Vet Med* 98:67, 2003.
116. Finkbeiner AE: Is bethanechol chloride effective in promoting bladder emptying? *J Urol* 134:443, 1985.
117. Labato MA: Disorders of micturition. In Morgan R, editor: *Handbook of small animal practice*, ed 5, St Louis, 2008, Churchill Livingstone.
118. Rosin AH, Ross L: Diagnosis and pharmacologic management of disorders of urinary continence in the dog, *Compend Contin Educ Pract Vet* 3:601, 1981.
119. El-Salmy S, Downie JW, Awad SA: Urethral function after chronic cauda equina lesions in cats: I. The contribution of mechanical factors and sympathetic innervation to proximal sphincter dysfunction, *J Urol* 144:1022, 1990.
120. Boyd IW, Rohan AP: Urinary disorders associated with cisapride, *Med J Aust* 160:579, 1994.
121. Carone R, Vercelli D, Bertapelle P: Effects of cisapride on anorectal and vesicourethral function in spinal cord injured patients, *Paraplegia* 31:125, 1993.
122. Coates: 2004. Neurogenic micturition disorders, Proc 22nd Am College of Vet Intern Med Forum, Minneapolis, 2004, pp.324–326.
123. Lappin MR, Barsanti JA: Urinary incontinence secondary to idiopathic detrusor instability: cystometrographic diagnoses and pharmacologic management in 2 dogs and a cat, *J Am Vet Med Assoc* 191:1439, 1987.

124. Lane IF: Disorders of micturition. In Osborne C, Finco DR, editors: *Canine and feline nephrology and urology*, Baltimore, 1995, Williams & Wilkins, p 693.
125. Wefer J, Truss MC, Jonas U: Tolterodine: an overview, *World J Urol* 19:312–318, 2001.
126. Lane IF: Use of anticholinergic agents in lower urinary tract disease. In Bonagura J, editor: *Kirk's current veterinary therapy XIII*, Philadelphia, 2000, Saunders, p 899.
127. Kruger JM, Osborne CA, Lulich JP: Management of nonobstructive idiopathic feline lower urinary tract disease, *Vet Clin North Am Small Anim Pract* 26:571, 1996.
128. Ling GV: Feline urologic syndrome. In Ling GV, editor: *Lower urinary tract diseases of dogs and cats: diagnosis, medical management, and prevention*, St Louis, 1995, Mosby, p 179.
129. Bacon NJ, Oni O, White AS: Treatment of urethral sphincter mechanism incompetence in 11 bitches with a sustained-release formulation of phenylpropanolamine hydrochloride, *Vet Rec* 151:373, 2002.
130. Tapp AJS: The effect of sex hormones on the female lower urinary tract. In Cardozo L, editor: *Update on drugs and the lower urinary tract*, London, 1988, Royal Society of Medicine Services, p 15.
131. Arnold S: Relationship of incontinence to neutering. In Kirk RW, editor: *Current veterinary therapy XI, small animal practice*, Philadelphia, 1992, Saunders, p 875.
132. Mandigers PJ, Nell T: Treatment of bitches with acquired urinary incontinence with oestriol, *Vet Rec* 149:765, 2001.
133. Angioletti A, DeFrancesco I, Vergottini M, et al: Urinary incontinence after spaying in the bitch: incidence and oestrogen-therapy, *Vet Res Comm* 28:153–155, 2004.
134. Hoeijmakkers M, Janszen B, Coert A, et al: Pharmacokinetics of oestriol after repeatd oral administration to dogs, *Res Vet Sci* 75:55, 2003.
135. Barsanti JA, Edwards PD, Losonsky J: Testosterone responsive urinary incontinence in a castrated male dog, *J Am Anim Hosp Assoc* 17:117, 1981.
136. Ling GV: Disorders of urination. In Ling GV, editor: *Lower urinary tract diseases of dogs and cats: diagnosis, medical management, and prevention*, St Louis, 1995, Mosby, p 192.
137. Richter KP, Ling GV: Clinical response and urethral pressure profile changes after phenylpropanolamine administration in dogs with primary sphincter incompetence, *J Am Vet Med Assoc* 187:605, 1985.
138. Byron JK, March PA, Chew DJ, et al: Effect of phenylpropanolamine and pseudoephedrine on the urethral pressure profile and continence scores of incontinent female dogs, *J Vet Intern Med* 21:47, 2007.
139. Arnold S, Arnold P, Hubler M, et al: Incontinentin urinae bei der kastrierten huendin: haeufigkeit und rassedisposition, *Schweiz Arch Tierheilkd* 131:259, 1989.
140. White RAS, Pomeroy CJ: Phenylpropanolamine: an α-adrenergic agent for the management of urinary incontinence in the bitch associated with urethral sphincter mechanism incompetence, *Vet Rec* 125:478, 1989.
141. Scott L, Leddy F, Bernay F, et al: Evaluation of phenylpropanolamine in the treatment of urethral sphincter mechanism incompetence in the bitch, *J Small Anim Pract* 43:493, 2002.
142. Burgherr T, Reichler I, Hung L, et al: Efficacy, tolerance and acceptability of Incontex in spayed bitches with urinary incontinence, *Schweiz Arch Tierheikd* 149:307–313, 2007.
143. Carofiglio F, Hamaide AJ, Farnir F, et al: Evaluation of the urodynamic and hemodynamic effects of orally administered phenylpropanolamine and ephedrine in female dogs, *Am J Vet Res* 67:723–730, 2006.
144. Nendick PA, Lark WT: Medical therapy of urinary incontinence in ovariectomized bitches: a comparison of the effectiveness of diethylstilbesterol and pseudoephedrine, *Aus Vet J* 64:117, 1987.
145. Reichler IM, Hubler M, Jochle W, et al: The effect of GnRH analogs on urinary incontinence after ablation of the ovaries in dogs, *Theriogenology* 60:1207, 2003.
146. Reichler IM, Jochle W, Piche CA, et al: Effect of a long acting GnRH analogue or placebo on plasma LH/FSH, urethral pressure profiles and clinical signs of urinary incontinence due to sphincter mechanism incompetence in bitches, *Theriogenology* 66:1227, 2006.
147. Reichler IM, Barth A, Piche C, et al: Urodynamic parameters and plasma LH/FSH in spayed Beagle bitches before and 8 weeks after GnRH depot analogue treatment, *Theriogenology* 66:2127, 2006.
148. Norton PA, Zinner NR, Yalcin I, et al: Duloxetine versus placebo in the treatment of stress urinary incontinence, *Am J Obstet Gynecol* 187(1):40–48, 2002.
149. Arnold S, Hubler M, Lot-Stolz G, Rusch P: Treatment of urinary incontinence in bitches by endoscopic injection of glutaraldehyde cross-linked collagen, *J Small Anim Pract* 37:163, 1996.
150. Barth A, Reichler IM, Hubler M, et al: Evaluation of long-term effects of endoscopic injection of collagen into the urethral submucosa for treatment of urethral sphincter incompetence in female dogs: 40 cases (1993-2000), *J Am Vet Med Assoc* 226:73, 2005.
151. Byron JB, Chew DJ, McLaughlin MA, et al: Transurethral collagen implantation for treatment of canine urinary incontinence, *ACVIM Forum*, 2005:Abstract 120.
152. Hoelzler MG, Lidbetter DA: Surgical management of urinary incontinence, *Vet Clin North Am Small Anim Pract* 34:1057, 2004.
153. Rawlings C, Barsanti JA, Mahaffey MB, et al: Evaluation of colposuspension for treatment of incontinence in spayed female dogs, *J Am Vet Med Assoc* 219:770, 2001.
154. Khanna OP, Gonick P: Effects of phenoxybenzamine on canine lower urinary tract, *Urology* 6:323, 1975.
155. Barsanti JA, Coates JR, Bartges JW: Detrusor-sphincter dyssynergia, *Vet Clin North Am Small Anim Pract* 26:327, 1996.
156. Lees GE: Management of voiding disability following relief of urethral obstruction. In August JR, editor: *Consultations in feline internal medicine 2*, Philadelphia, 1994, Saunders, p 365.
157. Wein AJ: Drug therapy for neurogenic and non-neurogenic bladder dysfunction. In Seidmon EJ, Hanna PM, editors: *Current urologic therapy*, Philadelphia, 1994, Saunders, p 291.
158. Fischer JR, Lane IF, et al: Urethral pressure profile and hemodynamic effects of phenoxybenzamine and prazosin in non-sedated male beagle dogs, *Can J Vet Res* 67:30, 2003.
159. Lulich JP: Managing functional urethral obstruction, Minneapolis, 2004, Proc 22nd Forum of the American College of Veterinary Internal Medicine, p. 514.
160. Ohtake A, Sato S, Sasamata M, et al: Effects of tamsulosin on resting urethral pressure and arterial blood pressure in anaesthetized female dogs, *J Pharm Pharmacol* 58(3):345–350, 2006.
161. Sato S, Ohtake A, Hatanaka T, et al: Relationship between the functional effect of tamsulosin and its concentration in lower urinary tract tissues of dogs, *Biol Pharm Bull* 30:481–486, 2007.
162. Sudoh K, Tanaka H, Inagaki O, et al: Effect of tamsulosin, a novel alpha 1-adrenoceptor antagonist, on urethral pressure profile in anaesthetized dogs, *J Auton Pharmacol* 16(3):147–154, 1996.
163. Witte DG, Brune ME, Katwala SP, et al: Modeling of relationships between pharmacokinetics and blockade of agonist-induced elevation of intraurethral pressure and mean arterial pressure in conscious dogs treated with alpha(1)-adrenoceptor antagonists, *J Pharmacol Exp Ther* 300(2):495–504, 2002.
164. Tatemichi S, Tomiyama Y, Maruyama I, et al: Uroselectivity in male dogs of silodosin (KMD-3213), a novel drug for the obstructive component of benign prostatic hyperplasia, *Neurourol Urodyn* 25:792–799, 2006.
165. Straeter-Knowlen IM, Knowlen GG, Speth RC, et al: Effect of succinyl choline, diazepam and dantrolene on the urethral pressure profile of healthy, sexually intact male cats, *Am J Vet Res* 55:1739, 1994.

166. Straeter-Knowlen IM, Marks SL, Rishniw M, et al: Urethral pressure response to smooth and skeletal muscle relaxants in anesthetized, adult male cats with naturally acquired urethral obstruction, *Am J Vet Res* 56:919, 1995.
167. Polzin DJ, Osborne CA: Diseases of the urinary tract. In Davis LE, editor: *Handbook of small animal therapeutics*, New York, 1985, Churchill-Livingstone, p 333.
168. Blackwell NJ: Reflex dyssynergia in the dog, *Vet Rec* 132:516, 1993.
169. Collins BK, Moore CP, Hagee JH: Sulfonamide-associated keratoconjunctivitis sicca and corneal ulceration in a dysuric dog, *J Am Vet Med Assoc* 189:924, 1986.
170. Gookin JL, Bunch SE: Detrusor-striated sphincter dyssynergia in a dog, *J Vet Intern Med* 10:339, 1996.
171. Lane IF, Fischer JR, Miller EM, Grauer G: Functional urethral obstruction in three dogs: urethral pressure profile results and response to alpha adrenergic antagonists, *J Vet Intern Med* 14:43, 1998.
172. Porpiglia F, Ghignone G, Fiori C, et al: Nifedipine versus tamsulosin for the management of lower ureteral stones, *J Urol* 172:568, 2004.
173. Forman MA, Francey T, Fischer JR, et al: Use of glucagons in the management of acute ureteral obstruction in 25 cats (abstr.), *J Vet Intern Med* 18:417, 2004.
174. Kalkstein TS, Kruger JM, Osborne CA: Feline idiopathic lower urinary tract disease. Part IV: Therapeutic options, *Compend Contin Educ Pract Vet* 21:497, 1999.
175. Buffington CAT: External and internal influences on disease risk in cats, *J Am Vet Med Assoc* 220:994, 2002.
176. Westropp J, Buffington CAT, Chew D: Feline lower urinary tract diseases. In Ettinger SJ, Feldman E, editors: *Textbook of veterinary internal medicine*, ed 6, St Louis, 2006, Saunders.
177. Cameron ME, Casey RA, Bradshaw JW, et al: A study of environmental and behavioural factors that may be associated with feline idiopathic cystitis,, *J Small Anim Pract* 45:144, 2004.
178. Buffington CAT, Chew DJ: Lower urinary tract disease in cats: new directions, *Vet Clin Nutr* 1:53, 1994.
179. Ching SV, Fettman MJ, Hamar DW, et al: The effect of chronic dietary acidification using ammonium chloride on acid-base and mineral and bone metabolism in adult cats, *Am J Vet Res* 53:2125, 1992.
180. Dow SW, Fettman MJ, LeCouteur RS: Potassium depletion in cats: renal and dietary influences, *J Am Vet Med Assoc* 191:1569, 1987.
181. Kirk CA, Ling GV, Franti CE, et al: Evaluation of factors associated with development of calcium oxalate urolithiasis in cats, *J Am Vet Med Assoc* 207:1429, 1995.
182. Maede Y, Hoshino T, Inaba M: Methionine toxicosis in cats, *Am J Vet Res* 48:289, 1987.
183. Osborne CA, Kruger JM, Lulich JP, et al: Prednisolone therapy of idiopathic feline lower urinary tract disease: a double-blind clinical study, *Vet Clin North Am Small Anim Pract* 26:563, 1996.
184. Ross LA: Treating FUS in unobstructed cats and preventing its recurrence, *Vet Med* 85:1218, 1990.
185. Barsanti JA, Shotts EB, Crowell WA, et al: Effect of therapy on susceptibility of urinary tract infection in male cats with indwelling urethral catheters, *J Vet Intern Med* 6:64, 1992.
186. Bernard MA: Feline urologic syndrome: a study of seasonal incidence, frequency of repeat visits and comparison of treatments, *Can Vet J* 19:284, 1978.
187. Barsanti JA, Finco DR, Shotts EB, et al: Feline urologic syndrome: further investigation into therapy, *J Am Anim Hosp Assoc* 18:391, 1982.
188. Marks SL, Straeter-Knowlen IM, Knowlen GG, et al: The effects of phenoxybenzamine and acepromazine maleate on urethral pressure profiles of anesthetized healthy male cats, *J Vet Intern Med* 7:122, 1993.
189. Mawby DI, Meric SM, Crichlow EC, et al: Pharmacologic relaxation of the urethra in male cats: a study of the effects of phenoxybenzamine, diazepam, nifedipine and xylazine, *Can J Vet Res* 55:28, 1990.
190. Lane IF, Bartges JW: Treating refractory idiopathic lower urinary tract diseases in cats, *Vet Med* 94:633, 1999.
191. Buffington CAT, Blaisdell JL, Binns SP, et al: Decreased urinary glycosaminoglycan in cats with idiopathic lower urinary tract disease, *J Vet Intern Med* 7:126, 1993.
192. Buffington CAT, Chew DJ, DiBartola SP: Interstitial cystitis in cats, *Vet Clin North Am Small Anim Pract* 26:317, 1996.
193. Gao X, Buffington CAT, Au JLS: Effect of interstitial cystitis on drug absorption from urinary bladder, *J Pharmacol Exp Ther* 271:818, 1994.
194. Baldessarini RJ: Drugs and the treatment of psychiatric disorders. In Gilman AG, Rall TW, Niew AS, et al: *Goodman and Gilman's the pharmacological basis of therapeutics*, ed 8, New York, 1990, Pergamon, p 383.
195. Miller WH, Scott DW, Wellington JR: Nonsteroidal management of canine pruritus with amitriptyline, *Cornell Vet* 82:53, 1992.
196. Marder A: Psychotropic drugs and behavioral therapy, *Vet Clin North Am Small Anim Pract* 21:329, 1991.
197. Chew DJ, Buffington CAT, Kendall MS, et al: Amitriptyline treatment for severe recurrent idiopathic cystitis in cats, *J Am Vet Assoc* 213:1282, 1998.
198. Kruger JM, Conway TS, Kaneene JB, et al: Randomized controlled trial of the efficacy of short-term amitriptyline administration for treatment of acute, nonobstructive, idiopathic lower urinary tract diseases in cats, *J Am Vet Med Assoc* 222:749, 2003.
199. Kraijer M, Fink-Gremmels J, Nickel RF: The short-term clinical efficacy amitriptyline in the management of idiopathic feline lower urinary tract disease: a controlled clinical study, *J Feline Med Surg* 5:191, 2003.
200. Virga V: Behavioral dermatology, *Vet Clin North Am Small Anim Pract* 33:231, 2003.
201. Gunn-Moore DA, Cameron ME: A pilot study using synthetic feline facial pheromone for the management of feline idiopathic cystitis, *J Feline Med Surg* 6:133, 2004.
202. Parson CL: The therapeutic role of sulfated polysaccharides in the urinary bladder, *Urol Clin North Am* 21:90–100, 1994.
203. Messing EM: Interstitial cystitis and related syndromes. In Walsh PC, Retik AB, Stamey TA, et al: *Campbell's urology*, ed 6, Philadelphia, 1992, Saunders, p 982.
204. Pressler B: Fungal urinary infections, Minneapolis, 2004, Proc 22nd Am Coll Vet Intern Med Forum, p. 555.
205. Barsanti JA, Finco DR, Brown SA: The role of dimethyl sulfoxide and glucocorticoids in lower urinary tract diseases. In Bonagura JD, editor: *Kirk's current veterinary therapy XII*, Philadelphia, 1995, Saunders, p 1011.
206. Laing EJ, Miller CW, Cochrane SM: Treatment of cyclophosphamide-induced hemorrhagic cystitis in five dogs, *J Am Vet Med Assoc* 193:233, 1988.
207. Friberg S: BCG in the treatment of superficial cancer of the bladder: a review, *Med Oncol Tumor Pharmacother* 10:31, 1993.
208. Knapp DW: Tumors of the urinary system. In Withrow SJ, editor: *Withrow and MacEwen's small animal clinical oncology*, ed 4, St Louis, 2007, Saunders.
209. Knapp DW, et al: Piroxicam therapy in 34 dogs with transitional cell carcinoma of the urinary bladder, *J Vet Intern Med* 8:273, 1994.

19 Gastrointestinal Pharmacology

Dawn Merton Boothe

Chapter Outline

DRUGS THAT TARGET APPETITE OR CALORIC BALANCE

Drugs that alter body weight play can be important in the the prevention or treatment of disease in dogs and cats. Targets of pharmacologic management of weight include decreased energy intake (e.g., appetite, caloric absorption), altered energy partitioning, and increased energy expenditure.

Appetite is controlled primarily, but not exclusively, by the ventral and lateral nuclei of the hypothalamus. The nuclei respond to both short- and long-term signals.[1] Hypothalamic directives are influenced by energy, which in turn is influenced by ingestion, absorption, metabolism, and storage. Chemical signals mediating these directives act locally or distantly, often balancing one another. Signals include hormones, neuropeptides, cytokines and neurotransmitters, several of which are pharmacologic targets.

Although a discussion of energy utilization is too complex and extensive for this text, understanding of the role of body fat in appetitic control and body weight has been markedly advanced in the last decade and warrants review of those aspects relevant to drug therapy. In the arcuate nucleus, primary neurons detect concentrations of metabolites and secondary neurons synchronize signals and coordinate vagally mediated responses. Among these neurons are two distinct populations of primary neurons and neuropeptides that control food intake and energy expenditure. Orexigenic peptides increase food intake and include neuropeptide Y (NPY) and agouti-related protein (AgRP); gamma amino butyric acid (GABA) is also released as an orexigenic signal. The NPY/AgRP neurons direct the effects of leptin and ghrelin and stimulate feeding during states of fasting. They also influence the anorexigenic peptides, which decrease food intake. Anorexigenic peptids include the pro-opiomelanocortin (POMC) neurons which produce alpha-melanocyte hormone (α-MSH), a powerful appetite suppressant, and the β-endorphins. . The POMC extensively communicates with hypothalamic neurons as well as other regions that regulate energy. Both orexigenic and anorexigenic neurons have receptors for balancing signaling molecules, which often cause opposing effects by interacting at the same ligand. NPY and α-MSH ,located in the ventromedial nucleus of the appetite center, are considered balancing hormones. Other stimulatory mediators include norepinephrine (α_2-receptors), dopamine (possibly D_1 receptors), and opiate and pancreatic polypeptides. Although GABA also stimulates appetite, its effect may vary with route of administration.[1] Other inhibitory mediators include serotonin (5-hydroxytryptamine [5-HT]), calcitonin, cholecystokinin, and corticotrophin-releasing factor. In addition to their central roles, several of these mediators influence energy metabolism peripherally.

Among the major target tissues for signals modulating energy metabolism is adipose tissue, which is now a recognized endocrine organ (Figure 19-1). Hormones play a critical role in energy homeostasis, insulin sensitivity, and lipid and carbohydrate metabolism. The system appears to be more sensitive to preventing starvation rather than obesity. Leptin and insulin appear to be the predominant mediators that signal adiposity: both circulate in proportion to body fat, enter the central nervous system (CNS) in proportion to plasma

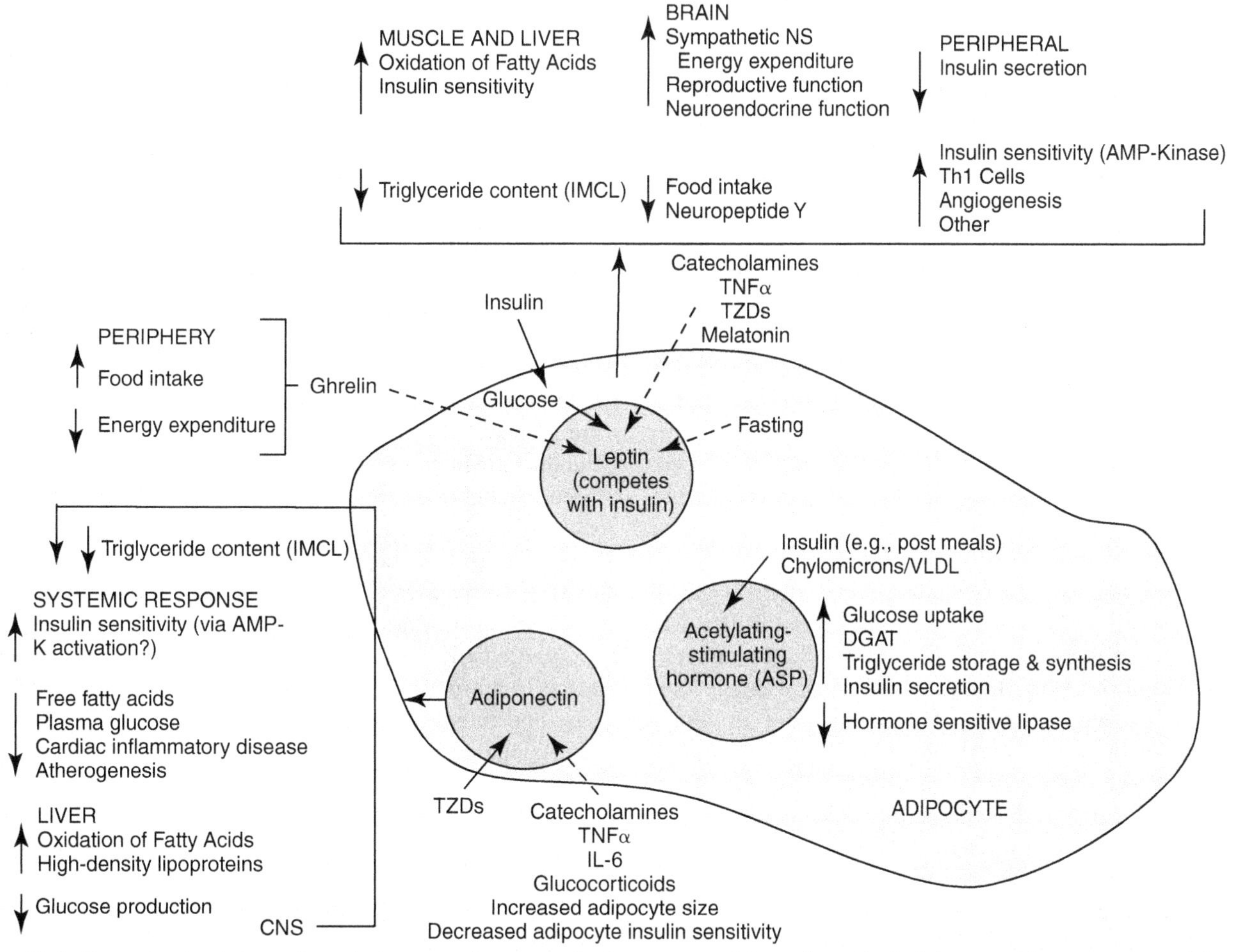

Figure 19-1 The complex interactions between adipose and other organs. The adipocyte is influenced by a number of factors and responds with paracrine, autocrine, and endocrine responses. Leptin is produced by many tissues, but particularly white adipose tissue. It inhibits food intake and increases energy expenditure while increasing insulin sensitivity (by way of activation of AMP kinase). Central influences include reproductive and neuroendocrine functions. In the adipocyte leptin is influenced by changes in adipocyte glucose metabolism as insulin secretion responds to food intake. Adiponectin also increases insulin sensitivity (through activation of AMP kinase), resulting in increased fatty acid oxidation in the muscle and liver and decreased hepatic triglycerides. Acetylation-stimulating protein also reduces hepatic glucose production. *Solid arrows,* stimulate; *dashed arrows,* inhibit; *DGAT,* diglycerol acyltransferase; *TZD,* thiazolidinediones.

concentrations, and interact with CNS receptors that influence energy regulation, as reviewed by Havel.[2] Other important peripheral mediators include acetylation-stimulating protein (ASP) and adiponectin, each being principally regulated by host nutritional status.

KEY POINT 19-1 Adipose tissue has emerged as one of the biggest endocrine organs, affecting appetite and energy homeostasis.

Leptin was discovered in obese mice that randomly emerged as mutants among normal populations. At least six leptin receptors ("LepR", *a* through *f*) are associated with the *ob* gene (Ob-R) (obesity gene), suggesting a complex role for this hormone. [3] Leptin receptors are similar to class I cytokine receptors, perhaps linking cytokines to diseases associated with obesity disorders.[3]

Currently, little information appears to be available regarding leptin content in dogs or cats and information must be drawn from other species. Although most organs produce leptin, white adipose tissue is the primary source, with the amount produced varying among species: more leptin is produced in subcutaneous compared with omental fat in humans, but the opposite is true in rats.[3] In humans, leptin content is greatest in the heart, liver, small intestine, prostate, and ovaries versus the lung and kidney in mice. Each tissue may have a particular receptor isoform, allowing differential roles among tissues. Leptin plays an important, albeit complex, role in the peripheral regulation of adipose tissues. Its primary function is as a lipostat, communicating to other tissues the current status of body fat reserves. As such, leptin mediates fuel movement and use (see Figure 19-1) and energy expenditure. [3] It is more effective in signaling deficient rather than excessive energy reserves.[2] Activated leptin receptors induce satiety in the appetite center (inhibition of NPY, stimulation of alpha-MSH neurons). Leptin also appears to influence thermogenesis. Peripherally, leptin appears to increase hematopoiesis, angiogenesis, wound repair, and puberty; its role in reproduction is particularly complex. Leptin is primarily regulated by food-induced responses to insulin, with influences being more dramatic during fasting and characterized by diurnal variation.[2] In normal animals, insulin appears to directly regulate leptin gene expression and excretion in adipose tissue; it also indirectly influences it through adipocyte glucose use and oxidative metabolism. Both hormones increase in concert.[3] Both leptin and insulin share inhibitory signal transduction pathways in response to food.[2] Leptin, in turn, appears to inhibit insulin secretion, and, peripherally competes with insulin; however conflicting results also suggest that leptin has no effect on insulin.[2,3] Glucocorticoids appear to stimulate leptin gene expression, although it is not clear if this effect is direct (gene expression) or indirect (altered food intake or insulin concentrations). Leptin is downregulated by melatonin at night; accordingly, humans with short sleep cycles may be predisposed to obesity. Depletion of body stores is not detected in hypoleptimemic animals, and as such, is more dangerous than hyperleptinemia. In humans, hypoleptinemia is associated with neuroendocrine, reproductive, metabolic, and immunologic imbalances,and in rodents, marked insulin reistance and hyperlipidemia.[2] Leptin concentrations in persons with eating disorders characterized by anorexia are similar to or lower than concentrations in persons without eating disorders.[3] . Its role in chronic liver disease increasingly is being recognized.[4] Many of these abnormalities can be normalized in humans with recombinant human leptin. Differences in genes (including mutations) regulating leptin also are linked to human obesity with hyperleptinemia indicating leptin resistance.

KEY POINT 19-2 Leptin acts as a lipostat, communicating to the tissue the status of fat reserves.

The second major hormone influencing energy metabolism, ASP, is produced from complement factor C. Locally, ASP paracrine actions in adipose tissue include increased glucose uptake and diacylglycerol acyltransferase activity and decreased hormone-sensitive lipase (see Figure 19-1). As such, adipocyte triglyceride synthesis and storage increase after eating, resulting in increased free fatty acids and triglyceride clearance. Serum ASP concentrations are increased by lipids, and increase in proportion to body fat in obese human patients; they decrease during states of fasting. Insulin may control ASP in reponse to eating or fasting; ASP in turn may directly stimulate insulin secretion.

Adiponectin, a large protein secreted by adiopocytes, is a third hormone influencing energy metabolism. Its biological effect varies with its state of diamerization.[2] Adiponectin appears to influence lipid and carbohydrate metabolism both directly and indirectly (see Figure 19-1). Adiponectin appears to be necessary for normal insulin actions. Concentrations are reduced in patients with type 2 diabetes compared with nondiabetic humans.[2] The effect of adiponectin on decreased circulating glucose are independent of fat content and occurs without influencing insulin secretion. Mechanisms may include decreased hepatic glucose formation and increased tissue glucose use by decreasing insulin resistance. Circulating adiponectin is negatively correlated with the content of body fat, particularly visceral (e.g., omental) rather than subcutaneous in humans.[2] Adiponectin may reduce ectopic fat in the liver and muscle through increased fat oxidation. Thus, low visceral fat may reduce adiponectin production, contributing to insulin resistance associated with obesity.[2] The impact of insulin on adiponectin is not clear. Among the emerging effects of adiponectin is protection against inflammatory cardiovascular disease (including atherosclerosis), which may explains the relationship between body fat and cardiac disease. Cytokines, catecholamines, and glucocorticoids decrease adiponectin production, which may contribute to their characteristic incease in insulin resistance.

KEY POINT 19-3 Adiponectin influences lipid and carbohydrate metabolism and is necessary for normal insulin action.

A final signal able to centrally influence energy metabolism is ghrelin. Located in peripheral tissues, ghrelin is released by an empty stomach, appears to oppose leptin in the hypothalamus, and has been shown to increase food intake and decrease energy expenditure.

Control of appetite through pharmacologic manipulation of orixogenic and anorexigenic signals has proven difficult. Obvious targets which might suppress appetite (e.g., α-MSH) have profound impacts in multiple body systems, increasing the risk of adverse reactions. The complexties of regulation contribute to the risk of adversity. For example, alternate pathways of synthesis or response tend to emerge with blockade of a target signal.

APPETITE STIMULANTS

Studies regarding the pharmacologic control of appetite have traditionally focused on decreased, rather than increased, food intake, particularly in humans. However, the role of cachexia associated with weight loss and anorexia in human patients with cancer has stimulated a renewed interest in appetite stimulants.[5] Drugs that inhibit gluconeogenesis, such as hydrazine sulfate, or promote gastric emptying, such as metoclopramide, have been used successfully to stimulate food intake in some human patients.[5] The use of steroids, including megestrol acetate, in treatment of cachexia is discussed later in this chapter.[5] Both glucocorticoids and B vitamins have been used to nonspecifically stimulate appetite in animals. Drugs used to treat depression and psychosis in human patients are associated with appetite increase and weight gain.[6] They antagonize a variety of receptors, although their clinical potency is often related to increased serotonin, which may, in fact, decrease appetite in some patients.

Mirtazapine is a piperazino-azepine antidepressant characterized by serotonergic activity as a result of 5-HT-$_1$ agonistic activity and inhibition of serotonin reuptake.[7] Sympathetic (norepinephrine) actions reflect antagonism of α -$_2$ autoreceptors as well as influences by other receptors. As a behavior-modifying drug, mirtazapine is discussed in greater depth in Chapter 26. Anecdotally, mirtazapine has been used to stimulate appetite in either dogs or cats, the latter at 3 mg/cat every 72 hours.

The benzodiazepines diazepam (Valium) and oxazepam, a metabolite of diazepam (Serax), have successfully induced appetite in cats, probably through gabaminergic effects and central inhibition of the satiety center in the hypothalamus (Table 19-1).[8] Diazepam is administered intravenously or orally, whereas oxazepam is administered orally. Of the two drugs, diazepam may be more effective, although sedation is greater. The benzodiazepines do not stimulate appetite in the dog as effectively as in the cat. Hepatotoxicity associated with diazepam therapy when used as an appetite stimulant has been reported in cats[9,10] and is discussed in more depth in Chapter 27. Toxicity appears to be idiosyncratic and thus may not be predictable; it is not likely to happen in a large percentage of animals receiving the drug.

Cyproheptadine, an antihistamine with antiserotonin properties, has caused weight gain in geriatric human patients and in adults and younger patients afflicted with eating disorders. Its mechanism probably reflects inhibition of serotonergic receptors that control appetite. Serotonin antagonists also increase food intake in cats,[1] and cyproheptadine has been used clinically to stimulate the appetite of some anorexic cats. Cyproheptadine kinetics have been reported in the cat. Oral bioavailability of the tablet is 100%, and the elimination half-life approximates 13 hours.[11] Cats tolerated a dose of 8 mg orally with no adverse effects, although impact on appetite was not described. Based on this study, once- to twice-daily dosing of 8 mg appears to be safe.

Cachexia

Cachexia is an involuntary state characterized by loss of more than 5% of body weight. In humans it occurs over a defined period, generally of 2 to 6 months. Ultimately, it is a condition of starvation characterized by depletion of body mass, particularly muscle, but to a lesser degree, adipose tissue.[12] Cachexia develops in 50% of human patients with cancer, contributing to substantially shortened survival times. Cachexia also is a manifestation of other chronic diseases, including (in humans), acquired immune-deficiency syndrome (AIDS), heart failure, rheumatoid arthritis, Crohn's disease, chronic obstructive pulmonary disease, and chronic renal disease.[12] It appears to be a cytokine-driven process, with key components including anorexia and a state of hypercatabolism. The principle cytokines appear to include TNF-alpha, interleukins 1 and 6, and interferon-γ Of these, TNF-alpha is presumed to stimulate mechanisms that lead to severe cachexia.[12] Muscle wasting may reflect inhibition of myogenic differentiation; an energy sink may result from increased concentrations of mitochondrial uncoupling proteins. Lipoproteinase activity is inhibited by TNF-alpha. Interleukins contribute to CNS-mediated anorexia and decreased albumin synthesis in the liver. Megestrol acetate is the only treatment approved by the Food and Drug Administration for cancer or AIDS-related cachexia syndromes in humans.[12] Other less commonly used drugs are glucocorticoids, anabolic steroids, antiseratonergic drugs, dronabinol, and prokinetic drugs.

Megestrol is a synthetic derivative of progesterone.[12] As such, megestrol acetate targets cachexia by directly and indirectly stimulating appetite and antagonizing the catabolic metabolic effects of cytokines. As with other steroidal hormones, the effects of megestrol (and progesterone) involve passive diffusion into the cell and binding to specific intracellular progesterone receptors A or B (PR-A or -B) and heat shock proteins. The drugs move into the nucleus, bind to progesterone response elements on target genes, and influence transcription through inhibition (PR-A) or stimulation (PR-B) of other steroid response elements. Although the majority of progesterone effects are genomic, nongenomic actions also occur. Metabolic effects of progesterone include increased basal insulin concentration and increased response to carbohydrate load; increased lipoprotein lipase with altered fat deposition, plasma lipid, and lipoprotein concentrations; and modulation of body temperature.[12] In humans and animal models of cancer, megestrol stimulates appetite, increases caloric intake, induces a sense

Table 19-1 Doses for Treatment of Gastrointestinal Disorders[161]

Drug	Indication	Dose	Route	Interval (hr)
6-aminosalicylic acid	See Mesalamine			
Activated charcoal	Gastrointestinal adsorbent	1 g/5-10 mL water. Administer 6-12 mL of slurry/kg; follow with 0.9% saline cathartic	PO	6 hr for several days
		1-8 g/kg (granules)	PO	6 hr for several days
Aluminum hydroxide	Phosphate binder	30-90 mg/kg	PO (with food)	8-24
Aluminum magnesium hydroxide	Laxative	2-10 mL	PO	2-4
		3 mg/kg (C)	PO	24
Aminopentamide	Antidiarrheal	0.1-0.4 mg	IM, PO, SC	8-12
		0.01-0.03 mg/kg	IM, PO, SC	8-12
		0.1 mg/cat	IM, PO, SC	8-12
Ammonium chloride	Ammonium tolerance test	0.1 mg/kg of 5% solution	Rectally	Once
		100 mg/kg. Maximum of 3 g	PO	Once
Apomorphine	Emesis	0.02-0.04 mg/kg (D)	IM, IV	Efficacy lost with subsequent doses
		0.08-0.1 mg/kg (D)	IM, SC	Efficacy lost with subsequent doses
		0.25 mg	Topical (conjunctival sac)	Flush once emesis begins; efficacy lost with subsequent doses
Aprotinin	Pancreatitis (protease inhibitor)	5000 kallikrein inhibitor units (KUI)/kg	IP (preferred), IV	6-8
Ascorbic acid	Copper-induced hepatotoxicity	500-1000 mg/day (D)	PO	24
	Feline infectious peritonitis	25 mg/kg or 125 mg (C)	PO	24
	Acetaminophen toxicosis	30 mg/kg (C)	PO, SC	6 hr × 7 treatments
	Urinary acidifier	100-500 mg (D)	PO	8-24
		100 mg (C)	PO	8-24
Atracurium besylate	Hypersialism	0.02 mg/kg	SC	As needed
Atropine	Hypersialism	0.02 mg/kg	SC	As needed
	Cholinergic toxins	0.2-2 mg/kg	Administer 0.25 of the total dose IV and the remaining dose SC, IM	To effect
Azathioprine	Myasthenia gravis	2 mg/kg (D)	PO	24 × 7 days then every 48
	Chronic atrophic gastritis	0.5 mg/kg (D)	PO	24-48
	Lymphocytic or eosinophilic enteritis	2-2.5 mg/kg (D)	PO	24-48
		0.2-0.3 mg/kg (C)	PO	24-48
	Chronic active hepatitis	2-2.5 mg/kg (D)	PO	24
Bisacodyl	Stool softener	5-20 mg/dog	PO	24 or as needed
		2-5 mg/cat	PO	24 or as needed
		1-3 suppositories	Rectally	24 or as needed
		1-2 mL enema	Rectally	24 or as needed
Bismuth subcarbonate	Gastrointestinal tract protectant	0.3-3 g	PO	4
Bismuth subsalicylate	Gastrointestinal tract protectant	175-524 mg/dog	PO	4-6
		4.4-52 mg/kg (D)	PO	6-8
		4.4 mg/kg (C)	PO	4-6
		18-52 mg/cat	PO	4-6
Bran	Bulk laxative	Approximately 15-30 mL (1-2 tbsp)/400 g food	PO	As needed

Table 19-1 Doses for Treatment of Gastrointestinal Disorders[161]—cont'd

Drug	Indication	Dose	Route	Interval (hr)
Budesonide	Inflammatory bowel disease	1 mg/small dog or cat	PO	24
		2 mg/large dog	PO	24
Calcium acetate (contains 0.235 mg elemental calcium)	Phosphate binder	60-100 mg/kg	PO	24
Calcium carbonate (contains 0.4 mg elemental calcium)	Antacid	0.5-5 g/dog	PO	As needed
Cascara sagrada	Laxative, stool softener	1-4 mL/dog	PO	12 to effect
		0.5-1.5 mL/cat	PO	12 to effect
Castor oil	Cathartic, stool softener	8-30 mL/dog	PO	12 to effect
		4-10 mL/cat	PO	12 to effect
Chlordiazepoxide–clidinium	Irritable colon syndrome	0.1-0.25 mg/kg (D). Based on clidinium dose	PO	8-12
Chlorpromazine hydrochloride	Antiemetic	0.5 mg/kg	IM, IV, SC	6-8
		0.05-0.5 mg/kg (D)	IM, SC	6-24
		1 mg/kg (D)	Rectally	8
		3.3 mg/kg (D)	PO	6-24
		1.1-6.6 mg/kg (D)	IM	6-24
	Irritable colon syndrome	0.5 mg/kg (D)	IM	8-24
		2 mg/kg (D)	PO	8-24
Cholestyramine	Short bowel syndrome	200-300 mg/kg	PO	12
		1-2 g/dog	PO	12
Cimetidine	Esophagitis, gastric ulceration, antiemetic, chronic gastritis, GI tract ulceration	5-15 mg/kg	IM, IV, PO	6-12 (D), 8-12 (C)
	Gastrinemia	5-15 mg/kg	IV, PO, SC	6
	Effects of mast cell tumors	5 mg/kg (D)	IV, PO	6-8
	Immunomodulator	6-10 mg/kg	IM, IV, PO	8
Cisapride	Prokinetic	0.1-0.5 mg/kg (D)	PO	8-12
		2.5-7.5 mg (C)	PO	8-12
Clindamycin	Stomatitis, acute pancreatitis	5-10 mg/kg	IM, IV	8
	Pancreatic exocrine insufficiency	5-10 mg/kg	PO	6-8, 30 min before meals
Clonidine	Refractory diarrhea, inflammatory bowel disease	1-10 μg/kg (C)	PO, SC	8-12
Codeine	Diarrhea	0.25-0.5 mg/kg (D)	PO	6 - 8
Colchicine	Chronic hepatic fibrosis	0.01-0.03 mg/kg (D)	PO	24
Cyanocobalamin	See Vitamin B_{12}		PO	24
Cyclizine	Antiemetic	4 mg/kg	IM	8
Cyproheptadine hydrochloride	Antihistamine	1.1 mg/kg (D)	PO	8-12
	Appetite stimulant	2-4 mg/cat	PO	12-24
Dexpanthenol (pantothenic acid)	Intestinal atony	11 mg/kg	IM	4-6
Diazepam	Irritable colon syndrome	0.15 mg/kg (D)	PO	8
	Appetite stimulant	0.05-0.4 mg/kg (C)	IM, IV, PO	24 or 48
		1 mg/cat	PO	24
Dicyclomine	Acute colitis, irritable colon	0.15 mg/kg (D)	PO	8
Dimenhydrinate	Motion sickness	25-50 mg/dog	PO	8-24
		12.5 mg/cat	PO	8
		4-8 mg/kg	PO	8

Continued

Table **19-1** Doses for Treatment of Gastrointestinal Disorders[161]—cont'd

Drug	Indication	Dose	Route	Interval (hr)
Dicyclomine	Detrusor hyperspasticity or urge incontinence	5-10 mg	PO	6-8
	Acute colitis, irritable colon	0.15 mg/kg (D)	PO	8
Dioctyl sulfosuccinate	Stool softener	25 mg/small dog or cat	PO	12-24
		50-100 mg/medium or large dog	PO	12-24
Diphenhydramine	Antihistamine	2-4 mg/kg	PO	6-8
	Mast cell disease, antiemetic	2 mg/kg	IM, IV (slowly)	12 or as needed
	Anaphylaxis, urticaria	2 mg/kg	IM, IV (slowly)	12 or as needed
	Angioneurotic edema	2 mg/kg	IM, IV (slowly)	12 or as needed
	Antipruritic, allergic skin disease	1-2 mg/kg (D)	PO	8-12
		5-50 mg	IM	12
Diphenoxylate (contains atropine)	Acute colitis, irritable colon syndrome	0.1-0.2 mg/kg (D)	PO	8
		0.05-0.2 mg/kg (C)	PO	12
	Antidiarrheal	2.5-10 mg (D)	PO	8
		0.6-1.2 mg (C)	PO	8-12
Dirlotapide	Weight loss	0.1 ml/kg (D)	PO	24 × 14 days
		0.2 ml/kg (D)	PO	24 × 14 days, then base on current weight (see package insert)
Docusate calcium, sodium	Stool softener	25-200 mg (D)	PO	12
		50 mg/cat	PO	12-24
Dolasetron mesylate	Antiemetic	0.6 mg/kg	IV, PO, SC	24
Domperidone	Prokinetic agent, antiemetic	2 mg/kg	PO	12-24
		0.1-0.3 mg/kg	IM, IV, PO	12
D-Penicillamine	Copper hepatopathy	10-15 mg/kg	PO (on an empty stomach)	12
		125 -250 mg/dog	PO (on an empty stomach)	12
Edrophonium	Tensilon test	0.11-0.22 mg/kg (D). Maximum of 5 mg	IV	Once
		0.1-0.5 mg/puppy	IV	Once
		0.25-0.5 mg/cat	IV	Once
Emetine	Emesis	1-2.5 mL/kg (D). Maximim of 6.6 mL/kg	PO	Once
		3.3 mL/kg, dilute 50:50 with water (C)	PO	Once
Famotidine	Gastric ulcers, esophagitis	0.5-1 mg/kg (D)	IM, IV, PO, SC	12-24
Flumazenil	Hepatic encephalopathy	0.01-0.02 mg	IV	As needed
Flurazepam	Appetite stimulant	0.5 mg/kg (D). Maximum of 30 mg/day	PO	4-7 days
Folic acid	Nutritional supplement	0.25-0.5 mg/kg (C)	PO	24
	Supplement to pyrimethamine	2.5 mg/cat	PO	24
Glucosamine sulfate	Gastrointestinal inflammation	0.5 g/kg	PO	24
Glycerin, enema	Constipation/obstipation	250 mg or 12 mL glycerin	Rectally	1; repeat once only
Glyceryl monoacetate	Hypersialism	0.01 mg/kg	SC	As needed
Glycopyrrolate	Hypersialism	0.01 mg/kg	SC	As needed
Granisetron	Antiemetic	0.01 mg/kg	IV, PO	As needed

Table **19-1** Doses for Treatment of Gastrointestinal Disorders[161]—cont'd

Drug	Indication	Dose	Route	Interval (hr)
Hydrogen peroxide 3%	Emetic	5-10 mL	PO	Repeat in 20-30 minutes one time only
Ipecac syrup	Emetic	1-2.5 mL/kg (D). Maximum of 15 mL	PO	Repeat once in 20 min
Isopropamide/prochlorperazine	Antiemetic, antidiarrheal	0.14-0.22 mg/kg (D)	SC	12
		0.5-0.8 mg/kg (C)	IM, SC	12
Kaolin/pectin	Gastrointestinal tract protectant	3-6 g/kg	PO	2-6
Lactitol	Stool softener, hepatic encephalopathy	250 mg	PO	12
Lactulose	Stool softener, hepatic encephalopathy	0.5 mL/kg (D)	PO	8 or to achieve 2-3 soft stools per day
		5-45 mL/dog	PO	8
		2.5-5 mL/cat	PO	8
		0.25-1 mL/cat	PO	12-24
		5-10 mL/cat (diluted 1:3 with water)	Rectally	To effect
	Constipation	1 mL/4.5 kg (D)	PO	8, to effect
Levodopa	Hepatic encephalopathy	6.8 mg/kg initially, then 1.4 mg/kg	PO	6
Lime water	Alkaline gastric lavage	5 mL/kg	PO	Once
Loperamide	Antidiarrheal, acute colitis	0.06-0.20 mg/kg (D)	PO	8-12
		0.1-0.3 mg/kg (C)	PO	12-24
		0.08-1.16 mg/kg (C)	PO	12
Magnesium citrate	Laxative	2-4 mL/kg	PO	12-24 or to effect
Magnesium hydroxide	Antacid	5-30 mL/dog	PO	12-24
		5-10 mL/cat	PO	8-24
	Cathartic	15-50 mL/dog	PO	24 or to effect
		2-6 mL/cat	PO	24
Magnesium oxide	Antacid, laxative	1-2 mEq/kg	PO	24
Magnesium salts	Cathartic, stool softener	0.75-1 mEq Mg^{2+}/kg	IV	Over 24 hrs; CRI thereafter
		0.3-0.5 mEq/kg	IV	24
Magnesium sulfate 25%	Hypomagnesemia	5-15 mL	IM, IV over 1-2 hr	Repeat as needed
Maropitant	Acute vomiting	1-2 mg /kg (D)	PO, SC	24
	Motion sickness	8 mg/kg (D)	PO	24 × 2 days
	Acute vomiting, motion sickness	1 mg/kg (C)	PO, SC	24
Meclizine	Antiemetic, motion sickness	25 mg/dog	PO	24, beginning 1 hr before riding in car
		4 mg/kg	PO	24
		12.5 mg/cat	PO	24, beginning 1 hr before riding in car
Megestrol acetate	Appetite stimulant/ anticachexia	0.25-5 mg/kg (C)	PO	24 × 3-5 days then every 48 to 72 hr
Mesalamine	Inflammatory bowel disease	10-20 mg/kg (D)	PO	6-8
Metamucil (psyllium)	Laxative	2-10 g/dog	PO (in moistened food)	12-24
		2-4 g/dog	PO (in moistened food)	12-24
Methscopolamine bromide	Antiemetic, decongestant	0.3-1 mg/kg	PO	8. Use cautiously in cats
Methylcellulose	Laxative	0.5-5 g/dog	PO	As needed
		1-1.5 g/cat	PO	As needed

Continued

Table **19-1** Doses for Treatment of Gastrointestinal Disorders[161]—cont'd

Drug	Indication	Dose	Route	Interval (hr)
Metoclopramide	Gastric motility disorders, antiemetic	0.2-0.5 mg/kg	IM, PO, SC	6-8
		5 to 20 μg/kg (0.005 - 0.02 mg/kg)	IV CRI	
	Gastric reflux	0.2-0.4 mg/kg	PO	8. Administer 30 min before meals and at bedtime
Metronidazole	Cholangitis	7.5 mg/kg	PO	8
	Bacterial overgrowth	10 to 15 mg/kg	PO	12
	Stomatitis	10 to 15 mg/kg	PO	12
	Giardia	10-30 mg/kg	PO	12-24
Milk thistle (silymarin)	Hepatoprotection	50-250 mg	PO	12-24
		30 mg/kg (D)	PO	24
Mineral oil	Laxative	5-30 mL (D)	PO, rectally	12
		1-2 mL/kg (D)	PO, rectally	12
		5-10 mL (C)	PO, rectally	12
Mirtazapine	Appetite stimulant	3.75 mg/cat (0.25 of a 15 mg tablet)	PO	As needed
Misoprostol	Gastric protectant	1-5 μg/kg (D)	PO	6-8
Nandrolone decanoate	Anabolic effects, appetite stimulant	5 mg/kg (D). Maximum of 200 mg/week	IM	2-3 weeks
	Bone marrow or appetite stimulant	1-3 mg/kg (D). Maximum of 200 mg per week	IM	Every 7 days
Neostigmine	Myasthenia gravis	<5 kg: 0.25 mg/dog	IM	6
		5-25 kg: 0.25-0.5 mg/dog	IM	6
		>25 kg: 0.5-0.75 mg/dog	IM	6
		40 μg/kg or 0.04 mg/kg (D)	SC	6-8
		40 μg/kg or 0.04 mg/kg (C)	SC	6-8
	Diagnostic aid for myasthenia gravis	40 μg/kg (D)	IM	Once
		20 μg/kg	IV	Once
Nizatidine	Gastric ulcers	5 mg/kg (D)	PO	24
	Prokinetic	2.5-5 mg/kg	PO	24
Omeprazole	Reflux esophagitis, gastrointestinal ulceration	0.7-2 mg/kg (D)	PO	24 × 10-14 days
		20 mg/dog	PO	24
		>20 kg: 1 capsule (20 mg)	PO	24
		<20 kg: 0.5 capsule (10 mg)	PO	24
		<5 kg: 0.25 capsule (5 mg)	PO	24
		0.5-1.5 mg/kg	PO	24
	Helicobacter (adjuvant)	0.7 mg/kg	PO	24
Ondansetron	Antiemetic	0.1-1 mg/kg	PO	12-24
		Loading dose: 0.5 mg/kg	IV	Once
		Followed by: 0.5 mg/kg	IV	1 h infusion
	Intractable vomiting	0.11-0.176 mg/kg	IV (slowly)	6-12
Olsalazine	Inflammatory bowel disease	10-20 mg/kg (D)	PO	8-12
Opium tincture	Antidiarrheal	0.01-0.02 mg/kg	PO	12
Oxazepam	Appetite stimulant	2-2.5 mg (C)	PO	12
Pancreatic enzyme	Pancreatic exocrine insufficiency	0.5- 2 tsp	PO (crush pills first)	Mix with food. If cat is intolerant, then dose orally. Mixing 20 min in advance may not be necessary.

Table 19-1 Doses for Treatment of Gastrointestinal Disorders[161]—cont'd

Drug	Indication	Dose	Route	Interval (hr)
Paregoric	Antidiarrheal	0.05-0.06 mg/kg (5 mL of paregoric corresponds to approximately 2 mg of morphine)	PO	8-12
Petrolatum, white	Laxative	1-5 mL/cat	PO	24
Phenobarbital	Irritable colon syndrome	2.2 mg/kg (D)	PO	12
Phosphate enemas	Constipation, obstipation	1-2 mL/kg (medium and large D)	Rectally	Once. Use cautiously
Polyethylene glycol	Colonscopic procedure	20-33 mL/kg	PO (volume may require orogastric or nasogastric tube)	In fasted (18-24 hr) animal, administer 2 doses 4-6 hr apart the day before the procedure. Follow with warm water enema before anesthesia.
		60 mL/kg	PO (volume may require orogastric or nasogastric tube)	In fasted (18-24 h) animal, administer 2 doses 4-6 h apart the day before the procedure. Follow with warm water enema before anesthesia.
	Preoperative mechanical cleansing	60 mL/kg	PO (volume may require orogastric or nasogastric tube)	The evening before surgery
Prednisolone/ Prednisone (++)	Eosinophilic ulcers, plasma cell gingivitis	1-2.2 mg/kg (D)	PO	24 × 7 days, then taper to every 48
	Eosinophillic gastritis, enteritis colitis	1-3 mg/kg (D)	PO	24, then taper to every 48
	Plasmacytic/lymphocytic enteritis	1-2 mg/kg	PO	12, then taper dose weekly
	Lymphocytic cholangitis, chronic active hepatitis, copper hepatopathy	0.25-2 mg/kg (D)	PO	12
	Myasthenia gravis	0.5 mg/kg (D)	PO	12 initially. Slowly increase to every 24 until remission then every 48.
Prochlorperazine	Antiemetic	1 mg/kg (D)	PO	12
		0.13-0.5 mg/kg (D)	IM	6-8
		0.1 mg/kg	IM	6
		0.13 mg/kg (C)	IM	12
		0.5 mg/kg (C)	PO	6-8
Promethazine hydrochloride	Antihistamine, antiemetic	0.2-0.4 mg/kg. Maximum of 1 mg/kg	IM, IV, PO	6-8
	Acute colitis, irritable colon syndrome, antiemetic	0.22-0.5 mg/kg	PO	8. Maximum of 3 days
	Antiemetic, antidiarrheal	0.25 mg/kg	PO	8
Propantheline bromide	Anticholinergic	0.25-1 mg/kg (D)	PO	8
		7-30 mg/dog	PO	8
		0.8-1.6 mg/kg (C)	PO	8
		7.5 mg/cat	PO	8
Prucalopride	Colonic motility	0.02-1.25 mg/kg (D)	IV, PO	Frequency not established
		0.64 mg/kg (C)	IV, PO	Frequency not established
Psyllium	Bulk laxative	3.4 g/5-10 kg (D)	PO (with food)	As needed

Continued

Table 19-1 Doses for Treatment of Gastrointestinal Disorders[161]—cont'd

Drug	Indication	Dose	Route	Interval (hr)
Pyridostigmine bromide	Myasthenia gravis	0.2-3 mg/kg (D)	PO	8-12. Administer anticholinergic first. Start at a low dose and increase as needed.
		0.3-0.5 mg/kg	PO	8-12
		7.5-30 mg/dog	PO	12
		<5 kg: 45 mg/dog	PO	6
		5-25 kg: 45-90 mg/dog	PO	6
		>25 kg: 90-135 mg/dog	PO	6
		0.02-0.04 mg/kg	IV	2
		Initial dose: 0.25 mg/kg (C)	PO	Once
		Followed by: 1-3 mg/kg (C)	PO	8-12
Ranitidine hydrochloride	Esophagitis, gastric reflux	1-2 mg/kg (D)	PO	12
	Chronic gastritis, gastrointestinal tract ulceration, gastrinoma	2-4 mg/kg (D)	PO	8-12
		0.5 mg/kg	IV, PO, SC	12
	Hypergastrinemia from chronic renal failure	1-2 mg/kg, or (D)	PO	12
		0.5 mg/kg (D)	IV, SC	12
		3.5 mg/kg (C)	PO	12
		2.5 mg/kg (C)	IV	12
Riboflavin (vitamin B_2)	Nutritional supplement	10-20 mg/day (D)	PO	24
S-adenyosyl methionine	Hepatopathy, behavioral disorders, degenerative joint disease	<5.5 kg: 90 mg	PO (on an empty stomach)	24
		5.5-11 kg: 180- 225 mg	PO (on an empty stomach)	24
		11-16 kg: 225 mg	PO (on an empty stomach)	24
		16-30 kg: 450 mg	PO (on an empty stomach)	24
		30-41 kg: 675 mg	PO (on an empty stomach)	24
		>41 kg: 900 mg	PO (on an empty stomach)	24
	Hepatitis	17-20 mg/kg	PO (on an empty stomach)	24
		200 mg/cat	PO (on an empty stomach)	24
Scopolamine hydrobromide	Antiemetic	0.03 mg/kg (D)	IM, SC	6
Selenium	Pancreatitis, acute	0.1 mg/kg	IV CRI	
Senna (granules)	Laxative	2.5 mL (0.5 tsp)/cat	PO (with food)	24
Senna (syrup)	Laxative	5 mL/cat	PO	24
Silymarin	See Milk thistle			
Simethicone	Antiflatulence	0.5-2 mg/kg	PO	6
Sodium sulfate (Glauber's salt)	Cathartic	1 g/kg (D)	PO	4 × 6
		50 mg/kg of a 1.5% solution made with water (C)	PO	4 × 6
		5-20 g/dog	PO	4 × 6
		2-5 g/cat	PO	4 × 6
Sorbitol	Laxative	3 mL/kg	PO	Once or to effect

Table 19-1 Doses for Treatment of Gastrointestinal Disorders[161]—cont'd

Drug	Indication	Dose	Route	Interval (hr)
Sucralfate	Gastrointestinal tract ulceration	0.5-1 g/dog	PO	6-8; maximum efficacy will occur if administered before antisecretory drugs
		0.25-0.5 g/cat	PO	8-12; maximum efficacy will occur if administered before antisecretory drugs
	Hemorrhagic pancreatits, vomiting with renal failure	0.5-1 g/dog	PO	8; maximum efficacy will occur if administered before antisecretory drugs
	Esophagitis, gastric reflux	0.5-1g, prepared as a slurry	PO	8
Sulfobromophthalein sodium	Hepatic function testing	5 mg/kg	IV	Once. Collect serum 30 minutes after injection
Tegaserod	Colonic motility	0.03-0.3 mg/kg (D)	IV	12
Tetramine	Copper hepatopathy	10-15 mg/kg (D)	PO	12
Thiamine, vitamin B_1	Nutritional supplement	1-2 mg/cat	IM	12 until resolution of signs
		100-250 mg/cat	IM, SC	12 until regression of symptoms
		4 mg/kg	PO	24
		Initial dose: 10-20 mg/kg (C)	IM, SC	8-12 until signs abate
		Followed by: 10 mg/kg (C)	PO	24 × 21 days
		5-50 mg/dog	IM, IV, SC	12-24
		1-2 mg	IM	12-24
		2 mg/kg	PO	24
		100-250 mg	SC	12 until regression of symptoms
Thiethylperazine	Antiemetic	0.2-0.4 mg/kg (D)	SC	8-12
		0.13-0.2 mg/kg	IM	8-12
Trimethobenzamide	Antiemetic	3 mg/kg (D)	IM	8-12
Tylosin	Inflammatory bowel disease	10-40 mg/kg (C)	PO	8-12
Ursodeoxycholic acid (ursodiol)	Hepatopathy	5-15 mg/kg	PO	24 or divide dose and administer every 12
Viokase	Pancreatic exocrine insufficiency	3 × 325 mg tablets or 2.2-4.4 g (1-2 tsp) of powder (D)	PO	With each meal
		1 × 325 mg tablet or 1.1-2.2 g (0.5-1 tsp) of powder (C)	PO	With each meal
Vitamin A	Nutritional supplement	400 IU/kg	PO	24 × 10 days
Vitamin B_{12}	Nutritional supplement	100-200 μg/dog	PO, SC	24
		50-100 μg/cat	PO, SC	24
	Inherited B_{12} malabsorption	0.25-1 mg/dog	SC, IM	7 days × 1 month, then every 3 months
Vitamin B_2, riboflavin	Nutritional supplement	10-20 mg/dog	PO	24
		5-10 mg/cat	PO	24
Vitamin E	Malabsorption syndromes	100-500 IU/dog	PO	24 × 4 wk
Vitamin K_1, phytonadione	Chronic liver disease	1-5 mg/kg	PO, SC	12. Recheck coagulation at 2 days and 3 weeks
		1 mg/kg/day	PO	24 x 4-6 weeks
		5 mg/kg (C)	IM	12-24
		Loading dose: 2.5 mg/kg (small D)	SC (several sites)	Once
		Followed by: 0.25-2.5 mg/kg	PO	Divide dose and administer every 8-12
		Loading dose: 5 mg/kg (large D)	SC (several sites)	Once
		Followed by: 5 mg/kg	PO	Divide dose and administer every 8-12

Continued

Table **19-1** Doses for Treatment of Gastrointestinal Disorders[161]—cont'd

Drug	Indication	Dose	Route	Interval (hr)
	Acute hepatopathy	2-3 mg/kg (small D)	SC	12, until coagulation normal
		5 mg/kg (large D)	SC	12, until coagulation normal
		15-25 mg/ small cat	IV	24 × 7 or until coagulation normal
		15-25 mg/large cat	IV	24 × 3-4 weeks until coagulation normal. Check 1-2 days after therapy discontinued
Xylazine	Emetic	0.44 mg/kg (C)	IM	To effect
Zinc acetate	Copper hepatotoxicosis	5-10 mg/kg (D)	PO	12
		Initial dose: 100 mg/dog	PO	12 × 3 months
		Maintenance dose: 50 mg/dog	PO	12
Zinc sulfate	Copper hepatotoxicosis	5-10 mg/kg (D)	PO	12

PO, By mouth; *C*, cat; *IM*, intramuscular; *SC*, subcutaneous; *D*, dog; *IV*, intravenous; *IP*, intraperitoneal; *GI*, gastrointestinal; *CRI*, constant-rate infusion.

of well-being, and causes weight gain, particularly of fat. Fat is the preferred weight gain because it provides more kilocalories per gram than proteins or carbohydrate and helps stabilize body temperatures.[12] Megestrol decreases the effects, sometimes by inhibiting formation of TNF-alpha, interleukin-1 (IL-1), and interleukin-6 (IL-6). Centrally, megestrol appears to modulate neurotransmitters responsible for appetite regulation such as NPY, which in turn stimulates the release of other mediators. Megestrol may also stabilize declining concentrations of β-endorphins in the cerebrospinal fluid.

KEY POINT 19-4 Megestrol acetate targets cachexia either directly and indirectly, stimulating appetite and antagonizing the catabolic metabolic effects of cytokines.

Effects of megestrol are dose and (particularly for fat gain) duration dependent. Initial weight gain requires high concentrations (>300 ng/mL) for more than 40% of a 24-hour dosing interval. In humans this requires administration of the tablet four times daily. Megestrol acetate is used rather than other progestationals, which must be given parenterally.[12] Bioavailabilty of megestrol acetate is variable, being greater with the oral solution compared to the tablet. With tablets, peak concentrations may vary 6 fold; variability is much less with the oral solution. Disposition is complex. Hepatic metabolism is necessary to free the steroid from acetate, with the steroids subsequently conjugated with glucuronic acid before elimination. Elimination also varies, with half-lives that range from 13 to 105 hours. In humans, a single daily dose of the suspension (800 mg) achieves peak concentrations between 1500 and 3000 ng/mL. Not surprisingly, the oral solution is associated with a much higher rate of response compared with the tablet. A micronized (nanocrystal) preparation is currently under investigation for human use.

Limited information is available regarding use of megestrol acetate in animals. The disposition of megestrol acetate has been described in Beagles as part of the preclinical assessment in humans. Four preparations were studied for 72 hours after administration of 10 mg/kg (by oral gavage) either in the fasted or the fed (high-fat meal) state. The preparations included two different nanocrystal oral solutions and two commercially available oral suspensions (Par Pharmaceutical and Bristol-Myers). After the high-fat meal, peak concentrations (1600 to 2200 ng/mL) and area under the curve (AUC) were higher with the nanocrystal oral suspensions compared with the commercially available oral suspensions (both approximating 300 ng/mL). Although the elimination half-life was not reported, the disappearance half-life of megestrol appeared to be between 10 and 20 hours.[12]

Megestrol acetate appears to be better tolerated in humans compared with animals. The primary adverse events in humans are thromobembolic, reflecting increased thrombin receptors in smooth muscles. Venous distention and capacitance increase, contributing to reduced blood flow and stasis. Addison's disease and glucose intolerance are sporadically reported, reflecting its intrinsic corticosteroid activities.[12]

Anecdotally, megesterol acetate has been effective in dogs to treat chemotherapy-induced nausea and inappetence. However, in humans a prospective randomized controlled clinical trial in cachectic human cancer patients compared the efficacy of an anabolic steroid (fluoxymesterone [10 mg, 0.142 mg/k] twice daily), megestrol acetate tablets (800 mg [11.4 mg/kg] once daily), and a glucocorticoid (dexamethasone, 0.75 mg [0.01 mg/kg] four times daily) as appetite stimulants. Of the three ,the anabolic steroid was least (significantly) and megestrol (nonsignificantly) most clinically effective. Glucocorticoids usually were discontinued because of side effects, although megestrol acetate was associated with the most thromboembolic events.[13]

APPETITE SUPPRESSANTS AND ANTI-OBESITY DRUGS

Obesity is a physiologic disorder of energy balance in which energy intake exceeds energy expenditures. Excessive energy is stored as fat. In rodent models and humans, leptin deficiency or leptin resistance can result in obesity caused by hyperphagia and decreased energy expenditure.[3] Other characteristics of obesity in humans include non–insulin-dependent diabetes mellitus, severe insulin resistance, hypothermia and cold intolerance, infertility, and decreased lean body mass.[3]

Anti-obesity drugs might target mediators of appetite or satiety. However, differences in response to drugs that affect appetite limit extrapolation of studies among species. Hypoleptinemia has been associated with obesity. However, obesity appears to be accompanied by resistance to leptin or leptin-like drugs. Alternative targets for treatment of obesity might include mediators of leptin actions, including NPY, Y1 and Y5 receptor agonists, and melanocortin MC4 receptors. Central chemical targets for drugs that might influence appetite include all mediators, their receptors, or upstream regulators of mediator release. These include anorexigenic signals such as α-MSH, opioids, and serotonin (specifically the 5-HT2C receptor) or mediators of satiety that emerge after food ingestion, such as cholecystokinin (CCK), glucagon-like peptide-1 (GLP-1), ghrelin, peptide YY (PYY), bombesin-like peptides, enterostatin, oxyntomodulin, and apolipoprotein IV (apoAVI).

Among the drugs studied for central suppressant effects are cannabinoids, the manipulation of which may influence consumption of highly palatable foods. For example, rimonabant is a cannabinoid receptor type 1 (CB1) receptor antagonist that decreases intake of palatable foods, leading to decreased body weight in rodents. However, dogs (and other species) respond differently to cannabinoids. For example, although CB1 antagonists decrease food intake, causing weight loss in dogs, appetite suppression is attenuated after several weeks. Dogs also appear more sensitive to side effects associated with CB1 antagonists, exhibiting vomiting, diarrhea, and pruritus at doses necessary to decrease appetite. Although cats tolerate antagonists better than dogs, they respond only at doses associated with severe pruritus, panting, agitation, and CNS stimulation.[14] Selective 5-HT_{2C} receptor antagonists appear to be effective in decreasing food intake in rodent models but not in dogs or cats. Higher doses that might be more effective are associated with adverse effects.[14] The human pancreatic lipase inhibitor orlistat is associated with modest weight loss in dogs. However, significant increase in food intake, presumably in response to caloric loss, is accompanied by markedly increased fecal fat, leading to uncontrolled leakage and perianal and abdominal soiling.[14]

KEY POINT 19-5 Anti-obesity drugs target mediators of appetite or satiety or alter energy intake, expenditure, or use.

Anti-obesity drugs might target altered energy intake. Dirlotapide is a selective microsomal triglyceride transfer protein inhibitor that blocks both assembly and release of lipoprotein particles into the bloodstream (package insert [PI]). However, the mechanism by which weight gain is controlled is not clear. Appetite suppression reflects local GI effects, including decreased fat absorption. Subsequent lipid filling of enterocytes appears to stimulate a satiety signal. Fecal fat is increased. Efficacy does not appear to correlate with serum concentrations. The impact of dirlotapide on serum or gastric mucosal leptin, ASP, or adiponectin apparently has not been addressed.

In dogs, dirlotapide (Slentrol) is systemically bioavailable after oral administration, although absorption is markedly variable. Elimination of absorbed drug reflects hepatic metabolism that follows nonlinear kinetics, with concentrations increasing disproportionately with dose. Mean half-life varies between 5 to 18 hours at the clinical dose but appears to increase with dose and duration of dosing ((package insert).

Safety of dirlotapide when administered in dogs for 1 year has been established in dogs. Adverse effects, should they occur, generally emerge within the first month of therapy. According to the package insert, the incidence of vomiting and diarrhea was greater in dirlotapide-treated (25% and 12%, respectively) compared with control-treated (corn oil) animals (22% and 7%, respectively). Serum chemistry changes occurred early, including mild to moderately increased serum hepatic transaminase, although concentrations remained within the normal range and decreased over the 4-month treatment period. Mean cholesterol and high-density lipoprotein also decreased (below reference range for cholesterol during the treatment period); however, triglycerides did not change. Serum total protein, albumin, and blood urea nitrogen levels also decreased compared with those of control animals, although all were within normal ranges. Enterocytes were characterized by lipid vacuolization and the liver by mild periportal fatty changes.

Absorption of fat-soluble vitamins might be affected by dilortapide. Plasma vitamins A and E concentrations were lower in treated compared with control dogs, but concentrations appeared to increase during weight stabilization (second through sixth months), reaching control concentrations after treatment was discontinued (PI). A study in 72 obese Labrador Retrievers (n = 48) receiving dilortapide at the labeled dose for 52 weeks was reported in materials obtained through the Freedom of Information Act. Weight loss during the initial and retraining phases was 18.4% and 5% to 6%, respectively. In addition to vomiting and diarrhea, ophthalmic abnormalities were found at study end. These included focal or multifocal retinopathies or diffuse retinal degeneration in eight dogs receiving the drug for 12 months and two dogs for 6 months. Generalized progressive retinal atrophy occurred in one dog treated for 12 months and one dog treated for 6 months, respectively. Cataracts were observed in four dogs receiving the drug for 12 months and one dog receiving the drug for 6 months. Pretreatment ophthalmic exams were not available, and abnormalities were not reported in control dogs, although it is not clear if they did not occur or simply were not recorded. However, a follow-up 9-month study of 34 dogs of different breeds, in which a different formulation was used that yielded pharmacokinetics similar to the commercial preparation, found no ocular lesions, leading investigators to conclude that previous ocular abnormalities reflected breed predisposition.

Use of dilortapide in dogs must be accompanied by a weight loss program. Loss of appetite will not last more than several days after therapy is discontinued. Dosing is complex and is

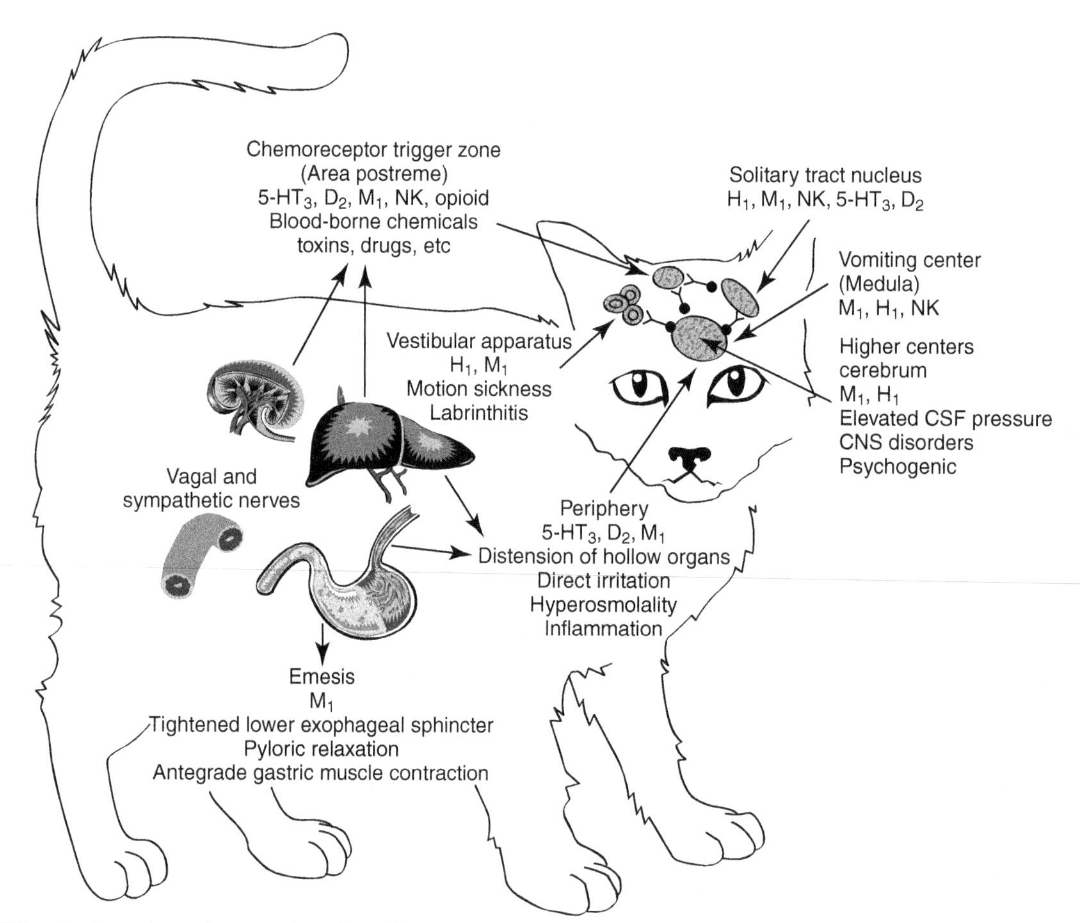

Figure 19-2 Sites that mediate the emetic reflex. The secondary neurotransmitters at each site are in parentheses. Stimuli that mediate emesis at each site are listed below the neurotransmitter. *CNS,* Central nervous system; *CTZ,* chemoreceptor trigger zone; *CSF,* cerebrospinal fluid; *LES,* lower esophageal sphincter.

based on body weight (see package insert). A total of 11% to 13% of body weight was lost in patients studied during drug approval (PI), an amount considered to contribute positively to animal health. At study end mean final dose was 0.26 to 0.56 mg/kg. Dilortapide should not be administered to humans or cats. Adverse reactions in humans include abdominal pain, distention, diarrhea, flatulence, nausea, and vomiting.

Several drugs may affect appetite secondary to their intended therapeutic effect. Propofol (1-2 mg/kg IV) was reported in a research abstract[15] to be an effective appetite stimulant, presumably through stimulation of GABA-A and NYP and inhibition of serotonin receptors. Anecdotally, omega-3 fatty acids (EPA and DHA) may stimulate appetite by inhibiting cytokines responsible for anorexia.

EMETICS AND ANTIEMETICS

The Vomiting Reflex

Emesis is a complex protective reflex that is not well developed in all species but does occur in both dogs and cats.[16-18] Although several afferent pathways may be responsible for initiating emesis, all signals are coordinated by the emetic center. Located in the lateral reticular formation in the mid brainstem, the emetic center is in close proximity to the nucleus tractus solitarius of the vagus nerve and the chemoreceptor trigger zone (CTZ), the latter of which is located adjacent to the area postrema in the bottom of the lateral ventricle. The latter coordinates vomiting associated with blood-borne chemicals (Figures 19-2 and 19-3). The emetic center coordinates vomiting associated with afferent peripheral and central (neural) signals. Among the signals coordinating vomiting is the tachykinin neuropeptid, ≥substance P. Drugs that cause or ameliorate vomiting generally do so by modifying afferent or efferent neurotransmitters responsible for transmission of the signal from various afferent sites. The emetic center is protected by the blood–brain barrier, whereas the CTZ is not; therefore, the CTZ is able to monitor the presence of emetics in the blood or cerebrospinal fluid. However, drug penetrability to each site varies, affecting both drug safety and efficacy.[16-20]

KEY POINT 19-6 Drugs that inhibit emetic signals at the vomition center have the potential to be the broadest in efficacy.

Several sites in the vomiting reflex are targeted by drugs. Ideally, drugs that target the emetic center would be characterized by the broadest spectrum and potentially the best efficacy. Historically, because such drugs must be able to penetrate

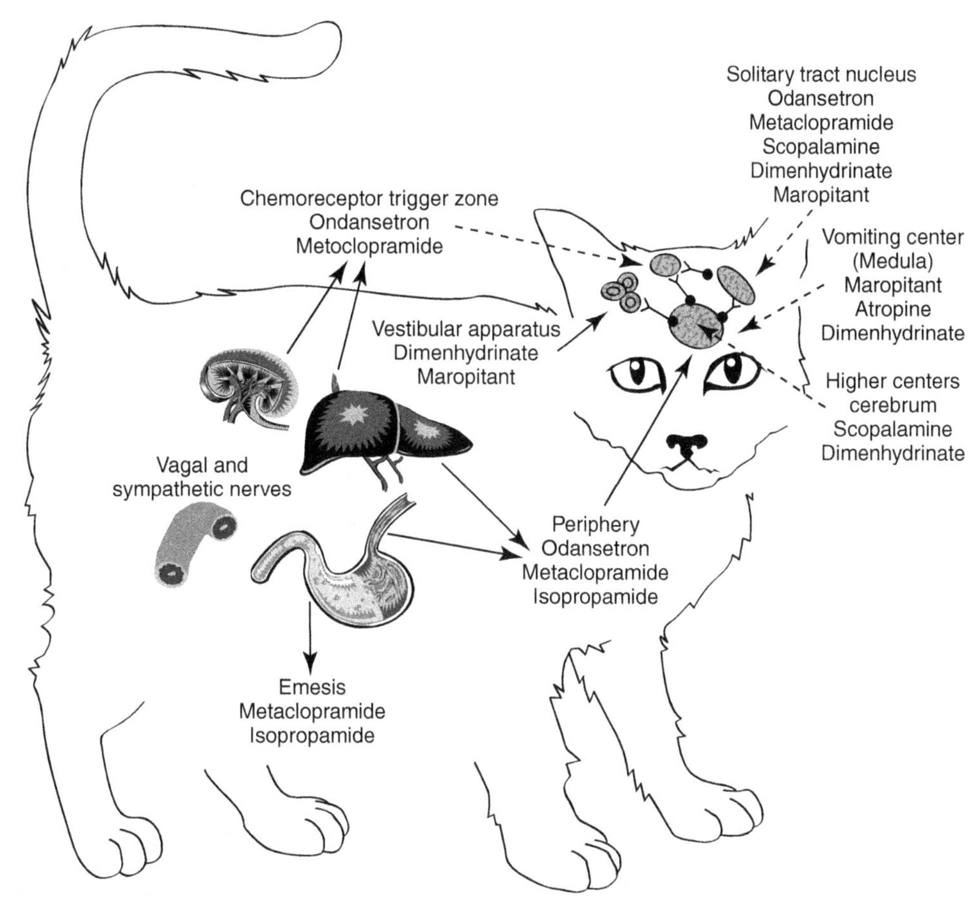

Figure 19-3 Antiemetic drugs effective at each site of the emetic reflex. *CTZ,* Chemoreceptor trigger zone.

the blood–brain barrier, they tend to be characterized by increased risk of side effects. This risk is minimized if the drug targets a mediator whose effects are limited to the vomiting center only. In addition to integration of the emetic reflex, impulses integrated by the center include afferent signals from higher centers such as the cerebral cortex and limbic system. For example, psychogenic vomiting, or vomiting induced by visual and olfactory stimuli, originates in the cerebral cortex, whereas head injuries and increased intracranial pressure initiate emesis by way of the limbic pathways. The solitarius nucleus contains receptors for enkephalin, histamine, serotonin (5-HT_3), and acetylcholine (ACh). ACh is a major afferent neurotransmitter in the higher centers, with histamine acting as a secondary transmitter by way of H_1 receptors.[19] However, substance P, a member of the tachykinin family of neuropeptides, has recently been identified as a key neurotransmitter associated with emesis in higher centers, including the emetic center.[21] Substance P targets neurokinin (NK_1) receptors located throughout the emetic center (as reviewed by Wu[20]), including the nucleus tractus solitarius, the area postrema, and the dorsal motor nucleus of the vagus.[22] The emetic center also involves cannabinoid receptors (also located in the CTZ), although their role is not clear.

Blood-borne chemical compounds stimulate the CTZ.[17,19] Examples include circulating toxins associated with disease (uremia, pyometra, liver disease, endotoxemia), radiation sickness, and drugs (e.g., opioids, cardiac glycosides, anticancer chemotherapeutic agents). Signals in the CTZ are mediated by dopaminergic (D_2)[19] and serotonergic (5-hydroxytryptamine; 5-HT_3) receptors[23] and neurokinin receptors. Histamine by way of H_1 receptors acts as a secondary neurotransmitter at the CTZ. Neurokinin receptors in humans are responsible for the delayed phase of vomiting associated with cisplatin anticancer chemotherapy. Alpha-2 receptors associated with the area postrema also induce emesis in dogs, cats, and other species.[24-26] The CTZ also is rich in opioid receptors. The safety of CTZ-active drugs may be increased by selectively targeting the subreceptor types for each neurotransmitter.

Emetic impulses originating from the semicircular canals of the vestibular apparatus are transmitted by the eighth cranial nerve to the vestibular nuclei and then by way of the CTZ and the uvula and nodulus of the cerebellum to the emetic center. This pathway, mediated by histaminergic (subtype H_1) receptors, is responsible for eliciting the emesis that accompanies motion sickness and labyrinthitis.[27]

Peripheral impulses cause emesis that arises from stimulation of the pharynx and fauces; the signals are transmitted by afferent nerves in the ninth cranial nerve to the emetic center. Other peripheral afferent pathways include those arising from stimulation (i.e., irritation or distention) of various visceral organs and tissues. Impulses may be carried by sympathetic or vagal afferents from the heart, stomach, duodenum, small intestine, liver, gallbladder, peritoneum, kidneys, ureter, urinary bladder, and uterus. ACh is the primary neurotransmitter mediating the afferent limb of the emesis reflex from peripheral causes. Muscarinic receptors initiate the impulse that travels to the emetic center by way of the vagus nerve.

Efferent signals that stimulate the emetic reflex travel back to the stomach by the tenth cranial (vagus) nerve. ACh also acts as the primary efferent neurotransmitter in the vagus and in the smooth muscle of the stomach. In the stomach, dopamine receptors (D_2) appear to inhibit gastric motility, during nausea and vomiting. In addition, dopamine receptors contribute to reflexes that allow relaxation of the upper stomach and delayed gastric emptying associated with gastric distention caused by food.[24] Finally, serotonin (by way of 5-HT_3 receptors) contributes afferent pathways from the stomach and small intestine.[24]

Emetics

Clinically, emesis is pharmacologically induced to empty the anterior portion of the digestive tract. Indications include preparation for induction of general anesthesia in animals that may have food in the stomach (e.g., use of hydromorphone) or treatment of ingested, noncorrosive poisons.

Peripherally Acting (Reflex) Emetics

Although their efficacy and safety vary, a number of substances induce emesis by either distending the pharynx, esophagus, stomach, or duodenum (hollow organs) or irritating the epithelium of the GI tract. Distention with warm water or saline can induce the emetic response. In addition, in the case of toxin ingestion, administration of warm water by stomach tube may help dilute poisons. Emesis can be induced in dogs by oral administration of a solution of warm saturated (strong) sodium chloride or pharyngeal placement of a small amount of plain table salt or neutral salt crystals, such as sodium carbonate. Orally administered hydrogen peroxide (3%) often induces emesis rapidly in cats and dogs, although fatal aspiration of hydrogen peroxide foam is possible. Ipecac syrup is an over-the-counter emetic commonly recommended to induce emesis in human pediatric patients. It contains the alkaloid emetine, which increases lacrimation, salivation, and bronchial secretions. Emesis usually, but not consistently, occurs as a result of both peripheral and central stimulation. If repeated use fails to induce emesis, however, gastric lavage may be indicated to remove potentially toxic doses of the drug. Although ipecac syrup or powder has been used as an emetic for many years for cats, adverse effects include death, and its use in cats is discouraged.

Centrally Acting Emetics

The central effects of ipecac were discussed in the previous section. Although a number of drugs are capable of stimulating the CTZ centrally, certain opiates, particularly apomorphine, are indicated for their emetic effect. Apomorphine hydrochloride is a synthetic derivative of morphine but is characterized with only marginal depressant activity. Its emetic activity reflects stimulation of dopamine receptors and more readily than other morphinelike actions. Emesis will occur regardless of the route of administration, although oral doses are higher than those by other routes to compensate for reduced oral bioavailability. Emesis generally occurs in 2 to 10 minutes after subcutaneous or conjunctival administration. Although apomorphine stimulates vomiting at the CTZ, it also directly depresses the emetic center, and subsequent doses are not likely to induce emesis if the first dose was not successful. Excessive doses of apomorphine can depress the CNS, particularly the respiratory center, and are contraindicated in the presence of existing central depression.Apomorphine is currently available as an injectable preparation.

Xylazine is an α_2-agonist historically used for sedative analgesia. Emesis in dogs is not as consistent as in cats. Emesis mediated by α_2 stimulation occurs in cats at doses lower than that recommended for sedation (0.05 mg/kg).[26] Emetogens were evaluated in cats in anticipation of an antiemetic clinical trial.[22] Three emetogens were tested, with xylazine (0.44 mg/kg intramuscularly) reliably causing emesis. In contrast, neither apomorphine (0.04 mg/kg intravenously) nor syrup of ipecac (0.5 mL/kg) predictably caused emesis. Syrup of ipecac causes anorexia for several days. The use of medetomidine to induce emesis has not been reported, although its actions are similar to those of xylazine.

Antiemetics

Antiemetics control emesis by either a central or a peripheral action (see Figures 19-2 and 19-3). Both actions depend on and can be correlated with blockade of neurotransmission at receptor sites.[27,28] Centrally acting antiemetics block impulses at higher centers and at the emetic center and include muscarinic anticholinergics and drugs that target neurokinin receptors; antidopaminergics and antiserotonergics, which block dopaminergic receptors at the CTZ; and antihistaminergics, which primarily block H_1 receptors at the vestibular apparatus but secondarily at multiple central centers. Antiemetic agents possess either a limited or a broad effect, depending on which signals and centers are inhibited.

Centrally Acting Antiemetics

Vomiting center. Maropitant (Cerenia) is a neurokinin (NK_1) receptor antagonist that blocks the actions of substance P in the area postrema and nucleus solatarius; Aprepitant is a human drug in the same classused as rescue anti-emetic therapy in cancer patients nonresponsive to $5HT_3$–dexamethasone combinations.[29] Approved as an oral or subcutaneous preparation for dogs for the prevention of acute vomiting and motion sickness, maropitant has proved efficacious in the control of vomiting associated with many central and peripheral causes (Table 19-2).

In dogs bioavailability is greater after subcutaneous (91%) compared with oral (24%) administration, probably because of first-pass metabolism (PI). Relevant pharmacokinetic parameters include C_{max} (ng/mL) of 92 and 81 ng/mL at 0.75 and 2 hours, respectively, after administration of 1 mg/kg subcutaneously and 2 mg/kg orally, respectively. It is highly (99.5%) bound to plasma proteins. Maropitant is metabolized in dogs by CYP2D15 and CYP3A12. Elimination half-life in

Table **19-2** Antiemetic Drug–Receptor Interactions

		Dopamine D_2	Histamine H_1	Muscarinic M_1	Neurokinin NK-1	Serotonin 5-HT_3
Chlorpromazine	Phenothiazine	4+	4+	2+	4+	1+
Cyclizine	Antihistamine	1+	4+	3+		
Dimenhydrinate	Antihistamine	1+	4+			
Diphenydramine	Antihistamine	1+	4+			
Dolasetron	Antiserotonergic					4+
Maropitant	Neurokinin-antagonist					
Meclizine	Antihistamine		4+			
Metoclopramide	Benzamide	3+				2+
Ondansetron	Antiserotonergic					4+
Prochlorperazine	Phenothiazine	4+		2+		2+
Promethazine	Antihistamine		4+	2+		
Scopolamine	Anticholinergic	1+		4+	1+	

dogs approximates 9 hours after subcutaneous administration and 4 to 5 hours after oral administration. However, saturation of drug-metabolizing enzymes (probably CYP2D15) results in nonproportional increases in drug concentrations as the dose is increased up to 16 mg/kg orally; proportionality returns at 20 to 50 mg/kg orally. The injectable product remains potent for 28 days when prepared and stored according to labeled directions (amber vial at room temperature). Pain on injection may be common. Side effects delineated on the package insert include bone marrow hypoplasia in puppies younger than 11 (but not greater than 15) weeks of age.

KEY POINT 19-7 As a neurokinin antagonist, the specificity of maropitant results in safe and effective control of motion sickness and vomiting associated with both central and peripheral causes of vomiting.

Maropitant kinetics have been described in the cat after single subcutaneous and oral dosing and multiple subcutaneous dosing.[22] The drug was well tolerated in cats (n = 6) during 15 days of subcutaneous administration at doses ranging from 0.5 to 5 mg/kg; one cat developed tremors at the 5 mg/kg dose. No changes occurred in clinical laboratory tests. Plasma maropitant concentrations increased proportionately with dose. After single intravenous dosing, the volume of distribution of maropitant in cats was 6.2 L/kg. Maximum drug concentration after oral and subcutaneous administration of 1 mg/kg in cats were 156 ng/mL and 269 ng/mL (with 50% coefficient of variabilility), respectively. The elimination half-life in cats was 13 to 17 hours; oral bioavailability varied from 50% to 117%. A dose of 1 mg/kg administered intravenously, orally, or subcutaneously prevented emesis induced by xylazine (0.44 mg/kg intramuscularly) and experimentally induced motion sickness.

Maropitant was approved for use in animals in Europe before the United States. It has proved effective for control of vomiting associated with drugs such as cisplatin, apomorphine, and morphine derivatives. Maropitant has been compared with metoclopramide (0.33 mg/kg every 8 hours subcutaneously in study one, 0.5 to 1 mg/kg/day in study two) in two multicenter, prospective, randomized, positively controlled clinical trials.[30] Dogs (n = 64 in study one, 77 in study two) were at least 8 weeks of age and had been vomiting for at least 24 hours. Maropitant as studied at 1 mg/kg once daily subcutaneously in study one, and 0.5 to 1 mg/kg subcutaneously in study two with oral dosing of either maropitant or metoclopramide continued in study two until vomiting stopped or for up to 5 days. Vomiting caused by toxin ingestion or in patients with clinical signs indicating the need for acute surgical treatment were excluded. Causes of vomiting were multiple, including metabolic disorders, neoplasia, drug-induced reactions, food intolerance, and parvovirus. In both studies, maropitant was associated with a greater antiemetic response (discontinuation of vomiting) compared with metoclopramide.[31]

The comparative efficacy and safety of maropitant have been recently described for dogs on the basis of manufacturer-sponsored studies. It was compared (1 mg/kg) to placebo, metoclopramide (0.5 mg/kg subcutaneously), chlorpromazine (0.5 mg/kg subcutaneously), or ondansetron (0.5 mg/kg intravenously) in prevention of apomorphine-induced (0.1 mg/kg intravenously) vomiting. Efficacy in controlling vomiting either central or peripheral in origin was superior to that of chlorpromazine or metoclopramide but did not differ from ondansetron.[32] Both safety and efficacy for prevention of emesis associated with motion sickness were assessed in dogs (n = 198) 16 weeks or older. Dogs received approximately 8 mg/kg orally. Data were collected from 26 different clinics in two different crossover randomized, placebo-controlled double-blinded trials with a 14-day washout period between trials. Vomiting was prevented in 86% or 77% of dogs dosed at 2 or 10 hours before a 60-minute car ride. No adverse events were described.

Vestibular Apparatus

Vomiting caused by motion sickness or inner ear disease is mediated by the vestibular apparatus (see Table 19-2). Motion sickness in dogs and cats can be controlled for several (8 to 12) hours by administration of antihistamines such as cyclizine hydrochloride, meclizine hydrochloride, or diphenhydramine hydrochloride (Figure 19-4; see also Figure 19-3). Effects may reflect, in part, sedative effects. In addition to direct effects on neural pathways arising in the vestibular apparatus, actions may also be independent of antihistaminic effects. These may include anticholinergic effects. Those drugs able to penetrate the blood–brain barrier may thus have effects at the vomiting center but generally only at higher doses. Drowsiness and xerostomia (dry mouth) are typical side effects that occur with use of this group of drugs in humans. Although phenothiazine antiemetics may be used to treat motion sickness (e.g., acepromazine), efficacy may reflect sedative rather than direct effects. Centrally active maropitant is approved for use in dogs to treat motion sickness (see preceding discussion) and has been used successfully in cats as well.

Drugs Active at the Chemoreceptor Trigger Zone

Phenothiazines. Phenothiazines are broad-spectrum antiemetics that control emesis induced by most central causes other than labyrinthine stimulation (see Figure 19-4). Their classification as broad reflects the variety of signals that serve as primary, secondary, and tertiary mediators. Phenothiazines block emesis mediated by the CTZ at low doses because of their antidopaminergic (D_2) and, secondarily, antihistaminergic effects. Several phenothiazines are also characterized by weak antiserotinergic activity (see Table 19-2).[24] At higher (perhaps nonpharmacologic) doses, their anticholinergic effects may also act at other central sites, including the vomiting center. A variety of phenothiazine derivatives (e.g., chlorpromazine, prochlorperazine, triflupromazine, perphenazine, trifluoperazine, and mepazine) are used in small animals as antiemetics. The primary adverse effects associated with their use as antiemetics are sedation (which contributes to their efficacy for motion sickness) and hypotension due to peripheral α-blockade. Selection of a particular phenothiazine may be based on avoidance of adverse reactions. Fluid replacement therapy should be instituted if necessary before use of a phenothiazine. The impact of phenothiazine derivatives on the seizure threshold and in epileptic dogs is discussed in more depth in see Chapter 27. In general, their use in epileptic animals may require caution but do not appear to be contraindicated.

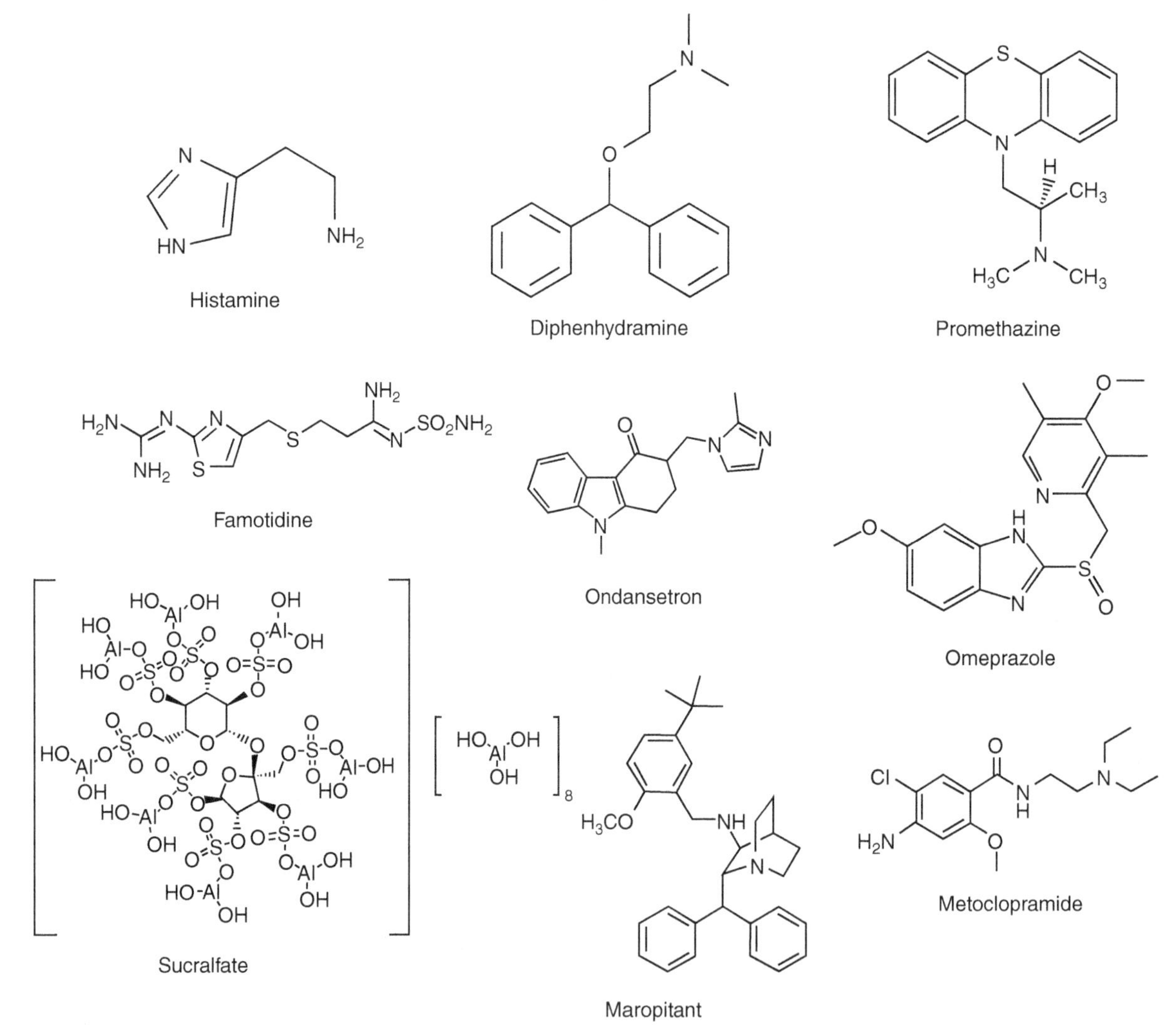

Figure 19-4 Chemical structures of selected gastrointestinal drugs.

KEY POINT 19-8 Drugs active at the CTZ are most effective for control of vomiting associated with drugs, toxins, and metabolic diseases.

Butyrophenone derivatives. Haloperidol (Haldol) and droperidol (Inapsine), which are also used as major tranquilizers, are potent antiemetics because of their antidopaminergic activity. These drugs are rarely used as antiemetics because of their side effects (similar to those encountered with the phenothiazine group but perhaps more profound).

Metoclopramide. Metoclopramide (see Figure 19-4) effectively blocks emesis mediated by the CTZ. Although its potent antagonism of dopamine was thought to be solely responsible for inhibition at the CTZ, metoclopramide is also a mixed 5-HT_3 receptor antagonist/5-HT_4 receptor agonist; emesis at high doses probably reflects 5-HT_3 receptor antagonism.[33] Metoclopramide effectively antagonizes apomorphine-induced emesis[34] and is 20 times as potent as phenothiazines (although differences in efficacy have not been documented).[35] The peripheral effects of metoclopramide on emesis resulting from prokinesis are discussed with the prokinetic drugs. Metoclopramide is indicated for control of emesis induced by a wide variety of blood-borne and peripheral causes.[36,37] High doses of metoclopramide, particularly when combined with dexamethasone, have been used to treat emesis associated with cancer chemotherapy in human patients.[38-40]

Serotonin antagonists. Serotonin antagonists are useful for their antiemetic effects mediated at the CTZ, particularly those induced by chemotherapeutic agents (see Table 19-2).[41] Unlike most other antiemetic drugs, antiserotonergics have no effects at other receptors, thus increasing the safety of those drugs selective for serotonin receptors. Ondansetron is a potent antiemetic and affects human cancer patients undergoing chemotherapy.[23,33,42] It has also been used in small animals suffering from refractory vomiting that have not responded to other antiemetics. The efficacy of ondansetron reflects, in part, its active metabolite dolasetron, which is also available as an orally administered as well as an intravenous product. Dolasetron also is metabolized (reduced) to a metabolite characterized by greater activity for 5-HT_3receptors compared with dolasetron.[43] The pharmacokinetics have been reported for dolasetron and its reduced metabolite in dogs ($n = 3$).[43] After intravenous administration of 2 mg/kg, clearance of the parent compound was 109 ± 41 mL/min/kg and volume of distribution was 0.83 ± 0.23 L/kg. After an oral dose of 5 mg/kg, C_{max} of the parent compound was 219 ± 149 ng/mL at 0.17 hours. The elimination half-life was 0.15 ± 0.11 hour. The active metabolite appears to potentially double the AUC of active compound. Although oral bioavailability of the parent compound is less than 10%, it is probable that first-pass metabolism results in formation of the active, reduced metabolite: oral administration of 5 mg/kg radioactive dolasetron results in a C_{max} of 700 ng/mL radioactivity (i.e., a combination of both radioactive parent and metabolite). Example uses of ondasetron include presurgical preparation, chemotherapy, and treatment of parvovirus infection; vomiting induced by hepatic lipidosis or GI irritation is less likely to respond. Ogilvie[44] has reviewed the use of dolasetron in dogs.

KEY POINT 19-9 Side effects of antiserotinergic antiemetics active at the CTZ are limited by their selectivity at the site.

Cyproheptadine is an anthistaminergic antiserotoninergic drug that has been used to control vomiting and diarrhea (the latter associated with spasticity) in humans. Its use in animals might be limited to more chronic control of vomiting when combined with other compounds or as part of combination therapy to treat vomiting and diarrhea associated with inflammatory bowel disease (IBD).

Miscellaneous Antiemetics

Sedatives such as the barbiturates (phenobarbital) and the benzodiazepines have been used to control psychogenic and behavioral vomiting. Glucocorticoids and in particular dexamethasone are characterized by antiemetic effects, although the antiemetic mechanism of action is not understood.[24] An antiinflammatory mechanism has been proposed. Glucocorticoids also appear to act in an additive or synergistic fashion when combined with other antiemetics. Both dexamethasone and methylprednisolone have been used in human patients to control vomiting associated with chemotherapy.

Natural extractions or synthesis of *Cannabis sativa* cannaboids inhibit vomiting, probably through stimulation of CB1 receptors. Dronabinol is an example of an antiemetic used in humans prophylactically to prevent chemotherapy-induced vomiting. It is characterized by complex kinetics that include high protein binding, extensive first pass metabolism to active and inactive metabolites. Side effects are similar to sympathomimetic drugs. Because dogs and cats respond differently to drugs which target cannanboid receptors, use should be based only on scientific evidence in the target species.

Peripherally Acting Antiemetics

Protectants. Drugs that locally protect the GI epithelium from further irritation may help prevent vomiting. Drugs that modulate gastric acid secretion might also provide antiemetic effects; these drugs are discussed later with the antiulcer drugs. Demulcents, antacids, and protectants such as kaolin, pectin, and bismuth salts are of limited benefit in the control of emesis that is gastric in origin. Distention or initial irritation of the stomach by these agents may exacerbate emesis. Antacids may be effective in certain cases. Other peripherally acting antiemetics include drugs that affect gastric motility, including anticholinergic drugs, and prokinetic drugs such as metoclopramide and domperidone (discussed later with modulators of GI motility).

Anticholinergics. Anticholinergic drugs that block muscarinic receptors in the emetic center also inhibit peripheral cholinergic transmission. Those anticholinergic drugs that do not cross the blood–brain barrier well are essentially peripheral in action and include glycopyrrolate, propantheline, isopropamide, and methscopolamine (which should not be used for cats). The ability of anticholinergics to suppress emesis is probably related to inhibition of afferent vagal impulses, relief of GI smooth muscle spasms, and inhibition of gastroenteric secretions. Delayed gastric emptying caused by these drugs may itself cause emesis, and anticholinergics should not be used for more than 3 days by the vomiting patient. Because of their anticholinergic properties, these drugs should not be used in combination with drugs whose actions depend on cholinergic activity in ganglion or smooth muscle. These include metoclopramide, cisapride, and the opioids.

KEY POINT 19-10 Centrally acting anticholinergic antiemetics are less ideal than other centrally acting drugs because they simultaneously act peripherally, increasing the risk of side effects.

Prokinetics. Prokinetics, and specifically metoclopramide, are peripherally acting antiemetics because of their prokinetic effects on the GI tract. Metoclopramide physiologically antagonizes emesis by virtue of its actions on the upper gastroduodenal area: increased esophageal sphincter tone, duodenal pyloric relaxation, and antegrade contraction of the gastric antrum. The prokinetic effects of metoclopramide are discussed later with other drugs that modify GI motility.

ANTIULCER DRUGS

Pathophysiology of Gastrointestinal Ulceration

Gastroduodenal Ulceration

The events leading to gastroduodenal ulceration are complex and reflect interactions between acid-secreting and defense mechanisms of the GI mucosa.[45,46] Regardless of the cause of GI erosion or ulceration, the basic pathologic mechanism is similar. Gastric acid secretion is a prerequisite for damage to the GI mucosa[46,47] with luminal damage not occurring unless luminal pH is less than 7. Pepsin and bile acids can contribute to mucosal damage. Even though these chemicals are inherently caustic, mucosal damage generally does not occur in the face of normal mucosal cytoprotective mechanisms. These include but are not limited to secretion of bicarbonate and mucus and rapid epithelial turnover. Deceased mucosal blood flow can have a profound effect on the ability of the injured mucosa to heal itself. Drugs used to control or treat GI erosion and ulceration include those that inhibit gastric acid secretion or provide or facilitate other cytoprotective effects. The role of *Helicobacter* sp. in the pathogenesis of gastroduodenal ulceration in human patients has been well established, but its role in disease in animals is less well documented (see later discussion; e.g., IBDs).

KEY POINT 19-11 Drugs that target mucosal damage either facilitate cytoprotection or decrease the effects of hydrochloric acid.

Physiology of Gastric Acid Secretion

Gastric acid secretion occurs in four phases. The first three phases—referred to as *cephalic, gastric,* and *intestinal*—are stimulated by food and mediated by gastrin, which is the most potent secretagogue.[48] Secretion is persistent during these phases, and gastric pH progressively decreases as nutrients traverse the GI tract. Gastrin secretion is inhibited as gastric pH declines to 3.5 and is completely inhibited at a pH of 1.5, to begin again only when pH approximates 3 to 3.5. The fourth phase of gastric acid secretion is basal and occurs in the absence of external stimuli. The amount of basal secretion varies among animals. In humans basal secretion follows a circadian rhythm, reaching a peak at midnight and a nadir at 7 AM.[49] As a model for the study of antisecretory drugs, information can be found regarding basal and responsive gastric acid secretion in dogs.[50,51] In fasted Beagle dogs (n = 8), gastric pH (collected by stomach tube) fluctuated from 2.7 to 8.3. Basal pH tended to be 7.0; treatment with a placebo (500 mg lactose) reduced pH almost the same magnitude as pentagastrin (3 and 2, respectively) at 1-2 hrs post treatment.50

Gastric acid secretion at the cellular level involves the generation and subsequent secretion of hydrogen ions by the parietal (oxyntic) cells of the gastric mucosa. Responses are controlled through chemical signals interacting with corresponding receptors located on the basolateral membrane of parietal cells. Central and peripheral signals stimulating gastric acid secretion include endocrine (gastrin: CCK), paracrine (histamine: H_2), and neuronal (ACh: M_3) (Figure 19-5).[49] In addition to its direct effects, acetycholine indirectly increases release of gastrin from G cells and histamine from enterochromaffin cells. Of the mediators increasing gastric acid secretion, gastrin is the most potent, although its effects are mediated indirectly through stimulation of histamine receptors, particularly on enterochromaffin cells.[48] Somatostatin, which inhibits gastric acid secretion, is released from D cells when gastric pH is less than 3. In humans the effects of *Helicobacter* spp. may reflect, in part, the ability of these organisms to decrease D cells. The hydrogen ion pump, located at the apical membrane and associated with the smooth endoplasmic reticulum, is unique in that it is a hydrogen–potassium ATPase exchange system. Three distinct pathways are capable of stimulating gastric acid. Each acts through chemical mediators that in turn interact with receptors on the parietal cell membrane.[49] H_2 receptors are linked to adenylyl cyclase and cyclic AMP.[48] Of these, the ACh pathway appears to be less important in small animals.

KEY POINT 19-12 Prevention and treatment of gastrointestinal ulceration focuses on prevention of hydrochloric acid secretion and promotion of cytoprotection.

Intracellular messengers mediating gastric acid secretion vary with the receptor stimulated. Histamine increases cAMP production, which subsequently activates the adenylyl cyclase cAMP-dependent protein kinases. Gastrin and muscarinic stimulation by cholinergic drugs increased cytosolic calcium, through inositol phosphate pathways. Both pathways activate

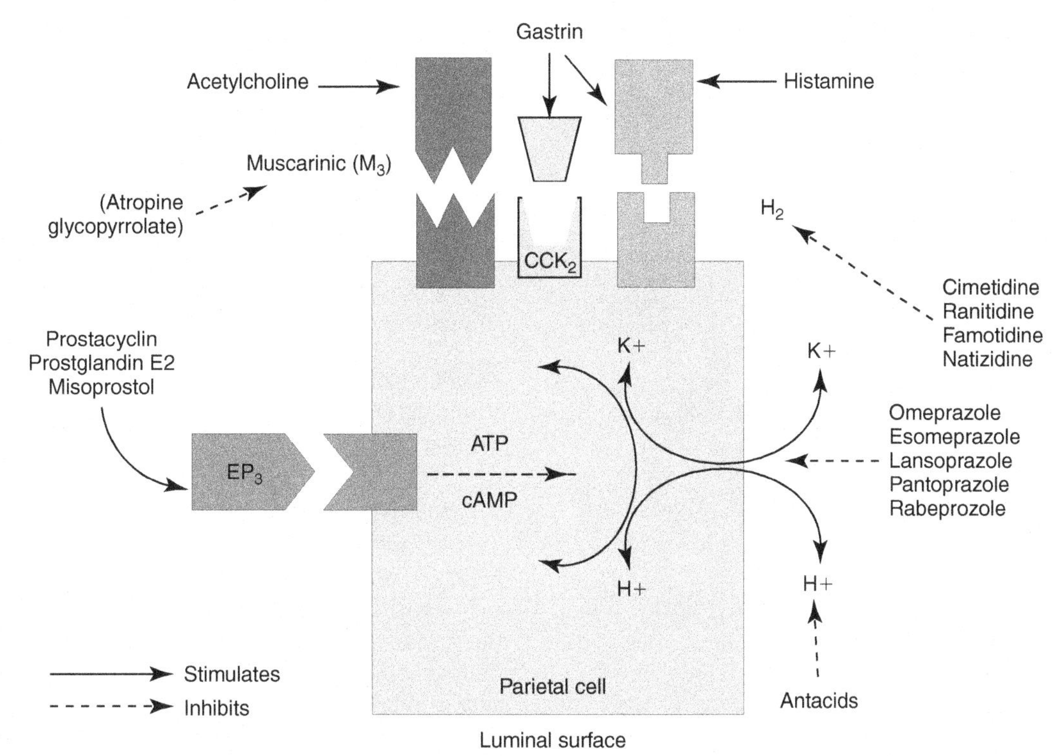

Figure 19-5 Receptor interactions that mediate gastric acid secretion by the parietal cell include acetylcholine with muscarinic receptors and histamine with H_2 receptors. Gastrin may interact with either receptor. Receptor stimulation activates the K^+, H^+-ATPase pump and exchange of potassium for hydrogen into the lumen. Prostaglandin E_1 (PGE) modulates gastric acid secretion by inhibiting cyclic adenosine monophosphate (cAMP). *ATP,* Adenosine triphosphate.

an H+, K+-ATPase proton pump that exchanges hydrogen and potassium across the parietal cell membrane. Prostaglandins of the E series serve to modulate these effects, inhibiting gastric acid secretion by blocking cAMP production through EP3 receptors, also on parietal cells.[48,49] The impact of opioid receptors on gastric acid secretion is discussed with drugs targeting intestinal secretion.

Mucosal Defenses

The primary mucosal defense of the esophagus reflects increased lower esophageal sphincter tone. Defenses of the GI mucosa require sufficient mucosal blood flow and act to prevent or repair GI ulceration (Figure 19-6).[52-54] These include (1) secretion of bicarbonate into the lumen and neutralization of hydrochloric acid in the lumen; (2) secretion of a thick, insoluble, alkaline mucus that traps and neutralizes inward-moving hydrogen ions and protects against macromolecules such as pepsin; (3) a gastric epithelial barrier composed of active phospholipids, a lipoprotein cell membrane, and tight junctional complexes, all of which prevent hydrogen ion back diffusion; (4) mucosal blood flow, which first provides nutrients and oxygen to mucosal cells and second removes hydrogen ions that have penetrated the gastric barrier; (5) rapid replication of mucosal epithelial cells; and (6) production of cytoprotective agents. Many of these effects reflect local secretion of prostaglandin E_2 and I_2, important defense mechanisms. They modulate hydrochloric acid secretion, increase bicarbonate and mucus production, and enhance mucosal blood flow and epithelialization.[55,56] Sulfhydryls also produced locally may act as scavengers of oxygen and other tissue-damaging radicals.[57]

Gastric Antisecretory Drugs

Drugs used to prevent or modulate gastric acid secretion include anticholinergics, H_2-receptor antagonists, proton pump inhibitors, and prostaglandin E_2.[49,55,58,59] Despite the role of muscarinic receptors in gastric acid secretion, anticholinergics have not proved effective for the control of GI ulceration in animals and are not discussed. Drugs that modify gastric acid (e.g., antisecretory drugs or antacids) are discussed with cytoprotectants. All drugs that modify gastric pH can cause complications of achlorhydria when used chronically. Although both gastric acid and pepsin are required for hydrolysis of proteins and other foods, achlorhydria is rarely accompanied by malabsorption unless bacterial overgrowth occurs. Achlorhydria can lead to malabsorption of certain nutrients, among them vitamin B_{12} and iron, as well as decreased absorption of some (weakly acidic) drugs. Although the advent of antihistaminergic antisecretory drugs represented a landmark change in the approach to medical management of GI ulcers in humans, their use is increasingly being replaced with proton pump inhibitors.

H_2-Receptor antagonists. H_2-receptor antagonists are reversible, competitive inhibitors that reduce both the amount and the hydrogen ion content of gastric secretion and the amount of pepsin[60] induced by a variety of secretagogues.[61] Secretion of intrinsic factor also is reduced, although this

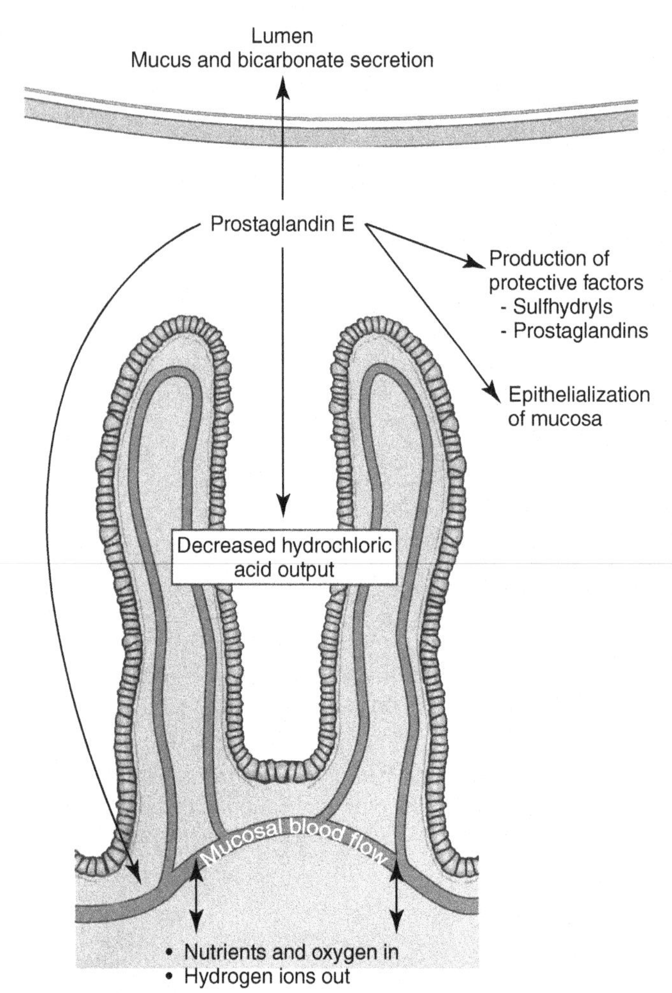

Figure 19-6 Protective mechanisms mediated by prostaglandin E against gastroduodenal ulceration provide targets for drug therapy. Bicarbonate secretion acts to neutralize gastric acid; mucus protects against hydrochloric and bile acids. The rapid turnover of epithelial cells is paramount for rapid healing if damage occurs. Mucosal blood flow not only provides critical oxygen and nutrients necessary for epithelialization but also removes H^+ ions that have penetrated the protective barrier. Other protective factors include mechanisms to control gastric hydrochloric acid secretion and the production of protective factors that scavenge mediators capable of cell damage.

effect does not appear to be clinically relevant.[24,48] Each antagonist is a congener of histamine, containing a bulky side chain (see Figure 19-4).[24,48] Cimetidine; ranitidine; and, to a lesser degree, famotidine have been used to control gastric acid secretion in animals. Nizatidine is the most recent of the approved drugs and has been used least in dogs and cats. Each drug varies in potency, duration of action, disposition, and drug interactions.[62] Ranitidine is 5 to 12 times more potent as an inhibitor of gastric acid secretion than cimetidine, whereas famotidine is nine times more potent than ranitidine and 32 times more potent than cimetidine. Famotidine (see Figure 19-4) has the longest duration of action.[40] In a cat model, famotidine was 4.5 times as potent as ranitidine; effects of famotidine were reversible at the highest dose studied (0.01-0.32 μmol kg/hr) supporting the need for higher doses or twice-daily dosing for conditions in which histamine-mediated high gastric acid output is mediated.[63] In animal models, including dogs, nizatidine is more potent than cimetidine.[64] In a Beagle model, ranitidine (50 mg IV) reduced resulted in a mean gastric pH of 7.8 by 1 hr; however, basal gastric pH was high as well. The pH was maintained for the 4-hour duration of the study.[50] Although the H_2-receptor antagonists have variable prokinetic actions, they appear to have inconsistent effects on the rate of gastric emptying or lower esophageal sphincter pressure.[48]

KEY POINT 19-13 Antihistaminergic antisecretory drugs are competitive inhibitors whose dose may need to increase as signals causing gastric acid secretion increase.

Disposition. The disposition of antisecretory antihistamines has not been well studied in animals, with information drawn largely from human data. Cimetidine, the oldest of the clinically used H_2-receptor antagonists, is rapidly absorbed from the GI tract, although food will delay the process. The drug undergoes hepatic metabolism and is about 70% bioavailable after oral administration. It is excreted in the urine in both the unchanged and conjugated forms. The plasma half-life is about 1 hour but may be prolonged in the presence of liver or kidney disease.

Ranitidine is less bioavailable (50%) than cimetidine after oral administration. Its elimination half-life is approximately 2.5 hours. Absorption is not impaired by food as with cimetidine. It is minimally protein bound (15%). Hepatic elimination is responsible for 30% of an intravenous dose and 73% of an oral dose.[65]

Famotidine is only 37% bioavailable after oral administration reflecting decreased oral absorption; however, this is compensated for somewhat by increased potency. In contrast, nizatidine is rapidly and completely absorbed.[60] Both drugs are largely eliminated unchanged in urine.[60] Nizatidine is almost exclusively eliminated by renal excretion, which suggests that it might be the preferred H_2-receptor antagonist for patients with hepatic disease. Its efficacy apparently has not been studied clinically in animals, although its safety has been established in healthy dogs.[62] Famotidine renal clearance appears to be saturable in the dog, albeit at suprapharmacologic doses.[66]

Drug interactions. The antisecretory antihistamines can be involved in a number of drug interactions, with cimetidine being best characterized.[48,67] Cimetidine, like all antisecretory drugs, impairs the oral absorption of a number of drugs (generally weak acids) through the alteration of GI pH. Cimetidine also directly impairs the absorption of many drugs by directly binding to the drugs. These effects might be balanced by competition for P-glycoprotein, for which cimetidine is a substrate. Cimetidine is a potent microsomal enzyme inhibitor and will decrease the hepatic metabolism of concurrently administered drugs.[68,69] Enzymes targeted in humans include CYP1A2, CYP2C9, and CYP2D6. Occasionally, this effect may be clinically useful, as in the prevention of acetaminophen intoxication in cases of accidental overdose.[70] However, impaired metabolism of other drugs can also lead to clinically relevant toxicity of other drugs metabolized by the liver. The impact of cimetidine on cyclosporine elimination has been studied in dogs. Although one study indicated a longer half-life, several other studies have demonstrated "no effect" of cimetidine on the disposition of cyclosporine (see Chapter 31). It is likely that the impact varies among animals, indicating a need to monitor. Cimetidine also reduces hepatic blood flow by about 20% and has been shown to reduce the clearance of flow-limited drugs such as propranolol and lidocaine.[71] Unlike cimetidine, the other antihistamines have limited to no effects on hepatic blood flow. Although ranitidine also inhibits CYP, its affinity for the enzymes is only about 10% of that for cimetidine. Famotidine and nizatidine have limited to no effect on the metabolism of other drugs (or endogenous compounds). Famotidine is a potent inhibitor of transport of cationic drugs, although the clinical relevance of this is not clear.

KEY POINT 19-14 Famotidine is the preferred antisecretory antihistamine because of its increased potency and fewer drug interactions

Adverse reactions. The side effects seen with any of the H_2-receptor antagonists are generally minor even at relatively high doses. Thrombocytopenia has been reported. Although there have been a number of reported side effects for ranitidine in humans, limited experience to date in animals has not indicated any serious toxic manifestations from ranitidine. Famotidine and nizatidine are devoid of many of the side effects of cimetidine.[64]

A clinically important disadvantage of H_2-receptor antagonists described in humans is relapse of gastroduodenal ulceration during or after H_2-receptor antagonist therapy is discontinued. Although several explanations for relapse have been offered, rebound hypersecretion of gastric acid appears to be most plausible.[72-74] Suppression of gastric acid by H_2-receptor antagonists results in increased plasma gastrin concentrations as early as 3 hours after a single dose. Subsequent stimulation of gastric mucosal G cells results in gastric acid hypersecretion that becomes evident when the drugs are discontinued. The likelihood of hypersecretion is compounded by increased parietal cell receptor sensitivity, which apparently characterizes (human) patients afflicted with ulcers.[75] Among the H_2 receptors studied, cimetidine seems to be the most likely and famotidine or nizatidine the least likely to cause rebound gastric acid hypersecretion.[74-76] Rebound hypersecretion can be minimized by tapering the dose as the drug is discontinued. Tolerance to the antisecretory effect of antihistaminergic antisecretory drugs also occurs, being well described in humans. Tolerance appears within 3 days of therapy and may not respond to increasing doses.[48]

KEY POINT 19-15 Rebound hypersecrtion can be minimized by use of famotidine and gradual discontinuation of any antisecretory drug.

Clinical use. The principal therapeutic uses of H_2-receptor antagonists include uremic gastritis, gastric and duodenal ulcers, stress-related erosive gastritis, and hypersecretory conditions such as gastrinoma or systemic mastocytosis. Although H_2-receptor antagonists can be used to treat drug-induced (e.g., nonsteroidal antiinflammatory drug [NSAID]) ulceration, their efficacy is controversial and other, more specific antidotes (e.g., PGE_1) or more effective antisecretory drugs (e.g., proton pump inhibitors) should first or also be administered.[77] On the other hand, the drugs have proved beneficial in providing protection against gastric ulceration induced by a number of etiologic agents, including aspirin and stress.[48] Their combination with proton-pump inhibitors is discussed in the following section. When treating drug-induced ulcers, antisecretory drugs that inhibit drug metabolizing enzymes should be avoided. H_2-receptor antagonists also appear to be effective in controlling upper GI bleeding when hemorrhage is not due to erosion of major blood vessels. H_2-receptor antagonists have also been used in gastroesophageal reflux disorders, esophagitis, and duodenal gastric reflux. In exocrine pancreatic insufficiency, cimetidine or ranitidine (and presumably famotidine), if given about 30 minutes before feeding, may decrease enzymatic and acid hydrolysis of replacement pancreatic enzymes added to food on their contact with gastric secretions, thus improving the efficacy and decreasing the cost of their use. Patients suffering from short bowel syndrome may benefit from long-term H_2-receptor therapy to decrease the hyperacidity associated with this syndrome. The H_2-receptor antagonists are sufficiently safe that high doses can be given to humans to maintain pharmacologic effects with once- to twice-daily dosing.[48] A meta-analysis in humans studied the impact of renal disease on the disposition of H_2-receptor blockers. Declining renal function is associated with a concomitant reduction in the renal clearance of those drugs renally eliminated. Appropriate dose reduction was associated with decrease in cost, as well as decrease in adverse events, with the major adversity being mentation disorders.[78]

KEY POINT 19-16 Proton pump inhibitors generally are more effective than antihistaminergic antisecretory drugs, but the lag time to efficacy may support initial therapy with both classes of antisecretory drugs.

Proton Pump Inhibitors

The substituted benzimidazole proton pump inhibitors are the most potent antisecretory drugs, reducing gastric acid secretion by 80% to 95%.[48] Each is a potent and irreversible antagonist of the H^+, K^+-ATPase proton pump, the final step in gastric acid secretion stimulated by any secretagogue. No differences in antisecretory efficacy have been demonstrated among these drugs. Omeprazole will be discussed as the model drug.

Mechanism of action. Omeprazole (Prilosec) (see Figures 19-4 and 19-5), was the first of the commercially available drugs. It is sold as a racemic mixture. Other proton pump inhibitors currently approved for use in the United States include esomeprazole (Nexium), the S-isomer of omeprazole (cleared more slowly than the R isomer in some species), lansoprazole (Prevacid), rabeprazole (Aciphex), and pantoprazole (Protonix). Omeprazole is approximately 30 times more potent as an antacid than is cimetidine.[79] Secretory volume is not as affected as is acidity.[79]

Pharmacokinetics. As a weak base, omeprazole is unstable in an acid environment and thus is formulated as encapsulated enteric-coated granules.[79] Drug dissolution occurs in the more alkaline environment of the small intestine. Acidity degrades (inactivates) the drug. Consequently, the drugs are generally prepared as enteric-coated products or combined with antacids (e.g., sodium bicarbonate). Compounded products must be made with attention to formulation, including pH, to ensure pharmaceutical efficacy. Oral bioavailability increases with environmental intestinal pH, and plasma drug concentrations tend to increase the first 4 to 5 days of therapy.[79] The complicated nature of proton pump inhibitors has limited the availability of parenteral preparations; however, pantoprazole and lansoprazole (and, in Europe, esomeprazole) are available for intravenous administration.

Once absorbed, the acidic environment (pH 0.8 to 1) of the GI tract causes omeprazole to selectively partition into the secretory canniculi of parietal cells compared with other cells (pH 5). In the acidic environment, the drug is protonated, trapped, and subsequently further transformed to the active inhibitor. As such, proton pump inhibitors are prodrugs. Ideally, the drugs are administered about 30 minutes before a meal; other antisecretory drugs do not appear to affect proton pump activity.[80] Indeed, antihistaminergic antisecretory drugs might be given in combination with proton pump inhibitors for a rapid response because of the slower onset of action of the proton pump inhibitors.[81] Once in the canniculi, omeprazole covalently and irreversibly binds to sulfhydryl groups of potassium-adenosine triphosphate (H^+, K^+-ATPase), thus inhibiting the energy source for the proton pump.[48,79] Because the enzyme is permanently inhibited, secretion of HCl will resume only after new molecules have been formed in the luminal membrane, which generally requires 24 to 48 hours.[48] Therefore the duration of action of proton pump inhibitors is much longer than their plasma half-life. Drug accumulation in parietal cells and alternating activity of parietal cells or pumps result in a lag time of up to 3 to 5 days before maximum effect (generally 70% of pumps are inhibited at steady state) is realized.[79,82] Consequently, alternative drugs may need to be considered if a rapid response is desired. In addition, efficacy will be maintained at low plasma drug concentrations and for some time after the drug is discontinued. Because of these characteristics, omeprazole can be administered once daily.[82] In humans omeprazole is highly (96%) bound to serum albumin and α_1-acid glycoprotein. Its apparent volume of distribution is 0.31 L/kg.[79] Clearance is accomplished through hepatic metabolism; in humans the major enzymes are CYP2C19, for which genetic polymorphisms have been reported (decreased activity in Asians), and CYP 3A4, an enzyme characterized by broad substrate specificity. Also in humans drug elimination depends on hepatic metabolism to inactive metabolites, and elimination half-life is short (52 minutes).[79] Omeprazole has been studied in dogs.[83] Oral bioavailability is reduced, although therapeutic concentrations can be achieved.

Dosing at 0.17 mg/kg orally once a day for five years was well tolereated in Beagles (n = 10). Changes in disposition were not detected across time. The AUC was similar to that measured in humans receiving 20 mg (approximately 0.28 mg/kg) daily. omeprazole daily. Mean inhibition of acid secretion by omeprazole 4-7 hours after dosing approximalted 50%.

Drug interactions. Partial inhibition of drugs eliminated by selected cytochrome P450 enzymes have been reported for omeprazole.[84] However, compared with cimetidine, omeprazole may be less likely to be involved in drug interactions. All proton pump inhibitors appear to inhibit a variety of CYPS (including CYP3A4), with clinically relevant drug interactions described for warfarin, cyclosporine, and diazepam. Omeprazole (more so than other proton pump inhibitors) appears to inhibit CYP2C19 and induce CYP1A2 (metabolism of several trycyclic or other behavior-modifying drugs); its S isomer is characterized by less in hibition. Other interactions are likely to exist, indicating caution when combining proton pump inhibitors with other drugs metabolized by the liver. Lansoprazole may be involved with fewer cytochrome P450–based drug interactions. Drug interactions appear to occur at the level of P-glycoprotein; omeprazole, lansoprazole, and pantoprazole appear to be substrates.[85] Because of the delay in onset of action, the use of more rapidly acting antihistaminergic drugs might be considered as proton pump therapy has begun. That the latter does not appear to have the efficacy of the former has been demonstrated.[80,81]

KEY POINT 19-19 The potential for inhibition of drug metabolism because of drugs or disease may result in longer drug half-lives of other drugs.

Adverse reactions. Adverse reactions caused by omeprazole are limited because the drug is selective for the H^+, K^+-ATPase pump. An exception is the sequelae of achlorhydria. Diarrhea and transient fluctuations in liver enzymes have been reported. Hypergastrinemia has been documented in human patients[79] after therapy with omeprazole, and is more severe compared with that associated with use of antihistaminergic antisecretory drugs and may be associated with gastric hyperplasia or an increase in gastric tumors. Rebound hypersecretion of gastric acid as described for antihistaminergic drugs should be anticipated, and discontinuation of proton pump inhibitors should occur gradually, with tapering or substitution of alternative drugs in at-risk patients.[48] Hypertrophy of gastric mucosa has been reported. A marked increase in gastric acid secretory capacity has been detected after omeprazole treatment, presumably owing to proliferation of an enterochromaffin-like cell mass.[86] However, in contrast to H_2-receptor blockers, proton pump inhibitors may not cause tolerance because their inhibition is distal to histamine-mediated secretion targeted by increased gastrin. Chronic use may decrease absorption of vitamin B_{12}, although clinical relevance is not clear.[48]

Clinical use. Proton pump inhibitors are indicated to support gastroduodenal healing, prevention or treatment of gastroesophogeal reflux, treatment of hypersecretory conditions, and other conditions that benefit from reduced hydrochloric acid secretion (e.g., IBDs). Omeprazole is the drug of choice for the treatment of the Zollinger–Ellison syndrome. Omeprazole has been used to control gastric acid secretion that has not responded to H_2-receptor antagonists, although its superiority to these and other antacid drugs has not been firmly established. Generally, however, studies support the superiority of omeprazole over cimetidine for treatment of GI ulceration, including response of pain.[79] Lansoprazole is often preferred in humans for prevention of NSAID-induced ulceration but does not appear to offer an benefit in terms of long-term efficacy.

Bersenas and coworkers[87] studied normal fasting and postprandial intragastric pH and its response to a variety of antisecretory drugs in Beagles (n = 12). Antisecretory drugs included ranitidine (2 mg/kg intravenously every 12 hours), famotidine (0.5 mg/kg intravenously every 12 hours), pantoprazole (1 mg/kg intravenously every 24 hours), and omeprazole (1 mg/kg orally every 24 hours), or saline placebo. Intragastric pH was recorded on days 0, 2, and 6. Outcome measures included median 24-hour intragastric pH, percentage of time pH was at or above 3, and percentage of time pH was at or above 4. All outcome measures were better (pH higher for longer) in the fasting compared with the postprandial state. Only famotidine, pantoprazole, and omeprazole suppressed gastric acid secretion, compared with placebo. The investigators also found that a suspension of omeprazole (1 mg/kg orally every 12 hours; n = 6) but not famotidine (0.5 mg/kg intravenously every 8 hours; n = 6) suppressed gastric acid secretion; information was not available regarding quality assurance of the suspensions. The authors concluded that only famotidine (at the doses and intervals studied), pantoprazole, and omeprazole significantly suppressed gastric acid secretion and the only suspension that was anticipated to be effective in treating gastric acid-related diseases (in normal dogs), based on outcome measures targeted in humans, was omeprazole; the power of the study may have impacted interpretation. This study suggests that ranitidine at 2 mg/kg, administered intravenously, is not an effective antisecretory drug in dogs, and famotidine is indicated at 12-hour intervals.

KEY POINT 19-20 Studies in the dog suggest that famotidine and omeprazole provide the most effective control of gastric acid secretion.

Prostaglandin Analogs

In addition to blockade of receptors that mediate secretion, gastric acid might also be modulated by prostaglandins of the E series. Their actions appear to be mediated by interaction with a basolateral membrane receptor. Intracellular concentrations of cAMP decrease, which in turn decreases protein kinase activity and hydrogen ion concentration (see Figure 19-6).[49] Misoprostol is a methyl ester analog of prostaglandin E_1. As such, it is pharmacologically active after oral administration, with effects lasting longer than those of endogenous prostaglandins.[88] Food delays its time of onset, which generally occurs within 30 minutes. Effects in humans tend to last for 3 hours, reflecting, in part, a short half-life of 20 to 40 minutes. The effects of misoprostol tend to be restricted to the local environment, with systemically absorbed drug rapidly metabolized by the liver.[89] Misoprostol does not appear to alter serum gastrin levels, and rebound acid hypersecretion has not been reported.[83] Basal, nocturnal, and food-induced gastric acid secretion is inhibited by misoprostol, which appears to be the primary cytoprotective effect. Although 75% to 85% of basal acid secretion may be inhibited, high doses at frequent intervals (four times daily in humans) may be necessary. The drug is not likely to be as effective as H_2-receptor or proton pump antagonists in decreasing intraluminal pH and appears less effective in controlling pain associated with hydrochloric acid secretion. Unabsorbed drug that reaches the intestine can cause intestinal secretion, smooth muscle contraction, and thus diarrhea (occurring in up to 30% of human patients), but these side effects may be resolved after several days.[88] Misoprostol can exacerbate clinical signs associated with inflammatory bowel disease and should be avoided in patients at risk.[48] Misoprostol can induce uterine contractions and is contraindicated in pregnancy; clients who are of childbearing age should be warned of this potential side effect. The primary indication for misoprostol is prevention or treatment of NSAID-induced ulceration, although more convenient drugs tend to be used for prevention. Its use might be considered in diseases associated with marked mast cell influx (e.g., mastocytosis) because of its inhibitory effect on mast cell degranulation.[90]

Cytoprotective Drugs

Antacids

Antacids have largely been replaced by drugs that more effectively prevent deleterious effects of gastric acid. Nonetheless, antacids continue to have a role in the treatment or prevention of mucosal disorders associated with gastric acid or other caustic agents. As with many GI-active drugs, information regarding the effects of antacids largely is extrapolated from data from studies on other species. Antacids chemically neutralize HCl present in the gastric lumen such that gastric luminal pH is increased to an acceptable level (pH of 3 or 4, at minimum) without causing systemic alkalosis.[91] Inactivation of pepsin and binding of bile salts by some products (e.g., aluminum hydroxide) are also important. Finally, some products (e.g., aluminum hydroxide) also induce the local synthesis of mucosal protectants (e.g., prostaglandins and sulfhydryls).[57,92] Some antacids are indicated for their impact on electrolyte (e.g., phosphorus) absorption. Factors influencing rational antacid therapy are rate of acid secretion, duration of time the antacid remains in the stomach, the potency of the antacid, and adverse effects.[93]

The relative efficacy of antacids is based on the number of milliequivalents of acid-neutralization available (the volume of 1N HCl, or milliequivalents of HCl, that can be titrated to a pH of 3.5 within 15 minutes). The major nonsystemic antacids used in veterinary medicine are salts of aluminum, magnesium, and calcium used either alone or in combination with each other or with various protectants, adsorbents, and astringent. In general, in vitro, 1 gram of these antacid compounds generally neutralize 20 to 35 mEq of acid. Neutralization of (reaction with) HCl generates chlorides, water, and carbon dioxide[48]; release of CO_2 from carbonates can cause abdominal distention and belching.[48] In the fasting state the action of gastric antacids is usually transient and lasts only 1 to 2 hours. In general, antacids are cleared from the stomach within 30 minutes. Neutralization of acid in the stomach antrum removes negative feedback control of gastrin release, which in turn leads to elevated gastrin levels and enhanced HCl secretion, with increased tone of the lower esophageal sphincter. In the past antacid administration was recommended at 4- to 6-hour intervals to minimize rebound hypersecretion. The presence of food, which increases gastric pH to about 5,[48] will prolong the effects of antacids for up to 2 to 3 hours. In human patients, however, administration with each meal has proved more convenient yet equally efficacious. Time to onset of action is different among antacids. Calcium and sodium carbonate are considered fast acting, magnesium salts moderate to rapid acting, and aluminum salts slow acting.

KEY POINT 19-21 Antacids containing a combination of aluminum and magnesium hydroxide provide the best balance in efficacy and avoidance of side effects.

Aluminum hydroxide is a good adsorbent (of bile acids and pepsin), as well as an antacid. Although slow in action, it tends to provide prolonged antacid effects.[48] Because it is slow acting, it is often combined with more rapidly acting magnesium salts. An advantage of aluminum hydroxide compared to other antacids is its stimulatory effect on local prostaglandin production in the intestinal mucosa.[92] Aluminum preparations tend to cause constipation and are often mixed with magnesium salts (laxative inaction) to prevent this side effect. However, this combination is not always effective, with emergence of constipation (because of aluminum) and diarrhea (because of magnesium) emerging in some patients. Aluminum hydroxide also decreases phosphate absorption by forming insoluble aluminum phosphates in the intestine and is used to control serum phosphorus in patients with renal disease. Note that prolonged administration with meals may cause hypophosphatemia in patients.

Magnesium-containing products can raise gastric pH higher than aluminum-containing antacids (as high as 9 versus 4).[91] Magnesium hydroxide is the most commonly used form of magnesium. Magnesium salts tend to be laxative and are often found in combination with aluminum and calcium salts. Their cathartic effects result from soluble but unabsorbed magnesium salts that remain in the intestine and retain water. The neutralizing effect of magnesium hydroxide is prompt and prolonged. Up to 20% of the magnesium is absorbed in normal circumstances, and in the presence of renal dysfunction repeated administration can result in hypermagnesia. Combination antacid products containing both aluminum and magnesium are often used to balance the adverse effects of each cation or bowel function.[93] Magaldrate is a hydroxymagnesium–aluminate hydroxide complex that rapidly dissociates in the gastric acid to magnesium or aluminum hydroxide, providing a sustained effect.

KEY POINT 19-22 Sucralfate must bind to damaged tissues and therefore is ineffective until damage occurs. However, prophylactic use should still be considered.

Calcium carbonate is a rapid-acting, potent antacid with a prolonged duration. Slowly developing metabolic alkalosis, gastric acid rebound, hypercalcemia, and calciuria with metastatic calcification and urolithiasis, hypophosphatemia, and constipation are, however, potential side effects that may occur after chronic administration of calcium carbonate.[93] In addition, interference with calcium-dependent processes may lead to excessive gastrin and HCl secretion.[48] Release of carbon dioxide may increase gastrin release owing to distention.

Antacids may be involved in a number of drug interactions, despite their largely local effects. Antacids may alkalinize the urine, generally increasing it 1 pH unit. The rate of elimination of renally eliminated weak acids will be increased (e.g., NSAIDs, phenobarbital), whereas that of weak bases is decreased.[48] Drug interactions of antisecretory drugs reflecting increased gastric pH may also occur with antacids. Oral absorption of a number of other drugs[94] may be affected as a result of changes in gastric pH. Further, magnesium and aluminum in particular are likely to chelate other drugs, precluding their absorption. Therefore antacids should be given approximately 2 hours before or after other orally administered drugs.

In addition to gastric distention (carbonates) and altered electrolytes that vary with each compound, side effects to antacids are not common. Antacids may increase the risk of food allergies based on a mouse model in which proteins extracted from caviar induced caviar-specific IgE antibodies, T-cell reactivity, and increased GI eosinophil and mast cells in mice simultaneously receiving ranitidine or sucralfate. The authors identified the aluminum hydroxide component of sucralfate as being responsible for the increased risk of allergic response. The rationale for the increased risk was incomplete protein digestion.[95]

Gastric hyperacidity, peptic ulcer, gastritis, reflux esophagitis, and chronic renal failure (uremia) are the more common indications for antacid preparations in veterinary medicine. Pyloric and duodenal peptic ulcers that may be related to gastric hyperacidity have been reported in dogs. Antacids intended to treat gastroduodenal ulceration generally are administered orally 1 and 3 hours after meals and at bedtime. For severe conditions or to treat uncontrolled reflux, doses in humans are repeated as often as every 30 to 60 minutes. Suspensions have greater neutralizing capacity than do powder or tablet dosage forms; in humans tables must be thoroughly chewed for maximum effect. A number of acid products

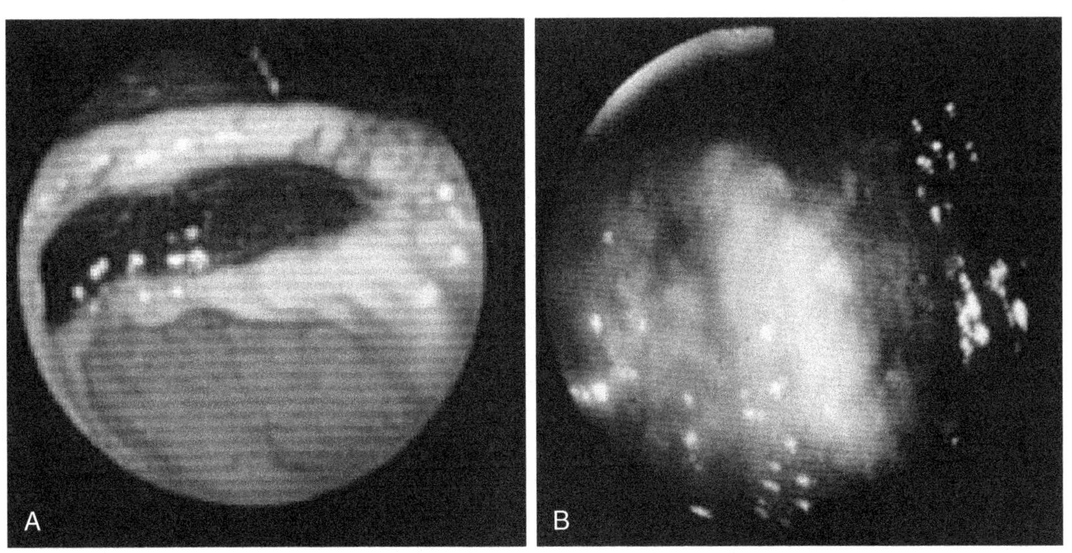

Figure 19-7 An endoscopic view of sucralfate bound to damaged gastrointestinal epithelium. Binding not only protects the damaged epithelium from further damage but also prevents loss of critical nutrients and fluids.

intended to treat "acid indigestion" in humans contain silmethicone (see the discussion of antiflatulence agents), a surfactant that decreases esophageal reflux. Whereas the choice of over-the-counter preparations containing a combination of antacids and silmethicone is reasonable, products that are combined with aspirin should be avoided.

Sucralfate

Sucralfate (see Figure 19-4) is an orally administered disaccharide (octasulfate of sucrose) aluminum hydroxide product that binds to and protects damaged epithelial cells from acid, bile, and pepsin activity.[96-99] In the acid environment of the stomach, sucrose is freed from aluminum hydroxide, cross-polymerizes, and binds to exposed (damaged) anions of GI epithelial cell membranes (Figure 19-7).[100] The maximum protective effects of sucralfate depend on an acid environment (pH <4) for activation; therefore it should be administered at least 30 minutes before antacids[100] and on an empty stomach, 1 hour before feeding.[48] Binding occurs in the base of ulcer craters and is greater in duodenal than in gastric ulcers. Sucralfate also binds to and inactivates bile acids, thus promoting its use in biliary disorders, and inhibits pepsin-mediated hydrolysis of mucosal proteins.[101] In addition to binding and protection of cells, the polymerized sucrose prevents exudation of protein and electrolytes into the gastric lumen. Effects of sucralfate may last up to 6 hours, supporting a four-times-daily dosing regimen.[48] The amount of aluminum hydroxide released from sucralfate may not effectively neutralize gastric acidity, although this may be controversial.[102] Sucralfate appears to stimulate production of local mediators that protect the gastric mucosa. These include prostaglandins[99,101,103] sulfhydryl ions or other oxygen radical scavengers, and epidermal growth factor.[104] Sucralfate effects on epidermal growth factor cause its accumulation in ulcerated lesions.[99,105] Sucralfate also increases mucosal blood flow either by inducing local nitric oxide or prostaglandin production[106] or by directly stimulating mucosal angiogenesis.[107]

KEY POINT 19-23 In addition to its mechanical protection, sucralfate also increases local prostaglandin protection and promotes angiogenesis and epithelialization.

Drug interactions with sucralfate are limited to local effects. Sucralfate binds to a number of drugs, with the prototypic example being cimetidine. Because cimetidine also increases gastric pH (thus potentially reducing activation of sucralfate), these two drugs probably should be alternated (i.e., administer sucralfate 1 to 2 hours before cimetidine) in patients receiving both drugs. In addition to direct binding to drugs, sucralfate may influence drug absorption through formation of a thick mucus layer. Thus, in general, other drugs should be administered at least 2 hours before sucralfate.

Sucralfate is minimally absorbed after oral administration and is associated with few, if any, side effects. Sucralfate is recognized to be the safest drug available for treatment of gastroduodenal ulcers.[101] Constipation occurs in up to 2% of humans. Currently, sucralfate is recommended for treatment of gastroduodenal erosion ulceration, regardless of the cause. Its prophylactic use is also recommended for illnesses associated with ulceration such as renal or liver disease, mastocytosis, and IBDs for which prolonged use of antiprostaglandin is indicated. However, sucralfate does not prevent the formation of the ulcer; rather, it protects damaged tissue once it occurs. Sucralfate appears beneficial prophylactically for stress-induced ulcers but is less effective prophylactically in patients receiving NSAID therapy.[100] Sucralfate is effective for treatment of acid-induced esophagitis,[108] although antisecretory drugs such as omeprazole or H_2-receptor antagonists are probably superior.[48] In critical patients at risk for nosocomial pneumonia, sucralfate may be preferred to antisecretory drugs such that increased gastric pH might be prevented.[48] Sucralfate has been administered rectally (in humans) for treatment of rectal ulcerative disease.

MODULATORS OF GASTROINTESTINAL MOTILITY

Normal Physiology

The GI tract functions to ensure the metabolic survival of the host and in doing so sorts ingested materials as to nutritional, toxic, or pathologic status. To accomplish its activities, the alimentary tract has its own enteric neurologic system (ENS) composed of vagal and sympathetic nerves (Figure 19-8). The network communicates through a large variety of chemicals, including neurotransmitters and neuropeptides. Primary signals include ACh, the tachykinins (substance P, neurokinin A), nitric oxide, adenosine triphosphate (ATP), vasoactive intestinal polypeptide, opioid peptides, neuropeptide Y, and 5-hydroxytryptamine.[109] Circuits of the ENS include intrinsic primary afferent neurons; interneruons; and either excitatory or inhibitory neurons that innervate effector motor, secretomotor, or vasodilator neurons. Additionally, the ENS integrates with the CNS, forming a brain–gut axis. The interactions of the integrated signals are complex and often not well characterized and thus are difficult to correct in the face of dysfunction, whether induced by disease or drugs.

Regulation of electrical and mechanical, activities of GI smooth muscle is a complex but ordered activity involving hormonal, myogenic, and neurogenic factors and sensory, relay and effector functions.[24] Integration occurs at the level of the CNS at both spinal and supraspinal levels[110] and locally through the ENS, including intrinsic and interneuronal nerves and ganglia are located between the longitudinal and smooth muscles and at least 10 different classes of receptors located on the smooth muscle cell. Intrinsic innervation includes the Auerbach (or myenteric) plexus, which forms a neural sympathetic and parasympathetic network connecting longitudinal and circular smooth muscle and the secondary Meissner (or submucosal) plexus, which parasympathetically innervates circular muscle. Both systems are secretory and motor in effect, although the Meissner plexuses predominantly modify mucosal absorption and secretion. Coordination of inhibitory and excitatory muscle movements results in two primary movements: mixing and aboral propulsion of liquefied contents. Mixing reflects rhythmic segmentations caused by simple nonprogressive contractions of circular muscle. Electrical activity for propulsion occurs initially as a "slow waves" whose crest is followed by "spike potentials." Slow waves keep the membrane potential in a constant state of fluctuation, with the frequency of contraction waves ranging between 10 to 20 times per minute, being fastest in the small intestine. Slow waves coordinate synchronous muscle contraction by releasing neurotransmitters from the myenteric plexus such

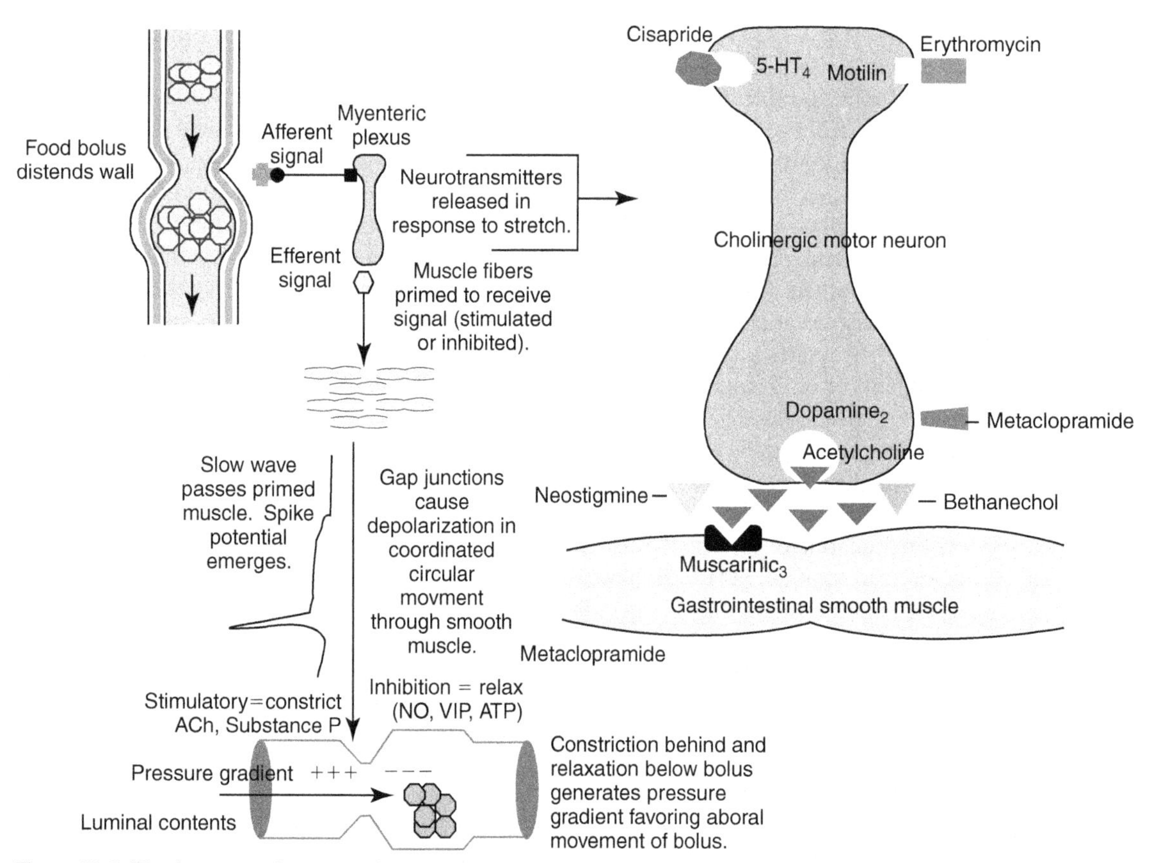

Figure 19-8 The integrated neurologic systems of the intestinal tract. See text for details. Metoclopramide antagonizes dopamine receptors, which antagonize release of acetylcholine. Cisapride is an agonist of 5-HT_4 receptors, which are excitatory in the enteric nervous system. Erythromycin acts as an agonist at excitatory motilin receptors. *Ach,* Acetylcholine, *NO,* nitric oxide; *VIP,* vasoactive intestinal peptide.

that smooth muscle fibers are "primed" to respond to the spike potential that follows. Gap junctions between circular and longitudinal fibers ensure that electrical stimuli (i.e., depolarization) spread outward in a circular fashion such that an entire ring of circular smooth muscle contracts in a coordinated fashion (Figure 19-9).

Peristalsis is the major propulsive movement, occurring principally in the esophagus and intestines, involving both longitudinal and circular smooth muscles and reflecting signals originating in the myenteric plexus without being influenced by signals peripheral to the ENS. Peristalsis reflects an ascending excitatory reflex of circular smooth muscle causing contraction on the oral side of a bolus, with ACh and substance P as the primary interneuronal mediators, and a descending inhibitory aboral reflex that causes relaxation, with nitric oxide, vasoactive intestinal peptide, and ATP as mediators.[24] Luminal contents follow the net pressure gradient. Contraction of longitudinal smooth muscle in the descending (aboral) phase and relaxation in the ascending oral phase facilitates peristaltic movements and aboral movement of intestinal contents.[111] Although peristaltic activity is mainly propulsive, it also ensures mixing and successful absorption. Wilson and coworkers review the physiology of the gastroesophageal sphincter.[112] Relaxation is mediated by noncholinergic and nonadrenergic signals. Absorption of luminal contents is facilitated as intestinal luminal contents are impeded by narrowing of the intestinal luminal diameter.

Receptors and Signals

Most smooth muscle activity ultimately reflects response to ACh through cholinergic receptors. However, activity of cholinergic receptors is modulated by a variety of other receptors (see Figure 19-8). Muscarinic (M_2) receptors regulate phasic bowel movements during fasting. Several types of muscarinic receptors have been identified pharmacologically (M_{1-4}) in the GI tract. Of these, M_1 or M_3 receptors interact with G protein and mobilize intracellular calcium; M_2 and M_{41} receptors inhibit adenylyl cyclase and regulate ion channels. M_1 receptors present in the myenteric plexus may inhibit motility by way of gabaminergic mechanisms. M_2 receptors, located presynaptically and postsynaptically, mediate presynaptic inhibition of ACh release. M_3 receptors appear to be located on smooth muscle cells, and although less abundant than M_2 by a ratio of 4:1, they are more important because they increase intracellular calcium.[24,110]

> **KEY POINT 19-24** Regulation of gastrointestinal motility is complex, with muscarininic (M_2 and M_3 subtypes) and 5-HT_4 being the major role players.

A number of other receptor types influence GI motility. Adrenergic receptors, including α_1, and α_2 postsynaptically and α_2, presynaptically regulate ACh release from the myenteric plexus. Generally, cholinergic neurons stimulate and

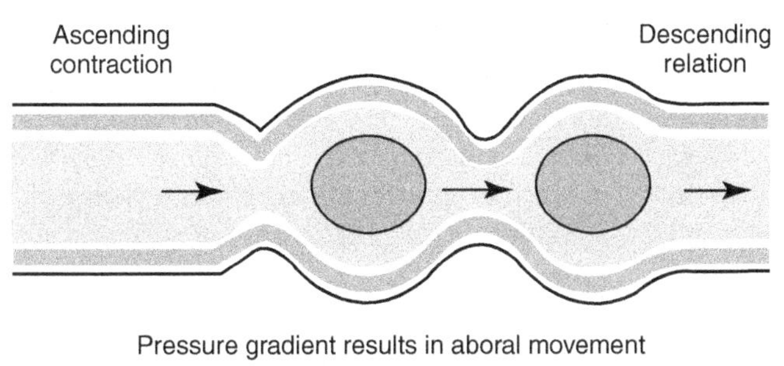

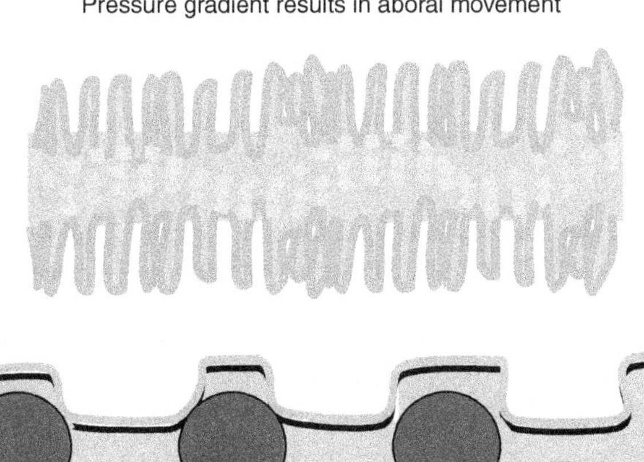

Figure 19-9 The sequelae of smooth muscle contraction in the intestines vary with the type of muscle. Longitudinal muscle contraction shortens the gastrointestinal tract; peristalsis thus forces expulsion of luminal contents. Contraction of circulatory muscle causes segmentation or resistance to outflow. This effect predominates with opioids. Anticholinergic drugs impair both types of muscle activity.

adrenergic neurons inhibit gastric motility. Both H_1 and H_2 receptors have been identified in the GI tract. They are located both prejunctionally, where they control ACh release, and postjunctionally. Stimulation of H_1 receptors induces, whereas H_2-receptors inhibit, smooth muscle contraction.[113] The role of dopamine and serotonin in gastric motility is complex and not well elucidated. Among the effects of dopamine are reduction in esophageal sphincter and intragastric pressures. Dopamine, by way of D_2 receptors, inhibits smooth muscle of the stomach, duodenum, and colon and has been implicated as a mediator of receptive relaxation in dogs (see Figure 19-8).[24,34] Dopamine exerts its inhibitory effect through inhibition of ACh at myenteric motorneurons.[34]

Over 90% of serotonin in the body is located in the GI tract, indicating its importance in this system. The majority of serotonin is produced by enterochromaffin cells that rapidly release serotonin in response to a variety of mechanical or chemical stimuli. Its effects generally are stimulatory by way of 5-HT_3 and 5-HT_4 receptors and inhibitory by way of 5-HT_{1P} receptors. The result is a peristaltic reflex, mediated by 5-HT_{1P} and 5-HT_4 receptors at the myenteric plexuses and 5-HT_3 receptors at extrinsic vagal and spinal sensory neurons.[24] Serotonin often exerts its effects through secondary chemicals. For example, the inhibitory effects of 5-HT_{1P} receptors reflect release of nitric oxide, which reduces muscle tone, whereas the stimulatory effects of 5-HT_4 receptors reflect enhanced ACh release. However, the effects of 5-HT_4 receptor stimulation appear to vary with species and origin. In the guinea pig ileum, effects are stimulatory, but in human and canine colons, 5-HT_4 receptor stimulation causes relaxation of smooth muscle.[114] In the dog, 5-HT_4 receptors appear to mediate relaxation in gastric cholinergic neurons where gastric contraction facilitates gastric emptying, and jejunal and ileal mucosa and circular colonic smooth muscle cells, where activation appears to cause relaxation. Conflicting studies may reflect the different roles that 5-HT_4 receptors have in stimulating contraction and peristalsis: a positive effect may occur with mucosal stimulation but not luminal distention.[114] 5-HT_4 receptors appear to be potent secretagogues in most species, again with effects variable among species and location. These differences among species and tissues suggest that extrapolation of therapeutic indications and doses should be based on scientific studies in the target species. The effects of serotonin are ameliorated, in part, by reuptake. However, uptake can be inhibited by CNS-active serotonin reuptake inhibitors, although the sequelae may cause diarrhea.

Other sites are targeted by motility-modifying drugs. Activation of the noncholinergic, nonadrenergic inhibitory neurons results in bowel relaxation.[113] Prostanoids and specifically prostaglandin E (PgE) receptors have been identified in the gastric fundus and ileum. PgE receptors may modulate motility from the esophagus to the colon.[113] Generally, PgE inhibits mechanical activity of circular smooth muscle, whereas prostaglandins of the D and F series are stimulatory. At high doses, PgE stimulates peristaltic activity, although this may represent mechanical response to excess watery fluid in the intestinal lumen stimulated by PgE.[113] Motilin is a peptide hormone located in M and enterochromaffin cells of the GI tract. Motilin appears to enhance and potentially induce phase III activity.

Smooth muscle activity in the large bowel varies from that in the small bowel. In the small bowel, slow waves generally occur continuously and propagate aborally. In the colon slow waves are sometimes absent, and propagation may be variable.[110]

Prokinetic Drugs

Prokinetics enhance the transit of intraluminal contents.[34] The mechanisms of action of these drugs are varied and are not completely understood. Their effects on intestinal functions generally reflect either promotion of an agonist, such as ACh by muscarinic drugs, or inhibition of an inhibitory signal, such as dopamine (see Figure 19-8).[34] Organ-specific and species-specific differences complicate our comprehension of these drugs.[34]

Cholinergics

Clinically, the use of cholinergics is limited by their tendency to cause systemic effects. Bethanechol is an ester derivative of choline that acts as a cholinergic agonist almost exclusively at muscarinic (M_2) receptors.[113] Bethanechol will enhance the amplitude of contractions throughout the GI tract, including the lower esophageal sphincter (Figure 19-10; see also Figure 19-8).[34,113] Its effects on the coordination of small intestinal contraction may be minimal, however, and thus it is often not considered to be a prokinetic agent.[34] Adverse effects reflect direct enhanced parasympathomimetic stimulation and include abdominal cramps, diarrhea, salivation, and bradycardia.[34]

Metoclopramide

Metoclopramide is a lipid-soluble derivative of para-aminobenzoic acid. It is structurally related to procainamide, a cardiac antiarrhythmic (see Figure 19-4).[34] In addition to its central antidopaminergic (antiemetic) effects, metoclopramide acts peripherally as both an antidopaminergic and as a direct and indirect stimulator of cholinergic receptors.[34,35]

The effect of metoclopramide on canine gastromotility was described as early as 1969.[115] Compared with saline, metoclopramide decreased transit time and volume but did not affect flow of intestinal contents. Clinically, its effects appear to be limited to the upper intestinal tract (see Figure 19-10).[35,37,116,117] The peripheral effects of metoclopramide apparently reflect enhanced release of ACh from intrinsic cholinergic neurons. These effects are completely inhibited by pretreatment with anticholinergics such as atropine.[34,37,118] The peripheral effects, however, appear to be mediated by effects on other (noncholinergic) local neurotransmitters, particularly dopamine. Serotonin receptors also may play a role.[34] The prokinetic activity of metoclopramide reflects muscarinic activity, D_2 receptor antagonist activity, and 5-HT_4 receptor agonist activity.[34] Because of its effects on the stomach, metoclopramide physiologically antagonizes emesis by increasing the tone in the lower esophageal sphincter, increasing the force and frequency of gastric antral contractions (gastrokinetic effect), relaxing the pyloric sphincter, and promoting peristalsis in the duodenum and jejunum, resulting in accelerated gastric emptying and upper intestinal transit.[35]

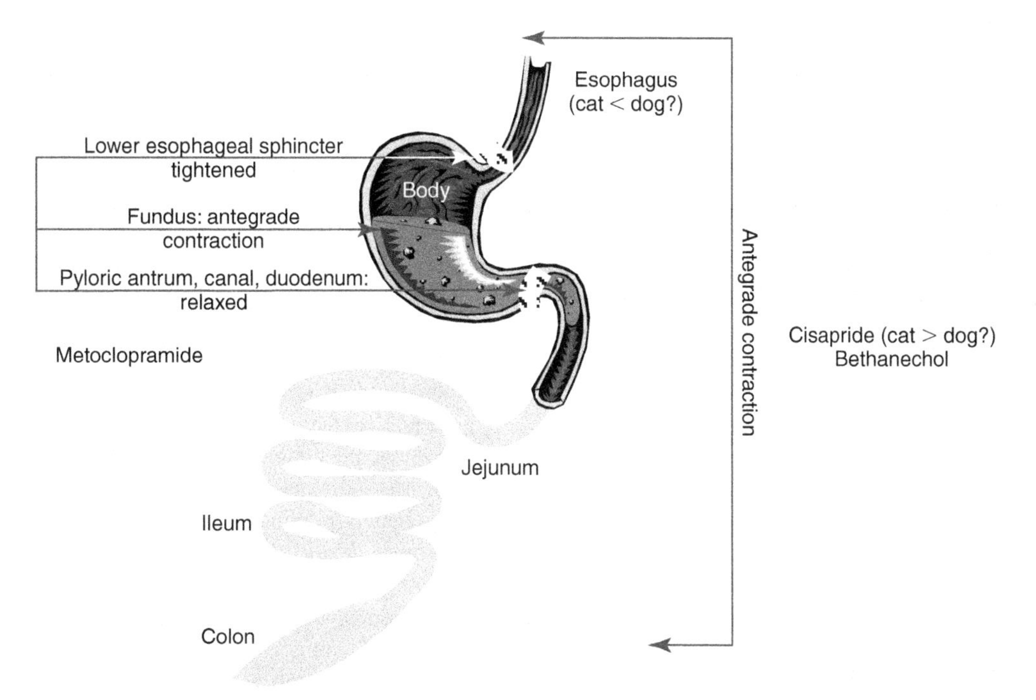

Figure 19-10 The sites of actions of two clinically useful prokinetic drugs. In vivo, at standard doses, metoclopramide's actions are limited to the lower esophagus (feline more than canine), stomach, and upper duodenum, where it physiologically antagonizes vomiting. Cisapride appears to increase motility throughout the gastrointestinal tract.

KEY POINT 19-25 Clinically, the prokinetic effect of metoclopramide is limited to the stomach, lower esophagus, and pylorus.

Metoclopramide is well absorbed orally but undergoes significant first-pass metabolism with a bioavailability in the 50% to 70% range. Tissue distribution is rapid, and excretion is both renal and hepatic. Because the plasma half-life in the dog is only 90 minutes, metoclopramide has a short duration of action.[35] Dose-dependent CNS side effects include nervousness, restlessness, listlessness, depression, and disorientation.[34,35,119] Extrapyramidal antidopaminergic effects include tremors and motor restlessness. Tremors in cats, particularly after intravenous administration, are not unusual. Gynecomastia caused by enhanced release of prolactin has been reported in humans.[34] GI disorders may also be observed, with constipation being common with long-term use.

Metoclopramide has a demonstrated impact on the oral bioavailability of several drugs, with the effect varying with the drug. For example, co-administration with the oral hypoglycemic agent ciglitazone decreased C_{max} by 16% and AUC 8%,[120] but co-administration with cephalexin increased cephalexin C_{max} by 21% and AUC by 36%.[121] It is not clear if the latter effect reflected increased gastric emptying or interference with intestinal transport proteins. As an antiemetic, the main indications for metoclopramide include severe and intractable emesis caused by chemotherapy or other blood-borne toxins as well as nausea and vomiting associated with delayed gastric emptying, gastroesophageal reflux, reflux gastritis, and peptic ulceration. As a prokinetic, metoclopramide is indicated for treatment of a variety of gastric motility disorders, including gastric dilation, volvulus, postoperative ileus, gastric ulceration, and idiopathic gastroparesis.[37] Metoclopramide is contraindicated in GI obstruction or perforation, potentially in epilepsy, and for patients receiving neuroleptics. Because of their anticholinergic effects, atropine and the opioid analgesics antagonize the action of metoclopramide.

KEY POINT 19-26 Anticholinergics and opioids decrease the prokinetic efficacy of metoclopramide.

Domperidone

Domperidone is a dopamine antagonist whose prokinetic properties are similar to those of metoclopramide.[122] However, unlike metaclopramide, it has no cholinergic activity and is not inhibited by atropine. Domperidone does not cross the blood–brain barrier as readily as metoclopramide. Like metoclopramide, however, domperidone can affect central dopamine receptors and thus modulate temperature control, prolactin secretion, and activity at the CTZ.[34] Extrapyramidal side effects are rare. Domperidone acts peripherally to coordinate antroduodenal contractions. Its peripheral effects accelerate small intestinal transit, but colonic activity is apparently unaffected.[119]

Cisapride

Cisapride has the broadest spectrum of action of the prokinetic agents.[123] It causes dose-dependent increased activity at all GI sites, including the esophagus, stomach, jejunum, ileum, small intestine, and colon[34] (see Figure 19-10). Because 75% of the feline esophagus is skeletal muscle, esophageal prokinetic effects are likely to be less in cats than in dogs. The prokinetic actions of cisapride appear to reflect indirect stimulation of cholinergic nerves. Serotonin appears to mediate this effect through 5-HT_4 receptors (see Figure 19-8). Stimulation of colonic contractions reflects 5-HT_{2a}. Because secretion is not enhanced, stimulation probably occurs at the level of the myenteric plexus.[34]

Well absorbed after oral administration, cisapride undergoes first-pass metabolism, with oral bioavailability in humans being 50%. Metabolites are apparently inactive. Volume of distribution is large (2.4 L/kg) in humans, and elimination half-life is 10 hours. Cisapride kinetics have been reported in the cat.[124] Oral administration is characterized by 30% bioavailability, and the elimination half-life approximates 5 hours. A dose of 1 mg/kg every 8 hours or 1.5 mg/kg every 12 hours is recommended on the basis of these data. Elimination may be prolonged in the presence of liver disease.[123] Indications for use of cisapride are similar to those for metoclopramide (excluding dopaminergic effects). Indications in humans include any disorder associated with impaired gastric emptying as well as gastroesophageal reflux. Unlike metacopramide, cisapride does not interact with central dopamine receptors, and its use is not associated with extrapyramidal side effects.[113] However, stimulation of 5-HT_4 receptors by cisapride (and other drugs) causes blockade of the rapid component of potassium influx through the delayed rectifier potassium channel. Prolongation of the QT interval results in torsades de pointes and the potential for sudden cardiac death. Subsequently, cisapride has been withdrawn from the human-medicine market, mandating the need for compounding for veterinary use. Myocardial side effects have not been reported in peer-reviewed literature but have been reported anecdotally. Further, in vitro studies have revealed a similar effect in the canine myocardium. The risk is greater when cisapride is combined with other drugs that inhibit the cytochrome P450 enzyme responsible for cisapride metabolism in humans (e.g., clarithromycin, itraconazole).[125]

Miscellaneous and Pending Prokinetic Drugs

Erythromycin stimulates GI motility at low doses not associated with antimicrobial effects (0.5-1 mg/kg every 8 hours). Its effects appear to mimic those of motilin (see Figure 19-8). Lower esophageal sphincter pressure will be increased. However, contraction in the stomach is not coordinated and may result in "dumping" of food from the stomach into the intestines before maceration is complete. Increased small bowel motility has led to its clinical use in humans with small bowel dysmotilities, but clinical use has not been reported in animals. Doses greater than 3 mg/kg may actually cause spastic contractions and cramps. The prokinetic effects of erythromycin may be responsible, in part, for GI disturbances that occur in up to 50% of patients receiving this drug. However, tolerance develops rapidly, probably because of downregulation of motilin receptors. Other macrolides will also stimulate motility to variable degrees.

Among the H_2- receptor antagonists, ranitidine and nizatidine inhibit anticholinesterase activity and thus are prokinetic at antisecretory doses.[126] Comparison between cisapride and ranitidine, an H_2-receptor antagonist, for the treatment of gastroesophageal reflux reveals both to be effective.[127] Nizatidine was demonstrated to have prokinetic effects similar to those of cisapride owing to noncompetitive inhibition of ACh at a level comparable to that of neostigmine.[128]

Misoprostol, a PgE analog, also is associated with prokinetic properties in the colons of dogs and cats. At least two prokinetic agents have been in various stages of approval in human medicine: prucalopride (R093877; Janssen Pharmaceutical) and tegaserod. Both are potent, partial agonists of 5-HT_4 receptors. Prucalopride (benzamide) is void of activity at other serotonin receptors or cholinesterase enzyme activity. Although pharmacokinetics have not been reported in dogs, prucalopride causes a dose-dependent (0.01-0.16 mg/kg [dog]) increase in gastric emptying and increased giant migrating contractions with defecation in dogs (0.02-1.25 mg/kg) or cats (0.64 mg/kg).[129] Fecal consistency does not appear to be affected. In contrast to prucalopride, tegaserod is a non-benzamide. In addition to effects at 5-HT_4 receptors, it acts as a weak agonist at 5-HT_{1D} receptors. Like prucalopride, tegaserod acts as a prokinetic in the canine colon, with effects apparent within 1 hour of an intravenous dose (0.03-0.3 mg/kg). Prokinesis also appears to occur in the intestine on the basis of normalization of transit time in opioid-induced bowel dysfunction in dogs (3-6 mg/kg orally). Because the colonic effects of tegaserod do not appear to be dose dependent, prokinetic effects in the colon may reflect an alternative mechanism of action. The impact of tegaserod on the canine stomach or in the cat have yet to be described. Tegaserod was approved for human use in the United States in 2002 (Zelnorm).

The Impact of Nongastrointestinal Drugs on Gastrointestinal Motility

Benzodiazepines influence gastrointestinal smooth muscle activity and secretion. In fasted dogs, the diazepam (0.5 mg/kg, IV) was associated with disruption of migrating myoelectric complexes and increased conctractility in the jejunum. In humans, diazepam (approximately 0.15 mg/kg PO) suppressed basal gastric acid secretion for 5 hours posttreatment.[129a,b] A variety of drugs alter esophageal sphincter function. Anesthetic drugs that reduce gastroesophageal sphincter tone include acepromazine, diazepam, morphine, halothane, isoflurane, xylazine, and atropine. The effect of intravenous morphine and butorphanol on GI motility has been studied in dogs. Morphine (0.1 mg/kg) was associated with a dose-dependent increase in duodenal smooth muscle activity and a dose-dependent decrease in bile duct flow, with the effects described as spasmogenic. In contrast, butorphanol administered at a dose described as equianalgesic (0.025 mg/kg intravenously) had little or no effect on the biliary or GI smooth muscle in dogs.[130]

The effect of xylazine (1 mg/kg) or the combination of acepromazine (0.1 mg/kg) and butorphanol (0.05, 0.2, or 1 mg/kg) on GI motility as it influenced GI radiocontrast studies was studied prospectively in healthy dogs (n = 6) using a randomized crossover saline–placebo-controlled design.[131] Total gastric emptying time (gastric and intestinal) was prolonged by xylazine and the combination of acepromazine and butorphanol (all doses). However, nonmanual restraint was facilitated and the combination protocol with butorphanol at 0.05 mg/kg provided sufficient chemical restraint to allow functional morphologic examination of the GI tract (within 5 hours).[131] It is unclear how this combination would affect the study in an animal with GI disease.

The impact of selected drugs on feline gastroduodenoscopy has been reported in normal cats receiving ketamine intramuscularly followed by isoflurane maintenance. Each of eight cats was studied four times, once per drug. No differences were detected in difficulty or time to pass the endoscope through the cardiac or pyloric sphincters for hydromorphone, with or without glycopyrrolate, medetomidine, or butorphanol. Passage into the stomach required only 16 seconds, and the drug took at most 2 minutes (generally 20 seconds) to pass into the duodenum. Although sample size may have precluded detection of significant differences among drugs, the authors concluded that none of the drugs impeded endoscopy.[132]

DRUGS AFFECTING THE INTESTINAL TRACT

Physiology, Pathophysiology, and Motility

The primary clinical sign reflecting intestinal disease is diarrhea; accordingly, drugs targeting the intestinal tract frequently are intended to control diarrhea. Drug therapy for diarrhea tends to be nonspecific, preferably targets the underlying disease rather than the GI tract, but occasionally might target the physiologic (rather than pathologic) cause of diarrhea. Diarrheas can be classified as inflammatory or infectious, osmotic (including malabsorption), and secretory. The goal of antidiarrheal therapy generally is to reduce the discomfort and inconvenience of frequent bowel movements and, when indicated, to replace fluids or electrolytes lost with diarrhea. Rehydration followed by oral replacement therapy often is the preferred treatment for diarrheas associated with infectious agents.[133] Suitable solutions contain K^+, HCO^+, Na^+, and glucose in sufficient quantities to replace stool losses.[133] Substantial evidence exists linking GI secretion with GI motility, with increased motility usually being accompanied by increased fluid and electrolyte secretion.[134] The physiology of intestinal motility was previously discussed.

Absorption and Secretion

Increased amounts of fecal water reflect either diminished absorption or a net secretion (accumulation) of fluid into the lumen of the intestine. In all diarrheal states, increased fecal water loss is associated with an overall secretion of electrolytes and water in selected segments of the GI tract. The absorptive capacity of the alimentary canal is overwhelmed distal to the site of secretion. Sodium-absorbing cells are present predominantly on the villi, and chloride-secreting cells are located primarily in the crypts.

Absorption in the small intestine occurs by passive sodium absorption across the luminal membrane and by active secretion of sodium across the basolateral membrane. Water follows the osmotic draw of sodium into the lateral intracellular space. The electrochemical gradient caused by sodium movement facilitates chloride diffusion into the cell.[133] A specific brush border carrier for NaCl co-transport accomplishes absorption. Nutrients such as glucose and other organic solutes, however, facilitate solvent drag of water and electrolytes as they enter cells.[133] Secretion in crypt cells of the intestinal epithelium is initiated by intracellular signaling (cAMP) or calcium. Increased chloride conductance into the lumen results in sodium recycling, first through the lateral intercellular space and second into the lumen. Although NaCl co-transport can be inhibited, NaCl movement can still occur as a result of solvent drag (i.e., that mediated by nutrients).[133]

Increased intestinal cell cyclic adenosine monophosphate, cyclic guanosine monophosphate, and Ca^{2+} (through calmodulin) all diminish sodium absorption and increase chloride secretion, with a net efflux of water into the lumen. Cholera enterotoxin is the best-known intestinal secretagogue,[133] but several hormones, including vasoactive intestinal peptide, gastric inhibitory peptide, CCK, secretin, glucagon, and PGE_1, and infectious agents (e.g., *Escherichia coli, Staphylococcus* spp.) are associated with net fluid accumulation.[133] Several laxative agents such as bile acids and ricinoleic acid may act through this mechanism. The exact role of intestinal motility in the alteration of fluid and electrolyte movement and the role of mucosal permeability or mucosal damage in the genesis of fluid accumulation within the gut lumen remain unclear.

Modulators of Intestinal Motility and Secretions

Anticholinergic Agents

Parasympatholytic or antimuscarinic agents diminish motor and secretory activity of the GI tract. Tone and propulsive movements are decreased (see Figure 19-9), and these agents will often relax spasm of visceral smooth muscle. Such antimuscarinic drugs are thus known as *antispasmodics* or *spasmolytics.* Although cholinolytic agents are commonly used as spasmolytics in antidiarrheal mixtures, the absence of segmentation may lead to severe forms of diarrhea with intestinal paralysis or ileus induced by the cholinergics. The main benefit of anticholinergic agents may be related to their ability to reduce intestinal secretions.

KEY POINT 19-27 A disadvantage of anticholinergic drugs is decreased gastrointestinal motility, loss of segmentation, and severe diarrhea.

Antimuscarinic agents used as spasmolytics include the belladonna alkaloids (atropine and hyoscine), their congeners (atropine methonitrate, homatropine methobromide, hyoscine butylbromide,), and synthetic cholinolytic drugs (aminopentamide, dicyclomine, glycopyrrolate, mepenzolate, oxyphenonium, propantheline). Many of the belladonna alkaloid derivatives are substituted tertiary amines and thus may have undesirable CNS and other systemic effects. The synthetic groups are mostly substituted quaternary amines and are devoid of CNS effects. Xerostomia, loss of lens accommodation, urinary retention, constipation, tachycardia, and CNS stimulation are potential side effects that may be encountered when parasympatholytics are administered.

Opioids

Receptors and peptides. Opiates have been used since antiquity to control diarrhea, and they remain the cornerstone of nonspecific antidiarrheal therapy for humans.[48] Opioids appear to influence normal GI physiology.[135] Opioids may stimulate GI motility both locally and by central effects in the brain or spinal cord.[113] Both opioid peptides and opioid receptors have been identified throughout the GI tract. The specific location of receptors has been based on the physiologic effects of opioid agonists and antagonists.[135-137] Both in vitro and in vivo preparations have been studied, often with conflicting results. Confounding interpretation is the variability in number and receptor type among species. High-affinity, reversible, and saturable binding of opioid receptors has been identified in longitudinal and circular smooth muscles and the myenteric and submucosal plexuses. Binding has also been noted in the muscularis mucosae. Although multiple opioid receptors have been identified, μ-type (OP_3) and δ-type (OP_1) opioid-binding sites appear to predominate among the species. Morphine acts to stimulate μ-receptors of the myenteric plexus, thus inducing migrating motor activity in the duodenum and jejunum. The relative importance of different receptor types in the control of intestinal peristalsis has not been established.

Not surprisingly, in addition to opioid recetpors, endogenous opioids are also present in high concentrations in the intestinal wall. Biosynthesis of enkephalins has been demonstrated in the myenteric plexus of some species. In addition, antral G cells are thought to be capable of synthesis of enkephalins or endorphins. β-endorphin and dynorphin have also been demonstrated. In cats enkephalin has been detected in both myenteric and submucosal plexuses. In contrast to other species, the predominant location of enkephalin neurons in dogs is the submucosal plexus. Opioid nerve fibers have also been documented in the lower esophagus, pyloric junction, and cardiac and ileocecal regions. Specific degradative enzymes for the opioid peptides have also been identified in similar locations.[135]

Impact of opioids on gastrointestinal motility. Much of the research regarding opioids and the GI tract reflects an attempt to understand the mechanisms of GI adversities resulting from opioid analgesic therapy. In vitro studies indicate that endogenous opioids in the GI tract modulate normal GI motility and gastrin release. Exogenous opioids depress the normal peristaltic reflex (see Figure 19-9), as has been repetitively demonstrated with the use of the pure antagonist naloxone, which consistently increases peristaltic activity. As such, among the side effects of opioids is constipation, associated with an inhibitory effect on smooth muscle motility. The intestinal opioid mechanism occurs in vitro throughout the intestinal tract, with function apparently increasing distally from duodenum to ileum. Endogenous opioids may thus be partially responsible for the *gradient of intestine,* a term that describes the oral to aboral phenomenon of decreasing frequency of peristaltic waves and decreasing sensitivity to distention stimuli.[135] GI opioids appear to be subject to feedback control.[135] The widely accepted mechanism of opioid actions in the GI tract is principally presynaptic inhibition of ACh (and potentially other mediators, such as serotonin) release.[109] Postsynaptic modulation of the effects of ACh already released may also be important for the effects of opioids on peristalsis. Intracellular mechanisms may involve increased calcium-dependent potassium conductance and hyperpolarization. Opioids also reduce calcium entry during the action potential and deplete neurons of calcium. In addition to inhibition of propulsion, tonic spasmogenic effects may occur in some species. The spasmogenic effect caused by opioids is antagonized by atropine. The effect of opioids on GI sphincters varies, with the effect appearing to vary with dose. For example, excitation (contraction) of the choledochoduodenal junction in dogs occurs with some drugs at low doses and inhibition at higher doses. Species differences in sites of action, receptor populations, and motility may be more quantitative than qualitative.[135]

KEY POINT 19-28 Opioids enhance retention of luminal contents facilitate absorption, rendering them very effective for treating diarrheas.

Impact of opioids on intestinal secretion. As with motility, the effects of opioids on gastric acid secretion vary with the study, species, and opioid. Opioids enhance gastric acid secretion mediated by histamine using in vitro studies, but the effect on ACh-induced secretion varies among in vivo studies. Dose dependence may account for some of the variability, with excitation or enhancement of basal secretion occurring at lower doses and inhibition at higher doses. A dual effect on stimulated gastric acid secretion appears to be mediated both peripherally and centrally.[135]

In contrast to gastric secretion, the effect of opioids on intestinal secretion appears to be consistent among the species.[135] Opioids stimulate the net absorption of water and electrolytes in enterocytes of both small and large intestines in a variety of species. In vitro studies indicate that these peripheral effects are mediated by δ-receptors. Receptor types may, however, vary with the site. These effects, which may reflect facilitated absorption or inhibited secretion, are largely responsible for the antidiarrheal properties of the opioids. Several mediators, acting centrally and peripherally, may mediate opioid antisecretory effects, with the impact varying with the chemical mediator. Presynaptic inhibition of ACh release and inhibition of prostaglandin-mediated adenylate cyclase activity have been implicated as the target signals, with sodium, but not chloride, the targeted ion that is negatively influenced. Opioids also centrally decrease intestinal secretions, perhaps through the sympathetic nervous system. Antisecretory effects may involve norepinephrine and its effects on vasoinhibitory peptide, PgE, or ACh.[113] Decreased intracellular free calcium also has been implicated as a possibility. In contrast to water and electrolyte secretion, opioids act to increase bicarbonate secretion from the gastric and duodenal mucosa.[135]

Drugs

Diphenoxylate hydrochloride is a meperidine derivative used specifically to control diarrhea. It is often administered in combination with atropine-like compounds, whose bitter taste and drying effect on salivary secretions are added as a deterrent to substance abuse. The actions of diphenoxylate largely depend on a direct peripheral effect on the GI wall. Because diphenoxylate can penetrate the blood–brain barrier, systemic opiate effects may occur. The potential for drug abuse has led to its designation as a Schedule V drug. The use of opioids in cats is generally reasonable, as long as accommodation is made for the increased sensitivity that appears to characterizes their response .

Loperamide hydrochloride, a butyramide derivative, is an orally active and effective antidiarrheal agent used for symptomatic control of acute and chronic nonspecific diarrhea. Unlike diphenoxylate, systemic opiate agonist effects do not appear to occur after oral administration of loperamide, and there are few side effects. Although loperamide has some structural similarities to diphenoxylate, it does not cross the blood–brain barrier, and it differs both qualitatively and quantitatively from diphenoxylate and difenoxin in its pharmacologic actions.[138] Intestinal transit time and intestinal luminal capacity increase after treatment with loperamide.[113]

KEY POINT 19-29 Because loperamide does not penetrate the blood–brain barrier, it has fewer side effects than diphenoxylate.

Miscellaneous Antisecretory Drugs

There are a number of potentially useful drugs that have not been extensively studied but for which there is some evidence of clinical benefit. Glucocorticoids have been found to be beneficial in treating refractory chronic diarrheal disease as well as chronic inflammatory diseases of the intestinal tract. Glucocorticoids stimulate active sodium absorption in the jejunum, ileum, cecum, and colon. However, because of many undesirable side effects when used chronically, the glucocorticoids should not be used on a routine basis to treat diarrhea.

Adrenergic agents appear to act predominantly by increasing basal fluid absorption and do so at very low concentrations. The mechanisms involved are unclear. Clonidine and other α_2-adrenergic agonists are potentially useful in this regard. Calcium/calmodulin antagonists may act by stimulating active absorption as well as by inhibiting intestinal secretion, but the precise mode of action of these drugs is not clear. Several drugs with this effect have been found to be useful in the control of certain forms of secretory diarrhea. Examples include chlorpromazine and trifluoperazine. NSAIDs such as aspirin, indomethacin, flunixin, and the subsalicylate of bismuth subsalicylate inhibit the cyclooxygenase pathway of arachidonic acid metabolism and thereby suppress the formation of prostaglandin mediators. The role of various prostaglandins in intestinal motility as well as in absorption and secretory processes is complex, and the inhibition of prostaglandin synthesis will not consistently influence secretory diarrheal states. The NSAIDs may, however, prove to be therapeutically beneficial in some acute and chronic diarrheal syndromes as long as care is taken regarding their gastrointestinal advesre effects.

Asulfidine (sulfasalazine) is a sulfapyridine-5-aminosalicylic acid (5-ASA; mesalazine) compound joined by a diazo bond that is broken by colonic microbes.[139] It is the 5-ASA component that is beneficial, with the sulfapyridine simply carrying the active drug to the colon.[139] This finding led to the development of 5-ASA products without the sulfonamide component. Compounds equally efficacious to sulfasalzine include osalazine, balsalazide, and mesalazine. An advantage of these products is efficacy above the colon (i.e., in the absence of microbial metabolic activation). A variety of preparations are available such that oral absorption is prevented and specific sites of delivery (e.g., jejunem versus ileum versus colon) might be targeted, with the intent of topical, rather than systemic, delivery. These include pH-dependent (e.g., Asacol) and slow continuous release (Pentasa) mesalazine (also known as mesalamine), diazo bond delivery (osalazine, a diamer of mesalazine), or balsalazide (a prodrug).[140] The exact mechanism of action of mesalazine is not known, but presumed activities include inhibition of cytokines, leukotrienes, and nuclear factor kappa B. Mesalazine is metabolized by both epithelial and hepatic acetylation. Although these newer 5-ASA products have not been proved to be more efficacious than sulfasalazine in treatment of IBD in humans, they are better tolerated. Because they are better tolerated than glucocorticoids, they are the cornerstone of therapy for some human IBDs.

As with all aspirin-containing compounds, caution is indicated when a sulfasalazine is used in the cat because salicylic acid released in the colon can be subsequently absorbed. For example, the aspirin component of mesalamine (and thus osalazine) may be 30% or more bioavailable (demonstrated in humans), and care should be taken to avoid aspirin toxicity, especially in cats. Mesalamine enema may contain sufficient sodium benzoate (as a preservative), which also should be used cautiously in cats (see Chapter 4).

GASTROINTESTINAL PROTECTANTS AND ABSORBENTS

Compounds that are not absorbed from the GI tract and either line the mucosal surface or adsorb toxic compounds are often incorporated into antidiarrheal mixtures. The protectants seemingly produce a coating of the GI epithelium that prevents irritation or erosion by potentially harmful substances. The adsorbents physically bind chemical compounds, which precludes their absorption, and they are then eliminated in the feces. Use of these two therapeutic classes is obviously directed at potentially harmful agents of either inorganic or organic nature. Adsorbents will also, however, bind concurrently administered drugs used for therapeutic purposes. Care must be taken with the use of over-the-counter products. Active ingredients may change under the same trade name. Although over-the-counter products often are safe, some may present a health risk to certain patients (e.g., bismuth subsalicylate and cats).

Many protectants and adsorbents possess both properties to varying degrees. Those most frequently used are magnesium trisilicate, hydrated magnesium aluminum trisilicate (activated attapulgite), kaolin (natural hydrated aluminum silicate), aluminum hydroxide and phosphate, bismuth salts, calcium carbonate, pectin (natural polygalacturonic acids), and activated charcoal.

The combination kaolin–pectin product is dissolved in 20 parts water. Described as a demulcent and adsorbent, the drug supposedly binds and removes bacteria and their metabolic products and toxins. These effects are controversial. Although stool consistency may improve, studies do not indicate that fluid and electrolyte imbalance is corrected, nor is the course of disease shortened.[141]

KEY POINT 19-30 Bismuth subsalicylate is an effective antidiarrheal because of its adsorptive capacity and effects on secretion.

The insoluble bismuth salts have been used for more than 400 years.[142] Products include bismuth subcarbonate, bismuth subnitrate, and bismuth subsalicylate. Bismuth subsalicylate is a crystalline 1:1 trivalent bismuth and salicylate compound. It is chemically transformed throughout the GI tract to bismuth and salicylate. The drug has been shown to have both antisecretory and antimicrobial effects in several species.[142] The subsalicylate fraction has been shown to have antiprostaglandin synthetase effects, which would enhance its action in controlling diarrheal syndromes.[133] In humans and cats, nearly all the salicylate is systemically available.[142,143] Caution is recommended in order to prevent salicylate toxicity in cats receiving this drug.

Activated charcoal has primarily adsorbent properties. Because of its broad spectrum of adsorptive activity and its rapidity of action, it is one of the most valuable agents for emergency treatment of certain cases of poisoning. It forms a stable complex with many substances and permits their evacuation from the body. Charcoal preparations vary according to the source of base material, surface area, capacity for drug binding and affinity, and avidity of drug binding.[144] Source materials are usually lignite, wood, or peat. Activation forms more pores and enlarges the surface area. Activation time is directly correlated with the molecular size of the compounds adsorbed. Because most drugs are of an intermediate molecular weight, charcoals with pore sizes between 10 to 20 Å are most appropriate.[141] Administration with a cathartic, such as sorbitol, is a common practice and facilitates rapid movement of the charcoal–toxin complex.[144] Activated charcoal loses its efficacy as the time interval between treatment and toxin ingestion increases. The optimal dose and interval for administration of activated charcoal have not been well established,[144] although a charcoal to toxicant ratio of 10:1 has been recommended.[141] One source suggests treatment at 6-hour intervals.[144] Powders are superior to tablets.[141] Food generally decreases the efficacy of these products. In the common domestic species, 20 to 120 mg/kg powered activated charcoal is usually administered as a drench after mixing with water. An activated charcoal suspension may be used for gas lavage in simple-stomached animals.

Cholestyramine is a basic anion exchange resin that binds to acidic side chains such as those occurring in bile acids. Endotoxin also is bound. To increase the number of basic binding sites, cholestyramine is attached to a polystyrene matrix that can act as a nonspecific adsorbent. As bile salts are bound in the GI tract, lipoproteins, cholesterol, and neutral fat absorption is also decreased. Although specifically indicated in humans for pruritis associated with increased bile acids (hypercholesterolemic syndromes) cholestyramine has also been used to symptomatically treat diarrhea, particularly that which is intractable. Nausea, constipation, steatorrhea, and decreased fat-soluble vitamin absorption are reported undesirable effects. The product should be administered in food or water.[141]

LAXATIVES AND CATHARTICS

Laxatives and cathartics promote defecation by increasing frequency of defecation or fecal volume or consistency.[119,145-147] Laxatives (or aperients) promote elimination of a soft-formed stool, whereas cathartics (or purgatives) tend to produce a more fluid evacuation. The difference between these two effects may be just a matter of dose, but in some instances laxatives are only capable of increasing the hydration or softness of the fecal mass without ever inducing catharsis. The enhanced intestinal transit times that occur with use of some of these cathartics are usually due to intrinsic local myenteric reflexes within the visceral smooth muscle or to stimulation of the cholinergic receptors of the extrinsic parasympathetic nervous system. Although a traditional classification of the group is presented here, it should be noted that many cathartics alter intestinal electrolyte transport to increase fecal water excretion, so the grouping of these compounds should perhaps more logically follow their effects on intestinal electrolyte movement.

A number of deleterious effects may occur with excessive or constant use of cathartics. Severe, continuous diarrhea and abdominal colic, leading to dehydration and even shock, may follow overdosage. Other potentially harmful effects include decreased sensitivity of the intestinal mucosa, megacolon, flatulence, loss of electrolytes (especially sodium, potassium, chloride, and bicarbonate), secondary aldosteronism, melanosis coli (anthraquinones), steatorrhea, protein-losing gastroenteropathy, excessive calcium loss with resultant osteomalacia, and exacerbation of inflammatory intestinal disease. Several drugs can also distribute into milk and adversely affect suckling young.

Emollient Laxatives

The emollient laxatives (lubricant laxatives, mechanical laxatives, fecal softeners) act unchanged. They are not absorbed to any appreciable extent and simply soften and lubricate the fecal mass, which in turn facilitates expulsion. Although not always reliable, particularly in the ruminant, they are used in all species.

Mineral oil (liquid paraffin) is a commonly used lubricant laxative. It is bland and generally safe, but chronic administration may impair absorption of fat-soluble vitamins, other nutrients, and co-administered therapeutic agents. Decreased irritability of the intestinal mucosa may develop with protracted use and, paradoxically, cause chronic constipation. White or yellow soft paraffins are used most commonly for small animals as lubricant laxatives (e.g., feline hairballs). Several anionic surfactants are employed as fecal softeners. Examples include docusate sodium, previously called *dioctyl sodium sulfosuccinate* and *dioctyl calcium sulfosuccinate.*

Simple Bulk Laxatives

The simple bulk laxatives are hydrophilic and not digested. As such, they adsorb water and swell, forming an emollient gel. Increased volume or bulk causes distention and reflex contraction, leading to peristaltic activity. Feces remain soft and hydrated. Methylcellulose, carboxymethylcellulose sodium, and plantago seed (psyllium seed) are examples of simple bulk purgatives. Wheat bran, prunes, and other fruits also belong in this group. In addition to their bulk action, celluloses and hemicelluloses will be fermented in the hind gut by bacteria to produce volatile fatty acids and other products that exert an osmotic effect, which enhances their laxative action. Meteorism and a very fluid stool often result from the use of simple bulk laxatives.

KEY POINT 19-31 Bulk laxatives cause reflex bowel contraction and softening of the stool.

Osmotic Cathartics

Osmotic cathartics (saline purgatives) consist of salts or compounds that are either partially and slowly absorbed or not absorbed. Water is osmotically retained or attracted into the intestinal lumen, although enhanced mucosal secretion of fluid may also occur. Drinking water must be freely available, and use is contraindicated with dehydration. Effects are realized in monogastric animals generally in 3 to 12 hours. Magnesium salts are frequently used as saline purgatives. Magnesium ions also cause release of CCK, which increases peristaltic activity. Magnesium sulfate (Epsom salts), isotonic in a 6% solution, magnesium hydroxide, magnesium oxide (milk of magnesia), and magnesium citrate are the magnesium salts most commonly employed. The solutions need not be hypertonic to produce an effect. About 20% of the magnesium ions are absorbed when magnesium sulfate is dosed orally, and if purgation does not occur, additional amounts of magnesium may be absorbed with subsequent depression of the excitable tissues in the body. This is more likely to occur if renal function is impaired. Salts such as sodium sulfate (Glauber's salt), sodium phosphate, potassium sodium tartrate (Rochelle salt), and even large quantities of sodium chloride are effective saline purgatives. Saline purgatives are often combined with polyethylene glycol (PEG) for whole bowel irrigation implemented for bowel preparation before lower bowel procedures such as surgery or colonoscopy.The safety and efficacy of sodium phosphate has been described in healthy dogs (n = 8) when used to prepare for colonoscopy. Orogastric sodium phosphate (1 mL/kg in 2 mL/kg water followed by 2 mL/kg) was less effective as a preparatory agent compared with PEG (66 mL/kg) and bisacodyl (10 mg/dog; dog weight not provided). Most (five of eight) dogs receiving sodium phosphate vomited during or after administration. In contrast, dogs receiving PEG tended to regurgitate. Sodium phosphate enemas were associated with transient hyperphosphatemia and hypocalcemia that were not considered clinically relevant in these normal dogs. Other electrolyte concentrations statistically varied but remained within normal limits. The protocols for colonoscopy preparation included 20 mL/kg warm water enemas; treatments were repeated at 4 hours and enemas at 24 hours (before procedures). Enemas may have contributed to vomiting because of distention. Dogs receiving PEG were also pretreated (20 minutes) with metoclopramide (0.3 mg/kg subcutaneously). The authors concluded that sodium phosphate enemas should not be considered as preparative agents for colonoscopy.[148]

The sugar alcohols mannitol and sorbitol will also induce an osmotic catharsis, as will the synthetic disaccharide lactulose, which is not digested in the small intestine because no specific enteric enzyme is present. It passes to the large intestine, where saccharolytic microflora ferment lactulose to produce acetic, lactic, and other organic acids, which in turn lower the pH of the colonic content and exert an osmotic effect. Water is attracted, the fecal mass softens, and colonic peristalsis ensues. Lactulose is used for chronic constipation and treatment of hepatic encephalopathy. Acidification of the contents of the large intestine favors a greater formation of the ionized and thus nonabsorbable ammonium ion rather than the readily absorbable ammonia molecule, which requires detoxification in the liver by the urea cycle. Hyperammonemia is thus decreased. Absorption of other toxic amines from the hind gut is also reduced by acidification of the contents. Some meteorism may be evident after administration of lactulose. Lactitol is an alternative osmotic cathartic. It is less sweet than lactulose and may be better tolerated.

Irritant Cathartics

Contact or irritant purgatives were thought to stimulate the mucosal lining of the GI tract and thereby initiate local myenteric reflexes that would enhance intestinal transit. However, they also activate secretion. Irritant cathartics act either directly or indirectly, depending on whether the compound must be metabolized to its active product. Some purgatives are so highly irritating that they may cause severe colic and superpurgation.

Several bland vegetable oils act as irritant purgatives. Their action is based on hydrolysis by pancreatic lipase in the small intestine and subsequent formation of sodium and potassium salts of the released fatty acids, which act as irritant soaps. They differ in potency depending on the oil used. Castor oil produces highly irritant ricinoleates; raw linseed oil leads to formation of less irritant linoleates; and olive oil leads to rather mild oliveates. The response to castor oil is prompt, and evacuation of the whole intestinal tract occurs, leading to an almost complete emptying. Moist bulky feeds are necessary after purgation with castor oil. It is used mainly in nonruminants and often employed in calves and foals. The effect occurs in 4 to 8 hours in small animals.

The diphenylmethane cathartics appear to have a greater effect on the large intestine. Their precise mechanism of action is unclear. An effect is usually seen within 6 to 8 hours, and excessive catharsis may occur with overdosage. Bisacodyl also is a diphenylmethane cathartic that inhibits glucose absorption and Na^+, K^+ ATP activity, as well as altering motor activity of the visceral smooth muscle. Only about 5% of any dose of bisacodyl is absorbed. This agent is used both orally and by enema.

Enemas

Introduction of solutions or suppositories into the rectum to initiate the defecation reflex is a useful and simple method to correct or prevent constipation. Many preparations have successfully served as enemas, including soapy water (soft anionic soap), isotonic or hypertonic sodium chloride solutions, sorbitol, glycerol, surfactants such as sodium lauryl sulfoacetate, mineral oil, and olive oil. Enema preparations that contain phosphate should not be used indiscriminately because they can precipitate potentially fatal hyperphosphatemia, hypocalcemia, and hypernatremia in cats[149] or debilitated animals.

AGENTS PROMOTING GASTROINTESTINAL FUNCTIONS

Several preparations are used therapeutically to control specific GI diseases by promoting digestive or other metabolic processes. These compounds generally consist of normal microbiota or digestive enzymes or related substances that are used for replacement therapy in deficiency states.

Digestive Enzymes

Pancreatic extracts that stimulate pancreatic exocrine secretions are of therapeutic benefit in cases of chronic pancreatitis and pancreatic hypoplasia, in which glandular function is diminished or destroyed. Pancreatin (Panteric, Stamyl, Viokase) obtained from hog pancreas is the major ingredient of most commercial pancreatic enzyme preparations. Enteric-coated preparations to prevent destruction of pepsin in the stomach are generally thought to be better than noncoated preparations. In a few instances, enteric-coated preparations are the most effective in dogs with pancreatic insufficiency; they are added to food and must be provided with each meal. Dosage is adjusted to obtain a normal stool. Simultaneous administration of nonsystemic alkalinizing agents to maintain an optimal pH range for enzyme activity has not proved successful clinically. However, the administration of cimetidine about half an hour before dosing with pancreatic extract does limit gastric inactivation of the enzymes. Proper dietary control is also essential for the successful management of animals suffering from pancreatic insufficiency. Premixing in food does not appear to be necessary for efficacy of these products.

Bile acids and their salts promote absorption of long-chain fatty acids and fat-soluble vitamins. They also act as choleretics (discussed previously). Examples include dehydrocholic acid (Decholin) and chenodiol (previously called *chenodeoxycholic acid*).

Diastases are amylolytic enzymes obtained from malt and *Aspergillus oryzae* and are used for replacement of pancreatic α-amylase and to control flatulence caused by gas produced from soluble carbohydrates by bacterial flora.

Antiflatulence Drugs

Simethicone is an inert over-the-counter mixture of siloxane polymers stabilized with silicon dioxide.[24] It acts as an antifoaming agent by covering bubbles with a thin layer that facilitates bubble collapse. Reduction in foam may reduce gas volume, although therapeutic efficacy is not clear.[24]

BIOTHERAPEUTICS: PREBIOTICS, PROBIOTICS, AND SYNBIOTICS

The concept that microbes might be beneficial rather than simply detrimental to health enjoys a long history of anecdotal evidence. Among the oldest observations is the Old Testament recording of Abraham ingesting sour milk (Genesis 18:8). The purported health benefits of microbial products are varied, but they are more often supported by testimonials than by scientific evidence. However, hypothesis-driven research is increasingly generating evidence-based examples of the therapeutic benefits of biotherapy.

KEY POINT 19-32 The normal intestinal microbiota plays an important role in nutrition, metabolism, pathogen control, and immunity.

Product Definitions

The term *probiotic* was originally coined in 1965 to refer to substances secreted by one microorganism that stimulate the growth of another.[150] The term has been modified at least five times and continues to vary with the author. Most recent modifications are intended to encompass nondairy products (e.g., plant-based products), recognizing the importance of organism load to ensure a therapeutic effect; to allow for transient, rather than prolonged, effects that would otherwise require transplantation (implying colonization), and to allow for multiple and diverse benefits, including those manifested beyond the GI tract.[150] Perhaps the easiest working definition of probiotics is that offered by the World Health Organization: live microorganisms that, when administered in adequate amounts, confer a health benefit on the host.[150]

In contrast to probiotics, *prebiotics* are nondigestible food ingredients (e.g., dietary fiber) that beneficially affect the bacterial population. They differ from other fermentable carbohydrates in that they interact with selective microorganisms.[151] They presumably are most beneficial to those microbes targeted for their therapeutic benefit, thus shifting the composition of the intestinal microbiota toward the beneficial organisms. Examples include fructooligosaccharides, inulin, transgalactosylated oligosaccharides, and soybean oligosaccharides that selectively promote the growth of bifidobacteria. Metabonomics is the scientific discipline that studies compounds formed from prebiotics. *Synbiotics* contain both prebiotics and probiotics, with the prefix *syn* implying a synergistic effect of the prebiotic on the probiotic portion of the combination products. To be a symbiotic, the prebiotic portion should have demonstrated positive effects on the specific probiotic component of the combination product.[150] Some products sold as probiotics are actually the fermentation products produced by target microbe; presumably, the products are those imparting the therapeutic benefits of the microbes.

Normal Microbiota

Normal Flora

Understanding the impact of biotherapeutics requires an appreciation of the normal GI microflora. The total body microbiota (human and presumably dogs or cats) outnumbers other cells by approximately tenfold. Up to 30% of dry fecal matter represents microbes. The number of microbial species in the GI tract (again in humans) is estimated to be between 400 and 500 based on 16S rRNA sequencing and metagenomic. However, only a fraction (approximately 10%) are conducive to cultures.[152,153] Whereas some of these unculturable microbes are closely related to those already identified, others represent totally new species. Therefore very little is known regarding the microbiota of the GI tract. To further complicate our understanding, the number and diversity of microbes increases with a number of factors. Differences owing to location in the GI tract reflect, in part, differences in pH and transit time. Peristalsis and low pH lower microbial counts in the stomach, duodenum, and jejunum,[152] whereas numbers and diversity increase in the ileum (10^{4-8} CFU or colony-forming units/mL) and colon. Rapid transit decreases numbers because bacteria colonizing sites with a high transit rate (e.g., lower ileum) must be able to effectively adhere to the mucosal epithelium; thus organisms such as lactobacilli must compete with pathogenic organisms for adherence receptors if they are to colonize these regions. Organisms that do not have to adhere are likely to be present in much higher numbers in the colon. Higher colonic pH (5 to 6) leads to slower epithelial turnover, which also increases bacterial counts. More rapid microbial growth results in a lower redox potential.

KEY POINT 19-33 The normal microbiota consists of close to 500 organisms, most of which have not been cultured or otherwise specifically identified.

Intestinal bacterial by-products produced under low redox conditions contribute to a higher short-chain fatty acid concentration. Even within the colon, bacterial growth and fermentation products are diverse among regions, with growth and carbohydrate fermentation greater proximally and protein fermentation greater distally. Diet has a profound impact on microbiota. Nondigestible foods are a source of energy and carbon for the microbiota and may influence metabolites that positively or negatively influence the population. Food also affects host GI function and health and thus indirectly affects the microbiota.[152]

The microbiota of the human GI tract was recently reviewed and may provide insight into the complexities of microbiota in other species.[152] The number of colony-forming units per mL increased from the stomach and duodenum (10^3) to the colon (10^{14}). The composition increases in complexity with age such that the microbiota is relatively simple in newborn and very old subjects. Nutritional and physical requirements are sufficiently sophisticated that the conditions for optimal growth simply are not known for up to 70% of the bacterial population.[151] However, four microhabitats have been described: the lumen; the mucous layer of epithelial cells; the surface of epithelial cells; and the crypts of the ileum, cecum, and colon (which generally are colonized with motile, spiral-shaped organisms). In humans a central core of microbiota might be partitioned into five bacterial groups: *Clostridium leptum; Clostridium coccoides; Bacteroides;* and, in smaller part, *Bifidobacterium*.[151]

The GI flora of dogs has been described and compared to that in humans,[154,155] (Table 19-3) and the microbiota of the cat has been described.[154] Selective media often do not support the growth of target microbes in dogs, contributing to the list of unculturable bacteria.[154] However, because the dog is a carnivore, its GI tract is shorter than that of humans. Similarities between human and dog include the proportion of gram-negative to anaerobic organisms, the makeup of gram-negative isolates, and floral behavior in response to probiotics or prebiotics.[154,156] Genera that are numerous in both the GI tract of restricted-access dogs and humans include *Lactobacillus, Bifidobacterium, Eubacterium, Bacteroides, and Peptostreptococcus.* The major difference between dogs and humans appears to be the proportion of bifidobacteria;[154] however, a study examining floral changes in response to different housing environments demonstrated that the number of bifidobacteria dramatically increase under conditions in which exposure to the environment is controlled.[156] Under such conditions major differences between the two species among culturable bacteria are limited and include the following: (1) *Bacteroides* and *Streptococcus* are the most common isolates in the ileum and colon of dogs; however, these isolates, although not the predominant isolate in humans, are present in a large proportion of humans; (2) *Fusobacterium* is not as numerous in dogs as in humans. In the cat, bifidobacteria appear to be even less numerous than in the dog.

Gastrointestinal Microbe–Host Interactions

The sophisticated interactions among the intestinal mucosa, host immune cells, the microbiota, and food have been described,[157] and the impact of probiotics on host immunity has been reviewed.[158] It is beyond the scope of this chapter to discuss the interactions, but it is notable that the mechanisms by which commensals are recognized as such and fail to stimulate an inflammatory response by the GI tract are not yet known. Interactions are modulated in part through pattern recognition receptors (PRRs) that recognize microbial motifs referred to as *pathogen-associated molecular patterns (PAMPs).* The PAMPs are evolutionarily highly conserved, not varying within microbes in the same class. Consequently, mammalian cells are able to recognize all microorganisms with only a few PRRs. Receptor families that identify PAMPS include Toll-like receptors located either on the cell surface or intracellularly and nucleotide-binding oligomerization domain

Table 19-3 Canine Normal Microbiota

Region	Human (%)	Dog (log CFU/g)
Gram-Negative Aerobes		
Escherichia coli		N/A
Enterobacter	1%	
Pseudomonas		N/A
Gram-Negative Rods		Jejunum (4)*
		Feces(6)*
Gram-Positive Aerobes		
Enterococcus		Colon (6-7)†
Streptococcus		Colon (8-9)†
Staphyloccoccus		Colon (8-9)†
Combined		Jejunum (3)*
		Feces (9)*
Gram-Positive Cocci		Jejunum (3)*
		Feces(4)*
Corynebacterium		N/A
Gram-Positive Rods		Jejunum (3)*
		Feces (4)*
Gram-Negative Anaerobes		
Bacteroides	20% to 42%	Colon (10+)
		Jejunum (2)*
		Feces (6)*
Porphyromonas		N/A
Prevotella	6%	
Fusobacterium		Colon (8-9)†
		Jejunum (3)*
		Feces (6)*
Bifidobacterium	1%-7%	Colon (6-8)†
Veillonellaceae		N/A
Gram-Negative Rods, other		Jejunum (3)*
		Feces (6)*
Gram-Positive Anaerobes		
Gram-Positive Cocci		Jejunum (3)*
		Feces (10)*
Peptostreptococcus		N/A
Peptococcus		N/A
Gram-Positive Rods		Jejunum (3)*
		Feces (7)*
Lactobacillus		Colon (7-10)†
Clostridium	22%-30%	Colon (6-8)†
		Jejunum (3)*
		Feces (10)*
Eubacterium		N/A

CFU, Colony-forming units. *Eubacterium* and *Corynebacterium* are pleomorphic.
*Data from Mentula S, Harmoinen J, Heikkilä M et al: Comparison between cultured small-intestinal and fecal microbiotas in beagle dogs, *Appl Environ Microbiol* 71(8):4169-75, 2005.
†Data from Rastall RA: Bacteria in the gut: friends and foes and how to alter the balance, *J Nutr* 134:2022S-2026S, 2004.

(NOD) receptors. Thus far, 11 mammalian Toll-like receptors have been identified.[157] Whether colonization is necessary for immunomodulation to occur is not clear.[158] However, microbial adhesion to the epithelial cells or mucus is generally recognized to be necessary. Activation of the immune system may reflect microbial alteration of epithelial tight junctions with subsequent bacterial translocation.

KEY POINT 19-34 The relationship between microbiota and the gastrointestinal immune system represents one of the most sophisticated communication systems in the body and its inadvertent or intended or manipulation is likely to contribute to disease or control, respectively.

Impact of Normal Flora on Gastrointestinal Health and Disease

In the last decade, the role of normal microbiota in GI physiology has been recognized as critical, protecting against invasion of pathogenic strains of bacteria, facilitating maturation and maintenance of the immune system, facilitating normal bowel smooth muscle function, supporting digestion of certain foods, and contributing to nutrition through the production of vitamins (vitamin K; vitamin B in some species) and other nutrients (e.g., short-chain fatty acids). Energy salvage is facilitated through conversion of nutrients to short-chain fatty acids.[152,159] Known effects of commensal intestinal bacteria include GI epithelial cell proliferation, energy capture, and production of metabolites; the latter, in particular, also can result in detrimental health effects.[152]

By-products of microbial metabolism may be either beneficial or detrimental. When included with probiotics, by-products are intended to support beneficial organisms or ameliorate negative effects of by-products. However, organisms themselves are chosen for their anticipated by-products. Among the organisms most commonly cited as beneficial are *Lactobacillus* and *Bifidobacterium* spp. Major sources of food for microbes include resistant starches; dietary fibers such as cellulose, hemicellulose, pectin, and inulin; and unabsorbed sugars and sugar alcohols. Substrates also include dietary protein (host or diet) and endogenous materials such as pancreatic enzymes, GI secretions, the mucoid layer, and sloughed GI epithelial cells. By-products of carbohydrates are formed primarily in the proximal colon; products include monosaccharides, disaccharides, and oligosaccharides. Further metabolism of these by-products results in short-chain fatty acids (including butyrate), as well as lactic, succinic, and formic acid. Butyrate is the major fuel source of colonic epithelial cells. However, butyrate purportedly also reduces the risk of colon cancer and inhibits proinflammatory cytokines. Intestinal microbes may metabolize other compounds into active or inactive metabolites, which may be subsequently absorbed. Examples include flavonoids, isoflavonoids and plant lignans.[152] Benefits of microbial fermentation of plant products include the production of enterolignans associated with estrogenic and antioxidant effects. *Oxalobacter formigenes* transforms oxalates; its absence increases the risk of oxalate stones in humans.[152] The production of potentially beneficial by-products often requires cooperative actions among different populations of microbes.

Bacterial by-products have a number of adverse effects. Protein by-products, produced primarily in the distal colon, include ammonia and amines resulting from deaminations; these products are associated with procarcinogenic effects (e.g., nitrosamines). Cysteine and methionine degradation yields sulfides, which inhibit colonic use of butyrate. Anaerobic colonic fermentation of aromatic amino acids tyrosine to phenols and tryptophan to indoles and their subsequent metabolism yield several procarcinogenic compounds. Many of these determinental compounds also play a role in hepatic encephalopathy. Bacterial deconjugation and dehydroxylation of bile acids contribute to their enterohepatic circulation; other compounds conjugated by compounds such as taurine, glycine, and sulfate may likewise be recycled. The general effect of recycling is longer exposure to potentially toxic compounds.

Probiotics as Therapeutic Agents

The science behind the use of probiotics is profoundly complicated by the unknown nature of the normal microbiota; the variables that influence it, including diets, diseases, and other patient factors such as breed, age, or gender; a lack of understanding of the pathophysiology of targeted disease; and issues regarding the quality of the products. Further hampering our understanding are the studies themselves. A variety of in vitro and in vivo models have been used (as reviewed by de Vrese and Schrezenmeir[160] and Lenoir-Wijnkoop and coworkers[151]), but poor scientific design mars the credibility of many.

KEY POINT 19-35 Evidence for the beneficial effects of probiotics will be difficult to establish because of the impact of multiple (including unknown) variables on response.

In humans probiotics have been demonstrated to have an impact on a large number of potential health problems (Table 19-4).[151] Although the data were drawn from humans, a review of those indications relevant to dogs and cats is reasonable; this discussion is limited to those indications for which sufficient evidence exists to support potential to probable therapeutic benefit. This review summarizes human reviews of well-designed clinical trials.[151,161, 162]

Gingival disease. Theoretically, probiotic microbes able to adhere to dental tissues occupy spaces that otherwise would be occupied by pathogens. For example, dairy products containing *Lactobacillus* or *Bifidobacerium*organisms might compete with cariogenic microbes such as salivary *Streptococcus mutans* or others. Several clinical trials have demonstrated a reduction in the number of dental caries in humans who ingest probiotics containing *Lactobacillus*.[151]

Antibiotic-induced diarrhea. Diarrhea as a side effect of selected commonly used antibiotics may reflect colonic overgrowth of *Clostridium difficile* or other organisms. Strategies for treatment (discontinuation of the inciting antibiotic, immediate retreatment with a new antibiotic) are not always successful, and one of the most commonly selected antibiotic in humans (oral vancomycin) to treat overgrowth of *Clostridium* organisms tends to be associated with adverse events. Although other antibiotics may be as effective as vancomycin, use of probiotics is a reasonable approach.

Based on a review of 10 clinical trials in close to 2000 children ranging in age from less than 1 year up to 18 years of age, probiotics were beneficial in the prevention of pediatric antibiotic-associated diarrhea.[162] Probiotic strains that showed the most promise included *Lactobacillus GG*, *Lactobacillus sporogenes*, and *Saccharomyces boulardii* when 5 to 40 billion colony-forming units were administered daily. Other organisms studied included members of *Lactobacillus* spp., *Bifidobacterium* spp., *Streptococcus* spp., and *S. boulardii* alone or in combination, including other treatments that might prevent antibiotic-associated diarrhea. The impact of age (e.g., infants versus older children) or duration of antibiotic therapy could not be assessed. Probiotics tended to be well tolerated after 2 to 12 weeks of therapy. Although the review concluded that routine treatment of probiotics for the prevention of pediatric antibiotic-associated diarrhea could not yet be recommended, further studies are warranted.

Infectious diarrhea. Probiotics also appear to be beneficial when used as an adjunct to rehydration fluids in the treatment of acute, infectious diarrhea in adults and children, although further research is indicated to determine the most effective probiotic and dosing regimen. In contrast, the use of probiotics as an adjunct to antibiotic therapy for *C. difficile* colitis could not be supported by a review of relevant clinical trials. However, the number of studies was small.

Liver disease. A review of clinical trials studying the use of probiotics for treatment of nonalcoholic fatty liver disease and nonalcoholic steatohepatitis found insufficient evidence to support or refute treatment. However, the use of probiotics and synbiotics to support liver function or treat liver disease has been reviewed by Lenoir-Wijnkoop and coworkers[151] and is discussed with regard to the management of liver disease.

Hyperlipidemia. Several species of *Lactobacillus* may bind to cholesterol in the presence of bile acids and low redox potential.[161]

Inflammatory bowel disease. Because of the complex relationship between the intestinal microbiota and the immune response, the use of probiotics as adjunct therapy for treatment of IBD is reasonable.[163] Probiotics have been used successfully to reduce *Helicobacter pylori* colonization in humans; severity of mucosal inflammation also is reduced in a mouse model. Clinical trials investigating the efficacy of probiotics in the treatment of *H. pylori* often are conflicting, ranging from ineffective as sole therapy to effective if used in conjunction with standard therapy antimicrobial and antiulcer therapy. One study in humans (n = 138) found that equal numbers of *Lactobacillus acidophilus*, *Lactobacillus bulgaricus*, *Streptococcus thermophilus*, and *Bifidobacterium lactis* (total of 10^9 organisms/mL) combined with quadruple therapy (amoxicillin, metronidazole, bismuth subcitrate, and omeprazole) eradicated infection in 85% of humans compared with 71% receiving quadruple therapy alone (as reviewed by Lenoir-Wijnkoop and coworkers[151]).

Table 19-4 Examples of Probiotic Indications for Treatment of (Human) Disease[161]

Organism	Specific Indications		Comments
Lactobacillus	2,4,7,8		
acidophilus	2,6,7,8,9,10	C	Decreased diarrhea of various causes
breve	7		Decrease *Clostridium* infection
bulgaricus	6,7	C, E	Microbial intereference
caseia		P	Decreased urogenical infection by *E. coli,* others
gasseria		E	Decreased *Candida* infection
GG	4		Decreased colon cancer
jonhsonii		L	Decreased cholesterol
lactis	7		Adjunct to antibiotics
paracaseia	3,7	U	Preservation of key nutrients
plantarum	3,7	C,U	Reduced inflammatory bowel disease
reuteri		L	Reduced irritable bowel syndrome
rhamnosus	7	L	Promotion of immunity
salivarius	7		Eradication of *Helicobacter pylori*
sporogenes	4,10		Reduction in hepatic encephalopathy
Bacillus		E or S	
Bifidobacterium	2, 4,7		Decreased neonatal necrotizing enterocolitis
bifidum		C	Decreased *Candida*
lactic		C	
longum		C	
breve		L	
infantis		L	
animalis			
lactis	6		
Enterococcus			
faecium		C	Decreased duration of acute diarrhea with gastroenteritis
faecalis		L	
Streptococcus			
salivarius		L	
thermophilus	6,7	A	
mutans	4		
Saccharomyces			Decreased *Candida*
boulardii	4	C	Decreased risk of antibiotic-induced diarrhea
			Decreased irritable bowel syndrome
			Source of microbial nutrients
Leuconostoc			
mesenteroides	3,7	A,U	
Lactococcus		E	
Oxalobacter			
formigenes			
Pediococcus			
pentasoaceus	3,7	U	

Key:
1 Allergic disease
2 Antibiotic-induced diarrhea
3 Bacterial translocation
4 Gingival disease
5 Infectious diarrhea
6 Inflammatory bowel disease
7 Liver disease
8 Urinary tract infection
9 Decreased *Clostridium* (Dog)
10 Lower cholesterol

E Enteric coating
P Patented with substantial research
C Evidence supported with clinical studies
L Limited evidence
S Spores
U Urease producer (useful in hepatic encephalopathy)
A Requires protection from acid

Probiotic therapy with conventional therapy does not appear to provide any benefit compared with conventional therapy alone in patients with mild to moderate ulcerative colitis. Although limited evidence suggests that probiotics may reduce clinical signs, support was not sufficient for recommendations. Likewise, evidence was not sufficient to support a role for probiotics in the treatment of Crohn's disease.

Probiotics do not appear to be effective for prevention of allergic diseases or food hypersensitivity in pediatric patients.

Urinary tract infection. The use of probiotics in the treatment of urinary tract infections in human patients was reviewed by Lenoir-Wijnkoop.[151] GI bacteria are a major source of urinary tract infections. As in animals, those causing UTI in humans are predominantly caused by uropathogenic *E. coli*, gram-negative organisms, and *Enterococcus faecalis*. In general, *Lactobacillus* sp. is the most common probiotic recommended for treatment of UTI. However, selected species are likely to emerge as more effective than others. A meta-analysis of 25 studies in human medicine found probiotics (lactobacilli) to be of benefit in treatment of bacterial vaginosis. However, a clear benefit could not be demonstrated for UTI (five studies); conclusions were difficult to draw because of limitations, including differences in study design and limited sample size.[163a]

Oxalate urolithiasis. The use of probiotics in the treatment of renal oxalate stones in human patients was reviewed by Lenoir-Wijnkoop and coworkers.[151] The absence of *O. formigenes* from fecal microbiota increases the risk of kidney stones. Both animal and human studies have documented that *O. formigenes* is able to become established in the GI tract, and establishment reduces urinary oxalate concentration. At least two studies have demonstrated a potential benefit of probiotics containing *O. formigenes* in the prevention or treatment of oxalate crystalluria.[164,165] Weese and coworkers[166] demonstrated that fecal samples containing lactic acid bacteria and several bacteria isolated from dogs or cats degraded oxalate in vitro. The addition of selected prebiotics (e.g., guar gum) increased the degradation.[166]

Allergic diseases. The use of probiotics in the treatment of allergic diseases (including atopic allergic disease and asthma in human patients) was reviewed by Lenoir-Wijnkoop and coworkers.[151] The rationale for efficacy reflects the immunomodulatory effects of probiotics. Based on clinical trials in humans, response has been limited to younger patients with severe disease. Similarly, probiotics have had only a limited, if any, effect on allergic rhinitis and asthma in humans.

Nosocomial infections. A meta-analysis examined the impact of probiotics on the prevention and treatment of nosocomial *C. difficile*–associated diarrhea and hospital-associated pneumonia in humans.[167] Although the prevention of antibiotic-induced diarrhea was a recognized beneficial effect, no evidence was found to support the theory that probiotics prevent nosocomial infection; clinical trials were recommended.

Irritable bowel syndrome. A meta-analysis[168] identified the limitations of drawing conclusions given differences in study design, including organisms, doses, and the definition of irritable bowel syndrome (IBS). Clinical efficacy was reported in several studies, with improvement manifested as decreased bloating, gas, and pain. *Lactobacillus* spp. and *Bifidobacterium* were targeted treatments.

Prebiotics (as opposed to probiotics) also have been associated with therapeutic benefits in humans with effects extending beyond local (GI) sites. The list is not much different than that for probiotics. Those conditions for which scientific evidence supports the potential use of prebiotics include allergies, immunomodulation (gut-associated lymphoid tissue as well as cellular Th1/Th2 ratio) that improves resistance to infections, constipation, irritable bowl syndrome, mineral metabolism (particularly strengthening of bone), prevention of cancer, and treatment of *H. pylori* infections. In addition, prebiotics have been scientifically associated with weight loss, presumably as a result of increased satiety mediated through GI suppression of ghrelin. Feed conversion efficiency has been described in food production animals. Interestingly, fermentation of prebiotics purportedly increases bacterial biomass in which nitrogen is fixed, thus decreasing the ammonia load in patients with hepatic encephalopathy.

Scientific data regarding the use of biotherapeutics in dogs and cats are slowly emerging. The use of prebiotics and probiotics in dogs has been reviewed by Rastall.[154] *L. acidophilus* DSM 13241 fed (2×10^9 colony-forming units daily per dog) in 15 healthy dogs decreased the number of culturable *Clostridum* spp. and was associated with an increase in indices indicative of immunomodulation (increased serum IgG and monocytes and decreased plasma nitric oxide). Prebiotics that have been studied[154] include lactosucrose and fructooligosaccharides. In their report, the authors noted that most prebiotics are enzymatically synthesized and that the technology can be modified such that enzymes are obtained from the target microbe, thus yielding highly specific probiotics.

Feeding 1.5 g lactusucrose daily for 2 weeks to healthy dogs (n = 8) increased bifidobacteria and decreased *Clostridium* spp. In another study, *Bifidobacterium* and *Lactobacillus* organisms also increased, and *Clostridium* and Enterobacteriaceae organisms decreased in cats receiving 0.75 g daily. A decrease in toxin levels and odor also was described for both dogs and cats. Fructooligosaccharides fed at a rate of 4 g/day to adult health dogs (n = 20) increased *Bifidobacterium* and *Lactobacillus* organisms and decreased *Clostridium* spp. Although both lactate and butyrate increased, ammonia, dimethylsulfide, and hydrogen sulfide also increased. Fructooligosaccharides at a rate of 0.75% in the diet of healthy adult cats for 2 weeks decrease *Clostridium* spp. and *E. coli*. Rastall[154] also described the formulation of a symbiotic containing *Lactobacillus* organisms cultured from one dog, following the tradition of probiotics being based on microbes isolated from the target species. Among the isolates cultured, *Lactobacillus mucosae, L. acidophilus,* and *Lactobacillus reuteri* were subjected to prebiotic carbohydrates. Baillon and coworkers[169] prospectively studied the viability of *L. acidophilus* added to a dry dog food at a concentration of 10(9) colony-forming units. Dogs (n = 15) were fed control and treated diet for 2 weeks each. Supplementation of the diet resulted in fecal recovery of organisms during but not after feeding of the treated diet, indicating colonization had occurred. The number of clostridial organisms was decreased.

Probiotics might comprise wild-type microbes associated with natural microbiota or genetically mutated forms of otherwise pathogenic but normal microbiota. Different strains of probiotic bacteria are presumed to impart differential effects, with variability representing habitat preferences of the microbe, specific capabilities of the microorganism, and differential enzymes. The number of colony-forming units ingested as probiotics is minor compared with the normal microbiota.[151] However, they travel through regions of the GI tract that are sparsely populated and therefore may transiently become the dominant microbe, potentially muting pathogens as a result of competitive exclusion. Rinkinen and coworkers[170] demonstrated the ability of lactic acid bacteria to competitively inhibit adhesion of selected canine pathogens (including *C. perfringens)* in vivo using isolated canine jejunal mucosa. However, *Enterococcus faecium* actually facilitated adhesion and colonization of *Campylobacter jejuni,* supporting the need for controlled clinical trials before assumptions are made regarding the impact of probiotics.

Probiotics and related compounds are not approved drugs and undergo no premarket approval with regard to efficacy, safety, or quality. Data, if available, represent efforts of the manufacturer or the scientific community. Consumer Laboratories (www.consumerlab.com) reviewed issues specifically related to quality assurance of a probiotic product. Many of these factors should be addressed on the label, including the following:

1. All types of bacteria or yeast, including genus and species, should be listed, with their correct spelling. The number of colony-forming units should also be included on the label. The number must be sufficient to allow adequate dosing in reasonable volumes. Generally 1 to 10 billion (10^9 to 10^{10}) colony-forming units are recommended (in humans) per day.
2. Viability of organisms, which may decrease during time that elapses from manufacture to purchase because of exposure to heat, moisture, and oxygen.
3. The presence of contaminating (potentially pathogenic) organisms including *E. coli, Salmonella* spp., *Staphylococcus aureus,* and *Pseudomonas aeruginosa* (according to Food and Drug Administration requirements).
4. The extent of enteric protection of selected organisms, including *L. bulgaricus, S. thermophilus,* and *Leuconostoc* and *Lactococcus* spp., varies (Table 19-4). Organisms that generally do not need protection include most *Lactobacillus, Bifidobacterium,* and *Streptococcus* organisms or organisms present as spores, including *Bacillus* and some *Lactobacillus* spp.

KEY POINT 19-36 Because probiotics and related compounds are not approved products, they undergo no premarket approval with regard to efficacy, safety, or quality; extra care should be taken to find a high-quality product.

Consumer Laboratories might also be solicited to identify superior products. Of 27 products (23 human, 4 pet) reviewed by Consumer Laboratories (as reviewed by the author January 2010), 10 (9 human, 1 pet) failed to contain the labeled amount of microbes and 5(2 human, 3 pet) failed to provide at least 10^9 colony-forming units per serving (although dogs and cats may require less than 1 billion). Marked variability was found in the dose delivered among pet products. No product failed as a result of microbial contamination (with mold). Weese and coworkers[166] also examined the quality of probiotics, including eight veterinary products. The contents of only two of thirteen products matched labeled descriptions, with five veterinary products not providing specific content information. Some products did not contain all labeled products while some products contained additional bacteria, some of which were potentially pathogenic. Organisms in several products were not viable. These studies emphasize the importance of selecting a probiotic that meets the standards of quality assurance reviews.

DRUGS AFFECTING THE LIVER

Cholagogues and Choleretics

Substances that cause contraction of the gallbladder are called *cholagogues.* The resistance of the sphincter of Oddi decreases as bile flows freely into the duodenum. Dietary fat and concentrated magnesium sulfate introduced directly into the duodenum through a tube exert a cholagogue effect through release of CCK/pancreozymin from the upper small intestine. Vagus stimulation also promotes contraction of the gallbladder.

Substances that increase secretion of bile by the hepatocytes are known as *choleretics.* A drug that stimulates the liver to increase output of bile of low specific gravity is called a *hydrocholeretic.*

Bile acids are synthesized from cholesterol and secreted into bile. Their production is increased by stimulation of the vagus nerves and by the hormone secretin, which increases the water and bicarbonate content of bile. Physiologically, however, bile acids are mainly responsible for the "bile salt–dependent" component of bile secretion and flow. Bile salts secreted with bile are almost complete (95%) resorbed, undergoing enterohepatic circulation. Reabsorption occurs principally in the terminal ileum. The primary bile acids are cholic and chenodeoxycholic acids; secondary acids include deoxycholic and lithocholic acid; lithocholic acid and ursodeoxycholic acid (UDCA) represent less than 5% of the total bile salt components. The major salts of bile acids are glycine and taurine. Bile acids induce bile flow, inhibit (by feedback) cholesterol synthesis, and promote dispersion and absorption of lipids and fat-soluble vitamins.

A number of natural bile salts and several partially synthetic derivatives are used therapeutically as choleretics, including dehydrocholic acid, which is the most potent hydrocholeretic agent. Naturally occurring bile acid conjugates such as glycocholate and taurocholate enhance bile flow to a lesser extent. Bile salts used therapeutically have a dual action in directly promoting fat absorption and stimulating biliary secretion after they have been absorbed. Overdosage with these compounds tends to cause diarrhea. UDCA is a natural bile acid constituting a very small portion of the bile acid pool. It is a degradation production of chenodeoxycholic acid. Among the bile acids, UDCA has the lowest hydrophobic–hydrophilic balance, the lowest capacity to make micelles, and the least potential for cholestatic or cellular membrane toxicity. Because cholestatic liver disease may be associated with accumulation of toxic bile acids, treatment with UDCA is appealing. Its efficacy in a variety of chronic liver diseases has been established. Its mechanism of action is not well understood but is probably related to bile acid metabolism.[171] The use of UDCA in dogs suffering from selected cholestatic liver diseases has been documented.[172] The disposition of UDCA has been studied in healthy cats.[173] Sporadic vomiting and diarrhea were reported, but otherwise the drug appears to be safe. Scientific studies establishing its safety and efficacy in diseased animals are indicated. Bile acids are effluxed from the canicular membrane into bial by a transport protein described as a "sister" to P-glycoprotein. However, selected bile acids, including UDCA, inhibit P-glycoprotein. [174] The therapeutic implications in patients with cholestasis or being treated with UDCA are not clear.

Liver Protectants and Hepatotropic Agents

A comprehensive review of the treatment and management of hepatic disease is beyond the purview of this chapter. However, a selection of the drugs for treatment of liver failure are listed and the rationale for their use noted. The major pharmacologic properties of many of these substances are discussed elsewhere in this volume. Hepatotropic agents are those having a special affinity for the liver or exerting a specific effect. Lipotropic agents hasten removal of fat or decrease its deposition in the liver. Use of lipotropic agents (choline, methionine, cysteine, betaine, lecithin, hydroxocobalamin) to increase mobilization of hepatic lipid is of proven value only in cases in which deficiencies of these substances exist. Deficiencies may be present in hepatic disease as a result of anorexia or insufficient dietary protein. Patients receiving and consuming a nutritious diet with adequate amounts of protein do not require supplementation with lipotropic agents, but their use has not been shown to be detrimental.

S-adenosyl-L-methionine

S-adenosyl-L-methionine (SAMe) is an endogenous coenzyme composed of ATP and the sulfur-containing amino acid methionine. The methyl group attached to the sulfur of methionine is chemically reactive such that it can be donated (i.e., transmethylation) to a number of acceptor substrates. Up to 80% of methionine in the body is used to form SAMe in the liver, which is the major, but not sole, site of methylation reactions. Regeneration of SAMe depends on vitamins B_6 and B_{12} and folic acid.[175] Transmethylation represents the primary function of SAMe, although sulfhydryl (transulfation) and aminopropyl (aminopropylation) groups also are donated. As such, SAMe is involved in more than 40 metabolic reactions in the body. Substrates are variable and include nucleic acids, proteins, and lipids. SAMe donates methyl groups to diverse compounds such as choline, creatine, carnitine, norepinephrine, DNA, and transfer RNA.

KEY POINT 19-38 Many hepatoprotectants either facilitate bile acid secretion or promote the activity of glutathione oxygen radical scavenging.

Aminopropylation yields compounds that affect cell and tissue repair. Transmethylation is important in detoxification, energy utilization, gene transcription and membrane functions that influence growth, and cellular signaling and adaptation. Transmethylation is necessary for formation of the phospholipid bilayer of outer cell membranes and membrane fluidity. After donating its methyl group, SAMe is converted to S-adenosylhomocysteine, the precursor to transsulfuration reactions. Transsulfuration also is important, resulting in the formation of sulfur and thiolated compounds, glutathione (GSH; one of the principle antioxidants of the liver), cysteine (the rate-limiting substrate for GSH formation), and sulfates. Each is particularly important in detoxification and conjugation reactions, including bile conjugation and bile flow. Glutathione has many additional effects on cellular biology, including gene transcription, triggering proinflammatory cell signaling and apoptosis, and also is important as an intracellular scavenger of oxygen radical.

The importance of SAMe in GSH synthesis suggested a possible role in liver disease. Studies in humans have demonstrated that SAMe is associated with an increase in hepatic GSH in chronic liver disease. Bile flow increases, presumably in response to increased sulfate bioavailability; sulfated bile acids are more soluble than others. Lieber[175] reviewed the role of SAMe in the body and its role in the treatment of liver disease in humans.[176] In an original research report, Center and coworkers[177] also reviewed the role of SAMe, with an emphasis in the liver. Multiple hepatic functions are dependent on GSH. Howver, SAMe formation from methionine decreases with severe liver disease as a result of downregulation of SAME synthetase. Sequelae include impairment of multiple hepatic functions as well as retention of methionine, which may contribute to hepatic insufficiency.

Because SAMe is unstable and is destroyed in the GI tract, it must be administered as an enteric-coated product. After absorption, oral bioavailability of SAMe is low on account of first-pass metabolism. Gender differences in oral bioavailability exist for SAMe in humans, with peak concentrations threefold to sixfold higher in women compared with men. SAMe is minimally bound to serum proteins (in humans) and is able to penetrate into and accumulate in cerebrospinal fluid.[174]

A case report[178] described the successful treatment of acetaminophen overdose (1 g/kg) in a dog with SAMe and supportive care; treatment was not begun until 48 hours after ingestion. Center and coworkers[177] examined the safety and effects of SAMe on the redox potential in red blood cells and the liver in normal, healthy cats (n=15) receiving 48 mg/kg of SAMe (Denosyl) orally once daily for 113 days. Plasma SAMe concentrations increased in concert with each dose. Peak concentrations approximating 1 to 1.5 μg/mL occurred between 2 to 4 hours after each dose; the disappearance half-life after oral dosing approximated 3 hours. Concentrations did not accumulate during the 113-day dosing period. Unmetabolized

SAMe appears to be eliminated almost equally in urine and feces. In humans and normal cats, SAMe was not associated with adverse events. In clinically normal cats, the redox status of both red blood cells and hepatocytes was increased after 113 days of SAMe administration. Further, red blood cells became more resistant to osmotic lysis. Hepatic cysteine, GSH, and protein increased, the latter attributed to an anabolic effect of SAME. Bile flow also increased, and histologic improvement was noted in the seemingly normal cats that had asymptomatic nonsuppurative portal inflammation.

SAMe is among the supplements for which comparison of labeled and actual contents may not match. The hygroscopic nature of SAMe contributes to quality assurance issues in that improper formulation and storage can result in the loss of active ingredient. The lack of premarket approval suggests that consumers should take a proactive approach to ensuring the quality of purchased products. Manufacturers appear to have improved the predictability of high-quality product in that eight of eight manufactured products tested by Consumer Laboratories and reported on its website in 2007 passed evaluation (as of January 2010). This compares to 2003, in which one product was found with only 30% of its listed amount, and in 2000, when close to 50% of tested products contained less than the labeled content (www.consumerlab.com). Enteric-coated products are available to protect SAMe from GI acidity; among the tests implemented by Consumer Laboratories is assurance of proper dissolution of enteric-coated products.

KEY POINT 19-39 The hygroscopic nature of SAMe may result in poor-quality product, and efforts should be taken to prescribe a product of known quality.

SAMe is available in several salt forms, each of which weighs a different amount and thus contributes variably to the total weight in mg. Care should be taken to dose on the active ingredient (i.e., SAMe). Salts include tosylate, disulfate tosylate, disulfate ditosylate, and 1,4-butanedisulfonate (Denosyl). For example, 200 mg of S-adenosyl-methionine disulfate tosylate contains only 100 mg of SAMe. The salt name should be included on the label as part of the chemical name, and the label should indicate the amount of active ingredient. SAMe also can be reviewed in the Herb and Plant Supplement at consumerlab.com[179]

SAMe may be involved in a number of drug–diet interactions. Because it inhibits uptake of serotonin, any other compound that does likewise should be avoided or used cautiously. This includes antidepressant behavior-modifying drugs such as monoamine oxidase inhibitors, selective serotonin reuptake inhibitors, tricyclics, tramadol, and selected herbs (such as St. John's wort).

Animal studies and clinical human studies indicate that SAMe improves biochemical parameters of liver function.[180]

Endogenous concentrations are reduced in patients with cirrhotic liver disease. Production of sulfated compounds and phosphatidylcholine subsequently is reduced. In animal studies SAMe improved bile secretion impaired by a variety of toxins and by pregnancy. Drug-induced hepatotoxicity and chronic liver disease were also reduced, without occurrence of serious side effects.[176] SAMe may act synergistically with UDCA for treatment of chronic progressive liver disease.[181] Although absorbed well after oral administration, SAMe undergoes extensive first-pass metabolism.[180] The compound is so hygroscopic that it is unstable unless protected; it might be most.

prudent to use products in bubble packets. Tablets cannot be broken without risking loss of efficacy. Caution is recommended when purchasing SAMe; an independent investigation that compared the content of SAMe with the labeled amounts found 6 of 13 products to be mislabeled. SAMe is marketed with silymarin (discussed in the next section) by Nutramax Laboratories for use in animals.

Milk Thistle

Silymarin has been reviewed by the Herb and Plant Supplement Encyclopedia at consumerlab.com. A member of the daisy family (Asteraceae), silymarin is one of the most important medical constituents of ripe seeds of the blessed milk thistle plant *(Silybum marianum)*. The name reflects the legend that attributes the white leaf veins to a drop of the Virgin Mary's milk and the location of the hidden infant Jesus during the family's flight from Egypt. Other synonyms for milk thistle include Marian thistle, Mary thistle, St. Mary's thistle, Lady's thistle, Holy thistle, sow thistle, thistle of the blessed virgin, Christ's crown, Venus thistle, heal thistle, variegated thistle, and wild artichoke.

Silymarin is a combination of seven flavonolignans (a flavanoid). The most prevalent is silybinin (silybin), which itself is two different compounds, with others including silychristin (or silicristin), and silydianin (also silidianin). Although all parts of the plant have been used medicinally,[182] the concentration of silymarin is highest in the seeds and leaves. Generally, the flavonoids are extracted. Silybin is often complexed with phosphatidylcholine, which improves its bioavailability. Dosing should be based on silybinin equivalents. As with flavonoids, the active ingredient of silymarin are potentially potent antioxidants, scavenging hydroxyl radicals, superoxide anions, and lipid oxygen radicals owing to lipid peroxidation.

Animal models (including tetrachloromethane hepatotoxicity in dogs and a variety of other hepatotoxicants) support a hepatoprotective effect. Its mechanism of hepatoprotection is not known. Suggested mechanisms include increased hepatic regeneration (by stimulating RNA polymerase, ribosomal RNA, and potentially DNA synthesis), scavenging of oxygen radicals, "stabilization of " hepatocyte cell membranes, and competitive inhibition of toxins that might otherwise bind to hepatic and damage cell membrane receptors (e.g., *Amanita phalloides)*. In rat and mice models of acetaminophen toxicosis, silymarin was associated with higher concentrations of hepatic glutathione and superoxide dismutase in experimental compared with control animals. Silymarin can also bind to steroid receptors, although the clinical relevance of this is not clear. Antifibrotic effects have been demonstrated in animal models. Finally, antinflammatory effects may reflect inhibition of lipoxygenase and subsequent leukotriene synthesis.[182]

KEY POINT 19-40 SAMe and milk thistle are among the few dietary supplements for which evidence of efficacy for treatment or prevention of liver disease exists.

Silymarin is poorly water soluble, and concentrated products are considered necessary for effective absorption. According to Consumer Laboratories, most studies involving silymarin are based on extract products that contain 70% to 80% silymarin on a weight basis. However, some products composed of seed powder contain only 1.5% silymarin. Quality assurance is likely to be an issue with silymarin: of eight products tested by Consumer Laboratories, only two contained the labeled amount. The remaining seven products ranged from 19% to 85% (median 64%). When properly labeled, the source of milk thistle (generally the seed) should be noted on the product. Care must be taken when dosing on the basis of label information; doses range from 15 to 1200 mg, reflecting in part the source and type of preparation. For example, pills made from seed powder contain about 9 to 15 mg of silymarin compared with 112 to 240 mg for pills made from dry extracts. Differences in doses may also reflect different salt preparations. In humans the phosphatidylcholine preparation may be more orally bioavailable, leading to a dose that is lower (1.5 to 3 mg/kg twice daily) compared with a 70% extract (3 mg/kg twice to thrice daily).

As a flavonoid, silymarin is an inhibitor of P-glycoprotein and should be used cautiously with drugs known to serve as substrates for the transport protein. Silymarin may also inhibit selected CYP450 (specifically P450 2C9) enzymes.

Milk thistle is used to prevent or treat a number of medical conditions, including hepatitis (acute or chronic), and to protect the liver from toxicants, including medications. Milk thistle is the most common alternative medicine used in humans for treatment of liver diseases, with more than 50% of users claiming efficacy. Other proposed health benefits of silymarin include improved diabetic control. An intravenous preparation of silybinin is available in Europe for treatment of mushroom poisoning caused by *A. phalloides.* Note that as of January 2010, of the 10 milk thistle products tested by Consumer Laboratories, nine did not pass, the primary reason being that the actual amount was less than the label claimed amount.

Miscellaneous Vitamins, Minerals, and Nutrients

Choline

Choline is an indispensable metabolite of the body. It forms part of a number of endogenous compounds, particularly phospholipids. Phosphatidylcholine, lysophospholipids, plasmalogens, and sphingomyelins are phospholipids that contain choline. The mode of action of choline as a lipotropic agent is unknown. It may promote conversion of liver fat into choline-containing phospholipids, which are more rapidly transferred from the liver into blood. Choline is also essential for synthesis of phospholipids that are used in intracellular membranes concerned with lipoprotein synthesis. It is thought that the lipotropic agents methionine, betaine, and lecithin are beneficial because they contain choline or promote choline synthesis. The requirement for choline is well recognized in all conditions predisposing to fatty infiltration of the liver, including diabetes mellitus, malnutrition, and cirrhosis. Greater than normal quantities of choline seem to be necessary for prevention of a fatty liver when the liver is already damaged. Choline deficiency is not the only cause of fatty liver in these conditions, nor will choline supplementation alone restore the liver to full functional competence. Choline is, however, extremely valuable in the multitherapeutic approach to prevention and cure of fatty liver.

Selenium and Vitamin E

Selenium is now known to be essential for tissue respiration and is protective against dietary hepatic necrosis. It is extremely active and is only required in minute amounts. Vitamin E enhances the action of selenium, but both are required.

Selenium is an essential component of glutathione peroxidase, which catalyzes oxidation of reduced glutathione:

$$\text{(2)Glutathione-SH} + H_2O_2 \text{ (reduced form)} \rightarrow$$
$$\text{Glutathione} - S - S \text{ glutathione} + 2H_2O \text{ (oxidized form)}$$

This glutathione peroxidase catalyzes removal of hydrogen peroxide and fatty acid hydroperoxides and thus exerts a protective effect on all cells but especially on muscle, liver, and erythrocytes. The essential substances required for removal of peroxides are reduced glutathione and glutathione peroxidase. Vitamin E maintains glutathione in the reduced form by preventing formation of hydroperoxides; it is an antioxidant and thus reduces the amount of glutathione peroxidase required. Cysteine (*N*-acetylcysteine) is required for the reduced sulfhydryl radical of glutathione and is generally present in adequate quantities. Selenium and vitamin E enhance each other's action and together protect cells, especially hepatocytes, against harmful buildup of peroxides.

Vitamins

In the presence of liver disease, the fat-soluble vitamin K should be supplemented because hepatic stores may be quite rapidly depleted. The water-soluble vitamins of the B-complex group are frequently employed in therapeutic regimens for hepatic insufficiency. Few controlled studies have been carried out in this regard, but the rationale behind their clinical use is based on ensuring an adequate supply of metabolic cofactors.

Hydroxocobalamin (previously called *vitamin* B_{12}) is stored in the liver, mainly in mitochondria, but there is also a microsomal fraction. This microsomal vitamin may be of importance in hepatic protein metabolism. Microsomal cell fractions from the livers of hydroxocobalamin-deficient animals are defective in the incorporation of methionine and alanine into protein. General liver protein synthesis is depressed in hydroxocobalamin deficiency.

Hydroxocobalamin has a lipotropic effect. It is involved in metabolism of labile methyl groups and in formation of choline. Hydroxocobalamin is also necessary for overall utilization of fat. When intake is low, however, the demand for this vitamin in hematopoiesis exceeds that for any other clinically recognizable physiologic function.

Glucose and Fructose

The liver resists many forms of injury when its stores of carbohydrate and protein are adequate; its efficiency is impaired when hepatocytes are laden with fat. Administration of a hypertonic solution of glucose and fructose produces favorable responses in a variety of hepatic abnormalities. A high glycogen content appears to protect liver cells from damage, and inhibition of gluconeogenesis (which occurs with administration of both insulin and glucose) may play an important role. Under the influence of insulin, hepatocytes undergo glycogen storage, hypertrophy, and hyperplasia. Insulin has a major anabolic effect on the liver.

TREATMENT OF SPECIFIC (NON-INFECTIVE) DISORDERS OF THE GASTROINTESTINAL TRACT

Treatment of gastrointestinal disorders frequently involves drugs that target the disease rather than the gastrointestinal tract. Enhanced discussion of such conditions or the drugs used to treat them might be found in their respective chapters (i.e., Treatment of Bacterial Infections [Chapter 8], Glucocorticoids [Chapter 30] or Immunomodulators [Chapter 31]). Treatment of specific infectious diseases also will be found in chapters that address treatment of the causative organisms.

Diseases of the Oral Cavity

The primary treatment for the *feline eosinophilic granuloma complex* is glucocorticoids,[183] given orally (prednisone, 1 to 2 mg/kg twice daily), subcutaneously (methylprednisolone acetate, 20 mg every 2 weeks), or intralesionally (triamcinolone, 3 mg weekly). Progestational compounds such as methylprogesterone may prove beneficial, but side effects associated with long-term use (including hyperadrenocorticism and diabetes mellitus) should limit their use to cases that have not responded to any other (properly administered) drug therapy. Up to 50% of treated cats may relapse. Because of the potential impact of leukotrienes on eosinophil trafficking (see the section on inflammatory bowel disease), leukotriene receptor antagonists might be considered. *Stomatitis* may be a reflection of an autoimmune skin diseases, renal disease, microbiologic infection (viral, bacterial, or fungal) or may be idiopathic. Antimicrobial therapy should be considered in cases of idiopathic stomatitis; therapy may be necessary on a chronic, intermittent basis. Drugs should target anaerobic organisms (e.g., metronidazole, a penicillin derivative, or clindamycin). Glucocorticoid therapy should be used cautiously in stomatitis unless an autoimmune disorder has been diagnosed or other causes (including infectious ones) have been ruled out.

Diseases of the Esophagus

Megaesophagus

Myasthenia gravis is the most common cause of secondary megaesophagus in dogs. It is diagnosed on the basis of response to edrophonium chloride, a short-acting anticholinesterase.[184] Effects of the drug on skeletal muscle occur within 1 minute of intravenous administration and last up to 10 minutes or longer in some myasthenic patients. Drug therapy of megaesophagus associated with myasthenia gravis targets improvement in muscular activity with anticholinesterase therapy (pyridostigmine bromide, 1 to 3 mg/kg orally every 12 hours) and suppression of the immune response with glucocorticoid or other immunosuppressive therapy (e.g., azathioprine). Pyridostigmine improves appendicular muscle strength but may not improve pharyngeal or esophageal function. Prednisone tends to be the preferred glucocorticoid but may contribute to muscle weakness. Azathioprine does not have many of the side effects of glucocorticoids, but remission takes longer to achieve (up to several weeks), and neutropenia may limit treatment. Mycophenolate mofetil is a lymphocyte-inhibiting immunomodulator used orally to prevent graft-versus-host rejection in human renal transplant patients. The drug inhibits purine synthesis but only in lymphocytes (both B and T lymphocytes), and side effects are limited to GI upset. The drug can be given orally, causing response within 4 hours of administration. The drug has proved efficacious for treatment of myasthenia gravis in dogs (5 to 10 mg/kg every 12 hours orally).[185] Thyroid hormone replacement (thyroxine) may also prove helpful. Treatment for megaesophagus for which an underlying cause cannot be found is difficult. A number of drugs that stimulate GI smooth muscle have been recommended, including metoclopramide and cisapride, with varying reports of success. Neither of these two prokinetic drugs are likely to be effective in the striated muscle of the esophagus; further, enhanced lower esophageal sphincter tone might impede esophageal emptying. Bethanechol may stimulate propagating contractions in selected dogs. Drugs that relax the lower esophageal sphincter (anticholinergics and calcium channel blockers) have not proved effective. A major focus for treatment of myasthenia gravis is prevention of aspiration pneumonia and treatment or prevention of esophagitis.

Esophagitis

Esophagitis should be treated by correction of the underlying etiology. It is commonly associated with ingestion of a corrosive or hot (thermally) material. The feline esophagus appears to be particularly susceptible to drug-induced esophagitis (discussed in the following section). Antibiotic therapy in such cases should be reserved for esophageal perforation. The mucosa can be protected by administration of sucralfate administered as a slurry (1 g in 10 mL warm water), 5 to 10 mL every 6 to 8 hours. Lidocaine solution (Xylocaine viscous solution) may be administered orally (2 mg/kg every 4 to 6 hours) to minimize pain. Esophagitis caused by gastroesophageal reflux should respond well to medical management. In addition to protecting the damaged mucosa with sucralfate, drug therapy targets increasing gastric pH and tightening the lower esophageal sphincter. Antisecretory drugs (e.g., famotidine, omeprazole) help minimize damage induced by gastric acid and pepsin. Among the antihistaminergic drugs, ranitidine and nizatidine have prokinetic activity in humans comparable to that of cisapride, an effect evident within 1 hour after administration.[128] Interestingly, a peppermint–caraway oil preparation induced relief from dyspepsia equal to that produced by cisapride in human patients.[186] Antacids may also prove beneficial; products containing alginic acid may provide additional protection of the esophagus by providing a barrier of foam. Prokinetic drugs should be administered to tighten the lower esophageal sphincter. Indeed, metaclopramide or cisapride is probably as effective as antisecretory drugs in preventing further esophageal damage associated with gastric reflux. Glucocorticoids can be used to minimize esophageal stricture formation resulting from damage to the esophagus that extends into the muscular layers. Therapy should include tapered doses of glucocorticoids followed by reevaluation at 2-week intervals. Pentoxifylline may be an alternative or adjuvant therapy, particularly for drug-induced esophagitis.[187]

Gastroesophageal Reflux

Up to 60% of humans are considered to be at risk for developing perioperative gastroesophageal reflux (GER), whereas GER was demonstrated in 17% to 55% of healthy dogs. The difference in incidence of GER between these studies might be attributable to differences in the anesthetic agents used.

Metaclopramide prevents GER in unanesthetized dogs, as was demonstrated experimentally.[188] Wilson and coworkers[189] also prospectively studied the effect of metoclopramide on GER (defined when esophageal pH to <4 or an increase to >7.5 that lasted more than 30 seconds) in anesthetized dogs. Animals were undergoing orthopedic surgical procedures; anesthetic protocols (morphine and acepromazine as premeds and thiopental for induction) and surgical positioning were the same in treatment and placebo (saline) groups. Blinded and randomization methods were not clear. The authors determined, after reviewing the medical records of dogs undergoing the same surgical procedures and anesthetic protocols, that 55% of dogs experienced GER. A high dose (1 mg/kg followed by constant-rate infusion [CRI] 1 mg/kg/hr) but not a low dose (0.4 mg/kg followed by 0.3 mg/kg/hr CRI) of metoclopramide reduced the relative risk of GER by 54%. The timing of metoclopramide administration in relation to anesthesia was not provided. Vomiting occurred preoperatively in 55% of animals but was not a predictive factor for the risk of GER. No adverse effects attributed to treatment were identified. Preoperative vomiting in response to preanesthetic agents was not a risk factor for GER in dogs, whereas the duration of surgery (but not anesthesia) tended to be a risk factor.[190] Wilson and coworkers[190] compared the effects of pre-anesthetic morphine to mepiridine with or without acepromazine in healthy dogs (n = 30) using a randomized design. When compared with morphine, treatment with meperidine alone or with acepromazine before anesthesia was associated with a 55% and 27% risk reduction in risk of developing GER. In this same study, GER was detected in 51 of 90 dogs within 36 minutes of induction isoflurane (n = 14), halothane (n = 19) or sevoflurane (n = 18).

Esophogeal Motility and Oral Medications

The association of doxycycline administration with esophageal lesions in cats[191, 191a] has led to several studies focusing on passage of medications through the feline esophagus. In one study, approximately 50% of capsules were retained in the midcervical esophagus of cats for longer than 240 seconds. Trapped capsules passed into the stomach if a small amount of food was administered.[192] A prospective study used fluoroscopy to document the esophageal transit of barium tablets (20 mg) or capsules (size 4) in cats.[193] The percentage of swallows needed for successful passage (movement of the medication into the stomach) of each medication was determined when administered with or without a follow-up bolus of water (6 mL). Success was only 36.7% 5 minutes after administration, compared with 90% at 30 seconds and 100% at 90 seconds if the medication was followed with a water bolus. The study was performed in a nonrandomized fashion, with the "wet" study always following 5 minutes after a "dry" study. Retention of dry medicaments was generally in the cervical esophageal region.[193] Treatment should consist of an antisecretory drug, sucralfate, and metoclopramide. An anti-inflammatory may be helpful; glucocorticoids have been used, but pentoxyfylline might also be considered.

Diseases of the Stomach

Acute Gastritis

Acute gastritis is best treated by resolution of the underlying cause, whether it is diet, infectious agents or chemicals (including drugs or toxins), or metabolic diseases (e.g., renal or liver disease). Chemicals, including hydrochloric acid and bile acids, can induce vomiting as a result of direct damage or hypertonicity. Inflammation, if allowed to progress, can result in erosion and ulceration. Although most patients with acute gastritis improve in 1 to 5 days, some patients require supportive therapy.[194] Depending on the patient, supportive therapy (in addition to nothing given orally) may include fluid therapy, antiemetics, and protectants or adsorbents. Fluid therapy with balanced crystalloids may require the addition of potassium. Bicarbonate is rarely indicated; glucose supplementation may be indicated in some patients. Any of the antiemetics previously discussed can be used, although phenothiazine derivatives should be withheld until volume replacement has begun. Metaclopramide is useful when given either peripherally or centrally; maropitant is likely to be very effective. Among the protectants, bismuth subsalicylate has proved most useful in decreasing vomiting associated with acute gastritis. However, gastric distention from the drug may cause the animal to vomit; therefore prudence is indicated in its use.

Gastric Ulceration and Erosion

There is no sensitive indicator of damage to the GI mucosa; damage may be quite extensive before hematemesis or melena is noted. Damage to the GI mucosa (erosion or ulceration) probably occurs more frequently than anticipated. For example, up to 25% of human patients admitted to intensive care units have gastric erosions; by the third day of hospitalization, this number increases to 90%. The risk of translocation of enteric pathogens is increased in these patients, suggesting an important role for prophylactic anti-ulcer therapy. Sucralfate has been recommended as the preferred method of prophylaxis in patients in whom enteral nutrition is not possible.[195] Diseases in which mucosal damage should be anticipated and treatment implemented include but are not limited to mast cell disease, renal disease, liver disease, and IBD. The underlying cause of ulceration must be resolved; additionally, antisecretory drugs and antacids are indicated for treatment of mucosal damage.

Nonsteroidal antiinflammatory drugs. The most commonly recognized cause of GI ulceration in dogs is probably use of NSAIDs. The primary mechanism of ulceration by NSAIDs is inhibition of both the constitutive and inducible forms of cyclooxygenase, the enzyme responsible for formation of the cytoprotective prostaglandin E (see Chapter 29). The latter (inducible) enzyme is particularly important for healing in the damaged gastrointestinal mucosa. Alteration of ion (probably hydrogen) transport across the mucosa also has a variable role in ulcer formation, depending on the NSAID used (e.g., aspirin).[196] Ulcerogenic drugs (e.g., glucocorticoids, which also inhibit the inducible cycclooxygenase) but potentiate ulceration caused by NSAIDs. Treatment of NSAID-induced GI ulceration includes discontinuation of the drug; replacement of missing prostaglandins by administration of cytoprotectants such as misoprostol; providing cytoprotection through sucralfate; and inhibiting acid secretion by administration of an antisecretory drug (e.g., ranitidine or omeprazole). Sucralfate, misoprostol, H_2-receptor antagonists and proton-pump blockers have been studied either as sole agents or in various combinations for their ability to prevent GI ulceration in patients requiring high doses or long-term NSAID therapy. Among them, misoprostol probably provides the most consistent protection, followed by sucralfate and then antisecretory drugs. Although famotidine was found to be equal in efficacy to misoprostol for treatment of NSAID-induced ulceration in humans,[197] the H_2-receptor blockers are described as having only limited efficacy, particularly for ulcers in the stomach, unless it is used at higher than (generally twice) recommended doses[198] Proton pump inhibitors have proved superior to H_2-receptor antagonists for treatment of NSAID-induced ulceration.[198]

KEY POINT 19-41 Sucralfate has been associated with effective prevention of ulcers associated with nonsteroidal antiinflammatory drugs and stress.

The effect of misoprostol (3 mg/kg orally every 8, 12, or 24 hours) on gastric injury induced by aspirin (25 mg/kg orally every 8 hours) was studied prospectively in normal dogs (n = 24; 6 dogs per group) using a parallel, placebo-controlled design. Animals were dosed with aspirin and either placebo or misoprostol, the latter at 8- or 12-hour intervals, for 28 days with gastroscopy performed on -9, 5, 14, and 28 days. Visible lesions were scored on a scale of 1 (mucosal hemorrhage) to 11 (perforating ulcer). Median total scores between the placebo or misoprostol at 24 hours were significantly greater than scores in the group receiving misoprostol at 8-or 12-hour intervals. In contrast, no differences were measured between placebo and misoprostol at 24-hour intervals. Differences were not detected among groups for vomiting, diarrhea, or anorexia.[199]

In cases of NSAID overdosing (including accidental ingestion), prophylactic administration of both sucralfate and misoprostol is recommended along with an antisecretory drug. The duration of antiulcer therapy depends in part on the elimination half-life of the drug and the amount of NSAID ingested. The elimination half-life of some of the drugs is several days, suggesting that toxic concentrations may remain in the bloodstream for some time (1 to 2 weeks). Omeprazole may prolong the half-life of the NSAID, suggesting that treatment duration should err on the side of too long rather than too short. Prevention of NSAID-induced ulceration in humans is best accomplished with proton pump inhibitors; omeprazole was superior to either ranitidine or misoprostol after 6 months of NSAID therapy for reducing the risk of either gastric or duodenal ulcer.[200] Omeprazole also may be the preferred choice in dogs; at least twice daily dosing also is recommended for famotidine. [87] Because of its potential to impair drug metabolism, omeprazole might be less desirable than the antihistaminergic antisecretory drugs when preventing ulcers in order to avoid prolonging NSAID half-life. Administration of cytoprotective agents for treatment of ulcers depends on the drug and the amount ingested. In general, treatment should extend at least 1-2 weeks after the inciting NSAID has been eliminated (i.e., at least 5 half-lives of the inciting NSAID or longer in the case of accidental ingestion that saturates drug metabolizing enzymes). Administration of cytoprotective antacids such as magnesium–aluminum hydroxide combinations with a meal may provide further protection.

Stress ulcers. A European meta-analysis (Mantel–Haenszel test) found that sucralfate was superior to H_2 antisecretory drugs and equal to antacids in the prevention of macroscopic stress bleeding in long-term ventilated patients in an intensive care unit. Further, the incidence of pneumonia (caused by nosocomial organisms) was less in those ventilated patients receiving sucralfate compared with antacids or antisecretory drugs.[201]

The efficacy of omeprazole (20 mg orally once daily) in prevention of exercise-induced gastric ulceration in Racing Alaskan Sled Dogs (three teams of 16) was tested using a randomized placebo design.[202] Response was based on endoscopic scoring of the gastric mucosa after completion of the race (0=least, 3=numerous bleeding ulcers). Mean score was significantly less (0.65) for treatment compared with placebo (1.09), although diarrhea was worse in the treatment group (54%) compared with placebo (21%). The percentage of animals that developed ulcers between the two groups was not reported. Williamson and coworkers[203] subsequently reported on the efficacy of famotidine in this study.

Helicobacter species. *H. pylori* infects over 50% of the global human population. Infection will persist for life, unless specifically treated. All infected persons develop gastritis, with 15% of infected persons developing peptic ulceration. Infection also is associated with an increased risk of gastric adenocarcionoma and mucosa-associated lymphoid tissue lymphoma; indeed, it is classified as a class 1 carcinogen by the World Health Organization.[209a] The role of *Helicobacter* species as causal agents in GI diseases in dogs and cats is being elucidated. It is likely that a causal relationship exists between the organism and the disease.

A causal relationship also has been suggested in ferrets, cheetahs, and cats. Clinical signs attributed to *Helicobacter* organisms in dogs and cats include chronic vomiting and diarrhea, inappetence, pica, and fever.[210] More than 70% of human patients with GI ulceration associated with *Helicobacter* organisms are cured of their ulcerative disease if *Helicobacter* is successfully eradicated. The pathophysiology of *Helicobacter* in part reflects urease-mediated conversion of urea to ammonia and bicarbonate. Ammonia causes local tissue damage, whereas bicarbonate appears to facilitate deeper colonization of the organism into the mucosa.[210] Cytokine production by the organism appears to be associated with inflammation and ulcerogenesis; biochemical changes in the mucosa also contribute to disease. Treatment includes a colloidal bismuth (i.e., bismuth subsalicylate), an antibacterial that targets *Helicobacter* (metronidazole, amoxicillin, or clarithromycin), and an antacid (an H_2-receptor antagonist or omeprazole). Bismuth accumulation causes cell wall damage and subsequent cell lysis. Among the antibacterials selected, amoxicillin is associated with the greatest and clarithromycin with the least amount of microbial resistance in humans. Resistance to metronidazole is also increasing. The duration of therapy in humans is several weeks. Reports of similar therapy in dogs and cats support but do not conclusively prove this approach may be beneficial in dogs and cats suffering from selected GI diseases. One study reported marked improvement in 90% of dogs and cats treated with a combination of metronidazole, amoxicillin, and famotidine for 3 weeks. Sucralfate may also be of benefit.

Gastric Dilatation–Volvulus

Therapy for gastric–dilatation volvulus (GDV) focuses on management of this acute and potentially life-threatening disease and long-term prevention. Medical management of the patient with acute disease focuses on resolution of the dilatation or volvulus and treatment of the sequelae of the syndrome. The sequelae of GDV that are most life-threatening are decreased cardiac preload (compression of the posterior vena cava and hepatic portal systems by the enlarged stomach), ischemia of the gastric wall (with loss of the mucosal barrier and increased risk of perforation), and congestion of abdominal viscera with subsequent endotoxemia and disseminated intravascular coagulation. Although they are potentially later in onset, cardiac arrhythmias also may become life-threatening. Shock should be treated with a balanced crystalloid electrolyte solution or hypertonic saline. Shock doses of glucocorticoids (methylprednisolone) may ameliorate some of the signs or clinical sequelae of endotoxemia although evidence for such use is lacking. Free radical scavengers (deferoxamine or allopurinol) may help reduce damage caused by reperfusion. Methylprednisolone may also be helpful in minimizing the effects of oxygen radicals The impact of prophylactic lidocaine on reperfusion injury was retrospectively studied in dogs (n = 51; 47 nontreated dogs served as control). Animals receiving lidocaine for cardiac arrhythmias were excluded from study. Dogs received either a loading dose (2 mg/kg intravenously) followed by CRI or a CRI alone (0.05 mg/kg/min) for at least 3 hours. No difference was detected in survival or complications between the two groups, although hospitalization was longer in the treatment group.[204]

Decompression of the dilated stomach can be facilitated by chemical restraint or sedation. Oxymorphone may be the drug of choice. Cardiac arrhythmias are most commonly ventricular in origin but may include atrial arrhythmias such as fibrillation. Intravenous lidocaine is the preferred drug for ventricular arrhythmias, administered initially as an intravenous bolus followed by a CRI (75 μg/kg/min). Procainamide can be used (intravenously, including CRI if lidocaine is ineffective; mexiletine) may be preferred. Amiodarone may also be used to acutely treat atrial fibrillation. Use of anti-secretory drugs is recommended to minimize the effects of hydrochloric acid on the already damaged mucosa. Although antimicrobials may be indicated, their use ideally is limited to situations in which contamination is known (i.e., surgical) or translocation is likely. Corrective surgery, including gastropexy, may be indicated. Medical management of chronic GDV has not been well established. Motility modifiers (metaclopramide, cisapride) and H_2-receptor antagonists may be indicated, particularly after an acute episode, to minimize the accumulation of gastric secretions. However, their efficacy has not been established.

Gastric Motility Disorders

Dietary management of delayed gastric emptying should precede pharmacologic management. Underlying causes, including electrolyte abnormalities, should be corrected, and use of concurrent drugs (e.g., anticholinergics, alpha-adrenergics, opioid antagonists) that might alter motility or response to prokinetic agents should be discontinued. Prokinetic agents can be added when dietary management fails; cisapride is preferred.

Vomiting

For many causes of vomiting, studies regarding the etiology, prevention or treatment in animals are lacking. Accordingly, much of the information is drawn from the human literature. The discussions are offered as points of consideration, recognizing that relevance to dogs or cats remains to be demonstrated.

Chemotherapy-induced Emesis

Ellebaek and Herrstedt[205] reviewed the prevention and treatment of nausea associated with chemotherapy in humans. The relative emetogenic potential of antineoplastic agents was described. In humans level 1 agents (lowest potential; <10% of patients) include chlorambucil, hydroxyurea, interferon α, tamoxifen, and vincristine; level 2 (10% to 30%): asparaginase, fluorouracil, gemcitabine, melphalan, paclitaxel, and thiopeta; level 3 (30% to 60%): cyclophosphamide (at <600 mg/m_2), doxorubicin, methotrexate (<1000 mg/m_2), and mitomycin; level 4 (60% to 90%): busulfan, carboplatin, cyclophosphamide (≥600 mg/m_2), doxorubicin (>60 mg/m_2), methotrexate (≥1000 mg/m_2), and mitoxantrone; and level 5, the highest (>90% incidence): cisplatin (≥60 mg/m_2), cyclophosphamide (1000 mg/m_2), pentostatin, and others.[205a]

Chemotherapy-induced vomiting appears to reflect the release of serotonin from enterochromaffin cells of the GI mucosa with subsequent stimulation of type 3 vagal afferent 5-HT_3 serotonin receptors in the mucosa, the nucleus tractus solitarius of the medulla oblongata, and the CRZ. At the CRZ, D_2, opioid, and 5-HT_3 receptors stimulate vomiting. Neurokinin receptors in humans are responsible for the delayed phase of vomiting associated with cisplatin anticancer chemotherapy. Maropitant appears to be effective for control of chemotherapy-induced emesis in dogs.[205a,b] Rau and coworkers demonstrated the efficacy of maropitant (2 mg/kg PO once daily) for control of vomiting associated with doxorubicin administration in dogs (n = 25) with cancer. Dogs were studied using a randomized, placebo-controlled study (n = 24) for 5 days posttreatment. Both vomiting and diarrhea were significantly less in the treatment group.[205a] D_2 antagonists, such as phenothiazines and butyrophenones, have limited efficacy in humans in preventing acute vomiting associated with chemotherapy, with their use limited primarily to combination therapy for breakthrough nausea and vomiting. In a comparative study of humans undergoing cisplatin chemotherapy, antiemetic efficacy of metoclopramide was evident at 0.54 mg/L with efficacy as an antiemetic being dose dependent.[206] Glucocorticoids, and specifically dexamethasone, improve the antiemetic efficacy of metoclopramide in humans; trials in dogs or cats are lacking. However, acute nausea induced by chemotherapeutic agents appears to be best prevented by the combination of dexamethasone (0.22 mg/kg intravenously) with serotonin antagonists. Among the antiserotinergic drugs, no differences in clinical efficacy appear to exist between ondansetron and dolasetron; however, granisetron, although not necessarily more effective, may last twice as long, perhaps because of its tighter affinity for serotonin receptors.

Postoperative Nausea and Vomiting

The use of antiemetics to prevent or treat postoperative nausea was reviewed by Ku and Ong.[207] The incidence of postoperative vomiting in humans receiving volatile anesthesia ranges from 20% to 30%. Risk or predictive factors include age, gender (greater in females), history of vomiting or motion sickness, and duration and type of surgery and anesthesia. Opioid preanesthetics increase and alpha-2 agonists decrease the risk. Intraoperative drugs that increase the risk in humans include nitrous oxide (especially in patients already vomiting), whereas the more potent volatile anesthetics are associated with less vomiting compared with the less potent anesthetics. Propofol as an inducing agent causes less vomiting than do thiopental, etomidate, and ketamine; propofol also may reduce vomiting associated with general anesthesia.[20] The impact of anticholinergics (atropine) or neuromuscular blockade antagonists (neostigmine) on postoperative emesis is less clear, although the incidence is reduced with the combination of the two agents. As with preoperative opioids, postoperative opioids increase the risk of nausea and emesis (due to direct stimulation of the CTZ and decreased GI motility) even if pain is effectively controlled. The incidence of vomiting associated with opioid-induced analgesia can be reduced by using those opioids associated with less emesis, and balanced analgesia.

Treatment of postoperative emesis is approached by either preventing or rescuing the patient. Drugs used as preventives include antagonists of H_1 receptors (dimenhydrinate), muscarinic receptors (scopolamine patch), and 5-HT_3 receptors (ondansetron or other carbazalone derivatives). Glucocorticoids (dexamethasone [0.11 to 0.14 mg/kg] and methylprednisolone), whose antiemetic mechanisms are unknown, also are recommended (administered intravenously) in patients with a high risk. Their use is more effective when combined with other antiemetics, particularly 5-HT_3 antagonists. The NK_1 receptor antagonists have recently undergone investigation, with early information in humans suggesting that NK_1 antagonists may be more effective than $5HT_3$ receptor antagonists; accordingly, maropitant is reasonable choice in dogs or cats. Combinations are recommended over single drugs when treating breakthrough vomiting or nausea. Examples include 5-HT_3 receptor antagonists with antihistaminergic drugs (e.g., ondansetron with cyclizine or promethazine) or combinations of droperidol, metoclopramide, or dimenhydrinate.[20] Combinations with an NK_1 receptor antagonist should be considered. Ideally, the combination would not include a drug that has already failed to control vomiting.

Postoperative Ileus

In humans, the time for gastric motility to recovery postoperatively ranges from 24 to 48 hours, the colon 48 to 72 hour. Thus, even with uncomplicated ileus, the time to recovery after surgery is 72 hours or less. The efficacy of metoclopramide in treating or preventing postoperative ileus has been studied in humans with conflicting results.[208] In an observational, prospective study design, Seta and Kale-Pradhan[208] found no difference in time to first bowel movement in intensive care unit patients that received metaclopramide postoperatively compared with those that did not. The drawbacks of this study include its design (nonrandomized, nonblinded, and non–placebo controlled) and very small sample size (n = 32; 16 per group). The authors reviewed the impact of metoclopramide on the effects of postoperative ileus in the report. Differences in dose, poor end points, and variability in study subjects (including surgical procedures) preclude consensus among the studies. Further, differences in opioid use among treatment groups generally has not been addressed. Time to reduction in oral feeding was a more frequent positive indicator of response to metoclopramide than was time to first bowel movement. However, the authors caution that the time to first bowel movement more likely reflects initiation of an oral diet, and studies using both outcome measures must address cause and effect. The review of the studies regarding the effect of metaclopramide on postoperative ileus are inconclusive.

The effect of lidocaine as a prokinetic for treatment of postoperative ileus after abdominal surgery has been the subject of a Cochrane Review of randomized clinical trials in humans.[209] A review of 39 trials found that the data were insufficient (generally owing to inconsistent outcomes, small sample size, or poor data-collection methods) to recommend the use of CCK-like drugs, cisapride, dopamine antagonists, propranolol, or vasopressin. The authors noted that cisapride has been withdrawn from the marked, and further consideration was not given. Fifteen trials had reviewed alvimopan, a peripheral mu receptor antagonist that currently is an investigational drug. The authors noted that alvimopan may prove effective but further information was needed to define the criteria for use. Erythromycin was found to be consistently ineffective. Of the drugs studied, only intravenous lidocaine or neostigmine were considered potentially effective, but further assessment based on clinically relevant outcomes was indicated. No major adverse events to any of the drugs was noted in the review.

For postoperative ileus induced by opioids, treatment options include stimulant laxatives, oral naloxone, prokinetic agents (metoclopramide should follow an opioid antagonist), and potentially alvimopan. Misoprostol (high dose; approximately 6 μg/kg in humans) also might be considered; because this dose might be associated with nausea (in humans), a lower dose, given more frequently, may be necessary. Therapy should begin early.

Small Intestinal Diseases

Diarrhea

Acute diarrhea. Like vomiting, diarrhea should be managed by providing supportive therapy, treating symptoms, and resolving the underlying cause with specific therapy.[210] Generally, intestinal causes of acute diarrhea include diet, toxins or drugs, and infections (including viral, microbial, and parasitic). A number of extraintestinal diseases include diarrhea as a manifestation. For many diarrheas rehydration and maintenance of hydration and electrolyte balance are the cornerstones of therapy Antiemetics should be used to control vomiting accompanied by acute diarrhea. Those antiemetics that cause hypotension (e.g., phenothiazine derivatives) should be withheld until fluid replacement has begun. Protectants and adsorbents are indicated for diarrheas associated with toxins (including "garbage enteritis") and may be used for nonspecific (undiagnosed) causes of acute diarrhea. Kaolin may be useful for its adsorbent properties. Bismuth subsalicylate provides both adsorbent and antiinflammatory effects and is the preferred antidiarrheal agent for toxin-associated diarrheas.

Motility modifiers must also be used with discretion for treatment of diarrhea. Hypomotility rather than hypermotility is the more likely abnormality, and most motility modifiers cause hypomotility. Further, such drugs are often associated with side effects. However, among the motility modifiers, opioid drugs such as loperamide increase resistance to outflow as well as provide antisecretory effects. As such, of the motility modifiers, the opioid derivatives are preferred for short-term use as long as toxins, drugs, or obstructive disease have been ruled out as causes. Anticholinergic motility modifiers are reserved for psychogenic causes of acute diarrhea.

Viral Enteritis

There is no specific treatment for diarrheas of viral origin. Fluid therapy, electrolyte replacement, and antiemetics are indicated, depending on the severity of clinical signs. Among the viral causes of diarrhea, canine parvovirus stands out for its severity and life-threatening nature. Intensive, aggressive care such as that offered at tertiary hospitals can increase survival rates to 96% compared with 67% at local practitioners. The rate of survival with no therapy may range from 64% to 79%.[211] Supportive therapy centers around the intravenous administration of balanced electrolytes (e.g., lactated Ringer's solution) with potassium replacement. Damage to the mucosal barrier and risk of bacterial translocation should be addressed with parenteral antibiotics. The use of the viral neuromidase inhibitor olstamavir may be helpful in this regard. Antibiotics should target both aerobes and anaerobes. *E. coli* was identified as an organism associated with septicemia in canine parvovirus[212,213]; however, *C. perfringens* may also play a role.[214] Because of the life-threatening nature of sepsis, combination therapy with a beta-lactam antibiotic (amoxicillin may be preferred to cephalexin because of a better anaerobic spectrum) and an aminoglycoside (gentamicin, amikacin) is recommended. Vomiting and the life-threatening nature of the illness preclude oral administration of antibiotics. Ceftiofur has been used by some clinicians because of its efficacy toward *E.coli*; however, its limited spectrum (toward anaerobes) might limit efficacy for treatment of parvovirus-associated bacteremia; adverse events also may be an issue. Fluorinated quinolones should be avoided if possible because of the risk of cartilage defects in young, growing animals. Because fluid therapy is likely to be intensive in these patients, and because most patients are pediatric, an increased volume of distribution should be anticipated and higher higher doses of antimicrobials, particularly water soluble, may be indicated. Treatment of septic shock may include drugs that target eicosanoids and other mediators of endotoxic shock. Prevention of endotoxemia or its effects, is reasonable, although reaching consensus regarding effect through randomized clinical trials is limited by study designs.[211] Glucose may be added when indicated by clinical signs consistent with septicemia. Glucocorticoids and flunixin meglumine have historically been advocated to ameliorate some of the negative sequelae resulting from endotoxemia, with benefits more likely if treatment occurs within 4 hours of the onset of endotoxemia. Shock doses of glucocorticoids should be used. Controversy regarding the use of flunixin meglumine centers primarily on the risk of GI damage. However, damage is generally so severe at the time of clinical presentation that it is reasonable to assume that the use of a single dose of flunixin meglumine is not likely to contribute to further damage. An additional benefit of flunixin meglumine is its potent visceral analgesic effect, which may be important is alleviating the marked pain and its negative pathophysiologic sequelae. Because cyclooxygenase 2 is the predominant eicosanoid mediating the sequelae of shock, any of the newer injectable NSAIDs that target cyclooxygenas 2 (e.g., carprofen, meloxicam, firocoxib) presumably should be equally effective in treatment or prevention of endotoxic shock. Opioids should be avoided because of their inhibitory effect on expelling luminal contents.

KEY POINT 19-43 Although gram-negative coliforms clearly should be targeted in patients with viral enteritis for which translocation is a concern, anaerobes also should be targeted.

Although currently experimental, compounds targeting endotoxin may prove to be an important adjuvant to patients suffering from sepsis. Examples include endotoxin serum or a bacterial toxoid (*Salmonella typhimurium*; 10 mL/kg). The latter is commercially available. Transfusions with fresh whole blood or plasma can be beneficial in some dogs, particularly those that are hypoproteinemic or anemic. The impact of a recombinant amino terminal fragment of bactericidal permeability-increasing protein ($rBPI_{21}$; an antimicrobial and endotoxin-neutralizing agent) was studied in dogs (n = 40) with viral enteris. Treatment (3 mg/kg intravenously over 30 minutes, followed by 3 mg/kg intravenously over 5.5 hours) was implemented using a randomized placebo (n = 9 dogs treated with canine plasma protein) controlled design. Outcome measures included plasma endotoxin concentration, severity of clinical signs, and survival of parvovirus. No treatment effect could be identified ; however, contributing factors were insufficient sample size and biased patient selection toward animals that are less ill than the average infected animal.[211]

Treatment of diarrhea associated with parvovirus is generally not indicated. Until the mucosa has had time to heal, drugs intended to prevent or resolve diarrhea are not likely to be effective.

Bacterial Enteritis

The role of antimicrobial therapy in the treatment of diarrhea should be closely examined. Bacterial infection is not a major cause of diarrhea, nor does infection appear to perpetuate small intestinal diseases. More important, use of antimicrobial agents does not appear to improve the course of most acute diarrheas. Antimicrobials (neomycin, ampicillin) may, in fact, worsen diarrhea, perhaps because of suppression of normal microflora. Use of antimicrobials for treatment of diarrhea should be based on a diagnosis of intestinal bacterial infection (overgrowth detection, based in part, on fecal gram staining) or in cases of mucosal damage sufficiently severe to allow bacterial translocation. In the latter case, clinical signs generally include hemorrhagic diarrhea, fever, and abnormal white blood cell counts. Systemic antimicrobial therapy is indicated for bacterial translocation.

Despite the low incidence (less than 4% of cases of acute diarrhea), bacterial infections have been associated with both acute and chronic enterotoxigenic diarrhea of both small and large intestines. Diagnosis and antibacterial treatment are best based on culture and susceptibility data when possible. The most likely therapy for each of the infecting organisms is enrofloxacin, trimethoprim–sulfonamide combinations, and chloramphenicol for *Salmonella*; erythromycin, enrofloxacin, furazolidone, doxycycline, neomycin, clindamycin, or chloramphenicol for *C. jejuni*; a prolonged course of trimethoprim–sulfonamide combinations, tetracycline, or chloramphenicol for *Yersinia enterocolitica* (prognosis is guarded); metronidazole for *C. difficile*; and amoxicillin, ampicillin, metronidazole, tylosin, or clindamycin for *C. perfringens*. For *E. coli* the role will be difficult to establish. *Clostridium piliformis* (formerly *Bacillus piliformis*: Tyzzer's disease) is a less common, although rapidly fatal, cause of acute hemorrhagic enterocolitis. The organism appears to be nonresponsive to antimicrobials, wih therapy being supportive in nature. Salmon poisoning (*Neorickettsia helminthoeca*) is an endemic, fatal cause of diarrhea in dogs in the Pacific Northwest. As with other rickettsial organisms, tetracycline (oxytetracycline, doxycycline) is the treatment of choice. Oral therapy (in the absence of vomiting) includes tetracycline, chloramphenicol, sulfonamides, and penicillins. Therapy should continue for 2 to 3 weeks; the trematode vector can be treated with fenbendazole for 10 to 14 days (50 mg/kg, once daily). Because bacterial infections as a cause of diarrhea are often associated with some type of toxin production, motility modifiers should be avoided. Bismuth subsalicylate may be beneficial for both its adsorbent and antiinflamamtory effects.

Hemorrhagic Gastroenteritis

This syndrome of uncertain etiology is characterized by a packed cell volume (PCV) that may be as high as 80%. Hemoconcentration rather than dehydration is the cause. Treatment requires prompt and rapid but appropriate volume replacement with a balanced electrolyte solution until the PCV falls below 50%. Fluid therapy should continue for an additional 24 hours to maintain the PCV at 50% or lower. Disseminated intravascular coagulopathy may develop if fluid therapy is not instituted rapidly.

Chronic Diarrhea

Treatment of chronic diarrhea should be based on removing the underlying causes. This is perhaps more important than in acute diarrhea because drugs used to symptomatically treat acute diarrhea should not be continued on a long-term basis. Chronic IBD is discussed later as a separate entity.

Bacterial overgrowth is increasingly being recognized as a cause of chronic intermittent small bowel diarrhea in dogs. Because no sensitive, specific, and widely available diagnostic test is available, diagnosis is difficult unless an underlying cause (e.g., partial intussusceptions, tumors, foreign body) can be identified. Oral treatment should include broad-spectrum antibiotics, such as tylosin (10 to 20 mg/kg every 12 hours) or metronidazole, a drug effective against anaerobes (10 to 20 mg/kg every 12 hours). The use of probiotics should be considered as previously discussed.

Intestinal **fungal disease** may also manifest as chronic diarrhea. Prognosis is generally poor to fair. Intestinal histoplasmosis should be treated with an orally administered azole drug. Itraconazole is the drug of choice (5 to 10 mg/kg every 12 hours) followed by ketoconazole (10 to 15 mg/kg every 12 hours); both drugs should be given 3 to 4 months after clinical signs of remission. Voriconazole also might be considered.

Amphotericin B can be given in addition to an azole drug, particularly for severe cases. Currently, no antifungal drug has been effective for treatment of pythiosis (previously phycomycosis). Surgical resection followed by imidazole therapy (itraconazole or ketoconazole) is indicated in animals in which the disease is diagnosed before tissue damage and infiltration.

Protozoal diseases of the small intestine include coccidioidomycosis, cryptosporidiosis, and giardiasis. *Pentatrichomonas hominis* also has been associated with diarrhea, particularly in puppies and kittens. Diagnosis of each infection is based on identification of the organism or of cysts in feces. Treatment of coccidioidomycosis includes sulfadimethoxine (50 to 65 mg/kg once daily orally for 10 days); trimethoprim–sulfonamide combinations (30 mg/kg orally once daily for 10 days), quinacrine (10 mg/kg orally once daily for 5 days), or amprolium (100 mg [small dogs] to 200 mg [large dogs] of 20% powder once daily in gelatin capsules, or 1 to 2 teaspoons of 9.6% amprolium per gallon of free-choice water for 1 to 2 weeks). There is no effective treatment of cryptosporidiosis in dogs. This infection is generally self-limiting in immunocompetent animals. A number of therapies can be used to treat giardiasis. Metronidazole (25 to 30 mg/kg orally twice daily for 5 to 10 days) is the treatment of choice, although up to a third of animals may not respond. Metronidazole benzoate has demonstrated efficacy in treatment of feline giardiasis based on a study in 26 chronically infected cats, 10 of which also were infected with *Cryptosporidium parvum*.[215] Cats were treated with 25 mg/kg orally twice daily for 7 days; the drug was prepared as a solution. It is not clear if the dose was based on active ingredient (i.e., metronidazole base) or total drug. All cats were negative for three consecutive fecal examinations (based on indirect immunofluorescence assay) for the 15 day after treatment study period. Albendazole (25 mg/kg orally every 12 hours for 2 days) can be used in dogs, but safety and efficacy have not been reported in cats. Fenbendazole (50 mg/kg orally once a day for 3 days) may also be effective. Furazolidone (4 mg/kg orally every 12 hours for 5 to 10 days) can be used in cats, although toxicity may limit its use. For nonresponsive cases in dogs, quinacrine (6.6 mg/kg orally every 12 hours for 5 days) can be used, although side effects (anorexia, lethargy, vomiting, and fever) are common. Ipronidazole (126 mg/L drinking water) is a poultry drug that can be used for treating groups of animals. Tinidazole (currently not available in the United States; 44 mg/kg once orally) may also be useful. Pentatrichomoniasis should respond to a 5-day course of metronidazole therapy; tinidazole for 3 days may also be useful. Both drugs can be used according to previously described dosing regimens.

Short Bowel Syndrome

Short bowel syndrome occurs after surgical removal of a large portion of the small intestine. Resultant malabsorption results in malnutrition and diarrhea. The impact of the resection on bowel function and the ability of the remaining bowel to adapt to the loss depend on the extent and site of resection. Dogs have functioned with an absence of clinical signs following resection of up to 85% of the small intestine. Preservation of the ileum is important because of its role in slowing transit and absorption of vitamin B_{12} and bile acids. Medical management focuses primarily on correction of secondary ill effects. Exocrine pancreatic insufficiency should be treated with enzyme supplementation. Gastric hypersecretion should be treated with H_2-receptor antagonists. Bacterial overgrowth should be treated with appropriate antimicrobial therapy (e.g., metronidazole, tylosin). Cholestyramine can be used to bind excessive bile acids that result in diarrhea. Occasionally, motility modifiers may be indicated to slow transit time. The opioids are preferred because of their effects on segmentation and thus retention of luminal contents.

Bacterial translocation. Bacterial translocation refers to the movement of gastrointestinal origin microbes or their products across the intact gastrointestinal tract into normally sterile tissues and subsequent direct infection or inflammation causing tissue injury, organ failure, and death. The treatment of subsequent sepsis is addressed in Chapter 8. Bacterial translocation ideally is prevented.[151a-c] Among the choices to prevent bacterial translocation are antimicrobials (selective gastrointestinal or digestive decontamination; SDD) and probiotics. The concept of SDD has been promoted and studied in the human critical care patient. Steinberg has reviewed the impact of bacterial translocation (in the surgical patient)[215a] and Schultz and co workers have reviewed the conclusions of several metaanalysis that focus on SDD in the critical care patient as part of their report of a clinical trial involving SDD with a favorable outcome. [215b] In general, scientific clinical evidence supporting SDD is lacking, and as such, SDD has not become a standard of care for the critical care patient. Nonetheless, Schultz has demonstrated a benefit of SDD in a population of critical care patients receiving ventilator support. In their review, the authors indicate that the risk of emergent resistance as a sequelae of SDD—a major antagonist argument against its routine implementation—did not occur in one clinical trial: indeed, SDD was associated with decreased resistance in this trial. This might be a reasonable expectation particularly if principles of judicious use are applied (see Chapter 6). Care must be taken when extrapolating the results of meta-analysis regarding SDD use in humans to the veterinary patient in that the applicability of the sample human populations may not represent the diseases with which veterinary criticalists are faced. Drug choices for SDD include oral drugs that target gram-negative coliforms but are not orally bioavailable, coupled with systemic antimicrobials targeting the same. However, Schulz and coworkers have also demonstrated that oral absorption of drugs normally characterized by no oral bioavailability may indeed occur in the critical care patient.[215c] As such, further caution is recommended when using SDD. There is a need for well-designed clinical trials that address SDD with antimicrobial therapy are lacking in the veterinary critical care patient.

The use of probiotics to prevent colonic bacterial translocation in human patients undergoing abdominal surgery was reviewed by Lenoir-Wijnkoop and coworkers.[151] The rationale targets the increased risk of bacterial translocation associated with surgical trauma, portal hypertension, decreased hepatic function and immunosuppression. Several controlled clinical trials have been implemented using synbiotics. One study in human liver transplant recipients found that the incidence of infection was much lower (3%) in patients receiving antibiotics plus a highly concentrated combination product of four fibers (2.5 g each of beta-glucan, resistant starch, inulin, and pectin) and four probiotics (10^{10} *Lactobacillus plantarum, Lactobacillus paracasei, Lactobacillus mesenteroides,* and *Pediococcus pentosaceu)* compared with those patients that received antimicrobials only (48%). A recent controlled clinical trial in humans undergoing pancreatic surgery found that the combination of probiotics and selective bacterial decontamination had no effect on bacterial translocation and other selective outcome measures.[215d]

Diseases of the Large Intestine

Diarrhea

Diarrhea associated with the large intestine should be approached in the same manner as diarrhea of the small intestine. Chronic IBD is discussed as a separate entity.

Irritable bowel syndrome. IBS, spastic colon, or nervous colitis is a poorly described functional disorder afflicting dogs and is diagnosed by ruling out other causes of large bowel diarrhea. Effective treatment is complicated by the intermittent nature of the syndrome.[216] Dietary management should be stressed for long-term management. Some large bowel diarrheas may respond to dietary fiber (psyllium). Intermittent bouts of diarrhea attributed to IBS can be managed with administration of short-term opioid antidiarrheals (1 week or less). Anticholinergics can be used to reduce intestinal spasms, particularly those associated with pain and tenesmus. Combination anticholinergics and sedatives (e.g., chlordiazepoxide and clidinium) also may prove useful.

Treatment of IBS in humans was reviewed by Spanier and coworkers.[217] Whereas the prevalence in humans is as high as 24%, the role of IBS as a cause of diarrhea in dogs or cats is not clear. In humans no specific therapy emerges as clearly effective, causing afflicted patients to seek out alternative therapies. A review of clinical trials reveals therapies of variable efficacy to include probiotics *(L. acidophilus, Candida* and others); herbal products such as aloe or peppermint oil; and nonmedicinal therapies such as colonic irrigation, acupuncture, psychotherapy, and meditation. None was well supported, but positive scientific evidence was greatest for Chinese herbal therapy and psychological therapy.[217]

***Clostridium* spp.** *C. difficile* has reached epidemic proportions in human medicine, with antimicrobial-induced suppression of normal flora as a major risk factor. Those drugs most commonly associated with its emergence included clindamycin, penicillins, and cephalosporins; fluoroquinolones have also been identified in humans (see Chapter 8). Environmental contamination and fecal-to-oral transmission are important, with hand carriage by health care personnel occurring in human patients in much the same way as with methicillin-resistant *Staphylococcus aureus.* In humans a new strain has emerged with increased virulence. Outbreaks have increased in the hospital setting, with community-acquired infections increasing in North America and Europe.[218] Clinical signs range from mild diarrhea to pseudomembranous colitis to toxic (and potentially fatal) megacolon. Clostridial toxins increase with deletion of the gene that downregulates production. Pathophysiology reflects binding of toxin by intestinal cells, disruption of epithelial tight junctions, and inflammation. Watery diarrhea is the clinical hallmark of infection. A seasonal pattern has been described for selected human hospitals.[220] Enterotoxicosis associated with *C. perfringens* is also emerging as a cause of large bowel diarrhea primarily in dogs (see Chapter 8). Diagnosis is based on a reverse latex agglutination test available in many human laboratories. Acute treatment includes metronidazole, ampicillin, or amoxicillin. Tylosin may be effective for cases requiring long-term treatment. High-fiber diets (or psyllium) may also be helpful. Other bacterial diseases of the large intestine were discussed as causes of diarrhea in the small intestine.

Clostridial resistance may have already emerged toward newer 8-methoxy fluoroquinolones used to treat the organism (e.g., gatifloxacin and moxifloxacin).[221]

Antibiotic-responsive diarrheas. Several chronic enteropathies afflicting dogs are reported to respond to a number of antibiotics, leading to the term *antibiotic-responsive diarrhea (ARD).* The distinction of antibiotic-responsive diarrhea from small bowel diarrheas associated with (idiopathic) small intestinal bacterial overgrowth is not clear.[222] Small bowel diarrhea of German Shepherd Dogs typifies the syndrome. Antibiotics to which animals have responded include tetracycline, metronidazole, ampicillin, tylosin, and enrofloxacin.

Tylosin-responsive chronic diarrhea was described in dogs (n = 14).[222] Middle-aged, large-breed dogs are more commonly affected with clinical signs referable to both the small and large bowels. However, the study is complicated by study design (e.g., all dogs were treated with tylosin 1 month before starting the study, and animals that responded to sequential therapies were dropped from the study). Nonetheless, the authors reported that all animals responded to tylosin (6 to 16 mg/kg orally once daily) within 3 days (most commonly within 24 hours), with clinical signs recurring within 30 days of discontinuing therapy in 86% of dogs. Other failed therapies attempted with recurrence included prednisone treatment (for 3 days; partial response) or *Lactobacillus rhamnosus* probiotics (no responders). On the basis of response to tylosin, potential pathogens have been proposed, including *C. perfringens,* campylobacters, and *Lawsonia intracellularis.* A proposed rationale for the syndrome is the existence of an as of yet to be identified specific enteropathogenic common to the canine GI tract that is susceptible to tylosin.

Several antimicrobials have beneficial immunomulatory effects in the GI mucosa (as reviewed by Westermarck and coworkers[222]). These include metronidazole and fluoroquinolones (ciprofloxacin and enrofloxacin). The use of enrofloxacin to treat inflammatory bowel disease is discussed later. Probiotics have been shown to be effective for pediatric antimicrobial diarrhea, but not that associated with *C. difficile. Trichomoniasis* is caused by *Entamoeba histolytica* and *Balantidium coli,* protozoal organisms associated with diarrhea of the large intestine in dogs and cats. Treatment of trichomoniasis was delineated in the section on diseases of the small intestine.

Treatment of *B. coli* infection has not been delineated in animals but, based on the response in humans, might include the use of tetracyclines or metronidazole.

Megacolon. Initial medical management of megacolon associated with mild constipation should include bulk laxatives and more active laxatives such as bisacodyl or docusate sodium suppositories. As constipation progresses to obstipation, enemas and evacuation under general anesthesia are implemented. In severe cases broad-spectrum antimicrobials may be indicated to decrease the potential for bacterial translocation across the damaged mucosa. Long-term medical management should be accompanied by dietary management. Laxatives and periodic enemas are indicated. Prokinetics such as cisapride have had variable success but should be tried. Earlier use is more likely to be prevent progression from constipation to obstipation in cats. Erythromycin demonstrated a prokinetic effect on colonic motility but did not provide a clinically evident benefit in human patients with postoperative colonic ileus.[183] Antisecretory drugs with anticholinesterase activity (e.g., ranitidine, nitazidine) might also be considered.

Inflammatory Bowel Disease

Pathophysiology

IBD is characterized by infiltration of inflammatory cells in the gastric or intestinal mucosa (or both).[194,223] Its emergence in predisposed animals is facilitated by the large immune system and its multivariate responses presented by the GI tract, coupled with the vast number of antigens from ingested microbes, parasites, food, toxins, endogenous microbes or their products, and other materials. Increased intestinal permeability to antigens probably plays a role, but it is not clear if this is an initiating event or a sequela. Disruption of the intricate balance between microbe and host leads to breakdown of mucosal tolerance. This key event leads to initiation, progression, and reemergence of disease.[223] Loss of mucosal tolerance generally requires a loss of the normal barrier, as might occur with loss of cadherins. Immunologic dysfunction largely reflects altered T-cell [CD-4] activity. High concentrations of IL-10 and 18, and TGF-β promote T cell differentiation to the Th-1 phenotypes, resulting in high concentrations of IL-2, INF-γ, and TNF-alpha.[224] A third factor in the loss of mucosal tolerance is the presence of endogenous microflora.

KEY POINT 19-44 Effective treatnment of of IBD is complicated by the complex interaction between microbes, the gastrointestinal tract, and the local immune response.

German and coworkers[223] reviewed IBD in dogs, and Allenspach and coworkers[225] described risk factors for therapeutic failure. Canine IBD is a group of diseases that are highly variable in cause and presentation. Manifestations and treatment depend on cell type (with lymphocytic–plasmacytic most common, followed by eosinophilic), region affected (any location but most commonly small intestine) and breed (e.g., histiocytic [large macrophages] ulcerative colitis of Boxers, protein-losing enteropathies of Soft Coated Wheaten Terriers, gluten sensitivity of Irish Setters, and immunoproliferative enteropathy of Basenjis).[223] The type of predominating cell (lymphocytic, plasmocytic, eosinophilic, or histocytic) that causes inflammation can serve as a basis of the classification and, to some degree, treatment of IBD.[226] Overgrowth of small intestinal bacteria in response to either a primary (e.g., idiopathic) or secondary (e.g., acquired) disorder has been studied as a potential cause, particularly in German Shepherd Dogs; IgA deficiency has been suggested.[223] Although commonalities exist between human and canine IBD, the most common forms in human include ulcerative colitis and Crohn's disease. Ulcerative colitis is diffuse and superficial, involving predominantly neutrophils, with some lymphocytes and plasma cells, particularly in the ileum. Crohn's disease is focal and segmental, characterized by chronic pyogranulomatous inflammation. When extrapolating therapeutic options between human and canine or feline IBD, considerations must also include differences in the pathophysiology of the diseases among species. Even within species, preferred therapies and extent of response is too variable among canine and feline populations to be predicted without supportive diagnostic (histopathologic) data. Accordingly, treatment should be approached individually (Table 19-5). A scoring system has been proposed for dogs to facilitate treatment.[226]

The "4-R's" approach to treatment of Crohn's disease in humans includes **r**emoval (underlying causes such as inappropriate diet), **r**eplacement (missing nutrients, such as vitamin B_{12}), **r**e-inoculation with "friendly" bacteria (*L. acidophilus* and *L. bulgaricus* along with fructose oligosaccharides), and **r**epair. Dietary considerations in the role of (human) IBD have been reviewed by Shah.[227] The role of gut flora, GI immunity, and IBD based on models and spontaneous disease has been reviewed in humans.[228,229] A series of studies using interleukin 10–deficient mouse colitis models demonstrated the influence of different bacterial substrates at different sites of inflammation. Inflammation best responded to a combination of vancomycin–imipenem or neomycin–metronidazole compared with ciprofloxacin and metronidazole. Response to the latter was effective for acute but not chronic colonic inflammation. Narrow-spectrum antimicrobials such as ciprofloxacin were more effective in preventing but not treating experimentally induced colitis[230] (see also the discussion of antibiotic-responsive diarrhea). Studies have demonstrated that inflammatory disease will not evolve experimentally in microbe-free environments but can be experimentally induced by transfer of T-cells reactive to bacterial antigens. In human patients with IBD, lesions are worse in those areas with highest microbial counts. Although the role of potential pathogens has been intensively studied, emerging data suggest that it is the commensal, rather than pathogenic, microbes that are contributing to the disease. As such, perpetuation of the disease may reflect abnormal signaling between host immune system and microbes and a loss of host tolerance for microbes. Accordingly, treatment for IBD targets not only suppression of the inflammatory response but also manipulation of the contributing microbiota with either antimicrobials or probiotics.

Table 19-5 Products for Treatment of Inflammatory Bowel Disease

Category	Product	Example Drug or Active Compound
	Undigested carbohydrates	
	Undigested proteins	
Supplement	Iron	
	Protein	
	Water- and fat-soluble vitamins	
	Cyanocobalamine	
	Trace elements	
	Electrolytes	
Antiinflammatories	Aminosalicylates	
	Mesalazine (5 aminosalicylic acid, 5 ASA)	Asacol (Mesalamine) Increased stability in acid medium; absorption slowed)
		Salofalk (coated with ethylcellulose)
	Sulfasalazine	Sulfapyridine diazotized to 5 ASA
	Pentoxyfylline	
	Leukotriene receptor antagonists	
Immunomodulators	Cyclosporine	
	Glucocorticoids	
	Systemic	
		Prednisolone (preferred to prednisone in cats and possibly some dogs)
		Prednisone
	Topical (oral)	Budesonide
		Fluticasone
		Tixocortol pivolate
	Topical (foams; rectal)*	Hydrocortisone acetate
		Prednisolone metasulphobenzoate
		Hydrocortisone sodium phosphate
		Prednisolone sodium phosphate
	Enema	Methylprednisolone
		Betamethasone valerate
		Beclometasone diproprionate
		Budesonide
Directed polypeptides	Role not yet elucidated	
Probiotics	*Lactobacilus acidophilus, bulgaricus*	With fructose oligosaccharide
	Bifidobacterium?	
	Others	
Antibiotics	Metronidazole	
	Fluoroquinolone	Enrofloxacin†
	Others (e.g., Tylosin)	
Protection	Sucralfate	
	Antisecretory drugs	Famotidines, proton pump inhibitors
	Polysulfated glycosaminoglycans	Glucosamine, chondroitin sulfates

*Foams adhere to mucosa and are for colonic disease. Administered at night.
†Histocytic ulcerative colitis.

Unfortunately, IBD is a diagnosis of exclusion and is made after other causes of inflammatory disease of the GI tract have been ruled out. Food allergies or intolerance; infections by fungal, bacterial, or parasitic organisms; and neoplasms must be ruled out or their role in the pathophysiology identified and treated accordingly. Confirmation of the diagnosis is based on biopsy, which also is necessary to identify the predominant inflammatory cell associated with the disease and the most appropriate therapy. For example, eosinophilic infiltrates may respond to dietary management alone. Monitoring response to therapy should include, in addition to clinical signs, serum folate and cyanocobalamin concentrations; serum albumin levels can be used as a monitoring tool in animals with protein-losing enteropathy. Allenspach and coworkers[225] retrospectively determined that hypocobalaminemia (<200 ng/mL), along with hypoalbuminemia, is a risk factor for therapeutic failure.

Initial medical management may vary with the severity and length of disease. In dogs, particularly, elimination of an irritating diet and antibiotic-responsive causes might be considered before biopsy. This is best accomplished by a well-designed clinical trial in the patient. The role of diet in human IBD has been well reviewed.[227] Feeding the animal an elimination diet containing novel or highly digestible protein foods or (particularly for colonic disease) a high-fiber diet (e.g., yams, sweet potatoes, pumpkin) might be considered first. The role of diets with altered n:3 to n:6 omega-fatty acid ratios or hydrolyzed diets (protein molecules are small and presumably nonantigenic) is not yet clear but may be promising.[223]

Antiinflammatories remain the cornerstone of therapy for IBD in dogs and cats. Use of glucocorticoids should be reserved for animals in which biopsy has confirmed a diagnosis of IBD. Indiscriminate use of glucocorticoids can be dangerous, particularly in areas in which fungal causes of GI disease are not uncommon. In addition, use of glucocorticoids in patients with GI lymphoma may render the neoplasia resistant to further glucocorticoid therapy used as part of a combination antineoplastic regimen. Glucocorticoids are indicated in dogs and cats with lymphocytic–plasmacytic IBD. Prednisolone (2.2 mg/kg/day orally) should result in clinical response within 1 to 2 weeks. Therapy should continue at the same rate for another 2 weeks (beyond clinical response) and then slowly be tapered. More severe cases of IBD or cases that do not initially respond to prednisolone may respond to dexamethasone (0.22 mg/kg/day orally).Because glucocorticoids impair healing in the gastrointestinal mucosa (by virtue of cyclooxygenase 2 inhibition), antisecretory and cytoprotectant drugs are indicated. Indeed, their use is indicated in general to facilitate healing development of multidrug resistance has been implicated as a cause of therapeutic failure with glucocorticoids in some human patients with IBD; expression of mucosal multidrug resistance may ultimately be used to determine response of IBD patients to therapy.[231] Several mechanisms of glucocorticoid resistance have been described in humans and may be relevant to dogs or cats.[232] These include heterogenicity of the disease process itself, overexpression of the MDR1 gene causing increased P-glycoprotein–mediated efflux of glucocorticoid from target cells; impaired glucocorticoid–receptor signaling; and activiation of epithelial proinflammatory mediators such as nuclear factor kappa B.

KEY POINT 19-45 Although glucocorticoids are the cornerstone of inflammatory bowel disease therapy, glucocorticoids also impair gastrointestinal healing, and gastroprotective therapies should simultaneously be implemented.

Humans generally do not tolerate systemic glucocorticoids as well as dogs or cats, leading to effective alternative therapies for IBD.[233] For example, 80% of human ulcerative colitis cases are successfully controlled with a variety of 5-aminosalicylic acid preparations. Rectal glucocorticoid foams have also proven useful for diseases involving the colon. "Topical" budesonide is as effective as systemic glucocorticoids and is better tolerated than systemic glucocorticoids. Glucocorticoids are the cornerstone of therapy for Crohn's disease; more severe disease responds to higher doses of steroids. The extrapolation of these treatments to dogs and cats is limited in part because colonic disease is not as common (limiting applicability of therapies targeting the colon). Further, the extent of first-pass metabolism of budesonide is not known. A number of therapies should be considered in dogs or cats that do not respond to initial therapy or for which glucocorticoids are not tolerated or contraindicated. Various immunomodulators should be considered. In humans, these have included cyclosporine and mycophenolate mofetil.. Allenspach and coworkers[234] reported on the use of cyclosporine for treatment of IBD in dogs (Chapter 19). Overall, cyclosporine was considered effective in 78% of the animals. In humans, long-term cyclosporine may facilitate long-term control when used in combination (but not alone) with other immunomodulating drugs. Leukotrienes appear to be involved in chronic allergic diseases such as IBD, atopy, and asthma. A role has been described in signaling and trafficking between eosinophils and lymphocytes in affected tissues, and in the IL-5 eotaxin induced differentiation, proliferation, and release of eosinophils at the level of the bone marrow. Accordingly, leukotriene receptor antagonists (e.g., zafirlukast or montelukast; see Chapter 29) might be considered as the sole agent in mild disease in those animals in which glucocorticoids are contradicted, in combination for nonresponders, or as dose-sparing agents. The role of TNF-alpha in Crohn's disease of humans has led to some scientific support for pentoxifylline (also referred to as *oxpentifylline)*.[235] It has proved useful in mouse models of colitis[236] and in humans as a dose-sparing agent when combined with glucocorticoids or directed polypeptide therapy.[237]

Sulfasalazine (20 mg/kg every 12 to 24 hours orally in cats; 50 mg/kg/day divided every 8 to 12 hours in dogs) may also be beneficial in cats and dogs with IBD. Response may take 1 to 2 weeks. As a sulfonamide, sulfasalazine may cause immune-mediated diseases ascribed to other sulfonamide antibiotics; use of the drug should be based on a histologic diagnosis whenever possible. Newer 5-aminosalicylate (sulfasalazine-like drugs) such as mesalazine and olsalazine (10 to 20 mg/kg every 12 hours) might be considered; both may decrease tear production in dogs. Omega fatty acid (fish oil) products also may be helpful for their antiinflammatory effects; response may take several weeks.

Animals that continue to be unresponsive to medical management of IBD may respond to azathioprine (0.3 mg/kg every other day, orally in cats; 2.2 mg/kg/day in dogs). Response may take up to 5 weeks. Side effects of azathioprine are sufficiently severe that a diagnosis of severe IBD should be confirmed (based on biopsy) before its use. White blood cell counts should be monitored weekly and the drug temporarily discontinued if neutrophil counts drop below 2000/uL.

The role of directed polypeptides in the management of refractory human IBD is emerging.[238,239] Emerging therapies are targeting co-stimulatory molecules which are responsible for initial interactions between T cell receptors and macrophage MHC antigen complexes.[224] Endotoxin and cytokines interact directly or indirectly with a variety of co-stimulatory molecules, including CD40-ligands (with T-cells) and B-7, an immunoglobulin that serves as a ligand for C28 (also a T cell co-stimulatory molecule). Because many of these therapies represent proteins foreign to dogs and cats and because animals are already affected by a dysfunctional immune system, caution is recommended with their use. Side effects can be profound in humans and may preclude adaptation to dogs or cats. Use in dogs and cats should be implemented only after collecting intensive scientific support.

Antibiotic therapy is intended to resolve bacterial overgrowth that might be contributing to the inflammatory process and either mimicking or contributing to IBD. However, response may just as likely reflect immunomodulation rather than antimicrobial therapy. Therapy for overgrowth in the large intestine should target clostridial organisms (metronidazole or ampicillin), whereas broader-spectrum drugs (tylosin, ampicillin) should be used for small intestinal disease. *C. perfringens* overgrowth in the small intestine may be difficult to detect; drug therapy that targets this organism includes tylosin and ampicillin. Metronidazole therapy in conjunction with glucocorticoids is indicated not only for its antibacterial effects but also because it appears to have immunomodulatory capabilities; indeed, this may explain why it may be effective as the sole therapy in some cases of IBD.

Nonhypoproteinemic dogs with lymphocytic–plasmacytic enteritis responded to a combination of oral antiinflammatory agents (prednisone, 1 mg/kg twice daily slowly decreased to 0.5 mg/kg every 48 hours) and antimicrobial agents (metronidazole 10 mg/kg twice daily for 21 days); most dogs also received oral cimetidine (0.5 mg/kg bid) and metaclopramide (0.5 mg/kg bid) for 90 days.[240] Treatment dogs (n = 16) received a prescription diet. A group of normal animals (n = 9) were studied as untreated controls. Dogs were studied for 120 days, with outcome measures including clinical signs, endoscopic lesions and histopathy of endoscopic biopies. After treatment, the mean activity index diminished from 7.3 at baseline to 1.7, 0.8, 0.5, and 0.19 at baseline, on days 30, 60, 90, and 120, respectively. Further, gastric and duodenal endoscopic lesions decreased in 75% of animals, although no significant reduction was detected histologically.

Hostutler and coworkers[241] have retrospectively described a series of cases (n = 9) of canine histoycytic ulcerative colitis responsive to antibiotics. The common drug among all nine dogs was enrofloxacin, with or without combinations of amoxicillin or metronidazole. Four of the dogs had failed to respond to antiinflammatory therapy that included combinations of prednisolone, azathioprine, or sulfasalazine, with or without other antibiotics, for a duration of 1 to 20 weeks. The remaining five dogs responded to antibiotics alone. Diarrhea resolved within 3 to 12 days of treatment with enrofloxacin at standard recommended doses. Although three dogs remained asymptomatic for 7 to 14 months, some dogs have required therapy for 2 to 21 months or longer.

Among the more promising approaches of therapy that do not directly suppress inflammation is the use of probiotics (see the earlier discussion of biotherapeutics). Probiotics are intended to replace the pathogens with healthy flora that have developed host tolerance. Their use in patients with IBD should be strongly considered; however, notably lacking is scientific evidence regarding their use. Necssary information ranges from characterization of the normal state of microbiota in the canine and feline gastrointestinal tract to its state in patients with IBD; the optimal replacement microbiota; and clinical trial evidence of response when used as either sole or combined therapy. Further, deficiencies in product quality may limit effective response. None the less, attention must be given to this approach to therapy. The role of probiotics in the treatment of IBD in humans has been reviewed.[228,229] Randomized controlled clinical trials in humans have demonstrated resolution or improvement of IBD compared with controls (placebo or 5-aminosalicylic acid) after treatment with probiotics containing bifidobacteria, lactobacilli, and streptococci as core microbes.[228,229] However, because the pathophysiology of IBD and endogenous microbiota (and presumed response to biotherapeutic) varies with site, age, diet, species, and other factors, scientific evidence of efficacy of biotherapeutics in IBD may be slow to emerge. Human and mice model data are not necessarily relevant to either dogs or cats; studies in target species are needed to support efficacy. Further, the microbiota of individuals with IBD is different from that in normal animals and (has been described as unstable). Accordingly, although biotherapeutics are largely safe in normal animals, the unknown impact of colonization of microbes in the diseased intestine mandates that discretion (and knowledge) accompany biotherapeutic use. Marteau and coworkers[228] reviewed the role of biotherapeutics in the treatment of IBD. Several studies suggest that *E. coli* and *Bacteroides vulgatus,* both normal flora, in particular, may be reasonable targets of therapy. Members of bifidobacteria and lactobacilli generally tend to be the most likely organisms to provide protection against IBD, but species differences in normal flora are likely to mandate clinical trials in target species as a basis of proof.

KEY POINT 19-46 The mechanism of efficacy of selected antimicrobials for treatment of inflammatory bowel disease may reflect immunomodulation more that antibacterial effects.

Associated clinical signs of IBD that may require medical management include vomiting, small or large bowel diarrhea, flatulence, and occasionally GER. Hematochezia may be present with colitis. Diarrhea is the primary presentation of IBD in dogs. Vomiting occurs less commonly with gastric and enteric IBD; hematochezia occurs consistently in colitis. Anorexia and weight loss occur to variable degrees in IBD. Use of antisecretory drugs is indicated, in part to provide GI protection; sucralfate likewise is indicated, particularly in the presence of erosive or ulcerative disease and glucocorticoid therapy.

Supplementation of cobalamin should be considered at least in cats with chronic inflammatory disase of the small intestine associated with hypocabalaminemia. Ruaux and coworkers[242] studied 19 cats severly deficient in cobalamine (based on serum concentrations) during and after treatment (250 units subcutaneously once weekly) for 4 weeks.

Treatment for *Helicobacter* spp. might also be considered. Leib and coworkers[216] demonstrated marked improvement in dogs with IBD when they were treated for *Helicobacter* spp. Chronically vomiting dogs with spirochetes and either normal or inflamed stomach or duodenum (based on biopsy samples) were studied. Dogs were assigned to receive twice daily for two weeks "triple" therapy (amoxicillin 15 mg/kg, metronidazole 10 mg/kg and bismuth subsalicylate at 13 to 26 mg/kg [0.25 to 2 262-mg tablets, depending on body size), either with or without famotidine (0.5 mg/kg). Potential therapeutic benefits of bismuth subsalicylate include antibacterial effects, altered microbial adhesion, protection agains ulcerative effects, and decreased resistance to metronidazole (as reviewed by Leib and coworkers[216]). Placebos apparently were not given and blinding was not ascribed; assignment to either group was by coin toss, and although other therapies were discouraged, some dogs did receive other antibiotics as well as antiinflammatory therapies. Dogs were reevaluated at 4 weeks and 6 months. No significant treatment effect emerged in the famotidine group, with the frequency of vomiting reduced by 86% and organisms eradicated in approximately 75% of dogs in both groups. On the basis of this study, the authors concluded that famotidine did not enhance response to therapy; however, caution is recommended in basing therapy on this conclusion, in part becausethe ability of the study to detect a famotidine effect was not identified. In humans eradication of *Helicobacter* might be expected in more than 90% of human patients receiving "quadruple" (i.e., with antisecretory drugs) therapy. As with other investigators, recrudescence or re-infection of dogs with *Helicobacter* after presumably successful eradiction (based on the presence of the organism rather than molecular techniques) is not unusual. In Leib's study[216] close to 50% of dogs negative for *Helicobacter* at 4 weeks were positive by 6 months, suggesting improved therapy is still needed.

Liver Diseases

With few exceptions, treatment of liver disease is nonspecific, being primarily supportive and symptomatic.[243] Feline hepatic lipidosis is largely a nutritionally managed disease and as such is not discussed in this chapter; however, future considerations should be made in the role of adipose hormones in the initiation or perpetuation of the syndrome. Recommended supplements include L-carnitine (250 to 500 mg/cat), taurine (250 mg), B vitamins at twice the standard recommended dose, vitamin C (30 mg/kg), vitamin E (100 to 400 mg/cat), and elemental zinc (7 to 8 mg/cat). Supplemenation with vitamin K (e.g., 0.5 to 1.5 mg/kg) also may be indicated.

Acute Hepatic Failure

Supportive therapy includes intensive fluid therapy with a balanced electrolyte solution to which potassium chloride, B vitamins, and (particularly in the presence of hypoglycemia or septicemia) glucose has been added. Coagulopathies are likely to reflect disseminated intravascular coagulopathy (stimulated by massive endothelial damage in the liver), impaired coagulation protein synthesis, or both. Clinical coagulopathies should be treated with heparin and replacement therapy (fresh whole blood or plasma or fresh frozen plasma). Rapid destruction of hepatic storage sites of vitamin K may also contribute to bleeding disorders, and replacement therapy may be indicated. Gastric ulceration should be anticipated and GI bleeding minimized by the use of antisecretory drugs. However, cimetidine is not recommended because of its negative effects on hepatic enzyme activity; omeprazole likewise might be used only cautiously. Antibiotics are indicated because of increased risk of bacteremia. Bacteria are likely to be gram-negative coliforms or anaerobes from the GI tract or *Staphylococcus* spp. Combination antimicrobial therapy is indicated for full antibacterial coverage. No documented studies have established the usefulness of drugs intended to support the liver as it heals or overcomes acute hepatic necrosis. Intrahepatic glutathione is an important scavenger of oxygen radicals, and its depletion probably contributes to inflammatory damage. Replacement in the form of acetylcysteine (e.g., Mucomyst) is certainly indicated for acetaminophen overdose but also might be considered in any case of acute hepatic necrosis. Cimetidine, a potent inhibitor of hepatic microsomal enzymes, might be considered in cases of acute hepatic failure associated with the formation of toxic drug metabolites, such as acetaminophen. However, its routine use in other cases of acute disease is discouraged because of its inhibitory effects.

KEY POINT 19-47 Acute drug hepatopathies might be treated with intravenous *N*-acetylcysteine.

Treatment for hepatic encephalopathy focuses on decreased absorption of encephalotoxins generated by microbes from protein and fat degradation. Medical management should be implemented in conjunction with dietary management. Lactulose is a semisynthetic disaccharide that is metabolized by colonic bacteria to lactic acid. In addition to the osmotic laxative effect, which causes evacuation of the luminal contents, acidification of the contents results in ionization of ammonia, precluding its absorption across the rectal mucosa. It can be administered either orally or, in severe cases of encephalopathy, as a retention enema (three parts lactulose to seven parts saline, administered at

20 mL/kg every 4 to 6 hours). The enema should be retained for 15 to 20 minutes. Lactitol is an alternative to lactulose that is less sweet and perhaps better tolerated. It is administered as a powder (500 mg/kg daily orally). Oral doses for long-term management with either lactulose or lactitol should generate two to three soft stools a day. Povidone–iodine (10%) given as an enema also acidifies luminal contents and provides some antibacterial activity. Selective microbial decontamination may reduce formation of encepahlotoxins. Neomycin (22 mg/kg orally twice daily or as an enema in water) also decreases bacteria responsible for formation of encephalotoxins. Other antimicrobials used for long-term management of hepatic encephalopathy include metronidazole (7.5 mg/kg orally every 8 to 12 hours) and ampicillin (22 mg/kg orally every 8 hours). With severe encephalopathy glucose-containing fluids may help prevent accumulation of ammonia in neurons.

Benzodiazepine receptors increase in patients with hepatic encephalopathy; use of benzodiazepine receptor antagonists such as flumazenil can be effective in human patients, but its efficacy is less well established in animals. If the drug is used, animals should be monitored for seizures. Intracranial pressures may increase in some patients; treatment should include mannitol (1 mg/kg of a 20% solution intravenously over 30 minutes, at 4-hour intervals) and furosemide. Glucocorticoids appear to offer no advantage to patients suffering from hepatic encephalopathy and may be contraindicated for treatment of increased intracranial pressure associated with hepatic encephalopathy.

Vomiting in patients with acute or chronic liver disease should be treated with antiemetics active at the CTZ or emetic center. Metoclopramide has been the first drug of choice, followed by a phenothiazine derivative; maropitant might reasonably replace either. Impaired hepatic function may increase the duration of action of the drug, whereas dehydration may increase plasma drug concentrations. Dosing regimens should take these changes into account. Volume replacement should take place before treatment with phenothiazine antiemetics in the dehydrated patient.

Chronic Hepatic Diseases

Halting hepatic inflammation. As with acute hepatic disease, treatment of chronic disease focuses on removal or correction of the inciting cause and supportive and symptomatic therapy. Long-term management should be accompanied by discontinuation of any drugs that are contributing to the chronic damage to the liver and dietary regimen. Drugs intended to remove the inciting cause are used in diseases for which the diagnosis is clear. For example, cecoppering agents are indicated in dogs predisposed to copper storage disease. However, Poldervaart and coworkers[244] retrospectively reviewed hepatitis in dogs and concluded that the role of copper as a cause or contributor to acute or chronic hepatitis may be underestimated. Drugs used to treat copper-related hepatic disease include D-penicillamine (10 to 15 mg/kg orally 30 minutes before a meal, every 12 hours; start with a lower dose and increase after the first week) and, for animals that cannot tolerate D-penicillamine, trientine (2,2,2-tetramine, 10 to 15 mg/kg orally twice daily). In Bedlington Terriers with copper hepatotoxicosis, 2,3,2-tetramine (7.5 mg/kg orally every 12 hours) may be used instead of trientine (and may result in greater copper elimination), but the drug must be reformulated. A more controversial treatment for copper storage disease focuses on decreased absorption of copper in the diet by treatment with zinc acetate (5 to 10 mg/kg or 100 mg for the first 3 months and 50 mg thereafter orally every 12 hours, 1 hour before each meal). This treatment should be started at a young age, before hepatic accumulation of copper has occurred. Monitoring plasma zinc concentrations every 2 to 3 months has been recommended to ensure therapeutic concentrations and to prevent toxic concentrations of zinc that might lead to hemolytic anemia (therapeutic range of zinc is 200 to 500 μg/dL; higher than 1000 μg/dL is considered toxic).

Suppression of hepatic inflammation in chronic liver disease is problematic but critical if the progression of chronic to cirrhotic disease is to be halted. Underlying causes should be identified and removed. Consideration should be given to the role that insulin resistance, adioponectin, and adiponectin have in perpetuating the inflammatory response.[4] Hepatic damage by drugs often is reversible if the drug is discontinued before fibrosis has occurred. Drug-induced hepatic disease is often dose and duration dependent, meaning that the risk of toxicity increases with higher doses (plasma drug concentrations) and long-term therapy. Consequently, single doses or short-term therapy with a hepatotoxic drug is not likely to lead to chronic hepatic disease. Examples of drugs associated with chronic liver disease in dogs are discussed in Chapter 4. Anticonvulsants (primidone, phenobarbital, and phenytoin) and heartworm preventive (oxibendazole–diethylcarbamazine) are among the most commonly used drugs associated with hepatic disease. However, any drug metabolized by the liver and to exposure is considerable (ie, large initial doses, or long duration of exposure) might be considered as a possible cause of liver disease.

Identifying the role of infection as a continued cause of liver disease may be difficult. However, with the exception of ascending chronic cholangiohepatitis, bacterial infection as a cause of chronic liver disease is uncommon. Because the liver is well perfused, any antimicrobial with a good gram-negative spectrum should be effective. However, as disease progresses and fibrosis deposition occurs, drugs that are more lipid-soluble should be considered Because of the loose but increasingly characterized association of *Helicobacter* spp. and cholangiohepatitis in cats,[245] treatment for helicobacter might be considered.

Idiopathic chronic hepatitis (chronic active hepatitis or chronic active liver disease) is generally detected by increases in serum alanine transferase activity (greater than 10 times normal) and alkaline phosphatase activity (greater than 5 times normal). Biopsy should provide a confirmation as well as a histologic description on which therapy and response to therapy can be based. Inflammation usually is controlled with immunosuppressant drugs; evidence of piecemeal necrosis, bridging necrosis, and fibrosis indicates their need.

Prednisolone (1 to 2 mg/kg orally a day) should be administered until clinical remission occurs (generally 7 to 10 days) and the dose then gradually tapered (decreased every 10 days) until a minimum effective dose has been established. Clinical signs, clinical pathologic changes (at 1- to 2-week intervals), and ultimately a repeat hepatic biopsy (at 2 to 3 months) should be monitored for response to therapy. Note that glucocorticoids can increase serum bile acids, and the failure of these to decrease is not necessarily indicative of continued damage. More aggressive immunosuppressive therapy is implemented if glucocorticoids cannot be tolerated or if the progression of hepatic disease cannot be halted with glucocorticoids. Azathioprine therapy is initiated (2 mg/kg/day or 50 mg/m^2 orally given every day for 7 days, then every other day), with prednisolone therapy continued for the first 7 days and then alternated with azathioprine thereafter. Weekly white blood cell counts should be performed to detect bone-marrow suppression by azathioprine; therapy should be suspended for 5 to 7 days if the neutrophil count drops below 2000 cells/μL or the platelet count below 50,000/μL. Lymphocytic or sclerosing cholangitis/cholangiohepatitis in cats may also respond to glucocorticoid therapy (2.2 mg/kg orally a day). In order to avoid the adverse events associated with azaothioprine or other anti-inflammatory drugs, alternative therapies might be considered. Pentoxifylline is among these alternative drugs for additional control of inflammatory disease.[246] The role of mycophenolate or cyclosporine in treating immune-mediated liver disease has not been addressed.

Ursodeoxycholic acid has proved beneficial in both dogs and cats with chronic liver disease, particularly if it is associated with a significant cholestatic component. The dose in patients with chronic hepatitis (8 to 10 mg/kg) is less than that in patients with primary biliary cirrhosis or sclerosing cholangitis (10 to 5 mg/kg/day). Note that more studies are needed to describe the clinical efficacy of ursodeoxycholic acid in dogs and cats. The drug appears to be safe; cats showed no evidence of adversity when dosed with 10 mg/kg orally for 8 weeks. Dehydrocholic acid (10 to 15 mg/kg orally every 12 hours) has also been recommended in cats with cholangiohepatitis and "ludged bile." Note, however, that less evidence is available to support the efficacy of this bile acid and that it is among the lipid-soluble and thus potentially hepatotoxic bile acids. A deletion in an efflux transport protein has been identified as the underlying cause of biliarly mucoceole in dogs; its role in feline diseases has yet to be identified. Ascorbic acid (25 mg/kg/day orally) has been suggested as supportive therapy in dogs with chronic hepatic disease because the liver is less able to produce this vitamin. Zinc therapy has also been suggested to reduce copper deposition in the damaged liver.

When the progression of disease cannot be halted and, specifically, fibrotic tissue deposition continues, antifibrotic drugs can be considered. Prednisolone provides some prevention of collagen deposition. Colchicine appears to improve (histologically) the progression of cirrhosis in human patients, but evidence is lacking in dogs because of lack of controlled trials. Adverse reactions have not been reported in dogs receiving colchicine (0.03 mg/kg/day orally) for 6 to 30 months.

Sequelae of Chronic Liver Disease

Management of GI ulceration was previously discussed. As disease progresses, the likelihood of ulceration increases not only because of impairment of the mucosal barrier but also because of increased risk of bleeding resulting from coagulopathies. Bleeding into the GI tract increases the risk of hepatic encephalopathy. Treatment of hepatic encephalopathy was discussed under acute hepatic failure.

Control of ascites can be difficult with chronic disease. Fluid accumulation is more likely to reflect increased sodium and water retention (stimulated by portal hypertension) rather than decreased albumin, although hypoalbuminemia may contribute to ascitic fluid formation. Dietary restriction of sodium should be the targeted method by which ascitic fluid formation is controlled. If this is insufficient, diuretic therapies should be instituted. Because ascites may be associated with high aldosterone concentrations, spironolactone (1 to 2 mg/kg orally every 12 hours) might be the first diuretic used. The dose may be doubled in 1 week if there has been little response. Note that its cardioprotective effects (see Chapter 15) may also potential contribute to control of inflammation in the liver. Because spironolactone is a potassium-sparing diuretic, potassium supplementation may not be necessary and may be dangerous. If the patient continues not to respond to spironolactone, furosemide therapy can be instituted (1 to2 mg/kg orally every 8 to 12 hours initially and then titrated to a minimum effective dose daily, every other day, or every third day). Care must be taken not to dehydrate the patient. Total eradication of ascitic fluid need not be the goal of diuretic therapy.

Animals with chronic (including cirrhotic) liver disease are increasingly susceptible to bacterial infections and specifically to septicemia. However, routine use of antimicrobials is not recommended in order to avoid advent of resistance; fluoroquinolones in particular should be avoided routinely. Previous exposure to antibials should be considered as drugs are empirically selected to treat septicemia. Both gram-negative coliforms and anaerobes should be targeted with antimicrobial therapy.

As hepatic disease progresses to end-stage disease, note that patients are more susceptible to disseminated intravascular coagulation. This syndrome should be anticipated in patients and managed accordingly.

A review of of 41 relevant articles regarding the use of SAMe in human patients with liver disease, including a focus on cholestasis.[179] Most studies enrolled only a small number of patients, and the quality of the studies were markedly variable. The review concluded that SAMe was more effective than placebo in reducing hyperbilirubinemia and pruritis associated with cholestasis, in studies comparing SAMe with traditional therapy (ursodeoxcycholic acid) for liver disease, although two clinical trials indicated that ursodeoxycholic acid was preferred to SAMe for cholestatic pruritis associated with pregnancy. The remaining studies were too diverse with regard to diagnosis to allow conclusions to be drawn.

Sixteen placebo-controlled clinical trials were reviewed in human patients with a variety of chronic liver diseases who were receiving milk thistle. As with the SAMe studies, poor study methods or reporting limited effective evaluation, causing reviewers to have difficulty with interpretation of results. In general, meta-analyses indicated small treatment effects, with some statistical significance favoring milk thistle for treatment of selected liver disorders based on improvements in aminotransferases and liver function tests. Milk thistle was associated with few adverse events, and these generally were considered minor.[247] Cholangitis and cholangiohepatitis in the cat are frequently associated with IBD or pancreatitis. In the cat, the common association may reflect the proximity of the bile duct to the pancreatic duct. Treatment is similar to that for chronic liver disease, including SAMe and silymarin, choleretics, and antimicrobials (to decrease bacterial and toxin load), which target gastrointestinal microflora. Immune suppression is indicated in nonsuppprative disease, particularly if associated with IBD. In the dog, the presence of fibrosis may indicate the need for antifibrotics (e.g., colchicine or elemental zinc).

PORTOSYSTEMIC SHUNTING

In his original report of cerebrospinal fluid concentrations of potential mediators of hepatic encephalopathy, Holt and coworkers[248] reviewed the pathophysiology of neurologic abnormalities associated with portosystemic shunting.

Among the proposed altered mediators, which might serve as targets of drug therapy, are monoamine and amino acid neurotransmitter systems, endogenous benzodiazepines and their receptors, and ammonia. Upregulation of genes encoding peripheral GABA-like receptors has been proposed as a cause of altered neurotransmission. Accumulation of potential neurotoxins, including GABA, has also been proposed. Others include include short-chain fatty acids, mercaptans, false neurotransmitters such as tyramine, octopamine, beta-phenylethanolamines; manganese, and ammonia. Ammonia is associated with increased cerebrospinal fluid tryptophan, possibly because of direct stimulation by way of the neutral amino acid transport proteins at the blood–brain barrier. In the absence of a urea cycle, CNS ammonia is removed by transamination of glutamate into glutamine, which occurs in astrocytes by way of a specific astroglial enzyme in rats. Glutamine, in turn, however, may competively inhibit blood–brain barrier transport proteins responsible for efflux of the large, neutral amino acids. Supporting this mechanism, clinical signs of hepatic encephalopathy resolved in rats with portosystemic shunting treated with methionine sulfoximine, an inhibitor of glutamine synthetase.

A Cochrane review of clinical trials studying the use of probiotics for treatment of nonalcoholic fatty liver disease and nonalcoholic steatohepatitis found insufficient evidence to support or refute treatment. However, the use of probiotics and synbiotics to support liver function or treat liver also disease has been reviewed by Lenoir-Wijnkoop and coworkers.[151] The rationale reflects the impact that these agents might have on the microbiota of the gut–liver axis, a term used in human medicine to refer to the impact that gut-derived endotoxins and active metabolites have on the liver. Upregulation of proinflammatory cytokines may contribute to inflammation progressing to fibrosis and lipid peroxidation. Theoretically, modulation of the gut microflora might reduce these detrimental microbiota effects. Again, in a mouse model, a probiotic containing three species of *Bifidobacterium,* four species of *Lactobacillus,* and *Streptococcus thermophilus* decreased the extent of (alcohol-induced) liver disease. In a human clinical trial, treatment of a synbiotic containing fructooligosaccharides, *Bifidobacterium,* and seven species of Lactobacillus (*L. acidophilus,L.. rhamnosus, L. plantarum, L. salivarius, L. bulgaricus, L. lactis, L. breve plus)* decreased liver enzymes and (in the alcoholic group) increased hepatic function in patients with nonalcoholic fatty liver disease and alcoholic cirrhosis. More intriguing, a prospective, randomized study in human patients with liver cirrhosis associated with minimal hepatic encephalopathy positively responded to a symbiotic containing four probiotic non–urease-producing strains (*L. plantarum, L. paracasei, Leuconostoc mesenteroides, Pediococcus pentosaceus*) and four fibers (beta-glucan, resistant starch, inulin, pectin). The fecal microbiota was recolonized with non–urease-producing *Lactobacillus* spp., urinary pH decreased along with serum ammonia and endocoxin. Hepatic encephalopathy was reversed in 50% of patients, and hepatic function improved in 50% of patients receiving the symbiotic.

Diseases of the Pancreas and Acute Pancreatitis

The combination of feline trypsinogen-like imunoreactivity and abdominal ultrasound findings appear to be able to diagnose feline pancreatitis with high sensitivity and specificity.[249] Steiner et al provides evidence that exocrine pancreatic insufficiency does occur in cats and can be diagnosed on the basis of feline trypsin-like immunoactivity.[250] Cobalamin but not folic acid absorption is impaired in exocrine pancreatic insufficiency. Decreased folic acid indicates concurrent intestinal disease.

Medical management of acute pancreatitis is supportive and symptomatic, allowing the pancreas to "rest" and heal. Drugs that may contribute to pancreatitis[251,252] should be discontinued. Suspected drugs include thiazide diuretics, furosemide, azathioprine, L-asparaginase, sulfonamides, and tetracyclines. Glucocorticoids, bromide, phenobarbital, and H_2-receptor antagonists have also been implicated. Glucocorticoids may impair macrophage clearance of alpha-macroglobulin complexes (protease inhibitors complexed with proteolytic enzymes), thus predisposing the pancreas to stimulation by CCK.

Animals should be fasted to prevent pancreatic stimulation. Fluid therapy consisting of balanced electrolytes should be administered for at least 3 to 4 days, depending on the severity of the case. Electrolytes and acid–base therapy should be monitored; hypokalemia should be anticipated and treated accordingly. Because of the risk of subclinical hypocalcemia, sodium bicarbonate should be used cautiously because alkalosis can precipitate a hypocalcemic episode in these patients. Antiemetics should be used in animals that continue to vomit. Ideally, a drug that acts both centrally and peripherally, such as metoclopramide, should be chosen.

Analgesic therapy is indicated in patients with moderate to severe pain. Opioid analgesics such as butorphanol or buprenorphine should be considered. Meperidine has been recommended as well, although its short duration of action may preclude effective use. Fresh whole blood or plasma may replace alpha macroglobulins responsible for clearing the pancreas of proteolytic enzymes and may increase plasma albumin. This may be important, particularly in the case of severe pancreatitis or that associated with disseminated intravascular coagulation. The advent of disseminated intravascular coagulationshould be treated accordingly.

Protease inhibitors such as aprotinin (250 mg or 1,500,000 kallikrein inhibitory units intraperitoneally every 6 to 8 hours) may be more effective in dogs than in humans because of differences in potency.[253] However, the drug may be prohibitively expensive. Alternatively, 5000 kallikrein inhibitory units/kg intravenously every 6 hours has been recommended but is not as preferred as intraperitoneal injection. Selenium (0.1 mg/kg every 24 hours by intravenous infusion administered as selenious acid [40 μg/mL]) may be helpful.

Because oxidative stress plays a major role in the early stage of acute pancreatitis, antioxidant therapy might be considered. Among the antioxidants studied is *N*-acetylcysteine, which intracellularly is converted to a reduced GSH provider, which directly scavenges reactive oxygen species. N-acetylcysteine (1000 mg/kg every 3 hours intraperitoneal [IP]) was effective in reducing outcome measures (cytokines, conjugated dienes, lung injury, survival) associated with acute pancreatic in a mice ceruline or diet model when administered prophylactically (1 hour before induction or with the diet).[253] Glucocorticoid therapy is controversial because of the potential for these drugs to contribute to pancreatitis. Even in patients suffering from shock, the role of glucocorticoids is not clear. However, it is unlikely that a very short-term administration of glucocorticoid therapy (i.e., one to two doses) will be harmful in patients with fulminating pancreatitis. Methylprednisolone succinate is probably preferred because of the oxygen-scavenging ability of this glucocorticoid compared to others. Inhibition of gastric secretions with H_2-receptor antagonists, proton pump inhibitors, antacids, or drugs targeting the pancreas and its secretion (e.g., atropine, calcitonin, and somatostatin) has not yet proved effective for the treatment of acute pancreatitis. With time, natural or synthetic enzyme inhibitors directed toward pancreatic secretions may become useful (and available). In very acute cases or repetitive cases, insulin therapy may be indicated in the presence of persistent hyperglycemia indicative of diabetes mellitus.

Manipulation of microflora may be a target of treatment for pancreatitis. The role of parenteral antibiotics is not clear in the treatment of acute pancreatitis, and caution is recommended because of the risk of emergent multidrug-resistant microorganisms. If the decision is made to use parenteral antimicrobials, a number of drugs will penetrate the pancreas effectively. As with any infection involving the abdomen, gram-negative coliforms should be the primary target, but anaerobes should not be overlooked. Trimethoprim–sulfonamide combinations have been suggested, although sulfonamides are one of the groups of drugs implicated in the cause of pancreatitis. Bacterial depopulation of the GI tract by antimicrobials decreases the risk of bacterial translocation, thus potentially reducing the incidence of systemic organ failure. However, the advent of multidrug-resistant bacteria is negatively affecting widespread implementation of antibacterial prophylaxis. The use of probiotics for treatment of pancreatitis was reviewed in humans.[151] Use targets that small proportion of patients for which acute pancreatitis shifts from mild to severe and life threatening. As reviewed by Lenoir-Wijnkoop and coworkers,[151] a clinical trial in humans found the incidence of pancreatic necrosis to be less (1 of 22, or 5%) in a group receiving a probiotic compared with a group that received a heat-inactivated probiotic (7 of 23, or 30%). A multicenter clinicial trial in Europe is further investigating the use of *B. bifidum* W23, *B. infantis* W52, *L. acidophilus* W70, *L. casei* W56, *Lactobacillus salivarius* W24, and *Lactococcus lactis* W58; these specific organisms were selected on the basis of their ability to survive in the GI environment associated with pancreatitis. In a rat model, probiotic use increased survival in acute pancreatitis. Although the use of probiotics in prevention of acute pancreatitis appears promising, the potential risk for (pathogenic) colonization of the necrotic pancreas with the probiotic microorganisms has not been effectively addressed. In human medicine the advent of pancreatitis actually has been associated with IBD. Chronic pancreatitis may reflect generation of autoantibodies toward pancreatic acinar cells, which may reflect hapten formation and drug allergies.[255]

A number of drugs used (in humans) to treat IBD have been associated with the advent of acute pancreatitis in those patients. These include mercaptopurine, azathioprine, coricosteroids, sulfasalazine, and 5-aminosalicylic acid products.[255] For the former, treatment of chronic pancreatitis should focus primarily on treatment of IBD, whereas the latter includes discontinuation of the inciting drug.

Exocrine Pancreatic Insufficiency

Clinical signs associated with exocrine pancreatic insufficiency (e.g., diarrhea, weight loss, polyphagia) reflect decreased intraduodenal concentrations of pancreatic enzymes and, to a lesser degree, bicarbonate or other materials. These deficiencies result in malassimilation of fats, carbohydrates, proteins, fat-soluble vitamins, and cobalamin. Additionally, the number and composition of the small intestinal bacterial flora may change, contributing to the clinical signs. Accordingly, supplementation of B vitamins and cobalamin and treatment with probiotics should be considered.

Medical management of exocrine pancreatic deficiency should be supported by dietary management. Enzyme replacement using commercially available products should be sufficient in most animals. Use of the powder in two daily feedings (two teaspoons of the nonenteric product per 20 kg) with each meal should resolve diarrhea within 3 to 4 days and promote weight gain. Because commercial dried pancreatic extracts are relatively expensive, chopped pig or cow pancreas (certified as healthy) can be used (3 to 4 ounces per 20 kg) in lieu of the commercial preparation. Fresh pancreatic tissue can be frozen for 3 to 4 months without apparent loss of pancreatic enzyme activity.

Commercial powders are not particularly efficient; much of the enzyme activity is rapidly lost due to inactivation by gastric acidity. For animals that do not respond to therapy initially, attempts can be made to improve the action of the enzymes. Of the methods suggested to improve efficiency or reduce gastric loss (including preincubation with food and addition of bile acids), inhibition of gastric acid secretions appears most useful. An H_2-receptor antagonist can be given with food or, to further improve efficacy, 30 to 60 minutes before feeding. Enteric coating not only does not appear to improve efficiency but may further decrease availability of the enzymes.

Supplementation of vitamin B_{12} (250 μg intramuscularly or subcutaneously once weekly for 1 month) and vitamin A (tocopherol; 400 to 500 IU once daily with food for 30 days) may be necessary for some patients and might be considered in animals in whom diarrhea persists despite enzyme replacement. Bacterial overgrowth may become a problem in some patients because of the presence of undigested nutrients that serve as a nutrient source for bacteria. Long-term antibiotic therapy is discouraged because of the risk of altered microflora and damage to the GI mucosa. Short-term therapy with oral metronidazole, tylosin, or oxytetracycline should prove beneficial in cases where bacterial overgrowth is causing malabsorption and diarrhea. Occasionally, animals may also have IBD, which contributes to clinical signs. Treatment with glucocorticoids may be indicated for 7 to 14 days.

REFERENCES

1. Sugrue MF: Neuropharmacology of drugs affecting food intake, *Pharmacol Ther* 32:145–182, 1987.
2. Havel PJ: Section IV: lipid modulators of islet function, update on adipocyte hormones, regulation of energy balance and carbohydrate/lipid metabolism, *Diabetes* 53(Suppl 1):S143–S151, 2004.
3. Margetic S, Gazzola C, Pegg GG, et al: Leptin: a review of its peripheral actions and interactions, *Int J Obes* 26:1407–1433, 2002.
4. Tsochatzis ET, Manolakopoulos S, Papatheodoridis GV, et al: Insulin resistance and metabolic syndrome in chronic liver diseases: old entities with new implications, *Scand J Gastroenterol* 44(1):6–14, 2009.
5. Spaulding M: Recent studies of anorexia and appetite stimulation in the cancer patient, *Oncology* 3(Suppl 8):17–23, 1989.
6. Bernstein JG: Psychotropic drug induced weight gain: mechanisms and management, *Clin Neuropharmacol* 11:S194–S206, 1988.
7. Timmer CJ, Ad Sitsen JM, Delbressine LP: Clinical pharmacokinetics of mirtazapine, *Clin Pharmacokinet* 38(6):461–474, 2000.
8. Macy DW, Gasper PW: Diazepam-induced eating in anorexic cats, *J Am Anim Hosp Assoc* 21:17–20, 1985.
9. Center SA, Elston TH, Rowland PH, et al: Fulminant hepatic failure associated with oral administration of diazepam in 11 cats, *J Am Vet Med Assoc* 209(3):618–625, 1996.
10. Hughes D, Moreau RE, Overall KK, et al: Acute hepatic necrosis and liver failure associated with benzodiazepam therapy in six cats, 1986-1995, *J Vet Am Crit Care* 6:13–20, 1997.
11. Norris CR, Boothe DM, Esparza T, et al: Disposition of cyproheptidine in cats after intravenous or oral administration of a single dose, *Am J Vet Res* 59:79–82, 1998.
12. Femia RA, Goyette RE: The science of megestrol acetate delivery, *Biodrugs* 19(3):179–187, 2005.
13. Loprinzi CL, Kugler JW, Sloan JA, et al: Randomized comparison of megestrol acetate versus dexamethasone versus fluoxymesterone for the treatment of cancer anorexia/cachexia, *J Clin Oncol* 17(10):3299–3306, 1999.
14. Miller KJ: Serotonin 5-ht2c receptor agonists: potential for the treatment of obesity, *Mol Interv* 5(5):282–291, 2005.
15. Long JP, Greco SC: The effect of propofol administered intravenously on appetite stimulation in dogs, *Contemp Top Lab Anim Sci* 39(6):43–46, 2000.
16. Johnson SE: Clinical pharmacology of antiemetics and antidiarrheals, *Proc Kal Kan Waltham Symp Treat Small Anim Dis* 8:7–15, 1984.
17. Johnson SE: Clinical pharmacology of antiemetics and antidiarrheals, *Gastroenterology* 80:1008, 1985.
18. Andrews PLR, Rapeport WG, Sanger GJ: Neuropharmacology of emesis induced by anti-cancer therapy, *Trends Pharmacol Sci* 9:334–341, 1988.
19. Merrifield KR, Chaffee BJ: Recent advances in the management of nausea and vomiting caused by antineoplastic agents, *Clin Pharmacol* 8:187–199, 1989.
20. Saito R, Takano Y, Kamiya HO: Roles of substance P and NK(1) receptor in the brainstem in the development of emesis, *J Pharmacol Sci* 91(2):87–94, 2003.
21. Diemunsch P, Grelot L: Potential of substance P antagonists as antiemetics, *Drugs* 60:533–546, 2000.
22. Hickman MA, Cox SR, Mahabir S, et al: Safety, pharmacokinetics and use of the novel NK-1 receptor antagonist maropitant (CereniaTM) for the prevention of emesis and motion sickness in cats, *J Vet Pharmacol Therap* 31:220–229, 2008.
23. Kohler DR, Goldspiel BR: Ondansetron: a serotonin receptor (5-HT3) antagonist for antineoplastic chemotherapy-induced nausea and vomiting, *Ann Pharmacother* 25:367–380, 1991.
24. Pasricha PJ: Treatment of disorders of bowel motility and water flux, antiemetics, agents used in biliary and pancreatic disease. In Brunton LL, Lazo JS, Parker KL, editors: *Goodman & Gilman's the pharmacological basis of therapeutics*, ed 11, New York, 2006, McGraw-Hill.
25. Hikasa Y, Ogasawara S, Takase K: Alpha adrenoceptor subtypes involved in the emetic action in dogs, *J Pharmacol Exp Ther* 261:746–754, 1992.
26. Hikasa Y, Takase K, Ogasawara S: Evidence for the involvement of alpha-adrenoceptors in the emetic action of xylazine in cats, *Am J Vet Res* 50:1348–1350, 1989.
27. Peroutka SJ, Snyder SH: Antiemetics: neurotransmitter receptor binding predicts therapeutic actions, *Lancet* 1:658–659, 1982.
28. Costall B, Naylor RJ: Neuropharmacology of emesis in relation to clinical response, *Br J Cancer Suppl* 19:S2–S8, 1992.
29. Hesketh PJ, Younger J, Sanz-Altamira P, et al: Aprepitant as salvage antiemetic therapy in breast cancer patients receiving doxorubicin and cyclophosphamide, *Support Care Cancer*, Dec 6, 2008.
30. Conder GA, Sedlacek HS, Boucher JF, et al: Efficacy and safety of maropitant, a selective neurokinin 1 receptor antagonist, in two randomized clinical trials for prevention of vomiting due to motion sickness in dogs, *J Vet Pharmacol Ther* 31(6):528–532, 2008.
31. de la Puente-Redondo VA, Siedek EM, Benchaoui HA, et al: The anti-emetic efficacy of maropitant (Cerenia™) in the treatment of ongoing emesis caused by a wide range of underlying clinical aetiologies in canine patients in Europe, *J Small Anim Pract* 48:93–98, 2007.
32. Sedlacek HS, Ramsey DS, Boucher JF, et al: Comparative efficacy of maropitant and selected drugs in preventing emesis induced by centrally or peripherally acting emetogens in dogs, *J Vet Pharmacol Ther* 31(6):533–537, 2008.

33. Tyers MB: Pharmacology and preclinical antiemetic properties of ondansetron, *Semin Oncol* 19(Suppl 10):1–8, 1992.
34. Reynolds JC: Prokinetic agents: a key in the future of gastroenterology, *Gastroenterol Clin North Am* 18:437–457, 1989.
35. Burrows CF: Metoclopramide, *J Am Vet Med Assoc* 183: 1341–1343, 1983.
36. Urbie M, Ballesteros A, Strauss R, et al: Successful administration of metoclopramide for the treatment of nausea in patients with advanced liver disease, *Gastroenterology* 88:757–762, 1985.
37. Albibi R, McCallum RW: Metoclopramide: pharmacology and clinical application, *Arch Intern Med* 98:86–95, 1983.
38. Shinkai T, Saijo N, Eguchi K, et al: Control of cisplatin-induced delayed emesis with metoclopramide and dexamethasone: a randomized controlled trial, *Jpn J Clin Oncol* 19:40–44, 1989.
39. Gralla RJ, Itri LM, Pisko SE, et al: Antiemetic efficacy of high-dose metoclopramide: randomized trials with placebo and prochlorperazine in patients with chemotherapy-induced nausea and vomiting, *N Engl J Med* 305:905–909, 1981.
40. Howard JM, Chremos AN, Collen MJ, et al: Famotidine, a new, potent, long-acting histamine H_2-receptor antagonist: comparison with cimetidine and ranitidine in the treatment of Zollinger–Ellison syndrome, *Gastroenterology* 88:1026–1033, 1985.
41. Aapro M, Johnson J: Chemotherapy-induced emesis in elderly cancer patients: the role of 5-HT3-receptor antagonists in the first 24 hours, *Gerontology* 51(5):287–296, 2005.
42. Burrows CF: Ondansetron: a new drug to control nausea and emesis in cancer patients, *Vet Clin Briefs* 8:3, 1990.
43. Dow J, Francesco GF, Berg C: Comparison of the pharmacokinetics of dolasetron and its major active metabolite, reduced dolasetron, in dog, *J Pharm Sci* 85(7):685–689, 1996.
44. Ogilvie GK: Dolasetron: a new option for nausea and vomiting, *J Am Anim Hosp Assoc* 36:481–483, 2000.
45. Robert A, Kauffman GL Jr: Stress ulcers, erosions and gastric mucosal injury. In Sleisenger MH, Fordtran JS, editors: *Gastrointestinal diseases: pathophysiology, diagnosis, management*, ed 4, Philadelphia, 1989, Saunders, pp 773–855.
46. Moreland KJ: Ulcer disease of the upper gastrointestinal tract in small animals: pathophysiology, diagnosis and management, *Compend Contin Educ Pract Vet* 10:1265–1279, 1988.
47. Kleiman RL, Adair CG, Ephgrave KS: Stress ulcers: current understanding of pathogenesis and prophylaxis, *DICP Ann Pharmacother* 22:452–460, 1988.

47a. Abelö A, Holstein B, Eriksson UG, et al: Gastric acid secretion in the dog: a mechanism-based pharmacodynamic model for histamine stimulation and irreversible inhibition by omeprazole, *J Pharmacokinet Pharmacodyn* 29(4):365–382, 2002.

48. Hoogerwerf WA, Pasricha PJ: Pharmacotherapy of gastric acidity, peptic ulcers, and gastroesophageal reflux disease. In Brunton LL, Lazo JS, Parker KL, editors: *Goodman & Gilman's the pharmacological basis of therapeutics*, ed 11, New York, 2006, McGraw-Hill, 2006.
49. Wolfe MM, Soll AH: The physiology of gastric acid secretion, *N Engl J Med* 319:1707–1715, 1988.
50. Akimoto M, Nagahata N, Furuya A, et al: Gastric pH profiles of beagle dogs and their use as an alternative to human testing, *Eur J Pharm Biopharm* 49(2):99–102, 2000.
51. Abelö A, Holstein B, Eriksson UG, et al: Gastric acid secretion in the dog: a mechanism-based pharmacodynamic model for histamine stimulation and irreversible inhibition by omeprazole, *J Pharmacokinet Pharmacodyn* 29(4):365–382, 2002.
52. Baker KJ: Binding of sulfobromophthalein sodium and indocyanine green by plasma alpha1 lipoproteins, *Proc Soc Exp Biol Med* 122:957–963, 1966.
53. Toutain PL, Alvinerie M, Ruckebusch Y: Pharmacokinetics of dexamethasone and its effect on adrenal gland function in the dog, *Am J Vet Res* 44:212–217, 1983.
54. Shorrock CJ, Rees WDW: Overview of gastroduodenal mucosal protection, *Am J Med* 84(Suppl 2A):25–34, 1988.
55. Miller TA: Protective effects of prostaglandins against gastric mucosal damage: current knowledge and proposed mechanisms, *Am J Physiol* 245:G601–G623, 1983.
56. Charlet N, Gallo-Torres HE, Bounameaux Y, et al: Prostaglandins and the protection of the gastroduodenal mucosa in humans: a critical review, *J Clin Pharmacol* 25:564–582, 1985.
57. Szelenyi I, Brune K: Possible role of sulfhydryls in mucosal protection induced by aluminum hydroxide, *Dig Dis Sci* 31:1207–1210, 1986.
58. Whittle BJR, Garner A: New targets for anti-ulcer drugs, *Trends Pharmacol Sci* 9:187–189, 1988.
59. Muir WW: Small volume resuscitation using hypertonic saline, *Cornell Vet* 80:7–12, 1990.
60. Krishna DR, Ulrich K: Newer H_2-receptor antagonists clinical pharmacokinetics and drug interaction potential, *Clin Pharmacokinet* 15:205–215, 1988.
61. Hirschowitz BI, Gibson RG: Effect of cimetidine on stimulated gastric secretion and serum gastrin in the dog, *Am J Gastroenterol* 70:437–447, 1987.
62. Bemis K, Bendele A, Clemens J, et al: General pharmacology of nizatidine in animals, *Drug Res* 39:240–250, 1989.
63. Coruzzi G, Bertaccini G, Noci MT, et al: Inhibitory effect of famotidine on cat gastric secretion, *Agents Actions* 19(3-4):188–193, 1986.
64. Price AH, Brogden RN: Nizatidine: a preliminary review of its pharmacodynamic and pharmacokinetic properties, and its therapeutic use in peptic ulcer disease, *Drugs* 36:521–539, 1988.
65. Brogden RN, Carmine AA, Heel RC, et al: Ranitidine: a review of its pharmacology and therapeutic use in peptic ulcer disease and other allied diseases, *Drugs* 24:267–303, 1982.
66. Boom SP, Hoet S, Russel FG: Saturable urinary excretion kinetics of famotidine in the dog, *J Pharm Pharmacol* 49(3):288–292, 1997.
67. Ames TR, Patterson EB: Pharmacokinetics of a long-acting oxytetracycline injectable in healthy and diseased calves, *Proc 13th World Cong Dis Cattle* 2:931–935, 1984.
68. Sedman AJ: Cimetidine-drug interactions, *Am J Med* 76: 109–114, 1984.
69. Gibaldi M: Drug interactions: part I, *Ann Pharmacother* 26:709–713, 1992.
70. Jackson JE: Cimetidine protects against acetaminophen toxicity, *Life Sci* 31:31–35, 1982.
71. Jackson JE: Reduction of liver blood flow by cimetidine, *N Engl J Med* 307:99–101, 1981.
72. Guharoy SR: Streptokinase versus recombinant tissue-type plasminogen activator, *DICP Pharmacother* 25:1271–1272, 1991.
73. el-Omar E, Banerjee S, Wirz A, et al: Marked rebound acid hypersecretion after treatment with ranitidine, *Am J Gastroenterol* 91:355–359, 1996.
74. Fullarton GM, MacDonald AMI, McColl KEL: Rebound hypersecretion after H_2-antagonist withdrawal: a comparative study with nizatidine, ranitidine and famotidine, *Aliment Pharmacol Ther* 5:391–398, 1991.
75. Marks IN, Johnston DA, Young GO: Acid secretory changes and early relapse following duodenal ulcer healing with ranitidine or sucralfate, *Am J Med* 91(Suppl 2A):2A-95S-2A-100S, 1991.
76. Yamaji Y, Abe T, Omata T, et al: Effects of successive doses of nizatidine, cimetidine and ranitidine on serum gastrin level and gastric acid secretion, *Drug Res* 41:954–957, 1991.
77. Larsen KR, Dajani EZ, Ives MM: Antiulcer drugs and gastric mucosal integrity effects of misoprostol, 16, 16-dimethyl PGE2, and cimetidine on hemodynamics and metabolic rate in canine gastric mucosa, *Dig Dis Sci* 37:1029–1037, 1992.

78. Boudville N: The predictable effect that renal failure has on H_2 receptor antagonists—increasing the half-life along with increasing prescribing errors, *Nephrol Dial Transplant* 20:2315–2317, 2005.
79. Lampkin TA, Ouellet D, Hak LJ, et al: Omeprazole: a novel antisecretory agent for the treatment of acid-peptic disorders, *DICP Ann Pharmacother* 24:393–402, 1990.
80. Tutuian R, Katz PO, Ahmed F, et al: Over-the-counter H(2)-receptor antagonists do not compromise intragastric pH control with proton pump inhibitors, *Aliment Pharmacol Ther* 16(3):473–477, 2002.
81. Fändriks L, Lönroth H, Pettersson A, et al: Can famotidine and omeprazole be combined on a once-daily basis? *Scand J Gastroenterol* 42(6):689–694, 2007.
82. Larsson H, Mattsson H, Carlsson E: Gastric acid antisecretory effect of two different dosage forms of omeprazole during prolonged oral treatment in the gastric fistula dog, *Scand J Gastroenterol* 23:1013–1019, 1988.
83. Säfholm C, Havu N, Forssell H, et al: Effect of 7 years' daily oral administration of omeprazole to beagle dogs, *Digestion* 55(3):139–147, 1994.
84. Andersson T: Omeprazole drug interaction studies, *Clin Pharmacokinet* 21:195–212, 1991.
85. Pauli-Magnus C, Rekersbrink S, Klotz U, et al: Interaction of omeprazole, lansoprazole and pantoprazole with P-glycoprotein, *Naunyn Schmiedebergs Arch Pharmacol* 364(6):551–557, 2001.
85a. Li XQ, Andersson TB, Ahlstron M, et al: Comparison of inhibitory effects of the proton pump-inhibiting drugs omeprazole, esomeprazole, lansoprazole, pantoprazole, and rebeprazole on human cytochrome P450 activities, *Drug Metabolism and Disposition* 32(8):821–827, 2004.
86. Waldon HL, Arnestad JS, Brenna E, et al: Marked increase in gastric acid secretory capacity after omeprazole treatment, *Gut* 39:649–653, 1996.
87. Bersenas AM, Mathews KA, Allen DG, et al: Effects of ranitidine, famotidine, pantoprazole, and omeprazole on intragastric pH in dogs, *Am J Vet Res* 66(3):425–431, 2005.
88. *Misoprostol Monograph: Misoprostol: Preclinical and Clinical Review*, Glenview, Ill, 1990, Physicians and Scientists Publishing Co.
89. Jones JB, Bailey RT Jr: Misoprostol: a prostaglandin E1 analog with antisecretory and cytoprotective properties, *DICP Ann Pharmacother* 23:276–282, 1989.
90. Babakhin AA, Nolte H, DuBuske LM: Effect of misoprostol on the secretion of histamine from basophils of whole blood, *Ann Allergy Asthma Immunol* 84:361–365, 2000.
91. Morrissey JF, Barreras RF: Drug therapy, antacid therapy, *N Engl J Med* 290:550–554, 1974.
92. Vergin H, Kori-Lindner C: Putative mechanisms of cytoprotective effect of certain antacids and sucralfate, *Dig Dis Sci* 35:1320–1327, 1990.
93. Siepler JK, Mahakian K, Trudeau WT: Current concepts in clinical therapeutics: peptic ulcer disease, *Clin Pharmacol* 5:128–142, 1986.
94. Steinberg WM, Lewis JH, Katz DM: Antacids inhibit absorption of cimetidine, *N Engl J Med* 307:400–404, 1982.
95. Untersmayr E, Schöll I, Swoboda I, et al: Antacid medication inhibits digestion of dietary proteins and causes food allergy: a fish allergy model in Balb/c mice, *J Allergy Clin Immunol* 112:616–623, 2003.
96. McCarthy DM: Sucralfate, *Drug Ther* 325:1017–1023, 1991.
97. Tarnawski A, Hollander D, Gergely H: The mechanism of protective, therapeutic and prophylactic actions of sucralfate, *Scand J Gastroenterol* 22(Suppl 140):7–13, 1987.
98. Hickey AR, Wenger TL, Carpenter VP, et al: Digoxin immune fab therapy in the management of digitalis intoxication: safety and efficacy results of an observational surveillance study, *J Am Coll Cardiol* 17:590–598, 1991.
99. Hollander D, Tarnawski A: The protective and therapeutic mechanisms of sucralfate, *Scand J Gastroenterol* 25(Suppl 173):1–5, 1990.
100. Konturek SJ, Brzozowski T, Drozdowicz D, et al: Role of acid milieu in the gastroprotective and ulcer-healing activity of sucralfate, *Am J Med* 91, 2A-20S-2A-29S, 1991.
101. Jensen SL, Jensen PF: Role of sucralfate in peptic disease, *Dig Dis* 10:153–161, 1992.
102. Furukawa O, Matsui H, Suzuki N: Effects of sucralfate and its components on acid- and pepsin-induced damage to rat gastric epithelial cells, *Jpn J Pharmacol* 75(1):21–25, 1997.
103. Slomiany BL, Piotrowski J, Tamura S, et al: Enhancement of the protective qualities of gastric mucus by sucralfate: role of phosphoinositides, *Am J Med* 91(Suppl 2A):2A-30S-2A-36S, 1991.
104. Wada K, Kamisaki Y, Kitano M, et al: Effects of sucralfate on acute gastric mucosal injury and gastric ulcer induced by ischemia-reperfusion in rats, *Pharmacology* 54(2):57–63, 1997.
105. Slomiany BL, Piotrowski J, Slomiany A: Cell cycle progression during gastric ulcer healing by ebrotidine and sucralfate, *Gen Pharmacol* 29(3):367–370, 1997.
106. Konturek SJ, Brzozowski T, Majka J, et al: Role of nitric oxide and prostaglandins in sucralfate-induced gastroprotection, *Eur J Pharmacol* 211:277–279, 1992.
107. Szabo S, Vattay P, Scarbough E, et al: Role of vascular factors, including angiogenesis, in the mechanisms of action of sucralfate, *Am J Med* 19(Suppl 2A):2A-158S-2A-160S, 1991.
108. Katz PO, Geisinger KR, Hassan M, et al: Acid-induced esophagitis in cats is prevented by sucralfate but not synthetic prostaglandin E, *Dig Dis Sci* 33:217–224, 1988.
109. Holzer P: Opioids and opioid receptors in the enteric nervous system: from a problem in opioid analgesia to a possible new prokinetic therapy in humans, *Neurosci Lett* 6;361(1-3): 192–195, 2004.
110. Crema A, De Ponti F: Recent advances in the physiology of intestinal motility, *Pharmacol Res* 21:67–73, 1989.
111. Grider JR: Reciprocal activity of longitudinal and circular muscle during intestinal peristaltic reflex, *Am J Physiol Gastrointest Liver Physiol* 284(5):G768–75, 2003.
112. Wilson DV, Evans AT, Mauer WA: Influence of metoclopramide on gastroesophageal reflux in anesthetized dogs, *Am J Vet Res* 67(1):26–31, 2006.
113. Demol P, Ruoff H-J, Weihrauch TR: Rational pharmacotherapy of gastrointestinal motility disorders, *Eur J Pediatr* 148:489–495, 1989.
114. Hedge SS, Eglen RM: Peripheral 5-HT-4 receptors, *FASEB J* 10:1398–1407, 1996.
115. Tinker J, Cox AG: Effect of metoclopramide on transport in the small intestine of the dog, *Gut* 10(2):986–989, 1969.
116. Hunt JM, Gerring EL: A preliminary study of the effects of metoclopramide on equine gut activity, *J Vet Pharmacol Ther* 9:109–112, 1986.
117. Wingate D, Pearce E, Hutton M, et al: Effect of metoclopramide on interdigestive myoelectric activity in the conscious dog, *Dig Dis Sci* 25:15–21, 1980.
118. Sojka JE, Adams SB, Lamar CH, et al: Effect of butorphanol, pentazocine, meperidine, or metoclopramide on intestinal motility in female ponies, *Am J Vet Res* 49:527–529, 1988.
119. Clark ES, Becht JL: Clinical pharmacology of the gastrointestinal tract, *Vet Clin North Am Equine Pract* 3:101–123, 1987.
120. Cox SR, Harrington EL, Capponi VJ: Bioavailability studies with ciglitazone in beagles. II. Effect of propantheline bromide and metoclopramide HCL on bioavailability of a tablet, *Biopharm Drug Dispos* 6(1):81–90, 1985.
121. Prados AP, Kreil V, Albarellos G, et al: Metoclopramide modifies oral cephalexin pharmacokinetics in dogs, *J Vet Pharmacol Therap* 30:127–131, 2007.

122. Takahashi T, Kurosawa S, Wiley JW, et al: Mechanism for the gastrokinetic actions of domperidone, *Gastroenterology* 101:703–710, 1991.
123. McCallum RW, Prakash C, Campoli-Richards DM, et al: Cisapride: a preliminary review of its pharmacodynamics and pharmacokinetic properties, and therapeutic use as a prokinetic agent in gastrointestinal motility disorders, *Drugs* 36:652–681, 1988.
124. LeGrange S, Boothe DM, Herndon S, et al: Pharmacokinetics and suggested oral dosing regimen of cisapride: a study in healthy cats, *J Am Anim Hosp Assoc* 33:517–523, 1997.
125. Piquett RK: Torsade de pointes induced by cisapride/clarithromycin interaction, *Drug Sat* 17:265–275, 1997.
126. Ueki S, Seiki M, Yoneta T, Aita H, et al: Gastroprokinetic activity of nizatidine, a new H_2-receptor antagonist, and its possible mechanism of action in dogs and rats, *J Pharmacol Exp Ther* 264(1):152–157, 1993.
127. Pouderoux P, Kahrilas PJ: A comparative study of cisapride and ranitidine at controlling oesophageal acid exposure in erosive oesophagitis, *Aliment Pharmacol Ther* 9(6):661–666, 1995.
128. Zarling EJ: Prokinetic activity of nizatidine: implications for the management of patients with gastroesophageal reflux disease, *Clin Ther* 21:2038–2046, 1999.
129. Briejer MR, Prins NH, Schuurke JAJ: Effects of the enterokinetic prucalopride (R093877) on colonic motility in fasted dogs, *Neurogastroenterol Motil* 13(5):465–472, 2001.
129a Fargeas MJ, Fioramonti J, Bueno L: Time-related effects of benzodiazepines on intestinal motility in conscious dogs, *J Pharm Pharmacol* 1984 36(2):130–132, 1984.
129b. Birnbaum D, Karmeli F, Tefera M: The effect of diazepam on human gastric secretion, *Gut* 12(8):616–618, 1971.
130. Roebel LE, Cavanagh RL, Buyniski JP: Comparative gastrointestinal and biliary tract effects of morphine and butorphanol (Stadol), *J Med* 10(4):225–238, 1979.
131. Scrivani PV, Bednarski RM, Myer CW: Effects of acepromazine and butorphanol on positive-contrast upper gastrointestinal tract examination in dogs, *Am J Vet Res* 59(10):1227–1233, 1998.
132. Smith AA, Posner LP, Goldstein RE, et al: Evaluation of the effects of premedication on gastroduodenoscopy in cats, *J Am Vet Med Assoc* 225:540–544, 2004.
133. Hughes S: Acute secretory diarrhoeas: current concepts in pathogenesis and treatment, *Drugs* 26:80–90, 1983.
134. Greenwood B, Davison JS: The relationship between gastrointestinal motility and secretion, *Am J Physiol* 252:G1–G7, 1987.
135. Kromer W: Endogenous and exogenous opioids in the control of gastrointestinal motility and secretion, *Pharmacol Rev* 40:121–162, 1988.
136. Allescher HD, Ahmad S, Kostka P, et al: Distribution of opioid receptors in canine small intestine: implications for function, *Am J Physiol* 256:G966–G974, 1989.
137. Shook JE, Lemcke PK, Gehrig CA, et al: Antidiarrheal properties of supraspinal mu and delta and peripheral mu, delta and kappa opioid receptors: inhibition of diarrhea without constipation, *J Pharmacol Exp Ther* 249:83–90, 1989.
138. Schiller LR, Santa Ana CA, Morawski SG, et al: Mechanism of the antidiarrheal effect of loperamide, *Gastroenterology* 86:1475–1480, 1984.
139. Ishaq S, Green JRB: Tolerability of aminosalicylates in inflammatory bowel disease, *Biodrugs* 15(5):339–349, 2001.
140. Sellin JH, Pasricha PJ: Pharmacotherapy of inflammatory bowel disease. In Brunton LL, Lazo JS, Parker KL, editors: *Goodman & Gilman's the pharmacological basis of therapeutics*, ed 11, New York, 2006, McGraw-Hill.
141. Wilcke JR, Turner JC: The use of absorbents to treat gastrointestinal problems in small animals, *Semin Vet Med Surg* 2:266–273, 1987.
142. DuPont HL: Bismuth subsalicylate in the treatment and prevention on diarrheal disease, *DICP Ann Pharmacother* 21:687–693, 1987.
143. Papich MG, Davis CA, Davis LE: Absorption of salicylate from an antidiarrheal preparation in cats and dogs, *J Am Anim Hosp Assoc* 23:221–228, 1987.
144. Watson WA: Factors influencing the clinical efficacy of activated charcoal, *DICP Ann Pharmacother* 21:160–166, 1987.
145. Dimski DS: Constipation: pathophysiology, diagnostic approach, and treatment, *Semin Vet Med Surg* 4:247–254, 1989.
146. Horn D: The impact of fecal impactions, *Cornell Fel Health Cent Info Bull* 2:1–8, 1987.
147. Burrows CF: Gastrointestinal pharmacology, *AAHA Ann Meet* 51:197–200, 1984.
148. Daugherty MA, Leib MS, Rossmeisl JH, et al: Safety and efficacy of oral low-volume sodium phosphate bowel preparation for colonoscopy in dogs, *J Vet Intern Med* 22:31–36, 2008.
149. Atkins CE, Tyler R, Greenlee P: Clinical, biochemical, acid-base, and electrolyte abnormalities in cats after hypertonic sodium phosphate enema administration, *Am J Vet Res* 46:980–988, 1985.
150. Schrezenmeir J, de Vrese M: Probiotics, prebiotics, and synbiotics: approaching a definition, *Am J Clin Nutr* 73:361S–364S, 2001.
151. Lenoir-Wijnkoop I, Sanders ME, Cabana MD, et al: Probiotic and prebiotic influence beyond the intestinal tract, *Nutr Rev* 65(11):469–489, 2007.
151a. Steinberg SM: Bacterial translocation: what it is and what it is not, *Am J Surg* 186(3):301–305, 2003.
151b. Schultz MJ, de Jonge E, Kesecioglu J: Selective decontamination of the digestive tract reduces mortality in critically ill patients, *Crit Care* 7(2):107–110, 2003.
151c. ol M, van Kan HJ, Schultz MJ, de Jonge E: Systemic tobramycin concentrations during selective decontamination of the digestive tract in intensive care unit patients on continuous venovenous hemofiltration, *Intensive Care Med* 34(5):903–906, 2008.
152. Blaut M, Clavel T: Metabolic diversity of the intestinal microbiota: implications for health and disease, *J Nutr* 137: 751S–755S, 2007.
153. Marchesi J, Shanahan F: The normal intestinal microbiota, *Curr Opin Infect Dis* 20:508–513, 2007.
154. Rastall RA: Bacteria in the gut: friends and foes and how to alter the balance, *J Nutr* 134:2022S–2026S, 2004.
155. Mentula S, Harmoinen J, Heikkilä M, et al: Comparison between cultured small-intestinal and fecal microbiotas in beagle dogs, *Appl Environ Microbiol* 71(8):4169–4175, 2005.
156. Davis CP, Cleven D, Balish E, Yale CE: Bacterial association in the gastrointestinal tract of beagle dogs, *Appl Environ Microbiol* 34:194–206, 1977.
157. Winkler P, Ghadimi D, Schrezenmeir J, et al: Molecular and cellular basis of microflora-host interactions, *J Nutr* 137: 756S–772S, 2007.
158. Corthesy B, Gaskins HR, Mercenier A: Cross-talk between probiotic bacteria and the host immune system, *J Nutr* 137:781S–790S, 2007.
159. Dethlefsen L, McFall-Ngai M, Relman DA: An ecological and evolutionary perspective on human–microbe mutualism and disease, *Nature* 449(7164):811–818, 2007:18.
160. de Vrese M, Schrezenmeir J: Probiotics, prebiotics, and synbiotics, *Adv Biochem Eng Biotechnol* 111:1–66, 2008.
161. Drisko JA: Probiotics in health maintenance and disease prevention—probiotics, *Altern Med Rev* 8(2):143–155, 2003.
162. Johnston BC, Supina AL, Ospina M, et al: Probiotics for the prevention of pediatric antibiotic-associated diarrhea, *Cochrane Database of Sys Rev* 2:CD004827, 2007. doi: 10.1002/14651858.CD004827.pub2.

163. Kwon JH, Farrell RJ: Probiotics and inflammatory bowel disease, *Biodrugs* 17(3):179–186, 2003.
163a. Abad CL, Safdar N: The role of lactobacillus probiotics in the treatment or prevention of urogenital infections–a systematic review, *J Chemother* 21(3):243–252, 2009.
164. Duncan SH, Richardson AJ, Kaul P, et al: *Oxalobacter formigenes* and its potential role in human health, *Appl Environ Microbiol* 68(8):3841–3847, 2002.
165. Lieske JC, Goldfarb DS, De Simone C, et al: Use of a probiotic to decrease hyperoxaluria, *Kidney Int* 68:1244–1249, 2005.
166. Weese JS, Weese HE, Yuricek L, et al: Oxalate degradation by intestinal lactic acid bacteria in dogs and cats, *Vet Microbiol* 101(3):161–166, 2004:Jul 14.
167. Isakow W, Morrow LE, Kollef MH: Probiotics for preventing and treating nosocomial infections, review of current evidence and recommendations, *Chest* 132:286–294, 2007.
168. Quigley EM, Flourie B: Probiotics and irritable bowel syndrome: a rationale for their use and an assessment of the evidence to date, *Neurogastroenterol Motil* 19(3):166–172, 2007.
169. Baillon MLA, Marshall-Jones ZV, Butterwick RF: Effects of probiotic Lactobacillus acidophilus strain DSM13241 in healthy adult dogs, *Am J Vet Res* 65:338–343, 2004.
170. Rinkinen M, Jalava K, Westermarck E, et al: Interaction between probiotic lactic acid bacteria and canine enteric pathogens: a risk factor for intestinal Enterococcus faecium colonization? *Vet Microbiol* 92(1-2):111–119, 2003.
171. Heller FR, Martinet JP, Henrion J, et al: The rationale for using ursodeoxycholic acid in chronic liver disease, *Proc Natl Acad Sci USA* 88:9543–9547, 1991.
172. Meyer DJ, Thompson MB: Bile acids: beyond their value as a liver function test, *Biochem J* 285:929–932, 1992.
173. Nicholson BT, Center SA, Rowland PJ, et al: Evaluation of the safety of ursodeoxycholic acid in healthy cats, *Mech Ageing Dev* 48:145–155, 1989.
174. Mazzanti R, Fantappié O, Kamimoto Y, et al: Bile acid inhibition of P-glycoprotein-mediated transport in multidrug-resistant cells and rat liver canalicular membrane vesicles, *Hepatology* 20(1 Pt 1):170–176, 1994.
175. Lieber CS: S-adenosyl-L-methionine: its role in the treatment of liver disorders, *Am J Clin Nutr* 76(5):1183S–1187S, 2002.
176. Lieber CS, Packer L: S-adenosylmethionine: molecular, biological, and clinical aspects:an introduction, *Am J Clin Nutr* 76(5):1148S–1150S, 2002.
177. Center SA, Randolph JF, Warner KL, et al: The effects of S-adenosylmethionine on clinical pathology and redox potential in the red blood cell, liver, and bile of clinically normal cats, *J Vet Intern Med* 19:303–314, 2005.
178. Wallace KP, Center SA, Hickford FH, et al: S-Adenosyl-L-Methionine (SAMe) for the treatment of acetaminophen toxicity in a dog, *J Am Anim Hosp Assoc* 38:246–254, 2002.
179. Herb and Plant Supplement, Consumerlab.com, reviewed October 2007 by EBSCO CAM Review Board. Accessed January 5, 2010, at www.consumerlab.com/tnp.asp?chunkiid=21460.
180. Osman E, Owen JS, Burroughs AK: Review article: S-adenosyl-L-methionine: a new therapeutic agent in liver disease, *Aliment Pharmacol Ther* 7:21–28, 1993.
181. Concari M, et al: S-adenosyl-L-methionine enhances hepatoprotective effects of ursodeoxycholic acid in HEPG2 cell line. AASLD abstract: *Hepatology* 29(4): pt 2, No. 196, 1996.
182. Lawrence V, Jacobs B, Dennehy C et al: Report on milk thistle: effects on liver disease and cirrhosis and clinical adverse effects, *AHRQ* Publication No. 01–E025 October 2000.
183. Smith AJ, Nissan A, Lanouette NM, et al: Prokinetic effect of erythromycin after colorectal surgery: randomized, placebo-controlled, double-blind study, *Dis Colon Rectum* 43:333–337, 2000.
184. Jergens AE: Diseases of the esophagus. In Ettinger SJ, Feldman EC, editors: *Textbook of veterinary internal medicine*, ed 6, St Louis, 2005, Saunders.
185. Dewey C, Boothe DM, Rinn KL, et al: Treatment of a myasthenic dog with mycophenolate mofetil, *J Vet Emerg Crit Care* 10(3):177–187, 2000.
186. Madisch A, Heydenreich CJ, Wieland V, et al: Treatment of functional dyspepsia with a fixed peppermint oil and caraway oil combination preparation as compared to cisapride. A multicenter, reference-controlled double-blind equivalence study, *Arzneimittelforschung* 49:925–932, 1999.
187. Apaydin BB, Paksoy M, Art T, et al: Influence of pentoxifylline and interferon-alpha on prevention of stricture due to corrosive esophagitis, *Eur Surg Res* 33:225–231, 2001.
188. Stanciu C, Bennett JR: Metoclopramide in gastrooesophageal reflux, *Gut* 14(4):275–279, 1973.
189. Wilson DV, Evans AT, Mauer WA: Influence of metoclopramide on gastroesophageal reflux in anesthetized dogs, *Am J Vet Res* 67:26–31, 2006.
190. Wilson DV, Tom Evans A, Mauer WA: Pre-anesthetic meperidine: associated vomiting and gastroesophageal reflux during the subsequent anesthetic in dogs, *Vet Anaesth Analg* 34(1):15–22, 2007.
191. Melendez LD, Twedt DC, Wright M: Suspected doxycycline-induced esophagitis with esophageal stricture formation in three cats, *Feline Pract* 28:10–12, 2000.
191a. German AJ, Cannon MJ, Dye C: Oesophageal strictures in cats associated with doxycycline therapy, *J Fel Med Surg* 7(1):33–41, 2005.
192. Graham JP, Lipman AH, Newell SM, et al: Esophageal transit of capsules in clinically normal cats, *Am J Vet Res* 61:655–657, 2000.
193. Westfall DS, Twedt DC, Steyn PF, et al: Evaluation of esophageal transit of tablets and capsules in 30 cats, *J Vet Intern Med* 15:467–470, 2001.
194. Simpson KW: Diseases of the stomach. In Ettinger SJ, Feldman EC, editors: *Textbook of veterinary internal medicine*, ed 6, St Louis, 2005, Saunders.
195. Marino P: *The ICU book*, ed 2, Philadelphia, 1997, Lippincott Williams & Wilkins.
196. La Corte R, Caselli M, Castellino G, et al: Prophylaxis and treatment of NSAID-induced gastroduodenal disorders, *Drug Saf* 20:527–543, 1999.
197. Wu CS, Wang SH, Chen PC, et al: Does famotidine have similar efficacy to misoprostol in the treatment of non-steroidal anti-inflammatory drug-induced gastropathy? *Int J Clin Pract* 52:472–474, 1998.
198. Brown GJ, Yeomans ND: Prevention of the gastrointestinal adverse effects of nonsteroidal anti-inflammatory drugs: the role of proton pump inhibitors, *Drug Saf* 21:503–512, 1999.
199. Ward DM, Leib MS, Johnston SA, et al: The effect of dosing interval on the efficacy of misoprostol in the prevention of aspirin-induced gastric injury, *J Vet Intern Med* 17:282–290, 2003.
200. Lazzaroni M, Bianchi Porro G: Non-steroidal anti-inflammatory drug gastropathy: clinical results with H_2 antagonists and proton pump inhibitors, *Ital J Gastroenterol Hepatol* 31(Suppl1):S73–S78, 1999.
201. Tryba M: Sucralfate versus antacids or H_2-antagonists for stress ulcer prophylaxis: a meta-analysis on efficacy and pneumonia rate, *Crit Care Med* 19(7):942–949, 1991.
202. Davis MS, Willard MD, Nelson SL, et al: Efficacy of omeprazole for the prevention of exercise-induced gastritis in racing Alaskan sled dogs, *J Vet Intern Med* 17(2):163–166, 2003.
203. Williamson KK, Willard MD, McKenzie EC, et al: Efficacy of famotidine for the prevention of exercise-induced gastritis in racing Alaskan sled dogs, *J Vet Intern Med* 21(5):924–927, 2007.

204. Buber T, Saragusty J, Ranen E, et al: Evaluation of lidocaine treatment and risk factors for death associated with gastric dilatation and volvulus in dogs: 112 cases (1997-2005), *J Am Vet Med Assoc* 230(9):1334–1339, 2007.
205. Ellebaek E, Herrstedt J: Optimizing antiemetic therapy in multiple day and multiple cycles of chemotherapy, *Curr Opin Support Palliat Care* 2(1):28–34, 2008.
205a. Vail DM, Rodabaugh HS, Conder GA, et al: Efficacy of injectable maropitant (Cerenia) in a randomized clinical trial for prevention and treatment of cisplatin-induced emesis in dogs presented as veterinary patients, *Vet Compar Oncol* 5:38–46, 2007.
205b. Rau SE, Barber LG, Burgess KE: Efficacy of maropitant in the prevention of delayed vomiting associated with administration of doxorubicin to dogs, *J Vet Intern Med* 24(6):1452–1457, 2010.
206. Brechot JM, Dupeyron JP, Delattre C, et al: Continuous infusion of high-dose metoclopramide: comparison of pharmacokinetically adjusted and standard doses for the control of cisplatin-induced acute emesis, *Eur J Clin Pharmacol* 40(3):283–286, 1991.
207. Ku CM, Ong BC: Postoperative nausea and vomiting: a review of current literature, *Singapore Med J* 44(7):366–374, 2003.
208. Seta ML, Kale-Pradhan PB: Efficacy of metoclopramide in postoperative ileus after exploratory laparotomy, *Pharmacotherapy* 21(10):1181–1186, 2001.
209. Traut U, Brügger L, Kunz R, et al: Systemic prokinetic pharmacologic treatment for postoperative adynamic ileus following abdominal surgery in adults, *Cochrane Database of Systematic Reviews*. Issue 1, Art. No: CD004930, 2008, doi: 10.1002/14651858. CD004930.pub3.
209a. Correa P, Houghton J: Carcinogenesis of *Helicobacter pylori*, *Astroenterology* 133(2):659–672, 2007.
210. Hall EJ, German AJ: Diseases of the small intestine. In Ettinger SJ, Feldman EC, editors: *Textbook of veterinary internal medicine*, ed 6, St Louis, 2005, Saunders.
211. Otto CM, Jackson CB, Rogell EJ, et al: Recombinant bactericidal/permeability-increasing protein (rBPI21) for treatment of parvovirus enteritis: a randomized, double-blinded, placebo-controlled trial, *J Vet Intern Med* 15:355–360, 2001.
212. Isogai E, Isogai H, Onuma M: *Escherichia coli* associated endotoxemia in dogs with parvovirus infection, *Nippon Juigaku Zasshi* 51:597–606, 1989.
213. Turk J, Miller M, Brown T, et al: Coliform septicemia and pulmonary disease associated with canine parvoviral enteritis: 88 cases (1987-1988), *J Am Vet Med Assoc* 196:771–773, 1990.
214. Turk J, Faks W, Miller M, et al: Enteric Clostridium perfringens infection associated with parvoviral enteritis in dogs: 74 cases (1987-1990), *J Am Vet Med Assoc* 200:991–994, 1992.
215. Scorza AV, Lappin MR: Metronidazole for the treatment of feline giardiasis, *J Feline Med Surg* 6:157–160, 2004.
215a. Steinberg SM: Bacterial translocation: what it is and what it is not, *Am J Surg* 186(3):301–305, 2003.
215b. Schultz MJ, de Jonge E, Kesecioglu J: Selective decontamination of the digestive tract reduces mortality in critically ill patients, *Crit Care* 7(2):107–110, 2003.
215c. ol M, van Kan HJ, Schultz MJ, de Jonge E: Systemic tobramycin concentrations during selective decontamination of the digestive tract in intensive care unit patients on continuous venovenous hemofiltration, *Intensive Care Med* 34(5):903–906, 2008.
215d. Diepenhorst GM, van Ruler O, Besselink MG, et al: Influence of prophylactic probiotics and selective decontamination on bacterial translocation in patients undergoing pancreatic surgery: A randomized controlled clinical trial, *Shock* , June 22, 2010:[Epub ahead of print] PubMed PMID: 20577144.
216 Leib MS, Duncan RB, Ward DL: Triple antimicrobial therapy and acid suppression in dogs with chronic vomiting and gastric Helicobacter spp, *J Vet Intern Med* 21:1185–1192, 2007.
217. Spanier JA, Howden CW, Jones MP: A systematic review of alternative therapies in the irritable bowel syndrome, *Arch Intern Med* 163:265–274, 2003.
218. Kuijper EJ, Coignard B, Tull P: Emergence of *Clostridium difficile*-associated disease in North America and Europe, *Clin Microbiol Infect* 12(Suppl 6):2–18, 2006.
219. Loo VG, Poirier L, Miller MA, et al: A predominantly clonal multi-institutional outbreak of Clostridium difficile–associated diarrhea with high morbidity and mortality, *N Engl J Med* 353:2442–2449, 2005.
220. Miller MA, Hyland M, Ofner-Agostini M, et al: Canadian Hospital Epidemiology Committee. Canadian Nosocomial Infection Surveillance Program. Morbidity, mortality, and healthcare burden of nosocomial *Clostridium difficile*–associated diarrhea in Canadian hospitals, *Infect Control Hosp Epidemiol* 23(3):137–140, 2002.
221. Drudy D, Quinn T, O'Mahony R, et al: High-level resistance to moxifloxacin and gatifloxacin associated with a novel mutation in gyrB in toxin-A-negative, toxin-B-positive, *Clostridium difficile*, *J Antimicrob Chemother* 58(6):1264–1267, 2006.
222. Westermarck E, Skrzypczak T, Harmoinen J, et al: Tylosin-responsive chronic diarrhea in dogs, *J Vet Intern Med* 19: 177–186, 2005.
223. German AJ, Hall EJ, Day MJ: Chronic intestinal inflammation and intestinal disease in dogs, *J Vet Intern Med* 17:8–20, 2003.
224. Maerten P, Liu Z, Ceuppens JL: Targeting of costimulatory molecules as a therapeutic approach in inflammatory bowel disease, *Biodrugs* 17(6):395–411, 2003.
225. Allenspach K, Wieland B, Gröne A, et al: Chronic enteropathies in dogs: evaluation of risk factors for negative outcome, *J Vet Intern Med* 21:700–708, 2007.
226. Jergens AE, Schreiner CA, Frank DE, et al: A scoring index for disease activity in canine inflammatory bowel disease, *J Vet Intern Med* 17:291–297, 2003.
227. Shah S: Dietary factors in the modulation of inflammatory bowel disease activity, *Med Gen Med* 9(1):60, 2007.
228. Marteau P, Lepage P, Mangin I, et al: Review article: gut flora and inflammatory bowel disease, *Aliment Pharmacol Ther* 20(Suppl 4):18–23, 2004.
229. Sheil B, Shanahan F, O'Mahony L: Probiotic effects on inflammatory bowel disease, *J Nutr* 137:819S–824S, 2007.
230. Hoentjen F, Harmsen HJM, Braat H, et al: Antibiotics with a selective aerobic or anaerobic spectrum have different therapeutic activities in various regions of the colon in interleukin 10 gene deficient mice, *Gut* 52:1721–1727, 2003.
231. Farrell RJ, Murphy A, Long A, et al: High multidrug resistance(P-glycoprotein 170) expression in inflammatory bowel disease patients who fail medical therapy, *Gastroenterology* 118:279–288, 2000.
232. Farrell RJ, Kelleher D: Mechanisms of steroid action and resistance in inflammation, *J Endocrinol* 178:339–346, 2003.
233. Schölmerich J: Review article: systemic and topical steroids in inflammatory bowel disease, *Aliment Pharmacol Ther* 20(Suppl 4):66–74, 2004.
234. Allenspach K, Rüfenacht S, Sauter S, et al: Pharmacokinetics and clinical efficacy of cyclosporine treatment of dogs with steroid-refractory inflammatory bowel disease, *J Vet Intern Med* 20:239–244, 2006.
235. Tilg H, Kaser A: Antitumour necrosis factor therapy in Crohn's disease, *Expert Opin Biol Ther* 2(7):715–721, 2002.
236. Murthy S, Cooper HS, Yoshitak H, et al: Combination therapy of pentoxifylline and TNF-α monoclonal antibody in dextran sulphate-induced mouse colitis, *Aliment Pharmacol Ther* 13:251–260, 1999.
237. Sands BE, Kaplan GG: The role of TNF-alpha in ulcerative colitis, *J Clin Pharmacol* 47(8):930–941, 2007.

238. Baumgart DC, Dignass AU: Current biological therapies for inflammatory bowel disease, *Curr Pharm Des* 10:4127–4147, 2004.
239. Kaser A, Tilg H: Novel therapeutic targets in the treatment of IBD, *Expert Opin Ther Targets* 12(5):553–563, 2008.
240. Garcia-Sancho M, Rodriguez-Franco F, Sainz A, et al: Evaluation of clinical, macroscopic, and histopathologic response to treatment in nonhypoproteinemic dogs with lymphocytic-plasmacytic enteritis, *J Vet Intern Med* 21:11–17, 2007.
241. Hostutler RA, Luria BJ, Johnson SE, et al: Antiobiotic-responsive histiocytic ulcerative colitis in 9 dogs, *J Vet Intern Med* 18:499–504, 2004.
242. Ruaux CG, Steiner JM, Williams DA: Early biochemical and clinical responses to cobalamin supplementation in cats with signs of gastrointestinal disease and severe hypocobalaminemia, *J Vet Intern Med* 19:155–160, 2005.
243. Johnson SE: Diseases of the liver. In Ettinger SJ, Feldman EC, editors: *Textbook of veterinary internal medicine*, ed 4, Philadelphia, 1995, Saunders, pp 1313–1357.
244. Poldervaart JH, Favier RP, Penning LC, et al: Primary hepatitis in dogs: a retrospective review (2002-2006), *J Vet Intern Med* 23(1):72–80, 2009.
245. Greiter-Wilke A, Scanziani E, Soldati S, et al: Association of Helicobacter with cholangiohepatitis in cats, *J Vet Intern Med* 20:822–827, 2006.
246. Tuncer I, Uygan I, Dülger H, et al: The comparative effects of pentoxifylline and ursodeoxycholic acid on IL-1β, IL-6, IL-8 and TNF-α levels in nonalcoholic fatty liver, *East J Med* 8(2):27–32, 2003.
247. *Milk Thistle: Effects on Liver Disease and Cirrhosis and Clinical Adverse Effects.* Summary, Evidence Report/Technology Assessment: Number 21, September 2000. Agency for Healthcare Research and Quality, Rockville, MD. Accessed January 5, 2010, at www.ahrq.gov/clinic/epcsums/milktsum.htm.
248. Holt DE, Washabau RJ, Djali S, et al: Cerebrospinal fluid glutamine, tryptophan, and tryptophan metabolite concentrations in dogs with portosystemic shunts, *Am J Vet Res* 63(8): 1167–1171, 2002.
249. Forman MA, Marks SL, De Cock HE, et al: Evaluation of serum feline pancreatic lipase immunoreactivity and helical computed tomography versus conventional testing for the diagnosis of feline pancreatitis, *J Vet Intern Med* 18(6): 807–815, 2004.
250. Steiner JM, Williams DA: Serum feline trypsin-like immunoreactivity in cats with exocrine pancreatic insufficiency, *J Vet Intern Med* 14:627–629, 2000.
251. Scarpelli DC: Toxicology of the pancreas, *Toxicol Appl Pharmacol* 101:543–554, 1989.
252. Simpson KW: Diagnosis and treatment of acute pancreatitis in the dog. In Ettinger SJ, Feldman EC, editors: *Textbook of veterinary internal medicine*, ed 4, Philadelphia, 1995, Saunders, pp 117–124.
253. Steiner JM: Canine pancreatitis. In Bonagura J, editor: *Kirk's current veterinary therapy*, ed 14, St Louis, 2009, Saunders.
254. Demols A, Van Laethem JL, Quertinmont E, et al: N-acetylcysteine decreases severity of acute pancreatitis in mice, *Pancreas* 20(2):161–169, 2000.
255. Inamura H, Kashiwase Y, Morioka J, Kurosawa M: Acute pancreatitis possibly caused by allergy to bananas, *J Invest Allergol Clin Immunol* 15(3):222–224, 2005.

Drugs Affecting the Respiratory System

20

Dawn Merton Boothe

Chapter Outline

NORMAL RESPIRATORY PHYSIOLOGY

Airway Caliber Changes

Nervous innervation to the smooth muscle of the respiratory tract is complex. The parasympathetic system provides the primary efferent innervation, with acetylcholine as the primary neurotransmitter.[1,2] Its fibers are responsible for the baseline tone of mild bronchoconstriction that characterizes the normal respiratory tract through M_3 muscarinic receptors. The effects are balanced by bronchodilation resulting from β_2-receptor stimulation.[3-5] In contrast, α-adrenergic stimulation can contribute to bronchoconstriction.[2,4,6] A third, largely understood nervous system, referred to as the *nonadrenergic, noncholinergic system* or the *purinergic system,* also innervates bronchial smooth muscle.[1,7] This system mediates bronchodilation by way of vagal stimulation. The afferent fibers of this system are probably irritant receptors, and although the neurotransmitter has not yet been conclusively identified, vasoactive intestinal peptide has been implicated in the cat.[8,9] Malfunction of this system has been associated with bronchial hyperreactivity, which often characterizes asthma.[7]

The intracellular mechanisms that transmit signals from the nervous system to smooth muscle depend in part on changes in the intracellular concentration of cyclic adenosine monophosphate (cAMP) and cyclic guanosine monophosphate (cGMP) (Figure 20-1). The effects of these two secondary messengers are reciprocal such that the increased intracellular concentration of one is associated with a decreased concentration of the other. Cyclic AMP-induced bronchodilation is decreased by α-adrenergic stimulation and increased by β_2-receptor stimulation.[3] In contrast, cGMP-induced bronchoconstriction is increased by stimulation of muscarinic (cholinergic) and, indirectly, histaminergic receptors (see Figure 20-1). The relative sensitivity of bronchial smooth muscle to histamine-induced

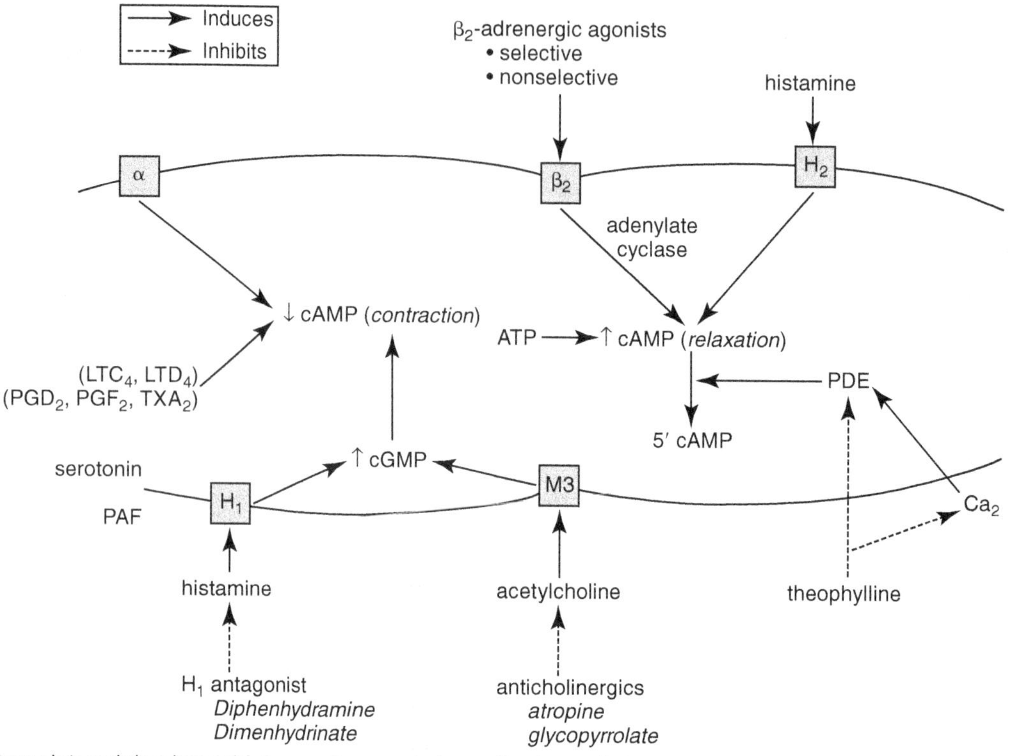

Figure 20-1 Factors determining bronchial smooth muscle tone. Reciprocal changes in cyclic adenosine monophosphate (cAMP) and cyclic guanosine monophosphate (cGMP) determine muscle tone. Contraction occurs when cAMP levels are decreased by events such as α-adrenergic stimulation or when cGMP levels increase in response to muscarinic receptor (M_3) stimulation by acetylcholine or H_1-receptor stimulation by histamine. Calcium (Ca^{2+}) and several mediators can also induce bronchoconstriction. Increased cAMP levels induced by β-adrenergic or histamine (H_2) receptor stimulation counteract muscle contraction. Inhibition of phosphodiesterase (PDE) also causes increase cAMP. Although the effects of most inflammatory mediators are best counteracted by preventing their release, several drugs may be used to antagonize smooth muscle contraction regardless of the etiology. *LTC,* Leukotriene C; *LTD,* leukotriene D; *PAF,* platelet-activating factor; *PGD_2,* prostaglandin D_2, *PGF_2,* prostaglandin F_2; *TXA_2,* thromboxane.

and acetylcholine-induced bronchoconstriction varies with the location and species.[5,10,11] Peripheral airways in dogs are more susceptible than in cats to acetylcholine; feline airways, in general, are more sensitive to acetylcholine and serotonin than histamine.[12] Smooth muscle receptors are also susceptible to stimulation by a variety of chemical mediators (see Figure 20-1), which may also modulate cAMP and cGMP.[13-15]

KEY POINT 20-1 The normal state of the airway is one of bronchoconstriction, mediated by the parasympathetic system (via cGMP). However, this is offset by sympathetic (via cAMP) bronchodilation.

Control of bronchial smooth muscle tone is very complex and depends on input from sensory receptors. At least five types of sensory receptors have been identified in cat lungs, all of which can be classified as irritant (or mechanoreceptor), stretch, or J-receptors.[7] All appear to be innervated by the parasympathetic system. Irritant receptors, located beneath the respiratory epithelium, occur in the upper airways[2] and, in cats, as far peripherally as the alveoli.[1] Physical, mechanical, or chemical stimulation of these receptors results in tachypnea, bronchoconstriction, and cough. As reviewed by Canning,[7a] rapidly adapting receptors (RARs) terminate in or below the epithelium primarily of intra-pulmonary, but to some degree, extra-pulmonary airways. They can adapt within 1 to 2 seconds to changes in airway mechanics and are subject to activation by multiple stimuli, including chemical mediators. In contrast, slowly adapting receptors (SARs) may be responsible for physiologic responses (i.e., termination of inspiration and initiation of expiration). SARS centrally inhibit respiration and decrease airway smooth muscle tone. However, they may facilitate cough. Cats have few SARS but many RARs.[7a] C-fibers represent the majority of fibers innervating the airways and lungs. They are physiologically similar to nociceptors of other tissues. They appear to synthesize neuropeptides (e.g., substance P) that influence the central and peripheral nerve terminals. Mediators stimulating C-fibers vary: in dogs, pulmonary subtypes do not (but bronchial subtypes do) respond to histamine, and in other animal models, they do not respond to serotonin or adenosine. C-fibers regulate airway defense reflexes, interacting with RAR, although the scientific description of these fibers is not clear. C-fibers and RARS interact with the spinal cord through central sensitization. Subsequent heightened reflex responsiveness may occur; tachykinins (including substance P) appear to play a role in hyperreflexia,

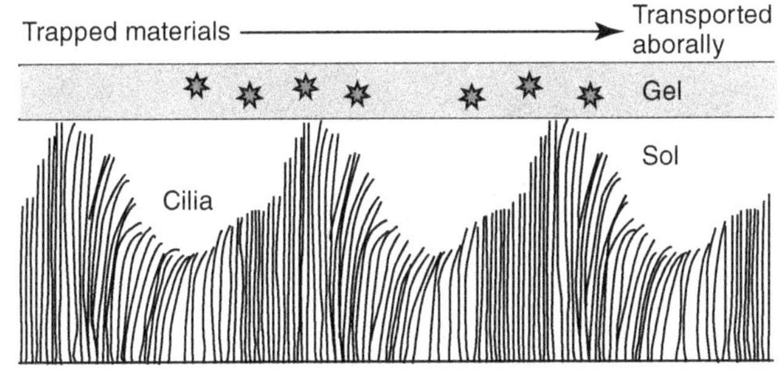

Figure 20-2 The mucociliary apparatus represents the first line of defense for pathogens entering the respiratory tract. Cilia are bathed in a water or sol layer. When the cilia beat in synchrony, the movements send forward (orally) the mucoid or gel layer that lies on top of the cilia. Materials trapped in this layer also move forward to be either swallowed or expectorated.

an effect prevented by neurokinin receptor antagonists. Convergence of vagal afferents in the nucleus of the solitary tract may explain in part the close relationship between vomiting and coughing. Receptors also converge in the ventral respiratory column of the medulla. Airflow velocity appears to be the most critical factor determining stimulation of irritant receptors in the upper airways.[1] Airway constriction sufficient to cause airflow velocity to exceed a specific threshold results in a vagally mediated cough reflex and bronchoconstriction. Airways can also be occluded by mucus and edema or by chemical mediators released during upper airway infections.[7]

In addition to the cough receptors, afferent nerves, efferent nerves and effector muscles, the cough reflex also consists of a poorly defined cough center.

Respiratory Defense Mechanisms

In addition to the cough and sneeze reflexes, two other systems provide the major defense of the respiratory tract against invading organisms or foreign materials: the mucociliary apparatus and the respiratory mononuclear phagocyte system.[2] The mucociliary apparatus (Figure 20-2) is the first major defense and consists of the ciliary lining of the tracheobronchial tree and the fluid blanket surrounding the cilia. Nervous innervation to the cilia has not yet been identified. Although ciliary activity increases with β-adrenergic stimulation, this may simply reflect the sequelae of β-adrenergic stimulation on respiratory secretions.[16] Two types of secretions form the fluid blanket of the respiratory tract.[17] The cilia must be surrounded by a low-viscosity, watery medium to maintain their rhythmic beat. A more mucoid layer lies on top of the cilia and serves to trap foreign materials inspired with air. The synchronous motion of the cilia causes the cephalad movement of the mucous layer and any trapped materials.

Changes in the viscoelastic properties of mucus such that it becomes either too watery or too rigid will result in mucus transport that is less than optimal.[2] Mucus released by goblet cells results from direct irritation[2] and is not amenable to pharmacologic manipulation. Surface goblet cells, which are uniquely prominent in feline bronchioles,[18] increase in number with chronic disease. Submucosal glands of the bronchi secrete both a serous and a mucoid fluid. The secretions tend to be more fluid than that of the goblet cells, but the degree varies with the stimulus. The normal consistency of the combined secretions of the tracheobronchial tree is 95% water, 2% glycoprotein, 1% carbohydrate, and less than 1% lipid.[2] Glycoproteins increase the viscosity of the secretions, providing protection and lubrication. Infection and chronic inflammatory diseases can have a profound effect on respiratory secretions. The glycoprotein component tends to be replaced by degradative products of inflammation such as DNA and actin.[17] Goblet cell numbers increase with a subsequent increase in the viscosity of respiration secretion. Parasympathetic, cholinergic stimulation increases mucus secretion, whereas β-adrenergic stimulation causes secretion of mucus, electrolytes, and water.[2,16]

KEYPOINT 20-2 The importance of the mucocilary escalator to treatment of respiratory disorders should not be underestimated. Its viscosity must be balanced if secretions and their entrapped materials are to be properly cleared from the airways.

The second major component of the pulmonary defense system is the respiratory mononuclear phagocyte system. In cats, calves, pigs, sheep, and goats, this includes both alveolar macrophages and the pulmonary intravascular macrophages (PIMs).[19] The PIMs are resident cells that are characterized by phagocytic properties and thus cause the release of inflammatory mediators. The clearance of blood-borne bacteria and particulate matter in these species is accomplished by PIMs rather than hepatic Kupffer cells and splenic macrophages as in most other species.[19] The pharmacologic significance of the mononuclear phagocyte system reflects their role in inflammation (Figure 20-3; see also Figure 20-1). A number of preformed (e.g., histamine and serotonin) and in situ (e.g., prostaglandins, leukotrienes, and platelet-activating factor [PAF]) mediators are released by inflammation cells.[13-15] Each is capable of inducing a variety of adverse effects that tend to decrease airway caliber size: edema, chemotaxis, increased mucus production, and bronchoconstriction (Table 20-1). The involvement of PIMs in both experimental and natural respiratory diseases of animals suggests that release of chemical mediators from these cells may be important in the pathogenesis of bronchial diseases.

KEYPOINT 20-3 The pulmonary intravascular macrophage system of cats may contribute to their predisposition to inflammatory respiratory diseases (compared with dogs).

SURFACTANT

The primary function of surfactant is to decrease surface tension in alveoli, affecting lung mechanics and gas exchange. However, pulmonary surfactant also affects pulmonary defense mechanisms.[20] Surfactant is a complex mixture of lipids and

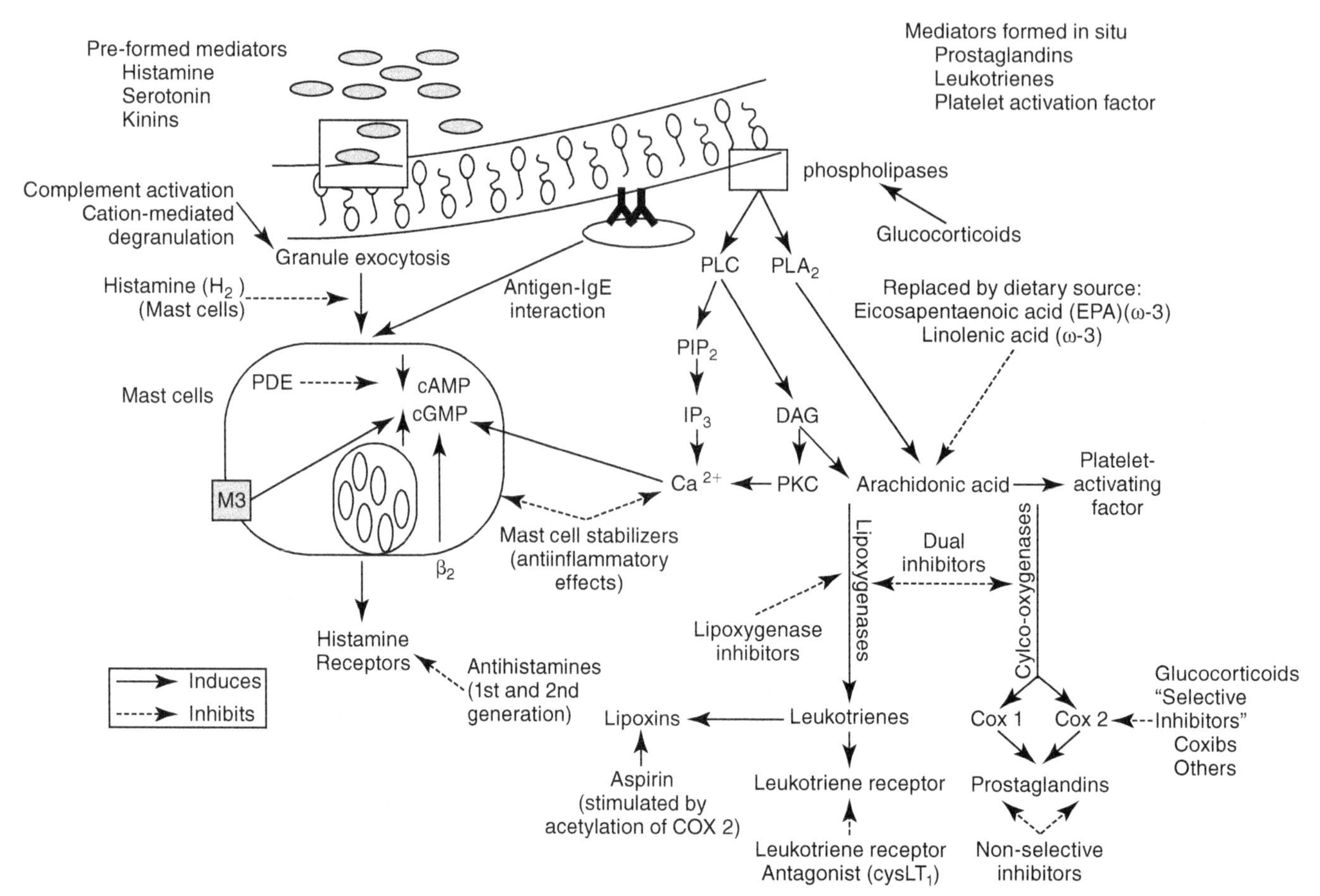

Figure 20-3 The formation of mediators important in the pathogenesis of respiratory disease. Leukocytes and other cells release arachidonic acid metabolites and platelet-activating factor (PAF) after activation of phospholipases by a variety of stimuli. Mast cell degranulation induced by both immune and nonimmune stimuli is also accompanied by arachidonic acid metabolism as well as by the release of preformed mediators that are stored in the granules. Intracellular mechanisms that induce mast cell degranulation include increased calcium (Ca^{2+}), increased cyclic guanosine nucleotide (cGMP) mediated by muscarinic (M_3) receptors, or decreased cyclic adenosine nucleotide (cAMP) mediated by α-adrenergic receptor stimulation. Drugs used to prevent mediator release include glucocorticoids, which are one of the few classes of drugs that can prevent activation of phospholipases (mediated by lipocortin) and thus release of arachidonic acid metabolites and PAF. Inhibition of prostaglandin synthesis by nonsteroidal antiinflammatory drugs may prove beneficial but also may lead to increased formation of leukotrienes by providing more arachidonic acid. Leukotriene actions can be blocked either by leukotriene receptor antagonists or by blockade of leukotriene receptors. Mast cell degranulation can be prevented by stimulation of β-adrenergic receptors, inhibition of calcium influx or phosphodiesterase (PDE), or prevention of M_3 receptor stimulation. Drugs that block β-adrenergic receptors are contraindicated in most respiratory diseases. *DAG,* diacylglycerol; *IP_3,* inositol triphosphate; *PIP_2,* phosphatidylinositol; *PKC,* protein kinase C; *PLC,* phospholipase C; *PLA_2,* phospholipase A_2.

proteins synthesized and secreted by alveolar type II cells with relative consistency among mammalian species.[20] In humans the proportion of components is predominantly phospholipids (80%) but includes proteins (12%) and other lipids (8%). The phospolipids principally comprise phosphatidylcholine (85%), the most important to reduction of surface tension being dipalmitoylated phosphatidylcholine (DPPC). Four surfactant-associated proteins (SP) are named A through D. Both SP-A and SP-D enhance phagycytosis of bacteria and viruses and regulate type II pneumocytes. The primary role of SP-B and SP-C is reduction of surface tension, particularly in terminal airways. A number of nonspecific host defense mechanisms have been attributed to surfactant.[20] Enhanced stability of the alveolar lining film allows it to serve as a nonspecific barrier to microorganism adhesion and subsequent pulmonary invasion. Muciliary transport is improved by its viscoelastic and rheologic properties. Particle clearance is enhanced, in part through an apparently stimulatory effect on chloride ion transport. Antiinflammatory effects reflect superoxide dismutase– and catalase-mediated oxygen radical scavenging and reduced neutrophil production of superoxide.[20,21] Direct antibacterial and antiviral properties have also been attributed to surfactant. Both SP-A and SP-D appear to provide a first line of defense by acting as collectins that target carbohydrate structures on a variety of pathogens. Alveolar macrophage response is increased by SP-A; SP-D enhances macrophage release of oxygen radicals. Cytokines (e.g., tumor necrosis factor [TNF]-α interleukin [IL]-1β, and IL-6) release is stimulated by SP-A.

Table 20-1 Inflammatory Mediators and Their Proposed or Known Role in Asthma

Class	Source	Targeted Therapy	Function
Lymphokines			**Cytokines of lymphocyte origin**
IL-2	CD4 (T_h2)	GLC	T cell growth and differentiation
IL-3*	CD4 (T_h2)	GLC	Hematopoietic growth factor
IL-4	CD4 (T_h2)	IL-4 antibodies; IL-4 receptor antagonists; GLC	T_h2 and eosinophil promotion; IgE synthesis; increased low affinity IgE receptor synthesis; increased VCAM-1
IL-5*	CD4 (T_h2)	IL-5 antibodies; IL-5 receptor antagonists; GLC	Eosinophil activation, maturation, and mobilization
IL-13	CD4 (T_h2)	GLC	Eosinophil activation, IgE synthesis
Chemokines			**Chemotactic cytokines**
IL-8	Epithelial cells	GLC	Inflammation amplification through neutrophil activation; histamine and LT release from basophils
RANTES†	Epithelial cells	CCR antibody	Inflammation amplification through eosinophil activation
MCP-1†, MCP-2, MCP-3†, MCP-4†		CCR antibody	Eosinophil chemoattraction
MIP-α			VCAM-1 upregulation
Eotaxin			Neutrophil activation; histamine and LT release from basophils; eosinophil mobilization (with IL-5)
Proinflammatory Cytokines			
IL-1	Macrophages	GLC	T-cell activation; T_h2 expansion; adhesion molecule (ICAM) upregulation
IL-6 T	Macrophages		T cell and B cell growth factor, IgE synthesis
TNF-alpha	Macrophages	Antibodies; inhibitors of TNF-converting enzyme inhibitors	Activation of antigen-presenting cells activated, epithelial cells and macrophages; increased airway hypersensitivity; adhesion molecule (ICAM-1) increase
GM-CSF*	Epithelial cells (and CD4 (T_h2)		Amplification of inflammation through antigen presentation; eosinophil activation;maturation and proliferation of hemopoietic cells; leukotriene induction
Antiinflammatory Cytokines			
IL-10	CD4 (T_h2)	Recombinant; GLC	Inhibition of proinflammatory cytokines (e.g., IL-2); promotion of T_h2 from T_h0 (in contrast to other antiinflammatory cytokines)
IL-12		Pending?	T_h1 promoted, T_h2 inhibited; IgE synthesis inhibited
IL-1ra	Monocytes, macrophages, epithelial cells	Pending (retinoic acid: decreased expression)?	T_h2 proliferation inhibited, IgE synthesis blocked
IFN-γ	Th1	Recombinant; GLC	Antigen presentation; T_h2 cells inhibited; eosinophil influx inhibited, macrophage and epithelial cells inhibited; Il-1-induced IgE synthesis inhibited
Adhesion Molecules			Cell-to-cell communication through integrin binding molecules
VCAM-1			Vascular (endothelial) adhesion to support eosinophil and lymphocyte movement
ICAM-1			Intracellular adhesion
MAdCAM-1			Mucosal adhesion molecule

Continued

Table 20-1 Inflammatory Mediators and Their Proposed or Known Role in Asthma—cont'd

Class	Source	Targeted Therapy	Function
Integrins			Cell-to-cell communication through binding of adhesion molecules
α4β1 (VLA-4)	Eosinophils	Receptor antibodies (natalizumab); receptor antagonists	Binds to VCAM-1; promotion of migration, activation, and increased survival of inflammatory cells.
α4β7	Eosinophils		Binds to VCAM-1 and MAdCAM; promotion of migration, activation, and increased survival of inflammatory cells.

IL, Interleukin; *CD*, cluster of differentiation 4; *GLC*, glucocorticoid; *IG*, immunoglobulin; *LT*, leukotriene; *MCP*, monocyte chemotactic protein; *MIP*, macrophage inflammatory protein; *CCR*, chemokine receptor; *VCAM*, vascular adhesion molecule; *ICAM*, intercellular adhesion molecule; *TNF*, tumor necrosis factor; *GM-CSF*, Granulocyte-macrophage colony-stimulating factor; *MAdCAM*, mucosal vascular cell adhesion molecule; *VLA:* very late antigen; *RANTES*, Regulated upon Activation Normal T-cell Expressed, and Secreted.
*Eosinophils also a possible source.
†CCR.

Changes in surfactant have been associated with a number of respiratory diseases. In humans acute respiratory distress syndrome (ARDS) is associated with changes in the biochemical and biophysical characteristics of surfactant. As a result, surface tension increases, and the phospholipid, fatty acid, and protein profiles change. Serum proteins and inflammatory mediators directly inhibit or degrade surfactant. Abnormalities in the amount and both the phospholipid and the protein composition of surfactant have been associated with infectious diseases of the lungs. The ability of surfactant to suppress immune-mediated lung injury has been interpreted as a possible role of surfactant dysfunction in asthma. Elastase-induced dysfunction and impaired SP-A and -D also may contribute to the surface destruction associated with chronic obstructive pulmonary disease (COPD) and emphysema.[20]

PATHOGENESIS OF INFLAMMATORY RESPIRATORY DISEASES

Although it is not the only chronic disease of the respiratory tract, feline bronchial asthma has offered a model for understanding pathophysiology and identifying targets of drug therapy. The interaction of sensory receptors and mediators of bronchial tone is intricately balanced in the normal lung. A series of pathologic disturbances, however, severely disrupts the balance in bronchial asthma.

Asthma is a pathologic state of the lungs characterized by marked bronchoconstriction and inflammation.[22-26] Although recent evidence is emerging that airway smooth muscle plays a role in asthma independent of inflammation,[27] the latter is an important contributor to disease and warrants a continued focus for drug therapy. Airways become hypersensitive to selected mediators (e.g., histamine and cholinergic stimulants).[5,10] The terms *allergy* and *atopy* are often used interchangeably; however, for this discussion *allergy* refers to an uncommitted biological response to an antigen. The pathophysiology of chronic allergic diseases is discussed in Chapter 31. *Atopy* refers to an allergic response characterized by immunoglobulin E (IgE)–mediated antibodies. Atopy generally reflects a genetic predisposition to IgE antibody production against environmental allergens. Most commonly, the allergic response is low grade and thus beneficial (removal of inciting allergen). However, in atopic patients the response, including IgE antibody production, is exaggerated. Asthma is one of several chronic atopic diseases characterized by an increasing incidence in human medicine; others include allergic rhinitis, atopic eczema, and inflammatory bowel disease.[28] Inflammatory mediators are the major contributors of the pathophysiology in asthma (see Table 20-1).[22,23,25,26,29,30] Studies in several species have shown that initial exposure to an allergen activate mast cells, macrophages, and other cells lining the airways, increasing mucosal epithelial permeability. Subsequent mediator release not only directly and intensely affects airway inflammation, contraction of smooth muscle, and capillary permeability but also initiates release of chemotactic factors, local infiltration of activated eosinophils, and activation of T cells.[31]

The critical role of T cells in the initiation and perpetuation of asthma has been well documented[32] and is supported by response in asthmatics to both glucocorticoids and cyclosporine.[32,33] The exaggerated response that characterizes the atopic patient appears to reflect an imbalance in T_h1 versus T_h2 helper cells. Researchers in human medicine have postulated that atopic individuals fail (possibly as infants) to transition from a T_h2-primary response (mediated by ILs 4, 5, and 13) to an "allergy protective" T_h1-mediated primary response. The T_h1 response is dominated by cell-mediated immunity, and delayed hypersensitivity (cytotoxic T cells) is initiated through macrophage production of IL-12 followed by production of interferon (IFN)-γ by T_h1 and natural killer cells. In normal infants the shift from T_h2 to Th1 might be stimulated by exposure to a variety of antigens, including microbes with cytosine and guanosine nucleotides (CpG repeats). The hygiene hypothesis suggests that atopy develops because subjects are not sufficiently exposed to allergens at a young age, perhaps as a result of early use of antimicrobials or lack of exposure to allergens (e.g., children exposed to one another at day care, or environmental factors [e.g., farms]).[28] The T_h2 response that characterizes inflammatory disease is associated with increased production of IL-4, IL-5, and IL-13. The IL-4 from T_h2 supports B-cell IgE synthesis. The T_h2 cells have a particular influence on eosinophils through IL-5, which regulates both differentiation and bone marrow release (mature and immature cells), and the chemokine eotaxin.[28] Subsequent accumulation of eosinophils in atopic tissue is influenced by continued recruitment by eotaxins, the presence of selective adhesion molecules, and delayed apoptosis.[28]

KEYPOINT 20-4 The inflammation associated with chronic allergic respiratory disease may reflect an imbalance between Th_1 and $T h_2$ cells.

The role of the bone marrow in the pathophysiology of atopy increasingly is emerging as potential target, leading to a systemic rather than local approach to therapy.[34] Signaling appears to occur between the lung and bone marrow, with IL-5 and/or eotaxin being the commonality.[35] Increased IL-3 may also play a role in eosinophil stimulation, whereas IL-18, IL-12, and INF-γ are inhibitory toward eosinophils.[28,36] In animal models of asthma, including the canine *Ascaris* model, allergen exposure is associated with an increase in bone marrow eosinophils and trafficking from the bone marrow to the lungs.[37] Interestingly, cysteinyl leukotrienes may influence eosinophil differentiation (in the presence of IL-3 or IL-5); leukotriene-receptor antagonists are able (in vitro) to suppress eosinophil differentiation.[37,38]

Eosinophils contribute to mucosal damage through release of basic amines, cysteinyl leukotrienes, and PAF.[28] Inhibitory muscarinic (M_2) receptors are damaged, which facilitates persistent bronchoconstriction. Mediators are released following binding of allergens with the α chain of high-affinity IgE receptor (Fc€ RIα) on the cell. Regulation of IgE, which is found both on and in eosinophils, offers another potential target of therapy. IL-4 and IL-13 are the most important inducers of IgE production.[28]

As permeability increases in response to inflammation, histamine and other inflammatory mediators are better able to reach and stimulate inflammatory cells located in the submucosa. The continued release of mediators is associated with stimulation of afferent nerve endings in the mucosa and reflex cholinergic bronchoconstriction. Mediators also increase microvascular permeability, induce chemotaxis, and stimulate mucous secretion. The release of cytotoxic proteins and toxic oxygen radicals further damages the respiratory epithelium, and the bronchial tree becomes hypersensitive. Mediators can also inhibit mucociliary function.[25] Mucus production increases as submucosal glands and goblet cells increase. The consistency of the mucus changes to become more viscous. Bronchial smooth muscle often hypertrophies and undergoes spasms.[39] Airway obstruction in chronic disease reflects bronchoconstriction, bronchial wall edema, and accumulation of mucus and cells. As the disease progresses, airways eventually become plugged and ultimately collapse. Chronic inflammation leads to fibrosis, which contributes to the collapse, and air trapped within the alveoli can result in emphysema. Asthma is a disease of central and large as well as small (<2 mm) airways.[40] Regarding the type of asthma previously considered "silent," studies in humans have revealed the importance of a therapeutic focus on airways beyond the eighth or ninth generation of the bronchial tree. In humans asthma and allergic rhinitis commonly, but not always, co-exist,[40] and allergens associated with rhinitis may be too large to penetrate the lower airways.[41]

The complex physiology of asthma is exemplified by the reparative role that eosinophils also have. Damage repair contributes to airway remodeling through release of growth factors and matrix metalloproteinases.

INFLAMMATORY MEDIATORS IN THE RESPIRATORY TRACT

Histamine

Histamine is a vasoactive amine stored in basophils and mast cells. Airway mast cells are located primarily beneath the epithelial basement membrane in dogs.[24] Histamine produces a variety of effects (see Table 20-1) by interacting with specific receptors on target cells.[12,42] At least four histamine receptors have been identified,[5,29,43,44] two of which have been found in the trachea of the cat.[5,6] Interaction with the H_1 receptor causes an increase in intracellular calcium, and ultimately in cGMP (see Figure 20-3).[29] Histamine also stimulates cholinergic receptors in the airway.[24,29] Histamine causes constriction in both central and peripheral airways in dogs and cats.[12,24] The effects of histamine so closely mimic the pathophysiology of early asthma that, for many years, histamine was considered the major cause of the syndrome.[29] Lack of clinical response to H_1-receptor antagonists, however, led to the realization that other factors are more important. In contrast to H_1 receptors, stimulation of H_2 receptors causes an increase in cAMP and bronchodilation.[29] Thus antihistamine drugs that block H_2 receptors may be contraindicated in asthma. Some studies have suggested that a defect in H_2 receptors may contribute to airway hyperreactivity.[29] Finally, recent evidence suggests that histamine regulates both T_h1 and T_h2 cells. Further, cells perpetuating the allergic response may be influenced by histamine through H_4 receptors located on eosinophils, basophils, mast cells, and dendritic cells.[43]

Histamine contributes to bronchial occlusion by mechanisms other than bronchoconstriction. Mucous secretion is mediated via H_2 receptors and by secretion of ions and water via H_1 receptors.[29] Microvascular leakage resulting from contraction of endothelial cells also follows H_1-receptor stimulation.[29] Histamine is chemotactic to inflammatory cells, particularly eosinophils and neutrophils. Interestingly, histamine stimulates T-lymphocyte suppressor cells by way of H_2 receptors,[5] a function that also may be depressed in human patients with asthma.[29] Histamine also has a negative feedback effect on further histamine release mediated by IgE.[29] Both of these latter effects are mediated by H_2 receptors and would be inhibited by H_2-receptor antagonists.[5]

Serotonin

Serotonin (5-hydroxytryptamine [5-HT]) is released during mast cell degranulation.[29] Although serotonin does not appear to be an important mediator of human or canine bronchial asthma, both the central and peripheral airways in cats are very sensitive to its bronchoconstrictive effects after aerosolization or intravenous administration.[12] Constriction may reflect interaction with serotonin receptors or enhanced release of acetylcholine. Serotonin may also cause profound vasoconstriction of the pulmonary vasculature and microvascular leakage.[29]

Prostaglandins and Leukotrienes

Prostaglandins (PGs) and leukotrienes (LTs) are eicosanoids that are formed when phospholipase A_2 is activated in the cell membrane in response to a variety of stimuli (see Figure 20-3). Arachidonic acid (AA) is subsequently released from phospholipids and enters the cell. In the cell it is converted by cyclooxygenases to inflammatory, but unstable, cyclic endoperoxides. The actions of various synthetases and isomerases on the endoperoxides result in the final PG products, including PGE_2, $PGF_{2\alpha}$, PGD_2, prostacyclin (or PGI_2), and thromboxane (TXA_2). The amount of each PG produced in the lung varies with the cell type and species. The effects of the various PGs tend to balance one another. PGD_2, $PGF_{2\alpha}$, and TXA_2 cause bronchoconstriction, whereas PGE_1 and, to a lesser extent PGI_1, cause bronchodilation.[1,29] Bronchoconstriction induced by PGD_2 is about 30 times as potent as that induced by histamine.

Imbalances between PGs may be important in the pathogenesis of bronchial disease. Both PGD_2 and TXA_2 have been implicated in immediate bronchial airway hyperreactivity.[29] Thromboxane A_2 appears to be the predominant AA metabolite produced by feline lungs,[45] although other PG mediators are also important.[45]

The role of LTs in atopy has been increasingly scrutinized in recent years. Lipoxygenases catalyze the conversion of AA to hydroperoxyeicosatetraenoic acid (HPETEs), which are further metabolized to several hydroxy acids (HETEs) and LTs (Chapter 29). Eosinophils have been known to be preferentially activated 5-lipoxygenase[29]; selective activation of lipoxygenase by antigenic challenge yields subsequent formation of the cysteinyl LTs (cystLTs: LTB_4 C_4, and D_4), recognized as the components of slow reactive substance of anaphylaxis.[29] However, both intermediate and end products of lipoxygenase are active in the respiratory tract (see Table 20-1).[29] Among these mediators are some of the most potent inflammagens known. For example, bronchial smooth muscle contraction and microvascular permeability mediated by LTC_4 and LTD_4 is 100- to 1000-fold more potent than that induced by histamine. Both LTs are potent stimulators of mucous release in the dog but appear to be less potent in the cat.[29] In humans airway allergen challenge increases LTs in urine and bronchoalveolar lavage (BAL) fluid with asthma and nasal secretions with allergic rhinitis.[35] Increases in LTs in plasma, BAL fluid, or urine of challenged cats is controversial, although cats experimentally infected with dirofilariasis likewise exhibited increased plasma as well as BAL fluid cysLT concentrations (unpublished data). The cysteinyl LTs exert biologic effects through cysLT1 and cysLT2 receptors.[35] Binding by LTs to eosinophilic cysL1 receptors (particularly LTD4) results in chemotaxis and prolonged survival, effects that are blocked by LT-receptor antagonists.[35] Further evidence suggests that cysteinyl LTs are also involved in the initial systemic atopic response that is mediated from the bone marrow.[35,46]

Platelet-Activating Factor

PAF is also formed after activation of phospholipase A_2 in cell membranes. It is a potent, dose-independent constrictor of human airways, and it is the most potent agent thus far discovered in causing airway microvascular leakage.[22,23] PAF is also a potent chemotactant for platelets and eosinophils, both of which are a rich source of PAF. The effects of PAF may be mediated through LTs. PAF has been implicated as the cause of the sustained bronchial hyperresponsiveness that characterizes asthmatics.[23] The role of PAF in feline and canine respiratory diseases has not been addressed. Eosinophils are, however, a major cell type associated with feline bronchial disease and some canine diseases, and it is likely that PAF is an important inflammatory mediator.

REACTIVE OXYGEN SPECIES

Reactive oxygen species (ROS) are constantly formed in the lung as part of pulmonary defense toward microorganisms and neoplasm.[21] Free oxygen radicals, hydrogen peroxide and hypochlorous acid are among the species formed. Their formation is mediated, in part, by other inflammatory mediators such as TNF, IL-1, IL-6, and IL-8, and AA derivatives (PGs, LTs, and PAF). Hyperoxia will enhance generation of ROS.[21] Normal cells are generally protected from ROS by a tightly controlled redox balance and formation of endogenous antioxidants; formation is enhanced by exposure to antioxidants. Those located primarily intraceullularly include catalase, superoxide dismutase, and glutathione redox compounds (glutathione, glutathione peroxidase, and glutathione reductase). Primarily extracellular antioxidants include fat-soluble compounds (vitamin E), water-soluble compounds (vitamin C, cysteine, reduced glutathione, taurine), and high-molecular-weight antioxidants (mucus and albumin).[21]

Neuropeptides

Several chemicals stimulate release of inflammatory neuropeptides from sensory neurons enervating smooth muscles. Cells stimulating neuropeptide release include macrophages, T-cells, eosinophils, and mast cells; example neuropeptides include substance P and, to a lesser degree, calcitonin gene-related peptide and neurokinin A.[47] As with other inflammatory mediators, neuropeptides are associated with vasodilation, increased permeability and mucus production, as well as histamine release.

Cytokines

The role of cytokines in the coordination and persistence of chronic airway inflammation is integral and, not surprisingly, very complex. The integrated nature of their actions renders them simultaneously ideal as targets of drug therapy but potentially a source of adverse events should therapy be successful. Four cytokine classes have been proposed: lymphokines, chemokines, and proinflammatory and antiinflammatory cytokines (see Table 20-1). The role of lymphokines was largely addressed with the discussion of T_h cell role in atopy. Initiation of T_h2 cells is not clear, but appears to involve presentation of restricted antigens in the presence of IL-4 and IL-10. Perhaps the most notable lymphokine of asmtha is IL-5.[48] Recruitment of eosinophils into the lungs—the hallmark of asthma—is IL-5 dependent. However, IL-5 also is integral to the differentiation, proliferation, and maturation of eosinophil progenitor cells in the bone marrow before recruitment into the lung.

Chemokines are cytokines that attract inflammatory cells, including eosinophils, monocytes, and T-lymphocytes. Two groups have been described based on proximity of cysteine residues to one another: CXC or α chemokines (separated by an amino-acid) and CC or β-chemokines (no separation; see Table 20-1). Chemokines exert their effects through rhodopsin-like G protein–coupled receptors (referred to as CXC-R or CC-R). Because certain cells express selected receptors, pharmacologic therapy increasingly will be designed to be selectively antiinflammatory.[31] Among the cells influenced by chemokines are eosinophils, which in turn release more chemokines. Among the most notable drugs targeting proinflammatory chemokines, and particularly their transcription, are glucocorticoids (see Chapter 30). Newer therapies take advantage of the presence of antiinflammatory cytokines; indeed, glucocorticoids facilitate restoration of antiinflammatory cytokines such as IL-10.

Communication Molecules: Adhesion Molecules and Integrins

Communication between cells is facilitated by adhesion molecules that interact, by way of ligand binding, with receptors on the surface of inflammatory cells known as *integrins*. Integrins are present on many cells, with receptor specificity occurring for selective cells. Integrins are absent on T_h1 cells but are particularly prevalent on T_h2 cells, mast cells, and eosinophils. Interaction between adhesion molecules and integrins promotes migration, activation, and increased survival of inflammatory cells. Drugs that target eosinophilic integrins ($\alpha 4\beta 1$ and 7) offer a possible mechanism whereby selective control of inflammation may limit side effects.[49]

DRUGS USED TO MODULATE THE RESPIRATORY TRACT

The syndrome of chronic bronchial disease is best treated by breaking the inflammatory cycle while immediately relieving bronchoconstriction. Thus antiinflammatory drugs and bronchodilators represent the cornerstone of therapy for many bronchial diseases. Other categories of drugs that are effective for the management of respiratory diseases, particularly in small animals, include antitussives, respiratory stimulants, and decongestants.

Bronchodilators and Anti-Inflammatory Drugs

Because of a shared intracellular mechanism of action, most drugs that induce bronchodilation also reduce inflammation. Bronchodilators reverse airway smooth muscle contraction by increasing cAMP, decreasing cGMP, or decreasing calcium ion concentration (see Figure 20-1). In addition, these drugs also decrease mucosal edema and are antiinflammatory because they tend to prevent mediator release from inflammatory cells (see Figure 20-3). Rapidly acting bronchodilators include β-receptor agonists, methylxanthines, and cholinergic antagonists.

β-Receptor Agonists

β-receptor agonists (Figure 20-4) are the most effective bronchodilators because they act as functional antagonists of airway constriction, regardless of the stimulus.[22,50,51] Few β-agonists generally have been sufficiently studied in animals to describe pharmacokinetics or pharmacodynamics.

Large numbers of β_2-receptors are located on several cell types in the lung, including smooth muscle and inflammatory cells.[3] The receptor is linked to a stimulatory guanine nucleotide-binding protein (G protein). The interaction between a β-agonist and receptor causes a conformational change in the receptor and subsequent activation of adenylyl cyclase on the inner cell membrane (see Figure 20-1).[52] Adenylate cyclase converts adenosine triphosphate to cAMP, a second messenger for activation of specific protein kinases that ultimately activate enzymes responsible for airway smooth muscle relaxation. β-receptor agonists are most effective in states of bronchoconstriction. Additional effects of β-adrenergic receptors include increased mucociliary clearance, which reflects a decrease in fluid viscosity (presumed to reflect movement of chloride and water into the lumen) and an increase in ciliary beat frequency. Additionally, they inhibit cholinergic neurotransmission, enhance vascular integrity, and inhibit mediator release from mast cells, basophils, and other cells (see Figure 20-3).[22,23,51,52] Eosinophil, but not lymphocyte, numbers appear to decrease, but long-term inflammation does not appear to be affected,[52] probably because inflammatory cell β receptors are rapidly desensitized (discussed later). As such, long-term β-adrenergic use should be accompanied by antiinflammatory therapy.[41]

As with many membrane-associated receptors, high doses or repeated exposure to β-adrenergic agonists results in desensitization.[51] The mechanism depends on the duration of therapy. Initial drug–receptor interaction causes phosphorylation, which interferes with G proteins. Longer exposure causes receptors to internalize such that they are not accessible by the drug; continued exposure causes downregulation of receptor mRNA such that the number of receptors is actually reduced.[52] Reduction develops over several weeks before stabilizing. Desensitization may contribute to acute exacerbations of bronchoconstriction associated with long-acting β-adrenergics. Bronchodilation will be less in the desensitized airway necessitating increased treatment frequency. However, frequent use may mask clinical signs associated with uncontrolled inflammation and care must be taken that long-acting β-adrenergics are not used instead of antiinflammatory therapy. Despite these shortcomings, β-adrenergics are the most the most effective bronchodilators.

The β-adrenergic agonists (see Figure 20-4) can be given by a variety of routes. In humans inhalation is preferred because it is equally effective to parenteral administration and is safer. However, drug delivery to the peripheral airways must be addressed as much as possible.

Nonselective β-Agonists

The nonselective β-agonists (i.e., capable of both β_1 and β_2 stimulation) such as epinephrine, ephedrine, and isoproterenol are used for acute and chronic therapy of respiratory diseases. Epinephrine and isoproterenol can be administered parenterally to achieve rapid effects, and drugs that can be given orally for chronic therapy include isoproterenol and ephedrine.[6] Both epinephrine and ephedrine cause α-adrenergic activity, which may cause vasoconstriction and systemic hypertension and *may* contribute to airway constriction.[4] Nonselective β-agonists may cause adverse cardiac effects as a result of β_1-receptor stimulation. Aerosolization reduces the adverse effects of nonselective β-adrenergic agonists by increasing β_2 specificity, because only these β-receptors appear to line the airways.

β_2-Selective Agonists

At appropriate doses, β-selective agonists are not generally associated with the undesirable effects of β_1-adrenergic stimulation. The more commonly used β-agonists are categorized as to their duration of action: intermediate (3 to 6 hours) and long-acting (>12 hours). The two long-acting bronchodilators, salmeterol and formoterol, both have extended side chains, are highly lipophilic, and are characterized by high affinity for the β-2 receptors. However, the long duration of salmeterol reflects binding to a specific site within the receptor, whereas that for formoterol reflects gradual release from the cell membrane lipid.[52] The long-acting nature of bitolterol reflects its pulmonary metabolism to an active metabolite. However, it has a rapid onset of action and generally is used for acute therapy.

KEY POINT 20-5 Beta-adrenergic agonists are such effective bronchodilators that they may mask signs of inflammation that indicate ongoing disease.

Short-acting drugs that have been used in animals include albuterol, metaprotereno (a derivative of isoproterenol), and its analog terbutaline.[41] Metaproterenol is less β-2 selective

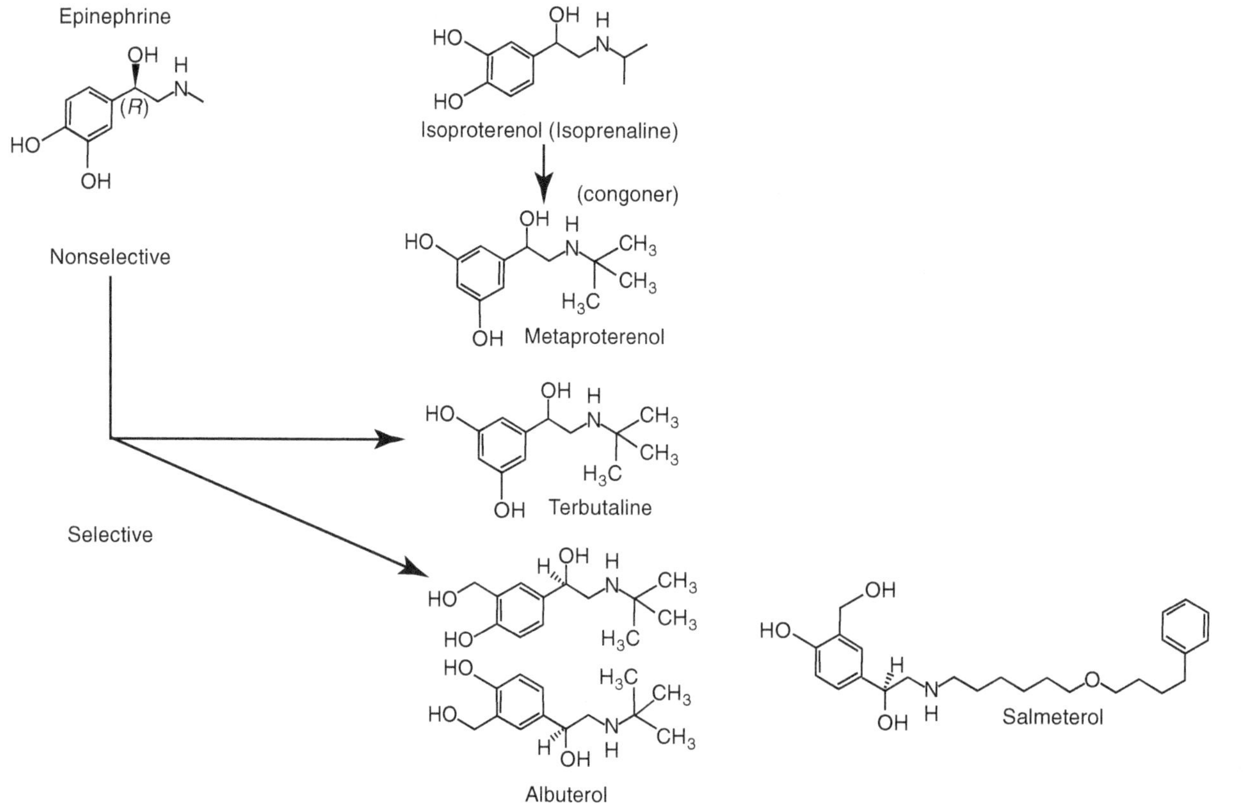

Figure 20-4 Structures of selected beta-adrenergic drugs used to induce bronchodilation. Epinephrine is the least and albuterol or terbutaline the most selective for β-2 receptors. Most β-adrenergic drugs are present as enantiomers, as is demonstrated here for albuterol.

than other agents and more apt to cause cardiac stimulation.[52] Therefore repetitive use should be pursued only cautiously. Albuterol, metaproterenol and terbutaline are available as oral preparations; each has been used apparently safely in dogs. Rapid first-pass metabolism reduces systemic bioavailability after oral administration; as such, oral doses are greater than parenteral doses. These drugs, but particularly metaproterenol, can cause β_1 side effects at high doses. Clenbuterol, also a β-2 selective agonist, is approved for use in horses. Although manufactured as the racemic mixture, pharmacologic effects are largely limited to the L-isomer.[53] Tachycardia occurs in dogs at 0.4 mg/kg, which is only half of the therapeutic dose recommended in horses. Further, cardiac necrosis occurs at 2.5 mg/kg, which represents only a threefold increase over the equine therapeutic dose. Consequently, use of clenbuterol in dogs may not be prudent. Albuterol and isoetharine are examples of β_2-selective agonists that have been administered by aerosolization to small animals.[30] Salbutamol is frequently used as a rescue bronchodilator in humans.[54]

Inhalant Devices

With the advent of metered doses inhalers in the 1960s, beta-adrenergics became a common therapy for treatment of human asthma. Short-acting β_2 agonists administered by aerosol (Figure 20-5) include albuterol and its R enantiomer levalbuterol, metaproteronol, pirbuterol, bitolterol, and terbutaline (see Figure 20-4). Longer-acting (in humans) beta-2 adrenergic drugs tend to be more lipophilic and thus remain in the presence of a receptor for a longer time. Examples include salmeterol and formoterol (see Figure 20-4).[40,41,55] The drugs differ in their effect and use. Short-acting products are associated with rapid symptomatic relief in human asthmatics when used at appropriate doses. However, use at high doses has been associated with an increase in mortality in humans, leading to their recommended use on an "only as needed" basis.[40,55] On the other hand, improvement in pulmonary function in humans was sustained with prolonged used of long-acting beta-adrenergics,[55] and thus such use was not associated with a decrease in symptomatic relief afforded by short-acting drugs. The duration of onset of long-acting beta-adrenergics may be 1 or more hours. Although minimally effective by themselves for control of inflammation, long-acting beta-adrenergics appear to enhance responsiveness to glucocorticoids. Rebound hyperresponsiveness does not appear to occur with rapid discontinuation of the long-acting drugs. The development of tolerance (desensitization) has been discussed and is probably more likely with long-acting drugs.[41] Because beta-adrenergics do not provide as much antiinflammatory control, their efficacy may be reduced in the presence of inflammation and combination therapy with an antiinflammatory drug (e.g., inhaled or systemic glucocorticoids), or use of theophylline may be indicated.[40,55]

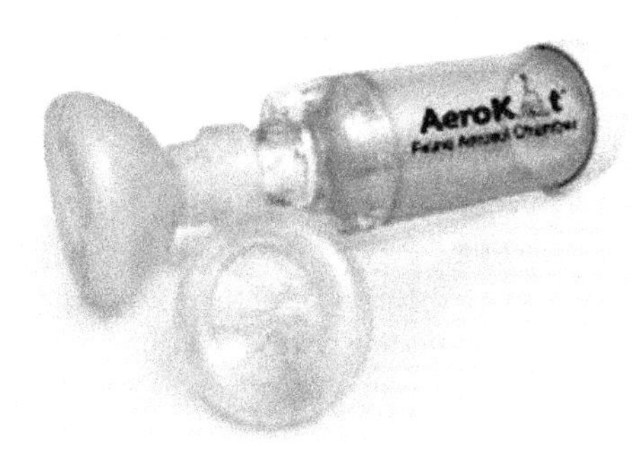

Figure 20-5 An example of a device commercially available, intended as an adapter for inhalant metered dose devices marketed for human use.

Drugs that block β_2-receptors such as propranolol are contraindicated in animals with bronchial disease. Inhalant devices are discussed more in depth in the following section.

Methylxanthine Derivatives

Pharmacologic Effects

Methylxanthines include caffeine, a potent respiratory stimulant, and theobromine, a recognized canine toxicant from chocolate and theophylline (Figure 20-6). Theophylline has been the cornerstone of long-term bronchodilatory therapy in animals,

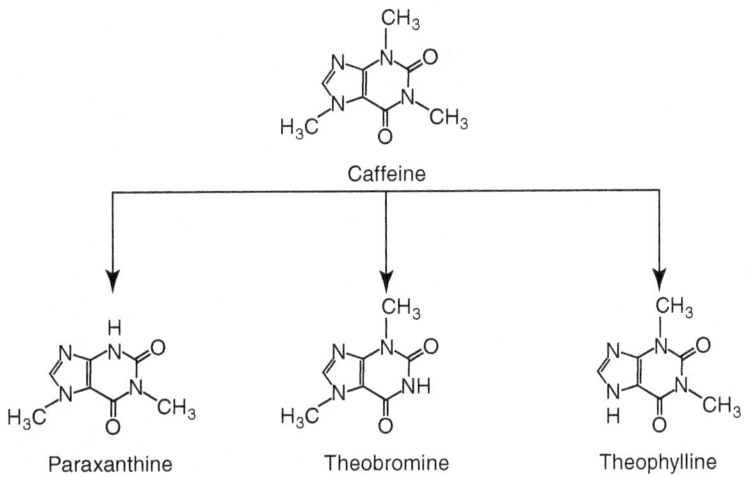

Caffeine

Paraxanthine Theobromine Theophylline

Figure 20-6 Caffeine, which is used as a respiratory stimulant in humans, is metabolized to other methylxanthines, theobromine, theophylline, and paraxanthine.

particularly dogs. Its mode of action has been attributed to nonspecific inhibition of phosphodiesterases (PDEs) and increased concentrations of cAMP and cGMP (see Figure 20-1).[41,56] This mechanism has been controversial, however, because theophylline does not inhibit PDE at therapeutic concentrations. However, this may reflect the existence of PDE as various isoenzymes (at least 11 members to this superfamily, each located in different sites within the cell, some of which are inaccessible to drugs).[22,23,41] Inhibition of PDE4 and PDE5 results in bronchodilation whereas inhibition of PDE4 contributes to its antiinflammatory effects.[41] The nonselective action of theophylline results in bronchodilation and inhibition of inflammation. Theophylline also is a competitive antagonist at adenosine receptors. The inhibitory neurotransmitter adenosine, which induces bronchoconstriction and during hypoxia and inflammation. Another mechanism by which theophylline induces bronchodilation, however, may be through interference of calcium mobilization.[22,23]

Compared to beta-2 agonists, theophylline is considered a weaker relaxant of airway smooth muscle.[40] As with β-agonists, theophylline is equally effective in large and small airways. Theophylline has other effects in the respiratory system that are important to its clinical efficacy.[22,23,56] In addition to its bronchodilatory effects, it inhibits mast cell degranulation and thus mediator release (see Figure 20-3)[57]; increases mucociliary clearance; and prevents microvascular leakage.[58] Its antinflammatory effects appear to include modulation of cytokines, particularly of macrophage origin.[59] Finally, antiinflammatory effects of theophylline may also reflect nuclear activation of histone deacetylase.[41] Decreased TNF-α and IFN-γ and increased IL-10 (antiinflammatory) have been reported. Pentoxifylline has similar antiinflammatory effects; its IV administration is addressed in Chapter 29. Increased mucociliary clearance has been reported in dogs.[60] In propofol-anesthetized cats (n = 6), no treatment effect could be detected in the mucociliary transport rate after oral administration of 25 mg/kg of a slow release (Slo-bid) product. The ability to detect a significant difference was not addressed. Further, the mucociliary the rate in untreated animals (22.2 ± 2.8 mm/min) was perceived to be maximal, leaving no room for theophylline-induced increase. The impact of propofol is not clear, and theophyllline concentrations were not measured to confirm adequate concentrations. Thus the lack of efficacy may not reflect theophylline as much as failed delivery or altered response.

In addition to its antiinflammatory effects, a major advantage of theophylline, compared with other bronchodilators, may be its increased strength of respiratory muscles and thus a decrease in the work associated with breathing.[56,62,63] This may be important to animals with chronic bronchopulmonary disease.

Disposition

Theophylline is one of the few drugs active in the respiratory tract whose disposition has been studied in animals. Because theophylline is not water soluble, it can be given only orally. Salt preparations of theophylline are available for either oral or parenteral administration. Dosing of the various salt preparations must be based on the amount of active theophylline (Table 20-2). Aminophylline, an ethylenediamine salt, is 80% theophylline, whereas oxtriphylline is 65% theophylline, and glycinate and salicylate salts are only 50% theophylline. Regular aminophylline is well absorbed (bioavailability of at least 90%) after oral administration in both dogs and cats.[64,65] In dogs peak plasma drug concentrations for the theophylline base (approximately 8 μg/mL after a dose of 9.4 mg/kg) occur 1.5 hours after oral administration.[64] The volume of distribution (L/kg) and clearance (mL/min/kg) in dogs are, respectively, 0.59 ± 0.045 and 0.78 ± 0.13. The extrapolated peak concentration after intravenous administration of 11 mg/kg aminophylline (8.6 mg/kg theophylline equivalent) was 22.94 ± 5.8 μg/mL.[66] In cats extrapolated concentrations after 10 mg/kg intravenous aminophylline approximated 10 μg/mL; volume of distribution (L/kg) and clearance (mL/min/kg) were 0.87 ± 0.07 and 0.87 ± 0.16, respectively.[67] Interestingly, peak concentrations after intravenous or oral (sustained-release) products are higher in cats when dosed in the evening compared with the morning.[68]

More than 30 slow-release preparations exist for use in humans. Although several products have been studied in dogs and cats,[68,69] their disposition is markedly variable and cannot be predicted on the basis of product name or description. Interchangability of products *cannot* be assumed, and monitoring is strongly encouraged to establish potential efficacy. For dogs, the rate of oral absorption of slow-release products is apparently faster than in humans. The extent of absorption varies with the preparation. Bioavailability of slow-release preparations varies from 30% (anhydrous theophylline 24-hour capsules; Theo-24, Searle Laboratories) to 76% (anhydrous theophylline tablets; TheoDur).[69] The least variation among animals occurs for oxtriphylline enteric-coated capsules (Choledyl-SA Tablets; Parke-Davis) and a 12-hour capsular anhydrous theophylline (Slo-Bid Gyrocaps), which are approximately 60% bioavailable. The minimum effective concenteration recommended for humans (10 μg/mL) may not be reached by all slow-release products. Plasma drug concentrations during a 12-hour dosing interval varies, by almost 120% for the oxtriphylline product but only 48% for the anhydrous tablet (Theo-Dur), suggesting it may be the best product for use in dogs.[69] However, neither Theo-Dur nor Slo-Bid Gyrocaps are currently available for use in the United States. Although the mean residence time of the slow-release preparation was significantly longer by 1 to 2 hours than that of the regular preparation in dogs, the clinical significance of this difference is questionable.[69] More recently, Bach and coworkers[66] described the disposition of a generic (Inwood Laboratories) extended-release theophylline tablet (Theochron) or capsule (TheoCap) in dogs (15.5 mg/kg orally; n = 6). The oral bioavailability (%) of the tablet and capsules was 98 ± 15.4 and 83.6 ± 18.5%, respectively. The C_{max} (μg/mL) was 17.4 ± 4.9 and 12.2 ± 2.8 for the tablet and capsule, respectively, whereas the elimination half-life was 10.9 ± 3.6 and 12.7 ± 2.7. Drug concentrations remained within the recommended therapeutic range for 12 hours. The authors concluded that 10 mg/kg every 12 hours would result in theophylline concentrations in the therapeutic range.

Table 20-2 Doses of Drugs Used To Treat Disorders of the Respiratory Tract

Drug	Indicators	Dose	Route	Interval (hr)*
Acetylcysteine	Respiratory inflammation	3-6 mL/hr for 30-60 min (D)	Nebulization	12
		125-500 mg	IV, PO	12
Albuterol	Bronchodilator	0.02-0.05 mg/kg	PO	8-12 × 10 days
		1-3 puffs	Metered dose inhaler	12 to 24
Aminophylline	Bronchodilator	5-11 mg/kg (D)	IM, IV, PO	8-12
		4-6.6 mg/kg (C)	PO	8-12
		2-5 mg/kg (C)	IV (slow)	12
Bitolterol	Bronchodilation	1-3 puffs	Metered dose inhaler	12 to 24
Butorphanol	Antitussive	0.05-0.12 mg/kg (D)	PO, SC	8-12
		0.55-1.1 mg/kg (D)	PO	6-12
Cetirizine	Antihistamine, allergies	0.15-5 mg/kg	PO	12
		5 mg/cat	PO	12
		2.5-10 mg/dog	PO	12-24
Chlorpheniramine maleate	Antihistamine	2-8 mg/dog	PO	8-12
		2-4 mg/dog	PO	12-24
	Behavioral disorders, excessive grooming, self-trauma	2-4 mg/dog	PO	12
	Mild sedation	0.22 mg/kg (D)	PO	8-12
		1-2 mg/kg (C)	PO	8-12
Clemastine	Antihistamine, allergic skin disease	0.05-0.5 mg/kg (D)	PO	12
		0.34-0.67 mg/cat	PO	12
	Atopy	0.15 mg/kg (C)	PO	12
Codeine	Cough	0.1-2 mg/kg (D)	PO	6-12
Cylcosporine	Chronic allergic diseases: asthma	4-6 mg/kg	PO	12 to 24; monitor
Cyproheptadine hydrochloride	Antihistamine	1.1 mg/kg (D)	PO	8-12
Dexamethasone	Asthma	Initial dose: 1 mg/kg	IV	Once
		Maintenance dose: 0.25-1 mg/cat	PO	8-24
Dextromethorphan	Antitussive	0.5-2 mg/kg (D)	IV, PO, SC	6-8
Diphenhydramine	Antihistamine	2-4 mg/kg	PO	6-8
Diphenoxylate (contains atropine)	Antitussive	0.2-0.5 mg (D)	PO	12
Doxylamine succinate	Antihistamine	1.1-2.2 mg/kg	IM, PO, SC	8-12
Doxapram	Respiratory stimulant	1-5 mg/kg	IV	As needed
	Neonate	1-2 drops	Sublingual	To effect
		0.1 mL or 10 mg/m^2	IV (umbilical vein)	To effect
Ephedrine	Bronchodilator, decongestant	2-5 mg/cat	PO	8-12
		1-2 mg/kg (D)	PO	8-12
Fexofenadine	Allergies, antihistamine	30 mg/kg (D)	PO	12
Fluticasone proprionate	Asthma	222 µg (1 puff)	Metered dose inhaler	12 to 24 or to effect
Formoterol	Bronchodilator	1-3 puffs	Metered dose inhaler	12 to 24
Hydrocodone bitartrate	Antitussive	0.25 mg/kg. Maximum of 1 mg/kg (D)	PO	6-8
		2.5-5 mg/cat	PO	8-12. Use with caution
Hydroxyzine hydrochloride or pamoate	Antihistamine, allergic skin disease	2.2 mg/kg (D)	PO	6-12

Continued

Table 20-2 Doses of Drugs Used To Treat Disorders of the Respiratory Tract—cont'd

Drug	Indicators	Dose	Route	Interval (hr)*
Hydroxyzine hydrochloride or pamoate		5-10 mg/cat	PO	12
		1-2 mg/kg	PO	8-12
Isopropamide/prochlorperazine	Bronchodilator	0.2 mg in 100 mL 5% D/W	IV	To effect at 8 hours
		0.004-0.006 mg/cat	IM	30 min as needed
		0.44 mg/kg (C)	PO	6-12
		0.5 mL of 1:200 dilution	Inhalant	4
Megestrol acetate	Asthma	5 mg/cat	PO	24 × 4 months, then once per week × 4 weeks
Metaproterenol sulfate	Bronchodilator	0.325-0.65 mg/kg	PO	4-6
Montelukast	Chronic allergic diseases (asthma, atopy, inflammatory bowel disease)	0.5-1 mg/kg	PO	24
Morphine SO_8	Antitussive	0.1 mg/kg (D)	SC	6-12
Morphine SO_9	Antitussive	0.05-0.1 mg/kg (C)	IM, SC	4-6
Noscapine	Cough, nonproductive	0.5-1 mg/kg	PO	6-8
Oxtriphylline	Bronchodilator	14 mg/kg (D)	PO	6-8
		30 mg/kg (D)	PO	12 (sustained-release formulation)
		6 mg/kg (C)	PO	8-12
		10-15 mg/kg	PO	6-8
		47 mg/kg (D). Equivalent to 30 mg/kg theophylline	PO	12
Pirbuterol	Bronchodilator	1-3 puffs	Metered dose inhaler	12-24
Prednisolone sodium succinate	Chronic allergic diseases (asthma, atopy, IBD)	2-4 mg/kg (D)	IV, IM	Repeat in 4-6 hrs
Prednisolone/prednisone (++)	Allergic bronchitis and rhinitis, asthma	0.5-2 mg/kg (D)	IM, PO	12
	Chronic bronchitis	0.1-0.5 mg/kg (D)	PO	12
	Pulmonary eosinophilic infiltrates	0.5-1 mg/kg	PO	24
Pseudoephedrine	Nasal decongestant	15-30 mg	PO	8-12
Salmeterol	Bronchodilator	1-3 puffs	Metered dose inhaler	12 to 24
Salmeterol/fluticasone	Asthma	1-3 puffs	Metered dose inhaler	See labeled instructions
Terbutaline	Bronchodilator	0.01 mg/kg	IM, SC	4
		0.312-0.625 mg/cat. Maximum of 1.25 mg/cat	PO	8
		1-3 puffs	Metered dose inhaler	12 to 24
Terfenadine	Antihistamine	2.5-5 mg/kg (D)	PO	12
Theophylline	Bronchodilator	5-11 mg/kg (D)	IM, IV, PO	6-8
		4 mg/kg (C)	IM, PO	8-12
Theophylline sustained-release	Bronchodilator	20-40 mg/kg (D)	PO	12; consider monitoring (see Chapter 5)
		20 mg/kg (C)	PO	24. Administer at night
Zafirlukast	Chronic allergic disease (asthma, atopy, IBD)	1-2 mg/kg	PO	12-24
		20 mg/dog	PO	24

D, Dog; *IV*, intravenous; *PO*, by mouth; *IM*, intramuscular; *C*, cat; *SC*, subcutaneous; *IBD*, inflammatory bowel disease.

KEY POINT 20-6 Oral bioavailability of slow-release theophyllines may markedly vary among products and patients, contributing to toxicity or therapeutic failure.

Cats also have been studied. Although it is not distributed to all body tissues, theophylline is characterized by a relatively large volume of distribution in dogs (0.7 to 0.8 L/kg) and a smaller volume in cats (0.41 L/kg).[64,69,70] Unlike human beings, distribution of theophylline is not limited by binding to serum proteins in dogs; serum protein binding is less than 12%.[71,72] Elimination of theophylline is not dose dependent in dose ranges of 3 to 15 mg/kg. Dye and coworkers[68,70] studied two sustained-release theophylline products (TheoDur and Slo-Bid Gyrocaps, William H. Rorer, Inc) in the cat. Although both products were reasonably (>75%) bioavailable in the cat, neither product is currently available in the United States. A more recent study addressed the disposition of a generic (Inwood Laboratories) extended-release theophylline tablet (Theochron; 15 mg/kg) and capsule (TheoCap; 19 mg/kg) in cats (n = 6).[67] The C_{max} (μg/mL) of the tablet and capsule was 17.8 ± 3.4 and 15.8 ± 3.1, respectively. Although bioavailability of both products was 100% or greater, the elimination half-life for the tablet and capsule was 13.6 ± 3.9 hour and 18.3 ± 8.0, respectively, compared with 11.7 ± 1.8 hour for the intravenous preparation (aminophylline), suggesting that the drugs did not always act in an extended-release manner in cats. Nonetheless, drug concentrations remained within the recommended therapeutic range for 24 hours. These data suggested that once-daily administration in cats should be sufficient to maintain concentrations within the therapeutic range. (see Table 20-2). A longer dosing interval might be acceptable if evidence supports an antiinflammatory effect at even lower concentrations. Based on a chronopharmacokinetic study of these sustained-release products, dosing in the evening rather than in the morning appears to be associated with better bioavailability and less peak plasma theophylline concentration fluctuation.[68] A disadvantage of the use of the slow-release products for small animals is the limited dose sizes available. The product cannot be divided for more accurate dosing without altering the kinetics of slow release.

Theophylline is metabolized by demethylation in the liver. Theobromine may be an active metabolite in some species. Different rates of metabolism result in variable clearance rates and drug elimination half-lives among animals, and doses consequently vary.[72] For example, the elimination rate constant of theophylline is less in cats (0.089/hr)[73] than dogs (0.12/hr), resulting in a longer half-life in the cat (7.8 hours) compared with the dog (5.7 hours),[64,65] thus necessitating a smaller dose in cats.[69] Theophylline concentrations can be affected—most commonly increased—by a number of drugs, including fluorinated quinolones,[74] erythromycin and its congeners,[75] and cimetidine.[76]

Adverse Reactions and Drug Interactions

Theophylline is associated with a wide range of adverse effects, including central nervous system excitation (manifested as restlessness, tremors, and seizures),[72] gastrointestinal upset (nausea and vomiting), diuresis, and cardiac stimulation (e.g., tachycardia). In a retrospective study of theophylline toxicity in human patients, clinical signs included severe vomiting (89%), seizures (21%), and cardiac arrythmias (16%).[77] Vomiting precluded treatment with oral charcoal but responded to metoclopramide. Therapy included mechanical ventilation, anticonvulsants or sedatives, and muscle relaxants. Because of the risk of toxicity, intravenous use should be limited to patients who have not responded to β-agonist therapy and are facing life-threatening disease. Compared with the salt preparations, theophylline is more irritating to the gastrointestinal tract than aminophylline.[30,56] Rapid infusions or infusions of undiluted aminophylline can cause cardiac arrhythmias, hypotension, nausea, tremors, and acute respiratory failure.[30]

Theophylline may be involved in a number of drug interactions; hepatic metabolism and potentially serious adverse effects should lead to cautious use with other drugs. Inhibition of drug-metabolizing enzymes by fluorinated quinolones has been described in human medicine and for both enrofloxacin and marbofloxacin in animals.[78] For enrofloxacin 5 mg/kg decreased theophyllline clearance by 43%[79]; a different study found a 26% decrease by marbofloxacin (5 mg/kg).[78] This translates to an increase in C_{max} by 31% for theophylline, sufficient to contribute to toxicity. Indeed, the author has measured peak theophylline concentrations above 70 μg/mL and an elimination half-life of 19 hours in a dog concomitantly given enrofloxacin at 5 mg/kg. Clinical signs of theophylline toxicity emerged within 24 hours of beginning enrofloxacin therapy. Theophylline–terbutaline interactions do not appear to be clinically relevant, as has been shown in humans,[80] supporting their combined use for patients not responding to a single bronchodilator.

The application of therapeutic drug monitoring to guide therapy would assist in identifying the most appropriate dosing regimen, particularly when using slow-release preparations whose bioavailability might vary among patients, in patients receiving drug combinations that increase the risk of drug interactions, and in patients with hepatic dysfunction. Although a therapeutic range has not been established for small animals, the range recommended for humans (10 to 20 μg/mL) can be extrapolated until a more definitive range has been established. Dogs are apparently more tolerant of theophylline toxicity than are humans. In one study toxicity manifested as tachycardia, central nervous system stimulation (restlessness and excitement), and vomiting did not occur until plasma theophylline concentrations reached 37 to 60 μg/mL. Doses of 80 to 160 mg/kg of a sustained-release preparation were required to induce toxicity.[81] In cats concentrations as high as 40 μg/mL do not induce adverse reactions, although salivation and vomiting are common after administration of more than 50 mg/kg, and seizures may occur at doses greater than 60 mg/kg.[82]

The side effects of theophylline are dose dependent and might be prevented to a large degree by appropriate dosing. Therapeutic drug monitoring should facilitate the design of proper dosing regimens to prevent toxicity.

Anticholinergic Drugs

Pharmacologic Effects

Anticholinergic drugs compete with acetylcholine at muscarinic receptor sites.[83] In the respiratory tract, they reduce the sensitivity of irritant receptors and antagonize vagally mediated bronchoconstriction. The site of action of these drugs in the respiratory tract is controversial. In some studies bronchodilation is reported throughout the airways in asthmatic human patients and cats, whereas other investigators believe that the effects are confined to large airways.[83] The route by which anticholinergic drugs are administered influences their bronchodilatory effects. Despite their effect on bronchial airways, the anticholinergic drugs have not proved clinically effective in the treatment of bronchial diseases in animals, and their use is limited to treatment of bronchoconstriction associated with organophosphate toxicity or in animals in status asthmaticus unresponsive to bronchodilator therapy. The lack of clinical efficacy of anticholinergics may reflect nonselective drug–receptor interaction.[22,23] Thus far, three types of muscarinic receptors have been identified in airways. M_3 receptors release acetylcholine, whereas M_2 receptors block its release. Nonselective blockade of muscarinic receptors by atropine and ipratropium may actually potentiate acetylcholine release by antagonizing the effects of M_2-receptor stimulation. Drugs specific for M_3 receptors may ultimately lead to successful treatment of bronchial disease with anticholinergics drugs.[22,23] As with beta-adrenergic drugs, use of inhaled anticholinergic drugs reduces systemic adverse effects.

Atropine

Aerosolized atropine, a prototype anticholinergic drug, affects predominantly the central airways, whereas both central and peripheral airways are affected if the drug is administered intravenously.[22,23] Because atropine is highly specific for all muscarinic receptors, it causes a number of systemic side effects, including tachycardia, meiosis, and altered gastrointestinal and urinary tract function.[64] In the respiratory tract, atropine reduces ciliary beat frequency, mucous secretion, and electrolyte and water flux into the trachea. The net effect is decreased mucociliary clearance, which is undesirable in patients with chronic lung disease.[64] Aerosolization of atropine does not reduce the incidence of respiratory adverse reactions. Atropine is well absorbed (in humans) after oral administration. In humans atropine has proved most useful for treatment of chronic bronchitis and emphysema, diseases that are characterized by increased intrinsic vagal tone.[83] Its adverse effects on respiratory secretions and ciliary activity, however, apparently negate its benefits to bronchial tone during long-term administration in animals. The primary indication for atropine in small animals is facilitation of bronchodilation in acutely dyspneic animals. It is the treatment of choice for life-threatening respiratory distress induced by anticholinesterases. A combination of atropine with either β-adrenergic agonists or glucocorticoids will cause better bronchodilation than either drug alone.[83]

Ipratropium Bromide

Ipratropium bromide is a synthetic anticholinergic that is pharmacodynamically superior to atropine. Although the two drugs are equipotent, ipratropium does not cross the blood–brain barrier. It is not well absorbed after aerosolization, which limits the likelihood of adverse effects. Ipratropium has been studied in the dog but not in the cat.[83] Of the anticholinergic drugs studied in dogs, ipratropium appears to cause the greatest bronchodilation (twice as much as atropine) with the least change in salivation.[83] When inhaled, it is more effective in preventing bronchoscopy-induced bronchoconstriction compared with intramuscular atropine.[54] Unlike atropine, it does not alter mucociliary transport rates.

Ipratropium bromide is generally not promoted as a bronchodilator in dogs or cats. However, with the advent of inhalant devices, this may change. The combination of salbutamol (120 mg, 1 puff) and ipratropium bromide (20 mg, 2 puffs) was found to be superior to either drug alone in the prevention of BAL-induced bronchoconstriction in experimentally induced allergen sensitive, conscious cats (n = 18).[54] Drugs were administered using a pressurized inhalant metered devices (pMDI). with a spacing chamber connected through an inspiratory valve to a face mask.

Glycopyrrolate

Glycopyrrolate can also be used as a bronchodilator in small animals. Although its onset of action is slower than that of atropine,[30] its half-life is 4 to 6 hours compared with 1 to 2 hours for atropine. The potency after systemic therapy has apparently not been compared between the two drugs, although glycopyrrolate is twice as potent when aerosolized. The systemic side effects of glycopyrrolate are minimal.

Mast Cell Stabilizers

Drugs that stabilize mast cells are most effective in syndromes associated with marked mast cell activity. Included in this category may be newer antihistamines, discussed later. The stabilizing effects of β-adrenergic agonists, methylxanthines, and glucocorticoids (see Chapter 30) on inflammatory cells have been discussed.

Cromolyn

Although the mechanism of action of cromolyn is not certain, it appears to inhibit calcium influx into mast cells, thus preventing mast cell degranulation and the release of histamine and other inflammatory mediators (see Figure 20-3).[22,23,84] At high concentrations, cromogylate inhibits IgE-triggered mediator release from mast cells.[85] Some studies suggest that the activation of inflammatory cells other than the mast cells (e.g., macrophages, neutrophils, eosinophils) is also inhibited by cromogylate.[28] Cromolyn is most useful as a preventive before activation of inflammatory cells. It is not significantly absorbed after oral administration and is characterized by a short half-life (=). Thus effective therapy depends on frequent aerosolization, which limits its utility in the treatment of small animal diseases. Currently, cromolyn is the safest drug used to manage asthma in humans.[84] It is associated with only minor side effects, and its discovery has revolutionized the management of bronchial asthma in people. Because of its wide therapeutic window and its apparent efficacy in the control of many inflammatory cells, its use in the control of small animal bronchial disease warrants further investigation.

Calcium Antagonists

The efficacy of calcium antagonists in the management of asthma has yet to be identified.[86] Their potential benefits include prevention of mediator release, smooth muscle contraction, vagus nerve conduction, and infiltration of inflammatory cells.[86,87] Most studies indicate that calcium antagonists have only a modest effect on airway smooth muscle contraction. Their antiinflammatory effects may ultimately prove of greater benefit.

Drugs that Target Inflammatory Mediators

Glucocorticoids

Glucocorticoid use in dogs and cats is addressed in Chapter 30. In 1997 the National Heart, Lung, and Blood Institute Expert Panel Guidelines recommended control of mild persistent asthma with a single, long-term control medication with antiinflammatory properties.[55] Accordingly, gluccocorticoids are the cornerstone of asthma therapy.[88] The antiinflammatory effects of glucocorticoids reflect an inhibitory effect on essentially all phases of inflammation. Airway infiltration with eosinophils, mast cells, and basophils is decreased, although the effect on T cell population in the lungs is less clear. Glucocorticoids differentially downregulate T_h2 cytokines, including IL-4, IL-5, and IL-13, but appear to upregulate T_h1 cytokines, including IFN-γ and IL-12. Most recently, glucocorticoids have been demonstrated to reduce eotaxin and other eosinophil-associated chemokines but have little effect on IL-8.[89] Glucocorticoids have little effect on cys-LTs.[90] Glucocorticoids have a "permissive" effect on β-adrenergic receptors and help prevent desensitization, which may accompany therapy with long-acting drugs.

KEY POINT 20-7 The role of glucocorticoids as the cornerstone of inflammatory lung disease reflects both their antiinflammatory effects as well as their permissive effects of beta receptors mediating bronchodilation.

Glucocorticoid efficacy for treatment of respiratory inflammatory disease depends on therapeutic concentrations in and below the epithelium of all diseased airways. However, whereas systemic therapy might provide the most consistent exposure to diseased airways, it also provides the greatest exposure to tissues other than the lungs, leading to adverse effects. A number of approaches have been taken to minimize adverse effects of systemic glucocorticoids when used to treat asthma. Although dogs and cats appear to tolerate glucocorticoids better than humans, making these approaches less important, they nonetheless may be beneficial to animals. These include selective gene targeting, increased potency for the glucocorticoid receptors (allowing administration in specialized [inhalant] drug delivery systems), and development

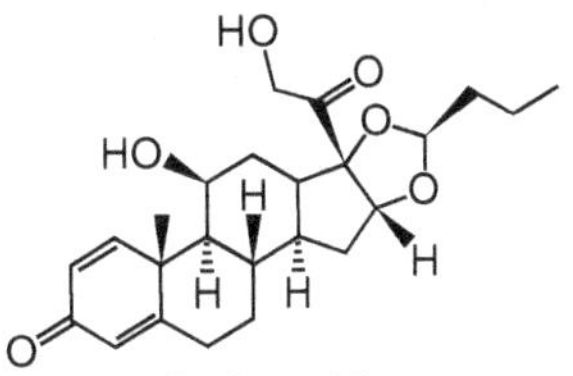

Budesonide

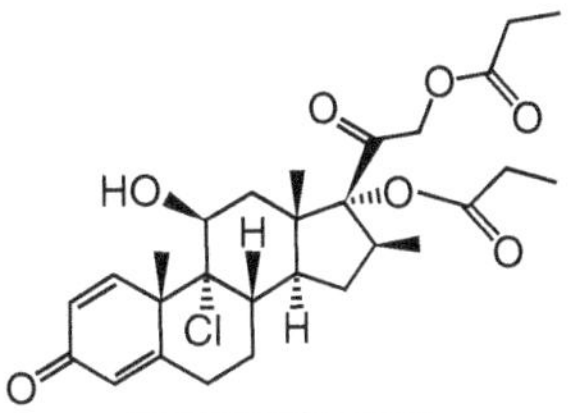

Beclomethosone

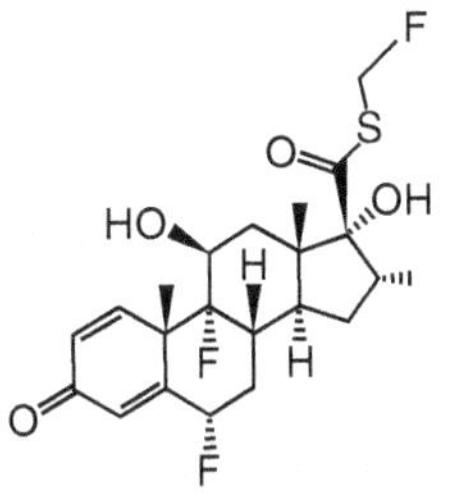

Fluticasone

Figure 20-7 Structures of selected "soft" glucocorticoids used in inhalant devices for the topical treatment of respiratory inflammatory diseases. These drugs are very potent and often are characterized by first-pass metabolism such that swallowed drug will be minimally absorbed.

of drugs that undergo first-pass metabolism. Aerosol administration minimizes many side effects. The preferred route in humans with mild disease is low-dose inhaled glucocorticoids.[55] Beclomethasone was among the first aerosol glucocorticoids developed for inhalant therapy.[40] Corticoisteroids marketed as inhalant metered devices (MDIs; see later discussion) in the United States include beclomethasone dipropionate (Beclovent), triamcinolone acetonide (Azmacort), flunisolide (Aerobid), budesonide (Pulmicort), fluticasone propionate (Flovent), and mometasone (Asmanex) (Figure 20-7).

Aerosolized glucocorticoids, such as occurs with MDIs, result in local delivery of higher concentrations. Although side effects are minimized, up to 90% of an inhaled dose is still deposited on the oral mucosa or pharynx and swallowed in humans; a similar or greater proportion might be anticipated in animals. Thus multiple methods have emerged to reduce adversities without decreasing efficacy. The delivery device may influence adverse effects. Systemic side effects associated with deposition of glucocorticoids on the pharynx and central airways and local side effects in the upper airway (e.g., dysphonia in up to 50% of the patients) led to the inclusion of "spacers" that removed larger particles before they penetrated the pharynx.[40]

Corticosteroid delivery of MDIs also has been improved by the advent of hydrocarbon fluoroalkyl (HFA)–propelled MDI. Beclomethasone dipropionate delivery to peripheral airways increases from 5% to 15% for the chlorofluorocarbon -propelled preparation to 50% to 60% with the HFA propellant.[91] Not only is total lung delivery increased, but the depth of penetration also is enhanced, a potentially critical improvement for controlling progression of the disease.

The glucocorticoid itself has been manipulated to decrease adversity. Corticosteroids marketed in MDI vary up to fivefold or more in potency. The relative potency of drugs marketed as MDI roughly follows the following order: monmetasone, which exceeds both fluticasone and budesonide, which, in turn, are 2 to 3 times more potent than beclomethasone; triamcinolone is the least potent of these drugs. While potency does allow administration of a small dose, it does not predict clinical efficacy of inhaled glucocorticoids.[91] Despite sixfold differences in potencies among inhaled glucocorticoids, comparative clinical trials in humans have failed to demonstrate differences in efficacy when drugs are administered at equipotent dosages.[91] Further, dose response curves for inhaled glucocorticoids tend to be flat, indicating that increasing doses is not likely to enhance efficacy.

Ultimately, differences in pharmaceutical (delivery) and pharmacokinetic properties largely determine variable responses to inhaled glucocorticoids. Inhaled corticosteroids generally are delivered as microcrystals, which must dissolve in the epithelial mucosal fluid. Crystals must be water soluble to ensure local delivery before the mucociliary tract removes the drug. However, alteration of dissolution times may also affect local delivery and thus local effects. For example, the dissolution time for budesonide is 6 minutes compared with beclomethasone dipropionate (5 hours) and fluticasone (8 hours). Lipophilicity of the drug enhances uptake and the duration of local effects. The addition of a halogen increases tissue retention compared with nonhalogenated drugs. Lipophilicity is greatest for beclomethasone and fluticasone followed by budesonide, with triamcinolone followed by dexamethasone and, finally, prednisolone as the least liphophilic. Not surprisingly, the most lipophilic of the drugs also is associated with the greatest number of side effects, including suppression of the hypothalamic pituitary adrenal axis. In humans, fluticasone is both the most potent and most lipophilic glucocorticoid. As such, it is characterized by the greatest evidence of systemic side effects. As such, recommendations for humans are that high-dose fluticasone propionate (>500 mg twice daily) be used only on the order of a physician and that the dose be titrated down to the lowest effective dose. Budesonide offers an example of a different type of manipulation that may allow longer dosing intervals while minimizing side effects. Because of its structure (a free C21 hydroxyl group) (see Chapter 30), excess intracellular budesonide complexes with long chain fatty acids. The complex is inactive but probably allows persistence of the drug at the site, much as a depot form would, with reversible esterification occuring as receptors are depleted of active drugs. Other drugs with a free C21 hydroxyl include triamcinolone, flunisolide, and ciclesonide, although long-chain fatty acid esterification has not been determined for them. Neither fluticasone, nor beclomethasone dipropionate, and probably mometasone, form fatty acid esters.[91]

Finally, although most devices require or allow twice- to four-times-daily dosing, those designed for once-daily administration also should enhance efficacy through improved compliance. Poor compliance with use of inhaled glucocorticoids in human patients also led to the development of combinations of steroids with long-acting β_2 agonists (e.g., salmeterol/fluticasone or formoterol/budesonide). Although compliance has improved, concern has arisen that the β_2 agonists will mask clinical signs that might otherwise indicate worsening of the disease.[40] Indeed, recent studies of the efficacy of inhaled beclomethasone diproprionate found improvements in clinical signs to be short-lived, probably because the inhaled drug does not control inflammation well.[40] Reduced airway caliber will further decrease efficacy by reducing drug delivery to the peripheral airways. Antiinflammatory therapy should target both large and small airways if inflammation is to be suppressed.[40] Thus systemic therapy should be considered (either as sole therapy or in addition to systemic therapy) in animals with moderate to severe disease. The peak effect of inhaled glucocorticoids may not occur for 1 to 2 weeks after therapy has begun.

Inhaled glucocorticoids have been recommended for use in cats with asthma,[39] although few studies have provided guidance. One abstract has reported a beneficial effect of flunisolide (250 μg/puff) but not zafirlukast (10 mg orally every 12 hours) in cats with experimental feline asthma.[92] Reinero and coworkers[93] compared the impact of inhaled flunisolide (250 μg puff twice daily) to that of oral prednisone (10 mg/day orally) and placebo on indices of inflammation and adrenal gland suppression in healthy cats (n = 6). No treatment effect was apparent with regard to serum immunoglobulin or cytokine activity. The inhaled glucocorticoid was associated with lower baseline cortisol compared with placebo and and lower cortisol after adrenocorticotropic hormone stimulation compared with oral and placebo therapy. A limitation of the study may have been the use of prednisone rather than prednisolone as is suggested by impact on cortisol concentrations, although oral therapy did impact both T and B cells. This study supports the potentially inappropriate use of prednisone in cats and suggests that topical flunisolide therapy may suppress the hypothalamic pituitary adrenal axis in cats with flunisolide.

Drugs that Target Leukotrienes

LTs are very potent causes of marked edema, inflammation, and bronchoconstriction.[94] Their role in the pathophysiology of inflammation and their inhibition are discussed in Chapter 30. Their inhibition by glucocorticoids may be limited, leaving a void in therapy.[90] The approval of drugs that specifically inhibit the formation of LTs or their actions have offered a new avenue of control of respiratory inflammatory disease (e.g., asthma) in human medicine. Two classes of drugs have focused on their impact on LTs: LT synthesis (5-lipoxygenase) inhibitors (zileuton) and LT-receptor antagonists (LRAs). The latter class has proved to be more effective (Figure 20-8). Currently, two LRAs are approved in the United States: zafirlukast, administered twice daily, and montelukast, administered once daily. The disposition of neither drug has been studied in dogs

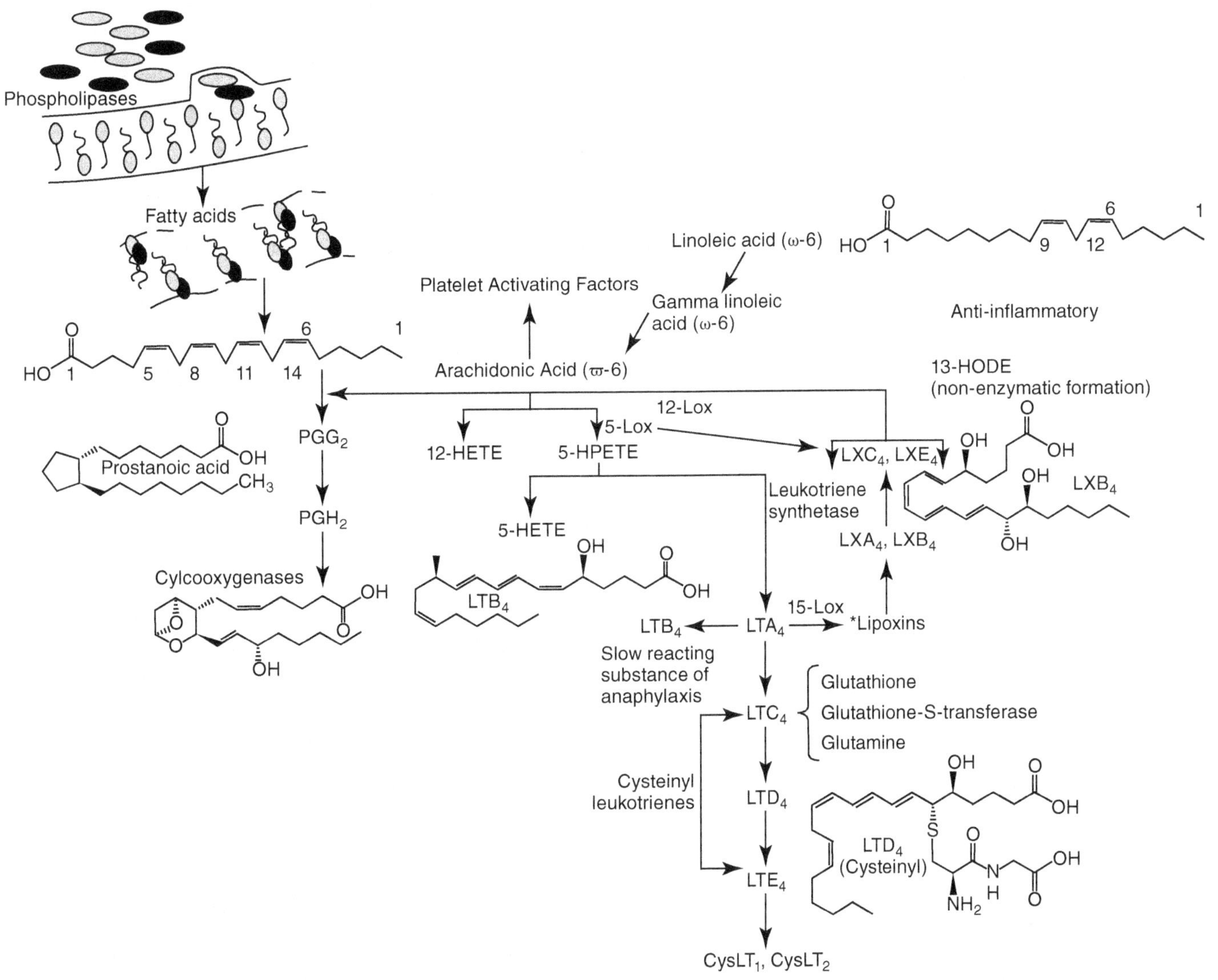

Figure 20-8 The arachidonic cascade and the formation of proinflammatory or antiinflalmmatory mediators catalyzed by lipoxygenases.

or cats; in humans the dosing intervals reflect a half-life of 5 and 10 hours, respectively.

KEY POINT 20-8 Leukotriene receptor antagonists should be considered for both local and peripheral control of respiratory inflammation in mild cases, as adjunct therapy in poor responders, and in patients intolerant to glucocorticoids.

In human clinical trials, LRAs inhibit early- and late-phase bronchoconstriction and increased bronchial hyperresponsiveness in response to allergens; accumulation of inflammatory cells and mediators in bronchial lavage fluid; and acute bronchospasms stimulated by exercise, cold air, and aspirin.[95] Their bronchodilatory effects are less than that of long-acting β-adrenergics, whereas the antiinflammatory effects are less than those of glucocorticoids.[90] However, response does occur to single doses. In contrast to β-adrenergics, tolerance does not develop toward LRA effects. Their use has been associated with improvement of asthma either as sole therapy (instead of low-dose inhaled glucocorticoids) in mild to moderate asthma or as add-on therapy regardless of disease severity in glucocorticoid nonresponders.[95] The LRAs are well tolerated, particularly compared with glucocorticoids. A subset of asthmatics treated with LRAs have developed Churg–Strauss syndrome, a state of systemic hypereosinophilia. However, its emergence may reflect decreased doses of glucocorticoids permitted once LRAs are begun rather than a toxic effect of LRAs.[90]

Recommendations regarding the role of LRAs in treatment of human asthma are dynamic. Currently, because they are less effective than glucocorticoids, their role as monotherapy is not recommended, even with mild disease. In contrast, LRAs have proved effective as monotherapy for treatment of allergic rhinitis in humans.[90] For asthma, because of their unique mechanism of action, LRAs have been combined with a number of other drugs used to treat asthma. For example, glucocorticoids minimally affect cys-LT; as such, combination with LRAs would be expected to have an additive effect, as has been demonstrated when combined with inhaled glucocortiocids. The combination of LRAs and glucocorticoids generally is as effective as glucocorticoids combined with β-adrenergic agonists. The use of an LRA as part of triple therapy (i.e., with corticosteroids, β-adrenergics) is a reasonable, albeit understudied, therapeutic approach in patients not responding to dual therapy. Finally, LRAs also have been recommended in the treatment of aspirin-sensitive asthma (discussed later).

The role of LTs in the treatment of feline asthma was previously discussed. Therapy with LRAs has had little scientific support, although this should not preclude their use, particularly in animals that have not sufficiently responded to or cannot tolerate (e.g., diabetics) corticosteroids. Receptors for LTs have yet to be identified in the smooth muscle of airways in cats; further, LTs have not been identified in the urine or plasma of cats with experimentally induced asthma.[92] However, LTs were associated with experimentally induced heartworm disease in cats.[96] The recent approach to asthma as a systemic response mediated at the level of the bone marrow warrants consideration of the use of LRAs for treatment of feline asthma, particularly in nonresponders or patients that cannot tolerate glucocorticoids. Other potential indications would include control of inflammation in dogs in which glucocorticoids are contraindicated or pulmonary diseases characterized by eosinophilic infiltrate. Anecdotally, LRAs appear to be safe in both dogs and cats, although no study has confirmed their safety.

Nonsteroidal Antiinflammatory Drugs

The role of nonsteroidal antiinflammatory drugs (NSAIDs) in the treatment of respiratory inflammatory diseases requires definition.[97,98] Both LTs and PGs are important in the pathophysiology of inflammatory diseases. Although NSAIDs effectively block PGs through inhibition of cyclooxygenase, they do not negatively affect lipoxygenase. Rather, in the aspirin-sensitive asthmatic (human) patient, aspirin and NSAIDs that selectively inhibit cyclooxygenase I shunt AA toward 5-lipoxygenas and the overproduction of cys-LTs.[90] They have no effect on other chemical mediators of inflammation. Additionally, NSAIDs nonselectively block all PGs, including those that provide some protection during periods of bronchoconstriction.[99] Some studies have shown that LT production increases in response to NSAID therapy, perhaps by providing more AA for lipoxygenase metabolism. Currently, labels include a contraindication for use in human patients with aspirin-induced asthma. However, although more studies are needed, thus far the newer NSAIDS generally are not associated with emergence of asthma.[100]

Currently, the use of NSAIDs for the treatment of respiratory diseases in small animals is limited to aspirin therapy as treatment for thromboembolism associated with heartworm disease.[101,102] Aspirin is the preferred NSAID because at low doses it irreversibly inhibits TXA_2, an important contributor to pulmonary arterial vasoconstriction that accompanies thromboembolism. Current efforts in NSAID research are oriented toward identifying drugs that successfully inhibit both arms of the AA metabolic cascade or specific PG or LT inhibitors. The use of selective TXA_2 inhibitors for selected feline respiratory diseases is an example.[45] Among the NSAIDs that might be considered, are the dual inhibitors, such as tepoxalin, which target both PGs and LTs.

Antihistamines

A number of nonantihistaminergic drugs act to ameliorate the effect of histamine (Figure 20-9). However, in general, histamine is not recognized to be a major contributor to clinical signs of asmtha based on the limited control of clinical signs afforded by antihistaminergic drugs. Those drugs that prevent histamine release may be of most benefit because they will also prevent release of other inflammatory mediators associated with asthma.

Drugs that interact with beta receptors and stimulate cAMP depress histamine release. Thus epinephrine can be used prior to or *early* during anaphylaxis to reduce histamine release. However, most of the histamine has already been released by the time treatment occurs, and in fact, most of the beneficial effects of epinephrine during anaphylaxis result from physiologic antagonism of histamine-induced bronchoconstriction. Glucocorticoids impair histamine release through their permissive effects on beta-adrenergic receptors. Additionally, glucocorticoids are lytic to neoplastic mast cells. The newer (but not older) antihistamines such as cetirizine or loratadine may inhibit histamine release from mast cells.[103] These newer products have not been widely used in animals, although the disposition of several is discussed in Chapter 29.

The use of H_1 blockers may be detrimental in animals with chronic disease because of their effects on airway secretions.[29] The role of H_2 receptors in bronchodilation, mucous secretion, and inflammation suggests that H_2-receptor blockers should also be used with caution.[5,29] Among the drugs for which anecdotal discussion suggests efficacy for treatment of tracheal collapse is doxepin, a tricyclic antidepressant that is also characterized by marked H_1 antagonism. Efficacy may be related to antiinflammatory effects or some level of central nervous system depression.[104] Alternatively, local anesthetic actions may be contributing to efficacy.[105] Although not yet clinically available, drugs that specifically target H_4 receptors may prove useful through control of signals mediating chronic allergic responses. Cyproheptadine is an antiserotinergic, antihistaminergic drug. Because feline airways are exquisitely sensitive to the constrictor effects of serotonin, this drug may prove particularly useful in cats either alone or as an adjunct to bronchodilators or glucocorticoids.[106] The disposition of cyproheptadine has been described in cats (n = 6).[107] It is characterized by 100% oral bioavailability, a volume of distribution of 1 ± 0.5 l/kg and an elimination half-life of 12.8 ± 9.9 hours, supporting a once- to twice-daily dosing interval. A single intravenous dose of 2 mg was well tolerated. An oral dose of 8 mg yielded a C_{max} of 419 ± 99 ng/mL. Both the intravenous and oral dose were well tolerated. Studies following transdermal administration are pending.

ANTITUSSIVES

The goal of antitussive therapy is to decrease the frequency and severity of cough without impairing mucociliary defenses (Figure 20-10). Whenever possible, the underlying cause should be identified and treated. Cough suppressants should be used cautiously and are contraindicated if the cough is productive.[2] Irritants and perhaps chemoreceptors and stretch

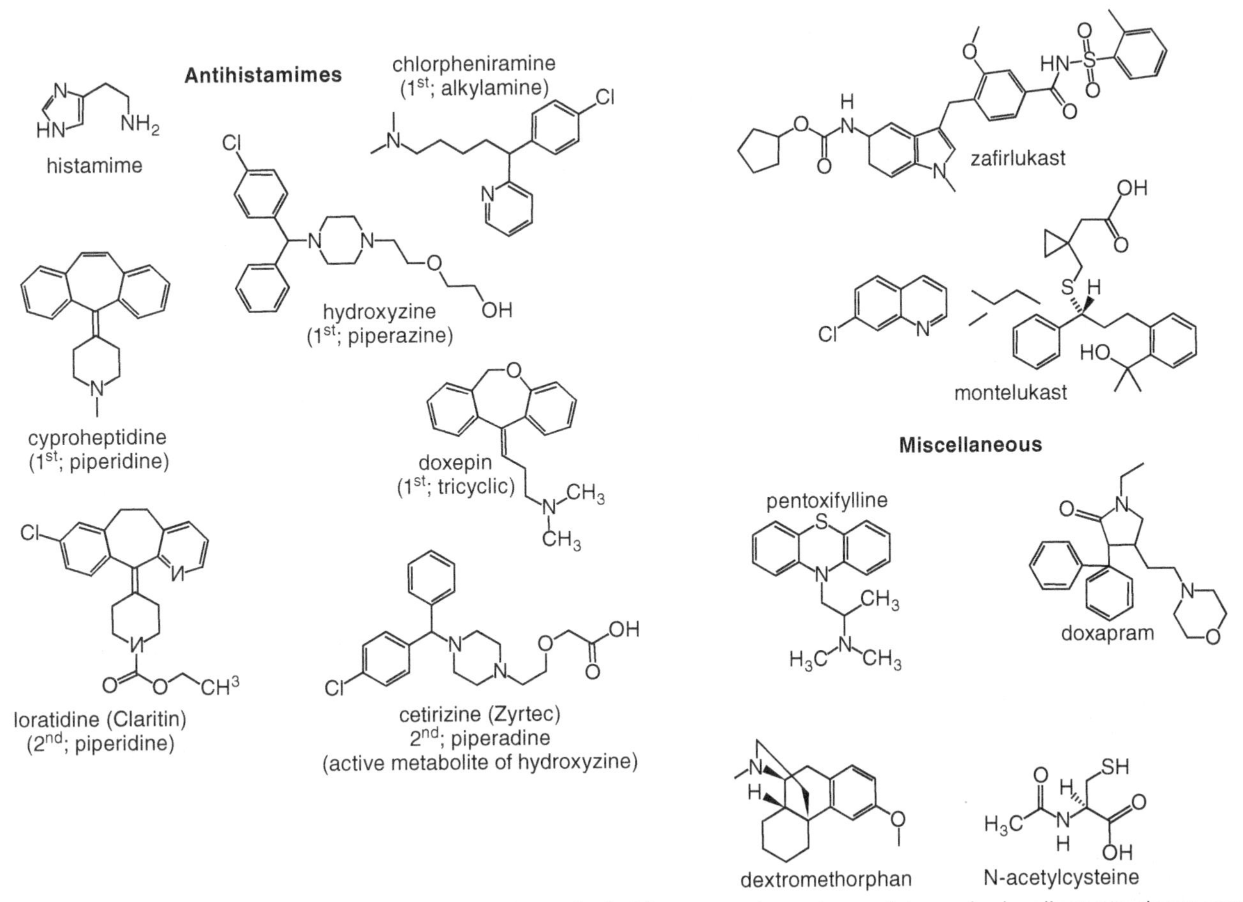

Figure 20-9 Structures of selected antihistaminergic drugs, leukotriene receptor antagonsists, and miscellaneous drugs used to treat disorders of the respiratory tract.

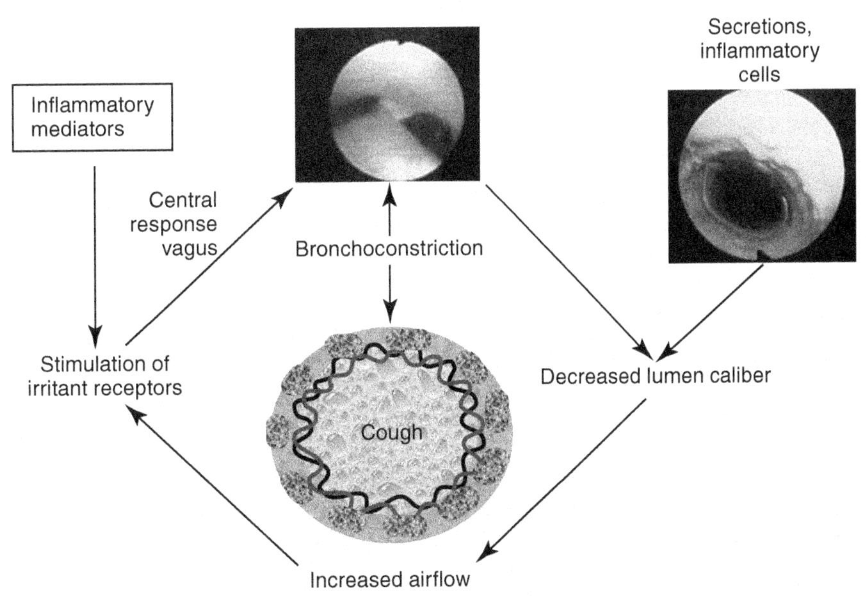

Figure 20-10 The most potent stimulus for the cough reflex is decreased airway caliber size. The subsequent increase in airflow velocity irritates stretch receptors. The vagus nerve serves as the afferent and efferent limbs of the cough reflex, which is mediated centrally by the respiratory center in the medulla. Accumulation of debris and inflammatory mediators can either irritate receptors or decrease airway luminal caliber. Cough is accompanied by bronchoconstriction, which can further exacerbate coughing.

receptors initiate the cough reflex.[2,73] Bronchoconstriction is probably the most frequent and important cough stimulus. The cough reflex can be blocked peripherally, either by facilitating removal of the irritant with mucolytics or expectorants or by blocking peripheral receptors to induce bronchodilation, or it can be blocked centrally at the cough center in the medulla (see Figure 20-4).[2,108] Mediators targeted for treatment of cough might be opioid, serotonin (5-HT1A), nociceptin, or gamma amino butyric acid-B agonists and neurokinin (NK-1 or NK-2) or N-methyl-D-aspartate (NMDA) antagonists.[7a-c]

KEY POINT 20-9 Cough might be reduced peripherally through therapies that increase airway caliber size. This includes bronchodilation or facilitating removal of intraluminal debris.

Centrally active antitussives are classified as narcotic and non-narcotic drugs.[108,109]

Opioid Antitussives

Opioid (narcotic) antitussives depress the cough center sensitivity to afferent stimuli. They can, however, be associated with strong sedative properties, as well as constipation, when administered chronically. Morphine, codeine, and hydrocodone are the narcotics most commonly used to control coughing. As class II drugs, each is subject to the Controlled Substances Act of 1970 and can be used for cough suppression in both dogs and cats. Other opioids may have antitussive actions but are generally not used for that indication. Examples include diphenoxylate, a drug to which powerful antitussive actions have been ascribed.

Codeine

Codeine is the prototype narcotic antitussive and one of the most effective drugs available to suppress the cough reflex. Codeine phosphate and codeine sulfate can be used either alone or in combination with peripheral cough suppressants or decongestants. Over-the-counter preparations are available for human use. Compared with morphine, codeine is equally effective as a cough suppressant but is less suppressing to other central centers and causes less constipation. Side effects of codeine include nausea and constipation. Codeine is also addressed in Chapter 28.

Hydrocodone

Hydrocodone is a more potent antitussive than codeine but causes less respiratory depression. It is probably the most commonly used antitussive for dogs. Hydrocodone bitartrate is a hydrolysis product of dihydrothebaine.

Butorphanol

Butorphanol tartrate is probably more commonly used as an analgesic. Reclassified as a Schedule IV drug, it is now subject to the Narcotics Act. It is approved for use as an antitussive for dogs. As an antitussive, it is 100 times more potent than codeine and 4 times more potent than morphine.[110] In dogs, after subcutaneous administration, butorphanol concentrations peak at 1 hour. Mean half-life is 1.7 hours, with a duration of activity of 4 hours or more. Butorphanol is characterized by a wide safety margin. The LD_{50} in dogs after intramuscular administration is 20 mg/kg.[111] Therapeutic concentrations cause minimal cardiac or respiratory depression. Side effects include sedation, which can be significant and desirable; nausea; some diarrhea; and appetite suppression. The narcotic agonist/antagonist butorphanol tartrate is a potent antitussive when given orally or parenterally in dogs and cats.

Non-Narcotic Antitussives

Non-narcotic antitussives commonly used in veterinary medicine include the narcotic agonist/antagonist butorphanol and dextromethorphan.

Dextromethorphan

Dextromethorphan hydrobromide (see Figure 20-9) is a semisynthetic derivative of opium. It is the d-isomer of the codeine analog of methorphan. Unlike its L-enantiomer, levomethorphan, it lacks narcotic, direct analgesic, or addictive properties. It is an acid receptor antagonist and as such is also discussed in Chapter 28. Antagonists of NMDA receptors are powerful antitussives in some species (including humans). Dextromethorphan's metabolite dextrorphan also is active. Because sedation is unusual after its use, it is classified as non-narcotic. Its antitussive mechanism is not certain; only the D-isomer has antitussive activity, which is similar to codeine in potency. Dextromethorphan interacts with sigma receptors (previously thought to be opioid receptors). Its onset of action is rapid, being fully effective within 30 minutes after oral administration. It is metabolized by CYP2D6, a drug-metabolizing enzyme found to be deficient in a significant proportion of the human population. Dextromethorphan is commonly found in over-the-counter cough preparations. It can be used safely in cats. In humans it can release histamine and therefore is not often recommended for atopic children. Its use with selective serotonin uptake inhibitors and monoamine oxidase inhibitors is discouraged. Studies in humans have shown that the combination of dextromethorphan with a bronchodilator is superior to dextromethorphan alone for the control of cough.[112]

Noscapine

Noscapine is a nonaddictive opium alkaloid (benzylisoquinoline) that has antitussive effects similar to those of codeine.[113] Its use for small animals appears to be limited.

Neurokinin Receptor Antagonists

The role of NK-antagonists in control of cough is being elucidated. Their appeal reflects, in part, the increasingly recognized role of tachykinins in mediating cough and hyper-reflexivity. A potential role of NK antagonists in control of asthma in humans was recognized in the 1990s, although their clinical role has not been recognized.[113a] Their role for control of cough is supported by a number of reviews.[113a,b] Although the antiemetic maropitant (see Chapter 19) has not been studied for treatment of cough in dogs, its anecdotal use is supported by response to other NK-1 antagonists.[113b] Cough (mechanical intrathoracic tracheal stimulation) was reduced by 52% in dogs receiving an experimental NK1 antagonist.

Peripheral Bronchodilators

Bronchodilators (previously discussed) are powerful peripheral antitussives because they relieve irritant receptor stimulation induced by mechanical deformation of the bronchial wall during bronchoconstriction. Ephedrine peripherally induces bronchodilation, and as both a bronchodilator and decongestant it is a common constituent of over-the-counter cough preparations. Theophylline and isoproterenol are also common ingredients found in some preparations. Other peripheral antitussives include mucokinetic agents and hydrating agents.[108]

Bronchodilators counteract irritant receptor stimulation induced by mechanical deformation of the bronchial wall during bronchoconstriction. Increased fluidity of secretions and ciliary action may facilitate removal of accumulated materials, thus decreasing airway caliber size, airflow velocity, and turbulence-induced receptor stimulation. As such, previously discussed bronchodilators can be effective peripheral antitussives. Several drugs classified as bronchodilators are found in over-the-counter cough preparations for their antitussive-effective effects. Ephedrine is both an α and a β agonist; additionally, it causes the release of norepinephrine from sympathetic neurons. It peripherally induces bronchodilation, and as both a bronchodilator and a decongestant, it is a common constituent of over-the-counter cough preparations. It is present in herbal agents as ma huang or ephedra. Ephedrine is a potent central nervous system and cardiac stimulant and can contribute to hypertension and dysuria as a result of its α-adrenergic effects. Theophylline and isoproterenol are also common ingredients found in some preparations. Other peripheral antitussives include mucokinetic agents and hydrating agents.[108]

MUCOKINETICS

Mucokinetic drugs facilitate the removal of secretions from the respiratory tree. They are indicated for conditions associated with viscous to inspissated pulmonary secretions such as are commonly associated with chronic bronchial diseases. Mucokinesis can be induced by drugs that improve ciliary activity (e.g., β-receptor agonists and methylxanthines) or by drugs that improve the mobility of bronchial secretions by changing viscosity. Viscosity of bronchial secretions can be decreased by hydration (e.g., sterile or bacteriostatic water or saline), increasing pH (e.g., sodium bicarbonate), increasing ionic strength (sodium bicarbonate and saline), or by rupturing sulfur (S-S) linkages in the mucus (e.g., acetylcysteine or iodine). Hydrating agents can be administered parenterally (i.e., isotonic crystalloids) or by aerosolization. Home aerosolization can be easily achieved with a humidifier or steamed bathroom or with a commercially available aerosolizer. The efficacy of aerosolization in liquefying airway secretions is controversial,[26] with the greatest benefit occurring in the upper airways. Bland aerosols such as water and saline can actually be detrimental to mucociliary function.[26] The efficacy of ionic solutions or alkaline solutions compared with that of water on enhanced mucous mobility is controversial.[26]

Bromhexine

Bromhexine is a mucolytic that acts at the level of the mucus-secreting gland, decreasing the formation of mucoid secretions. On the basis of product information, in humans it is rapidly absorbed after oral absorption but undergoes extensive first-pass metabolism, resulting in an oral bioavailability approximating 20%. It is highly bound to plasma proteins. Its distribution includes penetration of the blood–brain barrier. Metabolites are excreted in the urine mainly as metabolites, resulting in an elimination half-life of up to about 12 hours. Although characterized by low toxicity, the mucolytic effects will occur in other areas of the body. Accordingly, caution is recommended for use in patients with a history of gastrointestinal ulceration. The impact in the patient with a urinary tract infection is not known. A Cochrane review[114] that focused on the efficacy of mucolytics in human patients with bronchiectasis found that bromhexine facilitated removal of mucus associated with infection, but the number of clinical trials was too few to allow meta-analysis.

Acetylcysteine

Acetylcysteine (*N*-acetyl-L-cystein) (NAC) (see Figure 20-9) is the N-acetyl derivative of the naturally occurring amino acid L- cysteine. It is the mucolytic drug most widely used by humans.[26,115] Although it appears to be efficacious after aerosolization, oral administration has become the preferred route.[115] In Europe the drug is available in solid and powder dosing forms. Unfortunately, only the solution, which is unpalatable and malodorous, is approved for use in the United States. The powder is available as a chemical reagent from several chemical companies and application to food or as a capsule might be considered.

KEY POINT 20-10 The beneficial effects of *N*-acetylcysteine, which include control of inflammation as well as mucokinesis, can be realized with oral as well as inhalant therapy.

Regardless of the route of administration, the mechanism of NAC reflects destruction of mucoprotein of the disulfide bonds by a free sulfhydryl group. The subsequent smaller molecules are less viscid and less able to efficiently bind to inflammatory debris. As a thiol compound, NAC is a radical scavenger, able to directly interact with oxidants such as hydrogen peroxide, hydroxyl radicals, and hypochlorous acid.[21] In addition to these direct effects, as a cysteine, NAC appears to promotes cellular glutathione production, a critical intracellular scavenger of radicals.[116] Increased intracellular glutathione appears to contribute to the control of inflammation.[117] A number of animal studies indicate efficacy of NAC in the prevention and therapy of lung injury associated with oxygen radicals.[116,118] These effects may be additive with dexamethasone.[119] However, although NAC has an antiinflammatory effect, it has an apparent dose-dependent, paradoxical effect on polymorphonuclear cells. Respiratory burst is suppressed but phagocytosis is increased in humans receiving increasing doses of 6 to 18 g (60 to 180 mg/kg) of NAC by constant slow intravenous infusion.[116] In contrast, at a low mucolytic dose (300 mg or approximately 4.5 mg/kg three times daily in humans), respiratory burst is increased. The impact of high doses can be beneficial in the presence of inflammatory disease or syndromes associated with ischemia/reperfusion or endothelial cell activation but detrimental in the presence of infectious diseases; lower doses might be recommended in the presence of infectious disease dependent on leukocyte activity. Acetylcysteine appears to induce respiratory tract secretions, probably by way of a gastropulmonary reflex. Effects on bronchial secretions appear to be clinically relevant. Acetylcysteine improved gas exchange in a study of dogs with experimentally induced methacholine bronchoconstriction.[120] The effects of NAC in human patients with COPD is not conclusive, with study results ranging from no effect to clinical effect.

In humans acetylcysteine is rapidly absorbed from the gastrointestinal tract and extensively distributed to the liver, kidneys, and lungs, where it may accumulate. It is rapidly metabolized by the liver to the natural amino acids cysteine and cystine.[115,121]

The indications for oral acetylcysteine therapy for humans include toxic inhalants (including tobacco smoke), bronchitis, COPD, cystic fibrosis, asthma, tuberculosis, pneumonia and emphysema, and ARDS.[117] Installation of a 10% to 20% solution has also been used to clean and treat chronic sinusitis.[115] Physiotherapy will enhance the efficacy of acetylcysteine. For example, one study in humans with COPD (n = 523) could not establish a beneficial effect of NAC (4.5 mg/kg every 8 hours orally) for 3 years in prevention of deterioration of disease.[122] However, a potential beneficial effect was found in those patients not receiving inhaled steroids. In contrast, Sutherland[123] performed a meta-analysis from eight trials (randomized n = 2,214) and concluded that that NAC significantly reduced the odds of experiencing exacerbations, including in active smokers. This report also found a greater effect when persons using inhaled glucocorticoids were removed, suggesting that inhaled steroids attenuate the effect of NAC. Accordingly, the authors concluded that treatment with NAC may be beneficial in a subset of patients with COPD.

Acetylcysteine therapy is associated with few adverse affects. In humans doses as high as 500 mg/kg are well tolerated,[121] although vomiting and anorexia can occur. Kao and coworkers[124] retrospectively performed a meta-analysis to review the adverse events in humans receiving NAC intravenously for treatment of acetaminophen toxicity. Of the 187 patients receiving the drug, seven adverse events were reported, six of which were cutaneous and rapidly responded to antihistamines. The authors concluded that the rate of adversities was low. The median LD_{50} in dogs after oral use is 1 g/kg and parenterally 700 mg/kg. Because it is metabolized to sulfur-containing products, it should be used cautiously in animals suffering from liver disease characterized by hepatic encephalopathy. Aerosolization of NAC can cause reflex bronchoconstriction as a result of irritant receptor stimulation and should be preceded with bronchodilators.

No scientific support appears to exist for the use of NAC in animals with lung disease. Historical successful use focuses in treatment of acetaminophen toxicosis. The author has used these high doses (144 mg/kg intravenously followed by 70 mg/kg 12 hours later) in life-threatening pulmonic conditions, including pneumonia. Other conditions to consider include but are not necessarily limited to chronic bronchial diseases, chronic sinusitis, electrical-cord bites, and other respiratory syndromes associated with inflammation. Although NAC in the form of Mucomyst might be administered orally, an alternative method is procurement of a scientific-grade granule product (e.g., Spectrum Chemicals). Further, many health-food stores offer NAC in capsular form for reasonable prices, although the quality of the products may not be known.

EXPECTORANTS

Expectorants such as potassium iodide are common ingredients in over-the-counter cough preparations. Expectorants increase the fluidity of respiratory secretions through several mechanisms and are often used as adjuvants for the management of cough by facilitating removal of the inciting cause. Bronchial secretions are increased by vagal reflex after gastric mucosa irritation (iodide salts) and directly through sympathetic stimulation or by volatile oils that are partially eliminated by way of the respiratory tract. Although the combination of expectorants with antitussives in over-the-counter cough preparations may seem irrational, the antitussive drugs in these combination products do not appear to prevent stimulation of the cough reflex induced by liquefied secretions commonly included in over-the-counter cough preparations. Their mechanism of action is unknown, although they may be ineffective at the doses used in cough preparations.

Iodide Preparations

Potassium iodide is a saline expectorant capable of increasing secretions by 150%. Ethylenediamine dihydriodide, used as a nutritional source of iodine in cattle, may be useful for the treatment of mild respiratory diseases. Iodide preparations should not be used in pregnant or hyperthyroid animals or in milk-producing animals. Demulcent expectorants such as syrup are often used as the vehicle for cough medicaments but have no apparent expectorant value. They may, however, be useful for treatment of cough caused by pharyngeal irritation.

Stimulant Expectorants

Stimulant expectorants are used more commonly for coughing associated with chronic bronchial diseases. Guaiacol and its glyceryl ether guaifenesin (glyceryl guaiacolate) are wood tar derivatives. Neither the volume of viscosity nor respiratory secretions appear to change after treatment with guaifenesin, although airway particle clearance increases in bronchitic human patients.

Miscellaneous Expectorants

Among the chemicals that potentially contribute to COPD are DNA and actin.[17] The ability of bovine pancreatic deoxyribonuclease (DNase) to decrease the viscosity of lung secretions led to its approval in the early 1960s. However, adverse reactions (probably to contaminating enzymes) limited its use. Recombinant technology allowed the development of human DNase (rhDNase; dornase alfa) which is used in the treatment of cystic fibrosis. Expiratory volume increases and the incident of clinical exacerbations is reduced when used (2.5 mg by aerosolization) on an alternate-day basis.[17] rhDNase has been used for management of both acute and chronic disease, although time to response is longer in patients with the most severe disease. The effects of DNase may decrease with long-term therapy, and concerns have been raised that its effects may be merely cosmetic, masking clinical signs indicative of serious disease.[17] The cost of rhDNase may preclude use in animals, particularly if clinical effects with long-term use are not definitive.

Aerosolized hypertonic (5.85%) saline (10 mL twice daily) also have demonstrated efficacy in human patients with cystic fibrosis. Postulated mechanisms focus on osmotic draw of fluid into the airway lumen or cleavage of mucin bonds, either of which decreases mucus viscosity. Bronchodilators should be administered before aerosolization to prevent bronchoconstriction.

DECONGESTANTS

The indications for decongestants include sinusitis of allergic or viral etiologies and reverse sneezing or other complications of postnasal drip. Information regarding the use of decongestants in animals is largely based on extrapolation from human patients for which allergic rhinitis and the common cold are the more common indications. Often decongestants are administered as a single drug combined with expectorants.

The two major categories of drugs used as decongestants are the histamine (H_1) receptor antagonists (e.g., dimenhydrinate, diphenhydramine, chlorpheniramine, and hydroxyzine, as well as newer second-generation drugs such as loratadine and cetirizine) and the sympathomimetic drugs (i.e., α-adrenergic agonists) (such as ephedrine [EDE], pseudoephedrine [PSE], and phenylephrine [PNE]).[125-127] These drugs can be given topically to avoid the systemic effects associated with oral therapy.

Stimulation of α_2-receptors concentrated on precapillary arterioles results in vascular smooth muscle vasoconstriction. Blood flow to the nasal mucosal capillary bed is reduced; excess extracellular fluid associated with congestion and a "runny" nose is thus decreased. α-receptors are concentrated on the postcapillary venules; when stimulated, the venules act as capacitance vessels that reduce blood volume in the mucosa. Mucosal volume decreases, reducing congestion. Sympathomimetic drugs mimic norepinephrine. Direct-acting agents stimulate one (PNE: α_1) or both types of α-receptors, depending on drug chemistry. Indirect-acting agents (PSE) displace norepinephrine from nerve terminals and sometimes block its reuptake, effectively increasing its action on postjunctional α-receptors. Some drugs (e.g., PSE, EDE) are both direct and indirect in their actions. Prolonged use of agents that act indirectly (e.g., EDE) may deplete storage granules, and the animal may become refractory to its effects. Alternatively, downregulation of receptors (tachyphylaxis) may result in refractoriness.[126,127]

Topical agents containing sympathomimetic drugs (i.e., nasal sprays) act within minutes, with minimal side effects. In contrast, rebound hyperemia is common, particularly with extended use of the drugs. The mechanism of rebound hyperemia is not clear but may result from secondary β-adrenergic effects, as β-receptors upregulate or desensitize α-receptors. Regardless of the cause, repeated contraction of the vasculature can result in ischemia and mucosal damage, perhaps as a result of loss of nutrition. Oral treatment of sympathomimetic drugs can be associated with a number of adverse reactions. Systemic vasoconstriction may cause hypertension; cardiac stimulation may result in tachycardia or reflex bradycardia. Stimulation of the central nervous system may also prove problematic, particularly with lipid-soluble agonists such as ephedrine. Stimulation of urinary sphincter α-receptors may result in urinary retention. Mydriasis may decrease aqueous humor exit and can prove detrimental in patients with glaucoma. Because of their effects on endocrine and other organs associated with metabolic function, these drugs should not be used in patients with metabolic disorders, including thyroid disease and diabetes mellitus. The relationship between plasma drug concentration and nasal decongestant efficacy with the α-agonists appears to be minimal, suggesting that topical therapy is as efficacious. In addition, oral administration of some drugs (e.g., PNE) is limited by first-pass metabolism, which prevents therapeutic concentrations of the drug from being reached. Thus topical therapy may be the preferred route for sympathomimetic drugs. Note, however, that in the United States PSE is an "old drug" and as such is exempt from Food and Drug Administration regulation, which includes various topical formulations. However, issues regarding substance abuse have led to a Schedule III status for PSE (along with EDE and phenylpropanolamine) with the Drug Enforcement Agency.

Antihistamines are effective for the treatment of allergic rhinitis in human patients. In this scenario, they relieve and prevent itching and rhinorrhea but not nasal congestion. Thus antihistamines are frequently combined with sympathomimetic drugs. The efficacy of these drugs for the treatment of symptoms related to the common cold (and, presumably, unknown microbial causes in animals) has not been proved. Sedation is the most common side effect of the first-generation antihistamines (diphenhydramine). Newer antihistamines (e.g., chlorpheniramine) are associated with minimal sedation. In contrast to other causes of rhinitis, topical decongestants may be more of a risk for patients with allergic rhinitis because of the risk of drug reaction (rhinitis medicamentosa). This side effect does not occur with topical therapy. Because the antihistamines are safer than the sympathomimetic drugs after oral administration, this may be the preferred route for antihistamines.[125]

Formulations of topical preparations can influence drug efficacy. Controlled-release polymers can decrease the rate of drug dissolution (and thus its ability to reach cellular targets). Although these differences may not be clinically relevant, it is important to realize that bioequivalency of the topical decongestant products containing older drugs may vary. The major disadvantage of topical agents is their short duration of action.

Respiratory Stimulants

Caffeine, as previously noted, is a respiratory stimulant often used to treat premature infants. It appears not to affect dogs and cats in that capacity. Doxapram (see Figure 20-9) is a respiratory stimulant that acts indirectly by stimulating chemoreceptors of the carotid arteries, which in turn stimulates the respiratory center. It may be helpful in counteracting the depressant effects of opioids or other drugs. In humans high doses may be associated with hypertension and tachycardia. The effect of doxapram (2.2 mg/kg intravenously) on laryngeal function was studied in healthy dogs (n = 30) preanesthetized with butorphanol and acepromazine followed by propofol (4 mg/kg intravenously) induction. Improved respiratory effort and laryngeal motion led the authors to suggest routine use of doxapram during laryngoscopy.[128]

AEROSOLIZATION AS A ROUTE OF DRUG ADMINISTRATION

Aerosolization of drugs (inhalation therapy) is characterized by several advantages. Higher drug concentrations in target tissues leads to lower doses, thus enhancing efficacy while minimizing toxicity (e.g., anticholinergics, glucocorticoids, and beta-adrenergics). Additionally, response to therapy may be more rapid than that to systemic therapy. Hepatic first-pass metabolism after oral administration is circumvented, which serves to prolong the pharmacologic effect of selected drugs (e.g., β-adrenergic agonists and beclomethasone). In human medicine, with the development of more effective inhalant devices, asthma is predominantly treated with inhalant medications. The primary indications for aerosolization in small animals also has been direct delivery of drugs to the respiratory tract and to facilitate liquefaction and mobilization of respiratory secretions. However, the use of human inhalant devices designed to treat asthma is generally accepted for cats, although use in dogs is less common.

The success of patient response to aerosolized drugs is more likely to reflect adequate drug delivery rather than drug efficacy. Three factors determine the amount of drug reaching the airways: anatomy, ventilation, and aerosol characteristics.[129] The anatomy of the respiratory tract is designed to filter inhaled particles. Indeed, up to 90% of particles produced by pMDI are removed before they reach the airways in humans.[129] The more tortuous the airways traversed by an aerosol, the smaller the percentage delivered. Canine and feline anatomy is likely to contribute substantially to deposition in the oral pharynx and upper airways.

Variations in tidal volume; airflow rates; and respiratory rate, depth, and pattern also will affect the amount of drug delivery. In humans breath holding is particularly important to drug delivery.[129] With progression of chronic disease, or with moderate to severe acute disease, aerosol therapy may become less effective as the respiratory pattern becomes shallow and rapid. For stressed animals, tachypnea will further decrease depth of aerosol penetration decreases, with more drugs deposited in upper airways. The utility of aerosolization may be further limited because of stimulation of irritant receptors and reflex bronchoconstriction.[26,130] Resistance by the animal to aerosolization may further exacerbate respiratory distress and thus affect the site of particle deposition.

Among the characteristics of the aerosol that will influence airway deposition are diameter, shape, electrical charge (for particles less than 1 μm in size), density, mass, hygroscopicity, and preparation type (i.e., solution versus suspension).[2,113,129,131,132] The optimum particle size for particle (and drug) deposition in the trachea is 2 to 10 μm and in peripheral airways, 0.5 to 5.0 μm. Differences in methods, devices, diseases, and drugs have generated a number of contradictory reports regarding the best particle size for aerosolized drug delivery in diseased humans. Most studies suggest penetration of small airways is best accomplished with particles 1.5 μm or less in size, although others have found maximum improvement in lung function with an aerosol of 3 μm particles.[129,131] Jet and ultrasonic nebulizers (described later) tend to generate heterogenous particles of that range from 1.2 to 6.9 and 3.7 to 10.5 μm in size, respectively. Spinning disk nebulizers produce particles that range from 1.3 to 30 μm. For inhalant devices, particle size generated for MDIs varies from 1 to 35 μm, but particle size is dependent on (inspiratory) flow for dried-powder inhaler (DPI) devices.[129]

Aerosol deposition also will be affected by the technique of delivery (i.e., mask versus endotracheal tube and nose versus mouth). Larger particles generated by aerosol devices will be impacted on masks, pharynx, and in upper airways (or endotracheal tubes). Indeed, oral absorption of particles is sufficient that side effects to inhaled glucocorticoids in humans tend to reflect systemic response to the drugs. In animals grooming may increase the risk of systemic side effects to drugs deposited on the face during mask administration. One method whereby drug delivery is enhanced, thus increasing efficacy and safety, is the device used for drug delivery. Modern aerosol therapy is administered through one of three devices: nebulizers, MDIs, and DPIs.[131,133,134]

Two basic types of nebulizers have been developed: jet and ultrasonic.[131,133] The ultrasonic nebulizer is based on a high frequency (1-3 MHz) vibrating piezoelectric crystal that generates a fountain of liquid in the chamber. Droplet size decreases as vibration frequency increases. Jet nebulizers are based on the Bernoulli principle. Compressed gas (air or oxygen) is forced through a narrow orifice, creating a low-pressure area at the outlet of the adjacent liquid feed tube. Drug in solution is drawn from a fluid reservoir and shattered into droplets by the gas stream. Breath-enhanced jet nebulizers have an added valve system that directs inspired air to the well during inspiration. This second source of air optimizes the number and size of particles. Still, the amount of drug delivered by nebulizers to airways (in humans) can be as little as 10%. In humans adapters have been added that time drug release with the initial inspiratory effort, increasing the amount of drug delivery to airways to up to 69%; such adapters are not likely to be helpful in animals. Other factors particularly affecting nebulized drug delivery include solution viscosity, ionic strength, osmolarity, pH, and surface tension. Acidic and nonisotonic solutions increase the risk of bronchoconstriction, coughing, and irritation of the lung mucosa. High drug concentrations may also decrease the drug output; foaming is a particular problem with ultrasonic units.

A number of companies offer reasonably priced ($70 to $250 or above) portable compressor-based nebulizing units. Compressors that accompany the nebulizers can generate air at pressures (20 to 40 psi) and airflow velocities (7 to 10 mL) comparable to oxygen-based flow meters (e.g., Omron Healthcare Inc, www.omronhealthcare.com). Aerosol units are small enough to be placed in an aquarium of appropriate size or, for large dogs, can be adapted to a mask. For tracheostomized patients, infant or adult tracheostomy masks that deliver aerosol directly into the tracheostomy are available. Although aerosol units are generally reusable, attention must be made to keep units sterile; great care must be taken to ensure that nebulizers remain free of microorganisms between uses. Adherence to cleansing procedures after each use of nebulizing equipment should be strict. Cold sterilization agents should be effective against *Pseudomonas* spp. Manufacturers of reusable equipment recommend washing it in warm soapy water, rinsing it well, and soaking it (including the tubing) for 30 minutes in a solution of 1 part vinegar and 3 parts water. Disposable equipment should be replaced frequently; replacement after use in patients with infection is particularly encouraged.

The MDI has been described as a revolutionary change for aerosol therapy in humans; it is the most commonly used device. [88,133,134] The aerosol of an MDI is driven by a propellant. The more common older chlorofluorocarbons (CFCs) are being replaced by hydrofluoroalkanes (HFAs), which contain no chlorine and thus do not affect the ozone layer. The HFA-propelled MDIs also lack the "cold Freon" effect that causes human patients to fail to inspire completely. The drug in an MDI is emitted at a high velocity (>30 m/s) through a nozzle. However, as with nebulizers, only a small percentage of drug (10% to 20%) reaches peripheral airways, with most (in humans) being deposited in the oropharnyx. Surfactants enhance particle stability in the presence of CFC propellants; ethanol is similarly used for HFA propellants. For HFAs drugs are delivered as a solution rather than as a micronized suspension. As such, particles released by the device valve are much smaller; referred to as *extra fine,* the average size is 1.1 μm, compared with 3.5 to 4.0 μm in size for the CFC. The smaller size enhances deeper airway penetration.[40] Indeed, the pattern of particle deposition with HFA propellants (60% deposited in small airways rather than the oropharynx) is reversed compared with that for CFC propellants.[134] Spacer tubes, valved holding chambers, and mouthpiece extensions have been added to minimize the need for hand–breath–inhalation coordination, thus improving delivery. Spacers and holding chambers yield an aerosol that is more uniform in lung distribution and characterized by deeper penetration in peripheral airways. Breath-activated MDIs also have been developed, which, as with nebulizers, minimize the need for hand–breath–inhalation coordination. Despite these innovations, studies using radiolabeled aerosols in normal humans have documented that less than 20% (usually only 10%) of drug reaches the airways, even if the respiratory pattern is optimal.[40,134] The DPI was designed to eliminate the need for hand–inhalant coordination necessary for the MDI. Drug aerosol of DPI is generated by air forced through powder. Particles are aggregated and too large for effective delivery. However, dispersal into smaller particles is accomplished by turbulent airflow. In contrast to MDIs, DPIs do not require spacers. A number of types of DPIs are available, ranging from single-dose devices loaded by the (human) patient to multi-unit dose devices in a blister pack, blister strip, or reservoir. However, a major disadvantage of DPIs in veterinary medicine is the dependency of particle size on inspiratory effort. Each DPI is characterized by a different airflow resistance; finer particles require more resistance to air flow, which, in turn, requires greater inspiratory effort. Consequently, DPI application may be limited in animals. The use of nebulizers or inhalant devices in small animal patients is largely based on anecdotal reports. One study demonstrated that a radiopharmaceutical will be distributed to peripheral airways in cats using a simple face mask.[135] To maximize the site of particle deposition, animals to be aerosolized should be pretreated with a β-adrenergic or methylxanthine bronchodilator 10 minutes before aerosolization, or (potentially less preferable) a bronchodilator should be included in the aerosolized medicament (e.g., 100 mg aminophylline). Care should be taken not to overhydrate and flood the respiratory tract. Treatments of approximately 30 to 45 minutes should be repeated every 4 to 12 hours. In humans aerosolization is a well-established route of administration for bronchodilators and antiinflammatories[26,136] (Box 20-1) and is recommended for dogs for selected infectious tracheobronchitis.[137] In veterinary patients aerosolization is more commonly used for administration of antimicrobials and mucolytics. Indications include asthma, chronic bronchial disease, and infections of both lower and upper airways. The dose of drug to be nebulized is generally not scientifically derived. A general approach would be dilution of the calculated systemic dose in a sufficient volume of saline necessary for a 30-minute aerosol. Drugs prepared by the manufacturer in irritating solutions (e.g., NAC) should be diluted. The choice of antibiotic to be aerosolized should be based on efficacy against the targeted organism. Because the amount of drug that reaches the site can not easily be quantitated and minimum inhibitory concentrations based on aerosolized drug have yet to be defined, the use of culture data based on the minimum inhibitory concentration (a plasma-based target) is a reasonable approach.

Adaptations to inhalant devices for animals range from modifications in inhalant masks[39] with a one-way valve that limits drug movement to inhalation to simple administration through an empty toilet paper roll "spacer" that facilitates adequate exposure during inspiration. Cats breathe six to seven times after the medication is dispensed from the inhaler. Despite innovations designed to enhance small airway penetration with inhalant devices, the smallest airways

Box 20-1

Drugs Administered by Aerosolization*

Bronchodilators
Isoproterenol
Isoetharine
Albuterol
Atropine†
Glycopyrrolate†

Glucocorticoids
Beclomethasone
Triamcinolone

Mucokinetics
Water
Saline
Bicarbonate
N-acetylcysteine‡

Antimicrobials
Ceftriaxone (40 mg/mL in water or dimethylsulfoxide)
Chloramphenicol (13 mg/mL)
Enrofloxacin (10 mg/mL)
Gentamicin, amikacin (5 mg/mL)
Kanamycin
Polymyxin B (66,600 IU/mL)
Amphotericin B‡ (7 mg/mL in 5% dextrose)
Nystatin‡
Clotrimazole (10 mg/mL in polyethylene glycol)
Enilconazole (10 mg/mL in water)

Other
Alcohol‡

*In general, solutions can be made with injectable products (1 part) mixed with saline (9 parts). The concentration of specific drugs is noted in parentheses. The diluent for these drugs is saline, unless noted otherwise. Tris-EDTA might be used as a diluent when infections caused by *Pseudomonas aeruginosa* or other problematic gram-negative infections are being treated.
†In combination with other bronchodilators.
‡Drug-induced bronchoconstriction may be severe.

are likely to remain untreated. Additionally, aerosol therapy is limited to the epithelial surface of the airways. Finally, compliance in humans with inhaled therapy is poorer than with systemic therapy.[40] As such, the use of inhalant devices should be accompanied by frequent thorough monitoring. Inhalant antimicrobial therapy should not replace systemic therapy. The factors decreasing small airway drug delivery in animals are likely to be greater than in humans. As such, scientific support is paramount to guide the appropriateness of and indications for inhalant bronchodilator and antiinflammatory therapy as a replacement for systemic therapy.

DRUG THERAPY OF SPECIFIC DISEASES OF THE RESPIRATORY TRACT

Treatements of infectious diseases of the respiratory tract are discussed in Chapter 9; diseases associated with chronic inflammation are also addressed in Chapter 19.

Therapy of Fungal Infections of the Nose

Nasal aspergillosis in dogs is difficult to treat and generally most successful if medical management is accompanied by surgical débridement. Topical therapy includes flushing the nasal mucosa with povidone–iodine solutions (10%) every 8 hours for 6 to 8 weeks after surgery; a 10% solution of clotrimazole in polyethylene glycol, instilled in nasal tubes and administered twice daily or in direct contact for 1 hour during surgical exploration; or enilconazole (10%) at 5 mg/kg instilled into nasal tubes twice daily for 7 to 14 days. Topical therapy should be accompanied by systemic therapy with itraconazole. Treatment of fungal infections is discussed in greater depth in Chapter 11.

Therapy of Disorders of the Trachea

Tracheitis

Resolution of underlying causes is important to successful control of the inflamed trachea. Noninfectious causes (e.g., exposure to smoke, cough) are more common than infectious causes. In addition to resolution of the underlying cause, drug therapy should be implemented to control symptoms. Cough can be controlled with peripheral or central antitussives or a combination thereof. Over-the-counter preparations that contain expectorants can prove helpful. Humidifying secretions (liquefaction of mucoid material) becomes increasingly important with chronic tracheitis and may include nebulization four to six times a day or exposure in a steam-filled bathroom for 15 to 20 minutes three times daily. Physical therapy (coupage) should be implemented after liquefaction of secretions. Short-term therapy with short-acting glucocorticoids may help break the cough cycle, although care must be taken that glucocorticoids do not exacerbate the underlying condition.

Antibiotics are indicated for infectious tracheitis/tracheobronchitis. Infectious tracheobronchitis in dogs (kennel cough) is a complex syndrome caused by multiple organisms, including viruses, bacteria, and mycoplasma. This syndrome is discussed with bronchial diseases.

Structural Disorders of the Trachea

Pharmacologic management of structural disorders of the trachea focuses on supportive therapy.

Hypoplastic trachea. Slight or moderate tracheal hypoplasia may respond to bronchodilator therapy. Recurrent infections (bacterial) should be anticipated because of a poorly functioning mucociliary tract. Although prophylactic antibiotic therapy is discouraged to avoid emergence of resistance, antibiotic therapy during active infection should be anticipated. Culture and susceptibility data may be particularly important for these patients because recurrent infections are more likely to occur in them than in animals with a normal trachea. Drugs that facilitate mucociliary clearance should be considered on a daily basis; these might include mucokinetic drugs. More serious episodes of respiratory compromise might benefit from NAC therapy administered by any route. The use of bronchodilators should be considered; although the tracheal diameter may not be affected, the effects of these drugs on peripheral airways can be beneficial. Supportive actions should also include weight control, avoidance of smoke and other environmental contaminants, and avoidance of actions or drugs that can compromise the immune response.

Tracheal collapse. Tracheal collapse as a cause of respiratory distress can progress to a life-threatening situation. Early therapy may help decrease or slow the progression of the syndrome in some animals, simply by decreasing damage to the trachea as a result of paroxysmal coughing. Tracheal rings in afflicted animals lose their ability to remain firm, leading to collapse. The characteristic "goose honk" cough is dry and chronic. Most commonly afflicting smaller breeds, tracheal collapse is often associated with chronic valvular (cardiac) disease, and it is important to differentiate between the two. Diagnosis requires proper radiographic examination and motion studies with either a fluoroscope or a bronchoscope.

Drug therapy targets control of the cough with bronchodilators and centrally acting antitussives. Severe coughs may require narcotic antitussives associated with sedation (a desirable characteristic in some patients) until the cough is controlled. Mucokinetic drugs may also be helpful. Short-term glucocorticoid therapy may be important to minimize the inflammatory response to damage induced by paroxysmal coughing. Nebulization may be helpful, but pretreatment with bronchodilators is probably important. The use of bronchodilators should be considered for their effects on peripheral airways. Digitalization reportedly has been beneficial in some patients that do not respond to other therapies.[138]

Proteoglycan content and size of tracheal cartilage matrix changes that accompany age have been demonstrated in a number of species, including humans.[139,140] Hamaide and coworkers[140] suggested that age-related changes may lead to compliance changes that accompany tracheal ring collapse. Trachea collapse appears to reflect loss of rigidity associated with decreased glucosamine glycan chondroitin sulfate. A number of old studies have demonstrated uptake of labeled glucosamine by cartilage rings under in vitro conditions, suggesting cartilage turnover may be sufficiently rapid that supplementation may be beneficial. Accordingly, supplementation in the form of injectable and oral products as is recommended for osteoarthritis is a reasonable approach for preventing or supporting other therapies for tracheal collapse. The role of glutamine and chondroitin sulfates in supporting damaged or healing cartilage in osteoarthritis is addressed in Chapter 29. Response, if it is to occur, will be prolonged in onset, depending on the rate of tracheal proteoglycan turnover.

Bronchial Diseases

Diagnosis of bronchial diseases should be based on physical examination, thoracic radiography, tracheal or bronchial wash, and bronchoscopy. Examination for structural defects, cytologic studies, and microbial cultures are among the diagnostic tools of use for bronchial diseases.

Canine Infectious Tracheobronchitis

Bordetella bronchiseptica is the bacterial organism most commonly associated with kennel cough. Viral organisms include canine parainfluenza, canine herpes, and canine distemper viruses. The clinical syndrome is characterized by a dry, hacking, paroxysmal cough in an otherwise healthy animal. Clinical signs of this highly contagious syndrome generally appear 3 to 5 days after exposure. Tracheal cytology should reveal neutrophils and bacteria. Therapy of uncomplicated cases is supportive. Antitussives, in relative order of efficacy (least to most), include dextromethorphan (antitussives), butorphanol, and hydrocodone. Hydrocodone may be associated with sedation, which may be beneficial in cases of paroxysmal coughing. Antimicrobial therapy in uncomplicated cases (lasting 7 to 10 days) is discouraged; indeed, most antimicrobials used empirically (e.g., amoxicillin) generally do not penetrate bronchial secretions in sufficient quantities to be effective.

In contrast, antibiotic therapy (in addition to other supportive therapy) is indicated for complicated infections or for dogs whose coughing persists after 2 weeks and for which evidence exists of secondary bacterial infection. Other indicators of complications include any evidence of infection occurring lower than the upper bronchi or systemic signs of illness. Because of the complicated nature, and particularly if the patient has received previous antimicrobials, selection of the appropriate antibiotic should be based on a properly collected culture at the site of infection (not a pharyngeal or laryngeal swab). Selection of an antimicrobial empirically is complicated by the possibility of mycoplasma as a causative agent. Selection of antimicrobials for treatment of respiratory tract infections is discussed in Chapter 8.

Therapies intended to support mucociliary function should be continued. Because coughing associated with kennel cough can be paroxysmal, a single treatment with a short-acting glucocorticoid might be considered to ameliorate some of the effects of inflammation. In the immunocompromised animal, however, this may lead to spread of infection.

Feline Bronchial Diseases

Feline bronchial diseases include feline bronchial asthma as well as acute and chronic bronchitis and emphysema. It is characterized by damage or hypertrophy (or both) of the airway epithelium; increased production of airway secretions; and spasms of bronchial smooth muscle, which itself may become hypertrophied.[39] Causes of feline bronchial diseases have not been found, but a type I hypersensitivity reaction has been suspected as a cause of asthma. Initial contact between the allergen and bronchial mucosa may lead to the release of histamine and other mediators that allow penetration of the allergen into the submucosa. The resultant inflammatory response to the allergen leads to the characteristic disease. The source of inflammatory mediators includes essentially any cell of the respiratory tract, white blood cells, and platelets. Smooth muscle hypertrophy and increased mucus and inflammatory cell infiltrate (particularly eosinophils) characterize asthma and its clinical signs. Acute bronchitis is generally reversible and short in duration but can be life-threatening.

Should airway inflammation persist, bronchitis may become chronic. Inflammation lasting 2 to 3 months can lead to deposition of fibrous tissue; these lesions tend to be irreversible. Emphysema can occur as a result of chronic bronchitis and is characterized by enlarged airspaces with destruction of bronchiolar and alveolar walls and airway collapse. Cough is the most consistent clinical sign of bronchial disease in cats. Respiratory distress may be absent or episodic, particularly in the presence of bronchial asthma.

Diagnosis should be based on thoracic radiographs, a complete blood count (which may reveal eosinophilia), tracheal or bronchial wash (particularly if bacterial or parasitic causes are suspected), and fecal examination (for parasitic causes). Cultures of *Mycoplasma* species should be performed whenever possible, particularly in nonresponders. Treatment should include environmental management. In particular, exposure to smoke (e.g., cigarette, fireplace) should be avoided; other potential environmental allergens include litter dust, perfumes, household cleaning products, deodorants, and insulation products. Asthma in cats has been classified according to the severity (mild, moderate, and severe) of clinical signs in order to facilitate the need for treatment.[39] However, clinicians are urged not to become too complacent in their approach to the disease and to ensure that seemingly mild disease does not progress to a more severe state in the absence of therapy. The primary focus of therapy is control of inflammation. Control of inflammation in peripheral airways may be paramount to successful therapy.

Management of Acute Asthma

Acute respiratory distress resulting from bronchial disease should be handled as a medical emergency. Administration of drugs should be accompanied by oxygen therapy and rest. The hydration status of the patient should be assessed at presentation and corrected if indicated. Overzealous fluid therapy can prove detrimental, however, and should be avoided. Therapy should include bronchodilators, glucocorticoids (for their permissive effect on β-$_2$ adrenergic receptors) and as necessary, anticholinergics.

Glucocorticoid therapy should be initiated in conjunction with bronchodilators in cats with status asthmaticus. The permissive effects of glucocorticoids are likely to improve response to bronchodilator therapy. Rapidly acting drugs such as prednisone sodium succinate should be administered at presentation and again at 4 to 6 hours.[6,30] Prednisolone is preferred to prednisone; the latter should not be given orally (see Chapter 30). Alternatively, dexamethasone or dexamethasone phosphate may be administered because of its antiinflammatory potency. Oral bronchodilator and glucocorticoid therapy can begin when the patient is stabilized.

Among the bronchodilators, β_2-adrenergic agonists are preferred (although doses have not been well established for animals), but nonselective agonists can be equally effective in critical cases. Parenteral rather than oral administration will ensure the most rapid onset of action, although use of a short-acting inhalant beta-adrenergic also might be considered (see the discussion of inhalant devices). Note that epinephrine has marked β_1 (and α) effects and in the presence of hypoxemia can cause fatal cardiac arrhythmias. Aerosolization should not replace, but can be used in concert with, parenteral administration if the stress of aerosolization is not dangerous to severely dyspneic animals. Subcutaneous epinephrine can be administered at presentation and, if the patient responds, repeated every 30 minutes for several doses.[30] Terbutaline can also be administered subcutaneously either instead of epinephrine or for animals that fail to respond to epinephrine. Aminophylline can be infused intravenously (2 to 5 mg/kg in 5% dextrose or saline) in animals that fail to respond to β-agonists.[30] The addition of atropine or glycopyrrolate may facilitate bronchodilation. Exacerbation of hypoxia is a complication of bronchodilator therapy, particularly with theophylline, due to drug-induced pulmonary vasodilation, and the potential for ventilation-perfusion mismatching necessitates administration of humidified oxygen. The use of an anticholinergic (atropine preferred) also should be considered after therapy with beta-adrenergics and glucocorticoids.

Reinero and coworkers[141] addressed the impact of flunisolide (inhaled glucocorticoid), prednisone, zafirlukast, and cyproheptadine along with placebo on inflammatory mediators in an experimental model of feline asthma (n = 6) using a randomized crossover design. The only significant changes detected were a decrease in the percentage of eosinophils in bronchoalveolar lavage fluid for both prednisone and flunisolide compared with control and the content of allergen-(Bermuda grass) specific IGE in serum in cats receiving oral glucocorticoids. The power of the study to detect significant differences and the use of prednisone were limitations of the study.

Long-term management of feline asthma. Response to glucocorticoids in the acute management of respiratory distress in cats may indicate a favorable response to long-term management. Glucocorticoids are the preferred drug, particularly in cats with moderate to severe disease, for control of inflammation. Prednisolone is the most commonly preferred maintenance drug, although triamcinolone is acceptable, prednisone is discouraged. Initially, doses should be as high as 2 to 3 mg/kg divided two to three times a day. A 2- to 3-week trial may be indicated to establish efficacy and need. Maintenance doses are likely to markedly vary among animals and should be slowly tapered to a minimum effective dose 1 to 2 weeks after therapy is started. Doses as little as 1.25 mg/cat every 72 hours may be sufficient in some animals. Glucocorticoid therapy should be maintained for a minimum of 2 months; complete cessation of therapy may not be possible in selected cases. Therapy should be continued for several weeks after cessation of signs to resolve residual and clinically inapparent small airway disease. Tracheal cytology may be helpful in identifying the continued need for antiinflammatory therapy both before and after therapy is discontinued. Repositol forms of glucocorticoids might be avoided because of the risk of exacerbation of disease.[30]A study in humans found the repositol form of methylprednisolone just as effective as a tapering regimen of oral glucocorticoids upon hospital discharge that followed acute management of asthma;

however, the intent of the therapy was to slowly withdraw the drug with no continued therapy. Because remission of clinical signs appears to be more difficult in animals that have received these drugs, if therapy is anticipated to continue beyond the duration anticipated for reposital therapy, daily dosing should continue or care should be taken to avoid relapse. For animals for which daily glucocorticoids cannot be given consistently doses of 2 to 4 mg/kg can be given every 10 to 30 days to control clinical signs. In cases of exacerbation in patients receiving glucocorticoids, intermittent high doses of intravenously administered or aerosolized glucocorticoids, and particularly beclomethasone dipropionate, in conjunction with oral maintenance glucocorticoids can be used to treat animals whose disease worsens.[30] Alternatively, megestrol acetate has been recommended instead of intermittent high doses of glucocorticoids in cats with refractory bronchial asthma.[30]

Addition of bronchodilator therapy should be considered for animals that do not respond sufficiently to glucocorticoid therapy. Intermittent use may help during periods of exacerbation of disease, although long-term therapy may be necessary for some animals. Bronchodilators may decrease the amount of glucocorticoids necessary to control clinical signs. Oral theophylline is the bronchodilator most commonly used for long-term bronchodilator therapy in dogs and cats,[6,30] although terbutaline can be used as an alternative, particularly in animals refractory to theophylline. Alternating between theophylline and β-agonists may prevent the incidence of refractoriness owing to downregulation of β-receptors. Alternatively, the combination of the two should be considered, particularly in nonresponders; an additive response might be expected.[142] Monitoring serum theophylline concentrations is encouraged, particularly in animals that do not respond sufficiently or in animals receiving long-acting theophylline products. Theophylline, particularly long-acting products, might be given to cats in the evening to maximize therapeutic efficacy.

The use of cyclosporine, cyproheptadine, and LRAs as antiinflammatories should be considered in cats that have not sufficiently responded to or cannot tolerate glucocorticoid or bronchodilator therapy. The treatment of asthma as a chronic inflammatory disease is also addressed in Chapter 31. Cats suffering from *A. suum*–induced airway reactivity had decreased reactivity and remodeling after receiving CsA; differences were noted with 24 hours of therapy.[141b] Schooley and coworkers[143] examined the effect of cyproheptadine (8 mg orally twice daily) or cetirizine (5 mg orally twice daily) in cats (n = 9) with experimentally induced asthma (Bermuda grass allergen) using a randomized crossover design. Although no significant differences were detected, the percentage of eosinophils in bronchoalveolar lavage fluid was less in the cats treated with cyproheptadine (27 ± 16%) and cetirizine (31 ± 20%) compared with those in the placebo group (40 ± 22%).

The role of inhalant devices in treatment of feline asthma. Despite the paucity of well-designed, controlled clinical trials, the use of MDIs for the control of feline asthma is now a generally accepted method of administering glucocorticoids or bronchodilators to asthmatic cats.[39] Studies are emerging. For example, response to orally administered prednisone, inhaled flunisolide, zafirlukast, or cyproheptadine was studied using a controlled crossover design in cats (n = 6) with experimentally induced (Bermuda grass allergen) asthma.[141] Significant findings were limited to decreased eosinophils in bronchoalveolar lavage fluid for both glucocorticoid groups. On the basis of this study, response to inhaled glucocorticoids might be anticipated in the cat with spontaneous asthma, but the authors' conclusions that inhaled glucocorticoids might serve as an alternative to oral glucocorticoids should be applied to long-term management only with caution.

Drug delivery in cats using inhalant devices is anecdotally described.[39] Care must be taken to coordinate breath intake with drug administration, which is facilitated by the presence of spacer. In animals with mild disease, use of inhaled glucocorticoids (e.g., fluticasone propionate preferred, others include flunisolide, budesonide, and beclomethasone dipropionate) has been recommended twice daily.[39] Inhaled short-acting beta-adrenergics (e.g., albuterol preferred, others include pirbuterol, bitolterol) are used as needed to control exacerbations or in animals for which clinical signs do not occur every day. However, client compliance should be ensured when using inhalant devices as primary therapy. Additionally, control of small airway inflammation may remain a concern. For animals with moderate disease (clinical signs have affected daily life, but cough and wheeze are not persistent), oral glucocorticoids should be added short term (e.g., 5 days twice daily followed by 5 days once daily). Systemic effects of inhaled glucocorticoids should preclude the need for tapering oral glucocorticoid doses further as they are discontinued. For severe disease both systemic and inhaled glucocorticoid therapy should be considered. Systemic therapy may include intravenous dexamethasone during an acute crisis. Inhaled bronchodilators should be continued as needed up to 4 times a day. For cases that continue to be refractory, the addition of cyproheptadine has generally found more support than LRAs.

The small number of feline studies precludes drawing conclusions regarding the use of other drugs (e.g., cyproheptadine, antihistamines, LRAs) or combination therapies for treatment as asthma. Their sole use should not be considered in animals with moderate or severe disease, and caution is recommended even for mild disease that might be insidiously progressive. Oral bronchodilator therapy also should be considered in animals with moderate to severe disease or in animals for which inhalant therapy is not reasonable or effective because of poor drug delivery or other reasons.

Canine Chronic Bronchitis

Acute bronchitis is not as likely to present as a life-threatening situation in dogs and refers primarily to duration of clinical signs. Inflammation that persists more than 2 months may cause permanent damage to airways and is referred to as *chronic bronchitis*.[144] *Bronchiectasis* refers to irreversible dilation of the bronchi and can be a sequela of chronic bronchitis (inflammation) that does not resolve. The underlying cause is rarely identified but may include allergies; inhaled irritants (including cigarette smoke); viral, microbial, or parasitic infections; and heartworm disease. Bacterial infections are more difficult to diagnose, should be based on quantitative rather than qualitative assessment, and generally are not initiators of chronic disease.[144] Foreign bodies are a less common cause. As with cats, eradication of the underlying cause is paramount to halting the progression and therapeutic success. Diagnostic aids are the same as discussed for cats. Medical management of chronic airway disease in dogs is frustrating and should be approached as a perpetuating, slowly progressive, noncurable disease. As such, resolution of identifiable inciting causes (including triggers such as cigarette smoke) and conditions that confound success should accompany drug therapy. Owners may have to adjust their tolerance levels. Additionally, therapy should be accompanied by weight loss and physical therapy (mild exercise or coupage to facilitate movement of respiratory secretions).

Allergic bronchitis is not a common or easy diagnosis in dogs. The canine respiratory tract is probably more resistant to antigenic stimulation as a cause of cough compared with that of cats (and humans). Parasitic infections including heartworm disease must be ruled out. If airway cytology supports an allergic response and the underlying cause has not been identified or yet eradicated, glucocorticoids are indicated. A minimum effective dose should be rapidly established. Long-term glucocorticoid therapy may not be indicated for dogs unless the disease is associated with eosinophilic or mononuclear infiltrates; this is particularly true for patients with bronchiectasis.

Medical management of chronic bronchitis in dogs must be modified for the individual patient. Exposure to irritants such as secondary cigarette smoke must be avoided. Bronchodilator therapy provides the mainstay of medical management of chronic bronchitis in many dogs. Ideally, bronchodilators will also facilitate movement of secretions and control inflammation. Drugs used for cats can be used for dogs; the major difference is in frequency of administration, which will be more common in dogs. Response generally is based on improvement in clinical signs; therapeutic monitoring is encouraged for theophylline products, particularly for dogs that do not sufficiently respond and in dogs receiving delayed-release products intended for human use. Both terbutaline and albuterol can be used for dogs and might be considered in combination with theophylline for nonresponders for which therapeutic concentrations of theophylline have been maximized or on an alternating basis with theophylline.

Control of inflammation may be facilitated by the use of NAC; additionally, its expectorant and mucolytic effects also should prove beneficial. LRAs should be considered as well. Glucocorticoids should be used only if cytologic examination indicates a large mononuclear or predominantly eosinophilic component to the inflammation. Use should be implemented only after appropriate quantitative culture techniques have failed to yield microbes in the presence inflammatory cytology. However, the role of *Mycoplasma* also must be ruled out. Ideally, inhaled glucocorticoids are preferable to systemic. However, their role is less well established for dogs than for cats.

The routine use of antimicrobials for the treatment of chronic diseases is and potentially contraindicated. Distinction between infection and colonization should be made whenever possible. The risk of causing a resistant infection in the presence of a chronic progressive disease suggests that antimicrobial selection be based on quantitative culture ($> 2.7 \times 10^3$ colony-forming units/mL) based on a properly collected sample[144] and be designed such that microorganisms (and particularly first-step mutants) are killed (rather than inhibited). High doses for a shorter duration of time are preferred to doses that target the minimum inhibitory concentration of the infecting organism. Drugs that penetrate bronchial secretions well are preferred in the presence of adequate susceptibility. Selection of the antimicrobial should be based on culture and susceptibility data. Cytologic findings should be used to guide the need for antimicrobial therapy; culture data are likely to enhance therapeutic success. Antimicrobial therapy should target *Bordetella*. The potential of infection with *Mycoplasma* should not be overlooked. A trial course of antimicrobials is indicated if cytologic findings are supportive of microbial infection; care should be taken to use an antimicrobial effective against *Mycoplasma* before microbial infection is ruled out. In general, when possible, drugs that accumulate in phagocytic cells should be considered when treating pulmonary conditions. A more comprehensive discussion of antimicrobial therapy for respiratory tract infections can be found in Chapter 8.

The role of antitussives in the treatment of diseases depends on the character of the cough. Inflammation and infection can result in mediator release and cough without an increase in bronchial secretions. Narcotic antitussives are generally indicated if the cough is nonproductive and is paroxysmal and irritating in of itself. Use of glucocorticoids is indicated if airway inflammation is the major contributing factor (as opposed to accumulation of airway secretions). In the case of productive cough, the use of expectorants or mucolytic antitussives may exacerbate cough as is intended if accumulated debris is to be removed. Hydration of respiratory secretions is critical to effective mucociliary transport function. As such, diuretics are contraindicated, and daily water intake must be maintained. Exposure to humidified air (i.e., humidifiers, vaporizers, or a visit to the bathroom during family member showers) is likely to facilitate liquefaction of respiratory secretions.

Pulmonary Diseases

As with other regions of the respiratory tract, causes of pulmonary diseases include viral, microbial, and parasitic infections; allergic (hypersensitivity) or immune-mediated diseases; and, although rare, nonspecific causes of interstitial lung disease. Malignancy of the lungs is discussed elsewhere. Supportive therapy should include bronchodilators and a means to maintain airway hydration (mucokinetics or mucolytics). NAC should be considered for both its antiinflammatory and mucolytic actions. Pentoxifylline also should be considered. Bronchodilators should not be used indiscriminately. Although they can contribute to both bronchial relaxation and controlled inflammation, they may also be associated with ventilation–perfusion mismatching. Diuretics are contraindicated unless vascular overload has led to pulmonary edema.

Oxygen is a consistent supportive therapy for the hypoxic animal; positive pressure ventilation is indicated for patients with poor pulmonary compliance. Physical therapy (coupage) is indicated in conditions associated with accumulation of respiratory secretions. Glucocorticoids are indicated for selected acute and chronic inflammatory conditions. Use in acute conditions generally is intended to minimize the acute inflammatory response; methylprednisolone is often recommended for immediate short-term therapy because of its ability to scavenge oxygen radicals.

Immune-Mediated Diseases

Diseases of the respiratory tract associated with eosinophilic infiltrates of the bronchi were discussed earlier with chronic causes of tracheobronchitis. Eosinophilic infiltrates that target lung parenchyma, referred to as *pulmonary infiltrates with eosinophils,* are associated with a spectrum of conditions ranging from mild diffuse infiltrates to granulomatous responses characterized by nodular masses that are visualized radiographically.

As with bronchial diseases, medical management of immune-mediated diseases should be accompanied by removal of any suspected allergen. Immunosuppressive doses of glucocorticoids are indicated for animals that do not respond to environmental changes. An exception is made for eosinophilic granulomatosis, for which cytotoxic drugs (cyclophosphamide) are indicated. For nongranulomatous disease, glucocorticoid therapy may need to be long term. Adherence to general principles of glucocorticoid use is indicated (i.e., tapering to a minimum effective dose, alternate-day therapy, and slow withdrawal). Granulomatosis, whether eosinophilic or lymphoid, is accompanied by a poor prognosis. Combination therapy should include cyclophosphamide (50 mg/m^2 orally every 48 hours) and immunosuppressive doses (1 mg/kg every 12 hours) of prednisone. NAC and bronchodilators should be used as previously discussed.

Vascular Diseases

Pulmonary Hypertension

Because pulmonary hypertension is most commonly a secondary problem, treatment should focus on eradication of the underlying cause; its treatment is addressed in Chapter 14. Causes can be precapillary (alveolar hypoxia caused by lung disease or high altitude) or postcapillary (congenital heart disease with left to right shunting of blood or acquired heart disease). Dirofilariasis is probably the most common cause of pulmonary hypertension in dogs; bronchial asthma might be a cause in cats.

Pulmonary Edema

As in any tissue, excessive fluid accumulation in the lungs occurs as a result of increased hydrostatic pressure, decreased oncotic pressure, lymphatic blockage, or changes in vascular permeability. Increased hydrostatic pressure generally occurs as a result of volume (vascular) overload. In contrast to fluid dynamics in other tissues, hydrostatic pressure in the lungs is low, and lymphatic flow is high. Expansion of lymphatics, as well as fluid movement into the alveoli, can accommodate marked increases in capillary pressure. Thus capillary hydrostatic pressures must markedly increase for excessive fluid to accumulate in the lungs. Hypoalbuminemia is not a likely cause of pulmonary edema. Rather, vascular overload as a result of overcirculation is a common cause of pulmonary edema secondary to increased oncotic pressure. Left-sided heart failure is the most common cause of vascular overload. Regardless of the cause of pulmonary edema, oxygen therapy and actions that minimize stress and anxiety of the patient are indicated. Unless contraindicated, bronchodilators should be administered.

Diuretics are indicated for treatment of pulmonary edema associated with volume overload (increased hydrostatic pressure). Drugs that cause sodium and chloride excretion (i.e., furosemide) may be more effective, particularly in cases of sodium and water retention. Attention might be made to selection based on underlying cause (e.g., aldosterone antagonists in the presence of high aldosterone output). Diuretics are contraindicated for patients that are hypovolemic. Use in normovolemic animals should be cautious and the dose titrated to the minimum needed to control clinical signs associated with pulmonary edema. In life-threatening situations of pulmonary edema associated with volume overload, venous dilators can be used to increase the capacitance of the vascular system, thus "drawing" the increased volume into the veins, away from the heart and pulmonary system. Topically applied nitroglycerin or morphine sulfate (0.1 mg/kg intravenously as needed) can be used for this purpose. Morphine has the added advantage of sedating animals whose anxiety is contributing to hypoxia. Methylxanthines such as theophylline might be helpful in the short term because they also bronchodilate, and in the patient with heart failure they may improve contractility. They will also, however, increase oxygen demand by the heart, and their diuretic effects are short lived (2 to 3 days).

Pulmonary edema as a result of increased vascular permeability probably occurs more frequently than is anticipated. Any disorder that causes inflammation of the lungs will contribute to pulmonary edema of the lungs. The extreme manifestation of permeability-induced pulmonary edema is ARDS, which has been described in humans. The fluid contains protein that, as long as it is present, will continue to provide oncotic draw of fluid into the parenchyma. Pulmonary edema of this type is difficult to treat. Pulmonary wedge pressure is normal; vascular overload is not present. In this situation diuretics will serve to decrease fluid retention only at the cost of extracellular fluid volume and thus are not an effective treatment. Glucocorticoids might be indicated to decrease inflammation and support bronchodilation, although their use is controversial. Among the glucocorticoids, methylprednisolone should be considered because of its ability to scavenge oxygen radicals. Vasodilators might be used; the therapeutic intent of these drugs is not certain, but decreased delivery of blood to the lungs and a further decrease in wedge pressure may decrease movement of blood into the parenchyma. Vascular shunting and hypotension may, however, preclude their use. Newer therapies are likely to target mediators responsible for permeability, such as TNF or nitric oxide, or replace surfactant.

MISCELLANEOUS

Aspiration Pneumonia

Clinical signs resulting from aspiration pneumonia may result from mechanical obstruction in small or large airways, and the inflammatory response to foreign materials (including gastric acid or other chemicals), bacterial infection is. Decreased pulmonary compliance and bronchoconstriction are likely to be a source of some of the clinical signs. Oxygen therapy, bronchodilatory therapy, and positive pressure ventilation are indicated, the latter particularly for patients with poor pulmonary compliance. Bronchoscopy can be used to guide removal of visible foreign material. Glucocorticoids might be used to minimize the inflammatory response during the initial phase of therapy; methylprednisolone and NAC might be considered to minimize oxygen radical damage. Immunosuppression probably negates the advantages of controlled inflammation after 48 hours of therapy. Among the drugs to be considered is pentoxifylline. Its early use (immediately after aspiration) as a loading dose followed by infusion resulted in 17% mortality versus 67% mortality in placebo-controlled rats.[145] In another study involving rats and measurement of inflammatory mediators, pre-treatment was found to be superior to post-aspiration treatment, suggesting preventative therapy might be considered in patients at high risk for post-operative aspiration. [145] Routine antibiotic coverage should be avoided to minimize the risk of resistance until evidence of a bacterial component in the inflammatory process exists.

Near Drowning

Standard supportive therapy for near drowning includes oxygen, positive pressure ventilation, and therapy for shock. Bronchodilators may be of benefit. Using a rat model of hydrochloride-induced lung injury, pretreatment with pentoxifylline significantly reduced damage, with some benefit shown in animals whose treatment was withheld until post injury. Further, pentoxifylline administered as a continuous infusion significantly reduced lung injury in dogs in which near-drowning was experimentally induced.[145a] Therapies for treatment of inflammation associated with aspiration should be considered. Use of glucocorticoids is controversial; however, use of methylprednisolone is appealing because of its oxygen-scavenging abilities. NAC therapy may be useful for its oxygen radical–scavenging effects as well as other benefits. Short-term therapy may be of benefit. Use of antimicrobials should probably be reserved for evidence of infection. Supportive therapy should also target the advent of cerebral edema; an additional advantage of using methylprednisolone is minimizing oxygen radical damage in the event of cerebral hypoxia.

Smoke Inhalation

Oxygen therapy is critical for removal of carbon monoxide; the half-life of carboxyhemoglobin decreases from 4 to 0.5 hours in the presence of 100% oxygen. Other supportive therapy includes airway hydration (as needed), bronchodilators, and (if indicated) positive pressure ventilation, and drugs intended to control inflammation.[147] Short-term administration of glucocorticoids (methylprednisolone preferred) may be of benefit to minimize inflammation and oxygen radical damage and to facilitate bronchodilation. However, pentoxifylline should also be considered. Using an ovine model, pentoxifylline administered continuously after induction of smoke inhalation injury was associated with less hypoxia and ventilation perfusion mismatching, pulmonary hypertension and markers of inflammation.[147]

Chylothorax

The pathophysiology of chylothorax, or the accumulation of lymphatic fluid in the pleural cavity, is not well understood. Beyond repetitive drainage, both surgical and medical management arc limited in success. Rutin is a non-anticoagulant coumarin a flavone benzo-γ-pyrone plant fruit extract (bioflavonoid) from the Brazilian fava d'anta (*Dimorphandra*). It acts to stimulate macrophage removal of proteins and thus removes the oncotic flux of fluid into tissues. It has been used to treat selected causes of peripheral limb edema associated with protein exudation in human patients. It is available in health food stores as a supplement. Response may take several weeks to months. There appear to be no toxicities associated with the drug. Several case reports cite partial resolution of chylous effusion in cats receiving 50 mg/kg orally every 8 hours.[148-150] In humans, octrenotid is an octapeptide omatostatin-mimicking drug used to treat acromegaly. However, it also has been used (based on case reports) successfully with a medium chain triglyceride diet to control chylothorax associated with cardiac surgery.[151]

Diseases of the Pleura

A number of diseases are associated with pleural effusion, and successful management of the effusion largely depends on resolution of the underlying diseases. Thus pleural effusion resulting from cardiac failure, neoplastic disease, and other causes is treated by treatment of the cause; pleurodesis is used as needed to manage life-threatening effusion. Pleurodesis stimulated by lavage of irritating substances (with the intent of "closing" the pleural space by causing fibrosis) is strongly discouraged. An exception is made for empyema, which can be a primary disease.

Empyema

Empyema refers to the accumulation of infectious inflammatory material within the pleural space. Infection can be an extension of a primary pulmonary lesion,the result of direct penetrating trauma, or by way of a lymphatic or hematogenous route. Accumulation of inflammatory debris provides a continued colloidal draw of fluid into the cavity. Lymphatic obstruction by debris further worsens the ability of pleural fluid mechanics to resolve the accumulation. Thus chest drainage is critical to successful control. Microbiologic examination (including Gram stains initially pending culture and susceptibility data) should be the basis of initial antimicrobial selection. Subsequent daily cytologic studies with Gram staining should provide the basis for response to therapy. The fluid should be recultured if bacterial growth has not changed for 2 to 3 subsequent days or if the morphology of the organism changes. Note that absence of an organism on Gram stain does not necessarily indicate the absence of organisms at the site of infection. Because the incidence of anaerobic infections in empyema is high in dogs and cats, both aerobic and anaerobic cultures should be collected. Care must be taken to collect the anaerobic culture properly. Despite the presence of organisms on Gram stains, cultures often do not yield growth. Thus antimicrobial therapy often must be empirical.

Empirical therapy should include drugs effective against likely infecting organisms, including anerobic organisms (see Chapter 8).

REFERENCES

1. Moses BL, Spaulding GL: Chronic bronchial disease of the cat, *Vet Clin North Am Small Anim Pract* 15:929–949, 1985.
2. Slonim NF, Hamilton LH: Development and functional anatomy of the bronchopulmonary system. In Carson D, editor: *Respiratory physiology*, ed 5, St Louis, 1987, Mosby, pp 27–47.
3. Scott JS, Berney CE, Derksen FJ, et al: α-Adrenergic receptor activity in ponies with recurrent obstructive pulmonary disease, *Am J Vet Res* 52:1416–1422, 1991.
4. Gustin P, Dhem AR, Lekeux P, et al: Regulation of bronchomotor tone in conscious calves, *J Vet Pharmacol Ther* 12:58–64, 1989.
5. Chand N: Reactivity of isolated trachea, bronchus, and lung strip of cats to carbachol, 5-hydroxytryptamine and histamine: evidence for the existence of methylsergide-sensitive receptors, *Br J Pharmacol* 73:853–857, 1981.
6. Moise NS, Spaulding GL: Feline bronchial asthma: pathogenesis, pathophysiology, diagnostic, and therapeutic considerations, *Compend Contin Educ Pract Vet* 3:1091–1103, 1981.
7. Inque H, Masakazu I, Motohiko M, et al: Sensory receptors and reflex pathways of nonadrenergic inhibitory nervous system in feline airways, *Am Rev Respir Dis* 139:1175–1178, 1989.

7a. Canning BJ: Anatomy and neurophysiology of the cough reflex: ACCP evidence-based clinical practice guidelines, *Chest* 129(1Suppl):33S-47S, 2006.

7b. Bolser DC: Central mechanisms II: pharmacology of brainstem pathways, *Handb Exp Pharmacol* 187:203-217, 2009.

7c. Canning BJ, Chou YL: Cough sensors. I. Physiological and pharmacological properties of the afferent nerves regulating cough, *Handb Exp Pharmacol* 187:23-47, 2009.

8. Altiere RJ, Diamond L: Comparison of vasoactive intestinal peptide and isoproterenol relaxant effects in isolated cat airways, *J Appl Physiol* 56:986–992, 1984.
9. Altiere RJ, Szarek JL, Diamond L: Neuronal control of relaxation in cat airway's smooth muscle, *J Appl Physiol* 57:1536–1544, 1984.
10. Derksen FJ, Robinson NE, Armstrong PJ, et al: Airway reactivity in ponies with recurrent airway obstruction (heaves), *J Appl Physiol* 58:598–604, 1985.
11. Downes H, Austin DR, Parks CM, et al: Comparison of drug responses in vivo and in vitro in airways of dogs with and without airway hyperresponsiveness, *J Pharmacol Exp Ther* 237:214–219, 1986.
12. Colebatch HJH, Olsen CR, Nadel JA: Effect of histamine, serotonin, and acetylcholine on the peripheral airways, *J Appl Physiol* 21:217–226, 1966.
13. Townley RG, Hopp RJ, Agrawal DK, et al: Platelet-activating factor and airway reactivity, *J Allergy Clin Immun* 83:997–1011, 1989.
14. Soler M, Mansour E, Fernandez A, et al: PAF-induced airway responses in sheep: effects of a PAF antagonist and nedocromil sodium, *J Allergy Clin Immun* 67:661–668, 1990.
15. Gray PR, Derksen FJ, Robinson NE, et al: The role of cyclooxygenase products in the acute airway obstruction and airway hyperreactivity of ponies with heaves, *Am Rev Respir Dis* 140:154–160, 1989.
16. Blair AM, Woods A: The effects of isoprenaline, atropine, and disodium cromoglycate on ciliary motility and mucous flow in vivo measured in cats, *Br J Pharmacol* 35:P379–P380, 1969.
17. Suri R: The use of human deoxyribonuclease (rhDNase) in the management of cystic fibrosis, *BioDrugs* 19(3):135–144, 2005.
18. Gallagher JT, Kent PW, Passatore M, et al: The composition of tracheal mucus and the nervous control of its secretion in the cat, *Proc R Soc Lond* 192:49–76, 1975.
19. Winkler G: Pulmonary intravascular macrophages in domestic animal species: review of structural and functional properties, *Am J Anat* 181:217–234, 1988.
20. Frerking I, Günther A, Seeger W, et al: Pulmonary surfactant: functions, abnormalities and therapeutic options, *Intensive Care Med* 27:1699–1717, 2001.
21. Gillissen A, Nowak D: Characterization of N-acetylcysteine and ambroxol in anti-oxidant therapy, *Respir Med* 92:609–623, 1998.
22. Barnes PJ: The drug therapy of asthma: directions for the 21st century, *Agents Actions* 23(Suppl):293–313, 1988.
23. Barnes PJ: Our changing understanding of asthma, *Respir Med* 83(Suppl):17–23, 1989.
24. Gold WM, Meyers GL, Dain DS, et al: Changes in airway mast cells and histamine caused by antigen aerosol in allergic dogs, *J Appl Physiol* 43:271–275, 1977.
25. Norn S, Clementson P: Bronchial asthma: pathophysiological mechanisms and corticosteroids, *Allergy* 43:401–405, 1988.
26. Wanner A, Rao A: Clinical indications for and effects of bland, mucolytic, and antimicrobial aerosols, *Am Rev Respir Dis* 122:79–87, 1980.
27. An SS, Bai TR, Bates JH, et al: Airway smooth muscle dynamics: a common pathway of airway obstruction in asthma, *Eur Respir J* 29(5):834–860, 2007.
28. Kay AB, Walsh GM, Moqbel R, et al: Disodium cromoglycate inhibits activation of human inflammatory cells in vitro, *J Allergy Clin Immunol* 80:1–8, 1987.
29. Barnes PJ, Chung KF, Page CP: Inflammatory mediators and asthma, *Pharmacol Rev* 40:49–84, 1988.
30. Bauer T: Pulmonary hypersensitivity disorders. In Kirk RW, editor: *Current veterinary therapy IX*, Philadelphia, 1986, Saunders, pp 369–376.
31. Doshi U, Salat P, Parikh V: Cytokine modulators in asthma: clinical perspectives, *Indian J Pharmacol* 34:16–25, 2002.
32. Larché M, Robinson DS, Kay AB: The role of T lymphocytes in the pathogenesis of asthma, *J Allergy Clin Immunol* 111(3):450–463, 2003.
33. Umetsu DT, Akbari O: DeKruyff RH: Regulatory T cells control the development of allergic disease and asthma, *J Allergy Clin Immunol* 112:480–487, 2003.
34. Dorman SC, Sehmi R, Gauvreau GM, et al: Kinetics of bone marrow eosinophilopoiesis and associated cytokines after allergen inhalation, *Am J Respir Crit Care Med* 169(5):565–572, 2004.
35. Braccioni F, Dorman SC, O'Byrne PM, et al: The effect of cysteinyl leukotrienes on growth of eosinophil progenitors from peripheral blood and bone marrow of atopic subjects, *J Allergy Clin Immunol* 110(1):96–101, 2002.
36. Sterk PJ, Hiemstra PS: Eosinophil progenitors in sputum: throwing out the baby with the bath water? *Am J Respir Crit Care Med* 169:549–556, 2004.

37. Denburg JA: The bone marrow and airway inflammation: evidence for allergy as a systemic disease, *Clin Exp All Rev* 3:23-27, 2003.
38. Denburg JA: Haemopoietic mechanisms in nasal polyposis and asthma, *Thorax* 55(Suppl 2):S24-S25, 2000.
39. Padrid P: Feline asthma. Diagnosis and treatment, *Vet Clin North Am Small Anim Pract* 30(6):1279-1294, 2003.
40. Bjermer L: History and future perspectives of treating asthma as a systemic and small airways disease, *Respir Med* 95:703-719, 2001.
41. Undem BJ: Pharmacotherapy of asthma. In Brunton LL, Lazo JS, Parker KL, editors: *Goodman & Gilman's the pharmacological basis of therapeutics*, ed 11, New York, 2006, McGraw-Hill.
42. Eiser NM, Mills J, Snashall PD, et al: The role of histamine receptors in asthma, *Clin Sci* 60:363-370, 1981.
43. Dunford PJ, O'Donnell N, Riley JP, et al: The histamine H_4 receptor mediates allergic airway inflammation by regulating the activation of CD4+ T cells, *J Immunol* 176(11):7062-7070, 2006.
44. Skidgel RA, Erdös EG: Histamine, bradykinin, and their antagonists. In Brunton LL, Lazo JS, Parker KL, editors: *Goodman & Gilman's the pharmacological basis of therapeutics*, ed 11, New York, 2006, McGraw-Hill.
45. McNamara DB, Harrington JK, Bellan JA, et al: Inhibition of pulmonary thromboxane A_2 synthase activity and airway responses by CGS 13080, *Mol Cell Biochem* 85:29-41, 1989.
46. Inman MD, Denbrug JA, Parameswarn K, et al: The effect of cysteinyl leukotrienes on growth of eosinophil progenitors from peripheral blood and bone marrow of atopic, *J Allergy Clin Immunol* 110:96-101, 2002.
47. McKay IR, Rosen FS: Allergy and allergic disease, *N Engl J Med* 334:30-37, 2001.
48. Hogan JB, Piktel D, Landreth KS: IL-5 production by bone marrow stromal cells: implications for eosinophilia associated with asthma, *J Allergy Clin Immunol* 106:329-336, 2000.
49. Preventing migration of inflammatory cells. Dual integrin antagonists: a new approach to the treatment of asthma, 2001. Accessed October 26, 2009 at www.roche.com/pages/downloads/company/pdf/ om/pages/downloads/company/pdf/ rddpenzberg02 01e.pdf.
50. Daemen MJAP, Smits JFM, Thijssen HHW, et al: Pharmacokinetic considerations in target-organ directed drug delivery, *Trends Pharmacol Sci* 9:138-141, 1988.
51. Reed MT, Kelly HW: Sympathomimetics for acute severe asthma: should only beta2-selective agonists be used? *DICP Ann Pharmacother* 24:868-873, 1990.
52. Nelson HS: β-adrenergic bronchodilators, *New Eng J Med* 333(8):499-506, 1995.
53. Committee for Veterinary Medicinal Products: Clenbuterol Hydrochloride Summary Report. The European Agency for the Evaulatuion of Medicinal Products, *Veterinary Medicine and Information Technology Unit*, 2000.
54. Kirschvink N, Leemans J, Delvaoux F, et al: Bronchodilators in bronchoscopy-induced airflow limitation in allergen-sensitized cats, *J Vet Intern Med* 19:161-167, 2005.
55. Nelson HS: Combination therapy of bronchial asthma, *Allergy Asthma Proc* 22(4):217-220, 2001.
56. Hendeles L, Weinberger M: Theophylline: a state of the art review, *Pharmacotherapy* 3:2-44, 1983.
57. Mizus I, Summer W, Farrkuhk I, et al: Isoproterenol or aminophylline attenuate pulmonary edema after acid lung injury, *Am Rev Respir Dis* 131:256-259, 1985.
58. Short CE: Telazol: a new injectable anesthetic, *Cornell Fel Health Cent Info Bull* 2:1-3, 1987.
59. Mascali JJ, Cvietusa P, Negri J, et al: Anti-inflammatory effects of theophylline: modulation of cytokine production, *Ann Allergy Asthma Immunol* 77:34-38, 1996.
60. Sackner MA: Effect of respiratory drugs on mucociliary clearance, *Chest* 73(6):958-966, 1978.
61. Dunn ME, Taylor SM: Effects of theophylline on tracheal mucociliary clearance rates in healthy cats, *Am J Vet Res* 63:1320-1322, 2002.
62. Murciano D, Aubier M, Lecocguic Y, et al: Effects of theophylline on diaphragmatic strength and fatigue in patients with chronic obstructive pulmonary disease, *N Engl J Med* 311:349-353, 1984.
63. Viires N, Aubier M, Murciano D, et al: Effects of aminophylline on diaphragmatic fatigue during acture respiratory failure, *Am Rev Respir Dis* 129:396-402, 1984.
64. McKiernan BC, Davis CAN, Koritz GD, et al: Pharmacokinetics studies of theophylline in dogs, *J Vet Pharmacol Ther* 4:103-110, 1981.
65. McKiernan BC, Koritz GD, Davis LE, et al: Pharmacokinetics studies of theophylline in cats, *J Vet Pharmacol Ther* 6:99-104, 1983.
66. Bach JE, Kukanich B, Papich MG, et al: Evaluation of the bioavailability and pharmacokinetics of two extended-release theophylline formulations in dogs, *J Am Vet Med Assoc* 224(7):1113-1119, 2004.
67. Guenther-Yenke CL, McKiernan BC, Papich MG, et al: Pharmacokinetics of an extended-release theophylline product in cats, *J Am Vet Med Assoc* 231(6):900-906, 2007.
68. Dye JA, McKiernan BC, Jones SD: Sustained-release theophylline pharmacokinetics in cats, *J Vet Pharmacol Ther* 13:278-286, 1990.
69. Koritz GD, McKiernan BC, Davis CAN, et al: Bioavailability of four slow-release theophylline formulations in the beagle dog, *J Vet Pharmacol Ther* 9:293-302, 1986.
70. Dye JA, McKiernan BC, Neft Davis CA, et al: Chronopharmacokinetics of theophylline in cats, *J Vet Pharmacol Ther* 12:133-140, 1989.
71. Munsiff IJ, Koritz GD, McKiernan BC, et al: Plasma protein binding of theophylline in dogs, *J Vet Pharmacol Ther* 11:112-114, 1988.
72. Larsson CI, Kallings P, Persson S, et al: Pharmacokinetics and cardio-respiratory effects of oral theophylline in exercised horses, *J Vet Pharmacol Ther* 12:189-199, 1989.
73. McKiernan BC: Principles of respiratory therapy. In Kirk RW, editor: *Current veterinary therapy VIII: small animal practice*, Philadelphia, 1983, Saunders, pp 216-221.
74. Rybak MJ, Bowles SK, Chandrasekar PH, et al: Increased theophylline concentrations secondary to ciprofloxin, *Drug Intell Clin Pharmacol* 21:879-881, 1987.
75. Rodvold KA: Clinical pharmacokinetics of clarithromycin, *Clin Pharmacokinet* 37:385-398, 1999.
76. Cremer KF, Secor J, Speeg KV: The effect of route of administration on the cimetidine-theophylline drug interaction, *J Clin Pharmacol* 29:451-456, 1989.
77. Henderson A, Wright DM, Pond SM: Management of theophylline overdose patients in the intensive care unit, *Anaesth Intensive Care* 20(1):56-62, 1992.
78. Hirt RA, Teinfalt M, Dederichs D, et al: The effect of orally administered marbofloxacin on the pharmacokinetics of theophylline, *J Vet Med A Physiol Pathol Clin Med* 50(5):246-250, 2003.
79. Intorre L, Mengozzi G, Maccheroni M, et al: Enrofloxacin-theophylline interaction: influence of enrofloxacin on theophylline steady-state pharmacokinetics in the beagle dog, *J Vet Pharmacol Ther* 18(5):352-356, 1995.
80. Jonkman JH, Borgstrom L, van der Boon WJ, et al: Theophylline-terbutaline, a steady state study on possible pharmacokinetic interactions with special reference to chronopharmacokinetic aspects, *Br J Clin Pharmacol* 26(3):285-293, 1988.

81. Munsiff IJ, McKiernan BC, Davis CAN, et al: Determination of the acute oral toxicity of theophylline in conscious dogs, *J Vet Pharmacol Ther* 11:381–389, 1988.
82. Persson CGA, Ergefalt I: Seizure activity in animals given enprofylline and theophylline, two xanthines with partly different mechanisms of action, *Arch Int Pharmacodyn* 258:267–282, 1982.
83. Gross NJ, Skorodin MS: Anticholinergic, antimuscarinic bronchodilators, *Am Rev Respir Dis* 129:856–870, 1984.
84. Murphy S, Kelly HW: Cromolyn sodium: a review of mechanisms and clinical use in asthma, *DICP Ann Pharmacother* 21:22–35, 1987.
85. Holgate ST: Reflections on the mechanisms of action of sodium cromoglycate (Intal) and the role of mast cells in asthma, *Respir Med* 83(Suppl):25–31, 1989.
86. Massey KL, Hendeles L: Calcium antagonists in the management of asthma: breakthrough or ballyhoo? *DICP Ann Pharmacother* 21:505–508, 1987.
87. Creese BR: Calcium ions, drug action and airways obstruction, *Pharmacol Ther* 20:357–375, 1983.
88. Gupta R, Jindals PD, Kumar G: Corticosteroids: the mainstay in asthma, *Bioorg Med Chem* 12:6331–6342, 2004.
89. Hamid Q: Effects of steroids on inflammation and cytokine gene expression in airway inflammation, *J Allergy Clin Immunol* 112:636–638, 2003.
90. Currie GP, Srivasta VA, Dempsey OJ, et al: Therapeutic modulation of allergic airways disease with leukotriene receptor antagonists, *Q J Med* 98:171–182, 2005.
91. Kelly HW: Pharmaceutical characteristics that influence the clinical efficacy of inhaled corticosteroids, *Ann Allergy Asthma Immunol* 91:326–334, 2003.
92. Norris CA: Research Abstract Program of the 21st Annual ACVIM Forum, #22 Charlotte, NC, June 4-7, 2003.
93. Reinero CR, Brownlee L, Decile KC, et al: Inhaled flunisolide suppresses the hypothalamic-pituitary-adrenocortical axis, but has minimal systemic immune effects in healthy cats, *J Vet Intern Med* 20(1):57–64, 2006.
94. Hui Y, Funk CD: Cysteinyl leukotriene receptors, *Biochem Pharmacol* 64(11):1549–1557, 2002.
95. Tashkin DP: The importance of control in asthma management: do leukotreine receptor antagonists meet patient and physician needs? *Allergy Astham Proc* 22(5):311–319, 2001.
96. Boothe, 2006.
97. Parratt JR, Sturgess RM: The effect of indomethacin on the cardiovascular and metabolic responses to E. coli endotoxin in the cat, *Br J Pharmacol* 50:177–183, 1974.
98. Wasserman MA: Modulation of arachidonic acid metabolites as potential therapy of asthma, *Agents Actions* 23(Suppl):95–111, 1988.
99. Walker BR, Voelkel NF, Reeves JT: Pulmonary pressor response after prostaglandin synthesis inhibition in conscious dogs, *J Appl Physiol* 52:705–709, 1982.
100. Bennett A: The importance of COX-2 inhibition for aspirin induced asthma, *Thorax* 55(Suppl 2):S54–S56, 2000.
101. Keith JC: Pulmonary thromboembolism during therapy of dirofilariasis with thiacetarsamide: modification with aspirin or prednisolone, *Am J Vet Res* 44:1278–1283, 1983.
102. Rawlings CA, Keith JC, Lewis RE, et al: Aspirin and prednisolone modification of radiographic changes caused by adulticide treatment in dogs with heartworm infection, *J Am Vet Med Assoc* 183:131–132, 1983.
103. Chyrek-Borowska S, Siergiejko Z, Michalska I: The effects of a new generation of H_1 antihistamines (cefirizine and loratadine) on histamine release and the bronchial response to histamine in atopic patients, *J Invest Allergol Clin Immunol* 5:103–107, 1995.
104. Stahl SM: Selective histamine H_1 antagonism: novel hypnotic and pharmacologic actions challenge classical notions of antihistamines, *CNS Spectr* 13(12):1027–1038, 2008.
105. Sudoh Y, Cahoon EE, Gerner P, et al: Tricyclic antidepressants as long-acting local anesthetics, *Pain* 103(1-2):49–55, 2003.
106. Padrid PA, Mitchell RW, Ndukwu IM, et al: Cyproheptadine-induced attenuation of type I immediate hypersensitivity reactions of airway smooth muscle from immune sensitized cats, *Am J Vet Res* 56:109–115, 1995.
107. Norris CR, Boothe DM, Esparza T, et al: Disposition of cyproheptadine in cats after intravenous or oral administration of a single dose, *Am J Vet Res* 59(1):79–81, 1998.
108. Roudebush P: Antitussive therapy in small companion animals, *J Am Vet Med Assoc* 180:1105–1107, 1982.
109. Irwin RS, Curlye FJ, Bennett FM: Appropriate use of antitussives and protussives. A practical review, *Drugs* 46:80–91, 1993.
110. Gingerich DA, Rourke JE, Strom PW: Clinical efficacy of butorphanol injectable and tablets, *Vet Med Small Anim Clin* 78:179–182, 1983.
111. Christie GJ, Strom PW, Rourke JE: Butorphanol tartrate: a new antitussive agent for use in dogs, *Vet Med Small Anim Clin* 75:1559–1562, 1980.
112. Tukianinen H, Silvasti M, Flygare U, et al: The treatment of acute transient cough: a placebo-controlled comparison of dextromethorphan and dextromethorphan-beta2-sympathomimetic combination, *Eur J Respir Dis* 69:95–99, 1986.
113. Brain JD: Factors influencing deposition of inhaled particles, *Proc 3rd Annu Comp Respir Soc Symp* 3:232, 1983.
113a. Ichinose M, Miura M, Yamauchi H, et al: A neurokinin 1-receptor antagonist improves exercise-induced airway narrowing in asthmatic patients, *Am J Respir Crit Care Med* 153(3):936-941, 1996.
113b. Chapman RW, House A, Liu F, Celly C, et al: Antitussive activity of the tachykinin NK1 receptor antagonist, CP-99994, in dogs, Eur J Pharmacol 485(1-3):329-332, 2004.
114. Crockett A, Cranston JM, Alpers JH, et al: Mucolytics for bronchiectasis, *Cochrane Database of Systematic Reviews Issue 1. Art. No: CD001289* , 2001.
115. Ziment I: Acetylcysteine: a drug that is much more than a mucokinetic, *Biomed Pharmacother* 42:513–520, 1988.
116. Heller AR, Groth G, Heller SC, et al: N-acetylcysteine reduces respiratory burst but augments neutrophil phagocytosis in intensive care unit patients, *Crit Care Med* 29(2):272–276, 2001.
117. Tirouvanziam R, Conrad CK, Bottiglieri T, et al: High-dose oral N-acetylcysteine, a glutathione prodrug, modulates inflammation in cystic fibrosis, *Proc Natl Acad Sci U S A* 103(12):4628–4633, 2006.
118. Cuzzocrea S, Mazzon E, Dugo L, et al: Protective effects of n-acetylcysteine on lung injury and red blood cell modification induced by carrageenan in the rat, *FASEB J* 15(7):1187–2000, 2001.
119. Rocksen D, Lilliehook B, Larsson R: Differential anti-inflammatory and anti-oxidative effects of dexamethasone and N-acetylcysteine in endotoxin-induced lung inflammation, *Clin Exp Immunol* 122(2):249–256, 2000.
120. Ueno O, Lee L-N, Wagner PD: Effect of N-acetylcysteine on gas exchange after methacholine challenge and isoprenaline inhalation in the dog, *Eur Respir J* 2:238–246, 1989.
121. Ziment I: Acetylcysteine: a drug with an interesting past and a fascinating future, *Respiration* 50(Suppl 1):26–30, 1986.
122. DeCramer M, Rutten-van Mölken M, Dekhuijzen PN, et al: Effects of N-acetylcysteine on outcomes in chronic obstructive pulmonary disease (Bronchitis Randomized on NAC Cost-Utility Study, BRONCUS): a randomised placebo-controlled trial, *Lancet* 365(9470):1552–1560, 2005.

123. Sutherland ER, Crapo JD, Bowler RP: N-acetylcysteine and exacerbations of chronic obstructive pulmonary disease, *COPD* 3(4):195–202, 2006.
124. Kao LW, Kirk MA, Furbee RB, et al: What is the rate of adverse events after oral N-acetylcysteine administered by the intravenous route to patients with suspected acetaminophen poisoning? *Ann Emerg Med* 42(6):741–750, 2003.
125. Hendeles L: Selecting a decongestant, *Pharmacotherapy* 13:129S–134S, 1993.
126. Johnson DA, Hricik JG: The pharmacology of alpha-adrenergic decongestants, *Pharmacotherapy* 13:110S–115S, 1993.
127. Kanfer I, Dowse R, Vuma V: Pharmacokinetics of oral decongestants, *Pharmacotherapy* 13:116S–128S, 1993.
128. Miller CJ, McKinernan BC, Pace J, et al: The effects of doxapram hydrochloride (Dopram-V) on laryngeal function in healthy dogs, *J Vet Intern Med* 16(5):524-528, 2002.
129. Thompson PJ: Drug delivery to the small airways, *Am J Respir Crit Care Med* 157:S199–S202, 1998.
130. Malik SK, Jenkins DE: Alterations in airway dynamics following inhalation of ultrasonic mist, *Chest* 62:660–664, 1972.
131. Labiris NR, Dolovich MB: Pulmonary drug delivery. Part I: physiological factors affecting therapeutic effectiveness of aerosolized medications, *Br J Clin Pharmacol* 56(6):588–599, 2003.
132. Newhouse MT, Ruffin RE: Deposition and fate of aerosolized drugs, *Chest* 73(Suppl):936–943, 1978.
133. Labiris NR, Dolovich MB: Pulmonary drug delivery. Part II: the role of inhalant delivery devices and drug formulations in therapeutic effectiveness of aerosolized medications, *Br J Clin Pharmacol* 56:600–612, 2003.
134. Dolovich MB, Ahrens RC, Hess DR, et al: American College of Chest Physicians; American College of Asthma, Allergy, and Immunology. Device selection and outcomes of aerosol therapy: Evidence-based guidelines: American College of Chest Physicians/American College of Asthma, Allergy, and Immunology, *Chest* 127(1):335–371, 2005.
135. Schulman RL, Crochik SS, Kneller SK, et al: Investigation of pulmonary deposition of a nebulized radiopharmaceutical agent in awake cats, *Am J Vet Res* 65(6):806–809, 2004.
136. Johnson CE: Aerosol corticosteroids for the treatment of asthma, *Drug Intell Clin Pharmacol* 21:784–790, 1987.
137. Bemis DA, Appel MJG: Aerosol, parenteral, and oral antibiotic treatment of Bordetella bronchiseptica infections in dogs, *J Am Vet Med Assoc* 170:1082–1086, 1977.
138. Ettinger SJ, Kantrowitz B: Diseases of the trachea. In Ettinger SJ, Feldman E, editors: *Textbook of veterinary internal medicine*, ed 6, St Louis, 2005, Saunders.
139. Roberts CR, Pare PD: Composition changes in human tracheal cartilage in growth and aging, including changes in proteoglycan structure, *Am J Physiol* 261(2 Pt 1):L92–101, 1991.
140. Hamaide A, Arnoczky SP, Ciarelli MJ, et al: Effects of age and location on the biomechanical and biochemical properties of canine tracheal ring cartilage in dogs, *Am J Vet Res* 59(1): 18–22, 1998.
141. Reinero CR, Decline KC, Byerly JR, et al: Effects of drug treatment on inflammation and hyperreactivity of airways and on immune variables in cats with experimentally induced asthma, *Am J Vet Res* 66(7):1121–1127, 2005.
141a. Green SS, Lamb GC, Schmitt S, et al: Oral versus repository corticosteroid therapy after hospitalization for treatment of asthma, *J Allergy Clin Immunol* 95(1 Pt 1):15–22, 1995.
141b. Padrid PA, Cozzi P, Leff AR: Cyclosporin A inhibits airway reactivity and remodeling after chronic antigen challenge in cats, *Am J Respir Crit Care Med* 154:1812-1818, 1996.
142. Chow OK, Fung KP: Slow release terbutaline and theophylline for the long term therapy of children with asthma: a Latin square and factorial study of drug effects and interactions, *Pediatrics* 84:119–125, 1989.
143. Schooley EK, McGee Turner JB, Jiji RD, et al: Effects of cyproheptadine and cetirizine on eosinophilic airway inflammation in cats with experimentally induced asthma, *Am J Vet Res* 68(11):1265–1271, 2007.
144. McKiernan BC: Diagnosis and treatment of canine chronic bronchitis: twenty years of experience, *Vet Clin N Amer Small Anim Pract* 30(6):1267–1278, 2003.
145. Pawlik MT, Schreyer AG, Ittner KP, et al: Early treatment with pentoxifylline reduces lung injury induced by acid aspiration in rats, *Chest* 127(2):613–621, 2005.
145a. Ji Q, Zhang L, Wang L, et al: Pentoxifylline reduces indirect lung injury of fresh water drowning in canis, *Clin Chim Acta* 365(1-2):221-229, 2006.
146. Oliveira-Júnior IS, Maganhin CC, Carbonel AA, et al: Effects of pentoxifylline on TNF-alpha and lung histopathology in HCL-induced lung injury, *Clinics (Sao Paulo)* 63(1):77–84, 2008.
147. Ogura H, Cioffi WG, Okerberg CV, et al: The effects of pentoxifylline on pulmonary function following smoke inhalation, *J Surg Res* 56(3):242–250, 1994.
148. Thompson MS, Cohn LA, Jordan RC: Use of rutin for medical management of idiopathic chylothorax in four cats, *J Am Vet Med Assoc* 1;215(3):345-348, 1999.
149. Gould L: The medical management of idiopathic chylothorax in a domestic long-haired cat, *Can Vet J* 45(1):51-54, 2004.
150. Kopko SH: The use of rutin in a cat with idiopathic chylothorax, *Can Vet J* 46(8):729-731, 2005.
151. Barbetakis N, Xenikakis T, Efstathiou A, et al: Successful octreotide treatment of chylothorax following coronary artery bypass grafting procedure. A case report and review of the literature, *Hellenic J Cardiol* 47(2):118-122, 2006.

Drug Therapy for Endocrinopathies

21

Ellen N. Behrend, Tanya D. Civco, and Dawn Merton Boothe*

Chapter Outline

Hormones fall into two broad categories. The majority are peptides and amino acid derivatives, including complex polypeptides (e.g., thyroid-stimulating hormone [TSH]), intermediate-size peptides (e.g., insulin), small peptides (e.g., thyrotropin-releasing hormone [TRH]), dipeptides (e.g., T_4 and T_3), and derivatives of single amino acids (e.g., catecholamines). The remainder consists of steroid derivatives of cholesterol, of which there are two types: those with an intact steroid nucleus (e.g., adrenal and gonadal steroids) and those in which the B ring of the steroid has been cleaved (e.g., vitamin D). In general, the cellular effects of hormones are achieved either through interactions with cell membrane receptors, thus stimulating a cascade of intracellular reactions often involving secondary messenger systems, or through passive diffusion to the cellular nucleus, stimulation of protein synthesis, and subsequent formation of the effector protein(s). Protein hormones typically interact with cell membrane receptors, an exception being thyroid hormones, whereas steroidal hormones passively diffuse through the cell membrane to the nucleus.

Drug therapy for the endocrine system is implemented to either replace a deficient hormone or prevent or reduce the formation or effects of an overabundant hormone. Hormones may also be administered to provocatively test for the presence of an endocrine disease. Understanding the proper uses of the drugs depends on an appreciation of the normal physiology of each endocrine system, including mechanisms of control and behavior of target tissues (Table 21-1).

*A table is included in the chapter that lists drug doses for treating endocrine diseases. Please note that monitoring and tailoring of therapy is typically required in the treatment of endocrine diseases. The table contains starting doses only. Please see the text for details on monitoring and recommended dosage adjustment.

DISEASES OF THE THYROID GLAND

Synthesis of Thyroid Hormones

The protein thyroglobulin is synthesized by the endoplasmic reticulum and Golgi apparatus of thyroidal follicular cells and is released in vesicles into the colloid within follicular lumens. Iodine is accumulated by an active transport process in thyroidal follicular cells (Figure 21-1). Once in the follicular lumen, iodine is rapidly oxidized and combined with a tyrosine residue within thyroglobulin to form monoiodotyrosine. Monoiodinated tyrosines are then joined to form diiodinated tyrosines; further combinations yield triiodinated tyrosine (i.e., triiodothyronine [T_3] and thyroxine [T_4]), which contains four iodine molecules (Figure 21-2). The enzyme thyroid peroxidase mediates oxidation of iodine and formation of monoiodinated and diiodinated tyrosines as well T_3 and T_4. Four or more sites exist within the thyroglobulin molecule for the generation of thyroid hormones; generally, each molecule contains three or four molecules of T_4 and zero to one of T_3 (humans). The preformed hormones are released from the follicular colloid upon stimulation with TSH, with much greater quantities of T_4 being released than T_3. The hormones are transported bound to one of several transport proteins in the bloodstream and are delivered to target cells. At a target cell, both hormones are taken up. Intracellularly, T_4 is deiodinated on its outer ring to produce T_3, which is actually the active hormone that causes physiologic effects. In contrast, deiodination of the inner ring produces physiologically inactive reverse T_3 (rT_3). Thyroid hormones stimulate many metabolic processes, including activity of many enzymes; metabolism of vitamins and minerals; regulation of other hormones; and stimulation of calorigenesis, protein and enzyme synthesis, and carbohydrate and lipid metabolism.

Table 21-1 Endocrine Drugs and Recommended Doses*

Drug	Dose	Route	Interval (hr)
Drugs Used To Diagnose/Treat Hypothyroidism			
rhTSH	50-100 μg/dog (D)	IV	
Sodium levothyroxine	20 μg/kg (D)	PO	12
	5-10 μg/kg (D)	IV	12
	50-100 μg/cat (C)	PO	24
Sodium liothyronine	4-6 μg/kg (D)	PO	8
	4.4 μg/kg (C)	PO	8-12
Drugs Used To Treat Hyperthyroidism			
Atenolol	2 mg/kg or 6.25 mg/cat	PO	24
Methimazole	2.5-7.5 mg/cat	PO, transdermal	12[†]
Potassium iodide	1-2 drops SSKI/cat	PO (in gelatin capsule)	24
	50-100 mg/cat	PO	24
Propranolol	2.5-7.5 mg/cat	PO	8-12
Drugs Used To Treat Hypocalcemia/Hypoparathyroidism			
Calcitriol	Loading: 20-40 ng/kg	PO	24
	Maintenance: 5-15 ng/kg	PO	24
Calcium (oral)	1.0-4.0 g/d (D)[‡]	PO	
	0.5-1.0 g/d (C)	PO	
Calcium gluconate (10% solution)	5-15 mg/kg (0.5-1.5 ml/kg)	IV over 20 min	1-12
	5-15 mg/kg (0.5-1.5 ml/kg)	SC diluted in 2-4 parts saline[§]	1-12
Ergocalciferol	Loading: 4000-6000 U/kg	PO	24
	Maintenance: 1000-2000 U/kg	PO	24-168
Magnesium sulfate	1-2 mEq/kg	IV	24
Drugs Used To Treat Hypercalcemia			
Alendronate	10 mg/cat (C)	PO with butter and water	Once weekly
Dexamethasone[¶]	0.1-0.22 mg/kg	IV, PO, SC	12
Etidronate	5-15 mg/kg (D)	PO	12-24
Furosemide	5 mg/kg then 5 mg/kg/hr	IV	
	2-4 mg/kg	IV, PO, SC	8-12
Pamidronate disodium[‖]	1.3-2.2 mg/kg	IV, diluted in saline, over 2-4 hr	
Prednisone[¶]	1-2.2 mg/kg (D or C)	IV, PO, SC	12
	5-10 mg/cat (for idiopathic hypercalcemia)	PO	12
Salmon calcitonin	4-6 IU/kg	SC	8-12
Sodium bicarbonate	1-4 mEq/kg	IV slowly	
Drugs Used To Treat Hypoglycemia/Insulin Overdose			
Dextrose (50%)	0.5 g/kg diluted 1:4	IV	As needed
Drugs Used To Treat Diabetes Mellitus			
Acarbose	25-200 mg/dog (D)	PO with meals	12
	12.5-25 mg/cat (C)	PO with meals	12
Glipizide	2.5-5 mg/cat (C)	PO	12
Insulin			
Glargine	0.25 U/kg if BG <360 mg/dL (C)	SC	12
	0.5 U kg if BG >360 mg/dL (C)	SC	12
Lente	0.25 U/kg (D) 0.25 U/kg if BG <360 mg/dL (C)	SC	12-24
	0.5 U kg if BG >360 mg/dL (C)	SC	12
NPH	0.25 U/kg	SC	12-24
Regular[†]	1-3 U/cat	IV, IM, SC	
	See text		
	See text		

Table 21-1 Endocrine Drugs and Recommended Doses*—cont'd

Drug	Dose	Route	Interval (hr)
Drugs Used To Treat Diabetes Mellitus—cont'd			
Magnesium	0.75-1 mEq/kg/d	IV infusion in 5% dextrose for DKA	
Metformin	25-50 mg/cat (C)	PO	12
Phosphate	0.01-0.03 mMl/kg/hr 0.03-0.12 mMl/kg/hr	IV infusion for DKA IV infusion for DKA	
Vanadium	0.2 mg/kg (C)	PO	24
Drugs Used To Diagnose and Treat Hypoadrenocorticism			
ACTH	5 μg/kg (D) 125 μg/cat (C)	IM, IV IV	
Calcium gluconate	0.5-1.0 mg/kg	IV over 20 min.	
Desoxycorticosterone pivalate (DOCP)	2.2 mg/kg (D) 10-12.5 mg/cat (C)	IM, SC IM	25-28 days 28 days
Dexamethasone	0.5-2.0 mg/kg	IV	2-6
Fludrocortisone	0.01-0.02 mg/kg (D) 0.1 mg/cat (C)	PO PO	24 24
Hydrocortisone	2-4 mg/kg	IV over 2-4 min	8
Methylprednisolone acetate	10 mg/cat (C)	IM	28 days
Prednisone	0.1-0.22 mg/kg	PO	12-24
Prednisolone sodium succinate	1-2 mg/kg	IV over 2-4 min	2-6
Regular insulin	0.06 to 0.125 U/kg	IV, plus 20 mL of a 10% glucose solution	
Sodium chloride	0.1 mg/kg	PO	24 divided into 2-3 doses
Drugs Used To Diagnose or Treat Hyperadrenocorticism			
ACTH	5 μg/kg (D) 125 μg/cat (C)	IM, IVI V	
Dexamethasone	Low-dose test 0.01-0.15 mg/kg (D) 0.1 mg/kg (C) High-dose test 0.1-0.15 mg/kg (D) 1.0 mg/kg (C)	 IM, IV IM, IV IM, IV IM, IV	
Ketoconazole	5-20 mg/kg (D) 5-10 mg/kg (C)	PO PO	12 12
l-Deprenyl	1-2 mg/kg (D)	PO	24
Metyrapone	65 mg/kg (C) 30-70 mg/kg (C)	PO PO	8 12
Mitotane	Pituitary-dependent disease: Loading: 20-25 mg/kg (D) Maintenance: 40-50 mg/kg/wk (D) Adrenal tumor: Loading: 25-37.5 mg/kg (D) Maintenance: 50-100 mg/kg (D)	 PO PO PO PO	 12 Divided into 2-3 doses 12 Divided into 2-3 doses
Trilostane	2.2-6.7 mg/kg (D)**	PO	12-24 with food
Drugs Used To Treat Hyperaldosteronism			
Amlodipine	0.625-1.25 mg/cat	PO	12-24
Potassium gluconate	2-6 mEq	PO	24
Spironolactone	2-4 mg/kg	PO	12

Continued

Table 21-1 Endocrine Drugs and Recommended Doses*—cont'd

Drug	Dose	Route	Interval (hr)
Drugs Used To Treat Hormone Deficiency			
Growth hormone (porcine)	U/kg (D)	SC	3 times/wk
Medroxyprogesterone acetate	2.5-5 mg/kg (D)	SC	28 days
Proligestone	10 mg/kg (D)	SC	3 wk
Drugs Used To Treat Diabetes Insipidus			
Chlorothiazide	20-40 mg/kg (D)	PO	12
DDAVP	1-4 drops (intranasal preparation)	Ocular drop	8-12
	0.1 mg/dog	PO	8
Hydrochlorothiazide	2.5-5.0 mg/kg (D)	PO	12
	12.5 mg/cat (C)	PO	12

rhTSH, Recombinant human thyroid-stimulating hormone; *D,* dog; *IV,* intravenous; *PO,* by mouth; *C,* cat; *SSKI,* saturated solution of potassium iodide; *SC,* subcutaneous; *BG,* blood glucose concentration; *IM,* intramuscular; *ACTH,* adrenocorticotropic hormone; *DDAVP,* l-deamino-(8-D-arginine) vasopressin.

*This information is meant only to guide the reader toward choosing an initial drug dose for the various endocrine disorders discussed in this chapter. Endocrine diseases are by nature dynamic disorders, and the dose of any drug will certainly change over time. Concurrent diseases or medications, as well as individual variability toward response to and tolerance of a drug, must be a factor in drug selection and dose calculations. Please see the text for details on monitoring and recommended dosage adjustment.

†Alternative protocols possible; see text.

††Multiple forms exist; see text.

§Use cautiously; possibility of calcinosis cutis has been reported.

¶Should not be used to treat hypercalcemia until the cause is known.

‖Minumum 4-hour IV saline.

**Initiate as close to 2 mg/kg q24h or 1 mg/kg q12h as possible.

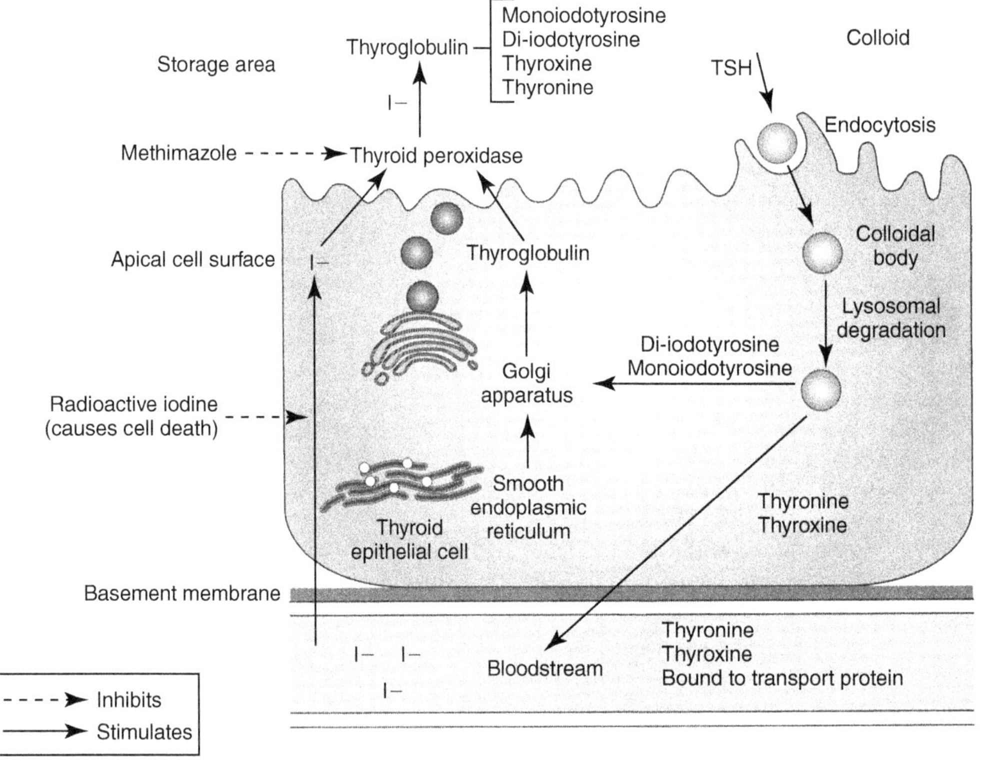

Figure 21-1 Synthesis of thyroid hormones. Iodine is concentrated in the apical cell colloid. At the same time, thyroglobulin is synthesized by the smooth endoplasmic reticulum and Golgi apparatus. At the apical cell surface, thyroglobulin and then tyrosine are iodinated, iodotyrosyl precursors are coupled to form thyronine and thyroxine, and all are stored in colloid. Thyroxine peroxidase mediates iodinization of the thyroglobulin–iodotyrosyl complexes. When signaled by thyroid-stimulating hormone (TSH), thyroglobin (as a colloid droplet) is engulfed by pinocytosis into the apical cell. Lysosomal degradation releases thyroxine and thyronine, which enter the blood stream, and the iodotyrosyl precursors, from which iodine is released and recirculated. The thyroid hormones reach target tissues bound to a circulating protein. Once inside the cell, thyroxine is converted to thyronine, the physiologically active thyroid hormone. Targets of thyroid hormone inhibition include administration of radioactive iodine, which is accumulated in active cells, ultimately leading to their destruction; methimazole, an inhibitor of thyroid peroxidase (controls but does not cure hyperthyroidism); and control of peripheral tissue response to excessive thyroid hormone release. *I,* Iodine.

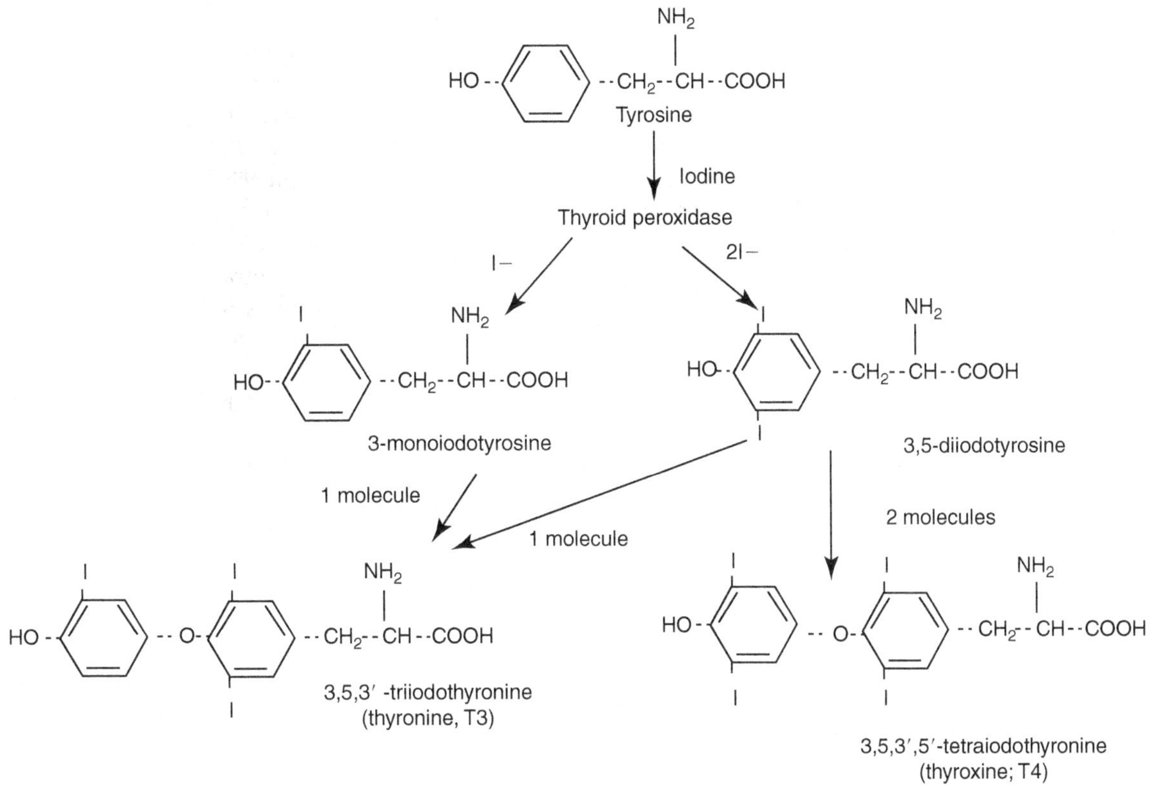

Figure 21-2 Iodination of tyrosine results in the formation of the monoiodinated and diiodinated precursors. Combinations of the two yield triiodothyronine and thyroxine. This reaction and the iodination of tyrosine are mediated by thyroid peroxidase.

They also have marked cardiac inotropic and chronotropic effects, stimulate erythropoiesis, and affect virtually every body tissue.

Hypothyroidism

Pathophysiology

Spontaneous hypothyroidism is a common endocrinopathy in dogs and exceedingly rare in cats. In primary hypothyroidism, which accounts for 99% of cases of spontaneous canine disease, the thyroid gland itself is affected. Cells are lost as a result of either lymphocytic thyroiditis or idiopathic atrophy; neoplastic destruction is rare. Secondary hypothyroidism results from a deficiency of pituitary TSH. Congenital secondary hypothyroidism can result from pituitary malformation or isolated thyrotroph (i.e., TSH-secreting cell) abnormalities. Acquired secondary hypothyroidism is rarely seen due to pituitary neoplasia. Tertiary hypothyroidism results from a lack of hypothalamic TRH and has not been reported in dogs. Congenital absence of the thyroid gland and iodine deficiency are rarer causes of hypothyroidism. Cats suffering from clinically evident hypothyroidism generally develop the disorder in response to iatrogenic removal or destruction of thyroidal tissue as treatment for hyperthyroidism. Congenital primary hypothyroidism occurs uncommonly in kittens, and iodine deficiency is even rarer.

The clinical signs of hypothyroidism refer to multiple body systems. Dermatologic signs include bilateral, nonpruritic, localized, or diffuse alopecia. The hair coat is dry, coarse, and slow to grow. Hyperkeratosis, scaling, or seborrhea may be present. Immunosuppression may lead to secondary pyoderma. Cardiac abnormalities may develop with severe hypothyroidism, including bradycardia and a weak apex beat. Various mild electrocardiographic and echocardiographic changes may be noted, such as increased left ventricular end-systolic diameter, decreased systolic left ventricular posterior wall thickness, and decreased fractional shortening. However, no substantiated reports of congestive heart failure secondary to canine hypothyroidism exist. Possible reproductive disorders include abnormal estrous cycles and lack of libido. Neuromuscular dysfunctions include weakness or stiffness, muscle wasting, neuropathies, and facial muscle weakness. Gastrointestinal signs are uncommon, but constipation is most likely to occur, if anything. Diarrhea may occur in hypothyroid dogs, but a cause-and-effect relationship has not been established. In cats lethargy and obesity are the most common clinical manifestations. Clinical laboratory abnormalities of hypothyroidism in dogs and cats include normocytic, normochromic, nonregenerative anemia and hypercholesterolemia with hypertriglyceridemia or hyperlipidemia.

Myxedema coma is a rare endocrine emergency resulting from decompensation of severe chronic hypothyroidism. *Myxedema* refers to dermal accumulation of glycosaminoglycans, which bind water and cause an increased skin thickness and nonpitting edema, mostly in the face, jowls, and distal extremities.[1] Myxedema coma is characterized by profound weakness, bradycardia, hypotension, hypoventilation, hypothermia without shivering, and altered mentation ranging from dullness and depression to stupor or coma. The actual mortality rate is not known but is thought to be high, primarily because myxedema coma is not widely recognized. The diagnosis should be made clinically, and therapy should be initiated without waiting for results of thyroid hormone concentrations.[1] In addition to the biochemical abnormalities typical of hypothyroidism, additional findings may include hypoxia, hypercarbia, hyponatremia, and hypoglycemia. Serum thyroid hormone concentrations are typically very low or undetectable.

In humans the presence of concurrent disease and altered mentation are essential features for supporting a diagnosis of myxedema coma. In one study of seven hypothyroid dogs for which intravenous levothyroxine therapy was deemed necessary, five dogs had altered mentation. Of those five, all had concurrent disease and four had myxedema. Because of the low incidence of myxedema coma, it is not known if there is a breed predilection, but in a study by Pullen and Hess,[2] three were Rottweilers, two were mixed breeds, one was a Cocker Spaniel, and one was a Shetland Sheepdog. Rottweilers were overrepresented. Treatment is with intravenous levothyroxine (discussed later).

Baseline and Provocative Testing of Thyroid Status

Diagnosis of hypothyroidism can be challenging. Hormones typically measured include T_4, free T_4, and TSH. If serum total T_4 concentration is normal, it is highly unlikely that the dog is hypothyroid.[3-6] Because nonthyroidal factors such as drugs, illness, and age affect T_4, if the T_4 concentration is below normal, the dog may or may not be hypothyroid,[3-5,7] and further testing is required. Breed may also affect reference ranges.[8,9,10]

Thyroid hormones are bound to plasma proteins. Approximately only 0.1%, of circulating hormone is unbound and thus available to cells and physiologically active. Most laboratories measure total (bound and unbound) T_3 and T_4 concentrations. A number of techniques purportedly quantify the fraction of unbound thyroxine (i.e., free T_4 [fT_4]), including equilibrium dialysis, the gold standard for comparison with other methods, and several immunoassays that indirectly detect fT_4. Currently, methods that depend on equilibrium dialysis are the most accurate measurements of fT_4; measurement of fT_4 by analog radioimmunoassay techniques offer no diagnostic advantage over measurement of total T_4. Regardless of the test, normal thyroid hormone concentrations will vary with the laboratory and the kit used; any test must be validated for the target species (i.e., dog or cat).

Because the pituitary-thyroid axis functions to maintain free, not total, T_4 within a certain range, fT_4 is less affected by nonthyroidal factors; therefore measurement of serum fT_4 concentration more accurately reflects thyroidal axis status. Accordingly, fT_4 is a more sensitive and more specific test for diagnosis of hypothyroidism, but it is also not as good a stand-alone test as once believed (discussed later). Measurement of serum fT_4 concentration can be the initial test for diagnosis of hypothyroidism or can be used in dogs found to have low total T_4 concentrations.

Serum TSH concentration can also be measured to help establish a diagnosis of canine hypothyroidism. In primary hypothyroidism TSH concentration should be elevated owing to lack of negative feedback of serum T_4 on the pituitary (i.e., in normal dogs T_4 feeds back and suppresses TSH secretion). Although 99% of canine hypothyroidism cases are believed to be due to primary thyroidal failure, only approximately 63% to 82% of hypothyroid dogs have elevated serum TSH concentrations.[11-14] The reason for the discrepancy is unknown but is likely due to inadequacy of currently available assays. Of the hormones measured to diagnose hypothyroidism, however, TSH measurement is the most specific—that is, it has the smallest chance of a false-positive result.

The effect of nonthyroidal illness on testing can be quite significant. Dogs that are ill because of a disease but that do not have hypothyroidism can have low T_4 and fT_4 concentrations; if the disease is severe (e.g., a dog is in intensive care), a 44% chance exists that the fT_4 concentration will be below normal even though the dog is not hypothyroid. Serum TSH concentration, however, is less affected by nonthyroidal factors. Therefore in sick dogs the first choice for diagnosis of hypothyroidism would be a combination of TSH, fT_4, and T_4; second choice a combination of TSH and fT_4; and third choice a combination of TSH and T_4. If the results are ambiguous (i.e., some parameters suggest hypothyroidism, and others do not), the ideal would be to resolve the nonthyroidal illness, if possible, and retest the dog at that time or possibly to perform a TSH stimulation test, if available.

Bovine TSH previously was used as the provocative agent for TSH stimulation testing but is no longer available. Thyrogen, recombinant human TSH (rhTSH), can be used instead. The optimal protocol for distinguishing normal and hypothyroid dogs, however, remains to be determined, although results of studies evaluating rhTSH in dogs are promising.[15-17] Doses of 50 to 100 μg/dog given intravenously with samples taken before and at 4 or 6 hours after injection are likely appropriate. Euthyroid animals should respond to TSH stimulation with increased T_4 concentration, whereas hypothyroid animals should not. Reconstituted rhTSH can be stored at 4°C for 4 weeks and at −20°C for 8 weeks without loss of biological activity.[18]

Measurement of serum T_3 concentration is not helpful for diagnosing hypothyroidism. Most T_3 is derived from intracellular metabolism or conversion by peripheral tissues of T_4 to T_3 and reverse T_3 (rT_3). Thus most body T_3 is located within cells, and serum T_3 concentration does not reflect total body levels. A previous argument for measuring serum T_3 concentration was the belief that some dogs were "poor converters" and could produce T_4 but not T_3. The theory was apparently substantiated by finding normal serum T_4 but nondetectable T_3 concentrations in a small percentage of dogs. Such discrepant results are now known, however, to be an artifact caused by the presence of T_3 autoantibodies. Insofar as poor conversion has never been proved and currently is not believed to exist, measurement of serum T_3 concentration is not recommended.

Autoantibodies made against T_4 or T_3 can be measured and can be a marker of immune-mediated destruction of the thyroid gland. Autoantibodies typically cause spurious elevations in serum T_3 or T_4 concentrations, so their presence should be suspected if either hormone is measured in a patient suspected to be hypothyroid and the concentration of either or both hormones is reported to be greater than the reference range. However, the clinical and prognostic significance of autoantibodies is unknown. The presence of autoantibodies does not mean a patient is hypothyroid. If autoantibodies are suspected, serum fT_4 concentration should be measured by equilibrium dialysis for the best assessment of function.[19] If the serum fT_4 concentration is within the reference range, thyroidal function is normal at that time but the patient should be reevaluated periodically (e.g., every 3 months) for development of hypothyroidism. If serum fT_4 concentration is low, the dog is likely hypothyroid. One study followed 234 dogs with normal T_4 and TSH levels and elevated antithyroglobulin antibodies (TGAA) for 1 year. Only 19% developed clinical signs of hypothyroidism or consistent laboratory values (or both). Another 57% remained TGAA positive without signs or laboratory evidence of hypothyroidism, 8% went from positive to borderline results, and 15% became TGAA negative.[20]

Calculation of the percentage of uptake of radioactive pertechnetate ($^{99m}TcO_4^-$) has proved to be a useful tool aiding in the diagnosis of thyroidal illness in humans and cats and may also be valuable for dogs with primary hypothyroidism. Normal lobes of canine thyroid glands are uniformly intense, symmetric ovals, slightly smaller than the parotid salivary glands, and have smooth and regular margins. The parotid glands also concentrate $^{99m}TcO_4^-$, and the normal uptake ratio between these the thyroid and parotid glands is 1:1. In 14 dogs with histologically confirmed primary hypothyroidism, the percentage of uptake of $^{99m}TcO_4^-$ distinguished hypothyroid dogs from dogs with nonthyroidal illness.[21] The dogs with nonthyroidal illness had $^{99m}TcO_4^-$ uptake ranging from 0.39% to 1.86%, similar to what has been described in healthy Beagles. The hypothyroid dogs had $^{99m}TcO_4^-$ uptake ranging from 0.03 to 0.26%. In fact, of the tests examined in the study (T_4, fT_4, TSH, and TSH and TRH stimulation tests), scintigraphy was the only one that did not have overlap between the two groups of dogs. Limitations of the test include requirement for specialized equipment and the fact that reference ranges have not been defined in a large number of dogs from a variety of breeds. Additionally, increased $^{99m}TcO_4^-$ uptake can occur with a diet high in iodine and has been reported in a hypothyroid dog with thyroiditis,[22] so false-negative results are possible. The final complicating factor is that in humans with thyroiditis, the $^{99m}TcO_4^-$ uptake pattern depends on disease stage. The role scintigraphy holds in aiding in the diagnosis of canine hypothyroidism remains to be defined.

Another area that has received recent attention as an ancillary test in the diagnosis of canine hypothyroidism is ultrasonography. In healthy dogs and dogs with nonthyroidal illness, the thyroid gland lobes are fusiform in the longitudinal plane and triangular in the transverse plane, have a smooth thyroid capsule, and homogenous echotexture, usually hyperechoic or isoechoic to the sternothyroid muscle.[23,24] The ultrasonographic description of the thyroid gland lobes of hypothyroid dogs is more variable. However, they tend to be either round or ovoid on the transverse view. Echotexture may depend on whether the animal has thyroglobin autoantibodies. Thyroid lobes from antibody-positive hypothyroid dogs were homogenously hypoechoic to the sternothyroid muscle, whereas the lobes of those that were antibody negative were heterogeneous in echotexture.[23] However, another study did not find a difference based on thyroglobin autoantibody status; thyroid lobes were reported to be hypoechoic to the sternothyroid muscle.[24] Additionally the volume of the glands is smaller in hypothyroid dogs. A thyroid volume of less than 0.05 mL/kg was reported to be 81% sensitive, 96% specific, and 91% accurate for the diagnosis of primary hypothyroidism.[23] Care should be taken with the use of this modality for diagnosing canine hypothyroidism because ultrasonography is highly user dependent and substantial interobserver variability exists when taking measurements.

Therapy of Hypothyroidism

Disposition of thyroid hormones. Thyroidal hormone disposition varies between preparations and species. Although thyroid hormones are bioavailable after oral administration, T_4 absorption can be decreased by a number of factors such as the type of preparation and intraluminal contents of the ileum or colon, where most absorption occurs. In humans bioavailability ranges from 40% to 80%. Because of differences among formulations, some authors recommend initiating therapy with a brand-name product.[25] However, the pharmacokinetics of T_4 is idiosyncratic; some dogs achieve higher postpill concentrations when treated with a generic brand. No evidence exists that a single brand is consistently better than another. Therapy can probably be started with any brand, but if a dog does not respond, another brand should be administered to see whether better results and higher postpill levels can be achieved; if the first brand tried is generic, the second should not be. In contrast to T_4, T_3 is well absorbed (95% in humans) from the gastrointestinal tract.

In dogs the half-life of T_3 and T_4 is 5 to 6 hours and 12 to 15 hours, respectively. However, the half-life of T_4 may be dose dependent.[26] The short half-life makes avoidance of fluctuations in serum concentrations during a 12- to 24-hour dosing interval difficult. However, the status of intracellular T_3 concentration is not well known; the impact of fluctuating T_4 may be minimized by physiologic conversion. Steady-state concentrations will occur at five drug half-lives (i.e., 75 hours for T_4 and 30 hours for T_3 in dogs). On the other hand, clinical response varies depending on the complication of hypothyroidism present. The first evaluation after starting supplementation should occur after about 4 weeks of therapy in order to judge blood levels as well as therapeutic response. Certain abnormalities (e.g., dermatological) can take up to 3 months to resolve once therapeutic blood levels have been achieved.

Preparations. Thyroid hormones can be supplemented as crude extracts of animal origin or as synthetic preparations. The biological activities of animal-origin products, such as desiccated thyroid and thyroglobulin, vary, however, and therapeutic failure with these products is not uncommon. Thus synthetic products are recommended.

Several synthetic thyroid hormone products are available as T_4 or T_3 individually or in combination. Sodium levothyroxine (T_4) is the drug of choice for most patients. If T_4 therapy has failed to achieve a response in a dog with confirmed hypothyroidism, T_3 can be administered, but failure of T_4 therapy is very rare. If no apparent response to T_4 is seen or inadequate blood levels are achieved with appropriate dosing, another brand of T_4 should be used first before prescribing T_3. The diagnosis of hypothyroidism should also be reevaluated if resolution of clinical signs does not occur with documentation of adequate blood concentrations and a sufficient duration of therapy. Combination products generally contain T_4 and T_3 at a ratio of 4:1, the proportion of thyroid hormones secreted in normal humans. Use of combination products is not recommended. The administration frequency of T_4 and T_3 should differ, orally absorbed T_4 is converted as needed to T_3 by target cells so therapy with T_4 alone usually achieves adequate T_3 concentrations, and use of combinations may result in serum T_3 concentrations that produce thyrotoxicosis.[1]

Plasma half-life of T_4 varies among dogs, and a marked variability in the dose necessary to achieve therapeutic concentrations exists. Beginning doses of T_4 should be 20 μg/kg every 12 hours for dogs and 50 to 100 μg once daily in cats. After resolution of clinical signs, approximately 25% of dogs maintain adequate blood levels and a good therapeutic response with once-daily dosing. Initial doses as low as 5 μg/kg may be indicated in dogs with concurrent illness, especially cardiac, to allow the body to slowly adapt to the increase in oxygen demand that may accompany thyroid hormone replacement. The dosage can then be increased over the following 3 to 4 weeks.

Pharmacokinetics of oral liquid levothyroxine suggest that once-daily dosing should be adequate,[27] and administration of liquid levothyroxine (Leventa Intervet/Schering-Plough) once daily in 35 hypothyroid dogs was recently evaluated.[28] Dogs were started at a dose of 20 μg/kg once daily and monitored every 4 weeks (adjustment phase). At the reevaluation visit, serum T_4 and TSH concentrations were obtained 4 to 6 hours after the pill was administered, and dose adjustments were made if the T_4 value did not fall within the target therapeutic range. Once clinical signs resolved and T_4 concentrations were within the target range, the adjustment phase ended and the maintenance phase began. To assess long-term efficacy, dogs were then reevaluated at 9 and 22 weeks, with the same parameters measured at each visit and dosages adjusted as needed.

The starting dose of 20 μg/kg was also the maintenance dose in 79% of the dogs. Maintenance doses for the remaining dogs were 10 μg/kg (3%), 15 μg/kg (3%), and 30 μg/kg (15%). In the maintenance phase, dose adjustments were required for 16% of dogs. The median dose was 24 μg/kg once daily. Clinical signs improved within 4 weeks in 90% of dogs and within 4 weeks in 100%. Body condition scores initially assessed as overweight or obese had normalized in 52% of dogs by week 22, and dermatologic abnormalities had resolved in 68%. Peak serum T_4 concentrations were within the target therapeutic range in 65% of dogs at the first follow-up visit after beginning the maintenance phase of the study and in 79% of dogs at the 22-week examination. The remaining dogs had clinical control of the disease, but transiently low T_4 concentrations. Reported adverse events included sudden death in one dog after 47 days of treatment, vomiting after administration of the solution in two dogs, and reddish discoloration of hair coat in one dog.

Intravenous levothyroxine is used in the treatment of dogs with myxedema coma. In 7 dogs given intravenous levothyroxine, the median dose was 7 μg/kg. Three of the seven dogs were given intravenous levothyroxine once. To resolve the neurologic issues, the remaining dogs received a total of 5, 6, 10, or 13 doses each. The injections were given every 12 hours in three of four dogs and every 8 hours in the remaining dog. The dogs were started on oral levothyroxine within 24 hours of the last intravenous dose.[2]

Sodium liothyronine (T_3) should be reserved for patients not responding to T_4 therapy. Dosing should start at 4 to 6 μg/kg every 8 hours for dogs and 4.4 μg/kg every 8 to 12 hours for cats. Clinical improvement may take 4 to 6 weeks; twice-daily administration can begin at that time.

Response to Therapy

Therapeutic Drug Monitoring. Variability in blood concentrations after oral administration of T_4 can be very large because of differences in disposition, including bioavailability, so monitoring is an important tool with which to guide therapy. Blood concentrations should not be monitored until steady-state concentrations of the hormone have been reached and sufficient time for a physiologic response to the new concentration has passed. Thus concentrations should be monitored 1 month after therapy has begun.

For monitoring a sample should be drawn 4 to 6 hours after the pill is administered. At that time, serum T_4 concentration should be in or slightly above the upper half of the reference range. TSH concentration can also be measured in the same sample and can be helpful. Increased values are associated with inadequate therapy, but TSH concentrations within the reference range are not interpretable; dogs with both adequate and inadequate control can have TSH concentrations within the reference range.[29] Measurement of fT_4 probably is unnecessary and does not add any more information, except in patients who have T_4 autoantibodies; in such patients T_4 concentration as measured by radioimmunoassay is falsely elevated. Whether measurement of prepill hormone concentrations is helpful remains controversial. If T_3 is the sole supplement, peak concentrations can be collected 3 hours after administration of the pill if an 8-hour dosing interval is being used. With subsequent retesting, samples should be collected at the same time as previously, so comparisons between tests across time in the same patient are more valid.

Interpretation of thyroid hormone concentrations must be made in the context of clinical signs. Animals should be supplemented for 1 to 3 months before clinical efficacy can be judged. Although no clinical signs of thyrotoxicosis may be present, whether increased serum T_4 concentrations without clinical signs of hyperthyroidism are detrimental has never been studied. In humans elevated postpill T_4 concentrations are strictly avoided. Low serum T_4 concentrations should also be interpreted with response to therapy. The effects of concurrent drug therapy or other diseases that might influence the metabolism of thyroid hormones must be considered. Drug dose can be changed to achieve the therapeutic range. However, the pharmacokinetics of T_4 are not linear—that is, to achieve a 15% change in serum T_4 level, a 25% change in dose, not a 15% change, may be required.[30]

Effects of other drugs on thyroid hormones. Numerous drugs can affect thyroid hormone concentrations. The reader is referred elsewhere for complete information.[31,32]

Glucocorticoids, phenobarbital, sulfa antibiotics, tricyclic antidepressants, and nonsteroidal antiinflammatory agents, among others, have been shown to decrease T_4, T_3, fT_4, and TSH.

Hyperthyroidism

Pathophysiology

Neoplasia of the thyroid gland, whether benign or malignant, is the most common cause of hyperthyroidism. In cats a benign tumor is the etiology in approximately 99% of cases, whereas in dogs a thyroid tumor leading to hyperthyroidism is almost always malignant. (Note, however, that most canine thyroid tumors do not cause hyperthyroidism; at least 90% of canine thyroid tumors are nonfunctional, and they can cause hypothyroidism as a result of the destruction of normal thyroidal tissue.) Occasionally, administration or accidental ingestion of thyroid hormones can cause thyrotoxicosis.

The clinical signs of hyperthyroidism reflect abnormalities in several body systems as a result of excessive concentrations of T_4 and T_3. Increased energy expenditure results in weight loss and polyphagia. As skin protein synthesis and blood flow increase, the hair coat changes. Increased renal blood flow, glomerular filtration rate (GFR), and renal tubular activity account for polydipsia and polyuria; loss of medullary interstitial tonicity can also contribute. Vomiting may reflect a direct effect on the chemoreceptor trigger zone, overeating, or gastrointestinal hypermotility. Malabsorption and hypermotility can cause diarrhea. Thyroid hormones may directly stimulate the central nervous system, causing behavioral changes that typify hyperthyroid cats (i.e., nervousness, hyperkinesis, agitation). Occasionally, hypokalemia develops, which may explain the weakness that affects some cats.

Heat and stress intolerance, panting, and respiratory distress may be related to decreased pulmonary vital capacity, decreased pulmonary compliance, slightly elevated body temperature, and cardiac stimulation (associated with catecholamine release). Cardiac disturbances include tachycardia, premature cardiac contractions, and gallop rhythms. Secondary cardiac hypertrophy can occur, which is distinct at a microscopic level from that seen with primary idiopathic hypertrophic cardiomyopathy. Thus cats with hypertrophy secondary to hyperthyroidism have thyrotoxic cardiac disease, not hypertrophic cardiomyopathy. Long-standing untreated thyrotoxic cardiac disease can progress to congestive heart failure. Thyroid hormones directly affect the cardiac muscle, as well as increase the needs of peripheral tissues, causing a high cardiac output state and an increase in myocardial oxygen demand. Peripheral resistance, on the other hand, is generally decreased. Catecholamines may contribute to the positive inotropic and chronotropic effects of thyroid hormones on the heart. Thyrotoxicosis probably increases the myocardial responsiveness to catecholamines by increasing the number of catecholamine receptors.

Baseline and Provocative Testing

Baseline serum T_4 concentration can be measured to diagnose hyperthyroidism and is sufficient in the majority of cases as it is elevated in approximately 91% of hyperthyroid cats.[33] (It is important to remember, however, that rare normal cats may have an elevated T_4.) The other 9% of cats represent those with early or mild hyperthyroidism where serum T_4 concentration can fluctuate in and out of the normal range[34] or cats with concomitant nonthyroidal illness. Nonthyroidal illness can suppress serum T_4 concentration,[35] so the serum T_4 concentration in hyperthyroid cats can be within the normal range.[36,37] As a result, resting serum T_4 concentrations obtained from cats must be critically evaluated and the possibility of further testing considered.

If the serum T_4 concentration of a hyperthyroid cat is within the reference range, it will typically be in the upper half of the range. If a serum T_4 concentration is in the lower half of the reference range, it is highly unlikely (but not impossible) that the cat is hyperthyroid, and another diagnosis should be considered. In sick, older cats with normal thyroidal function, serum T_4 concentration is usually low,[35] so the finding of a T_4 even in the upper half of the reference range in such a cat may indicate hyperthyroidism. If the T_4 concentration is in the upper half of the reference range but there hyperthyroidism is still suspected, further diagnostics should be pursued. Options for additional tests include the following: (1) measurement of serum fT_4 concentration by equilibrium dialysis; (2) repeat measurement of total T_4 concentration (Because serum T_4 concentration may fluctuate in and out of the normal range, on a second test the sample may be drawn by chance while the T_4 concentration is above normal and diagnostic. Unfortunately, there is no way to predict when this will occur.); (3) performance of a T_3 suppression test or TRH stimulation test. These latter two tests are valid, good tests, although they are more labor intensive and often not necessary.

As in dogs, serum fT_4 concentration in cats is less affected by nonthyroidal factors than is total T_4 concentration and is a more accurate reflection of thyroid function. For example, fT_4 concentration is elevated in 94% of mildly hyperthyroid cats, whereas total T_4 concentration is elevated in only 61%.[33] However, fT_4 concentration may also be elevated in 6% to 12% of sick, euthyroid cats.[33,38] To help discriminate between hyperthyroid and sick euthyroid cats, a total T_4 should be measured along with fT_4 concentration. Sick euthyroid cats with an elevated fT_4 typically have T_4 concentrations that are within the lower half of or below the reference range. Thus if the T_4 concentration is in the upper half of the normal range or above and the fT_4 concentration is elevated, this is consistent with a diagnosis of hyperthyroidism. If the T_4 concentration is in the lower half of the normal range or below and the fT_4 concentration is elevated, the cat is very unlikely to be hyperthyroid, and another diagnosis should be sought.

Measurement of serum T_3 is not very helpful for diagnosis and is not recommended. Overall, only 67% of hyperthyroid cats have an elevated T_3 concentration.[33] In cats with mild hyperthyroidism, only 21% actually have an elevated serum T_3 concentration.[33]

Performance of pertechnetate scans to diagnose hyperthyroidism is quite useful overall. Uptake of radioactive pertechnetate can confirm hyperthyroidism as well as delineate functional thyroid tissue, establish the extent of thyroid involvement, and possibly detect metastasis (some metastases, but not all, will concentrate radioiodine). For cats in which biochemical evidence of hyperthyroidism is clear, scans will clearly identify functioning tissue. However, false-positive results may occur;[39] in other words, nonhyperthyroid cats can have a scan suggesting the presence of hyperthyroidism, and timing of a scan after methimazole therapy may affect results.[40]

Relationship of Treatment for Feline Hyperthyroidism to Renal Disease

Treatment of hyperthyroidism can lead to decreases in GFR and unmask chronic renal disease,[41-45] and no therapy appears to be safer than another. However, how best to assess cats before definitive therapy (i.e., radioactive iodine [^{131}I therapy] or surgery) is unknown. Although one study determined that a GFR value of 2.25 mL/kg/min might represent a cutoff for deciding whether renal failure is a possibility,[43] measurement of GFR is not easily obtained and GFR measurements vary depending on the technique used,[46] with each laboratory needing to determine its own guidelines. Furthermore, in two studies, hyperthyroid cats with GFR greater than 2.25 mg/kg/min were azotemic 30 days after treatment;[42,44] whether this simply reflects a difference in methodology is unclear. Unfortunately, no readily available clinical indicators, including urine specific gravity, exist.[47,48] Cats with pretreatment urine specific gravity greater than 1.035 may develop azotemia with treatment.[48]

Therefore the best option is probably to treat cats transiently with methimazole until serum T_4 concentration is adequately controlled and then maintain euthyroidism for 30 days. When the serum T_4 concentration is maintained within the normal range, renal function and the effect of definitive therapy can be assessed. Many cats exhibit an increase in serum blood urea nitrogen (BUN) or creatinine concentration (or both) with therapy, but the clinical result must be assessed as the most important parameter. Most cats improve clinically despite the increased renal parameters when their hyperthyroidism is treated. If they improve and the renal failure is not clinically apparent, the hyperthyroidism can be definitively treated.

Whether all cats that are to undergo ^{131}I treatment or thyroidectomy need to have their kidney function evaluated with a methimazole trial remains to be determined. We prefer performing a trial on all cats before definitive therapy is undertaken. Certainly, if there is any question about the adequacy of renal function, trial therapy with methimazole is warranted. If renal failure becomes clinically apparent during the trial, methimazole administration should be stopped and therapy for renal failure instituted. Once the cat is stable again, the hyperthyroidism should be controlled as best as possible for life with methimazole and therapy for renal failure continued. Alternatively, if a trial is not performed and renal failure becomes overt because of definitive correction of hyperthyroidism, exogenous thyroid hormone can be supplemented in an attempt to support the kidneys, but the efficacy of such therapy is unknown and may be questionable.[49] A balance must then be struck between creating iatrogenic hyperthyroidism and maintaining renal function.

Drugs Used To Control Hyperthyroidism

Hyperthyroidism may be medically controlled with methimazole and ipodate. Both can be used as either the sole drug to manage hyperthyroidism or in preparation for surgery or radioiodine administration. Propylthiouracil administration is not recommended because of associated possible severe adverse effects. In general, methimazole blocks synthesis of thyroid hormones and, specifically, thyroid peroxidase activity necessary for coupling of tyrosine residues by acting as a preferential substrate for the enzyme. As a result, T_3 and T_4 are not secreted. Carbimazole is a methimazole prodrug currently used in Europe but not available in the United States. It appears to be equal in efficacy but safer than methimazole. Controlled-release carbimazole tablets are now available in Europe. Based on pharmacokinetics in normal cats the controlled-release formulation may be appropriate for once-daily dosing;[50] however, dosing has not been evaluated in hyperthyroid cats. Ipodate is a cholecystographic agent that acts primarily by inhibiting conversion of T_3 to T_4 but also has some direct inhibitory effects on thyroid hormone secretion.

Overall, methimazole is highly effective at reversing thyrotoxicosis and maintaining euthyroidism. In 262 spontaneously hyperthyroid cats, methimazole treatment lowered the serum T_4 in more than 99%.[51] A very small percentage of cats may be truly methimazole resistant. In the 262 cats, clinical side effects occurred, unrelated to the dose of methimazole used, in 18%, including anorexia (11%), vomiting (11%), lethargy (9%), excoriation of the face and neck (2%), bleeding (2%), and icterus (2%). Anorexia, vomiting, and lethargy typically happened during the first month of therapy and resolved despite continued drug administration. However, in eight cats, gastrointestinal side effects persisted and required cessation of therapy. Treatment with methimazole was also permanently stopped in cats that developed liver failure (e.g., vomiting, anorexia, and icterus), excoriated faces or necks, or a bleeding tendency.[51] Myasthenia gravis has been reported after treatment with methimazole in four cats. In two cats, prednisone was used to control the myasthenia.[52] Lymphadenomegaly, which resolved with discontinuation of methimazole administration, was reported in a single cat.[53]

On hematologic screening, eosinophilia, lymphocytosis, leukopenia, thrombocytopenia, and agranulocytosis may be noted. The milder adverse effects—eosinophilia, lymphocytosis, and leukopenia—are usually noted within 1 to 2 months of initiation of treatment and are transient despite continued therapy. The more serious complications (e.g., thrombocytopenia, agranulocytosis) occur in a minority of cats (≤3%) within the first 3 months of therapy and necessitate permanent discontinuation of methimazole administration.[51] The mechanism of hematologic disorders induced by methimazole is not understood. Interestingly, bleeding occurred in one cat without a decrease in platelet number, so thrombocytopenia is not the only mechanism that can cause a bleeding tendency. In human patients receiving propylthiouracil, vitamin K therapy reduced bleeding caused by hypoprothrombinemia; however, the benefits of vitamin K therapy have not been studied in cats receiving thyroid peroxidase inhibitors.[54] Immunologic effects, including induction of positive antinuclear antibodies (ANAs), can occur. The risk of developing a positive ANA result appears to increase with length of therapy and dose. However, clinical signs of a lupuslike syndrome (e.g., dermatitis, polyarthritis, glomerulonephritis, thrombocytopenia, fever) or hemolysis do not occur.[51]

A starting dose of 10 to 15 mg/day divided into two or three daily doses depending on the severity of the hyperthyroidism has been recommended. The goal for cats on methimazole is to have a serum T_4 concentration in the lower half of the reference range. Postpill timing does not matter. Although some cats require methimazole only once daily for adequate control, methimazole generally is more effective twice daily.[55] For the first 3 months, the period during which most adverse effects develop, cats receiving methimazole should be evaluated every 2 to 3 weeks with a complete physical examination, determination of serum T_4 concentration, complete blood count (CBC), and measurement of liver enzymes and bilirubin. Renal parameters should also be monitored to assess kidney function. Although cats with a subnormal serum T_4 concentration typically are not clinically hypothyroid, development of a positive ANA titer may be related to dose. Thus the minimal dose necessary to maintain serum T_4 concentration in the lower half of the reference range, and not below, should be used. If serum T_4 concentration remains high and poor compliance or difficulty in giving the medication has been ruled out as the cause of persistent hyperthyroidism, the methimazole dose should be increased in 2.5- to 5-mg increments to a maximum of 20 mg/day. If hepatopathy, facial excoriation, a bleeding tendency, or serious hematologic consequences occur, the medication should be halted permanently and alternative therapy used. After the first 3 months, serum T_4 concentration should be determined every 3 to 6 months to evaluate adequacy of therapy. Because blood dyscrasias are unlikely but not impossible after 3 months of therapy, a CBC need be performed only if clinical signs suggest agranulocytosis, hemolysis, or thrombocytopenia.[51]

To prevent development of adverse effects, other authors have recommended an initial dose of 2.5 mg twice daily for 2 weeks.[56] If after this period an owner observes no untoward side effects, the physical examination reveals no new problems, and a CBC (including platelets) is within normal limits, the dosage should be increased to 2.5 mg thrice daily for an additional 2 weeks. A similar recheck should then be completed, including measurement of a serum T_4 concentration. If serum T_4 concentration is within or near the normal reference range, the dose may be maintained for 2 to 6 weeks to determine the need for any further dosage adjustments. The dosage should be increased by 2.5 mg/day increments to a maximum of 20 mg/day (assuming correct methimazole administration) or until the hyperthyroidism is controlled.[56] Monitoring for adverse effects should be done as previously described.

Because of the relationship between hyperthyroidism and renal disease (as previously discussed), a third protocol has been advocated if abnormal renal parameters are present. Methimazole should be administered at a dose of 2.5 mg twice daily for 2 weeks, then 2.5 mg thrice daily for 2 weeks, then 5 mg twice daily for 2 weeks, and finally 5 mg thrice daily as needed. The serum T_4 concentration, BUN, creatinine, phosphate, and a CBC should be evaluated at the end of each 2-week period. The dose escalation should stop once serum T_4 concentration has normalized. If the serum T_4 can be decreased to within the reference range and the renal parameters remain stable or improve, antithyroid medications may be continued or a permanent therapy may be considered. If clinical signs of renal disease worsen with therapy, treatment of the hyperthyroidism should be reevaluated. Some cats may be healthier without treatment.[56] Alternatively, the dose of methimazole can be titrated to achieve the best control possible of the hyperthyroidism while maintaining adequate renal function.

Methimazole can be given transdermally. Although methimazole in pleuronic lecithin organogel (PLO) is absorbed poorly in healthy cats after a single dose,[57] it is likely that chronic dosing leads to improved absorption and resolution of hyperthyroidism as transdermal methimazole can be used to treat hyperthyroidism.[58-60] The transdermal route may take longer, however, to bring about remission. In a randomized, prospective study of hyperthyroid cats, owners dosed their cats with methimazole orally (tablets) or transdermally (in PLO; 50 mg/mL) at 2.5 mg every 12 hours.[59] Of cats treated transdermally 56% were euthyroid at 2 weeks, which was significantly fewer cats than the control rate in response to oral administration (88%); by 4 weeks the difference was no longer statistically significant (67% control with transdermal methimazole versus 82% for oral), but the lack of difference may have been due to a small number of cats remaining in the study at 4 weeks. Whether transdermal administration for a longer period of time would have controlled the hyperthyroidism in more cats was not evaluated. An advantage of transdermal methimazole is a significantly decreased rate of gastrointestinal adverse effects. However, the incidence of hepatopathy, facial excoriation, and blood dyscrasias is similar for both the transdermal and oral routes. Some cats develop erythema at the transdermal dosing site, but it is typically not severe enough to require drug discontinuation.[59]

Methimazole administration does not affect tumor size. Clinical signs will recur with discontinuation of the drug. Methimazole can be used before surgery to decrease serum T_4 concentrations to within the reference range to stabilize the patient. Discontinuation of methimazole 2 weeks before radionuclide scanning or therapy has been recommended.

Because radionuclide uptake is increased in normal tissue for 9 days after discontinuation of methimazole therapy,[40] treatment within that window may increase the risk of iatrogenic hypothyroidism with radioiodine administration.

In humans, use of cholecystographic agents for treatment of hyperthyroidism has been studied, and the radiopaque organic iodine agent ipodate has shown some success. Experience with ipodate in veterinary medicine has been limited. A single study of 12 spontaneously hyperthyroid cats was performed using calcium ipodate granules reformulated into 50-mg capsules.[61] Initial dosage was 50 mg/cat, administered orally twice daily. The dosage was increased to 150 mg (100 mg in the morning, 50 mg at night) and then 200 mg (100 mg orally twice daily) at 2-week intervals if serum T_3 did not normalize or if other abnormalities attributable to hyperthyroidism failed to resolve satisfactorily. (Because the main mechanism of action of ipodate is to inhibit conversion of T_4 to T_3, monitoring of serum T_3 concentrations is necessary to judge efficacy.) Only eight cats responded during the 14-week study period; seven of these were treated at a dosage of 100 mg/day, and one required 150 mg/day. Interestingly, serum T_3 concentration decreased in the responders and declined into the normal range in two nonresponders as well. No adverse clinical signs or hematologic abnormalities attributable to ipodate treatment were noted.[61] The reason for poor response in four cats was not apparent. Lack of efficacy of ipodate has been noted in human patients, especially those with Graves' disease and severe hyperthyroidism. The effect of ipodate may be transient in some cats, given that two cats clearly had relapsed at the end of the 14 weeks.

Thus cholecystographic agents may be a feasible alternative to methimazole for medical treatment of feline hyperthyroidism and may be a good option for cats that require medical treatment but cannot tolerate methimazole. The need for special formulation of capsules may limit availability. Unfortunately, efficacy of treatment cannot be predicted, although cats with severe hyperthyroidism are less likely to respond. If treatment is efficacious, serum T_3 concentrations will normalize and clinical signs will abate. Owners should also be warned that a positive response might be transient. Unfortunately, ipodate is no longer available. Iopanoic acid has been recommended for use at the same dosage, but no studies exist proving its efficacy.

Drugs Used To Cure Hyperthyroidism

Compared with medical therapy that simply controls hyperthyroidism, ^{131}I therapy provides a cure. The goal of ^{131}I therapy is to restore euthyroidism with a single dose of radiation without producing hypothyroidism. Surgery can also cure the disease, but ^{131}I is the definitive treatment of choice in cats with ectopic thyroid tumors that are not surgically accessible (e.g., intrathoracic). In addition, ^{131}I may be the best way to treat metastatic carcinoma. Radioactive iodine, like stable iodine, is actively taken up by and stored in thyroidal tissue. The emitted β particles cannot travel far, thus limiting damage to adjacent normal tissues. Because normal tissue has atrophied and is quiescent, ^{131}I will be concentrated within a thyroid tumor(s), and normal tissue is relatively spared from destruction by the radioactive particles.

The ^{131}I dose can be administered orally, subcutaneously, or intravenously but is usually given subcutaneously to avoid the stress of intravenous catheterization or injection and the possibility of vomition of radioactive material. The major disadvantages of radioactive iodine therapy include accessibility (a limited number of facilities are licensed to use radiopharmaceuticals, but this is changing), cost, and the possible extent of hospital stay while radioactivity decreases in the patient (potentially up to 2 weeks, depending on local radiation safety regulations). After discharge, cats will continue to excrete a small amount of radiation for 2 to 4 weeks, and close contact with the cat should be minimized during this time.

TSH increases ^{131}I uptake of the thyroid gland in humans, and rhTSH is routinely administered before ^{131}I treatment to lessen the ^{131}I dose and minimize irradiation of nonthyroidal tissues. Whether rhTSH would increase the uptake of ^{131}I in thyroid glands of hyperthyroid cats was recently examined.[62] Five hyperthyroid cats were given 25 μg rhTSH intravenously 1 hour before ^{123}I administration; ^{123}I can be used to visualize hyperfunctional tissue and will be handled by the body like ^{131}I but will not cure hyperthyroidism. The same cats were given another ^{131}I injection 8 days later without first receiving rhTSH. The rhTSH increased radioactive iodine uptake by the thyroid gland by 7.33%, which was statistically significant. Thus hyperthyroid cats undergoing ^{131}I therapy may require a lower radioactive iodine dose if given rhTSH before treatment, but further studies are needed to optimize the rhTSH dose and the interval between its administration and the ^{131}I injection.

Administration of ^{131}I by any route appears to be relatively safe. Pain or discomfort in the area of the thyroid gland presumably reflects radioactive thyroiditis and should resolve within several days of therapy. A transient voice change has been noted in one cat[63] and transient dysphagia in eight.[64] Although many cats develop a subnormal serum T_4 concentration following ^{131}I administration, a low serum T_4 concentration in itself does not mean hypothyroidism is present. Because nonthyroidal diseases can suppress serum T_4 concentration, nonthyroidal disease should always be excluded before a diagnosis of hypothyroidism is made. Supplementation is required only if clinical signs of hypothyroidism develop. Although 11% of cats have a low serum T_4 concentration after ^{131}I therapy, approximately only 2% require L-thyroxine supplementation.[64]

Clinical signs of euthyroidism generally occur within 1 to 3 weeks of ^{131}I administration; the first sign generally is normalization of appetite and weight gain. Therapeutic failure rate is approximately 2%. If T_4 is still elevated 3 to 6 months after ^{131}I administration, the hyperthyroid state is unlikely to resolve without further treatment. Most of these cats will respond to a second dose of ^{131}I.[63-67] In one study 2.5% of cats had a relapse of hyperthyroidism 1.1 to 6.5 years after initial radioiodine treatment.[64]

Percutaneous ultrasound-guided intrathyroidal injection of ethanol or percutaneous radiofrequency ablation of thyroidal tissue has been tried as a means of targeting and destroying thyroid tumors. After treatment of unilateral disease with percutaneous ethanol injection (PEI), resolution was obtained lasting at least 12 months.[68] However, only a small number of cats were studied. Bilateral PEI for bilateral disease led to mortality in one cat, likely because of laryngeal paralysis. Treating bilateral disease with staged injections has not shown long-term success, with the longest remission obtained being 27 weeks.[69] Adverse effects include mild gagging, voice change, Horner's syndrome, and laryngeal paralysis; are usually transient; and resolve in 8 weeks or less.[68,69]

Radiofrequency ablation was used to treat four cats with unilateral thyroid disease and five cats with bilateral disease.[70] The nine cats were administered 14 treatments. Of the cats with unilateral disease, three became clinically and biochemically euthyroid for 1, 6, and 18 months; the fourth cat became clinically euthyroid for 6 weeks, although the serum T_4 concentration remained slightly above the reference range. Interestingly, all cats with bilateral disease had treatments on one side and remission was obtained after 1 to 3 treatments for 1 to 6 months. Repeat therapy was used in some cats to induce a second or third remission when clinical signs returned. Transient Horner's disease was the sole clinical complication and was seen after 3 of the 14 treatments. Clinically inapparent laryngeal paralysis was noted in one cat during laryngeal examination.[70]

Neither ethanol injection nor radiofrequency ablation is currently widely available for treatment of feline hyperthyroidism, and both require considerable experience. Radiofrequency ablation also requires specialized equipment.

Drugs Used To Control Clinical Signs of Hyperthyroidism

Thyroid hormones may increase the number or sensitivity of β-receptors in the myocardium.[56] Tachycardia, myocardial hypertrophy, heart failure, and cardiac arrhythmias have been associated with thyrotoxicosis in hyperthyroid cats. Beta-adrenergic blockers (e.g., propranolol) have no effect on thyroid hormone concentration but decrease the neuromuscular and cardiovascular effects of hyperthyroidism, such as hyperexcitability, hypertension, and cardiac hypertrophy. These agents can be used in combination with an antithyroid drug such as methimazole or alone if a patient cannot tolerate antithyroid medications, and they may be helpful in preparing a patient for thyroidectomy or radioactive iodine by making the cat a better candidate for surgery or hospitalization. Nonselective β blockade by propranolol can reduce the hyperdynamic effects of thyroid hormones on the myocardium. In addition, propranolol inhibits conversion of T_4 to T_3 by peripheral tissues in hyperthyroid humans. Because propranolol does not directly affect the thyroid gland, however, patients are not returned to a euthyroid state. Propanolol dosing in cats suffering from cardiac disorders associated with hyperthyroidism should begin at 2.5 mg orally every 12 hours and be increased to 7.5 mg every 8 hours as necessary to control heart rate. If propranolol is being used to prepare a patient for surgery, therapy should continue for 14 days preoperatively. Care should be taken in patients with congestive heart failure because the negative chronotropic effects of propranolol may decrease myocardial reserve. In addition, as a nonselective β blocker, propranolol can cause bronchospasms, which may be lethal in cats with respiratory distress or may exacerbate feline asthma. Atenolol, a selective $\beta_1$blocker, might be used instead of propranolol (2 mg/kg or 6.25 mg/cat once daily).

Administration of large doses of iodide (e.g., sodium or potassium iodide) for a short time (1 to 2 weeks) will cause transient hypothyroidism in normal animals. Organification of thyroid hormones is prevented and hormone secretion is reduced. The clinical effects of high-dose iodine therapy will occur in 7 to 14 days in humans; however, refractoriness to these effects will develop in several weeks to months. In hyperthyroid cats, iodine (50-100 mg orally, once daily) has been used to prevent an acute thyroid crisis (i.e., a thyroid storm) in patients undergoing thyroidectomy. One to two drops of a saturated solution of potassium iodide can be administered in gelatin capsules beginning 10 days before surgery.[71]

DISEASES OF THE PARATHYROID GLANDS

Normal Calcium Homeostasis

Calcium balance is maintained by the integrated influences of parathyroid hormone (PTH) on calcium and phosphorus reabsorption in bone and distal renal tubular cells and by the intestinal absorption of calcium as mediated by vitamin D (Figure 21-3). Of the total calcium present in serum, approximately 40% is protein bound, 10% is bound to other factors such as citrate or phosphate, and 50% is ionized. Serum ionized calcium concentration, which is the biologically active portion, normally fluctuates less than 0.1 mg/dL. Secretion of PTH is exquisitely sensitive to changes in ionized calcium concentration. Decreases in serum calcium concentration stimulate PTH secretion, which in turn causes increased calcium resorption from urine (distal renal tubule), increased mobilization of calcium and phosphorus from bone, and increased vitamin D synthesis. Parathyroid hormone mediates the activation of vitamin D (see Figure 21-3).

The main function of vitamin D is to increase gastrointestinal calcium and phosphorus absorption. In humans vitamin D (cholecalciferol) can be ingested or made by irradiation of cutaneous 7-dehydrocholesterol; the serum half-life of vitamin D is 19 to 25 hours, although the vitamin is stored in fat depots. In dogs vitamin D must be ingested; what occurs in cats is unknown. Cholecalciferol is converted to 25-hydroxycholecalciferol (25-OHD, calcidiol) in the liver by hepatic microsomal enzymes (see Figure 21-3). Once in circulation, 25-OHD is bound to a binding globulin. In humans 25-OHD has an elimination half-life of about 19 days. Calcidiol is further hydroxylated to the most potent form, 1,25-dihydroxycholecalciferol (calcitriol), in the renal proximal tubules. The enzyme responsible for hydroxylation of 25-OHD is inhibited by calcitriol in a negative feedback manner and by hyperphosphatemia. On the other hand, conversion of 25-OHD to

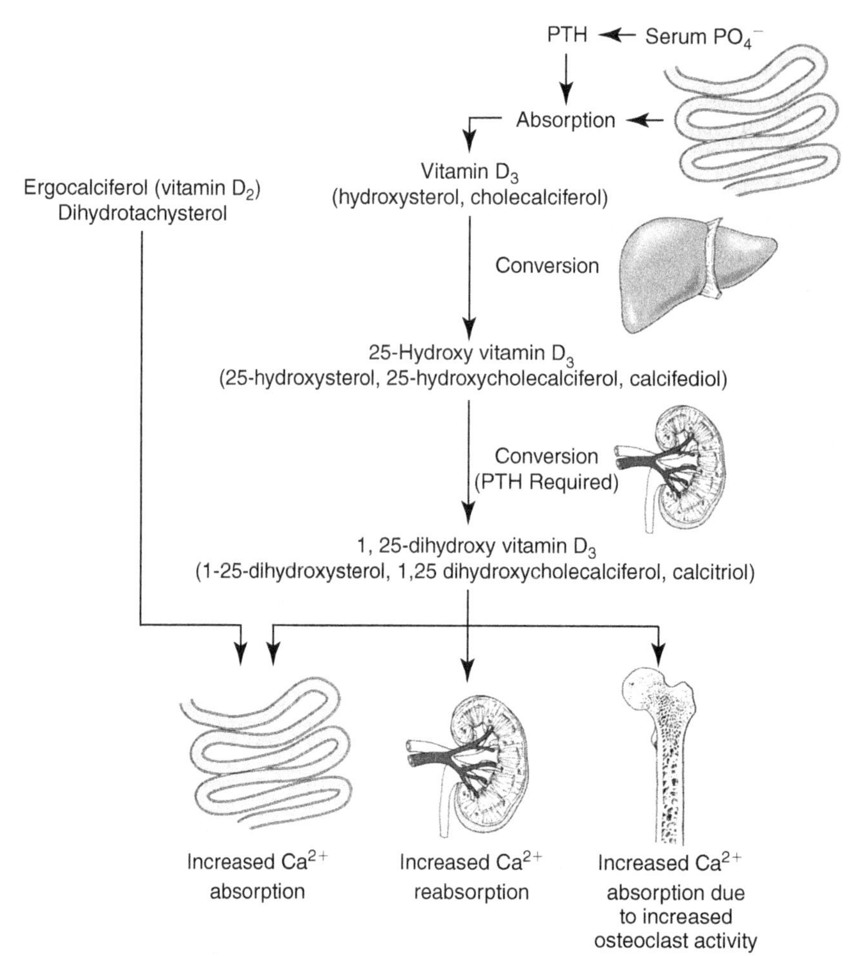

Figure 21-3 Calcium is very tightly regulated through the combined effects of parathyroid hormone (PTH), calcitonin, and vitamin D. The figure shows the activation of vitamin D and the way vitamin D and PTH act to increase serum calcium concentrations. Vitamin D must undergo several sequential activation steps before it is fully functional; calcitriol, the end product, acts to increase serum calcium concentrations and is essential for synthesis of PTH. Calcitonin, on the other hand, decreases serum calcium concentrations.

calcitriol requires PTH; thus without PTH, little to no calcitriol is made and there is practically no functioning vitamin D in the body. Renal and, to some degree, bone activities mediate the acute response to calcium homeostasis. Intestinal calcium reabsorption may take several days to occur, in part because of the time necessary for vitamin D synthesis or activation. Calcitriol is further hydroxylated to 1,24,25-(OH) 3-D_3 and subsequent metabolites that have variable activity.

Calcitonin, a polypeptide hormone secreted from thyroidal C (parafollicular) cells in response to hypercalcemia, is the least important regulator of calcium metabolism. It has a mild blood calcium–lowering effect by decreasing both the absorptive activity of osteoclasts and the formation of new osteoclasts. The main role of calcitonin may be to limit postprandial hypercalcemia. In normal animals the role of calcitonin is more important in juveniles. Calcitonin has minor effects on calcium handling by the gastrointestinal tract and at high doses promotes urinary calcium excretion.

Because ionized Ca is available to cells and is thus the biologically active form, it is critically important in the diagnosis of calcium disturbances. If ionized calcium is normal, even if total calcium is not, no further diagnostics are warranted. The correction formulas previously advocated and used to correct calcium concentration for serum albumin or protein concentration are no longer recommended.[72] To know a patient's calcium status, the clinician must measure ionized calcium concentration.

Hypoparathyroidism

Pathophysiology and Diagnosis of Primary Hypoparathyroidism

Primary hypoparathyroidism in dogs can reflect destruction of the parathyroid glands by disease (e.g., lymphocytic parathyroiditis) or trauma, including surgical removal. The most common cause in cats is injury or removal of the parathyroid glands during thyroidectomy. Hypomagnesemia can be a cause or effect of hypoparathyroidism in dogs and cats. Cessation of PTH secretion results in the loss of calcium mobilization from bone, of calcium retention by the kidneys, and of calcium absorption from the intestines. The primary clinical manifestation of hypoparathyroidism reflects decreased serum calcium concentration.

Hypoparathyroid patients may be hyperphosphatemic as a result of decreased renal phosphorus excretion. Measurement of serum PTH concentration is required to establish a diagnosis of hypoparathyroidism. Serum PTH concentrations below the reference range in hypocalcemic dogs and cats confirm the diagnosis, assuming the assay used is reliable and validated. Serum PTH concentrations in the low end of the reference range are not appropriate in hypocalcemic individuals, and a diagnosis of hypoparathyroidism can also be made.[73]

Hypocalcemia

Hypocalcemia and, in particular, decreased serum ionized calcium concentration leads to neuromuscular hyperexcitability as the stabilizing influence of calcium on neuronal sodium permeability is lost. Although both central and peripheral nerves are affected, clinical signs are usually peripheral, ranging from latent tetany (e.g., muscle cramping, lameness, irritability) to muscle fasciculations and stiff gait to tetanic seizures. The concentration of ionized calcium below which tetany develops depends on the rate at which hypocalcemia develops. Furthermore, cerebrospinal fluid concentrations may be more critical and may remain stable in the face of fluctuations in serum concentrations. Despite the importance of calcium in cardiac contractility, clinical evidence of cardiac dysfunction generally does not develop. Differential diagnoses for hypocalcemia include primary hypoparathyroidism, acute and chronic renal failure, acute pancreatitis, puerperal tetany (eclampsia), intestinal malabsorption syndromes, nutritional secondary hyperparathyroidism, ethylene glycol toxicity, administration of phosphate-containing enemas, congenital vitamin D receptor defects, and hypomagnesemia.

Treatment of Hypocalcemia and Hypoparathyroidism

No treatment fully compensates for the absence of PTH.[74] The need for calcium therapy is based on serum calcium concentrations and clinical signs. Total serum calcium concentrations of 6.5 mg/dL might be considered critical; below 6 mg/dL generally results in clinical tetany, and below 4 mg/dL may be fatal.

Hypocalcemic tetany is a life-threatening condition, requiring immediate intravenous replacement. Because calcium can be lethal, it must be administered slowly to effect over 20 to 30 minutes. The amount of calcium in both oral and intravenous preparations varies with the salt. Because it is much less caustic if administered perivascularly, the calcium gluconate salt (10% solution: 9.3 mg calcium /mL) is preferred to the chloride (10% solution: 27.2 mg calcium/mL) and glucoheptonate (22% solution: 18 mg calcium/mL) salts. The dose of calcium for intravenous administration is 5 to 15 mg/kg (i.e., for the 10% gluconate salt solution [0.5 to 1.5 mL/kg] given slowly and intravenously. An electrocardiogram should be monitored during infusion; if bradycardia, premature ventricular contractions, or shortening of the Q-T interval is seen, the infusion should be slowed or briefly discontinued. Fluids containing bicarbonate, lactate, acetate, or phosphate cannot be used to administer calcium because the calcium will precipitate out of solution. Although seizures will stop once eucalcemia is established, other signs, such as nervousness, panting, and behavioral changes, may persist for 30 to 60 minutes after normalization of serum calcium concentration.[73] Correction of tetany should help resolve hyperthermia that developed as a result of excess muscle activity. Life-threatening hyperthermia should be treated as an emergency.

Duration of response to a single dose of calcium varies from 1 to 12 hours. The type of future therapy required depends on the cause of hypocalcemia. If primary hypoparathyroidism is diagnosed, long-term treatment with oral vitamin D is required insofar as no suitable commercial PTH preparations exist. Oral calcium supplementation will also be needed in the long-term, but parenteral calcium administration is required in the short-term. Oral maintenance therapy with calcium should begin as soon as possible, but oral calcium is not absorbed from the gastrointestinal tract until vitamin D therapy begins to take effect, which is usually in 1 to 5 days. In the meantime, continuous calcium infusion is recommended (60-90 mg/kg/day elemental calcium) until oral medications provide control. If initial hypocalcemia was severe, the dose administered should be in the upper end of the range. The dose can be decreased as the oral medications begin to work and based on serum calcium concentration.[73] Intermittent intravenous infusions are not recommended because of the wide fluctuations in serum calcium concentrations that will occur.[74]

In theory, the gluconate salt can be given subcutaneously, diluted 1 part calcium to 2 to 4 parts saline, but this is not recommended. Although not fully conclusive that calcium gluconate was the cause, two case reports suggest that severe calcinosis cutis and subsequent sloughing resulted from subcutaneous administration of calcium gluconate.[75,76] Calcium carbonate solutions can never be given subcutaneously.

The daily oral calcium dose is 25 to 50 mg/kg, divided in several doses. Parenteral calcium administration can be slowly discontinued beginning 1 to 2 days after initiation of oral treatment; the rate will depend on serum calcium concentrations. Calcium salts available for oral administration include lactate (13% elemental calcium available), gluconate (10% elemental calcium available), carbonate (40% elemental calcium available [tablet form]), chloride (27% elemental calcium available) and citrate (21% elemental calcium available). The carbonate form has the highest percentage of calcium; does not cause gastric irritation, as do other forms; and is a phosphate binder, lowering serum phosphate, which has positive effects on endogenous calcitriol synthesis. Thus it is the preferred oral form. Other salts containing smaller amounts of calcium may require many tablets to be administered as a single dose. Over-the-counter preparations (e.g., Tums, which contains calcium carbonate) can also be used for oral maintenance therapy. As vitamin D therapy becomes effective, calcium supplementation should no longer be necessary (discussed later).

Vitamin D therapy (Figure 21-4) is necessary for both absorption of orally administered calcium and normalization of calcium homeostasis. Patients should be hospitalized during induction of vitamin D therapy, until serum calcium

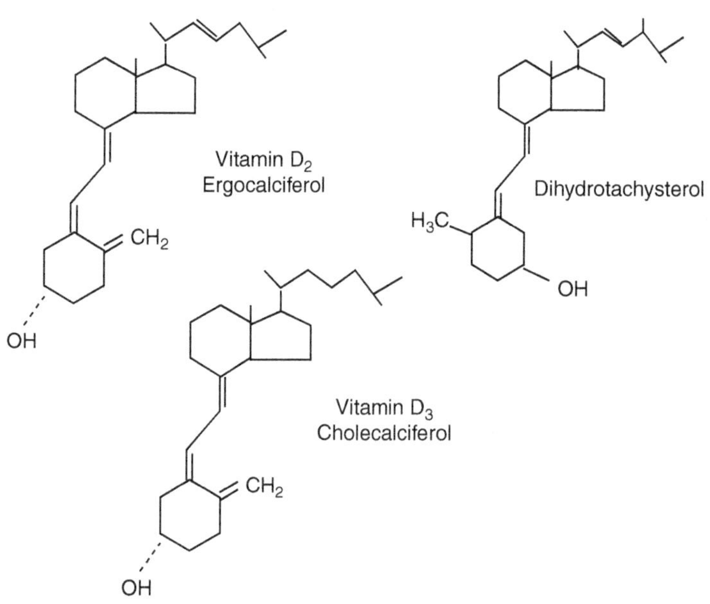

Figure 21-4 Structures of ergocalciferol, vitamin D_2, present in plants, and cholecalciferol, vitamin D_3, present in animals. Dihydrotachysterol is a congener of vitamin D_2, currently not available commercially.

concentrations remain between 8 and 10 mg/dL without parenteral support. Vitamin D preparations vary in potency, time to onset (time to steady-state concentrations), and cost. Vitamin D can be administered as ergocalciferol (vitamin D_2) and calcitriol (active vitamin D_3). Vitamin D_3 is likely, however, to be better absorbed orally than is ergocalciferol. Bile is essential for adequate oral absorption; the majority of absorbed vitamin D occurs in chylomicrons in the lymph. Dihydrotachysterol (DHT), a synthetic form of vitamin D previously used to treat hypoparathyroidism, is no longer available.

Ergocalciferol, or vitamin D_2 (4000 to 6000 U/kg per day), is inexpensive and widely available. Large doses are necessary, however, to compensate for decreased potency in hypoparathyroid patients—it is an inactive form, and conversion to the active form will be impaired by low PTH concentrations in the patient. Large doses are also required to saturate fat depots (vitamin D is a fat-soluble vitamin). The effect of the medication is usually obvious 5 to 14 days after beginning therapy, and parenteral calcium can usually be discontinued 1 to 5 days after starting oral treatment.[73] Once the serum calcium concentration is in the target range of 8 to 10 mg/dL, ergocalciferol can be administered every other day. Serum calcium concentration should be monitored weekly, with the ergocalciferol dose adjusted to maintain calcium in the target range.[73] The required maintenance dose is 1000 to 2000 U/kg once daily to once weekly.[73]

In patients in whom development of hypocalcemia can be anticipated (e.g., after parathyroid gland tumor removal), it may be necessary to start vitamin D supplementation preemptively. Guidelines exist, although they are unproven. If the serum calcium is below 14 mg/dL, vitamin D therapy is not recommended preoperatively. If calcium is above 15 mg/dL or a dog has more than one parathyroid mass, calcitriol therapy should be started the morning of surgery or immediately thereafter.[74]

Even after a pet appears stable, rechecks are recommended monthly for the first 6 months and then every 2 to 3 months for life.[73] Hypercalcemia must be avoided because it can cause renal and other organ damage and numerous other problems. A disadvantage of ergocalciferol therapy is that because of high lipid solubility and body fat–store saturation, serum calcium concentrations can take up to 4 weeks to decline once ergocalciferol administration has been discontinued. Hypercalcemia should be treated aggressively if it occurs. Because of the risk of hypercalcemia and the difficulty of treatment, ergocalciferol is not recommended for treatment of hypoparathyroidism.

Calcitriol is the vitamin D of choice for treatment of hypoparathyroidism. Although calcitriol is significantly more expensive than ergocalciferol, it is much safer. As calcitriol is already active, small doses may be used and the dose may be adjusted frequently because of its rapid onset of action (1 to 4 days versus 5 to 21 days for ergocalciferol) and brief biological effect. If hypercalcemia occurs, the effects of this drug abate quickly after stopping therapy or with dose reduction.[73] A loading dose of 20 to 30 ng/kg daily can be administered for 3 to 4 days and then decreased to a maintenance dose of 5 to 15 ng/kg daily.[74] Doses should be divided and given twice daily. Reformulation may be required for veterinary patients; alternatively, a liquid form can be used to facilitate dose adjustments.

When calcitriol is used, dose adjustments should be made in 10% to 20% increments and only after enough time has elapsed for a previous alteration to take effect. Total calcium measurement is recommended daily in the initial phase, weekly during maintenance until a satisfactory serum calcium concentration is obtained, and then quarterly thereafter. The target for total serum calcium concentration, regardless of the form of calcium or vitamin D used, is just below the reference range.

If hypomagnesemia is documented, magnesium sulfate (1 to 2 mEq/kg/day) should be administered. Correction of serum magnesium concentrations can decrease needed doses of vitamin D or calcium (or both).[74]

If hypoparathyroidism is due to surgical intervention and expected to be temporary (e.g., at least one parathyroid gland was left after the thyroidectomy in cats or a parathyroid tumor was removed in dogs), calcitriol can be discontinued over time. In cats parathyroid function usually recovers in 2 weeks but can take up to 3 months; after removal of a parathyroid tumor in dogs, return of function of the remaining gland (or glands) can take up to 12 weeks.[74] Tapering of the calcitriol dose can begin after 4 weeks. If hypocalcemia returns, the calcitriol dose should be increased to the previous level and attempts at tapering made again later. If tapering after 3 months still results in hypoparathyroidism, permanent therapy with calcitriol will likely be necessary.[74]

Oral calcium should be continued until serum calcium is maintained between 8 and 10 mg/dL, usually 1 to 2 days to several weeks after vitamin D therapy is started (depending on the vitamin D product used). Calcium can gradually be tapered over weeks as normal serum concentrations are maintained.

Because of potential nephrotoxic and other effects, hypercalcemia should be avoided. If hypercalcemia (>12 mg/dL) occurs at any time regardless of the product used, vitamin D administration should be discontinued until serum calcium concentration returns to normal. In addition, oral calcium supplements, if being given, also need to be ceased and the patient should be placed on a calcium-restricted diet.

Primary Hyperparathyroidism

Hypercalcemia

Multiple rule-outs for hypercalcemia exist. They can be remembered by the mnemonic *GOSHDARNIT:* **G**ranulomatous disease, **O**steolytic disease, **S**purious (e.g., sample lipemia or hemolysis), **H**yperparathyroidism, **D** toxicosis (i.e., vitamin D toxicosis), **A**ddison's disease, **R**enal failure, **N**eoplasia, **I**diopathic (only recognized in cats), and **T**emperature (hypothermia has been noted as a cause). The most common cause of hypercalcemia in dogs is malignancy.[77] Lymphosarcoma is most likely, but multiple myeloma and anal sac apocrine cell adenocarcinoma and others are possible. In cats idiopathic hypercalcemia is most likely, but neoplasia or renal failure are also possibilities. Squamous cell carcinoma and lymphosarcoma are the most common hypercalcemia-causing neoplasias in cats.[78]

Assessing the phosphorus levels can aid in ranking differential diagnoses. The net effect of PTH is to increase serum calcium but decrease phosphorus. In primary hyperparathyroidism (PHPTH) the normal feedback mechanism of calcium on the parathyroid glands is lost. With elevated PTH hypercalcemia occurs with a low normal or low serum phosphorus concentration. The most common cause of PHPTH is neoplasia (functioning adenoma) of the chief cells of the parathyroid glands.[79] Hyperplasia of the parathyroid gland(s), multiple endocrine neoplasia, and hereditary hyperparathyroidism are less common causes. Secondary hyperparathyroidism generally occurs as calcium and phosphorus homeostasis becomes unbalanced (e.g., renal or nutritional secondary hyperparathyroidism).

Most neoplasias cause hypercalcemia by secreting the hormone parathyroid hormone related–peptide (PTHrP), which binds to PTH receptors affecting serum calcium and phosphorus just as PTH does, mimicking PHPTH. Hematologic malignancies growing in the bone marrow or metastases of solid tumors to bone can also cause hypercalcemia.

Vitamin D toxicosis leads to elevations in both calcium and phosphorus and can result from ingestion of cholecalciferol-containing rodenticides or human antipsoriasis creams containing calcipotriene, a synthetic vitamin D_3 (e.g., Dovonex)[80] or from oversupplementation. Toxicity may not be evident until the drug has accumulated, which may take several weeks to months depending on the product. Granulomatous disease is an uncommon cause of hypercalcemia and may be due to the ability of macrophages to activate vitamin D independent of feedback mechanisms.

Unfortunately, the presence of renal failure can make interpretation of results difficult. Hypercalcemia can lead to renal failure and vice versa. If azotemia is present, phosphorus is likely to be elevated and cannot be used to help in ranking differential diagnoses. In addition, it can be hard to determine if the hypercalcemia or the renal failure came first. The clinician should be sure always to assess ionized calcium concentration. In the presence of azotemia, ionized calcium is often normal (and therefore not a cause for worry) when total serum calcium concentration is high. If ionized calcium is high, the diagnosis is likely PHPTH, whereas if the ionized calcium is normal to low, it is likely primary renal failure.

Clinical signs of hypercalcemia can be severe but are usually insidious and unnoticed. Polyuria and polydipsia are the most common in dogs. Hypercalcemia can cause secondary nephrogenic diabetes insipidus, initially increased and then decreased GFR, nephrocalcinosis, and soft tissue mineralization. Muscle weakness and atrophy, depression, anorexia, vomiting, shivering, bone pain, constipation, a stiff gait, and cardiac arrhythmias can also be seen. In cats presenting signs include vomiting, weight loss, dysuria, anorexia, inappropriate urination, lethargy, diarrhea, hematuria, pollakiuria, and stranguria. Signs of lower urinary tract disease may be seen in up to one third of hypercalcemic dogs and cats, which are prone to forming calcium-containing uroliths. Fibrous osteodystrophy of all bones, but particularly the skull, can occur with hyperparathyroidism.

Pathophysiology and Diagnosis of Primary Hyperparathyroidism

PHPTH results in hypercalcemia from autonomous PTH secretion from solitary or multiple parathyroid gland adenomas or hyperplasia or parathyroid gland carcinoma. Although no epidemiologic studies have been done, PHPTH is uncommon in dogs and rare in cats, primarily affecting older animals. It can occur in any breed, but it is an autosomal dominant, genetically transmitted disease in the Keeshond.[81] Because clinical signs tend to be absent to mild, hypercalcemia can be diagnosed on a serum biochemistry profile obtained for unrelated concerns. Given the numerous diseases that cause hypercalcemia, a minimum database of a hemogram, serum biochemistry profile, urinalysis, and urine culture should be obtained and a full, careful physical examination performed in all hypercalcemic animals.

If clinical signs are present, the most common ones involve the renal, gastrointestinal, or neuromuscular systems. Of the clinical signs reported in dogs with PHPTH, 81% had polyuria or polydipsia; 73% had either urinary tract calculi, a urinary tract infection, or both; 53% had decreased activity; and 37% had a decreased appetite; azotemia was documented in only 5%. The most commonly reported clinical signs in cats are anorexia, lethargy, and vomiting. In contrast to dogs, in which a parathyroid mass is rarely palpable, 11 of the 19 reported cats with PHPTH had a palpable mass.[79]

In uncomplicated PHPTH, the biochemistry profile usually demonstrates persistently elevated total and ionized calcium, decreased to low-normal phosphorus, and normal BUN and creatinine levels. Assays for PTH and PTHrP are relatively sensitive, readily available diagnostic tools to help identify the cause of hypercalcemia. In general, in animals with PHPTH, serum PTH levels are within the normal reference range or elevated, and PTHrP is usually undetectable. In the face of hypercalcemia, a PTH concentration within the upper half of the reference range is wholly inappropriate and consistent with a diagnosis of PHPTH. In the face of hypercalcemia, a PTH concentration in the lower half of the normal range should raise suspicion for PHPTH, although it does not confirm it diagnostically.

Although previous reports state that 90% of dogs and cats with PHTPH have a solitary adenoma,[79] in one recent study, 42% of dogs had multiglandular disease.[82] It is therefore important to identify all abnormal glands before or at the time of definitive treatment. Selective sampling and determination of serum PTH concentrations in both jugular veins have proved inconsistent in predicting the affected side, and this procedure is not recommended.[79,82] Cervical ultrasonography can be a useful diagnostic aid in locating and identifying abnormal parathyroid glands, with reported sensitivity rates ranging from 42% to 100% when performed by highly experienced ultrasonographers.[82,83] However, finding parathyroid glands with ultrasound requires a great deal of practice and skill.

Treatment of Primary Hyperparathyroidism

For PHPTH the only effective long-term therapy is ablation of the abnormal parathyroid tissue. Several methods of definitive treatment for PHPTH exist, but surgical excision is the most common, with cure rates up to 95% if all autonomously functioning tissue is removed.[83] In humans undergoing parathyroidectomy, PTH concentrations are measured preoperatively and intraoperatively 10 minutes after removal of the abnormal gland. A greater than 50% decrease in PTH concentration between the preexcision and postexcision samples is associated with successful removal of autonomously functioning tissue in humans. A minimum period of 6 months of normocalcemia postoperatively is considered curative in human medicine. With this in mind, a rapid intact PTH assay was recently validated in dogs. In 12 dogs the assay accurately detected increased serum PTH concentrations in all dogs with PHPTH preoperatively. A greater than 50% decrease in serum PTH levels between the preexcision and postexcision samples corresponded with a return to normocalcemia for at least 6 months in 92% of the dogs in the study.[82]

Ethanol injection[84] or application of radiofrequency[85] has been reported for treatment of PHPTH. In a retrospective study, ethanol injection had only a 72% efficacy rate, whereas radiofrequency ablation and surgery had success rates of 90% and 94%, respectively, for medians of approximately 560 days.[83] Thus chemical ablation is not recommended. Unfortunately, radiofrequency ablation is not widely available and requires considerable expertise. With bilateral disease, staged treatments are needed.

Treatment of Hypercalcemia

Because hypercalcemia is best treated by addressing the underlying disorder, the cause should be delineated as quickly as possible and appropriate therapy instituted. Hypercalcemia can be damaging, especially to the kidneys, with severity appearing to depend on the phosphorus concentration. If the product of multiplying the serum calcium concentration by the serum phosphorus concentration is above 60 to 80, nephrotoxicity is likely.[79] If the etiology cannot be identified rapidly and continuing hypercalcemia is judged to be deleterious, clinical signs are present, or the hypercalcemia is idiopathic, the hypercalcemia should be addressed directly.

If treatment is deemed necessary, intravenous fluid therapy should be initiated. Dehydration may be present and should be corrected because it decreases GFR and can perpetuate hypercalcemia. Saline (0.9%) is the fluid of choice. Fluid deficits should be replaced and then fluid rates maintained at 120 to 180 mL/kg daily to promote calciuresis. Potassium supplementation is usually required to prevent hypokalemia.[79]

Furosemide may be given to increase calcium excretion, but patients should be well hydrated first. Constant-rate infusion is typically recommended (5 mg/kg intravenously followed by a 5 mg/kg/hr infusion).[79] Lower doses (2-4 mg/kg 2 to 3 time daily, intravenously, subcutaneously, or orally) may produce a milder reduction in hypercalcemia. Thiazide diuretics are discouraged because they may increase renal calcium reabsorption.

Glucocorticoids have many beneficial effects; they decrease intestinal calcium absorption, reduce bone resorption, and increase renal calcium excretion. Prednisone (1-2.2 mg/kg twice daily, orally, subcutaneously, or intravenously) or dexamethasone (0.1-0.22 mg/kg twice daily, orally, subcutaneously, or intravenously) can be used. Steroid-sensitive hypercalcemias include lymphoma/leukemia, multiple myeloma, vitamin D toxicity, granulomatous disease, hypoadrenocorticism, and feline idiopathic hypercalcemia. Glucocorticoids should not be administered unless a definitive diagnosis is known. Even one dose can cause remission in a patient with lymphosarcoma.

Although this could be beneficial in the short-term, it will make diagnosis impossible until remission ends. Furthermore, if standard combination chemotherapy is started after remission from prednisone alone is lost, it will be less effective, and, accordingly, overall prognosis will be worse.

Calcitonin (salmon calcitonin, 4-6 IU/kg subcutaneously, 2 to 3 times daily) can be used if other treatments fail. It can be an effective treatment for vitamin D toxicosis or other diseases in which bone resorption is a major cause of the hypercalcemia. In dogs the response may be short-lived, and anorexia, vomiting, or allergic reactions may occur. Information in cats is lacking.

Bisphosphonates, "osteoclast poisons," are believed to act by interfering with hydroxyapatite crystal dissolution or by direct action on osteoclasts. They may also be used if bone resorption is a major source of the hypercalcemia. Pamidronate disodium has been used to treat vitamin D toxicosis secondary to calcipotriene ingestion at a dose of 1.3 to 2 mg/kg,[86,87] as well as hypercalcemia associated with nocardiosis (one cat), idiopathic hypercalcemia and renal failure (one cat), lymphoma (two dogs), thyroid carcinoma (one dog), and multiple endocrine neoplasia (one dog).[87] Given its potential nephroxicity, pamidronate should be diluted in saline and infused intravenously over a 4-hour period with a minimum of 4-hour diuresis both before and after the treatment.[87] Calcium and phosphorus normalize in 24 to 48 hours.[86,87] The decrease in total and ionized calcium concentration after treatment is proportional to the degree of hypercalcemia.[87] Treatment can be repeated if necessary, but may not be needed depending on the cause of the hypercalcemia. In one cat with idiopathic hypercalcemia, although a first treatment worked, a second and third did not. For the second and third treatments, previously frozen pamidronate was thawed and administered.[87] Whether lack of response was due to progression of the disease state or to instability of the pamidronate with freezing, storage, and thawing is unknown. Etidronate is an oral drug that has had limited use in dogs but may be helpful (5-15 mg/kg once to twice daily). Clodronate, which is not available in the United States, has been used successfully to treat experimentally induced vitamin D toxicity if given within 24 hours after vitamin D ingestion.[88] Clodronate toxicity and efficacy for treating accidental vitamin D overdose remain to be determined.

Sodium bicarbonate (1 to 4 mEq/kg intravenously by slow bolus) can be given during a hypercalcemic crisis. This does not always lower total serum calcium concentration but decreases the ionized portion, so adverse effects of the hypercalcemia are less common.

It is unclear whether therapy for treatment of feline idiopathic hypercalcemia is required. One guideline is to make the decision using the previously described guidelines for emergency treatment: Treat if calcium continues to rise, the calcium-phosphorus product is greater than 60 mg/dL, the ionized calcium concentration is greater than 1 mg/dL above the reference range, or clinical signs or azotemia are present.[89] The aggressiveness of therapy depends on the clinical status and parameters present. If treatment is not pursued at first, calcium concentrations should be monitored every 1 to 3 months and the need for therapy reevaluated. With any treatment, ionized calcium may not normalize even though total calcium does,[90] so measurement of the ionized form is required for accurate assessment of therapeutic success.

Dietary therapy with a high-fiber diet was reported to be successful in five cats based on measurement of total serum calcium and/or resolution of clinical signs.[91] Although dietary management was not effective in other cats,[90] the recommended first line of treatment for idiopathic hypercalcemia is to place an affected cat on a diet that is not designed to acidify the urine; urine-acidifying diets have been theorized to contribute to development of hypercalcemia. High-fiber, oxalate-prevention, or renal diets can be implemented. If ionized calcium has not normalized after 3 months, prednisone therapy should be added[89] and may be successful.[90] The recommended starting dose is 5 to 10 mg per cat per day, but it can be increased to 10 mg twice daily if needed. Prednisolone may be preferred to prednisone.[89] Bisphosphonates may be useful, and intravenous pamidronate has been used in one cat.[87] Although no peer-reviewed publications exist, use of alendronate (10 mg/cat/once weekly) has been successful for up to 1 year.[89] Because erosive esophagitis has been reported in women taking alendronate, the weekly pill should be followed with 6 mL of water given by a dosing syringe and then a small dab of butter on the cat's lips to increase licking and salivation.[89] Therapy for renal failure should be instituted as needed. Subtotal parathyroidectomy has not been successful.[90]

DISEASES OF THE PANCREAS: DIABETES MELLITUS

Normal Physiology

Glucagon stimulates glucose production from both hepatic conversion of glycogen and metabolism of noncarbohydrates, such as amino acids and lipids, into glucose or glucose precursors (e.g., lipids to fatty acids and glycerol). Low blood glucose concentrations increase glucagon secretion from pancreatic α cells. Should glucose concentrations become too high, insulin secretion is stimulated from pancreatic β cells. Insulin lowers blood glucose by stimulating formation of glycogen from glucose in the liver, inhibiting peripheral formation of glucose from amino acids and lipids, and facilitating diffusion of glucose into cells in insulin-dependent tissues such as muscle and adipose tissue. As a result, amino acids are synthesized in muscle, and adipocytes produce and store fat. Insulin secretion is regulated by a negative feedback mechanism sensitive to blood glucose concentrations. As the blood glucose concentration decreases, pancreatic β cells secrete less insulin and blood glucose does not decline further. With lower serum insulin concentrations, insulin-dependent cells can no longer utilize blood glucose, whereas insulin-independent cells such as neurons, which obtain glucose by simple diffusion, continue to use any glucose that remains in the blood.

Diabetes mellitus (DM) is a progressive disease resulting from an absolute or relative insulin deficiency caused by insufficient insulin secretion from pancreatic β cells and is characterized by four stages in human patients. Prediabetic patients are normal but subsequently develop the disease; subclinical DM can be diagnosed only by sophisticated provocative tests. In latent DM, patients are clinically normal but respond abnormally to a glucose load, and in overt DM, patients have persistent fasting hyperglycemia. The duration of progression from stage I to stage IV can be weeks to years, depending on the type of DM.

How best to classify DM in veterinary medicine is controversial, with the current classification scheme adapted from human medicine. Type 1 DM is characterized by β-cell destruction with progressive, eventually complete, insulin insufficiency. Genetic susceptibility plays a role, and β-cell destruction is usually due to immunologic processes. Causes of type 1 DM in animals may include hereditary factors and pancreatic destruction by pancreatitis, viruses, or autoimmune disease. Insulin resistance, dysfunctional β cells, and increased hepatic gluconeogenesis characterize type 2 DM. A classification of "other specific types of diabetes" also exists, formerly referred to as "secondary" DM. On the basis of pancreatic islet histology, lack of β-cell antibodies, risk factors, and clinical behavior of the disease, type II DM appears to be the most common form in cats.[92] Approximately 10% to 20% of diabetic cats have "other specific types of DM", which includes diseases that lead to β-cell loss, such as pancreatic neoplasia, and conditions such as hyperadrenocorticism or acromegaly that cause marked insulin resistance.[93] The remaining cats are believed to be type I diabetics. DM in dogs is believed to be mainly type 1.[94]

DM can also be classified as insulin-dependent DM (IDDM) or non-insulin-dependent DM (NIDDM), depending on the need for insulin therapy to control glycemia, prevent ketoacidosis, and survive. Individuals with IDDM must receive insulin to prevent ketoacidosis, whereas control of glycemia and avoidance of ketoacidosis can be accomplished through diet, exercise, and oral hypoglycemic drugs in patients with NIDDM.[95] At the time of diagnosis, all dogs are likely to be insulin dependent, as would be expected with type 1 diabetics, and at least 75% of cats with type 2 DM are insulin dependent.[93]

Management of persistent hyperglycemia is important to the progression of the syndrome, especially in cats. Cats may alternate between being insulin dependent and not, and the DM can go into remission for weeks to years with appropriate therapy. Persistent hyperglycemia can profoundly reduce insulin secretion and induce apoptosis in β cells, ultimately causing permanent DM in cats that at one point had a normal β cell mass,[96] a situation referred to as *glucose toxicity.* The effects begin within 2 days of onset of persistent hyperglycemia, and the impact on β cells increases with the magnitude of hyperglycemia.[97] Pancreatic βcell death by apoptosis occurs within 10 days of persistent hyperglycemia.[97] The impact of glucose toxicity is more severe in the presence of reduced β cell mass, underscoring the importance of effective control and βcell preservation. Control of blood glucose, ideally with insulin but potentially with oral hypoglycemic therapy, may allow β cells to regain insulin secretory capacity. As a result, the diabetic state is transient in 15% to 68% of cats[96,98-100] and can require as much as 20 to 52 weeks of insulin therapy before remission is achieved.[101,102]

Diagnosis

Presence of appropriate clinical signs (e.g., polyuria or polydipsia, polyphagia, and weight loss) and documentation of persistent fasting hyperglycemia (>200 mg/dL) and glycosuria are used to diagnose overt DM. Occasionally, a definitive diagnosis of DM may be difficult to make. Mild hyperglycemia, such as that induced by stress or certain diseases (e.g., hyperadrenocorticism), may uncommonly result in glycosuria. In nondiabetic cats, blood glucose concentrations may reach 400 mg/dL. Thus diagnosis of DM must be based on blood glucose and the presence of the classic signs. Unfortunately, the clinical signs are not unique to DM, and other differential diagnoses must be considered. On the other hand, some latent diabetic animals become overtly diabetic because of the presence of concurrent diseases; clinical signs of the precipitating disease may obscure the classic signs of DM. Hospitalization of a patient and reevaluation of blood glucose after the patient has adjusted to the new environment may help identify nondiabetic hyperglycemic states. Alternatively, urine can be monitored for the persistent presence of glucose at home. The presence of ketonuria strongly supports a diagnosis of DM. Identifying current drug therapy can also be important; progesterone or prolonged glucocorticoid therapy, which can precipitate DM, might support its diagnosis.

Measurement of glycosylated proteins can be used to corroborate a diagnosis of DM. Non-enzymatic, irreversible binding of glucose to hemoglobin results in the formation of glycosylated hemoglobin (GHb). *Fructosamine* refers to glycosylated serum proteins, mainly albumin, but glycated albumin (GA) also can specifically be measured in dogs and cats.[103,104] Glycosylated proteins form at a rate proportional to the average blood glucose concentration, so the higher the mean blood glucose concentration over time, the greater the glycosylated protein concentrations should be. Glycosylated protein levels are also affected by the half-life of the native protein; the shorter the half-life, the quicker the concentration of glycosylated protein falls after correction of hyperglycemia. Albumin has a short half-life compared with that of red blood cells. Thus in dogs and cats, GHb reflects glycemic control over the previous 2 to 3 months. In comparison, in dogs fructosamine reflects the previous 2 to 3 weeks and GA the previous 1 to 3 weeks.[104] In cats plasma proteins may be more rapidly metabolized, and fructosamine concentrations reflect the glucose concentrations in the previous 7 days.[105]

One study suggested that fructosamine might be more sensitive than GHb for monitoring control,[106] but measurement of either can be helpful. Both parameters are typically not affected by stress.[107-112] However, measurement of either is neither perfect nor absolute. Although in general, the higher the blood glucose concentration over time, the higher serum glycosylated protein concentrations should be, normal animals or well-controlled diabetics can have elevated concentrations of these substances, and, conversely, uncontrolled diabetic animals can have normal levels of either.[110,111,113] Thus the glycosylated protein concentration must be interpreted in conjunction with all other data.

Dietary Therapy

Dietary therapy is very important for treatment of DM. Through unknown mechanisms, dietary fiber can delay gastrointestinal glucose absorption, reducing postprandial fluctuations in blood glucose and enhancing glycemic control. High-fiber diets have been traditionally recommended for diabetics, but this is now being questioned. Insoluble fiber is beneficial in diabetic dogs.[114,115] However, the response of diabetic dogs to fiber varies between individuals. A recent study showed that high-fiber, moderate-starch diets were not advantageous for dogs with stabilized DM compared with a moderate-fiber, low-starch diet.[116] Insoluble fiber, the type present in commercial feline high-fiber diets, can also improve glycemic control in diabetic cats.[117] However, recent theories suggest that high-carbohydrate diets may lead to DM in cats, and high-protein diets may be more beneficial. The DM of cats on a high-protein, low-carbohydrate diet either resolved or was treatable with a reduced insulin dose.[118,119]

Although veterinary low-carbohydrate, high-protein prescription diets such as Purina DM or Hill's m/d are the first-choice dietary recommendation for most cats with DM, a carefully selected over-the-counter high-protein, low-carbohydrate diet can provide the same degree of effective glycemic control as prescription diets[120] when financial constraints dictate the less-expensive option or when a cat will not readily eat a veterinary diet. Many canned over-the-counter diets are relatively low in carbohydrate content (<5.0g/100kcal), but information must be obtained from the manufacturer on specific brands and flavors to ensure that the target nutrient composition is being met. Most dry over-the-counter diets are higher in carbohydrate content. Thus, if a prescription dry veterinary low-carbohydrate, high-protein diet is not an option, it may, unfortunately, be more difficult to identify a good-quality dry food with low carbohydrate content. Caution should be used in feeding diabetic cats with concurrent renal disease a high-protein diet; a high-fiber diet may be a better choice.

Drug Therapy

Insulin is the mainstay of therapy in diabetic dogs and cats. Its administration must be integrated with meals, exercise, owner's needs, and other characteristics of the patient or pet owner's lifestyle; these factors have been described elsewhere.[95,121-123] Although the ideal goal of insulin therapy is to maintain blood glucose concentrations as close to physiological as possible, this is difficult to do because exogenous insulin is administered as one or two large daily doses rather than in response to glucose concentrations. The realistic goal for insulin therapy, at least, should be elimination of the clinical signs of DM. Because secondary complications that dramatically alter the quality of health of human diabetics such as retinopathy or nephropathy appear to be rare in animals, near normalization of glucose concentrations may not be as important for diabetic dogs and cats as it is for human diabetic patients. Glucose concentrations should, however, be sufficiently controlled to prevent development of ketoacidosis and detrimental effects of hyperglycemia. Hyperglycemia is associated with an increased risk of bacterial infections; hepatic lipidosis; pancreatitis; and renal, hepatic, and pulmonary disease. Complicating problems that may alter response to insulin therapy must be identified in diabetics, as well as underlying diseases that led to the development of clinical signs in a covert diabetic.

Insulin Preparations

Insulin preparations are defined by modifications that alter time of onset and duration of action. They also vary in the source species and therefore in potential antigenicity. Chemical extracts of cattle and swine pancreases traditionally were the primary source. More recently, bacterially produced human recombinant products have been developed, but these are more expensive. More problematic, development of human products has led to discontinuation of several animal-source products that had been used successfully for controlling DM in dogs and cats.

The kinetics of individual insulin products vary markedly among species. Insulin products are generally classified as short-acting (e.g., regular insulin), intermediate-acting (e.g., neutral protamine Hagedorn [NPH], lente), or long-acting (e.g., PZI, Ultralente). The duration of action of regular insulin is the same in dogs and cats, but the duration of action of other insulins is typically shorter in cats than dogs. Intermediate- and long-acting insulins tend to be less bioavailable and thus less potent than short-acting insulins when given subcutaneously.

Regular insulin (zinc insulin crystals) is unmodified and acts the same whether crystalline or noncrystalline. Given intravenously, it begins working immediately, with maximal effects occurring at 0.5 to 2 hours and duration of effect being 1 to 4 hours. When insulin is given intramuscularly, time to effect is 10 to 30 minutes, time to peak effect is 1 to 4 hours, and duration of effect is 3 to 8 hours. When it is given subcutaneously, onset of effects occurs in 10 to 30 minutes, maximal effects occur at 1 to 5 hours, and duration is 4 to 10 hours. Inhaled insulin has recently been shown to be systemically bioavailable and physiologically active in dogs and cats, with an onset of action between 5 and 15 minutes[124] and a duration of action of 3 hours.[125] Neutral regular insulin will maintain its potency for as long as 18 months when stored at 5° to 25° C and will maintain 95% of its potency when stored at 37° C for 12 months.

Regular insulin is generally reserved for treatment of ketoacidosis. Use in daily maintenance therapy might include administration in combination with longer-acting products to provide a rapid onset with long duration of action; however, in general, such combinations are not needed or used. Insulin is available commercially in stable preparations of 70% NPH/30% regular or 50% NPH/50% regular (e.g., 70/30 or 50/50 insulin, respectively), but these are often quite potent, causing a rapid decrease in blood glucose concentration, and duration of effect is usually short.[95]

Protamine zinc insulin (PZI) was developed to prolong the effects of regular insulin. The preparation is formed by mixing insulin, zinc, and protamine, a fish protein, in a buffered solution such that it precipitates as a poorly soluble form. Poor solubility prolongs the absorption time after subcutaneous administration and provides a slower onset of activity and a longer duration of action. For PZI insulin the onset of action occurs at 1 to 4 hours, and maximum effect occurs at 3 to 12 hours. Duration is 12 to 24 hours in cats, and it may be necessary to administer the drug twice daily (in approximately 25% of cats). Use of PZI Vet (Idexx Pharmaceuticals) is limited to the existing supply; in April 2008 the manufacturer announced that after the sale of its existing inventory, it would no longer manufacture or sell animal-based insulin. Although many pharmacists can compound bovine PZI insulin, the authors do not recommend its use because the potency of compounded insulins varies between bottles.

To replace PZI Vet, a similar formulation based on recombinant human insulin (Prozinc) has recently been developed by Idexx. Limited data exist evaluating its efficacy and safety in diabetic cats, and no published pharmacodynamic studies of Prozinc in cats are available. One study compared glycemic control achieved with Prozinc with that of PZI Vet in diabetic cats. Fifty cats with stable glycemic control on PZI Vet were switched to Prozinc on day 0. Serum fructosamine concentrations, body weight, and insulin dose were measured on days 0, 15, and 30. On day 30, the cats were switched back to PZI Vet. Owners' subjective assessments of their cats' glycemic control were obtained at all time points. There were 47 cats completing the study; three were removed because of diabetic remission (n = 1), hypoglycemia (n = 1), and fractious behavior (n = 1). In the cats that completed the study, no difference in glycemic control between the insulin types was detected. The only adverse event reported was hypoglycemia in one cat.[126] A second study evaluated Prozinc in 126 newly diagnosed and 13 poorly controlled diabetic cats.[127] Control was assessed on days 7, 14, 30, and 45 by evaluating clinical response, body weight, serum fructosamine, and serial blood glucose concentrations over a 9-hour blood glucose curve. Based on the measured parameters, 84% of cats were judged to have good glycemic control by day 45. Thus Prozinc appeared safe and efficacious in diabetic cats. Prozinc has gained FDA approval for use in diabetic cats.

Isophane (NPH) insulin, developed as a compromise between short-acting regular insulin and slow-acting PZI, is made by manipulating the ratio between insulin and protamine. Isophane insulin is more potent and faster-acting than PZI but shorter in duration. For NPH administered subcutaneously, onset of action occurs in 0.5 to 3 hours and maximum effects occur at 2 to 8 hours. Duration of action is as little as 6 to as long as 12 hours in cats and 18 hours in dogs. Twice-daily administration is usually necessary for adequate diabetic control.

Lente insulin does not incorporate protamine but contains insulin and high concentrations of zinc (10 times greater than that in regular insulin) in an acetate rather than a phosphate buffer. Adjustment of pH causes insoluble precipitates to form that are longer-acting (i.e., ultralente) compared with soluble, shorter-acting (i.e., semilente) preparations. Lente insulin is a mixture of approximately 70% ultralente and 30% semilente, and its effects begin immediately. In dogs, time to maximum effect is 2 to 10 hours and duration is 8 to 20 hours. In diabetic cats, time to maximum effect for lente is 2 to 5 hours and duration of effects is 8 to 12 hours.[128] Human recombinant forms of lente and ultralente insulins are no longer available. The only veterinary preparation of lente insulin is Vetsulin (Intervet), which is porcine in origin. Vetsulin is currently approved in the United States by the Food and Drug Administration for use in both dogs and cats; it has been available for many years in other countries under the name Caninsulin. It is the only insulin approved for use in dogs. Currently, ultralente is not formulated as a veterinary preparation.

Lastly, "designer" recombinant insulins are made in which the amino acid structure of the protein has been altered slightly in order to change the pharmacokinetic profile. One of these products, glargine (Lantus), is used in veterinary medicine. Glargine differs from human insulin in that glycine is substituted for asparagine at position 21 in the α chain of insulin and by addition of two arginine residues to the βchain. Glargine is a clear aqueous solution with a pH of 4. The interaction of the acidic insulin and the relatively neutral pH of subcutaneous tissues causes microprecipitates to form and thus gives a relatively constant systemic absorption profile. As formation of microprecipitates depend on the solution's acidity, glargine cannot be mixed or diluted.[129] Although marketed as a "peakless" insulin in humans, it does have peaks and nadirs in healthy cats. In nondiabetic cats given 0.5 U/kg glargine insulin once daily, the mean time to the glucose nadir was 14 hours.[130] It is long-acting, with blood glucose concentrations suppressed below baseline at 24 hours in approximately half the cats studied, whether given once daily (0.5 U/kg) or twice daily (0.25 U/kg).[130,131] Another long-acting insulin analog, detemir, has lower within-subject variability compared with NPH and glargine in human type 1 or type 2 diabetics.[132,133] In one study of detemir using healthy cats, the findings suggest that glargine may have a more rapid onset then detemir, but the peak effect of detemir may be more predictable. It also appears that detemir may have a longer duration of action than glargine.[134] There are no published studies evaluating detemir insulin in diabetic cats or dogs at this time.

The species of origin of insulin products potentially plays a role in therapeutic efficacy. Canine and porcine insulin have identical amino acid sequences, so porcine insulin is less immunogenic in dogs.[135] Reduced antigenicity may, however, be undesirable (discussed later). Porcine insulin has a shorter duration of action than does beef insulin in dogs; human insulin appears more potent than beef–pork insulin in cats, thus requiring lower (25%) dosing.

Commercial insulins are available in concentrations of 40 (U-40), 100 (U-100), and 500 (U-500) U/mL. One unit of insulin is equal to 36 μg. Syringes are available for the corresponding insulin concentration. Accurate dosing requires that the appropriate syringe be used. For U-100 insulin, low-dose syringes are highly recommended for patients requiring low doses.

Insulin should be mixed before administration by gently rolling the bottle between the palms of one's hands; aggressive shaking may denature the product. Although refrigeration is not necessary, extreme sunlight and heat can destroy insulin. Refrigeration can protect the insulin.

Insulin Therapy

Individual response to insulin varies greatly. In cats, differences in required doses probably reflect, at least in part, availability of endogenous insulin. Both dose and frequency of administration should be designed for an individual patient; it may be necessary to base frequency on a compromise between meeting client needs and minimizing fluctuations in blood glucose. Although long-acting preparations can initially be tried every 24 hours, a 12-hour interval usually proves necessary; the authors prefer starting with twice-daily dosing to achieve control sooner. In one study 94% of dogs required twice-daily dosing regardless of insulin type used for adequate control.[136]

Regular insulin can be given by intravenous, intramuscular, or subcutaneous routes, but all other preparations should be given subcutaneously. Injection should occur in the lateral, not dorsal, thoracic or lumbar areas. The dorsum can be poorly vascularized, especially between the shoulder blades, and drug absorption can be erratic. Although some authors recommend a starting dose of 0.25 U/kg twice daily,[95] others recommend using 0.5 U/kg if the blood glucose is greater than 360 mg/dL and 0.25 U/kg if it is less than 360 mg/dL.[137] Dogs should be fed 50% of their daily food immediately before each injection to ensure appropriate caloric intake before administration of a full dose of insulin. Semimoist foods are discouraged.

The type of insulin to use is a matter of personal opinion and experience. For dogs, therapy should begin with an intermediate-acting insulin (e.g., NPH, lente). In one study, 53 dogs with uncomplicated diabetes were treated with Vetsulin for 60 days after a variable initial dose determination period. Therapy started once daily and was changed to twice daily as needed. The starting dose was 1 U/kg, with a supplemental dose depending on body weight (dogs below 10 kg received 1 U supplement, 10-11 kg 2 U, 12-20 kg 3 U, and above 20 kg 4 U), as formerly recommended in the package insert. (Note that the dosing scheme was based on the package insert at the time of the study, but recommendations are now different.) Efficacy and safety were evaluated at the end of the dose determination period (time 0) and 30 (time 1) and 60 days (time 2) later. At times 0, 1, and 2, 100%, 66%, and 75% of the dogs, respectively, were judged to be adequately controlled based on blood glucose concentrations and clinical signs. By day 60 66% were receiving twice-daily injections. The median number of days required to achieve adequate glycemic control was 35 (range 5-151). No unexpected side effects were observed, but 22 dogs had signs at some time that could have been caused by hypoglycemia and two died of presumed hypoglycemia. The owners of seven dogs reported swelling or pain (or both) at the injection site, but neither symptom was noted by the investigators.[138]

In cats, good options are glargine, PZI, and lente insulins. Ultralente is no longer available. Prozinc currently is an acceptable insulin choice for cats; detemir (discussed previously) may be a good option for the treatment of diabetic cats in the future, but because of the lack of availability and limited data, it cannot be recommended at this time.

One study evaluated use of PZI in 67 diabetic cats. Initial PZI dosage ranged from 0.2 to 0.6 U/kg twice daily. After 45 days, the mean dose was 0.9 U/kg (range 0.2 to 1.8). Mean blood glucose nadir occurred approximately 5 to 7 hours after insulin injection but ranged from 1 to 9 hours.[139] Overall, 90% of owners believed their cat improved. Clinical hypoglycemia occurred in five cats, and hypoglycemia without clinical signs occurred in another 21 (31%). Ten cats were not controlled by day 45. Whether longer treatment and more dosage adjustments would have achieved control is unknown. In general, cats with newly diagnosed DM had a better response than those with previously treated DM; perhaps the cats that failed previous treatment had an underlying cause of insulin resistance. Most diabetic cats will require PZI twice daily for adequate control, but once-daily injections may suffice in up to 25%. Initial PZI dosage should be low (e.g., 1 U/injection) to prevent hypoglycemia.[139] The initial reports on Prozinc also support initial low doses with this insulin. In one study one cat was removed because of documented hypoglycemia, and in another study 160 of 690 serial blood glucose curve values documented hypoglycemia in 87 of 139 diabetic cats. The reports do not state whether any episodes of hypoglycemia were clinically apparent.[126,127]

In diabetic cats, the use of glargine appears extremely promising. Glargine has a long duration of action and predictable blood glucose–lowering effects. In eight newly diagnosed cats treated with a high-protein, low-carbohydrate diet, the DM resolved in all cats within 4 months.[140] Glargine appears to be appropriate for use in any cat, providing control of blood glucose concentrations throughout most of the day. Long-term diabetic cats have been switched to and treated with glargine insulin as well with excellent results;[141] remission is less likely after long-term treatment with another insulin, but it may still occur.[120] In a study evaluating remission rates in diabetic cats initially treated with insulin, 55 diabetic cats were evaluated whose owners followed a highly intensive monitoring and blood glucose regulation (blood glucose concentrations maintained between 50-100mg/dL) protocol using insulin glargine and fed a low-carbohydrate diet. A total of 35 cats (64%) achieved remission. Cats that received glucocorticoid treatment within 6 months before diagnosis of DM, that required a lower maximum insulin dose, or that were intensively managed using glargine within 6 months of diagnosis were more likely to achieve remission, whereas cats with a peripheral neuropathy present at diagnosis (e.g., difficulty climbing stairs or a plantigrade stance) were less likely to do so. Other factors examined that were not predictors of entering remission were age at diagnosis, gender, obesity, evidence of diabetic ketoacidosis at diagnosis, development of azotemia during therapy, concurrent hyperthyroidism, and frequency of asymptotic hypoglycemia.[142] In the authors' opinion, glargine insulin is the current preferred insulin choice for diabetic cats, be they newly diagnosed or long-term diabetics with poor glycemic control on their current insulin regimen. It is also the only commercially available long-acting insulin that has been extensively studied in diabetic cats.

Cats should be started at a glargine dose of 0.5 U/kg if the blood glucose concentration is above 360 mg/dL or 0.25 U/kg if the blood glucose concentration is below 360 mg/dL. In either case, twice-daily administration is recommended. Compared with other types of insulin, with which dose adjustments are typically made based on the blood glucose nadir, for glargine dose adjustments should be made based on the fasting blood glucose value. Because the doses are typically small, 0.3 mL, low-dose syringes should be used for accurate dosing.

Lente insulin can be used in cats, but because it has a shorter duration of action than glargine or PZI, it almost always, if not always, must be administered twice daily.[128] A recommended starting dose is 0.25 U/kg twice daily if the blood glucose concentration is 216 to 360 mg/dL or 0.5 U/kg twice daily if the blood glucose concentration is above 360 mg/dL.[143] Alternatively, a dose of 1 U/cat twice daily for cats weighing less than 4 kg and 1.5 to 2 U/cat twice daily for cats weighing more than 4 kg can be used to initiate therapy.[144]

A multicenter study recently assessed the efficacy and safety of porcine lente insulin in 46 diabetic cats.[102] Therapy was initiated twice daily at a dose of 0.25 U/kg if the blood glucose concentration was 270 to 360 mg/dL and 0.5 U/kg if the blood glucose concentration was above 360 mg/dL. All cats were followed for a stabilization period of approximately 16 weeks, and 23 cats were followed for an additional variable period of up to 49 weeks. Diabetic remission was achieved in 15%; all were newly diagnosed diabetics, and time to remission ranged from 2 to 56 weeks. The mean insulin dose both at the end of the stabilization period (week 16) and the end of the study (week 49) was 2 U per cat twice daily. The authors concluded that lente insulin was safe and effective in diabetic cats; achieving diabetic stability with lente may take 3 to 4 months; cats were more likely to go into remission if they were newly diagnosed, compared with previously diagnosed, diabetics; and it could take as long as 56 weeks to achieve remission.

Long-term response to insulin was assessed in 54 diabetic cats that were evaluated numerous times over a minimum of 3 months.[145] Insulins used included beef/pork PZI (n = 14), beef/pork ultralente (n = 26), and beef/pork lente (n = 14). Response was based on resolution of clinical signs and mean blood glucose, with good, mediocre, and poor response considered to be a blood glucose concentration less than 200 mg/dL, between 200 and 300 mg/dL, and greater than 300 mg/dL, respectively. No difference was found among the types of insulin regarding therapeutic success, although this may reflect the small number of animals studied rather than variability of the outcomes.[145]

Interestingly, the percentage of cats that were judged to have responded was different depending on which criteria were used: clinical signs versus mean blood glucose concentration. For PZI and ultralente, 14% and 15% of cats achieved good control based on mean blood glucose, whereas no animals were considered well controlled for lente. If using clinical signs as the means to assess control, the percentage of good responders was greater for all treatment groups: 50% for PZI and ultralente and 79% for lente. Improvements in mean blood glucose were considered mediocre in 64% of the PZI group and 50% each for ultralente and lente, whereas improvements in clinical signs were considered mediocre in 50%, 42%, and 21% of the PZI, ultralente, and lente groups, respectively. Glycemic control was significantly better in the cats without concurrent disease compared with cats that did have it. Survival was evaluated in a total of 104 cats. Mean and median survival times in cats with good glycemic control (on the basis of mean blood glucose) for all treatment groups were 24 and 16 months compared with 17 and 20 months for cats with mediocre control, respectively.[145]

Monitoring of Therapy and Alteration of Insulin Dose

Marked variation in insulin kinetics—particularly in cats—makes monitoring diabetic control crucial. Options include performance of serial glucose curves either in a hospital or at home, measurement of serum glycosylated protein concentrations, monitoring of presence and degree of glycosuria, and assessment of the presence or absence of clinical signs of DM.

Performance of in-hospital blood glucose curves has long been the gold standard for assessing diabetic control. Glucose curves should establish the insulin effectiveness, time to peak effect, duration of effect, glucose nadir, and degree of fluctuation in blood glucose concentration and identify the Somogyi phenomenon (discussed later), if present. To construct a curve, blood glucose concentration is measured in general every 2 hours for one interval between injections (i.e., for 12 hours if insulin is administered twice daily or for 24 hours if insulin is given once daily). When blood glucose concentration is below 125 mg/dL, the concentration should be measured hourly. A normal insulin and feeding schedule *must* be maintained as much as possible. If a patient does not eat the normal amount of the normal food at the usual time, the serial glucose curve should probably not be performed. The patient should be fed its standard diet at the usual time and the insulin given by the owner at home or, if possible, in the hospital so a veterinarian or veterinary technician can assess the owner's injection technique. Obtaining a fasting blood sample for measurement of blood glucose concentration before insulin injection can aid in appraisal of glycemic control, but this may not be possible for the morning value if normal feeding time occurs before the hospital opens. Clearly, cooperation between client and veterinarian is necessary to maximize the information obtained with minimal disturbance to routine.

A curve should be performed the first day insulin therapy is initiated or changed. Glucose concentrations may be lower than expected after the first 24 to 48 hours of insulin therapy, especially in cats as stress hyperglycemia resolves.[146] The first curve is done solely to ensure that hypoglycemia does not occur. If hypoglycemia is found, the insulin dose should be decreased 25% and another curve done the following day to check for hypoglycemia. The insulin dose should not be increased based on the first day's curve. A patient requires 5 to 7 days on a dose of insulin to equilibrate and reach maximal effect. Another blood glucose curve should be performed 7 to 10 days after discharge. Based on assessment of the curve, the insulin dose can be increased or decreased as necessary.

The pattern of insulin effect should be used to determine dose, interval, and feeding schedule. Ideally, glucose concentrations should reach a nadir (i.e., the lowest point) of 80 to 150 mg/dL. The highest glucose concentration should be close to 200 to 250 g/dL in dogs or 300 mg/dL in cats. The actual nadir and peak concentrations in a patient will probably be lower or higher, respectively, than measured because the exact timing of nadir and peak effects of insulin are not known and can change day to day; therefore blood glucose concentration is not often measured exactly at those times. Changes in insulin dose can usually be made without affecting true (as compared to apparent) duration of effect. The glucose differential is the difference between the nadir and the blood glucose concentration before the next dose and can be a measure of insulin effectiveness.[147] If the curve is relatively flat (e.g., differential of 50 to 100 mg/dL), the insulin may not be having a desired effect. However, the glucose differential should be interpreted in conjunction with the absolute blood glucose concentrations obtained from the curve. If all blood glucose concentrations are less than 200 mg/dL, then the insulin is very effective. However, if all blood glucose concentrations are between 350 and 400 mg/dL, then the insulin is ineffective or stress hyperglycemia is present.

When assessing a glucose curve, whether it is the first curve performed on a patient or the last of many, the clinician should ask three basic questions. First, has the insulin succeeded in lowering the blood glucose? Second, if the insulin has lowered the blood glucose, what was the lowest blood glucose value? Third, how long has the insulin lasted? By answering these questions, logical changes in dosing regimen can be made if necessary. Results of a serial glucose curve should always be interpreted in light of clinical signs. Curves vary from day to day in dogs[148] and cats.[149] Stress hyperglycemia can falsely elevate results, and a patient's refusal to eat while hospitalized can falsely decrease results.[150] If a patient is not polyphagic or polydipsic and polyuric and body weight is stable or increasing, diabetic control is likely good.

The first aim in regulating a diabetic is to achieve an acceptable nadir, with blood glucose concentrations ideally falling between 80 and 150 mg/dL. In general, if an acceptable nadir is not achieved, the insulin dosage should be adjusted depending on the size of the animal and the degree of hypoglycemia or hyperglycemia. Usually, changes of approximately 10% are appropriate. Hypoglycemia should always be avoided. No matter what other blood glucose concentrations are during the day, if the nadir blood glucose concentration is below 80 mg/dL, decrease the dose by 25%. Blood glucose concentrations should be reevaluated 7 to 10 days after an insulin dose adjustment is made if hyperglycemia was the issue. If a dose is lowered because of the presence of hypoglycemia, a curve should be performed the next day to ensure that hypoglycemia does not recur.

Once an acceptable nadir exists, duration of action can be determined by a blood glucose curve. Duration of action is the time from the insulin injection through the lowest glucose concentration until the blood glucose concentration exceeds 200 to 250 mg/dL. If the insulin dose is inadequate and the target glucose nadir has not yet been achieved, the dose must be increased until the nadir is acceptable before duration of effect of the insulin can be determined.

If insulin with too short a duration of activity is used, obtainment of an acceptable glucose nadir may not be possible. In these patients, blood glucose concentration is typically quite high in the morning because control has been inadequate for most of the previous day. A blood glucose curve in this situation shows a noticeable but brief decrease in serum glucose concentration after the insulin injection. Increasing dosing frequency from once to twice a day or changing to a longer-lasting insulin type is indicated.

Based on duration of action, the following general recommendations can be made. If the duration is 22 to 24 hours, once-daily therapy is adequate. If the duration is 16 to 20 hours, a shorter-acting insulin should be used twice daily. If the duration is 13 to 16 hours, twice-daily insulin therapy can be tried, but the evening dose should be lower than the morning dose. If the duration is 10 to 12 hours, the patient should receive insulin twice daily. If the duration appears to be less than 8 hours, a blood glucose nadir higher than 80 mg/dL must be ensured. If blood glucose drops below 60 mg/dL at any time, the Somogyi phenomenon can occur. The Somogyi phenomenon or overswing, also called *hypoglycemia-induced hyperglycemia,* refers to a period of hypoglycemia followed by marked hyperglycemia. The phenomenon results from a normal physiologic response when blood glucose concentrations decline to less than 60 mg/dL in response to an insulin dose that is too high or when blood glucose concentration decreases rapidly regardless of the nadir.[95] In either case a number of reflexes are triggered that act to increase blood glucose. Counterregulatory hormones such as epinephrine, cortisol, glucagon, and growth hormone (GH) are secreted. The net effect of these hormones is to increase hepatic glycogenolysis and gluconeogenesis and to decrease peripheral tissue glucose utilization. Hyperglycemia usually occurs rapidly, thus preventing a hypoglycemic seizure. Insulin secretion does not occur in response to the rise in glucose, however, as would occur in normal dogs and cats, and diabetics become extremely hyperglycemic (400 to 800 mg/dL). If the Somogyi phenomenon is observed, the insulin dosage should be decreased so the nadir is above 80 mg/dL; counterregulatory hormones will no longer interfere with the action of the exogenous insulin, and the true duration of effect will become apparent. If the duration of insulin action is truly less than 8 hours, adequate therapy with that type of insulin requires injections more frequently than twice daily, which is impractical for most owners. A switch between different types of intermediate-acting insulin can also be beneficial. For example, a dog or cat may metabolize NPH insulin quickly, resulting in too short an effect, but lente insulin may have a longer duration.

Once control has been achieved, blood glucose curves should be performed every 3 to 6 months to assess adequacy of glycemic control or earlier if clinical signs suggest that control has been lost. The more precarious the control, the more frequently rechecks should be done. As during the initial curves, if the nadir is unacceptable, the insulin dose must be lowered or raised accordingly. If duration of action appears to have changed, then the same modifications as previously discussed can be made.

If using glargine insulin in cats, interpretation of blood glucose curves and dose adjustment is different than for other insulin types. For the first 3 days, 12-hour blood glucose curves should be performed (i.e., the curve should be performed for the interval between the morning and evening dose). The purpose of the blood glucose curve is to detect hypoglycemia, if present, and lower the glargine dose as needed. Many cats require dose reduction within the first 3 days. It is important to note that the insulin dose should not be increased regardless of the appearance of the curves. After the first 3 days, the cat should be sent home and then return for a curve 7 days later. Subsequent blood glucose curves should be performed at 1, 2, and 4 weeks and then as required.

Recommendations for dose adjustments are based on the pre-insulin blood glucose concentration, compared with other insulins for which dose is altered on the basis of the nadir. If at recheck the pre-insulin blood glucose concentration is higher than 290 mg/dL, the glargine dose should be increased by 1 U per cat. The dose should not be changed if the pre-insulin blood glucose concentration is 220 to 290 mg/dL. In either of these first two scenarios, a curve should be done to ensure that hypoglycemia does not occur. The dose should be decreased 0.5 to 1 U/cat if the pre-insulin blood glucose concentration is 80 to 180 mg/dL. If biochemical hypoglycemia is present (i.e., blood glucose concentration is below 80 mg/dL but no clinical signs of hypoglycemia are present), the dose should be decreased by 1 U per cat. If clinical signs of hypoglycemia are present, the glargine dose should be decreased 50%. Administration of glargine should not be discontinued within 2 weeks of starting treatment even if euglycemia is present; the clinician should decrease the dose if needed but should not stop the insulin.[151]

To determine if a cat is in remission, insulin administration should be continued until the cat is receiving 1 U twice daily. Then, if the pre-insulin blood glucose concentration is below 180 mg/dL, once-daily administration is appropriate. If the next day the pre-insulin blood glucose concentration is still below 180 mg/dL, the clinician should not administer insulin and should do a complete curve. If the pre-insulin blood glucose concentration is above 180 mg/dL when the cat is receiving once-daily insulin, the clinician can go back to twice-daily administration. An attempt to wean the cat can again be made in a couple weeks. Diabetic cats in remission should stay on a low-carbohydrate diet.

If performance of a curve is impossible because of the cat's temperament or the owner's financial constraints, the clinician may start glargine at 0.25 U/kg (with a maximum dose of 2 U/cat) subcutaneously twice daily and have the owner monitor urine glucose concentration or water intake. A cat well regulated on glargine should have trace urine glucose at most, and urine glucose should be negative most of the time. If after 2 weeks of receiving glargine, urine glucose is greater than trace, the dose should be increased 1 U per cat weekly until urine glucose is negative or water intake is below 20 mL/kg in a 24-hour period if the cat is eating canned food and below 60 mL/kg in a 24-hour period if the cat is eating dry food. At this point, the cat should be kept on the same dose for 2 weeks, and then the clinician can start decreasing the dose by 1 U per cat weekly until urine glucose is positive or the insulin has been discontinued.[152]

Performance of blood glucose curves has become controversial, insofar as they are certainly not perfect. Blood glucose curves can be affected by the stress of hospitalization, especially in cats, and deviation from normal routine, and they vary day to day. In one study, glucose curves were performed in diabetic dogs on 2 consecutive days, with all conditions being identical on both days (e.g., type and dose of insulin, amount and type of diet). Parameters such as minimum, maximum, and mean blood glucose concentration; fasting blood glucose concentration before the morning or evening injection (all dogs were treated twice daily); and time from insulin injection to nadir were significantly different between the two curves. In some dogs, the curve showed better control on day 1, whereas others showed better control on day 2. To examine the clinical implications of day-to-day variability of the curves, a theoretical recommendation for adjustment of the dog's insulin dose was based on the results of each curve. The researchers assessed 30 sets of paired 12-hour curves. Opposite theoretical recommendations for adjustment of a dog's insulin dose were made on day 2 compared with day 1 in 27% of occasions. For 17% of the curves, a different but not opposite recommendation resulted. The same dosage adjustment recommendation was made on both days in 57%. Given this variation, predicting the timing of a diabetic's nadir based on previous serial blood glucose curves and obtaining a single sample at that time is unlikely to give a reliable result—in other words, spot-checking does not provide helpful information.[148]

To avoid some of the problems associated with in-hospital curves, performance of glucose curves at home has taken on new importance. For glucose curves it is not necessary for venous blood to be collected. Capillary blood is suitable,[153] with the ear being the best site for blood collection. Two types of lancing device are available. If conventional automatic devices designed for pricking human fingertips are used, a device with a variable needle depth should be chosen and the appropriate depth for each patient used.[154] Warming of the ear with a hair dryer or a warm, wet washcloth inside a plastic bag may be necessary but not well tolerated, and it may take up to 2 minutes to obtain an adequate sample depending on the size of the drop required.[154] A device that creates a vacuum after the skin is lanced (e.g., Microlet Vaculance, Bayer) does not require warming of the ear and generates an adequate drop of blood within approximately 30 seconds,[154] but mastery may be a bit difficult and require repeated instruction.[155] Glucometers that require minimal amounts of blood as well as those that "sip" the blood into the strip are desirable. Studies support that owners are both willing and able to generate home serial glucose curves, although some owners may require additional demonstrations.[156-158]

Unfortunately, home-generated curves have not eliminated all the problems associated with serial glucose curves, because variability remains a problem. Interestingly, a study of diabetic cats compared four serial blood glucose curves generated at home and in the clinic.[158] Owners obtained a 12-hour glucose curve once monthly for 4 months. Within a week of obtaining the at-home curve, the cats were brought to the clinic, where the curve was repeated. The mean glucose concentrations tended to be lower in the clinic than at home. The mean glucose concentrations for each of the four clinic curves compared with the home-generated curves were 336 mg/dL versus 363 mg/dL, 316 mg/dL versus 381 mg/dL, 235 mg/dL versus 307 mg/dL, and 235 mg/dL versus 345 mg/dL. One explanation put forth for these findings was that the cats commonly refused to eat while in clinic. Theoretical treatment recommendations based on nadir glucose concentrations of the home-generated and in-clinic curves were compared, and decisions differed in 38% (14 of 37). In three of these instances, treatment decisions would have been completely contrary.[158] Additionally, day-to-day variability in curves persists, even if home-generated. In seven diabetic cats, paired glucose curves were generated on 2 consecutive days at home or in the clinic. Considerable day-to-day variability existed in both, with no greater agreement between home curves and clinic curves.[156] These findings augment the recommendation that changes in insulin dose be made on the basis of biochemical indicators of glycemic control (e.g., glucose concentration, fructosamine) as well as clinical support of glycemic control (e.g., weight gain, absence of polyuria or polydipsia).

Continuous monitoring of glucose concentrations has also received attention of late.[149,159,160] The CGMS (Continuous Glucose Monitoring System, MiniMed) is a device that can be strapped onto a patient and a small needle inserted into the subcutaneous tissue. Interstitial glucose concentrations are sampled every 5 minutes for up to 72 hours. Using such a device gives many more data points for evaluation and avoids the stress of multiple venipunctures or catheterization. Furthermore, a patient could wear the device at home if necessary.

The device has been assessed in normal and diabetic dogs and cats. Interstitial and blood glucose concentrations were highly correlated overall.[149,159,160] However, postprandial increases in blood glucose concentration may not be detected in the interstitial fluid.[160] Accuracy varied between patients, and the difference between blood and interstitial glucose concentrations was more marked in some patients than others. The greatest discrepancies occurred at higher glucose concentrations.[160] The working range of the CGMS is approximately 40 to 400 mg/dL—that is, blood glucose concentrations outside the range cannot be measured. In fact, if the device repeatedly detects values outside the range, it is interpreted as a machine error and the device shuts off. No irritation resulted from sensor placement.[149,159,160] Preliminary results suggest that the CGMS is useful for clinical management of insulin therapy.

Measurement of urine glucose concentration at home can aid in monitoring. First, urine glucose levels can be determined as needed to aid in assessment of glycemic control, especially when other data are conflicting. Consistently negative readings on urine glucose may indicate that insulin dosages are either adequate or excessive. A serial glucose curve will differentiate between adequate insulin therapy and use of excessive doses that could result in hypoglycemia. Uniformly high urine glucose readings coupled with unresolved clinical signs indicate that the insulin dose may be inappropriate. Negative urine glucose concentrations in the afternoon, followed by high urine glucose readings the following morning, may be indicative of the Somogyi phenomenon; however, documentation of the Somogyi phenomenon requires performance of a glucose curve. Second, urine glucose concentrations can be determined regularly (at least weekly) to help in the assessment of ongoing control. Changes in urine glucose levels may alert the owner and clinician to loss of glycemic control and the need for reevaluation. If a cat's urine cannot be collected, use of Glucotest (Purina), a product that is sprinkled in a litter box and changes color to reflect the urinary glucose concentration, may help.[161]

Monitoring of GHb or fructosamine may be helpful. Measurement of glycated proteins alone is probably not adequate for assessment of overall control, but looking at trends can be illuminating. Concentration of either glycated protein should be measured when a diabetic is first diagnosed, and then reassessed with every recheck examination. In general, if the concentration is increasing, control is deteriorating, and if the concentration is decreasing, control is improving. A study of healthy cats infused with intravenous glucose to maintain moderate or marked hyperglycemia (mean glucose 306 mg/dL and 522 mg/dL, respectively) found considerable overlap in fructosamine concentrations between the two groups.[105] Although elevated in the cats with marked hyperglycemia, fructosamine concentrations only intermittently exceeded the reference range in cats with moderate hyperglycemia.[105] Finally, to attribute a change in fructosamine concentration over time to altered glycemic control in the patient and not just inherent variability in the test, a critical difference of more than 33 μmol/L was identified.[105] Thus trends of sufficient magnitude in fructosamine concentrations of individual patients may be the best use of this tool to monitor glycemic control in diabetic patients.

Lastly, home monitoring of clinical signs has been advocated as a useful adjuvant tool in assessing glycemic control. (It should be emphasized, however, that home monitoring of clinical signs alone is not an appropriate means of monitoring a diabetic animal but should be one of several monitoring modalities employed. This is discussed later in this chapter.) One study evaluated the usefulness of a variety of different clinical and biochemical measurements in 23 cats treated with lente insulin.[162] The investigators compared subjective clinical control and water intake to biochemical markers of glycemic control (i.e., serial blood glucose, fructosamine, beta-hydroxybutyrate, cholesterol, triglycerides, glycerol, and urine glucose concentrations). No single measurement best correlated with the level of clinical control identified. The amount of water drunk over 24 hours, maximum blood glucose concentration, mean blood glucose concentration, and urine glucose were the most useful practical indicators of clinical control. Owners were often happy with the level of control in their cats despite not having laboratory evidence of tight glycemic control, emphasizing the importance that the long-term aim of treatment in diabetic cats is to control the clinical signs associated with hyperglycemia.

In one study of 53 dogs, control was judged to be good or poor based on clinical signs, physical examination findings, and body weight. Then, clinical determination of good or poor control was compared with fasting blood glucose, serial glucose curve, and serum fructosamine and GHb concentrations. Although all parameters of glucose control were significantly lower in dogs with good control, considerable overlap existed between the two groups for all. All blood glucose measurements and fructosamine and GHb concentrations were consistent with good glycemic control in 60% of dogs judged to have good clinical control or with poor control in only 39% of dogs judged to have poor clinical control. The initial fasting blood glucose was 100 to 300 mg/dL in 80% of dogs with good clinical control and in 21% of dogs with poor clinical control.[163]

Although the importance of home monitoring of clinical signs cannot be overemphasized, these authors believe that glucose curves should be performed periodically in all diabetic patients (for aggressive animals or those who experience stress hyperglycemia in the hospital, the curves are most appropriately performed at home, if possible). If diabetic control appears inadequate based on clinical signs, the only way to know how to adjust the dose is by performing a curve. Furthermore, hypoglycemia can be clinically nondetectable until a crisis is reached (e.g., the patient begins to have seizures). Performance of curves can demonstrate occurrence of hypoglycemia, and the insulin dose can be changed before clinical signs occur.

Complications of Insulin Therapy

Periods of hyperglycemia in otherwise well-controlled diabetics are difficult to avoid. Evaluation is indicated if hyperglycemia is present most of the time or clinical signs exist. Owner compliance regarding storage, mixing, and administration of insulin should be re-examined first in such a scenario, as well as patient management (e.g., diet, exercise). After these causes of poor control have been eliminated, a glucose curve should be performed to identify causes of poor control such as the Somogyi phenomenon (discussed previously), short duration of insulin action, or insulin resistance.

Interestingly, not every hypoglycemic event triggers the Somogyi phenomenon. The precise reason is not known, but it may have to do with how quickly the blood glucose concentration drops; the Somogyi phenomenon may be more likely to occur with a more rapid decline. Cats, in general, may be less likely to have a Somogyi phenomenon than dogs. In a recent study that evaluated intensive blood glucose control using glargine in 55 diabetic cats,[164] asymptomatic hypoglycemia (blood glucose concentration <50 mg/dL) was measured in most (93%) cats at least once. However, symptomatic hypoglycemia was rare, with only a single event in one cat that had mild signs of restlessness.[164] Despite the high number of hypoglycemic periods, only four single documented Somogyi events occurred in four cats.[165]

The Somogyi phenomenon can occur in dogs or cats receiving any insulin dose, but it should be particularly considered as a possibility in patients receiving more than 2.2 U/kg of insulin per dose in the face of persistent glycosuria (>1 g/dL) and clinical signs indicative of poor control (i.e., polyuria, polydipsia, and polyphagia). In addition, it may occur particularly when insulin dose adjustments are made based on early-morning urine glucose concentrations. Diagnosis of the phenomenon is based on documenting nadir and peak glucose concentrations of below 65 mg/dL and above 300 mg/dL, respectively, within a single dosing interval or a rapid decrease in blood glucose concentration followed by a rapid rise and a marked hyperglycemia, regardless of whether hypoglycemia occurred. Because the timing of the blood glucose nadir varies day to day,[148] the presence of the Somogyi phenomenon cannot be documented by measuring blood glucose concentration at a single time point.

Documenting the presence of the Somogyi phenomenon can be challenging. The hormones secreted (e.g., GH, cortisol) may induce insulin resistance that lasts for as long as 72 hours after a hypoglycemic episode. Depending on when a glucose curve is performed, the overswing may be seen; alternatively, if a curve is done on the day after the overswing, only consistently high blood glucose concentrations may be measured. If the presence of glucosuria is monitored, it may be absent or quite elevated, depending on when a sample is collected.

If a Somogyi overswing is present, the daily insulin dose should be decreased by at least 25% and by 50% if clinical signs of hypoglycemia are noted. A glucose curve should be performed immediately after the reduced insulin dose is administered to ensure that hypoglycemia is no longer occurring. Once hypoglycemia has been eliminated, another curve should be performed in approximately 5 to 7 days and the dose adjusted further if necessary. If the cause of the overswing is rapid lowering of blood glucose concentration and not hypoglycemia, a change in insulin type is required.

Rapid metabolism of insulin can result in a clinical situation that looks similar to the Somogyi overswing. With rapid insulin metabolism, the patient may become markedly hyperglycemic before the next insulin dose, but the hyperglycemia is not preceded by hypoglycemia or a rapid decline in blood glucose concentration, as with the Somogyi phenomenon. Morning urine glucose concentrations will be high, and clinical signs of DM generally persist. Increasing the insulin dose will only cause a lower nadir, not prolong duration of action, and hypoglycemia may result. The syndrome can be diagnosed only through construction of a curve. Treatment involves changing to a longer-acting insulin or increasing injection frequency. The vast majority of diabetic dogs require twice-daily insulin therapy for adequate control.[136] Evaluation of glycemic control should be done approximately 5 to 7 days after initiating a new insulin dose, and further dose adjustments made as needed.

Hypoglycemia. Hypoglycemia is the most common complication of insulin therapy in dogs and cats. Insulin overdose, failure to eat, presence of vomiting, and increased exercise raise the risk of hypoglycemia. Humans can suffer from hypoglycemic unawareness, a condition associated with poorly controlled DM, in which mild hypoglycemia is not sensed and clinical signs of hypoglycemia do not develop until the blood glucose concentration is quite low. Although not documented, the same may occur in dogs and cats.

Clinical signs of hypoglycemia are neurologic, and tissues with the highest metabolic activity are impaired first. Cortical signs include disorientation, weakness, and hunger followed by lethargy and ataxia. Seizures and coma ensue if hypoglycemia persists. Blindness may be a permanent sequela. Death can occur as a result of central respiratory and cardiac depression.

In a retrospective study, the most common clinical signs of hypoglycemia in diabetic dogs were seizures, ataxia, and weakness, occurring at a median of 3 months after initiation of insulin therapy; in cats seizures, recumbency, anorexia, shaking, vomiting, ataxia, and dullness occurred after a median duration of 8 months of therapy. Other clinical signs noted in dogs were anorexia, diarrhea, restlessness, pacing, blindness, and coma; in cats amaurosis, vocalization, circling, lethargy, weakness, diarrhea, urination, stupor, and coma were noted. Obese cats were considered at greater risk for overdosage.[166]

The development of hypoglycemia in a previously well-controlled animal suggests that a change has occurred either exogenously (e.g., use of an incorrect syringe, overly concentrated insulin because of improper mixing) or endogenously (e.g., DM was transient, patient is vomiting or anorectic, patient has developed maldigestion or malabsorption). Overlap of action of injections should also be considered (i.e., one injection is given when blood glucose concentration is still low from the previous injection).

Treatment of hypoglycemia varies according to the severity of signs. Mild hypoglycemia can be treated by feeding a normal meal; moderate signs may require treatment with sugar or syrup (e.g., Karo syrup) being fed to the animal or rubbed on the buccal membranes. Convulsions require intravenous administration of 50% dextrose. A slow intravenous bolus of 50% dextrose (0.5 g/kg diluted 1:4) should be administered, followed by a continuous-rate infusion of 5% dextrose until the patient can be fed. A single dose of dextrose may not be adequate. Dextrose doses from 0.25 to 19.2 g/kg and 0.2 to 6.3 g/kg were required in dogs and cats, respectively, to attain euglycemia after an insulin overdose, and continuaton of a dextrose drip may be necessary for up to 4 days to maintain normal blood glucose concentrations.[166] Insulin therapy should be discontinued until hyperglycemia is documented. Once the animal is sufficiently conscious, food can be offered.

Insulin resistance. Insulin resistance should be suspected in any pet in which marked hyperglycemia persists throughout the day despite insulin doses of more than 1.5 U/kg per injection or when large doses of insulin (i.e. >2.2 U/kg per injection) are needed to maintain adequate glycemic control. However, use of these doses does not mean that insulin resistance is present. The problem could lie with owner technique of insulin administration, patient management (e.g., exercise, diet), or insulin choice. Lack of response to high doses of one insulin type does not mean all insulins will be ineffective; for example, 20% of cats did not respond to high doses of ultralente insulin but could be effectively managed by twice-daily lente.[167] In addition, longer-acting insulin (PZI) will be more slowly absorbed and less bioavailable than shorter-acting insulin; thus slightly more than 2.2 U/kg of long-acting insulin may be required.

Before a thorough and costly workup for insulin resistance is initiated, factors that mimic insulin resistance should be ruled out. The owner's technique and insulin handling should always be evaluated first. Possible causes for an unsatisfactory response to insulin include inadequate mixing of insulin before withdrawal into the syringe; use of the incorrect syringe (e.g., using a U100 syringe with U40 insulin); misunderstanding of how to read the insulin syringe; problems with insulin injection technique; inactivation of insulin as a result of improper handling; and, if diluted insulin is being used, improper dilution. A bottle of insulin should be discarded after 2 to 3 months of use because activity may begin to decrease. If owner issues are suspected, a glucose curve should be performed after the owner administers insulin using a new, undiluted bottle and while being observed. Second, the owner should be questioned to ensure consistent and appropriate diet and exercise. If hyperglycemia is believed to be due to a postprandial surge from feeding a meal when the insulin's effects are waning, timing of meals should be adjusted. Alternatively, addition of an oral hypoglycemic agent such as acarbose can be considered. Third, if no response is seen to one type of insulin, then another should be tried to see if it might be effective. Fourth, absorption of insulin can vary among subcutaneous sites, so another injection site should be used; the lateral thorax or abdomen is recommended. Lastly, a glucose curve should be performed to eliminate other possible mimics of insulin resistance, such as the Somogyi phenomenon and inadequate duration of insulin action.

Once true insulin resistance has been documented, the following differential diagnoses should be considered.

Insulin antibodies are a commonly discussed cause of insulin resistance. The clinical significance of anti-insulin antibodies (AIAs) remains unclear at this time. Although antibodies may form against exogenous insulin, associated clinical insulin resistance appears rare. AIAs were measured in diabetic subjects after starting therapy with porcine lente insulin (n=100), bovine lente insulin (n=100), or bovine protamine zinc insulin (n=20); 12%, 56%, and 90%, respectively, developed AIA. No association was detected between AIA concentration and insulin dose or fructosamine concentrations.[135] If AIAs are believed to be a cause of resistance, a commercial assay for measurement of AIAs now exists. Alternatively, in pursuing this diagnosis for insulin resistance, use of a radioimmunoassay (RIA) for insulin may be helpful.[168] Circulating AIAs can interfere with measurement of serum insulin by RIA, causing spuriously high insulin concentrations, and the artifact can provide evidence of antibody presence. Typically, 24 hours after the last insulin injection in a diabetic pet, serum insulin concentration should be less than 50 μU/mL. In comparison, apparent serum insulin concentration is above 400 μU/mL if AIAs are present.[168] If AIAs are believed to be causing insulin resistance, the insulin source should be switched to a different one. Glycemic control should improve within 2 weeks of changing the species of insulin if insulin-binding antibodies are causing resistance.[168]

Infection, ketoacidosis, and concurrent illness can cause insulin resistance. The urinary tract and oral cavities are common sites of infection; a urinalysis and urine culture, regardless of urinalysis finding,[169] and complete oral examination should always be performed. Renal disease, hepatic insufficiency, cardiac insufficiency, pancreatitis, and starvation should be considered as possible causes of insulin resistance. Malnutrition can lead to insulin resistance and diminished insulin secretion. Obesity has been linked to glucose intolerance and abnormal insulin secretion in cats and dogs, but its role in creating insulin resistance is unclear insofar as obese diabetic pets generally remain insulin responsive. Hyperthyroidism, hypothyroidism, and hyperadrenocorticism can cause insulin resistance through diverse mechanisms.

Based on data from several recent studies, acromegaly may be a more common cause of insulin resistance in cats than previously recognized, and several reliable methods exist by which a diagnosis may be obtained, especially when the tests are used together. Computed tomography (CT) has proved useful in demonstrating the presence of a mass lesion in the region of the pituitary gland in insulin-resistant diabetic cats suspected of having acromegaly or hyperadrenocorticism, with a mass visualized on CT in all 16 such cats in one study.[170] In another study designed to screen diabetic cats for the presence of acromegaly, serum IGF-1 concentrations were measured in 184 variably controlled diabetic cats. Of the 184 cats screened, 59 had increased serum insulin-like growth factor I (IGF-I) concentrations—that is, greater than 1000ng/mL (reference range 208-443 ng/mL). Eighteen of the 59 cats underwent further examination, including intracranial CT, contrast-enhanced CT, or magnetic resonance imaging (MRI), and acromegaly was confirmed in 17. Contrast-enhanced CT allowed detection of most, but not all, pituitary masses, and one cat with a postmortem examination diagnosis of acromegaly did not have a visible mass on CT or MRI.[171] In another recent study, diabetic cats were screened for concurrent acromegaly by measuring plasma GH and IGF-1 concentrations and examining the pituitary fossa using MRI.[172] Of the 16 cats in the study, six required an insulin dosage at or above 1.5 U/kg per injection and had an enlarged pituitary gland on MRI; one cat receiving less than 1.5 U/kg of insulin per injection had an enlarged pituitary gland. Five of the six cats were diagnosed with acromegaly based on the enlarged pituitary gland on MRI and elevated plasma GH concentrations. Finally, a study evaluating the usefulness of IGF-I concentrations as a screening test for the diagnosis of acromegaly in diabetic cats found that 25.6% (19 of 74) of all diabetic cats and 47.5% (19 of 40) of poorly controlled diabetics had acromegaly.[173] Currently, no one test appears to be completely effective in diagnosing feline acromegaly, but a combination of serum IGF-1 concentrations, feline GH concentrations where available, and contrast-enhanced CT or MRI are options (see also the section on GH later in this chapter).

Certain drugs can cause insulin resistance, most notably progestogens and glucocorticoids. Although cats are resistant to development of many of the common adverse effects of glucocorticoids, such as polyuria and polydipsia, they may develop glucocorticoid-associated glucose intolerance readily. If possible, use of these medications should be slowly discontinued in diabetic patients. Otherwise, the patients may need to be treated as insulin-resistant. Neoplasia has been associated with insulin resistance in 5% to 10% of diabetic cats and dogs.[95] Hyperlipidemia should be considered as a possible cause of insulin resistance.

When a cause for insulin resistance is sought, the easiest causes to rule out and the most likely should be eliminated first, proceeding through to the least likely. The following order, in general, has been recommended in cats: concurrent drugs, obesity, concurrent disease (including infection and ketoacidosis), hyperthyroidism, acromegaly, hyperadrenocorticism, and insulin antibodies. The order to use in dogs, in general, is as follows: concurrent drugs, diestrus/acromegaly, obesity, concurrent disease (including infection and ketoacidosis), hyperadrenocorticism, hypothyroidism, hyperlipidemia, and insulin antibodies.[174] This order is not absolute. If strong evidence exists for a differential diagnosis lower in the order, that possibility should be ruled out first.

Management of insulin resistance requires correcting the underlying disorder, if possible. For causes such as a simple bacterial infection or concurrent administration of diabetogenic medications, eliminating the underlying problem can be relatively easy; other problems, such as acromegaly, may be more difficult to correct. If insulin antibodies are suspected, the insulin can be switched to a less antigenic form.

If the cause cannot be determined or eliminated, the following guidelines are suggested:[174] (1) Administer insulin at least twice daily. (2) Avoid long-acting insulins, unless regular insulin is added. Intermediate-acting insulins are more effective in overcoming insulin resistance and lowering blood glucose concentrations. (3) Consider using mixtures of short-acting and longer-acting insulins. (4) Administer insulin shortly before or at the time of feeding to help control postprandial hyperglycemia. Large insulin doses may be required, but it will be necessary to determine the actual dosage using serial blood glucose curves, as for any diabetic.

Oral Antidiabetic Agents

Oral antidiabetic agents, including the sulfonylureas (e.g., glipizide), biguanides (e.g., metformin), α-glucosidase inhibitors (e.g., acarbose), and the thiazolidinediones (e.g., darglitazone), are commonly used to treat human patients with

NIDDM. Mechanisms of action vary and, with the exception of acarbose, are directed toward the underlying abnormalities of type 2 diabetics (Figure 21-5).

Sulfonylureas stimulate pancreatic beta cells to secrete insulin and have been among the most popular oral antidiabetic agents in human medicine. Extrapancreatic effects include decreased hepatic gluconeogenesis and increased tissue sensitivity to insulin. Hypoglycemia is the main adverse effect of sulfonylureas in humans, although it may be least likely to occur with glipizide.[175]

Mechanisms of action of metformin, a biguanide, include decreased hepatic gluconeogenesis (perhaps the primary mechanism) and increased insulin sensitivity by hepatic and peripheral tissues.[175] Metformin appears more effective than glipizide in humans in resolving disorders associated with insulin resistance. Side effects occur in up to 20% of human patients and include diarrhea, abdominal discomfort, nausea, and anorexia. Lactic acidosis is a potentially severe adverse effect of biguanide antidiabetic agents in general but occurs rarely with metformin.[175] Among the oral hypoglycemic drugs, metformin is recommended as initial therapy in obese human diabetic patients because it may ameliorate insulin resistance and is less likely to be associated with weight gain.[175] As with glipizide, the initial dose of metformin in humans is low and is progressively increased on the basis of glucose monitoring. Both glipizide and metformin are given with meals in human diabetics.

The alpha-glucosidase inhibitors such as acarbose are complex oligosaccharides of bacterial origin that competitively inhibit small intestinal enzymes responsible for degradation of complex carbohydrates into absorbable monosaccharides.[175] Some of the antihyperglycemic effects of acarbose may be mediated through its effect on thyroid hormones.[176] When acarbose is ingested, the postprandial glucose concentration surge is delayed and diminished. The drug is not absorbed, so systemic effects are uncommon. Flatulence, soft stools, and diarrhea, however, occur because of the osmotic effect and bacterial fermentation of nondigested carbohydrates. The adverse effects appear to be transient, however, and are minimized in humans by starting therapy at a low dose. Acarbose is used in humans primarily to reduce postprandial glucose fluctuations and to improve glycemic stability when response to traditional oral antidiabetic agents is insufficient.[177]

The thiazolidinediones (e.g., rosiglitazone, darglitazone) bind to a novel receptor called the peroxisome proliferator-activated receptor-γ (PPAR-γ) and enhance insulin action and promote tissue glucose utilization. They are referred to as *insulin sensitizers* because they stimulate nuclear receptors that enhance the expression of proteins involved in glucose and lipid metabolism. Like metformin, troglitazone may target disorders associated with insulin resistance.

Clinical Use

Therapy of any disease is ideally aimed toward the underlying abnormality. In type 1 DM, insulin is lacking, so treatment provides an exogenous source. Type 1 diabetic patients do not have the metabolic abnormalities present in type 2 DM that are addressed by oral hypoglycemic agents (i.e., insulin resistance, dysfunctional β cells, and increased hepatic gluconeogenesis). Consequently, administration of these agents to type 1 diabetics is inappropriate, with the exception of acarbose. For type 2 DM, oral hypoglycemic drugs can be used initially, but as type 2 DM progresses, exogenous insulin injections will be required.

Because knowing the type of DM is helpful when choosing therapy, distinguishing between types 1 and 2 in cats and dogs would be extremely helpful. As dogs are mainly type 1 diabetics, oral hypoglycemics have not been used widely in this species. Cats are believed to be mainly type 2, at least initially. However, patients with advanced type 2 DM and glucose toxicity, a population likely to represent the majority of diabetic cats, will have totally lost insulin secretory ability. Accordingly,

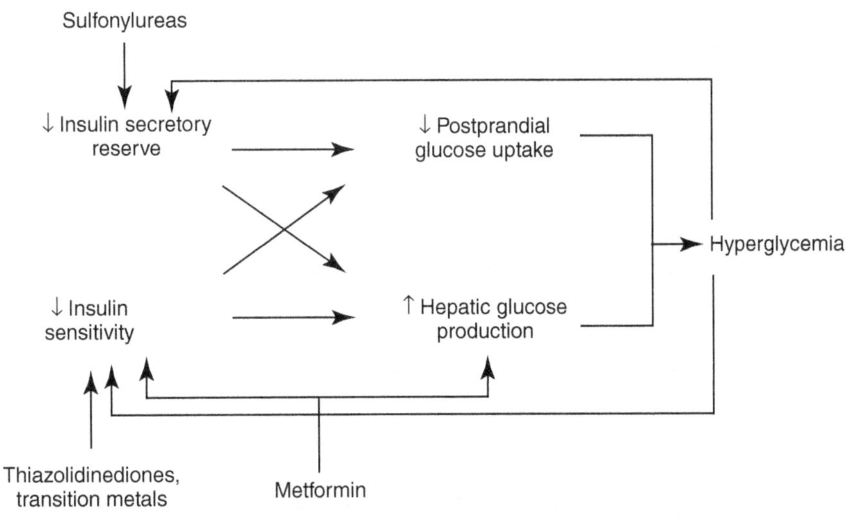

Figure 21-5 Diagram of main metabolic abnormalities underlying type 2 diabetes mellitus and the way they are targeted by the oral hypoglycemic agents. The abnormalities are shown in *red,* along with their accompanying minor abnormalities and consequences. The oral hypoglycemics are noted in *blue,* and the *blue arrows* show which of the main metabolic abnormalities they target.

some diabetic cats will respond to oral hypoglycemic agents, but most will require insulin therapy.

The most studied and used oral hypoglycemic agent in cats is the sulfonylurea glipizide. Because of the mechanism of action, the ability of sulfonylureas to further the progression of DM remains controversial. Beta cells normally co-secrete the hormone amylin with insulin. Amyloid deposits can be found in the pancreatic islets of more than 90% of human patients with type 2 DM and in 65% of diabetic cats, and in diabetic cats the deposits are associated with significant loss of islet beta cells.[178] Amylin is the precursor of the islet amyloid. Although the mechanisms underlying the transformation of amylin into amyloid fibrils are largely unknown, findings in one recent study support the hypothesis that islet amyloidosis results from prolonged beta cell stimulation. In this study, DM was induced in eight healthy domestic cats by a partial pancreatectomy, followed by induction of insulin resistance with corticosteroid and GH treatment. The cats were then treated with either glipizide (n = 4) or insulin (n = 4) for 18 months. All cats were negative for the presence of islet amyloid at the time of pancreatectomy. At the end of the study, all of the glipizide-treated cats and one of the four insulin-treated cats had pancreatic islet amyloid deposits. The glipizide-treated cats had threefold higher basal and fivefold higher glucose-stimulated plasma amylin concentrations than insulin-treated cats, suggesting an association between elevated amylin secretion and islet amyloidosis.[179] Whether this is a positive association between glipizide treatment and development of islet amyloidosis or a negative association between insulin treatment and the development of islet amyloidosis or whether similar events would occur in naturally occurring feline DM remains uncertain.

The long-term success rate with glipizide is estimated to be approximately 35%,[100,145] but which cats will respond cannot be predicted. The ideal patient for treatment with glipizide is a stable, nonketotic diabetic cat of optimal to obese body weight that has mild clinical signs with no complicating diseases. Patients that are emaciated, dehydrated, or debilitated or that have recently lost 10% or more of their body weight or have concomitant disease are not good candidates. Additionally, glipizide can be tried in any cat whose owners refuse to give injections.

Adverse effects are minimal. Vomiting is most common (approximately 15%).[99,100] Increased liver enzymes and icterus develop within 4 weeks of initiating therapy in approximately 10%. Hypoglycemia occurs in approximately 12% to 15% of responder cats; usually these cats are transient diabetics. Most cats that respond without continued adverse effects can be treated with glipizide for life, but glipizide loses effectiveness in at least 5% to 10%. The period from initiation of therapy until failure is unpredictable, ranging from weeks to more than 3 years.[121]

Glipizide therapy should be instituted at a dosage of 2.5 mg/cat orally twice daily with food, and the cat should be examined after 1 and 2 weeks. A history, complete physical examination, body weight, blood glucose concentration, and urine glucose and ketones test should be evaluated. If no problems occurred during the first 2 weeks, the dosage should be increased to 5 mg/cat twice daily. If ketonuria is found, the medication should be discontinued and insulin therapy initiated. If vomiting or icterus is present, the drug should be discontinued until the problem resolves. Most cats will tolerate the medication if started at a lower dosage and gradually increased. If hepatic enzyme elevation or icterus occurred, liver enzymes and serum bilirubin concentration should be checked periodically after reinitiation. If problems recur, drug administration should be stopped and the cat placed on insulin.

Once a dosage of 5 mg twice daily has been given for 2 weeks, the previously mentioned parameters and a 10- to 12-hour glucose curve should be checked every 4 weeks.[121] Response to therapy is demonstrated by resolution of clinical signs, blood glucose concentrations during the curve at or below 200 to 300 mg/dL, and lack of glycosuria. Time until response varies, so therapy at the full dosage should continue for 12 weeks unless a contraindication develops.[121]

If a cat becomes hypoglycemic while on glipizide therapy, discontinue drug administration and reevaluate the cat, potentially with a glucose curve, to assess if continued glipizide therapy is needed. If the cat becomes hyperglycemic after discontinuation of glipizide treatment, restart therapy with a 50% dose reduction and continue to monitor as described above.

If no response is seen after 12 weeks, glipizide administration should be stopped and insulin therapy instituted. If clinical signs and glycosuria resolve and blood glucose concentrations are at or below 200 mg/dL, glipizide therapy should be stopped and the blood glucose concentration reevaluated in 1 week. If hyperglycemia is present then, glipizide should be reinitiated. If euglycemia is present, no medication is warranted. Glipizide can be used again, however, at any time if hyperglycemia recurs. The patient should be rechecked every 3 months to ensure ongoing control.

Cats that have resolution of clinical signs according to the owner, stable body weight, and normal physical examinations but serial blood glucoses at or above 300 mg/dL present a clinical dilemma. Either the clinical signs have not truly resolved or the hyperglycemia is due to stress. Such cats should ideally be monitored by serum glycated protein concentrations and urine glucose concentrations to determine overall glycemic control. If glycosuria is absent and glycated protein concentrations are at a level or downward trend, glipizide therapy can proceed. If glycosuria is present or glycated protein levels are trending upward, insulin should be used instead.

Biguanides. Metformin doses of 25 to 50 mg/cat twice daily should attain plasma concentrations used for treating human DM,[180,181] but the use of the drug in diabetic cats is not promising.[180] In the single published study evaluating metformin use in diabetic cats, five newly diagnosed cats received metformin at a gradually increasing dosage, and only one achieved glycemic control after 8 weeks of therapy. In one nonresponder, serum alanine aminotransferase activity was within the reference range at the start of the study but had increased to 1440 U/L at week 7; 3 weeks after discontinuation of the medication, serum alanine aminotransferase activity was 95 U/L. One cat was found dead after 2 weeks, and no response was seen after 7 to 8 weeks in four cats. The responding cat was treated with 10 mg metformin daily for 1 week, then 10 mg twice daily for 2 weeks, followed by 25 mg twice daily for 5 weeks. Subsequently, the dose was increased to 50 mg twice daily, and 3 weeks later the owner reported resolution of clinical signs of DM. Metformin was used successfully for 4 months until pancreatitis developed, at which time therapy was changed to insulin. The serum insulin concentration was within or greater than the reference range in the responder diabetic cat and was undetectable or at the low end of the reference range in the nonresponders, suggesting that metformin may be beneficial only in diabetic cats with detectable serum insulin concentration at the time treatment is initiated. Adverse effects are common and include inappetence, weight loss, and vomiting. The size of pills commercially available is not amenable to cats, and use of this drug for felines requires compounding.[180]

Alpha-glucosidase inhibitors. In five dogs, a combination of acarbose and insulin provided better glycemic control over insulin alone. However, the final conclusion was that because of the expense and adverse effects, acarbose is primarily indicated for poorly controlled diabetic dogs in which the cause for the poor control cannot be identified.[182] Acarbose, in conjunction with a low-carbohydrate diet, was an effective means of decreasing exogenous insulin dependence and improving glycemic control in one group of diabetic cats,[118] but how much of the dose reduction in insulin was due to the diet and how much to acarbose is unclear. Acarbose may be helpful in cats with renal disease that cannot be placed on a low-carbohydrate diet because of the high protein content of these diets. Acarbose may be administered at a dosage of 25 to 200 mg/dog or 12.5 to 25 mg/cat twice daily with meals. Side effects include flatulence, semiformed stools, or diarrhea.

Thiazolidinediones. Although recent work suggests that darglitazone has beneficial effects in obese nondiabetic cats to decrease insulin secretion and glucose concentrations in a glucose tolerance test,[183] no work has been done in diabetic cats.

Transition metals. Transition metals are insulin mimetic. In healthy nonobese cats, dietary chromium supplementation causes a small but statistically significant, dose-dependent improvement in glucose tolerance.[184] The most commonly reported side effects are mild GI upset. Unfortunately, however, large clinical studies on the effect of vanadium or chromium in diabetic cats are lacking. In one study, chromium had no effect in concert with insulin treatment in diabetic dogs.[185]

Acute Metabolic Complications

Diabetic Ketoacidosis

Diabetic ketoacidosis (DKA) is a complex catabolic disorder caused by either relative or absolute insulin deficiency. Diabetogenic hormones (e.g., cortisol, progesterone, GH), probably contribute to its development. Thus any disease that increases the secretion of these stress hormones can predispose diabetic patients to the development of ketoacidosis, and insulin therapy may become ineffective.

Glycogen, protein, and fat, rather than glucose, are used by the body for energy in the absence of insulin. Glycogen is broken down into glucose. As a physiologic survival mechanism during starvation (insulin deficiency is perceived by the body as a state of starvation because glucose is not available for use by most cells), fatty acids formed from fat breakdown are transported into mitochondria and metabolized to ketone bodies to be used as a fuel source. The ketone bodies are acetone, acetoacetate, and β-hydroxybutyrate. The last is formed from acetoacetate and hydrogen ions. A lack of insulin decreases tissue utilization of ketone bodies. As ketones accumulate, the body's buffering systems become overwhelmed, and metabolic acidosis develops. Glucose formation continues unchecked and even accelerates. Glycosuria that accompanies hyperglycemia causes an osmotic diuresis with subsequent depletion of sodium, chloride, and potassium. If an animal is unable to ingest sufficient water to keep up with ongoing losses, dehydration and prerenal azotemia develop. Severe hyperosmolarity may result. Ketoacidosis can cause vomiting and diarrhea, further complicating acid–base and electrolyte disorders. Production of glucose counterregulatory hormones increases in response to the stress of illness, but the hormones antagonize insulin and worsen the hyperglycemia and ketonemia. Patients with DKA usually are ill when they are brought to the veterinarian, and 6% to 12% are dehydrated. Blood glucose concentration is generally greater than 300 mg/dL, and the patient may be severely acidotic (arterial bicarbonate <11 mEq/L).

Hypokalemia, hypophosphatemia, and hypomagnesemia may accompany DKA. Hypokalemia may develop because of decreased food intake or increased renal loss associated with osmotic diuresis. However, acidosis may cause intracellular potassium ions to shift extracellularly, thus masking total body potassium depletion. Rehydration, correction of acidosis, and insulin therapy may further decrease serum potassium concentrations. The risk of hypophosphatemia is similarly increased by diminished intake, urinary losses, fluid therapy, and translocation after insulin therapy. Energy (adenosine triphosphate [ATP]) depletion becomes evident in high-energy use cells such as skeletal muscle, brain, and red blood cells. Hemolytic anemia is the most common and serious sequela to hypophosphatemia but does not usually occur until serum phosphorus concentration is at or below 1 mg/dL.[186] Neuromuscular signs include weakness, ataxia, and seizures as well as anorexia and vomiting secondary to intestinal ileus. Lastly, osmotic diuresis may cause hypomagnesemia, and because of acid–base imbalances, magnesium may shift intracellularly. Clinical signs of hypomagnesemia (e.g., lethargy, anorexia, muscle weakness [including dysphagia and dyspnea], muscle fasciculations, seizures, ataxia, and coma) do not usually occur until serum total magnesium concentration is below 1 mg/dL.[186]

Diagnosis of DKA includes documentation of the presence of DM, ketone bodies, and acidosis. The existence of ketonuria establishes a diagnosis of ketosis; acidosis must be documented to differentiate ketosis from ketoacidosis. Urine test strips and nitroprusside reagents (e.g., Ketostix) do not detect β-hydroxybutyrate, which can be the predominant ketone present in the acidotic state. If ketoacidosis is suspected but a urine dipstick is negative, other means for detecting ketone bodies, such as Acetest tablets (Ames Division, Miles Laboratories, Elkhart, Ind.) should be used, if available. A commercially available hand-held ketone meter (PrecisionXtra, Abbott, Alameda, Calif.) will detect plasma β-hydroxybutyrate and can be used to aid in the diagnosis of DKA in dogs and cats if urine strips are negative for ketone bodies or urine cannot be obtained.[187]

Treatment of ill ketoacidotic patients should be aggressive, with the treatment goals being to restore water and electrolyte imbalances, provide sufficient insulin to begin normalization of metabolism, correct acidosis, identify precipitating factors for the DKA, and provide a carbohydrate substrate when required by the insulin treatment.[186] Care should be taken not to return blood glucose concentrations to normal too rapidly, because biochemical and osmotic problems could be created by overly aggressive therapy, as described in human "fragile" DKA patients that experience rapid changes in serum tonicity and develop cerebral edema. Cerebral cells of diabetic patients may accumulate sorbitol, an osmotically active polyol formed in response to excessive blood glucose concentrations. Thus as a hypertonic patient achieves normal tonicity and euglycemia with treatment, water may move into neurons that have become hypertonic relative to extracellular fluid.

The common use of isotonic, sodium-containing fluids may minimize large osmotic shifts by maintaining serum sodium concentrations as glucose concentrations decrease,[188] so development of cerebral edema may be uncommon, at least in diabetic cats. A recent retrospective study evaluated 13 diabetic ketotic cats treated in an intensive care unit and similarly managed with intravenous constant-rate infusions of regular insulin and 0.9% saline. The median change in glucose concentration was 122% (range 1% to 1230%). In cats with abnormal sodium concentrations, the median change in sodium (irrespective of direction) was 5.4% (range 1.3% to 11.6%). The median percentage change in serum tonicity (irrespective of direction) was only 2.9% (range 1.4% to 5.7%). At all time points examined, sodium was the major determinant of serum tonicity, with only minimal contributions from glucose. If sodium levels had not increased during treatment, the total decrease in serum tonicity owing to glucose alone would have been 13%. The minimal fluctuations in serum tonicity likely explain the low incidence of osmotic-mediated neurologic complications seen during treatment of diabetic cats.[188] Caution should still be exercised in treatment, especially of hyperglycemic, hyperosmolar, nonketotic diabetic patients. Blood glucose concentrations in hyperglycemic, hyperosmolar diabetics patients may be elevated to the point that they are a major determinant of serum tonicity; alternatively, a diabetic patient not managed with isotonic sodium-containing fluids may be lacking the sodium concentrations needed to buffer the changes in serum tonicity once measures are initiated to reduce the hyperglycemia. In either case, complications from too rapid a decrease in blood glucose concentrations could occur.

The first step in treating DKA should always be to initiate replacement and maintenance fluid therapy to enhance renal blood flow, promote urinary glucose excretion, and decrease the effects of diabetogenic hormones. Sodium chloride (0.9% saline) containing appropriate potassium supplementation is the fluid of choice. Because of the possible risk of cerebral edema formation, rapid fluid administration is indicated only in life-threatening situations. Fluid administration should be directed at gradually replacing hydration deficits over 24 hours while supplying maintenance fluid needs and matching ongoing losses. Once out of the critical phase, fluid replacement should be decreased in an effort to correct fluid imbalances in a slow but steady manner.[186] When serum sodium concentration is 140 to 155 mEq/L, Ringer's solution should be used; if serum sodium concentration increases to more than 155 mEq/L, 0.45% saline should be administered.

Ideally, potassium supplementation should be based on actual measurement of serum potassium concentration. If measurement is not available, 40 mEq potassium should be added to each liter of intravenous fluids.[186] Potassium supplementation should be adjusted every 6 to 8 hours, again ideally based on actual measurements, until the patient is stable and serum electrolytes are within the reference range. Total hourly potassium administration should not exceed 0.5 mEq/kg body weight. If the serum potassium concentration is greater than 5, 4 to 5.5, 3.5 to 4., 3 to 3.5, 2.5 to 3, 2 to 2.5, or less than 2 mEq/L, then no potassium, 20 to 30, 30 to 40, 40 to 50, 50 to 60, 60 to 80, and 80 mEq of potassium should be added to each liter of fluids administered, respectively.[186]

Phosphate therapy is indicated if clinical signs of hypophosphatemia or hemolysis are identified or if the serum phosphorus concentration is below 1.5 mg/dL. An intravenous constant-rate infusion of potassium phosphate (the solution contains 4.4 mEq/mL of potassium and 3 mM/mL of phosphate) should be a given at a rate of 0.03 to 0.12 mM phosphate/kg/hour. Administration of potassium must be taken into account when giving potassium phosphate for correction of hypophosphatemia.[189] Serum phosphate concentration must be measured to assess response and adjust the dose. Because adverse effects of phosphate administration include hypocalcemia, serum calcium concentration, preferably ionized calcium concentration, should also be monitored.

Whether magnesium supplementation is required is controversial. Hypomagnesemia is usually not treated unless persistent lethargy, anorexia, weakness, or refractory hypokalemia or hypocalcemia are encountered after 24 to 48 hours of therapy and another cause for the problem cannot be identified.[186] The initial intravenous dose for the first day is 0.75 to 1 mEq/kg administered by constant-rate infusion in 5% dextrose in water. The supplementation can be continued at half the initial dose for an additional 3 to 5 days if necessary. The dose should be decreased 50% to 75% in azotemic animals. Parenteral magnesium therapy can cause hypocalcemia, cardiac arrhythmias, hypotension, and respiratory depression.[186]

Bicarbonate therapy in the management of patients with DKA is contentious. Proponents point to potential deleterious effects of acidosis on cardiac hemodynamics, whereas opponents are concerned by possible creation of paradoxical central nervous system acidosis or a shift in the oxygen-hemoglobin dissociation curve resulting in tissue hypoxia. A prospective trial of human DKA patients with moderate to severe acidosis (pH 6.9 to 7.1) found no difference in outcome in patients treated with bicarbonate and those who were not.[190] Clinical presentation in conjunction with acid–base status should be used to determine the need. If plasma bicarbonate concentration is above 12 mEq/L, bicarbonate therapy is not indicated, especially if the patient is alert;[186] correction of dehydration and insulin administration usually eliminates acidosis. When plasma bicarbonate concentration is below 11 Eq/L (total venous CO_2 <12 mEq/L), specific therapy should be initiated. The amount of bicarbonate needed to correct acidosis to 12 mEq/L over 6 hours is calculated as

$$\text{mEq bicarbonate needed} = \text{Body weight(kg)} \times 0.4 \times (12 - \text{patient's bicarbonate}) \times 0.5$$

The factor 0.4 corrects for the extracellular fluid space in which bicarbonate is distributed (i.e., 40% of body weight). Using the factor 0.5 means that 50% of the full bicarbonate dose is infused, so a conservative dose is given. The bicarbonate should be infused intravenously over 6 hours (never as a bolus), then the serum bicarbonate concentration reassessed and a new dosage calculated and administered, if needed.[186]

Recommendations regarding insulin doses and routes vary for ketoacidotic patients, but authors agree that therapy should begin with low doses. Insulin therapy should be delayed at least 1 to 2 hours after the start of intravenous fluid therapy. At that time serum electrolytes should be measured; if hypokalemia is present, insulin therapy can be delayed an additional 1 to 2 hours to allow fluid therapy to replenish potassium.

The goal of insulin therapy is to lower the blood glucose concentration to 200 to 250 mg/dL over 6 to 10 hours. Regular insulin is used because it is short-acting and more easily regulated compared with longer-acting insulins. Blood glucose concentrations should be monitored hourly. The major risks associated with insulin therapy are hypoglycemia, hypokalemia, and hypophosphatemia.

The three techniques used are hourly intramuscular,[191] continuous low-dose intravenous infusion,[192] and intermittent intramuscular/subcutaneous.[193] An intermittent intravenous regimen is discouraged because the biologic effects of regular insulin administered intravenously last only 20 minutes. For the hourly intramuscular technique, an initial loading dose of 0.2 U/kg of regular insulin is given, followed by 0.1 U/kg every 1 to 2 hours. Lower doses can be used at first if hypokalemia is a concern. The rear legs are recommended sites for administration. If the blood glucose concentration declines at a rate greater than 75 mg/dL/hr, the dose should be decreased to 0.05 U/kg/hr. If the decrease is less than 50 mg/dL/hr, the dose should be increased to 0.2 U/kg/hr. When the blood glucose concentration is below 300 mg/dL, regular insulin can be given subcutaneously (0.1 to 0.3 U/kg, every 6 to 8 hours) and the dose altered as required. In addition, when blood glucose concentration is 250 to 300 mg/dL, 100 mL of 50% dextrose should be added to each liter of fluid to achieve a 5% dextrose solution. Blood glucose concentration should be maintained between 150 and 300 mg/dL until the patient is stable and eating. When the patient is no longer receiving fluids, is eating and drinking, has stopped vomiting, and is no longer ketoacidotic, maintenance insulin therapy with longer-acting insulin can be instituted.

For the constant-rate low-dose infusion technique, regular crystalline insulin (2.2 U/kg for dogs and 1.1 U/kg for cats) is added to 250 mL of 0.9% saline and initially administered at 10 mL/hr in a line separate from that used for fluid administration.[192] The first 50 mL of an insulin–electrolyte mixture run through intravenous tubing should be discarded because of adsorption of insulin to glassware and plastic. An intravenous infusion pump should be used to ensure a constant administration rate. The infusion rate can be slowed for 2 to 3 hours if hypokalemia is a concern and should be altered as needed so that blood glucose concentrations decline by approximately 50 mg/dL/hr. Once the blood glucose concentration reaches 250 mg/dL, the fluid should be changed to 0.45% saline with 2.5% dextrose. The insulin infusion can then be discontinued and regular insulin given every 6 to 8 hours, as previously described. Alternatively, the infusion rate can be slowed to maintain blood glucose concentrations between 150 and 300 mg/dL until the patient is stable enough to institute maintenance insulin therapy. If infusion is used, insulin should be added to the new fluid at the same concentration.

For the intermittent, intramuscular/subcutaneous insulin technique, the initial regular insulin dose is 0.25 U/kg intramuscularly every 4 hours. Once the patient is rehydrated, subcutaneous administration is substituted. Dose is adjusted based on serum glucose concentrations. This technique is not recommended, however. Blood glucose concentrations decrease rapidly, and the risk for hypoglycemia is great.

Hyperglycemic, Hyperosmolar, Nonketotic Syndrome

The true incidence of hyperglycemic, hyperosmolar nonketotic syndrome (HHNS) in the canine and feline diabetic pet population is unknown, but the condition is relatively uncommon. In one retrospective study of diabetic cats, HHNS constituted 6.4% of emergency room visits of diabetic cats.[194] However, it is associated with a high mortality rate in both humans with type 2 DM and feline diabetics.[194,195]

The pathogenesis of HHNS is not fully understood but may be a result of decreased insulin activity rather than a complete absence. Insulin deficiency causes excess glucagon secretion and decreased glucose use by peripheral tissues. As with DKA, decreased glucose utilization causes muscle and fat breakdown, thus supplying precursors needed for hepatic gluconeogenesis. Insulin deficiency in combination with excess glucagon promotes hepatic gluconeogenesis, and profound hyperglycemia develops. The insulin activity present prevents ketone bodies from forming.

Why some animals develop DKA and others HHNS is unclear. In both disorders patients commonly have concurrent diseases, so insulin resistance is likely to be important in both.[194] Interestingly, certain types of diseases may be more common in HHNS compared with DKA. In one study of cats with HHNS or DKA, overall presence of concurrent disease did not differ between the two groups but presence of specific diseases did. Chronic renal disease occurred in 58.8% of cats with HHNS but only 12.5% of those with DKA, and congestive heart failure was present in 29.4% of the HHNS cats but only 3% of cats with DKA.[194] Thus the presence of certain diseases may predispose one syndrome to develop over another, but this remains to be proven.

The diagnostic criteria for HHNS in veterinary medicine are the presence of severe hyperglycemia (>600 mg/dL) and serum hyperosmolarity (>350 mOsm/L). Severe dehydration causes hyperosmolarity, which leads to the central nervous system abnormalities such as dullness, circling, pacing, or unresponsiveness common with this disorder. Ketones are usually not present, but lactic acidosis often is.[194] The therapeutic goal is to correct the extreme volume depletion and hyperosmolarity. Despite the hyperosmolarity, the initial fluid of choice is isotonic (0.9%) saline.[186] Half the estimated dehydration deficit plus maintenance requirements should be replaced in the first 12 hours and the remainder in the following 24 hours. Potassium and phosphorus supplementation should occur as for patients with DKA. Insulin therapy should be delayed 4 to 6 hours until the positive benefits of fluid therapy are documented (e.g., correction of dehydration, stabilization of blood pressure, and improvement in urine production).[186] Insulin can be administered as for DKA, but the dosages should be decreased by 50% to dampen the decrease in blood glucose concentration and prevent a rapid decrease in extracellular fluid osmolarity.

Prognosis. To some degree, prognosis for a diabetic dog or cat depends on its owner's desire to treat, the presence and severity of underlying disorders, and how well the animal responds to therapy. One must also bear in mind that DM is most commonly diagnosed in the geriatric pet population. The mean survival time for diabetic dogs has been stated to be 3 years after diagnosis, with the highest mortality within the first 6 months.[95] A recent study assessing the incidence, survival, and breed distribution of insured dogs in the United Kingdom diagnosed with DM supports this estimation. Median survival time for 686 dogs was 57 days after the first insurance claim; if 223 dogs that survived less than 1 day were excluded from the analysis, median survival was 2 years. For dogs surviving at least 30 days (n=347), the median survival time was not reached by the end of the study.[196] Median survival times in newly diagnosed diabetic cats is reported to be 17 months,[145] and the life expectancy of diabetic cats that survive the first 6 months after diagnosis has been estimated to be 5 years.[121]

DISEASES OF THE ADRENAL GLANDS

Hypoadrenocorticism

Pathophysiology

Which hormones are deficient in hypoadrenocorticism (Addison's disease) varies according to the underlying pathophysiology. The most common form of hypoadrenocorticism is primary adrenal failure. Glucocorticoids (e.g., cortisol) alone or both glucocorticoids and mineralocorticoids (e.g., aldosterone) may be deficient, depending on which adrenocortical zones have been destroyed. Primary hypoadrenocorticism can be spontaneous or iatrogenic as a result of mitotane, ketoconazole, or trilostane administration. Secondary hypoadrenocorticism is due to pituitary failure to secrete adrenocorticotropic hormone (ACTH). Because ACTH has minimal effects on aldosterone secretion, ACTH deficiency causes isolated glucocorticoid insufficiency. ACTH deficiency can be idiopathic, caused by head trauma or neoplasia, or iatrogenic, secondary to chronic suppression of ACTH caused by administration of glucocorticoids[197] or progestins.[198,199] Exogenous glucocorticoids of any form, even topical, can feed back and turn off ACTH secretion. With chronic ACTH deficiency, adrenocortical atrophy occurs and cortisol secretion falls. Even though cats are considered to be relatively resistant to most side effects of glucocorticoids, they are just as susceptible as dogs to the adrenal suppressive effects. Administration of megestrol acetate (Ovaban) or other progestins to cats[200] can also suppress ACTH secretion. Certain breeds of dogs (e.g., Nova Scotia Duck Tolling retrievers, Standard Poodles, and Bearded Collies) can have a genetic component to development of hypoadrenocorticism.[201-203]

Hypoadrenocorticism can be a life-threatening condition requiring immediate life-saving therapeutic intervention. The acute life-threatening effects generally reflect mineralocorticoid deficiency and, less commonly, glucocorticoid deficiency. Glucocorticoids affect almost every tissue; many effects are critical to normal homeostasis and become more critical in stressed patients. Glucocorticoids stimulate gluconeogenesis and glycogenolysis by direct hepatic effects and by stimulating protein and fat catabolism peripherally. They also have a permissive effect on adrenergic receptors, enhancing tissue response to alpha- and beta-receptor stimulation. Mineralocorticoids are crucial to maintaining sodium, potassium, and water balance.

Lack of cortisol secretion may cause depression, lethargy, anorexia, vomiting, abdominal pain, shaking or shivering, and weight loss. In severe cases cardiovascular collapse may result. Clinical signs indicative of mineralocorticoid deficiency include collapse and bradyarrhythmias. On routine blood work in patients with mineralocorticoid deficiency, hyponatremia, hyperkalemia, and hypochloremia are usually present. Hypoadrenocorticoid patients often are azotemic. Hypoglycemia will be present due to glucocorticoid deficiency in a small percentage of cases. Hypercalcemia occurs in about 25% of patients. Mild to moderate metabolic acidosis may be present, particularly if mineralocorticoid secretion is impaired.

Diagnosis

Diagnosis of hypoadrenocorticism can be suspected or ruled out on the basis of a baseline cortisol but must be confirmed by performance of an ACTH stimulation test. In one study dogs with basal cortisol concentrations above 55 nmol/L (2 μg/dL) that were not receiving corticosteroids, mitotane, or ketoconazole were highly unlikely to have hypoadrenocorticism; however, if the basal cortisol concentration was less than 55 nmol/L, an ACTH stimulation test was needed for further evaluation.[204] Likely, the same applies to dogs receiving progestins or trilostane. The protocol for performance of an ACTH stimulation test is the same as for diagnosis of hypoadrenocorticism (discussed below). In patients with primary or secondary hypoadrenocorticism, baseline cortisol concentration will be low, with minimal to no response to ACTH stimulation. The test does not distinguish spontaneous from iatrogenic disease and only confirms cortisol insufficiency. In a cortisol-deficient patient, if moderate to marked hyponatremia or hyperkalemia are present, aldosterone is assumed to be lacking as well. Serum aldosterone concentrations can be measured, but this is often not necessary and interpretation can be problematic.[205]

To differentiate primary from secondary hypoadrenocorticism, plasma endogenous ACTH concentration can be measured, as described below (see section on hyperadrenocorticism). In primary hypoadrenocorticism, negative feedback on the pituitary is lost and endogenous ACTH concentrations will be greatly increased; secondary hypoadrenocorticism, by comparison, is, by definition, a lack of ACTH. Evaluation of endogenous ACTH concentration can be considered if a patient has glucocorticoid deficiency only. If aldosterone secretory ability is impaired, the disease must be primary to the adrenal glands. Distinguishing primary from secondary disease in patients with spontaneous isolated glucocorticoid deficiency can be prognostic. If the disease is primary, aldosterone secretion is likely to be lost in the future and serum electrolyte concentrations should be monitored regularly; if the hypoadrenocorticism is secondary, mineralocorticoid secretion will remain normal.

Therapy

Therapy for hypoadrenocorticism focuses first on acute management of a hypoadrenal crisis, if present, and then on long-term maintenance therapy. The goals of therapy for treatment of a crisis are to replace fluid volume and the needed hormones, correct cardiovascular collapse, and rectify electrolyte and acid–base imbalances. Once the acute crisis is resolved, patients with hypoadrenocorticism can lead normal lives as long as medication is used appropriately.

Before therapy is initiated, if hypoadrenocorticism is suspected and patient status permits, an ACTH stimulation test should be performed for diagnosis. If emergency care that includes glucocorticoid administration is required, dexamethasone is the first choice to use. Exogenous glucocorticoid administration can affect ACTH stimulation testing in two ways. First, certain glucocorticoids—prednisone, prednisolone, methylprednisolone, and hydrocortisone—cross-react on cortisol assays and, if present, will artificially elevate apparent cortisol concentrations. If any of these four glucocorticoids are administered, an ACTH stimulation test should not be performed for 12 hours, whereas if dexamethasone is given, an ACTH stimulation test can still be performed immediately. (If methylprednisolone acetate [e.g., Depo-Medrol] is administered, testing may need to be delayed much longer.) Second, any glucocorticoid can feed back and suppress ACTH and cortisol secretion. The degree of suppression and the length of duration depends on which glucocorticoid was administered, as well as the route, dose, and duration. For example, depending on the dose, a single dexamethasone injection given to treat an Addisonian crisis may, within a few days, completely suppress basal cortisol concentration and suppress post-ACTH cortisol concentrations up to 33%. However, such suppression is easily distinguishable from spontaneous hypoadrenocorticism in which serum cortisol concentration is nondetectable before and after administration of ACTH. Thus, if after a single dexamethasone injection, post-ACTH serum cortisol concentration is nondetectable, a diagnosis of hypoadrenocorticism is made; if the post-ACTH serum cortisol concentration is just below the reference range, the patient's suppressed adrenal function is likely due to administration of an exogenous glucocorticoid, not to hypoadrenocorticism.

For treatment of an Addisonian crisis, fluid therapy is paramount and the primary priority. Although use of 0.9% saline was once advocated, rapid correction of hyponatremia has now been recognized to lead to central nervous system dysfunction.[206,207] During chronic hyponatremia, the brain adapts to prevent cerebral edema. With rapid correction of serum sodium concentration, osmotic shifts and cerebral dehydration occur, with a possible resultant pontine myelinosis and neurologic signs such as disorientation, dysphagia, weakness, and quadriparesis. Thus, although balanced solutions such as Normosol-R or lactated Ringer's solution contain potassium, they are currently the fluid of choice, with the latter possibly being the best insofar as the sodium is the lowest. Hypertonic saline administration is contraindicated. For treatment of an Addisonian crisis, shock doses of fluids should be given initially and then rehydration corrected over 6 to 24 hours, depending on patient stability. Fluid therapy should be adjusted to increase serum sodium concentration at a rate of 0.5 mEq/L/hr. Frequent measurement of serum sodium concentration is important to ensure that the rate of correction of hyponatremia is appropriate. Fluid type and rate can be adjusted accordingly. If hypoglycemia is present, dextrose should be added to the fluids to make a 5% solution.

A rapid-acting glucocorticoid such as prednisolone sodium succinate (1 to 2 mg/kg over 2 to 4 minutes; can be repeated in 2 to 6 hours), dexamethasone or dexamethasone sodium phosphate (0.5 to 2 mg/kg intravenously, every 2 to 6 hours), or hydrocortisone hemisuccinate or hydrocortisone phosphate (2-4 mg/kg intravenously over 2 to 4 minutes, every 8 hours) should be administered. Alternatively, hydrocortisone sodium succinate can be infused at a rate of 0.5 to 0.625 mg/kg/hr intravenously. Although dexamethasone can be used to replace glucocorticoid deficiency, mineralocorticoid deficiency will not be affected; thus prednisolone, which has some mineralocorticoid activity, might be preferred, at least initially. However, the effect of glucocorticoid administration on diagnostic testing should also be considered (discussed previously). Mineralocorticoid therapy is needed only if aldosterone is deficient and is not recommended until serum sodium concentration is in the reference range or slightly below. Mineralocorticoid administration can correct serum sodium concentration fairly rapidly.

Dilutional effects and increased GFR secondary to fluid administration will begin to correct life-threatening hyperkalemia. Very rarely does hyperkalemia fail to respond rapidly to volume replacement. In such instances, or if the hyperkalemia is immediately life-threatening, 10% (100 mg/mL) calcium gluconate (0.5-1 mg/kg) can be given intravenously slowly. The calcium protects the myocardium from the effects of the potassium. An electrocardiogram must be monitored during calcium infusion and treatment stopped if new arrhythmias occur or bradycardia worsens. Alternatively, regular insulin (0.06-0.125 U/kg, plus 20 mL of a 10% glucose solution for every unit of insulin given) can be administered. Insulin causes glucose to move intracellularly, and potassium will follow. Glucose is infused in an attempt to prevent hypoglycemia. However, given the abnormal glucose metabolism in hypoadrenocorticism, hypoglycemia still often results. If a patient is already hypoglycemic, just giving dextrose alone is much safer and will also cause intracellular movement of potassium. Lastly, bicarbonate can be given to address acidosis but is rarely required because the other treatments usually resolve the acidosis.

Response to initial therapy of hypoadrenocorticism should occur in 1 or 2 hours in patients suffering from hypoadrenocorticism. In general, cats take longer to respond than dogs. Because sodium deficiency may result in a washout of the medullary interstitium, renal function may not return to normal quickly, and the patient may be diuresing for several days. Care must be taken to balance fluid input with excessive output.

Mineralocorticoid replacement therapy. Maintenance therapy for hypoadrenocorticism begins when vomiting, diarrhea, weakness, and depression have resolved. Mineralocorticoid replacement is needed only for patients that are aldosterone deficient and is available in oral or depot preparations. The initial recommended dose of fludrocortisone in dogs is 0.01 to 0.02 mg/kg orally daily[208] and in cats 0.1 mg/cat daily,[200,209] much higher doses than required in humans. Dosage adjustments, if necessary, are made on the basis of serum electrolyte concentrations. Ideally, sodium and potassium should be within reference ranges. Sodium and potassium should be monitored every 1 to 2 weeks after initiating therapy until a patient is stable. In dogs the daily dosage is adjusted by 0.05 to 0.1 mg increments. Once electrolyte concentrations have stabilized, a patient should be reevaluated monthly for the first 3 to 6 months and every 3 to 6 months thereafter, as long as no clinical signs are apparent. In cats timing of monitoring is the same, and adjustments are made in 0.05-mg increments. In the authors' experience, however, fludrocortisone fails to normalize sodium in a number of patients no matter how high the dose.

In dogs the final required fludrocortisone dose varies greatly between patients; in one study the median final required dose was 0.023 mg/kg/day (range approximately 0.008 to 0.75 mg/kg daily).[210] Required doses often increase over the initial 6 to 18 months of therapy,[205,210] possibly as a result of ongoing destruction of the adrenal cortex or changes in drug absorption or metabolism.

Overall, fludrocortisone therapy is effective. In 33 dogs, the response to treatment was considered good to excellent in 78.8%, fair in 9.1%, and poor in 12.1%.[211] The most common side effects are polyuria and polydipsia, but polyphagia, hair loss, and weight gain may be seen. Most of the adverse effects occur when prednisone and fludrocortisone are administered concurrently and resolve when glucocorticoid therapy is discontinued, but polyuria and polydipsia can be seen with fludrocortisone alone.[205,210,211] Although fasting hypercholesterolemia and hypertriglyceridemia have been noted with fludrocortisone administration,[211] the significance of these changes remain unknown.

The recommended starting dose of desoxycorticosterone pivalate (DOCP; Percorten, Novartis) for dogs is 2.2 mg/kg intramuscularly every 25 days. For cats the dose of DOCP is 10 to 12.5 mg/cat intramuscularly monthly.[209] The subcutaneous route, however, can be used, at least in dogs.[212] For the majority of dogs, the dosing regimen will be effective. Although one study initiated before a manufacturer's recommended dose was chosen found that some dogs did not need that high a dose, starting at 2.2 mg/kg is safe.[213,214]

To decrease cost, it may not be necessary to administer DOCP at the full label dose. With DOCP, clinicians typically assume a 28-day interval and start at a dose of 2.2 mg/kg. Electrolytes should be measured on days 14 and 28, and if they are within the reference range on day 28, the DOCP dose can be decreased 10%. When a dose is found that no longer maintains serum sodium and potassium concentrations in the reference range for the full 28 days, the lowest DOCP dose that lasted 28 days can be used. An alternative is to administer 2.2 mg/kg DOCP, lengthen the interval by 3 days with each injection until the interval is too long, and then use the longest interval during which serum electrolyte concentrations were in the reference range. However, it is probably harder for owners to remember the injections on a long interval, and the authors prefer lowering the dose and maintaining a 28-day interval instead.

A small percentage of dogs, however, do require either injections more frequently than every 25 days or more than 2.2 mg/kg to keep a 25-day or longer interval.[210,215] If the patient is hyponatremic or hyperkalemic at day 14, the next dose should be increased by 10%. If the electrolytes are normal on day 14 but abnormal on day 28, the interval between injections should be decreased by 2 days[205] or the dose increased 10%. In dogs that require DOCP more frequently than every 28 days, clinical signs of Addison's disease may recur before the recheck on day 28. If return of the hypoadrenal state is suspected, the dog should be seen immediately and serum electrolytes measured. If hyponatremia and hyperkalemia are documented, the DOCP injection can be given at that time. If the dosing interval is shortened, the timing of monitoring should be changed accordingly for the next treatment period. Two rechecks should be performed during each dosing interval until good control of the Addison's disease on the last day of the dosing interval is demonstrated.

DOCP is a highly efficacious treatment for hypoadrenocorticism with minimal side effects. Adverse effects reported include depression, polyuria, polydipsia, anorexia, skin and coat changes, diarrhea, vomiting, weakness, weight loss, incontinence, and pain on injection, but all are uncommon. Some of the adverse effects, such as polyuria and polydipsia, are more likely caused by concurrent glucocorticoid administration than by DOCP itself. Treatment failures also occur rarely.

Any recheck, whether monitoring fludrocortisone or DOCP therapy, should include a full physical exam, complete history, and determination of BUN concentration, as well as measurement of electrolytes. If at any recheck the serum electrolyte concentrations are within the reference range but problems, sometimes quite vague, such as anorexia, vomiting, diarrhea, or unwillingness to play exist, glucocorticoid deficiency is the likely cause, and the prednisone dose should be adjusted accordingly. An elevated BUN concentration can be a sign of dehydration caused by insufficient therapy.

Advantages and disadvantages exist with the use of either fludrocortisone or DOCP. For fludrocortisone the major advantage is the ease of diagnosing and adjusting an incorrect dosage because daily administration is easily altered. Daily therapy also constantly reminds owners that their pet is afflicted with a life-threatening disease and needs constant therapy and monitoring. Lastly, the medication is readily available at most pharmacies. However, fludrocortisone can be quite expensive despite the availability of a generic product, especially if higher doses are required; some patients may not be adequately controlled and side effects may occur, even when used without concomitant glucocorticoid therapy. If expense, existence of side effects, or lack of efficacy necessitates discontinuation of fludrocortisone, DOCP becomes the only choice.

For DOCP advantages include a low incidence of adverse effects if used alone, less common treatment failures than with fludrocortisone therapy, and need for infrequent administration. A subcutaneous injection can be given by owners if trained properly, but *great* care should be taken in selection of owners for this task. Missing an injection or giving one inappropriately and not realizing the mistake could be fatal for the patient. Apparent failures may be due to the owner's difficulty in providing injections; improper technique should always be ruled out. If a patient truly does not respond to DOCP, fludrocortisone therapy should be instituted.

Glucocorticoid replacement therapy. For all dogs and cats that have either iatrogenic or spontaneous secondary hypoadrenocorticism or primary Addison's disease without mineralocorticoid deficiency, only glucocorticoid replacement therapy is required. It should be remembered, however, that the disease of animals with primary glucocorticoid deficiency may progress to include mineralocorticoid insufficiency as well, and therapy must be adjusted accordingly. For an animal lacking both types of adrenocortical hormones, the need for daily maintenance glucocorticoid replacement therapy depends in part on which mineralocorticoid supplement is being administered. (For animals with hypoadrenocorticism under stress, excess glucocorticoids are always recommended; this is discussed later at more length.). Fludrocortisone has both glucocorticoid and mineralocorticoid activity, whereas DOCP has only mineralocorticoid properties. Thus approximately 50% of dogs receiving fludorocortisone may not require concomitant exogenous glucocorticoid administration.[205,208] Although some dogs on DOCP have not received glucocorticoid therapy,[211,215] this practice is not recommended[205] insofar as the patient will be glucocorticoid deficient on a daily basis.

All animals beginning maintenance therapy for spontaneous hypoadrenocorticism should receive prednisone or prednisolone at a "physiologic" dose of 0.1 to 0.22 mg/kg once daily; prednisolone may be the preferred form in cats. If the animal is on fludrocortisone, once a dose that maintains serum electrolyte concentrations within the reference range has been determined, the glucocorticoid can be tapered to alternate days and then discontinued to see whether continued glucocorticoid therapy will be required.[208] If the dog or cat is lethargic, dull, or unwilling to exercise or play or if clinical signs of hypocortisolism such as weakness, anorexia, vomiting, and diarrhea are apparent, glucocorticoids should be reinstituted at the lowest dosage that does not produce glucocorticoid-associated adverse effects and keeps the patient free of clinical signs. Patients receiving DOCP should always receive daily glucocorticoid replacement therapy, similarly at the lowest dosage possible. In cats methylprednisolone acetate (Depo-Medrol, 10 mg/month intramuscularly) can be administered if giving them pills is difficult,[209] but complications of glucocorticoid therapy such as DM may be more likely.[200] Depo-Medrol is not recommended for use in dogs.

In non-Addisonian patients receiving exogenous glucocorticoids chronically, every-other-day administration is recommended to minimize resultant adrenal atrophy. As patients with spontaneous hypoadrenocorticism already have significant adrenocortical destruction or atrophy, atrophy secondary to glucocorticoids is not a concern. Therefore, if a patient with spontaneous hypoadrenocorticism is deemed to need physiologic glucocorticoid replacement therapy, the medication should be given daily to make sure the patient is never glucocorticoid deficient.

During adverse periods such as illness, surgery or trauma, glucocorticoid requirements increase and additional glucocorticoid supplementation at 2 to 10 times the physiologic levels should be administered;[208] if the patient does not receive daily glucocorticoid supplementation, it should be given during such times. Working dogs such as hunters and field trial participants should be allowed to complete their usual activities, but owners must be instructed to monitor their pets more closely than normal and discontinue activity if a dog appears unduly fatigued. On days of planned increased exercise or stress, the daily glucocorticoid dose should be doubled,[205] or, if the animal is not receiving any glucocorticoids, a dose of 0.1 to 0.2 mg/kg can be given.

If the possibility of complete iatrogenic suppression of adrenal glucocorticoid secretion exists in patients receiving long-term exogenous glucocorticoids, the ideal way to assess adrenal reserve is by performing an ACTH stimulation test. If the response to an injection of ACTH is low, the patient should be tapered off the glucocorticoid supplementation until their adrenal gland function recovers. Once the decision to end steroid therapy is made, the dose of glucocorticoid should be decreased to physiologic doses of prednisone over 1 to 2 weeks.[205] If adrenal suppression is secondary to topical glucocorticoid administration, topical administration should be stopped and oral prednisone initiated at physiologic doses. If this dose of prednisone is tolerated for a week without clinical signs of cortisol deficiency, the dosage schedule should be reduced by administering the drug every other day. After 2 weeks at this dose, the dosage should be further reduced by giving the medication every third day. After 2 to 3 weeks, prednisone most likely can be discontinued.[205] Ideally, however, before discontinuation, an ACTH stimulation test should be performed 12 hours after the last dose of prednisone to ensure that the patient has a normal adrenal reserve. Cats should be placed on physiologic doses of prednisolone and tapered off as are dogs.

In older reference sources, salt supplementation was advocated for treatment of patients with mineralocorticoid deficiency,[216] but this may not be necessary for dogs being fed a standard diet.[205] Salt supplementation may still be helpful, however, in an occasional dog that requires large doses of an exogenous mineralocorticoid or that remains hyponatremic despite being normokalemic on an appropriate dose of mineralocorticoid.[205,210] If salt is administered, the initial dose should be 0.1 mg/kg/day, divided over two or three meals.[216] After initiating salt supplementation, serum sodium and potassium concentrations should be measured and the sodium chloride dose adjusted accordingly.

Prognosis

Prognosis for patients with Addison's disease is excellent. Median survival is approximately 5 years, and patients typically die as a result of other diseases. The cause of hypoadrenocorticism, the mineralocorticoid used for treatment (i.e., fludrocortisone versus DOPCP), and signalment do not affect survival.[210] Owners should be aware, however, that their pet has a potentially life-threatening disease when not treated appropriately and continuous, lifelong therapy for spontaneous hypoadrenocorticism and appropriate monitoring are essential. If the disease is iatrogenic, lifelong therapy may not be required, depending on the cause, but therapy is nonetheless important until adrenal function has recovered.

Hyperadrenocorticism

Pathophysiology

Canine and feline hyperadrenocorticism can be either pituitary or adrenal dependent. The pituitary form is more common in dogs and cats than the adrenal form, accounting for approximately 80% to 85% of cases of hyperadrenocorticism. In pituitary-dependent hyperadrenocorticism (PDH), a corticotroph tumor secretes ACTH. The excess ACTH secretion leads to increased release of cortisol from the adrenal glands. In adrenal-dependent hyperadrenocorticism, an adrenal tumor (AT) autonomously secretes cortisol. In dogs and cats, ACTH-secreting pituitary tumors are almost 100% benign, whereas cortisol-secreting ATs are approximately 50% benign and 50% malignant. In either form of the disease, the majority of the clinical signs are caused by hypercortisolemia. The pathophysiology leading to the clinical sequelae is complex because of the large number of body tissues influenced by endogenous glucocorticoids (see chapter on glucocorticoid therapy). Large tumors, either adrenal or pituitary, can also lead to clinical signs because of their mass-occupying effects.

Diagnosis

Diagnosis of hyperadrenocorticism is made on the basis of positive screening test results in patients with the appropriate history, clinical signs, and biochemical test results. Three screening tests are designed to help determine whether a patient has hyperadrenocorticism: the urinary cortisol:creatinine ratio (UCCR), the ACTH stimulation test, and the low-dose dexamethasone suppression test (LDDST). Measurement of a UCCR is a highly sensitive but very nonspecific test. Almost all (>95%) cats and dogs with hyperadrenocorticism have an elevated UCCR, but the ratio is very often elevated in dogs and cats that do not have hyperadrenocorticism (approximately 80% to 85%).[217] Thus the best use of the UCCR is as a means to rule out the diagnosis of hyperadrenocorticism. If a patient has a normal UCCR, it is highly unlikely to have hyperadrenocorticism; however, because of the very high rate of false-positive results, if a UCCR is elevated, another screening test must be done to confirm the presence of hyperadrenocorticism. One advantage of the UCCR is ease of testing: A single urine sample is required. As even the stress of being in a hospital can elevate a UCCR,[218,219] it should be measured on a sample collected at home.

The ACTH stimulation test is recommended for patients with minimal clinical signs of hyperadrenocorticism, patients that are receiving phenobarbital, or patients that have a nonadrenal illness present (e.g., a diabetic dog that is also suspected of having hyperadrenocorticism).[217] In addition, the ACTH stimulation test is the only screening test that can differentiate between spontaneous and iatrogenic hyperadrenocorticism. The recommended form of ACTH is cortrosyn (Cosyntropin, Amphastar Pharmaceuticals, Rancho Cucamonga, Calif.). To perform the test, the clinician injects cortrosyn at a dose in dogs of 5 μg/kg intravenously[220] or intramuscularly[221] or 125 μg in cats.[222] Blood samples are taken before and 1 hour after injection. In animals with spontaneous hyperadrenocorticism, the response to ACTH should be greater than in healthy patients.

Overall, the ACTH stimulation test will be positive in approximately 80% of dogs and cats with hyperadrenocorticism.[217,223] If the forms of hyperadrenocorticism are considered separately in dogs, for PDH the sensitivity is 87%, whereas for AT the sensitivity is 61%.[217] In PDH false-negative results may be attributable to early disease where adrenocortical hyperplasia is minimal. In AT the tumor tissue may not have ACTH receptors and therefore might not respond to an ACTH injection. Nonadrenal illness can affect the ACTH stimulation test in dogs and cats.[224,225] In one study 14% of dogs with nonadrenal illness had an ACTH stimulation test consistent with hyperadrenocorticismeven although they did not have the disease.[224] Infrequently, a subnormal ACTH response is seen in dogs with AT. A low baseline cortisol concentration with little to no response to exogenous ACTH suggests iatrogenic hyperadrenocorticism. The ACTH test also should be used to monitor patients receiving mitotane, ketoconazole, or trilostane therapy for treatment of hyperadrenocorticism.

Owing to issues related to the cost and availability of cortrosyn, interest has been raised in use of compounded ACTH. Two studies have assessed a total of five compounded forms in dogs. The gels studied appear to be effective in normal dogs.[226,227] However, the protocols recommended by the manufacturers may not be appropriate, and, if a compounded ACTH gel is being used, samples should be taken before injection and at both 60 and 120 minutes after injection, so the peak response is not missed.[227] Whether the gels are as effective at diagnosing hyperadrenocorticism as is cortrosyn has not been rigorously assessed; they may not be.[226]

In normal animals a low dose of dexamethasone suppresses ACTH secretion, and, as a result, blood cortisol concentration decreases. Patients with pituitary- or adrenal-dependent hyperadrenocorticism should continue to secrete cortisol despite being given a low dose of dexamethasone, and suppression will not occur. Overall, the LDDST shows inadequate suppression (i.e., is positive) in approximately 95% of dogs with hyperadrenocorticism.[217] In general, the LDDST is recommended in patients with moderate to severe clinical signs consistent with hyperadrenocorticism.[217] A disadvantage of the LDDST in dogs is that nonadrenal illness can cause the test to give false-positive results in a high percentage of dogs. As many as 56% of ill dogs that do not have hyperadrenocorticism may have a positive LDDST test result.[224] In cats 6 weeks of uncontrolled DM does not affect LDDST test results,[228] but whether longer or more severe illness may do so is unknown.

What is considered a "low-dose" test for screening varies between dogs and cats. In both species dexamethasone is administered with blood samples being taken before and 4 and 8 hours after injection. However, in dogs the dose used is 0.01 to 0.015 mg/kg, whereas in cats it is 0.1 mg/kg.

Which test is best, the ACTH stimulation test or LDDST, for diagnosing hyperadrenocorticism in cats is unknown. In one literature review, in cats with hyperadrenocorticism 81% of ACTH stimulation tests were positive (n=37), whereas 79% of cats (n=28) showed inadequate suppression at 8 hours after dexamethasone.[223] Interestingly, in three cats, two ACTH stimulation tests were performed, with one being negative and one positive. Other reports have not shown as high a sensitivity for the ACTH stimulation, and some authors prefer the LDDST.[229]

Once a diagnosis of hyperadrenocorticism is made, the underlying cause—pituitary or adrenal —must be delineated because this provides information on prognosis and treatment options. The UCCR or ACTH stimulation test can never be used to differentiate between PDH and AT. In up to 60% of dogs, the LDDST can provide the differentiation as well as the diagnosis of hyperadrenocorticism.[230] If the 8-hour postdexamethasone concentration is not fully suppressed (check with the laboratory for their definition of suppression; in most labs it is a serum cortisol concentration of less than approximately 30 nmol/L or 1 to 1.5 μg/dL), the results are consistent with a diagnosis of hyperadrenocorticism. If, in addition, the 4-hour postdexamethasone concentration is fully suppressed or if one or both postdexamethasone concentrations is less than 50% of baseline, PDH is present.[230] However, if the baseline cortisol is already below 30 nmol/L, these guidelines do not apply.[231] If both postdexamethasone concentrations are above 30 nmol/L and neither of these values is less than 50% of baseline, either PDH or AT is possible. In rare cases dogs with an AT may meet one of these criteria for diagnosing PDH.[231] Whether differentiation can be done with the LDDST in cats is not known.

If the LDDST was not done as the screening test or did not delineate the form of hyperadrenocorticism present, further tests available to differentiate between PDH and AT are measurement of plasma endogenous ACTH (eACTH) concentration; the high-dose dexamethasone suppression test (HDDST); and imaging such as abdominal ultrasound, CT, and MRI. An advantage of eACTH measurement is that only a single blood sample is required, but special handling is needed. Samples should be collected with EDTA and centrifuged within 15 minutes, and the plasma separated and placed in plastic tubes. Addition of aprotinin facilitates accuracy of measurement[232] as it prevents eACTH degradation. If aprotinin is used, the plasma sample must remain cool only until it arrives at a laboratory; if aprotinin is not used, the sample must remain frozen until analysis.

In dogs with PDH, eACTH concentration should be normal to elevated owing to secretion from the pituitary tumor. In dogs with an AT, the autonomous secretion of cortisol by the tumor will turn off pituitary ACTH secretion so eACTH should be below normal. Values to be used for test interpretation vary with the laboratory and assay used. An advantage of this test is that it can confirm the presence of an AT, whereas the HDDST can never do so. Unfortunately, nondiagnostic values exist. For example, at the Auburn University Endocrine Diagnostic Service, a concentration of less than 10 pg/mL is consistent with an AT, whereas one greater than 15 pg/mL is consistent with PDH. The area between 10 and 15 pg/mL is a "gray zone," in which differentiation is impossible. Although other laboratories may have different cutoffs, a similar gray zone will exist. Gray zone results occur in approximately 18% of canine submissions. However, with repeat testing when the initial result is in the gray zone, a definitive differentiation can be achieved in approximately 96% of dogs.[217] Unfortunately, there is no way to predict when a blood concentration will be in the diagnostic range.

The basis of the HDDST is that high doses of dexamethasone are generally sufficient to cause pituitary gland tumors to decrease ACTH secretion, and, as a result, cortisol concentration falls. In comparison, ATs secrete cortisol autonomously, and because eACTH concentrations are already low, dexamethasone administration does not suppress serum cortisol concentrations. After collection of a baseline cortisol concentration, 0.1 mg/kg dexamethasone is given intravenously in dogs and 1 mg/kg in cats, and then samples are collected 4 and 8 hours later. Suppression is defined as a 4- or 8-hour cortisol concentration less than approximately 30 nmol/L or 1.0 μg/dL (check with the laboratory for the specific ranges) or less than 50% of baseline. Because approximately 25% of dogs with PDH do not suppress on a HDDST, lack of suppression does *not* mean a patient has an AT. If the criteria for suppression are met, a patient has PDH. If the criteria are not met, a 50/50 chance still exists that the patient has PDH or AT. Thus the HDDST can *never* confirm the presence of an AT.

Imaging can be helpful in diagnosing hyperadrenocorticism but can never be used as a screening test. Changes associated with hyperadrenocorticism that may be seen on radiographs include hepatomegaly; a pendulous abdomen; calcinosis cutis; osteopenia; and dystrophic mineralization of bronchi, the renal pelvis, liver, gastric mucosa, and abdominal aorta. Abdominal radiography can be helpful in differentiation if an adrenal mass is found. Of 94 ATs in 88 dogs (six dogs had bilateral adenomas or carcinomas), 50 ATs (53%) were detected because of tumoral calcification (n=40) or visualization of a mass (n=17).[217] ATs can often be visualized by radiography in cats.[223] Both adenomas and carcinomas can contain mineral densities or appear as a mass cranial to the kidney. Mineralization itself, however, is not definitive for a tumor in either species, and as many as one third of normal cats can have adrenal calcification.

Ultrasonography may have more application as a differentiating tool than radiography because both adrenal glands can be visualized. Small or noncalcified ATs can be detected, and bilateral adrenal enlargement can be visualized in dogs with PDH. Ultrasonography defines location, size, and organ involvement of adrenal masses more precisely than radiography alone, but ATs are not always seen. A small degree of asymmetry exists normally. In 71 dogs, 68 of 79 (86%) tumors were found (eight had bilateral tumors).[217] Differentiation between an adrenal adenoma and carcinoma is unlikely with ultrasound insofar as they can have a similar appearance. Neither echogenicity nor the presence of mineralization can be used. Lesions suggestive of metastasis may be found, especially in the liver.[233] Evidence of invasion into the vena cava is suggestive of a carcinoma but can be difficult to judge by ultrasound. With ATs atrophy of the contralateral gland will not always be detectable by ultrasound.

Use of ultrasonography as a screening test for hyperadrenocorticism is not recommended. First, measurements of adrenal gland length and minimum and maximum diameter overlap between dogs with PDH and either dogs with nonendocrine disease or even normal dogs, so ultrasound cannot always distinguish between them. Second, the finding of an AT is not synonymous with hyperadrenocorticism. Ultrasonography cannot distinguish a functional adrenocortical tumor from a nonfunctional tumor, a pheochromocytoma, a metastatic lesion, or a granuloma.

Abdominal CT is an even more sensitive assessment of adrenal gland structure. Standard and dynamic CT can also be used for pituitary evaluation. Dynamic CT is more sensitive than conventional contrast-enhanced CT. If hypophysectomy is being considered for therapy, the extra sensitivity of dynamic CT may be helpful to ensure that the correct treatment is being provided. In other cases dynamic CT may not be warranted. MRI has been used not to differentiate but to assess the size of a pituitary mass in known cases of PDH. Biochemical testing cannot readily differentiate tumor size.

Although radiation therapy is not a great means of controlling hyperadrenocorticism,[234,235] radiation done for local control of a pituitary mass is more effective and provides a better outcome and prognosis the smaller the mass and with no or minimal neurologic signs present.[234,236] Compared with untreated dogs, radiation therapy for a pituitary mass, with or without the presence of hyperadrenocorticism or with or without the presence of neurologic signs, significantly increased survival. In one study median survival with treatment was not reached, but mean survival was 1405 days versus 359 for those not treated. Radiation also significantly increased control of neurologic signs.[237]

The true incidence of pituitary macroadenomas is unknown but has been estimated to be as high as 25% in dogs. The clinical progression of pituitary tumors is also widely unknown. Out of 21 dogs recently diagnosed with but untreated for PDH that had no neurologic signs, 11 had a pituitary mass visible on MRI.[238] At 1 year 13 of the 21 had follow-up imaging. Five had no visible tumor originally, whereas eight did of 4- to 11-mm greatest vertical height. One of the dogs with a visible mass had not been treated, whereas the rest had been treated with mitotane.[239] None of the five dogs with no visible mass originally had neurologic signs at follow-up; two had a visible pituitary tumor.[239] Of the eight dogs that had a visible mass at first imaging, four had no apparent change in their tumor size, whereas in four the tumor had enlarged. The untreated dog was in the latter group. Overall, four developed signs of central nervous system dysfunction (19% of the original 21 and 36% of the 11 dogs with tumors visible at the first scan). Tumor size appeared to correlate with the development of signs, insofar as no dog with a mass smaller than 10 mm had neurologic dysfunction. There was no apparent correlation between pituitary mass size before treatment and increase in size over the year. [239]

On the basis of this information, clinical experience, and theoretical considerations, recommendations for routine imaging of the pituitary in patients with hyperadrenocorticism have recently been formulated. With the recognition that the number of dogs studied is small, the suggestions are as follows: All dogs with PDH should have CT or MRI scans at the time of diagnosis. If no mass is visible, medical treatment should be implemented and no follow-up imaging is needed. If a mass 3 to 7 mm in greatest vertical height is seen, medical therapy should be implemented, with a repeat scan in 12 to 18 months. If a mass 8 mm or larger in greatest vertical height is seen, radiation therapy should be done and medical therapy used only if clinical hyperadrenocorticism fails to resolve within 3 to 6 months of finishing radiation. No studies have been performed to date to assess the validity of the guidelines.

Therapy for Canine Hyperadrenocorticism

Surgical and medical options exist for treatment of canine and feline hyperadrenocorticism. By whatever means, the ultimate goal of therapy is to eliminate hypersecretion of cortisol. In the United States, medical therapy is most often used for dogs with PDH. In Europe hypophysectomy is available and has been successful.[240,241] For cats with PDH, owing to the limited success of medical therapy, bilateral adrenalectomy may be the treatment of choice, followed by lifelong therapy for hypoadrenocorticism.[242] For dogs and cats with ATs, surgery is recommended.

Mitotane. Currently, there is no drug therapy that will cure PDH. Lifelong therapy should be anticipated. Mitotane, or o,p`-DDD (Lysodren) has long been the mainstay of medical therapy for canine PDH. A chlorinated hydrocarbon, mitotane is adrenocorticolytic, causing selective necrosis of the zona fasciculata and zona reticularis, the adrenocortical zones that secrete cortisol and sex hormones. The toxin is specific for the adrenal glands, particularly hyperplastic glands, with one exception. In normal animals mitotane has caused fatty degeneration and centrolobular atrophy of the liver, and hepatotoxicity secondary to mitotane therapy for hyperadrenocorticism has occurred.[243] Although the disposition of mitotane has not been well characterized in dogs, safety has been studied in a small number of animals. Normal animals tolerated the drug at 50 mg/kg administered 5 days out of 7 for months with no apparent adverse effects. Adrenocortical function was, however, impaired.

Therapy for hyperadrenocorticism with mitotane occurs in two phases: an induction (loading) phase and a maintenance phase. For treatment of PDH, a starting dose of 40 to 50 mg/kg divided twice daily (i.e., 20 to 25 mg/kg twice daily) and administered orally should be used.[244] In smaller dogs division may be impossible because of the 500-mg pill size, and the drug can be given in one dose. Doses higher than 50 mg/kg (administered daily) increase the risk of complete cortisol deficiency.[244] Mitotane should always be given with food because this increases the bioavailability of intact tablets.[245] Loading should end when appetite decreases, vomiting or diarrhea occurs, the patient becomes listless, water intake drops to less than 60 mL/kg daily (1 cup = 240 mL and 1 oz = 30 mL) or for a maximum of 8 days (Figure 21-6). Feeding twice-daily during loading allows better assessment of appetite, which may be the most common early sign that control has been achieved. To closely monitor the patient, best judge the endpoint, and impress on an owner the seriousness of overdosing, the clinician may find it helpful to make daily calls to the owner.[242] When signs suggest that loading is complete or at the end of 8 days if no changes have occurred, adrenal reserve is assessed by ACTH stimulation testing. If the signs of hyperadrenocorticism have not changed, daily therapy can continue until the results of the ACTH stimulation test are known; otherwise, mitotane should be discontinued while awaiting the laboratory report.[242]

The goal of the induction phase is to have serum cortisol concentrations before and after administration of ACTH stimulation in the normal resting range (e.g., cortisol concentration of 30 to 150 nmol/L or 1-5 μg/dL before and after ACTH). Dogs with PDH that continue to have responses to ACTH in the range for normal dogs (e.g., post-ACTH cortisol concentration of 220 to 560 nmol/L or 8 to 20 μg/dL) tend to have ongoing clinical signs. If pre- and post-ACTH cortisol concentrations are within the ideal range, maintenance therapy should begin. If cortisol concentrations are above the desired range, loading should continue for another 5 days or until clinical signs occur that suggest loading has

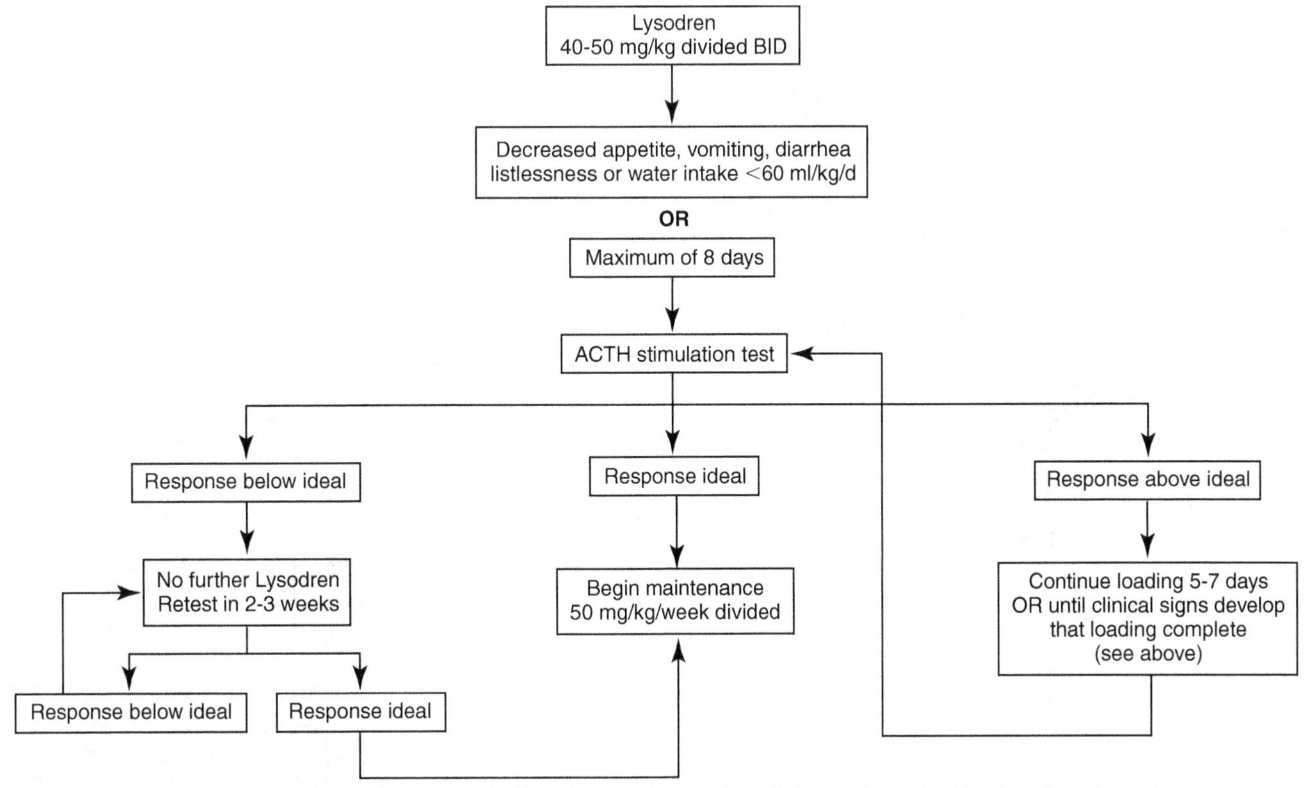

Figure 21-6 Protocol for mitotane induction therapy for canine pituitary-dependent hyperadrenocorticism.

been completed. The mean time required to achieve adequate control is 11 days, but up to 2 months is possible.[244] In general, smaller dogs (<12.5 kg) and those receiving phenobarbital may require greater than average induction times. Approximately 33% of dogs will have a serum cortisol concentration less than ideal (e.g., post-ACTH cortisol concentration <30 nmol/L) after induction; mitotane therapy should be discontinued and an ACTH stimulation test performed after 2 weeks to assess adrenal function. Prednisone should be administered at physiologic doses during that time, but none should be given in the 12 hours before performing an ACTH stimulation test. In most dogs serum cortisol concentrations will rise into the ideal range within 2 to 6 weeks, but up to 18 months may be required.[244]

Special consideration should be given to patients with concomitant hyperadrenocorticism and DM. If a diabetic has insulin resistance secondary to hyperadrenocorticism and requires large doses of insulin for adequate glycemic control, treatment with mitotane removes the cause of insulin resistance and can lead to a rapid decrease in daily insulin requirement. Consequently, insulin overdosage and hypoglycemia may occur if the insulin administration is not adjusted accordingly. To try to slow the return to insulin sensitivity and avoid hypoglycemia, the recommended induction dose for dogs with concurrent hyperadrenocorticism and DM is 25 mg/kg once daily. Furthermore, although administration of prednisone during induction therapy for PDH is discouraged in general by some authors, prednisone (0.4 mg/kg once daily) should be given to diabetics receiving induction phase mitotane, again to help avoid hypoglycemia. Even with these precautions, diabetic patients should be monitored more closely than usual during induction.

Adverse effects of mitotane are generally gastrointestinal or neurologic. One or more adverse effects occur in approximately 25% of dogs with PDH during loading and include weakness, vomiting, anorexia, diarrhea, and ataxia.[244] These develop as serum cortisol concentration falls rapidly and typically resolve quickly with appropriate therapy. If adverse effects occur, mitotane administration should be discontinued. Prednisone should be administered (0.2 to 0.5 mg/kg) until the dog can be examined, an ACTH stimulation test performed, and serum electrolytes measured. Most dogs show a clinical response to glucocorticoid administration within 2 to 3 hours. Persistence of apparent adverse effects may signify the presence of another medical problem.

If a dog does not respond to the induction protocol after 14 days, the following factors that could contribute to mitotane resistance should be considered:[242] (1) The patient may have an AT, which is more resistant to mitotane. (2) The patient may be inherently resistant to mitotane; some dogs with PDH have required as many as 30 to 60 days of daily therapy or doses of 100 to 150 mg/kg daily. (3) The induction dose is too low. Dogs receiving less than 40 mg/kg daily are less likely to be adequately controlled after 10 days. (4) The drug is not being absorbed well. Ensure that the medication is being given with food, preferably a fatty meal. (5) The diagnosis may be incorrect or the patient is suffering from iatrogenic hyperadrenocorticism. Neither an animal with iatrogenic hyperadrenocorticism nor one that does not have hyperadrenocorticism will respond to mitotane. (6) The owner may not be giving the medication as directed.

Maintenance therapy will be necessary for the remainder of the animal's life, although the dose and frequency vary among patients and can vary in an individual patient over time (Figure 21-7). In the absence of maintenance therapy, the

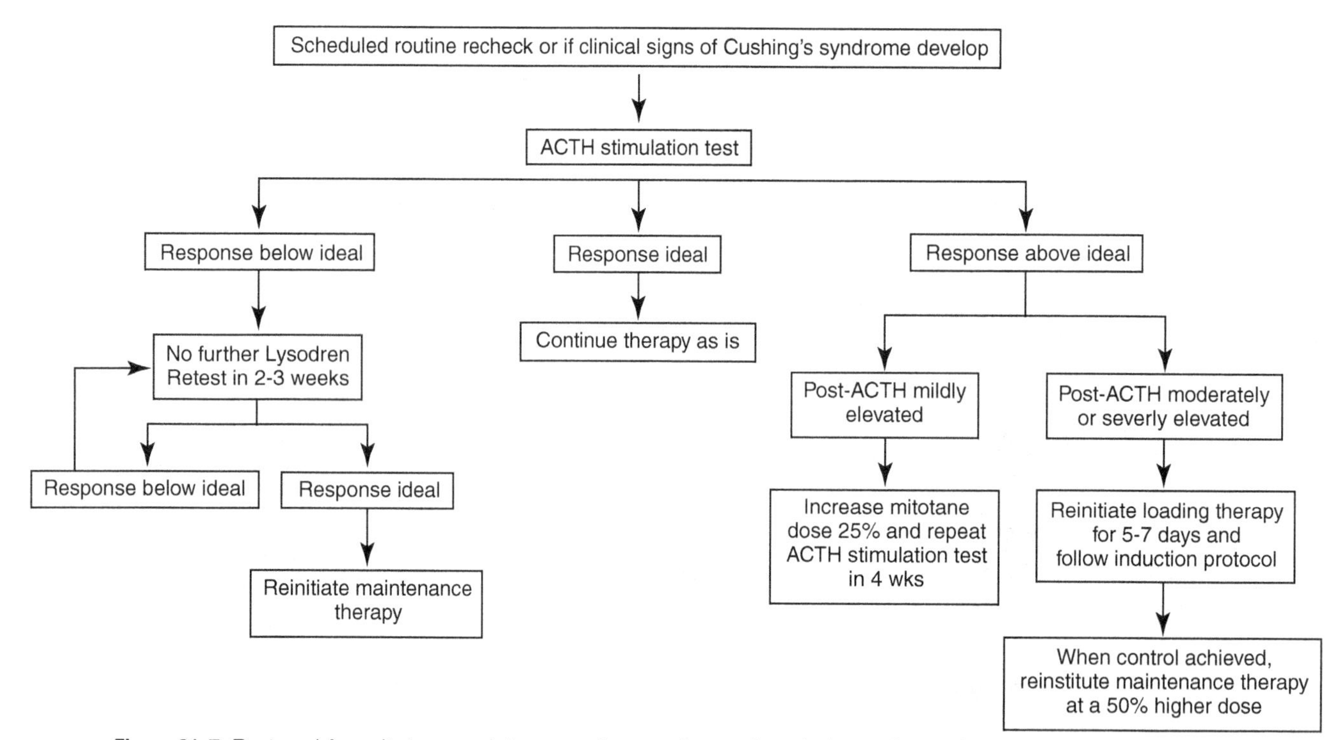

Figure 21-7 Protocol for mitotane maintenance therapy for canine pituitary-dependent hyperadrenocorticism.

adrenal glands will once again become hyperplastic in response to continued ACTH secretion from the pituitary gland. The maintenance phase uses a much lower overall mitotane dose of 50 mg/kg/week orally[244] given as 2 to 3 smaller fractions over the course of the week, if division is possible. Because approximately 60% of dogs with PDH on maintenance mitotane therapy, especially those receiving less than 50 mg/kg weekly, relapse within 12 months of starting therapy,[244] an ACTH stimulation test should be performed 1, 3, and 6 months after initiating maintenance therapy and approximately every 3 to 6 months thereafter to ensure continued control. If the pre- and post-ACTH serum cortisol concentrations are in the ideal range, therapy can remain as is. If the post-ACTH cortisol concentrations is mildly elevated (e.g., 150 to 250 nmol/L or 4-9 µg/dL), the maintenance dose can be increased by 25%, and the dog retested after 1 month to determine if adequate control has been achieved. If so, maintenance therapy should continue at the new dose. If serum cortisol concentrations are still above ideal, reinstitution of daily loading therapy for 5 to 7 days should be considered. If the post-ACTH cortisol concentration is moderately to greatly increased (e.g. greater than 250 nmol/L or 9 µg/dL), loading therapy should be reinstituted for 5 to 7 days. If induction therapy is reinitiated, the decision to end loading should be based on the same clinical signs as during the initial induction phase or should be done for a maximum of 7 days. Once the serum cortisol levels are again within the ideal range, maintenance therapy should be reinstituted at a 50% higher mitotane dosage.[246]

In 184 dogs with PDH treated with mitotane for a mean of 2 years, the final maintenance dosage required ranged from 27 to 330 mg/kg weekly, with the two highest doses required by dogs also receiving phenobarbital. Median survival time was 1.7 years (range 10 days to 8.2 years), with the response judged as excellent in 83%, fair in 16%, and poor in 0.6%.[244]

Approximately 33% of dogs on maintenance mitotane therapy will develop adverse effects including anorexia, vomiting, weakness, diarrhea, and ataxia, typically shortly after initiation of the maintenance dosage or during periods of relapse when daily therapy is reinstituted. If these develop, mitotane therapy should be discontinued, physiologic doses of prednisone administered, an ACTH stimulation test performed, and serum electrolyte concentrations measured. Presence of glucocorticoid deficiency with or without mineralocorticoid deficiency can be documented using these tests and differentiated from direct drug toxicity. If the clinical signs are due either to a hypoadrenal state or to a direct effect of mitotane, they should resolve quickly with prednisone administration. If the signs do not abate, presence of a nonadrenal illness should be suspected. If glucocorticoid deficiency is documented (e.g., before and after ACTH serum cortisol concentration <30 nmol/L or 1 µg/dL), mitotane therapy should be discontinued and physiologic prednisone replacement therapy continued until serum cortisol concentrations before and after ACTH increase into the ideal range, which usually requires 2 to 6 weeks. Complete mineralocorticoid and glucocorticoid deficiency is seen in approximately 6% dogs from 1 month to years after initiation of maintenance therapy and is usually permanent.[244] If mineralocorticoid and glucocorticoid deficiency is present, the patient needs to be treated for hypoadrenocorticism. Appearance of neurologic signs such as disorientation, dullness, or inappetence may be due to direct drug toxicity or may suggest the presence of a pituitary macroadenoma; CT or MRI is required to confirm the presence of a large tumor. Mitotane dose reduction may be necessary for animals that develop adverse reactions or an alternate dosing scheme can be used (e.g., the dose may be divided into smaller amounts to be given more frequently during the course of the week).

If therapy for hyperadrenocorticism is successful, most clinical signs of the disease or its complications resolve over time. Polyuria, polydipsia, and polyphagia should resolve as soon as cortisol secretion is adequately controlled. Resolution of some clinical signs (e.g., skin manifestations, nonhealing wounds, anestrus) may take 3 to 6 months or longer; calcinosis cutis may never fully resolve. Development of a puppy coat or a change in hair color may occur with mitotane treatment. Resolution of clinical laboratory changes (i.e., elevated liver enzyme activities and serum cholesterol concentration) may take up to 18 months.

An alternative protocol for treating PDH is aimed at nonselective adrenocorticolysis and complete destruction of adrenocortical tissue, with substitution therapy for ensuing adrenocortical insufficiency. Mitotane is given for 25 days at a dosage of 50 to 75 mg/kg daily and up to 100 mg/kg daily for toy breeds, divided into 3 or 4 approximately equal and equally spaced portions and given with food. Lifelong glucocorticoid and mineralocorticoid substitution is begun on the third day of mitotane administration. Prednisone should be initiated at a temporarily high dose of 1 mg/kg twice daily. Fludrocortisone (0.0125 mg/kg daily) and sodium chloride (0.1 mg/kg/day, divided over 2 or 3 meals) should also be administered.[216]

During the first month, owners should report by telephone at least weekly and as problems arise and should stop mitotane administration if any inappetence develops.[216] In this regimen appetite change, if seen, is a direct toxic effect of the medication; mild cortisol deficiency is offset by the glucocorticoid replacement therapy and should not cause any adverse effects. If mitotane therapy continues despite a diminished appetite, a hypoadrenocortical crisis can ensue. Glucocorticoid dosage may be increased temporarily if appetite diminishes. Usually, mitotane can be resumed after 4 or 5 days when the appetite returns without further problem.[216]

The first follow-up visit should be 1 week after completion of mitotane administration. Serum electrolytes should be measured to ascertain whether the fludrocortisone and salt doses are correct.[216] Performance of an ACTH stimulation test may be wise to ensure adequate control of the Cushing's syndrome. The original protocol recommends that patients be treated for hypoadrenocorticism with prednisone (1 mg/kg daily, divided either in 2 equal portions or two thirds in the morning and one third in the evening), fludrocortisone at a dosage that maintains normal serum electrolyte concentrations, and salt.[216] However, salt may not be necessary; lower prednisone and fludrocortisone doses may be sufficient (discussed later). Furthermore, DOCP may be used as an alternative to fludrocortisone.

The protocol was assessed in 129 dogs.[247] In 30% of the dogs, mitotane administration had to be stopped temporarily because of the development of anorexia, vomiting, weakness, neurologic abnormalities, depression, and diarrhea, but it could be resumed within days (median 7 days, range 1 to 63). Convincing signs of partial or complete remission of the hyperadrenocorticism such as hair regrowth, decreased water intake and appetite, and diminished abdominal size were noted in 86%. Relapse occurred in 33%; the median disease-free interval (time until recurrence, death, or last follow-up) was 450 days from the day therapy began (range 25 to 1885).[247] Adrenal testing (i.e., ACTH stimulation) is recommended only if clinical signs of hyperadrenocorticism recur, but routine measurement of serum urea nitrogen and electrolyte concentrations is required to ensure adequate control of the hypoadrenocorticism. Median survival time was 1.6 years (range 1 day to 6.1 years).[247] In another study that used a daily mitotane dose of 75 to 100 mg/kg daily in 46 dogs, median survival was approximately 2 years. Although recurrence rate of hyperadrenocorticism was only 29%, perhaps owing to a higher mitotane dose, 15 dogs suffered an Addisonian crisis at some point during therapy. Overall incidence of side effects was 24%.[248]

Although treatment of hypoadrenocorticism may appear easier than that of hyperadrenocorticism, two main disadvantages exist for the alternative protocol, and its use has not been strongly recommended. First, treatment of an Addisonian dog can be expensive, and mineralocorticoid with or without glucocorticoid replacement therapy will be required for life. Second, and more important, failure to give medication to an Addisonian patient can be fatal, whereas missing a dose of mitotane will not put a patient in life-threatening danger.[242]

If an AT is being treated, the mitotane protocol used is different from that for PDH; the goal is complete destruction of tumor tissue with serum cortisol concentrations before and after ACTH below the normal resting range (e.g., <10 nmol/L or 0.3 μg/dL on both samples).[249] Although approximately 20% of dogs with ATs respond to PDH induction protocols, higher induction dosages and longer induction times are generally required for control of an AT.[250,251] The cumulative induction dose of mitotane for PDH is usually 400 to 500 mg/kg, whereas that for dogs with an AT is often up to 10 times higher.[250]Thus initial mitotane induction dosage for treatment of an AT is 50 to 75 mg/kg daily. Because the goal is complete destruction of glucocorticoid-secreting tissue, physiologic doses of prednisone should be administered concurrently.[250] The same clinical signs can be used to judge the endpoint of induction as when treating PDH, with a maximum treatment span of 14 days. At the conclusion of a loading period, an ACTH stimulation test should be performed (Figure 21-8).

If a partial response is seen but adequate control has not been achieved (i.e., pre- and post-ACTH cortisol concentration are lower than before treatment but not in the ideal range), mitotane should be continued at the same dosage and an ACTH stimulation test repeated every 10 to 14 days until serum cortisol concentrations fall within the ideal range. If after the initial loading dose the ACTH response is unaltered, the daily mitotane dosage should be increased in 50 mg/kg increments daily every 10 to 14 days as necessary, until an ACTH stimulation test demonstrates a response to the medication or drug intolerance occurs. Therapy is then continued at the dosage at which a response was seen or at the highest tolerated dosage, and ACTH stimulation testing is again performed every 10 to 14 days or if clinical signs suggest an endpoint

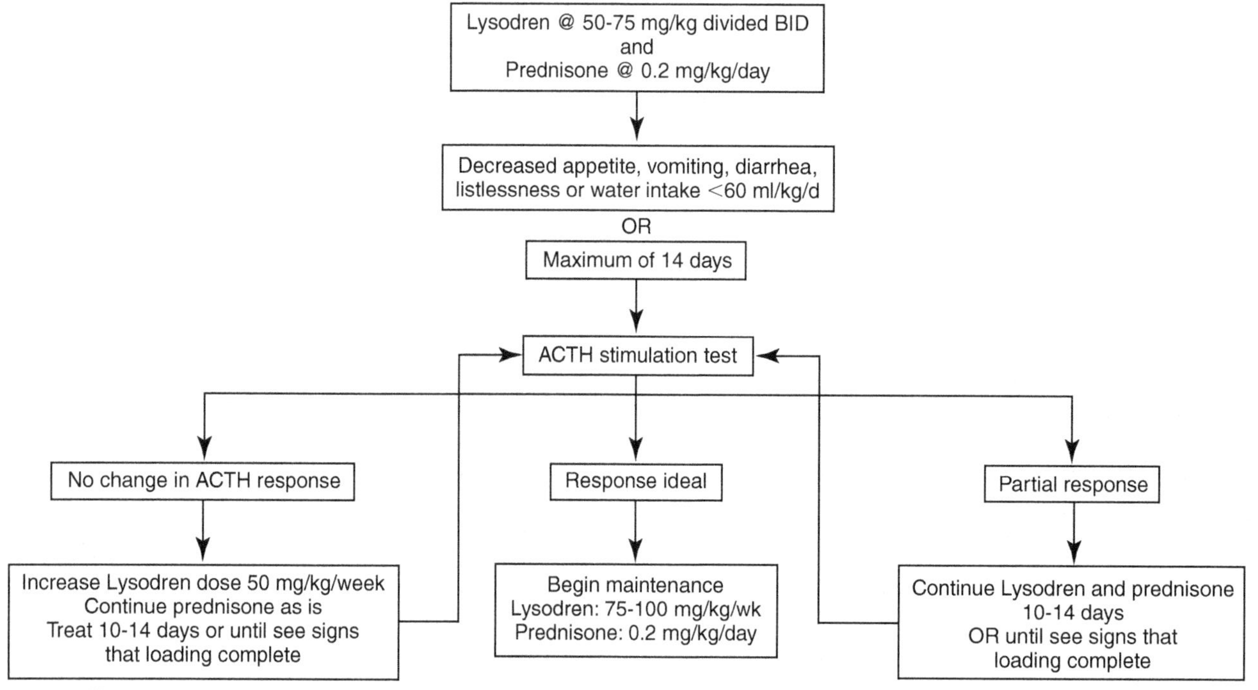

Figure 21-8 Protocol for mitotane induction therapy for canine adrenal-dependent hyperadrenocorticism.

has been reached. In 31 dogs with an AT, total induction time ranged from 10 days to 11 weeks with a mean of 24 days.[250]

Once cortisol concentrations before and after ACTH administration are within the ideal range, maintenance therapy should begin at an initial mitotane dosage of 75-100 mg/kg/week.[250] Daily physiological doses of prednisone should also be administered, as these dogs have subnormal basal serum cortisol concentrations. An ACTH stimulation test should be performed after 1 month of maintenance therapy to determine whether serum cortisol concentrations have remained adequately suppressed. If pre- or post-ACTH cortisol levels are within the normal resting range (i.e., 10 to 160 nmol/L or 1 to 4 μg/dL), the mitotane maintenance dose should be increased 50% and the dog retested in 1 month. If the cortisol levels are still above the resting range at that time, induction therapy should be reinstituted; once ideal cortisol levels are again achieved, maintenance should be restarted at a 50% higher dosage than previously used. An ACTH stimulation test should again be performed 1 month after a dose adjustment to assess control (Figure 21-9). Once ongoing successful therapy is documented, an ACTH stimulation test should be done every 3 to 6 months or if clinical signs recur. Relapse occurs during maintenance in approximately 66% of cases, usually because of either too low an initial maintenance dose or tumor growth.[250]

As are induction doses, maintenance doses required for adequate control of an AT are higher than for PDH. In 32 dogs with an AT, the final mean maintenance dose required was 159 mg/kg weekly, slightly more than double the average maintenance dose required to control PDH. Approximately 25% of dogs with ATs require maintenance doses greater than 150 mg/kg weekly. Adverse effects, as previously described, occur in approximately 60% of dogs with ATs treated with mitotane. They can develop as long as 16 months after initiation of therapy, are more common during the maintenance rather than the induction phase, and are due either to direct toxicity of medication or to adrenocortical insufficiency, with the former being approximately twice as likely.[250]

If severe side effects occur, mitotane should be stopped, the prednisone dose increased to 0.4 mg/kg daily, and the dog reevaluated as soon as possible with an ACTH stimulation test and measurement of serum electrolyte concentrations to determine whether complete mineralocorticoid and glucocorticoid deficiency exists. If serum electrolytes are normal but pre- and post-ACTH serum cortisol concentrations are below 10 nmol/L, it is likely that only glucocorticoids are deficient. Mitotane therapy should be restarted, and prednisone administration continued at a dosage of 0.4 mg/kg daily to exclude cortisol deficiency as the cause of the side effects. If adverse effects recur when mitotane is reinstituted despite an increased glucocorticoid dosage, direct drug toxicity is likely. If the adverse effects are due to the mitotane, its administration can be temporarily discontinued and then reinstituted at a 25% to 50% lower dosage once signs of toxicosis have resolved. If hyponatremia, hyperkalemia, and subnormal cortisol concentrations are present, both mineralocorticoids and glucocorticoids are deficient. Loss of both types of adrenocortical hormones is likely to be permanent. Replacement therapy for both hormones should be instituted, and mitotane should not be administered until adrenal recovery can be documented by an ACTH stimulation test.

Treatment of AT with mitotane can provide good results. Of 32 dogs with an AT treated with mitotane, 66%, 28%, and 6% were judged by their owners to have a good to excellent, fair, and poor response, respectively. Mitotane does not appear to arrest metastatic tumor growth, and the response in dogs without evidence of metastatic disease is better than that in dogs with metastases. Mean survival time of dogs with ATs treated with mitotane is approximately 16 months, with a reported range of 20 days to 5.1 years.[250]

Ketoconazole. Ketoconazole is a triazole antifungal drug widely used for the treatment of disseminated fungal diseases. The drug inhibits cytochrome P450 enzymes responsible for synthesis of gonadal and adrenal steroids and has been used to treat hyperadrenocorticism in people. In addition, ketoconazole may antagonize glucocorticoid receptors. In normal dogs

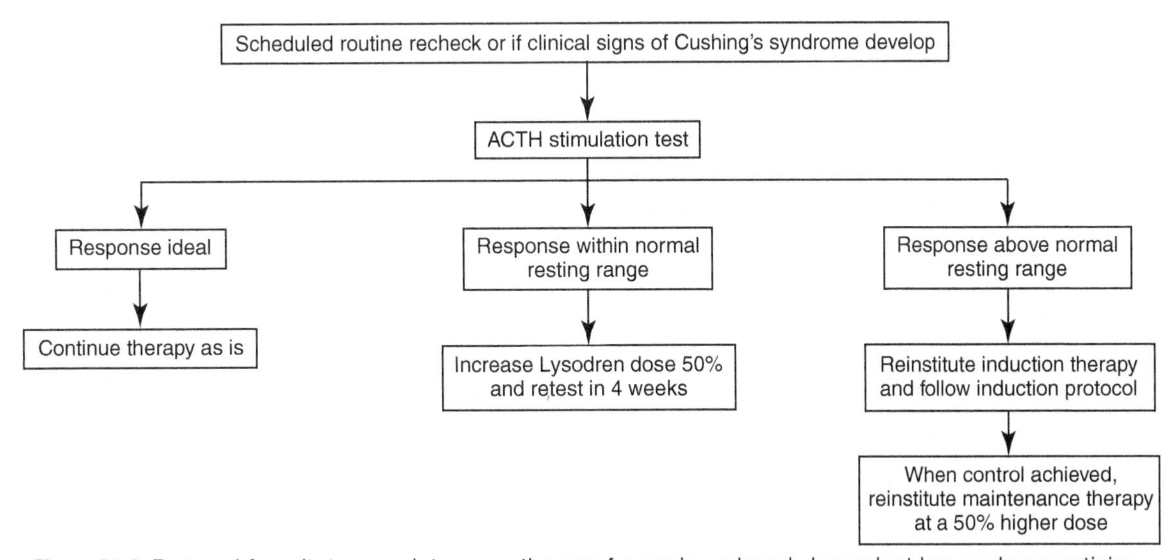

Figure 21-9 Protocol for mitotane maintenance therapy for canine adrenal-dependent hyperadrenocorticism.

ketoconazole administration decreases serum cortisol and testosterone, but not mineralocorticoid, concentrations.[252,253]

Dosing of ketoconazole should be initiated at 5 mg/kg orally twice daily for 7 days, a low dosage to allow an evaluation period for development of side effects such as gastroenteritis or hepatitis. Light feeding may ameliorate gastritis resulting from ketoconazole administration. If no ill effects are observed during the first week, the dosage should be increased to 10 mg/kg orally twice daily for 14 days, after which an ACTH stimulation test should be performed. The ideal ranges for serum cortisol concentrations before and after ACTH administration are the same as when mitotane is used. If serum cortisol concentrations are above ideal, the ketoconazole dosage should be increased to 15 mg/kg orally twice daily and the dog monitored every 14 to 60 days.[254] Dosages equal to or greater than 20 mg/kg twice daily may be required.[255,256] If no response is seen or the disease progresses despite therapy, ketoconazole should be discontinued and alternative therapy begun.

The efficacy of ketoconazole may be less than that of mitotane. After ketoconazole therapy, basal and post-ACTH cortisol concentrations may actually be higher than those pretreatment in some dogs.[242] Of 132 veterinary internists and dermatologists surveyed, specialists likely to treat Cushing's syndrome, 52% considered ketoconazole to be effective in less than 25% of cases, 19% reported effectiveness in 25% to 49% of cases, and 14% each believed ketoconazole to be efficacious in 50% to 74% and 75% to 100% of cases.[256] A recent report suggested a higher efficacy of 70% in 48 dogs,[257] but the follow-up on treated dogs was inconsistent and the ideal post-ACTH cortisol concentration was not as low as recommended by most authors. Thus, although ketoconazole may lower serum cortisol concentration in dogs with PDH and clinical improvement can be seen,[254,257] whether therapy is truly adequate in such a high percentage is unclear.

Ketoconazole appears to be relatively safe, with a low incidence of side effects. When seen, adverse effects may include anorexia, vomiting, elevated liver enzymes, diarrhea, and icterus.[256,257] Side effects believed to occur secondary to ketoconazole administration in a small number of cases include depression; weakness; lethargy and trembling; liver failure; polyuria and polydipsia; thrombocytopenia; and dermatologic changes such as altered coat color, poor coat condition, and scaling.[256] Lightening of the hair coat may also occur. The effect of ketoconazole on reproductive status has not been addressed, but it does decrease testosterone synthesis in healthy dogs[252] and should be used cautiously in male dogs intended for breeding.

Despite possibly limited efficacy and high cost compared with mitotane, ketoconazole therapy may occasionally be warranted. First, ketoconazole can be used in dogs that cannot tolerate mitotane. Second, it may be used as a diagnostic aid when the diagnosis of hyperadrenocorticism is unclear. If an ACTH stimulation test shows that ketoconazole therapy has adequately controlled cortisol secretion, then any clinical signs present that were caused by hyperadrenocorticism should resolve. If the disease is placed in remission and the diagnosis thus confirmed, mitotane treatment can be initiated instead. If no resolution of clinical signs is seen, hyperadrenocorticism can be ruled out as a diagnosis and ketoconazole discontinued. Ketoconazole provides a better alternative to trial therapy than mitotane or trilostane because the adrenolytic effects of mitotane or trilostane may be irreversible, whereas cortisol levels normalize within 24 hours of discontinuing ketoconazole.[254] Third, because ATs may be mitotane-resistant or the high doses of mitotane required to treat an AT may cause unacceptable side effects, ketoconazole may be used for medical treatment of ATs or before an adrenalectomy to prepare the patient for surgery. However, no study has evaluated ketoconazole efficacy in a large number of dogs with ATs.

Bromocriptine and selegiline. Dopamine clearly affects ACTH secretion from the pituitary; both elevated dopamine levels and dopamine agonism suppress ACTH secretion, at least from the intermediate lobe of the pituitary. Thus increasing dopamine concentrations or activity may inhibit ACTH oversecretion (Figure 21-10) and be useful for treatment of PDH. Raising dopamine levels can be effective only for PDH, however. Because endogenous ACTH secretion is suppressed in patients with an AT, dopamine agonism or alteration of dopamine metabolism would have little, if any, further effect on ACTH release. Moreover, because ATs function autonomously of ACTH, lowering ACTH levels would not alter cortisol secretion.

Bromocriptine, a dopamine agonist, has met with limited success for treating PDH. In one study bromocriptine was administered to seven dogs with PDH,[258] and 40 dogs were included in another.[259] Vomiting was a limiting side effect and cause for treatment discontinuation in a large proportion, and only 1 of the 47 responded clinically. Thus bromocriptine is not recommended for treatment of canine PDH.

Monoamine oxidase inhibitors, including selegiline (l-deprenyl), inhibit degradation of biogenic amines, most notably dopamine, and are used to treat dopamine-deficient conditions such as human Parkinson's disease. Unlike other monoamine oxidase inhibitors, selegiline is specific for cerebral forms (i.e., monoamine oxidase B). An important question in treating canine PDH, however, is whether the ACTH-lowering effect of dopamine is on the anterior or intermediate lobe of the pituitary (or both). If dopamine inhibits only intermediate lobe ACTH secretion, as is generally believed, then selegiline use would be efficacious only in cases of PDH caused by intermediate lobe tumors (i.e., approximately 20% of canine PDH cases). Indeed, one study of 10 dogs suggested a 20% response rate.[260] Unfortunately, only histopathology can differentiate anterior and pituitary lobe tumors. Furthermore, a more recent study found selegiline to be ineffective for treatment of PDH.[261]

If selegiline is used to treat PDH, as with other drugs, therapy must be for the lifetime of the animal.[262] Treatment should begin at 1 mg/kg orally once daily for 30 days. If no response is seen, the dose should be doubled for an additional 30 days. Failure to respond at that time indicates the need for an alternative therapy. Selegiline therapy is relatively safe. Side effects are uncommon and usually mild, including vomiting, diarrhea, and ptyalism.[260,261] Severe neurologic disturbances

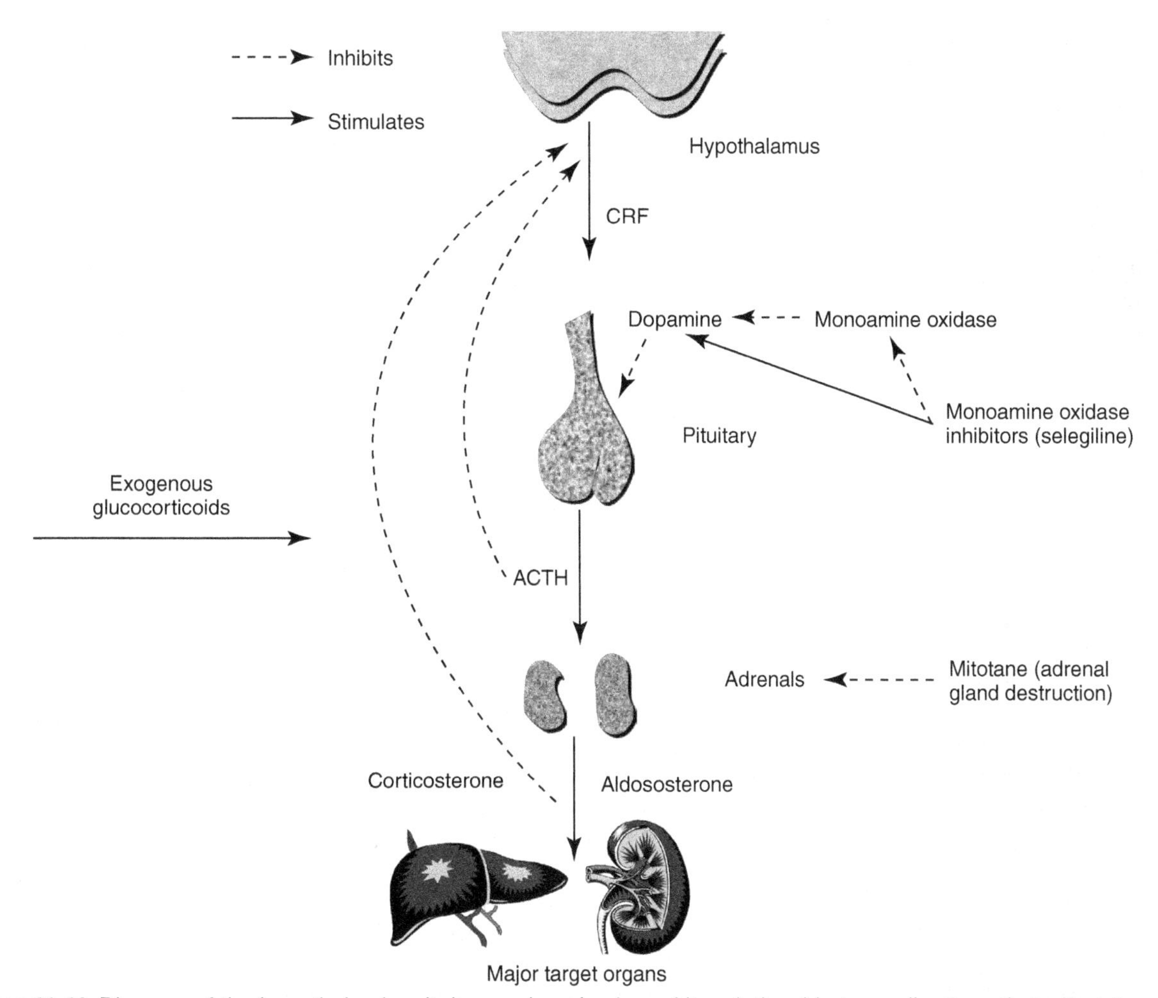

Figure 21-10 Diagram of the hypothalamic–pituitary–adrenal axis and its relationship to medications that affect the axis.

and pancreatitis possibly have been caused by selegiline therapy,[260] but the neurologic problems also may have been due to the presence of a large pituitary mass. Chronic selegiline therapy does not result in glucocorticoid insufficiency[263] and, based on its mechanism of action, would not be expected to affect aldosterone secretion. One disadvantage of selegiline is cost. Several generic versions are available, but although the bioequivalency of the generic preparations is the same among themselves, they are less bioavailable than the original product, l-deprenyl (Eldepryl); comparisons with the animal product Anipryl are not available. Thus, it may be wise to avoid the generic products until studies have established the appropriate canine dose. Another disadvantage of using selegiline for treating PDH is that monitoring of efficacy is based solely on relatively subjective findings. The results of the ACTH stimulation test do not change while dogs are receiving selegiline. Thus other objective measures of effect, such as quantification of water intake or measurement of urine specific gravity, should be used.

In general, use of selegiline to treat PDH is not recommended because of its low efficacy, but it could be tried in dogs with PDH that cannot tolerate mitotane and trilostane or as a diagnostic aid, as with ketoconazole. However, trial therapy with selegiline would be hard to judge. The sole measure by which to judge efficacy of therapy is resolution of clinical signs. If an animal does not respond clinically, it would be impossible to tell if the dog did not have hyperadrenocorticism or had an AT or l-deprenyl–resistant PDH. With ketoconazole therapy the ACTH stimulation test provides an objective measure of when adequate biochemical control has been achieved. If cortisol secretion is suppressed by ketoconazole and clinical signs continue, the diagnosis of hyperadrenocorticism can be ruled out.

Trilostane. Trilostane (Vetoryl) has been used to treat hyperadrenocorticism for a number of years in Europe and is now approved by the Food and Drug Administration for treatment of canine hyperadrenocorticism in the United States. A synthetic steroid analog that inhibits the adrenal enzyme 3β-hydroxysteroid dehydrogenase, trilostane suppresses production of progesterone and its end products, including cortisol and aldosterone. Additional enzymes such as 11β-hydroxylase and 11β-hydroxysteroid dehydrogenase may also be affected.[264] Trilostane appears to be highly effective in suppressing cortisol secretion and controlling clinical signs in the majority of patients.[248,265-270] As with mitotane, clinical signs of hyperadrenocorticism typically quickly resolve with control of cortisol concentrations, but certain ones such as dermatologic abnormalities can take up to 3 months. Other abnormalities such as calcinosis cutis or pseudomyotonia may not fully resolve. However, a small proportion of dogs with PDH (<10%) are not well controlled with trilostane.[267,270,271]

Trilostane is available as 10-, 30- and 60-mg capsules in the United States and may need to be compounded for smaller dogs. In approximately 50% of dogs, dosage adjustments, either up or down, will be required during the course of treatment. Authors of one study noted that in most dogs an initial sensitivity to the drug existed followed by a need for a dose increase. After time, the dose required often hit a plateau.[267] Interestingly, the final dose required for control has varied greatly between studies. Part of the discrepancy may relate to the differences in what was considered the ideal post-ACTH serum cortisol concentration. However, in one study the median final dose was 6.1 mg/kg,[270] and in another study it was 16 to 19 mg/kg.[267] In any case, each dog should be started on the recommended dose, and then the dose should be adjusted according to ACTH stimulation test results. The duration of survival is at least as good as that achieved with mitotane therapy.[268]

Reported adverse effects for the most part are relatively mild, including lethargy and vomiting, but fatality has occurred.[267,270,271] Although some studies found relatively low incidence of side effects, one non–peer-reviewed report described mild, self-limiting side effects such as diarrhea, vomiting, and lethargy in 63% of treated dogs.[272] Safety has not been evaluated in lactating dogs and males intended for breeding. Trilostane should not be given to pregnant females.

As with mitotane therapy, excessive adrenal gland suppression can occur and warrants discontinuing medication temporarily (discussed later) and lowering the dose. Trilostane can affect aldosterone secretion as well as cortisol, so a hypoadrenocortical crisis can occur. Caution should be used in administering trilostane with an angiotensin-converting enzyme inhibitor or an aldosterone antagonist (e.g., spironolactone) because the suppressive effect on serum aldosterone concentration may be cumulative.

Although, in theory, the effects of trilostane as an enzyme inhibitor should be rapidly reversible (e.g., within a couple days), suppression can last weeks to years.[266,267,273] One dog developed hypocortisolism after only 3 doses of trilostane; glucocorticoid replacement therapy was needed for at least 1 year.[273] Surprisingly, adrenal necrosis can occur secondary to trilostane administration as well.[274] The hypoadrenocorticism reported after complete adrenocortical necrosis in one dog lasted for at least 3 months but likely would be permanent.[274] How often acute iatrogenic hypoadrenocorticism will occur in dogs treated with trilostane is unknown but is likely more common than originally believed. In one study four of six dogs with PDH and one of one with AT treated with trilostane had some degree of adrenal necrosis at necropsy. In two dogs the damage was sufficiently severe to cause hypoadrenocorticism. Both dogs had received therapy with mitotane before trilostane but had been on trilostane for 15 and 22 months.[275] Thus the contribution of each drug is unclear. Adrenal rupture, possibly secondary to adrenal necrosis, may have occurred (see Vetoryl package insert).

Current guidelines are for a lower starting dose than previously recommended. The package insert states that therapy should be initiated at 2.2 to 6.7 mg/kg once daily with food. These authors recommend starting as close to the low end of the range as possible. If minor side effects are seen, drug administration should be stopped for 3 to 5 days until side effects resolve and then restarted, giving trilostane every other day for 1 week before continuing with the initial dosing scheme. It is important to differentiate minor adverse effects from hypocortisolism, and ACTH stimulation testing may be needed.

Postpill timing is crucial for dogs receiving trilostane, and the test should be initiated at 4 to 6 hours after the pill was administered. Keeping the timing consistent for each patient may also be important. The first scheduled recheck should be after 10 to 14 days of therapy. Lately, recommendations are being made to not increase the trilostane dose for at least 4 weeks after initiating therapy. An initial ACTH stimulation test should be performed after 10-14 days of therapy to ensure hypocortisolemia is not present. If at any time the post-ACTH cortisol concentration is below 40 nmol/L (1.45 μg/dL), the trilostane should be suspended and restarted at a decreased dose after 3 to 7 days (see package insert) or, ideally in the authors' opinion, after recovery of adrenocortical function has been demonstrated. At the 2-week recheck, the dose should only be raised in cases where the owner reports that no improvement has been seen, the clinical signs are still striking, and the post-ACTH cortisol concentration is markedly above ideal. Then, in such cases at 2 weeks or if waiting until the 4-week recheck, if the post-ACTH cortisol concentration is 40 to 150 nmol/L (1.45-5.4 μg/dL), the dose should continue as is. If the post-ACTH cortisol is 150 to 250 nmol/L (5.4-9.1 μg/dL), the dose can be continued if the dog is doing well clinically; if not, twice-daily therapy should be used. The same dose that was given once daily should be given twice (e.g., if the regimen is 60 mg once daily, it can be doubled to 60 mg twice daily), or a lower dose can be given in the evening (e.g., from 60 mg once daily to 60 mg in the morning and 30 mg in the evening). If the post-ACTH serum cortisol concentration is above 250 nmol/L (9.1 μg/dL), the trilostane dose should be increased. An ACTH stimulation test should be performed 10 to 14 days after every dose adjustment. Once the clinical condition of the dog and the dose have stabilized, an ACTH stimulation test should be performed 30 and 90 days later and then every 3 months thereafter. Size of dosage adjustment, either up or down, will likely be dictated by available capsule size but ideally should be approximately 25%.

Despite recommendations in the package insert for once-daily dosing, trilostane may begin to lose effectiveness 8 to 10 hours after the pill is given.[265,276,277] Indeed, trilostane has been administered twice daily.[248,265,266] In one study of 44 dogs with PDH, the initial dose of trilostane was 15 mg orally twice daily for dogs less than 5 kg, 30 mg twice daily for dogs 5 to 20 kg, 60 mg in the morning and 30 mg in the evening for dogs 20 to 40 kg, and 60 mg twice daily for dogs larger than 40 kg. At the first recheck (day 7), an ACTH stimulation test was performed starting at 4 to 6 hours after the pill was given. Good control was judged on the basis of clinical signs and a serum cortisol concentration before and after ACTH administration of 30 to 110 nmol/L. Dose was adjusted in 25% to 50% increments. On further rechecks, the ACTH stimulation test was initiated 8 to 12 hours after the pill was given. Good control was believed to be a post-ACTH cortisol concentration of 30 to 250 nmol/L.[266]

Mean initial dose of trilostane was 6.2 mg/kg (range 2.4 to 15) divided into twice-daily doses. The dose was not changed over the course of the study in 10 dogs, increased in 19, reduced in 5, and both increased and reduced at different times in 10. At all rechecks the mean dose was between 6 and 8 mg/kg divided into twice-daily doses, but the range was approximately 2 to 20. Adverse reactions were seen in 25% of cases related to low cortisol concentration. In 11% trilostane therapy was discontinued because of prolonged suppression of serum cortisol concentration. In four dogs adrenal function returned to normal and no further treatment was needed; one dog was treated as an Addisonian.[266]Another study using the same protocol found high efficacy with relatively few side effects, and survival times were longer compared with those of dogs treated with a nonselective adrenocorticolytic protocol.[248]

Special consideration should be given to twice-daily dosing in dogs in which breaks in control of the hyperadrenocorticism could be detrimental (e.g., in dogs with concurrent DM or dogs with pulmonary thromboembolism secondary to hyperadrenocorticism). The recommended starting dose is 1 mg/kg twice-daily. If using twice-daily therapy, although one study recommended performing an ACTH stimulation test 8-12 hrs post-pill,[266] such timing has not been critically evaluated.

An early paper suggested that monitoring of the urine cortisol:creatinine ratio (UCCR) before a trilostane dose could be an indication of duration of action.[261] However, two studies yielded conflicting results. In 22 dogs with HAC, a morning UCCR pre-dose was lower in dogs with good control compared to those with poor control (14.8 vs. 47.5); however, overlap existed between the 2 groups.[265] On the other hand, in 18 PDH dogs, the UCCR was measured in samples collected before or 6 hours after trilostane administration; a pair of urine samples was collected once weekly for 4 weeks. Although basal UCCRs were significantly higher than the 6-hour values, neither the basal nor the 6-hour samples were significantly different between dogs with adequate vs. inadequate control. Post-ACTH cortisol concentrations did not correlate with UCCR. Basal UCCRs in 13 dogs and 6 hours post-trilostane UCCRs in 12 were still above the reference range 8 weeks after the dose was judged to be optimal.[265a]

Interestingly, in one study, of 6 dogs that had UCCRs within the reference range most of the times, three developed hypocortisolism and in three hypocortisolism was suspected based on clinical signs but was not confirmed. The hypocortisolism was documented or suspected between 16 weeks and 21 months after the trilostane dose was judged to be optimal.[265a]

How best to switch a dog from mitotane to trilostane is unknown. According to the Vetoryl package insert, a post-ACTH cortisol concentration should be above 250 nmol/L (9.1 μg/dL) before giving trilostane. It may be ideal to wait at least 30 days after discontinuing mitotane, but if the clinical signs of hyperadrenocorticism are severe, trilostane can be started sooner as long as the post-ACTH cortisol concentration is high enough. Dogs previously treated with mitotane may have greater response to trilostane, so careful monitoring of adrenal function is required.

Trilostane has been used to treat five dogs with ATs.[278-280] Insufficient information is available to ascertain whether the treatment protocol or efficacy varies if treating dogs with PDH versus those with an AT. One dog did receive a maximum dose of 17.2 mg/kg.[280] Clinical signs were controlled, at least transiently, and survival prolonged. Survival in one dog was only 117 days.[278] In the other four dogs survival was at least 10 to 18 months; interestingly, in three trilostane therapy was initiated when an AT accompanied by pulmonary metastases was identified.[279,280] Response of ATs to trilostane, at least in these five dogs, compares favorably to that achieved with mitotane. However, in dogs with ATs mitotane theoretically may be the preferred treatment. Mitotane is truly a chemotherapeutic drug in this instance, killing primary neoplastic cells and, perhaps, metastatic cells as well. Trilostane simply would control tumoral secretion, not growth. In fact, in dogs with PDH and in one dog with an AT treated with trilostane, the size of the adrenal glands increased.[275,281]

Retinoic acid. 9-*cis* Retinoic acid has been used to treat a total of 27 dogs with PDH in two studies. Unfortunately, endogenous ACTH and α-melanocyte-stimulating hormone concentrations and UCCR were used to evaluate treatment, which makes the results difficult to interpret insofar as these tests are not typically used to monitor therapy. Interestingly, pituitary tumor size significantly decreased in 14 dogs that were treated for 180 days.[282,283] Although results were promising, much more work is necessary before retinoic acid therapy can be recommended, especially when proven therapies such as mitotane or trilostane are available. In addition, retinoic acid at the doses used in the study would likely be cost prohibitive to most owners.

Therapy for Feline Hyperadrenocorticism

Hypercortisolism. Medical therapy for feline classic hyperadrenocorticism (i.e., excessive cortisol as compared to excess of other adrenocortical hormones), appears not to be as successful as in dogs; however, very little information has been published. Unilateral adrenalectomy is the treatment of choice for an AT. Given the limited success of medical therapy, some authors believe bilateral adrenalectomy with subsequent lifelong therapy for hypoadrenocorticism is the treatment of choice for feline PDH. However, cats with severe hyperadrenocorticism may not be good surgical candidates because of the debilitating effects of the disease (e.g., thin skin, immunosuppression, poor wound healing), and medical control for stabilization before surgery would be ideal. Although not available in the United States, transsphenoidal hypophysectomy has been reported for treatment of PDH in seven cats.[284] Radiation therapy may be effective for aiding in the control of feline PDH.[285] (See also the section on acromegaly later in this chapter.)

Early reports suggested mitotane was not highly effective in cats at doses of 25 mg/kg or 50 mg/kg for up to 90 days,[286-288] but one case report suggested that mitotane therapy may be successful with higher doses and longer induction periods. A cat was treated with mitotane at 25 mg/kg once daily for 18 days with little effect. At 69 days, after a dose increase to 37.5 mg/kg once daily, there was still minimal effect, but by day 111 the hyperadrenocorticism was controlled.[289]

In one cat with an adrenocortical carcinoma, ketoconazole caused transient (3.5 months) resolution of polyuria and polydipsia and a reduction in the insulin dose required to control concurrent DM. Interestingly, although basal serum cortisol concentrations decreased during treatment, adrenocortical response to ACTH stimulation was not altered.[290] Other mechanisms of action of ketoconazole, such as antagonism of glucocorticoid receptors, may account for the clinical improvement, or it may have been coincidental. In four other cats with hyperadrenocorticism, two responded to ketoconazole doses of 5 mg/kg twice daily for 7 days, followed by 10 mg/kg twice daily indefinitely; one had no response after 2 months; and one developed severe thrombocytopenia after 7 days of treatment, necessitating withdrawal of therapy.[291]

Metyrapone affects cortisol synthesis by inhibiting the adrenal enzyme 11-β-hydroxylase. Clinical response without side effects other than hypoglycemia has been achieved in six cats using 30 to 70 mg/kg twice daily.[288,292,293] In two cats treated with an unknown dose, one had a slight clinical improvement (partial hair regrowth and slight resolution of polyuria and polydipsia) after 6 months, whereas the other showed no improvement after 1 month.[294] Although doses as high as 65 mg/kg three times daily have been used, a maximum of 70 mg/kg twice daily has been recommended to avoid gastrointestinal complications.[288] The ACTH stimulation test should be used to ensure adequate control of cortisol secretion with the same goal as for dogs treated with mitotane for PDH. Interestingly, however, one cat had clinical improvement without marked reduction in cortisol concentrations.[292] However, the availability of metyrapone varies.

In a total of six cats with PDH, trilostane administration reduced clinical signs and improved endocrine test results, but all continued to have some signs of hypercortisolemia, especially dermal changes.[295,296] In cats with PDH and DM treated by other means, the DM resolved in about 50% of cases;[223] however, insulin requirements did not change in four cats with PDH and DM treated with trilostane.[295,296] Thus trilostane ameliorates clinical signs of feline hyperadrenocorticism, but more research is needed before it can be recommended for treatment. Whether a higher dosage or longer duration of therapy will improve efficacy remains unclear.[295] Additionally, the ideal ranges for basal and post-ACTH serum cortisol concentrations and testing time (i.e., performance of ACTH stimulation tests beginning 4 to 6 hours after administration of the pill) for dogs were used. The pharmacokinetics and pharmacodynamics of trilostane are unknown in cats, and it may be necessary to optimize the testing protocols for cats.

Sex hormone excess. Progesterone-secreting adrenal masses have been reported in three cats.[288,297,298] Clinical signs are as those for hypercortisolism. With such a mass, the cortisol response to an ACTH stimulation test is blunted, suggestive of iatrogenic hypoadrenocorticism despite a lack of a history of exogenous glucocorticoid administration. Suppression is due to the ability of progestins to feed back on the pituitary and inhibit ACTH secretion as do glucocorticoids.[199] Measurement of sex steroids before and after ACTH stimulation should reveal marked hyperprogesteronemia. Abdominal ultrasonography may reveal an adrenal mass. Treatment of choice is unilateral adrenalectomy. Two cats with progesterone-secreting adrenal tumors were treated with aminoglutethimide, an inhibitor of adrenocortical steroid synthesis, preoperatively. One cat showed improvement at 2 weeks, but the response had diminished by week 6.[298] The second cat improved dramatically at first, but significant mammary gland enlargement ensued and aminoglutethimide administration was discontinued; the rapid decrease in progesterone potentially stimulated prolactin secretion.[288]

One spayed female cat with an AT secreting estradiol and testosterone has been identified, with the most notable clinical signs being aggression and male-type behavior, malodorous urine, and vulvar hyperplasia. Therapy with trilostane (30 mg once daily) was effective in reducing clinical signs; partial improvement was seen by day 28 and almost complete resolution by day 84. Interestingly, basal concentrations of both hormones as well as that of 17-hydroxyprogesterone and progesterone increased with therapy. Clinical signs returned by day 174 despite continued therapy. The reason for clinical improvement in the face of increased measured hormone concentrations is unknown.[299] Possibilities include a placebo effect (believed unlikely by the authors of the case report), false elevations of the apparent concentrations of the measured hormones by hormones that cross-react on the assays used,[299] or another nonmeasured hormone that did decrease in response to therapy and was responsible for causing the clinical signs. Although unlikely, the sex hormone elevations may have been false-positive test results for a state of excessive sex hormone secretion.

Hyperaldosteronism. Primary hyperaldosteronism can occur in cats from an aldosterone-secreting tumor or from idiopathic non-tumorous secretion of excess aldosterone. Although aldosterone-secreting AT were previously believed to be rare, the incidence may be increasing.[300] Affected cats are middle-aged to older, with no sex or breed predisposition. Clinical symptoms of hyperaldosteronism are typically nonspecific and result from potassium depletion, mainly causing hypokalemic myopathy. Historical complaints and physical examination findings include polyuria and polydipsia, nocturia, generalized weakness, collapse, anorexia, weight loss, a pendulous abdomen, and blindness.[300-303] One cat presented with respiratory distress; the respiratory failure was believed to be a manifestation of hypokalemic polymyopathy.[304] Some cats have bilateral retinal detachments and hypertension.[300,301] Adrenocortical tumors secreting more than one hormone (e.g., aldosterone and progesterone) have been reported,[305] and clinical signs associated with the other hormone (i.e., hyperprogesteronism) may also be present.

The hallmark of primary hyperaldosteronism is hypokalemia with an elevated serum aldosterone concentration but a normal or subnormal plasma renin activity. Measurement of an elevated serum aldosterone concentration alone is not truly adequate, but a feline plasma renin activity assay is not currently commercially available. In humans serum aldosterone concentration is measured after dietary intake of a specific sodium amount. Whether such standardization is necessary in veterinary medicine is unknown, making diagnosis of primary hyperaldosteronism more difficult. The presence of renal failure presents a particular dilemma, insofar as renal failure in and of itself can lead to hypokalemia and hyperaldosteronemia. The magnitude of aldosterone elevation may be the key. With primary hyperaldosteronism, serum concentrations were approximately 3000 pg/mL in two cats,[301] whereas it was a maximum of 518 pg/mL in azotemic cats.[306] Identification of an AT by radiography or ultrasonography in cats with appropriate clinical signs and laboratory results would also be highly suggestive of primary hyperaldosteronism. Until a feline plasma renin assay is available, diagnosis of primary hyperaldosteronism requires that all secondary causes of hyperaldosteronism (e.g., states associated with peripheral edema or liver failure) be ruled out.

Initial treatment of primary hyperaldosteronism is directed at controlling hypokalemia or hypertension (or both). Potassium supplementation using oral potassium gluconate at doses of 2 to 6 mmols twice daily has been used, and intravenous potassium chloride may be required in more severely hypokalemic cases. Amlodipine besylate (0.625 to 1.25 mg per cat once daily) is the initial treatment of choice for hypertension while test results are pending.[307] Spironolactone, a competitive aldosterone receptor antagonist, is also recommended (2 to 4 mg/kg once daily), assisting in the control of both hypokalemia and hypertension. Severe facial dermatitis has been reported in Maine Coon cats receiving spironolactone for management of hypertrophic cardiomyopathy.[308] Medical management may not be successful long-term or for normalization of serum potassium concentration. The role of antineoplastic chemotherapy has yet to be determined.

Treatment of choice for an AT is adrenalectomy. Given that these tumors are malignant in approximately 50% of cases, surgery may not be curative. In addition, the procedure has been associated with high perioperative mortality; approximately 33% of reported cases died intraoperatively or postoperatively, most commonly as a result of severe acute hemorrhage from the caudal vena cava.[307] Medical therapy preoperatively to stabilize a patient is ideal, especially if the tumor is secreting another hormone such as cortisol or progesterone that can create complications such as poor wound healing. A detailed description of perioperative and intraoperative management of an aldosterone-secreting adrenocortical carcinoma with attached caval thrombus has been recently reported.[309] Approximately 5% of human patients develop postoperative hyperkalemia, requiring transient administration of fludrocortisone; although not reported in the literature, the same may occur in cats.[307]

With medical management with combinations of potassium supplementation, amlodipine, and spironolactone, reported survival times in four of five cats with aldosterone-secreting AT ranged from 7 months to 984 days, with cats most commonly succumbing to chronic renal failure or a thromboembolic episode.[307] Poor response in the fifth cat may have been due to owner compliance issues. In some cases hypertension becomes refractory to medical management. For cases that undergo adrenalectomy and survive the immediate perioperative and postoperative periods, the prognosis is good; 8 of 17 adrenalectomized cats survived for at least 1 year, and two cats were alive 3.5 and 5 years postoperatively.[300] Cats with malignant tumors can do well; one cat with a carcinoma survived 1045 days after adrenalectomy.

An alternate form of hyperaldosteronism now recognized in cats is similar to the idiopathic or bilateral hyperplasia form in humans.[310] Clinical presentation is similar to the tumorous form with respect to signalment and presenting complaints, but retinal detachment and blindness, perhaps due to the presence of higher blood pressures in general, is more common with idiopathic hyperaldosteronism. Ultrasonography or CT examination of the adrenal glands reveals no changes or only subtle abnormalities such as an increase in adrenal echogenicity or areas of calcification and thickening or rounding of one pole of one or both adrenal glands. Therapy consists of medical management (as discussed previously), and affected cats tend to respond well.[307]

DISORDERS OF THE PITUITARY GLAND

Disorders of Growth Hormone

Normal Physiology

The primary function of GH is promotion of linear growth. The growth-promoting effects of GH are mediated by IGF-1 or somatomedin C. Growth hormone also stimulates protein synthesis. On the other hand, GH tends to decrease protein catabolism by directly promoting lipolysis and antagonizing the effects of insulin. In excess, GH decreases carbohydrate utilization and impairs cellular glucose uptake. The net effect is promotion of hyperglycemia; carbohydrate intolerance; and, with sustained increases in plasma GH, development of DM, which quickly becomes resistant to insulin treatment.[311]

Secretion of GH from the pituitary gland is controlled by releasing (GH-releasing hormone) and inhibiting (somatostatin) factors secreted by the hypothalamus in response to complex neurohumoral regulatory mechanisms. Other stimulators of GH release include the following: other hormones such as ghrelin;[312] neurogenic stimuli, including α-adrenergic, dopaminergic, and cholinergic factors such as clonidine and xylazine; and metabolic factors such as the presence of certain nutrient metabolites and hypoglycemia. Secretion of GH results in feedback inhibition to and subsequent release of somatostatin from the pituitary gland.

Hyposomatotropism

Conditions associated with GH deficiency include pituitary dwarfism and GH-responsive dermatosis. Congenital GH deficiency in dogs is most often encountered in German Shepherd dogs but has also been reported in cats and other canine breeds. In German Shepherd dogs, the defect is inherited through a simple autosomal recessive pattern, but the gene has yet to be identified.[313]

Clinical signs. Clinical signs of congenital GH deficiency include abnormal growth (i.e., proportional dwarfism), bilaterally symmetric truncal alopecia, and severe cutaneous hyperpigmentation. In adults with acquired hyposomatotropism, manifestations are purely dermatologic.

Diagnosis. Diagnosis of congenital pituitary dwarfism is made on the basis of signalment, history, physical examination, endocrine testing, and ruling out of other causes of small stature. Measurement of changes in GH concentrations in response to stimulation (e.g., administration of xylazine, clonidine, or ghrelin) can be used to diagnose disorders of GH secretion and would be ideal. In German Shepherd dogs, ghrelin-induced plasma GH concentrations above 5 μg/L likely exclude a GH deficiency. However, false-negative results may be encountered,[312] and validated GH assays are not commercially available in the United States. An alternative method of diagnosis of congenital GH deficiency is measurement of serum IGF-1 concentration, which should be low. Interpretation of results, however, must take into account the size of the breed, because smaller dogs have lower normal IGF-1 concentrations than larger breeds. Pituitary dwarves may also be hypothyroid, so appropriate testing should be undertaken.

Clinical manifestations of adult-onset GH deficiency are typically confined to the skin, causing bilaterally symmetric alopecia and hyperpigmentation. Hyposomatotropism may develop in adults in rare cases owing to pituitary gland destruction by inflammatory, traumatic, vascular, or neoplastic disorders.[311] An idiopathic form of acquired hyposomatotropism termed *adult-onset, GH-responsive dermatosis* was previously believed to occur in dogs, but its existence is now questioned. Dogs previously receiving this diagnosis likely had an idiopathic condition currently called *Alopecia X*. In addition, many other disorders can cause a similar clinical appearance (e.g., hyperadrenocorticism, Sertoli cell neoplasia, castration-responsive dermatosis, hyperestrogenism of intact female dogs, estrogen-responsive dermatosis of spayed female dogs, testosterone-responsive dermatosis, and telogen defluxion) and should be ruled out before a diagnosis of GH deficiency is sought in an alopecic dog. Although hair regrowth may occur with exogenous GH therapy, it is likely a nonspecific pharmacologic effect, and response to therapy does not prove a GH deficiency existed.

Therapy. Therapy for pituitary dwarfism relies on obtaining adequate serum GH concentrations, but no effective exogenous GH product is readily available for use in dogs. Recombinant human GH is expensive and can induce antibody formation that interferes with its effectiveness.[314] Although porcine and canine GH are structurally identical, the availability of porcine GH is variable. If obtainable, the recommended initial dose of porcine GH is 0.1 IU/kg subcutaneously 3 times weekly. Subsequent adjustments in dosage and administration frequency should be based on clinical response and plasma IGF-1 concentrations. The therapeutic goal is to maintain plasma IGF-1 concentration within the reference range for the breed. Hypersensitivity reactions, carbohydrate intolerance, and DM are the primary adverse effects; DM may become permanent if not detected early and the GH administration discontinued.[311]

Because progestins can cause mammary gland production and secretion of GH in dogs,[315,316] their administration is a potential therapy for canine GH deficiency. Two pituitary dwarves treated with medroxyprogesterone acetate (2.5 to 5 mg/kg initially at 3-week intervals and then at 6-week intervals) had an increased body size and growth of a complete adult hair coat. However, pruritic pyoderma, cystic endometrial hyperplasia with mucometra, and signs of acromegaly were noted in one or both dogs. The dogs were alive and healthy for at least 3 years after starting therapy.[317] Another three dogs were treated with proligestone (10 mg/kg subcutaneously every 3 weeks) and growth, increased IGF-1 levels, and improvement in hair coat were seen, but complications included development of clinical features of acromegaly, mammary development, and vulvar discharge in one intact female.[318] The dose of progestin used to treat GH deficiency must be altered to avoid side effects while maintaining a clinical response. Progestins can cause DM, however, as can GH, so appropriate monitoring must be done.

If treating GH-responsive dermatosis, if porcine GH is available, the recommended dose is 0.1 IU (0.05 mg)/kg subcutaneously 3 times per week for 4 to 6 weeks. Hypersensitivity reactions, carbohydrate intolerance, and overt DM are the primary adverse reactions. Hair regrowth and thickening of the skin are measures used to assess therapeutic response. The hair coat should improve within 4 to 6 weeks of the start of therapy. The hair that grows back consists primarily of secondary hairs, with variable regrowth of primary, or guard, hairs.[311] Duration of clinical remission in dogs that respond to therapy varies but may be up to 3 years. A 1-week course of GH treatment should be given if clinical signs begin to recur.[311] Some dogs with suspected GH-responsive dermatosis fail to respond adequately to GH treatment. A misdiagnosis, inactive GH, or the presence of GH antibodies should be considered.[311]

Hypersomatotropism

Acromegaly is caused by excessive GH secretion. Canine acromegaly is almost exclusively seen in intact bitches or in dogs receiving progestin therapy. In dogs progestins can induce GH production in foci of hyperplastic ductular mammary gland epithelium.[315,316] The progestin-induced mammary gland–derived protein is identical to GH from the pituitary gland and is biologically active.[315] In dogs a single case each of a GH-secreting pituitary tumor[319] and elevated serum GH concentrations secondary to an astrocytoma in a young dog have been reported.[320] Progestins do not cause GH secretion in cats. Feline acromegaly is due to GH-secreting pituitary tumors, predominantly in older, male castrated cats.

Clinical signs. Clinical signs of acromegaly reflect either anabolic or catabolic abnormalities. The most common in dogs is inspiratory stridor (due to soft tissue accumulation in the pharynx) and its accompanying sequelae. Increased body size can also be seen as a result of proliferation of connective tissues and flat-bone growth, particularly of the feet, head, and abdomen. Organomegaly is often present. Thickening of the skin and widening of interdental spaces may occur. In cats the most common observed clinical signs are organomegaly, prognathia inferior, broad facial features, and respiratory stridor, although some cats may not grossly appear to have any abnormalities.[171] Catabolic effects cause insulin antagonism; indeed, the presence of DM may be the first clinical problem noted. Cardiovascular abnormalities associated with acromegaly include the presence of systolic murmurs or gallop rhythms; radiographic evidence of cardiomegaly; echocardiographic changes such as left ventricular wall hypertrophy, intraventricular wall hypertrophy, and left or right (or both) atrial enlargement, and systolic anterior motion of the mitral valve;and, late in the course of the disease, congestive heart failure.[311,321] Lastly, in cases of acromegaly due to a pituitary tumor, neurologic signs may be observed.

Diagnosis. The diagnosis of acromegaly can be made on the basis of signalment, history, physical examination, and measurement of serum IGF-1 or GH concentrations. In dogs the vast majority of cases are due to progestin exposure, so they occur in middle-aged to older intact females or dogs receiving exogenous progestin therapy. In most cats the diagnosis is ultimately based on identification of conformational alterations (e.g., increased body size, large head, prognathia inferior, organomegaly) in a cat with insulin-resistant DM, a persistent increase rather than decrease in body weight in the face of poorly controlled DM, an increase in serum IGF-1 concentration in the face of insulin-resistant DM, and documentation of a pituitary mass by CT or MRI. Although nonacromegalic diabetic cats can have elevated IGF-1 concentrations,[322,323] measurement of IGF-1 is still helpful in diagnosis. The IGF-1assay is performed at only one laboratory in the United States (Michigan State University). The reference range for feline serum IGF-1 concentration is 5 to 70 nmol/L. An IGF-1 concentration above 100 nmol/L is consistent with acromegaly in cats with the appropriate clinical features; a concentration of 70 to 100 nmol/L is nondiagnostic. However, measurements repeated in 3 to 6 months are usually diagnostic as acromegalic or not.[311] An ovine GH assay was recently validated for measurement of feline GH, but it is not currently commercially available in the United States. Concentrations of GH ranged from 1.87 to 6.33 μg/L in healthy cats and from 8.45 to 33.2 μg/L in acromegalic cats.[324] Also, most cats have a tumor visible on CT or MRI at the time acromegaly is tentatively diagnosed.[311]

Therapy. Treatment for acromegaly caused by a pituitary tumor is aimed at decreasing tumor size as well as diminishing GH secretion. Transsphenoidal cryohypophysectomy has been described.[325] An effective medical option has not been reported; neither octreotide[321] nor l-deprenyl[326] has been successful in decreasing GH secretion or improving insulin sensitivity.

Radiation therapy is currently considered the best treatment option for feline acromegaly. In one study, eight cats with pituitary tumors were treated with radiation therapy.[327] Four cats had hyperadrenocorticism, three had acromegaly, and one tumor was nonsecretory. In six cats no acute adverse effects developed; in two cats transient early-delayed brain effects occurred in one and acute aural effects in the other. Reported late adverse effects included suspected radiation-induced hearing loss in two cats (mild in one, complete in another), bilateral cataracts 13 months after therapy in one, blindness in another (not clearly related to the radiation), and pharyngeal squamous cell carcinoma 16 months after radiation therapy in one. Other side effects of radiation therapy comprised transient, mild epilation and hair depigmentation in the treatment field. Clinical signs improved in all cats, but endocrine testing normalized in only one.[327] In another study of 14 acromegalic cats, adverse effects included personality change and seizures in one each and weight loss in two.[328]

Radiation therapy can help decrease insulin doses and improve insulin sensitivity. In six cats treated with radiation, three each with acromegaly and PDH, all had insulin-resistant DM before radiation therapy and became insulin sensitive after therapy. However, five required exogenous insulin administration for the rest of their lives.[327] In two cats with acromegaly, one had a slight reduction in insulin dose, and in the other the dose decreased 50%.[329] In 14 cats with acromegaly, 13 had improved diabetic control after radiation therapy that was sustained for variable, unpredictable lengths of time up to 60 months. Seven cats responded while still receiving radiation, but the mean time until improved control occurred was 5 weeks after therapy. Remission was achieved in six cats, at a mean of 3.6 months after therapy; three cats did not require insulin for at least 32 months, and three relapsed after 3, 17, and 24 months. In two cats, DM began to progress after 19 and 21 months. Interestingly, changes in IGF-1 concentrations did not appear to correlate with glycemic control.[328]

Of eight cats treated with radiation therapy, median survival time for all cats, those with an adenoma (n=6), and those with a carcinoma (n = 2) were 523, 587, and 252 days, respectively. For those with an adenoma, six were alive at 1 year and three at 2 years. In 14 cats, median survival was 28 months (approximately 840 days).[328] Euthanasia or death is often not related to the pituitary tumor, but in a few cases poor diabetic control can be a contributing factor.[327-329]

If acromegaly is due to progestin therapy in a dog, administration should be discontinued. Intact bitches should be spayed. With elimination of the endogenous or exogenous progestin exposure, the anabolically induced clinical signs (e.g., increased soft tissue mass) should resolve when GH concentrations return to normal.[311] On the other hand, if βcell activity of the pancreas has become impaired, DM may be permanent.

Despite lack of treatment options, prognosis is still good, given that GH-secreting tumors typically grows slowly. The concomitant DM, however, is ultimately very difficult to control because GH causes profound insulin resistance.

Diabetes Insipidus

Normally, vasopressin (antidiuretic hormone [ADH]) is secreted, along with oxytocin, from the posterior pituitary. The major stimuli for vasopressin release are an increase in plasma osmolality (≥2%) and volume depletion, but other stimuli such as nausea, pain, and hypoglycemia will stimulate its release.[330] Vasopressin has both pressor and antidiuretic effects. Arginine vasopressin is the predominant hormone in most animals (lysine vasopressin exists in pigs) and is associated with strong pressor actions. Vasopressin binds to the V_2 receptor on the basolateral surface of the principal cell of distal renal nephrons, causing increased water reabsorption. The binding leads to an increase in intracellular cAMP and activation of a cAMP-dependent protein kinase. The protein kinase phosphorylates a serine residue on vesicles containing water channels (aquaporins [AQPs]), beneath the luminal membrane. Ultimately, the AQPs fuse with the luminal membrane and increase tubular water permeability, allowing water and solutes to follow the concentration gradient into the hyperosmotic renal medullary concentrating gradient surrounding the ducts.[330,331] Up to 90% of the fluid filtered by the glomerulus that is not absorbed in the proximal nephron will be reabsorbed in the distal tubules under the presence of ADH. In the absence of ADH, the distal and collecting tubules become impermeable to movement of water or solutes (most notably urea). The hypotonic filtrate formed in the proximal nephron is eliminated unchanged, resulting in a water diuresis that is characterized by a large volume of urine with a low osmolality.

Diabetes insipidus results from either a complete or partial deficiency in ADH secretion (i.e., central diabetes insipidus [CDI]), or ADH interaction with its target receptors in the distal and collecting renal tubules (i.e., nephrogenic diabetes insipidus [NDI]). Causes of CDI include trauma, neoplasia, and hypothalamic–pituitary malformations or it may be idiopathic. Additionally, CDI is reported as a potential complication of transsphenoidal hypophysectomy in dogs.[241] NDI may be congenital or secondary to an acquired disease. In humans congenital NDI is most often secondary to an X-linked genetic mutation in a V_2 receptor gene that results in a mutation in the receptor.[332] Congenital NDI is rare in veterinary medicine and is not known to be a heritable defect. There are few published case reports of NDI in young dogs;[333,334] it has never been reported in cats. Documented causes of acquired NDI include drugs, such as amphotericin B; infections such as pyometra, neoplasia, hypercalcemia, and hypokalemia; endocrine disorders such as hyperadrenocorticism and hyperthyroidism; renal failure; and pregnancy.[335-337] Aging, in humans and rodents, is a cause of acquired NDI, likely mediated through interference with the aquaporin-2 water channels of the renal collecting ducts.[338,339]

Clinical signs. Polyuria and polydipsia are the clinical signs that tend to catch the attention of pet owners. Polyuria and polydipsia can also lead to worsening of urinary incontinence in dogs that are already are or predisposed to be incontinent and the incontinence may be the cause of presentation to a veterinarian. In patients with CDI secondary to a pituitary tumor, which may account for approximately 40% of cases of acquired canine CDI, neurologic signs may also be present.

Diagnosis. The modified water deprivation test is used to distinguish between CDI, NDI, and psychogenic polydipsia. The reader is referred elsewhere for an in-depth discussion on how to perform the test.[330] In working up dogs or cats with polyuria and polydipsia, the clinician should perform the modified water deprivation test *last*. All other causes of polyuria and polydipsia other than CDI, NDI, and psychogenic polydipsia should be ruled out before the test is performed.

Response to 1-deamino-(8-D-arginine) vasopressin (DDAVP) may be used diagnostically by evaluating response to therapy.[330,340] Although easier to perform than a modified water deprivation test, the results can be difficult to interpret. The patient's 24-hour water intake for 2 or 3 days should be measured while the patient is allowed free-choice water. A urine sample should also be collected at a given time each day to check urine osmolality and specific gravity. After these initial days, the patient should be treated with DDAVP by administering the intranasal preparation (1 to 4 drops placed in conjunctival sac) or the oral tablets (0.1 mg) every 12 hours for 5 to 7 days.[341] Water intake is monitored and a urine sample obtained on the fifth to seventh day of treatment at the same time of day as before treatment. A dramatic reduction in water intake or an increase in urine concentration (i.e. >50%) provides strong evidence for CDI. Moderate response is consistent with partial CDI.[330] A mild response is suggestive of psychogenic polydipsia. If no response is seen, NDI is present. Medullary washout initially may decrease response to DDAVP, but urine output should decrease nonetheless if CDI is the cause of the polyuria/polydipsia. Water intoxication is possible. Failure to respond to DDAVP indicates that treatment with DDAVP will not be successful.[330]

Therapy. In the ADH molecule, substitution of D-arginine for L-arginine (at amino acid 8) and modification of cysteine yields a powerful antidiuretic, DDAVP. Whereas AVP interacts with receptors in vascular smooth muscle (V_1 phosphatidylinositol-dependent receptors), thereby increasing blood pressure, and renal epithelial cells (V_2, c-AMP-dependent receptors), for the antidiuretic effects, DDAVP primarily interacts with V_2 receptors.

DDAVP is commercially available (Desmopressin) as a product approved for use in humans in three preparations: parenteral injection, nasal drops, or oral tablets. Because these products target primarily V_2 receptors, effects are essentially renal in action, with two exceptions. DDAVP can cause peripheral resistance and blood pressure to decrease.

For patients with complete CDI, the only therapeutic option is replacement therapy with DDAVP. This can be used for patients with partial CDI as well. If the intranasal drops available for humans are being used, administration may be more easily accomplished by transferring the nasal spray to a sterile eye-dropper bottle and placing the drops into the conjunctival sac. Duration of action of DDAVP is 8 to 24 hours, but it can vary even in the same individual, possibly because of discrepancies in drop size. The dose must be titrated to effect. Dosages in the range of 1 to 4 drops every 12 to 24 hours typically suffice,[342,343] but administration three times daily may be required.[340,344] Alternatively, DDAVP can be administered subcutaneously at 0.5 to 2 μg daily to twice daily.[330] Because nasal drops are less expensive than the parenteral preparation, subcutaneous administration of the intranasal drops has been reported. If the intranasal formulation is used, it should be passed through a bacteriostatic filter before injection. Lastly, oral DDAVP can be administered. A dose of 0.1 mg every 8 hours has been recommended, with a gradual increase as needed to effect if unacceptable polyuria and polydipsia persist 1 week after initiating therapy. Once clinical response is seen, a decrease in frequency to twice daily can be tried.[330] It should be noted that no controlled studies on efficacy or dose of oral DDAVP have been reported in veterinary medicine, and the recommendations are anecdotal.

DDAVP administration appears safe. Conjunctival irritation occasionally occurs because the solution is acidic.[330] In theory, water intoxication is a potential, serious complication. Given this possibility, it is recommended that DDAVP be administered only after polyuria and polydipsia recurs or only at night, when the need for control of polyuria and polydipsia is typically greatest so as to avoid nocturia. If DDAVP is given before polyuria and polydipsia is seen, the pet should ideally not be allowed free access to water immediately after each dose to prevent consumption of large amounts of water that the animal will not be able to excrete owing to the DDAVP effects. Although most owners do not do this, water intoxication has not been reported.

DDAVP therapy can be expensive. As an alternative, DDAVP may be administered only when polyuria and polydipsia is objectionable (e.g., to prevent nocturia or when guests are expected). As long as the pet always has unlimited access to water and an appropriate area for urination, therapy can be discontinued. A low-salt diet should be fed.[330]

Chlorpropamide is an oral hypoglycemic agent discovered to reduce urine output by 30% to 70% in humans with CDI. The exact mechanism of action is unknown, but chlorpropamide may raise the sensitivity of the renal collecting duct epithelium to low concentrations of ADH. Thus chlorpropamide is probably useful only for partial CDI in which the neurohypophysis has some residual secretory capacity.[330,344] Chlorpropamide has not been highly successful in veterinary medicine. No success was seen at 10 to 40 mg/kg in several cases, and severe hypoglycemia occurred in one patient.[344] Clinical signs resolved in one cat for 7.5 months (40 mg/day orally) until the cat died suddenly. Although the death was not believed to be due to the medication, the cause was unknown.[345] No adverse effects have been reported other than hypoglycemia. To prevent hypoglycemia, regular feeding schedules must be used.[330]

Paradoxically, thiazide diuretics are advocated for treatment of CDI and NDI. By inhibiting sodium reabsorption in the ascending loop of Henle, thiazides reduce total body sodium concentration, causing contraction of extracellular fluid volume and increasing salt and water reabsorption in the proximal tubule. As a result, the fluid reaching the distal renal tubule has a lower sodium concentration and exerts less osmotic pressure. The net effect is a slight increase in urine osmolality with a proportionate reduction in urine volume. Depending on sodium intake, polyuria is reduced by 30% to 50% in humans.[330]

No published reports exist for use of thiazide diuretics in dogs with CDI. Hydrochlorothiazide (2.5-5.0 mg/kg twice daily) and chlorothiazide (20-40 mg/kg twice daily) can be tried.[346] In two cats hydrochlorothiazide (12.5 mg/cat twice daily) and a sodium-restricted diet decreased water intake 35%.[340,347] A low-salt diet should be fed.[330] For spontaneous NDI, therapy is restricted to thiazide diuretics or a low-sodium diet (or both). In one dog chlorothiazide (approximately 35 mg/kg twice daily orally) and a low-sodium diet decreased water intake approximately fourfold, although it was still approximately 2 times normal.[333]

REFERENCES

1. Feldman EC, Nelson RW: Hypothyroidism. In Feldman EC, Nelson RW, editors: *Canine and feline endocrinology and reproduction*, ed 3, St Louis, 2004, Saunders.
2. Pullen WH, Hess RS: Hypothyroid dogs treated with intravenous levothyroxine, *J Vet Int Med* 20:32–37, 2006.
3. Ferguson DC: Update on diagnosis of canine hypothyroidism, *Vet Clin North Am Small Anim Pract* 24:515–539, 1994.
4. Miller AB, Nelson RW, Scott-Moncrieff JC, et al: Serial thyroid hormone concentrations in healthy euthyroid dogs, dogs with hypothyroidism, and euthyroid dogs with atopic dermatitis, *Br Vet J* 148:451–458, 1992.
5. Nelson RW: Use of baseline thyroid hormone concentrations for diagnosing canine hypothyroidism, *Canine Pract* 22:39–40, 1997.
6. Panciera DL: Hypothyroidism in dogs: 66 cases (1987-1992), *J Am Vet Med Assoc* 204:761–767, 1994.
7. Lawler DF, Ballam JM, Meadows R, et al: Influence of lifetime food restriction on physiological variables in Labrador retriever dogs, *Exp Gerentol* 42:204–214, 2007.
8. Geffen CV, Bavegems V, Duchateau L: Serum thyroid hormone concentrations and thyroglobulin autoantibodies in trained and non-trained healthy whippets, *Vet J* 172:135–140, 2006.
9. Gaughan KR, Bruyette D: Thyroid function testing in greyhounds, *Am J Vet Res* 62:1130–1133, 2001.
10. Lee JA, Hinchcliff KW, Piercy RJ, et al: Effects of racing and non-training on plasma thyroid hormone concentrations in sled dogs, *J Am Vet Med Assoc* 224:226–231, 2004.
11. Dixon RM, Graham PA, Mooney CT: Serum thyrotropin concentrations: a new diagnostic test for canine hypothyroidism, *Vet Rec* 138:594–595, 1996.
12. Bruner J, Scott-Moncrieff JC, Williams DA: Effect of time of sample collection on serum thyroid-stimulating hormone concentrations in euthyroid and hypothyroid dogs, *J Am Vet Med Assoc* 212:1572–1575, 1998.
13. Peterson ME, Melian C, Nichols R: Measurement of serum total thyroxine, triiodothyronine, free thyroxine, and thyrotropin concentrations for diagnosis of hypothyroidism in dogs, *J Am Vet Med Assoc* 211:1396–1402, 1997.
14. Ramsey IK, Evans H, Herrtage ME: Thyroid-stimulating hormone and total thyroxine concentrations in euthyroid, sick euthyroid and hypothyroid dogs, *J Small Anim Pract* 38:540–545, 1997.
15. Sauve F, Paradis M: Use of recombinant human thyroid-stimulating hormone for thyrotropin stimulation test in euthyroid dogs, *Can Vet J* 41:215–219, 2000.
16. Boretti FS, Sieber-Ruckstuhl NS, Willi B, et al: Comparisons of the biological activity of recombinant human thyroid-stimulating hormone with bovine thyroid-stimulating hormone and evaluation of recombinant human thyroid-stimulating hormone in healthy dogs of different breeds, *Am J Vet Res* 67:1169–1172, 2006.

17. Daminet S, Filetti S, Paradis M, et al: Use of recombinant human thyroid-stimulating hormone for thyrotropin stimulation test in healthy, hypothyroid and euthyroid sick dogs, *Can Vet J* 48:1273–1279, 2007.
18. De Roover K, Duchateau L, Carmichael N, et al: Effect of storage of reconstituted recombinant human thyroid-stimulating hormone (rhTSH) on thyroid-stimulating hormone (TSH) response testing in euthyroid dogs, *J Vet Int Med* 20:812–817, 2006.
19. Kemppainen RJ, Young DW, Behrend EN, et al: Autoantibodies to triiodothyronine and thyroxine in a Golden retriever, *J Am Anim Hosp Assoc* 32:195–198, 1996.
20. Graham PA, Lundquist RB, Refsal KR, et al: A 12-month prospective study of 234 thyroglobulin antibody positive dogs which had no laboratory evidence of thyroid dysfunction (Abstract), *J Vet Int Med* 15:298, 2001.
21. Diaz-Espineira M, Mol JA, Peeters ME, et al: Assessment of thyroid function in dogs with low plasma thyroxine concentration, *J Vet Int Med* 21:25–32, 2007.
22. Chastain CB, Young DW, Kemppainen RJ: Anti-triiodothyronine antibodies associated with hypothyroidism and lymphocytic thyroiditis in a dog, *J Am Vet Med Assoc* 194:531–534, 1989.
23. Reese S, Breyer U, Deeg C, et al: Thyroid sonography as an effective tool to discriminate between euthyroid sick and hypothyroid dogs, *J Vet Int Med* 19:491–498, 2009.
24. Bromel C, Pollard RE, Kass PH, et al: Ultrasonographic evaluation of the thyroid gland in healthy hypothyroid, and euthyroid golden retrievers with nonthyroidal illness, *J Vet Int Med* 19:499–506, 2005.
25. Refsal KR, Nachreiner RF: Monitoring thyroid hormone replacement therapy. In Bonagura JD, editor: *Kirk's current veterinary therapy XII: small animal practice*, Philadelphia, 1996, Saunders, pp 364–369.
26. Nachreiner RF, Refsal KR, Ravis WR: Pharmacokinetics of L-thyroxine after its oral administration in dogs, *Am J Vet Res* 54:2091–2098, 1993.
27. Le Traon G, Burgaud S, Horspool LJI: Pharmacokinetics of total thyroxine in dogs after administration of an oral solution of levothyroxine sodium, *J Vet Pharmacol Therap* 10:1–7, 2008.
28. Le Traon G, Brennan SF, Burgaud S, et al: Clinical evaluation of a novel liquid formulation of L-thyroxine for once daily treatment of dogs with hypothyroidism, *J Vet Int Med* 23:43–49, 2009.
29. Dixon RM, Reid SWJ, Mooney CT: Treatment and therapeutic monitoring of canine hypothyroidism, *J Small Anim Pract* 43:334–340, 2002.
30. Nachreiner RF, Refsal KR: Radioimmunoassay monitoring of thyroid hormone concentrations in dogs on thyroid replacement therapy: 2,674 cases (1985-1987), *J Am Vet Med Assoc* 201:623–629, 1992.
31. Daminet S, Ferguson DC: Influence of drugs on thyroid function in dogs, *J Vet Int Med* 17:463–472, 2003.
32. Gulikers KP, Panciera DL: Influence of various medications on canine thyroid function, *Compend Contin Educ Vet* 24:511–523, 2002.
33. Peterson ME, Melian C, Nichols CE: Measurement of serum concentrations of free thyroxine, total thyroxine, and total triiodothyronine in cats with hyperthyroidism and cats with nonthyroidal disease, *J Am Vet Med Assoc* 218:529–536, 2001.
34. Peterson ME, Graves TK, Cavanagh I: Serum thyroid hormone concentrations fluctuate in cats with hyperthyroidism, *J Vet Int Med* 1:142–146, 1987.
35. Peterson ME, Gamble DA: Effect of nonthyroidal illness on serum thyroxine concentrations in cats: 494 cases (1988), *J Am Vet Med Assoc* 197:1203–1208, 1990.
36. McLoughlin MA, DiBartola SP, Birchard SJ, et al: Influence of systemic nonthyroidal illness on serum concentration of thyroxine in hyperthyroid cats, *J Am Anim Hosp Assoc* 29:227–234, 1993.
37. Refsal KR, Nachreiner RF, Stein BE, et al: Use of the triiodothyronine suppression test for diagnosis of hyperthyroidism in ill cats that have serum concentration of iodothyronines within normal range, *J Am Vet Med Assoc* 199:1594–1601, 1991.
38. Mooney CT, Little CJL, Macrae AW: Effect of illness not associated with the thyroid gland on serum total and free thyroxine concentrations in cats, *J Am Vet Med Assoc* 208:2004–2008, 1996.
39. Tomsa K, Glaus TM, Kacl GM, et al: Thyrotropin-releasing hormone stimulation test to assess thyroid function in severely sick cats, *J Vet Int Med* 15:89–93, 2001.
40. Nieckarz JA, Daniel GB: The effect of methimazole on thyroid uptake of pertechnetate and radioiodine in normal cats, *Vet Radiol Ultrasound* 42:448–457, 2001.
41. Boag AK, Neiger R, Slater L, et al: Changes in the glomerular filtration rate of 27 cats with hyperthyroidism after treatment with radioactive iodine, *Vet Rec* 161:711–715, 2007.
42. DiBartola SP, Broome MR, Stein BS: Effect of treatment of hyperthyroidism on renal function in cats, *J Am Vet Med Assoc* 208:875–878, 1996.
43. Adams WH, Daniel GB, Legendre AM, et al: Changes in renal function in cats following treatment of hyperthyroidism using 131I, *Vet Radiol Ultrasound* 38:231–238, 1997.
44. Graves TK, Olivier NB, Nachreiner RF: Changes in renal function with treatment of hyperthyroidism in cats, *Am J Vet Res* 55:1745–1749, 1994.
45. Becker TJ, Graves TK, Kruger JM, et al: Effects of methimazole on renal function in cats with hyperthyroidism, *J Am Anim Hosp Assoc* 36:215–223, 2000.
46. van Hoek I, Lefebvre HP, Kooistra H, et al: Plasma clearance of exogenous creatinine, exo-iohexol and endo-iohexol in hyperthyroid cats before and after treatment with radioiodine, *J Vet Int Med* 21:879–885, 2008.
47. Rogers KS, Burkholder WJ, Slater MR, et al: Development and predictors for renal disease and clinical outcomes in hyperthyroid cats treated with 131-I (Abstract), *J Vet Int Med* 14:343, 2000.
48. Riensche MR, Graves TK, Schaeffer DJ: An investigation of predictors of renal insufficiency following treatment of hyperthyroidism in cats, *J Fel Med Surg* 10:160–166, 2008.
49. Graves TK: Hyperthyroidism and the kidneys. In August JR, editor: *Consultations in feline internal medicine*, ed 6, St Louis, 2010, Saunders, pp 268–273.
50. Frenais R, Burgaud S, Horspool LJI: Pharmacokinetics of controlled-release carbimazole tablets support once daily dosing in cats, *J Vet Pharmacol Therap* 31:213–219, 2008.
51. Peterson ME, Kintzer PP, Hurvitz AI: Methimazole treatment of 262 cats with hyperthyroidism, *J Vet Int Med* 2:150–157, 1988.
52. Shelton GD, Joseph R, Richter K, et al: Acquired myasthenia gravis in hyperthyroid cats on tapazole therapy, *J Vet Int Med* 11:120, 1997.
53. Niessen SJM, Voyce MJ, de Villiers L, et al: Generalised lymphadenomegaly associated with methimazole treatment in a hyperthyroid cat, *J Small Anim Pract* 48:165–168, 2007.
54. Trepanier L: Medical treatment of feline hyperthyroidism. In Bonagura JD, Twedt DC, editors: *Kirk's current veterinary therapy XIV: small animal practice*, St Louis, 2009, Saunders.
55. Trepanier LA, Hoffman SB, Kroll M, et al: Efficacy and safety of once versus twice daily administration of methimazole in cats with hyperthyroidism, *J Am Vet Med Assoc* 222:954–958, 2003.
56. Feldman EC, Nelson RW: Feline hyperthyroidism (thyrotoxicosis), *Canine and feline endocrinology and reproduction*, ed 3, St Louis, 2004, Saunders, pp 152-218.
57. Hoffman SB, Yoder AR, Trepanier LA: Bioavailability of transdermal methimazole in pluronic lecithin organogel (PLO) in healthy cats, *J Vet Pharmacol Therap* 25:189–193, 2002.

58. Lecuyer M, Prini S, Dunn ME, et al: Clinical efficacy and safety of transdermal methimazole in the treatment of feline hyperthyroidism, *Can Vet J* 47:131–135, 2006.
59. Sartor LL, Trepanier LA, Kroll MM, et al: Efficacy and safety of transdermal methimazole in the treatment of cats with hyperthyroidism, *J Vet Int Med* 18:651–655, 2004.
60. Hoffman G, Marks SL, Taboada J, et al: Transdermal methimazole treatment in cats with hyperthyroidism, *J Fel Med Surg* 5:77–82, 2003.
61. Murray LAS, Peterson ME: Ipodate treatment of hyperthyroidism in cats, *J Am Vet Med Assoc* 211:63–67, 1997.
62. van Hoek I, Daminet S, Vandermeulen E, et al: Recombinant human thyrotropin administration enhances thyroid uptake of radioactive iodine in hyperthyroid cats, *J Vet Int Med* 22:1340–1344, 2008.
63. Turrel JM, Feldman EC, Hays M, et al: Radioactive iodine therapy in cats with hyperthyroidism, *J Am Vet Med Assoc* 184:554–559, 1984.
64. Peterson ME, Becker DV: Radioiodine treatment of 524 cats, *J Am Vet Med Assoc* 207:1422–1428, 1995.
65. Meric SM, Rubin SI: Serum thyroxine concentrations following fixed-dose radioactive iodine treatment in hyperthyroid cats: 62 cases (1986-1989), *J Am Vet Med Assoc* 1990(197):621–623, 1990.
66. Mooney CT: Radioactive iodine therapy for feline hyperthyroidism: efficacy and administration routes, *J Small Anim Pract* 35:289–294, 1994.
67. Jones BR, Cayzer J, Dillon EA, et al: Radioiodine treatment of hyperthyroid cats, *New Zealand Vet J* 39:71–74, 1991.
68. Goldstein RE, Long CD, Swift NC, et al: Percutaneous ethanol injection for treatment of unilateral hyperplastic thyroid nodules in cats, *J Am Vet Med Assoc* 218:1298–1302, 2001.
69. Wells AL, Long CD, Hornof WJ, et al: Use of percutaneous ethanol injection for treatment of bilateral hyperplastic thyroid nodules in cats, *J Am Vet Med Assoc* 218:1293–1297, 2001.
70. Mallery KF, Pollard RE, Nelson RW, et al: Percutaneous ultrasound-guided radiofrequency heat ablation for treatment of hyperthyroidism in cats, *J Am Vet Med Assoc* 223:1602–1607, 2003.
71. Foster DJ, Thoday KL: Use of propranolol and potassium iodate in the presurgical management of hyperthyroid cats, *J Small Anim Pract* 40:307–315, 1999.
72. Schenck P, Chew DJ: Prediction of serum ionized calcium concentration by use of serum total calcium concentration in dogs, *Am J Vet Res* 66:1330–1336, 2005.
73. Feldman EC, Nelson RW: Hypocalcemia and primary hypoparathyroidism. In Feldman EC, Nelson RW, editors: *Canine and feline endocrinology and reproduction*, ed 3, St Louis, 2004, Saunders, pp 716–742.
74. Chew DJ, Nagode LA, Schenck PA: Treatment of hypoparathyroidism. In Bonagura JD, Twedt DC, editors: *Current veterinary Therapy XIV*, St Louis, 2009, Saunders.
75. Ruopp JL: Primary hypoparathyroidism in a cat complicated by suspect iatrogenic calcinosis cutis, *J Am Anim Hosp Assoc* 37:370–373, 2001.
76. Schaer M, Ginn PE, Fox LE, et al: Severe calcinosis cutis associated with treatment of hypoparathyroidism in a dog, *J Am Anim Hosp Assoc* 37:364–369, 2001.
77. Chew DJ, Carothers M: Hypercalcemia, *Vet Clin North Am Sm Anim Pract* 19:265–287, 1989.
78. Savary KCM, Price GS, Vaden SL: Hypercalcemia in cats: a retrospective study of 71 cases (1991-1997), *J Vet Int Med* 14:184–189, 2000.
79. Feldman EC, Nelson RW: Hypercalcemia and primary hyperparathyroidism. In Feldman EC, Nelson RW, editors: *Canine and feline endocrinology and reproduction*, ed 3, St Louis, 2004, Saunders, pp 660–715.
80. Volmer PA, Gwaltney-Brant SM, Albretson JC, et al: Severe hypercalcemia in dogs due to ingestion of Dovonex (calcipotriene) ointment (Abstract), *J Vet Int Med* 13:243, 1999.
81. Goldstein RE, Atwater DZ, Cazolli DV, et al: Inheritance, mode of inheritance, and candidate genes for primary hyperparathyroidism in keeshonden, *J Vet Int Med* 21:199–203, 2007.
82. Ham K, Greenfield CL, Barger A, et al: Validation of a rapid parathyroid hormone assay and intraoperative measurement of parathyroid hormone in dogs with benign naturally occurring primary hyperparathyroidism, *Vet Surg* 38:122–132, 2009.
83. Rasor L, Pollard R, Feldman EC: Retrospective evaluation of three treatment methods for primary hyperparathyroidism in dogs, *J Am Anim Hosp Assoc* 43:70–77, 2007.
84. Long CD, Goldstein RE, Hornof WJ, et al: Percutaneous ultrasound-guided chemical parathyroid ablation for treatment of primary hyperparathyroidism in dogs, *J Am Vet Med Assoc* 215:217–221, 1999.
85. Pollard RE, Long CD, Nelson RW, et al: Percutaneous ultrasonographically-guided radiofrequency heat ablation for treatment of primary hyperparathyroidism in dogs, *J Am Vet Med Assoc* 218:1106–1110, 2001.
86. Gwaltney-Brant SM, Albretson JC, Khan SA, et al: Use of pamidronate disodium in the treatment of hypercalcemia secondary to ingestion of calcipotriene in dogs (Abstract), *J Vet Int Med* 13:243, 1999.
87. Hotstutler RA, Chew DJ, Jaeger JQ, et al: Uses and effectiveness of pamidronate disodium for treatment of dogs and cats with hypercalcemia, *J Vet Int Med* 19:29–33, 2005.
88. Ulutas B, Voyvoda H, Pasa S, et al: Clodronate treatment of vitamin D-induced hypercalcemia in dogs, *J Vet Emerg Crit Care* 16:141–145, 2006.
89. Chew DJ, Schenck PA: Idiopathic feline hypercalcemia. In Bonagura JD, Twedt DC, editors: *Current veterinary therapy XIV*, St Louis, 2009, Saunders.
90. Midkiff AM, Chew DJ, Center SA, et al: Idiopathic hypercalcemia in cats, *J Vet Int Med* 14:619–626, 2000.
91. McClain HM, Barsanti JA, Bartges JW: Hypercalcemia and calcium oxalate urolithiasis in cats: a report of five cases, *J Am Anim Hosp Assoc* 35:297–301, 1999.
92. Rand JS: Current understanding of feline diabetes mellitus: part 1, pathogenesis, *J Fel Med Surg* 1:143–153, 1999.
93. Rand JS, Martin GJ: Management of feline diabetes mellitus, *Vet Clin North Am Sm Anim Pract* 31:881–914, 2001.
94. Hoenig M: Pathophysiology of canine diabetes, *Vet Clin North Am Sm Anim Pract* 25:553–561, 1995.
95. Feldman EC, Nelson RW: Canine diabetes mellitus. In Feldman EC, Nelson RW, editors: *Canine and feline endocrinology and reproduction*, ed 3, St Louis, 2004, Saunders, pp 486–538.
96. Rand JS: Pathogenesis of feline diabetes. In Reinhart GA, Carey DP, editors: *Recent advances in canine and feline nutrition, 1998 Iams Nutrition Symposium Proceedings*, Wilmington, Ohio, 1998, Orange Frazer Press, pp 83–95.
97. Zini E, Osto M, Franchini M, et al: Hyperglycaemia but not hyperlipidaemia causes beta cell dysfunction and beta cell loss in the domestic cat, *Diabetologia* 52:336–346, 2009.
98. Nelson RW, Griffey SM, Feldman EC, et al: Transient clinical diabetes mellitus in cats: 10 cases (1989-1991), *J Vet Int Med* 13:28–35, 1999.
99. Nelson RW, Feldman EC, Ford SL, et al: Effect of an orally administered sulfonylurea, glipizide, for treatment of diabetes mellitus in cats, *J Am Vet Med Assoc* 203:821–827, 1993.
100. Feldman EC, Nelson RW, Feldman MS: Intensive 50-week evaluation of glipizide administration in 50 cats with previously untreated diabetes mellitus, *J Am Vet Med Assoc* 210:772–777, 1997.
101. Sieber-Ruckstuhl NS, Kley S, Tschuor F, et al: Remission of diabetes mellitus in cats with diabetes ketoacidosis, *J Vet Int Med* 22:1326–1332, 2008.

102. Michiels L, Reusch CE, Boari A, et al: Treatment of 46 cats with porcine lente insulin—a prospective, multicentre study, *J Fel Med Surg* 10:439–451, 2008.
103. Mori A, Lee P, Takemitsu H, et al: Comparison of insulin signaling gene expression in insulin sensitive tissues between cats and dogs, *Vet Res Commun* 33:211–226, 2009.
104. Sako T, Mori A, Lee P, et al: Serum glycated albumin: potential use as an index of glycemic control in diabetic dogs, *Vet Res Commun* 33(5):473–479, 2009.
105. Link KR, Rand JSL: Changes in blood glucose concentration are associated with relatively rapid changes in circulating fructosamine concentrations in cats, *J Fel Med Surg* 10:583–592, 2008.
106. Reusch CE, Dlough U, Heusner AA: Evaluation of statistically significant changes in the level of glycosylated hemoglobin and serum fructosamine (Abstract), *J Vet Int Med* 9:186, 1995.
107. Jensen AL: Serum fructosamine in canine diabetes mellitus: an initial study, *Vet Res Commun* 16:1–9, 1992.
108. Kaneko JJ, Kawamoto M, Heusner AA, et al: Evaluation of serum fructosamine concentration as an index of blood glucose control in cats with diabetes mellitus, *Am J Vet Res* 53:1797–1801, 1992.
109. Reusch CE, Liehs MR, Hoyer M, et al: Fructosamine: a new parameter for diagnosis and metabolic control in diabetic dogs and cats, *J Vet Int Med* 7:177–182, 1993.
110. Lutz TA, Rand JS, Ryan E: Fructosamine concentrations in hyperglycemic cats, *Can Vet J* 36:155–159, 1995.
111. Crenshaw KL, Peterson ME, Heeb LA: Serum fructosamine concentration as an index of glycemia in cats with diabetes mellitus and stress hyperglycemia, *J Vet Int Med* 10:360–364, 1996.
112. Thoresen SI, Bredal WP: Clinical usefulness of fructosamine measurements in diagnosing and monitoring feline diabetes mellitus, *J Small Anim Pract* 37:64–68, 1996.
113. Elliott DA, Nelson RW, Feldman EC: Glycosylated hemoglobin concentration for assessment of glycemic control in diabetic cats, *J Vet Int Med* 11:161–165, 1997.
114. Nelson RW, Duesberg CA, Ford SL, et al: Effect of dietary insoluble fiber on control of glycemia in dogs with naturally acquired diabetes mellitus, *J Am Vet Med Assoc* 212:380–386, 2006.
115. Kimmel SE, Michel KE, Hess RS, et al: Effects of insoluble and soluble dietary fiber on glycemic control in dogs with naturally occurring insulin-dependent diabetes mellitus, *J Am Vet Med Assoc* 216:1076–1082, 2000.
116. Fleeman LM, Rand JS, Markwell PJ: Diets with high fiber and moderate starch are not advantageous for dogs with stabilized diabetes compared to a commercial diet with moderate fiber and low starch (Abstract), *J Vet Int Med* 17:433, 2003.
117. Nelson RW, Scott-Moncrieff C, Feldman EC, et al: Effect of dietary insoluble fiber on control of glycemia in cats with naturally acquired diabetes mellitus, *J Am Vet Med Assoc* 216:1082–1088, 2000.
118. Mazzaferro EM, Greco DS, Turner AS, et al: Treatment of feline diabetes mellitus using an a-glucosidase inhibitor and a low-carbohydrate diet, *J Fel Med Surg* 5:183–189, 2003.
119. Frank G, Anderson W, Pazak H, et al: Use of a high-protein diet in the management of feline diabetes mellitus, *Vet Ther* 2:238–246, 2001.
120. Hall TD, Mahony O, Rozanski EA, et al: Effects of diet on glucose control in cats with diabetes mellitus treated with twice daily insulin glargine, *J Fel Med Surg* 11:125–130, 2008.
121. Feldman EC, Nelson RW: Feline diabetes mellitus. In Feldman EC, Nelson RW, editors: *Canine and feline endocrinology and reproduction*, ed 3, St Louis, 2004, Saunders, pp 539–579.
122. Broussard JD, Wallace MS: Insulin treatment of diabetes mellitus in the dog and cat. In Bonagura JD, editor: *Kirk's current veterinary therapy XII: small animal practice*, Philadelphia, 1996, Saunders, pp 393–398.
123. Behrend EN, Greco DS: Feline diabetes mellitus: overview and therapy, *Comp Cont Educ Vet* 22:423–438, 2000.
124. DeClue AE, Leverenz E, Wiedmeyer CE, et al: Glucose lowering effects of inhaled insulin in healthy cats, *J Fel Med Surg* 10:519–522, 2008.
125. Edgerton DS, Cherrington AD, Neal DW, et al: Inhaled insulin is associated with prolonged enhancement of glucose disposal in muscle and liver in canine, *J Pharmacol Exp Ther* 328:970–975, 2009.
126. Norsworthy GD, Lynn RC: Clinical study to evaluate a new formulation of protamine zinc insulin for treatment of diabetes mellitus in cats (Abstract), *J Vet Int Med* 22:729–730, 2008.
127. Nelson RW, Henley K, Cole C: Efficacy of protamine zinc recombinant insulin for treating diabetes mellitus in cats (Abstract), *J Vet Int Med* 22:730, 2008.
128. Martin GJ, Rand JS: Pharmacology of a 40 IU/ml porcine lente insulin preparation in diabetic cats: findings during the first week and after 5 or 9 weeks of therapy, *J Fel Med Surg* 3:23–30, 2001.
129. Rand JS, Marshall RD: Insulin glargine and the treatment of feline diabetes mellitus, *Proc 22nd Ann Am Coll Vet Int Med Forum* 22:584–586, 2004.
130. Marshall RD, Rand JS, Morton JM: Glargine and protamine zinc insulin have a longer duration of action and result in lower mean daily glucose concentrations than lente insulin in healthy cats, *J Vet Pharmacol Ther* 31:205–212, 2008.
131. Marshall RD, Rand JS, Morton JM: Insulin glargine has a long duration of effect following administration either once daily or twice daily in divided doses in healthy cats, *J Fel Med Surg* 10:488–494, 2008.
132. Danne T, Datz N, Endahl L, et al: Insulin detemir is characterized by a more reproducible pharmacokinetic profile than insulin glargine in children and adolescents with type 1 diabetes: results from a randomized, double-blind, controlled trial, *Ped Diabetes* 9:554–560, 2008.
133. King AB: Once-daily insulin detemir is comparable to once-daily insulin glargine in providing glycaemic control over 24h in patients with type 2 diabetes: a double-blind, randomized crossover study, *Diabetes Obesity Metab* 11:69–71, 2009.
134. Gilor C, Keel T, Attermeier KJ: Hyperinsulinemic-euglycemic clamps using insulin detemir and insulin glargine in healthy cats (Abstract), *J Vet Int Med* 22:729, 2008.
135. Davison LJ, Walding B, Herrtage ME, et al: Anti-insulin antibodies in diabetic dogs before and after treatment with different insulin preparations, *J Vet Int Med* 22:1317–1325, 2008.
136. Hess RS, Ward CR: Effect of insulin dosage on glycemic response in dogs with diabetes mellitus: 221 cases (1993-1998), *J Am Vet Med Assoc* 216:217–221, 2000.
137. Fleeman LM, Rand JS: Management of canine diabetes, *Vet Clin North Am Sm Anim Pract* 31:855–880, 2001.
138. Monroe WE, Laxton D, Fallin EA, et al: Efficacy and safety of a purified porcine insulin zinc suspension for managing diabetes mellitus in dogs, *J Vet Int Med* 19:675–682, 2005.
139. Nelson RW, Lynn RC, Wagner-Mann CC, et al: Efficacy of protamine zinc insulin for treatment of diabetes mellitus in cats, *J Am Vet Med Assoc* 218:38–42, 2001.
140. Marshall RD, Rand JS: Insulin glargine and a high protein-low carbohydrate diet are associated with high remission rates in newly diagnosed diabetic cats (Abstract), *J Vet Int Med* 18:401, 2004.
141. Weaver KE, Rozanski EA, Mahony OM, et al: Use of glargine and lente insulins in cats with diabetes mellitus, *J Vet Int Med* 20:234–238, 2006.
142. Roomp K, Rand JS: Factors predictive of non-insulin dependence in diabetic cats initially treated with insulin (Abstract), *J Vet Int Med* 22:791, 2008.
143. Rand JS: Management of feline diabetes, *Aust Vet Pract* 27:68–76, 1997.
144. Reusch CE: Monitoring and treatment of the diabetic cat, *ECVIM-CA 15th Annual Congress*, 2005 pp 125–127.

145. Goossens M, Nelson RW, Feldman EC, et al: Response to insulin treatment and survival in 104 cats with diabetes mellitus (1985-1995), *J Vet Int Med* 12:1-6, 1998.
146. Rand JS: Understanding feline diabetes, *Proc 14th Ann Amer Coll Vet Int Med Forum*, 1996, pp 82–83.
147. Nelson RW: Disorders of the endocrine pancreas. In Nelson RW, Couto CG, editors: *Essentials of small animal internal medicine*, Philadelphia, 1998, Mosby Year Book, pp 734–774.
148. Fleeman LM, Rand JS: Evaluation of day-to-day variability of serial blood glucose concentration curves in diabetic dogs, *J Am Vet Med Assoc* 222:317–321, 2003.
149. Ristic JME, Herrtage ME, Walti-Lauger SMM, et al: Evaluation of a continuous glucose monitoring system in cats with diabetes mellitus, *J Fel Med Surg* 7:153–162, 2005.
150. Reusch CE, Kley S, Casella M: Home monitoring of the diabetic cat, *J Fel Med Surg* 8:119–127, 2006.
151. Rand JS, Marshall RD: Update on insulin glargine use in diabetic cats, *Proc 23rd Ann Am Coll Vet Int Med Forum*, 2005, pp 483–484.
152. Rand JS: Use of long acting insulin in the treatment of feline diabetes mellitus. In August JR, editor: *Consultations in feline internal medicine*, ed 6, St Louis, 2010, Saunders, pp 286–296.
153. Casella M, Wess G, Reusch CE: Measurement of capillary blood glucose concentrations by pet owners: a new tool in the management of diabetes mellitus, *J Am Anim Hosp Assoc* 38:239–245, 2002.
154. Reusch CE, Wess G, Casella M: Home monitoring of blood glucose concentration in the management of diabetes mellitus, *Comp Cont Educ Vet* 23:544–556, 2001.
155. Casella M, Wess G, Hassig M, et al: Home monitoring of blood glucose concentration by owners of diabetic dogs, *J Small Anim Pract* 44:298–305, 2003.
156. Alt N, Kley S, Haessig M, et al: Day-to-day variability of blood glucose concentration curves generated at home in cats with diabetes mellitus, *J Am Vet Med Assoc* 230:1011–1017, 2007.
157. Kley S, Casella M, Reusch CE: Evaluation of long-term home monitoring of blood glucose concentrations in cats with diabetes mellitus: 26 cases (1999-2002), *J Am Vet Med Assoc* 225:261–266, 2004.
158. Casella M, Hassig M, Reusch CE: Home-monitoring of blood glucose in cats with diabetes mellitus: evaluation over a 4-month period, *J Fel Med Surg* 7:163–171, 2005.
159. Wiedmeyer CE, Johnson PJ, Cohn LA, et al: Evaluation of a continuous glucose monitoring system for use in dogs, cats, and horses, *J Am Vet Med Assoc* 223:987–992, 2003.
160. Davison LJ, Slater LA, Herrtage ME, et al: Evaluation of continuous glucose monitoring system in diabetic dogs, *J Small Anim Pract* 44:435–442, 2003.
161. Fletcher JM, Behrend EN, Lee HP, et al: Accuracy of Purina Glucotest for monitoring of glucosuria in cats (Abstract), *J Vet Int Med* 20:770–771, 2006.
162. Martin GJ, Rand JS: Comparisons of different measurements for monitoring diabetic cats treated with porcine insulin zinc suspension, *Vet Rec* 161:52–58, 2007.
163. Briggs CE, Nelson RW, Feldman EC, et al: Reliability of history and physical examination findings for assessing control of glycemia in dogs with diabetes mellitus: 53 cases (1995-1998), *J Am Vet Med Assoc* 217:48–53, 2000.
164. Roomp K, Rand JS: Evaluation of intensive blood glucose control using glargine in diabetic cats (Abstract), *J Vet Int Med* 22:790, 2008.
165. Roomp K, Rand JS: The Somogyi effect is rare in diabetic cats managed using glargine and a protocol aimed at tight glycemic control (Abstract), *J Vet Int Med* 22:790–791, 2008.
166. Whitley NT, Drobatz KJ, Panciera DL: Insulin overdose in dogs and cats: 28 cases (1986-1993), *J Am Vet Med Assoc* 211:326–330, 1997.
167. Nelson RW, Feldman EC, DeVries S: Use of Ultralente insulin in cats with diabetes mellitus, *J Am Vet Med Assoc* 200:1828–1829, 1992.
168. Nelson RW: Diabetes mellitus. In Ettinger SJ, Feldman EC, editors: *Textbook of veterinary internal medicine*, ed 6, St Louis, 2005, Saunders, pp 1563–1591.
169. Forrester SD, Troy GC, Dalton MN, et al: Retrospective evaluation of urinary tract infection in 42 dogs with hyperadrenocorticism or diabetes mellitus or both, *J Vet Int Med* 13:557–560, 1999.
170. Elliott D, Feldman EC, Koblik PD, et al: Prevalence of pituitary tumors among diabetic cats with insulin resistance, *J Am Vet Med Assoc* 216:1765–1768, 2000.
171. Niessen SJM, Petrie G, Gaudiano F, et al: Feline acromegaly: an underdiagnosed endocrinopathy? *J Vet Int Med* 21:899–905, 2007b.
172. Slingerland LI, Voorhout G, Rijnberk A, et al: Growth hormone excess and the effect of octreotide in cats with diabetes mellitus, *Domest Anim Endocrinol* 35:352–361, 2008.
173. Berg IM, Nelson RW, Feldman EC, et al: Serum insulin-like growth factor-I concentration in cats with diabetes mellitus and acromegaly, *J Vet Int Med* 21:892–898, 2007.
174. Peterson ME: Diagnosis and management of insulin resistance in dogs and cats with diabetes mellitus, *Vet Clin North Am Sm Anim Pract* 25:691–713, 1995a.
175. Scheen A, Lefebvre P: Oral antidiabetic agents: a guide to selection, *Drugs* 55:225–236, 1998.
176. Rameshwar J, Anand K: Antihyperglycaemic and antiperoxidative roles of acarbose in type 2 diabetes mellitus are possibly mediated through changes in thyroid function, *Clin Exper Pharmacol Physiol* 33:1104–1106, 2006.
177. Lam K, Tiu STM: Acarbose in NIDDM patients with poor control on conventional oral agents, *Diabetes Care* 21:1154–1158, 1998.
178. Johnson KH, Hayden DW, O'Brien TD, et al: Spontaneous diabetes mellitus - islet amyloid complex in adult cats, *Am J Pathol* 125:416–419, 1986.
179. Hoenig M, Hall G, Ferguson DC: A feline model of experimentally induced islet amyloidosis, *Am J Pathol* 157:2143–2150, 2000.
180. Nelson RW, Spann D, Elliott D, et al: Evaluation of the oral antihyperglycemic drug metformin in normal and diabetic cats, *J Vet Int Med* 18:18–24, 2004.
181. Michels GM, Boudinot F, Ferguson DC, et al: Pharmacokinetics of the antihyperglycemic agent metformin in cats, *Am J Vet Res* 61:775–778, 1990.
182. Nelson RW, Robertson J, Feldman EC, et al: Effect of the α-glucosidase inhibitor acarbose on control of glycemia in dogs with naturally acquired diabetes mellitus, *J Am Vet Med Assoc* 216:1265–1269, 2000.
183. Hoenig M, Ferguson DC: Effect of darglitazone on glucose clearance and lipid metabolism in obese cats, *Am J Vet Res* 64:1409–1413, 2003.
184. Appleton DJ, Rand JS, Sunvold GD, et al: Dietary chromium tripicolinate supplementation reduces glucose concentrations and improves glucose tolerance in normal-weight cats, *J Fel Med Surg* 4:13–25, 2002.
185. Schachter S, Nelson RW, Kirk CA: Oral chromium picolinate and control of glycemia in insulin-treated diabetic dogs, *J Vet Int Med* 15:379–384, 2001.
186. Feldman EC, Nelson RW: Diabetic ketoacidosis. In Feldman EC, Nelson RW, editors: *Canine and feline endocrinology and reproduction*, St. Louis, 2004, Saunders, pp 580–615.
187. Hoenig M, Dorfman M, Koenig A: Use of a hand-held meter for the measurement of blood beta-hydroxybutyrate in dogs and cats, *J Vet Emerg Crit Care* 18:86–87, 2008.
188. Kotas S, Gerber L, Moore LE, et al: Changes in serum glucose, sodium, and tonicity in cats treated for diabetic ketosis, *J Vet Emerg Crit Care* 18:488–495, 2008.

189. Hess RS: Diabetic emergencies. In August JR, editor: *Consultations in feline internal medicine*, St Louis, 2009, Saunders, pp 297–303.
190. Morris LR, Murphy MB, Kitabchi AE: Bicarbonate therapy in severe diabetic ketoacidosis, *Annals Int Med* 105:836–840, 1986.
191. Chastain CB, Nichols CE: Low-dose intramuscular insulin therapy for diabetic ketoacidosis in dogs, *J Am Vet Med Assoc* 178:561–564, 1981.
192. Macintire DK: Treatment of diabetic ketoacidosis in dogs by continuous low-dose intravenous infusion of insulin, *J Am Vet Med Assoc* 202:1266–1272, 1993.
193. Feldman EC: Diabetic ketoacidosis in dogs, *Comp Cont Educ Vet* 11:456–463, 1980.
194. Koenig A, Drobatz KJ, Beale BA, et al: Hyperglycemic, hyperosmolar syndrome in feline diabetics: 17 cases (1995-2001), *J Vet Emerg Crit Care* 14:30–40, 2004.
195. Cochran JB, Walters S, Losek JD: Pediatric hyperglycemic hyperosmolar syndrome: diagnostic difficulties and high mortality rate, *Am J Pathol* 24:297–301, 2006.
196. Fall T, Hamlin HH, Hedhammar A, et al: Diabetes mellitus in a population of 180,000 insured dogs: incidence, survival and breed distributions, *J Vet Int Med* 21:1209–1216, 2007.
197. Behrend EN, Kemppainen RJ: Glucocorticoid therapy: pharmacology, indications and complications, *Vet Clin North Am Sm Anim Pract* 27:187–213, 1999.
198. van den Broek AHM, O'Farrell V: Suppression of adrenocortical function in dogs receiving therapeutic doses of megestrol acetate, *J Small Anim Pract* 35:285–288, 1994.
199. Court EA, Watson ADJ, Church DB, et al: Effects of delmadinone acetate on pituitary-adrenal function, glucose tolerance and growth hormone in male dogs, *Aust Vet J* 76:555–560, 1998.
200. Duesberg CA, Peterson ME: Adrenal disorders in cats, *Vet Clin North Am Sm Anim Pract* 27:321–347, 1997.
201. Hughes AM, Nelson RW, Famula TR, et al: Clinical features and heritability of hypoadrenocorticism in Nova Scotia Duck Tolling Retrievers: 25 cases (1994-2006), *J Am Vet Med Assoc* 231:407–412, 2007.
202. Oberbauer AM, Benemann KS, Belanger JM, et al: Inheritance of hypoadrenocorticism in bearded collies, *Am J Vet Res* 63:643–647, 2002.
203. Famula TR, Belanger JM, Oberbauer AM: Heritability and complex segregation analysis of hypoadrenocorticism in the standard poodle, *J Small Anim Pract* 44:8–12, 2003.
204. Lennon EM, Boyle TE, Hutchins RG, et al: Use of basal serum or plasma cortisol concentrations to rule out a diagnosis of hypoadrenocorticism in dogs: 123 cases (2000-2005), *J Am Vet Med Assoc* 231:413–416, 2007.
205. Feldman EC, Nelson RW: Hypoadrenocorticism. In Feldman EC, Nelson RW, editors: *Canine and feline endocrinology and reproduction*, ed 3, St Louis, 2005, Saunders, pp 394–439.
206. Brady CA, Vite CH, Drobatz KJ: Severe neurologic sequelae in a dog after treatment of hypoadrenal crisis, *J Am Vet Med Assoc* 215:222–225, 1999.
207. MacMillan KL: Neurologic complications following treatment of canine hypoadrenocorticism, *Can Vet J* 44:490–492, 2003.
208. Kintzer PP, Peterson ME: Primary and secondary canine hypoadrenocorticism, *Vet Clin North Am Sm Anim Pract* 27:349–358, 1997.
209. Peterson ME, Greco DS, Orth DN: Primary hypoadrenocorticism in ten cats, *J Vet Int Med* 3:55–58, 1989.
210. Kintzer PP, Peterson ME: Treatment and long-term follow-up of 205 dogs with hypoadrenocorticism, *J Vet Int Med* 11:43–49, 1997.
211. Melian C, Peterson ME: Diagnosis and treatment of naturally occurring hypoadrenocorticism in 42 dogs, *J Small Anim Pract* 37:268–275, 1996.
212. McCabe MD, Feldman EC, Lynn RC, et al: Subcutaneous administration of desoxycorticosterone pivalate for the treatment of canine hypoadrenocorticism, *J Am Anim Hosp Assoc* 31:151–155, 1995.
213. Chow E, Campbell WR, Turnier JR, et al: Toxicity of desoxycorticosterone pivalate given at high dosages to clinically normal Beagles for six months, *Am J Vet Res* 54:1954–1961, 1993.
214. Kaplan AJ, Peterson ME: Effects of desoxycorticosterone pivalate administration on blood pressure in dogs with primary hypoadrenocorticism, *J Am Vet Med Assoc* 206:327–331, 1995.
215. Lynn RC, Feldman EC, Nelson RW: Efficacy of microcrystalline desoxycorticosterone pivalate for treatment of hypoadrenocorticism in dogs, *J Am Vet Med Assoc* 202:392–396, 1993.
216. Rijnberk A, Belshaw BE: o, p'DDD treatment of canine hyperadrenocorticism: an alternative protocol. In Kirk RW, Bonagura JD, editors: *Current veterinary therapy XI: small animal practice*, Philadelphia, 1992, Saunders, pp 345–349.
217. Behrend EN, Kemppainen RJ: Diagnosis of canine hyperadrenocorticism, *Vet Clin North Am Sm Anim Pract* 31:985–1003, 2001.
218. van Vonderen IK, Kooistra HS, Rijnberk A: Influence of veterinary care on the urinary corticoid:creatinine ratio in dogs, *J Vet Int Med* 12:431–435, 1998.
219. Cauvin AL, Witt AL, Groves E, et al: The urinary corticoid: creatinine ratio (UCCR) in healthy cats undergoing hospitalisation,, *J Fel Med Surg* 5:329–333, 2003.
220. Kerl ME, Peterson ME, Wallace MS, et al: Evaluation of a low-dose synthetic adrenocorticotropic hormone stimulation test in clinically normal dogs and dogs with naturally developing hyperadrenocorticism, *J Am Vet Med Assoc* 214:1497–1501, 1999.
221. Behrend EN, Kemppainen RJ, Bruyette DS, et al: Intramuscular administration of a low dose of ACTH for ACTH stimulation testing in dogs, *J Am Vet Med Assoc* 229:528–530, 2006.
222. Peterson ME, Kemppainen RJ: Comparison of intravenous and intramuscular routes of administering cosyntropin for corticotropin stimulation testing in cats, *Am J Vet Res* 53:1392–1395, 1992.
223. Behrend EN, Kemppainen RJ: Adrenocortical disease. In August JR, editor: *Consultations in feline internal medicine*, ed 4, Philadelphia, 2001, Saunders, pp 159–168.
224. Kaplan AJ, Peterson ME, Kemppainen RJ: Effects of disease on the results of diagnostic tests for use in detecting hyperadrenocorticism in dogs, *J Am Vet Med Assoc* 207:445–451, 1995.
225. Zerbe CA, Refsal KR, Peterson ME, et al: Effect of nonadrenal illness on adrenal function in the cat, *Am J Vet Res* 48:421–454, 1987.
226. Hill KE, Scott-Moncrieff JCR, Moore GE: ACTH stimulation testing: a review and a study comparing synthetic and compounded ACTH products, *Vet Med* 99:134–146, 2004.
227. Kemppainen RJ, Behrend EN, Busch KA: Use of compounded adrenocorticotropic hormone (ACTH) for adrenal function testing in dogs, *J Am Anim Hosp Assoc* 41:368–372, 2005.
228. Kley S, Alt M, Zimmer C, et al: Evaluation of the low-dose dexamethasone suppression test and ultrasonographic measurements of the adrenal glands in cats with diabetes mellitus, *Schweiz Arch Tierheilkd* 149:493–500, 2007.
229. Kemppainen RJ: Answers to commonly asked endocrine diagnostic questions. In August JR, editor: *Consultations in Feline Internal Medicine*, ed 6, St Louis, 2010, Saunders, pp 251–253.
230. Feldman EC, Feldman MS, Nelson RW: Use of low- and high-dose dexamethasone tests for distinguishing pituitary-dependent from adrenal tumor hyperadrenocorticism in dogs, *J Am Vet Med Assoc* 209:772–775, 1996.
231. Norman EJ, Thompson H, Mooney CT: Dynamic adrenal function testing in eight dogs with hyperadrenocorticism associated with adrenocortical neoplasia, *Vet Rec* 144:551–554, 1999.
232. Kemppainen RJ, Clark TP, Peterson ME: Preservative effect of aprotinin on canine plasma immunoreactive adrenocorticotropin concentrations, *Domest Anim Endocrinol* 11:355–362, 1993.
233. Reusch CE, Feldman EC: Canine hyperadrenocorticism due to adrenocortical neoplasia, *J Vet Int Med* 5:3–10, 1991.
234. Goossens MMC, Feldman EC, Theon AP, et al: Efficacy of cobalt 60 radiotherapy in dogs with pituitary-dependent hyperadrenocorticism, *J Am Vet Med Assoc* 212:374–376, 1998.

235. Dow SW, LeCouteur RA, Rosychuk RA, et al: Response of dogs with functional pituitary macroadenomas and macrocarcinomas to radiation, *J Small Anim Pract* 31:287–294, 1990.
236. Theon AP, Feldman EC: Megavoltage irradiation of pituitary macrotumors in dogs with neurologic signs, *J Am Vet Med Assoc* 213:225–231, 1998.
237. Kent MS, Bommarito D, Feldman EC, et al: Survival, neurologic response and prognostic factors in dogs with pituitary masses treated with radiation therapy and untreated dogs, *J Vet Int Med* 21:1027–1033, 2007.
238. Bertoy EH, Feldman EC, Nelson RW, et al: Magnetic resonance imaging of the brain in dogs with recently diagnosed but untreated pituitary-dependent hyperadrenocorticism, *J Am Vet Med Assoc* 206:651–656, 1995.
239. Bertoy EH, Feldman EC, Nelson RW, et al: One-year follow-up evaluation of magnetic resonance imaging of the brain in dogs with pituitary-dependent hyperadrenocorticism, *J Am Vet Med Assoc* 208:1268–1273, 1996.
240. Meij BP: Transsphenoidal hypophysectomy for the treatment of pituitary-dependent hyperadrenocorticism in dogs, *Curr Res*, 2004.
241. Hanson JM, Van 't HM, Voorhout G, et al: Efficacy of transsphenoidal hypophysectomy in treatment of dogs with pituitary-dependent hyperadrenocorticism, *J Vet Int Med* 19:687–694, 2005.
242. Feldman EC, Nelson RW: Canine hyperadrenocorticism (Cushing's syndrome). In Feldman EC, Nelson RW, editors: *Canine and feline endocrinology and reproduction*, ed 3, St Louis, 2004, Saunders, pp 252–357.
243. Webb CB, Twedt DC: Acute hepatopathy associated with mitotane administration in a dog, *J Am Anim Hosp Assoc* 42:298–301, 2006.
244. Kintzer PP, Peterson ME: Mitotane (o, p'-DDD) treatment of 200 dogs with pituitary-dependent hyperadrenocorticism, *J Vet Int Med* 5:182–190, 1991.
245. Watson ADJ, Rijnberk A, Moolenaar AJ: Systemic availability of o, p'-DDD in normal dogs, fasted and fed, and in dogs with hyperadrenocorticism, *Res Vet Sci* 43:160–165, 1987.
246. Peterson ME, Kintzer PP: Medical treatment of pituitary-dependent hyperadrenocorticism, *Vet Clin North Am Sm Anim Pract* 27:255–272, 1997.
247. den Hertog E, Braakman JCA, Teske E: Treatment of pituitary-dependent hyperadrenocorticism in the dog by non-selective adrenocorticolysis with o, p'DDD, *Vet Quart* 19(Suppl 1):S17, 1997.
248. Clemente M, De Andres PJ, De Arenas C, et al: Comparison of non-selective adrenocorticolysis with mitotane or trilostane for the treatment of dogs with pituitary-dependent hyperadrenocorticism, *Vet Rec* 161:805–809, 2007.
249. Kintzer PP, Peterson ME: Diagnosis and management of cortisol-secreting adrenal tumors, *Vet Clin North Am Sm Anim Pract* 27:299–307, 1997.
250. Kintzer PP, Peterson ME: Mitotane treatment of 32 dogs with cortisol-secreting adrenocortical neoplasms, *J Am Vet Med Assoc* 225:54–61, 1994.
251. Feldman EC, Feldman MS, Farver TB: Comparison of mitotane treatment for adrenal tumor versus pituitary-dependent hyperadrenocorticism in dogs, *J Am Vet Med Assoc* 200:1642–1647, 1992.
252. Willard MD, Nachreiner R, McDonald R, et al: Ketoconazole-induced changes in selected canine hormone concentrations, *Am J Vet Res* 47:2504–2509, 1986.
253. DeCoster R, Beerens D, Dom J, et al: Endocrinological effects of single daily ketoconazole administration in male beagle dogs, *Acta Endocrinologica* 107:275–281, 1984.
254. Feldman EC, Bruyette DS, Nelson RW, et al: Plasma cortisol response to ketoconazole administration in dogs with hyperadrenocorticism, *J Am Vet Med Assoc* 197:71–77, 1990.
255. Feldman EC, Nelson RW: Use of ketoconazole for control of canine hyperadrenocorticism. In Kirk RW, Bonagura JD, editors: *Current veterinary therapy XI*, Philadelphia, 1992, Saunders, pp 349–352.
256. Behrend EN, Kemppainen RJ, Clark TP, et al: Treatment of hyperadrenocorticism in dogs: a survey of internists and dermatologists, *J Am Vet Med Assoc* 215:938–943, 1999.
257. Lien Y-H, Huang H- P: Use of ketoconazole to treat dogs with pituitary-dependent hyperadrenocorticism: 48 cases (1994-2007), *J Am Vet Med Assoc* 233:1896–1901, 2009.
258. Drucker WD, Peterson ME: *Pharmacologic treatment of pituitary-dependent canine Cushing's disease, Proceedings 62nd Annual Meeting Endocrine Society*, 1980, p 89.
259. Rijnberk A, Mol JA, Kwant MM: Effects of bromocriptine on corticotrophin, melanotrophin, and corticosteroid secretion in dogs with pituitary-dependent hyperadrenocorticism, *J Endocrinol* 118:271–277, 1988.
260. Reusch C, Steffen T, Hoerauf A: The efficacy of L-deprenyl in dogs with pituitary-dependent hyperadrenocorticism, *J Vet Int Med* 13:291–301, 1999.
261. Braddock JA, Church DB, Robertson ID, et al: Inefficacy of selegiline in treatment of canine pituitary-dependent hyperadrenocorticism, *Aust Vet J* 82:272–277, 2004.
262. Bruyette DS, Ruehl WW, Entriken T: Management of canine pituitary-dependent hyperadrenocorticism with 1-deprenyl (Anipryl), *Vet Clin North Am Sm Anim Pract* 27:273–286, 1997.
263. Bruyette DS, Ruehl WW, Smidberg TL: Canine pituitary-dependent hyperadrenocorticism: a spontaneous animal model for neurodegenerative disorders and their treatment with 1-deprenyl, *Prog Brain Res* 106:207–213, 1995.
264. Sieber-Ruckstuhl NS, Boretti FS, Wenger M, et al: Cortisol, aldosterone, cortisol precursor, androgen and endogenous ACTH concentrations in dogs with pituitary-dependent hyperadrenocorticism treated with trilostane, *Domest Anim Endocrinol* 31:63–75, 2006.
265. Vaughn MA, Feldman EC, Hoar BR, et al: Evaluation of twice-daily, low-dose trilostane treatment administered orally in dogs with naturally occurring hyperadrenocorticism, *J Am Vet Med Assoc* 232:1321–1328, 2008.

265a. Galac S, Buijtels JJCWM, Kooistra HS: Urinary corticoid: creatinine ratios in dogs with pituitary-dependent hypercortisolism during trilostane treatment, *J Vet Int Med* 1214-1219, 2009.

266. Alenza DP, Arenas C, Lopez ML, et al: Long-term efficacy of trilostane administered twice daily in dogs with pituitary-dependent hyperadrenocorticism, *J Am Anim Hosp Assoc* 42:269–276, 2006.
267. Braddock JA, Church DB, Robertson ID, et al: Trilostane treatment in dogs with pituitary-dependent hyperadrenocorticism, *Aust Vet J* 81:600–607, 2003.
268. Barker EN, Campbell S, Tebb AJ, et al: A comparison of the survival times of dogs treated with mitotane or trilostane for pituitary-dependent hyperadrenocorticism, *J Vet Int Med* 19:810–815, 2005.
269. Neiger R, Ramsey IK, O'Conner J, et al: Trilostane treatment of 78 dogs with pituitary-dependent hyperadrenocorticism, *Vet Rec* 150:799–804, 2002.
270. Ruckstuhl NS, Nett CS, Reusch C: Results of clinical examinations, laboratory tests, and ultrasonography in dogs with pituitary-dependent hyperadrenocorticism treated with trilostane, *Am J Vet Res* 63:506–512, 2002.
271. Neiger R, Ramsey IK: Trilostane therapy of canine hyperadrenocorticism, *Proc 20th Ann Amer Coll Vet Int Med Forum*, 2002, pp 544–546.
272. Neiger R: Hyperadrenocorticism: the animal perspective - comparative efficacy and safety of trilostane, *Proc 22nd Ann Vet Med Forum*, 2004, pp 699–701.
273. Ramsey IK, Richardson J, Lenard Z, et al: Persistent isolated hypocortisolism following brief treatment with trilostane, *Aust Vet J* 86:491–495, 2008.
274. Chapman PS, Kelly DF, Archer J, et al: Adrenal necrosis in a dog receiving trilostane for the treatment of hyperadrenocorticism, *J Small Anim Pract* 45:307–310, 2004.

275. Reusch CE, Sieber-Ruckstuhl N, Wenger M, et al: Histological evaluation of the adrenal glands of seven dogs with hyperadrenocorticism treated with trilostane, *Vet Rec* 160:219–224, 2007.
276. Witt A, Neiger R: Adrenocorticotropic hormone levels in dogs with pituitary-dependent hyperadrenocorticism following trilostane therapy, *Vet Rec* 154:399–400, 2004.
277. Bell R, Neiger R, McGrotty Y, et al: Study of the effects of once daily doses trilostane on cortisol concentrations and responsiveness to adrenocorticotrophic hormone in hyperadrenocorticoid dogs, *Vet Rec* 159:277–281, 2006.
278. Machida T, Uchida E, Matsuda K, et al: Aldosterone-, corticosterone- and cortisol-secreting adrenocortical carcinoma in a dog: case report, *J Vet Med Sci* 70:317–320, 2007.
279. Benchekroun G, DeFornel-Thibaud P, Lafarge S, et al: Trilostane therapy for hyperadrenocorticism in three dogs with adrenocortical metastasis, *Vet Rec* 163:190–192, 2008.
280. Eastwood JM, Elwood CM, Hurley KJ: Trilostane treatment of a dog with functional adrenocortical neoplasia, *J Small Anim Pract* 44:126–131, 2003.
281. Mantis P, Lamb CR, Witt A, et al: Changes in ultrasonographic appearance of adrenal glands in dogs with pituitary-dependent hyperadrenocorticism treated with trilostane, *Vet Radiol Ultrasound* 44:682–685, 2003.
282. Castillo V, Blatter C, Gomez NV, et al: Diurnal ACTH and plasma cortisol variations in healthy dogs and in those with pituitary-dependent Cushing's syndrome before and after treatment with retinoic acid, *Res Vet Sci* 86:223–229, 2009.
283. Castillo V, Giacomini D, Páez-Pereda M, et al: Retinoic acid as a novel medical therapy for Cushing's disease in dogs, *Endocrinology* 147:4438–4444, 2006.
284. Meij BP, Voorhout G, Ingh TSGAM van den: Transsphenoidal hypophysectomy for treatment of pituitary-dependent hyperadrenocorticism in 7 cats, *Vet Surg* 30:72–86, 2001.
285. Mayer MN, Treuil PL: Radiation therapy for pituitary tumors in the dog and cat, *Can Vet J* 48:316–318, 2007.
286. Nelson RW, Feldman EC, Smith MC: Hyperadrenocorticism in cats: seven cases (1978-1987), *J Am Vet Med Assoc* 193:245–250, 1988.
287. Zerbe CA, Nachreiner RF, Dunstan RW, et al: Hyperadrenocorticism in a cat, *J Am Vet Med Assoc* 190:559–563, 1987.
288. Feldman EC, Nelson RW: Hyperadrenocorticism in cats (Cushing's syndrome). In Feldman EC, Nelson RW, editors: *Canine and feline endocrinology and reproduction*, ed 3, St Louis, 2004, Saunders, pp 358–393.
289. Schwedes CJ: Mitotane (o, p'-DDD) treatment in a cat with hyperadrenocorticism, *J Small Anim Pract* 38:520–524, 1997.
290. Jones CA, Refsal KR, Stevens BJ, et al: Adrenocortical adenocarcinoma in a cat, *J Am Anim Hosp Assoc* 28:59–62, 1992.
291. Nelson RW, Feldman EC: Hyperadrenocorticism. In August JR, editor: *Consultations in feline internal medicine*, Philadelphia, 1991, Saunders, pp 267–270.
292. Moore LE, Biller DS, Olsen DE: Hyperadrenocorticism treated with metyrapone followed by bilateral adrenalectomy in a cat, *J Am Vet Med Assoc* 217:691–694, 2000.
293. Daley CA, Zerbe CA, Schick RO, et al: Use of metyrapone to treat pituitary-dependent hyperadrenocorticism in a cat with large cutaneous wounds, *J Am Vet Med Assoc* 202:956–960, 1993.
294. Peterson ME: Endocrine disorders in cats: four emerging diseases, *Comp Con Educ Vet* 10:1353–1362, 1988.
295. Neiger R, Witt AL, Noble A, et al: Trilostane therapy for treatment of pituitary-dependent hyperadrenocorticism in 5 cats, *J Vet Int Med* 18:160–164, 2004.
296. Skelly BJ, Petrus D, Nicholls PK: Use of trilostane for the treatment of pituitary-dependent hyperadrenocorticism in a cat, *J Small Anim Pract* 44:269–272, 2003.
297. Boord M, Griffin C: Progesterone-secreting adrenal mass in a cat with clinical signs of hyperadrenocorticism, *J Am Vet Med Assoc* 214:666–669, 1999.
298. Rossmeisl JH, Scott-Moncrieff JCR, Siems J, et al: Hyperadrenocorticism and hyperprogesteronemia in a cat with adrenocortical adenocarcinoma, *J Am Anim Hosp Assoc* 36:512–517, 2000.
299. Boag AK, Neiger R, Church DB: Trilostane treatment of bilateral adrenal enlargement and excessive sex steroid hormone production in a cat, *J Small Anim Pract* 45:263–266, 2004.
300. Ash RA, Harvey AM, Tasker S: Primary hyperaldosteronism in the cat: a series of 13 cases, *J Fel Med Surg* 7:173–182, 2004.
301. Flood SM, Randolph JF, Gelzer ARM, et al: Primary hyperaldosteronism in 2 cats, *J Am Anim Hosp Assoc* 35:411–416, 1999.
302. Eger CE, Robinson WF, Huxtable CRR: Primary aldosteronism (Conn's syndrome) in a cat; a case report and review of comparative aspects, *J Small Anim Pract* 24:293–307, 1983.
303. Mackay AD, Sparkes AH: Successful surgical treatment of a cat with primary aldosteronism, *J Fel Med Surg* 1:117–122, 1998.
304. Haldene S, Graves TK, Bateman S, et al: Profound hypokalemia causing respiratory failure in a cat with hyperaldosteronism, *J Vet Emerg Crit Care* 17:202–207, 2007.
305. DeClue AE, Breshears LA, Pardo ID, et al: Hyperaldosteronism and hyperprogesteronism in a cat with an adrenal cortical carcinoma, *J Vet Int Med* 19:355–358, 2005.
306. Jensen J, Henik R, Brownfield M, et al: Plasma renin activity and angiotensin I and aldosterone concentrations in cats with hypertension associated with chronic renal disease, *Am J Vet Res* 58:535–540, 1997.
307. Refsal KR, Harvey AM: Hyperaldosteronism. In August JR, editor: *Consultations in feline internal medicine*, ed 6, St. Louis, 2010, Saunders, pp 254–267.
308. MacDonald KA, Kittleson MD, Kass PH: Effect of spironolactone on diastolic function and left ventricular mass in Maine coon cats with familial hypertrophic cardiomyopathy, *J Vet Int Med* 22:335–340, 2008.
309. Rose SA, Kyles AE, Labelle P, et al: Adrenalectomy and caval thrombectomy in a cat with primary hyperaldosteronism, *J Am Anim Hosp Assoc* 43:209–214, 2007.
310. Javadi S, Djajadiningrat-Laanen SC, Kooistra HS, et al: Primary hyperaldosteronism, mediator of progressive renal disease in cats, *Domest Anim Endocrinol* 28:85–104, 2005.
311. Feldman EC, Nelson RW: Disorders of growth hormone. In Feldman EC, Nelson RW, editors: *Canine and feline endocrinology and reproduction*, St Louis, 2004, Saunders, pp 45–84.
312. Bhatti SFM, De Vliegher SP, Mol JA, et al: Ghrelin-stimulation test in the diagnosis of canine pituitary dwarfism, *Res Vet Sci* 81:24–30, 2006.
313. van Oost BA, Versteeg SA, Imholz S, et al: Exclusion of the lim homeodomain gene LHX4 as a candidate gene for pituitary dwarfism in German shepherd dogs, *Molec Cell Endo* 197:57–62, 2002.
314. van Herpen H, Rijnberk A, Mol JA: Production of antibodies to biosynthetic human growth hormone in the dog, *Vet Rec* 134:171, 1994.
315. Mol JA, van Garderen E, Selman PJ, et al: Growth hormone mRNA in mammary gland tumors of dogs and cats, *J Clin Invest* 95:2028–2034, 1995.
316. Selman PJ, Mol JA, Rutteman GR, et al: Progestin-induced growth hormone excess in the dog originates in the mammary gland, *Endocrinology* 134:287–292, 1994.
317. Kooistra HS, Voorhout G, Selman PJ, et al: Progestin-induced growth hormone (GH) production in the treatment of dogs with congenital GH deficiency, *Domest Anim Endocrinol* 15:93–102, 1998.
318. Knottenbelt CM, Herrtage ME: Use of proligestone in the management of three German shepherd dogs with pituitary dwarfism, *J Small Anim Pract* 43:164–170, 2002.

319. van Keulen LJM, Wesdorp JL, Kooistra HS: Diabetes mellitus in a dog with a growth-hormone producing acidophilic adenoma of the adenohypophysis, *Vet Pathol* 33:451–453, 1996.
320. Nelson RW, Morrison WB, Lurus AG, et al: Diencephalic syndrome secondary to intracranial astrocytoma in a dog, *J Am Vet Med Assoc* 179:1004–1010, 1981.
321. Peterson ME, Taylor S, Greco DS, et al: Acromegaly in 14 cats, *J Vet Int Med* 4:192–201, 1990.
322. Starkey SR, Tan K, Church DB: Investigation of serum IGF-1 levels amongst diabetic and non-diabetic cats, *J Fel Med Surg* 6:149–155, 2004.
323. Lewitt MS, Hazel SJ, Church DB, et al: Regulation of insulin-like growth factor-binding protein-3 ternary complex in feline diabetes mellitus, *J Endocrinol* 166:21–27, 2000.
324. Niessen SJM, Khalid M, Petrie G, et al: Validation and application of a radioimmunoassay for ovine growth hormone in the diagnosis of acromegaly in cats, *Vet Rec* 160:902–907, 2007.
325. Blois SL, Holmberg DL: Cryohypophysectomy used in the treatment of a case of feline acromegaly, *J Small Anim Pract* 49:596–600, 2008.
326. Abraham LA, Helmond SE, Mitten RW, et al: Treatment of an acromegalic cat with the dopamine agonist L-deprenyl, *Aust Vet J* 80:479–483, 2002.
327. Mayer MN, Greco DS, LaRue SM: Outcomes of pituitary tumor irradiation in cats, *J Vet Int Med* 20:1151–1154, 2006.
328. Dunning MD, Lowrie CS, Bexfield NH, et al: Exogenous insulin treatment after hypofractionated radiotherapy in cats with diabetes mellitus and acromegaly, *J Vet Int Med* 23:243–249, 2009.
329. Kaser-Hotz B, Rohrer CR, Stankeova S, et al: Radiotherapy of pituitary tumors in five cats, *J Small Anim Pract* 43:303–307, 2002.
330. Feldman EC, Nelson RW: Water metabolism and diabetes insipidus. In Feldman EC, Nelson RW, editors: *Canine and feline endocrinology and reproduction*, ed 3, St Louis, 2004, Saunders, pp 2–44.
331. Sands JM, Bichet DG: Nephrogenic diabetes insipidus, *Annals Int Med* 144:186–194, 2006.
332. Arthus MF, Lonergan M, Crumley MJ, et al: Report of 33 novel AVPR2 mutations and analysis of 117 families with X-linked nephrogenic diabetes insipidus, *J Am Soc Nephrol* 11:1044–1054, 2000.
333. Breitschwerdt EB, Verlander JW, Hribernik TN: Nephrogenic diabetes insipidus in 3 dogs, *J Am Vet Med Assoc* 179:235–238, 1981.
334. Takemura N: Successful long-term treatment of congenital nephrogenic diabetes insipidus in a dog, *J Small Anim Pract* 39:592–594, 1998.
335. Newman SJ, Langston CE, Scase TJ: Cryptococcal pyelonephritis in a dog, *J Am Vet Med Assoc* 222:180–183, 2003.
336. Earm J-H, Christensen BM, Frokiaer J, et al: Decreased aquaporin-2 expression and apical plasma membrane delivery in kidney collecting ducts of polyuric hypercalcemic rats, *J Am Soc Nephrol* 9:2181–2193, 1998.
337. Amlal H, Krane CA, Chen Q, et al: Early polyuria and urinary concentrating defect in potassium deprivation, *Am J Physiol Renal Physiol* 279:F655–F663, 2000.
338. Tian Y, Serino R, Verbalis JG: Downregulation of renal vasopressin V2 receptor and aquaporin-2 expression parallels age-associated defects in urine concentration, *Am J Physiol Renal Physiol* 287:F797–F805, 2004.
339. Combet S, Gouraud S, Gobin R, et al: Aquaporin-2 downregulation in kidney medulla of aging rats is post-transcriptional and is abolished by water deprivation, *Am J Physiol Renal Physiol* 294:F1408–F1414, 2008.
340. Kraus KH: The use of desmopressin in diagnosis and treatment of diabetes insipidus in cats, *Comp Cont Educ Vet* 209:168–173, 1987.
341. Nichols R: Clinical use of the vasopressin analogue DDAVP for the diagnosis and treatment of diabetes insipidus. In Bonagura J, editor: *Kirk's current veterinary therapy XIII: small animal practice*, Philadelphia, 2000, Saunders, pp 325–326.
342. Nichols R, Hohenhaus AE: Use of the vasopressin analogue desmopressin for polyuria and bleeding disorders, *J Am Vet Med Assoc* 205:168–173, 1994.
343. Harb MF, Nelson RW, Feldman EC, et al: Central diabetes insipidus in dogs: 20 cases (1986-1995), *J Am Vet Med Assoc* 209:1884–1888, 1996.
344. Schwartz-Porsche D: Diabetes insipidus. In Kirk R, editor: *Current veterinary therapy VII: small animal practice*, Philadelphia, 1980, Saunders, pp 1005–1011.
345. Rogers WA, Valdez H, Anderson BC: Partial deficiency of antidiuretic hormone in a cat, *J Am Vet Med Assoc* 170:545–547, 1977.
346. Nichols R: Diabetes insipidus. In Kirk R, editor: *Current veterinary therapy X: small animal practice*, Philadelphia, 1989, Saunders, pp 973–978.
347. Burnie AG, Dunn JK: A case of central diabetes insipidus in the cat: diagnosis and treatment, *J Small Anim Pract* 23:237–241, 1982.

22 Dermatologic Therapy

Robert A. Kennis and Dawn Merton Boothe

Chapter Outline

A major advantage of treating diseases of the skin is easy access to the site of disease. Drug delivery can be facilitated by topical therapy, and response can be based on visual examination (clinical signs) rather than solely on supportive diagnostic aids. The advent of topical drug therapy has also, however, led to a plethora of systems designed to deliver drug to the skin; its upper layers; through the skin; and, in some instances, into systemic circulation. The result is an innumerable list of products that vary in active and inactive ingredients. This chapter approaches treatment of skin diseases by first discussing drugs that are intended for topical administration and then drugs intended for systemic therapy. Finally, specific skin diseases are addressed.

KEY POINT 22-1 Successful dermatologic therapy is based on myriad factors. Dosages and frequency of administration should be modified to meet the needs of the individual patient.

ANATOMY AND PHYSIOLOGY OF THE SKIN AS THEY RELATE TO DRUG THERAPY

The skin is the largest organ of the body, accounting for 12% of body weight in the adult dog and 24% in the puppy.[1] Although structurally canine and feline skin markedly varies from human skin, some similarity is maintained among the species. Generally, skin is thickest on the head, dorsum, and plantar and palmar surfaces of the feet; thinner on the ventral abdomen, medial aspects of the limbs, and inner pinnae; and thinnest on the scrotum.[2] The skin is perforated by several appendages, the number and structure of which varies among the species. In cats and dogs, these include hair follicles, sebaceous and sweat glands, and nails.

Histologically, the skin is composed of the epidermis and dermis. Dermis is essentially composed of connective tissue, including collagen, elastin, and reticular fibers, and amorphous ground substance. It can be roughly separated into a dense, deeper reticular layer that connects the dermis to the hypodermis (composed mostly of fat) and a more superficial, loosely packed papillary layer. The dermis contains an arterial and venous network that provides nutrients to the epidermis and receives topically administered drugs able to penetrate this region, which distribute to the rest of the body.[2] Cutaneous blood flow rates can affect percutaneous absorption of drugs. Cutaneous blood flow in the dog and cat is greatest in the skin of the ventral abdomen and pinnea.[2] This fact, coupled with skin thickness, leads to these regions serving as the site of drug delivery for many topically applied drugs intended to have systemic effects.

The epidermis is composed of stratified squamous keratinized epithelium that undergoes sequential superficial differentiation. Five layers of the epidermis exist, with the stratum basale being deepest, followed by the stratum spinosum, stratum granulosum, stratum lucidum, and the stratum corneum (the most superficial layer). Among these layers the stratum corneum is the most important to topical drug therapy because it is the primary barrier. The stratum corneum consists of several layers of dead cells, which present a significant lipid barrier to drug penetration. The thickness varies with the area of the body. The cells are aligned to minimize water loss and are surrounded by a plasma membrane that serves as a barrier to movement into or out of the skin.[2]

The epidermis is anaerobic[2] because of the absence of capillaries that directly provide oxygen to the cells.[2] Despite the fact that 80% of the total energy requirements of the skin occur by anaerobic glycolysis, the skin is metabolically active. Drugs that are able to pass through the stratum corneum potentially are subjected to drug-metabolizing enzymes similar to those in the liver. The skin has a great capacity to synthesize lipids, which are located in the extracellular (intercellular) material, the primary barrier to drug penetration in this region of the epidermis.[2] Lipids are important to intercellular cohesion, permeability (barrier), function, and normal desquamation of mature corneocytes.[3] Epidermal lipids include both free and esterified fatty acids, sphingolipids, free and esterified cholesterol, and phospholipids.[3] The lipids form a bilipid layer, with the hydrophobic and hydrophilic ends aligning within themselves.[2] As the epidermis differentiates, the fatty acid component tends to increase. Alterations in the lipid layer result in the release of arachidonic acid and the subsequent formation of inflammatory mediators. Keratin is the major protein of the skin and is the foundation of the hair.[2]

PRINCIPLES OF TOPICAL DRUG THERAPY

Topical drug therapy is indicated as initial therapy until a definitive diagnosis can be made (i.e., while waiting for results from diagnostic tests), as an adjunct to systemic therapy, and as sole treatment for selected specific dermatologic diseases. A definitive diagnosis of the cause of the skin disease should be made if possible before any masking treatments have been initiated. Therapy may be based on the morphology of skin lesions if further diagnostics yield no useful data. The clinician must be able to distinguish between primary and secondary lesions. Primary lesions develop as a direct result of the underlying disease. Secondary lesions may evolve from the primary lesion, trauma (e.g., scratching) induced by patient response to the lesion, or medications. The clinician must also be able to recognize or discriminate between acute versus chronic, deep versus superficial, and benign versus malignant lesions.

Clinicians should be very familiar with one or two drugs from each class (e.g., one keratolytic, two topical antifungals). Lesions should be evaluated frequently to assess therapy and the need to modify treatment because of treatment failure or adverse effects. The clinician must know the adverse effects of each drug and anticipate and look for evidence of these effects. Clients must be well educated regarding topical drug agents and the need for compliance. Several principles can guide effective use of dermatologic agents.

Drug Movement and the Skin

The skin functions as a barrier to prevent loss of water, electrolytes, and macromolecules and to exclude external agents (chemical, physical, and microbiologic) from the internal environment. The stratum corneum is the layer of the epidermis that is primarily responsible for this physical barrier because of the abundance of keratin and the configuration and content of the intercellular lipids. Topically applied drugs can be absorbed by three routes; they are, in order of importance or magnitude, the stratum corneum (between rather than through the cells), hair follicles, and sweat or sebaceous glands that open into the hair follicle. Movement of drug through the stratum corneum occurs by passive diffusion. Only a very small proportion of topically applied drug penetrates the stratum corneum. Despite the alignment of the lipid layer, both lipid-soluble and water-soluble drugs can pass through the stratum corneum, although passage may occur through the appendages. In general, permeability of lipophilic drugs through intact skin is generally greater than that of polar drugs.[4] More drug is likely to pass through the skin of heavily haired animals because of the larger number of hair follicles.

Before a drug can move through the stratum corneum, it must first move out of the vehicle. Thus factors that affect percutaneous absorption are not limited to the drug but include factors involving the vehicle. Drug movement through the skin has been mathematically described (Fick's law)[2] to be directly proportional to the partition coefficient between the vehicle and the stratum corneum, the concentration of drug dissolved in the vehicle, the diffusion coefficient, and the surface area of the skin to which the drug is applied. Percutaneous absorption is inversely proportional to the depth of the stratum corneum (and additional layers). The driving force for absorption, as with any drug movement, is concentration of diffusible drug. The higher the concentration of the dissolved drug in the barrier (stratum corneum), the greater the diffusion "gradient." Drugs with a high degree of lipid solubility achieve higher concentrations in the stratum corneum because it is lipophilic. Large drug molecules are absorbed less readily.

Vehicles

A vehicle is a substance used in a medicinal preparation as the agent for carrying the active ingredient. Occasionally, the vehicle is therapeutic, but usually it is inactive. The vehicle of a topical agent can profoundly affect movement of drug into the skin. Two topical medications may have the same active ingredient at the same concentration but have different vehicles and thus markedly differ in efficacy. A drug must be sufficiently soluble in a vehicle such that it can distribute throughout the vehicle and thus come in contact with the skin in diffusible form. It cannot, however, be so soluble in the vehicle that it does not leave the vehicle and thus penetrate the skin. Vehicle selection is critical to effective topical therapy. A vehicle not only acts as a carrier but also can have a direct impact on the skin and thus on drug movement.

Characteristics of a Vehicle

The physical and chemical characteristics of the vehicle and the drug largely determine drug movement. The partition coefficient describes the relative affinity of a hydrophobic phase and a hydrophilic phase. The greater the partition coefficient, the greater the affinity between the drug and the lipid phase of the skin, which generally results in an increase in percutaneous absorption of the drug. Once the skin is penetrated, however, the drug must be able to leave the lipid phase of the skin if it is to reach systemic circulation. Drugs with very high partition coefficients tend to remain in the lipid layer, causing a reservoir effect. A partition coefficient of 1 is desired for topical medicaments.[2]

The rate of vehicle penetration through the stratum corneum also influences percutaneous absorption. If vehicle penetration of the stratum corneum is more rapid than penetration of the skin, the concentration of drug in the vehicle on the surface of the skin increases, perhaps to the point of precipitation, slowing absorption. Evaporation of the vehicle will cause the same effect.[2] Some vehicles are used to facilitate drug movement into the skin. For example, dimethylsulfoxide (DMSO) is so hygroscopic that it readily moves through the skin, carrying many drugs with it. The vehicle may contain ingredients (e.g., Tween) intended to facilitate percutaneous drug absorption by altering the integrity of the stratum corneum. Disruption of the composition or lipid orientation of the stratum corneum enhances drug penetrability. A vehicle that hydrates the corneum facilitates drug penetration. Occlusion of the skin increases hydration; vehicles can occlude by preventing skin transpiration, the passage of water vapor from the skin. Occlusive bandages also can be used to facilitate drug absorption. Water associated with hydration alters the compact structure of the corneum, decreasing resistance to drug movement. Dehydration of the stratum corneum decreases drug absorption; rehydration might be indicated before drug application.

Other patient factors that influence drug movement include the integrity of the barrier presented by the stratum corneum. Drug absorption dramatically increases if the skin has been traumatized, leading to the disruption of the stratum corneum. Absorption may also be enhanced by rubbing a medicament vigorously onto the skin. Prior removal of debris on the surface of the skin (e.g., dirt, blood, hair) can increase drug absorption, as can increasing the temperature of the skin (with sweats or water). Enhanced blood flow to the area might force drug into the hair follicles and through the stratum corneum. A warmer environmental temperature also might increase drug movement into the skin.

Many vehicles are represented in the commercial products for veterinary use. Compounding of dermatologic products is a relatively common practice in veterinary medicine. Although this can often provide a safe and effective therapeutic agent, it is important to remember that the effect of the vehicle on bioavailability of the active ingredient(s) can be profound. The resulting product may be entirely ineffective because of lack of absorption, or it may cause toxicity as a result of systemic absorption.

Types of Vehicles

Water itself can be therapeutic. Bathing with water vehicles (especially shampoos) contributes to dermatologic therapy by removing debris, including potential allergens, bacteria, and other organisms, from the skin surface and rehydrating and cooling the skin (if cool water is used).[5] The addition of other drugs (shampoos, soaks, and dips or rinses) to water, forming an aqueous solution, suspension, or lotion, can create other therapeutic effects. Aqueous medications are often the topical treatment of choice for acute exudative dermatoses.

Shampoos, a type of water vehicle, can be very effective adjuvants for the control of dermatoses.[5,6] In general, contact time should be at least 10 minutes. Shampoos generally are applied once to twice weekly. Examples of shampoos with therapeutic intent include hypoallergenic shampoos, which are cleansing and moisturizing; antipruritic shampoos, which often contain colloidal oatmeal along with antihistamines, anesthetics (pramoxine hydrochloride), or cortisone 1%; and insecticidal shampoos containing compounds such as pyrethrins, carbaryl, and permethrin. Application of rinses, sprays, or lotions can enhance the residual effect of shampoos.

Rinses generally are applied after a shampoo and are not necessarily intended to be completely rinsed from the coat. Incomplete rinses may increase the residual effect of the drug but also may leave the coat greasy to the touch and dull (especially on long-haired coats). Rinses include cream rinses (generally rinsed off the animal) and aqueous rinses (generally not rinsed off). Aqueous rinses also can be applied as a soak, which should last at least 10 to 15 minutes. Powders (colloidal oatmeal) intended to be applied as soaks can be placed in cheesecloth or nylon stockings before placement in water. Humectants such as Humilac (Virbac U.S.) may be applied as a spray directly onto the skin or diluted with water and applied as a rinse. Humectants are oil-free products that help draw moisture to the stratum corneum.

Lotions are liquid or semiliquid combinations of active ingredient with a water, alcohol, glycerin, or propylene glycol base. Often the liquid base evaporates, and a thin film of powder remains on the skin. For this reason lotions may have a drying effect on the skin. Examples include calamine lotion and the antifungal Resizole (Virbac U.S.). Lotions also are available with a variety of antipruritic and parasitic medications.

Both aerosol and pump sprays are available for many veterinary products. Those with alcohol bases may be drying to the target area. Clipping animals may be necessary to facilitate penetration of the hair coat. Foams consist of a mixture of finely divided gas bubbles interspersed in a liquid. These preparations provide an effective way of spreading a small amount of liquid over a large surface area. A potential drawback of sprays is the noise of the application, which may frighten the patient. Both sprays and lotions may be easier to use than creams and ointments, especially for dogs with long hair coats.

Creams and ointments are mixtures of grease or oil and water that are blended together into an emulsion. In general, ointments are greasy to the touch and form an occlusive layer over the skin, reducing water loss. Creams are smooth to the touch and, once applied to the skin, are rapidly absorbed or evaporate (i.e., there is no occlusive layer left on the surface of the skin). In general, ointments are contraindicated in exudative areas. Examples include triple antibiotic ointments and creams and hydrocortisone ointments and creams. Hydrocarbon bases are emollient, being composed of vegetable oils and animal fats. Examples include oleic acid, paraffin, petrolatum, and wax. They generally are hydrophobic and occlusive, causing the stratum corneum to hydrate. They are greasy, however, and cannot be washed off. Anhydrous absorption bases contain little to no water but readily accept large amounts of water while maintaining a thick consistency. Examples include hydrophilic petrolatum and anhydrous lanolin.

Emulsions are oil and water combinations. Water–oil emulsion bases are water-washable bases that are easily removed from the skin surface. The oil phase generally is petrolatum with an alcohol; the aqueous phase may be water, propylene glycol, polyethylene glycol, or glycerin. Oil-water emulsion bases are composed of an aqueous phase that is greater than the oil component. These tend to be water washable, nongreasy, and nonocclusive. Finally, water-soluble–based ointments have no hydrophobic lipid base. They are completely water soluble, do not hydrolyze, and do not support the growth of microorganism contaminants in the product. If the preparation is in a gelled medium, the product is a gel (e.g., a combination of propylene glycol, propylene gallate, methylcellulose, polyethylene glycol, and others). DMSO is commonly prepared as a gel.[2] Gels are clear, colorless, and water miscible. Gels are becoming more popular because they can be rubbed into the skin to completely disappear and do not leave a sticky feeling. Examples of gels in veterinary medicine are KeraSolv, OxyDex and Pyoben.

DMSO has the ability to allow some substances ordinarily unable to penetrate the skin to be carried through it. DMSO is a waste product of wood processing that has been used in a large number of topical medicaments. In addition to its hydrophilic actions, DMSO is characterized by bacteriostatic, antiinflammatory, fibrinolytic, and vasodilatory actions. Topical analgesia may reflect a thermal effect, which occurs with direct application.[2] At concentrations greater than 70%, however, DMSO can cause skin irritation. In concentrations greater than 50%, DMSO has been shown to enhance the percutaneous absorption of a large number of drugs, including glucocorticoids, antibiotics, hormones, and antiinflammatory agents. Absorption increases as DMSO concentration reaches 100%.[2] DMSO increases percutaneous absorption of fluocinolone (a potent glucocorticoid) by a factor of five and other compounds by as much as a factor of 25. DMSO is approved for use only in the horse (for traumatic musculoskeletal injuries) and in the dog (in Synotic, a commercial steroid ear preparation). Any other use for DMSO is considered extralabel use. Toxic effects that should be considered when DMSO is used include teratogenicity (contraindicated in pregnant animals); potential for inducing degranulation of mast cells in underlying skin; and, in cats, hemolysis with hemoglobinuria and methemoglobinuria. DMSO has been shown to induce lenticular changes in animals and humans. Rubber gloves should be worn when DMSO is handled.

Adsorbents act to bind potentially noxious agents, keeping them from damaging the skin. Protectants provide an occlusive layer that physically protects the skin from the external environment. Together these two classes of vehicles are represented by dusting powders and mechanical protectives (kaolin, lanolin, mineral oil, petrolatum, zinc stearate). Dusting powders generally are inert, composed of starch, calcium carbonate, talc, titanium dioxide, zinc oxide, and boric acid. Smooth-surfaced powders prevent friction, protecting abraded and raw skin. Rough or porous powder surfaces absorb water, tending to occlude the skin surface when wetted. Rough powders should be avoided on moist or exudative lesions because of the risk of secondary bacterial or fungal infections. Care should be taken to make sure that powders, and in particular talc, are not used within a body cavity because of the potential for a massive granulomatous response.

Demulcents are high-molecular-weight water-soluble compounds that reduce irritation. Like protectants, they can coat the surface of damaged skin, protecting the stratum corneum and its underlying structures, and they inherently reduce irritation. Examples include mucilages, gums, dextrins, starches, methylcelluloses, and polyvinyl alcohol.[2] Among those most commonly used in veterinary medicine are glycerin, propylene glycol, and polyethylene glycols. Glycerin, when used in high concentrations on the skin, can dehydrate and irritate it by increasing transepidermal water loss. Propylene glycol is miscible with water. Like glycerin, it is hygroscopic, is not occlusive, and also is bacteriostatic and fungistatic. As such, it might be considered the ideal vehicle. It spreads easily on the skin surface, has a low evaporation rate, is not greasy, and may hydrate rather than dehydrate the skin.[2] A mixture of one part propylene glycol to one part water has been used to treat canine sebaceous adenitis. Topical hypersensitivity occurs occasionally. Several polyethylene glycols are available. They differ markedly in molecular weight, with the number directly correlating with size and viscosity. Polyethylene glycols that are 900 or above tend to be semihard to waxy solids at room temperature; lower-molecular-weight products are liquid. These compounds are not easily hydrolyzed but are very water soluble and nontoxic.[2]

Astringents cause precipitation of proteins and prevent exudation. Because of their inability to penetrate the skin, their action is predominantly on the surface. Many astringents are also antiseptic. Astringents can arrest hemorrhage by coagulating plasma proteins (ferric chloride, silver nitrate). Burow's solution is available commercially as Domeboro (aluminum acetate powder or tablets) for use as an astringent in exudative dermatoses. Commercially available otic products containing Burow's solution (Bur-Otic, Virbac U.S.)) can be used to treat dogs that spend a lot of time in the water or after bathing to reduce the risk of secondary infection. Magnesium sulfate (Epsom salt) is not an astringent but acts to dehydrate or "draw" water from the tissues.

Emollients are fatty or oleaginous substances that soften, protect, and soothe the skin. They are often used to make the cream or ointment vehicle in many dermatologic preparations. Examples include mineral oil, petrolatum, glycerin, and vegetable and animal oils. In veterinary medicine emollients are commonly used as cream rinses after baths. Most of these chemicals have a characteristic medicinal odor that appeals to owners. Active ingredients can be added (pramoxine hydrochloride) to enhance therapeutic effect.

Classes of Topical Drugs

Many topical products are commercially available, and many have multiple effects. Some of these agents are also discussed in other chapters (e.g., those on parasitology, antibacterials, and antifungals).

Antiseborrheics

Antiseborrheic drugs include keratolytics and keratoplastics. The appropriate antiseborrheic depends on the patient's condition (seborrhea sicca versus seborrhea oleosa).

Sulfur is keratolytic (keratolytics hydrate and soften the stratum corneum, promoting its mechanical removal) and keratoplastic (keratoplastics normalize cornification). It has a mild follicular flushing action but is not a good degreaser. It also has antibacterial and antipruritic effects. Its keratolytic effects may reflect inflammation that ultimately causes sloughing of the stratum corneum. Keratoplastic effects probably reflect cytostatic effects.[2] Many commercially available products containing sulfur are available. Shampoo products containing sulfur may have additional active ingredients for enhanced therapy. Lime sulfur (LymDip) is used for its antifungal, antipruritic, and antiparasitic effects.

Salicylic acid is keratoplastic, bacteriostatic, and mildly antipruritic. It is frequently used in combination with sulfur products, including most of the sulfur products listed previously. When salicylic acid is combined with sulfur, a synergistic effect results. In stronger concentrations (6%) it acts as a keratolytic.

Coal tar is keratolytic and keratoplastic and has good degreasing action. It is also frequently used in combination with sulfur and salicylic acid. Commercial shampoos are frequently used in veterinary medicine and include Lytar, Allerseb-T, and Mycodex Tar & Sulfur. Straight tar lotions should not be used in veterinary medicine. Coal tar is toxic to cats. Coal tar preparations are potentially irritating, photosensitizing, carcinogenic, and staining. In general, these products are reserved for severe seborrheic disorders.

Benzoyl peroxide (2% to 5%) is keratolytic, bactericidal, degreasing, and follicular flushing. It also is a strong oxidizer, free radical generator (and therefore antibacterial), and antimicrobial.[2] Benzoyl peroxide is metabolized by viable epidermal cells in the skin to benzoic acid. In high concentrations it can irritate the skin. It may be too drying for some patients with seborrhea sicca. These products are not well tolerated by cats and should not be used on them. Commercial products available for veterinary patients include Oxydex, Pyoben, Derma Ben SS, and Benzoyl-Plus shampoos. A gel form of 5% is available for veterinary use, primarily for treatment of chin acne.[7] Other uses include fold pyodermas and local superficial or deep pyodermas. Benzoyl peroxide will bleach clothing.

Resorcinol is a keratolytic agent that also has bactericidal and fungicidal effects. It is a protein precipitant that promotes keratin hydration, acting as a keratolytic.[2] It often is combined with another keratolytic (e.g., sulfur, salicylic acid).[2]

Selenium sulfide is antiseborrheic, keratolytic, and keratoplastic by virtue of its antimitotic effects. Cell proliferation and sebum formation are slowed. It tends to be irritating, however, and can stain hair. Mucous membrane irritation may result if accidental contact occurs. A product for human beings is Selsun Blue. Fatty acids (e.g., undecylenic acid [Desenex]) are also keratolytic.

Retinoids

Retinoids are natural or synthetic derivatives of retinol (vitamin A) that exhibit vitamin A activity (Figure 22-1).[8] Dermatologic effects of vitamin A include epithelial differentiation. Vitamin A deficiency causes metaplasia of glandular epithelia; excessive vitamin A causes keratinizing epithelia to differentiate into a secretory epithelia.[9] The antikeratinizing effects are the target of drug therapy.[9] Retinoids tend to "normalize" the skin. Although natural retinoids have proved to be too toxic for clinical use, the synthetic products are characterized by specific effectiveness with decreased toxicity. They tend to vary in bioavailability, in metabolism to active versus inactive metabolites, and in tissue distribution patterns. First-generation compounds include retinol and its derivatives tretinoin and isotretinoin. The second-generation products are synthetic and include etretinate and acitretin, approved for treatment of human acne and psoriasis, respectively. The third-generation compounds, arytenoids, are in development.[8]

The effects of the retinoids include cellular proliferation and differentiation, immunomodulation, inflammation, and production of sebum. Their actions are mediated by retinoic acid receptors, members of the thyroid/steroid receptors.[8] Retinoids may influence genomic expression of cells by altering RNA synthesis, typical of other steroids. Tretinoin increases dermal thickness and granular layer thickness, decreases melanocytic activity, and increases the secretion of a polysulfated glycosaminoglycan intercellular matrix. In humans wrinkling is reduced. It is formulated as a 0.01% to 0.1% topical preparation. Therapy begins with lower concentrations and gradually increases. Adverse effects include erythema, peeling, burning, and stinging, which tend to decrease with time and are less likely to occur when the drug is prepared as an emollient.

Isotretinoin normalizes keratinization of the follicular epithelium and reduces sebum synthesis and, in human beings, *Proprionobacterium acnes.* It is administered orally, however, with cumulative doses being important to efficacy. Toxicity is manifested in the skin and mucous membranes; is dose dependent; and, in humans, may facilitate the growth of *Staphylococcus aureus.* Dermatologic manifestations include epistaxis, dry eyes, blepharoconjunctivitis, erythematous eruptions,

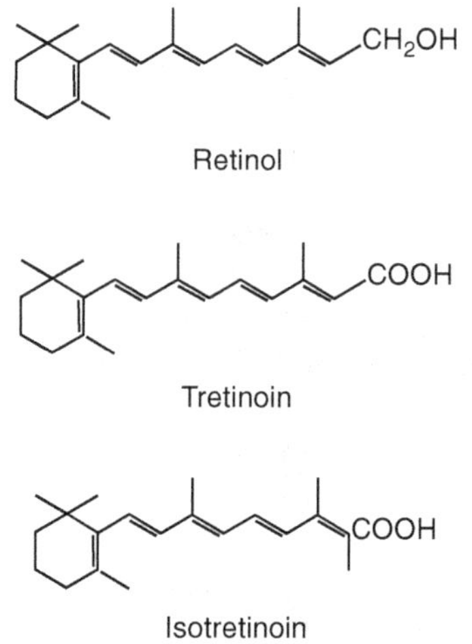

Retinol

Tretinoin

Isotretinoin

Figure 22-1 Stuctures of synthetic retinoids.

and dry mucous membranes.[8] Systemic manifestations can be minimized with short-term therapy and include increased liver enzymes, myalgia, and arthralgia. Teratogenicity occurs with all retinoids; the drugs generally are contraindicated in pregnancy. Isotretinoin was studied in dogs.[10] Four of 29 developed conjunctivitis, which resolved once therapy was discontinued. Cats may have a higher incidence of side effects, including periocular erythema, epiphora, and blepharospasm. The potential veterinary applications of isotretinoin include selected abnormalities of sebum production such as primary idiopathic seborrhea and comedo syndromes.

Etretinate is a synthetic aromatic retinoid that is effective for the treatment of inflammatory psoriasis. The retinoids are highly potent aromatic analogs of retinoic acid and represent the third generation. Etretinate is extremely lipophilic and is stored in adipose tissue. Accumulation is sufficient to allow detection of the drug in humans 2 to 3 years after its use is discontinued. It normalizes keratin expression in epidermal cells, suppresses chemotaxis, decreases stratum corneum cohesiveness, and may impair cytokine function.[8] It is less likely than isotretinoin to cause conjunctivitis, but hair loss, cutaneous exfoliation, bruising, and liver dysfunction are more common. Collection of a baseline minimum database is recommended for humans before its use. Its teratogenicity precludes use by women of childbearing age; owners of animals using the drug should be warned of its contraindications.[8] The drug may no longer be available because of its adverse effects. Acitretin has now replaced etretinate in the U.S. market. A dose of 0.5 to 1 mg/kg orally per day was suggested.[11]

The use of retinoids in clinical veterinary medicine has not been well established. Animals are not afflicted by skin diseases typical of those for which retinoids are indicated in human patients (e.g., psoriasis, acne). Use is limited by lack of known effects and indications, cost, and the risk of side effects. Dogs, however, appear to be more tolerant of the retinoids than human beings.[10,12] Side effects that have been reported in dogs include inappetence, vomiting, diarrhea, thirst, pruritis, conjunctivitis, cheilitis, stiffness, and hyperactivity.[12] Keratoconjunctivitis has been reported in dogs.[10,12] Tear composition is changed, leading to more rapid evaporation. Schirmer's tear test should be monitored monthly for the first 6 months of therapy. Clinical pathology changes are rare, but monitoring before and 30 days after the start of therapy is recommended for dogs receiving synthetic retinoid therapy.[12] In cats the most common side effect is anorexia. Teratogenicity is a likely problem, particularly with etretinate, when used for intact females.

The most common use of synthetic retinoids in dogs has been for treatment of keratinization disorders of dogs, particularly primary seborrhea of cocker spaniels. Etretinate has been evaluated in spaniels with idiopathic seborrheic dermatitis (approximately 10 mg or 0.75 to 1 mg/kg orally per day). Animals generally respond well with a decrease in scaling, a softening and thinning of seborrheic plaques, decreased pruritis, and reduction in odor. Response occurs within 2 months, and improvement continues for at least 2 more months.[12] The more severe the syndrome, the slower the time to response; discontinuation of therapy is likely to result in recrudescence of clinical signs within 3 to 12 weeks.[9] The drug was minimally effective in the treatment of ceruminous otitis associated with seborrhea.[12] Maintenance therapy ranges from 10 mg every other day to 10 mg daily, alternating 30 days on and 30 days off. Isotretinoin (1 and 3 mg/kg per day) appears to be much less effective.[9] Neither isotretinoin nor etretinate has proved to be effective in West Highland White Terriers, and etretinate was ineffective in Basset Hounds. Both etretinate and isotretinoin have proved effective in the treatment of Schnauzer comedo syndrome[9,12] and canine ichthyosis. Newer applications of the synthetic retinoids include hair follicle dysplasia (etretinate), which should respond in approximately 30 days, and selected dermatologic cancers. These include solar-induced squamous cell carcinoma (etretinate 2 mg/kg divided or once daily for 6 months), mycosis fungoides (etretinate or isotretinoin 3 to 4 mg/kg divided or once daily), and selected benign cutaneous neoplasms (multiple sebaceous adenomas, epidermal cysts, inverted papillomas, and infundibular keratinizing acanthomas).[12]

Isotretinoin for the treatment of disorders of the sebaceous glands has been variably successful; success may be breed dependent. It was proved effective in sebaceous adenitis of standard poodles in one study but ineffective in another.[9] A higher dose (2 to 3 mg/kg) has been recommended. Hair growth in poodles that do respond is abnormal, however, in that kinks are lost. Vizslas appear to respond to isotretinoin very well.[9] In contrast, neither isotretinoin nor etretinate appears to be effective in sebaceous adenitis of Akitas.

Retinoids appear to be safe for cats but do not appear to be effective for solar-induced squamous cell carcinoma. Either isotretinoin or etretinate (2 to 2.5 mg/kg) can, however, be beneficial for preneoplastic actinic disease. Cats tolerate retinoids well, although anorexia is more common in cats than in dogs.[12] Reducing treatment to every other day or every other week may limit this side effect. Topical tretinoin (0.025% cream) may be efficacious for treatment of feline acne. The product must be used very sparingly, however, so as not to incur severe tissue irritation.[12]

Although there are no reports of either acute or chronic toxicity in animals receiving retinoids, animals nonetheless should be closely monitored. Monitoring should begin with a physical examination before implementation of therapy, including measurement of tear production. These tests should be repeated at 4- to 6-month intervals. A complete blood count and serum chemistries, including triglycerides, should be monitored at baseline, at 1 and 2 months of therapy, and then every 4 to 6 months during therapy. Care should be taken to counsel clients regarding the cost, importance of compliance, and risk of accidental human ingestion.

Ceruminolytics

Ceruminolytics are topical products that emulsify, soften, and break up waxy debris and exudate. Generally, they are detergents or surfactants used for cleaning or flushing the ear. Examples include dioctyl sodium sulfosuccinate, which is water soluble (and perhaps less messy); squalene, which is an oil-based product; propylene glycol; glycerin; and oil.

Carbamide peroxide differs from most other ceruminolytics in that it is a humectant, releasing urea and oxygen to cause its foaming action. Ceruminolytics and drying products are often combined with alpha hydroxy acid such as lactic, salicylic, benzoic, and malic acids. These acids have the added advantage of decreasing local pH and are mildly antibacterial and antifungal, along with their keratolytic effects. These products need to be placed in the ear 3 to 15 minutes before flushing with water or saline.

Antipruritics

Antipruritics (topical)[5] are used to provide temporary relief of itching, but their efficacy is debatable. In general, antipruritics relieve itching by four mechanisms. (1) The itching sensation can be substituted with another sensation (such as heat or cold). Examples of agents with this mechanism of action include menthol, camphor, warm soaks or baths, and ice packs. (2) The skin can be protected from external factors such as scratching, biting, irritants, and changes in humidity or temperature. This can be accomplished with bandages or impermeable protective agents. (3) Peripheral sensory nerves can be anesthetized by local anesthetics (benzocaine, lidocaine). These drugs may, however, cause allergic sensitization. A new product in this category for small animals is pramoxine (Dermacool). (4) Biochemical agents used topically to treat pruritus include glucocorticoids and antihistamines. Despite the fact that the skin contains large numbers of mast cells, topical antihistamines do not seem to be efficacious. Systemic antihistamines, on the other hand, may be useful.

Topical glucocorticoids may not be as potent as their oral or injectable counterparts.[13] Like systemic glucocorticoids, however, the active ingredients vary in potency and risk of side effects. For topical glucocorticoids ointments provide greater efficacy than creams. Topical glucocorticoids can be absorbed through the skin and cause systemic effects. This is more likely to be a problem with the potent fluorinated agents (betamethasone, dexamethasone, triamcinolone, flumethasone, and flucinolone) and when combined with DMSO (Synotic). Gloves should be worn to apply these drugs. There are many forms of glucocorticoids available for topical use, including use on extensions of the skin such as the external ear canal and anal sacs. Once absorbed through the skin, topical corticosteroids are handled by the body in the same capacity as systemically administered glucocorticoids. The extent of percutaneous absorption of topical glucocorticoids depends on factors such as the vehicle, the ester form of the steroid (greater lipid solubility enhances percutaneous absorption), duration of exposure, surface area, and integrity of the epidermal barrier. A new product containing 0.015% triamcinolone (Genesis spray, Virbac U.S.) has been formulated to be applied topically to the entire skin surface for its antipruritic effect.[11] This product may also be used for spot treatment of pruritic regions. Ointment bases are occlusive and are therefore more likely to increase percutaneous absorption of the same glucocorticoid in a cream base. Highly potent preparations in any form should not be used on abraded skin.

Irritants

A number of products are used to inflame or irritate the skin to various degrees. Examples include those that cause hyperemia (rubefacients), inflammation (irritants), and cutaneous blisters (vesicants). Caustics are corrosive agents that destroy tissue after one or more applications. Examples include camphor, coal tar, creosote, menthol, methyl salicylate, iodine, mercuric iodide, alcohols, and pine tar. Among these, only coal tar is used to any degree in veterinary medicine. It is a by-product of bituminous coal distillation and, as an irritant, decreases epidermal synthesis of DNA.[2] Escharotics also are corrosives that precipitate proteins, causing the formation of a scab and eventually a scar. Examples include glacial acetic acid, aluminum chloride, gentian violet, phenol, salicylic acid, and silver nitrate. The uses in veterinary medicine are few.[2] Irritant products have been used empirically for many centuries. Their proposed mode of action is masking of moderate to severe pain by milder pain caused by the application. Another desired effect of irritants is to induce a healing action on chronic wounds. The idea is to heal chronic inflammation by converting it to acute inflammation. Chemicals used include phenol, formalin, mercuric iodide, and camphor. Menthol-containing products are sometimes used to treat acral lick dermatitis ("lick granuloma") in dogs but may be painful upon initial application. Capsaicin has been used topically on human beings for relieving arthritis pain. It also has been used to treat acral lick dermatitis in dogs.

Antimicrobials

Alcohols, iodine, chlorhexidine, iodophors, and hexachlorophene can be effective in the treatment of infectious skin diseases (see Chapters 10, 11, and 13).

Benzoyl peroxide, discussed with the antiseborrheics, is a potent broad-spectrum antibacterial agent. It is an excellent adjunctive treatment for pyoderma. In a clinical trial of four antibacterial shampoos (containing 3% benzoyl peroxide, 0.5% chlorhexidine, 1% available iodine in a povidone complex, and 0.5% triclosan combined with 2% salicylic acid and 2% sulfur), although each was effective prophylactically, the product containing benzoyl peroxide was most effective.[14] Use of the veterinary products (as opposed to the human proprietary products) is strongly recommended. Benzoyl peroxide is very irritating to cats and should be avoided.

Many antibiotics are available in topical form as ointments. Examples include neomycin, bacitracin, polymyxin B, gramicidin, and nitrofurazone. Often these drugs are available in combination with each other or with steroids.

Mupirocin is a compound produced by *Pseudomonas fluorescens* that is effective against superficial (topical) infections caused by *Staphylococcus* species. It is less active against gram-negative organisms and in humans is not active against normal skin flora. It inhibits protein synthesis by binding to bacterial tRNA synthetase. Prepared as an ointment, it often is used for prophylaxis of superficial infections resulting from wounds and injuries.[8] Veterinary products containing mupirocin recently have become available (Muricin ointment 2%, Dechra).

Treatment of otitis externa often involves a topical antibiotic–steroid combination such as Tresaderm or Panalog. Any of the agents contained in these products, neomycin in particular, can cause allergic sensitization or irritation. Cats appear to be more sensitive to topically applied otics than dogs.

In general, topical therapy of dermatophytoses in dogs and cats is not highly effective because of the thick hair coat and the location of the organisms deep in the hair follicle. The drugs are often unable to reach the site of the infection in adequate concentrations. Gentle clipping of the affected area(s) may aid in topical application, but whole body clipping is generally not recommended. Amphotericin B (Fungizone), available as 3% cream, lotion, or ointment, can be used for *Candida* infections. Chlorhexidine is a mild antifungal as well as antibacterial and is available as a rinse or shampoo (1% to 4% recommended). By itself it is not very effective for the treatment of dermatophytosis. New formulations combined with miconazole (Malaseb rinse, shampoo and spray DVM) or ketoconazole (Ketochlor, Virbac US)) shampoo can be used for *Malassezia* dermatitis or adjunct therapy for dermatophytosis. Clotrimazole 1% (Lotrimin, Veltrim) is effective against dermatophytes, *Candida,* and *Malassezia.* It may cause mild irritation. Miconazole is available as a 2% cream or 1% lotion (Conofite and Resizole 2%) and shampoo (Dermazole) and is effective against dermatophytes, *Malassezia,* and *Candida.* Nystatin (Panalog ointment or cream, nystatin cream) is effective against some yeast and some dermatophytes but not *Malassezia* species. Sulfur is effective against dermatophytes and therefore may be used for localized or generalized dermatophytosis (LymDyp, DVM). Cats may become ill if they groom after treatment so it is recommended that they wear an Elizabethan collar until the product is dry. Lime sulfur dip is also antiparasitic and antipruritc and very cost effective compared with other topical treatments. Lime sulfur dip may stain fabric and can tarnish jewelry. It is a very efficacious product, but because of the strong odor, owner compliance may be weak. Thiabendazole is effective for dermatophytes and some yeast, including *Malassezia.* Products including thiabendazole include Tresaderm, a combination product with neomycin and dexamethasone, which is best used for local lesions. In general, the use of a topical agent containing corticosteroid is not recommended when treating dermatophytosis.

Antiparasitics

Drug delivery systems. Antiparasitics are available as sprays, powders, shampoos, foams, spot-ons, tablets, and dips. The use of parasiticides is discussed in Chapter 15. Spot-on products are commonly used as broad-spectrum antiparasitic agents. Their ease of use and efficacy make them a preferred product for many circumstances. Powders are the safest formulation but must be frequently applied. They often are messy and must be applied deep into the coat to be effective. Sprays may have little residual effect depending on the active ingredient and concentration of the product, and the noise made during application often frightens the animal. Efficacy can be enhanced by ensuring adequate penetration of the hair. The hair should be brushed away from the skin so that the spray can reach the skin. The face can be treated by spraying into a glove and then rubbing the face. A water-based spray may cause less drooling than an alcohol-based spray.

Shampoos have little residual effect and must stay on the skin at least 10 minutes to kill fleas and ticks. The active ingredients (pyrethrin, pyrethroids, carbaryl) in these preparations are not intended to be absorbed systemically. Any factor that would increase the absorption of these drugs (see earlier discussion) may result in system toxicity. Because cats are especially susceptible to the toxicities of certain parasiticides, only those products specifically intended for use on cats should be used. Flea shampoos should not be used more than once weekly to avoid drying of the skin. A humectant rinse may help compensate for the drying effects. Shampoos remove flea eggs, flea feces, and other debris, facilitating other topical therapy and making the animal look and feel better. High-concentration pyrethrins may be effective as repellents for fleas and ticks. They are rapidly destroyed by ultraviolet light. Toxicity can follow ingestion (grooming) or percutaneous absorption. Toxicity is manifested as salivation, tremors, and seizures. Treatment is symptomatic but should include bathing.

A number of spot-on products act as adulticides and some are effective against the juvenile stages as well. They are applied to the infrascapular area from where they diffuse over the body. Some products are intended to be systemically absorbed for their antiparasitic effects. They can cause contact allergy and irritation. Examples include imidacloprid (Advantage, Bayer), fipronil (Frontline, Merial) selemectin (Revolution, Pfizer), metaflumazone (ProMeris, Fort Dodge), and dinotefuran (Vectra 3D, Summit).

In most cases flea collars have limited efficacy. Collars containing carbaryl, pyrethrin, or organophosphates are readily available in stores. Besides having limited efficacy, collars occasionally cause irritation reactions. Collars containing methoprene (Ovitrol) act to "sterilize" the fleas and are helpful in flea eradication. To keep clients from being disappointed with the results, clinicians should inform them that these products do not kill adult fleas. Collars containing amitraz (Preventic) are effective against ticks but not fleas. The feeding ticks will detach and die. Recent studies demonstrate that the tick will be killed before being able to transmit borreliosis, but other tick-borne diseases were not evaluated. This collar will not affect nonfeeding ticks. Ingestion of the collar is associated with acute toxicity. Yohimbine can be an effective antidote. Even though the active ingredient is amitraz, it has been shown to have many beneficial effects for the treatment of demodicosis.

Active ingredients. Pyrethrins are extracts from the chrysanthemum flower. Their mechanism of action involves disrupting neurologic function by prolonging Na^+ in nerve membranes. They rapidly kill fleas, flies, lice, cheyletiella, otodectes, and mosquitoes but have little residual activity. Although among the safest products for use in cats, only those products approved for cats should be used. Pyrethrin-containing products are available in many formulations. Both pyrethrins and permethrins have repellent properties, but their residual effects are not well documented.

Pyrethroids are synthetic analogs of pyrethrins with the same mechanism of action but greater ultraviolet stability and thus longer action. Microencapsulation of pyrethroids provides further residual activity. They have a slower knockdown than pyrethrins, and thus they are often combined with them. Toxicity and treatment thereof is the same as for pyrethrins. Permethrins are available as 0.05% to 25% flea sprays but also up to 65% as spot flea and tick products. A relatively new product (K9 Advantix) combines imidacloprid with permethrin for increased efficacy against ticks. Toxicities have been seen with this product when it was inadvertently applied to a cat.

Chlorinated hydrocarbons should not be used (if there happens to be any still on the market). There are two types of cholinesterase inhibitors available: carbamates and organophosphates.

Carbamates such as carbaryl are available in sprays, dips, collars, and premise-control sprays, and they are safe for dogs and cats. Toxicity of carbamates as well as organophosphates reflects overstimulation of the parasympathetic system and should be treated with atropine and 2-pyridine aldoxime methylchloride.

Organophosphates are the most toxic insecticides used in veterinary medicine. With one exception, these agents should not be used around cats. Care should be taken to avoid cumulative exposure if animals are exposed to this class of insecticide in lawn and garden preparations. Examples of commonly used organophosphates are chlorpyrifos (Dursban, Duratrol), used for flea sprays and dips; diazinon, used for environmental flea and tick control; malathion, used on both cats and dogs and often combined with other insecticides (noncholinesterase inhibitors); phosmet (Paramite Dip), useful for flea control and sometimes used for scabies; cythioate (Proban), a systemic insecticide; and fenthion (Pro-Spot), topically applied for a systemic effect. Organophosphates are disappearing from the market because of concerns of safety of animals and human beings.

Fipronil (Frontline) is a new synthetic molecule in the phenylpyrazole family. It acts at gamma-aminobutyric acid (GABA) receptors and inhibits GABA-regulated chloride flux into the nerve cell. It is a flea adulticide and has efficacy against ticks. It may also be effective in preventing scabies mite infestation. Preliminary studies indicate good residual activity even after bathing. This product is available as an on-animal spray or as a spot-on product. Frontline Plus contains fipronil and methoprene for its ovicidal properties.

Imidacloprid (Advantage and K9 Advantix) is a spot-on application product that kills adult fleas. It works by preventing postsynaptic binding of acetylcholine, leading to respiratory paralysis of the flea. This product may be removed by frequent bathing but is labeled as waterproof. It must be applied every 30 days to be effective. Advantage may be applied as frequently as every 7 days if needed to treat severe infestations of fleas. The addition of permethrin to the K9 Advantix provides efficacy against ticks and mosquitoes and repellent properties against mosquitoes and other parasites. Again, this product is to be used only on dogs.

A combination product containing imidacloprid and moxidectin (Advantage Multi) is available in a spot-on formulation for dogs and cats. The age restriction is 7 weeks and 9 weeks, respectively. This product is used to treat for fleas, heartworm prevention, intestinal worms, and ear mites. It is not approved for use in the United States for the treatment of sarcoptes (scabies) or demodicosis but may prove to be efficacious.

Selamectin (Revolution, Pfizer) is available as a spot-on formulation. It is approved for the treatment of fleas, heartworm prevention, tick (*Dermacentor* sp.) infestations, sarcoptes (scabies), and otodectes (ear mites) for dogs. The age restriction is 6 weeks. The formulation for cats has an age restriction of 8 weeks. It is approved for the treatment of fleas, heartworm prevention, otodectes, roundworms, and hookworms. Anecdotal reports indicate efficacy for feline scabies mites, Notoedres, though not approved for this use.

Nitenpyram (Capstar, Novartis) is an oral medication for the treatment of flea infestations in dogs and cats. The age restriction is 4 weeks, and the animal's body weight must be greater than 2 pounds. This product may be given daily but is often used in conjunction with other flea medications on an as-needed basis. Rapid and complete kill of adult fleas is the main reason for using this product. Anectotal reports indicate efficacy when inserted rectally (i.e., during a surgical procedure when fleas are discovered). It has also been used to treat subcutaneous maggot infestations of dogs and cats. Neither of these uses are licensed or approved by the Food and Drug Administration.

Amitraz (Mitaban) is a monoamine oxidase inhibitor. It is the only licensed product for treatment of generalized demodicosis. Mitaban is also efficacious against scabies and ticks, but this is considered an off-label use. This product rapidly oxidizes on exposure to light and air, and the breakdown product is more toxic than the parent compound. Mitaban should be mixed fresh each time, and the entire contents should be used to avoid toxicity. Side effects include sedation and lethargy (sometimes for 24 hours), pruritus, bradycardia, hypothermia, hypotension, and hyperglycemia. Hyperexcitability is an uncommon side effect. Amitraz is not appropriate for epileptic dogs and animals receiving behavior-modifying drugs. Yohimbine works as a reversing agent. The large animal form of amitraz (Taktic) should not be used on dogs. ProMeris for dogs (Fort Dodge) is a spot-on formulation containing amitraz and metaflumazone. It has recently been approved to treat localized and generalized demodicosis in dogs greater than 8 weeks of age. The recommended application rate is every 14 days until remission. Potential side effects include those associated with amitraz application. Anecdotal skin reactions have been noted.

Ivermectin (Ivomec 1%) is a GABA agonist that leads to parasite paralysis. In mammals GABA in the central nervous system is protected by the blood–brain barrier. Ivermectin is a large molecule that cannot pass the blood–brain barrier except in certain breeds. It is efficacious against scabies, lice, otodectes (ear mites), and cheyletiella. It is *not* approved for use in small animals for treatment of parasites other than as a heartworm preventive. Ivomec is rapidly absorbed orally or subcutaneously. The administration into the ear canal is not recommended except for the 0.01% ivermectin product Acarex. It should not be used in Collies, Border Collies, Shetland Sheepdogs, Australian Shepherds, Old English Sheepdogs, or any dog that looks like a Collie. Also, it is not recommended for any animal younger than 12 weeks of age. Daily ivermectin has been used to treat demodicosis. Enzodiazepines are contraindicated for concurrent use. Treatment of ivermectin toxicity is symptomatic and supportive. There is no good antagonist available.

Milbemycin (Interceptor) has a similar action to ivermectin. Its use in dermatology is confined to daily oral administration for the treatment of refractory demodicosis. Therapy may take 6 to 9 months, and relapses are common. Cost is a limiting factor. This drug is not approved for use for demodex treatment. Although not contraindicated in Collies and Collielike dogs, caution is advised for side effects. A new otic product containing milbemycin (Milbemite) is a very effective treatment for ear mites in dogs and cats.

Spinosad is the active ingredient in Comfortis (Eli Lilly). This is an oral tablet that is given monthly to control fleas on dogs only. The age restriction is 14 weeks. Safety in pregnant animals is not evaluated. Side effects have been noted when this medication has been used in conjunction with off-label usage of ivermectin; this is not recommended. This product has no efficacy against ticks. Vomiting was the most common adverse reaction noted. Absorption of the medication is adequate after 1 hour.

A combination product containing dinotefuran, permethrin, and pyriproxyfen (Vectra 3D, Summit VetPharm) has been approved for use on dogs older than 7 weeks of age. This spot-on product is effective against fleas and ticks and will repel and kill mosquitoes. It is recommended to apply this product monthly. The feline formulation does not contain permethrin. The age restriction is 8 weeks for kittens.

A combination product containing metaflumizone and amitraz (ProMeris, Fort Dodge) is a spot-on product approved for dogs older than 8 weeks of age. It is effective for fleas and ticks and has recently been approved for the treatment of localized and generalized demodicosis. ProMeris for cats (8 weeks or older) does not contain amitraz and is for the treatment of fleas only.

Flea insect growth regulators (IGRs) are endogenous chemicals in insects that control the early stages of their metabolism, morphogenesis, and reproduction. Synthetic compounds mimic the effects of the natural chemicals. Because IGRs maintain high levels of these chemicals during maturation and development of larvae, insects are prevented from developing. Natural levels decrease over time and allow normal maturation. IGRs have no effects on mammals and are very safe. They are combined with pyrethrins or pyrethroidsor fipronil to increase the spectrum of activity to include adults. Several products are available: Methoprene (Ovitrol spray) is a juvenile hormone analog available for on-animal and environmental use. It is degraded by ultraviolet light and hormone esterase. Pyriproxifen (Nylar) is a juvenile hormone mimetic for fleas. Preliminary studies indicate very long residual activity even when the animal is bathed and excellent environmental stability. This ingredient is available mixed with 2.5% permethrin (KnockOut spray) and is a very effective treatment for canine flea allergy. The high concentration of pemethrin precludes its use on cats. Pyriproxifen is also included in Vectra 3D (Summit Labs).

Lufenuron (Program) is a benzoylphenylurea that inhibits synthesis and deposition of chitin within the ova and larval exoskeleton of developing fleas. It is strongly lipophilic and stored in adipose tissue with slow release into the blood vasculature, providing long residual activity from a single dose. It does not affect adult fleas. Lufenuron is taken up by the feeding flea and incorporated into the developing egg. It is excreted in the flea feces. If the flea larvae consume flea feces containing lufenuron, they will be unable to mature into the pupal stage. Because of the slow absorption from the gastrointestinal tract, this product is given with food. Cats do not absorb this product as well as dogs, and therefore a higher dosage on a per-pound basis is needed for the same efficacy and duration of effect. This product is very safe and carries no contraindications.

Miscellaneous. Pennyroyal oil is a volatile oil extracted from plants in the mint family. Because of its limited efficacy and evidence of hepatotoxicity, this product is not recommended. D-limonene is from oils of citrus fruits. Toxicities have been noted in the cat, especially depression, ataxia, and toxic epidermal necrolysis. This product is not recommended. Tea tree oil contains various monoterpenes. Toxicities with this oil have been reported, and there is no scientific evidence to support claims of its efficacy as an antiparasitic agent.

SYSTEMIC DERMATOLOGIC THERAPY

Systemic dermatologic therapy is indicated for diffuse, serious, or chronic conditions (Table 22-1).

Antimicrobials

Antimicrobials indicated for the treatment of dermatologic disorders are discussed in Chapters 10 and 11. A number of antimicrobials are effective for the treatment of bacterial skin diseases (pyoderma). Care should be taken when using sulfonamides, often selected as first-choice therapy, because of their ability to suppress the synthesis of thyroid hormones (see Chapter 32). A study in 20 dogs receiving sulfamethoxazole (with trimethoprim) at 30 mg/kg every 12 hours for 6 weeks found marked suppression of thyronine concentrations and response to thyroid-stimulating hormone. Suppression did not occur with 15 mg/kg of sulfadiazine (trimethoprim) once daily for 4 weeks.[15] Thyroid function returned to normal within 3 weeks of discontinuing therapy. Suppression may result from inhibition of thyroid peroxidase by the amino group in the sulfonamide. The effect of sulfonamides on feline thyroid function has not been reported.

Antiinflammatory and Antipruritic Agents

Glucocorticoids

Glucocorticoids are discussed in Chapter 30. Glucocorticoids continue to be overused and abused for treatment of dermatologic diseases.[13,16] Scott[13] noted that more than 50% of

Table 22-1 Dosing Regimens of Systemic Dermatologic Drugs

Drug	Dose (mg/kg)*	Route	Frequency (hr)
Glucocorticoids			
Dexamethasone	0.11 (D)	PO	48
	0.2 (C)	PO	48
Methylprednisolone	0.25-0.55	PO	24-48
	0.88 (D)	PO	48
Prednisolone	1.1 (D)	PO	48
	2.2 (C)	PO	48
Triamcinolone	0.88 (D)	PO	48
Antihistamines			
Astemizole	1 (D)	PO	24
Cetirizine HCL	1.0	PO	24
Chlorpheniramine	0.22-0.8	PO	8-12 not to exceed 1 mg/kg every 24 hr
	2.4 mg/cat	PO	12-24
Cyproheptadine	0.25-0.5 (D)	PO	12
Clemastine	0.05-1.0 (D)	PO	12
	0.34-0.68 mg total (C)	PO	12
Diphenhydramine	2.2	PO	8
Hydroxyzine	2.2	PO	8
	10 mg total (C)		
Loratadine	0.5-1.0 (D)	PO	24
Trimeprazine	2.5-5 mg total (D)	PO	8
Behavior modifiers			
Amitriptyline	2.24.4 (D)	PO	24
	5-10 mg/cat	PO	24
Clomipramine	1-3 (D)	PO	24
Doxepin	0.5-1 (D)	PO	12
Fluoxetine	1 (D)	PO	24
Hydrocodone	0.25	PO	8
Imipramine	2.24.4	PO	12-24
Naltrexone	2.2	PO	12-24
Antimicrobials			
Enrofloxacin	2.5-5	PO	12
Clofazimine	2-3	PO	24 (feline leprosy)
	8-12	PO	24
Dapsone	1.1	PO	12
Griseofulvin			
Microsize	25-60	PO	Divided or every 24
Ultramicrosize	5-10	PO	Divided or every 24
Itraconazole	5-10	PO	12-24 (with food)
Terbinafine	10 (up to 30?)	PO	24
Antiparasitics			
Ivermectin			
Scabies	0.2 (D)	SC	Two or three doses, 14 days apart
	0.3 (D)	PO	Four doses, 7 days apart
Cheyletiellosis	0.3	SC	Two doses, 21 days apart
Ear mites	0.24.4	SC	One to two doses, 14-21 days apart
Demodectic mange	0.3-0.6 (D)	PO	24
Milbemycin			
Demodectic mange	1-2 (D)	PO	24

D, Dog; *PO*, by mouth; *C*, cat; *SC*, subcutaneous.

his referral cases are complicated by the excessive use of the drugs. Yet glucocorticoids remain an important and legitimate component of both acute and chronic treatment of a variety of skin diseases associated with pruritus or inflammation resulting from allergic diseases (e.g., atopy, flea bite, other insect- and arachnid-mediated hypersensitivity, food hypersensitivity, contact dermatitis), pyotraumatic dermatitis ("hot spots"), and acral lick dermatitis.[13] Note that glucocorticoids for acral lick dermatitis may largely be replaced with behavior-modifying drugs for this syndrome. Glucocorticoids also remain the cornerstone of therapy for many of the autoimmune diseases affecting the skin, including the eosinophilic granuloma complex, pemphigus complex, systemic lupus erythematosus, and discoid lupus erythematosus. Optimal therapy of each of these diseases varies, insofar as some may respond to glucocorticoids alone and some may require a combination of glucocorticoids and alternative immunosuppressive drugs such as azathioprine, chlorambucil, cyclosporine, or cyclophosphamide. Routes of administration vary with lesion and intent and include oral, topical, intralesional, and systemic (intravenous, subcutaneous, intramuscular). The use of topical glucocorticoids was previously discussed; note that side effects of glucocorticoids will not necessarily be prevented by limiting therapy to topical application. In general, oral administration is preferred for its convenience and ability to regulate dosage safely (including rapid withdrawal relative to other routes). Although some animals may appear to respond better to injectable rather than oral drugs, differences in response may reflect an insufficient oral dose. This is particularly likely to occur if the oral drug is one that is less potent than the injectable drug.[13]

The choice of glucocorticoid should be based on desired potency (e.g., dexamethasone is more potent than prednisolone and may be preferred for acute needs) balanced with avoidance of side effects (prednisolone is characterized by a smaller tendency to affect the hypothalamic–pituitary–adrenal axis negatively; see Chapter 30).[16] Personal preference among clinicians ultimately also will determine the selection of specific drugs: Whereas prednisolone may be efficacious for some situations, it may not be for others. In addition, an animal may develop intolerable side effects with one glucocorticoid but not another. The development of steroid tachyphylaxis may lead to deselection of a steroid that previously was efficacious.[13] Remission in the case of acute exacerbation of clinical signs might respond to a pulse-dose approach using the original antiinflammatory dose.[16]

Dermatologic conditions requiring glucocorticoid therapy range from mild to serious. Dermatoses associated with life-threatening conditions generally are limited to diseases that also are accompanied by diseases of multiple organs (e.g., immune-mediated disease). In such cases glucocorticoid therapy should be aggressive, with doses sufficiently high to control disease. Regardless of the indication of glucocorticoids, alternate-day therapy should be a goal of maintenance.[16] Not all conditions will, however, be sufficiently controlled with alternate-day therapy.[13] Because high doses of glucocorticoids are often required to adequately treat immune-mediated diseases, adverse effects are likely to occur. Concurrent administration of additional immunosuppressive drugs (azathioprine, chlorambucil, cyclosporine, or cyclophosphamide) may allow the glucocorticoid dose to be decreased. Dose reduction for patients with autoimmune diseases should be conducted gradually and should occur for at least 2 weeks (longer if time to clinical remission was prolonged), and the actual dose should be decreased by no more than half. Relapse may occur if the dosage is decreased too rapidly. Clinical reassessment should continue until a minimally effective dose is established for maintenance therapy.

Chronic inflammatory disorders (e.g., atopy or flea allergy dermatitis) should be treated less aggressively. A minimum effective dose should be determined by trial and error and reevaluated such that the dose is reduced when possible. Agents that are amenable to alternate-day administration include the first-choice drugs prednisone and prednisolone and the second-choice drug methylprednisolone.[16] The ideal alternate-day dose for these drugs is 0.22 to 0.55 mg/kg.[16] The durations of action of hydrocortisone and cortisone may be too short for effective alternate-day therapy. Although triamcinolone's duration of antiinflammatory action is longer than that of prednisolone and methylprednisolone, suppression of the hypothalamic–pituitary–adrenal axis is more likely but less typical of the long-acting agents such as dexamethasone and betamethasone.

All patients receiving long-term glucocorticoids should be monitored, with physical examinations occurring at least twice yearly. Urinalysis is recommended with a urine culture because of the risk of subclinical urinary tract infection.[16] In cases of relapse, the animal should be reevaluated for complicating diseases or conditions such as pyoderma, dermatophyte infection, and demodicosis.[13,16] Glucocorticoids should be discontinued whenever possible; however, discontinuation may not be possible for immune-mediated disorders.[13,16] Concurrent treatment with nonglucocorticoid antipruritics such as antihistamines or fatty acid supplements, either systemically or topically, should be attempted to reduce the glucocorticoid dose[16] Other agents being studied include misoprostol and cyclosporine.

Cyclosporine

Cyclosporine may be used to control pruritus in dogs and cats with atopic dermatitis.[17,18] It appears to be quite effective at 5 mg/kg orally once daily, and doses range from 2.5 to 6 mg/kg daily. Initially it should be given with food to decrease the likelihood of vomiting, but it is best given on an empty stomach for improved absorption. Food decreased the bioavailability by 22%.[19] The water-soluble forms should be selected (Atopica, Neoral). Long-term use of cyclosporine for the treatment of canine atopic dermatitis has been reviewed.[20] Laboratory abnormalities were detected in 25% of the dogs; 0.039% developed oral growths, and 0.058 % developed hirsutism. Many dogs were tapered to 2 to 3 times per week to control clinical signs. Interestingly, 24% of the dogs did not require ongoing therapy when cyclosporine was discontinued. In another report approximately 40% of dogs treated with cyclosporine for 4 months did not relapse during a 2-month follow-up.[19] There appears to be good evidence to support the beneficial response to cyclosporine therapy in atopic dogs.[21] A poor response to therapy, not due to side effects of cyclosporine, may indicate secondary skin infections, ectoparasitism, or non–atopy-related causes of the pruritus. Cyclosporine has also been used for treating canine perianal fistulae, erythema multiforme, sterile granuloma, pemphigus complex disease, and occasionally sebaceous adenitis.[22] Tacrolimus ointment (Protopic 0.1%) applied topically once daily for 4 weeks led to clinical improvement of localized lesions associated with atopic dermatitis in the dog.[23] Improvement was not noted in dogs with generalized lesions. Tacrolimus ointment may also be used for the treatment of autoimmune diseases with localized severity such as discoid lupus erythematosus confined to the planum nasale. This potent immunosuppressive agent is still in its infancy with respect to the uses in veterinary dermatology.

Dapsone

Dapsone is a sulfone product that has been used dermatologically for its antiinflammatory effects.[8] Prevention of myeloperoxidase respiratory burst impairs white blood cell activity, and blocking of integrin-mediated adherence impairs neutrophil migration. Antibody adherence to neutrophils also is blocked. Dapsone is approved for use in humans for a number of immune-mediated diseases. Dapsone is metabolized to a toxic compound (dapsone hydroxylamine) that depletes glutathione in cells with a glucose-6-phosphate dehydrogenase deficiency in people; the importance of this effect has not been documented in animals. The metabolite, however, causes rapid hemolysis. Cimetidine can be used to minimize toxicity by competing for drug-metabolizing enzymes.[8]

Antihistamines

Despite structural differences, all classes of H_1 antihistamines have similar antiinflammatory actions and side effects. The primary mechanism of action of these drugs reflects competitive inhibition of histamine at the receptor. Newer H_1 antagonists also block histamine release and have proved effective for treatment of atopy in humans (see the discussion of antihistamines in Chapter 31). However, differences in response among drugs, species, or disorders might also reflect impaired histamine release from mast cells or altered T-cell function. Side effects of these drugs also vary with the product and include gastrointestinal upset and neurologic manifestations, including drowsiness (the most common side effect) and hyperexcitability. Contraindications include central nervous system disorders (including epilepsy), glaucoma, and smooth muscle motility disorders such as might occur in the gastrointestinal or urinary tract. These products are generally used safely in human pregnancy, although safety has not been established in the pregnant or nursing cat and dog. Products with antihistamine activity only generally have fewer contraindications; the particular product should be reviewed before use and those with other pharmacologic effects avoided when appropriate.

Antihistaminergics can be beneficial in some cases of pruritus in dogs and cats. Because of varying effects among the drugs, each antihistaminergic should be tried for at least 1 week before an alternative medication is sought. Among the drugs tested in clinical trials, clemastine appears to be the most effective in stopping itching associated with pruritus in dogs and cats and is the antihistamine of choice.[24] Cost, however, can be prohibitive. A recent study found that after oral administration of clemastine, bioavailability was only 1% to 6%. It may be necessary to modify dose regimens for greater systemic effect.[25] Chlorpheniramine should be considered next for both dogs and cats.[7] The bitter taste of chlorpheniramine might be avoided by use of time-release capsules, which need to be administered only once daily. Diphenhydramine and hydroxyzine may be less efficacious; in addition, hyperexcitability may limit use in cats. A minimally effective dose may reduce the incidence of side effects. Astemizole is another recently approved human product. Although it appears safe (1 mg/kg), its efficacy has not been established in animals. In human medicine a combination of H_1 (the traditional antihistaminergic selection) and H_2 blockers has been recommended. The immunomodulating effects of H_2 blockers may benefit the dermatologic patient.[8] Newer H_1-blocking drugs (loratadine) do not cause anticholinergic effects and are not sedating. Caution should be taken when combining these products with H_2 receptors, however, because of an increased risk of cardiac arrhythmias, probably due to inhibition of drug-metabolizing enzymes.[8] Antihistamines may act synergistically with misoprostol in controlling pruritus. There is fair evidence for its efficacy in controlling pruritus in dogs with atopy[21]; studies currently are under way.

Omega-3 (Omega-6) Polyunsaturated Fatty Acids

Body fats are stored as either adipose tissue or structural fat. Adipose tissue is rich in triglycerides, which are composed of a glycerol backbone and three fatty acids. Structural fats are represented by phospholipids, also composed of a glycerol backbone; two fatty acids (at the 1 and 2 positions); and a phosphate group (at the 3 position). Fatty acids can be released from glycerol by phospholipase. Saturated fatty acids have no double bonds. Unsaturated fatty acids (UFAs) include monounsaturated fatty acids, which have one double bond, and polyunsaturated fatty acids (PUFAs), which have two or more double bonds. The shorthand identification system of PUFA reflects the number of carbon atoms, the number (n) of double bonds, and the position of the first double bond from the terminal or omega methyl group end of the molecule.[3] For example, the formula for linoleic acid, an essential fatty acid for mammals, is 18:2n-6; it contains 18 carbons and two double bonds, with the first double bond located between the sixth and seventh carbon. Alpha-linolenic acid (ALA) (18:3n-3) also contains 18 carbons but has three double bonds, with the first located between the third and fourth carbon (Figure 22-2).

Essential fatty acids (EFAs) are those fatty acids required for normal physiologic function that cannot be synthesized by the animal and thus must be obtained in the diet.[3] Among the functions of EFAs are serving as a structural component of cell

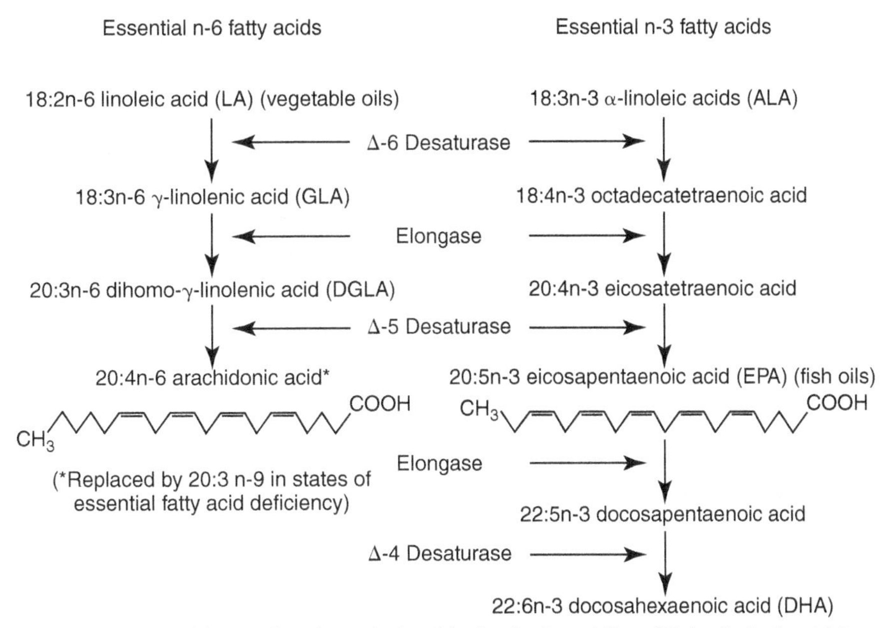

Figure 22-2 The three families of fatty acids are the plant-derived (α-linolenic acid) and fish oil-derived (eicosapentaenoic acid) n-3 family, the plant-derived n-6 family, and the de novo (nonessential) fatty acid family. Fatty acid biosynthesis includes desaturation, wherein a double bond is added, and elongation, wherein two carbon atoms are added. The same enzymes are used for fatty acid biosynthesis; the fatty acids in different families are not interconvertible.

membranes, primarily as arachidonic acid and in specialized tissues (retina and brain) as eicosapentaenoic acid (EPA) and docosahexaenoic acid.[3] The PUFA component is important in determining fluidity of the membrane, rendering it more stable, and maintaining cellular permeability. The epidermal water barrier of the skin depends on linoleic acid (LA) lipids located in the intercellular lamellar granules at the level of the stratum granulosum–corneum interface. EFAs are also the source of eicosanoids, from which are derived prostaglandins, leukotrienes, platelet-activating factor, and related compounds. Prostaglandins are notable for their protective effects in many body systems; both classes of eicosanoids also are potent inflammagens (see Chapter 16).

Two families of UFAs are essential for mammals (see Figure 22-2). Fatty acids of the n-3 (omega-3) series include ALA; EPA (20:5n-3) is a metabolic product of ALA found in fish oil. Fatty acids of the n-6 (omega-6) family include LA, the precursor to arachidonic acid (AA), a fundamental component of cell membranes and thus the most important of the EFAs in mammals.[3] Gamma-linolenic acid (GLA) is a product of LA found in certain plant oils. It is elongated to dihomo-gamma-linolenic acid, which is then converted to AA. Of the omega-3 series, ALA is elongated to EPA and then docosahexaenoic acid (DHA) (see Figure 22-2). Because of the absence of microsomal desaturase enzymes necessary to make double bonds, mammals are unable to synthesize LA and ALA.[3] Most mammals are, however, able to synthesize AA from dietary sources of LA, EPA, and DHA from dietary sources of ALA. Thus, although LA and ALA are EFAs, their products and end products are conditionally essential because their synthesis requires the precursor. However, cats cannot synthesize AA.[3] In addition, enzymes necessary for conversion of LA to AA apparently are not present; thus AA must be consumed in their diet. Dietary supplements contain

Table 22-2 Essential Free Fatty Acid Doses

	APPROXIMATE FATTY ACID DOSE (mg/9.1 kg BW)				
	LA	GLA	ALA	EPA	DHA
EPO	320	40			
MFO			90-360	60-240	
Product 1	269	10.2	0.4	10.3	6.8
Dermcaps	277.2	30.8			
Corn oil	1040	100			
GLA		63.7-354.9			
EPA				11.38-63.7	

BW, Body weight; *LA*, linolenic acid; *GLA*, gamma-linolenic acid; *ALA*, alpha-linolenic acid; *EPA*, eicosapentaenoic acid; *DHA*, docosahexaenoic acid; *EPO*, evening primrose oil; *MFO*, marine fish oil.
(From White PD: Essential fatty acids in veterinary medicine, Shawnee Mission, Kan, 1991, Veterinary Learning Systems for Bayer Corporation.)

PUFAs rich in LA and GLA (plant sources) and EPA (fish oil), although the quantity or ratio of plant and animal oils varies with the source (Table 22-2).

After ingestion from the diet, and metabolism and restructuring in the body, the end products of n-3 and n-6 PUFAs are EPA and AA, respectively. Both of these products are inserted as components of phospholipids into cell membranes. When the membrane is damaged, both EPA and AA are released into the cell, where they are converted by lipoxygenase and cyclooxygenase to various eicosanoid (leukotriene and prostaglandin) end products (see Chapter 16). The activities of these end products vary with the fatty acid: Those formed from EPA are much less inflammogenic than those formed from AA. The composition of PUFA in cell membranes can be nutritionally modified by replacing AA with either EPA or GLA.[3] These nutritional modifications can result in changes in inflammagen mediators. Inclusion of GLA (an n-6 EFA) in the diet specifically should reduce the formation of two inflammatory eicosanoids found in skin: leukotriene B_4 (LTB_4) and prostaglandin E_2 (PGE_2) because GLA may be elongated to DGLA, apparently increasing the concentrations of PGE_1, an antiinflammatory prostaglandin.[3] In addition, DGLA has a higher affinity for lipoxygenases than AA.

Inclusion of EPA and DHA (n-3 EFA) causes replacement of AA in the cell membrane; increasing the proportion of EPA or ALA also can decrease inflammatory responses by the cell. Because EPA has a high affinity for but is a poor substrate for cyclooxygenase, the generation of inflammatory prostaglandins is inhibited.[3] In addition, LTB_5, a leukotriene that is less chemotactic than LTB_4, is preferentially formed. Immunologic reactivity also may be modulated with fatty acid supplementation. Mobility of cell surface receptors and movement of materials between the inside and outside might be affected. The cell-mediated response can be reduced, especially at high doses.[26] Combinations of EFA of the n-3 (EPA) and n-6 (GLA) series appear to enhance control of inflammation, and the two should be given in combination for maximum effects.[3] Several combinations are available in commercial preparations (see Table 22-2). The most appropriate combination of n-3 versus n-6 fatty acids has not, however, been documented, but a ratio of 5 to 10:1 has been suggested on the basis of a study that found a decrease in LTB_4 and an increase in LTB_5 in the skin of dogs whose diets were supplemented with these ratios.[3]

Current therapeutic indications for EFA include pruritus caused by atopy and other disorders and keratinization disorders. EFAs may have steroid-sparing effects, but these products may take 12 weeks or longer for full therapeutic effect.[27] Newer inflammatory conditions being studied include lupus erythematosus, rheumatoid arthritis, hypothyroidism, and cancer cachexia and neoplasia.[3]

Noninflammatory prostaglandins also are affected by replacement of AA with EPA. The normal role of prostaglandins (reviewed in Chapter 16) can be modified with fatty acid supplementation, and this can account for some of their side effects. Side effects reported in humans include nose bleeds and hemoptysis; gastrointestinal distress; and decreased serum vitamin E, which could increase inflammation owing to increased oxygen radical. Side effects reported in dogs include lethargy, pruritus, vomiting, diarrhea, and urticaria. Use of fatty acids may increase the incidence of pancreatitis in dogs prone to that disease; fatty acid supplementation should begin with a low dose that is gradually increased over several weeks.

Behavior Modifiers

Tricyclic and other antidepressant drugs are used to treat stereotypic behaviors, including those resulting in skin lesions (see Chapter 25). The most common behaviors are related to grooming, such as acral lick dermatitis (lick granuloma) and hair chewing. Pruritus has also become a common indication for antidepressant therapy. Most behavior modifiers (psychotropic drugs) have the ability to alter multiple central nervous system neurotransmitters. Most notably affected are the biogenic amines, including serotonin and dopamine (and, to a lesser degree, epinephrine). Acetylcholine and histamine may also be affected. Because these neurotransmitters are affected centrally, they can affect many physiologic behaviors, including control of the endocrine system, motor control, appetite, and so forth. Because physiology varies markedly among animals, adverse reactions to the drugs should be anticipated on account of differences in response (i.e., pharmacodynamics) and differences in drug disposition. The behavior-modifying drugs should be used cautiously, and their use is best based on previous studies or experiences noted in the veterinary literature. Antidepressants interact with cholinergic, histaminergic, and α-adrenergic receptors and thus are associated with a variety of adverse effects. Adverse reactions have been noted in cats (central nervous system signs, gastrointestinal upset). Amitriptyline, imipramine, and clomipramine are tricyclic antidepressants that have been used in dogs and cats. Doxepin is a tricyclic antidepressant with potent antihistaminergic (H_1) effects that has also been used to treat pruritus. Fluoxetine is a nontricyclic antidepressant that specifically binds serotonergic receptors.

The behavioral aspects of the self-mutilation syndrome of acral lick dermatitis have been treated with tricyclic antidepressants, fluoxetine (Prozac), and narcotic antagonists. Narcotic antagonists are reportedly effective for humans and animals for the control of certain behavioral disorders. The mechanism of action of these drugs is unknown. Increased release of endogenous opioids has, however, been detected in self-mutilative behaviors in experimental animals. The use of chemical antagonists may be a reasonable alternative to the plethora of treatments recommended by various authors for this syndrome. Other postulated benefits of the opioid antagonists include eradication of endorphin-mediated "self-reward" and analgesia. Like naloxone, naltrexone appears to be a pure opioid antagonist. Naltrexone is, however, characterized by a higher oral efficacy and longer duration of action. The success of treatment with naltrexone varies; if there has been no response after 10 days, the dose is doubled. Treatment for 1 to 2 months will cause remission in up to 60% of animals with lick granulomas, although relapses are likely in some when the drug is discontinued. Response has also been reported with hydrocodone bitartrate (Hycodan).

Antiparasitic Drugs

A limited number of agents are administered systemically (orally or by injection) for control of dermatologic parasites. Milbemycin and lufenuron are two examples. These drugs are discussed in greater depth in Chapter 15.

Macrolide Antibiotics

Ivermectin. Ivermectin is used to treat a number of parasitic dermatoses in animals. The drug stimulates the release of the inhibitory neurotransmitter GABA at peripheral neuronal synapses, resulting in paralysis and death of the parasite (see Chapter 15). Selective activity in animals reflects a difference in the peripheral role (nematodes and arthropods) versus central role (mammals) of this neurotransmitter. In most mammals ivermectin does not penetrate the blood–brain barrier in sufficient concentrations to cause side effects. The drug is administered orally and parenterally; up to 3 weeks may elapse before the drug is totally eliminated in feces. The primary indication for ivermectin in small animals is mite infestation: feline and canine scabies, cheyletiellosis, and ear mites. The drug has also been used for mite infestations of guinea pigs and birds. Although clinical response may occur in several weeks, animals may remain skin-scrape positive for several to many months. Adverse reactions are idiosyncratic and have been reported primarily in herding breeds (Collies, Border Collies, Shetland Sheepdogs, Old English Sheepdogs, Australian Shepherds). Adverse reactions are associated with a mutation in the MDR1 gene. Testing is available at Washington State University for this mutation to help identify dogs at risk for life-threatening reactions. Reactions have ranged from mydriasis to tremors, hypersalivation, ataxia, coma, and death. The 1% bovine product may be diluted with propylene glycol to allow more accurate dosing in small animals. Ivermectin can be used (off-label) for the treatment of generalized canine demodicosis. Treatment is usually started at 0.1 mg/kg daily and gradually increased. The commonly used dosage ranges from 0.2 mg/kg daily to 0.6 mg/kg daily, but some clinicians recommend dosages as high as 0.8 mg/kg/day. Careful patient monitoring for side effects and response to therapy is warranted.

Milbemycin. Like ivermectin, milbemycin at 1.5 to 2 mg/kg daily is effective for the treatment of demodectic mange. Cost may be a limiting factor. Response to treatment is lengthy, and relapses may occur. The dosage may be modified if an inadequate response is seen after 1 month of therapy. Also like ivermectin, milbemycin can cause toxicity, particularly in Collie-type dogs, although this drug is slightly safer than ivermectin. Moxidectin also may be efficacious; Collies also appear to be more sensitive to its adverse effects. Moxidectin is not approved for the treatment of canine demodicosis in the United States.

Immunomodulators

Immunomodulators (biologic response modifiers) potentiate some facet of the immune response (see Chapter 19). Many compounds described as immunomodulators have been used to treat a variety of dermatologic conditions. Immunosuppressants used to treat immune-mediated dermatologic disorders include glucocorticoids, cytotoxic (antineoplastic) drugs, and selected hormones. Immunostimulants tend to be less effective (see Chapter 19).

Staphylococcus aureus phage lysate (Staphage Lysate) is a vaccine containing parts of *S. aureus*, a bacteriophage, and culture medium ingredients. It is indicated for treatment of canine staphylococcal pyoderma. Vaccination is intended to result in stimulation of antibacterial antibodies. There may also be a hyposensitizing effect. Concomitant antimicrobial therapy should be used for the initial 4 to 6 weeks. Staphage Lysate is administered subcutaneously once a week initially, and then the dosage interval is lengthened. The vaccine is relatively expensive. Possible side effects include allergic reactions and local redness and swelling at the injection site. This vaccine should be reserved for patients with recurrent staphylococcal pyoderma that responds to antimicrobial therapy but recurs when therapy is discontinued. It is extremely important that other causes of pyoderma (e.g., allergies, ectoparasites, endocrinopathies) are identified and treated.

Propionibacterium acnes killed suspension (Immuno-Regulin) is available as an adjunct to antimicrobial therapy in the treatment of canine pyoderma. It has been shown to induce cell-mediated immunity. This bacterium is the species associated with human acne. Treatment with Immuno-Regulin involves intravenous injections twice weekly initially and then once weekly. Potential adverse effects include anaphylactic reactions. Disadvantages include expense and the need for intravenous injections (client cannot administer at home). It is the author's opinion that use of this agent should be reserved for patients in which all other forms of therapy have failed.

Hyposensitization involves parenteral administration of allergens (antigens) in allergic patients. Although the mechanism of action of this therapy is unknown, the most appealing theory is that repeated exposure to the allergen may result in reduced cellular sensitivity (tolerance). Hyposensitization is one of best therapies for long-term management of the dog and cat. Patient and client selection are critical for success because therapy generally lasts as long as the patient is alive. Hyposensitization solutions may be based on intradermal allergy testing or serum allergy testing. Many protocols are available insofar as patient response may be quite variable.

TRANSDERMAL DELIVERY OF DRUGS

Most drugs in human and veterinary medicine that are applied to the skin are intended to provide their pharmacologic effect where they are applied. Systemic absorption is intended to be minimal so that systemic effects will not be encountered. There are, however, a small number of drug products that are designed to be applied to the skin and absorbed transdermally, whereupon they attain sufficiently high plasma concentrations to produce systemic effects. The same factors mentioned in the discussion of the principles of topical drug therapy affect drug absorption from cutaneous sites.

Transdermal drug delivery offers several advantages. It is easier to administer drugs transdermally, and drug delivery can be sustained, thus ensuring continued therapeutic effects. Drug input might be more precisely controlled over oral therapy because there are fewer factors complicating transdermal drug absorption, such as first-pass hepatic metabolism.

Not all drugs may be administered transdermally. The drug should not be irritating to the skin and should be transdermally bioavailable. Effective transdermal drug delivery formulations are very difficult to design, which is probably why so few products are available. Some products used in veterinary medicine, although not intended for transdermal absorption, can result in systemic absorption in the person treating the animal. Such drugs should be handled with nonpermeable gloves (e.g., DMSO, all anticancer drugs, nitroglycerin ointment, all antiparasitics [dips and shampoos], and altrenogest

[Regu-Mate]). Gloves might also be used when administering chloramphenicol, although percutaneous absorption in association with oral medication of small animals has not been documented.

Several products are used in veterinary medicine with the intent of achieving systemic therapeutic effects. Nitroglycerin ointment relaxes vascular smooth muscle primarily on the venous side and is used for dogs and cats to treat cardiogenic edema. The ointment is applied to glabrous areas (i.e., axillary, inguinal, or inside the ears). Onset of action is approximately 1 hour. Selemectin (Revolution, Fort Dodge) and other systemic insecticides (discussed previously) are applied topically. Scopolamine, nitroglycerin, and clonidine transdermal patches are available for use in human patients to treat motion sickness, angina, and hypertension, respectively. Fentanyl, a narcotic analgesic available in transdermal patches, has proved to be an effective and safe alternative to injectable opioid delivery for control of pain in dogs and cats (see Chapter 28).

TREATMENT OF SPECIFIC DERMATOLOGIC DISORDERS

Selected skin diseases are discussed in other chapters. Otitis externa, pyoderma, and other bacterial infections of the skin are discussed in Chapter 8. Fungal disorders are additionally discussed in Chapter 9, external parasites are additionally discussed in Chapter 13, immune-mediated diseases of the skin are discussed in Chapter 31, behavioral disorders of the skin are discussed in Chapter 26, and endocrinopathies affecting the skin are addressed in Chapter 21.

Chronic Pruritus

Pathophysiology

Pruritus is a cutaneous sensation that leads the animal to resolve the feeling by scratching, rubbing, licking, or chewing. The cause of the sensation is complex, as can be its resolution. Ideally, the underlying cause of the sensation is identified and treated, ultimately leading to resolution of the pruritus. Discussion of or even provision of a comprehensive list of the causes of pruritus is beyond the scope of this chapter.

Like pain, the sensation of pruritus consists of a peripheral signal, originating in the skin, and central perception, ending at the sensory cortex. A number of chemicals are responsible for signal generation and transmission in the skin, although the precise types that predominate in the dog and cat are not known. The chemicals largely are the same as those generating the inflammatory response and include both preformed chemicals (histamine, serotonin) and those synthesized in situ (prostaglandins, leukotrienes, proteases). The signal generated at the level of the skin can be modified by emotional, biochemical, or central factors, leading to behavior that appears to be disproportionate to the inciting cause (i.e., skin trauma induced in response to a single flea bite).[28] Drugs oriented toward control of pruritus can target either peripheral or central transmission. For chronic pruritus drugs with systemic effects generally are more effective.

Drug Therapy

Topical Therapy

A number of nonglucocorticoid topical preparations may control pruritus.[5,13] Care should be taken to select products that are not irritating or drying. Shampoos generally should be applied once to twice weekly. Cool water may be effective in some animals; antipruritic efficacy can be enhanced by the addition of moisturizing agents, colloids, antiinflammatories, or anesthetics. Preparations that can be applied in "spots" include Dermacool (hamamelis extract and menthol.[13] ResiSoothe (Virbac U.S.) and Relief cream rinse (DVM) are lotions that are also effective for spot treatment.

Other medications available in sprays that might be helpful for control of pruritus include local anesthetics such as lidocaine (Dermacool) or promaxine (with colloidal oatmeal: Relief Spray), 2% benzyl alcohol with 0.05% benzalkonium chloride, and hamamelis distillate (PTD). In addition to anthistaminergic medications, sprays also may contain glucocorticoids for treatment of localized pruritus such as pyotraumatic pruritus and allergic dermatitis.[5] More potent sprays intended for acute management contain 0.1% triamcinolone, 0.025% fluocinolone, or 0.1% betamethasone; "milder" glucocorticoid sprays for long-term maintenance contain 0.5% to 2.5% hydrocortisone. Sprays can be applied two to three times per day.[5] Sprays should be applied every 12 hours until inflammation and pruritus are controlled and then tapered to an as-needed basis. Systemic side effects may be seen with extended use. Localized adverse effects such as the development of thin skin or alopecia may also occur.

Glucocorticoid ointments and creams may be difficult to use because of lack of penetration through the hair coat into the skin. A hydrocortisone lotion that is not greasy or staining may be useful for treatment of large areas with some residual activity.[5] ResiCort (1% hydrocortisone) lotion (Virbac U.S.) is a formulation that is easier to apply to the skin surface than ointments and creams.

Total body application of moisturizing and hypoallergenic shampoos, or colloidal oatmeal soaks or shampoos with or without antihistamines, local anesthetics (Relief Shampoo DVM), or hydrocortisone (Cortisoothe, Virbac U.S.) are indicated for patients with generalized pruritus.[6,13] Colloidal shampoos containing pyrethrins, carbaryl, or pyrethrins and permethrin will facilitate control of pruritus associated with fleas.[5] Application of a rinse, spray, or lotion after a shampoo will provide some residual effect.[5] Cream rinses containing colloidal oatmeal with (pramoxine) or without a local anesthetic are available for control of pruritus. Incomplete rinsing of a cream rinse may facilitate residual activity in dogs with short hair coats (coats of long hair become greasy). Antipruritic cream rinses might also be applied locally for control of localized pyoderma (e.g., Relief lotion).[5] Several aqueous rinses also are available for control of pruritus. These include 100% colloidal oatmeal (Aveeno), oilated oatmeal with 43% colloid (Aveeno Oilated Bath) (for very dry skin and hair coats, also applied as a soak), and moisturizing bath oils or humectants (Humilac spray, Virbac U.S.). Aqueous rinses generally also can be applied as sprays, although efficacy is greater as a total body rinse.[5]

Topical shampoo therapy is an important component of treatment or prevention of superficial and deep pyodermas. Antibacterial shampoos containing benzoyl peroxide, chlorhexidine, or ethyl lactate are indicated as adjuvant therapy for pruritus associated with pyoderma (see Chapter 8). Those most effective contain benzoyl peroxide or chlorhexidine.[6] Following the shampoo with a chlorhexidine rinse (dilution of a 2% solution to 0.5%) further enhances antibacterial activity. Maximum ChlorhexiDerm HC shampoo (DVM), a new product containing 4% chlorhexidine and 1% hydrocortisone, has been developed to treat secondary pyoderma associated with an underlying pruritic disorder. Very few controlled and blinded studies exist to guide the selection and use of drugs for treatment of chronic pruritus in dogs or cats. In general, those that have provided support for selected drugs define success or response as a reduction in pruritus by 50%.There is good evidence, however, that glucocorticoids and cyclosporine are beneficial for the treatment of canine atopy.[21]

Antibiotics

Antibiotics may be indicated to control secondary infection (generally *Staphylococcus)* that can contribute to pruritus. The use of antibiotics for treatment of dermatologic disorders is discussed in Chapter 8. For some animals antibiotic therapy may be the sole therapy needed to control pruritus. Some antibiotics (e.g., erythromycin, tetracyclines) directly provide some relief from pruritus (rather than by controlling infection).[29] Tetracyclines in general are not, however, effective for treating pyoderma associated with staphylococcal infections. Erythromycin can be effective against *Staphylococcus* species, but it can cause gastrointestinal upset.

Glucocorticoids

Glucocorticoids remain the most effective drugs for control of chronic pruritus associated with allergies.[13,28] The principles of glucocorticoid therapy (see Chapter 30) must be closely observed when a glucocorticoid is used to control pruritus. Injectable products should be avoided when possible. Miller and coworkers[28] suggest that injections may be acceptable for animals in which a single injection provides pruritic relief for 3 to 4 months or more. The temptation to increase the frequency of administration of an injectable product to less than 3-month intervals should be resisted. Prednisone and prednisolone (0.55 to 1.1 mg/kg per day [dog]; 2.2 mg/kg per day [cat]) remain the glucocorticoids most commonly used for long-term treatment. The dose can be divided and given twice or once daily. The dose is titrated to a minimum effective dose defined by the point at which the animal is "tolerably itchy"—that is, the itch does not disrupt the animal's (or owner's) life or cause secondary trauma to the skin.[28] The lack of pruritus suggests that the dose is too high. Many animals cannot tolerate even an alternate-day regimen of glucocorticoids; other animals remain pruritic at doses associated with marked side effects. Long-term side effects will be seen with continued use. It has been suggested that alternative therapies should be sought for animals that require glucorticoid therapy for more than 3 months out of the year.

Some clinicians find glucocorticoids devoid of mineralocorticoid to be less frequently associated with polyuria and polydipsia[28]; however, the rationale behind this observation is not clear because this side effect is related to anti–antidiuretic hormone effects rather than to increased mineralocorticoid effects. Nevertheless, an alternative glucocorticoid might be tried; however, triamcinolone and dexamethasone have increasingly longer biologic effect times, and the risk of hypothalamic–pituitary–adrenal suppression increases with continued use. Methylprednisolone may be a viable alternative. If undesirable side effects occur with glucocorticoid use, combination therapy might be tried (e.g., antihistamines, bathing, fatty acid therapy) in an attempt to decrease the dose of glucocorticoids. In some animals, however, only continued use of glucocorticoids in the face of side effects will control pruritus sufficiently. In such patients the risk of therapy must be weighed carefully against the disadvantages of continued pruritus. Glucocorticoid-sparing drugs should be attempted before selecting glucocorticoids. If proved effective as sole drug therapy, then combined use should be considered to reduce the dose and thus likelihood of side effects. These include antihistamines, misoprostol, and omega series fatty acids.

Antihistamines

Antihistamines traditionally have been considered ineffective as a sole therapy for controlling pruritus in dogs or cats. However, with the advent of newer drugs and modification of the goal of therapy (e.g., reduction in the glucocorticoid dose), the following approaches may enhance the use of antihistamine therapy for control of pruritus. The clinician should wait at least 1 week before evaluating efficacy. If one drug does not work, an alternative should be tried. The clinician also should aim to reduce the itching sensation rather than eradicate it. The antihistamine also can be combined with other drugs that might decrease itching (e.g., fatty acids). Drugs most likely to be useful include diphenhydramine (Benadryl), hydroxyzine, chlorpheniramine, and clemastine. Cyproheptadine, also an antiserotinergic, and the tricyclic antidepressants amitriptyline and doxepine (both with antihistaminergic effects) also may be useful. It may be necessary to increase the dosage of doxepin to as high as 5 mg/kg for it to be effective in some dogs.

Few studies have properly evaluated the use of antihistamines for the treatment of pruritus in dogs. One study[30] provided support for a reduction in pruritus in allergic dogs treated with one of three antihistamines. In general, however, response occurred in at most 25% of animals treated. Thus response rates tend to be low. Response to chlorpheniramine was best, followed by diphenhydramine or hydroxyzine. Follow-up studies[28,31] found clemastine to be much more effective than astemizole or trimeprazine. Thus, of the antihistamines studied in clinical patients, clemastine appears to be the most effective. Because of low bioavailability when clemastine is given orally, a higher dose (1 mg/kg twice daily) may be more clinically effective.[32] Misoprostol may enhance the efficacy of antihistamines used to treat pruritus.

Cats appear to respond to antihistamines better than dogs. Chlorpheniramine can be used to treat cats without causing the excitement that often occurs with diphenhydramine (the latter effect probably reflects overdosing). One study found response to chlorpheniramine to be excellent in 73% of cats when dosed at 2 mg every 12 hours within 2 weeks. Other reports consistently have been favorable with doses of 2 to 4 mg/cat twice daily. Occasionally, a 24-hour dosing interval may be effective. The 8-mg time-release capsule (sprinkling one fourth to one half of the contents on food) may prove easier to administer than the bitter-tasting tablets. Alternatively, the 4-mg tablet can be broken in half and dipped in tuna fish.[7] It is generally recommended that the 4-mg tablet be administered unbroken, however. An over-the-counter solution is also available. Side effects reported in cats include vomiting, diarrhea, and hyperexcitability. Hydroxyzine and amitriptyline can cause adverse reactions in cats. Clemastine (0.34 to 0.68 mg every 12 hours orally) may be effective.

A combination of both H_1 and H_2 receptor antagonists has been recommended but has not proved useful in animals thus far.[28]

Fatty Acid Supplements

Studies that focus on the effects of dietary supplementation of EFA on canine atopy vary. Interpretation among clinical trials is complicated by the quantity and source of the PUFAs (GLA, EPA, and DHA), the lack of tissue fatty acid analysis, the duration of therapy (which probably was not sufficiently long), and differences in outcome measures and adjuvant therapy. In addition, many of the studies were not controlled or blinded.

White[3] provides a summary of the results of selected clinical trials implemented by various dermatologists. A study evaluating LA, linolenic acid, and EPA in dogs with atopy, flea allergy, and idiopathic pruritus (nonseasonal) found the response rate to the PUFA to be low (20% or fewer being controlled well; another 36% responding by a 50% reduction in pruritus). An open comparison of evening primrose oil, marine fish oil, and EFA products administered for 2 weeks found response in 25% of animals, but no product appeared more effective than the others. Responders worsened when supplementation was removed. Comparison of evening primrose oil alone or combined with marine fish oil found significant improvement with the sole product and increased (but not significant) efficacy with the combined product. A double-blind placebo-controlled crossover study with olive oil (placebo) or evening primrose administered for 9 weeks found clinical improvement with evening primrose oil. Two recent blinded studies have reported the benefits of EFA (EPA 180 mg and DHA 120 mg per 4.55 mg/kg) supplementation when administered for 6 weeks. Eleven of 16 dogs responded to fish oil, 3 of 16 responded better to corn oil, and 2 of 16 dogs responded to neither oil. A parallel study of 28 dogs supplemented with high doses of GLA (350 mg), EPA (250 mg), or linolenic acid (250 mg) and EPA (50 mg) found a benefit with all three supplements, suggesting that higher doses may be important to efficacy.

Cats seem to respond better than dogs, with up to 40% efficacy reported by some authors.[28] Again, however, results of clinical trials tend to be conflicting. Pruritic cats with miliary dermatitis and other nonlesional causes of pruritus responded to 2 and 6 weeks of therapy of a linolenic acid–EPA supplement. In contrast, 12 weeks of therapy with evening primrose oil (3.7 mg linolenic acid/kg) or olive oil did not improve feline skin disease in another study. A 6-week course of evening primrose alone or when combined with marine fish oil resulted in improvement in feline pruritus and dermatitis; in contrast, marine fish oil by itself caused worsening of the skin disease. A 12-week course of therapy with evening primrose and sunflower oil also improved the skin and coat of cats with miliary dermatitis.[3] White[3] suggests that atopy should be most responsive to EFAs that are low in LA and high in linolenic acid and/or EPA/DHA. Addition of vitamins to the EFA supplement may facilitate efficacy of the EFA product. The appropriate ratio (n-6:n-3) is not clear, nor is the duration of therapy. A ratio of 5 to 10:1 has been suggested on the basis of a study that found a decrease in LTB_4 and an increase in LTB_5 in the skin of dogs supplemented with diets containing these ratios.[3] Response has been reported in as few as 7 to 14 days or as many as 9 to 12 weeks.

The most appropriate use of EFA for control of pruritus may be in combination with antihistamines or glucocorticoids.[3] Success with fatty acid supplements also is most likely if an alternative product is tried if and when the first fails, adequate time is allowed to elapse before clinical assessment is complete, the goal is reduction rather than eradication of pruritus, or the goal is reduction of the dose of other drugs associated with adverse effects (e.g., glucocorticoids).

Behavior-Modifying Drugs

The use of behavior-modifying drugs is increasingly popular; the proper use and side effects associated with these drugs are discussed in Chapter 25. Among the behavior-modifying drugs, those that are characterized by antihistaminergic effects might be preferred (e.g., doxepin or amitriptyline).

Behavior-modifying drugs have been used to treat feline pruritus, particularly those associated with psychogenic alopecia.[7] Psychogenic alopecia also has responded to naloxone (1 mg/kg subcutaneously, one dose), although time to recurrence of the abnormal behavior ranged from as short as 1 week to as long as 6 months.[7] The dopamine antagonist haloperidol (2 mg/kg intravenously) did not appear very useful long term when compared with a control for treatment of psychogenic alopecia.[7] Cats did, however, respond within 48 hours. Buspirone does not appear to be effective for control of psychogenic alopecia.[7] Fluoxetine has been useful for chronic, idiopathic licking in cats.

Combination Therapy

Combinations of drugs that alter the sensation or response to the sensation through different mechanisms of action should be considered. The combinations that appear to be most effective include fatty acid supplements (Dermcaps) with glucocorticoids (leading to a 25% to 50% reduction in the glucocorticoid dose)[28]; antihistamines (trimeprazine) and glucocorticoids (an increase from 50% improvement with glucocorticoids alone to 76% improvement with the combination, with a 50% to 75% reduction in the glucocorticoid dose)[33]; and fatty acid supplements with antihistamines (chlorpheniramine and Dermcaps in combination caused a 35% response in animals that responded to neither drug alone).[28] Combination of misoprostol with antihistamines is being investigated. Assessment at weekly intervals should be accompanied by a change in therapy if response has not been sufficient.

Nonsteroidal Antiinflammatory Drugs

Nonsteroidal antiinflammatory drugs should be avoided in pruritic skin diseases. Inhibition of prostaglandin formation may result in greater synthesis of leukotriene and related compounds. Newer lipoxygenase-specific inhibitors (approved for use in the treatment of human bronchial asthma) may be beneficial, but these drugs have not been studied with the intent of controlling pruritus.

Future Therapies

Future therapies may focus on biologic response modifiers.[34] Products with potential efficacy for human patients with atopy include interferon-γ, thymopentin (an active pentapeptide of a thymic hormone that promotes differentiation of mature T lymphocytes), and interleukin-2.

Acral Lick Dermatitis

Acral lick dermatitis (lick granuloma) is a self-traumatizing syndrome that afflicts dogs, occurring almost exclusively in larger breeds. The cause is not known, but it has patterns similar to an obsessive–compulsive disorder. It is often considered psychogenic in origin; suggested behavioral causes include boredom, loneliness, and confinement.[35] Underlying bony pathology or allergy may also be the cause of the lesions. Chronic lesions are frequently infected with bacteria or fungal organisms, which can also contribute to the pruritic stimulation. Local irritation has, however, been suggested as a provoking cause. Not surprisingly, drugs used to treat obsessive–compulsive disorders in humans have proved effective. The proper use of these drugs is discussed in Chapter 26. In one clinical trial with 43 dogs, the drugs most effective were those that increase serotonin at the neurotransmitter. This is not surprising because the serotonin system has been implicated in a variety of abnormal behaviors.[35] Dose ranges of the drugs (orally per day) proven successful in clinical trials[36] include clomipramine (2.4 to 3.6 mg/kg),[36] fluoxetine (0.55 to 1.36 mg/kg), and sertraline (2.7 to 4.3 mg/kg). Of these, clomipramine followed by fluoxetine appeared to be most effective, causing response (50% or more reduction in behavior) in close to 50% of animals studied. Clinical response was not evident until the second week of therapy and continued to decline through the 5 weeks of one study.[35] Adverse effects occurred in approximately 25% of dogs in each treatment group, but they tended to be mild and subsided with time. Discontinuation of the behavior-modifying drug may cause recrudescence of clinical signs. Drugs to which there was little response included desipramine and fenfluramine. In most cases, secondary infection is present and must be treated. Glucocorticoid therapy is usually indicated in the early stage of treatment to decrease the inflammation. Antiinflammatory dosages rather than immunosuppressive dosages are recommended. Oral prednisone or prednisolone are the favored products. Additional topical therapy with Synotic applied twice daily may be selected instead of oral glucocorticoid therapy. Appropriate antibiotic therapy based on culture and susceptibility is indicated.

Both naloxone and naltrexone, both pure narcotic antagonists, have been used to resolve abnormal behavior in dogs with lick granulomas. Increased release of endogenous opioids has been detected in self-mutilating behaviors in experimental animals. Opioid antagonists may eradicate endorphin-mediated self-reward and analgesia. Like naloxone, naltrexone is a pure opioid antagonist but is characterized by a higher oral efficacy and longer duration of action. An uncontrolled study of the use of naltrexone in dogs with acral lick dermatitis reported a 64% success rate.[37] A dose of 2.2 mg/kg orally once daily (1 mg/kg subcutaneously) was increased to 2.2 mg/kg orally twice daily when there was no response after 10 days. Dogs were treated for 1 month; lesions returned when the drug was discontinued, and time of recurrence varied from 1 week to 3 years after the drug was discontinued. One animal that failed to respond to naltrexone responded to nalmefene, another narcotic antagonist. Chronic cases or those with a poor response to therapy should be biopsied to rule out neoplasia and cultured for infectious agents.

Canine Seborrhea

Canine idiopathic seborrhea is an inherited disorder of keratinization characterized by pruritus, epidermal thickening, and formation of dry or greasy crusts and seborrheic plaques.[3,38] The pathophysiology is not well understood, but hyperproliferation of the epidermis, hair follicle infundibulum, and sebaceous glands have been reported. Renewal time for the epidermis is reduced from 22 to 8 days.[38] Increased cutaneous concentrations of AA have been measured in affected dogs. Treatment controls but generally does not cure the condition. The production of increased scale can be caused by myriad diseases and problems. The search for the cause of the scale is more important than symptomatic therapy. Primary idiopathic seborrhea as a diagnosis is fairly uncommon.

Therapy for seborrhea oleosa should include shampoos that are keratolytic, keratoplastic, and degreasing. Ingredients that serve this purpose contain sulfur; salicylic acid; benzoyl peroxide; or, less commonly, coal tar. Among these, benzoyl peroxide is probably the preferred ingredient, although a sulfur salicylic shampoo might be tried first. Benzoyl peroxide activity is enhanced with the addition of sulfur (SulfOxydex, DVM). In general, products for human beings should not be used on dogs. Products also can be alternated.

Animals should be bathed twice a week until scaling, greasiness, and odor are controlled; the frequency of bathing is then decreased to the minimum necessary to control clinical signs. Contact with the shampoo (completely lathered) must occur for at least 10 minutes. For animals with an extremely thickened accumulation, bathing with a mild cleanser such as D-Basic (DVM) before a medicated shampoo is used may prove beneficial and will be sparing of the more expensive products. PUFAs have recently been used for treatment of seborrhea. Supplementation should begin as topical therapy is started. Corn, sunflower, or safflower oil (1.5 mL/kg every 24 hours orally) or commercial EFA products can be used.[38] It is possible that the skin of affected dogs cannot obtain or metabolize LA, suggesting that topical administration of EFA (LA) may be more appropriate than oral administration.[3]

Generalized Demodicosis

Therapy for generalized demodicosis should be accompanied by proper nutrition, minimization of stress, and control of accompanying pyoderma. Self-cure can be expected in 50% of dogs younger than 12 months of age, although no factors appear to be predictive of self-cure.[39] The most efficacious treatment for generalized demodicosis appears to vary in the literature. No single drug will cure all cases; up to 10% cannot be cured.[39] Amitraz (Mitaban)19.9%, and amitraz in ProMeris (Fort Dodge) are the only drugs approved by the Food and Drug Administration for treatment of demodicosis, although an Environmental Protection Agency–registered solution is available (Taktic). Amitraz (Mitaban)is labeled for treatment at 2-week intervals (diluted to 250 ppm or 10.6 mL in 7.6 L). Original reports regarding its efficacy using the approved protocol apparently were inappropriately optimistic (90% predicted cure rates). Long-term cure rates according to the approved treatment regimen range from as little as 0% to 50% (0.025% or 250 ppm dip).[40] Follow-up studies at greater concentrations have more favorable results.

Concentrations of 500 ppm (double strength) may be used for refractory cases. Weekly dips of 250 to 500 ppm are curative in 75% to 80% of cases, respectively.[40] Long hair coats should be clipped and animals bathed first. Treatment should continue until two dips have occurred after two negative skin scrapings, regardless of how many dips must occur. Weekly application may be implemented if biweekly therapy is not successful. Oral vitamin E therapy at 200 IU/dog five times daily may enhance efficacy of amitraz, although this has not been proved.[40] ProMeris (Fort Dodge) is to be applied every 14 days until a remission is reached. Adverse side effects similar to the those of of Mitaban have been reported. Immunomodulators such as Staphage Lysate, ImmunoRegulin, and levamisole appear to be ineffective.[40]

Should amitraz fail, a macrolide antibiotic should be considered. Milbemycin at 1 and 2 mg/kg daily appears to cure 50% to 90% of dogs, respectively. Duration of therapy in one study ranged from 90 to 300 days; treatment should occur for 60 days past multiple negative skin scrapings. Side effects should be limited as long as 2.5 mg/kg is not exceeded.[39] Ivermectin at 0.3 to 0.6 mg/kg per day orally (but not 0.2 to 0.4 mg/kg per week subcutaneously) also may be efficacious, with treatments being necessary for as long as 210 days. Because the drug is very bitter, administration in vanilla ice cream or apple sauce is recommended.[40] This dosing regimen is not safe for Collies and related breeds. Testing for reaction to ivermectin involves administration of 0.125 mg/kg per day for 7 days. Alternatively, hospitalization might occur for the initial period during which a starting dose of 0.1 mg/kg is gradually increased to the maintenance dose. Signs of pending toxicity include mydriasis and excessive salivation. Neurologic signs are also possible. Testing for the MDR1 gene mutation is available through Washington State University. This test will help identify those dogs that are sensitive to ivermectin toxicity.

Should relapse occur within 3 months, inadequate treatment is the most likely cause,[39] and the therapeutic protocol can be repeated but for a longer duration. Later relapses probably reflect recurrence; repetition of the initial treatment protocol is not likely to be effective,[39] and an alternative protocol should be selected. It is essential to resolve any complicating skin infections and to search for an underlying cause of refractory demodicosis. Also, underlying allergic disorders must be addressed.

Dermatophytosis

Treatment of dermatophytes is also addressed in Chapter 9. Establishment of the efficacy of selected treatment regimens is handicapped by the often self-resolving nature of the infection. Moriello[41] emphasizes that, as with pyoderma, topical therapy alone is not sufficient for effective treatment of dermatophytosis. Indeed, several disadvantages are associated with topical therapy. Hairs protect spores; in addition, many commonly used topical antifungal solutions and shampoos are not sporicidal. Among the more efficacious are lime sulfur (1:16) and enilconazole (bottle dilution, but not licensed for use in the United States).[41] Unfortunately, both of these topical products are associated with side effects: Enilconazole has caused death in some cats, and lime sulfur can be very irritating. Grooming after topical treatment increases the risk of toxicity in cats if they are allowed to groom while the product is wet. Pet owners are exposed to topical agents, increasing their risk. Occasionally, topical agents worsen infection, perhaps because of damage to the skin (mechanical scrubbing) during shampooing. The efficacy of topical ointments, creams, and gels is questionable. Among the topical ointments and creams, bifonazole is more effective than miconazole, but its efficacy also is questionable, particularly if infection involves haired skin. In addition, topical agents tend to be messy, are groomed by the animal, and encourage "spot" therapy. Nonetheless, topical therapy is an important adjuvant for treatment of dermatophytosis. Topical therapy will limit environmental contamination and contagion if spores on the hair coat are killed. The preferred topical product[41] is lime sulfur (4 to 8 oz/gallon); higher concentrations are potentially irritating and cause exfoliation. Gauze sponges should be used to pat, not rub, the dip onto the skin. An Elizabethan collar should reduce the risk of ingestion.

Five drugs are used to systemically treat dermatophytosis: griseofulvin, ketoconazole, itraconazole, and fluconazole and terbinafine (see Chapter 9). Even in infections that will be self-resolving (self-cure generally occurs in 60 to 100 days), systemic antifungal therapy will hasten the time to recovery and thus is beneficial, limiting environmental contamination and exposure to human beings. Griseofulvin remains the drug of choice because it is licensed and approved for use in dogs and cats. Either the microsize dose (25 to 50 mg/kg divided or once every 24 hours) or the ultramicrosize dose (5 to 10 mg/kg orally once daily) can be administered. Because many animals are intolerant to ketoconazole, itraconazole is the second drug of choice should an animal not tolerate griseofulvin therapy or fail to respond to it. Ketoconazole is significantly less expensive than itraconazole and is a reasonable choice for dogs. Although improvement should be evident within 2 to 3 weeks of therapy, several weeks (generally 30 to 70 days) must lapse before a cure is achieved. A comparison study in kittens infected with *Microsporum canis* found that time to resolution with griseofulvin (50 mg/kg orally divided or once every 24 hours) was 70 days versus 56 days with itraconazole (10 mg/kg orally once daily); the control group remained positive at 100 days. Therapy should be monitored by fungal cultures biweekly after 4 to 6 weeks of therapy and treatment continued until two or three consecutive weekly cultures are negative. Note that false-positive fungal cultures can occur after clinical recovery because of environmental contamination. Cats with questionable positive results should be isolated from the environment for 3 to 5 days and subsequently recultured. Griseofulvin should not be used in pregnant animals, those younger than 12 weeks of age, or those that test positive for feline immunodeficiency virus. This drug should be discontinued immediately if the cat becomes anorexic or lethargic or if gastrointestinal signs are seen. Terbinafine, a systemic antifungal approved for use in human beings for treatment of dermatophytosis, has not been studied for efficacy or safety in animals. However, an unpublished pharmacokinetic study with cats (in Europe) indicates that a dose of 10 mg/kg once daily is appropriate; 10 to 30 mg/kg orally once daily has been suggested in Internet resources. Fluconazole may also be effective when other treatments fail or are associated with side effects. The recent change to a generic drug has reduced the cost dramatically. Terbinafine has been shown to be effective for treating *Malassezia* and may be an alternative antidermatophyte treatment.

Cleansing of the environment is obviously critical in a cattery or kennel situation but can also be important in a single-animal household. Undiluted bleach and 1% formalin are the most effective products for resolving environmental contamination.[41] This regimen is likely to kill 100% of spores; residual activity is likely to be greatest with undiluted bleach, followed by 1% formalin, enilconazole (not available in the United States), and common household bleach diluted 1:10. Common household bleach is not as efficacious in killing spores as the other two products, but it is the least expensive and most readily available. Aqueous chlorhexidine is ineffective.

Canine Perianal Fistulae (Anal Furunculosis)

Very little has been written on the topic of canine perianal fistulae. Nonsurgical management is the new standard of therapy.[42] Cyclosporine orally at 5 mg/kg twice daily until a remission is reached is the treatment of choice. The available water-soluble forms should be selected (Neoral, Atopica).[43] Vomiting and diarrhea are common side effects. Additional side effects can include gingival hyperplasia and secondary infections. Tacrolimus ointment (protopic 0.1%) is a topical analog of cyclosporine. It has been shown anecdotally to be effective for the treatment of perianal fistulae when used as a sole treatment. In the author's experience, this product alone is not beneficial. Cyclosporine orally with or without tacrolimus ointment appears to be the current treatment of choice. Treatment may take several weeks to induce a remission before tapering off the dosage to every other day. Relapses are common. Secondary infections are common and should be treated on the basis of culture and susceptibility testing.

REFERENCES

1. Pavletic MM: Anatomy and circulation of the canine skin, *Microsurgery* 12:103–112, 1991.
2. Riviere JE, Spoo HW: Dermatopharmacology: drugs acting locally on the skin. In Adams HR, editor: *Veterinary pharmacology and therapeutics*, Ames, Iowa, 1995, Iowa State University Press, pp 1050–1089.
3. White PD: *Essential fatty acids in veterinary medicine, Shawnee Mission, Kansas*, 1995, Bayer Corporation and Veterinary Learning Systems, Bayer Corporation, Agriculture Division, Animal Health.
4. Millis PC, Magnusson BM, Cross SE: The effect of solute lipophilicity on penetration through feline skin, *J Vet Pharmacol Ther* 26:311–314, 2003.
5. Kwochka KW: *Topical antipruritic therapy. In Dermatology: 19th Annual Waltham/OSU for the treatment of small animal disease*, Waltham USA, 1995, Vernon, Calif, pp 41–45.
6. Rosenkrantz WS: Shampoo therapy. In Bonagura JD, Twedt DC, editors: *Kirk's current veterinary therapy XIV*, St Louis, 2009, Saunders.
7. Messinger LM: Therapy for feline dermatoses, *Vet Clin North Am Small Anim Pract* 25:981–1005, 1995.
8. Guzzo CA, Lazarus GS, Werth VP: Dermatologic pharmacology. In Hardman JG, Limberd LE, editors: *Goodman and Gilman's the pharacologic basis of therapeutics*, ed 9, New York, 1995, McGraw-Hill, pp 1593–1616.
9. Power HT, Ihrke PJ: Synthetic retinoids in veterinary dermatology, *Vet Clin North Am Small Anim Pract* 20:1525–1540, 1990.
10. Kwochka KW: Retinoids in dermatology. In Kirk RW, editor: *Current veterinary therapy X: small animal practice*, Philadelphia, 1989, Saunders, pp 553–560.
11. Kwochka KW: Treatment of scaling disorders in dogs, *Proceedings Atlantic Coast Veterinary Conference* , 2003.
12. Power HT, Ihrke PJ: The use of synthetic retinoids in veterinary medicine. In Bonagura J, editor: *Current veterinary therapy XII: small animal practice*, Philadelphia, 1995, Saunders, pp 585–590.
13. Scott DW: Rational use of glucocorticoids in dermatology. In Bonagura J, editor: *Current veterinary therapy XII: small animal practice*, Philadelphia, 1995, Saunders, pp 573–581.
14. Kwochka KW, Kowalski JJ: Prophylactic efficacy of four antibacterial shampoos against Staphylococcus intermedius in dogs, *Am J Vet Res* 52:115–118, 1991.
15. Hall JA, Campbell KL: The effect of potentiated sulfonamides on canine thyroid function. In Bonagura J, editor: *Current veterinary therapy XII: small animal practice*, Philadelphia, 1995, Saunders, pp 595–597.
16. Kunkle G: Steroid therapy for the skin. In *Dermatology: 19th Annual Waltham/OSU for the treatment of small animal disease*, Waltham USA, 1995, Vernon, Calif, pp 37–40.
17. Guaguère E, Steffan J, Olivry T, Cyclosporine A: a new drug in the field of canine dermatology, *Vet Derm* 15:61–74, 2004.

18. Olivry T, Steffan J, Fisch RD, et al: Randomized controlled trial of the efficacy of cyclosporine in the treatment of atopic dermatitis in dogs, *J Am Vet Med Assoc* 221(3):370–377, 2002.
19. Steffan J, Strehlau G, Maurer M, et al: Cyclosporin A pharmacokinetics and efficacy in the treatment of atopic dermatitis in dogs, *J Vet Pharmacol Ther* 27(4):231–238, 2004.
20. Radowicz SN, Power HT: Long-term use of cyclosporine in the treatment of canine atopic dermatitis, *Vet Derm* 16:81–86, 2005.
21. Olivry T, Mueller RS: Evidence-based veterinary dermatology: a systematic review of the pharmacotherapy of canine atopic dermatitis, *Vet Derm* 14:121–146, 2003.
22. Steffan J, Horn J, Gruet P, et al: Remission of the clinical signs of atopic dermatitis in dogs after cessation of treatment with cyclosporine A or methylprednisolone, *Vet Record* 154:681–684, 2004.
23. Marsella R, Nicklin CF, Saglio S, et al: Investigation on the clinical efficacy and safety of 0.1% tacrolimus ointment (Protopic) in canine atopic dermatitis: a randomized, double-blinded, placebo-controlled, cross-over study, *Vet Derm* 15:294–303, 2004.
24. Logas D: Systemic nonsteroidal therapy for pruritus: the North American experience. In *Dermatology: 19th Annual Waltham/OSU for the treatment of small animal disease*, Waltham USA, 1995, Vernon, Calif, pp 32–36.
25. Hansson H, et al: Clinical pharmacology of clemastine in healthy dogs, *Vet Dermatol* 15:152–158, 2004.
26. Campbell KL: Fatty acid supplementation and skin disease, *Vet Clin North Am Small Anim Pract* 20:1475–1486, 1990.
27. Saevik BK, Bergvall K, Holm BR, et al: A randomized controlled study to evaluate the steroid sparing effect of essential fatty acid supplements in the treatment of canine atopic dermatitis, *Vet Derm* 15:137–145, 2004.
28. Miller WH, Scott DW, Wellington JR: A clinical trial on the efficacy of clemastine in the management of allergic pruritus in dogs, *Can Vet J* 34:2–27, 1993.
29. White SD, Rosychuk RAW, Reinke SI, et al: Use of tetracycline and niacinamide for treatment of autoimmune skin diseases in 31 dogs, *J Am Vet Med Assoc* 200:1497–1500, 1992.
30. Scott DW, Buerger RG: Nonsteroidal antiinflammatory agents in the management of canine pruritus, *J Am Anim Hosp Assoc* 24:424–428, 1988.
31. Paradis M, Lemay S, Scott DW: The efficacy of clemastine, a fatty acid containing product (Dermcaps) and the combination of both products in the management of canine pruritus, *Vet Dermatol* 2:17–20, 1991.
32. Hansson H, Bergvall K, Bondesson U: Clinical pharmacology of clemastine in healthy dogs, *Vet Derm* 15:152–158, 2004.
33. Paradis M, et al: Further investigations on the use of nonsteroidal and steroidal anti-inflammatory agents in the management of canine pruritus, *J Am Anim Hosp Assoc* 27:44, 1991.
34. Cooper KD: New therapeutic approaches in atopic dermatitis, *Clin Rev Allergy* 11:543–559, 1993.
35. Rapoport JL, Ryland DH, Kriete M: Drug treatment of canine acral lick. An animal model of obsessive–compulsive disorder, *Arch Gen Psychiatry* 49:517–521, 1992.
36. Goldberger E, Rapoport J: Canine acral lick dermatitis: response to the antiobsessional drug clomipramine, *J Am Anim Hosp Assoc* 22:179–182, 1991.
37. Dodman N, Shuster L, White S, et al: Use of narcotic antagonists to modify stereotypic self-lick, self-chewing, and scratching behavior in dogs, *J Am Vet Med Assoc* 193:815–819, 1988.
38. Kwochka KW: Treatment of seborrhea in the American cocker spaniel. In Kirk RW, editor: *Current veterinary therapy XI: small animal practice*, Philadelphia, 1992, Saunders, pp 523–527.
39. Miller WH: Treatment of generalized demodicosis in dogs. In Bonagura J, editor: *Current veterinary therapy XII: small animal practice*, Philadelphia, 1995, Saunders, pp 625–628.
40. Scott DW: *Update on the treatment of generalized demodicosis in dogs. In Dermatology: 19th Annual Waltham/OSU for the treatment of small animal disease*, Waltham USA, 1995, Vernon, Calif, pp 77–81.
41. Moriello KA: Treatment of dermatophytosis in dogs and cats: an update. In *Dermatology: 19th Annual Waltham/OSU for the treatment of small animal disease*, Waltham USA, 1995, Vernon, Calif, pp 46–54.
42. Patricilli AJ, Hardie RJ, McAnulty JF: Cyclosporine and ketoconazole for the treatment of perianal fistulas in dogs, *J Am Vet Med Assoc* 220(7):1009–1016, 2002.
43. Patterson AP, Campbell KL: Managing anal furunculosis in dogs, *Compend Contin Educ Vet* 27(5):339–355, 2005.

Rational Use of Reproductive Hormones

23

Autumn P. Davidson, Janice L. Cain, and Sophie A. Grundy

Chapter Outline

The use of reproductive hormones as pharmaceuticals should be based on knowledge of both the reproductive physiology of the species under treatment and the pathophysiology of the disorder being treated. Too often, the use of hormonal therapies in small animal reproduction is based on their documented action in other species. Hormonal therapies are also used when the underlying reproductive disorder has not been fully studied nor understood in small animals. Although there are specific indications for the rational (evidence-based) use of reproductive hormones in small animal theriogenology, they are commonly used inappropriately. This chapter includes a review of the basic physiology of hormones used therapeutically in small animal theriogenology, a discussion of their clinical availability, their appropriate applications, and common misuses.

PHYSIOLOGIC PRINCIPLES OF REPRODUCTIVE HORMONES

Hypothalamic Hormones

Gonadotropin-Releasing Hormone and Its Analogs

Gonadotropin-releasing hormone (GnRH) is a highly conserved hypothalamic decapeptide with the same amino acid sequence in all mammals. After puberty GnRH is released in a pulsatile manner from the hypothalamus, traverses the hypothalamic–hypophyseal portal system, and activates anterior pituitary gonadotroph receptors. The pituitary responds by releasing luteinizing hormone (LH) and follicle-stimulating hormone (FSH) in a pulsatile pattern.[1] Stimulation of the pituitary by GnRH must be in pulsatile form for repeated release of LH and FSH; after receptor activation, GnRH is rapidly deactivated and cleared. The frequency and amplitude of GnRH pulses vary depending on the phase of the reproductive cycle. The frequency of GnRH pulsatile release in primates during folliculogenesis is every 70 to 90 minutes.[2] It is this natural *pulsatile* secretion of GnRH and its short biological half-life that cause difficulties when attempting to use GnRH as a pharmaceutical. Investigations with specialized infusion devices for pulsatile delivery have successfully augmented fertility in a variety of species,[3-5] but the clinical application of such a method lacks practicality for routine use in small animal patients.

GnRH analogs are synthetically prepared substances that differ from GnRH by various amino acid substitutions in the peptide sequence. Analogs with a few amino acid substitutions can act as GnRH agonists because of their increased binding affinity and decreased clearance compared with GnRH.

Heavily substituted analogs can cause receptor blockade and have an antagonist function. The result is a suppressive effect on the pituitary–gonadal axis. This axis is easily downregulated such that frequent or high dosing of a GnRH agonist will suppress the release of LH and FSH also.[6] GnRH agonists and antagonists thus may have the same ultimate physiologic effect.

Oxytocin

A nonapeptide hormone synthesized by neurons in the hypothalamus, oxytocin is transported axonally to the posterior pituitary, where it is stored. This peptide hormone is released from the posterior pituitary into the general circulation after appropriate neural stimulation. Its primary effects are on mammary tissue and the myometrium. The effects of oxytocin on the milk let-down reflex and parturition have been well described.[7] The ability of oxytocin to induce myometrial contraction is enhanced by prior estrogen sensitization to "prime" the myometrium for maximal response.[8] The half-life of oxytocin in the blood is short, approximately 1.5 minutes; thus secretion pulse frequency and amplitude are important for its physiologic effects. The release of neurotransmitters may alter the amplitude and frequency of oxytocin release; for example, dopamine enhances burst frequency and amplitude, whereas cholinergic antagonists may be inhibitory.[9]

Pituitary Gonadotropins

Luteinizing Hormone and Follicle-Stimulating Hormone

The pituitary gonadotropins LH and FSH are relatively large glycoproteins, each consisting of two covalently bound structural subunits (α and β). Within a species the amino acid sequence of the α-subunits are identical for all anterior pituitary glycoproteins, with high sequence homology existing across species. The β-subunits are specific for individual hormones (i.e., thyroid-stimulating hormone) and provide the functional specificity of each. The overall size of these glycoproteins precludes economic synthetic production of these hormones.[8]

The secretion patterns of these hormones differ depending on the species and the phase of the ovarian cycle. A unique pattern of LH secretion in the bitch has been documented[10] (Figure 23-1). Serum concentration of LH is at basal levels during anestrus. Significant increases in both the amplitude and frequency of LH pulsatile release occur before proestrus. The frequency of LH pulsatile release during anestrus is 3 to 7 hours; before proestrus LH pulse frequency is 60 to 120 minutes.[11] This increase in LH release before the onset of proestrus is likely involved with termination of the anestrus phase.[1] The factors that lead to the LH increase at that time are unknown. Serum estrogen concentration at that time also decreases; estrogen production inhibits LH release. What causes the relative decrease in estrogen production at that time is also unknown.

Serum LH concentration returns to basal levels for most of proestrus (i.e., folliculogenesis). The increase in serum estrogen concentration during folliculogenesis contributes to an inhibition of LH release during that phase.[1] When estrogen

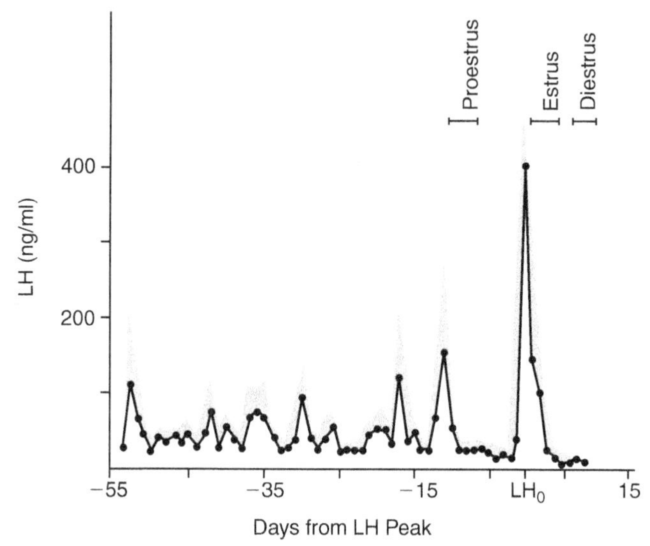

Figure 23-1 Concentrations of luteinizing (LH) hormone in canine serum throughout late anestrus, proestrus, estrus, and early diestrus. *Stippled area* is the standard error of the mean (*bars* indicate ranges of proestrus, estrus, and diestrus). (From Olson PN, Bowen RA, Behrendt MD et al: Concentrations of reproductive hormones in canine serum throughout late anestrus, proestrus, and estrus, *Biol Reprod* 27:1196, 1982.)

production decreases, the inhibition of LH release is discontinued. At that time a preovulatory surge in LH release (the preovulatory LH peak) occurs and is thought to trigger ovulation. The duration of the preovulatory LH peak is 1 to 3 days, after which LH secretion returns to a basal state in early diestrus. Additionally, LH is luteotrophic throughout most of the luteal phase in the bitch.

Similar to the pattern of LH secretion, FSH secretion also appears to be inhibited by relatively high concentrations of estrogen during proestrus. Inhibin, a modulary hormone released from the ovary during folliculogenesis, also inhibits FSH release during this phase. When estrogen secretion declines in late proestrus, FSH secretion surges to maximal levels before ovulation, in concert with the preovulatory LH peak[1,10] (Figure 23-2). After this FSH surge, serum FSH concentration remains relatively high during diestrus and pregnancy. Interestingly, the bitch is also unique with regard to the pattern of FSH secretion during anestrus. During anestrus serum FSH concentration can be 50% to 100% of the concentration found at the preovulatory FSH peak and is 5 to 10 times higher than during proestrus.[1] It is unclear why FSH produced during anestrus is unable to stimulate folliculogenesis. It has been postulated that perhaps the FSH measured during anestrus is in a biologically inactive form.[1]

The patterns of LH and FSH secretion in the queen have not been clearly determined. It has been documented that after adequate copulation LH release begins within minutes. Queens are induced ovulators; thus this response is expected. Apparent spontaneous ovulation, without copulation or other tactile stimulation, has been reported in the queen.[12] The pattern of LH secretion during the apparent spontaneous ovulation has not been determined, however.

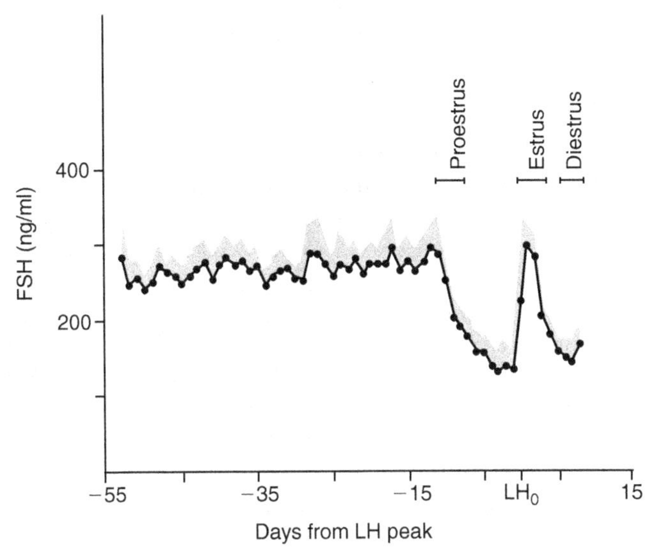

Figure 23-2 Concentrations of follicle-stimulating hormone (FSH) in canine serum throughout late anestrus, proestrus, and early diestrus. *Stippled area* is the standard error of the mean *(bars* indicate ranges of proestrus, estrus, and diestrus). (From Olson PN, Bowen RA, Behrendt MD et al: Concentrations of reproductive hormones in canine serum throughout late anestrus, proestrus, and estrus, *Biol Reprod* 27:1196, 1982.)

The release of LH and FSH is also pulsatile in response to GnRH in the male. Both glycoprotein hormones are necessary for spermatogenesis. Testicular interstitial cells bind LH and respond by increasing testosterone production. Activation of receptors on Sertoli cells by FSH promotes spermatogenesis and produces inhibin, a hormone that, as in the female, regulates FSH release by the pituitary. After neutering the loss of negative feedback inhibition causes serum FSH concentrations to increase dramatically.[13] This has also been documented in cases of infertility resulting from primary testicular degeneration.[14] Postcastration elevations in LH serum concentrations also occur, but overlap in measured values between intact and neutered dogs is possible.[13]

Some species also produce placental gonadotropins. A luteotrophic gonadotropin produced by the human placenta (human chorionic gonadotropin [hCG]) has a potent LH-like effect in many species. A gonadotropin produced by fetal trophoblastic cells in horses is referred to as equine *chorionic gonadotropin (eCG)* or *pregnant mare serum gonadotropin (pmSG)*. In most species eCG has a combination of FSH and LH activity. Additionally, eCG products commonly contain components of equine serum that can be antigenic when used as a pharmaceutical in another species.

Prolactin

A relatively large polypeptide produced by the anterior pituitary, prolactin is luteotrophic in the bitch and queen.[15,16] It is suspected that prolactin is also involved in the maintenance of the anestrus phase in the bitch.[1] Prolactin is under negative control by dopamine such that the administration of a dopamine agonist will inhibit prolactin secretion. Inhibition of prolactin secretion can promote luteolysis during the second half of diestrus or pregnancy in the bitch[15] and queen.[16] Various dopamine agonists have been investigated for inducing abortion and shortening anestrus (i.e., estrus induction). Bromocriptine is a dopaminergic drug that has been used in various protocols. Its use has not gained acceptance, however, because it commonly causes vomiting and diarrhea. The highly potent dopamine agonists cabergoline and metergoline have fewer or no apparent side effects, respectively. The effect of metergoline to decrease prolactin secretion may primarily result from blockade of central serotonin receptors and may function as a dopamine agonist only at higher doses.[17] Metoclopramide, more commonly used as a central serotonin antagonist, may be used to enhance prolactin release in the bitch and queen, and thus enhance milk let-down, through its central dopamine (D_2) agonist effects.

Gonadal Steroids

Estrogen

Produced by the ovary during folliculogenesis, estrogens affect target tissues, causing vulvar edema, vaginal mucosal hyperplasia, sanguineous vulvar discharge in the bitch, and sexual attraction in both the bitch and queen. The bitch uniquely exhibits sexual receptivity when estrogen production decreases; serum concentration of estrogen peaks 1 to 2 days before the end of proestrus. A concurrent increase in progesterone is required for complete expression of sexual receptivity. Estrogen acts synergistically with progesterone to stimulate growth of endometrial and mammary glands, and estrogen priming may be important before the natural effect of oxytocin on the myometrium during parturition.[8] Male production of estrogen occurs in both the Leydig and Sertoli cells, by way of de novo steroidogenesis in the Leydig cell and P450 aromatase conversion of testosterone alone in the Sertoli cell. Considerable interspecies variation occurs with respect to the relative ratios of estrogen produced by each cell. Excessive production of estrogens by Sertoli cell tumors and, less commonly, by other testicular or adrenal tumors results in male feminizing syndrome. Estrogens are involved in receptor sensitivity and feedback influence on the hypothalamic–pituitary–gonadal axis.

The adverse effects of estrogen (i.e., bone marrow aplasia, cystic endometrial hyperplasia/pyometra, infertility) have been documented in dogs after administration of any estrogen preparation.[18,19] The unique sensitivity of dogs to estrogen toxicity may be due to the relatively weak binding affinity of sex-steroid binding proteins for estrogen in the dog. The result is a decrease in the inherent buffering mechanism that would otherwise regulate the amount of free hormone available to penetrate cell membranes. Estrogen toxicity can occur with exogenous or endogenous estrogens (e.g., Sertoli cell tumors, ovarian follicular cysts, and ovarian neoplasia).

Progesterone

As the main progestational hormone in both bitches and queens, progesterone is produced by corpora lutea just before and after ovulation. The bitch continues to produce progesterone during nonpregnant diestrus; serum concentrations of progesterone are indistinguishable in concentration or duration of production from that of pregnancy. The decline of progesterone and increase in prolactin production at the termination of diestrus cause the clinical manifestations of pseudopregnancy in the nonpregnant bitch. This is a demonstration of a normal physiologic occurrence that should not be confused with a pathologic state and in fact suggests normal ovarian function. There is some variation among bitches regarding the maximum amount of progesterone produced in midgestation (or mid-diestrus), with levels reaching 80 to 100 ng/mL in some individuals. The minimum serum progesterone concentration necessary to maintain pregnancy appears to be 2 ng/mL.[20] The minimum amount of progesterone required to sustain pregnancy in the queen has not been determined; however, serum progesterone concentrations of less than 1 ng/mL for several days occurred before termination of pregnancy were observed in one study.[16]

Placental production of progesterone by the queen during the latter half of pregnancy had been suggested as a requirement to maintain pregnancy. It has been learned, however, that corpora lutea of the queen are necessary for progesterone production throughout pregnancy.[21] During pseudopregnancy in queens (i.e., nonfertile ovulation), peak luteal activity appears to occur at days 10 to 15 and then declines to basal values by days 35 to 40.[22]

In the bitch progesterone is produced before ovulation by follicular luteinization, approximately concurrent with the preovulatory LH peak. Serial evaluations of serum progesterone concentrations during proestrus and estrus can be used to indirectly determine the preovulatory LH peak and thus determine the time of ovulation in the bitch. This methodology, known as *ovulation timing,* is used to improve breeding management. The bitch typically exhibits sexual receptivity (behavioral estrus) when the serum concentration of estrogen is decreasing and progesterone is increasing.

Synthetic progestational compounds (progestagens) are commercially available. Megestrol acetate has been marketed as a drug to suppress estrus or inhibit ovulation, depending on the time and dose of administration. The method by which progestagens inhibit folliculogenesis and ovulation is not precisely understood. It appears that although megestrol acetate will not decrease the serum concentration of LH that is already at low basal levels, it may be able to prevent the increases in LH that normally occur at the end of anestrus.[1]

Testosterone

Produced by the interstitial cells of the testes, testosterone is necessary for gonadal development, spermatogenesis, and libido in the male. The normal function of Sertoli cells to promote spermatogenesis depends on an intratesticular testosterone concentration that greatly exceeds circulatory levels.[8] Pharmacologic administration of androgens, including testosterone, can induce infertility by negative inhibition of LH and FSH release, which are necessary for spermatogenesis. Testosterone is converted in the prostate to dihydrotestosterone (DHT), which promotes development of this gland and the eventually contributes to the anticipated formation of benign prostatic hyperplasia in mature dogs. DHT is an androgen with greater biological activity than testosterone.

Testosterone and the androgenic steroid mibolerone have been used to suppress ovarian activity and thereby prevent estrus cycles in the bitch. Mibolerone was specifically approved for this use, although the duration of time from discontinuing administration to the occurrence of the next estrous cycle was variable. Silent heats following mibolerone therapy were common. Persistent anestrus (i.e., lack of return to estrous cycles) has been a problem in some Greyhound bitches treated with injectable testosterone to prevent estrus cycles during racing.

Inhibitors of Gonadal Steroids

Tamoxifen is both an estrogen agonist and antagonist that has been used as adjunctive therapy for women with mammary carcinoma. The nature of its effect depends on tissue estrogen receptor type. Tamoxifen appears to have, at least in part, a direct estrogenic effect in the bitch. Some bitches treated with tamoxifen had observable vulvar edema; sanguineous vaginal discharge; and, in some cases, pyometra of the uterine stump.[23] Tamoxifen and clomiphene, another antiestrogenic compound, have been used to promote superovulation in women, possibly by promoting an increase in endogenous FSH release. Tamoxifen has been used in the bitch as a mismate therapy but was associated with pyometra, endometritis, and cystic ovaries in a high percentage of bitches; was reliably effective only when given during the first 14 days of diestrus; and is not advised.[24]

Antigestagens are agents that inhibit the effect of progesterone by binding to and altering the progesterone receptor and have been investigated as abortion agents in humans (i.e., mifepristone, RU-486). Preliminary studies have documented the effectiveness of mifepristone to terminate pregnancy in bitches.[25]

Finasteride is another useful inhibitor of gonadal steroids. Testosterone is converted to DHT in the prostate by the action of the enzyme 5α-reductase. Trophic in its effect, DHT induces benign prostatic hyperplasia as a dog ages. Finasteride inhibits the action of 5α-reductase, thereby reducing DHT concentrations in the prostate. Finasteride may also alter prostatic angiogenesis and reduce hemospermia through a change in microvessel density. Developed for use in men with prostatic hyperplasia, finasteride has been investigated for successful similar use in dogs.[26] Benign prostatic hyperplasia causing hemospermia can be detrimental to efforts to successfully freeze and thaw canine semen; otherwise, it is minimally problematic in the dog unless accompanied by infection or neoplasia.

Autacoids

Prostaglandin $F_{2\alpha}$

Prostaglandins, potent autacoids, have therapeutic indications in small animal theriogenology. Administration of prostaglandin $F_{2\alpha}$($PGF_{2\alpha}$) induces a direct luteolytic effect in bitches and queens during pregnancy or diestrus. Induction of luteolysis depends on dose, frequency of drug administration, and stage of diestrus that the drug is administered. After day 30 of diestrus, $PGF_{2\alpha}$ is reliably luteolytic in both the bitch[27] and queen.[22] Corpora lutea are relatively resistant to luteolysis by PGF_2-alpha during the first 5 days of diestrus in the bitch.[28] There is evidence that $PGF_{2\alpha}$ will cause either a transient decrease in progesterone production or complete luteolysis when administered during early diestrus after day 6.[28] In addition to a direct luteolytic effect, $PGF_{2\alpha}$ also has a stimulatory action on the myometrium, promoting evacuation of uterine luminal contents. The drug is therefore effective as an abortifacient and for the treatment of open cervix pyometra in the bitch and queen.

Additional effects of PGF_2-alpha administration include panting, nausea, vomiting, diarrhea, hypersalivation, and tachycardia in dogs and vocalization, mydriasis, and possibly vomition and diarrhea in cats. These adverse clinical signs usually stop within 20 to 30 minutes of drug administration. The drug is preferably administered after fasting in the dog and cat to decrease the incidence of vomiting. The adverse effects of $PGF_{2\alpha}$ are potentially dose related, although there is individual sensitivity, and signs usually abate after repeated dosing. Although extremely rare, cardiovascular collapse after PGF_2-alpha administration is possible.

Most protocols using $PGF_{2\alpha}$ are based on the formulation of dinoprost tromethamine. This product is not approved for use in dogs or cats in the United States. Informed owner consent is advised, although the use of $PGF_{2\alpha}$ is established in the veterinary literature. The more potent synthetic $PGF_{2\alpha}$ analogs (cloprostenol and fluprostenol) are now used clinically in both the dog and the cat; studies regarding the use of these compounds indicate efficacy with fewer side effects, owing to the increased specificity of the compounds for uterine smooth muscle.

KEY POINT 23-1 Both natural and synthetic hormonal products are available for the treatment of small animal reproductive conditions; the clinician should weigh the benefits of both before selecting therapy.

COMMERCIAL AVAILABILITY OF REPRODUCTIVE HORMONES

Gonadotropin-Releasing Hormone And Its Analogs

Lack of availability is a major hindrance to widespread use of GnRH analogs to control reproduction in humans and animals. Analogs are expensive to produce and are often available only as investigational products for research studies; availability also varies throughout the United States. One marketed GnRH analog (an antagonist) is leuprolide (Lupron, TAP Pharmaceuticals, Deerfield, Ill.). The native GnRH hormone (gonadorelin, Rhone Merieux) is commercially available (Cystorelin, or Factrel, Fort Dodge Laboratories, Fort Dodge, Iowa). Implant formulations of GnRH agonists such as deslorelin have been shown to be effective for reversible long-term suppression of reproductive function in the male and female dog and estrus suppression in the queen[29,30] and have been manipulated for estrus induction in the bitch.[31]

Gonadotropins

Currently, FSH is not available in the United States; hCG is readily available (Chorulon, chorionic gonadotropin, Butler, Columbus, Ohio). In the United States eCG is not commercially available but may be available in Canada (Equinex, Ayerst Laboratories, Quebec) and in some European countries. Purified canine LH is not commercially available, but human LH can be purchased in a 1:1 ratio with human FSH in a product used to treat human infertility (Repronex, menotropin, Serono Laboratories, Norwell, Mass.). Additionally, purified human FSH is available (Metrodin, Bravelle, Serono Laboratories). The use of human menotropins has not been extensively studied in small animal medicine, and these products are likely to be too costly for routine use.

Dopamine Agonists

Bromocriptine (Parlodel, Sandoz Pharmaceuticals, East Hanover, NJ) is available, as is the newer dopamine agonist cabergoline (Dostinex, Pharmacia and Upjohn); metergoline (Virbac Laboratories, Carros, France) is available in Europe.

Gonadal Steroids

Other than antigestagens, which are not available in the United States, gonadal steroids and their inhibitors are widely available in many formulations. Some hormones are available in repositol formulation (i.e., medroxyprogesterone acetate, Depo-Provera, Upjohn, Kalamazoo, Mich.), and others are available in esters that exert a more potent effect (i.e., esters of estradiol). Some commonly available products include compounded diethylstilbestrol (DES), progesterone in oil (Eli Lilly), and testosterone propionate (Steris Laboratories, Phoenix, Ariz.).

Inhibitors of Gonadal Steroids

Tamoxifen (Nolvadex, Zeneca Pharmaceuticals, Wilmington, Del.) and finasteride (Proscar, Merck and Co., West Point, Pa.) are commonly available through pharmacies for humans. One product that is available (but not recommended on account of the side effects of progesterone administration in intact bitches) for contraception (heat prevention) in bitches is megestrol acetate (Ovaban, Schering-Plough).

Antiprogestins

Progesterone-receptor blockers (antiprogestins), such as mifepristone and aglepristone, are clinically available for use only in humans, and they are not available in the United States at this time.

Miscellaneous

Other products commonly available include oxytocin (Butler), natural prostaglandin $F_{2\alpha}$ (Lutalyse, Upjohn), Cloprostenol (Estrumate, Cayman Pharma), misoprostol, and PGE, (Cytotec, G. D. Searle & Co., Chicago, Ill.).

INDICATIONS FOR THE RATIONAL (EVIDENCE-BASED) USE OF REPRODUCTIVE HORMONES

Some reproductive disorders are common and well described in the literature (e.g., pyometra, dystocia). Others are either incompletely understood or are less common (e.g., estrus induction, luteal insufficiency) such that information can be difficult for the practicing veterinarian to obtain. The discussion presented here is intended to provide an overview of several reproductive problems of dogs and cats that commonly require veterinary intervention (Table 23-1). Many of these disorders are topics of current research, which is needed to better understand and manage them.

KEY POINT 23-2 Medical management of reproductive conditions best treated surgically (i.e., neutering) should be reserved for individuals with good reproductive potential.

Estrus Induction

Induction of Estrus in the Bitch

A reliable, practical method to successfully induce fertile estrus in the bitch has long been sought. Protocols that are successful in other species usually do not produce the same effect in the bitch. This is primarily because of the unique reproductive physiology of the bitch and a lack of understanding of all the factors that initiate a new estrous cycle. Various protocols have been tested using all classes of reproductive hormones: GnRH, GnRH analogs, gonadotropins, dopamine agonists, and DES (Table 23-2). Some relatively successful protocols use compounds that are not commercially available at this time. It is important to thoroughly evaluate all potential causes of reproductive failure before estrus induction is attempted and realize that protocols are designed and tested using bitches that are reproductively normal. The outcome of estrus induction in bitches that have reproductive pathology is not known.

Investigation into the use of GnRH as an agent to induce estrus in the bitch resulted in seven of eight Beagle bitches that ovulated and conceived (GnRH 140 μg/kg per pulse every 90 minutes intravenously for 11 to 13 days).[5] This protocol used a programmable, portable pulsatile infusion device (Pulsamat, Ferring Laboratories, Ridgewood, N.J.) that delivered the GnRH from a reservoir within the pump to a jugular intravenous catheter. The pump, attached to a harness worn by the bitch, was well tolerated by laboratory Beagles. The pump and harness were not well tolerated by privately owned Labrador Retriever bitches, however. The fragility of the pump and its expense preclude its routine use in veterinary medicine.

Table 23-1 Uses of Reproductive Hormones for Dogs and Cats

Indication	Hormone Used	Considerations
Estrus induction	See Table 23-3	
Induction of ovulation		
Ovulatory failure	hCG or GnRH to induce ovulation	Difficult to accurately determine follicular maturity to administer at correct time
Ovarian cysts	hCG or GnRH to induce luteinization	Often ineffective, may require ovariectomy need to differentiate neoplasia
Vaginal hyperplasia	hCG or GnRH to hasten ovulation	Not proven to shorten time for spontaneous recovery
Luteal insufficiency	Progesterone to maintain gestation	Potentially teratogenic, inhibits lactation development, luteal insufficiency is rare; need diagnosis before treatment attempted
Estrus prevention	Mibolerone or megestrol acetate GnRH analogs (implant)	Mibolerone: unpredictable and unavailable, irregular return to estrus after withdrawal; megestrol acetate: potential for infertility, pyometra; requires compounding GnRH analogs are not available in all states
Signs of pseudocyesis, galactostasis, mastitis	Cabergoline	Mild GI side effects
Pyometra/postpartum metritis	PGF_2, cloprostenol	Transient side effects of PGF_2, need careful evaluation and supportive clinical care
Pregnancy termination	PGF_2, cloprostenol, dopamine agonists, dexamethasone.	Transient side effects of PGF_2; unavailability of some dopamine agonists, steroid side effects (transient)
Dystocia	Oxytocin 10 μ/ml	Can induce uterine tetany and fetal demise if overdosage occurs Use less concentrated solution
Mammary gland carcinoma	Tamoxifen	Controversy as to efficacy, possibly exacerbates condition
Urinary incontinence	DES	Phenylpropanolamine can be synergistic if ineffective alone
Cryptorchidism	hCG or GnRH	Ethical concerns, not proven to be effective
Benign prostatic hyperplasia	Finasteride	Costly, requires compounding in small dogs
Hypogonadism	Gonadotropins	Rare condition, difficult to document

hCG, Human chorionic gonadotropin; *GnRH,* gonadotropin-releasing hormone; *PGF_2,* prostaglandin F_2; *DES,* diethylstilbestrol.

GnRH analogs, many of which are not currently commercially available, have been investigated as agents to induce estrus in bitches. The advantage of GnRH analogs is their relatively longer bioavailability and increased potency. Concannon[32] reported the use of [D-Trp^{6}NmeLeu^{7}Pro^{9}NEt] GnRH administered by a constant-rate infusion device. Twenty-four bitches received 1.7 to 2.5 μg/kg/day subcutaneously for 14 days; nine bitches ovulated and whelped litters. In a preliminary report, the use of [D-Trp^{6}Pro^{9}NEt] GnRH was administered to bitches (1 μg/kg subcutaneously every 8 hours) by the following protocol: every 8 hours subcutaneous injections until the observation of behavioral estrus, after which treatment was continued for another 3 days at half the original dose (i.e., 0.5 μg/kg subcutaneously every 8 hours).[33] Four of six bitches treated with this protocol whelped litters as a result of an induced estrus.

Deslorelin implants have also been used successfully as vulval implants for 10 days to induce estrus in the bitch.[31] They must be removed before downregulation occurs.

The gonadotropins FSH and LH have been investigated with numerous protocols as agents to induce estrus in the bitch. Most protocols use either eCG or FSH to stimulate folliculogenesis and hCG to induce ovulation. Some protocols additionally use DES administered before gonadotropins; estrogen can increase the responsiveness to gonadotropins. Gonadotropin protocols are largely unreliable and can induce adverse effects (e.g., ovarian hyperstimulation with hyperestrogenism), and with some protocols an abnormal luteal phase was detected.[34] One report indicated great success with the currently unavailable product PLH (Burns-Biotech),[35] although it is unknown what the relative biopotency of FSH and LH was in the product marketed as PLH. That protocol was investigated using Greyhound bitches that had previously received testosterone to suppress estrus during racing. Those bitches had not received testosterone during the 12 months before inclusion in the study, and none of the bitches had an observed proestrus or estrus during that period of time.

The protocol was as follows: DES was administered (5 mg/bitch per day orally) until proestrus was evident and then for 2 days thereafter. If no signs of proestrus were observed by day 7 of DES treatment, the dose was doubled (10 mg/bitch per day orally) until a response was elicited (not to exceed 7 additional days of DES therapy). On day 5 of proestrus, PLH was administered (5 mg/bitch intramuscularly), and on days 9 and 11 of proestrus FSH was administered (10 mg/bitch intramuscularly).[35] All seven bitches in this report became pregnant when bred during an induced estrus. This method used gonadotropin administration in a reverse sequence to that of other reported studies. Because the LH used in this study was no longer available, an attempt to modify the protocol using hCG in place of LH was attempted, but results were disappointing.[36]

Subsequent studies into the use of DES as a sole agent to induce estrus may indicate that the DES used in other protocols was the primary active agent, and perhaps the administration of additional hormone products decreases the response. Fertile estrus has been induced in bitches by the sole administration of oral DES. In a preliminary report DES (5 mg/bitch orally) was administered daily until proestrus was observed and then for 2 days thereafter.[37] The DES therapy continued for 6 to 9 days and resulted in an induced proestrus lasting 0 to 2 days (range) and an estrus duration of 15 to 26 days (range). The preovulatory LH peak occurred 13.5 ± 3.7 days after the last day of DES treatment, although one treated bitch did not have a detectable preovulatory LH peak. All five treated bitches in this study became pregnant, four bitches whelped at term, and one bitch aborted. The lengths of proestrus and estrus and the sizes of the litters did not significantly differ between treated and control groups (n = 5 in each group). The bitches used in this study were treated during a defined

Table 23-2 Hormones Used to Induce Estrus in Bitches

Hormone Classification	Considerations	Drawbacks
GnRH	Leaves normal feedback mechanisms intact; drug is available, not expensive	Requires expensive, cumbersome pump for drug delivery
GnRH analogs	Success in preliminary reports; subcutaneous administration or delivery by implanted infusion devices	Leuprolide, lutrelin, deslorelin, lupron
Gonadotropins	Many different protocols proposed	Most successful protocol used PLH, which is no longer commercially available. Hormones that are available (eCG, hCG, FSH, LH) are less unsuccessful. Can cause hyperstimulation and hyperestrogenism
Estrogen	Oral administration of DES, readily available compounded	Reliably induces signs of proestrus, ovulation less predictable. Information available based on one study at this time. Better protocols exist.
Dopamine agonists	Shortened interestrous interval	Cost of the newer dopamine agonist cabergoline, which has decreased adverse effects, but usually requires compounding; bromocriptine available but associated with vomiting and diarrhea. Must allow 8 week anestrus period.

GnRH, Gonadotropin-releasing hormone; *eCG,* equine chorionic gonadotopin (also known as pregnant mare's serum gonadotropin [PMSG]); *hCG,* human chorionic gonadotropin; *FSH,* follicle-stimulating hormone; *DES,* diethylstilbestrol.

period of anestrus (95 to 129 days; mean 107 ± 13 days), which resulted in a shorter period of anestrus than is normal for the colony (175 ± 87 days). Additional investigation into the use of DES as an agent to induce fertile estrus is needed before client-owned bitches are treated. The optimum dosage schedule and potential for toxicity must be assessed. It may be necessary to adjust the dose in smaller bitches to avoid toxicity.

Another method to shorten the naturally long interestrus interval in the bitch is by the administration of a dopamine agonist to decrease prolactin secretion. Prolactin secretion may alter ovarian responsiveness to gonadotropins; the continued presence of prolactin during anestrus may be responsible for the duration of this phase of the estrous cycle. Decrease in prolactin secretion can shorten the length of anestrus and can induce estrus if treatment occurs during late anestrus. Recent work indicates that the effect of bromocriptine causing shortening of anestrus is due to a yet-undefined action other than its lowering of plasma prolactin concentration and can shorten either diestrus or anestrus to have this effect.[38] Bromocriptine (20 μg/kg twice daily administered 112 ± 4 days after the last onset of proestrus) was used in one study to decrease the interestrus interval in bitches.[39] Bromocriptine causes vomiting, and investigation into its use has been largely replaced by the dopaminergic drugs cabergoline and metergoline. Termination of anestrus and induction of fertile estrus with minimal side effects has been reported by several authors in dogs using cabergoline.[40,41] One protocol uses cabergoline at 5 μg/kg/day until the second cytologic day of proestrus. Treatment for up to 40 days has been reported as effective in inducing fertile estrus in 70% to 90% of normal bitches when started in late anestrus.[42] Ovulation timing and appropriate breeding management result in normal pregnancies. Two protocols using metergoline were reported in one study.[43] Bitches were treated with metergoline (12.5 mg/bitch intramuscularly every 3 days) until the onset of proestrus. Response to therapy was considered positive if proestrus was observed within 40 days after the first day of treatment; 18 of 20 bitches so responded. Ten of these bitches received no additional treatment and were bred, and nine produced litters. Eight other bitches responding to metergoline were additionally treated with hCG (500 IU/bitch intramuscularly) during late proestrus. Six of these bitches ovulated, and four achieved pregnancy. Overall, the metergoline protocol without hCG was more effective in producing pregnancy.

The administration of $PGF_{2\alpha}$ can also shorten the interestrus interval if administered during diestrus. Diestrus normally has a duration of 65 to 70 days in the bitch, and luteolytic therapy with $PGF_{2\alpha}$ abbreviates this phase of the estrous cycle. Bitches that have undergone luteolytic therapy will still enter a phase of anestrus for a variable period, but the return to proestrus or estrus can be sooner than expected, by 1 to 2 months.

Induction of Estrus in the Queen

The domestic cat has been used as a model for reproductive techniques that can apply to preservation of the nondomestic large felines.[44] Queens are apparently sensitive to effects of gonadotropins administered to induce folliculogenesis, but production of anovulatory follicles or cysts can result. The administration of eCG as a single bolus (100 IU) to anestrus queens, followed in 5 to 7 days by a single injection of hCG (50 IU), resulted in a pregnancy rate that was comparable with that produced by natural matings.[45] Daily administration of FSH-P (2 mg/queen per day intramuscularly) for 5 to 7 days results in 72% of queens that will mate and deliver normal offspring.[46]

Induction of Ovulation

Ovulatory Failure in the Bitch

Ovulation failure is rare in the bitch. Too often, bitches are suspected of ovulatory failure when they have seemingly long proestrous and estrous phases, produce small litters, or fail to conceive. Bitches can have signs of estrus, and a fully cornified vaginal smear, for up to 21 days before natural spontaneous ovulation. Also, bitches can have a split estrus: signs of proestrus or estrus without ovulation, a period of anestrus for several weeks, and then return to proestrus. Often the second estrus will be ovulatory and fertile. Split estrus is more common in pubertal bitches but can occur in mature bitches.

Ovulation can be reliably detected with ultrasonography but requires thrice-daily monitoring during the ovulatory period and technical expertise. Direct visualization by laparoscopy is not possible because of the ovarian bursa (it requires bursal resection and is done only experimentally); thus the determination of ovulation is usually attempted indirectly. Serum progesterone concentration can be measured in bitches that historically fail to conceive. The timing of the progesterone measurement is important. It is recommended to evaluate progesterone during the first few weeks of diestrus. Serum concentration of progesterone should be in excess of 5 ng/mL (and generally in excess of 20 ng/mL) at this time. A progesterone level of less than 2 mg/mL indicates either ovulation failure or luteal insufficiency. Values between 2 and 5 ng/mL are suspect and can indicate ovulatory failure, luteal insufficiency, or an uncommonly low progesterone production during diestrus.

Bitches that have normal proestrus and estrus but apparently do not ovulate can be given hormonal products in an attempt to induce ovulation. To mimic the preovulatory LH peak, either GnRH or hCG can be administered at the point of follicular maturation. The determination of follicular maturity is difficult. Incorrect administration (i.e., inappropriate timing) of either preparation can cause preovulatory luteinization of follicles without ovulation or the ovulation of immature, nonviable ova. It has been recommended to administer either GnRH (50 μg/bitch intramuscularly) or hCG (500 to 1000 IU/bitch intramuscularly) on either the day before or the day after the first breeding.[47] Bitches can begin sexual receptivity several days before or after spontaneous ovulation; therefore this protocol is questionable and not documented. It may be advisable to measure serum LH concentration daily during proestrus and estrus and administer either GnRH or hCG on the day of the natural preovulatory LH peak. This presumes that the bitch produces enough LH to measure a peak but either does not produce enough LH to cause ovulation or has another factor inhibiting ovulation. Bitches that fail to ovulate may not produce a measurable LH peak, in which case this recommendation would also fail. Clearly, more investigation is needed in this area.

Ovulatory Failure in the Queen

Queens can be sexually receptive before follicular maturation; sexual receptivity may not correlate with follicular development because estrogen may not return to baseline. Limited mating before the third to fourth day of estrus can result in an attenuated LH secretion and ovulatory failure.[48] Additionally, although an LH response after one effective mating will occur, a maximal LH response ensuring ovulation of all mature ova will more likely occur if numerous matings over a several-day period is allowed. In one report 10 of 48 queens ovulated after a single mating, whereas 30 of 36 ovulated after multiple matings.[49] Optimal breeding management includes mating three times per day at 4-hour intervals throughout estrus. Matings starting on the third day of estrus are advised.

If it is determined that a queen fails to ovulate despite appropriate management, induction of ovulation can be attempted. Protocols with either hCG or GnRH have been reported as follows: hCG 500 IU/queen intramuscularly on day 1 of estrus[50] and GnRH 25 μg/queen intramuscularly on day 2 of estrus.[51]

Treatment of Follicular and Luteal Ovarian Cysts in Bitches

Estrogen-producing follicular cysts can cause prolonged proestrus, nymphomania, estrogen toxicity, and resultant infertility. A luteinized follicular cyst producing progesterone can cause persistent diestrus and resultant infertility. Nonfunctional ovarian cysts can prevent normal cycling and result in infertility. Ovarian cysts are often detected during ovariohysterectomy of older bitches as incidental findings. The detection of a cystic ovarian structure by ultrasonography can be a significant finding. Normal ovarian follicles, luteal structures, and subepithelial cysts should be ruled out, often by sequential ultrasonographic examinations in concert with serum hormone (estradiol and progesterone) measurements. The possibility of a cystic ovarian neoplasm, which can produce clinical signs identical to those of benign cysts, must be considered and is more likely in bitches older than 5 years of age. The measurement of estrogen and progesterone concentrations from the fluid of percutaneously aspirated ovarian cysts can assist the diagnosis of a functional cyst; this will not, however, differentiate between a cyst and neoplasm.

Whether to attempt therapeutic pharmacologic intervention when an ovarian cyst is detected is controversial; ovarian cysts can spontaneously regress.[52] Estrogen-producing follicular cysts can be luteinized with GnRH (50 μg/bitch intramuscularly) or hCG (500 to 1000 IU/bitch intramuscularly). Either treatment can be used as a single injection or repeated daily for three treatments. Response to therapy is a termination of estrous behavior or decrease of estrogen and increase of progesterone serum concentrations. Efficacy of these regimens has not been reported, and surgical removal of the cyst by unilateral ovariectomy is usually required if aggressive intervention is deemed necessary. Similarly, lysis of luteal ovarian cysts with PGF_2-alpha can be attempted but is usually unrewarding in the authors' experience. Ovariectomy permitting histopathologic evaluation of both follicular and luteal ovarian cystic disorders is advised. Ultrasound-guided aspiration of follicular cysts has been advocated as a successful method of terminating prolonged proestrus or estrus in the bitch and deserves further controlled evaluation.

Treatment of Vaginal Hyperplasia and Prolapse

Estrogen produced during folliculogenesis normally causes a hyperplastic response of the vaginal mucosal epithelium and cornification of the vaginal epithelial cells, in preparation for the copulatory lock. The estrogen response can induce a hyperplastic vaginal periurethral papillary mass in some bitches that can prolapse through the vulvar cleft. Follicular luteinization can be attempted to prematurely decrease estrogen production with GnRH (50 μg/bitch intramuscularly) or hCG (500 to 1000 IU/bitch intramuscularly). It is doubtful that medical intervention is of benefit given that most bitches resolve this condition after ovulation. Successful surgical methods of amputating the hyperplastic tissues have been reported; the condition resolves in normal bitches when estrogen levels fall.[53] Prolonged vaginal hyperplasia or prolapse most commonly occurs with ovarian pathology (follicular ovarian cysts), requiring ovariectomy for resolution.

Diagnosis and Treatment of Premature Labor

Corpora lutea in both the queen and bitch produce progesterone during gestation. Evidence of spontaneous abortion or fetal reabsorption associated with serum progesterone concentrations below 1 to 2 ng/mL can suggest luteal insufficiency, which is usually associated with inappropriate myometrial contractility. By the time fetal death is observed clinically, progesterone secretion has likely decreased secondarily.[54] Also, a serum progesterone concentration below 1 to 2 ng/mL after estrus can indicate lack of ovulation rather than luteal insufficiency. Primary luteal insufficiency has not yet been documented in the bitch and queen.

Bitches with a documented history of fetal reabsorption (i.e., ultrasonographic confirmation with no other associated pathology) should be evaluated after the next breeding with both uterine monitoring, ultrasonography, and serum progesterone concentrations.[55] If inappropriate uterine contractility is determined with no contributory pathology evident, tocolytic therapy can be considered (terbutaline 0.03 mg/kg orally every 8 to 12 hours to effect). Serum progesterone concentration should be evaluated; if it is less than 3 to 5 ng/mL and viable fetal vesicles are detected, progesterone supplementation can be considered. Because excessive or inappropriate progesterone administration during pregnancy can cause masculinization of female fetuses and interfere with lactogenesis, it should be undertaken only when indicated (i.e., when tocolytic therapy alone is not effective). Progesterone administration will also prevent normal spontaneous parturition; therefore treatment must be discontinued 3 days before the calculated date of parturition. Therapeutic intervention in suspected hypoluteoidism can be accomplished with the administration of injectable natural progesterone or oral synthetic progestagens. Total serum levels of progesterone can be monitored only when supplemented with the natural product. Progesterone in oil is given intramuscularly at 2 mg/kg every 72 hours.[56] Altrenogest (Regu-Mate, Hoechst-Roussel), a synthetic progestagen manufactured for use in the mare, is dosed orally at 0.088 mg/kg every 24 hours.[57] Both forms of supplementation must be discontinued in a timely fashion so as not to interfere with normal parturition, within 24 hours of the due date with the oral synthetic product, and within 72 hours with the natural, injectable depot form. This requires accurate identification of gestational length using prior ovulation timing (parturition is expected to occur 64 to 66 days from the LH surge or initial rise in progesterone or 56 to 58 days from the first day of cytologic diestrus). Less accurate identification of gestational length can be made from breeding dates (58 to 72 days from the first breeding), radiography, or ultrasound.

Luteal insufficiency is also uncommon in the queen, although it is frequently suspected in queens that experience late-term abortion (i.e., day 50 to 55 of gestation). As in the bitch, luteal insufficiency is diagnosed by determination of viable pregnancy and inadequate progesterone secretion.

Evaluation of such queens early in gestation for inappropriate myometrial activity is advisable. Evaluation of protocols designed to cause medical abortion in queens has determined that a measured serum progesterone concentration of 1 ng/mL may be sufficient to support pregnancy, at least for a short time.[16] The criteria to diagnose luteal insufficiency in the queen, therefore, remains undetermined. Premature labor in an otherwise benign uterus can be effectively treated with tocolytics (terbutaline 0.03 mg/kg orally as needed), the exact dose based on response to therapy, as evaluated by uterine monitoring.

Prevention or Termination of Estrus

Megestrol acetate is the only substance currently licensed in the United States to delay or suppress estrus in bitches. There are no products currently licensed for this purpose in the queen. It is advised not to use progestational products to delay or suppress estrus in bitches intended for future breeding because of the predictable side effects of progesterone in the intact bitch. A progestagen hormone, megestrol acetate, promotes the development of endometrial gland proliferation and suppresses the local uterine immune response. These effects can increase the incidence of pyometra and infertility. Progestagens can cause pathologic changes in mammary glands, the endocrine pancreas, and prolactin-producing and growth hormone–producing cells of the pituitary gland.[58] The drug is contraindicated in cases of previous uterine or mammary gland disease or diabetes mellitus.

If megestrol acetate therapy is chosen despite potential adverse effects, the treatment protocol depends on the stage of the estrous cycle in which treatment is begun. To prevent estrus, megestrol acetate (0.55 mg/kg per day orally for 32 days) is given beginning at least 7 days before the onset of proestrus. After discontinuation of therapy, the bitch will likely begin an estrous cycle. Alternatively, megestrol acetate (2.2 mg/kg per day orally for 8 days) administration can be started during proestrus to abbreviate the signs of estrus and prevent ovulation. In addition to a dose-related effect, this high-dose protocol can be potentially more deleterious than the low-dose protocol because the uterine effects of megestrol acetate can be enhanced by endogenous estrogens increased during proestrus.

Although not yet commercially available in most of the United States, GnRH analogues in a repository form offer good options for preventing estrous cycles for approximately 6 months resulting from down regulation.

Prolongation of Interestrus Intervals in the Bitch

Synthetic androgen (previously available as mibolerone, the availability of which is currently variable) therapy was recommended as a therapeutic protocol to delay estrus in bitches that have interestrus intervals of less than 4 months and are infertile as a result of an abbreviated anestrus. Frequent ovulatory estrous cycles may not allow sufficient time for the endometrium to recover from the trophic influences of progesterone during a nonpregnant diestrus.[59] Synthetic androgen suppression of ovarian activity for 6 to 9 months was previously recommended after ruling out other causes of infertility in bitches with short interestrus intervals.[54] Fertility rates after the use of mibolerone for this purpose have not been reported; the benefit of this protocol have never been proved. As there is no documented effective therapy for abbreviated anestrus, breeding affected bitches at the earliest opportunity, before progesterone-mediated changes in the endometrium have occurred, is advised. The heritability of this tendency has not been established. Because of problems with human abuse of androgenic substances, the availability of such compounds is variable.

Treatment of Clinically Significant Pseudocyesis

The decrease in serum progesterone and increase in serum prolactin concentrations at the end of diestrus can cause overt signs of pseudocyesis (e.g., nesting, galactorrhea, reclusiveness, and possibly aggression) in some bitches. Because this is a normal phenomenon, clinical signs rarely warrant therapeutic intervention. Rarely, mastitis occurs during pseudocyesis. Cabergoline, a prolactin inhibitor, at 5 μg/kg orally every 24 hours for 3 to 5 days, alleviates the signs of pseudopregnancy if problematic.

Pyometra and Postpartum Metritis

The pathophysiology and diagnostic criteria of pyometra and postpartum metritis are well described.[54,60] Case selection must be considered carefully because medical therapy should be reserved for animals that are medically stable and have future reproductive potential. Ovariohysterectomy, after appropriate medical stabilization, remains the treatment of choice for bitches or queens older than 6 to 7 years of age or if signs of systemic sepsis are present.

Many protocols have been proposed for the effective treatment of open-cervix pyometra and postpartum metritis in the bitch and queen using PGF_2. These protocols use the natural hormone dinoprost tromethamine, marketed as Lutalyse or Prostin (Upjohn). Dosage recommendations range from 0.1 to 0.2 mg/kg body weight every 12 to 24 hours for 5 to 7 days. Alternatively, the synthetic prostaglandin cloprostenol has fewer side effects and appears to be equally effective, using doses of 1 to 3 μg/kg subcutaneously every 12 to 24 hours, to effect. Monitoring with ultrasonography aids in the documentation of disease resolution. Some individuals may require repeated or prolonged treatment if the initial regimen is unsuccessful. The administration of concurrent appropriate systemic antimicrobial therapy, either broad spectrum in anticipation of or based on culture and sensitivity results from a guarded sample of the cranial vaginal vault, is indicated.

Similar management of closed-cervix pyometra is problematic. Treatment can be attempted in the bitch with closed-cervix pyometra that is medically stable and carefully monitored during the treatment process. The use of a PGE_1 analog (misoprostol) intravaginally in conjunction with $PGF_{2\alpha}$ has been advocated as a method of establishing cervical patency.[61] Failure to respond to therapy or worsening of clinical signs indicates the need for ovariohysterectomy.

Pregnancy Termination

There are now several options for the management of an unwanted breeding (i.e., misalliance or mismating) of a bitch that has future reproductive potential. The administration of estrogen is no longer recommended because of potential toxicity, induction of a pyometra, or future infertility (see additional information in the later discussion of misuses of reproductive hormones). Besides allowing the pregnancy to proceed to term or performing an ovariohysterectomy during early gestation, there are safe, reliable methods to induce medical abortion in the bitch and queen.

Early Diestrus Protocol

Administration of $PGF_{2\alpha}$ (dinoprost tromethamine) to bitches in early diestrus can result in transient or permanent luteolysis and thus prevent continuation of pregnancy.[28] Fetal contents are reabsorbed, and outward signs of abortion are not detected. In one study the following protocol was successful for all 25 bitches treated with $PGF_{2\alpha}$: 0.25 mg/kg subcutaneously twice daily for 4 days between days 5 and 19 of diestrus.[28] Clinicians are advised to determine the onset of diestrus cytologically by evaluating sequential vaginal cytology after the mismating. The major drawback to this regimen is that treatment occurs before documentation of pregnancy can be performed. Because many mismatings (60%) do not result in pregnancy, bitches can be unnecessarily treated with this protocol.[27] This regimen can be performed on an outpatient basis, and its relatively short treatment period (i.e., 4 days) is favorable.

Midgestation Protocols

After day 30 of gestation, $PGF_{2\alpha}$ therapy induces luteolysis and myometrial contractions, resulting in fetal expulsion. Treatment is begun after documentation of pregnancy by ultrasonography. Ultrasonography is repeated during the treatment period to determine the end point of therapy because some bitches can partially abort their litter and carry the remaining pups to term. The following protocol has been reliably successful in bitches treated after day 30 of gestation: $PGF_{2\alpha}$ 0.1 mg/kg subcutaneously every 8 hours for 2 days and then increasing the dose to 0.2 mg/kg subcutaneously every 8 hours until the abortion is complete.[27] The range of therapy is from 3 to 9 days, with excellent subsequent reproductive capability in treated bitches. Queens have also been similarly treated with good results.[54] Cloprostenol can be substituted for $PGF_{2\alpha}$ with fewer undesirable physical side effects.

An adjunctive therapy to $PGF_{2\alpha}$ has been proposed to hasten the treatment period (i.e., the duration of treatment needed to produce effect). Administration of misoprostol, a prostaglandin E compound, intravaginally daily (1 to 3 μg/kg) concurrently with the previously described $PGF_{2\alpha}$ protocol was found to decrease the treatment period by 1 to 2 days.[61] The proposed action of the misoprostol in this regimen is to soften and open the cervix, thus permitting evacuation of uterine contents.

Dexamethasone has been used successfully to induce abortion and resorption in the bitch.[24] Dexamethasone administered at 0.2 mg/kg orally twice daily for 10 days initially is advised and effective. Pregnancies of less than 40 days generally are resorbed with minimal vaginal discharge. Successful pregnancy was reported in 18 of 20 bitches bred at the subsequent estrus. It is imperative that ultrasonographic evaluation of the pregnancy take place after the 10-day treatment period, insofar as fetal death occurs between 8 and 12 days, and additional days of treatment may be needed to complete termination. Progesterone levels, when measured, were below 1 ng/mL, suggesting luteolysis. Side effects include polydipsia, polyuria, polyphagia, and panting, which were tolerable for the treatment period and resolved when the drug was discontinued. Dexamethasone-induced abortion permits outpatient treatment of unwanted pregnancy with minimal expense.

Abortion can be induced in bitches and queens by the antiprolactin effect of dopamine agonists. Because bromocriptine is not well tolerated, studies investigating the use of cabergoline and metergoline to terminate pregnancy in the bitch and queen have been conducted.[15,16] Pregnancy termination with a dopamine agonist results in fetal reabsorption more commonly than the uterine evacuation that occurs with the $PGF_{2\alpha}$ regimen. The protocols appear to be effective and well tolerated; the availability and expense of the latter generation dopamine agonists are the major drawback.

Medical Management of Dystocia

Oxytocin is the most commonly used reproductive hormone in general veterinary practice. Its use in the medical management of uterine inertia has been well described elsewhere.[54] It is important to accurately assess the indication for the use of oxytocin and ensure that fetal malposition or obstruction is not present. Additionally, overuse of oxytocin can result in a tetanic uterus and can impede fetal (placental) blood supply and cause fetal compromise.[55] Judicious use of oxytocin to treat uterine inertia can be beneficial. Dose ranges are lower than previously reported, from 0.25 to 2 units subcutaneously or intramuscularly per dose, and can be repeated every 30 minutes to effect. Previously suggested doses of more than 1 U/kg are superphysiologic and contraindicated because they may induce tetanic contractions, compromise fetal (placental) blood supply, and cause uterine rupture. It has been recommended to administer calcium gluconate subcutaneously 10 to 15 minutes before the oxytocin therapy despite the typical eucalcemic status of bitches experiencing dystocia, suggesting that the benefit of exogenous calcium occurs at the cellular level. Calcium improves strength of uterine contractions, whereas oxytocin increases their frequency.[55] The use of uterine and fetal monitoring systems permitting insightful mediation (WhelpWise) is strongly advocated during the management of labor.

Adjunct Therapy for Mammary Gland Carcinoma

The use of the antiestrogen tamoxifen has been investigated as an adjunct in the treatment of mammary gland adenocarcinoma in the bitch.[62] Although the bitch exhibits direct estrogenic effects to the reproductive tract (i.e., vulvar edema, stump pyometra) after the administration of tamoxifen, this drug may have an antiestrogenic effect on mammary tissue. In one report tamoxifen therapy (mean dose 0.42 mg/kg orally twice daily) was effective for five of seven bitches with nonresectable or metastatic mammary carcinoma.[62] In another study tamoxifen was administered (0.7 mg/kg every 24 hours orally for 4 to 8 weeks) but had no observable effect in 10 bitches that had advanced mammary cancer.[62] The use of tamoxifen as an adjunct in the treatment plan for mammary neoplasia requires more investigation before it can be advised routinely.

Urinary Incontinence in Spayed or Neutered Dogs

Supplementation with reproductive hormones can be considered when a diagnostic evaluation for chronic urinary incontinence in a neutered dog detects decreased urethral sphincter tone with no other pathology evident. Supplementation with DES or testosterone in ovariectomized bitches or castrated dogs, respectively, can enhance the sensitivity of α-adrenergic receptors to endogenous α-agonists. Oral treatment with DES can be started at 0.1 to 1 mg/bitch per day for 7 days, after which the frequency is diminished to the lowest effective dose. If signs cannot be controlled with infrequent therapy (i.e., 1 mg or less every 3 to 5 days in a 30-kg bitch), alternative or adjunctive drug therapy with phenylpropanolamine should be considered. Potential side effects of DES treatment include estrogen-induced bone marrow toxicity (not reported with oral diethylstilbesterol), attraction of male dogs, and dermatologic disorders. Supplementation of incontinent male dogs with testosterone (testosterone cypionate 2.2 mg/kg intramuscularly every 30 days) can be considered.[63] Adverse effects include prostatic hyperplasia and behavioral changes such as inappropriate urination, aggression, and sexual excitability. When treating idiopathic urinary incontinence in either the neutered female or male dog, the clinician may prefer to consider a compounded α-agonist phenylpropanolamine. Essentially no side effects are expected with this type of therapy, but the owner may need to administer the drug multiple times per day for a consistent effect. The role of gonatotropins in idiopathic incontinence has been reported; a depot administration of GnRH has been used for the treatment of urinary sphincter incompetence in the bitch with good results, suggesting a future role for adjunct therapy of urethral sphincter incompetence in the bitch.[64]

Cryptorchidism

Cryptorchidism is an inherited congenital disorder for which bilateral castration is recommended. Medical treatment to cause descent of a retained testicle is unethical if performed for the purpose of enabling the dog to be shown or bred and likely ineffective. Alternatively, descent of a retained testicle before castration will allow a prescrotal surgical approach. Protocols using either GnRH or hCG have been recommended, although no controlled studies to document efficacy have been published. The precise method of action of these hormones to induce testicular descent is unknown. One protocol for GnRH is 50 to 100 μg/dog subcutaneously or intramuscularly, repeated after 4 to 6 days if no improvement is observed. An alternative protocol is to administer hCG 100 to 1000 IU/dog intramuscularly 4 times spaced over a 2-week period.[55] This protocol has been unsuccessful when used in dogs older than 16 weeks of age, and no actual controls existed in the study describing its use.[54]

Cryptorchidism is uncommon in cats. To the authors' knowledge, the medical treatment of this disorder in cats has not been investigated.

Benign Prostatic Hyperplasia

Chronic administration of a GnRH analog can cause downregulation, and serum testosterone concentrations can decline to castrate levels. This is the basis of therapy for the administration of leuprolide (a GnRH analog) to men with prostatic carcinoma. Prostatic carcinoma occurs with equal frequency in dogs castrated before puberty as in intact dogs, indicating that testicular androgens are not the sole inciting factor in the development of prostatic neoplasia in the dog.[65] Adrenal androgens may play a role in the development of prostatic neoplasia in dogs and in men refractory to downregulation therapy.

It is possible that downregulation therapy could successfully treat other androgen-dependent conditions in the dog (e.g., perianal adenoma, perineal hernia formation, benign prostatic hyperplasia). Factors such as cost, lack of appropriate dosing information, and the routine acceptance of surgical castration in the dog make treatment with GnRH analogs for such cases unlikely. The advantage of medical treatment versus surgical castration is the potential reversibility of infertility with cessation of downregulation therapy, although the androgen-dependent disorder would likely recur.

Successful treatment of benign prostatic hyperplasia using finasteride has been reported.[26] The advantage of finasteride administration is the maintenance of spermatogenesis, because finasteride decreases intraprostatic DHT concentrations and does not affect intratesticular or circulating testosterone concentrations. Recommendations have been to administer finasteride to dogs at the dosage currently used for men: 5 mg/dog orally once daily. Whether a lower or less frequent dosing regimen is possible remains to be investigated. The disadvantage of finasteride administration in men, as a potentially teratogen, is not of concern in dogs because of the minimal exposure associated with typical breedings. One problem resulting from the long-term use of finasteride is a reduction in the volume of the prostatic fraction of the ejaculate, perhaps necessitating the use of semen extenders. The impact of this lack of prostatic fluid on natural breedings (in which the volume of prostatic fluid forces semen into the uterus) is not known. The use of progestagens (i.e., medroxyprogesterone and megestrol acetate) has also been reported as a method to decrease prostatic hypertrophy and maintain sperm production. The potential adverse systemic effects of these compounds (i.e., effects on growth hormone production, liver function, insulin secretion, mammary gland disease) make this treatment less appealing.

Hypogonadism

Hypogonadotropic hypogonadism, a congenital condition in which the pituitary fails to produce gonadotopins, occurs in men. Affected men can respond to gonadotropin replacement therapy with resultant fertility. Hypothalamic or hypogonadotropic hypogonadism has not been documented to occur in a congenital form in dogs. Acquired pituitary dysfunction can occur in dogs with space-occupying neoplasms, but the diagnosis of hypogonadism is difficult. Lack of negative feedback inhibition causes dogs with primary testicular degeneration or atrophy to have high serum LH and FSH concentrations. If primary pituitary failure was the cause of azoospermia, the serum FSH and LH concentrations would be low. At present, FSH and LH assays are not readily available for the dog; a semiquantitative LH kit is available (Synbiotics). Because of the nature of LH secretion, challenge testing is recommended to evaluate pituitary function.

Treatment of this form of infertility depends on the etiology of the pituitary disease; fertility may be unimportant in view of the dog's general health. Although the prognosis for return to fertility is guarded, one protocol using gonadotropin replacement therapy is to administer 500 IU hCG biweekly (subcutaneously or intramuscularly) and FSH at either 1 mg/kg intramuscularly every 48 hours or 25 mg/dog subcutaneously once weekly.[54] Because spermatogenesis and spermatozoa maturation requires approximately 77 days in the dog, therapy must be continued for 3 months before the effectiveness of this protocol can be evaluated.

Management of Retrograde Ejaculation; Improvement of Ejaculate

Retrograde ejaculation causes semen to flow into the urinary bladder, reducing the effective ejaculate. Retrograde ejaculation is treated with pseudoephedrine hydrochloride (3 to 5 mg/kg given 3 hours and 1 hour before collection) or phenylpropanolamine (3 mg/kg every 12 hours).[42]

It is often desirable to increase the sperm quantity in an ejaculate to optimize the sample for freezing for shipping. In the dog it has been theorized that GnRH administration before ejaculation will induce an LH surge with a primary increase in testosterone and thus improve the total spermatozoa per ejaculate; however, a recent study evaluating eight mature mixed-breed dogs showed no objective improvement in semen parameters or libido. Interestingly, administration of PGF_2-alpha (0.1 mg/kg 15 minutes before collection) significantly increased the total number of sperm per ejaculate compared with control dogs and dogs receiving oxytocin and GnRH before collection. It is thought that administration of PGF_2-alpha before ejaculation facilitates the movement of spermatozoa from the epididymis to the ductus deferens, thus enhancing the ejaculatory output.[66]

MISUSES OF REPRODUCTIVE HORMONES

Some reproductive hormones have been misused for many years (Table 23-3). Assumptions based on incomplete information about canine reproductive physiology led to the development of these protocols in the past. Current knowledge and other alternatives (i.e., for mismating in bitches) have resulted in the discontinuation of these practices, which are now considered inappropriate.[67]

Table 23-3 Misuses of Reproductive Hormones

Disorder	Hormone Misused	Considerations	Alternatives
Female infertility	GnRH, gonadotropins	Alteration of feedback loop decreases fertility	Appropriate diagnostic evaluation; ovulation timing and optimal breeding management
Male infertility	GnRH, gonadotropins, testosterone	Lack of effect or decreased fertility; testosterone decreases spermatogenesis	Appropriate diagnostic evaluation
Mismating	Estrogens (DES or ECP)	Can cause bone marrow toxicity, infertility, pyometra	Early or late diestrus treatment with $PGF_{2\alpha}$, cabergoline, dexamethasone.
Benign prostatic hyperplasia	Estrogen (DES)	Can cause squamous metaplasia and increased risk of bacteria prostatitis	Castration; treatment with finasteride

GnRH, gonadotropin-releasing hormone; *DES*, diethylstilbestrol; *ECP*, estradiol cypionate; $PGF_{2\alpha}$, prostaglandin $F_{2\alpha}$.

Treatment of Idiopathic Infertility

Infertility in the Bitch

Physiologic processes that control folliculogenesis in the bitch are complex and involve precise, minute amounts of hypothalamic and pituitary hormones that are sensitively controlled by the ovarian feedback loop. To interrupt the hypothalamic–pituitary–ovarian axis pharmacologically leads to dysfunction, rather than an augmentation, of the system. The rational administration of GnRH requires pulsatile administration, the use of GnRH analogs results in downregulation, and the use of gonadotropins is largely unsuccessful to induce fertile estrus in *known* fertile bitches. There is no evidence to support the use of these hormones in bitches with a history of infertility or decreased fecundity. Careful evaluation of the underlying causes of infertility and optimal breeding management and husbandry with ovulation timing (i.e., serial evaluation of measured parameters to determine the time of ovulation) is recommended.

Infertility in the Stud Dog

Decreased production of sperm is usually the result of primary testicular degeneration and atrophy. Gonadotropin secretion is increased as a result of the lack of negative feedback inhibition. The administration of GnRH or gonadotropins in such cases is therefore inappropriate. Careful investigation to determine the cause of infertility (e.g., testicular atrophy, bacterial prostatitis, infectious or immune-mediated orchitis, spermatic tubular obstruction) is recommended.

As is true of GnRH and gonadotropins, the use of gonadal steroids to enhance fertility is contraindicated. The most common misuse of gonadal steroids to potentiate fertility is the administration of testosterone to heighten libido. Pharmacologic administration of testosterone inhibits steroidogenesis by interruption of the sensitive feedback mechanisms of the hypothalamic–pituitary–gonadal axis. The concentration of testosterone within the seminiferous tubules normally exceeds that found in circulation. An increase of circulating testosterone will serve to decrease output of FSH and LH and thereby decrease spermatogenesis. Additionally, many dogs with low libido have normal concentrations of serum testosterone but have a decrease in libido for other reasons (e.g., prostatic disease, behavioral issues).

Treatment of Mismating and Pregnancy Termination

Estrogens, in the form of either estradiol cypionate (ECP) or DES, have been used historically to prevent pregnancy after mismating in the bitch. The administration of estrogen in any form is no longer recommended for this condition because estrogens are either ineffective or unsafe to use. All bitches treated with estrogens are at risk for the development of bone marrow aplasia, pyometra, or infertility. Although most cases of estrogen-induced bone marrow toxicity have been associated with ECP administered at high doses (i.e., >1 mg), aplastic anemia has been observed in bitches receiving a lower dose. One study determining the efficacy of estrogens to prevent pregnancy found that DES (75 μg/kg orally for 7 days) was ineffective when treatment began in proestrus, estrus, or day 2 of diestrus.[19] Also, ECP (22 μg/kg intramuscularly) was ineffective when administered once during proestrus or estrus, preventing pregnancy in only 50% of treated bitches.[19] The administration of estrogens during diestrus increases the risk of the development of pyometra because the progesterone effect on the uterus to promote glandular secretion and decrease local uterine immunity is enhanced in the presence of estrogen. To prevent pregnancy in mismated bitches, protocols using $PGF_{2\alpha}$, dexamethasone, or dopamine agonists should be considered.

Treatment of Benign Prostatic Hyperplasia

The use of estrogens to treat benign prostatic hyperplasia in dogs is not recommended. In addition to potential toxicity with the administration of estrogens, estrogen-induced squamous metaplasia of the prostate gland may increase the risk of bacterial prostatitis and cyst formation.

KEY POINT 23-3 Hormonal therapy for reproductive conditions is best limited to protocols for which specific studies exist in the dog and cat; interspecific extrapolations are not reliable.

REFERENCES

1. Concannon PW: Biology of gonadotrophin secretion in adult and prepubertal female dogs, *J Reprod Fertil* (Suppl 47), 1993.
2. Hull ME, Kenigsberg DJ: Gonadotropin-releasing hormone function and clinical use, *Lab Manag* 25:51, 1987.
3. Leyendecker G, Wildt L, Hansmann M: Pregnancies following chronic intermittent (pulsatile) administration of GnRH by means of a portable pump (Zyklomat): a new approach to the treatment of infertility in hypothalamic amenorrhea, *J Clin Endocrinol Metab* 51:1214, 1980.
4. Johnson AL: Induction of ovulation in anestrous mares with pulsatile administration of gonadotropin-releasing hormone, *Am J Vet Res* 47:983, 1986.
5. Cain JL, Cain GR, Feldman EC, et al: Use of pulsatile intravenous administration of gonadotropin-releasing hormone to induce fertile estrus in bitches, *Am J Vet Res* 49:1988, 1993.
6. McRae GI, Roberts BB, Worden AC, et al: Long-term reversible suppression of oestrus in bitches with nafarelin acetate, a potent LHRH agonist, *J Reprod Fertil Suppl* 74:389, 1985.
7. Johnston SD: Parturition and dystocia in the bitch. In Morrow DA, editor: *Current therapy in theriogenology*, ed 2, Philadelphia, 1986, Saunders, p 501.
8. Carruthers TD: Principles of hormone therapy in theriogenology. In Morrow DA, editor: *Current therapy in theriogenology*, ed 2, Philadelphia, 1986, Saunders, p 3.
9. Delouis C, Richard P: Lactation. In Thibault C, Levasseur M, Hunter R, editors: *Reproduction in mammals and man*, Paris 1993, Edition Marketing, p. 503.
10. Olson PN, Bowen RA, Behrendt MD, et al: Concentrations of reproductive hormones in canine serum throughout late anestrus, proestrus, and estrus, *Biol Reprod* 27:1196, 1982.
11. Concannon PW, Whaley S, Anderson SP: Increased LH pulse frequency associated with termination of anestrus during the ovarian cycle of the dog, *Biol Reprod* 34:119, 1986.
12. Lawler DF, Johnston SD, Hegstad RL, et al: Ovulation without cervical stimulation in domestic cats, *J Reprod Fertil Suppl* 47:57, 1993.

13. Olson PN, Mulnix JA, Nett TM: Concentrations of luteinizing hormone and follicle-stimulating hormone in the serum of sexually intact and neutered dogs, *Am J Vet Res* 53:762, 1992.
14. Soderberg SF: Infertility in the male dog. In Morrow DA, editor: *Current therapy in theriogenology*, ed 2, Philadelphia, 1986, Saunders, p 544.
15. Onclin K, Silva LDM, Donnay I, et al: Luteotrophic action of prolactin in dogs and the effects of a dopamine agonist, cabergoline, *J Reprod Fertil Suppl* 47:403, 1993.
16. Verstegen JP, Onclin K, Silva LDM, et al: Abortion induction in the cat using prostaglandin F_2alpha and a new anti-prolactinic agent, cabergoline, *J Reprod Fertil Suppl* 47:411, 1993.
17. Krulich L, McCann SM, Mayfield MA: On the mode of the prolactin release-inhibiting action of the serotonin receptor blockers metergoline, methysergide and cyproheptadine, *Endocrinology* 108:1115, 1981.
18. Teske E: Estrogen-induced bone marrow toxicity. In Kirk RW, editor: *Current veterinary therapy IX: small animal practice*, Philadelphia, 1986, Saunders, p 495.
19. Bowen RA, Olson PN, Behrendt MD, et al: Efficacy and toxicity of estrogens commonly used to terminate canine pregnancy, *J Am Vet Med Assoc* 186:783, 1985.
20. Root MV, Johnston SD: Pregnancy termination in the bitch using prostaglandin F_{2alpha}. In Bonagura JD, editor: *Current veterinary therapy XII: small animal practice*, Philadelphia, 1995, Saunders, p 1079.
21. Verstegen JP, Onclin K, Silva LDM, et al: Regulation of progesterone during pregnancy in the cat: studies on the roles of corpora lutea, placenta and prolactin secretion, *J Reprod Fertil* (Suppl 47):165, 1993.
22. Shille VM, Stabenfeldt GH: Luteal function in the domestic cat during pseudopregnancy and after treatment with prostaglandin F_2-alpha, *Biol Reprod* 21:1217, 1979.
23. Kitchell BE, Fidel JL: Tamoxifen as a potential therapy for canine mammary carcinoma, *Proc Vet Cancer Soc Annual Forum* 12:91, 1992.
24. Eilts BE: Pregnancy termination in the bitch and queen. In Greco DS, Davidson AP, editors: *Clinical techniques in small animal practice: Reproductive techniques in small animals*, Philadelphia, 2002, Saunders, pp 116–123.
25. Concannon PW, Yeager A, Frank D, et al: Termination of pregnancy and induction of premature luteolysis by the antiprogestagen, mifepristone, in dogs, *J Reprod Fertil* 88:99, 1990.
26. Cohen SM, Taber KH, Malatesta PF, et al: Magnetic resonance imaging of the efficacy of specific inhibition of 5 alpha reductase in canine spontaneous benign prostatic hyperplasia, *Magn Reson Imaging Med* 21:55, 1991.
27. Feldman EC, Davidson AP, Nelson RW, et al: Prostaglandin induction of abortion in pregnant bitches after misalliance, *J Am Vet Med Assoc* 202:1855, 1993.
28. Romagnoli SE, Camillo F, Cela M, et al: Clinical use of prostaglandin F_{2alpha} to induce early abortion in bitches: serum progesterone, treatment outcome and interval to subsequent oestrus, *J Reprod Fertil Suppl* 47:425, 1993.
29. Trigg TE, Wright PJ, Armour AF, et al: Use of a GnRH analogue implant to produce reversible long-term suppression of reproductive function in male and female domestic dogs, *J Reprod Fert Suppl* 51:255, 2001.
30. Munson L, Bauman JE, Asa CS, et al: Efficacy of the GnRH analogue for suppression of oestrous cycles in cats, *J Reprod Fertil Suppl* 57:269, 2001.
31. Kutzler MA, Wheeler R, Volkmann DH: Serum deslorelin and progesterone concentrations in bitches after ovuplant administration. In *Proceedings Ann Meet Soc Theriogenology*, 2003.
32. Concannon PW: Induction of fertile oestrus in anoestrus dogs by constant infusion of GnRH agonist, *J Reprod Fertil Suppl* 39:143, 1989.
33. Cain JL, Davidson AD, Cain GR, et al: Induction of ovulation in bitches using subcutaneous injections of gonadotropin-releasing hormone analog (abstr), *Proc 8th Ann Vet Med Forum, ACVIM*, 1990, p 1126.
34. Cain JL: Induction of estrus and ovulation in the bitch. In Kirk RW, editor: *Current veterinary therapy X: small animal practice*, Philadelphia, 1989, Saunders, p 1288.
35. Moses DL, Shille VM: Induction of estrus in greyhound bitches with prolonged idiopathic anestrus or with suppression of estrus after testosterone administration, *J Am Vet Med Assoc* 192:1541, 1988.
36. Shille VM, Thatcher MJ, Lloyd ML, et al: Gonadotrophic control of follicular development and the use of exogenous gonadotrophins for induction of oestrus and ovulation in the bitch, *J Reprod Fertil Suppl* 39:103, 1989.
37. Bouchard GF, Gross S, Ganjam VK, et al: Oestrus induction in the bitch with the synthetic oestrogen diethylstilboestrol, *J Reprod Fertil Suppl* 47:515, 1993.
38. Beijerink NJ, Dieleman SJ, Kooistra HS, et al: Low doses of bromocriptine shorten the interestrous interval in the bitch without lowering plasma prolactin concentration. In *Proceedings Reproduction in Companion, Exotic and Laboratory Animals, 2nd Course: Pathology of Canine and Feline Reproduction, Physiology and Pathology of the Neonate* (1):112, 2003.
39. Van Haaften B, Vieleman SJ, Okkens AC, et al: Induction of a fertile oestrus in beagle bitches with PMSG and bromocriptine, *Proc 11th Int Congr Anim Reprod AI Dublin* 4:463, 1988.
40. Verstegen JP, Onclin K: Early termination of anestrus and induction of fertile estrus in dogs by the dopamine superagonist cabergoline, *Biol Reprod Suppl* 50(Abstr 14):12, 1989.
41. Gobello C, Castex G, Corrada Y: Use of cabergoline to treat primary and secondary anestrus in dogs, *J Am Vet Med Assoc* 11:1653, 2002.
42. Romagnoli SE: Aspermia/oligozoospermia caused by retrograde ejaculation in the dog. In Bonagura JD, Twedt DC, editors: *Kirk's current veterinary therapy XIV: small animal practice*, St Louis, 2009, Saunders.
43. Handaja Dusma PS, Tainturier D: Comparison of induction of oestrus in dogs using metergoline, metergoline plus human chorionic gonadotrophin, or pregnant mares' serum gonadotrophin, *J Reprod Fertil Suppl* 47:363, 1993.
44. Goodrowe KL, Howard JG, Schimdt PM, et al: Reproductive biology of the domestic cat with special reference to endocrinology, sperm function and in-vitro fertilization, *J Reprod Fertil Suppl* 39:73, 1989.
45. Cline EM, Jennings LL, Sojka NJ: Breeding laboratory cats during artificially induced estrus, *Lab Anim Sci* 30:1003, 1980.
46. Wildt DE, Kinney GM, Seager SWJ: Gonadotropin induced reproductive cyclicity in the domestic cat, *Lab Anim Sci* 28:301, 1978.
47. Burke TJ: Causes of infertility. In Burke TJ, editor: *Small animal reproduction and infertility: a clinical approach to diagnosis and treatment*, Philadelphia, 1986, Lea & Febiger, p 227.
48. Banks DH, Stabenfeldt GH: Luteinizing hormone release in the cat in response to coitus on consecutive days of estrus, *Biol Reprod* 26:603, 1982.
49. Wildt DE, Seager SWJ, Chakraborty PK: Effect of copulatory stimuli on incidence of ovulation and on serum luteinizing hormone in the cat, *Endocrinology* 107:1212, 1980.
50. Wildt DE, Seager SWJ: Ovarian response in the estrual cat receiving varying dosages of hCG, *Horm Res* 9:144, 1978.
51. Chakraborty PK, Wildt DE, Seager SWJ: Serum luteinizing hormone and ovulatory response to luteinizing hormone releasing hormone in the estrous and anestrous cat, *Lab Anim Sci* 29:338, 1979.
52. Davidson AP, Feldman EC: Ovarian and estrous cycle abnormalities in the bitch. In Ettinger SJ, Feldman EC, editors: *Textbook of veterinary internal medicine*, ed 6, St Louis, 2005, Saunders.

53. Schaefers-Okkens A: Vaginal oedema and vaginal fold prolapse in the bitch, including surgical management. In *Proceedings Reproduction in Companion, Exotic and Laboratory Animals, 2nd Course: Pathology of Canine and Feline Reproduction, Physiology and Pathology of the Neonate* (1):51, 2003.
54. Feldman EC, Nelson RW: *Canine and feline endocrinology and reproduction*, ed 3, St Louis, 2004, Saunders.
55. Davidson AP: Uterine and fetal monitoring in the bitch. In Davidson AP, editor: *Vet Clin North Am Small Anim Pract: Clinical Theriogenology* 31(2):305-313, 2001
56. Scott-Moncrieff JC, Nelson RW, Bill RL, et al: Serum disposition of exogenous progesterone after intramuscular administration in bitches, *Am J Vet Res* 51:893, 1990.
57. Eilts BE: Pregnancy maintenance in the bitch using Regumate, *Proc Ann Meet Soc Theriogenology* :144–147, 1992.
58. Concannon PW, Meyers-Wallen VN: Current and proposed methods for contraception and termination of pregnancy in dogs and cats, *J Am Vet Med Assoc* 198:1214, 1991.
59. Al-Bassam MA, Thompson RG, O'Donnell L: Normal postpartum involution of the uterus in the dog, *Can J Comp Med* 45:217, 1981.
60. Davidson AP: Medical treatment of pyometra with prostaglandin F2-alpha in the dog and cat. In Bonagura JD, editor: *Current veterinary therapy XII: small animal practice*, Philadelphia, 1995, Saunders, pp 1081–1083.
61. Davidson AP, Nelson RW, Feldman EC: Induction of abortion in 9 bitches with intravaginal misoprostol and parenteral PGF 2alpha (abstr), *Proc 15th Ann Vet Med Forum, ACVIM,* 1997, p 670.
62. Henry CJ: Mammary cancer. In Bonagura JD, Twedt DC, editors: *Kirk's current veterinary therapy XIV*, St Louis, 2009, Saunders.
63. Forrester SD: Urinary incontinence. In Ettinger SJ, Feldman EC, editors: *Textbook of veterinary internal medicine*, ed 6, St Louis, 2005, Saunders.
64. Reichler IM, Hubler M, Jochle W, et al: The effect of GnRH analogs on urinary incontinence after ablation of the ovaries in dogs, *Theriogenology* 60(7):1207–1216, 2003.
65. Orbradovich J, Walshaw R, Goullaud E: The influence of castration on the development of prostatic carcinoma in the dog, *J Vet Int Med* 1:183, 1987.
66. Kustritz MV, Hess M: Effects of administration of prostaglandin F2 alpha or presence of an estrous teaser bitch on characteristics of the canine ejaculate, *Theriogenology* 67(2):255–258, 2007.
67. Wiebe VJ, Howard JP: Pharmacologic advances in canine and feline reproduction. In Davidson AP, editor: Topics in Companion Animal Medicine, *Reproduction* 24(2):71, 2009.

Anesthetic Agents

Elizabeth A. Martinez

24

Chapter Outline

PREANESTHETIC MEDICATIONS

The use of preanesthetic medications before general anesthesia in dogs and cats has several advantages. The advantages include helping to decrease stress and anxiety, providing analgesia, decreasing the amount of subsequent anesthetic drugs used, and minimizing the cardiopulmonary depression associated with the commonly used anesthetic agents. Additionally, certain preanesthetic medications will facilitate recovery from anethesia.

The preanesthetic medications used routinely in dogs and cats include the anticholinergics, phenothiazine and benzodiazepine tranquilizers, opioids, and alpha$_2$-adrenergic agonists. Certain drugs discussed in this chapter are not labeled for use in dogs or cats or for the dose and route of administration suggested. Decisions regarding extralabel use should be based on the judgment of the veterinarian and the current laws governing extralabel use of drugs.

KEY POINT 24-1 Selecting an appropriate anesthetic regimen for the small animal patient requires a thorough understanding of the commonly used anesthetic premedication, induction, and maintainence agents, including their indications, contraindications, and potential adverse effects.

Anticholinergics

General Pharmacology

Anticholinergics competitively antagonize acetylcholine at postganglionic terminations of cholinergic fibers in the autonomic nervous system. They are used as preanesthetic medications to decrease salivary secretions, decrease gastric fluid acidity, and inhibit the bradycardic effects of vagal stimulation. Other effects include mydriasis, decreased tear formation, decreased intestinal motility, and bronchodilation. Atropine and glycopyrrolate are the two anticholinergic drugs used in dogs and cats.

Atropine Sulfate

Atropine sulfate (0.02 to 0.04 mg/kg) can be administered intramuscularly, subcutaneously, or intravenously. The duration of action is 60 to 90 minutes. Atropine may stimulate vagal nuclei in the medulla and cause an initial bradycardia before the desired effect is seen, particularly when the drug is administered intravenously. Other central effects of atropine include depression, restlessness, and delirium. Atropine administration may cause cardiac arrhythmias and sinus tachycardia. Atropine does cross the placental barrier and may lead to central and peripheral anticholinergic effects in the fetus when administered to the dam. Arrhythmias are more common after intravenous administration and include second-degree atrioventricular block, unifocal ventricular premature contractions, and ventricular bigeminy.[1] Atropine is contraindicated in animals with preexisting tachycardia.

Glycopyrrolate

Glycopyrrolate is a synthetic quaternary ammonium anticholinergic. Glycopyrrolate may be given intramuscularly, subcutaneously, or intravenously at a dose of 0.011 mg/kg. The duration of action of vagal inhibition is 2 to 4 hours, significantly longer than with atropine. The antisialagogue effect may persist for up to 7 hours. The cardiovascular effects of glycopyrrolate are similar to those of atropine. Because of its large structure, glycopyrrolate does not cross the blood–brain or placental barrier readily and therefore has minimal central or fetal effects.[2]

Tranquilizers

Acepromazine

Acepromazine (0.05 to 0.1 mg/kg intravenously, intramuscularly, or subcutaneously, not to exceed a total dose of 3 mg; oral dose is 1 to 2 mg/kg), a phenothiazine tranquilizer, is used commonly as a premedication before general anesthesia in dogs and cats to relieve anxiety. Through depression of the reticular activating system and antidopaminergic actions in the central nervous system (CNS), acepromazine produces mental calming, decreased motor activity, and increased threshold for responding to external stimuli. Acepromazine does not produce analgesia but may act synergistically when administered concurrently with other drugs with analgesic activity. Administration of acepromazine will decrease the dose of subsequent anesthetic agents. Other effects include antiemetic activity and antihistaminergic properties. Hypotension and hypothermia can result from depression of vasomotor reflexes. Acepromazine is metabolized by the liver and should not be used in patients with liver disease. Because of the potential for hypotension, acepromazine should be used cautiously in compromised patients, particularly those with significant cardiovascular disease. Acepromazine may inhibit platelet function and should be avoided in patients with coagulopathies.[2]

In many veterinary textbooks, authors cautioned against the use of acepromazine in animals at risk for seizures. Recently, this caution is being questioned on account of a lack of references. In two retrospective studies, no evidence was found that acepromazine lowered the seizure threshold in dogs with a history of seizure disorders.[3,4] It was further concluded that a controlled prospective study is necessary for a more thorough evaluation of the use of acepromazine both in this patient population and in the general canine population.

Diazepam

Diazepam (0.1 to 0.2 mg/kg intravenously) is a benzodiazepine tranquilizer that possesses muscle relaxant and anticonvulsant properties. Benzodiazepines exert their effect by enhancing the CNS inhibitory neurotransmitters gamma-aminobutyric acid (GABA) and glycine and by combining with CNS benzodiazepine receptors.[1] Diazepam may produce a mild calming effect in some patients, but agitation and excitement can also occur. Diazepam is solubilized by mixing with propylene glycol. Diazepam has minimal cardiovascular effects; bradycardia and hypotension may be seen after rapid intravenous administration. Propylene glycol is associated with pain on injection and incompatibility when mixed in the same syringe with other drugs. Clinical uses of diazepam in small animal anesthesia include providing muscle relaxation when given concurrently with dissociative anesthetics and as a co-induction agent with injectable anesthetics (thiopental, propofol, etomidate) to decrease their doses or side effects (or both). The effects of diazepam can be reversed with the benzodiazepine antagonist flumazenil.

Midazolam

Midazolam (0.1 to 0.2 mg/kg intravenously and intramuscularly) is a benzodiazepine tranquilizer with behavioral effects and clinical uses similar to those of diazepam. Midazolam is more potent and has a shorter duration of action than diazepam. Midazolam is water soluble at a pH of 3.5. At a pH above 4, the chemical structure changes to become lipid soluble.[5] Unlike diazepam, midazolam can be mixed with other anesthetic agents and can be administered intramuscularly without causing irritation. Flumazenil can be used to antagonize the effects of midazolam.

Midazolam is often used as a component of a total intravenous anesthetic technique (TIVA). The advantage of TIVA is that general anesthesia can be maintained without the use of inhalant agents, which can cause significant cardiovascular depression in certain high-risk patients. Midazolam, 8 μg/kg/min, combined with fentanyl, 0.8 μg/kg/min, are delivered as a constant-rate infusion (CRI) after induction of anesthesia. The dose can be adjusted as needed to produce a desirable level of anesthesia. Typically, the dose is lowered periodically during the anesthetic period, based on the judgment of the level of anesthesia. This technique makes recovery less prolonged. In certain patients a low concentration of inhalant (e.g., sevoflurane) may be added if the TIVA is inadequate to maintain a desirable level of anesthesia. This is particularly true in animals that are alert and active preoperatively. These patients have significant cardiovascular disease precluding a primary inhalant regimen but are asymptomatic or well-compensated. Examples include young dogs with valvular stenosis or patent ductus arteriosis without evidence of heart failure.

Opioids

Opioids act by combining with one or more specific receptors in the brain and spinal cord to produce analgesia, sedation, euphoria, dysphoria, and excitement. The mu receptors are thought to mediate supraspinal analgesia, respiratory depression, and euphoria. Kappa receptors mediate spinal analgesia, miosis, dysphoria, and sedation; the sigma receptors mediate hallucinations, psychomimetic activity, and respiratory and vasomotor stimulation. Delta receptors are thought to primarily modify mu receptor activity.[1] Opioids are classified as agonists, agonist–antagonists, or antagonists according to their receptor activity.

Opioids, agonists or agonist–antagonists, are used before, during, and after surgery in dogs and cats to provide analgesia. Certain opioids may produce sedation in some patients. The antagonists are used to reverse the effects of the agonists or agonist–antagonists. The opioid chosen is based on the degree and duration of expected pain and physical status of the patient. Understanding the differences between the commonly used opioids and their possible side effects are also important when choosing which drug to use. Dose, route, classification, and duration of action of the commonly used opioids in dogs and cats during the perioperative period are shown in Table 24-1.

The most common side effects of opioids preanesthesia include bradycardia and second-degree atrioventricular

Table **24-1** Commonly Used Opioids for Dogs and Cats

Opioid	Dose, mg/kg	Route	Duration of Action	Classification
Morphine	0.05-1.0	IM, SC	4 hrs	Agonist
Hydromorphone	0.1-0.2	IV, IM, SC	4 hrs	Agonist
Butorphanol	0.2-0.4	IV, IM, SC	2 hrs	Agonist–antagonist
Buprenorphine	0.005-0.020	IV, IM, SC	6-8 hrs	Agonist–antagonist
Fentanyl	0.005-0.01	IV, IM	20-40 min	Agonist
Nalbuphine*	1	IV to effect	NA	Agonist–antagonist
Naloxone	0.04-0.06	IV to effect	NA	Antagonist

IM, Intramuscular; *SC,* subcutaneous; *IV,* intravenous; *NA,* not applicable.
*Nalbuphine is used to reverse the sedative effects of opioid agonists, without affecting analgesia

blockade. These effects may be prevented or treated with an anticholinergic agent. When given as a preanesthetic medication, certain opioids may cause vomiting. It is more commonly seen after administration of a mu agonist (morphine, hydromorphone). Respiratory depression can also occur, especially at high doses. The respiratory depressant effects may be additive to those caused by inhalant anesthetic agents. The user should be prepared to assist or control ventilation if necessary. This is especially crucial in patients with suspected space-occupying masses or lesions of the brain. Hypercapnia resulting from respiratory depression causes cerebral vasodilation and can lead to a life-threatening increase in intracranial pressure. The opioids can cause histamine release and should not be used before intradermal skin testing for allergies.

CRIs of many of the opioids can be used both intraoperatively and postoperatively to provide analgesia and decrease the amount of inhalant anesthetic agent required. Fentanyl (2 to 5 μg/kg/hr intravenously), morphine (0.1 to 0.2 mg/kg/hr intravenously), hydromorphone (0.02 to 0.05 mg/kg/hr), and butorphanol (0.1 to 0.2 mg/kg/hr intravenously) will provide acceptable analgesia for most patients. Remifentanil (18 to 36 μg/kg/hr intravenously) is unique in that it is undergoes rapid hydrolysis by nonspecific tissue and plasma esterases. Therefore it has a rapid onset and offset and is noncumulative, and clearance is unaffected by decreased hepatic function.

Alpha$_2$-Adrenergic Agents

The alpha$_2$-adrenergic agonists are used to produce sedation, muscle relaxation, and analgesia in dogs and cats by stimulating presynaptic alpha$_2$-adrenoreceptors and causing a decrease in norepinephrine release both centrally and peripherally. This action leads to a decrease in both CNS sympathetic outflow and circulating catecholamines.[2] Cardiopulmonary effects can be significant with these drugs and include respiratory depression, bradycardia, first- or second-degree atrioventricular blockade, decreased cardiac output, and increased peripheral vascular resistance. Because of these effects, careful patient monitoring should be employed after administering these drugs in dogs and cats. Alpha$_2$-adrenergic agonists should not be used in compromised patients. Other effects seen with the use of alpha$_2$-adrenergic agonists include vomiting, hyperglycemia, decreased gut motility, and dieresis. The commonly used drugs are xylazine, medetomidine, and dexmedetomidine.

Xylazine

Xylazine (0.2 to 1 mg/kg intravenously and intramuscularly) can be given as a premedication agent alone or in combination with opioids to facilitate intravenous catheter placement and decrease dose requirements of subsequent injectable and inhalant anesthetic agents. It is also used commonly as an adjuvant with dissociative anesthetic agents to improve muscle relaxation and provide visceral analgesia for short surgical procedures.

Medetomidine

Medetomidine is an alpha$_2$-adrenergic agonist approved for use in dogs. Although the clinical effects are similar, medetomidine is more potent and possesses a higher alpha$_2$ receptor selectivity profile than xylazine. The preanesthetic dose in dogs is 5 to 10 μg/kg, intravenously and intramuscularly and up to 20 μg/kg for sedation. Medetomidine is not approved for use in cats. However, it has been used successfully, either alone or in combination with an opioid or dissociative agent, for immobilization or surgical anesthesia. The preanesthetic dose in cats is 10 to 15 μg/kg, but a dose range up to 40 to 80 μg/kg intramuscularly is reported.[6] This author recommends using the lowest dose needed to produce the desired effect. Combining medetomidine with an opioid may have a synergistic effect, allowing a lower dose of each drug to be used. The use of medetomidine (20 μg/kg intramuscularly) in feline hypertrophic cardiomyopathy patients with concurrent left ventricular outflow obstruction has been shown to improve the hemodynamics of these patients.[7]

When medetomidine is used as a preanesthetic medication, the dose of subsequent anesthetic agents will be markedly reduced. This includes both induction and inhalational agent requirements. The patients should be monitored carefully throughout the anesthetic period. Profound bradycardia is common after medetomidine administration but can be minimized by preemptive treatment with an anticholinergic agent. If severe bradycardia or hypotension occurs, the medetomidine can be reversed with atipamezole.

Failure to achieve adequate sedation, or no effect at all, can occur in stressed, agitated animals because of high levels of endogenous catecholamines. These animals should be allowed to rest before medetomidine is given. Repeat dosing is not recommended in dogs that do not respond satisfactorily to medetomidine. It is important to remember that sudden arousal and the potential for biting after minimal stimulation or handling can occur. To prevent harm, the user is warned against a false sense of security when handling animals sedated with medetomidine.[8]

Dexmedetomidine

Dexmedetomidine is the active, dextrorotary enantiomer of the racemic mixture medetomidine. The same indications for medetomidine apply to the clinical use of dexmedetomidine at equal pharmacologic doses. Dexmedetomidine has approximately twice the potency as medetomidine; therefore it is dosed at one half the amount of medetomidine to achieve the same level of sedation and analgesia. The pharmacologically inactive enantiomer levomedetomidine has no sedative, analgesic, or cardiorespiratory effects, but its absence may influence the pharmacokinetic and pharmacodynamic effects of dexmedetomidine. Differences would be expected in the drug metabolism of dexmedetomidine compared with medetomidine given that only half of the racemic mixture is administered and subsequently metabolized. One study in cats comparing medetomidine and dexmedetomidine before ketamine anesthesia reported that cats premedicated with dexmedetomidine recovered more quickly that the cats receiving medetomidine.[9]

Romifidine

Romifidine is the newest alpha$_2$-adrenergic agonist to be evaluated for use in small animal veterinary patients. It is not approved for use in small animals in the United States. Compared with xylazine, the onset of action is slower and the duration of action is longer. At equipotent doses the cardiovascular effects are similar to those of xylazine. In healthy dogs 10 to 20 µg/kg administered intramuscularly produced mild to moderate sedation with limited effects on cardiovascular function.[10] In healthy cats 40 µg/kg adminisered intramuscularly produced moderate sedation.[11]

Alpha$_2$-Adrenergic Antagonists

Reversal of the clinical effects of xylazine and medetomidine can be accomplished with specific alpha$_2$-adrenergic antagonists. Yohimbine (0.1 mg/kg intravenously), tolazoline (2 mg/kg IV), and atipamezole are most commonly used in dogs and cats. Atipamezole is used to reverse the effects of medetomidine. The dose of atipamezole is determined by the amount of the agonist given and the time elapsed since the agonist was administered. To prevent neurologic (excitement and muscle tremors), cardiovascular (hypotension and tachycardia), and gastrointestinal (salivation and diarrhea) side effects, atipamezole should be given intramuscularly and at the lowest dose needed to produce reversal of the CNS and cardiovascular effects of medetomidine.

INJECTABLE ANESTHETICS

Injectable anesthetic agents are used to rapidly produce unconsciousness. They usually are given before maintenance of general anesthesia with an inhalant anesthetic agent but may also be administered by repeated injection or infusion, alone or in combination with other injectable agents, to maintain anesthesia. The major disadvantage of injectable agents once administered is that the effects are not immediately eliminated, including any unwanted cardiopulmonary changes. The injectable agents used in veterinary patients include the barbiturates, dissociative agents, propofol, and etomidate.

Barbiturates

The barbiturates cause depression of the CNS by interfering with passage of impulses to the cerebral cortex. Barbiturates are categorized according to their duration of action. The ultrashort-acting barbiturates thiopental and methohexital are the two most commonly used in dogs and cats to produce a rapid induction of anesthesia. The transition to inhalant anesthesia is smooth, and recovery is relatively rapid because of redistribution. Methohexital is cleared from the body at a faster rate and is preferred in sighthounds, which have a more prolonged recovery with the thiobarbiturates.

The barbiturates decrease cerebral blood flow, cerebral metabolic rate of oxygen, and electrical activity of the brain.[2] Because of these CNS effects, anesthetic induction using a barbiturate is preferred in patients with certain neurologic diseases (seizure disorders, space-occupying lesion of the brain). Other organ system effects include cardiovascular and respiratory depression that is dependent on the dose and rate of administration. Cardiac arrhythmias may occur, with ventricular extrasystoles and bigeminy being the most common.[2]

Maximal effect from an intravenous injection of an ultrashort-acting thiobarbiturate is reached within 30 seconds. The duration of action depends on redistribution to lean body tissues. Barbiturates are primarily metabolized by the liver and eliminated by renal excretion. Care should be taken when administering barbiturates to patients with liver disease because the duration of action may be prolonged.

Thiopental

Thiopental can be used as a 2% to 5% solution in dogs and cats. More concentrated solutions may cause severe tissue damage if accidentally administered perivascularly. For induction of anesthesia, thiopental is administered in small increments, 2 to 6 mg/kg intravenously, until the desired effect is reached. A total dose of 10-12 mg/kg is usually sufficient for induction, before intubation and maintenance with an inhalant agent. Repeated injections of thiopental for maintenance of anesthesia have a cumulative effect and can cause a prolonged recovery.

Methohexital

Methohexital is similar in its effects to thiopental, except it is more rapidly metabolized and is not cumulative.[2] Methohexital is reconstituted as a 2.5% solution, and a calculated dose of 6 to 10 mg/kg is drawn up in a syringe. One half is administered initially and the remainder given to the desired effect. In patients that have not been premedicated, involuntary excitement or emergence delirium can be seen during the recovery period. Treatment is accomplished with intravenous administration of diazepam, 0.2 mg/kg .

Dissociative Agents

Dissociative anesthesia is an anesthetic state caused from interruption of ascending transmission from the unconscious to conscious parts of the brain.[12] This group includes ketamine and tiletamine. Tiletamine is a component of Telazol. Dissociative anesthesia is characterized by a catalepsy; somatic analgesia; and intact ocular, laryngeal, and pharyngeal reflexes. Because control of the airway may not be complete, intubation with a cuffed endotracheal tube is recommended. Visceral analgesia is poor. Muscle rigidity or reflexive skeletal muscle movements can also occur. Dissociative agents are commonly used for induction and maintenance of anesthesia in cats and dogs.

Ketamine

Both ketamine and tiletamine increase cerebral blood flow and intracranial pressure and therefore should be avoided in patients in which these effects could be detrimental.[12] Seizure activity may be seen particularly in dogs. As a result of sympathetic stimulation, the cardiovascular effects include an increase in heart rate and arterial blood pressure. The myocardium becomes sensitized to catecholamine-induced arrhythmias. Although ventilation and arterial oxygenation generally remain adequate, an apneustic or irregular breathing pattern may be observed after administration of a dissociative agent. Transient apnea may be seen after rapid intravenous administration. Excessive salivation may occur and is controlled by administration of an anticholinergic. Hallucinatory behavior, emergence delirium, or CNS excitement may be observed during the recovery period. Prior administration of a tranquilizer will attenuate these effects.

Whereas ketamine is metabolized primarily by the liver in the dog, it is excreted intact by the kidneys in the cat. Ketamine should be used with caution in animals with hepatic or renal disease. In cats with urethral obstruction, ketamine can be used if renal disease is absent and the obstruction is relieved. Tiletamine is excreted predominantly by the kidneys. Telazol is contraindicated in patients with pancreatic disease or impairment of renal function.

Ketamine can be administered intravenously (1-2 mg/kg) or intramuscularly (2-20 mg/kg) for induction or maintenance of anesthesia in cats and dogs. Intravenous administration is used for induction before intubation and maintenance with an inhalant agent or for anesthesia for short procedures. Intramuscular administration, in combination with agents providing analgesia and muscle relaxation (e.g., dexmedetomidine), is used for maintenance of anesthesia for surgical procedures. Duration of action is dose dependent. Recovery from large intramuscular doses of ketamine may be associated with prolonged recoveries. Ketamine should be combined with a tranquilizer, muscle relaxant, or opioid to provide muscle relaxation and additional analgesia and to smooth the recovery period. Using adjuvants is important when administering ketamine to dogs because when it is used alone, extreme muscle tone, spontaneous movements, violent recovery, and convulsions can occur.

Ketamine may also be administered as an intravenous CRI both intraoperatively and postoperatively to provide analgesia. At subanesthetic doses, ketamine blocks the *N*-methyl-D-aspartate (NMDA) receptor responsible for the transmission of painful stimuli from the peripheral nervous system to the CNS. Low-dose ketamine administered as a CRI helps to prevent "wind-up," an exaggerated and prolonged response to pain caused by NMDA receptor activation. In dogs undergoing forelimb amputation, an initial bolus of 0.5 mg/kg of ketamine administered intravenously, followed by a CRI dose of 10 μg/kg/min intraoperatively and 2 μg/kg/min for 18 hours after surgery, resulted in lower pain scores that dogs receiving saline infusions. Both groups also received a fentanyl CRI (1 to 5 μg/kg/hr) during the 18-hour postoperative period.[13]

Telazol

Telazol is a combination of tiletamine and zolazepam. Tiletamine has a longer duration of action and greater analgesic effect than ketamine. Zolazepam, a benzodiazepine tranquilizer, provides muscle relaxation and is an effective anticonvulsant. Telazol has been used intramuscularly (4 to 15 mg/kg), alone or in combination with xylazine or an opioid, for induction and maintenance of anesthesia for surgical procedures. Lower doses (2 to 4 mg/kg) can be given intravenously for induction before intubation and maintenance with an inhalant agent. Adverse responses to Telazol can occur during the recovery period, particularly in dogs. These responses include muscle rigidity, convulsions, and emergence delirium. Using the lowest dose of Telazol possible and treatment with a tranquilizer will minimize these effects.

Propofol

Propofol (2,6-diisopropylphenol) is classified as a nonbarbiturate sedative–hypnotic agent. It is an alkylphenol, poorly soluble in water, and is solubilized in a lecithin-containing emulsion (Intralipid). Because propofol emulsion is capable of supporting microbial growth, any unused propofol, in either an ampule or vial, should be discarded within 6 hours. The advantage of propofol over other injectable anesthetic agents is its rapid recovery profile.[14]

Propofol causes a decrease in both intracranial and cerebral perfusion pressures and therefore can be used in patients with neurologic disease. Propofol has cardiovascular effects similar to those of the thiobarbiturates, including a dose-dependent decrease of arterial blood pressure, cardiac output, and systemic vascular resistance. Heart rate may remain unchanged or increased. Ventricular arrhythmias may also be observed. Propofol should be used with caution in patients with severe cardiovascular disease. Propofol does cause a dose-dependent respiratory depression and may also cause transient apnea. Methods for ventilatory support should be available.

Propofol is noncumulative. Termination of the anesthetic effects from propofol is due to redistribution from vessel-rich tissues followed by rapid biotransformation by the liver. Propofol is rapidly cleared from the body by hepatic and extrahepatic metabolism.

Propofol can be administered as an intravenous bolus (4 to 6 mg/kg) for induction of anesthesia as well as maintenance of anesthesia by a CRI (0.4 mg/kg/min intravenously).

Propofol does not provide analgesia; therefore painful procedures should not be performed when given alone. Premedication with an opioid or alpha$_2$ agonist will provide analgesia, but dose requirements for propofol will be lowered. Propofol allows for a rapid recovery with little to no hangover effect compared with the thiobarbiturates. Side effects include excitement during induction or recovery in patients that have not been premedicated, pain on injection, and occasional muscle tremors or myoclonic activity.[15] The main disadvantages of propofol are cost and limited shelf-life.

Etomidate

Etomidate is an imidazole derivative classified as a rapid-acting, nonbarbiturate anesthetic agent.[16] Etomidate is not a good analgesic. Etomidate (1 to 3 mg/kg) is used as an intravenous induction agent before intubation and maintenance with an inhalant agent. The main advantage of etomidate over other injectable induction agents is its minimal cardiopulmonary depressant effects; therefore it is very useful in severely compromised patients.

Etomidate is a good induction agent for neurologic procedures insofar as it depresses cerebral blood flow and cerebral metabolic rate of oxygen. Administration of etomidate produces little change in heart rate, arterial blood pressure, and cardiac output. Transient apnea may be observed after induction. In patients that have not been premedicated, administration of etomidate may be associated with pain on injection, involuntary muscle movements, gagging, or retching.[16] Premedication with a tranquilizer or opioid will attenuate these effects. Etomidate causes transient adrenocortical suppression.[17] The effect may be seen for 2 to 3 hours after a single intravenous bolus. Although it is believed that this suppression is not clinically significant after a single dose, long-term infusion with etomidate is not recommended. Etomidate is noncumulative, is rapidly redistributed, and undergoes some ester hydrolysis.

INHALANT ANESTHETICS

Inhalant anesthetic agents are used to produce general anesthesia in dogs and cats. These drugs produce unconsciousness, muscle relaxation, and analgesia. Inhalant anesthetic agents are administered directly to the respiratory system, absorbed from the alveoli into the bloodstream, and passed to the brain. The advantage of using inhalant agents instead of injectable agents for maintenance of general anesthesia is the ability to adjust the depth of anesthesia by increasing or decreasing the amount of inhalant delivered to the patient. Also, the commonly used inhalant agents permit a rapid induction and recovery from anesthesia because of its elimination through the lungs. Delivering inhalant anesthetic agents requires the use of an anesthetic machine. A proper machine consists of a vaporizer for drug delivery, a source of oxygen, a patient breathing circuit, and methods for eliminating carbon dioxide and scavenging waste gases. Additionally, the patient is often intubated; therefore ventilation can be supported if necessary, and arterial oxygenation is improved because of the high levels of oxygen present in the breathing circuit.

Potency of inhalant anesthetic agents is expressed by its MAC value, which is the minimum alveolar concentration of anesthetic that produces no responses in 50% of patients exposed to a painful stimulus. MAC is measured as the end-tidal concentration of anesthetic. The lower the MAC value of the inhalant agent, the greater its potency. Surgical anesthesia is approximately 1.5 to 2 times the MAC. Several factors control the partial pressure of inhalant anesthetic in the brain. The brain tension mirrors the alveolar concentration of anesthetic agent, which depends on the amount delivered to the lungs and uptake from the lungs. Several factors determine uptake of anesthetic from the lungs. These include solubility (blood–gas partition coefficient), cardiac output, the alveolar–venous anesthetic tension difference, and the presence of shunts or any pathologic change in the alveoli that may cause a diffusion barrier. Elimination of inhalants is primarily by the lungs. Some anesthetic agents undergo varying degrees of biotransformation by the liver. Toxic metabolites are formed by several of the inhalant anesthetic agents. The most commonly used inhalant anesthetic agents in dogs and cats are nitrous oxide, isoflurane, and sevoflurane. Another inhalant agent, which is not used routinely in dogs and cats, is desflurane.

Nitrous Oxide

Nitrous oxide has a MAC value of greater than 100% in the dog and cat.[18] It is used as a mild analgesic or to add to the effects of other inhalant anesthetic agents. As it crosses the alveolar membranes, it will speed the uptake of the primary inhalant agent (second gas effect). A period of denitrogenation with 100% oxygen should be performed before nitrous oxide is introduced into the breathing circuit. Up to 70% nitrous oxide is then administered to the patient. Typically, nitrous oxide is administered as 1:1 or 2:1 N_2O:O_2 ratio. Care must be taken to prevent hypoxia by delivering a minimum of 30% oxygen and, when nitrous oxide is discontinued, delivering 100% oxygen for a minimum of 5 minutes before allowing the patient to breathe room air. Nitrous oxide is eliminated through the lungs rapidly after its discontinuation.

Nitrous oxide has minimal effects on the cardiopulmonary system. Because nitrous oxide is 30 times more soluble in blood than nitrogen, it diffuses into air containing cavities faster than nitrogen diffuses out. Therefore the administration of nitrous oxide is contraindicated in patients with pneumothorax, obstructed bowel, or other closed-air cavities. Nitrous oxide should not be used with closed-circuit or low-flow anesthesia because of the significant risk that a hypoxic mixture will be delivered.

Isoflurane

The MAC value for isoflurane is 1.28% in the dog and 1.63% in the cat.[19] Although isoflurane causes a dose-dependent increase in intracranial pressure, it can be used safely in patients with neurologic disease if less than 1 MAC is delivered and hypoventilation is avoided. Vasodilation caused by increased muscle and skin blood flow can be significant and result in hypotension. Isoflurane is a respiratory depressant; therefore it may be necessary to assist ventilation at higher anesthetic depths. Less than 1% of isoflurane undergoes biodegradation. The majority is eliminated unchanged by the lungs. The rapid recovery produced by isoflurane in patients that have not been premedicated may lead to emergence delirium. Treatment with a tranquilizer such as acepromazine may be required. Opioids are strongly recommended if the animal is thought to be in pain. Isoflurane is an excellent choice for either induction or maintenance of anesthesia in most small animal patients. As with any anesthetic technique, vigilant monitoring of the cardiopulmonary system is encouraged.

Sevoflurane

The MAC value of sevoflurane is 2.36% in the dog[20] and 2.58% in the cat.[21] The principle advantage of sevoflurane over isoflurane is its extremely rapid induction and recovery times. The cardiovascular and respiratory effects are similar to those produced by isoflurane. Sevoflurane does not sensitize the myocardium to catecholamine-induced arrhythmias. Sevoflurane undergoes minimal metabolism by the liver; the majority is eliminated unchanged by the lungs. Sevoflurane reacts with carbon dioxide absorbents and decomposes to compound A. Compound A is a vinyl halide that has been shown to be nephrotoxic in laboratory rats. There have been no case reports of compound A–associated renal injury in human or veterinary patients. Although compound A formation is an area of controversy among researchers, sevoflurane should not be used during low-flow or closed-circuit anesthesia to prevent the accumulation of the potentially nephrotoxic substance.

Because of its low lipid solubility, sevoflurane produces a rapid and smooth induction and a rapid recovery. As with isoflurane, patients that have not been premedicated may experience emergence delirium. Sevoflurane may be advantageous for outpatient procedures in which a rapid surgery-to-discharge time is desired. During the anesthetic management of critically ill patients, wherein it may be necessary to make rapid changes in the depth of anesthesia, sevoflurane may be preferred over isoflurane. Also, sevoflurane is preferred for maintenance of anesthesia for cesarean sections because the neonates, if ventilating adequately, will quickly eliminate residual inhalant agent. The primary disadvantages of using sevoflurane is the higher cost compared with isoflurane.

Desflurane

The MAC value of desflurane is approximately 7.2% in the dog[22] and 9.79% in the cat.[23] Desflurane has an extremely low blood–gas partition coefficient allowing for a very rapid induction and recovery from general anesthesia. A dose-dependent respiratory depression is seen. The cardiovascular depressant effects are similar to isoflurane. Desflurane is very pungent, which may make mask inductions difficult in some patients. Desflurane is eliminated from the lungs and has not been reported to cause hepatic or renal toxicity. Desflurane requires a special, electrically heated vaporizer for delivery because of its high vapor pressure. Desflurane is not used routinely in veterinary patients at this time.

REFERENCES

1. Thurmon JC, Tranquilli WJ, Benson GJ: Injectable anesthetics. In Thurman JC, Tranquilli WJ, Benson GJ, editors: *Lumb and Jones' veterinary anesthesia*, ed 3, Baltimore, 1996, Williams & Wilkins.
2. Muir WW, Hubbell JAE: *Handbook of veterinary anesthesia*, ed 4, St Louis, 2007, Mosby.
3. Garner JL, Kirby R, Rudloff E: The use of acepromazine in dogs with a history of seizures, *J Vet Emerg Crit Care* 14:S1, 2004.
4. Tobias KM, Marioni-Henry, Wagner R: A retrospective study on the use of acepromazine maleate in dogs with seizures, *J Am Anim Hosp Assoc* 42:283, 2006.
5. Ilkiw JE: Other potentially useful new injectable anesthetic agents, *Vet Clin North Am Small Anim Pract* 22(2):281, 1992.
6. Plumb DC: *Veterinary drug handbook*, ed 5, Ames, Iowa, 2005, Blackwell.
7. Lamont LA, Bulmer BJ, Sisson DD, Grimm, et al: Doppler echocardiographic effects of medetomidine on dynamic left ventricular outflow tract obstruction in cats, *J Am Vet Med Assoc* 221(9):1276, 2002.
8. Tranquilli WJ: α_2-agonists. In Greene SA, editor: *Veterinary anesthesia and pain management secrets*, Philadelphia, 2002, Hanley & Belfus.
9. McKusick BC, Westerholm FC, Väisänen M: Clinical evaluation of dexmedetomidine premedication prior to ketamine anesthesia in cats [abstract], *Proc Assoc Vet Anaesth Spring Meet* 66, 2005.
10. Lemke KA: Sedative effects of intramuscular administration of a low dose of romifidine in dogs, *Am J Vet Res* 60:162, 1999.
11. Selmi AL, Barbudo-Selmi GR, Moreira CF, et al: Evaluation of sedative and cardiorespiratory effects of romifidine and romifidine-butorphanol in cats, *J Am Vet Med Assoc* 221:506, 2002.
12. Lin HC: Dissociative anesthetics. In Thurman JC, Tranquilli WJ, Benson GJ, editors: *Lumb and Jones' veterinary anesthesia*, ed 3, Baltimore, 1996, Williams & Wilkins.
13. Wagner AE, Walton JA, Hellyer PW, et al: Use of low doses of ketamine administered by constant rate infusion as an adjunct for postoperative analgesia in dogs, *J Am Vet Med Assoc* 221:72, 2002.
14. Branson KR, Gross ME: Propofol in veterinary medicine, *J Am Vet Med Assoc* 204:1994, 1888.
15. Smith JA, Gaynor JS, Bednarski RM, et al: Adverse effects of administration of propofol with various preanesthetic regimens in dogs, *J Am Vet Med* 202:1111, 1993.
16. Muir WW, Mason DE: Side effects of etomidate in dogs, *J Am Vet Med* 194:1430, 1989.
17. Kruse-Elliott KT, Swanson CR, Aucoin DP: Effects on adrenocortical function in canine surgical patients, *Am J Vet Res* 48:1098, 1987.
18. Steffey EP, Gillespie JR, Berry JD, et al: Anesthetic potency (MAC) of nitrous oxide in the dog, cat, and stumptail monkey, *J Appl Physiol* 36:530, 1974.
19. Steffey EP, Howland D Jr: Isoflurane potency in the dog and cat, *Am J Vet Res* 38:1833, 1977.
20. Kazama T, Ikeda K: Comparison of MAC and the rate of rise of alveolar concentration of sevoflurane with halothane and isoflurane in the dog, *Anesthesiology* 68:435, 1988.
21. Doi M, Yunoki H, Ikeda K: The minimum alveolar concentration of sevoflurane in cats, *J Anesth* 2:113, 1988.
22. Doorley MB, Waters SJ, Terrell RC, et al: MAC of I-653 in beagle dogs and New Zealand white rabbits, *Anesthesiology* 69:89, 1988.
23. McMurphy RM, Hodgson DS: The minimum alveolar concentration of desflurane in cats, *Vet Surg* 24:453, 1995.

25 Muscle Relaxants

Elizabeth A. Martinez

Chapter Outline

Muscle relaxants may be chosen for use in veterinary patients for several reasons. Because of their muscle-relaxing effects, they are used during certain surgical procedures. Orthopedic procedures such as dislocation and fracture reductions can be performed more easily because of abolished skeletal muscle tone.[1] When a balanced anesthesia technique is used that combines opioids, nitrous oxide, and low-dose inhalant agents, muscle relaxation is greatly improved if a neuromuscular blocking agent is given. This technique is especially beneficial for critically ill patients in which high doses of inhalant agents may lead to unwanted cardiovascular depression.[2] During intraocular procedures or for patients with penetrating eye injuries requiring surgery, muscle relaxants may be beneficial by producing a central pupil, motionless eye, and soft globe. When used during induction and intubation, they can help prevent an increase in intraocular pressure that can occur during coughing or vomiting.[2]

KEY POINT 25-1 The use of muscle relaxants in anesthetized small animal patients can help facilitate the procedure being performed, but it is important to remember that these drugs do not provide analgesia or analgesia.

When using a muscle relaxant, the clinician must remember that these agents do not provide either anesthesia or analgesia. The patient must be adequately anesthetized, which may be even more difficult to determine because some of the usual indicators of depth of anesthesia is abolished. These indicators include purposeful movement, palpebral response, and degree of jaw tone. Owing to paralysis of the muscles of respiration, ventilation must also be controlled until neuromuscular function is restored.

NEUROMUSCULAR BLOCKING AGENTS

Anatomy and Physiology of the Neuromuscular Junction

The components of the skeletal neuromuscular junction include the somatic motor nerve terminal, synaptic cleft, and the motor end plate of the muscle fiber. The cell bodies of the somatic motor neurons are located within the spinal cord. The axon divides into multiple branches, each of which innervates a single muscle fiber in mammalian species. At each neuromuscular junction, the terminal portion of the axon loses its myelin sheath and forms an arborization that lies in close proximity to the motor end plate of the muscle fiber (Figure 25-1). The site of action of neuromuscular blocking agents is at the nicotinic cholinergic receptors located at the motor end plate of the muscle fiber.

The nicotinic receptors at the neuromuscular junction bind and respond to the endogenous neurotransmitter, acetylcholine (ACh). ACh is synthesized from the acetylation of choline by the enzyme choline acetyl transferase, using acetyl coenzyme A as the source of the acetyl groups. ACh is then packaged at high concentrations into synaptic vesicles by carrier-mediated transport. When a motor nerve is stimulated and action potential subsequently generated reaches the nerve terminal, ACh is released rapidly into the synaptic cleft by way of calcium-mediated exocytosis. One presynaptic nerve impulse releases 100 to 500 vesicles or approximately 3 million ACh molecules. ACh then diffuses across the synaptic cleft and, upon binding with a nicotinic cholinergic receptor, stimulates opening of an ion channel located on the muscle fiber membrane. This allows sodium ions to move and allow sufficient current through them that the resting membrane potential is shifted toward threshold, generating an action potential that triggers muscle contraction. Unbound ACh within the synaptic cleft is rapidly hydrolyzed by the enzyme acetylcholinesterase to choline and acetate. The choline is taken up by the nerve terminal and recycled for continued synthesis of ACh (this is the rate-limiting step in ACh synthesis).

Pharmacology

Neuromuscular blocking agents exert their effects by interfering with the postsynaptic action of ACh. They can be divided into two classes, depolarizing and nondepolarizing neuromuscular blocking agents. Nondepolarizing drugs produce muscle relaxation by preventing ACh from binding to its receptors on

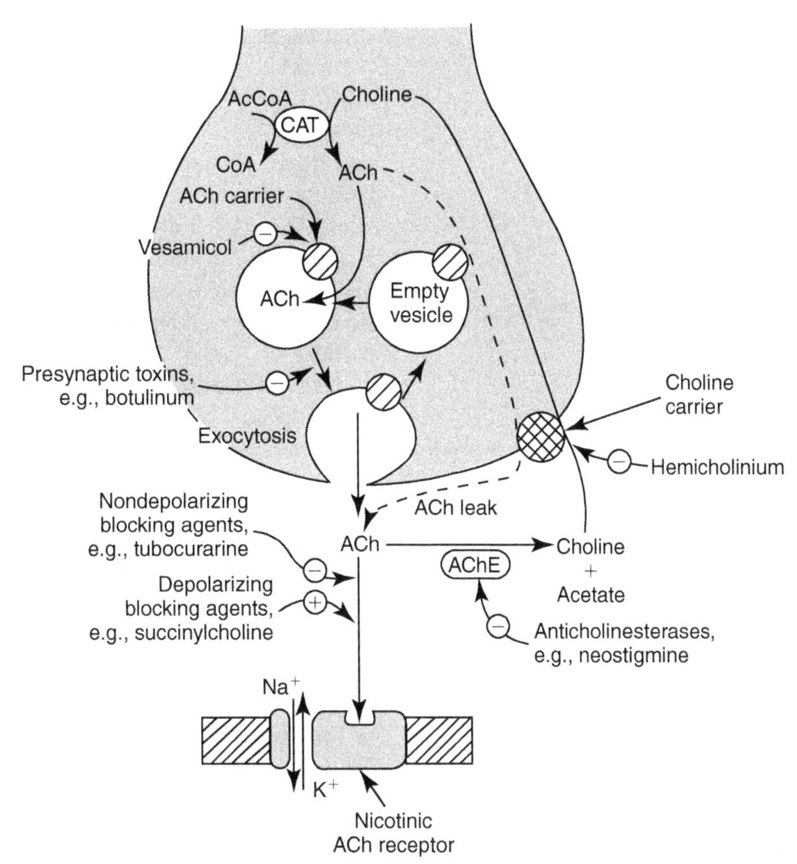

Figure 25-1 Neuromuscular junction with sites of drug action. *AcCoA,* Acetyl coenzyme A; *ACh,* acetylcholine; *AChE,* acetylcholinesterase; *CAT,* catecholamine; *CoA,* coenzyme A. (From Rang HP, Dale MM, Ritter JM et al: *Pharmacology,* New York, 1995, Churchill Livingstone.)

the motor end plate. As a result of this competitive antagonism, the ion channels will not open, no shift in the resting membrane potential will occur, the motor end plate will not depolarize, and the muscle becomes flaccid. Complete neuromuscular blockade will occur when approximately 90% to 95% of the receptors are occupied.[3]

Depolarizing drugs elicit their pharmacologic effect by binding to the ACh receptor in the same way ACh does, causing transient muscle fasciculations. Because these drugs are not immediately metabolized by acetylcholinesterase, however, they bind for a much longer period than ACh does, causing persistent depolarization of the muscle fiber endplate. In mammals the result of this maintained depolarization is a loss of electrical excitability by the postsynaptic muscle fiber, producing neuromuscular blockade.

Individual Agents

The development of newer muscle relaxants has given the practitioner many options when selecting which agent to use. These drugs differ in their onset and duration of action, recovery time, cardiovascular effects, and route of elimination. When making the decision on which muscle relaxant to use, it is important to consider the reason for neuromuscular blockade, the desired duration of action, and the physical status of the patient. Organ dysfunction and concurrent drug administration may alter the clinical effect of muscle relaxants. Doses for depolarizing and nondepolarizing neuromuscular blocking agents for dogs and cats are listed in Table 25-1.

Depolarizing Agents

Succinylcholine. Succinylcholine is the only depolarizing neuromuscular blocking agent in clinical use today. Succinylcholine has a rapid onset of action, and its short duration of action is primarily due to rapid hydrolysis by plasma cholinesterase.[4] For these reasons succinylcholine is used routinely to facilitate endotracheal intubation in human patients. Its use in small animal patients has been limited because the larynx of the dog and cat is easily visualized and does not routinely exhibit excessive laryngospasm, making neuromuscular blockade unnecessary for intubation.[5]

Because of the short duration of action of succinylcholine, frequent redosing or a constant-rate infusion is required if long-term neuromuscular blockade is desired. This may lead to tachyphylaxis (increased dose requirement) and change the character of the initial block (phase I block) to one similar to that produced with nondepolarizing blocking agents (phase II block), which may increase recovery time and require the use of a reversal agent (anticholinesterase therapy).[6]

Use of succinylcholine may be associated with significant side effects. A transient increase in serum potassium concentration occurs because of the leakage of potassium from the interior of cells. Severe, life-threatening hyperkalemia can occur after

Table 25-1 Doses of Neuromuscular Blocking Agents for Dogs and Cats

Drug	Dose (mg/kg IV)
Succinylcholine*	0.22 (dog) 0.11 (cat)
Atracurium*	0.22
Cisatracurium†	0.1
Vecuronium*	0.1
Pancuronium*	0.044-0.11
Mivacurium‡	0.01 - 0.05
Rocuronium§	0.18
Doxacurium¶	0.008

IV, Intravenous.
*Plumb DC: *Veterinary drug handbook*, Ames, Iowa, 2005, Blackwell.
†Adams WA, Robinson KJ, Senior JM: The use of the neuromuscular blocking drug cis-atracurium in dogs, *Vet Anaesth Analg* 28:156, 2001.
‡Smith LJ, Moon PF, Lukasik VM et al: Duration of action and hemodynamic properties of mivacurium chloride in dogs anesthetized with halothane, *Am J Vet Res* 60:1047, 1999.
§Cason B, Baker DG, Hickey RF et al: Cardiovascular and neuromuscular effect of three steroidal neuromuscular blocking drugs in dogs, *Anesth Analg* 70:382, 1990.
¶Savarese JJ, Wastila WB, Basta SJ et al: Pharmacology of BW A938U, *Anesth* 59(3):A274, 1987.

succinylcholine administration in patients with severe burns, trauma, nerve damage, neuromuscular disease, closed head injury, intraabdominal infections, and renal failure.[7] Succinylcholine should also be avoided in patients in which increases in intraocular, intracranial, and intragastric pressures are undesirable. Other side effects of succinylcholine administration include myalgia and cardiac arrhythmias (e.g., sinus bradycardia, catecholamine-induced ventricular arrhythmias).[7]

Any agent than inhibits plasma cholinesterase (organophosphates, procaine) will prolong the duration of action of succinylcholine. Certain disease states such as liver disease, malnutrition, and chronic anemia can decrease the plasma cholinesterase level. Succinylcholine must be used cautiously, if at all, in these patients.[4]

The current goal in the research and development of newer neuromuscular blocking agents is to find a drug that can be offered as an alternative to succinylcholine. This drug would have both a rapid onset and duration of action and possess minimal unwanted side effects. Although the ideal replacement has yet to be discovered, drugs such as rocuronium and mivacurium have proved useful in certain clinical situations. Both are discussed in detail later in this chapter.

Nondepolarizing Agents

Atracurium besylate. Atracurium is an intermediate-acting nondepolarizing agent with an onset of action of 3 to 5 min and a duration of action of 20 to 35 min.[8] It is metabolized primarily through Hofmann elimination and ester hydrolysis.[9] For this reason atracurium is the muscle relaxant of choice in patients with hepatic or renal disease. The rate of spontaneous degradation through Hofmann elimination is pH and temperature dependent. Both acidemia and hypothermia will prolong atracurium-induced neuromuscular blockade. Administration of atracurium can cause histamine release at higher doses, resulting in hypotension and tachycardia. Atracurium should be avoided in patients in which cardiovascular stability is desired. Administration of large doses slowly will attenuate these effects.[10] Repeated doses or an infusion of atracurium produces a consistent degree of block and duration of action because of its noncumulative effects, making it an attractive choice for a constant-rate infusion for long-term paralysis.[11,12] A metabolite of atracurium, laudanosine, can cause central nervous system (CNS) stimulation and cardiovascular depression, but this problem is rarely seen when clinical doses are used.[12]

Cisatracurium besylate. Cistracurium is the purified form of one of the 10 stereoisomers of atracurium. Because of this, the neuromuscular-blocking profile of cisatracurium is similar to that of atracurium. However, it is less likely to lead to histamine release. When administered to cats at up to 60 times the effective dose in 95% of cases (ED_{95}), plasma histamine levels were unchanged.[13] In human patients Hofmann elimination accounts for 77% and renal clearance accounts for 16% of total body clearance.[14] A study in anesthetized dogs reported the onset of action as 3.8 minutes and duration of action as 27.2 minutes.[15]

Vecuronium bromide. Vecuronium is an intermediate-acting nondepolarizing agent with an onset of action of 2 minutes and duration of action of 25 minutes.[8] The lack of cardiovascular or histamine-releasing effects, even at higher doses, is an advantage.[12] Vecuronium is the muscle relaxant of choice for patients when hemodynamic stability is needed. Recovery from vecuronium-induced muscle relaxation depends on hepatic elimination. Animals with hepatic disease may exhibit a prolonged duration of action. Vecuronium is noncumulative and is well suited for repeated doses or constant-rate infusions.[12]

Pancuronium bromide. Pancuronium is a long-acting nondepolarizing agent with an onset of action of 2 to 3 minutes and duration of action of 30 to 45 minutes.[8] It lacks histamine-releasing effects but does possess vagolytic and sympathomimetic effects, which can result in tachycardia, increased arterial blood pressure, and catecholamine-induced ventricular arrhythmias.[16] Pancuronium is mainly eliminated by the kidney, with the remainder undergoing hepatic metabolism; therefore is should be used with caution in patients with renal or hepatic disease.[17] Repeated doses or infusions of pancuronium are cumulative and can produce a delayed recovery.[18]

Mivacurium chloride. Mivacurium was recently developed as an alternative to succinylcholine for intubation in human patients. Its onset of action is 1 to 2 minute, with a duration of action of 15 to 20 minutes.[19] Because its metabolism is by way of plasma cholinesterase, prolonged recoveries are possible in patients with hepatic disease, renal disease, or organophosphate toxicity.[20] Mivacurium can cause histamine release, is noncumulative, and can be used for infusion administration.[19] In human patients the onset and depth of blockade has a high interpatient variability. Preliminary work in dogs suggested that the dose should be reduced below doses used in human patients.[21] In a later study, it was shown that one third of the human dose given to dogs resulted in a duration of action five times longer than that with human patients.[22] The species differences may be explained, in part, by the fact that normal plasma cholinesterase levels in dogs vary from 19% to 76% of human patients.[23] Also, the canine pseudocholinesterase enzyme may exhibit different affinity for the three primary isomers of mivacurium.[23] Mivacurium has not been available in the United States since 2006. It is listed on the Food and Drug Administration's Discontinued Drug Product List.

Rocuronium bromide. Like mivacurium, rocuronium was developed as an alternative to succinylcholine for intubation in human patients because of its rapid onset of action. In halothane-anesthetized dogs, rocuronium had an onset and duration of action of 1.1 ± 0.49 and 13.7 ± 0.49 minutes, respectively.[24] Rocuronium lacks significant cardiovascular and histamine-releasing effects.[25] It is metabolized primarily by the liver, with a small fraction eliminated by the kidney.[26] In small animal anesthesia, rocuronium may be chosen if a rapid onset of action without significant hemodynamic effects is desired.

Doxacurium chloride. Doxacurium is the most potent nondepolarizing agent available for use at this time.[19] It is a long-acting muscle relaxant with a slow onset of action and long duration of action in human patients. Doxacurium has minimal cardiovascular or histamine-releasing effects.[27] Because metabolism is through renal elimination, a prolonged or more variable duration of action is seen in patients with renal disease.[28] Doxacurium is not commonly used in veterinary medicine. Becaue of its long duration of action, doxacurium may not be suitable for routine clinical use in small animal patients, but it may be an attractive choice for researchers when long-term relaxation with minimal hemodynamic effects is desired.

Drug Interactions

Many medications that are given to veterinary patients during the perioperative period can alter the pharmacodynamics and pharmacokinetics of nondepolarizing agents, leading to an increased or decreased effect. Table 25-2 lists the medications and their effects on the muscle relaxant.

Table 25-2 Effect of Medication on Nondepolarizing Neuromuscular Blockade

Drug	Effects on Depth/ Duration	Comments
Antibiotics Aminoglycosides Lincomycin Clindamycin Tetracycline Polymixins	Increased	Calcium may reverse effect
Anticholinesterases	Decreased	
Anticonvulsants Phenytoin Carbamazine	Increased	After chronic therapy (>2 weeks)
Dantrolene	Increased	
Induction agents Thiopental Propofol Ketamine	Increased	Dose-dependent potentiation
Inhalational anesthetics	Increased	
Sedatives/ tranquilizers Benzodiazepines Chlorpromazine	Increased	
Steroids	Increased or decreased	Most likely to decrease but may also increase or exert no effect
Succinylcholine	Increased	When given before nondepolarizing agents
Theophylline	Decreased	

From Silverman DG, Mirakhur RK: Effects of other agents on nondepolarizing relaxants. In Silverman DG, editor: *Neuromuscular block in perioperative and intensive care*, Philadelphia, 1994, JB Lippincott.

Monitoring Neuromuscular Blockade

Whenever a muscle relaxant is administered, the neuromuscular junction should be monitored to allow the proper dose of relaxant and antagonist to be determined accurately. Also, the degree of residual blockade during the recovery period, if any, can be detected and treated appropriately. Evoked responses are used to evaluate neuromuscular blockade. This involves stimulating a peripheral motor nerve in order to evaluate the resultant motor response. Several hand-held peripheral nerve stimulators are available (Figure 25-2).

Sites of Stimulation

Sites for stimulation of peripheral motor nerves in dogs and cats include the peroneal and ulnar nerves; the more accessible is chosen (Figure 25-3).

Electrical Stimulus Characteristics

There are standard methods of stimulating peripheral motor nerves because the physical characteristics of electrical stimuli influence the motor response they evoke. The output from the peripheral nerve stimulator should be a square wave stimulus having duration of 0.2 to 0.3 milliseconds. Ideally, the output current is adjustable and should be sufficient to produce a supramaximal impulse.

After the two electrodes are placed over the nerve to be stimulated, the stimulus is adjusted to deliver a supramaximal current, slightly greater than that required to elicit a maximum motor response. This ensures that all neurons in the bundle are depolarized, which will cause the muscle fibers to contract in an all-or-none fashion. Any subsequent changes in the motor response are from effects at the neuromuscular junction.

Patterns of Stimulation

Peripheral nerve stimulators should provide single-twitch, tetanus of 50 Hz, and train-of-four stimulus patterns. Newer stimulators may also have the capability to deliver a double-burst pattern (Figure 25-4).

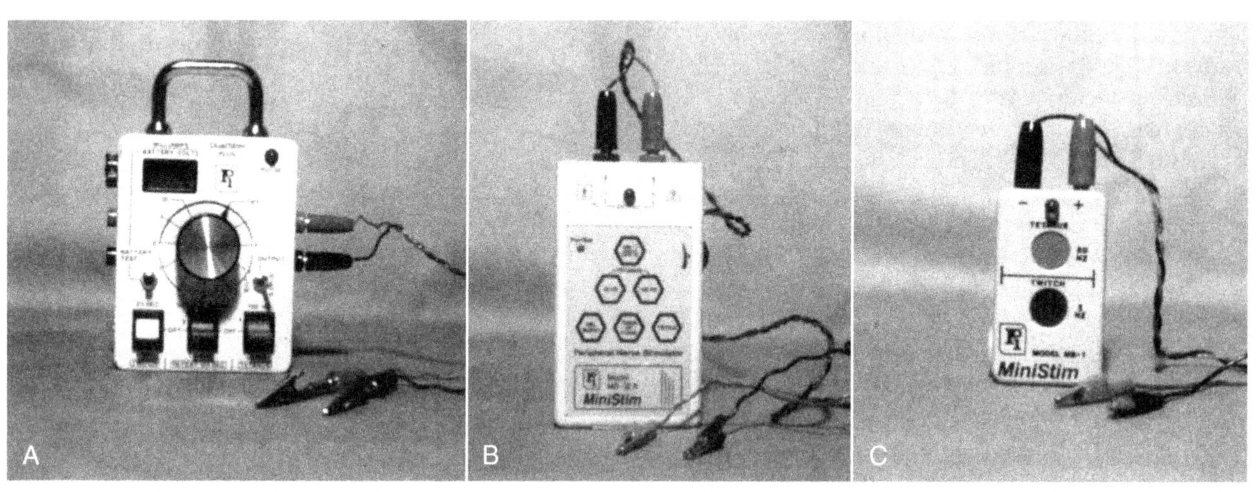

Figure 25-2 *A-C*, Several hand-held peripheral nerve stimulators available to monitor neuromuscular blockade in small animals.

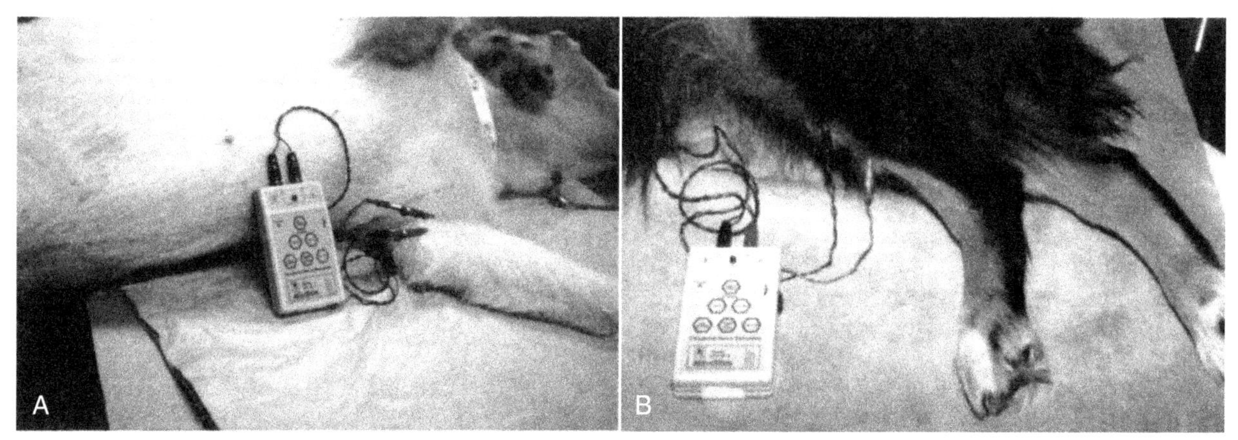

Figure 25-3 Sites for peripheral nerve stimulation in the dog. *A*, Ulnar nerve; *B*, superficial peroneal nerve.

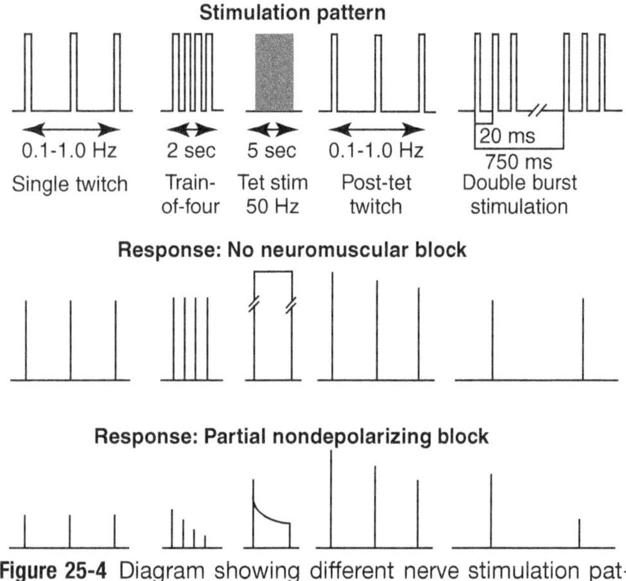

Figure 25-4 Diagram showing different nerve stimulation patterns for monitoring neuromuscular blockade. *Stim,* stimulation; *tet,* tetanic. (Courtesy Cullen LK: Muscle relaxants and neuromuscular block. In Thurman JC, Tranquilli WJ, Benson GJ, editors: *Lumb and Jones' veterinary anesthesia,* ed 3, Baltimore, 1996, Williams & Wilkins.)

Single-twitch method. The single-twitch method is used to evaluate the degree of relaxation by dividing the elicited response by the control response. The control response is taken before the administration of the relaxant. The frequency should not be greater than 0.15 Hz (1 twitch/7-10 seconds). This is due to the prejunctional effects of the relaxant, which greatly decreases the amount of ACh release.[29] The resultant motor response will be less than the baseline values, making accurate determination of the degree of relaxant difficult. The disadvantages of using the single-twitch method are that a baseline response is necessary before administration of the muscle relaxant and that it is insensitive for the detection of residual blockade.[30]

Train-of-four method. The train-of-four method consists of four supramaximal impulses delivered at a frequency of 2 Hz (2 twitches/second). The degree of blockade is evaluated by comparing the ratio of the fourth twitch to the first twitch (T_4/T_1 ratio). The train-of-four serves as its own control; therefore no baseline values before muscle relaxant administration are necessary. The train-of-four stimulus can be delivered intermittently or at regular intervals 10 to 20 seconds apart. In the absence of muscle relaxants, the T_4/T_1 ratio is approximately 1. Following the administration of a nondepolarizing muscle relaxant, the fourth, third, second, and first twitches disappear (fade) in that order as the block becomes more profound. The degree of fade, strength of the remaining twitches, and length of time that the twitches are absent depends on the dose of relaxant given. A T_4/T_1 ratio of 0.7 or higher correlates with clinical signs of adequate recovery from neuromuscular blockade.[31]

During phase 1 block with succinylcholine, there is a flat T_4 response (no fade). Repeated or prolonged infusions of succinylcholine changes the character of the block to phase 2, where fade during a train-of-four stimulus is seen.[32]

Tetanic stimulation. Serial supramaximal stimulation at high frequency, 50 Hz, for 5 seconds causes sustained muscle contraction.[32] After administration of a nondepolarizing muscle relaxant, fade is seen as the muscle is unable to maintain the strength generated by the tetanic stimulus.[18] Although it is a sensitive indicator of residual paralysis during the recovery period, this method is painful and will elicit a physiologic response (tachycardia, hypertension, movement) in the lightly anesthetized animal.[12]

Double-burst stimulation. Double-burst stimulation consists of the delivery of two minitetanic (50 Hz) bursts. Each burst consists of three impulses and is 750 milliseconds apart.[33] The ratio of the second burst compared with the first burst (D_2/D_1) correlates highly to the T_4/T_1 ratio and is preferable to train-of-four monitoring to some individuals because fade is more readily seen.[34,35] Another advantage is that D_1 is still detected at slightly deeper levels of block than is T_1.[36]

Quantifying Evoked Responses

During routine clinical use of muscle relaxants in veterinary patients, visual observation of the evoked response is used to detect the degree of block present. This method is unreliable, especially in detecting residual blockade.[37] With experience in using muscle relaxants in small animals, visual means are adequate in detecting clinical recovery, but more accurate methods are needed in research settings. The two methods most commonly used to accurately assess the motor response after peripheral nerve stimulation are mechanomyography (MMG) and electromyography (EMG). A third method, accelerography, has also been used in veterinary research patients but to a much lesser extent.

Mechanomyography. MMG measures the evoked contractile response of the stimulated muscle by force translation. This method is the most commonly used and has been well described in the cat, dog, and horse.[24,38,39] Simply put, the paw or hoof of the front or rear limb is immobilized, the stimulating electrodes (surface or needle) placed over the nerve supplying the muscle to be studied, and a force transducer attached to the paw or hoof perpendicular to the twitch angle. A resting tension of 100 to 300 grams is applied to provide maximum tension development. After supramaximal single-twitch, train-of-four, tetanic, or double-burst stimulation, the evoked response is recorded on a strip chart. Although this method is extremely accurate, use of MMG in the clinical setting is limited because the limb must be immobilized, and no movement can occur throughout the duration of recording period because it will affect resting tension and twitch angle.[37]

Electromyography. EMG involves the measurement of the compound action potential of the muscle fibers during a supramaximal stimulus of a peripheral motor nerve. Two stimulating electrodes are placed over the peripheral nerve. The active recording electrode is placed over the innervation zone of the muscle to be studied, usually midway between the origin and insertion. The reference electrode is placed over the insertion of the muscle. A ground electrode is positioned between the stimulating and recording electrodes to decrease stimulation artifact. Its advantages over MMG is that it requires no limb immobilization, no resting tension, and greater flexibility in the muscles monitored. Disadvantages are that proper skin preparation and electrode placement is crucial to obtain valid results.[37] Although used on human patients, this method has not been described for veterinary patients. This author has used EMG (Relaxograph, Datex) successfully on dogs and horses. In the dog the ulnar nerve is stimulated with recording electrodes placed over the abductor digiti quinti. In the horse the superficial peroneal nerve is stimulated with recording electrodes placed over the lateral digital extensor. Skin preparation involves shaving the hair with a single-edged razor, rubbing the skin vigorously with isopropyl alcohol, and allowing the skin to dry completely before surface electrode placement.

Mechanomyography Versus electromyography. Although MMG remains the gold standard for quantifying evoked responses in veterinary patients in the research setting, EMG may become an attractive choice for use in the clinical patients once the methodology is validated. In human patients differences exist between the two methods. Compared with MMG, the EMG method tends to show a lesser degree of relaxation with nondepolarizing agents and overestimates the degree of relaxation with depolarizing agents.[40,41] Future studies in veterinary patients will help in the development of different criteria for onset and reversal on neuromuscular blockade based on the type of monitoring used.

Accelerography. Accelerography is based on Newton's second law: Force equals mass times acceleration. In other words, acceleration is directly proportional to the force if the mass is constant. During electrical stimulation of a peripheral nerve, a piezoelectric sensor assesses the acceleration during an isotonic contraction of the innervated muscle. A study in human patients comparing accelerography with EMG concluded that the wide variations in individual patients and the differences in clinical duration and recovery index do not allow the two monitoring techniques to be used interchangeably.[42] Compared with MMG, published studies in human patients present inconsistent results. In one study accelerography showed good correlation and was considered a simple and reliable monitoring tool.[43] In two other studies, the limits of agreement were unacceptably wide.[44,45] A study in dogs comparing the neuromuscular effect of vecuronium during either propofol or sevoflurane anesthesia used accelerography to quantify neuromuscular function.[46] The fibular nerve was stimulated with the acceleration transducer fixed over the cranial tibial muscle.

Accelerography appeared to be an acceptable technique for quantifying neuromuscular blockade in anesthetized dogs. More studies are needed, both in dogs and other species, to determine if it can be used easily and reliably in clinical veterinary patients.

REVERSAL OF NEUROMUSCULAR BLOCKADE

Recovery from succinylcholine (phase 1 block) and mivacurium-induced neuromuscular blockade is usually rapid and spontaneous owing to rapid hydrolysis by plasma cholinesterases. Delayed recovery will be seen in patients with decreased plasma cholinesterase levels.

Residual neuromuscular blockade from nondepolarizing agents and phase 2 block from succinylcholine may be reversed at the conclusion of surgery to prevent potentially serious complications in the recovery period. Complications include muscle weakness and inadequate ventilation, which can lead to life-threatening hypoxia or respiratory acidosis.

Before reversal of blockade, it is desirable to have 3 to 4 twitches of the train-of-four visible. This is achieved by close monitoring of neuromuscular function throughout surgery and not redosing the patient close to the time of anticipated reversal.

The anticholinesterase drugs used clinically include neostigmine, pyridostigmine, and edrophonium. Doses are listed in Table 25-3. They reverse neuromuscular blockade by inhibiting the enzyme acetylcholinesterase, which is responsible for the hydrolysis of ACh. The effect is an accumulation of ACh at muscarinic and nicotinic receptor sites. Because nondepolarizing agents and ACh compete for the same receptor binding sites, anything that increases the concentration of ACh tips the balance of competition in favor of ACh and restores neuromuscular transmission. Reversal of neuromuscular blockade requires only the nicotinic cholinergic effects of anticholinesterase drugs; therefore the muscarinic effects are attenuated or prevented by concurrent administration of an anticholinergic such as atropine or glycopyrrolate.

Sugammadex is the first selective relaxant binding agent (SRBA). It is a novel agent used to reverse neuromuscular blockade produced by rocuronium and, to a lesser extent, other steroidal muscle relaxants (rocuronium > vecuronium > pancuronium). Sugammadex is a modified gamma cyclodextrin that binds and encapsulates the rocuronium molecule.

Table 25-3 Doses of Neuromuscular Reversal Agents for Dogs and Cats

Drug	Dose (mg/kg IV)
Neostigmine*	0.04
Edrophonium†	0.5
Pyridostigmine†	0.2

*Muir WW, Hubbell JAE,: *Handbook of veterinary anesthesia,* ed 4, St Louis, 2007, Mosby.
†Dose used at Veterinary Teaching Hospital, Texas A&M University.

Once bound within the lipophilic core of sugammadex, it is rendered unavailable to bind to the ACh receptor.[47] A significant advantage of sugammadex is the ability to reverse neuromuscular blockade without the use of anticholinesterase drugs. In addition, because there is no need to co-administer antimuscarinic drugs with sugammadex, its use is associated with greater cardiovascular and autonomic stability. Sugammadex is approved in the European Union but is not currently approved for use in the United States.

Monitoring neuromuscular function and support of ventilation must be continued until complete reversal has been accomplished. An adequate plane of anesthesia must be maintained while monitoring the degree of block with a peripheral nerve stimulator because this can cause the patient some discomfort, especially if tetanic stimulation is used. A T_4/T_1 ratio of 0.7 or greater correlates well to clinical recovery. Once reversal is complete and the use of the nerve stimulator is discontinued, the animal is allowed to recover from anesthesia. Although recurarization is uncommon after reversal, spontaneous respiratory efforts, sufficient to maintain adequate ventilation, should be present and monitored closely during the recovery period.

SKELETAL MUSCLE RELAXANTS (SPASMOLYTICS)

Although neuromuscular blocking agents are effective for skeletal muscle spasticity, these agents are too nonselective to be an appropriate choice for this purpose. Several other drugs are available and commonly used to reduce muscle tone without abolishing voluntary skeletal muscle contraction. Some of these drugs may also possess sedative effects, which may be beneficial to animals that are experiencing both anxiety and pain.

Physiology

Skeletal muscle spasticity may be due to an increase in tonic stretch reflexes originating from the CNS, with involvement of descending pathways, and results in hyperexcitability of motor neurons in the spinal cord. Several diseases involving increased muscle tone caused by defective neuronal control of muscle activity have been described in Scottish Terriers (Scotty cramp), Dalmatians, and Norwich Terriers.[48,49] These dogs are normal at rest and on initiation of exercise, but episodic muscle rigidity or cramping are seen during heavy exercise or excitement. Familial reflex myoclonus has been described in Labrador Retrievers. Symptoms appear in young puppies and are characterized by paroxysmal muscle spasms and progressive muscle stiffness. Either a defect in the major inhibitory neurotransmitter glycine or altered genetic regulation of the spinal cord glycine receptor is thought to be the basis for this condition.[50] Intervertebral disk disease in dogs may cause painful spasms of the neck and shoulder (cervical disk) or back (thoracolumber disk) muscles. In certain clinical cases, skeletal muscle relaxants are used as part of a conservative management protocol for animals with intervertebral disk disease.

Pharmacology

Skeletal muscle relaxants act in the CNS or directly on skeletal muscle to reduce muscle tone and relieve spasticity without abolishing voluntary motor control. Centrally acting muscle relaxants block interneuronal pathways in the spinal cord and in the midbrain reticular activating system. These drugs have little effect on the diaphragm and respiratory muscles at therapeutic doses. Dantrolene, a hydantoin derivative, is a peripherally acting muscle relaxants that acts by decreasing the amount of calcium released from the sarcoplasmic reticulum.

Individual Agents

Centrally acting skeletal muscle relaxants used in small animal veterinary medicine include guaifenesin, methocarbamol, and the benzodiazepines. The most common side effect seen with these drugs is CNS depression, which is manifested as sedation and lethargy. Ataxia and muscle weakness are also possible. Additive depression can occur when these drugs are given concurrently with other CNS depressant agents. Anticholinesterase agents given with either guaifenesin or methocarbamol may result in severe muscle weakness. Dantrolene is the only clinically used peripherally acting skeletal muscle relaxant.

Guaifenesin

Although more commonly used in large animals, guaifenesin is used in small animal veterinary patients to induce muscle relaxation as an adjunct to general anesthesia. The dose in dogs is 33 to 88 mg/kg adminstered intravenously. Guaifenesin has also been used in the treatment of strychnine intoxication in dogs.

Methocarbamol

Methocarbamol is labeled for adjunctive therapy of acute inflammatory and traumatic conditions of skeletal muscle and the reduction of muscle spasms in dogs and cats. The dose is 44 mg/kg intravenously or 61 to 132 mg/kg orally, initially divided every 8 to 12 hours. For muscle relaxation as a part of conservative management of intervertebral disk disease in dogs, methocarbamol is given at a dose of 15 to 20 mg/kg orally three times a day. To control the severe effects of strychnine and tetanus, the dose in dogs and cats is 55 to 220 mg/kg intravenously (not to exceed 330 mg/kg daily). Half of the dose is given rapidly, whereupon the clinician waits until the patient begins to relax and then continues administering the drug to effect.

Diazepam

Diazepam is the primary benzodiazepine used for the purpose of muscle relaxation. Although its clinical indications include seizure control, appetite stimulation, and sedation, only its use as a muscle relaxant will be discussed here. Diazepam may be effective in reducing skeletal muscle spasticity in dogs with episodic muscle cramping such as Scotty cramp or in certain myopathic syndromes. The dose range is 0.5 to 2 mg/kg intravenously or orally three times daily.

Diazepam is also used to treat intraurethral obstruction secondary to acquired lower urinary tract disease in male cats. It is believed that muscle spasms of the urethra, along with inflammation of the urethral tissue, make removal of the obstructing plug more difficult. Additionally, these factors may create a "functional" obstruction of the urinary tract even after the obstructing plug has been removed. Diazepam has been recommended for treatment of external urethral sphincter hypertonus at a dose of 2 to 10 mg/kg (total) orally every 8 hours. Because the urethral musculature contains a predominance of smooth muscle, it may be necessary to combine skeletal muscle relaxants (which affect only the external urethral sphincter) with smooth muscle relaxants, such as prazosin.

Dantrolene

The clinical indications for dantrolene include functional urethral obstruction resulting from increased urethral tone and treatment of malignant hyperthermia. For treatment of functional urethral obstruction, dantrolene is administered at a dose of 1 to 5 mg/kg orally every 8 hours (dogs) or 0.5 to 2 mg/kg every 8 hours (cats). Dantrolene has been shown to decrease urethral pressure in the postprostatic/penile urethral segment but has no effect on intraurethral pressures in the prostatic or preprostatic urethral segment.[51] Concurrent use of smooth muscle relaxants may be of benefit in relieving urethral obstruction. For treatment of malignant hyperthermia, the dose of dantrolene is reported in dogs at 0.29 and 0.69 mg/kg intravenously.[52,53] Dantrolene has moderate to poor oral bioavailability and is highly bound to albumin. Dantrolene undergoes hepatic metabolism with metabolites excreted in the urine. Adverse effects include hepatotoxicity, sedation, muscle weakness, and gastrointestinal effects.

REFERENCES

1. Hall LW, Clarke KW: Relaxation of skeletal muscles during anaesthesia. In Hall LW, Clarke KW, editors: *Veterinary anesthesia*, ed 8, London, 1983, Baillière Tindall.
2. Ilkiw JE: Advantages of and guidelines for using neuromuscular blocking agents, *Vet Clin North Am Small Anim Pract* 22(2):347, 1992.
3. Hunter JM: New neuromuscular blocking drugs, *N Engl J Med* 332:1691, 1995.
4. Benson GJ, Thurmon JC: Clinical pharmacology of succinylcholine, *J Am Vet Med Assoc* 176(7):646, 1980.
5. Hubbell JAE: Disadvantages of neuromuscular blocking agents, *Vet Clin North Am Small Anim Pract* 22(2):351, 1992.
6. Silverman DG, Donati F: Neuromuscular effects of depolarizing relaxants. In Silverman DG, editor: *Neuromuscular block in perioperative and intensive care*, Philadelphia, 1994, JB Lippincott.
7. Miller RD, Savarese JJ: Pharmacology of muscle relaxants and their antagonists. In Miller RD, editor: *Anesthesia*, ed 2, New York, 1986, Churchill Livingston.
8. Plumb DC: *Veterinary drug handbook*, ed 5, Ames, Iowa, 2005, Blackwell.
9. Fisher DM, Canfell PC, Fahey MR, et al: Elimination of atracurium in humans: contribution of Hofmann elimination and ester hydrolysis versus organ-based elimination, *Anesthesiology* 65:6, 1986.
10. Scott RPF, Savarese JJ, Basta SJ, et al: Atracurium: clinical strategies for preventing histamine release and attenuating the hemodynamic response, *Br J Anaesth* 57:550, 1985.

11. Hildebrand SV: Neuromuscular blocking agents, *Vet Clin North Am Small Anim Pract* 22(2):341, 1992.
12. Miller RD, Rupp SM, Fisher DM, et al: Clinical pharmacology of vecuronium and atracurium, *Anesthesiology* 61:444, 1984.
13. Wastila WB, Maehr RB, Turner GL, et al: Comparative pharmacology of cistracurium (51W89), atracurium, and 5 isomers in cats, *Anesthesiology* 85:169, 1996.
14. Kisor DF, Schmith VD, Wargin WA, et al: Importance of the organ-independent elimination of cisatracurium, *Anesth Analg* 83:1065, 1996.
15. Adams WA, Robinson KJ, Senior JM: The use of the neuromuscular blocking drug cis-atracurium in dogs, *Vet Anaesth Analg* 28:156, 2001.
16. Stoelting RK: *Pharmacology and physiology in anesthetic practice*, ed 3, Philadelphia, 1999, Lippincott-Raven.
17. Silverman DG, Mirakhur RK: Nondepolarizing relaxants of long duration. In Silverman DG, editor: *Neuromuscular block in perioperative and intensive care*, Philadelphia, 1994, JB Lippincott.
18. Hildebrand SV: Neuromuscular blocking agents in equine anesthesia, *Vet Clin North Am Equine Pract* 6(3):587, 1990.
19. Mirakhur RK: Newer neuromuscular blocking drugs: an overview of their clinical pharmacology and therapeutic use, *Drugs* 44(2):182, 1992.
20. Basta SJ: Clinical pharmacology of mivacurium chloride: a review, *J Clin Anesth* 4(2):153, 1992.
21. Lukasik VM: Neuromuscular blocking drugs and the critical care patient, *J Vet Emerg Crit Care* 5(2):99, 1996.
22. Smith LJ, Moon PF, Lukasik VM, et al: Duration of action and hemodynamic properties of mivacurium chloride in dogs anesthetized with halothane, *Am J Vet Res* 60:1047, 1999.
23. Smith LJ, Schwark WS, Cook DR, et al: Pharmacokinetic variables of mivacurium chloride after intravenous administration in dogs, *Am J Vet Res* 60:1051, 1999.
24. Cason B, Baker DG, Hickey RF, et al: Cardiovascular and neuromuscular effect of three steroidal neuromuscular blocking drugs in dogs, *Anesth Analg* 70:382, 1991.
25. Hudson ME, Rothfield KP, Tullock WC, et al: Haemodynamic effects of rocuronium bromide in adult cardiac surgical patients, *Can J Anaesth* 45:139, 1998.
26. Morris RB, Cahalan MK, Miller RD, et al: The cardiovadcular effects of vecuronium (ORG NC45) and pancuronium in patients undergoing coronary bypass grafting, *Anesthesiology* 58:438, 1983.
27. Faulds D, Clissold SP: Doxacurium: a review of its pharmacology and clinical potential in anaesthesia, *Drugs* 42(4):673, 1991.
28. Cook RD, Freeman JA, Lai AA, et al: Pharmacokinetics and pharmacodynamics of doxacurium in normal patients and in those with hepatic or renal failure, *Anesth Analg* 72:145, 1991.
29. Ali HH, Savarese JJ: Stimulus frequency and dose-response curve to d-tubocurarine in man, *Anesthesiology* 52:39, 1980.
30. Ali HH, Miller RD: Monitoring of neuromuscular function. In Miller RD, editor: *Anesthesia*, ed 2, New York, 1986, Churchill Livingstone.
31. Brand JB, Cullen DJ, Wilson NF, et al: Spontaneous recovery from nondepolarizing neuromuscular blockade: correlation between clinical and evoked response, *Anesth Analg* 56:55, 177.
32. Klein LV: Neuromuscular blocking agents. In Short CE, editor: *Principles and practice of veterinary anesthesia*, Baltimore, 1987, Williams & Wilkins.
33. Silverman DG, Brull SJ: Patterns of stimulation. In Silverman DG, editor: *Neuromuscular block in perioperative and intensive care*, Philadelphia, 1994, JB Lippincott.
34. Drenck NE, Ueda N, Olsen NV, et al: Manual evaluation of residual curarization using double-burst stimulation: comparison with train-of-four, *Anesthesiology* 70:578, 1989.
35. Saddler JM, Bevan JC, Donati F, et al: Comparison of double-burst and train-of-four stimulation to assess neuromuscular blockade in children, *Anesthesiology* 73:401, 1990.
36. Braude N, Vyvyan HAL, Jordan MJ: Intraoperative assessment of atracurium-induced neuromuscular block using double-burst stimulation, *Br J Anaesth* 67:574, 1991.
37. Law SC, Cook DR: Monitoring the neuromuscular junction. In Lake CL, editor: *Clinical monitoring*, Philadelphia, 1990, Saunders.
38. Forsyth SF, Ilkiw JE, Hildebrand SV: Effect of gentamicin administration on the neuromuscular blockade induced by atracurium in cats, *Am J Vet Res* 57(10):1675, 1990.
39. Hildebrand SV, Hill T: Interaction of gentamycin and atracurium in anaesthetized horses, *Equine Vet J* 26:209, 1994.
40. Kopman KF: The relationship of evoked electromyographic and mechanical responses following atracurium in humans, *Anesthesiology* 63:208, 1985.
41. Weber S, Muravchick S: Monitoring technique affects measurement of recovery from succinylcholine, *J Clin Monit* 3:1, 1987.
42. Dahaba AA, Rehak PH, List WF: Assessment of accelerography with the TOF-GUARD: a comparison with electromyography, *Eur J Anaesthesiol* 14:623, 1997.
43. Viby-Mogensen J, Jensen E, Werner MU, et al: Measurements of acceleration: a new method of monitoring neuron-muscular function, *Acta Anaesthesiol Scand* 32:45, 1988.
44. Harper NJN, Martlew R, Strang T, et al: Monitoring neuromuscular block by accelerography: comparison of the Mini-Accelerograph with the Myograph 200, *Br J Anaesth* 72:411, 1994.
45. Loan PB, Paxton LD, Mirakhur RK, et al: The TOF-Guard neuromuscular transmission monitor: a comparison with the Myograph 200, *Anaesthesia* 50:699, 1995.
46. Kastrup MR, Marsico FF, Ascoli FO: Neuromuscular blocking properties of atracurium during sevoflurane or propofol anaesthesia in dogs, *Vet Anaesth Analg* 32:222, 2005.
47. Naguib M: Sugammadex: Another milestone in clinical neuromuscular pharmacology, *Anesth Analg* 104:575, 2007.
48. Meyers KM, Clemmons RM: Scotty cramp. In Kirk RW, editor: *Current veterinary therapy VIII*, Philadelphia, 1983, Saunders.
49. Woods CB: Hyperkinetic episodes in two Dalmatian dogs, *J Am Anim Hosp Assoc* 13:225, 1977.
50. Furber RM: Cramp in Norwich terriers, *Vet Rec* 115:46, 1984.
51. Straeter-Knowlen IM, Marks SL, Rishniw M, et al: Urethral pressure response to smooth and skeletal muscle relaxants in anesthetized, adult male cats with naturally occurring urethral obstruction, *Am J Vet Res* 56:919, 1995.
52. Kirmayer AH, Klide AM, Purvance JE: Malignant hyperthermia in a dog: case report and review of the syndrome, *J Am Vet Med Assoc* 185:978, 1984.
53. Bagshaw RJ, Cox RH, Rosenberg H: Dantrolene treatment of malignant hyperthermia, *J Am Vet Med Assoc* 178:1029, 1981.

Drugs That Modify Animal Behavior

26

Dawn Merton Boothe

Chapter Outline

NEUROTRANSMITTERS AND THEIR ROLE IN ABNORMAL BEHAVIORS

Little is known about the cellular mechanisms of abnormal behavior in humans or animals. The most likely neurotransmitters (NTs) associated with abnormal behaviors might be identified based on the NTs targeted by drugs used to modify the behaviors. NTs identified for their role or potential role in abnormal behaviors include the biogenic amines serotonin and histamine (H_1 subtype), the monoamine dopamine, the catecholamine norepinephrine, acetylcholine, gamma-aminobutyric acid (GABA), and the excitatory amino acids such as glutamate.[1-3] Several of these neurotransmitters are discussed in Chapter 27.

Behavior also can be affected by other chemicals, including circulating hormones, opioids, and neurokinins.

The NT most commonly associated with abnormal behaviors is serotonin.[4] Accordingly, the more effective drugs for modification of behavior are those (e.g., fluoxetine, clomipramine) that tend to be selective for serotonin. Serotonin is synthesized in the brain from tryptophan. Serotonin receptors differ in anatomic location and behavioral roles, with the majority of 5-hydroxytryptamine (5-HT) receptors being located in the gastrointestinal tract. Receptors in the central nervous system (CNS) are located in the raphe nucleus, the basal ganglia, and the limbic area. At least nine 5-HT receptor subtypes have been identified, four of which appear to be particularly important to behavior or mood.[3] The 5-HT_1 receptors, located primarily in the brain, are predominantly inhibitory (toward adenylyl cyclase) both presynaptically (autoreceptors; 1A and 1D) and postsynaptically (1A, 1D, 2A, 2C, and 3 and 4). Regulation of serotonin action is complex, involving both presynaptic and postsynaptic mechanisms[3] with postsynaptic receptors regulating serotonin release from the presynaptic nerve endings. Serotonin may exert tonic inhibition on the dopaminergic system; drug-mediated increase may result in extrapyramidal effects.[4] Badino and coworkers[5] compared serotonergic and adrenergic receptor density in dogs neurologically normal except for aggressive behavior (n = 8) and normal, nonaggressive dogs (n = 8). The concentration of high affinity (serotonin) 5-HT receptors was increased in the thalamus, and low affinity 5-HT receptors were increased throughout the regions of the CNS studied (frontal cortex, thalamus, hypothalamus, hippocampus) in aggressive dogs compared with nonaggressive dogs. Riva and coworkers[6] demonstrated that plasma levels of serotonin and dopamine were higher in anxious dogs (n = 22) compared with control dogs (n = 13).

KEY POINT 26-1 Drugs that are among the most effective and safest for behavior modification are those that tend to be most selective for serotonin.

In addition to serotonin, dopamine is also increased in dogs with anxiety.[6] Dopamine is synthesized in neurons from L-DOPA in presynaptic vesicles. Synthesis begins with oxidation of the dietary amino acid tyrosine, followed by decarboxylation to L-DOPA.[3] Those neurons in which dopamine is found lack the enzyme that converts dopamine to norepinephrine. Dopamine is removed by monoamine oxidase (MAO) and catechol-*O*-methyltransferase (COMT). Dopamine receptors are distributed throughout the brain, although less so than norepinephrine receptors. Dopamine appears to be largely located in the midbrain, hypothalamus, and limbic system (the part of the brain thought to control emotions).[3] Dopamine receptors (at least five subtypes) are found in portions of the extrapyramidal system responsible for coordinated movement.[1,2] At least four dopamine receptors are affected by mood disorders and stereotypics; increased dopamine appears to stimulate these abnormal behaviors.[1,2] Because dopamine generally suppresses acetylcholine activity, blockade of dopamine receptors generally results in an increase in acetylcholine release.[4]

Norepinephrine is the end product of dopamine oxidation. Its inactivation occurs primarily by active transport or reuptake into presynaptic vesicles. The NT is then deaminated by mitochondrial monoamine oxidases or catechol-o-methyltransferase in the presynaptic nerve terminal. Norepinephrine is located predominantly in the gray matter of the pons and in the medulla; projections in the locus ceruleus into the limbic cortex regulate emotions. Norepinephrine interacts postsynaptically with α_1 receptors (G protein–mediated activation of phospholipase C and inositol triphosphate formation) and β receptors (activation of adenylyl cyclase) and presynaptically with α_2 receptors (G proteins).The behavioral effects of norepinephrine appear to affect arousal, functional reward systems, and mood. The latter effect may reflect a decrease in depression and an increase in mania.

GABA is a major inhibitory NT, being active at 30% of synapses in the human CNS, and particularly in the cortex and thalamus. Its precursor glutamate is widely distributed throughout the brain. As with norepinephrine, dopamine, and serotonin, GABA has a presynaptic transporter. Two primary receptor types, $GABA_A$ and $GABA_B$, appear to cause postsynaptic inhibition by facilitating chloride ion influx into the neuron. Several drugs, including the benzodiazepines and barbiturates (e.g., phenobarbital), interact with the $GABA_A$ receptor in an agonistic fashion, causing neuronal inhibition.[1] The physiologic and behavioral effects of GABA and its receptors have not yet been totally characterized (see Chapter 27).[3]

Several abnormal human behaviors have been associated with changes in excitatory NTs, including aggressive, impulsive, and schizophrenic disorders. Among the more important excitatory NTs is glutamate. Glutamate is preformed and stored in synaptic vesicles released by calcium-mediated endocytosis. Barbiturates and progesterone modulate behaviors, in part by inhibiting calcium uptake and thus release of glutamate at the NT.[1,2]

Acetylcholine, the most widely distributed NT in the brain,[3] is preformed from choline and acetyl coenzyme A and stored at the terminal end of the synapse in vesicles. Calcium stimulates its release by exocytosis into the synaptic cleft, where it is rapidly metabolized by acetylcholinesterase. Acetylcholine generally is an excitatory NT, interacting with nicotinic and muscarinic receptors. At least five muscarinic receptors are located in the CNS. Receptors (M_1) are also found in the gastrointestinal and cardiovascular systems, accounting for some of the adverse effects associated with several behavior-modifying drugs.[1]

NTs tend to be formed and degraded locally. Both formation and inhibition offer pharmacologic targets. A number of drugs result in an increase in the presence of NTs in the synaptic cleft by inhibiting either the metabolism (e.g., dopamine) or the reuptake (e.g., serotonin, norepinephrine) of the NT after release (Figure 26-1).

DRUGS USED TO MODIFY BEHAVIORS

Drugs that modify behavior are classified initially on the basis of their (human) therapeutic use, followed by their chemistry and neurochemical activity.[4] Included are the antipsychotic drugs (predominantly antidopaminergic in action), anxioselective drugs such as the azapirones (primarily antiserotonergic in action), drugs used to treat affective or mood disorders (antidepressants, lithium, and selected anticonvulsant drugs), and drugs used to treat anxiety and anxiety-related disorders (anxiolytics or minor tranquilizers, benzodiazepines). Other drugs include antihistamines, beta blockers, progestins, anticonvulsants, and opioid antagonists. Most of the drugs used to modify behaviors are used for treatment of other disorders, and as such may be discussed elsewhere in this volume. Only drugs that have veterinary application are discussed here. Table 26-1 provides dosing information about the use of these drugs.

KEY POINT 26-2 Drugs that modify the central nervous system should not be withdrawn suddenly. Extra precaution is indicated for drugs with short half-lives.

In general, the disposition of behavior-modifying drugs is complex, with characteristics that tend to be different among species. Oral absorption, first-pass metabolism, significant binding to serum proteins, profoundly large volumes of distribution, and metabolism to enantiomers and active metabolites (the latter potentially contributing to more activity than the parent compound) all contribute to these drugs' lack of predictable behavior when dosing regimens are extrapolated among species. Hepatic metabolism increases the risk of both hepatotoxicity and drug interactions. The former, although rarely reported in humans, appears to be increasing and warrants additional attention as the use of these drugs increases in animals. Many behavior-modifying drugs are inhibitors of cytochrome P450 (CYP). Drug interactions at the level of CYP are well known in human medicine and should be anticipated in animals, particularly if drugs are used in combination. However, differences in CYP distribution and activity preclude predictable extrapolation of reported drug interactions among the species. The potentially toxic nature of these drugs places the animal patient further at risk because many dosing regimens are extrapolated from humans. Exceptions include clomipramine, fluoxetine and selegiline, each of which has been approved for use in dogs. The disposition of several drugs also has been reported in cats.

Antipsychotic Drugs

Psychotic disorders in humans involve a severe disturbance of brain function characterized by thought and speech disruption and hallucinations or delusions.[3] Although psychotic disorders do not appear to occur in veterinary medicine, drugs developed for their management in humans have proved efficacious for a number of veterinary applications. Antipsychotic drugs (also called *neuroleptics* or *major tranquilizers)* are largely structurally dissimilar from one another, but the commonality among them is dopamine, and particularly D_2 receptors, as a target. Drugs include the phenothiazines, the thioxanthenes (structurally related to the phenothiazines), heterocyclic dibenzepines, the butyrophenones, and diphenylbutylpiperidines (Figure 26-2).[7]

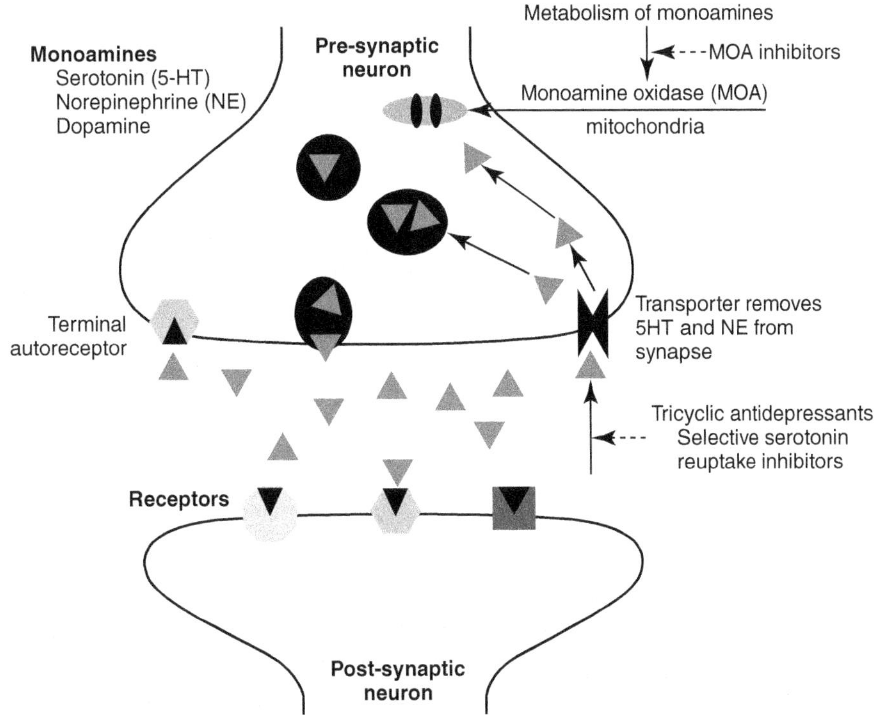

Figure 26-1 Mechanism of action of selected behavior-modifying drugs. Neurotransmitters responsible for behavior are released from the presynaptic neuron into the synaptic cleft and interact with postsynaptic receptors. Following exocytosis, inactivation of the transmitter occurs primarily by reuptake into the presynaptic neuron, the site of action of most behavior-modifying drugs. Activation also may involve metabolic degradation, as in the case of the monoamines (MOA).

Structure–Activity Relationships

Antipsychotic drugs are categorized by structure and by potency. Low-potency drugs (chlorpromazine, acepromazine, promazine) are characterized by greater sedation and cardiac and anticholinergic side effects compared with their high-potency counterparts. High-potency drugs (e.g., haloperidol, fluphenazine, trifluoperazine, prochlorperazine, and thiothixene) are administered at lower doses and are associated with less sedation and fewer anticholinergic and cardiac side effects. They do, however, have a greater incidence of extrapyramidal side effects.

The largest structural class of antipsychotics is the phenothiazines or tricyclic antipsychotics, which should not be confused with the tricyclic antidepressant drugs (discussed later). The tricyclic antipsychotic drugs are represented by phenothiazine, a three-ring structure containing a sulfur and nitro group in the ring connecting two benzene rings. Substitutions on one of the benzene rings yield different drugs (e.g., chlorpromazine, promazine), which differ in efficacy (see Figure 26-2). The pharmacology also is affected by substitutions of nitro groups such that potency (but not efficacy) is reduced by an aliphatic side chain (e.g., chlorpromazine, thorazine, acepromazine, and trifluopromazine).[7] The length of the side chain also determines antihistaminergic properties, with two-carbon side chains such as that occurring in promethazine being more antihistaminergic. Drugs with higher potency have a piperazine side chain, as can be found on fluphenazine and rifluoperazone. Esterification with long-chain fatty acids results in long-acting (due to slow hydrolysis and absorption) drugs (e.g., fluphenazine enanthate or decanoate).[7] The use of these latter drugs in small animal veterinary medicine has yet to be established. The butyrophenone neuroleptics include haloperidol (the prototype) and droperidol. The latter is very short acting and highly sedative; thus its use is limited to anesthetic regimens.[7]

Pharmacologic Effects

The pharmacologic effects of antipsychotic drugs generally are similar among humans and animals.[7] Phenothiazines are also categorized as tranquilizers. As tranquilizers, the phenothiazines are calming in nature, causing a decrease in spontaneous activity that generally decreases response to external stimuli.[1] The predominant antipsychotic action of the phenothiazines is *neuroleptic*, a term derived from the effect of the drugs on human psychiatric patients and intended to contrast with signs typical of CNS depression.[7] The neuroleptic effects are attributed, although not conclusively so, to the antidopaminergic effects at D_2 receptors.[7]

Some of the neuroleptics (e.g., the phenothiazines) have high affinity for and thus also antagonize D_1 dopamine receptors, although pharmacologic effects at these receptors appear to be minimal. Phenothiazines also block D_3 and D_4 (which are D_2-like) receptors. Selected "atypical" antipsychotic drugs (e.g., clozapine) have a low affinity for D_2 receptors and are not characterized by extrapyramidal effects. They are, however, characterized by α_2-adrenergic antagonism. Some of the antipsychotic drugs also have affinity for serotonergic (5-HT_2) receptors (e.g., clonazepam). Cholinergic and histaminergic

Table 26-1 Drugs Used To Modify Small Animal Behavior

Drug	Drug Class	Indication	Dose	Route	Interval (hr)
Acepromezine	Phenothiazine, low potency		1-2 mg/kg	PO	8
			0.05-0.1 mg/kg	IV, IM	8
Alprazolam	Benzodiazepine	Anxiolytic	0.125-0.25 mg/cat	PO	8-24
			0.01-0.1 mg/kg. Maximum of 4 mg/day	PO	As needed
			0.22-0.4 mg/kg	PO	4
			0.25-2 mg/dog	PO	6-12
Amitriptyline	Tricyclic antidepressant	Antidepressant	1-4.4 mg/kg (D)	PO	12-24. Taper withdrawal
		Behavioral problems, urine spraying, feline lower urinary tract disease	5-12.5 mg/cat	PO	24. Taper withdrawal
			1-2 mg/kg (C)	PO	12. Taper withdrawal
Buspirone	Azaperone	Anxioselective	2.5-15 mg/dog	PO	8-12
			1 mg/kg (D)	PO	8-12
			0.5-1 mg/kg (C)	PO	8-12
Chlordiazepoxide	Benzodiazepine	Anxiolytic	2.2-6.6 mg/kg	PO	As needed
			0.5-1 mg/kg (C)	PO	12-24
Chlordiazepoxide–clidinium		Irritable colon syndrome	0.1-0.25 mg/kg (D). Based on clidinium dose	PO	8-12
Clomipramine	Tricyclic antidepressant	Antidepressant	1-3 mg/kg (D)	PO	12-24
			1-5 mg/cat	PO	12-24
			0.5-1 mg/kg (C)	PO	24
Clonazepam	Benzodiazepine	Anxiolytic	0.05-0.25 mg/kg	PO	12-24
Clorazepate dipotassium	Benzodiazepine	Anxiolytic	0.5-1 mg/kg (D)	PO	8-12
Clorazepate, sustained release	Benzodiazepine	Anxiolytic	5.6 mg/small dog	PO	12-24
			11.25 mg/medium dog	PO	12-24
			22.5 mg/large dog	PO	12-24
			0.2- 2.2 mg/kg (D)	PO	12-24
			0.2-0.5 mg/kg (C)	PO	12-24
Diazepam	Benzodiazepine	Anxiolytic	1-2 mg/cat	PO	12
	Benzodiazepine	Anxiolytic	0.5-2.2 mg/kg (D)	PO	As needed
Diazepam, sustained delivery	Benzodiazepine	Anxiolytic	0.1-1 mg/kg	PO	12-24
Doxepin	Tricyclic antidepressant, antihistaminergic	Separation anxiety	3-5 mg/kg (D). Maximum of 150 mg	PO	12
Fluoxetine hydrochloride	Selective serotonin reuptake inhibitor	Antidepressant	1-3 mg/kg (D)	PO	24
			0.5-1 mg/kg (D)	PO	24
			0.5-5 mg/cat	PO	24

Fluvoxamine	Selective serotonin reuptake inhibitor	Antidepressant	0.5-2 mg/kg (D)	PO	12
			0.25-0.5 mg/kg (C)	PO	24
Haloperidol			0.5 to 4 mg/dog	PO	12 to 24
Hydrocodone	Opioid		0.25 to 1 mg/kg	PO	8
Imipramine	Tricyclic antidepressant	Separation anxiety	0.5-1 mg/kg (D)	PO	8
			2.2-4.4 mg/kg (D)	PO	12
			2.5-5 mg/cat	PO	12
Medroxyprogesterone acetate	Progestin	Aggressive masculine behavior	10 mg/kg (D)	IM, SC	As needed
		Urine marking, anxiety, intraspecies aggression	10-20 mg/kg (C)	SC	As needed. Maximim of 3 injections per year
		Male behavior disorders	Initial dose: 100 mg/cat	IM	Once
			Followed by: 50 mg/cat	IM	30 days
		Female behavior disorders	Initial dose: 50 mg/cat	IM	Once
			Followed by: 25 mg/cat	IM	30 days
Megestrol acetate	Progestin		1-2 mg/kg (up to 4 mg/kg)	PO	24 × 7-14, then decrease by 50% increments till discontinued by 3-4 wk
Methylphenidate		Narcolepsy	5-10 mg/dog	PO	8-12
Mirtazapine	Serotonin antagonist, indirect agonist				
Nalfemene	Opioid antagonist	Stereotypic behavior	1-4 mg/kg (D)	SC	
			1-4 mg/kg (D)	SC	
Naloxone hydrochloride	Opioid antagonist	Stereotypic behavior	20 mg	SC	12
Naltrexone (Trexan)	Opioid antagonist	Stereotypic behavior	1 mg/kg (D)	SC	12-24
			2.2-5 mg/kg	PO	12-24
			25-50 mg/cat	PO	12
	Opioid antagonist	Test dose	0.01 mg/kg	SC	Once
Nortriptyline	Tricyclic antidepressant	Separation anxiety	0.5-2 mg/kg	PO	12-24
Oxazepam	Benzodiazepine	Anxiolytic	0.2-1 mg/kg (D)	PO	12-24
	Benzodiazepine	Anxiolytic	0.2-0.5 mg/kg (C)	PO	12-24
Paroxetine	Selective serotonin reuptake inhibitor	Antidepressant	0.125-0.25 of a 10 mg tablet	PO	24
Phenobarbital	Anticonvulsant	Psychogenic alopecia, others	4-8 mg/cat	PO	12
Pimozide		Behavioral disorders, including dyskinetic disorders	0.025-0.1 mg/kg (D)	PO	24
Protriptyline		Narcolepsy	5-10 mg/dog	PO	24 at bedtime
Risperidone			0.5-1 mg/m(2)	PO	

Continued

Table 26-1 Drugs Used To Modify Small Animal Behavior—cont'd

Drug	Drug Class	Indication	Dose	Route	Interval (hr)
S-Adenyosyl methionine	dietary supplement	Miscellaneous behavior disorders	<5.5 kg: 90 mg	PO (on an empty stomach)	24
			5.5-11 kg: 180- 225 mg	PO (on an empty stomach)	24
			11-16 kg: 225 mg	PO (on an empty stomach)	24
			16-30 kg: 450 mg	PO (on an empty stomach)	24
			30-41 kg: 675 mg	PO (on an empty stomach)	24
			>41 kg: 900 mg	PO (on an empty stomach)	24
			17-20 mg/kg	PO (on an empty stomach)	24
			200 mg/cat	PO (on an empty stomach)	24
Sertraline	Selective serotonin reuptake inhibitor	Antidepressant	0.5-4 mg/kg (D)	PO	24
			0.5-1 mg/kg (C)	PO	24
Thioridazine		Stereotypic and aggressive behavior	1.1 mg/kg (D)	PO	12
Trifluoperazine		Miscellaneous behavior disorders	0.03 mg/kg	IM	12
		Hyperkinesis	2-4 mg/kg (D)	PO	As needed
		Stereotypic behavior	1 mg/kg (D)	SC	12-24
		Behavioral disorders, lick granulomas	2.2-5 mg/kg	PO	12-24
		Behavioral disorders, adjuvant	25-50 mg/cat	PO	12

PO, By mouth; *IV*, intravenous; *IM*, intramuscular; *D*, dog; *C*, cat; *SC*, subcutaneous.

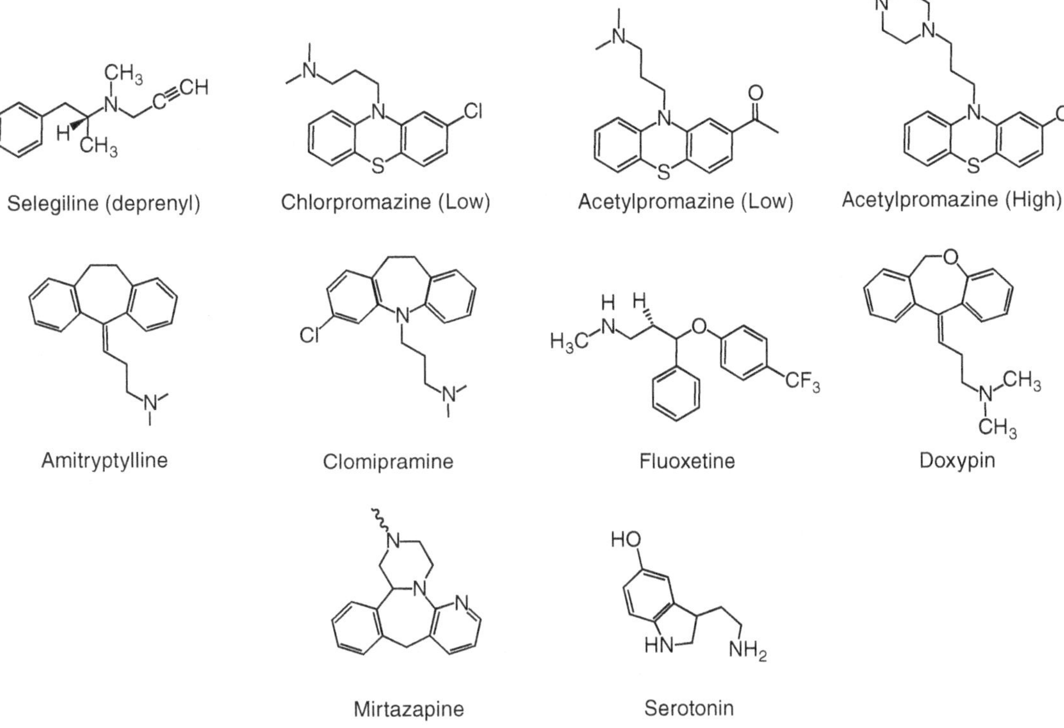

Figure 26-2 Structures of selected behavior-modifying drugs.

(H_1) receptors also are targeted by some of the drugs, resulting in unique pharmacologic effects among the neuroleptics. Variable interactions with different receptor types lead to unpredictable effects on the autonomic system. Among the neuroleptics, chlorpromazine has significant α-adrenergic antagonistic actions. In general, the antimuscarinic actions of neuroleptics are weak.

Neuroleptic effects include suppression of spontaneous movements or complex behaviors but minimal effects on spinal reflexes and unconditioned nociceptive avoidance behaviors. Interest in the environment is minimized (ataraxia), as are manifestations of emotion. Patients are easily aroused; ataxia or incoordination should not be evident at appropriate doses.[7] Aggressive or impulsive behavior should gradually diminish. As a result, conditioned avoidance (but not unconditioned escape or avoidance) behavior and exploratory behavior are minimized. Feeding and emesis also are inhibited. At high doses, cataleptic immobility is evident (particularly in cats[3]), resulting in increased muscle tone (and the ability to place animals in an abnormal posture) and ptosis. Akathisia, an increase in restless activity, is an undesirable side effect that occurs in humans but apparently not in animals. Akathisia occurs as an adaptive response to increased phenothiazines in extrapyramidal tissues.[7]

The effects of phenothiazines occur throughout the CNS. Cortical effects are responsible for many of the neuroleptic actions. Antagonism of D_2 receptors is largely responsible for the various extrapyramidal effects of the drugs. Many of these sites appear to be spared from the adaptive changes of tolerance.[7] Neuroleptics have been associated with an increased incidence of seizures.[8] Selected drugs lower seizure threshold as well as induce discharges typical of epileptic seizures. Aliphatic, low-potency phenothiazines are particularly characterized by this effect.[7] Although the effect is more likely to occur in patients who are epileptic or who are predisposed to seizures, the effect is also a dose-dependent characteristic of some drugs. These drugs are contraindicated in human epileptic patients or patients undergoing withdrawal from central depressants.[7] The relevance of this precaution to dogs is not clear. Both Tobias and coworkers[9] and McConnell and coworkers[10] retrospectively studied the frequency of seizures in epileptic dogs treated with low doses of acepromazine and found no increased risk (see also Chapter 27). Indeed, acepromazine was associated with decreased seizure activity in some of the patients that did not respond to other therapies. However, because the author experienced induction of seizures in a non-epileptic patient (lead poisoning) immediately after intravenous administration of acepromazine, caution is warranted when using phenothiazine derivatives in epileptic patients. Increasing doses slowly and accompanying with anticonvulsant therapy are indicated if the drugs must be used by epileptic patients.

The neuroleptic drugs have a number of effects in the limbic system. Although D_2 antagonism occurs in the limbic system, because D_3 receptor stimulation may be responsible for many of the behaviors targeted by neuroleptics, attempts are being made to identify D_3-selective drugs for treatment of psychoses.[7] Neuroleptics stimulate prolactin secretion in human beings. Indeed, the potency of neuroleptic action and ability to cause prolactin secretion are well correlated for most drugs. Pageat and coworkers[11] demonstrated that prolactemia correlates with response to selected behavior-modifying drugs. Tolerance is not likely to develop to this side effect. In humans prolactin secretion caused by neuroleptics also is responsible for breast engorgement and galactorrhea. Releases of growth hormone and corticotropin-releasing hormone occur in response to stress; neuroleptics (especially chlorpromazine) also interfere with the release of growth hormone, although apparently not sufficiently for treatment of acromegaly. Impaired release of serotonin may result in weight gain (particularly with low-potency drugs), and impaired glucose tolerance and insulin release may be impaired in "prediabetic" patients (especially with chlorpromazine).[7]

In the brainstem the neuroleptics have little effect, even in cases of acute overdosing. Life-threatening coma is rare. In contrast, most neuroleptics protect against nausea and emesis at the chemoreceptor trigger zone in the medulla. These effects occur at low doses. Potent piperazines and butyrophenones are also often effective against nausea stimulated by the vestibular system.[7]

Phenothiazines characterized by lower potency have a predominant sedative effect that is more apparent initially but tends to decline as tolerance develops. The phenothiazines are characterized by anxiolytic effects, but more specific anxiolytic drugs are available. In addition, the risk of either autonomic (e.g., low-potency drugs) or extrapyramidal (e.g., highly potent drugs) effects increases the likelihood of causing anxiety.[7]

The neuroleptic drugs impart physiologic (especially cardiovascular) effects through peripheral actions. The effects are complex because the neuroleptics interact with a number of receptor types that have cardiovascular effects. Hypotension induced by phenothiazines—low potency in particular—reflects direct effects on the blood vessels, indirect actions in the CNS and autonomic receptors, and a direct negative inotropic effect on the heart. Chlorpromazine also has antiarrhythmic effects on the heart, similar to quinidine.

Disposition

The antipsychotics are characterized by variable bioavailability, high lipophilicity, high protein binding, and accumulation in a number of tissues. Elimination occurs primarily through hepatic metabolism. In humans the elimination half-life is long, ranging from 20 to 40 hours. Biologic effects persist for more than 24 hours, allowing once-daily therapy in humans.[7] Metabolites can be detected in urine for several months.

Side Effects and Toxicity

The antipsychotic drugs tend to be very safe; lethal ingestion is rare in human patients. Side effects tend to reflect the pharmacologic actions of the drugs, including effects of the CNS and cardiovascular, endocrine, and autonomic systems.[7] In human patients other effects include dry mouth, blurry vision, and constipation. Urinary retention may occur in male patients with prostatitis. At high doses antipsychotics may cause catalepsy, characterized by immobility, increased muscle tone, and abnormal postures.[4] Extrapyramidal neurologic side effects reflecting inhibitionof dopamine occur in humans but have not been reported in animals. However, involuntary motor movements associated with extrapyramidal effects may be confused with seizures. The risk of seizures may be increased, but risk factors are not known (discussed previously). Some animals exhibit signs of hyperactivity after treatment with acepromazine.[3] In addition, at least one report cites increased agitation and irritability after treatment of aggression with acepromazine.[12] Jaundice has occurred in humans after taking chlorpromazine and may resolve despite continued treatment. Blood dyscrasias, including leukopenia, eosinophilia, and leukocytosis, occur but are less common with low-potency phenothiazines. Skin reactions tend to be common in people, again more commonly with low-potency phenothiazines. Small doses of acepromazine (0.1 mg/kg, given subcutaneously 30 minutes before testing) appear to have no effect on intravenous glucose tolerance testing in dogs.[13] Acepromazine sedation (0.03 mg/kg given intramuscularly 30 minutes before measurement) markedly increased peak latencies but minimally affected peak amplitude of middle-latency auditory-evoked potential in dogs (n = 12).[7,14]

Drug Interactions

Chlorpromazine is used in combination anesthetic regimens because of its ability to potentiate central depressants. Effects of analgesics and sedatives also can be enhanced. Interactions with antihypertensive drugs can be unpredictable and are more likely to be adverse with low-potency products.[7] Selected phenothiazines can antagonize the positive inotropic effects of digoxin.

Clinical Indications

In general, the use of phenothiazines for treatment of aggressive behavioral abnormalities is inappropriate because both normal and abnormal behaviors are blunted. Acepromazine is particularly problematic. Restraint of aggressive dogs with the drug renders dogs more likely to be reactive to noises and more easily startled.[1] In addition, because the degree and duration of tranquilization vary, reactions in dogs are unpredictable. Phenothiazines are not selective as antianxiety drugs but can reduce responsiveness in general, and thus they are useful in some cases of episodic anxiety.[3] Thioridazine has been used in one case of aberrant motor behavior.[15] Newer atypical antipsychotics (e.g., risperidone) may prove useful for treatment of selected abnormal behaviors (e.g., environmental-specific anxieties, impulsive explosive disorders).[4]

Antidepressant Drugs

Much of the information regarding the use of these mood-modifying drugs in animals has been extrapolated from human use. These drugs are characterized by clinical pharmacology and mechanisms of action that are likely to differ markedly among animals. Yet limited scientific information is available to guide their use in animals. Among the human mood-modifying drugs that are approved for their use for treatment of behavioral disorders in either dogs or cats are the tricyclic antidepressants (TCAs) (clomipramine), the MAO inhibitors (selegiline), and selective serotonin reuptake inhibitors (SSRIs; e.g., fluoxetine). Affective (behavior) disorders targeted by antidepressants in humans range from depression to manic-depressive disorders. In animals the list of targeted disorders is much greater and may be publically perceived to include any type of behavior deemed unacceptable by pet owners.

For a better understanding of the pharmacologic actions (intended and undesirable) of these drugs, it is necessary to appreciate the extent to which NTs targeted by these drugs are active in the brain. Among the most commonly targeted NTs is the biogenic amine system, with norepinephrine, 5-HT (serotonin), and dopamine serving as primary targets. Acetylcholine and histamine are common, although generally secondary, targets. In addition, α-adrenergic receptors may be stimulated by some of these drugs. The pharmacologic and side effects of these drugs vary with the NT targeted. Drugs that are more specific in their actions tend to be safer. Inability to predict the effect of antidepressant drugs on behavior reflects in part the inability to predict effects at the synapse as well as a lack of knowledge regarding the impact of neurotransmission on behavior. In general, blockade of dopamine transport appears to be stimulatory rather than antidepressant whereas inhibition of either serotonin or epinephrine reuptake appears to produce an antidepressant effect.

Tricyclic Antidepressants

Structure–Activity Relationships

The TCAs are among the most frequently prescribed drugs in human behavior medicine. Their name reflects their chemical structure (see Figure 26-2). The TCAs were identified as a group of potentially useful drugs for the modification of behavior in the 1940s after the generation of a number of drugs with antihistaminergic, sedative, analgesic, and antiparkinsonian effects. Imipramine was selected on the basis of its hypnotic and sedative effects. Imipramine differs from phenothiazine only by the replacement of sulfur with an ethylene bridge, yielding a seven-member ring. This compound proved ineffective in quieting agitated psychotic patients but very effective for selected mood disorders.[7]

The search for chemically related compounds yielded a number of additional drugs. Clomipramine, amitriptyline, and doxepin are all derivatives of imipramine.[7] Each contains a tertiary amine at one of the substitution sites on the seven-member ring. Desipramine, a major metabolite of imipramine, and nortriptyline, the *N*-demethylated metabolite of amitriptyline, are secondary amine tricyclics. Protriptyline and trimipramine are other TCAs with few veterinary applications.[3] Differences in the effects of NT reuptake vary with the different amine structures.[7]

Mechanism of Action

The mechanism of action of the TCAs (and MAO inhibitors and SSRIs) is blockade of the mechanisms of physiologic inactivation (see Figure 26-1). For the TCAs the mechanism is inhibition of reuptake at presynaptic biogenic amine NT receptors in the brain. As reuptake is inhibited, the concentration of NTs increases, prolonging their actions (CNS stimulation). Differences in NTs affected reflect, in part, the chemical structures.[7] Imipramine and its derivatives with a tertiary amine side chain block norepinephrine reuptake but have little effect on dopamine reuptake.

The secondary amine derivatives of imipramine are potent and highly selective inhibitors of norepinephrine reuptake; however, they are characterized by fewer autonomic and anticholinergic effects. Tertiary amines that are metabolized in the patient to secondary amines will have effects on norepinephrine reuptake. Clomipramine has marked effects on serotonin reuptake and minimal effects on other NTs or receptors, although a poorly understood dopaminergic effect has been described. Its active metabolite appears to inhibit norepinephrine uptake as well.[16] Doxepin is characterized by greater antihistaminergic actions (thus explaining its frequent recommendation for chronic pruritus). Although amitriptyline is the most commonly prescribed drug for animals, clomipramine has recently been approved for treatment of separation anxiety in dogs.

The effect of clomipramine (3 mg/kg once daily orally for 6 weeks) on the concentration of monoamines (5HIAA [5-hydroxyindoleacetic acid], HVI [homovanillic acid] and MHPG [methoxy4-hydroxyphenylglycol]) in the cerebrospinal fluid was compared with that of placebo using a randomized crossover design in otherwise behaviorally normal dogs (n = 6) with obsessive-compulsive disorders (OCDs).[16] The concentration of monoamines did not significantly differ (power of the study now known), leading the authors to conclude that clomipramine did not affect monoamine turnover in the brains of behaviorally normal dogs, further confirming the need for studies in affected dogs.

Pharmacologic Effects

Adaptation to pharmacologic effects. The effects of TCAs at presynaptic and postsynaptic receptors and autoregulation result in complex responses that are not well understood. Although inhibition of reuptake occurs very rapidly, peak effects still take several weeks. This prolonged time to maximal effect reflects in part disposition (e.g., time to steady-state for the parent compound and active metabolites; see later discussion of clinical pharmacology) but also appears to reflect adaptation in the CNS to changes in NT concentrations at the synapse. Administration of a TCA results in an immediate decrease in the synthesis and release of norepinephrine or serotonin (depending on the major target of the TCA) in selected areas of the brain. The effects appear to be mediated presynaptically through autoreceptors (α_2 or serotonin, respectively). Turnover, however, gradually normalizes within 1 to 3 weeks. Autoreceptors appear to be downregulated and become desensitized to the presence of the TCA.[7] The number and sensitivity of postsynaptic adrenergic receptors do not appear to be affected by continued use of a TCA.

Adaptive responses appear to influence the pharmacologic properties of TCAs at adrenergic receptor sites. The TCAs have a moderate affinity for α_1-receptors and only limited affinity for α_2-receptors and β-receptors. Changes in serotonin receptors after repeated treatment with TCAs are complex. Although the impact is not clear, the general effect appears to be increased sensitivity to serotonin. This may be an important component to the outcome of prolonged treatment.[7] The TCAs also appear to influence the effect of other NTs and their receptors, including GABA (unknown significance), and dopamine (D_2; desensitization of autoreceptors resulting in mood elevation). Other factors to consider regarding adaptation to TCA effects include changes in adenosine monophosphate–dependent protein kinases and potential changes at the level of gene expression.[7]

In addition to tolerance (to sedative and autonomic effects), physical dependence on the TCA can develop. Physical dependence after acute withdrawal is manifested in human patients as malaise, chills, coryza (head cold), and muscle aches.[7] Slow discontinuation of the drug is recommended.

Autonomic nervous system. The predominant effect of TCAs on the autonomic nervous system appears to reflect inhibition of norepinephrine transport into adrenergic nerve terminals and antagonism of muscarinic cholinergic and α_1-adrenergic responses to the NTs. Blurred vision, dry mouth, constipation, and urinary retention at therapeutic doses (documented in humans) appear to reflect anticholinergic effects.[7]

Cardiovascular system. Cardiovascular effects of TCAs occur at therapeutic doses and can become life threatening with overdose. Postural hypotension occurs in humans (unlikely in dogs or cats) as a result of α-adrenergic blockade. Mild sinus tachycardia results from inhibition of norepinephrine uptake and muscarinic (M_1) blockade.[7] Conduction time is prolonged, especially at concentrations above 200 ng/mL. The TCA can also directly suppress the myocardium.[7] The myocardial depressant effects are greater in the presence of underlying cardiac disease.

Clinical Pharmacology

The disposition of the TCA favors adverse reactions in that the characteristics of disposition are those that tend to vary greatly among animals, and extrapolation between species is complicated. Unfortunately, the disposition has not been scientifically studied in animals except for clomipramine, and information for other drugs or species is extrapolated from human or canine data. The TCAs are very lipophilic. As such, they are well absorbed after oral administration. They can, however, undergo marked first-pass metabolism. Typical drug concentrations achieved in humans at recommended doses are 100 to 250 ng/mL for amitriptyline, 150 to 500 ng/mL for clomipramine, and 200 to 300 ng/mL for imipramine.[7] High doses can cause anticholinergic effects on the gastrointestinal tract, slowing absorption or making it erratic. Absorption in humans can result in peak concentrations as rapidly as 2 hours or as long as 12 hours after administration.[7] The drugs are very highly protein bound, but unbound drug is characterized by a very large volume of distribution (10 to 15 L/kg in human patients), contributing to a long elimination half-life of the parent drug or its metabolites. Drug may bind avidly to selected tissues.

Drugs are eliminated by hepatic (oxidative) metabolism with the main reaction being N-demethylation to the active metabolite, desmethylclomipramine (DCMP). This reaction is catalyzed by CYP3A4, CYP2C19, CYP2C9, and CYP1A2. The parent and metabolite are hydroxylated by CYP2D6 and then glucuronidated.[17,18] Metabolism is variable among human and canine patients, accounting for plasma concentrations that differ by tenfold to thirtyfold. Species and gender differences in metabolism or pharmacokinetics have been demonstrated for clompramine.[17,18] Metabolism of TCA yields active and inactive metabolites. It is not clear what percentage of the antidepressant activity of the TCA is associated with the metabolites. Metabolites generally have an elimination half-life that is twice or more that of the parent compound.[7] Thus accumulation of the metabolites can result in a marked proportion of the pharmacologic effect of TCAs.

Clomipramine is approved for use in dogs for treatment of separation anxiety. After multiple oral administration in dogs, both clomipramine and its principal active metabolite, desmethylclomipramine, accumulate in a dose-dependent manner at doses ranging from 1 to 4 mg/kg.[19] Food does not appear to alter the rate or the extent of oral absorption,[20] with bioavailability of clomipramine being 20% and of the metabolite 140%. The ratio of metabolite to parent in dogs approximates 0.6, varying across time.[21] After a single dose of 3 mg/kg in normal dogs (n = 6), clomipramine C_{max} was quite variable for both clomipramine (16 to 310 ng/mL at 0.75 to 3.1 hr) and desmethylclomipramine (21 to 134 ng/mL at 1.4 to 8.8 hr).[22] After multiple dosing, (28 d) clomipramine C_{max} again was markedly variable at 43 to 222 ng/mL (at 3 to 8 hr), compared with 21 to 134 ng/mL at 1.4 to 8.8 hr, for desmethylclomipramine. Hewson and coworkers[21] reported trough concentrations of clomipramine ranging from 2 to 17 ng/mL and desmethylclomipramine ranging from 2 to 15 ng/mL following 26 days of dosing at 3 mg/kg; neither compound was detectable in three of six dogs at trough times (24 hr). Protein binding of both the parent compound and its metabolite are greater than 96%. Hepatic clearance of clomipramine in dogs is flow-limited; changes in hepatic blood flow, but not hepatic mass (i.e., CYP activity), should be expected to alter clomipramine elimination. However, rapid clearance is balanced by a very large volume of distribution. Despite this large volume, clomipramine elimination half-life is shorter and markedly variable in dogs ranging from 1.2 to 16 hours after a single oral dose in dogs (n = 6) compared to 20 in humans. After multiple (28 days) dosing, both variability and duration of half-life decreased to 1.5 to 9 hours.[21] An average half-life of 5 to 6 hours was reported for dogs in a subsequent study.[19] Half-life of the desmethyl clomipramine in dogs also is short (2 to 3.8 hours, compared to 36 hours in humans),[19,21] with total concentration of the metabolite being less than that of the parent compound. Steady-state concentrations are reached by 4 days or less, resulting in response within 1 to 2 weeks. Cats metabolize (based on in vitro hepatic microsomal studies) clomipramine more slowly than do dog or rats, with male cats being less efficient metabolizers.[17] The pharmacokinetics of clomipramine and its major metabolite desmethylclomipramine have been described in cats (n = 6) using a randomized crossover single-dose oral (0.5 mg/kg) and intravenous (0.25 mg/kg) administration study).[23] After oral administration, C_{max} (μg/mL) was

0.87 ng/mL at 6.2 hours. After intravenous administration, volume of distribution and clearance were 0.393 L/kg and 0.833 mL * min/kg, respectively, resulting in an elimination half-life of 12.3 hours. Area under the curve (AUC) of clomipramine and desmethylclomipramine after oral administration were 948 and 613 ng * min/mL, respectively. Oral bioavailability of clomipramine and its active metabolite approximated 30%. Variability among cats was marked. On the basis of these data, Lainesse and coworkers[18] found no correlation between either clomipramine or desmethylclomipramine concentrations and sleep scores. However, gender differences in metabolism may have contributed to the lack of correlation.

KEY POINT 26-3 For a number of the behavior-modifying drugs, slow elimination and formation of active metabolites complicate the design of dosing regimens.

Of the TCAs, only amitriptyline appears to have been studied after transdermal delivery in cats. Plasma drug concentrations were not detectable in cats (n = 6) receiving a single 5-mg transdermal (pluronic lecithin organo [PLO]) gel dose. This compared with a mean peak concentration of 61 ± 6.2 ng/mL after oral administration of 5 mg.[24] The author has demonstrated, using a randomized crossover, dummy-placebo controlled design, that although amitryptylline administered as a transdermal gel achieved detectable concentrations in 5/6 cats receiving 2 mg/kg twice daily for 3 weeks, bioavailability was very poor. After 3 weeks of dosing, serum drug concentrations were 46 to 101 ng/mL after gel administration compared to 1336 to 5230 ng/mL after oral administration at the same dose. The disappearance half-life in the cats receiving the oral drug (based on peak and trough dosing) was markedly variable among cats, ranging from 20 to approximately 85 hrs after 3 weeks. Two of the cats receiving the gel developed marked aural erythema and scaling. Despite the very high concentrations, 4/5 cats tolerated the oral administration well; the one cat with concentrations of 5230 ng/mL was depressed, with resolution occurring once the drug was discontinued. Interestingly, disappearance half-life of amitryptyilline was only 20 hrs in this cat, suggesting that oral bioavailabilitymay have been contributing to the high serum concentrations.

Side effects. Up to 5% of human patients receiving a TCA react adversely. Sedation is common with the TCAs.[3] The most common reactions reflect antimuscarinic effect or overdosing. Cardiac toxicity (reflecting a quinidine-like membrane-stabilizing effect) is a less frequently reported but serious effect, but not apparently with clomipramine administration in dogs. The effect may be lethal at 15 mg/kg.[4] Tachycardia may also reflect anticholinergic effects and must be differentiated from true cardiotoxicity. Other side effects include dry mouth, gastric distress, constipation, dizziness, tachycardia, or other arrhythmias, blurred vision, and urinary retention (particularly problematic in the presence of prostatic hypertrophy).[7] Weakness and fatigue reflect CNS effects. Cardiac toxicity is more likely in patients who start therapy with cardiac disease. In healthy patients the most likely cardiac response is hypotension as a result of α-adrenergic blockade.

An undesirable side effect of antidepressant drugs in humans is referred to as the "switch process." Patients undergo a transition from depression to hypomanic or manic excitement.[7] This effect has not been reported in animals. Confusion and delirium are behavior aberrations that occur commonly in human patients, with the incidence of 10% in all patients, increasing to more than 30% in elderly patients over age 50 years.[7] Miscellaneous toxic effects in human patients include leukopenia, jaundice, and skin rashes. Weight gain occurs, particularly with those drugs that are selective for serotonin reuptake. Isolated reports that address the side effects of TCAs in dogs are uncommon. Goldberger and Rapoport[25] reported side effects in 5 of 13 dogs receiving clomipramine for lick granuloma. Clinical signs included lethargy, anorexia, diarrhea, and growling.

Acute poisoning with TCAs is common in human patients (accidental or intentional) and appears to be a significant potential problem in animals.[26] Symptoms in humans vary and are complex. Excitement and restlessness may be accompanied by myoclonus or tonic–clonic seizures. Coma may rapidly develop, associated with depressed expiration, hypoxia, hypothermia, and hypotension.[7] Anticholinergic effects include mydriasis, dry mucosa, absent bowel sounds, urinary retention, and cardiac arrhythmias, including tachycardia. Clinical signs reported after accidental ingestion in animals[26] include hyperexcitement and vomiting as early manifestations, followed by ataxia, lethargy, and muscular tremors. Bradycardia and other cardiac arrhythmias occur later. These later signs occurred shortly before death in experimental animal models of TCA toxicosis.[26]

Treatment for TCA toxicosis is supportive, including respiratory (intubation) and cardiovascular support. Gastric lavage with activated charcoal can be used early. Emetics probably should be avoided because of the risk of aspiration pneumonia in seizuring animals (some antiemetics may further predispose the animal to seizures). Short-acting barbiturates (or similar drugs) without pre-administration of atropine are preferred for anesthetic control during gastric lavage. Cathartics (sorbitol or sodium sulfate–Glauber's salt) can be of benefit. Magnesium sulfate should not be used because impaired gastrointestinal motility can facilitate absorption of magnesium. Resolution of coma may require several days; the threat of cardiac arrhythmias likewise persists for several days. Pharmacologic interventions for cardiac arrhythmias have not been well established. Alkalinization (sodium bicarbonate sufficient to maintain blood pH above 7.5: 2 to 3 mEq/kg, administered intravenously over 15 to 30 minutes) may prevent death by increasing protein binding and increasing cardiac automaticity (as a result of potassium shifts).[26] Traditional cardiac drugs, including antiarrhythmics and digoxin, are contraindicated in human patients. However, phenytoin may provide safe antiarrhythmic effects and in human patients is useful for treatment of seizures.[7] Relevance to dogs or cats is not clear: phenytoin has a short half-life in dogs and is associated with adverse events when administered IV (see Chapter 27). Diazepam is indicated for acute management of seizures. β-adrenergic receptor antagonists and lidocaine may be useful.[7] The risk of tonic–clonic seizures is increased in human patients, particularly at high doses.

Clomipramine generally is associated with less sedation than with the other TCAs.[27] Systemic phospholipidosis (excessive accumulation of phospholipids in tissues) occurs with chronic administration of cationic, amphophilic drugs, including the TCAs, and fluoxetine.

Indications

The TCAs have been recommended among animal behaviorists for most abnormal behaviors manifested in dogs or cats. These include, but are not limited to, behaviors associated with fear and aggression,[27,28] stereotypics, OCDs or self-mutilation disorders, and excessive barking. The use of clomipramine is discussed later with specific disorders. However, using an open trial, Seksel and Lindeman[29] reported the efficacy and tolerance of clomipramine (1 to 2 mg/kg every 12 hours for the initial dose, increased up to 4 mg/kg twice daily) in a variety of behavioral disorders in dogs (n = 24). Included in the study were OCD (n = 9), separation anxiety (n = 14), and noise phobia (n = 4). Treatment included behavior modification and continued for at least 1 month after resolution of clinical signs. Resolution to marked improvement of clinical signs was reported in 67% of the dogs, whereas 21% reported slight to moderate improvement versus no change in 12.5% (3 of 24) animals. Clomipramine discontinuation (without return of the abnormal behavior) was described as successful in five of the nine animals in which it was attempted.

KEY POINT 26-4 The tricyclic antidepressants have been recommended among animal behaviorists for most abnormal behaviors manifested in dogs or cats. These include, but are not limited to, behaviors associated with fear and aggression, stereotypes, obsessive–compulsive or self-mutilation disorders, and excessive barking.

Contraindications

The TCAs are not recommended for animals with a metabolic disease. Specific contraindications include a history of cardiac or hepatic disease, seizures, glaucoma, hyperthyroidism, and thyroid hormone supplementation.[27,28]

Drug Interactions

The TCAs can interact with a number of other drugs. Competition for protein-binding sites with other highly protein-bound drugs can result in increased drug concentrations; however, this may be balanced by increased hepatic clearance. Drugs that affect drug-metabolizing enzymes, through either inhibition or induction, also affect the clearance of TCAs. The sequelae of the impact are difficult to predict because active metabolites similarly are affected. In general, however, drugs that inhibit metabolism are likely to result in greater drug accumulation and increased risk of toxicity. TCAs and other antidepressants also can compete with other compounds for metabolism. The drugs themselves may affect metabolism of other drugs. Clomipramine inhibits the metabolism of other drugs; but a more relevant interaction may be the impact of other drugs on the metabolism of clomipramine (e.g., cimetidine).[7] The antidepressants potentiate the effects of sedative drugs. The TCAs should not be used in combination with other drugs that modify CNS NTs. Included are MAO inhibitors and amitraz.[27,28] In human patients a potentially lethal interaction has been reported when a TCA, particularly one that inhibits serotonin uptake, is combined with an MAO.[7] The term *serotonin syndrome* has been applied to this interaction, which is characterized by restlessness, muscle twitches, hyperreflexia, shivering, and tremors.[30] Drugs or herbal products whose combination might result in the serotonin syndrome are indicated in Table 26-2.

Clinical Use

Most drugs take 2 to 3 weeks for clinical efficacy to be realized. The exception might be amitriptyline, which may cause a response in 3 to 5 days; however, maximum response may take longer, particularly in cats, for which the half-life may be long.[27] Dogs can respond to clomipramine in 1 to 2 weeks. In an approval study, clomipramine (Clomicalm) treatment

Table 26-2 Drugs or Supplements Whose Combined Use Increases the Risk of Serotonin Syndrome

Drug Class	Interacting Drug Class	Example Drugs
Monamine oxidase inhibitors	Tricyclic antidepressants	Amitriptyline
		Imipramine
		Clomipramine
	Miscellaneous	Isocarboxazid
		Phenelzine
Serotonin uptake inhibitors	SSRI	Fluoxetine
		Fluvoxamine
		Paroxetine
		Sertraline
		Citalopram
	Serotonin and norepinephrine uptake inhibitors	Trazazone
Bupriopion		Venlaflaxine
Opioids		Fentanyl
		Mepiridine
		Tramadol
		Dextromethorphan
Antimicrobials	Antibacterials	Linesolid
	Antivirals	Ritonavir
Antiemetics		Metoclopramide
		Ondansetron
		Granisetron
Herbals		St. John's wort
		SAMe
		Ginseng
Substances of abuse		MDMA
		Cocaine

with behavior modification improved separation anxiety in dogs compared with behavior modification alone (according to package insert). King and coworkers[31,32] (manufacturer sponsored studies) studied the efficacy of clomipramine for treatment of separation anxiety in dogs. Using a parallel, randomized, double-blinded design, researchers gave dogs with "hyper attachment" behavior (n = 97) either a low dose (0.5 to 1 mg/kg twice daily; n = 25), a standard dose (1 to <2 mg/kg twice daily; n = 28), or no dose of clomipramine (n = 32) along with behavior therapy for 12 weeks. At each of three assessment periods, treatment dogs responded better, and overall, to therapies three times more rapidly than nontreatment dogs in all behaviors (destructive or inappropriate elimination) with the exception of vocalization. Among the treatment dogs was an epileptic; this dog had no seizure episodes during the treatment period. Differences in the frequency of side effects among treatment groups were vomiting and gastritis, which occurred in 13/25 and 8/28 dogs in the low and standard group, respectively, compared with three in the placebo group, and lethargy or sleepiness in four of the standard group compared with two in the other two groups. Interestingly, one healthy dog collapsed with hyperthermia (111°F) and disseminated intravascular coagulopathy. No other underlying illness was reported; the dog survived the episode, but clomipramine was discontinued. In their follow-up questionnaire-based study,[32] 12 dogs continued to receive clomipramine long term (13 to 16 months or more), with 10 of these dogs improving further. No increases in adverse events were identified. Behavior changes were also studied in dogs for which the drug was either discontinued (n = 48) or had not been administered within 4 months of the questionnaire (n = 16). However, the data are confounded by the use of other behavior-modifying drugs. Behaviors worsened in the first 2 weeks after therapy was discontinued in three of ten dogs receiving low-dose clomipramine; however, no dogs in the standard-dose group exhibited clinical signs potentially consistent with withdrawal. For treatment groups, after 2 weeks behavior worsened in 13% to 15% of dogs compared with 23% of dogs receiving placebo. Six of nine dogs for which clinical signs worsened had not responded totally to therapy during the trial, whereas three of nine had been considered successes. The time to worsening was longest for the standard dose group. On the basis of response to clomipramine, the authors raised the possibility that treatment accompanied by behavioral therapy might allow permanent control.

Clomipramine has been studied for acute management of anxiety in dogs. Frank and coworkers[33] prospectively studied transport-induced stress in Beagles treated with clomipramine (2 mg/kg twice daily for 7 days). Compared with placebo, treatment only tended to reduce clinical signs of panting or drooling; however, cortisol concentrations increased less in treated versus untreated controls after three 1-hour trips.

Therapeutic drug monitoring may facilitate the safe and effective use of the drugs. In human patients plasma concentrations that range between 100 and 250 ng/mL are most likely to cause satisfactory antidepressant effects; toxicity can be expected at concentrations above 500 ng/mL, with fatal consequences likely as concentrations approach 1000 ng/mL.[7] Variability among human patients (and presumably among animals) supports the use of monitoring to guide therapy. Monitoring to avoid toxicity is, however, complicated by the recognition that serum concentrations by themselves are not reliable predictors of toxic responses. Because of the risk of withdrawal associated with physical dependence, discontinuation of TCAs should occur over a week or longer if therapy has been prolonged.[7]

Selective Serotonin Reuptake Inhibitors

Structure–Activity Relationships and Mechanism of Action

The SSRIs enhance CNS serotonin by blocking presynaptic neuronal uptake (see Figure 26-1). They may also increase postsynaptic receptor sensitivity.[3] Among the drugs currently approved for use in humans are fluoxetine, paroxetine, sertraline, and fluvoxamine. Of these, sertraline appears more potent (see the discussion of monitoring).[7] Potency of fluoxetine for 5-HT receptors is similar to that of amitriptyline, but much less than that of amitryptyline for adrenergic, histaminic, muscarinic, opiate, or dopaminergic receptors. Consequently, fluoxetine is considered selective for serotonin. Because of their selectivity for serotonin uptake, the diverse effects that characterize TCAs are generally absent with SSRIs. Fluoxetine is prepared as a 50:50 racemic mixture; enantiomers are equally potent for 5-HT receptors although it is not clear if this is true for all species. However, for the metabolite (also racemic), the S metabolite isomer is fourteenfold more potent than the R isomer for 5-HT receptors.[34]

The lag time described for maximal efficacy of fluoxetine may reflect, in part, its impact on serotonin reuptake: Initially, increased serotonin in the somatodendritic area leads to $5\text{-HT}_{(1A)}$ downregulation or desensitization. Aznavour and coworkers[35] described response of $5\text{-HT}_{(1A)}$ receptors in the brains of cats to acute and chronic administration of fluoxetine. Described as the primary target of SSRI, these receptors are autoreceptors that inhibit the firing and release of serotonin by the neurons they regulate. They are activated in response to increased serotonin concentrations in the synapse associated with SSRI treatment. Their ability to inhibit 5-HT neuronal firing and release, however, is muted by desensitization associated with acute SSRI (or other agonist) therapy. Although initially transient, in 2 to 3 weeks this desensitization allows a return to baseline firing and release and is paramount for successful therapy with SSRI. The acute desensitization probably reflects internalization of the autoreceptors. In cats therapy with 5 mg/kg fluoxetine intravenously resulted in a marked decrease in $5HT_{(1A)}$ binding in the nucleus raphe dorsalis but not other regions of the brain. However, with chronic administration (5 mg/kg subcutaneously per day for 3 weeks), binding was not altered in any region of the brain, indicating that 5-HT_1 autoreceptors are fully desensitized and 5-HT neuronal firing returns to baseline, at least in healthy cats.

KEY POINT 26-5 A lag time should be expected for the maximum effect of selective serotonin inhibitors, particularly for drugs (and their active metabolites) characterized by long elimination half-lives.

Clinical Pharmacology

As with the TCAs, the clinical pharmacology of the SSRIs is complicated. Plasma concentrations thought to be effective for human patients range from 100 to 300 ng/mL for fluoxetine (and its active metabolites). Effective concentrations for paroxetine and sertraline are 30 to 100 and 25 to 50 ng/mL, respectively.[7] Fluoxetine disposition is characterized by high protein binding, metabolism to an active compound, long elimination half-life of both parent and metabolite, a delayed onset of action, and drug interactions.[7] For both the dog and the cat, because the active metabolite norfluoxetine represents a substantial, if not dominant, portion of the AUC (exposure), response to therapy cannot be evaluated at least until both fluoxetine and its metabolite reach steady state (approximately 10 to 14 days).

Fluoxetine is available as a chewable tablet approved for use in dogs. A number of efficacy studies were implemented during the approval process. Pasloske[34] reviewed fluoxetine disposition in dogs and cat in abstract form. In Beagles, after administration of a single 1 mg/kg dose, oral bioavailability averaged 72%, yielding a C_{max} for fluoxetine of 49 ng/mL at 1.8 hours, and for norfluoxetine 79 ng/mL. As in humans, the volume of distribution for fluoxetine is large in dogs, averaging 39 L/kg, reflecting accumulation that approximates a 100-fold increase compared with plasma in some tissues. Despite the very large volume of distribution of fluoxetine, elimination half-life averaged between 6 and 10 hours in Beagles. Norfluoxetine is the major metabolite formed from hepatic metabolism, accounting for more than 56% of the total peak area in dogs. The volume of distribution of norfluoxetine is one third of that for fluoxetine, at 10.7 L/kg, yet the elimination half-life of 48 to 57 hours for the metabolite is much longer than that of fluoxetine. The shorter half-life of fluoxetine compared with that of its metabolite reflects, in part, fluoxetine clearance, which, at 6 mL/kg/min, is threefold higher that that for norfluoxetine at 2 mL/kg/min.[34] The AUC for the S-isomer of fluoxetine (14 times more potent than R) was threefold higher than that for the R-isomer.

The disposition of fluoxetine also has been reported in cats receiving 1 mg/kg. Oral bioavailability approximates 100%; C_{max} is 83 ng/mL (at approximately 2 hours), compared with 25 ng/mL (at 40 hours) for norfluoxetine. The elimination half-life (0.5 mg/kg intravenously) of fluoxetine in cats is 34 to 47 hours, which is much longer than that in dogs. The volume of distribution in cats is smaller (by 50%) than that in dogs (18 L/kg), whereas clearance is similar (6.4 L/kg). The metabolite has a much larger volume of distribution compared with the parent in cats (32.6 L/kg), resulting in a longer elimination half-life (51 to 55 hours) for the metabolite (although clearance is similar to the parent at 7.4 mL/kg/min).

Whereas gradual withdrawal may not be necessary for fluoxetine because of its long half-life (including the metabolite), the same is not true for paroxetine, sertraline, or fluvoxamine. Several weeks of decreasing dosing should follow chronic dosing.

Fluoxetine has been studied after administration of a single dose as a PLO transdermal gel in cats (n = 12) at either 5 or 10 mg/kg, compared with 1 mg/kg orally.[36] For oral administration C_{max} of 94.8 ± 34 ng/mL was achieved at 8.5 ± 2.9 hours, with AUC being 5.4 ± 2.4 μg*hr/mL. This compares to a C_{max} of 23 ± 20.2 at 51 ± 28 hours for 5 mg/kg transdermal (AUC = 2.9 ± 1.8) and 33 ± 9.1 (C_{max}) at 87 ± 34 hours (AUC of 5.4 ± 0.5 μg*hr/mL) at 10 mg/kg. Although this study demonstrated systemic absorption of fluoxetine that approximated oral administration after transdermal administration (at 10 times the oral dose), single doses may not have been sufficient to generate therapeutic concentrations. Further, the variability in drug concentrations achieved was substantial, suggesting that absorption may not be predictable among animals. Because both the parent compound and metabolite have a long half-life in the cat, accumulation to effective concentrations may increase the potential efficacy after transdermal administration. Monitoring of the parent compound to document drug absorption after transdermal delivery should be considered. Although cats in this aforementioned study tolerated a single 10 mg/kg transdermal dose well, a second study of multiple dosing was terminated because of substantial dermal irritation after several days of therapy.[7,36]

Drug Interactions

Fluoxetine may inhibit its own metabolism through inhibition (both parent and metabolite) of CYPIID6-mediated demethylation.[34] The SSRIs also can inhibit the metabolism of other drugs; the order of potency of inhibition is paroxetine>norfluoxetine>fluoxetine=sertraline. Because of the risk of drug interactions, SSRIs should not be used in combination with other antidepressants (see earlier discussion of serotonin syndrome and drug interactions of TCAs and MAO inhibitors).[7] Fluvoxamine minimally affects drug metabolism.

Side Effects

As a class, the SSRIs are generally considered safer than TCA in humans. Exceptions may occur for clomipramine in dogs. Unlike the TCAs, SSRIs have minimal effects on the cardiovascular system.[7] Their safety for patients with underlying cardiac disease has not, however, been established. Sedation is not a common side effect and is least likely with fluoxetine.[3] In humans gastrointestinal side effects are the most common, occurring in as many as 25% of patients receiving the drug.[3] Their incidence is minimized by starting with a low dose and gradually increasing the dose until efficacy is evident.

Toxicity of fluoxetine has been studied in both dogs and cats.[34,37] Steinberg and coworkers[37] found no adverse cardiovascular effects of fluoxetine in anesthetized dogs, concluding that it was thus safer than tricyclic antidepressants. Beagles survived up to 100 mg/kg when fluoxetine was administered as a single dose, although emesis, mydriasis, tremors, and anorexia occurred. In contrast, with multiple dosing dogs could not tolerate 10 to 20 mg/kg orally per day for 6 months.[34] Intolerance was manifested as tremors, anorexia, slow or incomplete pupillary response, mydriasis, aggressive behavior, nystagmus, emesis, hypoactivity, and ataxia. Aggressive behavior and anorexia also were evident. All of the physical signs of toxicity were reversible within 2 months of drug discontinuation. Tremors, slow or incomplete pupillary response, and occasional anorexia may be present at 1 mg/kg. Histologically, phospholipidosis occurred in the lung, liver, adrenals, lymph nodes, spleen, and peripheral leukocytes at 20 mg/kg and occasionally in the lung and leukocytes at 1 mg/kg. Cats receiving a single dose of 50 mg/kg also developed emesis, mydriasis, tremors, and anorexia. Oral administration to cats of 1 and 3 mg/kg once daily was well tolerated, although sporadic anorexia and vomiting occurred occasionally at 3 mg/kg. At 5 mg/kg daily, toxicity appeared at approximately 60 days and was manifested as body tremors, hypoactivity, convulsions, low food consumption, and dehydration. In contrast to dogs, for which cardiovascular depression did not occur, heart rates decreased in a non–dose-dependent manner in cats. Infiltration of alveolar macrophages, consistent with phospholipidosis, occurred at 3 and 5 mg/kg daily. At 5 mg/kg, centrilobular hepatocellular degeneration and decreased T-lymphocytes were detected.

Side effects also have been reported in animals after clinical use. In 4 of 14 dogs receiving fluoxetine for treatment of lick granuloma,[38] side effects included lethargy, anorexia, and hyperactivity. Another study[39] reported the same side effects as well as polydipsia, diarrhea, and increased or decreased appetite. At least 50% of animals appeared to develop some type of side effect, although side effects were described as mild. Side effects reported by owners in a study of fluoxetine for treatment of canine dominance-related aggression included fatigue, lethargy, and decreased appetite.[40]

A very early study[41] demonstrated that fluoxetine potentiates morphine hyperthermia in cats. Although SSRIs are considered stimulatory in the sense that serotonin increases and might thus be considered proconvulsant, Jobe and Browning[42] argued that they may, in fact, be anticonvulsant and that deficiencies in norepinephrine and serotonin contribute to proconvulsant tendencies.

Citalopram is the most recent SSRI to be approved for use in the United States. However, its approval was delayed after a study in which 50% of dogs receiving 8 mg/kg as part of a preapproval toxicity study (for humans) died as a result of cardiac side effects at 17 to 31 weeks of therapy. Therefore the drug probably should not be used in dogs. Diarrhea is a side effect reported for both paroxetine and sertraline. Paroxetine may be more likely than fluoxetine to cause anticholinergic side effects.[4] Initiating therapy with a low dose that is increased after the first week of therapy may prevent this side effect. Paroxetine also is associated with an idiosyncratic, dose-dependent increase in arousal, awakening, and rapid eye movement suppression in dogs.[4]

Clinical Indications and Use

Clinical use also is addressed with specific indications. Probably no behavior-modifying drug has received more attention in the veterinary and lay literature than fluoxetine.[43,44] Despite the plethora of opinions or testimonials regarding the efficacy of this drug for treatment of animal behavioral disorders, few scientific studies existed until its approval in dogs. Efficacy for treatment of lick granulomas is supported by a double-blind crossover study.[38] One third of the animals studied did not repeat the abnormal behavior when fluoxetine was discontinued. Fluoxetine also has been studied in an open (nonblinded) study of dogs with a variety of behavioral problems.[39] Approximately 65% of dogs with lick granuloma, 100% of animals with separation anxiety, and 85% of animals with tail mutilation disorders responded to fluoxetine. Unfortunately, data were not controlled for other treatments, making interpretation of the success of fluoxetine in this study difficult. The Freedom of Information Act file delineates several clinical trials of field studies that support its use. In a European study, doses of 1 to 4 mg/kg for 2 to 4 weeks were associated with improvement in 80% of dogs (n = 47) with separation anxiety. The most frequent adverse reactions were anorexia, weight loss, constipation, mydriasis and muscle tremors; clinical signs were considered unacceptable at 3 mg/kg. A field trial found improvement compared with control (n = 112) in dogs (n = 117) with separation anxiety treated for 56 days with fluoxetine therapy (1 to 2 mg/kg). All dogs received behavior modification. One dog in the control and three in the treatment groups developed seizures. Seizures developed 10 days after the end of therapy in one dog (this dog eventually died as a result of seizures), 45 days into therapy and 24 days into therapy. Simpson and coworkers[45] and Landsberg and coworkers[46] reported on the efficacy of fluoxetine for treatment of separation anxiety based on manufacturer-sponsored studies. A multicenter placebo-controlled, parallel double-blinded study was implemented in dogs (n = 208) with separation anxiety using fluoxetine (1-2 mg/kg) as a chewable tablet; treatment occurred for 6 weeks. At each week, dogs in the treatment group had improved compared with those receiving placebo; improvement occurred even in those dogs not receiving behavior modification. Destructive behavior and inappropriate urination were reduced. Seizures occurred in one dog in each group.

Fluoxetine also has been used successfully to treat psychogenic alopecia in a cat,[47] dominance aggression in dogs,[40] and inappropriate urination in cats.[48] As with TCAs, monitoring to guide therapy with SSRI is complicated. Effective concentrations have not been established in animals and must be extrapolated from human studies. The relationship between plasma drug concentrations and therapeutic efficacy has not been well established[3] and is complicated by the presence of the active metabolite, which cannot be predicted by the parent compound. Paroxetine and fluvoxamine have no active metabolites (in human patients). One advantage of paroxetine over fluoxetine in veterinary medicine is convenience in dosing with the availability of multiple tablet sizes and scored tablets.

Atypical Antidepressants

Trazodone is a mixed serotonergic agonist–antagonist used to treat sleep disorders and major depression in humans. It is characterized by a wide therapeutic range (typical drug concentrations in humans after administration of the recommended dose are 800 to 1600 ng/mL.[7] The likelihood of drug interactions appears to be limited, despite the fact that it is an inhibitor of CYP2D6 metabolism. It has been used in dogs to treat mild thunderstorm phobias either as sole therapy or in combination with a TCA or SSRI. It does not appear to be effective, even at high doses (10 mg/kg), for treatment of severe thunderstorm phobias in dogs. Side effects reported in dogs include vomiting, diarrhea, and sedation. Initiating therapy at a low dose with a gradual increase may minimize this side effect.

Monoamine Oxidase Inhibitors

Structure–Activity Relationships

The recognition that the antitubercular drug isoniazid tended to elevate the mood of patients receiving the drug for treatment of tuberculosis led to further discovery of drugs that inhibit MAO. The first drugs used were structurally related to hydrazine and were associated with marked hepatotoxicity. An attempt was made to synthesize CNS-stimulant compounds unrelated to hydrazine but similar to amphetamine. Ultimately, selegiline was a result of this later effort.[7]

The MAO inhibitors potentially affect a variety of monoamines by inhibiting mitochondrial MAO and the subsequent degradation of monoamines, most notably dopamine (see Figure 26-1). Most of the clinically relevant drugs are nonselective toward two major enzyme groups[7] that are characterized by different substrate specificities. MAO-A prefers serotonin and is inhibited by clorgyline, an MAO-A–selective inhibitor, whereas MAO-B prefers phenylethylamine and is inhibited by selegiline (deprenyl). Selegiline is the only currently used MAO inhibitor characterized by selectivity. The drug targets MAO-B and is relatively selective for dopamine. It is approved for use in dogs for treatment of pituitary-dependent hyperadrenocorticism (purported to be a dopamine deficiency) and cognitive dysfunctions. Binding to the MAO is irreversible, and recovery from effects requires synthesis of new enzyme. In human patients this appears to require 1 to 2 weeks. Metabolism occurs more slowly in geriatric patients.[7]

Pharmacologic Effects

The potential antiepileptic effects of selegilinle[49,50] are briefly addressed in Chapter 27. The behavioral effects of the MAO inhibitors occur on systems affected by sympathomimetic amines and serotonin. Although as a class the MAO inhibitors inhibit a number of enzyme systems other than MAO, generalizations to the class do not necessarily apply to selegiline. Selegiline potentiates dopamine in selected neurons and has been approved to treat Parkinson's disease in humans and cognitive dysfunctions in animals, conditions assumed to be associated with dopamine deficiency. Selegiline also scavenges oxygen radicals and reduces neuronal damage caused by reactive products of oxidative metabolism of dopamine or other compounds.[7] A delay in the therapeutic effect of up to 2 or more weeks characterizes the use of selegiline. Reasons for the delay are not known.[7]

Clinical Pharmacology

The MAO inhibitors are readily absorbed after oral administration. Maximal inhibition occurs within 5 to 10 days. Despite a long biologic activity, efficacy appears to decrease in human patients if the drugs are administered at an interval longer than 24 hours.[7] Selegiline is metabolized to L-amphetamine and L-methamphetamine in dogs and, along with an increase in CNS phenylethylamine, may contribute to clinical and side effects of selegiline.

Side Effects and Drug Interactions

Selective MAO inhibitors appear to be safe. Severe and potentially fatal interactions have, however, been described when MAO inhibitors were combined with other antidepressants. Particularly problematic is the combination of MAO inhibitors with drugs that inhibit the reuptake of serotonin (see earlier discussion of serotonin syndrome with TCAs). Amitraz also is an MAO inhibitor and should not be used concurrently with selegiline. Other drugs with which MAO inhibitors may interact include meperidine and precursors of biogenic amines. Selective MAOs such as selegiline are not necessarily safer than the older or nonselective inhibitors when combined with other drugs. Hypertensive crisis, a serious side effect that occurs when aged cheeses containing tyramine (a bacterial monoamine by-product) are ingested in the presence of nonselective MAO inhibitors, does not occur with selective MAO inhibitors such as selegiline.

KEY POINT 26-6 Although safe as sole agents, a number of drugs will interact with monoamine oxidase inhibitors, increasing the risk of toxicity.

Anxiolytics

Pharmacology

The primary anxiolytics used in veterinary medicine are the benzodiazepines (see Chapter 27 for more extensive discussion), including diazepam, its metabolite oxazepam, clorazepate (metabolized in the stomach to *N*-desmethyldiazepam, a major metabolite of diazepam), lorazepam, alprazolam, and clonazepam. Differences in the drugs largely reflect pharmacokinetic characteristics, although alprazolam is classified as a high potency drug. The assumed mechanism of action of these drugs is gabaminergic through interaction with the $GABA_A$ receptor. The anxiolytic effects are separate from the general CNS depressant effects caused by these drugs. Their central effects are somewhat dose dependent. Sedative effects occur at low doses; as a result, excitement is tempered. Antianxiety effects are evident at moderate doses, being beneficial to social interactions. At high doses hypnotic effects become evident. Sedation becomes profound at high doses, ataxia is evident and sleep is facilitated.[1] Decreased skeletal muscle activity—particularly of value in animals experiencing seizures—is central in nature and is independent of sedative effects. Cats appear to be more prone than dogs to muscle relaxation.[1] Benzodiazepines may distribute differently in cats, with extensive binding of diazepam and its major metabolite, desmethyldiazepam, in the brain.[51]

The disposition and tolerance to and withdrawal of most of the benzodiazepines are discussed in Chapter 27. The effects of the benzodiazepines reflect in part metabolism to active, inactive, and potentially toxic metabolites. If efficacy reflects formation of an active metabolite (e.g., desmethyldiazepam), accumulation may be necessary before maximum effects are seen. Accumulation will be more likely with twice-daily dosing. The elimination half-life of many benzodiazepines in general is short. Efficacy can be prolonged by metabolism to active metabolites (in humans). Shorter-acting compounds include clorazepate and midazolam. Intermediate half-life drugs such as oxazepam, lorazepam, chlordiazepoxide, and alprazolam have no active metabolites. Longer-acting benzodiazepines include diazepam and clonazepam. Alternatively, clorazepate is available as a sustained-release product that can be administered less frequently.

Tolerance develops to the anticonvulsant and sedative effects of many benzodiazepines (see Chapter 27). Tolerance appears less likely to develop to the anxiolytic effects of these drugs.[3] In contrast, withdrawal can accompany rapid discontinuation of the drug. Thus doses should be tapered gradually (e.g., 25% per week) as the drug is discontinued.[1,3]

The cat has served as a sleep model for studies investigating the effect of therapeutic agents on sleep cycles in humans. Accordingly, a fair amount of dated literature is available regarding the use of benzodiazepines in cats. Although routes (e.g., intraperitoneal, which avoids first-pass metabolism) and doses are not always relevant to therapeutic use in cats, some information might be gleaned from the studies. For example, whereas flurazepam (1.25 to 2 mg/kg intraperitoneally) depresses reticular formation activity for 72 hours or more,[52] tolerance develops even after one dose, and dependence (resulting in withdrawal signs) was maximal in 7 days.[53] Because of the diverse impact of benzodiazepines on CNS activity (including efficacy, tolerance, and withdrawal) and the variability that characterizes their disposition (e.g., variable first-pass metabolism, variability in the activity and half-life of metabolites), the use of this class of drugs, perhaps more so than others, should be based on scientific studies that establish not only pharmacokinetics but also acute and chronic pharmacodynamic responses.

Side Effects

In addition to changes in behavior, the benzodiazepines have been associated with a number of side effects in human patients. Reaction may be to the parent drug or a metabolite. Long-term use in human patients has been associated with neutropenia and liver disease. Acute fulminating hepatotoxicity has been reported in cats receiving diazepam orally.[54] Clinical signs include anorexia, vomiting, lethargy, hypothermia, and jaundice. The adversity appears to be dose dependent (and thus may be idiosyncratic), occurring in most animals within 5 to 11 days after therapy is begun. Mortality rates are high (8 of 11 cats in one report) despite intensive therapy. Histology revealed severe acute to subacute lobular to massive hepatic necroses, suppurative cholangitis, and biliary hyperplasia. Baseline hepatic function data might be collected from cats before therapy is begun and again 3 to 5 days after therapy is begun in order to minimize the damage induced by diazepam administered to cats at risk. Any evidence of illness (or evidence of prolonged elimination) should lead to discontinuation of the drug. Clorazepate used in combination with phenobarbital in dogs for control of seizures has, in the author's experience, also been associated with liver disease. Tolerance will generally develop toward ataxia and sedation, which may accompany initial therapy. Paradoxical hyperactivity may require transitioning to another class of anxiolytics.[4] Drug withdrawal should be gradually tapered for any benzodiazepine administered for more than 1 week, particularly for high-potency drugs such as alprazolam. The duration of withdrawal should be in proportion to the duration of therapy. Care should be taken not to miss doses, particularly with high-potency drugs such as alprazolam; twice-daily administration may be necessary to avoid clinical signs of withdrawal.

The Animal Poison Control Center of the American Society for the Prevention of Cruelty to Animals has reported alprazolam toxicity in dogs. Clinical signs developed within 30 minutes of ingestion and included ataxia/disorientation, depression, hyperactivity, vomiting, weakness, tremors, vocalization, tachycardia, tachypnea, hypothermia, diarrhea, and increased salivation. In addition to supportive treatment, flumazenil was suggested to counter severe CNS depression.[55]

Clinical Indications

The benzodiazepines are less desirable as behavior-modifying drugs because of their nonspecific nature.[1] Thus a notable disadvantage of the long-term use of benzodiazepines is their tendency to interfere with the ability to learn in animals undergoing behavior modification as part of their treatment program.[4,56] Animals may forget previous learned behaviors. An exception can be made for chlordiazepoxide, which appears to facilitate operant conditioning in nervous dogs (e.g., Pointer).[3] Paradoxical reactions may occur in some animals, including rage, hyperexcitability, and anxiety. In addition, the risk that pet owners may use the animal's drug should lead to close scrutiny of the animal's drug needs and use.

KEY POINT 26-7 The short half-life and nonspecific nature of benzodiazepines decrease their efficacy as behavior modifiers.

Benzodiazepines are indicated for the treatment of anxiety. Alprazolam and clonazepam may be associated with fewer side effects and might be preferred[1]; however, fewer reports exist regarding their use in animals. The benzodiazepines are contraindicated in aggressive patients.[1] Simpson and Simpson[3] noted that the contraindication may depend on the cause of aggression. If aggression is a manifestation of an underlying fear or anxiety, then the benzodiazepines may reduce aggression. If, however, anxiety or fear is masking aggression, the benzodiazepine may increase aggression. Other indications for benzodiazepines include treatment of inappropriate elimination,[1] noise phobias, and selected anxieties such as visits to the veterinarian.[1,3] Oxazepam and lorazepam are not metabolized to active metabolites; as such, their use might be preferred in patients with liver disease.

Anxioselective Drugs: Azapirones (Buspirone)

Structure–Activity Relationships

Buspirone also is referred to as a nonspecific anxiolytic. Members of this group were specifically developed for atypical depressions, nonspecific generalized anxiety disorders, and selected OCDs. Buspirone is the first nonsedating antianxiety drug to be marketed.[3] Its effects appear to reflect blockade of 5-HT_1 receptors at both presynaptic and postsynaptic sites. Presynaptic inhibition increases serotonergic activity when serotonin is low, whereas postsynaptic control reduces serotonin when it is high.[3] Buspirone will cause downregulation of 5-HT receptors. In addition, it will act as a dopamine agonist throughout the brain.[3] Maximum efficacy may require several weeks.[4]

Side Effects

In contrast to benzodiazepine anxiolytic drugs, buspirone has no sedative, muscle relaxant, or anticonvulsant actions. It does not impair motor performance.[3] Side effects to buspirone manifested in cats include increased aggressiveness (toward other household cats), increased affection toward owners, mild sedation, and agitation.[56] Vomiting and tachycardia also have been reported.[56] In contrast to the anxiolytic drugs and TCAs, buspirone is associated with a low abuse potential. Withdrawal symptoms after discontinuation of the drug apparently do not occur.[1] Because it is not metabolized by CYP enzymes, drug interactions are less likely compared with other behavior-modifying drugs.

Clinical Indications

Buspirone has been used to treat canine aggression, canine and feline stereotypic behaviors, self-mutilation, OCDs, thunderstorm phobias, and feline spraying.[1] Buspirone apparently has been particularly useful for treatment of anxiety associated with social situations such as aggression or marking behaviors.[1] One week of therapy may be sufficient to evaluate the drug. Buspirone might be used in combination with other drugs that target reuptake of serotonin, particularly if intraneuronal serotonin is depleted.[4]

Transdermal delivery of buspirone does not appear to be a reasonable method of administration in cats. Drug concentrations were not detectable in circulation in cats (n = 6) receiving a single dose of 2.5 mg transdermally as a PLO gel. This compared with a mean peak concentration of 3.5 + 5.5 ng/mL after oral administration of 2.5 mg.[24] Although a therapeutic range has not been established, typical drug concentrations after administration of a recommended dose in humans approximate 75 to 100 ng/mL.[7]

Miscellaneous (Nonspecific) Drugs Used To Modify Behavior

Progestins

Progestin interaction with GABA receptors is 10 to 50 times more potent than that of barbiturates.[1] This may account for the nonspecific calming effects of the drugs observed in veterinary medicine. The advent of newer behavior-modifying drugs (e.g., TCAs, SSRIs) and the incidence of side effects largely limit the use of progestins to animals that have failed other medications and are faced with euthanasia.

Several side effects have been well documented in animals receiving progestins for long periods. Among the more notable side effects, because of their magnitude or life-threatening nature, are gynecomastia, mammary gland neoplasia, diabetes mellitus, aplastic anemia, and pyometra.[27,28] Animals should be monitored frequently for evidence of adversities.

Progestins are most wisely reserved for adjuvant short-term therapy until the second drug takes effect (i.e., 4 to 6 weeks), and only the oral form is recommended. The progestins also are an alternative for animals in whom euthanasia is being considered; in such cases, a high dose (4 mg/kg orally every 24 hours) has been recommended in order to stimulate a rapid response.[27]

Anticonvulsants

A number of anticonvulsant drugs have been used to treat behavioral abnormalities. The most notable used for animals include the barbiturate phenobarbital (and its congener primidone) and phenytoin, a hydantoin derivative. Their use has been somewhat efficacious for treatment of overactive or aggressive behaviors (which actually may have been an expression of psychomotor epilepsy).[1] Efficacy is, however, generally dependent on administration of sedative (and, with long-term use, potentially toxic) effects. More notably, their use has largely been replaced by the TCAs or SSRIs. The side effects of these drugs (discussed in Chapter 27) limit their long-term use, although monitoring (as with anticonvulsant therapy) may help prevent toxicity.

Phenytoin has been useful for the treatment of explosive aggression in human patients. Phenobarbital may prove useful for controlling excessive feline vocalization during car travel[1] or canine aggression.[57] Carbamazepine (an iminodibenzyl derivative of imipramine) also has been used to treat explosive aggression in humans. Valproic acid may be useful for treatment of aggression.[57]

Opioid Agonists and Antagonists

The drugs are discussed more in depth for pain control (see Chapter 28). The antagonists in particular have proved useful in the treatment of selective OCDs in humans. Efficacy also has been reported to treat selected self-mutilation disorders in dogs (e.g., acral lick dermatitis or lick granuloma).[1,3,57] Pure antagonists, including naloxone and naltrexone, the latter an orally bioavailable product, and mixed agonists–antagonists such as pentazocine appear effective. These drugs block mu and kappa receptors. The assumed mechanism of action is blockade of self-reward mediated by endogenous opioid release that may accompany self-destructive behavior. Using a double-blind crossover study, a single dose of naloxone (1 mg/kg subcutaneously) decreased excessive grooming behavior in cats (n = 12) for 2.5 to 24 weeks (median 12 weeks). Likewise, a single dose of haloperidol (2 mg/kg intravenously) decreased grooming behavior, with effects lasting 16 weeks in 6 of 10 cats. The authors postulated that efficacy of naloxone might be limited only to recently developed stereotypic behaviors, whereas haloperidol might be effective for more chronic behaviors.[58] Hydrocodone (for destructive behaviors) and naloxone and haloperidone (for OCDs) have shown some efficacy for treatment of behavioral disorders. Dextromethorphan, a non-narcotic opioid, also is an N-meth-D-aspartate receptor antagonist (see Chapter 28) and has shown some efficacy for OCDs. Dodman and coworkers[59] prospectively compared the effect of dextromethorphan (2 mg/kg orally twice daily) with placebo for treatment of chewing or excessive grooming in dogs (n = 14) with chronic allergic dermatitis. A randomized double-blinded crossover design was used for each 2-week phase of the study. The percentage of time that abnormal behaviors and pruritus were observed was less in dogs in the treatment group.

Antihistamines

The mildly sedative (e.g., with hydroyzine) or hypnotic (e.g., with diphenhydramine) effects caused by H_1 receptor blockade can be of benefit for some behavioral disorders. These drugs are discussed in greater depth as antiinflammatories (see Chapter 29) and antiemetics at the vestibular apparatus (see Chapter 19). Indications as behavior-modifying drugs might include the treatment of chronic pruritus, late-night activity, car travel, and selected transient behaviors accompanied by pacing and vocalization.[1]

β-Blockers

β-adrenergic blockers (e.g., propranolol, pindolol) have been used in human medicine for the treatment of aggressive outbursts associated with self-mutilation or injury problems, intermittent explosive behaviors, conduct disorders, dementia, and schizophrenia.[1] The use of these drugs for similar disorders in animals has not, however, been very successful.[1] Nonselective β-blockers also have been used to treat anxiety in human beings. One animal behaviorist reports success with propranolol or pindolol (the latter also affecting serotonin receptors) for the treatment of fear aggression in dogs.[57]

Stimulants

Stimulants include dextroamphetamine, methylphenidate (Ritalin), and pemoline, a drug whose actions are similar to those of methylphenidate. Stimulants are characterized by paradoxical effects in that they cause excitement in the normal patient but a calming effect in the hyperactive patient. Their indication for human patients is for the treatment of attention deficits. Conditions of hyperactivity are rare in veterinary medicine. Proper diagnosis is imperative to successful therapy with stimulants.

They act to increase sympathomimetic stimulation. Side effects include increased heart and respiratory rate and anorexia. Tremors and hyperthermia may occur. The drugs are contraindicated for patients with cardiovascular disease, glaucoma, and hyperthyroidism. The drugs should not be used in combination with other behavior-modifying drugs.[1] Methylphenidate toxicosis was described in a 10-year-old cat treated with a 5-mg tablet. Plasma concentrations of 83 ng/mL (5 to 16 times the therapeutic range recommended in humans) were associated with restlessness, vocalizing, and circling. Treatment was environmental (external stimuli minimized); clinical signs resolved within 25 hours of ingestion.[60]

Others

Pheromones are increasingly becoming popular adjuvants for the treatment of behavioral and other disorders. Their use has been reviewed.[61] Pheromones used to modify behavior include Dog Appeasing Pheromone (DAP). A number of clinical trials have been performed with DAP, most showing some degree of improvement, regardless of the behavior studied. However, study design, including appropriateness of sample size, control, blinding, and randomization procedures, should be carefully critiqued as the validity of the conclusions and their application to clinical practice is considered. Taylor and Mills[62] studied the effect of DAP (assumed to be maternal appeasing pheromone) in newly adopted puppies. Based on the number of nights puppies cried, DAP reduced the time compared with placebo, but only in gun dog breeds. Incorporation of DAP into a collar was studied as a means to reduce travel-related problems in dogs (n = 62).[63] The study was neither controlled nor blinded. Response was based on assessment of 21 behavioral signs assessed every 3 weeks; dogs were subjected to car rides at least twice weekly for 9 weeks. Significant improvement occurred in nine of the signs, with reduction in fear intensity the most consistent. DAP was also studied for its ability to decrease aggressive behavior associated with veterinary examination (n = 15 dogs), but no significant effect was found regarding aggression. Dogs, however, were more relaxed compared with those in the placebo group.[64] Todd and coworkers[65]studied the effect on barking of DAP administered to shelter dogs treated for 7 consecutive days (n = 37 treated, 13 control). Mean barking amplitude and frequency were reduced. Responses toward strangers (e.g., sniffing frequency) also were reduced. DAP has been compared with clomipramine to treat separation anxiety[66] and noise phobias[67,68] (see later discussions), and feline facial pheromone (FFP) has been studied for inappropriate urination (see later discussions).[69]

Herbals

Several herbal products have been recommended in humans for treatment of behavioral problems. Hypercium and St. John's wort have been studied in controlled trials in humans, with variable activity. Hypercium contains at least 10 active agents, with hypericin and hyperforin identified as inhibitors of amine transport. Sceletium contains mesembrine, which may be clinically active. The mechanism is not clear but appears to be different than that of traditional SSRI s on the basis of neuronal discharge in cats.[70] S-Adenyosyl methionine has demonstrated mood elevation in humans, and ginkgo biloba extract has demonstrated some effects with mild dementia.[7] The risk of interactions between herbal products and drugs should not be ignored. The combination of herbal ingredients that target serotonin with one another or with drugs that share a similar pharmacologic effect may contribute to manifestations indicative of the serotonin syndrome.

KEY POINT 26-8 Care should be taken when combining drugs or supplements that target serotonin.

Other Considerations

Drug Combinations

For patients that are refractory to drug therapy, behavioral modification therapy, or environmental changes, combination drug therapy might be considered. Drugs should be selected on the basis of their having mechanisms that will complement one another. However, care must be taken to ensure that combined drugs do not result in adverse drug reactions as a result of drug interactions, particularly at the level of mechanism of action or drug metabolism. Particularly problematic will be the combinations of drugs and herbal agents that affect serotonin. Among the drugs most likely to be safe when combined with other modifying drugs are the benzodiazepines. Examples of combinations that may be reasonable include[4] neuroleptic phenothiazines with drugs that target serotonin for treatment of OCDs; buspirone with SSRIs or TCAs, and combined use of beta blockers.

Newer Drugs and Therapies

Treatment of human behavioral disorders continues to be a major focus of research and development. Newer agents are likely to focus on the noradrenergic or serotonergic pathways, with selectivity for either receptor or system to be expected. The plethora of serotonin receptor subtypes should lead to drugs with increasing selectivity (i.e., 5-$HT_{1A, 2A, 2C}$, or $_3$). Example drugs selectively targeting neuronal transport of norepinephrine include levoprotiline, and a tomoxetine. Drugs classified as mixed serotonin–norepinephrine transport antagonists such are venlafaxine coupled with serotonergic drugs (thus enhancing serotonergic properties beyond SSRIs or TCAs) has led to studies of duloxetine and milnacipran, the latter an analog of buspirone. Complex atypical antidepressants include the α-2 adrenergic receptors antagonists such as mianserin and mirtazapine. MAO inhibition continues to be a focus of development, although the risk of drug interactions remains high. Other drugs of interest for potential development include drugs that target GABA-A receptors, cerebral peptides (opioids, neurokinin K), and neuroactive steroids.[7]

Mirtazapine is a piperazino–azepine antidepressant that is structurally similar to serotonin (see Figure 26-2). It is characterized by blockade of 5-HT_2 and 5-HT_3 receptors and histamine (subtype 1) receptors. Sympathetic (norepinephrine) and serotonergic (5-HT_1) actions reflect antagonism of $alpha_2$ autoreceptors (similar to yohimbime) and heteroreceptors (receptors that alter release of mediators other than their ligand). In humans adverse events to mirtazapine tend to be limited in part because of its target selectivity. Its actions at 5-HT_1 receptors have been referred to as *indirect agonist.* Its antiserotonergic effects contribute to its efficacy as an antiemetic, with effects similar to ondansetron. Regarding its behavioral modification, a meta-analysis comparing mirtazapine and amitryptyline treatment for behavioral disorders in humans demonstrated equal efficacy. Mirtazapine has not yet been studied in animals. In humans disposition is complex, warranting scientific studies to support its use in dogs and cats. Oral bioavailability in humans is approximately 50%, largely owing to first-pass metabolism. In addition to plasma protein binding (approximately 85%), 40% of the drug is bound to erythrocytes. Hepatic metabolism is extensive, by way of CYP2D6 and CYP3A4.[71] Approximately 50% of the AUC of active drug reflects the demethylmirtazapine metabolite (CYP3A4). However, the potency of the metabolite is only 10% to 20% of the parent compound; as such, the active metabolite contributes to only 5% to 10% of bioactivity. Elimination half-life is both gender and age dependent, ranging from 14 to 32 hours in men and 30 to 40 hours in women. Time to steady state (in humans) is 4 days. The elimination half-life is increased 33% to 40% in the presence of either hepatic or severe (but not mild) renal disease. Not surprisingly, mirtazapine is involved in a number of pharmacokinetic drug interactions, involving selected behavior-modifying drugs, as a result of pharmacokinetic (e.g., cimetidine, risperidone, fluoxetine, and amitryptyline) and pharmacodynamic (behavior-modifying drugs, diazepam) effects. In humans behavior-modifying response does not correlate with plasma drug concentrations; mean concentrations associated with response range from 5.7 to about 111 at the lowest (0.21 mg/kg) and highest (0.64 mg/kg) effective doses, respectively. However, despite its complex disposition, mirtazapine is characterized by a wide therapeutic margin such that increased dosing is not associated with serious toxicity.[71]Anecdotally, mirtazapine has been used to stimulate appetite in dogs and cats.

TREATMENT OF SPECIFIC BEHAVIORAL DISORDERS

Care must be taken to distinguish behavior that is perceived to be abnormal by the pet owner and normal behavior. Pharmacologic management of abnormal behavior should be approached as an adjunct, and specifically as a facilitator, to normalizing behavior rather than as a cure. The treatment of disorders of veterinary behavior has been the topic of a 2008 Veterinary Clinics of North America conference.[72] A number of nondrug techniques have been recommended by many animal behaviorists.[3,73-77] Abnormal behaviors that require drug therapy should be simultaneously managed with behavior-modification training. For example, decreasing arousal and fear can facilitate learning a new behavior.[27,28] The evidence supporting use of behavior-modifying drugs is increasing, but well-designed clinical trials are still limited. Before a study involving pharmacologic control is accepted as guidance for management of behavioral disorders in animals, the study design must be closely scrutinized for evidence of randomization; placebo control; blinding procedures that minimize bias; equal handling of treatment groups; and perhaps most commonly overlooked, a sufficient number of animals to detect a significant difference. Outcome measures most appropriately support the study hypothesis or purpose. The inability of a study to prove a significant treatment effect should not be interpreted as no treatment groups or that the treatment groups are the same.

KEY POINT 26-9 Pharmacologic management of abnormal behavior should be approached as an adjunct, and specifically as a facilitator, to normalizing behavior rather than as a cure.

In addition to the lack of well-designed clinical trials, many of the drugs used to modify behavior can cause serious side effects, and the clinical pharmacology of the drugs increases the likelihood of adversity because of unpredictability of plasma or tissue drug concentrations. Many of the side effects may not be readily observed by the pet owner, further increasing the risk of side effects. Finally, slow response to therapy may lead to unsupervised manipulation of dosing regimens by the pet owner, again predisposing the animal to adverse reactions. Owners should be well counseled regarding the risks and benefits of behavior-modifying drugs, including potential changes in behavior that may be less desirable than the behavior targeted by the drug. Although many drugs recommended for use in dogs and cats are approved for human, but not veterinary, use, behavior-modifying drugs stand out as having potential risks of adversity.[26] Obtaining informed owner consent may be prudent before implementing therapy with these drugs. Caution should be taken to prevent substance abuse by pet owners.

Monitoring serum drug concentrations may be of benefit for selected drugs. Monitoring must, however, be performed in conjunction with clinical response, including both efficacy and safety. Antidepressants should be used cautiously or not at all for patients suffering from metabolic illnesses. Adequate time must be allowed before a drug or a dosing regimen is considered to fail. At least two drug elimination half-lives plus the time described to maximum efficacy for the particular drug should elapse. In general, combinations of behavior-modifying drugs should be avoided. One drug should be withdrawn, often slowly, before another is begun. A drug-free time of two drug elimination half-lives is recommended in humans before a new drug is begun. Generally, 10 to 20 days should elapse until a drug-free period has been sufficiently long for a short-acting drug and up to 6 to 8 weeks for longer-acting drugs.[1]

The following description of drug therapy for selected behaviors is not intended to be a "cookbook" approach to managing abnormal behavior in dogs and cats. Rather, clinicians should familiarize themselves with the assumed behavior and its proper nondrug behavioral modification management. Clinicians should be thoroughly familiar with the drug to be used. Because indications are less clear with these drugs, an emphasis should be placed on side effects, drug interactions, and contraindications. Consultation with a veterinary behaviorist is strongly recommended before implementing any drug therapy.

COGNITIVE DYSFUNCTION

The use of deprenyl to treat cognitive dysfunction in animals is supported by the efforts of Ruehl.[78] Reported in abstract, using a randomized, placebo-controlled design, dogs (n = 199) with cognitive dysfunction received either placebo or 0.2 mg/kg or 1 mg/kg daily of selegiline HCl (Anipryl). Response in the higher-dose group (1 mg/kg) significantly improved compared with the placebo group; response in the lower-dose group was not reported.

Among the postulated causes of cognitive dysfunction is age-related neuropathy. Among the leading causes of neuropathy is the progressive and accumulated changes in the neuron induced by reactive oxygen species generated through normal mitochondrial aerobic respiration. Damage reflects not only direct effects caused by the radicals but also mutations in DNA and formation of aldehydes and secondary toxins.[79] Accumulative damage coupled with limited regenerative capacity results in changes associated with age. A direct relationship between age and loss of oxidative scavenging ability supports the free radical theory of aging. As such, attenuation or reversal of the process might be achieved through treatment with compounds that facilitate maintenance of or an increase in radical scavenging ability. For example, Ikdea-Douglas and coworkers[79] demonstrated that 90 days of dietary antioxidant supplementation was associated with improved performance on landmark-discrimination tasks in aged (9 to 13 years) Beagles (n = 30). Improvements in behavior could be associated with concentrations of antioxidant supplementation, although the role of inflammation control could not be ruled out. Vitamin E (*all-rac-* α-tocopherol) was supplemented as a lipid-soluble antioxidant at low (83 ppm) to high (799 ppm) concentrations. Other supplements included vitamin C (an aqueous antioxidant), and L-carnitine and dl-α-lipolic acid as mitochondrial cofactors. Osella and coworkers[80] reported the efficacy of a neuroprotective nutraceutical (Senilife) that contains phosphatidylserine, ginkgo biloba extract, d-α-tocopherol, and pyridoxine in dogs (n = 8) with cognitive dysfunction. However, no placebo group was treated. The authors reported that animals were markedly improved, although none underwent complete remission. The use of other nutraceuticals for treatment of age-related diseases has been reviewed by others.[81] Finally, efficacy of deprenyl may reflect, in part, its neuroprotectant ability through scavenging of oxygen radicals.

Canine Behaviors

Dominance-Related Aggression

Aggression appears to be related to noradrenergic, dopaminergic, and serotonergic receptors; of these, the serotonergic appear most important. Consequently, drugs that are selective for serotonin receptors may be more effective for aggression. Among the TCAs, clomipramine might be preferred. One group[82] found no effect of amitriptyline for treatment of aggressive behaviors using both a prospective and retrospective approach. Prospectively, amitriptyline was compared with placebo using randomized, double-blind, placebo-controlled crossover design in 12 dogs; retrospectively, no treatment effect for amitriptyline was found in 27 dogs. The authors concluded, on the basis of both studies, that amitriptyline did not improve aggressive behaviors. However, their conclusion is likely to be limited by the power of the study. Variability in the underlying causes of aggression may have further limited interpretation. Hewson and coworkers[22] also reported no effect for clomipramine on dominance aggression in dogs (n = 29). Their study was well controlled and blinded, but again, the ability to detect a significant difference was not reported.

Fluoxetine, paroxetine, and sertraline are selective for serotonin uptake; among these, fluoxetine has been used in dogs for dominance aggression.[83] Fluoxetine (1 mg/kg orally every 24 hours) significantly decreased owner-directed aggression in eight of nine dogs in a single-blind crossover study; although "placebo controlled," placebo was administered only 1 of the 5 weeks of treatment. Behavioral modification was not included with drug therapy.[83]

Administration of tryptophan, a serotonin precursor, has been associated with reduced aggression. Other drugs that may reduce aggression include propranolol (episodic aggression in people), carbamazepine, lithium, and phenobarbital.[84] Long-term adverse effects outweigh the potential behavior-modifying effect of progestin administration for aggression. Anxiolytic drugs may reduce dominance-related aggression if aggression is a manifestation of fear or anxiety.[3,12] Aggression may worsen in some patients treated with benzodiazepine derivatives, however, especially if normal inhibitory mechanisms are suppressed.[3] In human patients anticonvulsants have been useful for treatment of "explosive" aggression. Phenytoin and carbamazepine both have been used. In animals carbamazepine is preferred for profound aggression that has not responded to other therapy.[1] Monitoring may facilitate successful therapy; concentrations known to be effective for control of seizures in human patients (6 to 10 μg/mL) may be effective for control of aggression in animals.[1]

Stereotypic Motor Behaviors, Obsessive Disorders, and Self-Mutilating Disorders

Luescher[85] has reviewed treatment of compulsive disorders in dogs and cats. Stereotypics are repetitive behaviors without an obvious goal and thus appear pointless and mindless to the observer.[57] They are usually derived from normal behaviors and may be a component of displacement behavior (reflecting an inability to perform more than one strongly motivated behavior) or a compulsive disorder. They are generally associated with chronic conflict, confinement, and sensory deprivation. OCDs are poorly defined in veterinary medicine. In humans OCDs are ritualistic and sufficiently invasive either cognitively or physically to interfere with normal function.[1,86] They may reflect a chronic state of conflict anxiety, leading to displacement. Abnormal behaviors in animals that might be considered OCDs include stereotypic, ritualistic circling, spinning, pacing, howling, flank sucking, and fly biting; selected ingestive behaviors; polydipsia; and self-mutilation or grooming behaviors, including acral lick granuloma.[1,2,86,87] In humans the disorders may reflect aberrant serotonin metabolism and possibly increased dopamine. Therefore treatment has focused on serotonergic metabolism. A similar approach seems to work for dogs with OCDs. A series of cases of obsessive–compulsive behaviors in dogs provides evidence of the potential efficacy of clomipramine but not amitriptyline.[1,86] Other reports support the use of clomipramine for treatment of OCDs.[25,89] One single-blind crossover study of lick granuloma found clomipramine but not desipramine to reduce licking by 50% in half of patients studied.[25] Another clinical report noted the efficacy of clomipramine, but not diazepam, naloxone, or phenobarbital, in a single dog affected with self-trauma.[88]

Well-designed controlled clinical trials supporting drug therapy for OCDs or stereotypics are increasing. One well-designed study (randomized, placebo-controlled, double-blinded, balanced crossover) in dogs (n = 51) with canine compulsive disorder (including spinning and acral lick dermatitis) were fourfold more likely to improve (although not be cured) after 4 weeks of treatment with clomipramine.[22] A retrospective study in dogs (n = 103) and cats (n = 23) with OCDs found first that compliance with behavior modification was high; second, that the combination of behavior modification and medication was associated with a marked decrease (>50%) in intensity and frequency of OCDs in most animals; and third, that clomipramine was significantly more efficacious than amitriptyline.[89]

Fluoxetine has been reported as useful for treatment of OCDs or self-mutilation, including acral lick granuloma[38,39,90] and tail mutilation.[39] Wynchank and Berk[90] studied the efficacy of fluoxetine (20 mg) using a randomized, double-blinded, placebo-controlled study in dogs (n = 63); dogs were treated for 6 weeks. Both owners and veterinarians reported improvement. Clomipramine also has been studied. In an open clinical trial, clomipramine (2 mg/kg orally once daily) was associated with marked healing of acral lick granuloma in 8 of 10 dogs within 3 weeks. Dogs were studied for 6 months, with response maintained in three dogs at least 3 months after therapy was discontinued.[91]

The phenothiazine derivative thioridazine was reported as useful in one case of aberrant motor behavior.[15]

Opioid antagonists also have been reported to be effective for stereotypic behaviors in dogs manifested as self-mutilation acral lick dermatitis. Release of endogenous opioids may serve as a reward system after mutilation. Breaking the reward cycle with antagonists may resolve the behavior.[57,87] Both naltrexone and nalmefene, pure opioid antagonists, were found to be useful. In one study self-mutilation activity significantly decreased in seven of eleven dogs and was partially effective in three more.[92] On the basis of accompanying pharmacokinetic studies, concentrations of 20 to 50 ng/mL of nalmefene were considered therapeutic. The short half-life of the drug (2 to 3 hours in dogs) may necessitate frequent dosing. Using a double-blind crossover study, a single dose of naloxone (1 mg/kg subcutaneously) decreased excessive grooming behavior in cats (n = 12) for 2.5 to 24 weeks (median 12 weeks). Likewise, a single dose of haloperidol (2 mg/kg intravenously) decreased grooming behavior, with effects lasting 16 weeks in six of ten cats. The authors postulated that efficacy of naloxone might be limited only to recently developed stereotypic behaviors, whereas haloperidol might be effective for more chronic behaviors.[58] Dextromethorphan inhibits the uptake of serotonin (see Table 26-2)[93] The successful use of dextromethorphan (2 mg/kg every 12 hours orally for 2 weeks) for treatment of self-licking, self-chewing, and self-biting associated with pruritus has been described in a series of dogs.[59] Pruritus scores also decreased in the dogs. Animals (n = 14) were studied using a placebo-controlled, randomized, double-blind crossover study. Dextromethorphan was administered as the pure drug substrate, with filler administered in a gelatin capsule. Two dogs were withdrawn because of side effects (lethargy and diarrhea, respectively).

Multiple-Animal Households

Abnormal behaviors sometimes accompanying the addition of a new pet to the household that already has one or more pets (generally dogs) include excessive barking, territorial defense, predatory aggression (exhibited in dogs allowed to roam unsupervised), or intraspecies aggression (aggression toward other dogs either within or outside the household). Drugs that modify anxiety or fearfulness should be considered as adjuvant therapy. Included are the TCAs amitriptyline[27] and clomipramine (fear or anxiety), the SSRIs fluoxetine and paroxetine, the azapirone buspirone (antianxiety), and progestins. Of these drugs, fluoxetine and clomipramine may be most preferred. Amitriptyline and buspirone in particular have been cited for a potential increase in aggressive tendencies[27] with interdog aggression. Care should be taken to adhere to previously stated concerns regarding progestin therapy.

Excessive Barking

Occasionally, excessive barking reflects an OCD. Most cases are conducive to behavioral modification. Surgical treatment (vocal cordectomy) is a less desirable alternative treatment. The use of behavior-modifying drugs should be reserved for cases in which fear, separation anxiety, or other compulsive component can be identified in association with the behavior.[28] Drugs should be administered for a short period (2 to 4 months) and in conjunction with behavior modification. Once the desirable behavior is achieved and maintained for 4 to 6 weeks, medication can be tapered gradually until it is discontinued. Occasional cases may require lifelong medication in conjunction with behavioral modification. Drugs recommended by animal behaviorists include clomipramine, amitriptyline, buspirone, and fluoxetine.[28] Thioridazine was reported useful in one case of excessive barking accompanied by tail biting.[15]

Destructive Behavior

Destructive behavior can be dangerous to the animal (e.g., when foreign or toxic material is ingested) and economically undesirable to the pet owner. Causes of the behavior may vary with age. The underlying cause of the behavior may reflect exploration and play; attention-seeking behavior; or expression of territory, fear, or separation anxiety. Cognitive dysfunction in geriatric animals also may be manifested as destructive behavior.[94] Although behavioral modification is an important component of therapy, drug therapy may be urgent for animals in which the behavior is potentially harmful and for animals whose owners are intolerant of the behavior. Treatment of specific causes of destructive behavior is addressed with those disorders.

Tranquilizers such as the phenothiazine derivatives (acepromazine) may seem appropriate for destructive behavior and occasionally might prove useful. However, sedative effects may cause the animal to sleep rather than interact with family members.[94] Likewise, use of anxiolytics (e.g., clorazepate, diazepam) can cause sedation. Although rapid acting, the anxiolytics must be administered frequently. In addition, they may interfere with the learning ability of the animal undergoing behavior modification.[94] The efficacy of buspirone is generally poor. In addition, it is costly and characterized by a slow onset of action. Because it is safe, however, its use may be warranted in some cases.[94] For animals whose destructive behavior reflects separation anxiety, a TCA (amitriptyline, clomipramine) or SSRI (fluoxetine) is indicated. As with buspirone, a long onset of action time and relatively high cost should be anticipated.

Anxieties and Noise Phobias

Sherman and Mills[95] reviewed anxieties and noise phobias. A common complaint of owners is that their dogs exhibit disruptive behavior when left alone.[74] Behaviors include urination, defecation, barking, howling, chewing, and digging. An Internet survey of owners of dogs with noise phobias indicated a high level of frustration regarding attempts to control the behavior pharmacologically. Of the 69 respondents, 38% attempted some type of therapy, including behavioral therapy, training, prescribed medications, herbal remedies, or some combination of these treatments. Of these, only five reported improvement.[96] Riva and coworkers[6] demonstrated that plasma serotonin and dopamine were increased in dogs (n = 22) with anxiety disorders compared with control animals; norepinephrine, L-DOPA, and selected other NTs did not differ.

Clomipramine has been approved for use in dogs for treatment of separation anxiety. Its use was reported in 1997 in abstract form[97] based on a placebo-controlled clinical trial in dogs (n = 77). In addition to placebo, dogs were administered a low (0.5 to less than 1 mg/kg twice daily; n = 24) or a high (1 to 2 mg/kg) dose of clomipramine every 12 hours. Response was based on changes in four behaviors (vocalization, destruction, defecation, or urination) monitored at 4, 8, and 12 weeks. Significant improvement was detected in the high-dose group at 8 and 12 weeks; side effects were limited to more frequent vomiting, which was nonetheless described as infrequent and mild. In contrast, Podberscek and Serpell[98] reported the lack of efficacy of clomipramine for treatment of separation anxiety in dogs (n = 49) following a placebo-controlled, double-blinded clinical trial. However, outcome measures in this study were based on owner-response questionnaires. The power of the study to detect a significant difference was not provided. Gaultier and coworkers[66] compared DAP (n = 30) to clomipramine (n = 27) for treatment of separation anxiety. The DAP was administered in paraffin oil by way of a reservoir electrical diffuser, which was placed in a room where the dog spent most of its time. The study design was a multicenter, randomized, positive-controlled, parallel clinical trial. Clomipramine (n = 27) was administered as a positive control at 1 to 2 mg/kg orally twice a day; the study was designed to confirm noninferiority rather than lack of differences between the two treatment groups. A placebo diffuser was placed in the home of positive control dogs. Animals were treated for 28 days. Efficacy outcomes did not differ between the groups; however, the lack of a negative control (because of ethical considerations) and the significant placebo effect that has been demonstrated by other studies[98] should lead to cautious interpretation. In contrast to efficacy, undesirable effects were greater in the clomipramine group (gastrointestinal: vomiting, appetite changes).

Melatonin is produced from serotonin in the pineal gland; its use as an adjuvant anticonvulsant is addressed in Chapter 27. Its use as an adjuvant for treatment of thunderstorm phobias is anecdotally promoted, although no scientific studies have been reported. A homeopathic treatment has been studied[99] for treatment of noise phobias in dogs (n = 15). Dogs were studied prospectively using a randomized, placebo-controlled (n = 15) design. All treated dogs and 14 of 15 placebo-treated dogs responded, resulting in no significant differences between the groups; this study exemplifies the importance of placebo-controlled studies.

Separation anxiety appears to respond well to fluoxetine; one open study reported a 100% response rate.[39] Benzodiazepines also may be effective for treatment of anxiety. Examples include chlordiazepoxide or diazepam.[100] An advantage of the latter group is rapid response.

Fear behaviors in dogs are also common.[75] Fear is commonly manifested toward loud noises such as thunderstorms and firecrackers, sudden movements, unfamiliar people, or novel environment. Before the advent of specific anxiolytic or antidepressant medications, tranquilizers such as phenothiazines or anticonvulsants such as phenobarbital were recommended for pharmacologic management of fear behaviors in dogs.[75] The efficacy of phenothiazine tranquilizers, however, reflects reduction of general responsiveness and is only likely for episodic anxieties.[3] Benzodiazepines (including diazepam, clorazepate, and other derivatives) have stood the test of time for treatment of noise phobias.[57,75] They have been used to treat thunderstorm or other noise phobias. They must, however, be administered before the inciting event. For thunderstorm phobias oral administration should occur at or before the first atmospheric sign,[1] such as changes in atmospheric pressure, wind, or ambient light conditions. Clorazepate (sustained-release form) may be preferred to diazepam, which requires more frequent administration. Alprazolam, characterized by a longer half-life, may also prove more beneficial.[1]

The combination of benzodiazepines with clomipramine has been anecdotally supported and subsequently studied.[101] Using an unblinded, uncontrolled design, dogs (n = 40; 32 completed the study) with storm phobias were treated with clomipramine (2 mg/kg orally every 12 hours for 3 months, then decreased to 1 mg/kg for 2 weeks and 0.5 mg/kg for 2 weeks) combined with alprazolam (0.02 mg/kg orally, as needed 1 hour before anticipated storms and every 4 hours as needed). Dogs also received counter conditioning. Improvement occurred in 94% of patients and was maintained at least 4 months after study completion. Although storm phobia was reported (by caregiver) to resolve in only two dogs, behaviors associated with the phobia (panting, pacing, trembling, remaining near the caregiver, hiding, excessive salivation, destructiveness, excessive vocalization, self-trauma, and inappropriate elimination) decreased significantly during treatment. Improvement was greater during true storms (rain, thunder, and lightning) than during rain only. Response to auditory simulation did not change. The authors concluded that the combination of clomipramine, alprazolam, and behavior modification effectively decreased but did not cure the phobia.[101]

Dodman and Shuster[57] reported that phobias can be palliatively treated but not eradicated with buspirone. Onset of action may, however, take up to 4 weeks.

Nonapproved mediations have been suggested for treatment of noise phobias. Two examples include DAP and melatonin. The pheromone is marketed as spray (VPL) and might prudently be used in combination with other therapies. It has been studied using either retrospective[68] or an open noncontrolled clinical trial of 30 dogs.[67] Owners rated changes in responses of 14 behavioral signs, with ratings improving in 9 of the 14. The use of melatonin for other behavior disorders and seizures has been variably addressed elsewhere, and noise phobias join other putative, albeit unproven, uses. Melatonin should not be combined with other drugs that increase synaptic serotonin.

Sexual Behaviors

Abnormal sexual behaviors are unusual. Both too "much" and too "little" behavior will benefit from a full reproductive workup, including serum sex steroidal hormone measurements. Behaviors that reflect "too much" generally are those targeted for behavioral modification, which might include drug therapy. Sexual behaviors that might be considered abnormal in uncastrated male dogs include house soiling and possessive or dominance aggression. Care must be taken to distinguish soiling from marking. Castration is the preferred treatment. Abnormal behaviors of castrated dogs include mounting, which may be accompanied by aggression, destructiveness, house soiling, and barking.[76,77] Previous discussions regarding these behaviors apply when the behavior is a manifestation of sexual behavior.

Psychogenic Dermatoses

Psychogenic dermatoses generally consist of both a dermatologic and a behavioral component. Discriminating between the two components is difficult but vital to successful therapy. Some psychogenic dermatosis will respond only to behavioral management, others only to dermatologic management, and some will require both behavioral and dermatologic therapy.[87] Dermatoses requiring medical management are discussed in greater depth in Chapter 22.

Clinical manifestations of psychogenic dermatoses include pruritus, acral lick dermatitis, OCDs (e.g., trichotillomania), and self-mutilation manifestations (see previous discussion of OCDs). Causes of psychogenic dermatoses are complex and may include boredom; endogenous opioid release (previously discussed); attention-seeking behavior; and, less commonly, separation anxiety.[87]

A number of drugs have been recommended for treatment of psychogenic dermatoses.[87] These include antihistamines such as hydroxyzine or chlorpheniramine; TCAs, in particular clomipramine and doxepin, followed by amitriptyline[102]; and opioid antagonists (especially for acral lick dermatitis) such as naltrexone. Doxepin stands out among the TCAs for its antihistaminergic effects.

Hyperactivity

Hyperactivity must be distinguished from overactivity. The former is a medical condition. Hyperactivity or hyperkinesia is a very rare behavior in dogs and cats. It has been reported in association with aggression in dogs.[57] Low doses of stimulant drugs, such as dextroamphetamine, may be useful. Dextroamphetamine can be used to provocatively diagnose the syndrome (2.5 to 5 mg orally in a medium-size dog). The patient should be calmed, and heart rate and respiratory rate should decrease.[57] Dextroamphetamine can be used to manage hyperactive dogs. The addition of β-blockers has proved useful for human patients, but this use has not been documented in animals.[57]

Narcolepsy

Narcolepsy is an incurable neurologic disease manifested as a disturbance in the normal sleep cycle. It is an inherited (autosomal recessive) disorder in several breeds. Treatment includes methylphenidate or a TCA. Protriptyline is a nonsedative TCA that has been used successfully in human narcoleptic patients. The drug has been used successfully in one dog in which narcolepsy manifested as hyperinsomnia.[103]

Feline Behaviors

Inappropriate Elimination

Inappropriate elimination (urinary or defecation) was the most commonly identified risk factor for relinquishment of pet cats to an animal shelter in one study.[104] Treatment of inappropriate elimination is highly individualized. Inappropriate elimination may reflect a marking behavior (generally identified by the location of urine on vertical surfaces). Abnormal or excessive marking behavior may reflect an increase in territorialism or anxiety.[56] Inappropriate elimination also is an abnormal behavior that frequently has a medical rather than a behavioral cause. Care must be taken to distinguish between the two causes so that correct medical care can be provided when indicated.[56] For abnormal behaviors, careful history taking should help identify the cause of the abnormal behavior. Care should be taken to discriminate an aversion to the litter box from a desire to eliminate elsewhere; the former might easily be managed by simply moving the litter box.[56] For all behavioral causes, environmental and behavioral modification should precede any type of pharmacologic management. Surgical castration is recommended in males. If inappropriate urination reflects a social behavior or anxiety, the use of a behavior-modifying drug may be indicated.[56]

Buspirone, diazepam, TCA, and progestins have been recommended for treatment of inappropriate elimination in cats. Male and female cats appear equally likely to respond. Buspirone is safe but costly. In an open clinical trial, marking decreased by at least 75% in approximately 55% of cats (n = 62); however, relapse occurred in 50% of the responders.[105] Cats that do respond generally do so within 1 week.[56] Cats that are the sole cat in a household appear to be less likely to respond to buspirone (compared with diazepam) than are cats from multiple-cat households.[106] Cats may, however, become more aggressive (or "assertive") when treated with buspirone.[1] Relapse of inappropriate urination appears less likely when the cat is treated with buspirone (approximately 50%) than with diazepam (approximately 75% to 91% relapse).[12,105,107]

Diazepam can be effective for treatment of inappropriate elimination in cats (55% to 75% success rates in two studies). As with buspirone, males and females appear to respond equally well, although spayed females are less likely to respond, whereas castrated males are more likely to respond.[1,56] However, a potential disadvantage of the benzodiazepines and, most notably, oral diazepam is acute hepatic failure.[54] In the report of 12 cases, acute hepatic disease occurred despite use of the drug according to recommended dosing regimens. Drugs within the class of benzodiazepines that are less likely to undergo oxidative metabolism (e.g., oxazepam) may be less likely to induce hepatic failure, although their efficacy for treating abnormal elimination has not been validated.[1,56] Cats treated with diazepam are likely to stagger for the first several days of therapy,[1] with spontaneous resolution occurring afterward. Chlordiazepoxide and clorazepate also have been useful for suppressing inappropriate elimination in cats,[1] although drug concentrations may be less predictable than in diazepam.

Among the TCAs, use of amitriptyline is reported most commonly, although evidence is anecdotal rather than scientific.[56] The incidence of adverse reactions may preclude use of amitriptyline. Clomipramine seems reasonable instead of amitriptyline on the basis of a nonrandomized, single-blinded, placebo-controlled crossover study in cats (n = 26) expressing inappropriate elimination behavior. Placebo was administered 5 days before and 3 days after a 7-day treatment period with 5 mg of clomipramine administered orally once daily. Based on the number of urine marks, the inappropriate behavior resolved in 35% of the cats, and a 75 % reduction in the number of marks occurred in 80% of the cats.[108] The findings of Landsberg and Horwitz,[72] reported in abstract form, were similar. Cats (n = 25) received 0.5 mg/kg daily in an open trial; 84% responded (at least a 75% reduction in marking behaviors), generally within 2 to 3 weeks.

Using a randomized, placebo-controlled multicenter clinical trial, King and coworkers[109] reported a response in neutered cats (n = 67) with clomipramine at either a low (0.125 to 0.25 mg/kg), medium (0.25 to 0.5 mg/kg), or high (0.5 to 1 mg/kg) dose when administered once daily for up to 12 weeks. Behavioral and environmental modifications were encouraged. Sedation was reported in 54% of the cats but was not sufficient to cause withdrawal from the study. This study supports the use of a low dose of clomipramine but also supports a gradual increase in dose in nonresponders if necessary.

Fluoxetine also has demonstrated efficacy for control of inappropriate urination. Using a randomized, placebo-controlled, double-blinded design, the effect of fluoxetine (1 mg/kg orally once daily) on urine spraying was studied in neutered cats (n = 17).[48] Drug therapy was accompanied by environmental management. Within 1 week of therapy, all but one cat had responded, with the last responding by week 2. Differences between the placebo and treatment group increased as drug therapy continued, supporting a lag time between initiation of therapy and maximal response time noted for fluoxetine in humans. Weekly episodes of spraying reduced from 8.6 ± 2 to 1.7 ± 0.6 compared with 5.5 ± 1.8 episodes in placebo-treated cats. Cats were treated for 8 weeks and monitored for an additional 4 weeks after therapy. Marking behavior returned in six of nine drug-treated cats, with those cats marking most before drug therapy also marking most at the end of the 4-week posttherapy monitoring period. Appetite decreased in four of nine cats receiving therapy; vomiting and lethargy were reported rarely.

FFP has been studied for treatment of urine spraying in cats using a double-blinded placebo-controlled design (n = 22).[69] Comparisons were made within each group to baseline but not to one another. Spraying decreased compared with baseline in the treatment but not the placebo group.

The use of progestins (discussed in Chapter 19) to treat inappropriate urination should be reserved for animals that have failed all other alternatives. A single case report cited the successful use of alprazolam (2.5 mg orally every 12 hours) for treatment of soiling. Response occurred within 1 week of therapy, with mild sedation the only reported side effect. The behavior returned after the alprazolam dose was discontinued over the next 6 weeks.[110]

The use of fluorescein has been recommended to detect the soiling culprit in multicat households. The injectable product is sold as a 10% (10 g/dL; 100 mg/mL) solution, which can be administered orally in the evening (50 mg once daily with food or 30 mg once daily without food) for 4 to 5 days.

Social Behaviors and Aggression

Disorders of aggression are the second most common cause of abnormal behavior in cats.[111] Causes associated with aggression include dominance; fear; defensive, territorial, or play aggression toward another cat; or play and fear aggression toward the owner or another person. Intolerance of petting often is manifested as an aggressive behavior. For many types of aggression (an exception being fear aggression), neutering may decrease the undesirable behavior.[111] Behavioral modification techniques are the preferred method of treatment. Pharmacologic management is indicated for cats that do not respond to behavioral modification or in conjunction with behavioral modification. Little information is available, however, regarding treatment of aggression in cats. Benzodiazepines have been used with variable results. Chlordiazepoxide or diazepam has been recommended for frustration or social anxiety in cats.[12,100,112] Diazepam may, however, increase predatory behavior in cats.[3]

Psychogenic Dermatoses

Feline psychogenic alopecia manifests as a traumatically induced regional alopecia. Underlying dermatologic causes include flea allergy, food allergy, and allergic inhalant dermatitis. Neurodermatitis also includes evidence of more damage (excoriations, crusting) and is more common in high-strung cats (e.g., Siamese, Burmese, Abyssinian). The lesions reflect overzealous grooming. Recommended treatments include TCAs (clomipramine and amitriptyline) or antihistamines.[87] Fluoxetine was successful in a report of a single cat[47] and clomipramine in another.[113]

Sexual Behaviors

Abnormal sexual behaviors in cats that may require management generally occur in toms and include urine spraying and mounting. Spraying by uncastrated cats is more appropriately treated by environmental management or according to previous discussions regarding inappropriate elimination; mounting that has not responded to behavioral modification techniques may respond to amitriptyline or another TCA.[76,77]

Depression

Among the classic signs of depression in the cat is anorexia; early intervention is important. Benzodiazepines should be used as appetite stimulants as early as possible. For depression, clomipramine hydrochloride or fluoxetine has been recommended (either drug at 0.5 mg/kg orally once daily).[114] Clomipramine is preferred if anorexia is intermittent and associated with endogenous or environmental stressors; fluoxetine is preferred for long-term management. Treatment may be required for 4 to 6 months and should be accompanied by behavior and environmental modification.

REFERENCES

1. Overall KL: Pharmacologic treatments for behavior problems, *Vet Clin North Am Small Anim Pract* 27(3):637–666, 1997.
2. Overall KL: Pharmacological treatment in behavioral medicine: the importance of neurochemistry, molecular biology and mechanistic hypotheses, *Vet J* 162(1):9–23, 2001.
3. Simpson BS, Simpson DM: Behavioral pharmacotherapy. In Voith VL, Borchelt PL, editors: *Readings in companion animal behavior*, Trenton, NJ, 1996, Veterinary Learning Systems, pp 100–115.
4. Simpson BS, Papich MG: Pharmacologic management in veterinary behavioral medicine, *Vet Clin North Am Small Anim Pract* 33(2):365–404, 2003.
5. Badino P, Odore R, Osella MC, et al: Modifications of serotinergic and adrenergic receptor concentrations in the brain of aggressive *Canis familiaris*, *Comp Biochem Physiol A Mol Integr Physiol* 139(3):343–350, 2004.
6. Riva J, Bondiolotti G, Michelazzi M, et al: Anxiety-related behavioural disorders and neurotransmitters in dogs, *Appl Anim Behav Sci* 114:168–181, 2008.
7. Baldessarini Ross J: Drug therapy of depression and anxiety disorders. In Brunton LL, Lazo JS, Parker KL, editors: *Goodman & Gilman's the pharmacological basis of therapeutics*, ed 11, New York, 2006, McGraw-Hill.
8. Lipka LJ, Lathers CM: Psyoactive agents, seizure production, and sudden death in epilepsy, *J Clin Pharmacol* 27:169–183, 1987.
9. Tobias KM, Marioni-Henry K, Wagner R: A retrospective study on the use of acepromazine maleate in dogs with seizures, *J Am Anim Hosp Assoc* 42:283–289, 2006.
10. McConnell J, Kirby R, Rudloff E: Administration of acepromazine maleate to 31 dogs with a history of seizures, *J Vet Emerg Crit Care* 17(3):262–267, 2007.

11. Pageat P, Lafont C, Falewee C, et al: An evaluation of serum prolactin in anxious dogs and response to treatment with selegiline or fluoxetine, *Appl Anim Behav Sci* 105(4):342-350
12. Marder AR: Psychotropic drugs and behavioral therapy, *Vet Clin North Am Small Anim Pract* 21:329–342, 1991.
13. Ionut V, Kirkman EL, Bergman RN: Investigation of the effect of acepromazine on intravenous glucose tolerance test in dogs, *Am J Vet Res* 66:1124–1127, 2004.
14. Murrell JC, de Groot HNM: Venker-van Haagen AJ: Middle-latency auditory-evoked potential in acepromazine-sedated dogs, *J Vet Intern Med* 18:196–200, 2004.
15. Jones RD: Use of thioridazine in the treatment of aberrant motor behavior in a dog, *J Am Vet Med Assoc* 191:89–90, 1987.
16. Hewson CJ, Luescher UA, Parent JM, et al: Effect of clomipramine on monoamine metabolites in the cerebrospinal fluid of behaviorally normal dogs, *Can J Vet Res* 64(2):123–129, 2000.
17. Lainesse C, Frank D, Beaudry F, et al: Comparative oxidative metabolic profiles of clomipramine in cats, rats and dogs: preliminary results from an in vitro study, *J Vet Pharmacol Ther* 30(5):387–393, 2007.
18. Lainesse C, Frank D, Beaudry F, et al: Effects of physiological variables on pharmacokinetic parameters of clomipramine in a large population of cats after a single oral administration, *J Vet Pharmacol Ther* 30(2):116–126, 2007.
19. King JN, Maurer MP, Hotz RP, et al: Pharmacokinetics of clomipramine in dogs following single-dose intravenous and oral administration, *Am J Vet Res* 61(1):74–79, 2000.
20. King JN, Maurer MP, Altmann BO, et al: Pharmacokineticis of clomipramine in dogs following single-dose and repeated-dose oral administration, *Am J Vet Res* 61(1):80–85, 2000.
21. Hewson C, Luescher A, Parent JM, et al: The pharmacokinetics of clomipramine and desmethylclomipramine in dogs: parameter estimates following a single oral dose and 28 consecutive daily oral doses of clomipramine, *J Vet Pharmacol Ther* 21(3):214–222, 1998.
22. Hewson CJ, Luescher A, Parent JM, et al: Efficacy of clomipramine in the treatment of canine compulsive disorder, *J Am Vet Med Assoc* 213(12):1760–1766, 1998a.
23. Lainesse C, Frank D, Meucci V, et al: Pharmacokinetics of clomipramine and desmethylclomipramine after single-dose intravenous and oral administrations in cats, *J Vet Pharmacol Ther* 29(4):271–278, 2006.
24. Mealey KL, Peck KE, Bennett BS: Systemic absorption of amitriptyline and buspirone after oral and transdermal administration to healthy cats, *J Vet Intern Med* 18:43–46, 2004.
25. Goldberger E, Rapoport JL: Canine acral lick dermatitis: response to the antiobsessional drug clomipramine, *J Am Anim Hosp Assoc* 27:179–182, 1991.
26. Johnson LR: Tricyclic antidepressant toxicosis, *Vet Clin North Am Small Anim Pract* 20(2):393–403, 1990.
27. Juarbe-Diaz SV: Social dynamics and behavior problems in multiple dog households, *Vet Clin North Am Small Anim Pract* 27(3):497–514, 1997.
28. Juarbe-Diaz SV: Assessment and treatment of excessive barking in the domestic dog, *Vet Clin North Am Small Anim Pract* 27(3):515–532, 1997.
29. Seksel K, Lindeman MJ: Use of clomipramine in treatment of obsessive-compulsive disorder, separation anxiety and noise phobia in dogs: a preliminary, clinical study, *Aust Vet J* 79(40):252–256, 2001.
30. Dvir Y, Smallwood P: Serotonin syndrome: a complex but easily avoidable condition, *Gen Hosp Psychiatry* 30(3):284–287, 2008.
31. King JN, Simpson BS, Overall KL, et al: Treatment of separation anxiety in dogs with clomipramine: results from a prospective, randomised, double-blinded, placebo-controlled, multi-centre clinical trial, *Appl Anim Behav Sci* 67:255–275, 2000.
32. King JN, Overall KL, Appleby D, et al: Results of a follow-up investigation to a clinical trial testing the efficacy of clomipramine in the treatment of separation anxiety in dogs, *Appl Anim Behav Sci* 89:233–242, 2004.
33. Frank D, Gauthier A, Bergeron R: Placebo-controlled double-blind clomipramine trial for the treatment of anxiety or fear in beagles during ground transport, *Can Vet J* 47(11):1102–1108, 2006.
34. Pasloske K: New therapeutic horizons: fluoxetine pharmacology and safety in dogs and cats and its role in behavior modification, *Proceedings of the American College of Veterinary Medicine*, 2003.
35. Aznavour N, Rbah L, Riad M, et al: A PET imaging study of 5-$HT_{(1A)}$ receptors in cat brain after acute and chronic fluoxetine treatment, *Neuroimage* 33(3):834–842, 2006.
36. Ciribassi J, Luescher A, Pasloske KS, et al: Comparative bioavailaibility of fluoxetine after transdermal and oral administration to healthy cats, *Am J Vet Res* 64:994–999, 2003.
37. Steinberg MI, Smallwood JK, Holland DR, et al: Hemodynamic and electrocardiographic effects of fluoxetine and its major metabolite, norfluoxetine, in anesthetized dogs, *Toxicol Appl Pharmacol* 82(1):70–79, 1986.
38. Rapoport JL, Ryland DH, Kriete M: Drug treatment of canine acral lick: an animal model of obsessive-compulsive disorder, *Arch Gen Psychiatry* 49:517–521, 1992.
39. Melman SA: Use of Prozac in animals for selected dermatological and behavioral conditions, *Vet Forum* 12:19–27, 1995.
40. Dodman NH, Mertens PA: Fluoxetine (Prozac) for the treatment of dominance-related aggression in dogs [abstract], *Newslett Am Vet Soc Anim Behav* 17:3, 1995.
41. French ED, Vasquez SA, George R: Potentiation of morphine hyperthermia in cats by pimozide and fluoxetine hydrochloride, *Eur J Pharmacol* 48(4):351–356, 1978.
42. Jobe PC, Browning RA: The serotonergic and noradrenergic effects of antidepressant drugs are anticonvulsant, not proconvulsant, *Epilepsy Behav* 7(4):602–619, 2005.
43. Kauffman S: Problem pets may now get Prozac, *Raleigh News-Observer August* 1:1B–5B, 1994.
44. Marder A: The promise of Prozac, *Vet Product News* 1(May/June) 45, 1995.
45. Simpson BS, Landsberg GM, Reisner IR, et al: Effects of reconcile (fluoxetine) chewable tablets plus behavior management for canine separation anxiety, *Vet Ther* 8(1):18–31, 2007.
46. Landsberg GM, Melese P, Sherman BL, et al: Effectiveness of fluoxetine chewable tablets in the treatment of canine separation anxiety, *J Vet Behavior* 3:12–19, 2008.
47. Hartmann L: Cats as possible obsessive-compulsive disorder and medications models [letter], *Am J Psychiatry* 152:1236, 1995.
48. Pryor PA, Hart BL, Cliff KD, et al: Effects of a selective serotonin reuptake inhibitor on urine spraying behavior in cats, *J Am Vet Med Assoc* 219:1557–1561, 2001.
49. Gupta M, Kulkarni SK: Studies on anticonvulsant actions of L-deprenyl, *Indian J Exp Biol* 38(4):332–337, 2000.
50. Loscher W, Honack D: Anticonvulsant and antiepileptogenic effect of L-deprenyl (selegiline) in the kindling model of epilepsy, *J Pharmacol Exp Ther* 274(1):307–314, 1995.
51. Placidi GF, Togoni C, Pacifici GM, et al: Regional distribution of diazepam and its metabolites in the brain of cats after chronic treatment, *Psychopharmacology* 48:133, 1976.
52. Novack GD, Owenburg KM: Flurazepam and triazolam: dose-response and time-response evaluation on cat sleep, *Electroencephalogr Clin Neurophysiol* 57(3):277–288, 1984.
53. Rosenberg HC, Chiu TH: Time course for development of benzodiazepine tolerance and physical dependence, *Neurosci Biobehav Rev* 9(1):123–131, 1985.
54. Center SA, Elson TH, Rowland PH, et al: Fulminant hepatic failure associated with oral diazepam in 11 cats, *J Am Vet Med Assoc* 190:618–625, 1996.
55. Wismer TA: Accidental ingestion of alprazolam in 415 dogs, *Vet Hum Toxicol* 44(1):22–23, 2002.
56. Cooper LL: Feline inappropriate elimination, *Vet Clin North Am Small Anim Pract* 27(3):569–600, 1997.

57. Dodman NH, Shuster L: Pharmacologic approaches to managing behavior problems in small animals, *Vet Med* 89:960–969, 1994.
58. Willemse T, Mudde M, Josephy M, et al: The effect of haloperidol and naloxone on excessive grooming behavior of cats, *Eur Neuropsychopharmacol* 4(1):39–45, 1994.
59. Dodman NH, Shuster L, Nesbitt G, et al: The use of dextromethorphan to treat repetitive self-directed scratching, biting, or chewing in dogs with allergic dermatitis, *J Vet Pharmacol Ther* 27:99–104, 2004.
60. Gustafson BW: Methylphenidate toxicosis in a cat, *J Am Vet Med Assoc* 208(7):1052–1053, 1996.
61. Pageat P, Gaultier E: Current research in canine and feline pheromones, *Vet Clin North Am Small Anim Pract* 33(2):187–211, 2003.
62. Taylor K, Mills DS: A placebo-controlled study to investigate the effect of dog appeasing pheromone and other environmental and management factors on the reports of disturbance and house soiling during the night in recently adopted puppies, *(Canis familiaris), Appl Anim Behav Sci* 105(4):358–368, 2007.
63. Gandia Estellés M, Mills DS: Signs of travel-related problems in dogs and their response to treatment with dog-appeasing pheromone, *Vet Rec* 159(5):143–148, 2006.
64. Mills DS, Ramos D, Estelles SG, et al: A triple blind placebo-controlled investigation into the assessment of the effect of dog appeasing pheromone (DAP) on anxiety-related behaviour of problem dogs in the veterinary clinic, *Appl Anim Behav Sci* 98:114–126, 2006.
65. Tod E, Brander D, Waran N: Efficacy of dog appeasing pheromone in reducing stress and fear related behaviour in shelter dogs, *Appl Anim Behav Sci* 93:295–308, 2006.
66. Gaultier E, Bonnafous L, Bougrat L, et al: Comparison of the efficacy of a synthetic dog-appeasing pheromone with clomipramine for the treatment of separation-related disorders in dogs, *Vet Rec* 156(17):533–538, 2005.
67. Sheppard G, Mills DS: Evaluation of dog-appeasing pheromone as a potential treatment for dogs fearful of fireworks, *Vet Rec* 152(14):432–436, 2003.
68. Mills DS, Gandia Estelles M, Coleshaw PH, et al: Retrospective analysis of the treatment of firework fears in dogs, *Vet Rec* 153(18):561–562, 2003.
69. Mills DS, Mills CB: Evaluation of a novel method for delivering a synthetic analogue of feline facial pheromone to control urine spraying by cats, *Vet Rec* 149(7):197–199, 2001.
70. Casimir A, Fornal CA, Metzler CW, et al: Effects of standardized extracts of St. John's wort on the single-unit activity of serotonergic dorsal Raphe neurons in awake cats: comparisons with fluoxetine and sertraline, *Neuropsychopharmacology* 25(6):858–870, 2001.
71. Timmer CJ, Sitsen JM, Delbressine LP: Clinical pharmacokinetics of mirtazapine, *Clin Pharmacokinet* 38(6):461–474, 2000.
72. Landsberg G, Horwitz D, editors: Practical applications and new perspectives in veterinary behavior, *Vet Clin North Am* 38(5):937-1172, 2008
73. Landsberg G: Products for preventing or controlling undesirable behavior, *Vet Med* 89(10):970–983, 1994.
74. Voith V, Borchelt PL: Separation anxiety in dogs, *Compend Contin Educ Small Anim Pract* 7:42–53, 1985.
75. Voith VL, Borchelt PL: Fears and phobias in companion animals, *Compend Contin Educ Small Anim Pract* 7:209–218, 1985.
76. Houpt KA: Sexual behavior problems in dogs and cats, *Vet Clin North Am Small Anim Pract* 27(3):601–616, 1997.
77. Houpt KA, editor: *Progress in companion animal behavior*, Philadelphia, 1997, Saunders.
78. Ruehl WW: *Anipryl treatment of canine cognitive dysfunction in a fully blinded, placebo-controlled trial for the Cognitive Study Group*, Reno, 1997, Presented at the AVSAB Meeting.
79. Ikdea-Douglas CJ, Zicker SC, Estrada J, et al: Prior experience, antioxidants and mitochondrial cofactors improve cognitive function in aged beagles, *Vet Ther* 5(1):1–16, 2004.
80. Osella MC, Re G, Odore R, et al: Canine cognitive dysfunction syndrome: prevalence, clinical signs and treatment with a neuroprotective nutraceutical, *Appl Anim Behav Sci* 105:297–310, 2007.
81. Head E, Zicker SC: Nutraceuticals, aging, and cognitive dysfunction, *Vet Clin North Am Small Anim Pract* 34(1):217–228, 2004.
82. Virga V, Houpt KA, Scarlett JM: Efficacy of amitriptyline as a pharmacological adjunct to behavioral modification in the management of aggressive behaviors in cogs, *J Am Anim Hosp Assoc* 37(4):325–330, 2001.
83. Dodman NH, Donnelly R, Shuster L, et al: Use of fluoxetine to treat dominance aggression in dogs, *J Am Vet Med Assoc* 209:1585–1587, 1996.
84. Reisner LR: Assessment, management and prognosis of canine dominance-related aggression, *Vet Clin North Am Small Anim Pract* 27(3):479–496, 1997.
85. Luescher AU: Diagnosis and management of compulsive disorders in dogs and cats, *Vet Clin North Am Small Anim Pract* 33(2):253–267, 2003.
86. Overall KL: Use of clomipramine to treat ritualistic stereotypic motor behavior in three dogs, *J Am Vet Med Assoc* 205: 1733–1741, 1994.
87. Shanley K, Overall K: Psychogenic dermatosis. In Kirk RW, Bonagura JD, editors: *Current veterinary therapy XI*, Philadelphia, 1992, Saunders, pp 552–558.
88. Thornton LA: Animal behavior case of the month, *J Am Vet Med Assoc* 206:1868–1870, 1995.
89. Overall K, Dunham AE: Clinical features and outcome in dogs and cats with obsessive-compulsive disorder: 126 Cases (1989-2000), *J Am Vet Med Assoc* 221(10):1445–1452, 2002.
90. Wynchank D, Berk M: Fluoxetine treatment of acral lick dermatitis in dogs: a placebo controlled randomised double blind trial, *Eur Neuropsychopharmacol* 6(3):70, 1996.
91. Mertens PA, Dodman NH: Canine acral lick dermatitis: clinical experiences regarding the pharmacological treatment of stereotypic behavior in dogs, Birmingham, England, 1997, *Proceedings of the First International Conference on Veterinary Behavioural Medicine*, p 227.
92. Dodman N, Shuster L, White SD, et al: Use of narcotic antagonists to modify stereotypic self-licking, self-chewing and scratching behavior in dogs, *J Am Vet Med Assoc* 193:815–819, 1988.
93. International Programme on Chemical Safety: Dextromethorphan. Accessed January 7, 2010, at http://www.inchem.org/documents/pims/pharm/pim179.htm.
94. Lindell EM: Diagnosis and treatment of destructive behavior in dogs, *Vet Clin North Am Small Anim Pract* 27(3):533–549, 1997.
95. Sherman BL, Mills DS: Canine anxieties and phobias: an update on separation anxiety and noise aversions, *Vet Clin North Am Small Anim Pract* 38(5):1081–1106, 2008.
96. McCobb EC, Brown EA, Damiani K, et al: Thunderstorm phobia in dogs: an internet survey of 69 cases, *J Am Anim Hosp Assoc* 37(4):319–324, 2001.
97. Simpson B: Treatment of separation-related anxiety in dogs with clomipramine. Results from a multicentre, blinded, placebo controlled clinical trial for the clomipramine in canine separation-related anxiety study group, Birmingham, England, 1997, *Proceedings of the First International Conference on Veterinary Behavioural Medicine,* pp 143-154.
98. Podberscek AL, Serpell JA: Evaluation of clomipramine as an adjunct to behavioural therapy in the treatment of separation-related problems in dogs, *Vet Rec* 145:365–369, 1999.

99. Cracknell NR, Mills DS: A double-blind placebo-controlled study into the efficacy of a homeopathic remedy for fear of firework noises in the dog, *(Canis familiaris), Vet J* 177(1):80–88, 2007.
100. Beaver B: *Feline behavior: a guide for veterinarians*, Philadelphia, 1992, Saunders.
101. Crowell-Davis SL, Seibert LM, Sung W, et al: Use of clomipramine, alprazolam, and behavior modification for treatment of storm phobia in dogs, *J Am Vet Med Assoc* 222(6):744–748, 2003.
102. Miller WH, Scott DW, Wellington JR: Nonsteroidal management of canine pruritus with amitriptyline, *Cornell Vet* 82:53–57, 1992.
103. Shores A, Redding RW: Narcoleptic hypersomnia syndrome responsive to protriptyline in a Labrador retriever, *J Am Anim Hosp Assoc* 23:455–458, 1987.
104. Neville P: Behaviour problems in the cat. In Fischer J, editor: *The behaviour of dogs and cats*, Ondon, 1993, Stanley Paul & Co, pp 130–148.
105. Hart BL, Eckstein RA, Powell KL, et al: Effectiveness of buspirone on urine spraying and inappropriate urination in cats, *J Am Vet Med Assoc* 203:254–258, 1993.
106. Overall KL: Commentary on "buspirone for use in treating cats," *Adv Small Anim Med Surg* 7:4, 1994.
107. Cooper L, Hart BL: Comparison of diazepam with progestin for effectiveness in suppression of urine spraying behavior in cats, *J Am Vet Med Assoc* 200:797–801, 1992.
108. Dehasse J: Feline urine spraying, *J Appl Anim Behav Sci* 52: 365–371, 1997.
109. King JN, Steffan J, Heath SE, et al: Determination of the dosage of clomipramine for the treatment of urine spraying in cats, *J Am Vet Med Assoc* 225(6):881–887, 2004.
110. Seibert LM: Case report, *J Am Vet Med Assoc* 224(10): 1594–1596, 2004.
111. Crowell-Davis SL, Barry K, Wolfe R: Social behavior and aggressive problems in cats, *Vet Clin North Am Small Anim Pract* 27(3):549–568, 1997.
112. Leuscher A: Behavioral disorders. In Ettinger SJ, editor: *Textbook of veterinary internal medicine*, ed 6, St. Louis, 2005, Saunders.
113. Swanepoel N, Lee E, Stein DJ: Psychogenic alopecia in a cat: response to clomipramine, *J South Afr Vet Assoc* 69(1):22, 1998.
114. Overall KL: Treating depression in a cat after it loses a companion, behavior Q & A, *Vet Med* 97(7):508–510, 2002.

27 Anticonvulsants and Other Neurologic Therapies in Small Animals

Dawn Merton Boothe

Chapter Outline

Successful control of seizures with anticonvulsant drugs reflects a balance in achieving seizure control and minimizing undesirable drug side effects. Variability in the disposition of anticonvulsants and interactions among them and other drugs are important confounders of successful therapy. This chapter reviews selected anticonvulsants, focusing on drugs most likely to control seizures in small animals However, drugs that have been used historically and selected drugs that are used in humans but for which information is available in dogs or cats are also discussed, in part to explain why they may be less than ideal choices.The proper use of anticonvulsants is discussed, with an emphasis on the differences in individual drug disposition, detection of these differences (e.g., therapeutic drug monitoring), and rational approaches to responding to these differences by dose modification. The primary topic of discussion is treatment of generalized, tonic–clonic seizures, the most common type afflicting small animals. Opinions regarding anticonvulsant therapy vary among clinicians. Treatment of behavioral disorders that might manifest as seizural type activity is discussed in Chapter 26. Some of the comments and recommendations offered in the discussions of selected drugs reflect personal observations obtained in the direction of a therapeutic drug monitoring service or through clinical trials that focus on the use of anticonvulsants either alone or in combination with phenobarbital.

It is important to approach epilepsy as a clinical manifestation of an underlying disease. Thus therapy is more likely to be effective if the underlying disease is treated. Such causes should be identified and appropriately treated—if possible, before chronic anticonvulsant therapy is instituted. Neutering of affected animals (male and female) is strongly encouraged not only for ethical reasons (i.e., precluding perpetuation of contributing genes) but also to minimize the potential adverse effect of circulating sex hormones on neuronal membrane stability. Unfortunately, the underlying cause of epilepsy often cannot be identified (idiopathic epilepsy) or, if identified, cannot be corrected such that seizures are adequately controlled. In such instances, regardless of the cause of seizures, management is based on control with anticonvulsant drugs. Undesirable side effects are often the limiting factor in the use of anticonvulsant drugs, and not all seizures necessarily require treatment.

KEY POINT 27-1 Long-term therapy with anticonvulsant drugs increases the risk of adverse reactions and drug interactions in the epileptic patient.

Certainly immediate, short-term anticonvulsant therapy is indicated for status epilepticus (see later definition) or cluster seizures. Chronic therapy is generally indicated for seizures that last more than 3 minutes, cluster seizures (for which there is no delineable interictal period), or seizures that occur more frequently than once a month. Seizures that are not sufficiently controlled can lead to additional seizuring (kindling) or to the development of a second "mirror" focus of seizure activity. This might be manifested as a decreasing interictal period or a worsening of seizure activity (including duration).

PHYSIOLOGY AND SEIZURE PATHOPHYSIOLOGY

Anatomy

Neurons are either layered or clustered (forming nuclei) and classified according to function (sensory, motor, or interneuron), location, or the neurotransmitter synthesized and released by the neuron.[1] Neurons are outnumbered by several orders of magnitude by other cells, including macroglia, microglia, and cells of the vascular elements. Microglia are related to macrophage/monocyte lineage and are either resident or recruited during inflammation. The macroglia are the most abundant of the supportive cells and include, among other cells, astrocytes and oligodendroglia. The latter are the myelin-producing cells, whereas astrocytes provide metabolic support and remove extracellular neurotransmitters.

Barriers to Drug Distribution

The blood–brain barrier and blood–cerebrospinal fluid (CSF) barrier form a permeability boundary, rendering the brain a sanctuary by limiting penetration of macromolecules. They also act as selective barriers to inflow and outflow of small, charged molecules, including drugs, neurotransmitters, and their precursors or metabolites. The blood–brain barrier is absent in selected locations, thus allowing the brain to monitor chemicals. These areas include but are not limited to the area postrema, median eminence of hypothalamus, and the posterior pituitary and pineal glands. Cerebral ischemia and inflammation modify the integrity and function of the barriers. The blood–brain barrier comprises blood capillaries that differ in structure compared to other tissues in that they lack fenestrae and are joined by tight junctions similar to the epithelium of other tissues. Microvessels comprise about 95% of the total surface area of the barrier. Astrocyte foot processes encapsulate the capillaries, forming the tight junctions (Figure 27-1). Because pinocytosis also is absent, compounds can enter the brain only by passive diffusion, limiting penetration to small, lipid-soluble, non-ionized molecules. In addition to the physical barrier, function mechanisms exist to preclude central nervous system (CNS) penetration. These include degradative enzymes, which target not only chemicals but also many peptides, and high concentrations of efflux transporters. These include adenosine triphosphate (ATP)–binding cassette proteins such as P-glycoprotein (among the most abundant and most well characterized) and others, resulting in a combined broad substrate specificity that targets many drugs.[2] The substrate specificity of the P-glycoprotein transporter is large; its role in breed susceptibility to CNS adverse drug reactions is discussed in Chapters 2 and 3. Interactions involving P-glycoprotein (or other efflux transporters) are among the drug interactions described at the level of the blood–brain barrier.[3] In the dog this protein is regulated by only one gene (ABCB1).[4]

The blood–CSF barrier prevents compounds moving from interstitial fluid into brain parenchyma.[5] This barrier is located in the epithelium of the choroid plexus, limiting movement of compounds from the blood into the CSF. The choroid plexus consists of the highly vascularized pia mater and cells with microvilli on the CSF side. The plexus dips into pockets formed by folding of ependymal cells onto themselves, forming a double layer structure between the dura and pia (i.e., the arachnoid membrane). This double layer contains the subarachnoid space. Although the capillaries of the choroid plexus are fenestrated, the adjacent choroidal epithelial cells form tight junctions, precluding movement of most macromolecules. Like the blood–brain barrier, the blood–CSF barrier contains organic acid transporters that preclude penetration of many therapeutic agents.[6] The role of efflux pumps and P-glycoprotein in particular is discussed later.

The formidable barrier presented to chemical penetration of the brain contributes to therapeutic failure when treating dysfunction of the CNS. A number of strategies have been described to enhance drug delivery to the brain.[6] These include manipulation of the drugs such that they are chemically more likely to penetrate the barrier, administration of prodrugs, the combination of drugs with compounds that decrease drug efflux, the design of vectors or other carriers that are able to penetrate, and temporary disruption of the barriers themselves. The use of nanotechnology offers potentially viable options.[7] Finally, alternative routes of delivery include intraventricular, intrathecal, olfactory, and direct interstitial routes. None thus far has proved consistently safe or relevant to all therapeutic agents.

Physiology of Neuronal Activation

Neuronal activity can be manipulated through molecular mechanisms at several levels: (1) ion channels, which mediate excitability; (2) neurotransmitters and their receptors; (3) auxiliary intramembranous or cytoplasmic transductive molecules that couple receptor signals to intracellular actions; and (4) neurotransmitter transporters that facilitate their conservation through reaccumulation into the terminal (plasma membrane proteins) and then synaptic vesicles (vesicular transporters) (Figure 27-2). The combined influence of these molecular entities regulate three major cations (Na^+, K^+ and Ca^{2+}) and the major anion (Cl^-). The cations are directly regulated through voltage-dependent Ca^{2+}, N^+, and K^+ channels, allowing for rapid changes in ion permeability, thus facilitating the excitation–secretion coupling necessary for transmitter release. They also are influenced by ligand-gated ion

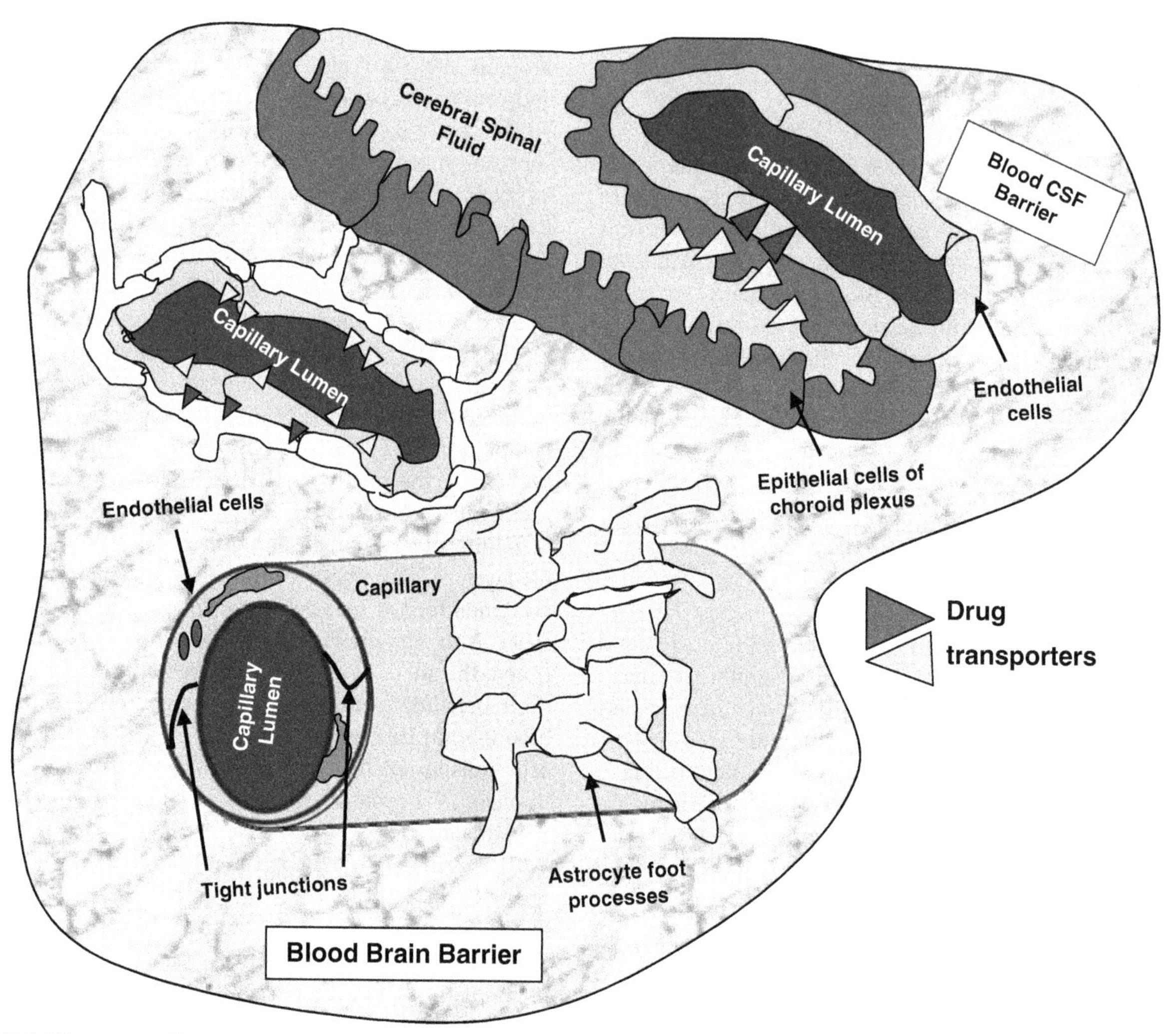

Figure 27-1 Diagrammatic representation of the blood brain *(left)* and blood–cerebrospinal fluid *(right)* barriers, structures that limit compound movement from blood into the interstitial fluids of brain parenchyma. The endothelium of the capillaries of the blood–brain barrier lack fenestrae, are joined by tight junctions, and are encapsulated by astrocyte foot processes. Only small, lipid-soluble, non-ionized molecules in the blood stream are likely to move through the endothelium into the brain. The blood–CSF barrier is formed from the epithelium of the choroid plexus, which forms tight junctions. The plexus dips into a double-celled structure made from folding of ependymals cells on themselves. (See text for other mechanisms by which drugs might be excluded from each of these sites.)

channels, which in turn are regulated by neurotransmitter binding. These include but are not limited to glutamate receptors and ionophore receptors for acetylcholine (nicotinic), $GABA_A$, and glycine.[1]

Neurons generally release the same substance at each synaptic terminal in which the neuron is involved. Neurotransmitters generally result in either excitation, reflecting an influx of positively charged ions, depolarizations, and reduced membrane resistance, or inhibition, resulting in hyperpolarization and decreased membrane resistance. Selected transmitters (e.g., monoamines and peptides) may enhance or suppress the classical neuronal response to the neurotransmitter. **Neurohormones** receive synaptic information from central neurons and respond by secreting transmitters into circulation. **Neuromodulators** originate from nonsynaptic sites but influence nerve cell excitability. Examples include CO_2; ammonia; circulating steroid hormones (neurosteroids); and locally released adenosine, eicosanoids, and nitric oxide. **Neuromediators** participate in the postsynaptic response and are exemplified by the secondary messengers cyclic AMP or GMP and inositol phosphates.

KEY POINT 27-2 Drugs that target the inhibitory neurotransmitter gamma-aminobutyric acid have traditionally been among the most effective anticonvulsant drugs.

Neurotransmitters

Amino acid neurotransmitters include the excitatory dicarboxylic amino acids glutamate and aspartate and the inhibitory monocarboxylic ω-amino acids glycine, **gamma-aminobutyric acid** (GABA), β-alanine, and taurine (Figure 27-3, Table 27-1). Because of their ubiquitous distribution in the brain and their rapid, reversible, and reduntant effects, amino acid

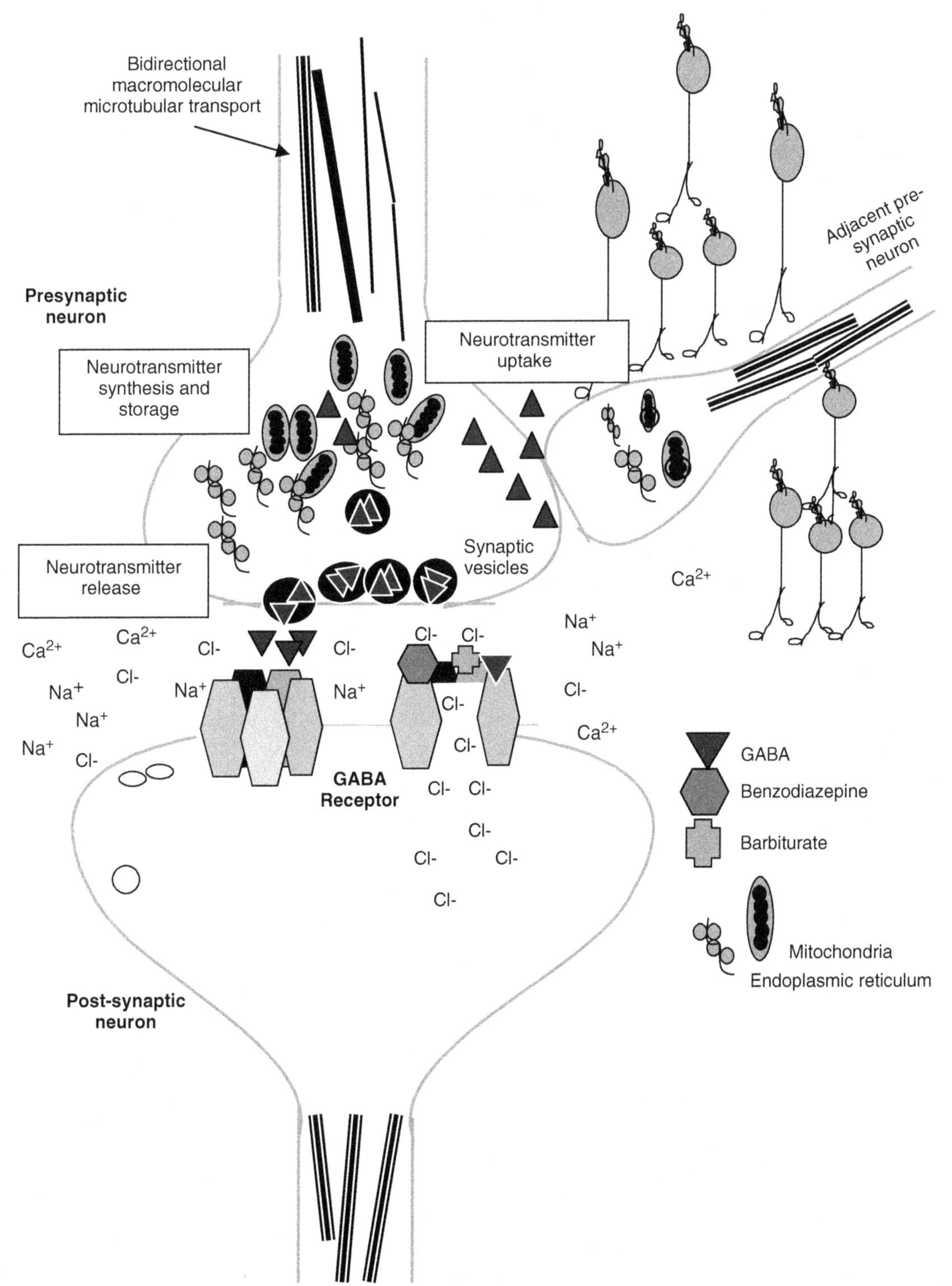

Figure 27-2 Potential therapeutic targets of anticonvulsant and behavior-modifying drugs include the presynaptic nerve terminal and the postsynaptic neuron. Presynaptically, microtubules allow for bidirectional transport of macromolecules to and from the neuronal cell body and distal processes; motors responsible for transport may be subject to drug action. Active uptake, synthesis, storage, and release of neurotransmitters may also be targeted. Postsynaptically, neurotransmitter-receptor interaction can be targeted. The receptor for gamma-aminobutyric acid (GABA) has binding sites for GABA, barbiturates, and benzodiazepines. Interaction between the drug and receptor causes a channel in the receptor to open to chloride flux. Increased chloride concentrations inside the cell increase electronegativity, thus hyperpolarizing the cell. Intracellular targets that express synaptic activity may also be targeted.

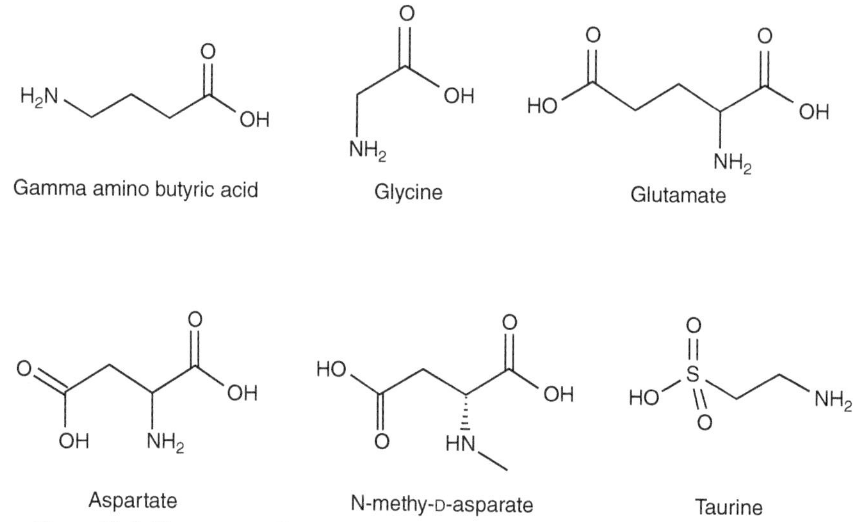

Gamma amino butyric acid

Glycine

Glutamate

Aspartate

N-methy-D-asparate

Taurine

Figure 27-3 Structures of selected amino acids that affect neurotransmission.

Table 27-1 Neurotransmitters Influential in the Treatment of Seizures

Neurotransmitter	Receptors	Target	Agonists	Antagonist	Transporter blocker	Comment
Acetylcholine	Nicotinic	Inotropic, fast excitatory, cationic channels				
	Alpha and beta isoforms	N/A				
	Muscarinic	GPCR modulatory				
Aspartate	GLU	Inotropic, fast, excitatory, cationic channels	Kainate, AMPA		None	
	KA					
	NMDA	Inotropic, slow, excitatory, Mg^{2+} gated	NMDA	Phencyclidine		
	NMDA 1,2 (A-D)		Glutamine, aspartate			
	mGLU	GPCR, second messengers	Multiple			
Dopamine	$D_{1\text{-}5}$	GPCR (Gs: D_1, D_5; Gi: $D_{2\text{-}4}$)	Bromocriptine (D_2)	Domperidone (D_2)	Cocaine	
GABA	$GABA_{(A)}$	Inotropic; fast, inhibitory, Cl^- channel	Barbiturates, Benzodiazepines	Picrotoxin, Penicillin, pentylenetetrazole		5 Isoforms
	$GABA_{(B)}$	Presynaptic and postsynaptic receptor actions	Baclofen			
	$GABA_{(C)}$	Inotropic; slow, sustained, inhibitor, Cl^- channel				
Glutamate	AMPA	Inotropic; fast, excitatory, cationic channel (as with aspartate GLU)				
Glycine	Alpha and beta	Inotropic; fast, inhibitory, Cl^- channels		Strychnine		
Histamine	H_3	Autoreceptor: inhibition of transmitter release				
Norepinephrine	Alpha ($_{1A\text{-}D}$)	GPCR			Cocaine	
	Alpha ($_{2A\text{-}C}$)	GPCR		Yohimbine		
Serotonin	$5\text{-}HT_{1\ (A\text{-}F)}$	GPCR		Clomipramine, fluoxetine		
	$5\text{-}HT_2$	GPCR				
	$5\text{-}HT_3$	Ligand gated				

N/A; Not applicable; *GPCR,* G protein–coupled receptor; *GLU,* glutamate; *AMPA,* alpha-amino-3-hydroxy-5-methyl-4-isoxazolepropionic acid; *KA,* kainic acid; *NMDA,* N-methyl-D-aspartate; *Mg^{2+}*, magnesium; *GABA,* gamma-aminobutyric acid; *5-HT,* 5-hydroxytryptamine.

neurotransmitters were precluded from initial inclusion as classical neurotransmitters. Glycine, glutamate, and GABA are now considered central neurotransmitters. GABA is enzymatically formed from glutamic acid by glutamic acid decarboxylase. The effects of GABA are experimentally identified in response to picrotoxin and bicuculline. These include inhibitory actions at the level of the local interneuron and potentially presynaptic inhibition in the spinal cord. Convulsant compounds that appear to act through GABA receptors include the selective antagonists penicillin and pentylenetetrazole. Nontherapeutic agents have also been identified that mimic GABA, inhibit its active reuptake, or alter its turnover. Three types of GABA receptors have been identified: A, B, and C, with type A being the most common. It is a ligand-gated, chloride channel ionotropic receptor and is the site of action of many drugs, including benzodiazepines, barbiturates, anesthetic steroids, and volatile anesthetics. The B type GABA receptor is a G protein–coupled receptor (GPCR) that interacts with Gi to inhibit adenylyl cyclase, activate K^+ channels, and reduce Ca^{2+} conductance. The B type receptors act presynaptically as autoreceptors, inhibiting GABA release. Type C GABA receptors are less common, but GABA is much more potent for this receptor. The type C receptor is distinguished by its lack of interaction with several compounds that interact with type A GABA receptors, including baclofen, benzodiazepines, and barbiturates.

Amino Acids

Glycine receptors are located primarily in the brainstem and spinal cord, where they are inhibitory in nature.

Glutamate and **aspartate** occur in very high concentrations and are powerful excitatory signals throughout the brain. Glutamate receptors are either ligand-gated ionotropic receptor channels or G protein coupled. Ligand-gated ion channels include N-methyl-D-aspartate (NMDA) and non-NMDA receptors (alpha-amino-3-hydroxy-5-methyl-4-isoxazolepropionic acid [AMPA] and kainic acid [KA]).[1,8,9] The NMDA receptors, derivatives of aspartic acid, are pH sensitive, and response to endogenous signals, including zinc ions, selected neurosteroids, arachidonic acid metabolites, redox regions, and selected polyamines. Although NDMA receptors are involved in normal synaptic transmission, they appear to be more closely involved with induction of synaptic plasticity. This includes long-term potentiation, which reflects an increase in the magnitude of the postsynaptic response to presynaptic stimulation of a specific strength. The activation of NMDA receptors requires simultaneous firing of at least two neurons, including binding of glutamate released from the synapse and simultaneous postsynaptic depolarization from different neurons. High concentrations of glutamate can cause neuronal death. The mechanism partially, but not solely, reflects excessive activation of NMDA or AMPA/KA receptors and calcium influx. For example, ischemia or hypoglycemia may be associated with massive glutamate release; when coupled with impaired cellular reuptake, cell death may occur. Depletion of Na^+ and K^+ and increased extracellular $Zn2^+$ may play a role in activation of necrotic or apoptotic cascades.[1] The role of these receptors in pain is discussed in Chapter 28.

Monoamines

Acetylcholine is an excitatory neurotransmitter for Renshaw interneurons and other CNS cells. Actions reflect interactions between nicotinic and muscarinic receptors.

Several catecholamines act as neurotransmitters in the CNS. **Dopamine** comprises more than 50% of CNS catecholamine and is found in high concentrations is selected areas. Its effect depends on the subreceptor targeted, with five thus far identified in the brain (see Table 27-1). **Epinephrine** is present only in limited areas, and its role has not yet been identified. However, **norepinephrine** is found throughout the brain but in very large concentrations in the hypothalamus, certain zones in the limbic system, and other regions. All three receptor types (alpha 1, alpha 2, and beta) and subtypes are located in the brain. The nonclassical electrophysiologic synaptic effects of norepinephrine vary with the state but are considered "enabling." Although excitatory in nature, the effects of norepinephrine (and serotonin) can be anticonvulsant, rather than proconvulsant.[10]

Biogenic Amines

Serotonin is one of two biogenic amines active in the CNS. Thus far 14 receptor (5-hydroxytryptamine [5-HT]) types or subtypes are found in CNS nuclei that are located in or adjacent to the midline regions of the pons and upper brainstem. Up to five different 5-HT_1 receptor subtypes inhibit adenylyl cyclase or regulate K^+ and Ca^{2+} channels. 5-HT_2 receptor subtypes (three) are linked to G proteins and phospholipase C. 5-HT_{2C} may modulate CSF production. 5-HT_3 receptors are located in the area postrema and solitary tract nucleus, where they cause emesis and antinociception. Members of the 5-HT_4 through 5-HT_7 receptor types have not yet been studied in the CNS.

Histamine is the second biogenic amine that serves as a neurotransmitter. Four subtypes have been described in the CNS, all acting through G proteins. Most neurons that synthesize histamine are located in the ventral posterior hypothalamus and extend throughout the entire CNS through ascending and descending tracts.[1]

Synaptic Vesicle Protein

The importance of the synaptic vesicle protein 2 (SV2) emerged as part of the research into the mechanism of action of levetiracetam. Levetiracetam, but not other anticonvulsants, binds to synaptic vesicle (SV) protein through the brain in a steroselective, concentration-dependent manner.[11] However, ethosuximide, pentobarbital, and pentylenetetrazole compete with levetiracetam for binding. The distribution of the protein does not follow any pattern consistent with classical receptors, and the protein is located in synaptic vesicled (SVs). Three isoforms exist (A, B, C), with SV2A the most widely distributed. Knockout mice without SV2A die within 3 weeks as a result of spontaneous seizures. The role of SV2A is not clear, but it may modulate exocytosis that precedes neurotransmitter release; disruption of activity appears to result in calcium accumulation and increased neurotransmitter release.[11]

The Action Potential

The normal resting membrane potential (RMP) of the neuronal cell is 70 mV. The electrical difference across the cell membrane is maintained by a Na^+, K^+-ATPase pump. Depolarization and the generation of an action potential occur when the RMP becomes sufficiently positive to reach threshold. As with other membranes, the RMP of a neuron is determined by the concentration of negative and positive ions across the membrane. Important ions include Na^+, K^+, Ca^{2+}, and Cl^-. The concentration reflects ion fluxes and thus permeability of the cell membrane to the ions. Fluxes resulting in an increase in positive ions inside the cell relative to the outside hypopolarize the RMP, bringing it closer to threshold and subsequent depolarization. The tendency of a neuron to depolarize reflects, in part, the sum total effect of neurotransmitters (NTs) that interact with the cell membrane. Inhibitory NTs such as GABA render the RMP more negative and less susceptible to depolarization (see Figure 27-2).[12] The principal postsynaptic receptor for GABA is the $GABA_A$ receptor; activation increases inflow of Cl- ions into the cell, hyperpolarizing the neuron. Glycine and serine are also inhibitory neurotransmitters. Excitatory neurotransmitters, such as acetylcholine and glutamate, elevate the RMP to a more positive status, rendering it more susceptible to reaching the threshold necessary for depolarization.[12]

Pathology

Conventional evidence indicates that neurons are terminally differentiated cells and do not respond to proliferate stimuli. The presence of neuronal stem cells may, however, offer an avenue of treatment for degenerative conditions or damage. In the absence of proliferation, neurons have developed adaptive functional and structural responses to injury.[1]

Several animal models have been used to study either seizures or epilepsy. Models intended to study epilepsy ideally include both seizure activity as well as chronic epileptiform behavior (i.e., spontaneous seizures).[13] The attributes of animal models are generally based on their relevance to human epilepsy in regard to electrophysiologic activity, etiology, pathologies, signalment, associated behavioral changes, and response to anticonvulsant drugs. That multiple models have been developed for study reflects the more than 100 human seizure or epileptic disorders. Chemical convulsants that cause seizures after systemic or direct administration include KA (a glutamate analog), pilocarpine, NMDA, and GABA antagonists, Pentylenetetrazole is among the most commonly used chemicals; repeated injections mimic electrical kindling. Injections of high doses consistently and predictably cause tonic–clonic seizures, allowing its use as a screen for new drugs. Lower doses induce absencelike seizures. Kindling models are considered epileptic models and involve periodic stimulation of low-intensity signals in the amygdala, resulting in tonic–clonic seizures. The animal remains sensitive to electrical stimulation, with the number of stimuli necessary to induce seizures quantifiable. Genetic models have been either developed or genetically designed;[13] for example, deletion of the gene encoding tyrosine kinase prevents the genesis of epilepsy in the kindling model administration of chemoconvulsants.[1]

Seizures are the clinical results of rapid, excessive neuronal discharge in the brain. Seizures are classified as primary (i.e., genetic) or acquired, and as generalized or focal. Generalized seizures are much more common in small animals; the incidence is greater in dogs than in cats. With seizure onset of a generalized character, convulsive electroencephalographic activity begins simultaneously in all brain regions.[14] Epilepsy is a disorder of the brain characterized by an enduring predisposition to generate seizures and by the neurobiologic, cognitive, psychological, and social consequences of this condition. The definition of epilepsy requires the occurrence of at least one epileptic seizure.[10]

KEY POINT 27-3 Epilepsy is a clinical manifestation of an underlying disorder and is not likely to be cured unless the cause is corrected.

Seizures in epileptic subjects often are attributed to a cortical origin. However, the brainstem, particularly the pontine reticular formation, also can manifest self-sustained seizure discharge and may be important in the generation and expression of generalized tonic convulsions.[15] Depression of reticular core activity is an essential characteristic of antiepileptic drugs, suggesting that the reticular formation is involved in the spread and generalization of clinical seizures.[16] In the dog the most common form of epilepsy is generalized tonic–clonic or grand mal seizures.[17] Epilepsy or seizure disorders of the CNS in the dog may be caused by an acquired organic lesion such as brain tumor, head trauma, toxicosis, electrolyte imbalance, hypoglycemia, renal failure, or hepatic disease (acquired or secondary epilepsy) or may be genetic or inherited ("true," idiopathic, or primary epilepsy). An autosomal gene associated with a sex-linked suppressor on the X chromosome may explain the higher incidence of seizures in male dogs. Interestingly, in human medicine the role of autoantibodies is emerging as a potential underlying cause of neurotoxicity and associated epileptic seizures.[18]

Status epilepticus (SE) refers to failure of the patient to recover to a normal alert state between repeated tonic–clonic attacks or episodes that last at least 30 minutes.[19] Convulsive or tonic–clonic SE is a medical emergency in which convulsive seizures must be terminated by treatment with anticonvulsant agents. In humans epileptic seizures must not be allowed to persist more than 60 minutes if severe, permanent neurologic injury or death is to be avoided.[19] The longer an epileptic seizure persists, the greater the incidence of mortality and morbidity. Hyperthermia caused by continuous muscle contraction may become life threatening during continued seizure activity. Brain damage resulting from hypoxia or the sequelae of hyperthermia is more likely if more than 30 minutes of uninterrupted seizures occur.

KEY POINT 27-4 Permanent neurologic damage may occur if seizures persist longer than 60 minutes.

During seizures individual neurons depolarize and fire action potentials at high frequencies. Increased excitability reflects increased extracellular potassium and decreased extracellular calcium. Once initiated, the seizure discharge may synchronize with other neurons and propagate or spread to surrounding areas in the brain. Seizures can be initiated by four general mechanisms:

1. Altered neuronal membrane function. Permeability changes may occur as a result of hypoxia, inflammation, trauma, or other disease. Changes may reflect altered voltage-gated ion channels (calcium, sodium, or potassium) or ion exchangers (e.g., sodium/hydrogen/potassium).
2. Altered receptor number, sensitivity, or function. Examples include nicotinic cholinergic or glutamate receptors. As an example, glutamate receptors initiate seizures experimentally with antagonism of NMDA receptors blocking the excitatory effects and AMPA/kainate.[3,20,21]
3. Altered neurotransmitter physiology, including changes in concentration, transporter, or function. Potential contributors include either decreased inhibitory neurotransmitters, such as GABA, the most potent inhibitory neurotransmitter in the CNS, or increased excitatory neurotransmitters, such as glutamate. The role of gabaminergic mechanisms in seizure activity has been well established in animal models, based on seizure activity caused by GABA agonists or drugs that impair GABA synthesis (e.g., glutamic acid decarboxylase) and eradication of seizure activity in response to GABA antagonists (as reviewed by Ellenberger and coworkers).[22] Altered neurotransmitters have been described in epileptic dogs, including increased glutamate concentrations and decreased GABA concentrations.[23] More recently, Ellenberger and coworkers[22] reported lower CSF concentrations of both GABA and glutamate in epileptic Labrador Retrievers (n = 35; 14 treated with phenobarbital ≤ 3 weeks) compared with other epileptic dogs (n = 94; 42 treated with phenobarbital <2 weeks) or non-epileptic controls (Beagles). Lower aspartate concentrations also were detected in all epileptic dogs compared with control dogs.
4. Changes in extracellular potassium and calcium concentrations might also contribute to seizure activity.[12,24]

PRINCIPLES OF ANTICONVULSANT THERAPY

Anticonvulsants block seizure initiation and propagation by blocking either abnormal events in a single neuron or the synchronization of related neurons. Thus a goal of therapy is reduction in the firing frequency. A common mechanism by which this goal might be achieved is prevention of sodium channel recovery from inactivation (i.e., prolongation of the refractory period) (Table 27-2). It is during this period that membranes are nonresponsive to other signals. Example drugs that target this mechanism include carbamazepine, phenytoin, valproic acid, toparimate, and zonisamide.[25] Another common mechanism is increased interaction between agonists and $GABA_A$, which facilitates hyperpolarization. Drugs that act as agonists at the $GABA_{(A)}$ receptor include the barbiturates, and the benzodiazepines. At high concentrations these drugs also may also inhibit high-frequency firing. Other drugs include tiagabine, which targets the GABA transporter, GAT-1, decreasing neuronal and glial uptake of GABA and levetiracetam, which targets SV proteins. In general, drugs that

Table 27-2 Indications for Anticonvulsants in Humans Based on Seizural Activity

	Partial	Generalized			Mode of Action
		Absence	Myoclonic	Tonic-Clonic	
Ameltolide					a
Bromide (Na^+, K^+)					d or e?
Carbamazepine	X			X	a,j,k,l,p
Clonazepam			X		e
Clorazepate					e
Diazepam					e
Ethosuximide	X	X			c
Felbamate	X			X	a,b,e,f,
Gabapentin	X				e
Lamotrigine	X	X	X	X	a,h,l,m
Leviteracetam	X	X	X	X	i
Oxycarbazepine	X				
Phenobarbital	X				b,e,h
Phenytoin	X			X	a,b,o,j,k
Primidone	X				
Tiagabine	X				
Topiramate	X	X	X	X	b,g,q,r
Valproic acid	X	X	X	X	e,f,a,b
Zonisamide	X		X	X	a,c,g,j,k,n,r,s

Key:

Inhibition of sodium channel of flux	a
Inhibition of calcium channels or flux	b
Inhibition of T-calcium channels	c
Increase GABA concentration	d
Increase or potentiate GABA receptors	e
Decrease NMDA receptor activity	f
Decreased glutamate receptors	g
Inhibition of glutamate release	h
Altered synaptic vesicle function	i
Enhanced serotonin	j
Enhanced dopamine	k
Decreased serotonin release	l
Decreased dopamine release	m
Altered acetylcholine release	n
Reduced aspartate	o
Decreased GABA	p
decrease carbonic anhydrase	q
Neuroprotection	r
Enhanced GABA transport	s

target more than one mechanism tend to be most effective. Alternatively, combination therapy with drugs that target different mechanisms of neuronal function may be effective in seizures that do not respond to single-drug therapy.

KEY POINT 27-5 Mechanisms of action should be complementary when combining anticonvulsant drugs.

Anticonvulsant drugs target seizures; antiepileptic drugs target epilepsy. For the remainder of this chapter, the terms may be used interchangeably, in part because most antiepileptic drugs are also anticonvulsant drugs. Because successful anticonvulsant therapy may depend on the maintenance of plasma drug concentrations within the therapeutic range, understanding the disposition of each anticonvulsant is paramount to therapeutic success.[26,27] Epilepsy is controlled, not cured, with historical rates of success in only 60% to 70% of the cases, although control might be improved to at least 85% if monitoring supports therapy (see later discussion).[28] Generally, but not always, treatment for epilepsy involves drug administration for the rest of the animal's life.[29] The most common anticonvulsant drugs that have been used in veterinary medicine are phenobarbital, diazepam, and potassium bromide (Figure 27-4). A number of newer (human) drugs are increasingly being used, including zonisamide, levetiracetam, several benzodiazepines (clorazepate, clonazepam), gabapentin, and (less frequently) felbamate. Older drugs whose historical use has declined include primidone, phenytoin, and valproic acid. Drugs commonly used in humans that are minimally used in dogs or cats include ethosuximide, lamotrigine, and topiramate. Scientific support of efficacy for each of these drugs in dogs or cats generally is limited; differences compared with humans should be anticipated, not only because of differences in the underlying pathophysiology of disease but also in the disposition of the drugs among species and pharmacodynamic response. Even if pharmacokinetic information is available, generally the data were generated in a small sample size of healthy, drug-free animals. Pharmacokinetic differences in anticonvulsant drugs among and within breeds and species can be profound, with drug disposition often affecting the efficacy of the drug. Studies in Beagles or other pure breeds may not reflect the canine population as a whole. Antiepileptic drugs are generally administered chronically. As such an understanding of the determinants of drug disposition (Chapter 1) is paramount to understanding their most effective use, particularly as it pertains to drug toxicity and avoidance of drug fluctuations during a dosing interval that might contribute to either therapeutic failure. The more important points are as follows.

PHARMACOKINETIC CONSIDERATIONS

Absorption determines the magnitude of, but also the time to, peak anticonvulsant effect. Most anticonvulsants are administered either orally or intravenously, although alternative routes such as nasal and rectal administration are proving increasingly useful for emergency administration (Table 27-3). Most of the anticonvulsants used as antiepileptic drugs are well absorbed after oral administration, with the notable exception of phenytoin. Because food may slow the absorption of anticonvulsant drugs, peak plasma drug concentrations may occur as late as 4 to 6 hours after administration. This generally is not a problem with chronic dosing for drugs that accumulate, but it may affect the time of peak sample collection. Fasting before sample collection might be prudent. Rectal administration has offered a clinically effective alternative for administration for several anticonvulsant drugs. The colonic absorption of anticonvulsant drugs can be predicted to some degree by hydrophilicity. For example, whereas gabapentin is poorly bioavailable compared with phenytoin, maximum plasma concentration of phenytoin after colonic administration equals that after oral administration.[30] A potentially emerging problem — suggested by the author's therapeutic drug monitoring service — are differences in oral bioavailability of human generic products prescribed for animals. The therapeutic equivalence (including bioavailability)

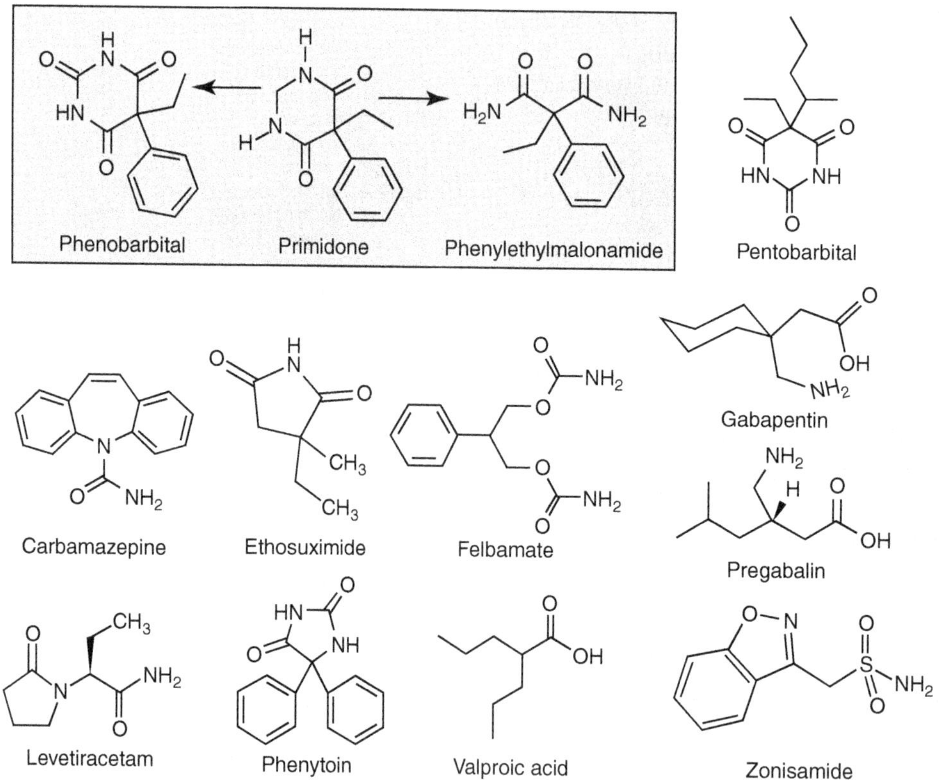

Figure 27-4 Structures of selected clinically useful anticonvulsant drugs. Note the similarities in structures of primidone and its active metabolite, phenobarbital.

Table 27-3 Doses of Drugs Used To Treat Disorders of the Peripheral or Central Nervous System

Drug	Indication	Dose	Route	Interval (hr)
Bethanechol	Urinary bladder atony, dysautonomia	2.5-25 mg/dog	PO	8
Bromide, potassium or sodium	Anticonvulsant	Loading dose: 90-150 mg/kg	PO (with food)	5 days for a total of 450-600 mg/kg
		Maintenance: 30-90 mg/kg	PO (with food)	24; monitor
Carbamazepine	Anticonvulsant	15-20 mg/dog	PO	12
		2-3 mg/kg (D)	PO	8-12
Chlorpromazine hydrochloride	Muscle relaxation during tetanus	0.5 mg/kg (D)	IM, IV	12
	Amphetamine poisoning	10-18 mg/kg	IV	Once
Clonazepam	Adjunctive anticonvulsant	0.5-1.5 mg/kg (D)	PO	8-12
	Status epilepticus	1-10 mg/dog	PO	6-24
		50-200 µg/kg (D)	IV	To effect
Clorazepate dipotassium	Behavioral disorders, anxiolytic drug	1-2 mg/kg (C)	PO	8-12
	Anticonvulsant	0.5-2 mg/kg (D)	PO	8-12
Diazepam	Behavioral disorders, psychogenic alopecia	1-2 mg/cat	PO	12
	Behavioral disorders, separation anxiety	0.5-2.2 mg/kg (D)	PO	As needed
	Restraint	0.2-0.6 mg/kg (D)	IV	To effect
		0.25 mg	PO	8
Diazepam	Sedation	0.5-2.2 mg/kg	PO	As needed
	Anticonvulsant	0.15-0.70 mg/kg (C)	PO	8
		2-5 mg/cat	PO	8
	Anticonvulsant (acute)	1-4 mg/kg (D)	PO	6-8
	Anticonvulsant	2-5 mg/kg	IV, PO	8
		1-2 mg/kg	Per rectum	As needed
	Status epilepticus, certain toxicoses	0.5-5 mg/kg	IV	As needed. Start with a lower dose and increase in increments of 5-20 mg.
	Strychnine-induced seizures	2-5 mg/kg	IV	As needed
	Acquired tremors	0.25 mg/kg (D)	PO	6-8
	Scotty cramps	0.5-2 mg/kg (D)	IV, PO	To effect or every 8
	Preanesthetic	0.1-0.2 mg/kg (D)	IV (slowly)	
		0.22-0.44 mg/kg. Maximum of 5 mg	IM, IV	To effect
		0.5 mg/kg	IV	To effect
	Irritable colon syndrome	0.15 mg/kg (D)	PO	8
	Reflex dyssynergia (urethral obstruction)	2.5-5 mg/cat	PO	6-8
		1.25-2.5 mg/cat	PO	8-12
		0.5 mg/kg	IV	To effect
	Appetite stimulant	0.05-0.4 mg/kg (C)	IM, IV, PO	24 or 48
		1 mg/cat	PO	24
	Functional urethral obstruction	2-10 mg	PO	8
Ethosuximide	Seizures	Loading dose: 40 mg/kg	PO	Once
		Maintenance dose: 20 mg/kg	PO	
Felbamate	Anticonvulsant	15-65 mg/kg (D). Maximum of 200 mg (small) and 400 mg (large)	PO	8-12 as needed
Flumazenil	Hepatic encephalopathy	0.01-0.02 mg	IV	As needed
Gabapentin	Analgesic adjuvant, cancer pain	3 mg/kg	PO	24
	Analgesic, neuropathic pain	10-30 mg/kg (D)	PO	8
	Anticonvulsant	10-30 mg/kg	PO	8

Continued

Table **27-3** Doses of Drugs Used To Treat Disorders of the Peripheral or Central Nervous System—cont'd

Drug	Indication	Dose	Route	Interval (hr)
Glyceryl monoacetate	Sodium fluoroacetate toxicosis	0.55 mg/kg. Maximum of 2-4 mg/kg	IM	Hourly until maximum dose reached
Levetiracetam	Anticonvulsant	20 mg/kg	PO	8; monitor
Lorazepam	Status epilepticus	0.2 mg/kg (D)	IV, intranasal	As needed
Methocarbamol	Controlling effects of strychnine and tetanus	55-220 mg/kg. Maximum of 330 mg/kg/day	IV	Give first half of dose rapidly until relaxation occurs then continue.
		Initial: 44-66 mg/kg (D)	PO	8-12
		Followed by: 20-66 mg/kg	PO	8-12
Methylprednisolone sodium succinate	Spinal trauma	Loading dose: 30 mg/kg (D)	IV	Once
		Followed by: 5.4 mg/kg	IV CRI	24-48
		Or followed by: 15 mg/kg	IV, SC	Once in 2, then every 6 × 2 days. Taper dose over 5-7 days.
4-Methylpyrazole 5%	Ethylene glycol toxicosis	Loading dose: 20 mg/kg (D)	IV	Once
		Followed by: 5 mg/kg (D)	IV	12 × 2 treatments
		Then: 5 mg/kg (D)	IV	Once (at 36 hours after initial injection)
Pentobarbital	Status epilepticus	5-15 mg/kg	IV	To effect
	Sedation	2-4 mg/kg	IV, PO	6 or to effect
	Anesthesia	10-30 mg/kg (D)	IV	Administer first half as a bolus, then to effect
		25 mg/kg (C)	IV	Administer first half as a bolus, then to effect
Phenobarbital	Status epileptic	Loading: 3-30 mg/kg (D)	IM, IV, PO	Increase by 3 mg/kg increments to effect
		3-6 mg/kg	IM, IV, PO	12-24; monitor
		Each 3 mg/kg increases plasma drug concentrations by approximately 5 μg/mL	IV, IM, PO	
	Maintenance antiseizure therapy	2-4 mg/kg	IV, PO	12; monitor
	Irritable colon syndrome	2.2 mg/kg (D)	PO	12
	Sedation	1-2 mg/kg (D)	PO	8-12
		1 mg/kg (C)	PO	12
Phenytoin	Tumor-induced hypoglycemia	6 mg/kg (D)	PO	8-12
	Anticonvulsant	20-40 mg/kg (D)	PO	8
		2-3 mg/kg (C)	PO	24
Physostigmine	Ivermectin toxicity	0.06 mg/kg	IV (slowly)	30-90 min, as needed
	Muscarinic mushroom intoxication	0.5-3 mg/dog	IM	30-90 min, as needed
Physostigmine 0.5%	Dysautonomia	Apply 0.3 cm (0.125 inches)/cat	Topical	8
Picrotoxin (use is controversial)	Ivermectin toxicity	1 mg/min	IV (over 8 min)	Once
Pilocarpine 1% ophthalmic solution	Dysautonomia	1 drop	Both eyes	6
Potassium permanganate (1:2,000)	Strychnine toxicosis	5 mL/kg	PO (gastric lavage)	As needed
Pregabalin	Chronic pain, anticonvulsant	4 mg/kg (D)	PO	8
Primidone	Anticonvulsant	Loading dose: 55 mg/kg (D)	PO	Once. Efficacy of primidone reflects metabolism to phenobarbital; monitor.
		Maintenance dose: 10-15 mg/kg (D)	PO	8 to 12

Table 27-3 Doses of Drugs Used To Treat Disorders of the Peripheral or Central Nervous System—cont'd

Drug	Indication	Dose	Route	Interval (hr)
		11-22 mg/kg (C)	PO	8. Not effectively converted to phenobarbital in cats.
		20 mg/kg (C)	PO	12
Propofol	Refractory status epilepticus	0.1-0.6 mg/kg	IV, CRI	To effect
Taurine	Anticonvulsant (adjuvant)	5 mg/kg (D)	PO	12
	Anticonvulsant (adjuvant)	500 mg/cat	PO	12
Tetanus toxoid	Tetanus treatment	0.2 mL (test dose)	SC	Once. Watch for anaphylaxis × 30 min.
Topiramate	Anticonvulsant	5-10 mg/kg	PO	12
Valproic acid	Anticonvulsant	25-65 mg/kg	PO	8 (monitor)
Zonisamide	Anticonvulsant	3-8 mg/kg	PO	12 (monitor)

PO, By mouth; *D*, dog; *IV*, intravenous; *C*, cat; *IM*, intramuscular; *CRI*, constant-rate infusion; *SC*, subcutaneous.

that characterizes human generic products may not translate to therapeutic equivalence when that product is used in animals. Pharmacies may change a generic product intermittently as product prices change. Dispensing pharmacists may not understand the potential risk of differences in bioavailability between animals and humans. The prudent client should query pharmacists regarding changes in products, and the discerning clinician might encourage monitoring with new prescriptions, particularly in patients at risk for life-threatening seizures.

Rectal availability of diazepam has been well demonstrated. Intranasal administration has also been demonstrated as an effective route for selected drugs, particularly benzodiazepines. However, the physical volume that can be administered intranasally may limit practical application.

KEY POINT 27-6 Bioequivalence required of human drugs may not translate to bioequivalence in animals.

Distribution into the CNS is important for all anticonvulsant drugs, although at steady state, each generally distributes sufficiently into the CNS. Indeed, most anticonvulsant drugs are sufficiently lipid soluble that they are distributed to a volume that exceeds total body water (i.e., more than 0.6 L/kg). In contrast to chronic use, for acute situations rate and amount of drug movement into the CNS may not be sufficient for the rapid response necessary to resolve life-threatening seizures. Drug binding to serum proteins may limit the amount and rate of drug moving into the CNS. However, diazepam is the most lipid-soluble anticonvulsant and very rapidly distributes in the CNS despite its 90% protein binding (see Figure 27-4). Phenobarbital is less lipid soluble and is 50% protein-bound, and therapeutic effects may take as long as 15 minutes to be achieved. Löscher and Frey[31] described the relative half-times to penetration of anticonvulsant drugs into the CSF of dogs. For diazepam its active metabolites desmethyldiazepam and oxazepam, clonazepam, and ethosuximide, the distribution half-time was 3 to 7 minutes, compared with 12 to 18 minutes for valproic acid, phenytoin, phenobarbital, and carbamazepine. In contrast, distribution half-time for primidone, its metabolite phenylethylmalonamide, and the active metabolite of carbamazepine (i.e., carbamazepine-10, 11-epoxide) was 40 to 50 minutes. Lipophilicity, rather than extent of protein binding or degree of ionization, was the major determinant of the rate of distribution.

The role of P-glycoprotein and other ABC transporters in CNS drug distribution is well recognized, being present at both the blood–brain and blood–CSF barriers. The efflux pumps, often accompanied by drug-metabolizing enzymes, contribute to the poor CNS drug penetrability. However, Mealey and coworkers[32] suggest that the impact of P-glycoprotein is very limited at the blood–CSF barrier compared with the blood–brain barrier in dogs, based on similar penetration of a radiolabeled P-glycoprotein substrate into the CSF, but not brain, of normal (wild-type) dogs compared with ABCB1 knockout dogs. The role that efflux pumps contribute toward epilepsy, particularly refractory, is emerging.[2] Increased concentrations of Ppg are associated with seizures and refractory in human patients. In animal models of refractory epilepsy, efflux pump inhibitors have been associated with an increase in drug response. Yet several studies have demonstrated that the anticonvulsant drugs often are not substrates for Ppg. Using a canine osteosarcoma cell line, West and Mealey[4] demonstrated that diazepam, gabapentin, lamotrigine, levetiracetam, and phenobarbital were weak substrates, whereas carbamazepine, felbamate, phenytoin, topiramate, and zonisamide were not substrates. However, other factors may affect the state of P-glycoprotein. For example, glutamate induces P-glycoprotein expression, which may contribute to a pre-epilpetic condition. Pekcec and coworkers[33] demonstrated upregulation of P-glycoprotein in dogs after an episode of SE. Furthermore, a number of other transporters may exist in the brain that might also affect anticonvulsant drugs.

Lipid solubility, which characterizes many anticonvulsants, necessitates hepatic metabolism if the drugs are to be eliminated. Metabolism of anticonvulsant drugs can have a profound effect on therapeutic success. The effect in part depends on the sequelae of phase I metabolism on the particular drug (i.e., inactivation, activation, or generation of toxic compounds). The rate of metabolism of anticonvulsants is variable: Phenobarbital is slowly metabolized, characterized by a long half-life, whereas diazepam is metabolized rapidly and is characterized by a short half-life (Table 27-4). The rate of metabolism

Table 27-4 Pharmacokinetics of Selected Anticonvulsant or Antiepileptic Drugs in Dogs or Cats

	Species	Dose mg/kg	Route	C_{max} µg/mL	T_{max} hr	Vd_{ss} L/kg	Cl mL/min/kg	k_e hr (-1)	HL hr	MRT	F
Bromide (Na+, K+)	Dog(n=4; 0.2%)	14	PO	80**	0.6				69±22 D		
	Dog (n=4; 0.4%)	14	PO	96	1				46±6 D		
	Dog (n=1.3%)	14	PO	85	0.7				24±7 D		
Carpamazepine[138]	Dog	40	PO-liquid	32 nmole/mL (30-64)				0.48(0.37-0.63)	1.45(1.1-1.9)		
			PO-tablet	16 (8.5-30)	1			0.43 (0.36-0.52)	1.6(1.3-1.9)		
(carpamazepine 10,11 epoxide)			PO-liquid	48(28-84)				0.255-0.45	2.2(1.6-3.1)		
			PO-tablet	29(14-60)	3.7(2.3-5.9)			0.099-0.25	2.8-7		
Clonazepam[105]	Dog	0.2	IV	0.110±0.26 (Co)	2.1(1-4.5)	2.15±0.66	19(12-90)	0.53+0.115	1.4±0.34		0.013
			PO	0.012(0.012-0.032)	4.2(2.9-6.3)			0.51+0.131	1.4±0.34		
Clorazepate[101]	Dog (n=3)	2	IV	0.1-0.54							
			PO	0.03-0.05	1 to 3						
Diazepam[96,97,99]	Dog	2	IV	2.4 (1-3) (Co)		5.6±1.3	19±4.2	0.22(0.14-0.33)	3.2 (2.1-4.9)		
Desmethyldiazepam			IV	1.1 (0.7-1.5)				0.19 (0.12-0.29)	3.6(2.4-5.6)		
Oxazepam			IV	0.1 (0.076-0.15)				0.12(0.094-0.16)	5.7(4.4-7.3)		
			PO	0.135(0.065-0.280)				0.33(0.21-0.51)	2.1(1.3-3.3)		0.01-0.03
Desmethyldiazepam			PO	1.2 (0.75-1.9)	0.7(0.2-2.4)			0.2(0.17-0.23)	3.4 (2.9-4.1)		
Oxazepam			PO	0.125(0.079-0.2)	2.2(1-4.6)			0.13(0.1-0.16)	5.3 (4.2-6.6)		
Ethosuximide[140]	Dog	40	IV	68±9 (Co)	0.75-1	0.59±0.066	0.42±0.09	0.042±0.12	17±3.9		
		40	PO	see text	1 to 2			0.04±0.008	18±5.1		91±2.8
Felbamate	Dog (n=20F)	60	PO	52.9±8.6	2 (1.6-2.5)	See text	See text		4.68±1.09		
	Dog (n=20M)			48.6±8.4		See text	See text		6.71±1.64		
Gabapentin [163]	Dog (n=4; Beagle)	600/dog	PO-IR	32.5±4.4				0.229±0.016	3.1±0.2		
			PO-SR	27.2±1.8	2			0.196±0.02	4.0±0.6		
Lamotrigine					4.7±1.6						
Levetiracetam[174,175]	Cat	20	IV	37.5±6.8	4,8±2.3	0.53±0.09	2.0±0.6		2.9±0.7	4.6±0.9	
		20	PO	25,5±8.0					2.95±1.0	5.65±1.25	1
	Dog	60	IV	254±81	2±0	0.48±0.08	1.4±0.28		4±0.82	6±0.9	
	Dog (Hound; n=6)	20	IV	37±5	N/A	0.55	55 mL/min		3±0.3		
		20	IM	30±3							113±13
		20	PO	30±4							100±7

Oxycarbazepine					2.3±0.3						
Phenobarbital[40, 44,43, 48]	Dog (n=8)	5.5	IV	8.25		0.7±0.15	5.6±2.3		96±23	124±34	
	Dog (n=8)	15	IV	19.75		0.69±0.15	6.7±0.8		72±15.5	106±23	
	Dog (n=8)	5.5	PO	7							0.88
	Dog (n=8)	15	PO	19.5							0.97
	Dog (n=6)	2 (tid) × 5 days	PO	13-24	1.67±1.73				53±15		
	Dog	15	IV	21± 2.1 (Co)		0.68±0.029	7.0±1.3	0.011±0.0028	64±15		
		10	PO	15(14-17)				0.014 (0.0112-0.0157)			91(86-96)
Phenytoin[188,190-192]	Dog (n=10)	11	IV	12.9 (Co)		0.85		0.212	3.65		
	Dog (Bassett; n=6)	15	IV								
		30	PO	2.66-7.9							
		10	PO	0.99-1.94							
	Dogs	15	IV	10±0.95 (Co)		1±0.91	2.8(2-3.8)		4.4±0.78		36 (19-68)
	Kitten	3	IV			1.1			41.5		
	Dog (Beagle, n=5)	12	IV X 5 d	Appr 12		1.14±0.15	0.42±0.03		1.89±0.11	2.6±0.12	
Primidone[83]	Dog	10	IV	12.6±3.6 (Co)		0.815±0.27		0.375	1.85		
	Dog	30	PO	10.5 (7.5-15)				0.058 (0.044-0.07)	10 (9.3-11.5)		
	Beagle	30	PO	17±4.7				0.138±0.02	5.1±0.81		
PEMA		10	IV	14±4.2	6(4-8)	0.73±0.2		0.0098	7.1		
Topiramate[201]	Dog (Beagle; n=1)	10	IV				1.1		6.5		
	Dog (Beagle; n=4)	10	PO (tablet)	9.2±1.8	2.4+2.5				3.7±0.2		33
		40	PO	45.4±10.8	1.4+0.3				2.6±0.3		
		150	PO	137.7±47.8	3.9±1.8				2.9±0.6		
Valproic acid[202]	Dog	20	IV	85 (Co)		0.31±0.97	3.03±0.74	0.35 to 0.46	1.5-2.8		
		20	PO (sol)	30-60	19						89±8.2
		40	PO (tablet)	30-75	42						78±17
Zonisamide[217,218]	Dog	6.9	IV	8.4±2.7		1.2±0.5	0.9±0.4		16.4±7.8	22.4±7.8	
		10.3	PO	13.2±2					17.4±4.9	26.8±6.6	68±12
		10 (bid) for 12 wk	PO	52±8.7	2.5±0.65			0.03±0.01	21.4±5.4		
	Cat	10	PO	13(13.1 (10.1-14.3)					31.5(21.3-22.8)		

C_{max}, Maximum concentration; T_{max}, maximum time; Vd_{ss}, volume of distribution at steady state; *Cl*, clearance; k_e, elimination rate constant, *HL*, half-life; *MRT*, mean residence time; *PO*, by mouth; *D*, dog; *IV*, intravenous; *F*, female; *M*, male; *N/A*, not applicable; *IR*, immediate release; *SR*, sustained release; *IM*, intramuscular.

*Multiple dose.

**Normally reported in mg/mL

may vary markedly among species: Phenytoin is metabolized slowly in humans but is characterized by a half-life of less than 2 hours in dogs. Phase I metabolism often yields an active compound; anticonvulsant efficacy of the metabolite may be equal, greater, or less than that of to the parent drug. Primidone must be metabolized to its active metabolite, phenobarbital before it is effective in dogs. Clorazepate, a benzodiazepine, is a prodrug derivative of a diazepam metabolite that is converted in the stomach to its active form (Figure 27-5). Although diazepam is rapidly metabolized, its duration of pharmacologic effect is prolonged because most of its metabolites have some degree of anticonvulsant effect. The half-life of the metabolites may also be longer than those of the parent compounds.

Hepatic metabolism affects both efficacy and safety, in part because of its influence on fluctuation of drug concentrations during the dosing interval. Although it is clearance (regardless of hepatic or renal) that physiologically affects drug concentrations throughout the dosing interval, half-life is the practical pharmacokinetic measure of its impact (Box 27-1; see also Chapter 1). Neither antiepileptic efficacy nor safety of an anticonvulsant drug should be evaluated until at least 87% of steady-state concentrations has been reached, plus one seizure interval (such that the brain is challenged; see Table 27-1). Every time a dosing regimen is changed, a new steady-state equilibrium should be reached before final reevaluation. The time that must elapse before steady-state concentrations and maximum therapeutic response can occur may be unacceptably long for patients suffering from severe, life-threatening seizures or from unacceptable adverse effects to the initial antiepileptic drug. For such patients a *loading dose* might be administered such that therapeutic antiepileptic drug concentrations are achieved rapidly. The amount of the loading dose necessary to achieve steady-state concentrations (not equilibrium) increases proportionately with the half-life of the drug to be loaded: The loading dose is a sum of all the daily doses that would have been administered before steady state occurs, less any drug that will be eliminated from the body during that time period. The major disadvantage of a loading dose is the sudden effect of therapeutic concentrations in the CNS; no time is allowed for adaptation, and adverse effects (sedation, ataxia) are more likely than with gradual increases in drug concentrations. The maintenance antiepileptic drug dose that follows the loading dose is designed to maintain concentrations achieved by the loading dose. Both loading and maintenance doses are based on population disposition parameters; monitoring should be used to ensure that dosing regimens achieve targets

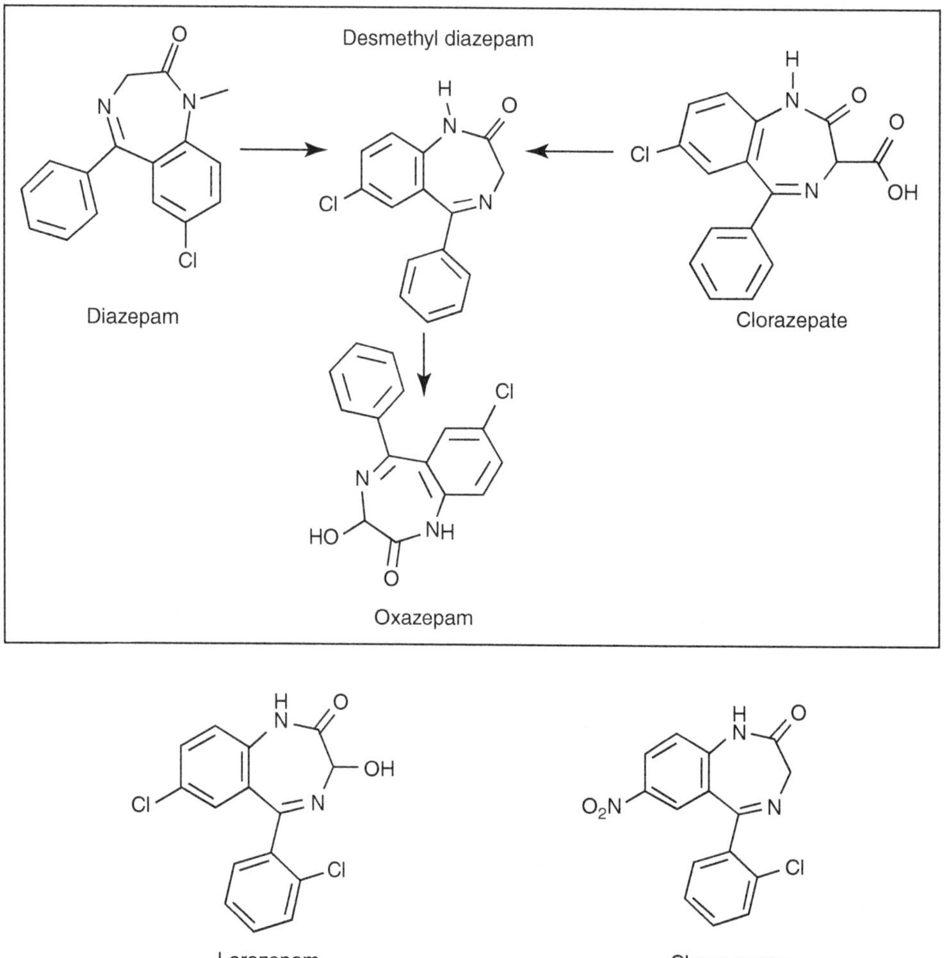

Diazepam

Desmethyl diazepam

Clorazepate

Oxazepam

Lorazepam

Clonazepam

Figure 27-5 Phase I metabolism of diazepam yields metabolites of active, although less potent, metabolites. Clorazepate is metabolized in the stomach. Desmethyl diazepam, nordiazepam.

Box 27-1

Impact of Dosing Interval and Half-Life

The shorter the half-life of the drug compared with the dosing interval, the more drug concentrations will fluctuate during a dosing interval; the longer the elimination half-life is compared to the dosing interval, the less fluctuation and the more accumulation across time. For example, if the half-life of phenobarbital approximates 72 hours in dogs, 50% of the first dose remains in the body by the sixth dose if the drug is given twice daily. Consequently, phenobarbital accumulates across time and will continue to do so until a steady-state concentration is reached. With a 72-hour half-life, only a small amount of each dose is eliminated during a 12-hour dosing interval—that is, before the next dose is administered. Accordingly, peak and trough concentrations will vary little during a 12-hour dosing interval, as long as the half-life does not dramatically shorten (i.e., due to induction). As steady-state equilibrium is reached (three to five drug half-lives), accumulated phenobarbital concentrations will be much greater than concentrations were after the first dose. The magnitude of accumulation (i.e., maximum drug concentration after the first dose compared with steady-state concentrations) increases as the difference between the dosing interval and half-life increases. Doses for such drugs are designed such that therapeutic concentrations are achieved at steady state. From a clinical standpoint, response to therapy should not be evaluated until steady state is reached; however, by one half-life, concentrations should be at 50% of maximum, which may be enough to affect seizure activity. For such drugs each daily dose contributes little to the total amount of drug in the animal, and therefore adding a single extra dose in a seizuring (or pre-ictal) patient will generally not affect drug concentrations. Rather, a "mini" loading dose generally must be given to rapidly increase drug concentrations sufficient to control seizures. On the other hand, should the patient miss a single dose (and for some drugs, multiple doses), the patient may be "protected" by the slow decline in drug concentrations reflecting the long half-life. In contrast, for drugs with a short half-life compared with the dosing interval, most of each dose is eliminated between doses. Fluctuation between peak and trough concentrations during a dosing interval can be dramatic and dangerous. For example, for a drug with a 12-hour half-life, concentrations will fluctuate 50% during a 12-hour dosing interval and 75% with a 24-hour dosing interval. For such drugs accumulation either does not occur or is minimal. Likewise, steady-state equilibrium does not really apply. Because each dose essentially achieves the maximum (and minimum) concentrations, response to therapy can be assessed rapidly. Likewise, should the patient need rapid control, an additional dose may be helpful because the total amount of drug in the body is generally provided with each dose. However, should a dose be missed for such drugs, a rapid decline in drug concentrations can precipitate seizures, including status epilepticus.

for the patient. Generally, antiepileptic drug monitoring is indicated immediately after the loading dose is completed (e.g., the next day). Patients should be monitored again one half-life later to ensure that the maintenance dose is able to maintain concentrations achieved with the loading dose. If the maintenance dose does not maintain what is achieved with the loading dose, the majority of the change as new steady state is reached with the new dose will occur during the first half-life of the drug.

KEY POINT 27-7 The impact of drug half-life on therapeutic efficacy may be profound. Attention to detail becomes more important for drugs with a short half-life.

SAFETY

The safety of anticonvulsant drugs is profoundly affected by metabolism, not only by virtue of short elimination half-lives (for some drugs) but also because of toxicity. Phase I metabolites, by their nature, are reactive. Although intended to progress to phase II metabolism (with subsequent detoxification, particularly by glutathione), some reactive metabolites can interact with and damage surrounding tissues; concentration in the liver can lead to predictable (type A or type I, also referred to as "intrinsic") hepatotoxicity. Thus the risk of hepatotoxicity is likely to be increased with dose and frequency of administration.However, idiosyncratic toxicity (i.e., neither dose nor duration dependent) may also be the sequelae of a metabolite. Although dogs receiving chronic anticonvulsant therapy often develop abnormalities in serum biochemistries and hepatic function tests,[34-36] only about 15% of dogs receiving long-term anticonvulsant therapy have been estimated to be at risk to develop serious hepatotoxicity. This risk is, however, greatly increased if drug concentrations approach the maximum therapeutic range. Primidone is probably most commonly associated with hepatotoxicity in dogs, followed by phenobarbital and then phenytoin in combination therapy.[34-36] One of the many reasons that phenytoin is no longer used as an anticonvulsant in dogs is hepatotoxicity. The risk of hepatotoxicity is discussed with each individual anticonvulsant. Toxicity may be enhanced by concurrent administration of drugs (e.g., phenobarbital) that induce drug-metabolizing enzymes and therefore increase the formation of potentially toxic (particularly phenytoin) intermediates.

Selected anticonvulsants (including phenytoin, phenobarbital, and zonisamide) can affect thyroid hormones; testing before initiation of anticonvulsant therapy might be prudent. Mechanisms include displacement from binding proteins (e.g., phenytoin), increased peripheral metabolism (e.g., phenobarbital), or decreased synthesis (e.g., zonisamide).These effects are discussed with the individual drug. Several anticonvulsants have been associated with changes in serum lipids (e.g., phenobarbital, carbamazepine, valproic acid) in both dogs[37] and humans.[38]

DRUG INTERACTIONS

Most drug interactions involving antiepileptic drugs occur at the level of hepatic drug-metabolizing enzymes. Hepatic metabolism increases the risk of drug interactions; use of any drug metabolized by the liver should be lead to a focus on potential drug interactions. For some anticonvulsants (especially phenobarbital), drug interactions and sequelae have been well described; both induction and inhibition of drug-metabolizing enzymes have been reported. Phenobarbital is the most potent hepatic drug-metabolizing enzyme inducer known and will increase the rate and extend of hepatic metabolism of many drugs, including phenobarbital. Combinations of anticonvulsants can lead to unpredictable effects on drug metabolism. Antiepileptic drugs metabolized by the liver likewise can be affected by other drugs that alter drug-metabolizing enzyme. Cimetidine, ketoconazole, and chloramphenicol are drugs that decrease drug metabolism and have the potential to profoundly increase concentrations of the anticonvulsant. Drug interactions may also involve P-glycoprotein or other efflux transporters.[2] The impact of these interactions is an emerging area of research for antiepileptic drugs.

KEY POINT 27-8 The clinician should anticipate that the risk of drug interactions and hepatotoxicity is directly proportional to the proportion of the antiepileptic drug metabolized by the liver.

Drug interactions also can occur for drugs renally excreted, as is exemplified by bromide and drugs that affect urine chloride. Drug–diet interactions also have been described for bromide.

THERAPEUTIC DRUG MONITORING

Therapeutic drug monitoring can be a critically impotant tool in the successful control of the difficult epileptic patient. However, not all anticonvulsant drugs can be nor need be monitored (see Chapter 5). For example, a therapeutic range must be established for the drug (and, if established in humans, be relevant for dogs or cats), and response must correlate with plasma drug concentrations. An easy, cost-effective assay that requires minimal sample handling must be available. Among the anticonvulsants to be discussed, automated assays are available for several anticonvulsants whereas more tedious and thus costly assays (e.g., high performance liquid chromoatography) must be implemented for others. Regardless of the methodology, clinician should confirm that the laboratory has validated any procedure used to quantitate drug in the target species and implements an external quality-assurance program.

In human medicine, the use of therapeutic drug monitoring for newer anticonvulsants (which tend to be safer) is not as well established compared with that for older drugs, in part because of the lack of generally accepted target ranges (Table 27-5). However, Bialer and coworkers[27] demonstrated a concentration–response relationship for antiepileptic drugs in humans, justifying monitoring. Controlled clinical trials establishing concentration–response relationships are needed in both human and animals to establish therapeutic ranges. Currently, the range in serum concentration associated with efficacy is large for some drugs and overlaps with toxicity in some patients.[39] Nevertheless, therapeutic drug monitoring

Table 27-5 Therapeutic Drug Monitoring Data for Drugs in Dogs or Cats

Drug	Dose[1] mg/kg	Route	Interval	Half-life	Time to SS[2]	MW	Therpeutic Range(3)					
							Low	High	Units	Low	High	Units
(+)Bromide	25-30	PO	12-24	21-24 d(D) 14 d (C) 4-6 (d); 5-10	2-3 mos	79	1405	3937	mmol/L	0.8-1[10,11]	3[11]	mg/mL
Clonazepam										70		
Clorazepate	0.5-1	PO	8 hrs	4-6 (d); 5-10	<24 hrs	409	367	978	nmol/L	150[3]	400	ng/mL
Diazepam	1-2	PO	8 hrs		<24 hrs	284	528	1408	nmol/L	150[3]	400	
	0.5-2[4]	IV	5-10 min									
	5 to 20[5] total	IV inf	60 min									
Felbamate	15	PO	divided	5-8(d)	<24 hrs	238.2	125	250	μ/L	30	60	mcg/mL
Gabapentin	10-30	PO	8-12	<14 hrs	2-3 days	171.25	70	120	μ/L	12	21	mcg/mL
Leviteracetam				2-3		170	32	120	μ/L	6	21	mcg/mL
Phenobarbital	2	PO	12 hrs	45-90 (D); 45(C)	2 to 3 wks[7]	232.2	86	194	μ/L	20	45	mcg/mL
	3-6	IM		(9-12; d)	2 to 3 days							
	3-16[6] total	IV inf	60 min									
	6-12[8]	IV slow										
Phenytoin				2.5 after multiple dosing	<24 hrs	252	40	80	μ/L	10	20	mcg/mL
Pregabalin	3-4	PO	8-12	7	<24 hrs	159				3	9.5	mcg/mL
Topiramate						212.2	15	60	μ/L	2	13	mcg/mL
Zonisamide	4-6	PO	8-12	16-44*	2-3 days	339	35	180	μ/L	10	40	mcg/mL

(+)Bromide (K+) 119
Bromide (Na+) 103
D= Dog

remains a recognized tool for individualization of drug therapy. The author suggests a "start-up", "follow-up", "check-up," and "what's-up" approach to monitoring (Box 27-2). Clearly, monitoring should be implemented to avoid toxic concentrations and to establish the minimum effective range for the epileptic patient This latter reason is particularly relevant for previously controlled patients suffering from breakthrough seizures (previously well controlled): a decrease in drug concentrations compared with baseline should lead to a focus on owner compliance, drug interactions, changes in disposition, and so forth, whereas seizures despite no change in concentrations might be interpreted as worsening of underlying disease and the potential need to control seizures more aggressively. therapy not be considered failed until trough concentrations are in the higher

Box 27-2

Therapeutic Drug Monitoring and Antiepileptic Drugs

When to monitor:

Start-up: To establish base-line concentrations, and ideally the minimum effective concentration for the patient. This is particularly important in the patient that subsequently has break-through seizures or a sudden change in clinical signs suggestive of side effects or adverse events. Start up monitoring should be designed to establish a minmum effective dose such that the patient is not exposed to higher than necessary concentrations. Start-up is also indicated to establish when a uncontrolled patient has exceeded the maximum therapeutic range and further increases in therapy are not likely to contribute significantly to seizure control. At that point (and ideally only at that point) is combination therapy implemented. Start-up monitoring also should be implemented within a day of a loading dose.

Follow-up: Every time a new dosing regimen is implemented the patient should be remonitored at steady-state (this might be withheld until response is realized). A new dosing regimen is defined by any change in dose or interval, or the appearance of a patient factor that might change drug disposition. This includes transitioning from a loading dose to a maintenance dose or adjusting a maintenance dose. Monitoring also should be implemented if a change is anticipated in the patient that might alter drug half-life and thus drug concentrations. Examples include the addition (or discontinuation) of one or more drugs (antiepileptic drugs or nonantiepileptic drugs that can influence the disposition of the antiepileptic drug), a change in the diet (e.g., for bromide), or a change in patient health such that disposition might change as disease progresses or responds to therapy. Determining the most appropriate time point for monitoring will be complicated in patients in which drug half-life has changed and is no longer predicted by sample population statistics. For such patients more frequent monitoring is suggested.

Check-up: Monitoring proactively is particularly important for patients at risk for therapeutic failure. Monitoring is also important as patients age, are placed on diets, etc. The interval of routine monitoring should be individually determined, ranging from 3 months in patients with proven history of variability in drug concentrations to yearly as part of the annual physical examination.

What's-up? Monitoring should be implemented if a previously controlled patient begins to experience seizures or clinical signs emerge suggested of side adverse events. Availability of baseline greatly facilitates interpretation. Monitoring helps identify factors which might cause drug concentrations to change (e.g., drug interactions, change in diet, poor owner compliance). Monitoring should also be implemented to help clarify the role of disease in clinical signs.

Loading dose: If a loading dose is used, drug concentrations should be monitored after a loading dose, one drug elimination half-life later and, to establish a new steady state, three to five drug half-lives later. The sample collected at one drug elimination half-life should be equivalent to the loading dose sample; if not, the maintenance dose must be adjusted accordingly. The collection of a sample one half-life after a loading dose is minimally useful unless a postload sample has been collected; because the patient is not yet at steady state with the maintenance dose, plasma drug concentrations are still in a state of flux. ***No loading dose:*** If a loading dose is not administered, and the drug is characterized by a long half-life (i.e., several weeks to months until steady state is reached), a sample can be collected at one half-life to allow proactive evaluation of the appropriateness of a chosen dosing regimen: doubling the concentration measured at one half-life predicts baseline steady-state concentrations. If the predicted concentrations are not on target, the maintenance dose can be adjusted. Otherwise, for most drugs, monitoring can begin with a baseline sample collected at three to five drug half-lives.

Number of samples: The need for peak, trough, or both samples depends on the half-life of the drug. If the half-life in the patient is substantially longer than the dosing interval (we recommend greater than 2 to 3 times), peak and trough concentrations will be very similar, and a single trough sample collected just before a dose is sufficient (e.g., bromide, and for the majority of patients, phenobarbital; zonisamide). The trough sample is preferred: not only does it reveal the lowest concentration to which the patient is exposed during a dosing interval, it also is not impact by absorption and distribution and thus is most likely to be consistent for across-time comparisons. For drugs that might fluctuate markedly during a dosing interval (e.g., levetiracetam, gabapentin, pregabalin, and zonisamide in some pateints), both a peak and trough sample should be taken to determine patient half-life. If the half-live is revealed to be long, then subsequent single trough samples are indicated.

Other considerations: Animals should be fasted before samples are collected, particularly for drugs that do not accumulate (i.e., those that are characterized by a short half-life). Special handling preparations generally are unusual, although each laboratory should be called to confirm special handling procedures. Serum separator tubes are contraindicated because the silicon separator can bind anticonvulsant drugs and falsely decrease serum drug concentrations. If used, serum should be immediately harvested after centrifugation.[149]

Interpretation of therapeutic drug monitoring results can be facilitated by a clinical pharmacologist. Monitoring should be used to identify the therapeutic range for the individual patient.Therapeutic failure should not be considered if a patient is having seizures simply because the therapeutic range has been achieved, nor should a drug be discontinued or the dose increased if a patient is not having seizures despite subtherapeutic concentrations. For a patient that is not sufficiently controlled, doses can be gradually increased until the maximum range has been reached and the risk of adverse affects becomes too great. Many patients require and can tolerate concentrations of less toxic drugs (e.g., bromide) that are well above the maximum.

end of the therapeutic range. Serum separator tubes should not be used for collection of samples intended for therapeutic drug monitoring.

KEY POINT 27-9 Among the most important reasons for monitoring antiepileptic drugs is to establish a baseline for comparison in the event of breakthrough seizures.

ANTICONVULSANT DRUGS

Phenobarbital

Mechanism of Action

Phenobarbital sodium (see Figure 27-4) specifically depresses the motor centers of the cerebral cortex, thus enhancing anticonvulsant properties. Electroshock experiments with cats and other species established phenobarbital as one of the most potent anticonvulsants available. It has the widest spectrum of activity in different convulsive seizure patterns. Many AED have been synthesized as structural variants of phenobarbital. For example, primidone is a close congener of phenobarbital.

Phenobarbital is the most effective anticonvulsant to delay progressive intensification of seizure activity that may accompany epilepsy. Phenobarbital both increases the seizure threshold required for seizure discharge and decreases the spread of discharge to surrounding neurons; its primary mechanism is enhancement of responsiveness to the inhibitory postsynaptic effects of GABA. Interaction of GABA opens a chloride channel, resulting in higher intracellular concentrations of chloride and hyperpolarization of the RMP (see Figure 27-3). Phenobarbital also, however, inhibits glutamate activity and probably calcium fluxes across the neuronal membrane. A study that compared CSF concentrations of GABA and glutamate in epileptic Labrador Retrievers versus non–Labrador Retrievers and in non-epileptic Beagles also compared concentrations in those epileptic dogs treated with phenobarbital and those not treated.[22] Within the non–Labrador Retriever phenobarbital-treated group, GABA, glutamate, and aspartate CSF concentrations were lower compared with those of their untreated counterparts. This difference was not detected in the Labrador Retrievers treated versus untreated groups; however, only 14 Labrador Retrievers were receiving phenobarbital, which may have limited the power to detect a significant difference.

Phenobarbital might be considered a broad-spectrum anticonvulsant. Despite introduction of new antiepileptic drugs, phenobarbital has generally been the anticonvulsant of choice for the cat and dog.[17] It is effective in all types of epileptic seizures observed in cats and dogs.

Disposition

As a weak acid (pK_a 7.3), phenobarbital is well absorbed after oral administration, although peak plasma concentrations may not be reached for 4 to 6 hours after administration. The absorption half-life in dogs is 1.27 ± 0.21 hours.[40] With an elimination half-life of 0.26 ± 0.18, about 6.4 hours may be required for near complete absorption of phenobarbital from the gastrointestinal tract. Absorption is 88% to 95% complete.[41] Phenobarbital is 45% bound to serum protein in dogs.[42] The volume of distribution of phenobarbital in dogs is 0.7 ± 0.15 L/kg and 0.7 ± 0.4 in cats.[43] Approximately 16 days (8 to 15.5 days) of multiple dosing is necessary to attain steady-state serum concentrations in the normal (uninduced) animal; however, induction may cause this period to be shorter after a change in the dosing regimen of an animal already receiving phenobarbital. Maintenance doses of 5.5 mg/kg daily (in one to three equal doses) administered orally are required to reach an average serum concentration of 20 μg/mL, according to one study.[44]

KEY POINT 27-10 The efficacy of phenobarbital must be balanced with the risk of liver disease, which increases as drug concentrations increase.

Through microsomal enzyme action, phenobarbital is metabolized by oxidative hydroxylation to form hydroxyphenobarbital. This metabolite has a weak anticonvulsant activity that does not contribute significantly to the action of phenobarbital. Hydroxyphenobarbital is rapidly eliminated from blood by conjugation with glucuronide and excretion in urine of the dog. Up to 25% of the parent drug is eliminated renally in dogs. Individual variability in the rate of phenobarbital elimination is marked owing to differences in hepatic metabolism. Half-life varies not only between and within species but also in the same animal, in part because of induction (discussed later).

Breed differences may exist in phenobarbital clearance. Frey and Löscher[42] reported a half-life of phenobarbital at 64 ± 15 hours in largely mongrel dogs, but 32 ± 4.8 in Beagles; clearance was 7.0 ± 1.3 and 13 ± 1.7 mL/kg/min, respectively. Alkalinization of urine (pH >7.5) accelerates excretion of unaltered phenobarbital by reducing back-diffusion (tubular reabsorption) through drug ionization.[45] Fukunaga and coworkers[46] demonstrated that a twice-daily fed diet containing either 0.6 gof potassium citrate (pH 7.8 to 8.2) or 0.2 g of ammonium chloride (pH approximating 5.9 to 6.5) increased urine clearance of a single dose of phenobarbital compared with a water vehicle (pH 6.8 to 7.5) in Beagles (n = 5; female). However, the effect did not significantly (statistically nor clinically)impact peak plasma drug concentrations (μg/mL: 3.25, 2.96, and 2.97 μg/mL for water placebo, ammonium chloride, or potassium citrate, respectively) or area under the curve. Yet, half-life was affected (52, 59.6, and 51.1 hours, respectively), and as such peak concentrations might be slightly affected if the drug is dosed to steady state.

Phenobarbital is a potent inducer of hepatic drug-metabolizing enzymes and is capable of increasing the rate of clearance of other drugs metabolized by the liver as well as increasing its own rate of metabolism.[47] In the dog phenobarbital (2 mg/kg) administered orally 3 times a day for 5 days results in an elimination half-life between 37 and 75 hours, with a mean elimination half-life of 53 ± 15 hours.[44] After a single 5-mg/kg intravenous dose, clearance is 5.6 to 6.6 mL/kg per hour, and elimination half-life is 92.6 ± 23.7 hours in dogs[40] and 47 ± 3 hours after oral administration (5 mg/kg) in cats. The effects of multiple doses of phenobarbital were documented by Ravis and coworkers.[48] After 90 days of treatment (5.5 mg/kg), mean elimination half-life decreased from 88.7 ± 19.6 hours to 47.5 ± 10.7 hours in dogs. In cats 21 days of oral phenobarbital at 5 mg/kg resulted in a half-life of 43 ± 3 hours.[43]

Preparations

Phenobarbital is available as either an oral or an injectable preparation. Oral tablets contain 0.25, 0.50, or 1 grain (15, 30, and 65 mg, respectively) phenobarbital. An elixir is also available (4 mg/mL) for treatment of very small animals. The injectable form is intended for intravenous use but can be given intramuscularly and rectally. Under the 1970 Controlled Substances Act, phenobarbital is classified as a Schedule IV drug.

Clinical Use

Phenobarbital is reportedly effective in 60% to 80% of canine patients suffering from epilepsy if serum concentrations of the drug are maintained within the recommended therapeutic ranges of 20 to 45 μg/mL.[49] This is consistent with the early work of Farnbach,[50] who reported that the concentrations of phenobarbital necessary to control seizures (control defined as interictal interval prolonged at least twice that of the pretreatment period). Concentrations considered effective (n = 22) ranged from extremes of 6.5 to 81.3 μg/mL, with others ranging from 14.2 to 46 μg/mL (mean 23 μg/mL); however, concentrations not associated with control (n=20) ranged from 4.7 to 42 μg/mL. Efficacy might be higher if therapeutic failure is not considered until the maximum end of the range (i.e., 35 to 45 μg/mL) has been reached (Figure 27-6.). The author has reported 85% efficacy in eradication of seizures in spontaneous canine epilepsy with phenobarbital concentrations at 25.4 ± 5.7 μg/mL with such an approach.[28] In this same study, phenobarbital was found to be superior to bromide for first choice control of seizures in dogs (see the discussion of bromide). Phenobarbital has been used successfully to treat hypersialosis.[51]

Patients should not considered refractory to phenobarbital therapy until plasma concentrations reach 35 to 40 μg/mL unless unacceptable side effects persist at lower concentrations. However, because of the potential for phenobarbital-induced hepatotoxicity, the author often recommends adjuvant therapy once phenobarbital concentrations exceed 25 μg/mL in an uncontrolled dog. The dose necessary to achieve target concentrations may vary dramatically among dogs and in the same dog across time because of differences or changes in drug disposition. Changes are likely to reflect, in part, induction of drug-metabolizing enzymes; monitoring should occur 1 to 2 months after baseline is established to detect the possible impact of induction. Measurement of both a peak and trough sample can detect a short half-life; for patients in which phenobarbital half-life is 24 hours or less, the same or a slightly higher (e.g., 25% increase) total dose divided into 8-hour rather than 12-hour intervals may minimize fluctuation of plasma drug concentrations. Clearly, once-daily dosing should be avoided in the face of induction that decreases half-life to 36 hours or less. Phenobarbital elimination half-lives of 9 to 12 hours have been documented in the author's laboratory in some dogs that have been receiving phenobarbital for several months.

Phenobarbital can be administered intravenously for acute control of seizures, although a lag time (i.e., 20 to 30 minutes) may be observed before control of seizures. An intravenous loading dose of 12 mg/kg is designed to achieve therapeutic concentrations (20 μg/mL) immediately; the dose can be decreased proportionately (on the basis of serum phenobarbital concentrations) if the patient is currently receiving phenobarbital. Alternatively, the calculated dose can be given in four to six equal hourly doses. Collection of a postload monitoring sample would be prudent once seizures are controlled; this sample can provide a target for maintenance therapy. A second sample 2 or 3 days later should be used to assess the oral maintenance dose. If used in combination with intravenous diazepam (for its more immediate effects) to prolong the control of seizures, the phenobarbital dose might be administered intramuscularly to avoid respiratory and cardiovascular depression. Once seizures are controlled with phenobarbital alone, monitoring should establish the target concentration for chronic therapy in the patient.

KEY POINT 27-11 The long half-life of phenobarbital precludes rapid response unless a mini "loading" dose is administered.

Limited information is available regarding the use of phenobarbital in cats. Phenobarbital administered at 6 mg/kg daily was useful in suppressing experimentally induced hippocampal generalized seizures in cats; drug concentrations ranged between 15 and 25 μg/mL. After-discharge was totally suppressed in 33% of cats at 35 to 50 μg/mL (12 mg/kg daily). However, phenobarbital was less effective for amygdaloid-kindled seizures.[52]

Drug Interactions

Hepatic microsomal enzyme activity, especially mixed-function oxidase (cytochrome P450 [CYP]) induction, is accelerated by phenobarbital.[53-56] Enzyme induction by phenobarbital appears to be dose related.[57] Long-acting barbiturates are better inducers of microsomal enzyme activity than are short-acting compounds. For example, compared on a molar basis, phenobarbital has been described as the most potent enzyme stimulatory agent known,[58] whereas pentobarbital and thiopental sodium are less potent inducers of microsomal enzyme activity, in part because duration of therapy dose, and thus impact, is limited. Enzyme induction may take weeks to months and may occur with each dose increase. Induction has been documented in dogs[59-62] but apparently not in cats. Although it may occur occur in the latter species, saturation of drug met. Phenobarbital was associated with a twofold increase in CYP protein and increased clearance of the hepatic metabolism marker antipyrine in Beagles treated with 5 mg/kg orally every 12 hours for 35 days. Among the CYP isoenzymes characterized by an increase in activity were CYP1A, CYP2B, CYP2C, and CYP3A; in contrast, CYP2D did not appear to increase.[63]

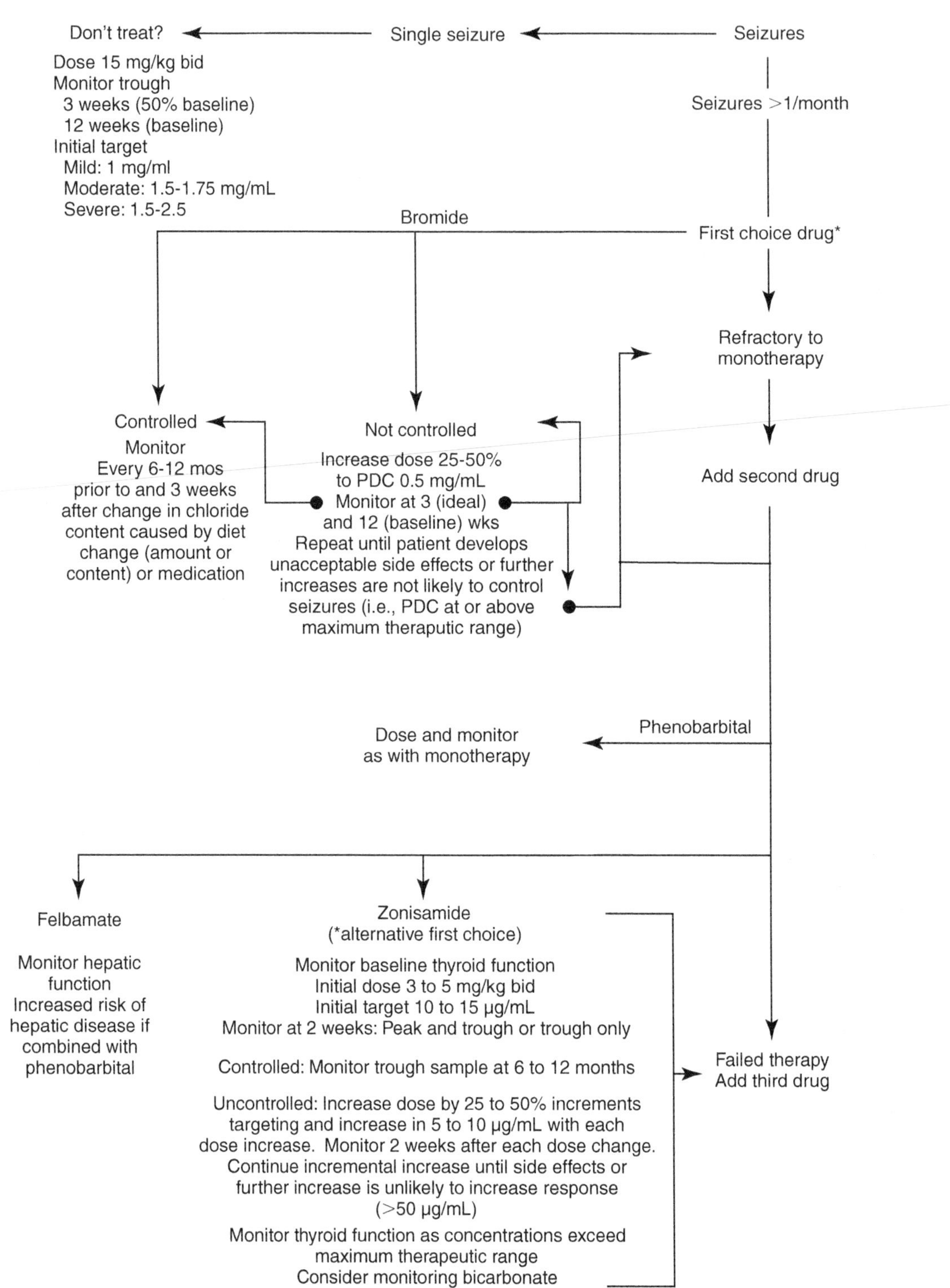

Figure 27-6 Algorithm for modification of anticonvulsant dosing regimens. The goal of monitoring in a stepwise fashion is to achieve adequate control of seizures with the lowest plasma drug concentration possible. This approach minimizes side effects and drug interactions and may allow for the least adaptation by the brain. The highest concentration is generally not initially chosen, particularly for drugs associated with side effects. Combination therapy generally should not be pursued until monotherapy fails (i.e., seizures remain unacceptable despite drug concentrations at the maximum end of the therapeutic range, or in the presence of unacceptable side effects). If initial combination therapy fails, a third drug may be necessary. If the patient responds to combination therapy and if seizure history warrants doing so, the drug that is least effective or associated with the most side effects might be gradually discontinued. Monitoring during withdrawal might be prudent to determine the minimum effective concentration necessary to control seizures should the patient develop breakthrough seizures. Should grogginess emerge with the addition of a second or third anticonvulsant drug, a 25% decrease in the drug most sedative and with the shortest half-life should be considered.

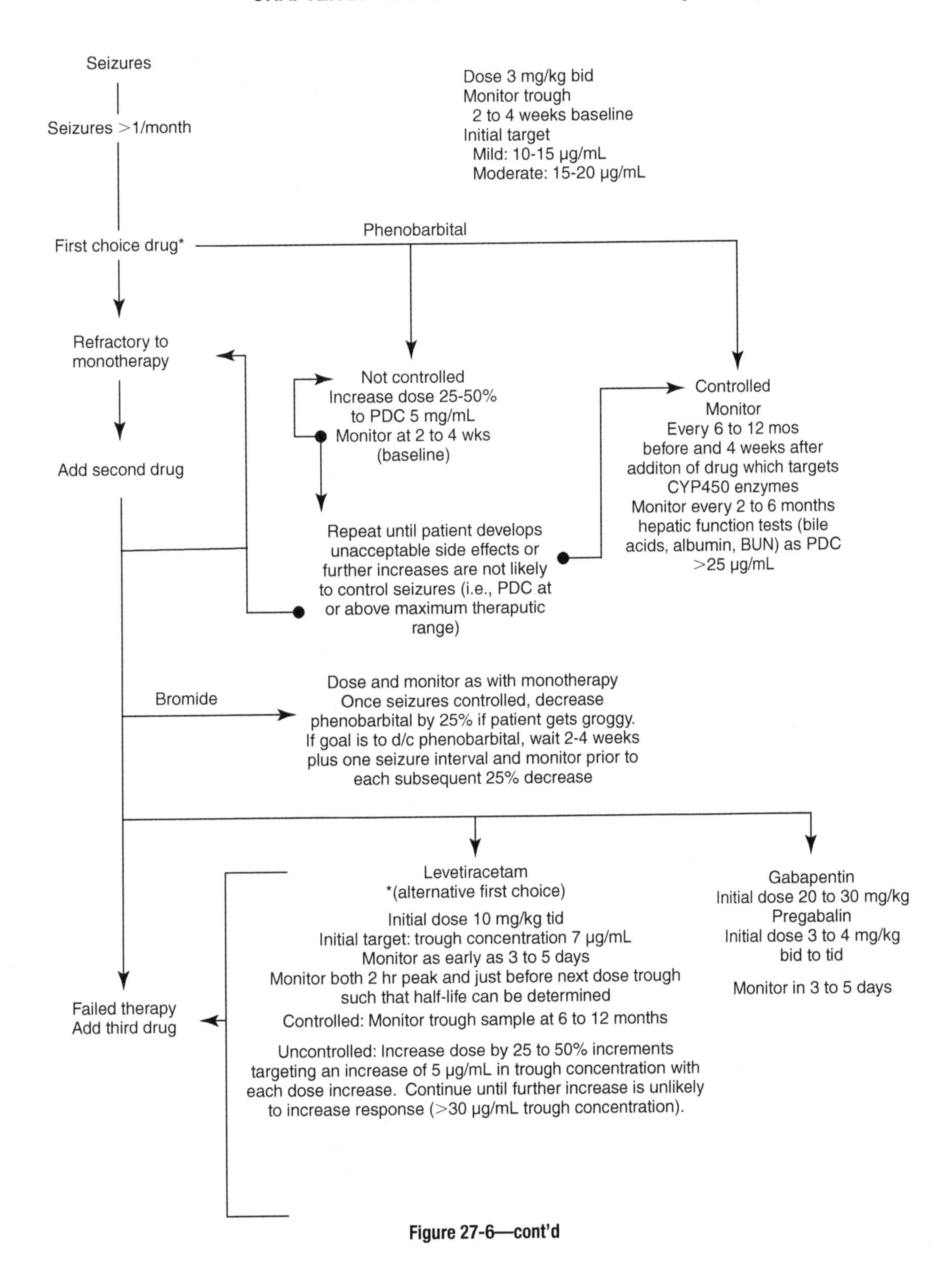

Figure 27-6—cont'd

Induction does not immediately resolve once a drug is discontinued: For example, once phenobarbital initiates induction, up to 7 months may be required for complete resolution in the dog. Fukunaga and coworkers[64] demonstrated that antipyrine clearance was increased in response to phenobarbital at 4 weeks but not 6 weeks in dogs receiving 5 mg/kg of phenobarbital twice daily. Clearance was increased by close to 60% during phenobarbital therapy. Interestingly, volume of distribution increased almost threefold, and half-life *increased*, as did mean residence time, despite the change in clearance. The investigators did not include a control group that did not receive phenobarbital, complicating interpretation. Clinically, as per the author's therapeutic drug monitoring laboratory, however, induction often decreases the elimination half-life and thus duration of therapeutic response to other drugs metabolized by those enzymes induced by phenobarbital (see Chapter 2). In the dog, experimental documentation includes digoxin and digitoxin[44,65,66] and thiopental.[67] However, induction does not appear to affect thiopentone (thiopental) dose requirements in the dog.[68] For drugs in which toxic metabolites are produced, the induced liver will produce more metabolites; therefore potentially hepatotoxic drugs should not be used with phenobarbital. *N*-Acetylcysteine should be used in cases of drug-induced acute hepatopathy, regardless of the cause (exceptions might be made in the presence of hepatic encephalopathy). Longer term support might include s-adenosyl methionine (SAMe) or milk thistle as well as other therapies.

Phenobarbital therapy (2.5 mg/kg orally every 12 hours for 30 days) was associated with a decrease in the peak concentrations of benzodiazepines (diazepam/oxazepam) after single-dose administration of 2 mg/kg either intravenously (about 10%, from 5963 to 5565 ng/mL) or rectally (about 60% decrease, from 630 to 270 ng/mL). However, the target associated with seizure control (150 ng/mL) was achieved in five of six dogs within 8 minutes of rectal administration.[69]

KEY POINT 27-12 Phenobarbital is among the most potent inducers of drug-metabolizing enzymes. Serum alkaline phosphatase also may be induced.

Side Effects

Behavior. Polyphagia, polydipsia, and polyuria are side effects that occur in animals receiving clinical dosages of phenobarbital. The polyuric effect is apparently due to an inhibitory action in the release of antidiuretic hormone. [70] Identical sedative side effects are observed in the dog after treatment with phenobarbital or primidone (discussed later).[17] Dogs appear fatigued and listless after receiving either drug; some are weak in the rear legs, and ataxia occurs. All of these effects may be long lasting and may persist in some cases for the duration of treatment; however, tolerance to these effects generally develops in most dogs 1 to 2 weeks after initiating the dosing regimens.

Bone marrow dyscrasias and others. Phenobarbital can cause what is an apparent allergic reaction manifested as a bone marrow dyscrasia in dogs. Pancytopenia or (more commonly) neutropenia is detected after a complete blood count in animals that presented with a variety of clinical signs. Bone marrow suppression generally resolves rapidly once phenobarbital is discontinued.[71] Bone marrow necrosis also has been associated with phenobarbital. [72] Care should be taken to begin an alternative anticonvulsant drug (e.g., bromide) in animals that are at risk for worsening of seizures should phenobarbital be rapidly discontinued. It is likely that a metabolite is the cause of the dyscrasia; as such, an anticonvulsant minimally metabolized by the liver may be a wiser choice for drug replacement. Phenobarbital-induced coagulopathy has been reported in the cat.[73] Superficial necrolytic dermatitis has been reported in dogs receiving phenobarbital.[74]

Thyroid. Phenobarbital can induce tissue (peripheral tissues and the liver) metabolism of thyroid hormones. Serum total thyroxine (T_4), total triiodothyronine (T_3), free T_4, and thyroid-stimulating hormone (TSH) concentrations were compared in epileptic dogs (n = 78) with seizure disorders and treated with phenobarbital (n = 55), phenobarbital and bromide (n = 15), and bromide (n = 8) and clinically normal dogs (n = 150). Whereas T_3 and TSH total did not differ among groups, total and free T_4 were lower in phenobarbital and phenobarbital plus bromide compared with concentrations in clinically normal dogs. Bromide-treated dogs did not differ from clinically normal dogs. Serum total and free T_4 concentrations were lower than normal (i.e., in the range typical for dogs with hypothyroidism) in the dogs treated with phenobarbital.[75] In a second study of experimental dogs (n = 12), Gieger and coworkers[76] demonstrated that phenobarbital at 4.4 to 6.6 mg/kg adminstered orally twice daily for 27 weeks resulted in significant decreases in serum T_4 and free T_4 and increased TSH. These changes persisted for up to 4 weeks after discontinuation of therapy.[76] Thyroid screens in apparently normal animals that yield results indicative of hypothyroidism do not necessarily indicate the need for treatment; indeed, overtreatment may result in undesirable CNS stimulation. On the other hand, if an animal presents with clinical signs consistent with hypothyroidism, replacement therapy may be indicated.

Osteomalacia. In humans long-term (more than 2 years) treatment of epileptic patients with selected anticonvulsants (phenobarbital and primidone but not phenytoin) has been associated with development of osteomalacia; subnormal serum calcium is seen in such patients. The mechanism is not clear, although accelerated conversion accelerated of vitamin D_3 to 25-hydroxycholecalciferol (25-OHD3) but not 25-OHD3 to 1,25-dihydroxycholecalciferol (1,25-(OH)2D3) is a documented effect of phenobarbital.[76]

Hepatotoxicity. At high plasma drug concentrations (i.e., more than 30 to 40 μg/mL), phenobarbital appears to be hepatotoxic.[77] Animals whose liver is induced and thus requires high doses of phenobarbital to maintain drug concentrations in the lower therapeutic range may also be more susceptible to toxicity because of increased formation of metabolites. Phenobarbital will also cause nonpathologic changes in hepatic clinical laboratory tests because of induction of enzymes. Serum alkaline phosphatase (SAP) and the transaminases are likely to increase with chronic therapy.[34,36,77-79] These are not necessarily indicative of liver disease. However, Gaskill and coworkers[79a] suggest that changes in SAP associated with phenobarbital are indicative of hepatopathy rather than hepatic disease. Changes associated with true hepatic pathology appear to be more likely with primidone (see later discussion). Moderate elevations in alanine transaminase and SAP, coupled with changes in hepatic function (e.g., serum bile acids, albumin, and serum [blood] urea nitrogen) are more indicative of hepatic pathology (i.e., liver disease). Hepatic function tests (e.g., serum bile acids) should be studied to monitor the development or progression of liver disease. Bilirubin has not been a sensitive indicator of liver disease induced by phenobarbital in the author's experience; indeed, it generally increases only with end-stage liver disease, if at all. Interestingly, decreased serum cholesterol levels have occurred relatively early. Liver enzymes should not be monitored until several days after a seizure to avoid the impact of hypoxia and other effects on hepatic leakage enzymes. Consistent increases in serum bile acids and decreased serum urea nitrogen and albumin concentrations are supportive of phenobarbital-induced hepatic disease and the need for rapid but cautious withdrawal of phenobarbital in concert with initiation of an alternative anticonvulsant. Toxicity can occur within several months but appears reversible if the drug is discontinued before fibrotic disease develops.[79] The incidence of serious liver toxicity might be reduced by avoiding combinations of drugs in which more than one is characterized by hepatic metabolism, using therapeutic drug monitoring to achieve adequate serum concentrations at the smallest dose possible,and evaluating clinical pathology changes every 4 to 6 months (or more frequently in animals at risk) while the patient is receiving therapy. Although liver disease associated with phenobarbital therapy has been occasionally noted at phenobarbital concentrations ranging from 12 to 25 μg/mL in patients being monitored in the author's laboratory, the direct cause and effect was not established.

KEY POINT 27-13 Hepatic function tests (serum albumin, urea nitrogen, and bile acids) should be the basis for diagnosis of phenobarbital hepatotoxicity.

Decreasing drug concentrations should also reduce the progression of chronic disease to cirrhotic disease, although what constitutes a safe target phenobarbital concentration in these patients has not been documented. Bromide therapy should be initiated for patients with liver disease (regardless of the cause) who must also receive anticonvulsant therapy. Despite its ability to cause hepatotoxicity, phenobarbital appears to be a safe and effective anticonvulsant if drug concentrations can be maintained well below the recommended maximum.

Hypertriglyceridemia. Phenobarbital is among several anticonvulsant drugs (others being carbamazepine and valproic acid) associated with serum lipid profiles in children.[38] Effects of phenobarbital are described as transient. Phenobarbital has been associated with hypertriglyceridemia in dogs.[37] Median fasting serum triglyceride (mmol/L) was 0.6 (range 0.9 to 1.6) for phenobarbital (n = 28) and 0.6 (range 1.2 to 3.6 mmol/L) for the combination of phenobarbital and bromide (n = 29); compared to non-epileptic control dogs at 0.4 (n = 57) (range 0.6 to 0.9) not receiving phenobarbital.[37] Of the 57 dogs studied, triglycerides were increased in 33% when compared with a reference range established in the non-epileptic dogs. Phenobarbital was higher and more variable in dogs receiving phenobarbital with bromide (109 ± 47 μmole/L) only compared with dogs receiving phenobarbital alone (83 ± 21 μmole/L). Body condition score was significantly related to increased triglycerides. Although no correlation was found between phenobarbital and triglyceride concentrations, a trend was identified between phenobarbital dose and triglycerides. However, the control group consisted of normal healthy animals rather than epileptics not receiving anticonvulsants, and an additional study is warranted to address the potential risk of higher triglycerides in epileptic dogs receiving phenobarbital compared to no phenobarbital.

Phenobarbital may be associated with pancreatitis. Although studies have focused on bromide , studies supporting this association have documented an increased risk in patients receiving both bromide and phenobarbital, as well as phenobarbital alone.[80,81]

Treatment of Acute Phenobarbital Toxicosis

Treatment of acute phenobarbital toxicosis is generally supportive. Dogs apparently can tolerate marked acute overdosing (in the author's experience, concentrations approximately 150 μg/mL) without persistent effects, once the drug has been discontinued. Sedation is the most detrimental effect. Artificial respiration with oxygen should be administered to prevent respiratory arrest induced. Although less effective than oxygen, doxapram or other analeptic drugs might stimulate the respiratory center. Alkalinization of the urine accelerates renal excretion of phenobarbital because of ion trapping in the urine, although this is not easily accomplished.[45] Activated charcoal effectively accelerates the body clearance of phenobarbital.[82] When charcoal is administered in the human, the biological half-life of phenobarbital is decreased from 110 ± 8 to 45 ± 6 hours; it increases the total body clearance of phenobarbital from 4.4 ± 0.2 to 12.0 ± 1.6 mL/kg per hour.[82] Assuming drug metabolizing enzymes are not saturated (threshold not known in the dog or cat), the time needed for phenobarbital concentrations to decline such that sedation is no longer present depends on the drug concentrations (i.e., the extent of overdose) and the elimination half-life of the drug in the patient. For example, at 150 μg/mL, approximately three half-lives must elapse before concentrations drop below 35 μg/mL; for a 72-hour half-life, 9 days must elapse. Both the magnitude and half-life (assuming saturation has not occurred) of phenobarbital can be monitored in an overdose patient; a sample should be collected on presentation and again 24 hours later. Timing of sample collections must accompany the samples if a half-life is to be calculated. A follow-up sample 2 or 3 days later can confirm that the original half-life was correct (i.e., saturation has not occurred). In cases indicative of acute hepatopathy, *N*-acetylcysteine should be administered, as for acetaminophen toxicosis.

Primidone

Primidone is metabolized in the liver to phenylethylmalonic acid (PEMA) and phenobarbital (see Figure 27-4).[83] Although all three compounds have anticonvulsant activities, phenobarbital is much more potent and has a longer half-life than primidone and PEMA (and thus accumulates). Thus phenobarbital contributes up to 85% of the anticonvulsant activity, and phenobarbital concentrations, not the parent drug, correlates with primidone efficacy.[49] Frey and Löscher[42] studied both primidone and PEMA after intravenous and oral administration in dogs and Beagles (see Table 27-4). Primidone is characterized by a short half-life (6 to 12 hours) compared with phenobarbital, although concentrations decrease, presumably as a result of induction, after 14 days of therapy. Phenobarbital reached approximately 65 mmol/mL (11 μg/ml) compared with 50 mol/mL for PEMA, with primidone at 14 mol/mL. The rate of entry into the CNS ranged from 0.01 to 0.023/min for primidone and 0.11 to 0.022/min for PEMA. In 15 epileptic dogs,[49] primidone administered at a range of 10.6 to 20.3 mg/kg every 8 hours yielded mean phenobarbital, PEMA, and primidone concentrations were (presumably at steady state) 31.9, 16.5, and 0.9 μg/mL, respectively. As such, phenobarbital should be monitored rather than primidone, using the phenobarbital therapeutic range. Further, all attributes and detractors previously discussed for phenobarbital generally apply to primidone. Primidone has been used in patients refractory to phenobarbital at the maximum therapeutic drug concentration (i.e., 40 μg/mL), but its efficacy in this scenario has not been proved.[17,84,85] Efficacy may simply reflect improved conversion to phenobarbital (i.e., animals that are induced may metabolize the drug to greater concentrations of phenobarbital than generated from administration of phenobarbital alone). Farnbach[50,86] reported that the concentration of phenobarbital associated with effective anticonvulsant therapy in dogs given primidone (n = 12) ranged from 4.8 to 70.7 μg/mL (median 27; dose 15.2 to 81 mg/kg daily), compared with ineffective concentrations (n = 11), which ranged from 0.3 to 52.8 (dose 5.5 to 83.3 mg/kg). According to Farnbach,[50,86] there is no advantage to using primidone rather than phenobarbital for control of epilepsy in most dogs.

The conversion ratio of primidone to phenobarbital is 3.8:1. A patient should receive approximately 65 mg (1 grain) of phenobarbital for each 250 mg of primidone. Because this rate does not reflect the potential effects of phenobarbital (i.e., primidone) induction, however, animals may convert primidone to phenobarbital at different rates. Baseline phenobarbital concentrations should be established before conversion. Conversion should probably be progressive (e.g., 25% change each month) in at-risk patients (i.e., those whose seizure history includes prolonged or cluster seizures). Cats do not metabolize primidone to phenobarbital as efficiently as dogs.[87] Phenobarbital, PEMA, and primidone concentrations (μg/mL) were 4.1, 11.5, and 5.1, respectively, in cats (n = 11) receiving 20 mg/kg primidone orally twice daily for up to 90 days. The elimination half-life was 7 hours. Although primidone was considered safe, anticonvulsant concentrations were not therapeutic. Thus the safety of primidone at effective concentrations has not been established in cats, and its use is not recommended for the treatment of feline seizures.

Side Effects

All side effects noted for phenobarbital are caused by primidone. Primidone may induce nystagmus, nausea, drowsiness, and ataxia. According to Schwartz-Porsche et al.,[17] polydipsia is more common in dogs treated with primidone. In humans it is recommended that therapeutic plasma concentrations of primidone and its metabolite phenobarbital not exceed 15 and 30 μg/mL, respectively. Megaloblastic anemia is one of the more serious adverse effects of primidone in humans. Pruritis characterized by alopecia, scaling, ulceration, pigmentation, and fissuring has been recorded in dogs.[86]

KEY POINT 27-14 The use of primidone, a prodrug for phenobarbital, is discouraged because of the increased risk of liver disease.

In the dog primidone induces progressive hepatic injury, as manifested by increases in liver enzyme values.[89] In a clinical study, signs of liver toxicity were reported in 14 of 20 dogs.[17] Hepatic cirrhosis associated with primidone and phenobarbital after 7 years of use has been reported in a dog.[90] Primidone-induced dermatitis has been reported in a dog.[88]

Drug Interactions

Drug interactions previously described for phenobarbital also occur with primidone. Primidone should not be used concurrently with chloramphenicol, which is a potent inhibitor of the microsomal enzyme system. Severe CNS depression and inappetence occur in the dog after concurrent use of these drugs.[91]

Pentobarbital Sodium

Pentobarbital sodium (pentobarbitone sodium; Nembutal Sodium), administered intravenously, is considered to be the most efficacious drug for abolishing refractory SE in the dog. Pentobarbital is a general anesthetic (not an anticonvulsant), but it is nonetheless an effective drug for control of nonresponsive seizures; extreme care is required not to overdose. An added advantage of pentobarbital is its ability to scavenge oxygen radicals and decrease cerebral oxygen consumption (see later discussion of increased intracranial pressure). The effective dose varies considerably from one animal to the next. Consequently, pentobarbital is carefully given to effect. Careful monitoring of the cardiovascular and respiratory systems is necessary. Prolonged treatment may be necessary for some patients; some human patients remain anesthetized for up to 9 days before seizures are controlled.

In humans tonic–clonic SE, which is refractory to phenobarbital, phenytoin, or diazepam, may respond to an intravenous infusion of pentobarbital given continuously for 3 days.[92] It is then discontinued, and oral phenobarbital, along with other anticonvulsants, is advocated to control recurring epileptic episodes.

Pentobarbital intoxication has been reported after ingestion of drug-tainted tissue. One case report[93] described a bitch that became intoxicated after consuming a puppy that had been euthanized with pentobarbital. Other reports have involved zoo animals ingesting food derived from barbiturate-contaminated horse meat.[94]

Benzodiazepines: Diazepam, Clorazepate, Clonazepam, and Lorazepam

Mechanism of Action

Benzodiazepines enhance the inhibitory effects of GABA in both the brain and spinal cord (see Figure 27-2). Thus they not only decrease seizure spread but also block arousal and centrally depress spinal reflexes (see Chapter 26 for additional discussion). In dogs, tolerance to the anticonvulsant activity of diazepam develops rapidly, within 1 week, and as such, diazepam is not an effective anticonvulsant for chronic therapy in dogs. Intravenous diazepam is, however, the drug of choice for the treatment of SE in both dogs and cats, in part because of its mechanism bt also because it rapidly crosses the blood–brain barrier into the CSF.

Disposition

Diazepam is the prototype benzodiazepine used in small animals. The drug is well absorbed after oral administration but undergoes rapid and extensive hepatic metabolism. Although only 1% to 3% of diazepam is orally bioavailable, 74% to 100% of the drug and all active metabolites are available.[42] Diazepam is generally administered intravenously but can also be administered intramuscularly, although absorption is not predictable using this route. In human pediatric and canine patients, diazepam has been administered rectally.[95,96]

The metabolites of diazepam (nordiazepam [desmethyldiazepam] and oxazepam) are active (see Figure 27-4), although less so (25% to 33%) than the parent compound. 3-Hydroxydiazepam also is a metabolite, although its anticonvulsant activity is not known.[96] Although less potent than the parent compound, the half-lives of the metabolites are slightly longer than that of diazepam (3.6 hours for desmethyldiazepam and 5.2 hours for oxazepam, compared with 15 minutes for diazepam).[94,96] After oral administration diazepam undergoes rapid first-pass metabolism, with diazepam representing only 1% to 3% of the total (parent and metabolite) area under the curve, compared with 7% to 21% after intravenous administration. Oral bioavailability of all compounds approximates 74% to 100%. After oral administration metabolite concentration surpasses that of the parent compound.[96] Using a crossover study in both mixed-breed dogs (n = 6) and Beagles (n = 4), intravenous (0.5 mg/kg) or rectal (2 mg/kg to mixed-breed dogs and 0.5 mg/kg to Beagles) administration, and high-performance liquid chromatography to detect either diazepam and its active metabolites, desmethyldiazepam (nordiazepam) and oxazepam, Papich and Alcorn[95] demonstrated that the sum total of metabolites will surpass the parent compound. Löscher and Frey[97] reported that the sum bioavailabililty (%) of parent compound and metabolites ranged from 74 to 100 (median 86). Although rectal bioavailaibity of diazepam was only 7.4 ± 5.9% and 2.7 ± 3.2 % for the high and low dose (or mixed breed and Beagles), respectively, bioavailability of diazepam and its two metabolites increased to 79.9 ± 20.7 and 66.0 ± 23.8 for the high dose and low dose, respectively. After intravenous administration, diazepam was characterized by an elimination half-life of approximately of 15 minutes, compared with approximately 2.5 hours disappearance half-life for desmethyldiazepam and 3.8 hours for oxazepam. Peak concentrations of both diazepam and desmethyldiazepam after intravenous administration (0.5 mg/kg) approximated 800 ng/mL; oxazepam peaked at approximately 350 ng/mL. However, whereas diazepam concentrations were below 100 ng/mL within 45 minutes of administration, concentrations were above 300 ng/mL (adjusting for 30% potency of diazepam) for desmethyldiazepam at 8 hours and oxazepam at 1.5 hours. Rectal administration of 2 mg/kg diazepam yielded peak diazepam concentrations of only 75 ng/mL; this compared to peak desmethyldiazepam and oxazepam concentrations of approximately 1600 and 550 ng/mL, respectively. Both desmethyldiazepam and oxazepam concentrations remained above 300 ng/mL at study end (8 hours). As such, rectal administration of diazepam can be expected to yield effective anticonvulsant activity, with concentrations remaining above the minimum recommended for about 8 hours for desmethyldiazepam.[95]

KEY POINT 27-15 Benzodiazepams tend to be the most rapidly acting anticonvulsants and thus are indicated for acute seizure management.

Diazepam has also been studied in dogs (n=6) after intranasal administration (0.5 mg/kg) either as drops or a commercially available atomizer. Bioavailability approximated 40%. Of the two routes, the atomizer was well tolerated. [98] Another study diazepam administered IN (0.5 mg/kg; drug measured as benzodiazepines) in dogs (n = 6, crossover design) reported mean peak plasma concentration of benzodiazepine was 448 ± 41 ng/mL at 4.5 minutes, compared with 1316 ± 216 at 3 minutes after intravenous administration. Intranasal bioavailability of benzodiazepine was 80 ± 9%. Plasma drug concentrations exceeded the recommended anticonvulsant therapeutic concentration (300 ng/mL).[99]

The generation of active metabolites complicates the utility of therapeutic monitoring for benzodiazepines as a guide to therapy because anticonvulsant activity is not necessarily correlated with concentration of the parent compound. For diazepam all metabolites and parent drugs should be measured. Methods based on polarized immunofluorescence appear to correlate with total activity relatively well but are likely to underestimate concentrations by 50% or more;[94,95] the amount of underestimation does not appear to be predictable but probably reflects failure to detect oxazepam.

Benzodiazepines enter the CSF rapidly, with peak concentrations usually occurring within 15 minutes of intravenous administration. The more lipophilic drugs enter CSF most rapidly. CSF to plasma drug ratios generally are less than unity, although concentrations may stay higher in CSF compared to plasma, prolonging the duration nof effect.[100] Both diazepam and desmethyldiazepam rapidly pass into the CSF.[96,101]

Diazepam and nordiazepam have been studied in cats after intravenous administration of 5, 10, and 20 mg/kg of diazepam and 5 and 10 mg/kg of nordiazepam. Elimination of both drugs was linear over the range of doses covered. Total body clearance of diazepam (4.72 ± 2.45 mL/min/kg) was sixfold greater than that of nordiazepam (0.85 ± 0.25 mL/min/kg). Approximately 50% of an administered dose of diazepam was biotransformed to nordiazepam in the cat.[102]

Clorazepate is metabolized in the stomach to its active metabolite, nordiazepam (desmethyl diazepam), which is also a major, although less efficacious, metabolite of diazepam. After oral administration of 2 mg/kg, clorazepate reaches peak benzodiazepine concentration of 446 to 1542 ng/mL in dogs; mean residence time was 8.5 hours. After multiple administration, mean residence time was significantly longer (approximately 12 hours).[103] Scherkl and coworkers[101] described the consequences of long-term use of clorazepate in dogs. After 2 hours of clorazepate infusion, only nordiazepam was detected in CSF. The elimination half-life of nordiazepam ranged from 7.2 to 12 hours and did not change with 6 weeks of oral therapy. Only nordiazepam and oxazepam were in plasma. Oral doses of 2 mg/kg were associated with ataxia and difficulty standing; these signs resolved 3 to 4 days after treatment. Concentrations of 0.180 to 0.780 μg/mL were associated with decreased seizure threshold. Tolerance was demonstrated in two of six dogs, with some, but not total, loss of anticonvulsant activity. Withdrawal also was demonstrated by manifestation of generalized tonic-clonic seizures in two of six dogs rapidly withdrawn from therapy; death occurred in one of the dogs. The remaining four dogs exhibited no signs of withdrawal.

KEY POINT 27-16 Dogs, but not cats, develop tolerance to diazepam and will become refractory to its anticonvulsant effects after approximately 2 weeks.

Clorazepate anecdotally is an alternative anticonvulsant in cats (3.75 to 7.5 mg/cat orally every 8 to 12 hours). However, because it is an active metabolite of diazepam in other species, its role in diazepam-induced hepatotoxicity cannot be ruled out and caution is probably indicated with its use in cats.

Lorazepam is a benzodiazepine derivative used as an anxiolytic in human medicine. It has been studied after intravenous and rectal administration in dogs,[104] although its role in the management of seizures has not been identified. After IV administration of 0.2 mg/kg IV, concentrations remained above 190 ng/mL for 20 min in two of three dogs, and above 30 ng/mL for 90 min in all dogs. However, lorazepam was not detectable after rectal administration of 1 mg/kg, presumably due to high first pass metabolism. Lorazepam also has been studied after intranasal administration. Lorezpam is absorbed almost 3 times as rapidly after intranasal administration compared with oral administration, yielding a relative bioavailability that approximates 2.5 times that after oral administration.[105] Mariami reported in abstract form that the IN administration of 0.2 mg/kg in dogs yielded peak plasma lorazepam concentrations of 106 ng/mL compared with 165 ng/mL following intravenous administration. Concentrations of lorazepam achieved 30 ng/mL (effective anticonvulsant target in humans) by 9 minutes after IN administration in six of six dogs and remained at or above the target for 60 minutes in three of six dogs. Midazolam also has been studied after IN administration with IN aadminsitration exceeding oral administration by 2.5 fold.[106]

Clonazepam (Klonopin) is a benzodiazepine derivative and chemically is 5-(*o*-chlorophenyl)-1,3-dihydro-7-nitro-2H-1,4-benzodiazepine-2-one (see Figure 27-4). It is more potent than diazepam and is used only in the emergency treatment of SE in the dog.[42] Clonazepam is given orally or intravenously (0.05-0.2 mg/kg; the intravenous preparation is not available in the United States). Accumulation occurs with continued administration. Tolerance develops within days to weeks after administration, however, as a result of hepatic enzyme induction. Consequently, clonazepam, like diazepam, is unsatisfactory for long-term control of epilepsy in dogs. However, it might be considered for long-term use in cats (0.016 mg/kg/day; target concentration 70 ng/mL). The relationship between clonazepam and liver disease has not been addressed in cats. The disposition of clonazepam has been described in the dog (see Table 27-4).[107,108]

Preparations

Diazepam is available as both an intravenous and an oral preparation; clorazepate is available as an oral preparation and a sustained-release preparation.[109] It is classified as a Schedule IV drug under the 1970 Controlled Substances Act. Clonazepam is available as an intravenous preparation (not in the United States) and as oral tablets.

Safety

Sedation is the most common direct side effect of the benzodiazepines. Adverse effects (sedation, ataxia, increased appetite, and in some cases hyperactivity) are likely to occur if concentrations reach 500 ng/mL. An 8-hour rather than a 12-hour dosing interval may be indicated to avoid both toxic and side effects. Care must be taken not to discontinue benzodiazepines abruptly because of the potential for SE.[110]

Diazepam may cause hepatotoxicity in cats.[111] Reports have focused on cats receiving diazepam as an appetite stimulant rather than as an anticonvulsant. Manifestations include vomiting, depression, jaundice, lethargy, and acute death. Clinical laboratory tests associated with toxicity include increased serum alanine transaminase, aspartate transferase, and alkaline phosphatase activities and increased bilirubin. Toxicity does not appear to be associated with the dose or duration. Toxicity has not been experimentally induced, suggesting that the reaction is idiosyncratic (i.e., nonpredictable).

Physical dependency toward benzodiapenes has been described in dogs, with the risk and severity of signs of withdrawal dependent on dose and drug. Studies that demonstrate dependency often are based on precipitation of clinical signs after administration of a benzodiazepine antagonist; the severity of withdrawal also appears to be dependent on the dose of flumazenil. Both diazepam and lorazepam can be associated with withdrawal in dogs, although only high doses (60 and 1000 mg/kg per day, respectively, for diazaepam and lorazepam) have been studied. Clinical signs included, but were not limited to, tremor, "hot foot walking," rigidity, and decreased food intake. Lorazepam withdrawal appears to be much less intense but has a shorter latency to onset than the diazepam in manifestation of abstinence syndrome. For diazepam, withdrawal signs include bi-phasic clonic and tonic–clonic convulsions, appearing at 24 and 48 hours. Diazapam syndrome was lethal in two dogs studied experimentally. Administration of diazepam can reduce but not obliterate the major signs of the diazepam withdrawal. The syndrome was worsened by the administration of a benzodiazepine antagonist, although tonic–clonic seizures were not precipitated[112] A follow-up study described withdrawal after oral administration of increasing doses of diazepam administered every 8 hours for 5 to 6 weeks: 0.05625, 0.225, 0.5625, 4.5, 9, or 36 mg/kg daily every 8 hours. Abstinence was precipitated by administration of a benzodiazepine antagonist, flumazenil, at 0.66, 2, 6, 18, 36, and 72 mg/kg, but included a placebo. Withdrawal intensity increased proportionately with the dose of diazepam and the dose of flumazenil. The pattern of withdrawal signs varied with dogs receiving high doses of diazepam more sensitive to flumazenil than those receiving lower doses. Seizure activity occurred only in dogs receiving 9 and 36 mg/kg/day of diazepam. Withdrawal signs increased linearly with plasma and brain concentrations of diazepam, oxazepam, and nordiazepam but not with free concentrations of diazepam alone.[113]

Although desmethyldiazepam (nordiazepam) has been theorized to be the metabolite causing physical dependence in dogs receiving diazepam (in part because the area under the curve for nordiazepam is much greater than that for diazepam),[114] follow-up studies using benzodiazepines whose area under the curve is not surpassed by nordiazepam suggest otherwise.[115,116]

The ability of flumazenil to induce clinical signs of withdrawal, including clonic seizures, in dogs, is well described.[114] Flumazenil precipitated withdrawal scores were higher in dogs receiving diazepam (and halazepam, which is converted to nordiazepam) compared with nordiazepam, although clonic seizures were greater in the diazepam- and nordiazepam-dependent dogs, compared with halazepam-dependent dogs. The magnitude of withdrawal does not appear to reflect a predominance of one parent compound or metabolite but rather a combined effect.[115] Oral flunitrazepam at 7.6 mg/kg per day caused more severe clinical signs of precipitated withdrawal, compared with diazepam (at 6 to 9 mg/kg every 6 hours) administered in four equally divided doses. However, precipitated signs persisted longer with diazepam than flunitrazepam, leading investigators to conclude that diazepam and flunitrazepam were equivalent in their ability to produce induced signs of withdrawal. Difference in kinetics, including protein-binding, among drugs and metabolites, as well as receptor interactions are likely to play a role in differences in response. For example, the estimated free plasma concentration of flunitrazepam and its metabolites was equal to or greater than that of diazepam and its metabolites; further, affinity of flunitrazepam for the benzodiazepine receptor is greater than that of either diazepam, nordiazepam, or oxazepam.[116] The disposition of flumazenil in dogs has been described after oral dosing. Rapid absorption is followed by rapid elimination with concentrations being essentially nondetectable in 4 hours.[117] Interestingly, benzodiazepine withdrawal induced by flumazenil was described in one study to occur particularly as plasma concentrations markedly decreased.[117]

Drug Interactions

Clinically important drug interactions resulting from chronic diazepam therapy have not been reported. Despite reports to the contrary,[118] interactions between clorazepate and phenobarbital appear to confound therapy. In our studies clorazepate consistently increases phenobarbital concentrations in patients that have been receiving long-term phenobarbital therapy if doses of clorazepate exceed 1 mg/kg every 8 to 12 hours. The increases are usually evident by the first month of therapy but may take longer. It may be necessary to decrease phenobarbital doses. Yet clorazepate concentrations tend to decrease across time despite no change in dose, presumably because of the inductive effects of phenobarbital. As clorazepate concentrations decrease, phenobarbital concentrations may also decrease, which may put an epileptic at risk, particularly if the dose of phenobarbital has been reduced.

Therapeutic Use

As in humans, efficacy, including rapidity of onset, coupled with lack of toxicity, leads to intravenous diazepam as the first drug of choice for control of SE in humans.[45] Likewise, diazepam is the drug of choice for emergency treatment of SE in dogs and cats.[42] However, because of its short half-life, diazepam is likely to have to be repeated once or twice during the first 2 hours of stabilization.[49] Not surprisingly, various methods of administration have been recommended in an attempt to maintain effective diazepam concentrations necessary to maintain efficacy. Intravenous doses vary, beginning at 5 to 20 mg or 0.5 to 1 mg/kg.[42] The dose can be repeated in 1 to 2 minutes if necessary; giving the same dose intramuscularly may provide longer therapeutic concentrations. If a response has not occurred after the second dose of the drug, an intravenous infusion can be implemented (note that the infusion line should first be flushed with the diazepam solution to allow diazepam binding to the polyvinyl). Alternative anticonvulsants might be considered in animals failing to respond (discussed later). Patients that respond to the first or second dosages of diazepam are carefully monitored, and if SE returns within 2 to 4 hours after the initial treatment, the diazepam regimen is repeated. Intravenous diazepam may be replaced with other benzodiazepines, such as clonazepam (0.05 to 0.2 mg/kg), toward which tolerance develops more slowly. For cats an intravenous dose (5 to 10 mg) generally is given to effect. The dose may need to be repeated; up to 20 mg may be necessary. High doses should be injected slowly. Diazepam (0.5 mg/kg using 5 mg/mL solution) has been used successfully by rectal administration for home control of cluster seizures.[119]

For chronic therapy rapid metabolism coupled with rapid development of tolerance precludes long-term treatment with diazepam and several other benzodiazepines in dogs.[29] However, compared with diazepam, tolerance does not appear to develop as readily to the anticonvulsant effects of clorazepate in dogs. Clorazepate has been studied when added to phenobarbital in dogs still seizuring despite phenobarbital concentrations that exceeded 32 μg/ml (author, unpublished data). Seizures were eradicated in about 35% of animals and reduced 50% or more in another 15%. However, its use in combination with phenobarbital was complicated by drug interactions (including marked fluctuations in nordiazepam disappearance half-life), and an apparent increased risk of hepatotoxicity. Drug interactions between phenobarbital and clorazepate may necessitate dose modification in response to changes in drug concentrations. The short half-life (which might be documented with sequential peak and trough plasma drug concentration measurements) may increase the risk of seizures if drug concentrations decrease below effective concentrations in the patient. The therapeutic range of benzodiazepines (including metabolites) in dogs has been extrapolated from human studies and does not reflect combination therapy. For efficacy, trough concentrations should be maintained at least above 100 ng/mL, although monitoring should establish each patient's range. Dogs receiving phenobarbital are likely to become groggy when peak clorazepate concentrations exceed 300 to 500 ng/mL (varying with the patient).

For chronic control in cats, diazepam can be given orally in doses of 2 to 5 mg 2 or 3 times daily; diazepam may be increased or decreased in increments of 2 mg with or without phenobarbital. Whereas distribution of diazepam in the cat brain reflects blood flow, nordiazepam accumulates to high concentrations throughout all brain matter, which may be the reason for its efficacy with long-term use.[120]

Bromide

Bromide is an old anticonvulsant that was used in the 1800s for control of seizures. However, it has enjoyed a resurgence in veterinary medicine, proving to be an effective add-on anticonvulsant for refractory (canine) seizures, as well as a sole anticonvulsant for some canine patients.

Mechanism of Action

Bromides mechanism of action is not completely understood.[121] The original proposed mechanism—replacement of negatively charged chloride with bromide in the neuron—is unlikely because bromide is less negatively charged than chloride.[122] In vitro, bromide enhances GABA-activated currents, leading the authors to conclude that bromide potentiates inhibitory postsynaptic potentials of GABA. Regardless of the mechanism, the anticonvulsant effects of bromide correlate with plasma concentration.[123]

Disposition

The pharmacokinetics of bromide have been described using either the sodium or potassium salt. In a small study, the half-life in dogs was reported as 21 to 24 days after oral administration, suggesting steady-state concentrations being achieved only at 2.5 to 3 months.[124] Distribution is to extracellular fluid,[125] yet sufficient quantities penetrate the CNS. Bromide is eliminated slowly (presumably as a result of marked reabsorption) in the kidney. Bromide appears to compete with chloride for renal elimination, with elimination appearing to decrease proportionately to the amount of chloride in the diet.[126,127]

KEY POINT 27-17 As a renally excreted compound, bromide is not likely to be involved in drug interactions. However, serum bromide concentrations will change proportionately and inversely with the amount of chloride consumed by the patient.

Bromide (20 mg/kg bromide; approximately 26 mg/kg sodium bromide) has been studied in Beagles as the sodium salt after intravenous (n = 4) and oral (n = 4) administration, but only at the daily maintenance dose (which is about 1/15 to 1/20 the loading dose).[128] Dogs received a diet containing 0.4% chloride on a dry-matter basis. Elimination half-life after intravenous administration was 39 ± 10 days and after oral administration, 46 ± 9 days; clearance (reported in ml/kg/day) was 9 ± 3.9, and apparent volume of distribution (Vd area) was 0.45 ± 0.07 L/kg. Oral bioavailability (calculated from mean area under the curve from intravenous and oral groups) was 46%. A study by the same investigators[127] in Beagles measured changes in bromide (sodium; 14 mg/kg orally) disposition in response to dietary chloride content (0.2, 0.4, and 1.3%, dry-matter basis). Mean apparent elimination half-life decreased from 69 ± 22 days (0.2%) to 24 ± 7 days (1.3%). Predicted maximum drug concentrations were quite variable within treatment groups but were profoundly influenced by dietary chloride content, ranging from 1.95 ± 1.1 mg/mL at 0.2% chloride, 1.27 ± 0.36 mg/mL at 0.4% chloride, to a low of 0.3 ± 0.15 mg/mL at 1.3% dietary chloride.

A study of potassium bromide (20 mg/kg per day bromide or approximately 30 mg/kg potassium bromide), mixed as a 20 mg/mL solution in canned dog food, in Beagles (n = 6) receiving 0.55 to 0.72% dietary chloride reported a median bromide concentration at 115 days of 2.45 mg/mL (low of 1.8 and high of 2.7 mg/mL); the time to steady state was not provided, but concentrations were within 90% of steady-state concentrations by 60 days.[129] The median elimination half-life, estimated from time to reach steady state, was 15 days (low of 12, high of 20 days). Renal clearance (based on 24-hour urine collection) ranged from 6 to 12 .6 mL/kg per day (median 8.2). The median ratio of bromide in CSF to serum at day 9 was 0.63; this improved to 0.86 (0.82 to 0.99) by day 120. An increase in dose sufficient to generate serum bromide concentrations 3.4 mg/mL (median; does not provide but designed to target 4 mg/mL) resulted in an increase in the CSF: serum ratio to 0.86, suggesting a greater risk than anticipated of CNS side effects. Whereas neurologic side effects were not described at the dose of 60 mg/kg per day, caudal paresis and ataxia developed in two of six dogs. Electrodiagnostic changes were mild even at the high dose; within individual dogs, latency shifts were mild and either progressively increased over time or appeared with doses designed to target 4 mg/mL.

Bromide was studied (report in progress by the author) after rectal administration in normal hound dogs after a loading dose (600 mg/kg) of sterile potassium bromide solution (concentration 250 mg/mL) over 24 hours, either by 6 intrarectal boluses of 100 mg/kg, each every 4 hours, or constant-rate infusion (CRI) throughout the 24-hour period. The average peak serum bromide concentration after intrarectal loading was 0.91 mg/mL (range: 0.81 to 1.11 mg/mL), compared with 1.10 mg/mL after intravenous loading (range: 0.89 to 1.22 mg/mL). The average peak serum K^+ concentration during potassium bromide loading was 5.80 mEq/L (range: 5.5 to 6.8 mEq/L) and 6.14 mEq/L (range: 5.6 to 7.7 mEq/L) for intrarectal and intravenous loading, respectively (normal range: 3.5 to 5.5 mEq/L). The mean half-life ($t_{1/2}$) of intrarectally administered bromide was 488.8 hours, or 20.4 days. A side effect of both intrarectal and intravenous potassium bromide loading was mild sedation, and of intrarectal loading was transient (24 to 48 hours) diarrhea. Bioavailability (F) of intrarectally administered bromide for the 24-hour loading period was calculated to be 107% for the five dogs. In two dogs overall bioavailability (F) of intrarectally administered bromide was calculated to be 57.7%. Results of this study indicate that potassium bromide is well absorbed rectally and that a 24-hour intrarectal loading protocol is safe to administer in normal dogs.

Bromide has been studied in cats after oral administration of the potassium salt at the lower end of the canine dose. After a dose of 30 mg/kg, maximum serum bromide concentration was 1.1 ± 0.2 mg/mL at 8 weeks. Mean disappearance half-life was 1.6 ± 0.2 weeks. Steady state was achieved at a mean of 5.3 ± 1.1 weeks.[129a] However, the use of bromide in cats is discouraged due to safety reasons.[129a]

KEY POINT 27-18 Bromide in cats may lead to signs consistent with bronchial asthma.

Preparations and Sources

Bromide is available as a potassium or sodium salt. Triple bromide salt preparations (Na, K, and NH_4) also may be available through some pharmacies. The accompanying cation does not appear to alter efficacy, although sodium bromide is more difficult to solubilize in water than is potassium bromide. In addition, because potassium weighs less than sodium, 1 g of sodium bromide contains more bromide (78% bromide, or 780 mg) than does 1 g of potassium bromide (67% bromide, or 670 mg). Thus the amount of sodium bromide used to make a solution should be less (211 mg/mL) than potassium bromide (250 mg/mL) to achieve equivalent amounts of bromide in the solution. At the time of publication, a commercial product of potassium bromide is being marketed as a chewable tablet and solution. The product contains B vitamins as well. This product has not been approved by the Food and Drug Administration. It is being marketed under the "generally recognized as safe" category reserved for food of food ingredients; however, this status does not apply to drugs It is important to recognize that the product has not undergone premarket evaluation by any regulatory agency for safety, efficacy, or quality and although its use is not necessarily discouraged, clinicians should be aware that this is a manufactured-compounded product.

Potassium bromide can be compounded by veterinarians or pharmacists on an individual-need basis. It can be purchased through chemical companies (request medicinal or ACS grade [Curtin Matheson]). Chemical companies have refused to sell bromide for medicinal purposes without an investigational new animal drug application (INADA). This application is no longer necessary, however, because the Food and Drug Administration (Division of Drug Compliance) will grant regulatory discretion.

Bromide can be compounded in a syrup or water solution or administered in a gelatin capsule. A number of compounding pharmacies now offer this service, although the compounded solution can be much more costly when compounded by a pharmacist compared with the cost of the ingredients. The solution can be compounded by the clinician with minimal equipment, particularly if monitoring is used to document maintenance of drug concentrations with compounded preparations. If purchased (1-kg bottle) from a chemical company, potassium bromide can be weighed and divided into 250-g (four equal) packets. A liter bottle of distilled water can be purchased from any grocery store. Before the bromide is mixed, a line should be drawn at the 1-L volume mark and approximately 50% of the water removed and set aside. One of the four 250-g packets of bromide is added to the bottle and the bottle shaken well to dissolve the bromide (this may require aggressive shaking and the addition of more water). Once the bromide is dissolved, the volume should be returned to 1 L with either water or a flavored syrup. The final solution will approximate 250 mg/mL. The solution should be stable for at least 6 months, and refrigeration should minimize microbial growth in the solution. Refrigerating the solution may cause the salt to crystallize; warming the solution should cause the drug to redissolve. Note that while this solution can be dispensed from a practice, it cannot legally be sold to others.

Side Effects

Adverse reactions to bromide tend to be dose dependent. They appear to be related to the anticonvulsant or other centrally acting effects of the drug and predominantly affect the CNS (e.g., ataxia, grogginess). This is supported by the recent retrospective report of Rossmeisl and Inzana,[130] which described signs of "bromism" in epileptic dogs (n = 31). Clinical signs included ataxia and stupor, with one dog being comatose. Other clinical signs included bilateral mydriasis; head pressing was evident in two dogs. Mean bromide concentration at time of admission was 3.7 ± 0.3 mg/mL compared with the most recent monitoring result before admission (1.9 ± 0.3 mg/mL) and compared with a control group of epileptic dogs without bromism at 1.7 ± 0.1 mg/mL. Of the 31 dogs, 26 dogs also were receiving phenobarbital at a mean concentration of 31 ± 12 μg/mL; control group phenobarbital was 26 ± 1 μg/mL. Causes for the increase in bromide were attributed to reduction in renal function, dosing error, shifting from potassium to sodium bromide, and exposure to bromide in drinking water or alternative medications. Changes in diets, the most common reason for increased bromide in the author's therapeutic drug monitoring laboratory, was not addressed. Diuresis was implemented in affected dogs (n = 27); four of these dogs had breakthrough seizures. Furosemide therapy was initiated in five dogs; however, it is not clear what impact furosemide has on bromide clearance.

Up to 3 months may be required for accommodation to the sedative effects of bromide. This reflects in part the time necessary to reach steady-state concentrations. Gradual reduction of phenobarbital in 25% increments may resolve some of the side effects and may be preferred to saline diuresis in those patients for which nonthreatening clinical signs of bromism emerge. Alternatively, the bromide dose can be decreased by 25%, although 1 to 2 weeks may elapse before a response is seen. Sodium bromide administered as a loading dose sufficient to achieve steady-state concentrations has been reported to be well tolerated in dogs.[131]

Fluids containing sodium chloride can be used to treat acute bromide toxicity; monitoring should occur immediately after saline treatment to establish a new baseline. Note that diuresis may increase the risk of breakthrough seizures and SE. Diuresis should be reserved for animals with profound sedation for which a decrease in phenobarbital (if on combination therapy) or bromide will not provide a sufficiently rapid response. Pruritic skin lesions may occur, particularly in patients that had pruritic disorders before starting therapy. A short period of glucocorticoid therapy may control pruritis.

Hyperactivity is an occasional side effect and may or may not be dose dependent. Like other anticonvulsants, bromide tends to increase the appetite of dogs. Vomition is not uncommon and appears to reflect the hypertonicity of the salt and direct gastric irritation. Solutions appear to be better tolerated than capsules, although this may vary. Dividing the daily dose into smaller, more frequent doses or feeding before or with medication may decrease gastrointestinal side effects. Sodium bromide may be more tolerated than other bromide salts.

Pancreatitis has been associated with the use of bromide when combined with phenobarbital. A retrospective report found 10% of dogs receiving a combination of potassium bromide and phenobarbital developed clinical signs consistent with pancreatitis, compared with 0.3% of dogs receiving phenobarbital alone.[80] Serum pancreatic lipase immunoreactivity was found to be increased in the serum of dogs receiving either bromide or phenobarbital, alone or in combination, indicating that the risk may occur with either drug. [81]

Although cats tolerated 8 weeks of oral potassium bromide dosing (experimentally) at 30 mg/kg, clinical patients do not appear to tolerate the drug as well. However, in a retrospective study, bromide (n = 4) or bromide and phenobarbital (n = 3) was associated with eradication of seizures in 7 of 15 cats (bromide dosage range, 1 to 1.6 mg/kg [0.45 to 0.73 mg/lb]); however, bromide administration was associated with adverse effects in 8 of 16 cats. Coughing developed in six of these cats, leading to euthanasia in one cat and discontinuation of bromide administration in two cats. Although somewhat effective in seizure control, the incidence of adverse effects may not warrant routine use of bromide for control of seizures in cats.

Because it is renally eliminated, bromide does not negatively interact with other anticonvulsants metabolized by the liver. However, dietary (or therapeutic) chloride will compete with bromide for renal excretion and can shorten bromide half-life, probably because the kidneys will selectively resorb chloride.[127] In addition, laboratory assays may not be able to distinguish among anions; for some, bromide may artificially increase serum chloride measurements.[132]

Therapeutic Use

Bromide has been used to treat seizures in dogs for over 15 years. Initially, it was used as an adjunct to phenobarbital therapy, an indication that persists.[133,134] However, it is increasingly being used as sole therapy.[28] Therapeutic ranges vary, with initial studies indicating 0.7 to 2 mg/mL.[134] More recently, dogs (n = 122; from 1992-1996) with major motor epilepsy were studied retrospectively to determine the therapeutic range of bromide, either alone or in combination with phenobarbital or primidone. Bromide successfully controlled seizures (≥50% reduction in seizure frequency) in 72% of animals. Phenobarbital or primidone could be discontinued in 19% of animals receiving the combination. For dogs that continued to receive both drugs, 45% remained controlled with a phenobarbital dose below 20 µg/mL. The concentration of bromide necessary to control seizures when given as sole therapy was higher (1.9 mg/mL) than when combined with either barbiturate (1.6 mg/mL). The authors concluded that the range for bromide depends on whether bromide will provide sole anticonvulstant support (0.8 to 2.4 mg/mL) or is combined with a barbiturate (0.88 to 3 mg/mL). If phenobarbital could not be discontinued, the range necessary for control was 9 to 36 µg/mL.[135] A distinction in therapeutic ranges as sole or combination therapy of bromide may not be necessary. Concentrations may fall outside or within a range of 1 to 3 mg/mL (based on the gold chloride method of detection) as needed to control the patient's seizures, regardless of concomitant therapy. Because the side effects of bromide apparently are not associated with cellular toxicity (unlike phenobarbital), the therapeutic range can be surpassed in animals, if tolerated and if necessary to control seizures. Drug concentrations can be increased beyond this concentration if there is no evidence of toxicity. Some animals will present with side effects at concentrations in the lower end of the range, particularly if a loading dose is administered. Therefore it is generally wise to avoid a loading dose if seizure history and drug safety (e.g., phenobarbital) is supportive. Bromide generally should be given once or twice daily, depending on the animal's gastric tolerance of the drug. Twice-daily administration of bromide offers no benefit over once-daily administration, with the potential exception of decreased gastric irritation. Indeed, an animal can miss several days of dosing with minimal impact on serum drug concentrations. Missed doses in such instances should be given when convenient. On the other hand, if bromide is better tolerated when broken into much smaller, more frequent doses, no disadvantages are apparent with this approach, other than inconvenience to the owner.

KEY POINT 27-19 The long half-life causes the loading dose of bromide (450 mg/kg) to be substantially higher than the daily maintenance dose (30 mg/kg).

In humans bromide has been used to treat intractable seizures in pediatric patients.[81,136,137] Bromide's initial introduction into veterinary medicine was as an add-on anticonvulsant, particularly combined with phenobarbital, for control of refractory seizures in dogs or in patients that have developed liver disease in association with phenobarbital therapy. Increasingly, however, bromide is proving efficacious as a first-choice antiepileptic drug for dogs. For example, bromide has been used as the sole drug for patients whose seizure history is limited to mild seizure episodes.[133] Because of its long half-life, bromide may be the drug of choice for dogs whose owners are noncompliant because the plasma drug concentrations are not easily manipulated. The author studied bromide as an add-on anticonvulsant in dogs with refractory epilepsy (n = 20) in which seizures continued despite phenobarbital concentations at 32 µg/ml or more. Bromide eradicated seizures in 60% of the patients and reduced seizure frequency by 50% or more in another 20%.

Two choices should be considered when starting bromide therapy: administration of a maintenance dose, which allows the body to gradually adapt to the presence of the drug, or administration of a loading dose. The maintenance dose approach is indicated when possible to minimize the advent of side effects. A targeted concentration should be selected (lower concentrations for milder seizures; higher concentrations may be necessary for severe seizures). In general, 30 mg/kg per day orally will achieve 1 mg/mL at steady state. For every 0.5 mg/mL increment above 1 mg/mL, another 15 mg/kg per day should be administered. To proactively monitor when using the maintenance dose approach to steady state, one sample should be collected at 3 weeks, or halfway to steady state. Doubling the measured concentrations provides an estimate of steady-state concentrations. However, because kinetics vary among animals, a steady-state sample should be collected to confirm baseline concentrations at 3 months.

The second option for beginning bromide therapy is implementation of loading dose. This approach is recommended in patients for which lack of seizure control can be life threatening (including the risk of euthanasia by a distraught owner), or in patients for whom serum phenobarbital concentrations must be rapidly decreased because of hepatotoxicity or bone marrow suppression. Both loading dose and maintenance dose must be established; the loading dose is designed to target steady-state concentrations, but the patient will not be at steady state until being on the same dose for 2 to 3 months. Thus as the loading dose is discontinued and the maintenance dose is begun, a new time to steady state begins. Drug concentrations may increase or decrease compared with the loading dose as steady-state concentrations are reached. Monitoring can ensure that the maintenance dose will maintain what the loading dose achieved. However, this requires a sample collected after loading (within 1 or 2 days) to document what loading achieved, and another sample one elimination half-life after the maintenance dose is started (about 3 weeks). This time is chosen because if concentrations are not maintained by the loading dose, the majority of change (50%) will occur in the first elimination half-life. If the two samples are not within about 10 to 15% of one another (i.e., postload and 3-week maintenance), the maintenance dose should be increased or decreased accordingly. Generally, an increase at the 3-week point is not problematic (and often is desirable), but a decrease is undesirable. If not curtailed by an increase in the maintenance dose, as steady state is reached, the decrease may be sufficient to lead to seizures 2 to 3 months after the loading dose successfully controlled seizures.

A loading dose should reflect all the doses that would have been given as steady state is reached, less drug eliminated by clearance. Thus the loading dose of bromide is substantially higher than the maintenance dose. To target the lower end of the therapeutic range (1 mg/mL), 450 mg/kg should be given as a loading dose. Thereafter, for every 0.5 mg/mL desired increase in bromide concentrations, the loading dose should be increased by approximately 225 mg/kg. Because animals may not tolerate the loading dose as a single oral dose, it generally is divided into 10 equal doses given twice daily for 5 days. However, note that the maintenance dose should be added to the loading dose if the targeted concentration is to be reached. For example, to target 1.5 mg/mL with a 5-day loading period, the patient should receive 675 mg/kg split over a 5-day period, plus a maintenance dose of 45 mg/kg/day. Thus for 6 days, the patient should receive approximately 135 mg/kg. On day 6 the maintenance dose of 45 mg/kg is begun and a postload sample is collected (assume the loading dose achieved 1.3 mg/mL). A second sample is collected 3 weeks later. Allowing for some variability in analytic error, then the maintenance dose can be adjusted in proportion to the difference between the postload and 3 week sample. For example, if the postload was 1.3 mg/ml, and a 3-week concentration is 0.8 mg/mL, the maintenance dose may need to be increased by about 25% to 30%). If a patient already is receiving bromide and an increase in concentrations is desired (e.g., 0.5 mg/mL), the maintenance dose can be increased 15 mg/kg/day. A third sample can be checked at 3 weeks to make sure drug concentrations are moving in the right direction. If a rapid response is desired in a patient already receiving bromide, a "mini" loading dose of 225 to 250 mg/kg total can be given along with an increase in maintenance dose.

The use of bromide as an add-on anticonvulsant to phenobarbital also is discussed later in this chapter. Monitoring in such patients is important if the goal of the additional bromide is to decrease or discontinue phenobarbital. If the goal is to replace phenobarbital, the bromide target should approximate the current phenobarbital concentration in the patient. For example, if the patient has phenobarbital concentrations of 20 μg/mL, (midtherapeutic range), then the bromide dosing regimen might approximate the midtherapeutic range (i.e., about 1.5 to 2 mg/mL). To prevent excessive grogginess, bromide should be initiated as a maintenance rather than loading dose. At least 3 weeks of dosing (i.e., halfway to steady state) should occur, ideally, to allow a halfway to steady-state sample that confirms the bromide dose is on target before phenobarbital is decreased. However, if the patient becomes unacceptably groggy at any point, assuming the seizure history is appropriate, phenobarbital rather than bromide should be decreased by 25% (not only is bromide safer, response will be more rapid for phenobarbital because its half-life is shorter). If all remains well as the new phenobarbital dose reaches steady state (about 2 weeks), assuming the patient has been challenged by a seizure (thus waiting at least one seizure interval is ideal), then an additional 25% decline in phenobarbital can be considered. Ideally, phenobarbital concentrations are measured at each step. This process can be repeated until phenobarbital is eradicated or the patient seizures again. A much more rapid approach will be necessary in animals that develop a life-threatening adversity to phenobarbital (including bone marrow dyscrasias). In such cases a loading dose is indicated, with immediate (6- to 7-day) and 3-week postload samples being critical to ensure maintenance of bromide concentrations in the targeted range. If the loading dose option is taken, phenobarbital probably can be decreased by 25% to 50% as little as 2 to 3 days into the loading dose. Ideally, phenobarbital concentrations should not be decreased completely unless the patient has a bromide concentration of 1.5 mg/mL. For some patients phenobarbital can be completely discontinued once bromide is begun. For others, a combination may be necessary to control seizures. Unfortunately, for a small percentage of animals, seizures may continue even if both drugs are at the maximum end of the therapeutic range or side effects are untenable.

For life-threatening seizures that have not responded to phenobarbital, bromide also can be given rectally as a loading dose (see the discussion of disposition). Efficacy and safety of bromide versus phenobarbital has been compared in spontaneously epileptic dogs (n=46)[28] using a parallel, randomized double-blinded study design. Enrollment was based on seizure history, physical and neurologic examinations, and clinical pathology. Dogs were loaded over a 7-day period to achieve the minimum end of the therapeutic range of the assigned drug phenobarbital (3.5 mg/kg), or bromide (15 mg/kg) was administered every 12 hours. Data (clinical pathology and drug concentrations) were measured at baseline and at 30-day intervals for 6 months. All but three patients completed the study. Seizures initially worsened in three dogs on bromide but not in any phenobarbital-treated patient. Compared with baseline, mean seizure number, frequency, and severity were reduced at 6 months for both drugs; seizure duration was shorter for phenobarbital but not bromide. Seizure activity was eradicated in a greater percentage of phenobarbital-treated patients (85%) compared with bromide-treated patients (65%), and the seizure duration decreased more for those on phenobarbital than for those on bromide, but successful control (at least 50% reduction in seizure number with no unacceptable adverse drug reactions) tended ($p = 0.06$) to be better only for those in the phenobarbital group. For patients in which seizures were eradicated, mean phenobarbital concentration was 25.4 ± 5.4 (95% confidence interval of 23 to 28 μg/mL) (see Table 27-4) but ranged from 12 μg/mL to 34 μg/mL (dose was 4.1 ± 1.1 mg/kg). For bromide mean concentration associated with eradication of seizures was 1.8 ± 0.5 mg/mL at a range of 0.9 to 3.3 mg/mL (dose of 31 ± 11 mg/kg). Both drugs caused abnormal behaviors. Weight increased by 10% in both groups. Changes in clinical pathology were limited to increased (but within normal) serum alkaline phosphatase and decreased (but within normal) serum albumin at 6 months for phenobarbital compared with baseline and compared with bromide at 6 months. Side effects at 1 month were greater for phenobarbital vs bromide and ataxia (55% vs 22%), polyuria (35% vs 13%), but greater for bromide vs phenobarbital for polyphagia (43% vs 30%), vomiting (57% vs 20%), and hyperactivity (43% vs 35%). At 6 months, most clinical signs had resolved to less than 15% of animals in either group with the exception of vomiting that continued in 21% of dogs in the bromide group (0% in the phenobarbital group). One dog failed phenobarbital therapy because of neutropenia; two dogs failed bromide due to vomiting. This study suggests that both phenobarbital and bromide are reasonable first choices for control of epilepsy in dogs, although phenobarbital may provide better control. Side effects can be expected to be greater in bromide following chronic dosing.

KEY POINT 27-20 If a loading dose is administered, monitoring should occur immediately and then again in 3 weeks. The two concentrations should match if the maintenance dose is correct.

Although bromide has been used in the cat successfully, adverse effects (consistent with bronchial asthma) are sufficiently common that an alternative anticonvulsant should be considered.[129a] While administration of bromide (n = 4) or bromide and phenobarbital (n = 3) was associated with eradication of seizures in 7 of 15 cats (serum bromide concentration range, 1.0 to 1.6 mg/mL); bromide coughing developed in 6 cats, leading to euthanasia in 1 cat and discontinuation of bromide administration in 2 cats.

Carbamazepine

Carbamazepine is approved for human use as an antiepileptic drug and currently is considered a primary drug for treatment of partial and tonic–clonic seizures. Further, it is a primary choice for treatment of trigeminal neuralgia; this and its efficacy for treatment of manic–depressive disorders may reflect its chemical similarity to tricyclic antidepressants.[25] Its mechanism appears to slow recovery of sodium channels, preventing repetitive firing. In humans pharmacokinetics are complex. Slow, erratic oral absorption may take as long as 8 hours and appears to be dose dependent. Carbamazepine is approximately 75% protein bound. Hepatic metabolism, principally by CYP3A4, includes production of an active metabolite, carbamazepine 10,11 epoxide, which may achieve up to 50% of the CNS concentrations of the parent compound. Other metabolites are mostly glucuronidated and excreted in the urine. Carbamazepine induces cytochrome P450 isoenzymes CYP2C and CYP3A. As such, carbamazepine is involved in a number of drug interactions, decreasing the concentrations of several drugs (e.g., valproate, lamotrigine, tiagabine, topiramate, and other nonanticonvulsants). It can in turn be influenced by inducers (phenobarbital, phenytoin, valproic acid) and inhibitors (e.g., erythromycin, cimetidine, fluoxetine) of drug-metabolizing enzymes. Adversities in humans include both acute toxicity (stupor and coma) and increased seizures. Other neurologic signs may emerge with long-term use, potentially reflecting neurotoxicity to which tolerance may develop. Bone marrow suppression and other evidence of hypersensitivity may occur. However, some cases of leukopenia or thrombocytopenia may be only transient, resolving after several weeks. Carbamazepine also reduces antidiuretic hormone but, paradoxically, may cause water retention, a potentially serious complication in patients with cardiac disease. A therapeutic range of 6 to 12 μg/mL (based on the parent compound) has been suggested, but the relationship between parent concentration and response is complex. Side effects have been reported at 9 μg/mL.

Description of the disposition of carbamazepine in dogs is limited, with one report comparing two oral pharmaceutical preparations (see Table 27-4).[138] Both the parent compound and active metabolite are characterized by a short half-life (3 hours), which will limit therapeutic use. Carbamazepine has been used intermittently in dogs. A case report[139] described successful long-term control of psychomotor seizures in one dog, although parent drug could not be detected in serum. The patient previously had been treated with a variety of anticonvulsants alone or in combination. However, the patient immediately responded to carbamazepine at 7 mg/kg twice daily. The dose was increased to 14 mg/kg. The drug was discontinued because the patient developed leukopenia. Although the leukopenia resolved, clinical signs returned. Therapy was reinstituted, clinical signs resolved, and leukopenia returned but resolved after 3 to 4 months of therapy. In his review Holland[139] notes that doses of carbamazepine in dogs have ranged from 4 to 40 mg/kg divided into 2 daily doses.

Oxcarbazepine is an antiepileptic drug that is a keto-analog of carbamazepine approved as a prodrug. Similar to carbamazepine in action, its induction of drug-metabolizing enzymes is less potent than that of carbamazepine, leading to its substitution with combination therapy.

Ethosuximide

Ethosuximide is a succinimide anticonvulsant used to treat absence seizures in humans. Its mechanism is reduced threshold of T-calcium channels in the thalamus. At therapeutic concentrations it is not effective against tonic hind limb extension of electroshock nor kindled seizures.[25] Side effects include CNS depression and gastrointestinal upset. Allergic skin reactions have been reported in humans. It has been studied in a limited number of dogs. A concentration of 50 to 70 μg/mL was maintained by oral administration of 15 to 25 mg/kg thrice daily after a loading dose of 40 mg/kg; recommended therapeutic concentrations range from 40 to 100 μg/mL.[42,140] The duration of dosing was not provided.

Felbamate

Felbamate was approved in the United States in the late 1990s for treatment of human epilepsy either as the sole drug or in combination with other anticonvulsants. Similar to meprobamate in chemistry, felbamate's mechanism of action appears to be inhibition of NMDA receptor–mediated calcium or sodium influx (inhibition of excitatory signals) as well as potentiation of GABA receptor–mediated chloride (negative) influx.[141] Thus the drug should have a broad mechanism of anticonvulsant activity with an action that might be considered complementary to phenobarbital.

The drug was proved very safe and efficacious in the treatment of partial and generalized seizures in experimental animals[142,143] and humans, particularly children.[144,145] Initially studied as monotherapy treatment of partial seizures, the drug has since proved useful as monotherapy for other seizures, including generalized seizures.[145-148] When added to phenobarbital in refractory canine epileptics in an unpublished clinical report by the author, it eradicated seizures in 35% and decrease seizure numbers by at least 50% or more in another 20%.[149]

Felbamate is well absorbed after oral administration, although bioavailability in pediatric animals may be as little as 30% of that in adult dogs, necessitating a higher dose.[15] The drug is eliminated by hepatic metabolism to metabolites that are largely inactive.[150] Initial preclinical toxicity studies in the dog revealed felbamate to be completely absorbed after oral administration of 1.6 to 1000 mg/kg. At each dose C_{max} was 12.6 to 168.4 μg/mL, respectively, in dogs with T_{max} occurring at 3 to 7 hours, respectively. Plasma elimination half-life was 4.1 to 4.5 hours at both doses. After multiple oral doses of 50 mg/kg, plasma concentrations did not appear to change, and much (at least 50%) of the drug (based on [14C] felbamate) was eliminated in the urine (58% to 87.7%), with at least 7% eliminated in feces and the remainder in bile.[151] Volume of distribution was 0.72 L/kg, and binding to plasma proteins was at most 36%. Plasma clearance was 108 mL*h/kg renal clearance of unchanged drug was between 20% and 35%, and hepatic clearance resulting from metabolism was between 65% and 80% of overall clearance.[151]

KEY POINT 27-21 The combination of phenobarbital with any other drug eliminated primarily by cytochrome P450 is likely to increase the risk of liver disease.

In adult dogs the half-life of felbamate is 4 to 8 hours (mean of 5.2 hours); the elimination half-life is shorter in pediatric (Beagle) dogs (mean of 2.5 hours) probably.[151,152] Felbamate also was studied in adult and pediatric dogs at 60 mg/kg orally once a day for 10 days. Oral bioavailability was less in pediatric dogs compared with adults, apparently because of more rapid clearance. Bioavailability also decreased by day 10 compared with day 1. Safety has been experimentally documented at doses ranging from 15 mg/kg divided twice daily (the starting therapeutic dose) to 300 mg/kg. Oral bioavailability is markedly variable. The oral disposition of felbamate has been described in adult and pediatric male and female dogs after single (see Table 27-4) and multiple dosing. [152] Felbamate was characterized by a lower C_{max} (33 and 37 μg/mL for males and females, respectively) and area under the curve and shorter half-life (2.87 ± 0.52 [males] and 2.93 + 0.33 [females] in pediatric animals compared with adults (see Table 27-4). Clearance increased to 0.98 - 0.11 L/hr/kg), resulting in a decrease in half-life from 8.48 and 6.17 hours (males and females, respectively) to 6.1 and 5.1 hr (males and females, respectively) after multiple dosing (10 days).

Sedation, polyuria, polyphagia, and polydipsia, side effects typical of most anticonvulsants, do not appear to occur in dogs. Aplastic anemia caused by bone marrow suppression, however, developed in 1 of 10,000 patients (human) receiving felbamate,[153] leading to marked curtailment of the use of the drug in humans. Felbamate has not been sufficiently used in dogs to detect a similar side effect, although it is probably as likely to occur in dogs as in humans. Hepatotoxicy has been reported in dogs receiving both phenobarbital and felbamate and has occurred in 3 of 15 patient treated with combination therapy by the author in an unpublished clinical trial. However, the author has administered felbamate to dogs also receiving phenobarbital at doses as high as 300 mg/kg divided daily for over 6 months with no apparent initial adverse effects. In one of 15 dogs receiving this regimen, progressive liver disease that ultimately proved fatal developed 1.5 years into the combination therapy. Because felbamate is a drug metabolized by the liver, prudence suggests not combining it with phenobarbital, particularly in patients requiring high serum concentrations of phenobarbital to control seizures. In humans interactions have led to increases in phenobarbital by felbamate,[154] although this appears to be due to selective inhibition of a cytochrome P450 enzyme in only 25% of the population. Phenobarbital concentrations should be measured to detect any drug interaction that might lead to an increase in drug concentrations and a subsequent increased risk of liver disease. Greater risk may reflect decreased felbamate concentrations resulting from induction by phenobarbital.[154] Currently, there is no easy, cost-effective means for assaying felbamate, although selected laboratories may offer the service. Human therapeutic concentrations range from 20 to 100 μg/mL, with trough concentrations ideally remaining in the range of 60 to 80 μg/mL for best efficacy.[155]

Gabapentin

Gabapentin is an anticonvulsant approved in 1994 for treatment of partial seizures with or without generalization in humans with epilepsy.[156-158] It has been used in dogs (and anectodally in cats). It appears to act by a novel mechanism promoting the release of GABA, although the actual mechanism of release is not known. Although gabapentin is absorbed well after oral administration, its absorption appears to be dose dependent, relying on a saturable transport process. This process has been cited as the reason that antiepileptic drug effects last longer than anticipated on the basis of drug half-life, potentially allowing twice-daily administration. The short half-life of gabapentin (in humans) results in steady-state concentrations within 24 to 48 hours. In humans the drug is eliminated entirely by renal elimination, thus avoiding some of the risks of hepatotoxicity and drug interaction. Because the drug is relatively safe, therapeutic drug monitoring is not necessary; rather, the dose is increased as needed to control seizures. Mild dizziness, nausea, and vomiting have occurred in a small percentage of human patients.

Gabapentin studies with animals are limited.[159-162] Gabapentin has been studied in the dog after oral administration of 50 mg/kg. Oral bioavailability was 80%, and plasma protein binding was below 3%. Mean intravenous elimination half-life of 2.9 hours has been reported in dogs. Repeated administration did not alter gabapentin pharmacokinetics, nor did gabapentin induce hepatic drug-metabolizing enzymes. In the dog 34% of the dose was metabolized to the inactive N-methyl form. The principal route of excretion was the urine.[161,162] A more recent study compared gabapentin (600 mg to Beagles) after oral administration of either an immediate or a slow-release product (see Table 27-4).[163] The sustained-release product did not disintegrate, but the release kinetics were not substantially different from those of the immediate-release product.

The addition of gabapentin (35 to 50 mg/kg divided every 8 to 12 hours) to either phenobarbital or bromide was studied in epileptic dogs (n = 17) using an open, uncontrolled design. The interictal period increased, but the number of seizures did not. However, seizures were eradicated in three dogs. Side effects that developed with the addition of gabapentin included sedation, which resolved within several days, and hind limb ataxia, which resolved with a reduction in the bromide dose.[164] One of the major disadvantages of this drug is its expense, although several generic preparations are now available. Gabapentin may not be effective for the control of epilepsy when used at doses extrapolated from human patients. Clinical trials are indicated to establish the most appropriate dosing regimen for dogs or cats. Gabapentin is among the drugs for which SE may occur during withdrawal.[165]

KEY POINT 27-22 The advantage of either gabapentin or pregabalin as adjuvant antiepileptic drugs is renal excretion and thus reduced risk of drug interactions or hepatotoxicity.

Pregabalin

Pregabalin is the *S* enantiomer of 3-(aminoethyl)-5-methylhexanoic acid, an analog of GABA. It is also structurally related to the amino acid leucine and gabapentin (Figure 26-4). Pregabalin has been developed for the treatment of neuropathic pain and as adjunctive therapy in the treatment of partial seizures. However, according to manufacturer-generated approval research, its mechanism of action is not clear.[166] It does not appear to involve gabaminergic transmission, does not alter binding or responses at GABA-A or GABA-B receptors, and is not a substrate or blocker of GABA transporter GABA transaminase. It decreases central neuronal excitability by binding to an auxiliary subunit (alpha$_2$-delta protein) of a voltage-gated neuronal calcium channel on neurons. It also reduces the release of multiple neurotransmitters (in vitro concentration of 1.6 ng/mL), glutamate, norepinephrine, substance P, and calcitonin gene-related peptide. It serves as a substrate of L-amino acid transporter in neuronal cell membranes, which facilitates pregabalin transport into the cell. In animal models pregabalin controls seizures induced by a variety of methods, including threshold clonic seizures from pentylenetetrazol, and behavioral and electrographic seizures in hippocampal-kindled rats.

Pregabalin appears to be well absorbed after oral administration, minimally bound to plasma proteins, and distributed well to tissues, including the brain. In dogs it is characterized by a volume of distribution of 0.6 L/kg. In most species (e.g., rodents, primates) studied, pregabalin is eliminated principally unchanged in the urine. However, in dogs, while ≥ 80% of a dose is excreted in the urine, approximately 45% of the dose excreted as the N-methyl metabolite. However, pregablin does not appear to affect cytochrome P450 drug-metabolizing enzymes. The disposition of pregabalin has been described in apparently healthy Labrador Retriever–Greyhound cross dogs (four female, two male) after a single oral dose of 4.mg/kg (Table 27-4). The duration that plasma drug concentrations were above the presumed minimum effective concentration of 2.8 μg/mL ranged from 7 to 14.5 hours.[167]

Dewey and coworkers described the use of pregabalin as an adjunct to anticonvulsant therapy in the control of epilepsy in 11 dogs using an uncontrolled clinical trial.[168] Animals had not responded sufficiently to either phenobarbital or bromide, or a combination of the two. Insufficient control was defined as two or more seizures per month despite concentration in the recommended therapeutic range of the appropriate drug. For phenobarbital concentrations ranged from 20 to 40 μg/mL and for bromide 0.2 to 2.81 mg/mL. Dogs whose bromide concentrations were subtherapeutic were receiving phenobarbital in the therapeutic range. Dogs were treated with 3 to 4 mg/kg pregabalin every 8 hours, yielding mean pregabalin concentrations of 6.4+ μg/mL. Therapy resulted in a reduction of seizures by at least 50% (range of 23% to 83%) in seven of nine dogs that completed the study. However, 10 of the 11 dogs developed adverse effects, including ataxia. Increases in liver enzymes were present during the study, but it is not clear if these increases were related to phenobarbital or pregabalin. Although the study provides support for the possible use of pregabalin as an add-on anticonvulsant, a controlled clinical trial is indicated in dogs to assess both efficacy and safety.

Levetiracetam

Levetiracetam is a single (S)-enantiomer acetamide-derivative antiepileptic drug. Its mechanism of action is novel and does not appear to involve any known neurotransmitter, ion channel protein, or receptor. Rather, it appears to interact with synaptic vesicles (SVA), and appears to impede conduction of impulses across the synapse. Levetiracetam was most useful experimentally in blocking seizures caused by pilocarpine and KA and in the kindling model of rats, both models for complex partial seizures with secondary generalization. Food does not impair the extent, but does impair the rate, of oral absorption. In humans close to 70% of the drug is renally excreted; hepatic metabolism of the remainder reflects acetamide hydrolysis, which is not CYP 450 dependent. Levetiracetam is metabolized by plasma B-esterases, which will continue once blood is drawn. As such, serum rather than plasma or whole blood is the desired test tissue of choice.[169] The elimination half-life in humans is approximately 7 hours. Drug interactions appear to be minimal; competition for renal tubular secretory proteins may occur.

KEY POINT 27-23 The novel mechanism of action of levetiracetam and its wide therapeutic margin are balanced by its very short half-life.

The disposition of levetiracetam has been described in mongrel dogs (n=6).[170,171] Intravenous administration of 20 mg/kg yielded a maximum concentration of approximately 44 μg/mL, volume of distribution of 0.45 ± 0.13 L/kg, clearance of 1.5 mL/min/kg, elimination half-life of 3.6 ± 0.8 hours and mean residence time of 5 ± 1 hours. In a diferent study[172] (male and female dogs), oral administration of 54 mg/kg yielded a C_{max} of 50 to 65 μg/mL (mean of 53 and 55 μg/mL in male and female dogs, respectively), and an elimination half-life of 2 to 3 hours. Dewey and coworkers[173] reported the disposition of levetiracetam in dogs (n = 6) after a single dose (60 mg/kg over 2 min) administered intravenously. The extrapolated peak plasma drug concentration (Co) was 254 ± 81 mg/mL, steady-state volume of distributionof 0.48 L/kg, and clearance of1.4 mL*min/kg. The elimination half-life was 4 ± 0.82 hours, and mean residence time was 6 ± 0.9 hours. The dose was well tolerated. Patterson and coworkers[174] studied levetiracetam after intravenous, intramuscular, and oral (19.5 to 2.6 mg/kg) administration in hound dogs (n = 6). Peak drug concentrations were 37 ± 5, 30.3 ± 3, and 30 ± 4 μg/mL after intravenous (Co:extrapolated peak plasma concentration), intramuscular, and oral administration, respectively. The volume of distribution (beta) was 0.55 L/kg, and clearance was 55 mL/min (not standardized to kg). Elimination half-life was 3 ± 0.3 hours. Bioavailability after intramuscular and oral administration were 113+13% and 100+7%, respectively. No pain was detected with intentional perivascular injection.

In dogs 1200 mg/kg administered intravenously or 2000 mg/kg administered orally was not lethal but was associated with salivation, vomiting, tachycardia, and restlessness; 1200 mg/kg per day for 13 and 52 weeks resulted in transient restlessness and tremor and centrally mediated salivation and vomiting.. Long-term administration (≥6 months) in some species was associated with enzyme induction (centrilobular hypertrophy) at 50 mg/kg per day. Liver weight increased, although histopathologic changes did not appear in the liver.

The disposition of levetiracetam has been described in cats (n=10) receiving 20 mg/kg either intravenously or orally as a single dose.[175] Cats tolerated dosing well, with no significant adverse effects noted. However, transient mild to moderate hypersalivation occurred with oral dosing. Median peak concentration after intravenous dosing was 37.52 μg/mL (range 28.05 to 51.86 μg/mL), with a median half-life of 2.86 hours (range 2.07 to 4.08 hours) and mean residence time of 4.57 hours (range 3.09 to 6). Clearance was 2 mL/kg/min (range 1.5 to 3.4 mL/kg/min) and steady-state volume of distribution was 0.52 L/kg (range 0.33 to 0.64 L/kg). After oral dosing therapeutic plasma concentrations were achieved in 7 of 10 cats within 10 minutes and remained within the therapeutic range for at least 9 hours. Median peak concentration (C_{max}) was 25.54 μg/mL (range 13.22 to 37.11 μg/mL), T_{max} was 1.67 hours (range 0.33 to 4 hours), $T_{1/2}$ was 2.95 hours (range 1.86 to 4.63 hours), and mean residence time was 5.65 hours (range 4.23 to 7.86). Mean oral bioavailabililty was 100%. When levetiracetam is monitored, because of its very short half-life (according to the author's measurements, as short as 1 hour in dogs and cats), the therapeutic range should be applied to trough rather than peak concentrations. Ideally, both a peak and trough should be measured at least once a year in the patient to determine drug half-life.

Response to levetiracetam of dogs (n=14) with refractory epilepsy was described prospectively.[176] Refractoriness was based on monitoring; eligibility required that drug concentrations be in the upper quartile of the recommended range (mean 32 ± 4.6 μg/mL). Levetiracetam was administered at 10 mg/kg orally every 8 hours; the dose was increased to 20 mg/kg thrice daily if seizures did not decline by at least 50%. At 2 months 8 of 10 dogs responded, with seizure number reduced by 73% and number of days or months reduced by 67%. At 6 months 6 of 11 dogs remained classified as responders. However, with long-term follow-up, only three animals remained responders, suggesting that efficacy of levetiracetam declined. Drug concentrations were not measured; as such, the cause of therapeutic failure (i.e., tolerance or worsening disease) was not distinguished from declining drug concentrations.[176]

The use of levetiracetam in cats has been reported.[175,177] Four cats with seizure disorders that were poorly controlled with phenobarbital alone were treated with oral levetiracetam as an add-on drug at a dose regimen of 20 mg/kg body weight, every 8 hours. Levetiracetam serum concentrations were within the reported therapeutic range for people (5 to 30 to 45 μg/mL) for all samples in all cats. The overall average serum levetiracetam level for all cats was 16.5 μg/mL (range: 6.9 to 24.3 μg/mL). The median serum disappearance half-life (t ½) of (based on peak and trough samples) was 5.3 hours. Seizure frequency was reduced by an average of 30.5% in three cats and increased by 33.3% in one cat. The results of this pilot study suggest that levetiracetam is a safe drug for cats that may provide some therapeutic benefit when used as an add-on to phenobarbital.

KEY POINT 27-24 Trough (rather than peak) concentrations of levetiracetam should target the recommended therapeutic range.

Phenytoin Sodium

Phenytoin sodium, previously named *diphenylhydantoin,* depresses motor areas of the cortex (antiepileptic action) without depressing sensory areas. It is approved by the Food and Drug Administration for control of epileptiform convulsions in dogs.

Phenytoin is a hydantoin derivative (see Figure 27-4);[45] others of lesser importance are mephenytoin and ethotoin. Hydantoins are five-member ring structures, whereas barbiturates are six-member structures. A major point of difference between the hydantoins and barbiturates is the absence of a C=O group. Phenytoin is not a general anticonvulsant, as is phenobarbital, and is not used for emergency treatment of poisoning by convulsant drugs or tetanic seizures. Oral preparations are available in suspension, capsule, and tablet forms. Phenytoin (50 mg/mL) is also available for human use in a special solvent for intravenous administration. Intravenous injection of the drug causes a marked drop in arterial pressure and is not advised in the dog.[178]

Phenytoin is no longer used to control seizures in the dog because of its lack of efficacy,[179] which may be related to decreased bioavailability and rapid clearance. Phenytoin is much less effective in the dog than either phenobarbital or primidone in the control of epileptic seizures.[50] The half-life of phenytoin is too short in the dog to permit maintenance of adequate drug concentrations in plasma and the CNS.[17] When administered alone, phenytoin cannot be considered a satisfactory drug for treatment of epilepsy in the dog.[29,180] Because of drug interactions and enhanced hepatotoxicity, a combination of phenytoin with phenobarbital is not a viable alternative.

KEY POINT 27-25 Phenytoin is not a preferred drug for treatment of epilepsy because of its short half-life, variability, poor oral bioavailability, and potential for toxicity.

In the cat phenytoin is relatively toxic and generally undesirable as an anticonvulsant.[70] The efficacy and safety of phenytoin in cats have not been determined.[29]

Pharmacologic Activity

Phenytoin produces a stabilizing effect on synaptic junctions that ordinarily allow nerve impulses to be readily transmitted at lower thresholds. Consequently, the level of synaptic excitability that permits impulses to be transmitted easily is reduced or stabilized or both. This effect appears to be associated with active extrusion of Na^+ from neurons and decreased posttetanic potentiation or spread of nerve impulses to adjacent neurons. Phenytoin may reduce calcium movement across cell membranes. Further, phenytoin may inhibit activation of protein phosphorylation by the calcium–calmodulin complex.[181] Phosphorylation and norepinephrine release in neurons requires calmodulin. Reduction in spread of the "burst" activity associated with epilepsy prevents genesis of the cortical seizure. Phenytoin stabilizes hyperexcitable neurons without causing general depression of the CNS.[45]

Disposition

Absorption of phenytoin is erratic after intramuscular administration. This may be related to crystallization of the drug at the injection site because of alteration in pH by tissues.[45] Administration of phenytoin by the intramuscular route is not advised because considerable necrosis and sloughing at the injection site occur.[178] Absorption of the drug from the gastrointestinal tract of the dog is rapid but erratic and incomplete.[179] Bioavailability of phenytoin from the tablet formulation averages 36% in the dog.[180] Poor oral absorption and differences in product bioavailability contribute to the difficulty in achieving effective serum levels of phenytoin. The generic preparations of phenytoin should not be used.[182] Dosing at 30 mg/kg thrice daily for 3 days resulted in concentrations of less than 8.5 μg/mL.[179] Dosing at 10 mg/kg thrice daily for 5 to 8 days yielded concentrations less than 2.5 μg/mL.

At therapeutic concentrations (10 to 20 μg/mL), phenytoin is highly bound (75% to 85%) to plasma proteins in animals and humans.[183] The high degree of phenytoin binding predisposes this acidic drug to interaction with other drugs by a displacing effect at protein (albumin) binding sites, although the relevance of this in the presence of increased clearance is not known. In uremic patients decreased plasma protein binding is associated with accelerated renal clearance or elimination of the drug. Phenytoin readily crosses the placenta.[184] High concentrations of phenytoin are attained in the maternal liver and maternal and fetal hearts. The brain (ostensibly the primary target organ) contains nearly the lowest concentration of the drug.

Phenytoin is metabolized via CYP2C9 and to a lesser degree CYP2C19[185] into metahydroxyphenytoin or parahydroxyphenytoin, which are conjugated with glucuronic acid. In humans approximately 60% to 75% of the daily dose of phenytoin is excreted in the glucuronide form;[45] the dog also converts a high percentage of phenytoin into this form. In addition, diphenylhydantoic acid, a minor metabolite in some laboratory animals, and dihydrodiol are formed in dogs. Interestingly, high concentrations of diphenylhydantoic acid are found in cat urine. The dihydrodiol metabolite is probably involved in formation of catechol metabolites; these are also formed in most animals.[186] Epoxide metabolites are also speculated to be formed in humans. Because phenytoin is not very soluble in water, little of the unmetabolized drug is excreted in urine.

In the dog, despite relatively large single daily oral doses (50 mg/kg), the plasma concentration of the drug is low, perhaps reflecting the short half-life of 6 to 7.8 hours[187] compared with 4 to 6 hours after an intramuscular injection (50 mg/kg) as well. The shorter half-life of the second study probably reflects induction after multiple dosing;[188] the half-life of phenytoin in the dog dramatically decreases after 7 to 9 days of treatment.[179,180.] A 2.5-hour half-life was predicted for phenytoin after 14 days of therapy compared with 3.3 hours with single dosing. Other studies have confirmed a short half-life for phenytoin in the dog: After a single intravenous dose (15 mg/kg), a value of 4.5 hours was obtained by Sanders and coworkers,[189] and a half-life of 3.65 hours was determined by Pedersoli and coworkers[190] after an intravenous bolus of 11 mg/kg. The clearance of phenytoin has been described as dose dependent in dogs.[179] More recently, using a parallel design, the disposition of phenytoin was described in Beagles (n=5) after 5 days of intravenuos administration of 12 mg/kg (see Table 27-5).[191]

After oral administration (10 mg/kg) in the cat, plasma half-life of phenytoin was 24 to 108 hours,[188,192] contributing to the prolonged effect of phenytoin observed in the cat more than in other species. This may reflect decreased glucuronide conjugation.

Clinical Use

In humans clinical therapeutic effects and intoxication are related to the blood concentration of phenytoin. A reduction in the number of seizures occurs when phenytoin blood concentrations exceed 10 μg/mL. Recommended therapeutic doses of phenytoin administered orally every 8 hours for control of seizure disorders in the dog indicate considerable variation: 6.6 to 11 mg/kg,[178] 11 mg/kg,[49] and 35 mg/kg.[179] However, oral administration of phenytoin (4.4 and 11 mg/kg) every 8 hours fails to reach serum concentrations of 10 μg/mL in the dog. Indeed, serum phenytoin after either single or repeated oral doses of 10 mg/kg does not exceed a concentration of 2 μg/mL.[179] To achieve a serum concentration of approximately 10 μg/mL phenytoin, it appears that an oral dose of at least 35 mg/kg given thrice daily is necessary for the adult dog.[49,179] According to Pedersoli and coworkers,[190] an oral dosage schedule of 20 mg/kg every 8 hours of the phenytoin microcrystalline suspension should be sufficient to reach a serum concentration of 10 μg/mL or higher. This dose, however, will maintain a plasma therapeutic level for only the first 2 or 3 days of treatment.[180] Farnbach[50] found that only 3 of 77 epileptic dogs receiving phenytoin were controlled; concentrations in all dogs ranged from 0.2 to 13 μg/mL, with a median of 2.3 μg/mL, despite doses ranging from 3 to 129 mg/kg per day (generally divided into twice-daily doses).

Drug Interactions

The combined use of phenytoin and phenobarbital or primidone may lead to increased formation of epoxide metabolites in animals. This could possibly result in cholestatic hepatic injury similar to that reported in three dogs.[36] The effect may also reflect induction by phenytoin. Phenytoin must be considered a potent inducer of the hepatic microsomal enzyme system in the dog.[180] Between 7 and 9 days after administration of phenytoin, its half-life may be reduced from 5.5 to 1.3 hours. In contrast, the half-life after oral administration in humans averages 22 hours, with a range of 7 to 42 hours. This contrasts to humans, in which phenytoin has a moderate inducing ability in the human. The differences between the two species may help explain the efficacy of phenytoin for control of epileptic seizures in humans compared to dogs. Further, although the combined use of phenytoin and phenobarbital is considered optimal therapy in humans,[55] use of both drugs is controversial because both induce hepatic microsomal enzyme activity. This combined induction complicates successful therapy because therapeutic concentrations are difficult to achieve and the increased production of potentially toxic metabolites.[178] Metabolism of a number of chemicals or drugs is enhanced by phenytoin. These include digitoxin, dexamethasone, and cortisol.[193] In humans the half-life of theophylline decreases by 50% with an increase in clearance of twofold.[194]

Phenytoin metabolism in humans is inhibited by other drugs prolonging their effect. Examples include dicumarol, chloramphenicol, phenylbutazone, and the phenothiazines. In vitro inhibition has been demonstrated by diazepam and propoxyphene hydrochloride. In the dog the serum half-life of intravenous phenytoin increased from 3 to 15 hours when administered with chloramphenicol, and signs of phenytoin toxicosis reversed within 24 hours after cessation of chloramphenicol treatment.[195] Phenylbutazone is also known to increase plasma concentration as a result of inhibition.[45] Despite predominant renal elimination, vigabatrin, a drug similar to gabapentin, deceased phenytoin clearance by 31% and increased phenytoin half-life by 45% in Beagles.[191] In contrast, gabapentin had no effect.

Serum phenytoin concentration declines in the presence of folic acid therapy, presumably because the hydroxylase enzyme that metabolizes phenytoin is folate dependent. Phenytoin may prolong the prothrombin time.[196] Blood coagulation defects similar to that induced by vitamin K deficiency can occur in neonates exposed to phenytoin in utero. The coagulation defect can be reversed by treatment with vitamin K.

Blood Concentrations and Associated Toxicity

In humans mild signs of intoxication such as nystagmus develop with blood levels of 20 μg/mL; patients with levels over 40 μg/mL have marked nystagmus and are uncoordinated and lethargic. Blood levels in the dog would probably have to increase a comparable 100% to 400% as in humans before serious signs of intoxication develop.

Hepatitis, jaundice, and death after clinical use of phenytoin have been reported in one dog that initially received primidone (500 mg daily).[197] Toxic hepatopathy and intrahepatic cholestasis associated with phenytoin administration in combination with phenobarbital or primidone (or both) have been reported in three dogs.[36,89] Two distinct forms of hepatotoxicity have been ascribed to reflect the sequelae of anticonvulsant phenytoin in dogs.[36] The first (type B reaction) is characterized by clinical signs after extended treatment at lower than recommended doses and may result from an (unpredictable) idiosyncratic reaction. Indications are that histologic changes with this form will progress from chronic hepatitis to cirrhosis. The second form is more frequently characterized by intrahepatic cholestasis and is associated with a poor prognosis. This form of liver disease has been associated with high doses of phenytoin in combination with primidone or phenobarbital and may represent an intrinsic hepatotoxicity. Induction of enzymes is likely to increase formation of toxic metabolites, which may contribute to hepatotoxicity. Hepatotoxicity resulting from phenytoin is more likely if the drug is used in combination therapy with either primidone or phenobarbital. Toxicity may be related to generation of toxic metabolites. Two forms of toxicity appear to occur with phenytoin therapy: a dose-independent chronic hepatitis that may progress to cirrhosis and that appears to be reversible after discontinuation of the drug early in the disease and a dose-dependent intrahepatic cholestasis that is accompanied by a poor prognosis.

Other Side Effects

The CNS side effects of phenytoin in the dog are moderate in part because of its action but also because it is rapidly metabolized.[49] Transient incoordination and oversedation may occasionally occur after administration of phenytoin. A moderate degree of polyphagia, polydipsia, and polyuria may be seen in animals medicated with this drug. Sialosis, weight loss, and vomiting have been reported after the use of phenytoin in the cat. Inhibition of release of antidiuretic hormone accounts for the polyuria that develops after administration of phenytoin. Insulin secretion also is inhibited.[45]

Displacement of T_4 by highly protein-bound drugs (e.g., phenytoin) from T_4-binding globulin increases T_4 concentrations, induction of hepatic drug-metabolizing enzymes results in increased clearance of both T_4 and T_3, and increased conversion of T_4 to T_3 by peripheral tissues further decreases T_4. The latter mechanism has been postulated as the reason that T_3 concentrations may remain normal despite increased T_3 clearance[198] in patients receiving phenytoin. Clinical signs of hypothyroidism may not be apparent in such cases. Note, however, that both serum T_4 and free T_4 may be decreased in some patients receiving anticonvulsants.

Fosphenytoin is a phosphate ester prodrug of phenytoin, with the latter being released after dephosphorylation by tissue (liver, red blood cells, and others) phosphatases.[199] Enzymatic conversion half-life is about 3 minutes in dogs, with equimolar concentrations of phenytoin emerging with fosphenytoin. Similar antiarrhythmic (antiseizure was not reported) effects occurred for fosphenytoin and phenytoin in dogs. Side effects are similar to phenytoin, although local irritation was less with intramuscular administration of fosphenytoin compared with phenytoin. No information could be found regarding use of fosphenytoin in dogs.

Topiramate

Topiramate is a monosaccharide D-fructose anticonvulsant derivative developed in the 1980s.[200] Its mechanism of action is not entirely understood but includes enhanced gabaminergic actions at the GABA-A receptor. Sodium channel blockade may also be involved (package insert). Its effects are similar to those of diazepam but are not blocked by flumazenil, suggesting actions through a novel, non-benzodiazepine (BDZ)–sensitive binding site on the GABA-A receptor. It may also inhibit the kainite/AMPA (but not NMDA) glutamate receptor. Topiramate appears to increase the seizure threshold and prevent seizure spread. In selected studies potency is similar to phenytoin and phenobarbital. However, while useful in kindled and ischemia-induced epilepsy, it has variable efficacy for prevention of pentylenetetrazole (a GABA-A receptor antagonist) or picrotoxin-induced seizures. In humans it has been predictably effective in controlling partial and secondary seizures but not absence seizures.

In humans topiramate is eliminated primarily through the kidneys as the parent compound, although up to eight metabolites have been identified.

Topiramate inhibits isoenzymes of carbonic anhydrase; this mechanism appears to be more relevant to side effects than control of seizures. Binding to the enzyme results in a large proportion of the drug being located in erythrocytes at low concentrations. Its oral disposition has been reported in male and female Beagles; intravenous data are available for one dog (see Table 27-4).[201] Based on comparison of the area under the curve after 10 mg/kg intravenously and orally, oral bioavailability appears to be about 35% for tabular form but is increased twofold when administered as a solution. Dogs treated with up to 400 mg/kg experienced no lethal side effects, although acute toxicity associated with ataxia, decreased motor activity, tremors, and clonic convulsions occurred. Dosing for 3 and 12 months was not associated with overt indicators of toxicity in dogs. However, increased liver weights (indicative of induction), increased serum gastrin levels and gastric mucosal hyperplasia, and renal and urinary epithelial hypertrophy have been associated with long-term use in other species. Topiramate is available as a sprinkle formulation. Its use apparently has not been reported in dogs or cats.

Valproic Acid

Valproic acid is a vehicle used for other drugs that was serendipitously found to have anticonvulsant properties. It is a simple branched-chain carboxylic acid (see Figure 27-4). Valproic acid is effective against a variety of seizures, including absence seizures. Its mechanism of action appears to be similar to that of phenytoin in that it prolongs recovery of voltage-activated Na^+ channels from inactivation. It may also affect Ca^{2+} fluxes but does not appear to impair GABA. The drug is rapidly absorbed, highly protein bound, and in humans has a half-life of 10 to 15 hours. The half-life can, however, be shortened in the presence of other (inducing) anticonvulsant drugs.

The difficulty in using this drug in dogs probably reflects an inability to achieve therapeutic concentrations. Valproic acid is metabolized in the liver; metabolites can be as potent as the parent compound in controlling seizures, although only one of them enters the CNS to any appreciable extent. Valproic acid can alter liver enzymes (up to 40% of human); increases can be associated with toxicity. Hepatotoxicity is likely to be increased when used in combination with other drugs. It also causes gastrointestinal upset and, like other anticonvulsants, CNS side effects (e.g., sedation, ataxia). Valproic acid has not proved very useful for controlling seizures in dogs. It might be considered in combination with phenobarbital, although drug interactions may complicate therapy.

The disposition of valproic acid has been reported for dogs by several authors (reviewed by Frey and Löscher)[42] (see Table 27-4). Peak serum concentration after oral absorption is markedly variable and appears to be greater with solution (30 to 60 μg/mL at 20 mg/kg) compared with tablets (30 to 75 μg/mL at 40 mg/kg). However, bioavailability is not as divergent, reaching 89 ± 8.2 for solution compared with 78 ± 17 for tablets.[42] Löscher[202] demonstrated that therapeutic drug concentrations could be maintained in part because of decreased protein binding in dogs compared with humans. Half-life of valproic acid did not change over 14 days of treatment at 168 to 180 mg/kg (divided into three equal doses). Löscher attributed some antiepileptic efficacy of valproate to its metabolites, which appear to accumulate in dogs (n = 3). In a study of multiple oral dosing (60 mg/kg thrice daily for 14 days), mean plasma concentrations of valproic acid, 2-en- valproic acid, 3-hydroxy-valproic acid, 3 keto-valproic acid, and "total equivalents" of valproic acid were 20, 3.1, less than 0.4, and 3.7 (23 equivalents) on day 1 of dosing, compared with 8, 16, 0.7, and 9.1 (18 equivalents) at day 14.

The use of valproic acid for treatment in idiopathic epileptic dogs (27 female and 40 male), 29 of which were considered refractory to anticonvulsant drugs was described by Nafe and coworkers.[203] The addition of valproic acid (25 to 40 mg/kg per day) resulted in improvement in six of eleven dogs already receiving phenytoin or phenobarbital and one of six dogs receiving primidone (dog was tapered off of primidone). Valproic acid (25 to 105 mg/kg per day) alone markedly improved seizures in 7 of 16 dogs, and the combination of valproic acid and phenobarbital resulted in marked improvement in 14 of 24 dogs. One dog developed noninflammatory alopecia.

Zonisamide

Developed in Japan, zonisamide, 3-sulfamoylmethyl-1,2 benzisoxazole, is a synthetic sulfonamide-based anticonvulsant approved for use in the United States in 1998 for treatment of seizures related to human epilepsy.[204] The efficacy of zonisamide for treatment of human epilepsy is similar to phenobarbital and superior to other classic drugs, including valproic acid and phenytoin. Its mechanism is not clear, but it appears to inhibit neuronal voltage-dependent sodium and T-type calcium channels.[205,206] It also modulates the dopaminergic system and accelerates the release of GABA from the hippocampus.[207,208] An additional potential advantage of zonisamide is free radical scavenging, which protects against the destructive nature of radicals, especially in neuronal membranes.[209] Finally, zonisamide blocks the propagation of seizures from cortex to subcortical areas of the brain. Its antiepileptic efficacy has been described as similar to that of phenytoin or valproic acid, thus minimally affecting normal neuronal activity. These multiple mechanisms of action may translate to improved efficacy compared with other anticonvulsant drugs.

The clinical pharmacology of zonisamide has been investigated in humans with similar characteristics in dogs.[210-212] Disposition is complicated. Oral absorption tends to be rapid, complete, and minimally impaired by food. After 12 hours of dosing, zonisamide concentrations in the brain are twofold that in plasma. The extent of protein binding is not sufficient to limit the rapid movement into the brain. Binding of zonisamide to erythrocytes (red blood cells) and plasma proteins contributes to complex kinetics. Erythrocyte concentrations in whole blood tend to be twice as high as plasma and serum in humans and are characterized by binding that is both saturable and nonsaturable;[213] the saturable portion may reflect binding to carbonic anhydrase in epileptic patients. Accumulation of drug in red blood cells is reversible, and the complex relationship between zonisamide and red blood cells may make therapeutic drug monitoring of plasma or serum advantageous. Metabolism of zonisamide involves both phase I and phase II hepatic metabolism, with cytochrome P450 3A4 being the major isozyme and a glucuronidated compound the major metabolite.[214] Enzymes CYP3A4, CYP3A5, and CYP2C19 contribute to metabolism in humans.[215] Renal elimination and recovery of zonisamide indicate parent drug recovery of 35%. Using radiolabeled (carbon) zonisamide administered to dogs, 83% of the drug was excreted in 72-hour urine as the either the parent compound or metabolites. The remaining proportion was recovered in feces.[210] The terminal half-life of zonisamide in the dog after a single oral dose (20 mg/kg) administration differed depending on the tissue studied, with the shortest being 15 hours for plasma and the longest 42 hours for red blood cells.[210] The longer elimination half-life allows a convenient dosing interval while minimizing dramatic fluctuations in zonisamide concentrations that might cause recurrence of seizures. Recommended therapeutic concentrations for zonisamide initially were 10 to 70 μg/mL, with 16.5 to 49.6 μg/mL also suggested when dosed twice daily.[216] The author recommends the more commonly accepted 10 to 40 μg/mL; however, monitoring should be based on patient need. Nonlinear pharmacokinetics have been reported in some human patients, particularly with chronic dosing, resulting in disproportionate, and thus unexpected, increases in drug concentrations compared with changes in dose. In dogs undergoing toxicity studies, plasma concentrations never reached steady state over the course of 13 weeks of dosing at 75 mg/kg, compared with proportional steady-state concentrations by week 13 at 10 to 30 mg/ kg.[212]

KEY POINT 27-26 Its unique mechanism of action, reasonable half-life, and wide therapeutic margin render zonisamide an increasingly useful drug for control of epilepsy in dogs and cats.

Clinical pharmacokinetics of zonisamide have been described in normal dogs (n = 8), four male and four female, ranging from 3 to 4 years of age, using a randomized crossover design after single intravenous and oral administration,

6.85 and 10.25 mg/kg, respectively.[217] Zonisamide concentrations differed among blood compartments after single dosing, with oral maximum concentration (C_{max}) being greatest in red blood cells (28.73μg/mL) and least (14.36 μg/mL) in plasma. Clearance of zonisamide was 57.55 mL/hr/kg from plasma and 5.06 mL/hr/kg from red blood cells. However, zonisamide concentrations did not differ among blood compartments at the end of multiple dosing, suggesting any blood component can be monitored. The fraction of unbound drug was 60.48 ± 13.4%. Elimination half-life in plasma was 16.4 hours in serum and 57.4 hours in red blood cells. Volume of distribution also differed, being greater (1 L/kg) in plasma and least in (0.4 L/kg) red blood cells. Bioavailability was 126.8% for red blood cells and 189.6% for plasma. After multiple dosing (10.17 mg/kg) twice daily for 8 weeks, the accumulation ratio of zonisamide was 3.5 (plasma) and 4.3 (red blood cells). The resulting mean C_{max} at steady state was 56 ± 12 μg/mL, suggesting a beginning dose of 2 to 3 mg/kg twice daily to target the low end of the therapeutic range. The half-life at 8 weeks was 23 ± 6 hours. Plasma drug concentrations varied by 17.2% between 12-hour dosing intervals, which suggests that a 12-hour dosing interval is appropriate. Differences in clinical pathology data occurred at the end of the 8-week study period, although all results remained within normal limits. Serum alkaline phosphatase and calcium increased above baseline, whereas total serum protein and albumin both decreased below baseline.

Zonisamide pharmacokinetics have been described in cats (n = 5) after a single dose of 10 mg/kg (see Table 27-4).[218] Safety and adverse reactions were studied during chronic (9 weeks) dosing at 20 mg/kg once daily. Zonisamide was not well tolerated at this dose; 50% of cats exhibited vomiting, diarrhea, and anorexia. Mean peak and trough concentration with chronic dosing in all cats were 46 and 59 μg/mL, respectively, with concentration at 42, 59, and 79 in cats with adversities. Zonisamide appears to be minimally involved in drug interactions typicalof highly protein-bound drugs.[210] However, it is involved with interactions involving CYP enzymes. Nakasa and coworkers[215] demonstrated that clearance was decreased 31%, 23%, and 17% by ketoconazole, cyclosporine A, and miconazole, respectively; fluconazole inhibited clearance to a lesser degree, but itraconazole appeared to have no effect.

Oral bioavailability of human generic preparations should not be assumed to act similarly in dogs and cats. Accordingly, clinicians and owners both should request that dispensing pharmacists inform the owner or veterinarian if the dispensing pharmacy has changed to a different generic preparation since the last prescription.

Zonisamide does not appear to affect its own metabolism nor the metabolism of other drugs in animals or humans. Phenobarbital will shorten zonisamide half-life. The impact of 35 days of dosing phenobarbital on the disposition of zonisamide was studied in dogs. Unfortunately, all data were pictorially represented, limiting assessment of changes in disposition.[219] After 35 days of phenobarbital administration, concentrations appeared to decrease to about 2.75 μg/mL, returning to 3.5 only after approximately 12 weeks after phenobarbital was discontinued. The decrease in half-life appeared to be about 3 hours, or approximately 30%. Phenobarbital shortened the half-life of zonisamide from 27 to 36 hours in humans, resulting in lower plasma drug concentrations.[220] The impact of phenobarbital does not appear to be profound, but monitoring is warranted, and collection of both a peak and a trough sample might be warranted in patients receiving phenobarbital with zonisamide. The effect does not appear to warrant starting the drug at higher doses in patients on phenobarbital unless monitoring has confirmed the need.

Dogs appear to tolerate zonisamide well; concentrations in samples submitted for monitoring at the author's laboratory indicate concentrations that exceed 60, 80, and in some dogs, 100 μg/ml well. Dose increases for zonisamide in dogs may cause disproportionate increases in plasma drug concentrations based on data in the author's laboratory. It is possible this may reflect saturation of acetylation enzymes in the dogs.

As a sulfonamide, zonisamide inhibits thyroid synthesis of thyroid hormones. Anticonvulsants (phenytoin) may also have a direct negative effect on TSH response to thyrotropin-releasing hormone. Drug-induced changes in T_4-binding globulins have also been documented in human patients taking anticonvulsants. Boothe and Perkins[217] demonstrated that zonisamide dosed for 8 weeks was associated with a decrease in total T_4 below normal limits. Free T_4 and TSH were also decreased from pretreatment concentrations, although both were within normal limits. Zonisamide concentrations were higher than the recommended therapeutic range. Thyroxin and TSH concentrations might facilitate diagnosis of hypothyroidism in animals receiving zonisamide.[198] Note that thyroid supplementation suppresses response to TSH, and testing should not be performed until supplementation has been discontinued for 4 to 6 weeks. As with carbonic anhydrase inhibitors, zonisamide has been linked to metabolic acidosis in humans. The FDA recommends that bicarbonate be measured before and intermittently during therapy. Renal calculi have formed in a very small number of human patients receiving zonisamide for long periods. Because it does not contain an aryl-amine, allergic responses associated with sulfonamide antimicrobials may not occur in dogs.

Clinical reports of zonisamide use in animals are limited. In one report zonisamide was effective in reduction of seizures in patients with epilepsy that had not sufficiently responded to one or more anticonvulsants (including phenobarbital and/or bromide) in 7 of 12 dogs at doses designed to achieve 10 to 40 μg/mL. Dose reduction or discontinuation of concurrent anticonvulsant was possible in 8 of 12 dogs. Mean concentrations approximated 20 μg/mL; mean dose was 9 mg/kg every 12 hours.[221] A second open clinical trial studied zonisamide for treatment of refractory seizures in dogs (n = 13).[222] Mean reduction in seizure was 70%, with three dogs relapsing. Drug concentrations were not measured.

KEY POINT 27-27 At high concentrations, zonisamide will inhibit thyroid gland synthesis. Therapy should be initiated at a low dose and concentrations increased as needed to control seizures.

ACUTE MANAGEMENT OF SEIZURES

Status Epilepticus

The leading cause of SE in humans is inappropriate low concentrations, with noncompliance with prescribed medications among the most common reasons. Accordingly, the application of the principles of pharmacology to anticonvulsant therapy should facilitate effective control and the avoidance of SE. A number of proepileptic drugs are also cited as causes for SE (discussed later).[223]

Early therapeutic intervention is more important than drug choice; in humans intervention within the first 30 minutes was associated with an 80% response to first-choice drugs, whereas 60% of patients in SE for more than 2 hours did not respond to first-line therapy. Physiologic responses of concern include fever, cardiac arrhythmias, changes in systemic (initially hypertension and later hypotension) and pulmonary blood pressures, and altered blood chemistries.[223]

In humans[223] the traditional definition of SE as continuous or repetitive seizures lasting 20 minutes or more has been challenged; therapy for SE is recommended for two or more generalized convulsions without full recovery of consciousness between seizures, or continuous convulsive activity lasting more than 10 minutes. However, recommendations have been reduced to 5 minutes because few seizures last this long.

Benzodiazepines tend to be more effective early but not later, whereas NMDA receptor antagonists (e.g., ketamine) tend to be effective later but not early. In humans, drugs of choice vary with the duration of SE. The suggested approach is 6 to 10 minutes: intravenous lorazepam, followed by diazepam or midazolam (intranasally, or intramuscularly); 10 to 20 minutes: fospheyntoin for 10 to 60 min followed by midazolam by CRI or phenobarbital IV if no response,propofol by CRI or valproate if no response, and finally, the addition or alternative of pentobarbital or midazolam if no response. For seizures greater than 60 minutes in duration, pentobarbital is indicated. Despite ketamine's potential efficacy as an anticonvulsant drug, antagonism of NMDA may result in severe neurotoxicity, and its use in SE should be reserved until scientific data support its efficacy.

In dogs or cats, treatment for more than one seizure per hour is a medical emergency.[49] The use of drugs for acute management of seizures is addressed in detail with individual drugs. In general, however, acute therapy of seizures (e.g., SE) is preferentially implemented with diazepam (intravenous bolus to effect). Diazepam has a short half-life, and it may be necessary to repeat the dose once or twice during the first 2 hours to stabilize the dog.[49] To terminate the seizures, various methods of administration have been recommended. Diazepam is recommended in an intravenous dose of 5 to 20 mg. Frey and Löscher[42] recommended an intravenous dose of 0.5 to 1 mg/kg. Control by diazepam can be prolonged by continued administration as a CRI (2 to 5 mg/hr of 5% dextrose; the infusion line should first be flushed with the diazepam solution to allow diazepam binding to the polyvinyl), or coadministration of phenobarbital (2 to 6 mg/kg intramuscularly to avoid respiratory or cardiac depression). Clonazepam (0.05 to 0.2 mg/kg intravenously) may provide antiepileptic efficacy that lasts longer (but is not necessarily any more efficacious) than that of diazepam. Unfortunately, an intravenous preparation is not available in the United States.Alternatively, phenobarbital can be administered as the first choice (intravenous bolus to effect, as a loading dose). Note that for each 3 mg/kg of phenobarbital given intravenously, serum concentration increases approximately 5 μg/mL. For a patient not receiving phenobarbital at the time that therapy is begun, up to 18-mg/kg total dose (given in 3- to 6-mg/kg increments at 15- to 30-minute intervals) may be necessary to achieve the midtherapeutic range (30 μg/mL). Drug distribution of phenobarbital into the CNS may take 15 to 30 minutes. Failure to control seizures may indicate the need for pentobarbital. As such, the risk of cardiovascular or respiratory depression is great. An advantage to the use of pentobarbital, however, is its protective effects on the brain during periods of hypoxia induced by the seizure.

KEY POINT 27-28 Although diazepam is very effective, its short duration of action may require alternative drugs or methods of administration.

Alternative routes of anticonvulsant therapy might be considered for clients attempting to control life-threatening seizures without immediate access to veterinary medical assistance. Phenobarbital (5 mg/kg), diazepam, and bromide are partially to completely bioavailable after rectal administration.[94,95] The risk of potassium overload can be minimized by administration of the loading dose over a 12- to 24-hour period in 5- to 15-mL increments.

A small number (20) of human patients with refractory epilepsy were treated with either propofol (14) or midazolam (6) in a retrospective study. For each drug seizures were eradicated in about 65% of patients. However, overall mortality, although not statistically significant, was higher with propofol (57%) compared with midazolam (17%).[224]

General gas anesthesia generally is not recommended in the patient with SE because of the risk of hepatotoxicity induced by the anesthetic that may occur with prolonged therapy. If the clinician decides that general gas anesthesia is necessary, anesthetics that are minimally hepatotoxic are preferable. Discontinuation of therapy should be undertaken cautiously to minimize the risk of seizures. Propofol and etomidate are two chemical restraining agents that, are characterized by anticonvulsant effects, although these drugs are expensive. Of the two, etomidate (a human drug only) may be characterized by CNS-protective effects. These drugs can be administered as intravenous infusions to effect (see later discussion regarding brain trauma).

Diazepam can be used in the cat to control acute epileptic disorders regardless of etiology Generally, an intravenous dose (5 to 10 mg) is given to effect. A dose as high as 20 mg may be necessary; if high dosages are used, they must be injected slowly. The procedure commonly followed is to administer 2 to 10 mg intravenously and then wait 10 minutes. If seizures persist, phenobarbital sodium can be administered (5 to 60 mg). Caution must be taken not to oversedate or depress the animal when these drugs are administered in close succession. Should the animal manifest refractoriness to diazepam and phenobarbital, as in SE, pentobarbital anesthesia is then carefully administered to effect.

SE may require management of cerebral edema (see later discussion of brain trauma and injury).

CHRONIC CONTROL OF SEIZURES

Use of selected antiepileptic drugs to control seizures has been discussed with regard to individual drugs. What constitutes successful anticonvulsant therapy will vary among clinicians and may be defined by client satisfaction. Eradication of seizures may be an unachievable goal; decreased frequency, severity, or duration of the seizure episode may be considered a success for many animals. Indeed, close counseling of clients and reorientation to what constitutes successful control may be important techniques to successfully treating an epileptic dog. Chronic control of epilepsy is likely to be a balancing act for many patients: controlling seizures without putting the patient's health at excessive risk. Because patients are likely to need drug therapy for the rest of their lives, establishing a minimum effective dose for any anticonvulsant drug is prudent. Monitoring is important to prevent toxic concentrations, or to confirm ineffectiveness at high concentrations, even for newer, safer drugs. Monitoring should be used to determine the minimum effective dose for each patient. In the case of breakthrough seizures, monitoring can help the clinician determine whether the seizures reflect a decrease in drug concentrations (which should lead the clinician to confirm owner compliance, addressing potential drug or diet interactions, and so forth) or a change in the underlying pathophysiology (leading to further diagnostics and potential treatment).

KEY POINT 27-29 Ideally, long-term control of therapy should begin with a single drug, with combination therapy initiated only after the first drug fails. Failure should be assumed only as drug concentrations approach the maximum end of the therapeutic range.

If manipulation of a dosing regimen is the focus of successful control, a chosen therapeutic regimen should not be abandoned until steady-state plasma drug concentrations have been reached. Thus an animal should not be considered refractory to a drug simply because it is receiving more than the recommended dose or its serum concentrations are within the therapeutic range. A drug should not be abandoned until serum concentrations in the maximum therapeutic range (and, in some circumstances, exceeding it if the drug is sufficiently safe) have been documented or unacceptable adverse side effects occur. Regardless of the anticonvulsant used, therapy should never be stopped suddenly, and drug concentrations should not be allowed to drop precipitously during a dosing interval. SE may occur. Cautious exceptions might be made for drugs with a very long half-life (e.g., bromide) that naturally gradually decline (as long as chloride content in the animal has not increased).

The thyroid and liver status of patients should be determined before initiation of therapy. Anticonvulsant-induced liver disease should be distinguished from hepatic induction for several anticonvulsant drugs; unnecessary discontinuation of a drug that is controlling seizures might thus be avoided. Moderate elevations in the serum transaminases and SAP activity and abnormalities (more than 50 mmol/L) in fasting bile acids and serum albumin are indicative of hepatic pathology. The incidence of serious liver toxicity can be reduced by avoiding combination therapy with more than one drug metabolized by the liver; using therapeutic drug monitoring[225] (see Chapter 5) to achieve adequate serum concentrations at the smallest dose possible; and evaluating hepatic function every 6 months or more, depending on the magnitude of phenobarbital serum concentrations. The higher the plasma drug concentration, the more important hepatic monitoring becomes. Seizure-induced hypoxia can result in liver damage; thus evaluation of the liver should not occur in association with a seizure episode. Hepatotoxicity induced by anticonvulsants is often reversible if the drug dose is sufficiently decreased before cirrhotic changes occur.

Phenobarbital has remained the first-choice anticonvulsant for chronic control of seizures in both dogs and cats because of its efficacy and, as long as drug concentrations do not approach the maximum therapeutic concentration, safety. However, increasingly evidence is emerging that other anticonvulsants may be effective. Therapeutic drug monitoring should be used to ensure that adequate serum drug concentrations have been achieved before the patient is considered refractory. As concentrations of phenobarbital approach the maximum end of the therapeutic range, an alternative regimen should be considered. The addition of a second anticonvulsant is the most likely next step.

Combination Therapy

Use of combination therapy appears to be popular in veterinary medicine, on the basis of therapeutic drug monitoring information in the author's laboratory. Although combination therapy is a reasonable approach for control of seizures in patients that fail to reasonably respond to first-choice anticonvulsants (e.g., plasma drug concentrations approach or enter the high end of the therapeutic range, or unacceptable side effects emerge), many of these patients are on two or more drugs, each of which is in the subtherapeutic to low-therapeutic range. The American Epilepsy Society notes that most human patients can be controlled with single-drug therapy and that higher concentrations of a single drug are preferred to lower concentrations of multiple drugs. Single-drug therapy should be considered prudent for several reasons. The most obvious is avoidance of side effects (the combined side effects of a drug might, like efficacy, be worse than either drug by itself), fewer drug interactions, better owner compliance, and reduced cost (because multiple drugs require more than one prescription and additional monitoring). Other reasons to limit combination therapy to patients with proven need are likely to be less obvious. However, no drug therapy is likely to be innocuous. Drugs that affect the CNS may be problematic because of the sophisticated mechanisms that exist to minimize the effects of CNS drugs. These include efflux proteins, receptor downregulation, and desensitization. In the author's opinion, because the CNS does not *want* drugs in the CNS, an attempt should be made to respect the body's attempt to limit exposure of the brain to drugs. Accordingly, the author recommends that single-drug therapy be targeted and combination therapy be instituted only in patients that have failed initial therapy.

Bromide increasingly is recommended as a first-choice antiepileptic drug. Although Boothe and Dewey[28] demonstrated that it is not as efficacious as phenobarbital for control of seizures in dogs, its lack of drug interactions and improved safety compared with phenobarbital warrant consideration as first choice, particularly in older dogs for which the risk of drug interactions and liver disease might be decreased.

Bromide also has been recommended as the first combination drug of choice for dogs should phenobarbital therapy fail. However, as newer predominantly renally excreted drugs become available in generic preparations, their use should be considered so as to avoid the gastrointestinal side effects of bromide. Bromide increasingly is being used as the sole anticonvulsant, although a severe seizure history may warrant using a more accepted and predictable first-choice drug (e.g., phenobarbital).

Controlling refractory seizures with any anticonvulsant drug might be facilitated using a stair-step approach. Using bromide as an example, increase concentrations in 0.5-mg/mL increments. If the patient develops seizures at one concentration, the concentration is increased to the next level. This is continued until the patient is acceptably controlled or sedation becomes untenable. In the latter case, decreasing phenobarbital concentrations by 25% may help resolve grogginess. If the goal of bromide therapy is to wean the patient off an anticonvulsant (using phenobarbital as an example), concentrations should be confirmed before implementing a stair-step decrease. For example, bromide concentrations ideally are at least 1.5 mg/mL before phenobarbital is decreased by 25%. Every time the dose of an anticonvulsant is changed, at least 3 drug half-lives, plus one seizure interval (to assure the patient is challenged by a seizure at the new concentration), must lapse before the impact of the dose change can be fully assessed. For phenobarbital, at least 2 to 4 weeks should lapse before a second decrease is implemented. Ideally, the anticonvulsant is monitored at each decrease in dosage so that a target has been identified, should seizures return. Deciding what concentration to target with the second anticonvulsant can be difficult. If the goal is to simply add a second anticonvulsant, targeting in the lower therapeutic range of the new drug is reasonable. If the goal is to reduce the first anticonvulsant, the target of the second drug might be a little higher. If the goal is to eradicate the original anticonvulsant, at the very least, the second drug concentration should be at the same level of the therapeutic range (if not higher) than the first. For example, if a patient's phenobarbital dose is 25 μg/mL (midtherapeutic range), bromide should be at least 2 mg/mL before a decrease is considered. Some animals will require higher concentrations: for example, for bromide, higher than 2.5 mg/mL before phenobarbital can be lowered to less than 20 μg/mL (the standard goal). It may not be possible to decrease the first anticonvulsant in some patients, despite the addition of a second drug at concentrations that are in the high therapeutic range. On the other hand, some patients can be completely weaned off the first anticonvulsant (e.g., phenobarbital).

Diazepam has been the second drug of choice for chronic control of seizures in cats. However, its use may be limited by the concern for hepatic disease. In the author's monitoring laboratory, either zonisamide or levetiracetam appear to be well tolerated and effective, with gabapentin a third viable alternative.

Discontinuing Therapy

Whether anticonvulsant therapy facilitates remission of spontaneous seizures is not clear, although a tendency for contemporary anticonvulsant therapy to be associated with epileptic cure has been described in humans.[226] In human medicine, antiepileptic drugs can be withdrawn in 60% of patients that remain seizure free for 2 to 4 years. A similar statistic is not available in veterinary medicine. The likelihood of success can be somewhat correlated with the underlying cause or type of seizure, with the best chance occurring in the nonjuvenile patient with idiopathic generalized epilepsy. Such patients should have a normal neurologic exam, and the absence of a structural brain lesions. The author recommends that therapy might be discontinued in those patients whose drug concentrations are substantially below the recommended therapeutic range. Should the decision be made to discontinue therapy, concentrations might first be monitored (to provide a target to which concentrations can be returned if the patient has a seizure) and then the antiepileptic drug be slowly discontinued over several months (e.g., 25% each month). Note that with each decrease, the response should be assessed after the drug has reached steady state plus one seizure interval (i.e., ensure, to the extent possible, that the patient is challenged by a seizure before the next decrease is implemented).

Alternative Therapies

Melatonin is described as having demonstrated anticonvulsant activity in many animal models.[225] A study in gerbils demonstrated greater survival in animals treated with melatonin (25 μg subcutaneously daily). Anticonvulsant activity of melatonin may reflect antioxidant activity and subsequent free radical scavenging.[228] In an open, uncontrolled study in epileptic children refractory to standard therapy, melatonin (3 mg at bedtime), seizure activity decreased and sleep improved in five of six patients.[228]

Deprenyl was associated with reduction in experimentally induced seizures in a rat kindling seizure model after multiple intraperitoneal dosing.[229] L-Deprenyl (and to a lesser degree, D-deprenyl) was effective in controlling electroshock-induced seizures in mice when administered at 1 to 40 mg/kg intraperitoneally, with the highest reduction (44%) occurring at the highest dose. Although less potent, D-deprenyl also reduced seizures but was toxic at doses higher than 10 mg/kg.

Pentylenetetrazol nduced clonic and myoclonic, but not tonic, seizures. Seizures also were decreased by L-deprenyl at 5 mg/kg intraperitoneally (but not subcutaneously); 10 mg/kg did not provide further control. The spectrum of anticonvulsant activity was described as comparable to that of phenobarbital (and levetiracetam), including breadth of seizure type controlled. A proposed mechanism is inhibition of norepinephrine and dopamine metabolism. Other proposed mechanisms include modulation of NMDA receptor activity and stimulation of melatonin synthesis in the pineal gland. In his review, Löscher[229] notes that tricyclic antidepressants provide some anticonvulsant effects through inhibition of norepinephrine uptake.

The role of phenothiazines, and acepromazine in particular, in epileptic dogs is controversial. Although phenothiazines are connected with seizures in humans,[230] the contraindication for phenothiazines, and specifically acepromazine, in epileptic animals is less clear. The author has personally induced seizures in a dog suffering from lead poisoning that developed acute respiratory distress syndrome. Treatment with acepromazine was immediately followed by severe seizures. However, Tobias and coworkers[231] retrospectively studied the use of acepromazine in epileptic dogs (n = 47; 15 with idiopathic epilepsy) with seizures that received acepromazine for diagnostic testing, anesthetic premedication, to facilitate postoperative recovery, or to decrease excitatory behavior; acepromazine was given with the intent of reducing seizures in 11 of the dogs. Acepromazine also was administered to 11 of the 47 dogs in order to decrease seizure activity, with either seizures stopping for 1.5 to 8 hours (n = 8) or not recurring (n = 2). Chlorpromazine has been used (2 to 4 mg/kg orally every 8 to 12 hours) to treat SE, with 9 of 10 dogs responding (as reviewed by Tobias and coworkers).[231] McConnell and coworkers[232] also retrospectively studied the medical records of 31 dogs experiencing no seizures (n = 3) or a history of acute or chronic seizures, including SE (n = 3) or cluster seizures (n = 22). Fifteen of 22 dogs with a history of seizures were receiving AED medication. Dogs were treated with a median of 2 but up to 5 doses of acepromazine during hospitalization; the intravenous dose ranged from 0.008 to 0.057 mg/kg. Seizures (n = 23) occurred in 11 of 31 dogs during hospitalization; 15 before and 8 (n = 4 dogs) after treatment with acepromazine. The dose of acepromazine in dogs that experienced seizures after administration ranged from 0.019 to 0.036 mg/kg, with seizures occurring at 18 minutes to 10 hours after administration. It is the author's opinion that these retrospective studies support the potential use of acepromazine in epileptic dogs as adjuvant therapy—and potentially as anticonvulsant therapy, but only after well-designed placebo or other controlled randomized clinical trials in epileptic patients have determined the impact in epileptic dogs or cats.

DRUGS CONTRAINDICATED FOR EPILEPTIC PATIENTS

A number of medications are associated with decreased seizure threshold and an increased risk of SE in humans (Table 27-6). Several anticonvulsant drugs may be proepileptic at suprapharmacologic doses (e.g., phenytoin).[223] The impact of phenothiazines was discussed with alternative drugs. Drugs inducing seizures in selected patients include fluorinated quinolones, lidocaine, and possibly metoclopramide. Seizures induced by lidocaine should be treated with a benzodiazepine (e.g., diazepam).[233] Morphine sulfate and related compounds as well as CNS stimulants such as the methylxanthines and behavior-modifying drugs should be avoided. Chloramphenicol also activates the CNS and should not be used in dogs known to have epileptiform seizures. Glucocorticoids may also decrease seizure threshold, although they stabilize neuronal membranes. Long-term effects on the neuronal membrane, however, may reflect downregulation of glucocorticoid receptors and thus loss of the stabilizing effect. Long-term use of glucocorticoids might be minimized for epileptic patients. Behavior-modifying drugs are CNS stimulants and, accordingly, might be associated with an increased risk of seizures. Cocaine acts on monoamine transporters to block the reuptake of dopamine, norepinephrine and serotonin from synapses following their release. Activity at dopamine, adrenergic and serotonin receptors will increase, although the major effects of cocaine are thought to be reflect actions on dopaminergic systems. Cocaine will also increase motor activity by increasing dopamine in the striatum, and at high doses can cause psychosis. Finally, cocaine also acts as a sympathomimetic, increasing

Table 27-6 Potentially Proconvulsant Drugs[10,223]

Drug Class	Drug
Analgesics	fentanyl meperidine tramadol
Antiarrhythmics	digoxin lidocaine mexiletine
Antibiotics	cefazolin imipenem fluoroquinolones metronidazole
Anticonvulsants at Supraphysiologic Doses	
Immunomodulators	chlorambucil cyclosporine interferons tacrolimus
Tranquilizers	butyrophenones phenothiazines (see text)
Others	baclofen reserpine theophylline
Behavior-modifying drugs	amitriptyline clomipramine nortriptyline imipramine doxepin bupropion

activity of the sympathetic nervous system, due to its action on norepinephrine transport.

Drugs associated with seizures in nonhuman animal models have included but are not limited to the tricyclic antidepressants, bupropion, and doxepin. However, increased concentration of serotonin or norepinephrine by transport inhibitors are likely to be associated with anticonvulsant rather than proconvulsant effects in epileptic patients, despite the fact that overdose may be associated with seizures.[10] Finally, drugs for which CNS derangements or seizures are a listed side effect generally should be avoided in epileptic animals.

TREATMENT OF OTHER NEUROLOGIC CONDITIONS

Brain Trauma or Injury

Pathophysiology of Brain Injury

After head trauma, secondary injury occurs in both contused and adjacent tissues.[234] A cascade of events begins with massive depolarization and ion fluxes that initiate increased energy expenditure by the sodium/potassium adenosine triphosphatase (ATPase) pump, the main regulator of cell volume and electrochemical gradient. Systemic hypotension and disrupted cerebral blood flow exacerbate ATP depletion. Brain tissue is extremely sensitive to decreased oxygenation. Glutamate, an excitatory neurotransmitter that allows calcium influx into the neuron, appears to play an important role in the early stages of secondary brain injury caused by head trauma. Normal intracellular concentrations are approximately 1500-fold greater than extracellular concentrations. Well-developed energy-requiring mechanisms exist to maintain very low extracellular glutamate concentrations; this system becomes overwhelmed as a result of the combined effects of efflux of intracellular glutamate and decreased energy. As a result, calcium influx causes uncontrolled release of intracellular calcium and subsequent cytotoxic events, including uncoupling of oxidative phosphorylation necessary for ATP. Enzyme systems activated included protein kinase C, the phospholipases (and thus arachidonic acid cascades and platelet-activating factor), and nitric oxide synthase. Oxygen radicals are released, leading to irreversible cell injury and death.[234]

Blood flow to the CNS is well autoregulated through a combination of metabolic, vascular pressure, and oxygen-related mechanisms. Cerebral vasculature and intracranial pressure (ICP) must, however, be functioning normally. Metabolic demands of the brain appear to affect regional blood flow through the effects of pH and adenosine on vascular tone. Increased metabolic activity decreases vascular tone, causing vasodilation. Arterial P_{CO_2} has global control of the brain such that increases result in increased cerebral blood flow (and increased ICP), whereas decreases cause decreased cerebral flow. The potential exists for these reflex responses to exceed (in the case of increase) or to be insufficient (in the case of decrease) for the metabolic needs. Response to P_{CO_2} is regional, complicating the use of hyperventilation as a treatment for increased ICP.[234] Local nitric oxide synthesis plays a role in regional blood flow and can contribute to secondary brain injury.

The cerebral ischemic response is global and depends on an intact vasomotor center. It occurs relatively late in response to poor perfusion. Increased ICP decreases cerebral perfusion. Increased P_{CO_2} causes the vasomotor center to increase heart rate and intense systemic vasoconstriction in an attempt to support cerebral blood flow. Clinically, the increase in systemic blood pressure may cause a decrease in heart rate, an indicator that increased ICP is limiting cerebral blood flow. The lack of the ischemic response does not, however, indicate that ICP increase is not severe; rather, it may reflect vasomotor damage.

Causes of Severe Brain Injury

Primary brain injury occurs as a result of direct brain trauma.[234-236] Secondary brain injury reflects damage to the brain as a result of increased metabolic demands, inadequate cerebral blood flow, or both. Epilepsy causes the former by increasing metabolic demands (oxygen and glucose). Hyperthermia increases ICP (several millimeters of increase for each degree of increase in body temperature) by increasing metabolic demands. Head trauma tends to cause the latter by increasing ICP. Systemic hypotension also can cause secondary brain injury. Because the patient with severe head injury is less tolerant of derangements in metabolism, both hyperglycemia and hypoglycemia can contribute to secondary damage. Hypoglycemia contributes to decreased ATP production, whereas hyperglycemia can lead to anaerobic glycolysis and cellular acidosis in cells with impaired mitochondrial function.

Cerebral Edema

Cerebral edema can be categorized into a number of forms, each of which can occur after head trauma.[237] Vasogenic edema reflects increased permeability of the blood–brain barrier and may be exemplified by focal cerebral contusion and hemorrhage. Water, sodium, and protein increase in the interstitial space. In addition to trauma, causes of vasogenic edema include loss of the tight endothelial junctions (as might occur during infusion of hyperosmotic solutions), tumors, hyperthermia, and epileptic seizures. Mediators associated with vasogenic edema include bradykinin, serotonin, histamine, and the eicosanoids (especially leukotrienes), as well as free oxygen radicals. Drugs that increase cerebral blood flow will increase the rate of cerebral edema. White matter has more compliance, and most of the edema accumulates there.

Cytotoxic edema occurs intracellularly when membrane sodium/potassium ATPase pump mechanisms fail because of a lack of energy. Energy loss can reflect decreased cerebral blood flow (i.e., ischemia). Potassium accumulation occurs in the extracellular space. Calcium influx initiates a cascade of events that are lethal to astrocytes. The remaining types of edema might be considered a variation of either vasogenic or cytotoxic edema. Hydrostatic edema reflects accumulation of protein-free fluid in the interstitial tissues. Hydrostatic edema probably results from an abrupt increase in the hydrostatic pressure gradient between the intravascular and extravascular spaces. Osmotic brain edema occurs as serum osmolality (generally caused by hyponatremia) declines below a critical threshold. The use of 5% dextrose can contribute to osmotic brain edema. Interstitial edema is exemplified by high-pressure hydrocephalus associated with increased hydrostatic pressure in the ventricular CSF. Water infiltrates into the periventricular tissues. This type of edema occurs rarely after CNS trauma.

At the cellular level, traumatic brain injury is associated with loss of the axonal cytoskeleton and subsequent irreversible of axonal division with 12 hours. This damage is associated with very high concentrations of glutamate.[238] Traumatic depolarization, characterized by a massive influx of ions at the moment of injury, may reflect excitatory neurotransmitters and is among the most important mechanisms of cellular injury leading to cerebral edema and increased ICP. Cerebral edema and axonal swelling are sequelae; these may respond to interventions intended to block oxidative or nitrosative stresses.[238] The blood–brain barrier also is disrupted with severe injuries, perhaps in response to vascular endothelial growth factor and subsequent release of nitric oxide. Secondary neuronal damages reflect the neuroinflammatory response, resulting in production of reactive oxygen species and inflammatory cytokines. Cyclophilin (targeted by cyclosporine) appears to be among the mediators contributing to postinjury inflammation.[238]

Treatment of traumatic brain injury focuses on control of brain edema and ICP. This includes reversal of the underlying cause, medical management, and surgical decompression.

Increased Intracranial Pressure

The control of increased ICP is paramount in the treatment of head trauma. In humans approximately 40% of those losing consciousness after a traumatic episode will develop intracranial hypertension, and mortality will parallel increases in ICP. Indeed, ICP is a strong predictor of outcome, and monitoring ICP in human medicine has become a safe and effective tool for monitoring both the need for and efficacy of treatment.

Early and aggressive treatment has been shown to improve outcome.[235,236] The pressure at which ICP is maintained is not clear, but humans maintained at 15 mm Hg (normal being 20 mm Hg) had an improved outcome compared with those managed at 25 mm Hg. This may reflect the fact that herniation after lesions in some areas can occur despite ICP being normal (20 mm Hg). Recommendations in human medicine are to treat ICP when increased above 20 mm Hg for more than 15 minutes. Hypotension (systolic blood pressure <90 mm Hg) and hypoxia (Pao_2 <60 mm Hg) also commonly occur in patients with head trauma and can contribute to increased ICP. Of the two, however, hypotension is more devastating and is predictive of a poorer outcome of severe head injury. Thus hypotension should be prevented and immediately treated when present.

KEY POINT 27-30 Treatment of increased cranial pressure should be early and aggressive.

Surgical removal of brain volume is the easiest method (in humans) of lowering ICP. Removal of CSF is another method.[239] Medical management is facilitated by discriminating the cause of ICP. Omeprazole may be useful for long-term management of increased CSF production. Although the mechanism is not clear, in an experimental rabbit model, 0.2 mg/kg reduced production by 35%.[239a]

Medical Management

Because little information is known regarding the direct treatment of damaged neuronal tissue, treatment focuses on maintaining as normal an environment as possible to support neuronal regeneration. Supportive management focuses on maintaining normal physiologic homeostasis. Blood pressure, arterial oxygenation (pulse oximetry and arterial blood gases), body temperature, and fluid and electrolyte balance should be maintained. Electrocardiographic monitoring also is indicated. Hypotension in particular must be avoided in the patient with increased ICP; the hyperdynamic state (physiologic responses compensating for hypovolemia) will complicate control of ICP. Hyperglycemia can increase metabolism and should be avoided and aggressively managed in the patient with head trauma. Fluids containing dextrose should be avoided in such patients.

Adjuvant Nonpharmacologic Management

Elevation of the head 30 degrees above heart level appears to be beneficial in decreasing ICP.[235,236,240] Hypercapnia must be avoided in patients with head trauma; this includes hypercapnia that may be iatrogenically induced during procedures intended to support the respiratory system. Hyperventilation to maintain a $Paco_2$ of 27 to 30 mm Hg can decrease cerebral blood flow and help lower ICP. It is, however, dependent on intact autoregulation. Hyperventilation can decrease the metabolic activities of the brain and induce or potentiate cerebral ischemia. Its effectiveness in diminishing cerebral blood volume decreases with time (at 72 to 96 hours), and a rebound effect with restoration to normocapnia may potentially increase ICP.

Hypocarbia is easy to induce. Its use in the management of increased ICP might be reserved for the initial stages. Later use should be accompanied by strict monitoring of ICP, especially as hyperventilation is discontinued. Profound hyperventilation should be avoided. Hypothermia currently is being investigated for use in the prevention of CNS ischemia associated with severe head injuries.[239] It has been used experimentally in dogs. Mild degrees of hypothermia (between 31° and 35°C) are recommended to prevent cardiovascular instability.[240]

Diuretics

Osmotic diuretics are commonly used to treat intracranial hypertension.[235,236,239,241] Both mannitol and urea have been used, although mannitol has largely replaced urea. Mannitol is a 6-carbon sugar, similar in structure to glucose, but it is not able to cross the normal blood–brain barrier.[239] Thus it remains in the extracellular and intravascular spaces of the brain, where it will cause an osmotic draw toward the extravascular tissues, and intracranial fluid will move into the vascular space. The effect of mannitol on increased ICP are severalfold. Reversal of the blood–brain osmotic gradient decreases extracellular fluid volume in both the normal and damaged brain. This effect is delayed for 15 to 30 minutes but can continue for up to 6 hours. Blood viscosity is lowered, causing reflex vasoconstriction and lowered ICP. This effect, however, requires that mannitol be administered as a bolus, not slowly.[235,236,239]

Doses of 0.25 mg/kg appear to be as effective as larger doses (1 mg/kg) in lowering ICP. Repeated administration of mannitol can induce hyperosmolar states, rendering it ineffective and subjecting the patient to the risk of renal failure. Additionally, continuous administration of mannitol can lead to increased penetration of the blood–brain barrier in the injured brain, resulting in a rebound ICP increase. For these reasons, serum osmolality should not be allowed to increase above 320 mOsm/L. Additionally, this effect is more likely if mannitol is give as a CRI rather than as a rapid bolus.[239]

A Cochrane Review has addressed the efficacy of mannitol for treatment of acute brain injury in humans.[242] Four clinical trials were eligible for review. Among these, mannitol (1 g/kg generally over 5 minutes) was compared with standard care, with pentobarbital (10 mg/kg intravenous bolus followed by CRI of 0.5 to 3 mg/kg such that ICP remained less than 20 torr), with hypertonic saline (2.5 mL/kg of a 7.5% solution over 20 minutes) and with placebo (5 mL/kg 0.9% saline), with treatment occurring before hospitalization. Treatment consisted of 5 mL/kg of a 20% (1 g/kg) mannitol solution; placebo groups were given saline. The review concluded that no evidence existed to support prehospitalization treatment, evidence showed that mannitol might be preferred to pentobarbital but hypertonic saline might be preferred to mannitol. The overall conclusion of the review is that reliable evidence on which recommendations might be made for the use of mannitol in patients with traumatic brain injury was lacking. The review further concluded that randomized clinical trials were clearly indicated.

Benefits of nonosmotic diuretics in the treatment of increased ICP are less clear. Furosemide is not as effective as mannitol, but it may prolong its effects.[237] It may interact synergistically with mannitol to decrease ICP.[235,236] However, it also may exacerbate the dehydrating effects of mannitol and complicate the maintenance of normovolemia.

KEY POINT 27-31 Clear evidence supporting the efficacy of mannitol for treatment of intracranial pressure is lacking.

Neuroprotection

Jain[238] reviewed neuroprotection associated with traumatic brain injury. Drugs that may be relevant include immunomodulators and antiinflammatory compounds. The observation that cyclophilin (an inducer of micochondrial permeability) concentrations increase and appear to contribute to secondary neurodegeneration after traumatic brain injury provides a basis for use of cyclosporine.[238] Cyclosporine is available or being developed in a neuroprotective formula for military personnel subjected to brain injury or gas poisoning. Erythropoietin has demonstrated several potential mechanisms of neuroprotection. This includes inhibition of apoptosis, reduction of cerebral edema, and possibly reduction of glutamate concentrations. A variety of neurotrophic factors are under investigation.[238] Phase II or III clinical trials examining the effect of darbepoietin or human recombinant erythropoietin are currently under way. Other pharmacologic approaches have included NMDA or AMPA-receptor antagonists; a phase II clinical trial examining the effects of ketamine is under way in children. Several antiepileptic drugs also have demonstrated oxygen radical scavenging or other neuroprotectant effects.

KEY POINT 27-32 Among the drugs to be considered for neuroprotection are cyclosporine and methylprednisolone.

Glucocorticoids

Naturally occurring neurosteroids allosterically modulate the $GABA_{(A)}$ receptors, protecting against NMDA overactivation and ischemia associated with injury. Endogenous examples include progesterone and its metabolite, alloprenanolone. Interestingly, progesterone appears to facilitate repair of the blood–brain barrier, as well as decreasing edema and muting the inflammatory response.[238] A phase II clinical trial involving progesterone is apparently under way in human medicine.[238] In contrast to endogenous neurosteroids, the role of glucocorticoids in traumatic brain injury is less clear. Kamano[243] reviewed the earlier evidence supporting their use, and particularly megadose of methylprednisolone in human patients with severe brain injury. Although such dosing may be appropriate for acute spinal cord injury, the same is not true for acute head injury.

The use of steroids to treat increased ICP is generally ineffective, with the possible exception of increases associated with tumors.[239] The potential beneficial effects support consideration of their use in patients with increased ICP. Damaged vascular permeability might be restored in areas of damage, rendering them particularly useful for vasogenic edema (e.g., such as that caused by tumors). Decreased CSF production has been documented in dogs.[239,244] Oxygen-mediated free radical lipid peroxidation can be reduced by glucocorticoids, particularly methylprednisolone.[245]Despite these potential therapeutic effects, however, clinical studies have failed to show a therapeutic benefit of glucocorticoids for patients with head trauma.[239] Jain[238] notes that a phase III corticoisteroid clinical trial in humans failed to show efficacy. However, a phase II clinical trial (in humans) involving prednisone showed some efficacy .

The use of glucocorticoids may increase the risk of a poor outcome in patients with traumatic brain injury.[235,236] Their effects on metabolism (increasing peripheral glucose and cerebral glutamate) and immunosuppression contribute to their potential detrimental effects. Among the glucocorticoids, methylprednisolone appears to have the greatest radical-scavenging ability and, should glucocorticoids be used in CNS trauma, would be preferred to others. If there is to be a positive benefit, it will be realized only with early administration. Steroids that have no glucocorticoid activity, such as the lazaroids, provide oxygen radical–scavenging effects without many of the detrimental effects of glucocorticoids. These products are not yet commercially available.

Barbiturates

Although their use is very labor intensive (and thus reserved for critical care environments), barbiturates (pentobarbital, human dose 10 mg/kg over 30 minutes, followed by 1 to 1.5 mg/kg per hour) have been shown to be beneficial for human patients with severe head injury who have not responded to other therapies. Thus barbiturates may be indicated for patients with sustained, refractory intracranial hypertension. Barbiturates decrease cerebral metabolism, alter vascular tone, and inhibit lipid peroxidation mediated by free radicals.[239] Lowered metabolism decreases the cerebral ischemia threshold, allowing lower cerebral oxygenation and thus cerebral blood flow (without ischemic damage).[239] Barbiturates also may decrease intracellular calcium.[240] Although they appear to rapidly lower ICP, barbiturates place the patient in a coma and thus can cause complications resulting from hypotension, hypothermia, and hypercapnia.

In human medicine the use of barbiturates is accomplished in conjunction with intubation and ventilation, fluid administration, and monitoring of arterial blood pressure (pulmonary artery catheter) and temperature. In human patients support of the pulmonary system is rigorous to prevent pneumonia or atelectasis. Electroencephalographic monitoring accompanies barbiturate therapy in order to document a dose sufficient for burst suppression. Serum barbiturate concentrations are measured (ideally maintained between 30 and 50 mg per day). The efficacy of the barbiturates in lowering ICP are less likely in patients with cardiovascular complications (e.g., hypotension). Once ICP control has been satisfactory for 24 to 48 hours, the drug can be gradually tapered (e.g., 50% per day) to prevent uncontrolled rebound hypertension. Mannitol may be helpful during this period to control ICP. Prophylactic control with barbiturates appears to offer no therapeutic advantage.[239]

Fluid Therapy

Crystalloids, colloids, and blood may be indicated for treatment of brain trauma or injury. Physiologic crystalloids containing saline or saline and glucose, with or without the addition of potassium, generally can be administered as necessary to prevent hypovelemic shock. Whereas glucose is essential as an energy substrate, under anaerobic conditions it can be converted to lactate, contributing to neurotoxic acidosis.[241] Albumin and other colloids are indicated for acute volume expansion, although subsequent metabolism to smaller molecules can contribute to disruption of ion balance. Blood remains the best resuscitative fluid in patients that are hypovolemic and hypotensive.[241] Infusion of plasma protein (50 to 100 mL) after mannitol administration also has been recommended to prevent hypovolemia.[235] Colloidal products such as hetastarch or Oxyglobin may be similarly effective.

Anticonvulsants

Prophylactic use of anticonvulsants has been recommended for patients with head trauma to minimize the risk of posttraumatic seizure disorders. Seizures increase ICP and may be masked by unconsciousness. Indeed, electroencephalography is recommended for patients with unexplained autonomic dysfunction or increased ICP to detect possible SE. Seizures are more likely when treating for intracranial hypertension. Because the risk of seizures is high, neurologists frequently recommend anticonvulsant therapy for their human patients.

Analgesics, Sedatives, Paralytics, and General Anesthetics

Pain or agitation will exacerbate ICP hypertension, and analgesia is recommended. Human patients (even those subjected to pharmacologic paralysis) are often routinely treated with a reversible opioid analgesic (e.g., morphine). Pharmacologic paralysis is a therapeutic modality that is more applicable to human patients or veterinary patients in a critical care environment. Paralysis is used to prevent muscle activity (particularly in intubated patients, such as those on ventilators), which can contribute to increased ICP. Paralysis is often, however, combined with sedation; the latter can preclude effective neurologic evaluation.[235,236] The impact of phenothiazine tranquilizers was previously discussed with regard to epilepsy.

Armitage-Chan and coworkers have reviewed the use of anesthetic agents in canine patients with traumatic brain injuries.[246] A number of anesthetic agents have been cited for protective effects in patients with head trauma. Althesin is a rapidly acting steroidal anesthetic that, during CRI, can decrease ICP while maintaining cerebral perfusion pressure. Its tendency to cause anaphylaxis in human patients led to its removal from the market in the United States.[239] Propofol can provide protective effects when used at a rate of infusion that induces coma.[241] Etomidate is an imidazole anesthetic agent somewhat similar to barbiturates in action. It causes electroencephalography burst suppression, decreased cerebral blood flow, and decreased ICP in human patients with severe head injury.[235,236,239] Etomidate may provide some cytoprotective effects induced by hypoxia. Finally, it appears to have antiseizural effects induced through gabaminergic actions (see earlier discussion of anticonvulsants). For humans, however, a single report of interference with the adrencortical axis and stress response after CRI led to its exclusion as recommended therapy for increased ICP. Controlled clinical studies regarding the efficacy of etomidate for the patient with increased ICP have yet to be performed.

Miscellaneous Drugs or Compounds

Lidocaine decreases CNS synaptic transmission (either directly or as a result of the blockade of sodium channels) and may cause vasoconstriction. The net result is a decrease in cerebral oxygen and glucose consumption. Lidocaine appears to be effective in minimizing increased ICP caused by intubation and surgical stimulation and, in dogs, decreases hypertension after acute cerebral ischemia. Risks associated with lidocaine include myocardial depression and lowering of the seizure threshold. Thus it is generally recognized to be ineffective in treating patients with increased ICP.

Acute Thoracolumbar Disk Extrusion

Chondrodystrophoid breeds of dogs are predisposed to disk extrusion. The intervertebral disks of these breeds contain more collagen, fewer proteoglycans, and hence less water in the nucleus pulposus. Poor biomechanics of the degenerating disk result in disruption of the annulus fibrosus and the eventual eruption of calcified disk material into the spinal cord. Demyelination and necrosis of the spinal cord develop as a result of the secondary injury mechanisms. These include decreased spinal cord flow, increased intraneuronal calcium, and increased free radical formation. Despite predilection for the chondrodystrophoid breeds, acute disk extrusion can occur in a large number of nonchondrodystrophoid breeds as well. The clinical manifestations vary with the severity of extrusion. Medical management is indicated for animals with grades 1 and 2 thoracolumbar disk protrusion. This includes animals with spinal hyperesthesia and ataxia that is mild enough to allow weight bearing.[247] Surgical intervention is indicated for animals that cannot ambulate, regardless of the perception of pain. The loss of deep pain sensation for more that 24 hours is, however, associated with a poor prognosis.[247] Smith and Jeffery[248] described spinal shock as a component of severe spinal injury. A common manifestation in humans, the pathophysiology may be sufficiently different in dogs that it is often overlooked. However, unexplained neurologic abnormalities caudal to the anatomic localization may support the diagnosis. Further research may be warranted to identify differential therapies targeting the pathophysiology in animals that endure spinal shock.

Medical Management

Nonpharmacologic therapy of thoracolumbar disk extrusion is appropriate for mild to moderate cases of prolapse and focuses on strict immobilization (i.e., cage or crate) for at least 3 weeks.[249,250] This time is intended to allow resolution of spinal cord inflammation, reabsorption of extruded disk material, and fibrosis of the ruptured annulus fibrosus. Physical therapy with both passive and active exercises is indicated. Urinary catheterization may be necessary for some dogs. Pharmacologic therapy should focus on control of the inflammatory response to the extruded disk material. Muscle relaxants (e.g., methocarbamol; see Chapter 25) may be helpful. For thoracolumbar disk protrusion, the success rate in ambulatory dogs treated with medical management ranges from 82% to 100%; the success rate in nonambulatory dogs ranges from 43% to 51%.[249] Because the intervertebral disk function depends on glycosaminoglycans, compounds used as disease-modifying agents (e.g., glucosamine, chondroitin sulfates) might be considered for long-term prevention or treatment.

KEY POINT 27-33 Pharmacologic therapy of disk protrusion focuses on control of accompanying inflammation.

Among the drugs to control inflammation are glucorticoids and nonsteroidal antiinflammatory drugs (NSAIDs). Mann and coworkers[251] reviewed some of the advantages and disadvantages of each. Low doses of corticosteroids (0.5 mg/kg prednisolone or prednisone orally twice daily) are intended to control spinal cord edema, inflammation, and pain and improve spinal cord blood flow. Methylprednisolone at high doses (30 mg/kg intravenously, repeated at 2 and 6 hours at 15 mg/kg intravenously, if indicated) presumably provides the additional advantage of free radical scavenging generated by lipid peroxidation (see Chapter 29). However, some drugs may impair healing of the annulus fibrosus. Both glucocorticoids and newer NSAIDs are more potent toward cyclooxygenase-2, the cyclooxygenase isoform more consistently associated with promotion of healing. Thus both classes of drugs might be associated with a adverse effect. However, an advantage to glucocorticoids might be inhibition of collagen contraction, which has been demonstrated for dexamethasone and hydrocortisone. Timing of drug therapy is important, with neurologic recovery greater in humans for which methylprednisolone was initiated within 8 to 12 hours of recovery. However, this and other recommendations in human medicine are complicated by limitations in supportive study designs.[251a]

A number of prospective or retrospective studies have addressed the role of glucocorticoids in the treatment of intervertebral disk disease. Bush and coworkers[252] prospectively studied the functional outcome of 51 nonambulatory dogs weighing less than 15 kg. Dogs had undergone hemilaminectomy. By 10 days after the operation, 90% were ambulatory, 98% pain free, and 82% continent. The numbers improved to 100%, 94%, and 86% by 6 weeks based on phone interviews. All dogs had received a myelogram as part of their presurgical diagnostics. Levine and coworkers[253] demonstrated that 20% of dogs receiving no glucocorticoid and 69% receiving dexamethasone developed urinary tract infection (UTI) in association with hospitalization and surgical correction of disk prolapse. Factors other than immunosuppression that may have contributed to UTI were not addressed. The incidence associated with long-term management is less clear. Wyndaele[254] and Igawa and coworkers[255] reviewed the role of catheterization in the cause or prevention of UTI in humans with spinal injuries; much of the information may be relevant to dogs. In humans UTI is among the complications associated with long-term intermittent catheterization.[254] Identifying the need for antibacterial treatment is difficult in humans because of differences in evaluation, prophylactic antibiotics, and other methods. However, asymptomatic bacteriuria is not necessarily an indication for treatment. The incidence of bacteriuria in human ranges from 11% to 25% asymptomatic to 53% symptomatic (3% with major symptoms). Indwelling catheters increased the risk of infection both during acute and chronic phases of treatment and increase the risk of sepsis. Trauma associated with catheterization (which is not unusual, particularly if someone other than the patient is catheterizing) does not appear to lead to long-term complications. Prophylaxis is helpful and does not necessarily include antibiotics. Indeed, antimicrobials should be reserved for symptomatic patients: Use of ciprofloxacin eradicated susceptible organisms from the urinary tract in humans, only to be replaced shortly thereafter by resistant gram-positive isolates.

Controversy exists regarding the best methods of UTI prevention. Urine can be kept sterile for 15 to 20 days during acute stages of spinal cord injury without prophylaxis and up to 55 days if prophylaxis is implemented. Predictive factors for infection in humans include gender (female), age (young), and neurogenic bladder dysfunction; in male patients low frequency of catheterization was a risk factor. Prostatitis may also be present and increases the risk of recurrent infections. Increased residual volume also is a risk factor; the incidence of infections increased in humans when the frequency of catheterization was reduced from sixfold to threefold. Bacteriuria was a risk factor for clinical infection. Use of dipsticks to detect bacturia other than pyuria alone is recommended to detect bacturia. *E. coli* is the predominant infecting organisms. Technique and materials, but particularly education of the catheter team, were the most important factors associated with prevention of complications. The use of hydrophilic catheters has been proposed to lower the risk of urinary strictures or false passages (more likely if urethra bleeding has occurred), complications associated with intermittent catheterization. Instillation of colistin–kanamycin at the end of catheterization decreased the incidence of bacteriuria by 50% in humans. Alternatives to standard antimicrobial use also include intravesicular administration of kanamycin–colistin coupled with low-dose nitrofurantoin therapy. The role of adjuvant therapies, including vitamin C, cranberry juice, and polysulfated glycosaminoglycans, are not supported by convincing evidence but warrant consideration in lieu of or in addition to antimicrobial therapy.

KEY POINT 27-34 Glucocorticoid therapy (particularly dexamethasone) for intervertebral disk disease may be associated with a higher risk of urinary tract infection.

Mann and coworkers[251] retrospectively examined the recurrence rates of dogs with Hansen type I intervertebral disk disease managed medically with either glucocorticoids or NSAIDs. Dogs were scored according to the level of spinal hyperpathia and neurologic defects; recurrence occurred at least 4 weeks after the initial episode and was identified through communication with owners. Of the 78 dogs studied, 39 (50%) experienced recurrence. Schnauzers were less likely to experience recurrence than any other breed. Recurrences were less likely with methylprednisolone (n = 12; four recurrences) or NSAIDs (n = 36; 12 recurrences) compared with with other glucocorticoids (n = 30; 23 recurrences). The specific NSAIDs or alternative glucocorticoids were not delineated. Timing of methylprednisolone therapy was not an important risk factor; however, only 16 dogs were treated with methylprednisolone, and it is not clear whether the sample size was sufficiently large to detect a difference. The study supports a clinical trial that compares NSAIDs and methylprednisolone.

Levine and coworkers retrospectively reviewed the medical management of cervical and thoracolumbar disk disease.[256,257] One veterinary teaching hospital and several emergency clinics in the same state were involved. Inclusion criteria focused on ensuring that presentation and clinical condition were related only to intervertebral disk disease. A prospective client questionnaire was included in assessment. Animals were classified as to success, recurrence, or failure in regard to initial therapy. For thoracolumbar disease (n = 223),[256] response to NSAIDs and glucocorticoids was studied. Antiinflammatory drugs used included deracoxib (n = 25), carprofen (n = 42), and others (n = 80) versus 143 dogs receiving none. Glucocorticoids used (n = 105 compared with none in 118) included prednisone (51), dexamethasone (n = 46), and methylprednisolone (n = 8). Glucocorticoids were associated with a lower quality-of-life score, contributing to a lower success score in animals that did, versus did not, receive glucocorticoids. No predictive factor for success could be identified with regard to the specific drug chosen, dose, or duration. In contrast, NSAIDs were associated with a higher quality-of-life score; the success rate between treatment and no treatment with NSAIDs did not differ. For cervical disease (n = 88),[257] use of NSAIDs (n = 43, compared with n=45 receiving no treatment) was associated with success. The most common drugs used included deracoxib (n = 21) and carprofen (n = 18). Glucocorticoids (30 receiving, 58 not) did not influence success or quality of life.

KEY POINT 27-35 Further clinical studies are indicated for comparison of nonsteroidal antiinflammatory drugs versus glucocorticoids for treatment of disk protrusion.

Glucocorticoids and Other Antiinflammatory Drugs

Glucocorticoids have been used extensively to control the inflammatory response to disk extrusion. Additional potential benefits include reduction of edema and improved spinal cord blood flow. Controversy, however, surrounds efficacy, the proper drug, and the proper dosing regimen (including route, dose, interval, and duration of therapy). Dexamethasone stands out among the glucocorticoids as the one most likely to be associated with severe and potentially fatal gastrointestinal complications when used to treat dogs with disk extrusion.[258] Potential complications include gastrointestinal hemorrhage, ulceration, pancreatitis, and colonic ulceration and perforation.

Methylprednisolone may be the preferred glucocorticoid for treatment of disk extrusion. At high doses (30 mg/kg intravenous bolus followed by 5.4 mg/kg per hour), it inhibits oxygen radical formation and thus inhibits lipid peroxidation.[259] In humans neurologic function appears to improve after treatment with methylprednisolone within 8 hours of the injury (compared with placebo). At higher doses (60 mg/kg), however, lipid peroxidation appears to be promoted. Cats with experimentally induced spinal damage underwent neurologic recovery more rapidly with methylprednisolone than with other drugs.[260] A more recent study using a similar model in dogs failed to show a significant difference in neurologic improvement with administration of either methylprednisolone or lazaroids, but the model of spinal cord damage may not have been sufficient for evaluation of the drug.[261]

Levine and coworkers[253] reported on a retrospective comparison of the adverse events associated with dexamethasone (n = 49) versus no treatment (n = 80) and other glucocorticoid therapy (primarily methylprednisolone sodium succinate but also prednisone [n = 23]) for treatment of acute thoracolumbar intervertebral disk herniation in dogs. Two teaching hospitals were involved in the study. All treatments were implemented by the referring veterinarian within 48 hours of admission, and dogs treated with glucocorticoids within the month preceding the episode were excluded. Episode duration was less than 7 days, and surgeries were performed within 36 hours of admission. Of the 161 dogs studied, 87 were dachsunds. No signalment differences occurred among treatment groups. Median duration was less at 5 days for the dexamethasone group compared with the other treatment groups at 6 days, but this difference was not significant when corrected for confounding factors. Likewise, client cost was least (by just under 20%) for the alternative glucocorticoid group compared with the no-treatment group (most expensive), but the differential was negated by confounding factors. The mean dexamethasone dose was 2.25 mg ± 4.28 m/kg (range 1 to 30 mg/kg; dose was not associated with adversity, although the power to detect a relationship was not clear). Doses of the other glucocorticoids were not provided. The dexamethasone group tended to be characterized by a smaller proportion of immediate improvement compared with the other groups, but no difference was found among groups in short-term outcome (29-day follow-up). Adversities that were greater in the dexamethasone group compared with the no-treatment group (with the alternate group generally tending to differ) included vomiting and diarrhea (packed cell volume was lower, but patients were not anemic). UTIs also were more frequent in the dexamethasone-treated patients (11 of 16 that were evaluated); not all patients were tested for infection. Female dogs were more likely to develop UTIs. Less than 20% of dogs examined were positive for UTIs in the other groups. Overall, the dexamethasone group was 3.4 times more likely to develop an adverse effect compared with other groups, with 45 of 49 developing complications compared with 53 of 80 for the no-treatment group. Interestingly, dogs at one institution were 6 times as likely to develop an adverse effect compared with those at the other institution. It is not clear if this was a reporting differential or a true effect.

Side effects associated with methylprednisolone may be rare unless animals have previously been treated with NSAIDs or glucocorticoids.[262] Methylprednisolone should be administered after disk extrusion, including before surgical decompression (assuming other antiinflammatory drugs have not been administered), by way of slow intravenous injection within 8 hours of spinal trauma. The initial dose of 30 mg/kg should be followed at 2 and 6 hours with 15 mg/kg intravenously.[262]

Other drugs that have been recommended for treatment of disk extrusion include prednisolone sodium succinate, dimethylsulfoxide, NSAIDs, and narcotic antagonists. Clinical studies have not been performed with these drugs. Mannitol is not recommended for animals with disk extrusion because of its risk of increased hemorrhage in the gray matter of the spinal cord.

In animals with severe spinal hyperesthesia, 3 to 5 days of oral prednisolone *or* (not *and)* NSAIDs can accompany confinement therapy. The risk of gastrointestinal ulceration is a cause for concern. In addition, decreased inflammation may lead to increased activity, with subsequent need for surgical intervention.[262]

Postoperative analgesics should include opioids. NSAIDs can be used for 3 to 5 days postoperatively; carprofen may be the drug of choice because of its apparent relative cyclooxygenase-2 specificity. The use of drugs that decrease bladder sphincter hypertonicity (phenoxybenzamine, 5 to 15 mg every 24 hours) are discussed elsewhere.

Miscellaneous drugs. A phase I trial in dogs (n = 39) with naturally occurring traumatic paraplegia or paraparesis investigated the ability of 4-aminopyridine (4-AP) to restore conduction in (presumed) demyelinated nerve fibers. Injuries generally (77%) reflected thoracolumbar degenerative disk disease resulting in chronic, complete paraplegia. Treatment (0.5 to 1 mg/kg intravenously) of 4-AP generally improved hind limb (n = 18) increased response to pain (n = 10) and partial recovery of the cutaneous trunci muscle reflex (n = 9). Effects became evident in 15 to 45 minutes but reversed within a few hours of administration. Remaining animals (36%) either did not improve or exhibited slightly improved hind limb reflex tone. Although higher doses led to more dramatic improvement, side effects, including diazepam-responsive seizures and hyperthermia, occurred.[263] *N*-acetylcysteine (NAC) is among the drugs studied for its impact on oxygen radicals. Baltzer and coworkers[264] found no effect of pretreatment with intravenous NAC in dogs (n = 70) with acute spinal injury on urinary concentrations of 15F2t isoprostane, a prostanoid metabolite, or neurologic function 42 days after surgery, when compared with placebo.

OCULAR PHARMACOLOGY

Relevant Anatomy, Physiology, and Drug Preparations

Treatment of ocular disease can be implemented both locally and systemically. Local administration includes both topical (cornea or conjunctival sac) and directed therapy, the latter including intraocular (aqueous [anterior] or vitreal [posterior] chamber), subconjunctival (targeting anterior chamber and its associated structure), and retrobulbar (targeting the posterior chamber or choroids) routes. Although movement into the eye from topical or local delivery is facilitated by the ability to use higher drug concentrations in the vehicle, delivery might be offset, regardless of the route of administration, by intraocular pressure (IOP), which causes consistent outflow of fluid and any drug that it contains. Although inflammation will facilitate drug penetration in both the anterior and posterior ocular chambers, resolution of inflammation (or, potentially, severe inflammation) may be associated with reduced drug penetrability. Inflammation also may alter penetrability by virtue of its impact on pH (discussed later).

Directed (local) ophthalmic therapy is appealing for three reasons: (1) As with other sites, topical therapy allows use of drugs at concentrations that are likely to be therapeutic but likely to be associated with adverse effects if the drug is applied topically, thus limiting the effective use of the drug. (2) Adversity is reduced with topical administration. Examples include the antimicrobials polymyxin B, bacitracin, and neomycin, each of which is characterized by a high incidence of nephrotoxicity with systemic administration. Drugs that cause agonistic or antagonistic sympathetic or parasympathetic effects in the eye can cause profound cardiovascular and other systemic side effects when given systemically at doses necessary to cause a therapeutic ocular response. The safe use of antiinflammatories such as NSAIDs and glucocorticoids is facilitated with topical delivery. However, even if glucocorticoids are topically applied, sufficient drug may reach systemic circulation to affect the adrenal axis. (3) Ophthalmic delivery avoids the blood–eye barrier at both the ciliary and retinal epithelium presented to systemically delivered drugs. However, as with the skin, drugs applied topically with the intent of intraocular effects must penetrate a protective barrier. Most drug is absorbed through the corneum; this is balanced by drug flow from the sclera in response to a constant outward pressure. The cornea comprises several layers that vary in their chemical nature and thus drug penetrability. The lipid-soluble epithelium is several layers thick and presents the major barrier to penetration of topically applied drugs. Ingredients added to ophthalmic preparations with the intent to facilitate drug delivery include surfactants that increase the permeability of the corneal epithelium. The next deepest layer is the water-soluble stroma, followed by the innermost lipid-soluble endothelium. Topically applied vehicles and the drugs they carry must balance water and lipid solubility to ensure not only dissolution of the drug but also its movement into and through the different layers of the cornea. Drug pKa and environmental pH directly influence drug ionization as well as drug dissolution (and, as discussed later, drug stability), both of which will alter drug penetrability; changes in vehicle or local pH may change drug penetrability. Inflammation may change the slight alkalinity of the tears (7.4) to become more acidic, which will ionize and thus reduce penetrability of the drug.

Drugs intended for ophthalmic preparations are most commonly prepared as either solutions (drops) or ointments. Although easier to administer (facilitating owner compliance) and more rapid in onset (greater immediate contact over a larger surface area), the effect of drops is reduced by a shorter contact time; solutions are characterized by rapid dilution with tears. The volume of the subconjunctival sac, which acts as a reservoir for the drug, can expand to 30 to 50 μl. The optimal drop size for ophthalmic delivery is 20 μl. Whereas tear turnover is 15% in the nonirritated or untreated eye, it becomes 30% with drug delivery or in the inflamed eye; 80% of tears containing diluted drug exiting through the lacrimal duct. As such, a 5-minute contact time can be expected with drops applied 4 times or more a day (recommended). Further, the optimum time before adding a second drop is 5 minutes. Contact time of the drug with the cornea can be prolonged by increasing the concentration of the drug (often prepared as 1% or 100 mg/dL), preparation viscosity, or addition of surfactants that increase corneal epithelial permeability. Drug movement into the eye also can be facilitated by manipulation of the pH: Because tears are slightly alkaline (7.4), increasing the pH such that it is slightly basic will decrease the un-ionized and thus absorbable proportion of a basic drug. Devices such as canulas allow more effective topical subpalpebral or nasolacrimal administration of solutions in selected species. Ointments allow a longer contact time and thus thrice-daily administration. Less drug enters the lacrimal passages, which may be an advantage for some drugs. However, disadvantages of ointments include the potential for reduced owner compliance (more difficult to administer compared with solution) and slower onset of action. Indeed, drug movement through the ointment into the cornea may be so slow that concentrations may remain subtherapeutic. Other disadvantages of ointments include impaired vision, impaired penetration of other drugs simultaneously administered ophthalmic ally (particularly solutions), and potentially impaired corneal healing.

The advantages of topical ophthalmic drug delivery are offset to some degree by drug safety considerations. More so than other topically applied drugs, the vehicle of ophthalmic preparations must be formulated such that adverse (ophthalmic) drug reactions are minimized. Considerations include tonicity (must be similar to tears, such as 1.4% NaCl; reasonable range is 0.7 to 2%), which is often accomplished using phosphate buffer. The pH (generally buffered at 3.5 to 10.5) must be appropriately balanced, yet altering pH for safety considerations may alter drug delivery. Not only might lipid solubility (because of changes in ionization) be affected (see previous discussion), but dissolution and stability also may be affected, with positive changes in one often causing negative changes in the other. As with many drugs in solution, ophthalmic preparations may lose potency with storage, and strict adherence to expiration dates is indicated. Tonicity and pH are less important for drugs prepared as ointments. Although stability tends to be better overall in ointments, stability may nonetheless be reduced, particularly in water-based ointments. In contrast to solutions, a disadvantage of ointments is their potential to cause inflammation should the vehicle (not the drug itself) penetrate intraocular tissues. In contrast to drugs administered on the skin, ophthalmic preparations generally should be sterile. All should be prepared aseptically, although this does not ensure sterility. Methods that might facilitate sterility include autoclaving, filtering, and adding preservatives (e.g., benzalkonium chloride, phenol, and merbromin); however, each can be irritating to intraocular tissues and may interfere with diagnostic (culture) procedures. A major disadvantage of compounded ophthalmic preparations is the absence of quality-control procedures documenting product stability, potency, and sterility.

Drugs Targeting Ocular Tissues

Anesthetics

General anesthetics, with the exception of ketamine, generally lower IOP. In contrast, opioids generally increase IOP. Local anesthetics block sodium channels, thus impeding impulse conduction through nerve fibers. Their duration is variable and is affected by pH as well as manipulation of chemical structure. The presence of an ester in topically applied preparations shortens duration of action, whereas the addition of an amide prolongs anesthetic effects. Esters include proparacaine (0.5%; 15-second onset; 20-minute duration), tetracaine (longer-acting but more toxic), whereas amides, which are generally applied as local (rather than topical) drugs, include lidocaine (5-minute onset, 2- to 4-hour duration) and bupivacaine

(≥20-minute onset, 6- to 8-hour duration). Other topical products include benoxinate, butacaine, phenocane, dibucaine, and piperocaine. All local anesthetics inhibit blood vessel formation and corneal epithelialization and may cause minute punctate corneal ulcers. Some can actually cause systemic toxicity with topical administration because of rapid (i.e., conjunctival) absorption. The loss of sensation removes protective reflexes; therefore these drugs should be used only under direct veterinary supervision (i.e., not sent home with clients).

Autonomic Nervous System

Autonomic drugs are generally, but not exclusively, used to treat glaucoma and control associated ocular pain through paralysis of ciliary muscles.

Stimulation (contraction) of the constrictor muscle of the iris is mediated by the parasympathetic (cholinergic; acetylcholine) system, leading to miosis. Flow of aqueous humor is subsequently facilitated. The cholinergic system also controls formation of aqueous humor at the level of the ciliary body. Longitudinal contraction of the ciliary body also occurs and may help lower IOP (e.g., glaucoma) possibly by distending the trabecular meshwork; some miotics may actually decrease outflow by effects on other ciliary sites. Parasympathomimetic drugs include **pilocarpine** (0.5 to 6%), which directly interacts with cholinergic receptors as well as stimulates secretory glands (which is why it is used for treatment of keratitis sicca); echothiophate (0.03 to 0.25%) or demecarium bromide (0.125 and 0.25%; the most toxic) and isoflurophate (0.025%) are parasympathomimetics are irreversible inhibitors of acetylcholinesterase. The use of these drugs in animals wearing anticholinergic flea preparations should be done cautiously. Echothiophate is among the most effective drugs, in part because it is irreversible and therefore can be used only twice daily. Carbachol (3%) is both act both directly and indirectly, with a longer duration of action than pilocarpine (allowing thrice-daily treatment). Pilocarpine must be given several times a day and may cause pain on application. The use of a 4% pilocarpine gel in dogs has not been reported. Miotics should not be used in the presence of inflammation of the anterior chamber (i.e., anterior uveitis) because of the risk of anterior synechia.

Parasympatholytic drugs relax the cilary body, causing cycloplegia and mydriasis. Drugs include **atropine** (1%; up to 4% to 5% in horses; longest acting), homatropine (0.5% and 2%; intermediate acting), scopolamine (0.3 to 0.5%; used primarily before intraocular surgery), and **tropicamide** (1%). Topical anticholinergics are much more effective than systemic drugs. These drugs are not used to treat glaucoma and, in fact, are contraindicated in some types of glaucoma. Rather, because these drugs cause cycloplegia, they are useful in the relief of pain associated with spasms of the ciliary muscle, which often accompany anterior uveitis. Tear production may be decreased by parasympatholytic drugs. Tropicamide is rapid in onset and of short duration (2 to 3 hours, although mydriasis and cyclopegia may last up to 12 hours in some cats and dogs); therefore it is often used for ocular examinations.

Contraction of the dilator muscle is mediated by the sympathetic (epinephrine) system by way of alpha receptors, leading to mydriasis (dilation) and, as with parasympathomimetic drugs, as a result of constriction of ciliary body vasculature, decreased formation of aqueous humor and decreased IOP.

Sympathomimetic drugs include epinephrine (which does not penetrate the eye well), which directly interacts with alpha more than beta receptors (used as a 1:1,000 dilution to control conjunctival or scleral hemorrhage or to prolong effects of local anesthetics), phenylephrine (0.125% solution for vasoconstriction; 10% as mydriatic; onset of action in 1 hour, duration up to 24 hours), largely limited to alpha receptor stimulation (30- to 60-minute onset with 4-hour duration), and dipivefrin, a lipid-soluble drug that acts indirectly by causing epinephrine release (used to decrease IOP; 30 to 60 minutes to onset). Sympatholytics include alpha antagonists (thymoxamine) which inhibits the dilator muscle, causing miosis. Beta antagonists, represented by timolol (0.5%) (others include Optimpranolol, 0.3% and Betagan, 0.5%), act to decrease IOP by decreasing aqueous humor production. These drugs may be limited in their usefulness although may be effective for treatment of ocular hypertension.

Prostaglandins

The newest class of drugs developed to treat glaucoma are the topically applied prostaglandins. These drugs target the trabecular meshwork or collagen of the ciliary body such that outflow obstruction is decreased. Examples include bimatoprost and travoprost.

Direct Impact on Aqueous Humor

In addition to the impact of drugs targeting the autonomic nervous system, reduced production of aqueous humor can be accomplished by carbonic anhydrase inhibitors, which also have diuretic effects (the latter probably has limited effect on aqueous humor formation). Topical products include dorzolamide and brinzolamide. Systemic drugs include acetazolamide and the newer drugs, methazolamide and dichlorphenamide. These drugs can reduce aqueous humor production by up to 50% and are often used in combination with autonomic drugs. Aqueous humor production is also rapidly decreased by osmotic diuretics, including mannitol and glycerin. Mannitol (given intravenously) is limited to emergency therapy (two treatments) of glaucoma or to reduce IOP before surgery. Additional potential benefits of osmotic agents include reduction in vitreous humor volume (a potential advantage with lens disruption) and resolution of corneal edema (topical only). Glycerol has the disadvantage of being less effective than mannitol but can be administered (orally) at home by the pet owner; care must be taken to avoid emesis.

Antiinflammatory and Immunomodulatory Ophthalmic Preparations

Drugs used to treat ocular inflammation include glucocorticoids (systemic and local) and NSAIDS (topical). Drugs that act to modulate the immune system (e.g., cyclosporine; topical or systemic) also control the inflammatory response. Glucocorticoids target in situ mediators (eicosanoids: prostaglandins and leukotrienes), preformed biogenic amines (histamine, serotonin), and the immune system (macrophage processing, T-cell expansion). Additionally, glucocorticoids are antiangiogenic (inhibit vascularization). Glucocorticoids are indicated for any inflammatory condition of ocular tissues (e.g., conjunctivitis, blepharitis, episcleritis, keratitis, iridocylitis). Glucocorticoids inhibit healing, increase the potential for infection, and also stimulate collagenase. Collagen breakdown in the stroma can result in corneal perforation, and therefore glucocorticoids are contraindicated in the presence of an ulcer. Topical glucocorticoids are available in solution, suspension, and ointment. Preparations include hydrocortisone, 0.1% dexamethasone, and 1% prednisolone acetate (generally the drug of choice).

In contrast to glucocorticoids, NSAIDs principally target eicosanoids and thus are more limited in their control of inflammation (although they may have other effects). However, topically applied NSAIDs also can decrease inflammation; examples include flurbiprofen (0.03%) and diclofenac (0.1%), which are available as topical preparations. Cyclosporine specifically targets T-helper cells and thereby controls the immune response. Available as a 2% solution, cyclosporine is indicated for the treatment of keratitis sicca, pigmentary keratitis, and other ocular immune-mediated disorders.

Antihistamines rarely are useful topically, although systemic therapy may be helpful with allergic ocular reactions.

Antiprotease Drugs

Proteases responsible for tissue destruction and perpetuation of inflammation are produced by ocular epithelial and stroma cells as well as inflammatory cells and select bacteria (e.g., *Pseudomonas*). Acetylcysteine is an effective protease inhibitor that also is monolithic; consequently, it is useful for treatment of keratoconjunctivitis sicca. The low pH must be buffered before topical administration (7 to 7.5); although it can be used as a 20% solution, 5% would be less irritating.

Antiinfective Drugs

Because of the ability to administer high concentrations of antibiotics, traditional classification of bacteriostatic versus bactericidal (fungistatic or fungicidal, virostatic or virucidal) may not be relevant to antiinfective drugs.

Topical antibacterial drugs are available as single or multiple antibiotic agents. Drugs that target gram-negative organisms include the water-soluble, weakly basic aminoglycosides (also effective against *Staphylococcus* spp.) tobramycin (0.3%; drug of choice for treatment of *Pseudomonas)*, gentamicin (available with the glucocorticoid betamethasone), and neomycin (generally available only in combination with other antibiotics). Polymyxin B also is a water-soluble drug that is notable for its nephrotoxicy when given systemically. The fluorinated quinolones also target gram-negative organisms, including *Pseudomonas* as well as *Staphyloccoccus*. In contrast to the aminoglycosides, the fluorinated quinolones are lipid soluble. Drugs include ciprofloxacin and ofloxacin and its congener levofloxacin. Note that systemic fluorinated quinolone has been associated with retinal degeneration in cats; a similar finding has not been reported after topical use. Drugs that target gram-positive organisms include the lipid-soluble erythromycin (0.5%; bacteriostatic), the efficacy of which is limited by resistance, and the water-soluble bacitracin, which, like polymyxin B, is most known for its nephrotoxicity associated with systemic therapy. Triple antibiotic combinations include neomycin, polymyxin B, and bacitracin. Broad-spectrum topical antibiotics include chloramphenicol (prohibited for use in food animals), tetracyclines (drugs of choice for ocular *Mycoplasma* or *Chlamydia*), and the sulfonamides. Each is lipid soluble.

Topical antifungal antimicrobials include the polyene natamycin. Its spectrum includes all fungal agents except dermatophytes. The imidazoles (i.e., miconazole, fluconazole, and itraconazole) must be compounded from intravenous solutions. Their spectrum includes opportunistic, dimorphic fungi and dermatophytes.

Antiviral drugs are indicated for treatment of herpes keratitis. Drugs indicated for acute therapy include trifluridine (1%; probably the most effective); idoxuridine (0.1%; intermediate efficacy; must be compounded), and vidarabine (least effective and least irritating). These drugs tend to be irritating but must be administered no less than 5 times a day. For chronic therapy (chronic carrier state), betadine can be diluted (1:30); failure to dilute may be caustic to the eye.

Protectants and Lubricants

Aqueous solutions may be insufficient for replacement of tears because they cannot adhere to the epithelium. Polyvinylpyrrolidone (1.67%) is an artificial mucin that replaces mucopolysaccharides in the precorneal tear film and thereby stabilizes the film. Bicarbonate-based buffer will normal maintain pH, thus facilitating healing. Artificial tears are indicated to compensate for insufficient tear production, decrease loss of fluid from the cornea resulting from evaporation, and facilitate penetration of water-soluble drugs. Other protectants include methylcellulose (0.5 to 1%); hydroxyethyl cellulose; hydroxypropyl methylcellulose; and polyvinyl alcohol (1.4%), which may be too irritating.

Solutions that might be used for intraoperative flushing (rinsing or a wetting agent) include eye washes (commercial formulas preferred), povidine–iodine (2% to 4% in saline), and benzalkonium chloride (1:5000; incompatible with fluoresceine, nitrates, salicylate, and sulfonamides). Zinc sulfate (0.2% and 0.25% solution; 0.5% ointment) is a mild astringent and antiseptic that can be used for mild conjunctivitis.

REFERENCES

1. Bloom FE: Neurotransmission and the central nervous system. In Brunton LL, Lazo JS, Parker KL, editors: *Goodman & Gilman's the pharmacological basis of therapeutics*, ed 11, New York, 2006, McGraw-Hill.
2. Robey RW, Lazarowski A, Bates SE: P-glycoprotein: a clinical target in drug-refractory epilepsy? *Mol Pharmacol* 73(5):1343–1346, 2008.
3. Eyal S, Hsiao P, Unadkat JD: Drug interactions at the blood–brain barrier: fact or fantasy? *Pharmacol Ther* 123(1):80–104, 2009.
4. West CL, Mealey KL: Assessment of antiepileptic drugs as substrates for canine P-glycoprotein, *Am J Vet Res* 68(10): 1106–1110, 2007.

5. Ambikanandan M, Ganesh S, Aliasgar S: Drug delivery to the central nervous system: a review, *J Pharm Pharm Sci* 6(2): 252–273, 2003.
6. Misra A, Ganesh S, Shahiwala A, et al: Drug delivery to the central nervous system: a review, *J Pharm Pharm Sci* 6(2):252–273, 2003.
7. Jain KK: Nanobiotechnology-based drug delivery to the central nervous system, *Neurodegener Dis* 4(4):287–291, 2007.
8. Sagratella S: NMDA antagonists: antiepileptic-neuroprotective drugs with diversified neuropharmacological profiles, *Pharmacol Res* 32(1-2):1–13, 1995.
9. Chapman A: Glutamate and epilepsy, *J Nutr* 130:1043S–1045S, 2000.
10. Jobe PC, Browning RA: The serotonergic and noradrenergic effects of antidepressant drugs are anticonvulsant, not proconvulsant, *Epilepsy Behav* 7(4):602–619, 2005.
11. Lynch BA, Lambeng N, Nocka K, et al: The synaptic vesicle protein SV2A is the binding site for the AED drug levetiracetam, *Proc Natl Acad Sci U S A* 101(26):9861–9866, 2004.
12. Watanabe M, Maemura K, Kanbara K, et al: GABA and GABA receptors in the central nervous system and other organs, *Int Rev Cytol* 213:1–47, 2002.
13. Sarkisian MR: Overview of the current animal models for human seizure and epileptic disorders, *Epilepsy Behav* 2(3): 201–216, 2001.
14. Faingold CL, Hoffmann WE, Caspary DM: Mechanisms of sensory seizures: brain-stem neuronal response changes and convulsant drugs, *Fed Proc* 44(8):2436–2441, 1985.
15. Browning RA: Role of the brain-stem reticular formation in tonic-clonic seizures: lesion and pharmacological studies, *Fed Proc* 44:2425–2431, 1985.
16. Fromm GH: Effects of different classes of AED drugs on brain-stem pathways, *Fed Proc* 44(8):2432–2435, 1985.
17. Schwartz-Porsche D, Löscher W, Frey HH: Therapeutic efficacy of phenobarbital and primidone in canine epilepsy: a comparison, *J Vet Pharmacol Ther* 8:113–119, 1985.
18. Ganor Y, Godberg-Stern H, Lerman-Sagie T: Autoimmune epilepsy: distinct subpopulations of epilepsy patients harbor serum autoantibodies to either glutamate/ AMPA receptor GluR3, glutamate/NMDA receptor subunit NR2A or double-stranded DNA, *Epilepsy Res* 65:11–22, 2005.
19. Delgado-Escueta AV, Wasterlain C, Treiman DM, et al: Current concepts in neurology: management of status epilepticus, *N Engl J Med* 306:1337–1340, 1982.
20. Rogawski MA: The NMDA receptor, NMDA antagonists and epilepsy therapy, *Drugs* 44:279–292, 1992.
21. Whetsell WO: Current concepts of excitotoxicity, *J Neuropathol Exp Neurol* 55:1013, 1996.
22. Ellenberger C, Mevissen M, Doherr M, et al: Inhibitory and excitatory neurotransmitters in the cerebrospinal fluid of epileptic dogs, *Am J Vet Res* 65(8):1108–1113, 2004.
23. Podell M, Hadjiconstantinou M: Cerebrospinal fluid, gamma-aminobutyric acid, and glutamate concentrations in dogs with epilepsy, *Am J Vet Res* 58:451–456, 1997.
24. Stringer JL: Treatment of seizure disorders. In Wecker L, editor: *Brody's human pharmacology: molecular to clinical*, ed 5, St Louis, 2010, Mosby.
25. McNamara JO: Pharmacotherapy of the epilepsies. In Brunton LL, Lazo JS, Parker KL, editors: *Goodman & Gilman's the pharmacological basis of therapeutics*, ed 11, New York, 2006, McGraw-Hill, New York.
26. Brown SA: Anticonvulsant therapy in small animals, *Vet Clin North Am Small Anim Pract* 18(6):1197–1215, 1988.
27. Bialer M, Twyman RE, White HS: Correlation analysis between anticonvulsant ED_{50} values of AED drugs in mice and rats and their therapeutic doses and plasma levels, *Epilepsy Behav* 5(6):866–872, 2004.
28. Boothe DM, Dewey C: Comparison of phenobarbital and bromide as first choice antiepileptic drug rherapy for treatment of canine epilepsy; Submitted to, *J Am Vet Med Assoc*, August 2009.
29. Frey HH: Use of anticonvulsants in small animals, *Vet Rec* 118:484, 1986.
30. Stevenson CM, Kim J, Fleisher D: Colonic absorption of AED agents, *Epilepsia* 38(1):63–67, 1997.
31. Löscher W, Frey HH: Kinetics of penetration of common AED drugs into cerebrospinal fluid, *Epilepsia* 25(3):346–352, 1984.
32. Mealey KL, Greene S, Bagley R, et al: P-glycoprotein contributes to the blood-brain, but not blood-cerebrospinal fluid, barrier in a spontaneous canine p-glycoprotein knockout model, *Drug Metab Dispos* 36(6):1073–1079, 2008.
33. Pekcec A, Unkrüer B, Stein V, et al: Over-expression of P-glycoprotein in the canine brain following spontaneous status epilepticus, *Epilepsy Res* 83(2-3):144–151, 2009.
34. Bunch SE, Baldwin BH, Hornbuckle WE, et al: Compromised hepatic function in dogs treated with anticonvulsant drugs, *J Am Vet Assoc* 184(40):444–448, 1984.
35. Bunch SE, Castleman WL, Baldwin BH, et al: Effects of long-term primidone and phenytoin administration on canine hepatic function and morphology, *Am J Vet Res* 46(1):105–115, 1985.
36. Bunch SE, Conway MB, Center SA, et al: Toxic hepatopathy and intrahepatic cholestasis associated with phenytoin administration in combination with other anticonvulsant drugs in three dogs, *J Am Vet Med Assoc* 190(2):194–198, 1987.
37. Kluger EK, Malik R, Ilkin WJ, et al: Serum triglyceride concentration in dogs with epilepsy treated with phenobarbital or with phenobarbital and bromide, *J Am Vet Med Assoc* 233(8): 1270–1277, 2008.
38. Verrotti A, Basciani F, Domizio S, et al: Serum lipids and lipoproteins in patients treated with AED drugs, *Pediatr Neurol* 19(5):364–367, 1997.
39. Johannessen SI, Battino D, Berry DJ, et al: Therapeutic drug monitoring of the newer AED drugs, *Clin Pharmacokinet* 38(3): 191–204, 2000.
40. Pedersoli WM, Wike JS, Ravis WR: Pharmacokinetics of single doses of phenobarbital given intravenously and orally to dogs, *Am J Vet Res* 48(4):679–683, 1987.
41. Tahan FA, Frey HH: Absorption kinetics and bioavailability of phenobarbital after oral administration to dogs, *J Vet Pharmacol Ther* 8:205–207, 1985.
42. Frey HH, Löscher W: Pharmacokinetics of anti-epileptic drugs in the dog: a review, *J Vet Pharmacol Ther* 8(3):219–233, 1985.
43. Cochrane SM, Parent JM, Black WD: Pharmacokinetics of phenobarbital in the cat following multiple oral administration, *Can J Vet Res* 54:309–312, 1990.
44. Ravis WR, Pedersoli WM, Turco JD: Pharmacokinetics and interactions of digoxin with phenobarbital in dogs, *Am J Vet Res* 48(8):1244–1249, 1987.
45. Flomenbaum N, Goldfrank L, Hoffman R, et al: *Goldfrank's Toxicologic Emergencies*, ed 8, New York, 2006, McGraw-Hill, p 568.
46. Fukunaga K, Saito M, Muto M, et al: Effects of urine pH modification on pharmacokinetics of phenobarbital in healthy dogs, *J Vet Pharmacol Ther* 31(5):431–436, 2008.
47. Graham RA, Downey A, Mudra D, et al: In vivo and in vitro induction of cytochrome P450 enzymes in Beagle dogs, *Drug Metab Dispos* 30:1206–1213, 2002.
48. Ravis WR, Pedersoli WM, Wike JS: Pharmacokinetics of phenobarbital in dogs given multiple doses, *Am J Vet Res* 50(8): 1343–1347, 1989.
49. Cunningham JG, Haidukewych D, Jensen HA: Therapeutic serum concentrations of primidone and its metabolites, phenobarbital and phenylethylmalonamide in epileptic dogs, *J Am Vet Med Assoc* 182(10):1091–1094, 1983.

50. Farnbach GC: Serum concentrations and efficacy of phenytoin, phenobarbital, and primidone in canine epilepsy, *J Am Vet Med Assoc* 184(9):1117–1120, 1984.
51. Stonehewer J, Mackin AJ, Tasker S, et al: Idiopathic phenobarbital-responsive hypersialosis in the dog: an unusual form of limbic epilepsy? *J Small Anim Prac* 41(9):416–421, 2000.
52. Sumi T: Different effects of chronically administered phenobarbital on amygdaloid- and hippocampal-kindled seizures in the cat, *Hokkaido Igaku Zasshi* 68(2):177–189, 1993.
53. Greenlee WF, Poland A: An improved assay of 7-ethoxycoumarin o-deethylase activity: induction of hepatic enzyme activity in C57BL/6J and DBA/2J mice by phenobarbital, 3-methylcholanthrene and 2,3,7,8-tetrachlorodibenzo-p-dioxin, *J Pharmacol Exp Ther* 205(3):596–605, 1978.
54. Kutt H: Interactions between anticonvulsants and other commonly prescribed drugs, *Epilepsia* 24(Suppl 2):S118–S131, 1984.
55. Morselli PL, Rizzo M, Garattini S: Interaction between phenobarbital and diphenylhydantoin in animals and in epileptic patients, *Ann NY Acad Sci* 179:88–107, 1971.
56. Nossaman BC, Amouzadeh HR, Sangiah S: Effects of chloramphenicol, cimetidine and phenobarbital on and tolerance to xylazine-ketamine anesthesia in dogs, *Vet Hum Toxicol* 32(3):216–219, 1990.
57. Waxman DJ, Azaroff L: Phenobarbital induction of cytochrome P-450 gene expression, *Biochem J* 281(Pt 3):577–592, 1992.
58. Valerino DM, Vesell ES, Aurori KC, et al: Effects of various barbiturates on hepatic microsomal enzymes. A comparative study, *Drug Metab Dispos* 2(5):448–457, 1974.
59. Aldridge A, Neims AH: The effects phenobarbital and beta-naphthoflavone on the elimination kinetics and metabolite pattern of caffeine in the beagle dog, *Drug Metab Dispos* 7(3):378–382, 1979.
60. Bekersky I, Maggio AC, Mattaliano V Jr, et al: Influence of phenobarbital on the disposition of clonazepam and antipyrine in the dog, *J Pharmacokinet Biopharm 5(5)*:507–512, 1977.
61. Ciaccio PJ, Halpert JR: Characterization of a phenobarbital inducible dog liver cytochrome P450 structurally related to rat and human enzymes of the P450IIIA (steroid-inducible) gene subfamily, *Arch Biochem Biophys* 271:284–299, 1989.
62. McKillop D: Effects of phenobarbitone and beta-naphthoflavone on hepatic microsomal drug metabolizing enzymes of the male beagle dog, *Biochem Pharmacol* 34(17):3137–3142, 1985.
63. Hojo T, Ohno R, Shimoda M, et al: Enzyme and plasma protein induction by multiple oral administrations of phenobarbital at a therapeutic dosage regimen in dogs, *J Vet Pharmacol Therap* 25:121–127, 2002.
64. Fukunaga K, Saito M, Matsuo E, et al: Long-lasting enhancement of CYP activity after discontinuation of repeated administration of phenobarbital in dogs, *Res Vet Sci* 87(3):455–457, 2009.
65. Breznock EM: Effects of phenobarbital on digitoxin and digoxin elimination in the dog, *Am J Vet Res* 36(4):371–373, 1975.
66. Pedersoli WM, Ganjam VK, Nachreiner RF: Serum digoxin concentrations in dogs before, during, and after concomitant treatment with phenobarbital, *Am J Vet Res* 41(10):1639–1642, 1980.
67. Sams RA, Muir WW: Effects of phenobarbital on thiopental pharmacokinetics in greyhounds, *Am J Vet Res* 49(2):245–249, 1988.
68. Dugdale AH, Lakhani KH, Brearley JC: Thiopentone induction dose requirement in dogs is little influenced by co-administration of diazepam or prior treatment with phenobarbitone or corticosteroids, but is reduced in the presence of brain pathology, *Vet J* 161(1):93–97, 2001.
69. Wagner SO, Sams RA, Podell M: Chronic phenobarbital therapy reduces plasma benzodiazepine concentrations after intravenous and rectal administration of diazepam in the dog, *J Vet Pharmacol Therap* 21:335–342, 1998.
70. de Bodo C, Prescott KF: The antidiuretic action of barbiturates (phenobarbital, amytal, pentobarbital) and the mechanism involved in this action, *Pharmacol Exp Ther* 85:222–233, 1945.
71. Jacobs G, Calvert C, Kaufman A: Neutropenia and thrombocytopenia in three dogstreated with anticonvulsants, *J Am Vet Med Assoc* 212(5):681–684, 1998.
72. Weiss DJ: Hemophagocytic syndrome in dogs: 24 cases (1996-2005), *J Am Vet Med AssocMar* 230(5):697–701, 2007:1.
73. Solomon GE, Hilgartner MW, Kutt H: Phenobarbital-induced coagulation defects in cats, *Neurology* 24(10):920–924, 1974.
74. March PA, Hillier A, Weisbrode SE, et al: Superficial necrolytic dermatitis in 11 dogs with a history of phenobarbital administration (1995-2002), *J Vet Intern Med* 18:65–74, 2004.
75. Kantrowitz LB, Peterson ME, Trepanier LA, et al: Serum total thyroxine, total triiodothyronine, free thyroxine, and thyrotropin concentrations in epileptic dogs treated with anticonvulsants, *J Am Vet Med Assoc* 214(12):1804–1808, 1999.
76. Gieger TL, Hosgood G, Taboada J, et al: Thyroid function and serum hepatic enzyme activity in dogs after phenobarbital administration, *J Vet Intern Med* 14(3):277–281, 2000.
77. Dayrell-Hart B, Steinberg SA, VanWinkle TJ, et al: Hepatotoxicity of phenobarbital in dogs: 18 cases, *J Am Vet Med Assoc* 199(8):1060–1066, 1991.
78. Muller PB, Taboada J, Hosgood G, et al: Effects of long-term phenobarbital treatment on the liver in dogs, *J Vet Intern Med* 15:165–171, 2000.
79. Bunch SE: Hepatotoxicity associated with pharmacologic agents in dogs and cats, *Vet Clin North Am Small Anim Pract* 23(3):659–670, 1993.
79a. Gaskill CL, Miller LM, Mattoon JS, et al: Liver histopathology and liver and serum alanine aminotransferase and alkaline phosphatase activities in epileptic dogs receiving phenobarbital, *Vet Pathol* 42(2):147–160, 2005.
80. Gaskill CL, Cribb AE: Pancreatitis associated with potassium bromide/phenobarbital combination therapy in epileptic dogs, *Can Vet J* 41(7):555–558, 2000.
81. Steiner JM, Xenoulis PG, Anderson JA, et al: Serum pancreatic lipase immunoreactivity concentrations in dogs treated with potassium bromide and/or phenobarbital, *Vet Ther* 9(1):37–44, 2008.
82. Berg MJ, Berlinger WG, Goldberg MJ, et al: Acceleration of the body clearance of phenobarbital by oral activated charcoal, *N Engl J Med* 307:642–644, 1982.
83. Frey HH, Göbel W, Löscher W: Pharmacokinetics of primidone and its active metabolites in the dog, *Arch Int Pharmacodyn Ther* 242(1):14–30, 1979.
84. Schwartz-Porsche D, Löscher W, Frey HH: Treatment of canine epilepsy with primidone, *J Am Vet Med Assoc* 181(6):592–595, 1982.
85. Frey HH, Löscher W: Is primidone more efficient than phenobarbital? An attempt at a pharmacological evaluation [author's translation], *Nervenarzt* 51(6):359–362, 1980.
86. Farnbach GC: Efficacy of primidone in dogs with seizures unresponsive to phenobarbital, *J Am Vet Med Assoc* 185(8):867–868, 1984.
87. Sawchuk SA, Parker AJ, Neff-Davis C, et al: Primidone in the cat, *J Am Anim Hosp Assoc* 21:647–650, 1985.
88. Henricks PM: Dermatitis associated with the use of primidone in a dog, *J Am Vet Med Assoc* 191(2):237–238, 1987.
89. Meyer DJ, Noonan NE: Liver tests in dogs receiving anticonvulsant drugs (diphenylhydantoin and primidone), *J Am Anim Hos Assoc* 17:261–264, 1981.
90. Poffenbarger EM, Hardy RM: Hepatic cirrhosis associated with long-term primidone therapy in a dog, *J Am Vet Med Assoc* 186(9):978–980, 1985.

91. Campbell CL: Primidone intoxication associated with concurrent use of chloramphenicol, *J Am Vet Med Assoc* 182(9): 992–993, 1983.
92. Young RS, Ropper AH, Hawkes D, et al: Pentobarbital in refractory status epilepticus, *Pediatric Pharmacol* 3(2):63–67, 1983.
93. Fucci V, Monroe WE, Riedesel DH, et al: Oral pentobarbital intoxication in a bitch, *J Am Vet Med Assoc* 188(2):191–192, 1986.
94. Martin HD, Mallock A: Management of barbiturate intoxication in cougars (Felis concolor), *J Zoo Anim Med* 18(2-3): 100–103, 1987.
95. Papich MG, Alcorn J: Absorption of diazepam after its rectal administration in dogs, *Am J Vet Res* 56(12):1629–1636, 1995.
96. Löscher W, Frey HH: Pharmacokinetics of diazepam in the dog, *Am J Vet Res* 56(12):1629–1636, 1995.
97. Löscher W, Frey HH: Pharmacokinetics of diazepam in the dog, *Arch Int Pharmacodyn Ther* 254(2):180–195, 1981.
98. Musulin SE, Mariani SL, Papich M: Diazepam pharmacokinetics after nasal drop and atomized nasal administration in dogs, *J Vet Pharm Ther*, 2010:in press.
99. Platt SR, Randell SC, Scott KC, et al: Comparison of plasma benzodiazepine concentrations following intranasal and intravenous administration of diazepam to dogs, *Am J Vet Res* 61(6):651–654, 2000.
100. Arendt RM, Greenblatt DJ, deJong RH, et al: In vitro correlates of benzodiazepine cerebrospinal fluid uptake, pharmacodynamic action and peripheral distribution, *J Pharmacol Exp Ther* 227(1):98–106, 1983.
101. Scherkl R, Kurudi D, Frey HH: Clorazepate in dogs: tolerance to the anticonvulsant effect and signs of physical dependence, *Epilepsy Res* 3(2):144–150, 1989.
102. Cotler S, Gustafson JH, Colburn WA: Pharmacokinetics of diazepam and nordiazepam in the cat, *J Pharm Sci* 73(3): 348–351, 1984.
103. Forrester SD, Brown SA, Lees GE, et al: Disposition of clorazepate in dogs after single- and multiple-dose oral administration, *Am J Vet Res* 51(12):2001–2005, 1990.
104. Podell M, Wagner SO, Sams RA: Lorazepam concentrations in plasma following its intravenous and rectal administration in dogs, *J Vet Pharmacol Ther* 21(2):158–160, 1998.
105. Mariami CL, Clemmons RM, Lee Ambrose L: A comparison of intranasal and intravenous lorazepam in normal dogs, *American College of Veterinary Internal Medicine Annual Forum* 2003.
106. Lui CY, Amidon GL, Goldberg A: Intranasal absorption of flurazepam, midazolam, and triazolam in dogs, *J Pharm Sci* 80(12):1125–1129, 1991.
107. Al-Tahan F, Löscher W, Frey HH: Pharmacokinetics of clonazepam in the dog, *Arch Int Pharmacodyn Ther* 268(2):180–193, 1984.
108. Kaplan SA, Alexander K, Jack ML, et al: Pharmacokinetic profiles of clonazepam in dog and humans and of flunitrazepam in dog, *J Pharm Sci* 63(4):527–532, 1974.
109. Brown SA, Forrester SD: Serum disposition of oral clorazepate from regular-release and sustained-delivery tablets in dogs, *J Vet Pharmacol Ther* 14(4):426–429, 1991.
110. Gatzonis SD, Angelopoulos EK, Daskalopoulou EG, et al: Convulsive status epilepticus following abrupt high-dose benzodiazepine discontinuation, *Drug Alcohol Depend* 59(1):95–97, 2000.
111. Elston TH, Rosen D, Rodan I, et al: Seven cases of acute diazepam toxicity, *Proc Am Anim Hosp Assoc*, October, 1993, pp 343–349.
112. McNicholas LF, Martin WR, Cherian S: Physical dependence on diazepam and lorazepam in the dog, *J Pharmacol Exp Ther* 226(3):783–789, 1983.
113. Sloan JW, Martin WR, Wala E: Effect of the chronic dose of diazepam on the intensity and characteristics of the precipitated abstinence syndrome in the dog, *J Pharmacol Exp Ther* 265(3):1152–1162, 1993.
114. Löscher W, Honack D, Fassbender CP: Physical dependence on diazepam in the dog: precipitation of different abstinence syndromes by the benzodiazepine receptor antagonists Ro 15-1788 and ZK 93426, *Br J Pharmacol* 97(3):843–852, 1989.
115. Sloan JW, Martin WR, Wala E, Dickey KM: Chronic administration of and dependence on halazepam, diazepam, and nordiazepam in the dog, *Drug Alcohol Depend* 28(3):249–264, 1991.
116. Sloan JW, Martin WR, Wala EP: A comparison of the physical dependence inducing properties of flunitrazepam and diazepam, *Pharmacol Biochem Behav* 39(2):395–405, 1991.
117. Wala E, McNicholas LF, Sloan JW, et al: Flumazenil oral absorption in dogs, *Pharmacol Biochem Behav* 30(4):945–948, 1988.
118. Forrester SD, Wilcke JR, Jacobson JD, et al: Effects of a 44-day administration of phenobarbital on disposition of clorazepate in dogs, *Am J Vet Res* 54:1136–1138, 1993.
119. Podell M: The use of diazepam per rectum at home for the acute management of cluster seizures in dogs, *J Vet Intern Med* 9(2):68–74, 1995.
120. Placidi GF, Tognoni G, Pacifici GM, et al: Regional distribution of diazepam and its metabolites in the brain of cat after chronic treatment, *Psychopharmacology (Berl)* 48(2): 133–137, 1976.
121. Wuth O: Rational bromide treatment, *J Am Med Assoc* 88:2013–2017, 1927.
122. Suzuki S, Kawakami K, Nakamura F, et al: Bromide, in the therapeutic concentration, enhances GABA-activated currents in cultured neurons of rat cerebral cortex, *Epilepsy Res* 19(2):89–97, 1994.
123. Grewal MS: Correlation between anticonvulsant activity and plasma concentration of bromide, *J Pharmacol Exp Ther* 112:109–115, 1954.
124. Schwartz-Porsche D, Jurgens N, May T, et al: Pharmacokinetics of bromide and bromide therapy in canine epilepsy, *Proceedings of the 4th Annual Symposium of the European Society of Veterinary Neurology*, Bern, 1990, Switzerland, pp 32–34.
125. Wallace GB, Brodie BB: The distribution of administered bromide in comparison with chloride and its relation to body fluids, *J Pharmacol Exp Ther* 65:214–219, 1939.
126. Rauws AG, van Logeten MJ: The influence of dietary chloride on bromide excretion in the rat, *Toxicology* 3:29–32, 1975.
127. Trepanier LA, Babish JG: Effect of dietary chloride content on the elimination of bromide by dogs, *Res Vet Sci* 58:252–255, 1995.
128. Trepanier LA, Babish JG: Pharmacokinetic properties of bromide in dogs after the intravenous and oral administration of single doses, *Res Vet Sci* 58:248–251, 1995.
129. March PA, Podell M, Sams RA: Pharmacokinetics and toxicity of bromide following high-dose oral potassium bromide administration in healthy Beagles, *J Vet Pharmacol Ther* 25: 425–432, 2002.
129a. Boothe DM, George KL, Couch P: Disposition and clinical use of bromide in cats, *J Am Vet Med Assoc* 221(8):1131–1135, 2002.
130. Rossmeisl JH, Inzana KD: Clinical signs, risk factors, and outcomes associated with bromide toxicosis (bromism) in dogs with idiopathic epilepsy, *J Am Vet Med Assoc* 234(11): 1425–1431, 2009.
131. Podell M, Fenner WR: Bromide therapy in refractory canine idiopathic epilepsy: combination therapy in epileptic dogs, *Can Vet J* 41:555–558, 2000.

132. Rossmeisl JH Jr, Zimmerman K, Inzana KD, et al: Assessment of the use of plasma and serum chloride concentrations as indirect predictors of serum bromide concentrations in dogs with idiopathic epilepsy, *Vet Clin Pathol* 35(4):426–433, 2006.
133. Pearce LK: Potassium bromide as an adjunct to phenobarbital for the management of uncontrolled seizures in dogs, *Prob Vet Neurol* 1(1):95–101, 1990.
134. Schwartz-Porsche D, Jurgens U: Effectiveness of bromide in therapy resistant epilepsy of dogs, *Praxis* 19(4):395–401, 1991.
135. Trepanier LA, Van Schoick A, Schwark WS, et al: serum drug concentrations in epileptic dogs treated with potassium bromide alone or in combination with other anticonvulsants: 122 cases (1992-1996), *J Am Vet Med Assoc* 213(10):1449–1453, 1998.
136. Ernst JP, Doose H, Baier WK: Bromides were effective in intractable epilepsy with generalized tonic-clonic seizures and onset in early childhood, *Brain Dev* 10(6):385–388, 1988.
137. Woody RC: Bromide therapy for pediatric seizure disorder intractable to other AED drugs, *J Child Neurol* 5:65–67, 1990.
138. Frey HH, Löscher W: Pharmacokinetics of carbamazepine in the dog, *Arch Int Pharmacodyn Ther* 243(2):180–191, 1980.
139. Holland CT: Successful long term treatment of a dog with psychomotor seizures using carbamazepine, *Aust Vet J* 65(12): 389–392, 1988.
140. el Sayed MA: Löscher W, Frey HH: Pharmacokinetics of ethosuximide in the dog, *Arch Int Pharmacodyn Ther* 234(2): 180–192, 1978.
141. Rho JM, Donevan SD, Rogawski MA: Mechanism of action of the anticonvulsant felbamate: opposing effects on N-methyl-D-aspartate and gamma aminobutyric acid receptors, *Ann Neurol* 35:229–234, 1994.
142. Palmer KJ, MacTavish D: Felbamate: a review of its pharmacodynamic and pharmacokinetic properties, and therapeutic efficacy in epilepsy, *Drugs* 45:1041–1065, 1993.
143. White SH, Wolf HH, Swinyard EA: A neuropharmacologic evaluation of felbamate as a novel anticonvulsant, *Epilepsia* 33:564–572, 1992.
144. Ritter FJ: Efficacy of felbamate in childhood epilepetic encephalopathy (Lennox-Gastaut syndrome), *N Engl J Med* 328:29–33, 1993.
145. Carmant L, Holmes GL, Sawyer S, et al: Efficacy of felbamate in therapy for partial epilepsy in children, *J Pediatr* 125:481–486, 1994.
146. Burgeois B, Leppik IE, Sackellares JC, et al: Felbamate: a double-blind controlled trial in patients undergoing presurgical evaluation of partial seizures, *Neurology* 43:693–696, 1993.
147. Sachdeo R, Kramer LD, Rosenberg A: Felbamate monotherapy: controlled trial in patients with partial onset seizures, *Ann Neurol* 32:386–392, 1992.
148. Faught E, Sachdeo RD, Remler MP, et al: Felbamate monotherapy for partial onset seizures: an active control trial, *Neurology* 43:688–692, 1993.
149. Boothe DM: Anticonvulsant therapy in small animals, *Vet Clin North Am Small Anim Pract* 28(2):411–448, 1998.
150. Adusumalli VE, Yang JT, Wong KK, et al: Felbamate pharmacokinetics in the rat, rabbit, and dog, *Drug Metab Dispos* 19(6):1116–1125, 1991.
151. Yang JT, Morris M, Wong KK, et al: Felbamate metabolism in pediatric and adult beagle dogs, *Drug Metab Dis* 20:84–88, 1992.
152. Adusumalli VE, Gilchrist JR, Wichmann JK, et al: Pharmacokinetics of felbamate in pediatric and adult beagle dogs, *Epilepsia* 33:955–960, 1992.
153. Theodore WH: Felbamate. In Engel J, Pedley TA, editors: *Epilepsy: a comprehensive textbook*, Philadelphia, 1997, Lippincott-Raven, pp 1508–1514.
154. Reidenberg P, Glue P, Banfield CR, et al: Effects of felbamate on the pharmacokinetics of phenobarbital, *Clin Pharmacol Ther* 58:279–287, 1995.
155. Graves N: Felbamate, *Ann Pharmacother* 27:1073–1081, 1993.
156. Goa KL, Sorkin EM: Gabapentin. A review of its pharmacologic properties and clinical potential in epilepsy, *Drugs* 46(3): 409–427, 1993.
157. McLean MJ: Clinical pharmacokinetics of gabapentin, *Neurology* 44:S17–S22, 1994.
158. Ramsay RE: Clinical efficacy and safety of gabapentin, *Neurology* 44:S23–S30, 1994.
159. Vollmer KO, von Hodenberg A, Kolle EU: Pharmacokinetics and metabolism of gabapentin in rat, dog and man, *Drug Res* 34(1):830–839, 1986.
160. Cochran S: Update on seizures in cats. World Small Animal Veterinary Conference; Australia, 2007. Accessed January 20, 2010, at http://www.ivis.org/proceedings/wsava/2007/pdf/84_20070520165138_abs.pdf.
161. Radulovic LL, Turck D, von Hodenberg A, et al: Disposition of gabapentin (neurontin) in mice, rats, dogs, and monkeys, *Arzneimittelforschung* 36(5):830–839, 1986.
162. Vollmer KO, von Hodenberg A, Kolle EU: Pharmacokinetics and metabolism of gabapentin in rat, dog and monkeys, *Toxicol Sci* 45(2):225–232, 1998.
163. Rhee YS, Park S, Lee TW, et al: In vitro/in vivo relationship of gabapentin from a sustained-release tablet formulation: a pharmacokinetic study in the beagle dog, *Arch Pharm Res* 31(7):911–917, 2008.
164. Govendir M, Perkins M, Malik R: Improving seizure control in dogs with refractory epilepsy using gabapentin as an adjunctive agent, *Aus Vet J* 83(10):602–608, 2005.
165. Barrueto F Jr, Green J, Howland MA, et al: Gabapentin withdrawal presenting as status epilepticus, *J Toxicol Clin Toxicol* 40(7):925–928, 2002.
166. European Medicines Agency. Accessed January 10, 2010, at http://www.ema.europa.eu/humandocs/PDFs/EPAR/lyrica/084504en6.pdf.
167. Salazar V, Dewey CW, Schwark W, et al: Pharmacokinetics of single-dose oral pregabalin administration in normal dogs, *Vet Anaesth Analg* 36(6):574–580, 2009.
168. Dewey CW, Cerda-Gonzalez S, Levine JM, et al: Pregabalin as an adjunct to phenobarbital, potassium bromide, or a combination of phenobarbital and potassium bromide for treatment of dogs with suspected idiopathic epilepsy, *J Am Vet Med Assoc* 235(12):1442–1449, 2009.
169. Patsalos PN, Ghattaura S, Ratnaraj N, et al: In situ metabolism of levetiracetam in blood of patients with epilepsy, *Epilepsia Nov* 47(11):1818–1821, 2006.
170. Benedetti MS, Coupez R, Whomsley R: Comparative pharmacokinetics and metabolism of levetiracetam, a new AED agent, in mouse, rat rabbit and dog, *Xenobiotica* 34(3):281–300, 2004.
171. Isoherrranen N, Yagen B, Soback S, et al: Pharmacokinetics of levetiracetam and its entantiomer (R)-α-ethyl-2-oxo-pyrrolidine acetamine in dogs, *Epilepsia* 42(7), 2001:825–230.
172. Benedetti MS, Coupez R, Whomsley R, et al: Comparative pharmacokinetics and metabolism of levetiracetam, a new anti-epileptic agent, in mouse, rat, rabbit and dog, *Xenobiotica* 34(3):281–300, 2004.
173. Dewey CW, Bailey KS, Boothe DM, et al: Pharmacokinetics of single-dose intravenous levetiracetam administration in normal dogs, *J Vet Emerg Crit Care* 18(2):153–157, 2008.
174. Patterson EE, Goel V, Cloyd JC, et al: Intramuscular, intravenous and oral levetiracetam in dogs: safety and pharmacokinetics, *J Vet Pharmacol Ther* 31(3):253–258, 2008.
175. Carnes MB, Boothe DM, Axlund TX: Disposition of Levetiracetam in cats, Annual American College of Veterinary Internal Medicine (ACVIM) Forum, San Antonio, Tex, June 4-7, 2008. Abstract published in, *J Vet Int Med* 22(3):215, 2008.

176. Volk HA, Matiasek LA, Luján Feliu-Pascual A, et al: The efficacy and tolerability of levetiracetam in pharmacoresistant epileptic dogs, *Vet J* 176(3), 2008:310–309.
177. Bailey KS, Dewey CW, Boothe DM, et al: Levetiracetam as an adjunct to phenobarbital treatment in cats with suspected idiopathic epilepsy, *J Am Vet Med Assoc* 232(6):867–872, 2008.
178. Pasten LJ: Diphenylhydantoin in the canine: clinical aspects and determination of concentrations of phenytoin in the dog, *J AmAnimHosp Assoc* 13:247–254, 1977.
179. Sanders JE, Yeary RA: Serum concentrations of orally administered diphenylhydantoin in dogs, *J Am Vet Med Assoc* 172: 153–156, 1978.
180. Frey HH, Löscher W: Clinical pharmacokinetics of phenytoin in the dog: a reevaluation, *Am J Vet Res* 41(10):1635–1638, 1980.
181. Marx JL: Calmodulin: a protein for all seasons, *Science* 208(4441):274–276, 1980.
182. Overduin LM, van Gogh H, Mol JA, et al: Pharmacokinetics of three formulations of diphenylhydantoin in the dog, *Res Vet Sci* 46(2):271–273, 1989.
183. Baggot JD, Davis LE: Comparative study of plasma protein binding of diphenylhydantoin, *Comp Gen Pharmacol* 4:399–404, 1973.
184. Mirkin BL: Perinatal pharmacology: placental transfer, fetal localization, and neonatal disposition of drugs, *Anesthesiology* 43:156–170, 1975.
185. Bajpai M, Roskos LK, Shen DD, et al: Roles of cytochrome 4502C9 and cytochrome P4502C19 in the stereoselective metabolism of phenytoin to its major metabolite, *Drug Metab Dispos* 24:1401–1403, 1996.
186. Glazko AJ: Diphenylhydantoin metabolism. A prospective view, *Drug Metab Dispos* 1:711–714, 1973.
187. Dayton PG, Cucinell SA, Weiss N, et al: Dose-dependence of drug plasma level decline in dogs, *J Pharmacol Exp Ther* 158:305–316, 1967.
188. Roye DB, Serrano EE, Hammer RH, et al: Plasma kinetics of diphenylhydantoin in dogs and cats, *Am J Vet Res* 34:947–950, 1973.
189. Sanders JE, Yeary RA, Powers JD, et al: Relationship between serum and brain concentrations of phenytoin in the dog, *Am J Vet Res* 40:473–476, 1979.
190. Pedersoli WM, Redding RW, Nachreiner RF: Blood serum concentrations of orally adminsitered diphenylhydantoin in dogs and pharmacokinetic valures after an intravenous injection, *J Am Anim Hosp Assoc* 17:271, 1981.
191. Matar KM, Nicholls PJ, Bawazir SA, et al: Effect of vigabatrin and gabapentin on phenytoin pharmacokinetics in the dog, *Pharmacol Res* 42(6):517–521, 2000.
192. Tobin T, Dirdjosudjono S, Baskin SI: Pharmacokinetics and distribution of diphenylhydantoin in kittens, *Am J Vet Res* 34:951–954, 1973.
193. Conney AH, Burns IJ: Metabolic interactions among environmental chemicals and drugs, *Science* 178:576–586, 1972.
194. Marquis J-F, Carruthers SG, Spence JD, et al: Phenytoin-theophylline interaction, *N Engl J Med* 307:1189–1190, 1982.
195. Sanders JE, Yeary RA, Fenner WR, et al: Interaction of phenytoin with chloramphenicol or pentobarbital in the dog, *J Am Vet Med Assoc* 175:177–180, 1979.
196. Keith DA, Gundberg CM, Japour A, et al: Vitamin K-dependent proteins and anticonvulsant medication, *Clin Pharmacol Ther* 34:529–532, 1983.
197. Nash AS, Thompson H, Bogan JA: Phenytoin toxicity: a fatal case in a dog with hepatitis and jaundice, *Vet Rec* 100:280–281, 1977.
198. Senuty P, Baker DE, Yuen GJ: Assessment of thyroid function during phenytoin therapy, *DICP Ann Pharmacother* 22: 609–610, 1988.
199. Browne TR: Fosphenytoin (Cerebyx), *Clin Neuropharmacol* 20(1):1–12, 1997.
200. Michelucci R, Passarelli D, Riguzzi P, et al: The preclinical and therapeutic activity of the novel anticonvulsant topiramate, *CNS Drug Reviews* 4:165–186, 1998.
201. Streeter AJ, Stahle PL, Holland ML, et al: Pharmacokinetics and bioavailability of topiramate in the beagle dog, *Drug Metab Dispos* 23(1):90–93, 1995.
202. Löscher W: Plasma levels of valproic acid and its metabolites during continued treatment in dogs, *J Vet Pharmacol Ther* 4(2):111–119, 1981.
203. Nafe LA, Parker A, Kay WK: Sodium valproate: a preliminary clinical trial in epileptic dogs, *J Am Anim Hosp Assoc* 17: 131–133, 1981.
204. Masuda Y, Ishizaki M, Shimizu M: Zonisamide: pharmacology and clinical efficacy in epilepsy, *CNS Drug Review* 4:341–360, 1998.
205. Suzuki S, Kawakami K, Nishimura S, et al: Zonisamide blocks T-type calcium channel in cultured neurons of rat cerebral cortex, *Epilepsy Res* 12:21–27, 1992.
206. Biton V: Clinical pharmacology and mechanism of action of zonisamide, *Clin Neuropharmacol* 30(4):230–240, 2007.
207. Okada M, Kaneko S, Hirano T, et al: Effects of zonisamide on dopaminergic system, *Epilepsy Res* 22:193–205, 1995.
208. Ueda Y, Doi T, Tokumaru J, et al: Effect of zonisamide on molecular regulation of glutamate and GABA transporter proteins during epileptogenesis in rats with hippocampal seizures, *Brain Res Mol Brain Res* 116:1–6, 2003.
209. Mori A, Noda Y, Packer L: The anticonvulsant zonisamide scavenges free radicals, *Epilepsy Res* 30:153–158, 1998.
210. Matsumoto K, Miyazaki H, Fujii T, et al: Absorption, distribution and excretion of 3-(sulfamoyl[14C]methyl)-1,2-benziosoxazole (AD-810) in rats, dogs and monkeys and of AD-810 in men, *Arzneimittelforschung* 33:961–968, 1983.
211. Nishiguchi K, Ohnishi N, Iwakawa S, et al: Pharmacokinetics of zonisamide; saturable distribution into human and rat erythrocytes and into rat brain, *J Pharmacobiodyn* 15:409–415, 1992.
212. Walker RM, DiFonzo CJ, Barsoum NJ, et al: Chronic toxicity of the anticonvulsant zonisamide in beagle dogs, *Fundam Appl Toxicol* 11:333–342, 1988.
213. Ieiri I, Morioka T, Kim S, Nishio, et al: Pharmacokinetic study of zonisamide in patients undergoing brain surgery, *J Pharm Pharmacol* 48(12):1270–1275, 1996.
214. Stiff DD, Zemaitis MA: Metabolism of the anticonvulsant agent zonisamide in the rat, *Drug Metab Dispos* 18:888–894, 1990.
215. Nakasa H, Nakamura H, Ono S, et al: Prediction of drug-drug interactions of zonisamide metabolism in humans from in vitro data, *Eur J Clin Pharmacol* 54(2):177–183, 1998.
216. Sackellares JC, Donofrio PD, Wagner JG, et al: Pilot study of zonisamide (1,2-benzisoxazole-3-methanesulfonamide) in patients with refractory partial seizures, *Epilepsia* 26:206–211, 1985.
217. Boothe DM, Perkins J: Disposition and safety of zonisamide after intravenousand oral single dose and oral multiple dosing in normal hound dogs, *J Vet Pharmacol Ther* 31(6):544–553, 2008.
218. Hasegawa D, Kobayashi M, Kuwabara T, et al: Pharmacokinetics and toxicity of zonisamide in cats, *J Feline Med Surg* 10(4):418–421, 2008.
219. Orito K, Saito M, Fukunaga K, et al: Pharmacokinetics of zonisamide and drug interaction with phenobarbital in dogs, *J Vet Pharmacol Ther* 31(3):259–264, 2008.
220. Mimaki T: Clinical pharmacology and therapeutic drug monitoring of zonisamide, *Ther Drug Monit* 20:593–597, 1998.

221. Dewey CM, Guiliano R, Boothe DM, et al: Zonisazmide therapy for refractory idiopathic epilepsy in dogs, *J Am Anim Hosp Assoc* 40:285–291, 2004.
222. von Klopmann T, Rambeck B, Tipold A: Prospective study of zonisamide therapy for refractory idiopathic epilepsy in dogs, *J Small Anim Pract* 48(3):134–138, 2007.
223. Abou Khaled KJ, Hirsch LJ: Updates in the management of seizures and status epilepticus in critically ill patients, *Neurol Clin* 26(2):385–408, 2008.
224. Prasad A, Worrall BB, Bertram EH, et al: Propofol and midazolam in the treatment of refractory status epilepticus, *Epilepsia* 42(3):380–386, 2001.
225. Neff-Davis CA: Therapeutic drug monitoring in veterinary medicine, *Vet Clin North Am Small Anim Pract* 18(6):1287–1307, 1988.
226. Eadie MJ: Can anticonvulsant drug therapy 'cure' epilepsy? *CNS Drugs* 15(9):679–690, 2001.
227. Champney TH, Hanneman WH, Legare ME, et al: Acute and chronic effects of melatonin as an anticonvulsant in male gerbils, *J Pineal Res* 20(2):79–83, 1992.
228. Peled N, Shorer Z, Peled E, et al: Melatonin effect on seizures in children with severe neurologic deficit disorders, *Int J Neurosci* 90(3-4):223–232, 1997.
229. Löscher W, Lehmann H: Anticonvulsant efficacy of L-deprenyl (selegiline) during chronic treatment in mice: continuous versus discontinuous administration, *Neuropharmacology* 37(12):1587–1593, 1998.
229a. Lindvall-Axelsson M, Nilsson C, Owman C, et al: Inhibition of cerebrospinal fluid formation by omeprazole,, *Exp Neurol* 115(3):394–399, 1992.
230. Lipka LJ, Lathers CM: Psyoactive agents, seizure production, and sudden death in epilepsy, *J Clin Pharmacol* 27:169–183, 1987.
231. Tobias KM, Marioni-Henry K, Wagner R: A retrospective study on the use of acepromazine maleate in dogs with seizures, *J Am Anim Hosp Assoc* 42:283–289, 2006.
232. McConnell J, Kirby R, Rudloff K: Administration of acepromazinemaleate to 31 dogs with a history of seizures, *J Vet Emerg Crit Care (San Antonio)* 17(3):262–267, 2007.
233. Sawaki K, Ohno K, Miyamoto K, et al: Effects of anticonvulsants on local anaesthetic-induced neurotoxicity in rats, *Pharmacol Toxicol* 86(2):59–62, 2000.
234. Proulx J, Dhupa N: Severe brain injury. Part I, Pathophysiology, *Compend Contin Educ Small Anim Pract* 20:897–905, 1998.
235. Chesnut RM, Marshall LF, Marshall SB: Medical management of intracranial pressure. In Cooper PR, editor: *Head injury*, ed 3, Baltimore, 1993, Williams & Wilkins, pp 225–247.
236. Chesnut RM: The management of severe traumatic brain injury, *Emerg Med Clin North Am Neurol Emerg* 15:581–604, 1997.
237. Miller JD: Traumatic brain swelling and edema. In Cooper PR, editor: *Head injury*, ed 3, Baltimore, 1993, Williams & Wilkins, pp 331–354.
238. Jain KK: Neuroprotection in traumatic brain injury, *Drug Discov Today* 13(23-24):1082–1089, 2008.
239. Allen CH, Ward JD: An evidence-based approach to management of increased intracranial pressure, *Crit Care Clin Evidence Based Crit Care* 14:485–495, 1998.
240. Bagley RS: Intracranial pressure in dogs and cats, *Compend Contin Educ Small Anim Pract* 18:605–621, 1996.
241. Gruen P, Liu C: Current trends in the management of head injury, *Emerg Med Clin North Am Contemp Issues Trauma* 16:63–83, 1998.
242. Wakai A, Roberts I, Schierhout G: Mannitol for acute traumatic brain injury, *Cochrane Database of Systematic Reviews* 2007, Issue 1 Art. No: CD001049. DOI: 10.1002/14651858.CD001049.pub4.
243. Kamano S: Are steroids really ineffective for severely head injured patients? *Neurosurg Focus* 8:1–7, 2000.
244. Weiss MH, Nulsen FE: The effect of glucocorticoids on CSF flow in dogs, *J Neurosurg* 32:452–458, 1970.
245. Topsakal C, Erol FS, Ozveren MF, et al: Effects of methylprednisolone and dextromethorphan on lipid peroxidation in an experimental model of spinal cord injury, *Neurosurg Rev* 25(4):258–266, 2002.
246. Armitage-Chan EA, Wetmore LA, Chan DL: Anesthetic management of head trauma patient, *J Vet Emerg Crit Care* 17(1):5–14, 2007.
247. Jerram RM, Dewey CW: Acute thoracolumbar disk extrusion in dogs, Part I, *Compend Contin Educ Small Anim Pract* 21(10):922–930, 1999.
248. Smith PM, Jeffery ND: Spinal shock: comparative aspects and clinical relevance, *J Vet Intern Med* 19(6):788–793, 2005.
249. Coates JR: Intervertebral disk disease, *Vet Clin North Am Small Anim Pract* 30(1):77–110, 2000.
250. Griffin JF, Levine J, Kerwin S, et al: Canine thoracolumbar invertebral disk disease: diagnosis, prognosis, and treatment, *Compend Contin Educ Vet* 31(3):E1–E14, 2009.
251. Mann FA, Wagner-Mann CC, Dunphy ED`, et al: Recurrence rate of presumed thoracolumbar intervertebral disc disease in ambulatory dogs with spinal hyperpathia treated with anti-inflammatory drugs: 78 cases (1997-2000), *J Vet Emerg Crit Care* 17(1):53–60, 2007.
251a Pandya KA, Weant KA, Cook AM: High-dose methylprednisolone in acute spinal cord injuries: proceed with caution, *Orthopedics* 33(5):327–331, 2010.
252. Bush WW, Tiches DM, Kamprad C: Functional outcome following hemilaminectomy without methylprednisolone sodium succinate for acute thoracolumbar disk disease in 51 non-ambulatory dogs, *J Vet Emerg Crit Care* 17(1):72–76, 2007.
253. Levine JM, Levine GJ, Boozer L, et al: Adverse effects and outcome associated with dexamethasone administration in dogs with acute thoracolumbar intervertebral disk herniation: 161 cases (2000-2006), *J Am Vet Med Assoc* 232(3):411–417, 2008.
254. Wyndaele JJ: Complications of intermittent catheterization: their prevention and treatment, *Spinal Cord* 40(10):536–541, 2002.
255. Igawa Y, Wyndaele JJ, Nishizawa O: Catheterization: possible complications and their prevention and treatment, *Int J Urol* 15(6):481–485, 2008.
256. Levine JM, Levine GJ, Johnson SI, et al: Evaluation of the success of medical management for presumptive thoracolumbar intervertebral disk herniation in dogs, *Vet Surg* 36(5):482–491, 2007.
257. Levine JM, Levine GJ, Johnson SI, et al: Evaluation of the success of medical management for presumptive cervical intervertebral disk herniation in dogs, *Vet Surg* 36(5):492–499, 2007.
258. Toombs JP, Collins LG, Graves GM, et al: Colonic perforation in corticosteroid treated dogs, *J Am Vet Med Assoc* 188:145–150, 1986.
259. Bracken MB, Shepard MJ, Collins WF, et al: A randomized controlled trial of methylprednisolone or naloxone in the treatment of acute spinal injury, *N Engl J Med* 322:1405–4111, 1990.
260. Horlein BF, Redding RW, Hoff EJ, et al: Evaluation of naloxone, crocetin, thyrotropin releasing hormone, methylprednisolone, partial myelotomy and hemilaminectomy in the treatment of acute spinal cord trauma, *J Am Anim Hosp Assoc* 21:67–77, 1985.
261. Coates JR, Sorjonen DC, Simpson ST, et al: Clinicopathologic effects of a 21 aminosteroid compound (U74389G) and high dose methylprednisolone on spinal cord function after simulated spinal cord trauma, *Vet Surg* 24:128–139, 1995.

262. Jerram RM, Dewey CW: Acute thoracolumbar disk extrusion in dogs, Part II, *Compend Contin Educ Small Anim Pract* 21:1037–1046, 1999.
263. Blight AR, Toombs JP, Bauer MS: The effects of 4-aminopyridine on neurological deficits in chronic cases of traumatic spinal cord injury in dogs: a phase I clinical trial, *J Neurotrauma* 8(2):103–119, 1991.
264. Baltzer WI, McMichael MA, Hosgood GL, et al: Randomized, blinded, placebo-controlled clinical trial of N-acetylcysteine in dogs with spinal cord trauma from acute intervertebral disc disease, *Spine* 33(13):1397–1402, 2008.

28 Control of Pain in Small Animals: Opioid Agonists and Antagonists and Other Locally and Centrally Acting Analgesics

Dawn Merton Boothe

Chapter Outline

DEFINITION OF PAIN AND ITS RECOGNITION

Classification of Pain

The International Association for the Study of Pain (IASP) defines *pain* as an unpleasant sensory and emotional experience associated with actual or potential tissue damage.[1] During the past several decades, the importance of pain has evolved from being underestimated, to being recognized for its contributions to morbidity and mortality. In 2000 the Joint Commission on Accreditation of Healthcare Organizations[2] mandated that hospitals for humans consider pain as the fifth vital sign, thus ensuring its inclusion in the routine evaluation of all patients.

Pain has been classified in several ways. Severity (mild, moderate, and severe) is among the most common, but this categorization also includes an emotional component of pain. As such, in veterinary medicine this classification requires interpretation by either the clinician or owner. Pain also is classified according to its source. Physiologic pain is a protective mechanism, leading the animal to withdraw from a potentially damaging stimulus. In contrast, pathologic pain reflects tissue damage. Unresolved physiologic pain eventually can lead to pathologic pain by causing neurologic damage (also classified as neuropathic pain). Neuropathic pain is also classified according to the location at which the damage occurs (e.g., neurologic damage), with nociceptive pain reflecting tissue damage. Pain might also be localized to the body site: visceral pain is associated with abdominal or thoracic pain, whereas somatic pain originates from musculoskeletal damage. Either of these locations can be further divided as superficial or deep. Pain also is described by duration. Acute pain is abrupt in onset and resolves in 24 to 72 hours, whereas chronic pain is slow in onset and generally persists for several weeks to months. Acute pain is more protective in nature (compared with chronic pain) and indicates that something is going wrong, whereas chronic pain reflects disturbed homeostasis. Acute pain results from traumatic, surgical, or infectious events and generally is conducive to resolution with analgesics. In contrast, chronic pain is a long-standing physical disorder or emotional distress and includes pain associated with degenerative joint disease and some types of cancer. Chronic pain may not respond to traditional analgesic therapy, with tranquilizers or behavior-modifying drugs combined with environmental manipulation and behavioral conditioning commonly implemented. The transmission of chronic pain increasingly is being understood, with knowledge regarding neural pathways elucidating possible targets of therapy. Accordingly, newer drugs are increasingly being identified for their potential efficacy.[3]

KEY POINT 28-1 Whereas physiologic pain is protective, pathologic pain indicates tissue damage and if unresolved can lead to neurologic damage or neuropathic pain.

KEY POINT 28-2 Chronic pain may be more amenable to nontraditional analgesic therapy.

Transmission of Pain

Nociceptive Pain

Nociception refers to a neural response of nociceptors to a noxious stimulus.[1] Nociception is a normal nervous system function that serves as a warning of danger or credible threat. The nociceptive response comprises a nociceptor and three neuron chains, originating in the peripheral tissues and ending in the cerebral cortex. Nociception is unique among sensory nerves because nocicpetors must detect a wide range of stimuli, including physical and chemical signals, heat and cold, and acid and mechanical pressure. Nociceptors are located in every tissue of the body, originating from a group of neuronal bodies in the dorsal root ganglia (Figure 28-1). Nociception varies with location (peripheral versus central) and organ. Nociception in the skin occurs at the surface (i.e., is somatic), resulting in sharp, defined, localized, and limited pain. In contrast, internal, or visceral, nociception is generally diffuse, dull, and often referred.[4] The action potential stimulated by a nociceptor crosses the synapse in the dorsal horn and stimulates the second order neurons in the gray matter of the spinal cord. There the signal is transmitted to the brain, where it is processed and interpreted. The transmission of pain from nociceptors is carried by either small, myelinated A delta fibers, smaller unmylelinated C fibers, or A a fibers. A delta fibers are fast, being responsible for sharp and acute pain, and transmit somatic and parietal pain. Because these receptors are discrete,

Pathophysiology of neuropathic pain

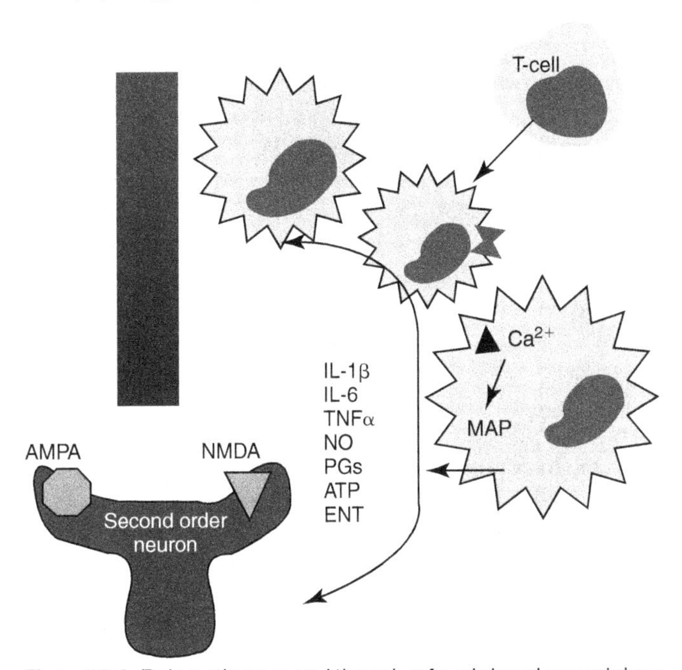

Figure 28-1 Pain pathways and the role of peripheral nerve injury in the emergence of neuropathic pain. See text for the transmission and perception of pain *(left).* The *right* side demonstrates mechanisms whereby neuropathic pain might emerge. The lower left diagram delineates the impact of peripheral nerve injury on sensory neurons. Injury is followed by recruitment and proliferation of non-neuronal elements (including Schwann cells, mast cells, macrophages, and T cells). Cells release pro-inflammatory and other chemicals (TNFα tumor necrosis factor-alpha] , IL[interleukin]-1, IL-6, CCL2, PGs (prostaglandins) and NGF [nerve growth factor]). Sensory abnormalities are initiated and maintained either locally at the site of damage or with retrograde transport to cell bodies in the dorsal root ganglion, where neuronal gene expression is influenced. Increased intracellular calcium results in activation of the p38 and MAPK/ERK pathway. Perpetuation of the response is maintained through recruitment of inflammatory cells in general and T-cells in particular. In the spinal cord *(upper right),* microglia surrounding primary afferent neurons contribute to self-propogation of neuropathic pain after activation by chemicals or the influence of other primary afferent neurons. Subsequent mediator release may presynaptically or postsynaptically modulate pain. Examples include but are not limited to TNF-α, IL-1 , IL-6, nitric oxide (NO), ATP, and PGs and excitatory neurotransmitters (ENT). *AMPA,* amino-3-hydroxy-5-methyl-4-isoxazole propionic acid; *NMDA, N*-methyl-D-aspartate; *MAP,* mitogen-activated protein kinases.

animals can localize this pain. In contrast, C fibers are slow, transmitting dull, aching, burning, or throbbing pain that is difficult to localize. A fibers also are slow, transmitting stimuli associated with vibration, stinging, or tickling. However, because they are not able to discriminate between painful versus nonpainful stimuli, they are not pure nociceptor neurons.

Chemical mediators are important components of the nociceptor reflex and offer a target of pharmacologic modulation. These include but are not limited to adrenocorticotropic hormone, glucocorticoids, vasopressin, oxytocin, brain opioids, catecholamines, angiotensin II, endorphins/enkephalins, vasoactive intestinal peptides, substance P (centrally), eicosanoids (prostaglandins, leukotrienes), tissue kininogens (bradykinin), histamine, serotonin, potassium, and proteolytic enzymes.[6] Several of these mediators are also associated with stress. Several neurotransmitters associated with nociception and transmission of peripheral pain also function in the dorsal horn, the first site of signal processing. Spinal neurotransmitters include but are not limited to peptides (e.g., substance P, calcitonin gene-related peptide), excitatory and inhibitory amino acids (aspartate, glutamate, gamma-aminobutyric acid [GABA]), nitric oxide, prostaglandins, adenosine-5'-triphosphate (ATP), endogenous opioids, monoamines (serotonin, norepinephrine), protons (acids), and neurotrophins. Opioid peptides are synthesized by interneurons in the superficial dorsal horn; they regulate further neurotransmitter release, probably through decreased calcium conduction. Glutamate, the primary excitatory nociceptor neurotransmitter, is released in response to calcium, following depolarization. Subsequent postsynaptic binding to N-methyl-D-aspartate (NMDA) receptors influences pain transmission, hyperalgesia, allodynia, and neurotoxicity, thus providing the rationale for combination analgesic therapy that includes NMDA-receptor antagonists.

KEY POINT 28-3 N-methyl-D-aspartate receptors and products of cyclooxygenase activity promote several aspects of neuropathic pain.

The IASP definition of pain includes both a sensory and emotional component.[2] Indeed, of all the sensory systems, the nociceptive system is most able to elicit an arousal response in the brain. The emotional portion of pain occurs at the level of the limbic system (emotional), cortex (cognitive appraisal), and frontal lobes. Stimulation in the reticular formation results in emotional reaction to pain (anxiety, depression, suffering), whereas stimulation in the cerebral cortex leads to conscious perception and interpretation of pain. Transmission of central pain reflects a "gate control" phenomenon. The dorsal horn cells modulate the patterns of incoming information transmitted to the brain, which ultimately produces response and perception. The brain, in turn, can enhance or counter nociception. For example, when pain is sustained, released opioid peptides bind mu receptors in the brain and spinal cord, decreasing pain. Modulation regulates pain response, thus maintaining homeostasis.[7] In addition to central transmission of pain, the first-order neuron can also synapse with neurons that cause a local reflex. The reflex can be myoneural or sympathetic in action (e.g., release of norepinephrine, smooth muscle spasm, vasoconstriction). Voluntary reflexes require conscious pain perception, whereas nociceptive reflexes do not.

Not surprisingly, a variety of mechanisms transduce nociceptive signals.[8] At least two classes of channels are involved: One class detects noxious stimuli or products of tissue damage, and another sets the threshold necessary for a nociceptor action potential. Channels that detect noxious stimuli include transient receptor potential (TRP) channels, acid-sensing ion channels (ASICs), and the ATP-gated P2X receptor family. Of these, the TRP channels are emerging as the dominant channels transmitting nociceptor signals. The TRP channels are general receptors, able to sense multiple types of noxious stimuli. Their actions are complex, with channels having different roles in different tissues. Further, each channel is able to respond to more than one stimulus and with overlapping sensitivities. Four of the nine currently described nociceptive TRP channels respond to heat. The TRP receptors are regulated through a number of kinases (e.g., kinase C, kinase A, calcium/calmodulin–dependent kinase). In contrast to the general TRP channels, ASIC channels are specialists, able to detect only acidity, as might occur with bone cancer (high levels of acid leak into surrounding tissues), inflammation (local pH can drop to 5.5), and ischemia (resulting from metabolites such as lactic acid). Because extracellular ATP is a major product of inflammation, P2X channels are also drawing interest for their potential role in inflammatory pain, particularly visceral pain.[7]

The second type of channels that transmit nociceptor signals set thresholds and include newly discovered voltage-dependent sodium channels. Unlike other sodium channels, these channels are resistant to blockade by tetrodotoxin (TTX), which serves as a method of identifying and classifying the channels. Normally, these channels set the nociceptor threshold very high. However, in the presence of pathology, thresholds are decreased such that nociceptors respond to much weaker stimuli. Thus, unlike most sensory systems, channels responsible for nociception become more sensitive, rather than less sensitive, to stimuli. The TTX-resistant sodium channels tend to be redistributed after tissue injury.

Neuropathic Pain

Pathophysiology. Nociception is not limited simply to transmission of acute (nociceptive) pain; it also contributes to neuropathic pain. Both acute and unrelieved chronic pain can shift from nociceptive to neuropathic pain. Neuropathic pain includes hyperalgesia (overreaction or increased sensitivity to painful stimuli), allodynia (reaction to an innocuous stimulation), or reflex sympathetic dystrophy. The latter is a complex disorder of pain, sensory abnormalities, abnormal blood flow, sweating, and trophic changes in superficial and deep tissues.[7] Failure to control development of acute pain and hyperalgesia can lead to chronic pain; progressive and prolonged stimulation can lead to a "wind-up" phenomenon that reflects increased excitation of neurons in the dorsal horn. The wind-up phenomenon is manifested as a pain response outside the site of injury and can persist beyond resolution of the inciting cause (pathologic pain). Dysesthesia is another example of neuropathic pain characterized by an unpleasant spontaneous or provoked sensation. Dysesthesia has been described in humans as a burning or shooting sensation reflecting damage to peripheral nerves. Excess stimulation of pain fibers, or reduced activity of non-nociceptive sensory pathways contribute to an imbalance between painful and nonpainful inputs to the central nervous system (CNS).[9] Examples include phantom pain, a centrally mediated pain manifested as an intense burning sensation at the nerve ending of a damaged, paralyzed, or missing extremity. Another example is "stump" pain, a peripheral neuropathic pain secondary to neuroma formation at the site of amputation. These are examples of pain without any obvious noxious input. Further, for some chronic or persistent pain disorders, pain does not necessarily originate at the periphery.[4]

Heightened pain sensitivity is probably a protective response, reducing tissue exposure to further risk of tissue damage, and normally resolves when the tissue is healed. Both local and spinal changes contribute to neuropathic pain. Tissue damage intensifies the sensation of pain by recruitment of otherwise silent receptors. Chemical mediators are produced and released by both neuronal and non-neuronal cells (e.g., fibroblasts, mast cells, neutrophils), increasing nociceptor sensitivity. Local injury causes release of inflammatory mediators (cyclooxygenase-2 [COX-2], interleukins [ILs], leukotrienes [LTs], H+, K+, histamine, bradykinin), generating a slightly acidic inflammatory milieu that lowers threshold sensitivity (allodynia) by facilitating chemical binding to nociceptors. Activation of the nociceptors initiates neurogenic inflammation, leading to the release of substance P and peptides, which in turn perpetuate inflammation.[5] Dysesthesia may reflect spontaneous activity originating in the regenerating, primary, nociceptive neurons (myelinated, small afferent fibers). Changes in dorsal root Na+ channels also have been reported. Dysesthesia may thus reflect a focal inflammatory process as opposed to axonal damage. Further, potential involvement of (fast) Na+ channels that generate ectopic discharges supports the use of local anesthetics (Na+ channel blockers) as part of a combined analgesic approach.[9]

Heightened sensitivity also involves retrograde signals from the site of injury to the neuronal cell body; signals alter neurotransmitter release and receptor transcription and expression. Among the mediators of hypersensitivity are mitogen-activated protein kinases (MAP: p38, ERK and JNK), which may initiate changes in the microglia of the dorsal horn.[6] These changes may persist for weeks. Other mediators released and associated with hypersensitivity in the spinal cord include but are not limited to the proinflammatory cytokines tumor necrosis factor (TNF), IL-1 and IL-6, prostaglandins, and reactive oxygen species. Microglial cell bodies also hypertrophy and multiply, a reaction that, along with release of proinflammatory cytokines, may be inhibited by minocycline. Interestingly, chronic morphine administration may activate microglial cells and thus exacerbate hypersensitivity, an effect that might be reversed by minocycline or pentoxifylline, exemplifying the complexities of hyperalgesia.[10]

A role for NMDA receptors has not yet been identified in normal spinal cord transmission. However, a role might be suggested in transmission of pain. Both glutamate and aspartate are major excitatory neurotransmitters in the CNS that bind to NMDA receptors. After tissue injury, impulses from sensitized nociceptors of C fibers stimulate glutamate and other chemical release (e.g., neurokinins) in the primary afferent in the spinal cord. Calcium influx and activation of early genes leads to the development and maintenance of hypersensitivity or the wind-up phenomenon and hyperalgesia. Hyperalgesia associated with opioid use may involve NMDA receptors (see later discussion). Another mediator group that may be involved with changes in response to pain is prostaglandins (PGs). Induced COX-2 prostaglandin E (PGE) has been associated with hyperalgesia in either the spinal cord (primary hyperalgesia) or peripherally at nociceptors (secondary hyperalgesia).[11] Induction of spinal COX-2 in the dorsal horn has been associated with central sensitization.[11-13] Finally, PGs may potentiate the effects of other chemical mediators involved in pain or inflammation (e.g., histamine, bradykinin, substance P, nitric oxide), neurotransmitters (e.g., inhibition of glycine or potentiation of glutamate), or other receptors (e.g., NMDA), although this role in central sensitization and hyperalgesia has yet to be determined.

Nociception may awaken long dormant processes. For example, GABA is normally inhibitory, but it becomes excitatory in the spinal cord after peripheral nerve injury.[7] Further, if the inciting cause is sufficient, quiescent nociceptors will be recruited; output of non-nociceptive neurons (e.g., touch receptors) may be interpreted as nociception by second-order neurons in the spinal cord.[5]

Preemptive control. Successful preemptive analgesia prevents the development of increased central nociceptive pathway responsiveness that is triggered by intense afferent neural activity. Surgery involving limbs exemplifies the importance of preemptive analgesia. For example, local anesthetic blockade of exposed nerves before transaction presumably protects the spinal cord from a sudden, massive impulse surge from nociceptors. Further, ghost phantom pain can be reduced through epidural analgesia or adequate prevention of postoperative pain, particularly during the first 72 hours after surgery.

KEY POINT 28-4 Effective preemptive analgesia decreases the emergence of neuropathic pain.

Meta-analyses of human studies that focused on timing of analgesia in surgical patients warrant review for their implications with regard not only to timing but also to the importance of effective pain control.[14,15] One meta-analysis examined randomized, double-blinded, controlled trials that addressed either preemptive or postoperative analgesia for acute or chronic postoperative pain relief. Analgesic protocols that were reviewed studied the following: Twenty of the clinical trials reported the analgesic efficacy of NSAIDs (n=20; diclofenac, ketorolac, ketoprofen, ibuprofen, flurbiprofen, and naproxen [endodontal]), opioids (n=8; morphine, fentanyl, alfentanil, sufentanil, meperidine), and NMDA antagonists (n=8; ketamine, dextromethorphan). Further, epidural, caudal, or intrathecal (n=20) or local anesthetics (n=20) were considered. Outcome measures included comparison of pain scores before and 24 hours after surgery, time to the need for analgesics, and the need for supplemental analgesic therapy.

In general, meta-analysis concluded that pre-emptive timing did not alter the magnitude of postoperative pain, although the consumption of analgesia and the time to request additional analgesics were reduced. For NMDA antagonism, preemptive use of ketamine (as part of combination analgesic therapy, generally with opioids) uniformly did not cause a statistical difference in postoperative pain (a finding substantiated by both meta-analyses), whereas dextromethorphan did, although only two trials were reviewed. For epidural analgesia 7 of 11 trials using opioids indicated potential benefits, although the authors concluded that clinical relevance would be improved if epidural analgesia continued for a longer postoperative period. In general, preemptive nonsteroidal antiinflammatory drug (NSAID) therapy provided no difference in pain relief, leading the authors to conclude that the risks associated with preemptive NSAID therapy (e.g., bleeding, renal compromise) may not be justified; the power of the study to detect a significant difference is not known. Only one of the trials addressed the advent of chronic (6 months) pain after a surgical procedure. This trial found chronic pain to be significantly reduced in patients receiving preemptive analgesia. The overall conclusions by the authors was that preemptive analgesia may not be an effective method for reducing postoperative pain. However, the authors also suggested that future studies should not focus on the timing so much as on the approach to prevention of postoperative pain. Specifically, studies might address the importance of aggressive control, including the use of combinations designed to prevent neuropathic pain. Indeed, the lack of evidence of effective preemptive analgesia for control of postoperative pain reported in this study may reflect failed actions that occur in clinical patients. Because even abbreviated sensory events may initiate events leading to central sensitization, effective prevention may be dependent on continuous sensory blockade—that is, throughout the presence of the stimulating nociceptive event. Further, the success of afferent blockade may depend on blockade of input from small nonmyelinated C fibers or spinal, rather than peripheral, analgesia. Indeed, the meta-analysis indicated that neither systemic morphine nor small doses of intrathecal opioids had an effective preemptive impact. However, larger intrathecal doses of morphine were effective. Thorough regional blockade may also be paramount to the success of preemptive operative analgesia.

PHARMACOLOGIC CONTROL OF PAIN

Analgesia reflects the selective interruption of the transmission of injury signals (real or potential) between primary sensory neurons, the spinal cord dorsal horn, the rostroventral medulla, and the cortex opioids.[5] The paradigm for the approach of pain control in both human and veterinary medicine has been shifting with the increasing realization that uncontrolled pain is not only bad but also avoidable.[16,17] Appropriate pain management is part of the practice of good medicine: For human patients, analgesic control is associated with more rapid clinical recovery, shorter hospital stays, fewer readmits, and improved quality of life.[1]

CONTROL OF PAIN

Assessing Response to Pain and Stress

One of the more difficult aspects of acceptable control of pain for the clinician is detection or recognition of pain.[19-21] Scientists agree that all animals feel pain, although the level of nociception may vary between vertebrates and invertebrates and among classes of animals.[22] Animals may feel pain as easily as human patients; any stimulus that is likely to cause pain in a person will cause pain in animals. Animals differ from people, however, in their response to pain. Indeed, the laws of behavior in wild animals require that abnormal behavior associated with pain be avoided. Avoidance, escape, or control of pain and distress are responses to pain that are important for (wild) animal survival and allow animals to adapt to a new or changed environment. Animals showing weakness, pain, and distress become targets for predators. Ill or injured animals tend to be abandoned by others so that an entire stock is not jeopardized. This evolutionary process makes clinical recognition of pain in animal patients difficult. For example, a critical patient is often unable to manifest pain and unwilling to care for itself; the clinician must be diligent to recognize the likelihood of an underlying disorder in causing pain. Increase in heart rate usually is caused by the underlying pathology, not in response to pain. The more severe the illness, the more important the need for analgesics.

Response to acute and chronic pain varies and includes both physiologic and behavioral changes. If pain is too severe for the animal to accommodate, a state of distress can develop.[23] Beyond protection, pain rarely has any useful function and is associated with dramatic and potentially life-threatening physiologic changes.[24-26] Physiologic responses to distress include gastrointestinal lesions, immunosuppression, and hypertension. In human patients failure of response to treatment, hospitalization duration, and hospitalization costs can be positively correlated with failure of effective pain control. The sensation of pain can be associated with a marked adrenergic (catecholamine) release, which may cause life-threatening hypertension or cardiac arrhythmias. Response to acute pain includes physiologic changes such as tachycardia, tachypnea, mydriasis, and salivation and behavioral responses such as guarding, protection, vocalization (especially with movement or palpation of painful area), licking, biting or scratching, shaking, restlessness or insomnia, and recumbency.

Failure to control acute pain can stimulate changes at the level of the nociceptor and CNS; nociceptive pain may progress to neuropathic pain. Neuroplastic changes such as hypersensitization or allodynia worsen the stress response that often follows surgery. The response is adaptive and is mediated by behavioral, neural, endocrine, immune, hematologic, and metabolic changes that attempt to restore homeostasis. However, the combined effects can prove detrimental to the patient. Potential sequelae include cardiovascular instability, hypercoagulability, insulin resistance, increased metabolic rate and protein catabolism, and immunosuppression. As such, effective control of pain is paramount in the postoperative or otherwise stressed patient.

Responses to chronic pain include limping; licking, perhaps to the point of self-mutilation (of an associated region if an animal can reach it, an unassociated one if not); reluctance to move; loss of appetite; changes in personality; physiologic dysfunctions such as dysuria, tenesmus, and diarrhea; changes in appearance of hair coat and degree of eye brightness; failure to groom; discharges from eyes and nose; decreased food and water intake; and behavioral changes such as aggression or docility, agitation, cringing, and extreme submissiveness. The well-trained clinician or pet owner can detect subtle changes in gait or posture.

Variability among animals in response to stress also makes diagnosis of pain difficult (Box 28-1).

The American Veterinary Medical Association reviewed the major consensus concepts generated by the Cross-species Approach to Pain and Analgesia workshop that took place in 2002.[22] In addition to recommendations regarding the use of animals in research involving pain, the review provides guidelines for development of a pain assessment tool. The guidelines stipulate that a numeric (1-10) scale, based on observable behaviors and quantifiable biological markers, be used. Factors that are likely to alter assessment include animal factors such as species (and strain), stage of development (including prepartum and postpartum development), gender, previous experience to pain; environmental factors; and the type of pain. Other factors, such as nutrition, drugs, concurrent disease, and owner social status, should also be considered. The American Society of Anesthesiologists developed a pain-scoring system (for humans) based on several categories, each scored from 1 to 15. Included are behavior (depressed = 1, normal = 3, apprehensive = 5, and excited or aggressive = 10), preexisting pain (none = 1, minimal = 5, moderate = 10, and severe = 15), surgically induced trauma or pain (minimal = 5, moderate = 10, and severe = 15), duration of surgery (less than 1 hour = 5, 1 to 2 hours =10, and >3 hours = 15), and patient health (normal = 1, mild disease = 2, severe disease = 3, moribund = 4, and life-threatening = 5).

Appropriate analgesic combinations for any pain group, regardless of score, include opioids, local analgesics, NSAIDS and (for surgical candidates) epidural analgesic therapy. For opioids scores less than 20 might warrant less aggressive control of pain (i.e., mixed agonists–antagonists or partial agonist opioids), whereas scores of 20 to 30 might require more aggressive analgesia (pure opioids) and scores of 30 the most aggressive therapy (e.g., constant-rate infusion [CRI] of pure opioids). The use of NMDA-receptor antagonists should be considered for members of the latter two groups. The prudent clinician might consider assessing pain using a numeric scale at intervals appropriate for the management of the pain and reassess therapy as indicated by the scale. This may be particularly important for prevention or treatment of chronic pain.

Box 28-1

Types of Biologic Response to Pain

Types of biologic response to pain vary with genetic, age, or physiologic state or makeup:

1. Age: Young animals may exhibit reduced tolerance to acute or physical pain. Lack of learned or conditioned responses thus may be less likely to lead to emotional stress or anxiety associated with anticipated painful experience.
2. Sex: Females appear to be less sensitive than males to pain.
3. Health: Healthy patients are less sensitive to pain, and severely debilitated animals are less able to respond to pain.
4. Species variation: Compared with cats, dogs tend to be stoic. Interestingly, however, cats appear to be treated with analgesics less commonly,[23] perhaps out of concern for adverse reactions.
5. Breed differences: Working and sporting breeds of dogs tend to be more stoic than other breeds.

Levels of Consciousness

Marked species differences exist in response to drugs intended to control or help control pain. *Analgesia* is defined as the absence of pain. This may be harder to define in animals than in people. *Tranquilization* (ataxia, neurolepsis) is a state of behavioral change in which the patient is relaxed and unconcerned by surroundings. Generally, the state is not accompanied by drowsiness, analgesia, or unconsciousness. Targets of tranquilizers include the hypothalamus and reticular activating system. The tranquilized animal feels pain but frequently is indifferent to minor pain. Tranquilizers may act synergistically with analgesics in the control of pain. *Sedation* reflects a mild degree of central depression. Sedated animals are calm, awake, and possibly drowsy. Sedatives target the cerebral cortex. With *anesthesia,* light to complete unconsciousness is realized and is accompanied by loss of feeling or sensation. *General anesthesia* is both a loss of consciousness and a loss of pain; it is also characterized by muscle relaxation, hyporeflexia, and amnesia. However, the loss of pain induced by general anesthesia may not be sufficient to preclude the intraoperative use of analgesics.

Two other states of consciousness may be associated with drugs that also provide analgesia. *Hypnosis* is a state of artificially induced unconsciousness (sleep) from which the patient can be easily aroused. *Akinesia* is simply the absence of muscle movements and is generally induced by neuromuscular blocking drugs. Pain may best be controlled with a balanced combination of drugs, each of which targets a different site in the nociception pathway.

Endogenous and Exogenous Pain Control

Endogenous opiates (opiopeptins) provide analgesia when released in high concentrations in selected regions of the brain. These include enkephalins, dynorphins, and endorphins (Figure 28-2). Each opiopeptin is derived from a larger precursor molecule. Each of the precursor molecules has a characteristic anatomic distribution that is not limited to the CNS. The precursor for endorphin (β-endorphin) is pro-opiomelanocortin, which is also the precursor of melanocyte-stimulating hormone as well as adrenocorticotropic hormone and beta-lipotropin, suggesting a strong link between the opioid system and stress hormones.[27] Endogenous recognition sites for these chemicals are also the targets of the exogenous drugs. A variety of other neuropeptides also have been implicated in endogenous analgesia

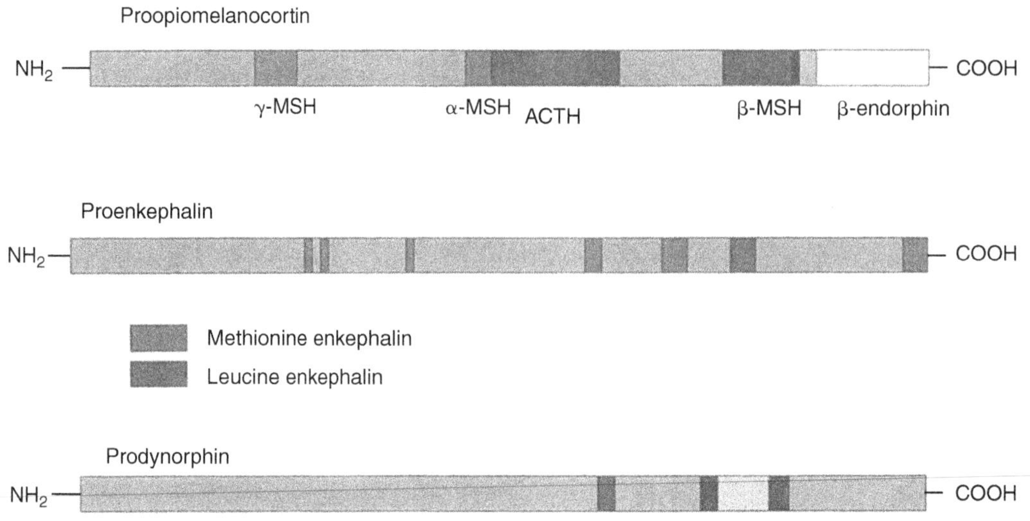

Figure 28-2 Endogenous opiopeptins that provide analgesia (endorphins, enkephalins, and dynorphins) are synthesized from precursor molecules. Each opiopeptin is derived from a larger precursor molecule. Each of the precursor molecules has a characteristic anatomic distribution that is not limited to the central nervous system The precursor for endorphin (β-endorphin) is proopiomelanocortin, which is also the precursor of melanocyte-stimulating hormone (MSH). Endogenous recognition sites for these chemicals are also the targets of the exogenous drugs.

(e.g., vasopressin, neurotensin, cholecystokinin, substance P). Some of these act in concert with other chemicals to stimulate nociceptors. Most notable are the eicosanoids (PGs, LTs), substance P, and bradykinin. The inflammatory process involves the release of a number of these chemical mediators either from the tissues at the site of infection or from the inflammatory cells themselves. Control of pain caused by these mediators is often largely dependent on controlling the inflammatory process. Nociceptin (NC, orphanin FQ, or OFQ) is a novel endogenous opioid peptide named for its ability to lower some pain thresholds. The NC/OFQ system is non-opioid, characterized by behavioral and pain modulator actions that differ from the classical opioids.[27] Nocistatin is a related protein of the NC/OFQ system.

KEY POINT 28-5 Exogenous opioids target receptors for endogenous compounds.

Factors such as emotional state, expectation, attention, blood pressure, stress, counterirritation, and drugs can modulate pain, possibly by activating analgesia systems. In humans national, religious, and cultural backgrounds and ethnicity also influence pain. Emotions also modify pain: Human patients function better when they believe that they have some control over pain, an aspect that may be lost or is difficult to assess in animals.[2]

Pain may be relieved or its intensity reduced by environmental (e.g., soft bedding) or behavioral (e.g., petting) manipulation and by the administration of drugs (Table 28-1).[28] With environmental control, emphasis is placed on the well-being of the animal. For dogs with osteoarthritis, this has centered on controlled exercise, although this method may be an inappropriate anthropomorphism. The single action for dogs most responsible for stress relief appears to be socialization (with humans). Factors such as emotional state, blood pressure, stress, and drugs can modulate pain, possibly by activating endogenous analgesia systems such as the opiates. The endogenous opiates, such as the enkephalins and endorphins, provide analgesia when released in high concentrations in selected regions of the brain.

The best treatment for pain is removal of the underlying cause. Control of pain often includes nonpharmacologic modalities. For example, the goal of pain control with chronic wounds in humans includes availability of both local and systemic analgesics but also removal of all nonviable, locally infected tissue and elimination of cellulitis, identification of wound pathogenesis, and assessment of objective improvement through the periodic use of an analgesic scale. Notably, the most important aspect of pain control in humans is objective assessment coupled with assuring the patient that pain will be resolved. The importance of the latter in animals is not known, nor is the ability of veterinary clinicians to provide such assurance.

At one time analgesics were categorized by their major site of action—that is, whether they acted centrally or peripherally. This categorization is limited because of the shared signals between the two locations (see Figure 28-1). Multiple target sites are available for drugs in both the peripheral nervous system and CNS; additionally, a large number of specialized receptors exist in the skin and other tissues that signal chemical, thermal, and mechanical changes. However, redundancies in their activation generally lead to compensatory effects by one system on blockade of another. This is particularly true for TRP channels and ASICs. As such, targeting sites of signal convergence may be more effective. Examples include sodium channels specific to the peripheral nociceptive afferents, glutamate receptors in the spinal cord, and their homologs in the trigeminal system (e.g., NMDA receptors that are uniquely activated by persistent input).[4]

Table 28-1 Doses of Selected Analgesic Drugs in Dogs and Cats

Drug	Indication	Dose	Route	Interval (hr)
Alfentanil	Preanesthetic	5 μg/kg	IV	To effect
	Analgesic supplement	2-5 μg/kg	IV	20 min
Amantadine	Combination analgesia	1.25 to 4 mg/kg (D)	PO	12-24
Amitriptyline	Behavioral problems, pruritis, neuropathic pain	1 to 4.4 mg/kg (D)	PO	12-24. Taper withdrawal
Atipamezole	Reversal agent for medetomidine	Volume equivalent to medetomidine	IV	As needed
Bupivacaine hydrochloride	Epidural analgesia	0.22 to 0.3 mL of 0.5% (max 6 mL/dog) (preservative free, methylparaben acceptable)	Epidural	Once
	Local anesthetic	0.5 to 1 mL of 0.25% solution	Topical, local	Once
		0.22 mL/kg	Intraarticular	Once
		1.5 mg/kg in 10 to 15 mL saline	Intrathoracic, intraabdominal	Once
Buprenorphine	Analgesia	<11 kg: 15 μg/kg (D)	IM, IV, SC	4-8
		11 to 23 kg: 10 μg/kg (D)	IM, IV, SC	4-8
		>23 kg: 5 μg/kg (D)	IM, IV, SC	4-8
		5 to 30 μg/kg (D)	IM, IV, SC, epidural	4-8
		5 to 30 μg/kg (C)	IM, IV, SC, topical (buccal)	12
Butorphanol	Antitussive	0.05 to 0.12 mg/kg (D)	PO, SC	8-12
		0.55 to 1.1 mg/kg (D)	PO	6-12
	Preanesthetic	0.05 to 0.4 mg/kg	IM, IV, SC	To effect
	Analgesia, sedation	0.1 to 1 mg/kg	IM, IV, SC	1-6
		0.55 to 1.1 mg/kg	PO	6-12
	Antiemetic	0.2 to 0.6 mg/kg	IM, SC	Once before chemotherapy
Cetacaine		Topical anesthetic		Topical to effect
Codeine	Cough	0.1 to 2 mg/kg (D)	PO	6-12
	Pain	0.5 to 4 mg/kg	PO	6-12
		1 mg with each 5 mg acetaminophen (dog only)	PO	8-12
	Diarrhea	0.25 to 0.5 mg/kg (D)	PO	6-8
Acetaminophen with codeine	Analgesic	10 to 15 mg/kg (D) (based on acetaminophen)	PO	8-12
Dimethyl sulfoxide 40%	Spinal cord trauma	0.5 to 1 g/kg (D). Dilute to a 10% solution	IV (over 45 min)	6-8
Dextromethorphan	Antitussive	0.5 to 2 mg/kg (D)	IV, PO,SC	6-8
	Combination analgesia, pruritis	2 mg/kg	IV, PO,SC	6-8
Fentanyl citrate	Analgesia	Loading dose: 5 μg/kg (D)	IV	Once
		Maintenance dose: 3 to 10 μg/kg (D)	IV, CRI	To effect
		Loading dose: 2 to 3 μg/kg (C)	IV	Once
		Maintenance dose: 2 to 3 μg/kg (C)	IV, CRI	To effect
		Maintenance dose: 2 to 3 μg/kg (C)	IV	20 minutes
	Perioperative pain	5 -10 μg/kg (D)	IM, IV, CRI, SC	To effect
		2.5-5 μg/kg (C)	IV, IV CRI	To effect
	Induction	1-5 μg/kg (D)	IV	To effect
		1-2 μg/kg (C)	IV	To effect

Continued

Table 28-1 Doses of Selected Analgesic Drugs in Dogs and Cats—cont'd

Drug	Indication	Dose	Route	Interval (hr)
Fentanyl citrate		0.01 mg/kg	Transdermal	2-5 days (approximate)
		25 μg/hr (C)	Transdermal	2-5 days (approximate)
		<10 kg: 25 μg/hr	Transdermal	2-5 days (approximate)
		10-20 kg: 50 μg/hr	Transdermal	2-5 days (approximate)
		20-30 kg: 75 μg/hr	Transdermal	2-5 days (approximate)
		>30 kg: 75 μg/hr	Transdermal	2-5 days (approximate)
Fentanyl/droperidol	Tranquilization	>25 kg: 75 μg/hr	IV	To effect
		0.3 to 0.5 mL/55 kg (D)	IV	To effect
		0.04 to 0.09 mL/kg (D)	IM	To effect
		0.01 to 0.14 mL/kg (D)	IM	To effect
	Preanesthetic	0.11 mL/kg (C)	IM	To effect
Gabapentin	Analgesic adjuvant, cancer pain	3 mg/kg	PO	24
	Analgesic, neuropathic pain	10 to 30 mg/kg (D)	PO	8
	Anticonvulsant	10 to 30 mg/kg	PO	8
Hydromorphone	Analgesia	0.05 to 0.3 mg/kg	IM, IV, SC	2-6
	Preoperative medication	0.1 mg/kg	IM, IV, SC	To effect
	Alternative induction medication	0.1 to 0.2 mg/kg	IV infusion	To effect
Ketamine hydrochloride	Sedation	7 to 11 mg/kg in combination with 1.1 to 2.2 mg/kg xylazine	IV	To effect
		22 mg/kg in combination with 1.1 mg/kg xylazine	IM	To effect
		5.5 to 10 mg/kg in combination with 0.3 to 0.5 mg/kg diazepam	IV	To effect
		6.6 to 11 mg/kg in combination with 0.066-0.22 mg/kg midazolam IM or IV	IM	To effect
		33 mg/kg in combination with 0.22 acepromazine	IM	To effect
		16 mg/kg in combination with 0.66 mg/kg acepromazine	IM	To effect
		5.5 to 22 mg/kg (adjunctive sedative or tranquilizer treatment recommended) (D)	IM, IV	To effect
	Anesthesia	22 to 33 mg/kg (C)	IM	To effect
		2.2 to 4.4 mg/kg (C)	IV	To effect
	N-methyl-D-aspartate antagonist (analgesia)	0.1 to 1 mg/kg	IM, PO, SC	4-6
	Systemic analgesia	Analgesia, with morphine and lidocaine	IV, CRI	To effect
Ketorolac tromethamine	Analgesia	0.5 mg/kg (D)	IM, IV, PO	12 × 2 doses
		0.25 mg/kg (C)	IM, IV, PO	8-12 × 2 doses
Levallorphan	Narcotic antagonist	0.02 to 0.2 mg/kg	IV	As needed
Levorphanol tartrate	Analgesia	22 μg/kg (D)	SC	As needed
Lidocaine	Dental nerve block	7 mg/kg (D)	At site	Once

Table 28-1 Doses of Selected Analgesic Drugs in Dogs and Cats—cont'd

Drug	Indication	Dose	Route	Interval (hr)
Lidocaine		2 mg/kg (C)	At site	Once
	Decreased cerebral blood flow	2.2 mg/kg	IV	Once
	Intraarticular intraoperative block	0.22 mL of 2% solution, max 5 mL	At site	Once
	Epidural analgesia	4.4 mg/kg (D)	Epidural	Once
		1 to 2 mg/kg (C)	Epidural	Once
		0.2 mL/kg of 2% (maximum 6 mL/dog; preservative free; methylparaben acceptable) (D)	Epidural	Once
	Analgesia with ketamine, morphine		IV, CRI	To effect
	Decreased cerebral blood flow			
Lignocaine	See Lidocaine			
Medetomidine hydrochloride	Chemical restraint, sedation, analgesia, muscle relaxant	0.75 to 1 mg/m^2	IM, IV	To effect
Meperidine hydrochloride	Analgesia, acute pancreatitis	3 to 10 mg/kg (D)	IM	As needed
	Sedation	5 to 10 mg/kg (D)	IM, IV (slowly)	As needed
		1 to 5 mg/kg (C)	IM	As needed
	Preanesthetic	2.5 to 6.5 mg/kg (D)	IM	To effect
		2.2 to 5 mg/kg (C)	IM, SC	To effect
Mepivacaine	Local anesthetic	Local infiltration as needed	Local infiltration	To effect
		0.2 mL/kg of 2%. Maximum 6 mL/ dog; preservative free; methylparaben acceptable) (D)	Epidural	Every 30 seconds until reflexes absent
Methadone	Analgesia	0.5 to 2.2 mg/kg (D)	SC, IM, IV	3-6
		0.2 to 0.5 mg/kg (C)	SC, IM	3-6
		0.05 to 0.2 mg/kg (C)	IV	3-6
	Preoperative	0.2 to 0.5 mg/kg (D)	IM, SC	Once
		0.1 to 0.2 mg/kg (C)	IM, SC	Once
Morphine SO_4	Supraventricular premature beats	0.2 mg/kg (D)	IM, SC	2-12 (determine dose and interval per patient)
	Analgesia	0.5 to 1 mg/kg (D)	IM, SC	2-12 (determine dose and interval per patient)
		1.5 to 15 mg/kg (D)	PO	12; variable dose reflects very erratic absorption
	Preanesthetic	0.1 to 0.2 mg/kg (D)	SC	To effect
	Antitussive	0.1 mg/kg (D)	SC	6-12
		0.05 to 0.1 mg/kg (C)	IM, SC	4-6
	Cardiogenic edema	0.1 mg/kg (D)	IV	As needed to effect
		0.25 mg (D)	SC	As needed
	Hypermotile diarrhea	0.25 mg/kg (D)	PO	4-6
	Spinal analgesia	0.3 mg/kg (D)	Epidural	Once
		0.1 mg/kg (C)	Epidural	Once
Nalbuphine hydrochloride	Analgesia	0.03 to 0.10 mg/kg (D)	IV	1-6, to effect

Continued

Table **28-1** Doses of Selected Analgesic Drugs in Dogs and Cats—cont'd

Drug	Indication	Dose	Route	Interval (hr)
Nalbuphine hydrochloride	Analgesia	0.2 to 0.5 mg/kg (D)	SC	8-12
		0.2 to 0.3 mg/kg (C)	SC	6-8
		0.75 to 1.5 mg/kg	IV	1-6, to effect
Nalmefene	Stereotypic behavior	1 to 4 mg/kg (D)	SC	
Nalorphine hydrochloride	Narcotic antagonist	0.1 mg/kg (D). Maximum of 5 mg	IV	To effect, repeat as needed
		0.1 mg/kg (C). Maximum of 1 mg	IV	To effect, repeat as needed
		0.44 mg/kg	IM, IV, SC	To effect, repeat as needed
		1 mg for every 10 mg of morphine	IM, IV, SC	To effect, repeat as needed
Naloxone hydrochloride	Stereotypic behavior	20 mg	SC	12
	Shock	2 mg/kg	IV infusion	Over 1 hour. Repeat hourly as needed to effect
	Opioid reversal	0.002 to 0.04 mg/kg	IM, IV, SC	To effect, repeat as needed
		0.04 mg/kg (D)	IM, IV, SC	To effect, repeat as needed
		0.02 to 0.1 mg/kg (C)	IV	To effect, repeat as needed
Naltrexone (Trexan)	Test dose	0.01 mg/kg	SC	Once
	Stereotypic behavior	1 mg/kg (D)	SC	12-24
	Behavioral disorders, lick granulomas	2.2 to 5 mg/kg	PO	12-24
	Behavioral disorders, adjuvant	25 to 50 mg/cat	PO	12
Oxymorphone	Sedation	0.05 to 0.1 mg/kg (D)	IM, IV, SC	To effect
		0.1 to 0.2 mg/kg (D)	IM, SC	To effect
	Preanesthetic	0.1 to 0.4 mg/kg	IM, IV	Once, to effect in combination with acepromazine, glycopyrrolate, or atropine
	Intraoperative analgesia	0.025 to 0.066 mg/kg (D)	IV	As needed
	Postoperative analgesia	0.05 to 0.1 mg/kg (D). Maximum of 4 mg	IM, IV, SC	1-6
		0.05 to 0.15 mg/kg (C)	IM, IV, SC	1-6. Tranquilizer may be necessary
		0.05 to 0.1 mg/kg (D) if cardiovascular disease	IV, IM, SC	2-4
	Analgesia	0.1 to 0.4 mg/kg (C)	IV	2-4 or to effect
	Restraint/sedation	0.02 to 0.1 mg/kg (C)	IV, IM, SC	Once, to effect. Tranquilizer may be necessary
	Anesthesia, during gastric dilation	0.1 to 0.2 mg/kg (D). Maximum of 3 mg	IM, IV	Once, to effect
Pentazocine	Analgesia	2.2-3.3 mg/kg (C)	IM, IV, SC	Maximum of every 4. May cause unacceptable dysphoria in cats
		1.65-36 mg/kg (D)	IM, IV, SC	

Table 28-1 Doses of Selected Analgesic Drugs in Dogs and Cats—cont'd

Drug	Indication	Dose	Route	Interval (hr)
Pregabalin	Chronic pain, anticonvulsant	4 mg/kg (D)	PO	8
Ropavacaine 0.5%	Analgesia	0.2 mL/kg of 0.5% solution (D). Maximum of 6 mL/dog; preservative free; methylparaben acceptable	Epidural	Once
Tramadol	Analgesia	1 to 4 mg/kg	PO	8-12
		2.5 to 5 mg/kg (D)	PO	4-6
		2 mg/kg (C)	PO	12
Xylazine	Sedation, analgesia, muscle relaxation	1.1 mg/kg (D)	IV	To effect
		1.1 to 2.2 mg/kg	IM, SC	To effect
	Hypoglycemic crisis	1.1 mg/kg (D)	IM	To effect
	Emetic	0.44 mg/kg (C)	IM	To effect
Xylocaine	See Lidocaine			
Yohimbine	Narcolepsy, xylazine reversal	50 to 100 μg/kg (D)	SC	8-12
		0.11 mg/kg (D)	IV	To effect
		0.25 to 0.5 mg/kg	IM, SC	12
		0.5 mg/kg (C)	IV	To effect

IV, Intravenous; D, dog; PO, by mouth; IM, intramuscular; SC, subcutaneous; C, cat; CRI, constant-rate infusion.

OPIATES

Among the most effective and potent drugs used for controlling pain in animals, particularly acute pain, are the centrally and peripherally acting opioid analgesics.

Definitions

Opiates, including morphine, codeine, and a number of semisynthetic or synthetic derivatives, are drugs derived from opium. A number of drugs are derived from thebaine, a component of opium. Opioids include all drugs that exhibit morphinelike activity, as either agonists or antagonists (Figure 28-3).[27] This includes all naturally occurring and synthetic drugs. The term *narcotic,* from the Greek word for *stupor,* is most appropriately used for any drug that induces sleep. The term has, however, become more associated with powerful opioid analgesics (which are more likely to be associated with sedation). Interestingly, endogenous opioid peptides exist in many animals, where they act as neurotransmitters and appear to act as modulators of neurotransmission or neurohormones. Their complete physiologic role has yet to be described; however, their existence was demonstrated in part by the ability of naloxone to reverse endogenous analgesia.[27] In addition to the endogenous opioids, several opium derivatives found in nature are also found in mammalian cells, usually conjugated or bound to proteins. These include morphine, codeine, and some related compounds.[29]

Mechanism of Action

Receptors

The existence of multiple opioid receptors was postulated on the basis of in vivo canine studies.[30] The pharmacologic effects result from interaction with one or more of three major opioid receptors named based according to the first letter of the first compound that bound to each receptor: mu (μ; morphine), kappa (κ; ketocyclazocine), and delta (δ). Receptors are similar in structure, expressing at least 40 homologies.The NC/OFQ receptor is a fourth member of the class whose similarity to opioid receptors is based on receptor homology. As with sigma receptors, they do not bind to classical opioid ligands. However, changes in as few as four amino acids would allow the nociceptin receptors to bind to classical opioids. Sigma receptors are no longer considered opioid receptors; they bind to and are activated by drugs completely unrelated to opioids. Opioid receptors also are chronologically classified, with OP-1 (δ) discovered first, followed by OP-2(κ), and OP-3 (μ) (the most recently discovered). The Committee on Receptor Nomenclature and Drug Classification has indicated a final designation: MOP, DOP, and KOP, reflecting mu (μ), delta (δ), and kappa (κ) opioid receptors, respectively.[27] This latter classification will predominate in this chapter. Nociceptor receptors are classified as OP4 or NOP. Other opioid receptors (e.g., epsilon) may reflect splice variants or diamers.

Each of the opioid receptors is subtyped: μ-1, μ-2, κ 1-3, and δ1 and δ-2, with differences in structure probably generated after translation. Receptors vary in several characteristics that complicate predictive responses. The μ-1 or MOP_1 receptors are described as very high affinity receptors that do not discriminate well between μ and δ. Dimerization among the receptors may play a role in their differential effects; thus far, both δ κ and δμ diamers have been identified. Differential affinity of the heterodiamerized receptors compared to homodiamers for selected ligands (endogenous peptides or drugs) markedly alters the pharmacologic response. Further, binding

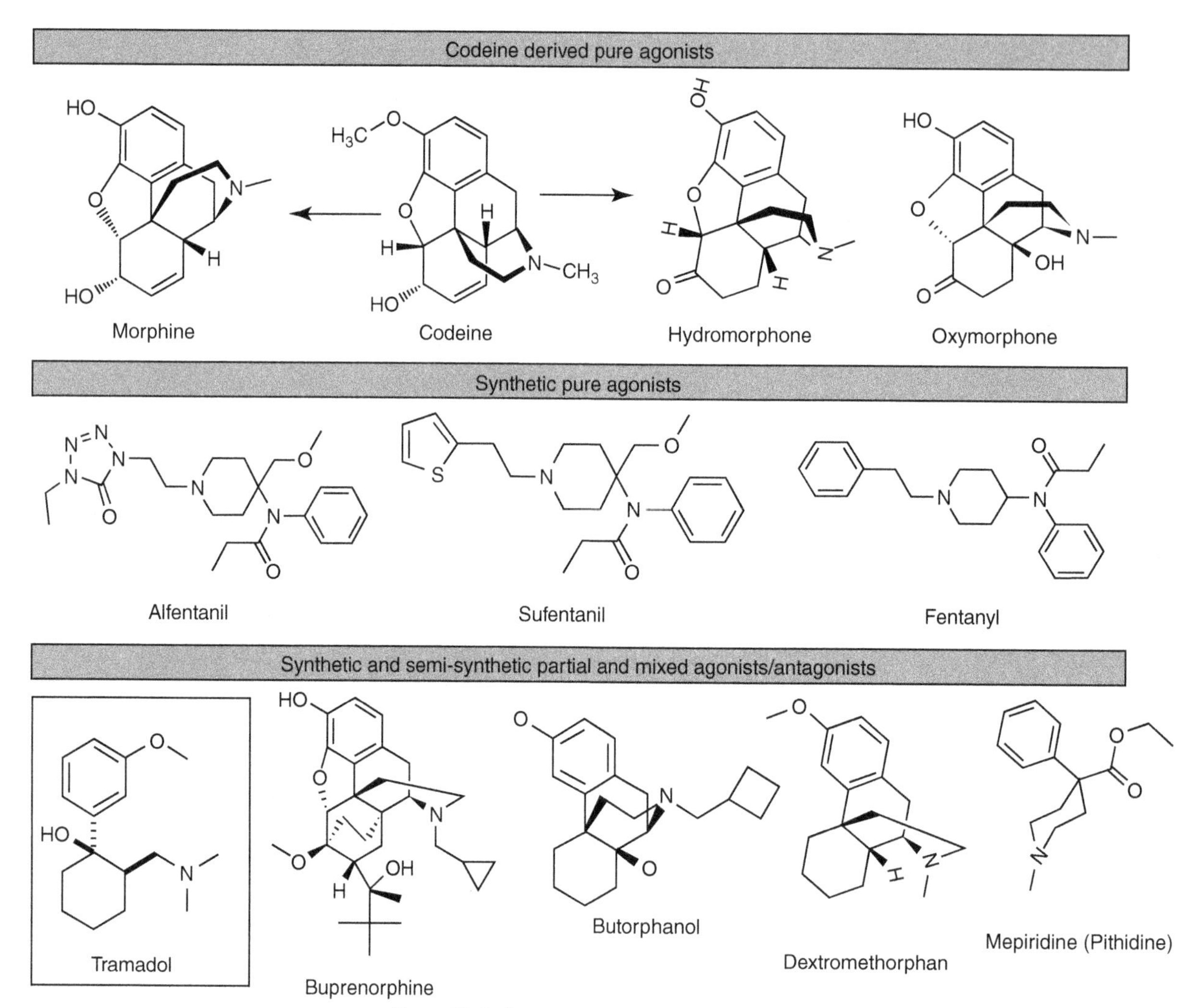

Figure 28-3 Structures of selected opioids.

sites of peptides are different from those of alkaloids (drugs): The latter appear to fit completely inside or at the mouth of the receptor core, whereas peptides appear to bind to extracellular loops. Differential binding sites allows for differential ligand effects, influencing conformation and subsequent responses. Opioid receptors differ from many other receptor systems in that a large number of endogenous ligands interact with a small number of receptors, potentially limiting the precise control that characterizes most systems.[27] However, mechanisms whereby distinct responses to endogenous opioids might occur despite the lack of apparent substrate specificity include differences in duration of action, activation of multiple receptors or their heterodimers, production of endogenous opioids with unique activation profiles (perhaps in part through differential responses at the level of intracellular signaling), and differences in intracellular trafficking of the receptors themselves (see the discussion of adaptation). These mechanisms offer means by which pharmacologic interventions might be designed to generate the desired opioid response.

Opiate receptors occur throughout the body but are in high density in the dorsal horn of the spinal cord, where they are responsible for modulating pain reception. The NC/OFQ system is distributed in the hippocampus, cortex, and selected sensory sites and is responsible for complex behavior.[27] Peripherally, receptors also are located in the spleen, kidney, intestine, vas deferens, and retina.[31] These include effects on drug reward and reinforcement, stress responsiveness, and feeding behavior. The system is closely related to stress processes. Lester and Traynor[32] demonstrated in vitro that the effect of commonly used opioids correlated to their binding of opioid or NOP receptors throughout the brain and spinal cord of dogs.

Pharmacodynamics

It is likely that species differences in receptor number, location, and specificity or sensitivity to the various drugs are important to differences in response to the opiates. Additionally, the type of interaction between ligand and opioid receptor influences the response. Ligands may act as *agonists* (which bind and stimulate) or *antagonists* (which block and inhibit the effect). Endogenous antagonists generally have no direct effect but occasionally may inhibit normal functions (e.g., appetite or release of selected hormones). For example, agonists increase whereas antagonists decrease appetite effects of endogenous opioids. *Mixed agonists* exhibit variable binding specificities at each receptor type, with some sites being agonistic and other sites antagonistic (e.g., butorphanol is a KOP agonist and MOP antagonist). *Partial agonists* do the same as mixed agonists, but their positive interaction with the receptors occurs with less than full activity at some of the receptors. The magnitude of each ligand–receptor interaction is likely to vary among species.

KEY POINT 28-6 Predictability in opiod response is confounded by receptor subtype and species differences in receptor type or subtype, tissue distribution, and receptor–drug interactions.

The cellular mechanism and the pharmacologic effects of the opioids probably reflect several different effector mechanisms. All three opioid receptors are coupled to G proteins. Accordingly, they inhibit adenylyl cyclase activity and activate receptor-linked potassium currents while decreasing voltage-gated calcium currents. The proposed, but as yet unproven, analgesic mechanism thus may reflect hyperpolarization of the neuronal resting membrane potential. Further complicating the understanding of their mechanism is their potential to affect other secondary messenger systems. They may activate MAP kinases and phospholipase C (PLC) mediated cascades that lead to formation of inositol triphosphate and diacylglycerol. Other actions include inhibition of neurotransmitter release (acetylcholine, glutamic acid, dopamine, serotonin, substance P [particularly peripherally], norepinephrine), or modulation of a potassium channel. Control of pain appears to occur without diminution of other senses. The NC/OFQ receptors also are linked to G proteins, as has been demonstrated in dogs.[31]

The pharmacologic effects of opioid derivatives, including the degree of analgesia, depends on the receptor bound, the location of receptor and drug in the body, and the type of interaction between the opioid and the receptor (Table 28-2).[29] Opioids act centrally to elevate the pain threshold and alter the psychologic response to pain. The opioids also act peripherally. The primary pharmacologic effects of all opioids are analgesia, euphoria, and sedation (without loss of consciousness).[29] MOP receptors give rise to analgesia and sedation above the spinal cord (MOP_1) or in the spinal cord (MOP_2); interaction with central MOP receptors might provide greater analgesia than interaction with spinal MOP receptors. For example, morphine causes analgesia primarily by way of MOP_1 receptors when given systemically.[29] However, administration of morphine at both spinal and supraspinal sites results in synergistic analgesic effects, with a tenfold reduction in the total dose of morphine necessary at either site alone.[29]

KEY POINT 28-7 Analgesia, euphoria, and sedation reflect interaction with MOP or KOP receptors.

Table 28-2 Opioid Receptors, Their Pharmacodynamic Effects, and the Impact of Drug–Receptor Interaction

Receptor Type	Target	Agonist	Antagonist	Drug	Effect
MOP	Spinal Analgesia (MOP-1)	Increase	NE	Methadone	3+
	Supraspinal Analgesia (MOP-2)	Increase	NE	Morphine	3+
	Sedation	Increase	NE	Fentanyl	3+
	Appetite	Increase	Decrease	Sufentanil	3+
	Respiratory function	Decrease	NE	Etorphine	3+
	Gastrointestinal	Increase	NE	Oxymorphone	3+
	Acetylcholine	Decrease	NE	Butorphanol	Partial
	Dopamine	Decrease	NE	Buprenorphine	Partial
	Prolactin release	Increase	Decrease	Pentazocine	Partial
	Growth hormone release	Increase	NE	Naloxone	3-
	Physical dependence	Increase	NE	Naltrexone	3-
				Nalorphine	3-
KOP	Spinal analgesia	Increase		Etorphine	3+
	Supraspinal analgesia	Increase		Butorphanol	3+
	Sedation	Increase		Sufentanil	1+
	Appetite	Increase		Morphine	1+
	Gastrointestinal	Increase		Buprenorphine	2-
				Naloxone	2-
				Naltrexone	2-
DOP	Spinal analgesia	Increase		Etorphine	3+
	Supraspinal analgesia	Increase		Sufentanil	1+
	Appetite	Increase		Naloxone	1-
	Dopamine	Decrease		Naltrexone	1-
	Growth hormone release	Increase			

MOP, KOP, DOP, are mu, kappa, and delta opioid receptors, respectively. *NE,* No effect.

Interaction with MOP receptors also causes euphoria, respiratory depression, and physical dependence.[33] MOP receptors located in the gastrointestinal tract mediate the pharmacologic effects characteristic of opiates in this body system. KOP receptors (three subtypes) are responsible for analgesia that is spinal in origin and stimulate miosis and sedation. Interestingly, stimulation of KOP receptors appears to cause effects antagonistic to MOP receptors, including analgesia, tolerance, and reward.[33] DOP receptors (two subtypes) are located on smooth muscle and lymphocytes, in addition to the CNS. Interaction with DOP receptors appears to modulate, among other effects, emotional behavior and immunomodulation (see Chapter 26). Sigma receptors interact with a selected synthetic opioids; positive interactions between drugs and these receptors provide no analgesia but do cause adverse events including dysphoria, hallucinations, respiratory stimulation, and some of the vasomotor responses.

The pharmacologic effects of opioids extend beyond control of pain. For example, nonanalgesic pharmacologic effects account for many of the side effects associated with the use of these drugs for control of pain. The effect of opioids on the immune system is discussed in Chapter 31. The cardiovascular system in particular offers an example of the nonanalgesic pharmacodynamic effects of opioids. Opioid receptors regulate the cardiovascular system centrally (hypothalamus and brainstem) and peripherally (cardiac myocytes and blood vessels). In the heart both KOP and DOP, but not MOP, receptors have been identified.[34] Appetite is influenced by all three receptor types, with agonists increasing and antagonists decreasing response (see Chapter). DOP opioid receptors interact (by way of the G protein) with several K+ cardiac channels, and KOP opioid receptors interact with calcium cardiac channels.[34] Opioid receptors appear to be involved both in the physiology of the normal myocardium and pathophysiology of disease. DOP receptors appear to attenuate adrenergic response and decrease cardiac performance yet also inhibit acetylcholine-induced vagal bradycardia; suppress baroreceptor responses; and increase inotropy, chronotropy, and blood pressure. In contrast, KOP have been associated with arrhythmias. The impact of opioids on the myocardium is, not surprisingly, complex. On the one hand, opioids appear to facilitate arrhythmias and other disturbances associated with circulatory shock, congestive heart failure, and myocardial ischemia and reperfusion injuries. Yet, opioids appear to protect the heart (and several other organs) from hypoxic or ischemic insults. For example, large amounts of endogenous opioids are released in the heart in response to a number of stimuli, including ischemia, leading to a cardioprotective effect. During acute myocardial ischemia, morphine attenuates neutrophils and endothelial activation and reduces adhesion molecules.[34] Indeed, opioids (endogenous) appear to be involved in ischemic preconditioning. This phenomenon involves the protective effect of coronary artery occlusion before a prolonged ischemic insult; irreversible tissue damage is prevented, and ATP depletion is reduced.[34]

Administration of nociceptin (FOQ ligand) causes a broad range of physiologic changes, with the often contradictory responses depending on the site of administration. These include antinociception or pronociception, anxiousness, altered appetite and cardiovascular effects (depression).[31] Nociceptin also influences transmission at GABA receptors.[35]

Pharmacokinetics

Most opiates are well absorbed after oral, subcutaneous, or intramuscular administration (see Table 28-4 later in this chapter). In an attempt to reduce side effects without loss of analgesic activity, while improving the convenience of opioid administration, a number of alternative routes of administration have been studied. Oral, transmucosal (transbuccal), and rectal routes are examples discussed with individual drugs. Additionally, intranasal administration of opioids has been reviewed in humans.[36] First-pass metabolism precludes oral as a reasonable route of administration for most opiates. Oral administration can be facilitated with a higher dose (if safe), slow-release products, or generation of active metabolites. For example, morphine is only 25% bioavailable in humans after oral administration. However, it is used effectively through oral administration for control of cancer pain in humans.[29] In veterinary medicine use of oral opioids has been limited to codeine (60% bioavailability), hydrocodone, and (at high doses) butorphanol but more recently includes morphine. Morphine is also available as a slow-release oral (and limited injectable) preparation. Buprenorphine (including compounded products) has been used successfully after oral administration. Naltrexone is a pure antagonist, similar in actions to naloxone, which is also orally bioavailable. Selected drugs, including morphine, are available as rectal suppositories.

Drugs for which intranasal pharmacokinetics have been described include fentanyl, pethidine, butorphanol, oxycodone, and buprenorphine. In contrast to other mucosal routes of administration, lipophilicity does not appear to be a major determined of drug absorption through the nasal mucosa; indeed, nasal bioavailability of the opioids studied in humans ranges from a low of 46% for buprenorphine to a high of 71% for fentanyl and butorphonal, with the time to maximum concentrations generally being as little as 5 minutes and less than 50 minutes. Adverse effects were drug- (opioid-) related effects, rather than damage to the nasal mucosa. Limitations to this route of administration include the volume (limited to 150 μl per nostril) and pharmacokinetic variability, which tended to exceed that for intramuscular and subcutaneous administration. Both of these limitations may have reflected the use of the intravenous preparations: administration of an appropriate dose at times required a volume that exceeded that recommended, leading to pharyngeal delivery and subsequent swallowing (oral administration). Current interest in this route as a method of patient-delivered analgesia may lead to approval of products prepared with the intent of intranasal administration.

Transdermal preparations are available for systemic delivery of selected very lipid-soluble products (e.g., fentanyl patch.). In general, transdermal gels have not been successful in the systemic delivery of opioid analgesics, although limited efficacy may ultimately be demonstrated for selected lipid-soluble opioids (e.g., buprenorphine: unpublished work by the author). Epidural or intrathecal administration results in penetration of the spinal cord with limited systemic effects. Drugs that are more lipid soluble (e.g., fentanyl) tend to move rapidly across the dura into the spinal tissue and thus have a rapid, albeit local response. Drugs that are less lipid soluble, such as morphine, do not distribute rapidly into the spinal cord. Therefore they are more likely to diffuse up or down the spinal cord, potentially providing a larger area of analgesia. However, the use of epidural opioids alone for control of postoperative analgesia might be reconsidered for some patients. In children continuous epidural infusion of fentanyl and bupivacaine was found to be superior to intermittent epidural morphine in children undergoing major abdominal or genito-urologic surgery, as is supported by other human studies.[37]

KEY POINT 28-8 First-pass metabolism that precludes oral absorption of most opioids and a desire to avoid intravenous administration have led to a number of alternative routes of opioid delivery.

Distribution of the opioids from blood into the CNS varies. Most opiates are sufficiently lipid soluble to distribute into the CNS, although the rate into and out of the CNS is variable. Generally, onset of action occurs most rapidly for the highly lipid-soluble drugs (heroin, codeine) but is countered by rapid movement out of the CNS and thus resolution of pharmacologic response. The amphoteric opioids such as morphine move less rapidly, take longer to be effective, and generally act longer. Some opiates, such as loperamide, are designed to poorly penetrate the CNS with the intent of having peripheral (e.g., gastrointestinal) effects only. In the developing fetus, opioid derivatives pass more easily into the CNS because the blood–brain barrier is not fully developed. In humans the developing fetus can suffer severe depression induced by opiates, despite no evidence of depression in the pregnant mother.

Most of the opioids are biotransformed by the liver. Glucuronide conjugation is a common metabolic pathway. In some species metabolitesmay be active, including glucuronide metabolites. Cats may be deficient in some of these pathways, contributing to the increased risk of overdose that occurs with this species. Hepatic elimination for many drugs is "flow limited," meaning that hepatic blood flow determines the rate of elimination. Thus liver disease, particularly that associated with portal to systemic vascular shunting, renders a patient susceptible to adverse reactions (toxicity). Hepatic metabolites are renally excreted. Elimination of the bile and enterohepatic circulation for some drugs may, however, prolong pharmacologic effects. In general, the opioids are very rapidly eliminated in normal animals, with elimination half-lives ranging from 30 minutes to 2 hours and duration of action being less than 2 hours in many animals for many of the drugs. For selected drugs (morphine, oxymorphone, buprenorphine), pharmacologic effects may remain for up to 6 hours, depending on the type of pain, species, and route of administration. Formation of active metabolites also affects (prolongs) duration of effect. Adherance to receptors may play a role in duration of affect of some drugs (e.g., buprenorphine).

Altered response to the opioids should be expected among species, in very young and very old patients,[38] and in patients suffering from hepatic, cardiovascular, or respiratory disease; hypotension; cranial trauma; and (in cats) hyperthyroidism. The duration, but not the extent, of analgesia increases with age in human patients,[29] presumably because of changes in hepatic metabolism and hepatic blood flow. Doses are decreased up to 75% in some patients, particularly geriatric patients or those with liver disease. However, prolonging the interval, rather than decreasing the dose, should be a more effective means of compensating for the effects of opioids normally characterized by a short half-life unless volume of distribution changes result in higher plasma concentrations as well. An exception is with CRI, for which doses should be decreased. Both liver disease and renal disease can alter the disposition of opioids, leading to adverse effects. Renal disease affects the elimination of morphine, codeine, and meperidine, in part because of the accumulation of active metabolites.[29]

Adverse Effects

Central Nervous System

The major disadvantages of opioids reflect general CNS depression, including dose-related respiratory depression and, to a lesser degree, cardiac depression. CNS depression tends to preclude the use of opioids in syndromes such as shock, severe cranial trauma, and diseases associated with respiratory compromise. Synthetic opioids were designed to induce analgesia with minmal undesirable side effects (i.e., sedation, respiratory depression).

Sedation is common with opioid use, depending on the drug and its target receptors, and the species (i.e., MOP and to a lesser degree KOP receptor stimulation in the dog) and can be a disadvantage or an advantage, depending on the clinical situation. Species differences in response to the sedative effects of opioids can be profound. "Morphine mania," typical of that described in cats is manifested as dysphoria and psychomotor activity. It may reflect sigma receptor stimulation for selected opioids or simply may reflect overdosing. Opioids tend to cause release (rather than inhibition) of some neurotransmitters (e.g., dopamine, acetylcholine), and this may occur in cats with high doses. When opioids are used in combination with phenothiazine derivatives (which block many of the neurotransmitter actions), the incidence of adverse effects appears to be reduced in cats. Dogs also are subject to dysphoria, as is exemplified by a series of three cases reported by Hofmeister and coworkers.[39] Dysphoria was manifested as vocalization that began within 5 minutes of administration of either hydrocodone, morphine, or fentanyl in association with postoperative analgesia. Clinical signs abated with administration of naloxone.

KEY POINT 28-9 Synthetic opiods are designed to minimize cardiovascular or respiratory adverse effects without sacrificing analgesic efficacy.

Respiratory depression usually is the cause of death in humans who succumb to opioids. The mechanism is reduction in the responsiveness of the brainstem respiratory centers to carbon dioxide, the primary stimulation for respiration. Centers that regulate respiratory rhythm are also depressed.[29] Depression, manifested as a slow respiratory rate, is discernible at doses lower than those associated with sedation and increases as the dose increases. Rate, tidal volume, and minute volume all decrease. Respiratory depression is, however, rarely a clinical concern except in cases of overdose or in the presence of pulmonary dysfunction in cases of standard doses.[29] Opioids should be used cautiously in patients with compromised respiratory function. Patients may appear to be handling the drugs well but in fact may be using compensatory mechanisms such as increased respiratory rate.[29] Concentrations of CO_2 may be increased, and respiratory centers may already be less sensitive to CO_2. The administration of an opioid may be dangerous in such situations. Use of opioids in the pregnant animal can lead to marked respiratory depression in the developing fetus, with little to no effect on the mother, because of the underdeveloped blood–brain barrier in the fetus.[29]

KEY POINT 28-10 "Morphine mania" in cats may simply reflect neurotransmitter release at relatively higher doses.

Opioids have precipitated attacks of asthma in human anesthetized patients, probably as a result of histamine release. The importance of this in animals is not clear.

Opioids increase intracranial pressure as a result of increased concentrations of CO_2 and cerebral vasodilation. Cerebrospinal fluid (CSF) pressure also increases.[29] These effects may be exaggerated after head injury. The effects on intraocular pressure are not clear and may vary with the species. In humans accommodation is increased, with a decrease in intraocular pressure. Opioids cause miosis in humans, and mydriasis occurs in some species. Mydriasis may impede vision in cats; cats will be sensitive to light until mydriasis resolves.[43]

Convulsions occur in some species when opioids are administered in high doses. Mechanisms probably include inhibition of GABA and may be more likely with morphinelike drugs.[29] The convulsant effects of some opioids can be reversed by naloxone,[29] suggesting that drugs with antagonistic actions (e.g., butorphanol, buprenorphine) at some receptors might be preferred in the patient having seizures. The impact of opioids on epileptic patients is not clear.

Morphine and related opioids directly depress the cough center at concentrations lower than that required for analgesia. Respiratory depression and cough suppression do not appear to be related. Thus antitussive opioids do not necessarily cause respiratory depression.[29]

KEY POINT 28-11 Morphine and related drugs directly suppress cough without causing respiratory depression.

In contrast to depression, opioids directly stimulate the chemoreceptor triggering zone and thus may cause nausea and vomiting. Individual differences in the emetic response to opioids are marked in humans, but the amount of variability is not clear in animals.[29] In human patients in whom opioids cause emesis, after subsequent administration, opioids act as antiemetics, blocking further response by the chemoreceptor trigger zone to opioids. Actions at the vestibular apparatus may also be responsible for emesis. The emetic effects that typify administration of opioids as sole agents do not typically occur in the postoperative, sick, or pain-ridden patient. Butorphanol has been used in some species as an antiemetic to control vomiting induced by cisplatin.[44] In the awake dog, at doses associated with sedation, MOP agonists (morphine, fentanyl, and methadone) prevent emesis induced by apomorphine and copper sulfate. At lower doses morphine was able to cause emesis. KOP agonists also blocked the apomorphine emetic response at sedative doses. Antiemetic effects were blocked by naloxone. In contrast, DOP agonists did tend to cause emesis, leading the authors to conclude that delta receptor stimulation is associated with emesis, but MOP and KOP receptor stimulation with antiemesis.[45] Nausea, vomiting, and salivation are associated with morphine or hydromorphone administration in cats. Buprenorphine, butorphanol, or meperidine are unlikely to be associated with these side effects.[43,46] Decreased appetite may occur after several days of continuous opioid treatment in cats.[43] Urinary retention has been described for MOP-active opioids in animals, although effects may vary with species.[47] Mechanisms may reflect a centrally mediated vasopressin effect on the kidneys. Alternative mechanisms may include opioid-induced hypotension, which is probably more likely with morphine. Anderson and Day[47] demonstrated that both fentanyl and morphine decreased urine output in normal and traumatized dogs.

Both long- and short-term use of opioids has paradoxically been associated with hyperalgesia. A biphasic, dose-dependent effect has been described and may reflect an initial increase in excitatory neurotransmitters. The hyperalgesic effects of opioids may involve NMDA receptors. Opioids appear to increase NMDA neural currents, providing a rationale for the combination of opioids with NMDA antagonists for enhanced analgesia. Several types of opioid hyperalgesia have been described both experimentally and clinically. At low doses, probably a reflection of disinhibition, intrathecal opioids induce an excitatory effect, which is otherwise masked with the sedation typical of larger doses. In contrast, very high intrathecal doses stimulate allodynia. With single-dose opioids, increased nociception may appear as the opioid effect diminishes. This may be manifested as an increased postoperative need for analgesia in patients receiving short-acting opioids intraoperatively. Reversal of opioids with naloxone often produces marked hyperalgesia. Hyperalgesia has also been associated with chronic use; among the clinical sequelae might be marked hyperalgesia with opioid withdrawal.[48-50]

Changes in body temperature reflect altered thermoregulatory response. Hypothermia is more common in dogs, whereas hyperthermia is more common in cats.[56] Opioids most commonly associated with hyperthermia in the cat include hydromorphone (at 3 times the dose) and meperidine;

buprenorphine is unlikely to be associated with hyperthermia in cats.[43,57,58] Experimentally, hydromorphone (1 mg/kg intravenously) increased body temperature (range 104° to 108° F) 1 to 5 hours after anesthesia. Doses at or less than 0.05 mg/kg had no effect, whereas 0.1 mg/kg was associated with increased skin temperature.

Prolonged exposure of opioid receptors to ligands results in adaptation to their presence at multiple cellular levels.[30] Cellular tolerance is translated to animal adaptation manifested as tolerance, physical dependence, sensitization, and withdrawal. However, their emergence is not a reason to forgo opioid use. *Tolerance* refers to a decrease in drug efficacy associated with repeated administration. Acute tolerance (i.e., tachyphylaxis) may reflect short-term receptor desensitization, perhaps owing to phosphorylation of MOP or KOP receptors. Long-term administration of MOP ligands causes superactivation of adenylyl cyclase, the mechanism traditionally assumed to be associated with long-term tolerance. Different ligands appear to initiate acute or chronic tolerance through different mechanisms. Examples include internalization of receptors (MOP or DOP but not MOP), truncation of receptors or other changes. Adaptation by one response may mitigate adaptation by downstream responses; indeed, this sequela (i.e., failure to initiate downstream adaptations) has been proposed as a mechanism of failed desensitization that characterizes some drugs.[27] Accordingly, the ability of different ligands to initiate tolerance differs. Changes in nitric oxide or neurotransmitters or their pathways have been implicated as contributors to the development of tolerance.[29] Tolerance will most likely develop for analgesia, euphoria, sedation, respiratory depression, nausea or vomiting, and suppression of cough.

KEY POINT 28-12 Opioid therapy may be associated with both tolerance and physical dependence in animals, leading to controlled status for many of the drugs.

Physical dependence occurs when continued administration is necessary to prevent clinical signs characteristic of withdrawal. Physical dependence on opioids occurs as exogenous opioids replace endogenous opiates. Opioids affect numerous physiologic systems that become imbalanced before drug administration. A new balance or equilibrium is established in the presence of the drug,[27] and abrupt discontinuation of the drug requires rapid readjustment to a new equilibrium, predisposing the patient to withdrawal. Care must be taken to discriminate between dependence, which is associated with physical withdrawal, and addiction.

Addiction to opioids may reflect attenuation of the inhibition of dopamine release in the nucleus accumbens. This region of the brain has a central role in the reward circuit; dopamine promotes desire. The prevalence of addiction in humans using opoids is high. [51] Abrupt discontinuation of opioids after chronic dosing leads to symptoms of withdrawal, with the severity and duration reflecting the rate of onset and clearance of the opioid. Withdrawal is generally manifested as sign opposite to the original effects caused by the drug and reflects CNS hyperarousal as readaptation to the absence of the drug occurs.[27] Symptoms in humans include nausea and diarrhea, coughing, tearing, yawning, sneezing, rhinorrhea, profuse sweating, twitching muscles, abdominal and muscle pain and cramps, piloerection, and dysphoria. Hyperthermia, tachypnea, tachycardia and hypertension also may occur. Pharmacokinetic variables may be helpful in the prediction of withdrawal.[27] Morphine dependence has been described in dogs.[52] Mixed agonists–antagonists or partial agonists are associated with the least risk of dependence; among the opioids studied, buprenorphine appears to be the least likely to cause dependence in dogs.[53] Opioids can be discontinued in drug-dependent human patients without causing signs typical of withdrawal by decreasing the dose 25% to 50% every couple of days. In human patients suffering from withdrawal, clonidine, an α_2-adrenergic agonist, minimizes the autonomic symptoms of opioid withdrawal.[27]

It is the advent of tolerance and physical dependence that has led to the scheduling or classification of most opioids as potential substances of abuse. The actual class designated varies among the states. Pure agonists tend to be scheduled in class II or III; mixed or partial agonists tend to be scheduled in class IV or V, depending on the abuse potential. Both butorphanol and burpenorphine have been rescheduled from class V to class IV.

Cardiovascular System

The effects of opioids in the myocardium have been described. Cardiac depression (particularly bradycardia) is caused by selected opioids; pretreatment with atropine can reduce the incidence. The risk of hypotension is increased with drugs that also cause histamine release.

Those opioids most likely to be associated with histamine release are morphine (but not oxymorphone) and meperidine.[40,41] Histamine release caused by buprenorphine has been demonstrated only in vitro; fentanyl, oxymorphone, and butorphanol do not cause histamine release in dogs (as reviewed by Guedes and coworkers).[41] Hydromorphone was associated with an apparent type I allergic reaction when used preoperatively in a dog (Chapter 2). However, species differences should be anticipated. Histamine antagonists (H_1) partially block morphine-induced hypotension; naloxone completely blocks it in human patients.[29,42] Fentanyl and its congeners are less likely to cause hypotension associated with surgery in part because they do not cause histamine release.[29] Volume replacement should be instituted before administration of morphine derivatives that causes histamine release in patients that are at risk for hypovolemia. Allergic phenomena in general (including bronchoconstriction) and those manifested in skin may be exacerbated with opioid use if morphinelike drugs are used. In humans opioids cause vasodilation of cutaneous vessels, probably because of histamine release. Pruritis may occur, in part because of histamine but also because of direct effects on neurons.[29]

Gastrointestinal Tract

In addition to effects at the chemoreceptor trigger zone, opioids have direct effects in the gastrointestinal tract. Hydrochloric acid secretion is generally decreased but occasionally may be increased.[29] Tone of smooth muscle in the antral portion of the stomach and upper duodenum will increase, despite decreased gastric peristaltic motility. Passage of endoscopic or other equipment through the stomach can be precluded for up to 12 hours after administration. Drug or food movement through the stomach likewise can be delayed.[29] In the small intestine, and particularly in the upper small intestine, resting tone (segmental) is increased, and propulsive activity is markedly decreased.[29] Initial stimulation of gastrointestinal motility may result in defecation; subsequent depressed gastric motility may cause constipation with prolonged use.

Opioids also decrease small intestinal secretions, and water absorption increases. In the presence of secretory diarrheas, morphinelike opioids inhibit movement of electrolytes and water into the lumen, probably through inhibition of the stimulatory effects of PGE_2, acetylcholine, or vasoactive intestinal peptide.[29] Because of increased transit time allowing more complete absorption of luminal contents, opioids may be contraindicated in patients suffering from obstructive gastrointestinal diseases and those associated with bacteria or toxin production. Opioids also decrease biliary and pancreatic secretions.[29] Morphinelike opioids, however, cause contraction of the sphincter of Oddi and increased bile duct pressure.[29,54,55]

KEY POINT 28-13 Mechanisms that cause opioids to be effective for treatment of diarrhea may also cause constipation.

Other Effects

Ureteral tone may increase and the voiding reflex of the bladder may be diminished as a result of the increased tone of the external sphincter and increased volume of the urinary bladder. Morphine appears to have antidiuretic effects.[29] Inhibitory effects on uterine tone may prolong labor; hyperactivity induced by oxytocin can be normalized with morphine. Neonatal health may be impaired by use of morphinelike drugs during parturition; the neonate appears to be particularly susceptible to respiratory depression induced by opioids, in part because of a poorly developed blood–brain barrier.[29]

Opioids appear to inhibit cytotoxic activity of natural killer cells. Selected opioid compounds, however, appear to enhance macrophage and killer cell activity, possibly through a novel opioid receptor (see Chapter31).[29]

Drug Interactions

The depressant effects of opioids can be exacerbated by other CNS depressants. Several CNS depressants prolong the effects of opioids, including the phenothiazines and tricyclic antidepressants (TCAs). Although some phenothiazines may reduce the amount of opioid necessary for analgesia, others may increase the amount of opioid.[29] Among the drug interactions associated with opioids are those at the receptor level (pharmacodynamic) – a interaction often intended for the purposes of reversal of undesireable clinical effect. These interactions are discussed with antagonists.

Drugs. Improvements have altered the state of the interaction between the opioid and the receptor. A useful categorization largely reflects the potency of the opioids at receptors whose ligands control pain: The more powerful drugs tend to be those interacting principally with MOP; as such, they provide the most effective analgesia but the greatest incidence of side effects. Drug companies have attempted to improve the effects of opioids by enhancing the desired pharmacologic effect while minimizing undesirable effects through chemical alteration of the natural opioids. Semisynthetic drugs are made from simple chemical changes of morphine (codeine) or thebaine (e.g., oxycodone, etorphine, and naloxone). Other morphine derivatives include apomorphine (an emetic), hydrocodone, and oxymorphone.[29] These changes have allowed for differential effects, perhaps by rendering a full agonist to a partial agonist or antagonist.

POWERFUL PURE AGONISTS

Morphine

Morphine is considered the prototypic narcotic. A class II drug, morphine targets primarily MOP and to a lesser degree DOP and KOP receptors. Morphine frequently is studied as morphine sulfate, for which 1 mg will provide 0.76 mg active base.

Morphine causes profound sedation and analgesia for up to 6 hours in the dog. Its effects are reversed with narcotic antagonists. Morphine can cause cardiac depression;[59] in addition, hypotension may reflect histamine release or CNS (vasomotor) depression.[40,60] Morphine can cause respiratory depression,[61] particularly in neonates,[62] and can cause acute pulmonary edema resulting from histamine release.[60] Therapeutic uses include premedication for surgical anesthesia (reducing the amount of other potentially irreversible CNS depressants) and analgesia. Morphine is also used in cases of acute, fulminating pulmonary edema because of its ability to reduce cardiac preload through hepatic venous constriction and splanchnic pooling.

KEY POINT 28-14 Profound sedation and analgesia associated with morphine is amenable to reversal in the dog.

The minimum effective concentration of morphine associated with analgesia is variable: in humans, it ranges from from 9.1 to 40 ng/mL, but increases to as high as 364 ng/mL with chronic administration (as reviewed by Kunakinch et al).[66] A common target for pharmacokinetic studies in dogs is 20 ng/ml. Establishing the minimum target concentration is complicated by the formation of active metabolites. Morphine-6-sulfate (M6S) is metabolite characterized by a thirtyfold greater potency compared with morphine in mouse models, similar to the active morphine metabolite morphine-6 beta-glucuronide (M6G). Its analgesia also is reversed by 3-methoxynaltrexone.[63] However, the major metabolite of morphine with clinical significance is morphine-6-β-glucuronide (M6G). It is characterized by pharmacologic activity equal to that of the parent compound in some species.

Table 28-3 Drugs with Potential Epidural Use in Dogs or Cats[227]

Drug	Dose	Onset (min)	Duration (hr)	Comments
Morphine	0.1	20 to 6	16 to 24	62-hour duration has been reported for a sustained-release encapsulated product
Meperidine			1 to 4	
Methadone	0.7 to 1	Rapid	4	
Oxymorphone	0.1		10	
Fentanyl				Only as adjunct to other epidural analgesics
Butorphanol	0.25		3	No advantage to epidural
Buprenorphine	0.0125	60		
Xylazine		30	3	Large animal information available only
Medetomidine	0.01 to 0.015		4 to 8	Lower dose for cats; cats are likely to vomit
Ketamine	0.4		1.5	Dog; must be preservative free
Lidocaine 2%	0.22 mL/kg	10 to 15	1 to 2	with 1:200,000 epineprhine. Lower dose (0.17 ml/kg) for Ceasarean section
Bupivacaine 0.5%	0.2 ml/kg	20 to 30	4 to 6	

Jones 2001

Although more potent than morphine, the metabolite cannot cross the blood–brain barrier as effectively.[29] However, with chronic morphine dosing, drug concentrations will accumulate, and the metabolite is likely to contribute more than the parent compound to control of pain in humans. It appears to be associated with fewer gastrointestinal side effects.[64]

A role for M6G in analgesic efficacy of morphine in dogs is not clearly evident. A study of morphine disposition in dogs[66] demonstrated that M6G was not detected (<25 ng/mL) after either intravenous (0.5 mg/kg) or oral (approximately 1.5 mg/kg, extended release) administration of morphine in normal Beagles (n = 6). This is in contrast to Jacqz and coworkers,[67] who did detect glucuronidated morphine in dogs. They described a significant (but not exclusive) role of extrahepatic tissues in the formation of the metabolite, which appeared within 5 minutes of administration. Garrett and Jackson[68] also detected formation and renal excretion of morphine monoglucuronide in dogs. The differences in metabolite detection between these studies may reflect differences in the actual metabolite itself, and particularly the position of the glucuronide. The impact of the glucuronidated metabolite to analgesic control in dogs may not be clear.

Disposition of Morphine

In contrast to cats, parenteral and epidural administration of morphine is generally well established in dogs and multiple studies are available to describe its disposition; several studies also address its metabolites (Tables 28-3 and 28-4; see also Table 28-1). Numerous studies using variable preparations, routes and doses in dogs are summarized in Table 28-4 and below. [65-75] Multiples studies have focused on more convenient routes of administration (other than IV), including oral (including extended release products), rectal and epidural. Much of the IV data has been generated in studies that focus on alternate routes of delivery or in the context of determining analgesic concentrations.

Peak morphine concentration has been determined in several studies after intravenous, IM and SC administration. Morphine clearance appears to be dose dependent in the dog, with an elimination half-life of 83 ± 8 minutes at doses ranging from 7.2 to 7.7 mg/kg versus 37 ± 13 minutes at 0.019-0.07 mg/kg intravenously.[68] Bioavailability of intramuscular morphine is high (119%) but variable (57% to 161%), and elimination half-life approximates 90 minutes.

Studies focusing on the nociceptive concentration of morphine revealed an effective 50% concentration of 29.5 ± 5.4 ng/mL in dogs.[72] The authors indicated that an intravenous infusion of 0.15 mg/kg/hr or multiple doses of 0.5 mg/kg every 2 hours for 3 doses provided significant nociception. The short half-life of morphine may require administration as a CRI in dogs. Because steady state may require 3 to 5 hours, a loading dose may be indicated. No differences in either analgesia or adverse reactions were detected in dogs undergoing exploratory laporatomy treated with morphine administered either intramuscularly (1 mg/kg at induction and extubation and every 4 hours thereafter) or CRI (0.12 mg/kg/h). Steady-state serum morphine concentration after CRI was 30 ± 2 ng/mL. The power to detect a significant difference was not addressed.

Morphine has been studied in dogs subcutaneously prepared as a solution and as a sustained-release gel (N,O-carboxymethylchitosan polymer) product[69] given either subcutaneously or orally[70] (it is not clear if the sustained oral preparation is the same as that approved for use in humans). After subcutaneous injection at 1.2 mg/kg, peak concentrations for the solution and sustained product were 488 and 180 ng/mL, respectively, with time to peak concentrations being 10 and 55 minutes, respectively. Variability among animals was large. Elimination half-life was 79 (solution) and 108 (gel) minutes. The duration of analgesia was reported to be between 1 and 2 hours but appeared longer clinically. Emesis should be anticipated.[56]

Oral administration of morphine in humans generates effective systemic concentrations, although first-pass metabolism

Table 28-4 Pharmacokinetic Data for Selected Opioids in Dogs or Cats*227

Drug	Species (n)	Route	Dose mg/kg	C_{max} (1) μg/mL	T_{max} hr	AUC μg/mL/hr	Vd_{ss} L/kg	CL mL/min/kg	Half-life (2) h	MRT h	F %	Ref
Buprenorphine	Cat(n=5)	IV	0.01		3 min		7.1	16.7	6.93	6.97		158
	Cat (n=6)	IM	0.01	0.0036 to 0.0018 (or 0.0087)					6.33	6.83		
	Cat (n=6)	IV	0.01	0.0071 to 0.0267								
	Cat (n=6)	IV	0.02	0.003 to 0.059 (or 0.093)								
	Cat (n=6)	TM	0.01	0.0054 to 0.012	15 to 30						113	
	Cat (n=6)	TM	0.02	0.0026 to 0.019								
	Dog (n=6)	IV	0.015	0.014±0.003		3.08±1.05	1.6±0.3	5.4±1.9	4.5±2.1	264 (199 to 600)(4)		161
	Dog (n=6)	IV	0.01									160
	Dog (Beagle, n=6)	IV	0.02				26 L/dog	330±62 mL/min/dog	16.5±3.7			159
		TM	0.12									
Butorphanol	Cats (n=6)	IM	0.4	0.132	0.35							141
		TM		0.034	1.1							
	Dogs	SC	0.25	33.3±16/9	26.6±13				1.7±0.4			132
		IM	0.25	25.1±6/7	42±13				1.5±0.23			
	Dogs (n=3)	IV(8)	0.052	8.2±5.6			27±10	137±19	3.4±1.8			133
Dextromethorphan	Dog (6)	IV	2.2	1.14±0.47 (Co)		1.2± 0.37	5.1±4.4	33.8±16.5	±±0.6	2.6±0.9	11	187
		PO	5	0.09±0.03	1							
Fentanyl	Cat (n=6)	IV	0.01	4.7-8.3 ng/mL		9.12±2.0	2.6	19.8±2.7	2.4±0.6			101
	Cat (n=6)	TD-Patch	25 μg/hr (full)	3.55±0.77	44±10	193±21.6						
	Cat (n=16)	TD-Patch	25 μg/hr (full)	2.22±0.64 ng/mL								
			25 μg/hr (50% expoure)	1.14±0.86 ng/mL	36							
	Cat	PO	0.002	0.96 ng/mL	0.03 (2 min)							
		IN	0.002	1.5 ng/mL	0.08 (5 min)							
	Dog						10.65 ± 5.53	27.9±9.2	6.03			
	Dogs (Hound; n=?)	IV	0.01	0.0015					2.5			65
			0.02	0.0028					2.5			65

Fentanyl	Dog (n=14)	IV	0.01	0.0015(B)		8.2±2.5	4.9±0.85 (area)	78±22	0.77			104
		IV, CRI	0.01	1.1 to 1.25	1 to 3				2.5 to 3			
			0.01 hr									110
	Dog (n=6)	IV										108
		TD-Patch	50 μg/hr	(C_{ss})1.6 ng/mL								
	Dog (n=6)	TD-Patch	50 μg/hr	(C_{ss}) 0.7±0.2 ng/mL	24				3.6±1.2			109
			75 μg/hr	(C_{ss})1.4±0.5 ng/mL	24				3.4±2.7			
			100 μg/hr	(C_{ss}) 1.2±0.5 ng/mL	24				2.5±2.0			
Hydromorphine	Beagle (n=8)	IV	0.5				12.5	129				100
Liposomal		SC										
	Beagle (n=4) (5)	IV	0.1	0.032 & 0.032 (Co)		0.014 & 0.014	4.24 & 4.1	106 & 111	0.57 & 0.63	0.66, 0.73		99
	Beagle (n=4)	IV	0.5	0.157 & 143 (Co)		0.123 & 0.135	4.41 & 4.7	60 & 55	1 & 1	1.2&1.2		
	Beagle (n=6)	SC	0.1	0.033 & 0.034	0.19 & 0.12	0.026 & 0.025			0.66 0.67	0.9 & 0.95		
	Beagle (n=5)	SC	0.5	0.149 & 0.159	0.3 & 0.25	0.20 & 0.21			1.1 & 1.1	1.4 & 1.4		
	Dog (n=5)	IV	0.1	0.29±0.39(Co); 0.016±0.006 (B)		94.4±0.44**	4.5±2.4	68±20.4	1.1±0.3	1.6±0.5		94
			0.2	0.41±0.51(Co); 0.025±0.012 (B)		169±43**	7.2±3.1	74.7±0.19	1.76±1.18	1.3±0.87		
	Cat (n=6)	IV	0.1	0.025 (0.008 to 0.035) (B)(3)		244 (170-257)** (4)	3.0 (2.4-4.3)	25(23-35)	1.7 (1-2.3)	1.85 (0.1-2.53)		95
Ketamine	Dog	IV	15				1.9	32	1.00			
Methadone	Greyhounds (n=6)	IV	0.5	0.097±0.023		151±22	7.3±1.8	56±9.4	1.53±0.18	2.1±0.2		124
	Beagles (n=6)	IV	1	0.389±0.150		742±250	3.5±1.1	25±0.2	1.75±0.25	2.4±0.3		125
		PO	2	Not detected								
Morphine (6)	Dog (n=6)	IV	0.5	0.135±0.007(Co); 0.061±0.010 (B)		0.113±15.9	4.6±1.7	62.5±10	1.6±1.5 h	1.36±0.19		66
		PO (ER)	1.6	0.005	2	0.0151			1.39	3.34	5.31	
	Dog (n=6)	IV	0.5	0.092 (7)		5.8 (3.76-11.84)	7.3(5.9-9.0)		1.6 (1.1-2.2)			75
		IM	1	0.185		12.3 (9.5-12.2)			1.4 (0.97-2.23)		119(58-161)	
		Rectal solution	2	0.029		3.9 (2.1-5.5)			1.1 (0.67-1.67)		16.5 (11-27)	
		Rectal suppository	1	0.02		2.2 (1.8-3.1)			1.51 (1.41-2.1)		23 (8.6-31)	

Continued

Table 28-4 Pharmacokinetic Data for Selected Opioids in Dogs or Cats*[227]—cont'd

Drug	Species (n)	Route	Dose mg/kg	C_{max} (1) µg/mL	T_{max} hr	AUC µg/mL/hr	Vd_{ss} L/kg	CL mL/min/kg	Half-life (2) h	MRT h	F %	Ref
		Rectal suppository	2	0.021		3.4 (2.8-5.4)			1.18 (0.7-1.83)		16.5 (7.6-28)	
		Rectal suppository	5	0.053		8.7 (6.2-11.5)			1.65 (0.98-2.6)		19 (7.6-21)	
	Cat(6)	IV	0.2		0.25		2.6	24	1.22	1.75		
	Cat (4)	IM	0.2						1.55	2		
Oxymorphone	Dog (n=6)	IV	0.1	0.026-0.061		0.018-0.044	2.8-9.3	33-82	0.4-1	1-1.9		92
		SC		0.014-0.042	0.08-0.33	0.02-0.04	N/A	N/A	0.7-1.3		0.8-1.5	
Pethidine	Cat (6)	IM	5		0.12				3.60	5.12		
Tramadol	Cat	IV	2	0.46±23 (B); 1.32±0.92 (C_{max})(3)		1.65±0.2	3.0±0.1	20.8±3.2	2.23±0.3			177
(ODM-Tramadol) (9)		N/A		0.37±0.031	0.91±0.28	2.247±0.30			4.35±0.46			
Tramadol	Cat	PO	5.2	0.80±0.16 (B); 0.91±0.23 (Co)		4.1±0.05			3.4±0.13		93±7	
(ODM-Tramadol)		N/A		0.655±0.77	0.83±0.21	4.42±0.314			4.82±0.32			
Tramadol	Dog (n=6)	IV	4	1.7±0.4 (Co); 0.31±0.26 (B)		1.2±0.18	3.0±0.45	54.6±8.2	1.8±1.2	0.93±0.12		176
(ODM-Tramadol)		N/A		0.147±0.040	0.4±0.2	0.362±0.072			1.69±0.45	2.59±0.67		
		PO	11.2±2	1.4±0.7		3.9±2.2			1.7±0.12	3±0.4	65±38	
		N/A		0.45±0.21	0.5±0.2	1.1±0.38			2.18±0.55	3.2±0.8		
	Dog (3)	IV	1	0.53±0.029 (Co)		0.48±0.07	2.57±0.02	34.9±5.53	0.94±0.09			

AUC, Area under the curve; *Vd_{ss}*, volume of distribution at steady state; *CL*, clearance; *MRT*, mean residence time; *F*, bioavailability; *Ref*, reference; *IV*, intravenous; *IM*, intramuscular; *TM*, transmucosal; *SC*, subcutaneous; *PO*, by mouth; *TD*, transdermal; *IN*, intranasal; *C_{ss}*, concentration at steady state; *ER*, extended release; *N/A*, not applicable, *B*, y intercept extrapolated from the terminal phase of plasma drug concentration vs time curve; C_{max}, maximum drug concentration at T_{max} (time to maximum concentration).

*See text for additional information.

**Note that units in table have been standardized for each drug and may not necessarily match units described in the text.

1 Elimination or terminal
2 C_{max} was reported after IV administration.
3 C_{max} = oral; for IV, Co=Y intercept of initial phase; B=Y intercept of terminal phase
4 Median (low-high)
5 Mean and median
6 Administered as morphine sulfate (76% morphine base)
7 Median at 5 minutes post injection
8 Based on parent compound and norbutorphanol metabolite
9 ODM is the o-demethylated metabalite of tramadol.
CO *y* intercept extrapolated from initial phase of plasma drug concentration vs time curve initial phase
ER Extended release
F Bioavailability
L Liposome encapsulated

requires oral doses that are two to six times parenteral doses. A sustained-release oral morphine preparation (Morphelan) has been approved for use in humans in the United States. The product is designed for both immediate and extended release. Because several days are required for steady-state kinetics to be reached, an initial loading dose of twice the intended subsequent daily dose has been recommended to achieve steady-state concentrations within 2 days of initiation of therapy.[71] However, the role of oral administration of morphine in providing effective analgesia in dogs is not clear. The formation of M6G after oral administration of approximately 1.6 mg/kg, morphine sulfate extended release in dogs was previously discussed. In their study, KuKanich and coworkers [66] compared the disposition of intravenous morphine (morphine sulfate 0.5 mg/kg) and orally administered morphine as a commercially available extended-release tablet (1.6 ± 0.1 mg/kg) in Beagles (n=6) (see Table 28-4). One dog vomited after oral administration. Oral absorption of the extended-release tablet was poor (5%) and erratic, achieving a C_{max} of morphine of 5.0 ng/ml (variability not provided); this low concentration presumably reflects poor oral absorption rather than high first pass metabolism in that M6G was not detected. This compares to an extrapolated (after distribution) peak concentration of 60 ± 10 ng/ml after IV administration of 0.5 mg/kg. Accordingly, for effective analgesia, a dose of 0.5 mg/kg intravenously every 2 hours was recommended.

More recently, Aragon and coworkers[74] reported the disposition of morphine (1 and 2 mg/kg) as either an immediate or oral sustained-release product in dogs (n=14). Although drug concentrations were detectable for 24 hours, concentrations were considered too low and too variable to be of clinical use.

Rectal administration may be a viable alternative route of of administration in dogs. After rectal administration in dogs, morphine is approximately 20% bioavailable,[75] achieving peak concentrations of 28 ng/mL when 2 mg/kg is administered as a solution and 20, 21, and 51 ng/mL when administered as a suppository at 1, 2, and 5 mg/kg, respectively. Elimination half-life (minutes) ranged from 65 (solution) to 98 (suppository) (see Table 28-4). Vomiting was common (five of six animals) with a 5-mg/kg rectal suppository.

Morphine was studied in dogs after intramuscular and rectal administration, the latter as either a solution or suppository (see Table 28-4). Median peak concentrations were reported at 5 minutes. The duration that drug concentrations were above a target of 20 ng/mL were 120 minutes for the intramuscular dose, 5 to 30 minutes for the rectal solution, less than 40 minutes for the low (1 mg/kg) and medium (2 mg/kg) suppository dose, and 120 minutes for the high suppository dose (5 mg/kg morphine sulfate).[75]

Morphine also has been studied in dogs after epidural administration of the solution (0.1 mg/kg)[76] and as a sustained-release encapsulated preparation (experimental; 10 and 30 mg in 3 mL saline).[77] Both appear to prolong analgesia while avoiding side effects. King and coworkers[78] demonstrated that epidural morphine (0.07 mg/kg, containing 0.1% sodium metabisulfate) was not associated with histologic damage to the spinal cord in dogs (n=16). Morphine has been studied in Beagles after repetitive epidural administration (30 mg at 10 mg/mL) as a sustained-release multivesicular liposome preparation (DepoFoam drug delivery system).[79] Adverse reactions were limited to moderate, transient behavioral and physiologic changes, consistent with morphine administration, at each injection. A modest effect on cord histopathology was not associated with changes in CSF or neurologic signs.[79]

Morphine also has been studied intravaginally in humans. When this route was used, pain was effectively reduced in one patient, although close monitoring was necessary.[80] Morphine has been studied in both dogs and cats after transdermal administration as a pluronic lethicin organo (PLO) gel. Drug was not quantifiable in either species when administered at 1.6 to 2 mg/kg.[65]

Adverse Events and Drug Interactions

Adversities of morphine were discussed as a class. Morphine appears to cause more sedation than transdermal fentanyl when used as a postoperative analgesic.[76] Guedes and coworkers[41] demonstrated that morphine was associated with variable histamine release in conscious dogs at 0.3 and 0.6 mg/kg load followed by 0.17 or 0.34 mg/kg/hr, although the difference from placebo was statistically significant only for the higher dose. Flushing of the skin occurred within 5 minutes of 60% and 100% of dogs receiving the lower and higher dose, respectively. Although no adverse cardiovascular events were detected, adversities might be anticipated in at-risk patients.

Intrathecal administration of morphine at 0.15 mg/kg has been associated with a number of adverse effects in dogs, including bradycardia, hypotension, myoclonus, and urinary retention (as reviewed by Novello and coworkers).[81] However, Novello and coworkers[81] demonstrated in clinical cases undergoing cervical or thoracolumbar laminectomy that a low intrathecal dose of morphine (0.023 to 0.034 mg/kg) administered at the lumber level 25 to 65 minutes before surgery reduced the dose of fentanyl (1.2 μg/kg/hr) needed to maintain a steady-state heart rate and arterial blood pressure when compared with a placebo group (4.2 μg/kg/hr fentanyl infusion). Ketamine was also administered to all animals (0.5 mg/kg every 60 minutes starting 10 minutes before surgery). Induction and fentanyl protocols differed among animals in the study; it is not clear if both methods were distributed similarly among treatment groups.

Vomiting is relatively consistently associated with morphine administration in dogs. Vomiting occurred after intravenous (0.5 mg/kg) or intramuscular (1 mg/kg) administration in one study (five of six dogs) at a mean morphine concentration of 66 ng/mL, and heart rates were significantly lower.[75]Drug interactions with morphine appear to be limited. KuKanich and Borum[73] found morphine disposition in Greyhounds was not affected by ketoconazole. The simultaneous combination of morphine with the pure antagonists naltrexone did not affect the disposition of either drug in dogs.[82]

Therapeutic Use

Morphine has been used in the dog and cat effectively as a premedicant or a perioperative analgesic[56] using a variety of routes. Lucas and coworkers[83] found no differences in the analgesic efficacy of morphine when administered as a CRI (0.12 mg/kg/hr) or intramuscularly at intubation, extubation, and every 4 hours in dogs (n=20) undergoing exploratory laparotomy. Morphine can be administered safely epidurally, although preparations made specifically for epidural administration are preferred. Epidural administration appears to be effective when given either epidurally[84,85] or locally (intraarticularly)[84] for control of some orthopedic pains.

The postoperative analgesic effects of epidural morphine (0.1 mg/kg) or morphine combined with medetomidine (0.005 mg/kg) have been compared in dogs (n=6/group) undergoing cranial cruciate repair. No differences were detected in control of pain (power of the study not reported), although the combination drug consistently had a lower numeric score. Increasing sample size may have resulted in statistical signification. Likewise, no differences were detected in plasma morphine concentrations between the two treatment groups (peak concentrations of approximately 4 ng/mL).[86] The effect of morphine on healing corneal ulcers has been studied in dogs after administration of an ophthalmic preparation. Both MOP and DOP receptors have been identified in the canine cornea. Topical 1% (but not 0.5%) morphine provided good corneal analgesia with no apparent adverse effects.[87]

Morphine (0.2 mg/kg subcutaneously) was compared with buprenorphine (0.02 mg/kg subcutaneously) and methadone (0.2 mg/kg subcutaneously) in cats (n=8) subjected to mechanical and thermal stimulation. Morphine provided the best analgesia.[126]

Oxymorphone

Oxymorphone is a semisynthetic drug (class II) that has been used in both dogs and cats, It is characterized with 10 times the potency of morphine. Receptor interaction is similar to that of morphine. Unlike morphine, however, it does not appear to be associated with histamine release in dogs.[40] It has been a common component of neuroleptic analgesia. Oxymorphone is effectively antagonized by naloxone and partially antagonized by butorphanol.[56,88] Its duration of action is 4 to 6 hours, which may exceed that of its reversal agent, naloxone.[89] Like fentanyl, it is associated with marked auditory sensitization, altered thermoregulation, and bradycardia (pretreat with atropine). Decreased heart rate may still occur with epidural administration.[90] Oxymorphone is used primarily to induce neuroleptanalgesia or reduce the amount of barbiturate needed for surgical anesthesia. It also, however, has been commonly used to control postoperative pain in small animals, although use has been curtailed by limited availability and increased use of alternative opioids.[23] Oxymorphone has been studied with and is approved for use in the dog[91] and cat. It remains an excellent analgesic for both young and old patients and for debilitated patients.

Oxymorphone has been studied in normal dogs after intravenous and intramuscular use (Table 28-4).[92] Oxymorphone also has been studied in Beagles after administration as a subcutaneously administered slow-release liposome-encapsulated [LE] preparation.[93] A dose of 0.5 mg/kg LE preparation yielded concentrations comparable to 0.1 mg/kg of standard morphine achieving a (plasma C_{max} of approximately 37 μg/mL using an enzyme-linked immunosorbent assay (ELISA) that measures both parent compound and glucuronide metabolite; however, the elimination phase appeared to be similar (elimination half-life not reported). Sedation and physiologic scores were comparable at these two doses, suggesting no benefit in pharmacologic effects when morphine or its metabolite are delivered as LE preparations compared with standard preparations.

Hydromorphone

Hydromorphone is a pure MOP agonist with a potency (in humans) 5 to 7 times that of morphine suggesting effective concentrations to be 2 to 3 ng/mL. A minimum effective concentration of 4 ng/mL has been suggested (as reviewed by Guedes and coworkers).[94] It has been administered for control of pain by a number of routes in humans, including parenteral, transmucosal, and epidural. Hydromorphone (0.1 mg/kg intravenously) disposition and its association with analgesia have been described in the cat.[95] Peak plasma concentration was of 94.25 ± 8.40 ng/mL after intravenous administration of 0.1 mg/kg; median concentrations extrapolated from the terminal phase were 25 ng/mL (range 8 to 35). Despite a short elimination half-life (median 100 minutes; range approximately 60 to 140) leading to nondetectable concentrations (less than 1 ng/mL) by 6 hours, analgesia as measured by thermal threshold was maintained for 7.5 hours.[95] No behavioral side effects were reported; most cats became nauseated, but none vomited. Mydriasis and "tail tucking" were observed in all cats.

The impact of hydromorphone on nociception has been studied in cats. Hydromorphone at 0.1 mg/kg provided thermal antinociception for 230 minutes (as reviewed by Guedes and coworkers.)[94] A dose-dependent effect was evident between 0.025 and 0.1 mg/kg. In contrast to dogs, hyperthermia is associated with hydromorphone treatment in cats. Analgesic effects, based on thermal thresholds, of hydromorphone (0.1 mg/kg intramuscularly), butorphanol (0.4 mg/kg intramuscularly), or the combination have been studied in cats.[96] The duration of analgesia was approximately 3 hours for butorphanol, 6 hours for hydromorphone, and 9 hours for the combination. However, the initial intensity of hydromorphone and, to a lesser degree, butorphanol analgesia was substantially reduced when the combination was used. Side effects included dysphoria (butorphanol only) and vomiting (hydromorphone only).[97]

The pharmacokinetics of hydromorphone have been described in Beagles at 0.1 and 0.5 mg/kg intravenously or subcutaneously (see Table 28-4).[99] The short half-life (30 to 60 minutes) led the authors to recommend that treatment should occur at 2-hour dosing intervals for either route of administration or that a CRI be used. Hydromorphone was also studied in Beagles after administration in a controlled-release LE product at 0.5 intravenously or, 1, 2, and 3 mg/kg subcutaneously using a randomized design with a 14- to 28-day washout.[100] Serum drug concentrations corrected for dose ranged from 19.41 to 25 ng/mL at 0.19 to 0.27 hour. Concentrations approximated 4 ng/mL for 6 to 72 hours at 2 mg/kg; at 3 mg/kg, concentration exceeded 4 ng/mL for 96 hours.

Guedes and coworkers[94] also described the pharmacokinetics (see Table 28-4) and pharmacodyanmics of intravenous hydromorphone (0.1 or 0.2 mg/kg) in dogs (n=5; 2 Beagles) and coupled their studies with pharmacodynamic assessment of analgesia. Antinociceptive effects (based on towel clamp–induced withdrawal) and sedation were compared with those of morphine (0.5 and 1 mg/kg). Hydromorphone clearance surpassed hepatic blood flow reported for dogs, leading the authors to suggest extrahepatic clearance. Both drugs were associated with more antinociception and sedation compared with placebo, but differences were not detected between doses or drugs. The authors suggested that lack of dose dependency may reflect achievement of the maximum effect at the low dose. The lack of differences between drugs was interpreted as confirmation of the potency of hydromorphone compared with morphine. However, the power of the study to detect significant differences was not reported. Analgesic concentrations of 0.5 to 4 ng/mL were suggested on the basis of their work as well as that of others, including studies of humans. Other differences compared with placebo were increased respiratory rate, with return to baseline occurring more rapidly for the hydromorphone compared with morphine group. Body temperature decreased in a dose-dependent manner for both drugs, although changes were significantly different only when compared with placebo. Hydromorphone provided clinically relevant antinociception for at least 2 hours.

Fentanyl

Fentanyl is a synthetic opioid (class II) with a potency 100 times that of morphine and 500 times that of meperidine. Doses are cited in μg/kg rather than mg/kg. Fentanyl is a pure MOP agonist, but it also positively interacts, although to a lesser degree, with DOP and KOP receptors. In contrast to morphine, fentanyl is associated with minimal hemodynamic changes or cardiac suppression. Historically, fentanyl has been recognized as a drug used to induce neuroleptanalgesia (when combined with droperidol). After parenteral administration, however, it causes profound sedation and respiratory depression. Auditory sensitization and altered thermoregulation (leading to panting) may occur. Pretreatment with atropine is indicated when administering the drug parenterally. Because it undergoes redistribution (as with thiobarbiturates), repetitive administration may result in accumulation of the drug in fat and prolonged duration of effect.

Pharmacokinetics and Pharmacodynamics

Fentanyl has been studied in dogs and cats using several different methods of delivery. Using a thermal threshold response, fentanyl concentrations greater than 1 ng/mL have been recommended for therapeutic analgesic effects in cats.[101] A dose of 10 μg/kg intravenously provided analgesia (measured by thermal response) for approximately 2 hours in cats.

In normal dogs the elimination half-life approximates 3 hours and the volume of distribution 10 L/kg (see Table 28-4); μg/kg was 1.5 and 2.8 ng/mL, respectively; elimination half-life was approximately 2.5 hours.[65] In normal cats the elimination half-life also approximates 3 hours, but volume of distribution appears to be smaller.[102]. A half-life approximating 2.5 to 3 hours in either species potentially supports the use of a CRI, although a loading dose is indicated. An infusion rate of 0.4 μg/kg/min after a loading dose of 5 μg/kg is recommended in cats. For dogs, fentanyl has been studied after an intravenous loading dose, and an intravenous loading dose (10 μg/kg) followed by CRI (10 μg/kg/hr) for 1 to 3 hours (see Table 28-4).[103] Concentrations declined to below 1 ng/mL by 20 minutes after the intravenous loading dose and reached 1 ng/mL again by about 2 hours, with steady-state concentrations at 1, 3, and 4 hours of infusion being 1.0 ± 0.7, 1.11 ± 0.4, and 1.25 ± 0.7 ng/mL, respectively. Variability in concentrations was marked. The elimination half-life of fentanyl after the CRI was discontinued was 151 ± 61 (2.51+1 hours) to 182 ± 68 (3+1 hours).

Fentanyl is among the drugs for which alternative routes of administration have been developed,[104] several of which have been studied in dogs and cats. Transdermal delivery of 10 or 30 μg/kg as a PLO gel yielded no detectable plasma fentanyl nor any analgesia in cats in one study.[101] However, a second study (unpublished data by author) found a C_{max} of 8.8 ± 5 ng/mL at 10 ± 19 hours after transdermal delivery of a PLO gel (5 mg/mL) to cats (n=3) at a mean dose of 0.08 ± 0.03 mg/kg (80 ± 30 μg/kg). Potentially therapeutic concentrations persisted throughout the duration of the study: concentrations of 4 ± 5 ng/mL were measured at 61 hours. In contrast to cats, fentanyl was not detected in dogs after administration of 0.88 mg/kg (880 μg/kg) as a transdermal PLO gel.[65]

KEY POINT 28-15 Fentanyl is such a potent pure MOP agonist that it is dosed in micrograms rather than milligrams.

Fentanyl (2 μg/kg) has been studied after oral and intranasal administration in cats. C_{max} (ng/mL) 5 minutes after oral administration was 0.96 and 2 minutes after intranasal administration, 1.48 ng/mL.[101] Although not yet studied in dogs or cats, nn humans, after administration as an aerosol (50 μg/mL solution aerosolized for 5 minutes), fentanyl concentrations were approximately 25% of that achieved after 100 μg intravenously (1.4 ng/mL versus 4.4 ng/mL, respectively), suggesting aerosolization as a possible route of administration.[105]

Fentanyl has been available for about 10 years as a transdermal drug delivery system intended for control of pain (Figure 28-4). Issues surrounding transdermal drug delivery in animals have been well reviewed. [106] The transdermal patch system has proved safe and effective for delivery of fentanyl to both dogs and cats. The transdermal drug delivery system provides slow, continuous drug delivery that is intended to provide a fairly constant plasma fentanyl concentration. Peak and trough concentrations, which might cause toxicity and therapeutic failure, respectively, are thus avoided. The fentanyl transdermal patch system has been approved for control of cancer pain in humans. The system consists of a patch with an adhesive layer that attaches to the skin. A "release" membrane controls the rate of release of drug from the reservoir. Because the amount of drug that is released is proportional to the size

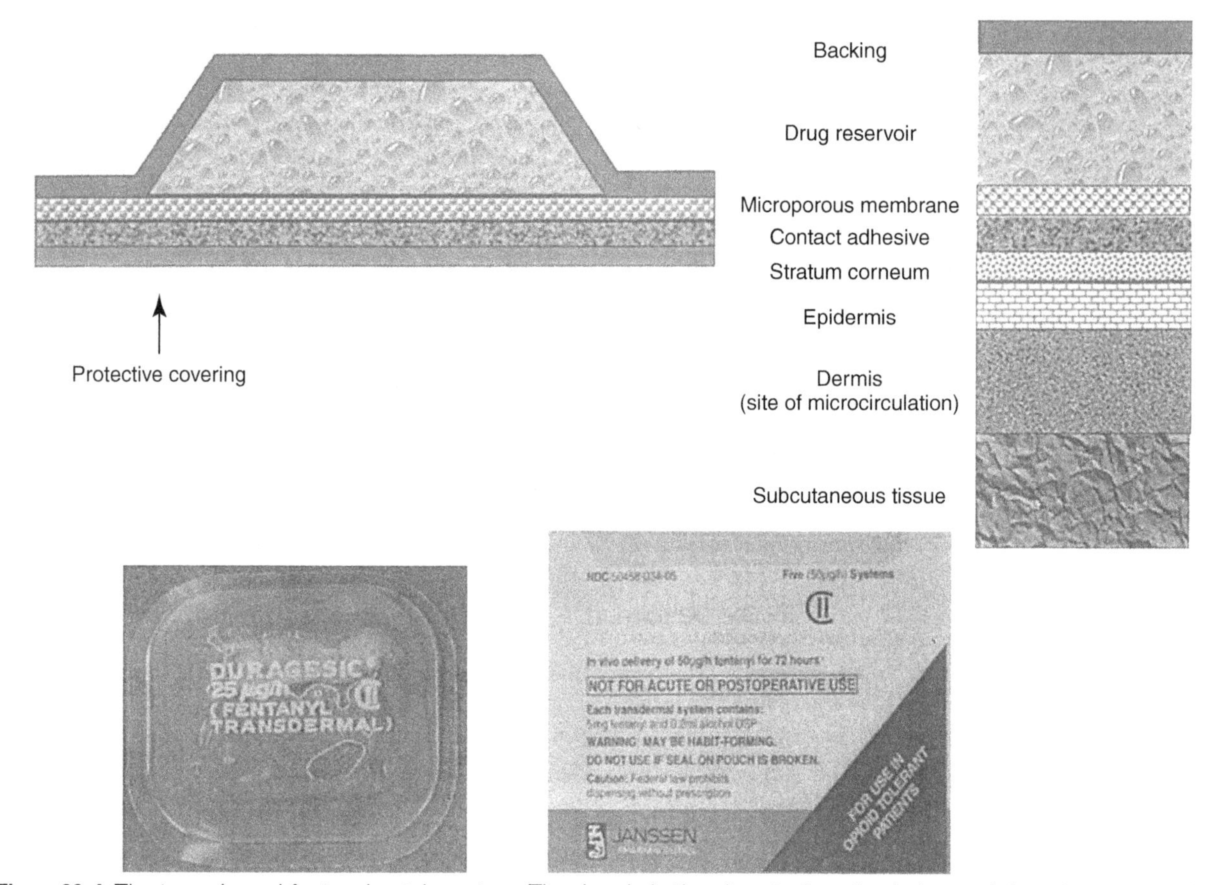

Figure 28-4 The transdermal fentanyl patch system. The dermis is the site of microcirculation and thus drug absorption.

(area) of the patch,[107] the dose delivered is the amount of drug (in μg) released per unit time (hour). The system is available in four sizes: 25, 50, 75, and 100 μg/hr. Drug delivery through the stratum corneum can be influenced by a number of factors that vary among patients. These include thickness of the stratum corneum and epidermal layer, skin appendages (e.g., number of sweat glands), body temperature, hydration status, and diseases that might alter the permeability of the stratum corneum.

Species difference mandate that the fentanyl patch system be studied in the target species before use. Peak concentrations occur within 24 hours in the dog and can occur in as few as 3 to 5 hours in the cat. The commercially available fentanyl patch has been studied in both dogs[102, 108,109] and cats.[110] With the 50 μg/hr patch, drug delivery approximated 37 μg/hr (range of 13.7 to 59.8 μg/hr) in dogs, and the patch was found to be an effective means of constant, slow drug delivery.[108] A comparison of drug delivery from different patch sizes found the average fentanyl concentration from 24 to 72 hours to be 0.7 ng/mL (50 μg/hr), 1.4 ng/mL (75 μg/hr), and 1.2 ng/mL (100 μg/hr) in dogs weighing approximately 20 kg.[109] The elimination (disappearance) half-life ranged from 3.6 hr (50 μg/hr) to a low of 2.5 hr (100 μg/hr). Variability among dogs was marked, making duration of analgesia difficult to predict in individual animals.

Fentanyl delivery has been studied after administration of a 25 μg/hr patch in cats.[102] Delivery was approximately 8.5 μg/hr (36% of the predicted) with mean steady-state concentrations of 1.58 ng/mL being achieved at 12 to 100 hr; the maximum concentration of 3.6± 0.8 was achieved at 44±12 hr. Concentrations dropped below 1 ng/mL in four of six cats within 12 hours of patch application and in all cats within 36 hours. The amount of drug delivered through a fentanyl transdermal patch can be reduced by decreasing the surface area contact with the skin. The most accurate approach probably is removal of only a portion of the protective lining cover of the patch, although the proportion of drug delivery will not be exactly proportional to the amount of lining removal. Folding half of a 25 μg/hr patch in cats yielded mean peak concentrations of 1.14 ± 0.9 ng/mL compared with 1.8 ± 0.9 ng/mL (38% reduction) for full patch exposure. [110]

Robertson and coworkers[101] determined the pharmacodynamic response of fentanyl either intravenously or as a PLO (10 μg/kg) applied to the inner pinna. Plasma fentanyl concentrations greater than 1 ng/mL were required for effective analgesia. The only value reported in the study was C_{max} (rather than extrapolated γ intercept) for fentanyl after intravenous administration. However, mean concentrations appeared to be above 1 ng/mL for approximately 60 minutes after intravenous administration. Elimination half-life estimated from the plasma drug concentration versus time curve approximated 15 to 30 minutes. Cats tolerated fentanyl administration well, with most cats exhibiting euphoria. Fentanyl was not detected after PLO administration when administered at 30 μg/kg.

In this same study, Robertson and coworkers[101] studied fentanyl after oral or intranasal administration of 2 μg/kg, yielding C_{max} values of 0.96 and 1.48 ng/mL at 5 and 2 minutes, respectively. Cats receiving the drug orally or intranasally salivated profusely and were difficult to restrain. Thermal antinociception differed from saline control for approximately 2 hours.

The rate of drug release from the patch and skin can vary with environmental factors that alter delivery through the stratum corneum. Most notable is temperature; fever or a heating pad will increase drug movement. Body temperature was shown to influence fentanyl concentrations when delivered using a fentanyl as a transdermal patch in cats undergoing isoflurane anesthesia. Peak concentrations were 1.8 ± 0.6 ng/mL in normothermic patients compared with 0.6 ± 0.3 ng/mL in hypothermic cats.[114] In another study, experimentally induced hypothermia (35°C) was associated with a decline in plasma fentanyl concentrations of 33% (0.6 ng/mL) compared with that at baseline (1.8 ng/mL).[117] Patches had been applied 24 hours before anesthesia. In contrast, hyperthermia may increase the risk of fentanyl overdose.[115]

Therapeutic Use

Only a few clinical trials have compared non-transdermal fentanyl to alternative opioids. Anderson and Day[47] compared the effects of morphine (0.12 mg/kg/hr), fentanyl (3 μg/kg/hr) administered by CRI with those of placebo on urine output in healthy (n = 23) and traumatized (n = 18) patients. All animals received a similar rate of fluid infusion. Both fentanyl and morphine decreased urine output in both the trauma and healthy groups (approximately 0.7 to 0.76 mL/kg/hr in all groups compared with 1.2 mL/kg/hr in the untreated group).

Several studies have demonstrated efficacy of the fentanyl transdermal patch system in cats.[110,111,113] Fentanyl administered as a 25 μg/hr patch was effective on controlling pain associated with ovariohysterectomy in cats.[111] Fentanyl was more effective than butorphanol (0.4 mg/kg intravenously) in cats undergoing ovariohysterectomy or onychectomy.[113] A number of studies have documented analgesic efficacy of transdermal fentanyl in dogs. Analgesia did not differ from produced by intramuscular oxymorphone (0.05 mg/kg), but fentanyl was associated with less sedation when used in canine patients undergoing ovariohysterectomy.[112] Robinson and coworkers[76] compared the efficacy of transdermal fentanyl (100 μg/hr; placed 24 hours before surgery) with that of epidural morphine (0.1 mg/kg) at induction of anesthesia in dogs (n=10) undergoing major orthopedic surgery. Fentanyl provided superior analgesia. The fentanyl patch system was equal to or better than epidural morphine (0.1 mg/kg) in canine patients undergoing orthopedic surgery[76].

KEY POINT 28-16 The transdermal fentanyl patch system has proved to be an effective method of analgesia delivery in dogs and cats.

The fentanyl transdermal patch appears to be a reasonable alternative to pain management for dogs and cats, but with several caveats. Patches can cause irritation. Because the time to peak therapeutic concentrations of the drug may be up to 24 hours,[109] the need for shorter-term control of pain (e.g., for postoperative pain) should be anticipated. Patches should be applied 12 to 24 hours before the anticipated need for analgesia. Likewise, after the patch is removed, a similar 12- to 24-hour period must elapse before the drug is no longer detectable in the patient. Analgesia is provided for 24 to 72 hours, although variability among animals can be marked, making use of the patch for the individual animal less predictable. Intravenous fentanyl (30 μg/kg has been recommended for dogs) can be given at the time of patch application as a loading dose for patients in need of immediate analgesia. Other opioids also can be given intravenously, intramuscularly, or subcutaneously until the patch is effective. Although a pure opioid (morphine, oxymorphone) is probably preferable, a mixed or partial drug (butorphanol or buprenorphine, respectively) can be given. Because both of the latter drugs have some MOP antagonist effects, however, the MOP effects of fentanyl from the patch will be blocked until the antagonist is eliminated. This may be more problematic with buprenorphine, which has a very tight affinity for MOP receptors.[113a]

The transdermal delivery of fentanyl appears to be very useful in small animals experiencing pain, including postoperative pain, cancer pain, and pain associated with trauma. The patches can be dosed as follows on the basis of body weight: 5 to 10 kg: 25 μg/hr; 10 to 20 kg: 50 μg/hr; 20 to 30 kg: 75 μg/hr; and more than 30 kg: 100 μg/hr.[115] The dose of fentanyl administered by a transdermal patch can be decreased in animals ≤5 kg by folding the adhesive membrane such that only a portion of the patch is exposed to the skin or by cutting away half of the seal (but not the patch itself). However, variability in concentrations will complicate effective use. Exposure of the second half of the patch may not provide equivalent analgesia if applied to a different cat or after all fentanyl has been eliminated. For animals larger than 30 kg, multiple patches can be applied. Patches can be used on an outpatient basis. Heating pads should not be placed at the site of a patch. Patches generally are placed on the dorsum of the neck, which first must be clipped and dried. The patch must come in close, snug contact with the skin. A bandage should be applied to keep the patch in place and prevent the animal or people (especially children) from disturbing the patch.

If the patch is prescribed, veterinarians should apply the patch to, and on completion of analgesia remove it from, the animal rather than allow the client to do so. Clients should be warned that the patches are not approved for use in animals. Patches that are sent home with the patient should be collected when removed from the animal to minimize the risk of drug abuse by pet owners.[116] Animals occasionally remove the patch and swallow it; however, the risk of drug toxicity is minimized because it is unlikely that the close contact necessary for drug delivery will occur between the mucosa and the patch. In addition, first-pass metabolism of any fentanyl that is absorbed will limit the amount of drug that reaches systemic circulation. This will not be true if the patch is chewed such that absorption through the buccal mucosa occurs.

Sufentanil

Sufentanil is a thiamylal derivative of fentanyl. It is 5 to 10 times as potent as fentanyl but is apparently associated with fewer cardiac or respiratory side effects. Its half-life is shorter than that of fentanyl, but its onset of action is much more rapid. It has been used as an effective analgesic in dogs.[118]

Meperidine (Pethidine)

Meperidine (pethidine) (2 to 10 mg/kg intramuscularly every 2 hours [dogs]; 2 to 4 mg/kg intramuscularly every 2 hours [cats]; class II) induces analgesia that is about one fifth that of morphine and lasts approximately 1 to 2 hours. Its sedative properties, however, are useful for preanesthesia. It undergoes marked first-pass metabolism and is eliminated rapidly in dogs. Meperidine reduces the heart rate and systemic arterial pressure in dogs partly through peripheral vasodilation. Bronchoconstriction also occurs in the dog. It is a potent initial stimulant of the gastrointestinal tract. Rapid intravenous injection can cause peripheral vasodilation. Diphenoxylate (the active opioid ingredient in Lomotil) is a derivative of meperidine. In a randomized, blinded, multicenter clinical trial, meperidine (postoperatively, 3.3 mg/kg intramuscularly; n = 57) provided analgesia equal to that of carprofen (preoperatively, 4 mg/kg subcutaneously; n = 59) in cats.[119] However, the duration of analgesia was longer for the carprofen group. Millette and coworkers[120] studied the effects of meperidine (5 mg/kg intramuscularly) on various nociceptive thresholds in cats (n = 8). Both thermal and mechanical thresholds changed with meperidine.

KEY POINT 28-17 The short duration of action of meperidine largely limits use to preanesthesia.

MILD TO MODERATE PURE AGONISTS

Codeine

Codeine is 60% bioavailable in humans after oral administration. Although effective concentrations reach circulation after oral administration, the potency of codeine as an analgesic is less than that of morphine. Codeine has a very low affinity for opioid receptors, and its analgesic effects are primarily due to metabolism (demethylation) to morphine.[29] Only a small percentage (10%) of morphine is formed, however, and its antitussive effects probably reflect direct interaction with codeine receptors.[29] In dogs, even less codeine appears to be converted to morphine. Its antitussive effects require lower plasma drug concentrations than expected for analgesia. Currently, its primary indication for small animals is as a cough suppressant (2.2 mg/kg [dogs]) or antidiarrheal. Outpatient use of this drug as an analgesic, particularly when combined with a non-narcotic analgesic (i.e., NSAIDs or acetaminophen) is increasing. Codeine is scheduled as class II.

The disposition of codeine (20 mg/kg) after subcutaneous administration was briefly described in dogs.[121,122] The elimination half-life of the free form approximated 2.5 hours, and the conjugated form 4 hours. Urinary excretion was the major route of elimination (approximately 50% to 70% of total dose) as either the conjugated (approximately 50% of total dose) or free form (up to 11%). Morphine was not detected.

Methadone

Methadone is an MOP receptor agonist similar to morphine in action. Analgesia is largely due to the l-methadone isomer, which is eightfold to fiftyfold more potent than the d-isomer. The -d-isomer is characterized by antitussive activity.[27] Its extended duration of action is useful for its suppressant effects on withdrawal in physically dependent humans. Further, effects persist with repeated administration. Its ability to block tolerance induced by morphine may reflect its mild antagonism of NMDA receptors, also a function of the d isomer.[123] In humans it is characterized by an elimination half-life of 15 to 40 hours, resulting in its designation as a long-acting drug. Side effects are similar to those produced by morphine; tolerance develops to the gastrointestinal (including anorexia), sedative, miotic, and cardiac and respiratory effects but not to the constipative effects. Its overall abuse potential is similar to that of morphine in humans.

Methadone has been used as an analgesic in dogs. The disposition of methadone (0.5 mg/kg; 0.45 mg/kg free base) has been described in Greyhounds[124] and Beagles.[125] Interestingly, the disposition is different between the two breeds. A larger volume of distribution in Greyhounds (Table 28-4) was attributed by the authors to potentially reflect pH partitioning of methadone (pKa of 7.4) from plasma (pH 7.39) into muscles (pH 6.9). Methadone was well tolerated in Greyhounds at the dose, although dogs panted and defecated shortly after administration. Because clearance is twice the volume in Greyhounds compared with Beagles, elimination half-life is similar between the two breeds despite the larger volume of distribution in Greyhounds. The antinociceptive effects of methadone apparently have not yet been determined in dogs. The impact of the CYP and P-glycoprotein inhibitors ketaconazole and omeprazole on the disposition of oral methadone (2 mg/kg) was studied in Beagles.[125] Oral methadone was not detected in any dogs, with the exception of one that was also receiving ketaconazole. Methadone (0.2 mg/kg subcutaneously) was compared with buprenorphine (0.02 mg/kg subcutaneously) and morphine (0.2 mg/kg) in cats (n = 8) subjected to mechanical and thermal stimulation.[126] Analgesia associated with methadone was better than that associated with buprenorphine and compared favorably with that produced by morphine, although it was not quite as effective.

Miscellaneous Drugs

Oxycodone (Percodan, class II), *hydrocodone* (Hycodan, class III), and *propoxyphene* (Darvon, class IV) are used to varying degrees in veterinary medicine. Among them, hydrocodone is most commonly used for suppression of cough. *Diphenoxylate* (class II as a sole agent; when combined with atropine to control substance abuse as Lomotil, class V) is used to control diarrhea because of its effects on the gastrointestinal tract.

Loperamide is similar to diphenoxylate, but it does not penetrate the blood–brain barrier as effectively and therefore is associated with no CNS side effects.

MIXED AGONISTS AND ANTAGONISTS

Butorphanol

For decades, butorphanol had a nonscheduled designation by the Food and Drug Administration, but it has since been redesignated as class IV. Butorphanol (0.4 to 0.8 mg/kg intramuscularly, subcutaneously, intravenously every 3 to 6 hours [dogs, cats]; oral [antitussive in dog]: 0.5 to 1 mg/kg every 12 hours) is a KOP agonist and a MOP antagonist, although it may have moderate MOP agonistic actions. It is three to five times more potent (KOP agonist) than morphine and about 50 times *less* potent than naloxone as an antagonist. Butorphanol has been used as both a preanesthetic and a perioperative analgesic in dogs and cats. Historically, it has been one of the three most commonly used opioids for control of postoperative pain in small animals,[127,128] the other two being buprenorphine and oxymorphone.[23] However, the short duration of analgesia provided by butorphanol increasingly is limiting its use to pre-operative in nature. Butorphanol also is approved in dogs for use as an antitussive.[129]

The duration of analgesia after intravenous or subcutaneous administration in dogs is 30 to 45 min at 0.4 mg/kg[130,131] although analgesic effects can last up to 4 to 6 hours in some animals. The duration of analgesia is shorter than sedation.[130] Limited information is available regarding pharmacokinetics in dogs (see Table 28-4).[132,133] In dogs the elimination half-life is 1.65 hours.[132] At high doses butorphanol provides some relief of somatic pain. Butorphanol may be an effective analgesic for mild to moderate pain. For postsurgical pain, butorphanol should be administered 10 minutes before the end of surgery. In general, the efficacy of butorphanol as an analgesic in dogs does not compare favorably with that of NSAIDs. For example, butorphanol (0.2 mg/kg intravenously) was less effective than carprofen, etodolac, or meloxicam for control of pain associated with experimentally induced acute synovitis in Beagles despite the small sample size (four dogs per treatment group).[134] In this study butorphanol was different from control only at 3 and 4 hours after treatment of the 6-hour study period. Butorphanol (0.4 mg/kg) was ineffective as an analgesic in dogs (n = 22) undergoing laparotomy or shoulder arthotomy.[135] The intent of the study was to compare butorphanol with ketorolac or flunixin meglumine; oxymorphone was subsequently substituted.

KEY POINT 28-18 The short duration of efficacy of butorphonal limits its use as a primary analgesic.

The oral preparation of the drug has been dispensed for 1 to 2 days in patients released from the hospital; higher oral doses compared with parenteral doses are required because of its reduced bioavailability after oral administration (0.5 to 1 mg/kg every 12 hours). However, there is no evidence that this is an effective analgesic dose.

Butorphanol may act synergistically when combined with acetaminophen (dogs only) for control of pain.[136] Although safe, epidural administration of butorphanol does not provide sufficient duration of action to be clinically useful.[137, 138] As such, the short duration of action (and mechanism of action of butorphanol) should be questioned with regard to efficacy in most cases of pain control.

An advantage of butorphanol is its MOP antagonistic effects. Butorphanol (0.4 mg/kg) can be used to partially reverse the sedative or respiratory depressant effects of oxymorphone[88] (and presumably other pure opioid agonists). Some of the analgesic effects of the pure opioid will also, however, be reserved. An advantage of butorphanol as a reversal agent is its apparent efficacy as a reversal agent in cats, which is in contrast to naloxone. For example, the initial intensity of hydromorphone and, to a lesser degree, butorphanol analgesia was substantially reduced when the two drugs were used in combination. Side effects included dysphoria (butorphanol only) and vomiting (hydromorphone only).[97]Although butorphanol does cause respiratory depression, a ceiling apparently is reached beyond which additional dosing does not cause further depression (a MOP antagonist).[139] Butorphanol causes less biliary spasm than does morphine, supporting the postoperative use of butorphanol.[54]

Butorphanol appears to be safe in cats if used cautiously, although again, its analgesic efficacy is questionable.[140] Butorphanol has been studied in cats (n = 6) after intramuscular and buccal transmucosal administration of 0.4 mg/kg.[141] The relative bioavailability of butorphanol transmucosally compared with intramuscularly was 38%. The duration of potential antinociception was quite variable at 155 ± 130 minutes based on the duration that concentrations were at or above 45 ng/mL. The latter was the target concentration based on a review of the literature. The antinociceptive potential of butorphanol was studied in cats (n = 6) at 0.2, 0.4, or 0.8 mg/kg.[142] No dose–response relationship was detected, although this likely reflected the small number of cats in the face of small changes in dose. Analgesia began at 15 minutes and persisted for 90 minutes after injection. Mydriasis and dysphoria were frequent. Lascelles and Robertson[96] demonstrated that hydromorphone prolonged the antinociceptive effects of butorphanol (or vice versa).

Johnson[143] compared the antinociceptive potential of intramuscular butorphanol, buprenorpine, or the combination in cats (n = 6). Marked variability was recorded in terms of duration of response: 1 to 8 hours for butorphanol, 0.5 to 5 hours for buprenorphine, and 1 to 8 hours with the combination. This variability contributed to the lack of significant differences among the opioid treatment groups.

Buprenorphine

Buprenorphine (0.005 to 0.03 mg/kg intravenously, intramuscularly, subcutaneously, epidurally [dogs]) is a class IV thebaine derivative with potent analgesic effects 25 or more times greater than those of morphine.[144] It is a KOP antagonist and a MOP partial agonist–antagonist.[145] It is metabolized to norbuprenorhpine, which, as with buprenorphine, is then glucuronidated. The metabolite has approximately 1/50 the analgesic effect of the parent compound (in rats) inpart because of poor penetration of the blood–CSF or blood–brain barrier as well as low intrinsic activity compared with buprenorphine.[146] Buprenorphine has a long duration of activity which reflects, in part, tight adherence to its target receptors.[146]

Buprenorphine is one of the three most commonly used opioids for control of pain in small animals,[127,128,147] and it has been recommended as the most generally useful analgesic for controlling pain in laboratory animals (including dogs).[148] Although its onset of action is longer than that of morphine, its effects last much longer (in humans). In dogs buprenorphine appears to have a 42-hour half-life.[149] Because of its high lipophilicity, buprenorphine has a very high volume of distribution (33 L/kg) and appears to be sequestered in tissues. The long half-life may contribute to its longer duration of action compared with butorphanol. It is metabolized by CYP3A4.

KEY POINT 28-19 Buprenorphine may be the most generally useful analgesic in dogs and cats.

Several studies have addressed the disposition of buprenorphine via alternative routes of administration. Sublingual use has been noted as impossible because of local pH inactivation. However, buprenorphine is approved as a sublingual product in the United Kingdom; sublingual bioavailability in humans ranges from 16% to 94% compared with 40% to 90% after intramuscular administration.[157] Greater doses are claimed to be associated with longer duration of analgesia with no increase in sedation, yet increased doses have been associated with lethal respiratory depression in humans. The intravenous disposition has been reported in cats[158] and dogs by a number of investigators (see Table 28-4).[159-161] Among them are oral and transmucosal routes. Abbo and coworkers[160] described the disposition of buprenorphine (20 and120 μg/kg) in dogs (n=6) after oral transmucosal administration. The bioavailability was 38 ± 12 % and 47 ± 16%, respectively, for the two doses. Robertson and coworkers[138] described the disposition of buprenorphine after oral transmucosal (transbuccal) administration (0.01 mg/kg administered as 0.033 mg/kg) in cats. Peak concentrations of 7.5 mg/mL were achieved at 15 minutes.

Like morphine, buprenorphine induces dose-dependent respiratory depression, which may be delayed in onset. Like butorphanol, a ceiling is reached in respiratory depression but not analgesia in humans.[150] The differential effect may reflect full agonistic actions at analgesic receptors and partial agonism at receptors controlling respiratory depression. The differences may also reflect differences in receptor number. Although respiratory depression has not been a problem in human patients receiving the drug, it is noteworthy that these effects are not fully reversible with antagonists such as naloxone. The risk of respiratory depression associated with buprenorphine is markedly increased when used in combination with other CNS-active drugs. Adversities, including deaths, have been reported in humans simultaneously taking opioids (drug addicts taking buprenorphine as substitution therapy),[151] fentanyl,[152] or ketorolac as part of balanced analgesia and diazepam;[153] only mild interactions have been reported with amitriptyline.[154]

Cardiovascular side effects of buprenorphine are limited. The cat may respond to buprenorphine with mydriasis and agitation at doses exceeding 0.2 mg/kg. An added advantage of buprenorphine is its ability to reverse opioid-induced sedation while maintaining analgesia. It has been recommended as the reversal agent of choice (i.e., instead of naloxone) for human patients receiving neuroleptanalgesics.

Naloxone, when combined with buprenorphine at a 1:4 ratio, has no antagonistic effect when administered sublingually in humans.[155] However, it causes withdrawal signs in humans physically dependent on opioids and is combined for such purposes to prevent abuse.

Buprenorphine has proved to be a very effective analgesic. For example, in humans buprenorphine (intravenously) was found to provide superior analgesia and improved hemodynamic indices compared with fentanyl (intravenously) in human patients undergoing spinal surgery.[156] A plethora of anectodal information exists regarding the use of buprenorphine in animals.

Buprenorphine is the most popular opioid used in small animal practice in the United Kingdom.[138] It may provide 6 hours of analgesia after intramuscular administration (0.01 mg/kg), although onset of action may take 2 hours.[138] Robertson and coworkers[138] a determined the analgesic threshold of buprenorphine in cats after intravenous or transmucosal administration of 20 μg/kg. Bioavailability of the transmucosal route was 113%. Thermal thresholds did not differ by route; peak effect occurred at 90 minutes. The authors concluded that transmucosal was as effective as intravenous administration, providing analgesia for 6 hours. Buprenorphine also has been studied in cats (n = 6) after administration as a transdermal patch.[162] Peak buprenorphine was 10 ± 0.81 ng/mL, but thermal thresholds did not change throughout the 72-hour test period. Steagall[163] evaluated the antinociceptive response of IV buprenorphine in cats using both thermal and mechanical stimulation. Cats (n = 8) were treated with 0.01, 0.02 or 0.04 mg/kg using a randomized three-way crossover design with a week washout period between treatments. Response among cats was markedly variable and was not correlated with coat color or group. Cats (1 in the middle dose and 2 in the high dose) exhibited marked euphoric behavior. Thermal antinociceptive response was noted within 15 minutes at any dose, lasting from 2 to 4 hours at the low and middle dose and 8 hrs at the high dose. The medium and high doses were associated with greater MT antinociception. Slingsby and coworkers[166] compared the difference between a 4-hour 10 μg/kg dose or a second 6-hour 20 μg/kg postoperative dose of buprenorphine in dogs (14 dogs per group) undergoing castration; both groups received buprenorphine (10 or 20 mg/kg) preoperatively. Dogs were studied using a parallel randomized design. Pain scores were low for both groups, decreasing again with the second dose. A trend towards better analgesia occurred with the higher dose and longer interval. Sedation was also effective in both groups. Three dogs at the low dose and 1 dog at the high dose required carprofen rescue analgesia.

A number of prospective clinical trials have examined the analgesic efficacy of buprenorphine compared with other drugs. Changes in thermal threshold for buprenorpine (0.01 mg/kg) was compared with those for morphine (0.2 mg/kg), butorphanol (0.2 mg/kg), and placebo.[46] For butorphanol the threshold increased at 5 minutes but decreased by 2 hours. The duration for morphine was 4 to 5 hours and for buprenorphine 4 and 12 hours. Johnson and coworkers[143] compared the antinociceptive response of intramuscular buprenorphine, butorphanol, or the combination thereof to placebo in cats using a thermal threshold method. Each treatment provided analgesia greater than that in the control group, but no differences could be demonstrated among treatment groups (power of this study not addressed). Duration of analgesia was from 35 minutes to 5 hours for buprenorphine and 50 minutes to 8 hours for butorphanol or the combination. Steagall and coworkers[126] also compared the analgesic efficacy of methadone (0.2 mg/kg subcutaneously), morphine (0.2 mg/kg subcutaneously), and buprenorphine (0.02 mg/kg) in cats (n=8). Cats were studied using a four-way crossover design; mechanical and thermal antinociception was studied. Response to buprenorphine provided the least analgesia, which was attributed in part to subcutaneous administration. Bosmans and coworkers[164] compared the combination of tepoxalin and buprenorphine to buprenorphine alone during the 24-hour period after cruciate repair in dogs (n=20; 10 per group). Animals were studied using a parallel randomized, blinded design. Pain was assessed using visual analog scales and a multifactorial pain scale. No statistical differences were found in either control of pain or side effects. However, the ability to detect a difference is likely to have been limited by the small sample size. Shih and coworkers[165] compared the analgesic efficacy of buprenorphine (0.02 mg/kg) alone, carprofen (4 mg/kg) alone, and carprofen combined with buprenorphine in dogs (n=20 per group) undergoing ovariohysterectomy. A randomized parallel design was used. Anesthetic protocols were the same for all animals. Efficacy was based on a dynamic visual analog scale, and wound swelling was assessed. The carprofen-treated group required more propofol for induction compared with the other two groups. All three treatments provided effective analgesia at 6 and 24 hours, but the pain and wound management scores were superior for the groups treated with carprofen. Buprenorphine also has been compared to local analgesics (e.g., bupivacaine) (see later discussion).

The partial receptor effects of buprenorphine have proved therapeutically beneficial in the detoxification and maintenance treatment of heroin and methadone addicts. The potency of buprenorphine complicates kinetic studies because the low concentrations associated with analgesia are difficult to detect and thus difficult to characterize. The role of buprenorphine as a reversal agent in dogs or cats apparently has not been studied.

Pentazocine

Pentazocine (2 to 3 mg/kg intramuscularly every 2 hours [dogs] or every 4 to 5 hours [cats]) induces analgesia that is one third as potent as that induced by morphine. It is not, however, associated with as severe cardiovascular and respiratory depression. It is effective only as a visceral analgesic. Its utility is limited by its short duration of activity (30 minutes) and its tendency to cause undesirable behavior.[140]

Nalbuphine

Nalbuphine is a nonscheduled opioid that was at one time used as an analgesic for small animals. It is an MOP receptor antagonist and KOP receptor agonist with minimal cardiovascular effects. Butorphanol and buprenorphine have largely replaced the use of this drug.

NARCOTIC ANTAGONISTS

Antagonists are used to provide quick reversal in the event of an overdose or serious respiratory depression or if ambulation is desirable after use of an opiate. Depending on the antagonist and the receptors with which it interacts, analgesia will be reversed along with the undesirable side effects. This is particularly true of pure antagonists. Like agonists, antagonists can be considered pure or partial in their effects. The use of butorphanol as an antagonist was previously discussed. Antagonists generally are not scheduled. The use of MOP opioid antagonists as behavior-modifying drugs is addressed in Chapter 26.

Naloxone

Naloxone (is a pure antagonist with 30 times the potency of nalorphine and 50 times the potency of butorphanol. It is approved for use in the dog but not the cat. As a pure antagonist (0.04 mg/kg intramuscularly, subcutaneously, intravenously every 2 hours or as needed [dogs, cats]; dilute dose in 10 mL of saline and administer to effect intravenously; give remaining dose subcutaneously), it is not regulated by the Controlled Substances Act. Its ability to block each of the opioid receptor types varies; indeed, receptor type can be based somewhat on response to naloxone. MOP receptors are the most sensitive to naloxone antagonism, sigma receptors the least. High doses of naloxone will reverse both DOP and KOP receptors. Reversal with naloxone also depends on the affinity for naloxone and the target receptor being greater than that of the drug to be reversed and on the receptor. Among the opioids, buprenorphine is characterized by a very high affinity for receptors that exceeds that of naloxone; thus buprenorphine is not reversible by naloxone.[155]

After successful reversal with naloxone, respiratory, sedative, and cardiovascular effects of opioids are reversed for 1 to 4 hours. Repeat administration may be indicated, depending on which opioid agonist was used. For example, the effects of oxymorphone may last longer than those of naloxone.[89] Reversal of undesirable opioid side effects with naloxone can be accomplished while maintaining opioid analgesia by mixing 0.1 to 0.25 mL/kg of 0.4 mg/mL naloxone with 10 mL saline. The diluted solution is then administered at 1 mL/minute until unwanted affects are eliminated.[167] Dosing may need to be repeated at 30-minute intervals.

KEY POINT 28-20 MOP receptors are most conducive to antagonism, and in dogs more so than in cats.

Naloxone should be administered slowly when given as an intravenous bolus because of possible cardiovascular stimulation that manifests as increased sympathetic nervous system activity.[168] The increased sympathetic nervous system activity presumably reflects the sudden reversal of analgesia and thus the perception of pain. In human beings this increased sympathetic nervous system activity may be demonstrated as tachycardia, hypertension, pulmonary edema,[169,170] and cardiac dysrhythmias (including ventricular fibrillation). Naloxone induces hyperglycemia in cats, similar to that caused by morphine.[171] Naloxone antagonizes the effects of nonopiate depressants and alters dopamine and GABA actions in the CNS.[56] It has also been studied for its ability to alter detrimental physiologic response in circulatory and septic shock; however, this therapeutic use, which was once considered a benefit, appears to provide no decrease in mortality rates and may cause detrimental effects. Diltiazem may impair the pharmacologic actions of naloxone (statement in abstracts of drug interactions with buprenorphine). Naloxone is not approved as a reversal agent in cats, and cats do not appear to react predictably to reversal with naloxone. Recovery and survival were not improved in kittens in which opioids were reversed.[172]

Nalorphine

Nalorphine is a partial agonist and as such is a class III drug. Sedation and analgesia are maintained, and CNS (including respiratory) depression is reduced.

Nalbuphine

Nalbuphine (Nubain) (1 mL of 20 mg/mL solution to 9 mL saline, as with naloxone) is discussed as a mixed agonist–antagonist. Like butorphanol and buprenorphine, nalbuphine has been used as a partial antagonist to induce reversal of CNS depression but not as an analgesic.

Naltrexone

Naltrexone is an orally bioavailable pure antagonist that has been used to treat lick granulomas in dogs (see Chapter 26).

THERAPEUTIC USE OF OPIOID ANALGESICS

Opioids are used in veterinary medicine to control pain; as adjuvant anesthesia, emetics (apomorphine), antitussives, and antidiarrheals; and for chemical restraint. In 1954 the optimum dose of opioids as defined in human medicine was described as "that which provided the desired therapeutic effects with a minimum of undesirable side effects".[173] Yet caution was encouraged when opioids were used to control pain because of their unpleasant, dangerous side effects and the risk of addiction. Hence a 4- to 6-hour dosing interval has largely been followed, even though subsequent studies in humans have shown this approach to be largely ineffective. For human patients suffering from pain, a sophisticated method of opioid self-administration (patient-controlled analgesia [PCA]) is available; interesting observations have been generated from users of PCA regarding the effectiveness of opioids to control pain; many of these observations can be applied to the control of pain in animals.[173,174]

In patients using PCA, the method preferred by patients, the dose varies eightfold to tenfold among those within a given age group. Additionally, the analgesic needs of any patient are rarely constant; rather, temporary increases in the dosage of opioids are necessary for "incident" pain such as that caused by ambulation and wound dressing. As expected, the dose declines each day after the surgery. The use of visual analogs reduces the risk of underdosing. The sedative effects of the opioid that occur at high doses appear to prevent the risk of self-overdose. Excessive sedation is an earlier and better indicator of respiratory depression; reduced respiratory rate is a late and unreliable indicator of overdosage. Older patients require less drug than younger patients. Indeed, age is a better predictor of the initial dose than is body weight, although this likely reflects similarities in weight among people, a characteristic that would be more variable in animals. Opioid addiction occurs very rarely when these drugs are used to control postoperative pain.[173]

Comparisons of opioids have been based on potency, with morphine generally serving as the prototypic drug for comparison. Interestingly, the thermal threshold for a variety of opioids in cats approximates 50 ng/mL.[135] Factors determining potency include lipid solubility (and movement into and out of the CNS), affinity for receptor sites, and other factors. As such, fentanyl and its congeners and buprenorphine are among the most potent drugs and thus are dosed in μg/mL as opposed to mg/mL. In contrast to potency, efficacy is affected by relationship to receptors and pharmacokinetics that describe absorption, distribution (including rate and extent), and elimination. Therefore elimination half-life will play a role in the selection of the drug. Generally, lipophilic drugs move rapidly into the CNS, but duration is short because of rapid movement from the CNS.[173] In human patients the plasma elimination of the opioids varies from twofold to fourfold. Uptake and elimination from the CNS also may vary. Thus differences among patients should be anticipated, underscoring the importance of a visual pain-scoring system when evaluating patient need for opioid dosing.

Pain is generally best controlled with sufficient fixed doses at short intervals (generally 2 to 4 hours).[23,29] Intramuscular doses will usually prolong the duration of analgesia. However, a transdermal patch or CRI can be used to provide prolonged analgesia without peak and trough effects of marked fluctuation in the plasma drug concentration. Epidural administration achieves analgesia at doses that are a fraction of parenteral doses.

Indications of opioid analgesics include but are not limited to trauma, postoperative pain, and thermal injuries. Postoperative analgesia is best achieved if the drug is administered before anesthetic recovery; preanesthetic administration may be indicated if postoperative analgesia is anticipated. Control of chronic pain with opioids may be difficult in part because tolerance and physical dependence may complicate therapy. Although long-term opioid therapy may be very effective, alternative therapies such as local nerve blocks, acupuncture, and behavioral modification also are implemented for human patients. Other drugs that might be used include antidepressants and NSAIDs. NSAIDs should also be considered in combination with opioids, particularly for orthopedic pain associated with cancer. For example, butorphanol and acetaminophen appear to act synergistically for control of pain.[136] Constipation should be anticipated with chronic use of opioids, and mild laxatives or stool softeners may be necessary.

Rotation of opioids remains a therapeutic option for control of pain in humans.[175] Drugs most commonly used are morphine, fentanyl, 1-methadone, and buprenorphine. The most common indications for change included insufficient control of pain (most common at 43%) and intolerable side effects or both. Change is successful in controlling pain in 65% of patients for which initial opioid choice failed. Intolerable side effects tend to reflect individual differences in response rather than dose dependency. Unpredictable and incomplete cross-tolerance among the drugs requires careful titration whenever one opioid replaces another.[175]

OTHER CENTRALLY ACTING DRUGS

Tramadol

Structure Activity Relationship

Tramadol (Ultram) is a synthetic analog of codeine currently marketed as a racemic (1:1) mixture of ± enantiomers. Tramadol appears to have multiple mechanisms of analgesia, with interaction among the pathways perhaps contributing to its efficacy. Opioid analgesia reflects agonistic interaction with MOP receptors; additionally, tramadol enhances spinal pain inhibitory pathways through inhibition of neuronal reuptake of serotonin (5-HT) and noradrenaline (NA) and release of 5-HT. As such, tramadol might be indicated for a broad array of conditions associated with pain, including chronic pain: Studies suggest that the analgesia associated with 5-HT_{1A} receptor agonists increases with chronic or repeat administration.[48]

KEY POINT 28-21 Tramadol has multiple mechanism of analgesic efficacy. However, its metabolite may provide most of the efficacy, contributing to variability in response among animals.

Both tramadol stereoisomers are associated with analgesia, although receptor interactions appear to differ between the isomers. Tramadol is de-ethylated by CYP2D6 to an active metabolite, O-desmethyltramadol (ODT, M1). Opioid MOP receptors are bound by both tramadol (low affinity) and ODT (higher affinity). Studies in CYP2D6 deficient or inhibited states suggest that the majority of analgesic activity (at different receptor types) reflects ODT. In animal models ODT is 200 times as potent as tramadol in MOP-opioid binding and up to 6 times more potent as an analgesic (sponsor information). However, the potency of ODT is still 6000 times less than that of morphine. Differences in enantiomer and receptor interactions with opioid and nonopioid drugs have been described for both tramadol and ODT. (+)-Tramadol and ODT interact with opiate (MOP, KOP, and DOP) receptors, alpha $_{(2)}$ receptors, and (tramadol) serotonin reuptake and receptors, whereas (-)-tramadol and ODT interact with norepinephrine uptake and alpha $_{(2)}$ receptors.[176] Although ODT may be responsible for the majority of analgesic activity, tramadol appears to act synergistically with ODT, which may explain its apparent efficacy in dogs despite the apparently small contribution of ODT to tramadol metabolism.[176]

Minimum effective plasma concentrations for tramadol and ODT are quite variable, ranging from 298 (± 171) to 590 (± 410) for tramadol and 39.6 (± 29.5) to 84 (± 34 ng/mL) for ODT in postoperative human patients.[176] The efficacy of tramadol as an analgesic is dose dependent, with efficacy described as being between that of codeine and morphine and similar to that of meperidine (pethidine), or about 10% to 20% of that of morphine.

Disposition

The volume of distribution of tramadol in humans (and dogs; discussed later) is large, and in rat models the drug crosses the blood–brain barrier. Hepatic metabolism of tramadol produces a number of metabolites. As noted, hepatic demethylation of tramadol by CYP2D6 (an enzyme characterized by polymorphism in humans) yields ODT (M1), which also exists as a racemic mixture. Tramadol also is metabolized by CYP3A4 and CYP2B6, with parent drug and metabolites excreted renally.

The disposition of tramadol and its active metabolite ODT have been studied in normal Beagles;[176] ODT was studied after both intravenous and oral administration of tramadol or ODT (1 mg/kg IV) (see Table 28-4). The proportion of tramadol metabolized to ODT in dogs is approximately 15% after intravenous administration. After an oral dose of 11 mg/kg, plasma C_{max} (ng/mL) of the parent compound is 1403 ± 695 occurring at 1.04 ± 0.51 hours. Oral bioavailability of tramadol is of 65 ± 38%. Elimination half-life of tramadol is approximately 2 hours (1.8 ± 1.2). The volume of distribution of tramadol appears to be larger than that of ODT. However, clearance also is faster for the parent compound compared with that for the metabolite, resulting in an elimination or disappearance half-life that is similar for both. Although the volume of distribution of tramadol is similar in humans compared with dogs, the elimination half-life of both tramadol and ODT is shorter in dogs compared with humans (approximately 6 and 7 hours, respectively for humans), suggesting that a more frequent dosing interval is indicated for tramadol in dogs. Simulated oral dosing regimens based on kinetics determined in the dog indicate that 5 mg/kg every 6 hours or 2.5 mg/kg every 4 hours should yield tramadol and M1 plasma concentrations associated with analgesia in humans. After intravenous administration of ODT (1.1 mg/kg), nausea and sedation occurred in all dogs (n=3), probably reflecting the MOP 1 agonistic properties. However, even though the area under the curve for ODT after intravenous administration of 1.1 mg/kg approximated that achieved after tramadol at 11 mg/kg, no side effects to tramadol were reported.

The disposition of tramadol and ODT after either intravenous (2 mg/kg) or oral (5 mg/kg) administration of tramadol also has been described in cats (n=6 see Table 28-4).[177] The area under the curve of active metabolites is equal to or surpasses that of the area under the curve of the parent compound compared with dogs, for which it reaches about 30% of the parent compound in dogs (see Table 28-4). The elimination half-life of both parent and ODT is approximately twofold higher in cats. Cats tolerated tramadol by either route, although they exhibited euphoria for several hours. A 5 mg/kg oral dose achieves for tramadol and well exceeds for ODT the minimum effective analgesic concentrations suggested in humans. It is not clear if a similar level of analgesia would be expected in cats, but based on the higher concentrations of ODT in cats, a dose of 2 mg/kg twice daily is a reasonable starting dose.

Adverse Events and Drug Interactions

Side effects of tramadol appear to be unusual and generally reflect either overzealous use or overdosage. The risk of overdosage is increased in both renal and hepatic disease owing to prolonged elimination of both parent and metabolite. Cirrhosis is associated with a threefold to fourfold increase in elimination time in humans (sponsor information); the impact in the dog—in which the half-life is shorter—is not known. Dosage adjustment is recommended if hepatic or renal function is significantly impaired; for dogs prolongation of the interval may be more appropriate than reduction of the dose. Gender and age differences do not appear to play a major role in overdosing. Overdosage in humans is associated with significant neurologic clinical signs, including seizures, coma, and respiratory depression. Internet resources addressing safety of tramadol for human use indicate that seizures generally reflect overzealous use of tramadol, are of short duration, and are easily treated. Inappropriate (overzealous) administration of naloxone (an appropriate antidote to toxicity) may increase the risk of seizures. CNS side effects may emerge when tramadol is combined with other drugs or compounds that increase serotonin (e.g., behavior modifying drugs, s-adenosyl methionine [SAMe] or silymarin; see also Chapter 26).[177a] Cardiovascular signs, even with overdosage, tend to be limited to mild tachycardia and hypertension. Respiratory depression is unusual, although the risk may be increased with renal disease, with retention of ODT implicated as a cause in review references. Gastrointestinal motility disturbances typical of opioids, such as postoperative ileus and constipation (including that associated with chronic use), generally are not associated with tramadol. The incidence of nausea and vomiting appears to be similar to that of opioids in humans. However, vomiting did not occur in Beagles (n = 6) receiving tramadol intravenously, whereas it did in those treated with ODT;[176] ODT may have a greater presence in humans compared with dogs, thus explaining the potential lack of this side effect in dogs.

Despite its widespread use, clinical trials demonstrating efficacy of tramadol as an analgesic are lacking in dogs and cats. Steagall and coworkers[178] studied the antinociceptive effects of tramadol (1 mg/kg subcutaneously) with or without acepromazine (0.1 mg/kg) in cats (n=8) subjected to thermal stimulation. Animals had only a limited response to tramadol, although the effect was increased when tramadol was combined with acepromazine.

N-methyl-D-aspartate Agonists

Ketamine

Ketamine is a noncompetitive antagonist of NMDA receptors in the spinal cord and consequently may help prevent or reduce neuropathic pains such as hyperalgesia or wind-up pain. Norketamine is an active metabolite that also binds to NMDA receptors.[179] Three "levels" of ketamine use can be discriminated in dogs or cats: a high dose associated with anesthetic effects, a low dose that targets analgesia and prevention of wind-up pain (hyperalgesia), and a subanalgesic dose that, when combined with other analgesics, provides analgesic dose-sparing effects. Ketamine combined with opioids appear to provide superior analgesia compared with either drug alone.[180] Ketamine and other NMDA-receptor antagonists may impart a neuroprotective effect after reperfusion of ischemic tissues. The local anesthetic effects of ketamine are described later.

After intravenous ketamine (15 mg/kg) administration in dogs,[181] the volume of distribution of the central and peripheral compartments were 0.52 and 1.95 L/kg, respectively; clearance was 32 mL/min/kg. Elimination half-life was 61 minutes. The drug was 53% protein bound. Ketamine was converted to ketamine I (62%) and II (11%). The N-demethylketamine metabolites were measured and determined not to accumulate sufficiently to interfere with anesthesia.

A number of studies have examined the efficacy of ketamine as an analgesic when included in combination therapy. The targeted minimum anesthetic concentration is 3 μg/mL. The addition of ketamine or magnesium enhanced tramadol analgesia in humans undergoing major abdominal surgery.[182] Subanesthetic doses of ketamine were useful in controlling complex regional pain syndrome in humans. Complete resolution of pain occurred in 76% of 33 patients; partial pain relief occurred in another 18%. Side effects included a feeling of inebriation, hallucinations, and light-headedness.[183] The analgesic benefits of ketamine have been demonstrated in dogs. Dogs presenting for elective forelimb amputation associated with neoplasia and receiving fentanyl (2 μg/kg intravenous bolus followed by 2 μg/kg/hr intravenously) and ketamine by intravenous infusion (0.5 mg/kg before surgery and 2 μg/kg/hr at 12 and 18 hours postoperatively) had lower pain scores and more rapid return to activity postoperatively compared with dogs receiving fentanyl and a saline infusion.[180] Administration of a subanesthetic dose of ketamine (2.5 mg/kg intramuscularly) preoperatively or postoperatively delayed the onset of postoperative wound hyperalgesia in dogs undergoing OHE compared with dogs receiving no ketamine.[184] The use of subanesthetic doses offers the advantage of minimal side effects. The same is true when administered as a CRI (an initial loading dose of 0.25 to 0.5 mg/kg of ketamine, followed by an infusion of 10 mg/kg/min for dogs). Because ketamine can be given by essentially any route, including oral administration,[185] consideration might be given to its oral use in the control of neuropathic pain. A variety of dosing regimens are described for ketamine when used in combination with other analgesics such as lidocaine, morphine, and fentanyl.

KEY POINT 28-22 Combination analgesia might reasonably include a drug that targets N-methyl-D-aspartate receptors.

Amantadine

According to its package insert, amantadine is an antiviral drug with an unknown mechanism of antiviral replication action. It is approved to treat influenza A virus, but it also is useful for treatment of Parkinson's disease in humans and drug-induced extrapyramidal effects. Its mechanism of action in Parkinson's disease is not known, but proposed mechanisms included increased extracellular concentrations of dopamine (increased release or decreased uptake) at presynaptic neurons, direct simulation of dopamine receptors, or increased sensitivity of the receptors. Additionally, at concentrations considered to be in the low range, amantadine inhibits NMDA-receptor–mediated stimulation of acetylcholine release (rat striatum; probably at the MK-801 site). Although a dose of 31.5 mg/kg in dogs (equivalent to an approximate human dose of 15.8 mg/kg based on body surface area conversions) is not associated with anticholinergic actions, it nonetheless does cause anticholinergic-like side effects, including dry mouth, urinary retention, and constipation.

The drug is well absorbed in humans, with peak concentrations of about 0.22 mg/mL occurring at 3 hours after an oral dose of 100 mg (about 1.4 mg/kg). In humans saturation kinetics occur at 200 mg; after 15 days at this dose, C_{max} doubled in healthy human patients. Volume of distribution is large and variable in humans (3 to 8 L/kg), indicating tissue binding. The acetylated metabolite accounts for up to 80% of a dose in about 40% of humans, with the metabolite not occurring in the remainder; only 5% to 15% of this metabolite occurs in the urine. It is not known if this metabolite is active or toxic. Because the dog is deficient in metabolic reactions involving acetylation, extrapolation of human kinetics to dogs is questionable. The drug is cleared as either the parent compound or its metabolite in the urine. The half-life of the drug in adult humans is approximately 15 hours but 29 hours in elderly patients because of smaller clearance; the reason for the differences in clearance is not known. Renal clearance was also higher in human male patients compared with that in human female patients. Renal disease results in at least a proportional decrease in amantadine clearance. Acidification of urine pH is likely to increase renal clearance of amantidine.

Amantadine has been associated with lethal acute intoxication in humans, with the lowest reported acute lethal dose being 1 gram (approximately 14 mg/kg) in humans. However, anticholinergic effects do not occur in dogs receiving 31.5 mg/kg (package insert). Acute toxicity may be attributable to the anticholinergic effects of amantadine. Drug overdose has resulted in cardiovascular (arrhythmias, including tachycardia, and hypertension), respiratory, renal, or CNS (behavioral changes, seizures) toxicity. A less common but life-threatening manifestation is neuroleptic malignant syndrome, which is characterized by fever or hyperthermia, muscle rigidity, involuntary movements, and altered consciousness or other mental status changes. Other disturbances, such as autonomic dysfunction, tachycardia, tachypnea, hypertension, or hypotension may occur; clinical pathology changes include increases in serum creatine phosphokinase activity, leukocytosis, myoglobinuria, and increased serum myoglobin. Treatment of acute intoxication has included dopamine agonists (e.g., bromocriptine) and muscle relaxants (e.g., dantrolene), but their efficacy has not been scientifically demonstrated. Doses should be adjusted for both liver and renal disease. The drug should not be used in conjunction with other anticholinergics, and extra precautions should be taken when combining with any other CNS-active drugs. Anecdotally, amantadine has been used safely in both dogs and cats as part of combined analgesic therapy.

Using a randomized, placebo controlled, blinded design, Lascelles and coworkers[186] prospectively studied the efficacy of amantadine (3 to 5 mg/kg once daily) when combined with meloxicam (0.2 mg/kg followed by 0.1 mg/kg per day orally) in clinical canine cases (n=31) of pelvic limb lameness associated with osteoarthritis. Animals had not sufficiently responded to NSAIDs alone. Amantadine resulted in more activity compared with NSAIDs alone.

Dextromethorphan

Dextromethorphan is a semisynthetic derivative of opium (the d-isomer of the codeine analog of methorphan) that lacks narcotic, analgesic, or addictive properties. Sedation is unusual after its use. Its antitussive mechanism is not certain. Its onset of action is rapid, being fully effective within 30 minutes after oral administration. Dextromethorphan, which is sold in over-the-counter cough preparations, also is an NMDA-receptor antagonist. It has increased the analgesic effects of opiates and NSAIDs.[14] The elimination half-life of dextromethorphan in dogs is approximately 2 hours.[187] After intravenous administration of 2.2 mg/kg, an approximate extrapolated C_{max} (Co) of 800 ± 400 and 360 ± 150 occurred before and after the distributive phase, respectively. This compares to a C_{max} of 89.8 ± 47.2 at approximately 1 hour after oral administration, yielding an oral bioavailability of 11% or less. Dextromethorphan is metabolized by CYP2D6 to dextrorphan, which is characterized by pharmacodynamics that are similar to, albeit less potent (25% to 30%) than, that of dextromethorphan. Dextrorphan is a metabolite produced in dogs, although it was detected only as the glucuronide metabolite by KuKanich and Papich.[187] After intravenous administration of 2.2 mg/kg in dogs, adverse reactions to dextrorphan were consistent with NMDA antagonism, ranging from lateral recumbency to nonresponsiveness, including ataxia, sedation, muscle rigidity, urination, and ptyalism. Changes in cardiovascular indices did not occur. Clinical signs resolved within 90 minutes, at concentrations of approximately 100 ng/mL. Oral administration was associated with vomiting in one dog. The role of dextromethorphan as an NMDA antagonist in either dogs or cats is not clear but is worth consideration. Dodman and coworkers[188] reported the potential usefulness of dextromethorphan (2 mg/kg orally) for 2 weeks in dogs (n=12) with chronic allergic dermatitis using a double-blinded crossover placebo-controlled design. The percentage of time abnormal behaviors (self-licking, chewing and biting) were observed and the overall pruritis score were significant lower than that in the placebo group; global assessment improved in 11 of 12 dogs.

Other Tranquilizers and Sedatives

Tranquilizers generally are not analgesic, but they alter animals' response to pain. They are most commonly used in combination with opioid analgesics, with which they may act. Some also may provide muscle relaxation. The common tranquilizers and sedatives are the phenothiazine derivatives (which may also provide antiemetic effects), such as chlorpromazine, promazine, and acetylpromazine, and the benzodiazepine derivatives, such as diazepam and midazolam. Phenothiazines (see Chapter 26) should be used cautiously for hypotensive patients or for patients with cardiovascular disease. The benzodiazepines (see Chapter 27) are particularly useful for geriatric and debilitated animals. Agents from either group can be combined with opioid analgesics.

α_2-Agonists

Canine $alpha_{2a}$ receptors in the brain appear to be closely related to those in humans.[189] $Alpha_2$ agonists such as xylazine and medetomidine warrant special consideration because they are potent analgesics at doses that do not cause sedation. (see Chapter 24). Xylazine's duration of analgesia is short (0.5 hours), and it has profound cardiovascular effects. Its CNS-depressant effects, however, can be reversed with yohimbine or tolazoline. In addition, xylazine can be used in combination with opioid agonist–antagonists such as butorphanol and as an epidural just before surgery or surgical recovery. Newer α_2 agonists such as medetomidine (0.75 mg/m^2 intravenously or 1 mg/m^2 intramuscularly [dogs]) are associated with fewer cardiovascular effects and longer duration of activity than xylazine. Medetomidine provides both sedation and analgesia and is labeled for use in dogs for clinical procedures that require short-term chemical restraint. The effects can be reversed with atipamezole, an α_2-antagonist, and as such, the drug may be useful for incident pain, such as bandage change. Like xylazine, medetomidine can cause vomiting and cardiovascular suppression. Medetomidine has proved to be an equal or better analgesic than buprenorphine for control of pain in dogs. The safety of the two drugs has not, however, been compared.[190]

In dogs the DEX enantiomer of medetomidine appears to be largely responsible for analgesia, sedation, and cardiovascular side effects of medetomidine.[191] Although the LEV enantiomer appears to be pharmacologically inactive, it may be involved in drug interactions. The sedative or analgesic (based on withdrawal) effects of medetomidine appear to be characterized by a ceiling effect.[191] Plasma concentrations associated with analgesia vary, ranging from 1 to 5 ng/mL, although 9.5 ng/mL was not associated with pain-induced withdrawal in dogs.[191] The combination of epidural medetomidine and morphine offered only minimal analgesic benefits compared with epidural morphine alone.[86]

ANTICONVULSANTS AND BEHAVIOR-MODIFYING DRUGS

Anticonvulsants (see Chapter 27) such as carbamazepine, phenytoin, valproic acid, and clonazepam, and more recently, gabapentin and pregabalin have been used by humans to control selected neuralgias.[5] TCAs (see Chapter 26) have also been used by humans for the treatment of chronic pain. Efficacy of TCAs, anticonvulsants, and antiarrhythmics requires several weeks and generally requires dose titration.[9] Amitriptyline and imipramine are considered first-line drugs, particularly for pain that is continuous and aching. Their use for pain control has not been documented in animals, although they have been used successfully for behavioral problems. The sedative and anticholinergic side effects of these drugs may be undesirable. Not all TCAs—and particularly the newer products—appear to have analgesic properties. Neuropathic, myofascial, and arthritic pains appear to be most conducive to control. These drugs are contraindicated for patients suffering from urinary retention, heart block, or narrow-angle glaucoma.

Gabapentin and Pregabalin

Both gabapentin and pregablin were initially developed as human antiepileptic drugs. Pregabalin was approved for use for treatment of neuropathic pain in humans, most recently that associated with fibromyalgia. Both are structurally related to GABA; gabapentin is a molecule of GABA covalently bound to a lipophilic cyclohexane ring (Figure 28-5).[192] Although their mechanism of action was intended to be a GABA agonist, pharmacologically, they do not bind to any portion of the GABA receptor, nor do they appear to interfere with degradation or other aspects of GABA receptor activity. Rather, their mechanism of analgesic action appears to occur through binding to $Ca_v\alpha_{2d}$ proteins on voltage-gated calcium channels.[193] Decreased calcium influx prevents release of neurotransmitters otherwise stimulated by a variety of chemical signals.

A Cochrane review of the ability of gabapentin to control pain covered 14 studies in human medicine, one of which was for management of acute pain.[194] The remaining causes of pain included herpes, diabetic neuropathy, cancer, phantom limb, and spinal cord injury. Gabapentin offered no benefit for control of acute pain. However, for chronic pain 42% of participants improved compared with 19% of patients receiving placebo. Side effects necessitating withdrawal were not considered significant.

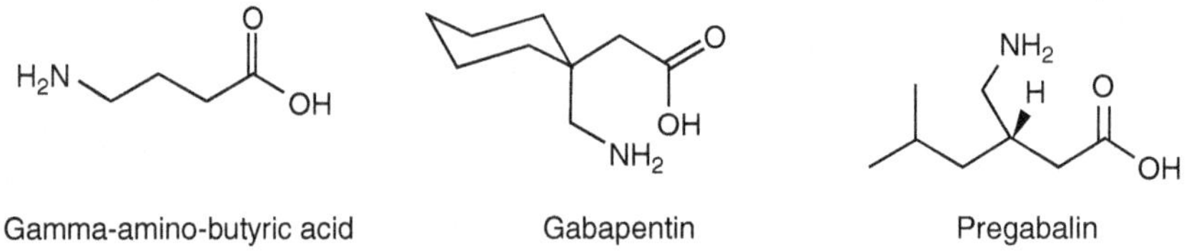

H2N OH O — Gamma-amino-butyric acid
O OH NH2 — Gabapentin
NH2 H O OH — Pregabalin

Figure 28-5 The structure of anticonvulsant-analgesics and gamma-aminobutyric acid.

A study comparing the impact of gabapentin on analgesia provided by morphine in humans found gabapentin to have no analgesic effects by itself (concentrations approximating 3.5 mcg/mL) compared to placebo, but morphine analgesia was markedly enhanced (at gabapentin concentrations of about 5.5 mcg/ml). The disposition of gabapentin was altered by morphine, with an increased in AUC by more than 40%. The effect was posulated to reflect increased oral absorption.[194a] Dosing for control of pain is instituted at approximately 1.25 mg/kg once to three times daily and gradually increased every 1 to 3 days to a dose of approximately 15 to 50 mg/kg total daily dose. The gradual increase is intended to allow accommodation to the drug. Doses were reduced in the presence of renal disease.

Wagner and coworkers194b were not able to detect a significant difference between placebo or gabapentin 10 mg/kg followed by 5 mg/kg bid PO for 3 days prior to forelimb amputation in dogs (n = 30, 15 each group). Other analyses were also used, which along with a small sample size, limited detection of a significant effect.

KEY POINT 28-23 Increasingly, gabapentin and pregabalin are proving to be effective alternatives for long-term neuropathic pain control.

LOCAL ANESTHETICS

Local anesthetics act by binding reversibly to a target receptor located in the pore of voltage-gated sodium channels in nerves. Ion movement is subsequently blocked, preventing conduction of the action potential in any nerve fiber. In general, sensation of pain disappears first, followed by loss of the sensations of temperature, touch, deep pressure, and finally motor function. In addition to effects in the periphery, selective central blockade of afferent evoked activity in the spinal cord also has been suggested as a mechanism of local anesthetics. Further, selected drugs (e.g., lidocaine) may interact with (activate) the endogenous opioid system (as reviewed by Joad and coworkers).[9] Local anesthetics also bind to other membrane proteins, including potassium, but generally at higher concentrations.

Local anesthetic effects were recognized for cocaine, an ester of benzoic acid. Safety concerns led to the development of synthetic alternative drugs. Local anesthetics generally consist of a lipid-soluble, aromatic component; an amide (e.g., lidocaine) or ester (e.g., procaine) link; and a water-soluble amine (usually tertiary) component (Figure 28-6).[195] Whereas esters tend to be rapidly metabolized by esterases, amides are more resistant to clearance and generally are characterized by longer duration of effect.

The potency, onset of action, and duration of local anesthetic actions depend on lipid solubility, pK_a, and protein binding, respectively. Highly lipid-soluble molecules are more potent and have a longer duration of effect because of their ability to penetrate cell membranes, thus accessing the receptor while avoiding clearance. However, lipophilic drugs also tend to be associated with more side effects. Larger drugs tend to have a longer duration of effect because they are less able to leave the site of action, an important characteristic for rapidly firing cells. Bupivacaine is more lipid soluble and 10 times

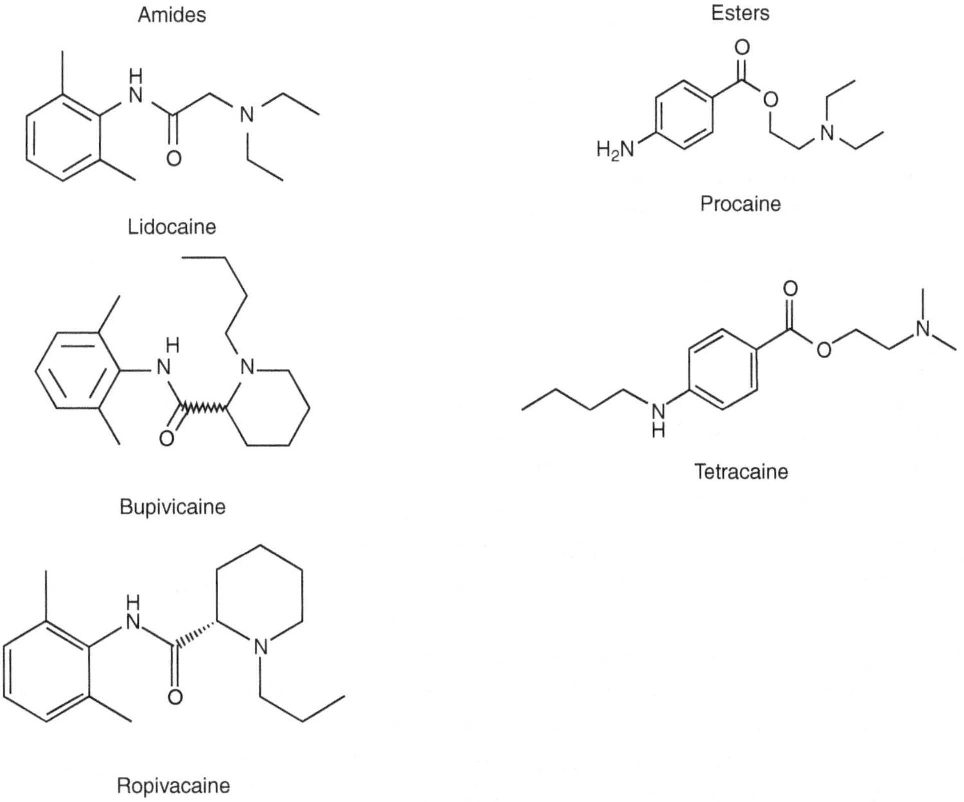

Amides

Lidocaine

Bupivicaine

Ropivacaine

Esters

Procaine

Tetracaine

Figure 28-6 The structure of selected amide *(left)* and ester *(right)* local or topical anesthetics.

more potent than lidocaine. Likewise, tetracaine is more lipid soluble and 40 times more potent than procaine (an aromatic ring is added).

KEY POINT 28-24 The analgesic effect of local anesthetics vary with lipid solubility, pKa, and protein binding.

Drug pK_a also influences drug movement by determining the amount of un-ionized and thus diffusible drug. Local anesthetics are weak bases with pK_as of 7.7 to 9. In pharmaceutical preparations the pH of the solution tends to be acidic; thus most of the drugs are present in ionized form. Although penetration of tissues is decreased, once penetrated, it is the protonated (cationic) form that preferentially interacts with the receptor. Thus the higher the pK_a, the more drug present in ionized form and the longer the onset of action.

Local anesthetics that are more highly protein bound tend to be attracted to receptors and remain within sodium channels longer. Thus bupivacaine, which is highly protein bound, has a longer duration of activity than procaine. Duration of activity is also affected by the effect of the drugs on local vasculature or the presence of vasoconstrictors (e.g., epinephrine; discussed later).

Local anesthetics should contact the tissue for at least 20 minutes to be effective. Methods include splash blocks or direct infiltration at the surgical site to enhance intraoperative or postoperative analgesia (orthopedic procedures, lateral ear resections or total ear canal ablation, dew claw removal, onychectomy, and ear trims), infiltration of nerves before transection during amputation, regional nerve blocks (e.g., intercostal); intraarticular filtration (analgesic effect may last up to 24 hours), intrapleural infiltration, and epidurals. Lidocaine and bupivacaine are the agents most commonly used (nonophthalmically) in dogs and cats. Lidocaine is characterized by a rapid (5- to 10-minute) onset but a short (1- to 2-hour) duration; the pharmacologic (analgesic) action appears longer than its half-life. The lidocaine dose should not exceed 4 to 7 mg/kg. Side effects at 11 mg/kg include restlessness, muscle tremors, cardiac depression, and seizures.

All local anesthetics cause vasodilation, which decreases the duration of action and prolongs the onset of action. Lidocaine is available as a commercial preparation combined with epinephrine designed to prolong anesthetic effects. In humans, after intraperitoneal administration, the time to maximum absorption of lidocaine varies in proportion to the amount of epinephrine (reviewed by Wilson and coworkers).[196] Maximum concentrations occur in approximately 30 minutes when epinephrine is not included. When epinephrine is included, the time ranges from 45 to 60 minutes when epinephrine is added at 1:320,000 (epinephrine) to up to 3 hours when present at 1:500,000. Maximum lidocaine concentrations likewise vary with both the dose of lidocaine and epinephrine; in humans at 400 mg (approximately 3.8 mg/kg), C_{max} ranged from 2.7 to 4.3μg/mL with no epinephrine but approximated only 1.9 μg/mL at 1:800,000 and 2.3 μg/mL at 1:320,000.

Lidocaine (2% lidocaine, with 1:200,000 epinephrine commercial preparation, diluted to a volume of 0.8 mL/kg) has been studied after local (incisional: 2 mg/kg, final epinephrine 1:400,000) and intraperitoneal (8 mg/kg; final epinephrine 1:200,000) administration in normal dogs undergoing ovariohysterectomy.[196,197] Administration occurred during abdominal closure. The combined administration yielded peak concentrations of lidocaine (n-acetyl metabolite not studied) of 1.45 ± 0.36 μg/mL at approximately 40 minutes after administration; disappearance half-life was 1.17 ± 0.11 hour. No clinical signs of toxicity occurred.

The addition of sodium bicarbonate with lidocaine (9:1) has been recommended to minimize pain on injection (one part sodium bicarbonate [1 mEq/L] to nine parts 1% to 2% lidocaine). Bupivacaine likewise can be diluted at a rate of 0.5 mL bupivacaine (0.5%) to 0.025 mL bicarbonate. Alkalinization may affect local anesthetic effect, although impact is likely to vary with the drug. Local analgesia may also potentially be enhanced, perhaps because of either an increase in the un-ionized local anesthetic or accelerated conversion of local anesthetic from un-ionized to ionized form, with intracellular acidification caused by bicarbonate.[198] However, the risk of precipitation of anesthetic also should be considered and products modified with alkalinizers carefully monitored for changes in anticipated efficacy.

Lidocaine can be applied topically for local effects. A cream approved for use in humans containing 2.5% of lidocaine and prilocaine (eutectic mixture of local anesthetics [EMLA] cream) was found to be effective in awake cats undergoing percutaneous jugular catheterization.[199] The cream (1 mL at 1 g/mL, yielding a 5 mg/kg dose of each anesthetic for a 5 kg cat) was applied to a 2 × 5-cm region on the skin at the site of anticipated catheter placement and covered with an occlusive bandage for 1 hour. Six of ten cats were successfully intravenously catheterized without the addition of chemical restraint; struggling was attributed to fear rather than pain. Neither anesthetic was detectable in the plasma of any cat, and methemoglobinemia did not deviate from baseline. The disposition of lidocaine after administration of a liposomal gel (equivalent to 15 mg/kg lidocaine) was studied in cats (n = 6).[200] Absorption was negligible in two cats. In the remaining four cats, peak concentrations reached approximately 150 ng/mL at a median time of 2 hours.

Lidocaine is available in a transdermal patch. Lidocaine is contained in a polymer matrix; the amount of drug moving into the system is proportional to the covered skin surface. Weil and coworkers[201] reviewed their use in dogs or cats. In contrast to fentanyl patches, lidocaine patches can be cut to size. Weiland and coworkers[202] described the pharmacokinetics of one 5% lidocaine patch applied to the lateral thorax of Beagles (n = 6). Dogs were either clipped or treated with a depilatory agent. Peak concentrations (ng/mL) of lidocaine were 63 ± 24 and 103 ± 34 respectively (well below the concentration recommended for antinociception, see later discussion), with or without the depilatory. The areas under the curve were 517 and 1128 ng/hr/mL, respectively. The time to maximum concentration was approximately 10 hours for both groups. Ko[203] also reported the impact of two 5% lidocaine patches, each containing 700 mg of lidocaine, applied to the ventral abdominal area of dogs weighing between 18 to 23 kg. Concentrations (ng/mL) increased from 18.5 ± 29.4 at 12 hr to 72.8 ± 65.8 at 24 hrs. Concentrations remained at steady-state for another 24 hrs; at 48 hrs, concentrations declined, reaching to 21.4 ± 24.7 ng/mL by 60 hour and remained detectable (30 ± 26 ng/mL) at 78 hour but were not detectable by 80 hour. The concentrations approximated 1/10th of that achieved when dogs are given 2 mg/kg IV (as reviewed by Weil).[201] Ko and coworkers[204] also studied the impact of a 700-mg lidocaine patch applied to the lateral thorax of cats (n = 8). Cats were also given lidocaine intravenously at 2 mg/kg. The overall bioavailability of lidocaine in the patch was 6.3 ± 2.7%, with 56% of the patch dose being systemically absorbed. Lidocaine was detectable within 3 hours of patch application and reached steady-state concentration was 103 ± 0.037 (which was approximately 10% of the peak concentration reached with intravenous administration). Peak concentrations occurred at 64 ± 4 hours. Plasma concentrations were still at steady state when the patch was removed at 72 hours.

Toxicity associated with cream preparations has been reported in humans but generally reflects inappropriate administration that facilitates increased rate or amount of absorption. Actions to be avoided include application to a larger-than-recommended surface area, longer contact time, increased body temperature, or application to surfaces not protected by an intact stratum corneum (diseased skin, mucosal membranes).

The use of lidocaine for prevention of reperfusion injury and thus a systemic inflammatory response associated with multiorgan dysfunction syndrome has been reviewed.[205] Lidocaine has received considerable attention for its efficacy as a general analgesic when administered systemically. Concentrations of 0.620 to 5.7 µg/mL are recommended for antinociception.[206] In human patients 5 mg/kg/hr was used effectively to control cancer pain associated either with the tumor itself or its treatment (e.g., surgery, radiation therapy). Interestingly, general sensation of pain and dysaesthetic, preanesthesia, and nightly exacerbations of pain were significantly decreased in the majority (70% for most symptoms) of patients studied (n=10) for up to 2 weeks.[9] Unfortunately, the clinical trial was not controlled, and a placebo effect was not assessed. Systemic lidocaine has decreased halothane MAC at antiarrhythmic concentrations in dogs.[207] Serum concentrations of 3 to 6 µg/mL have decreased halothane requirements in dogs by 10% to 28%,[208] as reviewed by Wilson.[196] In another study[209] lidocaine CRI (2 mg/kg intravenously followed by 50 µg/kg/min as low dose and 200 µg/kg/min as high dose) significantly reduced, in a dose-dependent manner, the MAC of isoflurane in dogs (n=10). The MAC was reduced 19% at the low dose. Lidocaine and metabolite concentrations were (µg/mL) 1.5 µg/mL (lidocaine), 0.11 (glycinexylidide), and 0.18 (monoethylglycinexylidide). For the high dose MAC was reduced 43% at concentrations of 1.5, 0.18, and 0.47 µg/mL for lidocaine and its metabolites, respectively. No significant cardiovascular effects were observed. Smith and coworkers[210] prospectively compared the efficacy of systemic lidocaine (1 mg/kg intravenously followed by 0.025 mg/kg/min CRI) to morphine (0.15 mg/kg intravenously followed by 0.1 mg/kg/hr CRI) or saline placebo for control of postoperative ocular pain. Morphine rescue was necessary in all placebo-treated dogs and in 50% of the dogs treated with lidocaine and morphine. The incidence of measures of ocular inflammation did not differ among groups.

Lidocaine pharmacokinetics pharmacodynamics were determined in cats after intravenous administration of 2 mg/kg. Pharmacodynamics were then based on thermal antinociception.[206] Lidocaine at 0.250 to 4.32 µg/mL did not affect the thermal threshold in cats. However, the authors noted that the power of the study was sufficient to detect a thermal difference of 3.75° C as opposed to other studies. Pypendop and Ilkiw[211] also demonstrated that, when used to decrease isoflurane dose, lidocaine (dosed to achieve 3 to 11 µg/mL) was associated with unacceptable adverse cardiac effects in cats. The authors recommended that lidocaine not be used with the intent to lower isoflurane MAC. This may reflect, in part, marked changes in the disposition (particularly reduced clearance) of lidocaine associated with anesthesia compared with awake cats.[212]

Bupivacaine can be a very effective analgesic. However, in contrast to lidocaine, bupivacaine needs approximately 20 minutes to take effect but provides 4 to 6 hours of analgesia. The bupivacaine dose should not exceed 2.2 mg/kg. Side effects typical of lidocaine occur at 4 mg/kg.[115] Diazepam appears to enhance the cardiodepressant effects of bupivicaine.[213] When administered locally (around five intercostal nerves), it was equal to epidural morphine for control of pain associated with lateral thoracotomy in dogs.[85] Another prospective study in dogs (n=26) undergoing intercostal thoracotomy compared buprenorphine (10 µg/kg intravenously every 6 hours) with bupivicaine (1.5 mg/kg of 0.5% intrapleurally, by slow injection through a pediatric feeding tube placed dorsally, every 4 hours). Dogs were treated for 24 hours, starting 10 minutes before tracheal extubation. Significant changes from preoperative values in pain scores and cardiovascular assessment occurred in the buprenorphine group but not the bupivicaine group.[214]

KEY POINT 28-25 Bupivacaine requires approximately 20 minutes to become effective.

Cardiotoxicity of bupivacaine led to the development of ropivacaine, a nonracemic product consistent of the less toxic S isomer compared with the R isomer. Like bupivicaine, it is long acting, but it is less cardiotoxic. The incidence of arrhythmias and death is lower in animals given toxic doses of intravenous ropivacaine than those given bupivacaine.

A toxicity study in dogs demonstrated better safety for ropivacaine in dogs. Intravenous lidocaine (8 mg/kg/min), bupivacaine (2 mg/kg/min), and ropivacaine (2 mg/kg/min) were administered intravenously. Two of the lidocaine-treated dogs developed lethal hypotension and respiratory arrest. All bupivacaine-treated dogs developed ventricular arrhythmias, with death occurring in five of these, whereas only two of six (one death) dogs developed arrhythmias in the ropivacaine group.[215] The C_{max} of drugs in nonsurvivors were 469, 70 ± 14, and 72 µg/mL for lidocaine, bupivacaine, and ropivacaine, respectively.

The use of ketamine as an NMDA antagonist was previously discussed. However, ketamine has local anesthetic effects by blockade of Na+ and K+ channels, stabilizing cellular membranes and reducing nerve transmission, similar to that of other local anesthetics. The alkalinization of 5 mL of 1% ketamine solution with 0.5 mEq bicarbonate produced a more consistent and longer-lasting local analgesia (sesamoid block) in horses compared with 1% ketamine solution alone.[216] However, a greater amount of sodium bicarbonate was associated with precipitation.

MISCELLANEOUS AGENTS

Conotoxins

Conotoxins represent a new class of natural compounds produced by the marine mollusks of the *Conus* genus. Investigations regarding their therapeutic use in a variety of diseases, including control of pain, are under way. More than 500 species of *Conus* exist, each capable of producing 100 or more conotoxins (conopeptides); thus more than 50,000 pharmacologically active compounds may be investigated for potential therapeutic use. In their natural environment, conotoxins are used for prey capture (paralysis of fish), defense, and competitor deterrence.[217] The molecular targets of conopeptides are functionally diverse; some target G protein–coupled receptors, others neurotransmitter transporters; and others are characterized by enzymatic activity. Most of the currently described conopeptides are small, structured peptides that target either ligand-gated or voltage-gated ion channels. Targets identified thus far include Na+, K+, Ca^{2+} or nicotinic acetylcholine channels, serotonergic receptors, and norepinephrine transporters. Most conotoxin families target specific structures: for example, ω-conotoxins target Ca channels, whereas α-conotoxins target nicotinic receptors. Different conotoxins may target the same structure but generally at different sites (e.g., μ and δ conotoxins target different sites on sodium channels). In December of 2004, the Food and Drug Administration approved ziconotide (Prialt), a synthetic peptide that mimics a conotoxin produced by *Conus magus*. The venom is used by the sea snail to paralyze fish; its analgesic mechanism of action is not clear but appears to reflect blockade of N-type calcium channels. Use is currently limited to intrathecal administration and thus is largely indicted for relief of pain that does not respond to all other options. Currently, because of their ability to discriminate among molecularly similar ion channels, the conotoxins are also being studied for their potential to identify and characterize the role of sodium channels isoforms in diseases, including pain.[218]

Others

Nicotine (e.g., that available in over the counter smoking-cessation products) increasingly is being investigated for its ability to relieve pain. Its mechanism appears to target nicotinic acetylcholine receptors, and specifically heteropentameric ion channels activated by acetylcholine. Nicotine may act synergistically with opioids.[218] Nicotine poisoning as a result of tobacco ingestion has been reported in dogs. Clinical signs in one report were primarily CNS in origin but also include hypersalivation, vomiting, diarrhea, tachycardia, tachypnea, hypertension, and hyperthermia. Animals may present in total collapse, with dilated pupils, slow and shallow respirations, hypotension, tachycardia, and a weak and irregular pulse.[219]

The analgesic effects of marijuana appear to reflect its interaction with cannabinoid (CB) receptors in the CNS, peripheral nervous system, or other tissues. Current efforts are focusing on methods whereby the psychoactive effects, reflecting interaction with CB_1 receptors, are avoided without minimizing interaction with CB_2 receptors (not present in the CNS) associated with acute, inflammatory, and neuropathic pain.[218]

SPECIAL CONSIDERATIONS FOR CONTROL OF PAIN IN ANIMALS

Neuropathic Pain

The use of drugs for treatment of neuropathic pain are also addressed under preemptive analgesia. The most comprehensively studied class of drugs for treatment of neuropathic pain in humans are the TCAs, although anticonvulsants are probably most commonly used.[220] These drugs interact with a number of transporters, receptors, and channels associated with pain. In addition to their impact on synaptic serotonin and norepinephrine, TCAs modulate both sodium and potassium channels and NMDA and ATP receptors. The efficacy of TCAs for treatment of neuropathic pain may reflect closing of sodium channels that inappropriately remain active in response to injury. However, drugs that increase serotonin or other neurotransmitters in the synapse also minimize neuropathic pain, suggesting that multiple mechanisms of action may be important.[218]

Other classes of drugs used to treat neuropathic pain in humans include mexiletine, capsaicin, NMDA inhibitors, clonidine, tramadol, and lidocaine patches. Each has been used with variable success.[220]

Gabapentin appears to target neuropathic pain by binding calcium channels, specifically at the $alpha_2$ $delta_1$ subunit. As a result, neurotransmitter release appears to be altered.[218]

Cancer Pain

The pathophysiology of cancer-induced bone pain (CIBP) has been reviewed and includes both inflammatory (nociceptive) and neuropathic pain.[221] Among the drugs used to control CIBP are the opioids, the mainstay of analgesic control; the NSAIDS, therapeutically appealing in part because of their recently recognized antitumor effects; and the bisphosphonates, which were originally used to treat hypercalcemia.[221] Bisphosphonates inhibit the recruitment and activation of osteoclasts, increase osteoprotegerin, induce apoptosis, inhibit cancer cell proliferation, and reduce cytokine production and metalloproteinase secretion. The analgesic effect is delayed several weeks to months.[221]

Pregnant, Neonate, and Pediatric Animals

In her review, Matthews[167] indicates that opioids are the analgesic of choice in pregnant animals. However, care should be taken in that the fetal blood–brain barrier is permeable to these drugs (see previous discussion). Chronic use (beyond several weeks) is likely to have a negative impact on the fetus, causing lower birth weights and behavioral deficits. The latter may reflect decease nervous system plasticity as a result of opioid effects on neuronal development. In contrast, short-term use is not considered to present a significant problem. Methadone appears to be safe in humans. Buprenorphine also should be safe, at least with single dosing, because the placenta serves as a depot site from which less than 10% of the drug is transferred to the fetus. In contrast, fentanyl rapidly crosses the placenta. An advantage to opioid use for cesarean section is its reversibility and general responsiveness of neonates to reversal. Repetitive dosing (e.g., 30 minutes) may be indicated if the status of the neonate indicates opioid depression. Animals should respond to sublingual administration. Ketamine also rapidly crosses the placenta. It may contribute to uterine contraction and potentially to discomfort of the mother. The risk of increased uterine tone, respiratory depression in the mother, and altered muscle tone in the fetus warrants careful consideration regarding ketamine use in the pregnant animal. Opioids also are preferred for analgesic control in the nursing mother. Some accumulation should be anticipated in the milk, particularly for the more lipid-soluble drugs. As weak bases, drugs with higher pKa levels may be accumulated to a higher degree. Nursing might be coordinated just before administration of doses. In humans butorphanal concentrations in milk approximated those in serum, whereas little hydromorphone was distributed to milk. Neonates might be observed for evidence of opioid-induced sedation.

NSAIDs should be avoided in pregnant animals for several reasons (see Chapter 29). Fetal defects may occur with administration in the first trimester of pregnancy. The impact of NSAIDs on the reproductive system may adversely affect the pregnancy itself by altering fetal circulation. If administered during labor, they may cause its cessation. Further, the impact of prostaglandin inhibition on the developing fetus (e.g., fetal kidneys) is being elucidated. Postoperatively, a single dose of NSAIDs is acceptable,[167] but unless such administration is demonstrated to offer advantages over opioids, alternative analgesics (e.g., opioids) should be considered in the nursing bitch or queen. Likewise, because of their diffuse effects in the reproductive system, NSAIDs are not recommended for breeding animals.

Analgesic therapy should not be avoided in pediatric patients for fear of adversities. Again, opioids are preferred, although lower doses should be anticipated, particularly in the first 5 weeks of life. Higher volumes of distribution may require higher doses; longer intervals should be anticipated because of both the larger volume of distribution and decreased clearance. Transdermal patches are generally not recommended because of the unpredictable disposition in pediatric patients. NSAIDs should not be used in animals younger than 3 to 6 months unless safety for that particular drug has been demonstrated (see Chapter 29). The package insert for firocoxib states that the drug is not tolerated in juvenile animals, and similar responses might be anticipated for other NSAIDs. Local anesthetics can be used in both neonatal and pediatric patients, although a lower dose is recommended in neonates because of the immaturity of the nervous system.[167] Buffering procedures might be used to reduce pain associated with injection. Topically applied gels might be considered as well.

Geriatric Patients

Because opioids are active in the CNS, the geriatric patient is predisposed to adverse reactions to opioid analgesics.[38,222,223] Cardiac disease increases the risk of toxicity to opioids or any other CNS-active drug because of increased drug delivery to the brain. On the other hand, decreased receptor sensitivity may result in a reduced response to opioid analgesics. The mentation status of the geriatric animal may complicate interpretation of clinical response to opioids; CNS depression may be difficult to identify. The opioid analgesics decrease central response to increased PCO_2, which is already impaired in the geriatric patient. The opioid analgesics are eliminated from the body by hepatic clearance. Both hepatic blood flow and hepatic metabolism are decreased in geriatric patients. Thus changes in hepatic clearance of these drugs renders the geriatric patient more susceptible to toxicity. Increased response of human geriatric patients to opioid analgesics (who require 60% to 75% less drug than younger patients) has been attributed to changes in drug elimination. Use of opioids that cause minimal sedation (e.g., butorphanol, buprenorphine) should be considered. Alternatively, opioid analgesics that are reversible are indicated for geriatric patients. Buprenorphine essentially is not reversible, as are most other opioid analgesics.

Surgical Pain

Pain associated with surgery is acute, but if it is insufficiently controlled, it can lead to neuropathic pain. The use of preemptive analgesia has been reviewed (see earlier discussion).[14] To effectively prevent neuropathic pain, effective analgesics should be administered as long as the cause of the pain remains. Surgical pain should be managed with a combination of local anesthetics, NSAIDs, opioids, and NMDA antagonists; routes should include local, systemic, and epidural. α_2 agonists are also indicated, although sedative and cardiovascular effects limit their use to epidural administration or as part of combination therapy. General anesthesia alone may not be sufficient to control intraoperative analgesia.

Several opioid analgesics are useful for the control of surgical pain. For animals suffering pain before surgical induction, oxymorphone or butorphanol administered as part of a preanesthetic or anesthetic regimen can both control pain and reduce the amount of general anesthetic. Likewise, animals to be subjected to a surgical procedure that will induce pain that is not likely to be successfully controlled with general anesthetics will also benefit from presurgical administration. Meperidine is generally used as a preanesthetic to minimize the amount of general anesthetic needed for a geriatric or debilitated (e.g., poor cardiovascular system) animal rather than to control pain. In addition, a fentanyl patch can be applied the day before surgery. Opioids might also be given intraoperatively if cardiovascular signs indicate the perception of pain despite a general anesthetic. Agents that can be reversed or those with a ceiling effect should be used to minimize the risk of respiratory or cardiovascular depression.

Postoperatively, any of the opioids can be administered, and the selection should be based on the degree of analgesia desired balanced with the risk of sedation in the postoperative patient (see the section on assessing pain). Those most commonly selected by small animal practitioners include oxymorphone, buprenorphine, and butorphanol, although the indications for butorphanol should be limited.[23,127,128] Severe pain indicates the need for pure agonists such as fentanyl, morphine, hydormorphone, or oxymorphone. Fentanyl transdermal patches can be applied postoperatively, but it is likely that the analgesic effects of the patch will need to be supplemented over the short term. Less severe pain may sufficiently respond to buprenorphine or (less ideal) butorphanol. Of the two, buprenorphine can be expected to consistently provide a longer period of analgesia (about 4 to 6 hours). Acepromazine can be combined with either butorphanol or buprenorphine for sedation. Pulse oximetry can be used to evaluate tissue oxygenation and the potential risk associated with a sedating drug, including a pure agonist opioid.

The sedative effects of the opioid may be desirable for some patients but undesirable for others. An advantage of these drugs is that the sedating effects can be reversed if necessary. Note, however, that repeated administration of the reversing agent may be necessary (e.g., naloxone). Alternatively, if a sedating opioid has been used and reversal of the sedating effects is desirable, butorphanol or buprenorphine can be used. A portion of the analgesic effect will also be reversed (because of antagonistic actions at MOP receptors for both of these drugs), but KOP receptors will mediate some analgesia.

NSAIDs can be very effective postoperatively; in addition to their peripheral antiinflammatory effects, NSAIDs may have central actions. Care should be taken with the use of NSAIDs; drugs that are selective for COX-2 are preferred (see Chapter 29). However, the impact of COX-2 inhibition on healing and other physiologic response must be addressed. The availability of several approved COX-1 protective drugs in the dog and meloxicam (COX-protective status unknown in cats) calls into question the wisdom of using alternative NSAIDs. Further, the efficacy of NSAIDs as preemptive analgesics coupled with their inherent risks mandates caution when used perioperatively or intraoperatively, particularly in the unhealthy patient. Fluid therapy during surgery is important to prevent renal complications, and excessive bleeding may occur as a result of the inhibition of thrombogenesis. Combinations of opioids (codeine, butorphanol) and NSAIDs or acetaminophen should be considered to avoid the side effects associated with NSAID use.

Critically Ill Patients

Stress that is too severe can complicate the care of the critically ill patient. Invasive procedures intended to support the patient produce pain that can be severe, requiring use of sedation, local analgesics, or central analgesics. Procedures that require some type of analgesic therapy include placement of urinary, nasal, and nasogastric catheters; bone marrow aspiration; and drainage or lavage of body cavities. Opioid sedation, or a combination of ketamine (100 mg/mL) and diazepam (5 mg/mL) mixed 1 to 1 and administered at 0.05 to 0.1 mL/kg may limit stress associated with these procedures.[25,224]

Among the opioids most commonly used to control pain beyond that associated with supportive procedures are morphine, oxymorphone, and butorphanol.[23] Side effects of most concern include respiratory and cardiac depression. Most animals can, however, tolerate mild respiratory depression associated with opioids, and respiratory disease or trauma is not a contraindication for opioid use in animals. For example, morphine can be used for the patient with pulmonary edema secondary to heart failure. In addition to splanchnic pooling and decreased preload to the heart, sedation decreases struggling and oxygen use. Morphine can be given to effect at 0.1 mg/kg every 3 minutes until light sedation has been achieved. Oxymorphone may be the preferred opioid of choice for animals for which systemic hypotension can be life threatening because it is less likely to cause histamine release. Fluid therapy is indicated if hypotension occurs.[25,224]

The use of local anesthetics for the critically ill patient should not be ignored. The short duration of action of lidocaine leads to its usefulness for short invasive procedures. It has been used intravenously in human patients as a centrally acting analgesic, but in animals it should be administered in conjunction with another analgesic if used centrally (1 to 2 mg/kg loading dose followed by CRI at 25 to 40 μg/kg per minute). The longer duration of action of bupivacaine lends itself to control of pain associated with surgery or trauma. Bupivacaine can be infiltrated in the proximal intercostal nerves for surgical procedures or infiltrated through a chest tube (0.25% to 0.5%, up to 1 to 2 mg/kg every 6 hours) for control of thoracic pain. Sufficient drug can be absorbed to induce toxicity after local administration. Bupivacaine is more cardiotoxic than lidocaine, and cardiac depression is more likely with repeated administration. CNS reactions include depression and stupor, which may precede seizures. Epinephrine can be used to slow absorption of drug into systemic circulation, although this should be used only with extreme caution in critically ill patients.[25,224]

The use of NSAIDs to control pain in the critically ill is risky because of the gastrointestinal, hematopoietic, and renal and other (often unknown) side effects of these drugs. Until data are available to support their use, however, all NSAIDs, including COX-2 preferential drugs, probably should not be used in the critically ill patient. An exception might be made for patients suffering from endotoxic shock.[25,224]

Assessment of the patient with cranial trauma can be difficult, complicating the monitoring of analgesic use. Clinical signs vary with the site and extent of brain injury (e.g., concussion, laceration, contusion). Brain trauma can lead to extracranial or intracerebral hemorrhage days after the injury (with clinical signs varying depending on exactly where the hemorrhage occurs), as well as edema (intracellular, extracellular, interstitial, or vasogenic), hypoxia (or ischemia), and increased intracranial pressure. Marked neuronal ion flux (sodium influx, potassium efflux) can lead to anaerobic glycolysis and marked cerebral acidosis. Calcium influx may lead to production of inflammatory mediators; edema is among the consequences of inflammation. The lipid nature of brain tissue renders it prone to damage by oxygen radical generation, which can contribute markedly to neuronal damage. Decreased cerebral blood flow can cause cessation of normal homeostasis, leading to cellular swelling. Loss of autoregulatory mechanisms for blood flow can persist for several days, further contributing to ischemic damage.[225] Cerebral ischemia increases with intracranial pressure. Cerebral arterial PCO_2 increases and PO_2 decreases, causing increased cerebral blood flow. Cerebral blood flow also increases with cerebral metabolism, such as that associated with response to excitement, fear, and pain.[225,226]

After cranial trauma the blood–brain barrier becomes permeable to small molecules normally excluded by the brain.[225] Maximal permeability occurs several days after the injury. Not only is the patient further predisposed to damage induced by metabolites, but also greater drug distribution into the brain increases the risk of neurologic adverse drug reactions. Conditions that might exacerbate the pathophysiologic sequelae of cranial trauma include systemic hypoxia (associated with pneumothorax, aspiration pneumonia, and adult respiratory distress syndrome), hyperglycemia (increases neuronal damage), and hyperthermia (exacerbating neuronal damage).

Control of pain in the patient with cranial trauma is controversial.[225,226] Whether or not injury to the brain causes the sensation or perception of pain, the physiologic consequences of pain or the release of endogenous opioids is not clear. Trauma to the brain alone may not be an indication for analgesic therapy. In contrast, the indication for analgesics in patients with other injuries in conjunction with cranial trauma is clear in part because the physiologic consequences of pain may worsen the cranial trauma. For example, hypertension may facilitate cranial bleeding, as might lowered arterial PCO_2 induced by tachypnea. Thus analgesic therapy is indicated for injuries sustained beyond cranial trauma. Among the analgesics, for such injuries the opioid analgesics tend to be preferred because of their efficacy, reversibility, and (compared with the NSAIDs) safety. The physiology of the damaged brain is not, however, well elucidated. Current knowledge has caused neurologists to reconsider traditional therapies such as the use of glucocorticoids (risk of hyperglycemia) and mannitol (increased risk of hemorrhage) for patients with cranial trauma. Even standard therapies such as resuscitative fluid therapy (increased risk of cerebral edema) can worsen damage induced by cranial trauma, and it is likely that neither the positive nor the negative sequelae of analgesics on the traumatized brain have been fully described. Thus caution is recommended not only in the selection of the analgesic but also in the supportive care provided to the patient with cranial trauma.

A number of known disadvantages are associated with the use of opioids in patients with cranial trauma. Altered mentation induced by cranial trauma and neurologic dysfunction associated with damage to the respiratory and cardiovascular systems are the major concerns. Failure to stabilize the patient and masking of worsening mentation induced by trauma with a sedating drug can lead to life-threatening depression. Because of their sedative effects, opioids selected for control of pain in the patient with cranial trauma should be either minimally depressive or reversible if there is risk of life-threatening sedation or continued loss of mentation caused by trauma. The time to maximal detrimental (as well as beneficial) effects of an opioid varies with the route of administration, occurring in most cases within 10 minutes after intravenous administration but up to 30 minutes after intramuscular administration in human patients. Administration of opioids in low doses and titrating the dose to match the patient's response to pain and physical status can minimize the risk of opioid-induced complications.[225,226]

Opioids have both direct and indirect effects on the brain. Opioids may directly increase cerebrospinal pressure, which may contribute to neurologic damage induced by trauma and its consequences. This may not be reversible with opioid antagonists, and thus increased CSF pressure should be avoided by reserving use of opioids until the CNS status of the patient has stabilized; repetitive, close monitoring is needed after drug administration. The blood–brain barrier is likely to be damaged in the patient suffering from cranial trauma, facilitating drug movement into the brain. Doses of drugs, including opioids, may need to be decreased. In addition, drugs that induce seizure activity, such as meperidine, are not recommended.[225,226]

All of the opioids are associated with some degree of CNS depression. Pure opioid agonists that act at the MOP receptors are associated with the greatest CNS depressant effect. Drugs predominantly active at KOP receptors (located usually in the spinal cord), such as butorphanol and buprenorphine, are characterized by less sedation. As such, these drugs may be more appealing for the patient with cranial trauma. Buprenorphine, however, has both MOP (supraspinal) agonistic and antagonistic effects, whereas butorphanol only antagonizes MOP receptors. In addition, buprenorphine is not fully reversible at MOP receptors and therefore should probably be avoided until the traumatized patient has been completely stabilized. Once the risk of degrading mental status is minimal, buprenorphine will be safer. Pure opioid agonists such as morphine and oxymorphone can be used, but these drugs are more likely to contribute to CNS depression induced by trauma. An advantage to either of these drugs, however, is their full reversibility by opioid antagonists. Should reversal be indicated, extra caution should be taken to ensure slow reversal, thus avoiding a hyperanalgesic response and its physiologic sequelae. In addition, care should be taken to assess the need for repeated administration of the reversal agent.[225,226]

KEY POINT 28-26 An advantage of pure opioids as choice drugs for control of pain in special-needs population is their reversibility in dogs.

Direct depression of the respiratory centers, coupled with decreased responsiveness to arterial PCO_2, are likely to be exacerbated in the patient with cranial trauma. Lung volume decreases in the normal patient, and depression of the cough reflex (especially morphine) increases aspiration of accumulated secretions and development of atelectasis owing to retention of respiratory secretions. Respiratory rate, depth, and rhythm should be closely monitored during opioid administration. Blood gases should be monitored in patients at risk for respiratory depression. Although pulse oximetry can confirm tissue oxygenation, tissue PCO_2 drives respiratory rate and cerebral vascular responses. Respiratory acidosis may develop despite normal tissue oxygenation. Increased PCO_2 can lead to increased cerebral blood flow, which may exacerbate cerebral hemorrhage. In addition to effects of cerebral vasculature, the respiratory rate may be altered (slowed). In a patient whose respiratory center is threatened as a consequence of cranial trauma, further suppression of the respiratory center by an opioid can be life threatening. Drugs characterized by a ceiling effect on respiratory depression (e.g., butorphanol and buprenorphine) will decrease, but not exclude, the risk of opioid-induced CNS respiratory depression. The use of continuous epidural opiate infusions is recommended for human patients who have sustained multiple pulmonary trauma.[225,226]

Cardiovascular depression is also a concern in the patient with cranial trauma receiving opioid analgesics. Depression can be mediated through the central centers, directly on the myocardium, or through peripheral effects (particularly opioids such as morphine that mediate histamine release). Again, close monitoring of rate, rhythm, and pulse is indicated during the initial stages of opioid use. Oxymorphone and fentanyl, which are not associated with as much histamine as is morphine, might be preferred over morphine.[225,226]

Epidural Analgesia

Epidural analgesia was reviewed by Jones.[227] Epidural administration of analgesics can be used to facilitate anesthesia for surgery or provide prolonged postoperative analgesia (see Table 28-3). The efficacy of epidural opioids and local anesthetics in the preemptive control of pain in humans also was reviewed (Jones[227] and Møiniche and coworkers[15]). For analgesic effects, opioids, particularly at high doses, are most useful. Opioids cause selective spinal analgesia by binding to opioid receptors in the dorsal horn of the spinal cord segments. The processing of signals sent by nociceptors is modulated. Thus central effects are absent. Opioids most commonly administered epidurally include morphine, oxymorphone, buprenorphine, and fentanyl. Opioids must cross through the dura and pass into the dorsal horn to be effective with epidural use.[227] Bernards[228] reviewed the factors that govern the rate and extent of opioid redistribution from epidural and intrathecal spaces such that target opioid receptors are reached. The specific opioid to be used depends on the targeted region. Pelvic analgesia can be provided by a number of opioids; for abdominal or thoracic analgesia, a drug with a low lipid solubility (e.g., morphine) is indicated to allow more time for cranial diffusion (after lumbosacral administration) before the dura is penetrated. Morphine also has the longest onset of action (up to 90 minutes) but provides the longest duration of analgesia (up to 24 hours) (see Table 28-3). When used to control postoperative pain, it should be administered before surgery. Sibanda and coworkers[229] demonstrated that the combined extradural administration of bupivacaine (up to 1.5 mg/kg) with morphine (0.1 mg/kg) in dogs reduced concentrations of measures of stress, including cortisol and acute phase proteins, in clinical animals undergoing surgical procedures.[229] Fentanyl is very lipid soluble. Its analgesia is very rapid in onset but does not extend more than one to two spinal cord segments from the injection site. Its central effects are more common than those of other analgesics because of its high lipid solubility and rapid absorption into systemic circulation. It can be combined with morphine to provide analgesia as the morphine penetrates the dura.

Pruritus is a common side effect in human patients receiving opioids epidurally. Delayed respiratory depression is a complaint in a much smaller percentage of the human population. Neither of these side effects has been reported in animals. Because opioids cause no paralysis, there is little to no loss of skeletal muscle (motor) function. Weakness of the detrusor muscle and urine retention are not, however, unusual. Among the opioids, buprenorphine appears the least likely to cause urinary retention. Catheterization may be necessary in some patients.

Local anesthetics have been used epidurally in dogs.[230] Local anesthetics provide direct anesthesia at any nerve root with which the drug comes in contact. This effect is spinal if the drug is administered into the CSF. Bupivacaine is more potent and lipid soluble than lidocaine yet has a slower onset of action and longer duration of effect. Motor blockade should be anticipated but can be minimized by use of dilute concentrations (0.0625% to 0.125%). An opioid can be used for diluting bupivacaine 1 to 1 up to 1 to 3 (by volume).

Epidural administration of analgesics is contraindicated for patients with neurologic deficits or injuries and coagulopathies, bacteremia, and severe systemic infections. Despite the lack of reported toxicity, drugs that contain preservatives (e.g., multiple-dose vials) should be avoided because they may contain preservatives that are neurotoxic. The risk of toxicity increases with multiple injections. Products containing sodium metabisulfite should not be administered intrathecally. The use of epinephrine in combination with local anesthetics and particularly bupivacaine also should be avoided because of very prolonged (24 to 48 hours) muscle weakness. Potential complications of epidural analgesia include epidural or intrathecal hemorrhage, spinal nerve root trauma, motor blockage (particularly with local anesthetics), central effects as the drug diffuses to the brain, and weakness or ataxia.

REFERENCES

1. *Pain terminology.* International Association for the Study of Pain, IASP Council in Kyoto, November 29-30, 2007.
2. Lanser P, Gesell S: Pain management: the fifth vital sign, *Healthc Benchmarks* 8:68–70, 2001.
3. Stein C, Clark JD, Oh U, Vasko MR, et al: Peripheral mechanisms of pain and analgesia, *Brain Res Rev* 60(1):90–113, 2009.
4. Dubner R: The neurobiology of persistent pain and its clinical implications, *Suppl Clin Neurophysiol* 57:3–7, 2004.
5. Heinricher MM, Tavares I, Leith JL, et al: Descending control of nociception: specificity, recruitment and plasticity, *Brain Res Rev* 60(1):214–225, 2009.

6. Hulsebosch CE, Hains BC, Crown ED, et al: Mechanisms of chronic central neuropathic pain after spinal cord injury, *Brain Res Rev* 60(1):202–213, 2009.
7. Christianson JA, Bielefeldt K, Altier C, et al: Development, plasticity and modulation of visceral afferents, *Brain Res Rev* 60(1):171–186, 2009.
8. Hwang SW, Oh U: Current concepts of nociception: nociceptive molecular sensors in sensory neurons, *Curr Opin Anaesthesiol* 20(5):427–434, 2007.
9. Joad ASK, Burad J, Mehta C: Intravenous lignocaine infusion for neuropathic pain in cancer patients-A preliminary study, *Indian J Anesth* 46(5):360–364, 2002.
10. Wawrzczak-Bargiela MJ, Osikowicz A, Makuch M, et al: Attenuation of morphine tolerance by minocycline and pentoxifylline in naive and neuropathic mice, *Brain Behav Immun* 23(1):75–84, 2009.
11. Kiefer W, Dannhardt G: Novel insights and therapetuical applications in the field of inhibitors of COX-2, *Curr Med Chem* 11:3147-3161, 2004.
12. Jain NK, Ishikawa TO, Spigelman I, et al: COX-2 expression and function in the hyperalgesic response to paw inflammation in mice, *Prostaglandins Leukot Essent Fatty Acids* 79(6):183–190, 2008.
13. Finnoff J: Differentiation and treatment of phantom sensation, phantom pain, and residual-limb pain, *J Am Podiatr Med Assoc* 91(1):23–33, 2001.
14. Ong CK, Lirk P, Seymour RA, et al: The efficacy of preemptive analgesia for acute postoperative pain management: a meta-analysis, *Anesth Analg* 100(3):757–773, 2005.
15. Møiniche S, Kehlet H, Dahl JB: A qualitative and quantitative systematic review of preemptive analgesia for postoperative pain relief, *Anesthesiology* 96:725–741, 2002.
16. Hogan QH: No preemptive analgesia: is that so bad? *Anesthesiology* 96(3):526–527, 2002.
17. Hellyer PW: Editorial: a new look at pain, *J Vet Intern Med* 18:461–462, 2004.
18. Phillips DM: JCAHO pain management standards are unveiled, *J Am Med Assoc* 284:428–429, 2000.
19. Johnson JA: The veterinarian's responsibility: assessing and managing acute pain in dogs and cats, Part I, *Comp Contin Educ Pract Vet* 13:804–807, 1991.
20. Kitchell RL: Problems in defining pain and peripheral mechanisms of pain, *J Am Vet Med Assoc* 191:1195–1199, 1987.
21. Sackman JE: Pain. Part II. Control of pain in animals, *Comp Contin Educ Pract Vet* 13:181–192, 1991.
22. Paul-Murphy J, Ludders JW, Roberson SA, et al: The need for a cross-species approach to the study of pain in animals, *J Am Vet Med Assoc* 224:692–696, 2004.
23. Hansen B, Hardie E: Prescription and use of analgesics in dogs and cats in a veterinary teaching hospital: 258 cases (1983-1989), *J Am Vet Med Assoc* 202(9):1485–1494, 1993.
24. Cousins MF: Management of postoperative pain, *Int Anesth Res J* 60:32–39, 1986.
25. Anthony C: Acute pain in the intensive care unit. In Shoemaker WC, Ayers SM, Grenvic A, et al: *Textbook of critical care*, ed 3, Philadelphia, 1995, Saunders, pp 1486–1498.
26. Potthoff A: Pain and analgesia in dogs and cats, *Comp Contin Educ Pract Vet* 11:887–896, 1989.
27. Gutstein HB, Akil H: Opioid analgesics. In Brunton LL, Lazo JS, Parker KL, editors: *Goodman and Gilman's the pharmacological basis of therapeutics*, ed 11, New York, 2006, McGraw-Hill, pp 547–590.
28. Wright EM, Marcella KL, Woodson JF: Animal pain: evaluation and control, *Lab Anim* 20–36, 1985:May/June.
29. Reisine T, Pasternak G: Opioid analgesics and antagonists. In Hardman JG, Limbird LE, editors: *Goodman and Gilman's the pharmacologic basis of therapeutics*, ed 9, New York, 1996, McGraw-Hill, pp 521–555.
30. O'Brien CP: Drug addiction and drug abuse. In Brunton LL, Lazo JS, Parker KL, editors: *Goodman and Gilman's the pharmacological basis of therapeutics*, ed 11, New York, 2006, McGraw-Hill, pp 607–627.
31. Johnson EE, Gibson H, Nicol B, et al: Characterization of nociceptin/orphanin FQ binding sites in dog brain membranes, *Anesth Analg* 97(3):741–747, 2003.
32. Lester PA, Traynor JR: Comparison of the in vitro efficacy of MOP, delta, KOP and ORL1 receptor agonists and non-selective opioid agonists in dog brain membranes, *Brain Res* 16:1073–1074, 2006:290-296.
33. Pan ZZ: MOP-opposing actions of the KOP-opioid receptors, *Trends Pharmacol Sci* 19:94–98, 1998.
34. Schultz JEE, Gross GJ: Opioids and cardioprotection, *Pharmacol Ther* 89:123–137, 2001.
35. Roberto M, Siggins GR: Nociceptin/orphanin FQ presynaptically decreases GABAergic transmission and blocks the ethanol-induced increase of GABA release in central amygdala, *Proc Natl Acad Sci USA* 103(25):9715–9720, 2006.
36. Dale O, Hjortkj ÆR: Nasal administration of opioids for pain management in adults, *Acta Anaesthesiol Scand* 46:759–770, 2002.
37. Kart T, Walther-Larsen S, Svejborg TF, Feilberg V, Eriksen K, Rasmussen M: Comparison of continuous epidural infusion of fentanyl and bupivacaine with intermittent epidural administration of morphine for postoperative pain management in children, *Acta Anaesthesiol Scand* 41(4):461–465, 1997.
38. Cooper JW: Reviewing geriatric concerns with commonly used drugs, *Geriatrics* 44:79–86, 1989.
39. Hofmeister EH, Herrington JL, Mazzaferro EM: Opioid dysphoria in three dogs, *J Vet Emerg Crit Care* 16(1):44–49, 2006.
40. Robinson EP, Faggella AM, Henry DP, et al: Comparison of histamine release induced by morphine and oxymorphone administration in dogs, *Am J Vet Res* 49(10):1699–1701, 1988.
41. Guedes AGP, Rude EP, Rider MA: Evaluation of histamine release during constant rate infusion of morphine in dogs, *Vet Anaesth Analg* 33:28–35, 2006.
42. Muldoon S, Otto J, Freas W, et al: The effects of morphine, nalbuphine, and butorphanol on adrenergic function in canine saphenous veins, *Anesth Analg* 62(1):21–28, 1983.
43. Robertson SA: Managing pain in feline patients, *Vet Clin Small Anim* 35:129–146, 2005.
44. Schurig JE, Florczyk AP, Rose WC, et al: Antiemetic activity of butorphanol against cisplatin-induced emesis in ferrets and dogs, *Cancer Treat Rep* 66(10):1831–1835, 1982.
45. Blancquaert JP, Lefebvre RA, Willems JL: Emetic and antiemetic effects of opioids in the dog, *Eur J Pharmacol* 128(3):143–150, 1989.
46. Robertson SA, Taylor PM, Lascelles BD, et al: Changes in thermal threshold response in eight cats after administration of buprenorphine, butorphanol and morphine, *Vet Rec* 153(15):462–465, 2003.
47. Anderson MK, Day TK: Effects of morphine and fentanyl constant rate infusion on urine output in healthy and traumatized dogs, *Vet Anaesth Analg* 35(6):528–536, 2008.
48. Xu Xao-Jun: Colpert F, Wiesenfeld-Hallin Z: Opioid hyperalgesia and tolerance versus 5-HT1A receptor-mediated inverse tolerance, *Trends Pharmacol Sci* 24(12):634–639, 2003.
49. Allen CP, Zissen MH: Mechanical allodynia and thermal hyperalgesia upon acute opioid withdrawal in the neonatal rat, *Pain* 110:269–280, 2004.
50. Sweitzer SM, Allen CP, Zissen MH, Kendig JJ: Mechanical allodynia and thermal hyperalgesia upon acute opioid withdrawal in the neonatal rat, *Pain* 110(1-2):269–280, 2004.
51. Martell BA, O'Connor PG, Kerns RD, et al: Systematic review: opioid treatment for chronic back pain: prevalence, efficacy, and association with addiction, *Ann Intern Med* 146(2):116–127, 2007.

52. Martin WR, Eades CG, Thompson JA, et al: The effects of morphine- and nalorphine-like drugs in the nondependent and morphine-dependent chronic spinal dog, *J Pharmacol Exp Ther* 197(3):517–532, 1976.
53. Jacob JJ, Michaud GM, Tremblay EC: Mixed agonist-antagonist opiates and physical dependence, *Br J Clin Pharmacol* 7(Suppl 3):291S–296S, 1979.
54. Roebel LE, Cavanagh RL, Buyniski JP: Comparative gastrointestinal and biliary tract effects of morphine and butorphanol (Stadol), *J Med* 10(4):225–238, 1979.
55. Vieira ZE, Zsigmond EK, Duarte B, et al: Double-blind comparison of butorphanol and nalbuphine on the common bile duct by ultrasonography in man, *Int J Clin Pharmacol Ther Toxicol* 31(11):564–567, 1993.
56. Branson KR, Gross ME, Booth NH: Opioid agonists and antagonists. In Adams HR, editor: *Veterinary pharmacology and therapeutics*, ed 7, Ames, Iowa, 1996, Iowa State University Press, pp 274–310.
57. Robertson SA, Taylor PM: Pain management in cats—past, present and future. Part 2. Treatment of pain—clinical pharmacology, *J Feline Med Surg* 6(5):321–333, 2004.
58. Robertson SA, Taylor PM, Sear JW: Systemic uptake of buprenorphine by cats after oral mucosal administration, *Vet Rec* 152(22):675–678, 2003.
59. Napier LD, Stanfill A, Yoshishige DA, et al: Autonomic control of heart rate in dogs treated chronically with morphine, *Am J Physiol* 275(6 Pt 2):H2199–H2210, 1998.
60. Hakim TS, Grunstein MM, Michel RP: Opiate action in the pulmonary circulation, *Pulm Pharmacol* 5(3):159–165, 1992.
61. Cullen LK, Raffe MR, Randall DA, et al: Assessment of the respiratory actions of intramuscular morphine in conscious dogs, *Res Vet Sci* 67(2):141–148, 1999.
62. Luks AM, Zwass MS, Brown RC, et al: Opioid-induced analgesia in neonatal dogs: pharmacodynamic differences between morphine and fentanyl, *J Pharmacol Exp Ther* 284(1):136–141, 1998.
63. Zuckerman A, Bolan E, de Paulis T, et al: Pharmacological characterization of morphine-6-sulfate and codeine-6-sulfate, *Brain Res* 842(1):1–5, 1999.
64. Osborne R, Thompson P, Joel S, Trew D, Patel N, Slevin M: The analgesic activity of morphine-6-glucuronide, *Br J Clin Pharmacol* 34(2):130–138, 1992.
65. Krotscheck U, Boothe DM, Boothe HW: Evaluation of transdermal morphine and fentanyl pluronic lecithin organogel administration in dogs, *Vet Ther* 5(3):202–211, 2004.
66. KuKanich B, Lascelles BDX, Papich MG: Pharmacokinetics of morphine and plasma concentrations of morphine-6-glucuronide following morphine administration to dogs, *J Vet Pharmacol Ther* 28:371–376, 2005.
67. Jacqz E, Ward S, Johnson R, et al: Extrahepatic glucuronidation of morphine in the dog, *J Pharmacol Exp Ther* 117(1):117–125, 1986.
68. Garrett ER, Jackson AJ: Pharmacokinetics of morphine and its surrogates. III: Morphine and morphine 3-monoglucuronide pharmacokinetics in the dog as a function of dose, *J Pharm Sci* 68(6):753–771, 1979.
69. Tasker RA, Ross SJ, Dohoo SE, et al: Pharmacokinetics of an injectable sustained-release formulation of morphine for use in dogs, *J Vet Pharmacol Ther* 20(5):362–367, 1997.
70. Dohoo S: Steady-state pharmacokinetics of oral sustained-release morphine sulphate in dogs, *J Vet Pharmacol Ther* 20(2):129–133, 1997.
71. Eliot L, Cato A, Geiser R, et al: Evaluation of two loading-dose regimens of Morphelan™ in healthy volunteers, *Journal of Applied Research in Clinical and Experimental Therapeutics*, 2000-2003. Accessed November 24, 2009, at http://www.jarcet.com/articles/Vol2Iss1/Eliot.htm.
72. KuKanich B, Lascelles BD, Papich MG: Use of a von Frey device for evaluation of pharmacokinetics and pharmacodynamics of morphine after intravenous administration as an infusion or multiple doses in dogs, *Am J Vet Res* 66(11):1968–1974, 2005.
73. KuKanich B, Borum SL: Effects of ketoconazole on the pharmacokinetics and pharmacodynamics of morphine in healthy greyhounds, *Am J Vet Res* 69:664–669, 2008.
74. Aragon CL, Read MR, Gaynor JS, et al: Pharmacokinetics of an immediate and extended release oral morphine formulation utilizing the spheroidal oral drug absorption system in dogs, *J Vet Pharmacol Ther* 32(2):129–136, 2009.
75. Barnhart MD, Hubbell JA, Muir WW, et al: Pharmacokinetics, pharmacodynamics, and analgesic effects of morphine after rectal, intramuscular, and intravenous administration in dogs, *Am J Vet Res* 61:24–28, 2000.
76. Robinson TM, Kruse-Elliott KT, Markel MD: A comparison of transdermal fentanyl versus epidural morphine for analgesia in dogs undergoing major orthopedic surgery, *J Am Anim Hosp Assoc* 35(2):95–100, 1999.
77. Yaksh TL, Provencher JC, Rathbun ML, et al: Pharmacokinetics and efficacy of epidurally delivered sustained-release encapsulated morphine in dogs, *Anesthesiology* 90(5):1402–1412, 1999.
78. King FG, Baxter AD, Mathieson G: Tissue reaction of morphine applied to the epidural space of dogs, *Can Anaesth Soc J* 31(3):268–271, 1984.
79. Yaksh TL, Provencher JC, Rathbun ML, et al: Safety assessment of encapsulated morphine delivered epidurally in a sustained-release multivesicular liposome preparation in dogs, *Drug Deliv* 7(1):27–36, 2000.
80. Ostrop NJ, Lamb J, Reid G: Intravaginal morphine: an alternative route of administration, *Pharmacotherapy* 18(4):863–865, 1998.
81. Novello L, Corletto F, Rabozzi R, et al: Sparing effect of a low dose of intrathecal morphine on fentanyl requirements during spinal surgery: a preliminary clinical investigation in dogs, *Vet Surg* 37:153–160, 2008.
82. Langguth P, Khan PG, Garret ER: Pharmacokinetics of morphine and its surrogates. XI: Effect of simultaneously administered naltrexone and morphine on the pharmacokinetics and pharmacodynamics in the dog, *Biopharm Drug Dispos* 11(5):419–444, 1990.
83. Lucas AN, Firth AM, Anderson GA, et al: Comparison of the effects of morphine administered by constant-rate intravenous infusion or intermittent intramuscular injection in dogs, *J Am Vet Med Assoc* 218(6):884–891, 2001.
84. Day TK, Pepper WT, Tobias TA, et al: Comparison of intra-articular and epidural morphine for analgesia following stifle arthrotomy in dogs, *Vet Surg* 24(6):522–530, 1995.
85. Pascoe PJ, Dyson DH: Analgesia after lateral thoracotomy in dogs. Epidural morphine vs. intercostal bupivacaine, *Vet Surg* 22(2):141–147, 1993.
86. Pacharinsak C, Greene SA, Keegan RD, et al: Postoperative analgesia in dogs receiving epidural morphine plus medetomidine, *J Vet Pharmacol Therap* 26:71–77, 2003.
87. Stiles J, Honda CN, Krohne SG, et al: Effect of topical administration of 1% morphine sulfate solution on signs of pain and corneal wound healing in dogs, *Am J Vet Res* 64:813–818, 2003.
88. Dyson DH, Doherty T, Anderson GI, et al: Reversal of oxymorphone sedation by naloxone, nalmefene, and butorphanol, *Vet Surg* 19(5):398–403, 1990.
89. Copeland VS, Haskins SC, Patz J: Naloxone reversal of oxymorphone effects in dogs, *Am J Vet Res* 50(11):1854–1858, 1989.
90. Torske KE, Dyson DH, Conlon PD: Cardiovascular effects of epidurally administered oxymorphone and an oxymorphone-bupivacaine combination in halothane-anesthetized dogs, *Am J Vet Res* 60(2):194–200, 1999.

91. Cone EJ, Darwin WD, Buchwald WF, et al: Oxymorphone metabolism and urinary excretion in human, rat, guinea pig, rabbit, and dog, *Drug Metab Dispos* 11(5):446–450, 1983.
92. KuKanich B, Schmidt BK, Krugner-Higby LA, et al: Pharmacokinetics and behavioral effects of oxymorphone after intravenous and subcutaneous administration to healthy dogs, *J Vet Pharmacol Ther* 31(6):580–583, 2008.
93. Smith LJ, Krugner-Higby L, Trepanier LA: Sedative effects and serum drug concentrations of oxymorphone and metabolites after subcutaneous administration of a liposome-encapsulated formulation in dogs, *J Vet Pharmacol Ther* 27:369–372, 2004.
94. Guedes AGP, Papich MG, Rude EP, et al: Pharmacokinetics and physiological effects of intravenous hydromorphone in conscious dogs, *J Vet Pharmacol Therap* 31:334–343, 2008.
95. Wegner K, Robertson SA, Kollias-Baker C, et al: Pharmacokinetic and pharmacodynamic evaluation of intravenous hydromorphone in cats, *J Vet Pharmacol Ther* 27(5):329–336, 2004.
96. Lascelles BD, Robertson SA: Antinociceptive effects of hydromorphone, butorphanol, or the combination in cats, *J Vet Intern Med* 18(2):190–195, 2004.
97. Duncan B, Lascelles X, Robertson SA: Antinociceptive effects of hydromorphone, butorphanol, or the combination in cats, *J Vet Intern Med* 18:190–195, 2004.
98. Briggs SL, Sneed K, Sawyer DC: Antinociceptive effects of oxymorphone-butorphanol-acepromazine combination in cats, *Vet Surg* 27(5):466–472, 1998.
99. KuKanich B, Hogan BK, Krugner-Higby LA, et al: Pharmacokinetics of hydromorphone hydrochloride in healthy dogs, *Vet Anaesth Analg* 35(3):256–264, 2008.
100. Smith LJ, KuKanich B, Hogan BK, et al: Pharmacokinetics of a controlled-release liposome-encapsulated hydromorphone administered to healthy dogs, *J Vet Pharmacol Ther* 31(5):415–422, 2008.
101. Robertson SA, Taylor PM, Sear JW, et al: Relationship between plasma concentrations and analgesia after intravenous fentanyl and disposition after other routes of administration in cats, *J Vet Pharmacol Ther* 28:87–93, 2005.
102. Lee DD, Papich MG, Hardie EM: Comparison of pharmacokinetics of fentanyl after intravenous and transdermal administration in cats, *Am J Vet Res* 61(6):672–677, 2000.
103. Sano T, Nishimura R, Kanazawa H, et al: Pharmacokinetics of fentanyl after single intravenous injection and constant rate infusion in dogs, *Vet Anaesth Analg* 33:266–273, 2006.
104. Committee on Drugs: Alternative routes of drug administration—advantages and disadvantages (subject review), *Pediatrics* 100:143–152, 1997.
105. Paut O, Lang P, Massias L: Pharmacokinetics of aerosolized fentanyl in healthy volunteers, *Anesthesiology* 99:A490, 2003.
106. Riviere JE, Papich MG: Potential and problems of developing transdermal patches for veterinary applications, *Adv Drug Deliv Rev* 50(3):175–203, 2001.
107. Grond S, Radburch L, Lehmann KA: Clinical pharmcokinetcis of transdermal opioids, *Clin Pharmacokinet* 38:50–89, 2000.
108. Kyles AE, Papich M, Hardie EM: Disposition of transdermally administered fentanyl in dogs, *Am J Vet Res* 57(5):715–719, 1996.
109. Egger CM, Duke T, Archer J, et al: Comparison of plasma fentanyl concentrations by using three transdermal fentanyl patch sizes in dogs, *Vet Surg* 27(2):159–166, 1998.
110. Davidson C, Pettifer GR, Henry JD: Plasma fentanyl concentrations and analgesic effects during full or partial exposure of transdermal fentanyl patches in cats, *J Am Vet Med Assoc* 224:700–705, 2004.
111. Glerum LE, Egger CM, Allen SW, et al: Analgesic effect of the transdermal fentanyl patch during and after feline ovariohysterectomy, *Vet Surg* 30(4):351–358, 2001.
112. Kyles AE, Hardie EM, Hansen BD, et al: Comparison of transdermal fentanyl and intramuscular oxymorphone on postoperative behaviour after ovariohysterectomy in dogs, *Res Vet Sci* 65(3):245–251, 1998.
113. Franks JN, Boothe HW, Taylor L, et al: Evaluation of transdermal fentanyl patches for analgesia in cats undergoing onychectomy, *J Am Vet Med Assoc* 217(7):1013–1020, 2000.
114. Hofmeister EH, Egger CM: Transdermal fentanyl patches in small animals, *J Am Anim Hosp Assoc* 40:468–478, 2004.
115. Paddleford RR: *Manual of small animal anesthesia*, ed 2, Philadelphia, 1999, Saunders.
116. Barrueto F Jr, Howland MA, Hofman, et al: The fentanyl tea bag, *Vet Hum Toxicol* 46(1):30–31, 2004.
117. Pettifer GR, Hosgood G: The effect of rectal temperature on perianesthetic serum concentrations of transdermally administered fentanyl in cats anesthetized with isoflurane, *Am J Vet Res* 64(12):1557–1561, 2003.
118. Carroll G: *Personal communication*, 1992, Texas A&M University.
119. Balmer TV, Irvine D, Jones RS, et al: Comparison of carprofen and pethidine as postoperative analgesics in the cat, *J Small Anim Pract* 39(4):158–164, 1998.
120. Millette VM, Steagall PV, Duke-Novakovski T, et al: Effects of meperidine or saline on thermal, mechanical and electrical nociceptive thresholds in cats, *Vet Anaesth Analg* 35(6):543–547, 2008.
121. Yeh SY, Woods LA: Excretion of codeine and its metabolites by dogs, rabbits and cats, *Arch Int Pharmacodyn Ther* 191(2):231–242, 1971.
122. Woods LA, Meuhlenbeck HE, Mellett LB: Plasma levels and excretion of codeine and metabolites in the dog and monkey, *J Pharmacol Exp Ther* 117(1):117–125, 1956.
123. Davis AM, Inturrisi CE: d-Methadone blocks morphine tolerance and N-methyl-D-aspartate-induced hyperalgesia, *J Pharmacol Exp Ther* 289(2):1048–1053, 1999.
124. KuKanich B, Borum SL: The disposition and behavioral effects of methadone in Greyhounds, *Vet Anaesth Analg* 35(3):242–248, 2008.
125. KuKanich B, Lascelles BD, Aman AM, et al: The effects of inhibiting cytochrome P450 3A, p-glycoprotein, and gastric acid secretion on the oral bioavailability of methadone in dogs, *J Vet Pharmacol Ther* 28(5):461–466, 2005.
126. Steagall PV, Carnicelli P, Taylor PM, et al: Effects of subcutaneous methadone, morphine, buprenorphine or saline on thermal and pressure thresholds in cats, *J Vet Pharmacol Ther* 29(6):531–537, 2006.
127. Dohoo SE, Dohoo IR: Postoperative use of analgesics in dogs and cats by Canadian veterinarians, *Can Vet J* 37(9):546–551, 1996.
128. Hubbell JA, Muir WW: Evaluation of a survey of the diplomates of the American College of Laboratory Animal Medicine on use of analgesic agents in animals used in biomedical research, *J Am Vet Med Assoc* 209(5):918–921, 1996.
129. Christie GJ, Strom PW, Rourke JE: Butorphanol tartrate: a new antitussive agent for use in dogs, *Vet Med Small Anim Clin* 75(10):1559–1562, 1980.
130. Houghton KJ, Rech RH, Sawyer DC, et al: Dose-response of intravenous butorphanol to increase visceral nociceptive threshold in dogs, *Proc Soc Exp Biol Med* 197(3):290–296, 1991.
131. Sawyer DC, Rech RH, Durham RA, et al: Dose response to butorphanol administered subcutaneously to increase visceral nociceptive threshold in dogs, *Am J Vet Res* 52(11):1826–1830, 1991.
132. Pfeffer M, Smyth RD, Pittman KA, et al: Pharmacokinetics of subcutaneous and intramuscular butorphanol in dogs, *J Pharm Sci* 69(7):801–803, 1980.

133. Vaugh D: *Pharmacokinetics of albuterol and butorphanol administered intravenously and via buccal patch (Thesis)*, May 2003, Texas A&M University, p 86.
134. Borer LR, Peel JE, Seewald W, et al: Effect of carprofen, etodolac, meloxicam, or butorphanol in dogs with induced acute synovitis, *Am J Vet Res* 64(11):1429–1437, 2003.
135. Mathews KA, Paley DM, Foster RA, et al: A comparison of ketorolac with flunixin, butorphanol, and oxymorphone in controlling postoperative pain in dogs, *Can Vet J* 37(9):557–567, 1996.
136. Pircio AW, Buyniski JP, Roebel LE: Pharmacological effects of a combination of butorphanol and acetaminophen, *Arch Int Pharmacodyn Ther* 35(1):116–123, 1978.
137. Troncy E, Cuvelliez SG, Blais D: Evaluation of analgesia and cardiorespiratory effects of epidurally administered butorphanol in isoflurane-anesthetized dogs, *Am J Vet Res* 57(10):1478–1482, 1996.
138. Robertson SA, Lascelles BD, Taylor PM, et al: PK-PD modeling of buprenorphine in cats: intravenous and oral transmucosal administration, *J Vet Pharmacol Ther* 28(5):453–460, 2005.
139. Hosgood G: Pharmacologic features of butorphanol in dogs and cats, *J Am Vet Med Assoc* 196:135–136, 1990.
140. Sawyer DC, Rech RH: Analgesia and behavioral effects of butorphanol, nalbuphine and pentazocine in the cat, *J Am Anim Hosp Assoc* 23:439–446, 1987.
141. Wells SM, Glerum LE, Papich MG: Pharmacokinetics of butorphanol in cats after intramuscular and buccal transmucosal administration, *Am J Vet Res* 69(12):1548–1554, 2008.
142. Lascelles BD, Robertson SA: Use of thermal threshold response to evaluate the antinociceptive effects of butorphanol in cats, *Am J Vet Res* 65(8):1085–1089, 2004.
143. Johnson JA, Robertson SA, Pypendop BH: Antinociceptive effects of butorphanol, buprenorphine, or both, administered intramuscularly in cats, *Am J Vet Res* 68(7):699–703, 2007.
144. Heel RC, Brogden RN, Speight TM, et al: Buprenorphine: a review of its pharmacological properties and therapeutic efficacy, *Drugs* 17:81–110, 1979.
145. Romero DV, Partilla JS, Zheng QX, et al: Opioid peptide receptor studies. 12. Buprenorphine is a potent and selective MOP/KOP antagonist in the [35S]-GTP-gamma-S functional binding assay, *Synapse* 34(2):83–94, 1999.
146. Ohtani M, Kotaki H, Sawada Y, et al: Comparative analysis of buprenorphine- and norbuprenorphine-induced analgesic effects based on pharmacokinetic-pharmacodynamic modelling, *J Pharamcol Exp Ther* 272(2):505–510, 1995.
146a. Boas RA, Villiger JW: Clinical actions of fentanyl and buprenorphine. The significance of receptor binding, *Br J Anaesth.* 57(2):192–196, 1985.
147. Watson AD, Nicholson A, Church DB, et al: Use of anti-inflammatory and analgesic drugs in dogs and cats, *Aust Vet J* 74(3):203–210, 1996.
148. Flecknell PA: The relief of pain in laboratory animals, *Lab Anim* 18(2):147–160, 1984.
149. Garrett ER, Chandran VR: Pharmacokinetics of morphine and its surrogates. X: analyses and pharmacokinetics of buprenorphine in dogs, *Biopharm Drug Dispos* 11(4):311–350, 1990.
150. Dahan A, Yassen A, Romberg R, et al: Buprenorphine induces ceiling in respiratory depression but not in analgesia, *Br J Anesth* 96(5):627–632, 2006.
151. Tracqui A, Tournoud C, Flesch F, et al: Acute poisoning during substitution therapy based on high-dosage buprenorphine, 29 clinical cases—20 fatal cases, *Presse Med* 27(12):557–561, 1998.
152. Zanette G, Manani G, Giusti F, et al: Paediatric respiratory depression following administration of low dose buprenorphine as postoperative analgesic after fentanyl balanced anaesthesia, *Anaesth* 6(5):419–422, 1996.
153. Gaulier JM, Marquet P, Lacassie E, et al: Fatal intoxication following self-administration of a massive dose of buprenorphine, *J Forensic Sci* 45(1):226–228, 2000.
154. Saarialho-Kere U, Mattila MJ, Paloheimo M, et al: Psychomotor, respiratory and neuroendocrinological effects of buprenorphine and amitriptyline in healthy volunteers, *Eur J Clin Pharmacol* 33(2):139–146, 1987.
155. Orman JS, Keating GM: Buprenorphine/Naloxone: a review of its use in the treatment of opioid dependence, *Drugs* 69(5):577–607, 2009.
156. Tabuchi Y, Takahashi S: A comparison of fentanyl and buprenorphine in total intravenous anesthesia using propofol during spinal surgery, *Masui* 49(7):745–749, 2000.
157. Bullingham RE, McQuay HJ, Dwyer D, et al: Sublingual buprenorphine used postoperatively: clinical observations and preliminary pharmacokinetic analysis, *Br J Clin Pharmacol* 12(2):117–122, 1981.
158. Taylor PM, Robertson SA, Dixon MJ, et al: Morphine, pethidine and buprenorphine disposition in the cat, *J Vet Pharmacol Ther* 24(6):391–398, 2001.
159. Andaluz A, Moll X, Abellán R, et al: Pharmacokinetics of buprenorphine after intravenous administration of clinical doses to dogs, *Vet J* 181(3):299–304, 2009.
160. Abbo LA, Ko JC, Maxwell LK, et al: Pharmacokinetics of buprenorphine following intravenous and oral transmucosal administration in dogs, *Vet Ther* 9(2):83–93, 2008.
161. Krotscheck U, Boothe DM, Little AA: Pharmacokinetics of buprenorphine following intravenous administration in dogs, *Am J Vet Res* 69(6):722–727, 2008.
162. Murrell JC, Robertson SA, Taylor PM, et al: Use of a transdermal matrix patch of buprenorphine in cats: preliminary pharmacokinetic and pharmacodynamic data, *Vet Rec* 160(17):578–583, 2007.
163. Steagall PV, Mantovani FB, Taylor PM, et al: Dose-related antinociceptive effects of intravenous buprenorphine in cats, *Vet J* 182(2):203–209, 2009.
164. Bosmans T, Gasthuys F, Duchateau L, et al: A comparison of tepoxalin-buprenorphine combination and buprenorphine forpostoperative analgesia in dogs: a clinical study, *J Vet Med A Physiol Pathol Clin Med* 54(7):364–369, 2007.
165. Shih AC, Robertson S, Isaza N, et al: Comparison between analgesic effects of buprenorphine, carprofen, and buprenorphine with carprofen for canine ovariohysterectomy, *Vet Anaesth Analg* 35(1):69–79, 2008.
166. Slingsby LS, Taylor PM, Waterman-Pearson AE: Effects of two doses of buprenorphine four or six hours apart on nociceptive thresholds, pain and sedation in dogs after castration, *Vet Rec* 159(21):705–711, 2006.
167. Mathews KA: Analgesia for the pregnant, lactating and neonatal to pediatric cat and dog, *J Vet Emerg Crit Care* 15(4):273–284, 2005.
168. Michalis LL, Hicker PR, Clark TA, et al: Ventricular irritability associated with the use of naloxone, *Ann Thorac Surg* 18:608–614, 1974.
169. Flacke JW, Flacke WE, Williams GD: Acute pulmonary edema following naloxone reversal of high dose morphine anesthesia, *Anesthesiology* 47:376–387, 1977.
170. Tanaka GY: Hypertensive reaction to naloxone, *J Am Med Assoc* 228:25–26, 1974.
171. Feldberg W, Pyke DA, Stubbs WA: Hyperglycaemia, a morphine-like effect produced by naloxone in the cat, *J Physiol* 340(1):121–128, 1983.
172. Faggella AM, Aronsohn MG: Anesthetic techniques for neutering 6- to 14-week-old kittens, *J Am Vet Med Assoc* 202(7):1040–1041, 1993.
173. Upton RN, Semple TJ, Macintyre PE: Pharmacokinetic optimisation of opioid treatment in acute pain therapy, *Clin Pharmacokinet* 33:225–244, 1997.

174. Tranquilli WJ, Fikes LL, Raffe MR: Selecting the right analgesics: indications and dosage requirements, *Vet Med* 84:692-697, 1989.
175. Kloke M, Rapp M, Bosse B, et al: Toxicity and/or insufficient analgesia by opioid therapy: risk factors and the impact of changing the opioid. A retrospective analysis of 273 patients observed at a single center, *Support Care Cancer* 8(6):479–486, 2000.
176. KuKanich B, Papich MG: Pharmacokinetics of tramadol and the metabolite O-desmethyltramadol in dogs, *J Vet Pharmacol Ther* 27:239–246, 2004.
177. Pypendop BH, Ilkiw JE: Pharmacokinetics of tramadol, and its metabolite *O*-desmethyl-tramadol, in cats, *J Vet Pharmacol Ther* 31:52–59, 2007.
177a. Sansone RA, Sansone LA: Tramadol: seizures, serotonin syndrome and co-administered antidepressants, *Psychiatry* 6: 17-21, 2009.
178. Steagall PV, Taylor PM, Brondani JT, et al: Antinociceptive effects of tramadol and acepromazine in cats, *J Feline Med Surg* 10(1):24–31, 2008.
179. Ebert B, Mikkelson S, Thorkildsen C, et al: Norketamine, the main metabolite of ketamine, is a non-competitive NMDA receptor antagonist in the rate cortex and spinal cord, *Eur J Pharmacol* 333:99–104, 1997.
180. Wagner AE, Walton JA, Hellyer PW, et al: Use of low doses of ketamine administered by constant rate infusion as an adjunct for postoperative analgesia in dogs, *J Am Vet Med Assoc* 221:72–79, 2002.
181. Kaka JS, Hayton WL: Ketamine is a non-competitive NMDA receptor antagonist, *Biopharm Drug Dispos* 11(5):419–444, 1990.
182. Unlügenç H, Gündüz M, Ozalevli M, et al: A comparative study on the analgesic effect of tramadol, tramadol plus magnesium, and tramadol plus ketamine for postoperative pain management after major abdominal surgery, *Acta Anaesthesiol Scand* 46(8):1025–1030, 2002.
183. Correll GE, Maleki J, Gracely EJ, et al: Subanesthetic ketamine infusion therapy: a retrospective analysis of a novel therapeutic approach to complex regional pain syndrome, *Pain Med* 5(3):263–275, 2004.
184. Slingsby LS, Waterman-Pearson AE: The post-operative analgesic effects of ketamine after canine ovariohysterectomy-a comparison between pre- or post-operative administration, *Res Vet Sci* 69(2):147–152, 2000.
185. Anonymous: Committee for Veterinary Medicinal Products, Ketamine: summary report, The European Agency for the Evaluation of Medicine Products Veterinary Medicine Evaluation Unit, December, 1997.
186. Lascelles BDX, Gaynor JS, Smith ES, et al: Amantadine in a multimodal analgesic regimen for alleviation of refractory osteoarthritis pain in dogs, *J Vet Intern Med* 22:53–59, 2008.
187. KuKanich B, Papich MG: Plasma profile and pharmacokinetics of dextromethorphan after intravenous and oral administration in healthy dogs, *J Vet Pharmacol Ther* 27:337–341, 2004.
188. Dodman NH, Shuster L, Nesbitt G, et al: The use of dextromethorphan to treat repetitive self-directed scratching, biting, or chewing in dogs with allergic dermatitis, *J Vet Pharmacol Ther* 27(2):99–104, 2004.
189. Schwarz DD, Jones WG, Hedden KP: Molecular and pharmaoclogical characterization of canine brainstem alphat 2A adrenergic rectpors, *J Vet Pharmacol Ther* 22:380–386, 1999.
190. Vainio O, Ojala M: Medetomidine, an alpha 2-agonist, alleviates post-thoracotomy pain in dogs, *Lab Anim* 28(4):369–375, 1994.
191. Kuusela E, Raekallio M, Anttila M, et al: Clinical effects and pharmacokinetics of medetomidine and its enantiomers in dogs, *J Vet Pharmacol Ther* 23:15–20, 2000.
192. McNamara JO: Pharmacotherapy of the epilepsies. In Brunton LL, Lazo JS, Parker KL, editors: *Goodman & Gilman's the pharmacological basis pf therapeutics*, ed 11, New York, 2006, McGraw-Hill, pp 501-525.
193. Taylor CP: Mechanisms of analgesia by gabapentin and pregabalin-calciumchannel alpha2-delta [Cavalpha2-delta] ligands, *Pain 142(1-2)* :13–16, 2009.
194. Wiffen PJ, McQuay HJ, Edwards JE, et al: Gabapentin for acute and chronic pain, *Cochrane database of systematic reviews*, 2005:Issue 3. Art. No: CD005452. DOI:10.1002/14651858. CD005452.
194a. Eckhardt K, Ammon S, Hofmann U, et al: Gabapentin enhances the analgesic effect of morphine in healthy volunteers, *Anesth Analg* 91(1):185–191, 2000.
194b. Wagner AE, Mich PM, Uhng SR, et al: Clinical evaluation of perioperative administration of gabapentin as an adjunct for postoperative analgesia in dogs undergoing amputation of a forelimb, J Am Vet Med Assoc 236:751-756, 2010.
195. Catterall WA, Mackie K: Local anesthetics. In Brunton LL, Lazo JS, Parker KL, editors: *Goodman & Gilman's the pharmacological basis of therapeutics*, ed 11, New York, 2006, McGraw-Hill, pp 369-386.
196. Wilson DV, Barnes KS, Hauptman JG: Pharmacokinetics of combined intraperitoneal and incisional lidocaine in the dog following overiohysterectomy, *J Vet Pharmacol Ther* 27:105–109, 2004.
197. Carpenter RE, Wilson DV, Evans AT: Evaluation of intraperitoneal and incisional lidocaine or bupivacaine for analgesia following ovariohysterectomy in the dog, *Vet Anaesth Analg* 31:46–52, 2004.
198. Ibusuki S, Katsuki H, Takasaki M: The effects of extracellular pH with and without bicarbonate on intracellular procaine concentrations and anesthetic effects in crayfish giant axons, *Anesthesiology* 88(6):1549–1557, 1998.
199. Gibbon KJ, Cyborski JM, Guzinski MV, et al: Evaulation of adverse effects of eMLA (lidocaine/prilocaine) cream for the placement of jugular catheters in healthy cats, *J Vet Pharmacol Ther* 26:439–441, 2003.
200. Fransson B, Peck K, Smith J, et al: Transdermal absorption of a liposome-encapsulated formulation of lidocaine following topical administration in cats, *Am J Vet Res* 63:1309–1312, 2002.
201. Weil AB, Ko J, Inoue T: The use of lidocaine patches, *Compend Contin Educ Vet* 29(4):208–210; 214–216, 2007.
202. Weiland L, Croubels S, Baert K, et al: Pharmacokinetics of a lidocaine patch 5% in dogs, *J Vet Med A Physiol Pathol Clin Med* 53(1):34–39, 2006.
203. Ko J, Weil A, Maxwell L, et al: Plasma concentrations of lidocaine in dogs following lidocaine patch application, *J Am Anim Hosp Assoc* 43(5):280–283, 2007.
204. Ko JC, Maxwell LK, Abbo LA, et al: Pharmacokinetics of lidocaine following the application of 5% lidocaine patches to cats, *J Vet Pharmacol Ther* 31(4):359–367, 2008.
205. Cassutto BH, Gfeller RW: Use of intravenous lidocaine to prevent reperfusion injury and subsequent multiple organ dysfunction syndrome, *J Vet Emerg Crit Care* 13(3):137–148, 2003.
206. Pypendop BH, Ilkiw JE, Robertson SA: Effects of intravenous administration of lidocaine on the thermal threshold in cats, *Am J Vet Res* 67(1):16–20, 2006.
207. Muir WH III, Weise AJ, March PA: Effects of morphine, lidocaine, ketamine and morphine-lidocaine-ketamine drug combination on minimum alveolar concentration in dogs anesthetized with isoflurane, *Am J Vet Res* 64:1156–1160, 2003.
208. Himes RS Jr, DiFazio CA, Burney RG: Effects of lidocaine on the anesthetic requirements for nitrous oxide and halothane, *Anesthesiology* 47(5):437–440, 1977.

209. Valverde A, Doherty TJ, Hernández J, et al: Effect of lidocaine on the minimum alveolar concentration of isoflurane in dogs, *Vet Anaesth Analg* 31(4):264–271, 2004.
210. Smith LJ, Bently E, Shi A, et al: Systemic lidocaine infusion as an analgesic for intraocular surgery in dogs: a pilot study, *Vet Anaesth Analg* 31(1):53–63, 2004.
211. Pypendop BH, Ilkiw JE: Assessment of the hemodynamic effects of lidocaine administered IV in isoflurane-anesthetized cats, *Am J Vet Res* 66(4):661–668, 2005.
212. Thomasy SM, Pypendop BH, Ilkiw JE, et al: Pharmacokinetics of lidocaine and its active metabolite, monoethylglycinexylidide, after intravenous administration of lidocaine to awake and isoflurane-anesthetized cats, *Am J Vet Res* 66(7):1162–1166, 2005.
213. Gerard JL, Edouard A, Berdeaux A, et al: Interaction of intravenous diazepam and bupivacaine in conscious dogs, *Reg Anesth* 14(6):298–303, 1989.
214. Conzemius MG, Brockman DJ, King LG, et al: Analgesia in dogs after intercostal thoracotomy: a clinical trial comparing intravenous buprenorphine and interpleural bupivacaine, *Vet Surg* 23(4):291–298, 1994.
215. Feldman H, Arthur G, Pitkanen M, et al: Treatment of acute systemic toxicity after the rapid intravenous injection of ropivacaine and bupivacaine in the conscious dog, *Anesth Analg* 73:373–384, 1991.
216. López-Sanromán J, Cruz J, Santos M, et al: Effect of alkalinization on the local analgesic efficacy of ketamine in the abaxial sesamoid nerve block in horses, *J Vet Pharmacol Ther* 26(4):265–269, 2003.
217. Terlau H, Olivera BM: Conus venoms: a rich source of novel ion channel-targeted peptides, *Physiol Rev* 84(1):41–68, 2004.
218. Livett BG, Sandall DW, Keays D, et al: Therapeutic applications of conotoxins that target the neuronal nicotinic acetylcholine receptor, *Toxicon* 48(7):810–829, 2006.
219. Vig MM: Nicotine poisoning in a dog, *Vet Hum Toxicol* 32(6):573–575, 1990.
220. Freeman G, Entero H, Brem H: Practical treatment of pain in patients with chronic wounds: pathogenesis-guided management, *Am J Surg* 188(Suppl to July):31S–35S, 2004.
221. Urch C: The pathophysiology of cancer-induced bone pain: current understanding, *Palliat Med* 18:267–274, 2004.
222. Portenoy RK, Farkash A: Practical management of non-malignant pain in the elderly, *Geriatrics* 43:29–47, 1989.
223. Wall RT: Use of analgesics in the elderly, *Clin Pharm* 6:345–364, 1990.
224. Murtaugh RJ, Kaplan PM: *Veterinary emergency and critical care medicine*, St Louis, 1996, Mosby.
225. Bullock R, Ward JD: Management of head trauma. In Shoemaker WC, Ayers SM, Grenvic A, et al: *Textbook of critical care*, ed 3, Philadelphia, 1995, Saunders, pp 1449–1456.
226. Dewey CW, Budsberg SC, Oliver JE: Principles of head trauma management in dogs and cats: parts I and II. In Drobatz K, editor: *Emergency medicine in small animal practice: the compendium collection*, Trenton, NJ, 1997, Veterinary Learning Systems, pp 63–83.
227. Jones RS: Epidural analgesia in the dog and cat, *Vet J* 161:123–131, 2001.
228. Bernards CM: Recent insights into the pharmacokinetics of spinal opioids and the relevance to opioid selection, *Curr Opin Anaesthesiol* 17(5):441–447, 2004.
229. Sibanda S, Hughes JM, Pawson PE, et al: The effects of preoperative extradural bupivacaine and morphine on the stress response in dogs undergoing femoro-tibial joint surgery, *Vet Anaesth Analg* 33(4):246–257, 2006.
230. Hendrix PK, Raffe MR, Robinson EP, et al: Epidural administration of bupivacaine, morphine, or their combination for postoperative analgesia in dogs, *J Am Vet Med Assoc* 209(3):598–607, 1996.

Antiinflammatory Drugs

29

Dawn Merton Boothe

Chapter Outline

THE PATHOPHYSIOLOGY OF INFLAMMATION

Inflammation can occur in any vascularized tissue. Initiated as a protective mechanism intended to remove the underlying cause, be it chemical, physical, or biological, the acute inflammatory process facilitates return of the inflamed tissue to normal function.[1,2] With time, however, its unfettered actions can lead to chronic inflammation, which can contribute to harm to the patient. The sequelae of inflammation are manifested as five cardinal signs: redness, heat, swelling or edema, pain, and loss of function. The initial response to vascular damage is vasoconstriction of small vessels in the area of injury, which serves to control hemorrhage within 5 to 10 minutes; however, vasodilation and increased vascular permeability of small venules are evident. Leukocytes, platelets, and erythrocytes in the injured vessels become "sticky," adhering to the endothelium. Leakage of cells and plasma-derived protein-rich fluid is followed by platelet aggregation and fibrin formation. Initially, the predominant cell type infiltrating damaged tissues is the polymorphonuclear leukocyte (PMN), in part because it predominates in circulation. These cells provide a protective response by removing chemicals or other materials that may have initiated the inflammatory response. As the short-lived PMNs die, macrophages become the predominant cell type. The migration and concentration of PMNs to the site of injury is facilitated by chemical mediators that act as chemotactic agents. As PMNs die, the contents of the lysed cells accumulate to form the component of inflammatory exudate commonly referred to as *pus*.

THE ROLE OF CHEMICAL MEDIATORS IN THE INFLAMMATORY RESPONSE

Released mediators perpetuate the inflammatory response (Table 29-1 and Figures 29-1 and 29-2) and are responsible for the clinical signs associated with inflammation, including pain and fever.[3] Mediators (see Table 29-1) are derived from both the cells (both preformed and formed in situ) and fluid that reach the site of tissue damage by way of the bloodstream. Although quantitative differences between species and tissue concentrations of the mediators vary, the effect on and role in the pathophysiology of inflammation that each mediator has are predominantly the same. Leukocytes are a rich source of a variety of chemical mediators of inflammation. These cells, as well as cells of the injured tissues (either at the time of damage or after subsequent damage), perpetuate the inflammatory

Table 29-1 Mediators Important in the Course of Inflammation

Mediator	Source	Action	Pharmacologic Modulator
Lysosomal contents	Phagocytes	Vessel permeability Membrane degradation Chemotactic factors Collagen, fibrin, cartilage (etc.) degradation	Glucocorticoids Dimethylsulfoxide Organic gold compounds
Histamine	Granulocytes	Vasodilation Capillary permeability Pain	Antihistamines (particularly H_{1+} and possibly H_2 blockers)
Serotonin	Platelets	Vasodilation and constriction Capillary permeability	
Eicosanoids Prostaglandins Leukotrienes Lipoxygenases	All cells	Chemotaxis Vascular permeability Vasodilation Pain	Glucocorticoids Nonsteroidal antiinflammatory drugs
Platelet-activating factor	Platelets	Platelet aggregation Chemotaxis	Glucocorticoids
Oxygen radicals	Damaged tissues Leukocytes	Highly destructive to a number of cellular constituents, particularly lipid membranes	Superoxide dismutase Vitamin E Ascorbic acid Dimethylsulfoxide Xanthine oxidase inhibitors
Kinins	Plasma	Vasodilation Capillary permeability Pain	Nonsteroidal antiinflammatory drugs
Complement	Plasma	Lysis of cells Histamine release Vascular permeability Release of lysosomal contents Chemotaxis	Glucorticoids Dimethylsulfoxide Antihistamine
Fibrinopeptides	Plasma	Enhance kinins Vascular permeability Chemotaxis	Nonsteroidal antiinflammatory drugs(?)
Cytokines		Proinflammatory: Control direction, magnitude, duration of immune response; local effects in general but may become systemic	Multiple: nonsteroidal antiinflammatory drugs, glucocorticoids, others
Tumor necrosis factor-alpha (cachectin)	Macrophages		
Tumor necrosis factor-beta (lymphotoxin)	Lymphocytes		
Interleukins (esp. IL-1)			
	Lymphocytes (T)	Antiiflammatory: downregulate immune response	
Chemokines (chemotactic cytokines)	Leukocytes, others	Second-order cytokines, induced by above; leukocyte migration	Multiple: nonsteroidal antiinflammatory drugs, glucocorticoids, others
Neutrophil-activating protein			

Table 29-1 Mediators Important in the Course of Inflammation—cont'd

Mediator	Source	Action	Pharmacologic Modulator
Platelet-activating factor			
IL-1			
Stress proteins			
Heat shock	Molecular chaperones (cytoprotection, protein) manipulation		
Superoxide dismutase			
Lipoxins	As with leukotrienes; lipoxygenase 15.	Antiinflammatory,	Aspirin (increases)
		Antiplatelet	Nonsteroidal antiinflammatory drugs (vary in impact)
		Vasodilatory	Not dual-acting nonsteroidal antiinflammatory drugs
		Regulates myelopoiesis	
EETs, HETEs, EpOMEs	As with eicosanoids; formation catalyzed by cytochrome P450	Modulate vascular tone; antiinflammatory	Soluble epoxide hydroxylase inhibitors
NFk-B	Cells producing proinflammatory mediators	Induces transcription of genes that control inflammatory mediators	Emerging; see text
Metzincins	Extracellular matrix	Cleavage of proteins, including adhesion molecules, cytokines, chemokines, growth factors; tissue remodeling. May be proinflammatory or antiinflammatory	
Metalloproteinases			
Tissue inhibitors of metalloproteinases	Extracellular matrix	Control of inflammation	

EETs, Epoxyeicosatrienoic acids; *HETEs,* hydroxyeicosatrienoic acids; *EpOMEs,* epoxyoctadecenoic acids; *NFk-B,* nuclear factor kappa-B.

response and become potential targets of antiinflammatory drugs. Preformed mediators include those located in granules (e.g., histamine and serotonin) and lysosomes and other enzymes. Their release occurs in the earliest stages of inflammation, to be followed by the release of mediators formed in situ. This latter group includes products of arachidonic acid (AA) metabolism, including eicosanoids (prostaglandins [PGs], leukotrienes, and related compounds), and platelet-activating factor, as well as oxygen radicals, and cytokines. The role each of these mediators varies. Although most mediators are proinflammatory in action, antiinflammatory mediators also are formed. Examples include lipoxins, epoxyeicosatrienoic acids (EETs), hydroxyeicosatetranoic acids (HETEs), and epoxyoctadecenoic acids (EpOMEs), selected cytokines, and possibly cyclooxygenase-2 (COX-2)–generated PGs formed in later stages of inflammation (see Table 29-1).[1,2] The induction of genes responsible for the generation of proinflammatory mediators is an emerging target of interest for antiinflammatory drugs. Among the inducible transcription factors that control inflammatory gene expression, nuclear factor NFκB is of particular interest because of its ability to coordinate soluble proinflammatory mediators such as cytokines and chemokines as well as leukocyte adhesion molecules. Normally, this factor is trapped in the cytosol by an inhibitory protein that hides the signal necessary for nuclear localization. However, in the face of proinflammatory cytokines (e.g., tumor necrosis factor-alpha [TNF-alpha], interleukin-1 [IL-1]), the inhibitory protein is phosphorylated and degraded, thus allowing movement of NFκβ to the nucleus.[4] The role of matrix metalloproteinases (MMPs) in the inflammatory process is being increasingly recognized.[5] The extraceullar matrix has long been recognized as a substrate for these proteolytic tissue-remodeling enzymes. However, other molecules serve as substrates, including cytokines and chemokines. As such, MMPs may act to control or perpetuate inflammation, and the sequelae of their inhibition may lead to adverse reactions as well as therapeutic benefits.

KEY POINT 29-1 The inappropriate inflammatory response reflects an imbalance between proinflammatory and antiinflammatory mediators.

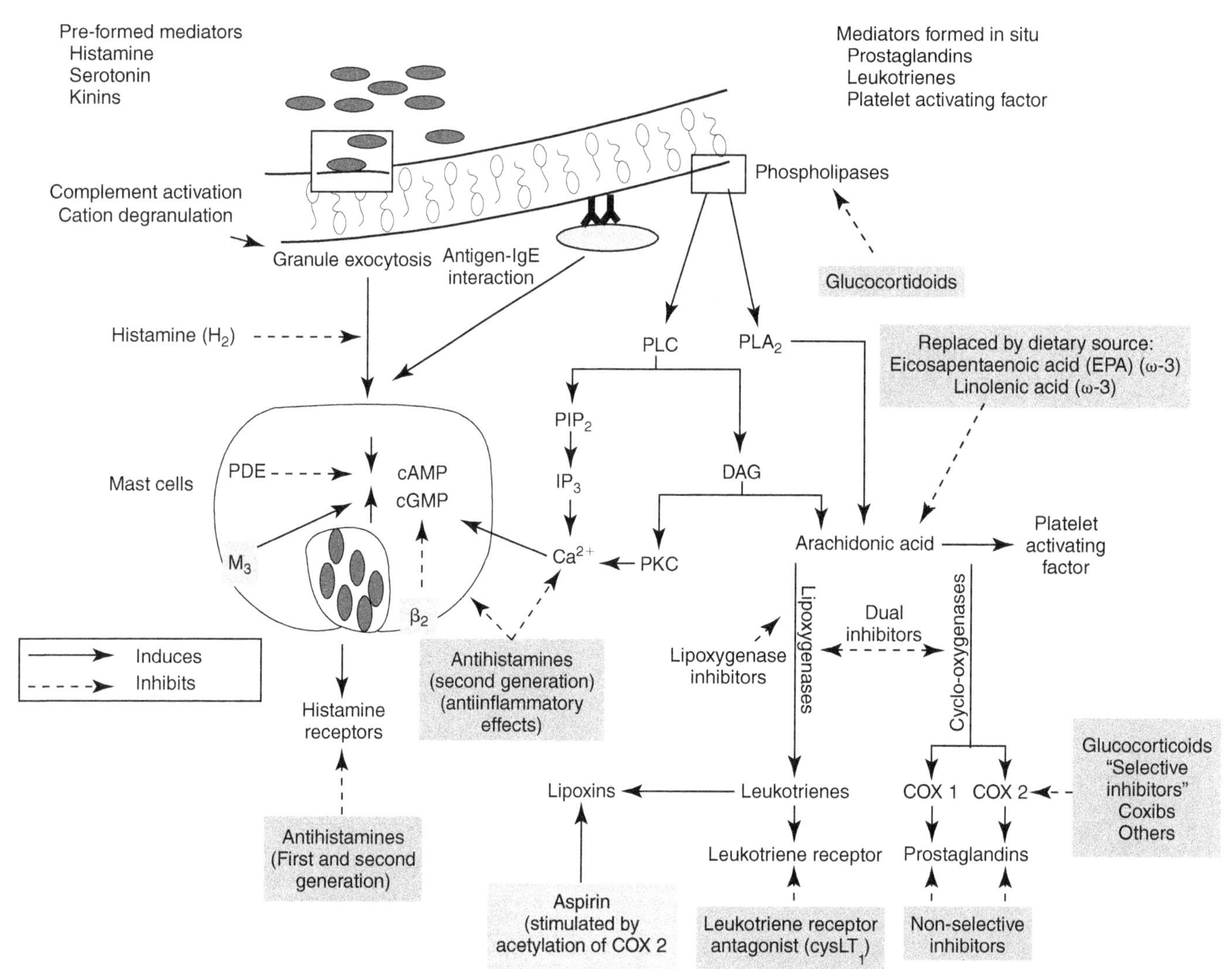

Figure 29-1 Leukocytes are an important source of inflammatory mediators that perpetuate the inflammatory response. Cellular mediators of inflammation include those preformed in granules or lysosomes, such as histamine and serotonin, and those formed in situ from arachidonic acid released by phospholipases in the cell membrane. Muscarinic receptors (M_3) stimulate, and β-adrenergic receptors ($_2$) inhibit, inflammatory mediator release. Although the phagocytic cell is intimately involved in the inflammatory reaction, it is not the only cell type capable of generating mediators of inflammation. The mediators of cellular origin interact with plasma-derived mediators, further compounding the response. Drugs used to control inflammation generally target specific mediators *(see boxes)* (see Table 29-1). *cAMP,* Cyclic adenosine monophosphate; *cGMP,* cyclic guanosine monophosphate; *DAG,* diacylglycerol; *IP_3,* inositol triphosphate; *PAF,* platelet-activating factor; *PDE,* phosphodiesterase; *PIP_2,* phosphatidylinositol; *PLA_2,* phospholipase A_2; *PLC,* phospholipase C.

Plasma-derived mediators also are important contributors to the inflammatory process. These include the kinins (e.g., bradykinin), released from their precursor form after appropriate physiologic or pathologic stimulation; complement and complement-derived peptides, released after activation of either the classic or the alternative pathway; and fibrinopeptides, released during the conversion of fibrinogen to fibrin during the clotting process and subsequent proteolysis of fibrin by plasmin.

Acute inflammation can cause severe organ or life-threatening damage. Monocytes, which follow neutrophils to the site of inflammation several hours later, release collagenases and elastases, softening local tissues. Interleukin release draws fibroblasts to the area, which in turn deposit collagen at the site. The collagen is gradually remodeled, and new blood vessels continue to form until oxygen tension is normal. If the cause of inflammation is removed, healing is complete. Failure to remove the inciting cause leads to persistent, chronic inflammation. Pharmacologic control of inflammation is oriented toward preventing the release of various chemical or plasma mediators, inhibiting their actions and treating pathophysiologic responses to them. Drugs useful for modulating the activity of chemical mediators derived from cells, plasma, or both are summarized in Table 29-1. Among the most important and frequently used drugs are the nonsteroidal antiinflammatory drugs (NSAIDs), all of which control fever; pain; and, to varying degrees, inflammation. A number of drugs and novel ingredients target inflammation particularly associated

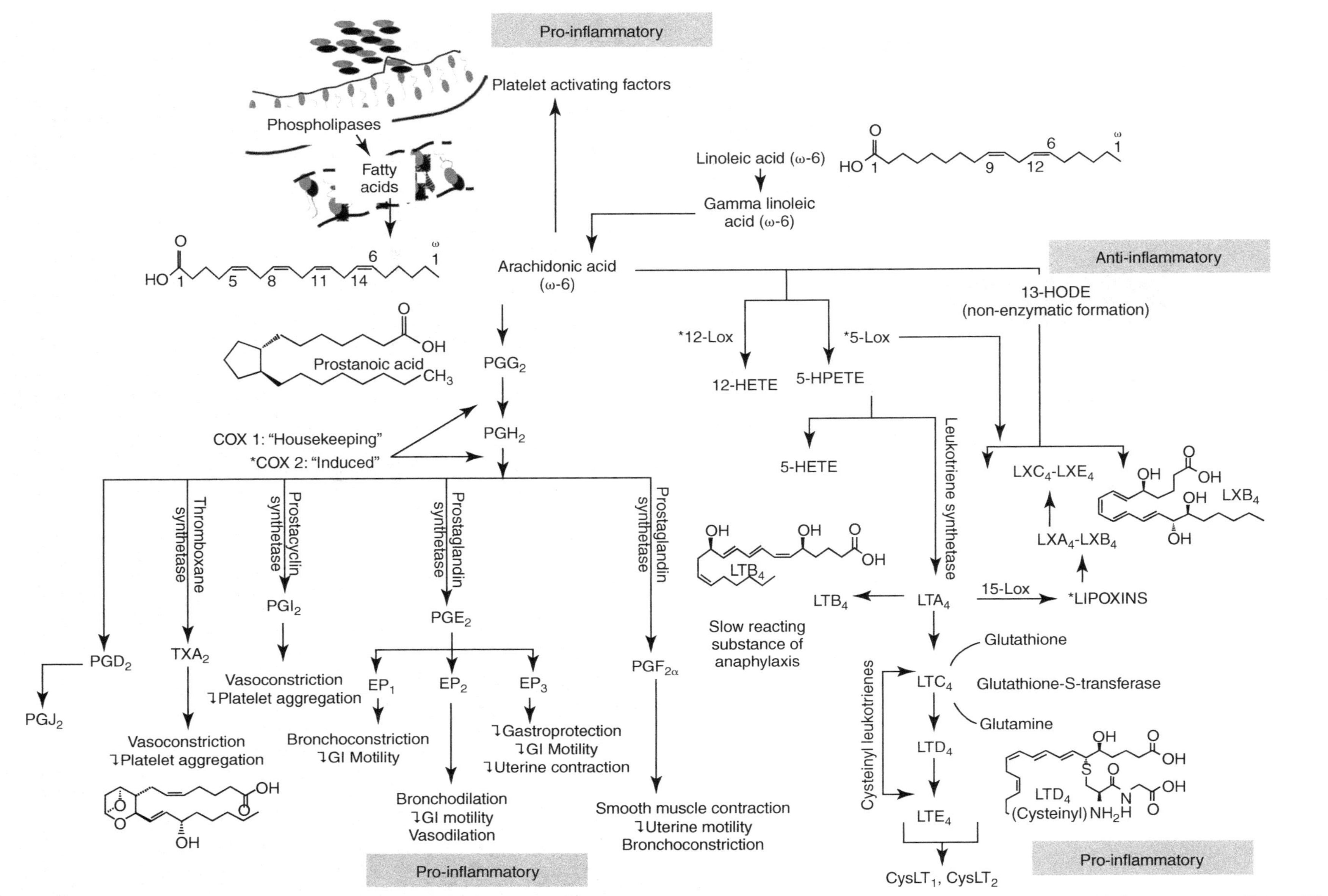

Figure 29-2 The release of arachidonic acid from the phospholipids in cell membranes leads to a cascade of events resulting in the formation of inflammatory mediators. The family of cyclooxygenases (COX) results in the formation of constitutive prostaglandins (COX-1) and inducible prostaglandins (COX-2). The inducible prostaglandins contribute to all cardinal signs of inflammation. Selectivity of nonsteroiodal antiinflammatory drugs (NSAIDs) for COX-2 ultimately may result in marked safety of the NSAIDs. Lipoxygenases result in the formation of leukotrienes, which, along with their precursors, are potent inflammagens in a number of tissues. However, among these products are antiinflammatory lipoxins. The cysteinyl leukotrienes play a major role in type I hypersensitivity and potentially in chronic inflammatory diseases as well (see Chapter 19). Platelet-activating factor also is a potent inflammagen, although some of its actions may be mediated through leukotriene activity.

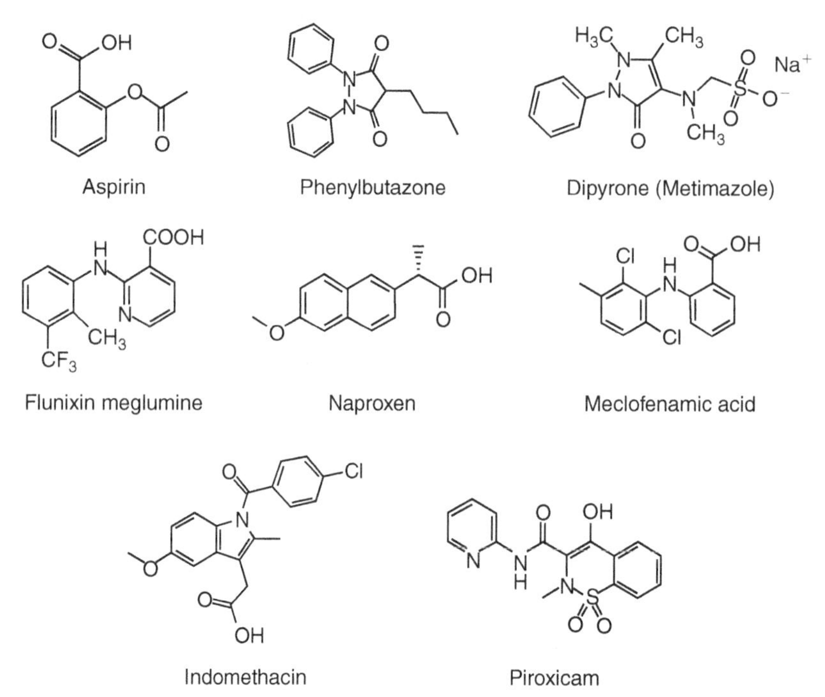

Figure 29-3 Structures of selected "traditional" nonsteroidal antiinflammatory drugs.

with specific conditions including osteoarthritis and septic shock; these are discussed separately. Glucocorticoids engage such a substantial role in the contribution, prevention, and treatment of inflammation that their discussion warrants a separate chapter.

SHARED PHARMACOLOGY OF NONSTEROIDAL ANTIINFLAMMATORY DRUGS

Chemistry

Although NSAIDs have been variably defined, the name is used to describe compounds that are not steroidal and that suppress inflammation. Generally, the classification is restricted to those drugs that inhibit one or more steps in the metabolism of AA, generally at the COX side of the cascade.[6] The NSAIDs vary in their ability to influence inflammation. The mechanism of action of some of these drugs is not limited to inhibition of AA metabolism.[7]

Aspirin, one of the earliest components of herbal therapy, is the progenitor NSAID, and terms such as *aspirinlike* and *aspirin and related drugs* have been used to refer to NSAIDs,[6] although this older terminology may become obsolete with approval of newer NSAIDs. Structurally, NSAIDs can be broadly classified as either the salicylate or carboxylic acid derivatives, including the indoles (indomethacin), propionic acids (carprofen, ibuprofen, and naproxen), fenamates (mefenamic acid), oxicams (piroxicam), and pyrazolones or enolic acids (phenylbutazone and dipyrone)(Figures 29-3 and 29-4).[6] Functionally, NSAIDs increasingly are being categorized by the enzymes they target: conventional (COX-1 and COX-2); newer COX-2–selective (COX-1 protective), which includes the coxibs as well as similarly acting drugs; more appropriate and dual inhibitors (tepoxalin) (see Figure 29-2). The coxibs include the sulfones and the sulfonamides. However, the term *coxib* refers to a chemical structure (see Figure 29-4) and not pharmacologic action and should not be used to refer to all drugs that might preferentially target COX-2 compared with COX-1. The coxibs are not arylamine sulfonamides (see Chapter 4), and therefore allergic reactions typical of sulfonamides antibiotics (see Chapter 7) may not occur. Nonetheless, several of these drugs are associated with keratitis sicca or suppression of thyroid gland activity.

KEY POINT 29-2 Although all nonsteroial antiinflammatory drugs share a common mechanism of action through inhibition of cyclooxygenase, the drugs vary in the isoform targeted, as well as in nonprostaglandin-mediated effects.

Mechanism of Action

Prostaglandins

Prostaglandin Formation. Eicosanoids, such as PGs and leukotrienes, are 20-carbon chain derivatives of cell membranes. Eicosanoids are potent mediators of inflammation and are particularly important in the later stages.[3,8] These compounds are synthesized when oxygen reacts with the polyunsaturated fatty acids of cell membrane phospholipids (see Figures 29-1 and 29-2). The most important of these fatty acids is AA, an omega-6 fatty acid, which is released into the cell from phospholipids of the damaged cell membranes. Release reflects activation of phospholipase A_2 (dependent on calcium and calmodulin) located in the cell membrane.[9] Once inside the cell, AA serves as a substrate for enzymes that generate intermediate and ultimately the final eicosanoid end product.[8,10] The formation of lipoxygenases and their subsequent

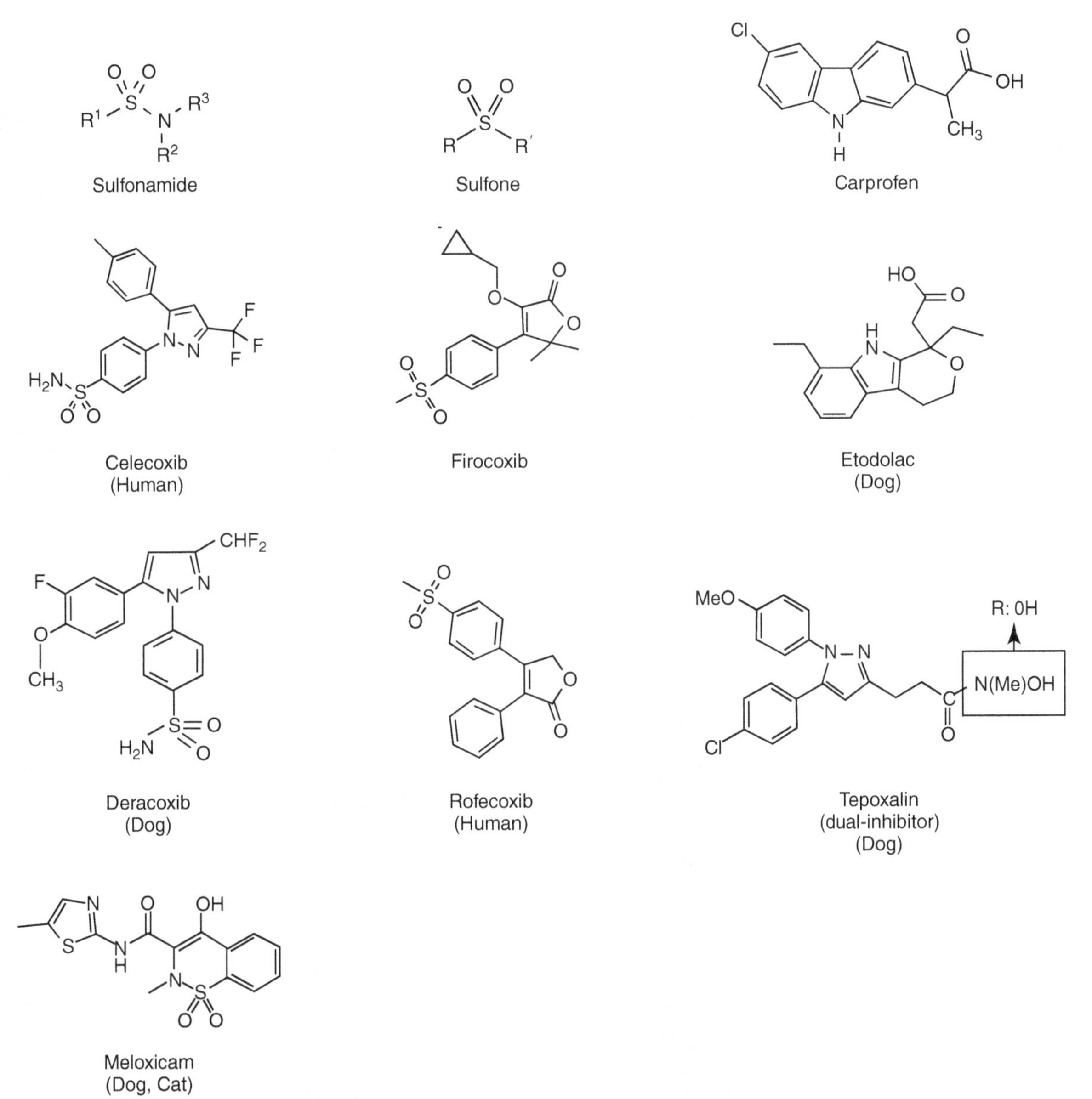

Figure 29-4 Structures of selected newer nonsteroidal antiinflammatory drugs that are more potent toward COX-2 compared with COX-1.

inhibition is discussed under "Miscellaneous Antiinflammtories." COX PG synthase or prostaglandin H (PGH) synthase, located in all cells except mature red blood cells, add oxygen to AA, generating unstable PG endoperoxides (PGG_2). Subsequent peroxidase reactions convert PGG_2 to PGH_2, the precursor of all PGs and thromboxane. The final PG end product depends on the presence of specific isomerase reductase or synthetase enzymes, some of which may be inducible.[8,9]

The direct effects of PGs are mediated through cell membrane–spanning G protein receptors located on target tissues and cells. At least nine subtypes have been identified, corresponding to each of the COX metabolites: DP1-2 (PGD_2), EP1-4 (PGE_2), FP A, B ($PGF_2\alpha$), IP (PGI_2), and TP α, β (TXA_2) (G&G);[11] another four have been characterized for PGE_2, opening the potential for selective drug activity.[9] In addition to their receptor interactions, PGs also act indirectly by enhancing other mediators such as histamine and bradykinin.

The role of PGs in normal physiology as well as in disease might best be understood by considering them as protective in nature, even those associated with inflammation. Their formation is mediated by one of at least two isoforms of cyclooxygenases (see Figures 29-1 and 29-2), located on different genes in humans.[12-14] COX-1, the "housekeeping" isoform,[14] mediates the formation of constitutive PGs produced by many tissues, including gastrointestinal cells, platelets, endothelials cells, and renal cells. PGs generated from COX-1 are constantly present, providing homeostasis through a variety of normal physiologic effects. These include protection of the gastrointestinal mucosa, hemostasis, and the kidney when subjected to hypotensive insults. COX-2 is the product of an "immediate-early" gene that is rapidly inducible and tightly regulated.[14] Regulation of COX expression is complex, with more sites present on the COX-2 compared with the COX-1 gene. Its expression is tightly restricted (but not absent) under basal conditions, but it is dramatically upregulated in the presence of inflammation or other diseases.[9] Diseases associated with increases include (in humans) rheumatoid arthritis, seizures, ischemia, and (posttranslational) cancer.[9] Proinflammatory cytokines such as TNFα and the interleukins stimulate the expression of COX-2 in many cell types, such as synovial cells, endothelial cells, chondrocytes, osteoblasts, and monocytes and macrophages.[14] COX-2 catalyzes the formation of inducible PGs, which are needed only intermittently or under specific situations.[12,13,15,16] A third COX isoform has been suggested, but it appears to be a variant of COX-1. Originally identified in high concentrations in canine cerebral cortex (hence the term used by some investigators, "canine COX-3"),[17] it is inhibited by acetaminophen (and other NSAIDs). Its inhibition may influence central analgesic effects of NSAIDs.[1,2] Differential or selective inhibition of COX-2 clearly offers potential some safety benefits by avoiding loss of homeostatic PGs; however, loss of COX-2 activity is also associated with adversities.[14] It is important to note that COX-2 is ofttimes constitutively expressed: in the kidney and brain it mediates a cytoprotective effect in damaged or inflamed gastrointestinal mucosa.

KEY POINT 29-3 Cyclooxygenase-2 is consistently, but not exclusively, associated with signals associated with inflammation, pain, and fever. However, it also plays a substantial role in noninflammatory diseases such as cancer and central nervous system diseases

Cyclooxygenases in health and disease. An appreciation of both efficacy and safety of COX inhibition (e.g., NSAIDs) is facilitated by an understanding of the role of COX in healthy and diseased tissues. COX has been described as the most common target of drug therapy with NSAIDs. In general, inhibition of COX-2 is responsible for efficacy, whereas inhibition of COX-1 is responsible for side effects.[9] However, strict adherence to this simplistic approach will lead to therapeutic failure and increased morbidity with NSAID use. Although COX-1 does indeed appear to be the predominant constitutive enzyme responsible for housekeeping, both COX-1 and COX-2 are constitutively expressed in many tissues. Further, although COX-2 clearly is more active in the promotion of inflammation, COX-1 does appear to have some role.

Inflammation. PGs, and primarily PGE2, induce vasodilation, capillary permeability, and chemotaxis. As such, PGs cause the cardinal and clinical signs of inflammation, including pain and fever.[8] PGE also modifies both T-cell and B-cell function, in part by inhibition of IL-2 secretion.[8] Other inflammatory effects of PGE include its regulation IL-6, macrophage colony-stimulating factor, and vascular endothelial growth factor. In general, research consistently indicates that it is COX-2 that predominantly mediates formation of PGE associated with inflammation, pain and fever. For example, whereas COX-1 is largely absent in normal synovial cells, COX-2 is induced in most types of arthritis, including inflammatory arthritis in animals and rheumatoid arthritis in humans. In cartilage COX-2 is associated with IL-1 degradation of proteoglycan and apoptosis of synovial cells.[18] However, not all of the inflammatory actions of COX-2 are undesirable in that COX-2 induction in response to inflammation contributes to tissue healing. For example, COX-2 is associated with healing in ligaments, bone, the gastrointestinal tract, and other tissues. The importance of COX-2 to dermal healing is not yet known.[9]

Central Nervous System. Both COX-1 and COX-2 are consitutively expressed in the brain and spinal cord. Constitutive COX is very responsive to ischemia, immunomodulation, cytokines, toxins, brain damage, and maturation processes.[17] However, although both isoforms are present, COX-2 predominates. PGs of the central nervous system (CNS) play a major role in pain; howevever increasingly they are recognized for roles in other disorders. Among them is the role of COX in the pathogenesis of Alzheimer's disease (AD). Extracellular deposition of fibrillar amyloid β (Aβ), intracellular accmumulation of abnormally phosphorylated tau protein, and subsequent formation of Aβ plaques mediating neurodegeneration and dementia in AD are associated with inflammation and COX-2.[19] Mediators of inflammation are present throughout all stages of the disease, whereas COX-2 is absent in normal astrocytes or microglial cells. Further, COX-2 is upregulated in acute brain injury and in animal models of AD.[9,19] Finally, the connection between AD and COX is supported by a lower incidence of AD in patients with rheumatoid arthritis, presumably because of the use of NSAIDs for its treatment.[19] The protective effects of NSAIDs in the AD patient may reflect the antiplatelet properties of NSAIDs; aspirin in particular may decrease the risk of ischemic damage induced by blocked capillaries of the brain. Decreased formation of amyloid β protein also has been proposed,[9] suggesting a possible role in other diseases associated with amyloid β protein deposition. Finally, COX-2 appears to be involved in the loss of glutamate-induced apoptotic cell death.[19] Because N-methyl-D-aspartate (NMDA) receptors stimulate the arachidonic acid cascade, NSAIDs mute the role of NMDA receptors in pain. NSAIDs may also inhibit NMDA–mediated neuronal cell death by preventing increased extraceullar glutamate.[19a]

Pain. PGs have been implicated in causing increased pain perception (allodynia) in damaged compared with normal tissues.[1,2] Induced COX-2 PGE as been associated with hyperalgesia (exaggerated response to pain) at the level of the spinal cord (primary hyperalgesia) or nociceptors (secondary hyperalgesia).[17] Induction of COX-2 in the dorsal horn has been associated with central sensitization, manifested as a change in excitability threshold.[9,17,18] Currently being descriped is the ability of PGs to contribute indirectly to neuropathic pain through influence on chemical mediators (e.g., histamine, bradykinin, substance P, nitric oxide [NO]), neurotransmitters (e.g., glycine inhibition or glutamate stimulation), or modulation of other receptors (e.g., NMDA).

Gastrointestinal and Other Healing. Both COX-1 and COX-2 are constitutively expressed in the gastrointestinal tract. However, constitutive expression of COX-1 has a predominant role in the protection of the gastrointestinal tract. COX-1 PGs decrease hydrochloric acid secretion, increase mucosal bicarbonate and mucus production, and increase epithelial cell proliferation and mucosal blood flow

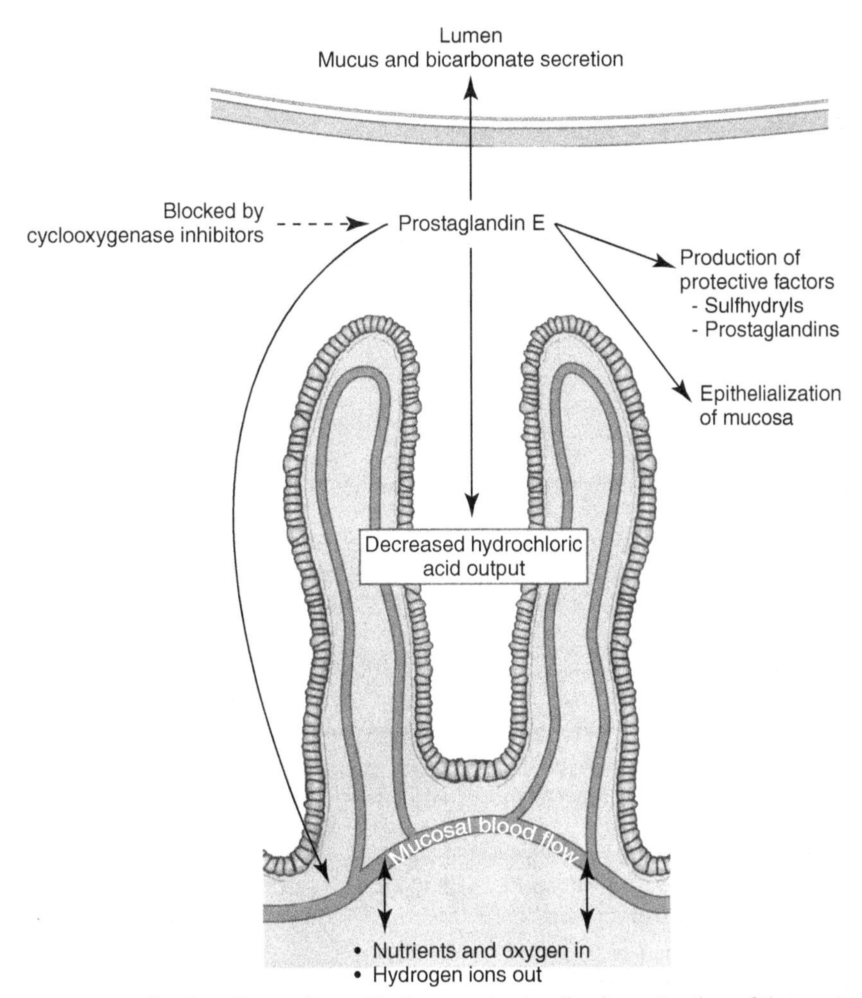

Figure 29-5 Among the many protective functions of constitutive prostaglandins is protection of the gastrointestinal mucosa from acid and other mediator-induced damage. Protective mechanisms include production of mucus and bicarbonate and inhibition of hydrogen ion secretion; epithelial turnover, which ensures rapid replacement of damaged cells; and increased mucosal blood flow, which ensures provision of oxygen and nutrients to the rapidly dividing epithelial cells as well as removal of hydrogen ions that are able to pass into the cells.

(Figure 29-5). The latter effect facilitates delivery of oxygen and nutrients to proliferating cells as well as rapid removal of damaging hydrogen ions that make their way into the mucosa. Drugs that express preferential potency for COX-2 PGs generally are associated with fewer gastrointestinal side effects compared to those targeting both COX isoforms, although the relative protection varies with the drugs. Protection appears to be more important in the presence of high drug concentrations (e.g., high doses).[20] COX-2 is critically important to the gastrointestinal tract as well, being important for healing of gastrointestinal damage: COX-2 appears within 1 hour of gastrointestinal damage. Newer coxib PGs will inhibit gastrointestinal healing as has been demonstrated in dogs receiving firocoxib (see the discussion of tepoxalin).[21] Interestingly, in the pancreas, constitutive COX-2 expression dominates, although the clinical relevance of this is not yet known.[20] The impact of NSAIDS on bone healing is an emerging concern. COX influences osteoblast and osteoclast; experimental studies have demonstrated impaired bone healing.[20a] Their use in controlling pain and limiting ectopic bone growth must be balanced with the increased risk of impaired fracture healing; conventional NSAIDs might be preferred compared to newer NSAIDs. The impact of NSAID on soft tissue healing (or ligaments) remains to be confirmed; whereas short term use may have minimal negative (and potentially a positive) impact, long term used might be approached cautiously. A recent meta-analysis in humans found no advantage in terms of return to function for coxibs, but recommended caution with long term use.[20b] A strong association has been reported between NSAIDs and severe necrotizing soft tissue infections.[20c]

Cardiovascular Disease. The role of PGs in the cardiovascular system is largely beneficial, and the relationship between COX-1 and COX-2 and their respective PG end products exemplifies the complex "ying–yang" balance that characterizes them (Figure 29-6). Platelets contain thromboxane, a synthase, which catalyzes the formation of thromboxane from AA. Thrombosis reflects platelet aggregation and vasoconstriction. The formation of a thrombus is kept in check by the presence of prostacyclin synthase in vascular endothelial cells. This enzyme catalyzes metabolism of AA to prostacyclin

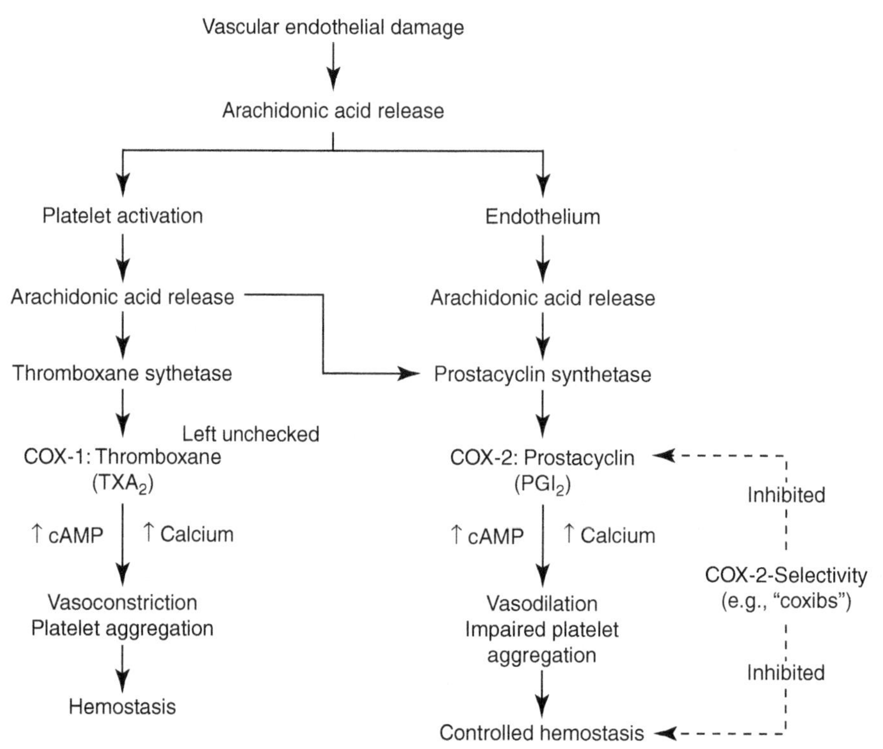

Figure 29-6 The role of constitutive prostaglandin products in hemostasis exemplifies the "ying-yang" relationship that often characterizes their action. Platelet activation in response to the damage is accompanied by the release of arachidonic acid, which is catalyzed by thromboxane synthetase, present in platelets, to thromboxane. Thromboxane causes platelet aggregation and local vasoconstriction. Excessive hemostasis is kept in check, however, by the simultaneous release of arachidonic acid from the damaged endothelial cell surface. Prostacyclin synthetase, located in the endothelial cells, results in the formation of prostacyclin, which is vasodilatory and inhibits platelet aggregation. *cAMP,* Cyclic adenosine monophosphate.

(PGI2), a vasodilatory and platelet-inhibiting PG end product. However, whereas thromboxane A2 (TXA2) is associated with COX-2, prostacyclin synthase co-localizes with COX-1. Thus, whereas drugs that target both COX isoforms will potentially allow the balance to be maintained, drugs that preferentially target only one isoform risk disruption of the balance. Such may be the case with COX-2 selective NSAIDs. Their preferential inhibition of COX-2 may allow thrombus formation to go unchecked, increasing the risk of thromboembolic disorders. Indeed, in a meta-analysis of human clinical trials, two coxib drugs (rofecoxib and valdecoxib) were associated with an increased risk of stroke (see "Adverse Events").[20d]

Kidney. In the kidney both COX-1 and -2 are constitutively expressed. Both are formed in the macula densa of humans and animals, but COX-2 may have a more important role than COX-1 (Figure 29-7). In animals, inhibition of COX-2 causes sodium and potassium retention in salt-depleted, but not normal, animals. However, in humans COX-2 appears to influence renal vasculature and podocytes. The role of COX in the kidney requires further elucidation before safety can be assumed for any NSAID; sparing COX-1 and targeting COX-2 can be expected to alter renal function. For example, kidneys do not develop in the embryos of COX-2–null knockout mice.[22] The role of COX differs among tissues and species; their impact on adverse reactions are addressed under "Adverse Reactions."[9]

Lungs. The role of PGs in the lungs does not appear to be as important as that of leukotrienes; the impact is primarily in disease, rather than health, for both eicosanoids. However, inflammatory diseases, such as asthma, are associated with smooth muscle proliferation, which is inhibited by COX-2. Thus, as in the gastrointestinal tract, COX-2 appears to have a protective role in the diseased lung. An interesting complication regarding eicosanoids in general is exemplified in the lungs: the increased formation of leukotrienes (LTs) in the presence of NSAIDs, presumably because of the increase availability of AA in the face of decreased PG synthesis.

Reproductive tract. Both COX-1 and -2 play a significant role in the normal reproductive tract. Induction of COX-2 is associated with ovulation, fertilization, implantation, and decidualization, as well as induction of labor.[22] Female knockout mice devoid of COX-2 are largely infertile.[22]

Cancer. In the 1990s a reduced risk of colon cancer was associated with consistent aspirin use. Subsequent studies demonstrated a marked increase in COX-2 in a variety of soft-tissue tumors in humans and in transitional cell carcinoma in dogs.[23] These studies suggest that benefits of NSAIDs in cancer may reflect inhibited COX-2.[9] Mechanisms by which COX-2 may facilitate cancer growth or spread include impaired apoptosis, transactivation of epidermal growth factors or receptors and promotion of angiogenesis.[9,17] Depending on the model, inhibition of COX-2 by NSAIDS reduces cell proliferation,

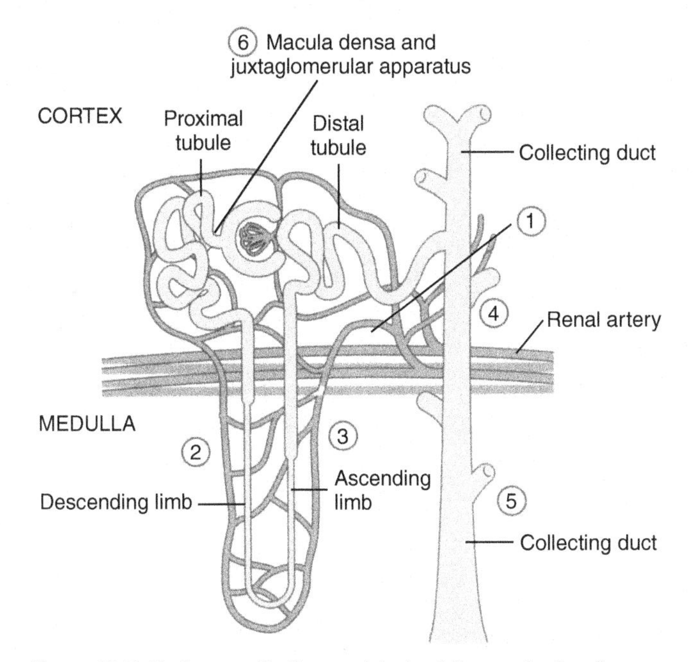

Figure 29-7 Both constitutive and inducible prostaglandins are important to renal blood flow, with the specific effect of each product varying among species. Renal prostaglandins ensure that intramedullary renal blood flow and urine formation will continue in the presence of decreased renal perfusion. Sites of action are noted by numbers and include shunting of blood from the cortices to the medullary intersitium, stimulation of natriuriesis, and inhibition of antidiuretic hormone. The nephrotoxicity of selected drugs reflects inhibition of renal prostaglandins.

increases apoptosis, and reduces metastasis. COX-2 inhibition may also enhance antitumor effects of radiation, although host toxicity also will be increased. Not surprisingly, gastrointestinal toxicity of anticancer drugs is also increased, presumably reflecting a combined toxic effect on the gastrointestinal tract.[9] COX-1 may also have a role in cancer as is suggested by a decrease in colon cancer in COX-1 knockout mice.[24]

Cycloloxygenase and nonsteroidal antiinflammatory drugs. NSAIDs (Table 29-2) act to block PG synthesis by binding to and inhibiting cyclooxygenase (see Figures 29-1 and 29-2).[8] This action is both dose and drug dependent. The planar form that characterizes these drugs is thought to facilitate their binding to COX.[6,25] Several investigators have shown that some drugs (e.g., phenylbutazone and flunixin meglumine) also reduce later steps of the formation of PGE_2 in inflammatory exudate at therapeutic doses.[26] However, both the major therapeutic and toxic effects of NSAIDs have been correlated extensively with their ability to inhibit PG synthesis, with antiinflammatory potency related to potency of impaired PG synthesis.[8]

The differential effect of NSAIDs on the isoforms of COX presumably contribute to clinical differences in efficacy and safety, .[17,27] Whereas as a class, NSAIDs appear to inhibit both COX-1 and COX-2, the ratio of the concentration of a NSAID necessary to inhibit the same level of COX-1 vesrus COX-2 activity (e.g., inhibition of 50% or 80% activivity [IC_{50} or IC_{80}]) compares the potency each drug toward each isoform, and as such, provides a basis for screening predicted relative safety

Table 29-2 Dosages of Nonsteroidal Antiinflammatory Drugs in Cats and Dogs

Drugs	Dose (mg/kg)	Route	Interval (hr)
Acetaminophen			
Dogs	10-15	PO	6-8
	20-30	PO	Sustained release 8-12
Adequan			
Dogs	5		Every other day × 3/week for 5-6 weeks
Cats	2	IM	3-7 days
Aspirin			
Dogs	10	PO	12-8
	10	PO	24 (endarteritis)
	10		12 (antipyresis)
	25-35		8
	25	PO	12 (autoimmune diseases)
	25-35	PO	24 (preoperative ocular surgery)
	40		18 (antiinflammatory)
	3		6 (antithrombotic)
Cats			
	10	PO	48
	10		24 (antithrombotic)
	15		24 (antiinflammatory)
	10		12 (antipyresis and analgesia)
	25-42		24 (antiinflammatory)
	25-35		8 (antiinflammatory)
	75		48 (antithrombotic)

Continued

Table 29-2 Dosages of Nonsteroidal Antiinflammatory Drugs in Cats and Dogs—cont'd

Drugs	Dose (mg/kg)	Route	Interval (hr)
Carprofen			
Dogs	4.4	SC or PO	24
	2.2	SC or PO	12
	4.4	SC or PO	One dose (2 hours before surgery)
Cats	4.4	SC, PO	One dose
	2.2	PO	24
Deracoxib			
Dog	1-2	PO	24 (osteoarthritis)
	3-4	PO	24 (postoperative analgesia)
Dipyrone			
Dogs	25	IM, SC	8-12
Cats	10-25	IM, SC	24
Etodolac			
Dogs	10-15	PO	24
Firocoxib			
Dogs	5	PO	24
Flunixin meglumine			
Dogs	0.5-1	IV, IM	24 × 1-3 (analgesic)
	0.25	IV	24 × 5 (uveitis)
Hyaluronic acid			
Dogs	20	IV	As needed
Ketoprofen			
Dogs	0.5-2.2	PO	12
Cats	2.2 initial dose followed by 1 every other day		
Ketorolac			
Dogs	0.3-0.5	IV, IM	8-12 × 2
Cats	0.25	IM	8-12
Meclofenamic acid			
Dogs	1.1-2.2	PO	24
Dogs	1-2	PO	24-72
Meloxicam			
Dogs	0.2	PO	Once day 1
	0.1	PO	24
Cats	0.03 or 0.1 mg/cat	PO	24*
	0.3	SC	Perioperative
Pentosan polysulfate			
Dogs	3	IM	7 days
Phenylbutazone			
Dogs	10	PO	8-12
	10-15	IV	12 (not to exceed four doses)
	22	PO	8 (not to exceed 800 mg)
Piroxicam			
Dogs	0.3		48
Tepoxalin			
Dogs	10 to 20	PO	Day 1
	10	PO	24
Cats	3	PO	24
Vedaprofen			
Dogs	0.5 mg/kg	PO	24

PO, By mouth; *IM*, intramuscular; *SC*, subcutaneous; *IV*, intravenous.
Note: Dogs weighing less than 5 kg cannot be accurately dosed.
*The FDA has indicated that meloxicam treatment should not extend beyond a single injectable

and efficacy of each. Thus, a COX-1 to COX-2 ratio greater than 1 (or a COX-2 to COX-1 ratio of less than 1) indicates greater potency for COX-2 which is desirable in that formation of inflammatory PGS should be inhibited preferentially to the housekeeping PGs.[12,13,15,16] Inhibition of platelet activity is commonly used to measure in vitro COX-1 inhibition whereas inhibition of PGs released from macrophages stimulated with endotoxin is used to measure COX-2. A number of drugs associated with *in vitro* COX-2 selectivity in humans, including rofecoxib (Vioxx) and celecoxib (Celebrex); others include etodolac, meloxicam, and nimesulide; the newest drugs are valdecoxib, etoricoxib, and (soon to be approved) lumiracoxib.[9] Drugs approved for use in animals include carprofen (the first) followed by etogesic; deracoxib; meloxicam; and, most recently, firocoxib.

Although the gene for COX-1 is about 3 times as large as that for COX-2, the two COX proteins, which are membrane bound, share about 60% homology.[9] Differences in NSAID selectivity for these two enzymes reflects smaller amino acids at two positions in COX-2 compared with larger amino acids at the same site in COX-1. The result is a larger and more flexible "pocket" into which the newer drugs insert and inhibit the COX-2 isoform.[9] For example, "coxib" drugs contain a sulfonamide group that interacts through hydrogen bonding to arginine of COX-2 but not histidine in the same position in COX-1.[28] Despite the usefulness of the COX-1:COX-2 ratio in screening drugs for safety or efficacy, its applicability to clinical use is questionable. Further, comparing results among studies is difficult. For example, whereas some studies focus on the $IC_{50,}$ others determine the IC_{80}, the latter probably being more clinically relevant. Assay methods contribute to variability in ratios among investigators for the same drug in the same species (Table 29-3). In vitro assasys based on cell culture or recombinant enzymes are easier to perform, but it is the ex vivo whole blood assays (as opposed to in vitro cell culture assays) that generally are recognized as the most representative of the clinical patient.[1] However, even whole blood assays do not take into account different distribution patterns to different tissues.[18,22] Extrapolation among species should be avoided.[29] For example, wherease the COX-1 to COX-2 ratio of etodolac is much better than that for carprofen in humans,[20,30] the opposite is true in dogs. Indeed, Wilson and coworkers[31] have demonstrated that, wherease critical residues in the active sites of canine COXs are identical with human homologs, amino acids differ (up to 54) at in active sites and may contribute to differences in activity that preclude extrapolation among species (see Table 29-3). Further complicating extrapolation among and within species is the fact that NSAIDs generally exist and are largely marketed as enantiomers (see Chapter 1), each with a possible different ratios. For example, Ricketts and coworkers[32] found the COX-1:COX-2 ratio of carprofen to be 129 for the racemic mixture but 181 for the S isomer and only 4.19 for the R isomer. Little information is available regarding COX selectivity in cats.[33,34] Much of the information that is available is based on manufacturer-sponsored studies and as such might potentially reflect reporting bias. For example, in Table 29-3, drugs that generally performed best in each study tended to be the drug manufactured by the sponsor of the study. As such, COX ratios might be considered a screening procedure[1,2]

KEY POINT 29-4 The markedly diverse role of multiple prostaglandins in normal physiology and the balance among prostaglandins that maintain homeostasis mandate extra caution when using nonsteroidal antiinflammatory drugs in unhealthy animals.

KEY POINT 29-5 Cyclooxygenase-1 to cyclooxygenase-2 ratios that assess potency of a nonsteroidal antiinflammatory are to be species specific and may not reflect clinical efficacy.

Other Mechanisms of Action

Inhibition of eicosanoid formation is not the sole antiinflammatory mechanism of action of NSAIDs. The NSAIDs also appear to alter cellular and humoral immune responses and suppress inflammatory mediators other than PGs.[7] As a group, all NSAIDs are planar and anionic, thus able to partition into lipid environments, including neutrophil cell membranes. As a result, cell membrane viscosity is altered, even at low concentrations.[10] At higher concentrations, NSAIDs appear to uncouple protein–protein interactions within the plasma membrane and thus interfere with a variety of cell membrane processes. Examples include oxidative phosphorylation and cellular adhesion.[10] Response of inflammatory cells to extracellular signals is impaired by affecting signal transduction proteins (G proteins).[10] Neutrophil adherence and activation is inhibited, as is subsequent release of inflammatory cellular enzymes, including collagenase, elastase, hyaluronidase, and others.[7] The extent of these effects varies with the drug. Whereas piroxicam inhibits superoxide ions and lysosomal enzymes release, ibuprofen does neither.[10] All NSAIDs appear to inhibit neutrophil adhesion. Some NSAIDS directly block PG receptors. Inhibition of nuclear transcription factor NF- B, is responsible for expression of many genes linked to inflammation. Modulation of peroxisome proliferator-activated receptors (PPARs), heat shock proteins (HSPs) and mitogen-activated protein kinases (MAPK cascades), and impaired induction of nitric oxide synthase (iNOS) are among the COX-independent effects of the class of NSAIDs.[2,28,35] Selected drugs (e.g., celecoxib but not rofecoxib) directly inhibit signaling needed to promote angiogensis, invasiveness, and proliferation of neoplasias.[28] Interestingly, sulfone coxibs (see Figure 29-4) are pro-oxidant, whereas sulfonamide coxibs are not.[28] Connective tissue metabolism may also be affected.[7]

NSAIDs are immunomodulators by virtue of their effect on several PGs and LTs as immunomodulators.[8] Nonsteroidal antiinflammatory cells indirectly influence lymphocyte activity through altered PG formation.[7] Selected NSAIDs appear to enhance cellular immunity by inhibiting PGE_2, a mediator that dampens the immune response.[7] This effect appears to be more important in the immunosuppressed animal.

Table 29-3 COX-1 to COX-2 Ratios for Selected Nonsteroidal Antiinflammatory Drugs in the Dog by Different Investigators

Author	Ricketts[32]	Warner[20] (3)	Brideau[33]	Kay-Mugford[219]	Lees[2]	Toutain[242]	Streppa[29]	Gierse[206]	McCann[213]	Wilson (4) [31]	Giraudel[34]
Year	1998	1999	2001	2000	2000	2001	2002	2002	2004	2004	2004
Method (1)	CC	WB	WB	CC		WB	WB	Cloned	WB	WB	WB
Drug	Ratio (2)										
Aspirin		0.25					0.39			0.37	
Carprofen (6)	129 (S:181; R:4.2)	<0.25	6.5 (D) 5.5 (C)	1.7	S:25; R:2.4		17/101 (7)	65	7/6 (7)	5.56	(C)3/21(5)
Celocoxib		10	9								
Deracoxib								1275	12		
Etodolac (6)	0.52	25					0.5	3.4		6.25	
Firocoxib									384		
Flunixin	0.64										
Ibuprofen (6)		0.5					0.7				
Ketoprofen (6)	0.23	0.15	0.6	0.36			0.17			0.57	
Meclofenamic acid	15	3.98					5			4.76	(C)26/65(5)
Meloxicam	2.9	12.5	10	12.3							
Naproxen		0.4									
Nimesulide		5.62				12.9+3.4				8.30	
Phenylbutazone	2.6		0.6				9	<1			
Piroxicam		1.99					2			1.89	
Rofecoxib		100									
Tolfenamic acid	15									14.29	

(1) WB= whole blood, cc = cell culture, D= dog, C=cat; S= S isomer; R = R isomer
(2) IC_{50} for all unless otherwise indicated
(3) *Humans*
(4) Inverse ratios reported in publication
(5) For S isomer only, IC_{50} and IC_{80}, respectively.
(6) Chiral compounds; data for racemic unless otherwise noted
(7) IC_{50} and IC_{80}, respectively

Pharmacokinetics

Shared Pharmacokinetic Properties

Each drug will be discussed in depth; however, the NSAIDs share a number of pharmacokinetic properties as a class. Package insert data for dog and cat contains selected information for some drugs, although the information often is not comprehensive, with content tending to vary, in part based on the requirements implemented by the FDA at the time of drug approval. The United States Pharmacopeia has provided a series of monographs providing pharmacokinetic information regarding the use of NSAIDS in species; information will be addressed for individual drugs. As weak acids, the NSAIDs tend to be well absorbed after oral administration. Bioavailability can vary between animals but has not been established for many drugs because of the lack of intravenous preparations.[36] Solutions of selected injectable preparations tend to be alkaline and can cause necrosis or pain if perivascular leakage occurs Food can impair the oral absorption of some NSAIDs or contribute to drug interactions.[37,38] The drugs are lipid soluble. Whereas the volume of distribution tends to be small (approximating 10%) when based on total drug as a result of ≥ 90% binding to serum albumin[39] the volume of distribution of unbound drug is consistent with distribution to extracellular fluid (Table 29-4). Only a small portion of pharmacologically active drug reaches peripheral tissues. Displacement from albumin (e.g., due to competition with other substrates for binding sites or from decreased serum albumin concentrations) may result in higher than expected concentrations of pharmacologically active drug and thus predispose the patient to drug-induced adverse effects. Although this increase is likely to be transient as the elimination of of unbound drug increases,[36,40] adversities might yet emerge particularly in patients at risk (e.g, decreased hepatic or renal function). Clearance of unbound drug is likely to be reduced in geriatric patients. The volume of distribution of unbound drug in pediatric animals is twice that in adults, which will contribute potentially to longer half-life.[36] For this and other reasons, (see metabolism), NSAIDs should not be used in the pediatric patient.

Most NSAIDs are eliminated primarily by both phase I and II hepatic drug-metabolizing enzymes. Clearance differs in both rate and extent among drugs and species. Differences in clearance are largely responsible for differences in drug half-life among animals.[36] Failing to anticipate these differences may contribute to adverse reactions. Conjugated parent drug or metabolites are eliminated through the bile or urine, depending on the drug. Stereoselective metabolism plays a profound role in species, gender and age differences. Saturation of drug metabolizing enzymes may occur at doses higher than recommended clinically for some drugs as has been demonstrated for phenylbutazone and derocoxib (package insert). Genetic polymorphism has been described in dogs for at least one NSAID (celecoxib)[41] and is likely to occur for others. Several drugs, or their enantiomers, undergo extensive enterohepatic circulation, again with differences among species (e.g., naproxen, meclofenamic acid, and the S enantiomer of carprofen in dogs), increasing the risk of gastrointestinal toxicity.[42] Renal active tubular secretion occurs for some parent drugs. Naproxen, carprofen, ketoprofen, and celecoxib are among the drugs which exemplify pharmacodynamics and pharmacokinetics differences in safety and efficacy among species.[36] Whereas allometric scaling generally can accurately predict systemic clearance and volume of distribution (based on body weight) of NSAIDs, allometric scaling generally cannot predict differences in pharmacodynamic indices (e.g., inhibition of TXB2 and PGE_2 synthesis).[43]

KEY POINT 29-6 Predicting nonsteroidal antiinflammatory drugs half-life is complicated by enantiomers and differences in rates of metabolism among animals.

Integration of Pharmacokinetics and Pharmacodynamics

Pharmacologic Effects

The pharmacologic effects of this class of drugs include analgesia, antipyresis, and control of inflammation. Antithrombosis also occurs, but this effect is variable, being the greatest for aspirin and the least to absent for newer COX-2 selective drugs. The effects are dose and drug dependent and include antithrombosis (when present), which occurs at the lowest concentrations (relatively lower for aspirin compared to all others); followed by antipyresis, analgesia and antiinflammation, with the latter occurring at the highest concentrations, although an exception appears to occur again for aspirin.[10,43d] Studies that compared efficacy and safety traditional or newer NSAIDs are generally are based on *in vitro* or *ex vivo* methods, with clinical trials limited. Yet, differences should be anticipated even among the newer NSAIDs. The mechanisms by which NSAIDs inhibit (interact with) COX are responsible, in part, for the variable antiinflammatory effects that characterize these drugs. Although several NSAIDs are characterized by a short plasma elimination half-life, the clinical response may last for over 24 hours after a single dose or up to 72 hours after multiple doses. These differential durations reflect, in part, drug-receptor interactions,with irreversible binding to COX most likely contribute to a longer biologic response.[44] Lees and co-workers have reviewed the relationship of NSAID effect and dose, emphasizing the advantages of PK-PD modeling as a basis of dose design.[44a] Inhibition of COX-1 has been described as simple competitive inhibition, whereas that for COX-2 has been described as a slowly reversible, contributing to a longer biologic versus plasma half-life.[45] Aspirin binds reversibly to the COX activity site on PGH synthase and then irreversibly inactivates the enzyme by acetylating a serine residue.[10] Both thromboxane and prostacycline synthase are impacted. However, platelets cannot produce additional thromboxane synthase; as such, platelet activity depends on new platelet production in the absence of aspirin. In contrast, endothelial cells are able to synthesize more prostacyclin synthetase and are less susceptible to the inhibitory effects of low dose aspirin.[10] In contrast to irreversible binders of COX, ibuprofen binds reversibly with COX and thus competes with AA for binding. In laboratory

Table 29-4 Pharmacokinetic Data for Selected Antiinflammatory Drugs in Dogs and Cats

Drug	Species	Route	Dose mg/kg	C_{max} (1) μg/mL	T_{max} hr	Bioavailability (%)	Clearance (2) mL/min/kg	Vd (3) L/kg	$F_{unbound}$ (%)	Half-life (hr)	MRT
Aspirin	Cats[127]	PO	2.5							27-45	
	(n=5)	IV	20	118			0.088±0.13	0.17±0. 01		22±3	35±4.5
			44				0.065	0.21	40	37.6	
	Dog[127]	PO	35	96	2	100					
		IV	44				0.255	0.19	40	8.6	
		IV	17.5				0.68	0.29 (ss)		4.5	
Carprofen	Dog[127,182]	PO	2	16.9	1	> 99				4.95±1.32	
			4	35±2.7	1.25±0.25						
			7.5	57.3±9.7	0.1±0.5						
		SC	2	8	2.6			0.14±0.02 (ss)		7.1±2.3	
				8			0.28±0.05			8 to 12	
R (−)							0.28±0.07	0.12±0.02			
S (+)							0.47±0.16	0.19±0.05			
	Cat[128] (n=5)	IV	4	24±9.7			0.1±0.03	0.14±0.05 (ss)		20.1±16.6	23±16
R (−)	Cats[199]						0.13±0.03	0.24±0.05 (ar)		21.3±9.1	
S (+)							0.32±0.07	0.35±0.1 (ar)		14.6±5.8	
Celexocib[41]	Dog (EM)	PO	5	0.23±0.04	1.5	27.4±14.6					
	Dog (PM)	PO	5	0.40±0.1	7.5±5.3	42.2±4.9					
	Dog (EM)	IV	5					1.9±0.08		1.3±0.02	21.8±2.3
	Dog (PM)	IV	5					2.3±0.06		5.1±0.05	7.4±0.5
Deracoxib	Dog (PI)		2.35		2	> 90	5		<10	3 (5)	
			20				1.7			19	
	Cat[206]	PO	1	0.28±1.3	3.6±3.2					8	
Etodolac	Dog (PI)[127]					Complete			<5	14	
										9.7±0.98	
			12 to 17	22±6.4	1					7.6±2	
			12 to 17	16.9±8.4	1					12±5.5	
Firocoxib[212]		PO	8	6.1 μM		100		2.9	3	5.9	
		PO	5	0.5(0.9 to 1.3)	1 to 5	38	6.7	4.6	4	7.8	
Flunixin	Dog[141]	IV	1.1				1.1±0.2	0.18±0.08 (ss)		3.67±1.2	
	Cat[60] (n=4)	IV	2	12.5/0.11 (9)			1.39	0.75±0.3 (ss)		6.6±2.4	4.6±2
Ibuprofen[148]	Dog	PO			0.5-3	60-80	0.49	0.164		4.6±0.8	
Ketoprofen	Dog[127]					Complete				5	
	Cat					Complete				1.5	
Ketorolac	Dog[162] (n=6)	PO	0.34	1.6±0.3	0.85±0.75	100±47					
		IV	0.34	8.26±8.54			1.25±1.13	0.33±1 (ss)		6.43 (2.5-18)	
Meloxicam	Dog (PI)[127]	PO	0.2	0.46	7.5	about 100			3	23.7±7.1	

		SC	0.2	0.73	2.5					23.7±4.3	
		IV					0.17±0.02	0.32±0.07		24±6.3	
	Cat (PI)	SC	0.3	1.5±0.9						15.1±5	
Nimesulide	Dog(4) [242]	PO		10.1±2.7 (8)	6.1±1.6	47±12 (8)					12.8±3.7
		IM		6.5±1.5	10.9±2.1	69±22				14±5.3	29.1±8.3
		IV					15.3±4.2	0.18±0.01 (ss)		8.5±2.1	12.6±3.8
Naproxen	Dog[163]	PO	5	40-50		68-100	0.021	0.13	1	45-92 (IV)	
Phenylbutazone	Dog[164]	PO	15	49-75						7.3-18	
Piroxicam	Dog[177]					80		0.34		40-50	
	Cat (8) [178]	IV	0.3				5±0.1	0.48±081.		11	
	Cat (8)	PO	0.3	0.52±0.2	3.2±2.4	89±21				13	19±1.7
Robenacoxib	Dog[235]	IV	1	5.5±0.9 (1)			14±3.2	0.24±0.04 (ss)	2	0.63±0.2	0.3±0.04
		PO, fasted	1	0.95±0.52	0.5	84±20				0.81±0.3	
		PO, fed	1	0.83±0.4	0.25	62±10				1+0.7	
		SC	1	0.7±0.2	0.5	88±15	10.5±4.8			0.8±0.2	
	Cat	IV	2	1.7±0.4						1.1	
Rofecoxib	Dog[241]	PO	5		1.5	26					
		IV	5				3.6	1.0		2.6	
Tepoxalin	Dog [127]	PO	20	0.8±0.5	2.3±1.4				2	2.0±1.2	
metabolite				0.8±0.4	4.7±6.2				2	13.7±10.7	
	Cat[127]	PO	10	2.3±1.8	8.8±4.3					4.7±0.8	
				1.8±1.2	2.8±4.2					3.5±0.4	
Vedaprofen	Dog (4) [236]	PO	0.5	2.74±0.3	0.63±0.14	86±7			1	12.7±2.1	
R (−)				1.6±0.4	0.7±0.2	124±28					
S (+)				1.3±0.3	0.7±0.2	91±17					
		IV		4.6±0.7 (10)						16.8±0.2	
R (−)							1.6±0.83				
S (+)							2.1±0.58				

Vd, Volume of distribution; *F*, fraction unbound; *MRT*, mean residence time; *PO*, by mouth; *IV*, intravenous; *ss*, steady state; *SC*, subcutaneous; *EM*, efficient metabolizer; *PM*, poor metabolizer; *PI*, package insert;
(1) extrapolated to Y intercept for IV
(2) time units indicated
(3) Vd source indicated: ss= steady state; ar = area
(4) Beagles
(5) Saturation kinetics have been reported; see text
(6) Median
(7) C_{max} was 8.1+3 and F was 58+ 16% following 5 days of once-daily dosing
(8) Median
(9) C_{max} following extrapolation of distribution and elimination phase, respectively
(10) C at 5 minutes; all results for vedaprofen are mean + standard error of the mean
(11) As the hydrochloride salt, equivalent to 1.7 mg/kg of hydroxyzine base
(12) The active metabolite of hydroxyzine
(13) Predicted by author from plasma drug concentration versus time curve

animals and humans, a relative potency (not to be confused with efficacy) has been established for selected conventional NSAIDs and COX: meclofenamic acid >indomethacin >naproxen >phenylbutazone >aspirin.[44] However, differential potency for COX-1 versus COX-2 varies among the NSAIDs and their enantiomers. In addition to drug-receptor interaction, prolonged elimination of NSAIDs from inflammatory exudate compared with plasma may also result in differential effects among the drugs and species.[37,44]

Along with inhibition of PGs, disruption of cellular signaling is responsible for all three pharmacologic effects (antipyresis, analgesia, anti-inflammation) that characterize all NSAIDs.[10] The antipyretic effect of NSAIDs may or may not be of benefit. Indeed, in human medicine little scientific support exists for the use of antipyretics for relief of discomfort or reduction of morbidity and mortality associated with fever.[47] Fever may have a beneficial effect on the outcome of bacterial or viral infections and often inversely correlates with the severity of lesions or the time to resolution. Thus the antipyretic effects of NSAID may be of most benefit when increased metabolism induced by fever might prove detrimental, such as with septicemia.[47] Central analgesic effects have been suggested for some but not all NSAIDs because NSAIDs can provide analgesia at very low intrathecal doses.[15,16,46]

The impact of COX on disease has led to a number of new applications for NSAIDs. The antiendotoxic effect of selected NSAIDs has been known (see the discussion of flunixin), but newer mechanisms are being examined. For example, several NSAIDs (carprofen, flunixin meglumine, and phenylbutazone) may specifically inhibit activation of the proinflammatory transcription factor nuclear factor kappa B (NF-κB) and on lipopolysaccharide (LPS) induction of iNOS. Using a mouse macrophages line, carprofen and flunixin, but not phenylbutazone, inhibited iNOS, whereas carprofen and, to a lesser degree, flunixin, inhibited NF-kappaB activation.[35]

Because NSAIDs are commonly first-choice treatments for arthritis, a focus on the effects of NSAIDs on cartilage is warranted. NSAIDs have been shown to inhibit proteoglycan synthesis in vitro, and for the salicylates this is supported by in vivo studies.[48] This effect has been attributed to inhibition of uridine diphosphate glucose dehydrogenase, an enzyme important in proteoglycan synthesis.[48] Hyaluronic acid synthesis, also dependent on this enzyme, does not appear to be as affected. The clinical effects of NSAIDs on cartilage are controversial. Some NSAIDs may, in fact, favorably modify the metabolism of proteoglycans, collagen, and matrix and may decrease the release of proteases or toxic oxygen metabolites.[48] This may reflect, in part, control of inflammation. Thus, whereas several NSAIDs have documented adverse effects on normal cartilage, ranging from decreased proteoglycan synthesis (e.g., aspirin) to chondrocyte death (phenylbutazone), others (e.g., naproxen, piroxicam, ketoprofen, and possibly carprofen) are recognized for their chondroprotective effects. Dual inhibitors have been noted for their potential efficacy to slow the progression of arthritis.[48b]

KEY POINT 29-7 Newer nonsteroidal antiinflammatory drugs are less destructive to the cartilage at therapeutic concentrations than older nonsteroidal antiinflammatory drugs.

The use of NSAIDs in the control of acute pain is evolving. Preemptive use (just before and immediately after surgery) has been demonstrated in humans to be more effective than either placebo or control,[17] and similar findings have been reported in the clinical use of COX-1–sparing drugs in animals. Drugs that target COX-2 (NSAIDs) offer a morphine-sparing effect for control of postoperative pain.[17] Their use in multimodal analgesia is increasing.

NSAIDs are currently being investigated for their potential antitumor effects. Knapp and coworkers[50] found piroxicam to be clinically useful in reducing tumor size and increasing survival time in dogs with transitional cell tumors of the urinary bladder. The result does not appear to reflect direct cytotoxic effects.[49-51] NSAIDs may be beneficial when combined with other anticancer drugs.[52] The effects of drugs inhibiting COX-2 cancerogenesis may be dose dependent: At least for aspirin, the maximum anticancer effect occurs at a dose less than that associated with control of inflammation but similar to that associated with antiplatelet effects.[9] Mechanisms other than COX inhibition contribute to NSAID antitumor effects.[51a] In addition to the inhibition of cancer growth, the use of COX-1–sparing drugs may improve gastrointestinal tolerance of anticancer drugs.

Drug Interactions

The NSAIDs can be involved in a variety of drug interactions during any phase of drug disposition (see the discussion of individual drugs). Trepanier[53] has reviewed some of these interactions. Displacement of only a small percentage of bound drug from albumin can increased the concentration of pharmacologically active drug in tissues. Few, if any, adverse reactions resulting from drug displacement have been reported, in part because of the failure to recognize the combination as problematic. In addition, the increase in pharmacologically active drug is only transient: Clearance of the unbound drug by both the liver and kidneys will increase.[36,40] However, the impact of changes in protein binding in patients with altered liver function may be problematic; accordingly, attention to the possibility that protein-binding drug interactions may worsen risks associated with liver disease might be prudent. Several NSAIDs can induce or inhibit drug-metabolizing enzymes and thus the clearance and half-life of other drugs cleared by the liver.[36] Phenylbutazone can both increase and inhibit selected drug-metabolizing enzymes depending on the second drug, whereas salicylates increase metabolism.[36] Renal competition with other organic acids for active renal tubular secretion in the proximal tubule has been documented for aspirin and other drugs, although the clinical relevance of this is not clear.

KEY POINT 29-8 Among the less appreciated drug interactions involving nonsteroidal antiinflammatory drugs are pharmacodynamic interactions that impair normal physiologic responses.

KEY POINT 29-9 Nonsteroidal antiinflammatory drug–induced gastrointestinal adversities should be anticipated and clients counseled regarding their advent.

Drug interactions also occur at the level of pharmacodynamics and may increase the risk of adversities. Most notable is the combinations of NSAIDs or glucocorticoids, which increase the risk of gastrointestinal toxicity (discussed later). Also notable are those drugs that, like NSAIDs, alter renal blood flow, and potentially renal autoregulation, thus increasing the risk of nephrotoxicity (e.g., aminoglycosides, angiotensin-converting enzyme inhibitors, amphotericin B). NSAIDs, in turn, may blunt response to diuretics and hypertensive drugs. NSAIDs may also block endogenous responses to hypertensive drugs (e.g., alpha adrenergics such as phenylpropanolamine), thus increasing the risk of hypertension, although this is more likely a risk only in animals for which primary hypertension is a concern.[54] The impact of combining NSAIDs with other drugs that affect platelet function or coagulation proteins is complicated by the differences in mechanisms of action between nonselective and preferentially selective drugs. Nonselective drugs would be expected to potentiate platelet function defects or deficiencies, whereas preferentially selective drugs would not. Prudence dictates that NSAID use ideally be avoided in patients with metabolic, hematologic, cardiovascular, or other disorders that put the patient at risk. NSAIDs are more likely to cause CNS effects if combined with fluorinated quinolones with unsubstituted piperazinyl rings (ciprofloxacin) at position 7.[55] It is not clear if the interaction occurs at the level of CNS (at the level of the gamma-aminobutyric acid receptor) or as a result of altered clearance.[56]

Selective serotonin reuptake inhibitors increase the risk of upper gastrointestinal hemorrhage based on a meta-analysis of the human-medicine literature.[57] The risk is greater in elderly patients; those drugs most selective for reuptake are associated with a higher risk. Among the proposed mechanisms is depletion of platelet serotonin and loss of platelet aggregation.

Adverse Reactions

All NSAIDs induce undesirable and potentially life-threatening side effects. In general, side effects tend to be predicted by toxicity studies implemented during the approval process,[58] although the small number of animals tends to limit their prediction to only the most common side effects. The role of drug interactions in causing adverse events was previously described. Accidental poisoning has been described for several NSAIDs, with the most common among the conventional drugs being ibuprofen, acetaminophen, aspirin, and indomethacin;[59] decreased use of these drugs as newer NSAIDs are used decreases relevancy. The most common clinical signs of toxicosis were vomiting and diarrhea followed by CNS depression, and circulatory manifestations.[59] Most adverse reactions reflect the inhibitory effects of NSAIDs on PG activity. Acute intoxication by selected drugs can be fatal; the more common adverse drug events are discussed along with their prevention and treatment below.

The adverse event reporting site of the Food and Drug Administration (FDA) is publically acceptable and can be reviewed for adverse drug events associated with NSAIDs in animals.[59a] However, effective epidemiologic assessment is limited and cause and effect between drug and adverse drug event may not exist. Further, the FDA is not provided information regarding the number of units sold precludes standardizing incidence of adverse drug events among drugs. Among the greatest contributing limitations to the adverse event reporting site may be failure of veterinarians or clients to report adverse events.

Transitioning from one NSAID to another in an attempt to reduced toxicity (or improve efficacy) should be based on elimination half-life (plasma or biological, whichever is longer). For those that reversibly impair COX, 3 to 5 elimination half-lives of the current NSAID should elapse prior to initiating the second (see Table 29-4). Prudence dictates that prophylactic measures be implemented during transition for at-risk patients.

Toxicity as a result of overdosing should be treated as with other overdoses (i.e., removal of ingested drug, supportive therapy). Treatment generally should continue for at least 3 to 5 half-lives of the ingested NSAID; longer may be necessary, particularly if the intoxicating amount is sufficient to saturate drug metabolizing enzymes. The risk of saturation kinetics is greater in age extremes, for selected drugs (e.g., phenylbutazone, deracoxib), and in the presences of liver disease. For NSAIDs characterized by enterohepatic circulation, administration of cholestyramine should be considered. The drug binds to at least several NSAIDs, thus preventing enterohepatic circulation, decreasing half-life as well as gastrointestinal exposure.[60] Treatment of other specific disorders is addressed with the adverse drug events.

Gastrointestinal

Mechanism of Gastrointestinal Adverse Events

Gastrointestinal damage is the most common and serious side effect of the NSAIDs. Dogs are described as being "exquisitively sensitive" (see package insert for meclofenamic acid, Fort Dodge) to NSAID-induced gastrointestinal ulceration. The incidence of gastrointestinal side effects associated with NSAID use in dogs (or cats) is not known. However, essentially every NSAIDs (conventional and new) used in the dog has been cited literature, at the FDA adverse event reporting site, in manufacturing package inserts, or other sources as causing gastrointestinal adverse drug events.[61-66] Gastrointestinal ulceration should be anticipated in dogs receiving these drugs, and clients should be counseled regarding the side effects and potential treatments for ulcerative injury. The incidence of side effects associated with new NSAIDs approved for use in animals has led the inclusion of client information sheets (as part of package inserts) to be distributed to clients when NSAIDs are dispense to animals for at home therapy.

The mechanism of gastrointestinal damage is not completely understood. A review of the FDA-CVM adverse event website reveals gastrointestinal adversities to be the most common for most, if not all, NSAIDs for which adversities are reported. In the cat, gastrointestinal adversities are the first, or more commonly second, adverse event reported for most NSAIDs. It is likely that several mechanisms act in concert to cause adversities; the mechanisms and risks as they are perceived in human medicine have been reviewed.[67-69] Several mechanisms offer a target for prevention and treatment. Gastroduodenal erosion and ulceration reflect, in part, inhibition of COX-1–stimulated PGE_2-mediated bicarbonate and mucous secretion, epithelialization, and increased blood flow.[70-71] Breakdown of small blood vessels resulting from a deficiency of mucus may be the initiating lesion.[72] Enhanced LT synthesis from AA shunted from the COX pathway to the lipoxygenase pathway exacerbates damage: due to vasoconstriction-induced mucosal damage as well as platelet aggregation and neutrophil activation. Dual inhibitors which target LTs as well as PGs may be less ulcerogenic. Direct irritation contributes to gastrointestinal mucosal damage for acidic drugs: [70] ion trapping in the mucosa precipitates hydrogen ion diffusion from the lumen of the stomach to the mucosa.[70,73] The lack of a sensitive indicator of gastrointestinal damage complicates assessment of gastrointestinal adverse drug events caused by NSAIDs. Boston and coworkers[74] as others could not find a relationship appears between the presence of gastric lesions and positive fecal occult blood. A method based on sucrose absorption in the gastrointestinal tract may be successful for detecting NSAID-induced gastrointestinal damage.[75] Some investigators have gone so far to suggest that endoscopic presence of erosive lesions is not necessarily indicative of ulcerogenic effects of NSAIDs.[76] The lack of well-designed clinical trials assessing detection, risk, prevention or treatment is problematic. Some studies continue to inappropriately ascribe the lack of statistical differences among treatment groups as evidence of no treatment (diagnostic) effect. Yet, failure to detect a significant difference (type II statistical error) often reflects the small sample size characterizing these clinical trial and caution is recommended to not overinterpret "lack of significant difference" as "sample populations are similar".

Prevention and Treatment of Gastrointestinal Adverse Events

Prevention of gastrointestinal toxicity is based on identifying those patients at greatest risk; avoiding NSAIDs drugs, if possible, in these patients; and if this is not possible, selecting the safest drug (i.e., COX-1–sparing drugs) and using it in a dosing regimen that results in the lowest exposure necessary for efficacy. Prevention also includes co-treatment with prophylactic drugs, including those that prevent gastric acid secretion or those that replace PGs.[73] The use of other therapies that might decrease the need for NSAIDs (e.g., combination analgesic therapy, cartilage-supportive disease-modifying agents) also is indicated.

KEY POINT 29-10 Patients at risk for nonsteroidal antiinflammatory drug–induced gastrointestinal adversities should be identified before implementation of therapy, and preventive measures should be taken, if warranted.

Risk factors for NSAID-induced gastrointestinal adverse events. Several risk factors for NSAID-induced gastrointestinal adverse events identified in humans are applicable to animals. No chemical characteristic predicts the likelihood of gastrointestinal toxicity by a particular conventional NSAID.[70,72] Drugs that undergo enterohepatic circulation (e.g., naproxen, carprofen, etodolac) may be associated with a greater incidence of gastrointestinal upset. Other risk factors include advanced age (altered disposition coupled with decreased ability to protect damaged mucosa),[77] concurrent use of glucocorticoids (increasing the risk 4.4-fold in humans) or other NSAIDs (the exception might be low-dose aspirin, as discussed later), or anticoagulants. Comorbidity (renal, cardiovascular, or liver disase) is also a risk factor.[73]

The combination of steroids and NSAIDs causes worse lesions than either drug alone, as has been demonstrated for flunixin meglumine or dexamethasone.[74,78,79] Further, the FDA adverse drug events site indicates that the risk of gastrointestinal toxicity is greater when drugs are given with glucocorticoids. In a restrospective study of gastrointestinal perforation associated with deracoxib, a risk factor was combination with glucocorticoids (or other NSAIDs) within the past 24 hours.[80] Other NSAIDs appear to shift use of AA from the COX pathway to the production of cysteinyl LTs and LTB4, eicosonoids that promote leukocyte migration, break down the mucosal barrier, and stimulate gastric acid secretion. Inhibition of COX-2 may preclude angiogenesis critical to the healing ulcer.[81] Persons with previous history of gastric ulcer disease also are predisposed to NSAID-induced gastrointestinal adverse drug events. Although peptic ulcer disease is unusual in animals, prudence dictates that evidence of any gastrointestinal disease associated with mucosal damage (e.g., inflammatory bowel disease) that might require COX-2–mediated healing be considered a potential risk factor.

Dose-dependent toxicity has been demonstrated during the approval process essentially for all NSAIDs as is indicated by product package inserts (Table 29-5). The single most common cause of NSAID-induced toxicity found by a review of NSAID-induced adverse drug event reports by the FDA is overdosing, in particular failure to adhere to the recommended dosing regimen. Overdosing was associated with an increased risk of NSAID-induced gastrointestinal perforation in dogs.[80] Drugs for which low-concentration preparations are not available increases the risk of toxicity because of inaccurate dosing. Use of compounded preparations (for which oral bioavailability is not known) should be implemented with extreme cautions; increasing bioavailability will result in a proportional increase in drug concentrations. The risk for overdosage is greater for selected drugs for which higher doses may result in zero-order elimination (e.g., deracoxib, phenylbutazone). For such drugs half-life is no longer germane, and the risk of drug accumulation dramatically increases.

The relationship between dose and risk of toxicity remains complex, even for NSAIDs, as is exemplified by aspirin. At low doses (concentrations), aspirin blocks COX activity and thus shunts AA into the lipoxygenase pathway. Although gastrotoxic LTs are produced (cysteinyl LTs and LTB4), aspirin also simultaneously triggers lipoxin (aspirin-triggered lipoxin [ATL]) formed by lipoxygenase-15. Lipoxin is antiinflammatory and thus inhibits the gastrotoxic leukocyte recruitment and activation caused by cysteinyl LTs, as well as mediates the antiadhesive platelet effects of aspirin. As such, low-dose aspirin tends to be both cardioprotective as well as safe to the gastrointestinal tract. However, at higher doses production of LTs is sufficient that the protective effects of lipoxin are masked and gastrotoxicity emerges. Interestingly, COX-1–sparing (COX-2

Table 29-5 Safety Data for Selected NSAIDs in Dogs and Cat Based on Target Safety Studies and Clinical Trial Field Studies

	TARGET SAFETY STUDIES						FIELD TRIAL STUDIES				
	Magnitude of Dose increase	Duration (weeks)	N	Gastrointestinal Lesions	Renal Lesions	Source	Dosing Regimen†	Clinical sign	Emesis	Diarrhea	Anorexia
Drug								N	%	%	%
Carprofen	3	6	NR	Hematachezia (1/6)	NR	PI	4.4/24/NR		ND	ND	ND
	5	6	NR	NSF	NR	PI	2.2/12/14	297	ND	ND	ND
	5.7	13		NSF	NR	PI	4.4/24/14	252	ND	ND	ND
	5.7	52	6	NSF	NR	PI	4.4/preop then	331	ND	ND	ND
	5.7	52	6	NSF	NR	PI	4.4/24/2 or 3		ND	ND	ND
	10	2		Blood in stool (1/8)	NR	PI					
	20*	6	8	Blood in stool (1/8)	NR						
Deracoxib	1-4-4	3	NR	NSF	NSL	PI	1-2/24/43	194	ND	ND	ND
	1.5-6	3	NR	NSF	NSL	PI	3-4/24/6	207	10	ND	ND
	2-8	3	NR	NSF	NSL	PI					
	1-8	26	NR	NSL	Increased BUN; focal renal papillary necrosis	PI					
	*1-5	2	NR	Jejunal erosions or ulcers	Increased BUN; focal renal papillary necrosis	PI					
Etodolac	1.5	26	NR	GI erosions		PI	10/24/8	116	4.3		
	2.7	NR	NR	Vomiting, GI ulceration		PI					
	5.3	12	8	Death (6/8 dogs; one at 3 weeks, others at 3 to 9 months)	Renal tubular necrosis (1/8) at 52 wk	PI					
Firocoxib*	3	26	8	Vomiting, diarrhea (1/8)		PI	5/24/30	128	ND	ND	ND
	5	26	8	Vomiting, diarrhea; ulcer (1/8)		PI					
	3	26	6	One dog euthanized (poor clinical condition)		PI					
	5	26	12	One dog died (82 days), three euthanized because of anorexia, vomiting, moribund status*		PI					
	10	22	4	Vomiting, diarrhea, intestinal erosion or ulceration (3/4)		PI					

Continued

Table 29-5 Safety Data for Selected NSAIDs in Dogs and Cat Based on Target Safety Studies and Clinical Trial Field Studies—cont'd

	TARGET SAFETY STUDIES						FIELD TRIAL STUDIES				
	Magnitude of Dose increase	Duration (weeks)	N	Gastrointestinal Lesions	Renal Lesions	Source	Dosing Regimen†	Clinical sign	Emesis	Diarrhea	Anorexia
Drug								N	%	%	%
Meloxicam	3	6	6	Gastric mucosal petechiae (2/6)	Renal enlargement (2/6)	PI	0.2 followed by 0.1/24/13	147	25	12	3
	5	6	6	Gastric mucosal petechiae (1/6)	Renal enlargement (2/6) and papillary necrosis (3/6)	PI					
	3	26		Gastrointestinal distress (vomiting, diarrhea) 6/6	NR	PI					
	5	26		Gastrointestinal distress (vomiting, diarrhea) 6/6	NR; increased BUN	PI					
	3 (IV)	3 days		Superficial hemorrage, erosions, other	Histologic lesions	USP[127]					
	5 (IV)	3 days		Superficial hemorrage, erosions, other	Histologic lesions	USP[127]					
	10 (IV)	3 days		See above	Renal compromise	USP[127]					
Tepoxalin	2	26	14	Gastric irritation (2/14)	PI	Technical mono-graph	20 then 10/24/6	101	ND	ND	ND
	10	26	14	Gastric ulceration (2/8)	PI	Technical mono-graph	20 then 10/24/28	107‡	20	21	1
	30	26	14	Gastric ulcer (3/14)	PI	USP[127]					
	2	52	8		PI	USP[127]					
	10	52	8	Vomiting, gastric irritation (2/8)	PI	USP[127]					
	30	52	8			USP[127]					

N, animal number; *PI*, package insert; *ND*, no difference from placebo; NR: not reported; *NSF*, no significant findings; *NSL*; no significant lesions; *BUN*, blood urea nitrogen; *GI*, gastrointestinal; *IV*, intravenous; *USP*, United States Pharmacopeia.
*See text for explanation: micronized preparation (not approved version) studied for deraxocib; dosing occurred in juvenile dog for firocoxib.
†Dose regimen listed as mg/kg/frequency (hr)/number of days.
‡No placebo reported.

preferential drugs) inhibit the formation of lipoxin, contributing to the toxicity of the newer drugs when combined with low-dose aspirin.[81] Theoretically, whereas COX-inhibiting drugs should not be combined with low-dose aspirin, dual-acting NSAIDs, which do not target lipoxygenase-15 (see the discussion of dual-acting NSAIDs), should not inhibit lipoxin and thus should maintain the low-dose aspirin gastroprotective and cardioprotective effects.[81]

In general, conventional NSAIDs are associated with a greater risk of gastrointestinal adverse drug events in humans, but exceptions may occur. For example, in humans (but not dogs) ibuprofen, which is essentially equivalent in its COX-1 versus -2 selectivity, is ranked as low risk, along with the COX-1–sparing drugs celecoxib, rofecoxib, meloxicam, and etodolac.[73] Comparison in dogs of gastrointestinal safety among newer NSAIDs, including both COX-1–sparing drugs and dual-acting NSAIDs, might be based on toxicity data generated during the approval process and available on package inserts. This latter source includes both targeted safety studies (the dose is multiplied by 3, 5, or 10) and field studies (clinical trials at recommended doses under conditions of anticipated use) (see Table 29-5).

Comparison of clinical safety among NSAIDs ideally should reflect nonmanufacturer-sponsored, well-designed clinical trials involving a sufficient number of animals such that the power is sufficient to detect a significant difference. Placebo controls are imperative; positive responses have been reported in 40% or more of placebo-treated animals.[82] However, such studies in veterinary medicine are few and far between. Data that do exist thus far support the safety of the newer drugs compared with conventional NSAIDs. For example, using a placebo-controlled, parallel, randomly assigned design in dogs (n = 6/group), Reimer and coworkers[83] found that buffered aspirin caused endoscopic gastric lesions within 5 days of starting therapy compared with no or minimal lesions in animals treated with carprofen or etodolac (sample size may have limited the ability to discern a difference between the two groups); all drugs were administered at mid-recommended doses. Endoscopic lesions followed the same relative pattern among drugs throughout the 28-day study period, indicating that aspirin is more commonly associated with lesions in the canine gastrointestinal tract compared with the COX-1–sparing drugs. A separate study found no differences in gastrointestinal lesions in animals receiving ketoprofen (nonselective), carprofen, meloxicam, or placebo. However, the power of this latter study to detect a significant difference was not reported.

Pharmacologic prevention and treatment. Future pharmaceutical manipulations designed to deliver NSAIDs by alternative routes may decrease risk of gastrointestinal adverse drug effects, although their application to veterinary patients should not necessarily be assumed. For example, formation of nitroso derivatives of conventional NSAIDs may improve the safety margin of these drugs as a result of in vivo release of NO that provides gastroprotection while improving antiinflammatory and analgesic potency.[2] However, NO also has been associated with the pathogenesis of osteoarthritis, thus exemplifying the continuously complicated nature of designing safe NSAIDs (see later discussion).[22] In contrast to current drugs that only slowly dissociate with COX-1, newer NSAIDs appear to be weak and rapidly reversible binders of COX-1, thus enhancing safety.[17,45]

Topical (including transdermal) NSAID administration is appealing because it avoids direct contact between the drug and target tissue. Indeed, a meta-analysis of clinical trials comparing topical NSAIDs to placebos and oral NSAIDs in humans found this route to be effective, with no difference in response compared with oral. Topical administration was safe, although not necessarily safer than oral. Of the NSAIDs reviewed, ketoprofen was described as the best.[84] Thus far, topical NSAID administration has not proved to be a vital means of avoiding gastrointestinal adverse drug events in small animals, primarily because of failed drug delivery. Because the amount of drug delivered cannot be predicted, administration of NSAID in novel drug delivery systems offered by compounding pharmacists is not recommended unless the amount of drug delivered by that system has been scientifically demonstrated, as would occur for an approved drug. Enteric coatings, combination drugs (e.g., with gastroprotectants), and other approaches may be of some benefit for some drugs (e.g., aspirin) and, if currently available, are discussed with the individual drugs.

Both the prevention and treatment for gastrointestinal toxicity focus on, in order of priority, control of gastric acid secretion, replacement of the missing PGs, and (for treatment) protection of the damaged mucosa.[64,85] The two major categories included antisecretory drugs and the PG analog misoprostol; cytoprotectants, such as sucralfate, also play a role in treatment.

Among the antisecretory drugs, proton pump inhibitors (PPIs) generally have proved more effective than H_2 receptor blockers for prevention and treatment of NSAID-induced gastrointestinal adverse drug events. An exception has been demonstrated in humans for famotidine, but only when it is administered at higher than recommended doses (40 mg twice rather than once daily).[73] Boulay and coworkers[86] demonstrated that cimetidine did not protect the gastric mucosa from developing lesions in dogs receiving nonbuffered aspirin (35 mg/kg every 8 hours). PPIs appeared to be more effective, as well as better tolerated, compared with misoprostol. In one human study, close to 30% of persons reciving misoprostol could not tolerate the full dose.[76] Omeprazole generally is the PPI of choice, although lansoprazole may also be a reasonable choice. Although lansoprazole was not found to be superior to misoprostol for prevention of gastrointestinal adverse drug events in humans, improved compliance and better tolerance made it the preferred PPI drug in humans. However, the use of PPI will not prevent ulcers in all patients, as has been demonstrated in humans. Symptoms of GI side effects still occur in 20% of human patients receiving omeprazole.[73] Although routine use of PPI in nonrisk animals receiving NSAIDs is not indicated, strong consideration should be given to their use in at-risk animals. As a class, the PPIs are inhibitors of drug-metabolizing enzymes, and care should be taken to review drug interactions before their use. Among them, esomeprazole may be the least likely to impact metabolizing enzymes.[86a]

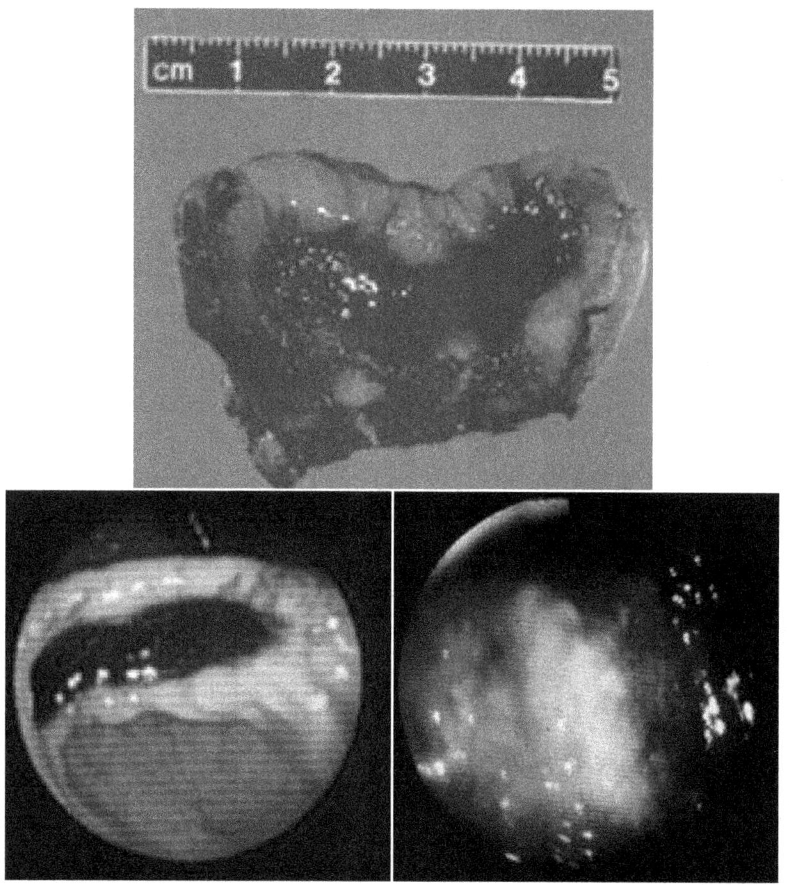

Figure 29-8 A gross (top) and endoscopic view of two gastric ulcers in dogs treated with aspirin and glucocorticoids. The bottom ulcer responded to treatment with misoprostol, sucralfate, and ranitidine.

However, PPI also have been shown to induce selected CYP45O enzymes (P45OIA1 and A2) but this impact appears to be most clinically relevant to (human) poor metabolizers that are deficient in enzymes.[86b]

KEY POINT 29-11 Among the antisecretory drugs, proton pump inhibitors generally have proved more effective than H_2 receptor blockers for prevention and treatment of nonsteroial antiinflammatory drug–induced gastrointestinal adversities.

Misoprostol is a synthetic PPGE analog that both prevents and helps heal gastrointestinal ulceration caused by NSAIDs.[87] The efficacy of misoprostol has been well established in human patients suffering from NSAID-induced ulceration,[71] and studies support similar benefits in dogs.[88,89] Combination NSAID–misoprostol products have been approved for use by human patients,[90] supporting its their combined use. Interestingly, misoprostol, when combined with an NSAID, also appears to enhance the antiinflammatory effect of the NSAID.[90] Indeed, misoprostol inhibits IL-1, TNF, and thromboxane release from macrophages, and it is the most potent inhibitor of histamine release from human mast cells.[90] Misoprostol has potentiated the antiinflammatory effect of a variety of compounds in animalsand appears to have analgesic effects, although at high concentrations, acting synergistically with other NSAIDs.[90] Finally, misoprostol may be more effective in the presence of agents that decrease gastric acid secretion.[64]

Gastroprotective drugs include sucralfate and potentially glucosamine–chondroitin products (Figure 29-8). The benefits of sucralfate in the treatment of NSAID-induced adverse drug events include binding to and thus protecting damaged mucosa, as well as increasing PG synthesis, angiogenesis, and sulfhydryl (oxygen radical scavenger) production at the site of damage. Despite the fact that sucralfate binds only to damaged mucosa, it nonetheless consistently performs better than placebo in the prevention of gastric or duodenal ulcers in human patients receiving NSAIDs. Sucralfate is minimally effective than antisecretory drugs in preventing stress ulcers (e.g., critical care patients).[90a] The combined use of NSAIDs and disease-modifying agents (glucosamine and chondroitin sulfates) for treatment of osteoarthritis is discussed later. An added advantage of their combined use is the potential gastroprotection that might be realized because of enhanced mucopolysaccharide production.[91] Interestingly, metronidazole has been ascribed a protective effect on the gastrointestinal tract when combined with NSAIDs, presumably through removal of the microbial impact on neutrophil chemoattractant.[92]

KEY POINT 29-12 Although sucralfate will not prevent gastrointestinal ulceration, it can protect and facilitate healing of damaged mucosa once it emerges.

The Canadian Agency for Drugs and Technologies in Health (CADTH) sponsored an in-depth analysis of the literature in an attempt to identify the most cost-effective gastroprotective strategies in persons receiving NSAIDs.[93] In their report, based on Monte-Carlo modeling, investigators considered patients receiving a nonselective NSAID (diclofenac) alone, a COX-2 preferentnial NSAID alone (celexocib); or either group of the NSAIDS with misoprostol, an H_2 receptor blocker (ranitidine), or a proton pump inhibitor (omeprazole). In their 2007 report, they found that no prophylaxis and treatment with a traditional NSAID; but no gastroprotection was least costly but least effective in avoiding adverse events. Of the combinations, PPI consistently was more effective than no prophylaxis; further, the most cost-effective strategy was the combination of nonselective NSAIDs with PPIs. Combination of nonselective NSAIDs with H_2 receptor antagonists also reduced the risk of gastrointestinal complications, but at a higher cost (25%). Use of Cox-2 selective drugs or combination with misoprotol were effective (but more costly) alternatives, although combination with misoprostol was associated with increased adversity because of its PG effects. The CADTH investigators further observed the need for a large, prospective, multicentered clinical outcome study that directly compares the efficacy of PPIs with H_2 receptor antagonists to prevent NSAID-associated gastrointestinal adversities.

The use of 5-lipoxygenase inhibitors for prevention of NSAIDs gastrointestinal toxicity might be considered. Lis facilitate ulcer formation by virtue of their effect on platelets and blood vessels; these effects and others also might be inhibited by LT receptor antagonists (see later discussion). Among the approaches in reducing gastrointestinal toxicity associated with NSAIDs is the development of NO-NSAIDs.[69] NO has been recognized as an important gastroprotectant. Its mechanism appears, in part, to reflect inhibition of neutrophil adherence to vascular endothelium, which is necessary for mucosal damage to occur. Whereas adverse reactions are likely to preclude use of drugs that promote NO release systemically, NSAIDs that facilitate local release of NO (COX-inhibiting NO donors; NO-NSAIDs) are currently being developed. The drugs contain a NO-releasing moiety; their continuing development has been reviewed.[69] For example, the addition of the moiety to naproxen has yielded naproxcinod. The gastric mucosa also is protected by the formation of hydrogen sulfide (H_2S) when produced in appropriate quantities. Accordingly, NSAIDs are being designed with a moiety that allows local, limited release of H_2S. In either case (NO- or H_2S-releasing moiety), the antiinflammatory potency of the drug may also be improved as gastric adversity is decreased.

Liver disease should be an anticipated sequela of long-term use of any drug extensively concentrated or metabolized by the liver, including NSAIDs (see Chapter 4).[94] All NSAIDs approved for use in dogs have been associated with increased liver enzymes; most have been reported scientifically or anecdotally to cause hepatitis. Although their occurrence is discussed with individual NSAIDs, hepatic function tests (e.g., serum bile acids, albumin, urea nitrogen) should be implemented throughout drug exposure in patients at risk (discussed previously). The use of hepatoprotectant drugs (e.g., *N*-acetylcysteine, *S*-adenosylmethionine [SAMe]) should be considered for both prevention and treatment.

Clinical signs indicative of gastrointestinal ulceration may be exacerbated by an increased risk of bleeding induced by NSAIDs. In addition to their antiplatelet effects, selected NSAIDs (e.g., phenylbutazone) have also been associated with bone marrow dyscrasias.[95-98] Gastrointestinal bleeding is probably the most common sign of bleeding dyscrasias, in part because of the ulcerogenic properties of these drugs. Epistaxis has also been reported. Because prostacyclin is mediated largely by COX-2, use of COX-2–selective drugs may increase the risk of thrombosis.[99]

Renal

Analgesic nephropathy is a relatively common adverse effect of NSAIDs in human beings.[100] In the kidney both COX-1 and COX-2 mediate renal effects of PGs. Vasodilatory and tubuloactive PGs are protective, ensuring that medullary vasodilation and urinary output continue during states of renal arterial vasoconstriction (see Figure 29-7). The loss of this protective effect becomes important in patients with compromised renal function.[100] NSAIDs inhibit the synthesis of renal PGs and may lead to deterioration of renal function in patients whose kidneys are physiologically stressed.[100,101] However, some side effects reflect mechanisms other than PG inhibition. Renal side effects include both acute and chronic renal disease, nephrotic syndrome, interstitial nephritis, hyperkalemia, and disturbances in water and sodium movement.

Two different forms of renal disease associated with NSAIDs are generally described: hemodynamically mediated ischemic nephropathy and acute interstitial nephritis.[102] Nephrotoxicity is more common in human patients than in veterinary patients, probably because therapy with NSAIDs is prolonged in the human patient and often occurs without physician supervision. NSAID therapy is also more common in geriatric patients, which is more likely to have reduced renal function as well decreased nephroprotective function. As such, animals that are likely to be predisposed to developing analgesic nephropathy are those that are geriatric, afflicted with conditions that impair renal blood flow (e.g., cardiac, renal, or cirrhotic liver disease), subjected to a hypotensive state (e.g., prolonged anesthesia without fluid support), and receiving nephroactive or nephrotoxic drugs in addition to the NSAID. Patients receiving more than one NSAID, aminoglycosides, amphotericin B, and possibly angiotensin-converting enzyme inhibitors are potential candidates for analgesic nephropathy.[103] Interstitial nephritis, a less common syndrome associated with NSAID use in human patients, apparently has not been reported in dogs or cats. The cause of this syndrome appears to be a cell-mediated allergic response. Loss of renal PGs may potentiate the disease as inflammation progresses unchecked.

In contrast to gastrointestinal adverse drug events, the risk of renal adverse drug events may not necessarily be reduced with use of newer COX-2-selective drugs compared with conventional NSAIDs. In human medicine clinical trials have demonstrated that the renal effects of COX-1–protective (COX-2–selective) drugs are similar to those of conventional

NSAIDs. A low-salt diet may increase the risk: Elderly human patients on a low-sodium diet receiving either single or multiple doses developed reductions in glomerular filtration rate, creatinine clearance, and sodium renal clearance.[104] Acute changes in renal function in humans generally occur within 24 hours, with return to normal by 48 hours.[105]

KEY POINT 29-13 The newer nonsteroial antiinflammatory drugs may offer no advantage to older nonsteroial antinflammatory drugs in preventing nephrotoxicity; cats in particulary may be predisposed to adverse renal effects.

A number of studies have focused on the impact of perioperative NSAID use on renal function in dogs. Lobetti and Joubert[106] studied the effects of ketoprofen (1 mg/kg) and carprofen (4 mg/kg) as well as ketorolac (0.5 mg/kg) and morphine (0.1 mg/kg; "control group") on renal function as assessed by serum urea and creatinine concentrations, urine γ-glutamyltransferase, fractional renal clearance of sodium, and urinalysis. Measurements were collected before and 24 and 48 hours after ovariohysterectomy in dogs (n=40; four per group, with no placebo control). Fluids were not administered during the surgical procedure, which ranged between 1 and 5 hours in duration. Although all dogs remained clinically normal, transient azotemia was detected in two dogs each (2/4) in the ketoprofen and ketorolac groups, and changes in fractional clearance were detected in all three NSAID groups. Urine specific gravity increased in carprofen-treated dogs, although the clinical relavence of this is not clear.

In their study of carprofen safety in cats, Steagall and coworkers[107] cite a report from the European Union that indicates 50% of the surveyed cases of acute renal failure in cats were associated with NSAID therapy. Gunew and coworkers[108] prospectively studied the effects of long-term (approximately 6 months) treatment of cats with osteoarthritis (n = 46) meloxicam at 0.01 to 0.03 mg/kg using a case-controlled design. Cats were approximately 13 ± 4 years for both groups. Unfortunately, indices of renal dysfunction were compared between groups only at 1 month; no differences were detected at that time. The author has summarized adverse events reported for carprofen and meloxicam in dogs versus cats at the FDA adverse event reporting site for reported after 2006 but before 2009. (Figure 29-9). Although direct numbers of adverse events cannot be compared (no information on units or doses sold for each drug), the proportion of each advent might be compared among drugs. The percent of adverse events related to the kidney suggest that the incidence is clinically relevant in both the dog and cat. However, the data also suggests that the incidence of renal adverse events is generally higher for the cat compared to the dog. Further, the data suggests that the risk of increased BUN and serum creatinine is greater for meloxicam (45 and 46%, respectively) compared to carprofen (24 and 22%, respectively). However, assessment of the more recent data suggests a broader implication. For more recent data, the number of animals for which each specific adverse event occurs has been removed from the site. As such, current comparisons must be limited to ranking of adversities. The rank of increased BUN or serum creatinine is

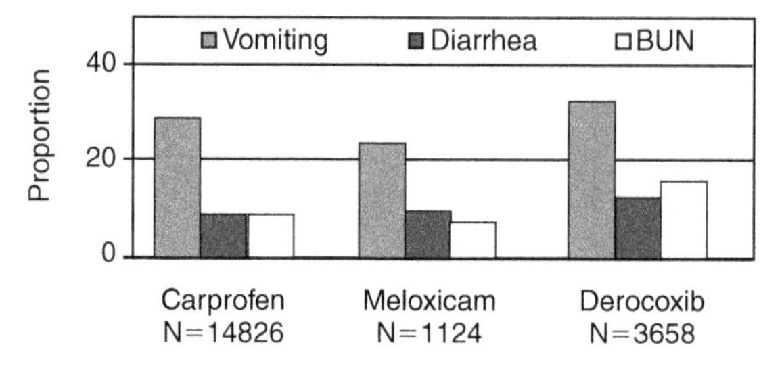

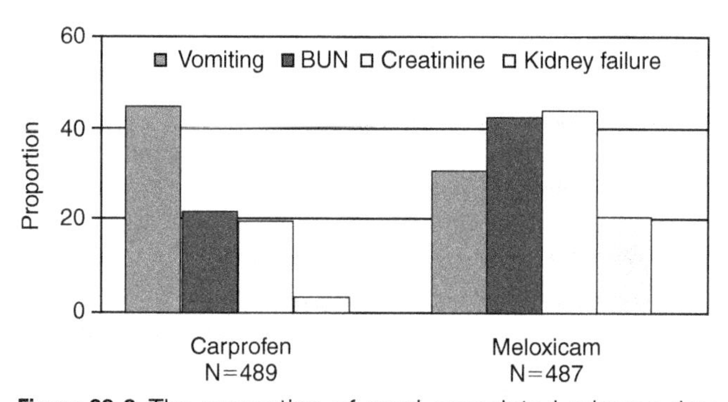

Figure 29-9 The proportion of renal-associated adverse drug events drug for nonsteroidal antiinflammatory drugs (NSAIDs) reported in either dogs or cats. The proportion comes from the total number of adverse events reported for that drug. The total number of adverse events should not be directly compared among drugs because the data cannot be adjusted for the number of units sold or animals treated. For example, a greater number of adverse events in dogs should be expected for carprofen compared with other NSAIDs because carprofen has been approved for a longer time. Further, veterinarians may be less inclined to report adverse events for newly approved NSAIDs if the event is one that is expected of the class. The cause-and-effect relationship for the adverse event and the NSAID was not confirmed but reflects cumulative adverse events reported to manufacturers or directly reported to the Food and Drug Administration (FDA) at the time the data were studied (2007–2008). The data were collected from the FDA's adverse event reporting site from 2006 to 2008 (data were no longer available at time of publication).

higher in cats for each NSAID (approved or not approved) compared to dogs. This includes both meloxicam and ketoprofen (Table 29-6). Accordingly, caution is recommended to not over estimate renal safety of these products in either dogs or cats; further, monitoring of renal function might be indicated in cats receiving NSAIDs long term, particularly if other risk factors for renal disease are present.

Studies have attempted to identify methods to prevent or treat NSAID-induced analgesic nephropathies. Despite some studies supporting its role,[109] misoprostol does not have a recognized role in the prevention or treatment of NSAID-induced nephrotoxicity. Its impact on other drug-induced nephropathies associated with vasoconstriction has been variable (e.g., cyclosporine[110, 111]). Misoprostol has been used clincally in human patients suffering from clinical conditions

Table 29-6 Post-Market Surveillance Data Ranking for Selected Renal-Related Adverse Events Reported for Orally Administered NSAIDs in Dogs and Cats*

	CARPROFEN (Po)		DEROCOXIB (Po)		MELOXICAM (Po)		FIROCOXIB (Po)		KETOPROFEN (Inj)	
Species	Dog (17,585)	Cat (542)	Dog (5006)	Cat (44)	Dog (2112)	Cat (1132)	Dog (2437)	Cat (13)	Dog (113)	Cat* (41)
Vomiting	1	1	1	1	1	5	1	1	1	NR
BUN	9	4	5	2	5	3	3	4	3	2
Creatinine	11	5	6	4	7	2	7	5	4	3

From the Food and Drug Administration Center for Veterinary Medicine Cumulative Adverse Event website: fda.gov/AnimalVeterinary/SafetyHealth/ProductSafetyInformation/ucm055394.htm), accessed January 2011. The rank for each adverse event (vomiting, increased BUN or serum creatinine) indicates the frequency of reports citing that adverse event for that drug in dogs or cats, where a ranking of 1=most frequent. Numbers in parentheses indicate the number of animals for which adverse events were reported. The absolute number of adverse events should not be directly compared among drugs because it is not correctable for the number of units sold.
NR, Not reported; *PO*, oral; *Inj*, injectable.

associated with peripheral or renal vasoconstriction; however, its effects may be dose related, with natriuresis, diuresis, and vasodilation occurring at low doses and vasoconstriction and impaired salt and water excretion occurring at high doses. Currently, preventive measures, including therapy with sodium-containing fluids, minimizing of drug interactions, and avoidance of use in patients at risk, appears to be the best method of avoiding the nephrotoxic effects of NSAIDS.

N-acetylcysteine has been studied experimentally for the prevention or treatment of NSAID-induced nephrotoxicity.[102,112] Proposed mechanisms include vasodilation, although other mechanisms may be relevant. However, although animal models have indicated potential efficacy, clinical trials, including meta-analyses, have thus far failed to provide conclusive evidence of efficacy.[113] Nonetheless, in the absence of effective therapies, *N*-acetylcysteine is generally recommended (approximately 10 mg/kg or more orally twice daily) preventively for drug-induced toxicity.

Cardiovascular

All conventional NSAIDs are able to impair platelet activity as a result of impaired PG (thromboxane) synthesis, a COX-1–selective action (see Figure 29-6). At pharmacologic doses aspirin selectively and irreversibly acetylates a serine residue of a platelet COX.[114] The platelet form of this enzyme is up to 250-fold more sensitive to acetylation by aspirin compared with COX (prostacyclin synthetase) in vascular endothelial cells. Although platelets cannot regenerate more COX, endothelial cells apparently are able to rapidly synthesize and replace impaired COX.[114] Platelet aggregation defects caused by aspirin will last until platelets can be replaced, generally 1 to 2 weeks.

KEY POINT 29-14 Cyclooxygenase-2–preferential drugs should be expected to increase the risk of thrombosis rather than hemostasis.

The effect of newer NSAIDs differs from that of conventional NSAIDs. The loss of COX-2–mediated formation of prostacyclin and its antithrombotic effects in the vascular endothelium predisposes (human) patients to COX-1–mediated platelet aggregation, leukocyte activation, and adhesion and accumulation of cholesterol in vascular cells. The potential association of COX-2 inhibitors and an increased risk of thromboembolic disease evolved in the analysis of side effects in treatment groups receiving selected COX-2 preferential drugs (e.g., rofecoxib or celecoxib compared with placebos or conventional NSAIDs) as part of clinical trials evaluating their use for treatment of cancer, treatment of AD, or association with gastrointestinal side effects. The trials initially were not designed to compare cardiovascular events, and initial evaluation could not discern whether it was treatment with rofecoxib or lack of treatment with naproxen (and thus loss of a cardioprotective effect) that led to the increased risk.[115] Subsequent studies that have focused specifically on the risk of thromboembolic events have yielded conflicting results, ranging from a clear increased risk to no detectable increase in risk. The results of these studies have been reviewed,[115] but conclusions are complicated by the presence of aspirin. However, neither conventional nor COX-selective NSAIDs are as likely to impair platelet aggregation as well as aspirin does. For platelet aggregation to be impaired, TXA2 must be inhibited by at least 95%, an impact that competitive TXA2 inhibitors cannot achieve; the possible exception is naproxen because of its long half-life. In contrast, aspirin irreversibly acetylates TXA2. Accordingly, both aspirin and naproxen tend to be associated with cardioprotective effects. However, aspirin has the added advantage of stimulating lipoxin, which provides antiplatelet effects.[20] A number of NSAIDs, including naproxen, block aspirin's cardioprotective effect, in part by physically binding the serine site of TXA2 acetylation by aspirin. Although this is less likely for newer NSAIDs, they may impair lipoxin, thus impairing antiplatelet effects through a different mechanism. This complicates interpretation of these studies, particularly if groups are not controlled for aspirin dose, duration, and timing. However, in general, review of these clinical trials indicate that COX-2–selective drugs do increase the risk of cardiovascular adverse events, particularly in patients already suffering from disease.[115]

The impact of COX-2 selective drugs on hemostasis in veterinary medicine is not clear, but preferential COX-2 inhibition by endogenous glucocorticoids may help explain the increased risk of thrombogenesis in dogs suffering from hyperadrenocorticism. In a canine model of coronary vessel occlusion, celecoxib decreased the vasodilatory response to AA, leading the authors to conclude that a potential risk exists for acute vascular events in animals suffering from inflammatory disorders and receiving COX-2–selective drugs.[116] However, celecoxib also prevents the cardioprotective effects provided by low dose aspirin, contributing to the increased risk of thromboembolic events in some human patients.[116a] The lack of unequivocal information regarding COX selectivity of the various NSAIDs in either dogs or cats complicates assessment of risk. As such, NSAIDs should be used only with great caution in animals with comorbidity influencing hemostasis (e.g., heart worm thromboembolis). This may be particularly problematic in the cat (e.g., hypertrophic cardiomyopathy) for which little information regarding COX selectivity among drugs is available.

Miscellaneous

Thyroid

A number of NSAIDs adversely affect thyroid function, primarily through competition for or impairment of binding to carrier proteins. Displacement appears to cause plasma concentrations to rapidly increase, leading to decreased thyroid-stimulating hormone; however, with time, increased clearance of the hormone should alter the balance in the opposite direction. The impact of NSAIDs on the thyroid gland may reflect the sulfur moiety present on many of the drugs (see Figures 29-3 and 29-4); it is possible that displacement from protein-binding sites might increase clearance. Using a randomized crossover design, Daminet and coworkers[117] reported that aspirin reduced total T_4 within 24 hours of administration of 25 mg/kg twice daily; thyroid-stimulating hormone and free T_4 were not affected. Ketoprofen at 1 mg/kg once daily had no effect compared with placebo. Whereas etodolac appears to have minimal impact on thyroid function.[118] Ferguson (as reviewed by Sauve)[119] reported slightly decreased serum T_4 and cTSH in dogs receiving carprofen for 2 to 5 weeks. Sauve and coworkers[119] prospectively studied in osteoarthritic dogs (n=62) the effect of meloxicam (n=14; 0.2 mg/kg load followed by 0.1 mg/kg daily for 60 days total), carprofen (n=14; 1.7 to 2.3 mg/kg twice daily for 60 days) and chondroitin sulfate–glucosamine–manganese combinations (n=18; 1 to 3 capsules daily for 60 days) compared with placebo on thyroid function. The study was randomized and placebo (n=16) controlled. Thyroid function did not significantly differ among any treatment group across time or between groups; however, free T_4 declined 20% in the meloxicam group. Sample size may have limited the ability to detect differences in other groups.

Lungs

The "allergy" to aspirin described for human asthmatics is generally recognized to reflect increased production of LTs, although the loss of the inhibitory effect on LT production by PGs also has been suggested. Drugs that are COX-1 sparing do not appear to precipitate asthma as do conventional NSAIDs and aspirin in particular, suggesting that the newer drugs are safe in asthmatic patients.[20] The impact of low-dose aspirin (which would allow the production of aspirin-induced lipoxin) on pulmonary inflammatory diseases has not been addressed.

Other

Miscellaneous side effects associated with the use of NSAIDs include aseptic meningitis,[120-122] diarrhea, and CNS depression.[59]

CONVENTIONAL NONSTEROIDAL ANTIINFLAMMATORY DRUGS

Aspirin: The Prototypic Nonsteroidal Antiinflammatory Drug

The discovery of the mechanisms of aspirin and its elucidation of COX enzyme isoforms was recently reviewed.[122a]

Structure–Activity and Preparations. Aspirin, the salicylic acid ester of acetic acid, is the prototype of the salicylate drugs, which includes sodium salicylate, bismuth subsalicylate, and others. In addition to inhibition of COX enzyme activity, salicylates inhibit the formation and release of kinins, stabilize lysosomes, and remove energy necessary for inflammation by uncoupling oxidative phosphorylation. Among the traditional NSAIDs, aspirin stands out for its impact on the AA cascade. Its effect on thromboxane synthetase was previously described. Additionally, at low doses, aspirin triggers the formation of lipoxins and their 15-epimers, epoxins.[123, 123a] The latter are antiinflammatory mediators that counter the proinflammatoroy mediators of the cascade (see Figures 29-1 and 29-2). Aspirin is available in several different preparations, including plain, film-coated, buffered, time-release, and enteric-coated tablets. Capsules and suppositories are also available.[70] Oral salicylates are also available in preparations intended to treat inflammatory bowel disease.

Disposition. The oral bioavailability of aspirin products may vary because of differences in disintegration, drug formulation, stomach content, and gastric pH.[124] Although buffered aspirin is more soluble than plain aspirin, a larger proportion is ionized and less rapidly absorbed. The rate of absorption of both products is the same.[70] Aspirin undergoes rapid metabolism to the hydrolyzed active product salicylic acid by plasma esterases. This metabolite is not as potent an analgesic or antiinflammatory drug because of the loss of the acetyl group, which is able to acetylate key proteins.[70] Salicylic acid is between 50% and 70% bound to serum albumin among species.[125] Hypoalbuminemia may result in transient increases in plasma drug concentrations associated with adverse effects. Distribution of salicylic acid into extracellular fluid is rapid and includes synovial and peritoneal fluids, saliva, and milk. Salicylic acid is eliminated by hepatic conjugation with glucuronide and glycine, renal excretion by glomerular filtration, and tubular secretion.[125,126] Species differences in the biotransformation and elimination of salicylates are dramatic. Excretion is more rapid in alkaline urine, which might be used therapeutically to treat acute aspirin intoxication. Salicylate can achieve substantial concentrations in milk. Elimination occurs more slowly in pediatric patients.[127]

The disposition of acetyl salicylate appears to be the only salicylate for which data is available in dogs or cats.[127, 128] Other oral salicylates such as sulfasalazine have been used to treat chronic inflammatory conditions of the bowel (see Chapter 19). Although their mechanism of action is unclear, splitting of the diazo bond by colonic bacteria to yield sulfapyridine and 5-aminosalicylic acid (5-ASA) may be involved. The 5-ASA is considered to be the active moiety.[129] Both the sulfapyridine and sulfasalazine (up to 25%) are absorbed from the small intestine, but most of the 5-ASA remains in the colon. That absorbed (approximately 20% in humans) is rapidly acetylated and inactivated by either the colonic mucosa or liver. Newer products composed principally of 5-ASA are being investigated for the treatment of chronic inflammatory bowel diseases.[129] Alternative methods of delivery of these compounds such that side effects are minimized are also being studied.[130]

Adverse reactions. Aspirin is theoretically characterized by a wide safety margin in most species. The recommended therapeutic range in humans ranges from 100 to 250 μg/mL,[131] with higher concentrations necessary to control inflammation, particularly that associated with immune-mediated disease.[5] Analgesia and antipyresis generally require concentrations of 20 to 50 μg/mL,[70] whereas control of inflammation may require concentrations that exceed 50 μg/mL. Response of rheumatoid arthritis in human beings requires concentrations approximating 200 μg/mL. Although the drug concentration necessary to achieve an antithrombotic effect has not been established for aspirin in animals, smaller doses have proved efficacious (e.g., 3 mg/kg). These studies did not effectively evaluate safety (gastrointestinal changes). Studies based on gastrointestinal permeability demonstrate that aspirin alters gastrointestinal permability.[7]

Clinical signs of aspirin toxicity may be present at concentrations necessary for clinical response, but they worsen as serum salicylate concentrations exceed 300 μg/mL. The effects of NSAIDs on cartilage are largely detrimental. Hepatotoxicity and decreased renal function have been reported at 250 μg/mL. Decreased prothrombin time, deafness, and hyperventilation occur at 300 to 350 μg/mL, with severe toxicity, including metabolic acidosis, occurring at doses above 400 μg/mL.[127]

Treatment of acute aspirin toxicity is largely supportive, including increasing elimination. Toxicity (acute) is usually manifested as depression, vomiting, hyperthermia, electrolyte imbalances, convulsions, coma, and death. Toxicity is more likely in cats because of slow metabolism with accumulation. Acute toxicity includes serious acid–base disturbances resulting from uncoupling of oxidative phosphorylation. Hyperventilation resulting from direct stimulation of the respiratory center may be followed by depression at high doses. Bleeding disorders may also be evident,[70,132] as might dose-dependent hepatotoxicity. Salicylate markedly suppresses augmented proteoglycan synthesis in osteoarthritic cartilage and permeates the damage joint more than the undamaged joint.[133]

Dogs. In dogs aspirin is distributed to a volume ranging from 0.4 to 0.6 L/kg. Bioavailability probably varies with the manufacturer as well as the preparation and ranges from 68% to 76%.[134] The bioavailabilities of plain, buffered, and enteric-coated aspirin (25 mg/kg) do not appear to vary markedly, although plasma salicylate concentrations were most variable for the enteric-coated preparation.[135] Concentrations of 91 to 120 μg/mL are achieved at 25 mg/kg administered at 8-hour intervals.[127] After several doses of 25 mg/kg at 12-hour intervals, the biological half-life of aspirin is 7.5 hours in dogs. This time increased to a mean of 12.2 hours, however, when the dosing interval was decreased to 8 hours.[136] In another study the elimination half-life of aspirin varied after intravenous injection of 36 to 60 mg/kg, ranging from 2.2 to 8.7 hours.

One study in clinical patients found that plasma salicylate concentrations correlated with response.[134] The dose necessary to maintain clinical control of various lamenesses in dogs in one study ranged from 23 to 86 mg/kg twice daily, resulting in plasma drug concentrations ranging from 71 to 281 μg/mL.[137] Marked individual variability in drug elimination among animals suggests that therapeutic drug monitoring may be useful to ensure that therapeutic drug concentrations have been achieved and that toxic concentrations (>300 μg/mL) are avoided.[134] However, when 25 mg/kg is administered at 8-hour intervals, therapeutic concentrations can be expected to be maintained throughout the dosing interval. Gastrointestinal side effects of aspirin in dogs also appear to be dose and preparation related[62,135] and may be decreased by using special preparations. Doses of 25 mg/kg of plain aspirin caused mucosal erosions in 50% of dogs that received plain aspirin, whereas minimal damage occurred in animals receiving buffered and coated preparations.[135]

Cats. As a phenol, aspirin is a compound for which glucuronidation is generally deficient in cats compared with other species.[132,138] Its plasma elimination half-life may be dose dependent.[139] The half-life is 22 to 27 hours after doses of 5 to 12 mg/kg but 45 hours after administration of 25 mg/kg.[7,128] No clinical signs of toxicosis occurred in one study in which cats were treated with 25 mg/kg every 48 hours.[138] Clinical signs of aspirin toxicity in cats are similar to those seen in human patients.[140] Subtle changes in liver function may reflect nonspecific hepatitis, the primary histologic lesion.

Flunixin Meglumine

Structure–activity relationship. Flunixin meglumine is a nicotinic acid derivative approved for use in the horse. Described as a potent analgesic agent, it has been used to control pain that might otherwise respond only to opioids. It is particularly useful for visceral pain. In addition to its analgesic effects, flunixin meglumine has been studied and cited for its antiendotoxic effects in experimental models of septic shock in several species.[141-145]

Disposition. The disposition of flunixn has been studied in dogs and cats (see Table 29-4).[60,146] Flunixin appears to undergo enterohepatic circulation in cats. Its half-life differs considerably depending on the study, with more recent studies perhaps being more accurate because of a lower limit of detection that allows description of the true elimination phase.[60] However, because therapeutic concentrations are not known, the true elimination phase may reflect concentrations that are subtherapeutic and may not be clinically relevant. At least two transport systems appear to be involved in the disposition of flunixin in cats (one being organic anion transporter polypeptide-2 in the liver, the other renal in origin),[60] which may subject the drug to drug interactions.

Therapeutic use. Although the mode of action has not been documented, flunixin is specifically recommended as an analgesic in the treatment of colic in horses and has been useful for control of visceral pain in dogs (e.g., parvovirus) or postoperative pain.[66] It also has been useful for the treatment (and especially pretreatment) of endotoxic shock.[44] It prevents many of the adverse effects caused by administration of endotoxin, TXA2, and PGI2.[146] Flunixin meglumine appears to modulate response to septic shock in dogs.[141,145,147] In dogs a dose of 1.1 mg/kg flunixin meglumine blocks PGI2 production, and 2.2 mg/kg improves survival times of septic dogs.[146] Newer COX-2–targeting NSAIDs might be similarly effective in the treatment or prevention of endotoxemia. Pharmacokinetics of flunixin in septic dogs does not appear to differ from that of control dogs.[146] Toxicity, most commonly manifested as gastrointestinal upset, limits use of this drug in dogs to 2 to 3 days. Doses at three to five times those recommended caused gastrointestinal disturbances in one study.

Ibuprofen

Ibuprofen is a propionic acid derivative that has been used in dogs. Ibuprofen may be less effective as an analgesic than aspirin, perhaps on account of differences in binding of COX (reversible for ibuprofen and irreversible for aspirin). Ibuprofen remains a popular and effective antiinflammatory drug in humans. The disposition of ibuprofen has been studied in dogs (see Table 29-4). Pharmacokinetics are similar at doses of 5 and 10 mg/kg.[148] A dose of 12 to 15 mg/kg is, however, necessary to achieve therapeutic concentrations, as reported in humans.[148] After repetitive administration of this dose, plasma drug concentrations decrease despite no change in drug half-life.[148]

KEY POINT 29-15 Ibuprofen and naproxen should be considered as contraindicated in the dog just as acetaminophen is contraindicated in the cat.

In humans ibuprofen is associated with a low incidence of gastrointestinal side effects and has been compared favorably with even the newer COX-2–selective drugs.[73] This may lead clients to assume the same is true for dogs or cats. However, ibuprofen is among the least safe NSAIDs in dogs. Vomiting commonly occurs after several (2 to 6) days of ibuprofen therapy in dogs with either the gelatin- or enteric-coated capsules.[148] Gastrointestinal inflammation and gastric erosions have been documented after administration of 8 mg/kg daily despite the lack of clinical signs of toxicity.[148,149] Death associated with gastrointestinal hemorrhage occurred in one dog given 3 mg/kg every other day for 6 weeks.[149] These effects occur despite a short half-life for ibuprofen in dogs (less than 5 hours). The COX-1 to COX-2 ratio apparently has not been determined for ibuprofen in dogs. Because gastric lesions occur at doses less than those necessary to achieve therapeutic concentrations, ibuprofen is not recommended for use in dogs.

Ketoprofen

Structure–activity relationship and mechanism of action. Ketoprofen is a propionic acid NSAID approved for use in humans and horses. Because ketoprofen is a strong inhibitor of COX, it has been ascribed powerful antiinflammatory, analgesic, and antipyretic properties. Although not firmly established, the efficacy of ketoprofen has been attributed to its ability to inhibit some lipoxygenases and thus formation of LTs.[150] Ketoprofen is also a powerful inhibitor of bradykinin.[150]

Disposition. Ketoprofen is rapidly absorbed from the gastrointestinal tract. Although peak plasma drug concentrations are lower in dogs after oral than intravenous administration, mean residence times (4.59 versus 3.81 hours, respectively) were not different.[151] Bioavailability does not seem to be impaired by food. As with other NSAIDs, ketoprofen is approximately 99% protein bound, principally to albumin. Elimination reflects metabolism to inactive metabolites by the liver and excretion as the glucuronide conjugate in the urine.[150] Ketoprofen has a slightly shorter half-life in cats compared with dogs (see Table 29-4). Ketoprofen is sold as a racemic mixture. The R and S isomer are handled differently by the body and induce different pharmacodynamic and pharmacokinetic responses, with variability expected among and within species. Disposition is further complicated by the potential conversion that occurs between isomers, with the extent and sequelae also varying among and within species.[127] Conversion of the R to S isomer, but not the S to R isomer, has been documented in dogs and cats. Cats may convert up to 37% of the R to the S isomer. Not surprisingly, species differ as to which isomer predominates after administration of the racemic mixture. In dogs the S isomer represented 91% of the peak plasma drug concentration 3 hours after administration of the R isomer.

Drugs that are similar in structure may be markedly different in their pharmacokinetic and pharmacodynamic description, as is exemplified by ketoprofen and a similar drug, fenoprofen, in cats.[152] For ketoprofen the R and S isomers behave similarly: Respective clearance was 235 and 216 mL/hr/kg, and half-life of each was 0.5 hour. For the structurally similar fenoprofen, clearance for the R isomer was ninefold greater compared with that for the S isomer (980 versus 112 mL/hr/kg), leading to a shorter half-life (0.53 hour) for the R isomer compared with the S isomer (3 hours). Further, 93% of R-fenoprofen was converted to the S-isomer, compared with only 37% of R-ketoprofen.[152] As such, at least for the cat, exposure to either isomer of ketoprofen may be largely equivalent (based on area under the curve) but is approximately sixfold higher for S-fenoprofen (the COX-active isomer) compared with R-fenoprofen.[152] As with disposition, the pharmacodynamic impact of each ketoprofen isomer on inflammation and analgesia is variable among species. The anti-COX effect of ketoprofen (and fenoprofen) reflects the S-enantiomer in cats.

Drug interactions specific for ketoprofen have not yet been documented.[153] However, in humans adverse reactions to ketoprofen occur in approximately 30% of the patients studied.[154,155] The most frequent complaint was upper gastrointestinal upset. Other commonly encountered side effects include CNS reactions, such as headaches and dizziness, and nephritis. Side effects were severe enough in one report that therapy was discontinued in approximately 13% of patients.[153] Alternative preparations, such as rectal suppositories, have been formulated for ketoprofen to reduce the incidence of gastrointestinal toxicity.[151]

KEY POINT 29-16 Ideally, the preferred nonsteroidal antiinflammatory drug for perioperative use will be one approved for use in the target species and known to be cyclooxygenase-2 preferential in action.

Ketoprofen is not approved for use in small animals in the United States but is approved for both dogs and cats in Canada and Europe. It has proved to be an efficacious NSAID in humans and animals. In human patients suffering from rheumatoid arthritis, ketoprofen has been shown to be as efficacious as aspirin, naproxen, aspirin, indomethacin, ibuprofen, diclofenac, and piroxicam.[156] Similar results occurred in cancer patients receiving either aspirin–codeine combinations or ketoprofen.[155] For control of postoperative pain, ketoprofen has proved as effective as pentazocine and meperidine[156] and equally effective but longer in duration than acetaminophen–codeine combinations.[157] In dogs analgesia provided by ketoprofen has been reported to last between 12 and 20 hours.[127]

The use of ketoprofen as an analgesic and antipyretic has been studied in cats. The antipyretic effect of ketoprofen (2 mg/kg subcutaneously followed by 1 mg/kg once daily orally) in febrile cats was rapid, being evident in 4 hours with temperatures normalized at that time.[158] Temperatures did not change in the cats treated with antibiotics only. The use of ketoprofen as an analgesic is variable.[159] In cats subjected to ovariohysterectomy, ketoprofen (2 mg/kg subcutaneously) compared favorably with buprenorphine (0.006 mg/kg or 6 μg/kg intramuscularly) and meperidine as gas anesthesia was discontinued. Response was based on visual analog scores and overall clinical assessment. Response was equal to that of buprenorphine at 4 hours and better at 8 hours. Response was better for both drugs compared with the control at both 4 and 8 hours but still present for buprenorphine only compared with control at 18 hours.

Ketorolac

Ketorolac is an NSAID approved for use in human patients. In contrast to many NSAIDs, ketorolac is only moderately effective as an antiinflammatory.[160] It is a potent analgesic, however, that has been described as equivalent to morphine. As such, it has been used as a perioperative analgesic in dogs.[161] Ketorolac appears to be superior to butorphanol and equal to flunixin meglumine for control of postoperative pain. The disposition of ketoralac is quite variable in in dogs (see Table 29-4) after single intravenous or oral dosing (0.34 mg/kg), although investigators indicate that the disposition was similar to humans.[162] In humans ketorolac causes gastrointestinal upset, and similar side effects occur in dogs. In one study 1 of 21 dogs developed gastrointestinal ulceration after a single dose.[66] Therefore recommendations are to limit use to one to two treatments, or 3 days. Other side effects reported in human patients include dizziness, headache, nausea, and pain at the site of injection.[160] Caution should be taken particularly in the perioperative patient, which is more likely to be dependent on renal PGs during the surgical procedure.

Meclofenamic Acid

Meclofenamate is an anthranilic NSAID available as a palatable granular preparation intended to be mixed with food for large animals and as a tablet. It is approved for use in dogs in the United States. Among the NSAIDs, it is noted for its slow onset of action. The package insert associated with the label of this drug describes dogs as being exquisitely sensitive to the gastrointestinal ulcerogenic effects of these drugs. Meclofenamic acid appears to have no clear advantage to other drugs for treatment of osteoarthritis in dogs and may be more likely to cause gastrointestinal upset.

Naproxen

Naproxen is approved for use in humans and is available in over the counter preparations. Although it contains a chiral carbon, it is sold as the pure S isomer. Its disposition has been studied in dogs and, notably, it varies from that in humans. Compared with 12 to 15 hours in humans and 5 hours in horses, the elimination half-life of naproxen after intravenous administration in dogs ranges from 45 to 92 hours.[163] Peak concentrations in dogs after oral administration of 5 mg/kg were 40 to 50 μg/mL. Tissue concentrations paralleled plasma concentrations, with a peak of 20 to 30 μg/mL; concentrations declined over a period of 200 hours.[164] Extensive enterohepatic circulation has been credited as the cause for prolonged elimination in dogs. Because of its long half-life, naproxen need be given only once daily to every other day. Although a loading dose has been recommended, the gastrointestinal toxicity of this drug in dogs suggests that a loading dose be avoided to minimize the risk of toxicity.

The dog has been described as the animal most sensitive to naproxen.[163] Its use in dogs does not seem prudent. Gastrointestinal toxicity occurs at doses of 5 mg/kg daily.[165] Toxicity appears most likely when plasma drug concentrations exceed 50 μg/mL. If this NSAID must be used in dogs, doses initially should be low (1 to 2 mg/kg) and subsequently titrated to the animal's need. Animals should be watched closely for evidence of gastrointestinal upset. Bleeding dyscrasias have also been reported in dogs receiving large doses of naproxen.[163,165,166]

Naproxen has been cited for a positive protective effect on articular cartilage. In a canine experimental model of osteoarthritis, naproxen decreased the loss of proteoglycans and suppressed metalloproteinase activity.[167]

Phenylbutazone

Phenylbutazone is a weakly acidic, lipophilic NSAID approved for use in dogs. Inhibition of the AA cascade by phenylbutazone occurs after conversion to reactive intermediates at the level of PGH synthase and prostacyclin synthase. Prostanoid-dependent swelling, edema, erythema, and associated pain are reduced by phenylbutazone.[37] Phenylbutazone has been associated with some attenuation of some clinical signs associated with endotoxic shock in experimental models.[142,144]

Bioavailability after intramuscular administration of phenylbutazone is less than that after oral administration in most species studied because of precipitation in the neutral pH of muscle.[37,168] Phenylbutazone is metabolized by the liver, with less than 2% of the drug being excreted as a parent compound in the urine in some species. Its major metabolites are oxyphenylbutazone, which is less active than phenylbutazone, and inactive γ-hydroxyphenylbutazone.[37,169,170] Dose-dependent zero-order kinetics has been reported in dogs.[127] Reported adverse reactions caused by phenylbutazone include bleeding dyscrasias, hepatopathy, and nephropathy (primarily in horses).[37,96,171,172] Phenylbutazone has chondrodestructive effects.[173,174]

Dogs. Despite approval of the oral preparation for use in dogs, there is little information regarding the use of phenylbutazone in dogs. The half-life in plasma (7.3 to 18 hours) is shorter than that in tissues (20 hours), although peak concentrations in tissues (13 to 20 μg/mL) were approximately one third of those in plasma (49 to 75 μg/mL)[164] after a dose of 15 mg/kg orally. The elimination half-life (in Greyhounds) is 6 to 7 hours.[169,170] Dogs apparently are more tolerant of phenylbutazone than are humans. When used to treat racing greyhounds, phenylbutazone should be used with caution because of routine drug testing. One study[175] has documented that phenylbutazone can be detected in the urine of Greyhounds after topical administration in a commercially available cream.

Toxicity manifested as hemorrhage, biliary stasis, and renal failure has been reported in one dog receiving close to recommended doses.[97,172,176] For reasons not explained, the package insert notes a total maximum dose and requires the drug to be discontinued slowly. Bone marrow dyscrasias (including neutropenia) also have been reported.

Cats. Although phenylbutazone has been used in cats, a high incidence of toxicity suggests extreme caution. One hundred percent of cats treated with 44 mg/kg daily became anorectic at 2 to 3 days, with 80% mortality at 2 to 3 weeks. Toxicity occurs primarily in the bone marrow and is characterized by decreased erythroblastic activity and possible interference with myeloid maturation. Gastrointestinal damage, nephrotoxicity, and hepatotoxicity also occur.[96]

Piroxicam

Piroxicam is an oxicam NSAID approved for humans that has been used to treat osteoarthritis in dogs. More recently, it has received attention for its ability to reduce the size of tumors (transitional cell tumors and others) in dogs.[49,50-52] Piroxicam may interact by an additive or synergistic action with anticancer drugs to cause tumor cell death. Piroxicam is a potent antiinflammatory in musculoskeletal conditions. The disposition of piroxicam has been studied in both the dog[177] and cat.[178] Notably, the half-life of the drug is much shorter in cats (12 hours) compared with dogs (40 to 50 hours). Although the LD_{50} of piroxicam is greater than 700 mg/kg in dogs, gastric lesions and renal papillary necrosis have occurred in dogs receiving 0.3 to 1 mg/kg daily.[49,177] The ratio of COX-2 to COX-1 suggests that gastrointestinal toxicity occurs. Little evidence of toxicity (gastrointestinal or bleeding), however, was noted after administration of 0.3 mg/kg every other day.[49,177] Extrapolation of human use to dogs should be done cautiously because of possible differences in volume of distribution, therapeutic concentrations, or safety margin.

Tolfenamic acid. Tolfenamic acid (Tolfedine) is a nonselective NSAID approved for use in Canada for long-term use in dogs and short-term use in cats. The half-lives in dogs and cats are, respectively, 6.5 hours and 8 hours. The drug appears to undergo enterohepatic circulation.

CYCLOOXYGENASE-1–SPARING NONSTEROIDAL ANTIINFLAMMATORY DRUGS

Because the extent of COX-1 and COX-2 inhibition for many of the newer NSAIDs is not clear, particularly in dogs and cats, the term *preferential COX-2 inhibitors* is preferred in this text to *selective COX-2 inhibitors,* with the former reflecting the potential for inhibition of both isoforms. COX-1 sparing is intended to mean the same. Bergh and Budsberg[179] reviewed the use of coxib NSAIDs in veterinary medicine.

Carprofen

Dogs. Carprofen is a proprionic acid–derived NSAID approved in the United States for use in dogs for the treatment of osteoarthritis.[180] The drug is approved for use in dogs and cats in selected countries outside of the United States. Like other NSAIDs, carprofen has antipyretic, analgesic, and antiinflammatory effects.[180] Its potency is equal to that of indomethacin and surpasses that of aspirin or phenylbutazone,[180] and doses consequently are smaller for carprofen than for these NSAIDs.

The mechanism of action of carprofen is not certain, but, unlike other members of its class (e.g., ibuprofen, ketoprofen, naproxen), it may be relatively selective for inhibition of COX-2. McKellar and coworkers[181] reported that it does not inhibit thromboxane activitiy in platelets, PGE_2 (isoform not identified) nor 12-HETE in inflammatory cells. With canine platelet-derived COX-1 and macrophage-like cell COX-2, the ratio of COX-1 to COX-2 IC_{50} (concentration that caused 50% inhibition) for the racemic mixture (that available in the commercial preparation) was 129; the ratio was 181 for the S isomer (thus the "antiinflammatory" enantiomer) but only 4.19 for the R isomer (see Table 29-3).[32] These differences in COX inhibition may explain the apparent safety of carprofen compared with conventional NSAIDs in dogs and with safety in the dog compared to that in humans, for whom the ratio is less than 1.

Pharmacokinetics. Carprofen has been studied in dogs after oral and subcutaneous administration (see Table 29-4). Increases in oral doses generally result in proportional increases in C_{max}, with peak concentrations occurring at approximately 1 hour. Peak concentrations appear to occur more slowly with subcutaneous than with oral administration; the former route may prolong onset of efficacy. Although C_{max} differed between oral and subcutaneous administration, the area under the curve did not, indicating bioequivalence among the two routes after both single and multiple dosing.[182] Like other NSAIDs, carprofen is highly protein bound. Carprofen is metabolized by the liver and in dogs is characterized by a half-life of approximately 10 hours, which is sufficiently long that it has been approved for once-daily administration. Between 70% and 80% of carprofen metabolites are excreted in the feces, with the remainder in the urine.

The dispositions of the two carprofen enantiomers have been studied in dogs.[181,183] Administration as a racemic mixture yields a C_{max} of the R isomer at 18 μg/mL versus 14 μg/mL for the S isomer. Conversion apparently does not occur between the R or S isomer in dogs. Both the R isomer (72%) and the S isomer (92%) are extensively excreted in the bile, but enterohepatic circulation appears to be relatively specific for the S isomer (the isomer characterized by a very favorable COX-2 specificity), probably owing to greater glucuronidase-resistant isoglucuronides for the R isomer.[183] Up to 34% of the S isomer is recirculated.[127] Because both the clearance and the volume of distribution of the S isomer are greater than those of the R isomer, the mean residence times and half-lives of the two isomers do not differ.[183] After a single subcutaneous dose of 4 mg/kg either preoperatively or postoperatively, duration of analgesia ranged from 18 to 24 hours.[127]

Adverse reactions. On the basis of toxicity data, carprofen appears to be among the safest of the new NSAIDs approved for use in dogs (see Table 29-5). According to the package insert, dogs dosed with more than 10 times the amount necessary to achieve therapeutic concentrations did not develop gastrointestinal side effects when dosed for 2 weeks or when dosed at almost six times the recommended dose for 52 weeks. In a clinical trial of 70 dogs, 6 of 36 carprofen-treated dogs (2.2 mg/kg orally every 12 hr) developed clinical signs indicative of gastrointestinal upset; three dogs that received placebo also developed gastrointestinal signs.[184]

KEY POINT 29-17 On the basis of toxicity and field trial data on package inserts, carprofen appears to be among the safest of the newer nonsteroidal antiinflammatory drugs approved for use in dogs.

Forsyth and coworkers[185] compared the gastrointestinal side effects of carprofen (2 mg/kg orally twice daily for 7 days followed by 2 mg/kg once daily), meloxicam (0.2 mg/kg orally once daily), and ketoprofen (1 mg/kg orally every 24 hours) with those of placebo after 28 days of therapy in dogs. The fewest and least severe gastroduodenal lesions apparent endoscopically were in the carprofen-treated and control group, but there was no statistical significance between the three NSAIDs and the control group, making interpretation difficult. No animals revealed clinical signs associated with gastrointestinal upset. Reimer and coworkers[83] found etodolac and carprofen to not differ from the placebo and all three to cause fewer gastric lesions than aspirin when dosed at labeled doses for 28 days. Craven and coworkers[186] also prospectively compared the effects of carprofen (n = 10 dogs; 4 mg/kg days 1 and 2, 2 mg/kg daily thereafter) to meloxicam (n = 10 dogs; 0.2 mg/kg daily, 1 then 0.1 mg/kg daily) on gastrointestinal epithelium as measured by sugar permeability tests. Dogs were dosed for at least 7 days and studied for 8. Significant changes across time occurred within the carprofen-treated group but resolved by study end; further, although not significant, changes also appeared to have occurred for at least one sugar test for meloxicam. No significant changes were detected in urinary recovery of any sugar between the two treatment groups; placebo controls were not studied. The impact of this comparison is somewhat limited by the absence of untreated controls, large number of comparisons made (two treatment groups, 3 times, seven sugars; potentially, 42 comparisons), and the small number of dogs studied in the face of the variability of the data; the power of the study to detect significant differences was not reported.

Hepatotoxicity reflecting acute hepatic necrosis has been reported as an unexpected adverse effect of carprofen in dogs.[187] Toxicity studies supporting carprofen approval found only mild changes in liver enzymes when the drug was administered at 25 mg/kg for 13 to 52 weeks (package insert data); serum alanine transaminase (SALT) increased with a dose of 80 to 160 mg/kg per day. However, approximately 1 year after its approval, reports of gastrointestinal toxicity led Pfizer to address concerns regarding side effects in a technical report.[188] Of the 1 million dogs receiving carprofen, an incidence of 0.2% suspected side effects was reported, with 0.02% involving the liver. Although 33% of animals affected in initial studies were Labrador Retrievers, this number was not corrected for the prevalance of this species. Hepatopathy has been diagnosed in all breeds of dogs receiving carprofen clinically. At least 70% of afflicted animals were considered geriatric, suggesting that this age group is predisposed, perhaps because of decreased hepatoprotective function (e.g., glutathione scavenging of metabolites). Although death has occurred in some animals, timely discontinuation of the drug can lead to complete resolution of biochemical abnormalities. Animals with liver disease in one study also had evidence of renal tubular disease.[187] MacPhail and coworkers[187] studied 21 animals and reported clinical signs of anorexia, vomiting, lethargy, diarrhea, polyuria, polydipsia, and hematuria occurring between 5 and 30 days; however, clinical signs did not occur until as long as 60 and 180 days for two dogs. In this study 13 of the 21 dogs were Labrador Retrievers, with dogs ranging in age from 4 to 15 years. The most common clinical laboratory abnormalities included increased activities of SALT, aspartate transaminase (SAST), alkaline phosphatase (SAP), and bilirubin. Histologic lesions in the liver ranged from mild to severe and consisted of hepatocellular necrosis. Four of the 21 dogs died; those remaining that were hospitalized were treated with supportive therapy, including gastrointestinal protectants.

Hepatic disease associated with carprofen might be minimized by pretreatment evaluation because lesions appear to occur within the first several weeks of therapy. Consequently, monitoring (clinical laboratory tests) for hepatic damage and hepatic function (bile acids) at weekly or biweekly intervals for the first month is recommended, particularly in predisposed (e.g., geriatric) animals. Monitoring should continue at intervals of 2 to 4 weeks for 3 months and perhaps longer in patients at risk for liver disease. Animals receiving phenobarbital have been anecdotally reported to be more susceptible to hepatotoxicity. Induction of hepatic drug-metabolizing enzymes (e.g., phenobarbital, others) may increase the risk of toxicity if associated with toxic metabolites. Use of hepatoprotective agents such as *N*-acetylcysteine (a glutathione precursor) or SAMe may be beneficial during initial or continued hepatic damage.

The potential for carprofen-induced nephrotoxicity also has been studied in dogs. Crandell and coworkers[105] found no changes compared with saline placebo in renal function (glomerular filtration rate, serum urea, and creatinine) in young healthy dogs (n = 12) receiving placebo, meloxicam (0.2 mg/kg), or carprofen (4 mg/kg) after 30 minutes of electrically stimulated pain. Dogs were studied using a randomized crossover design; anesthesia consisted of butorphanol and acepromazine as preanesthetics, ketamine and diazepam for induction, and isoflurane for maintenance.[105] The study was designed such that power was sufficient to detect a change in glomerular filtration rate of 0.5 mL/kg/min, suggesting that the two treatment groups were the same. This is in contrast to the results of Forsyth and coworkers,[189] who found that creatinine clearance was significantly less in dogs 24 hours after undergoing routine castration and receiving either carprofen (4 mg/kg intravenously), ketoprofen (2 mg/kg intravenously) compared to placebo or saline (0.2 mL/kg intravenously) at induction of anaesthesia. The anesthetic protocol is this study differed among animals (drugs included morphine, thiopental, and halothane).[189] Bostrom and coworkers[190] investigated the effect of carprofen (4 mg/kg intravenously) administered either 30 minutes before or 30 minutes after induction of anesthesia (acepromazine–thiopentone–isoflurane) on renal function (glomerular filtration rate) in dogs (n = 6) after experimentally induced decrease in blood pressure to 65 mm Hg. Significant adverse effects were not detected, although the power of the study to detect a significant difference was not assessed.

The impact of carprofen on hemostasis has been studied. Although carprofen was associated with decreased platelet aggregation and increased partial thromboplastin time in one study, all values were within normal limits. Neither buccal mucosal bleeding time nor complete blood count parameters changed after 12 days of dosing at 2.2 mg/kg twice daily.[191] Other investigators have found no changes in in vitro indices of platelet function.

The effect of carprofen on cartilage physiology appears to be biphasic.[192] In vitro studies with canine chondrocyte cell cultures revealed that carprofen increases the rate of polysulfated glycosaminoglycans (PGAG) synthesis at synovial fluid concentrations (≤10 μg/mL) achieved in human patients receiving a therapeutic dose of carprofen. The S-isomer stimulated PGAG synthesis at a tenfold higher rate compared with the R isomer (United States Pharmacopeia [USP]).[127] Inhibition of PGAG synthesis, however, occurs at concentrations of 20 μg/mL or more.[192] Concentrations that occur in dog synovial fluid after administration of a therapeutic dose of carprofen have not been determined.

Carprofen is approved for use in dogs for control of perioperative pain and treatment of osteoarthritis. It is available as either an oral preparation or an injectable solution intended for subcutaneous injection. Carprofen solution is stable for 1 month if not refrigerated. A chewable table is available, although the risk of accidental overdose may be greater with this product. Although approved for subcutaneous use, injectable carprofen has been given intravenously (4.4 mg/kg) as a single dose with no adverse effects.[190]

Carprofen appears to be equally or more effective than many other NSAIDs studied for the control of inflammation, and it has proved effective for control of the pain associated with the inflammation of osteoarthritis[184] and postoperative pain[193-195] when administered preoperatively. Because carprofen was the first COX-1–protective NSAID approved for use in dogs, approval of subsequent similar-acting NSAIDs generally used it as a positive control. As such, several studies have compared the efficacy of carprofen with that of other NSAIDs, although these studies tend to be manufacturer sponsored. Using a non–placebo-controlled randomized crossover design, Borer and coworkers[196] compared single-dose carprofen (0.2 mg/kg intravenously or 4 mg/kg, orally), etodolac (17 mg/kg, orally), or meloxicam (0.2 mg/kg, orally); (n = 12; studied in groups of four at 3-week intervals) in dogs with experimentally induced acute synovitis (monosodium urate injection). Outcome measures included kinetic gait analysis (force plate), orthopedic evaluation, and serum C-reactive protein (CRP) (n = 6). Lameness was assessed on a biomechanical force platform and by orthopedic evaluations of the stifle joints; blood was collected to monitor serum CRP concentration. All dogs in the treatment groups had improved indices of lameness compared with control animals. Although greatest improvement occurred in carprofen-treated dogs, onset was fastest in etodolac-treated animals. Both carprofen and etodolac were associated with lower pain compared with butorphanol, although the authors concluded that meloxicam also was more effective than butorphanol. Serum CRP was not different among groups.[196]

Carprofen or meloxicam also were compared with a combination glucosamine–chondroitin sulfate (Cosequin) product using a prospective, double-blinded study in dogs (n = 71) with osteoarthritis; the study was supported by the manufacturers of meloxicam. Treatment continued for 60 days, and response was based on force plate analysis and subjective evaluation by owners. Although animals responded to both meloxicam and carprofen, only meloxicam was associated with a return to baseline function. Side effects were minimal, although one dog receiving carprofen developed hepatopathy and one dog receiving meloxicam withdrew from the study because of vomiting.[197]

Finally, Aragon and coworkers[198] evaluated the quality of evidence of NSAIDs, including carprofen, or supplements used to treat osteoarthritis in dogs. The FDA's evidence-based ranking was applied to scientific data collected from a review of the literature before 2006. Studies were ranked on the basis of study design, quality, and total body of evidence (quantity of studies or study subjects, consistency among the different reports, and the likelihood that the magnitude of the response was physiologically meaningful). The evidence was then ranked according to strength (high, moderate, low, or extremely low level of comfort). Only 16 clinical trials met the inclusion criteria. Of the compounds studied, the evidence for meloxicam was accorded a high level of comfort (i.e., that efficacy is scientifically valid), and the evidence for carprofen, etodolac, PGAG, and glucosamine –chondroitin–manganese was ranked as moderate. Hyaluronan was ranked extremely low. Care must be taken not to overinterpret this data because of the limited number of studies reviewed

Cats. Carprofen is approved for use in cats in certain countries outside the United States. The disposition of the drug and its enantiomers has been studied in cats at the dose associated with control of inflammation (4 mg/kg; Table 29.4).[128,199-201] The smaller clearance for carprofen in cats results in an elimination half-life that is at least twice as long in cats as in dogs. The S isomer is cleared almost 3 times as rapidly as the R isomer, resulting in a shorter half-life for S compared with R in the cat

The relative COX-2 selectivity of carprofen that occurs in dogs has not been well documented in cats, although data from Brideau and coworkers[33] suggests relative selectivity similar to that in dogs (see Table 29-3). Clinically, however, this may not be true. The gastrointestinal effects of single-dose carprofen (4 mg/kg intravenously) or aspirin (20 mg/kg intravenously) were studied in cats (n = 5) using endoscopy and a randomized crossover design. Lesions in the stomach and duodenum 8 hours after injection were limited to minor pinpoint erosion in one cat. Clinical laboratory tests were not affected by either drug.[128] Duodenal perforation has been reported in cats receiving oral carprofen (2.2 mg/kg twice daily for 7 days) after ovariohysterectomy.[202] The ulceration may have been exacerbated by the flunixin meglumine and dexamethasone with which the cat was treated before referral.

Parton and coworkers[128] prospectively compared the gastrointestinal effects of carprofen (4 mg/kg intravenously) and salicylate (20 mg/kg intravenously) in cats using a crossover design. Only a single dose was studied; gastric lesions were scored endoscopically 8 hours after dosing. No differences were found between treatment groups or times, with one exception in the salicylate group for which pinpint erosive lesions were found. Steagall and coworkers[107] also prospectively studied the adverse effects of carprofen, after multiple doses (6 days) of decreasing doses (4 mg/kg on day 1 to 1 mg/kg on day 6). A randomized, blinded crossover, placebo-controlled design was used, with a 4-week washout. Endoscopic lesions were scored before and 7 days after treatment. Changes in biochemistry profiles included decreased albumin but no other abnormalities, including gastrointestinal lesions or changes in renal dysfunction.

As a postoperative analgesic in cats, carprofen compares favorably with pethidine (meperidine), providing equal but longer analgesia (at least 24 hours) when administered at 4 mg/kg subcutaneously postoperatively.[201] In a clinical trial of cats undergoing ovariohysterectomy, the analgesic effects of carprofen, ketoprofen, meloxicam, or tolfenamic acid were compared. Outcome was based on the visual analog scale and a nociceptive threshold at the incision site, as well as clinical response. No difference was found between treatment groups in providing analgesia. With nine of ten cats responding, all responses were described as good, although none prevented wound tenderness.[203] Taylor and coworkers[204] prospectively compared the efficacy of carpofen (4 mg/kg) and buprenorphine (0.01 mg/kg) as preventives for hyperalgesia in an experimental model of inflammatory pain in cats. Cats (n = 8) were studied using a randomized, crossover, placebo-controlled design. Drugs were administered before (3 hours for carprofen, 1 hour for buprenorphine) anesthesia. Carprofen completely prevented inflammation, and buprenorphine almost completely did so, although hypoalgesia was not realized.

Deracoxib

Deracoxib is approved for use as an oral chewable preparation in dogs. As a coxib, deracoxib would be expected to be COX-1 sparing, which appears to be true on the basis of studies using cloned canine COX enzymes (see Table 29-3). However, specificity is lost at higher concentrations. Deracoxib undergoes extensive hepatic metabolism. At 8 mg/kg (approximately 2 to 8 times the recommended dose [1 to 4 mg/kg]), nonlinear kinetics emerge, increasing the risk of toxicity. As with other NSAIDs, gastrointestinal toxicity occurs with increased doses. The package insert indicates that toxicity occurs at 3 times the dose when a micronized (which differs from the approved product) compound was administered (in a rapidly dissolving capsule) but not when the commercial preparation was administered at the same dose (see Table 29-5). Whether or not derocoxib is more likely than other NSAIDs to reach saturation kinetics is not known. The difference in preparations may have resulted in much more rapid exposure of the gastrointestinal mucosa to drug. The gastrointestinal lesions associated with the micronized material were attributed to a local effect (osmotic, pH, pharmacologic, others) rather than a systemic effect.[205] Dose-dependent increases in blood urea nitrogen were reported when dogs received deracoxib at 3, 4, and 5 times the recommended dose (2 mg/kg); variable renal histologic lesions were reported. The disposition of deracoxib has been described in cats after a single oral dose (see Table 29-4).[206] Safety information in cats was not available at the time of this publication other than at the FDA CVM site (Table 29-6).

As a sulfonamide, deracoxib might be expected to be associated with adverse reactions (but not those typical of antimicrobial sulfonamides), including keratitis sicca.

In a study at least partially funded by the manufacturer, efficacy of deracoxib administered as a single dose (0.3, 1, 3, or 10 mg/kg) was compared with that of carprofen (2.2 mg/kg) in 24 hound dogs. Drugs were administered 30 minutes before induction of chemically induced (urate crystal) synovitis, and lameness indices (including clinical scores, force plate analysis, and joint fluid analysis) were measured for 24 hours after induction. Deracoxib was found to be somewhat more effective at 3 mg/kg (determined to be the minimum effective dose) and more effective than carprofen at 10 mg/kg (not a recommended dose) on the basis of outcome measures for lameness which included lameness scores, pain joint effusions, and pain threshold response[207]; no significant differences were found between carprofen or the placebo group.

Lascelles and coworkers[80] described a series of cases of gastrointestinal perforation associated with deraxocib administration in dogs (n = 29). The mean age was 6.4 ± 3.2 years. Among the more important points of the report was that 55% of the dogs received a dose higher than recommended on the label; and 59% had received, within the previous 24 hours, either a different NSAID or a glucocorticoid. A total of 90% of the dogs had received one or the other and a total of 20% had received both. Of the dogs, 68% either died or were euthanized. The mean dose in dogs receiving the drug for long-term pain management was 3± 1.1 mg/kg/day, ranging from 2.3 to 6.2 mg/kg.

The safety of deracoxib (1.5 mgkg daily) was prospectively compared with that of buffered aspirin and placebo (25 mg/kg orally every 8 hours) in dogs (placebo controlled) based on gastroscopy and clinical scores assessing vomiting and diarrhea.[208] Aspirin-related gastric lesions and vomiting were higher than similar lesions in the deracoxib-treated and placebo-treated groups, beginning with the first endoscopic exam at 6 days.

Etodolac

Etodolac is a pyranocarboxylic acid that has shown potent NSAID activity by inhibiting chondrocyte and synoviocyte biosynthesis of PGE_2 COX-1 to COX-2 ratios vary among studies. The ratio using human cells appears to favor safety,[209] although studies using canine cells[32] reveal the opposite. Ricketts and coworkers[32] reported a COX-1 to COX-2 ratio of only 0.517 compared with 129 for carprofen (study sponsored by carprofen manufacturer). In dogs the drug is rapidly absorbed, with food slowing absorption. Its elimination half-life is approximately 14 hours,[210] which is sufficiently long to allow once-daily dosing. Food may prolong elimination (see Table 29-4). The drug is extensively metabolized, with the majority eliminated in the bile and up to 10% excreted in the urine; enterohepatic elimination is extensive, potentially increasing the risk of gastrointestinal toxicity.[127] Etodolac is marketed as a racemic mixture, although the disposition of the enantiomers has not been well described in animals. Because it is approved for use in humans, much information is available regarding possible side effects in humans. However, in vitro studies indicate pharmacodynamic effects may differ in animals, and extrapolation of information may be inappropriate. Because of its longer half-life and enterohepatic elimination, etodolac may be associated with a greater risk of gastroduodenal ulceration than other COX-2 preferntial drugs. Toxicity studies also suggest that etodolac may not be as safe as other newer NSAIDs, which might be supported by COX ratios in the dog (see Table 29-3). According to the package insert, six of eight dogs developed gastrointestinal erosions and subsequently died after etodolac was administered at five times the recommended dose for 6 to 9 months (see Table 29-5). Five of six dogs developed excessive bleeding when receiving etodolac at the recommended dose, although the duration of therapy was not clear from the package insert. However, clinically, based on field studies, etodolac does not appear to be less safe than the other COX-2 preferential drugs.

Liver disease in dogs such as that associated with carprofen has not been reported in the literature but has been anecdotally reported and has been seen by the author. Etodolac (mean dose of 13.7 mg/kg orally every 24 hours for 28 days) administration did not significantly affect serum T_4, T_3, fT_4, or cTSH concentrations or serum osmolality in healthy random-source mixed breed dogs (n = 19). However, plasma total protein, albumin, and globulin concentrations were decreased by day 14 of administration; decreases were still evident by day 28 of administration, although all concentrations were within normal limits.[118] The effect of etodolac on cartilage metabolism has not been well documented, although one study found it to be associated with more cartilage damage than carprofen.[211] Etodolac has been associated with keratitis sicca. [211a] In a series of cases collected from the manufacturer or surveyed veterinary ophthalmologists, lesions were commonly considered severe, occurred in both eyes more than 50% of the time, with remission occurring in 10 to 15% of animals. Remission was 4 times more likely if treatment duration was less than 6 months.

Etodolac is available of an oral capsule prepration for use in dogs. Despite potential gastrointestinal adverse drug events, when dosed at 10 to 15 mg/kg once daily, etodolac was effective yet safe for controlling lameness associated with hip dysplasia.[212] A clinical trial comparing carprofen and etodolac was previously discussed (see carprofen).[196] Aragon and coworkers[198] ranked etodolac as moderate with regard to scientific evidence of efficacy claims.

Firocoxib

Firocoxib has recently been approved for use in dogs in a chewable tablet form. Its disposition was reported before its approval by McCann and coworkers,[213] who reported on COX-2 selectivity (canine whole blood), pharmacokinetic properties (2 mg/kg intravenously and 8 mg/kg orally) in healthy male and female mixed-breed dogs (n = 21). The IC_{90} for COX-2, according to the monograph, is 0.3 µg/mL, compared with a C_{max} of about 0.5µg/mL at the recommended dose in dogs (Table 29-4). In the manufacturer sponsored study, the COX-1 to COX-2 ratio using canine blood was 384, compared with 6 for carprofen and 12 for deracoxib. Although the volume of distribution is larger than for most NSAIDs, clearance also is rapid, resulting in a relatively short half-life compared with that of other NSAIDs (see Table 29-4). Nonetheless, the drug is administered once a day. The oral bioavailability of firoxocib as listed on the package insert at 5 mg/kg is 38% (variability not reported); as such, care may be indicated in anticipating potential differences in oral bioavailability among animals.*

Firocoxib is approved for use in dogs greater than 3.2 kg (smaller dogs cannot be accurately dosed) as a chewable tablet. The package insert overdose data and its impact on gastssrointestinal toxicity for firocoxib are indicated in Table 29-5. The manufacturer of firocoxib was interested in avoiding an age limit to drug administration, and accordingly, studied firoxocib in juvenile Beagle dogs (Table 29-5). Fatty livers were consistent findings in drug-treated juvenile dogs. In addition to the gastrointestinal effects, one juvenile dog given a dose 3 times that recommended developed juvenile polyarthritis, thrombocytopenia, decreased albumin, and elevated liver enzymes. In a separate study, one dog receiving 3 times the dose was euthanized because of poor clinical condition, although no indication was given as to whether adversity was

*Data on package insert provided among the NSAID may differ depending, in part, on requirements of the FDA. As such, bioavailability data may not be available for all drugs. This may preclude accurate comparisons among drugs.

related to the drug. However, 4 of 12 juvenile dogs receiving 5 times the dose either died (n = 1) or were euthanized (on account of a moribund status) as early as day 38 and as late as day 79; two of the dogs had gastrointestinal ulceration. This data should not be interpreted as a greater risk of toxicity to firocoxib as much as a potential indication that NSAIDs should be avoided in animals 6 months or younger.

For the approval process, efficacy of firocoxib was compared at 8 mg/kg with carprofen (2.2 mg/kg) as the positive control in healthy male Beagles (n = 24; eight per group) using chemically induced (urate) synovitis. The drugs were administered either prophylactically (administration 2 hours before induction of synovitis) or therapeutically (administration 1 hour after induction). Both drugs were effective in controlling pain and inflammation when administered either prophylactically or therapeutically; failure to find a difference between the two NSAIDs was attributed to the variability in the data compared to animal numbers studied. Although a treatment effect was found across time for firocoxib compared with carprofen, superiority of firocoxib compared with carprofen was not sufficient to allow label claims as such. Pollmeier and coworkers,[214] in a manufacturer-sponsored study, reported the results of a multicenter field trial that compared firocoxib (5 mg/kg/day) to carprofen (4 mg/kg/day) using a double-blinded, randomized design in dogs (n = 218) with osteoarthritis. Efficacy was assessed by both owners and veterinarians. Reponse was slightly better for firocoxib at 96% compared with 92% for carprofen.

Meloxicam

Dogs

Structure–activity relationship. Meloxicam, like piroxicam, is a member of the oxicam group of NSAIDs. It is approved for use in tablet and oral suspension forms in the United States, Canada, and Europe in dogs and cats (the injectable form [subcutaneous] only is approved for one time use in cats in the US). The COX-2 to COX-1 ratio for meloxicam, unlike that for piroxicam, favors selective COX-2 inhibition in humans, suggesting that it has a wider margin of safety than most other NSAIDs.[215-218] The drug is more potent (although not necessarily more efficacious) than aspirin, indomethacin, and piroxicam; hence its dose is smaller. In a study partially funded by the manufacturer of meloxicam, using in vitro methods, Kay-Mugford and coworkers[219] determined the ratio of COX-1 and COX-2 activity of meloxicam, tolfenamic acid, carprofen, and ketoprofen using a canine monocyte–macrophage cell line. In this cell line, expression of COX-1 is constitutive, but COX-2 is induced in response to LPS. The COX-1 to COX-2 ratios were more favorable for meloxicam than carprofen (see Table 29-3), which suggests that meloxicam is COX-1 protective in the dog.

Disposition. The plasma concentration–time profile for meloxicam in dogs was described as being comparable to that in humans, in contrast to that of selected other species.[219] Although oral bioavailability is close to 100% in dogs (according to package insert), time to peak concentration is approximately 7 to 8 hours, one of the longest of NSAIDs in dogs (see Table 29-4). Likewise, the elimination half-life is long compared with that of other NSAIDs (both conventional and new) in the dog, with a minimum of 3 days expected before steady state is achieved. A loading dose of 0.2 mg/kg is suggested in dogs, followed by a maintenance dose of 0.1 mg/kg. Cautious clinicians might consider administering the loading dose themselves rather than allowing the client to do so; this reduces the risk that the client will continue to administer the drug at a dose that is higher than appropriate. The package insert also indicates that disposition of meloxicam changes with chronic dosing, with elimination half-life becoming longer. As with most drugs, the selectivity enjoyed with the mechanism of action of this or any selective NSAID is likely to be lost at high doses.[220]

Adverse reactions. The safety profile of meloxicam, as indicated on the package insert, supports its safe use in dogs, although direct comparison with other newer NSAIDs is limited by differences in doses studied (see Table 29-5). Interestingly, in field studies the incidence of vomiting in dogs receiving meloxicam was among the highest of the newer NSAIDs. The safety of meloxicam has been compared with that of carprofen (see the discussion of carprofen). Meloxicam-induced hepatotoxicity has been reported in humans.[221]

The impact of meloxicam (0.1 mg/kg subcutaneously once daily), dexamethasone (0.25 mg/kg subcutaneously twice daily), or the combination of the two on the gastrointestinal mucosa was prospectively compared with that of saline after 3 days of therapy in Beagles (n = 20). Outcome measures included scores collected from five regions of the gastroduodenal region. Scores were greater for the combination-treated group than for the other groups; additionally, dexamethasone was associated with higher scores than either meloxicam or saline. No significant differences in histologic findings were found among groups, although this may reflect a low power for the study. However, the lack of correlation between gross and histologic gastroduodenal lesions is not unusual. Lesions associated with NSAIDs were greater in the pylorus and pyloric antrum compared with other regions, a finding also consistent with other studies.[74]

Gastrointestinal perforation associated with the administration of meloxicam was reported in a series of cases (n = 5).[222] Ages ranged from 2.5 to 11 years. Doses associated with vomiting ranged from a single postoperative dose of 0.1 mg/kg (on day 8) to a high dose of 0.2 mg/kg orally as a single or divided daily dose. Onset of vomiting ranged from as early as day 2 to as late as day 8. Predisposing factors such as glucocorticoid or NSAID administration were not evident. Unidentified underlying gastrointestinal disorders were postulated as possible risk factors.

A single case report has described cutaneous and ocular lesions in a 10-year-old 25-kg mixed-breed dog with a history of atopy receiving meloxicam.[223] Meloxicam (0.1 mg/kg orally once daily) was administered in anticipation of surgery. The patient returned after 3 days of therapy with cutaneous clinical signs consistent with a potential drug reaction and corneal edema. Skin biopsies were collected several days after initial lesions emerged; the patient was treated with glucocorticoids. Skin lesions had resolved by 6 weeks, and ocular lesions persisted.

Therapeutic Use. Meloxicam has been demonstrated to be both safe and effective for treatment of osteoarthritis in dogs.[82,224] The efficacy of meloxicam in treatment of locomotor disorders in dogs compares favorably with that of other NSAIDs in studies supported by the manufacturer.[218,225] In their evidence-based review of clinical trials addressing treatment of osteoarthritis, Aragon and coworkers[198] found meloxicam to be the only drug worthy of the highest level of confidence reported in the study in regards to scientific validity of efficacy claims. Several studies have demonstrated efficacy of meloxicam compared to placebo. Doig and coworkers[224] studied 40 dogs (manufacturer sponsored), and Peterson and Keefe[82] studied 217 dogs with spontaneous osteoarthritis. Duration of therapy was 7 to 14 days, respectively. Placebo effects were reported in up to 38% of animals, underscoring the importance of placebo controls.[82] Meloxicam (0.2 mg/kg every 24 hours) and aspirin (25 mg/kg every 12 hours) were compared in a clinical trial using a crossover (randomization not indicated) design in dogs (n = 12) with experimentally induced (cranial cruciate rupture) osteoarthritis of the stifle. Animals were treated for 21 days; outcome measures included measurement of PGE_2, thromboxane B2 (TXB2) in blood and synovial fluid, and endoscopically collected gastric mucosa. Both aspirin and meloxicam administration significantly suppressed PGE_2 concentrations in blood and synovial fluid. Aspirin, but not meloxicam, suppressed TXB2 concentration in blood and PGE_2 in gastric mucosa, leading the authors to conclude that meloxicam behaves in vivo as COX-1 sparing.[226]

KEY POINT 29-18 The Food and Drug Administration has indicated that meloxicam should not be administered in cats more than as a single dose.

Meloxicam also has been compared with opioid analgesics for control of perioperative pain. Mathews and coworkers[229] compared the safety and efficacy of preoperative administration of a single dose of meloxicam, ketoprofen, and butorphanol in dogs (n = 36; 12 per group) undergoing abdominal surgery. The butorphanol-treated group received a second dose immediately after surgery. Overall efficacy was rated as good or excellent in 9 of 12 dogs that received either meloxicam or ketoprofen compared with only 1 of 12 that received butorphanol. Analgesic effects of meloxicam were maintained for 20 hours postoperatively. Budsberg and coworkers[230] compared the analgesic effects of meloxicam (0.2 mg/kg intravenously) and butorphanol (0.1 mg/kg) administered immediately after surgery (at incision closure) for control of postoperative pain in client-owned dogs (n = 40) presenting with rupture of the cranial cruciate ligament. Outcome was based on evidence of pain (visual analog scale) and serum cortisol concentrations for a 24-hour period. Differences in pain response did not emerge between the treatment groups until 8 hours later, with the meloxicam-treated group exhibiting less pain 8 to 11 hours after extubation. Failure to detect a significant difference between treatment groups earlier than 8 hrs may have reflected low overall scores for both groups coupled with low animal numbers (i.e., poor power of the study). Overall serum cortisol was less in the meloxicam-treated group compared with butorphanol group. Otherwise, significant differences could not be demonstrated. Using a model of acute inflammation (intraarticular injection of calcium pyrophosphate dehydrate), the effects of meloxicam (0.2 mg/kg intravenously for 3 doses) on proteoglycan biosynthesis in vitro and ex vivo were compared with indomethacin (0.5 mg/kg intravenously for 3 doses). Indomethacin is known to contribute to joint injury in humans in part by inhibiting sulphated proteoglycans., Neither drug contributed to joint damage, but pain and exudates were decreased more by meloxicam than indomethacin.[231]

Cats

The disposition of meloxicam has been studied in cats. Meloxicam is among the NSAIDs characterized by a shorter half-life in cats than in dogs (see Table 29-4). It is one of the few NSAIDs that appear to be well tolerated in cats. Its use in Canada for several years predated its approval for use in cats in the United States. Meloxicam is the only NSAID approved for use in cats in the United States, with the approved use limited to perioperative single dosing. Meloxicam is approved in cats outside the United States for single dose administration as both an injectable and oral product.

Despite its apparent safety compared with other NSAIDs, the therapeutic margin of meloxicam is relatively narrow. The association between renal disease and NSAIDs, including meloxicam, in cats was discussed previously. Cats do not tolerate multiple doses greater than or equal to 0.3 mg/kg, and gastric ulceration and death have occurred at three to six times the normal dose for 10 days. Several studies support the efficacy of meloxicam in cats. In one study the optimal dose of meloxicam to prevent endotoxin-induced fever in cats was 0.3 mg/kg.[232] The need for a long-term safe yet effective analgesic in cats was supported by a symposium that focused on osteoarthritis in cats.[233] The safety of meloxicam in cats in regards to renal disease was previously addressed (Table 29-6). A prevalence of degenerative joint disease was found in 34% of cats (n = 218), with previous reports placing the prevalence as high as 90%.

A number of clinical trials have addressed efficacy of meloxicam in cats. In cats subjected to ovariohysterectomy, meloxicam, carprofen, ketoprofen, and tolfenamic acid all were effective in controlling postoperative pain, with 10% of cats in each group requiring opioid rescue.[203] In a comparison of carprofen (4.4 mg/kg subcutaneously) and meloxicam (0.3 mg/kg subcutaneously) in 80 cats undergoing ovariohysterectomy, no difference was found in control of postoperative pain; one cat in the carprofen group and two in the meloxicam group required opioid rescue.[228]

The efficacy of meloxicam for treatment of osteoarthritis in cats was reported in abstract form[233] on the basis of a prospective crossover pilot study (n = 7; mean age 14 years). Cats were treated with either 0.05 mg/kg meloxicam orally for 5 days (first dose 0.1 mg/kg) or placebo (neither washout period nor randomization described). A tendency toward improvement has been described. Lascelles and coworkers[227] prospectively compared the efficacy of meloxicam (0.3 mg/kg orally, followed by 0.1 mg/kg for 4 days orally) to ketoprofen (1 mg/kg orally once daily for 5 days) for treatment of acute or chronic pain associated with locomotor disease in cats (n =69). Although both drugs were effective in reducing clinical signs associated with pain, meloxicam was considered more palatable.

Robenacoxib

Robenacoxib is approved for use in companion animals outside the United States.[45,234] The disposition of robenacoxib has been described in dogs after single-dose administration of 1 mg/kg either orally (fasted or fed), intravenously, or subcutaneously[235] (see Table 29-4). Isoform preference in studies supported by the manufacturer indicate a COX-1 to COX-2 ratio (95% inhibition) of 450 using whole blood assays in cats.[45] The disposition of robenacoxib in cats at 2 mg/kg intravenously has been reported.[45] Data from the ex vivo and pharmacokinetic studies were subsequently integrated with a model of inflammation in cats (n=10), resulting in a recommended dose 2 mg/kg dose every 12 hours.

Vedaprofen

Vedaprofen is marketed outside the United States for use in dogs as an oral gel preparation. A document provided by the manufacturer indicates that the racemic mixture is approximately 8 times more potent toward COX-2 than COX-1, with the majority of activity exihibited by the S enantiomer. The pharmacokinetics of vedaprofen, including its enantiomers, are available in the dog (see Table 29-4)[236] after administration either intravenously or as an oral gel preparation. Although volume of distribution was not provided, the elimination (disappearance) half-life was 12 to 17 hours, depending on oral versus intravenous administration. Bioavailability of the gel preparation was near complete. The S and R enantiomers are present generally at a ratio of 1:1, with variability ranging as low as 0.5 (toward the end of the 24-hour dosing interval) and as high as 3.10 (at 2 to 3 hours) after single dosing. After oral multiple dosing for 14 days, the R:S ratio averaged about 1.8 throughout the 24-hour dosing interval. The higher concentration of the R enantiomer appears to reflect more rapid clearance of the S enantiomer (see Table 29-4). The dispositionof vedaprofen did not appear to change substantially with 14 days of dosing.[236] The efficacy and safety of vedaprofen were compared with that of meloxicam, which was used as the control during the approval process. Differences could not be detected for either safety or efficacy. Gastrointestinal side effects were reported in approximately 11 to 12% for both groups despite treatment for approximately 15 days (acute) and 40 days (chronic). Both drugs were effective in both acute (approximately 88%) and chronic (approximately 67%).[237]

CYCLOOXYGENASE-1–SPARING DRUGS APPROVED FOR USE IN HUMAN MEDICINE

Celecoxib

Celecoxib appears to be COX-1 sparing in the dog (see Table 29-3).Its disposition has been studied in Beagles after single and multiple oral dosing, using different (a solution and solid) dosing forms, with and without food.[238] Celecoxib metabolism in dogs is characterized by polymorphism: Paulson and coworkers[41] described dogs that metabolize the drug poorly (poor metabolizers [PMs]) compared with efficient metabolizers (EMs). The elimination half-life of the drug in PMs is approximately 4 times as long as that in EMs (see Table 29-4). The drug is normally extensively metabolized (principally hydroxylation followed by oxidation). In both EMs and PMs, approximately 80% of the drug is eliminated in the feces. In EMs disposition does not appear to change with chronic (1-year) dosing. Administration of the drug with a fatty meal increased both the C_{max} and the bioavailability. The disposition of celecoxib also has been studied in normal Greyhounds after single (12.5 mg/kg) and multiple dosing. Decreases occurred in C_{max} (22%), elimination half-life (shorter), and area under the curve (40%) after 10 days of dosing at 12.5 mg/kg per day.[239] The pharmacodynamic and toxic effects of celecoxib have not been well studied in the dog.

Rofecoxib

Rofecoxib is described as a COX-2–selective drug in humans, but no information is available regarding its selectivity in dogs. Its disposition has been studied in dogs (see Table 29-4).[241] The drug is cleared after oral administration primarily by biliary excretion after extensive hepatic metabolism to hydroxyl and glucuronide metabolites, with some urinary excretion.[241] The effects of rofecoxib (0.5 mg/kg/day orally) on the canine gastrointestinal tract were compared endoscopically to those of the dual-acting NSAID licofelone (2.5 mg/kg orally twice daily) and placebo after 56 days of dosing.[240] Whereas no endoscopic lesions were evident for either the placebo or licofelone, rofecoxib was associated with lesions in both the gastric (six of seven) and duodenal (four of seven) areas. This occurred despite a progressive decline in mean plasma drug concentrations for rofecoxib across time: Baseline concentrations were 110.1 ± 85.8 (2 days) compared with study end concentrations of 65.3 ± 49.1 ng/mL (56 days). Concentrations of licofelone also decreased: 761.0 ± 413.8 at baseline compared with 307 ± 106.5 ng/mL at study end.[240]

Nimesulide

Nimesulide is a COX-2–selective drug approved for use in humans that also appears to act as a COX-1–sparing drug in dogs.[31,242] The disposition of nimesulide has been studied in dogs (n = 8-10) after single-dose administration of 5 mg/kg intravenously, intramuscularly, and orally and after 5 days of once-daily administration of the same dose (see Table 29-4).[242] The terminal elimination half-life after intramuscular administration was longer than that after intravenous administration, indicating a flip-flop model for this route. On the basis of the integration of pharmacokinetics and pharmacodynamics, the authors determined an effective concentration (EC_{50}) to be 2 to 6 μg/mL, which would be achieved at the studied dose, with some inhibition of COX-1 also occurring.[243] However, the study was performed on Beagles, which may not be generally applicable to the canine population at large. The safety of nimesulide has not apparently been studied in dogs.

MISCELLANEOUS NONSTEROIDAL ANTIINFLAMMATORY DRUGS

Indomethacin

Indomethacin is an NSAID that was developed specifically to abate the inflammatory response to the indolic hormones serotonin and tryptophan.[6] As a powerful antiinflammatory, it became a standard for comparison with other drugs. In humans toxicities are not serious, but CNS side effects are undesirable.[6] The incidence of gastrointestinal hemorrhage after administration of indomethacin at doses of 2 to 5 mg/kg precludes its clinical utility in dogs. In one study all dogs developed melena within 1 week of receiving 2 mg/kg daily; 60% of these animals had gastric ulcers.[244] Interestingly, pretreatment with pure 5-lipoxygenase inhibitors prevents the ulcerogenic effects of indomethacin.[2]

Acetaminophen

Acetaminophen (paracetamol) is a coal tar analgesic used in human medicine as an effective alternative to aspirin for control of fever and pain. Classically, it is recognized to have poor antiinflammatory activity, although this view has become more controversial.[245] Although often classified as an NSAID, its mechanism does not involve inhibition of COX. Rather, acetaminophen interferes with the endoperoxide intermediates (PGG_2, PGH_2) of AA conversion. Inhibition of a new isoenzym, COX-3, has been suggested, but studies suggest that this isoform is actually a variant of COX-1.[9] Concentrations necessary to inhibit this variant are high, leading some investigators to suggest that its efficacy as an analgesic and antipyretic (but not antiinflammatory) reflect its effects on PGH synthases and glutathione-dependent PGE_2 synthases.[17] The relatively weak antiinflammatory activity of acetaminophen has been attributed to the high concentrations of peroxides that occur in peripheral inflammatory lesions but may reflect limited COX enzyme activity. Acetaminophen may be more effective against inflammatory conditions in the CNS.

The major disadvantage of acetaminophen use in veterinary patients is the narrow safety margin in cats.[140] The drug is normally conjugated with glucuronide and to a lesser degree with sulfate. Drug that is not conjugated is metabolized by phase I microsomal enzymes to cytotoxic oxidative metabolites (see Chapter 4). Intracellular glutathione normally scavenges the metabolites, but in the case of overdose or glucuronide deficiency (as with the cat), the formation of toxic metabolites overwhelms the glutathione-scavenging system. In cats methemoglobinemia is the most common indication of toxicity, although centrolobular hepatic necrosis may also occur. Treatment of acetaminophen toxicity includes administration of antioxidants, including *N*-acetylcysteine, a precursor of glutathione, and ascorbic acid (vitamin C).[246-248] The administration of cimetidine, a microsomal enzyme inhibitor, will reduce the formation of toxic metabolites and will result in clinical improvement if given within 48 hours of acetaminophen administration.[249,250] The use of SAMe has been demonstrated scientifically and has been reported as clinically effective in a case report.[251] A potential advantage of SAMe is response despite late administration.

Acetaminophen toxicity in cats has been retrospectively described in a series (n = 17) of cases.[252] Treatments consisted of emesis induced by apomorphine or xylazine, activated charcoal, intravenous balanced crystalloids, intravenous *N*-acetylcysteine (140 mg/kg, followed by 70 mg/kg every 3 to 6 hours), and ascorbic acid (30 to 100 mg/kg orally or parenterally every 4 to 6 hours). Cimetidine was administered to three cats and methylene blue with dexamethasone to one. The survival rate was 82%. Responding cats were normal within 48 hours of treatment. Median acetaminophen dose in surviving animals was 170 mg/kg (highest 400 mg/kg) versus 100 mg/kg in nonsurvivors (highest dose 170 mg/kg), suggesting dose was not a determinant of outcome.Ten of 12 surviving cats were treated within 14 hours of ingestion. In four of the five deaths, *N*-acetylcysteine was not begun until 17 hours after acetaminophen exposure, emphasizing the importance of early treatment.

Acetaminophen can interfere (false increase) with glucose determination on certain bedside glucometers.[253]

In humans, according to the American College of Rheumatology, acetaminophen remains the first choice for treatment of patients with osteoarthritis because of its efficacy, safety, and cost. NSAIDs are recommended only after acetaminophen has failed. Among the NSAIDs, it is characterized as among the most able to penetrate the CNS, thus potentially providing better analgesia. Acetaminophen (15 mg/kg every 8 hours) may be as effective as aspirin for the control of postoperative pain and inflammation in dogs. An extended-relief formulation has proved useful (20 to 30 mg/kg every 8 to 12 hours) at a longer interval.[254] Acetaminophen also can be combined with opioids,with a commercial preparation available with codeine (dose based on codeine at 1 to 2 mg/kg orally every 8 to 12 hours). Acetaminophen appears to be safe in dogs. At daily doses of 0.5 g every 8 hours (average weight 18 kg, or 28 mg/kg), acetaminophen causes no clinical signs of adverse drug effects.[245] Other studies, however, have shown that adverse reactions (e.g., depression, methemoglobinemia, vomiting) can occur at higher (100 mg/kg) doses.[255, 256] In another study, 900 mg/kg intravenously caused fulminant hepatic failure in dogs.[257]

Leukotrienes and Their Inhibition

Leukotriene Formation

Although COX has been the primary target of NSAIDs, the complex role of lipoxygenases in the inflammatory process increasingly is being recognized and targeted. Further, improved gastrointestinal safety as a result of inhibition of leukotrienes supports their potential use. Goodman and coworkers[258] recently reviewed the role of LTs and their inhibition in dogs and cats.

Lipoxygenase enzymes located within cells can also metabolize AA to inflammatory mediators, with lipoxygnases 5, 12, and 17 apparently being the most clinically relevant.[7,8,17,259] Lipoxygenase enzymes are not as ubiquitous in the body as the COX enzymes, but the enzymes do vary in tissues location. Lipoxygenase-5 enzymes are found primarily in cells of myeloid origin, including macrophages (and all tissues in which they are found) as well as B-lymphocytes. The initial product formed

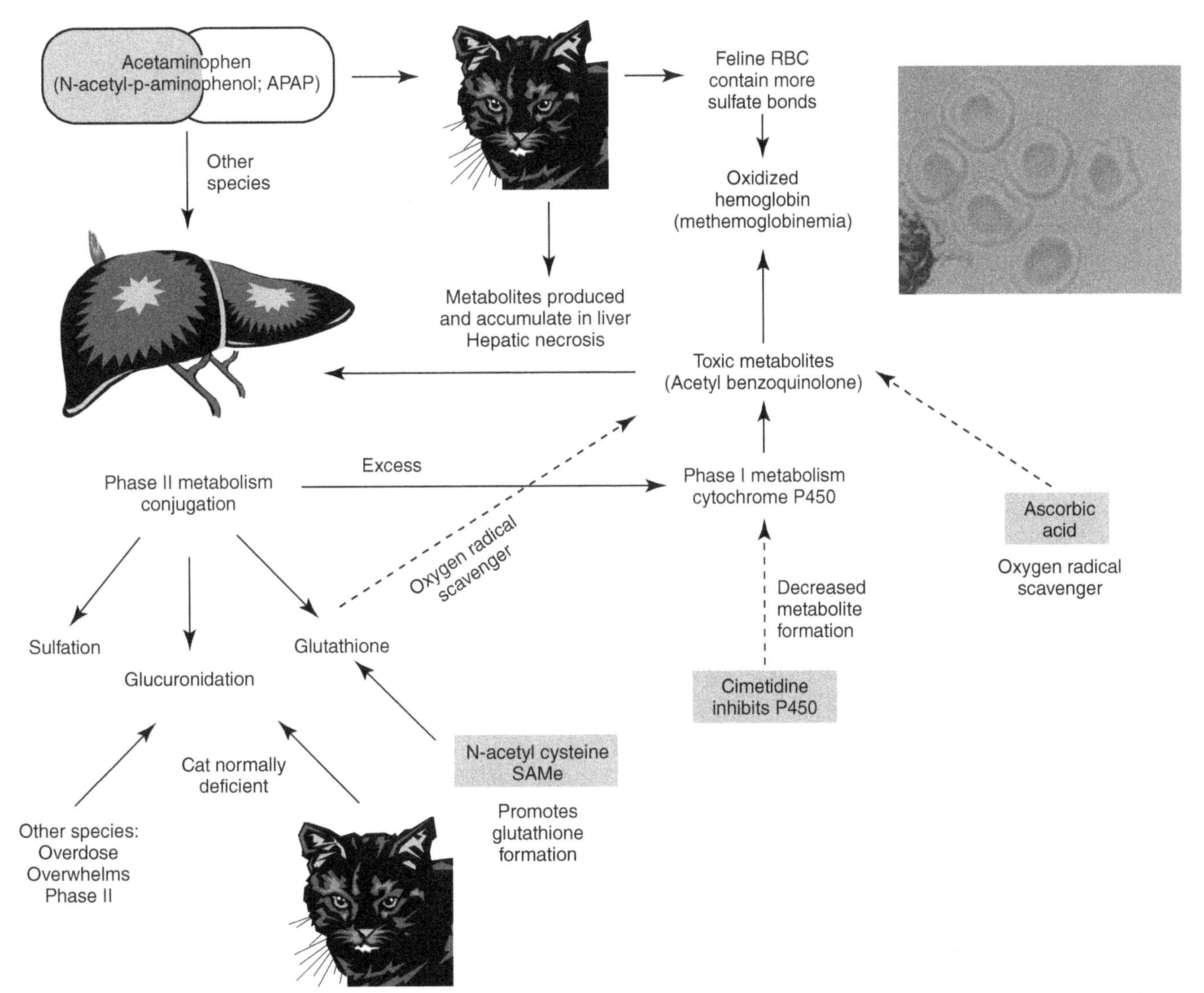

Figure 29-10 Acetaminophen toxicity reflects a cytotoxic type A adverse reaction. Because cats are deficient in glucuronidation, phase II metabolism is easily overwhelmed, and drug is shunted more aggressively back into phase I metabolism. The same process occurs in dogs after an overdose. The products of phase I metabolism are reactive and cause destruction of tissues (liver and red blood cells). Glutathione, an important phase II scavenger, prevents damage but is easily depleted in cats. Supplementation in the form of *N*-acetylcysteine can decrease damage. Cimetidine is useful because it decreases phase I metabolism and thus the formation of phase I metabolites.

from its action on AA is HPETE, followed by LT A4 (Figure 29-10; see also Figures 29-1 and 29-2). Further conversion (by way of hydroxylase) of LTA4 produces LTB4, a very potent chemotactant, and LTC4 (by way of reduced glutathione) or LTD4 (γ-glutamyltranspeptidase). From these, LTD4 is further converted to LTE4. LTs C, D, and E are referred to as cysteinyl-LTs (see Figure 29-2).[22] A second lipoxygenase enzyme, lipoxygenase-12, occurs in platelets, where it catalyzes the formation of 12-HPETE.[7,22] A third enzyme, lipoxygenase-15, catalyzes the formation of lipoxins. In contrast to LTs, lipoxins (LXA_4 and LXB_4) are characterized by *anti-inflammatory* activity.[260] Lipoxin formation can occur when 5-lipoxygenase products interact with 12- lipoxygenase or 15- lipoxygenase.[261] Lipoxins are described as counterregulatory, with a particular focus on those inflammatory responses that resolve inflammation.[260] LTs act through membrane receptors located on inflammatory and other cells. Receptors are linked to G proteins, increasing intracellular calcium and decreasing cAMP (see Figure 29-1). For example, LTB4 binds to BLT1 and 2 subreceptor types located in inflammatory cells, whereas cysteinyl LTs (C-E) bind to CysLT1 and 2 subreceptor types located in eosinophils, macrophages, and bronchial smooth muscle.

Leukotrienes in Health and Disease

With the exception of lipoxins, each of the lipoxygenase-catalyzed products is a potent mediator of inflammation. At picomolar concentrations, they are effective in the activation, recruitment, migration, and adhesion of immune cells.[22] LTs and other selected lipoxygenase products modulate lymphocyte function.[8] LTB4 increases production and release of inflammatory cytokines, including activation of NF-kB (transcription factor responsible for expression of proinflammatory cytokins), and expression of TNF-alpha and IL-1β. In the cartilage these cytokines increase expression of MMPs.[18] Inhibition of 5-lipoxygenase reduces expression of the cytokines, including TNF-alpha.[22] In addition to their effect on leukocytes, the cysteinyl LTs are extremely spasmogenic, causing bronchoconstriction (being 100 times more potent than histamine) in the lungs and exacerbation of ulcerogenic effects in the gastrointestinal tract. The cysteinyl LTs are important mediators in hypersensitivity reactions. They are particularly effective chemoattractants for eosinophils; as such, they play important roles in a number of inflammatory and allergic diseases.[258] LTB4 most common is associated with inflammation associated with inflammatory bowel lesions; colonic epithelials cells are able to produce LTB4. A potential role for lipoxygenase in cancer also is emerging: Lipoxygenase-5 is overexpressed in cancer cells; upregulation in pancreatic cancer suggests a potential therapeutic role for lipoxygenase inhibitors.[24,258,262] The role of LTs in eosinophil signaling and chronic (allergic) inflammatory diseases is discussed in Chapter 31.

KEY POINT 29-19 Although less ubiquitous in the body, leukotrienes also represent a balance of proinflammatory and antiinflammatory signals.

A potential sequela of COX blockade by NSAIDs is shunting of unused AA to the lipoxygenase pathway, resulting in increased production of LTs from AA that would have otherwise been metabolized to PG products.[8] For example, aspirin hypersensitivity has been associated with the diversion of AA from the PG to the LT (5-lipoxygenase) pathway and the production of mediators that are more inflammatory than the products of PGH synthetase.[10,22] Aspirin hypersensitivity also has been attributed to the loss of PGs that might otherwise have specifically inhibited the formation of LTs. The adverse reactions of NSAIDs thus reflect not only loss of PGs but also augmentation of LT synthesis.[8] Examples include exacerbation of bronchoconstriction and increasing ulcerogenicity of NSAIDs. Newer NSAIDs that preferentially target COX-2 are not characterized by aspirin hypersensitivity, presumably because AA can yet be metabolized to PGs by way of COX-1.

Lipoxygenase Inhibition

Originally, studies indicated that NSAIDs were not capable of inhibiting LT synthesis. However, the antiinflammatory efficacy of some of the NSAIDs (e.g., ketoprofen)[263] has been attributed, in part, to inhibition of lipoxygenase and thus prevention of LT formation.[6] However, the ability of NSAIDs to inhibit 5-lipoxygenase is controversial.[8] More recently, dual-acting NSAIDs, which impair COX-1 and -2 and lipoxygenases, have been approved. These include tepoxalin, which was initially studied in humans, but approved only for use in dogs. The class of di-tert-butylphenol antiinflammatory agents have the added advantage of antioxidant (phenolic properties) and radical-scavenging properties.[22] These include tebufelone, darbufelone, and licofelone. Finally, the effects of LTs can be inhibited at the level of the receptor. LT-receptor antagonists include zafirlukast and montelukast (Figure 29-11).

Lipoxygenase Inhibitors

Zileuton is a potent, selective 5-lipoxygenase inhibitor. It is the only drug of this class approved for use in the United States. Use of these drugs has largely been limited by hepatotoxicity; further, efficacy has been limited.

Dual-Acting Nonsteroidal Antiinflammatory Drugs

Despite the advantages of NSAIDs that COX-1–sparing drugs offer, the need for improved gastrointestinal tolerance continues. Because the formation of LTs from AA that might otherwise have been metabolized to PGs appears to contribute to the toxicity (gastrointestinal, repiratory, and other) of NSAIDs (conventional more so than newer drugs), a drug with both COX and lipoxygenase inhibitory effects has been the target of the pharmaceutical industry for some time. However, the presence of an iron atom in the structure of COX or lipoxygenase required that such drugs be redox active in their mechanism. Therefore these drugs tended to inhibit other redox-active enzyme systems, including those in the liver. Consequently, hepatotoxicy has limited the use of dual-acting drugs. Two drugs have been studied in human medicine for their dual actions: tepoxalin and licofelone. The latter is an AA substrate and as such acts as a competitive inhibitor of COX and lipoxygenase without redox activity;[81] it is not clear whether tepoxalin similarly avoids redox activity. Neither drugs target lipoxygenase-12 or -15, and thus minimally affect lipoxin formation, further improving potential gastrointestinal tolerance. Further, in the cardiovascular system, because both COX-1 and COX-2 (prostacyclin and thromboxane formation) are inhibited, thrombembolic balance should not be disrupted.

In addition to enhanced safety, enhanced efficacy of dual-acting NSAIDs toward inflammatory diseases should be anticipated. As such has been demonstrated for licofelone in experimentally induced osteoarthritis in dogs. Not only are LT and PG formation decreased, but also formation of proinflammatory cytokines is decreased. Their ability to inhibit both COX and lipoxygenase may result in synergistic activity in the control of inflammation.[264] Preliminary data suggest that dual inhibitors may slow the progression of osteoarthritis.[265] Because of their potential enhanced efficacy and safety, dual inhibiting NSAIDs have been referred to as a class of breakthrough NSAIDs.[22] Indications for dual inhibitors include osteoarthritis, the chronic inflammatory allergic diseases asthma and atopy, and chronic inflammatory bowel disease.

Tepoxalin. Among the dual-acting NSAIDs, only tepoxalin has been approved for use in animals. This drug was being investigated in humans, but pharmacokinetics (not safety) precluded further development.[17] It is a potent antiinflammatory and analgesic pyrazole derivative that also inhibits production of IL-1 and suppresses NFkB activation and dependent gene expression.[17] Its dual inhibitory effect has been demonstrated in dogs. For example, tepoxalin inhibited COX-1, COX-2, and lipoxygenase-5 in synovial fluids (stifle) of dogs with osteoarthritis.[266,267] Tepoxalin, but not firocoxib or meloxicam, inhibited TXA2 in canine blood compared with baseline.[267] Its disposition has been reported in both dogs and cats (see Table 29-4). In dogs tepoxalin is approved

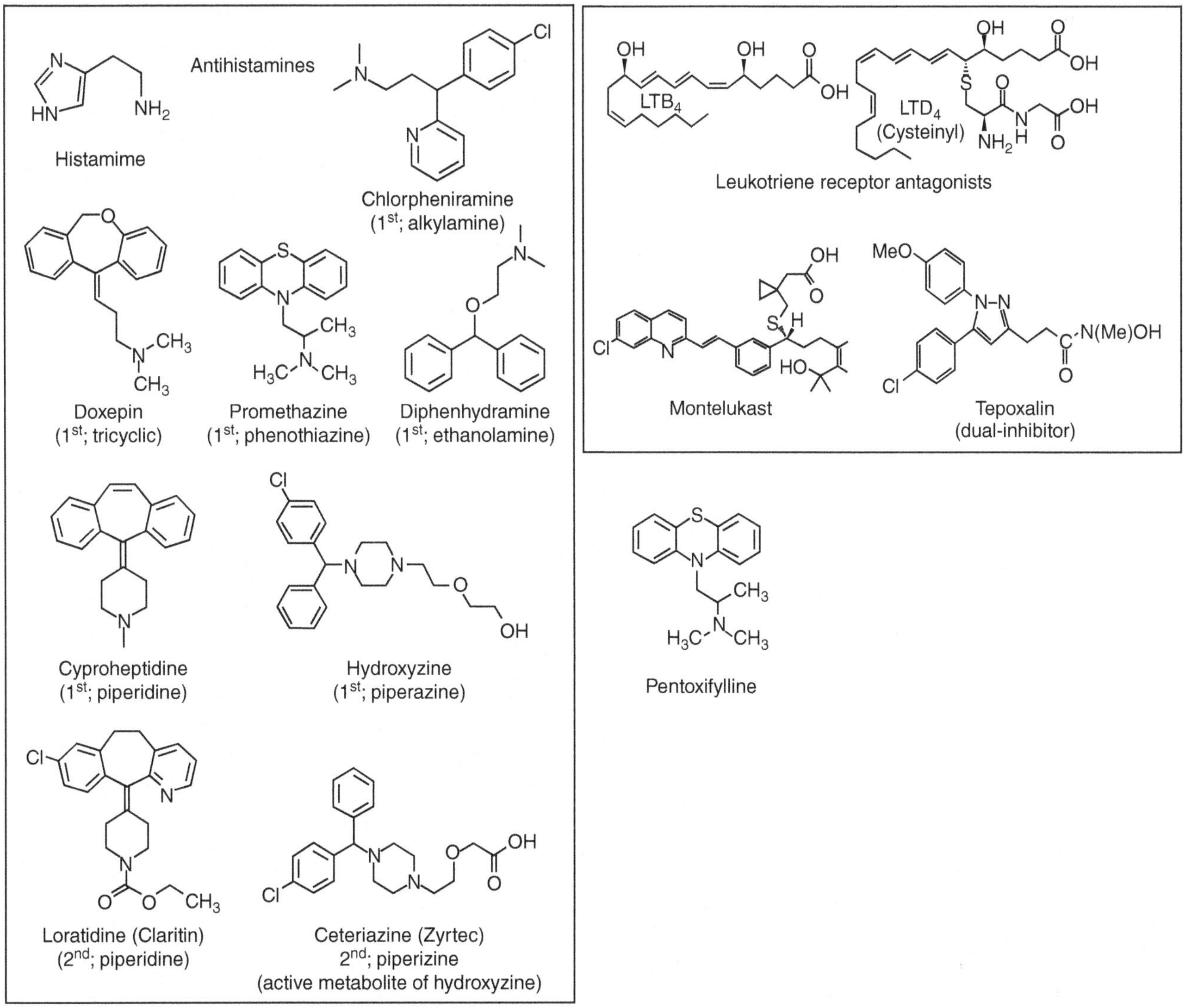

Figure 29-11 Structures of selected drugs used to treat various aspects of inflammation. Antihistamines are generally structurally similar to histamine (upper left).

as a tablet that rapidly disintegrates in the oral cavity, with absorption nonetheless occurring in the intestinal tract. Food enhances oral absorption.[127] Tepoxalin undergoes hepatic metabolism. It is converted to at least one major metabolite whose activity contributes substantially to its clinical effect in part because its half-life is substantially longer than that of the parent compound. Both the parent compound and its active metabolite are highly protein bound. Chronic administration does not appear to alter either the C_{max} or the elimination half-life of either the parent compound or the active metabolite (USP).[127] Essentially all drugs or metabolites, either as parent compound or metabolites, are eliminated in the feces. Feeding appears to increase absorption. The toxicity data generated for the approval of tepoxalin suggest that it should be among the safest of the NSAIDs recently approved for use in dogs (see Table 29-4), although gastrointestinal toxicity can occur. Its safety is supported by the study of Goodman and coworkers.[21] Gastric and pyloric ulcers were monitored endoscopically in dogs (n = 6) treated with tepoxalin, firocoxib, or placebo for 7 days. Animals were studied using a randomized crossover design. Eicosanoids were determined in plasma and lesion margins, and lesions were scored. The firocoxib lesions were larger than placebo or tepoxalin lesions despite the fact that tepoxalin prostaglandin concentrations in the mucosa were lower than in either group. Safety appears to reflect blockade of LTs whose vasoconstrictive and neutrophil chemotaxis, adhesion, and degranulation effects are necessary for mucosal erosion.[258] Agnello and coworkers[266] demonstrated tepoxalin inhibition of PGE_2 and LTB4 in the gastric mucosa of dogs. Despite its impact on both COX pathways, in a manufacturer-sponsored study, tepoxalin did not cause significant changes in hemostatic or renal function tests when administered (10 mg/kg orally) to young, healthy dogs (n = 8; 4 placebo) before surgery. Tests of renal function (serum blood urea nitrogen, creatinine and urine gamma glutamyl transferase [GGT] creatinine ratios) were studied for 48 hrs. Hemostatic tests included buccal mucosal bleeding time, as well as bleeding at the site of (experimental) surgical incision. The power of the study was not addressed. In a different study, tepoxalin did not alter renal function when administered with with angiotensin-converting enzyme inhibitors for up to 28 days.[258]

KEY POINT 29-20 Dual-acting inhibitors might be expected to be more efficacious toward some inflammatory conditions, particularly those associated with allergies, compared with nonsteroidal antiinflammatory drugs.

Tepoxalin also has been studied in cats. Whereas tepoxalin was well tolerated in cats when administered at 100 mg/kg once daily for 3 consecutive days, saturation kinetics occurred with two doses of 60 mg/kg 4 hours apart. Signs suggestive of CNS adverse drug events occurred (drunkenlike state), a response not recorded in any other species. Tepoxalin is a potent antipyretic agent in cats at doses between 5 and 10 mg/kg and provides analgesia at least equivalent to that of butorphanol at 10 mg/kg for onychectomy.[268]

The action of tepoxalin as a dual inhibitor might render it useful for control of pain or inflammation typical of other NSAIDs. This includes a potential added advantage for treatment of chronic allergic diseases for which LTs play a role in cellular signaling. However, preoperative use of tepoxalin may not be prudent, particularly in animals at risk for hemostasis problems. Its postoperative use might be considered. Bosmans and coworkers[269] compared the combination of tepoxaline and buprenorphine to buprenorphine alone during the 24-hour period after cruciate repair in dogs (n = 20; 10 per group). Animals were studied using a parallel randomized, blinded design. Pain was assessed using visual analog scales and a multifactorial pain scale. No statistical differences could be demonstrated for either control of pain or side effects.

Licofelone. Licofelone impairs PGE production in a similar manner to conventional NSAIDs, but unlike other NSAIDs, it also prevents the formation of LTB4. Although licofelone has not been approved for use in dogs, its pharmacodynamic effects have been studied in dogs.[240] Licofelone appears to have potent antioxidative properties.[269a] Its effects on the canine gastrointestinal tract (2.5 mg/kg orally twice daily) as measured endoscopically were negligible to those of rofecoxib (see the discussion of rofecoxib) after 56 days of treatment with either drug. In that study, as with rofecoxib, concentrations of licofelone also decreased across time. Baseline concentrations were 761.0 ± 413.8 compared with 307 ± 106.5 ng/mL at study end.[240] The drug's safety was explained in part because of decreased bioavailability at high doses but also because of prevention of lipoxygenase.[2] Licofelone has been found effective in the treatment of experimentally induced arthritis in the dog.[264]

Leukotriene Receptor Antagonists

Zafirlukast and montelukast are competitive cysLT-1 receptor antagonists (LAR) approved for use to treat human asthma. However, their use increasingly is being expanded to treatment of a variety of chronic allergic inflammatory diseases. Interestingly, their use might be considered in combination with NSAIDs to reduce the risk of gastrointestinal toxicity. The currently available LARs are available only for oral administration. Disposition information is not available for dogs or cats. In humans the drugs are rapidly and nearly completely absorbed. Metabolism of zafirlukast is by CYP2C9 and for montelukast by CYP3A4 and CYP29C. Metabolites are not active. Half-lives in humans are 10 hours (zafirlukast) and 3 to 6 hours (montelukast). Maximum efficacy may require 2 to 4 weeks, although an initial response may be evident within several days. The drugs are generally very safe, probably reflecting the limited effects of LTs in the body.[270]

Pentoxifylline

Pentoxifylline is a methylxanthine derivative of theobromine with minimal bronchodilator activity but with clinically apparent rheologic effects.[271] It is used to treat human patients with claudication associated with chronic occlusive arterial disease. Mechanisms do not include vasodilation or cardiac stimulatory effects. Its rheologic effects appear to reflect increased flexibility of red blood cells and reduced blood viscosity.[272]

The disposition of pentoxifylline is complex, with hepatic metabolism to at least seven metabolites, two of which (I and V) are responsible for most of the pharmacologic effects.[273] Pentoxifylline inhibits the complement cascade, neutrophil degranulation, and cytokine production. Among the cytokines, inhibition of TNF-alpha may be particularly important to its efficacy.[274] IL-1 and IL-6 also are inhibited, as is expression of adhesions molecules. Pentoxifylline also increases fibroblast collagenases, decreases collagen, fibronectin, and glycosaminoglycan production.[274] Inhibition of phosphodiesterase contributes to its antinflammatory effects.

The disposition of the drug has been studied in normal dogs.[275] After a dose of 30 mg/kg orally and 8 mg/kg intravenously (n = 5 dogs), pentoxifylline and its metabolites are characterized by an elimination half-life of 125 ± 192 and 450 ± 533 minutes, respectively, suggesting slow absorption. Peak concentrations were 41 ± 46 and 40 ± 32 µg/mL for intravenous and oral administration, respectively. Bioavailability was 76 ± 78%. No side effects occurred in any dog at this dose. Although therapeutic concentrations have been recommended in humans, this is based on the parent compound. However, therapeutic ranges should be based on both the parent drug and its most active metabolites.

In human patients inflammatory conditions for which pentoxifylline has been used include contact dermatitis, systemic vasculitis, and sepsis syndromes.[271] However, for the latter indication (septic shock), one study demonstrated increased risk of mortality in septic dogs treated with pentoxifylline as a constant intravenous infusion, presumably because of decreased endotoxin clearance.[276] Pentoxifylline was able to decrease the extent of esophageal stricture induced by erosive esophagitis.[277] Pentoxifylline increasingly is being used to treat dermatolgic disorders in humans.[274] The drug has been used to treat Collie dermatomyositis, although animals probably benefit as much from the antiinflammatory effects as from the rheologic effects.

KEY POINT 29-21 The anti–tumor necrosis factor effects of pentoxifylline warrant consideration of its use for treatment or prevention of a variety of inflammatory conditions, ranging from life-threatening septic shock to nonresponsive inflammatory bowel disease.

Antihistamines

Histamine in Health and Disease

Histamine is a low-molecular-weight amine, synthesized from histidine by its decarboxylation. Histidine decarboxylase is ubiquitous in the body, occuring in the CNS, gastric parietal cells, mast cells, and basophils. Upon its formation histamine is stored. Most histamine is stored bound to heparin in granules located in either mast cells or their circulatory counterparts, basophils. Histamine is not the sole mediator of clinical relevance located in mast cells. Because histamine release occurs by mast cell degranulation, it is accompanied by the release of other mediators, including those preformed and stored in granules (e.g., serotonin) and those synthesized in situ (e.g., AA products). Currently, four histamine subreceptors have been identified. The H_1 receptors couple to G proteins, activating the PLC–IP3–Ca^{2+} pathway [G&G].[278] H_2 receptors link to Gs, activating the adenylyl cyclase cAMP pathway. Both H_3 and H_4 receptors are inhibitory toward adenylyl cyclase; 35% or more homology between the two complicates pharmacologic distinction.

The impact of antihistamines is complex but somewhat predictable based on the location and impact of each receptor. For example, H_1 receptors on vascular endothelium activate calcium mobilization and nitric oxide production (eNOS), causing local vascular smooth muscle relaxation. In contrast, activation of H_1 receptors in smooth muscle will cause *contraction* (e.g., bronchoconstriction), which is balanced by stimulation of H_2 receptors in the same cells that mediate *relaxation.* Both H_1 and H_2 receptors are distributed throughout the peripheral nervous system and CNS, whereas H_3 receptors are limited to the CNS. The H_3 receptors serve as autoreceptors. In general, their stimulation promotes sleep, and antagonism is manifested as wakefulness. H_4 receptors are located primarily in cells of hematopoietic origin.[278] These include granulocytes. Stimulation of H_4 receptors on eosinophils induces a change in the shape of the cell, chemotaxis, and upregulation of adhesion molecules; antagonists therefore may be particularly useful for treatment of chronic allergic diseases.

The effects of histamine on H_1 and H_2 receptors vary with the site and extent of release. In general, histamine affinity for H_1 receptors is probably greater than that for H_2 receptors. In the vasculature both H_1 and H_2 receptor activation causes relaxation of arteriolar smooth muscle (resistance vessels), resulting in vasodilation. Whereas H_1-mediated responses are rapid, H_2- mediated response are slow and prolonged. In contrast to its effect on smaller vessels, histamine may cause contraction of the smooth muscle, causing hypertension in some species. In the heart contractility and automaticity increase, primarily through H_2 receptors. Endothelial cells of venules contain more histamine receptors than other tissues. In postcapillary venules, H_1 receptors cause endothelial cells to contract and separate, regulating cell-to-cell cytoskeleton interactions.[278a] The loss of the endothelial barrier results in increased permeability, typical of edema. Passage of inflammatory cells into tissues is facilitated. In nonvascular smooth muscle, H_1 receptors cause contraction, whereas H_2 receptor activation causes relaxation. Thus in the bronchi the predominant effect of smooth muscle contraction is bronchoconstriction; in the gastrointestinal tract, diarrhea may occur. Species sensitivity to these effects vary; for example, histamine does not appear to play a major role in bronchoconstriction associated with asthma in the cat. Release of histamine from mast cells and basophils causes H_2-mediated inhibition of further histamine release. Gastric acid secretion is mediated by H_2 receptors. The H_1 receptors also stimulate sensory nerve endings; for example, pruritis reflects, in part, stimulation of type C nerve fibers.

The manifestation of the vascular effects of histamine varies depending on the magnitude of response. Local effects in the skin are manifested as the typical wheal and flare response; in contrast, systemic release, if sufficient, may be manifested as hypotensive shock, typical of anaphylactic or anaphylactoid response. The clinical signs vary with the species, depending on the "shock" organ, which in turn generally reflects the tissue with the greatest number of mast cells (lungs in cats, gastrointestinal tract in dogs).

Prevention or treatment of the effects of histamine can be accomplished in several ways: preventing histamine release (e.g., inhibition of mast cell degranulation), targeting the histamine receptor itself, or antagonizing (modulating) tissue response to histamine (e.g., the use of beta antagonists to blunt histamine-induced bronchoconstriction). Of these, the most comprehensive response is likely to occur if mast cell degranulation is prevented. This reflects the fact that histamine is not the only mediator released with degranulation. Others simultaneously released include those stored with histamine, such as serotonin (to which feline bronchial smooth muscle has been described as very sensitive), and those mediators formed in situ (e.g., eicosanoid mediators such as PGs, LTs [LTB4], or slow-reactive substance of anaphylaxis), platelet activating factor, and related compounds (see Figure 29-1)

Inhibitors of histamine release (mast cell degranulation) (see Figure 29-1), are exemplified by cromolyn sodium. It prevents calcium-dependent release of histamine from mast cells (but not basophils). Its mechanism of action may involve inhibition of calcium flux into the mast cell. Because degranulation is prevented, the release of other autacoids released with histamine is also prevented. However, the drug is poorly absorbed orally and can be given only by inhalation. Thus its use is limited to respiratory disease associated with mast cells. Because it prevents degranulation, it is useful only when administered prophylactically.

Structure–Activity Relationship

Anthistamines historically refer to those drugs specific for H_1 receptors. Some of the drugs also inhibit muscarinic, serotonin, or alpha-adrenergic receptors. All H_1 receptor blockers or antagonists are structurally similar to histamine; however, the primary amine of histamine is replaced by a tertiary amine (see Figure 29-11). Previously referred to as *competitive antagonists* at histamine receptors, they are now described as *inverse agonists.* They preferentially bind to the receptor in its inactive state, maintaining the conformation of the inactive state, thus prolonging the state of inactivity.[205] Antihistamines are among the most used drugs in human medicine, with over 40 different drugs available worldwide, many of them nonprescription.

Traditional categorization results in six chemical groups: ethanolamines, ethylenediamines, alkylamines, piperazines, piperidines, and phenothiazines. Alternatively, another classification is based on sedative potential, with first-generation drugs being sedating and second-generation drugs being nonsedating.

Pharmacologic Effects

The effects of the H_1 receptor blockers are similar and predictable regardless of the preparation. Specific effects include smooth muscle inhibition in the gastrointestinal tract and respiratory tract; inhibition of histamine-induced vasodilation of resistance vessels in the vasculature (residual vasodilation may require H_2 blockers); and strong antagonism of capillary and venule permeability. In the CNS both stimulation and depression may occur, depending on the drug. However, second-generation drugs (particularly cetirizine or fexofenadine, but less so loratadine) do not penetrate the blood–brain barrier and are less likely to be associated with CNS side effects.[279] The difference appears to reflect, in part, whether the drugs are substrates for P-glycoprotein, with second-generation drugs more likely. Effects on anaphylactic (or anaphylactoid) shock vary with species and tissues. Inhibition of motion sickness may actually reflect anticholinergic activity (promethazine). Antiallergic effects of the newer drugs in particular may reflect inhibition of mediator release,[205] probably by way of direct inhibition of inward calcium flux through calcium ion channels.

KEY POINT 29-22 The central nervous system–related side effects of antihistamines reflect their ability to penetrate and remain in the brain, a characteristic more consistent among the first-generation drugs than the newer second-generation drugs.

Example drugs include doxepin (marketed as a tricyclic antidepressant), diphenhydramine (antimuscarinic and sedating ethanolamine), chlorpheniramine (first-generation alkylamine; such drugs as a class are very potent and less sedating), hydroxyzine, cyclizine, and meclizine (a first generation piperazines), cetirizine (a second-generation piperazine and active metabolite of hydroxyzine), promethazine (a phenothiazine), cyproheptadine (a first-generation piperazine that also has antiserotonergic effects), and terfenadine (a second-generation piperazine). Dimenhydrinate (Dramamine) and diphenhydramine (Benadryl) are characterized by marked sedation and significant antimuscarinic effects. Tripelennamine is one of the most specific H_1 antagonists and is associated with less sedation but more gastric side effects. Chlorpheniramine is one of the most potent H_1 blockers and also is associated with less sedation but more CNS stimulation. Promethazine is the most potent inhibitor of motion sickness. Piperazines are very effective for motion sickness and may have more prolonged action (cyclizine and meclizine). Phenothiazines (promethazine as the prototype) are characterized by considerable anticholinergic activity and prominent sedation but are the most effective for motion sickness.

Pharmacokinetics

Few antihistamines have been studied in animals. Species differences are likely to preclude extrapolation of dosing regimens among species, and particularly between humans and dogs. This reflects, in part, differences in pH of the human skin (4.8) versus canine skin (similar to plasma). As weak bases, antihistamines are likely to accumulate in skin.[280] In the ionized form, the accumulated drug will be inactive in human skin. However, the skin may serve as a depot, allowing slow release as the unionized, active form. This may either prolong elimination half-life from plasma or, if concentrations are too low to be detected in plasma, may allow a local pharmacodynamic effect that exceeds the duration indicated by pharmacokinetics. These benefits may not be realized in dogs.

Hydroxyzine is a piperazine antihistaminergic drug that is further metabolized to cetirizine, the active ingredient in Zyrtec. Its disposition has been described in dogs (n = 6) after oral and intravenous administration of 2 mg/kg hydroxyzine, using a randomized crossover design (14-day washout between routes).[281] The pharmacokinetic study was accompanied by pharmacodynamic response based on immunoglobulin E (IgE) cutaneous wheal formation. Dogs tolerated each dose well. The maximum response to hydroxyzine occurred during the first 8 hours, correlating with plasma cetirizine concentrations that exceeded 1.5 μg/mL, with response attributed almost exclusively to cetirazine. Accordingly, the authors recommended cetirizine at 2 mg/kg twice daily.

In cats the disposition of cetrizine has been described after an oral dose of 0.9 ± 0.2 mg/kg (see Table 29-4).[282] Despite the high proportion of bound drug, the effective concentration in humans of 10.5 to 27.3 ng/mL was achieved (based on calculation of free drug) and maintained during a 24-hour dosing period. Cats tolerated the single dose well, despite drug concentrations that are higher than those generally achieved in humans (human dose 10 mg/person).

Clemastine is an ethanolamine antihistaminergic drug. Its disposition and pharmacodynamic response have been described in dogs (Table 29-7).[280] Target concentrations in human approximate 0.7 ng/mL. After oral administration bioavailability of clemastine was less than 5%. Although not reported, plasma drug concentrations versus time curves indicate that 0.7 ng/mL is achieved but maintained for less than 3 hours in dogs after oral absorption. Poor oral absorption contributed to poor response to antigen challenge, whereas intravenous administration inhibited wheal formation entirely for 7 hours. Accordingly, the oral dose of the drug should be at least 1 mg/kg every 12 hours or more; in contrast, the intravenous dose of 0.1 mg/kg would be effective twice daily.

Drug Interactions

Antihistamines generally are substrates for P-glycoprotein and other drug transport systems; therefore competition should be expected when they are used in concert with other P-glycoprotein substrates. Selected drugs may also cause the induction or inhibition of drug-metabolizing enzymes.

Table **29-7** Pharmacokinetic Data for Selected Antihistamines In Dogs and Cats

Drug	Species	Route	Dose mg/kg	C_{max} µg/ml	T_{max} hr	Bioavailability Percentage	Clearance mL/min/kg	L/kg	$F_{unbound}$ (%)	Half-Life (hr)
Cetirizine[282]	Cat	PO	0.9±0.2	3.3±1.2	3.1±3.3	NA	NA	NA	88±1.5	10.1±4
Hydroxyzine[281]	Dog	IV	2	1.1±0.1			5.3±3.5	12.6±7		59±58
		PO	2	0.16±0.05	3±1.1				71±39	17.1±7
[Cetirizine] [281*]	Dog	IV	(2)	2.41±0.9	2.4±0.8					11.4±1.8
			(2)	2.2±0.53	3.5±0.4					10.1±2.4
Clemastine[280]	Dog	IV	0.1				35 (25 to 60) (8)	13.4 (11-21)	2	7.9(3.1-13.6)
		PO	0.5	1.75 (13)		2.9 (1.1-5.8)				

F, fraction of drug unbound *PO*, by mouth; *NA*, not applicable; *IV*, intravenous.
*Cetirizine formed from hydroxyzine.

Adverse Drug Reactions and Side Effects

Because side effects to first-generation drugs are problematic, alternative drugs were developed. For example, diphenhydramine adversely affects learning in children and alters cognition and mood. Several drugs cause a level of intoxication similar to that produced by alcohol; chlorpheniramine causes a hangover effect. Gastrointestinal side effects include anorexia, nausea and vomiting, constipation, and diarrhea. Other effects, such as a dry respiratory tract and urinary retention or dysuria, can be attributed to atropine-like (anticholinergic), antiadrenergic, and antiserotonin effects. Newer antihistamines (H_1) do not interact with muscarinic receptors as effectively as did the first-generation drugs, thus avoiding many of these side effects. Side effects in the CNS are not unusual at therapeutic doses. However, they are rarely serious, and adaptation occurs with chronic use. Sedation is affected by pH, lipophilicity, and activity of transport proteins such as P-glycoprotein.[283] Lack of sedation in the newer drugs has been attributed to transport proteins that mediate active efflux from the CNS and thus limit CNS distribution. Collies and related breeds deficient in P-glycoprotein might be expected to manifest more CNS reactions with newer drugs compared with other dog breeds.

Two early second-generation H_1 antihistamines, astemizole and terfenadine, were associated with cardiotoxicity (prolongation of the QT interval: torsades de pointes) as a result of blockade of the rapid component of the delayed rectifier potassium current. More recent drugs, including loratadine, desloratadine (a metabolite of loratadine), cetirizine, and fexofenadine (a metabolite of terfenadine), are not associated with this effect.

Acute poisoning is not uncommon in humans; its occurrence in dogs and cats is not known. There is no specific therapy. Signs include ataxia, incoordination, convulsions, dry mouth, and fever, with treatment being supportive.

Therapeutic Use

Indications for antihistamines include the prevention or treatment of anaphylactic shock (IgE-mediated histamine release) or anaphylactoid response (e.g., cationic drug-induced histamine release), motion sickness (see the discussion of the gastrointestinal tract), particularly dimenhydrinate, piperazines, and promethazine, and allergic disease, including that affecting the skin. These indications are addressed in the relevant chapters. Antihistaminergic drugs have proved variably useful in the control of small animal allergic diseases.[284-286] This no doubt reflects differences in receptors and drug receptor interactions. However, profound differences also are likely in the disposition of the drugs, including oral bioavailability (e.g., clemastine in dogs). Part of the lack of efficacy also reflects limited actions: Although the effects of histamine at H_1 receptors may be blocked, limited to no effects on mast cell degranulation will result in inflammatory response to other mediators.

TREATMENT OF OSTEOARTHRITIS

Physiology and Pathophysiology

Osteoarthritis Defined

Degenerative joint disease, or *osteoarthritis,* is defined as a loss of articular cartilage and chondrocyte death. In its primary form, it is considered a disease of "wear and tear," and inflammation does not play a significant role in the onset of the disease process.[287] Although the role of inflammation in the pathogenesis of the disease is also limited compared with that of other joint disorders (i.e., sepsis or immune-mediated diseases), the role of inflammation is sufficiently important that drugs modifying inflammation have become important in the management of degenerative joint disease. However, the concept of chondroprotection in the damaged joint has become a focus for therapy, as have agents that modify the disease process.

Degenerative joint disease is a progressive disease characterized by degeneration and destruction of articular cartilage.[288,289] Certain conditions are predisposed to cause secondary degenerative joint disease, although it can occur as the primary disorder. Secondary degenerative joint disease can develop as a result of abnormal joint mechanics (e.g., instability) or direct trauma.

Cartilage Physiology and Pathophysiology

In order to understand the potential role of disease-modifying agents in the treatment of osteoarthritis, a discussion of normal and diseased cartilage is warranted. Normal cartilage is avascular and tightly adheres to cortical bone.[290,291] A load-bearing and gliding surface of the joint is formed such that

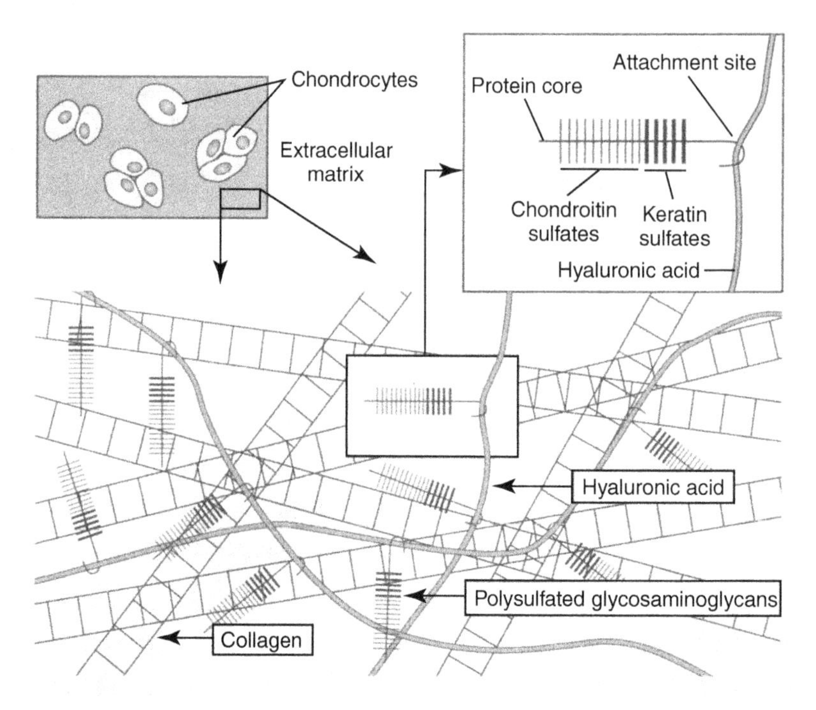

Figure 29-12 Hyaline articular cartilage is characterized by highly metabolic chondrocytes surrounded by an extracellular matrix that they secrete *(inset, top left)*. The matrix is composed of collagen, which provides strength to the joint, and polysulfated glycosaminoglycans (PGAGs). The PGAGs cause retention of water, thus providing a cushion to joint stresses. The PGAGs are composed of a central protein core *(inset, top right)* to which is attached keratin sulfates (base) and chondroitin sulfates. The PGAG attaches to hyaluronic acid.

a frictionless surface occurs throughout the range of motion of the joint. The fibrous capsule of the joint contains a layer of synovial cells that are very vascular and serve as a selective membrane, precluding passage of molecules greater than 12,000 molecular weight. Synovial fluid produced by the cells lubricates and nourishes cartilage. Hyaline cartilage contains a small number of chondrocytes that synthesize the matrix in which they are embedded. The matrix is composed of collagen fibers interspersed in a well-structured manner with proteoglycan aggregates of varying molecular weights (Figures 29-12 and 29-13). Proteoglycans comprise glycosaminoglycans encircling a core protein. The proteoglycan complex in turn is bound (by a link protein) to hyaluronic acid. Chondroitin sulfate is the principal proteoglycan of mature cartilage, with other sulfates (e.g., keratin, dermatan) making up the remainder. Chondroitin sulfates are glycosaminoglycans composed of alternating sulfated residues of a glucuronic acid and a galactosamine. Sources of chondroitin sulfate for commercial purposes include bovine trachea, nasal septum, and shark cartilage. Proteoglycans are large, hydrophilic (containing oxygen, nitrogen, and sulfur) molecules that trap water, thus maintaining the gel-like consistency of cartilage, and act as an elastic shock absorber. Chondrocytes are very metabolically active, constantly breaking down and resynthesizing proteoglycan and collagen. The substrates and energy for these activities are transported to, and waste material from, the cartilage by a synovial "pump" mechanism.

The initial insult leading to cartilage degeneration may vary (i.e., injury, congenital malformation, chronic overload, age), but the sequence of events is similar. The changes occur well before clinical (including radiographic) signs are evident. The initial lesion in osteoarthritis occurs in cartilage. Chondromalacia (softening of the cartilage) occurs early in the course of disease. Collagen turnover is markedly increased by the chondrocytes; reparation may not yield the appropriate (type II) collagen. Ultimately, collagen loss may predominate. Species differences in the repair of collagen are likely to exist. Proteoglycans are also lost as degenerative joint disease progresses. Initially, proteoglycan synthesis is markedly increased, but the normal ratios of high-molecular-weight versus low-molecular-weight proteoglycans may not be maintained. Eventually, proteoglycan synthesis markedly decreases. Hyaluronic acid concentrations also decrease.

The loss of cartilage matrix is mediated, in part, by proteolytic enzymes such as metalloproteinases, including collagenases, stromelysin, and aggrecanases, and lysosomal enzymes released (stimulated by IL-1 or TNF) by synovial cells or chondrocytes.[287] IL-1 and IL-6, TNF, and nitric oxide also act as cellular or molecular mediators.[287,292-295] Mediators (eicosanoids, IL-1, and TNF) act to upregulate catabolic enzymes of destruction while downregulating mediators that inhibit catabolic actions.[293] The catabolic process of cartilage degradation worsens as these enzymes are released. Chondrocyte death may occur early in the process of degenerative joint disease. Synovial cells phagocytize the products of degradation and initiate a (chemical) inflammatory process. Collagen is exposed; fissures develop in the cartilage. Local tissue degradation increases, and leukocytes are activated, eventually leading to a viscous cycle of degradation and inflammation. Synovial fluid amount is increased, which reduces the content of hyaluron.[287]

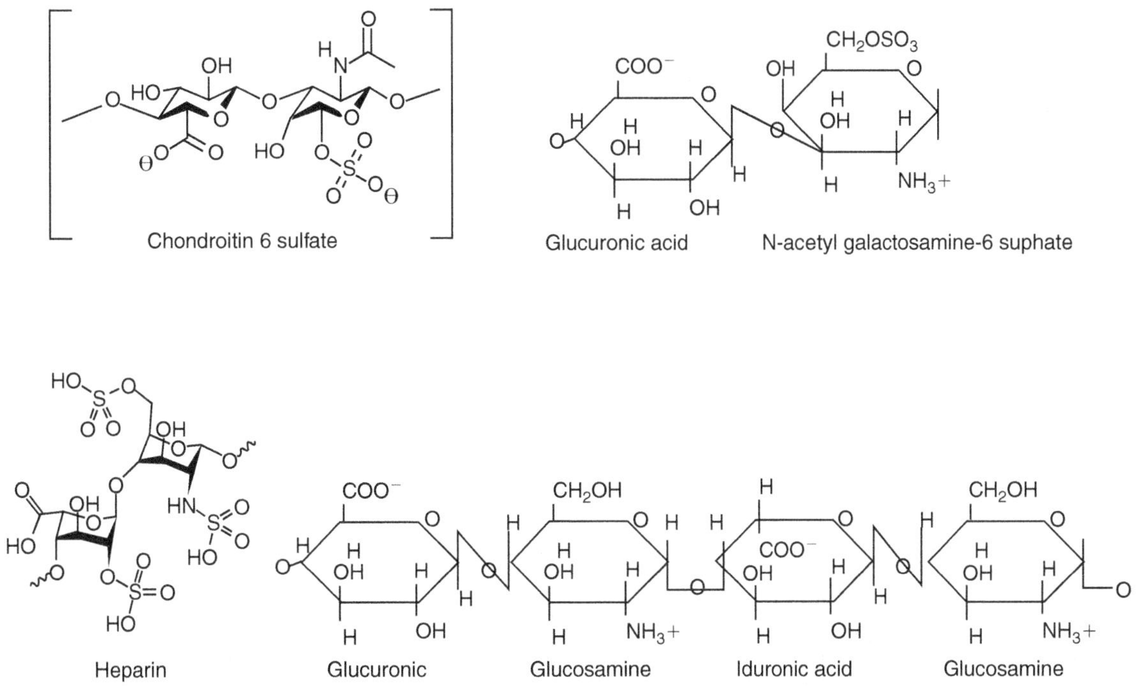

Chondroitin 6 sulfate Glucuronic acid N-acetyl galactosamine-6 suphate

Heparin Glucuronic Glucosamine Iduronic acid Glucosamine

Figure 29-13 Chondroitin sulfates structurally are very similar to heparin and hyaluronic acid (not shown). The negative charges of the repeating units cause retention of water. Inappropriate chemical configuration of the chondroitin sulfates contributes to abnormal stresses on the joint and ultimately continued articular damage.

As cartilage continues to bear weight, mechanical destruction and physiologic changes continue. The damaged cartilage cannot bear weight appropriately, and subchondral bone is exposed to forces that normally would be dampened. Subchondral sclerosis occurs, and apposing articular surfaces become eburnated. Cartilage homeostasis is interrupted, limiting access to fluid-containing nutrients. Fluid released into the synovial joint may not be efficiently absorbed. In addition, mediators of inflammation are released by both chondrocytes and synovial cells. The joint becomes painful as a result. Microfractures and fissures allow synovial fluid to penetrate into the bone, with resulting subchondral cyst formation. The damaged cartilage attempts to repair the damage as it occurs by synthesizing new proteoglycan and collagen. Osteoarthritis probably occurs when the catabolic process overwhelms the repair process.

Therapy with Drugs and Other Agents

The goals of drug therapy for degenerative joint disease should be (1) to control pain, (2) to increase mobility, (3) to prevent continued degradation of the joint, and (4) to provide support to reparative processes. In addition to drug therapy, dietary management (i.e., weight control) and exercise control should be implemented, and surgical options should be considered when appropriate. Mechanisms of therapeutic drugs designed to retard the deterioration of degenerative joint disease include inhibition of synovial cell–derived cytokines and chondrocyte-derived degradative enzymes, inactivation of superoxide radicals, stimulation of matrix synthesis, and enhancement of synovial fluid lubrication.[296,297]

Advances in the pathophysiology of degenerative joint disease (osteoarthritis) have provided new therapeutic foci. The progressive degeneration of articular cartilage that characterizes this disease reflects an imbalance between cartilage matrix synthesis and breakdown. The role of inflammation in the pathophysiology of degenerative joint disease is controversial. The impact of NSAID therapy can be a double-edged sword: The effects may be either harmful or beneficial, depending on the drug. The primary effect of NSAIDs in the disease may be analgesic rather than antiinflammatory.[296] A number of other antiinflammatory drugs have been studied for their efficacy in the treatment of degenerative joint disease, and clinical trials addressing their use for treatment of osteoarthritis has been previously discussed with each drug. The dose of NSAID needed to control pain associated with osteoarthritis may vary greatly among animals. Drugs can control pain not associated with inflammation at doses lower than those necessary to control pain associated with inflammation. On the other hand, for some animals pain may be controlled only if inflammation is successfully controlled. The choice of the most appropriate NSAID should be based on both efficacy and safety.

Until relatively recently, little justification existed for the selection of one NSAID over another for treatment of osteoarthritis in dogs. Approval of the newer class of NSAIDs, which are more selective for COX-2 in their inhibition compared with COX-1, has, however, provided a realistic first-choice drug. Of the conventional NSAIDs, aspirin has been the second drug of choice simply because it is a known entity; phenylbutazone may also be used because it is approved for use in dogs in the US. In countries in which ketoprofen is approved, it may be the second choice. Chondroprotection by the NSAID also should be considered. Differential effects on healthy or damaged cartilage among the newer NSAIDs are likely to exist. For example, etodolac appears to contribute to damage, whereas carprofen appears to facilitate its repair at therapeutic concentrations.[211] Caution is recommended with use of all drugs (or supplements) whose action targets COX, with relative potential toxicity likely being greatest for conventional NSAIDs, less for COX-1–protective (often referred to as COX-2–selective) and least for dual-acting (COX- and lipoxygenase- inhibiting) drugs. Ideally, NSAID use for treatment of osteoarthritis is limited to "rescue" situations in animals with mild to moderate disease, with maintenance therapy focusing on disease-modifying agents (discussed later). NSAIDs might be reserved in such patients for short term treatment of acute conditions (or "flare-ups") . If NSAIDs are required for maintenance therapy, simultaneous use of disease-modifying agents should be considered so that the animal may benefit from any synergistic effect the combination of therapies might have,[298] as well as to decrease the amount of time that an NSAID is necessary, to protect the cartilage from any NSAID damage that might occur, and to potentially protect the gastrointestinal tract.[91] Selection of an NSAID for treatment of osteoarthritis in cats is confounded by the lack of data identifying COX-1 protection. Meloxicam and ketoprofen each are characterized by shorter half-lives in the cat (compared with the dog), which may or may not contribute to the relative tolerance the cat has to these drugs compared with other NSAIDs. Further, meloxicam is approved in the U.S. for use in cats. As such, meloxicam might be a first choice for treatment of pain or inflammation associated with osteoarthritis in the cat. However, concerns regarding renal disease indicate the need for pre- and during treatment evaluation of renal function. The FDA has led the manufacturer of meloxicam to state that meloxicam should not be used beyond a single dose in cats, increasing the risk of liability for veterinarians that use the drug off label. Signed informed consent is recommended if meloxicam is used off-lable. Care must be taken that the daily dose does not exceed 0.03 mg/kg (or 0.1 to 0.15 mg/cat). Time may reveal dual inhibitors to be well tolerated by cats. Although used safely as a platelet inhibitor, the use off aspirin at doses necessary to control pain in cats is likely to be unsafe. Disease-modifying agents also should be used in cats.

The use of glucocorticoids alone for the treatment of osteoarthritis is discouraged. In general, these drugs should not be used for prolonged periods because of their chondrodestructive effects, which are likely to occur at clinically used doses. Rather, use, including intraarticular injections, should focus on short-term management or in patients for which other therapies have failed. The combination of NSAIDs with drugs that control inflammation through mechanisms other than COX inhibition should be strongly considered. These include disease-modifying agents (discussed later). For acute flare ups in animals already receiving the maximum dose of a chosen (safe) NSAID, the use of opioids, tramadol, or NMDA receptor inhibitors (e.g., amantadine) should be considered. Although scientific evidence is needed, gabapentin increasingly is being used based on anecdotal recommendations for control of chronic pain.

DISEASE-MODIFYING AGENTS: CHONDROPROTECTANTS

A number of compounds are able to modify the progression of osteoarthritis, most commonly by supporting the cartilage. These products help achieve the goals of preventing further degradation and providing support for the reparative cartilage.Although variable, evidence exists that supports the use of these products as sole or adjuvant therapy in the treatment of the damaged joint (see the discussion of recommendations regarding the use of disease-modifying agents in the treatment of joint disease). Care should be taken to not overinterpret studies that fail to demonstrate a statistical difference between treatment groups (including placebo); such studies do not demonstrate a lack of treatment effect, but rather, are unable to demonstrate a treatment effect. Commonly, treatment design fails to effectively address the complex nature of the conditions being treated, particularly in terms of sample size.

Injectable Products

Polysulfated Glycosaminoglycans

Efforts to treat osteoarthritis have focused on drugs that favorably shift the balance from degradation to synthesis of cartilage matrix. Two compounds composed of PGAGs are available in the United States and Canada: Adequan and pentosan polysulfate. Hyaluronic acid (e.g., Legend) is also a PGAG but differs in structure sufficiently to be addressed separately. Because of similarities in structure, however, the disposition of these drugs (at least as much as is understood) and their assumed mechanism of action are similar. On the one hand, subtle differences in chemical structure may impact physiologic function (e.g., water retention in cartilage), and thus change efficacy.On the other hand, for products with demonstrated efficacy but presumed different mechanisms of action, combination therapy in the damaged joint. Their use should not be limited to osteoarthritis, but should include any conditions associated with of joint damage—trauma, immune-mediated diseases, septic or drug-induced damage, surgery (including prophylaxis) and others. Further, prophylactic use should be considered in animals predisposed to joint damage (e.g., conformation predisposing to joint damage or intensive sports training). Because PGAGs are responsible for normal functions in a variety of body tissues, their potential applications include disorders other than osteoarthritis (e.g., interstitial cystitis and glomerulonephritis).

Chemistry. A PGAG s a polymeric chain of repeating units of hexosamine and hexuronic acid. Considered a hypersulfated compound, approximately 14% of the drug is sulfated. It is extracted and purified from bovine tracheal tissues.[299] Normal cartilage matrix is composed of proteoglycan complexes, collagen, and water. Side chains of glycosaminoglycans (keratin and chondroitin) are attached to the core protein of the proteoglycan molecule by a strand of hyaluronate (see Figures 29-12 and 29-13). Water trapped between these complexes accounts for the resiliency of cartilage. PGAGs closely mimic the proteoglycan complexes found in normal articular cartilage.

Pharmacologic effects. PGAGs appear to be chondroprotective in both in vitro and in vivo models. In vivo models have included chemically and traumatically induced cartilage damage.[300,301] Cartilage degradation is retarded in the presence of PGAG. Although the mechanisms of these protective actions are not known, chondrocyte proliferation and matrix biosynthesis appear to be important.[301] Collagen, proteoglycan, and hyaluronic acid syntheses increase.[302] In addition, proteolytic enzymes such as collagenase,[302,303] leukocyte elastase,[304] proteases,[299,305] and lysosomes are inhibited,[305] although these actions are likely to be complex.[302] Complement activity is also inhibited; the degree of inhibition appears to be related to the sulfate load of the chondroitin sulfate matrix.[306] PGAGs appear to have no effect on the ability of IL-1 to stimulate metalloproteinase activity in cartilage.[307]

Disposition and safety. Deposition of PGAG in normal and damaged cartilage has been demonstrated after parenteral administration. Drug that is not retained in cartilage is excreted primarily by the kidneys with minimal degradation of the parent compound. Toxicity is limited in all species studied. In dogs the LD_{50} is 1000 mg/kg.[299] Heparin and PGAG are chemically similar. Adverse effects related to the anticoagulant activity of PGAG have been suggested. One study found coagulation times to be prolonged after administration (see below). This suggests that PGAGs should not be administered at the time surrounding a surgical procedure. Heparin-associated thrombocytopenia, a presumed immunologically mediated decrease in circulating platelet numbers, has been reported in human patients receiving PGAGs.[308]

At the time of this publication, several injectable PGAG products are being marketed as "generic" Adequan. These products (e.g., Chondroprotec for horses) are not "generic" in that they have undergone no FDA approval process. That such products contain the same ingredients and will provide the same level of response as approved products cannot be assumed without inbiased scientific evaluation. Although a peer review paper disputing the efficacy of such products could not be identified at the time of this publication, a review of the internet reveals testimonial based evidence of the lack of efficacy of these products and the lack of understanding regarding their approval status. Although veterinarians might be legally empowered to prescribe or recommend such products, liability and standard of care concerns should lead to caution regarding their use. Differences in chemistry may be very subtle but may impact efficacy both safety and efficacy. Among the biggest concerns might be the impact of adulteration, as has occurred for heparin, also a PGAG (see Chapter 17). That these products can become unsafe if composed of improper PGAGs has been recently demonstrated.

Clinical use. Adequan has been approved for use in dogs for the treatment of osteoarthritis. The drug might, however, be considered in any situation in which the joint has been or will be injured. This includes trauma, elective surgical procedures, and arthritis associated with immune-mediated or infectious conditions. Additionally, PGAGs should be considered in conjunction with NSAIDs for their chondroprotective effects, as well as with the intent to potentially discontinue the NSAID. Disease-modifying agents including PGAG or its precursors (see later discussion of nutraceuticals) might also be considered as preventive therapy in animals that are likely to develop osteoarthritis for whatever reason, including conformation problems. Use of these drugs before clinical signs of osteoarthritis develop may prolong the time until NSAIDs are necessary. In patients with osteoarthritis, the time to clinical response is likely to be directly related to the severity of disease. Treatment that is begun before the joint is markedly damaged is more likely to be successful. Adequan may negatively impact hemostasis. Dogs treated at 10 times the recommended dose develop hemotomas and prolonged protime (package insert). Surgical candidates probably should not be treated with Adequan on the day of or prior to surgery unless coagulation studies indicated no effect. Care should be taken to not use Adequan in patients with bleeding disorders (see package insert), which might include patients receiving aspirin. The impact on patients receiving COX-2 preferential drugs is not clear.

KEY POINT 29-23 Injectable polysulfated glycosaminoglycans should be anticipated to act more rapidly than orally administered products.

Pentosan Polysulfate

Pentosan polysulfate (PPS) is isolated from beechwood hemicellulose and synthetically modified by adding sulfates to its repeating units of xylan pyranoses. Thus, unlike Adequan, it is not derived from animal sources. It is available as an injectable product, and an oral product has been approved in the United States for people with interstitial cystitis, a syndrome that may reflect a quantitative and qualitative defect in bladder mucosal glycosaminoglycans.[309,310] It is approved for use under the market name Cartrophen for treatment of osteoarthritis in dogs in Canada and Europe, where it has been marked for at least 15 years.

PPS has a number of pharmacologic effects. Response of interstitial cystitis (based on resolution of pain in humans) ranges from 6% to 20%. In Europe PPS is used to treat thrombosis and hyperlipidemia, and an application for its use in treatment of osteoarthritis is pending. For cartilage PPS may improve subchondral and synovial membrane blood flow. In addition, it modulates cytokine actions, stimulates hyaluronic acid synthesis, and maintains PGAG content in joints.[302,311] When PPS was administered intramuscularly (2 mg/kg once weekly) in a model of osteoarthritis in dogs, cartilage damage was significantly decreased. In a double-blind clinical trial in 40 dogs, after 3 mg/kg intramuscularly per week, lameness, body condition, pain on joint manipulation, and willingness to exercise were improved at 4 weeks.[312] The work of Budsberg and coworkers[313] supports the efficacy of PPS in selected surgeries. The investigators prospectively studied the efficacy of PPS in dogs (n = 40; 10 per group) with spontaneous cranial cruciate rupture using a parallel, randomized, blinded, placebo-controlled design. Dogs were divided into four groups on the basis of radiographic score (low versus high) and a partial meniscectomy was performed. Within each group animals were randomly assigned to receive either placebo or 3 mg/kg PPS weekly for 4 weeks after surgery. Animals were evaluated for 48 weeks, with biomarkers of collagen cleavage, aggrecan activity, and osteocalcin activity measured in serum. Radiographs and gait analysis were included in the postoperative evaluation. A total of 10 response variables were compared among the groups. Although lameness scores did not differ, PPS-treated dogs generally improved faster than placebo-treated dogs, and in those dogs with partial meniscectomies, biochemical markers were reduced compared with placebo-treated dogs. An oral dose has not been established for dogs.

PPS appears to be safe, but like other PGAG-like compounds, it appears to prolong clotting times and may cause thrombocytopenia. Safety information from the manufacturer available online[314] indicated an adverse event reporting incident of 0.01% with no signalment predisoposition. Clinical signs considered to be "probably related" to the drug, based on their appearance within 10 to 15 minutes of administration, included vomiting (78% of those reports, or 0.0047% of animals dosed) and a change in demeanor (i.e., quiet, etc; 0.0062% of animals). Experimentally, at 3 mg/kg, PPS increased partial thromboplastin time (PTT) and thrombin time (TT) but not prothrombin time (PT) above baseline in dogs, with the peak effect at 2 hours and resolution by 8 hours. Although hemorrhage has been reported in clinical cases using PPS, few of those reports have been designated as probable cause. Local reactions at the injection site did not occur in experimental studies, even at 30 mg/kg. The posibility that PPS and similar products worsens gastrointestinal hemorrhage induced by NSAIDs has not been addressed; indeed, evidence suggests a protective nature is imparted by related products in the gastrointestinal tract. It should be noted that information provided by the manufacturer of Cartrophen indicates that generic products are not therapeutically equivalent because they differ both chemically and thus in their interation with target proteins. As such, differences in therapeutic response among these products in general might be anticipated.

The use of this product for syndromes other than osteoarthritis in humans (e.g., interstitial cystitis, thrombosis) potentially might lead to similar uses in animals. For example, a study of mouse mesangial cells found that PPS decreased proliferation and net extracellular matrix production, mechanisms that may explain its apparent ability to slow the progression of glomerular sclerosis.[315,316] PPS inhibits calcium oxalate crystallization in vitro[317] and is being studied for possible use in vivo. The compound is being studied for its apparently clinically beneficial effects for the treatment of acquired immune deficiency syndrome–related Kaposi's sarcoma in human patients.[318]

Hyaluronic Acid

Hyaluronic acid is a linear polydisaccharide (glucuronic acid combined with glucosamine) that is an essential component of synovial fluid, where it is chemically linked to proteoglycans in articular cartilage. As such, it helps to form large, aggregating proteoglycans in articular cartilage (Figure 16-12).[296] Its mode of action is not certain, but it is assumed to function as a lubricant by increasing viscosity of synovial fluid. It may also act as an antiinflammatory. Studies in horses support its efficacy in the treatment of osteoarthritis. After intraarticular injection, the drug persists in joints for several days. The drug also has been given intravenously; the half-life in horses is 96 hours, but no studies could be found regarding dogs. Hyaluronic acid exists in variable molecular weights. High-molecular-weight hyaluronic acid inhibits phagocytosis, lymphocyte migration, and synovial permeability and stimulates hyaluronic acid synthesis.[319] Prior treatment with glucocorticosteroids or bony changes limits response. Hyaluronic acid appears to be very safe; side effects tend to be associated with administration of the drug. The drug has been used with variable success after intraarticular injection in horses[320] and dogs.[321]

The role of viscosupplementation in the treatment of human osteoarthritis has been reviewed.[322] A meta-analysis of 22 studies of hyaluron use in humans found it to have a small effect compared with placebo, but the study also found publication bias.[322] Accordingly, as with glucocorticoids, intraarticular administration of hyaluron tends to be limited in humans to patients who have not responded to other therapies.

Oral Disease-Modifying Agents

Veterinary Nutraceuticals

The use of oral disease-modifying agents (slow-acting disease-modifying agents)[323,324] for the treatment of damaged joints remains controversial despite increasing evidence regarding their potential contributions. Currently, with the exception of oral PPS (for which an approved drug version exists), these products can be classified as veterinary nutraceuticals.[323-327] The North American Veterinary Nutraceutical Council (no longer active) defined a veterinary nutraceutical as "a [non-drug] substance that is produced in a purified or extracted form and administered orally to a patient to provide agents required for normal body structure and function and administered with the intent of improving the health and well-being of animals."[325,326]

Regulatory considerations. Neither human nor veterinary nutraceuticals, botanicals, herbs or other novel ingredients (including botanicals or biological) undergo any mandated federal approval process, and therefore neither quality, safety nor efficacy necessarily have been documented before they are marketed. Chapter 4 addressed some of the safety issues associated with these products, and particularly those of plant origin. Unfortunately, clients may not realize the lack of regulation of these products, and counseling by veterinarians regarding the implications may be important.

The issues relating to quality, safety, and efficacy of disease-modifying agents have been reviewed,[327] but the complexity of their nature and the impact the lack of regulation has on products warrant a short review. The FDA historically has held dietary supplements to the same standards applied to foods, requiring evidence of safety as well as evidence that labeling was truthful and not misleading. In 1994 the dietary supplement industry was successful in lobbying Congress to pass the Dietary Supplement Health and Education Act of 1994

(DSHEA), which amends the Food, Drug and Cosmetic Act such that it addresses these products. The amendment, which legally defines a dietary supplement, effectively restricts the FDA's ability to regulate dietary supplements. Various label claims that refer to effects on structure or function of the body are now allowed on these products. Premarket safety evaluation is no longer required; rather, the manufacturer is responsible for ensuring safety, However, the FDA is responsible for monitoring the safety, despite the lack of a mandated mechanism for adverse event reporting. Rather, all adverse event reporting is voluntary, which may preclude effective safety assessment of products by the FDA. Consequently, the burden of proof that a product is unsafe rests with the FDA. Since DSHEA passage, the FDA has been able to require that manufacturers of hebal products include proper herbal names, and when relevant, the generic drug name for the product (e.g., ma guang for caffeine), and to indicate the part of the plant (e.g, stem, leaf, flower), from which the ingredient is derived.

The Center for Veterinary Medicine (CVM) of the FDA has determined that DSHEA does not apply to animals or animal feeds, including veterinary nutraceuticals. Therefore the term *dietary supplements* does not apply to veterinary products and theoretically should not be used when referring to products marketed for veterinary use. The term animal dietary supplements will nonetheless be used in this document. The CVM believes that public health is better served if the special concessions given to human dietary health supplements by the DSHEA do not apply to those given to food-producing animals. This reflects their goal of ensuring that harmful residues from either the compound or its metabolite do not reach food intended for human consumption and their concern that extrapolation of information among species receiving novel ingredients is complex and difficult. Most notably, the CVM is concerned that current "production drugs" (i.e., those that increase the production of food) might be considered by manufacturers or users of these products to fall under the lax guidelines of DSHEA, thus increasing the risk of human exposure to unapproved products. Thus, unlike human products, the FDA-CVM has retained its ability to regulate animal dietary supplements, although the lack of resources necessary to adequately regulate their sale will limit regulation. However, in contrast to dietary supplements, states can and do restrict the sale of products for animals through an alternative mechanism. Federal and state feed officials have organized the American Association of Feed Control Officials (AAFCO),[328] whose stated goal is to "provide a mechanism for developing and implementing uniform and equitable laws, regulation, standards, and enforcement policies for regulating the manufacture, distribution, and sale of animal feeds" such that the use of these products is "safe, effective and useful." Although nonregulatory, the AAFCO nonetheless influences state regulation and thus the marketing of oral products administered to animals in many (although not all) states. For those states that follow the AAFCO's guidelines, a manufacturer seeking the sale of an unapproved oral product in a state must provide information necessary for the product to be recognized as an "ingredient" that has been "defined" by the AAFCO. Sale of a product that is not a drug, food, or feed additive is more likely to be denied by a state feed official if the product is not listed as a defined ingredient in the AAFCO publication.

The dramatic increase in veterinary nutraceutical use in the last 15 years led the AAFCO to focus more aggressively on the regulation of these products. The National Animal Supplement Council (NASC),[329] based in the United States, has taken an active approach in working with the AAFCO to implement voluntary actions among nutraceutical manufacturers that will cause the AAFCO to respond to their products positively, thus allowing their sale. Veterinarians should be reminded that because DSHEA specifically applies only to human beings and neither dietary supplements (humans) nor novel ingredients (other animals) are not approved drugs, the use or prescription of these products is *not* protected by the Animal Medical Drug Use Clarification Act of 1994, which otherwise legalizes veterinary extralabel drug use.

Quality assurance. Several sources of scientific information indicate the need to focus on those products whose quality assurance can be verified. Chondroitin sulfate products (CDS) offer an example of consistent mislabeling. A University of Maryland study, funded in part by Nutramax Laboratories, found deviations from label claims for CDS in 84% (9 of 11) of the products studied; the amount by which products were mislabeled ranged from 0% to 115%.[329a] Further, the study found that products costing less than or equal to $1 per 1200 mg of CDS were seriously deficient (less than 10% of the label claim), which suggests that cheaper products should be avoided. Costliness did not guarantee accuracy, however. Several of the most expensive products also were found in this study to be mislabeled. In contrast to CDS, the glucosamine of only 1 of 14 products was mislabeled in this study. However, another study found glucosamine sulfate to vary 60% to 140% of the label claim.[329b] ConsumerLab[330] (www.Consumerlabs.com) is a for-profit laboratory (with income based largely on subscription to their site) that offers a seal of "validation" for dietary supplements that are appropriately labeled. The efforts of the laboratory are two fold in origin: dependent, based on requests from a sponsoring manufacturer or independent, that is, an unsponsored investigation. In either case, the products to be tested are obtained from commercial sites (grocery or health food stores) rather than from the manufacturer, thus avoiding manufacturer-induced bias through product selection. The samples are subjected to ingredient analysis by independent laboratories. The "pass" criteria vary for each ingredient but are based on comparing content as determined from ingredient analysis to the labeled ingredients. Criteria include labeling of ingredients by proper name (for herbs, this includes the part of the plant and herbal names); a misatch between the listed and measured ingredients; and lack of contaminants, including toxicants (heavy metals, cleaning agents, and [particularly for herbs] pesticides or insecticides), metabolites, and other degradative products of the active ingredient. Products that pass analysis are allowed to place the ConsumerLab seal on the product label. Members of the public can read selected information on the ConsumerLab website for a fee ($23 annual fee at the time of this printing) for ingredients that have been tested. Criteria for passing and failing and reasons for failure for specific ingredients can be viewed, as can a list of proprietary products that have passed. Animal products have just recently been included in the review. A review of the website reveals that an important proportion of both human and animal products fail quality assessment; in general, animal products have fared more poorly than products marketed to humans. Among the passing products are those manufactured by Nutramax Laboratories, although a number of other human products also have passed. The USP[127] has also recently implemented the Dietary Supplement Verification Program (DSVP), a voluntary standards assessment program for human dietary supplements; veterinary products have not yet been included in their review. Although its activities are nonregulatory, the USP criteria are recognized in the Food, Drug and Cosmetic Act and its amendments, including the DSHEA. The NASC Compliance Plus program offers a potential mechanism for ensuring the accuracy in labeling of veterinary products; however, it is not clear if their program is is based on independent product analysis or if their criteria include the the use of ingredients that meet USP standards.

KEY POINT 29-24 Because they undergo no premarket approval process, dietary supplements for animals or humans often lack in quality.

Assessing Quality. Veterinarians and consumers should fully evaluate a product under consideration.[327] First, the user should establish whether the product has been manufactured according to good manufacturing practices. The label should include the exact amount of each active ingredient; labels that combine metric and apothecary systems may be intentionally misleading because conclusions regarding product content are more difficult to determine. Each product listed on the label should contain a specific dosage. The source of each compound should be noted on the label. Note that products based on whole body tissues (e.g., mussel-containing glycosaminoglycans) will lack milligram contents of specific compounds (e.g., chondroitin sulfate). When individual products are listed, the purity of the compounds is likely to vary among and within products. The stated purity may not be the actual purity, particularly if good manufacturing procedures are not followed. Anderson[324] noted that 70% of products analyzed for glucosamine and chondroitin sulfate did not meet the labeled claims.

Safety and Efficacy Considerations. The lack of efficacy data should not lead to the assumption that the benefits of these products are negligible. Establishing efficacy for many novel ingredients, including disease-modifying agents targeting cartilage, may be very difficult because of the complex nature of their actions and the dependence of their actions on other endogenous molecules.[326] For example, the disease-modifying agents accumulate in tissues and have a carryover effect that requires a minimum of 6 to 8 weeks of therapy, necessitating long studies.[331] A placebo effect of more than 40% mandates the need for controls. Studies that do not demonstrate a significant difference between treatment groups should not be considered evidence of "no effect" unless the power of the study to demonstrate an effect is sufficient. Establishing safety may be easier simply because many adverse events are dose and duration dependent. It should be noted, however, that with poorly manufactured products, harm may occur not only because of the compounds themselves but also because of possible contaminants. Additional harm may occur if the client neglects traditional therapies in the belief that the nutraceutical agent will be sufficiently effective.

Nutraceutical Disease-Modifying Agents

Nutraceutical products that contain various forms of glycosaminoglycans or their component parts (aggregates form proteoglycans, the major constituent of cartilage matrix), such as glucosamines or chondroitin sulfates, appear most promising for treatment of osteoarthritis according to studies supporting their efficacy[332-340] and safety.[341] Presumably, as precursor nutrients, chondroitin sulfates, glucosamines, and other ingredients that comprise these will be extracted from the serum by chondrocytes and used to synthesize proteoglycans. During periods in which cartilage degradation exceeds cartilage formation, the need for precursor molecules may exceed availability, inhibiting the repair process. The availability of orally administered compounds not only increases the efficiency of the ability of the chondrocytes to repair damaged cartilage, as is demonstrated by increased synthesis, but also leaves less opportunity for formation of inappropriate molecules. The role of glucosamine and chondroitin sulfate, the major component of oral disease-modifying agents, in veterinary medicine has recently been reviewed.[342, 342a]

Glucosamine

Glucosamine is an amino sugar that is among the aminosugars necessary for synthesis of mucopolysaccharides such as chondroitin, heparin and hyaluronic acid. As such, it is important in chondrocyte synthesis of PGAG. A deficiency of the compound has been implicated as a cause of decreased PGAG synthesis in early osteoarthritis. Alternatively, glucosamine also may stimulate synovial production of hyaluronic acid.[339]

Glucosamine is not available in foods. It is derived from either bovine cartilage or chitin, the hard outer shells of shrimp, lobsters, and crabs. Several glucosamine salts are available, including sulfate, hydrochloride, N-acetyl, and hydroiodide; although it is glucosamine that is active, the oral absorption of the salts varies.

After intravenous injection of radiolabeled (at a carbon atom) glucosamine sulfate, about 10% appears in plasma, with the rest rapidly disappearing from plasma as it is incorporated into plasma globulins. After oral administration, at least 88% of the compound is absorbed, with oral bioavailability being only 44%, due to first-pass extraction. Radioactivity remains in the body, with a half-time of approximately 95 hours. Radioactivity rapidly appears in multiple tissues, including articular cartilage. After intravenous administration, 49% of the dose is excreted in the lungs as radiolabled CO_2, presumably after hepatic or other peripheral tissue metabolism. However, another 29% is excreted in the urine.[344] A meta-analysis of studies on glucosamine in humans concluded that the compound is well absorbed after oral administration; first-pass metabolism due to incorporation into proteins reduced oral bioavailability to 26%.[340,343] Glucosamine sulfate kinetics have been studied in dogs as well and appear to resemble that in humans.[344,345] After oral administration, absorption was rapid and nearly complete in dogs (87%). Glucosamine hydrochloride also is well absorbed in dogs, with peak concentrations occurring in 1.5 to 2 hours; bioavailability after a single dose is 12% although bioavailability is likely to increase, as it does with chondroitin sulfates, after multiple dosing.[331] Glucosamine hydrochloride exhibits a dose-dependent effect on plasma glucosamine concentrations, although, unlike chondroitin sulfates, glucosamine does not appear to accumulate in dogs with multiple dosing.[331]

KEY POINT 29-25 If only a single disease-modifying agent is chosen, glucosamine is a reasonable first choice because it is the rate-limiting step in polysulfated glycosaminoglycans synthesis; its oral absorption and safety have been demonstrated; and among the supplements, it tends to be one that is labeled appropriately.

The safety and efficacy of glucosamine have been well reviewed in human medicine.[287, 342a, 343] Glucosamine appears to be safe; an LD_{50} value cannot be established in mice or rats, even at doses of 5000 mg/kg orally or 3000 mg/kg intramuscularly, or 1500 mg/kg IV. Safety has been established both in the dog and cat after medium to high doses for 30 days.[341,346] Oral doses ranging from 160 to 2000 mg/kg for up to 180 days were associated with no adverse effects in dogs.[343] Safety in animals with comorbidity may be a concern. The impact of glucosamine on glucose metabolism, particularly through the hexosamine pathway,[343] has led to concern regarding diabetic control. However, glucosamine metabolism follows a different path than radiolabeled glucose,[344] and glucosamine does not appear to interact with glucose disposition.[347] Diabetes could not be induced in rats genetically predisposed to sugar-induced diabetes mellitus after treatment with glucosamine, chondroitin sulfate, or the combination of the two at 3 to 7 times the recommended dose.[348] In a separate series of studies in humans, glucose concentrations did not change and histologic lesions could not be identified as a result of glucosamine administration.[343] Using a placebo-controlled, double-blinded, randomized clinical trial, human patients requiring medical management of type 2 diabetes mellitus and receiving Cosequin (1200 mg CDS, 1500 mg glucosamine) for 90 days were monitored in an outpatient clinic. Diabetic control did not change in either group during the study period, and concentrations of glycosylated hemoglobin did not differ between treatment or placebo groups.[349] With rare to no exceptions, reviews of clinical trials in humans reveal that the use of glucosamine is not associated with adverse effects in humans.[343] Indeed, some trials find fewer adverse effects associated with glucosamine than with placebo.[343]

The use of glucosamine for treatment of osteoarthritis remains controversial despite in vitro and in vivo studies supporting its efficacy in improving lameness scores and mobility in human and animal models of degenerative joint disease. Some of the controversy probably reflects poor design of selected clinical trials.[340] However, several meta-anlayses and reviews of clinical trials generally find glucosamine (hydrochloride or sulfate) moderately effective for treatment of osteoarthritis in humans.[342a, 343] A prospective study found glucosamine to be highly cost effective in the treatment of human osteoarthritis.[343a]

All glucosamine salts appear to be equally effective,[336] although one in vitro study suggests that the *N*-acetyl salt may be less efficacious, perhaps owing to less absorption. This is in contrast to galactosamine salts (also found in PGAGs) and glucuronide salts, which do not appear to be effective in damaged joints.[336] Dosing differences should be expected among the glucosamine products. The differences reflect, in part, the different salts, with the molecular weight of the salts being hydrochloride (36.5), *N*-acetyl (58), and sulfate (96). This compares to a molecular weight of 192 for glucosamine. Thus approximately 16% of the molecular weight of glucosamine hydrochloride is represented by the (hydrochloride) salt, compared with 24% of the *N*-acetyl salt and 33% of the sulfate salt. Consequently, on the basis of weight alone (of the total salt), the dose of glucosamine sulfate should be 15% higher. An additional adjustment must be made for differences in bioavailability. Some glucosamine salts, including sulfate, are accompanied by sodium or potassium, whose molecular weight also may be included with the active moiety. Sulfate has been proposed as the active moiety responsible for efficacy of glucosamine sulfate insofar as it is required for glycosaminoglycan synthesis. Because sulfate, but not glucosamine, increases in plasma and sulfate concentrations appear in the joint, some investigators believe that it is the sulfate moiety of glucosamine sulfate that is responsible for its effects.[350] Therefore the sulfate salt might be the preferred form, but clinical trials comparing the salts are warranted. An injectable glucosamine preparation is available, and the acetyl salt is available as an enema preparation.

A number of studies support the use of glucosamine for treatment of osteoarthritis. In 2001 Reginster and coworkers[351] reported on the success of glucosamine sulfate in the treatment of knee osteoarthritis in humans in a non–manufacturer-sponsored study. The placebo-controlled, blinded study encompassed 3 years, a sample size that exceeded 200, and included outcome measures that were less subjective to bias (radiographic measurements) compared with clinical assessment. The investigators have since published additional studies[352] in different sample populations, with similar success. Glucosamine has been compared to NSAIDs as well. A meta-analysis[353] comparing ibuprofen and glucosamine for treatment of osteoarthritis pain found glucosamine to be a reasonable alternative to or adjuvant with ibuprofen or other NSAIDs.

Chondroitin Sulfate

Chondroitin sulfates are glycosaminoglycans (repeating units of galactosamine sulfate and glucuronic acid) that can be found in many tissues (see Figure 29-13). In cartilage matrix they bind to and support collagen. Differences in molecular weight result in variable oral bioavailability with lower weight molecules being more bioavailable. Chondroitin 4-sulfate is mammalian in origin, and it is the most abundant chondroitin in growing mammalian cartilage. Chondroitin sulfate generally is derived from bovine trachea. Processing is costly and variable, with differences in fractionation, particle size, molecular weight, location, purity (presence of other PGAGs, such as keratan or dermatan sulfate), and degree of sulfation evident among products. As such, products containing CDS are more likely to be mislabeled with regard to CDS content compared with glucosamine, which is less expensive to manufacture.

With age, chondrocyte secretion of chondroitin 4-sulfate may decline, contributing to the initiation of degenerative joint disease. Chondroitin 6-sulfate is derived from shark cartilage and conceptually may be less ideal than chondroitin 4-sulfate. Chondroitin sulfates appear not only to increase synthesis of PGAGs but also to competitively inhibit the actions of metalloproteases in cartilage matrix. They have a variety of other in vitro and in vivo effects on cartilage. In humans (dosed at 1 to 1.5 g/day) they decrease the need for NSAIDs.

Despite its large molecular size, 70% of CDS is absorbed in various sizes ranging from intact chains to monomer subunits after oral administration. In humans more than 70% of radioactivity was absorbed and distributed to urine and tissues after oral administration of radiolabled low molecular weight (14,000) CDS.[347,354] The presence of intestinal chondroitinases in carnivorous and omnivorous animals has been postulated as the reason for absorption.[336] In contrast to glucosamine, chondrotin sulfate accumulates after multiple dosing (for 7 days); bioavailability of 200% was reported, indicating that a carryover or residual effect might be expected after dosing is discontinued.[331]

In dogs oral chondroitin increases serum glycosaminoglycans. Because of its ubiquitous location in the body, indications other than joint disease should be considered for chondroitin sulfates, including cardiovascular diseases associated with thrombogenesis and indications previously noted for PPS. Attention should be paid to the source of chondroitin sulfates in nutraceuticals. Syndromes such as interveterbral disc disease (discs are comparised of CDS), tracheal collapse (a hyaline cartilage related problem), and chronic urinary (cystitis) infection may be rationale indications. Purified preparations are expensive, but the amount of chondroitin in whole animal tissues (mussel, shark cartilage, sea cucumber, or sea algae) cannot be determined from the label. Bioavailability of the chondroitin sulfates in such products is not known.

Efficacy of Glucosamine–Chondrotin Sulfate Combination

Glucosamine by itself might be expected to be the most effective of the oral nutraceuticals for the following reasons: (1) It is the rate-limiting step in PGAG synthesis; (2) it is generally labeled more accurately than chondroitin sulfate; and (3) clinical trials have demonstrated a clinical effect using glucosamine alone. However, the combination product might offer some advantages. A number of studies support the efficacy of the combination of chondroitin sulfate and glucosamine.[355,356] Many are sponsored by the manufactuer, most commonly Nutramax Laboratories. This should not be surprising insofar as this company holds the patent for their glucosamine–chondrotin sulfate product (Cosamin for humans and Cosequin for animals) and strives to ensure product quality and safety. In a single-center study sponsored by the manufacturer, humans with mild to moderate radiographic damage in the knee improved more when receiving Cosamine compared with placebo after 6 months of therapy.[357] Some evidence supports the possible efficacy of combination products in lower-back degenerative diseases. Leffler and coworkers[358] reported improvement in Navy personnel (n = 34) afflicted with knee or lower-back cartilage degeneration osteoarthritis after 16 weeks of Cosamin therapy compared with control. A European meta-analysis of studies found a large treatment effect in persons receiving chondroitin sulfate (of similar molecular weight to the Nutramax products Cosamin or Cosequin) and a moderate treatment effect for glucoasmine.[359] Fajardo and Di Cesare[360] reviewed meta-analyses examining the effect of glucosamine and chondroitin on treatment of human osteoarthritis. In general, the studies revealed that glucosamine provides significant effects on most outcome measures, including structural efficacy (based on radiography of joint spaces), whereas effects of chondroitin tend to be significant for symptomatic outcome measures.

Clegg and coworkers[361] reported the results of a large multicenter double-blinded clinical trial that compared placebo (negative control), celecoxib (positive control), glucosamine (1500 mg), chondroitin sulfate (1200 mg), and the combination of glucosamine and chondroitin sulfate in humans (n = 1583), with osteoarthritis graded as mild (n = 1229) and moderate and severe (n = 354). The primary outcome measure was a 20% decrease in knee pain by week 24 of treatment. The only treatment that significantly reduced pain compared with placebo was celecoxib; however, the placebo effect was 60%, underscoring the importance of negative control groups. More important, the group receiving the combination therapy tended to respond better than the placebo group ($p = 0.09$). Further, within the subgroup of patients with moderate to severe pain, the combination product, but no other treatment, was significantly more effective than placebo.

Efficacy also has been demonstrated in dogs using a variety of models, including in vitro studies and experimental and spontaneous disease. Most of these studies also have been manufacturer sponsored. With use of in vitro methods, biosynthetic activity was greater in canine cartilage cores incubated in serum collected from dogs receiving Cosequin for 1 month compared to incubation in serum collected from the same dogs before Cosequin administration.[362] Under experimental conditions, in surgically induced instability in rabbits, the combination product was found to be superior to placebo, glucosamine hydrochloride, chondroitin sulfate, or manganese

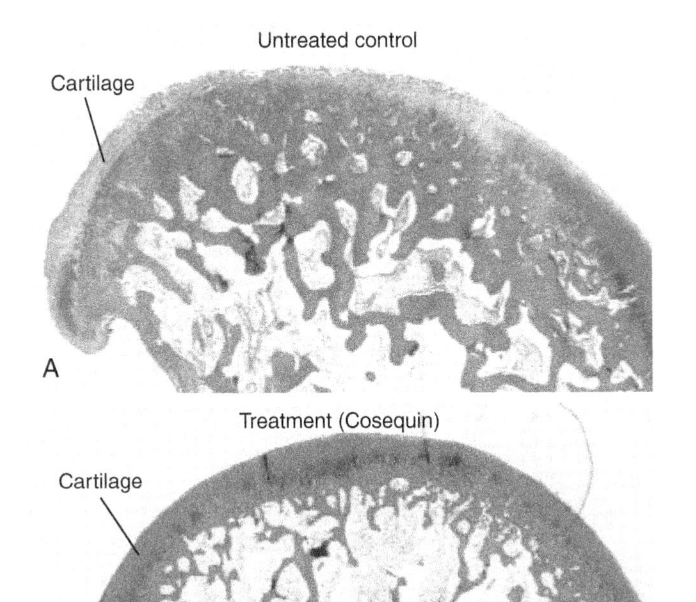

Figure 29-14 Histologic evidence of the clinical efficacy of disease-modifying agents. A surgically induced instability model of osteoarthritis was induced in rabbits. Treated rabbits received 0.38 g glucosamine hydrogen chloride and 0.304 g sodium chondroitin sulfate (Cosequin, Nutramax Laboratories, Inc., Edgewood, Md.) per kilogram body weight per day. Histologic samples were collected at 16 weeks from the center of the medial condyle. Differences in lesions between the groups were significant ($p < 0.02$). (Photographs courtesy Nutramax Laboratories.)

alone (Figure 29-14). The results of this study led investigators to suggest that the combination product Cosequin was more effective (and perhaps acted synergistically) than individual ingredients. However, the dose that animals received was higher than that recommended. Using an experimental model in dogs, Canapp and coworkers[363] demonstrated a protective effect of Cosequin in dogs when administered 21 days before induction of chemical synovitis. These studies do not reflect a comprehensive review of the literature but nonetheless provide evidence of efficacy.

Other Oral Supplements

Nutritional products for treatment of osteoarthritis were scientifically reviewed in human medicine.[364] These studies were randomized (human or animal) clinical trials that focused on osteoarthritis, published in peer-reviewed journals, and based on nonsynthesized (i.e., natural) orally administered products. Because it is considered synthetic, SAMe was excluded (it is not stable in its endogenous form), whereas chondroitin sulfates and glucosamine were excluded because they were already well reviewed. Surprisingly, only of 52 of 2026 potential studies met all criteria. Each was then scored on a scale of −2 (evidence of no efficacy) to 2 (very good evidence of efficacy). Funding sponsorship for the trial as a possible source of bias was not addressed. No positive effects were found in 11 of 52 trials. An example of some of the major nutrients that emerged from the review and their respective scores are as follows: avocado soybean unsaponifiables ([ASU] score 1.58); methylsulfonylmethane (MSM) (1.21), vitamins B_3 or C (0.75); lipids from green-lipped mussels (0.58); boron (a nonmetallic trivalent chemical whose concentration is less in femoral osteoarthritis than in normal osteoarthritis; score of 0.50); cetyl myristoleate (a lipid of sperm whale and beaver gland origin; score of 0.58); ginger [0.42], vitamin E (0.17); hyperimmune milk (−0.9); and collagen hydrosylate (−0.17).

Avocado Soybean Unsaponifiable Lipids

The term *ASU lipids* refers to the residue left behind after the lipids associated with avocados and soybeans are saponified (ie "soapafied"). Saponification occurs through the addition of an alkali. For ASU the primary ingrediants associated with the beneficial effects are phytosterols. They appear to inhibit cholesterol absorption and endogenous cholesterol biosynthesis.[365] Among those present in ASU are beta-sitoseterol, which is particularly potent as an antiinflammatory. Among the anabolic, anticatabolic, and antiinflammatory effects cited for ASU are increased collagen and aggrecan synthesis, decreased collagenase, aggrecanase and matrix metalloproteinase activity, and decreased production of IL-6 and IL-8 and PGE_2 activity. ASU increases transforming growth factor in normal canine synovial fluid. The most common avocado to soybean ratio studied was 1:2; it was the most effective, followed by products with a ratio of 1:1; products with a ratio of 2:1 were less effective. In general, ASU appears to improve symptoms of osteoarthritis after several months and may slow down joint space loss. However, further studies are needed to confirm structure-modifying effects and long-term effects.

KEY POINT 29-26 A variety of nutraceutical ingredients target inflammation. The ideal supplement or supplement combination, however, should always include orally bioavailable glucosamine and chondroitin sulfates.

S-Adenosylmethionine

S-Adenosylmethionine (also addressed in Chapter 19) also is a nutraceutical product, but its mechanism for treatment of osteoarthritis is less clear and probably reflects antiinflammatory effects. It is synthesized in the body from methionine and is responsible for a number of biological reactions, serving as a methyl donor. In the joint it may act to transulfate glycosaminoglycans. Its precursor (methionine) cannot be administered during states of deficiency without toxicity. The product must be prepared as a salt because it is unstable; it is extremely hygroscopic, and the tablet cannot be broken without loss of efficacy. In human clinical trials (controlled and uncontrolled), SAMe has improved lameness scores and mobility. In vitro studies suggest that SAMe increases proteoglycan synthesis and protects the cartilage.[323] This is being studied in dogs. The human dose is 600 mg daily for the first 2 weeks, followed by 400 mg daily. Clinical response may not be evident for 1 or 2 months.

The efficacy of SAMe for treatment of osteoarthritis in humans compared with placebo or an NSAID was studied through meta-analysis.[366] Eleven studies (controlled clinical trials) met the critiera of the study. The authors concluded that SAMe was as effective as NSAIDS in reducing pain and improving function, without the adverse effects traditionally associated with NSAIDs. Limitations of the studies included higher than recommended doses for some studies; a short intervention for most studies (28 to 30 days), which may have underestimated NSAID efficacy; and, in general, study of only osteoarthritis of the knee or hip, which limited extrapolation of data to osteoarthritis of other joints. The mechanisms and other aspects of SAMe are addressed in greater depth in Chapter 19.

Phycocyanin

Phycocyanin (PC) is a phycobiliprotein chromoprotein that is a major pigment of the microalgae Spirulina. Among its function in algae is to harvest light, which also serves to protect the organism from undue damage associated with oxygen radical formation produced by exposure to ultraviolet light. Like many other light-harvesting pigments, it is an effective antioxidant compound. Structurally, it is similar to bilirubin, which also has antioxidant activities.[367] Romay and coworkers[367] reviewed the evidence supporting PC as a selective COX-2 inhibitor. First, antioxidant properties in general have been demonstrated in vitro, including scavenging of hydroxyl, alkoyl, peroxyl, and peroxynitrite radicals. Lipid peroxidation has been demonstrated, also in vitro. Neutrophil activation is decreased. Antiinflammatory effects have been demonstrated using inflammatory rodent models in a dose-dependent model. Because the models are also used to demonstrate inhibition of COX or lipoxygenase activities, the antiinflammatory effects of PC were considered to potentially reflect inhibition of AA metabolism, as well as prevention of lipid peroxidation. Separating out the direct inhibitionof COX or lipoxygenase from inhibition of fatty acid (i.e., AA) release from cell membranes is difficult. Studies in human whole blood have supported COX-2 inhibition, although selectivity was not demonstrated. However, a subsequent in vitro study using cloned human COX-1 and COX-2 does demonstrate selectivity.[367] The appropriateness of using COX-1 to COX-2 ratios as indicators of efficacy or safety has already been discussed. By virtue of its antioxidant effects, largely through animal models, PC has demonstrated potential efficacy as a hepatoprotectant and a treatment for arthritis and inflammatory bowel disease. Because efficacy has been demonstrated after oral absorption, it is possible that it is not active as the intact compound. Although its combined use as an antiinflammatory with disease-modifying agents containing glucosamine and chondroitin sulfates is reasonable, issues associated with dietary supplments in general should be addressed, including species differences, safety, and quality assurance of the product. This is particularly true if PC is an inhibitor of COX; its safety should be confirmed in target species, particularly when combined with NSAIDs.

OTHER ANTIINFLAMMATORY DRUGS

Orgotein

Orgotein, or superoxide dismutase, is a copper- and zinc-containing metolloprotein that can be an effective antiinflammatory. As an endogenous intracellular enzyme, it occurs at very low concentrations in many tissues, but particularly the liver, where it scavenges tissue-damaging oxygen radicals. Phagocytic cells (neutrophils and macrophages) generate large amounts of cytotoxic superoxides during the inflammatory process. Among the radicals apparently scavenged by orgotein is peroxynitrite, a long-lasting radical that can contribute to chondrocyte death.[323] The half-life of phagocytic cells is prolonged in the presence of superoxide dismutase.[369,370] Approximately 2 to 6 weeks of therapy may be required before therapeutic benefits are realized.

Orgotein is characterized by a wide margin of safety, with the lethal dose being over 40,000 times the therapeutic dose. As a large molecule, efficacy by any route other than intraarticular is questionable owing to poor absorption. The drug has, however, also been administered clinically both intramuscularly and orally.[371] Absorption of the oral preparation has not been documented. Molecular size limits renal elimination of the drug. After intraarticular administration, orgotein was 94% effective in horses lame for less than 2 months, compared with only 49% efficacy in horses lame for longer than 2 months before treatment.[372] The use of orgotein in combination with disease-modifying agents is a rational approach for control of inflammation; however, other antiinflammatories may be necessary for effective control of inflammation.

Dimethylsulfoxide

Dimethylsulfoxide (DMSO) is a hygroscopic solvent derived from wood pulp. It is used as a drug vehicle because of its ability to dissolve drugs that are not soluble in water.[373,374]

Pharmacologic Effects

As an antiinflammatory, DMSO is a scavenger of free oxygen radicals. Antiinflammatory effects have been reported in acute musculoskeletal injuries and CNS inflammatory processes and after trauma.[375,376] Chronic diseases are less responsive to the antiinflammatory effects of DMSO. Immunomodulation may be responsible for some of the antiinflammatory effects of DMSO. The drug inhibits white blood cell migration and antibody production. Fibroblast proliferation is also inhibited. The analgesic effects of DMSO have been compared with those of narcotic analgesics. Analgesia has been reported in a variety of situations, including acute and chronic musculoskeletal disorders and postoperative pain. Although nerve blockade has been reported in vitro, it is unlikely that concentrations occur in vivo sufficient to affect this response. Opiate receptors also do not seem to be involved. Other pharmacologic effects include inhibition or stimulation of enzymes, vasodilation (due to either histamine release or anticholinesterase effects), inhibition of platelet aggregation, radioprotection, cryopreservation, and antimicrobial (antifungal, bacterial, and viral) activity.[373,375] Diuresis occurs after topical, oral, or parenteral administration, probably because of its hygroscopic nature and ability to pull water into the tubules. DMSO (3 mg/kg in 20% solution) has been reported to protect the kidneys against ischemic insults. A sedative effect has also been reported in several species.[373]

Disposition

After oral administration of 1 g/kg, peak plasma drug concentrations occur within 4 to 6 hours, and detectable levels persist in the plasma for 400 hours.[375] Within 20 minutes of topical application, DMSO penetrates the skin and can be detected in all organs of the body.[373] Peak plasma drug concentrations occur 2 hours after topical administration.[375] Its ability to penetrate the skin is believed to reflect exchange and interchange with water in biologic membranes. Mucous membranes, lipid membranes of cells and organelles, and the blood–brain barrier are similarly penetrated without irreversible membrane damage.[373] Tooth enamel and keratin appear to be the only tissues that DMSO does not penetrate.[375] DMSO facilitates penetration of other substances across membranes; cutaneous penetration of steroids, sulfadiazine, phenylbutazone, and other drugs has been documented.[373,374] Enhanced absorption of therapeutic drugs can lead to toxicity, particularly for anesthetic, cardioactive, and anticholinesterase drugs.

DMSO is partially metabolized by hepatic microsomal enzymes,[373] but the primary route of elimination appears to be in the urine as the parent compound.[375] Although a significant amount of DMSO may be eliminated in the bile, most undergoes enterohepatic circulation.[375] Hepatic metabolism of a small amount of DMSO (3% to 6%) to dimethylsulfide and subsequent pulmonary excretion of this metabolite accounts for the halitosis that occurs regardless of the route of administration.[375]

Adverse Effects

DMSO is characterized by a large safety margin. Signs associated with near lethal intravenous doses include sedation, diuresis, intravascular hemolysis, and hematuria. Death is preceded by hypotension; prostration; convulsions; and respiratory distress characterized by dyspnea, tachypnea, and pulmonary edema. Phlebitis and venous obstruction may occur with intravenous dosing. Intravascular hemolysis is concentration and rate dependent, and concentrations less than 10% are recommended for intravenous administration. Susceptibility to hemolysis will vary with species on account of differences in erythrocyte fragility. Nephrotoxicity has been reported in some species. Necropsy lesions include hematuria, hemoglobinuria, and mild tubular nephrosis. Chronic toxicity studies in laboratory animals have documented hepatotoxicity, which may be due to its metabolism by the liver to toxic metabolites. DMSO may also enhance hepatotoxicity of other drugs, as well as hepatic binding and metabolism of selected carcinogens.

Teratogenicity has also been reported in some animals. Ocular toxicity occurs with daily, long-term administration and develops more rapidly in young animals. Lesions occur in the lens and appear as altered lucency, making animals myopic. Histologic abnormalities are not apparent. Such a response was reported in one horse that received 0.6 g/kg daily cutaneously for 2 months. Skin reactions are common, particularly at higher concentrations, and are manifested as erythema, warmth, and local vasodilation. A wheal and flare response and pruritus may also occur. Repeated application may result in drying and desquamation of the epithelium.[373]

Clinical Use

DMSO is approved for topical application in horses suffering from acute swelling caused by trauma and in the treatment of acute or chronic otitis. In humans DMSO is approved for interstitial cystitis. Although not approved, DMSO has been recommended for therapy in male cats suffering from urinary tract obstruction.[373] Other reported applications of DMSO include facilitation of healing of skin wounds (including habronemiasis of horses), acral lick dermatitis in dogs, postoperative fibrous adhesions, acute CNS trauma, inflammation, edema or ischemia, intervertebral disc disease, fibrocartilaginous embolization, ischemic insults, postoperative myositis, rheumatic diseases, myasthenia gravis, and chronic musculoskeletal conditions. DMSO also inhibits alcohol dehydrogenase and thus has been recommended for the treatment of ethylene glycol toxicity.[373]

Methylsulfonylmethane

Methylsulfonylmethane is a naturally occurring metabolite of DMSO that has also received attention as a food additive for control of musculoskeletal inflammation. Limited data[364] are available to support the use of this compound for therapy of osteoarthritis.

USE OF MODULATORS OF INFLAMMATION IN THE TREATMENT OF SHOCK AND CENTRAL NERVOUS SYSTEM TRAUMA

A number of drugs that modulate the inflammatory response have been studied for their effect in the patient suffering from shock, particularly that associated with the release of bacterial toxins such as endotoxin (septic shock). Because of the oxygen radical scavenging ability of some of these drugs, studies have also focused on their use in treatment of damage to the CNS.

Pathophysiology of Septic Shock

The pathophysiology of septic shock is addressed in Chapter 8. This discussion focuses on the inflammatory mediators associated with the syndrome. Increasingly, sepsis is recognized to reflect an exaggerated systemic inflammatory response to infectious organisms. Mediators of the response include lipopolysaccharide of gram-negative bacteria, lipoteichoic acid of gram-positive bacteria, and peptidoglycan from both. Cytokines released by host cells (macrophages and circulating monocytes) play a pivotal role in the pathyophysiology.

Gram-positive bacteria appear to secrete superantigens, which bind to both major histocompatibility complex molecules and T-cell receptors, initiating massive cytokine production. Lipoteichoic acid and endotoxin both stimulate cytokine production. The lipid A component of lipopolysaccharide, endotoxin, found on the surface of gram-negative organisms, is a highly conserved molecule responsible for the sequelae of endotoxic shock. The manifestation begins as endotoxin released from dying gram-negative organisms interacts with receptors on cells of the host defense system: macrophages, neutrophils, platelets, and lymphocytes. Endotoxin also directly interacts with vascular endothelial cells. In response, cells either release the mediators of endotoxic shock or render other cells more reactive to cellular signals and subsequent mediator release. Mediators of endotoxic shock are grouped as cytokines, lipid mediators, or secondary mediators.[377,378] Cytokines are small polypeptides released from inflammatory cells, especially macrophages. TNF and IL-1 are the two cytokines that appear to be primarily responsible for the cascade of endotoxemia. Their effects in turn are often mediated by nitric oxide. Lipid mediators are derived from AA, located in the phospholipids of cell membranes, particularly those of neutrophils, platelets, vascular endothelium, and vascular smooth muscle. Examples include PGs (including thromboxane), LTs, and platelet-activating factor.

Both cytokines and the lipid mediators act as signaling mechanisms among inflammatory cells, platelets, and the vascular endothelium through negative and positive feedback mechanisms. When the positive feedback loops overwhelm the negative feedback loops, the pathophysiology of endotoxic shock becomes a clinical reality. The pathophysiology reflects, in part, the direct effects of endotoxin (e.g., it directs activation of Hageman factor and complement components) and the combined or individual effects of the mediators. Secondary mediators (e.g., histamine, serotonin, vasopressin, angiotensin II, catecholamines, and opioids) are released in response to cytokines and lipid mediators, resulting in the general signs of endotoxic shock. Adhesion molecules, selectins, and leukocyte integrins are among the humoral mediators associated with the pathophysiology. Disruption in hemostasis balance also is affected by inflammatory cytokines. Interleukins 1α, 1β, and TNF-α activate tissue factor and subsequent coagulation; endotoxin also increased the activity of fibrinolytic inhibitors, contributing to an imbalance in the coagulation cascade. Changes in peripheral vasculature (i.e., constriction and dilation) coupled with activation of clotting factors and inhibition of fibrinolysis, results in widespread coagulopathy, microbembolization, and vascular endothelial damage.The clinical signs associated with each stage of shock depend on the mediators released during that stage and vary among species. The complex interactions of these mediators, however, if allowed to progress, can result in multiple organ failure in any species simply because of the cumulative effects of hypoxia: oxygen radical, lysosomal enzymes, thrombosis, and metabolic derangements.

Drug therapy is most likely to be successful when initiated early during the course of endotoxic shock. The role of steroidal compounds in the treatment of shock in animals was reviewed by Howe.[379] A number of investigators have recently reviewed the role of mediator-specific antiinflammatory agents in the prevention and treatment of septic shock.[380,381] Examples of these drugs include antibiodies to TNF, soluble TNF receptors, agonists of IL-1or platelet activating receptors, and drugs that target bradykinin or PGs. Thus far, these drugs appear to have demonstrated efficacy in clinical trials. Meta-analyses indicate that their use should be associated with clinical benefits in the individual patient.[381] However, because the targets of these drugs play complex roles in the pathophysiology of septic shock, their general use should be discouraged; rather their use should be matched to patient conditions that are more likely to benefit from treatment.

Role of Lipid Peroxidation in Tissue Injury

Lipid peroxide formation is the result of free radical–mediated cell and tissue injury caused by lipid peroxides within cell membranes and organelles. Both structure and function of the membranes and organelles are disrupted by lipid peroxide formation. Lipid peroxidation is a potentially geometrically progressing reaction that spreads over the surface of cell membranes, impairing phospholipid-dependent enzymes; ionic gradients across the cell membrane,;and, if sufficiently severe, membrane lysis (Figure 29-15). Its importance, along with the generation of oxygen radicals, is evident early in the pathophysiology of CNS trauma. Lipid peroxidation is only one of several sources of oxygen radial formation. Other sources include the AA cascade; catecholamine oxidation; mitochondrial "leak"; oxidation of extravasated hemoglobin; and, as the inflammatoryprocess proceeds, infiltrating neutrophils.

Lipid peroxidation is initiated by a reactive oxygen molecule. After CNS trauma, the generation of oxygen radicals during the normal reduction of oxygen overwhelms normal control mechanisms. Xanthine/xanthine oxidase, PG synthetase, and other mechanisms result in superoxide anion formation. Although superoxide anion is not in itself very reactive, it becomes more so by accepting a proton, thereby becoming more able to penetrate cell membranes. Other sources of superoxide anion include catecholamines; ascorbic acid and glutathione act to inhibit superoxide anion. The superoxide anion can also become more dangerous by conversion by way of superoxide dismutase to hydrogen peroxide. Inflammatory cells are an important source of hydrogen peroxide, as is degradation of monoamines mediated by monoamine oxidase. Mitochondria contain high concentrations of superoxide dismutase. Although hydrogen peroxide is not very damaging to intact tissues, it can easily penetrate cell membranes unless destroyed first by catalase. In the cell membrane, hydrogen peroxide interacts with iron to yield the highly reactive hydroxyl radical.

Normally, the conversion of oxygen to water is well controlled by the presence of superoxide dismutase, catalase, and endogenous antioxidants, with vitamin E being one of the most important membrane-bound antioxidants. After CNS trauma, normal control mechanisms are lost, and lipid peroxidase formation begins. Iron plays a crucial role in this process. Free iron released from hemoglobin, transferrin, or ferritin in the presence of a lowered tissue pH or oxygen radicals catalyzes radical-initiated peroxidation (see Figure 29-15). Iron–oxygen complexes probably initiate lipid peroxidase formation; damage during ischemic injury from

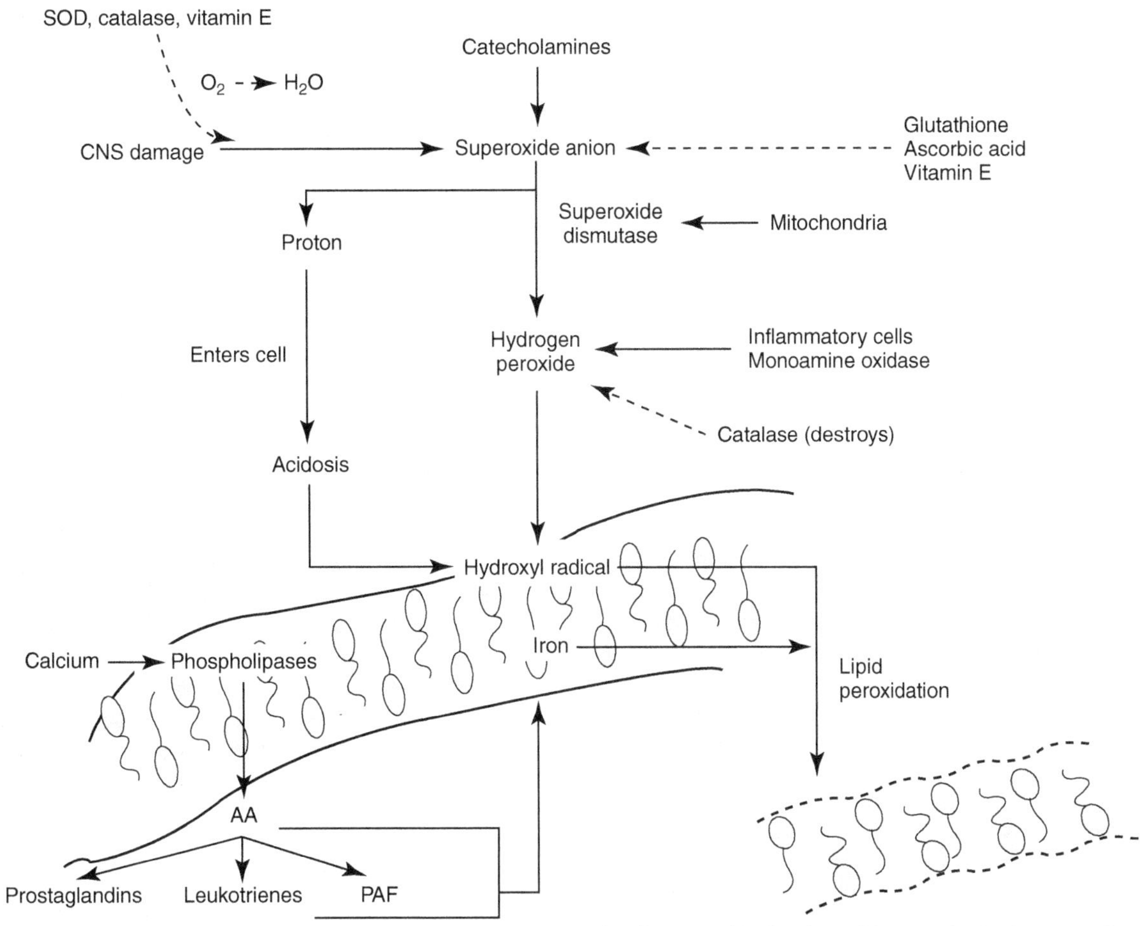

Figure 29-15 Lipid peroxidation of cell membranes reflects a cascade of events that begins with neurologic damage. Oxygen radical formation is potentiated in the presence of iron and is inhibited by endogenous protectants such as superoxide dismutase (SOD) (which converts the superoxide radical to hydrogen peroxide) and catalase. Catecholamine release can contribute to damage. The ability of the radicals to move down the cell membrane is facilitated by the fluidity of the membrane. Calcium influx accompanying cell membrane damage contributes to the formation of arachidonic acid metabolites and subsequent inflammation. *AA,* Arachidonic acid; *CNS,* central nervous system; *PAF,* platelet-activating factor.

radicals will be affected by the amount and location of iron (and copper) ions. Unfortunately, these ions become more available during injury. Acidosis, which often accompanies ischemia (anaerobic environment and lactic acidosis), increases the solubility of iron. Free calcium released during the injury stimulates phosopholipase A_2 and the AA cascade. Metabolites of AA are important sources of reactive oxygen species. Inflammatory cells become an important source of continued AA metabolism. Decreased concentrations of vitamin E, ascorbic acid, and glutathione (induced by scavenging of oxygen radicals) predicate the occurrence of lipid peroxidation.

Drugs That Impair Mediators of Sepsis

Nonsteroidal Antiinflammatory Drugs

A number of NSAIDs have been studied for their ability to block response to mediators of endotoxic shock. Indomethacin and ibuprofen have shown efficacy in human patients.[380,382] Flunixin meglumine has been studied in horses and dogs.[141,383] As with glucocorticoids, however, the effects of NSAIDs must be realized within the first 2 hours of the onset of endotoxic shock—that is, before mediators have been able to stimulate response. The use of NSAIDs may shunt AA substrate to the lipoxygenase pathway, which may cause detrimental effects. Thus drugs that impair both arms of the AA cascade may prove more useful. The efficacy of ketoprofen, an NSAID that appears to inhibit both PGs and LTs, has been shown to ameliorate many of the effects of endotoxin infusion.[384] The combined use of NSAIDs with LT antagonists apparently has not been reported in endotoxic shock, but the advent of dual inhibitors warrants further studies. Prolonged therapy with NSAIDs is not advisable because of toxic effects. Although gastrointestinal toxicity is the major concern in most animals, the patient suffering from endotoxic shock may be more predisposed.

Glucocorticoids

Glucocorticoids are discussed in Chapter 17. Glucocorticoids inhibit the enzyme phospholipase A_2 and the release of TNF and IL-2 from activated macrophages.[385] Glucocorticoids also alter synthesis of and biologic response to collagenase, lipase, and plasminogen activator. The immunosuppressive actions of glucocorticoids are more pronounced on the cellular arm than the humoral arm of the immune system. Glucocorticoids have minimal effects on plasma immunoglobulin concentrations but can modulate immunoglobulin function. Immunosuppressive actions of glucocorticoids, like their antiinflammatory actions, involve disruption of intercellular communication of leukocytes through interference with lymphokine production and biological action; however, these effects are largely transrepressive (see Chapter 17). Glucocorticoids block the effects of macrophage-inhibiting factor and interferon-γ (IFN-γ) on macrophages. IFN-γ, which is released from activated T cells, plays an important role in facilitating antigen processing by macrophages. Glucocorticoids inhibit the synthesis and release of IL-1 by macrophages, thereby suppressing the activation of T cells. Glucocorticoids also inhibit IL-2 synthesis by activated T cells. Interleukin-2 plays a critical role in amplification of cell-mediated immunity. Additionally, glucocorticoids suppress the bactericidal and fungicidal actions of macrophages.

Septic shock. Earlier experimental models of septic shock in animals indicated that glucocorticoids can be of benefit but only if administered before or concurrently with endotoxin administration—that is, within the first 2 hours. In canine models severe mesenteric vasoconstriction within the first 15 minutes can lead to irreversible shock. Thus glucocorticoids provided no beneficial effects when administered 30 to 60 minutes after administration of the endotoxin. Rapid-acting, water-soluble agents such as dexamethasone sodium phosphate (4 to 8 mg/kg intravenously), prednisolone sodium succinate or sodium phosphate (30 mg/kg intravenously), or methylprednisolone sodium succinate (30 mg/kg intravenously) have been recommended, at shock doses, which are 5 to 10 times the immunosuppressive dose. However, more recent data suggest that the use of glucocorticoids in patients with sepsis is controversial. Multiple meta-analyses of randomized human studies have demonstrated that high doses of glucocorticoids (e.g., methylprednisolone at 30 mg/kg) invariably do not prevent septic shock, reverse the shock state, or improve the 14-day mortality rate, despite theoretical and experimental animal evidence to the contrary. Indeed, mortality rates were greater in one study, presumably because of immunosuppression and secondary infection.[381] In contrast, stress-dose (or physiologic dose) glucocorticoids (e.g., hydrocortisone at 200 mg/day; approximately 3 mg/kg) intended to replace deficient corticosteroids (due to adrenal suppression) in patients with severe and refractory shock may be of benefit (see Chapter 17). Patients with persistent vasopressor-dependent shock should be targeted,[381] although controversies continue regarding this indication as well.[380] In human patients use of glucocorticoids is controversial, with no improvement in survival in some studies.[386]

Hemorrhagic shock. The use of glucocorticoids for treatment of hemorrhagic shock is controversial. Some studies in dogs suggest that dexamethasone sodium phosphate (5 mg/kg intravenously) may improve blood flow to the kidneys, lungs, and gastrointestinal tract. Other supportive measures, particularly aggressive fluid therapy, must also be instituted. Appropriate fluid replacement therapy will ensure adequate drug distribution to target tissues.

Oxygen radical scavengers. A neuroprotective role has been recognized for certain glucocorticoids and, most notably, methylprednisolone. Interest stemmed from the observation that the ability to inhibit CNS lipid peroxidation and influence other pathophysiologic processes strongly correlated with neurologic recovery. The neuroprotective effects have been separated from the glucocorticoid activity by the discovery of nonglucocorticoid steroids that are able to equal or surpass the antioxidant effects of methylprednisolone (see later discussion of lazaroids).

In a feline model of spinal injury, methylprednisolone (30 mg/kg) attenuates posttraumatic lipid peroxidation. In addition, perhaps because of the inhibitory effect on lipid peroxidation, methylprednisolone supports energy metabolism, reduces or prevents posttraumatic ischemia and neurofilament degradation, reduces intracellular calcium accumulation (resulting in the AA cascade), and inhibits vasoactive PGs ($PGF_2\alpha$ and thromboxane). In addition, like other steroids, methylprednisolone may increase spinal neuronal excitability, which may also be important to neurophysiologic recovery. Several pertinent points must be appreciated regarding these effects of methylprednisolone on spinal cord injury. First, these effects occur only at a high concentration (i.e., that achieved with an intravenous dose of 30 mg/kg). Second, the effects are biphasic, with loss at 60 mg/kg. As with many protective mechanisms, the drug must be administered early in the pathophysiologic process because spinal uptake of methylprednisolone decreases rapidly with time after injury. Loss of effect may reflect a decrease in blood flow to damaged tissues or the irreversible nature of lipid peroxidase. Finally, the time course of neuroprotection of methylprednisolone follows the disappearance of the drug from plasma or tissue—that is, it lasts only 2 to 6 hours (the half-life of the drug in feline spinal tissue). Thus the drug must be administered frequently to preserve tissues and maximize the potential for recovery. The role of glucocorticoids in treatment of intervertebral disc disease is addressed in Chapter 27).

Lazaroids

After the unique protective effect of methylprednisolone among the glucocorticoids in damaged nerve tissue was recognized, attempts were made to refine the structure of the steroidal molecule such that the neuroprotective (anti lipid peroxidase) effects would be maintained but the glucocorticoid effects minimized.[393] The result of these efforts was the synthesis of the 21-aminosteroids or lazaroids. Tirilazad mesylate is the prototypic drug (Figure 29-16). Lazaroids have been specifically designed to localize in cell membranes and inhibit (iron-mediated) lipid peroxidase. Although initial investigations were oriented toward acute trauma, because inhibition of lipid peroxidase may decrease neuronal degeneration, these drugs may also be useful for chronic neurodegenerative processes.

Tirilazad mesylate is a very lipophilic drug that preferentially distributes to the lipid components of cell membranes.

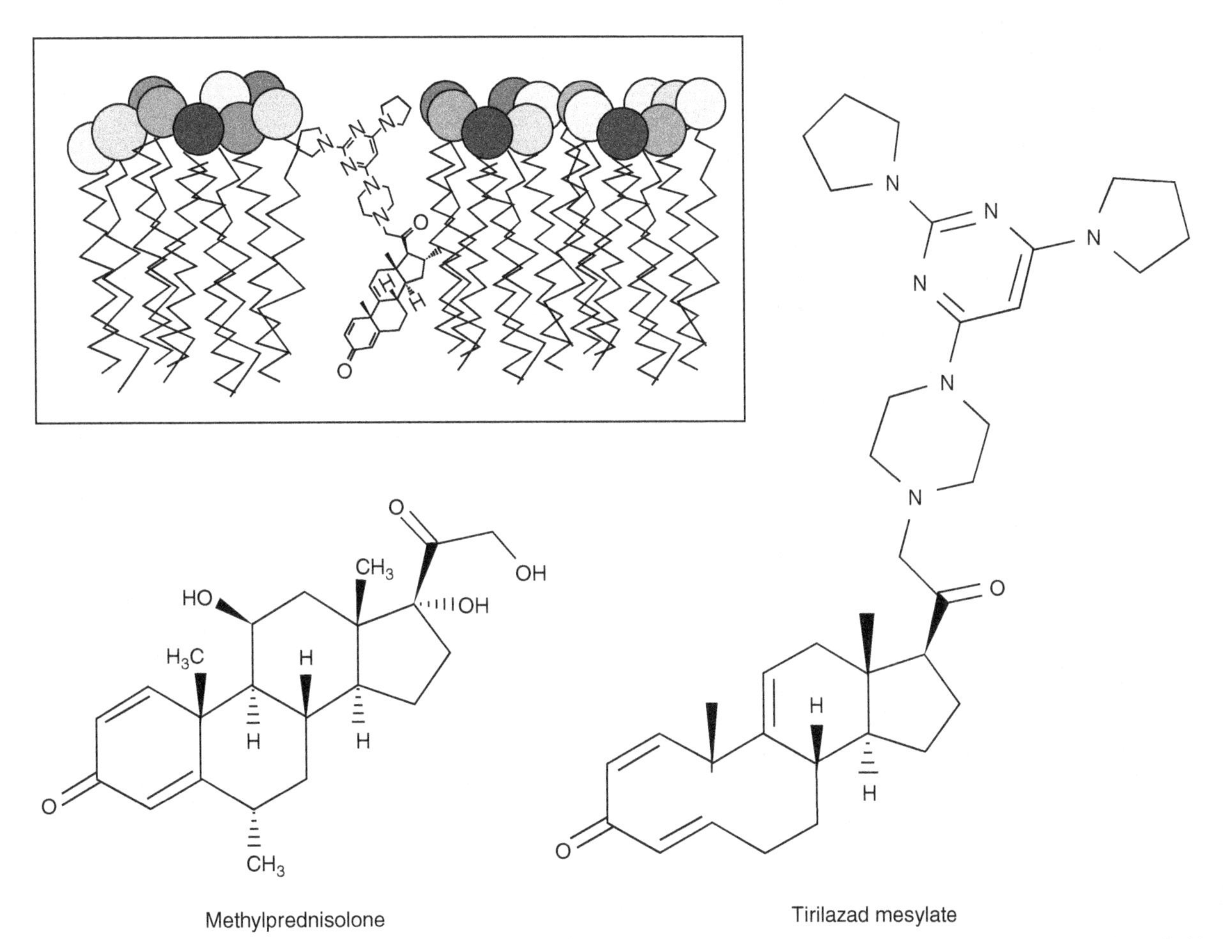

Figure 29-16 Tirilazad mesylate is an example of a lazaroid (a 21-aminosteroid). Compared with methylprednisolone *(left),* a glucocortiocoid capable of scavenging oxygen radicals, the 21-aminosteroids are devoid of steroidal activity. Their ability to inhibit lipid peroxidation and provide a neuroprotective effect occur in part by insertion into the lipid bilayer of the cell membrane. Cell membrane fluidity is decreased, thus impairing the ability of oxygen radical formation to cascade across the lipid layer. Lipid peroxidation is thus minimized.

Because neuronal tissue is composed of a greater proportion of lipid components, these drugs preferentially accumulate in neuronal tissue. Its pharmacologic actions are complex and include a radical scavenging–antioxidant effect and a physiochemical interaction with the cell membrane such that the fluidity of the membrane is decreased (see Figure 29-16). Although action against iron-mediated lipid peroxidase was sought for these drugs, they will in fact inhibit lipid peroxidase in iron-free systems as well. Tirilazad has proved to be an effective inhibitor of lipid peroxidase in all in vitro models studied. It also acts to reduce hydroxyl radicals by either direct scavenging abilities or decreased lipid peroxidase. Stabilization of cell membranes is considered an important part of its protective action. The nitrogen component of the steroid is thought to interact with the phosphate of the "head" groups (hydrophilic portion) of the bilipid layer by way of ionic interactions. The steroidal component localizes in the lipophilic portion of the membrane, compressing the phospholipid groups. Restriction of the movement of the cell membrane reduces the potential for lipid peroxidase by restricting the movement of lipid peroxyl and alkoxyl radicals in the membrane.

Tirilazad also has a high affinity for vascular endothelium. It appears to be able to protect vascular endothelium from damage by reactive oxygen species, possibly by preserving endothelium-derived relaxing function. It also appears to protect the blood–brain barrier against traumatically or chemically induced permeability. Tirilazad may protect other endothelial cells during trauma or hypoxic damage, such as the hepatic endothelium during hemorrhagic shock.

Animal models used to study the effects (not safety) of tirilazad have been primarily rats and monkeys. A few studies have focused on dogs or cats. Models of CNS damage have included that induced by cardiac arrest, altered cerebral blood flow, and subarachnoid hemorrhage. The clinical pharmacology of tirilazad has been studied in humans. It appears to be a flow-limited hepatically cleared drug. In humans there is a discrepancy in the elimination half-life of approximately 4 hours in one report and, after steady state, 35 hours. The difference appears to be a longer terminal phase after multiple dosing compared with single dosing; it is likely that volume of distribution cannot be accurately assessed after single dosing. The disposition of tirilazad is linear and does not appear to change with plasma drug concentration. Safety studies in humans have revealed the drug to be safe. Pain occurs at the site of injection, but this has been overcome by dilution of the drug, a change in the site of injection, and frequent catheter changes. Tirilazad does not appear to adversely affect the heart, blood pressure, or hepatic or renal function. Tirilazad has no glucocorticoid activity and will not alter parameters indicative of glucocorticoids (i.e., glucose, hematologic indices, adrenocorticotropic hormone, or cortisol). Apparent indications for tirilazad in humans include acute head or spinal injury, subarachnoid hemorrhage, and ischemic stroke.

The lazaroids have also demonstrated efficacy in traumatic shock,[387] hemorrhagic shock,[388] and endotoxemia.[389,390] Lazaroids decrease neutrophil accumulation, maintain arterial pressure, decrease myocardial injury, and increase survival. Lazaroids decrease formation of the eicosanoid mediators and production of TNF. When administered to dogs within 30 minutes of endotoxin infusion, lazaroids attenuated the effects of endotoxin.[391] Further studies are indicated before the use of lazaroids is confirmed. Currently, no lazaroid is approved for use in the United States.

Recombinant Human Activated Protein C

Activated protein C (APC) is an endogenous protein that simultaneously promotes fibrinolysis and inhibits thrombosis and inflammation, thus potentially modulating some of the negative sequelae of sepsis. In septic patients concentrations of protein C are decreased and conversion of protein C to activated protein C is inhibited. The role of protein C in septic shock led to the development and subsequent approval of a recombinant product, drotrecogin-activated, used in the treatment of human septic shock. In humans clinical trials largely support the safety and efficacy of the drotrecogin-alfa, activated, as indicated by decreased mortality rates.[380] Its efficacy has been attributed to effects beyond those on the coagulation cascade, with antiapoptotic effects on endothelial cells suggested. The use of APC may be of most benefit in patients with a high risk of death but may be harmful in patients with a low risk of death.[381,392] Consequently, the use of this product in small animals should be based on scientific studies that establish the optimal pharmacokinetic–pharmacodynamic relationship.

Inhibitors of Soluble Epoxide Hydrolase

The role of cytochrome P450 in the production of biologically active compounds, including the patient with septic shock, is largely overlooked. However, EETs or HETEs and EpOMEs are among the chemicals derived from the vascular endothelium that mediate vascular relaxation responses, as well as antiinflammatory effects in septic shock. Proposed mechanisms by which EETs modify the response of septic shock include inhibition of transcription factor nuclear factor-κB and IB kinase, thus preventing amplification resulting from macrophage production of proinflammatory proteins, such as TNF-α, IL-6, iNOS, and COX-2. Once formed, EETs and EpOMEs are further metabolized by soluble (in the cytoplasm) epoxide hydrolase (SEH). Persistence of these mediators by inhibition of SHE is being investigated as a therapeutic target in the patient in septic shock.[261] Drugs that target SHE not only facilitate EETs but also may facilitate the antiendotoxic effects of lipoxin.

REFERENCES

1. Lees P, Landoni MF, Giraudel J: Pharmacodynamics and pharmacokinetics of nonsteroidal anti-inflammatory drugs in species of veterinary interest, *J Vet Pharmacol Ther* 27(6):479–490, 2004.
2. Vane J, Botting R: Inflammation and the mechanism of action of antiinflammatory drugs, *FASEB J* 1:89–96, 1987.
3. Botting R: Inhibitors of cyclooxygenase: Mechanisms, selectivity and uses, *J Phys Pharm* 57(5):113–124, 2006.
4. D'Acquisto F, May MJ, Ghosh S: Inhibition of nuclear factor kappa B (NFκB): an emerging theme in anti-inflammatory therapies, *Mol Interv* 2:22–35, 2002.
5. Mohammed FF, Smookler DS, Khokha R: Metalloproteinases, inflammation, and rheumatoid arthritis, *Ann Rheum Dis* 62: 43–47, 2003.
6. Boynton CS, Dick CF, Mayor GH: NSAIDs: an overview, *J Clin Pharmacol* 28:512–517, 1988.
7. Hochberg MC: NSAIDs: mechanisms and pathways of action, *Hosp Pract* 15:185–198, 1989.
8. Robinson DR: Eicosanoids, inflammation, and antiinflammatory drugs, *Clin Exp Rheumatol* 7:155–161, 1989.
9. Warner TD: Cyclooxygenases: new forms, new inhibitors, and lessons from the clinic, *FASEB J* 18(7):790–804, 2004.
10. Weissmann G: The actions of NSAIDs, *Hosp Pract* 15:60–76, 1991.
11. FitzGerald GA, Burke A, Smyth E: Recent developments with traditional NSAIDs and COX-2 inhibitors" (Update). In Brunton LL, Lazo JS, Parker KL, editors: *Goodman & Gilman's the pharmacological basis of therapeutics*, ed 11, New York, 2006, McGraw-Hill.
12. Griswold DE, Adams JL: Constitutive cyclooxygenase (COX-1) and inducible cyclooxygenase (COX-2): rationale for selective inhibition and progress to date, *Med Res Rev* 16(2):181–206, 1996.
13. Williams CS, DuBois RN: Prostaglandin endoperoxide synthase: why two isoforms? *Am J Physiol* 270(3 Pt 1):G393–G400, 1996.
14. Crawford LJ: COX-1 and COX-2 tissue expression: implications and predictions, *J Rheumatol* 49(Suppl 24):15–19, 1997.
15. Cashman JN: The mechanisms of action of NSAIDs in analgesia, *Drugs* 52(Suppl 5):13–23, 1996.
16. Donnelly MT, Hawkey CJ: Review article: COX-II inhibitors: a new generation of safer NSAIDs? *Alimentary Pharmacol Ther* 11(2):227–236, 1997.
17. Kiefer W, Dannhardt G: Novel insights and therapeutical applications in the field of inhibitors of COX-2, *Curr Med Chem* 11:3147–3161, 2004.
18. Hinz B, Brune K: Pain and osteoarthritis: new drugs and mechanisms, *Curr Opin Rheumatol* 16(5):628–633, 2004.
19. Krause DL, Müller N: Neuroinflammation, microglia and implications for anti- inflammatory treatment in Alzheimer's disease, *Int J Alzheimers Dis* , 2010:Jun 14;2010. pii: 732806. PubMed PMID: 20798769; PubMed Central PMCID: PMC2925207.

19a. Izarraga I, Chambers JP, Johnson CB: Synergistic depression of NMDA receptor-mediated transmission by ketamine, ketoprofen and L-NAME combinations in neonatal rat spinal cords in vitro, *Br J Pharmacol* 153(5):1030–1042, 2008.

20. Warner TD, Giulano F, Vojnovic I, et al: Nonsteroid drug selectivities for cyclo-oxygenase-1 rather than cyclo-oxygenase-2 are associated with human gastrointestinal toxicity: a full in vitro analysis, *Proc Natl Acad Sci U S A* 96(13):7563–7568, 1999.

20a. Jones P, Lamdin R: Oral cyclo-oxygenase 2 inhibitors versus other oral analgesics for acute soft tissue injury: systematic review and meta-analysis, *Clin Drug Investig* 30(7):419–437, 2010.

20b. Vuolteenaho K, Moilanen T, Moilanen E: Non-steroidal anti-inflammatory drugs, cyclooxygenase-2 and the bone healing process, *Basic Clin Pharmacol Toxicol* 102(1):10–14, 2008.

20c. Souyri C, Olivier P, Grolleau S, et al: Severe necrotizing soft-tissue infections and nonsteroidal anti-inflammatory drugs, *Clin Exp Dermatol* 33(3):249–255, 2008.
20d. Roumie CL, Choma NN, Kaltenbach L, et al: Non-aspirin NSAIDs, cyclooxygenase-2 inhibitors and risk for cardiovascular events-stroke, acute myocardial infarction, and death from coronary heart disease, *Pharmacoepidemiol Drug Saf* 18(11): 1053–1063, 2009.
21. Goodman L, Torres B, Punke J, et al: Effects of firocoxib and tepoxalin on healing in a canine gastric mucosal injury model, *J Vet Intern Med* 23(1):56–62, 2009.
22. Bertolini A, Ottan A, Sandrini M: Dual-acting antinflammatory drugs: a reappraisal, *Pharm Res* 44(6):437–450, 2001.
23. Knapp DW: Expression of cyclooxygenase-1 and -2 in naturally occurring canine cancer, *Prostaglandins Leukot Essent Fatty Acids* 70(5):479–483, 2004.
24. Hennig R, Grippo P, Ding XZ, et al: 5-Lipoxygenase, a marker for early pancreatic intraepithelial neoplastic lesions, *Cancer Res* 65(14):6011–6016, 2005.
25. Higgins AJ: The biology, pathophysiology and control of eicosanoids in inflammation, *J Vet Pharmacol Ther* 8:1–18, 1985.
26. Lees P, Taylor JBO, Higgins AJ, et al: Phenylbutazone and oxyphenbutazone distribution into tissue fluids in the horse, *J Vet Pharmacol Ther* 9:204–212, 1986.
27. Laudanno OM, Cesolari JA, Esnarriaga J, et al: In vivo selectivity of nonsteroidal anti-inflammatory drugs on COX-1–COX-2 and gastrointestinal ulcers, in rats [in Spanish], *Acta Gastroenterol Latinoam* 28(3):249–255, 1998.
28. Little D, Jones SL, Blikslager AT: Cyclooxygenase (COX) inhibitors and the intestine, *J Vet Intern Med* 21:367–377, 2007.
29. Streppa HK, Jones CH, Busberg SC: Cyclooxygenase selectivity of nonsteroidal anti-inflammatory drugs in canine blood, *Am J Vet Res* 63:91–94, 2002.
30. Kawai S, Nishida S, Kato M, et al: Comparison of cyclooxygenase-1 and -2 inhibitory activities of various nonsteroidal anti-inflammatory drugs using human platelets and synovial cells, *Eur J Pharmacol* 347(1):87–94, 1998.
31. Wilson JE, Chandrasekharan V, Westover KD, et al: Determination of expression of cyclooxygeans 1 and 2 isoenzyme in canine tissues and their differential sensitivity to nonsteroidal anti-inflammatory drugs, *Am J Vet Res* 65:910–918, 2004.
32. Ricketts AP, Lundy KM, Seibel SB: Evaluation of selective inhibition of canine cyclooxygenase 1 and 2 by carprofen and other nonsteroidal anti-inflammatory drugs, *Am J Vet Res* 59(11):1441–1446, 1998.
33. Brideau C, Van Staden C, Chan CC: In vitro effects of cyclooxygenase inhibitors in whole blood of horses, dogs, and cats, *Am J Vet Res* 62(11):1755–1760, 2001.
34. Giraudel JM, Toutain PL, Lees P: Development of in vitro assays for the evaluation of cyclooxygenase inhibitors and predicting selectivity of nonsteroidal anti-inflammatory drugs in cats, *Am J Vet Res* 66(4):700–709, 2005.
35. Bryant CE, Farnfield BA, Janicke HJ: Evaluation of the ability of carprofen and flunixin meglumine to inhibit activation of nuclear factor kappa B, *Am J Vet Res* 64(2):211–215, 2005.
36. Braten DC: Clinical pharmacology of NSAIDs, *J Clin Pharmacol* 28:518–523, 1988.
37. Kenyon CJ, Hooper G, Tierney D, et al: The effect of food on the gastrointestinal transit and systemic absorption of naproxen from a novel sustained release formulation, *J Contro Release* 34(1):31–36, 1995.
38. Munsiff IJ, Koritz GD, McKiernan BC, et al: Plasma protein binding of theophylline in dogs, *J Vet Pharmacol Ther* 11: 112–114, 1988.
39. Galbraith EA, McKellar QA: Protein binding and in vitro serum thromboxane B_2 inhibition by flunixin meglumine and meclofenamic acid in dog, goat and horse blood, *Res Vet Sci* 61(1):78–81, 1996.
40. Toutain PL, Bousquet-Mélou A: Free drug fraction vs. free drug concentration: a matter of frequent confusion, *J Vet Pharmacol Ther* 25:460–463, 2002.
41. Paulson SK, Engel L, Reitz B, et al: Evidence for polymorphisn in the canine metabolism of the cyclooxygenase 2 inhibitor, celecoxib, *Drug Metab Dispos* 27:1133–1142, 1999.
42. Aitken MM, Sanford J: Plasma levels following administration of sodium meclofenamate by various routes, *Res Vet Sci* 19:241–244, 1975.
43. Lepist E-I, Jusko WJ: Modeling and allometric scaling of s(+)-ketoprofen pharmacokinetics and pharmacodynamics: a retrospective analysis, *J Vet Pharmacol Ther* 27:211–218, 2004.
43a. Morris T, Stables M, Hobbs A, et al: Effects of low-dose aspirin on acute inflammatory responses in humans, *J Immunol* 183(3):2089–2096, 2009.
44. Lees P, Higgins AJ: Clinical pharmacology and therapeutic uses of non-steroidal anti-inflammatory drugs in the horse, *Equine Vet J* 17:83–96, 1985.
44a. Lees P, Giraudel J, Landoni MF, et al: PK-PD integration and PK-PD modelling of nonsteroidal anti-inflammatory drugs: principles and applications in veterinary pharmacology, *J Vet Pharmacol Ther* 27(6):491–502, 2004.
45. Giraudel JM, King JN, Jeunesse EC, et al: Use of a pharmacokinetic/pharmacodynamic approach in the cat to determine a dosage regimen for the COX-2 selective drug rebenacoxib, *J Vet Pharmacol Ther* 32:18–30, 2008.
46. Laird JM, Herrero JF, Garcia de la Rubia P, et al: Analgesic activity of the novel COX-2 preferring NSAID, meloxicam in mono-arthritic rats: central and peripheral components, *Inflamm Res* 46(6):203–210, 1997.
47. Greisman LA, Mackowia PA: Fever: beneficial and detrimental effects of antipyretics, *Curr Opin Infect Dis* 15:241–245, 2002.
48. Brandt KD: The mechanism of action of nonsteroidal antiinflammatory drugs, *J Rheumatol* 18:120–121, 1991.
48a. Martel-Pelletier J, Lajeunesse D, Reboul P, et al: Therapeutic role of dual inhibitors of 5-LOX and COX, selective and non-selective non-steroidal anti-inflammatory drugs, *Ann Rheum Dis* 62(6):501–509, 2003.
49. Knapp DW, Richardson RC, Bottoms GD, et al: Phase I. Trial of piroxicam in 62 dogs bearing naturally occurring tumors, *Cancer Chemother Pharmacol* 29:214–218, 1992.
50. Knapp DW, Richardson RC, Chan TC, et al: Piroxicam therapy in 34 dogs with transitional cell carcinoma of the urinary bladder, *J Vet Intern Med* 8:273–278, 1994.
51. Knapp DW, Chan TC, Kuczek T, et al: Evaluation of in vitro cytotoxicity of nonsteroidal anti-inflammatory drugs against canine tumor cells, *Am J Vet Res* 56(6):801–805, 1995.
51a. Martinez JM, Sali T, Okazaki R, et al: Drug-induced expression of nonsteroidal anti-inflammatory drug-activated gene/macrophage inhibitory cytokine-1/prostate-derived factor, a putative tumor suppressor, inhibits tumor growth, *J Pharmacol Exp Ther* 318(2):899–906, 2006.
52. Braun DP, Bonomi PD, Taylor SG, et al: Modification of the effects of cytotoxic chemotherapy on the immune responses of cancer patients with a nonsteroidal, antiinflammatory drug, piroxicam. A pilot study of the Eastern Cooperative Oncology Group, *J Biol Response Mod* 6:331–345, 1987.
53. Trepanier LA: Potential interactions between non-steroidal anti-inflammatory drugs and other drugs, *J Vet Emerg Crit Care* 15(4):248–253, 2005.
54. Hulisz D, Lagzdins M: Drug-induced hypertension, *US Pharamcist* 33(9):HS11–HS20, 2008.
55. Fillastre J, Leroy A, Borsa-Lebas F, et al: Effects of ketoprofen (NSAID) on the pharmacokinetics of pefloxacin and ofloxacin in healthy volunteers, *Drugs Exp Clin Res* 18:487–492, 1992.
56. Jayaraman L, Sood J: An unusual cause of convulsions following general anesthesia, *J Anaesth Clin Pharmcol* 21(3):333–334, 2005.

57. Loke YK, Trivedi AN, Singh S: Meta-analysis; gastrointestinal bleeding due to interaction between selective serotonin uptake inhibitors and non-steroidal anti-inflammatory drugs, *Aliment Pharmacol Ther* 27(1):31–40, 2008.
58. Woodward KN: Veterinary pharmacovigilance. Part 6. Predictability of adverse reactions in animals from laboratory toxicology studies, *J Vet Pharmacol Ther* 28:213–231, 2005.
59. Jonnes RD, Baynes RE, Nimitz CT: Nonsteroidal anti-inflammatory drug toxicosis in dogs and cats: 240 cases, *J Am Vet Med Assoc* 201:475–477, 1992.
59a. http://www.fda.gov/AnimalVeterinary/SafetyHealth/ProductSafetyInformation/ucm055394.htm (accessed November 22, 2010).
60. Horii Y, Ikenaga M, Shimoda M, et al: Pharmacokinetics of flunixin in the cat: enterohepatic circulation and active transport mechanism in the liver, *J Vet Pharmacol Ther* 27(2):65–69, 2004.
61. Ellison GW: NSAIDs: How ulcerogenic are they? *Proc Am Coll Vet Int Med* :445–446, 1995.
62. Shaw N, Burrows CF, King RR: Massive gastric hemorrhage induced by buffered aspirin in a greyhound, *J Am Anim Hosp Assoc* 33(3):215–219, 1997.
63. Dye TL: Naproxen toxicosis in a puppy, *Vet Hum Toxicol* 39(3):157–159, 1997.
64. Giannoukas AD, Baltoyiannis G, Milonakis M, et al: Protection of the gastroduodenal mucosa from the effects of diclofenac sodium: role of highly selective vagotomy and misoprostol, *World J Surg* 20(4):501–506, 1996.
65. Vonderhaar MA, Salisbury SK: Gastroduodenal ulceration associated with flunixin meglumine administration in three dogs, *J Am Vet Med Assoc* 203:92–95, 1993:Published erratum appears in *J Am Vet Med Assoc* 203:869, 1993.
66. Mathews KA, Paley DM, Foster RA, et al: A comparison of ketorolac with flunixin, butorphanol, and oxymorphone in controlling postoperative pain in dogs, *Can Vet J* 37(9):557–567, 1996.
67. McCormack K, Brune K: Classical absorption theory and the development of gastric mucosal damage associated with the non-steroidal anti-inflammatory drugs, *Arch Toxicol* 60: 261–269, 1987.
68. Peura DA, Goldkind L: Balancing the gastrointestinal benefits and risks of nonselective NSAIDs, *Arthritis Res Ther* 7(Suppl 4):S7–S13, 2005.
69. Wallace JL: The 21st Gaddum Memorial Lecture, Building a better aspirin: gaseous solutions to a century-old problem, *Br J Pharmacol* 152:421–428, 2007.
70. Chastain CB: Aspirin: new indications for an old drug, *Compend Small Anim* 9:165–170, 1987.
71. Silverstein FD: Improving the gastrointestinal safety of NSAIDs. The development of misoprostol—from hypothesis to clinical practice, *Dig Dis Sci* 43:447–458, 1998.
72. Mazué G, Richez P, Berthe J: Pharmacology and comparative toxicology of non-steroidal anti-inflammatory agents. In Ruckebusch Y, Toutain PL, Koritz GD, editors: *Veterinary pharmacology and toxicology*, Boston, 1983, MTP Press Limited, pp 321–331.
73. Dickman A, Ellershaw J: NSAIDs: gastroprotection or selective COX-2 inhibitor? *Palliative Medicine* 18(4):275–286, 2004.
74. Boston SE, Moens NM, Kruth SA, et al: Endoscopic evaluation of the gastroduodenal mucosa to determine the safety of short-term concurrent administration of meloxicam and dexamethasone in healthy dogs, *Am J Vet Res* 64(11):1369–1375, 2003.
75. Meddings JB, Kirk D, Olson ME: Noninvasive detection of nonsteroidal anti-inflammatory drug-induced gastropathy in dogs, *Am J Vet Res* 56(8):977–981, 1995.
76. Neiger R: NSAID-induced gastrointestinal adverse effects in dogs—can we avoid them? *J Vet Intern Med* 17(3):259–261, 2003.
77. Palmer RH, DeLapp R: Gastrointestinal toxicity in elderly osteoarthritis patients treated with NSAIDs, *Inflammopharmacology* 8(1):19–30, 2000.
78. Dow SW, Rosychuk RA, McChesney AE, et al: Effects of flunixin and flunixine plus prednisone on the gastrointestinal tract of dogs, *Am J Vet Res* 51:1131–1137, 1990.
79. Kietzmann M, Meyer-Lindenberg A, Engelke A, et al: Pharmacokinetics and tolerance of an orally administered combination preparation containing phenylbutazone and prednisolone in the dog, *Deutsche Tierarztl Wochenschr* 103(1):14–16, 1996.
80. Lascelles BD, Blikslager AT, Fox SM, et al: Gastrointestinal tract perforation in dogs treated with a selective cyclooxygenase-2 inhibitor: 29 cases (2002-2003), *J Am Vet Med Assoc* 227: 1112–1117, 2005.
81. Brune K: Safetyof anti-inflammatory treatment—new ways of thinking, *Rheumatology* 43(Suppl 1):i16–i20, 2004.
82. Peterson KD, Keefe TJ: Effects of meloxciam on severity of lameness and other clinical signs of osteoarthritis, *J Am Vet Med Assoc* 225:1056–1060, 2004.
83. Reimer ME, Johnston SA, Leib MS, et al: The gastroduodenal effects of buffered aspirin, carprofen, and etodolac in healthy dogs, *J Vet Intern Med* 13(5):472–477, 1999.
84. Mason L, Moore RA, Edwards JE, et al: Topical NSAIDs for acute pain: a meta-analysis, *BMC Family Practice* 5:10, 2004.
85. Collins LG, Tyler DE: Experimentally induced phenylbutazone toxicosis in ponies: description of the syndrome and its prevention with synthetic prostaglandin E_2, *Am J Vet Res* 46:1605–1615, 1985.
86. Boulay JP, Lipowitz AJ, Klausner JS: Effect of cimetidine on aspirin-induced gastric hemorrhage in dogs, *Am J Vet Res* 47(8):1744–1746, 1986.
86a. Watkins P: Omeprazole induction of cytochrome P45O1A2: the importance of selecting an appropriate human model, *Hepatology* 17:748–750, 1993.
86b. Li XQ, Andersson TB, Ahlström M, et al: Comparison of inhibitory effects of the proton pump inhibiting drugs omeprazole, esomeprazole, lansoprazole, pantoprazole and rabeprazole on human cytochrome P45O activities, *Drug Met Rev* 32:821–837, 2004.
87. Bowersox TS, Lipowitz AJ, Hardy RM, et al: The use of a synthetic prostaglandin E_1 analog as a gastric protectant against aspirin-induced hemorrhage in the dog, *J Am Anim Hosp Assoc* 32(5):401–407, 1996.
88. Murtaugh RJ, Matz ME, Labato MA, et al: Use of synthetic prostaglandin E_1 (misoprostol) for prevention of aspirin-induced gastroduodenal ulceration in arthritic dogs, *J Am Vet Med Assoc* 202:251–256, 1993.
89. Johnston SA, Leib MS, Forrester SD, et al: The effect of misoprostol on aspirin-induced gastroduodenal lesions in dogs, *J Vet Int Med* 19:32–38, 1995.
90. Shield MJ: Diclofenac/misoprostol: novel findings and their clinical potential, *J Rheumatol* 25(Suppl) 51:31–41, 1998.
90a. Cook D, Guyatt G, Marshall J, et al: A comparison of sucralfate and ranitidine for the prevention of upper gastrointestinal bleeding in patients requiring mechanical ventilation, *N Engl J Med* 338, 1998:791–791.
91. Cho C-H, Liu ES, Shin VY: Polysaccharides: A new role in gastrointestinal protection. In Cho C-H, Wang J-Y, editors: *Gastrointestinal mucosal repair and experimental therapeutics, Front Gastrointest Res* 25:180-189, 2002.
92. Bjarnason I, Hayliar J, Smethurst P, et al: Metronidazole reduces intestinal inflammation and blood loss in non-steroidal anti-inflammatory drug induced enteropathy, *Gut* 33:1204–1208, 1992.
93. Canadian Agency for Drugs and Technologies in Health (CADTH): Preventing NSAID induced GI complications: an economic evaluation of alternative strategies in Canada, 2007. Accessed November 9, 2009, at cadth.ca/media/compus/pdf/compus_economic_evaluation_pud_model_e.pdf.
94. Lewis JH: Hepatic toxicity of nonsteroidal anti-inflammatory drugs, *Clin Pharmacol* 3:128–138, 1984.

95. Martin K, Andersson L, Stridsberg M, et al: Plasma concentration, mammary excretion and side-effects of phenylbutazone after repeated oral administration in healthy cows, *J Vet Pharmacol Ther* 7:131–138, 1984.
96. Carlisle CH, Penny RHC, Prescott CW, et al: Toxic effects of phenylbutazone on the cat, *Br Vet J* 124:560–566, 1968.
97. Watson ADJ, Wilson JT, Turner DM, et al: Phenylbutazone-induced blood dyscrasias suspected in three dogs, *Vet Rec* 107:239–241, 1980.
98. Markel MD: What is your diagnosis? *J Am Vet Med Assoc* 188:307–308, 1986.
99. Wallau JL: Distribution and expression of cyclooxygenase (COX) isoenzymes, their physiologic role, and the categorization of nonsteroidal antiinflammatory drugs (NSAIDs), *Am J Med* 107:11S–16S, 1999.
100. Dunn JM, Simonson J, Davidson EW, et al: Nonsteroidal anti-inflammatory drugs and renal function, *J Clin Pharmacol* 28:524–529, 1988.
101. Angio RG: Nonsteroidal antiinflammatory drug-induced renal dysfunction related to inhibition of renal prostaglandins, *Drug Intell Clin Pharmacol* 21:954–960, 1987.
102. Efrati S, Berman S, Siman-Tov Y, et al: N-acetylcysteine attenuates NSAID-induced rat renal failure by restoring intrarenal prostaglandin synthesis, *Nephrol Dial Transplant* 22:1873–1881, 2007.
103. Selig CB, Maloley PA, Campbell JR: Nephrotoxicity associated with concomitant ACE inhibitor and NSAID therapy, *South Med J* 83:1144–1148, 1990.
104. Swan SK, Rudy DW, Lasseter KC, et al: Effect of cyclooxygenase-2 inhibtion on renal function in persons receiving a low salt diet, *Ann Intern Med* 133:1–9, 2000.
105. Crandell DE, Mathews KA, Dyson DH: Effect of meloxicam and carprofen on renal function when administered to healthy dogs prior to anesthesia and painful stimulation, *Am J Vet Res* 65(10):1384–1390, 2004.
106. Lobetti RG, Joubert KE: Effect of administration of nonsteroidal anti-inflammatory drugs before surgery on renal function in clinically normal dogs, *Am J Vet Res* 61(12):1501–1506, 2000.
107. Steagall PVM, Moutinho FQ, Mantovani FB, et al: Evaluation of the adverse effects of subcutaneous carprofen over six days in healthy cats, *Res Vet Sci* 86:115–120, 2009.
108. Gunew MN, Menrath VH, Marshall RD: Long-term safety, efficacy and palatability of oral meloxicam at 0.01-0.03 mg/kg for treatment of osteoarthritic pain in cats, *J Fel Med Surg* 10:235–241, 2008.
109. Fullerton T, Sica DA, Blum RA: Evaluation of the renal protective effect of misoprostol in elderly, osteoarthritic patients at risk for nonsteroidal anti-inflammatory drug-induced renal dysfunction, *J Clin Pharmacol* 33:1225–1232, 1993.
110. Pouteil-Noble C, Chapuis F, Berra N, et al: Misoprostol in renal transplant recipients: a prospective, randomized, controlled study on the prevention of acute rejection episodes and cyclosporin Anephrotoxicity, *Dial Transplant* 9(5):552–555, 1994.
111. Boers M, Bensen WG, Ludwin D, et al: Cyclosporine nephrotoxicity in rheumatoid arthritis: no effect of short term misoprostol treatment, *J Rheumatol* 19(4):534–537, 1992.
112. Aitio M-L: N-acetylcysteine—passe-partout or much ado about nothing? *Br J Clin Pharmacol* 61(1):1–15, 2006.
113. Levin A, Pate GE, Shalansky S, et al: N-acetylcysteine reduces urinary albumin excretion following contrast administration: evidence of biological effect, *Nephrol Dial Transplant* , 2007.
114. Jackson ML: Platelet physiology and platelet function: inhibition by aspirin, *Compend Contin Educ Pract Vet* 9:627–638, 1987.
115. Konstantinopoulos PA, Lehmann DF: The cardiovascular toxicity of selective and nonselective cyclooxygenase inhibitors: comparisons, contrasts, and aspirin confounding, *J Clin Pharmacol* 45(7):742–750, 2005.
116. Hennan JK, Huang J, Barrett TD, et al: Effects of selective cyclooxygenase-2 inhibition on vascular responses and thrombosis in canine coronary arteries, *Circulation* 104(7):820–825, 2001.
116a. Rimon G, Sidhu RS, Lauver DA, et al: Coxibs interfere with the action of aspirin by binding tightly to one monomer of cyclooxygenase-1, *Proc Natl Acad Sci USA 5* 107(1):28–33, 2010.
117. Daminet S, Croubels S, Duchateau L, et al: Influence of acetylsalicylic acid and ketoprofen on canine thyroid function tests, *Vet J* 166(3):224–232, 2003.
118. Panciera DL, Johnston SA: Results of thyroid function tests and concentrations of plasma proteins in dogs administered etodolac, *Am J Vet Res* 63(11):1492–1495, 2002.
119. Sauve F, Paradis M, Refsal KR, et al: Effects of oral administration of meloxicam, carprofen, and a nutraceutical on thyroid function in dogs with osteoarthritis, *Can Vet J* 44:474–479, 2003.
120. Clemmons RM, Meyers KM: Acquisition and aggregation of canine blood platelets: basic mechanisms of function and differences because of breed origin, *Am J Vet Res* 45:137–144, 1984.
121. Berliner S, Weinberger A, Shoenfeld Y, et al: Ibuprofen may induce meningitis in (NZB X NZW) mice, *Arthritis Rheum* 28:104–107, 1985.
122. Syvlia LM, Forlenza SW, Brocavich JM: Aseptic meningitis associated with naproxen, *DICP Ann Pharmacother* 22: 399–401, 1988.
122a. Botting R: Vane's discovery of the mechanism of aspirin changed our understanding of its clinical pharmacology, *Pharmacol Rep* 62:518–525, 2010.
123. Romano M: Lipid mediators: lipoxin and aspirin-riggered 15-epi-lipoxins, *Inflamm Allergy Drug Targets* 5:81–90, 2006.
123a. Morris T, Stables M, Hobbs A, et al: Effects of low-dose aspirin on acute inflammatory responses in humans, *J Immunol* 183(3):2089–2096, 2009.
124. Conlon PD: Nonsteroidal drugs used in the treatment of inflammation, *Vet Clin North Am Small Anim Pract* 18: 1115–1131, 1988.
125. Davis LE, Westfall BA: Species differences in biotransformation and excretion of salicylate, *Am J Vet Res* 33:1253–1262, 1972.
126. Short CR, Hsieh LC, Malbrough MS, et al: Elimination of salicylic acid in goats and cattle, *Am J Vet Res* 51:1267–1270, 1990.
127. USP: Veterinary pharmaceutical information monographs, anti-inflammatories anonymous, *J Vet Pharmacol Therap* 27(Suppl 1), 2004.
128. Parton K, Balmer TV, Boyle J: The pharmacokinetics and effects of intravenously administered carprofen and salicylate on gastrointestinal mucosa and selected biochemical measurements in healthy cats, *J Vet Pharmacol Ther* 23(2):73–79, 2000.
129. Robinson MG: New oral salicylates in therapy of chronic idiopathic inflammatory bowel disease, *Gastroenterol Clin North Am* 18:43–50, 1989.
130. Takaya T, Sawada K, Suzuki H, et al: Application of a colon delivery capsule to 5-aminosalicylic acid and evaluation of the pharmacokinetic profile after oral administration to beagle dogs, *J Drug Targeting* 4(5):271–276, 1997.
131. Beasley VR, Buck WB: Acute ethylene glycol toxicosis: a review, *Vet Hum Toxicol* 22:255, 1980.
132. Larson EJ: Toxicity of low doses of aspirin in the cat, *J Am Vet Med Assoc* 143:837–840, 1963.
133. Palmoski MJ, Colyer RA, Brandt KD: Marked suppression by salicylate of the augmented proteoglycan synthesis in osteoarthritic cartilage, *Arthritis Rheum* 23(1):83–91, 1980.
134. Morton DL, Knottenbelt DC: Pharmacokinetics of aspirin and its application in canine veterinary medicine, *J S Afr Vet Assoc* 60:191–194, 1989.
135. Lipowitz AJ, Boulay JP, Klausner JS: Serum salicylate concentrations and endoscopic evaluation of the gastric mucosa in dogs after oral administration of aspirin-containing products, *Am J Vet Res* 47:1586–1589, 1986.

136. Konturek SJ: Physiology and pharmacology of prostaglandin, *Dig Dis Sci* 31:6S–19S, 1986.
137. Jezyk PF: Metabolic diseases: an emerging area of veterinary pediatrics, *Compend Contin Educ Pract Vet* 5:1026–1031, 1983.
138. Yeary RA, Swanson W: Aspirin dosages for the cat, *J Am Vet Med Assoc* 163:1117–1178, 1973.
139. Davis LE, Westfall BA, Short CR: Biotransformation and pharmacokinetics of salicylate in newborn animals, *Am J Vet Res* 34:1105–1108, 1973.
140. Oehme FW: Aspirin and acetaminophen. In Kirk R, editor: *Current veterinary therapy (small animal practice) X*, Philadelphia, 1986, Saunders, pp 188–190.
141. Hardie EM, Kolata RJ, Rawlings CA: Canine septic peritonitis: treatment with flunixin meglumine, *Circ Shock* 11:159–173, 1983.
142. Moore JN, Hardee MM, Hardee GE: Modulation of arachidonic acid metabolism in endotoxic horses: comparison of flunixin meglumine, phenylbutazone, and a selective thromboxane synthetase inhibitor, *Am J Vet Res* 47:110–113, 1986.
143. Templeton CB, Bottoms GD, Fessler JF, et al: Endotoxin-induced hemodynamic and prostaglandin changes in ponies: effects of flunixin meglumine, dexamethasone, and prednisolone, *Circ Shock* 23:231–240, 1987.
144. Jarlov N, Andersen PH, Haubro P, et al: Pathophysiology of experimental bovine endotoxicosis: endotoxin induced synthesis of prostaglandins and thromboxane and the modulatory effect of some non-steroidal anti-inflammatory drugs, *Acta Vet Scand* 33:1–8, 1992.
145. Davidson JR, Lantz GC, Salisbury SK, et al: Effects of flunixin meglumine on dogs with experimental gastric dilatation-volvulus, *Vet Surg* 21:113–120, 1992.
146. Hardie EM, Hardee GE, Rawlings CA: Pharmacokinetics of flunixin meglumine in dogs, *Am J Vet Res* 46:235–237, 1985.
147. McKellar QA, Galbraith EA, Bogan JA, et al: Flunixin pharmacokinetics and serum thromboxane inhibition in the dog, *Vet Rec* 24:651–654, 1989.
148. Scherkl R, Frey HH: Pharmacokinetics of ibuprofen in the dog, *J Vet Pharmacol Ther* 10:261–265, 1987.
149. Dunayer E: Ibuprofen toxicosis in dogs, cats, and ferrets, *Vet Med* 7:580–586, 2004.
150. Williams RL, Upton RA: The clinical pharmacology of ketoprofen, *J Clin Pharmacol* 28:S13–S22, 1988.
151. Schmitt M, Guentert TW: Biopharmaceutical evaluation of ketoprofen following intravenous, oral, and rectal administration in dogs, *J Pharm Sci* 79:614–616, 1990.
152. Castro E, Soraci A, Fogel F, et al: Chiral inversion of R(-) fenoprofen and ketoprofen enantiomers in cats, *J Vet Pharmacol Therap* 23:265–271, 2000.
153. Cailleteau JG: Ketoprofen in dentistry: a pharmacologic review, *Oral Surg Oral Med Oral Pathol* 66:620–624, 1988.
154. Beaver WT: Ketoprofen: a new nonsteroidal anti-inflammatory analgesic, *J Clin Pharmacol* 28:S1, 1988.
155. Stambough J, Drew J: A double-blind parallel evaluation of the efficacy and safety of a single dose of ketoprofen in cancer pain, *J Clin Pharmacol* 28:S34–S39, 1988.
156. Avouac B, Teule M: Ketoprofen: the European experience, *J Clin Pharmacol* 28:S2–S7, 1988.
157. Turek MD, Baird WM: Double-blind parallel comparison of ketoprofen, acetaminophen plus codeine, and placebo in postoperative pain, *J Clin Pharmacol* 28:S23–S28, 1988.
158. Glew A, Aviad AD, Keister DM, et al: Use of ketoprofen as an antipyretic in cats, *Can Vet J* 37:222–225, 1996.
159. Slingsby LS, Waterman-Pearson AE: Comparison of pethidine, buprenorphine and ketoprofen for postoperative analgesia after ovariohysterectomy in the cat, *Vet Rec* 143:185–189, 1998.
160. Insel PA: Analgesic, antipyretic and anti-inflammatory agents and drugs employed in treatment of gout. In Hardman JG, Limbird LD, editors: *Goodman and Gilman's the pharmacological basis of therapeutics*, ed 9, New York, 1996, McGraw-Hill, pp 617–659.
161. Paddleford RR: Analgesia and pain management. In Paddleford RR, editor: *Manual of small animal anesthesia*, ed 2, Philadelphia, 1999, Saunders, pp 227–246.
162. Pasloske K, Renaud R, Burger J, et al: Pharmacokinetics of ketorolac after intravenous and oral single dose administration in dogs, *J Vet Pharmacol Ther* 22:314–319, 1999.
163. Frey HH, Rieh B: Pharmacokinetics of naproxen in the dog, *Am J Vet Res* 42:1615–1617, 1981.
164. Zech R, Scherkl R, Hashem A, et al: Plasma and tissue kinetics of phenylbutazone and naproxen in dogs, *Arch Int Pharmacodyn Ther* 325:113–128, 1993.
165. Gfeller RW, Sandors AD: Naproxen-associated duodenal ulcer complicated by perforation and bacteria- and barium sulfate-induced peritonitis in a dog, *J Am Vet Med Assoc* 198:644–646, 1991.
166. Roudebush P, Morse GE: Naproxen toxicosis in a dog, *J Am Vet Med Assoc* 179:805–806, 1981.
167. Ratliffe A, Rosenwasser MP, Mahmud F, et al: The in vivo effects of naproxen on canine experimental osteoarthritic articular cartilage: composition, metalloproteinase activity and metabolism, *Agents Actions* 39(Suppl):207–211, 1993.
168. De Backer P, Braeckman R, Belpaire F, et al: Bioavailability and pharmacokinetics of phenylbutazone in the cow, *J Vet Pharmacol Ther* 3:29–33, 1980.
169. Mills PC, Ng JC, Hrdlicka J, et al: Disposition and urinary excretion of phenylbutazone in normal and febrile greyhounds, *Res Vet Sci* 59(3):261–266, 1995.
170. Mills PC, Ng JC, Skelton KV, et al: Phenylbutazone in racing greyhounds: plasma and urinary residues 24 and 48 hours after a single intravenous administration, *Aust Vet J* 72(8):304–308, 1995.
171. Murray MJ: Phenylbutazone toxicity in a horse, *Compend Contin Educ Pract Vet* 7:S389–S394, 1985.
172. Tandy J, Thorpe E: A fatal syndrome in the dog following administration of phenylbutazone, *Vet Rec* 81:398–399, 1967.
173. Kalbhen DA: The influence of NSAIDs on morphology of articular cartilage, *Scand J Rheumatol Suppl* 77:13–22, 1988.
174. Jolly WT, Whittem T, Jolly AC, et al: The dose-related effects of phenylbutazone and a methylprednisolone acetate formulation (Depo-Medrol) on cultured explants of equine carpal articular cartilage, *J Vet Pharmacol Ther* 18(6):429–437, 1995.
175. Thomas AD, Bowater IC, Vine JH, et al: Uptake of drugs from topically applied anti-inflammatory preparations applied to racing animals, *Aust Vet J* 75:897–901, 1997.
176. Weiss DJ, Klausner JS: Drug associated aplastic anemia in dogs: eight cases (1984-1988), *J Am Vet Med Assoc* 196:472, 1990.
177. Galbraith EA, McKellar QA: Pharmacokinetics and pharmacodynamics of piroxicam in dogs, *Vet Rec* 128:561, 1991.
178. Heeb HL, Chun R, Koch DE, et al: Single dose pharmacokinetics of piroxicam in cats, *J Vet Pharmacol Ther* 26(4):259–263, 2003.
179. Bergh MS, Budsberg SC: The coxib NSAIDs: potential clinical and pharmacologic importance in veterinary medicine, *J Vet Intern Med* 19(5):633–643, 2005.
180. Fox SM, Johnston SA: Use of carprofen for the treatment of pain and inflammation in dogs, *J Am Vet Med Assoc* 210(10):1493–1498, 1997.
181. McKellar QA, Delatour P, Lees P: Stereospecific pharmacodynamics and pharmacokinetics of carprofen in the dog, *J Vet Pharmacol Ther* 17(6):447–454, 1994.
182. Clark TP, Chieffo C, Huhn JC, et al: The steady-state pharmacokinetics and bioequivalence of carprofen administered orally and subcutaneously in dogs, *J Vet Pharmacol Therap* 26:187–192, 2003.

183. Priymenko N, Garnier F, Ferre JP, et al: Enantioselectivity of the enterohepatic recycling of carprofen in the dog, *Drug Metab Dispos* 26(2):170–176, 1998.
184. Vasseur PB, Johnson AL, Budsberg SC, et al: Randomized, controlled trial of the efficacy of carprofen, a nonsteroidal anti-inflammatory drug, in the treatment of osteoarthritis in dogs, *J Am Vet Assoc* 206:807–811, 1995.
185. Forsyth SF, Guilford WG, Haslett SJ, et al: Endoscopy of the gastroduodenal mucosa after carprofen, meloxicam and ketoprofen administration in dogs, *J Small Anim Pract* 39(9):421–424, 1998.
186. Craven M, Chandler ML, Steiner JM, et al: Acute effects of carprofen and meloxicam on canine gastrointestinal permeability and mucosal absorptive capacity, *J Vet Intern Med* 21:917–923, 2007.
187. MacPhail CM, Lappin MR, Meyer DJ, et al: Hepatocellular toxicosis associated with administration of carprofen in 21 dogs, *J Am Vet Med Assoc* 212(12):1895–1901, 1998.
188. Pfizer Carprofen Technical Report: 1998; Pfizer Animal Health.
189. Forsyth SF, Guilford WG, Pfeiffer DU: Effect of NSAID administration on creatinine clearance in healthy dogs undergoing anaesthesia and surgery, *J Small Anim Pract* 41(12):547–550, 2000.
190. Bostrom IM, Nyman GC, Lord PE, et al: Effects of carprofen on renal function and results of serum biochemical and hematologic analyses in anesthetized dogs that had low blood pressure during anesthesia, *Am J Vet Res* 63(5):712–721, 2002.
191. Hickford FH, Barr SC, Erb H: Effect of carprofen on hemostatic variables, *Am J Vet Res* 62:1642–1646, 2001.
192. Benton HP, Vasseur PG, Broderick-Villa A, et al: Effect of carprofen on sulfated glycosaminoglycan metabolism, protein synthesis and prostaglandin release by cultured osteoarthritic canine chondrocytes, *Am J Vet Res* 58:286–291, 1997.
193. Lascelles BD, Butterworth SJ, Waterman AE: Postoperative analgesic and sedative effects of carprofen and pethidine in dogs, *Vet Rec* 134(8):187–191, 1994.
194. Lascelles BD, Cripps PJ, Jones A, et al: Efficacy and kinetics of carprofen, administered preoperatively or postoperatively, for the prevention of pain in dogs undergoing ovariohysterectomy, *Vet Surg* 27(6):568–582, 1998.
195. Welsh EM, Nolan AM, Reid J: Beneficial effects of administering carprofen before surgery in dogs, *Vet Rec* 141:251–253, 1997.
196. Borer LR, Peel JE, Seewald W, et al: Effect of carprofen, etodolac, meloxicam, or butorphanol in dogs with induced acute synovitis, *Am J Vet Res* 64(11):1429–1437, 2003.
197. Moreau M, Dupuis J, Bonneau NH, et al: Clinical evaluation of a nutraceutical, carprofen and meloxicam for the treatment of dogs with osteoarthritis, *Vet Rec* 152(11):323–329, 2003.
198. Aragon CL, Hofmeister EH, Budsberg SC: Systematic review of clinical trials of treatments for osteoarthritis in dogs, *J Am Vet Med Assoc* 230(4):514–521, 2007.
199. Taylor PM, Delatour P, Landoni FM, et al: Pharmacodynamics and enantioselective pharmacokinetics of carprofen in the cat, *Res Vet Sci* 60(2):144–151, 1996.
200. Lascelles BD, Cripps P, Mirchandarin S, et al: Carprofen as an analgesic for postoperative pain in cats: dose titration and assessment of efficacy in comparison to pethidine hydrochloride, *Small Anim Prac* 36:535–541, 1995.
201. Balmer TV, Irvine D, Jones RS, et al: Comparison of carprofen and pethidine as postoperative analgesics in the cat, *J Small Anim Pract* 39(4):158–164, 1998.
202. Runk A, Kyles AE, Downs MO: Duodenal perforation in a cat following the administration of nonsteroidal antiinflammatory medication, *J Am Anim Hosp Assoc* 35:52–55, 1999.
203. Slingsby LS, Waterman-Pearson AE: Postoperative analgesia in the cat after ovariohysterectomy by use of carprofen, ketoprofen, meloxicam or tolfenamic acid, *J Small Anim Pract* 41(10): 447–450, 2000.
204. Taylor PM, Steagall PVM, Dixon MJ, et al: Carprofen and buprenorphine prevent hyperalgesia in a model of inflammatory pain in cats, *Res Vet Sci* 83:369–375, 2007.
205. Simmons K: Personal communication, Novartis Animal Health, October, 2004.
206. Gierse JK, Staten NR, Casperson GF, et al: Cloning, expression, and selective inhibition of canine cyclooxygenase-1 and cyclooxygenase-2, *Vet Ther* 3(3):270–280, 2002.
207. Millis DL, Weigel JP, Moyers T, et al: The effect of deracoxib, a new COX-2 inhibitor, on the prevention of lameness induced by chemical synovitis in dogs, *Vet Ther* 3(4):7–18, 2002.
208. Sennello KA, Leib MS: Effects of deracoxib or buffered aspirin on the gastric mucosa of healthy dogs, *J Vet Intern Med* 20: 1291–1296, 2006.
209. Glaser KB: Cyclooxygenase selectivity and NSAIDS: Cyclooxygenase-2 selectivity of etodolac (Lodine), *Inflammopharmacology* 3:335–345, 1995.
210. Cayan MN, Kraml M, Gerdinandi ES, et al: The metabolic disposition of etodolac in rats, dogs, and man, *Drug Metab Rev* 12:339, 1981.
211. Lippiello L, Han MS, Henderson T: Protective effect of the chondroprotective agent CosequinDS on bovine articular cartilage exposed in vitro to nonsteroidal antiinflammatory agents, *Vet Ther* 2(3):128–135, 2002.
211a. Klauss G, Giuliano EA, Moore CP, et al: Keratoconjunctivitis sicca associated with administration of etodolac in dogs: 211 cases (1992-2002), *J Am Vet Med Assoc* 230(4): 541–547, 2007.
212. Budsberg S, Johnston S, Schwarz P, et al: Evaluation of etodolac for the treatment of osteoarthritis of the hip in dogs: a prospective multicenter study (abstract), *Vet Surg* 25:420, 1996.
213. McCann ME, Andersen DR, Zhang D, et al: In vitro effects and in vivo efficacy of a novel cyclooxygenase-2 inhibitor in dogs with experimentally induced synovitis, *Am J Vet Res* 65(4): 503–512, 2004.
214. Pollmeier M, Toulemonde C, Fleishman C, et al: Clinical evaluation of firocoxib and carprofen for the treatment of dogs with osteoarthritis, *Vet Rec* 159:547–551, 2006.
215. Engelhardt G, Bogel R, Schnitzer C, et al: Meloxicam: influence on arachidonic acid metabolism, Part 1. In vitro findings, *Biochem Pharmacol* 51:21, 1996.
216. Engelhardt G, Bogel R, Schnitzer C, et al: Meloxicam: influence on arachidonic acid metabolism, Part II. In vivo findings, *Biochem Pharmacol* 51:29, 1996.
217. Engelhardt G, Homma D, Schlegel K, et al: General pharmacology of meloxicam, Part II. Effects on blood pressure, blood flow, heart rate, ECG, respiratory minute volume and interactions with paracetamol, pirenzepine, chlorthalidone, phenprocoumon and tolbutamide, *Gen Pharmacol* 27(4):679–688, 1996.
218. Hare JE, Darling H, Doig PA: *Metacam oral suspension: current safety data,* Boehringer Ingelheim Vetmedica, Toronto, Ontario, 1998, c/o Jonathan Hare, Janssen Animal Health, 19 Green Belt Drive.
219. Kay-Mugford PA, Grimm KA, Weingarten AJ, et al: Effect of preoperative administration of tepoxalin on hemostasis and hepatic and renal function dogs, *Vet Ther* 5:120–127, 2004.
220. Busch U, Schmid J, Heinzel G, et al: Pharmacokinetics of meloxicam in animals and the relevance to humans, *Drug Metab Dispos* 26(6):576–584, 1998.
221. Staerkel P, Horsmans Y: Meloxicam-induced liver toxicity, *Acta Gastroenterol Belg* 62(2):255–256, 1999.

222. Enberg TB, Braun LD, Kuzman AB: Gastrointestinal perofration in five dogs associated with the administration of meloxicam, *J Vet Emerg Crit Care* 16(1):34–43, 2006.
223. Niza NM, Felix N, Vilela CL: Cutaneous and ocular adverse reactions in a dog following meloxicam administration, *Vet Dermatol* 18:45–49, 2007.
224. Doig PA, Purbrick KA, Hare JE, et al: Clinical efficacy oand tolerance of meloxicam in dogs with chronic osteoarthritis, *Can Vet J* 41:296–300, 2000.
225. Van Bree H, Justus C, Quirke JF: Preliminary observations on the effects of meloxicam in a new model for acute intra-articular inflammation in dogs, *Vet Res Commun* 18(3):217–224, 1994.
226. Jones CJ, Streppa HK, Harmon BG, et al: In vivo effects of meloxicam and aspirin on blood, gastric mucosal, and synovial fluid prostanoid synthesis in dogs, *Am J Vet Res* 63(11):1527–1531, 2002.
227. Lascelles BD, Henderson AJ, Hackett IJ: Evaluation of the clinical efficacy of meloxicam in cats with painful locomotor disorders, *J Small Anim Pract* 42(12):587–593, 2001.
228. Slingsby LS, Waterman-Pearson AE: Comparison between meloxicam and carprofen for postoperative analgesia after feline ovariohysterectomy, *J Small Anim Pract* 43(7):286–289, 2002.
229. Mathews KA, Pettifer G, Foster R, et al: Safety and efficacy of preoperative administration of meloxicam, compared with that of ketoprofen and butorphanol in dogs undergoing abdominal surgery, *Am J Vet Res* 62(6):882–888, 2001.
230. Budsberg SC, Cross AR, Quandt JE, et al: Evaluation of intravenous administration of meloxicam for perioperative pain management following stifle joint surger in dogs, *Am J Vet Res* 63:1557–1563, 2002.
231. Rainsford KD, Skerry TM, Chindemi P, et al: Effects of the NSAIDs meloxicam and indomethacin on cartilage proteoglycan synthesis and joint responses to calcium pyrophosphate crystals in dogs, *Vet Res Commun* 23(2):101–113, 1999.
232. Justus C, Quirke JF: Dose-response relationship for the antipyretic effect of meloxicam in an endotoxin model in cats, *Vet Res Commun* 19(4):321–330, 1995.
233. Metacam Symposium on Arthritic Disease in Cats, Seville, Spain, June 1-3, 2007.
234. Giraudel JM, Toutain PL, King JN, et al: Differential inhibition of cyclooxygenase isoenzymes in the cat by the NSAID robenacoxib, *J Vet Pharmacol Ther* 32(1):31–40, 2009.
235. Jung M, Lees P, Seewald W, et al: Analytical determination and pharmacokinetics of robenacoxib in the dog, *J Vet Pharmacol Therap* 32:41–48, 2008.
236. Hoeijmakers M, Coert A, van Helden H, et al: The pharmacokinetics of vedaprofen and its enantiomers in dogs after single and multiple dosing, *J Vet Pharmacol Ther* 28:305–312, 2005.
237. Nell T, Bergman J, Hoeijmakers M, et al: Comparison of vedaprofen and meloxicam in dogs with musculoskeletal pain and inflammation, *J Small Anim Pract* 43(5):208–212, 2002.
238. Paulson SK, Zhang JY, Jessen S, et al: Comparison of celecoxib metabolism and excretion in mouse, rabbit, dog, cynomolgus monkey and rhesus monkey, *Xenobiotica* 30(7):731–744, 2000.
239. Hunter RP, Radlinsky M, Koch DE, et al: Single and multiple dose pharmacokinetics and synovial fluid concentrations of celecoxib in greyhound dogs, *Proc ACVIM* #286, 2003.
240. Moreau M, Daminet S, Martel-Pelletier J, et al: Superiority of the gastroduodenal safety profile of licofelone over rofecoxib, a COX-2 selective inhibitor, in dogs, *J Vet Pharmacol Therap* 28:81–86, 2005.
241. Halpin RA, Geer LA, Zhang KE, et al: The absorption, distribution, metabolism and excretion of rofecoxib, a potent and selective cyclooxygenase-2 inhibitor, in rats and dogs, *Drug Metab Dispos* 28(10):1244–1254, 2000.
242. Toutain PL, Cester CC, Haak T, et al: Pharmacokinetic profile and in vitro selective cyclooxygenase-2 inhibition by nimesulide in the dog, *J Vet Pharmacol Ther* 24(1):35–42, 2001.
243. Toutain PL, Cester CC, Haak T, et al: A pharmacokinetic/pharmacodynamic approach vs. a dose titration for the determination of a dosage regimen: the case of nimesulide, a Cox-2 selective nonsteroidal anti-inflammatory drug in the dog, *J Vet Pharmacol Ther* 24(1):43–55, 2001.
244. Ewing GO: Indomethacin-associated gastrointestinal hemorrhage in a dog, *J Am Vet Med Assoc* 161:1665–1668, 1972.
245. Mburu DN, Mbugua SW, Skoglund LA, et al: Effects of paracetamol and acetylsalicylic acid on the post-operative course after experimental orthopaedic surgery in dogs, *J Vet Pharmacol Ther* 11:163–171, 1988.
246. St. Omer VV, McKnight ED: Acetylcysteine for treatment of acetaminophen toxicosis in the cat, *J Am Vet Med Assoc* 176: 911–913, 1980.
247. Cullison RF: Acetaminophen toxicosis in small animals: clinical signs, mode of action, and treatment, *Compend Contin Educ* 6:315–321, 1984.
248. Savides MC, Oehme FW, Leipold HW: Effects of various antidotal treatment on acetaminophen toxicosis and biotransformation in cats, *Am J Vet Res* 46:1485–1489, 1985.
249. Jackson JE: Cimetidine protects against acetaminophen toxicity, *Life Sci* 31:31–35, 1982.
250. Ruffalo RL, Thompson JF: Cimetidine and acetylcysteine as antidote for acetaminophen overdose, *South Med J* 75:954–958, 1982.
251. Wallace KP, Center SA, Hickford FH, et al: S-Adenosyl-L-Methionine (SAMe) for the trestment of acetaminophen toxicity in a dog, *J Am Anim Hosp Assoc* 38:246–254, 2002.
252. Aronson LR, Drobatz K: Acetaminophen toxicosis in 17 cats, *J Vet Emerg Crit Care* 6(2):65–69, 1996.
253. Cartier L-J, Leclerc P, Pouliot M, et al: Toxic levels of acetaminophen produce a major positive interference on glucometer elite and accu-check advantage glucose meters, *Clin Chem* 44(4): 893–894, 1998.
253a. Flood AR: The role of acetaminophen in the treatment of osteoarthritis, *Am J Manag Care* 16:S48–S54, 2010.
254. Johnston SA, Budsberg SC: Nonsteroidal anti-inflammatory drugs and corticosteroids for the management of canine osteoarthritis, *Vet Clin North Am Small Anim Pract* 27:841–862, 1997.
255. Hjelle JJ, Grauer GF: Acetaminophen induced toxicosis in dogs and cats, *J Am Vet Med Assoc* 188:742–746, 1986.
256. Savides MC, Oehme FW: Acetaminophen and its toxicity, *J Appl Toxicol* 3:96–111, 1983.
257. Francavilla A, Makowka L, Polimeno L, et al: A dog model for acetaminophen-induced fulminant hepatic failure, *Gastroenterology* 96:470–478, 1989.
258. Goodman L, Coles TB, Budsberg S: Leukotriene inhibition in small animal medicine, *J Vet Pharmacol Ther* 31:387–398, 2008.
259. Newcombe DS: Leukotrienes: regulation of biosynthesis, metabolism, and bioactivity, *J Clin Pharmacol* 28:530–549, 1988.
260. Parkinson JF: Lipoxin and synthetic Lipoxin analogs: an overview of anti-inflammatory functions and new concepts in immunomodulation, *Inflamm Allergy Drug Targets* 5:91–106, 2006.
261. Schmelzer R, Kubala L, Newman JW, et al: Soluble epoxide hydrolase is a therapeutic target for acute inflammation, *Proc Nat Acad Sci* 102(28):9772–9777, 2005.
262. Ding XZ, Hennig R, Adrian TE: Lipoxygenase and cyclooxygenase metabolism: new insights in treatment and chemoprevention of pancreatic cancer, *Mol Cancer* 2:10–22, 2003.
263. Daffonchio L, Rossoni G, Clavenna G, et al: Protective activity of ketoprofen lysine salt against the pulmonary effects induced by bradykinin in guinea-pigs, *Inflammation Res* 45(5):259–264, 1996.

264. Martel-Pelletier J, Lajeunesse D, Reboul P, et al: Therapeutic role of dual inhibitors of 5-LOX and COX, selective and non-selective non-steroidal anti-inflammatory drugs, *Ann Rheum Dis* 62:501–509, 2003.
265. Jovanovic DV, Fernandes JC, Martel-Pelletier J, et al: In vivo dual inhibition of cyclooxygenase and lipoxygenase by ML-3000 reduces the progression of experimental osteoarthritis: suppression of collagenase 1 and interleukin-1 b synthesis, *Arthritis Rheum* 44:2320–2330, 2000.
266. Agnello KA, Reynolds LR, Budsberg SC: In vivo effects of tepoxalin, an inhibitor of cyclooxygenase and lipoxygenase, on prostanoid and leukotriene production in dogs with chronic osteoarthritis, *Am J Vet Res* 66(6):966–972, 2005.
267. Punke JP, Speas AL, Reynolds LR, et al: Effects of firocoxib, meloxicam, and tepoxalin on prostanoid and leukotriene production by duodenal mucosa and other tissues of osteoarthritic dogs, *Am J Vet Res* 69(9):1203–1209, 2008.
268. Hall G: Personal communication, Technical Service Veterinarian, *Schering-Plough* , April, 2009.
269. Bosmans T, Gasthuys F, Duchateau L, et al: A comparison of tepoxalin-buprenorphine combination and buprenorphine for postoperative analgesia in dogs: a clinical study, *J Vet Med A Physiol Pathol Clin Med* 54(7):364–369, 2007.
269a. Gupat A, Kumar A, Kulkarni S: Licofelone attenuates MPTP-induced neuronal toxicity: behavioral, biochemical and cellular evidence, *Inflammopharmacology* 18:223–232, 2010.
270. Undem BJ: Pharmacotherapy of asthma. In Brunton LL, Lazo JS, Parker KL, editors: *Goodman & Gilman's the pharmacological basis of therapeutics*, ed 11, New York, 2006, McGraw-Hill, pp 717–736.
271. Serafin WE: Drugs used in the treatment of asthma. In Hardman JG, Limbird LD, editors: *Goodman and Gilman's the pharmacological basis of therapeutics*, ed 9, New York, 1996, McGraw-Hill, pp 659–682.
272. Ambrus JL, Anain JM, Anain SM, et al: Dose-response effects of pentoxifylline on erythrocyte filterability: clinical and animal model studies, *Clin Pharmacol Ther* 48:50–56, 1990.
273. Ambrus JL, Stadler S, Kulaylat M: Hemorrheologic effects of metabolites of pentoxifylline (Trental), *J Med* 26:65–75, 1995.
274. Zargari O: Pentoxifylline: a drug with wide spectrum applications in dermatology, *Dermatology Online Journal* 14(11):2, 2008:Accessed February 12, 2009, at http://dermatology.cdlib.org/1411/reviews/pentoxy/zargari.html:(1 of 10).
275. Rees C, Boothe DM, Boeckh A, et al: Dosing regimen and hemotologic effects of pentoxifylline and its active metabolites in normal dogs, *Vet Ther* 4(2):188–196, 2003.
276. Quezado ZMN, Hoffman WD, Banks SM: Increasing doses of pentoxifylline as a continuous infusion in canine septic shock, *J Pharmacol Experiment Therapeut* 288:107–113, 1999.
277. Apaydin BB, Paksoy M, Arb T, et al: Influence of pentoxifylline and interferon-alpha on prevention of stricture due to corrosive esphagitis, *Eur Surg Res* 33:225–231, 2001.
278. Skidgel RA, Erdös EG: Histamine, bradykinin, and their antagonists. In Brunton LL, Lazo JS, Parker KL, editors: *Goodman & Gilman's the pharmacological basis of therapeutics*, ed 11, New York, 2006, McGraw-Hill, pp 629–651.
278a. Moy AB, Winter M, Kamath A, et al: Histamine alters endothelial barrier function at cell-cell and cell-matrix sites,*Am J Physiol Lung Cell Mol Physiol* 278(5):L888–L898, 2000.
279. Obradovic T, Dobson GG, Shingaki T, et al: Assessment of the first and second generation antihistamines brain penetration and role of P-glycoprotein, *Pharm Res* 24(2):318–327, 2007.
280. Hansson H, Bergvall K, Bondesson U, et al: Clinical pharmacology of clemastine in healthy dogs, *Vet Dermatol* 15(3):152–158, 2004.
281. Bizikova P, Papich MG, Olivry T: Hydroxyzine and cetirizine pharmacokinetics and pharmacodynamics after oral and intravenous administration of hydroxyzine to healthy dogs, *Vet Dermatol* 19(6):348–357, 2008.
282. Papich MG, Schooley EK, Reinero CR: Pharmacokinetics of cetirizine in healthy cats, *Am J Vet Res* 69(5):670–674, 2008.
283. Devillier P: Comparing the new antihistamines: the role of pharmacological parameters, *Clin Exp Allergy* 36:5–7, 2006.
284. Cook CP, Scott DW, Miller WH Jr, et al: Treatment of canine atopic dermatitis with cetirizine, a second generation antihistamine: a single-blinded, placebo-controlled study, *Can Vet J* 45(5):414–417, 2004.
285. DeBoer DJ, Griffin CE: The ACVD task force on canine atopic dermatitis XXI: antihistamine pharmacotherapy, *Vet Immunol Immunopathol* 81:323–329, 2001.
286. Scott DW, Miller WH Jr: Antihistamines in the management of allergic pruritus in dogs and cats, *J Small Anim Pract* 40:359–364, 1999.
287. Fajardo M, Di Cesare PE: Disease-modifying therapies for osteoarthritis: current status, *Drugs Aging* 22(2):141–161, 2005.
288. Gardner DL: The nature and causes of osteoarthrosis, *Br Med J* 286:418–424, 1983.
289. Jones AC, Doherty M: The treatment of osteoarthritis, *Br J Clin Pharmacol* 33:357–363, 1992.
290. Vaughan-Scott T, Taylor JH: The pathophysiology and medical management of canine osteoarthritis, *J S Afr Vet Assoc* 68(1):21–25, 1997.
291. Kelly GS: The role of glucosamine sulfate and chondroitin sulfates in the treatment of degenerative joint disease, *Altern Med Rev* 3(1):27–39, 1998.
292. Pelletier JP, DiBattista JA, Roughley P, et al: Cytokines and inflammation in cartilage degradation, *Rheum Dis Clin North Am* 19:545–568, 1993.
293. Pelletier JP, Mineau F, Ranger P, et al: The increased synthesis of nitric oxide induced by IL-1 in human chondrocytes markedly reduced the synthesis of IL-1 receptor antagonists: a possible role in osteoarthritic cartilage degradation, *Osteoarthritis Cartilage* 4(1):77–84, 1996.
294. Mitchell PG, Yocum SA, Lopresti LL, et al: Collagenase 1 and collagenase 3 expression in IL 1 treated cartilage explants: regulation of net activity by endogenous produced inhibitors, *Trans ORS* 459, 1997.
295. Singer II, Scott S, Kawka DW, et al: Aggrecanase and metalloproteinase specific aggrecan neo-epitopes are induced in the articular cartilage of mice with collagen 11 arthritis, *Osteoarthritis Cartilage* 5(6):407–418, 1997.
296. Pinals RS: Pharmacologic treatment of osteoarthritis, *Clin Ther* 14:336–346, 1992.
297. Altman RD, Kapila P, Dean DD, et al: Future therapeutic trends in osteoarthritis, *Scand J Rheumatol Suppl* 77:37–42, 1989.
298. Kelly GS: The role of glucosamine sulfate and chondroitin sulfates in the treatment of degenerative joint disease, *Altern Med Rev* 3(1):27–39, 1998.
299. White GW: Adequan: a review for the practicing veterinarian, *Vet Rev* 8:463–467, 1988.
300. Francis DJ, Forrest MJ, Brooks PM, et al: Retardation of articular cartilage degradation by glycosaminoglycan polysulfate, pentosan polysulfate, and DH-40J in the rat air pouch model, *Arthritis Rheum* 32:608–616, 1989.
301. Hannan N, Ghosh P, Bellenger C, et al: Systemic administration of glycosaminoglycan polysulphate (arteparon) provides partial protection of articular cartilage from damage produced by meniscectomy in the canine, *J Orthop Res* 5:47–59, 1987.
302. Nethery A, Giles I, Jenkins K, et al: The chondroprotective drugs, arteparon and sodium pentosan polysulphate, increase collagenase activity and inhibit stromelysin activity in vitro, *Biochem Pharmacol* 44:1549–1553, 1992.
303. Halverson PB, Cheung HS, Struve J, et al: Suppression of active collagenase from calcified lapine synovium by arteparon, *J Rheumatol* 14:1013–1017, 1987.

304. Rao NV, Kennedy TP, Rao G, et al: Sulfated polysaccharides prevent human leukocyte elastase-induced acute lung injury and emphysema in hamsters, *Am Rev Respir Dis* 142:407–412, 1990.
305. Montefiori DC, Robinson WE, Modliszewski A, et al: Differential inhibition of HIV-1 cell binding and HIV-1-induced syncytium formation by low molecular weight sulphated polysaccharides, *J Antimicrob Chemother* 25:313–318, 1990.
306. Biffoni M, Paroli E: Complement in vitro inhibition by a low sulfate chondroitin sulfate (matrix), *Drugs Exp Clin Res* 27:35–39, 1991.
307. Arsenis C, McDonnell J: Effects of antirheumatic drugs on the interleukin-1a induced synthesis and activation of proteinases in articular cartilage explants in culture, *Agents Actions* 27: 261–264, 1989.
308. Greinacher A, Michels I, Schäfer M, et al: Heparin associated thrombocytopenia in a patient treated with polysulphated chondroitin sulphate: evidence for immunological crossreactivity between heparin andpolysulphated glycosaminoglycan, *Br J Haematol* 81:252–254, 1992.
309. Jepsen JV, Sall M, Rhodes PR, et al: Long-term experience with pentosan polysulfate in interstitial cystitis, *Urology* 51(3): 381–387, 1998.
310. Barrington JW, Stephenson TP: Pentosan polysulphate for interstitial cystitis, *Int Urogynecol J Pelvic Floor Dysfunct* 8(5): 293–295, 1997.
311. Ghosh P, Hutadilok N: Interactions of pentosan polysulfate with cartilage matrix proteins and synovial fibroblasts derived from patients with osteoarthritis, *Osteoarthritis Cartilage* 4(1):43–53, 1996.
312. Read RA, Cullis-Hill D, Jones MP: Systemic use of pentosan polysulphate in the treatment of osteoarthritis, *J Small Anim Pract* 37(3):108–114, 1996.
313. Budsberg SC, Bergh MS, Reynolds LR, et al: Evaluation of pentosan polysulfate sodium in the postoperative recovery from cranial cruciate injury in dogs: a randomized, placebo-controlled clinical trial, *Vet Surg* 36(3):234–244, 2007.
314. Hannon RL, Smith JG, Cullis-Hill D, et al: Safety of Cartrophen Vet in the dog: review of adverse reaction reports in the UK2003, *J Small Anim Pract* :202–208, 2003.
315. Elliot SJ, Striker LJ, Stetler WG, et al: Pentosan polysulfate decreases proliferation and net extracellular matrix production in mouse mesangial cells, *J Am Soc Nephrol* 10:62–68, 1999.
316. Striker GE, Lupia E, Elliot S, et al: Glomerulosclerosis, arteriosclerosis, and vascular graft stenosis: treatment with oral heparinoids, *Kidney Int Suppl* 63:S120–S123, 1997.
317. Senthil D, Malini MM, Varalakshmi P: Sodium pentosan polysulphate—a novel inhibitor of urinary risk factors and enzymes in experimental urolithiatic rats, *Ren Fail* 20(4):573–580, 1998.
318. Schwartsmann G, Sprinz E, Kalakun L, et al: Phase II study of pentosan polysulfate (PPS) in patients with AIDS-related Kaposi's sarcoma, *Tumori* 82(4):360–363, 1996.
319. Suzuki Y, Yamaguchi T: Effects of hyaluronic acid on macrophage phagocytosis and active oxygen release, *Agents Actions* 38(1-2):32–37, 1993.
320. Asheim A, Lindblad G: Intra-articular treatment of arthritis in race-horses with sodium hyaluronate, *Acta Vet Scand* 17: 379–394, 1976.
321. Campos JFA: Efficacy of sodium hyaluronate in the treatment of hip dysplasia in dogs, *Ahora Vet* 17:59–61, 1998.
322. Fajardo M, Di Cesare PE: Disease-modifying therapies for osteoarthritis; current status, *Drugs Aging* 22(2):141–161, 2006.
323. Anderson M: Oral chondroprotective agents, part I: common drugs used today, *Compend Contin Educ Small Anim Pract* 21(7):601–609, 1999.
324. Anderson M: Oral chondroprotective agents, Part II: evaluation of products and future compounds, *Compend Contin Educ Small Anim Pract* 21(9):861–865, 1999.
325. Boothe DM: Nutraceuticals in veterinary medicine: Part I. Definitions and regulatory considerations, *Compend Contin Educ Pract Vet* 19:1248–1255, 1997.
326. Boothe DM: Nutracueticals in veterinary medicine: Part II. Evaluating safety and efficacy, *Compend Contin Educ Pract Vet* 20:15–21, 1997.
327. Deal CL, Moskowitz RW: Nutraceuticals as therapeutic agents in osteoarthritis. The role of glucosamine, chondroitin sulfate, and collagen hydrolysate, *Rheum Dis Clin North Am* 25(2):379–395, 1999.
328. American Association of Feed Control Officials (AAFCO). Accessed November 9, 2009, at www.aafco.org.
329. National Animal Supplement Council (NASC). Accessed November 9, 2009, at www.nasc.cc.
329a. Adebowale AO, Cox DS, Liang Z, et al: Analysis of glucosamine and chondroitin sulfate content in marketed products and the Caco-2 permeability of chondroitin sulfate raw materials, *J Am Nutr Assoc* 3:37–44, 2000.
329b. Russell AS, Aghazadeh-Habashi A, Jamali F: Active ingredient consistency of commercially available glucosamine sulfate products, *J Rheumatol* 29(11):2407–2409, 2002.
330. ConsumerLab. Accessed November 9, 2009, at www.Consumerlabs.com.
331. Adebowale A, Du J, Liang Z, et al: The bioavailability and pharmacokinetics of glucosamine hydrochloride and low molecular weight chondroitin sulfate after single and multiple doses to beagle dogs, *Biopharm Drug Dispos* 23(6):217–225, 2002.
332. Hanson RR, Smalley LR, Huff GK, et al: Treatment with an oral glucosamine-chondroitin sulfate compound for degenerative joint disease in horses: 25 cases, *Proc Vet Orthoped Soc* 24:5, 1996.
333. Hanson RR: Oral glycosaminoglycans in treatment of degenerative joint diseases in horses, *Equine Pract* 18:18–22, 1997.
334. White GW, Sanders T, Jones EW, et al: Efficacy of an orally administered sulfated glycosaminoglycan supplement in an induced equine carpitis model, *Proc Am Assoc Equine Practitioners* 42:139–141, 1996.
335. Anderson MA, Slater MR, Hammad TA: Results of a survey of small-animal practitioners on the perceived clinical efficacy and safety of an oral nutraceutical, *Prev Vet Med* 38:65–73, 1999.
336. Bucci LR: Chondroprotective agents: glucosamine salts and chondroitin sulfates, *Townsend Letters for Doctors* :52–55, 1994:January.
337. McNamara PS, Barr SC, Idouaraine A, et al: Effects of an oral chondroprotective agent (Cosequin) on cartilage metabolism and canine serum, *Proc Vet Orthoped Soc* 24:35, 1997.
338. Phillipi AF: Glucosamine, chondroitin and manganese ascorbate for degenerative joint disease of the knee or low back: a randomized, double-blind, placebo-controlled pilot study, *Mil Med* 164:85–91, 1999.
339. McCarty MF: Enhanced synovial production of hyaluronic acid may explain rapid clinical response to high-dose glucosamine in osteoarthritis, *Med Hypoth* 50(6):507–510, 1998.
340. Barclay TS, Tsourounis C, McCart GM: Glucosamine, *Ann Pharmacother* 32(5):574–579, 1998.
341. McNamara PS, Barr SC, Hollis NE: Hematologic, hemostatic and biochemical effects in dogs receiving an oral chondroprotective agent for thirty days, *Am J Vet Res* 57:1390–1394, 1996.
342. Neil KM, Caron JP, Orth MW: The role of glucosamine and chondroitin sulfate in treatment for prevention of osteoarthritis in animals,*J Am Vet Med Asoc* 226:1079–1089, 2005.
342a. Reginster JY, Bruyere 0, Neuprez A: Current role of glucosamine in the treatment of osteoarthritis, *Rheumatology* 46(5):730–735, 2007.

343. Anderson JW, Nicolosi RJ, Borzelleca JF: Glucosamine effects in humans: a review of effects on glucose metabolism, side effects, safety considerations and efficacy, *Food Chem Toxicol* 43(2): 187–201, 2005.
344. Setnikar I, Rovati LC: Absorption, distribution, metabolism and excretion of glucosamine sulfate. A review, *Arzneimittelforschung* 51(9):699–725, 2001.
345. Setnikar I, Giacchetti C, Zanolo G: Pharmacokinetics of glucosamine in the dog and man, *Pharmatherapeutica* 3:538–549, 1984.
346. McNamara PS, Barr SC, Erb HN, et al: Hematological, hemostatic, and biochemical effects in cats receiving an oral chondroprotective agent for thirty days, *Vet Ther* 1(2):108–117, 2000.
347. Volpi N: Oral bioavailability of chondroitin sulfate (Condrosulf) and its constituents in healthy male volunteers, *Osteoarthritis Cartilage* 10(10):768, 2002.
348. Echard BW, Talpur NA, Funk KA, et al: Effects of oral glucosamine and chondroitin sulfate alone and in combination on the metabolism of SHR and SD rats, *Mol Cell Biochem* 225(1-): 85–91, 2001.
348a. Scholtissen S, Bruyère O, Neuprez A, et al: Glucosamine sulphate in the treatment of knee osteoarthritis: cost-effectiveness comparison with paracetamol, *Int J Clin Pract* 64(6):756–762, 2010.
349. Scroggie DA, Albright A, Harris MD: The effect of glucosamine-chondroitin supplementation on glycosylated hemoglobin levels in patients with type 2 diabetes mellitus: a placebo-controlled, double-blinded, randomized clinical trial, *Arch Intern Med* 163(13):1587–1590, 2003.
350. Hoffer LJ, Kaplan LN, Hamadeh MJ, et al: Sulfate could mediate the therapeutic effect of glucosamine sulfate, *Metabolism* 50(7):767–770, 2001.
351. Reginster JY, Deroisy R, Rovati LC, et al: Long-term effects of glucosamine sulphate on osteoarthritis progression: a randomised, placebo-controlled clinical trial, *Lancet* 357(9252):251–256, 2001.
352. Bruyere O, Pavelka K, Rovati LC, et al: Glucosamine sulfate reduces osteoarthritis progression in postmenopausal women with knee osteoarthritis: evidence from two 3-year studies, *Menopause* 11(2):138–143, 2004.
353. Ruane R, Griffiths P: Glucosamine therapy compared to ibuprofen for joint pain, *Br J Community Nurs* 7(3):148–152, 2002.
354. Conte A, Volpi N, Palmieri L: Biochemical and pharmacokinetic aspects of oral treatment with chondroitin sulfate, *Arzneimittelforschung* 45(8):918–925, 1995.
355. Gregory S, Kelly ND: The role of glucosamine sulfate and chondroitin sulfates in the treatment of degenerative joint disease, *Altern Med Rev* 3:27–39, 1998.
356. Leffler CT, Philippi AF, Leffler SG, et al: Glucosamine, chondroitin and manganese ascorbate for degenerative joint disease of the knee or low back: a randomized, double-blind, placebo-controlled pilot study, *Mil Med* 164(2):85–91, 1999.
357. Das AK, Hammad TA: Efficacy of a combination of FCHG49 glucosamine hydrochloride, TRHI22 low molecular weight sodium chondroitin sulfate and manganese ascorbate in the management of knee osteoarthritis, *Osteoarthritis Cartilage* 8(5):343–350, 2000.
358. Leffler CT, Philippi AF, Leffler SG, et al: Glucosamine, chondroitin, and manganese ascorbate for degenerative joint disease of the knee or low back: a randomized, double-blind, placebo-controlled pilot study, *Mil Med* 164(2): 85–91, 1999.
359. McAlindon T, LaValley M, Gulin J, et al: Glucosamine and chondroitin for treatment of osteoarthritis - a systematic quality assessment and meta-analysis, *J Am Med Assoc* 283(11): 1469–1475, 2000.
360. Fajardo M, Di Cesare PE: Disease-modifying therapies for osteoarthritis: current status, *Drugs Aging* 22(2):141–161, 2005.
361. Clegg DO, Reda DJ, Harris CL, et al: Glucosamine, chondroitin sulfate, and the two in combination for painful knee osteoarthritis, *N Engl J Med* 354(8):795–808, 2006.
362. Lippiello L, Idouraine A, McNamara PS, et al: Cartilage stimulatory and antiproteolytic activity is present in sera of dogs treated with a chondroprotective agent, *Canine Pract* 24(1):18–19, 1999.
363. Canapp SO, McLaughlin RM, Hoskinson JJ, et al: Scintigraphic evaluation of glucosamine HCl and chondroitin sulfate as treatment for acute synovitis in dogs, *Am J Vet Res* 60(12):1552–1557, 1999.
364. Ameye LG, Chee WSS: Osteoarthritis and nutrition. From nutraceuticals to functional foods: a systematic review of the scientific evidence, *Arthritis Res Ther* 8:R127, 2006.
365. Lippiello L, Nardo JV, Harlan R, et al: Metabolic effects of avocado/soy unsaponifiables on articular chondrocytes, *Evid Based Complement Alternat Med* 5(2):191–197, 2008.
366. Soeken KL, Lee W-L, Bausell RB, et al: Safety and efficacy of S-adenosylmethionine (SAMe) for osteoarthritis, *J Family Pract* 51:425–430, 2002.
367. Romay Ch, Gonzalez R, Ledon N, et al: C-Phycocyanin: a biliprotein with antioxidant, anti-inflammatory and neuroprotective effects, *Curr Protein Pept Sci* 4:207–216, 2003.
368. Reddy CM, Bhat VB, Kiranmai G, et al: Selective inhibition of cyclooxygenase-2 by C-Phycocyanin, a biliprotein from Spirulina platensis, *Biochem Biophys Res Commun* 277:599–603, 2000.
369. Salin M, McCord JM: Free radicals and inflammation: protection of phagocytosing leukocytes by superoxide dismutase, *J Clin Invest* 56:1319–1323, 1975.
370. Tobin T: Pharmacology review: the nonsteroidal anti-inflammatory drugs. II. Equiproxen, meclofenamic acid, flunixin and others, *J Equine Med Surg* 6:298–302, 1979.
371. Breshears DE, Brown CD, Riffel DM, et al: Evaluation of orgotein in treatment of locomotor dysfunction in dogs, *Mod Vet Pract* 55:85–93, 1974.
372. Ahlengard S, Tufvesson G, Pettersson H, et al: Treatment of traumatic arthritis in the horse with intra-articular orgotein (Palosein), *Equine Vet J* 10:122–124, 1978.
373. Brayton CF: Dimethyl sulfoxide (DMSO), *Cornell Vet* 76:61–90, 1986.
374. Alsup EM: Dimethyl sulfoxide, *J Am Vet Med Assoc* 185: 1011–1014, 1984.
375. Wong LK, Reinertson EL: Clinical considerations of dimethyl sulfoxide, *Iowa State Univ Vet* 46:89–95, 1984.
376. Spitzer WO: Drugs as determinants of health and disease in the population, *J Clin Epidemiol* 44:823–830, 1991.
377. Olson NC, Hellyer PW, Dodam JR: Mediators and vascular effects in response to endotoxin, *Br Vet J* 151:489–522, 1995.
378. Whittle BJR: Nitric oxide in physiology and pathology, *Histochem J* 27:727–737, 1995.
379. Howe LB: Treatment of endotoxic shock: glucocorticoids, lazaroids, nonsteroidals and others, *Vet Clin North Am* 28:249–267, 1998.
380. Vincent JL: Evidence-based medicine in the ICU: important advances and limitations, *Chest* 126:592–600, 2004.
381. Minneci P, Deans K, Natanson C, et al: Increasing the efficacy of anti-inflammatory agents used in the treatment of sepsis, *Eur J Clin Microbiol Infect Dis* 22:1–9, 2003.
382. Kettelhut IC, Fiers W, Goldgerg AL: The toxic effects of tumor necrosis factor in vivo and their prevention by cyclooxygenase inhibitors, *Proc Natl Acad Sci USA* 84:4273, 1987.
383. Shuster R, Traub-Dargatz J, Baxter G: Survey of diplomates of the American College of Veterinary Internal Medicine and the American College of Veterinary Surgeons regarding clinical aspects and treatment of endotoxemia in horses, *J Am Vet Med Assoc* 210:87–92, 1997.

384. Sigurdsson GH, Youssef H: Amelioration of respiratory and circulatory changes in established endotoxic shock by ketoprofen, *Acta Anesthesiol Scand* 38:33–39, 1994.
385. Boumpas DT, Chrousos GP, Wilder RL, et al: Glucocorticoid therapy for immune-mediated diseases. Basic and clinical correlates, *Ann Intern Med* 119:1198–1208, 1993.
386. Bone RC, Fisher CJ, Clemmer TP, et al: A controlled clinical trial of high dose methylprednisolone in the treatment of severe sepsis and septic shock, *N Engl J Med* 317:653–658, 1987.
387. Aoki N, Lefer AM: Protective effects of a novel non-glucocorticoid 21 aminosteroid (U74006F) during traumatic shock in rats, *J Cardiovasc Pharmacol* 15:205–210, 1990.
388. Hall ED, Yonkers PA, McCall JM: Attenuation of hemorrhagic shock by the non-glucocorticoid 21-aminosteroid U74006F, *Eur J Pharmacol* 147:299–303, 1988.
389. Semrad SD, Rose M, Putnam ML: Efficacy and toxicity of lazaroid (U74006F) in neonatal endotoxemia, *Circ Shock* 27: 358–359, 1989.
390. Semrad SD, Rose ML, Adams JL: Effects of tirilazad mesylate (U74006F) on eicosanoid and tumor necrosis factor generation in healthy and endotoxic neonatal calves, *Circ Shock* 40:235–242, 1993.
391. Zhang H, Spapen H, Minikis P, et al: Tirilazad mesylate (U-74006F) inhibits effects of endotoxin in dogs, *Am J Physiol* 286:H1847–H1855, 1995.
392. Morris PE, Light RB, Garber GE: Identifying patients with severe sepsis who should not be treated with drotrecogin alfa (activated), *Am J Surg* 184:19S–24S, 2002.
393. Kavanagh RJ, Kam PC: Lazaroids: efficacy and mechanism of action of the 21-aminosteroids in neuroprotection, *Br J Anaesth* 86(1):110–119, 2001.

Glucocorticoids and Mineralocorticoids

30

Dawn Merton Boothe and Katrina A. Mealey

Chapter Outline

Glucocorticoids (GLCs) are among the most frequently used and misused drugs in veterinary medicine. Optimal therapy with GLCs requires a thorough understanding of their actions on all body systems and knowledge of the pharmacodynamic and pharmacokinetic differences of the synthetic GLC derivatives. The physiologic and pharmacologic effects of GLCs, beyond suppression of the hypothalamic–pituitary–adrenal axis, have not been extensively studied in the dog or cat; therefore much of the information presented represents data extrapolated from human patients or rodent studies. Whenever possible, information specific to the dog or cat has been included and is indicated as such.

PHYSIOLOGY: CONTROL OF ENDOGENOUS GLUCOCORTICOID SECRETION

The adrenal cortex comprises three zones, each of which synthesizes steroidal hormones. From superficial to deep, these include the zonas glomerulosa, the source of mineralocorticoids (predominantly aldosterone but also corticosterone); reticularis, a source of (weak) androgens; and fasciculata, the source of GLCs (cortisol and cortisone). As with many hormones, the secretion of corticosteroids reflects a balance between positive and negative feedback pathways. Corticotropin-releasing hormone (previously corticotropin release factor, CRH) is secreted by the hypothalamus and travels through the hypophyseal portal system to the adenohypophysis, where it stimulates the synthesis and secretion of adrenocorticotropin (ACTH) from the basophilic cells of the adenohypophysis (Figure 30-1). In addition to its role in promoting ACTH secretion, CRF appears to be involved in the autonomic, immunologic, and behavioral response to stress independent of the hypothalamopituitary axis. Administration of CRF to dogs results in a decrease in gastric acid secretion by activation of the sympathetic nervous system, an immediate decrease in mean arterial blood pressure accompanied by reflex tachycardia, and a marked increase in plasma vasopressin concentrations.[1] These actions of CRF are independent of GLCs.

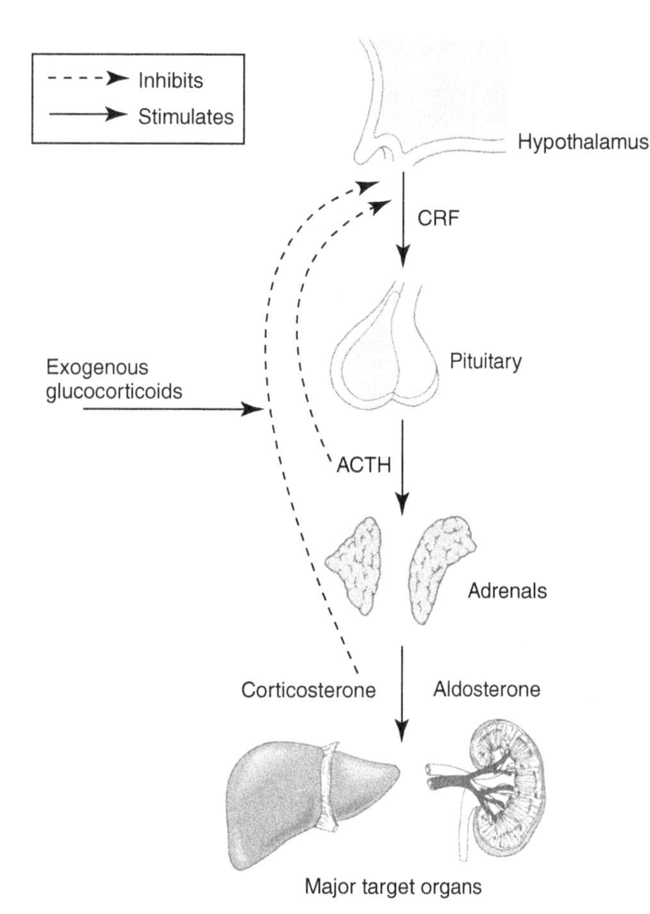

Figure 30-1 The relationship between the hypothalamus, pituitary, and adrenal glands. Release of corticotropin-releasing factor (CRF) is prevented by feedback inhibition of corticosteroids (exogenous or endogenous). Release of adrenocorticotropic hormone (ACTH) is subsequently inhibited, and further synthesis, primarily of glucocorticoids, is inhibited. The primary target organ of mineralocorticoids is the kidney; the liver and cardiovascular system are important targets of glucocorticoids.

In addition to CRF, ACTH also is stimulated by arginine vasopressor (AVP), which is a weak stimulator of ACTH but a strong stimulator of CRH and catecholamines; angiotensin II; serotonin; and vasoactive intestinal peptide. Other stimulators include the inflammatory cytokines interleukin (IL) -1, -2, and -6 and tumor necrosis factor-α(TNF-α).[2] Most stimulators of ACTH also stimulate CRH.[2] The primary short-term effects of ACTH are stimulation of the adrenal cortex synthesis and secretion of cortisol, corticosterone, aldosterone (the effect of ACTH on mineralocorticoid secretion is minimal), and weak androgenic substances. Long-term effects of ACTH increase the production of enzymes and cofactors necessary for cortisol production and cause an increase in adrenal receptors for low-density lipoprotein cholesterol.[2]

Cortisol and corticosterone concentrations in plasma subsequently influence CRF and ACTH secretion such that increased concentrations inhibit release of CRF and ACTH and reduced concentrations stimulate release of CRF and ACTH. Exogenous factors, such as trauma, heat, stress, surgery, and neural impulses, also mediate CRF and ACTH secretion. Exogenous corticosteroid administration can also suppress CRF and ACTH release. The degree of suppression depends on the particular drug used. For example, the synthetic drug dexamethasone is 50 to 100 times more potent in suppressing ACTH secretion than is the endogenous compound, cortisol.[3] The diurnal variation in GLC secretion that occurs in humans has not been well documented in dogs or cats. Nonetheless, morning dosing (in dogs) is among the strategies used to minimize the risk of adrenocortical suppression that might result from exogenous glucocorticoid therapy. These approaches thus include: 1. Determining a minimum effective dose; 2. Alternate day dosing; 3. Use of a "short-acting" glucocorticoids whose effects are 24 hrs or shorter in duration; 4. Dosing in the morning (and potentially dosing at nights for cats); and 5. Tapering the dose over days to weeks as therapy is discontinued, thus facilitating readaptation of the adrenal gland to secretion.

MECHANISM OF ACTION

The myriad physiologic effects of GLCs result from interaction of the drugs with the glucocorticoid receptor (GR), one member of a nuclear hormone receptor superfamily that also includes receptors for thyroid hormone, mineralocorticoid, estrogen, and progesterone.[4] Other activities may also reflect nonreceptor mechanisms.

Mineralocorticoid and Glucocorticoid Receptors

Two primary types of corticosteroid receptors exist. Type I, or mineralocorticoid receptors (MRs), bind both endogenous GLCs and aldosterone. Type II, or GRs, bind endogenous and exogenous GLCs but have a poor affinity for mineralocorticoids. The GRs and MRs are sufficiently similar that drugs may bind to both, causing similar responses. In human medicine, the cause and effect relationship between hypertension, heart failure, and MRs has led to a reassessment of the relationship between GLC and mineralocorticoid as well as androgen and progesterone receptors.[5] The distinction among the receptors, including the sequence of their evolution, becomes important when assessing the selectivity or lack thereof of therapeutic agents on each receptor type. In human medicine this is particularly germane to the impact of GLCs on the MRs and its implication in patients with cardiovascular disease.

Every cell appears to have GRs, although the liver is the primary target. The type and concentration of GRs varies between species and tissue. Type II receptors are more ubiquitous in the brain. The degree to which GLCs bind to each receptor type varies with the circulating concentration. At basal levels type I receptors are preferred, but as cortisol concentrations increase (e.g., during stress), type II receptors increasingly are activated.[6]

Within a given tissue, GR numbers appear to fluctuate with changing cell cycles and age and in response to a variety of endogenous or exogenous compounds. More than 15 endogenous regulators have been identified for GLC receptors.[7] Response to GLCs reflects receptor density or GLC concentration, depending on the tissue. GR density is autoregulated; increased receptor density associated with hypoadrenocorticism can be reversed with GLC replacement.[8] Likewise, chronic GLC therapy will result in downregulation of receptor density. However, autoregulation is tissue specific, and in some tissues the concentration of GLC is a more important determinant of response than is the number - or even type - of receptors. For example, as noted, the MR acts similarly to the GR and is sufficiently similar in structure that responses to substrates are also likely to be similar.[8,9] Any steroid with a ketone group at position 11 (Figure 30-2) will interact positively with either the MR or GR.[2] However, GLCs generally are present in concentrations that exceed those of mineralocorticoids by 1000-fold or more,[2] which suggests the potential for GLC response to predominate in any tissue exhibiting either GRs or MRs. The ability of receptors to respond to mineralocorticoids despite differences in concentration reflects a combination of conditions: (1) binding of glucocorticoids by globulins, which effectively sequesters the hormone, precluding interaction with GRs or MRs; (2) activation of discrete sets of target genes, perhaps reflecting a difference in repression of transcriptional induction (e.g., aldosterone activates the expression of several genes, with that of Na^+, K^+-ATPase in the basolateral membranes of tubular cells being the best characterized); (3) restrictive expression of MRs only, with the principle sites occurring in the renal cortical distal tubules and collecting ducts, colon, salivary and sweat glands, and hippocampus[8]; (4) differing rates of GLC inactivation, which allows mineralocorticoids to predominate and stimulate response. For example, tissues differ in their expression of 11 β-hydroxysteroid dehydrogenase type 2 (11 β-HSD2), the enzyme that inactivates cortisol to corticosterone. Tissues with high concentrations of 11 beta-HSD2are those that typically respond to mineralocorticoids—kidney, colon, salivary gland—allowing mineralocorticoid effects to predominate.[8,10] In the presence of 11 β-HSD2, GLC expression occurs only if present in concentrations several magnitudes higher than mineralocorticoids.

> **KEY POINT 30-1** Similarities in the mineralocorticoid and glucocorticoid receptors and steroid structures contribute to the shared action of drugs.

Certain disease conditions may reflect aberrations in methods allowing differential substrate response such as an absence of 11 β-HSD2 such that tissues respond to the inappropriate steroid.[9] The importance of renal metabolism of cortisol is implied in the impact renal failure has on prolongation of plasma cortisol half-life in human patients; half-life increased 30% in one study.[10] Impaired 11 β-HSD2 accompanying renal disease contributes to the pathophysiology of salt and water retention and hypertension in renal failure and therefore could contribute to selected consequences of renal disease (hypertension, sodium retention, hyperkalemia, and decreased glomerular filtration rate). Inhibition of 11β HSD2by selected compounds (licorice, selected angiotensin-converting enzyme inhibitors [ramipril]) contributes to pharmacologic or adverse events as well as drug interactions. Ramipril causes decreased ACTH-induced hypertension in the rat.[10] Inhibition allows GLCs to excessively stimulate MRs such that hyperaldosteronism emerges. Such interactions also can be favorable:

Nuclear and Non-nuclear Mechanisms of Action of Corticosteroids

The molecular description of the GR as it relates to its mechanism of interaction has been described.[11-14] The GR consists of at least two isoforms.[11] The α isoform binds to GLCs, DNA, and transcription factors and thus modulates transcription activity. The α isoform may also act through nongenomic mechanisms. In contrast, although the β isoform binds to DNA, it does not bind other ligands, fails to activate transcription, and appears to be able to interfere with the activities of α isoforms.[12] Corticosteroid receptors are located in the cytoplasm of the target cell complexed with heat shock proteins (Hsp 70 and Hsp 90) that act as chaperones, proteins which in non-functional activities (e.g., folding, assembly) of macromolecules, and an immunophilin, an intracellular protein that binds other immunosuppressive compounds.[9,11] The complexed receptor is inactive until bound to a steroid ligand.[9] Steroids enter the cells by passive diffusion, although a rate-limited active transport mechanism may also exist (Figure 30-2) Once in the cell, the GLC binds to the receptor, causing the heat shock protein and other molecules to dissociate. Intracellular GLCs impart their effects in one of three ways: The steroid–receptor complex moves into the nucleus and (1) binds to specific DNA sequences causing the regulation of genes (for example, lipocortin or genes responsible for gluconeogenesis) (referred to as a "cis" or element, resulting in transactivation), (2) interacts with other transcription factors (e.g., AP-1, NFκB), generally at lower concentrations, that prevent the transcription of targeted genes (e.g., TNFα, IL-1B, IL-4 and 5; referred to as a "trans element" resulting in transrepression); or (3) through non-genomic mechanisms involving membrane-associated GR and secondary messenger systems.[2, 12a] Non-genomic responses are rapid in onset, and includes

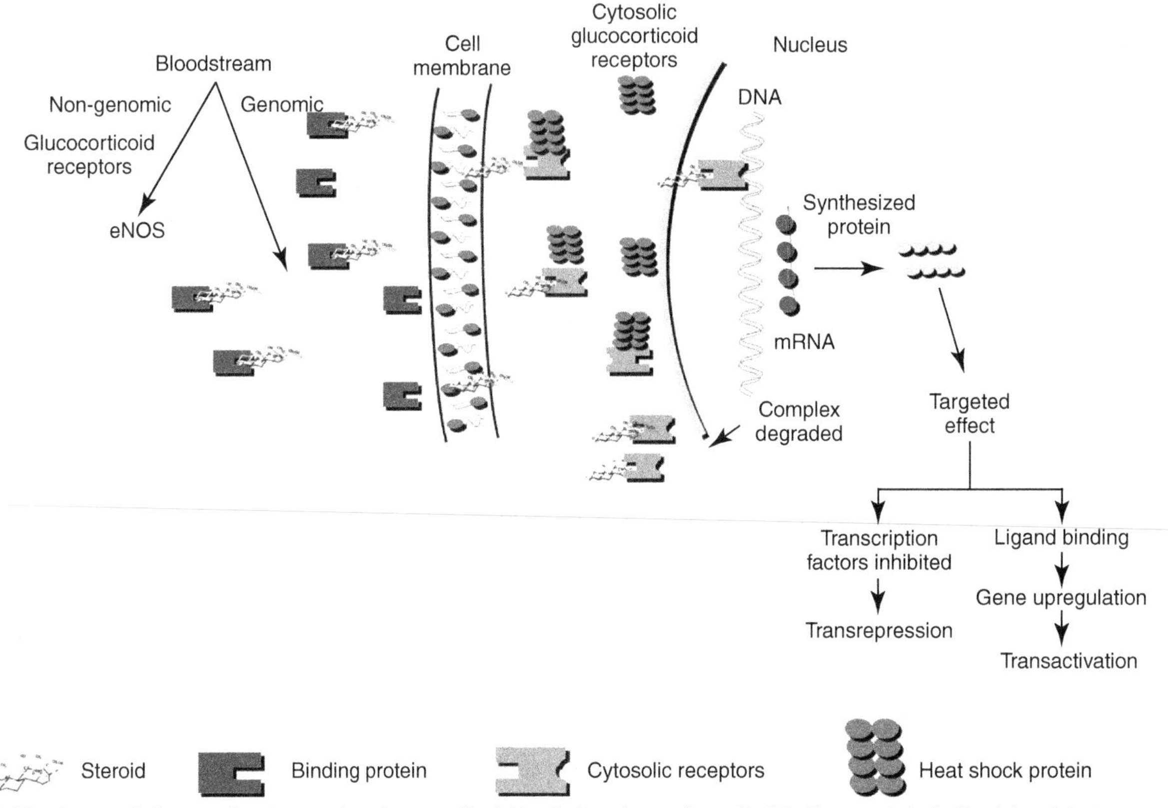

Figure 30-2 The intracellular mechanisms of a glucocorticoid include release from its binding protein in the bloodstream, passive diffusion of the drug through the cell membrane, movement through the cytosol in association with a receptor and chaperone heat shock protein, translocation to the nucleus, binding to DNA, transcription, either stimulation or inhibition of protein synthesis, and degradation of the protein–steroid complex.

vascular responses (eNOS activation), lymphocytolysis, and possibly, induction of inflammatory prostaglandins. "Permissive" effects of GLC may reflect non-genomic responses.

Because the effect of older, current and future GLC reflects the molecular relationship between drug and cellular macromolecules, a brief review or molecular interactions is warranted. Genomic effects of GLCs are initiated by translocation of the activated receptor–GLC complex to the nucleus (Figure 30-2). In the nucleus the complex binds to regulatory proteins of target genes. The short DNA sequences recognized by the activated GR are referred to as *glucocorticoid responsive elements* (GREs). It is through these GREs that specificity of GLC-modulated gene transcription is controlled.[4] Transcription of the gene and subsequent formation of the targeted protein is either induced (transactivated) or inhibited (transrepressed). The receptor and GLC are eventually metabolized (the exact location or timing is not documented). The cellular half-life of the activated complex is about 10 hours.[15] It is not known whether the rate of metabolism of the GLC–receptor complex is dependent on the specific GLC involved. Some of the proteins that are regulated by GLCs are listed in Table 30-1. The proteins encoded by these genes are responsible for some of the physiologic (pharmacologic) effects of GLCs.

KEY POINT 30-2 As with all steroids, corticosteroids cause their primary effects by inducing or inhibiting the synthesis of target proteins at the level of the gene.

Once activated, the activated ligand receptor influences gene expression by binding to specific GREs in the promoter regions of GLC-regulated genes. However, in addition to this classical transactivation mechanism, also referred to as positive GRE (pGRE), genes may also be negatively targeted, or transrepressed, through negative GRE (nGRE). The GR generally has a lower affinity for nGRE than pGRE. Transrepression involves protein–protein coupling to other transcription factors (e.g., nuclear factor kappa-B [NFκB], activator protein-1 [AP-1], STAT-5 (signal transducer and activator of transcription) or nuclear factor of activated T-cells [NFAT]) such that their activity is modulated. The importance of these different GR interactions results in differential physiologic (and pharmacologic) effects and ultimately provides a basis for directed drug therapy. The largely undesirable metabolic effects of long-term GLC therapy appear to be mediated by pGRE interaction (i.e., transactivation gene expression). In contrast, the desirable antiinflammatory effects appear to reflect modulation of transcription factors (i.e., transrepression through interaction with nGREs).[16,17] Indeed, nGREs contribute to the regulation of the hypothalamic–pituitary–adrenal axis (targeting pro-opiomelanocortin [POMC] and CRH), bone metabolism (through osteocalcin), skin function, inflammation (IL-1β), angiogenesis (proliferin), and lactation (prolactin).[17] Trans (protein-coupling) effects, and repression in particular, appear to occur at concentrations lower than that necessary for cis (transactivation)

Table 30-1 Immunomodulatory Actions of Glucocorticoids

Actions	Mechanism
Interference with cytokine production	1
Interleukin-1	
Interleukin-2	
Interleukin-6	
Interleukin-8	
Tumor necrosis factor-alpha	
Interferon-gamma	
Downregulation of cell adhesion molecules	1
Intercellular Adhesion Molecule 1 (ICAM-1)	
E-selectin	
Inhibition of chemokine synthesis	
Interference with leukocyte function enzymes	1
Inducible nitric oxide synthase	
Granzyme B	
Upregulation of cytokine receptors	
Interleukin-1	
Interleukin-6	
Induction of lymphocyte apotosis	
CD4+CD8+	
Inhibition of cyclooxygenase-2 expression	
Inhibition of wound healing	2
Epithelial cells	
Fibroblasts	
Induction of acute phase proteins (permissive effect)	3
Serum amyloid A	
Serum amyloid P	
AP-1	
NFk-B	
Stat proteins	

1=protein-protein interaction with transcription factors
2=Direct gene activation
3=Direct gene activation

effects,[18] providing another mechanism of directed therapy. "Designer" GLC might be developed such that potency for protein coupling (trans) repression is greater than DNA interaction, leading to cis or trans activation. Dexamethasone and prednisolone are examples of a "symmetric" GLC, characterized by equal binding affinity for both actions. Interestingly, medroxyprogesterone acetate exhibits a preponderance of transrepression activity rather than transactivation.[16] Newer GLCs are likely to have a preponderance of activity for either activation or repression. The recognition of this dual mechanism of GLC action will also facilitate the development of GR antagonists, which might be useful for the treatment of Cushing's disease.[16] Another term that has emerged is "Dissociated GLCs" which target GLC-dependent transactivation or alternatively act as inhibitors of NFκB-dependent transcription, thus retaining their in vivo antiinflammatory activity but avoiding their undesirable metabolic effects.[19]

KEY POINT 30-3 The desired inhibitory effects of glucocorticoids reflect indirect repression of transcription factors, whereas undesirable effects reflect direct interaction with DNA.

Differences in GR affinity for nGREs versus pGREs may also offer a mechanism for differential targeted drug response based on dose (or concentration). Treatment with low, rather than high, doses of GLCs appears to minimize undesirable side effects.[20] Using a retrospective analysis of published literature (meta analysis precluded by method variability) coupled with a prospective study, researchers found that most adverse effects to GLCs in humans were associated with high, rather than low, doses (7.5 mg prednisolone equivalent in humans [approximately 0.1 mg/kg]) of GLC (see the section on adverse events).

Glucocorticoid Resistance

Failure to respond to steroid therapy is observed in human patients being treated for a variety of diseases. Poor compliance and low bioavailability must be ruled out before other factors are considered. The documented phenomenon of GLC resistance (both familial and iatrogenic or drug induced forms have been reported in humans) may reflect, among other causes, reduced receptor numbers or affinity for GLC.[21] Cellular response to GLCs has been directly correlated with receptor numbers. Reversible downregulation of receptor numbers and a subsequent decrease in biological effect are documented sequelae of GLC treatment.[7] Such effects have been demonstrated on lymphocyte receptors.[22] GLC failure in patients receiving long-term GLC therapy for treatment of host-versus-graft rejection has been attributed to downregulation of cytoplasmic GRs in T lymphocytes. GLC doses subsequently must be increased.[23] Pulsing of high doses of GLCs may overcome this relative resistance (see the section on therapeutic use).[24] The relative balance of the α and β isoforms of GR appear to influence cell sensitivity to GLCs; higher concentrations of β contribute to GLC resistance.[12] Treatment of inflammatory bowel disease offers an example of potential mechanisms of GLC resistance. Some human patients with severe disease are nonresponsive to even high doses of GLCs. Lack of response has been associated with poor antiproliferative effects on blood T lymphocytes, in contrast to near-complete inhibition of responders. A similar relationship has been demonstrated for other chronic allergy-based diseases, such as asthma or rheumatoid arthritis, and renal allograft rejection. A relatively fast in vitro T lymphocyte proliferation assay has been useful in identifying nonresponders before treatment.[25] Several molecular mechanisms have been proposed to account for poor control of T cell proliferation by GLCs. These include overexpression of the multidrug resistance gene (MDR1 polymorphism), resulting in increased P-glycoprotein–mediated efflux of cytoplasmic (see relevant discussion in the section on neoplasia). This mechanism might be reversible by co-administration of cyclosporine, an inhibitor of P-glycoprotein. Other mechanisms include impaired GLC signaling by the GR and increased activation by epithelial cells of proinflammatory mediators that directly inhibit GR transcription. This latter mechanism (post-receptor failure) is supported by the presence of clinical signs consistent with Cushing's disease in humans with poor inflammatory control.[25] Differences in activation patterns of NFκB have been associated with GLC resistance in human patients with chronic inflammatory bowel disease.[19] Ultimately, differences in response at the molecular level may also be shown .

KEY POINT 30-4 Glucocorticoid resistance is a recognized contributor to therapeutic failure and reflects several potential mechanisms, some of which might be avoided with proper use.

PHYSIOLOGIC EFFECTS

Physiologic effects of GLCs required for the "normal" day-to-day function of the animal can be easily appreciated when GLCs are absent, as in the case of adrenocortical insufficiency (hypoadrenocorticism or Addison's disease), or present in excessive concentrations, as in hyperadrenocorticism. The primary role of aldosterone, the major mineralocorticoid, is regulation of sodium homeostasis. Interestingly, the effects of GLCs and mineralocorticoids can be directly antagonistic at some sites. For example, in some tissues aldosterone stimulates and GLCs inhibit sodium resorption.[8] Likewise, cortisone can have different and opposing effects, depending on whether it interacts with MRs or GRs. Cortisone inhibits microglial proliferation through GRs but stimulates proliferation through MRs.[26] Dexamethasone also inhibits microglial cell proliferation at concentrations lower than those for cortisone.[26]

Effects on Intermediary Metabolism: Carbohydrates, Proteins, and Lipids

The natural function of GLCs is to protect glucose-dependent cerebral functions by stimulating the formation of glucose by the liver, decreasing its peripheral utilization and promoting its storage as glycogen.[27] Teleologically, these effects protect glucose-dependent tissues, the brain and heart, from starvation.[9] The hyperglycemic effect of GLCs, as seen in the stressed patient, is due to an increase in gluconeogenesis and insulin antagonism. Gluconeogenesis is the result of an increase in precursors necessary for gluconeogenesis as well as induction of hepatic enzymes that catalyze reactions of glucose synthesis. Increased breakdown of proteins, particularly skeletal muscle and collagen, provides gluconeogenic precursors (e.g., amino acids and glycerol). This effect is exhibited clinically as muscle wasting, delayed wound healing, and thinning of the skin. The anti-insulin effect of GLCs is a result of decreased peripheral tissue utilization of glucose and reduced affinity of cellular receptors for insulin. Utilization appears to be decreased by translocation of insulin receptors from the cell membrane to an intracellular location inaccessible by insulin.[9]

KEY POINT 30-5 The physiologic effects of glucocorticoids reflect their underlying physiologic intent: maintenance of the body, particularly during states of stress.

Metabolism of lipids is also affected by GLCs. Specifically, GLCs promote lipolysis, generating the free fatty acids that, along with amino acids, serve as substrates for hepatic glycogen synthesis and inhibit long-chain fatty acid synthesis. Effects of GLCs on lipid metabolism reflect, in part, a permissive effect of the steroids on other agents, including growth hormone and β-adrenergic receptors. One sequela of these effects is redistribution of body fat (such as is typified by Cushing's disease). Differences in adipocyte sensitivity to insulin and the facilitating effects of GLCs may explain the redistribution phenomenon.[9]

Water and Electrolyte Balance

Cortisol appears to be essential for the maintenance of renal blood flow and glomerular filtration rate. Volume repletion alone is not sufficient to return renal function to normal in states of hypoaldosteronism. GLCs also generally increase the filtration fraction; impact on renal vascular resistance is not clear, varying with the method studied.[10] Aldosterone is the most potent natural corticosteroid that affects fluid and electrolyte balance. Mineralocorticoids act to enhance sodium reabsorption in exchange for potassium (from the distal renal tubules and collecting ducts) or hydrogen (the intercalated cells), resulting in a positive sodium balance, expansion of extracellular fluid volume, and an increase in glomerular filtration rate. Sodium reabsorption is enhanced by increasing the number of open Na^+ and K^+ pores; Na^+, K^+-ATPase activity at the basolateral membrane also is increased, causing sodium to be returned to the circulation. The ratio of exchange of these mono-charge cations may be greater than than 11:1.

KEY POINT 30-6 Actions of glucocorticoids will maintain blood glucose, blood pressure, cardiac output, and vascular volume. Accordingly, their absence can result in life-threatening cardiovascular collapse.

Effects of mineralocorticoids are not limited to renal tissues but also include the colon, ileum, ciliary apparatus, salivary, and (in human beings) sweat glands. GLCs influence water and electrolyte balance through mineralocorticoid actions. Differences in tissue response to various corticosteroids was addressed previously. Cortisol and the synthetic GLCs possess varying degrees of mineralocorticoid activity, but all have less than 1% of the mineralocorticoid activity of aldosterone. GLCs also impart a permissive effect on tubular mechanisms that maintain the glomerular filtration rate. GLCs have an inhibitory effect on antidiuretic hormone and may decrease permeability of the distal renal tubules to water through a direct action. The polyuria and polydipsia commonly observed in dogs (but not cats) receiving GLCs may result from a combination of mineralocorticoid and GLC effects.

Other reported renal actions of GLC include downregulation of sodium–phosphate co-transport and sulfate co-transport, upregulation on sodium–bicarbonate co-transport, modulation of the effects of sodium on amino acid transport, and other effects on acid–base balance.[10] GLCs also influence several aspects of calcium movement. In the renal tubular cells, calcium excretion is increased, and in the small intestine its absorption is impaired. GLCs also increase parathormone secretion, which in turn increases osteoclast-mediated bone resorption. The net effect of GLCs on calcium homeostasis is a decrease in total body calcium stores.

Hemolymphatic System

GLCs tend to increase the red blood cell content of the blood by retarding erythrophagocytosis. Lymphopenia, eosinopenia, and monocytopenia caused by cellular redistribution and neutrophilia caused by increased release from bone marrow, demargination, and a reduction of their removal from the circulation are all associated with GLC administration.[9] This blood cell profile represents the "stress leukogram" seen clinically in patients with increased concentrations of endogenous GLCs. The acute effects of GLCs on circulating lymphocytes are due to sequestration from the blood rather than lymphocytolysis, although cells of lymphocytic malignancies are destroyed by GLCs. In addition to reducing the number of circulating lymphocytes, GLCs also alter the responses of lymphocytes to mitogens and antigens. T lymphocytes are inhibited to a greater degree than B lymphocytes (see following discussion of immunomodulation). GLCs also induce lymphocyte apoptosis.[28] GLCs also have direct inhibitory effects on eosinophils, including eosinophil migration.[29] GLCs directly induce eosinophil and lymphocyte apoptosis.[30]

Antiinflammatory and Immunosuppressive Effects

GLCs are most frequently used in clinical medicine for their antiinflammatory and immunosuppressive actions (see Table 30-1).[31] Because the antiinflammatory and immunosuppressive effects of GLCs reflect specific actions on white blood cells, these effects are inextricably linked. They generally occur only when the amounts of steroid are present in concentrations greater than those found in the normal physiologic state (i.e., pharmacologic concentrations). The effects of GLCs on leukocyte numbers were discussed earlier. GLCs also profoundly affect white blood cell function. Ultimately, both the humoral and cell-mediated arms of the immune response are affected. The antiinflammatory effects of GLCs reflect all three mechanisms of GLC action (genomic transcription and transactivation; nongenomic membrane receptor signaling).[12]

GLCs upregulate or downregulate as many as 2000 genes involved in the regulation of the immune response (Table 30-4).[2] GLCs inhibit early and late phases of the inflammation. Responses that are inhibited include edema formation, fibrin deposition, leukocyte migration, phagocytic activity, collagen deposition, and capillary and fibroblast proliferation. Many of these processes involve lymphokines and other soluble mediators of inflammation, and it is through these mediators that GLCs exert their antiinflammatory actions. GLCs induce annexin I (also known as lipocortin), which inhibits phospholipase 2, thus blocking the release of arachidonic acid and its subsequent conversion to eicosanoids (i.e., prostaglandins, thromboxanes, prostacyclins, and leukotrienes). (Figure 30-3). GLCs also preferentially inhibit transcription of cyclooxygenase-2 (COX-2), the inducible form of cyclooxygenase.[12,32,33] Interestingly, recent evidence indicates that under some circumstances, GLCs may actually induce COX-2.[34] The net effect of specificity to inhibit COX-2 may be inhibition of inflammatory prostaglandins without negatively affecting the protective effects of prostaglandins in other body systems (e.g., gastrointestinal, renal, hemostasis). GLCs induce the protein MAPK phosphatase 1, which through various actions inactivates a number of proteins important in the signaling of cytokines.[12] Through physical interaction, transcription of NFκB is inhibited by GLCs. Many of the antiinflammatory effects of GLCs occur rapidly, apparently independently of changes in gene expression (nongenomic). Examples include activation of endothelial nitric oxide synthetase,[12] offering an alternative mechanism of action of a new class of more selective antiinflammatory drugs.[35]

KEY POINT 30-7 Glucocorticoids inhibit essentially every phase of the inflammatory response, including the immune response and wound healing.

Among the sequelae of these mechanisms, GLCs inhibit release of TNFα and IL-2 from activated macrophages. TNFα induces cytotoxicity and can enhance neutrophil and eosinophil function.[27] The release of platelet-activating factor from leukocytes and mast cells is inhibited by GLCs. Platelet-activating factor induces vasodilation, platelet and leukocyte aggregation, smooth muscle contraction (especially in the bronchi), and increased vascular permeability.[36]

The immunosuppressive actions of GLCs, like their antiinflammatory actions, involve disruption of intercellular communication of leukocytes through interference with lymphokine production, biological action, or both. GLCs inhibit the synthesis and release of IL-1 by macrophages, thereby suppressing the activation of T cells. GLCs also inhibit IL-2 synthesis by activated T cells. IL-2 plays a critical role in amplification of cell-mediated immunity. GLCs block the effects of the migration inhibitory factor-γ (causing macrophages to migrate away from the affected area) and interferon-γ (IFN-γ) on macrophages.[27] IFN-γ, which is released from activated T cells, plays an important role in facilitating antigen processing by macrophages. Additionally, GLCs suppress the bactericidal and fungicidal actions of macrophages. GLCs also alter synthesis of and biologic response to collagenase, lipase, and plasminogen activator. The antiinflammatory effects of GLCs also may reflect inhibition of the inducible form of nitric oxide synthase (iNOS).[37] Synovial macrophage nitric oxide production and iNOS synthesis are inhibited by dexamethasone. The inhibitory effect appears to be mediated by lipocortin.The immunosuppressive actions of GLCs are more pronounced on the cellular arm than the humoral arm of the immune system (Figure 30-4). GLCs have minimal effects on plasma immunoglobulin concentrations but can modulate immunoglobulin function. For example, opsonization of bacteria is inhibited. Therapeutic doses of GLCs do not significantly decrease an animal's antibody response to antigenic challenge (e.g., vaccinations). The immunosuppressive effects

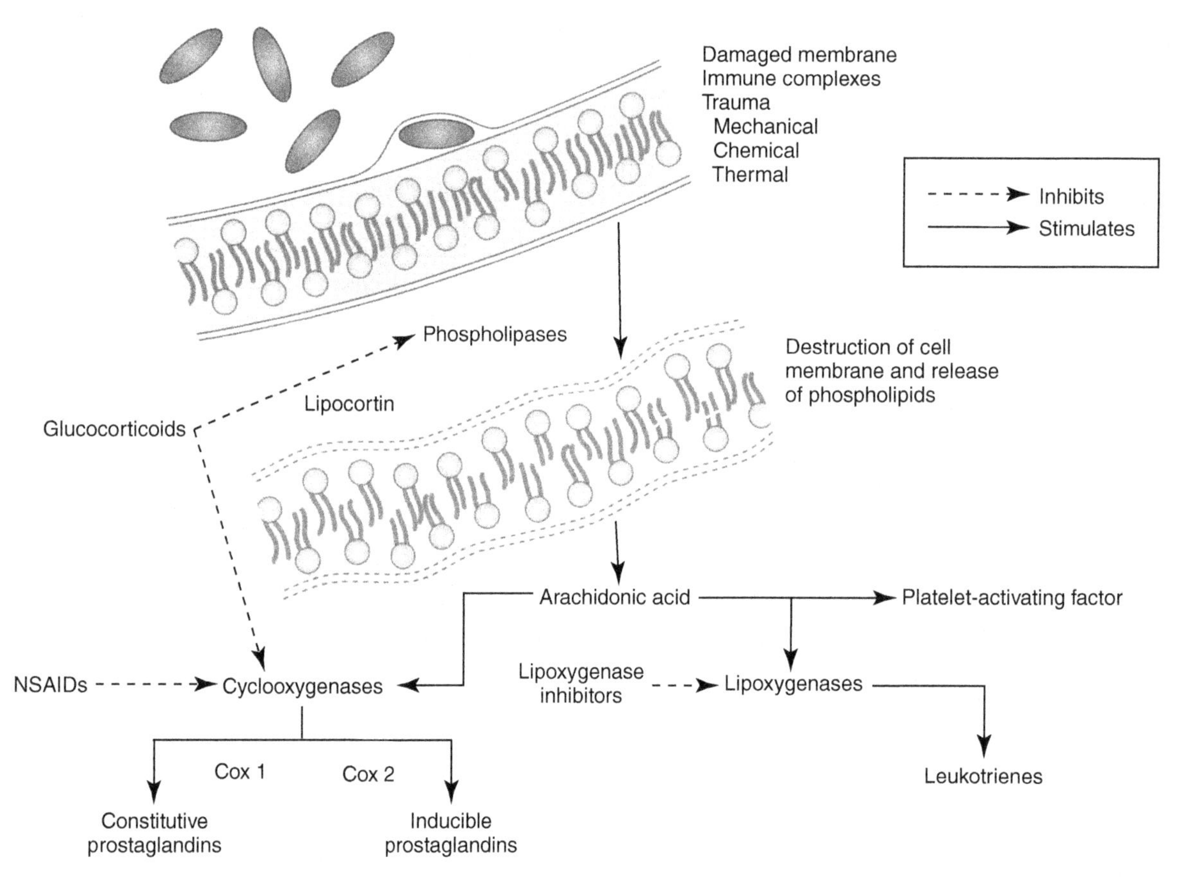

Figure 30-3 Site of glucocorticoid action in the arachidonic acid cascade. Glucocorticoids inhibit phospholipase and its subsequent degradation of cell membrane phospholipids to mediators of inflammation (platelet-activating factor, leukotrienes, and prostaglandins). Lipocortin is the effector protein whose synthesis is stimulated by glucocorticoids. In addition, glucocorticoids selectively inhibit cyclooxygenase-2. *NSAIDs,* Nonsteroidal antiinflammatory drugs.

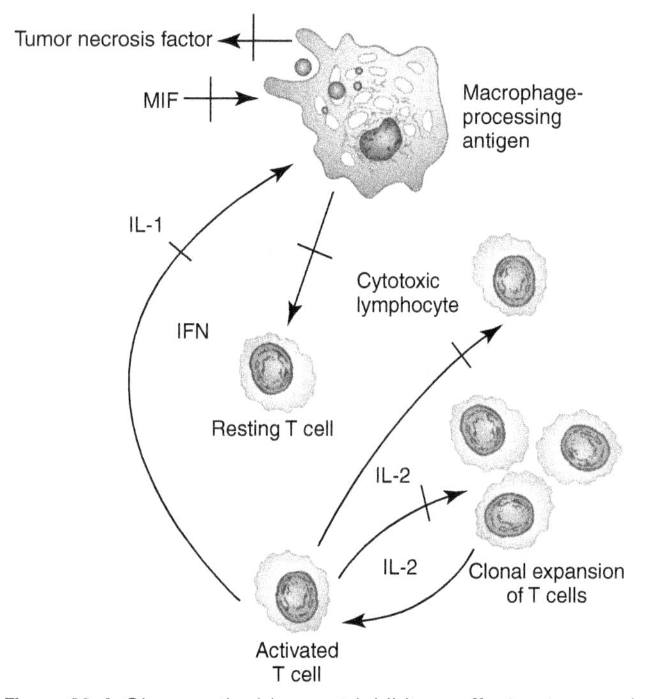

Figure 30-4 Glucocorticoids exert inhibitory effects at several sites in the cell-mediated response. Both macrophages and T cells are targeted. *IFN,* interferon; *IL,* interleukin; *MIF,* migration inhibitory factor.

of GLCs may also reflect actions on the hypothalamic–pituitary–adrenal axis. Multiple cytokines appear to regulate this axis. Specifically, IL-1 appears to stimulate the release of CRH and directly increase the release of ACTH, and it may cause the adrenals to release GLCs. These interactions appear to be important to modulation of stress and thus maintenance of homeostasis.[9]

Cardiovascular System

Corticosteroids have two major effects on the cardiovascular system. Mineralocorticoids and, to a lesser extent, GLCs affect the maintenance of extracellular fluid volume, as described previously. Interestingly, mineralocorticoids also appear to have direct actions on cardiovascular tissues; increased cardiac fibrosis has been induced experimentally in rats by administration of excessive mineralocorticoids, suggesting an indication for spironolactone as a diuretic in congestive heart failure associated with myocardial disease.[9] In addition, corticosteroids (predominantly GLCs) enhance vascular reactivity to other vasoactive substances (e.g., norepinephrine, angiotensin II).[9] Mechanisms appear to include increased receptor numbers in the vascular wall or other tissues. Other proposed mechanisms of GLC-induced hypertension include reduced activity of depressor systems (e.g., kallikrein-kinin, prostaglandins, and nitric oxide) and increased responsiveness to angiotensin II and norepinephrine.[38] In humans, Cushing's syndrome or prolonged administration of synthetic GLCs is associated with hypertension characterized by sodium chloride retention and volume expansion. However, hypertension may be independent of these effects; rather, downregulation of nitric oxide synthetase may be a more plausible explanation.[39] In contrast, in patients with insufficient concentrations of GLCs, negative sequelae include increased capillary permeability, decreased cardiac output, and inadequate vasomotor response of the smaller blood vessels to catecholamines. In humans, glucocorticoids are associated with worsening of cardiovascular disease. Hypertension appears to reflect increased glucocorticoid-mediated peripheral vascular resistance rather than aldosterone-mediated rather than sodium retention. The latter mechanism, along with myocardial remodeling, has been associated with worsening congestive heart failure.[39b]

Bone and Cartilage

GLCs antagonize the effects of vitamin D_3, accelerate bone resorption, and decrease bone formation (through direct action on osteoblasts), resulting in osteoporosis. This phenomenon is well documented in human patients after chronic GLC therapy, but to the authors' knowledge it has not been observed in animals.[40] At physiologic doses, glucocorticoids stimulate collagen. At supraphysiologic doses GLCs inhibit collagen synthesis by fibroblasts; depress chondrocyte metabolism; and decrease the proteoglycan content of cartilage, resulting in morphologic changes in articular cartilage.[41,42]

Skeletal Muscle

The permissive effects of GLCs include their influence on the ability of skeletal muscle to function normally. Too little will result in muscle wasting (generally resulting from hypokalemia). Likewise, and paradoxically, too much also will result in muscle wasting. Increased use of amino acids from muscle proteins is likely to contribute to this effect. Although the exact mechanisms of muscle wasting are unknown, the term *steroid myopathy* has been coined to reflect this condition in human patients and is used to refer to similar manifestations in small animals with hyperadrenocorticism.[9]

Central Nervous System

In the central nervous system (CNS), the highest concentration of MRs is in the limbic system, whereas GRs are more ubiquitous in the brain.[6] Indirectly, GLCs maintain adequate plasma concentrations of glucose for cerebral functions, maintain cerebral blood flow, and influence electrolyte balance in the CNS. GLCs decrease formation of cerebrospinal fluid, which results in a reduction of intracranial pressure. In human beings GLCs are believed to influence mood (e.g., producing euphoria), behavior, and brain excitability.[9] The euphoric effect commonly recognized in dogs also is likely to reflect differences in GRs. Steroids, including GLCs, also appear to regulate neuronal excitation, with differential effects occurring for some drugs. For example, dexamethasone inhibits microglial cell proliferation; cortisone also will inhibit proliferation at higher doses through GRs, but stimulate proliferation through MRs.[26] GLCs appear to have a protective effect in the CNS through induction of glutamine synthetase in both the CNS and peripheral nervous system; the enzyme adds an amine to and thus removes glutamate.[43] Increased glutamate has been associated with CNS pathology, although the relationship between the two remains controversial.[44,45] However, efficacy reflects regulation through transcription, which takes at least 24 hours. Glutamine has several roles in the CNS; in the presence of hyperammonia (e.g., liver disease) increases formation of glutamine in brain cells and the potenetial for cerebral edema.[45b] The use of glucocorticoids for treatment of cerebral edema might be avoided in situations in which increased glutamine increases the risk of cerebral edema.

Interestingly, GLC concentrations appear to be directly related to the severity of memory impairment in animals, including humans.[6] Learning is impaired in animals exposed to prolonged reductions in circulating concentrations of GLCs; conversely, memory also appears to be impaired if GLC concentrations are too high.

Respiratory System

GLCs are reported to have "permissive" effects (increased receptor number or affinity have been proposed) on β_2-receptors, promoting bronchodilation.[46] Other mechanisms are likely to evolve as non-genomic effects are understood. The effects of GLCs on leukotrienes, platelet-activating factor, and other mediators important in the pathogenesis of respiratory inflammatory diseases were discussed earlier and also are addressed in Chapters 20 and 29.

Alimentary Tract

GLCs decrease the absorption of calcium and iron from the gastrointestinal tract and increase the absorption of fats. Secretion of gastric acid, pepsin, and trypsin are increased by GLCs. Gastric mucosal cell growth and renewal are reduced by GLCs, and mucus production is decreased, resulting in compromise of the protective barrier of the gastric mucosa. Collectively, these effects contribute to increased susceptibility to gastric ulceration. A retrospective study in humans found that 5% developed gastric mucosal lesions while receiving GLCs, particularly patients with rheumatoid arthritis and collagenosis.[47] It is not clear whether the effects of GLCs on the gastric mucosa occur as a result of impaired mucosal prostaglandin synthesis, although failure of misoprostol (prostaglandin E) to protect against GLC-induced ulceration indicates that they do not. Indeed, some studies have shown that GLCs provide a gastroprotective effect during stress-induced ulceration.[48] Deposition of glycogen in the liver, resulting in hepatomegaly in animals chronically treated with GLCs, is a consequence of increased glycogen synthesis, as described previously. Excessive cortisol levels can induce pancreatic ductule hyperplasia.

Reproduction

GLCs can induce parturition during the latter stages of pregnancy in ruminants and horses, but their effect in dogs and cats has not been determined. GLC administration in pregnant dogs has been associated with cleft palate and abortion.

GLCs have been shown to inhibit cell division, DNA synthesis, or both in the developing liver, lung, brain, and thymocytes.

STRUCTURE–ACTIVITY RELATIONSHIP

There are close to 50 generic corticosteroid products approved for human use and several approved for use in small animals. These drugs differ primarily in their duration of action, mineralocorticoid activity, and antiinflammatory potency (Table 30-2). As the antiinflammatory potency of a particular agent increases, its biological half-life and duration of action also tend to increase. Antiinflammatory properties also parallel the effects on metabolism, that is, carbohydrate and protein metabolism, but mineralocorticoid effects can be altered independently by changing the molecular structure of the steroid (Figure 30-5). The 4,5 double bond and the 3-ketone are necessary for mineralocorticoid and GLC effects. Synthetic modifications of cortisol increase the antiinflammatory activity, decrease protein binding, and decrease hepatic metabolism, thus prolonging activity. First-generation GLCs formed with the addition of a 1,2 double bond increased the ratio of GLC to mineralocorticoid effects (prednisolone, prednisone, and methylprednisone) and duration of action. The second-generation steroids were fluorinated at the C-9 position, increasing potency. Methylation at the C-16 position eliminates mineralocorticoid activity (dexamethasone, betamethasone, and triamcinolone).

KEY POINT 30-8 In general, as exogenous glucocorticoid effects become more potent, mineralocorticoid effects become less potent.

The effects of GLCs are generally recognized to be dose dependent. Indeed, GLCs can be classified on the basis of their potency, generally relative to hydrocortisone. For example, dexamethasone is 30 times and prednisolone 4 times as potent as hydrocortisone in impairing glucose metabolism (Table 30-2).[20] Daily doses of glucocorticoids used therapeutically have been variably referred to as physiologic, which generally reflects 0.1 to 0.25 mg/kg predniosolone or equivalent, and a pharmacologic or supraphysiologic, ranging, for prednisolone, 0.8 mg/kg IV, to 1 to 2 mg/kg/day, and a high dose of approximately 10 mg/kg orally (or 4 to 60 mg/m^2/day). Some references refer to very high supraphysiologic doses (in dogs: hydrocortisone at 2-4 mg/kg, IV every 6 to 8 hrs, 4 to 20 mg/kg prednisolone IV every 2 to 6 hrs, 0.5 to 2.0 mg/kg dexamethasone, or 30 to 100 mg/kg methylprednisolone), which also might be referred to as a "shock" dose.

CLINICAL PHARMACOLOGY

Absorption

Several products are well absorbed orally. Differences between oral absorption occur, for example between prednisone and prednisolone in both the dog and cat (see below). For intramuscular or subcutaneous administration, the duration and onset of action of a particular GLC can be altered by the addition of an ester, usually bound to C-21. The GLC esters must be hydrolyzed – often by esterases located at the site of administration - to release the active, free form of the drug. However, the sodium phosphate and sodium succinate esters are water soluble, can be administered intravenously, and are rapidly hydrolyzed. These characteristics make them ideal for treatment of acute conditions. The acetate, acetonide, valerate, and dipropionate esters are water insoluble and release of the active steroid is very slow, providing GLC activity for days to weeks (i.e., repositol, or depot, products). The major advantage of these esters is convenience of administration. Administration at 2- to 6-week intervals, depending on the preparation used and disease being treated, has been recommended.

Table 30-2 Comparison of Glucocorticoid Free Bases

Glucocorticoids	Glucocorticoid Potency*	Mineralocorticoid Effect	Equivalent Dose	Duration of Effect on HPA
Cortisol	1	1	20	12 (S)
Cortisone	0.8	0.8	25	12 (S)
Hydrocortisone	1	0.8	20	12 (S)
Prednisone–Prednisolone	3.5–4	0.8	6	12–36 (I)
Methylprednisolone	5	0.5	4	12–36 (I)
Triamcinolone	5	0	4	12–36 (I)
Betamethasone	25	0	0.8	>48 (L)
Dexamethasone	30	0	0.7	>48 (L)
Mineralocorticoids		**Mineralocorticoid Potency**		
Fludrocortisone	10	125–200		12–36 (I)
Deoxycorticosterone	0	20		
Aldosterone	0	200–1000		

HPA, Hypothalamic–pituitary–adrenal axis, *I* = intermediate, *L* = long acting, *S* = short
*Both glucocorticoid and antiinflammatory potency.

Disadvantages include unpredictability of blood concentrations, chronic suppression of the hypothalamic–pituitary–adrenal axis (up to 12 weeks or more after administration of a single dose), possible induction of steroid resistance (mediated by receptor downregulation), and the fact that the drug cannot be withdrawn should adverse reactions develop. For these reasons the authors recommend the use of short- to intermediate-acting preparations administered daily or on alternate days over repositol steroid preparations.

KEY POINT 30-9 The slow-release salts of glucocorticoids preclude advantages of alternate-day dosing that occur with administration of short- or intermediate-acting base drugs.

There are many forms of GLCs available for topical use, including extensions of the skin such as the external ear canal and anal sacs. Once absorbed through the skin, topical corticosteroids are handled by the body in the same capacity as systemically administered GLCs. The extent of percutaneous absorption of topical GLCs depends on factors such as the vehicle, the ester form of the steroid (greater lipid solubility enhances percutaneous absorption), duration of exposure, surface area, and the integrity of the epidermal barrier. Ointment bases are occlusive and are therefore more likely to increase percutaneous absorption of the same GLC in a cream base. Highly potent preparations in any form should not be used on abraded skin.

GLCs are absorbed and can achieve physiologic and possibly pharmacologic concentrations after local administration. This includes the skin, as previously noted, synovial spaces, conjunctival sac, and the respiratory tract.[9] Suppression of the hypothalamic–pituitary–adrenal axis has been documented after ocular,[50] otic,[51] and topical[52] administration for several weeks. The impact of dexamethasone and betamethasone administered as a topical commercial otic preparation on

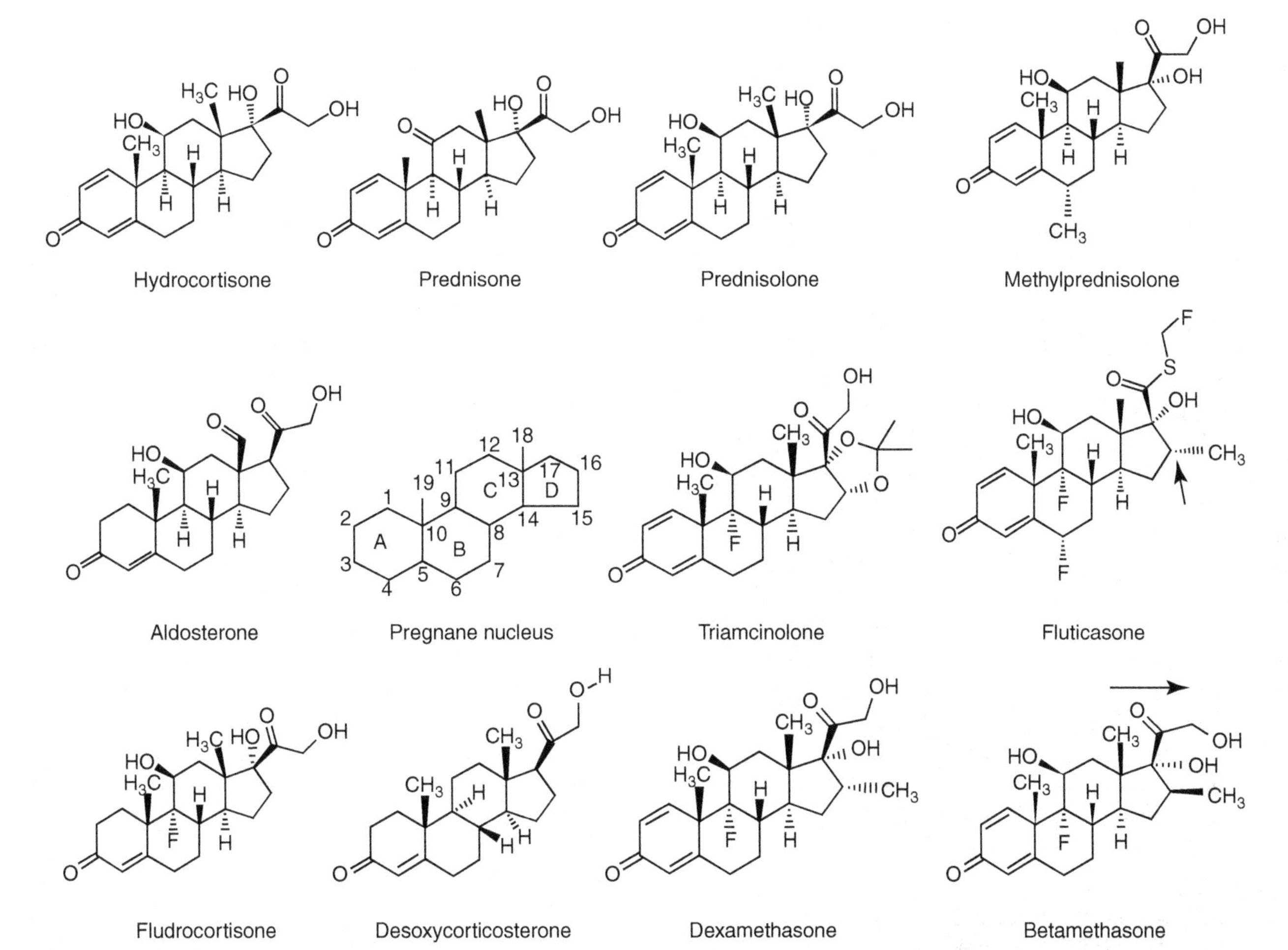

Figure 30-5 Chemical structures of selected adrenocorticosteroids. The pregnane nucleus provides the skeletal structure of corticosteroids. Corticosteroid activity depends on the double bond at position 4,5 and the keto group in the 3 position. Compounds with a double bond at position 1,2 have increased glucocorticoid activity (e.g., prednisone versus hydrocortisone) as well as a longer duration of action. Prednisolone differs from the prodrug prednisone only by the presence of a hydroxyl rather than a ketone group on the C ring. A methyl group at the C-16 position *(arrow)* eradicates mineralocorticoid activity (e.g., dexamethasone). Fluorination at the C-9 position enhances corticosteroid potency. The difference between betamethasone and dexamethasone is the orientation of the methyl group at position 16. The addition of acetate rather than succinate esters *(not shown)* to the various compounds also prolongs duration of action.

adrenal function was studied in normal dogs (with normal ears). Drugs were administered twice daily for 2 weeks according to the package insert: dexamethasone at 10 drops (0.223 mg) and betamethasone at 4 drops (0.1193) per ear. For the betamethasone-treated group (n = 7), ACTH response tests were normal at the end of the treatment period, which was in contrast to the dexamethasone-treated group, for which the adrenal gland was suppressed in 71% (five of seven) of animals. Response normalized in 1 to 2 weeks for all animals. No animal exhibited signs of hyperadrenocorticism.[53] Ginel and coworkers[54] prospectively examined the effect of 2 weeks of topical betamethasone administration (4 to 8 drops, depending on body weight, of 0.88 mg betamethasone/mL, Otomax) compared with placebo using a randomized crossover design with a 4-week washout period. Although adrenal gland suppression did not occur, serum alkaline phosphatase increased (but remained within normal limits) and response to intradermal testing was muted by day 14 of treatment.

Using a prospective parallel approach, Aniya and Griffin[55] recently compared the effect of vehicle and concentration of dexamethasone applied topically in the normal (not inflamed) ear of dogs (n = 21). Dexamethasone was applied as either 0.01% or 0.1% in saline (n = 7 each) and 0.1% in the commercially available product (Tresaderm; n = 7), for which propylene glycol is the carrier. Animals were treated for 2 weeks with 10 drops in each ear twice daily, resulting in a dose of approximately 0.89 mg dexamethasone for the 0.1% product (0.07 to 0.25 mg/kg). On the basis of ACTH stimulation, four of seven dogs in each 0.1% treatment group, but no dogs in the 0.01% treatment group, experienced adrenal gland suppression. Further, serum alkaline phosphatase was increased in one of seven dogs in the 0.1% propylene glycol treatment group. Finally, Reeder and coworkers[56] compared four GLC-containing otic preparations in dogs with otitis externa using a randomized, double-blinded parallel design. Drugs studied included 0.007 to 0.02 mg/kg once daily of mometasone (Mometamax; n = 9), 0.002 to 0.03 mg/kg twice daily of triamcinolone (Panalog; n = 12), 0.004 to 0.024 mg/kg twice daily of dexamethasone (Tresaderm; n = 8), and 0.006 to 0.03 mg/kg twice daily of betamethasone (DVMax; n = 11). Dogs were treated for 7 days. Mometasone was described to have 1.5 times the potency of fluticasone and 22 times that of dexamethasone.[56] Plasma cortisol was suppressed at 7 days in 0%, 9%, 17%, and 50% of the animals receiving Mometamax, betamethasone, triamcinolone, and dexamethasone, respectively.

KEY POINT 30-10 With few exceptions, it should be assumed that topical administration of glucocorticoids will result in drug absorption sufficient to affect the hypothalamic–pituitary–adrenal axis.

Selected steroids have been studied after transdermal administration in cats. Using a randomized crossover design, Willis-Goulet and coworkers[57] measured dexamethasone in the serum of cats (n = 6) after single-dose oral or transdermal administration of 0.05 mg/kg. Although drug was detected after oral administration (peak 30 μg/mL), drug was not detected after transdermal administration. A similar finding was reported by other investigators.[59] Oral absorption of GLCs may be affected by P-glycoprotein, depending on the specific drug.[58] Cortisol, aldosterone, and dexamethasone are demonstrated substrates. Even in dogs, oral absorption of prednisone may not result in prednisolone concentrations comparable to that achieved with oral prednisolone.

Distribution, Metabolism, and Excretion

In humans (and presumably many animals), endogenous (and exogenous) cortisol is bound to corticosteroid-binding globulin (transcortin). The two main binding proteins are cortisol-binding globulin and albumin.[2]

Transcortin is an α-globulin secreted by the liver. Whereas it has a high affinity for steroids, it has a relatively low binding capacity. Albumin, which has a low affinity but large binding capacity, also binds GLCs. Corticosteroids compete with one another (endogenous and exogenous) for binding sites and at high concentrations will displace one another. Steroidal hormones tend to be eliminated by oxidation or reduction followed by conjugation (generally glucuronide or sulfate) and excretion (principally renal). Metabolism occurs at both hepatic and extrahepatic (including the kidney) sites. Prednisone is the prodrug form of prednisolone; it is assumed, but not proven, that no barrier exists to formation of the latter Cortisol is metabolized by the liver by phase I and II enzymes. Metabolism to inactive corticosterone is mediated by 11 beta-hydroxysteroid dehydrogenase, particularly in the kidney.[2] Renal expression of this enzyme is one means whereby aldosterone response predominates; elimination of cortisol in human patients with renal disease may be prolonged as much as 30%.[60] Cortisol is metabolized by the liver by phase I and II enzymes and in the kidney, where it is converted to the inactive metabolite cortisone by 11 beta-hydroxysteroid dehydrogenanse.[2]

Biliary and fecal elimination of corticosteroids do not appear to be that significant.[9]

DRUGS AND PREPARATIONS

Knowledge of a few commercial preparations is sufficient for most clinical purposes (Tables 30-3 and 30-4). Selection is most commonly based on balancing the need for efficacy with the risk of adverse effects. Some distinct characteristics of selected steroids are presented in the following sections.

Hydrocortisone

Hydrocortisone is identical to cortisol, the most important endogenous GLC for most species. Extrahepatic elimination of hydrocortisone contributes substantially to clearance in the dog. Elimination is flow limited, with clearance being greatest in organs with greatest blood flow.[61] Elimination of hydrocortisone from the plasma is biphasic in dogs, with an elimination half-life of the terminal phase of 50 minutes. The volume of distribution in dogs is greater than 1 L/kg. Because of its short duration of action (<12 hours) and low potency,

Table **30-3** Preparations

Base	Oral	Intravenous Rapid IM, SC Absorption	Intralesional Slow IM, SC Absorption	Topical	Trade Name Products*
Beclomethasone				Dipropionate, inhalant (1)	(1) Beclovent, Vanceril
Betamethasone	Free base (2)	Na phosphate (31V)	Acetate (32V); Diproprionate (V)	Free base, benzoate, diproprianate (3); Valerate: otic (33V), ointment (34V), Topical Spray (35V)	(2) Celestone; (3) Diprolene; (30V, 31V: Betavet); (32V) Gentocin; (33V): Topagen; (34V) Gentocin, Otomax
Budesonide	Free base (4)		Diacetate	Free base: Inhalant (5), also with formeterol and fumerate (6); Nasal Spray (7)	(4) Entocort, (5) Pulmicort (6), Symbicort (7)Rhinocort
Desoxycorticosterone			Pivalate (35V)		(35V) Percorten
Dexamethasone	Free base (36V)	Na phosphate (37V)	Acetate	Free base: ophthalmic (8), otic (38V)	(8) Maxidex; (36V) Azium, Pet-Der III; (37V) Dex-A-Vet, Dexium SP; (38V) Tresaderm
Fludrocortisone	Acetate (9)				(9) Florinef
Fluticasone				Fumorate: nasal spray (10); fumarate: inhalant (11), also with salmeterol (12) Proprionate spray (13), cream	(10) Veramyst (11) Flovent HFA; (12) Advair, (13) Flonase
Hydrocortisone	Free Base, Acetate (14), cypionate	Na succinate (19)	Acetate	Free base: ointment (with multiple drugs), cream (15), lotion, spray (39V, with oxytetracycline); Acetate: rectal spray (16), Ointment with antibiotics (40V); Valerate: cream (17) Otic suspension; Butyrate: cream (18)	(14) Cortef; (15) Ala-cort, Synacort; (16) Cortifoam; (17) Locoid; (18) Westcort; (19) Solu-Cortef; (39V) Liqua-Cortril; (40V) Neo-Cortef, Amphoderm, Corticosporin
Methylprednisolone	Free base (20), (41V), with aspirin, methylprednisolone (42V)	Na succinate (21)	Acetate (22), (43V)	Acetate	(20) Medrol; (21) Solu-Medrol; (22) Depo-Medrol; (41V) Medrol, (42V) Cortaba; (43V) Depo-Medrol
Prednisolone	Free base; Acetate (23), (44V) and with trimeprazine (45V); sodium phosphate (24)	Sodium phosphate (46V), sodium succinate (47V)	Acetate (48V), tebutate, Sodium phosphate, Acetate	Free base; Acetate: Ophthalmic ointment (25) and with sulfacetamide (26); with antibiotics (49V) and ophthalmic solution (50V); Sodium phosphate: ophthalmic; Sodium succinate	(23) Flo-Pred; (24) Orapred; (25) Pred Mild, Pred Forte; with sulfacetamide (26); (44V) Delta Albaplex, PredniSTab; (45V)Temaril P; (46V) Prednis-A-Vet;(47V) Solu-Delta-Cortef; (48V) Meticortelone; (49V) Optisone, Chlorasone; (50V) Neo-Delta-Cortef;
Prednisone	Free base (51V)				(51V) Meticorten

Continued

Table 30-3 Preparations—cont'd

Base	Oral	Intravenous Rapid IM, SC Absorption	Intralesional Slow IM, SC Absorption	Topical	Trade Name Products*
Triamcinolone	Free base; acetonide (52V), diacetate		Acetonide (27) and (V), intraarticular or intravitreal (28), diacetate, hexacetonide	Free base; acetonide: ointment (53V), dental paste (29), nasal spray (30), cream (54V)	(27) Kenalog; (28) Trivaris; (29)Ora-cort, (30) Nasacort); (52V) Vetalog Tab; (53V) Panalog Ointment; (54V) Vetalog Cream

IM, Intramuscular; *SC*, subcutaneous; *V*, veterinary product.
*Example products. Other trade name products may be available, and many preparations are available as uncited generic preparations. Numbers refer to different preparation; *V* indicates the preparation is a veterinary-approved preparation.

Table 30-4 Dose

Drug	Indication	Dose	Route	Interval (hr)
Beclomethasone dipropionate (1)	Antiinflammatory	200 mg/cat	MDI	As needed
Betamethasone (3)	Pannus, episcleritis	1-2 mg/dog	Topical (subconjunctivally)	Decreasing dose (4)
		0.15 mg/kg (D)	IM	Once
		0.1-0.2 mg/kg	PO	12-24
Budesonide (1, 3)	Inflammatory bowel disease	1 mg/small dog or cat	PO	24
		2 mg/large dog	PO	24
Cortisone acetate (5)	Hypoadrenocorticism	1 mg/kg	IM, PO	24
Dexamethasone (3,6)	Adrenocortical collapse	0.1-0.5 mg/kg	IV, SC	
	Asthma	Initial dose: 1 mg/kg	IV	Once
		Maintenance dose: 0.25-1 mg/cat	PO	8-24
	Cerebral edema, spinal cord	Initial dose: 2-3 mg/kg	IV	Once
		Maintenance dose: 0.1 mg/kg	IV	8-12
	Hydrocephalus	0.25 mg/kg	IM, IV, PO	6-8
	Immune thrombocytopenia	Initial dose: 0.25-0.3 mg/kg (D)	IV, SC	Once
		Maintenance dose: 0.25-1.25 mg/kg	PO	12-24
		0.10-0.15 mg/kg	PO, SC	12 × 5-7 days, then taper dose
	Shock, anaphylaxis	4-6 mg/kg	IV (slowly)	Once
	Trauma, fibrocartilaginous disk, other CNS trauma	Loading dose: 1-2.2mg/kg	IV, SC	Once
		Maintenance dose: 0.1 mg/kg	IV, PO, SC	8-12
Dexamethasone $NaPO_4$ (7)	Shock	4-6 mg/kg	IV	Once
Flumethasone	Antiinflammatory	0.06-0.25 mg/kg	PO, SC, IM, IV	24
Fluticasone propionate (1)	Asthma	222 μg (1 puff)	MDI	12-24 or to effect
Hydrocortisone (8)	Replacement therapy	0.5-1 mg/kg	PO	24
	Antiinflammatory	2.5-5 mg/kg	PO	12
Hydrocortisone acetate	Hypoadrenocorticism	0.1-0.2 mg/kg	IM	8-12
	Immune-mediated hemolytic anemia	2-4 mg/kg	IM	12-24
Hydrocortisone sodium succinate	Antiinflammatory	5-8 mg/kg	IV	12-24
	Shock	50-150 mg/kg	IV	8 × 2 treatments
	Hypoadrenocortical crisis	5-20 mg/kg (D)	IV	2-6

Table **30-4** Dose—cont'd

Drug	Indication	Dose	Route	Interval (hr)
Methylprednisolone (9)	Antiinflammatory	0.5-2.0 mg/kg	PO	6-12
Methylprednisolone acetate (3)	Antiinflammatory	1 mg/kg	IM, SC	14 days
		1-5.5 mg/kg (C)	IM, SC	7 days-6 months
	Eosinophilic, linear granulomas	10-40 mg/cat	IM, SC, intralesional	2 weeks × 2-6 treatments
	Pannus, episcleritis	4-12 mg/dog	Subconjunctival	Once, then follow with topical therapy
Methylprednisolone sodium succinate (10)	Spinal trauma	Loading dose: 30 mg/kg (D)	IV	Once
		Followed by: 5.4 mg/kg	IV CRI	24-48 (see Appendix H)
		Or followed by: 15 mg/kg	IV, SC	Once in 2, then every 6 × 2 days. Taper dose over 5-7 days
	Shock	30-35 mg/kg (D)	IV	Once
Prednisolone/Prednisone (9,11)	Physiologic dose	0.25 mg/kg	PO	24
	Adrenal gland removal (replacement therapy)	102 mg/kg	IV	At induction
	Allergic bronchitis and rhinitis, asthma	0.5-2 mg/kg (D)	IM, PO	12
	Allergy	0.5-1 mg/kg (C)	IM, PO	12
	Angioedema, urticaria	2 mg/kg (D)	IM, PO	12
	Antiinflammatory	0.5-1 mg/kg (D)	IM, IV, PO	12-24, then taper to every 2 days
		2.2 mg/kg (C)	IM, IV, PO	12-24, then taper to every 2 days
	Blepharitis, episcleritis, uveitis	0.5-2 mg/kg	PO	12
	Brain tumors	0.5-1 mg/kg	PO	24-48
	Canine atopy, contact allergy, flea allergy, acanthosis nigricans	0.5 mg/kg (D)	PO	12 × 5-10 days, then taper
	Cerebral edema from brain tumors	0.5-1 mg/kg (D)	PO	24-48
	Chronic bronchitis	0.1-0.5 mg/kg (D)	PO	12
	Chronic therapy	2-4 mg/kg	PO	48
	Eosinophilic ulcers, plasma cell gingivitis	1-2.2 mg/kg (D)	PO	24 × 7 days, then taper to every 48
		1-2 mg/kg (C)	PO	24
		0.5-1.5 mg/kg	PO	12-24, then taper over 3 months
	Eosinophillic gastritis, enteritis colitis	1-3 mg/kg (D)	PO	24, then taper to every 48
	Feline infectious peritonitis	4 mg/kg	PO	24 (with cyclophosphamide)
	Food allergy, parasite hypersensitivity	0.5 mg/kg (D)	PO	12 to 24
	Heartworm disease, including hemoptysis, coughing, or pneumonitis	0.5-1 mg/kg	PO	12, taper over 14 days; prednisolone may increase heartworm resistance to treatment

Continued

Table 30-4 Dose—cont'd

Drug	Indication	Dose	Route	Interval (hr)
	Hydrocephalus, acquired tremors	0.5 mg/kg (D)	PO	48
Prednisolone/ Prednisone (9, 11)	Hypercalcemia	1-2.5 mg/kg (D)	PO	12
	Hyperinsulinism	0.25 mg/kg	PO	12
	Hypoadrenocorticism	0.2-0.4 mg/kg (D)	PO	24-48
	Hypoadrenocorticism	1 mg/kg (C)	IM, PO	12
	Hypoglycemia	0.25-3 mg/kg	PO	12
	Idiopathic or immune-mediated meningitis, reticulosis, granulomatous meningoencephalitis	1-2 mg/kg (D)	PO	12-24
	Immune-mediated hemolytic anemia	0.5-2 mg/kg (D)	PO	12
	Immune polymyositis, masticatory myositis	2 mg/kg	IM, PO	24
	Immune skin diseases	1.1-2.2 mg/kg	PO	12
	Immune thrombocytopenia	0.5-1.5 mg/kg (D)	PO	12
	Immune-mediated orchitis	1-2 mg/kg (D)	PO	24
	Immunosuppression	2 mg/kg (D)	IM, PO	12
		3 mg/kg (C)	IM, PO	12
		2-5 mg/kg	IM, PO, SC	12 to 24
		Initial dose: 2.2-6.6 mg/kg (C)	IM, IV, PO	24
		Then taper to 2-4 mg/kg (C)	IM, IV, PO	48
	Intervertebral disk disease, spondylopathy, cauda equina syndrome	Initial dose: 0.5 mg/kg (D)	PO	12 × 3 days
		Followed by 0.5 mg/kg (D)	PO	24 × 3-5 days
	Juvenile cellulitis	2.2 mg/kg (D)	PO	24
	Lymphocytic cholangitis, chronic active hepatitis, copper hepatopathy	0.25-2 mg/kg (D)	PO	12
	Lymphomas	Initial dose: 40 mg/m^2 (D)	PO	24 × 1 week
		Followed by 20 mg/m^2 (D)	PO	48
	Lymphosarcoma, myeloproliferative disorders, eosinophillic leukemia	1 mg/kg	PO	24, then every 48 as part of a protocol
		30-40 mg/m^2	PO	24, then every 48
	Mast cell tumors, mastocytosis	30-40 mg/m^2 (D)	PO	24 × 4 weeks, then every other 48
		40 mg/m^2 (C)	PO	24 × 4 weeks, then every other 48
	Multiple myeloma, macroglobulinemia	0.5 mg/kg (D)	PO	24 as part of a protocol
	Myasthenia gravis	0.5 mg/kg (D)	PO	12 initially; slowly increase to every 24 until remission, then every 48
		2 mg/kg (D)	PO	12-24
	Panosteitis, hypertrophic osteopathy	0.5 mg/kg (D)	PO	12-24
	Plasmacytic–lymphocytic enteritis	1-2 mg/kg	PO	12, then taper dose weekly
	Pulmonary eosinophilic infiltrates	0.5-1 mg/kg	PO	24

Table **30-4** Dose

Drug	Indication	Dose	Route	Interval (hr)
Prednisone/ Prednisone (9, 11)	Replacement therapy (hypoadrenocorticism) acute	Initial dose: 4-20 mg/kg	IV (over 2-4 min)	Once
	Replacement therapy (hypoadrenocorticism) acute	Followed by 0.2-0.4 mg/kg	PO	24
	Shock	15-30 mg/kg (D)	IV	Repeat in 1, 3, 6, or 10
	Sterile pyogranulomas	2-4 mg/kg (D)	PO	24
	Systemic lupus erythematosus	1.5-2 mg/kg	PO	12-24, then taper to <1 mg/kg every 48
	Urethritis, persistent hematuria	2.5-5 mg/cat	PO	24-48
Prednisolone acetate	Hypoadrenocorticism	0.1-0.2 mg/kg	IM	12
Prednisolone sodium phosphate (12)	Shock	11 mg/kg	IV	Repeat in 4-6
Prednisolone sodium succinate (13)	Chronic allergic diseases (asthma, atopy, IBD)	2-4 mg/kg (D)	IV, IM	Repeat in 4-6
		1-3 mg/kg (C)	IV, IM	Repeat in 4-6
	CNS trauma	Initial dose: 15-30 mg/kg	IV	Once
		Maintenance dose: 1-2 mg/kg	IV	12
	Hypoglycemia	1-2 mg/kg	IV	Repeat in 4-6
	Shock	11-30 mg/kg (D)	IV	Repeat in 4-6
Triamcinolone (3)	Antiinflammatory	0.25-2 mg (D)	PO	24
		0.25-0.5 mg/cat	PO	24 × 7 days
		0.11-0.22 mg/kg	IM, PO, SC	24-48
	Esophogeal dilation to prevent restricture	1-2 mg	In the esophageal submucosa	Infiltrate at 4 circumferential points
	Feline plasmacytic pharyngitis, pododermatitis	2-4 mg/cat	PO	24-48
	Feline polymyopathy	0.5-1 mg/kg	PO	24
Triamcinolone acetonide (3)	Glucocorticoid effects	0.1-0.2 mg/kg	IM, SC	24
	Anticancer	1.2-1.8 mg or 1 mg for every diameter of tumor	Intralesional	Every 2 weeks
Triamcinolone ophthalmic solution	Pannus, eosinophilic keratitism, episcleritis	4-8 mg ophthalmic solution (D)	Subconjunctivally	Once; follow with topical therapy
		4 mg ophthalmic solution (C)	Subconjunctivally	Once; follow with topical therapy

MDI, Metered dose inhalant; *D,* dog; *IM,* intramuscular; *PO,* by mouth; *IV,* intravenous; *CNS,* central nervous system; *SC,* subcutaneous; *C,* cat; *CRI,* constant-rate infusion; *IBD,* inflammatory bowel disease.

1 Potency facilitates topical efficacy.
2 Decreasing dose: every 5 × 5 days, every 6 × 4 days, every 8 × 3 days, every 12 × 2 days, then every 24 × 1 day.
3 Long-acting and thus not indicated for alternate-day use.
4 Increased risk of gastrointestinal toxicity may occur with oral use.
5 Rapid onset, short-acting, low potency; activity requires conversion to hydrocortisone.
6 Propylene glycol vehicle of intravenous solution may cause cardiac arrhythmias and sudden death with rapid administration.
7 Rapid onset reflects enhanced cell penetration.
8 Low potency not recommended for alternate-day use.
9 Acceptable for alternate-day use.
10 Choice for CNS damage.
11 Glucocorticoids generally are dosed to remission, then tapered to a minimum effective dose for maintenance. Doses should be tapered as drugs are discontinued. Prednisolone is generally preferred to prednisone in cats.
12 Efficacy in shock requires early and aggressive intervention.
13 50 mg/mL solution for IM injection is irritating.

hydrocortisone is not frequently used for systemic therapy. Hydrocortisone is available in creams and ointments for topical use.

Prednisolone and Prednisone

Prednisone is rapidly metabolized by the liver to prednisolone (C-11 ketol reduction). Liver disease probably has minimal effect on activation. Prednisone elimination in dogs is biphasic, with apparent half-lives of 15 and 82 minutes for each phase after intravenous administration.[62] However, prednisolone has an intermediate duration of action (12 to 36 hours) and is therefore considered appropriate for alternate-day administration.

Prednisone and prednisolone generally are considered equivalent in terms of therapeutic dosing in both dogs and cats. However, the two are not necessarily equivalent, as has been demonstrated in dogs and cats. Colburn and coworkers[63] demonstrated in Beagles (n = 16) that relative bioavailability is greater for prednisolone. After 5 mg orally of either drug, the C_{max} was twice as high and the area under the curve 40% higher for prednisolone compared with prednisone. All dogs received either 5 mg prednisolone or prednisone orally using a randomized crossover design. Both steroids were measured with each study. The pertinent pharmacokinetic parameters differed between the two drugs and were as follows: AUC (area under the curve; ng*mL/hr), C_{max}, (ng/mL), T_{max} (hour), and elimination half-life (hour). After administration of 5 mg prednisolone, the data for prednisolone was 986, 273, 0.9, and 1.8; and for prednisone, 855, 205, 1.3, and 1.6. After oral administration of 5 mg prednisone, the numbers were for prednisolone: 638, 111, 2, and 2.2; and for prednisone: 694, 132, 1.2, and 2.3. These data suggest rapid interconversion between both steroids, regardless of which is administered, in the dog but also about a 65% relative bioavailability for prednisolone (or prednisone) when prednisone is administered compared to prednisolone. Prednisolone also has been studied after IV administration but only in a single Beagle.[63a] The dog was dosed at 1.8 and 3.6 mg/kg. Clearance was 34 ml*kg/min and volume of distribution was 0.7 L/kg. Elimination half-live was 0.3 hour. The oral bioavailability of prednisolone solution or tablet approximated 50% but this was increased to essentially 100% when administered as a slurry. This study, although in one dog, supports a dose-dependent disposition of prednisolone.

That the two are not equivalent in cats was demonstrated by Graham-Mize and Rosser.[59] Disposition of prednisolone in cats after oral administration was as follows: area under the curve 3230.55 ng/mL/hr and C_{max} 1400.81 ng/mL, with a half-life for excretion of 1 hour. This compares to an area under the curve of 672.63 ng/mL/hr and C_{max} of 122.18 ng/mL after oral administration of prednisone. The half-life of prednisone was longer at 2.46 hours. According to these data, the dose of prednisone must be at threefold to fivefold higher than that of prednisolone to achieve equivalent activity. Boothe has studied the efficacy of drug delivery of prednisone and prednisolone after multiple (3 weeks) transdermal administration. Cats were studied using a random crossover design. Cats received prednisone and prednisolone (2 mg/kg) either orally or transdermally twice daily. At the end of each 3-week dosing period, and a 1-week washout, cats were rotated to the next randomly assigned treatment. Two-hour peak and 12-hour trough serum samples were assayed for the presence of prednisone and prednisolone. After 3 weeks of dosing (n = 6), neither prednisone nor prednisolone concentrations were detectable after oral or gel administration of prednisone. Prednisolone was not detectable after gel administration of prednisolone, but prednisolone reached therapeutic concentrations after oral administration of prednisolone. The use of prednisolone rather than prednisone might be more prudent for both species. Liver disease does not appear to impact conversion of prednisone to prednisolone as was demonstrated in human patients with chronic active liver disease (n = 10) compared to healthy volunteers (n = 7).[63b]

Methylprednisolone

Methylprednisolone possesses lipid antioxidant activity that has been shown to be beneficial in the treatment of experimental spinal cord trauma in cats and experimentally induced *Escherichia coli* bacteremia.[65,66] In contrast, methylprednisolone did not appear clinically beneficial in a canine model of spinal trauma, although the model may have caused insufficient damage for effective evaluation.[67] Although some other GLCs (dexamethasone, prednisolone) are efficacious as lipid antioxidants, methylprednisolone is the most potent. Methylprednisolone has an intermediate duration of action (12 to 36 hours) and is also a good candidate for alternate-day administration. The disposition of methylprednisolone succinate was described in normal dogs and then again after induction of hemorrhagic shock (n = 5).[68] The drug is characterized by a clearance of 1.6 ± 0.5 L*kg/hr and half-life 15.3 ± 3.8 minutes. During states of hemorrhagic shock, the clearance is reduced to 0.5 ± 0.2 L*kg/hr and half-life was prolonged to 41 ± 23 minutes.

Dexamethasone

Dexamethasone is a highly potent GLC, but it has virtually no mineralocorticoid activity. It possesses some lipid antioxidant activity. The disposition of dexamethasone in dogs exhibits dose dependency. Greco and coworkers[69] studied the disposition of dexamethasone after a low (0.01 mg/kg) and high (0.1 mg/kg) dose using a randomized crossover disease. The relevant pharmacokinetic parameters at each dose were A and B, (the Y intercept extrapolated from the initial and terminal components of the plasma drug concentration versus time curve, respectively; ng/mL), elimination half-life (hour), mean residence time (hour), and volume of distribution (L/kg). At 0.01 mg/kg, the data were: 22 ± 13.5, 5.3 ± 4.11, 192, 174 ± 42, and 1.9 ± 1.2. At 0.1 mg/kg, the data were 118 ± 74, 9.0 ± 5.7, 412, 324, and 6.41 ± 2. In addition to dose-dependent differences in clearance, the authors suggested that saturation of plasma protein-binding sites at the higher dose might explain the marked increase in volume of distribution. Elimination half-life is longer at a higher (0.1 mg/kg) compared with lower (0.01 mg/kg) dose, despite an increase in clearance; the differences presumably reflects the increase in the volume of distribution of dexamethasone at the higher dose.[69] The disposition of dexamethasone did not differ in the presence of simultaneous administration of ACTH (0.5 U/kg intravenously), although the power of the study was not addressed. The prolonged duration of action (biological half-life approximately 48 hours) of dexamethasone makes it inappropriate for alternate-day administration.

Betamethasone

Betamethasone is a very potent GLC that varies from dexamethasone only in the orientation of a side chain. Thus, like dexamethasone, it has virtually no mineralocorticoid activity. It has a long duration of action (biological half-life approximately 48 hours) and is therefore not appropriate for alternate-day administration.

"Soft" Glucocorticoids

Among the mechanisms whereby undesirable side effects of GLCs can be minimized is topical administration of drugs that are potent for GRs but also rapidly metabolized should the drug be absorbed into systemic circulation via the oral route. These efforts generally reflect manipulation of chemical groups on the D ring of the GLC. Examples include beclomethasone, budesonide, and fluticasone propionate, steroids designed specifically for use in inhalant metered doses. Their potency when inhaled varies in clinical trials, with fluticasone propionate being most potent and budesonide and beclomethasone dipropionate approximately equipotent. Time of onset in humans to budesonide is approximately 10 hours based on evidence of clinical improvement at that time. Improvement can be expected over the next 1 to 2 days, with maximum effects potentially not being evident until 2 weeks after therapy has begun.

KEY POINT 30-11 The use of topical "soft" glucocorticoids for treatment of asthma or inflammatory bowel disease may reduce side effects in humans but not necessarily in dogs or cats.

Budesonide is rapidly metabolized in the liver by CYP3A4, with affinity of metabolites of the GCR being less than 1% of the parent. Essentially 100% of topically (inhalant) administered drug in humans appears as metabolites in the urine, indicating that systemic absorption of the drug does occur.[70] Indeed, inhaled drug is generally considered to be absorbed, and as much as 25% of the inhaled dose in humans circumvents hepatic metabolism before entering systemic circulation. Because the potency that characterizes enhanced topical activity can similarly lead to peripheral effects, further development has focused on minimizing peripheral effects of topically administered GLCs that avoided hepatic metabolism.[18] Budesonide represented one of the first successful products of those efforts, with local receptor binding of the drug being greater than peripheral binding. Intracellular fatty acid esterification inactivates the drug. As such, esterification serves as a storage site, with esterified drug being rereleased as the concentration of free drug declines with clearance. The ability to esterify varies among tissues, with pulmonary tissue apparently having a much higher capacity compared with other tissues, leading to greater storage in airways than in peripheral tissues.

Topical GLCs combine enhanced efficacy with some reduction in systemic exposure. Because lipophilicity increases transcutaneous movement, GLC esters are the most effective choices in human medicine for treatment of atopic dermatitis and other inflammatory skin diseases. The 17-esters, in particular, are characterized by high activity, presumably because of tighter GR binding (i.e., increased potency). However, greater potency may lead to irreversible skin atrophy. This contrasts with 21-esters, whose lower potency may decrease the risk. Combination 17, 21-double esters such as prednicarbate, a prednisolone double ester, offers the advantages and minimizes the disadvantages of both ester types and therefore is characterized by an improved benefit–risk ratio.[71]

The side effects of GLCs might be reduced but probably will not be eliminated by topical therapy. Drugs that impaired CYP3A4 may increase the plasma drug concentration of budesonide over sevenfold. Even by itself, budesonide appears to suppress the hypothalamic–adrenal–pituitary axis in dogs based on a clinical trial in dogs (n = 6) with inflammatory bowel disease. Endogenous ACTH and baseline and post-ACTH–stimulated cortisol were decreased after treatment with budesonide (30 days at 3 mg/m^2) compared with baseline.[72] Although no differences were described in serum alkaline phosphatase activity, urine specific gravity or the incidence of side effects typical of GLCs (polyphagia, polyuria), the power to detect these indicators of hyperadrenocorticism was not described. Anecdotally, dogs receiving budesonide for prolonged periods to treat inflammatory bowel disease do develop clinical signs associated with iatrogenic hyperadrenocorticism.

Tirilazad Mesylate

Tirilazad mesylate is a novel, non-GLC, 21-aminosteroid (lazaroid) that possesses potent antioxidant activity (i.e., it protects against oxygen-derived free radicals). Unlike the GLCs, this agent does not inhibit phospholipase A_2, but it does inhibit lipid peroxidation-induced arachidonic acid release.[73] The mechanism appears to reflect, in part, insertion into the cell membrane. These products are discussed in depth in Chapter 29.

Fludrocortisone

Fludrocortisone is a synthetic steroid hormone with mineralocorticoid activity. In humans, although it has tenfold activity at the GR compared with cortisone, it has no appreciable GLC effect at standard human doses. Its mineralocorticoid activity is 125-fold greater than cortisol and is used for mineralocorticoid replacement therapy.[9] Fludrocortisone acetate is administered orally at 24- to 48-hour intervals for treatment of hypoadrenocorticism.

Desoxycorticosterone Pivalate

Desoxycorticosterone pivalate (DOCP) is an ester salt of a synthetic steroid hormone with mineralocorticoid (no GLC) activity. This form of desoxycorticosterone has a 20- to 30-day duration of action after intramuscular injection. Addisonian patients who have failed to completely respond to fludrocortisone may respond to therapy with DOCP.

THERAPEUTICS

Unless GLCs are being administered for replacement therapy in a deficiency state (i.e., hypoadrenocorticism), GLC therapy is not directed at the inciting agent. GLC therapy is intended to reduce the physiologic processes that are activated in response to the disease. Despite the adverse events associated with their use, GLCs continue to be heavily used in veterinary medicine, potentially at doses that exceed those recommended. Indeed, in human medicine the use of GLCs clearly exceeds that recommended in textbooks and review papers.[20] The advantages of low versus high doses have been previously discussed and are addressed again in the section on adverse reactions. In general, an antiinflammatory dose is considered to be 10 times the physiologic dose, and immunosuppressive doses are twice the antiinflammatory dose. Shock doses of GLCs have been reported at 5 to 10 times the immunosuppressive dose; however, the disadvantages of this high dose and the advantages of low-dose therapy in shock patients are discussed later. When treating a patient for an immediately life-threatening condition such as immune-mediated hemolytic anemia, the clinician should institute aggressive therapy, with a minimum effective dose determined after response has been achieved. Because high doses of GLCs are often required to adequately treat immune-mediated diseases, adverse effects are likely to occur and should be anticipated. Tapering of doses not only helps prevent side effects associated with long-term therapy but may also prevent the antibody rebound that has been associated with abrupt withdrawal of GLCs in human patients treated for prevention of graft-versus-host transplant rejection. Dose reduction in patients with autoimmune diseases should be conducted gradually. The reduced dose should be continued for at least 2 weeks before the next attempted dose reduction, and the actual dose should be decreased by no more than half. It is essential to assess the patient's status frequently for recurrence of clinical signs. Concurrent administration of additional immunosuppressive (azathioprine, cyclophosphamide) or antiinflammatory drugs other than NSAIDs (antihistamines, omega fatty acids) may allow the GLC dose to be decreased (dose-sparing effect; see Chapters 29 and 31).[74] High-dose pulse therapy has been reported in human patients with acute relapse of chronic graft-versus-host disease. In an open-design study, patients receiving no immunosuppressive therapy or patients that failed (a median of two failures) current therapy (mean prednisolone dose of 0.2 mg/kg per day, range of 0 to 2.5 mg/kg per day) were treated with methylprednisolone at 10 mg/kg intravenously or orally for 4 days. The rationale behind the high dose is based on the lympholytic properties of this dose, thus causing destruction of lymphocytes that otherwise would cause irreversible organ damage. The high dose is assumed to target the (nongenomic) metabolic processes necessary for sustained activity of lymphocytes, as opposed to the low (genomic) doses that target lymphocyte replication. Additionally, the high dose is considered to overcome GR saturation associated with GLC therapy, causing significant GLC downregulation. Induction of T lymphocyte apoptosis may also occur. Standard infection prophylactic therapy also was begun on day 1, consisting of fluconazole, levofloxacin, and valacyclovir (days 1 to 7) and a sulfadiazine–trimethoprim combination (continued until evidence of immunosuppression resolved). On day 5 a new immunosuppressive therapy (which varied with the hospital) was started using standard doses of standard immunosuppressive drugs. With use of this protocol, 75% of patients responded (48% classified as major response, indicating resolution of unequivocal improvement). During a 2-year follow-up, patients tolerated the therapy well, with no major life-threatening effects occurring in the first three months after treatment. However, three patients developed infections after completion of the therapy, suggesting profound immunosuppression. Yet the median time to progression of disease was 2 years after treatment, leading the authors to conclude that high-dose pulse steroid therapy is an effective and well-tolerated treatment for progressive graft-versus-host disease.[24] The author (Boothe) has used this approach in a single case of lymphosarcoma in a dog whose sole treatment was GLC therapy. After the first relapse at 5 weeks, a high dose of dexamethasone (1 mg/kg intravenously) was followed by a second remission, with relapse occurring 3 weeks later. Should this approach be considered as a "rescue" scenario, antimicrobial (and possibly antifungal) treatment might be anticipated along with prophylactic antiulcer therapy.

Long-term use should strive to identify the smallest dose of GLC that will achieve the desired effect, particularly for relatively benign, chronic inflammatory conditions such as atopy or flea allergy dermatitis. Optimum doses (initial and maintenance) for the variety of syndromes responsive to GLCs are largely based on trial and error, with intermittent reevaluation. Eventually, anti-inflammatory GLCs with minimal metabolic effects will be associated with a lower risk. An every-other-day dosage regimen with a short- or intermediate-acting agent can achieve therapeutic effects without untoward effects in many patients. Agents that are ideal for alternate-day administration include prednisone, prednisolone, and methylprednisolone. The duration of action of hydrocortisone and cortisone may be too short for effective alternate-day therapy. Although triamcinolone's duration of action is similar to those of prednisolone and methylprednisolone, its ability to suppress the hypothalamic–pituitary–adrenal axis is more typical of the long-acting agents such as dexamethasone and betamethasone. Side effects can occur if withdrawal of a GLC occurs too rapidly. In human patients receiving GLCs, the most frequent problem encountered with rapid withdrawals is recrudescence of the underlying condition for which the GLC was indicated.[9] The most severe but rare complication, however, is acute adrenal insufficiency. Because of variability in GLC impact on the hypothalamic–pituitary–adrenal axis and variability within and between animals, predicting which animal is likely to develop insufficiency is difficult. In general, iatrogenic Addison's disease is not common, but even this risk can be minimized by gradual withdrawal of the GLC. In human patients those who receive supraphysiologic doses for 2 weeks within the preceding year are considered to have some level of hypothalamic–pituitary–adrenal suppression.[9]

THERAPEUTIC INDICATIONS*

Dermatologic

GLCs are the cornerstone of therapy of many of the autoimmune diseases affecting the skin, including the pemphigus complex, systemic lupus erythematosus, and discoid lupus erythematosus. Optimal therapy for each of these diseases varies, insofar as some may respond to GLCs alone and some may require a combination of GLCs and alternate immunosuppressive drugs such as azathioprine or cyclophosphamide.

The long-term management of canine atopy (allergic inhalant dermatitis) frequently requires the use of GLCs. If at all possible, hyposensitization and avoidance therapy should be attempted before medical management. Although GLCs are the most effective antiinflammatory–antipruritic medication currently available for the atopic patient, alternate forms of therapy, as previously noted (e.g., antihistamines, misoprostol, omega fatty acids, and combinations thereof), should be attempted before sentencing a patient to chronic GLC therapy. Initial treatment with prednisolone at an antiinflammatory induction dose of 0.5 to 1 mg/kg per day is recommended. After resolution of clinical signs, the therapy should be switched to an alternate-day regimen. An effective alternate-day dose can be achieved by taking the lowest effective daily dose and increasing it by 50%.[75] Some dogs may require medication every 3 to 4 days. The use of injectable repositol forms of GLCs is not recommended for treatment of canine atopy.

Atopy is also believed to exist in the cat. There is little information regarding the efficacy of antihistamines and fatty acid supplements as antipruritics in the cat. GLCs are the therapy of choice for treatment of atopic pruritis in the cat.[76] As with dogs, short-acting to intermediate-acting compounds (prednisolone 1 to 2 mg/kg per day) are recommended, and alternate-day therapy should be the goal.

Otic

Otitis externa, often occurring as a component of atopy, is frequently responsive to topical GLC therapy (see Chapters 8 and 9 for discussion of antimicrobial drugs). Products usually contain an antibiotic and antifungal in addition to the GLC, and these agents can help resolve secondary infections. It is important to note that topically administered GLCs can be absorbed systemically.[51] Efforts to remove or resolve the inciting factors should be made in cases of chronic otitis externa. More severe otitis externa, such as idiopathic hyperplastic otitis externa of Cocker Spaniels, may require systemic GLC treatment (prednisolone at 0.5 to 1 mg/kg per day).[77] Follow-up examinations, usually at 2-week intervals, should include otoscopic and cytologic examinations to identify potential complications (otitis media, secondary yeast or bacterial infection, parasites, and so forth). It should be stressed that GLC therapy is *not* a substitute for thorough cleaning and drying of the ear.

Respiratory

GLCs have a pivotal role in the treatment of selected respiratory conditions (see Chapter 20). Their efficacy as bronchodilators (through their permissive effects on β_2-receptors) and as antiinflammatory agents has been well documented in patients with asthma. Among clinically used antiinflammatory drugs, GLCs alone inhibit prostaglandins, leukotrienes, and platelet-activating factor. Their effects on macrophage processing are well documented. These mediators have important roles in the pathophysiology of chronic bronchial disease. In human patients inhaled GLCs (beclomethasone, triamcinolone) tend to be first-line drugs. In cats suffering from bronchial asthma, GLCs are administered acutely and are the cornerstone of long-term therapy. Preference for the particular drug varies among clinicians. In patients suffering from status asthmaticus, water-soluble preparations of prednisolone tend to be used for their rapid effects, whereas dexamethasone may be preferred because it is more potent and provides a more prolonged effect. A combination of both products might be considered for immediate effects, followed by the more prolonged effects. Long-term therapy generally consists of oral forms of prednisolone, although some clinicians may prefer triamcinolone because of its enhanced potency. Alternate-day therapy may, however, be of no benefit for this intermediate- to long-acting GLC. As with other conditions requiring prolonged therapy, a higher dose is administered initially, with tapering of the dose to a minimal acceptable level. Lifelong therapy may be necessary for some cats. The use of repositol steroid preparations is controversial. Although they are convenient, the lack of predictability regarding retreatment may preclude their effective use. In cases of relapse, intravenous administration of dexamethasone or nebulized steroid therapy may be of benefit. Greater discretion is indicated for long-term use of GLCs in chronic respiratory diseases in dogs. Noninfectious diseases associated with eosinophilic or macrophage infiltrates are indications for GLC therapy, usually in conjunction with bronchodilator therapy. Short-acting GLCs can be used on a short-term basis (<48 hours) to break a cough cycle in patients with upper respiratory syndromes associated with inflammation (i.e., tracheobronchitis).

The design of topically administered inhalant GLCs and their use is also discussed with regard to "soft steroids" and adverse events, as well as in Chapter 20.

Musculoskeletal

Understanding the implications of GLC use for the treatment of osteoarthritis requires appreciation of the pathophysiology of osteoarthritis and the effects of GLCs on normal joint

*Among the difficulties in identifying a scientific basis for the recommended use of glucocorticoids in dogs or cats is the limited number of clinical trials. Further, many of the clinical trials base response on prednisone, rather than prednisolone. Caution is recommended in overinterpreting studies that fail to detect a response to prednisone (rather than prednisolone) because of evidence of poorer absorption of the former compared to the latter in both dogs and cats.[59,63]

physiology. GLCs have variable and opposite effects on joint physiology, depending on the dose used.[78] Low concentrations appear to be chondroprotective, whereas higher concentrations are chondrodestructive.

The term *steroid arthropathy* was coined to refer to the destructive condition that occurs in joints after multiple intraarticular injections of GLCs in human patients.[78] In animal models (including dogs), the detrimental effects of GLCs can occur after administration of a single intraarticular injection or multiple systemic doses. In addition to the destruction induced by GLCs on cartilage, indirect damage may occur because of failure to rest an injured joint. Finally, GLCs negatively affect subchondral bone by inhibiting osteoblastic activity.

Despite the obvious role GLCs have in preventing cartilage catabolism and controlling inflammation, their use for the treatment of osteoarthritis is controversial. Although short-term use is generally accepted for acute conditions or trauma, long-term use is less acceptable. Much of the controversy might be resolved if a physiologic dose could be defined. In a canine model of osteoarthritis, an oral dose of 0.2 to 0.25 mg/kg per day of prednisone or an intraarticular dose of 5 mg per month of triamcinolone hexacetonide significantly reduced the incidence and severity of cartilage lesions and osteophyte formation[79] The advantages of intraarticular administration include minimization (but not total elimination) of systemic effects. Disadvantages include the potential need for chemical restraint and the risk of sepsis.

Newer GLCs characterized by increased antiinflammatory potency yet decreased negative effects on cartilage may resolve the controversy regarding the use of GLCs in the treatment of osteoarthritis. Until these drugs are available or a physiologic dose has been established, the authors recommend reservation of GLCs in the treatment of osteoarthritis to animals that have failed to respond to chondroprotective agents or nonsteroidal antiinflammatory agents that are chondroprotective. Concurrent use of GLCs and nonsteroidal antiinflammatory agents enhances the risk for gastrointestinal ulceration and is not recommended. Finally, if GLCs are used, low doses (as noted previously) should be administered, and the simultaneous use of disease-modifying chondroprotective agents should be considered.

In humans suffering from osteoarthritis, intraarticular treatment with triamcinolone, methylprednisolone, and prednisolone are used to treat symptoms associated with osteoarthritis. Contraindications for such use include evidence of infection (e.g., bacteremia, adjacent osteomyelitis, or overlying skin) and joint prostheses. In humans corticosteroid injections are considered relatively safe, with long-term concerns focusing on the risk of long-term joint damage or infection.[80] The use of GLCs for treatment of osteoarthritis reduces the number of GRs in treated patients, leading to a decrease in responsiveness. Subsequent activation of metalloproteinases may contribute to joint degeneration, although long-term (>1 year) therapy was associated with a trend toward improvement in humans with osteoarthritis of the knee. However, because the long-term effects of GLC therapy are not clear, their use is generally limited to patients who have not responded to other therapies.

Central Nervous System

GLCs are used for treatment of both brain and spinal cord disease. Their beneficial effects include protection from free radicals, reduction in intracranial pressure (decreased production of cerebrospinal fluid), and maintenance of normal microvasculature integrity. GLCs appear to be beneficial in reducing or preventing cerebral edema associated with neoplasia; however, cerebral edema caused by trauma is thought to be less responsive to GLC therapy.

There is increasing evidence that lipid peroxidation and resultant formation of oxygen-derived free radicals play an important role in tissue damage subsequent to brain or spinal cord trauma. Several GLCs, including methylprednisolone (most potent), dexamethasone, and prednisolone, are capable of inhibiting lipid peroxidation.[73] Their ability to inhibit phospholipase A_2 may also protect injured nervous tissue. For treatment of acute CNS injury, the water-soluble salts should be used. Recommended dosage regimens for these agents in the treatment of CNS injury in dogs and cats are methylprednisolone sodium succinate 30 mg/kg intravenously, followed by 15 mg/kg 2 and 6 hours later, and then 2.5 mg/kg per hour for the first 48 hours; prednisolone sodium succinate 60 mg/kg intravenously, followed by 30 mg/kg 2 and 6 hours later, and then 5 mg/kg per hour for the first 48 hours; and dexamethasone sodium phosphate 4 mg/kg intravenously every 6 hours for the first 48 hours.[73] In studies involving cats with spinal cord injury, methylprednisolone sodium succinate–treated cats had significantly improved neurologic outcome, whereas the neurologic outcome of cats treated with dexamethasone was not significantly different than that of cats receiving placebo.[81,82]

Noninfectious, or so-called steroid-responsive, meningitis and granulomatous meningoencephalitis are diseases that frequently respond dramatically to GLC therapy. Prednisolone at a dose of 2 to 4 mg/kg per day has been recommended. The use of glucocorticoids for treatment of intervertebral disk disease is addressed in Chapter 28.

Inflammatory Bowel and Liver Disease

Inflammatory bowel disease in cats (especially those with lymphocytic–plasmacytic infiltrates) is frequently responsive to prednisolone at 2.2 mg/kg per day[83] (see Chapter 19). For more severe cases, dexamethasone at 0.22 mg/kg per day plus metronidazole may be effective. In either case, the initial dose should be maintained for 2 weeks beyond the time that the cat's clinical signs begin to resolve. Cats that respond immediately should receive the initial dose for at least 4 weeks before dose reduction is attempted.

Inflammatory bowel disease in dogs may be less responsive to GLC therapy than is the case in cats (canine patients with eosinophilic infiltrates are an exception). Initial treatment of lymphocytic–plasmacytic enteritis and colitis is with 2.2 mg/kg of prednisolone per day. Frequently, additional therapy is necessary (metronidazole, azathioprine). In all cases dietary modification should accompany pharmacologic therapy.

Alimentary lymphosarcoma should be ruled out before steroid therapy is initiated (especially in cats). The use of GLC for treatment of inflammatory bowel disease is also discussed in Chapter 19.

Corticosteroid therapy for liver disease remains somewhat controversial. Clinical studies in human medicine have shown that steroid therapy in chronic active hepatitis improves survival rates. Nonsuppurative cholangitis–cholangiohepatitis may respond to immunosuppressive GLC therapy.

Gingivitis and Stomatitis

The eosinophilic granuloma complex in cats is usually responsive to high-dose GLC therapy such as methylprednisolone acetate 20 mg intramuscularly every 2 to 3 weeks for three treatments. Lymphocytic–plasmacytic gingivitis and stomatitis in cats may respond to GLC therapy (prednisone 2 to 4 mg/kg orally every 24 hours).

Septic Shock and Functional Adrenocortical Deficiency

The antibacterial treatment of septic shock is addressed in Chapter 8, and the antiinflammatory component also is addressed in Chapter 29. A number of bacterial and viral infections activate the HPAA such that GLC release increases. The mechanism probably reflects cytokines or other inflammatory mediators.[4] It is likely that activation reflects both a direct effect on the adrenal glands or the hypothalamus or pituitary. Other proteins (e.g., *Staphylococus, Clostridium, Mycoplasma*) can also stimulated the response. A number of viruses have similar capability. However, although both bacterial and viral infections affect the hypothalamic–pituitary–adrenal axis such that GLC release is increased, other factors in the infected patient, such as pain, psychological stress, and the debilitating effects of infection, likewise activate the hypothalamic–pituitary–adrenal axis[4] and will modulate response to infection.

The use of GLCs in septic shock has been controversial, although their potential benefits were recognized as early as 1951[84,85] (see Chapter 29). Evidence varies with experimental versus clinical studies. Earlier experimental models of septic shock showed GLCs to be beneficial if administered before or concurrently with endotoxin administration (i.e., within the first 2 hours). In canine models, severe mesenteric vasoconstriction within the first 15 minutes can lead to irreversible shock. Thus GLCs are unlikely to provide beneficial effects if they are administered 30 to 60 minutes after administration of the endotoxin.[86] One of the differences between results of experimental versus clinical (spontaneous) models of septic shock may be the choice of outcome measures. Survival rates in experimental models are often based on short-term analysis (i.e., survival for several hours). In addition, the likelihood of knowing the time of onset of endotoxemia or sepsis in a clinical setting is extremely low.

The use of GLCs in human patients suffering from sepsis and septic shock was addressed in a large meta-analysis of human clinical trials.[84] In this study 10 of 49 published reports investigating the effects of corticosteroids in human patients experiencing septic shock were considered to be superior on the basis of scientific design (e.g., controlled study, blinding techniques). Even within these 10 studies, however, differences in experimental design, definition of septic shock, drugs, dosing regimens, timing of steroid administration, and other design considerations limited the number of conclusions that could be made. Mortality rates often were the basis of analysis; however, mortality was not determined at the same time in all 10 studies. Of the 10 studies examined, only one study offered a significant positive effect for patients receiving GLCs. Most studies show a beneficial effect of steroids during the first few hours after the initiation of shock. Patients with sepsis associated with gram-negative infections demonstrated a slightly better outcome. The most common or severe side effects after steroid treatment was gastrointestinal bleeding (reported in five studies), generally associated with administration for 6 or more days or months. Superinfection (secondary infection) was reported in 7 of the 10 studies. The authors made the following conclusions: (1) The broad use of corticosteroids in patients with sepsis or septic shock is not beneficial, and the authors went so far as to suggest that a new trial would not be indicated. (2) Short-term, high-dose treatment did not increase the risk of complications. (3) Very early initiation (or prophylactic use) of steroid therapy in gram-negative infections might reduce the generalized inflammatory response to infection.[84] The results of this and other studies led to a decline in the use of GLCs in septic shock in the early 1990s, only to be followed by a re-examination of the question in the late ‘90s and early 2000s. Renewed interest reflected the recent recognition that sepsis and septic shock are aggravated by transient adrenal failure and negative cardiovascular sequelae associated with adrenal insufficiency.[2] Mortality rates are increased in acutely septic patients in which corticotropin stimulation is attenuated.[87] In humans bilateral adrenal hemorrhage or necrosis is present in as many as 30% of patients dying as a result of septic shock, and peripheral ACTH resistance has been described in close to 20% of humans with septic shock. Predisposition to acute renal failure in septic shock may be facilitated by underlying pituitary or adrenal pathology, or co-treatment of drugs that impair cortisol synthesis (e.g., ketoconazole) or increase cortisol metabolism (e.g., phenobarbital).[2]

In contrast to early studies that focused on high doses of GLCs for treatment of septic shock, the realization of the potential role of adrenal insufficiency led to a physiologic approach to adrenal hormone replacement. A recent meta-analysis[88] concluded that the dose of GLC used in the patient experiencing septic shock affected risks associated with increased mortality. Whereas clinical trials reported before 1989 (n = 8) found decreased survival in patients treated with GLCs, analysis studies after 1997 (n = 5) consistently found beneficial effects on survival if physiologic doses were used, even if longer than 6 days. The mean *total* hydrocortisone equivalent reported in the later trials was 1209 mg, or 300 mg per day (approximately 4 mg/kg/day), compared with a mean total dose of 20 times that amount in the earlier studies. The impact of secondary bacterial infections was considered a contributing factor to increased mortality rates in trials before 1989. Although the incidence of secondary bacterial infections did not differ between the two time periods, the time to resolution of the secondary infection was shorter after 1997, presumably because of less immunosuppression and fewer deaths associated with secondary infection. The authors concluded that whereas short courses of high-dose GLCs decreased sepsis survival, a 5- to 7-day course of physiologic hydrocortisone doses, with subsequent tapering of doses, increased survival. The impact of physiologic GLCs appears to reflect reversal of vasopressor-dependent septic shock, including improved response to vasoactive drugs.[88] Other investigators have described decreased body temperature and heart rate when subjects are treated with low-dose GLCs. Improved survival rates in septic human patients treated with low-dose GLC therapy have led to the development of criteria intended to aid in the recognition of adrenal failure so that low-dose GLC therapy might be initiated. Basal cortisol concentration below 15 μg/dL are considered indicative of adrenal insufficiency in humans; for dogs, concentrations are < 2 μg/dL pre and post ACTH response (see also Chapter 21).[2] Treatment for adrenal failure in humans focuses on replacement therapy with hydrocortisone (200 to 300 mg/kg per day [for a 70-kg patient]) combined with fludrocortisone (50 μg per day) for up to 7 days.

Septic shock is not the only acute illness for which functional ACTH deficiency may occur. Deficiency associated with acute illnesses in humans has been reviewed.[89] Acute situations such as severe infection, trauma, burns, and surgery may cause up to a sixfold increase in cortisol secretion, with the increase proportional to the illness. Secretion may be impaired, however, for a variety of reasons, including preexisting disease affecting the hypothalamic-pituitary-adrenal axis, drug-impaired synthesis (e.g., imidazole antifungals, etomidate), adrenal necrosis, or hemorrhage as might accompany coagulopathies, or iatrogenic suppression such as that which may occur with exogenous GLC therapy. Cytokines associated with systemic inflammation may cause tissue GLC resistance; indeed, human patients with the most severe illness may have the highest cortisol concentrations, making "spot checks" of cortisol less helpful in the diagnosis of these patients.[89] The deficiency is generally transient but is difficult to diagnosis. In humans, hyponatremia, hyperkalemia, hypoglycemia, and eosinophilia may be present. A corticotropin stimulation test might be used to detect an incremental response. Deficiency, once diagnosed, is treated in humans differentially, depending on the severity of illness. No treatment is indicated for mild illness. A moderate illness or condition may be treated with approximately 0.2 mg/kg per day, with discontinuation (or return to predeficiency doses in those patients receiving GLCs) within 24 hours of resolution. Severe illness or major surgery is treated with approximately 0.7 mg/kg cortisone every 6 hours; on resolution, the dose is tapered 50% every day. Septic shock is treated similarly with the addition of 0.7 μg/mL of fludrocortisone daily; treatment continues for 7 days.[89]

The final word on the role of GLCs in critical patients has yet to be determined. A meta-analysis of controlled clinical trials (n = 5) evaluating the efficacy of GLC therapy in patients experiencing septic shock. The analysis found that a short course of high-dose hydrocortisone decreased survival rates, whereas a longer course (5 to 7 days) of low-dose hydrocortisone increased survival rates.[88] However, a recent multicenter clinical trial in humans (n = 251) with persistent hypotension despite fluid and resuscitation therapy found no significant response to corticotropin in patients that received low-dose hydrocortisone (approximately 0.72 mg/kg; n = 251) compared with saline placebo (n = 248) every 6 hours. Although time to reversal of shock was shorter in the treatment group, no difference in mortality rates was detected between groups or between responders and nonresponders within each treatment group.[90] Factors that may have led to the lack of difference, as opposed to other studies that have reported treatment success, included lack of fludrocortisone treatment, patients that were less severely ill compared with those in other studies, and continued therapy for up to 11 days (as opposed to 7 or fewer days for other studies). The authors concluded that corticotropin response does not seem to be a viable test for predicting the need for steroid therapy. Interestingly, perioperative glucocorticoid supplementation in the surgical patient has been a point of controversy for more than half a century.[90a] The rationale is based on the recognition of surgery-associated adrenal insufficiency. The need for use and guidelines for administration were reviewed by Salem and coworkers in 1994. In 2008, Jung and Inder revisited the issue, recognizing that no consensus exist regarding dosing regimens or duration. However, high doses (>200 mg hydrocortisone equivalent, or approximately 2.75 mg/kg a day) beyond 2 to 3 days clearly are to be avoided in the uncomplicated case.[90b]

Neoplasia

Prednisolone is often included in combination chemotherapy protocols for treatment of lymphoma and multiple myeloma for their cytotoxic actions. The impact of GLC treatment alone in patients with GLC-responsive cancer, before implementation of combination chemotherapy, is controversial. In general, use of GLCs before chemotherapy is generally discouraged because of the clinical perception that such use is associated with a decreased duration of survival, which presumably reflects rapidly developing resistance to GLCs. Indeed, Price and coworkers[91] demonstrated a significant decrease in the median duration of remission in dogs receiving GLCs before chemotherapy (134 days) compared with that of dogs not receiving GLCs (267 days). Proposed mechanisms whereby this might occur include the advent of multidrug resistance (e.g., by way of P-glycoprotein or related proteins) or a decrease in GLCs receptors. The use of GLCs as a single agent for treatment of lymphoma theoretically may rapidly induce multidrug resistance in neoplastic cells, causing the cell to be less responsive to not only GLCs but also other anticancer drugs, such as doxorubicin and vincristine. However, an in vitro study using canine cancer cells demonstrated dexamethasone resistance to cisplatin and methotrexate, but the resistance did not appear to reflect the multidrug resistant genes studied.[92] Because of the controversy surrounding single-agent chemotherapy of lymphoma with prednisolone, this approach is generally not recommended except under certain circumstances, such as in the presence of life-threatening or organ (kidney) hypercalcemia.

The impact of GLCs on drug–receptor interaction may be a more likely cause for the development of resistance. Failure has been correlated to receptor density, with cells (e.g., T lymphocytes) characterized by low density being less responsive to chemotherapeutic drugs in general.

GLCs are often used in patients with mast cell tumors to decrease the inflammatory response associated with mast cell degranulation. Additionally, GLCs may induce a partial or complete remission in some canine patients with mast cell tumors.[93]

Ophthalmic

Topical GLC therapy is efficacious for treatment of noninfectious conjunctival, scleral, corneal, and anterior uveal inflammatory diseases.[94] Before topical corticosteroid use, however, the corneal epithelium should be examined (using fluorescein dye) for signs of ulceration. The effects of glucocorticoids on corneal epithelial cells is biphasic, stimulating growth at low (physiologic) concentrations and inhibiting it at higher concentrations (supraphysiologic or pharmacologic).[94a] The presence of corneal ulceration precludes the use of topical corticosteroids. Prednisolone acetate penetrates the intact corneal epithelium and is therefore effective for treatment of intraocular inflammation.[94] Systemic absorption of topical ophthalmic corticosteroids has been documented in dogs. Systemic GLC therapy is necessary for treatment of noninfectious posterior segment inflammatory conditions.

Hematopoietic

GLCs are the mainstay, first-line therapy for both immune-mediated hemolytic anemia and thrombocytopenia. Some anecdotal evidence suggests that initial treatment with dexamethasone may be superior to prednisone therapy, but no controlled studies have substantiated this claim. This may, reflect, however, poor bioavailability of prednisone. Prednisone (2 to 4 mg/kg per day) or dexamethasone (0.3 to 0.6 mg/kg per day) therapy should be continued until erythrocyte or platelet numbers steadily increase. Subsequently, the dose should be slowly (over 3 to 6 months) tapered. Addition of GLCs is also beneficial for treatment of immune-mediated neutropenia and for treatment and prevention of transfusion reactions.

Hypoadrenocorticism

Replacement corticosteroid therapy for treatment of hypoadrenocorticism is discussed in Chapter 21. An Addisonian crisis requires treatment with rapid-acting GLCs and mineralocorticoids. Not all synthetic GLCs are effective for replacement of mineralocorticoid deficiency. Dexamethasone, methylprednisolone, triamcinolone, and betamethasone are virtually devoid of mineralocorticoid activity. For treatment of acute hypoadrenocorticism, if a mineralocorticoid such as fludrocortisone (Florinef) or DOCP is unavailable, prednisolone or cortisone may provide adequate mineralocorticoid activity.

ADVERSE EFFECTS

Adverse reactions resulting from GLC therapy can occur through either cessation of therapy or prolonged use. Acute adrenal insufficiency results from rapid withdrawal of GLCs after prolonged treatment (see earlier discussion of clinical use). Termination of GLC therapy in a chronically treated patient should be performed gradually over several months. Complete recovery of the hypothalamic–pituitary–adrenal axis may require 9 months. During this time, patients may need supplemental GLCs during "stressful" situations (e.g., surgery).

Complications of GLCs related to prolonged therapy are described later. In general, dogs are more susceptible to these complications than are cats. The incidence of adverse effects resulting from GLC administration is frequently related to the dose and duration of treatment. Alternate-day therapy with short-acting preparations can significantly reduce the incidence of adverse reactions.

The avoidance of GLC side effects is a focus of intense research in human medicine. The critical role that GLCs play in human asthma has directed much research in the design and development of the ideal GLC: one that combines marked efficacy and long-term safety, a convenient delivery device, and a reasonable price. Among the current methods by which risks are reduced is the design of drugs that target transrepression and through manipulation of the pharmacokinetic properties of GLC. This includes the administration of "soft" GLCs (previously discussed).[18] Another mechanism by which systemic effects of GLC might be reduced is activation of a prodrug at the site of action. For example, ciclesonide is a novel, inhaled corticosteroid approved or treatment of asthma. The drug is activated in the lungs to the potent drug desisobutyryl–ciclesonide (*des*-CIC) in the lungs. The metabolite exhibits 100-fold affinity for GR in the lungs compared with the parent compound, and thus is comparable to fluticasone in potency. Further, the drug is characterized by low bioavailability, in part because of its high first-pass metabolism.[95]

The use of low rather than high doses may prevent some undesirable side effects, although the impact varies with the adverse event in human medicine.[20] Osteoporosis persists, whereas osteonecrosis might be reduced. Myopathy is rare with low doses, whereas endocrinopathies, including glucose intolerance, fat redistribution, and weight gain, remain present with low doses; however, diabetes mellitus rarely occurs with low doses. Cardiovascular adverse events (e.g., atherosclerosis, sodium and water retention) tend to be minimized at low doses, whereas dermatologic events consistent with iatrogenic Cushing's syndrome persist, albeit at a lower level. Psychologic disturbances, including steroid psychosis, are largely absent at low doses. Ophthalmic events such as glaucoma and cataracts are largely reduced with low doses, as are gastrointestinal events, including gastroduodenal ulceration (generally associated with concomitant use of nonsteroidal antiinflammatory drugs) and pancreatitis. Immunosuppression resulting in increased susceptibility to infectious disease also is largely reduced but still remains for some pathogens (e.g., *Pneumocystis carinii)* at low doses. The impact of dose dependency on the use of GLCs for treatment of septic shock was previously discussed.

Steffan and coworkers[96] compared adverse events associated with cyclosporine A (n = 119; 5 mg/kg per day induction followed by tapering doses) versus methylprednisolone (n = 59; 0.5 to 1 mg/kg per day for 1 week, then every other day for 3 weeks, then tapered) in dogs with atopic dermatitis. The incidence of adverse events was similar between groups. The incidence of vomiting was significantly less in the methylprednisolone-treated group compared with the cyclosporine A–treated group (vomiting, 37% versus 5%). Whereas infections occurred with similar frequency in the two treatment groups, they were more likely to be classified as severe or very severe in the methylprednisolone-treated group, leading to more dropouts. Polyuria and polydipsia were more common in the methylprednisolone-treated group (25%) versus the cyclosporine A–treated group (4.3%); increased appetite and weight gain were also greater in the methylprednisolone-treated group (12% versus 3%). Serum chemistries indicative of renal function did not change from baseline levels. Potassium decreased approximately 0.7 mg/dL (and increased in the cyclosporine A–treated group) but was within normal values.

Levine and coworkers[97] retrospectively compared the adverse events associated with dexamethasone (n = 49) compared with no treatment (n = 80) and other GLC therapy (primarily methylprednisolone sodium succinate) for treatment of acute thoracolumbar intervertebral disk herniation in dogs. The mean dose was 2.25 mg ± 4.28 m/kg (range 1 to 30 mg/kg). Adversities that were greater in the dexamethasone-treated group included vomiting, diarrhea, and anemia. Urinary tract infections also were more frequent in the dexamethasone-treated patients, although not all patients were tested for infection.

Central Nervous System

GLCs act as centrally active appetite stimulants to induce polyphagia in dogs and, to a lesser degree, in cats. This may contribute to the development of obesity in some patients, but it also may stimulate the appetite of an anorexic patient. Changes in mood or behavior have been noted in human patients treated with GLCs. Although these are more difficult to document in veterinary patients, most clinicians have noted positive attitude changes in patients being treated with GLCs.

Musculoskeletal

Muscle weakness and muscle atrophy are commonly observed in dogs with hyperadrenocorticism and dogs receiving large doses of GLCs (see previous discussion). These effects in part reflect muscle wasting that may result from the catabolic gluconeogenic effects of GLCs.

GLCs are associated with osteoporosis and vertebral compression in 30% to 50% of human patients receiving the drugs chronically. Mechanisms include direct inhibition of osteoblasts (decreased bone formation); inhibition of calcium absorption from the intestines; increased parathormone secretion, which in turn increases osteoclast-mediated bone resorption; and increased calcium excretion.[9] Osteoporosis is not a clinically recognized entity in small animals receiving GLCs, in part because of differences in body posture as well as duration of therapy. Prudence is indicated, however, when GLCs are used in the face of conditions that facilitate or are facilitated by the negative sequelae of GLCs on bone formation. Aseptic necrosis has been reported in human patients after a short course of high doses of GLCs.[9]

Gastrointestinal and Liver

The likelihood of GLCs causing gastrointestinal ulceration is controversial. In general, patients that develop ulceration are predisposed to ulceration because of stress or are receiving other drugs that contribute to gastrointestinal damage, most notably nonsteroidal antiinflammatory drugs. In stressed animals peripheral effects of centrally or peripherally mediated norepinephrine may be important to the manifestation of gastrointestinal ulceration mediated by GLCs.[98] Colonic perforation in dogs with spinal cord injuries has been associated with the use of dexamethasone, perhaps in part because of modulation of local blood flow. Pancreatitis has been associated with the use of GLCs alone and in combination with azathioprine. GLCs can induce hepatocellular swelling as a result of fat, perivascular glycogen, or water accumulation. Centrilobular vacuolization is common, and focal necrosis occasionally occurs. Clinically, these changes are seen as hepatomegaly and elevated liver enzyme activity. In dogs induction of a steroid-induced alkaline phosphatase isoenzyme occurs in patients receiving GLCs. The effects of GLCs on the liver are slowly reversible, persisting 1 to 1.5 months after therapy is discontinued.

Metabolic

Glucose intolerance, insulin resistance, overt diabetes mellitus, and hyperlipidemia can be induced in canine patients receiving GLC therapy.

Hepatic

GLCs consistently cause diffuse to centrilobular vacuolization and perivascular glycogen accumulation in hepatocytes.[99,100] Focal necrosis has been occasionally described in clinical cases. Similar lesions result with hyperadrenocorticism. In addition to serum biochemical changes consistent with liver disease, GLCs also cause elevations in a steroid-specific alkaline phosphatase isoenzyme, which can be discerned with the levamisole test. This increase (induction) is not considered indicative of liver disease if other indicators of liver disease are absent. The pathologic changes associated with GLCs are slowly reversible over 1 to 1.5 months after discontinuation of therapy.

Endocrine

Exogenous administration of GLCs suppresses the hypothalamic–pituitary–adrenal axis through feedback inhibition on the anterior pituitary and the hypothalamus. Chronic suppression of the axis can result in iatrogenic hypoadrenocorticism on discontinuation of exogenous GLCs.

GLCs cause a decrease in plasma concentrations of total triiodothyronine, thyroxine, and thyroid-stimulating hormone, with a normal free triiodothyronine and thyroxine concentration.[101] Therefore, when assessing thyroid function in animals receiving GLCs, the clinician should keep in mind their influence on total thyroid hormone concentrations. GLC administration does not result in clinical hypothyroidism because the free hormone concentration is minimally affected. GLCs increase parathormone secretion.

Renal

Polyuria and polydipsia are classically associated with excessive GLC (either endogenous or exogenous). Several factors probably contribute to this effect, including increased glomerular filtration rate resulting from increased vascular volume, increased renal calcium excretion, inhibitory actions on antidiuretic hormone, and direct actions decreasing permeability of the distal tubule. Glucocorticoids may increase the risk of azotemia in patients with renal disease because of their catabolic effects, particularly in the presence of metabolic acidosis.

Cardiovascular

Many human patients receiving GLCs develop hypertension as a result of sodium retention. Hypertension occurs in dogs with hyperadrenocorticism and presumably could also occur in veterinary patients receiving exogenous GLCs. Postulated mechanisms for hypertension in canine hyperadrenocorticism include increased activation of angiotensin I, increased vascular responsiveness to catecholamines, and reduction of vasodilator prostaglandins.

Immune Function

Although the intent of GLC therapy generally reflects suppression of some facet of immune function, such use generally is associated with an increased risk of bacterial, viral, and fungal infection, although this effect is dose dependent, as was previously discussed with regard to treatment of septic shock. It is generally recognized that a single dose of a short- to intermediate-acting GLC is unlikely to significantly suppress immune function, but caution with this approach is prudent, particularly for infectious diseases. Chronic administration of GLCs can result in recurrent cystitis, septicemia, and endocarditis. Causes for these effects are multiple, including immune suppression and, potentially, upregulation of P-glycoprotein (see the discussion of neoplasia). Ihrke and coworkers[102] demonstrated as early as 1985 that close to 40% of dogs receiving immunosuppressive GLC therapy (mean of 0.8 mg/kg) also had a urinary tract infection. In a study of close to 200 dogs with pruritic skin disease, those receiving GLCs (either prednisone [70%] or methylprednisolone [30%]) for longer than 6 months had a higher incidence of urinary tract infections compared with dogs that did not receive GLCs.[103] Doses ranged from 0.12 to 1 mg/kg, with a mean of 0.28 ± 0.14, generally administered every 48 hours. The overall incidence was lower than that of the earlier study, at 12% for treated dogs compared with 0% for untreated dogs, when based on the first urine sample collected for each dog. However, the number increased to 23% when subsequent samples were included in the analysis, indicating the need for repetitive culturing in animals receiving GLCs. This study provided evidence that clinicians should perform routine cultures for patients with hyperadrenocorticism rather than rely on clinical signs or urinalysis. No dog with bacteriuria manifested clinical signs of urinary tract infection. Whereas the presence of bacteriuria and pyuria consistently indicated the presence of a urinary tract infection, the absence of bacteruria did not rule out urinary tract infection: Bacteriuria was not detected in 24% of urine samples that subsequently yielded bacterial growth. Female, but not male, dogs receiving GLCs were predisposed to infection, although this finding may have been biased by the limited number of male dogs treated with GLCs. Although *E. coli* was the most common organism isolated (14 of 34), a total of 10 different organisms were isolated. This study might be interpreted as justification of the routine use of antimicrobials. However, only 6 of 52 urine samples collected in patients receiving antibiotics were positive on culture. Particularly problematic was the fact that isolates cultured in dogs receiving cephalexin were resistant to the drug. Indeed, 51% of all isolates were resistant to cephalexin (a pattern typical of *E. coli* in general) and 22% were resistant to enrofloxacin, emphasizing the need for selection of an antimicrobial on the basis of susceptibility testing (see Chapter 8). Presumably, achieving bactericidal concentrations of a drug at the site of the urinary tract infection is paramount, should the decision be made to treat the infection. Dogs with intervertebral disk disease have an increased risk of UTI when treated with glucocorticoids (see Chapter 27).

Wound Healing

The impact of glucocorticoids on wound healing has been generally recognized for decades.[103a] The impact of exogenous glucocorticoids largely reflects their antiinflammatory effects and down regulation of pro-inflammatory cytokines (as reviewed by Grose et al, 2002).[103a] However, these effects occur at supraphysiologic (i.e., pharmacologic) doses. The effects of endogenous glucocorticoids (physiologic concentrations) also appear to be suppressive, but these latter effects may actually be beneficial in the control of late would healing.[103a]

Immune Reactions

Paradoxically, despite their immunomodulatory effects, GLCs have been associated with allergic reactions in humans, albeit rarely. Types I, III, and IV reactions have been reported, with reactions more common in patients treated chronically (e.g., asthmatics, transplant recipients) and patients receiving either hydrocortisone or methylprednisolone intravenously.[49,104] In addition to the active ingredient, reaction to (sulfate) excipients or to succinate salts has also been suspected. Vasculitis reactions have been reported after oral administration of either prednisone or prednisolone. Nakamura and coworkers[105] reported anaphylaxis that occurred after intravenous administration of succinate-containing GLCs (hydrocortisone or methylprednisolone) in severely atopic asthmatic humans. In this retrospective study, phosphate-containing drugs appeared to be safe. The authors recommended slow intravenous drip administration in patients with severe allergic disease who have been previously exposed to GLCs. Erdmann and coworkers[106] reported an anaphylactic reaction in an atopic person receiving oral prednisone; skin testing revealed reaction to prednisolone, prednisolone hydrogen succinate, prednisone, and betamethasone but not methylprednisolone or dexamethasone. Accordingly, anaphylaxis should be suspected with any GLC if clinical signs are supportive. Allergic reactions may not be limited to type 1. Finally, reactions may not be limited to active drug but may involve vehicles or salt forms. One case of anaphylaxis has been reported in a dog receiving dexamethasone.[107] The dog had been previously treated with dexamethasone in propylene glycol as well as oral prednisone therapy for immune-mediated hemolytic anemia. The vehicle contained methylparaben and propylparaben as well as benzyl alcohol. No occurrences of anaphylaxis or anaphylactoid reactions were cited in a review of adversities associated with dexamethasone treatment in dogs with thoracolumbar disease (n = 161).[97] In a review of the literature, Schaer and coworkers[107] noted that anaphylactoid reactions also have been reported.

Respiratory

Pulmonary thromboembolism is a potential complication of hyperadrenocorticism and presumably also can occur with excessive exogenous GLC. The exact pathophysiologic mechanism is unknown but may be a result of obesity, hypertension, increased hematocrit level, or hypercoagulability. In addition, because of the myopathic effect of GLCs, muscles of respiratory function may be weakened in animals receiving high doses of GLCs.[9]

Growth Retardation

The administration of small doses of GLCs to children has been associated with retardation of growth. The mechanism may reflect changes in collagen synthesis but is likely to be much more complex. Prepartum exposure to GLCs can predispose experimental animals to malformations (e.g., cleft palate).

CONTRAINDICATIONS

GLCs produce profound actions on virtually all systems of the body. Many of these effects can be tolerated by a healthy animal, but in certain disease states the use of GLCs may be deleterious. Diseases and conditions that the authors consider to be major, moderate, and minor contraindications to GLC therapy are mentioned in the subsequent sections.

Infectious Disease

Infectious diseases are a major contraindication. GLCs can exacerbate viral, bacterial, and fungal infections because of their immunosuppressive properties (although a single antiinflammatory dose of a short-acting agent is unlikely to be harmful).

Diabetes Mellitus

Diabetes mellitus is a major contraindication. GLC-mediated gluconeogenesis and general anti-insulin effects make regulating diabetic patients difficult.

Renal Failure

Renal failure is a moderate contraindication. Increased protein catabolism induced by GLCs results in increased quantities of nitrogenous waste products to be excreted. Additionally, patients with renal failure are already immunocompromised. Further immunosuppression would greatly increase their risk of developing pyelonephritis.

Corneal Ulceration

Corneal ulceration is a major contraindication. Topically administered GLCs delay healing of the cornea and may lead to corneal perforation.

Pancreatitis

Pancreatitis is a moderate contraindication. GLCs are believed to aggravate pancreatitis by increasing fatty acid circulation.

Gastrointestinal Ulceration

Gastrointestinal ulceration is a moderate contraindication. GLCs promote progression of ulcerative disease by delaying healing, increasing acid and pepsin secretion, and reducing the rate of mucosal cell proliferation in the gastrointestinal tract. Patients with eosinophilic enteritis, lymphocytic–plasmacytic enteritis, and certain ulcerative and granulomatous enteritides are potential exceptions. Colonic ulceration is a significant risk in animals with spinal trauma that are receiving dexamethasone. Concurrent administration of a nonsteroidal antiinflammatory drug greatly increases the likelihood of gastrointestinal ulceration and is *not* recommended. Misoprostol, a prostaglandin E_2 analog, may provide protection against GLC-induced gastric ulceration.

Pregnancy

Pregnancy is a moderate contraindication. GLC administration has been associated with abortion and cleft palate in the dog. Additionally, GLC administration to a bitch within 24 hours of parturition reduces neonatal intestinal permeability of immunoglobulins, thereby reducing colostrum absorption.[108]

Epilepsy

Epilepsy is a moderate contraindication. Endogenous GLCs suppress neuronal excitability, perhaps by potentiating the inhibitory effects of the neurotransmitter γ-aminobutyric acid. Chronic GLC use has been reported to be associated with lowering the seizure threshold. The mechanism for this possible effect is not clear. Exogenous GLCs may; however, downregulate steroid receptors, resulting in increased neuronal excitability.

REFERENCES

1. Mol JA, van Wolferen M, et al: Predicted primary and antigenic structure of canine corticotropin-releasing hormone, *Neuropeptides* 27:7, 1994.
2. Prigent H, Maxime V, Annane D: Clinical review: corticotherapy in sepsis, *Crit Care* 8(2):122–129, 2004.
3. Feldman EC, Nelson RW: Hypoadrenocorticism (Addison's disease). In Feldman EC, Nelson RW, editors: *Canine and feline endocrinology and reproduction*, ed 3, St Louis, 2004, Saunders, pp 394–439.

4. Webster JI, Sternberg EM: Role of the hypothalamic–pituitary–adrenal axis, glucocorticoids and glucocorticoid receptors in toxic sequelae of exposure to bacterial and viral products, *J Endocrinol* 181:207–221, 2004.
5. Funder JW, Mihailidou AS: Aldosterone and mineralocorticoid receptors: Clinical studies and basic biology, *Mol Cell Endocrinol* 301(1-2):2–6, 2009.
6. Alderson AL, Novack TA: Neurophysiological and clinical aspects of glucocorticoids and memory: a review, *J Clin Exp Neuropsychol* 24(3):335–355, 2002.
7. Burnstein KL, Cidlowski JA: The down side of glucocorticoid receptor regulation, *Mol Cell Endocrinol* 83:C1, 1992.
8. Rashid S, Lewis GF: The mechanisms of differential glucocorticoid and mineralocorticoid action in the brain and peripheral tissues, *Clin Biochem* 38:401–409, 2005.
9. Schimmer BP, Parker KL: Adrenocorticotropic hormone: adrenocortical steroids and their synthetic analogs; inhibitors of the synthesis and actions of adrenocortical hormones. In Brunton LL, Lazo JS, Parker KL, editors: *Goodman & Gilman's the pharmacological basis of therapeutics*, ed 11, New York, 2006, McGraw-Hill, pp 1587–1612.
10. Mangos GJ, Whitworth JA, Williamson PM: Glucocorticoids and the kidney, *Nephrology* 8:267–273, 2003.
11. Gupa BBP, Lalchhandama K: Molecular mechanisms of glucocorticoid action, *Curr Sci* 83(9):1103–1111, 2002.
12. Rhen T, Cidlowsk JA: Inflammatory action of glucocorticoids—new mechanisms for old drugs, *N Engl J Med* 353:1711–1723, 2005.
12a. Haller J, Mikics E, Makara GB: The effects of non-genomic glucocorticoid mechanisms on bodily functions and the central neural system. A critical evaluation of findings, *Front Neuroendocrinol* 29(2):273–291, 2008.
13. Reutner W, Smith CL: In vitro glucocorticoid receptor binding and transcriptional activation by topically active glucocorticoids, *Arzneimittelforschung* 48(9):956–960, 1998.
14. Kumar R, Thompson EB: Gene regulation by the glucocorticoid receptor: structure: function relationship, *J Steroid Biochem Mol Biol* 94:383–394, 2005.
15. Bodine PV, Litwack G: The glucocorticoid receptor and its endogenous regulators. In Litwack G, editor: *Receptor*, Clifton, N.J, 1990, Humana, p 83.
16. Schulz M, Eggert M: Novel ligands: fine tuning the transcriptional activity of the glucocorticoid receptor, *Curr Pharm Des* 10:2817–2826, 2004.
17. Dostert A, Heinzel T: Negative glucocorticoid receptor response elements and their role in glucocorticoid action, *Curr Pharm Des* 10:2807–2816, 2004.
18. Brattsand R: The ideal steroid, *Curr Pharm Des* 9:956–1964, 2003.
19. Bacher S, Schmitz LM: The NFκB pathway as a potential target for autoimmune disease therapy, *Curr Pharm Des* 10:2827–2837, 2004.
20. da Silva JAP, Jacobs JWG, Kinwan JR, et al: Low-dose glucocorticoid therapy in rheumatoid arthritis. A revew on safety: published evidence and prospective trial data, Ann Rhem Dis *online* , Aug 26, 2005:Downloaded from ard.Bmjournals.com:10-10-2005.
21. Lamberts SWJ, Koper JW, et al: Familial and iatrogenic cortisol receptor resistance, *J Steroid Biochem Mol Biol* 43:385, 1992.
22. Shipman GF, Bloomfield CD, Gajl-Peczalska KJ, et al: Glucocorticoids and lymphocytes. III. Effects of glucocorticoid administration on lymphocyte glucocorticoid receptors, *Blood* 61(6):1086–1090, 1983.
23. Reding R, Webber SA, Fine R: Getting rid of steroids in pediatric solid-organ transplantation, *Pediatr Transplant* 8:526–530, 2004.
24. Akpek G, Lee SM, Anders V, et al: A high dose pulse steroid regimen for controlling active chronic graft-versus-host diseases, *Biol Blood Bone Marr Transpl* 7:495–501, 2001.
25. Farrell RJ, Kelleher D: Mechanisms of steroid action and resistance in inflammation: glucocorticoid resistance in inflammatory bowel disease, *J Endocrinol* 178:339–346, 2003.
26. Tanaka J, Fujita H, Matsuda S, et al: Glucocorticoid and mineralocorticoid receptors in microglial cells: the two receptors mediate differential effects of corticosteroids, *Glia* 20(1):23–37, 1997.
27. Haynes RC Jr: Adrenocorticotropic hormone: adrenocortical steroids and their synthetic analogs; inhibitors of the synthesis and actions of adrenocortical hormones. In Gilman AG, Rall TW, et al, editors: *The pharmacological basis of therapeutics*, ed 8, New York, 1990, Pergamon, p 1445.
28. Planey SL, Litwack G: Glucocorticoid-induced apoptosis in lymphocytes, *Biochem Biophys Res Commun* 279(2):307, 2000.
29. Sugimoto Y, Ogawa M, Tai N, et al: Inhibitory effects of glucocorticoids on rat eosinophil superoxide generation and chemotaxis, *Int Immunopharmacol* 3(6):845–852, 2003.
30. Druilhe A, Létuvé S, Pretolani M: Glucocorticoid-induced apoptosis in human eosinophils: mechanisms of action, *Apoptosis* 8(5):481–495, 2003.
31. Reichardt HM: Immunomodulatory activities of glucocorticoids: insights from transgenesis and gene targeting, *Curr Pharm Des* 10:2797–2805, 2004.
32. Ristimaki A, Narko K, Hla T: Down-regulation of cytokine-induced cyclo-oxygenase-2 transcript isoforms by dexamethasone: evidence for post-transcriptional regulation, *Biochem J* 318(Pt 1):325–331, 1996.
33. Crofford LJ: COX-1 and COX-2 tissue expression: implications and predictions, *J Rheumatol Suppl* 49:15–19, 1997.
34. Pujols L, Benitez P, Alobid I, et al: Glucocorticoid therapy increases COX-2 gene expression in nasal polyps in vivo, *Eur Respir J* 33:502–508, 2009.
35. Pfeilschifter J, Eberhardt W, Hummel R, et al: Therapeutic strategies for the inhibition of inducible nitric oxide synthase—potential for a novel class of anti-inflammatory agents, *Cell Biol Int* 20(1):51–58, 1996.
36. Campbell WB: Lipid-derived autocoids: eicosanoids and platelet activating factor. In Gilman AG, Rall TW, et al: *The pharmacological basis of therapeutics*, ed 8, New York, 1990, Pergamon, p 600.
37. Yang YH, Hutchinson P, Santos LL, et al: Glucocorticoid inhibition of adjuvant arthritis synovial macrophage nitric oxide production: role of lipocortin 1, *Clin Exp Immunol* 111:117–122, 1998.
38. Saruta T: Mechanism of glucocorticoid induced hypertension, *Hypertens Res* 19:1–8, 1996.
39. Wallerath T, Witte K, Schafer SC, et al: Down-regulation of the expression of endothelial NO synthase is likely to contribute to glucocorticoid-mediated hypertension, *Proc Natl Acad Sci U S A* 96(23):13357–13362, 1999.
39b. Ng MK, Celermajer DS: Glucocorticoid treatment and cardiovascular disease, *Heart* 90(8):829–830, 2004.
40. Seale JP, Compton MR: Side-effects of corticosteroid agents, *Med J Aust* 144:217, 1989.
41. Glade MJ, Krook L, et al: Morphologic and biochemical changes in cartilage of foals treated with dexamethasone, *Cornell Vet* 73:170, 1983.
42. Adams ME: Cartilage research and treatment of osteoarthritis, *Curr Opin Rheumatol* 4:552, 1992.
43. Shirasawa N, Yamanouchi H: Glucocorticoids induce glutamine synthetase in folliculostellate cells of rat pituitary glands in vivo and in vitro, *J Anat* 194(Pt 4):567–577, 1999.
44. Vardimon L: Neuroprotection by glutamine synthetase, *Isr Med Assoc J* 2(Suppl):46–51, 2000.
45. Obrenovitch TP: High extracellular glutamate and neuronal death in neurological disorders. Cause, contribution or consequence, *Ann NY Acad Sci* 890:273–286, 1999.
45b. Albrecht J, Sonnewald U, Waagepetersen HS, et al: Glutamine in the central nervous system: function and dysfunction, *Front Biosci* 12:332–343, 2007.

46. Barnes PJ: Our changing understanding of asthma, *Respir Med* 83(Suppl):217, 1989.
47. Horcicka V, Linduskova M, Vykydal M: Injury to gastric mucosa due to cortisonoid therapy, *Acta Univ Palacki Olomuc Fac Med* 126:151–155, 1990.
48. Filaretova L, Mattcev N, Bogdanov A, et al: Role of gastric microcirculation in the gastroprotection by glucocorticoids released during water restraint stress in rats, *Clin J Physiol* 42:145–152, 1999.
49. Ventura MT, Muratore L, Calogiuri GF, et al: Allergic and pseudoallergic reactions induced by glucocorticoids: a review, *Curr Pharm Des* 9(24):1956–1964, 2003.
50. Roberts SM, Lavach JD, Macy DW, et al: Effect of ophthalmic prednisolone acetate on the canine adrenal gland and hepatic function, *Am J Vet Res* 45:1711–1713, 1984.
51. Meyer DJ, Moriello KA, et al: Effect of otic medications on liver function test results in healthy dogs, *J Am Vet Med Assoc* 196:743, 1990.
52. Zenoble RD, Kemppainen RJ: Adrenocortical suppression by topically applied corticosteroids in healthy dogs, *J Am Vet Assoc* 191:685–688, 1987.
53. Ghubash R, Marsella R, Kunkle G: Evaluation of adrenal function in small-breed dogs receiving otic glucocorticoids, *Vet Dermatol* 15:363–368, 2004.
54. Ginel PJ, Garrido C, Lucena R: Effects of otic betamethasone on intradermal testing in normal dogs, *Vet Dermatol* 18:205–210, 2007.
55. Aniya JS, Griffin CE: The effect of otic vehicle and concentration of dexamethasone on liver enzyme activities and adrenal function in small breed healthy dogs, *Vet Dermatol* 19:226–231, 2008.
56. Reeder CJ, Griffin CE, Polissar NL, et al: Comparative adrenocortical suppression in dogs with otitis externa following topical otic administration of four different glucocorticoid-containing-medications, *Vet Ther* 9(2):111–121, 2008.
57. Willis-Goulet HS, Schmidt BA, Nicklin CF, et al: Comparison of serum dexamethasone concentrations in cats after oral or transdermal administration using Pluronic Lecithin Organogel (PLO): a pilot study, *Vet Dermatol* 14:83–89, 2005.
58. Ueda K, Okamura N, Hirai M, et al: Human P-glycoprotein transports cortisol, aldosterone, and dexamethasone, but not progresterone, *J Biol Chem* 267(34):24248–24252, 1992.
59. Graham-Mize CA, Rosser EJ: Bioavailability and activity of prednisone and prednisolone in the feline patient, Plenary Session Abstracts, *Vet Dermatol* 25(Suppl 1):1–19, 2004.
60. Rohatag S, Appajosyula S, Derendorf H, et al: Risk-benefit value of inhaled glucocorticoids: a pharmacokinetic/pharmacodynamic perspective, *J Clin Pharmacol* 44:37–47, 2004.
61. McCormich JR, Herman AH, Lien WM, et al: Hydrocortisoine metabolism in the adrenalactomized dogs: the quantitative significance of each organ system in the total metabolic clearance of hydrocortisone, *Endocrinology* 94:17–26, 1974.
62. El Dareer SM, Struck RF, White VM, et al: Distribution and metabolism of prednisone in mice, dogs, and monkeys, *Cancer Treat Rep* 61(7):1279–1289, 1977.
63. Colburn WA, Sibley CR, Buller RH: Comparative serum prednisone and prednisolone concentrations following prednisone or prednisolone administration to beagle dogs, *J Pharm Sci* 65:997–1001, 1976.
63a. Tse FLS, Welling PG: Prednisolone bioavailability in the dog, *J Pharm Sci* 66:1751–1754, 1977.
64. Boothe DM, Bockelman A: Absorption of prednisolone and prednisone after transdermal versus oral administration in cats, In preparation, 2011.
64a. Uribe M, Summerskill WH: Comparative serum prednisone and prednisolone following administration to patients with chronic active liver disease, *Clin Pharmacokinet* 7:452–459, 1982.
65. Arvidsson S, Falt K, Haglund U: Feline *E. coli* bacteremia—effects of misoprostol/scavengers or methylprednisolone on hemodynamic reactions and gastrointestinal mucosal injury, *Acta Chir Scand* 156:215–221, 1990.
66. Means ED, Anderson DK, Waters TR, et al: Effect of methylprednisolone in compression trauma to the feline spinal cord, *J Neurosurg* 55:200–208, 1981.
67. Coates JR, Simpson S, Wright J, et al: Clinicopathologic effects of a 21 aminosteroid compound (U743894) and high dose methylprednisolone on spinal cord function after simulated spinal cord trauma, *Vet Surg* 24:128–139, 1995.
68. Toutain PL, Autefage A, Oukessou M, et al: Pharmacokinetics of methylprednisolone succinate, methylprednisolone, and lidocaine in the normal dog and during hemorrhagic shock, *J Pharm Sci* 76(7):528–534, 1987.
69. Greco DS, Brown SA, Gauze JJ, et al: Dexamethasone pharmacokinetics in clinically normal dogs during low- and high-dose dexamethasone suppression testing, *Am J Vet Res* 54(4):580–585, 1993.
70. Astra Zeneca, Budesonide (Rhinocort) package insert.
71. Hammer S, Spika I, Sippl W, et al: Glucocorticoid receptor interactions with glucocorticoids: evaluation by molecular modeling and functional analysis of glucocorticoid receptor mutants, *Steroids* 68:329–339, 2003.
72. Tumulty J, Broussard J, Steiner JM, et al: The influence of budesonide on the pituitary-adrenal axis in dogs with inflammatory bowel disease (IBD), *ACVIM* , 2003.
73. Brown SA, Hall ED: Role of oxygen-derived free radicals in the pathogenesis of shock and trauma, with focus on central nervous system injuries, *J Am Vet Med Assoc* 200:1849, 1992.
74. Miller WH, Scott DW: Medical management of chronic pruritus, *Compend Contin Educ Pract Vet* 16(4):449, 1994.
75. Bevier DE: Long term management of atopic disease in the dog, *Vet Clin North Am* 20:1486, 1990.
76. Gilbert S: Feline pruritis therapy. In Bonagura JD, Twedt DC, editors: *Kirk's current veterinary therapy XIV: small animal practice*, St Louis, 2009, Saunders.
77. Royschuk RA: Otitis externa part II: an update on management, *ACVIM Proc* 145, 1994.
78. Chunekamrai S, Krook LP, et al: Changes in articular cartilage after intra-articular injections of methylprednisolone acetate in horses, *Am J Vet Res* 50(10):1733, 1989.
79. Pelletier J-P, Martel-Pelletier J: Protective effects of corticosteroids on cartilage lesions and osteophyte formation in the Pond-Nuki dog model of osteoarthritis, *Arthritis Rheum* 23:181, 1989.
80. Fajardo M, Di Cesare PE: Disease-modifying therapies for osteoarthritis: current status, *Drugs Aging* 22(2):141–161, 2005.
81. Hoerlein BF, Redding RW, et al: Evaluation of dexamethasone, DMSO, mannitol, and solcoseryl in acute spinal cord trauma, *J Am Anim Hosp Assoc* 19:216, 1983.
82. Hoerlein BF, Redding RW, et al: Evaluation of naloxone crocetin, thyrotropin releasing hormone, methylprednisolone, partial myelotomy, and hemilaminectomy in the treatment of acute spinal cord trauma, *J Am Anim Hosp Assoc* 21:67, 1985.
83. Parnell NK: Chronic colitis. In Bonagura JD, Twedt DC, editors: *Current veterinary therapy XIV*, St Louis, 2009, Saunders, pp 515–520.
84. Lefering R, Neugebauer EA: Steroid controversy in sepsis and septic shock: a meta-analysis, *Crit Care Med* 23:1294–1303, 1995.
85. Hardie EM, Kruse-Elliott K: Endotoxic shock. Part II: a review of treatment, *J Vet Intern Med* 4:306–314, 1990.
86. Haskins SC: Management of septic shock, *J Am Vet Med Assoc* 200:1915, 1992.
87. Annane D, Sébille V, Trochée G, et al: A 3-level prognostic classification in septic shock based on cortisol levels and cortisol response to corticotropin, *J Am Med Assoc* 283:1038–1045, 2000.

88. Minneci PC, Deans KJ, Banks SM, et al: Meta-analysis: the effect of steroids on survival and shock during sepsis depends on the dose, *Ann Intern Med* 141:47-56, 2004.
89. Cooper MS, Stewart PM: Corticosteroid insufficiency in acutely ill patients, *N Eng J Med* 348:727-734, 2003.
90. Sprung CL, Annane D, Keh D, et al: Hydrocortisone therapy for patients with septic shock, *N Engl J Med* 358:111-124, 2008.
90a. Salem M, Tainish RE, Bromberg J, et al: Perioperative glucocorticoid coverage. A reassessment 42 years after emergence of a problem, *Ann Surg* 219:416-425, 1984.
90b. Jung C, Inder WJ: Management of adrenal insufficiency during the stress of medical illness and surgery, *The Med J Aust* 188:409-413, 2008.
91. Price G, Page R, Fischer B, et al: Efficacy and toxicity of doxorubicin/cyclophosphamide maintenance therapy in dogs with multicentric lymphosarcoma, *J Vet Int Med* 5:259-262, 1991.
92. Mealey KL, Bentjen SA, Gay JM, et al: Dexamethasone treatment of a canine, but not human, tumour cell line increases chemoresistance independent of P-glycoprotein and multidrug resistance-related protein expression, *Vet Comp Oncol* 1:67-75, 2003.
93. McCaw DL, Miller MA, et al: Response of canine mast cell tumors to treatment with oral prednisone, *J Vet Intern Med* 8(6):406, 1994.
94. Hollingsworth SR: Ocular immunotherapy. In Bonagura JD, Twedt DC, editors: *Kirk's current veterinary therapy XIV*, St Louis, 2009, Saunders, pp 1149-1153.
94a. Bourcier T, Forgez P, Bordene V, et al: Regulation of human corneal epithelial cell proliferation and apoptosis by dexamethasone, *Invest Ophthamol Vis Sci* 41:4133-4141, 2000.
95. Belvisi MG, Bunchschuh DS, Stoeck S, et al: Preclinical profile of ciclesonide, a novel corticosteroid for the treatment of asthma, *J Pharmacol Exp Ther* 314(2):568-574, 2005.
96. Steffan J, Alexander D, Brovedani F, et al: Comparison of cyclosporine A with methylprednisolone for treatment of canine atopic dermatitis: a parallel, blinded randomized controlled trial, *Vet Dermatol* 14:11-22, 2003.
97. Levine JM, Levine GJ, Boozer L, et al: Adverse effects and outcome associated with dexamethasone administration in dogs with acute thoracolumbar intervertebral disk herniation: 161 cases (2000-2006), *J Am Vet Med Assoc* 232:411-417, 2008.
98. Bakke HK, Murison R, Walther B: Effect of central noradrenaline depletion on corticosterone levels and gastric ulcerations in rats, *Brain Res* 368(2):256-261, 1986.
99. Badylak SE, Van Fleet JF: Sequential morphological and clinic pathologic alterations in dogs with experimentally induced glucocorticoid hepatopathy, *Am J Vet Res* 42:1310-1318, 1981.
100. Fittshen C, Bellamy JE: Prednisone-induced morphologic and chemical changes in the liver of dogs, *Vet Pathol* 21:399-406, 1984.
101. Feldman EC, Nelson RW: Hypothyroidism. In Feldman EC, Nelson RW, editors: *Canine and feline endocrinology and reproduction*, ed 3, St Louis, 2004, Saunders, pp 86-151.
102. Ihrke PJ, Norton AL, Ling GV, et al: Urinary tract infection associated with long-term corticosteroid administration in dogs with chronic skin diseases, *J Am Vet Med Assoc* 186:43-46, 1985.
103. Torres SM, Dias SF, Nogueir SA, et al: Frequency of urinary tract infection among dogs with pruritic disorders receiving long-term glucocorticoid treatment, *J Am Vet Med Assoc* 227:239-243, 2005.
103a. Grose R, Werner S, Kessler D, et al: A role for endogenous glucocorticoids in wound repair, *EMBO Reports* 3:575-582, 2002.
104. Calogiuri GF, Muratore L, Nettis E, et al: Anaphylaxis to hydrocortisone hemisuccinate with cross-sensitivity to related compounds in a paediatric patient, *Br J Dermatol* 151(3):707-708, 2004.
105. Nakamura H, Matsuse H, Obase Y, et al: Clinical evaluation of anaphylactic reactions to intravenous corticosteroids in adult asthmatics, *Respiration* 69:309-313, 2002.
106. Erdmann SM, Abuzabra F, Merk HF, et al: Anaphylaxis induced by glucocorticoids, *J Am Board Fam Pract* 18:143-146, 2005.
107. Schaer M, Ginn PE, Hanel RM: A case of fatal anaphylaxis in a dog associated with a dexamethasone suppression test, *J Vet Emerg Crit Care* 15(3):213-216, 2005.
108. Gillette DD, Filkins M: Factors affecting antibody transfer in the newborn puppy, *Am J Physiol* 210(2):419, 1966.

31 Immunomodulators or Biological Response Modifiers: Introduction and Miscellaneous Agents*

Dawn Merton Boothe

Chapter Outline

THE IMMUNE RESPONSE

Immunomodulators, or biological response modifiers, are agents or drugs that act to regulate or modify the host's immune response to a microbe, neoplasm, or inflammatory response. It is beyond the scope of this chapter to provide a comprehensive review of the immune system. The following is a general review only. Cytokine biology can also be reviewed elsewhere,[1,2] as can interferon (IFN) biology.[3]

Immune Defenses

Immune defenses are composed of the innate and adaptive systems. The innate systems are nonspecific in their response and are best exemplified by barriers provided by the integument; the gastrointestinal environment (acid pH, mucosal and epithelial barriers, microbiota); the mucociliary tract of the respiratory system; and the intimate vasculature of selected organs such as the placenta, brain, and prostate. Other nonspecific defense mechanisms are exemplified fever and the antimicrobial actions of many secretions. White blood cells also represent innate immunity. These include neutrophils, eosinophils, basophils, macrophages, and dendritic cells, and unconventional T-cell subsets bearing T-cell receptors (TCR), natural killer (NK; CD1d) cells and gamma/delta (γδ) T-cells. Natural killer (NK) cells are innate (non conventional) cytotoxic T cells that work in concert with the adaptive arm of immunity, targeting compromised host cells such as tumor or virally infected cells. Released in the vicinity of a cell slated for destruction, it is stimulated by macrophage cytokines. They recognize targeted cells which containing abnormally low concentrations of major histocompatibility complex [MHC] class I antigen ("missing self"). Materials that induce apoptosis enter the target cell through the pores, thus avoiding cellular lysis, which is of benefit in the presence of virally-infected cells that might release viral materials causing host re-infection. NK cells exhibiting the FrC receptor interact with the humoral arm of adaptive immunity, causing antibody-dependent cell cytotoxicity. Gamma-delta

*The author and publisher wish to acknowledge the original contributions of S. Kruth for the Regressin-V and Acemannan sections of this chapter.

T cells contain characteristics of both the innate and adaptive systems.

The adaptive immune system provides the host an ability to recognize and, with subsequent presentation, remember specific pathogens (B and T memory cells), and increasingly stronger responses each time the pathogen is presented. These capabilities reflect both hypermutability and irreversible genetic recombination in cells that are carried forward in subsequent progeny. The system is composed of two major arms, cell-mediated immunity and humoral immunity, each accompanied by a variable number of cells and their chemical mediators. Some of the nonspecific components are also part of the innate immune system, including phagocytic circulating leukocytes and tissue macrophages, and secretions or body fluids such as IFN, complement, and leukocyte substances such as lysozyme. The adaptive arm of the immune system provides the primary targets of pharmacologic manipulation. The adaptive response recognizes both non-self and missing-self antigens. As such, MHC plays a major role in the adaptive arm of the immune system. This large gene complex encodes proteins unique to the individual. Expression on the cell surface allows recognition of self by relevant cell types. At least two subgroups of MHC are important in adaptive immunity. All cells, save non-nucleated cells, generally express MHC class I peptides on the cell surface. They are derived from the cytosol and contain other cytosolic proteins. Abnormalities in MHC class I expression that initiate an adaptive response generally result in interactions exclusively with CD8+ cells, inducing apoptosis. The MHC class II complexes are located on antigen-presenting cells, including dendritic, macrophage, activated T cells, and B cells. These peptides generally are associated with presentation of extracellular pathogens, and presentation that results in an adaptive response generally reflects interactions only with CD4+ cells (T helper or T_h cells).

KEY POINT 31-1 The primary targets of pharmacologic manipulation of the immune system are the adaptive arms of the immune system.

Both cell-mediated and humoral immune mechanisms are characterized by specificity toward antigenic epitopes expressed as molecular components of infectious organisms, foreign (transplanted) cells, or transformed (malignant) cells. Cytokines, including soluble growth and activation factors (Table 31-1), are a vital component of the adaptive response and are released and subsequently mediate the response of the various cell populations involved in both cell-mediated and humoral immunity.[4] In addition to cytokines, a number of other molecules (e.g., adhesion or accessory molecules) are necessary as "second signals" for antigen processing, recognition, or response.[4]

Effectors

The following is a brief synopsis of the events following infection to implementation of the immune response (Figure 31-1). The antigen is exposed to an antigen-processing or presenting cell (APC), which includes dendritic cells (the principle APC), macrophages, and activated B cells.[4] The antigen is identified by the APC as foreign and is subsequently phagocytized by the APC. The APC "processes" the antigen and "exhibits" it on the cell surface in a groove made by the MHC molecule. Peptides derived from endogenous cytosolic proteins synthesized within the cell complex (including those synthesized in response to viral stimuli) are expressed with class II MHC molecules on the cell surface, whereas exogenous intracellular proteins are expressed bound to a class I MHC groove for presentation.[4]

A single APC surface may have tens of thousands of MHC molecules, each containing a different peptide; a single animal may have more than 10^8 APCs. The APC migrates to the T cell area of a lymph node and presents the antigen to naïve CD4 T cells. If the APC comes into contact with a CD4 T cell with a TCR that recognizes the antigen associated with the MHC, it becomes activated. The release of adhesion molecules causes the two cells to stick together, which facilitates interaction between the APC and the CD4. Cytokines move between the two cells, and production of interleukin-1 (IL-1) by the APC and interleukin-2 (IL-2) from the activated CD4 cell itself amplifies the sequelae of CD4 activation. The activated CD4 cell differentiates, proliferates, and produces a number of cytokines (see Table 31-1), which results in recruitment of other leukocytes, initiation of B cell production of immunoglobulins (Igs), and formation of other T cell colonies, including "memory" cells (see Figure 31-1).[4,5]

Cellular Components

Efficient pathogen elimination depends on the adaptive immune response. Two classes of lymphocytes are responsible for adaptive immunity (see Figure 31-1). B lymphocytes must be programmed to respond to antigen exposure and, after activation to plasma cells, are responsible for the production of specific Igs (humoral response). T lymphocytes provide the primary regulation of the immune response. T cell activity begins with specific antigen recognition by a receptor on the surface of the cell.[4] T cells are further subdivided into several populations of cells depending on their role in immunoregulation (see Figure 31-1). Helper cell (CD4 T cells; T_h cells) receptors recognize and bind to the peptide–MHC class II complex of APC cells. In response to IL-1, CD4 cells consequently proliferate and become primed as either T_h1 or T_h2 CD4 cells, which modulate further responses in both the cell-mediated and humoral arms (see Figure 31-1). Migration of activated lymphocytes from lymph nodes to tissues is facilitated by adhesion molecules expressed by endothelial cells in tissues. Whether a T cell becomes T_h1 or T_h2 reflects the stimulating cytokine: IL-12 activates signal transducer and activator of transcription 4 (STAT-4), which regulates T_h1 differentiation, whereas IL-4 activates STAT-6 and T_h2 differentiation.[5]

KEY POINT 31-2 T lymphocytes provide the primary regulation of the immune response, whereas B lymphocytes must be programmed to respond to antigen exposure.

Table 31-1 Immune Modulatory Functions of Cytokines

Chemokine	Produced by	Target Cells	Effect
GM-CSF	Macrophages	Myeloid stem cells	Differentiation to granulocytes and monocytes
IFN-alpha	Leukocytes	Normal cells	Antiviral, MHC I expression
IFN-β	Fibroblasts	Multiple	Antiviral, MHC I expression
IFN-γ	T_h1	Multiple	Antiviral, MHC I expression
	Tc	Macrophages	MHC expression, elimination of pathogen; possible T_h2 antiproliferation
	NK	T_h2	Antiproliferation
		Activated B cells	Switch to IgG2a
IL-1	Monocytes	T_h	Activation; fever (endogenous pyrogen)
Aβ precursors)	T	B cells	Maturation, expansion
	B cells	NK cells	Activation
IL-2	T_h1	Activated T, B, NK cells	Induce proliferation, activation
IL-3	T_h1	Stem	Suppress IL-1 production
	NK	Mast cells	Proliferation, degranulation
		B (antigen primed)	Activation, differentiation, IgG and IgE synthesis
IL-4*	T_h2	B (activated)	Proliferation
		Macrophages	Class switching (MHC class II)
		T cells	Proliferation
IL-5	T_h2, most cells	Activated B cells	Differentiation, IgA synthesis
		Eosinophils	Colony-stimulating factor
IL-6	T_h2	Proliferating B cells	Differentiation to plasma cells
	Monocytes	Plasma cells	Antibody secretion
	Macrophages	Myeloid stem cells	Differentiation
	Stromal cells	Myeloid stem cells	Differentiation
		Various	Acute phase response
IL-7	Marrow stroma	Stem cells	Differentiation into T, B progenitor
	Thymus stroma		
IL-8	Connective tissue	T	Chemoattractant
	Macrophage	PMN	
IL-9*	T cells	Hemopoietic cells	Cell proliferation, apoptosis
IL-10*	T_h2	Macrophages (lymphocytes)	Suppress IL-1 production, suppress TNF-α
		B cells	Survival, activation, antibody production
IL-12	Macrophages	Activated Tc	Differentiation to Tc; production of TNF-α, IFN-γ
	B cells	T_h1	Proliferation
IL-13*	Overlap with IL-4		
MIP1-alpha	Macrophages	Monocytes, T cells	Chemoattractant
MIP1β	Lymphocytes	T cells, monocytes, macrophages	Chemoattractant
TGF-β*	T cells, monocytes	Macrophages, monocytes, activated B cells	Differentiation to granulocytes and monocytes
TNF-alpha	Macrophages, NK	Tumor cells	Cytotoxic
TNF-β	T_h1, B	Tumor cells	Cytotoxic
C3a, C5a		Mast cells	Chemoattractant

GM-CSF, Granulocyte-macrophage colony stimulating factor; *IFN,* interferon; *MHC,* major histocompatibility complex; *T_h1, 2,* helper T cells (CD4); *Ig,* immunoglobulin; *NK,* natural killer cells (a subset of cytotoxic T cells); *PMN,* polymorphonuclear leukocytes; *TNF,* tumor necrosis factor; *Tc,* killer T cells, cytotoxic (CD8); *MIP,* macrophage inflammatory factor; *TGF,* transforming growth factor; *C,* complement.
*Antiinflammatory signals included in actions.

The T_h1 subsets of CD4 produce primarily proinflammatory cytokines such as IFN-γ (IFN-γ) and tumor necrosis factor-alpha (TNF-α) (cachexin; see Figure 31-1). As such, T_h1 cells regulate signals that promote cell-mediated immunity and control intracellular pathogens. T_h1 response is paramount to successful resistance to most microbial pathogens, including bacteria, intracellular protozoa, and fungal organisms. Additionally, T_h1 cells mediate organ-specific autoimmunity and as such are crucial to the pathogenesis of autoimmune diseases. The cell-mediated response occurs when activated CD4 (T_h1) cells attract other cells (polymorphonuclear leukocytes, eosinophils, and monocytes) to support cellular killing; the result is referred to as *delayed hypersensitivity.* Activated CD4 cells also yield, in response to IL-2, helper T cells that contain the glycoprotein CD8 and are responsible for the T cell–mediated cytotoxic response. Receptors of the CD8 T cells recognize

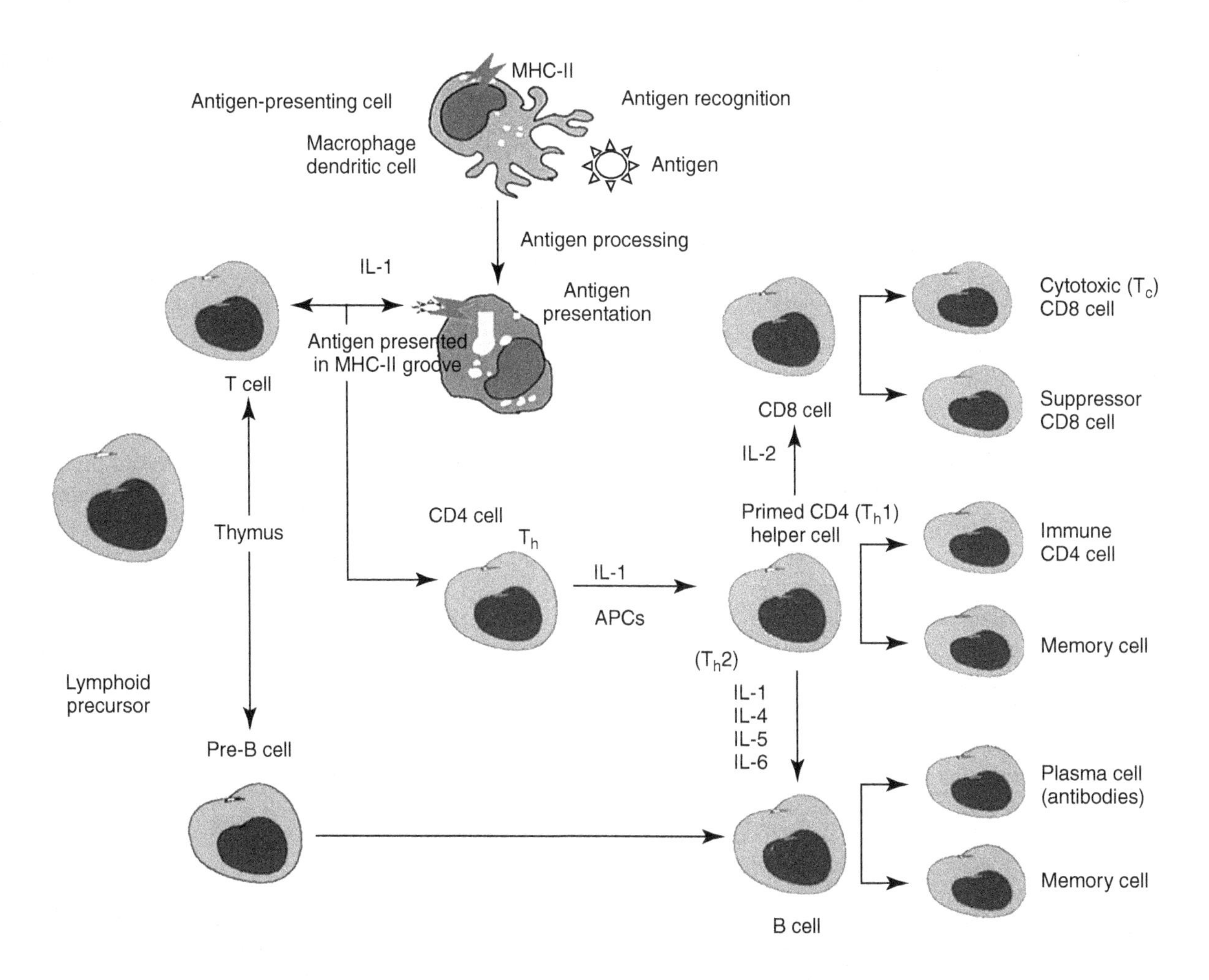

Figure 31-1 Overview of the immune response to antigen presentation. The antigen is presented to an antigen-presenting cell (APC), which processes the antigen and expresses its peptides in a groove located on the major histocompatibility complex (MHC) molecule. When presented to naïve CD4 T cells with appropriate receptors, the helper cell becomes primed to form CD8 cells, capable of directly killing cells presently containing the antigen; T_h1 cells, which result in the formation of memory T cells and T cells that attract other leukocytes (type IV hypersensitivity); or T_h2 cells, which stimulate B cell production of antibodies. A number of interleukins signal the activities; adhesion molecules (not shown) facilitate communication between cells as well as movement from lymph nodes through vascular endothelial cells into tissues. *IL*, Interleukin; *T_h*, T helper cell.

peptide–MHC class I complexes (generally associated with endogenous peptides present on all nucleated cells) on APCs. Recognition of the CD8 receptor and subsequent interaction with CD4 cells result in the generation of cytolytic (CTL) or cytotoxic T cells (T_C; killer T cells). Cytotoxic T cells are capable of directly (without further interaction with CD4 cells) causing lysis of cells expressing the targeted specific peptide–MHC complex.[4] This includes normal but otherwise damaged (include virally infected or cells damaged by TNF-β or lymphotoxin) cells. CD8 cells release several different cytotoxins which cause pores in the target cell membrane. Cytotoxic T cells also undergo clonal expansion, resulting in prepared effector cells. In contrast to T_h1 cells, T_h2 cells secrete *antiinflammatory* cytokines (IL-4, IL-9, IL-10, IL-13) (in additional to pro-inflammatory cytokines) and support the humoral immune response, including host defense against intestinal helminths. Because of their antiinflammatory effects, T_h2 cytokines can decrease autoimmune diseases associated with cell-mediated immunity; however, an imbalance toward T_h2 cells have been implicated in the pathogenesis of asthma and allergy (see below).[5] Dysregulation of the influence of STAT-4 and STAT-6—which have contrary effects—has been associated with immune-mediated diseases. For example, each STAT is reported to be involved in systemic lupus erythematosus: STAT-6 contributes to the development of glomerulosclerosis and antibody production, which is exacerbated in the absence of STAT-4.[5]

In contrast to immune-mediated diseases, in which T_h1 cells play key roles, key effector cells in all chronic allergic diseases include eosinophils, basophils, and T_h2 cells.[6] Their involvement occurs through release of preformed, or formed in situ, granule proteins and cytokines.[7] A focus on eosinophil regulation may offer targeted therapy for chronic allergic diseases. Cysteinyl leukotrienes appear to have an important role in the regulation of human eosinophil hematopoiesis, recruitment, and activation.[7] Eosinophils are generated from CD34+ progenitors in the bone marrow upon stimulation by cytokines such as IL- 5. A single dose of IL-5 antibody profoundly inhibited circulating eosinophils and allergen-induced sputum eosinophils but not airway hyperreactivity in humans. In a follow-up study, eosinophil numbers in blood and bronchoalveolar lavage were reduced 80% or more after 3 months of anti–IL-5 therapy numbers in bone marrow and bronchial biopsies were reduced 50% to 60%. This suggests that IL-5 antibody therapy effectively reduces circulating and airway luminal eosinophils, but less so bone marrow and lung parenchymal eosinophils.[8] Cys-leukotrienes (LTs) may also play a role in eosinophil regulation.Circulating eosinophil counts in humans decrease by almost 20% after treatment with cyst-LT-receptor antagonists. These effects may reflect actions at the level of the bone marrow. Eosinophil–basophil colony-forming units increase in number, adhesion, and function, including production of IL-4 when exposed in vitro in the presence of LTD4. These responses are blocked by the presence of cysLT1 antagonists.

Activation of the humoral system occurs when naïve B lymphocytes with appropriate receptors (Igs) recognize an epitope in the intact foreign antigen. The antigen binds to the Ig, is ingested, and is processed such that it is expressed on the surface of the B cell in association with the same MHC (class I or II) that presented the antigen initially.[4] Binding of the Ig receptor with the peptide and subsequent interaction with a CD4 cell that recognizes the antigen in its MHC complex stimulates proliferation of B cells, their differentiation into plasma cells, and the secretion of antibodies able to bind the epitope. Ig production is stimulated by IL-1, IL-4, IL-5, and IL-6 in B lymphocytes. The complete sequence occurs over 8 to 14 days and results in an anamnestic, or secondary, response. Generation of "memory" B and T cells provides a long-term mechanism for a rapid immune response on reexposure to the epitope (antigen).[4]

KEY POINT 31-3 The T_h1 subsets of CD4 produce primarily proinflammatory cytokines such as interferon-γ (IFN-γ) and tumor necrosis factor-alpha (TNF-α).

KEY POINT 31-4 In contrast to T_h1 cells, T_h2 cells secrete antiinflammatory cytokines and support the humoral immune response, including host defense against intestinal helminths.

Soluble Components

Soluble components of the immune response include the cytokines previously described, Igs described later, and the complement cascade.

Cytokines

More than 13 chemokine receptors are associated with rheumatoid arthritis, and at least 16 chemokines interact with these receptors.[9] Both constitutive (responsible for physiologic trafficking and homing of the adaptive immune response) and inducible (responsible for effector white blood cell recruitment, including lymphocytes) responses are involved. A number of the chemicals also are responsible for angiogenesis. The inappropriate production of chemokines is associated with formation of an ectopic germinal center, which contributes to an uncontrolled immune response. Consequently, drugs directed toward chemokine receptors offer a therapeutic approach to control.

TNFα induces a broad spectrum of activity. Cytotoxicity of multiple cell types, including tumors, reflects both apoptosis and necrosis. A large number of proteins are targeted, along with other central mediators of the inflammatory process and immune activation. Examples include nuclear factors (e.g., NFκB), nitric oxide synthetase (NOS), cell-surface molecules, MHC classes I and II, and secreted proteins such as IL (e.g., -l, -6, -8), IFN, granulocyte-macrophage colony-stimulating factor, platelet-derived growth factor, urokinase plasminogen activator, and TNF-α itself. When administered exogenously, high concentrations of TNFα causes a toxic syndrome similar to septic shock. Bacterial lipopolysaccharide is the most potent stimulator of macrophage TNFα production. TNFα appears to mediate ischemia–reperfusion injury after transplantation of the liver, kidney, intestine, heart, lung, and pancreas and is a marker cytokine during organ rejection. Inhibitors have proved useful in human medicine for treatment of a number of autoimmune diseases, including Crohn's disease, rheumatoid arthritis, psoriasis, and ankylosing spondylitis. Indications included corticosteroid-resistant graft-versus-host disease after bone marrow transplantation.[10]

KEY POINT 31-5 TNFα plays a pervasive role in the inflammatory response, interacting with a number of other cytokines and other mediators and has been identified as a major role player in the "cytokine storm" associated with some syndromes.

Not surprisingly, the pervasive role of TNFα has led to the development of drugs that inhibit its actions. Included are glucocorticoids, pentoxifylline, and monoclonal immunoglobulin G (IgG) antibodies (e.g, infliximab, etanercept and the "humanized" adalimumab) etanercept, a humanized soluble TNFα receptor (TNFR) construct, and onercept, a TNFα-binding protein.[10] A variety of other drugs targeting TNFα or its receptors are currently under investigation, as well as metalloproteinase inhibitors such as TNFα-converting enzyme (TACE). The use of these drugs, not surprisingly, is associated with a number of side effects. These include immunosuppresion, acute infusion reactions, delayed-type hypersensitivity reactions, autoimmune diseases, cardiovascular and neurologic adverse events, malignancies and lymphomas, and infectious complications.

Complement

The complement cascade is a major effector mechanism of the immune response. The cascade results in highly amplified events that interact with other physiologic cascades, including the coagulation pathway, kinin formation, and fibrinolysis.[11] Consequences of complement activation include opsonization, the release of biologically vasoactive peptides, and cellular lysis. Cell-mediated cytotoxicity is implemented by cytotoxic T lymphocytes, NK cells and antibody-dependent cell-mediated cytotoxicity (ADCC), mediated by a variety of cells that express surface Fc receptors. Effector cells of ADCC include monocytes, neutrophils, eosinophils, selected cytotoxic T cells, and NK cells.

Immunoglobulins

Five classes of Igs are recognized in animals. IgM is the largest, forming up to 15% of the total Ig present. IgM exists as a monomer or a large polymeric form. IgM is responsible for the primary Ig response; in animals, for some infections, it is the only defense.[11] The availability of five binding sites renders IgM efficient at antigen binding and agglutination, virus neutralization, and opsonization. IgM also is a potent activator of complement. Because it is such a large molecule, unless vascular permeability is altered, most IgM stays in circulation.

IgG (with multiple subclasses) makes up the majority of total Ig. It is the most soluble of the Igs and thus is able to reach extravascular spaces. Its primary biological functions are to facilitate the removal of microorganisms; neutralize toxins; and bind to microorganisms or infected cells, initiating effector mechanisms. IgG activates complement or initiates Fc-bearing effector cells (ADCC) and promotes removal of Ig-coated cells by ADCC.

IgE has a major role in the response to parasites and in the pathogenesis of allergic diseases in part because of its unique ability to bind by way of the Fc portion of the IgE molecule to specific receptors on mast cells and basophils. Cross-linkage of two IgE molecules results in calcium-mediated mast cell degranulation and the release of a number of preformed (e.g., histamine and serotonin) and synthesized (e.g., metabolites of arachidonic acid) mediators.

IgA is produced in submucosal lymphoid tissues and regional lymph nodes. After secretion outside of the cell, it travels to epithelial cells, where the secretory component of the IgA acts as a receptor, binding to IgA and stimulating its endocytosis. The two components are eventually exocytosed and attach to the mucosal surface, where they provide a protective component, neutralize toxins, adhere to bacteria and viruses, and interact with parasites.[11]

Each Ig molecule monomer comprises two heavy chains and two light chains attached by covalent bonds. The number of bonds varies with the Ig; the number of dimers varies with the class. A number of fragments (generated by enzymatic cleavage) can be described, including Fab, the antigen-combining fragment, and Fc, the crystallizable fragment, which binds to Fc receptors found on cells of the innatue immune system (e.g., NK cells, macrophages, neutrophils and mast cells).[11]

Mucosal Immunity

The common mucosal immune system (CIMS) has evolved as a system separate from the general systemic immune system. It includes the mucosa-associated lymphoid tissue (MALT), a complex network of tissues, lymphoid- and mucous membrane–associated cells and their effector molecules. Components include gut-associated lymphoid tissue (GALT) or nasal-associated lymphoid tissue (NALT), the mucosa of the genitourinary tract, the mammary and salivary glands, and draining lymph nodes. MALT differs from systemic lymphoid tissues in its characteristic lymphoid architecture, an epithelium that is unique in its uptake of antigen, and unique APCs (e.g., dendritic cells). Most notable among the differences is the predominance of IgA and the return of immune effector cells to either the originating mucosal sites or distant mucosal sites. Innate components of the CIMS include epithelial cells and antimicrobial peptides (AMP; see later discussion), the latter being exemplified by defensins; lactoferrin; lysozyme; the lactoperoxidase, secretory phospholipase A2, and cathelin-associated peptides. Adaptive components include IgA antibody and CD4+ T cell responses, and mechanisms that impart mucosal (oral) tolerance.

Effective mucosal immunity depends on induction of effective mucosal immune responses. Oral tolerance refers to the prevention of unwanted immune reactions to food or environmental antigens; such tolerance also can be induced nasally. Integral to mucosal tolerance are Toll-like receptors (TRC). Key molecules of the innate immune system, these receptors recognize conserved microbial molecules, alerting the system to their presence when physical barriers are breeched. The term "toll" refers to effect that toll gene mutations have on the physical appearance of Drisophila flies (making them appear "toll", the German translation meaning "wild"). Toll receptors are a type of pattern recognition receptor, able to distinquish host from microbial pathogen associated molecular patterns (PAMPS).

Induction of nasal mucosal tolerance can be manipulated, leading to mucosally induced immune therapy against selected infectious diseases (e.g, in *Escherichia coli* in human medicine). Mucosal tolerance has the advantage of inducing local and thus targeted T_h1- or T_h2- type immune responses, thus avoiding the negative sequelae of systemic cytokine injection. Mucosal adjuvants co-administered with antigens include cytokines (e.g., IL-1 and IL-12), or chemokines which promote specific CD4+ T helper cell cytokine responses (e.g., RANTES, lymphotactin, macrophage inhibitory protein–1 [MIP-1]). Therapeutic modulation of mucosal immunity generally targets unique T_h cells and cytokine responses. For example, inflammatory bowel diseases (IBDs) appear to reflect failure of oral tolerance to luminal antigens, resulting in an imbalance of regulatory cytokines involving both T_h1 and T_h2 cell–mediated inflammation.[12] Differences exist between orally and nasally induced immune responses. For example, aging more negatively influences GALT compared to NALT immunity. Nasal vaccines are more effective than oral vaccines in the promotion of protective immunity in the genitourinary tract. That these differences exist suggests that pharmacologic therapies might also be manipulated to locally target systemic effects or to limit therapy to local effects only, thus increasing benefits versus risks of treatment and that these therapies are likely to differentials, affect the different CIMS.

Antimicrobial and Host Defense Peptides

Antimicrobial peptides (AMPs, also called host defense peptides;) are evolutionarily ancient yet essential small cationic molecules found in animals, plants, and bacteria. Because they exhibit antimicrobial activity against a wide range of bacteria, fungi, and viruses, they are considered part of mucosal immunity. AMPs primarily act as cations, interacting with the anionic structure of and thus disrupting microbial membranes.[13] Phosphatidylcholine in eukaryotic cell membranes is thought to be more positive compared to that in prokaryotic membranes, thus decreasing attraction to (or repelling) positively charged AMPs. However, in addition to antimicrobial actions, AMPs also serve as multifunctional mediators of immunity, inflammation, and wound repair. The importance of AMP or HDP in veterinary medicine has been reviewed by Linde and coworkers.[14]

KEY POINT 31-6 Antimicrobial peptides are an ancient evolutionary arm of the mucosal immune system that act to disrupt microbial membranes.

Three major classes of antimicrobial molecules have been described: defensins, cathelicidins, and the four-disulfide core proteins, secretory leukocyte proteinase inhibitor (SLPI) and elafin. Cathelicidins are produced and stored inactive yet capable of exhibiting broad-spectrum killing activity. The number of cathelicidins among species ranges from multiple (pigs and cows) to one (humans and mice). The SLPI and elafin exhibit antimicrobial activity toward a number of bacteria (e.g., *E. coli, Pseudomonas aeruginosa, Staphylococcus aureus, Staphylococcus epidermis,* and group A *Streptococcus*); fungi (e.g., *Aspergillus fumigatus* and *Candida albicans*); and selected viruses (e.g., human immunodeficiency virus). In addition to their antimicrobial properties, SLPI and elafin are potent antiproteases, neutralizing potentially harmful proteases (e.g, human neutrophil elastase) and inhibiting proinflammatory microbial products (e.g., lipopolysaccharide). Many are chemotactic for white blood cells, including T lymphocytes. Other activities include, but are not limited to stimulation of angiogenesis or inhibition of signals which activate B cells (e.g., NFκB).

The AMPs are extensively integrated into other defense systems. They are stimulated by a number of signals (e.g, macrophage cytokines such as IL-β and TNF-α). In contrast, microbes may protect themselves by downregulating AMP expression. Microorganisms have other protective mechanisms, including changes in cell wall or membrane composition, secretion of factors that block AMP action, or manipulation of host cells such that AMP activity is decreased.

It is likely that the ability of AMP to modulate inflammation, immunity, and tissue repair processes contributes to a central role in numerous essential host defenses. Pharmacologic modulation of AMP is a focus of investigation for a treatment and prevention measures for a variety of disease, including as adjuvants for tumor or infectious vaccines.

Hypersensitivity Reactions and Cytokine Storm

An imbalance in the activities of CD4 T_h1 and T_h2 subsets may be responsible for the onset or exacerbation of immune-mediated diseases. Increased concentrations of T_h1 (and decreased T_h2) are associated with response to viral and fungal infections, whereas increased concentrations of T_h2 (and decreased T_h1) are associated with increased production of IgE and IgA antibodies. Autoimmune diseases are associated with a predominance (reflecting an imbalance) of T_h1. Imbalances also have been associated with resistance to infectious disease and malignancy.[15] In contrast, allergic inflammatory diseases (eg., atopy, inflammatory bowel disease, asthma) may reflect an imbalance that favors T_h2.

KEY POINT 31-7 An imbalance in the activities of CD4 T_h1 and T_h2 subsets may be responsible for the onset or exacerbation of immune-mediated diseases.

Multiple novel mechanisms have been identified for their underlying role in the pathogenesis of immune-mediated diseases. Most, if not all, involve transcription factors, each providing potential current of future opportunities for manipulation. Among the prominent immune-mediated diseases being intensely studied in an attempt to understand the molecular mechanisms of immune mediated diseases are diabetes type 1, rheumatoid arthritis, multiple sclerosis, IBDs, psoriasis, and systemic lupus erythematosus (SLE).[16]

Four types of reactions result from activation of immunologic pathways. Type I hypersensitivity results from antigen–IgE interaction (Figure 31-2). IgE that has previously interacted with the antigen binds to the surface of a basophil or mast cell. Subsequent interaction with the same antigen causes mast cell degranulation and the release of a number of mediators associated with *immediate hypersensitivity.* Mediator release can be instantaneous (e.g., anaphylaxis); delayed for 2 to 4 hours; or biphasic, with both an immediate and a delayed reaction. Systemic release of mediator results in systemic anaphylaxis; localized mediator release limits reaction to the site of release (eg, swelling, redness, pain). Atopy is an inherited predisposition to develop IgE antibodies to environmental antigens and is characterized by constant high levels of IgE. An *anaphylactoid* reaction may be similar to anaphylaxis in presentation but reflects nonimmune-mediated mast cell degranulation (e.g., cationic drug-induced) (see Chapter 4).

Type II hypersensitivity occurs when ADCC occurs after antibody binds to a cell or to an exogenous antigen associated with a cell surface or a basement membrane. Complement may be activated and contribute to the damage. Examples of type II hypersensitivity include drug hypersensitivities, autoimmune hemolytic anemia, immune-mediated thrombocytopenia, immune-mediated endocrinopathies, and immune-mediated dermatologic disorders such as bullous pemphigus.[11]

Type III hypersensitivity results from the formation of antigen–antibody or immune complexes that either circulate or are deposited as microprecipitates in vascular beds or

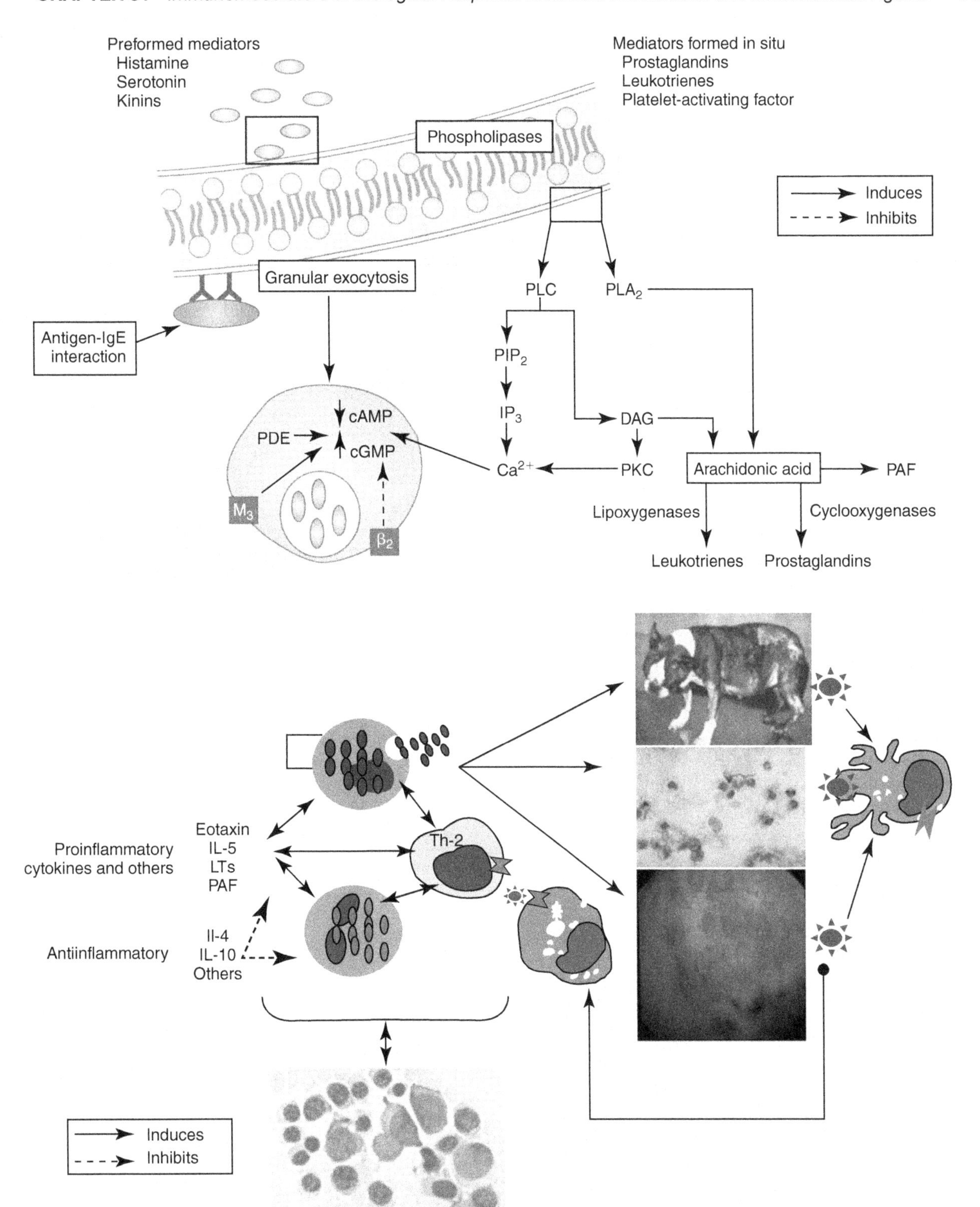

Figure 31-2 The shared pathophysiology of chronic allergic inflammatory disease begins with antigen processing at the tissue (e.g., skin, airways, gastrointestinal tract). Presentation and subsequent T_h2 helper cell acitivity results in signaling to basophils and eosinophils. Their release of inflammatory mediators at the site may perpetuate the response by increasing tissue permeability, allowing access of the antigen to deeper tissues. The chemotactant cytokine eotaxin and its interaction with interleukin-5 plays a major role in stimulating local responses as well as bone marrow production of eosinophils; leukotrienes may serve as signals for these interactions. Ultimately, cells released from the bone marrow perpetuate the response at the tissue. Accordingly, therapy might target not only the affected tissue (including adjuvant therapy) but also the bone marrow itself. *Inset:* Diagrammatic representation of a type I hypersensitivity reaction involving antigen bound to immunoglobulin E and calcium-mediated degranulation. Degranulation results in the release of both preformed mediators and mediators formed in situ (e.g., from arachidonic acid). Stimulation of muscarinic (M_3) receptors supports exocytosis, which is inhibited by stimulation of beta$_2$-adrenergic receptors. *cAMP,* Cyclic adenosine monophosphate; *cGMP,* cyclic guanosine monophosphate; *DAG*, diacylglycerol; *IP_3,* inositol triphosphate; *PAF,* platelet-aggregating factor; *PDE,* phosphodiesterase; *PIP_2,* phosphatidylinositol; *PKC,* protein kinase C; *PLA_2,* phospholipase A_2; *PLC,* phospholipase C.

basement membranes. The Arthus reaction occurs 2 to 4 hours after IgG interacts with an antigen in the vessel wall. Serum sickness occurs when circulating immune complexes develop as a result of intravascular injection of the antigen. Microprecipitates in circulation deposit in basement membranes and the vascular endothelium, resulting in immune complex diseases. The risk of serum sickness increases with the persistence of antigen. The size of the immune complex also determines the degree of damage because larger complexes are more likely to deposit and initiate inflammation. Complement both contributes to and protects against damage caused by immune complex disease.[11]

Type IV hypersensitivity involves sensitized T cells that initiate a cell-mediated reaction on interaction with the appropriate class II MHC antigen. Lymphocyte and macrophage influx to the site occurs over a 24- to 72-hour period. Allergic contact dermatitis is an example of a type IV hypersensitivity.[11]

The term *cytokine storm,* or *hypercytokinemia,* has been used to describe the inappropriate systemic reaction resulting from the release of cytokines (more than 150) from a healthy and reactive immune system. Its importance emerged in response to the impact that swine flu to have in some, but not all afflicted human patients.[17] The immune system appears to lose the control normally provided through a system of checks and balances involving both inflammatory signals (e.g., TNFα, IL-1, and IL-6) and antiinflammatory signals (e.g., IL-10), as well as coagulation factors, and oxygen free radicals. The impact of these signals on body tissues and organs can be profound and is exemplified by acute respiratory distress syndrome (particularly that associated with influenza or flu), sepsis, and systemic inflammatory response syndrome. Inhibiting T cell response has been proposed as a potential mechanism of treatment or prevention. Drugs that alter production or the impact of TNFα are among those studied for possible efficacy.

Regulation of the Immune Response

Transcription Factors

Regulation of the immune response reflects a balance of the integrated actions of proinflammatory and antiinflammatory cytokines that act to trigger signaling pathways. The pathways, in turn, modulate gene expression program in the cells. Transcription factors targeted by cytokines include NFκB (proinflammatory),[18] activator protein 1 (AP-1), SMAD proteins (responsible for transfer of extracellular signals from transforming growth factor to intracelluar nuclear TGF-ß gene transcription), glucocorticoid receptors (antiinflammatory)[19, 20] (see Chapter 30), and members of the STAT protein family (proinflammatory and antiinflammatory).[5]

NFκB is a transcription factor that, upon induction by a number of inflammatory agents, participates in the expression of a large number of target genes, many of which regulate both innate and adaptive immunity. Because a number of the target genes activate NFκB, signal amplification may occur at very low concentrations of the inciting antigen, causing profound effects. Regulatory failure has been associated with a number of autoimmune diseases, including IBDs such as Crohn's disease and ulcerative colitis.[18] NFκB appears to play a key role in rheumatoid arthritis in humans. Metalloproteinase-1 (MMP-1) and TNF-α are among the molecules it regulates.[16] The NFκB system is vital to survival, but regulatory activity is very complex, and undirected inhibition may result in undesirable immune suppression. For example, pharmacologic interference with a potentially therapeutic aspect (e.g., inactivation in enterocytes such that a systemic inflammatory response is avoided) often is accompanied by potentially lethal parallel effects (e.g., severe apoptotic damage to the reperfused intestinal mucosa). Pharmacologic manipulation is most likely to succeed only when tissue- or organ-targeted inhibition is possible. Another major role player is activator protein 1 (AP-1), a transcription factor with major proinflammatory effects. It regulates gene expression stimulated by cytokines, growth factors, stress, and bacterial and viral infections, thus controls diverse cellular processes such as differentiation, proliferation, and apoptosis.

KEY POINT 31-8 Nuclear factor kappa B (NFκB), a transcription factor induced by a number of inflammatory signals, is involved in the expression of genes that regulate both innate and adaptive immunity.

Patients with glucocorticoid-sensitive versus glucocorticoid-resistant chronic inflammatory disease exhibit different cellular activation of NFκB, and AP-1 and upstream kinases; activation occurs in macrophages of the lamina propria in steroid-responsive patients but predominantly in epithelial cells of steroid resistant patients. Thus directed therapy for steroid-resistant patients might focus on inhibition of NFκB activation in epithelial cells.[18]

The Janus kinase (JAK)–STAT pathway is a major signaling pathway by which cytokine signals lead to the expression of genes that regulate immune cell proliferation and differentiation. The JAK–STAT signaling pathway is activated in response to cytokines (e.g., ILs and IFNs) as well as certain peptide hormones. The binding of the signaling molecules to the receptors causes activation (phosphorylation) of JAKs (e.g., JAK-1 through -3), which provide docking sites on the JAK protein for STAT proteins. The STAT proteins are then activated (phosphorylation) and translocated to the nucleus, where they bind to their response elements in the promoter of target genes. Transactivation cannot occur without coactivation by proteins such as acetyl transferase binding protein (e.g., CREB, a cyclic adenosine monophosphate [cAMP]–responsive element binding protein that increases MMP production in the synoviocytes of patients with rheumatoid arthritis).[16]

Cytokines that promote immune and inflammatory responses (e.g., IL-6, IFN-γ, IL-12, and IL-18) as well as those that suppress the immune response (e.g., IL-4, IL-10, IL-13) mediate cellular responses through the JAK–STAT signaling pathway. Up to seven STAT (including STAT-1 through -4, 5a and 5b, and STAT-6) proteins have been identified in mammals, each with a specific function in the immune response that modulates either proinflammatory or antiinflammatory responses. For example, STAT-3, originally discovered as an acute-phase response factor activated by IL-6, is also activated by many other cytokines and appears to be a constitutive protein that influences chronic inflammation. However, its embryonic deletion is lethal.[5]

Immunomodulatory Effects of Opioids

The potential of opioids to influence the immune system was first recognized close to 100 years ago when the effects of opium on phagocytic function were observed.[21] Heroin addicts are more susceptible to infection. Rodent studies indicate increased mortality and morbidity rates when opioid-treated animals are exposed to infectious agents. The presence of opioid receptors on cells of the immune system has been recognized since the late 1970s.[21,22] Although further studies are needed to fully elucidate the effect of opioids on immune function, thus far both the cellular and humoral immune reactions are believed to be affected.

Effects of opioids on the immune system are variable but are directed centrally, rather than peripherally, and involve primarily, but not exclusively, supraspinal mu receptors. Effects (inhibitory versus stimulatory) are dose dependent but occur at clinically relevant doses in animal models. Multiple central opioid receptors and endogenous opioids appear to be involved in complex immune responses. NK cytolytic activity and mitogen-stimulated T-cell proliferation are reduced by centrally administered morphine by way of mu receptors, whereas antibody production is both increased and decreased by met-enkephalin, which probably reflects interaction with multiple receptors. Effects can occur with single or multiple administration of exogenous opioids. Both the neuroendocrine system and the autonomic nervous system may serve as the efferent mechanisms mediating central opioid modulation of the immune system.[21] Tolerance appears to develop to some of the immunomodulatory effects, but this remains controversial. The clinical implications regarding the role of opioids in modulating the immune response are not clear.

Immunomodulatory Effects of Vitamin D

Increasingly, vitamin D (1,25, dihydroxyvitamin D_3) is recognized to have a noncalcemic role. Among the proposed activities is support of the immune system, particularly T cell–mediated immunity.[23] Both T lymphocytes and macrophages are characterized by a high density of vitamin D receptors, particularly in immature immune cells and mature CD8 cells. Vitamin D compounds have been demonstrated in animal models to selectively immunosuppress, effectively preventing or modulating autoimmune diseases, including systemic lupus erythematosus, encephalomyelitis, rheumatoid arthritis, and IBD. Suppression or prevention of transplant rejection has been demonstrated in animal models. Mechanisms may include stimulation of the antiinflammatory mediators transforming growth factor beta 1 (TGF-β 1) and IL-4. These effects appear to occur without negatively affecting normal immune defense mechanisms. Therapeutic use may be limited by the advent of hypercalcemia, leading to investigations of noncalcemic analogs; indeed, some suggestion exists that hypercalcemia may be required for immunosuppression.

CLASSIFICATION OF IMMUNOMODULATORY DRUGS

Immunomodulators often are classified according to their source: microbial, animal, or synthetic. Immunomodulators can also be classified by either an inhibitory or a stimulatory effect on the immune system. Prohost agents augment the cellular immune response either by facilitating a normal response in the face of immunosuppression (immunorestoratives) or by stimulating the immune response (immunostimulants). Immunostimulants can be used either before antigenic challenge to protect immunocompromised patients at risk or after exposure to potentially virulent agents has occurred. Immunosuppressant agents are used to manage hypersensitivity reactions, including autoimmune diseases, and as anticancer drugs. Many immunomodulatory drugs are target specific in their effects. However, many also have nonspecific effects that affect several to many arms of the immune response. Immunostimulants may in fact inhibit components of the immune response in some instances. Care should be taken when selecting an immunomodualtory drug, particularly if all the effects of the drug are not known or anticipated. For example, selective depression of some virally induced immune reactions is beneficial if the host's immune response to the infecting virus threatens the host's survival. Drugs that inhibit B lymphocyte activity (e.g., cyclophosphamide) often lower the mortality risk associated with some human influenza viruses and presumably should prove beneficial in the treatment of feline viral diseases associated with poorly controlled Ig production (i.e., feline infectious peritonitis).

The major indications for pharmacologic modulation of the immune system in animals are treatment of autoimmune diseases; prevention or treatment of infections, particularly in immunocompromised hosts; and prevention and therapy of malignancies. A less common but increasingly growing use of immunomodulators in small animals is treatment of graft-versus-host reactions after organ transplantation.

IMMUNOMODULATION IN VIRAL AND NEOPLASTIC DISEASES

Biologica l response modifiers are discussed in Chapter 32. Their primary indications are for treatment of viral or neoplastic disease or (generally their antagonism) for treatment of immune-mediated disease.

Viral Diseases

Biological response modifiers potentially offer a logical and unique approach to the treatment of viral diseases because (1) viruses are capable of immunosuppression and (2) the immune response is an important determinant in the host's ability to overcome viral infection.[24,25] Resistance against and recovery from viral infections in mammals depend on three components of the immune system. The mononuclear phagocytic (reticuloendothelial) system represents the first barrier to viral infections, but it is nonspecific and not always efficient. Sensitized T lymphocytes provide specific cell-mediated immunity, which is followed later by humoral events, either narrowly specific (antibodies) or nonspecific (IFN). Multiple interactions occur among these systems. Unfortunately, several systems also contribute to the pathogenesis of viral disease. Viruses may cause immunosuppression by several mechanisms: They may directly injure or impair all classes of lymphocytes; cause the production of soluble immunosuppressing chemicals (e.g., IFN, p15[E] of feline leukemia virus [FeLV]) damage all three cell systems by infection, or cause an imbalance in immunoregulation, thus leading to overactivity of suppressor T cells.

Neoplastic Diseases

Many tumors have surface antigens toward which specific antibodies can be directed. Biological response modifiers can alter response to tumor antigen at one or several of these points, depending on the drug. Some biological response modifiers augment or restore normal host effector mechanisms by acting as either a mediator or an effector of the antitumor response. Transformation of tumor cells may be decreased or maturation of tumor cells may be increased by biological response modifiers. Host tolerance of damage caused by cytotoxic chemotherapeutic drugs also may be increased by biological response modifiers. Finally, biological response modifiers have been used to alter patient response to FeLV viremia and thus the subsequent associated neoplasms.[26,27]

IMMUNOMODIFYING DRUGS

The sequelae of immunomodulation are not always beneficial; alteration of the immune response can impair many aspects of the host's normal defense system. The use of immunomodulators remains in its early stages despite advances; this remains particularly true for veterinary medical applications. Because of the many facets of the immune system susceptible to regulation, the dose, timing, and route of administration of these drugs are important if undesired effects are to be avoided (Table 31-2). In addition, host effects such as age and nutritional status and the nature of the disease may be important determinants in the patient's response to these drugs.

Marked advances have been made in the use of drugs that target the adaptive immune response. For the purposes of this text, drugs used to modify the immune response will include drugs whose actions are relatively nonspecific in their immunomoldulatory effect and those products of biological (animal) origin that target specific mediators of the immune response or their receptors, the latter is the focus of Chapter 32.

The role of P-glycoprotein in drug-induced immunomodulation is an emerging area of interest.[28] The protein is expressed on peripheral blood mononuclear cells. It influences the secretion of cytokines secreted from antigen-presenting cells and selected T cells, and it has been shown to influence lymphocyte survival and antigen-presenting cell differentiation. These actions appear to contribute to the immunomodulatory actions of selected drugs capable of inhibiting P-glycoprotein (e.g., verapamil, progesterone, tamoxifen) and may account for the therapeutic immunomodulatory functions of these drugs. Eventually, these effects might be redirected for therapeutic benefit in allograft rejection and cell-mediated autoimmune disorders.

Immunosuppressant Drugs

Four major classes of immunosuppressive drugs are described in human medicine: glucocorticoids (discussed in Chapter 30), calcineurin inhibitors, antiproliferative–antimetabolic drugs, and biological agents.[4] The latter includes biological response modifiers (Chapter 32).

Several principles should guide use of immunosuppressant drugs.[4] First, suppression of the primary immune response is more easily accomplished than is suppression of the secondary (amnestic) response. Second, successful inhibition or suppression is easier if therapy begins before exposure to the inciting immunogen (antigen). Third, immunosuppressive drugs do not cause the same effect on all aspects of the immune system. Often, opposite effects are concentration dependent. Thus failure to achieve the desired response should not necessarily lead to an increase in dose. Finally, patients often require lifelong therapy, which increases the risk of adverse effects.

Two major limitations characterize immunosuppressive therapy. Patients receiving immunosuppressive therapy are predisposed to infections of any type. In addition, the risk of lymphomas and related malignancies is increased. This latter risk is more problematic in human patients because, in part, of their longer life span, but has proven a risk in dogs or cats receiving cyclosporine. Events that immunosuppressive drugs tend to target include antigen recognition, stimulation of IL-1, synthesis and release of IL-2 or other cytokines, and lymphocyte proliferation and differentiation.[4] Secondary signal molecules are also becoming increasingly important as targets of immunosuppressive therapy.

Immunosuppressive drugs are used to treat immune-mediated disease, which in this chapter include autoimmune diseases (e.g., immune-mediated anemias or thrombocytopenias) as well as chronic allergic inflammatory diseases (e.g., atopic dermatitis and asthma, IBD). A third, less common indication in veterinary medicine is prevention of organ rejection in renal transplant patients. Autoimmune diseases are characterized by sensitization to endogenous proteins that are perceived to be foreign. Both cell-mediated and humoral responses can be directed toward the protein. Many immune-mediated disorders afflicting dogs and cats respond sufficiently well to glucocorticoids (discussed in Chapter 30) and, when necessary (in severe cases), cytotoxic drugs. These include immune-mediated autoimmune hemolytic anemia or thrombocytopenia, acute glomerulopathies, and many dermatologic disorders with an immune-mediated basis. However, the approval of cyclosporine (CsA) for chronic allergic dermatitis has increased its use for autoimmune diseases, providing an alternative to cytotoxic drugs as a second tier.

Calcineurin Inhibitors

Calcineurin is a protein phosphatase that dephosphorylates and thus activates the transcription factor nuclear factor of activated T cell (NFATc). Upon activation, NFATc translocates to the nucleus and upregulates IL-2 expression of regulatory proteins.

Table 31-2 Dosing Regimens of Immunomodulating Drugs

Drug	Dose	Route	Interval
Acemannan	2 mg	Intratumorally	Weekly for 6 weeks
	1 mg/kg	Intraperitoneally	Weekly for 6 weeks
Aurothioglucose			
Test dose	1 mg < than 10 kg, 5 mg ≥ 10 kg	IM	Twice, 1 week apart
	1 mg/kg (D)	IM	Weekly until remission; then alternate weeks
With prednisolone	1 to 2 mg/kg	PO	12 to 48 hr
	0.5 to 1 mg/kg (C)	IM	7 days
Auranofin	0.1 to 0.2 mg/kg	PO	12 hr
Azathioprine (dog)	2 mg/kg	PO	24 hr
With prednisolone	1 mg/kg	PO	12 hr
Chlorambucil	0.1 to 0.2 mg/kg	PO	48 hr
Cyclophosphamide	100 to 250 mg/m^2	IV bolus	Once
	50 mg/m^2	PO	48 hr
With prednisolone	1 mg/kg	PO	12 hr
Cyclosporine	4 to 6 mg/kg	IV infusion	Over 4 hr
Perianal fistulae	5 to 10 mg/kg	PO	12 hr
Renal allografts	7.5 mg/kg	PO	12 hr
With prednisolone	0.125-0.25 mg/kg	PO	12 hr
Danazol	2-5 mg/kg	PO	24 hr
Dexamethasone	0.1 to 0.2 mg/kg	IV	
Dimercaprol	4 mg/kg	IM	4 hr
Fibronectin	0.5 to 2.0 mg/kg	IV	24 hr
Human gammaglobulin	0.5 to 1.5 g/kg	IV infusion	Over 12 hr
Leflunomide (dog)	3 to 8 mg/kg	PO	24
Levamisole	2.5-5 mg/kg	PO	3 times weekly
Megestrol acetate			
Induction	2.5 to 5 mg/cat	PO	48 hr, every other day
Maintenance	2.5 mg/cat	PO	7 to 14 days
Methylprednisolone acetate	2 mg/kg, minimum of 20 mg	Intralesional	14 days
Niacin	5 to 12 mg/kg	PO	8 hr
Pentoxifylline	30 mg/kg (D)	PO	8 to 12 hr
Prednisolone, prednisone			
Immunosuppressive	1 to 3 mg/kg	IV, SC, PO	12 hr
Alternate-day target	0.25-0.5 mg/kg	IV, SC, PO	48 hr
Promodulin	50 mg/kg up to 200 mg	IV	24 × 5days
Tetracycline	5 to 12 mg/kg	PO	8 hr
Vitamin E acetate or succinate	400 IU	PO	12 hr; 2 hr before or after a meal
Vinblastine	0.1 to 0.4 mg/kg	IV	7 to 14 days
	2 mg/m^2 (C)	IV	7 to 14 days
	1 to 3 mg/m^2 (D)	IV	7 days (in a protocol)
Vincristine	0.010 to 0.025 mg/kg (D)	IV	7 to 10 days
Immune-mediated thrombocytopenia			
Neoplasia	0.5 to 0.75 mg/m^2	IV	7 to 14 days

IM, Intramuscularly; *D*, dog; *PO*, by mouth; *C*, cat; *IV*, intravenous; *SC*, subcutaneous.

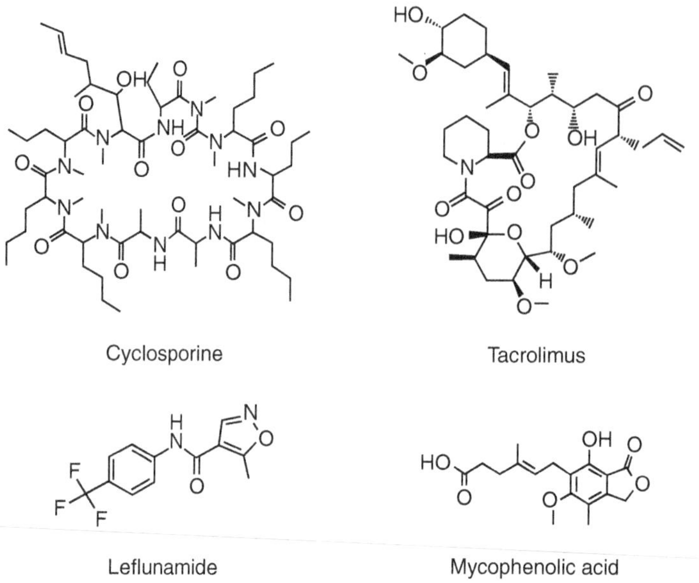

Cyclosporine

Tacrolimus

Leflunamide

Mycophenolic acid

Figure 31-3 The chemical structure of selected immunomodulating drugs.

Cyclosporine A

Chemistry–Structure Relationship

Cyclosporin A (CsA), now known as *cyclosporine,* is the most important immunosuppressive drug for human transplantation and the treatment of selective autoimmune disorders.[4,30] CsA is one of nine cyclosporins (A through I), each a cyclic peptide drug (Figure 31-3) isolated from the fungi *Cylindrocarpon lucidum* and *Trichoderma polysporum.* An M designation, when present, indicates a metabolite. The drug is both very lipophilic (hydrophobic) and must be solubilized before administration.[4] The oral preparation is a soft gelatin capsule (Sandimmune) or a (newer) microemulsion formulation (Neoral). The intravenous preparation is an ethanol–polyoxyethylated castor oil mixture. Historically, CsA has been formulated in peanut oil (for treatment of ophthalmic ocular disorders in dogs); however, an approved product formulated for topical use is now available.

Mechanism of Action

CsA is a unique immunosuppressant in that it specifically inhibits T_h cells (both T_h1 and T_h2) early in their immune response to antigenic and regulatory stimuli[4] without affecting suppressor cells. Suppression occurs as CsA binds to cyclophilin, a cytoplasmic receptor protein, forming a heterodimeric complex. This complex then binds to calcineurin. Binding of calcineurin inhibits calcium-stimulated phosphatase that dephosphorylates the regulatory protein. As such, CsA prevents transcription of T cell genes enhanced in response to T cell activation. Transcription mediated by IL-2, certain proto-oncogenes, and selected cytokine receptors are particularly affected.[4] IL-2 production (and thus T cell proliferation and antigen-specific cytotoxic T lymphocyte generation) also is attenuated because the expression of TGF-β, a potent inhibitor of IL-2, is increased.[4] B cells are not affected. The drug is most effective when administered before T cell proliferation has occurred. In addition to these immunomodulatory effects, CsA also affects other inflammatory cells. CsA inhibits skin mast cell numbers, survival, and response (secretory and histamine release) as well as secretion of IL-3, IL-4, IL-5, IL-8, and TNFα. Similarly, eosinophile response (release of granules and cytokines) and recruitment to allergic sites is impaired. CsA prevents TNFα-mediated late phase reactions, thus inhibiting IgE and mast cell–dependent cellular infiltration in the skin and bronchial mucosa. However, CsA does not inhibit IgA secretion or IgG and IgM formation in dogs and has no apparent effect on serum allergen-specific IgE levels, intradermal tests, or vaccination.

KEY POINT 31-9 Cyclosporine A specifically inhibitits T helper cells; however, little information is available regarding its impact on immune response in dogs or cats.

Surprisingly little information is available regarding immunomodulatory effects of CsA in dogs or cats. Using dermal microdialysis, Brazis and coworkers[31] demonstrated that CsA at 5 mg/kg per day for 15 and 30 days decreased histamine, but not prostaglandin D_2, release in sensitized Beagles challenged with *Ascaris suum.*

Preparations

CsA is available in a variety of preparations, two of which are approved in the United States for use in animals. CsA was first formulated for oral use in humans as vegetable oil. Oral absorption in this preparation depends on emulsification by bile acids. Poor oral bioavailability led to the formulation of a microemulsion preparation (modified CsA, ME), which, on contact with gastrointestinal fluids, disperses into a homogeneous monophasic microemulsion that mimics the mixed micellar phase of the standard formulation. In dogs the ME formulation offers a 35% bioavailability (Novartis Animal Health data on file).

Atopica is the veterinary-approved microemulstion preparation of CsA intended for systemic use in both capsules and solutions. A 0.2% ophthalmic ointment (Optimmune) is also available. A number of human-approved drugs are available, including an injectable solution, an oral solution (100 mg/mL), an ophthalmic emulsion (0.05%), and a variety of capsule sizes for the standard and the microemulsion-modified preparation. Included are a number of generic-modified CsA products. However, the therapeutic equivalence that has been established for these products in humans should not be assumed to be therapeutically equivalent to Atopica in animals. Indeed, one preparation made by IVAX Pharmaceuticals and sold by selected chain pharmacies appears to result in much higher concentrations in dogs compared with other preparations on the basis of samples submitted through the author's laboratory. Monitoring should be the basis for assessing the appropriate dose–concentration relationship for oral human CsA products used in dogs or cats; owners might need to be aware if and when a pharmacy switches from one human generic to another such that prophylactic monitoring might be implemented.

Clinical Pharmacology

The pharmacokinetic behavior of CsA is complex, resulting in marked variability in the relationship between dose and blood concentrations.[32] Variability reflects not only differences in both hepatic and intestinal metabolism (by CYP3A4) but also differences in P-glycoprotein among various tissues.[32] The disposition of CsA has been well reviewed in the dog.[33] Absorption after oral administration is slow and incomplete. The complex lipid nature of CsA complicates absorption by being dependent on bile acids, which generate a microemulsion. In humans oral bioavailability of the capsule ranges from 20% to 50% but is improved by 10% to 20% in the microemulsion form which is not dependent on bile acids.[4,34] Peak concentrations occur 1 to 4 hours after oral administration in human beings. When the capsule—but not the microemulsion—is administered with a fatty meal, absorption is slowed. Studies suggest that decreased bioavailability of CsA after oral administration may reflect activity of drug-metabolizing enzymes of the intestinal epithelium[35] or P-glycoprotein–mediated drug efflux.

KEY POINT 31-10 The kinetics of cyclosporine A are complicated by its large, liphophilic molecular structure.

The oral bioavailability of microemulsion in dogs is 35% compared with the 20% of the oral preparation.[33] Bioavailability of orally administered CsA is approximately 25% to 30% after multiple oral administration in cats (n = 6). Food may impair the absorption of CsA; peak concentrations in fasted dogs were 20% higher than in nonfasted dogs in one study, although time to peak (approximately 1.5 hours) was the same.[33] The drug is not predictably absorbed topically after transdermal administration (unpublished data, Boothe 2007). CsA is widely distributed, characterized by a large volume of distribution (13 L/kg in humans). The drug accumulates in erythrocytes (accounting for 50% or more of the drug in humans), and leukocytes (accounting for 10% to 20% of circulating drug in humans).[4] Consequently, monitoring of whole blood rather than plasma or serum is recommended. Remaining circulating drug is bound to plasma lipoproteins. Further, concentrations in skin are up to tenfold higher than in blood, although this is based on homogenate data (as reviewed by Guaguère and coworkers[33]). In contrast, largely because of the influence of adenosine triphosphate–binding transporters P-glycoproteins, especially the ABCB1 cassette (P-glycoprotein, MDR1 gene product), little CsA crosses the blood–brain barrier.

KEY POINT 31-11 In addition to its chemistry, the oral absorption of cyclosporine A is affected by a number of factors, resulting in marked variability. Differences in absorption of human generic or compounded preparations should be anticipated.

CsA is metabolized to a large number of metabolites predominantly by the liver, although sufficient metabolism occurs by intestinal enterocytes that oral bioavailability is affected. Microflorae also may contribute to metabolism.[37] CYP3A4 (commonly associated with P-glycoprotein or other efflux pumps) plays a major role in metabolism; many of the drug interactions involving CsA also involve CYP3A4 or associated glycoprotein. More than 25 to 30 metabolites have been documented in humans and dogs.[32,38,39] Metabolism is targeted primarily toward the side chains rather than the ring structure and reflects hydroxylation, demethylation, sulfation, and cyclization. The major hydroxylated metabolites (AM1 and AM9) are further metabolized, contributing to the complex metabolic profile. Both AM1 and AM9 may contribute 10 to 20% of CsA activity, with AM1 contributing 27% of trough activity.[40] In humans AM1 accumulates with chronic dosing and ultimately may surpass CsA, and monitoring assays might ideally detect the active compounds.[39] They are detected to variable degrees by selected immunoassays based on a monoclonal antibody (e.g., Abbott TdX, Architect systems, Seimens Dimension).[41,42] Selected laboratories may also offer a high-performance liquid chromatography (HPLC)–based system that, may or may not (generally not) quantitate the metabolites.[39] Ultimately metabolism continues until the drug is totally inactivate the drug, although this has not been proved conclusively.[4] Metabolites are excreted in bile and feces, with less than 2% of unchanged drug eliminated in the kidneys of dogs. CYP3A4 is largely responsible for metabolism.

The half-life of CsA in dogs is quite variable, depending on the investigator and assay. In blood the half-life ranges from a low of 5 hours (HPLC) to a high of 18 hours (using fluorescent polarized immunoassay [FPIA]); 29 hours was reported for serum.[43] That reported for Atopica, the product approved for use in dogs, is 4.5 hours, a length more consistent with that measured in the author's therapeutic drug monitoring laboratory using FPIA. In a manufacturer-sponsored affinity colony-mediated immunoassay (ACMIA) study, Steffan and coworkers[44] reported the disposition of CsA (5 mg/kg) after single-dose oral administration of either capsules or solution in fasting or fed conditions using a randomized crossover design with a 1-week washout between studies (Table 31-3); food decreased peak concentrations and area under the curve by 22%.

Table 31-3 Disposition of Cyclosporine Reported By Various Investigators

Species (n)	Dose mg/kg	Route	Preparation	Sample	Method	CsA ng/mL*	Timing (T_{max} in hr)	T_{max} (hr)	$T_{1/2}$ (hr)	DUR	State
Cat (n=5)(1)[56]	4	IV	Not provided	WB	HPLC	1410± 188	Peak (B)		10.7±0.86	SI	HN
						26,000	AUC (ng*hr/mL)				
Cat (n=6)(2)[45]	1	IV	Sandimmune	WB	HPLC	474± 112	Peak (B)			SI	HN
						7413±4268	AUC (ng*hr/mL)		9.7±5		
Cat (n=6)[45]	3	PO	Neoral	WB	HPLC	480±147	C_{max} (peak)	1±0.62	8.2±3.3	M (14 d)	HN
						301±250	C_{min} (12 hr trough)				
						6243±2746	AUC (ng*hr/mL)				
Cat[104]	1	IV				7413	C_{max} (peak)			SI	HN
	3	PO				480	C_{max} (peak)			SI	
	3	PO				740	C_{max} (peak)			M	
	3	PO				321	C_{min} (trough)			M	
	3	PO				450-1088				SI	
	3	OU				288-648				SI	
Dog (n=8)[77]	5	PO	Atopica	WB	FIPA	699±326	Peak	1.50±0.5	5.6±1.2	SI	Severe IBD
						34±26	C_{min} (24-hr trough)				
						4,770±2,672	AUC(0-24)				
Dog (n=16)[77]	5	PO		WB	FIPA	878±131	Peak	1.6±0.4	7.8± 1.1	SI	H, N
						50±22	C_{min} (24-hr trough)				
							AUC(0-24)				
Beagle (n=8)[44]	5	PO, C,F		WB	FIPA	1059±207	Peak	1.3±0.5		SI	H, N
						6386±2079	AUC(0-24)				
		PO, C, N		WB	FIPA	845±582	Peak	1.36±2.9		SI	H, N
						5453±1905	AUC(0-24)				
		PO, S,F		WB		1287±180	Peak	1		SI	H, N
						75233±17	AUC(0-24)				
		PO, S,N		WB		949±725	Peak	0.65±0.26		SI	H, N
						5396±2615	AUC(0-24)				
Beagle (n=16)[44]	5		Atopica	WB	HPLC	577±128	Peak	1.4±0.3	9.4±1.2	14 d	H, N
						34±12	Trough				
						3997±1108	AUC (infinity)				
				WB	FIPA	878±131	Peak	1.6±0.4	7.8±1.1	14 d	
						50± 22	Trough				
						6729±1587	AUC (infinity)				

CsA, Cyclosporine A; *DUR*, duration; *IV*, intravenous; *WB*, whole blood, *HPLC*, high-performance (pressure) liquid chromatography; *S*, solution; *H*, healthy; *N*, normal; *AUC*, area under the curve; SI: single dose; *M*, Multiple dose; *PO*, by mouth; *OU*, both eyes *FPIA*, polarized immunofluorescence assay; *IBD*, inflammatory bowel disease; *C*, capsule, F, fasted *C*, capsule; *N*, fed;
(1) Volume of distribution 2.06±0.14 L/kg; clearance 2.71+0.3 (ml*min/kg)
(2) Volume of distribution 1.71±0.3L/kg; clearance 0.20+0.154 L/kg*hr

In cats elimination half-life of CsA is 8 hours, which was similar to that after intravenous administration. Liver disease will decrease clearance of CsA substantially. However, for the nonmicroemulsion form, decreased oral absorption in the face of decreased bile may balance decreased clearance. Monitoring is recommended in the presence of hepatic or gastrointestinal disease.

Mehl and coworkers[45] reported the disposition of CsA in cats (n = 6 male) after single-dose intravenous (1 mg/kg) and multiple-dose (14 days; 3 mg/kg twice daily) as Neoral (see Table 31-3). Variability in plasma drug concentrations among cats and across time underlines the importance of monitoring if treating life-threatening conditions. After multiple-day (7 to 14 days) oral administration (3 mg/kg), mean (peak) plasma concentrations at 2 hours were 740 ± 326 (7 days) and 655 ± 285 ng/mL (14 days), whereas trough concentrations were 332 ± 237 and 301.5 ± 250 ng/mL, respectively. Oral bioavailability was only 25% to 29%.

Because cats may find the oral preparation unpalatable, the oral solution can be given diluted in olive oil. The intravenous preparation (4 to 6 mg/kg as a 4-hour intravenous infusion) can be given to animals for which oral administration is not possible.[46] Ocular administration might serve as an alternative route for systemic delivery of CsA in cats.[47] After ocular administration of either an oral preparation or an ocular preparation of CsA in olive oil, (5 mg/kg in each eye as a 10% solution) peak concentrations of 450 to 1033 ng/mL (oral preparation) and 288 to 648 ng/mL (ocular) were achieved, with an absorption lag time ranging from 0 to 1.34 hours for the oral solution and 0.27 to 1.2 hours for ocular preparation. The elimination half-life ranged from 2.41 to 10.04 hours (oral), and 3.09 to 15.75 hours (ocular), respectively. Blood concentrations were sufficient to inhibit lymphocyte activity as measured in vitro, leading the authors to conclude that ocular administration of CsA in an olive oil vehicle might be a reasonable alternative to oral, or even intravenous, administration in cats intolerant to the latter.

Drug Interactions

Novartis[48] provides a transplant drug interactions monograph that cites more than 600 references and delineates cyclosporine interactions involving more than 300 drugs. The list of drugs that might interact with CsA is extensive. The manual is available on the Novartis website at no charge and should be consulted when treating patients receiving additional drugs. Selected interactions can be found in Table 31-4. This review will focus on some of the more common interactions, including those used intentionally.

KEY POINT 31-12 Cyclosporine A is involved with a large number of drug interactions that might cause higher or lower than anticipated plasma drug concentrations.

The enzyme that metabolizes CsA (CYP3A4) is responsible (in humans) for approximately 30% of all drug metabolism; many of CsA drug interactions occur with this enzyme. Further, CsA is a target of P-glycoprotein, another site characterized by a substantial number of CsA–drug interactions.[4,49] The risk of drug interactions is another indication of the need for therapeutic drug monitoring as a guide to proper dosing regimens. CsA elimination is accelerated, probably in part because of the induction of drug-metabolizing enzymes, by phenytoin, phenobarbital, rifampin, and sulfamethoxazole–trimethoprim combinations, and others. Dexamethasone also is an inducer of CsA.[32] Its elimination is decreased by amphotericin B, erythromycin, and ketoconazole.[4] CsA also appears to alter the oral absorption of other drugs.[35] CsA use with other immunosuppressive drugs may benefit from these interactions, including glucocorticoids.[4]

The inhibitory effect of ketoconazole on intestinal epithelial and hepatic drug metabolism and on P-glycoprotein efflux may be of therapeutic benefit in patients receiving CsA by decreasing hepatic clearance and increasing oral bioavailability.[35,50-53] Ketoconazole may also decrease the lipoprotein that binds CsA, resulting in higher concentrations of free CsA.[51] Studies with ketoconazole in humans found the dose of CsA to be reduced by approximately 70% to 85%.[54] The use of ketoconazole in conjunction with CsA as a means of decreasing drug cost has been well accepted in human transplant patients.[51] The two drugs have been used safely for up to 47 months in one study reducing the CsA dose as much as 88%.[51] Although the effects emerge rapidly, with 62% of the effect is apparent by day 7, the maximum inhibitory effect may not be present for 12 months. This has implications regarding monitoring and supports the need for collection of peak and trough samples such that the impact of ketoconazole on drug elimination half-life might be determined.

The effect of combining ketoconazole with CsA has been studied in dogs.[55] Ketoconazole was studied at doses ranging from 1.25 to 20 mg/kg per day, with the magnitude of inhibition increasing with the dose of ketoconazole above but not below 2.5 mg/kg.[55] Clearance was reduced by 85% at 10 mg/kg per day. Differences in clearance did not result in significant differences in oral bioavailability. In their review, McNaulty and Lensmeyer[56] indicated that in dogs, CsA half-life will increase over twofold and decrease the concentration of active metabolites in response to 2.5 to 10 mg/kg ketoconazole. Up to 75% of the CsA dose could be reduced experimentally in Beagles concurrently receiving a dose of ketoconazole of 13.6 mg/kg per day.[57] In a study in dogs with perianal fistulae, Mouatt[58] examined the impact of ketoconazole (10 mg/kg once daily) on CsA concentrations (1 mg/kg twice daily). Samples were collected 12 hours after the last dose (duration not clear). Data were not provided on all dogs, but the author noted that at 1.1 mg/kg twice daily of CsA, all dogs exceeded 200 ng/mL at through (12 hours); nine dogs exceeded 900 ng/mL, and two dogs exceeded 1500 ng/mL. Concentrations varied by 10% to 40% in the same dog despite no dose change. This may have reflected variability in time to steady state, which took 2 to 4 weeks. A trough concentration of 200 ng/mL was targeted. Although 8 dogs maintained concentrations of 220 to 520 ng/mL with CsA doses as little as 0.35 to 0.55 mg/kg twice daily, one dog required only 0.16 mg/kg twice daily to maintain 159 to 225 ng/mL, whereas three others required 0.95 to 1.1 mg/kg twice daily to maintain 120 to 235 ng/mL.

Table 31-4 Cyclosporine Drug Interactions

Drug	Impact
ACE inhibitors	Increased nephrotoxicity
Acyclovir	Falsely increased CsA
Allopurinol	Increased toxicity
Aluminum	Increased nephrotoxicity and CsA bioavailability
Aminoglycosides	Increased nephrotoxicity
Amlodipine	Increased gingival hyperplasia
Antacids	Increased aluminum toxicity
Azithromycin	Increased gingival hyperplasia
	Increased CsA
Bile acids	Increased bioavailability
Chloramphenicol	Decreaesed clearance, increased CsA
Cimetidine	Delayed absorption
	No effect (?) on metabolism or absorption
Ciprofloxacin	Antagonizes CsA immunosuppression
Cisapride	Increased absorption
Clarithromycin	Decreased clearance, increased CsA
Cyclophosphamide	Increased hepatotoxiciy
Danazol	Decreasd metabolism, increased absorption
Dexamethasole	Increased CsA metabolism; synergistic immunosuppression
Digoxin	Increased digoxin toxicity
Diltiazem	Increased gingival hyperplasia, increased CsA
Erythromycin	Increased hepatotoxicity (decreased metabolism?)
Famotidine	Decreased clearance, increased CsA
Fluconazole	Oral: increased bioavailability
Fluoxetine	Decreased clearance, increased CsA
Furosemide	Decreased nephrotoxicity
Glucocorticoids	Increased metabolism, decreased CsA
Itraconazole	Decreased clearance, increased CsA
	Increased absorption(?)
Ivermectin	Increased neurotoxicity
Ketamine	Combined proconvulsant effects
Ketaconazole	Decreased clearance, increased CsA
	Increased absorption
	Increased toxicity
Leflunomide	Synergistic immunosuppression
Loperamide	Altered absorption
Methotrexate	Decreased clearance, increased CsA
	Increased methotrexate toxicity
Metoclopramide	Increased absorption, increased CsA
Metoprolol	Beneficial hemodynamics
Mitoxantrone	Increased mitoxantrone concentrations
Mycophenolic acid	Synergistic immunosuppression
Norfloxacin	Decreased CsA clearance?
Omeprazole	Delayed CsA absorption, decreased CsA clearance?
Pancuronium	Prolonged duration of pancuronium effect
Pentoxifylline	Synergistic inhibition of TNF and other immunosuppression
Phenobarbital	Increased CsA clearance, decreased CsA
Phenytoin	Increased CsA clearance, decreased CsA
Prazosine	Increased afterload
Prednisone	Increased risk of hepatotoxicity, hyperlipidemia
Primidone	Increased CsA clearance, decreased CsA
Propranolol	Antagonism of CsA immunosuppression
	Decreased propranolol clearance
Ranitidine	Increased risk of hepatotoxicity, thrombocytopenia
Rifampin	Increased CsA clearance, decreased CsA
Sirolimus	Synergistic immunosuppression
	Synergistic risk of toxicity
Spironolactone	Hyperkalemia
Sucralfate	Increased aluminum
Sulfadiazines	Interference with HPLC assay results in increased CsA
Tacrolimus	Decreased CsA clearance, increased CsA
Terbinafine	Inceased CsA metabolism
Ticlopidine	Altered CsA metabolism
Trimethoprim	Increased CsA clearance, decreased CsA
Ursodeoxycholic acid	Decreased T_{max}
Vasopressin	Enhanced vasopressin effects
Verapamil	Gingival hyperplasia, synergistic immunosuppression
Vitamin D_3	Additive suppressive effects
Voriconazole	Decreased metabolism?

ACE, angiotensin-converting enzyme; *CsA*, cyclosporine A.
From Neoral and Sandimmune Drug Interactions, Novartis package insert, 2007

This marked variability in response to ketaconozole appears to occur in clinical patients as is suggested by samples submitted to the author's therapeutic drug monitoring laboratory. Marked variability occurs not only in concentrations, but in the time to steady-state, which in turn determines when monitoring should be implemented. For example, the author's laboratory has demonstrated prolongation of the half-life of CsA in a patient from 4 hours (as reported in normal dogs) to over 150 hour. Steady state was not achieved in this patient until approximately 4 weeks, causing CsA concentrations to continue to increase despite a decrease in dose that was based on monitoring at 1 week. Yet, in other patients, half-life has been less than 12 hours, despite ketoconazole therapy. Detecting these diffrences requires collection of peak and trough samples such that half-life and time to steady-state can be determined in each patient.

The simultaneous administration of ketoconazole with CsA also has been studied in cats. McNaulty and Lensmeyer[56] prospectively studied the impact of a two doses of ketoconazole (10 mg/kg at 24 and 0.5 hr) before a single dose of CsA (4 mg/kg intravenously) in cats (n = 5) using a randomized crossover design with a 14-day washout. Concentrations of CsA were detected using HPLC. Clearance was reduced from 2.73 ± 0.3 to 1.22 ± 0.18 mL*kg/min, resulting in an elimination half-life prolongation from 10 ± 0.9 to 21 ± 3 hours.

Several studies have examined the impact of cimetidine, an inhibitor of CYP3A4, CYP2D6, and CYP1A2 on CsA concentrations. Cimetidine also is a substrate for P-glycoprotein. The results of the studies are contradictory, perhaps reflecting differences in duration of therapy and species. D'Souza and coworkers[59] found that 5 days of cimetidine therapy significantly decreased CsA clearance, increased volume of distribution (perhaps by impacting P-glycoprotein in distribution tissues) and prolonged elimination half-life in rabbits, whereas Bar-Meir and coworkers[60] found that short-term administration of cimetidine had no effect on CsA metabolism in rats. Shaefer and coworkers[61] found that 7 days of dosing with cimetidine or famotidine did not affect CsA pharmacokinetics in healthy men. Daigle[62] explored the impact of cimetidine (15 mg/kg orally every 8 hours for 8 days) on the disposition of CsA (5 mg/kg orally per day; the last 3 days of cimetidine administration) in dogs using a randomized crossover design with a 14-day washout. Significant differences could not be demonstrated for C_{max} or area under the curve the power to detect a significant change was not addressed. The author's therapeutic drug monitoring laboratory has identified some patients for which a cimetidine–CsA interaction may be present, but, other patients for which no effect could be measured.

Among the other drugs that impair CsA elimination or compete with efflux pumps include itraconazole, the calcium channel blockers such as diltiazem, and the macrolide antibacterial erythromycin.[50] In humans, diltiazem decreases the CsA dose by approximately 30% to 50%.[54] Other drugs that influence CYP activity should be expected to potentially affect CsA. For example, in the author's laboratory, a cat receiving azithromycin (5 mg/kg once daily) along with CsA (5 mg/kg twice daily), exhibited peak concentrations exceeded 4500 ng/mL, presumably in part resulting from an elimination half-life that exceeded 150 hours. Azithromycin also competes for P-glycoprotein. Other drugs that induce P-glycoprotein might decrease CsA concentrations. For example, P-glycoprotein is upregulated in the duodenum of dogs receiving glucocorticoids.[62a]

KEY POINT 31-13 Drugs intended to increase cyclosporine A concentrations are likely to differentially affect animals; both peak and trough concentrations should be measured to determine the full impact.

Side Effects

CsA is characterized by a narrow therapeutic index in human patients, with renal toxicity the primary adverse effect. Renal tubular cells develop hyperuricemia (worsened by diuretics) and hyperkalemia (a renal tubular and erythrocyte ion channel effect).[63] Hepatic injury also occurs. Although less common than renal dysfunction, the risk of severe hepatic damage is markedly increased when CsA is used in combination with cytotoxic drugs. CsA also increases the incidence of gallstones in human patients. However, in contrast to humans, renal and hepatic toxicities do not appear to be in dogs and cats. Risk factors, such as concurrent administration of nephroactive or nephrotoxic drugs, or renal transplantation have not been addressed in dogs or cats. Hyperlipidemia also has been a reported side effect in humans, particularly in patients receiving glucocorticoids. Other side effects reported in humans include neurotoxicity, gastrointestinal upset, and hypertension.[4] Development of B cell lymphoma also has been reported in humans; an incidence 10% has been reported in cats undergoing renal transplantation, with mean time to onset of 9 months. [63a] Side effects in dogs include gastrointestinal upset and dermatologic or mucosal abnormalities. Vomiting may occur in up to 40% of dogs, although it may be intermittent and short in duration. Diarrhea occurs less commonly (16% to 18%).Vomiting may be more likely when CsA is combined with ketoconazole, but this may reflect higher CsA concentrations. Dermatologic abnormalities reported in dogs include hair loss (possibly reflecting hair growth and pushing of hair from follicles), gingival hyperplasia, and gingivitis in up to 33% of dogs.[58] In one study,[58] hair loss resolved by 7 weeks, although hairy coats were thinner at study end (see Therapeutic Use). Hyperplasia may reflect an imbalance of fibroblast formation and collagen degradation by collagenase, although stimulation of TGF-β also has been suggested.[33] Stimulation of TGF-β also stimulates extracellular matrix and decreases degrading proteases. Treatment with antimicrobials (metronidazole, spiramycin) may be useful for treating hyperplasia.[58] Skin healing might be supported rather than inhibited, as occurs with glucocorticoids.[67]

At the doses used to treat atopy, risk of infection does not appear to be increased in dogs. However, the risk apparently has not been assessed at the higher doses used to treat immunosuppressive diseases. A report of central nervous system (CNS) toxoplasmosis has been reported in two cats receiving CsA (3 mg/kg twice daily for approximately 5 weeks and 6 mg/kg twice daily for approximately 8 weeks, respectively); presenting signs were respiratory in nature. Both had have previously been treated with glucocorticoids for a substantial time before diagnosis. A fatal case of toxoplasmosis was reported in a cat afflicted with eosinophilic granuloma complex receiving CsA at 5 mg/kg per day for a month, which was reduced because of anorexia to every other day. After 6 months of therapy, the patient developed fatal acute hepatic failure when the dose was increased to once daily. Toxoplasmosis was detected histologically in a number of tissues.[67] CsA apparently inhibits insulin secretion in a dose-dependent manner in humans.[33] Although this does not appear to be true in dogs, prudence dictates close monitoring of insulin needs in diabetic animals receiving CsA. [63b] In rare cases neurotoxocity, characterized by reversible cortical blindness, has been reported in human patients receiving CsA after bone marrow transplantation.[64]

KEY POINT 31-14 Cyclosporine A is much safer in dogs and other animals than in humans.

Mouatt[58] reported that 11 of 16 dogs receiving ketoconazole with CsA (Neoral solution) developed hair loss manifested as excessive shedding; five animals also developed metronidazole-responsive gingivitis with hyperplasia. Steffan[65] compared adverse events associated with CsA (n = 119; 5 mg/kg per day induction followed by tapering doses) versus methylprednisolone (n = 59; 0.5 to 1 mg/kg/day for 1 week, then every other day for 3 weeks, then tapered) in dogs with atopic dermatitis. The incidence of selected adverse events differed between groups. The most common in the CsA group were gastrointestinal, for a total of 55%. Among these, the most common was vomiting at 37%, which was significantly more than the methylprednisolone group (5%), followed by soft stools and diarrhea (18%). Infections occurred with similar frequency between groups but were more likely to be classified as severe or very severe in the methylprednisolone-treated group and led to more dropouts in that group. Polyuria, polydipsia, and increased appetite were more common in the methylprednisolone-treated group. Gingival hyperplasia was reported in 3% of CsA patients (none in the methylprednisolone-treated group). Serum chemistries indicative of renal function did not change from baseline. Potassium increased by approximately 0.6 mg/dL in the CsA-treated group (and decreased in the methylprednisolone-treated group) but was within normal values.

In their meta-anlysis of clinical trials evaluating the efficacy of CsA for treatment of atopic dermatitis in dogs (10 trials, 672 dogs treated with CsA for a duration of 0.5 to 6 months), Steffan[66] and coworkers reported that vomiting occurred in 25% of animals and soft stools or diarrhea in 15%. Remaining side effects occurred in less than 3% of the patients. The incidence of infection was not any greater for CsA-treatment groups and may have decreased in the skin and ear.

The commercial form of CsA intended for intravenous use has been associated with anaphylactoid reactions in the dog. The reactions appear to reflect the solubilizing agent. The vehicle of the intravenous preparation is very irritating and must not extravasate.

Monitoring

Monitoring of CsA concentrations can be an important tool to guide effective yet safe CsA regimens. The intent of monitoring should be to establish and maintain the therapeutic range for the patient, and to avoid toxicity or therapeutic failure, including that associated with drug interactions (see Chapter 5). Several points of controversy exist regarding monitoring. Reasons for monitoring in humans include, but are not necessarily limited to, avoiding nephrotoxicity; minimizing the risk of infection; and avoiding therapeutic failure, for which host-versus-graft rejection is the most important. In veterinary medicine monitoring might be implemented for the same reasons, but the need to avoid toxicity might take second stage to the need to assure effective concentrations in the face of marked variability in blood concentrations versus dose relationships. Identifying the intent of monitoring may influence down timing.

KEY POINT 31-15 The laboratory that will provide monitoring should be consulted regarding their therapeutic range. Therapeutic ranges should not be extrapolated from one laboratory to another.

Peak, trough, or midinterval samples are variably collected by veterinarians using the author's laboratory. Yet, the elimination half-life of CsA is short (approximately 5 to 8 hours). Accordingly, the drug generally does not accumulate or only minimally accumulates with multiple dosing. Therefore in most patients, no single sample can accurately predict the concentration throughout the dosing interval to which the patient is exposed. As such, the more critical the maintenance of effective doses throughout a dosing interval, the more helpful both a peak and trough sample might be. Detecting variability in absorption is best accomplished with peak concentrations whereas trough concentrations are influenced by both variability in absorption and elimination. Peak concentrations might be targeted if toxicity is of concern; trough concentrations might be targeted if a minimum effective dose must be maintained. However, trough concentrations run the risk of being nondetectable and failing to predict the marked variability that characterizes CsA absorption particularly with once daily dosing. The least useful sample is that collected mid-interval unless the patient is known to have a very long half-life. Note that if concentrations are to be compared across time (for example, to confirm that a dose increase resulted in higher concentrations), then care must be taken to collect subsequent samples at the same time point in the dosing interval. A difference of two hours can cause concentrations to fluctuate by 25% or more. The farther apart subsequent samples are and the shorter the elimination half-life of CsA in the patient, the less relevant are comparisons between samples collected across time.

KEY POINT 31-16 In addition to toxicity and efficacy, monitoring should be used to monitor drug interactions and to determine a patient's therapeutic range once a response has been realized.

Among the important determinants of whether a peak or trough sample is collected is knowing which concentration most accurately predicts response: peak (generally collected at 2 hrs to assure absorption and distribution have been largely completed), trough (just before the next dose, indicating the lowest concentration to which the patient is exposed during an interval) or area under the curve. Timing of sample collection (peak versus trough) is an area of investigation in human medicine. Monitoring traditionally has focused on trough concentrations (discussed later). However, trough (C_0, indicating the lowest concentration) correlates poorly to both graft rejection and acute nephrotoxicity.[68] Thus peak concentrations (C_2, indicating the highest concentrations anticipated at 2 hours) increasingly are becoming more relevant in humans, not only to predict efficacy but also to avoid toxic effects.[69] Because toxicity is a lesser concern in animals, trough concentrations might reasonably be preferred to ensure that drug concentrations stay above a minimum effective range throughout the dosing interval. Indeed most animal-based recommendations are based on trough concentrations (see later discussion). However, with the short half-life which characterizes most patients, reaching target concentrations will be easier if a peak sample is consistently collected. This is particularly true if a 24 hour dosing interval is used, for example, when treating atopy. Yet, a half-life of less than 8 hours often results in 24-hour concentrations that are minimally or not detectable. As such, although dose labeled for chronic allergic inflammation (e.g., atopy, asthma), it should not be assumed to be appropriate for autoimmune disorders or graft versus host rejection. For animals in which the CsA half-life is longer than 24 hours, concentrations may not be at steady state. If so, monitoring to establish baseline clearly must be withheld until steady-state concentrations are achieved; monitoring both a peak and trough, however, may be necessary to establish when steady state will occur (see previous discussion).

The impact of drug interactions is another reason for CsA monitoring. If altered clearance is anticipated, elimination half-life is the most likely outcome measure to be impacted that can be monitored. In such instances both a peak and a trough concentration are recommended; if a drug interaction is anticipated (e.g., the addition of ketoconazole), monitoring ideally will occur prior to and approximately 1 week after the inhibiting drug is administered. If a peak and trough concentration cannot be collected, then consistent timing (either a peak or a trough) should be targeted, with a sample before and 1 week after the other drug is changed. Note, however, that if the impact of the drug is to prolong the elimination half-life more than 48 hours, concentrations may not be at steady state at 1 week. The only means by which the duration of time that must elapse before steady state is reached (and thus baseline can be established) is determination of half-life (i.e., both a peak and trough sample). Monitoring should be implemented each time a drug that might alter the disposition of CsA is added or subtracted from the drug armamentarium for the patient.

KEY POINT 31-17 Recommendations for cyclosporine A concentrations are generally based on either a 2-hour peak or 12-hour trough; mid-interval samples are least helpful. Timing of sample collection should be consistent across time for the patient.

A second point of concern is the length of time after CsA therapy has begun that monitoring should be implemented. In general, the half-life of CsA is short enough that monitoring can be determined in 3 to 5 days. However, response to CsA may not occur that rapidly. Accordingly, if the goal of monitoring is to establish a therapeutic range in a responding animal, then monitoring is best implemented once a clinical response has been realized This is particularly relevant in the absence of concentration-response data in dogs or cats. The time to response (not resolution) is less clear, but several days to 2 weeks might be reasonable for most targets of therapy. However, some disease may require a longer period for maximum response (e.g., 4 months for perianal fistulae).

Among the limitations in CsA use in dogs and cats is evidence for the the actual concentration to be targeted, which in turn is closely related to timing of sample collection as well as the method used to detect CsA and the sample submitted. Guidelines offered in human medicine have served as targets for veterinary patients,[63] although the appropriateness of extrapolation has not been addressed. The impact of the assay reflects the presence of active metabolites (AM1, AM9) which may contribute up to 10 to 20% of activity in humans (more at trough concentrations); the concentration may be even greater if the metabolites accumulate. Several methods are available for measuring CsA concentrations, including HPLC, which generally detects only the parent compound. However, the contribution of active (and potentially toxic) metabolites has led to methods that detect both parent and metabolites.[39] The more common methods are immunoassays based on antibodies directed toward the parent (monoclonal) or parent and metabolites (polyclonal). These include radioimmunoassays (RIAs) and polarized immunofluorescence, which detect parent drug and metabolites. Immunoassays that are monoclonal (e.g., FPIA by Abbott TDx or ACMIA by Seimens) are less likely to detect in activemetabolites compared with polyclonal antibody-based assays. Either type of assay (HPLC versus antibody based) is acceptable; the choice might depend on cost or availability. The advantages of antibody-based assays are enhanced quality assurance and rapidity of turnaround time. The cost also should be lower. Each assay appears to be clinically useful. However, the target concentrations will vary with the methodology as well as the timing of the sample (i.e., peak or trough) and the sample collected (e.g., whole blood, plasma, or serum). Antibody-based assays will be accompanied by higher concentrations, with polyclonal concentrations higher than monoclonal. For example, in dogs blood concentrations measured by TDx assay are 1.5 to 1.8 times higher than those measured with HPLC assay.[33,44] However, this increase reflects, in part, detection of active metabolites; as such, monoclonal antibody-based assays that detect the metabolites might be the preferred type. Assays based on HPLC that determine the parent only will have the lowest therapeutic range; HPLC assays that include the metabolites will be higher. A disadvantage of HPLC assays is variability in results among laboratories. Even if similar methods are applied, variability in conditions can result in different concentrations. Thus the importance of using external quality-control programs will be particularly important for laboratories that use HPLC methods.

The sample submitted for CsA quantitation will also influence the concentrations and the therapeutic range. Most CsA in whole blood is located in red blood cells. Accordingly, whole blood is generally the preferred sample. Concentrations based on whole blood will be higher than those measured in plasma or serum. The most important point to be made regarding recommended therapeutic ranges is that they are laboratory specific, varying with sample timing, tissue collection, and assay method. If the laboratory is using an automated system, then the therapeutic ranges of that laboratory will be those established for the instrument. If the laboratory is using HPLC, then the ranges may be specific for that laboratory and only that laboratory. As an example of what might be expected, in humans recommended trough (before next dose) CsA concentrations (ng/mL) are as follows: for HPLC 100 to 300 (whole blood); RIA, monoclonal antibody methodology 150 to 400 (whole blood) or 50 to 125 (plasma or serum); RIA, polyclonal antibody methodology 200 to 800; fluorescent polarized immunoassay 250 to 1000. These numbers are offered as examples of therapeutic ranges. However, therapeutic ranges might also vary with the disease being targeted. A longitudinal replicate study examining differences between laboratories found marked variability within laboratories,[70] suggesting that intralaboratory variability is a major contributor to overall variability. Because of these reasons, care should be taken not to extrapolate results based on the methodology unless the laboratory fails to do so. However, the most important point to be made regarding therapeutic ranges is that this population statistic is a guide only. Monitoring should be used to determine the patient's therapeutic range. Once response has been realized, a sample should be collected, the concentration identified, and subsequent samples collected at that same time during the dosing interval.

Monitoring is generally based on 12 hour dosing. The dosing regimen recommended for treatment of atopy[71] should not be assumed to be effective for treatment of immune-mediated diseases. In humans, for which CsA is usually administered by mouth every 12 hours, estimates of drug exposure using the area under the time concentration curve appear to be the most accurate pharmacokinetic measure on which to based dosing in human patients subject to acute rejection episodes. However, the description of area under the curve requires multiple sample collection, which is not only inconvenient but also costly. Two established therapeutic drug-monitoring protocols have been used in humans: the traditional approach, based on trough blood concentrations (C_0), and the newer strategy, based on a sample taken 2 hours after oral administration (C_2). Because the greatest contributor to interindividual variability in CsA area under the curve in humans is absorption, monitoring that focuses on peak concentrations is evolving as more predictive for CsA. As was noted previously, the risk of graft-versus-host rejection was markedly reduced when CsA dosing was based on peak rather than trough concentrations in humans. However, the use of this parameter as a predictor of CsA exposure is based on a 12-hour dosing interval.[72] These recommendations are made regardless of the method of CsA detection (mRIA, EMIT, AxSym, CEDIA, or TDx/Architect) (Abbott FPIA). Mehl and coworkers[45] investigated the relationship between peak and trough plasma drug concentrations and area under the curve in cats receiving CsA. After 14 days of dosing, 2-hour peak concentrations correlated better than the 12-hour trough concentration with area under the curve during that same time period, which suggests that a 2-hour peak sample is the preferred sample for monitoring.[45] However, this study was based on predicting blood CsA concentrations and not predicting response.

A plethora of literature is dedicated to determining the best peak or trough target concentrations in humans receiving CsA, primarily for transplant patients but also for those with certain chronic allergic inflammatory disorders. For example, 12-hour concentrations, which probably do not accurately predict either rejection or toxicity but are reasonable for maintenance, range from 500 to 800, depending on the author. A review of the literature reveals that the range might also vary during the stage of disease, with initial concentrations for immune-mediated diseases being substantially higher, whereas lower concentrations are acceptable as targets for maintenance once response has been realized. Most recommendations in humans are based on monoclonal antibody assays.[72]

The consensus among most investigators is that area under the concentration versus time curve is the best predictor of acute or chronic graft rejection and toxicity.[69] Mahalati and coworkers[68] demonstrated that the initial area under the concentration-time curve (C_0 and C_4 ; or AUC_{0-4}) was a useful tool: ranges between 4400 and 5500 ng/mL per hour for the first 4 hours of dosing significantly reduced the risk of acute rejection and nephrotoxicity in humans. This parameter is more useful with newer microemulsion products because CsA disposition is more predictable with these products. For this study samples were collected at 0 (just before the next dose), 1,2, 3, and 4 hours. A similar approach might be considered for animals during the early, critical stages of immune-mediated disease, with sample collection at 0 and 4 hours. However, collection of sufficient samples to describe the curve completely is generally not practical in either human or veterinary patients. For single point prediction, 2-hour posttreatment (C_2) collection has repeatedly been demonstrated to be the most accurate predictor of area under the curve in humans, although even this time point is controversial. However, Einecke and coworkers[69] demonstrated that C_2 concentrations were not helpful in identifying patients at risk for rejection, but ranges between 500 and 600 ng/mL (whole blood, CEDIA antibody-based assay) were useful to maintain patients for long periods and avoid toxicity. This study suggests that the target range should vary as treatment moves from the induction to the maintenance mode.

Studies correlating CsA concentrations with efficacy are limited in animals. Perhaps the most supportive is with regard to perianal fistulae. Mouatt[58] found that dogs with perianal fistulae (n = 14) responded more rapidly if trough concentrations exceeded 600 ng/mL, but time to resolution (generally 4 weeks) could not be predicted by concentrations in this small group of dogs.

Use of monitoring for atopic dermatitis is less clear. In a manufacturer-sponsored study, Steffan[44] and coworkers investigated the relationship between CsA concentrations and response in dogs (n = 97) with atopic dermatitis. Concentrations were measured between 2 and 24 hours of the last dose at 28 days, and this single point concentration was used to predict the time course of CsA, based on a model generated from normal dogs (n = 16). Patients were then grouped into one of five categories of CsA exposure, ranging from very low to very high CsA. Clinical response to therapy was based on scoring of skin lesions (canine atopic dermatitis extent and severity index [CADESI]) and pruritis. Response to therapy (CADESI and pruritis scores) was then compared (not correlated) among groups. The study could not demonstrate a differenc in response among the groups, leading the authors to conclude that concentrations did not correlate with response and monitoring was not indicated. However, this study should not necessary be considered evidence against monitoring in dogs with atopic dermatitis. First, a single time point of CsA was used to predict 24-hour exposure of CsA for clinical patients. Second, the model used to predict CsA was based on normal Beagles, of which only eight had received multiple dosing of CsA. Third, variability in the clinical patients was greater than in normal animals, and the predicted model differed from the observed. The variability in peak CsA, in particular, found in this study is profound, and its impact on therapeutic success should be examined. Variability also occurred in pruritis scores, being equal or greater than the median, which may have impacted the power to detect a significant difference was likely low. Because peak concentrations appear to occur in most animals between 1 and 2 hours, a study that correlates actual peak concentrations with scores might be prudent before the use of CsA monitoring for anticipating response of atopic animals to therapy is set aside. Studies are indicated to determine the best sampling time for dogs receiving CsA. Because concentrations are so low at 24 hours and often undetectable, it is likely that some other sampling period is appropriate for 24-hour dosing intervals.

It is important to emphasize that studies that fail to correlate CsA concentrations with therapeutic response do not prove the lack of or preclude the usefulness of monitoring. In ability to demonstrate a significant difference does not equate to "no treatment" effect. Studies may fail to find a connection because of limitations in study design. In the event that a sufficiently well-designed study (or several studies) should fail to find a correlation, the clinician must remember that the most important reason for monitoring is to establish a therapeutic range for the patient. Once the patient has responded, monitoring might be most useful to maintain that concentration in the patient.

In summary, our laboratory offers the following recommendations for monitoring of patients treated every 12-hours: a 2-hr peak and just before the next dose trough sample is recommended within 3 to 5 days of initiating therapy; the more life threating the target disease, the more important a peak and trough sample may be. For less serious situations, or as treatment shifts from induction to maintenance, a singe 2-hr peak sample or, assuming bid dosing, a single 12 hour trough concentration may be sufficient for establishing and maintaining a target. If therapy is initiated such that CsA disposition might change (whether intentional, such as the addition of ketoconazole, or inadvertent, such as co-treatment with diltiazem or azithromycin or others), a peak and trough sample prior to and 1 week after therapy is initiated is suggested. In situations in which alternatve generic preparations are initiated, a single 2-hr peak concentration before and 3 to 5 days after the switch is recommended. For atopy (24 hr and beyond dosing), a single peak sample should be collected. Likewise, if toxicity is a concern, a single peak sample is indicated. However, in patients with a long half-life, both a peak and trough sample may be necessary to fully assess the risk of toxicity. Monitoring is recommended weekly to biweekly in critical patients, then monthly for the first several months of therapy or until concentrations are stable. For long-term maintenance, the frequency of samply may vary with the stability of the patient but should range from 3 to 6 months. Target concentrations vary with the condition but generally, based on a 12-hr dosing interval using a monoclonal antibody-based assay (i.e., as in the author's laboratory), a peak concentration of 800 to 1400 ng/mL and a trough concentration of 400 to 600 ng/mL (monoclonal based assay) is recommended for immune mediated diseases. For renal transplantation, trough concentrations of 750 ng/mL are suggested for the first month and 350 to 400 ng/mL, thereafter. For chronic allergic inflammatory disorders, lower concentrations are recommended: 250 ng/mL trough concentrations for chronic inflammatory bowel disorders, and for perianal fistulae, 12 hour trough concentrations at 100 to 600 ng/mL (the higher for induction, the lower for maintenance).

Therapeutic Use

Chronic Allergic Inflammatory Disorders

Atopy and other dermatologic conditions. The use of CsA for treatment of veterinary dermatologic syndromes has been reviewed.[73] Olivry and Mueller[74] reviewed treatment of atopic dermatitis in dogs in general and found good evidence for efficacy of glucocorticoids and CsA compared with fair evidence for topical triamcinolone, topical tacrolimus, oral pentoxifylline, and oral misoprostol. In the manufacturer-sponsored study, Steffan and coworkers[65] prospectively compared the efficacy of CsA (n = 119) and methylprednisolone (n = 59) in dogs with atopic dermatitis using a randomized, blinded (investigators but not owners) parallel study. Dosing began with an induction phase for both drugs, followed by a tapering phase, with the dose determined by CADESI scores. Dosing for CsA was 5 mg/kg once daily for 4 weeks, then tapered on the basis of the CADESI score, and for methylprednisolone, 0.5 to 1 mg/kg daily for 1 week, followed by every other day for 3 weeks, and then tapered on the basis of the CADESI score. Washouts were required for drugs that might influence response. At the end of the 4-month study period, the percentage of reduction in CADESI scores was approximately 45% in both groups. The proportion of responders (CADESI scores reduced by ≥ 50%) was approximatey 58% for methylprednisolone and 66% for CsA; a significant difference could not be demonstrated. Scores worsened in approximately 15% of both groups.

More recently, Steffan and coworkers[66] reviewed clinical trials evaluating the efficacy of CsA for treatment of atopic dermatitis in dogs. Ten trials met their standards; 799 dogs were treated with either CsA (n = 672 for a duration of 0.5 to 6 months), placebo (n = 160), oral glucocorticoids (n = 74), or antihistamines (n = 23). Further, safety data were available for 660 dogs. Among the concerns the authors addressed well was publication bias (the study was sponsored by the manufacturer). Treatment success was defined as a 50% or higher reduction in lesion scores after the 4- to 6-week induction period (denoted as high responders). Compared with placebo, but not oral glucocorticoids, the effects of CsA were highly significant. Dosing intervals generally could be prolonged to 48 hours in 40% to 50% of responders after 4 weeks and to twice weekly in 20% to 26% of dogs after 12 to 16 weeks. Predictors of success could not be identified, although initial response was predictive of long-term response. Feeding, age, and body weight did not appear to affect success; the influence of breed could not be assessed. The dose ranged from 2.5 mg/kg twice daily to 5 mg/kg twice weekly. Doses generally begin at 5 mg/kg once daily. The treatment induction period was considered 4 to 6 weeks, although not all studies reviewed treated for that time period. The authors identified those aspects of the meta-analysis that were relevant for clinical practice. They concluded that the severity of skin lesions can be expected to decrease by at least 40% during the initial 4 to 6 weeks of induction therapy at 5 mg/kg. The benefits may be less pronounced in dogs that previously received glucocorticoids. The dose can be reduced, generally by prolonging the interval, after this reduction period if a response has been realized. If clinical signs worsen, the previous dose should be reinstituted. A further reduction in clinical signs may be realized after the 4- to 6-week induction period, with a plateau of 50% to 70% reduction occurring at 2 to 4 months. Unacceptable adverse events (most notably vomiting) should respond to dose reduction if related to the drug. What was not resolved by this meta-analysis is the impact of long-term therapy, as well as the sequelae of discontinuing therapy; response in animals that have not responded to glucocorticoids; and the impact of combination therapies, including topical agents.

Radowica and Power[71] retrospectively studied the efficacy of CsA (5 mg/kg per day) when used for a minimum of 6 (range 6 to 30) months for treatment of atopic dermatitis in dogs (n = 51). Continued therapy was necessary to control clinical signs in at least 55% of dogs, with most of these animals receiving the drug 2 to 5 times weekly, but one out of five requiring daily therapy. Therapy could be discontinued in 24% of animals after 6 to 24 months as a result of clinical response. Adverse events occurred in 22% of animals, including oral growths or gingival hyperplasia and hirsutism.

Other dermatologic indications for CsA include, but are not limited to, perianal fistulae, atopy, and eosinophilic granuloma complex. Mathews and coworkers[75] found that CsA was effective in eradicating or markedly reducing the size or number of perianal fistulae in 10 of 10 dogs. Initial dosing began at 10 mg/kg orally every 12 hours but was reduced to 5 to 7.5 mg/kg after 1 week because of excessive trough concentrations. Doses were adjusted to a trough measurement of 400 to 600 ng/mL. Duration of therapy ranged from 8 to 12 weeks; remission required another 4- to 6-week trial of therapy in 3 dogs. Remission was persistent in all dogs for at least 6 months and up to 18 months at the time the report was published. A follow-up study of a randomized controlled trial in 20 dogs[76] found that fistulae recurred in 7 of 17 dogs treated with CsA and required subsequent treatment or surgical excision. CsA was, however, beneficial presurgically to reduce the extent of excision. The investigators also found that trough CsA concentrations between 100 and 300 ng/mL (HPLC) were effective for treatment of perianal fistulae. The most frequently reported side effect in this study was shedding of hair, which was noticeable by 16 weeks. Older hair coats tended to be replaced with a softer coat.

Dogs (16) with perianal fistulae were prospectively evaluated for the efficacy of CsA (1 mg/kg orally twice daily; administered as Neoral liquid administered in a gelatin capsule) when combined with ketoconazole (10 mg/kg orally once daily); blood concentrations of CsA (based on HPLC) were monitored to maintain trough concentrations above 200 ng/mL (FPIA 300 ng/mL). All dogs showed clinical signs of improvement within 2 weeks of therapy; animals whose concentrations were above 600 ng/mL responded more rapidly, but efficacy did not seem to differ, although the power of the study to detect a relationship between cure rates and drug concentrations was not addressed. Lesions resolved in 93% of the animals within the 16-week treatment period, with 50% of the animals remaining cured at 12 months. Recurrence in the remaining dogs occurred within 1 month (21%) or between 8 and 12 months (21%). Although both medications appeared to be well tolerated, 67% of dogs exhibited excessive hair loss that started at 2 weeks but stopped at 7 weeks; hair coats thinned but were normal by study end. Further, 31% of the dogs developed gingival hyperplasia and gingivitis, which responded to metronidazole and spiramycin.[58]

Inflammatory bowel disease. Allenspach and coworkers[77] studied the efficacy of CsA (Atopica; 5 mg/kg once daily for 10 weeks) for treatment of canine IBD (n = 14) refractory to steroid therapy (prednisolone, the majority receiving 2 mg/kg orally per day for 6 to 14 weeks or more). CsA concentrations were measured in eight dogs with severe disease during a 24-hour period after the first dose; CsA was detected in whole blood using FPIA; a cohort of healthy dogs was available from a previous study (see Table 31-3). Animals were scored (canine IBD activity index [CIBDAI] criteria) on the basis of clinical signs and histopathologic lesions. Of the 14 dogs studied, eight completely responded within 4 weeks and three partially responded (posttreatment score of 2 to 4). Two failed to respond. Five of the 14 dogs with protein-losing enteropathy partially responded (posttreatment median score of 5). Although body weight increased, histopathologic lesions (nine dogs had repeated biopsies) did not. Overall, CsA was considered effective in 78% of the animals. Concentrations of CsA varied more in the diseased dogs (peak occurring at 1-2 hours of 699 ± 326 ng/mL compared ot 878 ± 131 ng/mL in healthy dogs), leading the authors to speculate on the role of previous glucocorticoid therapy, which may have increased P-glycoprotein, thus decreasing absorption. Elimination half-life in the respective diseased versus healthy populations was 5.6 ± 1.2 and 7.8 ± 1.1 hr, respectively. However, the authors did not describe the CsA concentrations in all nonresponders, although one of them had the highest peak and trough concentrations measured in the study. Adverse events not evident before initiation of therapy were vomiting, anorexia (improved by administering with food), gingival ulceration (one dog; resolved after 7 weeks), and alopecia followed by hypertrichosis (full replacement of the hair coat) in the first 2 weeks of therapy.

CsA appeared to act synergistically with dexamethasone for the treatment of IBD in human patients. Each drug appears to target through different mechanisms the chemokines responsible for migration of white blood cells to the site of inflammation.[78] In humans a 12-hour trough concentrations of 150 to 250 ng/mL has been recommended for CsA when treating IBD. [79]

Asthma. Other potential indications for CsA warrant further investigation. Cats suffering from *A. suum*–induced airway reactivity had decreased reactivity and remodeling after receiving CsA; differences were noted with 24 hours of therapy.[80]

CNS Disorders. Adamo and O'Brien[84] reported on the successful use of CsA for treatment of granulomatous meningoencephalitis (GME) in a series of three cases. The initial dose of 3 mg/kg twice daily was increased to 6 mg/kg twice daily. Concentrations of CsA (ng/mL) were 235, 337, and 592 (unfortunately, sample timing not provided); variability was assumed to reflect, in part, differences in sampling times, which were not provided. In one dog, the initial dose of 3 mg/kg twice daily yielded CsA of 82 ng/mL (timing not provided); the dose was increased to 10 mg/kg twice daily. This dog did not sufficiently respond, developed azotemia and an *E. coli* urinary tract infection; on necropsy, disseminated GME was diagnosed. A different dog also was initiated at 3 mg/kg twice daily; CsA was 117 ng/mL, and the dose was increased to 6 mg/kg twice daily, which was subsequently decreased back to 3 mg/kg after 7 months, resulting in CsA at 215 ng/mL. The dose was tapered to 3 mg/kg once daily, yielding CsA at 63 ng/mL. Several attempts to detect CsA in cerebrospinal fluid revealed no detectable drug; however, its large size and the presence of P-glycoprotein is likely to preclude CNS penetration by CsA. However, efficacy of CsA is not likely to depend on penetration of the CNS. On the basis of this series, 6 mg/kg twice daily might be considered until animals with GME are in remission, with the dose tapered to 3 mg/kg twice daily on response. In humans, CsA has proven useful for treatment of chronic inflammatory demyelinated polyradiculoneuropathy; concentrations were not provided.[84a]

Immune-Mediated Disease

Systemic use of CsA increasingly is being used for treatment of autoimmune disorders, particularly in those that have not responded to traditional immunosuppressive therapy. However, the labeled doses for atopy should not be assumed to be relevant for other immune-mediated diseases, including dermatologic.

Noli and Toma[81] reported the successful use of CsA for treatment of immune-mediated adnexal skin disease in a series of cases (n = 3; two cats, one dog). In each case response occurred within 1 month of administration at 5 mg/kg once daily, CsA therapy was successful in treating aplastic anemia in three of four dogs[82] when dosed at 5 to 10 mg/kg every 12 hours (unfortunately, CsA concentrations were not provided).

Font and coworkers[83] reported a single case of cutaneous lupus erythematosus that was successfully treated with 4 mg/kg CsA once daily along with ketoconazole (4 mg/kg) once daily. Prednisone therapy was continued at 0.2 mg/kg for 10 days. Lesions resolved in 2.5 months of CsA therapy. Concentrations of CsA associated with response at 10 days was 139 ng/mL; the timing of sample collection was not indicated, although it is possible in the presence of ketoconazole, that this concentration did not vary substantially during the dosing interval. Concentrations were 279 ng/mL at the time ketoconazole was stopped. The dog remained in remission at the end of the 18-month report period, receiving 2 mg/kg daily. The use of glucocorticoids, ketoconazole, and lack of information regarding the collection of samples complicates correlating concentratiosn to response. A randomized placebo-controlled study on the use of CsA for treatment of spontaneous glomerulonephritis in dogs[46] failed to document a a significant improvement in treatment groups; the power of the study was not addressed. Packed cell volume was lower in the CsA-treated group; in addition, clinical signs compatible with decreasing renal function appeared to be more severe in animals receiving CsA.

With the availability of renal transplantation at several facilities, CsA is increasingly being used to prevent graft-versus-host rejections. Cats respond better than dogs, with renal allografts being maintained at 7.5 mg/kg every 12 hours coupled with prednisolone (0.125 to 0.25 mg/kg every 12 hours).[46] Trough concentrations of whole blood should be maintained at 500 ng/mL (HPLC; approximately 750 ng/mL should be expected for FPIA) the first month after transplantation but can be reduced to 250 (375 to 400 FPIA ng/mL) thereafter.

Topical CsA has been used with some success for localized immune-mediated diseases, including pemphigus foliaceus. An ophthalmic preparation is approved for use in dogs to treat keratitis sicca..[85] Benefits include both immunomodulation and an increase in tear production. A 0.2% CsA compound in a petrolatum–corn oil ointment is commercially available (Schering-Plough) for keratitis sicca in dogs. Application of one drop of the commercial preparation twice daily should be effective in up to 80% of dogs. The frequency of administration can be decreased to every other day for most dogs.

When compared with dexamethasone and indomethacin, topical CsA was equal in suppressing arachidonic acid–induced inflammation,[86] and studies are under way to evaluate its use in canine dermatologic diseases.

Tacrolimus and Related Drugs

Tacrolimus, like CsA, is a macrolide antibiotic, produced by *Streptomyces.* Like CsA, it inhibits T cell activation, but rather than binding to cyclophilin, it binds to and inhibits an alternative cytosolic protein, FKPB12. Calcineurin-dependent activation of lymphokine expression, apoptosis, and degranulation is inhibited.[4] The intracellular receptors for tacrolimus are distinct from those for CsA and it is 500 fold more potent than CsA in its effects. This may reflect, in part, a 3-fold greater uptake in lymphocytes for tacrolimus compared to CsA (however CsA uptake in RBC is 10-fold higher than tacroliumus).[86a] The drug is available for both oral and intravenous systemic administration. Toxicities are similar to those of CsA in humans, although gingival hyperplasia may be less prevalent. The drug may be more toxic than CsA in dogs, and its systemic use has not been recommended.[87] Tacrolimus disposition has been reported in male Beagle dogs receiving 1 to 4 mg/kg.[87a] Peak and trough concentrations (ng/mL), respectively, ranged from 0.8 to 1.8 ng/mL (at 1 mg/kg) to 3.2 to 5.3 ng/mL (2 mg/kg) and 0.25 to 0.8 ng/mL (1 mg/kg) to 0.2 to 2.3 ng/mL (2 mg/kg). For tacrolimus and sirolimus, trough (before the next 12-hour dose) rather than peak concentrations more effectively predict area under the curve.[72] Tacrolimus is also available as a topical ointment. The 0.1% preparation has been used in dogs to treat localized lesions associated with discoid lupus erythematosus as well as two cases of pemphigus erythematosus either as a sole therapy or adjunctive treatment.[88] No side effects were reported, and all animals improved after 8 weeks of topical application, with adjuvant therapy being discontinued in the majority of animals. Tacrolimus ointment also has been used effectively for the treatment of canine atopy.[89] Using a double-blinded, placebo controlled, cross-over study, dogs (n = 12) were treated with topical 0.1% tacrolimus (maximum dose of 0.1% mL/kg/day) applied topically at sites considered most pruritic for 4 weeks. Following a 2-week washout (based on a 9-hr half-life of tacrolimus in dogs), animals were switched to the alternative treatment. The randomization procedure was not robust (alternating treatment assignments). The mean clinical score improved in both the placebo and the treatment group at 4 weeks compared to baseline, but response was significant for the tacrolimus group. Tacrolimus was detectable in patients (peak concentration at 4 weeks of 1.4 ± 0.2 ng/mL). However, peak concentration of 0.6 ng/mL was also detected at week 4 in the placebo group calling into question the credibility of the report. Tacrolimus may impact intradermal skin testing in dogs, with an effect on the late phase, but not the immediate response. [89a]

Griffies and coworkers[88] reported on the successful use of tacrolimus (0.1%) topically in a series of cases in dogs. The drug was used as either sole agent or as an adjuvant topically for treatment of localized lesions associated with discoid lupus erythematosus or pemphigus erythematosus. Improvement required approximately 8 weeks of therapy, and adjuvant therapy could be discontinued in some dogs.

In contrast to tacrolimus, sirolimus and its derivative, everolimus, do not inhibit calcineurin; rather, they interact downstream from IL-2, targeting the immunophilin with FKBP12. This complex then inhibits mTOR (mammalian target of rapamycin), which prevents progression from the G1 to S phase transaction in the cell cycle, in a manner that prevents cytokine receptors from activating the cell cycle and subsequent signaling.[90] Its use is primarily replacement of CsA to protect renal function in humans.

Mycophenolate Mofetil

Mycophenolate mofetil (MMF) is the morpholinoethyl ester prodrug of mycophenolic acid (MPA), which is a product of several *Penicillium* species that possess antibacterial, antifungal, antiviral, antitumor, and immunosuppressive properties. MPA is a potent, selective, noncompetitive, reversible inhibitor of inosine monophosphate dehydrogenase (IMPDH). This enzyme is critical for the production of the guanine triphosphate precursor guanine monophosphate, which in turn is necessary for the de novo synthesis of purine nucleotides. As such, the drug is an antimetabolite. Two isoforms of human IMPDH exist. Type I is constitutively expressed in normal, nonreplicating cells, and type II is upregulated in replicating (including neoplastic) cells to the point that it is the predominanting isoform. As IMPDH is inhibited, guanine triphosphate is depleted; failure to make mRNA precludes synthesis of proteins, including cytokines, necessary for cell proliferation. Unlike other anticancer antimetabolites, MMF and its active metabolite MPA are relatively selective for lymphocytes because they are solely dependent on de novo synthesis of purines for DNA synthesis.[91,92] MMF is the first drug since CsA to be approved in the United States for prevention of renal allograft rejection; it has proved useful for treatment of steroid-resistant acute liver rejection.[93] In addition to its antiproliferative properties toward lymphocytes, MPA also impairs proliferation in nonimmune cells, including smooth muscle cells, renal tubular cells, mesangial cells, and dermal fibroblasts.[94] Consequently, MMF might be indicated for non–immune-mediated diseases associated with fibrosis.

A bilateral nephrectomized dog model has been used to study MMF.[91] The disposition appears to be characterized by marked variability in dogs. After doses of either 20 or 40 mg/kg, mean peak concentrations of MPA were, respectively, approximately 90 and 130 μg/mL, yet peak concentrations did not statistically differ between the two groups. Based on canine lymphocytes exposed to whole blood containing MPA, 200 μg/mL MPA is necessary to inhibit baseline activity of IMPDH by 50%. The elimination half-life of the drug ranged from 1.45 to 11.09 hours, with a mean of approximately 7 hours, regardless of the dose. The drug also has been studied in normal dogs at approximately 20 mg/kg, Maximum concentrations of MPA after intravenous (2-hour infusion) and oral administration, respectively, were 21 ± 3.6 and 11.8 ± 6.6 μg/mL; oral bioavailability was 54%.[95] The elimination half-life of MPA was about 45 minutes, and mean resistance time was approximately 2 hours. The half-life is substantially shorter than that reported in humans (17 to 19 hours). However, suppression of IMPDH lasted for a mean of about 6.5 hours,[96] suggesting an 8-hour dosing interval might be appropriate. In human monitoring of trough concentrations has been recommended: trough (predose) concentrations less than 1 μg/mL were associated with acute liver transplantation rejection, whereas concentrations greater than 3.5 μg/mL were associated with a threefold increase in the risk of leukopenia or pneumonia. Therefore trough concentrations between 1 and 3.5 μg/mL are recommended.[90] It may be necessary to increase the dose of MMF in patients with low albumin; the dose had to be increased in human patients by approximately twofold if serum albumin was less than 3.5 gm/dL. However, the dose could be decreased by approximately 40% in the presence of renal dysfunction.[90]

KEY POINT 31-18 Mycophenolic acid targets both T and B lymphocytes and accordingly should be associated with greater immunosuppression compared with cyclosporine A.

The primary side effects in human patients receiving the drug for allograft rejection are leukopenia, gastrointestinal upset, and cytomegalovirus disease. The incidence is, however, small. Gastrointestinal upset is characterized by nausea, diarrhea, vomiting, and abdominal cramping. Gastrointestinal toxicity (and bone marrow suppression) may reflect the need for IMPDH II because of the normally replicating nature of these tissues.[97] The drug also appears to be relatively safe in dogs, on the basis of renal and hepatic indices of damage, even when dosed at 80 mg/kg twice daily. At that dose, transient increases in hepatic damage enzymes occurred.[98] However, when used chronically at 30 mg/kg orally every 12 hours, severe diarrhea, anorexia, and weight loss occurred in dogs[95]; at 20 mg/kg orally every 12 hours, signs recurred, although the were less severe, within 1 week of initiating therapy. One dog died acutely with necrotizing pneumonia 7 days after initiation of therapy.[96] Dysgranulopoiesis, characterized by pseudo Pelger–Huet anomaly has been reported in a series of human cases receiving MMF for heart–lung transplantation; resolution occurred only after the drug was reduced in dose or discontinued.[99]

Among the indications for MMF is dose sparing of CsA, which probably is more clinically relevant in humans compared with dogs or cats.[100] Initial induction with CsA is followed by the addition of MMF and down titration of CsA. MMF has been used therapeutically in dogs both clinically and experimentally. Clinically, the drug has been used successfully to treat myasthenia gravis,[101] although review articles offer anecdotal support for use in other immune-mediated disorders. Experimentally, MMF (10 mg/kg subcutaneously every 12 hours) in combination with CsA (15 mg/kg orally every 12 hours) has been used in dogs to prevent renal allograft rejection.[102]

Leflunomide

Leflunomide is a recently approved immunomodulatory drug that inhibits dihydroorotate dehydrogenase, an enzyme responsible for the de novo synthesis of pyrimidine. Both T and B cell proliferation is inhibited; accordingly, both cell-mediated and humoral responses are targeted. Cell adhesion also impaired. Other proposed mechanisms are inhibition of cytokine and growth factors mediated by tyrosine kinase. Like MMF, it is a prodrug, with its activity reflecting a malononitrile metabolite (A77 1726). It has been studied for the treatment of rheumatoid arthritis in humans.[103] The half-life of the active compound is long in humans, ranging from 1 to several weeks, indicated a long time to steady state. However, a recent disposition study in dogs reveals the elimination half-life of the metabolite to be 14 hrs in the dog. Limited information is available regarding its use in dogs.[104] Anecdotal reports suggest that the drug is effective for treating a number of immune-mediated disorders, including immune-mediated hemolytic anemia (IMHA), immune-mediated thrombocytopenia, canine cutaneous histiocytosis, and pemphigus foliaceus (2 to 4 mg/kg orally every 24 hours). Side effects that reportedly occur in dogs include leukopenia, thrombocytopenia, and gastric ulceration. Gregory and coworkers[104] reported on the use of the drug (1.5 mg/kg twice daily to 2 to 4 mg/kg once daily) in dogs (n = 29) afflicted with various immune-mediated disorders. These include idiopathic thrombocytopenic purpura (n = 3; good to excellent response), IMHA with idiopathic thrombocytopenic purpura (Evans syndrome), systemic histiocytosis (n = 3; one failure and two total remissions), multifocal nonsuppurative encephalomyelitis (n = 5; good to excellent response), and a variety of other immune-mediated disorders that had not responded to glucocorticoids or azathioprine. Most of the animals had not responded to first- or second-tier immunosuppressants. Side effects included decreased appetite, mild anemia, and bloody vomitus or stools (n = 3). Leflunomide was studied at doses ranging from 2 to 16 mg/kg/day as sole therapy or in combination with CsA (10 mg/kg/day) in dogs undergoing experimental reanl transplantation[104a] Rejection occurred at 4 mg/kg; mean survival time increased from 9 days (non-immunesuppressed dogs) to 16 days at 4 mg/kg, 28 days at 8 mg/kg. The addition of CsA at 10 mg/kg to leflunomide at 4 mg/kg increased survival time to 68 days. Mean trough leflunomide concentrations ranged from 10 μg/mL (2 mg/kg) to 55 μg/mL (16 mg/kg).[104b] A recent retrospective study examined the efficacy of leflunomide for treatment of naturally occurring immune-mediated polyarthritis in dogs. [104c] At an initial starting dose of 3.0 ± 0.5 mg/kg orally once a day for 1 to 6 weeks, 8 of 14 dogs had complete resolution, and 5 partial resolution. No animal exhibited adverse reactions.

Emerging Drugs

The sphingosine-1-phosphate receptor (S1PR)[105] antagonists are a new class of drugs that decrease recirculation of lymphocytes from the lymphatic system to blood and peripheral tissues. These drugs will not be used as monotherapy, but they have shown efficacy in human medicine when combined with CsA, glucocorticoids, and other drugs. Lymphopenia is the most common side effect and is reversible when the drug is discontinued. However, it may also act as a negative chronotrope.

Hormones

Glucocorticosteroids (see Chapter 30) possess both antiinflammatory and immunomodulatory capabilities. Immunomodulation results in actions at a variety of targets in acquired immunodeficiency syndrome. Selected progestational compounds (e.g., megestrol acetate) have been used for their general immunosuppressive effects. Megestrol acetate (discussed in Chapter 19) may have longer and more potent antiinflammatory effects compared with glucocorticoids[106]; however, in the cat, the species for which these products tend to be used, side effects can be dramatic and life threatening. Thus their use is recommended only for conditions that will not or have not responded to glucocorticoids. Medroxyprogesterone exhibits glucocorticoid-like effects, which reflect, in part, actions at the level of DNA transcription. The impact of glucocorticoids on DNA transcription was previously reviewed (see Chapter 30); those glucocorticoids that target trans (rather than cis) repression (rather than activation) are directed toward desirable effects, avoiding many undesirable metabolic effects. Medroxyprogesterone appears to potentially focus on undesirable effects inflammatory responses, being characterized by a preponderance of transrepression activity rather than transactivation or cis activity.[19]

Danazol (5 mg/kg 2 to 3 times orally per day) is classified as an androgen but is characterized by weak androgenic activity. In human patients danazol has proved effective in stimulating increased concentrations of complement inhibitor and thus is indicated for treatment of angioneurotic edema.[107] Danazol also has immunomodulatory effects that are of benefit in type II immune complex diseases. Danazol apparently decreases the expression of or blocks Fc receptors on macrophages; initial displacement of glucocorticoids owing to competition of binding sites is less likely to be effective as glucocorticoid clearance increases.[108-111] The drug has proved useful in a number of type II immune-mediated diseases, including IMHA (autoimmune hemolytic anemia) and immune-mediated thrombocytopenia.[11,108,112,113]

Cytotoxic Drugs: Antimetabolites and Other Antineoplastic Agents

Antimetabolite and alkylating antineoplastic agents (see Chapter 33) are also used as chemical immunosuppressants by virtue of their effects on actively dividing cells.[114,115] Their effects should, however, be regarded as nonspecific. Macrophages, activated T and B cells, and NK cells are the targets of most of the drugs. Those most commonly used for their immunomodulatory effects are cyclophosphamide and azathioprine. In general, neither drug is sufficiently immunomodulatory and safe for use as the sole agent.

Cyclophosphamide is a nitrogen mustard. Its immunomodulatory effects reflect the same mechanism of action as its anticancer effects. Cyclophosphamide alkylates DNA in both proliferating and nonproliferating cells; proliferating cells are more susceptible to alkylation. Both B and T cells are impaired. Because B cells recover more slowly, however, cyclophosphamide inhibits the humoral response more than the cell-mediated response.[4] Note that at very high doses cyclophosphamide can actually induce tolerance to an antigen to which the patient has been exposed. Toxicities of cyclophosphamide are typical of drugs that target proliferating cells. In addition, hemorrhagic cystitis has been reported in dogs receiving the drug. Cyclophosphamide therapy should be discontinued if the neutrophil or platelet counts decrease less than 2000/L or less than 100,000/L, respectively.

Azathioprine interacts with nucleophils to form 6-mercaptopurine, which is converted to nucleotides. The nucleotides interfere with purine synthesis or cause DNA damage. The drug is available for both oral and intravenous administration. Co-administration with allopurinol increases the risk of toxicity. Toxicity results from inhibited growth of rapidly growing cells, including cells of the bone marrow and gastrointestinal tract. The association of thiopurine methyltransferase (TPMT) activity and risk of azathioprine-induced neutropenia in dogs is not clear. Difficulty in identifying a relationship is compounded by the low incidence of deficiency (not detected in 470 dogs). The lack of relationship is supported by the finding of severe azathioprine-associated myelosuppression (marked leukopenia, neutropenia, or thrombocytopenia) in six clinically ill dogs classified as nondeficient. Further, an intermediate classification of TPMT (14 to 38 nmol/gHb/hr) in hunting dogs was associated with a decrease in white blood cells after 30 days of azathioprine therapy (2.2 mg/kg orally once daily) but not severe clinical signs of bone marrow depression. As such, a TPMT deficiency may predispose to azathioprine toxicity, but other factors appear to play an important role.[116] Cats are much more sensitive to the toxic effects of azathioprine. Although the drug has been used in cats (0.3 mg/kg daily), reformulation may be necessary for accurate dosing. Care must be taken to ensure that the dose is compounded accurately.

Chlorambucil (starting oral dose of 0.1 to 0.2 mg/kg/day) is also a nitrogen mustard, and its cytotoxic effects are similar to those of cyclophosphamide. The drug is available in an oral preparation that allows accurate dosing in cats.[106] In contrast to cyclophosphamide, chlorambucil's myelosuppression is only moderate and gradual. Toxicities are rare in cats.[106] The incidence of gastrointestinal side effects can be reduced by alternate-day dosing. In human patients, however, excessive doses can cause hypoplastic bone marrow. Its effects (e.g., in chronic lymphocytic leukemia) are gradual in onset.[117] Therapeutic indications include chronic, refractory immune-mediated disorders, including pemphigus foliaceus and refractory cases of feline granuloma complex.

Vincristine is used to treat immune-mediated thrombocytopenia because of its ability to cause the maturation and release of mature thrombocytes from the bone marrow by stimulation of megakaryocyte endomitosis. Other anticancer drugs used for immunomodulatory effects include methotrexate, and vinblastine. The nonspecific effects of anticancer drugs on the immune system and other rapidly dividing cells limit their use on account of host toxicity (primarily bone marrow and gastrointestinal). A major indication for immunomodulation of these drugs is combination with glucocorticoids for treatment of autoimmune diseases. Vinblastine is another vinca alkaloid that has been used to treat type II hypersensitivities, specifically IMHA. Like danazol, vinblastine appears to decrease expression of Fc (IgG) receptors on macrophages.[110,111] The effects of vinblastine (weekly doses during induction followed by monthly doses during maintenance) when combined with danazol (given at 2 to 3 up to 10 mg/kg daily) proved effective for treatment of 63% of human patients with chronic idiopathic thrombocytopenic purpura.[110]

Gold Therapy

Gold has been used for centuries as an elemental agent for the control of pruritis.[118] Gold compounds are characterized by gold attached to sulfur (aurothio group) and include the more water-soluble compounds aurothioglucose and gold sodium thiomalate and the lipid-soluble compound auranofin. These compounds suppress or prevent inflammation of the joint and synovium associated with a number of infectious or chemical causes. The mechanism of action is not clear but may be inhibition of the maturation and function of mononuclear phagocytes and T cells. Gold is sequestered in mononuclear phagocytic cells. Other proposed but not generally accepted mechanisms include inhibition of prostaglandin synthesis, collagen linkage, complement activation, and a variety of lysosomal and other enzymes.[118]

The disposition of the gold compounds has not been studied in animals other than humans; these data provide the basis of discussion. Disposition varies with water solubility. Water-soluble compounds (not prepared in oil) are rapidly absorbed after intramuscular administration, with peak concentrations occurring in 2 to 6 hours. Oral absorption is erratic and not predictable for the water-soluble compounds but is more predictable for auranofin, the hydrophobic compound. Distribution varies with the compound and duration of therapy. The gold is bound (95%) to albumin in blood, but eventually concentrations in selected tissues (inflamed synovium) approximate 10 times that in plasma. For the water-soluble gold compounds, elimination rate constants and half-lives also vary with dose. In humans the plasma half-life is 7 days at a 50-mg total dose, but it increases to several weeks to months with prolonged therapy. Concentrations can be detected in the blood for 60 to 80 days after therapy is discontinued and for up to 1 year in the urine. Concentrations probably are detectable in the liver and skin several to many years after therapy is discontinued. Excretion is predominantly (60% to 90%) renal, with the remaining eliminated in the feces. For auranofin plasma concentrations tend to be lower, and accumulation is much less (20%) than that of the water-soluble compounds, probably because of less tissue binding. Auranofin is eliminated principally in the feces.

Toxicity, manifested as skin or mucocutaneous lesions, occurs in 15% of human patients. Lesions include stomatitis, pharyngitis, tracheitis, colitis, gastritis, and vaginitis. Gray to blue pigmentation may occur in the skin. The likelihood of toxicity is concentration dependent but not based on gold concentration. Whereas proteinuria occurs in up to 50% of human patients receiving gold therapy, renal dysfunction (as a result of proximal tubular damage or gold-induced glomerulonephritis) occurs in 10% or less. Lesions tend to be resolvable if therapy is discontinued before damage is too severe. Thrombocytopenia, which is thought to reflect increased destruction, occurs in a very small percentage of human patients. A number of miscellaneous side or toxic effects that resolve when therapy has been discontinued also have been reported. These include encephalitis, peripheral neuritis, hepatitis, and pulmonary infiltrates. In general, although auranofin is better tolerated than the water-soluble compounds, the incidence of gastrointestinal disturbances (diarrhea, abdominal cramping) is greater. The incidence of side effects and their seriousness can be minimized by regular physical examination. In addition, therapy should be initiated with a small dose that is gradually increased to the maintenance dose. As the dose is increased, treatment should temporarily cease until clinical signs of moderate to severe toxicity resolve. The risk of restarting therapy should be balanced with the need for therapy. Antihistamines or glucocorticoids might decrease the incidence. Dimercaprol, a heavy metal chelating compound, can be used if severe side effects persist after therapy has been discontinued.

The major indication for chrysotherapy in human patients is rheumatoid or other arthritis that has not responded to nonsteroidal antiinflammatory drugs or other therapy. The compounds slow the progression but do not cure disease. The usual human dose is 10 mg of the water-soluble compounds the first week followed by 25 mg the third and fourth weeks and 25 to 50 mg weekly thereafter to a cumulative 1-g dose. Response may take several months. The standard human dose for auranofin is 3 to 6 mg up to 9 mg divided in two to three doses or given once daily. Small animal doses are discussed with dermatologic disorders in this chapter. Wolheim[119] has discussed mechanisms by which rheumatic human patients become refractory to gold therapy. Induction of the efflux protein P-glycoprotein appears to play a major role.

Immunostimulant Drugs

Immunostimulants are indicated for immunodeficient animals. As with immunosuppressants, immunostimulants can target either humoral or cell-mediated immunity. The lack of specificity has limited the widespread use of immunostimulants. In general, response to immunostimulants is mild.

Immunostimulants of Microbial Origin

Bacteria and fungal microbes generally nonspecifically stimulate several aspects of the immune response. Macrophage, cytotoxic T cell, T_h cell, and B cell activities are enhanced, whereas T cell suppressor activity is decreased. Enhanced activity reflects, in part, increased activity of chemical mediators such as TNFα and IFN. The nonspecific enhancement of immune function can be used therapeutically. Adverse effects can be minimized by administration of killed organisms or selected microbial fractions, which stimulate the response while avoiding infection. A variety of mycobacterial products have been used to nonspecifically stimulate the immune system.[23,120] The classic biological response modifiers include Bacillus Calmette–Guérin (BCG) and *Propionibacterium acnes (Corynebacterium parvum).*

Bacillus Calmette–Guérin

BCG is a live, attenuated strain of *Mycobacterium bovis.*[4] Components of the bacterial cell wall of this organism activate B and primarily T cells; macrophage and neutrophil recruitment in response to lymphokine release results in a granulomatous reaction. The antiviral state induced by BCG appears to be essentially a nonspecific expression of a more or less prolonged stimulation of the immune system. The most likely mechanism for its antiviral activity is direct stimulation of the mononuclear phagocytic system; however, specifically sensitized T lymphocytes that further activate macrophages are generated after a period of time. Stimulated macrophages release colony-stimulating factor, which contributes to macrophage regulation, and IL-1, which promotes lymphocyte proliferation. The antiviral state is thus an indirect benefit of an essentially pathologic, although temporary, situation; the host is characterized by an increased ability to handle viral infections. BCG requires at least 10 days after inoculation to enhance resistance against viral infections. The state of enhanced resistance is, however, long-lasting; repeated administrations (of nonliving product) may lead to a more prolonged and marked effect.[120]

BCG has been used as an adjuvant in combination with tumor vaccines for dogs and cats. Tumors that undergo remission after BCG therapy may do so as a result of the release of tumor-specific antigens during nonspecific tumor lysis. The use of BCG has been studied in combination with a tumor vaccine. In human patients use of BCG as an adjuvant for anticancer therapy has focused primarily on intravesicular administration in bladder cancer.[4]

Muramyl Dipeptide

Muramyl dipeptide is a peptidoglycan and represents the smallest immunologically active component of the *Mycobacterium* cell wall. Like BCG, it nonspecifically enhances B cell, T cell, and macrophage activities. Because it is rapidly eliminated from the body, it is biologically modified to prolong its actions by incorporation into liposomes or conjugation with glycoproteins. Synthetic production has increased accessibility for clinical use.

Mycobacterium

Regressin-V. An emulsion of mycobacterial cell wall fractions, Regressin-V is licensed for the treatment of mixed mammary tumors and mammary adenocarcinoma in dogs and sarcoidosis in horses. The following information was supplied by the manufacturer. Regressin-V contains trehalose dimycolate and muramyl dipetide, which induce IL-1 and tumor necrosis factor-α secretion from monocytes and macrophages and activate T lymphocytes in a variety of species. In a study of seven dogs with mammary adenocarcinoma, complete remission was induced in five, with tumor-free survival times of 3 to 19 months; dogs were then lost to follow-up. There are no data suggesting that Regressin-V had any effect on metastatic disease.

The manufacturer recommends treating canine mammary tumors once 2 to 4 weeks before surgical excision. Fever and malaise may occur after injection. Surgical removal of the tumor creates cosmetic improvement (necrosis and draining of the tumor may be present for weeks); however, survival time is not significantly improved with surgery. If surgery is not performed, therapy can be repeated every 1 to 3 weeks for up to four treatments.

Mycobacterium vaccae

Ricklin Gutzwiller and coworkers[121] prospectively studied the impact of a single intradermal injection of heat-killed *Mycobaterium vaccae* on the severity of atopic dermatitis in dogs (n = 62). A double-blinded, placebo-controlled, parallel multicenter study design was used. Dogs were evaluated for 3 months. Skin lesions were scored on the basis of CADESI. The treatment was well tolerated. Treatment was effective in patients with mild or moderate dermatitis but did not affect animals classified as severe. Interestingly, the CADESI scores decreased by 22% in the placebo group (versus 33% in the treatment group).

Propionibacterium acnes

A killed suspension containing *P. acnes* (formerly *C. parvum:* Immunoregulin) has been approved for veterinary use (15 μg/kg intravenously biweekly for two to three treatments). Like BCG, it causes complex, nonspecific immunostimulation. Macrophage and cytotoxic T cell activities are enhanced, as is antibody production by both thymus-dependent and thymus-independent antigens. Cell-mediated immunity is also stimulated. It is indicated for the treatment of clinical signs associated with virus-induced and bacteria-induced immunosuppression, such as that caused by FeLV. The efficacy of *P. acnes* in the treatment of feline infectious peritonitis virus is questionable. One study was unable to demonstrate a difference in survival rate or mean survival time between untreated and treated animals experimentally infected with a high dose of feline infectious peritonitis virus. Studies investigating the antitumor effects of *Propionibacterium acnes* in dogs do not support its efficacy against early neoplasia, although it may be more effective in advanced disease when used in combination with other drugs.[25] Cats infected with FeLV and afflicted with various non-neoplastic diseases showed some signs of response to treatment with *P. acnes* (Immunoregulin), although no cat reverted to an FeLV-negative status.[23] Studies regarding the efficacy of *P. acnes* in FeLV-induced tumors apparently have not been done.[25]

Staphylococcal Protein A

Staphylococcal protein A (SpA) is a cell wall polypeptide of *S. aureus* Cowan I (SAC) that binds rapidly and with great affinity to immune complexes. Other regions of the molecule initiate T lymphocyte and B lymphocyte proliferation as well as secretion of soluble lymphocytic products such as IFN. Circulating immune complexes have been incriminated as "blocking factors" that aid in a tumor's escape from immunologic control. Therapeutic trials of the efficacy of SpA have been based on the hypothesis that removal of specific or nonspecific immunosuppressive molecules such as blocking factors will enhance host immune response to the tumor. Other regions of the SpA molecule initiate T lymphocyte and B lymphocyte proliferation and secretion of soluble lymphocyte products such as IFN. Treatment with SpA is achieved by extracorporeal perfusion of host plasma over whole SAC organisms or through filters containing purified SpA. Studies have shown that SpA or SAC treatment reduces tumor size, decreases levels of circulating immune complexes, and induces the appearance of cytotoxic antibodies directed toward neoplastic cells. A study in which SpA was used to treat FeLV-infected cats found that 50% of cats with FeLV-associated disease improved, and 33%

of cats afflicted with malignant disease responded with reductions in tumor size as well as in bone marrow and peripheral blood neoplastic cells.[23,25,122,123] Viremia was cleared in 28% of treated cats. Circulation of a γ-like IFN was demonstrated in some cats that responded to SpA and was followed by the appearance and rising titer of complement-dependent cytotoxic antibody. The antibody reacted with FeLV-infected cells and was specific for the major viral envelope glycoprotein gp70. The ability of cats to persistently remain FeLV negative appeared to correlate with the magnitude of FeLV antibody titer.[25]

Mixed Bacterial Vaccines

Mixed bacterial vaccines composed of *Streptococcus pyogenes* and *Serratia marcescens* have been studied in cats with malignant mammary tumors. Although not statistically significant, survival time was greater (875 days) when surgery was combined with mixed bacterial vaccines versus surgery alone (450 days).

Immunostimulants of Natural Origin

Cytokines

Biological response modifiers of natural original also are discussed in Chapter 32. A number of cytokines produced by leukocytes and related cells actively regulate the immune system. Recombinant DNA technology has led to widespread production and greater application of drugs that modulate cytokines or their receptors or transcription factors in the treatment of immunologically based disease. The cytokines most likely to be used for immunostimulatory effects include the IFNs and selected interleukins.

Passive Immunotherapy: Antibodies

Passive immunotherapy with monoclonal or polyclonal antibodies has been investigated for both the diagnosis and therapy of cancers. Antibodies are directed toward surface antigens expressed by tumor cells. Specificity of antibodies (as long as Igs are derived from the species intended to be treated) should limit host toxicity to those cells expressing the antigen (i.e., tumor cells), thus avoiding systemic toxic effects. The antibodies themselves may be directly toxic to the cell or induce complement-dependent cytotoxicity. In addition, antibodies can be conjugated to drugs, toxins, or radioisotopes toxic to tumor cells, thus limiting the specificity of a variety of pharmaceuticals for tumor cells.

Igs available in plasma obtained from donors generally contain detectable antibodies against bacterial, fungal, and viral pathogens.[4] Passive transfer of resistance to the immunodeficient patient can be accomplished with intramuscular or intravenous administration. In human patients the half-life of transferred Igs is approximately 3 weeks.[4] Indications for human patients have included congenital or acquired states of immunodeficiency, selected hematologic disorders such as autoimmune hemolytic anemia, infectious viral diseases, and selected neoplastic diseases such as chronic lymphocytic leukemia and multiple myeloma. Potential adverse reactions include anaphylaxis and transfer of infectious organisms.[4]

Studies investigating the efficacy of passive immunotherapy on feline lymphosarcoma have thus far been limited to the use of polyclonal FeLV-neutralizing antibodies, feline oncornavirus-associated cell membrane antigen (FOCMA) antibodies, or both in cats afflicted with lymphosarcoma and leukemia. In one study five of seven cats treated with both antibodies and six of eight cats treated with FOCMA antibodies alone underwent partial or complete regression of their disease.[25] Additional studies by Cotter and coworkers[124] suggest that polyclonal anti-FOCMA therapy combined with previously established chemotherapeutic regimens may improve remission time. Monoclonal antibodies have been used to treat canine lymphosarcoma.

Human intravenous immunoglobulin (hIVIG) has been studied in dogs using in vitro (lymphocytes and monocytes) and in vivo (spontaneous immune-mediated diseases) methods. Prepared from plasma of healthy donors, it contains polyspecific IgG and is intended to treat primary immunodeficiencies. In vitro studies[125] have shown hIVIG to bind to canine lymphocytes and monocytes and to inhibit through Fc-mediated binding monocyte phagocytosis, including that of antibody-coated red blood cells. It is administered as an intravenous infusion (0.5 to 1.5 g/kg) over 6 to 12 hours, and animals must be closely monitored for signs of anaphylaxis or other adverse reactions (e.g., thromboembolism). Clinical evidence of efficacy exists for treatment of IMHA,[126-128] with treated dogs developing an increased hemoglobin and hematocrit concentration up to 4 weeks after therapy. However, 50% of treated animals developed thrombocytopenia and five of seven dogs that died had evidence of thromboembolism. Only 3 of 10 dogs were alive at 12 months, suggesting that long-term survival was not improved. The combination of IgG with IFN α resulted in greater improvement in human patients with hepatitis C.[129]

Abetimus is a synthetic molecule consisting of four double-stranded oligodeoxyribonucleotides attached to polyethylene glycol (PEG). The nonimmunogenic PEG serves as the carrier. Abetimus induces tolerance to B cells by cross-linking surface antibodies directed toward double-stranded DNA (dsDNA). These antibodies appear to be associated with nephritis associated with systemic lupus erythematosus in humans.[130] In a preapproval clinical trial, the number of renal "flares" in patients receiving the drug was less than half of that encountered in patients not receiving the drug. The response was so dramatic that the trial was discontinued before its completion, and the FDA granted orphan drug status in 2000.[130]

Allergen-Specific Immunotherpy

Allergen-specific immunotherapy (ASIT) involves the administration of gradually increasing amounts of an allergen extract to patients allergic to the allergen to resolve symptoms associated with subsequent exposure to the allergen.[131] In their review Colombo and coworkers[131] note that when success is defined as a 50% (or greater) increase in the improvement of clinical signs after 4 months or more of therapy, ASIT is successful in 50% to 100% of cases of canine atopic dermatitis. They prospectively evaluated the effect on canine atopic dermatitis of low (1/10 the standard) dose induction followed by maintenance ASIT therapy (n = 27) to standard therapy (n = 13). Both groups responded, and neither group emerged as responding better at 9 months. Secondary infections were treated, and use of glucocorticoids was allowed to control severe clinical signs, except during the last 3 months of the study.

Miscellaneous Blood Components

Selective destruction of malignant lymphocytes occurs in several species in response to infusion of blood or blood components.

Antileukemic activity. Antileukemic activity (ALA) of humoral factors in serum, heparinized plasma, and whole blood has been documented in several species.[25] Evidence suggests that ALA of blood constituents may be present in high concentrations in cryoprecipitates prepared from heparinized plasma. Physicochemical constituents of the cryoprecipitate that might be the source of ALA include cold-insoluble globulin, fibronectin, cell surface protein, large external transformation-sensitive protein, and opsonic factor.[25] A study in 32 cats revealed that of 24 treated with either normal cat serum or whole blood (20 mL/kg), 14 had a complete antileukemic response and 8 had a partial response. Of 10 treated with cryoprecipitate, two completely responded and six had a partial response.[132]

Fibronectin. Fibronectin injections have resulted in the regression of leukemic nodes in mice, suggesting that fibronectin may be the source of ALA. Fibronectin, a glycoprotein dimer, is a major protein of both blood and tissues; its most important function appears to be tissue remodeling during embryogenesis and wound healing. Antitumor activity may result from immunomodulation and modification of metastasis. Enhancement of opsonization increases the phagocytic ability of macrophages and monocytes, thus enhancing their tumoricidal activity. MacEwen[26] studied the efficacy of fibronectin (0.5 to 2 mg/kg intravenously once daily) in 18 cats afflicted with lymphosarcoma. A 50% response rate was reported; one FeLV-positive cat converted to a negative status after treatment.[25] A single case of mycosis fungoides in a cat responded to a combination of intravenous and intralesional fibronectin. Intralesional injections caused local epithelial necrosis, which reduced the tumor load by 75% and may have prevented systemic involvement.[133]

Tumor cell vaccines. Tumor cells are thought to stimulate an immune response. This view is supported by the recognition that some tumors spontaneously regress; tumors are infiltrated with cells of the immune system, and the risk of cancer increases in the patient that is immunosuppressed. The antigenic potential of tumor cells is also the basis for the use of tumor cell vaccines. Tumor cell vaccines are most effective in the presence of residual disease and when combined with nonspecific immunomodulators. Parodi and co workers [133a] could not find a statistical improvement in cumulative survival rates in dogs with mammary tumors receiving BCG intralesionally alone (n = 51) or *Corynbacterium parvum* (killed) (n = 120) Jeglum and coworkers have treated cats afflicted with mammary adenocarcinoma using a combination of an autogenous tumor vaccine and BCG. Although not significantly different, the mean survival time for each treatment group was least for those treated with surgery, BCG, and tumor cell vaccine compared with animals treated with either surgery alone or surgery with BCG. Additional studies with tumor cell vaccines are necessary before their efficacy can be established.

Non-steroidal hormonal agents. Hormonal agents may offer a unique avenue of immunomodulation in viral diseases.[23,134] Hormones investigated for their immunomodulatory effects include prostaglandins and thymic proteins. Prostaglandins are local hormones that modulate both T and B lymphocytes. Prostaglandins, however, particularly prostaglandin E_2, are also immunosuppressants, and their role in immunopotentiation is limited. Thymosins are a group of endogenous substrates released from the thymus that stimulate the release of several pituitary neuropeptides. Thymic hormones induce maturation of T cell precursors, promote differentiation and proliferation of mature T cells, and thus restore rather than potentiate the immune system. Several synthetic thymic peptides have been synthesized by either chemical means or genetic engineering techniques. The primary clinical application of these proteins is restoration of the immune system in the immunoincompetent (including virally induced) patient.

Acemannan. Acemannan (Acemannan Immunostimulant) is a long-chain polydispersed $\beta_{1,4}$-linked mannan-based polysaccharide derived from the aloe vera *(barbadensis Miller)* plant. It stimulates the release of IL-1, IL-6, TNF-α, IFN-γ, and nitric oxide from macrophages, leading to tumor apoptosis and necrosis.[135,136] Other actions include enhancement of macrophage phagocytosis and cytotoxicity and interference with glucosidase I activity, leading to the production of abnormal glycoproteins by neoplastic cells, which appears to be associated with tumor cell death. Direct antiviral activity is associated with modified glycosylation of both virus-infected cells and glycoprotein coats of viruses, leading to inhibition of virus infectivity and replication.

Acemannan is licensed for the treatment of fibrosarcoma in dogs and cats. Intratumoral injection induces tumor encapsulation and necrosis, facilitating surgical excision. The recommended dosage is 2 mg intratumorally and 1 mg/kg intraperitoneally weekly for 6 weeks. No adverse effects of acemannan have been reported at the recommended dosage. In one report eight dogs and five cats with fibrosarcomas were treated with acemannan, surgical excision, and radiation therapy. Seven animals remained tumor-free at 440 to 603 days, with a median survival time of 372 days.[137] In an earlier clinical report, a variety of other carcinomas and sarcomas were also reported to respond.[138] It is not known what effect acemannan has on feline vaccine-associated sarcomas.

Acemannan has been used to treat cats with FeLV and feline immunovirus infections. Clinically affected cats treated with acemannan had improved quality of life and longer survival times than historical controls. Interestingly, oral administration of acemannan appeared to have the same efficacy as parenteral administration of acemannan, which is similar to cats treated with low-dose oral recombinant human IFN-α.

Synthetic Immunostimulants

Levamisole

Levamisole, a phenylimidazothiazide anthelmintic, has been the subject of intense and controversial research as a biological response modifier.[23,120] It is difficult to summarize the experimental and clinical data regarding the immunomodulating capabilities of levamisole. Levamisole has been regarded by some as a chemical agent capable of mimicking hormonal regulation of the immune system. It appears to stimulate recruitment and function of macrophages and T cells but only within a narrow range of doses and duration of administration in either the normal or immunoincompetent patient. Levamisole appears to alter cyclic nucleotide phosphodiesterases, decreasing cyclic guanosine monophosphate degradation and increasing cyclic adenosine monophosphate degradation. Elevated cyclic guanosine monophosphate in lymphocytes enhances proliferation and secretory responses. Chemotaxis, phagocytosis, lymphokine synthesis, and the ratio of helper to suppressor T cells are increased. Levamisole does not appear to have any effect in immunocompetent animals. The modulatory effects of levamisole range from enhancement to inhibition with much strain, sex, age, and antigen variability. T cell stimulation may be mediated by a soluble serum factor. Experimental studies generally have not supported the benefits of levamisole as have clinical studies. Levamisole (2 to 15 mg/kg) was frequently tested prophylactically in experimental trials, however, as opposed to therapeutically (i.e., in infected patients) in clinical trials, suggesting that potential benefits of levamisole result from restoration of immunocompetence after virally induced immunosuppression. Indications for levamisole in human medicine include Hodgkin's disease and rheumatoid arthritis and as an adjuvant chemotherapy of colorectal cancer.[4] The use of levamisole for treatment of cancer in animals is not supported. In two studies involving more than 130 cats with malignant mammary tumors, levamisole (5 mg/kg orally on 3 alternate days per week) did not increase survival time or decrease recurrence rate.[139] Levamisole causes adverse reactions typical of excessive cholinergic stimulation.

Cimetidine

Histamine exerts immunomodulatory effects, including suppression of cytotoxic T lymphocytes, downregulation of cytokines, and activation of suppressor T lymphocytes.[140] Cimetidine is a histamine (H_2) receptor antagonist that experimentally enhances a variety of immunologic functions. Suppressor T lymphocytes possess H_2 receptors, which, when blocked, result in potentiation of cell-mediated immunity. Although more studies are indicated, cimetidine may be useful in a variety of conditions associated with immunosuppression. Because it selectively inhibits suppressor function, however, cimetidine also may prove deleterious to patients with autoimmune disorders.

The anticancer effects of cimetidine have been studied in selected human cancers. The H_2 receptor blockers have been studied for their effects on gastric cancer cells. Cimetidine, but not famotidine, exhibits antiproliferative effects on gastric cancer cells. Ranidītine showed some inhibitory effects.[140] Cimetidine also appears to inhibit the growth of colorectal carcinoma;[141] lymphocyte infiltration increases in the cancers and is associated with an improved survival rate in patients receiving the drug.

Miscellaneous Immunostimulants

A variety of compounds are capable of inducing IFN; however, the immunomodulating effects of the inducers are variable. For example, double-stranded IFN-inducing polyribonucleotides (poly I:C) cause immunostimulation, whereas tilorone, a simple synthetic IFN inducer, enhances antibody production while depressing cell-mediated immune responses. Many other drugs are in the experimental phases of drug development. The following sections address some of the drugs that may or may not ultimately become approved.

ABPP (Bropirimine)

ABPP (2-amino-5-bromo-6-phenyl-4[^{3}H]-pyrimidinone), approved for use in humans, is a potent inducer of IFN in several species. Hamilton and coworkers[142] characterized the kinetics of ABPP and induced IFN in several species. They found that serum levels of IFN after treatment correlated well with serum concentrations of ABPP in the cat. ABPP was lethal in three of eight cats, however, at doses required to achieve minimal detectable levels of IFN. The authors postulated that the toxicity resulted from conversion of ABPP to phenolic derivatives that the cat excretes inefficiently.

Isoniplex

Isoniplex is an antiviral drug (see Chapter 10) that may also be used as an immunopotentiator in viral diseases.[23,120] Isoniplex enhances immune responses, including promotion of mitogen-stimulated T-lymphocyte proliferation and augmentation of antibody production and delayed-type hypersensitivity. The suggested mechanism of immunopotentiation by isoniplex begins with penetration of lymphocytes and suppression of viral RNA synthesis. It appears to support lymphocyte function by promoting RNA synthesis and translational ability. Further investigations regarding the use of isoniplex in viral infection should be anticipated because its efficacy results from an ideal combination of antiviral activity and immunopotentiation.

Promodulin

Promodulin is an experimental immunomodulating agent that has been subjected to clinical therapeutic trials for the treatment of cats concurrently infected with FeLV and feline infectious peritonitis.[23] Cats were treated with 50 mg/kg (up to 200 mg maximum dose) intravenously once daily for 5 consecutive days. Although promodulin induced rapid remission of clinical signs associated with feline infectious peritonitis, (e.g., anorexia, fever, and serosal effusions), it did not appear to be effective in the treatment of concurrent FeLV infections. Cats that responded did so within 2 weeks of the final injection; the duration of clinical remission appeared to vary between 1 and 3 months. Clinical signs after exacerbation of disease did not respond to a second treatment regimen. Promodulin also was not effective in treating FeLV-induced solid tumors.

Topical immunomodulators. Topical immunomodulators often are characterized by unique mechanisms. These include topical contact sensitizers (e.g., diphencyprone or dinitrochlorobenzene) and induction of mononuclear cell cytokines (IL-12, TNF-α) secretion (imidazoquinolines imiquimod and resiquimod). These latter drugs lead to T_h1-domination and a cell-mediated response used in humans to treat local viral infection and cancers.

Imidazoquinolines

Imiquimod and resiquimod (R-848) are members of the family imidazoquinolines. These drugs have proven antiviral and antitumor effects in a variety of animal models. Their immune actions appear to reflect stimulation of several arms of both innate and adaptive immunity, ultimately resulting in an indirect T_h-1 dominant response. Their ability to enhance cutaneous-adaptive responses and innate immunologic responses are key to their usefulness. Resiquimod is 10- to 100-fold more potent than imiquimod and is also capable of stimulating granulocyte and macrophage colony-stimulating factors and other mediators. Antigen processing also is improved. Indications include cutaneous viral infections and potentially nonmelanoma skin cancers, with the latter having potential therapeutic applications in animals.[143]

TREATMENT OF SPECIFIC IMMUNE-MEDIATED DISEASES

See also discussion of each syndrome in the appropriate chapter.

Chronic Allergic Diseases

Atopy refers to a genetic tendency toward certain hypersensitivity or allergic diseases. Atopic diseases include asthma, rhinitis, and dermatitis. Chronic allergic disease are generally complex in pathophysiology, with inflammatory disease manifested in the organ in which antigen–tissue interactions are initiated. For example, for asthma, inflammation causes airway narrowing associated with contraction and hypertrophy of bronchial smooth muscle, swelling of mucous membranes, and excessive production of mucus.

Mediators released during inflammation are the major contributors to the pathogenesis of pulmonary disease, particularly feline asthma. Mediators important in the pathogenesis of asthma include preformed mediators histamine and serotonin (particularly in cats); mediators formed in situ, including prostaglandins, leukotrienes, and platelet-activating factor; and reactive oxygen species.

The three atopic syndromes are characterized by common cell and mediators of inflammation in humans (see Figure 31-2).[121,144-147] A similar pathophysiology should be anticipated for other allergic diseases. The role of T (CD4+ helper) cells has been well described in the initiation and maintenance of allergic diseases, particularly asthma. In contrast to systemic immune-mediated diseases, in which T_h1 cells appear to be the biggest contributors of inappropriate response, T_h2 cells appear to be particularly important to allergic diseases. Their cytokines include interleukins and chemotactants that contribute to the inflammatory process. These include IL-4, which increases IgE synthesis; IL-5, which stimulates eosinophil growth and differentiation; IL-9, which causes mast cell differentiation; and in the lungs IL-13, which causes production of mucus and airway hyperactivity. Of these, IL-4, IL-10, and IL-13 in particular, have antiinflammatory activity. Previously, T_h1cells were thought to be beneficial by downregulating T_h2 cells. However, they are probably proinflammatory and, along with IFN (IFN) γ, contribute to the inflammatory process. The role of leukotrienes, and particularly cyst-LTs, are increasingly being described in atopic diseases.[148] In the lungs they are very potent (being 1000 times more so than histamine), causing marked edema, inflammation, and bronchoconstriction. In the gastrointestinal tract, their effects on neutrophils are necessary for ulcer formation; vasoconstriction and platelet aggregation probably contribute further. Senter and coworkers[149] found that 50% of atopic dogs responded to zafirlukast, supporting the possible role of leukotrienes as targets of treatment for atopy.

Treatment of inflammatory allergic diseases focuses on control of inflammation and clinical signs at the level of the target tissue. However, treatment of all three atopic disorders increasingly focuses on systemic rather than simply a local allergic disease. In particular, the bone marrow response to allergens and subsequent release of eosinophils are recognized to be an important systemic process in allergic inflammation. A central role of eotaxin and IL-5 has been suggested. Eotaxin released from local tissue cells stimulates, exclusively through CC chemokine receptor 3 (CCR3), flux of eosniophils into the target tissue.[150] Both IL-4 and TNF-α stimulate its release. T_h2 cells release IL-5; other sources include mast cells and eosinophils. In response to IL-5, eotaxin is released. In human patients with allergic diseases, both are increased in serum. The effects of these signals are not limited to the affected tissue. Rather, the primary significance may be their effects at the level of the bone marrow stroma, another source of IL-5. Among the functions of IL-5 are differentiation and maturation of progenitor cells to eosinophils and basophils, release of mature eosinophils, promotion of their survival, and inhibition of apoptosis. Activated eosinophil progenitor cells contain granulocyte-macrophage colony-stimulating factor and IL-5. Their circulation increases in allergic human patients and in dogs rendered hypersensitive to *A. suum*.[151]

Cysteinyl-LTs are necessary for accumulation of eosinophils in target tissues. However, in addition to their local effects, cyst-LTs may also have a role in bone marrow perpetuation of allergic disease. Cyst-LT receptors are expressed on a number of bone marrow progenitor cells and appear to be involved (based on effects of antagonists) in eosinophil– basophil progenitor differentiation. They appear to stimulate eosinphil proliferation in the presence of stimulatory cytokines.[152]

The commonalities of atopic diseases offer several targets of therapy. The efficacy of glucocorticoids can be appreciated from several aspects, their use is discussed in Chapter 30.

However, a number of "second tier" drugs might be used for their glucocorticoid dose-sparing effect or in animals intolerant to or minimally responsive to glucocorticoid therapy (e.g., CsA). Further, the involvement of T_h cells supports the potential role of CsA in their treatment. The role of leukotrienes supports use of receptor antagonists or other drugs (e.g., dual-inhibitor nonsteroidal antiinflammatory drugs) that modify their release. In human medicine drugs that target eotaxin, the CCR3, or particularly IL-5 are being explored. Finally, pentoxifylline might be considered for its ability to target TNF. These therapies might be considered for other atopic diseases, including allergic rhinitis and sinusitis perianal fistulae, and others.

Type I Hypersensitivities

Anaphylaxis and Anaphylactoid Reactions

Clinical signs of systemic anaphylaxis include nausea, vomiting, diarrhea, pale mucous membranes, coolness to peripheral extremities, tachycardia, and tachypnea. Localized "anaphylaxis" results in clinical signs referable to the site of localized mast cell degranulation. Examples include angioneurotic edema resulting in swelling of lips, eyelids, and conjuctiva and urticarial lesions (or hives). Treatment is oriented toward preventing further mast cell degranulation, blocking the interaction between histamine (or other mediator) and tissue receptors, and antagonizing the physiologic response to mediators. Drugs that antagonize physiologic response also tend to further decrease mast cell degranulation. The goals of therapy for systemic anaphylaxis include cardiovascular and ventilatory support. Epinephrine is indicated to antagonize bronchoconstriction and provide cardiovascular support. Glucocorticoids (prednisolone sodium succinate) facilitate adrenergic receptor responses and decrease further mast cell mediator release. Histamine 1 (H_1) receptor antagonists (e.g., diphenhydramine) are of benefit only in preventing interaction of histamine and its receptors, not in preventing further mast cell degranulation. Therapy may be more effective if administered in anticipation of mast cell degranulation, although this is somewhat controversial. Perioperative anaphylaxis, including drugs, risk factors, and therapies in humans, has been recently reviewed.[153]

Type II Hypersensitivities: Antigen- and Antibody-Dependent Cytotoxicity

Immune-Mediated Hemolytic Anemia

IMHA occurs as a result of increased red blood cell destruction mediated by the presence of an antibody on the membrane surface. The antigen to which the antibody binds is either of the red blood cell membrane or an exogenous antigen (e.g., drug or microbe) that has adhered to the surface. Igs associated with IMHA in dogs generally are IgG or, less commonly, both IgG and IgM. In cats IgM tends to be more common, with IgG alone causing IMHA in approximately 25% of cases. Complement activation is more likely with IgM-mediated IMHA. Antibody adherence and complement activation that are insufficient to cause erythrocyte lysis will result in damage and subsequent erythrophagocytosis of the deformed red blood cell (e.g., spherocyte). Intravascular hemolysis occurs when complement activation is extensive, leading to erythrocyte lysis. Released hemoglobin binds to serum haptoglobin, preventing glomerular filtration. If haptoglobin becomes saturated, however, free hemoglobin can be filtered. Renal toxicity can accompany intravascular IMHA as a result of antigen–antibody deposition or reaction in the basement membrane; free hemoglobin may also contribute to nephrotoxicity. Direct red blood cell agglutination or intravascular hemolysis increases the risk of thromboembolic disease.

Medical treatment of IMHA focuses on reducing phagocytosis of damaged or antibody-coated erythrocytes by reducing or blocking receptors on phagocytic cells, reducing or preventing the formation of more antibodies, and providing supportive therapy for complications associated with IMHA. Any likely inciting (exogenous) antigen (e.g., drug, microbe) should be removed. Treatment of IMHA is confounded by low survival rates (which range from 10% to 50% discharge survival, with continued patient loss after discharge) and the lack of scientifically based evidence supporting preferred therapies. Several of the clinical trials that address various therapeutic regimens unfortunately are biased in population selection, generally focusing on the worse cases and thus complicating extrapolation of results to less severe cases. Immunosuppressive therapy with glucocorticoids is the cornerstone of therapy; use of immunosuppressants for immune-mediated disorders is reviewed in Chapter 30. Differences of opinion exists regarding the initial route of administration of glucocorticoids, with oral proponents observing that response to glucocorticoids requires 5 to 7 days regardless of route. Although this observation may have some merit (many mechanisms of glucocorticoid require nuclear transcription and protein synthesis; time must elapse before inflammatory cell numbers and function are reduced), many mechanisms (e.g, non-genomic) of glucocorticoid action may occur immediately. Indeed, the importance of glucocorticoid supplementation in shock patients offers support for administration designed to cause immediate response (see Chapter 30). For rapid response dexamethasone (0.1 to 0.2 mg/kg intravenously) or methylprednisolone (11 mg/kg daily for up to 3 days) every 12 to 24 hours is administered initially, followed by oral prednisolone (1 mg/kg every 12 hours) as the animal responds. Choice of prednisone versus prednisolone is addressed in Chapter 30; the latter is strongly encouraged in dogs with life-threatening conditions, and the former should not be used in cats. Further reduction of red blood cell destruction may require administration of CsA, leflunomide or MMF, or their combination; continued failure may require cyclophosphamide or (dogs only) azathioprine. Combination therapy might be considered initially in patients with severe disease (see Chapter 30). Leflunomide doses as high as 8 mg/kg were necessary to prevent renal transplant rejection in dogs.[104a] Safety of anticancer drugs can be increased by dosing based on body surface area. Cyclophosphamide can be given as a single intravenous bolus (100 to 250 mg/m^2) in patients suffering from intravascular lysis or direct autoagglutination.[108] This regimen also is particularly useful for patients that require a blood transfusion.

However, efficacy of cyclophosphamide may not be realized until antibodies decline as a result of normal catabolism (generally 1 to 2 weeks).[11] Oral administration (50 mg/m^2 every 48 hours) is indicated in dogs that do not respond to glucocorticoids or might be considered as part of initial therapy, particularly in severe cases. Using a randomized prospective design, Mason and coworkers[154] investigated the impact of cyclophosphamide (50 mg/m^2) when combined with prednisone (1 to 2 mg/kg orally every 12 hours; n = 8) compared with prednisone alone (1 to 2 mg/kg orally every 12 hours; n = 10) for treatment of severe (based on clinical signs, less than 1 week in duration and packed cell volume less than 20%) idiopathic IMHA in dogs. The mortality rate did not differ between groups, but the power of the study was limited. Reticulocytosis appeared, and spherocytosis resolved more rapidly in the prednisone-only–treated group (within 1 week), leading the investigators to conclude that the addition of cyclophosphamide offered no advantage to prednisolone alone. Long-term cyclophosphamide will increase the risk of thrombocytopenia and neutropenia.[11]

Human gammaglobulin (0.5 to 1.5 g/kg intravenously over 6 to 12 hours) may prove useful for dogs that fail to respond to therapy.[127,128] Cost may, however, be prohibitive, and use may be limited by development of thrombocytopenia or thrombosis (see previous discussion). CsA may be of benefit in controlling the sequelae of IMHA that reflect tissue (and thus T cell–mediated) damage.[11] Blood transfusions are not recommended for patients with IMHA. Dogs with IMHA are predisposed to destruction of transfused red blood cells. Blood substitutes (oxyhemoglobin) may offer a viable alternative to blood transfusion. Although splenectomy should be considered as a surgical adjunct to medical management, removal of the spleen may also result in removal of an important site of extramedullary hematopoiesis. As with glucocorticoids, danazol (5 to 10 mg/kg orally every 12 hours) may block Fc receptors on phagocytic cells, reducing red blood cell destruction.[111] However, response may be slow, rendering danazolol lower on the list.

Response to therapy is based on daily hematocrit or platelet counts (or both); initial therapy should be continued or, as needed, improved until the packed cell volume is 15% or more in cats and 20% in dogs or the platelet count is 100, 000/μL or more. Drug therapy should be gradually tapered to avoid relapse or rebound; for example, prednisolone and azathioprine tapered to 0.5 to 1 mg/kg every second day is a reasonable target, with monitoring every 2 weeks as a basis of response. Therapy should be continued for another 3 months or so, with gradual tapering off attempted in animals that have been in remission for 3 to 6 months. For nonresponders, supportive therapy may include transfusions, which are more likely to be effective in patients whose disease reflects bone marrow rather than peripheral cellular targets.

Other supportive therapy should be considered. Anemia and reduced oxygen delivery to the gastrointestinal tract may predispose the patient to gastrointestinal induced ulceration. The importance of cyclooxygenase-2 in gastrointestinal healing warrants consideration of gastroprotectants, particularly in the face of glucocorticoid therapy. As such, antisecretory drugs (e.g., H_2-receptor antagonists, omeprazole) and gastroprotectants (e.g., sucralfate) should be considered as long as concerns regarding drug interactions are addressed. The use of heparin, including fractionated products, is controversial but might be considered (Chapter 15).

Immune-Mediated Thrombocytopenia

Immune-mediated thrombocytopenia is a syndrome that occurs more commonly in dogs than cats and in males than females. It can occur in concert with other immune-mediated disorders, including IMHA.[11] Thrombocyte numbers can decline as a result of destruction (i.e., antibody/complement-mediated phagocytosis) or, less commonly, decreased formation of mature thrombocytes as a result of antibody/complement-mediated destruction of megakaryocytes.[11] As with IMHA, antibody can be directed to an endogenous or exogenous antigen adhered to the platelet or megakaryocyte. The primary clinical signs, which include and reflect inappropriate bleeding, generally do not occur until thrombocyte numbers have dropped below 30,000/μL. Bleeding is more likely with a rapid, as opposed to a gradual, decline.

Medical treatment focuses on prevention of bleeding, decreased destruction of thrombocytes, and restoration of thrombocyte numbers (see also Chapters 15 and 30). Any likely inciting (exogenous) antigen (e.g., drug, microbe) should be removed. Glucocorticoids (dexamethasone, methylprednisolone, or prednisolone) are often the first choice of therapy (see earlier discussion of IMHA) and, in general, cause thrombocyte counts to normalize within 1 week. Use of cyclosporine and leflunoamide should be considered as suggested for other immune-mediated disease. Danazol also can be administered to reduce phagocytosis.[112,113] Vincristine (0.75 mg/m^2 intravenously) can be administered if platelet numbers fail to increase to sufficient numbers. Once platelet numbers increase, vincristine should be discontinued and glucocorticoids continued for several more weeks.[11] Vincristine may also be given after incubation with platelet-rich plasma in cases refractory to glucocorticoids, danazol, and vincristine. Presumably, incubation allows vincristine to bind to platelets. Subsequent phagocytosis destroys the phagocytic cell, causing an overall reduction in platelet destruction.[155] If successful, the treatment may need to be repeated as new macrophages are generated. Platelet-rich plasma also can be administered in an attempt to restore platelet numbers to a concentration that is not life threatening (>50,000/μL). The likelihood of relapse of immune-mediated thrombocytopenia also may be reduced after infusion of platelet-rich plasma.[11] The use of vinblastine might be considered in relapsing patients (see discussion of cytotoxic drugs) on the basis of its effectiveness in human patients. Splenectomy is a surgical alternative or adjunct therapy that should be considered in refractory cases. Because of the risk of relapse, patients should be monitored periodically. Surgical neutering, particularly of females, may be indicated once platelet numbers have normalized.

Immune-Mediated Neutropenia

As with other immune-mediated hematopoietic diseases, glucocorticoids are indicated for neutropenia.[156] Treatment can continue as described for IMHA.

The use of recombinant bone marrow growth factors (see Chapters15 and 32) to increase bone marrow production of deficient cells is probably not wise unless the factor is derived from the species to be treated. Even in those situations, studies should confirm a lack of immune-mediated reactions when used in patients affected with an immune-mediated disorder.

Dermatologic Disorders

A number of immune-mediated skin diseases reflect a type II hypersensitivity. Included are pemphigus (foliaceus, erythematosus, vulgaris, vegetans), bullous pemphigoid, and dermatomyositis.

Pemphigus Disorders and Bullous Pemphigoid. Pemphigus disorders reflect the reaction of autoantibodies directed toward antigens located in the intercellular spaces between epidermal cells. The definitive antigen is not known but apparently is located in or near the cytoplasmic membrane.[11] The various types may reflect variants, crossovers, or altered presentations of the different forms of the disease. In all variants antibody deposition causes the loss of adhesion between epidermal cells, leading to acanthosis. Complement activation results in local mast cell degranulation and an infiltration of inflammatory cells. Clinical signs vary within and among the variants and include visculobullous eruptions, cutaneous ulcerations, exfoliative lesions, and verrucous proliferations of the skin.[11] Bullous pemphigoid results from the generation of antibodies toward the lamina lucida of the basement membrane zone. As with pemphigus, complement activation may worsen the inflammatory response. Clinical signs include vesiculobullous lesions at mucocutaneous junctions; in the oral cavity; on footpads; and on the skin of the trunk, groin, axillae, and abdomen.[11]

Glucocorticoids can be expected to be effective in 40% of canine cases[11] of pemphigus. The initial dose should be high (2 to 3 mg/kg orally every 12 hours for 10 to 14 days); the dose can gradually be reduced over 4 weeks (targeting 1 mg/kg orally every 48 hours) if an adequate response has occurred. Failure to respond or inability to decrease the dose of glucocorticoids is an indication for the addition of a second immunosuppressive drug. Generally, azathioprine (2 mg/kg orally every 24 hours) has been the first choice to combine with prednisolone (1 mg/kg orally every 12 hours). Response within 10 to 14 days will allow alternating the drugs each day at the same dose. Continued remission will allow a gradual reduction in the doses of both drugs to 1 mg/kg orally every other day, alternating the drugs daily.[11] Cyclophosphamide (50 mg/m^2 orally every 24 hours) can be combined with prednisolone (1 mg/kg orally every 12 hours) for 4 consecutive days each week for 2 to 3 weeks. If remission occurs, doses are gradually reduced to 1 mg/kg orally, alternating drugs daily. Chlorambucil (0.1 mg/kg orally every 48 hours) can be used in place of cyclophosphamide; leukopenia and thrombocytopenia are potential side effects of this drug. Use of cyclosporine and leflunoamide should be considered as suggested for other immune-mediated disease.

The third alternative for immunosuppressive chemotherapy is use of aurothioglucose initially in combination with prednisolone (1 to 2 mg/kg orally every 12 to 48 hours). Chrysotherapy should be initiated only after administration of an intramuscular test dose (1 mg for animals less than 10 kg; 5 mg for animals 10 kg or larger) twice, 1 week apart. Toxicity will be manifested as dermatitis, stomatitis, nephrotic syndrome, blood dyscrasias, eosinophilia, thrombocytopenia, and manifestations of allergic reactions. Therapy can be continued at 1 mg/kg weekly intramuscularly until remission; however, continued therapy should be based on an acceptable complete blood count. At that time, the interval is decreased to alternate weeks and finally monthly. Prednisolone therapy might be gradually phased out.

Pemphigus foliaceus in cats can be treated with chlorambucil as the first choice.[106] Daily therapy (0.1 to 0.2 mg/kg/day) should be continued until lesions have markedly reduced, which may take 4 to 8 weeks. Alternate-day therapy should be implemented when approximately 75% improvement occurs and continued for several weeks. Complete blood counts should be monitored every 2 weeks of chlorambucil therapy.[106]

Dermatomyositis. Dermatomyositis might be classified as an inflammatory muscle syndrome. Unlike polymyositis, which appears to involve a cell-mediated, antigen-specific response, dermatomyositis appears to reflect an abnormality of the humoral response, resulting in vasculitis. In human patients treatment with low-dose methotrexate has proved beneficial[114,115] Dermatomyositis in veterinary medicine is an inherited idiopathic inflammatory syndrome affecting Collies, Shetland Sheepdogs, and their crosses. Skin lesions include erythema, scaling, and crusting, particularly around the eyes, tips of the ears and tail, digits, and carpal and tarsal regions. Pentoxifylline, a methylxanthine derivative, has been recommended[157,158] on the basis of its potential efficacy in humans.[159] Studies of the drug in dogs suggest a higher dose than that for humans, and a twice- to thrice-daily dosing interval should be used. Clinically, response may take several weeks. The drug appears to be well tolerated by dogs. Clinical trials in Collies with dermatomyositis are currently under way.

Feline Eosinophilic Granuloma Complex. Eosinophilic granulomas may respond to glucocorticoids. Direct lesional injection of methylprednisolone acetate (2 mg/kg, minimum of 20 mg) every 2 weeks is the preferred method of administration. High oral doses of prednisolone may be an effective alternative.[160] Drugs that target leukotrienes should be considered. Response to chlorambucil has been reported[104] within 6 weeks of therapy (0.1 to 0.2 mg/kg per day). Response to therapy should be followed by a 12-week period during which the dose of chlorambucil is decreased until discontinued. Megestrol acetate is an undesirable alternative unless the patient has proved refractory to other modalities, including chlorambucil. Urine should be monitored for glucose to detect the development of diabetes mellitus. Levamisole (2.2 mg/kg orally every 48 hours) has been reported to cause some (but incomplete) remission in certain cases.[160,161] Additionally, accurate dosing is difficult because of the large tablet size (184 mg). Cats often react adversely, with transient anorexia, vomiting, and hypersalivation being the most common side effects. Bone marrow suppression can be marked and is characterized by a long recovery period.

Type III Hypersensitivities: Immune Complex Disease

Systemic Lupus Erythematosus

The deposition of circulating autoantibodies or autoantibody–antigen complexes in the endothelium, particularly that of the glomerulus, appears to initiate complement-mediated inflammation. The inflammatory site is infiltrated by immune cells. In the glomerulus response includes proliferation of capillary cells, thickening of the basement membrane, and scarring. Other vascular beds affected include the skin, serous membranes, synovial tissues, and cutaneous and visceral blood vessels.[114,115] Soluble immune complexes are more problematic than large immune complexes, which precipitate and are rapidly phagocytized. Soluble complexes are able to penetrate deep into vascular endothelial channels, activate complement, and stimulate an inflammatory response. In humans intravenous cyclophosphamide has been established as the treatment of choice for lupus-induced nephritis. Bolus cyclophosphamide has also, however, proved effective for lupus affecting other body systems, including the CNS, lungs, and arteries. Azathioprine and weekly methotrexate are effective for treating human lupus that does not involve major organs, such as rashes, serositis, and arthritis, or in combination with glucocorticoids to reduce the glucocorticoid dose. CsA apparently has not been studied for treatment of systemic lupus erythematosus, although clinical response has been reported.[114,115]

Because systemic lupus erythematosus can be polysystemic in its presentation, the sequelae of immune complex deposition associated with systemic lupus erythematosus can affect a number of body systems, resulting in the need for medical management of secondary disease. Examples include but are not limited to glomerulonephritis, arthritis, and vasculitis. The reader is referred to the chapters that address these specific body systems for information on management of the sequelae of inflammatory disease. Treatment for the immune-mediated aspect of the disease is the same as for pemphigus skin disorders. Use of cyclosporine and leflunoamide should be considered as suggested for other immune-mediated disease.

Cutaneous Discoid Lupus Erythematosus

Considered a mild form of systemic lupus erythematosus, cutaneous discoid lupus erythematosus is not accompanied by systemic involvement. The most common form presents as a nasal dermatitis; skin surrounding the eyes, pinnae, lips, and feet may also be involved. Treatment includes immunosuppressive doses of glucocorticoids, as described for other immune-mediated diseases, although a lower initial dose may be effective (1 mg/kg orally twice daily). Vitamin E (400 IU orally 2 hours before or after a meal every 12 hours; acetate or succinate) may be effective as the sole agent; however, a 30- to 60-day lag time to efficacy mandates that initial therapy include glucocorticoids. Topical glucocorticoids may be effective in mild cases. Minimizing exposure to the sun, including use of topical sunscreen, or other ultraviolet light also will be helpful, particularly in animals with depigmentation. Niacin or tetracycline (5 to 12 mg/kg orally every 8 hours) was reportedly effective in 70% of cases in one study. Use of cyclosporine and leflunoamide should be considered as suggested for other immune-mediated disease; tacrolimus also might be considered.

Rheumatoid Arthritis and Other Arthritides

The rheumatoid factor is an antibody that reacts with IgG that has bound to antigen and subsequently undergone a conformation change. The reason for selectivity in joints is not understood. In humans drugs used to treat rheumatoid arthritis include gold compounds or penicillamine and cytotoxic drugs, including azathioprine, cyclophosphamide, and methotrexate. Since the late 1980s, low-dose weekly methotrexate has become the preferred medication.[114,115] Methotrexate has proved more rapid in onset. Because it is safer than traditional cytotoxic drugs, treatment generally can progress for a longer period of time. Because functional disabilities and progress of the disease occur rapidly in the first years of disease in humans, cytotoxic drugs are begun early. Drug combinations have been advocated because of the possibility of synergistic effects. Examples include methotrexate with sulfasalazine, CsA, or biological agents. Treatment in animals has not been as well investigated and focuses on control of inflammation with glucocorticoids and, if necessary, aspirin. The use of glucocorticoids is supported by the rapid clinical improvement and decrease in IL-6 activity documented in dogs with juvenile polyarthritis syndrome.[162] The use of other immunosuppressive drugs in animals (azathioprine, cyclophosphamide) has been reserved for severe cases. On the basis of findings in humans, however, a more aggressive approach may be warranted. Disease-modifying agents (e.g., glucosamine and chondroitin sulfates) should be used to support cartilage repair.

Feline chronic progressive polyarthritis is associated with feline leukemia virus and feline syncytium-forming virus and most commonly presents as osteopenia and periosteal bone proliferation around affected joints. Less commonly, joints are characterized by subchondral marginal erosions similar to those of rheumatoid arthritis. Rheumatoid factor cannot be identified, however. Treatment includes immunosuppressive doses of corticosteroids (1 to 3 mg/kg orally every 12 hours). Nonresponders may require treatment with chlorambucil, cyclophosphamide, or azathioprine. As previously suggested, disease-modifying agents may prove beneficial.

In a retrospective study of dogs (n = 39) with immune-mediated polyarthritis, 56% of dogs were cured after drug therapy. Response to prednisolone alone was 50% (overall 33%), although response to prednisolone (1 to 2 mg/kg every 24 hours or divided every 12 hours) by itself or combined with another drug was 81%. Duration of therapy was generally 4 to 16 weeks, although continuous medication was necessary in 10% to 18%. Response of animals to leflunomide was previously discussed.[104a] Drugs combined with prednisolone to which animals responded included antimicrobials and immunosuppressive drugs such as cyclophosphamide or azathioprine.[161] Treatment with levamisole or CsA as sole therapy generally was not successful.

Type IV Hypersensitivities: the Delayed Response

Allergic Contact Dermatitis

Allergic contact dermatitis is the most common type IV hypersensitivity recognized in small animals, being responsible for up to 10% of dermatologic cases.[11] The syndrome is initiated when the skin comes in contact with the inciting antigen or chemical. Actual chemicals that cause contact dermatitis are not known, but it is likely that the chemical acts as a hapten that subsequently covalently bonds to a protein. The location of the protein is not clear but is probably associated with the class II molecule of an APC, which in the skin is the Langerhans cell. Sensitization generally requires 4 to 10 days; subsequent exposure to the chemical results in a marked T cell–mediated response.[11] Treatment is best implemented by removal of the inciting antigen and short-term (7-day) administration of prednisolone (0.5 to 1 mg/kg every 12 to 24 hours).

Inflammatory Myopathies

In humans polymyositis appears to reflect cell-mediated, antigen-specific cytotoxicity, with azathioprine being the only cytotoxic drug to be of benefit in controlled studies. Low-dose methotrexate or azathioprine with high-dose glucocorticoid therapy has become the standard therapy. Combinations of methotrexate and either cyclophosphamide or CsA may be effective and are being studied.[114,115]

Inflammatory Bowel Disease

Inflammatory bowel disease also is discussed in Chapter 19. The use of immune-modifying therapy for human patients with IBD became popular only in the 1990s.[114,115,164,165] Controlled clinical trials in humans have focused on azathioprine, 6-mercaptopurine, CsA, and methotrexate. Azathioprine or 6-mercaptopurine has been effective for treatment of Crohn's disease, although efficacy depends on duration of therapy; at least 13 and more often 17 weeks of therapy is required before the drugs reach their full effects.

Intravenous administration of azothioprine may decrease the time to response. CsA has been studied at low doses (<1 mg/kg per day) or high doses (>5 mg/kg per day) to minimize the risk of nephrotoxicity (less of a concern in veterinary patients), but this has proved of little benefit in Crohn's disease. It has been more effective for treatment of ulcerative colitis at high doses (8 to 10 mg/kg per day), although only a few patients have been studied. CsA concentrations in responding patients were above 250 ng/mL. Methotrexate appears to be useful for both induction of remission and steroid sparing in patients with Crohn's disease and ulcerative colitis. Combinations of drugs also have been studied. Azathioprine and 6-mercaptopurine should not be used in combination with methotrexate because of the increased risk of toxicity. CsA and methotrexate have been used in human patients with IBD with some success. Drugs that target leukotrienes should be considered. Pentoxyfylline for treatment of human IBD is discussed in Chapter 19.

Amyloidosis

Primary (or AL) amyloidosis reflects the extracellular deposition of abnormally formed protein associated with a clonal plasma cell dyscrasia.[166] The protein is a monoclonal Ig light chain fragment secreted in an abnormal insoluble fibrillar form; the underlying plasma cell dyscrasia is generally insidious and nonproliferating. The AL amyloid fibrils are derived from the N-terminal region of monoclonal Ig light chains and consist of the whole or part of the variable (VL) domain. The propensity for Igs to form amyloid fibrils is inherent to their structure; unfortunately, they cannot be identified. Those able to form myeloid are capable of existing in partially unfolded states because of the loss of tertiary or higher structure. Aggregation and retention of b-sheet secondary results in the formation of protofilaments and fibrils; initiation of the process, or seeding, appears to facilate exponential progress of the amyloid template by "capturing" precursor molecules. Amyloid deposits exist in a state of dynamic turnover. Accumulation of amyloid progressively disrupts the normal tissue structure and ultimately leads to organ failure, frequently including, but not limited to, the kidneys, heart, liver, and peripheral nervous system. Hereditary forms of amyloidosis also exist, as do secondary forms (e.g., chronic immunologic stimulation). Treatment of the latter is best based on removal of the inciting cause. Because no therapy has successfully targeted amyloid deposition, therapy targets suppression of the underlying plasma cell dyscrasia as well as treatment intended to preserve organ function. A variety of low- and high-dose drug therapies, sometimes as sole agents but more commonly as combinations, have been recommended in humans. Low-dose single agents include melphalan or cyclophosphamide, (with or without prednisolone). However, clinical benefit occurred in only about 20% to 30% of human patients, after a median of 12 months' treatment. Intermediate dose regimens consist of a monthly course of VAD (vincristine, adriamycin, dexamethasone) or similar regimes or intravenous intermediate-dose melphalan 25 mg/m^2 with or without dexamethasone. High-dose therapy consists of intravenous melphalan (100 to 200 mg/m^2) but with stem cell rescue. Other approaches include a pulsed high-dose dexamethasone or thalidomide (with or without dexamethasone). However, thalidomide is a drug of restricted distribution in the United States and therefore cannot be prescribed by veterinarians. In veterinary medicine colchicine has been recommended for prevention in dogs predisposed to amylodids. Presumably, colchicine may block the deposition of amyloid. The dose is based on that used to treat hepatic fibrosis (0.03mg/kg every 24 hours for 2 weeks) with an increase (0.025 to 0.03mg/kg orally every 12 hours) if the drug is well tolerated during the initial therapy. In patients with renal amyloidosis, dimethyl sulfoxide has been recommended, although its efficacy is unsubstantiated.

REFERENCES

1. Aggarwal BB, Puri RK: Common and uncommon features of cytokines and cytokine R eceptors: an overview. In Aggarwal BB, Puri RK, editors: *Human cytokines: their role in disease and therapy*, Cambridge, 1995, Blackwell Science, p 3.
2. Hilton DJ: An introduction to cytokine receptors. In Nicola NA, editor: *Guidebook to cytokines and their receptors*, Oxford, England, 1994, Oxford University Press, p 8.
3. Tizard IR: Interferons. In Myers MJ, Murtaugh MP, editors: *Cytokines in animal health and disease*, New York, 1995, Marcel Dekker, p 1.
4. Krensky AM, Vincenti F, Bennett WM: Immunosuppressants, tolerogens, and immunostimulants. In Brunton LL, Lazo JS, Parker KL, editors: *Goodman & Gilman's the pharmacological basis of therapeutics*, ed 11, New York, 2006, McGraw-Hill, pp 1405–1431.
5. Pfitzner E, Kliem S, Baus D, et al: The role of STATs in inflammation and inflammatory diseases, *Curr Pharm Des* 10:2839–2850, 2004.
6. Feizy V, Ghobadi A: Atopic dermatitis and systemic autoimmune diseases: a descriptive cross-sectional study, *Dermatol Online J* 12(3):3, 2006.
7. Bochner BS, Hamid Q: Advances in mechanisms of allergy, *J Allergy Clin Immunol* 111:S819–S823, 2003.
8. Menzies-Gow A, Flood-Page P, Sehmi R, et al: Anti-IL-5 (mepolizumab) therapy induces bone marrow eosinophil maturational arrest and decreases eosinophil progenitors in the bronchial mucosa of atopic asthmatics, *J Allergy Clin Immunol* 111:714–719, 2003.
9. Shadidi KR: New drug targets in rheumatoid arthritis: focus on chemokines, *Biodrugs* 18(3):181–187, 2004.
10. Pascher A, Klupp J: Biologics in the treatment of transplant rejection and ischemia/reperfusion injury: new applications for TNFα inhibitors? *BioDrugs* 19(4):211–231, 2005.
11. Gorman N, Immunology: In Ettinger SJ, Feldman EC, editors: *Textbook of veterinary internal medicine*, ed 4, Philadelphia, 1995, Saunders, pp 1978–2002.
12. Boyaka PN, Tafaro A, Fischer R, et al: Therapeutic manipulation of the immune system: enhancement of innate and adaptive mucosal immunity, *Curr Pharm Des* 9:1965–1972, 2003.
13. Hiemstra PS, Ferni-King BA, McMichael PJ, et al: Antimicrobial peptides: mediators of innate immunity as templates for the development of novel anti-infective and immune therapeutics, *Curr Pharm Des* 10:2891–2905, 2004.
14. Linde A, Ross CR, Davis EG, et al: Innate immunity and host defense peptides in veterinary medicine, *J Vet Intern Med* 22(2):247–265, 2008.
15. Rabin BS: Measurement of immune function in PNI research: relevance of immune measures to health and disease, *Proc PNI Workshop*, May 1998.
16. Eggert M, Klueter An Zetta UK, et al: Transcription factors in autoimmune diseases, *Curr Pharm Des* 10:2787–2796, 2004.
17. Gibbons M: A Cytokine storm? Why are younger people who usually fight off flu succumbing to swine flu? *Advance for Nurses*, May 27, 2009. Accessed January 28, 2010, at http://nursing.advanceweb.com/Editorial/Content/Editorial.aspx?CC=200143.
18. Bacher S, Schmitz LM: The NF-B pathway as a potential target for autoimmune disease therapy, *Curr Pharm Des* 10:2827–2837, 2004.
19. Dostert A, Heinzel T: Negative glucocorticoid receptor response elements and their role in glucocorticoid action, *Curr Pharm Des* 10(23):2807–2816, 2004.
20. Schulz M, Eggert M: Novel ligands: fine tuning the transcriptional activity of the glucocorticoid receptor, *Curr Pharm Des* 10:2817–2826, 2004.
21. Mellon RD, Bayer BM: Evidence for central opioid receptors in the immunomodulatory effects of morphine: review of potential mechanisms of action, *J Neuroimmunol* 83:19–28, 1998.
22. Carr D, Rogers TJ, Weber RJ: The relevance of opioids and opioid receptors on immunocompetence and immune homeostasis, *Proc Soc Exp Biol Med* 213:248–257, 1996.
23. Deluca HF, Cantorna MT: Vitamin D: its role and uses in immunology, *FASEB J* 15(14):2579–2585, 2001.
24. Ford RB: Biological response modifiers in the management of viral infection, *Vet Clin North Am Small Animal Prac* 16:1191–1204, 1986.
25. Carrasco L: In Shugar D, editor: *Viral chemotherapy, The replication of animal viruses*, vol 1, New York, 1984, Pergamon, pp 111–148.
26. MacEwen EG: Approaches to cancer therapy using biological response modifiers, *Vet Clin North Am Small Anim Pract* 15:667–688, 1985.
27. Theilen GH, Hills D: Comparative aspects of cancer immunotherapy: immunological methods used for treatment of spontaneous cancer in animals, *J Am Vet Med Assoc* 181:1134–1137, 1982.
28. Pendse S, Sayegh MH, Frank MH: P-glycoprotein: a novel therapeutic target for immunomodulation in clinical transplantation and autoimmunity? *Curr Drug Targets* 4:469–476, 2003.
29. Krensky AM, Vincenti F, Bennett WM: Immunosuppressants, tolerogens, and immunostimulants. In Brunton LL, Lazo JS, Parker KL, editors: *Goodman & Gilman's the pharmacological basis of therapeutics*, ed 11, New York, 2006, McGraw-Hill.
30. Halloran PF: Immunosuppressive drugs for kidney transplantation, *N Engl J Med* 351:2715–2729, 2004.
31. Brazis P, Barandica L, Garcia F, et al: Dermal microdialysis in the dog: in vivo assessment of the effect of cyclosporin A on cutaneous histamine and prostanglandin D_2 release, *Eur Soc Vet Derm* 17:169–174, 2006.
32. Kelly P, Kahan BD: Review: metabolism of immunosuppressant drugs, *Curr Drug Metab* 3:275–287, 2002.
33. Guaguère E, Steffan J, Olivry T, Cyclosporin A: a new drug in the field of canine dermatology, *Vet Dermatol* 15:61–74, 2004.
34. Friman S, Backman L: A new microemulsion formulation of cyclosporin: pharmacokinetic and clinical features, *Clin Pharmacokinet* 30:181–193, 1996.
35. Gomez DY, Wacher VJ, Tomlanovich SJ, et al: The effects of ketoconazole on the intestinal metabolism and bioavailability of cyclosporine, *Clin Pharmacol Ther* 58:15–19, 1995.
36. Takaya S, Iwatsuki S, Nogughi T, et al: The influence of liver dysfunction of cyclosporine pharmacokinetics: a comparison between 70 percent hepatectomy and complete duct ligation in dogs, *Jpn J Surg* 19:49–56, 1989.
37. Ohta K, Agematu H, Yamada T, et al: Production of human metabolites of cyclosporin A, AM1, AM4N and AM9, by microbial conversion, *J Biosci Bioeng* 99(4):390–395, 2005.
38. Vickers AEM, Fischer V, Connors S, et al: Cyclosporine A metabolism in human liver, kidney and intestine slices: comparison to rat and dog slices and human cell lines, *Drug Metab Dispos* 120:802–809, 1992.
39. Khoschsorur G, Erwa W, Fruehwirth F, et al: High-performance liquid chromatographic method of the simultaneous determination of cyclosporine A and its four major metabolites in whole blood, *Talanta* 65:638–643, 2005.
40. Maurer G, Loosli HR, Shreier E, et al: Disposition of cyclosporine in several animal species and man I. Structural elucidation of its metabolites, *Drug Metab Dispos* 12:120–126, 1984.
41. Wallemace PE, Alexandre K: Evaluation of the new AxSYM cyclosporine assay: comparison with TDx monoclonal whole blood and emit cyclosporine assays, *Clin Chem* 45(3):432–435, 1999.
42. Yatscoff RW, Copeland KR, Faraci CJ: Abbott TDx monoclonal antibody assay evaluated for measuring cyclosporine in whole blood, *Clin Chem* 36(11):1969–1973, 1990.
43. Sangalli L, Bortolotti A, Jiritano L, et al: Cyclosporine pharmacokinetics in rats and interspecies comparison in dogs, rabbits, rats, and humans, *Drug Metab Dispos* 16(5):749–753, 1988.

44. Steffan J, Strehlau G, Maurer M, et al: Cyclosporin A pharmacokinetics and efficacy in the treatment of atopic dermatitis in dogs, *J Vet Pharmacol Ther* 27(4):231–238, 2004.
45. Mehl ML, Kyles AE, Craigmill AL, et al: Disposition of cyclosporine after intravenous and multi-dose oral administration in cats, *J Vet Pharmacol Therap* 26:349–354, 2003.
46. Vaden SL: Cyclosporine. In Bonagura JD, editor: *Kirk's current veterinary therapy small animal practice (XII)*, Philadelphia, 1995, Saunders, pp 73–77.
47. Gregory CR, Hietala SK, Pedersen NC, et al: Cyclosporine pharmacokinetics in cats following topical ocular administration, *Transplantation* 47(3):516–519, 1989.
48. Novartis: Transplant Drug Interactions Monograph, 2007. (http://www.novartis-transplant.com/hcp/about/interactions.jsp?usertrack.filter_applied=true&NovaId=7852773784371409923)
49. Terao T, Hisanaga E, Sai Y, et al: Active secretion of drugs from the small intestinal epithelium in rats by P-glycoprotein functioning as an absorption barrier, *J Pharm Pharmacol* 48:1083–1089, 1996.
50. McLachlan AJ, Tett SE: Effect of metabolic inhibitors on cyclosporine pharmacokinetics using a population approach, *Drug Monit* 20:390–395, 1998.
51. Keogh A, Spratt P, McCosker C, et al: Ketoconazole to reduce the need for cyclosporine after cardiac transplantation, *N Engl J Med* 333:628–633, 1995.
52. Lown KS, Mayo RR, Leichtman AB, et al: Role of intestinal P-glycoprotein (MRD1) in interpatient variation in the oral bioavailability of cyclosporine, *Clin Pharmacol Ther* 62:248–260, 1997.
53. Daigle JC: More economical use of cyclosporine through combination drug therapy, *J Am Anim Hosp Assoc* 38:205–208, 2002.
54. Martin JE, Daoud AJ, Schroeder TJ, et al: The clinical and economic potential of cyclosporin drug interactions, *Pharmacoeconomics* 15(4):317–337, 1999.
55. Myre SA, Schoeder TJ, Grund VR, et al: Critical ketoconazole dosage range for cyclosporine clearance inhibition in the dog, *Pharmacology* 43:233–241, 1991.
56. McNaulty JF, Lensmeyer GL: The effects of ketoconazole on the pharmacokinetics of cyclosporine A in cats, *Vet Surg* 28: 448–455, 1999.
57. Dahlinger J, Gregory C, Bea J: Effect of ketoconazole on cyclosporine dose in healthy dogs, *Vet Surg* 27:64–68, 1998.
58. Mouatt JG: Cyclosporin and ketoconazole interaction for treatment of perianal fistulas in the dog, *Aust Vet J* 80(4):207–811, 2002.
59. D'Souza MJ, Pollock SH, Solomon HM: Cyclosporine-cimetidine interaction, *Drug Metab Dispos* 16(1):57–59, 1988.
60. Bar-Meir S, Bardan E, Ronen I, et al: Cimetidine and omeprazole do not affect cyclosporine disposition by the rat liver, *Eur J Drug Metab Pharmacokinet* 18(4):355–358, 1993.
61. Shaefer MS, Rossi SJ, McGuire TR, et al: Evaluation of the pharmacokinetic interaction between cimetidine or famotidine and cyclosporine in healthy men, *Ann Pharmacother* 29(11):1088–1091, 1995.
62. Daigle JC, Hosgood G, Foil CS, et al: Effect of cimetidine on pharmacokinetics of orally administered cyclosporine in healthy dogs, *Am J Vet Res* 62(7):1046–1050, 2001.

62a. Allenspach K, Bergman PJ, Sauter S, et al: P-glycoprotein expression in lamina propria lymphocytes of duodenal biopsy samples in dogs with chronic idiopathic enteropathies, *J Comp Pathol* 134(1):1–7, 2006.

63. Kahan BD: Optimization of cyclosporine therapy, *Transplant Proc* 25:5–9, 1993.

63a. Wooldridge JD, Gregory CR, Mathews KG, et al: The prevalence of malignant neoplasia in feline renal-transplant recipients, *Vet Surg* 31(1):94–97, 2002.

63b. Kneteman NM, Marchetti P, Tordjman, et al: Effects of cyclosporine on insulin secretion and insulin sensitivity in dogs with intrasplenic islet autotransplants, *Surgery* 111(4):430–437, 1992.

64. Edwards LL, Wszolek ZK, Normand MM: Neurophysiologic evaluation of cyclosporine toxicity associated with bone marrow transplantation, *Acta Neurol Scand* 92(5):423–429, 1995.
65. Steffan J, Alexander D, Brovedani F, et al: Comparison of cyclosporine A with methylprednisolone for treatment of canine atopic dermatitis: a parallel, blinded, randomized controlled trial, *Vet Dermatol* 14:11–22, 2003.
66. Steffan J, Favrot C, Mueller R: A systematic review and meta-analysis of the fficacy and safety of cyclosporin for the treatment of atopic dermatitis in dogs, *Vet Dermatol* 17:3–16, 2006.
67. Last RD, Suzuki Y, Manning T, et al: A case of fatal systemic toxoplasmosis in a cat being treated with cyclosporin A for feline atopy, *Vet Dermatol* 15:194–198, 2004.
68. Mahalati K, Belitsky P, West K, et al: Approaching the therapeutic window for cyclosporine in kidney transplantation: a prospective study, *J Am Soc Nephrol* 12:828–833, 2001.
69. Einecke G, Mai I, Fritsche L, et al: The value of C_2 monitoring in stable renal allograft recipients on maintenance immunosuppression, *Nephrol Dial Transplant* 19:215–222, 2004.
70. Steele BW, Wang E, Soldin SJ, et al: A longitudinal replicate study of immunosuppressive drugs, *Arch Pathol Lab Med* 127:283–288, 2003.
71. Radowica SN, Power HT: Long-term use of cyclosporine in the treatment of canine atopic dermatitis, *Vet Dermatol* 16:81–86, 2005.
72. Levy GA: C2 monitoring strategy for optimising cyclosporin immunosuppression from the Neoral-1 Formulation, *BioDrugs* 15(5):279–290, 2001.
73. Robson DC, Burton GG: Cyclosporin: applications in small animal dermatology, *Vet Dermatol* 14:1–9, 2003.
74. Olivry T, Mueller RS: Evidence-based veterinary dermatology: a systematic review of the pharmacotherapy of canine atopic dermatitis, *Vet Dermatol* 14:121–146, 2003.
75. Mathews KA, Ayres SA, Tano CA, et al: Cyclosporin treatment of perianal fistulas in dogs, *Can Vet J* 38:39–41, 1997.
76. Mathews KA, Sukhiani HR: Randomized controlled trial of cyclosporine for treatment of perianal fistulas in dogs, *J Am Vet Med Assoc* 211:1249–1253, 1997.
77. Allenspach K, Rufenacht S, Sauter S: Pharmacokinetics and clinical efficacy of cyclosporine treatment of dogs with steroid-refractory inflammatory bowel disease, *J Vet Intern Med* 20:239–244, 2006.
78. van Deventer SJ: Review article: chemokine production by intestinal epithelial cells: a therapeutic target in inflammatory bowel disease? *Aliment Pharmacol Ther* 11(Suppl 3):116–120, 1997:discussion, 120-121.
79. Pham CQ, Efros CB, Berardi RR: Cyclosporine for severe ulcerative colitis, *Ann Pharmacother* 40(1):96–101, 2006.

80 Padrid PA, Cozzi P, Leff AR: Cyclosporin A inhibits airway reactivity and remodeling after chronic antigen challenge in cats, *Am J Respir Crit Care Med* 154:1812–1818, 1996.

81. Noli C, Toma S: Three cases of immune-mediated adnexal skin disease treated with cyclosporin, *Vet Dermatol* 17:85–92, 2006.
82. Barth T, Mischke R, Nolte I: Cyclosporin A in aplastic anemia in dogs: first results, *Berl Munch Tierarztl Wochenschr* 110:60–67, 1997.
83. Font A, Bardag M, Mascort J, et al: Treatment with oral cyclosporin A of a case of vesicular cutaneous lupus erythematosus in a rough collie, *Eur Soc Vet Derm* 17:440–442, 2006.
84. Adamo FP, O'Brien RT: Use of cyclosporine to treat granulomatous meningoencephalitis in three dogs, *J Am Vet Med Assoc* 225(8):1211–1216, 2004.

84a. Visudtibhan A, Chiemchanya S, Visudhiphan P: Cyclosporine in chronic inflammatory demyelinating polyradiculoneuropathy, *Pediatr Neurol* 33(5):368–372, 2005.
85. Williams DL: A comparative approach to topical cyclosporine therapy, *Eye* 11(Pt 4):453–464, 1997.
86. Puignero V, Queralt J: Effect of topically applied cyclosporin A on arachidonic acid (AA)- and tetradecanoylphorbol acetate (TPA)-induced dermal inflammation in mouse ear, *Inflammation* 21:357–369, 1997.
86a. Takada K, Katayama N, Kiriyama A, et al: Distribution characteristics of immunosuppressants FK506 and cyclosporin A in the blood compartment, *Biopharm Drug Dispos* 14(8):659–671, 1993.
87. Vaden SL: Cyclosporine and tacrolimus, *Semin Vet Med Surg Small Anim* 12:161–166, 1997.
87a. Venkataramanan R, Watty VS, Zemaitis MA, et al: Biopharmaceutical aspects of FK-506, *Transplant Proc* 19(5 Suppl 6):30–35, 1987.
88. Griffies JD, Mendelsohn CL, Rosenkrantz WS, et al: Topical 0.1% tacrolimus for the treatment of discoid lupus erythematosus and pemphigus erythematosus in dogs, *J Am Anim Hosp Assoc* 40(1):29–41, 2004.
89. Marsella R, Nicklin CF, Saglio S, et al: Investigation on the clinical efficacy and safety of 0.1% tacrolimus ointment (Protopic) in canine atopic dermatitis: a randomized, double-blinded, placebo-controlled, cross-over study, *Vet Dermatol* 15:294–303, 2004.
89a. Marsella R, Nicklin CF, Saglio S: Investigation on the effects of topical therapy with 0.1% tacrolimus ointment (Protopic) on intradermal skin test reactivity in atopic dogs, *Vet Dermatol* 15:218–224, 2004.
90. Tredger JM, Brown NW, Adams J: Monitoring mycophenolate in liver transplant recipients: toward a therapeutic range, *Liver Transpl* 10(4):492–502, 2004.
91. Langman LJ, Shapiro AMJ, Lakey JRT, et al: Pharmacodynamic assessment of mycophenolic acid-induced immunosuppression by measurement of inosine monophosphate dehydrogenase activity in a canine model, *Transplantation* 61:87–92, 1996.
92. Pirsch JD, Sollinger HW: Mycophenolate mofetil: clinical and experimental experience, *Ther Drug Monit* 19:357–361, 1996.
93. Pfitzmann R, Klupp J, Langrehr JM, et al: Mycophenolate mofetil for immunosuppression after liver transplantation: a follow-up study of 191 patients, *Transplantation* 76(1):130–136, 2003.
94. Morath C, Zeier M: Review of the antiproliferative properties of mycophenolate mofetil in non-immune cells, *Int J Clin Pharmacol Ther* 41(10):465–469, 2003.
95. Boothe DM, Dewey C, Neerman M: Disposition and oral bioavailability of mycophenolic acid following administration of mycofenolate mofatil in normal dogs, *Proc ACIM* , 2003.
96. Boothe: Unpublished Data.
97. Neerman MF, Boothe DM: A possible mechanism of gastrointestinal toxicity posed by mycophenolic acid, *Pharmacol Res* 47(6):523–526, 2003:(Review. No abstract available. Erratum in: *Pharmacol Res* 48(4):415, 2003.)
98. Platz KP, Sollinger HW, Hullett DA, et al: RS-61443—a new, potent immunosuppressive agent, *Transplantation* 51:27–31, 1991.
99. Kennedy GA, Kay TD, Johnson DW, et al: Neutrophil dysplasia characterised by a pseudo-Pelger-Huet anomaly occurring with the use of mycophenolate mofetil and ganciclovir following renal transplantation: a report of five cases, *Pathology* 34(3):263–266, 2002.
100. Angermann CE, Störk S, Costard-Jäckle A, et al: Reduction of cyclosporine after introduction of mycophenolate mofetil improves chronic renal dysfunction in heart transplant recipients—the IMPROVED multi-centre study, *Eur Heart J* 25(18):1626–1634, 2004.
101. Dewey CW, Boothe DM, Rinn KL, et al: Treatment of a myasthenic dog using mycophenolate mofetil, *J Vet Emerg Crit Care* 10:177–187, 2000.
102. Zaucha JM, Yu C, Zellmer E, et al: Effects of extending the duration of postgrafting immunosuppression and substituting granulocyte-colony-stimulating factor-mobilized peripheral blood mononuclear cells for marrow in allogeneic engraftment in a nonmyeloablative canine transplantation model, *Biol Blood Marrow Transplant* 7(9):513–516, 2001.
103. Smolen JS, Kalden JR, Scott DL, et al: Efficacy and safety of leflunomide compared with placebo and sulphasalazine in active rheumatoid arthritis: a double-blind, randomised, multicentre trial, European Leflunomide Study, *Lancet* 353:259–266, 1999.
104. Gregory CR, Stewart A, Sturges B, et al: Leflunomide effectively treats naturally occurring immune-mediated and inflammatory diseases of dogs that are unresponsive to conventional therapy, *Transplant Proc* 30:4143–4148, 1998.
104a. McChesney LP, Xiao F, Sankary HN, et al: An evaluation of leflunomide in the canine renal transplantation model, *Transplantation* 57(12):1717–1722, 1994.
104b. Colopy SA, Baker TA, Muir P: Efficacy of leflunomide for treatment of immune-mediated polyarthritis in dogs: 14 cases (2006-2008), *J Am Vet Med Asso* 236(3):312–338, 2010.
105. Marsolais D, Rosen H: Chemical modulators of sphingosine-1-phosphate receptors as barrier-oriented therapeutic molecules, *Nat Rev Drug Discov* 8(4):297–307, 2009.
106. Rhodes KH: Feline immunomodulators. In Bonagura JD, editor: *Kirk's current veterinary therapy small animal practice (XII)*, Philadelphia, 1995, Saunders, pp 581–584.
107. Snyder PJ: In Androgens. Brunton LL, Lazo JS, Parker KL, editors: *Goodman & Gilman's the pharmacological basis of therapeutics*, ed 11, New York, 2006, McGraw-Hill, pp 1573–1585.
108. Ward H: Immune-mediated hematopoietic diseases. Oncology and hematology, *20th Annual Waltham/OSU Symposium for the Treatment of Small Animal Diseases* 99–104, 1996.
109. Stadtmauer EA, Cassileth PA, Edelstein M, et al: Danazol treatment of myelodysplastic syndromes, *Br J Haematol* 77:502–508, 1991.
110. Choudhry VP, Kashyap R, Ahlawat S, et al: Vinblastine and danazol therapy in steroid resistant childhood chronic idiopathic thrombocytopenic purpura, *Int J Hematol* 61:157–162, 1995.
111. Schreiber AD, Chien P, Tomaski A, et al: Effect of danazol in immune thrombocytopenic purpura, *N Engl J Med* 316:503–508, 1987.
112. Bloom JC, Meunier LD, Thiem PA, et al: Use of danazol for treatment of corticosteroid-resistant immune-mediated thrombocytopenia in a dog, *J Am Vet Med Assoc* 194:76–78, 1989.
113. Holloway SA, Meyer DJ, Mannella C: Prednisolone and danazol for treatment of immune-mediated anemia, thrombocytopenia, and ineffective erythroid regeneration in a dog, *J Am Vet Med Assoc* 197:1045–1048, 1990.
114. Langford CA, Klippel JH, Balow JE, et al: Use of cytotoxic agents and cyclosporine in the treatment of autoimmune disease. Part I: rheumatologic and renal diseases, *Ann Intern Med* 128:1021–1028, 1998.
115. Langford CA, Klippel JH, Balow JE, et al: Use of cytotoxic agents and cyclosporine in the treatment of autoimmune disease. Part II: Inflammatory bowel disease, systemic vasculitis and therapeutic toxicity, *Ann Intern Med* 129:49–58, 1998.
116. Rodriguez DB, Mckin A, Easley R, et al: Relationship between red blood cell thiopurine tethyltransferase activity and myelotoxicity in dogs receiving azathioprine, *Vet Intern Med* 18:M339–M345, 2004.
117. Chabner BA, Amrein PC, Druker BJ, et al: Antineoplastic agents. In Brunton LL, Lazo JS, Parker KL, editors: *Goodman & Gilman's the pharmacological basis of therapeutics*, ed 11, New York, 2006, McGraw-Hill, pp 1315–1403.

118. Burke A, Smyth E, FitzGerald GA: Analgesic-antipyretic and antiinflammatory agents; pharmacotherapy of gout. In Brunton LL, Lazo JS, Parker KL, editors: *Goodman & Gilman's the pharmacological basis of therapeutics*, ed 11, New York, 2006, McGraw-Hill, pp 671–715.
119. Wollheim FA: *Multiple drug resistance and rheumatology*, Cutting Edge, 2003, Novartis Pharma Basel.
120. Werner GH, Zerial A: In Shugar D, editor: *Viral chemotherapy, Immunopotentiating substances with antiviral activity*, vol 1, New York, 1984, Pergamon, pp 511–559.
121. Ricklin Gutzwiller ME, Reist M, Peel JE, et al: Intradermal injection of heat-killed Mycobacterium vaccae in dogs with atopic dermatitis: a multicentre pilot study, *Vet Dermatol* 18:87–93, 2007.
122. Engelman RW, Trang LQ, Good RA: Clinicopathologic responses in cats with feline leukemia virus–associated leukemia-lymphoma treated with staphylococcal protein A, *Am J Pathol* 118:367–378, 1985.
123. Engelman RW, Good RA, Day NK: Clearance of retroviremia and regression of malignancy in cats with leukemia-lymphoma during treatment with staphylococcal protein A, *Cancer Detect Prevent* 10:435–444, 1987.
124. Cotter SM, Essex M, McLane MF, et al: Chemotherapy and passive immunotherapy in naturally occurring feline mediastinal lymphoma. In Hardy WD, Essex M, McClelland AJ, editors: *Feline leukemia virus*, Holland, 1980, Elsevier North Holland, pp 219–225.
125. Reagan WJ, Scott-Moncrieff JC, Christian J, et al: Effects of human intravenous immunoglobulin on canine monocytes and lymphocytes, *Am J Vet Res* 59:1568–1574, 1998.
126. Scott-Moncrieff Reagan WJ, Glickman LT, et al: Treatment of nonregenerative anemia with human gamma globulin in dogs, *J Am Vet Med Assoc* 206:1895–1900, 1995.
127. Scott-Moncrieff JC, Reagan WJ, Snyder PW, et al: Intravenous administration of human immune globulin in dogs with immune-mediated hemolytic anemia, *J Am Vet Med Assoc* 10:1623–1627, 1997.
128. Scott-Moncrieff JC, Reagan WJ: Human intravenous immunoglobulin therapy, *Semin Vet Med Surg* 12:178–185, 1997.
129. Malaguarnera M, Guccione N, Musumeci S, et al: Intravenous immunoglobulin plus interferon-in autoimmune hepatitis C, *Biodrugs* 18(1):63–70, 2004.
130. Anonymous: ADIS research and development profile: Abetimus, Abetimus sodium, LJP 394, *Biodrugs* 17(3):212–215, 2003.
131. Colombo S, Hill PB, Shaw DJ, et al: Effectiveness of low dose immunotherapy in the treatment of canine atopic dermatitis: a prospective, double-blinded, clinical study, *Vet Dermatol* 16:162–170, 2005.
132. Hayes AA, MacEwen EG, Matus RE, et al: Antileukemic activity of plasma cryoprecipitate therapy in the cat. In Hardy WD, Essex M, McClelland AJ, editors: *Feline leukemia virus*, Holland, 1980, Elsevier North Holland, pp 245–251.
133. Caciolo PL, Hayes AA, Patnaik AK, et al: A case of mycosis fungoides in a cat and literature review, *J Am Anim Hosp Assoc* 19:505–512, 1983.

133a. Parodi AL, Misdorp W, Mialot JP, et al: Intratumoral BCG and Corynebacterium parvum therapy of canine mammary tumours before radical mastectomy, *Cancer Immunol Immunother* 15(3):172–177, 1983.

134. Rosenthal RC: Hormones in cancer therapy, *Vet Clin North Am Small Anim Pract* 12:67–77, 1982.
135. Marshall GD, Gibbone AS, Pamell LS: Human cytokines induced by acemannan, *J Allergy Clin Immunol* 91:295, 1993.
136. Ramamoorthy L, Kemp MC, Tizard IR: Acemannan, a beta-(1,4)-acetylated mannan, induces nitric-oxide production in macrophage cell-line Raw-264.7, *Mol Pharmacol* 50:878, 1996.
137. King GK, Yates KM, Greenlee PG, et al: The effect of acemannan immunostimulant in combination with surgery and radiation therapy on spontaneous canine and feline fibrosarcomas, *J Am Anim Hosp Assoc* 31:439, 1995.
138. Harris C, Pierce K, King G, et al: Efficacy of acemannan in treatment of canine and feline spontaneous neoplasms, *Mol Biother* 3:207, 1991.
139. MacEwen EG, Hays AA, Mooney S, et al: Evaluation of effect of levamisole on feline mammary cancer, short communication, *J Biol ResponseModif* 5:541–546, 1984.
140. Hahm KB, Park IS, Kim HC, et al: Comparison of antiproliferative effects of 1-histamine-2 receptor antagonists, cimetidine, ranitidine, and famotidine, in gastric cancer cells, *Int J Immunopharmacol* 18:393–399, 1996.
141. Adams WJ, Morris DL: Pilot study—cimetidine enhances lymphocyte infiltration of human colorectal carcinoma: results of a small randomized control trial, *Cancer* 80:15–21, 1997.
142. Hamilton RD, Wynalda MA, Fitszpatick FA, et al: Comparison between circulating interferon and drug levels following administration of 2-amino-5-bromo-6-phenyl-4(3H)-pyrimidone (ABPP) to different animal species, *J Interferon Res* 2:317–327, 1981.
143. Hengge UH, Benninghoff B, Ruzicka T, et al: Topical immunomodulators-progress towards treating inflammation, infection, and cancer, *Lancet Infect Dis* 1:189–198, 2001.
144. Denburg JA, Schmi R, Saito H, et al: Systemic aspects of allergic disease: bone marrow responses, *J Allergy Clin Immunol* 106(Suppl 5):S242–S246, 2000.
145. Menzies-Gow AN, Flood-Page PT, Robinson DS, et al: Effect of inhaled interleukin-5 on eosinophil progenitors in the bronchi and bone marrow of asthmatic and non-asthmatic volunteers, *Clin Exp Allergy* 37(7):1023–1032, 2007.
146. Simon D, Braathen: Simon H-U: Eosinophils and atopic dermatitis, *Allergy* 59:561–571, 2004.
147. Al-Haddad S, Riddell RH: The role of eosinophils in inflammatory bowel disease, *Gut* 54(12):1674–1675, 2005.
148. Kanaoka Y, Boyce JA: Cysteinyl leukotrienes and their receptors: cellular distribution and function in immune and inflammatory responses, *J Immunol* 173:1503–1510, 2004.
149. Senter DA, Scott DW, Miller WH Jr: Treatment of canine atopic dermatitis with zafirlukast, a leukotriene-receptor antagonist: a single-blinded, placebo-controlled study, *Can Vet J* 43(3):203–206, 2002.
150. Pease JE, Williams TJ: Eotaxin and asthma, *Curr Opin Pharmacol* 1:248–253, 2001.
151. Denburg JA: Bone marrow in atopy and asthma: hematopoietic mechanisms in allergic inflammation, *Immunol Today* 20(3):111–113, 1999.
152. Braccioni F, Dorman SC, O'Byrne PM, et al: The effect of cysteinyl leukotrienes on growth of eosinophil progenitors from peripheral blood and bone marrow of atopic subjects, *J Allergy Clin Immunol* 110:96–101, 2002.
153. Dewachter P, Mouton-Faivre C, Emala CW: Anaphylaxis and anesthesia: controversies and new insights, *Anesthesiology* 111(5):1141–1150, 2009.
154. Mason N, Duval K, Shofer FS: Cyclophosphamide exerts no beneficial effect over prednisone alone in the initial treatment of acute immune-mediated hemolytic anemia in dogs: a randomized controlled clinical trial, *J Vet Intern Med* 17:206–212, 2003.
155. Helfand S, Jain NC, Paul M: Vincristine-loaded platelet therapy for idiopathic thrombocytopenia in a dog, *J Am Vet Med Assoc* 185:224, 1984.
156. Brown CD, Parnell NK, Brown D, et al: Steroid responsive neutropenia in dogs: 11 cases (1990-2002), *ProcAm Coll Vet Int Med abstract* :226, 2003.
157. Rees CA, Boothe DM, Boeckh A, et al: Dosing regimen and hematologic effects of pentoxifylline and its active metabolites in normal dogs, *Vet Ther* 4(2):188–196, 2003.

158. Rees CA, Boothe DM: Therapeutic response to pentoxifylline and its active metabolites in dogs with familial canine dermatomyositis, *VetTher* 4(3):234–241, 2003.
159. Asanuma Y, Yamada H, Matsuda T, et al: Successful treatment of interstitial pneumonia with lipo-PGE1 and pentoxifylline in a patient with dermatomyositis, *Ryumachi* 37:719–726, 1997.
160. Rosenkrantz WS: Eosinophilic granuloma confusion. In August JR, editor: *Consultations in feline internal medicine*, Philadelphia, 1991, Saunders, pp 121–124.
161. Messinger LM: Therapy for feline dermatoses, *Vet Clin North Am Small Anim Pract* 25:981–1005, 1995.
162. Hogenesch H, Snyder PW, Scott-Moncrieff JC, et al: Interleukin-6 activity in dogs with juvenile polyarteritis syndrome: effect of corticosteroids, *Clin Immunol Immunopathol* 77:107, 1995.
163. Clements DN, Grear RN, Tattrsall J, et al: Type I immune-mediated polyarthritis in dogs: 39 cases (1997-2002), *J Am Vet Med Assoc* 224:1323–1327, 2004.
164. Sandborn WJ: Cyclosporine therapy for inflammatory bowel disease: definitive answers and remaining questions, *Gastroenterology* 109:1001–1003, 1995.
165. Sandborn WJ: A review of immune modifier therapy for inflammatory bowel disease: azathioprine, 6-mercaptopurine, cyclosporine, and methotrexate, *Am J Gastroenterol* 91:423–433, 1996.
166. Bird J: Guidelines on the diagnosis and management of AL amyloidosis, *United Kingdom Myeloma Forum* 125(6):681–700, 2005.

Biologic Response Modifiers: Interferons, Interleukins, Chemokines, and Hematopoietic Growth Factors*

32

Paul R. Avery

Chapter Outline

KEY POINT 32-1 Natural or synthetic biological response modifiers are being developed as therapeutic mediators to increase the effectiveness of the immune response directed toward a pathogen or neoplasm, to stimulate the proliferation of hematopoietic progenitor cells (e.g., in the treatment of chemotherapy-associated neutropenia), or to decrease a chronic inflammatory response (e.g., chronic inflammatory bowel disease).

BIOLOGICAL RESPONSE MODIFIERS AND CYTOKINES

Natural or synthetic preparations given with the intent of altering the response of the host to a pathogen, neoplasm, or inflammatory process have been termed *biological response modifiers.* The goal of therapy may be to increase the effectiveness of the immune response directed toward a pathogen or neoplasm, to stimulate the proliferation of hematopoietic progenitor cells (e.g., in the treatment of chemotherapy-associated neutropenia), or to decrease a chronic inflammatory response (e.g., chronic inflammatory bowel disease). Biological response modifiers are not usually specific in an immunologic sense; rather, they alter physiologic systems through changes in regulatory pathways. They range from bacterial cell wall extracts to molecularly cloned cytokines. As mediators of physiologic processes, interferons, interleukins, and chemokines are candidates for therapeutic manipulation or even for use as drugs. Several recombinant human, feline, and canine cytokines are commercially available in pharmacologic quantities and are available for veterinary use (Box 32-1). Some generalizations about cytokine biology follow. See the reviews by Oppenheim and Feldman,[1] Nicola,[2] and Oppenheim and coworkers[3] for general discussions of cytokine, growth factor, and chemokine biology and the article by Gangur and coworkers[4] for a review of chemokines of veterinary relevance.

Cytokines are polypeptides that regulate cell growth and differentiation, apoptosis, inflammation, immunity, and repair. They are of fundamental importance in the pathogenesis and treatment of disease. They transmit information to target cells regarding the physiologic status of the animal, resulting in a biologic response in the target tissue. More than 50 distinct human cytokines and their receptors have been described. Cytokine nomenclature can be bewildering, with several historical names attached to the same molecule (e.g., *stem cell factor, c-kit ligand,* and *mast cell growth factor* are all the same cytokine). Cytokines Online Pathfinder Encyclopaedia (COPE) is a useful Internet resource with a large amount of information concerning cytokine, chemokine, and growth factor biology (www.copewithcytokines.de/cope.cgi). Cytokines can be categorized into families on the basis of homology in primary amino acid sequence, three-dimensional structure, induction mechanisms, chromosomal location, similarities in receptor type, and functional homology. Families that are currently clinically relevant in companion animal medicine include interferons (IFNs), which have antiviral and immunoregulatory functions; interleukins (ILs), which have a wide variety of functions; chemokines, which have to do

*From Kruth SA: Biological response modifiers: interferons, interleukins, recombinant products, liposomal products, *Vet Clin North Am Small Anim Pract* 28:269-295, 1998.

Box 32-1

Commercially Available Recombinant Canine and Feline Cytokines, Chemokines, and Growth Factors

Canine
Interferon-γ (R and D Systems)
Interleukin-1β 2, 4, 5, 6, 8, 10, 12, 23 (R and D Systems)
Interleukin-6 (Pierce, Genway Biotech)
CCL2 (MCP1) (R and D Systems)
CXCL8 (R and D Systems)
GM-CSF (R and D Systems)
Stem cell factor (R and D Systems)
TNF-a (R and D Systems, Pierce)

Feline
Interferon-α (R and D Systems, Pierce)
Interferon-g (R and D Systems)
Interleukin-1 β 2, 4, 5, 6, 8, 10, 12, 23 (R and D Systems)
Interleukin-6 (Pierce, Genway Biotech)
TNF-a (R and D Systems, Pierce)
CXCL8 (R and D Systems)
CXCL12 (SDF-1) (R and D Systems)
CCL5 (RANTES) (R and D Systems)
FLT-3 ligand (R and D Systems)
Stem cell factor (R and D Systems)
GM-CSF (R and D Systems)

with chemotaxis and organ development; and hematopoietic growth factors.

Most cytokines are not constitutively produced but are secreted after activation of cells by viral, bacterial, and parasitic infections. The cellular sources of most cytokines are diverse, with production occurring in many types of cells. Production is normally short lived, usually for hours to a few days. Normally, they have autocrine and paracrine (rather than endocrine) effects, with little to no detectable circulating levels. Because of high cytokine–receptor affinity, cytokines are effective in the picogram to nanogram per mL range.

Cytokines typically have pleiotropic and redundant actions. The same activity may be induced by several structurally distinct cytokines acting at unrelated cell surface receptors. For example, IL-1, tumor necrosis factor-alpha (TNF-alpha),* and IL-6 are all mediators of the acute inflammatory response; induce fever and the synthesis of acute-phase proteins in the liver; increase vascular permeability; and induce adhesion molecules, fibroblast proliferation, platelet production, IL-6 and IL-8, and T and B cell activation. Gene deletion experiments reveal that few individual cytokines are absolutely essential to life or even to individual cell function, with notable exceptions such as TNF-alpha and transforming growth factor-β (TGF-β). Also, the cellular response of most cytokines is modulated by other cytokines, with synergistic, additive, and antagonistic interactions described. Cytokines form a complex feedback network by either inducing or suppressing the expression of other cytokines, forming cascades similar to the blood coagulation cascades.

Structurally, most cytokines consist of a single glycosylated polypeptide chain. They interact with cells by binding to specific high affinity cell surface receptors. The intracellular signal transduction cascade initiated by binding of a cytokine to its receptor eventually results in the production of DNA-binding proteins that influence transcription of various genes. In addition to cell surface receptors, soluble receptors have been described for many cytokines. Soluble receptors may be involved in cytokine transport or inhibit cytokine activity.

A number of proteins that inhibit the activity of cytokines have been reported. One of the best characterized is the IL-1 receptor antagonist (IL-1RA), which binds to receptor but fails to activate the cell. IL-1RA is currently being investigated as a therapy for rheumatoid arthritis in humans and may have a role in the treatment of other inflammatory disorders if appropriate delivery systems can be developed. Peptide antagonists of chemokines have shown promise in breaking the cycle of inflammation in experimental models of disease. A second way in which a cytokine can be inhibited is by binding of soluble cytokine receptors that are able to bind the cytokine and neutralize its activity, as discussed earlier.

Recombinant DNA technology has been used to produce cytokines, many of which are now commercially available. The recombinant process involves cloning the cDNA encoding the protein of interest and placing it into an expression system (bacterial, yeast, insect, mammalian cell culture) under conditions that permit large amounts of the protein to be produced. By convention, these products are designated by an "r" preceding the name of the cytokine and a designation of the species of origin (e.g., *rhIL* indicates recombinant interleukin of human origin, and *rfeIFN* indicates a recombinant interferon of feline origin). Many cytokines are conserved in the evolutionary sense, and biological effects occur when some human recombinant products are administered to companion animals.

It is tempting to administer cytokines in pharmacologic doses; however, several points should be considered. Perhaps most important, systemic levels of a given cytokine will perturb many cytokine cascades, with resultant side effects and toxicity. The use of IL-12 as a therapeutic agent, as discussed later, has been limited by potentially severe hematopoietic and hepatic toxicities in animals and man and was associated with two deaths in a phase 1 trial in humans.[5] Dosing may be critical; for example, low doses of IFN appear to be immunostimulatory, whereas higher doses are immunosuppressive, and the specific type of IFN influences these effects. This concept of increasing doses of immunostimulatory cytokines leading to depression of the immune response has been demonstrated with IL-12 as well and appears to be due to the magnitiude of downstream IFN-γ and nitric oxide that is produced.[6] Currently, recommended cytokine doses are empirically derived. With the exceptions of rfeIFN-α (in cats) and rhIL-1 (in dogs),

*Tumor necrosis factor-alpha (TNF-alpha) is a multifunctional cytokine with biological activities that include modulation of tumor growth, infections, septic shock/systemic inflammatory response syndrome, and autoimmunity. The TNF family of cytokines is distinct from the IL and IFN families. Canine and feline TNF-alpha have been cloned. They are not discussed in this chapter.

the pharmacokinetics of cytokines in dogs and cats have not been well characterized.

The safety and efficacy of cytokines as biological response modifiers may be improved if they can be delivered directly to target cells. Delivery systems, such as liposomes and replication-defective adenoviruses, have been reported in the literature, with encouraging results. In some cases the cDNA for the cytokine of interest can be delivered (using a variety of methods) directly to the tissue of concern (usually a neoplasm), and controlled expression of the gene may confer clinical benefits. Both agonistic and antagonistic peptides have been sought for various cytokines in attempts to achieve systemic oral administration or suppress harmful effects.

INTERFERONS

Interferon Biology

Interferons are cytokines secreted by virus-infected cells and were originally characterized by their nonspecific antiviral activity. Interferons bind to receptors on other cells and induce antiviral proteins, protecting those cells from infection. It is now known that IFNs induce a wide range of pleiotropic effects, including antiviral, antitumor, antiparasitic, and immunomodulatory effects.

Two distinct classes of IFNs have been described. Class I interferons are subdivided into alpha, omega, and beta interferons (a subclass of omega interferons, the tau interferons, has been described in ruminant embryos and is important in maintaining pregnancy). Class II interferons are composed of a single protein, IFN-γ. IFN-α and IFN-ω were originally described as being secreted by leukocytes, but they are likely produced by all nucleated cells. Humans have at least 24 different alpha and omega genes, dogs have two alpha genes and no omega genes, and the genetic complement of cats has not been reported. Feline IFN-α cDNA has been cloned and the cytokine produced in a silkworm-recombinant baculovirus system, and its pharmacokinetic properties have been studied.[7-10] The pharmacokinetic data suggest that rfeIFN has similar pharmacokinetic properties to human IFNs and that it is distributed primarily to the liver and kidneys, is rapidly catabolized mainly in the kidneys, and is excreted in the urine without residual accumulation in the body. Since feline IFN-α was initially cloned, 14 additional subtypes have been described.[11,12] IFN-β is classically described as being produced by fibroblasts; however, many other cells can be stimulated to secrete the cytokine. Humans and dogs have one IFN-β gene. Synthesis of IFN-α and IFN-β can be induced by live or inactivated viruses, bacterial cell walls, synthetic oligonucleotides, IL-1, IL-2, and TNF-alpha. IFN-α and IFN-β compete for similar receptors. IFN-γ is produced by activated T and natural killer (NK) cells and is structurally and functionally distinct from IFN-α/β. All mammals investigated have only one IFN-γ gene. IFN-γ binds to a receptor distinct from the α/β receptor. Canine IFN-γ has been characterized, the cDNA and chromosomal gene have been cloned, and production and characterization of recombinant canine from *Escherichia coli* has been described.[13-15] Feline IFN-γ cDNA has also been cloned.[16,17]

After receptor binding, IFNs induce the transcription of a set of genes called *IFN-stimulated genes* (ISGs). Nearly 30 different ISGs have been identified. Induction of ISGs by IFN-α/β is rapid and transient, lasting for 3 to 4 hours. IFN-γ requires several hours of exposure before gene induction occurs. After the initial induction, ISG transcription declines and returns to basal levels.

IFNs inhibit the growth of almost all known viruses by interfering with viral RNA and protein synthesis. IFNs are induced by viral nucleic acid and bind to the receptors of nearby cells. The development of resistance to virus infections occurs within a few minutes and peaks within a few hours. Several proteins are induced, including RNase L (which cleaves viral RNA); nitric oxide synthetase (nitric oxide has antiviral activity); a protein kinase that phosphorylates an initiation factor called elL-2 (which inhibits viral protein synthesis by preventing the elongation of viral double-stranded RNA); and the Mx protein, which inhibits translation of viral mRN.[18] IFN-γ inhibits viral replication by stimulating the release of other IFNs. IFNs are also induced by bacteria, fungi, and some protozoa, and the activation of phagocytic cells is important in the host response to these pathogens.

IFNs induce increased expression of class I and class II major histocompatibility complex (MHC) molecules on antigen-presenting cells, leading to enhanced antigen presentation. They increase phagocytosis and intracellular and extracellular killing by macrophages and neutrophils. The IFNs also modulate T, B, and NK cell function, with IFN-γ having the most potent immunomodulating activity.

IFNs have several effects on neoplastic cells, including modulation of oncogene expression. Downregulation of c-myc, c-fos, c-Ha-ras, c-mos, and c-src have been described in various models. IFN-α augments NK cell cytotoxicity against neoplastic cells and acts synergistically with IL-2 to increase NK activity. Antiangiogenic activity has also been described.

Large-scale production of IFNs is accomplished by culturing stimulated cells, leading to the production of "natural" or "native" IFN (denoted by *N)* products. Alternatively, IFNs can be produced by recombinant methods. Human IFNs from both sources are commercially available, and recombinant feline and canine IFN-α and IFN-γ are commercially available (see Box 32-1). Natural IFNs are less concentrated and may contain a mixture of IFN types with other cytokines.

Interferons as Therapeutic Agents

In humans IFN-α has been approved for the treatment of hairy cell leukemia, melanoma, chronic myelogenous leukemia, Kaposi sarcoma, basal cell carcinoma, renal cell carcinoma, and genital warts. Effects on metastatic melanoma, endocrine–pancreatic tumors, metastatic colorectal and ovarian carcinoma, and bladder cancer have also been reported. IFN-β is also licensed for the treatment of chronic hepatitis B and hepatitis C infections. IFN-γ bound to polyethylene glycol (peg-IFN) has an increased circulating half-life and has shown improved efficacy in treating hepatitis C infections.[19] IFN-β has been approved for the treatment of multiple sclerosis and IFN-γ for the treatment of chronic granulomatous disease.

Experience using IFN therapy has generally shown that these products are most effective when combined with other antiviral or cytotoxic treatment modalities.[20]

Using a feline in vitro system, Weiss and Oostrom-Ram[21] showed that low levels of rhIFN-α had no effect on lymphocyte blastogenesis, whereas higher levels significantly suppressed blastogenic responses. In vivo, cats given 10^2 or 10^4 IU/kg had significantly enhanced blastogenesis, whereas cats given 1×10^6 IU/kg had depressed lymphocyte stimulation. In cats the immunomodulating effects of rhIFN-α appeared to be dose dependent.

Five feline IFN-α subtypes have been recently cloned, expressed, and characterized in feline cell lines.[11,22] All subtypes were shown to have antiviral effects on feline calicivirus and vesicular stomatitis virus in vitro. Additionally, they showed a species-specific antiproliferative effect on a feline tumor cell line. The IFN-α inducible Mx gene was upregulated 24 hours after administration to cats, demonstrating in vivo efficacy. In vitro work has also demonstrated the antiviral activity of IFN-α against feline herpesvirus-1 in the absence of any cytopathic effect on the cultured corneal cells.[23] Activity of rfeIFN-ω, a closely related cytokine to rfeIFN-α against rotavirus, feline panleukopenia virus, feline calicivirus, and feline infectious peritonitis coronavirus, was documented in cell cultures of feline origin. The antiviral effect was more pronounced when the cell cultures were treated continuously than when they were pretreated only before challenge. RfeIFN-ω did not have activity in canine cells challenged with vesicular stomatitis virus, implying species specificity of action,[24] yet de Mari and coworkers[25] described clinical benefits of another rfeIFN-ω preparation in dogs with parvoviral infection (discussed later). Recombinant feline IFN-ω is marketed in Japan as Intercat[R] (Toray Industries, Tokyo, Japan), and a second rfeIFN-ω product is licensed in Europe as Virbagen omega (Laboratory Virbac, Carros, France).

Feline Infectious Peritonitis

Parenterally administered rhIFN-α and IFN-β, with or without *Propionibacterium acnes* (which enhances IFN responses and augments T and NK cell activities) given prophylactically or therapeutically, did not significantly reduce the mortality rate of experimentally induced feline infectious peritonitis virus (FIPV) infection. Cats treated with high-dose IFN, 10 U/kg daily for 8 days and then on alternate days for an additional 2 to 3 weeks, however, had temporary suppression of clinical signs and decreased serum antibody responses to FIPV, and the mean survival time of cats treated with high-dose rhIFN-α was increased by a few weeks over that of untreated cats. IFN-related toxicities were not reported.[26] It is possible that the benefits of the high-dose protocol were due to the dose-dependent immunosuppressive effects of IFN. The increase in survival times in this study using experimental challenge was only 2 to 3 weeks, and there are few data documenting the response of cats with naturally occurring disease. There are anecdotal reports of orally administered low-dose rhIFN-α therapy (as described later) inducing remissions from clinical FIP, but there is currently no published data. A study of subcutaneous rfeIFN-ω administered to 12 cats clinically diagnosed with FIP demonstrated long-term survival in 4 animals.[27] As the authors acknowledge, this was not a case-controlled study and histologic confirmation of the disease was available only for those animals that died during the study. A recent placebo-controlled, double-blind trial in which rfeIFN-ω was administered subcutaneously to cats naturally infected with FIPV did not demonstrate any clinical, hematopoietic, or survival benefits to the therapy; conventional therapy with cytotoxic drugs and corticosteroids remains the treatment of choice.[28,29]

Feline Leukemia Virus and Feline Immunodeficiency Virus

Recombinant hIFN-α has been shown to inhibit the production or release (or both) of feline leukemia virus (FeLV) in tissue culture systems.[30] The parenteral administration of rhIFN-α alone or in combination with zidovudine (AZT) beginning 12 weeks after exposure to FeLV resulted in significant and sustained decreases in circulating virus levels. The anti-FeLV effect was limited by the production of anti–rhIFN-α antibodies detected 7 weeks after the start of therapy. IFN-associated toxicity was not observed.[31] In a subsequent study, treatment of FeLV-infected cats with AZT, IFN-α, and adoptive transfer of lectin/IL-2–activated lymphocytes resulted in clearance of circulating virus in four of nine cats despite the appearance of anti-rhIFN-α antibodies. Combination therapy appeared to reconstitute antiviral humoral immunity, counteracted immunosuppression, and induced the reversal of retroviremia.[32] Unfortunately, because of the problem of antibody induction, parenteral rhIFN-α appears to have little clinical utility as a monotherapy for FeLV infections. In vitro work supports the antiviral effects of rfeIFN-α and rhIFN-α but not rfeIFN-γ on feline immunodeficiency virus (FIV) replication.[33] Ovine IFN-τ has demonstrable effects on the in vitro replication of both FIV and human immunodeficiency virus (HIV).[34] A study of subcutaneous rfeIFN-α therapy in cats naturally infected with FeLV or co-infected with FeLV and FIV showed significant decreases in clinical scores and mortality rate during the 12 months of follow-up in the treated cats.[35] Recently, low-dose oral IFN-α (as described later) was shown to improve clinical condition and survival in cats naturally infected with FIV.[36]

Canine Parvovirus

Two studies, one with experimental infection and one with naturally occurring infection, have examined the efficacy on rfeIFN-ω (Virbagen, Laboratory Virbac, Carros, France) on the outcome of canine parvoviral enteritis. Ten 8- to 9-week-old dogs inoculated with parvovirus were divided into rfeIFN-ω or placebo treatment groups and received three daily injections. All five of the placebo-treated dogs succumbed to fulminant enteritis, whereas four of five rfeIFN-ω–treated dogs survived and eventually recovered fully.[37] In the second study of naturally occurring disease, 43 dogs were assigned to receive three daily intravenous injections of rfeIFN-ω, and 49 dogs received placebo treatment. There was a significant improvement in clinical signs and a significant decrease in mortality in the dogs receiving IFN therapy.[25]

Low-Dose Oral Recombinant Human Interferon-α

In 1988 Cummins and coworkers [38] reported that after experimental infection with the Rickard strain of FeLV, the administration of 0.5 or 5 U of natural hIFN-α orally once daily for 7 consecutive days on alternate weeks for 1 month was associated with survival in 70% of IFN-treated cats, whereas 100% of placebo-treated control cats died. However, 12 of 13 cats treated with IFN did develop persistent viremia. In another report, four cats with FeLV-associated nonregenerative anemia were treated with 100,000 U bovine IFN-β orally for 5 consecutive days on alternate weeks. General clinical improvement, reduction in circulating antigen levels, and normalization of hematocrit levels were reported in all cats,[39] and one cat cleared its viremia. Similar findings were reported by Steed,[40] who treated four FeLV-infected cats with low-dose natural hIFN-α or bovine IFN-β. Weiss and coworkers[41] reported on 69 FeLV-infected cats with clinical signs treated orally with either low-dose rhIFN-α or bovine IFN-β. Cats treated with rhIFN had significantly higher survival rates than did cats given bovine IFN; both groups had increased survival rates compared with historical controls. In general, clinical responses were observed within the first or second week of oral IFN administration, with increased appetite, greater activity, weight gain, resolution of fever, improved hemogram and leukocyte counts, and quicker recovery from secondary bacterial infections when antibiotics were administered. Most cats remained viremic.

In contrast to the aforementioned reports, Kociba and coworkers[42] reported that low-dose oral hIFN-α had no significant effects on viremia, course of the disease, or differential leukocyte counts in experimental FeLV infection. In their system the Kawakami–Theilen strain (A, B, and C subgroups, which consistently induce fatal erythroid aplasia) was administered to 12-week-old kittens. Methylprednisolone acetate was also given the day of inoculation. Neither rhIFN-α nor human natural IFN-α induced any significant benefit compared with placebo. A second study administering low-dose oral rhIFN-α showed a similar lack of benefit clinically or biochemically in naturally infected, clinically ill FeLV-positive cats.[43]

Pedretti and coworkers[36] recently reported that FIV-infected cats given a daily oral dose of 10 IU/kg rhIFN-α had a significantly prolonged survival rate compared with placebo-treated cats. In addition, clinical remission of many of the typical immunopathologic lesions occurred despite no significant reduction in circulating viral levels. This study selected FIV-infected cats that presented with evidence of immunosuppression and clinical signs of acquired immunodeficiency syndrome (AIDS) and utilized a mixture of multiple human IFN-α subtypes. Two large, double-blind, placebo-controlled trials of low-dose oral IFN-α failed to show any efficacy in ameliorating clinical signs, increasing CD4+ T cell counts, or decreasing mortality rates in HIV-infected humans.[44,45]

If orally administered low-dose human IFN-α has any effect in cats with retroviral infections, a direct systemic antiviral effect is unlikely. It may be possible that IFN may be acting as a biological response modifier after binding to cellular receptors in the oral cavity/pharynx, triggering cytokine cascades that have systemic immunomodulatory effects. Appetite stimulation may be due to direct central nervous system effects. When it was used orally in cats, adverse effects have not been reported, and anti-rhIFN-α neutralizing antibodies do not appear to develop.

Interferons as Therapy for Cancer

IFNs inhibit cell proliferation of both normal and malignant cells and have numerous immunomodulating effects. Several human cancers respond to IFN therapy. At present, there are only preclinical data suggesting that IFNs may have some utility in the treatment of cancer in companion animals. When canine mammary tumor and melanoma cell lines were incubated with canine IFN-γ, significantly increased expression of MHC antigen class I and II antigens and tumor-associated antigens were observed.[46] Increased expression of these antigens may be of benefit in tumor cell recognition and rejection by the immune system. Pretreatment of canine macrophages with rcIFN-γ resulted in increased in vitro tumor cell killing in canine models of melanoma and osteosarcoma.[47,48] In another study growth of canine and feline tumors was inhibited by rhIFN-α and rhIFN-γ in vitro. Sensitivity to IFN varied according to the type of neoplasm, with round cell tumors being most sensitive.[49] Recombinant rfeIFN was found to have a dose-dependent inhibitory effect on cell growth and colony formation on cell lines derived from canine acanthomatous epulis, benign mixed mammary tumor, squamous cell carcinoma, and malignant melanoma.[50] Recent work has demonstrated that intratumoral injection of rfeIFN-ω in cats with fibrosarcomas is safe and feasible; subsequent studies will be necessary to determine efficacy.[51]

INTERLEUKINS

Interleukin Biology

There are currently 35 defined ILs, named in order of discovery and classified into groups according to their structure, function, or both. ILs are a diverse group of cytokines, with functions including enhancement or suppression of various cells of the immune system (e.g., IL-1, IL-2, IL-4, IL-9, IL-10, IL-12, IL-13, IL-17, IL-23, IL-27), hematopoietic growth factor activity (e.g., IL-3, IL-11, IL-17, IL-32, IL-34), and the regulation of leukocyte function (e.g., IL-5 modulates eosinophil function; IL-8 is chemotactic for neutrophils). Some are growth factors for cells of the immune system (e.g., IL-7, IL-11, IL-14, IL-15), whereas others enhance the acute phase response (e.g., IL-1, IL-6). Most ILs have multiple effects on various cells and are part of complex regulatory cascades. Depending on the specific IL, they are produced by T and B lymphocytes, macrophages, dendritic cells (DCs), fibroblasts, and other stromal cells.

Examples Of Interleukin Therapy in Dogs and Cats

Interleukin-1

Human rIL-1α was shown to be chemokinetic and chemotactic for canine neutrophils in vitro and to cause dose-dependent and selective neutrophil infiltration after intradermal administration.[52] The pharmacokinetics of a single dose of human IL-1 has been studied in the dog. IL-1 was rapidly distributed, with a volume of distribution approximately twice that of the total body water of a lean dog. The terminal half-life was less than 30 minutes. Within approximately 1 hour after dosing,[53] IL levels were below the quantifiable limit of the enzyme-linked immunosorbent assay (ELISA). As IL-1 is a central mediator of inflammation, these data are useful for studying the physiology of IL-1; however, pharmacologic efforts will focus on inhibition of IL-1 activity, with applications in the therapy of acute and chronic inflammatory disorders and septic shock. The canine IL-1 receptor antagonist, which functions as a competitive inhibitor of IL-1, has been cloned.[54]

Interleukin-2

IL-2 synthesis is triggered by antigen-induced activation of T lymphocytes, and its most important activity is the promotion of clonal expansion of antigen-specific T cells. In NK cells and macrophages, IL-2 also promotes proliferation, production of IFN-γ, and cytolytic activity. It also induces growth of B cells as well as immunoglobulin secretion. An important clinical consideration is the observation that NK cells cultured in the presence of IL-2 have enhanced cytotoxic activity, with increased capability for lysis of neoplastic cells. These activated cells are called *lymphokine-activated killer (LAK) cells*. IL-2 is thus an attractive agent for the therapy of neoplastic disorders; however, parenteral administration of IL-2 is associated with significant hepatic, hematopoietic, and vascular toxicity, which appears to be largely due to the secondary release of TNF-alpha and nitric oxide.[55-57]

IL-2 was licensed in the United States in 1992 for the treatment of metastatic renal cell cancer, becoming the first biological agent approved for treatment of any cancer in humans. The availability of recombinant IL-2 spurred the development of *adoptive immunotherapy*, which refers to the transfer to the tumor-bearing patient immune cells that mediate antitumor effects. Adoptive immunotherapy has been performed with LAK cells and tumor-infiltrating lymphocytes. IL-2 is necessary for the generation of these cells in vitro and in vivo and is also administered systemically along with these cells in an effort to keep them functioning in the patient. More recently, IL-2 gene therapy for various cancers has been developed.

Several in vitro studies have demonstrated that rhIL-2 has activity in companion animals similar to the activity recognized in humans. Feline lymphocytes responded appropriately to the cytokinetic action of systemically administered rhIL-2,[58] and adoptive immunotherapy of FeLV-infected cats with lectin/rhIL-2–activated lymphocytes, IFN-α, and AZT led to reconstitution of antiviral humoral immunity, counteracted immunosuppression, and induced the reversal of retroviremia in a subset of treated cats.[32] Feline IL-2 cDNA was cloned, and the recombinant protein was shown to promote proliferation of feline, but not human, cells.[59,60] Helfand and coworkers[61] demonstrated that the immunobiology of IL-2 in the dog is similar to that of humans. Tumor cytotoxicity was induced in vitro in canine lymphocytes with rhIL-2, demonstrating that functional and morphologic changes compatible with LAK cells could be obtained in dogs.[62-64]

Infusion of rhIL-2 into normal dogs resulted in lymphocytosis and enhanced in vitro lysis of a canine tumor cell line. Side effects included vomiting, diarrhea, and inactivity.[65] Recombinant human TNF and rhIL-2 were administered in a sequential schedule to 30 dogs with a variety of spontaneous neoplasms. Objective tumor responses were seen in dogs with oral melanomas and cutaneous mast cell tumors. Dose-limiting toxicities were primarily gastrointestinal.[66]

In an effort to develop a delivery system that would be associated with less toxicity, Khanna and coworkers[67] nebulized free rhIL-2 and rhIL-2–containing liposomes into normal dogs. Free IL-2 resulted in increased peripheral blood mononuclear cell activation compared with saline-treated control dogs. IL-2 liposomes resulted in significantly increased bronchoalveolar lavage (BAL) effector leukocyte numbers and activation compared with empty liposomes. In dogs with primary and metastatic lung cancer, nebulized IL-2 increased the total number of BAL macrophages, eosinophils, and lymphocytes compared with pretreatment levels, and there was increased expression of CD3 on BAL lymphocytes. Mean BAL cytolytic activity increased compared with pretreatment activity during therapy to a maximum at day 15, and then it decreased (despite continued aerosol therapy) to pretreatment levels at day 30. Antibodies reacting with hIL-2 developed in the serum of all treated dogs, possibly accounting for the decrease in BAL cytolytic activity at day 30 compared with day 15. Toxicity was not recognized with either IL-2 preparation. Complete regression of pulmonary metastases in two of five dogs with metastatic osteosarcoma was maintained at greater than 370 and 700 at day 68. A phase I trial of liposome-complexed canine IL-2 administered parenterally to dogs with chemotherapy-resistant, metastatic osteosarcoma was recently completed.[69] The liposome formulation resulted in preferential expression of the IL-2 within the lung. The weekly injections were well tolerated, and 3 of the 14 dogs completing the 12-week therapy had partial or complete radiographic regression of metastases, with an additional four dogs showing stable disease. Despite the limitations in interpreting efficacy in a phase I pilot study, there was a significant increase in overall survival times in the treated dogs compared with historic controls with similar tumor staging.

Quintin-Colonna and coworkers[70] reported that dogs with oral melanoma treated with local resection, 45-Gy radiation therapy, and repeated local injections of xenogeneic Vero cells transfected with an hIL-2–expressing plasmid had longer median survival times than did dogs treated with resection and radiation therapy alone; dogs treated with surgery, radiation therapy, and nonengineered Vero cells; or dogs treated with surgery, radiation therapy, and injection of rhIL-2 into the tumor bed. Similar results were seen in cats with fibrosarcomas. An unexpected observation was the development of metastatic fibrosarcoma in three of five cats that relapsed in the group treated with engineered cells. Complications seen in some dogs and cats included anaphylaxis associated with injection of Vero cells and local inflammatory reactions.[70]

Canarypox virus and attenuated vaccinia virus vectors have been used to deliver rfIL-2 and rhIL-2, respectively, to cats with soft tissue sarcomas.[71] The injections were well tolerated, and there was a significant reduction in tumor recurrence rate with either of the virus delivery systems compared with controls 12 months after treatment.

IL-2 therapy appears to have a place in the immunotherapy of feline and canine cancers, particularly when administered in a manner that concentrates expression within the tumor, thereby limiting systemic toxicity. Adenoviral delivery and incorporation into liposomes appear to be particularly promising modes of therapy. Canine and feline IL-2 cDNA have been cloned[59,72,73] and are commercially available (see Box 32-1).

Interleukin-12

IL-12 is a proinflammatory cytokine that has shown great promise as a therapeutic agent in experimental models of infectious disease and cancer. Multiple lines of evidence indicated that IL-12, a heterodimer produced in response to endotoxins, intracellular parasites, and CD40 ligation, is pivotal in initiating a cell-mediated immune response.[74-76] Direct contact with microbial products or activated T cells can prompt antigen-presenting cells (e.g., macrophages, DCs) to release IL-12. In turn, IL-12 induces the synthesis of IFN-γ by T and NK cells. This early IL-12 generation is critical to early host containment of many intracellular pathogens, including *Toxoplasma gondii*,[77] *Listeria monocytogenes*,[78] *Leishmania major*,[79] and *Mycobacterium tuberculosis*.[80] To date, most veterinary studies using IL-12 have been designed to characterize the adjuvant effect of IL-12 in boosting the cell-mediated immune response to FeLV, FIV, and FIPV vaccination. Two studies administering intradermal FIV DNA showed protection from FIV infection in three of four cats when IL-12 was included in the vaccination, whereas all four cats that received the DNA vaccine alone became infected.[81,82] Similar DNA vaccinations protocols against FeLV challenge showed increased protection only when IL-12 was co-administered with IL-18, another cytokine known to enhance cell-mediated immunity.[83] Vaccination of cats against FIPV in combination with co-delivery of feline IL-12 encoding plasmids did not enhance protection and may have actually potentiated the infection.[84] There is precedence for the inhibition of cell-mediated immunity when IL-12 is administered at high doses,[6,85] and this may have played a role in the outcome of this study. Lasarte and coworkers[6] demonstrated that the depression of cell-mediated immunity at high IL-12 doses was related to the generation of large amounts of nitric oxide.

IL-12 is one of the most widely studied cytokines in cancer immunotherapy and has been found to eradicate experimental tumors, elicit long-term antitumor immunity,[86-88] and possess antiangiogenic properties.[89,90] The role of IL-12 as chemotherapeutic agent has been limited because of its toxicities. In mice, daily administration of 0.1 to 10 μg of recombinant murine IL-12 for up to 2 weeks resulted in liver function abnormalities; gastrointestinal toxicity; and hematopoietic changes, including anemia, neutropenia, lymphopenia, and thrombocytopenia.[91-93] In humans the toxic effects include fever, anemia, neutropenia, lymphocytopenia, thrombocytopenia, liver function test abnormalities, rhinitis, stomatitis, and colitis.[94] In a phase II clinical trial in renal carcinoma using rhIL-12, two deaths were reported.[5] The authors have seen dose-dependent hematopoietic toxicities (anemia, neutropenia, and thrombocytopenia) in preclinical trials of systemic administration of a replication-defective adenovirus encoding murine IL-12 in cats.[94a]

One approach that can be used to avoid the systemic toxicity of IL-12 is to use local intratumoral IL-12 gene therapy. A replication-defective adenovirus containing feline IL-12 under the control of the heat-shock promoter has been developed and characterized in vitro.[95] An added advantage of employing the heat-shock promoter is that IL-12 expression can be temporally induced by providing external hyperthermia to the tumor. A phase I dose escalation trial with feline soft tissue sarcomas was recently completed. A maximum tolerable dose was reached, although all cats completed the treatment regimen. At the highest dose of adenovirus, fever, anemia, and thrombocytopenia were reported.[96] Further follow-up and expanded studies will be required to determine clinical efficacy of this cytokine treatment. Intramuscular injection of a plasmid DNA expression vector of canine IL-12 induced enhanced peripheral blood mononuclear cell production of IFN-γ in treated dogs.[97] Recombinant mIL-12 has been shown to significantly inhibit the growth of a canine hemangiosarcoma cell line transplanted into mice.[98] It is unclear whether the growth inhibition was mediated mainly through antiangiogenic mechanisms, NK cell activation, or a combination of both.

IL-12 is a potent immunostimulant that holds tremendous promise as a vaccine adjuvant or cancer immunotherapeutic. The very potency of this cytokine contributes to its limitations, and continued studies designed to diminish systemic toxicities will be necessary before it can be commonly employed. Both feline and canine IL-12 have been cloned and expressed,[99,100] and the recombinant proteins are currently commercially available (see Box 32-1).

Other Interleukins

IL-6 is a proinflammatory cytokine (along with IL-1 and TNF-α) with pleiotropic activity, including effects on B and T cells and induction of acute phase proteins. Elevated levels of IL-6 have been reported in Chinese Shar-Peis with recurrent febrile illnesses, and IL-6 dysregulation has been postulated to play an etiologic role in the syndrome.[101] Systemic inflammatory response syndrome (SIRS) and sepsis are associated with increased IL-6 production, and high plasma IL-6 levels are negatively correlated with outcome in canine SIRS patients.[102] Cranial cruciate ligament rupture in dogs results in increased levels of synovial fluid IL-6.[103] Dogs with juvenile polyarteritis syndrome were also found to have increased levels of serum IL-6 activity during acute illness but undetectable levels during convalescence. Treatment of acutely ill dogs with prednisone resulted in rapid clinical improvement accompanied by a decrease in IL-6 activity; withdrawal of prednisone resulted in reappearance of signs and high serum IL-6 activity. Clinically, the most important inhibitors of IL-6 expression are glucocorticoids.[104] Specific blockade of IL-6 or the IL-6 receptor (or both) is a potentially promising means of controlling clinical disease in chronic inflammatory conditions.[105] IL-6 also has marked effects on megakaryocyte and platelet physiology. In dogs 80 μg/kg per day of rhIL-6 increased platelet counts modestly and enhanced the sensitivity of platelets to activation in response to thrombin and platelet-activating factor.[106] Other investigators have shown that IL-6 promoted increases in plasma fibrinogen and von Willebrand factor (vWF) and a decrease in free protein S concentrations.[107] These effects on the clotting mechanism may result in an overall prohemostatic tendency, which may prove beneficial for the amelioration of bleeding associated with a variety of conditions. Additional investigation is required to determine if IL-6–mediated alterations of hemostasis may lead to pathologic thrombosis. The cDNAs for feline and canine IL-6 have been cloned, the recombinant proteins have been described,[108-110] and they are commercially available (see Box 32-1).

IL-11 is a pleiotropic cytokine that enhances the activity of primitive, erythroid, and megakaryocyte progenitor cells and the production of hepatic acute phase proteins, and it supports growth of the intestinal epithelium. In animal models rhIL-11 has been shown to be effective in reconstituting platelet levels after the administration of chemotherapy or radiation therapy and in protection against radiation- or drug-induced damage to the intestinal epithelium. IL-11 has also been shown to increase circulating levels of vWF and rhIL-11 increases vWF in dogs with von Willebrand disease (vWD) with kinetics that are more gradual and sustained than desmopressin.[111] Unlike the release of preformed vWF from platelets induced by desmopressin, administration of IL-11 results in the increased production of vWF RNA. Phase II trials of IL-11 in human patients with vWD have recently been completed.[112] Clinically, rhIL-11 has also been used to support platelet levels in human cancer patients and in the management of Crohn's disease and ulcerative colitis. A side effect that limits the administration of rhIL-11 is plasma volume expansion, resulting in edema, a fall in hematocrit levels, and cardiac arrhythmias. In dogs rhIL-11 increased platelet counts, platelet size, ploidy, and the number of megakaryocytes in marrow and peripheral blood. Pneumonitis may be a dose-limiting side effect in dogs.[113]

CHEMOKINES

Chemokine Biology

Chemokines are largely responsible for leukocyte chemotaxis, mediating inflammation and coordinating the host response to infection. The chemokines can be divided into two large and two small subfamilies on the basis of the pattern of cysteine residues found at the amino terminal end. The two large groups consist of the CXC subfamily, in which one amino acid is interspersed between the two cysteines, and the CC subfamily, in which the two cysteines are directly apposed. The two minor subfamilies consist of chemokines in which a single cysteine is found at the amino terminal end (XC) and ones in which the cysteines are separated by three amino acids (CX_3C). Chemokines bind to one or more seven transmembrane, G protein–coupled receptors that, again, fall into two major and two minor subfamilies. In an attempt to standardize the nomenclature, the chemokines are grouped as CCL, CXCL, XCL, and CX_3CL, and the receptors as CCR, CXCR, XCR, and CX_3CR, where *L* denotes ligand and *R* denotes receptor and numbers are added in the order in which they have been described.[114] In this chapter chemokines are referred to according to the standard nomenclature with their former names provided in brackets if they have been commonly used in the literature. Currently 46 chemokines and 19 chemokine receptors have been identified.[115] Canine and feline CXCR4 and CCR5 have been isolated and demonstrate significant sequence homology and tissue distribution with their murine and human counterparts.[116-118]

Chemokines play a central role in inflammatory and allergic diseases. In response to signals such as lipopolysaccharide (LPS) from gram-negative bacteria or some of the inflammatory cytokines described earlier, such as IL-1 or TNF-α, chemokines are released at the site of injury, setting up a chemotactic gradient. Fibroblasts, smooth muscle cells, and epithelial cells have all been shown to be significant sources of chemokines. Neutrophils will move toward high levels of the chemokines CXCL1-3, CXCL6,7 and CXCL8 (IL-8); eosinophils respond to CCL5 (RANTES), CCL11,24,26 (eotaxin-1,2,3), CCL13 (MCP-4), and CCL28; and monocytes, DCs, and lymphocytes are attracted to CCL6 (C10), CCL2 (MCP-1), CCL3 (MIP1-α), and CCL4 (MIP1-β). There is a high level of overlap and promiscuity in the types of cells recruited by a particular chemokine based, in part, on the ability of some chemokines to bind multiple receptors and some receptors to bind multiple chemokines.

In addition to directing leukocytes to the site of inflammation or injury, chemokines provide the necessary gradients for DC trafficking to lymph nodes. Immature DCs circulate and act as sentinels for pathogens. In the immature state, they express a chemokine receptor repertoire that is poised to respond to many of the inflammatory chemokines. After recruitment to the site of inflammation, DCs encounter antigen and associated inflammatory cytokines and undergo maturational changes, including the expression of the chemokine receptor CCR7. The ligands for CCR7 are CCL19 (MIP3β) and CCL21 (6Ckine), which are expressed within the T cell–rich areas of lymphoid follicles. The end result is that the antigen-loaded, mature DC is preferentially drawn to the draining lymph node, where it will encounter T lymphocytes, thereby activating a specific cell-mediated response to the pathogen.

To describe chemokines in terms of leukocyte recruitment only would be to ignore their other important physiologic roles. The normal development of lymphoid organs depends on signals derived from chemokines, as does structural development of the fetal neurologic system[119,120] and intestinal vascular networks.[121] Chemokines have been proposed to play a role in embryo implantation and menstruation.[122] Many tumors express chemokine receptors, and they have been shown to play a role in tumor growth and in directing organ-specific metastasis.[123,124] The discovery that HIV uses the chemokine receptors CCR5 and CXCR4 as co-receptors for viral entry into target cells has helped highlight the way in which some pathogens exploit chemokine pathways.[125,126]

Therapeutic Manipulation of Chemokines

Inflammatory Diseases

Elevated chemokine levels have been demonstrated in a variety of inflammatory and autoimmune diseases in humans, including asthma, inflammatory bowel disease, rheumatoid arthritis, and sepsis. Because much of the pathology associated with these diseases is due to the cascade of effects caused by the ongoing chemotactic stimulus, chemokine antagonists have emerged as potential therapeutics.[127] The CC chemokine receptor CCR1 and its ligands CCL3 (MIP1-α) and CCL5 (RANTES) have been shown to be important in the pathology of models of rheumatoid arthritis, respiratory syncytial virus infection and sepsis. Serum levels of both CCL3 and CCL5 are elevated in septic humans,[128] and mice lacking CCR1, the receptor for these chemokines, were significantly more likely to survive experimental sepsis.[129] Limiting viral replication is clearly important in virally mediated pneumonia, but blocking chemokine-mediated recruitment of inflammatory cells has also shown dramatic benefits in experimental systems. In a murine model of respiratory syncytial virus infection, either blocking CCR1 signaling or deleting CCR1 expression in conjunction with antiviral treatment dramatically enhances survival compared with antiviral treatment alone.[130] Antagonists of CCR1 have been developed, and despite the species specificity of some antagonists,[131] cross-species efficacy has been demonstrated for other compounds. Liang and coworkers[132] have developed a selective peptide antagonist of CCR1 that has efficacy in both human and rat systems, although the binding affinity of the peptide is significantly lower in rats. Additionally, this peptide was shown to have good oral bioavailability in dogs. Relatively minor modifications of antagonist structure have been shown to improve activity across divergent species.[133]

CXCL8 (IL-8)–induced neutrophil influx into tissues by way of CXCR1 and CXCR2 is clearly beneficial in controlling the early stages of bacterial infection. There are other instances in which CXCL8 expression potentiates the pathology of diseases such as sepsis/peritonitis, acute respiratory distress syndrome, exacerbations of human chronic obstructive pulmonary disease and bovine pneumonic pasteurellosis.[134-137] CXCL8 is expressed in increased levels in several bacterial diseases of ruminants and in equine chronic obstructive pulmonary disease.[4] Li and coworkers[138] generated a potent CXCL8 antagonist that blocks signaling through both CXCR1 and CXCR2 in bovine neutrophils. They have shown efficacy in vitro against the neutrophil chemotactic activities of fluids from bovine pasteurella pneumonia and endotoxin- induced mastitis and in vivo against intradermal neutrophil influx in response to endotoxin.[139] Because this antagonist also effectively blocks human CXCL8 activities on human neutrophils, it may have uses in feline and canine inflammatory diseases.

Neoplasia

Introducing chemokines into tumors could be advantageous in recruiting immune effector cells to help destroy the tumor, and this has been shown to be true in murine cancer models. CCL16, CCL20, MIP3α, CCL21 (6Ckine) expression within murine tumors all resulted in increased infiltration of DCs, increased tumor immunogenicity, and decreased tumor growth.[140-143] Bringing DCs and T lymphocytes into the tumor is not always sufficient, and providing a simultaneous activation stimulus helps overcome the otherwise immunosuppressive tumor microenvironment. This has been accomplished by delivering the chemokines in adenoviral vectors where the virus itself provides an immune stimulus[140] or by simultaneously blocking immunosuppressive cytokines or providing innate immune system stimuli.[143,141] Because there is significant cross-species sequence homology in many of the chemokines[144] and precedence for cross-species efficacy between mice and humans with chemokines such as CCL20,[140] some of the currently available murine and human chemokines may prove useful in veterinary cancer applications.

The converse to the potentially beneficial aspects of tumor chemokine expression is the documented role that chemokines and tumor chemokine receptor expression play in the natural course of tumor progression. Chemokines can act as tumor growth factors either directly or through the recruitment of leukocytes. Some tumor cells both express the chemokine receptor and produce its ligand, allowing autocrine enhancement of proliferation and survival. Melanoma cells expressing CXCR2 and producing CXCL1 and CXCL8 (IL8) are one such example.[143] Macrophages recruited to tumors can elaborate tumor cell growth factors and increase angiogenesis within the tumor.[144] Chemokine receptor expression by tumor cells has also been shown to play a substantial role in metastasis. Tumor cells expressing chemokine receptors will move toward chemokine gradients, resulting in metastasis to draining lymph nodes or distant sites. CCR7 expression by melanoma cells is correlated with metastasis to draining lymph nodes.[145,146] It appears that the tumor cells are taking advantage of the normal chemokine gradient for activated, CCR7-expressing DC homing to draining lymph nodes. CXCR4 is expressed by a wide variety of tumors, including mesenchymal, epithelial, and hematopoietically derived cancers.[147] Malignant mammary tumors have been shown to express high levels of CXCR4, and its ligand, CXCL12 (SDF1), is preferentially expressed in common target tissues for mammary tumor metastasis such as lung, liver, bone marrow, and lymph nodes.[148] Oonuma and coworkers[149] have demonstrated increased expression of feline CXCR4 in metastatic mammary tumors of cats and high levels of CXCL12 production in feline lymph node, lung, and liver. Additionally, they demonstrated increased in vitro tumor cell migration toward CXCL12 gradients and inhibition of this migration when CXCR4 peptide antagonists were added. The same CXCR4 antagonist has shown efficacy in inhibiting the number of lung metastases in a mouse model of mammary carcinoma.[132] Some cases of canine osteosarcoma have been shown to express CXCR4 and migrate toward CXCL12 in vitro.[150] Selective chemokine receptor antagonists hold promise as potential in vivo therapeutics to minimize cancer metastasis, and feline mammary tumors appear to be an appropriate system to apply these compounds. The documented role of chemokine receptor expression in human squamous cell carcinoma,[151] melanoma,[152,153] and prostate carcinoma[154] awaits exploration in dogs and cats.

Retroviral Infections

The discovery that HIV uses the chemokine receptors CXCR4 and CCR5 as co-receptors for viral entry[125,126,155] has prompted the search for and development of drugs to inhibit virus binding. Subsequent work has shown that FIV uses CXCR4, but apparently not CCR5, as a co-receptor as well.[156] Bicyclams are potent CXCR4 antagonists, and one such compound, AMD3100, has been shown to inhibit in vitro replication of FIV.[157,158] Antagonists of feline CXCR4 have been developed and tested successfully in vitro.[159] The number of CXCR4 antagonists is continually expanding,[160] and FIV-infected cats may well benefit from these compounds in the future.

Rapid advances in the understanding of chemokine biology have allowed the exploration of ways to manipulate these factors in a wide variety of diseases. Whether they are used to recruit immune effector cells to tumors or their actions are blocked in an attempt to minimize inflammation or viral infection, manipulation of chemokines has the potential to be a powerful therapeutic tool.

HEMATOPOIETIC GROWTH FACTORS

In humans the hematopoietic system produces in the order of 10^{11} cells daily and is able to rapidly increase production even further when stimulated by hematopoietic growth factors. Hematopoietic growth factors include erythropoietin (EPO), granulocyte colony-stimulating factor (G-CSF), granulocyte/macrophage colony-stimulating factor (GM-CSF), monocyte colony-stimulating factor (M-CSF), thrombopoietin, stem cell factor (SCF), and most of the ILs. Hematopoietic growth factors act synergistically at various levels in the hematopoietic developmental system, and their actions are rarely restricted to a given lineage. The cDNAs for all of the known human factors, and some of the canine and feline factors, have been cloned. Recombinant hG-CSF (filgrastim), rhGM-CSF (sargramostim), and rhEPO (epoetin) are commercially available. For humans this has led to significant advances in the management of a variety of hematologic and neoplastic disorders. Canine and feline G-CSF, GM-CSF, and SCF have all been cloned and expressed,[161-165] and canine and feline GM-CSF and SCF are commercially available (see Box 32-1).

Recombinant Erythropoietin

In dogs EPO is secreted by cells adjacent to the proximal convoluted tubules in response to renal hypoxia. EPO stimulates the proliferation and maturation of erythroid progenitor cells, primarily colony-forming unit erythroid cells. Megakaryocytes are also stimulated by EPO. Recombinant human EPO was the first commercially available hematopoietic growth factor released for clinical use in humans and is indicated for the treatment of anemia secondary to chronic renal failure, anemia secondary to the treatment of HIV with AZT, and anemia secondary to cancer chemotherapy. The use of recombinant human, feline, and canine EPO in small animals is addressed elsewhere in this text (see Chapters 15 and 18).

Growth Factors Affecting Myeloid Lineages

Granulocyte Colony-Stimulating Factor

G-CSF is produced by fibroblasts and endothelial cells stimulated by IL-1 or TNF and by macrophages stimulated by bacterial endotoxins. Its major effects are on neutrophils and neutrophil progenitors. Recombinant hG-CSF is commercially available and for humans is indicated to decrease the incidence of infection in patients with nonmyeloid malignancies receiving myelosuppressive chemotherapy with or without bone marrow transplantation, congenital neutropenia, and cyclic neutropenia.

In normal dogs rhG-CSF induces rapid and marked neutrophilia but, similar to the situation with rhEPO, also induces antibodies that react with both rhG-CSF and endogenous canine G-CSF, leading to chronic but reversible neutropenia.[166,167] Whether dogs with cancer receiving immunosuppressive chemotherapy are able to mount an immune response to rhG-CSF has not yet been determined. In dogs treated with total body irradiation, rhG-CSF therapy was associated with earlier recovery of neutrophils and platelets and reduced the lethality of the hematopoietic insult compared with untreated irradiated controls.[16] In gray Collies with cyclic hematopoiesis, rhG-CSF eliminated neutropenic episodes but did not correct abnormalities in platelet aggregation or serotonin content or decreased neutrophil myeloperoxidase activity.[167,169] Recombinant hG-CSF has also been used to treat drug-induced pancytopenia in a dog.[170]

Canine G-CSF has been cloned but is not commercially available. In normal dogs rcG-CSF was shown to induce rapid and marked increases in neutrophils, moderate increases in lymphocyte and monocyte counts, and bone marrow hyperplasia. For example, five normal dogs were given 5 μg/kg rcG-CSF per day subcutaneously for 4 weeks. The mean neutrophil counts increased from 6537/μL to 26,330/μL within 24 hours after the first injection to a maximum of 72,125/μL by day 19. Blood counts returned to normal within 5 days after discontinuation of rcG-CSF, and clinically significant toxicoses were not associated with rcG-CSF administration. The induction of neutrophilia was induced again on repeated administration.[171-173] Recombinant cG-CSF prevented neutropenia and associated clinical signs in cyclic hematopoietic dogs but did not completely eliminate the cycling of neutrophils in cyclic hematopoietic dogs. Also, the time to bone marrow reconstitution was not decreased in dogs treated with rcG-CSF after autologous bone marrow transplantation, emphasizing that rcG-CSF action depends on the presence of progenitor cells in the bone marrow.[174]

To evaluate the utility of rcG-CSF in the management of chemotherapy-induced neutropenia, myelosuppression was induced with mitoxantrone in normal dogs and then treated with daily rcG-CSF for 20 days. None of the dogs receiving rcG-CSF developed serious neutropenia, whereas four of five untreated dogs did. These findings demonstrate that rcG-CSF is capable of reducing the duration and severity of mitoxantrone-induced myelosuppression.[175] The optimal cost-effective timing and duration of treatment for the management of therapy-induced myelosuppression has not been determined for canine or human origin cytokines, and it may only be necessary to treat when neutrophil counts fall below 1000 cells/µL, and only a few days of therapy may be necessary.[176] In addition to cancer treatment–induced neutropenia, rcG-CSF has been used to accelerate the rate of recovery from neutropenia in dogs with parvovirus. It has not been useful in dogs without neutrophil progenitors, such as those with aplastic anemia secondary to ehrlichia infections or estrogen toxicity.[177] Historical and bone marrow evaluations are important in determining which animals are likely to respond to therapy with any hematopoietic growth factor.

Recombinant G-CSFs of both human and canine origin have been studied in normal cats. In one study, 5 µg/kg rcG-CSF per day was administered to healthy cats for 42 days. Mean neutrophil counts increased from 10,966 cells/µL to 30,688 cells/µL within 24 hours after the first dose. Neutrophil counts increased and remained elevated until cytokine administration was discontinued at 42 days. No adverse effects were reported.[178] Normal cats given rhG-CSF developed neutropenia before the end of 3 weeks of therapy, presumably because antibodies developed against the growth factor.[179] Neutropenia has not been observed in cats given rcG-CSF, likely because of greater homology between the cat and dog cytokines.[178] It is not known if cats with immunosuppressive disorders or cats receiving antineoplastic chemotherapy are able to form antibodies that react with human-derived cytokines. Cats with Chédiak–Higashi syndrome treated with rcG-CSF had increased neutrophil counts and improvement in neutrophil function.[180] Recombinant G-CSF (of any species origin) may also be useful in the management of feline panleukopenia, neutropenia associated with FeLV and FIV infections, and sepsis.

Granulocyte/Macrophage Colony-Stimulating Factor

GM-CSF is produced by the bone marrow stroma and T and B cells and is a regulator of the intermediate stages of hematopoiesis. It supports the expansion and growth of both granulocytic and macrophage lineages and also enhance the function of mature macrophages and neutrophils.[181] In humans rhGM-CSF is indicated for the acceleration of hematopoietic reconstitution after autologous bone marrow transplantation in lymphoproliferative disorders. Recombinant hGM-CSF induces leukocytosis (primarily neutrophils but also eosinophils and monocytes) in normal dogs. In dogs undergoing total body irradiation and supported with rhGM-CSF, there was decreased severity and shortened duration of neutropenia, indicating that rhGM-CSF can be effective monotherapy for radiation-induced bone marrow failure in dogs. Anti–rhGM-CSF antibodies developed in 1 to 2 weeks and persisted for at least 150 days. Another potential concern with rhGM-CSF is that platelet counts dropped to nadirs of 20% to 30% normal levels.[182,183]

Canine GM-CSF has been cloned and its activity investigated in normal dogs, where it induced significant increases in neutrophil and monocyte levels. As with the human recombinant product, mean platelet counts decreased significantly. Further investigation into the mechanism of thrombocytopenia suggested that GM-CSF activates hepatic macrophages, with resultant increases in phagocytosis of platelets.[184,185] After otherwise lethal total body irradiation, rcGM-CSF was not effective in promoting hematopoietic recovery or improving survival.[186] In studies of partial body irradiation in dogs, 7 days of treatment with rhG-CSF resulted in a more efficient and rapid reconstitution of neutrophil numbers than similar treatment with rhGM-CSF.[187] It is thought that G-CSF results in an increase in the production of migratory hematopoietic progenitors from the protected marrow sites and an enhanced seeding of these progenitors into the regions of damaged marrow. These results suggest that, in situations of severely limited stem cell response, G-CSF may be more effective than GM-CSF in eliciting a rapid neutrophil recovery.

In an effort to avoid daily systemic administration of recombinant GM-CSF, direct intramarrow injection of adenoviral vector–cGM-CSF constructs (AdcGM-CSF) in normal dogs has been carried out.[188] Replication-deficient adenoviral vectors efficiently transduce marrow stromal cells and induce high levels of cytokine production. In vivo, high levels of protein production are found in bone marrow aspirates 72 hours after direct intramarrow administration of AdcGM-CSF. Localized myeloid expansion of marrow and significant peripheral leukocytosis have been identified in all treated dogs, and peripheral blood changes last for up to 3 weeks after a single intramarrow injection. It appears that adenoviral-mediated cytokine expression from the marrow of a single large bone (ileum) leads to compartmentalized expression of GM-CSF and an increase in hematopoiesis. Recent studies have demonstrated that intravenous administration of canine GM-CSF ligated to silica nanoparticles results in detectable GM-CSF for up to 10 days and prevented or restored vinblastine-induced neutropenia in dogs.[189,190] None of the dogs had detectable anti–GM-CSF antibodies 28 days after injection.

GM-CSF has been used to expand DC precursors from peripheral blood and bone marrow for potential therapeutic purposes. Ex vivo expanded DCs have been stimulated with antigen and reintroduced in experimental models of infectious and neoplastic diseases.[191,192] Both human and feline GM-CSF have been used to culture myeloid DCs from feline peripheral blood and bone marrow,[193,162,194] and canine GM-CSF has been used with canine peripheral blood and bone marrow.[195,196] In vitro culture, antigen stimulation, and reintroduction of bone marrow–derived DCs from three dogs with melanoma have been performed.[197] These cells were cultured with a combination of rhGM-CSF, SCF, and FLT3 ligand, matured with rhTNF-α and administered in conjunction with radiation therapy. One dog developed antigen-specific cytotoxic T cell activity and remained tumor free 48 months after therapy. It is likely that more studies employing DC vaccination will be carried out in canine and feline patients in the near future.

GM-CSF is a mediator of antibody-dependent cellular cytotoxicity and increases MHC expression, giving GM-CSF potential utility as a modulator of antitumor immunity. A vaccine consisting of irradiated hGM-CSF transfected canine melanoma cell line has been reported to produce GM-CSF at the site of intradermal injection for extended periods in normal dogs.[198] A phase I clinical trail using autologous tumor cells in dogs with melanoma and soft tissue sarcomas showed significant tumor infiltration of neutrophils and macrophages in treated tumors.[199]

Stem Cell Factor

SCF (c-kit ligand, mast cell growth factor) is produced primarily by bone marrow stroma, with effects on a wide range of precursor cells at different stages of differentiation, including primitive hematopoietic stem cells. It has little activity as a single agent; however, it is a potent co-stimulatory molecule when administered in combination with other hematopoietic growth factors. Canine SCF cDNA has been cloned and studied in long-term bone marrow cultures. Alone, rcSCF was nonstimulatory for committed marrow precursors. Synergistic stimulation of granulocyte/macrophage colony-forming units was demonstrated between rcSCF, rhGM-CSF, and rhIL-6.[200] In vivo, rcSCF induced neutrophilia in normal dogs and supported hematopoietic recovery in normal dogs undergoing total body irradiation without marrow transplant; however, results were similar to those obtained with rcG-CSF.[201] Recombinant canine SCF also prevented neutropenic periods in gray Collies with cyclic hematopoiesis.[202]

Hematopoietic growth factors have proved quite useful in small animal veterinary medicine for managing cytopenias and anemias. The recent cloning and expression of canine- and feline-specific reagents will help alleviate the problem of antibody generation with repeated use. Additional uses of factors such as GM-CSF in cancer chemotherapy and in the in vitro generation of DCs will expand the clinical utility of this class of growth factors.

SUMMARY

The concept of enhancing the normal immune response against infections and tumors has been considered for decades. The administration of various natural and synthetic products to simulate systemic infections has largely given way to the idea that specific cytokines can be used effectively when administered locally or systemically. IFNs, ILs, chemokines, and hematopoietic growth factors may offer substantial clinical benefit in chronic viral infections and in cancers. EPO has been shown to have great utility in the management of chronic renal failure. The recent increase in the commercial availability of canine and feline reagents allows for increased exploration of their efficacy in diseases of dogs and cats. These products may have significant clinical impact on several highly fatal disorders of dogs and cats. When administered systemically, cytokines perturb complex regulatory pathways, and serious side effects may occur. Innovative delivery methods, such as liposomes, adenoviral delivery, and even oral administration, may increase the therapeutic index of these molecules. Biological response modification, cytokine biology, and associated delivery systems are rapidly changing fields, and the small animal veterinarian will need to watch for significant advances in these areas over the next several years.

REFERENCES

1. Oppenheim J, Feldman M: Introduction to the role of cytokines in innate host defense and adaptive immunity. In Oppenheim J, Feldman M, editors: *Cytokine reference volume 1: ligands*, London, 2001, Academic Press, p 3.
2. Nicola N: Hematopoietic growth factors. In Oppenheim J, Feldman M, editors: *Cytokine reference volume 1: ligands*, London, 2001, Academic Press, p 849.
3. Oppenheim J, Howard O, Goetzl E: Chemotactic factors, neuropeptides and other ligands for seven transmembrane recptors. In Oppenheim J, Feldman M, editors: *Cytokine reference volume 1: ligands*, London, 2001, Academic Press, p 985.
4. Gangur V, Birmingham NP, Thanesvorakul S: Chemokines in health and disease, *Vet Immunol Immunopathol* 86:127–136, 2002.
5. Cohen J: IL-12 deaths: explanation and a puzzle, *Science* 270:908, 1995.
6. Lasarte JJ, Corrales FJ, Casares N, et al: Different doses of adenoviral vector expressing IL-12 enhance or depress the immune response to a coadministered antigen: the role of nitric oxide, *J Immunol* 162:5270–5277, 1999.
7. Nakamura N, Sudo T, Matsuda S, et al: Molecular cloning of feline interferon cDNA by direct expression, *Biosci Biotechnol Biochem* 56:211–214, 1992.
8. Sakurai T, Ueda Y, Sato M, et al: Feline interferon production in silkworm by recombinant baculovirus, *J Vet Med Sci* 54:563–565, 1992.
9. Ueda Y, Sakurai T, Yanai A: Homogeneous production of feline interferon in silkworm by replacing single amino acid code in signal peptide region in recombinant baculovirus and characterization of the product, *J Vet Med Sci* 55:251–258, 1993.
10. Ueda Y, Sakurai T, Kasama K, et al: Pharmacokinetic properties of recombinant feline interferon and its stimulatory effect on 2',5'-oligoadenylate synthetase activity in the cat, *J Vet Med Sci* 55:1–6, 1993.
11. Wonderling R, Powell T, Baldwin S, et al: Cloning, expression, purification, and biological activity of five feline type I interferons, *Vet Immunol Immunopathol* 89:13–27, 2002.
12. Nagai A, Taira O, Ishikawa M, et al: Cloning of cDNAs encoding multiple subtypes of feline interferon-alpha from the feline epitherial cell line, *J Vet Med Sci* 66:725–728, 2004.
13. Devos K, Duerinck F, Van Audenhove K, et al: Cloning and expression of the canine interferon-gamma gene, *J Interferon Res* 12:95–102, 1992.
14. Fuller L, Fernandez J, Zheng S, et al: Immunochemical and biochemical characterization of purified canine interferon-gamma. Production of a monoclonal antibody, affinity purification, and its effect on mixed lymphocyte culture and mixed lymphocyte kidney culture reactions, *Transplantation* 53:195–202, 1992.
15. Zucker K, Lu P, Asthana D, et al: Production and characterization of recombinant canine interferon-gamma from Escherichia coli, *J Interferon Res* 13:91–97, 1993.
16. Argyle DJ, Smith K, McBride K, et al: Nucleotide and predicted peptide sequence of feline interferon-gamma (IFN-gamma), *DNA Seq* 5:169–171, 1995.
17. Schijns VE, Wierda CM, Vahlenkamp TW, et al: Molecular cloning and expression of cat interferon-gamma, *Immunogenetics* 42:440–441, 1995.
18. Tizard IR: Resistance to viruses. In Tizard IR, editor: *Veterinary immunology: an introduction*, ed 6, Philadelphia, 2000, Saunders, p 267.

19. Zeuzem S, Heathcote JE, Martin N, et al: Peginterferon alfa-2a (40 kDa) monotherapy: a novel agent for chronic hepatitis C therapy, *Expert Opin Investig Drugs* 10:2201–2213, 2001.
20. Kirkwood J: Cancer immunotherapy: the interferon-alpha experience, *Semin Oncol* 29:18–26, 2002.
21. Weiss RC, Oostrom-Ram T: Effect of recombinant human interferon-alpha in vitro and in vivo on mitogen-induced lymphocyte blastogenesis in cats, *Vet Immunol Immunopathol* 24:147–157, 1990.
22. Baldwin SL, Powell TD, Sellins KS, et al: The biological effects of five feline IFN-alpha subtypes, *Vet Immunol Immunopathol* 99:153–167, 2004.
23. Sandmeyer LS, Keller CB, Bienzle D: Culture of feline corneal epithelial cells and infection with feline herpesvirus-1 as an investigative tool, *Am J Vet Res* 66:205–209, 2005.
24. Mochizuki M, Nakatani H, Yoshida M: Inhibitory effects of recombinant feline interferon on the replication of feline enteropathogenic viruses in vitro, *Vet Microbiol* 39:145–152, 1994.
25. de Mari K, Maynard L, Eun HM, et al: Treatment of canine parvoviral enteritis with interferon-omega in a placebo-controlled field trial, *Vet Rec* 152:105–108, 2003.
26. Weiss RC, Cox NR, Oostrom-Ram T: Effect of interferon or Propionibacterium acnes on the course of experimentally induced feline infectious peritonitis in specific-pathogen-free and random-source cats, *Am J Vet Res* 51:726–733, 1990.
27. Ishida T, Shibanai A, Tanaka S, et al: Use of recombinant feline interferon and glucocorticoid in the treatment of feline infectious peritonitis, *J Feline Med Surg* 6(2):107–109, 2004.
28. Ritz S, Egberink H, Hartmann K: Effect of feline interferon-omega on the survival time and quality of life of cats with feline infectious peritonitis, *J Vet Intern Med* 21(6):1193–1197, 2007.
29. Hartmann K: Feline infectious peritonitis, *Vet Clin North Am Small Anim Pract* 35:39–79, 2005.
30. Collado VM, Gómez-Lucía E, Tejerizo G, et al: Effect of type I interferons on the expression of feline leukaemia virus, *Vet Microbiol* 123(1-3):180–186, 2007.
31. Zeidner NS, Myles MH, Mathiason-DuBard CK, et al: Alpha interferon (2b) in combination with zidovudine for the treatment of presymptomatic feline leukemia virus-induced immunodeficiency syndrome, *Antimicrob Agents Chemother* 34:1749–1756, 1990.
32. Zeidner NS, Mathiason-DuBard CK, Hoover EA: Reversal of feline leukemia virus infection by adoptive transfer of lectin/interleukin-2-activated lymphocytes, interferon-alpha, and zidovudine, *J Immunother* 14:22–32, 1993.
33. Tanabe T, Yamamoto JK: Feline immunodeficiency virus lacks sensitivity to the antiviral activity of feline IFN-gamma, *J Interferon Cytokine Res* 21:1039–1046, 2001.
34. Pontzer CH, Yamamoto JK, Bazer FW, et al: Potent anti-feline immunodeficiency virus and anti-human immunodeficiency virus effect of IFN-tau, *J Immunol* 158:4351–4357, 1997.
35. de Mari K, Maynard L, Sanquer A, et al: Therapeutic effects of recombinant feline interferon-omega on feline leukemia virus (FeLV)-infected and FeLV/feline immunodeficiency virus (FIV)-coinfected symptomatic cats, *J Vet Intern Med* 18:477–482, 2004.
36. Pedretti E, Passeri B, Amadori M, et al: Low-dose interferon-alpha treatment for feline immunodeficiency virus infection, *Vet Immunol Immunopathol* 109(3-4):245–254, 2006.
37. Martin V, Najbar W, Gueguen S, et al: Treatment of canine parvoviral enteritis with interferon-omega in a placebo-controlled challenge trial, *Vet Microbiol* 89:115–127, 2002.
38. Cummins JM, Tompkins MB, Olsen RG, et al: Oral use of human alpha interferon in cats, *J Biol Response Mod* 7:513–523, 1988.
39. Tompkins M, Cummins J: Response of FeLV-induced non-regenerative anemia to oral administration of a bovine interferon-containing preparation, *Feline Pract* 12:6, 1982.
40. Steed V: Improved survival of four cats infected with feline leukemia virus after oral administration of interferon, *Feline Pract* 17:24, 1987.
41. Weiss RC, Cummins JM, Richards AB: Low-dose orally administered alpha interferon treatment for feline leukemia virus infection, *J Am Vet Med Assoc* 199:1477–1481, 1991.
42. Kociba G, Garg R, Khan K: Effects of orally administered interferon-alpha on the pathogenesis of feline leukemia virus-induced erythroid aplasia, *Comp Hematol Int* 5:79, 1995.
43. McCaw DL, Boon GD, Jergens AE, et al: Immunomodulation therapy for feline leukemia virus infection, *J Am Anim Hosp Assoc* 37:356–363, 2001.
44. Katabira ET, Sewankambo NK, Mugerwa RD, et al: Lack of efficacy of low dose oral interferon alfa in symptomatic HIV-1 infection: a randomised, double blind, placebo controlled trial, *Sex Transm Infect* 74:265–270, 1998.
45. Alston B, Ellenberg JH, Standiford HC, et al: A multicenter, randomized, controlled trial of three preparations of low-dose oral alpha-interferon in HIV-infected patients with CD4+ counts between 50 and 350 cells/mm(3). Division of AIDS Treatment Research Initiative (DATRI) 022 Study Group, *J Acquir Immune Defic Syndr* 22:348–357, 1999.
46. Whitley EM, Bird AC, Zucker KE, et al: Modulation by canine interferon-gamma of major histocompatibility complex and tumor-associated antigen expression in canine mammary tumor and melanoma cell lines, *Anticancer Res* 15:923–929, 1995.
47. Soergel SA, MacEwen EG, Vail DM, et al: The immunotherapeutic potential of activated canine alveolar macrophages and antitumor monoclonal antibodies in metastatic canine melanoma, *J Immunother* 22:443–453, 1999.
48. Kurzman ID, Shi F, Vail DM, et al: In vitro and in vivo enhancement of canine pulmonary alveolar macrophage cytotoxic activity against canine osteosarcoma cells, *Cancer Biother Radiopharm* 14:121–128, 1999.
49. Kessler M, Hammer A, Nailey M: Effects of human interferons and (60) cobalt radiation on canine and feline tumor cells-preclinical studies, *J Vet Med Series A* 43:599, 1996.
50. Tateyama S, Priosoeryanto BP, Yamaguchi R, et al: In vitro growth inhibition activities of recombinant feline interferon on all lines derived from canine tumours, *Res Vet Sci* 59:275–277, 1995.
51. Hampel V, Schwarz B, Kempf C, et al: Adjuvant immunotherapy of feline fibrosarcoma with recombinant feline interferon-omega, *J Vet Intern Med* 21(6):1340–1346, 2007.
52. Thomsen MK, Thomsen HK: Effects of interleukin-1 alpha on migration of canine neutrophils in vitro and in vivo, *Vet Immunol Immunopathol* 26:385–393, 1990.
53. Gray JE, Peterman V, Newton R, et al: ELISA determination and preliminary pharmacokinetics of modified human rIL-1 beta in dogs, *Res Commun Chem Pathol Pharmacol* 81:233–241, 1993.
54. Campbell SE, Nasir L, Argyle DJ, et al: Cloning of canine IL-1ra, TNFR and TIMP-2, *Vet Immunol Immunopathol* 78:207–214, 2001.
55. Nakagawa K, Miller FN, Sims DE, et al: Mechanisms of interleukin-2-induced hepatic toxicity, *Cancer Res* 56:507–510, 1996.
56. MacFarlane MP, Yang JC, Guleria AS, et al: The hematologic toxicity of interleukin-2 in patients with metastatic melanoma and renal cell carcinoma, *Cancer* 75:1030–1037, 1995.
57. Carey PD, Wakefield CH, Guillou PJ: Neutrophil activation, vascular leak toxicity, and cytolysis during interleukin-2 infusion in human cancer, *Surgery* 122:918–926, 1997.
58. Gonsalves SF, Landgraf BE, Ciardelli TL, et al: Early toxicity of recombinant interleukin-2 in cats, *Arch Int Pharmacodyn Ther* 310:175–185, 1991.
59. Cozzi PJ, Padrid PA, Takeda J, et al: Sequence and functional characterization of feline interleukin 2, *Biochem Biophys Res Commun* 194:1038–1043, 1993.

60. Cozzi PJ, Padrid P, Tompkins MB, et al: Bioactivity of recombinant feline interleukin-2 on human and feline leukocytes, *Vet Immunol Immunopathol* 48:27–33, 1995.
61. Helfand SC, Modiano JF, Nowell PC: Immunophysiological studies of interleukin-2 and canine lymphocytes, *Vet Immunol Immunopathol* 33:1–16, 1992.
62. Helfand SC, Soergel SA, Modiano JF, et al: Induction of lymphokine-activated killer (LAK) activity in canine lymphocytes with low dose human recombinant interleukin-2 in vitro, *Cancer Biother* 9:237–244, 1994.
63. Mitchell DH, Withrow SJ, Johnston MR, et al: Cytotoxicity against autologous, allogeneic, and xenogeneic tumor targets by human recombinant interleukin-2-activated lymphocytes from healthy dogs and dogs with lung tumors, *Am J Vet Res* 52:1132–1136, 1991.
64. Raskin RE, Holcomb CS, Maxwell AK: Effects of human recombinant interleukin 2 on in vitro tumor cytotoxicity in dogs, *Am J Vet Res* 52:2029–2032, 1991.
65. Helfand SC, Soergel SA, MacWilliams PS, et al: Clinical and immunological effects of human recombinant interleukin-2 given by repetitive weekly infusion to normal dogs, *Cancer Immunol Immunother* 39:84–92, 1994.
66. Moore AS, Theilen GH, Newell AD, et al: Preclinical study of sequential tumor necrosis factor and interleukin 2 in the treatment of spontaneous canine neoplasms, *Cancer Res* 51:233–238, 1991.
67. Khanna C, Hasz DE, Klausner JS, et al: Aerosol delivery of interleukin 2 liposomes is nontoxic and biologically effective: canine studies, *Clin Cancer Res* 2:721–734, 1996.
68. Khanna C, Anderson PM, Hasz DE, et al: Interleukin-2 liposome inhalation therapy is safe and effective for dogs with spontaneous pulmonary metastases, *Cancer* 79:1409–1421, 1997.
69. Dow S, Elmslie R, Kurzman I, et al: Phase I study of liposome-DNA complexes encoding the interleukin-2 gene in dogs with osteosarcoma lung metastases, *Hum Gene Ther* 16(8):937–946, 2005.
70. Quintin-Colonna F, Devauchelle P, Fradelizi D, et al: Gene therapy of spontaneous canine melanoma and feline fibrosarcoma by intratumoral administration of histoincompatible cells expressing human interleukin-2, *Gene Ther* 3:1104–1112, 1996.
71. Jourdier TM, Moste C, Bonnet MC, et al: Local immunotherapy of spontaneous feline fibrosarcomas using recombinant poxviruses expressing interleukin 2 (IL2), *Gene Ther* 10:2126–2132, 2003.
72. Dunham SP, Argyle DJ, Onions DE: The isolation and sequence of canine interleukin-2, *DNA Seq* 5:177–180, 1995.
73. Knapp DW, Williams JS, Andrisani OM: Cloning of the canine interleukin-2-encoding cDNA, *Gene* 159:281–282, 1995.
74. Trinchieri G: Interleukin-12: a cytokine produced by antigen-presenting cells with immunoregulatory functions in the generation of T-helper cells type 1 and cytotoxic lymphocytes, *Blood* 84:4008–4027, 1994.
75. Macatonia SE, Hosken NA, Litton M, et al: Dendritic cells produce IL-12 and direct the development of T_h1 cells from naive CD4+ T cells, *J Immunol* 154:5071–5079, 1995.
76. Cella M, Scheidegger D, Palmer-Lehmann K, et al: Ligation of CD40 on dendritic cells triggers production of high levels of interleukin-12 and enhances T cell stimulatory capacity: T-T help via APC activation, *J Exp Med* 184:747–752, 1996.
77. Gazzinelli RT, Wysocka M, Hayashi S, et al: Parasite-induced IL-12 stimulates early IFN-gamma synthesis and resistance during acute infection with Toxoplasma gondii, *J Immunol* 153:2533–2543, 1994.
78. Hsieh CS, Macatonia SE, Tripp CS, et al: Development of TH1 CD4+ T cells through IL-12 produced by Listeria-induced macrophages.[see comment], *Science* 260:547–549, 1993.
79. Heinzel FP, Rerko RM, Ahmed F, et al: Endogenous IL-12 is required for control of T_h2 cytokine responses capable of exacerbating leishmaniasis in normally resistant mice, *J Immunol* 155:730–739, 1995.
80. Cooper AM, Roberts AD, Rhoades ER, et al: The role of interleukin-12 in acquired immunity to Mycobacterium tuberculosis infection, *Immunology* 84:423–432, 1995.
81. Boretti FS, Leutenegger CM, Mislin C, et al: Protection against FIV challenge infection by genetic vaccination using minimalistic DNA constructs for FIV env gene and feline IL-12 expression.[see comment], *AIDS* 14:1749–1757, 2000.
82. Leutenegger CM, Boretti FS, Mislin CN, et al: Immunization of cats against feline immunodeficiency virus (FIV) infection by using minimalistic immunogenic defined gene expression vector vaccines expressing FIV gp140 alone or with feline interleukin-12 (IL-12), IL-16, or a CpG motif, *J Virol* 74:10447–10457, 2000.
83. Hanlon L, Argyle D, Bain D, et al: Feline leukemia virus DNA vaccine efficacy is enhanced by coadministration with interleukin-12 (IL-12) and IL-18 expression vectors, *J Virol* 75:8424–8433, 2001.
84. Glansbeek HL, Haagmans BL, te Lintelo EG, et al: Adverse effects of feline IL-12 during DNA vaccination against feline infectious peritonitis virus, *J Gen Virol* 83:1–10, 2002.
85. Lee K, Overwijk WW, O'Toole M, et al: Dose-dependent and schedule-dependent effects of interleukin-12 on antigen-specific CD8 responses, *J Interferon Cytokine Res* 20:589–596, 2000.
86. Brunda MJ, Luistro L, Hendrzak JA, et al: Role of interferon-gamma in mediating the antitumor efficacy of interleukin-12, *J Immunother Emphasis Tumor Immunol* 17:71–77, 1995.
87. Golab J, Zagozdzon R: Antitumor effects of interleukin-12 in pre-clinical and early clinical studies (Review), *Int J Mol Med* 3:537–544, 1999.
88. Colombo MP, Trinchieri G: Interleukin-12 in anti-tumor immunity and immunotherapy, *Cytokine Growth Factor Rev* 13:155–168, 2002.
89. Voest EE, Kenyon BM, O'Reilly MS, et al: Inhibition of angiogenesis in vivo by interleukin 12.[see comment], *J Natl Cancer Inst* 87:581–586, 1995.
90. Duda DG, Sunamura M, Lozonschi L, et al: Direct in vitro evidence and in vivo analysis of the antiangiogenesis effects of interleukin 12, *Cancer Res* 60:1111–1116, 2000.
91. Eng VM, Car BD, Schnyder B, et al: The stimulatory effects of interleukin (IL)-12 on hematopoiesis are antagonized by IL-12-induced interferon gamma in vivo, *J Exper Med* 181:1893–1898, 1995.
92. Tare NS, Bowen S, Warrier RR, et al: Administration of recombinant interleukin-12 to mice suppresses hematopoiesis in the bone marrow but enhances hematopoiesis in the spleen, *J Interferon Cytokine Res* 15:377–383, 1995.
93. Car BD, Eng VM, Lipman JM, et al: The toxicology of interleukin-12: a review, *Toxicol Pathol* 27:58–63, 1999.
94. Atkins MB, Robertson MJ, Gordon M, et al: Phase I evaluation of intravenous recombinant human interleukin 12 in patients with advanced malignancies, *Clin Cancer Res* 3:409–417, 1997.

94a. Lehman TL, O'Halloran KP, Bielefeldt Ohmann H, et al: Adverse effects of adenoviral il-12 administration in the cat, unpublished data.

95. Siddiqui F, Li CY, Zhang X, et al: Characterization of a recombinant adenovirus vector encoding heat-inducible feline interleukin-12 for use in hyperthermia-induced gene-therapy, *Int J Hyperthermia* 22(2):117–134, 2006.
96. Siddiqui F, Li CY, Larue SM, et al: A phase I trial of hyperthermia-induced interleukin-12 gene therapy in spontaneously arising feline soft tissue sarcomas, *Molecular Cancer Therapeutics* 6(1):380–389, 2007.
97. Saldarriaga OA, Perez LE, Travi BL, et al: Selective enhancement of the type 1 cytokine response by expression of a canine interleukin (IL)-12 fused heterodimeric DNA, *Vet Immunol Immunopathol* 110(3-4):377–388, 2006.
98. Akhtar N, Padilla ML, Dickerson EB, et al: Interleukin-12 inhibits tumor growth in a novel angiogenesis canine hemangiosarcoma xenograft model, *Neoplasia* 6:106–116, 2004.

99. Okano F, Satoh M, Yamada K: Cloning and expression of the cDNA for canine interleukin-12, *J Interferon Cytokine Res* 17:713–718, 1997.
100. Imamura T, Maeda H, Eda Y, et al: Cloning of full length cDNA, high-level expression and biological characterization of feline IL-12, *J Vet Med Sci* 62:1079–1087, 2000.
101. Rivas AL, Tintle L, Kimball ES, et al: A canine febrile disorder associated with elevated interleukin-6, *Clin Immunol Immunopathol* 64:36–45, 1992.
102. Rau S, Kohn B, Richter C, et al: Plasma interleukin-6 response is predictive for severity and mortality in canine systemic inflammatory response syndrome and sepsis, *Vet Clin Pathol* 36(3):253–260, 2007.
103. Hay CW, Chu Q, Budsberg SC, et al: Synovial fluid interleukin 6, tumor necrosis factor, and nitric oxide values in dogs with osteoarthritis secondary to cranial cruciate ligament rupture, *Am J Vet Res* 58:1027–1032, 1997.
104. Hogenesch H, Snyder PW, Scott-Moncrieff JC, et al: Interleukin-6 activity in dogs with juvenile polyarteritis syndrome: effect of corticosteroids, *Clin Immunol Immunopathol* 77:107–110, 1995.
105. Adachi Y, Yoshio-Hoshino N, Nishimoto N: The blockade of IL-6 signaling in rational drug design, *Curr Pharmacol Des* 14(12):1217–1224, 2008.
106. Peng J, Friese P, George JN, et al: Alteration of platelet function in dogs mediated by interleukin-6, *Blood* 83:398–403, 1994.
107. Burstein SA: Effects of interleukin 6 on megakaryocytes and on canine platelet function, *Stem Cells* 12:386–393, 1994.
108. Bradley WG, Gibbs C, Kraus L, et al: Molecular cloning and characterization of a cDNA encoding feline interleukin-6, *Proc Soc Exp Biol Med* 204:301–305, 1993.
109. Ohashi T, Matsumoto Y, Watari T, et al: Molecular cloning of feline interleukin-6 cDNA, *J Vet Med Sci* 55:941–944, 1993.
110. Shin IS, Kim HR, Nam MJ, et al: Studies of cocktail therapy with multiple cytokines for neoplasia or infectious disease of the dog I. cDNA cloning of canine IL-3 and IL-6, *J Vet Sci* 2:115–120, 2001.
111. Olsen EH, McCain AS, Merricks EP, et al: Comparative response of plasma VWF in dogs to up-regulation of VWF mRNA by interleukin-11 versus Weibel-Palade body release by desmopressin (DDAVP), *Blood* 102:436–441, 2003.
112. Ragni MV, Jankowitz RC, Chapman HL, et al: A phase II prospective open-label escalating dose trial of recombinant interleukin-11 in mild von Willebrand disease, *Haemophilia* 14(5):968–977, 2008.
113. Nash RA, Seidel K, Storb R, et al: Effects of rhIL-11 on normal dogs and after sublethal radiation, *Exp Hematol* 23:389–396, 1995.
114. Zlotnik A, Yoshie O: Chemokines: a new classification system and their role in immunity, *Immunity* 12:121–127, 2000.
115. Rot A, von Andrian UH: Chemokines in innate and adaptive host defense: basic chemokinese grammar for immune cells, *Annu Rev Immunol* 22:891–928, 2004.
116. Tsuchida S, Kagi A, Takahashi T: Characterization of cDNA and genomic sequences encoding a canine chemokine receptor, CXCR4 and its ligand CXCL12, *Vet Immunol Immunopathol* 116(3-4):219–225, 2007.
117. Kovacs EM, Baxter GD, Robinson WF: Feline peripheral blood mononuclear cells express message for both CXC and CC type chemokine receptors, *Arch Virol* 144(2):273–285, 1999.
118. Mosley M, Pullen S, Botham A, et al: The molecular cloning and functional expression of the dog CCR5, *Vet Immunol Immunopathol* 113(3-4):415–420, 2006.
119. Reiss K, Mentlein R, Sievers J, et al: Stromal cell-derived factor 1 is secreted by meningeal cells and acts as chemotactic factor on neuronal stem cells of the cerebellar external granular layer, *Neuroscience* 115:295–305, 2002.
120. Luo Y, Cai J, Xue H, et al: Functional SDF1 alpha/CXCR4 signaling in the developing spinal cord, *J Neurochem* 93:452–462, 2005.
121. Ara T, Tokoyoda K, Okamoto R, et al: The role of CXCL12 in the organ-specific process of artery formation, *Blood* 105:3155–3161, 2005.
122. Jones RL, Hannan NJ, Kaitu'u TJ, et al: Identification of chemokines important for leukocyte recruitment to the human endometrium at the times of embryo implantation and menstruation, *J Clin Endocrinol Metab* 89:6155–6167, 2004.
123. Zlotnik A: Chemokines in neoplastic progression, *Semin Cancer Biol* 14:181–185, 2004.
124. Arya M, Patel HR, Williamson M: Chemokines: key players in cancer, *Curr Med Res Opin* 19:557–564, 2003.
125. Feng Y, Broder CC, Kennedy PE, et al: HIV-1 entry cofactor: functional cDNA cloning of a seven-transmembrane, G protein-coupled receptor[see comment], *Science* 272:872–877, 1996.
126. Dragic T, Litwin V, Allaway GP, et al: HIV-1 entry into CD4+ cells is mediated by the chemokine receptor CC-CKR-5[see comment], *Nature* 381:667–673, 1996.
127. Johnson Z, Schwarz M, Power CA, et al: Multi-faceted strategies to combat disease by interference with the chemokine system, *Trends Immunol* 26:268, 2005.
128. Cavaillon JM, Adib-Conquy M, Fitting C, et al: Cytokine cascade in sepsis, *Scand J Infect Dis* 35:535–544, 2003.
129. Ness TL, Carpenter KJ, Ewing JL, et al: CCR1 and CC chemokine ligand 5 interactions exacerbate innate immune responses during sepsis, *J Immunol* 173:6938–6948, 2004.
130. Rosenberg HF, Bonville CA, Easton AJ, et al: The pneumonia virus of mice infection model for severe respiratory syncytial virus infection: identifying novel targets for therapeutic intervention, *Pharmacol Ther* 105:1–6, 2005.
131. Gladue RP, Tylaska LA, Brissette WH, et al: CP-481,715, a potent and selective CCR1 antagonist with potential therapeutic implications for inflammatory diseases, *J Biol Chem* 278:40473–40480, 2003.
132. Liang Z, Wu T, Lou H, et al: Inhibition of breast cancer metastasis by selective synthetic polypeptide against CXCR4, *Cancer Res* 64:4302–4308, 2004.
133. Onuffer J, McCarrick MA, Dunning L, et al: Structure function differences in nonpeptide CCR1 antagonists for human and mouse CCR1, *J Immunol* 170:1910–1916, 2003.
134. Walley KR, Lukacs NW, Standiford TJ, et al: Elevated levels of macrophage inflammatory protein 2 in severe murine peritonitis increase neutrophil recruitment and mortality, *Infect Immun* 65:3847–3851, 1997.
135. Goodman RB, Strieter RM, Martin DP, et al: Inflammatory cytokines in patients with persistence of the acute respiratory distress syndrome, *Am J Respir Crit Care Med* 154:602–611, 1996.
136. Qiu Y, Zhu J, Bandi V, et al: Biopsy neutrophilia, neutrophil chemokine and receptor gene expression in severe exacerbations of chronic obstructive pulmonary disease [see comment], *Am J Respir Crit Care Med* 168:968–975, 2003.
137. Caswell JL, Middleton DM, Sorden SD, et al: Expression of the neutrophil chemoattractant interleukin-8 in the lesions of bovine pneumonic pasteurellosis, *Vet Pathol* 35:124–131, 1998.
138. Li F, Zhang X, Gordon JR: CXCL8((3-73))K11R/G31P antagonizes ligand binding to the neutrophil CXCR1 and CXCR2 receptors and cellular responses to CXCL8/IL-8, *Biochem Biophys Res Commun* 293:939–944, 2002.
139. Li F, Zhang X, Mizzi C, et al: CXCL8((3-73))K11R/G31P antagonizes the neutrophil chemoattractants present in pasteurellosis and mastitis lesions and abrogates neutrophil influx into intradermal endotoxin challenge sites in vivo, *Vet Immunol Immunopathol* 90:65–77, 2002.
140. Fushimi T, Kojima A, Moore MA, et al: Macrophage inflammatory protein 3alpha transgene attracts dendritic cells to established murine tumors and suppresses tumor growth, *J Clin Invest* 105:1383–1393, 2000.

141. Furumoto K, Soares L, Engleman EG, et al: Induction of potent antitumor immunity by in situ targeting of intratumoral DCs [see comment], *J Clin Invest* 113:774–783, 2004.
142. Vicari AP, Ait-Yahia S, Chemin K, et al: Antitumor effects of the mouse chemokine 6Ckine/SLC through angiostatic and immunological mechanisms, *J Immunol* 165:1992–2000, 2000.
143. Guiducci C, Vicari AP, Sangaletti S, et al: Redirecting in vivo elicited tumor infiltrating macrophages and dendritic cells towards tumor rejection, *Cancer Res* 65:3437–3446, 2005.
144. Basu S, Schaefer TM, Ghosh M, et al: Molecular cloning and sequencing of 25 different rhesus macaque chemokine cDNAs reveals evolutionary conservation among C, CC, CXC, AND CX3C families of chemokines, *Cytokine* 18:140–148, 2002.
143. Dhawan P, Richmond A: Role of CXCL1 in tumorigenesis of melanoma, *J Leukoc Biol* 72:9–18, 2002.
144. Balkwill F, Mantovani A: Inflammation and cancer: back to Virchow? *Lancet* 357:539–545, 2001.
145. Takeuchi H, Fujimoto A, Tanaka M, et al: CCL21 chemokine regulates chemokine receptor CCR7 bearing malignant melanoma cells, *Clin Cancer Res* 10:2351–2358, 2004.
146. Wiley HE, Gonzalez EB, Maki W, et al: Expression of CC chemokine receptor-7 and regional lymph node metastasis of B16 murine melanoma, *J Natl Cancer Inst* 2093:1638–1643, 2001.
147. Balkwill F: The significance of cancer cell expression of the chemokine receptor CXCR4,, *Semin Cancer Biol* 14:171–179, 2004.
148. Muller A, Homey B, Soto H, et al: Involvement of chemokine receptors in breast cancer metastasis, *Nature* 410:50–56, 2001.
149. Oonuma T, Morimatsu M, Nakagawa T, et al: Role of CXCR4 and SDF-1 in mammary tumor metastasis in the cat, *J Vet Med Sci* 65:1069–1073, 2003.
150. Fan TM, Barger AM, Fredrickson RL, et al: Investigating CXCR4 expression in canine appendicular osteosarcoma, *J Vet Intern Med* 22(3):602–608, 2008.
151. Wang J, Xi L, Hunt JL, et al: Expression pattern of chemokine receptor 6 (CCR6) and CCR7 in squamous cell carcinoma of the head and neck identifies a novel metastatic phenotype, *Cancer Res* 64:1861–1866, 2004.
152. Scala S, Ottaiano A, Ascierto PA, et al: Expression of CXCR4 predicts poor prognosis in patients with malignant melanoma, *Clin Cancer Res* 11:1835–1841, 2005.
153. Murakami T, Cardones AR, Hwang ST: Chemokine receptors and melanoma metastasis, *J Dermatol Sci* 36:71–78, 2004.
154. Arya M, Patel HR, McGurk C, et al: The importance of the CXCL12-CXCR4 chemokine ligand-receptor interaction in prostate cancer metastasis, *J Exp Ther Oncol* 4:291–303, 2004.
155. Deng H, Liu R, Ellmeier W, et al: Identification of a major co-receptor for primary isolates of HIV-1, *Nature* 381:661–666, 1996.
156. Willett BJ, Picard L, Hosie MJ, et al: Shared usage of the chemokine receptor CXCR4 by the feline and human immunodeficiency viruses, *J Virol* 71:6407–6415, 1997.
157. Egberink HF, De Clercq E, Van Vliet AL, et al: Bicyclams, selective antagonists of the human chemokine receptor CXCR4, potently inhibit feline immunodeficiency virus replication, *J Virol* 73:6346–6352, 1999.
158. Richardson J, Pancino G, Merat R, et al: Shared usage of the chemokine receptor CXCR4 by primary and laboratory-adapted strains of feline immunodeficiency virus, *J Virol* 73:3661–3671, 1999.
159. Mizukoshi F, Baba K, Goto-Koshino Y, et al: Inhibitory effect of newly developed CXC-chemokine receptor 4 antagonists on the infection with feline immunodeficiency virus, *J Vet Med Sci* 71(1):121–124, 2009.
160. Fujii N, Nakashima H, Tamamura H: The therapeutic potential of CXCR4 antagonists in the treatment of HIV, *Expert Opin Investig Drugs* 12:185–195, 2003.
161. Shin IS, Nam MJ, Park SJ, et al: Cloning of canine GM-CSF and SCF genes, *J Vet Sci* 2:159–166, 2001.
162. Dunham SP, Onions DE: Isolation, nucleotide sequence and expression of a cDNA encoding feline granulocyte colony-stimulating factor, *Cytokine* 14:347–351, 2001.
163. Dunham SP, Bruce J: Isolation, expression and bioactivity of feline granulocyte-macrophage colony-stimulating factor, *Gene* 332:97–106, 2004.
164. Dunham SP, Onions DE: The cloning and sequencing of cDNAs encoding two isoforms of feline stem cell factor, *DNA Seq* 6:233–237, 1996.
165. Yamamoto A, Iwata A, Tuchiya K, et al: Molecular cloning and expression of the cDNA encoding feline granulocyte colony-stimulating factor, *Gene* 274:263–269, 2001.
166. Hammond WP, Csiba E, Canin A, et al: Chronic neutropenia. A new canine model induced by human granulocyte colony-stimulating factor, *J Clin Invest* 87:704–710, 1991.
167. Lothrop CD Jr, Warren DJ, Souza LM, et al: Correction of canine cyclic hematopoiesis with recombinant human granulocyte colony-stimulating factor, *Blood* 72:1324–1328, 1988.
168. MacVittie TJ, Monroy RL, Patchen ML, et al: Therapeutic use of recombinant human G-CSF (rhG-CSF) in a canine model of sublethal and lethal whole-body irradiation, *Int J Radiat Biol* 57:723–736, 1990.
169. Pratt HL, Carroll RC, McClendon S, et al: Effects of recombinant granulocyte colony-stimulating factor treatment on hematopoietic cycles and cellular defects associated with canine cyclic hematopoiesis, *Exp Hematol* 18:1199–1203, 1990.
170. Holland M, Stobie D, Shapiro W: Pancytopenia associated with administration of captopril to a dog, *J Am Vet Med Assoc* 208:1683–1686, 1996.
171. Kurzman ID, MacEwen EG, Broderick C, et al: Effect of colony-stimulating factors on number and function of circulating monocytes in normal dogs, *Mol Biother* 4:29–33, 1992.
172. Obradovich JE, Ogilvie GK, Powers BE, et al: Evaluation of recombinant canine granulocyte colony-stimulating factor as an inducer of granulopoiesis. A pilot study, *J Vet Intern Med* 5:75–79, 1991.
173. Zinkl J, Cain G, Jain N: Hematological response of dogs to canine recombinant granulocyte colony stimulating factor (Rcg-csf), *Comparative Clin Pathol* 2:151, 1992.
174. Mishu L, Callahan G, Allebban Z, et al: Effects of recombinant canine granulocyte colony-stimulating factor on white blood cell production in clinically normal and neutropenic dogs, *J Am Vet Med Assoc* 200:1957–1964, 1992.
175. Ogilvie GK, Obradovich JE, Cooper MF, et al: Use of recombinant canine granulocyte colony-stimulating factor to decrease myelosuppression associated with the administration of mitoxantrone in the dog, *J Vet Intern Med* 6:44–47, 1992.
176. Hammond WP, Boone TC, Donahue RE, et al: A comparison of treatment of canine cyclic hematopoiesis with recombinant human granulocyte-macrophage colony-stimulating factor (GM-CSF), G-CSF interleukin-3, and canine G-CSF, *Blood* 76:523–532, 1990.
177. Ogilvie GK: Hematopoietic growth factors: frontiers for cure, *Vet Clin North Am Small Anim Pract* 25:1441–1456, 1995.
178. Obradovich JE, Ogilvie GK, Stadler-Morris S, et al: Effect of recombinant canine granulocyte colony-stimulating factor on peripheral blood neutrophil counts in normal cats, *J Vet Intern Med* 7:65–67, 1993.
179. Fulton R, Gasper PW, Ogilvie GK, et al: Effect of recombinant human granulocyte colony-stimulating factor on hematopoiesis in normal cats, *Exp Hematol* 19:759–767, 1991.
180. Colgan SP, Gasper PW, Thrall MA, et al: Neutrophil function in normal and Chédiak-Higashi syndrome cats following administration of recombinant canine granulocyte colony-stimulating factor, *Exp Hematol* 20:1229–1234, 1992.
181. Vose JM, Armitage JO: Clinical applications of hematopoietic growth factors [see comment], *J Clin Oncol* 13:1023–1035, 1995.

182. Mayer P, Werner FJ, Lam C, et al: In vitro and in vivo activity of human recombinant granulocyte-macrophage colony-stimulating factor in dogs, *Exp Hematol* 18:1026–1033, 1990.
183. Nothdurft W, Selig C, Fliedner TM, et al: Haematological effects of rhGM-CSF in dogs exposed to total-body irradiation with a dose of 2.4 Gy, *Int J Radiat Biol* 61:519–531, 1992.
184. Nash RA, Schuening F, Appelbaum F, et al: Molecular cloning and in vivo evaluation of canine granulocyte-macrophage colony-stimulating factor, *Blood* 78:930–937, 1991.
185. Nash RA, Burstein SA, Storb R, et al: Thrombocytopenia in dogs induced by granulocyte-macrophage colony-stimulating factor: increased destruction of circulating platelets, *Blood* 86:1765–1775, 1995.
186. Nash RA, Schuening FG, Seidel K, et al: Effect of recombinant canine granulocyte-macrophage colony-stimulating factor on hematopoietic recovery after otherwise lethal total body irradiation, *Blood* 83:1963–1970, 1994.
187. Nothdurft W, Kreja L, Selig C: Acceleration of hemopoietic recovery in dogs after extended-field partial-body irradiation by treatment with colony-stimulating factors: rhG-CSF and rhGM-CSF, *Int J Radiat Oncol Biol Phys* 37:1145–1154, 1997.
188. Foley R, Ellis R, Walker I, et al: Intramarrow cytokine gene transfer by adenoviral vectors in dogs, *Hum Gene Ther* 8:545–553, 1997.
189. Choi EW, Shin IS, Chae YJ, et al: Effects of GM-CSF gene transfer using silica-nanoparticles as a vehicle on white blood cell production in dogs, *Exp Hematol* 36(7):807–815, 2008.
190. Choi EW, Koo HC, Shin IS, et al: Preventive and therapeutic effects of gene therapy using silica nanoparticles-binding of GM-CSF gene on white blood cell production in dogs with leukopenia, *Exp Hematol* 36(9):1091–1097, 2008.
191. Banchereau J, Palucka AK: Dendritic cells as therapeutic vaccines against cancer, *Nat Rev Immunol* 5:296–306, 2005.
192. Moll H: Antigen delivery by dendritic cells, *Int J Med Microbiol* 294:337–344, 2004.
193. Bienzle D, Reggeti F, Clark ME, et al: Immunophenotype and functional properties of feline dendritic cells derived from blood and bone marrow, *Vet Immunol Immunopathol* 96:19–30, 2003.
194. Sprague W, Pope M, Hoover E: Culture and comparison of feline myeloid dendritic cells vs macrophages, *J Comp Pathol* 133(2-3):136–145, 2005.
195. Catchpole B, Stell AJ, Dobson JM: Generation of blood-derived dendritic cells in dogs with oral malignant melanoma, *J Comp Pathol* 126:238–241, 2002.
196. Ibisch C, Pradal G, Bach JM, et al: Functional canine dendritic cells can be generated in vitro from peripheral blood mononuclear cells and contain a cytoplasmic ultrastructural marker, *J Immunol Methods* 298:175–182, 2005.
197. Gyorffy S, Rodriguez-Lecompte JC, Woods JP, et al: Bone marrow-derived dendritic cell vaccination of dogs with naturally occurring melanoma by using human gp100 antigen, *J Vet Intern Med* 19:56–63, 2005.
198. Hogge GS, Burkholder JK, Culp J, et al: Preclinical development of human granulocyte-macrophage colony-stimulating factor-transfected melanoma cell vaccine using established canine cell lines and normal dogs, *Cancer Gene Ther* 6:26–36, 1999.
199. Hogge GS, Burkholder JK, Culp J, et al: Development of human granulocyte-macrophage colony-stimulating factor-transfected tumor cell vaccines for the treatment of spontaneous canine cancer, *Hum Gene Ther* 9:1851–1861, 1998.
200. Shull RM, Suggs SV, Langley KE, et al: Canine stem cell factor (c-kit ligand) supports the survival of hematopoietic progenitors in long-term canine marrow culture, *Exp Hematol* 20:1118–1124, 1992.
201. Schuening FG, Appelbaum FR, Deeg HJ, et al: Effects of recombinant canine stem cell factor, a c-kit ligand, and recombinant granulocyte colony-stimulating factor on hematopoietic recovery after otherwise lethal total body irradiation, *Blood* 81:20–26, 1993.
202. Dale DC, Rodger E, Cebon J, et al: Long term treatment of canine cyclic hematopoiesis with recombinant canine stem cell factor, *Blood* 85:74–79, 1995.

33 Chemotherapy

Heather Wilson and Claudia Barton

Chapter Outline

Throughout the centuries the sufferers of this disease have been the subject of almost every conceivable form of experimentation. The fields and forests, the apothecary shop and temple have been ransacked for some successful means of relief from this intractable malady. Hardly any animal has escaped making its contribution in hide or hair, tooth or toenail, thymus or thyroid, liver or spleen in the vain search for a means of relief. — Bainbridge, The Cancer Problem, *1914*

Before appropriate treatment for a particular cancer can be instituted, the tumor must first be diagnosed by cytology or histopathology. Testing is then conducted to allow staging of the tumor—to determine if there is clinically visible evidence of metastatic spread. Lymph node cytology or biopsy, radiographs, ultrasound examinations, and computed tomography or magnetic resonance imaging scans may be used as staging procedures. The biological behavior typical for the cancer must be considered. If, as a rule, the tumor tends to remain localized, surgery or radiation therapy—or a combination of the two—may be the best way to obtain cure or control. If the tumor is likely to metastasize by lymphatics or hematogenously, however, some form of systemic therapy must be added to make a cure more likely. Systemic therapy involves the administration of biological agents, hormones, or cytotoxic chemotherapy. Theoretically, cancer chemotherapy is given to kill or suppress the growth of malignant cells without killing normal cells; in fact, however, most of the commonly used drugs are capable of killing both normal and malignant cells, depending on the dose administered. To be useful in clinical practice, an antineoplastic drug must possess selective toxicity—that is, it should be more toxic to cancer cells than to normal host cells at conventional doses. Finally, the clinician must determine whether the patient has concurrent diseases, with a complete blood count (CBC), biochemical panel, urinalysis, and possibly testing for feline leukemia virus and feline immunodeficiency virus. This section of the chapter addresses the principles of chemotherapy and the side effects seen in dogs and cats.

Drugs used in chemotherapy cause their anticancer effects by interacting with important substrates or enzymes that are related to DNA synthesis or function. Therefore most anticancer drugs are ineffective against cells that are not actively proliferating. Tumors with a high mitotic index (e.g., lymphoma) are much more likely to be sensitive to chemotherapy than those in which mitotic activity is low. Because chemotherapeutic drugs are effective principally on cells that are actively replicating, it is important to have an understanding of the phases of the cell cycle before discussion of individual drugs (Figure 33-1). The part of the cell cycle in which active mitosis occurs has been termed the *M phase;* it is quite short in all cells, generally lasting less than 1 hour. The period during which DNA synthesis occurs for chromosome doubling in preparation for mitosis is called the *S phase* and ranges from 8 to 30 hours. When scientists began to learn about cell division, they realized that there were other phases in the cell cycle; because they initially did not understand what was occurring in the cell at these times, the phases were called *G* (G_1 and G_2) for *gap.* G_1 follows mitosis, and protein synthesis and RNA transcription occur during this phase. G_1 is extremely variable in length depending on the cell type, ranging from 7 to 170 hours. G_2 precedes the next mitotic event and is usually brief, ranging from 1 to 4 hours. G_0 has been used to describe those cells that are not actively cycling. Certain cell types, such as myocytes and neurons, enter G_0 and never cycle again. Other cell types, such as hepatocytes, proliferate in young animals and then cease cycling at maturity but are capable of beginning to cycle again if cell replacement is necessary. Fibroblasts become terminally differentiated in connective tissue, but stem cells remain in the tissue. These can become reproductively active again to repopulate the tissue if a wound occurs.

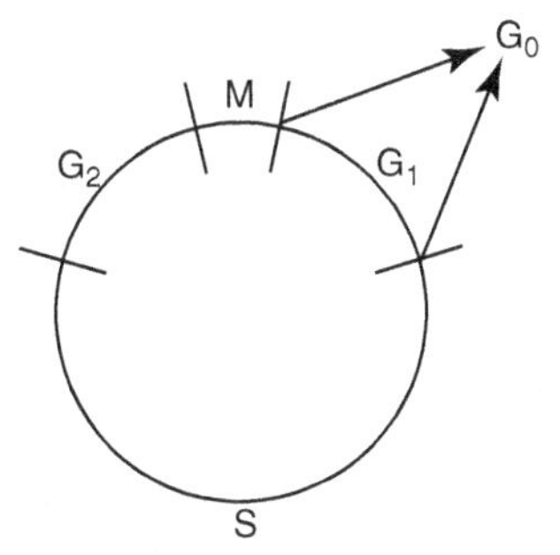

Figure 33-1 Cell generation cycle: M—mitosis; S—DNA content is being doubled in preparation for mitosis; G_1 and G_2—gaps. Protein synthesis and RNA transcription are occurring in these phases; G_0—cells that are not actively cycling.

Chemotherapeutic drugs can be classified into three groups on the basis of their activity in the phases of the cell cycle (Box 33-1). Agents that are considered to be lethal to cells in all phases of the cell cycle, with resting cells as sensitive as proliferating cells, are called *cycle nonspecific.* Examples include nitrogen mustard (the first chemotherapy agent; its activity was discovered in 1919 with the effects of mustard gas on the troops in World War I) and high-dose cyclophosphamide. Agents that are capable of damaging both resting and cycling cells (although cells in cycle are much more sensitive) include conventional-dose cyclophosphamide and doxorubicin. These drugs spare resting cells and are called *cycle specific.* Agents that are *phase specific* exert their lethal effects exclusively or primarily during one phase of the cell cycle, usually S or M; resting cells and cells in the other phases of the cell cycle are not killed. Examples include methotrexate, cytosine arabinoside, vincristine, and vinblastine.

There are three phases in the development of a new chemotherapeutic drug (Box 33-2). Many artificial chemicals and naturally occurring compounds are screened (generally by the National Cancer Institute or by industry) for cytotoxicity, first in cultures of cancer cells and then in mice or rats. If a particular compound looks promising, a *phase I* trial is conducted, providing an initial pharmacologic evaluation. The appropriate mode of administration is established for the drug, and common side effects are discovered. Patient tolerance of increasing dosage is also determined. Phase I trials are conducted on very small numbers of patients, generally with advanced and ultimately terminal cancers for which no conventional treatment is available, and doses tolerated by these patients may be below the ultimate therapeutic range. If the compound shows no prohibitive toxicity and shows even slight efficacy (a partial response in a few patients), the *phase II* trial begins. In this phase screening for efficacy of the drug against a variety of tumors is conducted. After the spectrum of activity is determined, dose-response relationships are determined. The *phase III* trial is then used to determine drugs that work effectively together, and the new combination protocol is ultimately compared with the existing best treatment. *Phase IV* trials are known as postmarketing surveillance trials. They involve safety surveillance after the necessary authorities permit the drug to be sold. This surveillance may be required by

Box 33-1

Sites of Action of Chemotherapeutic Drugs

Class I: *Cycle nonspecific* —Agents lethal to cells in all phases of the cell cycle. Resting cells are as sensitive as proliferating cells. Examples: radiation, nitrogen mustard

Class II: *Phase specific*—Agents that exert their lethal effects exclusively or primarily during one phase of the cell cycle, usually S or M. Resting cells are spared. Examples: methotrexate, cytosine arabinoside, vincristine

Class III: *Cycle specific*—Agents that are capable of damaging both resting and cycling cells, although cells in cycle are much more sensitive. Examples: cyclophosphamide, doxorubicin

Box 33-2

Development Phases for New Chemotherapeutic Drugs

Phase I Trial
Initial pharmacologic evaluation
Establishment of mode of administration
Establishment of tolerance of a schedule at increasing dosage

Phase II Trial
Screening for efficacy of a drug against a variety of tumors

Phase III Trial
Determination of effective drug combinations
Comparison of new protocol to existing "best" treatment

Phase IV Trial
Postmarketing safety surveillance to detect rare or long-term adverse effects

regulatory authorities. The chemotherapy agent may not have been tested for interactions with other drugs, for example. The safety surveillance is designed to detect any rare or long-term adverse effects over a much larger patient population and longer time period than was possible during the phase I through phase III clinical trials. Harmful effects discovered during phase IV trials may result in a drug being removed from the market.

Most cancers in animals and humans are diagnosed only after they are well advanced. In the 1960s, Skipper and coworkers[1] used the rodent L1210 leukemia to illustrate this point and determine cell kill kinetics in tumors. The L1210 leukemia is a rapidly growing tumor with a growth fraction of 100% and a doubling time of only 12 hours. At this rate of growth, a billion cells would accumulate in the rodent only 19 days after injection of a single cell. After treatment of the leukemia with chemotherapy, the investigators determined that cytotoxic drugs kill by log kill kinetics—that is, a given dose of an effective drug kills a constant fraction of cells and not a constant number, regardless of the number of cells present. This principle is known as the fractional kill hypothesis. For example, if a certain drug is known to kill 90% of the tumor cells present, it will kill 90% of the cells whether the beginning

Table 33-1 Tumor Depopulation Related to Successive Drug Cycles Assuming a 90% Fractional Cell Kill in a Model System

Drug Treatment Number	Number of Tumor Cells	Number of Tumor Cells Surviving	
1	10,000,000,000 (10^{10})	1,000,000,000	Clinical
2	1,000,000,000 (10^9)	100,000,000	Disease
	Complete Clinical Remission		
3	100,000,000 (10^8)	10,000,000	Subclinical
4	10,000,000 (10^7)	1,000,000	Disease
5	1,000,000 (10^6)	100,000	
6	100,000 (10^5)	10,000	
7	10,000 (10^4)	1,000	
8	1,000 (10^3)	100	
9	100 (10^2)	10	
10	10 (10^1)	1	
11	1 (10^0)	0	

number is 10 cells or 10 billion cells (Table 33-1). Thus it should be theoretically possible to cure with chemotherapy, with rapid successive administration of chemotherapy drugs. In fact, antineoplastic drugs kill an extremely variable fraction of cells, ranging from a very small fraction to a maximum of 99.99%; for many tumors the fractional kill is disappointingly small. What prevents theoretical "cures" with chemotherapy is (1) the inability to give drugs in rapid succession, because of host toxicity, and (2) the development of a drug-resistant population of tumor cells during the course of treatment.

Tumors as small as 1 g (10^9 tumor cells—a billion) *may* be detected in the body, especially if they are located in areas such as the skin or mouth. However, it is far more common for tumors to escape detection until they are 10 g (10^{10} tumor cells) or more. The maximum malignant tumor mass compatible with human life is about 1 kg (10^{12} tumor cells). If it is assumed that a given tumor originates from a single cell, then a 1-g tumor (10^9 cells) has gone through 30 doublings from the original cell. To get to 1 kg, only about 10 more doublings will take place.[2] It should be clear from these sobering numbers that a large, unresectable tumor burden with only modest sensitivity to chemotherapy cannot be cured or, in many cases, even palliated with conventional chemotherapy administration protocols. The average volume doubling time for various human solid (e.g., nonleukemic) tumors is about 2 months. However, for certain rapidly growing tumors such as embryonal nephroma, seminoma, lymphoma, and leukemia, the volume-doubling time is less than 1 month. For other tumors the volume-doubling time is as long as 1 year. Because chemotherapy affects rapidly dividing cells, tumors with short volume-doubling times are generally chemotherapy sensitive, whereas tumors with long volume-doubling times are generally chemotherapy resistant.

With regard to the efficacy of chemotherapeutic drugs, criteria have been described for measuring response; these are called RECIST (*R*esponse *E*valuation *C*riteria *i*n *S*olid *T*umors). To evaluate a tumor's response to treatment, the clinician must have a marker lesion, a repeatably measurable tumor mass or parameter that can be periodically rechecked and remeasured (preferably with the same person doing the repeat measurements). This may be a lymph node or nodes that can be measured with calipers, a liver lesion measured by ultrasound, nodules visible on a radiograph, a biochemical value such as the calcium level, and so forth. The evaluation as to efficacy of treatment is conventionally made after two cycles of chemotherapy or an appropriate trial of another agent has been administered:

Complete response (CR)—Resolution of all measurable neoplastic disease (or return of marker to normal, if there is no measurable disease), with appearance of no new lesions. A chemotherapeutic drug that can cause a CR in a significant number of animals with a specific cancer is quite likely to increase disease-free survival, especially when used as an adjuvant agent.

Partial response (PR)— Reduction in measurable tumor dimensions of 30% or greater, with no appearance of new lesions. Although a temporary PR may provide the patient with some decrease in discomfort from the cancer, it is unlikely to have a significant effect on survival. However, this drug might be useful in other patients at an earlier stage of disease or in patients in which the tumor can be surgically removed before chemotherapy. A PR proves that the drug does have *some* activity against the tumor that is being treated.

Stable disease (SD)—No significant change is noted in measurable tumor dimensions, or a response is seen that is less than a PR. Actual values are less than a 30% decrease in marker lesion size and less than a 20% increase in marker lesion size.

Progressive disease (PD)—The tumor is clearly growing (20% or greater increase in lesion size), or new lesions appear.

Certain criteria may be useful for declaring a treatment protocol ineffective or unsafe in a specific patient. Progressive growth (usually greater than 20%) in a measurable tumor lesion or the appearance of new lesions after two cycles of chemotherapy would suggest that the drug or protocol is not at all useful for the tumor being treated. Severe toxicity with irreversible, cumulative, or unpredictable manifestations also generally suggests that the drug should no longer be used in this particular patient. If symptoms from the cancer cause the patient's condition to deteriorate, with the only response to drug treatment being SD or PR, the drug should be discontinued and another treatment selected if possible.

The common cancers in dogs and cats can be broadly divided into three categories:

(1) *Tumors in which the cells are exquisitely sensitive to chemotherapy.* In these tumors CR can usually be obtained, and chemotherapy is therefore the accepted treatment of choice. Cure or solid long-term remission can be expected, and surgery or radiation therapy will not generally be necessary to decrease cell numbers before chemotherapy is administered. An example is the transmissible venereal tumor, in which an extremely high cure rate is possible with vincristine administration even when metastatic disease is

present. Another example is lymphoma, in which rapid and complete response is seen with chemotherapeutic treatment. In most patients with lymphoma, however, remission lasts only for only months (generally 12 months or less), insofar as a drug-resistant population of tumor cells develops during treatment. For this reason chemotherapeutic treatment of canine and feline lymphoma is generally considered to be palliative, not curative.

(2) *Tumors in which the cells are only modestly sensitive to chemotherapy.* PR may be obtained in some of these tumors, whereas in others response to drug treatment may be minimal. Chemotherapy may play a part in management of these cancers but only with previous or concurrent surgery or radiation therapy. An example of this type of tumor is canine osteosarcoma, in which carboplatin or doxorubicin are often used as an adjuvant treatment after amputation. Some soft tissue sarcomas with a high mitotic rate are also considered good candidates for chemotherapy treatment. *Adjuvant chemotherapy* is given along with or after another treatment modality, such as surgery or radiation therapy, to increase the percentage of curative resections or long-term responses; in other words, it is used in hopes of converting a palliative treatment to a cure. *Neoadjuvant chemotherapy* is administered before surgery or radiation therapy in an attempt to shrink the tumor and make it more amenable to removal or irradiation. Neoadjuvant treatment with chemotherapy drugs also allows an assessment as to whether the drugs that are available will produce a response; if so, then more chemotherapy treatments are given *after* surgery or radiation is completed, in hopes to "clean up" remaining microscopic tumor cells. Realistically, however, cures may occur but are rare in tumors with only modest sensitivity to chemotherapy. Palliation with some prolongation of life is generally the best result that can be expected.

(3) *Tumors in which chemotherapy is only rarely of any value for palliation or cure.* Progression of the cancer despite chemotherapeutic treatment will be the outcome for most of these cancers. Many carcinomas and some sarcomas of dogs and cats fall into this category.

In principle, all cells that are actively cycling in the body should be sensitive to chemotherapy; however, the fact that chemotherapy is generally only modestly effective speaks to the fact that this is not entirely true. In many cancers the tumor cells are actually less sensitive to cytotoxic drugs than are the hematopoietic cells within the marrow cavity. This forces the clinician to give a chemotherapeutic drug and wait to evaluate the toxic effects produced before another course of treatment can be administered. During the interval of time in which the patient's neutrophil or platelet count is too low to give another drug, endogenous hematopoietic growth factors are being produced, mediating proliferation of stem cells, the bone marrow recovers, and peripheral cell counts return to normal. Return of blood cell counts to normal after chemotherapy is the usual point at which another course of treatment may be given. It is important not to give another cycle of chemotherapy when peripheral blood counts are extremely low because stem cells are actively proliferating at this time; treatment with cytotoxic drugs administered when stem cells are actively dividing increases the chance that the stem cell population may be killed and recovery may never occur. In humans this is the point at which bone marrow or stem cell transplantation is performed.

Unfortunately, tumor cells may recover from chemotherapeutic injury and begin to proliferate again before the animal's marrow recovers. Even when a tumor is exquisitely sensitive to drug treatment and an apparent complete response is obtained, a line of drug-resistant cells often develops. It is a common clinical experience to find that a tumor may respond quite well to the first treatment with a drug, with progressively less impressive responses as the drug is given repeatedly. Classically, multidrug resistance occurs when large numbers of the cells in a tumor overexpress a gene (the MDR1 gene) that encodes P-glycoprotein, a transmembrane protein important in cell transport. This protein pumps chemotherapeutic drugs from the inside of the cell to the extracellular environment so that they cannot act within the cell; P-glycoprotein is a transmembrane drug efflux pump. Other mechanisms leading to acquired drug resistance include (1) the development in the tumor cell of alternative metabolic pathways to avoid the chemotherapeutic drug's mechanism of action; (2) the fraction of tumor cells actively dividing decreases after several cycles of treatment, thus protecting the remaining noncycling cells against damage; and (3) tumor cells may enter a biological "sanctuary site" in which they are protected from injury because of a lack of drug diffusion into that area (e.g., brain, eye, testicle, spinal cord).

Delaying administration of chemotherapy because of hematopoietic or gastrointestinal toxicity often results in a patient appearing to be in remission, with no visible neoplastic disease but with large amounts of microscopic tumor. Thus drug resistance sometimes develops as a result of chemotherapy being administered in a regimen that is "too little, too late." The highest possible doses of chemotherapy given as frequently as can be tolerated by the patient, early in the course of the neoplastic disease (when smaller numbers of cells are present), should have a much higher chance of producing a cure or long-term remission than chemotherapy given after a large number of tumor cells have infiltrated various organs. In human patients the wait for marrow recovery has been overcome with the use of bone marrow or stem cell transplants, performed after chemotherapy treatment is given in doses high enough to kill tumor cells as well as ablate normal marrow cells. The extreme expense, technical difficulty, and high morbidity rates associated with this procedure do not allow for its use in dogs and cats as a routine clinical procedure, at least at this time. In veterinary oncology in the early twenty-first century, clinicians are usually limited to palliation of tumors; only rarely can they expect to cure their patients.

A regimen of chemotherapy treatment can be divided into several phases. The period of *induction* is the initial intensive chemotherapy intended to produce remission. *Remission* is defined as the point at which no measurable tumor mass can be found; for lymphoma remission is declared when the enlarged lymph nodes, liver, and spleen have returned to normal size and malignant cells have disappeared from the peripheral blood and bone marrow. This does not mean that all (or even most) tumor cells have been killed, however, and *consolidation* therapy with different drugs may be given after apparent clinical remission to produce a larger tumor cell kill. For some tumors such as lymphoma, the animal may be given "pulse" doses of drugs after induction and consolidation to maintain the gains obtained with the induction protocol; this is called the *maintenance* phase of chemotherapy. Recently, *intensification* protocols have been described for tumors in which drug resistance is common. These protocols are administered during the maintenance period, when the patient is in apparent remission, and are an attempt to kill developing drug-resistant clones of cells by using one or two new drugs at high doses.

Combination chemotherapy is, in general, more effective than single-agent therapy. Using multiple drugs sequentially provides additive antitumor effects without greatly increasing host toxicity, especially if drugs are selected carefully for different toxicities. Combination chemotherapy may delay tumor resistance to drugs compared with single agents. Selecting different drugs that have effects on more than one cell cycle phase may also result in a greater fractional cell kill per cycle of chemotherapy.

Traditionally, in estimating the appropriate dose of a drug to administer to a patient, clinicians have used body weight of the patient as the main criterion; the dose has been figured as the number of mg/kg to be given. In a series of studies begun in the 1880s, however, it was demonstrated that many physiologic parameters could better be estimated on the basis of body surface area (BSA). Basal metabolic rate, blood volume, cardiac output, and renal function parameters were found to correlate much more closely to the individual's BSA than to weight. It was then found that drug doses calculated per unit of body weight were greater in smaller animals and children than in larger animals and adults, whereas doses calculated per unit of surface area were similar for all species and ages. On the basis of the findings in these studies, researchers concluded that BSA might be useful as a standard for calculating drug doses in cancer chemotherapy. The calculation for determining BSA for a given species is made by using the following formula:

$$\text{BSA in m}^2 = \frac{K_m \times W^{2/3}}{10^4}$$

In the preceding formula, K_m is a factor based on the different metabolic rate of each species; for the cat it is 10, and for the dog it is 10.1. *W* is the body weight in grams. Because the *K* values for dogs and cat are quite close, a table has been formulated that permits quick estimation of the BSA on the basis of the animal's weight in kilograms. The appropriate dose of the chemotherapeutic agent to be administered is calculated by multiplying the dose/m^2 by the patient's BSA (m^2) taken from the table. A serious and potentially fatal mistake made by some clinicians when using a nomogram or table to estimate the BSA has been to use the animal's weight in *pounds* rather than in kilograms. To avoid this error, a good rule is to calculate the dose of a chemotherapeutic drug and then ask another person to calculate it again separately before the drug is administered.

More recently, the use of BSA as a means of calculating doses for all chemotherapeutic agents has been questioned. For many chemotherapy drugs, myelosuppression is the most common toxicity and is dose limiting; it has been found that BSA does not correlate well with either stem cell number in the bone marrow or with resulting hematopoietic toxicity. In fact, correlation is highly significant between bone marrow effects of the cytotoxic drugs and body weight. A phase I study in dogs was performed to evaluate toxicity of doses of intravenous melphalan calculated by BSA. A significantly greater number of small dogs experienced significant toxicity than did large dogs. Another study compared marrow toxicity induced by doxorubicin given at 30 mg/m^2 to that induced by the drug given at doses calculated at 1 mg/kg. It was found that a disproportionately greater number of dogs weighing less than 10 kg developed severe myelosuppression at the 30 mg/m^2 dose than at the 1 mg/kg dose.[3] Limited toxicosis was seen in dogs weighing more than 10 kg with either of the dosing schemes, however. Plasma doxorubicin concentrations were less after treatment at the 1 mg/kg dose in both large and small dogs than in those given 30 mg/m^2, and it is possible that 1 mg/kg may be an inappropriately low dose for treatment of animals with cancer. For drugs that may produce severe myelosuppression, measurement of hematopoietic stem cell numbers for each individual patient would clearly provide the most information to prospectively calculate doses for chemotherapeutic agents. Until such a test is available, however, clinicians must use the doses available in the literature, always carefully taking into account the individual animal's response to the previous drug dose before administering the next treatment. If a doxorubicin dose of 1 mg/kg is well tolerated by a dog or cat weighing less than 10 kg, the next dose may be increased slightly, gradually approaching the dose calculated by BSA; this is called *dose escalation*. In daily clinical practice veterinarians judge the adequacy of therapy by measuring the response of visible, measurable masses; only much later are they able to evaluate the results of their treatment by survival results. In a rodent model for osteosarcoma, reduction in the dose intensity of melphalan and cyclophosphamide caused a marked decrease in the cure rate *long before there was a reduction in the rate of complete clinical remission*. On average, it is estimated that a dose reduction of approximately 20% leads to a loss of 50% in the cure rate. A positive relationship between dose intensity and response rate has been demonstrated in many human tumors, including lymphoma and ovarian, colon, and breast cancers. Clinicians should administer the highest dose of a chemotherapeutic drug that can be tolerated by the patient if they are attempting to cure; if palliation is the only goal, a dose that will produce clinical remission without dose escalation may be appropriate, however. Careful patient monitoring for therapeutic response and toxicity is still the best way to titrate the drug dose for each individual patient (Box 33-3).

Box 33-3

Timing of Chemotherapy (Dose–Schedule Relationships)

1. Intermittent high-dose ("pulse") therapy with cycle-specific and phase-specific agents produces more therapeutic benefit with less cumulative toxicity.
2. Intermittent therapy permits repair of normal tissues in the drug-free interval between doses.
3. Greater tumor cell kill may result from high drug gradients produced by intermittent high-dose therapy.
4. Timing of one drug in relation to another may permit some degree of tumor cell synchronization, followed by increased killing of such cells by a subsequent pulse of another phase-specific drug.
5. Pulse therapy is generally used in rapidly growing tumors, whereas continuous therapy using agents that kill at the resting phase is recommended for tumors that have a low growth fraction.
6. Continuous therapy is most effective with phase-specific drugs (cytosine arabinoside is often given by continuous ambulatory infusion for acute leukemias in humans), and pulse therapy is most commonly used for cycle-specific drugs.

Because chemotherapeutic drugs are quite toxic, the following guidelines for making the decision to begin chemotherapy are critically important:

1. Use chemotherapeutic agents only when a diagnosis of malignancy has been established definitively, either by cytology or histopathology.
2. Determine whether the particular tumor is known to respond to the treatment in a reasonable percentage of cases, with toxicities that will be tolerated by the patient and its owner.
3. Follow objective measurements of the tumor or its markers (e.g., hyperglobulinemia, hypercalcemia) if at all possible to determine whether the chemotherapy being administered is of benefit or should be discontinued.
4. Do not use chemotherapy in a patient unless proper supportive facilities are available for monitoring and treatment of any complications.
5. Do not use chemotherapy unless the animal's owner is likely to be compliant with instructions for drug administration and monitoring and will be observant of early signs of complications.

METRONOMIC CHEMOTHERAPY

Most chemotherapy targets rapidly dividing cells (preferably tumor cells, but inevitably some normal cells are also affected), and it is given at maximum tolerated doses (MTDs). Chemotherapy drugs also have another target: endothelial cells that form the lining of newly formed blood vessels, such as those whose creation is orchestrated by tumors to fuel their growth. There is a considerable body of evidence that even very low, almost nontoxic doses of chemotherapy drugs, when delivered frequently for a prolonged period of time, can retard tumor blood vessel growth (or angiogenesis) by destroying endothelial cells. Treatment approaches along these lines are now being tested in clinical trials, and they have been coined *metronomic chemotherapy.*

The treatment targets endothelial cell precursors (endothelial progenitor cells) that are recruited from the bone marrow and circulate to various sites in the body. Metronomic chemotherapy is given in very low doses repetitively (usually daily) over a long period of time compared with the MTD therapy that has been traditionally used. These repetitive low doses of chemotherapy drugs (cyclophosphamide at 10 mg/m^2 per day has been used most often in veterinary medicine) are designed to minimize toxicity and target the endothelium or tumor stroma, as opposed to targeting the tumor. Thus the treatment is theoretically useful to stabilize or slow tumor growth rather than kill tumor cells. Studies conducted in cell lines and animal models have also suggested that combining metronomic chemotherapy with targeted antiangiogenesis agents (e.g., piroxicam) is more effective than metronomic chemotherapy alone.

Metronomic chemotherapy will probably be most useful in slow-growing, indolent tumors, such as soft tissue sarcomas with a low mitotic index and well-differentiated carcinomas, particularly after debulking to microscopic disease. There is a low incidence of side effects, and the treatment is relatively inexpensive. The hope is that this treatment will allow some cancers to be treated as manageable chronic conditions.

COMMON SIDE EFFECTS OF CHEMOTHERAPY

Most clients are extremely satisfied with their experience with chemotherapeutic treatment of their pet's cancer. Fewer than one in four animals are reported to have significant side effects of chemotherapy, and only 5% will have a serious event that requires hospitalization. However, if a pet does experience a serious reaction, there are certainly adverse consequences. The animal's quality of life is decreased, at least for a time; there may be unexpected expenses for the owner associated with hospitalization and costly treatments; and it may be necessary to delay the next scheduled chemotherapy session, which sometimes allows the cancer to visibly return in the delayed interval between treatments. All this is likely to result in clients who are less enthusiastic about the idea of chemotherapy for their pet than they were before the occurrence of the unexpected side effect.

Many adverse effects of chemotherapy can be minimized or prevented by careful management, but some animals experience unanticipated side effects that no amount of care or forethought could have prevented. Certain breeds, especially Collies and rarely Australian Shepherds and Shetland Sheepdogs, are carriers of a mutation of the P-glycoprotein multidrug resistance 1 (MDR1) gene. If dogs that are homozygous for this gene are given anthracyclines or vinca alkaloids, the cellular excretion of the drugs is diminished, and they have increased drug exposure and thus increased toxicity. It is estimated that 70% of Collies in the United States are heterozygous for this mutated gene, and 31.2% of Collies are homozygous, with much lower percentages for Australian

Box 33-4

Three Growth Classes of Body Tissue

Static: Highly differentiated and have lost capacity to divide (e.g., nerve, muscle)

Expanding: Differentiated cells that survive for the lifetime of the organism and do not require replacement. With injury, however, the organ can replace lost cells (e.g., liver).

Renewing: Differentiated with a short life span requiring constant renewal (e.g., bone marrow, gastrointestinal mucosa, hair follicle)

Shepherds, Shetland Sheepdogs, and other herding dogs. A test for the mutation status of this gene is available through the Veterinary Clinical Pharmacology Laboratory at the College of Veterinary Medicine, University of Washington (http://www.vetmed.wsu.edu/depts-vcpl/). If this test is not performed, dogs of these breeds with cancer should be given conservatively low doses of anthracyclines and vinca alkaloids, or the drugs should not be given at all.

Cells of normal tissue are damaged by chemotherapy; most, given time, will recover. Tissues that are especially affected include those in which the cells have a short life span and require constant renewal (e.g., bone marrow, gastrointestinal mucosa, gonads, hair follicles). Box 33-4 provides a brief overview of the classes of body tissue and, if applicable, typical renewal properties.

Myelosuppression

Myelosuppression and subsequent infection are the most common dose-limiting toxic effects of chemotherapy. Drugs that can be particularly myelosuppressive in dogs and cats include lomustine (CCNU), cyclophosphamide, carboplatin, doxorubicin (particularly when used in combination with another chemotherapeutic agent), and vinblastine. In some cats vincristine has been noted to produce a marked and prolonged neutropenia.

Many mechanisms contribute to infection after chemotherapy. Certain chemotherapeutic agents prevent phagocyte mobilization or impair function of these cells. Some cancers infiltrate the bone marrow, producing myelophthisis and contributing to cytopenias. Suppression of leukopoiesis by chemotherapy drugs may lead to associated barrier disruptions of the skin, oral cavity, and alimentary tract mucus, and the normal pulmonary "mucociliary elevator" may not function effectively to clear bacterial organisms. Endogenous bacterial infections may develop, caused by the host's native microbial flora; these are commonly due to aerobic and anaerobic gram-negative bacteria from the gastrointestinal tract or *Staphylococcus* organisms from the skin. In addition, hospitalized patients frequently develop catheter-related bacteremias, often caused by microbes transmitted to the susceptible patient from the hospital environment or from another animal; these organisms may be antibiotic resistant. Patients with absolute neutrophil numbers greater than 1500/μL are generally protected against endogenous infections. If the number is between 1000 and 1500/μL, the owner is advised to monitor the animal's condition and report any fever or anorexia. If the number is between 500 to 1000/μL, prophylactic antibiotics are generally dispensed unless the period of neutropenia is anticipated to be very short. When the absolute neutrophil number is less than 500/μL, treatment with granulocyte colony-stimulating factor (G-CSF, filgrastim, Neupogen, Amgen) or granulocyte/macrophage colony-stimulating factor (GM-CSF, sargramostim, Leukine, Berlex) may be considered (discussed later), although many patients recover without the administration of one of these cytokines—of course, antibiotics should also be administered. If the patient is *not* febrile, it should probably not be hospitalized because its likelihood of acquiring a hospital-acquired resistant bacterial infection is high. If the patient is febrile, however, it should usually be hospitalized for blood cultures and intravenous antibiotic administration. In general, antibiotics should not be given prophylactically for neutropenia unless they are necessary, because they increase the risks for development of bacterial resistance and fungal infection in these immunocompromised patients. When necessary, choice of an empirical antibiotic regimen should take into account the type of infection the patient is likely to have: home acquired (probably endogenous) or hospital acquired (likely to be exogenous and possibly antibiotic resistant). Appropriate antibiotic combinations for use in the febrile neutropenic patient would be an aminoglycoside (e.g., amikacin) plus an antipseudomonal penicillin (ticarcillin, carbenicillin, piperacillin) or cephalosporin (cephalothin, cefazolin, cefoxitin). The third-generation cephalosporin ceftazidime is an antibiotic with an excellent spectrum of efficacy against gram-negative bacteria and *Pseudomonas,* and it is moderately effective for treatment of *Staphylococcus* infections. Because it has poor efficacy against anaerobic organisms, it must be combined with a drug such as clindamycin, metronidazole, or an antipseudomonal penicillin; these combinations are very useful in treating infections in neutropenic cancer patients. Imipenem is useful as a single agent in these patients, with excellent efficacy against enteric gram-negative bacteria, *Pseudomonas*, anaerobes, and *Staphylococcus*, but the high cost of this antibiotic limits its use in veterinary medicine at this time. It is also an antibiotic that should probably be reserved for use in humans with antibiotic-resistant infections.

If myelosuppression is severe and life-threatening, recombinant G-CSF or GM-CSF is often administered. These products are human glycoproteins that regulate production of neutrophils within the bone marrow; they are produced in *Escherichia coli* bacteria. Both stimulate neutrophil progenitor proliferation, differentiation, and functional activity with minimal toxicity. Long-term (i.e., longer than 30 days) use of human G-CSF in the dog or cat results in antibody formation, however, with significant and prolonged decreases in neutrophil counts. At a daily dose of 5 μg/kg subcutaneously, the effects of canine G-CSF on the normal canine bone marrow are rapid and predictable: Mean neutrophil counts in normal dogs increased to 26,330/μL after one injection, with a maximum count of 72,125/μL by day 19 of administration. The neutrophil counts returned to normal in these dogs within 5 days after daily therapy was discontinued.[4] Canine G-CSF is not commercially available, but recombinant human G-CSF has resulted in similar elevations of neutrophil counts in the dog. In cats 10 to 14 days of human G-CSF resulted in maximum neutrophil counts ranging from 20,370 to 61,400/μL.[5] Thus a short course of G-CSF may be used in dogs or cats either *before* aggressive chemotherapy, in an attempt to ameliorate or prevent myelosuppression, or as a rescue *after* chemotherapy has induced significant neutropenia.

Gastrointestinal Side Effects

Another frequent side effect of chemotherapy relates to the gastrointestinal toxicity of these drugs; anorexia, vomiting, and diarrhea may be noted in some individuals treated with cytotoxic agents. These side effects are not noted in dogs and cats as predictably as in humans, but they can occur in sensitive individuals with most of the commonly used drugs. Agents with a high potential for acute nausea after administration include cisplatin, dacarbazine, and high-dose cyclophosphamide; those with a moderate potential include carboplatin, conventional-dose cyclophosphamide, doxorubicin, mitoxantrone, and occasionally vincristine. In animals with only mild to moderate nausea, metoclopramide (0.2 to 0.5 mg/kg orally or subcutaneously thrice daily), or prochlorperazine (0.3 mg/kg orally or subcutaneously thrice daily) may be effective. Premedicating with subcutaneous administration of butorphanol at 0.4 mg/kg will sometimes block the postadministration vomiting caused by cisplatin. In animals with severe nausea and vomiting caused by chemotherapy (which is rare, fortunately), one of the serotonin 5-hydroxytryptamine (5-HT) receptor antagonists may be given either orally, subcutaneously, intramuscularly, or rectally. The most commonly available member of this class of drugs is ondansetron, but several newer antiemetics of the class are now also available (e.g., dolasetron), and the price of the drugs has dropped to make them reasonable to use now that ondansetron is available as a generic. The dose of ondansetron in the dog is 0.1 to 0.3 mg/lb intravenously or subcutaneously twice daily (oral dose is 0.5 to 1 mg/kg every 12 to 24 hours), and the dose of dolasetron is 0.5 to 0.6 mg/kg subcutaneously or intravenously every 24 hours. The serotonin receptor antagonists act more specifically than other antiemetics to prevent the vomiting induced by chemotherapy or radiation. Serotonin receptors of the 5-HT type are located on vagus nerve terminals and in the chemoreceptor trigger zone. Serotonin is released from enterochromaffin cells in the small intestine when they are severely damaged. The released serotonin stimulates vagal afferents through the 5-HT receptors, and nausea and vomiting ensue. Ondansetron and dolasetron block the 5-HT receptor site, which prevents the serotonin effect.

A new antiemetic that is proving to be very effective in the control of chemotherapy-induced nausea and vomiting is maropitant (Cerenia). It is a neurokinin-1 (NK-1) receptor antagonist and is available both in injectable form and as tablets; the dose is 1 mg/kg subcutaneously once daily or 2 mg/kg orally once daily. The NK-1 receptor antagonists drugs work at NK-1 receptors in the emetic center to block both peripheral and central stimuli that cause emesis, by inhibiting the binding of substance P. Substance P is found in significant concentrations in the nuclei that make up the emetic center and plays a central role as a neurotransmitter in the afferent pathways of the emetic reflex.

Other gastrointestinal side effects may also occur as sequelae to chemotherapy drug administration. Diarrhea occurs much less often than vomiting and nausea and is generally readily treated with loperamide (0.08 mg/kg orally thrice daily). Doxorubicin sometimes produces a severe hemorrhagic colitis in dogs, for which hospitalization and symptomatic treatment with antibiotics and intravenous fluids may be necessary; rarely, this side effect caused by doxorubicin can be life-threatening. Anorexia may be noted with several drugs, especially in cats with doxorubicin or vincristine administration. Appetite stimulation with drugs such as cyproheptadine may help in these cats, but enteral feeding is sometimes necessary.

Phlebitis and Necrosis

Several commonly used chemotherapeutic drugs will produce phlebitis or local necrosis (or both) at the site of administration if extravasated. Drugs that can be expected to produce severe reactions include the vinca alkaloids, doxorubicin, and dactinomycin; moderate reactions may be seen with bleomycin, cisplatin, dacarbazine, and mitoxantrone. These cytotoxic drugs may irritate the lining of access veins during administration, producing phlebitis, or may escape the cutaneous vasculature and spread throughout the surrounding tissues, causing a local inflammatory reaction (chemical cellulitis). Alternatively, some of the drugs will produce local tissue necrosis if extravasated. Doxorubicin produces the most dramatic and severe reactions. Extravasation will produce marked epidermal hyperplasia, with mitosis of many epidermal cells at the margins of the lesion; the reaction will contain individual necrotic keratinocytes, lobular panniculitis, and reactive fibroblasts and endothelial cells. No inflammatory reaction will be seen. In the area of direct extravasation, pan-epidermal, dermal, and subcutaneous tissue necrosis will be present. This necrosis begins 1 to 2 weeks after the drug is extravasated and may continue for up to 4 months. With all these drugs, extreme precautions should be taken to prevent extravasation, particularly with venipuncture and catheter placement. A "first-stick" catheter should always be used; infusion through a preexisting catheter is not advised. The animal should be observed closely (and possibly restrained) during the entire time of the infusion, in case movement should dislodge the catheter.

Infusion of the chemotherapy drug should be terminated immediately if the patient shows signs of pain during drug administration or if there is blebbing at the catheter or needle entrance site. If the catheter or needle is still present, the clinician should aspirate any fluid from the extravasated area. A continuing dilemma in the management of extravasation injuries is the absence of evidence-based management strategies. Almost all the recommendations in the literature are (of course) based on anecdotes; even knowing for sure that an extravasation occurred is sometimes difficult, so assessing whether there has been a positive response to a particular treatment is also questionable. However, the current recommendations for vinca alkaloid extravasation are to inject 150 units of hyaluronidase (if available; hyaluronidase has become difficult to obtain) through the patent catheter or needle and then apply local heat for 15 to 30 minutes four times daily for 48 hours. For anthracycline extravasation, the clinician should apply an ice pack for 15 to 30 minutes four times daily and 90% dimethyl sulfoxide (DMSO) topically several times daily for 7 to 14 days; surgical removal should be considered if the area of extravasation is confined. DMSO is a free radical scavenger that causes potent vasodilation and has pain reduction and antiinflammatory mechanisms. Dexrazoxane is a drug that has been used to prevent anthracycline-induced cardiotoxicity. It may also decrease free radical formation, and when given intravenously immediately after extravasation (1000 mg/m^2 intravenously, repeated at the same dose the next day), it appears to prevent the tissue necrosis associated with anthracycline extravasation. Growth factors regulate and coordinate wound healing, and they may also be helpful in altering damage from chemotherapy drug extravasation. In animal models both G-CSF and GM-CSF have been shown to be significantly better than saline or no treatment in decreasing the severity and extent of necrosis with doxorubicin extravasations. In one human patient who did not respond to injected dexrazoxane, GM-CSF injected into an ulcerated area of extravasation led to tissue granulation and complete healing within 8 weeks. With any luck, clinicians will never have to use the following protocol: A 1-mL vial of GM-CSF was diluted with saline. Several small injections were then given within the borders of the ulcer. As new granulation tissue formed, GM-CSF injections were given three times weekly for 2 weeks, then twice a week for 2 weeks. Because treatment of extravasation injuries is not yet uniformly effective in preventing the local irritation and necrosis caused by extravasation of these drugs, prevention is the best answer.

Alopecia

Alopecia is common in certain breeds of dogs after chemotherapy, particularly after administration of doxorubicin or cyclophosphamide. Hair loss is predictable in Poodles and in mixed-breed dogs of Poodle lineage; it is also commonly seen in Terriers and Old English Sheepdogs. Occasionally, it may be noted in other breeds as well. It is common for cats to lose their whiskers during chemotherapy. For some owners the alopecia induced by chemotherapy is very distressing, and owners of breeds in which this is likely to occur should be prepared for this possibility. Hair regrowth begins 1 to 2 months after chemotherapy is discontinued. However, an alteration in the color or texture of the new hair may be noted; the regrown hair may be a lighter or darker shade and may be softer or curlier than the animal's previous hair.

Reproductive Side Effects

Although generally less important in dogs and cats with cancer than in humans, the effects of chemotherapy on gonadal function should be explained to owners considering treatment, particularly if the animal is shown or has been used for breeding. Most chemotherapy drugs will cause hypofertility or infertility by impairing production of sperm and oocytes. In the male animal, loss of libido may result from Leydig cell dysfunction and decreased testosterone levels, especially with corticosteroid treatment for lymphoma. Owners should consider cryostorage of sperm from the dog before beginning chemotherapy. However, it is common to find on semen evaluation that general debility from the cancer itself has resulted in poor semen quality even before chemotherapy drugs have been given. Reversibility of gonadal dysfunction produced by chemotherapy is variable depending on the agent administered, the dose intensity of the protocol used for treatment, and the age of the patient itself. During chemotherapy and for a variable period after the treatment is completed, a male dog or cat should not be used for breeding and a female should not become pregnant because congenital malformations may result in the offspring.

Palmar–Plantar Erythrodysesthesia

Palmar–plantar erythrodysesthesia (PPES), also known as hand–foot syndrome in humans, has been seen with constant-rate infusions of doxorubicin, cyclophosphamide, ifosfamide, 5-fluorouracil, and other agents in humans. In dogs PPES has been most commonly associated with the administration of liposome-encapsulated doxorubicin (Doxil).[6] PPES is a primarily a dermal toxicity characterized by reddening of the skin. It is followed by edema and eventual ulceration of the skin. PPES tends to occur in areas of friction, such as the weight-bearing portions of the feet and the axillary regions. Histologically, these lesions are described as focal areas of parakeratosis, acantholysis, and chronic active inflammation of the skin and underlying dermis. PPES often resolves quickly after discontinuation of the drug but may recur if the drug is reinstituted. Oral pyroxidine may help ameliorate some of the side effects, although it will not completely prevent PPES.[7]

Human Health Hazards

Exposure of hospital personnel and owners to carcinogenic, mutagenic, and teratogenic drugs and drug-containing animal waste must be considered. In the days before clinicians took appropriate precautions when mixing and administering chemotherapy, there were many reports in the human literature of fetal loss and birth of infants with congenital defects among nurses and pharmacy staff members who were frequently exposed to chemotherapy drugs.[8,9] Proper storage, preparation, and administration of chemotherapeutic agents, as well as proper disposal of cytotoxic drug waste and urine and stool of the animal being treated, should be a concern of every clinician who treats an animal for cancer.[8,9] Reviews on proper handling of chemotherapy in the workplace are available; the Occupational Safety and Health Administration (OSHA) publication "Controlling Occupational Exposure to Hazardous Drugs" may be downloaded from OSHA's website (www.osha.gov/dts/osta/otm/otm_vi/otm_vi_2.html).

DRUGS USED IN CANCER CHEMOTHERAPY

The following sections cover drugs commonly used in veterinary oncology for the treatment of canine and feline neoplasia (Table 33-2). Included are cautionary comments regarding administration, toxicity, and effectiveness. Note that dosages for chemotherapy drugs vary greatly depending on tumor type and protocol used. It is extremely important that a clinician considering the use of one of these drugs as a single agent or in a combination protocol carefully consider all of the drug's possible toxicities rather than merely look up a dose from a chart or formulary.

Alkylating Agents

Nitrogen Mustards

Cyclophosphamide

Mechanism of action. Cyclophosphamide is a classic alkylating agent that is extensively metabolized in the liver to the active cytotoxic metabolites phosphoramide mustard and acrolein. The metabolite phosphoramide mustard is responsible for most of the antineoplastic effects of the drug. Cyclophosphamide is cell cycle specific at normal dosing schedules but may be cell cycle nonspecific at extremely high doses. Resistance to treatment with cyclophosphamide does develop in tumor cells, probably related to increased ability of the tumor cells to produce glutathione and obtain protection from oxidative damage. Excretion takes place principally by the kidneys, and modification of dose and dose interval should be considered when a patient has significant renal disease.

Preparations. Cyclophosphamide is available as 25-mg and 50-mg tablets for oral administration as well as an intravenous preparation in vials containing 100 mg, 200 mg, or 500 mg. The drug is equally effective when given orally or parenterally. Cyclophosphamide cannot be used for intracavitary treatment because it must be metabolized to its active form in the liver.

Side effects. Cyclophosphamide has the potential for extremely dangerous marrow suppression as well as nausea and vomiting. Of all the chemotherapeutic drugs in common use in veterinary oncology, neutropenia occurs most predictably with cyclophosphamide. As a result, the drug must initially be administered with great caution; the degree of myelosuppression varies from patient to patient but may be early and profound. For this reason neutrophil counts must be carefully assessed whenever the drug is used for the first time in a patient. Some animals will develop myelosuppression after a week of cyclophosphamide; in others the drug will have to be discontinued after 3 to 5 days because of severe neutropenia or thrombocytopenia. A baseline total white blood cell count, differential, and platelet estimate should be taken before the drug is administered. Usually, depression in the absolute neutrophil count begins on the third day of administration, so the next blood count is taken on that day. From that day on during the first cycle of cyclophosphamide therapy, a total leukocyte count, differential, and platelet estimate are obtained every day until the cycle of cyclophosphamide therapy is completed. If the absolute neutrophil count drops below 3000/μL, the drug is discontinued entirely for that cycle; on the next cycle, it is reinstituted at a dose 25% less than the initial daily dose. If the neutrophil count drops to less than 1500/μL, the drug is stopped and reinstituted on the next cycle at a dose 50% less than the initial dose. If the number of neutrophils drops to less than 1000/μL and fever ensues, empirical antibiotic therapy should be begun. Recombinant human G-CSF may also be given for several days if necessary until the animal's neutrophil count returns to normal. After the animal's individual tolerance for cyclophosphamide is determined, fewer CBCs will need to be checked during therapy. In maintenance protocols one CBC per cycle before administration of the drug begins is generally adequate.

Hemorrhagic cystitis may result from cyclophosphamide administration, usually after long-term use; however, it has been reported after one intravenous administration.[10] It is caused by the metabolite acrolein, which is excreted in urine and reaches a urine level of 100 to 200 times the serum concentration; this metabolite is extremely irritating to the bladder mucosa and produces necrosis of smooth muscle. Chronic cystitis leading to bladder fibrosis may occur with long-term use. Affected dogs and cats will present with clinical signs of gross hematuria, often with blood clots, and will be reported to be straining to urinate. Concurrent treatment with prednisone decreases the incidence of hemorrhagic cystitis, probably by causing polydipsia and polyuria. Lymphoma patients rarely develop this complication, insofar as prednisone administration is generally a part of the treatment protocol. Any animal that is to receive cyclophosphamide should have a urinalysis performed before the drug is administered to rule out preexisting hematuria caused by bacterial cystitis or prostatitis. The client should be warned to watch for hematuria during the course of treatment with cyclophosphamide, and administration should cease immediately if the problem is noted. Several precautions can help prevent this problem while an animal is receiving cyclophosphamide. The animal should be encouraged to drink more fluids; salting food and offering beef or chicken bouillon may help increase fluid intake. Because the cystitis is caused by acrolein producing local irritation on the bladder mucosa, the owner should encourage frequent urination by walking his or her dog more frequently and should make sure that the dog is allowed to urinate before retiring for the night. It is better not to administer cyclophosphamide in the evening because acrolein will then concentrate in the urine overnight. Although the free radical scavengers acetylcysteine and mesna have been reported to prevent cyclophosphamide-induced hemorrhagic cystitis in humans treated with high-dose cyclophosphamide before bone marrow transplantation, it is not clear that they are necessary in dogs and cats treated with standard chemotherapy protocols. The incidence of this side effect seems to be low with most current cyclophosphamide dosing regimens, which use intermittent "pulse" doses of cyclophosphamide rather than continuous daily dosing of the drug.

Alopecia occurs in susceptible dogs as another side effect of cyclophosphamide. When cyclophosphamide is used in

Table 33-2 Commonly Used Chemotherapy Agents

Drug	Indications	Dose	Route	Common Side Effects
Alkylating Agents				
Cyclophosphamide	LSA, MCT, carcinoma, sarcoma	Given orally divided over 4 days or intravenously at 200-250 mg/m^2 Metronomic: 10 mg/m^2 per day	PO or IV	Myelosuppression, gastrointestinal upset, alopecia, sterile hemorrhagic cystitis
Chlorambucil	Small cell LSA, CLL, thymoma, MCT, IBD, in place of cyclophosphamide	20 mg/m^2 PO every 14 days 15 mg/m^2 per week divided into 3 doses 0.8 mg/kg in COP protocol 1.4 mg/kg in the CHOP protocol	PO	Myelosuppression, gastrointestinal upset, alopecia
Dacarbazine	LSA rescue	200 mg/m^2 IV slow push daily for 5 days; 1000 mg/m^2 IV over several hours every 3 weeks	IV	Vesicant, myelosuppression, vomiting during administration, gastrointestinal upset, alopecia
Lomustine	LSA rescue, cutaneous LSA, MCT, histiocytic neoplasia, brain tumors, GME	50-70 mg/m^2 PO every 21 days	PO	Severe myelosuppression, hepatotoxicity, possible renal toxicity
Mechlorethamine	LSA rescue	3 mg/m^2 IV in the MOPP protocol	IV	Vesicant, myelosuppression, gastrointestinal upset, alopecia
Melphalan	Multiple myeloma, plasma cell tumors, anal sac adenocarcinoma, melanoma	For multiple myeloma dose 0.1 mg/kg daily for 10 days, then decrease to 0.05 mg/kg daily every other day. Pulse dosing: 7 mg/m^2 daily for 5 days every 3 weeks	PO	Myelosuppression (can be severe), mild gastrointestinal upset, alopecia.
Antimetabolites				
5-Fluorouracil	Carcinomas and sarcomas, gastrointestinal tumors	150 mg/m^2 once weekly	IV, topically	Fatal to cats, myelosuppression, neurotoxicity, alopecia, gastrointestinal upset
Cytosine arabinoside	LSA, GME, renal LSA in cats	150 mg/m^2 SC bid for 2 days (consecutively) or 600 mg/m^2 IV once weekly	SC, IM or IV	Myelosuppresion, gastrointestinal upset, alopecia
Methotrexate	LSA, OSA	0.8 mg/kg in combination with other chemotherapy drugs	IV or PO	Myelosuppression and gastrointestinal upset
Antitumor Antibiotics				
Doxorubicin	LSA, various sarcomas and carcinomas	30 mg/m^2 IV every 14-21 days (dogs); 1 mg/kg IV every 14-21 days (cats and small dogs)	IV	Vesicant, myelosuppression, cardiovascular (dogs), nephrotoxic (cats), hypersensitivity-like reactions, hemorrhagic colitis, alopecia, gastrointestinal upset
Mitoxantrone	TCC, Prostatic carcinoma, in place of doxorubicin, malignant effusions	Dogs: 5-5.5 mg/m^2 IV every 21 days; Cats: 6 mg/m^2 IV every 21 days	IV or IC	Myelosuppression, alopecia, gastrointestinal upset, blue color to urine, sclera or saliva
Actinomycin D	LSA, in place of doxorubicin	0.75-0.8 mg/m^2 IV every 21 days	IV	Vesicant, myelosuppression, alopecia, gastrointestinal upset
Antitubululin Agents				
Vincristine	LSA, MCT, TVT, ITP,	0.5-0.7 mg/m^2	IV	Vesicant, peripheral neuropathies, myelosuppression, alopecia, gastrointestinal upset
Vinblastine	MCT, in place of vincristine	2-2.3 mg/m^2 IV weekly or every other week	IV	Vesicant, alopecia, gastrointestinal upset
Vinorelbine	Primary lung tumors	12-15 mg/m^2 weekly or every other week	IV	Vesicant, alopecia, gastrointestinal upset

Table 33-2 Commonly Used Chemotherapy Agents—cont'd

Drug	Indications	Dose	Route	Common Side Effects
Paclitaxel	Carcinomas	Dogs: 132 mg/m² every 21 days; Cats: 80 mg/m² every 21 days	IV	Not recommended in cats because of hypersensitivity reactions (also seen in dogs, but less severe), arrhythmias, myelosuppression, alopecia, gastrointestinal upset
Docetaxel	Carcinomas	1.25 mg/m² IV every 21 days	IV	Hypersensitivity, acceptable in cats, arrhythmias, myelosuppression, alopecia, gastrointestinal upset.
Platinum Agents				
Cisplatin	OSA, seminoma, thyroid carcinoma, SCC, malignant effusions	70 mg/m² IV every 21 days	IV or IC	Fatal to cats, nephrotoxicity, immediate emesis, myelosuppression, gastrointestinal upset, alopecia, ototoxicity
Carboplatin	OSA, carcinomas	250-300 mg/m² every 21 days (dogs); 200-250 mg/m² every 21 days (cats)	IV	Myelosuppression, dose reduction in animals with renal insufficiency, gastrointestinal upset, alopecia
Miscellaneous Drugs				
Hydroxyurea	Polycythemia vera, brain tumors, myelodysplastic disease	50 mg/kg per day tapering to every other day once in remission (dogs); 10 mg/kg/day tapering to every other day once in remission (cats)	PO	Toe nail sloughing, myelosuppression, alopecia, gastrointestinal upset (mild)
L-Asparaginase	LSA	400 IU/kg or 10,000 IU/m²	SC, IM, or IP	Myelosuppression when given with vincristine, hypersensitivity
Procarbazine	LSA	50 mg/m² daily for 14 days with the MOPP protocol	PO	Myelosuppression and gastrointestinal toxicity
Receptor Tyrosine Kinase Inhibitors				
Toceranib	MCT, various other tumors	3.25 mg/kg every other day or Monday/Wednesday/Friday schedule	PO	Myelosuppression, proteinuria, gastric ulceration, diarrhea, vomiting, rash, muscle pain
Masitinib	MCT, various other tumors	12.5 mg/kg daily	PO	Myelosuppression, proteinuria, gastric ulceration, diarrhea, vomiting, skin rash

LSA, Lymphosarcoma; *MCT,* mast cell tumor; *IV,* intravenously; *PO,* by mouth; *CLL,* chronic lymphocytic leukemia; *IBD,* inflammatory bowel disease; *COP,* cyclophosphamide, vincristine, prednisone; *CHOP,* cyclophosphamide, doxorubicin, vincristine, prednisone; *GME,* granulomatous meningoencephalitis; *MOPP,* mechlorethamine, oncovin, procarbazine, and prednisone; *SC,* subcutaneously; *IM,* intramuscularly; *OSA,* osteosarcoma; *TCC,* transitional cell carcinoma; *IC,* intracavitary; *TVT,* transmissible venereal tumor; *ITP,* immune-mediated thrombocytopenia; SCC, squamous cell carcinoma; IP, intraperitoneally.

combination with doxorubicin or dactinomycin, cardiotoxicity of these compounds may be potentiated.

Dosing regimen. Cyclophosphamide is usually given in doses from 50 to 100 mg/m² daily orally for 4 to 7 days per week according to the particular tumor protocol. It may also be given intravenously at 200 mg/m² once weekly, but this protocol is likely to be dangerously myelosuppressive in some dogs.

Melphalan (phenylalanine mustard)

Mechanism of action. Melphalan is an alkylating agent that is a phenylalanine derivative of mechlorethamine, the first chemotherapeutic agent discovered. In World War I, it was noted that troops who had received poisoning with mustard gas often had aplastic anemia and severe lymphopenia, with depletion of lymphocytes in the spleen and lymph nodes. This finding caused clinicians to study the effects of nitrogen mustard on lymphoma, first in the mouse and later in humans. Many derivatives of this original compound have been discovered, but melphalan remains one of the most useful.

Spectrum of activity. In dogs and cats, melphalan is generally used for the treatment of plasma cell tumors, either plasma cell myeloma or extramedullary plasmacytoma.[11]

Preparations. Melphalan is available for oral use as a scored 2-mg tablet and for intravenous injection as a 50-mg vial. In dogs and cats, the drug is conventionally used orally.

Side effects. Myelosuppression is the most common side effect of melphalan, but it is not generally severe. Monitoring of a CBC should be done every 2 weeks during induction and then monthly during maintenance.

Dosing regimen. The recommended dose for melphalan is 0.1 mg/kg daily for 7 to 10 days, then 0.05 mg/kg daily until remission is achieved. The drug is then given as a maintenance agent for 7 days out of every month at 0.1 mg/kg per day. Because food can apparently decrease the oral absorption of the drug, it should be given several hours before the animal is fed.

Mechlorethamine

Mechanism of action. Mechlorethamine (Mustargen), is the prototypical nitrogen mustard. These drugs alkylate DNA by initially losing a chlorine molecule and allowing the β-carbon to react with the nucleophilic nitrogen atom to form the cyclic, positively charged, and very reactive aziridinium moiety. The reaction between this aziridinium ring and the electron-rich nucleophile creates the initial alkylated product. Cross-linking of the DNA occurs when a second aziridinium ring is formed by the remaining chloroethyl group, allowing for a second alkylation.

Spectrum of activity. In dogs it is used as a rescue agent in the MOPP protocol (*m*echlorethamine, *o*ncovin, *p*rocarbazine, and *p*rednisone) for high-grade lymphoma.

Preparations. Mechlorethamine is available in 5-g and 25-g bottles for reconstitution. It is also available in a topical preparation for mycosis fungoides; however, because of the risk of human exposure, the topical preparation is not recommended for veterinary use.

Side effects. Myelosuppression is the most common side effect of this drug; however, it is a potent vesicant and is irritating topically. The gastrointestinal side effects appear to be more severe with this drug than the other nitrogen mustards. A CBC should be performed 7 to 10 days after each dose and before each dose.

Dosing regimen. In the MOPP protocol, this drug is dosed at 3 mg/m^2 on days 1 and 7 of the 28-day protocol.

Chlorambucil

Mechanism of action. Chlorambucil is another of the derivatives of nitrogen mustard; it is the slowest acting and least toxic of the alkylating agents commonly used in veterinary medicine. The drug is easily absorbed by passive diffusion when administered orally, so any food given with it may interfere with its absorption.

Spectrum of activity. Chlorambucil is used as a mainstay for treatment of chronic lymphocytic leukemia,[12] small cell lymphoma, Waldenström's macroglobulinemia, and thymoma in dogs and cats. It has been substituted in combination chemotherapy protocols for cyclophosphamide when hemorrhagic cystitis has ensued but is not especially effective for maintenance therapy of high-grade lymphomas. Activity may also be seen against plasma cell myeloma and ovarian carcinoma.

Preparations. Chlorambucil is available as a 2-mg tablet for oral administration only.

Side effects. Marrow suppression is quite late, gradual in onset, and rapidly reversible in dogs and cats but may be profound if it is not discovered sufficiently early. In general, myelosuppression is not seen until the drug has been given daily for at least 1 month; it is recommended that a CBC be obtained once every 2 weeks during induction. As soon as remission occurs, the drug should be administered only intermittently as a maintenance protocol (i.e., alternate weeks or 1 week out of 4). Chlorambucil should not be administered with food.

Dosing regimen. The dose for chlorambucil is 0.1 to 0.2 mg/kg orally per day for 4 to 7 days, then 0.1 mg/kg daily until remission occurs. Alternatively, the drug may be given once every 2 weeks at a dose of 0.4 mg/kg. After remission is obtained, a maintenance protocol may be started, with the drug administered intermittently as indicated by the tumor treated (e.g., 0.1 mg/kg daily for 7 consecutive days, followed by 21 days off).

Nitrosoureas

Mechanism of action. CCNU (lomustine) and BCNU (carmustine) are drugs that are very lipid soluble and cross the blood–brain barrier with ease. Excretion is primarily renal, so dose modification must be considered if the patient has renal disease.

Spectrum of activity. Although CCNU and BCNU are used in humans to treat certain lymphomas, the drugs find their principal use in veterinary medicine for treatment of central nervous system (CNS) neoplasia.[13,14] The two drugs are unique in their ability to attain therapeutic levels in brain tissue. Recent information suggests that CCNU may also have some efficacy in treatment of canine mast cell tumor.

Preparations. BCNU is available in a 100-mg vial for intravenous administration; CCNU is given orally and is available as 10-, 40-, and 100-mg capsules.

Side effects. Both the nitrosoureas may be quite emetogenic immediately after administration. The vomiting and nausea usually last less than 24 hours after administration, and the animal's discomfort can generally be ameliorated with butorphanol given subcutaneously at 0.4 mg/kg thrice daily. In some cases, ondansetron will be necessary to relieve symptoms.

Prolonged bone marrow suppression is common with both of the nitrosoureas. Neutropenia may be noted as early as 1 week after administration but may persist for up to 6 weeks. In some cases neutropenia is severe enough to adversely affect the animal's quality of life, and treatment with intravenous antibiotics and recombinant human G-CSF may be necessary if the animal becomes febrile.

Dosing regimen. BCNU must be given intravenously. The product is reconstituted with alcohol and then added to saline or 5% dextrose in water to be given as an intravenous infusion over 1 to 2 hours. Severe pain may be seen at the injection site even if no extravasation is occurring; a longer infusion time may help decrease discomfort from the administration. The conventional dose of BCNU is 50 mg/m^2 given intravenously once every 6 weeks. CCNU is available as an oral preparation, and it is given as a single oral dose of 75 to 100 mg/m^2 once every 6 to 8 weeks.

Dacarbazine

Mechanism of action. The major mode of action of dacarbazine against tumor cells appears to be alkylation of nucleic acids. Its complete chemical name is 5-(3,3-dimethyl-1-triazeno)-imidazole-4-carboxamide, which is why it is also called *DTIC.* Dacarbazine is cycle specific.

Spectrum of activity. Dacarbazine is not often used in veterinary oncology. At one time, it was suggested as a treatment for canine melanosarcoma, but results were disappointing.

Dacarbazine has its major use for treatment of relapsed lymphoma in combination with doxorubicin.[15]

Preparations. Dacarbazine is available for intravenous administration in vials of 100, 200, and 500 mg.

Side effects. Local pain is often seen during administration; concentrated solutions of the drug are very irritating to veins, and extravasation will produce severe phlebitis. Myelosuppression is mild and does not occur until the second or third week after treatment, but a CBC should be checked before each subsequent treatment is administered. Vomiting and nausea are common during the first few days of treatment but can usually be blocked by prior administration of chemoreceptor trigger zone–blocking antiemetics. These gastrointestinal symptoms may be lessened by using a lower dose initially and gradually escalating the dose during the course of treatment, but the signs seem to subside after 1 or 2 days of treatment despite continued therapy with dacarbazine.

Dosing regimen. Dosage is 150 to 250 mg/m^2 given slowly intravenously for 5 days. Treatment is repeated every 3 weeks.

Mitotic Inhibitors

Vinca Alkaloids

Mechanism of action. The vinca alkaloids are extracted from the common periwinkle plant, *Vinca rosea.* This plant was originally investigated by pharmacologists because of its reported ability to lower blood glucose levels in several native populations. Although its efficacy as a hypoglycemic agent proved unimpressive, it was discovered that extracts of the plant had cytotoxic effects. Eventually, vincristine and vinblastine came into common clinical use as anticancer agents; the two compounds differ only slightly, with vincristine having a formyl side chain and vinblastine having a methyl side chain on the larger parent molecule. A third vinca alkaloid has recently become more popular in the veterinary market. Vinorelbine (Navelbine) acts similarly to the other vinca alkaloids, with the exception that it achieves very high concentrations within the lung parenchyma. All of the drugs appear to act as spindle poisons by binding to microtubular proteins within cells. The spindles are thus unable to act during mitosis, leading to arrest of the cell in metaphase. Generally, vincristine is thought of as a phase-specific drug effective only in the M phase of the cell cycle. Vinblastine, however, also blocks the cell's utilization of glutamic acid, thus inhibiting purine synthesis. For this reason vinblastine acts against cells in active mitosis but also in other phases of the cell cycle.

Spectrum of activity. Vincristine and vinblastine have their major use in veterinary medicine in combination chemotherapy protocols for treatment of lymphoma and lymphoid leukemias. Some efficacy of vincristine may be seen either as a single agent[16] or in combination with doxorubicin and cyclophosphamide for treatment of soft tissue sarcomas,[17] and vincristine is the drug of choice for treatment of transmissible venereal tumors.[18,19] Although it was previously suggested that vincristine might be effective in the treatment of mast cell tumor in the dog, a recent report has discounted the drug's role in management of this tumor; only 2 of 27 dogs with mast cell tumors had even a partial response to vincristine given at 0.75 mg/m^2.[20] The principal use of vinblastine in veterinary oncology at this time is in the treatment of mast cell tumors. It has been shown to be much more effective than vincristine at treating this disease, with reported response rates of 40% when combined with prednisone.[21] It may also be used as a substitute for vincristine in a combination chemotherapy protocol when a vincristine-induced neuropathy has been noted. Vinorelbine has been used primarily against primary lung tumors, especially well-differentiated ones such as bronchogenic carcinomas and bronchoalveolar carcinomas.

Preparations. Vincristine is available for intravenous use in 1-mg, 2-mg, and 5-mg vials. Vinblastine is also for intravenous administration only and is supplied in 10-mg vials. Vinorelbine comes in 10-mg or 50-mg vials of a 10 mg/mL solution.

Side effects. Because of its phase-specific effects, vincristine is not generally myelosuppressive in the dog; occasionally, it may produce significant neutropenia in the cat.[22] Anorexia and nausea are sometimes seen in both dogs and cats treated with vincristine, especially at the higher levels of the dose range. Unlike vincristine, vinblastine is quite myelosuppressive, and the interval between doses is often prolonged because of the duration of neutropenia produced by the drug. Vinorelbine is similarly myelosuppressive to vinblastine.

Local phlebitis and severe pain occur if any of the vincas is extravasated. Although a catheter may be placed, conventionally a butterfly needle is used to administer vincristine, vinorelbine, or vinblastine. The vein is punctured with the butterfly needle in the usual fashion, and blood flow is observed into the tubing. Several mL of saline are infused into the vein so that leakage may be observed. The vinca alkaloid is then given as a bolus injection and is followed by several more mL of sterile saline to ensure that not a drop of the drug remains on the tip of the needle.

One of the principal limitations of long-term treatment with vincristine in clinical practice is the development of a drug-induced sensory and motor neuropathy, the pathogenesis of which is poorly understood. The cat may be more sensitive to the development of this phenomenon than the dog.[23] Severe nerve fiber degeneration may be seen, as well as focal axonal swellings with secondary demyelination of peripheral nerves.[24,25] Vincristine administration should be discontinued immediately as soon as any signs of neuropathy are noted because further treatment may produce severe, generalized motor weakness. The neurotoxicity will generally improve within several months after the drug is discontinued, but some of the signs may be irreversible. Although neurologic problems are rare with vinblastine administration, they may rarely occur with this drug as well.

Dosing regimen. The appropriate dose of vincristine is 0.5 to 0.75 mg/m^2 intravenously once weekly according to the treatment protocol used. Treatment with vinblastine should begin at 2 mg/m^2 by intravenous injection once every 2 weeks. At each cycle, the clinician should increase the vinblastine dose in increments of 0.25 mg/m^2 until myelosuppression is seen (absolute neutrophil count less than 3000/μL). Then a maintenance dose of vinblastine, which is *one increment smaller than the dose that produced leukopenia,* should be administered.

Because vinblastine is so myelosuppressive, the clinician should not administer the drug when the animal's absolute neutrophil count is less than 3000/μL. The dose range for vinorelbine is 10 to 12.5 mg/m^2 intravenously, using the same dosing schedule as vinblastine.

Taxanes

Mechanism of action. The taxanes are one of the most significant additions to the anticancer arsenal added during the twentieth century. Paclitaxel, the parent drug, was discovered by a National Cancer Institute program in which extracts from thousands of plants were evaluated for anticancer activity. Paclitaxel is derived from the bark of the Pacific yew tree *(Taxus brevifolia)*. Paclitaxel and its semisynthetic analog, docetaxel, have demonstrated significant antitumor activity in humans. Both drugs have a unique mechanism of action compared with other microtubule inhibitors. The taxanes bind to the interior surface of the microtubule lumen at the N-terminal 1-31 amino acids and residues 217-233 of the β-tubulin subunit. Binding to this site does not interfere with the binding of other microtubule inhibitors to their respective sites. Ultimately, the taxanes disrupt microtubule dynamics by suppression of microtubule instability and treadmilling. Like the vinca alkaloids, these drugs are considered to be cell cycle specific for the M phase; however, the majority of cell death occurs in the S phase.

Spectrum of activity. In humans these drugs have been used primarily as anticarcinoma agents with Food and Drug Administration approval for carcinomas of the breast, ovarian carcinomas, prostatic carcinoma, head and neck carcinomas, gastric carcinoma, Kaposi's sarcoma, and non–small cell lung cancer. In dogs paclitaxel has been reported to have activity against mammary tumors, squamous cell carcinoma, transitional cell carcinoma, osteosarcoma, and malignant histiocytosis.[26,27] In vitro, paclitaxel has shown activity against a number of feline vaccine–associated cell lines; however, no in vivo information exists. Docetaxel has similar uses but is safer for cats. Paclitaxel has also been used with some success as an inhalation chemotherapy agent, although administration is difficult and not routinely available.[28]

Preparations. Paclitaxel is available in various sizes of a 20 mg/mL solution available for intravenous administration (30-mg, 100-mg and 300-mg multidose vials). This drug is not water soluble and therefore must be dissolved in a specific carrier, Cremophor. Docetaxel is available in various sizes of a 40 mg/mL solution for intravenous administration (20-mg and 80-mg single dose vials). Docetaxel must also be dissolved in a carrier solution of Polysorbate 80. These carriers are responsible for a number of the side effects seen, including hypersensitivity reactions. This drug is available in the United States only in an injectable form. It has low oral bioavailability on account of the high numbers of ABC transporters and P-glycoprotein efflux pumps within the intestinal lumen cells, as well as significant first-pass metabolism by the liver. Nonetheless, oral fomulations available in Europe have shown real promise against high-grade mast cell tumors. These formulations are given in conjunction with oral modulators of ABC transporters or cytochrome P-450 (or both).

Side effects. Side effects in dogs are fairly consistent with those seen in humans. Myelosuppression is common and typically occurs 5 to 7 days after injection. Gastrointestinal upset, including anorexia, nausea, diarrhea, and vomiting, can be seen as well. Alopecia has not been reported in the dog with this particular drug, although it stands to reason that this could be a possible sequela of drug administration. Peripheral neuropathies are more common with the vinca alkaloids, but they can be seen with administration of the taxanes as well. In humans arrhythmias are a common side effect of this drug. Indeed, the *Taxus* species of plants are known for causing arrythmias in cattle who ingest their bark. Though this has not been a reported side effect in the dog, it is recommended that an electrocardiogram be performed before administration. If underlying arrhythmias are noted, the clinician is advised not to use the taxanes in these patients. One of the most significant side effects of these drugs is hypersensitivity. This is related to the carriers (Cremophor and Polysorbate 80) that are necessary to keep these drugs in solution. Careful administration and monitoring during drug administration are recommended. Because of the severe hypersensitivity reaction of cats to paclitaxel, it is recommended that this drug be avoided in the species all together. Docetaxel has been safety administered to cats and is the preferred taxane for this species. This drug is not extremely myelosuppressive, and its myelosuppression is typically resolved at the next dose, 3 weeks later. The dose should be delayed if the mature neutrophil count is less than 2000 cells/μL.

Dosing regimen. The dose for paclitaxel is 165 mg/m^2 intravenously every 3 weeks. The dose range for docetaxel is 25 to 30 mg/m^2 given intravenously every 3 weeks. A specific premedication protocol is necessary to prevent severe hypersensitivity reactions. Animals are premedicated the night before treatment with 1 mg/kg of prednisone. Approximately 30 to 60 minutes before injection, diphenhydramine (4 mg/kg) is given intramuscularly, cimetidine (4 mg/kg) is given intravenously, and dexamethasone SP (1.5 to 2 mg/kg) is given intravenously. The diluted taxol (diluted 10:1 0.9% saline to drug) is started at a rate of 30 mL/hr for 30 minutes. If no allergic reaction is seen at that time, then the rate is increased to 60 mL/hour. The catheter is flushed with 25 to 30 mL of 0.9% saline afterwards. If signs of a hypersensitivity reaction do occur, the clinician should stop the infusion, medicate if necessary, and then restart at a slower rate. Therapy should be discontinued if severe hypersensitivity reactions occur.

Antitumor Antibiotics

Doxorubicin

Mechanism of action. Doxorubicin is an anthracycline glycoside derived from *Streptomyces peucetius*. It is directly cytotoxic, binding irreversibly with DNA and preventing both RNA and DNA synthesis. Cellular damage caused by doxorubicin results in enzyme-catalyzed, iron-mediated free radical formation, which produces further tissue damage. Ultimately, these effects result in induction of apoptosis in both normal and neoplastic cells. After intravenous administration doxorubicin is metabolized in the liver to active and inactive metabolites. The drug is excreted primarily in the bile but persists in plasma for prolonged periods.

Spectrum of activity. Doxorubicin has been proved effective in the treatment of a number of tumors of the dog and cat, including lymphoma, leukemias, and certain sarcomas and carcinomas.[29-33] It appears that doxorubicin may be synergistic with cyclophosphamide in the treatment of some sarcomas,[34] and it is combined with cytosine arabinoside as an extremely effective (although very myelosuppressive) protocol for leukemia.

Preparations. Doxorubicin is available for intravenous use only in vials of 10, 20, and 50 mg.

Side effects. Cardiotoxicity is generally the dose-limiting factor for doxorubicin administration in dogs.[35] It results from free-radical damage to the myocardium, with oxidation and death of myocardial cells in the presence of iron. Doxorubicin is an active iron chelator, and the resulting iron–doxorubicin complex catalyzes free radical reactions, leading to myocardial damage. Acute cardiac toxicity may occur at any time and after any dosage; it commonly takes the form of an arrhythmia, which resolves with time in most animals. Arrhythmias are more common if there is previous cardiac disease, previous or concurrent thoracic irradiation, or concurrent cyclophosphamide administration. The second form of cardiac toxicity induced by doxorubicin is congestive heart failure, with myocardial degeneration and cardiac muscle fibrosis leading to heart failure; this generally occurs with cumulative doses greater than 240 mg/m^2. Once congestive heart failure induced by doxorubicin is present, patients may respond to aggressive therapy for heart failure, but some patients will die despite all treatment. Many attempts have been made in humans to diagnose incipient cardiac toxicity before clinical manifestations of heart failure begin, but it remains impossible to predict which patients will develop these changes. Echocardiographic measurement of ventricular fractional shortening and serial electrocardiography are probably the best methods to monitor dogs and cats that are receiving treatment with doxorubicin.

Both humans and dogs have shown a great deal of individual variation in susceptibility to doxorubicin-induced cardiotoxicity. Even though clinical cardiac disease may not be evident after treatment with doxorubicin, subclinical damage to the heart is common. In a study of 115 children with lymphoblastic leukemia treated with doxorubicin and followed for many years, 57% had abnormal cardiac function later in life.[36] The EDTA-derivative drug ICRF-187 (dexrazoxane), given at 0.8 mg/kg 30 minutes before doxorubicin administration, apparently decreases cardiotoxicity without reducing cancer cell cytotoxicity,[37] but no large clinical trials of this compound in dogs or cats with cancer have been reported. Dexrazoxane acts as a cardioprotectant by chelating iron, helping to prevent the free radical–induced damage caused by doxorubicin; the product is not commercially available at this writing.

Although cats do not generally show clinical cardiac disease associated with doxorubicin treatment, histologic and echocardiographic evidence of damage to the myocardium occurs in cats treated with cumulative doses of 170 to 240 mg/m^2.[38] Renal damage also occurs in cats after chronic treatment with doxorubicin; this is manifested by azotemia, dilute urine, and gradually decreasing creatinine clearance values during the course of administration.[39] Another serious side effect in cats is the profound anorexia that may accompany administration of doxorubicin at the conventional dose given to dogs (30 mg/m^2); cats given this dose do not act as though they are nauseated, but they may not eat voluntarily for weeks, sometimes requiring placement of a feeding tube. Small dogs weighing less than 10 kg may also experience unexpected nausea and anorexia at this treatment dose. For cats and small dogs, a doxorubicin dose of 1 mg/kg has proved to be much better tolerated.

Myelosuppression may occur several days after administration, usually beginning on day 4. Peak action on the bone marrow occurs from days 10 to 14. Because doxorubicin has a high affinity for mast cells, causing them to degranulate, anaphylaxis, urticaria, generalized erythema, and head shaking have been seen in the dog. To prevent this, the patient may be premedicated with antihistamines and steroids before administration. Alopecia may also occur in susceptible breeds of dogs.

Extreme phlebitis and necrosis occur if doxorubicin is extravasated. This necrosis begins 1 to 2 weeks after the drug is extravasated and continues for 1 to 4 months. Doxorubicin also produces an unusual "radiation recall" effect; if previous radiation damage has occurred, even years before, doxorubicin administration will cause its recurrence. This is not likely to be a problem in dogs and cats, given that radiation therapy to the thorax is rarely performed in these species, but it is often a serious complication of doxorubicin treatment in humans. Radiation to the thoracic cavity (when the heart is in the radiation field) may also potentiate the cardiotoxicity of doxorubicin, which could be an important consideration for dogs and cats with thymoma or mediastinal lymphoma.

Dosing regimen. Although the conventional dose of doxorubicin in medium-size to large dogs is 30 mg/m^2 given every 3 weeks, in very small dogs or cats this dose may produce profound myelosuppression and anorexia. For this reason the dose in very small animals (less than 10 kg) should be reduced to 1 mg/kg every 3 weeks. Doxorubicin should be administered slowly into the tubing of a freely running intravenous infusion of saline or 5% dextrose solution. The tubing should be attached to a catheter that was placed on the first stick to prevent any leaking of drug through holes in the vein. *At least* 5 minutes should be taken to give the drug. Alternatively, doxorubicin may be mixed in a small volume of saline (50 to 100 mL) and dripped intravenously over 20 to 30 minutes. Because doxorubicin is physically incompatible with many other drugs, including heparin, aminophylline, cephalothin, dexamethasone, diazepam, hydrocortisone, and furosemide, care should be taken not to give other drugs through the same line during the doxorubicin infusion.

Doxorubicin Analogs

Mechanism of action. Because doxorubicin is so cardiotoxic, much effort has been devoted to development of analogs that might have less toxicity but that would maintain the level of tumor response. Epirubicin (4′-epidoxorubicin) is an analog that has been claimed to be less cardiotoxic in humans for equivalent doses. The mechanism of this drug is similar to that of doxorubicin. Idarubicin (4-demethoxydaunorubicin) is another anthracycline glycoside that is unusual in that it is the only antitumor antibiotic that can be given orally.

Spectrum of activity. The spectrum of canine and feline tumors that will respond to epirubicin therapy is probably similar to that for doxorubicin. Epirubicin's principal use has been as a single agent in dogs with canine lymphoma; response rate and duration of response are not significantly different from what would be expected with doxorubicin therapy.[40] Idarubicin has been used orally in cats for maintenance therapy of lymphoma after remission is obtained with other drugs.[41]

Preparations. Epirubicin is not commercially available at this time. Idarubicin is commercially available only in an injectable form, in 5-mg, 10-mg, and 20-mg vials.

Side effects. The claim that epirubicin has an advantage over doxorubicin in lessened toxicity has not proved to be particularly persuasive. Myelosuppression is similar, with the neutrophil nadir seen 10 days after administration. A significant number of dogs treated with epirubicin still show evidence of cardiotoxicity, as measured by ventricular fractional shortening on echocardiography. Idarubicin may produce gastrointestinal signs and myelosuppression in treated cats, and dose modification may be necessary. Because idarubicin is very cardiotoxic in humans, it presumably has the same effect in dogs and cats; appropriate precautions and monitoring should be considered.

Dosing regimen. Epirubicin is given intravenously at a dose of 30 mg/m^2 for dogs weighing more than 10 kg and 1 mg/kg for dogs less than 10 kg. Similar precautions for administration to those taken with doxorubicin should be followed. Idarubicin has been given orally at 2 mg/cat daily for 3 days once every 3 weeks; injectable doses of idarubicin for dogs and cats have not been reported.

Dactinomycin (Actinomycin D)

Mechanism of action. Dactinomycin is one of the actinomycins, a group of antibiotics produced by various species of *Streptomyces.* The drug binds to DNA by intercalation and causes single-strand DNA breaks. Ultimately, dactinomycin causes apoptosis in susceptible tumor cells. As with doxorubicin, drug resistance to dactinomycin is caused by overexpression of P-glycoprotein; it is therefore unlikely that response to dactinomycin will be seen in lymphomas in which the tumor cells have become resistant to doxorubicin.

Spectrum of activity. Dactinomycin has chemotherapeutic activity against canine lymphoma; activity has been seen in some drug-resistant lymphomas but generally only when the tumor is not yet doxorubicin resistant. Partial responses have been seen with dactinomycin treatment of nephroblastoma and botryoid rhabdomyosarcoma in the dog. Certain carcinomas may also respond, including anal sac adenocarcinoma, squamous cell carcinoma, thyroid carcinoma, and transitional cell carcinoma.[42] The principal use of dactinomycin, however, is as a substitute for doxorubicin when a potentially cardiotoxic cumulative dose of doxorubicin has been reached and it is desirable to continue administration of an antitumor antibiotic.

Preparations. Dactinomycin is administered intravenously and is supplied in vials containing 0.5 mg.

Side effects. Dactinomycin is extremely necrotizing when extravasated, similar to the effects produced by doxorubicin; it must be given through a "first-stick" catheter. Minimal myelosuppressive activity is noted when the drug is given as a solitary agent. Nausea and vomiting may occasionally occur during the first few hours after administration but may be partially prevented by administration of chemoreceptor trigger zone–blocking antiemetic agents. As with doxorubicin, dactinomycin potentiates the effects of radiation therapy and has a radiation-recall effect. Cardiotoxicity is extremely rare with this drug.

Dosing regimen. Dactinomycin is given intravenously at a dose of 0.5 to 1 mg/m^2 once every 3 weeks. Because it is extremely corrosive to soft tissue, catheter placement should be meticulous. The calculated dose should be mixed with normal saline or 5% dextrose in water and dripped intravenously over 20 to 30 minutes.

Bleomycin

Mechanism of action. Bleomycin is an antitumor antibiotic derived from a strain of *Streptomyces* first isolated from the soil of a Japanese coal mine. Its cytotoxic effect is mediated by DNA binding and fragmentation, with single- and double-strand breaks. Interestingly, bleomycin seems to be more damaging to nonproliferating cells than to those actively proliferating. It has a unique lung toxicity in most animal species studied.

Spectrum of activity. Bleomycin is most effective for treatment of squamous cell carcinoma in cats and dogs;[43] remissions are usually partial and of short duration, however. Recently, impressive results were obtained with intralesional injections of bleomycin into acanthomatous epulides in three dogs.[44] These benign oral tumors are generally treated with surgical removal, sometimes involving a partial mandibulectomy or maxillectomy. The tumors were markedly smaller after three weekly bleomycin injections and had disappeared by 8 to 10 injections. No recurrence was noted in any of the cases during the follow-up periods, which ranged from 1 to 2 years. Bleomycin is also effective in humans as a sclerosing agent in the treatment of malignant pleural effusion, but there are no reports of this use in dogs or cats.

Preparations. Bleomycin is given intravenously or by intralesional or intracavitary injection; it is supplied in 15-mg or 30-mg vials.

Side effects. Unlike the other antitumor antibiotics, myelosuppression is unlikely with bleomycin. Chronic administration of bleomycin to dogs every other day for more than 8 months resulted in the development of a pneumonitis, which progressed to pulmonary fibrosis.[45] The earliest symptom was dyspnea, with patchy opacities of the lung fields noted on radiographs. Microscopic changes included squamous metaplasia of the bronchiolar epithelium, fibrinous edema, and a diffuse interstitial fibrosis. Cutaneous ulceration and loss of nails also occurred in these dogs. Because bleomycin in clinical patients is principally used for short-term palliation of tumors, none of these chronic changes is likely to occur in clinical patients.

Dosing regimen. Bleomycin is given subcutaneously at a dose of 10 to 20 U/m^2 once weekly.

Mitoxantrone

Mechanism of action. Mitoxantrone is a derivative of anthracene and is related to doxorubicin and daunorubicin. It intercalates into DNA and causes cross-linking, with inhibition of both DNA and RNA synthesis. It is cell cycle specific but phase nonspecific.

Spectrum of activity. Partial and complete remissions have been reported when mitoxantrone is used as a solitary chemotherapeutic agent in lymphoma.[46] Because the drug is very expensive, it is not generally used for induction or maintenance therapy. Its principal use is in lymphomas in which the tumor cells are resistant to other drugs; a response rate of 26% can be expected.[47] Rare partial remissions and even rarer complete remissions are associated with administration of mitoxantrone to dogs and cats with various carcinomas and sarcomas, but the use of this drug in tumors other than lymphoma has been generally disappointing.

Preparations. Mitoxantrone is supplied in 20-, 25-, and 30-mg vials for intravenous use only.

Side effects. Side effects of mitoxantrone administration are mild to moderate gastrointestinal toxicity and myelosuppression. Although the myelosuppression associated with mitoxantrone is generally not marked, some dogs and cats will develop dangerously low neutrophil and platelet counts; for this reason it may be prudent to begin treatment at the lower end of the dose range, with gradual escalation of the dose as treatment proceeds. Extravasation of the drug may result in severe local reactions, including ulceration and cellulitis. Although mitoxantrone is a relative of doxorubicin, its cardiotoxicity in dogs appears to be much less; no clinical evidence of cardiac effects was noted in a study of mitoxantrone administration in 129 dogs with different malignancies.[48] However, because mitoxantrone does induce both acute and chronic congestive heart failure in humans, it probably is not a good choice for dogs or cats in which the maximum safe dose of doxorubicin has been reached or in patients with preexisting cardiac disease. A blue-green color may be noted in the sclera and urine of treated animals after therapy.

Dosing regimen. The dose of mitoxantrone in dogs and cats is 5 to 6.5 mg/m^2 given once every 3 weeks. The drug is diluted to at least 0.5 mg/mL in sterile saline and is given through a catheter over at least 3 minutes.

Antimetabolites

Methotrexate

Mechanism of action. Methotrexate is one of the antimetabolites, which as a class act as structural antagonists of normal metabolites or as cofactors of nucleic acids, generally having their greatest effect on cells in the S phase of the cell cycle. Methotrexate exerts its cytotoxic effect by competing for a binding site on the enzyme dihydrofolate reductase. This reversible binding prevents the synthesis of folate, which is important in production of the purine nucleotides and thymidine. An "antidote" for methotrexate cytotoxicity is leucovorin (citrovorum factor), which provides folate for biochemical activity in the cell. Methotrexate is principally eliminated in urine; in humans 80% to 90% of the administered dose is excreted unchanged in the urine within 24 hours. Assessment of renal function is important before administration of methotrexate, and dose modification in patients with compromised renal function may be necessary to prevent toxicity caused by delayed drug clearance. Because the antimetabolites have a short half-life in the body, they are most effective when given by constant-rate infusion, thus killing cells as they enter the S phase; however, a protocol for safe and effective constant-rate infusion of methotrexate has not been published for the dog.

Spectrum of activity. Although methotrexate has been widely used in human oncology, often at very high doses with "leucovorin rescue," it has found only limited use in veterinary medicine as a part of combination protocols for lymphoma.

Preparations. Methotrexate sodium may be administered intramuscularly, subcutaneously, or intravenously; the product for injection is available in 20-mg, 50-mg, 100-mg, 200-mg, 250-mg, and 1-g vials. For oral administration it is supplied as 2.5-mg scored tablets. Leucovorin calcium is available in vials of 100 mg for parenteral administration as well as 5- and 15-mg tablets for oral administration.

Side effects. Gastrointestinal side effects are the most important toxicities produced by methotrexate, with nausea occurring commonly. Oral ulceration and diarrhea may also be seen, and methotrexate should be used with great caution or not at all in patients with ulcerative colitis. Myelosuppression is mild at low-dosage ranges. With long-term, low-dose therapy, hepatic dysfunction is a significant problem in humans, and methotrexate hepatotoxicity has been reported in the dog.[49] Because nonsteroidal antiinflammatory drugs and aspirin may decrease renal excretion of methotrexate and thus increase its toxicity, these drugs should not be given along with methotrexate. Concurrent administration of methotrexate with a trimethoprin–sulfa antibiotic would be likely to lead to severe folate deficiency and therefore increase the severity of myelosuppression.

Dosing regimen. The oral dose of methotrexate is 2.5 mg/m^2 given daily for 5 days, followed by a 2-day rest period. This is repeated weekly until remission is achieved; 10 mg/m^2 given twice weekly followed by a 7-day rest period would be another acceptable protocol. Toxic hematopoietic effects may be reversed by 6 to 12 mg of leucovorin given subcutaneously four times a day for 4 doses.

Cytosine Arabinoside (Cytarabine, ara-C)

Mechanism of action. Cytosine arabinoside is highly specific for the S phase of the cell cycle, and its effectiveness is therefore dependent on maintaining constant drug levels; constant-rate infusion or frequent, closely-spaced doses are necessary for successful treatment of tumors using this drug. Cytosine arabinoside is transported into the cell and metabolized to

5′-triphosphate ara-C, which inhibits DNA polymerase. The metabolite is then incorporated into DNA, preventing templating from DNA and inhibiting DNA repair. Cytosine arabinoside is one of the few chemotherapeutic drugs that crosses the blood–brain barrier easily, and it can therefore be used to treat CNS lymphoma, as well as to kill leukemic cells in the cerebrospinal fluid.

Spectrum of activity. In veterinary oncology cytosine arabinoside is generally used in combination protocols for treatment of canine and feline lymphoma. It may also be used to treat acute leukemias of both lymphoid and nonlymphoid types.[50]

Preparations. Cytosine arabinoside is available for intravenous or subcutaneous injection in vials containing 100 mg, 500 mg, 1 g, or 2 g.

Side effects. Because of its specificity for cycling cells in the S phase, cytosine arabinoside will usually cause myelosuppression, with the degree of myelosuppression increasing with the frequency and duration of administration. When large intravenous doses are given by bolus injection intravenously rather than by infusion, nausea and vomiting are common.

Dosing regimen. For lymphoma single-agent cytosine arabinoside may be given at a dose of 600 mg/m^2 intravenously once a week; lower doses of 200 to 300 mg/m^2 weekly should be used if cytosine arabinoside is part of a combination drug protocol. For treatment of acute leukemias, 100 mg/m^2/day given by constant-rate infusion or divided into 4 daily subcutaneous injections repeated for 5 days will produce the greatest response against leukemic cells. It is important to note that cytosine arabinoside, especially when used with doxorubicin, is extremely effective in clearing the bone marrow of tumor cells in leukemia patients. In general, patients will have a period of severe bone marrow aplasia for 7 to 21 days after the cycle is completed, often with neutrophil numbers less than 1000/μL and platelet counts less than 50,000/μL. Infection or hemorrhage may ensue during this period, and treatment with recombinant human G-CSF should ideally be used daily along with chemotherapy.

5-Fluorouracil

Mechanism of action. 5-Fluorouracil is a pyrimidine analog that exerts its cytotoxic effect by inhibiting thymidylate synthetase and thus DNA synthesis and, to a lesser extent, RNA synthesis. The cytotoxic effects of 5-fluorouracil are greatest on cells in the G_1 and S phases; with longer periods of exposure to the drug, cells in other phases of the cell cycle may also be killed. Because the drug is erratically absorbed from the gastrointestinal tract, it is generally given intravenously. It is also available as a topical cream.

Spectrum of activity. In humans 5-fluorouracil is the drug of choice for gastrointestinal carcinomas; it is effective in the palliative management of carcinoma of the colon, rectum, stomach, and pancreas. In the dog and cat, however, it has found limited usage because of neurotoxicity.

Preparations. For injection 5-fluorouracil is available in 500-mg vials. For topical use it is supplied in 25-g tubes.

Side effects. 5-Fluorouracil treatment in dogs is often accompanied by CNS reactions (behavior changes such as barking incessantly, running in circles, aggressiveness)[51-53]; continuing administration of the drug in the face of such neurologic signs may lead to seizures and death.[54] Mild myelosuppression and nausea are sometimes noted. Stomatitis and mucositis resembling pemphigus vulgaris may be seen in dogs receiving several weeks of treatment. Because unprovoked rage, extreme dementia, and sudden death may occur in cats treated with 5-fluorouracil, it should not be used in this species.[55]

Dosing regimen. 5-Fluorouracil may be given intravenously at 150 to 200 mg/m^2 for 3 days, then 100 mg/m^2 on the fifth, seventh, and ninth days. No drug is given on the fourth, sixth, and eighth days. Blood count should be monitored at the end of the cycle and before the next cycle begins. If gastrointestinal signs, stomatitis, neurologic signs, or falling white blood cell count (less than 4000/μL) are noted, the drug should be discontinued. Generally, cycles of 5-fluorouracil are repeated monthly. In the dog 5-fluorouracil is useful for small skin carcinomas or solar keratosis as a topical cream. This is applied twice daily until there is an erosive inflammatory response with ulceration (usually 2 to 4 months), at which time use of the drug should be stopped. Healing may take several months after the topical treatment is discontinued. Owners should wear gloves while administering the cream. *5-Fluorouracil should not be used in cats.*

Hydroxyurea

Mechanism of action. Hydroxyurea inhibits ribonucleotide reductase, leading to depletion of essential DNA precursors; cells accumulate in the S phase of the cell cycle.

Spectrum of activity. Hydroxyurea is used for the palliative treatment of chronic myelogenous leukemia,[56] eosinophilic leukemia–hypereosinophilic syndrome in cats,[57] and basophilic leukemia in dogs.[58] It is also effective for management of polycythemia vera in the dog and cat.[59]

Preparations. Hydroxyurea is available in 500-mg capsules for oral administration.

Side effects. Side effects of hydroxyurea are generally mild and well tolerated and include nausea and myelosuppression. In the dog loss of toenails may occur with chronic hydroxyurea administration, and a seborrhea sicca–like syndrome may be noted.

Dosage regimen. Hydroxyurea is given orally at a dose of 35 to 50 mg/kg once daily for 7-10 days, then every other day until remission. After remission is obtained (leukemic cell counts are reduced in leukemia patients, or packed cell volume is normal in patients with polycythemia vera; neutrophil and platelet counts are in the normal range), a dose of hydroxyurea is determined that will maintain remission. In some patients daily administration of hydroxyurea will continue to be necessary, but at a lower dose—20 mg/kg/day, for example. In other patients administration of a higher dose (such as 50 to 75 mg/kg) twice weekly will be adequate. The dose of hydroxyurea is titrated to the patient's CBC results.

Platinum Drugs

Cisplatin

Mechanism of action. Cisplatin is a very useful drug in human and veterinary oncology. Its complete chemical name is *cis*-dichlorodiammineplatinum (DDP), reflecting the fact that it is formed by platinum surrounded by chlorine and ammonia atoms in the *cis* position of the horizontal plane. Its cytotoxic effects are thought to be due to alkylation of DNA.

Spectrum of activity. Cisplatin has been shown to produce objective responses in many types of carcinomas in the dog.[60-63] Administration of cisplatin as an adjuvant agent with amputation in canine osteosarcoma has produced significantly longer survival times than seen with amputation alone.[64,65] Complete remission has also been seen in dogs with metastatic seminoma. Intracavitary cisplatin has resulted in complete and durable palliation of pleural effusion resulting from mesothelioma and carcinomatosis of unknown origin[66]; intraperitoneal treatment with cisplatin for patients with carcinomatosis caused by ovarian carcinoma would also be reasonable.

Preparations. Cisplatin is available for parenteral injection in 50-mg and 100-mg vials.

Side effects. *Treatment of cats with cis-platinum is contraindicated*; dyspnea and death with pulmonary edema occur within 48 and 96 hours after cisplatin administration, even with only one treatment.[67] Cisplatin is *extremely* nephrotoxic in the dog, especially if prehydration is not performed with treatment. Before each treatment, blood urea nitrogen (BUN) and creatinine evaluations and a urinalysis should be performed; elevation of BUN and creatinine in the face of a dilute urine should signal the onset of renal toxicity, and additional treatments of cisplatin should not be given. Carboplatin, which is much less nephrotoxic, may be substituted for cisplatin.

Acute gastrointestinal toxicosis with nausea, anorexia, and vomiting is common after cisplatin administration, usually beginning 2 to 4 hours after treatment (most dogs will vomit for less than 6 hours); the severity of the emesis can be decreased with administration of butorphanol or ondansetron. Hypomagnesemia, hypocalcemia, hyponatremia, hypokalemia, and hypophosphatemia may occur after repeated doses of cisplatin, probably as a result of renal tubular damage. Myelosuppression is generally mild but lengthy, with a double neutrophil nadir at 6 and 15 days after treatment. A CBC should be performed before administration of each cisplatin treatment; neutropenia may persist as long as 28 days after a single treatment, causing delay in the administration of the next course of therapy.

Dosing regimen. The dose for cisplatin in dogs is 60 to 70 mg/m^2 given once every 21 days. An antiemetic such as butorphanol (0.4 mg/kg) is generally given before beginning the treatment; another dose may be given 2 hours later if vomiting becomes a problem. Intravenous saline solution should be given to prehydrate the patient at the rate of 25 mL/kg per hour for 3 hours (18.3 mL/kg per hour for 4 hours in dogs that might become volume overloaded), followed by a 20-minute intravenous infusion of cisplatin mixed in saline. This is followed by additional fluids given for an additional hour (2 hours for a heart failure patient because the fluid rate is lower) at the same rate. Needles or intravenous sets containing aluminum parts that may come into contact with cisplatin should not be used for preparation or administration because a precipitate will form, causing loss of potency. For intracavitary treatment of mesothelioma or carcinomatosis, the animal is prehydrated with intravenous saline, as previously described. For intraperitoneal therapy 50 mg/m^2 of cisplatin is diluted in 0.9% NaCl to a total volume of 1 L/m^2; for intrapleural delivery the dose is 250 mg/m^2 . The solution is warmed to body temperature and instilled through an aseptically placed catheter over 15 minutes, and posttherapy hydration is performed in the manner previously described. Treatments are repeated once every 4 weeks as needed to maintain remission. *Cisplatin must not be given to cats.*

Carboplatin

Mechanism of action. Because of the effectiveness of cisplatin in the treatment of many tumors, great interest developed in the search for another platinum compound that would maintain the same level of cytotoxicity without being as toxic to the patient. Carboplatin was developed at Michigan State University to fulfill these requirements; it is similar to cisplatin in pharmacology and antitumor effects. The major route of elimination of carboplatin, like cisplatin, is renal excretion; however, carboplatin causes significantly less renal toxicity, so fluid diuresis before and after administration is not required.

Spectrum of activity. In the treatment of human cancers, carboplatin and cisplatin appear to share the same spectrum of activity; this is presumed to be the case also in the dog. Because of its very different level of toxicity compared with cisplatin, carboplatin is a logical alternative to cisplatin for patients with renal disease or in patients with cardiac disease, in which the large amount of fluids administered with cisplatin treatment might be dangerous. Carboplatin is also safe to use in cats, unlike cisplatin, and intralesional injections of a carboplatin–oil emulsion into squamous cell carcinomas of the nasal planum in cats have resulted in objective responses and apparent cures in some cats.[68]

Preparations. Carboplatin is available for intravenous infusion in 50-, 150- and 450-mg vials.

Side effects. Carboplatin is significantly less nephrotoxic than cisplatin and only rarely produces nausea and vomiting. However, dose-dependent neutropenia and thrombocytopenia are common, and the myelosuppression produced by the drug may be prolonged. In general, carboplatin treatment should not be repeated until neutrophil and platelet counts are in the normal range. Toxicity in the cat is principally associated with myelosuppression, as in the dog.[69] Although carboplatin has limited renal toxicity, concomitant treatment with aminoglycosides may result in enhanced kidney toxicity as well as hearing loss.

When carboplatin in purified sesame oil has been used to treat squamous cell carcinomas in cats intralesionally, systemic toxicosis was not observed in any of the cats. Plasma concentrations of carboplatin did not significantly increase during the course of treatment. Water in sesame oil emulsions have been shown to be effective carriers for intratumor administration of antineoplastic agents, preserving drug activity and enhancing concentration of drug locally by allowing slow release into tissues. This allows for intensification of carboplatin chemotherapy without dose-limiting adverse effects.

Dosing regimen. Carboplatin is given as a 15- to 20-minute intravenous infusion at a dose of 250 to 300 mg/m^2 once every 3 to 4 weeks for dogs; unlike cisplatin, intravenous carboplatin is safe for cats at a dose of 150 to 200 mg/m^2 once every 3 to 4 weeks. As with cisplatin, aluminum reacts with carboplatin, causing a precipitate; needles with aluminum parts should not be used for the preparation or administration of carboplatin.

For intralesional injection of the nasal planum in cats with squamous cell carcinoma, treatments should be done with the animal under general anesthesia because of the pain that the injection procedure is likely to produce. Carboplatin is prepared in a water–oil emulsion that includes 10 mg of carboplatin in 1 mL of water mixed with 2 mL of sterile, purified, medical-grade sesame oil; a viscous, yellowish liquid is created by this mixture. The emulsion is injected into the tumor and surrounding borders so that approximately 1.5 mg of carboplatin is injected per cubic centimeter of tumor tissue. Four weekly doses are given.

Miscellaneous Drugs

Receptor Tyrosine Kinase Inhibitors

Mechanism of action. A new class of drugs, receptor tyrosine kinase inhibitors (RTKIs), has now entered the veterinary market. Receptor tyrosine kinases are a family of receptors expressed on the surface of all cells. These receptors play a large role in normal cell signal transduction and, when functioning normally, are tight regulators of cellular growth and differentiation. The ligands for these receptors are typically growth factors that are secreted by the cells themselves, released from the extracelluar matrix, or are secreted by other cells in the vicinity.[70] Once activated, these receptors work by phophorylating proteins on tyrosine residues using adenosine triphosphate (ATP) in the process. They can activate tyrosine residues on themselves or other proteins as part of the initiation of a cell signaling process that will eventually lead to alterations in gene transcription. Small molecule inhibitors such as the RTKIs inhibit the phosphorylation of tyrosine residues, thereby stopping the signal transduction process. In many neoplastic cells these receptors are overexpressed, mutated to be constitutively turned on, or both. In most cases these small molecule inhibitors competitively bind the ATP binding site on the receptor, preventing the binding of ATP that is necessary to drive the phosphorylation of tyrosine residues.[70] Two RTKIs are currently available or will soon be available to the veterinary market: toceranib (Palladia) and masitinib (Kinavet) has been recently approved by the FDA and will be available soon in the United States.

Spectrum of activity. Toceranib has been shown to have activity against members of the split kinase family of RTKs and inhibits vascular endothelial growth factor receptor, platelet-derived growth factor receptor, and c-kit (CD117).[71] This drug is thought to have antiangiogenic and antitumor effects. It is labeled for use against mast cell tumors in dogs; however, anecdotal reports suggest that it may be useful against other tumors as well (anal sac adenocarcinomas, osteosarcomas, and soft tissue sarcomas). Masitinib has been shown to have activity against c-kit and platelet-derived growth factor receptor. This drug has been approved in Europe for canine mast cell tumors and is currently undergoing approval by the Food and Drug Administration for use in the United States.

Preparations. Toceranib is available in 10-mg, 15-mg, and 50-mg oral tablets. Masitnib is available in 50-mg tablets, although smaller formulations may be available soon. Currently, toceranib is available only to board-certified veterinary pathologists; however, Pfizer plans to release the drug to general practitioners sometime in 2011.

Side effects. Although RTKIs have relatively targeted mechanisms of action, they also produce quite a few toxicities. It is important to remember that these drugs are still considered chemotherapy and should be treated with as much care and respect as other oral chemotherapy drugs.

Procarbazine

Mechanism of action. The mechanism of action of procarbazine is not clearly understood, although it is thought to work through DNA alkylation and methylation, thereby decreasing DNA and RNA synthesis. The drug is metabolized by the liver and excreted almost entirely in the urine.

Spectrum of action. Procarbazine is typically used as a part of the MOPP rescue protocol for lymphoma (see the section on mechlorethamine).

Preparations. Procarbazine is available in nonscored, unbreakable 50-mg tablets. It may be necessary to compound for smaller sizes in small dogs and cats.

Side effects. Myelosuppression is the primary side effect associated with procarbazine. Gastrointestinal side effects may also be seen. As with all chemotherapy drugs, alopecia is an additional possible side effect.

Dosing regimen. This drug is used at 50 mg/m^2 daily for 14 days.

L-Asparaginase, Pegaspargase

Mechanism of action. L-asparaginase, an enzyme derived from *E. coli,* exploits a qualitative biochemical defect found in some tumor cells. In acute lymphoid leukemia and lymphoma, most malignant cells depend on an extracellular source of asparagine for survival. Normal cells, however, are able to synthesize asparagine and thus are affected less by the rapid extracellular depletion of asparagine produced by L-asparaginase. Although most susceptible tumors respond with dramatic reduction in size with the first administration of L-asparaginase, drug resistance of these cells develops quickly; a population of tumor cells is selected for in which the enzyme asparagine synthetase is present, asparagine can be made intracellularly, and the tumor cells are therefore unaffected by the enzyme's administration. Pegaspargase is modified from L-asparaginase by covalently conjugating monomethoxypolyethylene glycol to the enzyme, forming the active ingredient PEG-L-asparaginase; pegaspargase produces fewer hypersensitivity reactions with administration than does conventional L-asparaginase.

Spectrum of activity. L-asparaginase is principally useful in the treatment of lymphoma and lymphoid leukemia. Because hypersensitivity and drug resistance develop relatively rapidly, L-asparaginase is a useful agent for induction of remission or in relapsed lymphoid malignancies, but it should not be employed as part of a maintenance protocol.

Preparations. L-asparaginase is available in vials containing 10,000 IU for parenteral administration. Pegaspargase is supplied in vials containing 3750 IU.

Side effects. Because asparaginase is a foreign protein, severe allergic reactions may be seen on repeated administration. In humans this is a significant problem, and it is recommended that an intradermal skin test be performed if the drug is to be given repeatedly; in the dog, however, anaphylactoid reactions are rare.[72] Extreme facial edema and swelling or pain at the site of injection have been noted in some dogs within 24 hours after L-asparaginase administration, however, presumably as a manifestation of an allergic reaction to the drug. Pegaspargase was developed in an attempt to decrease the allergic reactions associated with administration of the drug; it is conjugated with polyethylene glycol and is indicated when L-asparaginase therapy is necessary despite a hypersensitivity reaction to previous treatment. Studies with the polyethylene glycol–modified enzyme in dogs have indicated that it is also active against lymphoma.[73] The necessity for its use in veterinary medicine is limited because of the comparative rarity of allergic drug reactions with the use of conventional L-asparaginase.

Side effects associated with the administration of L-asparaginase in the dog are quite rare. Hyperamylasemia occurs in some patients and may progress to acute necrotizing pancreatitis.[74] L-asparaginase administration in humans causes a temporary but fairly dramatic inhibition in protein synthesis by the liver, resulting in reduced levels of clotting factors. Levels of antithrombin III and fibrinogen in dogs with lymphoma after L-asparaginase administration have not been found to be abnormal, however, and other clotting parameters were not significantly affected either.[75,76] Clinically important bleeding or thrombosis may occur in the dog but is extremely rare.[77] L-asparaginase deaminates extracellular asparagine to L-aspartic acid and ammonia. In patients with preexisting hepatic disease or significant liver function abnormalities related to tumor infiltration, treatment with L-asparaginase may result in a syndrome resembling ammonia encephalopathy, with confusion and stupor. If serum ammonia levels are found to be high in these patients, treatment with lactulose should be instituted until signs abate.

Dosing regimen. Dosage is 10,000 to 20,000 IU/m^2 or 400 IU/kg (maximum dose is 10,000 IU) weekly or as part of a combination protocol. The drug may be given subcutaneously, intramuscularly, or by intravenous administration. If L-asparaginase is given intravenously, the drug should be given over a period of not less than 30 minutes through the side arm of an already running infusion of sodium chloride or 5% dextrose.

Piroxicam

Mechanism of action. Piroxicam is a nonsteroidal antiinflammatory agent that has antiinflammatory, analgesic, and antipyretic properties in animals; edema, erythema, and tissue proliferation can be inhibited by the administration of the drug. Piroxicam inhibits the generation of thromboxane B2 in the blood of dogs by more than 70%, and more than 50% inhibition was maintained in most of the dogs for 48 hours.[78] The drug has also been reported to have antitumor activity in animal models and in metastatic tumors in humans. The exact mechanism for the role of piroxicam in cancer treatment is not established at this time, but it is unlikely that the effects can be attributed to a direct cytotoxic effect.[79]

Spectrum of activity. Piroxicam has produced objective responses in several types of carcinomas, including transitional cell carcinoma,[80] squamous cell carcinoma, mammary adenocarcinoma, and pulmonary metastatic carcinoma.[81] Its principal use is in palliation of transitional cell carcinoma of the urinary tract; relief of stranguria and hematuria often associated with transitional cell carcinoma may be seen for 4 to 11 months after the beginning of treatment.

Preparations. Piroxicam is supplied as 10-mg and 20-mg capsules for oral administration.

Side effects. Serious gastrointestinal toxicity with mucosal ulceration and bleeding, sometimes with perforation, may occur with piroxicam administration, especially if the drug is given daily. If daily administration of piroxicam is necessary, concurrent misoprostol at a dose of 5 μg/kg orally thrice daily should be considered to prevent gastrointestinal ulceration. Nephrotoxicity with renal papillary necrosis has also been reported with higher doses.

Dosing regimen. Dose is 0.3 mg/kg given orally once daily for 5 days, then every other day indefinitely, as long as efficacy is noted.

Corticosteroids

Mechanism of action. Several glucocorticoid hormones are used in the treatment of patients with cancer. In increasing order of potency, these are hydrocortisone, prednisone, and dexamethasone. The antiinflammatory effects of these hormones may help control pain in patients with terminal disease. Reduction of edema in the CNS with primary brain tumors or brain metastases occurs, especially with dexamethasone; barrier permeability within the tumor is decreased, thus reducing the rate of edema formation.

Corticosteroids are effective in lymphoid tumors by producing a direct lymphocytotoxic effect, apparently binding to intracellular receptors and inducing apoptosis. However, a population of steroid-resistant tumor cells (possibly lacking steroid receptors) develops rapidly if the steroid is used as a single agent, usually within 3 to 4 months after treatment of lymphoma begins. Because glucocorticoids are transported out of the cell by the multidrug resistance gene product P-glycoprotein, remission may be shorter and more difficult to achieve with certain other chemotherapeutic agents after steroid resistance develops.[82]

Spectrum of activity. Corticosteroids are most useful for their direct cytotoxicity in the management of lymphomas, lymphoid leukemias, thymomas, and plasma cell tumors. They are also important in the symptomatic management of mast cell tumors, shrinking these tumors by decreasing edema and inflammation and by reducing the eosinophilic and neutrophilic infiltrate commonly seen in these tumors. Whether neoplastic mast cells are actually killed by corticosteroid administration has not been determined. Corticosteroid administration may produce a dramatic improvement in clinical signs when used in patients with intracranial and spinal cord neoplasms, relieving signs of compression temporarily. These hormones are also useful in relieving the general debility, fever (noninfectious), and anorexia of cancer. Because corticosteroids produce a kind of euphoria, their administration to animals with terminal metastatic disease may improve quality of life transiently, even though tumor growth is not inhibited by the drug.

Preparations. Prednisone and dexamethasone are available for oral and parenteral use in a variety of tablet and solution strengths. The drugs are also available in preparations for ophthalmic administration.

Side effects. Side effects associated with the high doses of corticosteroids used in cancer treatment are numerous. For most dog owners, polydipsia and polyuria are the side effects of lymphoma or mast cell tumor treatment that are most difficult to accept; methylprednisolone, although much more expensive, may produce less polydipsia and polyuria. Owners should also be warned of the ravenous appetite often associated with steroid administration in dogs and cats. Temporal muscle atrophy, gastrointestinal ulceration and perforation, impaired wound healing, endocrine alopecia, increased incidence of bacterial infections, acute necrotizing pancreatitis, and personality changes are all occasional side effects seen with steroid administration, especially in dogs. Owners should be warned not to discontinue steroid treatment suddenly if their pet has been receiving corticosteroids for longer than 2 weeks because the hypothalamic–pituitary–adrenal axis is probably suppressed at the high doses being given.

Dosing regimen. Steroids may be administered orally, subcutaneously, intramuscularly, or intravenously, depending on the patient's condition. A conventional dose of prednisone for treatment of lymphoma would be 30 to 40 mg/m^2 orally once daily through induction, then on alternate days during maintenance. Edema induced by intracranial or spinal neoplasia may be treated with prednisone at the aforementioned dose or with dexamethasone at 0.1 mg/kg twice daily.

Monoclonal Antibodies

In humans, monoclonal antibody (Mab) therapy has been used successfully to treat non-Hodgkin's lymphoma (NHL) and colon cancer. Monoclonal antibodies such as rituximab (an anti-CD20 antibody) and bevicizumab (an anti-VEGF antibody) have been used successfully and are approved for use in human oncology. However, in the dog, these humanized antibodies do not have broad enough specificity to cross species. Two studies in the dog have evaluated the ability of rituximab to bind to canine CD20, a B-cell marker. However, in both studies, this antibody failed to bind CD20 and no tumor cell killing was identified.[83,84] Canine CD20 is not similar enough to human CD20 for cross reaction. Likewise, a study evaluating the efficacy of bevacizumab in canine mast cell tumors failed to show down regulation of VEGF and failed to decrease proliferation in this cell line.[85] Therefore, specific canine monoclonal antibodies for these receptors will have to be developed before these therapies will be made available for veterinary oncology.

Immunotherapy

Currently, only one FDA-approved anti-cancer immunotherapy is available for dogs, and no therapies are approved for cats. The Merial ONCEPT melanoma vaccine is the first DNA-based vaccine for canine cancer.

Mechanism of action. The canine melanoma vaccine uses a plasmid with DNA for a non-canine tyrosinase protein inserted. Tyrosinase is a protein found ubiquitously in melanocytes and functions in the packaging of melanin granules within the cells. The foreign tyrosinase produced by the vaccine is different enough from canine tyrosinase that it can break tolerance and be recognized by the dog's immune system as a foreign protein inducing an active immune response.[86,87] Cross-reactivity between the foreign tyrosinase response and canine tyrosinase can occur leading to destruction of neoplastic melanocytes.

Spectrum of activity. This drug is only approved for canine melanoma in the microscopic disease setting. Therefore, ideally, it should be combined with more local therapies such as radiation or surgery to delay or prevent the development of metastasis. This vaccine is often used in an extra-label fashion in the gross disease setting; however, long-term survival analyses, and response rates are not available. There are anecdotal reports of the vaccines use in other species such as horses and cats with no noted adverse events, however, efficacy data in these species is lacking.

Preparations. The melanoma vaccine is available in single dose vials and is administered at a total volume of 0.4 mL per dog intradermally using the specific applicator, the Canine Transdermal Device. The vaccine is administered initially once every other week for a total of 4 doses at induction and then a booster is administered once every 6 months for the remainder of the dog's life.

Side effects. The side effects of this immunotherapy are very minimal. A local pain reaction with vaccine administration may be seen in some dogs. The area may also appear red for 24 to 48 hours after vaccination. Additionally a transient low-grade fever may be seen in some dogs.

Other Immunotherapy

Many experimental treatments using immunotherapeutic principles are being explored including autologous T cell infusions, bone marrow transplantation, and dendritic cell vaccines. These therapies are only in the earliest stages of canine clinical trials and will likely not be commercially available for several years to come.

SUMMARY

Chemotherapeutic drugs can become common place in any general practice as long as the proper safety and handling precautions are instituted. These drugs can be dangerous to the veterinary hospital staff as well and the patient if handled or administered incorrectly. No one should ever administer a chemotherapy drug that they are uncomfortable handling for any reason. These drugs have varied clinical uses and side effects and a good understanding of each and every drug is necessary before administration. That being said, clinicians at veterinary hospitals who do not administer chemotherapy still need a basic knowledge of the side effects and their management for patients whom they have referred for chemotherapy elsewhere. Many clients will come to their general practitioner first for these conditions. Additionally, clients often seek advice from a trusted general practitioner regarding their options about cancer treatment in animals. The decision to treat their pet is often an emotional one, and a good understanding of the drugs and therapies that can be offered to them will put an owner at ease.

Cancer chemotherapy is a field that is constantly changing. New information is available almost daily and new drugs are approved every year. Indeed, cancer therapy is one of the most dynamic research fields. It is recommended that a practitioner who commonly uses chemotherapy frequently review the literature for new administration techniques, new drugs, and new uses for conventional chemotherapy drugs.

REFERENCES

1. Skipper HE, Schabel FM Jr, Wilcox WS: Experimental evaluation of potential anticancer agents: XII. On the criteria and kinetics associated with "curability" of experimental leukemias, *Cancer Chemother Rep* 35:1–111, 1964.
2. DeVita VT: Principles of chemotherapy. In DeVita VT, Hellman S, Rosenberg SA, editors: *Cancer: principles and practice of oncology*, Philadelphia, 1993, JB Lippincott, pp 276–292.
3. Arrington KA, Legendre AM, Tabeling GS, et al: Comparison of body surface area-based and weight-based dosage protocols for doxorubicin administration in dogs, *Am J Vet Res* 55:1587–1592, 1994.
4. Obradovich JE, Ogilvie GK, Cooper MF, et al: Effect of increasing dosages of canine recombinant granulocyte colony-stimulating factor on neutrophil counts in normal dogs, *Proc Vet Cancer Soc 10th Ann Conf* 5, 1990.
5. Fulton R, Gasper PW, Ogilvie GK, et al: Effect of recombinant human granulocyte colony-stimulating factor on hematopoiesis in normal cats, *Exp Hematol* 19:759–767, 1991.
6. Amantea M, Newman MS, Sullivan TM, et al: Relationship of dose intensity to the induction of palmar-plantar erythrodysesthesia by pegylated liposomal doxorubicin in dogs, *Hum Exp Toxicol* 18(1):17–26, 1999.
7. Vail DM, Chun R, Thamm D, et al: Efficacy of pyridoxine to ameliorate the cutaneous toxicity associated with doxorubicin containing pegylated (Stealth) liposomes: a randomized, double-blind clinical trial using a canine model, *Clin Cancer Res* 4(6):1567–1571, 1998.
8. Swanson LV: Potential hazards associated with low-dose exposure to antineoplastic agents. Part I. Evidence for concern, *Compend Cont Educ Pract Vet* 10:293–300, 1988.
9. Swanson LV: Potential hazards associated with low-dose exposure to antineoplastic agents. Part II. Recommendations for minimizing exposure, *Compend Cont Educ Pract Vet* 10: 616–624, 1988.
10. Peterson JL, Couto CG, Hammer AS, et al: Acute sterile hemorrhagic cystitis after a single intravenous administration of cyclophosphamide in three dogs, *J Am Vet Med Assoc* 201:1572–1574, 1992.
11. Trevor PB, Saunders GK, Waldron DR, et al: Metastatic extramedullary plasmacytoma of the colon and rectum in a dog, *J Am Vet Med Assoc* 203:406–409, 1993.
12. MacEwen EG, Hurvitz A, Hayes A: Hyperviscosity syndrome associated with lymphocytic leukemia in three dogs, *J Am Vet Med Assoc* 1977(170):1309–1312, 1977.
13. Dimski DS, Cook JR: Carmustine-induced partial remission of an astrocytoma in a dog, *J Am Anim Hosp Assoc* 26:179–182, 1990.
14. Fulton LM, Steinberg HS: Preliminary study of lomustine in the treatment of intracranial masses in dogs following localization by imaging techniques, *Semin Vet Med Surg* 5:241–245, 1990.
15. Van Vechten M, Helfand SC, Jeglum KA: Treatment of relapsed canine lymphoma with doxorubicin and dacarbazine, *J Vet Intern Med* 4:187–191, 1990.
16. Hahn KA: Vincristine sulfate as single-agent chemotherapy in a dog and a cat with malignant neoplasms, *J Am Vet Med Assoc* 197:504–506, 1990.
17. Hammer AS, Couto CG, Filppi J, et al: Efficacy and toxicity of VAC chemotherapy (vincristine, doxorubicin, and cyclophosphamide) in dogs with hemangiosarcoma, *J Vet Intern Med* 5:160–166, 1991.
18. Calvert CA, Leifer CE, MacEwen EG: Vincristine for treatment of transmissible venereal tumor in the dog, *J Am Vet Med Assoc* 181:163–164, 1982.
19. Singh J, Rana JS, Sood N, et al: Clinico-pathological studies on the effect of different antineoplastic chemotherapy regimens on transmissible venereal tumours in dogs, *Vet Res Commun* 20: 71–81, 1996.
20. McCaw DL, Miller MA, Bergman PJ, et al: Vincristine therapy for mast cell tumors in dogs, *J Vet Intern Med* 11:375–378, 1997.
21. Vickery KR, Wilson H, Vail DM, Thamm DH: Dose-escalating vinblastine for the treatment of canine mast cell tumour, *Vet Comp Oncol* 6(2):111–119, 2008.
22. Hahn KA, Fletcher CM, Legendre AM: Marked neutropenia in five tumor-bearing cats one week following single-agent vincristine sulfate chemotherapy, *Vet Clin Pathol* 25:121–123, 1996.
23. Todd GC, Griffing WJ, Gibson WR, et al: Animal models for the comparative assessment of neurotoxicity following repeated administration of vinca alkaloids, *Cancer Treat Rep* 63:35–41, 1979.
24. Cho ES, Lowndes HE, Goldstein BD: Neurotoxicology of vincristine in the cat. Morphological study, *Arch Toxicol* 52:83–90, 1983.
25. Hamilton TA, Cook JR, Braund KG, et al: Vincristine-induced peripheral neuropathy in a dog, *J Am Vet Med Assoc* 198: 635–638, 1991.
26. Poirier VJ, Hershey AE, Burgess KE, et al: Efficacy and toxicity of paclitaxel (Taxol) for the treatment of canine malignant tumors, *J Vet Intern Med* 18(2):219–222, 2004.
27. Simon D, Schoenrock D, Baumgärtner W, Nolte I: Postoperative adjuvant treatment of invasive malignant mammary gland tumors in dogs with doxorubicin and docetaxel, *J Vet Intern Med* 20(5):1184–1190, 2006.
28. Hershey AE, Kurzman ID, Forrest LJ, et al: Inhalation chemotherapy for macroscopic primary or metastatic lung tumors: proof of principle using dogs with spontaneously occurring tumors as a model, *Clin Cancer Res* 5(9):2653–2659, 1999.
29. Berg J, Weinstein MJ, Springfield DS: Results of surgery and doxorubicin chemotherapy in dogs with osteosarcoma, *J Am Vet Med Assoc* 206:1555–1560, 1995.
30. Moore AS, Cotter SM, Frimberger AE, et al: A comparison of doxorubicin and COP for maintenance of remission in cats with lymphoma, *J Vet Intern Med* 10:372–375, 1996.
31. Valerius KD, Ogilvie GK, Mallinckrodt CH, et al: Doxorubicin alone or in combination with asparaginase, followed by cyclophosphamide, vincristine, and prednisone for treatment of multicentric lymphoma in dogs: 121 cases (1987-1995), *J Am Vet Med Assoc* 210:512–516, 1997.

32. Ogilvie GK, Reynolds HA, Richardson RC, et al: Phase II evaluation of doxorubicin for treatment of various canine neoplasms, *J Am Vet Med Assoc* 195:1580–1583, 1989.
33. Jeglum KA, Wheareat A: Chemotherapy of canine thyroid carcinoma, *Compend Contin Educ Pract Vet* 5:96–98, 1983.
34. Sorenmo KU, Jeglum KA, Helfand SC: Chemotherapy of canine hemangiosarcoma with doxorubicin and cyclophosphamide, *J Vet Intern Med* 7:370–376, 1993.
35. Mauldin GE, Fox PR, Patnaik AK, et al: Doxorubicin-induced cardiotoxicosis, *J Vet Intern Med* 6:82–88, 1992.
36. Lipshultz SE, Colan SD, Gelber RD, et al: Late cardiac effects of doxorubicin therapy for acute lymphoblastic leukemia in childhood, *New Eng J Med* 324:808–815, 1991.
37. Imondi AR, Torre PD, Mazue G, et al: Dose-response relationship of dezrazoxane for prevention of doxorubicin-induced cardiotoxicity in mice, rats, and dogs, *Cancer Res* 56:4200–4204, 1996.
38. O'Keefe DA, Sisson DD, Gelberg HB, et al: Systemic toxicity associated with doxorubicin administration in cats, *J Vet Intern Med* 7:309–317, 1993.
39. Cotter SM, Kanki PJ, Simon M: Renal disease in five tumor-bearing cats treated with Adriamycin, *J Am Anim Hosp Assoc* 21:405–409, 1985.
40. Vonderhaar MA, Morrison WB, Glickman NW, et al: Comparison of efficacy of doxorubicin and epirubicin as single agent therapy for canine multicentric malignant lymphoma, *Proc Vet Canc Soc Ann Mtg* 13:46, 1993.
41. Moore AS, Ruslander D, Cotter SM, et al: Efficacy of, and toxicoses associated with, oral idarubicin administration in cats with neoplasia, *J Am Vet Med Assoc* 206:1550–1554, 1995.
42. Hammer AS, Couto CG, Ayl RD, Shank KA: Treatment of tumor-bearing dogs with actinomycin D, *J Vet Intern Med* 8:236–239, 1994.
43. Buhles WC Jr, Theilen GH: Preliminary evaluation of bleomycin in feline and canine squamous cell carcinomas, *Am J Vet Res* 34:289–291, 1973.
44. Yoshida K, Watarai Y, Sakai Y, et al: The effect of intralesional bleomycin on canine acanthomatous epulis, *J Am Anim Hosp Assoc* 34:457–461, 1998.
45. Schaeppi U, Phelan R, Stadnicki SW, et al: Pulmonary fibrosis following multiple treatment with bleomycin (NCS-125066) in dogs, *Cancer Chemother Rep* 58:301–310, 1974.
46. Ogilvie GK, Obradovich JE, Elmslie RE, et al: Efficacy of mitoxantrone against various neoplasms in dogs, *J Am Vet Med Assoc* 23:587–596, 1991.
47. Moore AS, Ogilvie GK, Ruslander D, et al: Evaluation of mitoxantrone for treatment of lymphoma in dogs, *J Am Vet Med Assoc* 205:1903–1905, 1994.
48. Ogilvie GK, Obradovich JE, Elmslie RE, et al: Toxicoses associated with administration of mitoxantrone to dogs with malignant tumors, *J Am Vet Med Assoc* 198:1613–1617, 1991.
49. Pond SM: Effects on the liver of chemicals encountered in the workplace, *West J Med* 137(6):506–514, 1982.
50. Hamilton TA, Morrison WB, DeNicola DB: Cytosine arabinoside chemotherapy for acute megakaryocytic leukemia in a cat, *J Am Vet Med Assoc* 199:359–361, 1991.
51. Harvey HJ, MacEwen EG, Hayes AA: Neurotoxicosis associated with use of 5-fluorouracil in five dogs and one cat, *J Am Vet Med Assoc* 171:277–278, 1977.
52. Hammer AS, Carothers MA, Harris CL, et al: Unexpected neurotoxicity in dogs receiving a cyclophosphamide, dactinomycin, and 5-fluorouracil chemotherapy protocol, *J Vet Intern Med* 8:240–243, 1994.
53. Dorman DC, Coddington KA, Richardson RC: 5-Fluorouracil toxicosis in the dog, *J Vet Intern Med* 4:254–257, 1990.
54. Okeda R, Kimura S, Toizumi S, et al: Neuropathologic study on chronic neurotoxicity of 5-fluorouracil and its masked compounds in dogs, *Acta Neuropath* 63:334–343, 1984.
55. Theilen G: Adverse effect from use of 5% fluorouracil, *J Am Vet Med Assoc* 191:276, 1987.
56. Leifer CE, Matus RE, Patnaik AK, et al: Chronic myelogenous leukemia in the dog, *J Am Vet Med Assoc* 183:686–698, 1983.
57. Hamilton TA: The leukemias. In Morrison WB, editor: *Cancer in dogs and cats*, Baltimore, 1998, Williams & Wilkins, pp 721–729.
58. MacEwen EG, Dragner FH, McClelland AJ, et al: Treatment of basophilic leukemia in a dog, *J Am Vet Med Assoc* 166:376–380, 1975.
59. Peterson ME, Randolph JF: Diagnosis of canine primary polycythemia and management with hydroxyurea, *J Am Vet Med Assoc* 180:415–418, 1982.
60. Fineman LS, Hamilton TA, de Gortari A, et al: Cisplatin chemotherapy for treatment of thyroid carcinoma in dogs: 13 cases, *J Am Anim Hosp Assoc* 34:109–112, 1998.
61. Himsel CA, Richardson RC, Craig JA: Cisplatin chemotherapy for metastatic squamous cell carcinoma in two dogs, *J Am Vet Med Assoc* 189:1575–1578, 1986.
62. Shapiro W, Kitchell BE, Fossum TW, et al: Cisplatin for treatment of transitional cell and squamous cell carcinomas in dogs, *J Am Vet Med Assoc* 193:1530–1533, 1988.
63. Knapp DW, Richardson RC, Bonney PL, et al: Cisplatin therapy in 41 dogs with malignant tumors, *J Vet Intern Med* 2:41–46, 1988.
64. Thompson JP, Fugent MJ: Evaluation of survival times after limb amputation, with and without subsequent administration of cisplatin, for treatment of appendicular osteosarcoma in dogs: 30 cases (1979-1990), *J Am Vet Med Assoc* 200:531–533, 1992.
65. Kraegel SA, Madewell BR, Simonsen E, et al: Osteogenic sarcoma and cisplatin chemotherapy in dogs: 16 cases (1986-1989), *J Am Vet Med Assoc* 199:1057–1059, 1991.
66. Moore AS, Kirk C, Carcona A: Intracavitary cisplatin chemotherapy experience with six dogs, *J Vet Intern Med* 5:227–231, 1991.
67. Knapp DW, Richardson RC, DeNicola DB, et al: Cisplatin toxicity in cats, *J Vet Intern Med* 1:29–35, 1987.
68. Theon AP, Van Vechten MK, Madewell BR: Intratumoral administration of carboplatin for treatment of squamous cell carcinomas of the nasal plane in cats, *Am J Vet Res* 57:205–210, 1996.
69. Hahn KA, McEntee MF, Daniel GB, et al: Hematologic and systemic toxicoses associated with carboplatin administration in cats, *Am J Vet Res* 58:677–679, 1997.
70. London CA: Tyrosine kinase inhibitors in veterinary medicine, *Top Companion Anim Med* 24(3):106–112, 2009.
71. London CA, Malpas PB, Wood-Follis SL, et al: Multi-center, placebo-controlled, double-blind, randomized study of oral toceranib phosphate (SU11654), a receptor tyrosine kinase inhibitor, for the treatment of dogs with recurrent (either local or distant) mast cell tumor following surgical excision, *Clin Cancer Res* 15(11):3856–3865, 2009.
72. Ogilvie GK, Atwater SW, Ciekot PA, et al: Prevalence of anaphylaxis associated with the intramuscular administration of L-asparaginase to 81 dogs with cancer: 1989-1991, *J Am Anim Hosp Assoc* 30:62–65, 1994.
73. MacEwen EG, Rosenthal RC, Fox LE, et al: Evaluation of L-asparaginase: polyethylene glycol conjugate versus native L-asparaginase combined with chemotherapy. A randomized double-blind study in canine lymphoma, *J Vet Intern Med* 6:230–234, 1992.
74. Hansen WE, Schulz G: The effect of dietary fiber on pancreatic amylase activity in vitro, *Hepatogastroenterol* 29(4):157–160, 1982.
75. Mandell C: Antithrombin III concentrations associated with L-asparaginase administration, *Vet Clin Pathol* 21:68–70, 1992.
76. Rogers KS, Barton CL, Benson PA, et al: Effects of single-dose L-asparaginase on coagulation values in healthy dogs and dogs with lymphoma, *Am J Vet Res* 53:580–584, 1992.
77. Swanson JF, Morgan S, Green RA, et al: Cerebral thrombosis and hemorrhage in association with L-asparaginase administration, *J Am Anim Hosp Assoc* 22:749–755, 1986.

78. Galbraith EA, McKellar QA: Pharmacokinetics and pharmacodynamics of piroxicam in dogs, *Vet Rec* 128:561–565, 1991.
79. Knapp DW, Chan TC, Kuczek T, et al: Evaluation of in vitro cytotoxicity of nonsteroidal anti-inflammatory drugs against canine tumor cells, *Am J Vet Res* 56:801–805, 1995.
80. Knapp DW, Richardson RC, Chan TC, et al: Piroxicam therapy in 34 dogs with transitional cell carcinoma of the urinary bladder, *J Vet Intern Med* 8:273–278, 1994.
81. Knapp DW, Richardson RC, Bottoms GD, et al: Phase I trial of piroxicam in 62 dogs bearing naturally occurring tumors, *Cancer Chemother Pharmacol* 29:214–218, 1992.
82 Price G, Page R, Fischer B, et al: Efficacy and toxicity of doxorubicin/cyclophosphamide maintenance therapy in dogs with multicentric lymphoma, *J Vet Intern Med* 5:259–262, 1991.
83. Impellizeri JA, McKeever KP, Crow SE: The role of rituximab in the treatment of canine lymphoma: an ex vivo evaluation, *Vet J* 171(3):556–558, 2006.
84. Jubala CM, Valli VE, Getzy DM, et al: CD20 expression in normal canine B cells and in canine non-Hodgkin lymphoma, *Vet Pathol* 42(4):468–476, 2005.
85. Rebuzzi L, Sonneck K, Gleixner KV, et al: Detection of vascular endothelial growth factor (VEGF) and VEGF receptors Flt-1 and KDR in canine mastocytoma cells, *Vet Immunol Immunopathol* 115(3-4):320–333, 2007.
86. Bergman PJ, et al: Development of a xenogeneic DNA vaccine program for canine malignant melanoma at the Animal Medical Center, *Vaccine* 24:4582–4585, 2006.
87. Bergman PJ, et al: Long-term survival of dogs with advanced malignant melanoma after DNA vaccination with xenogeneic human tyrosinase: a phase I trial, *Clin Cancer Res* 9:1284–1290, 2003.

Appendix 1

Regulatory Issues

Appendix Outline

THE FOOD AND DRUG ADMINISTRATION

The Food and Drug Administration (FDA) is one of several agencies that regulate the use of drugs, biologics, and medical devices in humans and nonhuman animals (Table 1). The FDA focuses its activities on ensuring the efficacy and safety of drugs to animals (including humans), drug handlers, and the environment. As such, the FDA develops and enforces regulations and written policies for statutory responsibilities in protecting public health through public hearings, public notices, and consultants. The history of the FDA begins in the mid-1800s, although the United States Pharmacopeia (USP) was established earlier by 11 physicians in 1820. The USP was the first organization to address drugs through the formulation of the first compendium of drug standards in the United States, which is one of many activities it continues to do today. The activities of the FDA began when the Bureau of Chemistry was formed as part of the newly created US Department of Agriculture (USDA) during Abraham Lincoln's presidency. Its primary function was analysis of agricultural products. The regulatory activities of the FDA were formalized to include prohibition of interstate commerce of misbranded or adulterated drugs with the passage of the Pure Food and Drug Act of 1906. In 1927, the agency was named the Food, Drug and Insecticide Administration, and its current name was acquired in 1930. In 1937, 107 persons, including many children, died after ingestion of the antibiotic sulfanilamide prepared in a diethylene glycol vehicle. In response to this incident, Congress empowered the FDA to assure safety of drug products with passage of the Federal Food, Drug, and Cosmetic Act in 1938. In 1962, in response to birth defects associated with the sleeping pill thalidomide, Congress passed the Kefauver-Harris Drug Amendment, which not only empowered the FDA to have greater input regarding drug safety but also provided regulation for assurance of drug efficacy. It was not until 1968, with passage of the Animal Drug Amendment, that animal drugs were defined and placed under the regulatory actions of the FDA. The current offices of the FDA are delineated in Figure 1. Other acts involving the FDA's oversight of veterinary or human issues can be found at the FDA website (see Table 1).

Laws regarding food and drugs are not passed by the FDA; rather, they are passed by Congress and enforced by the FDA through its regulations. Current activities of Congress, including those related to drugs, are noted in the *Federal Register.* FDA regulations (Table 2) also are printed in Title 21, Code of Federal Regulations (21CFR), which is updated on April 1 of each year. These books can be purchased from the US Government Printing Office. To facilitate implementation of its regulations by field officers, the FDA also publishes compliancy policy guidelines. Although not legally binding, they do provide insight into the Agency's current thinking.

The Center for Veterinary Medicine (CVM) identifies itself as a consumer protection agency that fosters public and animal health by approving safe and effective products for animals and by enforcing other applicable provisions of the Federal Food, Drug, and Cosmetic Act and other authorities. The organization of the FDA reveals that only a fraction of its efforts are directed toward the CVM. The organization of the CVM is shown in Figure 1. The CVM website at the

Table 1 Federal Regulatory Agencies Dealing with Animal Drugs, Biologics, and Medical Devices

Agency	Function
Department of Interior: Environmental Protection Agency (EPA)	Regulates human drugs, biological devices, radiation products and issues, and food safety
Food and Drug Administration (FDA)	Regulates human drugs, biological devices, radiation products and issues, food safety, cosmetics, and veterinary drugs (through the Center for Veterinary Medicine [CVM])
US Department of Agriculture: Animal and Plant Health Inspection Service	Regulates animal biologics, helps the FDA monitor proper use of drugs in animals, prohibits repackaging and relabeling of veterinary biologics for over-the-counter (OTC) sale or distribution
Department of Justice: Drug Enforcement Agency (DEA)	Regulates and enforces the Controlled Substances Act of 1970
Department of Interior	Controls licensing of topical animal pesticide use and distribution under the Federal Insecticide, Fungicide, and Rodenticide Act

time of printing was http://www.fda.gov/AnimalVeterinary/default.htm. A publication, *FDA and the Veterinarian*, is available at the FDA website.

Several publications define the FDA's laws and regulations: *Requirements of Laws and Regulations Enforced by the U. S. Food and Drug Administration*, which can be obtained from the US Department of Human Health Services, and *Code of Federal Regulations* (CFR). A more user-friendly account of the laws regulating veterinarians can be found in *FDA and the Veterinarian*. The most recent issue was published in 1989, but a newer version is being prepared. Finally, James E. Wilson, DVM, JD, has written a book, *Law and Ethics of the Veterinary Profession*, that provides a more focused perspective on the use of drugs in animals.

Keeping abreast of changes in the FDA's response to veterinary use of drugs can be difficult. Generally, the *Journal of the American Veterinary Medical Association* and the American Veterinary Medical Association (AVMA) have done an excellent job in putting together and publishing symposia that delineate and discuss the implications of FDA actions. In addition, the American College of Veterinary Clinical Pharmacology and the American Academy of Veterinary Pharmacology and Therapeutics provide guidance through publications and consultation. Finally, the FDA appears to be willing to answer any questions or concerns one might have regarding the use of drugs in animals. In the CVM, the Office of New Animal Drug Evaluation consists of the Division of Therapeutic Drugs for Non-Food, which in turn contains a section for Companion and Wildlife Drugs. Note that there are other federal agencies that regulate the use of drugs in animals, including the Environmental Protection Agency (EPA), the Animal and Plant Health Inspection Service, and others (see Table 1).

Drugs Defined

A drug is well defined by the FDA (see Table 1). It must be recognized as such (e.g., by the USP); intended for diagnosis, cure, mitigation, or prevention of disease in humans or other animals (note that the FDA defines humans as animals); intended to affect body structure or function; or a component of any of these. In 1968, the FDA first made a distinction between human and veterinary-labeled drugs. As with most regulations since that time, the distinction reflected a concern for human food safety. At that time, an animal drug was adulterated if used in an extralabel fashion. Thus a veterinarian could not modify a dosing regimen, therapeutic intent, and so on of a drug without being liable in both criminal and civil courts. Currently, a new animal drug (NAD) is "any drug intended for use in animals other than man … not recognized … as safe and effective under conditions on the label." A drug's label includes the label on the product, as well as any accompanying material (see Box 1). A prescription drug is defined by whether or not adequate directions can be prepared for use of the drug by a layperson. Any drug for which this is possible must be sold as an over-the-counter (OTC) preparation; any other product is a prescription (Rx) product that must bear the phrase: "Caution: Federal law restricts this drug to use by or on the order of a licensed veterinarian." Trying to identify the approval status of a drug can be difficult. Obviously, if the label has this cautionary statement, a new animal drug application (NADA) exists for the drug and it can be used legally *according to the label specifications*. Determining whether an NADA exists for a drug can, however, be difficult. If the drug is listed in the veterinary versions of the *Physician's Desk Reference* (i.e., the *Veterinary Drugs and Biological Products*, published by Medical Economics, or the *Compendium of Veterinary Products*, published by Bayer Animal Health [both basically are copies of package inserts]), then the drug has an NADA. Note that drugs listed in veterinary textbooks, including formularies, pharmacology texts, internal medicine texts, and so on, do not necessarily have an NADA. Other sources include members of the American College of Veterinary Clinical Pharmacology, the FDA *Green Book* (http://www.fda.gov/AnimalVeterinary/Products/ApprovedAnimalDrugProducts/ucm042847.htm, last accessed May 25, 2010), or the *Handbook of New Animal Drugs*, published by Shotwell and Carr.

The Drug Approval Process

From discovery of a new compound (including isolation and synthesis) through its development (including establishing safety and efficacy) to its marketing involves researchers and clinicians and a consortium of regulatory, industrial, and often academic investigators.

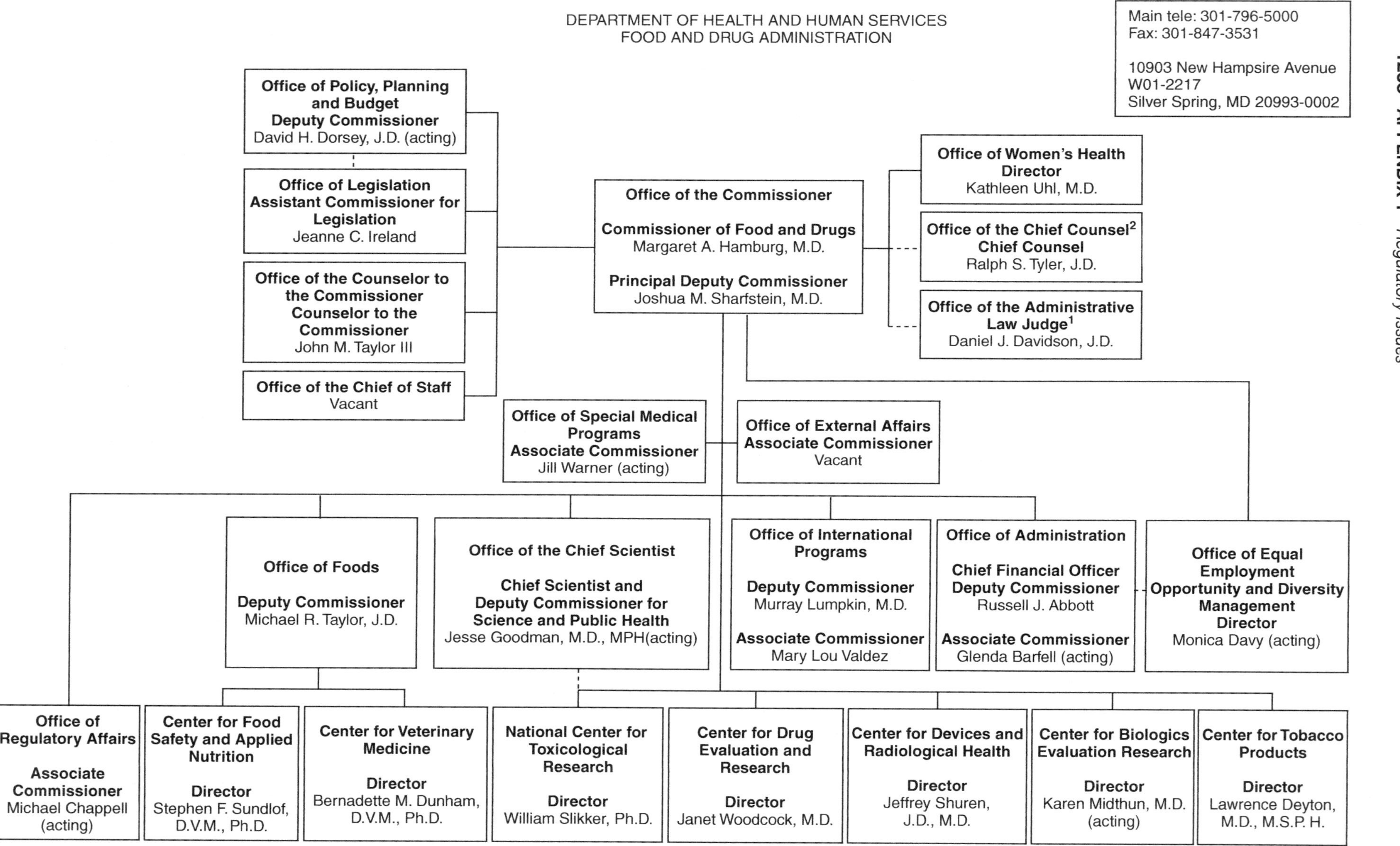

Figure 1 Extralabel drug use algorithm offered by the Food and Drug Administration (FDA) to veterinarians. *Record requirements include animal identification (individuals or as group; species; number treated; condition; drug name and active ingredient; dosing regimen; duration; and specified withdrawal, withholding, or discard time(s) (both label and that specified by veterinarian) when applicable (meat, milk, eggs, or animal-derived food). **Label requirements include name and address of prescribing veterinarian, name of drug, specified direction for use (class/species; identification of the animal or group; dosing regimen including route; and duration of therapy), and cautionary statements. ***The compounding of preparations from bulk drugs is generally considered by the FDA to be illegal.

Table 2 Drug Laws or Guidelines Affecting the Use of Human and Veterinary Drugs

Law or Guideline	Year	Action
Federal Pure Food and Drug Act	1906	Established standards for safety and purity.
Federal Food, Drug, and Cosmetic Act	1938	Prohibited marketing of new drugs until adequately tested under label conditions for safety.
Durham-Humphrey Amendment to the Food, Drug, and Cosmetic Act	1952	Defined over-the-counter (OTC) products by distinguishing them from prescription-only products.
Kefauver-Harris Amendment to the Food, Drug, and Cosmetic Act	1962	Required scientific proof of efficacy and safety before marketing of a drug and that the Food and Drug administration (FDA) be notified before testing of drugs in humans. Investigational new drug (IND) applications established. Safety and efficacy data needed retroactive to all drugs introduced between 1938 and 1962. Drugs introduced before 1938 are considered "grandfather" drugs as long as labeled use does not change (e.g., phenobarbital, levothyroxine, digoxin).
Animal Drug Amendments to the Food, Drug, and Cosmetic Act	1968	Animal drug regulations placed under one section of the Food, Drug, and Cosmetic Act; the use of animal drugs is restricted to the species and usage as specified on the label.
Poison Prevention Packaging Act	1970	Required that hazardous substances be dispensed in child-resistant containers.
Comprehensive Drug Abuse Prevention and Control Act (Controlled Substances Act)	1970	Controlled the manufacture and prescription of habit-forming drugs.
Orphan Drug Act	1983	Addressed the development of drugs indicated for rare diseases.
Compliance Policy Guidelines	1984	Addressed extralabel use of new animal drugs in food-producing animals and distribution and use of human-labeled drugs for animals. Note, however, that the policies and guidelines were in contradiction to the Food, Drug, and Cosmetic Act. Created the legal veterinary prescription.
Drug Price Competition and Patent Restoration Act	1984	Addressed new drug applications for generic drug products.
Generic Animal Drug and Patent Term Restoration Act (GAPTRA)	1988	Extended to veterinary products the right of companies to produce and sell generic versions of animal drugs approved after October 1962 without duplicating research done to prove them safe and effective.
Compliance Policy Guides	1991	Same as the 1984 Guidelines.
Animal Medicinal Drug Use Clarification Act (AMDUCA)	1994	Legalized extralabel drug use of certain approved animal drugs and approved human drugs for animals as long as specified criteria are met. Final act effective in 1996.
Dietary Supplement Health and Education Act	1994	Established specific labeling requirements, provided a regulatory framework, and authorized FDA to promulgate good manufacturing practice regulations for dietary supplements. This act defined "dietary supplements" and "dietary ingredients" and classified them as food. The act also established a commission to recommend how to regulate claims. The Center for Veterinary Medicine (CVM) subsequently determined that this act does not apply to products intended for use in animals.
Animal Drug Availability Act (ADAA)	1996	Provided additional legislation to address the lack of legally available animal drugs. Facilitated approval of new animal drugs through flexibility in the approval process.
Food and Drug Administration Modernization Act (FDAMA)	1997	Enhanced FDA's mission in ways that recognized the Agency would be operating in a twenty-first century characterized by increasing technologic, trade, and public health complexities. Many issues were addressed in the ADAA.

Human Drugs

The approval process for human drugs in the United States has been described as the most vigorous in the world, costing on average $359 million to move a drug from the laboratory to the patient. After identification and isolation of a compound, its safety is established in laboratory animals. *Preclinical testing* studies include acute and chronic toxicity studies focusing on the reproductive status, mutagenicity, and carcinogenicity of the drug. A safe dosing range is established, requiring both pharmacokinetic and pharmacodynamic (dose-response) studies. At this point, if the compound is considered a potential candidate for approval, an investigational new drug (IND) is filed by the sponsor, with protocols for clinical testing. This phase requires approximately 5 to 8 years, and generally only 1 drug in 5000 evaluated succeeds in this phase. At this point, if the compound is considered a potential candidate for approval, an IND is filed by the sponsor, along with protocols for clinical testing. Approximately 2000 INDs are filed with the FDA each

Box 1

Package Drug Inserts/Labels

Defined

The drug package insert (DPI) is a legal document that accompanies a finished dosing form of an approved drug product. As such, it applies only to the approved product that it accompanies. The DPI for a product includes the label on the product itself as well as any and all accompanying materials (i.e., inside the package. All information included must be approved by the Food and Drug Administration). The label does not include technical monographs or advertisements that might be distributed by a manufacturer. Although the manufacturer may sponsor post-market surveillance studies that can be cited in and provide the basis for information in monographs used for promotion of the product, care must still be taken not to promote a use not stated on the label. Changes to labels that might accommodate new findings regarding the disease targeted by the drug or its use require approval by regulatory agencies, a cost the manufacturer may not want to pursue. Any use of the product beyond that specifically delineated in the label constitutes extra label drug use (EDLU). Data provided in current drug package inserts (DPIs) might be categorized as Product Description, Product Efficacy, or Product Safety with some overlap among the categories.

Product Description: Drug or Drug Product Name

1. **Finished dosing form:** The approved product includes the combined presentation of the (a) active pharmaceutical ingredient (API; often referred to as the drug substance, which may or may not include the salt [co-ion] or ester modification); (b) the route (which may not be included if implied by the dosing form); the dosage form (tablet, solution, topical); and release characteristics (e.g., extended-release tablets), if appropriate. Each drug label provides three names to the product: a generic name for the drug product, which includes the generic name for the API, and the trade name for the specific drug product (see Box 2). In addition to the API, the product description includes any excipients, including fillers, stabilizers, or preservatives. These should be assessed as well for components that may contribute to allergies (i.e., meat flavoring) or adversities (benzyl alcohol as preservatives for cats, xylitol as flavoring agent or carrier in dogs).
2. **Dosage and administration:** USA dosing units for veterinary products have not been standardized to kilogram (kg) and thus are often offered in terms of pounds (lbs) and kg. Attention should be given to the basis of dosing for API modified as salts or esters: is the dose based on the total weight or the active ingredient? Newer drugs generally are named and dosed based on the active ingredient. However, older drugs may be described and dose on either the active ingredient or the salt/ester.
3. **Preparation for use and storage conditions:** Any variation beyond that stated on the label may increase the risk of loss of activity. The impact of freezing, refrigeration, or other storage conditions should not be assumed; queries should be directed toward the manufacturer. Products provided in protective packaging generally should be assumed to need the packaging to remain stable.
4. **Expiration date:** Generally, the expiration date should be respected, although the manufacturer may have additional information and may be willing to share this if specifically queried.
5. **Indications:** The approved indication often is not the applied indication. However, any deviation from the approved indication reflects ELDU. Efficacy and to a lesser degree, safety information can be used to support an ELDU indication.

Product Efficacy

1. **Mechanism of action (MOA):** The FDA requires scientific support for the MOA that is claimed on the DPI. As such, a MOA may not be provided.
2. **Clinical pharmacology:** As important as it may be to understanding the proper use of a drug in healthy and unhealthy animals, important pharmacokinetic information may not be provided on the package insert: studies may not have been performed and may not have been required by the FDA. Example of information that may or may not be included follows: *bioavailability, non-linear clearance or kinetics* **(a) Absorption:** Both *rate* and *extent*, C_{max}, (the maximum plasma drug concentration) that occurs at T_{max}; area under the curve (AUC); oral bioavailability (F = fraction); the impact of food (or other factors) on absorption; first pass metabolism; the potential impact of P-glycoprotein. **(b) Distribution:** volume of distribution (Vd); fraction of drug not bound to plasma proteins (f_{ub}); tissue drug concentrations (note that tissue homogenate data can be misleading because it includes both intracellular and interstitial tissue). **(c) Elimination:** Clearance (Cl, the organ of clearance should be identified, including the role of hepatic metabolism; and non-linear clearance identified); elimination half-life ($t_{1/2}$), or elimination rate constant, k_{el}). The mean elimination half-life may be arithmetic, harmonic (mean is determined from the inverse of half-life, which is averaged and then inversed again) or geometric (for numbers that increase non-linearly).
3. **Microbiology:** Pharmacodynamic data (MIC) should be based on an adequate sample of the target population (i.e., >100 isolates). The FDA may not allow microbiologic data for organisms not included in the approved use. Data generally includes the range, the MIC 50 (median) or MIC 90 (90th percentile).
4. **Effectiveness: field trials:** Efficacy field trials focus on the approved indication, reflect use as intended in target animals, and must be controlled. Controls may be, negative placebos, for which superiority must be demonstrated and accompanied by ethical constraints or positive controls for which non-inferiority is generally the target.

Product Safety

1. **Adverse reactions:** Adverse drug reactions in the medical literature generally refer to reactions that can cause harm to a patient and as such, may require a therapeutic intervention. This includes *all* side effects observed in all studies of the drug **Side effects** generally are not associated with harm but may be undesirable and may be sufficient to cause the drug to not be used. **Foreign marked adverse reaction information** reflects information that may have emerged as a result of the study or use of the drug in foreign markets.
2. **Safety information:** Three sources of safety data may be present on a package insert. **(a) Toxicity studies:** Collected in normal animals, as directed for each drug by the FDA, generally reflecting several magnitudes of the dose (i.e., 3, 5, or 10 X) and a duration several magnitudes beyond that recommended. Sample size is small. The FDA may compel inclusion of studies implemented but not necessarily in support of the approved indication. **(b) Field studies:** The drug is studied in animals with spontaneous disease, for the approved indication, under expected conditions. Sample size often exceeds 100 to 200 for each indication;

Box 1
Package Drug Inserts/Labels—Cont'd

response generally is compared to negative control (placebo) or positive control. **(c) Post-market surveillance:** This process may be added after approval if warranted sufficiently important by the FDA.

3. **Contraindications** represent the strongest warning and are established situations under which the drug should not be used. Such use should be expected to result in an adverse even. These might include, medical conditions such as kidney problems or known or anticipated allergies.
4. **Warnings** cover possible serious side effects that may occur.
5. **Precautions** explain how to use the medication safely, including physical impairments and potential drug interactions.
6. **Information for the owner** is not included for all drugs, but may emerge during post market surveillance in an attempt to reduce the risk of adversity. This information may be provided as a separate document that may be sent home with the client.
7. **Drug Interactions** may or may not be included; the absence of described drug interactions should not be interpreted as the lack of clinically relevant interactions.

Box 2
What's in a (Drug) Name?

A drug by any other name may not be the same. The name of the *active moiety* (AM; drug substance) must be distinguished from the *drug product name*. The AM will have a *chemical name* (determined by the Chemical Analytical Society [CAS] based on its structure) and a *generic name*. In contrast, the drug product will have a *non-proprietary (established) name* and *proprietary (brand) name*. In the United States, the generic AM is initially named by the United States Adopted Name [USAN] Council. Ideally, the name will also be approved by the International Nonproprietary Name (INN) Expert Committee, such that the generic name is globally applicable. As such, only one generic name should exist for any AM, although exceptions exist (e.g., epinephrine versus adrenaline; acetaminophen versus paracetamol, and occasional differences in spelling [alfa versus alpha]).

The generic AM name consists of three parts that logically apply to the AM activity. The *stem*, generally located at the end of the name, is the most important. It indicates an action unique to and shared by all drugs with the same stem. The stem can be based on a chemical relationships (e.g., azepams, cefalosporins), therapeutic activity (*terone* for antiandrogens or *poietins* for erythropoiten), or mechanism of action (*statin* for cholesterol-lowering drugs). Currently more than 300 stems exist. The *prefix* of a generic AM is used to discriminate among members having the same stem (e.g., ***dia***zepam, ***clon***azepam). The importance of racemates in the past decade has led to the use of logical prefixes indicating the enantiomer status of an AM. These include dextrorotatory (***dex***tromethorphams) or R (***ar***formeterol), and levorotatory (**levo**floxacin, **lev**atiracetam) or S (**es**molol). The *infix* of the drug name is irrelevant unless further subclassification is necessary. Because many approved drug products may have the same AM, it is the generic AM that is preferred for general use in order to facilitate the flow of scientific information within and among nations.

Some drug substances are accompanied by a salt or ester. In such cases, USAN will also provide an API that contains the AM (e.g., zonisamide, pancuronium, triamcinolone, or penicillin) is added to the associated salt (e.g., ***sodium*** zonisamide or pancuronium ***bromide***) or ester (e.g., triamcinolone ***acetate*** or ***procaine*** penicillin). The AM (or API) becomes part of the *established (non-proprietary) drug product name*, which is established nationally (e.g., the United States Pharmacopeia) and approved by the regulatory agency (e.g., the FDA). Generally, the non-proprietary drug product name includes the USAN generic AM or API (with the choice by USP depending on how important the salt or ester is to drug use), the route of administration (e.g., oral [excluded if implied by the dosing form], topical, ophthalmic) and the dosage form (e.g., tablet, solution, lotion, suspension, aerosol).

Other descriptors (e.g., altered release rate [e.g., delayed, extended release] or delivery system [e.g., transdermal patch) may be included. It is the USP generic drug product name (e.g., carprofen tablet, enrofloxacin otic solution) that is generally on the package insert of the drug product approved by the Food and Drug Administration. The USAN names and the possible options for drug product names can be found in the United States Pharmacopeia Dictionary and National Formulary (USP-NF), respectively, each published annually by the USP. Note that the AM (API) is likely to be only one of several ingredients found in the finished drug product that is approved by the regulatory agency (e.g., the Food and Drug Administration [FDA] in the United States); other ingredients might be excipients intended as filler, stabilizers or antibacterial.

The *proprietary* or *brand name* of the approved drug product (e.g., Rimadyl, Baytril Otic) belongs to the manufacturer, although the FDA offers guidelines that are intended to avoid inappropriate public perceptions of drug action or safety based on the brand name. A *generic drug product* that has been demonstrated by the manufacturer to be therapeutically equivalent to the pioneer *proprietary drug product* may be subsequently approved by the FDA. The two products will have the same USP established drug product name. However, the generic drug product must either not have a brand name or have a brand name that differs from the pioneer drug product (e.g., Novox as a generic Rimadyl). Finally, it is important to note that a manufacturer may actually change the AM (or API) associated with a brand name product; this is particularly common to over-the-counter products (e.g., Kaopectate). For other information that may be found on a package drug inserts, see Box 1.

year. Long-term safety studies continue in animals as the drug enters Phase I clinical trials in humans.

The *clinical phase* of drug approval involves three distinct phases of clinical trials that provide the basis of the drug label. *Phase I* is conducted on a small number of normal volunteers (generally 20 to 80; most commonly, young adult Caucasian males are studied) to determine a safe dosing range and the disposition of the drug (pharmacokinetics). *Phase II* begins studies in clinical effectiveness and safety in several hundred persons with target illnesses. In *Phase III,* the number increases to several thousand to establish risk:benefit ratios. Phases I through III last approximately 3 to 10 years; if the drug demonstrates a favorable risk:benefit ratio, the sponsor can submit a new drug approval (NDA). A typical NDA is approximately 100,000 pages or more in length. The FDA, by law, must review the NDA within 6 months, although generally this time period is exceeded. During this phase, the sponsor and FDA determine the detailed information that will accompany the label, including contraindications, precautions, side effects, dosages, routes of administration, and frequency of administration. Only one of five drugs studied for human use receives FDA approval.

After *approval,* the manufacturer can promote the drug, but large-scale clinical trials will continue to further define the safety profile. Additional *Phase IV* studies may be required. Once the drug is in widespread use, adverse effects previously undetected may be recognized. Occasionally, if the adversities are serious (fatal), the drug may be withdrawn from the market. Postmarket studies also may identify efficacy for indications not previously identified during the approval process. New information from postmarket studies are used to update the NDA. During this time period, reports of adverse reactions, particularly those not previously recognized or unexpected, are important to evaluating the safety of the drug. For human drugs, reports can be made on the Drug Experience Form, through MedWatch (a voluntary reporting program), and through the sponsoring pharmaceutical company.

Animal Drugs

The approval process for new animal drugs is not as clear cut as for human drugs. This reflects in part the variabilities presented by species differences, economic considerations, and the importance of food (human) safety. Thus, although the legal standards for safety and efficacy data are the same for both human and animal drugs, design of safety and efficacy studies and the criteria for approval differ, and the approval process for an NAD generally is tailored to the particular drugs. The differences are most marked for food animal drugs for which efficacy and safety data in the target species must be weighed in the context of economic considerations. The path of human drug approval does not apply to animals, although many of the same data are collected. The regulations for the approval of an animal drug can be found in 21CFR 514.1; however, several recent drug laws (e.g., the FDA Modernization Act and the Animal Medicinal Drug Use Clarification Act) and the Generic Drug Law of 1988 have impacted several aspects of this law, which is currently being updated by the FDA.

The approval process for animal drugs is changing but currently occurs in two distinct phases. (http://www.fda.gov/AnimalVeterinary/GuidanceComplianceEnforcement/GuidanceforIndustry/ucm123821.htm; last accessed May 25, 2010). During the investigational new animal drug (INAD) phase, five technical areas are reviewed by the FDA. These include composition, manufacturing, and chemistry (CMC, basic manufacturing data); target animal safety; evidence of clinical efficacy; environmental considerations; and human food safety, which includes tissue residue data, for animal tissues intended for human consumption. During this phase, the FDA, in concert with the sponsor, determines product development plans, reviews protocols for the study design, implements the studies, and generates the raw data intended to support approval; the FDA then decides whether the data are sufficient to address concerns. The protocols for toxicology and tissue residue chemistry studies are straightforward, but more creative and innovative approaches are taken for target animal safety and efficacy because of the diverse issues surrounding new animal drugs.

Once the technical sections are completed, the second phase, the NADA is filed. This phase is in transition and represents a new approach to drug approval by the FDA (an "administrative" NADA) in that the majority of data supporting the approval of a drug may have already been reviewed by the time this phase is begun. The drug may be known to be approvable before this phase is reached because of the phased INAD review. The review process becomes largely interactive through the phased review process (http://www.fda.gov/downloads/AnimalVeterinary/GuidanceComplianceEnforcement/GuidanceforIndustry/UCM052464.pdf).

Orphan Drugs

The Orphan Drug Act of 1983 provided incentive for development of drugs used to treat rare diseases, which did not present sufficient economic incentive for a sponsor to undergo the traditional approval process because they benefit only a small number of patients. The added incentives include tax advantages and marketing exclusivity to the sponsoring company. The National Institutes of Health often participates in the development of orphan drugs. Examples of the 300 human drugs given orphan status include erythropoietin, α_1-antitrypsin, and human growth hormone. Criteria that a drug must meet to become an orphan drug include intent to treat a serious or life-threatening disease; lack of a comparable or satisfactory alternative; involvement in a clinical trial as an IND; and active pursuit of full approval by the sponsor. If these criteria are not met, the drug may still be obtained for *compassionate use.* The clinician in essence becomes the investigator by submitting a treatment IND.

Generic Drugs

Pharmacists can dispense an equivalent, less expensive, nonproprietary (generic) drug without prescriber approval. An exception occurs if a state has a mandatory substitution law or if the brand name product is dispensed along with a Dispensed as Written (DAW.) order. Generics may be pharmaceutically equivalent but may not be therapeutically equivalent. Those tested by the FDA and found to be therapeutically equivalent are listed in *Approved Drug Products with Therapeutic Equivalence Evaluations*, known as the *Orange Book* (http://www.accessdata.fda.gov/scripts/cder/ob/default.cfm; last accessed May 25, 2010). Generic products not only contain the same active ingredient as the proprietary drug but also meet bioequivalence standards. Substitutions of generic drugs for proprietary drugs are recommended only for those drugs shown to be therapeutically equivalent. Examples of drugs that are not therapeutically equivalent to their brand name counterparts include digoxin, phenytoin, conjugated estrogens, and slow-release theophyllines. The Orange Book addresses therapeutic equivalence in human medicine. Veterinary clinicians should not mistake therapeutic equivalence established in humans to be the same in animals.

The Drug Availability Crisis

In the mid-1990s, the Animal Health Institutes focused on an issue they termed the *drug availability crisis*. It is based on the fact that veterinarians are faced with the need and desire for improved veterinary care for their patients; there is a great availability of human-labeled drugs but fewer NADA applications. Simplistically, the FDA requirements of NAD approval have not allowed for flexibility in keeping up with the scientific advancements in the diagnosis, treatment, and prevention of animal diseases. For example, in 1994, for dogs, there were only 369 Rx drug products and 67 OTC drug products. For cats, there were only 169 Rx and 40 OTC drug products. For cats, these 209 products reflect only 84 drugs, many of which are no longer used. Approximately 15% of drugs discussed by the author used to treat or prevent illnesses in dogs are approved for that use; the number is even smaller for cats (less than 10%).

Two potential reasons preclude pharmaceutical companies pursuing the approval of human drugs for animals. First, adverse reactions that may occur in animals receiving the drug may impact the human market even if the adverse reaction is not likely to occur in humans. The second detractor is economic recovery. The cost of approving drugs has progressively increased, in part because of the "moving target" presented by the FDA to pharmaceutical companies. Requirements are constantly changing, and it is often difficult for the company to predict or keep up with changes. All changes are costly. A common misconception is that veterinary drugs do not have to undergo the same intensive scrutiny for approval as do human drugs. In fact, the opposite might be considered true. Because of the concern with tissue residues, far more time and effort might be put into animal drug approval, particularly food animal approval, than human drug approval. Environmental impact studies may also be more intense. Thus the cost for approval of an animal drug is disproportionately higher than of a human drug, particularly when the cost is compared with the recovery of costs. The animal market is very small compared with the human pharmaceutical market (millions compared with billions). The time for development of a drug (from identification of a potential compound to its final FDA approval) is 5 to 10 years, and the cost is approximately 1 to 2 million dollars per year (the longer time for food animals). As drug approval costs increase, the number of NADAs may decline. Extralabel use of human generic versions of animal-approved drugs or compounding in lieu of prescribing approved drugs are also disincentives for manufacturers to pursue approval of a veterinary drug.

Extralabel Drug Use

If a new NADA exists for a drug, to use the drug in a legal manner the veterinarian must adhere to the specifications noted on the label (which includes both the label adhered to the medication and the accompanying package insert). Otherwise, an NAD is used in an *extralabel* manner. In 1994, Congress passed the Animal Medicinal Drug Use Clarification Act (AMDUCA), which legalized extralabel drug use (ELDU) by veterinarians as long as specific criteria or restrictions are met (see Table 2). ELDU, whether actual or intended, occurs when the drug is used in a manner that is not in accordance with the approved label directions. This includes but is not limited to a different dose, interval, route, indication, or species. Veterinary ELDU is legalized by AMDUCA (see Table 2) only for approved drugs (human or animal) and not for products intended for use as drugs but are not approved drugs. The latter substances are perceived by the FDA to be unapproved drugs and as such, fall under their regulatory jurisdiction. This includes novel ingredients, such as herbs and nutraceuticals, as well as products compounded outside the stipulations of AMDUCA. However, the FDA recognizes that there are diseases in animals for which there is no approved drug treatment and that strict enforcement of their law precludes the practice of veterinary medicine. To address these concerns, in 1984 and 1991, the FDA published Compliance Policy Guidelines for ELDU, including ELDU of animal drugs (Compliance Policy Guideline 7125.06) and ELDU of human drugs in animals (Compliance Policy Guideline 7125.35). The guidelines focused on ELDU in food animals and have been updated (http://www.fda.gov/AnimalVeterinary/ResourcesforYou/FDAandtheVeterinarian/ucm077390.htm).TheseincludeEDLU is permitted only by or on the order of a veterinarian; it is allowed only for FDA-approved animal and human drugs (which excludes compounded products; see Compounding); it must be implemented in the context of an existing valid veterinary-client-patient relationship (VCPR; (Box 3). For food animals,

Box 3

Requirements of a Valid Veterinary-Client-Patient Relationship (VCPR) as Defined by the Food and Drug Administration (FDA)

1. The veterinarian has assumed responsibility for making clinical judgments about the health of the animal.
2. The client has agreed to follow the veterinarian's instructions.
3. The veterinarian has sufficient knowledge to initiate a preliminary diagnosis of the animal's medical condition.
4. The veterinarian has examined the patient and is personally acquainted with the keeping and care of the animal.
5. The veterinarian is readily available for follow-up evaluation in the event of an adverse reaction to the treatment or therapeutic failure.

further restrictions apply. An interactive algorithm is available from the AVMA that directs the veterinarian using ELDU (http://www.avma.org/reference/amduca/amduca1.asp).

Compounding

The guidelines regarding the compounding of pharmaceuticals under the direction of a veterinarian are delineated in Compliance Policy Guideline 7125.40. Conditions under which compounding is legal are specified in the AMDUCA. Compounding includes any manipulation of the drug beyond that stipulated on the label (such as reconstitution of a powdered drug) (Table 4). Conditions under which compounding is not subject to regulatory actions include a legitimate practice (pharmacy or veterinary; includes licensure), operation within the conformity of state law, for pharmacists in response to a prescription, and for veterinarians in response to a valid VCPR. Compounding is likely to result in conversion of an approved animal drug into one that is unapproved. Compounding of human drugs and occasionally bulk drugs into appropriate dosage forms may be acceptable in certain circumstances (e.g., combinations of anesthetics to titrate administration, dilution of drugs for pediatric or small exotic animals). A legitimate medical need must be identified (e.g., health or life of the animal is threatened or suffering may occur). Additionally, there must be no marketed, approved animal or human drug, regardless of whether it is used in a labeled or extralabeled fashion that may be substituted for the compounded agent. Occasionally, other rare circumstances may be considered.

The compounded product must be dispensed by a veterinarian or prescribed and subsequently dispensed by a pharmacist. For companion animals, the safety and efficacy of the compounded drug must be consistent with current standards, appropriate steps should be taken to minimize the risk of human exposure to harmful ingredients, patient records must be kept, and the compounded drug must bear labeling information to ensure adequate and proper use of the product (including name and address of the veterinarian; the active ingredient; date dispensed and expiration date; directions for use; cautionary statement; and if dispensed by the pharmacist, appropriate pharmacist information). The compounded preparation cannot be sold to another veterinarian or pharmacist.

A number of pharmacists throughout the United States compound drugs for veterinarians. The Professional Compounding Center of America (PCCA) is a resource for education in compounding drugs for both human and veterinary medicine. Veterinarians seeking compounded products would be prudent to work with a pharmacist who is a member of the PCCA to be more certain of quality control concerns. The PCCA can be reached at 800-331-2498.

Compounded products are not regulated; assurance of quality, safety and efficacy is incumbent on the prescribing veterinarian. Because compounded products may be less safe that an approved product (other than increase accuracy in dosing), attention to patient response is important. Therapeutic failure may be a common adverse event that is easily forgotten with compounded products. Care must be taken to not misinterpret the availability of a compounded product as evidence of safety or efficacy. The discerning clinician should ensure, through contact with the pharmacist, that state pharmacy laws are followed. Sources of drugs should be confirmed with regard to quality. Manufactured products should be avoided for both ethical and safety reasons. The Pharmacy Compounding Accreditation Board (http://www.pcab.info/) offers accreditation to pharmacies willing to meet a robust set of criteria that ensure products meet both quality and ethical standards as intended by both the Food and Drug Administration and the pharmacy associations. Veterinarians are encouraged to identify those pharmacies that are PCAB accredited.

Alternative Mechanisms for Use of Human Drug in Animals

There are two other mechanisms by which a practitioner can legally use a human drug. *Regulatory discretion* (discretionary enforcement) has been applied by the FDA to selected drugs with no NAD. Recommendations for regulatory discretion of a drug are made by the Division of Drug for Non-Food Animals to the Division of Compliance. Digoxin is an example for which regulatory discretion has existed for a long time; labeling for animal use is even allowed for this product because it is so old. Newer regulations, however, prevent labeling for animals without an NADA. If a drug has been shown through illegal use to be safe and efficacious for the treatment of a disease in animals, the FDA will allow its use without an NADA (notification by letter). Examples include potassium bromide for treatment of refractory seizures, 4-methylpyrrazole for treatment of ethylene glycol toxicity, and calcium ethylene diaminetetra-acetic acid for treatment of lead poisoning. To obtain regulatory discretion, the practitioner needs to contact the Division of Compliance (see Box 3).

An alternative route to using a drug in an extralabel fashion legally for an animal is to procure an INAD application from the Division of Drug for Non-Food Animals (301-594-1722). The INAD provides statutory authority to exempt the drug from the NADA requirement. It limits the use of the drug to experts qualified by training and experience. A compassionate use INAD can be obtained in 1 day by calling the previous telephone number to treat an animal whose life is threatened. Note that the INAD is not necessary if the drug is approved for use in any species. The INAD is needed only if the drug is *unapproved,* meaning that there is no approved version for humans or animals (i.e., a drug approved in Canada, Mexico, or Europe but not the United States). Occasionally, the FDA may recommend that an INAD be obtained for the use of a drug recently approved for use in humans because data regarding the safety of the drug are probably still being collected for humans. An INAD may also be recommended if the drug is toxic (especially carcinogenic) or it is scheduled (regulated by the Drug Enforcement Agency). If an INAD is obtained, veterinarians must keep records regarding the use of the drug and must notify the FDA every time a shipment is requested or an adverse reaction occurs.

Extrapolation of human drugs to animals should be accompanied, whenever possible, by scientific studies that support proper dosing regimens. Recommendations regarding the extrapolation of dosing regimens among species is addressed in Chapter 2.

Schedule Drugs

Drug (substances) considered to be associated with a potential for abuse or physical dependence are restricted (controlled) by the FDA. The Controlled Substances Act delineates requirements that must be met when such drugs are administered, dispensed, or prescribed. The Drug Enforcement Agency (DEA) is charged with enforcement of the act, its amendments, and their regulations. The act includes federal requirements regarding the purchase, storage, prescription, and record keeping for controlled substance use. States may have additional requirements regarding purchase, dispensing, inventory, record keeping, and storage. Requirements are likely to vary from state to state (http://www.legislature.state.al.us/CodeofAlabama/1975/50719.htm).

Requirements for controlled substance use vary for practitioners, researchers, teachers, and pharmacists. Practitioners dispensing or prescribing Class I and II substances annually must obtain both federal and state registration; an exception is made if done in the confines of an employer (hospital)/employee (student) relationship and the employer is registered. Federal registration occurs through the DEA. For practitioners, use of Classes III to V must be preceded by a notice of intent to the DEA, although registration also may be required for Classes III to V, if certain conditions are not met (www.dea.gov). Registering practitioners must submit evidence of a professional degree. Licensure must be voluntarily surrendered on retirement. Mechanisms for state registration also vary; in the state of Alabama, registration of veterinarians occurs through the State Board of Veterinary Medical Examiners.

The DEA publishes a *Practitioner's Manual* (http://www.deadiversion.usdoj.gov/pubs/manuals/pract/index.html; last accessed May 25, 2010), which delineates requirements for the use of these substances. Among the major requirements, selected states require a special prescription blank (and often multiple copies). Generally, both state controlled substance registration (SCSR) and federal (DEA) numbers must appear on prescriptions. Purchase of controlled substances also requires a special triplicate form obtained from the DEA. All actions with controlled substances must be within the confines of a veterinary client–patient relationship. Containers must be designed such that children under the age of 5 cannot open the product, and a label stating "This Package for Households Without Young Children" must be applied when a childproof container is not used. Specific requirements also vary with the class or schedule of the controlled substance.

The classification of controlled substances reflects the perceived level of potential abuse or physiologic or psychological dependence (Table 3). The schedule of a controlled substance is indicated on the label of the product. Schedule I drugs have the highest potential of abuse and physical dependence. These drugs have no acceptable or safe medical use in the United States and are not to be prescribed, but they can be obtained for research purposes. Heroin is the most notable example. Schedule II drugs, exemplified by cocaine and morphine, are considered to have a high potential for abuse and dependence but have some medicinal worth. These drugs must be stored in a securely locked, well-constructed cabinet or safe. Loss or theft requires immediate contact of the nearest DEA field office. Prescription refills are not allowed for these drugs, and they cannot be prescribed by telephone unless in an emergency (with a follow-up written prescription provided within 72 hours). Schedule III drugs, exemplified by selected opioids and barbiturates, have an accepted therapeutic use. Although abuse of the substance may lead to moderate or low physical dependence, the risk of abuse is less than that of Schedule I or II drugs. Schedule IV drugs, exemplified by diazepam and butorphanol, are considered to present a low potential for dependence or abuse. These drugs can be refilled but only to a maximum of five times; the prescription is effective only for 6 months. Schedule V drugs, such as diphenoxylate, have the lowest potential of abuse or dependence. Restrictions for drugs in this schedule are limited to age (humans), distribution by a pharmacist, and purchase in limited quantities. Schedule V

Table 3 Scheduled Drugs

Schedule	Definition	Drugs (lists are NOT inclusive)
I	Highest risk of abuse and dependence and no medicinal use	Heroin, hallucinogens (LSD, mescaline, marijuana), amphetamines
II	High risk of abuse and dependence and limited medicinal use	Carfentanil, cocaine, codeine, diprenorphine, etorphine, fentanyl, hydrocodone, hydromorphone, methylphenidate, morphine, meperidine, opium extracts and so on, oxymorphone, pentobarbital, sufentanil, thebaine
III	Moderate potential for abuse and dependence, but accepted therapeutic use	Anabolic steroids, barbiturates, buprenorphine, codeine combinations, hydrocodone combinations, ketamine, morphine combinations, pentobarbital combinations, thiamylal, thiobarbiturate, tiletamine-zolazepam
IV	Low potential for abuse or dependence	Alprazolam, butorphanol, chloral hydrate, chlordiazepoxide, clonazepam, clorazepate, diazepam, flurazepam, lorazepam, midazolam, oxazepam, pentazocine, phenobarbital, propoxyphene
V	Lowest potential for abuse	Diphenoxylate; selected (low strength) codeine preparations; hydrocodone and so on, as part of drug combination product; low-strength opium preparations

From http://www.justice.gov/dea/pubs/scheduling.html (last accessed May 25, 2010); note that the list of drugs may vary with some states.

drugs include narcotics in Schedules II to IV included as part of a combination with other drugs (e.g., antitussives, antidiarrheals) with restrictions, including the concentration of the substance in the final product.

Reporting Adverse Drug Reactions

Adverse drug reactions are described in Chapter 3. Report of adverse reactions is an important means of monitoring the safety of products, as well as communicating unexpected adversities. In addition to the vehicles listed here, letters to the editors or case reports in veterinary journals or continuing education programs can be effective tools for reporting adverse drug reactions. Additionally, the adversity should be reported to the pharmaceutical company. Note that adverse events to biologics and pesticides should be reported to the respective agency (see Table 1). The steps to reporting an adverse event include contacting the technical services of the appropriate pharmaceutical manufacturer, if it is an animal-approved drug. If it is not an FDA-approved product for animals or if direct reporting to the FDA is desired, a report may be submitted via telephone at 1-888-FDA-VETS, or more appropriately, to the FDA on Form 1932a: Veterinary Adverse Drug Reaction, Lack of Effectiveness, Product Defect Report (postage prepaid and preaddressed). The form can be downloaded at the CVM website (http://www.fda.gov/downloads/AboutFDA/ReportsManualsForms/Forms/AnimalDrugForms/UCM048810.pdf; last accessed May 25, 2010) or can be obtained by written request at ADE Reporting System, Center for Veterinary Medicine, US Food & Drug Administration,7500 Standish Place, Rockville, MD 20855-2773.

Prescription Writing

Prescriptions are intended to provide direction to the pharmacist regarding the dispensing of a specific medication to a specific patient and must be written for all legend drugs. Specific guidelines regarding who may legally issue a prescription vary among states; however, licensed professionals may prescribe only within the profession in which they are licensed. Prescriptions must be issued only in the context of a valid VCPR (see Box 3). Prescriptions should be written in ink (includes typewritten and computer-generated forms) and must be signed by the prescriber. Pharmacies are not likely to stock veterinary drugs but may be willing to order them or infrequently used human products. The basic elements of a prescription (Box 4) may vary among states. Common mistakes made in prescription writing that can lead to mismedication include the inappropriate use of decimal points (a decimal point with a zero [e.g., 1.0] should not be used after a whole number because the decimal may be missed; a zero is always used to designate a fraction [e.g., 0.5] because the decimal may be missed) and the use of abbreviations that are similar (e.g., use of U for units [easily mistaken for a 0]). Writing numbers as words in lieu of or in addition to numerals may facilitate safety, particularly with toxic drugs.

Labels for prescription drugs should include the name, address, and phone number of the prescriber; the patient and owner's name (and for controlled substances, address and phone number); animal name (if appropriate) and species; dispensing date; drug name, quantity, and strength; instructions for use; and appropriate precautionary statements. State regulations regarding the contents of the drug label may vary. Drugs should be dispensed in a childproof container unless requested otherwise by the owner; a signed request should be kept in the record if so requested.

Box 4

Basic Elements of a Prescription

Standard Prescription

Prescriber name (legible), address, phone number
Animal owner name, address
Animal description, name (if appropriate)
Date written
Drug name, dosage form (e.g., tablet, capsule, suspension, injection), strength
Quantity to dispense
Directions for use: how much, how often, route, special instructions (e.g., with food, before food)
Signature of prescriber, with professional degree
Refills if appropriate
Other: indication for generic substitution, treatment indication

Controlled Substances

All scheduled drugs
- Owner address
- Quantity written as word and number

Schedules III-IV
- Drug Enforcement Agency (DEA) number of prescriber

Schedule II
- May require specific prescription form
- Check regarding duration that records must be kept

ETHICAL CONSIDERATIONS IN CLINICAL TRIALS*

Assurance of Ethical Use of Animals

The use of animals in prospective research studies is becoming increasingly controversial. In this section, considerations for client-owned animals are contrasted with experimental animals that are owned by the research facility. Included in this latter group are animals that have been donated by clients. This section also discusses ethical consideration for humans, experimental animals, and client-owned animals in clinical trials. General ethical considerations for all clinical trials are also be presented.

Rights of Human Subjects

It is not unreasonable to expect the same concern and consideration for veterinary patients that is given human patients used as clinical research subjects. Human patients involved in clinical research are very well protected against inhumane use. The Nuremberg Code of Ethics in Medical Research (1948)

*Excerpted from Boothe DM, Slater M: Proper implementation of clinical trials. In Dodds WJ (ed): *Veterinary medical specialization: bridging science and medicine,* vol 39 *(Advances in Veterinary Science),* Orlando, 1995, Academic Press.

emphasizes the rights of the experimental human subject. The Declaration of Helsinki (1964) as adopted by the World Medical Association went further and mandated the following:

1. Such research must conform to scientific principles.
2. Design and performance of the research must be clearly formulated in a protocol and transmitted to a specially appointed, independent committee.
3. Publication of results should accurately reflect the results of the study.

The Declaration emphasized the right of informed consent and specifically addressed human medical research that is combined with professional patient care. Research facilities, such as academic institutions that direct clinical research in humans, are guided by Institutional Review Boards whose primary charge is to ensure compliance with the Nuremburg Code and Declaration of Helsinki. With minor modifications, most of the guidelines delineated in these two documents also are applicable to the veterinary patient (client-owned animal) used in clinical research. Like human medical counterparts, veterinary clinical research facilities should institute a mechanism by which adherence to these guidelines is assured.

Welfare of Experimental Animals

Experimental animals are protected by guidelines offered by the Animal Welfare Act of 1966 and its subsequent amendments. The Public Health Service (PHS) Policy on Humane Care and Use of Laboratory Animals (i.e., the National Institutes of Health Policy) requires compliance with this act of all institutions receiving PHS funds. Most research facilities (academic institutions) have laboratory animal care committees that assure compliance by individual investigators with the PHS policy. However, these committees are not necessarily charged with the care of client-owned animals and often (as at Texas A&M University) agree that research involving client-owned animals does not fall under their purview.

Welfare of Client-Owned Animals

To protect the welfare of client-owned animals, some type of review board should be in place. In a university setting, a Hospital Review Committee evaluates clinical trials and other types of clinical research. The term *Health Review Committee* (HRC) is used in this manuscript to distinguish from Institutional Review Boards (IRB) that address human subjects in clinical research. The goals of an HRC should be to protect the patient, client, institution and attending veterinarian(s) from the intended or inadvertent application of investigations that are inhumane or unethical and to promote the advancement of science through clinical research. The HRC functions to safeguard the welfare of the patient through the approval of proposals involving clinical research. Although its mission is not to provide rigorous review of the scientific merits of a proposed study, decisions regarding the ethical nature of a proposed clinical trial may require the HRC to question the scientific basis and the scientific and statistical design of any proposals.

General Ethical Considerations

General considerations on the ethical use of animals in clinical trials arise from the human research guidelines. Some of the following considerations are most applicable for clinical trials using client-owned animals. An over-arching truth is that it is more ethical to perform a randomized clinical trial than to use treatments of unproven efficacy. The patient's best interest cannot be forsaken for the sole purpose of "therapeutic progress"; rather, treatment of the patient is the priority. Completion of the trial must not be rushed if it creates risks to the patient. In the study design phase, protocols should be developed for use in the situation where the risk:benefit ratio of the therapeutic intervention becomes too high during the course of therapy (e.g., the trial will be terminated, the currently recommended therapy will be used, and so on). Trials should include methods to evaluate the incidence, frequency, type, and severity of side effects of test treatments. This is especially important if client-owned animals are used.

In determining the treatment protocol, if periodic therapeutic withdrawal or use of a placebo is planned, assurance must be provided that the subjects' life or comfort is not threatened. The use of an inactive placebo is not appropriate (except in very unusual, experimental situations) if there is a standard treatment protocol for the disease to be investigated. The double-blind technique (defined here as blinding of the investigator and client or caretaker) should be abandoned if one treatment can be clearly recognized by the investigators to be preferred because of its beneficial effects, or if a treatment entails any risks that prove to be unreasonable. The code indicating a subject's treatment must always be available to appropriate participants in case of an emergency. For trials using client-owned animals, if a client withdraws an animal from the study, assurance should be given that patient care will remain available. There should be a system of verification of results that avoids the possibility of manipulating results after the study.

Additional questions regarding the scientific merits of the study that should be answered by the investigator include the following:

1. Is there a need for the study? The answer to this question includes evaluation of the importance and clarity of the primary objective without unnecessary duplication of previous studies (in target or other species). Consideration of the applicability of the results is also important.
2. What is the justification for the study? Considerations include the inclusion of appropriate numbers of patients and controls, explicit inclusion/exclusion criteria, and ethical risk:benefit ratios.
3. Are the risks to the subject reasonable in relation to the possible benefits to the subject and/or the importance of the knowledge that may be reasonably realized from the study? A sound research design that does not unnecessarily expose subjects to risk is critical to address this question. Currently accepted or proven procedures that are already available for diagnostic or therapeutic purposes should be applied when available.

4. Has informed consent been obtained? The legal client representatives of the animal patients must be informed regarding the study and allowed voluntary choices. Informed consent should be sought from each prospective animal patient's legally authorized representative and should be properly documented.

Guidelines for Completing an Informed Consent

The informed consent should be perceived as a document that provides information to the owner, in layman's terms. The information should be pertinent to the study and should include anything that is likely to be important to the animal owner. This recommendation might seem nebulous and needlessly all-inclusive. However, the intent of the consent form might best be appreciated by answering the following questions: If you (or your child) were the subject of this study, what would you want to know about it? Is there anything left out of the consent form that the client is likely to get mad about when he/she finds out? The informed consent should be succinct, clear, and above all else informative to the animal owner. Bolding might be used to emphasize points that the investigator feels are particularly important to the client.

The following consent form is organized for purposes of discussion. The organization should be tailored to the study in a manner that is not confusing to the animal owner. Use of lay terminology that the client can understand is paramount to an appropriate informed consent. Information should be clear and succinct.

Suggestions regarding generation of an informed consent follow. The first paragraph identifies the animal and animal owner. The reason for the animal's inclusion should be stated. Additional information might be included in a brochure, which should be submitted along with the protocol. Note that information in the brochure is not part of the informed consent and cannot replace the information required in the consent document. The second paragraph should provide information about the experimental protocol. The following information should be included:

1. The study name and study location (this might include both the central location and the site where the animal is to be studied).
2. Statement that the study constitutes research; an explanation of its purposes and the expected duration of involvement.
3. Description of the procedures to which the animal will be subjected.

Those that are experimental should be noted as such. Additional information might include the funding agency and the number of animals to be studied.

The third paragraph might focus on the risks and benefits associated with the study. The following must be included:

1. A description of the risks and discomforts that are reasonably foreseeable (this should include the clinical signs that the animal owner will recognize).
2. A description of the possible benefits to the animal and animal owner, as well as other animals.
3. A description of appropriate alternative treatments.

If a placebo or negative control is included in the study, it must be clear to the animal owner that there is a possibility that the animal may receive no therapeutic benefit from the study.

Additional information that might be included in this section is as follows:

1. A statement regarding the approval status of the drugs/therapies/tests to be studied.
2. A statement that unforeseen risks may occur.
3. A statement about the safety of the test intervention.
4. A description of the costs of the study assumed by the investigators (e.g., 50% of all clinical laboratory tests).
5. A description of the obligations of the animal owner.

This last statement might include costs to be incurred by the owner for participating in the study, the number of follow-up visits to a veterinarian, record-keeping, and telephone calls.

The fourth paragraph may focus on client options should an adverse reaction occur or client withdrawal be desired. Relevant information that should be included in this section is as follows:

1. An explanation of whether compensation or treatment will be available if injuries occur.
2. A statement regarding the client's right to withdraw at any time with no change in patient care.
3. Who is to be contacted in the event of an adverse reaction/injury or if questions regarding the study arise.
4. Conditions that might lead the investigators to withdraw a patient from the study (e.g., noncompliance, poor record keeping or "escape criteria," such as a worsening of the disease being tested).
5. A statement regarding financial obligations of the client should his or her animal be withdrawn from the study.
6. A statement allowing the client to seek a second opinion regarding the cause of death should his or her animal die while participating in the study.

The fifth paragraph ensures the confidentiality of the study. Points to be included are as follows:

1. A statement that assures that the data collected from the animal will be kept confidential.
2. A statement regarding notification of findings that might affect the willingness of the client to continue participation.
3. A statement regarding notification of the results of the study on its completion.
4. A statement verifying that the client has participated in this study willingly.

Each page of the informed consent should be numbered and accompanied by a place for the client's initials next to the number.

Informed consent may be *waived* under extenuating circumstances if the investigator and an unbiased clinician (one not participating in the study) certify in writing all of the following:

1. The patient is confronted with a life-threatening situation that necessitates the use of the intervention being tested.
2. Informed consent cannot be obtained from a legal representative of the patient (i.e., stray animals).

3. There is not sufficient time to obtain informed consent from the patient's legal representative.
4. There is no alternative method of approved or generally recognized therapy that provides an equivalent or greater likelihood of saving the patient's life.

REPORTING AND REVIEWING CLINICAL TRIALS

Data Reporting

A clinical trial is not complete until the information is disseminated. Publications of results should be prepared and made available as soon as possible. Although most manuscripts are prepared after closeout, in certain instances, interim publications are prepared.

Interim publications provide access to study results as they occur. Additional benefits might include easier preparation of the final manuscript and greater exposure of the study to the public. However, there are several disadvantages to interim reporting (Meinert, 1986). Results that are inconclusive may be confusing. If the results are discouraging, investigator enthusiasm may wane. Most critical is the possibility of bias in subsequent treatment assignment and data collection. Finally, data analysis and presentation may differ from and thus diminish the impact of the final report. Results of the study can be disseminated through publications in peer-reviewed journals and presentations at national meetings. Some journals (those that focus predominantly on human medicine) do not publish papers that have been presented nationally. The time gap between presentation and publication should be minimal. The choice of journal should be limited to referred journals that are covered in *Index Medicus* and *Index Veterinarius*. Unreferred journals should be avoided if they lack a critical review process. Such journals may reach a smaller public and thus may be more difficult for other investigators to identify or retrieve. A specialty journal (i.e., *Internal Medicine, Neurology,* or *Surgery*) might be considered if the results are of primary interest to the specialty group.

The potential importance of many veterinary clinical trials is not realized because of failure to publish the appropriate information. The goal of the publication should be to provide a clear, concise description of the study. Studies that report statistically insignificant findings should also be published. The clinical trial may only result in a single manuscript that is published on completion of the trials. The organization of the manuscript varies with the targeted journal. Typical components include the following.

The *title* is one of the most important components of the publication. It should be concise and as short as possible while indicating the main thrust of the paper. The term *clinical trial* should be included in the title. The title section should also include the authors, source of financial support, acknowledgements, and address for reprints. Finally, a list of key words selected by the author should be included to allow for retrieval.

The *abstract* is often the only part of a paper that is read and as such should provide a summary of the paper. The abstract will be included in Medline, the computerized version of *Index Medicus*, or other computerized databases. The abstract should include the study purpose or objective, primary outcome measure, intervention; type of control, method of allocation, blinding procedures, number of animals enrolled and studied, and conclusions.

The *introduction* should be short and succinct. Its purpose is to provide a historic background for the study. Included is a literature review, what led to the initiation of the study, the study objectives, and the rationale for the study. This might include a rationale for the study design, intervention, or outcome measurements.

The *methods section* should be sufficiently detailed to allow readers to make informed judgments regarding the quality of the methods. Citation of a previously published paper describing the methods can reduce the content if the paper was devoted primarily to the design and methods of the trial.

The *results section* is generally the longest. The crux of the paper should be represented by tables, charts, and figures, which should be understandable without reference to the text.

The *discussion* should highlight the important findings of the study. Positive and negative findings should be reported. The clinical implications of these results and consistency with previous findings should be discussed.

The *conclusion* may either stand alone or complete the discussion. The conclusions must be drawn from the results of the trial. If appropriate, the statistical power of the study should be noted if the conclusion favors the null hypothesis. Finally, a statement regarding the extent of generalization should be included.

References should be limited to those that support the rationale of the objectives and document methods of data collection and analysis. The journal of publication will dictate the organization of the references. Original articles should be referenced whenever possible. Secondary sources are acceptable if the primary cannot be found; if the primary is published in a foreign language; or if the secondary expands on information provided by the primary paper. Checks of accuracy of title name, spelling of author's name, and so on should be based on the article itself and not on citations listed in other bibliographies (e.g., Medline).

The *appendix section* is optional and may not be allowed by some journals. Contents should be limited to information regarding methods that is too technical or detailed to include in the body of the text. Examples of information to be contained in the appendices are details of sample size calculations; sample data forms; data collection schedules; special charts, figures, and equations; consent statements; and data listings.

The submission process can be facilitated if the manuscript is reviewed before submission. Authors should review the paper for inconsistencies in format and style (including tables and figures), for redundancy, and for reporting deficiencies. Figure and table numbers should match text citations. Citations should be reviewed to ensure that information cited is correct. Colleagues should provide the second review. Their primary function is to identify confusing aspects of the manuscript. Total rewrites may result from this internal review. The final review by the authors should focus on the format of the journal to which the manuscript is to be submitted. The number of copies and prints submitted, title page, style and format, and so on should match the specifications set forth in the journal's "Instructions to Authors." After publication, the primary authors should establish an archive consisting of all documents related to the paper, beginning with raw data and finishing with a copy of the printed manuscript. This information should be kept at least 3 years (Meinert, 1986).

Reviewing a Clinical Trial

When reviewing a manuscript that reports the results of a clinical trial, the reviewer should be unbiased regarding the results. The reviewer's opinion should be based on the merits of the study rather than on the opinions and critiques of others. The purpose of the clinical report should be strongly considered, particularly if sponsor support was critical to the study and the sponsor stands to gain financially from it. The information provided in the report should allow adequate review of methodology so that critical aspects of the report can be evaluated. Reproducibility of results and generalization of results to a large population (rather than a small subset) should be assessed. Exclusion of patients should be well justified. The study design should be well safeguarded against biases during the assignment and administration of the intervention and during data collection and analysis. Methods used to edit the data for errors or inadequacies should be cited. Statistical methods should be appropriately sophisticated. Major differences in baseline group comparability, dropout rates, or compliance should be evaluated for a possible role in treatment differences.

Appendix 2

Conversions, Equivalents, and Abbreviations

Table 1 Metrologic and Pharmaceutical Weights and Measures*

The Metric System of Weight
1 microgram (mcg) = 0.000,001 gram (g) (μg)
1 milligram (mg) = 0.001 g = 1000 mcg (μg)
1 gram (g) = 1.0 g = 1000 mg
1 kilogram (kg) = 1000.0 g
The Metric System of Liquid Measure
1 milliliter (mL) = 0.001 L
1 liter (L) = 1000 mL
The Avoirdupois System of Weights
437.5 grains (gr) = 1 ounce (oz)
16 oz = 1 pound (lb) = 7000 gr
Apothecaries' System of Weights
20 gr = 1 scruple
3 scruples (ε) = 1 dram = 60 gr
8 drams = 1 oz = 480 gr
12 oz = 1 lb = 5760 gr
Apothecaries' System of Liquid Measures (U.S. Wine Measure)
60 minims = 1 fluid dram
8 fluid drams = 1 fluid ounce (fl oz)
16 fl oz = 1 pint
8 pints = 1 gallon (cong.)

Remarks:
The avoirdupois system of weights is used in buying and selling in commerce. This includes drugs.
The apothecaries' system is used *only* for writing, compounding, and dispensing prescriptions.
The grain is identical in both the avoirdupois and apothecaries' systems, but the ounce and pound are not.
One minim does not weigh 1 grain, and 1 fluid ounce does not weigh 1 ounce, and 1 pint does not measure 1 pound.
The scruple and apothecaries' pound may be disregarded insofar as they are seldom used. When *pound* is used, it usually means an avoirdupois pound. When *ounce* is used, it usually means an apothecaries' ounce.
*See also Jag's Apothecary at http://www.ourworld.compuserve.com/homepages/jbaluri/home.HTM

Table 2 Equivalents (Approximate)

1 grain (gr)	64.8 milligram (mg)	60 mg
1 ounce (oz)	28.35 gram (g)	30 g
1 pound (lb)	453.6 g	454 g
1 dram (60 gr)	3.9 g	4 g
1 apothecary ounce (480 gr)	31.1 g	30 g
1 minim	0.06 (mL) milliliter	0.06 mL
1 fluid dram	3.7 mL	4 mL
1 fluid ounce	29.573 mL	30 mL
1 pint	473.1 mL	480 or 500 mL
1 gallon	3785.4 mL	4000 mL
1 mg	$\frac{1}{64.8}$ gr	$\frac{1}{65}$ or $\frac{1}{60}$ gr
1 g	15,432 gr	15 gr
1 kilogram (kg)		2.2 pounds (lb)
1 gallon (water)	8.337 lb (8 lb approx.)	3.8 kg (approx.)
1 gallon occupies 231 cubic inches		
1 mL	1.000027 cubic centimeters	
1 pint	473 mL	500 mL
1 quart	946 mL	1000 mL
1 drop	0.06 mL	1 minim
1 dessertspoonful		8 mL
1 teaspoonful (tsp)		5 mL
1 tablespoonful (Tb)		15 mL

Table 3 Conversions for Calculating Dosage

w/v%*	mg/mL	µg/mL (mcg/mL)	Dilution g to mL
10%	100	100,000	1:10
5%	50	50,000	1:20
2%	20	20,000	1:50
1%	10	10,000	1:100
0.1%	1	1,000	1:1,000
0.2%	0.2	200	1:5,000
0.01%	0.1	100	1:25,000
0.004%	0.04	40	1:25,000
0.002%	0.02	20	1:50,000
0.001%	0.01	10	1:100,000
0.001%	0.001	1	1:1,000,000

*The definition of w/v is grams/dL (see Table 6).

Table 4 Dry Weight and Volume Conversions

1 pound (lb)	453.6 grams (g)
1 gram (g)	0.0022 pound (lb)
1 gram (g)	1000 milligrams (mg)
1 gram (g)	1,000,000 micrograms (µg)
1 kilogram (kg)	1000 grams (g)
1 kilogram (kg)	2205 pounds (lb)
1 milligram (mg)	0.001 gram (g)
1 milligram (mg)	1000 micrograms (µg)
1 microgram (µg)	0.001 milligram (mg)
1 microgram per gram (µg/g)	1 part per million (ppm)
1 part per million (ppm)	0.454 milligram/pound (mg/lb)
1 part per million (ppm)	0.907 gram per ton (g/T)
1 liter (L)	1000 milliliter (mL)
1 milliliter (mL)	1000 microliter (µL or lambda)

Table 5 Abbreviations

Abbreviation	English Translation
ac	before meals
AD	right ear
ad lib	as desired
AS	left ear
AU	both ears
bid	twice a day (every 12 hours)
Ċ	with
cap	capsule
d/c	discontinue
ft	make
h	hour
hs	at bedtime
m	mix
OD	right eye
OS	left eye
OU	both eyes
pc	after meals
po	by mouth
PR	rectally
PRN	as needed
pulv	powder
PV	vaginally
qam	every morning
qd	every day
QD (SID)	once a day
QH	every hour
qid	four times a day (every 6 hours)
qpm	every evening
qod	every other day
qs	as much as needed
Rx	recipe, Latin for "take thou"
Š	without
sig	directions, Latin for "to label"
SL	sublingual
SOL	solution
ss	one half
stat	now, immediately
supp	suppository
tab	tablet
tid	three times a day (every 8 hours)
ud	as directed
ung	ointment

Table 6 Common Units and Conversion Factors

Common Units of Measure

Unit	Abbreviation
Concentration of solutions	
grams per deciliter	g/dL*
grams per liter	g/L
international units per liter	IU/L
micrograms per deciliter	μg/dL
micromoles per liter	μmol/L
microunits per milliliter	μU/mL
milliequivalents per liter	mEq/L
milligrams per deciliter	mg/dL
millimoles per kilogram	mmol/kg
millimoles per liter	mmol/L
milliosmoles per kilogram	mOsm/kg
parts per million	ppm
percent	g/dL
units per liter	U/L
Distance	
centimeter	cm
meter squared	m{2}
millimeter	mm
Fluids	
deciliter (10^2 mL)	dL
liter (10^3 mL)	L
microliter (10^{-6})	μL
milliliter (1 mL or 10^{-3} L)	mL
Pressure	
centimeters of water	cm H_2O
millimeters of mercury	mm Hg
Time	
every	q
hour	hr
minute	min
month	mo
second	sec
week	wk
year	yr
Weights	
grain (1 gr = 65 mg)	gr
gram (1 g or 10^{-3} kg)	g
kilogram (10^{-3} g)	kg
microgram (10^{-6} g)	μg

*Also known as % wv.

Continued

Table 6 Common Units and Conversion Factors—cont'd

milligram (10^{-3} g)	mg
nanogram (10^{-9} g)	ng
pictogram (10^{-12} g)	pg
Common Conversions	
Volume or Weight	**Equivalent**
1 dram	3.9 grams
1 drop (gt)	0.06 milliliter
15 drops	1 milliliter (1 cc)
1 fluid dram	3.7 milliliters
1 glass	240 milliliters (8 ounces)
1 grain	0.065 gram or 65 milligrams
1 gram	15.43 grains
1 kilogram	2.20 pounds (avoirdupois)
1 kilogram	2.65 pounds (Troy)
1 liter	1.06 quarts
1 liter	33.80 fluid ounces
1 measuring cup	240 milliliters (½ pint)
2 measuring cups	500 milliliters (1 pint)
1 milligram	1/65 grain
1 milliliter	16.23 minims
1 minim	0.062 milliliter
1 ounce	31.1 grams
1 ounce	30 milliliters or 28.35 grams
1 pint	473.2 milliliters
1 quart	946.4 milliliters
1 tablespoon	15 milliliters
2 tablespoons	30 milliliters
1 teacup	180 milliliters (6 ounces)
1 teaspoon	5 milliliters
1 unit (e.g., penicillin)	0.000625 mg
Temperature Conversions	
°Celcius to °Fahrenheit: (°C) (9/5) + 32°	
°Fahrenheit to °Celsius: (°F-32°) (5/9)	

Appendix 3

Sample Pharmaceutical Calculations

Dawn Merton Boothe and E. Murl Bailey, Jr.

Appendix Outline

DOSE CALCULATIONS

Dose may be calculated by the following formula:

$$\frac{\text{Dose per unit of body weight} \times \text{Total wt}^{*}}{\text{Unit of drug per mL}} = \text{Total dose in mL}$$

To convert pounds to kilograms, divide by 2.2 or multiply by 0.454.

$$\frac{20 \times 0.454 \times 10}{20} = 4.54$$

Example: If an animal weighs 20 lb and the clinician wants to administer 10 μg/kg of 1:50,000 solution, what is the dose in mL?

SOLUTIONS

Concentration of an analyte in solution is routinely generally is expressed as percent solution, molarity, molality or normality.

See also: DoseCalcu Online http://www.meds.com/Dchome.html

Percent Solutions

Definitions

Percent solutions are equal to parts per hundred or the amount of solute per 100 total units of solution. Three expressions of percent solution are as follows:

1. Percent weight in weight (w/w) expresses the number of grams of active constituent in 100 grams of solution.
2. Percent weight in volume (w/v) expresses the number of grams of an active constituent in 100 cubic centimeters of solution and is used in prescription practice regardless of whether water or some other liquid is the solvent.
3. Percent volume in volume (v/v) expresses the number of cubic centimeters of an active constituent in 100 cubic centimeters of solution.

When *percent* is used in prescriptions without qualification, it means the following: for mixtures of solids, percent weight in weight; for solutions of solids in liquids, percent weight in volume; for solutions of liquids in liquids, percent volume in volume; and for solutions of gases in liquids, percent weight in volume. For example, a 1% solution is prepared by dissolving 1 gram of a solid or 1 cubic centimeter of a liquid in sufficient solvent to make 100 cubic centimeters of the solution. A solution of approximately the same strength may be prepared by apothecary weight and measured by dissolving 4.5 grains of a solid or 4.8 minims of a liquid in sufficient solvent to make 1 fluid ounce of the solution.

Calculation of Percent Concentrations

The following formula may be used to calculate percent composition:

$$\frac{\text{The part}}{\text{The total}} \times 100 = \% \quad \text{or} \quad (x/y) \times 100 = z$$

If any two quantities are known, the third can be easily calculated by the preceding formula.

Consider the following examples:

1. What is the w/v strength of a solution made by dissolving 6 grams of a drug in sufficient water to make 300 mL?

$$6/300 \times 100 = x \qquad (x = 2)$$

2. How many mL of a 5% w/v solution can be made with 10 grams of drug?
3. How many grams of a drug are needed to make 200 mL of a 6% w/v solution?

$$10/x \times 100 = 5 \qquad (x = 200)$$

$$x/200 \times 100 = 6 \qquad (x = 12)$$

4. What is the w/v percentage strength of a solution containing 50 mg per mL?

$$50\ \text{mg}/1\text{mL} = 0.05\text{g}/\text{mL} = 5\text{g}/100\text{mL}$$

$$5/100 \times 100 = 5\%$$

*Can be substituted for body surface area or m^2 using conversion factor found in Appendix 2.

Dilute with a pure diluent

Example: Dilute a 5% solution to a 2% solution.

Take two parts of 5% solution, and dilute to 5 parts. This will yield a 2% solution.

$$\text{Proof}: 2 \text{ parts} \times 0.05 = 0.1;\ 0.1/5 \times 100 = 2\%$$

Mixing of two solutions or solids of unequal concentrations.

Example: Mix a 10% and a 25% solution in proper portions to make a 15% solution.

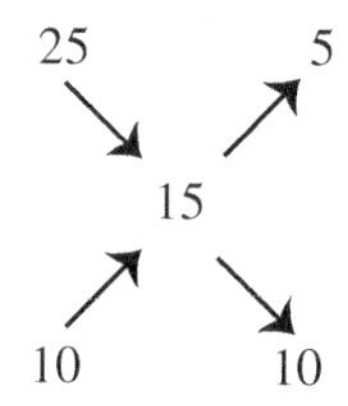

Solution by Pearson's Square

= 1 part of 25% 3 total

= 2 part of 10% 15 Total 3 Total

Subtract 10 from 15 to determine parts of 25% solution.

Subtract 15 from 25 to determine parts of 10% solution.

Proof: 1 parts 25% = 25

2 parts 10% = 20

3 parts 15% = 45

Algebraic solution:

let a = parts of 25%

b = parts of 10%

15(a+b) = parts of 15%

$$25 + 10b = 15a + 15b$$
$$10a = 5b$$
$$2a = b$$

Mixing of three or more solutions or solids of unequal concentrations:

Example: Mix 14%, 12%, 6%, and 4% solutions to make a 10% solution.

14 = 6 = 3 parts of 14%

12 = 4 = 2 parts of 12%

6 = 2 = 1 parts of 6%

4 = 4 = 2 parts of 4%

8 parts of 10%

Proof: 3 parts × 14% = 42

2 parts × 12 = 24

1 parts × 6 = 6

2 parts × 4 = 8

8 parts × 10 = 80

Algebraic solution:

let a = parts of 14%

b = parts of 12%

c = parts of 6%

d = parts of 4%

$$10(a + b + c + d) = \text{parts of } 10\%$$
$$14a + 12b + 6c + 4d = 10a + 10b + 10c + 10d$$
$$4a + 2b = 4c + 6d$$
$$2a + b = 2c + 3d$$

By substituting values for any of three, the fourth can be found. This formula can give a great number of possible combinations. For example, if a = 3 parts, b = 2 parts, and c = 1 part, then d = 2.

Concentration Terms

A *dilute* solution is one with relatively little solute, whereas a *concentrated* solution contains a large amount of solute in solution. A *saturated* solution contains an excess of undissolved solute particles, whereas a *supersaturated solution* has an even greater concentration of undissolved solute particles and therefore is thermodynamically unstable. The *density* of a substance is expressed in terms of mass per unit volume and often is referred to as *specific gravity* (usually expressed as gm/mL). Temperature and the presence of other ions can influence the solubility constant for a given solution and thus the saturation. Thus, in dispensing prescriptions, slight changes in volume owing to variations in room temperatures may be disregarded.

Molarity

Molarity (M) refers to the number of moles *per liter* of solution (i.e., the compound is added and the volume is brought up to 1 liter total), with one mole equaling the gram molecular weight of the compound. The traditional molar concentration of the solution is moles of solute per volume of solution, with volume generally given in terms of liters: mol/L, mmol/L (millimol), µmol/L (micromol), and nmol/L (nmol).

Example: How may grams are needed to make 1 liter of a 1.5 M solution of hydrochloric acid (HCl)?

$$\text{GMW HCl} = 1 + 35.5 = 36.5$$

$$1\text{M} = 1\text{GMW/L}$$

$$1.5\text{M} = 1.5\ \text{GMW/L} = 1.5 \times 36.5\ \text{g HCl} = 54.75\ \text{gm HCl}$$

added to sufficient solvent to make 1 liter

Molality

Molality (m) is the *amount of solute per kg* of solvent (i.e., the total amount of solution might exceed 1 liter compared with molarity). It is distinguished from molarity in that it is always expressed as weight per weight, or moles per 1000 gm of solvent. The preferred expression for molality is moles per kilogram (mole/kg).

Example: What is the equivalent weight, in grams, of NaCl, HCl, and H_2SO_4?

NaCl	HCl	H_2SO_4
Na = 23	H = 1	H_2 = 2
C = 35	Cl = 35	SO_4 = 32 + 4(16) = 96
Total = 58	Total = 36	Total = 98
Valence = 1	Valence = 1	Valence = 2
Equivalent weight = 58	Equivalent weight = 36	Equivalent weight = 49

Normality

Normality (N) is the number or gram equivalent weights per liter of solution. An equivalent of an electrolyte is the amount that produces one mole of either positive or negative charges when dissolved. The number of equivalents of an electrolyte is calculated by multiplying the number of moles of electrolyte by the total number of positive charges produced when one formula unit of the electrolyte dissolves. Alternatively, an equivalent weight is equal to the molecular weight of a substance divided by its valence. The valence of a molecule is the number of units that can combine with or replace one mole of hydrogen ions. *Normality* is not a commonly used expression; rather, milliequivalents per liter (mEq/L) or millimoles per liter (mmol/L) are used to express electrolyte concentrations.

Osmolarity

Osmolarity (Osm) is the total number of solute particles in a liter of solution (rather than relative weights of the specific solutes). It is calculated from the number of moles of solute particles that are present when 1 mole of the solute dissolves. Nonelectrolytes (glucose, etc.) do not dissociate, thus n=1 (i.e., molarity = osmolarity). However, electrolytes dissociate and their osmolarity is greater than their molarity, the magnitude depending on the number of ions produced upon dissociation (e.g., the Osm CaCl2 = 3 × M).

Table 1

Molecule	Abbrev.	Valence	GMW
Barium	Ba		137
Bromide	Br	1	79
Carbon	C		12
Calcium		2	40
Chloride	Cl	1	35.5
Copper	Cu		63.5
Fluoride	F		19
Gold	Au		108
Hydrogen	H	1	1
Iron	Fe	transition	55.8
Lead	Pb		207
Lithium	Li		6.9
Magnesium	Mg	2	24
Nitrogen	N		14
Oxygen	O	1	16
Phosphorus	P	3	31
Potassium	K	1	39
Sodium	Na	1	23
Sulfur	S		32
Zinc	Zn		65

Appendix 4

Nutrition and Pharmacology

Table 1 Essential Fatty Acids

Essential Amino Acids	Nonessential Amino Acids	Essential Fatty Acids*
Arginine (cats)	Arginine, asparagine	Linolenic (omega-3 or n-3 family)
Histidine	Alanine	
Isolecithin	Aspartic acid, cysteine	Linoleic (omcga-6 or n-6 family)
Leucine	Glutamic acid	
Lysine	Glutamine	
Methionine	Glycine, proline	
Phenylalanine	Serine	
Taurine (cats)	Tyrosine	
Threonine		
Tryptophan		
Valine		

*See also Chapter 33.
Adapted from Atkinson RL: Nutrional aspects of pharmacology. In Brody TM, Larner JL, Minneman KP, editors: *Human pharmacology: molecular to clinical,* Mosby, St. Louis, 1998, Mosby, pp 843-860.

Table 2 Role of Vitamins in Pharmacology

Vitamin	Forms	Role	Comments
Vitamin B_7, biotin (water-soluble vitamin)		Cofactor for enzymes that catalyze incorporation of bicarbonate into carboxyl groups. Substrates include pyruvate, acetyl coenzyme A (CoA), propionyl CoA, and β-methylcrotonyl CoA. Critical for fat and carbohydrate metabolism.	Bound tightly to avidin in raw egg white. Clinical deficiency rare due to microbial formation.
Vitamin B_9, folic acid (a water-soluble B vitamin)	Folates: all containing pterolglutamic acid	Transfer of methyl groups; DNA and protein synthesis.	Deficiencies in cells with rapid turnover, with macrocytic anemia most common followed by atrophy of intestinal mucosa. Supplementation may reduce homocysteine (humans), leading to atherosclerosis.
Vitamin B_3, niacin (or niacinamide) (a water-soluble B vitamin)	Nicotinic acid Nicotinamide	Present as nicotinamide dinucleotide (NAD) or nicotinamide adenine dinucleotide phosphate (NADP) serving as cofactor for enzymes catalyzing oxidation-reduction reactions needed for cellular electron transfer; electron carrier for enzymes oxidizing fuel substrates (NAD); transfer of adenosine triphosphate–ribosyl moieties to proteins; hydrogen donor for reduction reactions such as fatty acid synthesis (NADP).	Deficiency results in pellagra ("raw skin" [humans]), seen in predominantly grain diets. Marked oversupplementation can cause toxicity.

Table 2 Role of Vitamins in Pharmacology—cont'd

Vitamin	Forms	Role	Comments
Vitamin B_5, pantothenic acid (a water-soluble B vitamin)	Pantoic acid linked to β-alanine	Synthesized to acyl carrier protein CoA, which is a cofactor for enzyme-catalyzed transfer of acetyl. Acetyl CoA is necessary for oxidative metabolism of carbohydrates, gluconeogenesis, fatty acid metabolism, synthesis of steroids and porphyrins, and posttranslational modifications of proteins.	
Vitamin A (fat soluble)	All-*trans*-retinol (parent); acid form: retinoic acid; aldehyde form: rentinal Plant precursors: carotenoids Synthetic forms: etretinate (no longer available?), arotinoids	Retinol: gene expression of facial structures and limb buds Retinoic acid: epithelial tissues, bone, embryologic development, cell differentiation Retinal: retinal function	Carotenoids have antioxidant properties and have been advocated for prevention of cancer and heart disease. β-carotene may promote certain types of cancer. Doses 100-fold may produce acute toxicity (nausea, vomiting, vertigo, muscular incoordination), while 10 times the dose may cause chronic toxicity (skin changes, hepatomegaly, bone and joint disease).
Vitamin B_1, thiamine	Purimidine and thiazole nucleus linked by methylene bridge	Carbohydrate metabolism; in phosphorylated form, active as coenzymes, particularly in nonoxidative decarboxylation of α-ketoacids.	Deficiency referred to as *beri beri* (humans) leading to cardiac disease (hypertrophy and dilation of right heart); profound neurologic deficiencies, including polyneuropathy, ophthalmic disorders.
Vitamin B_2, riboflavin	Precursor to flavin mononucleotide and flavin adenine dinucleotide	Act as coenzymes for flavoprotein enzymes catalyzing oxidation-reduction reactions critical for energy production; participates in cytochrome P450 metabolism (dehydrogenations, hydroxylations, oxidative decarboxylations, reductions, and so forth).	Deficiency associated with increased lipid peroxidation, altered metabolism of other B vitamins (folic acid, pyridoxine, niacin) and vitamin K leading to liver disease, anemia, stomatitis, glossitis, seborrheic dermatitis, and, with prolonged deficiency, neuropathy.
Vitamin B_6	Pyridoxine Pyridoxal Pyridoxamine	Cofactors for over 100 enzymes, especially aminotransferases, decarboxylases, decarboxylations with carbon–carbon bond formation, side-chain cleavages, dehydratases, and racemoses.	Deficiency results in seborrheic skin rash, glossitis and stomatitis. High doses may cause peripheral neuropathy.
Vitamin B_{12}, various cobalamins (cyanocobalamin) (minimally absorbed)	Dietary form (must be activated)	DNA synthesis; facilitates folic acid metabolism	Cyclical structure similar to hemoglobin, with cobalt rather than iron in center. Deficiencies rare (see text) but result in *combined systems disease* or pernicious anemia that targets gastrointestinal tract, blood cells, and neurologic system.
Vitamin C (water soluble), ascorbic acid		Reducing agent, serving as an electron donor for enzymatic reactions, especially hydroxylation and amidation. Synthesized in most mammals (exceptions: humans and other primates, guinea pigs). Particularly important for collagen synthesis, conversion of lysine to carnitine, and folic acid to folinic acid; converts ferric iron to ferrous iron, assisting iron absorption from gastrointestinal tract. Antioxidant	Few scientific studies support claims regarding prevention or treatment of cardiac disease or cancer.

Continued

Table 2 Role of Vitamins in Pharmacology—cont'd

Vitamin	Forms	Role	Comments
Vitamin D (fat soluble)	Ergocalciferol: vitamin D_2 cholecalciferol: vitamin D_3 25-Hydroxycholecalciferol: calcifediol 1,25-Dihydroxycholecalciferol: calcitriol (vitamin D_2) Dihydrotachysterol (isomer of vitamin D_2)	Calcium metabolism, hemataopoiesis, cell differentiation, regulation of insulin secretion	Excessive consumption may result in hypercalcemia, anorexia, nausea, vomiting, polyuria, thirst, muscular weakness, joint pain, and bone demineralization
Vitamin E (fat soluble)	Tocopherols (alpha and gamma) and tocotrienols	Free radical scavenger, preventing oxidation of polyunsaturated fatty acids and thiol-rich proteins in cell membranes; T lymphocyte maturation; decreased oxidation of low-density lipoproteins; protects against free radical damage to retina and nervous system	Overdosing may interfere with vitamins A and K absorption; bleeding disorders may occur
Vitamin K	Phylloquinone (chlorophyll-containing plants) Menaquinones (bacteria)	Activates clotting factors VII, IX, and X	

Data from Atkinson RL: Nutritional aspects of pharmacology. In Brody TM, Larner JL, MinnemanKP, editors: *Human pharmacology: molecular* Mosby, St Louis, 1998, pp 843-860.

Table 3 Role of Microminerals* in Pharmacology

Microminerals	Role	Comments
Chromium	Glucose and insulin homeostasis; RNA synthesis (?)	Ubiquitous nature renders deficiency rare.
Copper	Red blood cell production; cofactor for enzymes, especially monoamine oxidase (inactivates catecholamines), cytochrome-*c*-oxidase; needed to incorporate iron into hemoglobin.	Anemia; increased sensitivity of cardiac muscle to catecholamines; collagen and elastin synthesis impaired: capillary fragility, weak arterial walls.
Iron	Critical for hemoglobin structure and promotion of electron transfer in cytochromes and other iron-dependent enzymes, especially NADH dehydrogenase.	Most common nutritional deficiency (in humans); characteristic microcytic anemia due to iron depletion of red blood cells. See text.
Selenium	Antioxidant; component of several enzymes, most notably glutathione peroxidase.	Deficiency results in muscle degeneration, liver necrosis, growth retardation, reproductive failure.
Zinc	Component of more than 50 metalloenzymes; stabilization of RNA, DNA, and ribosomes; productive binding of hormone receptor complexes; tubulin. polymerization; necessary for growth and reproductive function; participates in smell and taste; critical for night vision.	One of the most important trace elements. Deficiency causes growth retardation, failure of sexual maturity, fetal deformities, immunosuppression, corneal opacities, loss or impaired smell and taste, impaired glucose tolerance. Interrelated with vitamin A.

*Sodium, potassium, calcium, and magnesium are considered macrominerals and are important in the ionic movement across cell membranes. All macrominerals function in energy metabolism, membrane transport, and the maintenance of membrane potential by Na^+, K^+ -ATPase. Calcium is critical to the skeletal system, neuromuscular transmission, cellular signaling, and blood coagulation. Magnesium is critical in more than 300 enzymatic reactions; deficiency results in osteomalacia (humans), neuromuscular disorders, seizures, and cardiac dysrhythmias.

Data from Atkinson RL: Nutritional aspects of pharmacology. In Brody TM, Larner JL, Minneman KP, editors: *Human pharamacology: molecular to clinical,* St. Louis, 1998, Mosby, pp. 843-860.

Appendix 5

Clinical Toxicology

E. Murl Bailey, Jr.

Appendix Outline

INTRODUCTION

I. Toxicants are just another etiology of a disease process.
II. Toxicants are capable of mimicking bacterial or viral processes.
III. History is very important in diagnosing toxicoses.
IV. With few exceptions, it is more important to treat the animal than worry about the diagnosis (i.e., the diagnosis is important, but saving the animal's life is more important).
V. Do not let the client or anything else make the diagnosis for you.
VI. Important toxicants in veterinary clinical practice:
   A. Rodenticides
   B. Insecticides
   C. Organic compounds, such as antifreeze, halogenated hydrocarbon
   D. Inorganics: metals
   E. Plants

MANAGEMENT AND TREATMENT OF TOXICOSES

When the task at hand is treatment of intoxications, the primary emphasis should be on prevention, not treatment. Therefore client education is at the top of the list, whether the client is a producer or an individual animal owner. Client education should emphasize proper handling as well as storage techniques.

Primary Goals of Therapy

I. Emergency intervention and prevention of further exposure
   A. Removal of the animal from the toxicant, or the toxicant from the animal; washing the animal
   B. Maintenance of normal respiratory and cardiac function
II. Establishment of a tentative diagnosis on which to base rational therapeutic measures
III. Delaying of further absorption
IV. Application of specific antidotes and remedial measures
V. Hastening the elimination of the absorbed toxicant
VI. Supportive therapy
VII. Determination of the source of the toxicant
VIII. Client education

Telephone Instructions

The owner should do the following until the animal is taken to the veterinarian or until the veterinarian sees the animal(s).

I. Do not waste time.
II. Protect the animal from injuring itself, and protect the people and other animals in the vicinity. It is important that the animal owner protect himself or herself if externally applied chemicals (pesticides) are involved.
III. Bring suspect material, with original container, if possible along with any vomitus. Clean glass containers are best. This is especially important if medical/legal aspects are involved.
IV. If there will be a time delay, and if the owner is insistent about treating the animal with some "medication" and if the animal is not sedated or unconscious, then the owner can be advised to do the following:
  A. Administer milk.
  B. Administer activated charcoal if available.
  C. Administer water.
  D. The owner may be advised to wash dermally exposed animals with soap and water, but the owner should use proper precautions.
  E. 5 mL of hydrogen peroxide (1 tsp) on base of tongue or ½ to 1 tsp of syrup of ipecac; clinician must explain precautions about vomition as well as toxicity of syrup of ipecac.

TREATMENT AFTER THE ANIMAL IS SEEN

Emergency Intervention: Keep the Animal Alive

I. Establish patent airway.
II. Assess and maintain myocardial activity.

Delay Absorption

I. Remove external contaminants
II. Induce emesis
  A. Of little value after 2 to 4 hours of ingestion
  B. Syrup of ipecac
    1. 1 to 2 mL/kg, maximum of 15 mL for largest dog
    2. Only 50% effective in dogs, may repeat after 20 minutes. If emesis does not occur after second dosage, the syrup of ipecac must be removed by gastric lavage.
    3. Syrup of ipecac must not be used when activated charcoal will be used in the treatment regimen.
  C. Copper sulfate —dangerous
  D. Table salt —dangerous
  E. Hydrogen peroxide —5mL on base of tongue
  F. Apomorphine —Lilly
    1. Most reliable
    2. Most effective
    3. 0.04 mg/kg intravenously or
    4. 0.08 mg/kg intramuscularly
    5. Disadvantages
      a) Protracted emesis
      b) May deepen respiratory depression, but if respiration is depressed, then central nervous system depression is also present; therefore induction of emesis would be contraindicated.
      c) May be effectively controlled by appropriate narcotic antagonists administered intravenously
        (a) Narcan —0.04 mg/kg
        (b) Lorfan —0.02 mg/kg
        (c) Nalline —0.1 mg/kg
      d) It is a *Schedule II* drug that *is no longer manufactured.* It may be rereleased at some unspecified time in the future. Even though it is no longer being marketed, it is still found in many clinics.
III. Contraindications for INDUCTION OF EMESIS
  A. Unconsciousness or central nervous system depression (respiratory depression)
  B. Intoxication of petroleum distillates?
  C. Use of tranquilizers or antiemetics
  D. If > 2 to 4 hours since ingestion
  E. Ingestion of acids or alkalis: weakened stomach wall, retching may rupture, also reinjure esophagus and oral cavity.
IV. Activated charcoal may be used with emetics to increase the efficiency of both techniques.
V. Vomitus should be saved.

Gastric Lavage

I. Animal is unconscious: light anesthesia, with endotracheal tube (cuffed) extended beyond teeth.
II. Lower head and thorax.
III. Measure oral–gastric tube from muzzle to xiphoid cartilage and mark.
IV. Use same size oral–gastric tube as endotracheal tube 1 mm = 3 French; use as large a tube as possible.
V. Use 5 to 10 mL/kg of lavage solution for infusion.
VI. Aspirate solution from stomach using a large aspirator bulb or 50-mL syringe.
VII. Repeat cycle 10 to 15 times; activated charcoal will increase efficiency.
VIII. Precautions:
  A. Use low pressures; do not force fluid.
  B. Reduce volume in obviously weakened stomachs.
  C. Do not rupture esophageal or gastric walls.

Adsorbents

I. Activated charcoal
  A. Vegetable or petroleum origin, not animal origin
  B. Activated by increasing surface area and heating
  C. Sources:
    1. SUPERCHAR —Gulf Biosystems, Dallas (This is currently off the market (as of early 1991). A Japanese company has purchased it and is considering rereleasing it in the future.
    2. TOXIBAN —Vetamix, Shenandoah, Iowa
    3. Use a bathtub or another easily cleaned area
    4. Make a slurry with water, 1 gm/5-10 mL water
    5. Dosage = 2 to 8 g/kg BW
    6. Administer by oral–gastric tube using funnel or large syringe

7. Administer a saline cathartic 30 minutes after charcoal.
8. For best results, activated charcoal should be re-administered qid for several days after an intoxication.

D. *Remember:* Do not use with syrup of ipecac

E. Universal Antidote — not effective
1. Activated charcoal —2 parts
2. Magnesium oxide —1 part
3. Tannic acid —1 part
4. “Burnt” toast —not effective

Cathartics

I. Saline cathartic —best
   A. Sodium sulfate —1 g/kg best
   B. Magnesium sulfate

II. Mineral oil and/or vegetable oil may be contraindicated; always follow with a saline cathartic.

Colonic Lavage or High Enema

I. Sources of activated charcoal —see Table 1

II. Locally acting antidotes —see Table 2

III. Systemic antidotes —see Table 3

ELIMINATION OF ABSORBED TOXICANTS

General

I. Kidneys—easiest to manipulate

II. Bile, feces

III. Lungs

Renal Elimination

I. Requires adequate renal function: minimum of 0.1 mL/kg/min of urine production

II. May require hydration: fluid therapy

III. Diuretics
   A. Furosemide —Lasix - 5 mg/kg, every 6-8 hours
   B. Mannitol —2 gm/kg/hr
   C. Manipulation of pH
      1. For an acid, $pH = pKa + \log \frac{I}{U}$
      2. For a base, $pH = pKa + \log \frac{U}{I}$
      3. Many chemicals are weak acids or bases.
      4. Degree of ionization depends on pH of medium and pKa of compound.

IV. Facts about pKas of compounds
   A. Acid with low pKa = strong acid
   B. Acid with high pKa = weak acid
   C. Base with low pKa = weak base
   D. Base with high pKa = strong base
   E. At pHs above pKa
      1. Acids = ionized
      2. Bases = un-ionized
   F. At pHs below pKa
      1. Acids = un-ionized
      2. Bases = ionized
   G. Compounds that are un-ionized at physiologic pHs could be expected to traverse membranes if the compound is lipid soluble.
   H. The gastrointestinal tract and the kidney are the organs where clinicians can take advantage of the pH differences. “ION TRAPPING”
      1. Drugs are readily absorbed from the gastrointestinal tract if the non-ionized form is lipid soluble and if:
         a) an acid with pKa > 2
            or
         b) a base with pKa < 11
   I. Exceptions:
      1. 2-PAM —completely ionized, absorbed from stomach but will not readily cross blood–brain barrier
   J. Examples of “ION TRAPPING”
      1. Acid—Acetylsalicylic acid (aspirin) and some barbiturates remain more ionized in alkalinized urine.
      2. Bases—amphetamines and other basic compounds remain more ionized in acidic urine.
   K. Urinary acidifying agents
      1. Ammonium chloride — 200 mg/kg per day in divided doses
      2. Ethylenediamine dihydrochloride, Chlorethamine —1-2 tabs, tid
      3. Physiological saline (PSS) intravenously
   L. Urinary alkalinizing agents
      1. Sodium bicarbonate —5 meq/kg/hr

Peritoneal Dialysis

I. For use when kidneys do not function

II. Time consuming

III. Infusion of dialyzing fluids into peritoneal cavity, allowing the fluid to stay there for 30 to 60 minutes before removal

IV. May insert dialysis catheter, or just use 18-gauge needle

V. May alter pH of dialyzing fluids if type of offending agent is known (e.g., acid or base, pKa)

SUPPORTIVE MEASURES IN THERAPY OF INTOXICATIONS

I. Body temperature control

II. Respiratory support measures
   A. Analeptics
      1. Doxapram (Dopram): 3 to 5 mg/kg
      2. Short acting
      3. May induce convulsions
   B. Respirate: “GRAB THE CHEST”
      1. Patent airway—cuffed endotracheal tube
      2. Tracheotomy
      3. Respirator

III. Cardiovascular support
   A. Requirements
      1. Adequate circulating volume
      2. Adequate cardiac function

3. Adequate tissue perfusion
4. Adequate acid–base balance

B. Immediate concern - blood volume and cardiac activity
1. Hypovolemia: give whole blood if there loss of cells and volume
2. Hypovolemia: fluid loss—lactated Ringer's, plasma expanders
3. Cardiac activity - massage, pharmaceutical agents

IV. Acid–base balance

V. Pain

VI. Central nervous system disorders
A. Depression: see respiratory depression
B. Hyperactivity: managed by central nervous system depressants
1. Pentobarbital sodium —agent of choice for convulsions and hyperactivity (precautions)
2. Inhalant anesthetics: disadvantages and advantages
3. Skeletal muscle relaxants
a) Glyceryl guaiacolate, Guaiafenison
b) Methocarbamol, Robaxin
c) Diazepam, Valium: 0.5-1.5 mg/kg, intravenously or intramuscularly
4. Place in quiet, dark room to cut visual and auditory stimuli.

RODENTICIDES

Strychnine

I. Spinal convulsant
A. Competes with glycine
B. Reduces inhibitory postsynaptic potential

II. Signs occur 10 minutes to 2 hours after ingestion.

III. Apprehension, nervousness, tenseness, stiffness, tetanic convulsions with intermittent relaxation.

IV. Animal may die after 1 convulsion or may convulse for 1 to 2 hours before death occurs.

V. Affected animals almost never vomit. (i.e., full stomach at necropsy).

VI. Treatment:
A. After ingestion, before convulsions, with some signs:
1. Diazepam 2-5 mg/kg intravenously
a) Apomorphine intravenously, 0.04 mg/kg
b) Pentobarbital as needed
2. After onset of convulsions
a) Pentobarbital to effect
b) Gastric lavage
c) Place in quiet room
d) Animal should be observed for several days after apparent recovery.

Sodium Fluoroacetate (Compound 1080)

I. Biotransformed to fluorocitrate, blocks aconitase

II. Convulsant toxicant, not induced by external stimuli

III. Attempts to vomit, micturate, and defecate after onset of early nervous signs

IV. Convulsions can be controlled by pentobarbital, but it is extremely difficult to prevent death.

Anticoagulant Rodenticides

I. Competes with vitamin K, causes deficiencies in clotting factors II, VII,IX, X

II. Signs: hypovolemic shock, bleeding from body orifices, subcutaneous hemorrhages, pale mucous membranes, blood in body cavities

III. Treatment
A. Handle animals carefully.
B. Blood transfusion: whole blood or plasma blood transfusion, 25 mL/kg.
C. Use small needles.
D. Vitamin K_1 (Aqua-MEPHYTON, 5-mg caps, Merck & Co.)(Vita K_1, Eschar, 25-mg caps). Give 3-5 mg/kg/day with canned food. Treat 7 days for warfarin-type, treat 21 to 30 days for second-generation anticoagulant rodenticides. Oral therapy is more efficacious than intravenous therapy.

Cholecalciferol (Vitamin D_3) Quintox[R], True Grit Rampage[R], Ortho Rat-B-Gone[R]

I. Active ingredient: cholecalciferol, 0.075% baits

II. Mechanism of action: mobilizes calcium from bones into the blood, causing a "calcium-like" toxicity to the heart. Lower dosages over a long time can cause an actual vitamin D toxicoses.

III. Toxicity: mice = 84 mg/kg (lethal dose); rats = 50 mg/kg (lethal dose); dogs = >100 g/kg.

IV. Clinical signs: cessation of eating, lethargy, nausea, vomiting, diarrhea, polyuria, profuse sweating, polydipsia, and neurologic disturbances. Vasoconstriction and hypertension may be seen along with a shortened QT interval and prolonged PR interval. Serum calcium >11.5 mg/dL with increased BUN, creatine, and phosphorus.

V. Lesions: Acute = heart stops in systole; chronic = calcium deposits in soft tissues, aorta, tendons, muscle

VI. Reported by pest control personnel as safe around pets.

VII. No good antidotes; potassium chloride can be used if ECG monitoring is undertaken. No antidote for calcification

VIII. Treatment: Induce vomiting, and administer activated chrcoal. A saline cathartic should be used in cases of recent (within 3 hours) exposure. Moniter the serum calcium after 24 hours to determine if further therapy is necessary. Fluid therapy should include normal saline (intravenous) and furosemide as a diuretic. Thiazide diuretics are contraindicated. Corticosteroids have several beneficial effects and should be used. Also, calcitonin can be administered in microgram quantities (4-6 IU/kg) subcutaneously every 2 to 3 hours initially. Treatment with diuretics and cortisone should continue until serum calcium level remains normal. Check the serum calcium level 24 hours after treatment is stopped. Long-term therapy, for 2 weeks or more, may be required.

INSECTICIDES

Chlorinated Hydrocarbon Insecticides

I. Not as common, but still in use
II. Signs:
  A. Abnormal posture
  B. Fine tremors to gross convulsions
  C. Salivation
III. Treatment
  A. General treatment
  B. Control convulsions: pentobarbital, might try diazepam (intravenous) first

Rotenone

I. Botanical insecticide: *Derris* spp.
II. Low toxicity: 1 to 3 grams/kg
III. Signs: vomiting caused by gastric irritation
  A. Incoordination
  B. Muscle tremors
  C. Clonic convulsions
  D. Respiratory failure
IV. Treatment: General treatment

Pyrethrum and Synthetic Pyrethroids

I. Names: allethrin, cyfluthrin, cypermethrin, deltamethrin, decamethrin, fenpropathrin, fenvalerate, flumethrin, kadethrin, permethrin, resmethrin, terallethrin, tetramethrin (*-rin* suffix)
II. Low toxicity, except in fish and some tropical birds
III. Increased sensitivity to external stimuli: fine tremors to gross tremors to prostration
IV. Pawing, burrowing, salivation to writhing, convulsions
V. Treatment = diazepam

Diethyltoluamide (DEET)

I. History: DEET was synthesized in 1954 and used as an insect repellent. It is effective against mosquitoes, biting flies, gnats, chiggers, ticks, and fleas. The content of DEET in various products has ranged from 5% to 100%. The Hartz Company used DEET in dog and cat flea collars in their Blockade product line. Hartz withdrew its Blockade products from the market primarily because of consumer pressure and negative publicity. Some pets were reported to have died after exposure to Blockade.
II. Clinical signs and symptoms: In animals and humans, DEET is absorbed through the skin. It has been known to produce blisters, skin necrosis, erythema, central nervous system disturbances, and death in animals. In humans it also produces blisters, skin necrosis, a burning sensation, erythema, ulcerations, slurred speech, confusion, convulsions, and (without treatment) even death. It seems to be more toxic to female humans than male humans. This may be an occupational phenomenon of female association with dipping and spraying animals.
III. Although neurologic signs in animals and humans may resolve, the parent compound and its metabolites are detectable for up to 2 weeks after an episode.

Organophosphates and Carbamates

I. Signs: overstimulation of parasympathetic nervous system (cholinergic, nicotinic, central nervous system)
  A. Salivation, lacrimation, sweating
  B. Muscular involvement
  C. Constricted pupils
  D. Respiratory involvement
  E. Gastrointestinal involvement
  F. Urinary incontinence
  G. Central nervous system signs
II. Treatment organophosphates = Atropine + 2-PAM
  A. Atropine: 0.2-0.4 mg/kg (¼ intravenously, remainder subcutaneously)
  B. 2-PAM: 20-50 mg/kg intramuscularly (of no value after enzyme has "aged".
  C. Neither atropine nor 2-PAM will control all of the signs: *do not overtreat*
III. Treatment of carbamates: atropine only; some carbamates are just as toxic as organophosphates; extensive treatment not required, as with organophosphates
IV. Diazepam may be used to control some of the central nervous system signs.

ORGANIC COMPOUNDS

Ethylene Glycol (Antifreeze)

I. Biotransformed---> glycolic acid ---> oxalic acid ----> calcium oxalate (alcohol dehydrogenase)
II. Antifreeze = 95% ethylene glycol
III. Toxic dose = 2 to 10 mL/kg
IV. Early signs = depression, central nervous system signs, nausea, vomiting, polydipsia, polyuria, dehydration
V. May return to normal within 12 hours
VI. Signs return within 24 hours, with more severe, metabolic acidosis. Animals surviving 24 hours will have renal problems: signs of uremia, progressive increase in BUN, hyperkalemia, and acidosis; urine sediment may have birefringent crystals.
VII. Lesions: hemorrhages in gastrointestinal mucosa, swollen and congested kidneys, hyperemia and edema of lungs
VIII. Treatment:
  A. Activated charcoal (if within 8 hours)
  B. 20% ethanol, 5 mL/kg intravenously every 5-8 hours for 48-72 hours (causes central nervous system depression)
  C. 5% sodium bicarbonate, 8 mL/kg, every 8 hours as needed > 48 hours.
  D. 4-Methylpyrazole (5% solution) may be used *instead of* ethanol. It is better than ethanol because it does not induce central nervous system depression. As with ethanol, best results are obtained if treatment is initiated within 4 to 6 hours. *Do not use in cats.*
    1. Initial dosage 20 mg/kg
    2. 15 mg/kg 12 and 24 hours after ingestion
    3. 5 mg/kg 36 hours after ingestion.

Polyhalogenated compounds

I. Polyhalogenated biphenyls
  A. Induce enzymes
  B. "Multiple Diseases"
    1. Chick edema disease, reduced hatchability embryotoxic
    2. Acneiform dermatitis
    3. Interferes with poryphrin metabolism
    4. "Cola-colored" babies in Japan, "Yusho"
    5. Tolerances in food for human consumption
II. Dioxins
  A. Common contaminant in chlorinated hydrocarbons
  B. Extremely toxic in laboratory animals, not as toxic in humans
  C. Diseases
    1. Liver
    2. Rapidly proliferating tissues
    3. Spermatogenesis
    4. Gastrointestinal mucosa
    5. Cancer
    6. Teratogenesis: animals, humans
  D. Episodes
    1. Seveso, Italy
    2. Missouri (several episodes)
    3. Oregon
    4. Michigan

INORGANICS

Lead

I. Most common heavy metal toxicant in the world
II. Animals affected: cattle, young dogs, exotic birds
III. Age: Nursing animals are more susceptible
  A. Dogs: 2 to 8 months usually
  B. Bovine: any age
  C. Birds: any
IV. Signs:
  A. Gastrointestinal disturbances: vomiting, abdominal pain, anorexia
  B. Neurologic signs: 3 to 4 days after lead colic in dogs, abnormal behavior, pica, hysteria convulsions; cattle and birds: neurologic signs.
  C. Laboratory
    1. Hematopoietic: late in syndrome nucleated red cells, other red blood cell abnormalities
    2. Radiographic
      a) Gastrointestinal tract
      b) Lead line in Bones
    3. Blood lead > 0.6 ppm, 0.05-0.25 = normal
V. Treatment:
  A. Remove lead from gastrointestinal tract
  B. Calcium disodium EDTA: 75-100 mg/kg per day, intravenously or intramuscularly
  C. Penicillamine 100 mg/kg per day if owner refuses to hospitalize
  D. Bronchoalveolar lavage 4 mg/kg qid with EDTA w/ severe nervous signs
  E. Thiamine HCl: 5 mg/kg, intravenously bid for 1 to 2 weeks

Mercury (Possible Problem in Grains or Dog Food)

I. Inorganic and organic forms
  A. Inorganic absorbed through gastrointestinal tract, lungs
  B. Organic: also through skin
  C. Aryl and methoxyethyl forms produce signs similar to inorganic
  D. Alkyl = typical signs + neurologic signs
II. "Typical" signs
  A. Gastrointestinal, abdominal pain, weakness, anorexia, central nervous system depression, renal signs
  B. Proteinuria = common
III. Alkyl mercurial signs
  A. Sudden onset, ataxia, stumbling, hyperesthesia, convulsions, prostration
  B. Young born with neurologic deficits
  C. Focal central malacia, cord not affected.
IV. Treatment:
  A. Acute, "typical"—bronchoalveolar lavage
  B. Chronic—penicillamine
  C. No treatment for alkyl mercurial intoxications

Arsenical Intoxication

I. Inorganic and organic forms
II. Extremely important in some areas of United States, equal to lead in some cases
III. Many sources: herbicides (old and new), insecticides, tonics, heartworm treatment, growth promotants
IV. Clinical signs: gastrointestinal, abdominal pain, depression, diarrhea; chronic: rough hair coat, unthrifty, cattle may have enlarged joints
V. Clinical signs (phenylarsonic): central nervous system, paresis, incoordination (drunk pig syndrome), alert and will continue to eat, blindness (not constant); signs are reversible unless nerve damage has developed; just remove from source
VI. Treatment: "typical"
  A. Early = general treatment, sodium thiosulfate, orally
  B. Late = bronchoalveolar lavage 2.5 to 5 mg/kg, 2 to 4 times per day for 10 days or until recovery
  C. No treatment for phenylarsonic compounds.

Copper and Molybdenum

I. A "toxicity" of one means a deficiency of the other.
II. Copper toxicoses occurs primarily in sheep, although Bedlington Terriers have a congenital problem with copper accumulation.
III. Molybdenum toxicoses (molybdenosis) occurs primarily in cattle but may cause a problem in young lambs.
IV. Ideal ratio is Cu:Mo = 6:1 in the diet, total intake if the ratio is outside 2:1 to 10:1, problems can be expected.
V. Copper toxicoses
  A. An acute disease can occur; typical heavy metal along with intravascular hemolysis
  B. Usual disease = chronic accumulation in liver with a subsequent massive release of copper, > 150 ppm Cu, wet weight = potential problems

C. Usual sign = a sudden hemolytic crisis leading to anemia and jaundice (not always)
D. Course of disease = 24 to 48 hours

VI. Molybdenum toxicoses
A. Usually a chronic disease: "poor doers," chronic diarrhea, appear hypoproteinemic, achromotrichia, poor reproductive performance, anemia, joint problems
B. Sheep may develop wool problems, produce lambs with incoordination ("swayback")

VII. Treatment:
A. Copper toxicoses = penicillamine –chelating agent, ammonium tetrathiomolybdate, change diet
B. Molybdenosis = copper glycinate, change diet

Table 1 Some Available Activated Charcoal Products

Commercial Trade	Ingredients	Manufacturer or Distributor	Address
Activated charcoal gel	Activated charcoal, 100 mg/mL with electrolytes	Vets Plus, Inc 800-468-3877	102 3rd Ave Knapp, WI 54749
D-TOX-BESC	Activated charcoal, 100 mg/mL	Agripharm 901-366-4442	4869 E. Raines Road Memphis, TN 38175
Toxiban	Granules 47% activated charcoal, 10% kaolin, 42% wetting and dispensing agents, 5 kg-pail, Suspension, 10.4% activated charcoal, 6.25% kaolin in an aqueous dose; 240-mL bottle	Vet-A-Mix 800-831-0004	604 W. Thomas Ave. Shenandoah, IA 51601
UAA Universal Animal (Antidote Gel)	Activated charcoal, 100 mg/mL	Vedco 888-708-3326	5503 Corporate Dr. St. Joseph, MO 64507

Table 2 Locally Acting Antidotes Against Unabsorbed Poisons and Principles of Treatment

Toxicant	Antidote and Dose or Concentration
Acids, corrosives	Weak alkali-magnesium oxide solution (1:25 warm water) internally. *Never give sodium bicarbonate!* Milk of magnesia—1 to 15 mL. Flush externally with water. Apply paste of sodium bicarbonate.
Alkali, caustic	Weak acid—vinegar (diluted 1:4), 1% acetic acid, or lemon juice given orally. Dilute albumin (4 to 6 egg whites to 1 qt warm water) or give whole milk followed by activated charcoal and then a cathartic because some compounds are soluble in excess albumin. Local—flush with copious amounts of water and apply vinegar.
Alkaloids	Potassium permanganate (1:5000 to 1:10,000) for lavage or oral administration. Tannic acid or strong tea (200 to 500 mg in 30 to 60 mL of water) except in cases of poisoning by cocaine, nicotine, physostigmine, atropine, and morphine. Emetic or purgative should be used for prompt removal of tannates.
Arsenic	Sodium thiosulfate—10% solution given orally (0.5 to 3 g for small animals), followed by lavage or emesis. Protein—evaporated milk, egg whites. Tannic acid or strong tea (see specific antidote in Table 3).
Barium salts	Sodium sulfate and magnesium sulfate (20% solution given orally) Dosage: 2 to 25 gm.
Bismuth salts	Acacia or gum arabic as mucilage.
Carbon tetrachloride	Empty stomach, give high-protein and carbohydrate diet; maintain fluid and electrolyte balance. Hemodialysis is indicated in anuria. Epinephrine is contraindicated (ventricular fibrillation).
Copper	Albumin (see Alkali, above). Sodium ferrocyanide in water (0.3 to 3.5 g for small animals). (See specific antidote in Table 3.) Magnesium oxide (see Acids, above).
Detergents, anionic (Na, K, NH_4^+salts)	Milk or water followed by demulcent (oils, acacia, gelatin, starch, egg white)
Detergents, cationic (chlorides, iodides)	Soap (castile) dissolved in 4 times its bulk of hot water. Albumin (see Alkali, above).
Fluoride	Calcium (milk, lime water, or powdered chalk mixed with water) given orally.

Continued

Table 2 Locally Acting Antidotes Against Unabsorbed Poisons and Principles of Treatment—cont'd

Toxicant	Antidote and Dose or Concentration
Formaldehyde	Ammonia water (0.2% orally) or ammonium acetate (1% for lavage). Starch—1 part to 15 parts hot water, added gradually. Gelatin soaked in water for 30 min. Albumin (see Alkali, above). Sodium thiosulfate (see Arsenic, above).
Iron	Sodium bicarbonate—1% for lavage. (See specific antidote in Table 3.)
Lead	Sodium or magnesium sulfate given orally. Sodium ferrocyanide (see Copper, above). See specific antidote. Albumin (see Alkali, above).
Mercury	Protein—milk, egg whites (see Alkali, above). Magnesium oxide (see Acids, above). Sodium formaldehyde sulfoxylate—5% solution for lavage. Starch (see Formaldehyde, above). Activated charcoal—5 to 50 g. (See specific antidote in Table 3.)
Oxalic acid	Calcium—calcium hydroxide as 0.15% solution. Other alkalis are contraindicated because their salts are more soluble. Chalk or other calcium salts. Magnesium sulfate as cathartic. Maintain diuresis to prevent calcium oxalate deposition in kidney.
Petroleum distillates (aliphatic hydrocarbons)	Olive oil, other vegetable oils, or mineral oil given orally. After 30 min, sodium sulfate as cathartic. Emesis and lavage are contraindicated for ingested volatile solvents, but petroleum distillates are used as carrier agents for more toxic agents.
Phenol and cresols	Soap and water or alcohol lavage of skin. Sodium bicarbonate (0.5%) dressings. Activated charcoal and/or mineral oil given orally.
Phosphorous	Copper sulfate (0.2 to 0.4% solution) or potassium permanganate (1:5000 solution) for lavage. Turpentine (preferably old oxidized) in gelatin capsules or floated on hot water. Give 2 mL 4 times at 15-minute intervals. Activated charcoal. Do not give vegetable oil cathartic. Remove all fat from diet.
Silver nitrate	Normal saline for lavage. Albumin (see Alkali, above).
Unknown (e.g., toxic plants or other materials)	Activated charcoal (replaces universal antidote). For small animals: through stomach tube, as a slurry in water. Follow with emetic or cathartic and repeat procedure.

Table 3 Specific Systemic Antidotes and Dosages

Toxic Agent	Systemic Antidote	Dosage and Method for Treatment
Acetaminophen	B-acetylcysteine (Mucomyst, Mead Johnson)	150 mg/kg loading dose, PO or IV, then 50 mg/kg every 4 hours for 17-20 additional doses.
	Cimetidine	5 mg/kg, orally, every 6-8 hours for 2-3 days. To prevent biotransformation of acetaminophen.
Amphetamines	Chlorpromazine	1 mg/kg IM, IP, IV; administer only half dose if barbiturates have been given: blocks excitation. Higher doses (10-18 mg/kg IV) may be beneficial if large volumes are consumed. Treatment of increased intracranial pressure may be indicated (mannitol, furosemide)
	Urinary alkalinization: Ammonium chloride	100 to 200 mg/kg per day divided every 8 to 12 hours (contraindicated with myoglobinuria, renal failure of acidosis).
Amitraz	Atipamezole	50 g/kg IM. Signs should reverse in 10 minutes. Repeat every 3-4 hours as needed. Can follow with 0.1 mg/kg yohimbine IM every 6 hours.
	Yohimbine	Dogs 0.11 mg/kg IV slowly Cats 0.5 mg/kg IV slowly

Table **3** Specific Systemic Antidotes and Dosages—cont'd

Toxic Agent	Systemic Antidote	Dosage and Method for Treatment
Antitussives	Naloxone	If narcotic (e.g., hydrocodone, codeine)
Arsenic, mercury and other heavy metals except cadmium, lead silver, selenium, and thallium	Dimercaprol (BAL, Hynson, Wescott & Dunning)	10% solution in oil; give small animals 2.5 to 5 mg/kg IM every 4 hours for 2 days, bid for the next 10 days or until recovery. NOTE: In severe acute poisoning, 5 mg/kg dosage should be given only for the first day.
	D-Penicillamine (Cuprimine, Merck & Co.)	Developed for chronic mercury poisoning, now seems most promising drug; no reports on dosage in animals. Dosage for humans is 250 mg orally, every 6 hours for 10 days (3 to 4 mg/kg).
Aspirin	No specific antidote (see also, nonsteroidal antiinflammatory drugs)	Acute toxicosis: urinary alkalinization, other supportive therapy; doses of 50 mg/kg per day (dog) and 25 mg/kg/day (cat); 7 mL/kg per day of bismuth subsalicylate (dogs and cats) may be toxic.
Atropine, Belladonna alkaloids	Physostigmine salicylate	0.1 to 0.6 mg/kg (do not use neostigmine).
Barbiturates	Doxapram (Dopram)	2% solution: Give small animals 3 to 5 mg/kg IV only (0.14 to 0.25 mL/kg) repeated as necessary.
Barium, bismuth salts	Sodium sulfate/magnesium sulfate	20% solution given orally, 2 to 25 g.
Bleach	Treat as alkali	Use of emetics is controversial; treat as an alkali poisoning. Therapies have included milk or water (large volumes), milk of magnesia (2-3 mg/kg), egg whites, or powdered milk slurry. Sodium bicarbonate is *not* recommended.
Borates (roach killers, fleas products, fertilizers, herbicides, antiseptics, disinfectants, contact lens solutions)	No specific antidote	Supportive therapy includes emetics and gastric lavage, fluid therapy and diuresis, treatment of seizures and hyperthermia as indicated.
Botulism	Antitoxin	Use is controversial. Supportive care may be sufficient. Supportive therapy may include penicillin, physostigmine or neostigmine, and atropine.
Bromethalin	No specific antidote	Supportive care may include treatment of cerebral edema.
Bromides	Chlorides (sodium or ammonium salts)	0.5 to 1 g daily for several days; hasten excretion.
Caffeine/chocolate	No specific antidote	General treatment, diazepam (2 to 5 mg/kg) for tremors, treat arrhythmias as indicated.
Carbon monoxide	Oxygen	Pure oxygen at normal or high pressure; artificial respiration; blood transfusion.
Cholinergic agents	Atropine sulfate	0.02 to 0.04 mg/kg, as needed.
Cholinesterase inhibitors	Atropine sulfate	Dosage is 0.2 - 0.4 mg/kg, repeated as needed for atropinization. Treat cyanosis (if present) first. Blocks only muscarinic effects. Atropine in oil may be injected for prolonged effect during the night. *Avoid atropine intoxication!*
	Pralidoxime chloride (2-PAM) (organophosphates, some carbamates; but not carbaryl, dimethan, or carbam piloxime)	5% solution; five 20 to 50 mg/kg IM or by slow IV (0.2 to 1.0 mg/kg) injection (maximum dose is 500 mg/min), repeat as needed. 2-PAM alleviates nicotinic effect and regenerates cholinesterase. Morphine, succinylcholine, and phenothiazine tranquilizers are contraindicated.
	Diphenhydramine	1-4 mg/kg IM, PO every 8 hours to block nicotinic effects.
Cocaine	No specific antidote	Chlorpromazine (up to 15 mg/kg; may lower seizure threshold, use cautiously); butylcholinesterase may convert cocaine to inactive metabolites (currently under investigation); fluids metoprolol or isopropanolol to treat cardiac arrhythmias (see methylxanthines); phentolamine or sodium nitroprusside if beta blockers cause hypertension; lidocaine (instead of beta blockers) to control cardiac arrhythmias; see methylxanthines.
Crayons (aniline dyes)	Ascorbic acid	20-30 mg/kg PO or 20 mg/kg IV slowly

Continued

Table 3 Specific Systemic Antidotes and Dosages—cont'd

Toxic Agent	Systemic Antidote	Dosage and Method for Treatment
	Methylene blue (if ascorbic acid fails)	Dogs: 3-4 mg/kg IV Cats: 1.5 mg/kg.(Methylene blue may cause Heinz body formation in the absence of methemoglobinemia, and sometimes in the presence of methemoglobinemia.)
Copper	D-Penicillamine (Cuprimine)	52 mg/kg for 6 days (also see Arsenic)
	Ammonium molybdate Sodium thiosulfate	50 to 500 mg, PO, once a day 300 to 1000 mg, PO, once a day
	Ammonium tetrathiomolybdate	100 to 500 mg, PO on alternate days for 3 treatments
Coumarin-derivative anticoagulants	Vitamin K_1 (Aqua-MEPHYTON, 5 mg caps, Merck & Co.) (Vita K_1, Eschar, 25 mg caps) Whole blood or plasma	Give 3-5 mg/kg/day with canned food. Treat 7 days for warfarin-type, treat 21 to 30 days for second-generation anticoagulant rodenticides. Oral therapy is more efficacious than IV. Blood transfusion, 25 mL/kg.
Curare	Neostigmine methylsulfate	Solution: 1:5000 for 1:2000. (1 mL = 0.2 or 0.5 mg/mL). Dose is 0.005 mg/5 kg, SC. Follow with IV injection of atropine (0.04 mg/kg).
	Edrophonium chloride (Tensilon, Roche) Artificial respiration	1% solution; give 0.05 to 1.0 mg/kg IV.
Cyanide	Methemoglobin (sodium nitrite is used to form methemoglobin) Sodium thiosulfate	1% solution of sodium nitrite, dosage is 16 mg/kg IV (1.6 mL/kg). Follow with sodium thiosulfate 20% solution at dosage of 30 to 40 mg/kg (0.15 to 0.2 mL/kg) IV. If treatment is repeated, use only sodium thiosulfate. NOTE: The above may be given simultaneously as follows: 0.5 mL/kg of combination consisting of 10 g sodium nitrite, 15 g sodium thiosulfate, distilled water quantity sufficient 250 mL. Dosage may be repeated once. If further treatment is required, give only 20% solution of sodium thiosulfate at level of 0.2 mL/kg.
Decongestants	No specific antidote	Treat symptomatically.
Detergents: anionic (Na, K, NH_4^+)		Milk or water followed by demulcent (oils, acacia, gelatin, starch, egg white.)
Detergents: cationic (chlorides, iodides		Castile soap dissolved in 4 times bulk of hot water. Albumin, see Alkali above.
Diatomaceous earth		No treatment indicated unless pulmonary, then supportive.
Digitalis glycosides, oleander, and ***Bufo*** toads	Potassium chloride	Dog: 0.5 to 2.0 g, orally in divided doses, or in serious cases as diluted solution given IV by slow drip (ECG control is essential).
	Diphenylhydantoin Propranolol (ß -blocker)	25 mg/minute IV control is established. 0.5-1.0 mg/kg IV or IM as needed to control cardiac arrhythmias (ECG control is essential).
	Atropine sulfate	0.02 to 0.04 mg/kg as needed for cholinergic control.
		2 to 5 mg/kg, control convulsions
	Diazepam (Valium, Roche)	(2 to 5 mg/kg) in the case of *Bufo* toads, must treat convulsions first.
Ethylene glycol	Ethanol	See methanol and ethylene glycol. Minimal lethal dose of ethylene glycol is 4.2 to 6.6 mL/kg (4.5 ounces in 20-lb dog) and 1.5 mL for cats. Give IV, 1.1 g/kg (4.4 mL/kg) of 25% solution. Give 0.5 gm/kg (2.0 mL/kg) every 4 hours for 4 days. To prevent or correct acidosis, use sodium bicarbonate IV, 0.4 g/kg. Activated charcoal: 5 g/kg orally if within 4 hours of ingestion.
	4-Methylpyrazole	20 mg/kg, 15 mg/kg at 12 and 24 hours, 5 mg/kg at 36 hours
	Sodium bicarbonate 5%	8 mL/kg (dog) or 6 mg/kg (cat) IP every 4 hours for five treatments, then every 6 hours for four more treatments.
Fertilizer	No specific antidote	Supportive therapy may include treatment for electrolyte disorders, vomiting, H_2 receptor blockers for gastritis, (sucralfate and analgesics as needed)
Fluoride	Calcium borogluconate	3 to 10 mL of 5% to 10% solution.

Table 3 Specific Systemic Antidotes and Dosages—cont'd

Toxic Agent	Systemic Antidote	Dosage and Method for Treatment
Fluoracetate (Compound 1080®, Sigma)	Glyceryl monoacetin	0.1 to 0.5 mg/kg IM hourly for several hours (total 2 to 4 mg/kg); or diluted (0.5 to 1%) IV (danger of hemolysis). Monoacetin is available only from chemical supply houses.
	Acetamide	Animal may be protected if acetamide is given before or simultaneously with Compound 1080 (experimental).
	Pentobarbital NOTE: All treatments are generally unrewarding.	May protect against lethal dose (experimental).
Formaldehyde		Ammonia water (0.2% orally) or ammonium acetate (1% for lavage). Starch—1 part to 15 parts hot water, added gradually. Gelatin soaked in water for 30 minutes. Albumin (see Alkali, above). Sodium thiosulfate (see Arsenic, above).
Garbage	No specific therapy.	Supportive therapy may include antiemetics (metoclopramide or phenothiazines) and treatment of endotoxemia.
Hallucinogens (LSD, phencyclidine[PCP])	Diazepam (Valium, Roche)	As needed—avoid respiratory depression (2 to 5 mg/kg).
Heparin	Protamine sulfate	1% solution; give 1 to 1.5 mg to antagonize each 1 mg of heparin; slow IV injection. Reduce dose as time increases between heparin injection and start of treatment (after 30 minutes give only 0.5 mg).
Iron salts	Deferoxamine (Desferal, Ciba)	Dose for animals not yet established. Dose for humans is 5 g of 5% solution given orally, then 20 mg/kg IM every 4 to 6 hours. In case of shock, dose is 40 mg/kg by IV drip over 4-hour period; may be repeated in 6 hours, then 15 mg/kg by drip every 8 hours.
Ivermectin	Physostigmine	0.06 mg/kg IV very slowly; actions should last 30 to 90 minutes.
	Picrotoxin (GABA antagonist)	Use is controversial. May cause severe seizures. Other treatment may include epinephrine and, if the product causing toxicosis is Eqvalan, an antihistamine to counteract polysorbate 80 (releases histamine in dogs), and atropine.
Lead	Calcium disodium edetate ($CaNa_2EDTA$)	Dosage: Maximum safe dose is 75 mg/kg/24 hours (only for severe case). EDTA is available in 20% solution; for IV drip, dilute in 5% glucose to 0.5%; for IM, add procaine to 20% solution to give 0.5% concentration of procaine.
Lead (cont.)	EDTA and BAL	BAL is given as 10% solution in oil. Treatment: 1. In severe case (CNS involvement w/> 100 ug Pb/100 gm whole blood) give 4 mg/kg. BAL only as initial dose; follow after 4 hours, and every 4 hours for 3 to 4 days, with BAL and EDTA (12.5 mg/kg) at separate IM sites; skip 2 or 3 days, and then treat again for 3 to 4 days. 2. In subacute case w/< 100 ug Pb/100 g whole blood, give only 50 mg EDTA/kg/24 hours for 3 to 5 days.
	Penicillamine (Cuprimine, Merck & Co.)	3. May use after treatments either *1* or *2* with 100 mg/kg/day orally for 1 to 4 weeks.
	Thiamine HCl	Experimental for nervous signs; 5 mg/kg, IV, bid, for 1 to 2 weeks; give slowly and watch for untoward reactions
	Succimer (Chemet)	Oral human dose = 10 mg/kg every 8 hours for 5 days, then 10 mg/kg bid for 2 weeks (total of 19 days of therapy) Animal dosages have not been established. (Used if blood lead levels > 45 ppm.)
Local anesthetics	See treatment for methemoglobinemia	Particularly cats.
Marijuana	No effective antidotes	Protein—milk, egg whites (see alkali, above). Magnesium oxide (see acids, above). Sodium formaldehyde sulfoxylate—5% solution for lavage. Starch (see Formaldehyde, table 2) Activated charcoal—5-50 g.
Metaldehyde	Diazepam (Valium, Roche)	2 to 5 mg/kg IV to control tremors.

Continued

Table 3 Specific Systemic Antidotes and Dosages—cont'd

Toxic Agent	Systemic Antidote	Dosage and Method for Treatment
	Triflupromazine	0.2 to 2 mg/kg IV.
	Pentobarbital	To effect.
	Note: Should monitor liver function and treat accordingly	
Methanol and ethylene glycol	Ethanol	Give IV, 1.1 g/kg (4.4 mL/kg) of 25% solution. Give 0.5 g/kg (2 mL/kg) every 4 hours for 4 days. To prevent or correct acidosis, use sodium bicarbonate IV, 0.4 g/kg. Activated charcoal: 5 g/kg orally if within 4 hours of ingestion.
	4 - Methyl Pyrazole	20 mg/kg, 15 mg/kg at 12 and 24 hours, 5 mg/kg at 36 hours
Methemoglobinemia-producing agents (nitrites, chlorates)	Methylene blue	1% solution (maximum concentration), give by *slow* IV injection, 8.8 mg/kg; (0.9 mL/kg); repeat if needed. To prevent fall in blood pressure in case of nitrite poisoning, use a sympathomimetic drug (ephedrine or epinephrine). (Not recommended for cats.)
	Ascorbic acid	20 to 30 mg/kg PO or 20 mg/kg IV slowly; methylene blue; dog 3-4 mg/kg IV slowly if ascorbic acid not effective; cats 1.5 mg/kg.
Morphine and related drugs	Naloxone chloride (Narcan, Endo)	0.1 mg/kg IV. Do not repeat if respiration is not satisfactory.
	Levallorphan tartrate (Lorfan, Roche)	Give IV, 0.1 to 0.5 mL of solution containing 1 mg/mL. NOTE: Use either of the above antidotes only in acute poisoning. Artificial respiration may be indicated. Activated charcoal is also indicated.
Mothballs (naphthalene, paradichlorobenzene)	No specific antidote	Supportive care includes fluid therapy and maintenance of renal and hepatic function.
Narcotics	Naloxone	Emesis—indicated only if patient is sufficiently alert. Dog: 0.02 to 0.04 mg/kg IV; repeat as needed. Cat: 0.05 to 0.1 mg/kg IV; repeat as needed. Supportive therapy may include anticonvulsants (especially for meperidine), fluid therapy.
Nicotine	No specific antidote	Emesis—indicated only within 60 minutes and in absence of clinical signs. Atropine indicated to control parasympathetic signs.
Nonsteroidal antiinflammatory drugs	Sucralfate	500-100 mg PO every 8 hours.
	Misoprostol	3 to 5 μg/kg every 8 to 12 hours
	Omeprazole	0.7 mg/kg every 24 hours (dog); alternative, ranitidine or famotidine (dog and cat)
Oxalates	Calcium	Treatment: 23% solution of calcium gluconate IV. Give 3 to 20 mL (to control hypocalcemia). Or Ca hydroxide as 0.15% solution or chalk or other calcium salts. Magnesium sulfate as cathartic. Other alkalines are contraindicated because their salts are more soluble. Maintain diuresis to prevent calcium oxalate deposition in kidney.
Onion/garlic	No specific antidote	Supportive therapy should address methemoglobinemia and hemoglobinuria. Avoid acidic urine.
Organic solvents: acetone, benzene, benzol, methanol, methylene chloride, naphtha, trichloroethane, acetonitrile, chloroform, trichloroethylene, tuolulene, xylene, xylol	No specific antidote	Emesis contraindicated. Supportive therapy includes treatment of cardiac arrhythmias, methemoglobinemia, renal failure, chemical pneumonia.
Petroleum distillates (aliphatic hydrocarbons)		Olive oil, other vegetable oils, or mineral oil given orally. After 30 minutes, sodium sulfate as cathartic. Emesis and lavage are contraindicated for ingested volatile solvents, but petroleum distillates are used as carrier agents for more toxic agents.
Phenols and cresols		Soap and water or alcohol lavage of skin. Sodium bicarbonate (0.5%) dressings. Activated charcoal and/or mineral oil given orally.
Phenothiazine	Methylamphetamine (Desoxyn, Abbott)	0.1 to 0.2 mg/kg IV; also transfusion. Only available in tablet form.

Table 3 Specific Systemic Antidotes and Dosages—cont'd

Toxic Agent	Systemic Antidote	Dosage and Method for Treatment
	Diphenhydramine HCl	For CNS depression, 2 to 5 mg/kg IV for extrapyramidal signs.
Phytotoxins and botulin	Antitoxins not available commercially except with botulism.	As indicated for specific antitoxins. Examples of phytotoxins: ricin, abrin, robin, crotin.
Plants		Treat signs as necessary.
Red squill	Atropine sulfate, propranolol, potassium chloride	As for digitalis and oleander
Scorpion sting	Ativenin (may not be recommended)	Supportive therapy includes analgesia to control pain (morphine and meperidine but not butorphanol are contraindicated because of potential synergy with scorpion venom); methocarbamol (if muscle spasms evident) and fluid therapy.
Smoke inhalation	Supportive therapy	Supportive therapy should target the respiratory system and treatment of carbon monoxide intoxication. Oxygen therapy; intermittent positive pressure ventilation with positive end-expiratory pressure with positive inotropic support, bronchodilators, treatment for cyanide poisoning if indicated, and treatment for cerebral edema.
Snake bite Rattlesnake Copperhead Water moccasin	Antivenin (Wyeth) (Trivalent Crotalidae)(Fort Dodge)	Caution: equine origin. Administer 1 to 2 vials, IV, slowly, diluted in 250 to 500 mL of saline or lactated Ringer's. Also administer antihistamines. *Corticosteroids are contraindicated.*
Coral snake	(Wyeth)	Caution: equine origin. May be used as with pit viper antivenin.
Spider bite Black widow	Antivenin (Merck & Co.)	Caution: equine origin. Administer IV undiluted. Supportive therapy should include muscle relaxants (dantrolene or methocarbamol) analgesics, calcium gluconate for severe muscle cramping.
	Dantrolene sodium (Dantrium, Norwich-Eaton)	1 mg/kg IV. Followed by 1 mg/kg PO every 4 hours.
Brown Recluse	Dapsone	1 mg/kg, bid for 10 days
Strontium	Calcium salts	Usual dose of calcium borogluconate.
	Ammonium chloride	0.2 to 0.5 g orally 3 to 4 times daily.
	Potassium chloride	Give simultaneously with thiocarbazone or Prussian blue, 2 to 6 g orally daily in divided doses.
Strychnine and brucine	Pentobarbital	Give IV to effect; higher dose is usually required than that required for anesthesia. Place animal in warm, quiet room.
	Amobarbital	Give by slow IV infusion; inject to effect. Duration of sedation is usually 4 to 6 hours.
	Methocarbamol (Robaxin, Robins)	10% solution; average first dose is 149 mg/kg IV (range: 40 to 300 mg). Repeat half dose as needed.
	Glyceryl guaiacolate (Guaiafenison, Summit Hill Labs)	110 mg/kg IV, 5% solution. Repeat as necessary.
	Diazepam (Valium, Roche)	2 to 5 mg/kg, control convulsions, induce emesis, then use other agents.
Thallium	Prussian blue	0.2 gm/kg orally in 3 divided doses daily.
	Potassium chloride	Give simultaneously with Prussian blue, 2 to 6 gm orally daily in divided doses.
Theobromine	See caffeine/chocolate poisoning	
Toad poisoning (*Bufo alvarius, Bufo marinus*)	Propranolol (*Bufo* poisoning only)	1.5-5 mg/kg IV; repeat in 20 minutes if ECG does not normalize; supportive therapy includes fluid therapy.
	Atropine	0.04 mg/kg IV to control hypersalivation or asystole.
	Lidocaine	Dogs: 1-2 mg/kg IV followed by continuous infusion of 25 to 75 µg/kg/min; cats: 0.25 to 1 mg/kg IV bolus followed by 5 to 40 µg/kg/min continuous IV infusion.

Continued

Table 3 Specific Systemic Antidotes and Dosages—cont'd

Toxic Agent	Systemic Antidote	Dosage and Method for Treatment
	Diazepam (Valium, Roche)	(2 to 5 mg/kg) in the case of *Bufo* toads, must treat convulsions first.
Tricyclic antidepressants	No specific antidote	Supportive therapy should target seizures (diazepam, phenobarbital, or general anesthesia with pentobarbital or short-acting thiobarbiturates; or, if unsuccessful, neuromuscular blockade with pancuronium (0.03 to 0.06 mg/kg IV) or vercuronium (10 to 20 µg/kg IV in dogs or 20 to 40 µg/kg in cats]); cardiotoxicity (see toad poisoning): propanolol, lidocaine (quinidine, procainamide and disopyramide are contraindicated); sodium bicarbonate (1-3 meq/kg).
Unknown (e.g., toxic plants or other materials)	No specific antidote	Activated charcoal 2-5 gm/kg (replaces universal antidote). For small animals: through stomach tube, as a slurry in water. Follow with emetic or cathartic, and repeat procedure.
Vitamin D_3 rodenticides	Treatment of hypercalcemia	Supportive therapy should target treatment of hypercalcemia (0.9% saline solution); control of seizures and treatment of hyperthermia. Calciuria can be promoted with furosemide (1 to 5 mg/kg every 6 to 12 hours for 2 to 4 weeks); prednisolone; calcitonin (4 to 6 IU/kg every 6 to 12 hours if calcium > 18 mg/dl; sodium bicarbonate if severe metabolic acidosis.
	Amphogel, Basagel	As phosphate binders (aluminum hydroxide 30 to 90 mg/kg PO every 8 to 24 hours for 2 weeks).
Xylitol		Hypoglycemia: 1-2 mL of 25% dextrose followed by 2.5%-5% dextrose infusion as needed to maintain normoglycemia. Add potassium to fluids to maintain serum potassium (treat for 12 to 24 hours). Hepatic necrosis: 140 to 280 mg/kg *N*-acetylcysteine IV followed by 70 mg/kg qid IV or PO; S-adenosylmethionine 17-20 mg/kg/day PO, silymarin 20 to 50 mg/kg/day PO.
Zinc	Chelation therapy (see lead)	CaEDTA, Succimer. Other supportive therapy includes fluid therapy and antisecretory drugs such as ranitidine, famotidine, or omeprazole to decrease oral absorption of zinc.

PO, By mouth; *IV*, intravenous; *IM*, intramuscular; *IP*, intraperitoneal; *SC*, subcutaneous; *ECG*, electrocardiogram; *CNS*, central nervous system.

Appendix 6

Generic and Trade Names*

Provision of proprietary names is not intended to be comprehensive. Generics are generally human unless noted otherwise. The absence of a proprietary name for a particular product generally indicates that only a generic form of the drug exists in the United States. Note that oral bioavailability of human generics should not be assumed to be equally bioavailable in dogs or cats. Whenever possible, a drug approved for dogs or cats should be used in preference to a human generic, in part because of the risk that bioavailability will differ among human generics in animals. The absence of the word *generic* does not rule out the availability of a generic version of a particular product. The absence of a number in general indicates the drug is approved for use in humans; most of the drugs are approved in the United States, although occasionally a drug (and its trade or brand name) reflects approval in a different country. For both generic and trade names of human drug products, and for approved drugs (but not biologics), the FDA Orange Book can be consulted at http://www.accessdata.fda.gov/scripts/cder/ob/docs/queryai.cfm; for veterinary-approved products. For information regarding animal-approved drugs (but not biologics), the FDA Green Book can be consulted at http://www.fda.gov/AnimalVeterinary/Products/ApprovedAnimalDrugProducts/UCM042847.

Generic	Proprietary
2-Mercaptopropionyl glycine	Tipronine
4-Methylpyrazole 5% (fomepizole)	Antizol-Vet
5-Fluorouracil	Adrucil
6-Mercaptopurine	Purinethol
Acarbose	Precose
Acemannan	Carrisyn (1)
Acepromazine maleate	Generic (1)
Acepromazine maleate	PromAce (1, 2)
Acetaminophen	Tylenol, generic (5)
Acetazolamide	Diamox
Acetohydroxamic acid	Lithostat
Acetylcysteine	Acetylcysteine (6)
Acetylcysteine	Mucomyst
Acetylcysteine	Acetadote
Acetretin (see etretinate)	
Acetylsalicylic acid	Aspirin, generic
Actinomycin D (dactinomycin)	Cosmegen
Activated charcoal	Actidose-Aqua (5)
Activated charcoal	CharcoCaps (5)
Activated charcoal	ToxiBan, generic
Acyclovir	Zovirax
Acyclovir (valacyclovir hydrochloride)	Valtrex
Adequan: see Polysulfated glycosoaminoglycans	Adequan
Albendazole	Valbazen (3)
Albendazole	Albenza
Albuterol	Proventil
Albuterol	Ventolin
Albuterol	Generic
Albuterol (levalbuterol hydrochloride)	Xopenex
Alfentanil (opioid)	Alfenta (10-II)
Allopurinol	Generic
Aloe vera cream	Dermaide, Aloe (7)
Alpha Keri	Keri, others (7)
Alprazolam	Xanax (10-IV)
Alprazolam	Xanax XR (10-IV)
Alprazolam	Niravam (10-IV)
Alprazolam	Alprazolam (10-IV)
Altrenogest	Regu-Mate, Matrix
Aluminum carbonate gel	Basaljel
Aluminum hydroxide	Amphojel
Aluminum hydroxide	Foamcoat
Aluminum magnesium hydroxide	Maalox, Mylanta
Amantadine	Symmetrel
Amikacin	Amikin (1)
Aminocaproic acid	Amicar
Aminopentamide	Centrine (1, 2)
Aminophylline	Aminophylline, others

1, Approved in dogs; *2*, approved in cats; *3*, approved in other animal; *4*, no longer available: if need is appropriate, may be available through a compounding pharmacist; *5*, OTC (human or animal); *6*, dietary supplement (human or animal), also indicates an OTC designation; *7*, human cosmetic product, also indicates an OTC designation; *8*, EPA-approved product; *9*, biological (if animal, may not be approved; if animal approved, approval is likely through US Department of Agriculture and generally is based only safety, not efficacy); *10*, distribution controlled by the Drug Enforcement Agency, Schedule status (I-V) indicated; *11*, obtain through chemical or other company, compounding pharmacist may assist; *12*, product may not be available from manufacturer; *13*, animal generic available; *14*, special restrictions.

Continued

Generic	Proprietary
Aminophylline	Truphylline
Aminopromazine	Jentone (1, 2, 4)
Aminopropazine	see aminopromazine
Amiodarone	Cordarone
Amiodarone	Amiodarone HCL
Amiodarone	Pacerone
Amitraz	Mitaban (1)
Amitriptyline HCI	generic
Amlodipine	Norvasc
Ammonium chloride	Ammonium chloride in plastic container
Amoxicillin trihydrate	Amoxi-Tabs, generic (1, 2)
Amoxicillin trihydrate	Amoxi-Drops (1, 2)
Amoxicillin trihydrate	Amoxi-Inject (1, 2)
Amoxicillin clavulanic	Augmentin, generic
Amoxicillin/clavulanic acid	Clavamox (1)
Amphetamine SO4	Adderall
Amphetamine SO4	Adderall XR
Amphotericin B	Fungizone
Amphotericin B lipid complex	Abelcet
Amphotericin B lipid complex	Amphotec
Amphotericin B liposome	AmBisome
Ampicillin	Omnipen, generic (1)
Ampicillin	Principen
Ampicillin	Princillin
Ampicillin sodium salt	Generic
Ampicillin–sulbactam	Unasyn
Ampicillin trihydrate	Poly-Flex (1, 2)
Amprolium	Corid (3)
Amrinone	Inocor
Antazoline	
Antimony	Pentostam
Antivenin to coral snake (Elapidae family)	Coral (Micrurus fulvius) (9, 12)
Antivenin to U.S. pit vipers	Crotalidae (polyvalent) (9, 12)
Apomorphine	Apomorphine, generic
Aprindine	Generic (4)
Aprotinin	Trasylol
Ascorbic acid	Ascorbicap (6)
Ascorbic acid	Cebion (6)
Ascorbic acid	Cecon (6)
Ascorbic acid	Vitamin C (6)
Asparaginase	Elspar (6)
Aspirin (see Acetylsalicylic acid)	
Astemizole	Hismanal (4)
Atenolol (See beta-adrenergic antagonists)	Tenormin
Atipamezole	Antisedan (1)

Generic	Proprietary
Atovaquone	Mepron
Atracurium besylate	Tracrium
Atropin	AtroPen, generic
Auranofin	Ridaura
Aurothioglucose	Solganal
Azathioprine	Imuran
Azrithromycin	Zithromax
Aztreonam	Azactam
Baclofen	Lioresal
BAL (see Dimercaprol)	
Baquiloprim–sulphamethoxine	Sulphadimidine (4)
Baquiloprim–sulphamethoxine	Generic (4)
Beclomethasone dipropionate (glucocorticoids)	Beconase AQ
Beclomethasone dipropionate	Qvar 40/80
Benazepril	Fortekor
Bendroflumethiazide; Nadolol (thiazide diuretics)	Corzide
Benzocaine	Cetacaine, generic
Benzoyl peroxide	Benzoyl Plus (5)
Betamethasone	Celestone
Betamethasone	Diprolene AF
Betamethasone	Diprolene
Betamethasone	Celestone Phosphate
Betamethasone Acetate and NaP	Celestone Soluspan
Bethanechol	Urecholine
Bisacodyl	Dulcolax
Bismuth salicylate	Pepto-Bismol (5)
Bitolerol	Tornalate
Bleomycin	Blenoxane
Boldenone	Equipoise, Verboal (3, 10-III)
Bromide, potassium or sodium	KBro Vet (4, 6)
Bromocriptine mesylate	Parlodel
Budesonide	Entocort EC, Entocard
Bunamidine	Scolaban (1, 2)
Bupivacaine hydrochloride	Marcaine
Buprenorphine (opiates)	Buprenex (10-III)
Buspirone	Buspar
Busulfan	Myleran
Busulfan	Busulfex
Butamisole	Styquin
Butorphanol	Torbutrol (10-IV)
Butorphanol	Torbugesic (10-IV)
Butorphanol	Dostinex (10-IV)
Butorphanol	Miacalcin (10-IV)
Cabergoline	Dostinex
Calcitonin (salmon)	Calcimar
Calcitriol (vitamin D_3)	Calcijex

1, Approved in dogs; *2*, approved in cats; *3*, approved in other animal; *4*, no longer available: if need is appropriate, may be available through a compounding pharmacist; *5*, OTC (human or animal); *6*, dietary supplement (human or animal), also indicates an OTC designation; *7*, human cosmetic product, also indicates an OTC designation; *8*, EPA-approved product; *9*, biological (if animal, may not be approved; if animal approved, approval is likely through US Department of Agriculture and generally is based only safety, not efficacy); *10*, distribution controlled by the Drug Enforcement Agency, Schedule status (I-V) indicated; *11*, obtain through chemical or other company, compounding pharmacist may assist; *12*, product may not be available from manufacturer; *13*, animal generic available; *14*, special restrictions.

Generic	Proprietary
Calcitriol	Rocaltrol
Calcium carbonate	Tums (5)
Calcium chloride	Calcium chloride, generic (5)
Calcium acetate	PhosLo (5)
Calcium acetate	PhosLo Gelcaps (5)
Calcium citrate	Citracal (5)
Calcium EDTA	Versenate
Calcium gluconate 10%	Neocalglucon
Calcium lactate	Calphosan, generic
Captan powder, 50%	Orthocide (11)
Captopril	Capoten
Carbamazepine	Epitol
Carbamazepine	Generic
Carbamazepine	Tegretol
Carbenicillin	Geocillin
Carbenicillin indanyl	Geopen
Carbimazole	NeoMercazole
Carboplatin	Paraplatin
Carmustine	BiCNU
L-Carnitine	Generic (6)
Carprofen	Rimadyl
Carvedilol	Coreg, generic
Cascara sagrada	Nature's Remedy, generic (5)
Castor oil	Emulsoil, Neoloid, Purge (5)
Cefaclor	Ceclor
Cefaclor	Ceclor CD
Cefaclor	Raniclor
Cefadroxil	Ceta-Tabs (1)
Cefamandole	Mandol (4)
Cefazolin sodium	Ancef
Cefazolin sodium	Kefzol, generic
Cefdinir	Omnicef
Cefepime	Maxipime
Cefixime	Suprax
Cefmetazole	Zefazone
Cefoperazone	Cefobid
Cefoperazone	Cefobid
Cefotaxime	Claforan
Cefotetan	Cefotan, generic
Cefotetan	Generic
Cefoxitin sodium	Mefoxin in Dextrose 5% in Plastic Container
Cefoxitin sodium	Mefoxin
Cefpodoxine	Simplicef (1)
Cefpodoxime	Vantin
Ceftazidime	Ceptaz
Ceftiofur	Naxcel
Ceftizoxime	Cefizox
Ceftizoxime	Cefizox In Plastic Container
Ceftriaxone	Rocephin

Generic	Proprietary
Cefuroxime	Generic
Cefuroxime	Cefuroxime Axetil
Cefuroxime	Zinacet
Cefuroxime	Ceftin
Cephalexin	Keflex, generic
Cephaloridine	Generic (4)
Cephalothin Na	Keflin
Cephalothin Sodium	Cephalothin Sodium
Cephamandole	See Cetamandole
Cephapirin	Cefadyl
Cephradine	Anspor
Cetirizine	Generic
Cetirizine HCl	Zyrtec
Cetirizine HCl (Pseudoephedrine HCl)	Zyrtec-D 12 Hour
Chlorambucil	Leukeran
Chloramphenicol	Chloromycetin
Chloramphenicol	Chloromycetin Hydrocortisone
Chloramphenicol sodium succinate	Chloramphenicol sodium succinate, generic
Chlordiazepoxide–clidinium	Librax
Chlorhexidine	Nolvasan
Chlorothiazide	Diuril
Chlorpheniramine	Chlor-Trimeton Allergy 8 and 12 Hour
Chlorpheniramine	Generic
Chlorpheniramine	Aller-Chlor
Chlorpromazine	Thorazine
Chlorpromazine	Thorazine Spansules
Chlorpropamide	Diabinese
Chlortetracycline	Phichlor
Cholecalciferol	Fosamax Plus D
Cholestyramine	Questran Light
Chondroitin sulfate/glucosamine/ascorbate/manganese	Cosequin, generic
Chorionic gonadotropin	Follutein
Chromium	Generic (6)
Cilastatin Na; Imipenem	Primaxin
Cimetidine	Tagamet, generic
Cimetidine	Tagamet
Ciprofloxacin	Cipro
Ciprofloxacin	Cipro HC
Cisapride	Propulsid (4)
Cisplatin	Platinol-AQ
Clarithromycin	Biaxin
Clemastine	Tavist
Clenbuterol	Ventipulmin (3)
Clidinium	Generic
Clindamycin	Antirobe (1)
Clindamycin	Antirobe Aquadrops

Continued

Generic	Proprietary
Clindamycin	Cleocin Phosphate
Clindamycin	Cleocin Pediatric
Clindamycin	Cleocin
Clofazimine	Lamprene
Clomiphene citrate	Clomid
Clomipramine	Anafranil
Clomipramine	Clomicalm (1)
Clonazepam	Klonopin, generic (10-IV)
Clonidine	Duraclon
Clonidine	Catapres
Cloprostenol	Estrumate
Clorazepate	Tranxene (10-IV), generic
Clotrimazole	Veltrim
Clotrimazole	Otomax
Clotrimazole	Lotrimin AF
Clotrimazole	Gyne-Lotrimin 3
Clotrimazole	Gyne-Lotrimin Combo Pack
Cloxacillin	Cloxapen
	Orbenin-DC / Dariclox
Coal tar shampoos	
Cobalamine (see Vitamin B_{12})	
Cod liver oil	
Codeine/acetaminophen	Generic (10-III)
Codeine	Generic (10-II)
Coenzyme Q10 (Ubiquinone)	Coenzyme Q
Colchicine	ColBenemid, generic
Colloidal dispersion	
Colony-stimulating factor	Leukine, granulocyte
	Neupogen
Corticotropin gel	Generic (1)
Corticotropin	ACTH gel (1)
Cortisone acetate	Cortisone acetate
Cortisone acetate	Cortone
Cosyntropin	Cortrosyn
Cromolyn sodium 4%	Opticrom
Cromolyn sodium	Intal
Cromolyn sodium	Gastrocrom
Cyanocobalamin (see Vitamin B_{12})	Cyanocobalamin/Vibisone
Cyanocobalamin	Nascobal
Cyclizine	Marezine
Cyclophosphamide	Lypholized Cytoxan
Cyclophosphamide	Cytoxan
Cyclothiazide	Anhydron
Cyclosporine	Atopica (1, 2)
Cyclosporine	Generic
Cyclosporine	Sandimmune
Cyclosporine ophthalmic	Optimmune (1)
Cyclosporine	Neoral
Cyproheptadine hydrochloride	Periactin
Cytarabine	Cytosar
Cyothicate	Proban
Cytosine arabinoside (AKA Cytarabine)	Cytosar-U
Dacarbazine	DTIC-Dome
Dactinomycin	Cosmegen
Dalteparin	Fragmin
Danazol	Danocrine
Dantrolene	Dantrium
Dapsone	Dapsone, generic
Decoquinate	Deccox
Deferoxamine Mesylate	Desferal
Dehydrocholic acid	Decholin
Demeclocycline (Tetracyclines)	Declomycin
Deprenyl (selegiline)	Anipryl (1)
Deprenyl (selegiline)	Eldipryl
Deracoxib	Deramaxx (1)
Derm-Caps	Generic (6)
Desmopressin acetate	DDAVP
Desoxycorticosterone acetate	
Desoxycorticosterone pivalate	Percorten-V (1)
Dexamethasone	Azium, generic
Dexamethasone	Azium Solution (1, 2)
Dexamethasone Sodium Phosphate	Dexasone sodium, generic (3)
Dexamethasone	Generic
Dexamethasone	Decadron
Dexpanthenol (see Pantothenic acid)	D-panthenol (1, 2)
Dexrazoxane	Zinecard
Dextran 40	Rheomacrodex
Dextran 70	Macrodex
Dextroamphetamine	Dexedrine
Dextromethorphan	Tussin, generic (5)
Dextrose, 5%	D5W
Dextrose, 50%	Cartose
Diazepam	Diazepam intensol (10-IV)
Diazepam	Diastat (10-IV)
Diazepam	Valium, generic (10-IV)
Diazoxide	Proglycem
Diazoxide	Hyperstat
Dichlorphenamide	Daranide
Dichlorvos	Task (1, 2)
Dicloxacillin	Dycill

1, Approved in dogs; *2*, approved in cats; *3*, approved in other animal; *4*, no longer available: if need is appropriate, may be available through a compounding pharmacist; *5*, OTC (human or animal); *6*, dietary supplement (human or animal), also indicates an OTC designation; *7*, human cosmetic product, also indicates an OTC designation; *8*, EPA-approved product; *9*, biological (if animal, may not be approved; if animal approved, approval is likely through US Department of Agriculture and generally is based only safety, not efficacy); *10*, distribution controlled by the Drug Enforcement Agency, Schedule status (I-V) indicated; *11*, obtain through chemical or other company, compounding pharmacist may assist; *12*, product may not be available from manufacturer; *13*, animal generic available; *14*, special restrictions.

Generic	Proprietary
Dicloxacillin	Dynapen
Dicoumarol	
Dicyclomine	Bentyl
Diethylcarbamazine	Hetrazan (4)
Diethylcarbamazine	Nemacide, generic (4)
Diethystilbestrol	Stilphostrol (4)
Difloxacin	Dicural (1)
Digitoxin	Crystodigin (4)
Digoxin	Lanoxin (1)
Digoxin	Lanoxicaps
Dihydrostreptomycin	(4)
Dihydrotachysterol	Hytakerol
Dihydrotachysterol	DHT
Dihydrotachysterol	DHT Intensol
25-Dihydroxy vitamin D[3] (see Vitamin D_3)	
Diltiazem	Cardizem CD
Diltiazem	Cardizem
Diltiazem XR, Cardiazem CD	Dilacor XR
Dimenhydrinate	Dramamine (5)
Dimenhydrinate	Dinate (5)
Dimercaprol	BAL in oil
Dimethyl sulfoxide 40%	Domoso (1, 2)
Dimethyl sulfoxide 50%	Rimso-50
Diminazene aceturate	Berenil
Dioctyl sulfosuccinate	Surfak (5)
Diphemanil methylsulfate	
Diphenhydramine HCl	Benadryl, generic
Diphenoxylate HCl w/ atropine	Lomotil (10-II, IV)
Diphenylhydantoin	Dilantin-125
Diphenylhydantoin (see Phenytoin)	Dilantin
Diphenylhydantoin (see Phenytoin)	Phenytoin Sodium
Diphenylthiocarbazone	Dithizone
Dipyridamole w/ Aspirin	Aggrenox
Dipyridamole	Dipyridamole
Dipyridamole	Persantine
Dipyrone	Novin (3, 4)
Dirlotapide	Slentrol (1)
Disodium EDTA	Disotate
Disophenol	D.N.P.
Disopyramide PO4	Norpace / Norpace CR
Dithiazanine iodide	Dizan (1)
Divalproex sodium (Valproate)	See Valproic acid
DL-Methionine (Methionine)	Methio-Form, others (6)
DL-Methionine	(6)
Dobutamine HCl	Dobutrex
Docusate calcium	Surfak Liquigels (5)
Docusate sodium	Colace (5)
Docusate sodium	Ex-Lax Stool Softener (5)
Docusate sodium	Bloat Release (5)
Docusate sodium	Dioctynate (5)
Docusate sodium	Enema-DSS (5)
Docusate sodium	Therevac-SB (5)
Docusate sodium	Colace, generic (5)
Dolasetron mesylate	Anzemet
Domperidone	Motilium
Dopamine HCl	Inotropin
Dopamine HCl in 5% Dextrose for infusion	Generic
Doramectin	Dectomax
Doxapram	Dopram-V (1, 2)
Doxepin HCl	Sinequan
Doxorubicin HCl	Adriamycin PFS
Doxorubicin HCl	Doxil
Doxycycline HCl	Doxirobe (1)
Doxycycline (hyclate)	Vibramycin, generic
Doxycycline (monohydrate)	Monodox
Doxycycline (hyclate)	Doryx
Doxycycline (monohydrate)	Vibramycin
Doxycycline (calcium salt)	Vibramycin
Doxycycline (hyclate 10%)	Atridox
Doxycycline (hyclate)	Doxy 100 and 200
Doxylamine succinate	AH Tablets (1)
Doxylamine succinate	AH Injection (1)
D-Penicillamine	Cuprimine
D-Penicillamine	Depen
Edetate calcium disodium (Calcium EDTA)	Calcium Disodium Versenate
Edrophonium Cl	Tensilon
Edrophonium Cl (w/ atropine sulfate)	Enlon-Plus
Emetine	Generic
Enalapril	Enacard (1)
Enalapril	Vasotec
Endotoxin antisera	Generic (9)
Enflurane	Ethrane
Enilconazole	Clinafarm EC
Enoxaparin	Lovenox, generic
Enrofloxacin	Baytril (1, 2)
Enrofloxacin	Baytril 100 (3)
Ephedrine	Ephedrine Sulfate (5, 14)
Ephedrine + phenobarbital theophylline	Tedrigen, Theophan
Epinephrine	AmTech Epinephrine Injection USP, generic
Epinephrine	EpiPen
Epinephrine	EpiPen Jr
Epinephrine	Epinephrine
Epinephrine with marcaine	See Marcaine
Epinephrine with lidocaine	See Lidocaine
Epoetin (see Erythropoietin)	Epogen
Epostane	Generic (4)

Continued

Generic	Proprietary
Epsiprantel	Cestex (1, 2)
Ergocalciferol (vitamin D_2)	Drisdol
Erythromycin	Gallimycin (3)
Erythromycin	Gallimycin Injection (3)
Erythromycin	Gallimycin Dry Cow (3)
Erythromycin	Gallimycin -36 (3)
Erythromycin	Ery-Tab, generic
Erythromycin	Erythromycin Filmtabs
Erythromycin	PCE Dispertab
Erythromycin	Eryc
Erythromycin (estolate)	Generic
Erythromycin (stearate)	Erythromycin Stearate
Erythromycin (ethylsuccinate)	EES 400
Erythromycin (ethylsuccinate)	EES Granules
Erythromycin (ethylsuccinate)	EES 200
Erythromycin (ethylsuccinate)	EES 400
Erythromycin	Ilotycin
Erythromycin (ethylsuccinate)	EryPed Drops
Erythromycin (lactobionate)	Eythrocin
Erythromycin (gluceptate)	Ilotycin Gluceptate
Erythromycin	Generic
Erythropoietin, human recombinant Epoetin alpha	Epogen, Procrit
Erythropoietin, human recombinant beta	Darbepoietin
Esmolol	Brevibloc
Essential fatty acids	DermCap (6)
Essential fatty acids	EFAVet-20 (6)
Estradiol	Gynodiol (3)
Estradiol (cypionate)	ECP
Estradiol (cypionate)	Depo-Estradiol
Estradiol	Climara
Ethacrynic acid	Edecrin
Ethacrynic acid (ethacrynate sodium)	Edecrin Sodium
Ethambutol	Myambutol
Ethanol 20% (alcohol)	Thunderbird
Ethosuximide	Zarontin
Ethoxzolamide	Cardrase
Ethylisobutrazine HCl	Generic (3, 4)
Etidronate disodium	Didronel
Etidronate disodium	Didronel IV
Etodolac	EtoGesic (1)
Etodolac	Lodine
Etodolac	Lodine XL
Etomidate	Amidate
Etretinate (acitretin)	Soriatane
Euthanasia solution (pentobarbital sodium)	Beuthanasia-D-Special (1)
Euthanasia solution (pentobarbital sodium)	Fatal-Plus Powder (1, 2)
Euthanasia solution (pentobarbital sodium)	Sleepaway (1, 2)
Euthanasia solution (pentobarbital sodium)	Socumb-6 gr (1, 2)
Euthanasia solution (pentobarbital sodium)	Fatal-Plus Solution (1, 2)
Famotidine	Pepcid AC
Famotidine	Pepcid RPD
Famotidine	Pepcid
Febantel	Rintal
Febantel	Vercom (1)
Felbamate	Felbatol
Fenbendazole	Panacur Granules 22.2% (3, 5)
Fenbendazole	Panacur Granules 22.2% (3, 5)
Fenbendazole	Panacur Suspension (3, 5)
Fenbendazole	Panacur Paste (3, 5)
Fenbendazole	Safe-Guard Sweetlix (3, 5)
Fenbendazole	Safe-Guard 0.96% Scoop Dewormer (3, 5)
Fenbendazole	Safe-Guard Free-choice Cattle Dewormer (3, 5)
Fenbendazole	Safe-Guard 0.5% Cattle Top Dress (3, 5)
Fenbendazole	Safe-Guard 1.96% Scoop Dewormer Mini Pellets (3, 5)
Fenbendazole	Safe-Guard Premix (3, 5)
Fentanyl citrate	Sublimaze, generic (10)
Fentanyl	Duragesic - 25,50,75,100 (10)
Fentanyl	Actiq (10-II)
Fenthion	Spotton (1)
Ferric cyanoferrate	Prussian Blue (5)
Ferrous sulfate (iron)	Feosol (5)
Ferrous sulfate	Fer-In-Sol (5)
Ferrous sulfate	Slow Fe (5)
Fexofenadine	Allegra
Filgrastim (see colony-stimulating factor granulocyte)	
Filgrastim	Neupogen
Finasteride	Propecia
Fipronil	Frontline Top Spot
Firocoxib (nonsteroidal antiinflammatory)	Previcox (1)
Flavoxate (HCl)	Urispas

1, Approved in dogs; *2*, approved in cats; *3*, approved in other animal; *4*, no longer available: if need is appropriate, may be available through a compounding pharmacist; *5*, OTC (human or animal); *6*, dietary supplement (human or animal), also indicates an OTC designation; *7*, human cosmetic product, also indicates an OTC designation; *8*, EPA-approved product; *9*, biological (if animal, may not be approved; if animal approved, approval is likely through US Department of Agriculture and generally is based only safety, not efficacy); *10*, distribution controlled by the Drug Enforcement Agency, Schedule status (I-V) indicated; *11*, obtain through chemical or other company, compounding pharmacist may assist; *12*, product may not be available from manufacturer; *13*, animal generic available; *14*, special restrictions.

Generic	Proprietary
Florfenicol	Nuflor (3)
Fluconazole	Diflucan in Dextrose 5% in plastic container
Fluconazole	Diflucan in Sodium Chloride 0.9%
Fluconazole	Diflucan in NaCl 0.9% in plastic container
Fluconazole	Diflucan
Flucytosine	Ancobon
Fludrocortisone	Florinef
Flumazenil	Romazicon
Flumethasone	Flucort Solution (1, 2)
Flunixin meglumine	Banamine (3)
Flunixin meglumine	Banamine Paste (3)
Flunixin meglumine	Banamine Granules (3)
Flunixin meglumine	Banamine Granules (3)
Fluorouracil	5-fluorouracil
Fluoxetine HCl	Prozac Pulvules
Fluoxetine HCl	Prozac
Fluoxymesterone	Generic (10-III)
Flurazepam	Dalmane (10-IV)
Flurbiprofen	Ocufen
Flurbiprofen	Ansaid
Fluticosone proprionate	Flovent
Fluvoxamine maleate	Luvox
Folic acid	Folicet (6)
Folinic acid	See Leucovorin
Follicle-stimulating hormone	Super-OV
Formoterol	Foradil
Formoterol	Perforomist
Foscarnet sodium	Foscavir
Furazolidone	Furoxone
Furosemide	Lasix, generic
Furosemide	Lasix Injection 5%, generic
Gabapentin	Neurontin
Gamma globulin	Generic (9)
Gemfibrozil	Lopid, generic
Gentamicin SO4 0.1%	Gentocin
Gentamicin sulfate	Gentocin Otic
Gentamicin sulfate	Garamycin
Glargine	
Glimeperide	Amaryl
Glipizide	Glucotrol XL
Glipizide	Glucotrol
Glucagon	GlucaGen
Glucosamine	Generic (6)
Glucosamine with chondroitin sulfate	Cosequin
Glucose 40% ophthalmic	Glucose-40
Glutamine	Generic (6)
Glyburide–metformin HCl	Glucovance

Generic	Proprietary
Glycerin	Osmoglyn, others
Glyceryl guaiacolate	Gecolate (3)
Glycerol monoacetate	Generic
Glycopyrrolate	Robinul-V (1, 2)
Glycopyrrolate	Robinul
Gold sodium thiomalate	Myochrysine
Gonadotropin-releasing hormone (synthetic)	Gonadorelin (3)
Gonadotropin, chorionic (See Chorionic gonadotropin)	
Granisetron HCl	Kytril
Granulocyte colony-stimulating factor (Filgrastim)	Neupogen
Griseofulvin	Fulvicin (1)
Griseofulvin	Fulvicin-U/F Tablets (3)
Griseofulvin	Ultramicrosize Gris-PEG
Growth hormone	See Somatotropin
Guaifenesin	Guailaxin (3)
Guaifenesin	Robitussin (5)
Guaifenesin	Guaifenesin Injection
Haloperidol	Generic
Haloperidol (Decanoate)	Generic
Haloperidol (Lactate)	Generic
Haloperidol (Lactate)	Haldol
Halothane (Inhalant anesthetic)	Fluothane
Halothane	Generic
Hemoglobin (see Oxyglobin)	Polymerized bovine, Oxyglobin (1, 3)
Heparin sodium	Heparin Sodium
Heparin sodium (w/ 0.9% sodium chloride)	Generic
Heparin sodium (w/ 0.45% sodium chloride)	Generic
Heparin sodium (Lock Flush Solution)	Hep-Lock
Hetacillin	Hetacin-K (1, 2)
Hetastarch (see Hydroxyethyl starch)	Hextend, generic
Human gamma globulin (see Gamma globulin)	
Hyaluronate = Hyaluronan	Hyalovet
Hyaluronate (sodium)	Legend (3)
Hyaluronate (sodium)	Hyvisc (3)
Hyaluronate (sodium)	Hylartin (3)
Hyaluronate (sodium)	HyCoat (3)
Hydralazine	Apresoline, generic
Hydrochlorothiazide	HydroDiuril, generic
Hydrochlorothiazide; metoprolol tartrate	Lopressor
Hydrochlorothiazide; spironolactone	Aldactazide
Hydrochlorothiazide; triamterene	Dyazide
Hydrocodone bitartrate	Hycodan (10-III)

Continued

Generic	Proprietary
Hydrocodone bitartrate	Hycodan Syrup (10-II)
Hydrocortisone acetate	Generic
Hydrocortisone Na succinate	Solu-Cortef
Hydrocortisone	Acticort 100, generic
Hydrocortisone	Cortef, generic
Hydrocortisone (acetate)	Hydrocortone Acetate
Hydrocortisone (cypionate)	Cortef
Hydrocortisone (sodium phosphate)	Hydrocortone Phosphate
Hydrogen peroxide 3%	Hydrogen peroxide 3%, generic (5)
Hydromorphone	Dilaudid, generic (10-II)
Hydromorphone	Dilaudid-HP (10-II)
Hydromorphone	Dilaudid-5 (10-II)
Hydroxyethyl starch (Hetastarch)	Hetastarch
Hydroxyurea	Droxia
Hydroxyurea	Mylocel
Hydroxyzine	Atarax
Hydroxyzine	Vistaril
Hydroxyzine (pamoate)	Vistaril
Hypertonic saline	Generic
Ibuprofen	Motrin, Advil
Ibuprofen	Ibuprofen, generic
Idarubicin	Idamycin PFS
Idarubicin hydrochloride	Idomycin, generic
Idoxuridine	Dendrid, Herplex
Ifosfamide; Mesna	IFEX/Mesnex Kit
Imidocarb dipropionate	Imizol (1)
Imidacloprid	Advantage (1, 2)
Imipenem–cilastatin (beta-lactam antibiotics)	Primaxin IV
Imipenem–cilastatin (beta-lactam antibiotics)	Primaxin IM
Imipramine	Tofranil
Imipramine	Tofranil-PM
Inamrinone lactate	Amrinone
Indomethacin	Generic
Indomethacin	Indomethegan
Indomethacin	Indocin
Indomethacin	Indocin IV
Pork insulin regular,	Vetsulin (1, 2)
Insulin, lente	Humulin L
Insulin, NPH	Humulin N
Insulin, PZI	PZI Insulin (2)
Insulin, Ultralente	Humulin U
Insulin Lispro recombinant	Humalog
Insulin glusiline recombinant	Apidra
Insulin Regular Humunin R	
Insulin Aspart recombinant	Novolog
Insulin detemir recombinant	Levemir
Insulin glargine recombinant	Largine
Interferon, α2	Roferon-A
Iodine	Lugol's Solution (3)
Iodine sodium, potassium	Generic
Iohexol	Omnipaque 140
Iohexol	Omnipaque 180
Iohexol	Omnipaque 240
Iohexol	Omnipaque 300
Iohexol	Omnipaque 350
Iopamidol	Isovue-200
Iopamidol	Isovue-250
Iopamidol	Isovue-300
Iopamidol	Isovue-370
Iopamidol	Isovue-M 200
Iopamidol	Isovue-M 300
Ipecac syrup	Generic (5)
Ipodate	Oragratin
Ipronidazole	Ipropran (3)
Iron dextran	Dexferrum
Isoflupredone	Predef (3)
Isoflurane (inhalant anesthetic)	IsoFlo
Isometheptene	Generic
Isoniazid	Generic
Isoniazid	Laniazid
Isopropamide, iodide	Darbid (4)
Isopropamide/prochlorperazine	Darbazine (1, 2)
Isopropamide, prochlorperazine, neomycin	Neodarbazine (1)
Isoproterenol	Isuprel
Isosorbide dinitrate	Isordil
Isosorbide dinitrate	Dilatrate-SR
Isosorbide mononitrate	Generic
Isosorbide mononitrate	Monoket
Isotretinoin	Accutane
Isoxsuprine	Vasodilan
Itraconazole	Sporanox
Ivermectin	Heartgard (1, 2, 13)
Ivermectin–pyrantel	Heartgard-Plus (1, 2, 13)
Ivermectin	Heartgard (1)
Ivermectin	Ivomec (1)
Kanamycin	Kantrex
Kaolin–pectin	Kaopectate (5)
Kaolin–pectin	Kaolin Pectin Plus (5)
Ketamine HCl	Ketaset (1, 10-III)
Ketamine HCl	Ketalar (1, 10-III)

1, Approved in dogs; *2*, approved in cats; *3*, approved in other animal; *4*, no longer available: if need is appropriate, may be available through a compounding pharmacist; *5*, OTC (human or animal); *6*, dietary supplement (human or animal), also indicates an OTC designation; *7*, human cosmetic product, also indicates an OTC designation; *8*, EPA-approved product; *9*, biological (if animal, may not be approved; if animal approved, approval is likely through US Department of Agriculture and generally is based only safety, not efficacy); *10*, distribution controlled by the Drug Enforcement Agency, Schedule status (I-V) indicated; *11*, obtain through chemical or other company, compounding pharmacist may assist; *12*, product may not be available from manufacturer; *13*, animal generic available; *14*, special restrictions.

Generic	Proprietary
Ketamine HCl–aminopentamide–promazine	Ketaset-Plus (1, 10-III)
Ketoconazole	NizOral
Ketoprofen	Orudis
Ketoprofen	Ketofen (5)
Ketoprofen	Orudis KT
Ketoprofen	Oruvail
Ketorolac tromethamine	Acular (PF)
Ketorolac tromethamine	Toradol
Lactated Ringer's solution	LRS
Lactitol	Lacty (5)
Lactoferrin	Generic (6)
Lactoferrin, human recombinant	Activin (6)
Lactulose	Cephulac
Lactulose	Chronulac
L-Aspariginase (see Aspariginase)	
L-Carnitine (Levocarnitine)	Carnitor (6)
L-Deprenyl	Anipryl (1, 2, 13)
Lenperone	Elanone V
Leucovorin	Wellcovorin
Leucovorin Ca	Generic
Levallorphan	Lorfan (10-V)
Levamisole	Ergamisol
Levamisole	Tramisol Injectable (3)
Levamisole	Totalon
Levarterenol	See Norepinephrine
Levetiracetam	Keppra
Levoamphetamine	Levo-amphetamine
Levocarnitine	See L = Carnitine
Levodopa	Carbidopa and Levodopa
Levorphanol tartrate	Levo-Dromoran (10-II)
Levorphanol tartrate	Generic (10-II)
Levothyroxine, T_4 (thyroid hormones)	Thyroxine-L tablets (1)
Levothyroxine, T_4	Synthyroid
Levothyroxine, T_4	NutriVed T-4 Chewable Tablets (1)
Levothyroxine, T_4	Throxine-L Powder
Lidocaine	Anestacon
Lidocaine	Generic
Lidocaine	Xylocaine, generic
Lidocaine	Xylocaine Viscous
Lidocaine	LTA Kit
Lime sulfur suspension	Sulfa dip
Lime water	Vlemasque
Lincomycin	Lincocin (1, 2)
Lincomycin	Lincocin Aquadrops (1, 2)
Linezolid	Zyvox
Liothyronine, T_3 (thyroid hormones)	Cytomel
Liothyronine, T_3 (thyroid hormones)	Triostat
Lisinopril	Prinivil
Lithium carbonate	Lithium
Lobaplatin	
Lomustine	CeeNU
Loperamide HCl	Imodium A-D, generic (5)
Loperamide HCl	Imodium (5)
Loperamide HCl simethicone	Imodium Advanced (5)
Loratadine	Claritin, others
Lorazepam	Ativan (10-IV)
Lufenuron	Program (1, 2)
Lufenuron	Program Suspension (2)
Lufenuron–milbemycin	Sentinel (1)
Luteinizing hormone	LH
Lysine	Generic (6)
Lysine-8-vasopressin	Diapid
Mafenide acetate	Sulfamylon cream
Magnesium chloride	Generic (5)
Magnesium citrate	Evac-Q-Mag (5)
Magnesium hydroxide	Milk of Magnesia, Mylanta (5)
Magnesium oxide	Generic
Magnesium salts	Generic (5)
Magnesium sulfate	Generic
Mannitol 20%	Osmitrol
Marbofloxacin	Zeniquin (1, 2)
Maropitant	Cerenia (1, 2)
Mebendazole	Telmintic (1)
Meclizine	Dramamine Less Drowsy Formula (5)
Meclizine	Antivert (5)
Meclofenamic acid	Meclofen, Arquel (1)
Mechlorethamine HCl	Mustine
Medetomidine hydrochloride	Domitor (1)
Medium-chain triglycerides	MCT in oil (5)
Medroxyprogesterone acetate (Progestins)	Depo-Provera
Medroxyprogesterone acetate	Provera, generic
Megestrol acetate	Megace
Megestrol acetate	Ovaban (1)
Meglumine antimonate	Glucantime
Melarsomine HCl	Immiticide
Melatonin	Circadin, generic (6)
Meloxicam	Mobic
Meloxicam	Metacam (1, 2)
Melphalan	Alkeran
Menadiol	Adaprin
Meperidine HCl	Demerol (10-II)
Mephenytoin	Mesantoin
Mepivacaine	Carbocaine

Continued

Generic	Proprietary
Mercaptopurine	Purinethol, generic
Meropenem	Merrem IV
Mesalamine	Pentasa, Asacol
Mesalamine	Canasa (1)
Mesna	Mesnex
Metaproterenol sulfate	Alupent
Metaproterenol sulfate	Generic
Metyrapone	Metopirone
Metaraminol bitartrate	Aramine
Metformin HCl	Glucophage
Metformin HCl	Glucophage XR
Methadone	Methadose, generic (10-II)
Methazolamide	Glauctabs
Methenamine Hippurate	Urex
Methenamine mandelate	Mandelamine
Methenamine mandelate	Generic
Methicillin	Staphcillin
Methimazole	Tapazole
(DL)-Methionine	See DL-Methionine
Methocarbamol	Robaxin V (1, 2)
Methohexital sodium	Brevital (10-IV)
Methohexital sodium	Brevital Sodium (10-IV)
Methscopolamine	Pamine
Methscopolamine bromide	Generic
Methotrexate sodium	Generic
Methotrexate sodium	Trexal
Methoxamine HCl	Vasoxyl
Methoxyflurane (inhalant anesthetic)	Metofane
Methylcellulose	Citrucel
Methylene blue	Generic (5)
Methylene blue	Urolene Blue
Methylphenidate	Ritalin
Methylphenidate	Generic (10-II)
Methylphenidate	Ritalin-SR
Methylprednisolone	Medrol
Methylprednisolone acetate	Depo-Medrol (1, 2)
Methylprednisolone acetate/aspirin	Cortaba (1)
Methylprednisolone Na succinate	Solu-Medrol
Methyltestosterone	Android, generic (10-III)
Metoclopramide	Reglan
Metoclopramide	Metoclopramide Intensol
Metoprolol	Lopressor
Metoprolol	Toprol XL
Metronidazole	Flagyl IV
Metronidazole	Flagyl, generic
Metronidazole	Flagyl ER
Mexiletine	Mexitil
Mibolerone	Cheque (1, 10-III)
Miconazole	Monistat-Derm
Miconazole	Monistat 3
Midazolam	Versed (1, 10-IV)
Mifepristone	Mifeprex
Milbemycin oxime	Interceptor (1, 2)
Milbemycin oxime	Sentinel (1)
Milk thistle (Silymarin)	Generic (6)
Milrinone lactate	Primacor
Milrinone lactate	Primacor in Dextrose 5% in Plastic container
Mineral oil	Generic (5)
Minocycline	Minocin
Mirtazapine	Remeron, generic
Misoprostol	Cytotec
Mithramycin	Mithracin
Mitotane (o,p-DDD)	Lysodren
Mitoxantrone	Novantrone
Monensin	Rumensin (3)
Montelukast sodium	Singulair
Morphine SO4	Astramorph PF (10-III)
Morphine SO4	Generic (10-III)
Morphine SO4	MS Contin (10-III)
Morphine SO4	Avinza (10-III)
Moxidectin	ProHeart (1)
Moxidectin/imidacloprid	Advantage Plus (1, 2)
Mycobacterial cell wall extract	Urocidin (9)
Mycophenolate mofetil	CellCept
Nadolol	Corzide
Nafcillin	Nafcillin Sodium
Nalbuphine	Nubain
Nalmefene HCl	Revex
Nalorphine HCl	Nalline (10-III)
Naloxone HCl	Narcan
Naltrexone	Revia
Nandrolone decanoate	Deca-Durabolin (10-III)
Nandrolone phenylpropionate	Durabolin (4, 10-III)
Naphazoline HCl	Opcon A
Naproxen	Naprosyn (5)
Naproxen	EC-Naprosyn (5)
Naproxen	Aleve, generic (5)
Natamycin	Natacyn
Neomycin	Biosol (5)
Neomycin	Neomix AG 325 Soluble Powder (5)

1, Approved in dogs; *2*, approved in cats; *3*, approved in other animal; *4*, no longer available: if need is appropriate, may be available through a compounding pharmacist; *5*, OTC (human or animal); *6*, dietary supplement (human or animal), also indicates an OTC designation; *7*, human cosmetic product, also indicates an OTC designation; *8*, EPA-approved product; *9*, biological (if animal, may not be approved; if animal approved, approval is likely through US Department of Agriculture and generally is based only safety, not efficacy); *10*, distribution controlled by the Drug Enforcement Agency, Schedule status (I-V) indicated; *11*, obtain through chemical or other company, compounding pharmacist may assist; *12*, product may not be available from manufacturer; *13*, animal generic available; *14*, special restrictions.

Generic	Proprietary
Neomycin	Neomycin 325 (5)
Neomycin	Neo-Sol 50 (5)
Neomycin	Generic (5)
Neomycin	Neo-Fradin (5)
Neostigmine	Prostigmin (5)
Niacinamide (see Nicotinamide)	
Niclosamide	Yomesan (1, 2)
Nicotinamide (vitamin B_3)	Niacin (6)
Nifedipine	Procardia
Nifedipine	Adalat CC
Nifurtimox	Lampit (4)
Nikethamide	Coramine
Nitenpyram	Capstar
Nitrofurantoin	Dantafur (1)
Nitrofurantoin	Macrobid
Nitrofurantoin	Furadantin
Nitroglycerin	Nitro-Bid
Nitroglycerin 2% ointment	Nitro-Bid
Nitroglycerin	Minitran
Nitroprusside	Nitropress
Nitroscanate	Lopatol (1)
Nizatidine	Axid AR
Nizatidine	Axid
Norepinephrine bitartrate	Levophed
Norfloxacin	Noroxin
Nortriptyline	Aventyl
Noscapine	Generic
Novobiocin, tetracycline	Prednisolone, Delta Albaplex (3)
Nystatin	Mycolog
Nystatin	Nilstat
Nystatin	Mycostatin
Octreotide acetate	Sandostatin
Ofloxacin	Oflaxacin
Ofloxacin	Floxin Otic
Olsalazine	Dipentum
Omega fatty acid	Derm Caps (6)
Omeprazole	Prilosec, generic
Omeprazole	Gastrogard
Ondansetron	Zofran
Opium preparations	(10-II, V)
Opium tincture	Generic (10-III)
Orbifloxacin	Orbax (1, 2)
Orgotein	Palosein (6)
Ormetoprim (see Sulfadimethoxine/ ormetoprim)	Primor
Osalazine sodium	Osalmid
Oxacillin	Bactocill
Oxazepam	Serax (10-IV)
Oxfendazole	Synanthic
Oxtriphylline	Choledyl SA
Oxybutinin	Ditropan
Oxybutinin chloride	Ditropan XL
Oxyglobin (bovine hemoglobin glutamer 200)	Oxyglobin
Oxymetholone	Anadrol -50 (10-III)
Oxymetholone	Anadrol (10-III)
Oxymorphone	Numorphan (10-II)
Oxytetracycline	Terramycin
Oxytocin	Pitocin, others
Paclitaxel	Taxol
Pamidronate	Aredia
Pancreatic enzyme (see Viokase)	Viokase
Pancreatin	Kreon
Pancuronium bromide	Pavulon
Pantoprazole	Protonix
Paregoric	Corrective mixture (4)
Paromomycin (aminosidine)	Humatin
Paroxetine	Paxil
Paroxetine	Paxil CR
D-Penicillamine	Depen
D-Penicillamine	Cuprimine
Penicillin G aqueous (K or Na) (Penicillins)	Pfizerpen
Penicillin G benzathine	Bicillin L-A
Penicillin G benzathine	Bicillin
Penicillin G benzathine	Permapen
Penicillin G procaine	Penicillin G Procaine (5)
Penicillin G procaine	Crysticillin 300 A.S. (3)
Penicillin G, benzathine and procaine (Penicillins)	Ambi-Pen (3)
Penicillin G, benzathine and procaine	Bicillin C-R (3)
Penicillin G, benzathine and procaine	Bicillin C-R 900/300 (3)
Penicillin V, phenoxymethyl potassium	Generic
Penicillin V, potassium	Pen-Vee K
Pentamidine isethionate	Pentam
Pentamidine isethionate	Nebupent
Pentazocine	Talwin (10-IV)
Pentobarbital Na	Pentobarbital Injection (1, 2, 10-II)
Pentobarbital Na	Sodium Pentobarbital Injection (10-II)
Pentobarbital Na	Generic (10-II)
Pentobarbital Na	Nembutal (10-II)
Pentobarbital, phenytoin	Euthanasia III, Eutanol (1, 2, 10-III)
Pentosan polysulfate	Elmiron
Pentoxifylline	Trental, generic
Perphenazine	Generic

Continued

Generic	Proprietary
Petrolatum, white	Vaseline, generic (5)
Phenamidine isethionate	Fenamiphos (4)
Phenobarbital	Solfoton, generic (10-IV)
Phenobarbital	Luminal (10-IV)
Phenobarbital	Luminal Sodium (10-IV)
Phenoxybenzamine HCI	Dibenzyline
Phentolamine mesylate	Regitine
Phenylbutazone	Bizolin 100 (1)
Phenylbutazone	Amtech Phenylbutazone 20% Injection (1)
Phenylephrine	Neo-Synephrine (5)
Phenylephrine	AH-chew D
Phenylpropanolamine HCl	Proin 50 (1, 5, 14)
Phenylpropanolamine HCl	Cystolamine (1, 5, 14)
Phenylpropanolamine HCl	Proin Drops (1, 5, 14)
Phenytoin	Dilantin
Phenytoin	Dilantin Kapseals
Phenytoin	Phenytoin Sodium
Phenytoin	Dilantin-125
Phenytoin	Generic
Phenytoin	Beuthanasia-D-Special (1)
Pheromones	Dog Appeasing Phermone, Feliway
Phosphate, potassium	Generic
Phosphate, sodium	Generic
Physostigmine	Antilirium
Physostigmine	Eserine Salicylate
Physostigmine	Eserine Sulfate
Phytomenadione (Vitamin K_1)	Aquamephyton
Phytomenadione (Phytonadione)	Mephyton
Phytomenadione (Phytonadione)	K-Caps
Phytomenadione (Phytonadione)	Generic
*Picrotoxin (use is controversial)	Cocculin
Pilocarpine HCl	Pilopine HS
Pilocarpine HCl	Salagen
Pimobendan	Vetmedin (1)
Pimozide	Orap
Piperacillin sodium	Pipracil
Piperacillin (w/ tazobactam)	Zosyn
Piperazine	Pipa-Tabs, generic
Piperazine Citrate	Generic
Pirbuterol Acetate	Maxair
Piroxicam	Feldene, generic
Plicamycin	Mithracine
Polyethylene glycol electrolyte solution	Miralax, generic
Polymyxin B	Aerosporin
Polysulfated glycosaminoglycans	Adequan I.A.
Ponazuril	Marquis Paste (3)
Potassium chloride	Kaon (6)
Potassium chloride	Kaon -Cl (6)
Potassium chloride	KayCiel (6)
Potassium citrate	Urocit-K (6)
Potassium gluconate	Tumil-K, others
Potassium iodide	SSKI Solution
Potassium permanganate (1: 2,000)	Potassium permanganate-$KMnO_4$ (4)
Potassium phosphate	K-Phos, generic
Povidone–iodine	Betadine
Pralidoxime Cl	2-PAM
Praziquantel	Droncit (1)
Prazosin HCl	Minipress
Prednisolone acetate	Prednisolone acetate (1, 2)
Prednisolone acetate	Meticortelone acetate (1)
Prednisolone acetate	Optisone (1, 2)
Prednisolone Na phosphate	Prednis-A-Vet (1)
Prenisolone Na succinate	Solu-Delta-Cortef (1)
Prednisolone	Generic
Prednisolone, trimeprazine tartrate	Temanip (1)
Prednisone	Meticorten (1, 2)
Prednisone	Generic
Pregabalin	Lyrica
Primaquine phosphate	Primaquine
Primidone	Mysoline
Primidone	Generic
Procainamide	Pronestyl, generic
Procaine	Novocaine
Procarbazine	Matulane
Prochlorperazine	Compazine
Prochlorperzine/isopropamide (1) (see Isopropamide)	
Promazine HCl	See Acepromazine
Promethazine hydrochloride	Phenergran
Propantheline bromide	Pro-Banthine
Propiopromazine	Largon
Propionibacterium acnes	ImmunoRegulin (9)
Propofol	Rapinovet (1, 2)
Propofol	PropoFlo (1)
Propranolol hydrochloride	Inderal LA
Propranolol hydrochloride	Inderal
Propylthiouracil (PTU)	PTU, generic
Prostaglandin $F_{2\text{-alpha}}$	Lutalyse, Dinoprost (3)
Protamine sulfate	Generic
Protopam chloride	Pralidoxime
Protriptyline	Vivactil
Prucalopride	Resolor (4)

1, Approved in dogs; *2*, approved in cats; *3*, approved in other animal; *4*, no longer available: if need is appropriate, may be available through a compounding pharmacist; *5*, OTC (human or animal); *6*, dietary supplement (human or animal), also indicates an OTC designation; *7*, human cosmetic product, also indicates an OTC designation; *8*, EPA-approved product; *9*, biological (if animal, may not be approved; if animal approved, approval is likely through US Department of Agriculture and generally is based only safety, not efficacy); *10*, distribution controlled by the Drug Enforcement Agency, Schedule status (I-V) indicated; *11*, obtain through chemical or other company, compounding pharmacist may assist; *12*, product may not be available from manufacturer; *13*, animal generic available; *14*, special restrictions.

Generic	Proprietary
Pseudoephedrine	Sudafed, generic (5, 14)
Psyllium	Fiberall (6)
Psyllium	Metamucil (6)
Pyrantel pamoate	Nemex (1)
Pyridostigmine bromide	Mestinon
Pyrilamine maleate	Nisaval
Pyrimethamine	Daraprim
Pyrimethamine / sulfadoxine	Fansidar
Quinacrine	Atabrine
Quinidine gluconate	Generic
Quinidine polygalacturonate	Cardioquin
Quinidine sulfate	Generic
Racemethionine (see DL-Methionine)	
Ranitidine HCl	Zantac
Retinol (vitamin A)	Retin A
Ribavirin	Virazole, Rebetol
Riboflavin (vitamin B_2)	Vitamin B_2
Rifampin	Rifadin
Ringer's solution (see Lactated Ringer's solution)	
Roxithromycin	Azuril (4)
Rutin	Rutin (6)
S-adenosyl methionine	Denosyl (6)
Scopalamine	Donnatal (5)
Scopalamine	Generic (5)
Scopolamine	Transderm Scop
Selamectin	Revolution (1, 2)
Selegiline	Anipryl (1)
Selenium	Generic (6)
Selenium Sulfide	Selenium sulfide (6)
Senna	Senokot (6)
Sertraline hydrochloride	Zoloft
Sevelamer	Renagel
Sevoflurane	SevoFlo
Sevoflurane	Ultane
Silver nitrate solution 0.5%	Silvadene
Silver sulfadiazine	Silvadene
Silymarin (see Milk thistle)	
Simethicone	Flatulex
Skin So Soft (SSS)	(7)
Sodium aurothiomalate	Generic, Myochrysine
Sodium bicarbonate	Baking Soda, others
Sodium chloride	Adsorbonac
Sodium chloride	Ayr
Sodium chloride 5%	Muro 128
Sodium chloride 7.5%	Generic
Sodium iodide, 20% solution	Iodopen, generic
Sodium phosphate p-32	Phospho-Soda
Sodium polystyrene sulfonate	Generic
Sodium stibogluconate; antimony	Pentostam

Generic	Proprietary
Sodium sulfate	Glauber's salts (5)
Sodium thiopental	Pentothal (10)
Sodium thiosulfate 10%	Sodium thiosulfate
Somatotropin	Nutropin
Sorbitol	Sorbitol
Sotalol	Betapace
Spectinomycin	Spectinomycin
Spiramycin	Foromacidin, Rovamycin (4)
Spironolactone	Aldactone (4)
Spironolactone/ hydrochlorothiazide	Aldactazide
Stanozolol	Winstrol (1, 10-III)
Staphage lysate	SPL-Serologic Types I and III (9)
Staphylococcal A	Generic (9)
Streptokinase	Streptase
Streptomycin, dihydro	Streptomycin, dihydro
Streptozocin	Zanosar
Styrylpyridium/DEC	Styrid Caracide
Succimer	Chemet
Succinylcholine	Anectine
Sucralfate	Carafate
Sufentanil	Sufenta (10-II)
Sulfadiazine	Sulfadiazine
Sulfadiazine–trimethoprim	Tribrissen (1)
Sulfadimethoxine	Albon (1, 2)
Sulfadimethoxine	Bactrovet (1, 2)
Sulfadimethozine–ormetoprim	Primor (1)
Sulfamethoxazole	Gantanol
Sulfamethoxazole; trimethoprim (Sulfonamides)	Bactrim
Sulfasalazine	Azulfidine
Sulfisoxazole	Pediazole
Sulfobromophthalein sodium	(BSP)
Suprofen 1% ophthalmic solution	Profenal
Tamoxifen	Nolvadex
Taurine	Taurine (6)
Tegaserod	Zelnorm (14)
Teicoplanin	Tarsocid investigational drug
Telazol (See Teletamine + Zolazepam)	
Teletamine HCl (w/zolazapam)	Telazol (1, 2, 10-III)
Tepoxalin	Zubrin
Terbinafine HCl	Lamisil
Terbutaline	Brethine
Testosterone cypionate	Depo-Testosterone (10-III)
Testosterone ethanate	Delatestryl (10-III)
Testosterone propionate	Test Pro (10-III)
Testosterone, methyl (see Methyltestosterone)	Android (10-III)
Tetanus toxoid	Tetanus Toxiod (9)

Continued

Generic	Proprietary
Tetracycline HCl	Achromycin
Tetracycline HCl	Achromycin V, generic
Tetracycline HCl	Panmycin, generic (1, 2)
Tetracycline hydrochloride, novobiocin sodium and prednisolone	Delta-Albaplex (1)
Tetramine	Syprine
Tetramisole	Anthelvet
Thenium closylate	Canopar
Theophylline	Theophylline
Theophylline	Slo-Phyllin
Theophylline sustained-release	Slo-Bid Gyrocaps
Theophylline sustained-release	Theo-Dur
Thiabendazole	Tresaderm (1, 2)
Thiacetarsamide	Caparsolate (4)
Thiacetarsamide	Filaramide (4)
Thiamine	Vitamin B_1 (6)
Thiamylal sodium	Biotal (1, 2, 10-III)
Thiamylal sodium	Surital (1, 2, 10-III)
Thiethylperazine	Torecan
Thioguanine	Thioguanine Tabloid
Thiopental sodium	Pentothal (10-III)
Thioridazine	Mellaril
Thiotepa	Thiotepa, generic
Thyroid Stimulating Hormone/ Thyrotropin (Thyroid Hormones)	Thyrogen Dermathycin (1)
L-Thyroxine, T[4] (see Levothyroxine)	
Ticarcillin	Ticar
Ticarcillian–clavulanate	Timentin
Tiletamine HCl/Zolazepam (see Telazol)	Telazol (1, 2, 10-III)
Tilmicosin	Micotil
Tinidazole	Tindamax
Tiopronin	Thiola
Tobramycin	Nebcin
Tobramycin	Tobrex
Tocainide	Tonocard
Tolazoline	Priscoline hydrochloride
Tolfenamic acid	Generic (4)
Toltrazuril	Baycox
Topiramate	Topamax
Tramadol	Ultram, others
Tramadol, acetaminophen	Ultracet
Tretinoin	Retin-A
Triamcinolone	Vetalog
Triamcinolone acetonide	Generic (1, 2)
Triamcinolone, ophthalmic	Generic
Triamterene	Dyrenium
Trientine HCl	Syprine
Trifluoperazine	Stelazine, others
Triflupromazine	Vetame
Trifluridine ophthalmic solution	Viroptic
Triiodothyronine, T_3 liothyronine (Thyroid hormones)	Cytobin
Trilostane	Vetoryl (1)
Trimeprazine	Temaril-P (1)
Trimethobenzamide	Tigan, generic
Trimethoprim	Trimethoprim
Trimetrexate glucuronate	Neutrexin
Tripelennamine	Recovr, generic (1)
Trypan blue	VisionBlue
Tylosin	Tylan (3)
Tylosin tartrate	Tylan (3)
Tylosin with vitamins	Tylan Plus (3)
Urea	Generic (6)
Urofollitropin	Fertinex
Ursodiol (ursodeoxycholic acid)	Actigall
Valproic acid (valproate)	Depakene
Vanadium	trace element (supplement) (6)
Vancomycin	Vancocin
Vasopressin, aqueous	Pitressin
Vasopressin, tannate in oil	Pitressin tannate
Vecuronium bromide	Norcuron
Verapamil HCl	Calan
Verapamil HCl	Calan SR
Verapamil HCl	Isoptin SR
Verapamil HCl	Isoptin
Vidarabine	Vira-A
Vinblastine	Velban
Vincristine sulfate	Oncovin, generic
Vitamin A	Aquasol A (6)
Vitamin B complex	Becotin (6)
Vitamin B complex	Betalin complex (6)
Vitamin B_1 (Thiamine)	Thiamine HCl (6)
Vitamin B_{12}	Vitamin B_{12}(6)
Vitamin B_2 (Riboflavin)	Vitamin B_2 (riboflavin) (6)
Vitamin C (Ascorbic Acid)	Ascorbic acid (6)
Vitamin D (Dihydrotachysterol)	Dihydral, Hytakerol
Vitamin D_2 (see Vitamin D)	Calciferol
Vitamin D_3	Calcitriol
Vitamin E	Aquasol E (6)
Vitamin E	Eprolin (6)
Vitamin E	Natopherol (6)

1, Approved in dogs; *2*, approved in cats; *3*, approved in other animal; *4*, no longer available: if need is appropriate, may be available through a compounding pharmacist; *5*, OTC (human or animal); *6*, dietary supplement (human or animal), also indicates an OTC designation; *7*, human cosmetic product, also indicates an OTC designation; *8*, EPA-approved product; *9*, biological (if animal, may not be approved; if animal approved, approval is likely through US Department of Agriculture and generally is based only safety, not efficacy); *10*, distribution controlled by the Drug Enforcement Agency, Schedule status (I-V) indicated; *11*, obtain through chemical or other company, compounding pharmacist may assist; *12*, product may not be available from manufacturer; *13*, animal generic available; *14*, special restrictions.

Generic	Proprietary
Vitamin K_1 (phytonadione)	AquaMEPHYTON
Voriconazole	Vferd, generic
Warfarin	Coumadin
Xylazine	Rompun (1, 2)
Yohimbine	Yobine
Zafirlukast	Accolate
Zidovudine	AZT, Retrovir, generic
Zinc acetate (Zinc)	Generic (5)
Zinc methionine (Zinc)	Zinpro (5)
Zinc sulfate (Zinc)	Vi-Zac, others (5)
Zolazepam HCl (see Tiletamine)	Telazol (1, 2, 10)
Zonisamide	Zonegran

Appendix 7

Conversions of Weight to Body Surface Area

Conversions* of Weight to Body Surface Area (in Square Meters) for Dogs and Cats

Weight (lb)	Weight (kg)	K = 9.9 (m^2)	K = 10.0 (m^2)	K = 10.1 (m^2)	K = 10.4 (m^2)	K = 12.3 (m^2)
1.10	0.50	0.062	0.063	0.063	0.065	0.077
2.21	1.00	0.099	0.100	0.101	0.104	0.123
3.31	1.50	0.130	0.131	0.133	0.136	0.161
4.41	2.00	0.158	0.159	0.161	0.165	0.196
5.52	2.50	0.183	0.185	0.187	0.192	0.227
6.62	3.00	0.207	0.209	0.211	0.217	0.257
7.72	3.50	0.229	0.231	0.234	0.241	0.285
8.83	4.00	0.251	0.253	0.256	0.263	0.311
9.93	4.50	0.271	0.274	0.277	0.285	0.337
11.03	5.00	0.291	0.294	0.297	0.306	0.362
12.14	5.50	0.310	0.313	0.316	0.326	0.385
13.24	6.00	0.329	0.332	0.335	0.345	0.409
14.34	6.50	0.347	0.350	0.354	0.364	0.431
15.45	7.00	0.365	0.368	0.372	0.383	0.453
16.55	7.50	0.382	0.386	0.390	0.401	0.474
17.65	8.00	0.399	0.403	0.407	0.419	0.495
18.75	8.50	0.415	0.419	0.424	0.436	0.516
19.86	9.00	0.431	0.436	0.440	0.453	0.536
20.96	9.50	0.447	0.452	0.456	0.470	0.556
22.06	10.00	0.463	0.468	0.472	0.486	0.575
23.17	10.50	0.478	0.483	0.488	0.503	0.594
24.27	11.00	0.494	0.499	0.504	0.519	0.613
25.37	11.50	0.509	0.514	0.519	0.534	0.632
26.48	12.00	0.523	0.529	0.534	0.550	0.650
27.58	12.50	0.538	0.543	0.549	0.565	0.668
28.68	13.00	0.552	0.558	0.563	0.580	0.686
29.79	13.50	0.566	0.572	0.578	0.595	0.703
30.89	14.00	0.580	0.586	0.592	0.609	0.721
31.99	14.50	0.594	0.600	0.606	0.624	0.738
33.10	15.00	0.608	0.614	0.620	0.638	0.755
34.20	15.50	0.621	0.627	0.634	0.652	0.772
35.30	16.00	0.634	0.641	0.647	0.666	0.788
36.41	16.50	0.648	0.654	0.661	0.680	0.805
37.51	17.00	0.661	0.667	0.674	0.694	0.821
38.61	17.50	0.674	0.681	0.687	0.708	0.837
39.72	18.00	0.687	0.693	0.700	0.721	0.853
40.82	18.50	0.699	0.706	0.713	0.735	0.869
41.92	19.00	0.712	0.719	0.726	0.748	0.884
43.03	19.50	0.724	0.732	0.739	0.761	0.900
44.13	20.00	0.737	0.744	0.752	0.774	0.915
45.23	20.50	0.749	0.757	0.764	0.787	0.931
46.34	21.00	0.761	0.769	0.777	0.800	0.946
47.44	21.50	0.773	0.781	0.789	0.812	0.961
48.54	22.00	0.785	0.793	0.801	0.825	0.976
49.64	22.50	0.797	0.805	0.813	0.838	0.991
50.75	23.00	0.809	0.817	0.825	0.850	1.005
51.85	23.50	0.821	0.829	0.837	0.862	1.020
52.95	24.00	0.832	0.841	0.849	0.875	1.034

Conversions* of Weight to Body Surface Area (in Square Meters) for Dogs and Cats—cont'd

Weight (lb)	Weight (kg)	K = 9.9 (m^2)	K = 10.0 (m^2)	K = 10.1 (m^2)	K = 10.4 (m^2)	K = 12.3 (m^2)
54.06	24.50	0.844	0.853	0.861	0.887	1.049
55.16	25.00	0.856	0.864	0.873	0.899	1.063
56.26	25.50	0.867	0.876	0.885	0.911	1.077
57.37	26.00	0.878	0.887	0.896	0.923	1.091
58.47	26.50	0.890	0.899	0.908	0.935	1.105
59.57	27.00	0.901	0.910	0.919	0.946	1.119
60.68	27.50	0.912	0.921	0.930	0.958	1.133
61.78	28.00	0.923	0.932	0.942	0.970	1.147
62.88	28.50	0.934	0.944	0.953	0.981	1.161
63.99	29.00	0.945	0.955	0.964	0.993	1.174
65.09	29.50	0.956	0.966	0.975	1.004	1.188
66.19	30.00	0.967	0.976	0.986	1.016	1.201
67.30	30.50	0.977	0.987	0.997	1.027	1.214
68.40	31.00	0.988	0.998	1.008	1.038	1.228
69.50	31.50	0.999	1.009	1.019	1.049	1.241
70.61	32.00	1.009	1.020	1.030	1.060	1.254
71.71	32.50	1.020	1.030	1.041	1.072	1.267
72.81	33.00	1.030	1.041	1.051	1.083	1.280
73.92	33.50	1.041	1.051	1.062	1.093	1.293
75.02	34.00	1.051	1.062	1.073	1.104	1.306
76.12	34.50	1.062	1.072	1.083	1.115	1.319
77.23	35.00	1.072	1.083	1.094	1.126	1.332
78.33	35.50	1.082	1.093	1.104	1.137	1.344
79.43	36.00	1.092	1.103	1.114	1.148	1.357
80.53	36.50	1.102	1.114	1.125	1.158	1.370
81.64	37.00	1.113	1.124	1.135	1.169	1.382
82.74	37.50	1.123	1.134	1.145	1.179	1.395
83.84	38.00	1.133	1.144	1.156	1.190	1.407
84.95	38.50	1.143	1.154	1.166	1.200	1.420
86.05	39.00	1.153	1.164	1.176	1.211	1.432
87.15	39.50	1.162	1.174	1.186	1.221	1.444
88.26	40.00	1.172	1.184	1.196	1.231	1.456
89.36	40.50	1.182	1.194	1.206	1.242	1.469
90.46	41.00	1.192	1.204	1.216	1.252	1.481
91.57	41.50	1.202	1.214	1.226	1.262	1.493
92.67	42.00	1.211	1.223	1.236	1.272	1.505
93.77	42.50	1.221	1.233	1.245	1.282	1.517
94.88	43.00	1.230	1.243	1.255	1.293	1.529
95.98	43.50	1.240	1.253	1.265	1.303	1.541
97.08	44.00	1.250	1.262	1.275	1.313	1.552
98.19	44.50	1.259	1.272	1.284	1.323	1.564
99.29	45.00	1.268	1.281	1.294	1.333	1.576
100.39	45.50	1.278	1.291	1.304	1.342	1.588
101.50	46.00	1.287	1.300	1.313	1.352	1.599
102.60	46.50	1.297	1.310	1.323	1.362	1.611
103.70	47.00	1.306	1.319	1.332	1.372	1.623
104.81	47.50	1.315	1.329	1.342	1.382	1.634
105.91	48.00	1.325	1.338	1.351	1.391	1.646
107.01	48.50	1.334	1.347	1.361	1.401	1.657
108.12	49.00	1.343	1.357	1.370	1.411	1.669
109.22	49.50	1.352	1.366	1.379	1.420	1.680
110.32	50.00	1.361	1.375	1.389	1.430	1.691
111.42	50.50	1.370	1.384	1.398	1.440	1.703
112.53	51.00	1.379	1.393	1.407	1.449	1.714
113.63	51.50	1.389	1.403	1.417	1.459	1.725
114.73	52.00	1.398	1.412	1.426	1.468	1.736
115.84	52.50	1.407	1.421	1.435	1.478	1.747
116.94	53.00	1.415	1.430	1.444	1.487	1.759

Continued

Conversions* of Weight to Body Surface Area (in Square Meters) for Dogs and Cats—cont'd

Weight (lb)	Weight (kg)	K = 9.9 (m^2)	K = 10.0 (m^2)	K = 10.1 (m^2)	K = 10.4 (m^2)	K = 12.3 (m^2)
118.04	53.50	1.424	1.439	1.453	1.496	1.770
119.15	54.00	1.433	1.448	1.462	1.506	1.781
120.25	54.50	1.442	1.457	1.471	1.515	1.792
121.35	55.00	1.451	1.466	1.480	1.524	1.803
122.46	55.50	1.460	1.475	1.489	1.534	1.814
123.56	56.00	1.469	1.483	1.498	1.543	1.825
124.66	56.50	1.477	1.492	1.507	1.552	1.836
125.77	57.00	1.486	1.501	1.516	1.561	1.846
126.87	57.50	1.495	1.510	1.525	1.570	1.857
127.97	58.00	1.504	1.519	1.534	1.580	1.868
129.08	58.50	1.512	1.528	1.543	1.589	1.879
130.18	59.00	1.521	1.536	1.552	1.598	1.890
131.28	59.50	1.530	1.545	1.560	1.607	1.900
132.39	60.00	1.538	1.554	1.569	1.616	1.911
133.49	60.50	1.547	1.562	1.578	1.625	1.922
134.59	61.00	1.555	1.571	1.587	1.634	1.932
135.70	61.50	1.564	1.580	1.595	1.643	1.943
136.80	62.00	1.572	1.588	1.604	1.652	1.953
137.90	62.50	1.581	1.597	1.613	1.661	1.964
139.01	63.00	1.589	1.605	1.621	1.670	1.975
140.11	63.50	1.598	1.614	1.630	1.678	1.985
141.21	64.00	1.606	1.622	1.639	1.687	1.995
142.31	64.50	1.615	1.631	1.647	1.696	2.006
143.42	65.00	1.623	1.639	1.656	1.705	2.016
144.52	65.50	1.631	1.648	1.664	1.714	2.027
145.62	66.00	1.640	1.656	1.673	1.722	2.037
146.73	66.50	1.648	1.665	1.681	1.731	2.047
147.83	67.00	1.656	1.673	1.690	1.740	2.058
148.93	67.50	1.664	1.681	1.698	1.749	2.068
150.04	68.00	1.673	1.690	1.706	1.757	2.078
151.14	68.50	1.681	1.698	1.715	1.766	2.088
152.24	69.00	1.689	1.706	1.723	1.774	2.099
153.35	69.50	1.697	1.714	1.732	1.783	2.109
154.45	70.00	1.705	1.723	1.740	1.792	2.119

*A formula for more precise values follows: BSA in m^2 $(K \times W^{2/3})/100$ where *BSA*, body surface area; *m^2*, square meters; and *W*, weight in kilograms. The constant *K* varies with the body shapes: smaller values apply to small compact animals. The most common *K* value used for cats tends to be 10.1 (up to 10.4), and the most common value for dogs is 10.1 (ranging from 9.9 to 12.3).

From Ettinger, SJ: *Textbook of veterinary internal medicine,* vol 1, Philadelphia, Saunders, 1975, p.146.

Index

Page references followed by "f" indicate figures, "b" indicate boxes, and "t" indicate tables.

D

Q

R

S

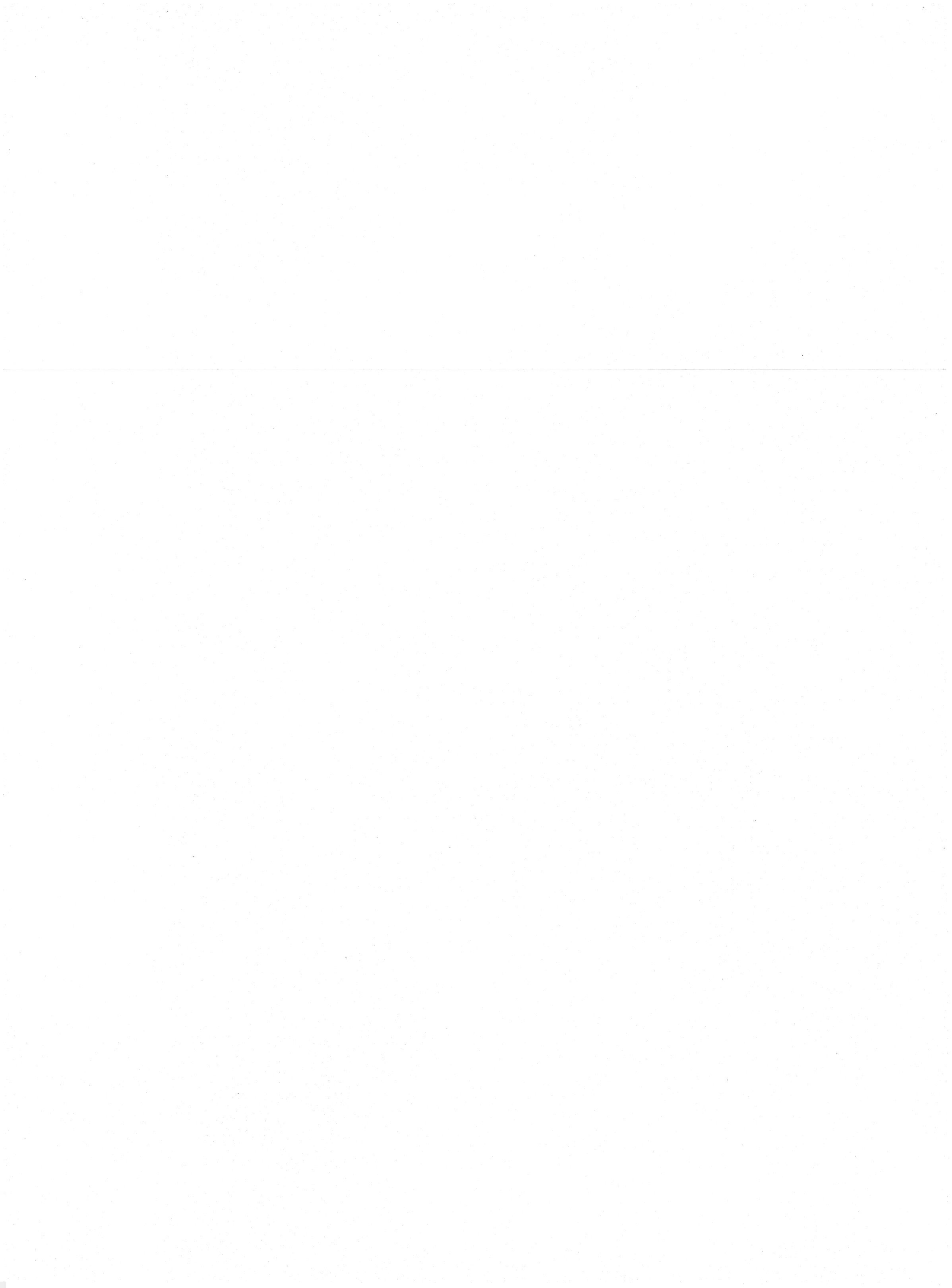